PRINCIPLES AND METHODS OF TOXICOLOGY

Fourth Edition

PRINCIPLES AND METHODS OF TOXICOLOGY

Fourth Edition

Edited by

A. Wallace Hayes
Vice President
Corporate Product Integrity
The Gillette Company
Boston, Massachusetts

TAYLOR & FRANCIS
ALERE FLAMMAM
Founded 1798

USA	Publishing Office:	TAYLOR & FRANCIS 325 Chestnut Street Philadelphia, PA 19106 Tel: (215) 625-8900 Fax: (215) 625-2940
	Distribution Center:	TAYLOR & FRANCIS 7625 Empire Drive Florence, KY 41042 Tel: 1 (800) 634-7064 Fax: 1 (800) 248-4724
UK	TAYLOR & FRANCIS	11 New Fetter Lane London EC4P 4EE Tel: +44 171 583 9855 Fax: +44 171 842 2298

PRINCIPLES AND METHODS OF TOXICOLOGY, Fourth Edition

2 3 4 5 6 7 8 9 0

Printed by Edwards Brothers, Ann Arbor, MI, 2001.
Cover design by Curtis Tow Graphics.

A CIP catalog record for this book is available from the British Library.
∞ The paper in this publication meets the requirements of the ANSI Standard Z39.48-1984 (Permanence of Paper).

Library of Congress Cataloging-in-Publication Data

Principles and methods of toxicology / [edited] by A. Wallace Hayes. – 4th ed.
p. ; cm.
Includes bibliographical references and index.
ISBN 1-56032-814-2 (alk. paper)
1. Toxicology. I. Hayes, A. Wallace (Andrew Wallace), 1939-
[DNLM: 1. Toxicology–methods. 2. Poisoning. 3. Poisons. 4. Toxicity Tests. QV 600 P957 2000]
RA1211 .P74 2000
615.9–dc21

00-037719

ISBN 1-56032-814-2 (case)

Contents

Part II: Agents of Toxicity

Part III: Methods of Toxicology

Contributing Authors

Melvin E. Andersen, Ph.D., D.A.B.T.
Center for Environmental Toxicology and Technology
Colorado State University
Foot Hills Campus
Fort Collins, Colorado 80523

Linda Baldwin, B.A.
Department of Environmental Health Sciences
School of Public Health
University of Massachusetts
Box 35712
Amherst, Massachusetts 01003-5712

Barbara D. Beck, Ph.D., D.A.B.T., FATS
Gradient Corporation
238 Main Street
Cambridge, Massachusetts 02142

William O. Berndt,, Ph.D., D.A.B.T., FATS
University of Nebraska Medical Center
986810 Nebraska Medical Center
Omaha, Nebraska 68198-6605

Joseph F. Borzelleca, Ph.D., FATS
Professor Emeritus
Virginia Commonwealth University-Medical College of Virginia Campus
Pharmacology & Toxicology
410 North 12th Street
PO Box 980613
Richmond, Virginia 23229-7319

Charles B. Breckenridge, Ph.D.
Manager of Human Safety Assessment
Syngenta
410 Swing Road
Greensboro, North Carolina 27409

David Brusick, Ph.D., FATS
Covance Laboratories Inc.
9200 Leesburg Pike
Vienna, Virginia 22182

Gary D. Byrd, Ph.D.
Research and Development
Targacept, Inc.
P. O. Box 1487
Winston-Salem, North Carolina 27102-1487

Edward J. Calabrese, Ph.D., FATS
Department of Environmental Health Sciences
School of Public Health
University of Massachusetts
Box 35712
Amherst, Massachusetts 01003-5712

William S. Caldwell, Ph.D.
Research and Development
Targacept, Inc.
P. O. Box 1487
Winston-Salem, North Carolina 27102-1487

Michel Charbonneau, Ph.D.
Human Health Research Center
INRS-Institut Armand-Frappier
Université du Québec
245 Hymus Boulevard
Pointe-Claire, Québec
Canada H9R 1G6

Mildred S. Christian, Ph.D., FATS
Primedica Argus Research Laboratories, Inc.
905 Sheehy Drive
Horsham, Pennsylvania 19044

Eric D. Clegg, Ph.D.
U.S. Army Center for Environmental Health Research
Fort Detrick, Maryland 21702-5010

Lorris G. Cockerham, Ph.D., DABFE
Phenix Consulting & Services, Ltd.
3006 Hinsen Road
Little Rock, Arkansas 72212-2712

Ralph R. Cook, M.D.
RRC Consulting, LLC
1401 Harwood Court
Midland, Michigan 48640-2765

Deborah A. Cory-Slechta, Ph.D.
University of Rochester
Department of Environmental Medicine
School of Medicine
575 Elmwood Avenue, Box EHSC
Rochester, New York 14642

Peter A. Crooks, Ph.D.
University of Kentucky
College of Pharmacy
Room 501A
Rose Street
Lexington, Kentucky 40536-0082

Cham E. Dallas, Ph.D.
Director, Interdisciplinary Toxicology Program
University of Georgia
Athens, Georgia 30602

Mary E. Davis, Ph.D.
West Virginia University Health Sciences Center
Department of Pharmacology and Toxicology
P. O. Box 9223
Morgantown, West Virginia 26506-9223

Jack H. Dean, Ph.D., D.A.B.T.
Sanofi-Synthelabo Research
A Division of Sanofi-Synthelabo, Inc.
9 Great Valley Parkway
Malvern, Pennsylvania 19355

J. Donald deBethizy, Ph.D., D.A.B.T.
Targacept, Inc.
P. O. Box 1487
Winston-Salem, North Carolina 27102-1487

Louis C. DiPasquale, M.S.
The Gillette Company
Gillette Medical Evaluation Laboratories
401 Professional Drive
Gaithersburg, Maryland 20879

Michael A. Dorato, Ph.D., D.A.B.T.
Director, Toxicology Projects and Environmental Sciences
Lilly Research Laboratories
A Division of Eli Lilly and Company
P. O. Box 708
Greenfield, Indiana 46140

Anne Fairbrother, D.V.M., Ph.D.
Parametrix, Inc.
Corvallis, Oregon 97333

Bruce A. Fowler, Ph.D., FATS
University of Maryland
Toxicology Program
1450 South Rolling Road
Baltimore, Maryland 21227

Shayne C. Gad, Ph.D., D.A.B.T.
Gad Consulting Services
1818 White Oak Road
Raleigh, North Carolina 27608

David W. Gaylor, Ph.D.
Sciences International Inc.
1800 Diagonal Road
Suite 500
Alexandria, VA 22314-2808

F. Peter Guengerich, Ph.D.
Department of Biochemistry and Center in Molecular Toxicology
Vanderbilt University School of Medicine
Nashville, Tennessee 37232-0146

Mary L. Haasch, Ph.D.
Chesapeake Biological Laboratory
University of Maryland
One William Street
P. O. Box 38
Solomons, Maryland 20688-0038

Robert L. Hall, Ph.D., D.V.M.
Covance Laboratories, Inc.
3301 Kinsman Boulevard
Madison, Wisconsin 53704

Jerry F. Hardisty, D.V.M.
Experimental Pathology Laboratories, Inc.
PO Box 12766
Research Triangle Park, North Carolina 27709

A. Wallace Hayes, Ph.D., D.A.B.T., FATS, C.N.S., FIBiol
Corporate Product Integrity
The Gillette Company
Prudential Tower Building
Boston, Massachusetts 02199

Johnnie R. Hayes, Ph.D., D.A.B.T., FATS
RJR Tobacco Company
Bowman Gray Technical Center
P. O. Box 1487
Winston-Salem, North Carolina 27102-1487

Robert V. House, Ph.D.
Covance Laboratories, Inc.
3301 Kinsman Boulevard
Madison, Wisconsin 53704

Michael J. Iatropoulos, M.D., Ph.D., FATS
Research Professor of Pathology
New York Medical College
Department of Pathology
Basic Science Building
Valhalla, New York 10595

Gerald L. Kennedy, Jr., B.S., D.A.B.T.
E. I. DuPont de Nemours & Co.
Haskell Laboratory
P. O. Box 50
1090 Elkton Road
Newark, Delaware 19714

Gary R. Klinefelter, Ph.D.
National Health and Environmental Effects Research Laboratory
Office of Research and Development
U.S. Environmental Protection Agency
Research Triangle Park, NC 27711

Kevin M. Kleinow, D.V.M., Ph.D.
Associate Professor
Veterinary Physiology, Pharmacology & Toxicology
School of Veterinary Medicine
Louisiana State University
Baton Rouge, Louisiana 70803-8420

Louis Andrew Koman, M.D.
Wake Forest University School of Medicine
Department of Orthopaedic Surgery
Medical Center Boulevard
Winston-Salem, North Carolina 27157

Kannan Krishnan, Ph.D.
Département de sante environnementale et sante au travail
Faculté de médecine
Université de Montréal
2375 Cote Ste Catherine, Office 4105
Montréal, Québec, Canada H3T 1A8

Michael R. Landauer, Ph.D.
Department of Radiation Pathophysiology & Toxicology
Armed Forces Radiobiology Research Institute
8901 Wisconsin Avenue
Bethesda, Maryland 20889-5603

Michael A. Lewis, Ph.D.
USEPA
Gulf Ecology Division
National Health and Environmental Effects Research Laboratory
Gulf Breeze, Florida 32561

Michael I. Luster, Ph.D.
NIOSH
Toxicology & Molecular Biology Branch
1095 Willowdale Road
Morgantown, West Virginia 26505-2888

Howard Maibach, M.D., FATS
University of California, San Francisco
Department of Dermatology
Surge 110
San Francisco, California 94143

Harihara M. Mehendale, Ph.D., D.A.B.T.
Department of Toxicology
College of Pharmacy
The University of Louisiana at Monroe
Monroe, Louisiana 71209-0470

Robert E. Menzer, Ph.D.
USEPA
National Center for Environmental Research
Washington, DC 20460

Jill C. Merrill, Ph.D., D.A.B.T.
The Gillette Company
Gillette Medical Evaluation Laboratories
401 Professional Drive
Gaithersburg, Maryland 20879

G. Andrew Mickley, Jr., Ph.D.
Department of Psychology
Baldwin-Wallace College
275 Eastland Road
Berea, Ohio 44017

Gary B. Morris, M.S., CIH, CSP
The Gillette Company
Occupational Hygiene Department
Gillette Medical Evaluation Laboratories
Gaithersburg, Maryland 20879

Joseph J. P. Morton, Ph.D., D.A.B.T.
The Gillette Company
Gillette Medical Evaluation Laboratories
401 Professional Drive
Gaithersburg, Maryland 20879

Arnold T. Mosberg, Ph.D., D.A.B.T.
Vice President, Toxicology and Product Assessment
RJR Tobacco Company
95 West 32nd Street
Winston-Salem, North Carolina 27102

Esther Patrick, Ph.D., D.A.B.T.
Director, Corporate Toxicology
L'Oréal, USA
111 Terminal Avenue
Clark, New Jersey 07066

Dennis J. Paustenbach, Ph.D., C.I.H., D.A.B.T.
Exponent
149 Commonwealth Drive
Menlo Park, California 94025

Sally D. Perreault, Ph.D.
National Health and Environmental Effects Research Laboratory
Office of Research and Development
U.S. Environmental Protection Agency
Research Triangle Park, North Carolina, 27711

Gabriel L. Plaa, Ph.D., D.A.B.T., FATS
Département de pharmacologie
Faculté de médecine
Université de Montréal
C.P. 6128
Succursale Centre-ville
Montréal, Québec, Canada H3C 3J7

Chada S. Reddy, B.V.Sc., Ph.D
Department of Veterinary Biomedical Sciences
College of Veterinary Medicine
University of Missouri
Columbia, Missouri 65211

Andrew Gordon Renwick, O.B.E., Ph.D., D.Sc.
Professor of Biochemical Pharmacology
University of Southampton
Biomedical Sciences Building
Bassett Crescent East
Southampton S016 7PX
United Kingdom

Joseph V. Rodricks, Ph.D., D.A.B.T.
The Life Sciences Consultancy, LLC
750 17th Street, NW
Suite 1100
Washington, DC 20006

Ruthann Rudel, M.S.
Silent Spring Institute
29 Crafts Street
Newton, Massachusetts 02458

Tracey M. Slayton, M.S.
Gradient Corporation
238 Main Street
Cambridge, Massachusetts 02142

Thomas L. Smith, Ph.D.
Wake Forest University School of Medicine
Department of Orthopaedic Surgery
Medical Center Boulevard
Winston-Salem, North Carolina 27157

Stephen D. Soileau, Ph.D., D.A.B.T.
The Gillette Company
Gillette Medical Evaluation Laboratories
401 Professional Drive
Gaithersburg, Maryland 20879

Robert C. Spiker, Jr., Ph.D., CIH
The Gillette Company
Occupational Hygiene Department
Gillette Medical Evaluation Laboratories
Gaithersburg, Maryland 20879

Katherine S. Squibb, Ph.D.
University of Maryland
Program in Toxicology
100 North Greene Street
Baltimore, Maryland 21201

James T. Stevens, Ph.D., D.A.B.T., FATS
Senior Science Advisor
Sygenta
410 Swing Road
Greensboro, North Carolina 27409

John A. Thomas, Ph.D., FATS
Professor Emeritus
Department of Pharmacology
University of Texas Health Science Center
San Antonio, Texas 78284-7722

Michael J. Thomas, M.D., Ph.D.
Department of Internal Medicine
(Division of Endocrinology)
University of North Carolina School of Medicine
Chapel Hill, North Carolina 27599-7000

Duncan Turnbull, D.Phil., D.A.B.T.
The Life Sciences Consultancy, LLC
750 17th Street, NW
Suite 1100
Washington, DC 20006

Rudolph Valentine, Ph.D., D.A.B.T.
E.I. DuPont de Nemours & Co.
Haskell Laboratory
P. O. Box 50
1090 Elkton Road
Newark, Delaware 19714

Mary Jo Vodicnik, Ph.D.
Lilly Research Laboratories
Director, Pharmaceutical Projects Management
Eli Lilly and Company
Lilly Corporate Center
Indianapolis, Indiana 46285

Thomas L. Walden, Jr., M.D., Ph.D.
Department of Radiation Oncology
Cape Fear Valley Medical Center
Fayetteville, North Carolina 28302

Carol T. Walsh, Ph.D.
Department of Pharmacology and Experimental Therapeutics
Boston University School of Medicine
715 Albany Street, R-608
Boston, Massachusetts 02118

Bernard Weiss, Ph.D.
University of Rochester
Department of Environmental Medicine
575 Elmwood Avenue, Box EHSC
Rochester, New York 14642

William J. White, V.M.D., M.S.
Charles River Laboratories
251 Ballardvale Street
Wilmington, Massachusetts 01887

Gary M. Williams, M.D., D.A.B.T.
Professor of Pathology
New York Medical College
Department of Pathology
Basic Science Building
Valhalla, New York 10595

Nelson H. Wilson, B.S., D.A.B.T.
Experimental Pathology Laboratories, Inc.
PO Box 474
Herndon, VA 20172

Acknowledgments

Appreciation is warmly expressed to the many people who contributed knowingly and otherwise to the Fourth Edition of this book. The editor most heartily thanks the contributors, who revised chapters or prepared new chapters, for keeping in mind that thoughtfully worded information is greatly appreciated by the reader. I am also indebted to the contributors for their combined expertise making a volume of this breadth possible. I thank Colleen Pritchard, Sandra Smith, Judith Curran, Mary Beth Gannon and Dana Pedersen for their skillful editing of the manuscript. Appreciation also is expressed to the staff of Taylor & Francis both in Philadelphia and London.

Foreword to the Third Edition

Until 1982 when the First Edition of this book was published, there was no specific source to which a student or an investigator could turn for a comprehensive presentation of the methods used in modern toxicology. For anyone who was trying to teach the subject, the book filled a great void for both the teacher and the student. The book appeared at a time when technical achievements in the field related to toxicology were undergoing tremendous refinements. Techniques and the tools of experimental biology, pathology, mathematics, engineering, physics, and analytical/biological chemistry, which had been barely conceived 20 years earlier, were in common use. The rapid growth of toxicology at that same time created a need for scientists from all of the above fields to apply their expertise to the science of toxicology. Toxicology borrowed freely from these related sciences so that a developing, modern, scientifically acceptable body of procedures became identified as the methods of toxicology. Prior to the span of a single human life, the methods of toxicology consisted of some general, short term test for the determination of the lethal and irritant qualities of chemicals on animals. The First Edition of this book was truly the first to chronicle the overall aspects of this difficult area of toxicology. The expotential rate of growth of toxicology continues and the Third Edition of the book continues to be an authoritative and comprehensive source of the methods that are currently used in this science.

It toxicology can be appropriately defined as the study of the harmful effects of chemicals on biologic systems, it must then embody a systemized knowledge of the effects of chemicals which are introduced into the simplest, as well as the most complex, of all biologic systems and methods must be available to accomplish these experiments. The availability of methods to detect the harmful effects of chemicals allows for the creation of data, but those data become useful in toxicology only after they are suitably interpreted. An additional link toward understanding the subject to toxicology is the placing of results obtained from the available methods in their proper relation and perspective to the whole picture of the role that toxicology can play for the improvement of mankind. In order to accomplish this function, the toxicologist must develop not only an understanding of the methods used but also determine the significance or insignificance of their data in the complete picture of the toxicity of each compound. My graduate school mentor, Dr Roger Hubbard, once told me that no scientifically valid experiment creates erroneous results, but inappropriate or application of those results can create erroneous conclusions. An understanding of the principles together with the methods involved in the science of toxicology prepares the critical scientist for developing an insight in regard to proper application of experimental results. Results that are properly obtained by acceptable methodology and that are suitably weighted for the conditions under which they were obtained certainly contribute to the development of proper conclusions. In this book, very highly qualified toxicologists present the procedures in detail that are currently used and accepted in the science of toxicology. Discussions of each procedure or category of procedures enable the reader to formulate an educated opinion about the limitations of interpretation of experimental results. Proper, critical conduct of acceptable toxicologic tests creates the body of systematized knowledge essential to the science of toxicology. Properly applied, that knowledge serves to protect mankind and the biologic realm in general from sudden, as well as delayed, insidious chemical induced harm.

Ted Loomis, M.D., Ph.D.
Professor Emeritus
University of Washington
Seattle, Washington

Foreword to the Fourth Edition

Publishing a toxicology book on the entrance into the third millennium is an appropriate time to reflect on the progress that has been made in that discipline since its inception. Almost five hundred years ago Paracelsus published a treatise based on his intuitive observations; he merely argued that these observations should convince one that the dose makes the poison. Now science has advanced enough so that we can prove that Paracelsus was correct, because the law of mass action tells us that the degree of perturbation of a system is proportional to the chemical potential of a substance in that system. We still, however, must rely heavily on observational epidemiology to determine the details of exactly what dose effects what change in humans.

The fourth edition of this book is a magisterial, state of the art compilation of the principles and methods that toxicologists must use to identify whether a causal relationship exists between specific doses of a chemical and an alleged adverse effect, observed primarily in humans. Proper integration of principles and methods of toxicology is extremely important since the primary purpose of toxicology is to predict human toxicity. Previous editions of this book have delincated in a very useful detail the methods of toxicology and how these methods have been perfected steadily and rapidly in the last few decades. The necessarily heavy reliance on animal experimentation for determining causality in humans is obvious and certainly warranted.

This book was the first to chronicle the overall aspects of the use of animal experiments in toxicology. The expediential rate of growth of toxicology continued to be reflected in further editions of the book as the authoritative and comprehensive source of methods used in this science. Proper and critical conduct of acceptable toxicological tests still continue to create the body of systematized knowledge essential to the science of toxicology.

The current edition continues this tradition, but adds some very significant new chapters. These chapters are on epidemiology, exposure assessment, and a chapter on repeat dosing that combines previous chapters that subdivided multiple dosing into arbitrary intervals. It is remarkable that we have returned, almost in full circle, to emphasis on direct exposure and effects in human population after finally, firmly establishing the basic scientific foundations of toxicology. This thorough, complete compendium is a necessary addition to the library of everyone interested in this subject.

William J. Waddell, M.D.,
Professor and Chair, Emeritus
Department of Pharmacology and Toxicology
University of Louisville, Kentucky

Preface to the Second Edition

The First Edition of this textbook was designed primarily for courses dealing with an evaluation of toxicologic data with a particular emphasis on those methodologies used in toxicology. This Second Edition has been expanded to include a more systematic approach to toxicology without losing its methodological basis. This edition describes current testing procedures, offers useful guidelines on data interpretation, and highlights major areas of controversy. Every effort has been made to keep the book simple and suitable for use as a textbook for graduate teaching.

Since toxicology is the study of the harmful action of chemicals on biologic tissues, it necessitates an understanding of biologic mechanisms as well as the methods employed to examine these mechanisms. However, the vastness of the field of toxicology and the rapid accumulation of data preclude the possibility of any one individual absorbing and retaining more than a fraction of these techniques. There are, however, specific methods that are applicable to a large number of chemicals. An understanding of the principles underlying these methods is not only manageable but essential. Thus, individuals who are not directly involved with the day-to-day activity of toxicology, or who have not yet entered a specialized field in toxicology, will find this book a valuable resource in acquiring a broad understanding of toxicological approaches available.

This volume has been designed to serve as a textbook for, or adjunct to, courses in general as well as advanced toxicology. The overall framework of the Second Edition follows that of the initial volume with the exception that major sections or principles related to toxicology have been added. A number of new authors have been added to this edition to broaden input and provide coverage of the ever-changing field of toxicology. New chapters have been added on metabolism, food-borne toxins, solvents, pesticides, and on the regulatory process as it relates to toxicology.

The only true "facts" in biology are the results of individual experiments carried out under control conditions by carefully defined methodology. Although it is not the purpose of this volume to catalog or to discuss these biologic "facts," it is the purpose of this book to present those methodologies which can generate these facts. Achievement of this goal requires the more or less arbitrary resolution to select methods and testing protocols from the current literature. The bibliography of each chapter will carry the reader beyond the techniques and methods presented in the book.

This volume has been organized to best facilitate its use. The first section covers basic toxicologic principles including the philosophies underlying testing strategies. The second section covers basic toxicologic testing methods and includes most of the testing procedures now required to meet regulatory standards. The third section deals with specific organ systems and contains chapters on kinetics and effects on cellular organelles and target organs. Each method or procedure is discussed from the standpoint of technique and interpretation of data. A state-of-the-art approach is emphasized as are the various problems and pitfalls encountered. Each chapter contains information that allows a person to perform an experiment or test a protocol, and also provides insight into the rationale behind the experiment.

Principles and Methods of Toxicology, Second Edition, will be useful as both a text for introductory courses in toxicology and as a valuable, timely review for the practicing toxicologist. Research scientists who have used the first edition as a reference source will find updated material in areas of their special or peripheral interest.

Preface to the Third Edition

The First Edition of *Principles and Methods of Toxicology* was designed for courses dealing with an evaluation of toxicological data with a particular emphasis on methodologies used in toxicology. The Second Edition was expanded to include a more systematic approach to toxicology without loosing its methodological basis. This Third Edition, as did the First and Second Editions, describes current testing procedures, offers useful guidelines on data interpretation, and highlights major areas of controversy. In addition, the Third Edition has been expanded and revised to reflect current needs and issues in toxicology. Every effort has been made to keep the book simple and suitable for use as a textbook for graduate teaching.

Since toxicology is the study of harmful effects of chemicals and physical agents on living systems, it necessitates an understanding of biologic mechanisms, as well as the methods employed to examine these mechanisms. However, the vastness of the field of toxicology and the rapid accumulation of data preclude the possibility of any one individual absorbing and retaining more than a fraction of these techniques. There are, however, specific methods that are applicable to a large number of chemicals. An understanding of the principles underlying these methods is not only manageable but essential. Thus, individuals who are not directly involved with the day-today activity of toxicology, or who have not yet entered a specialized field in toxicology, will find this book a valuable resource in acquiring a broad understanding of toxicological approaches available.

This volume has been designed to serve as a textbook for, or adjunct to, courses in general as well as advanced toxicology. The framework of the Third Edition follows that of earlier editions with the exception that several major sections on principles related to toxicology have been added, including chapters on environmental toxicology, pharmaceuticals and biotechnology products, metals, radiation, and risk assessment. New chapters on methods involving cellular and molecular techniques, instrumentation in toxicology, and physiologically based pharmacokinetics are included in the Third Edition. A number of new authors have been added to this edition to broaden input and provide coverage of the ever-changing field of toxicology. The history of toxicology now opens the book.

The only true "facts" in biology are the results of individual experiments carried out under controlled conditions by carefully defined methodologies. Although it is not the purpose of this volume to catalog those biologic—facts,- it is the purpose of this book to present those methodologies which can generate these facts. Achievement of the broad goal requires the more or less arbitrary resolution to select methods and testing protocols from the current literature. The bibliography of each chapter will carry the reader beyond the techniques and methods presented in this book.

This volume has been organized to best facilitate its use. As Abraham Lincoln so ably stated, "None seemed to think the injury arose from the use of a bad thing but from the abuse of a very good thing." The sixteenth century physician, Paracolsas, further pointed out that all substances can be poisonous with the difference between safe use and toxicity being the dose. Such often is the case in toxicology. The first section covers basic toxicological principles, including the history of toxicology and the philosophies underlying testing strategies. The second section covers agents of toxicity including food-borne toxicants, solvents and vapors, pesticides, metals, and radiation. The third section covers basic toxicological testing methods and includes many of the testing protocols now required to meet regulatory standards. Specific organ systems also are dealt with in this section. Each method or procedure is discussed from the standpoint of technique and interpretation of data. A state-of-the-art approach is emphasized as are various problems and pitfalls encountered with the various methodologies. Each chapter contains information that allows a person to perform an experiment or test a protocol and also provides insight into the rationale behind the experiment. Consideration is given in a number of the chapters to the need for, and yet the lack of acceptable, validated alternative methods to animal testing.

The Third Edition of *Principles and Methods of Toxicology will* be useful as both a text for introductory courses in toxicology and as a valuable, timely review for practicing toxicologists. Research scientists who have used earlier editions as reference sources will find updated materials in areas of their special or peripheral interests.

A. Wallace Hayes, Ph.D, D.A.B.T., FATS

Preface to the Fourth Edition

The First Edition of *Principles and Methods of Toxicology* was written to deal with evaluation of toxicological data. It described many of the testing procedures available at that time. The Second Edition included a more systematic approach to toxicology without loosing its methodological origin. It described not only current testing protocols but offered useful guidance for data interpretation. The Third Edition was expanded and revised to reflect current needs in toxicology. This Edition continues the tradition of earlier editions by providing detailed testing procedures but with an expanded insight regarding evaluation of data. The Fourth Edition has new chapters on epidemiology for toxicologists, on exposure assessment, and a chapter on repeat dosing that combines chapters that previously subdivided multiple dosing into arbitrary intervals. As before, every effort to reflect the needs and issues in toxicology and to keep the book suitable for use as a textbook in graduate education has been made.

Classically, toxicology is the study of adverse effects of chemicals and physical agents on living systems. Nonetheless, it should be remembered that Paracelsus said, "It is the dose that determines what is not a poison." Based on this important observation, toxicology must look beyond such a simple definition and focus its attention on determining a safe dose from a harmful or detrimental dose. In order to determine the safe use of a chemical or physical agent, it is necessary to have a sound understanding of biologic mechanisms and the methods employed to define these mechanisms. The vastness of the field of toxicology and the rapid accumulation of data preclude the possibility of absorbing and retaining more than a fraction of these techniques and information. However, an understanding of the principles underlying these methods is not only manageable but essential.

This tome was designed for courses in general and advanced toxicology. The framework of the Fourth Edition follows that of earlier editions. The history of toxicology opens the book and is followed by a section which covers basic toxicological principles. Chapters in this section include metabolism, toxicokinetics, physiologically based pharmacokinetic modeling, statistics, exposure assessment, quantitative aspects of interspecies extrapolation, and a chapter on epidemiology for the toxicologist. Also included in this section are chapters on the regulatory process and the toxicologic assessment of pharmaceutical and biotechnology products. The next section covers agent to toxicity including food-borne toxicants, solvents and vapors, pesticides, metals, and radiation. The third section covers basic toxicological testing methods including many of the test protocols now required to meet regulatory standards. Organ systems, tissue culture, and cell systems are dealt with in this section. Each method or procedure is discussed from the standpoint of technique and interpretation of data. A state-of-the-art approach is emphasized as well as discussions involving various problems and pitfalls that may be encountered in performing each procedure. Each chapter contains information that allows one to perform an experiment or test a hypothesis and provides insight into the rationale behind the experiment. Consideration is given in a number of the chapters to the need for validated alternative methods to animal testing. The last section contains a glossary of terms important in toxicology. The organization of the book should facilitate its use both by the student of toxicology and the more advanced researcher. A number of new authors allowed us to provide a broader coverage of the ever-changing field of toxicology.

The Fourth Edition of *Principles and Methods of Toxicology* will be useful as a text for courses in toxicology and as a valuable, timely review for practicing toxicologists. Research scientists who have used earlier editions as a reference source will find updated materials in areas of their special or peripheral interests.

A. Wallace Hayes, Ph.D., D.A.B.T., FATS, FIBiol

Principles and Methods of Toxicology,
Fourth Edition, edited by A. Wallace Hayes.
Taylor & Francis, Philadelphia © 2001.

Chapter 1

The Art, the Science, and the Seduction of Toxicology: An Evolutionary Development

Joseph F. Borzelleca

"We can never be fully in possession of a science until we know the history of its development." (Charles Greene Cumston)

"Continuity with the past is a necessity, not a duty." (Oliver Wendell Holmes, Jr.)

"History is bunk." (Henry Ford)

Toxicology! What an exciting word with interesting connotations. It initially evoked thoughts of poisons, poisoners, intrigue, cloak-and-dagger, villains, victims and perpetrators, and plants and chemicals as instruments of ill. What does the word conjure up today? Polluted water, air laden with noxious gases and particulates, foods contaminated with pesticides, soil loaded with heavy metals permanently handicapping children. There are still victims and perpetrators. In earlier times, the act of poisoning was deliberate and usually involved one or several people. Today, exposure to agents/chemicals is often unintentional (e.g., a spill), although it may be deliberate (e.g., suicide attempts) and may involve one or several individuals (e.g., in the workplace) or larger numbers of people (e.g., a community as a result of a spill). It is unfortunate that the same term, *poisoning*, is used whether exposure is deliberate or not. Poisonings in earlier times were probably not well reported for several reasons, including the inability to identify the poisoners or even that the cause of death was due to a poison, and to limited means of communication. Today, due to the significant advances in analytical chemistry and to better and faster means of communication, there is a faster and greater dissemination of information. Unfortunately, there is also a profusion of misinformation, and this is unnecessarily creating problems for the public. Industry is usually portrayed as the villain (by the media), and the unsuspecting public as the victim. Industry is also portrayed as profiting at the expense of the public health. If only the truth could be presented to the public in an unbiased manner! This is a challenge for modern toxicologists. Let those of us capable (by training and/or experience) of interpreting relevant data do so objectively and fairly. We must accept this challenge lest the public perish in a cesspool of media-fabricated hype. Will toxicologists rise to the occasion? The dedicated and concerned ones will.

How did we arrive at the present situation? What has happened as humans evolved from nomadic hunter-gatherers and cave dwellers to a relatively stable society of workers involved in many and varied activities? How can we explain the change from the direct use of poisons by individuals to kill one or several to the insidious exposure to presumed poisons to large groups by industry or other groups? An appreciation of the evolution of toxicology may be helpful.

Without definitions, meaningful discourse and science are impossible. "In the right definition of names lies the first use of speech, which is the acquisition of science; and in the wrong, or no definitions, lies the first abuse, from which proceed all false or senseless tenets" (Thomas Hobbes).

What is toxicology and how has it evolved to the eminent position it now enjoys? *Toxicology* is the study of the adverse effects of chemical or physical agents on biological systems; it is the science of poisons. A poison is any substance (chemical, physical, or biological) that is harmful or destructive to a biological (living) system. A poison derived from a biological source is a *toxin*, and the study of toxins is *toxinology*.

"Toxin" was originally *tekw*, a word meaning to run or flee, later becoming *toxsa* in Persian and *toxon* in Greek, meaning bow and arrow; the toxin meaning may have come from the poison used to tip the arrows, or, as Robert Graves suggested, from the yew tree *taxus*, from which arrows were best made and whose berries were long known to be poisonous. The word for poison came by a devious route, like a long-delayed afterthought. It derives from *poi*, to drink, becoming *potare* in Latin, whence "potion" (and also "symposium" from *sym*, together, plus *posis*, to drink). The venomous meaning did not come until the notion of love potions evolved, and the idea of poison came to consciousness. There is the same strange history behind the word "venom." This began as the simple word *wen* meaning to wish or will, leading more or less directly to "win." Along the way, a fork led to "venus," "venery" and "venerate," all indicating varieties of love. The love potion was called venin, and somehow this gradually acquired today's sense of venom. Nobody can explain why "poison" and "venom" come from love potions. Perhaps it was because the pharmacology of the day was primitive and chancy, a very fine line from toxicology. Or maybe there was a commonsense consensus that any sort of chemical additive intended to induce false love, is by nature, a fundamental poison. It tells something important about the good taste of earlier human beings that venom and poison were taken resentfully out of the hands of artificial lovers and transferred to the stings of insects and the fangs of serpents.

"Noxious," incidentally, came from *nek* meaning death, by way of *necare* and *nocere* in Latin, providing "necropsy" and cognate words for us; nectar was the drink of the gods because it prevented death (*tar*, meaning to overcome). Chance (origin is cadence). "Cadence" comes from *kad*, meaning to fall. Kad led to *cadere* in Latin and *cad* in Sanskrit, also meaning to fall, sometimes to die. Incidentally, "hazard" also came from *dice*, by way of Old French *hasard* and Spanish *azar*, from the Arabic *yasara*, to play at dice (55).

The development of toxicology reflects the history of the development of society; that is, a progression from simplicity to sophistication, from crude to cultured, from elemental to elegant. Consider killing. Killing animals for sustenance and survival predates recorded history. The biblical directive to Adam is clear. "Then God said: 'Let us make man in our image, after our likeness. Let them have dominion over the fish of the sea, the birds of the air, and the cattle, and over all the wild animals and all the creatures that crawl on the ground'" (Genesis 1:26). "God blessed them saying: 'Have dominion over the fish of the sea, the birds of the air, and all living things that move on the earth.'" God also said: "See, I give you every seed-bearing plant all over the earth and every tree that has seed-bearing fruit on it to be your food; and to all the animals of the land, all the birds of the air, and all the living creatures that crawl on the ground, I give all the green plants for food. And so it happened" (Genesis 1:28–30). Animals, including humans, were, and still are, born with a strong basic instinct for survival (and control) that involves eating and drinking. It became (and still is) necessary to kill plants and animals in order to survive. Humans also have an instinct to control their own destinies. Occasions arose when it became necessary to remove (i.e., to kill) other humans (for control, not nutritional survival). The methods used to kill humans were the same as those used to kill animals. The usual instruments of kill were clumsy physical weapons that required strength for effectiveness. Small and less powerful humans were at a great disadvantage. Even though later developments, such as the bow and arrow, required more skill and less physical strength, something more (an equalizer) was needed for the less physically endowed.

Early humans probably learned through experience about the harmful properties of insects and animals (including venoms). The women studied plants and determined which were beneficial and which were poisonous. The poisonous ones were then used by the men as aids in hunting (e.g., arrow poisons). Poisons proved to be very useful in killing animals. Could they be the equalizer needed by the less powerful to solve other problems? Could humans be dispatched as readily as animals with the use of poisons? It was worth testing. Killings were sometimes performed for reasons other than for survival, such as control, frustration, anger, or convenience. For example, to satisfy their lust for power, wealth, pleasure, and new excitements, the "power class" (wealthy landowners, rulers) found it necessary to kill other humans, but killing other humans was not limited to the "power class." In general, genteel, subtle, and undetectable means of killing were desirable (such as dispensing with a spouse to be able to enjoy a new lover), but these were not available until professional poisoners appeared on the scene. When used properly, poisons could be (and often were) the perfect solution to difficult problems and detection was impossible.

Once the value of poisons was recognized, they became very attractive as "fit instruments of ill." Humans then and now are seduced by things attractive (and useful). Poisoning as a solution to difficult problems was very appealing and had a great deal to recommend it; it could be fast or slow, painful or painless, poisons were inexpensive and readily available; and, as noted earlier, defied detection. The seduction of toxicology had begun! Once the need had been established, suppliers and practitioners were needed for proper implementation. The amateur or do-it-yourself poisoners were soon replaced by professional poisoners (early applied toxicologists), who offered advice and/or performed the required services. The agents used were initially naturally occurring; these were supplemented by new agents developed by alchemists/chemists. Thus, toxicology evolved into an art and then into a science.

The popularity of poisoning grew until it reached epidemic proportions in some countries. This popularity was enhanced by the inability to detect poisons and to prove that poisoning had occurred. However, once the chemists turned their skills from developing new poisons to detecting poisons, the popularity of poisons as killer agents began to wane. Poisoners could now be identified. Although poisons are still used today, more subtle and ingenious means of killing are available. Today, poisoning conjures up images of large groups of individuals unintentionally exposed to chemicals; however, detection and source/cause identification of the exposure are possible and responsible party (parties) identified. In earlier times, the poisoner was usually an individual; today, poisoning/pollution may involve a corporation.

> A man without a sense of history, without memory of the past, who is forced to reconsider his place in the world, a man deprived of the historic experience of his own and other peoples lacks any perspective and can only live in the present. (Chingiz Aitmatou, 1983)

POISONS ARE IN!

With respect to the art of poisoning, de Quincey wrote:

> The bowl needs for its effective management a scientific precision of plan and a subtlety of execution that place it in a different category from the vulgar methods of the knife, the bullet, or the bludgeon. The process can be almost indefinitely prolonged, giving large opportunities for the exercise of skill, resourcefulness, craft, and daring; and with allowing time for the enjoyment of the full passion of deliberate crime, which finds imperfect gratification in the hasty thrust of the knife. There have been persons who poisoned, not out of covetousness or hatred or wanton cruelty, but for the pleasure of the thing. They were true artists, practicing their art for its own sake, with a proper scorn for the limitations which an irrelevant morality would impose in its exercise.

Do poisons have any redeeming value; in other words, are there uses for poisons beyond killing? Very definitely! Poisons have contributed to the health and safety of humankind and to the advancement of biological sciences (including medicine) in a number of ways. In 1878, Claude Bernard, an outstanding early physiologist and probably the first and foremost mechanistic toxicologist wrote:

> Poisons can be used as agents for the destruction of life or as means to cure disease; but in addition to these uses—there is a third which particularly interests the physiologist. For him the poison becomes an instrument which dissociates and analyses the most delicate phenomena of the living machine and by careful study of the mechanism of death in different poisonings, he can gain knowledge, indirectly, of the physiological mechanism of life. (i.e. poisons can be used to explain physiological events). (translation of P. N. Mage, 1865)

For interesting discussions of these artist-poisoners, including Locusta, Toffana, the Marquise de Brinvilliers, Ezra Wharton, Florence Maybrick, the Borgias, Catherine de Medici, Sainte Croix, and Catherine Deshayes (La Voisine), the reader is referred to articles by Gallo and Doull, Decker, Thompson, and Osius.

Claude Bernard used curare to study the physiology of the neuromuscular junction. Radiation, a "physical poison," has been an invaluable tool in elaborating some of the basic events in mutagenesis and carcinogenesis. Identifying the role of mixed-function oxidases (MFOs) and cytochrome P450 (P450) and exploring hepatic mechanisms at the molecular level would have been delayed had it not been for hepatotoxins. Low doses of certain toxins may be useful in therapeutics: for example, botulinum toxin in the management of strabismus, blepharospasm, and spasmodic torticollis. Poisons are not all bad!

Farming (food production) has evolved from a very primitive but necessary human activity to feed a few people to a very sophisticated process that feeds multitudes. In earliest times, it involved the use of simple tools, few crops, and primitive methods. With the introduction of power (animal, then mechanical), larger areas could be cultivated. More crops were developed. Efficiency improved but there was considerable room for improvement. Enriching the soil resulted in increased yields, but pests competed with humans for crops thereby reducing effective availability. Pesticides are chemicals (usually) that are used to kill unwanted subhuman organisms. The judicious use of these materials has resulted in increased food production and storage and subsequently in better health and prolonged life expectancy. The introduction of genetically modified plants that are disease- and pest-resistant and have a better nutrient profile and improved organoleptic properties has resulted in diminished exposure to chemical agents. There is every reason to believe that this trend will continue.

With the introduction of chemical power to enrich the soil, treat the seeds, and eliminate pests, unprecedented yields were realized. Humans began to manipulate, to control, part of their environment; they worked with Nature to their benefit. But there were occasions when the interaction with Nature was not symbiotic—when air, water and/or soil were abused, often due to ignorance but sometimes to greed.

Food preparation and storage evolved in a similar manner. Prior to the introduction of heat (fire power), food was eaten raw. Cooking provided an opportunity to broaden one's choices and to improve the bioavailability of certain nutrients. Heat (sun, fire) was also used to preserve food by drying. Chemical power (e.g., salt) was also used to preserve food. Add to drying and chemical preservation the power of radiation and food could be maintained safe for human consumption for unbelievably long periods of time. In addition, chemicals (e.g., flavors and colors) could be used to enhance the organoleptic properties of foods. Again, humans were controlling the immediate environment to their benefit. The preparation of food (a renewable resource) for consumption was/is usually less destructive of nature.

And the need for safe drinking water! It took a long time to associate contaminated water with disease. Or did it? The Egyptians used a physical method (sand bag) to purify water, a technique used today (sand banks). But it was not until chemical power was introduced in the form of chlorine gas that waterborne diseases were finally eliminated.

Other natural products have played a role in the cultural/sociological/hedonistic aspects of human activities. These include sugar, salt, coffee, tea, rosemary, garlic, pepper, opium, digitalis, alcohol, and tobacco.

Toxicology is an evolving discipline: from art to science, from using chemicals that hurt to chemicals that help, or at least prevent hurting, and from taking lives to saving lives. It is not precisely known when the first human used a plant toxin, a phytotoxin (plant poison), to kill another human, but it probably did not require too great a leap of faith to extrapolate from effects in animals to humans. The age of poisoning, of practical toxicology, had begun. As poisoning developed into an art, its practitioners became famous/infamous. Identification of the culprit was extremely difficult since determination of the cause of death (proof of poisoning) required yet-to-be-developed analytical techniques.

Natural products were used (and are still used) to prevent and/or to treat disease. Women were the original naturopaths; they learned the biological properties (effects) of plants and used plants and/or their constituents with appropriate activity in the management of disease (to heal), while those with poisonous properties were used by the men in hunting (to kill). (The adverse effects of venomous insect stings and animal bites were probably also noted, but the practical utility of these venoms was limited.)

Interest in plant poisons (phytotoxins) and animal poisons (venoms), as nuisances to health and as tools for vindication, continued to grow. Lists (catalogs) of poisons and their effects in humans began to appear. Each culture/civilization appears to have had a list or lists of these. The use of plants, including herbs, for medicinal purposes also continued to evolve. The cures (healing or killing) for the problems of humankind were to be found in nature (a concept that has again found favor with many)! With time, the lists began to include detailed descriptions of preparation, use, and effects of biologically active plant materials. Understandably, concerns about prevention and treatment of poisoning began to emerge. Prevention of poisoning was accomplished by the use of appropriate bioassays (e.g., official tasters of prepared food and drink) and by the development of tolerance/adaptation through the repeated ingestion of small doses of toxins. Initially, treatment (antidotes) was shrouded in folklore and mysticism. Only when mechanisms of toxicity were understood and toxicology became a recognized science did treatment have a rational, scientific basis.

Advances in chemistry led to the development of analytical chemistry. The application of analytical techniques to the detection of poisons was the beginning of the science of forensic toxicology. This had a chilling effect on the use of poisons. Now poisoning could be proved. Practitioners became more sophisticated in attempts to avoid detection, but they were no match for the dedicated chemists who continued to develop exquisitely sensitive and specific analytical methods. Perpetrators/villains could now be identified and appropriate action taken. The development of ultrasensitive analytical methods has continued into the present. Contaminants in soil, air, and water are now easily identified and quantified. The origins and the originators can be identified and appropriate action taken. Ultrasensitive analyses continue to challenge toxicologists to assess the biological/health significance of the presence of chemicals at parts per billion or parts per trillion in body fluids or tissues. Dose-response relationships were established as correlations between the level of the chemical in blood and/or in tissues and biological activity were made. Concomitant with advances in analytical/forensic toxicology were efforts to elucidate the mechanisms of action of chemical agents. This was followed by the development of rational therapy for poisonings, including the development of specific antidotes.

POISONS ARE OUT!

In light of this scientific onslaught, the deliberate use of poisons to kill declined rapidly. The practitioners of the art of poisoning disappeared to be replaced by a new breed of toxicologist, the scientist who understood the basis of toxicity from the whole animal to the molecular level, could appreciate all of its ramifications, and could extrapolate to the human situation. Quantification of the responses to toxic agents and the relationship of structure to biological activity became, and still is, the basis for a great deal of scientific activity.

When it became known that nondeliberate exposure to chemicals could produce adverse health effects (e.g., in the workplace), efforts were directed to the prevention of the adverse effects of chemicals by defining safe conditions of exposure to protect humans and other life forms from chemical and physical injury. This was followed by the identification and quantification of the risk of adversity following exposure (risk identification, assessment, and management). Quantifying a risk, assigning a number to it, tends to decrease the uncertainty of extrapolation and to provide a comfort factor.

In maturing to a scientific discipline, toxicology passed through a number of phases, including observation/phenomenology (lists of poisons and antidotes), experimentation/deduction/mechanisms/analytical (including dose-response), and application (TLV, ADI, safety/uncertainty factor) and quantification (quantitative risk assessment)/prognostication). A transition from using chemicals to kill to finding uses for chemicals/poisons that would benefit humankind (e.g., pesticides and therapeutic agents) to identifying, quantifying, and preventing adverse effects of chemicals (e.g., establishing safe exposure conditions in the workplace and safe levels of chemicals in foods and water) occurred. Toxicology had evolved to another stage wherein it became a respected member of the scientific biomedical community.

The toxicologist was needed when poisons were in and continues to be needed now that poisoning is out. From supplying poisons to studying their mechanisms of action to developing analytical methods to identifying and quantifying poisons in body fluids and tissues to developing rational antidotes to establishing safe limits of exposure from carefully designed and executed studies to quantifying and predicting adverse effects—the toxicologist continues to play a critical role in the advancement of humankind.

AGE OF OBSERVATION/RECORDING OF PHENOMENA

Biblical

Although most of the references to poisons in the Bible appear to be limited to venoms, chemicals and food regulations are also mentioned. In the Book of Genesis, God is portrayed as the Supreme Regulator and protector; God proscribed certain foods. The regulated were Adam and Eve. Had they blindly accepted the regulations imposed upon them (had they had more faith in their Regulator), there would have been no dire consequences. Is there a lesson here for us today? The bitter water to test the fidelity of a wife suspected of unfaithfulness is described in Numbers 5:11. Venoms and plant poisons appear in Deuteronomy 32:24, "with the venom of reptiles gliding in the dust," and 32:31, "poisonous are their grapes and bitter their clusters." Arrow poisons are mentioned in Job 6:4, "for the arrows of the Almighty pierce me, and my spirit drinks in their poison," and in 20:16, "The poison of asps he shall drink in; the viper's fangs shall slay him." "The venom of asps lies behind their lips" appears in Romans 3:13. In Psalms 58:5, "theirs is poison like a serpent's, like that of a stubborn snake that stops its ears," and Psalms 140:4 "they make their tongues sharp as those of serpents; the venom of asps is under their lips." Jeremiah mentions chemical and biological poisons, "he has given us poison to drink" (8:14) and "I will send against you poisonous snakes against which no charm will work when they bite you" (8:17). In James 3:8, we find "the tongue no man can tame. It is restless evil, full of deadly poison." There appears to be an awareness of the natural occurrence of poisons and the effects produced, but no mention of the deliberate use of them. Antidotes are not mentioned, only charms. There is no list of poisons in the Bible, although there are proscriptions about foods and food practices (e.g., Deuteronomy 14, Leviticus 11, 17, 19), apparently based on potential adverse health effects.

Egyptian

The first list of poisons and antidotes appears in Egyptian writings. This is not unusual since the Egyptians were the intellectual leaders of the world and Egyptian medicine was reputed to be the most advanced. Menes (Mena, Meni, Min), the first king of unified Egypt and the founder of Memphis, the capital, was reported in the Egyptian papyri to have had an interest in poisons. He cultivated and studied the effects of poisonous and medicinal plants somewhere between 3500 and 3000 BC. Unfortunately, there is no detailed written history of these activities. His son Athothis, a physician, wrote a textbook on medicine in which sanitation was stressed.

A papyrus discovered in Thebes (Luxor) in 1872 by the German egyptologist Georg Moritz Ebers (1837–1898), named appropriately in his honor the Ebers Papyrus, was written between 1553 and 1500 BC. It is more than 20 m long and contains 110 columns of hieratic (priestly) script (about 110 pages). More than 700 drugs (medicinal substances) are identified in about 875 to 900 formulas (quantitative recipes). The formulas also contain specific indications and dosages, together with appropriate spells and/or incantations. Forty-seven case histories are presented. Modes of administration include snuffs, inhalations, gargles, pills, troches, suppositories, enemas, fumigations, lotions, ointments, and plasters. Drugs were identified on the basis of origin as plant (e.g., acacia, castor bean, wormwood, fennel, garlic), animal (e.g., milk, excrement) or mineral (e.g., alum, iron oxide, limestone, sodium bicarbonate, salt, sulfur). Vehicles used included beer, wine, milk, and honey. There is also a great deal of information on the toxicity of opium, hellebore, aconite, hyoscyamus, hemlock, lead, antimony, and copper. Insect and animal venoms were described. Antidotes, including incantations, were also mentioned. To assure recovery, Egyptian physicians used combination therapy: chemical and or biological materials (rational therapy) plus mysticism (requests for assistance from the gods; irrational therapy?). Today, some pray for assistance only after conventional therapy has been unsuccessful. Perhaps simultaneous is more effective than sequential!

There are other papyri detailing medical practices in early Egypt. The Edwin Smith Papyrus was discovered at the same time and place as the Ebers Papyrus, but it was probably written earlier. The Hearst Papyrus was written about 1400 BC and was discovered in upper Egypt in 1899. The Kahun Papyrus was written between 2000 and 1800 BC and was discovered by Sir Flinders Petrie in the Faiyum. It deals primarily with gynecology. The Berlin Papyri (two, the same period as Ebers Papyrus) and the Brugsch Papyrus were the latest to be discovered.

For example, the Egyptians used chemicals in the administration of justice. The Penalty of the Peach involved having the accused ingest the distillate from crushed pits of peaches (high in hydrocyanic acid); if the accused died, it was a presumption of guilt; if the accused lived, it was a presumption of innocence. This practice of using chemicals in the administration of justice was used by other cultures (e.g., Greek) and persists to the present; lethal injections of chemicals are used for executions in the United States.

Egyptian practitioners of medicine believed that respiration was the most important function of the body followed by circulation (blood and heart); that most diseases were caused by parasites (which is not surprising considering conditions in Egypt); that personal and social hygiene were very important in maintaining good health; and that therapeutics should be both rational and mystical. They covered all bases! The Egyptian contribution to toxicology includes lists of poisons and antidotes.

Chinese

On the other side of the world, the Chinese were also developing a culture that was advanced for the period. The second of China's mythical emperors, Shen Nung, is considered the father (founder) of Chinese medicine, materia medica, and agriculture. He is credited with inventing the cart, the plow, and the yoking of horses. He taught the Chinese how to clear land with fire to increase farmland. Shen Nung wrote a 40-volume herbal entitled *Pen Ts'ao or Pun Tsao* (the Great Herbal or Chinese Materia Medica) around 2735 BC. It contained lists of poisonous plants, plants with medicinal value (365), and drugs (265, 240 of which are vegetable in origin). The effects of plants and drugs and appropriate antidotes were described. Included among the drugs were iodine, aconite (also used as an arrow poison), opium, cannabis, rhubarb, alum, camphor, iron, sulfur, and mercury. He was also reputed to have discovered a number of drugs and experimented upon himself. Phytotoxicology appeared to be well developed. Here is the second list of poisons and antidotes. Like the Egyptians, drugs and poisons were presented together. (Pharmacology and toxicology joined together at this early age! Did this presage the development of toxicology?) Another emperor, Hwang Ti (2650 BC), wrote *Nei Ching*, the Book of Medicine, the basis for most Chinese medical writings.

In addition to the lists of drugs and poisons and their effects (the early Chinese contribution to toxicology and pharmacology), the Chinese made other significant contributions to medicine. These include discovering the circulation of blood; the yang and yin principles (two opposing forces that control everything including ebb and flow, male and female, life and death, moon and sun, heat and cold, strength and weakness (parasympathetic and sympathetic, cholinergic and adrenergic nervous systems?); the five elements of the human body (earth, fire, water, wood, metal); the five organs of the body (heart, liver, spleen, lung, kidney); five colors, and five heavenly bodies—five appeared to be a magic number in this culture. Other cultures had magical numbers; for the Greeks, it was four or seven. Health was the result of balance between the forces and elements, a concept that still has its adherents.

Hindu

The most significant contribution of the Hindus to medicine was in the field of surgery. Like the Chinese and the Egyptians, they also had their list of poisons and antidotes. The Rig-Veda, a Sanskrit document written between 1500 and 1200 BC, is the earliest written account of Hindu medicine. It contains many references to alchemy and science and magic in the treatment of disease. Included are discussions of many diseases including cough, fever, diarrhea, seizures, tumors, and skin diseases. There are treatments for specific diseases. These treatments, like the Egyptian, include spells and incantations, again the combination of rational and mystical therapies! Medicinal and poisonous plants and antidotes (e.g. for snake bites) are listed. The influence of gold as a therapeutic agent and on longevity is discussed. A later work, the Ayur-Veda, the Veda of long life, a Sanskrit document written about 700 BC, discussed medicine and all its branches in eight parts; drugs and poisons were also mentioned.

> "He who knows only one branch of his art is like a bird with one wing". (Susruta)

Susruta, a Hindu surgeon, authored a medical/surgical text called Susruta-Samhita, in the last centuries of the pre-Christian period. The text was divided into six sections. He identified 1120 diseases and gave fever great importance. He stressed the importance of hygiene and presented many surgical procedures in great detail. The section on drugs listed 760 indigenous medicinal plants, of which many were used externally as ointments, baths, sneezing powders, inhalations; it also listed animal and mineral remedies. The fifth section, the Kalpa Sthana, was the section on toxicology and contained mostly antidotes. The Hindus were keenly interested in poisons and antidotes, especially for bites and stings and aphrodisiacs (interesting; any message here?). Other topics discussed included malaria and the role of the mosquito and plague and the influence of rats.

Greek

There are many Greek legends and myths involving gods and goddesses concerned with poisons and poisoning. For example, Hecate used aconite; Medes, colchicine; and Hercules was poisoned with cantharidin applied to his shirt. Like other cultures, the Greeks also had their lists of poisons, lists that were consulted by citizens and by the government. Other and more significant contributions to the advancement of toxicology were made, including detailed descriptions of the effects of various agents in humans, antidotes, and principles for the management of poisonings.

The Greeks made many significant contributions to the advancement of humankind. For example, they developed a system of philosophy (*philos*, friend; *sophia*, wisdom) that defined the place of humans in nature; they attempted a rational explanation for nature and natural phenomena including medicine and the healing arts; and they believed that there exists a single fundamental principle, a prime force, from which everything in nature developed. The Greeks perceived medicine as both an art, the careful examination and accurate observation of the patient, and a science, part of the science of humans and their place/role in nature. The Greeks had a great deal of knowledge about poisons (especially plant poisons), metals (especially arsenic, antimony, mercury, gold, copper, and lead), and antidotes (e.g., hot oil and vomiting). The Greeks also executed criminals with poisons (e.g., hemlock, which was the state poison), which presaged the use of lethal injections in the United States today. Suicide by poisoning was not uncommon since poisons were readily available.

The father of the Pythagorean theorem (proposition), Pythagoras (580–489 BC), was born in Samos, and lived in southern Italy (Crotona) for many years. He was a mathematician who developed the theory of numbers and became known as the father (founder) of arithmetic, a physician and scientist who was especially interested in procreation and animal physiology, an astronomer, a philosophical-religious leader who tried to reform the political, social, and moral ills of the time, and a numerologist who considered the number seven highly significant. He believed the earth was a sphere, that animals possessed souls, and that both animal and human souls were immortal and transmigrated. His doctrine of numbers was probably the basis for the four elements and four humors and the four critical days in illness described by Hippocrates (this is surprising since he valued the number seven). His theory of harmony may be the basis for the theory that health is the result of a balance among the various elements and humors. He believed that health is perfect harmony and disease is a disruption of this harmony. His most significant contribution to medicine and to toxicology was the importance of causality and the need for critical thinking. His other contributions to toxicology include his studies of the effects of metals (e.g., tin, iron, mercury, silver, lead, gold, copper) in the body. Since he left few, if any, writings, all of his teachings have come through his disciples.

Empedocles of Agrigentum (490–430 BC) was the son of Meto, an activist politician; he was born in Sicily and died in Peloponnese, Greece. He was of the Pythagorean school, a physiologist, physician, philosopher, religious teacher, poet, and politician who believed in the unity of things. He also believed that all matter consisted of four elements (the Chinese believed in five), earth, fire, air, water; that nothing is destroyed (accord/love holds things together, discord/strife [stress?] tends to dissociate things). These two forces, one internal (accord) and one external (discord), are antagonistic (yang and yin?). His teachings became the basis for the four body humors—blood, phlegm, yellow bile (choler), black bile (melancholy)—and for the theory that health was the result of harmony among these humors and among the four elements (cf. Pythagoras). He was a strong advocate of hygiene, personal and social, and of public health measures to prevent epidemics (e.g., draining of swamps). Although Aristotle is often credited with identifying the four elements, he was merely a strong proponent of the four elements and not the first to identify them.

Empedocles believed the heart was the most important organ since it distributed the "pneuma" throughout the body. (Egyptians considered respiration most important.) He established the basis for sense perception. He was considered a wonder worker due to his great healing skills and to his abilities to prophesy. According to tradition, he cast himself into the crater of Mt. Etna to prove something or other.

> "There is only one good, knowledge; there is only one evil, ignorance." (Socrates)

Socrates (470–399 BC), son of Sophroniscus, a sculptor who was dispatched with hemlock, the state poison, is probably the most famous victim of poisoning in history. He developed the Socratic method of inquiry, a series of questions designed to elicit clear expressions or answers. He had a strong contempt for conventional ideas and life-styles that ultimately led to his demise. His idealistic philosophy was passed on through the writings of Plato, his most famous student; Socrates left no writings of his own.

> "Life is short, and the Art long; opportunity fleeting; experiment dangerous, and judgment difficult." (Hippocrates; was he thinking of toxicologists when he wrote this?)

Hippocrates (460–355 BC), the father of medicine, was born on the island of Cos, the son of Heraclides, a physician, and Phenarete. It is said that he was a member of the family of Asclepiadae. He was well educated and traveled extensively. He was a contemporary of Sophocles, Euripedes, Aristophanes, Pindar, Socrates, Plato, Herodotus, Thucydides, Phidias, and Polygnotus. He had two sons, Thessalus and Dracon, and many pupils. His contributions to the advancement of medicine are legendary, due in great measure to his belief that the causes of diseases were natural and not supernatural. In addition, he stressed the importance of nutrition/diet and believed that too little or too much food was equally harmful. What he lacked in instrumentation was more than compensated for by his use of the scientific method, sound observation, and logical reasoning. He is the presumed author of a number of significant texts and treatises characterized by advanced scientific and practical thinking and skillful clinical observation. Like other Greek physicians, he believed that health was the result of an equilibrium or balance in the body among the humors (blood, black bile, yellow bile, and mucus) and that disequilibrium resulted in ill health.

He apparently was the first physician of record (a clinical ecologist?) who believed that environmental factors should be considered as probable causes of disease. For example, in his book *Airs, Waters and Places*, he argued that environmental factors (overall weather, local weather conditions, and drinking water) can influence health. "Every disease has its own nature and arises from external causes, from cold, from the sun, or from changing winds." According to Hippocrates, the first step in treating disease, including poisonings, should be to purify the body of disease-producing humors by purgation (catharsis, purification) by diet or by drugs. This cleansing is the first step in restoring equilibrium (including the management of poisoning). Hippocrates probably foreshadowed the current practice of the clinical ecologists, who espouse thorough cleansing of xenobiotics from the body as the first step in restoring health.

Hippocrates taught that the body is maintained by air and nutriments, that it is nature that heals, and that the role of the physician is to assist nature in the healing process by increasing nature's healing forces ("help nature to help herself"; was he portending the current "back-to-nature" movement?). This can best be done by diet and modifying one's life-style, usually to get more rest and appropriate exercise. The key to good health is proper diet, sufficient exercise, and adequate rest (makes a great deal of sense even today!). Drugs may be used to assist the dietetic cure.

Hippocrates identified about 400 drugs, mostly of plant origin, that included narcotics (e.g., poppy, henbane, mandragora), purgatives, and sudorifics. He also advocated the use of emetics and enemas (as part of the cleansing process). The patient is a unit and must be treated as such (that is, as an individual), there must be very careful observation (good case history and physical examination?), and the approach to treatment should be appropriate, simple, and rational. Mysticism was not a part of his therapeutic regimen. His advice to physicians is summarized in his *Aphorisms*, which include being prepared "to do the right thing at the right time." He also established a code of medical ethics, the Hippocratic oath, which has survived to the present. His contributions to toxicology include the use of the scientific method, sound observation, logical reasoning ("the scientific method"), and basic approaches to the management of intoxication (decrease absorption; if ingested, induce vomiting) and the use of proper antidotes. He died in Thessaly in 355 BC.

> "For where there is the love of man [humans], there is also love of the art." (Hippocrates)

The second most famous Greek physician, Diocles of Carystus (375–300 BC), was loved for his kindness toward his fellow humans and greatly admired for his oratorical skills. He wrote a number of famous texts including *Anatomy* (the first systematic textbook on animal anatomy), *Dietetics, Physiology, Embryology*, and *Rhizotomikon* (considered to be the first work on botany that included the names of the plants, their habitat, means of collection, and medical uses). His second book on plants described those used for food and his third book dealt with poisonous plants. His works indicate that serious studies on the pharmacology and toxicology of plants had begun. Another famous book by Diocles was one that dealt with personal and social hygiene.

Diocles' recommendations for good health included cleaning teeth, massaging gums, walking and exercising before breakfast (which was a light meal), drinking water before meals, napping in the afternoon, exercising before dinner (just before sunset and followed by white wine diluted with water and honey), walking, and early retiring. Good advice!

Hippocrates and Diocles extended toxicology beyond merely listing poisons and antidotes. Rational methods for the study of the effects of poisons and the treatment of poisoning were proposed. Experimental studies to assess the biological effects of plants had begun.

"Nature does nothing without a purpose." (Aristotle)

Aristotle (384–322 BC) was the son of the court physician to Amyntas II, a student of Plato, a teacher of Alexander the Great, and a philosopher and scientist (though not a physician) who stressed the importance of biology as a science (pre-med curriculum?) and thereby influenced medicine. A scientific genius, he established the foundations for comparative anatomy and embryology. His "Ladder of Nature" was the beginning of the concept of evolution (presaging Darwin). Like other Greek scientists and physicians of his day, he believed that the human body possessed four qualities—hot, cold, dry, and moist; that it was composed of four humors—blood, phlegm, yellow bile, and black bile; and that disease resulted from an imbalance of these. His contributions to toxicology are related to his contributions to science, especially biology.

Theophrastus (372–287 BC), one of Aristotle's most famous pupils, was a philosopher and scientist (probably the most famous Greek botanist/herbalist) who wrote *Theoretical Botany* and *De Historia Plantarum* in 300 BC (two volumes, inquiry into plants and growth of plants). They included the natural history and descriptions of medicinal and poisonous plants and are considered the beginning of modern botany and an excellent medical botany text. Indications for the use of medicinal plants were presented. He was also the first to record adulteration of food. He was interested in food preservation and found that certain soils preserved wheat but in so doing it became adulterated. Others adulterated wheat with soil to increase its weight. His contributions to toxicology include a list of poisonous plants and the recognition of adulteration of food (might he be considered the founder of food toxicology?).

Cato (234–149 BC) was interested in food preservation (salting) and in detecting adulterations, expecially of wine.

Nicander of Colophon (185–135 BC) was a Greek physician, poet, and grammarian who wrote, among other things, two hexameter poems, *Alexipharmaca* (properties of poisonous substances and antidotes) and *Theriaca* (bites and stings of venomous animals and antidotes). Although there were some fanciful parts, much was accurate and reflected upon his powers of observation and his experiences. Theriac has come to mean antidote against poisons. It survived into the 19th century and was considered by some to be a tonic and a means of maintaining good health. His contribution to toxicology is his list of poisons and antidotes.

King Mithridates VI Eupator the Great, king of Pontus, polyglot king (120–63 BC), was considered a military genius and a dabbler in poisons. He evaluated poisons and potential antidotes in slaves and in prisoners (without implied consent or institutional review boards and to eliminate the need for extrapolation!). He was a student of toxicology but was obsessively possessed with a fear of poisons. To provide protection, he took daily doses of poisons (beginning with very small doses and increasing the amounts ingested) to develop polyvalent tolerance (the first recorded successful case); he drank the blood of ducks fed toxic chemicals and took mixtures of antidotes. Mithridatium, his universal antidote, which was presumably invented by one of his physicians, Zopyrus, consisted of 20 leaves of rue, one walnut, a grain of salt, and two dried figs and was to be taken each morning before breakfast to effectively prevent poisoning. The Mithridaticum of Celsus consisted of 36 ingredients, Pliny's 54, and Galen's 73; each pill was the size of a grape and 10 had to be taken before and after food. Mithridates was captured and tried to commit suicide by self-poisoning but proved immune to the actions of the various poisons. He was eventually killed with a sword (a throwback). The term *mithridatics*, antidotes or preventives for poisoning containing many ingredients, immortalizes his contribution to toxicology. He was probably the first to systematically study poisons in humans and thus became the first clinical toxicologist (could be considered the founder of clinical toxicology except for the nature of his clinical studies).

Heraclides Pontius of Tarentum (240 BC), a philosopher and student of Plato, was reported to have spent a great deal of time studying poisons and antidotes, but little remains of his contributions. He used opium to induce sleep and was concerned with cosmetology. His greatest contribution to science was probably his contention that the earth rotated on its own axis.

Andromachus the Elder (ca. 60 AD) was an archiater, the public physician who treated the poor, and the royal physician to Nero. He added squills, viper's flesh, and opium to the mithridatium and administered it, in honey, to Nero. This became known as the Theriaca of Andromachus, Theriaca Andromachi, or Venice Treacle; it contained 70 substances and was used until the 18th century. Interestingly, he wrote 175 Greek iambic verses describing it.

Dioscorides (Pedanius Dioscorides) (40–90 AD), was born in Anazarbia in Cilicia. He was a Greek physician and pharmacologist, physician and surgeon to Nero's army, and the originator of materia medica. He is the author of many texts, including one of the greatest works (if not the greatest) on materia medica of ancient times (77–78 AD). He took advantage of his military travels to study medicinal properties of plants and minerals, which he described in a five-volume series, *De Materia Medica, De Universa Medica*, the leading text in pharmacology for 16 centuries. Included are descriptions of about 600 plants and 1000 simple drugs. His approach differed from that in Eber's Papyrus, in which each disease had listed all the remedies for that disease. Dioscorides described a plant and then listed all the diseases it might cure. Also discussed are the dietetic and therapeutic value of animal products (e.g., milk, honey) and mineral drugs (e.g., mercury, arsenic, lead acetate, calcium hydrate, copper oxide). He also described a surgical anesthetic made from opium and mandragora and one made from an alcoholic extract of mandrake. He was the first to recognize the toxicity of mercury. His contributions to toxicology include classifying poisons into three major classes (animal, plant, mineral), identifying antidotes, and recommending decreasing absorption to control intoxication (for example, by inducing vomiting or purgation; cf. Hippocrates).

Galen of Pergamum (129–199 AD), considered by some to be the greatest Greek physician and surgeon, was the son of an engineer (Nicon) and was very well educated. He traveled widely to increase his knowledge of medicine (as did many others), studied philosophy, and began to write. He eventually became the most celebrated ancient medical writer and influenced medicine for 1500 years. His fame as an outstanding healer in Rome began with the successful treatment of the Aristotelian philosopher Eudemus, an influential Roman, who was dying despite the care of the best physicians in the city. Galen's practice flourished and his patients included the most influential Romans of the period. At this time, he was given a dissecting room in which to study comparative anatomy (using the bodies of slain gladiators). His benefactor, Flavius Boethus, also provided him with secretarial assistance, and several anatomy books followed. Galen is considered the founder of experimental physiology. He was the first to prove that the arteries carried blood and not air and conducted other experiments involving the nervous system, heart, and liver. He taught and practiced that it is essential to select the right drug for the right condition for the right patient; he introduced rationality into drug therapy.

Galen argued that although apothecaries knew drugs, only the physician understood both the drug and the patient, and further, that drugs are tools only for physicians (hence, few experimental nonphysician pharmacologists in Greece). He recommended mixtures of drugs for treating disease, which is the basis for the term *galenicals*. The foundation of his writings was the teachings of Hippocrates. Galen tried to amalgamate the various doctrines espoused by Hippocrates, including qualities, four humors, pneuma, and physis. Galen also believed, as did many early physicians, that health depended upon a balance of the various bodily humors (phlegm, blood, yellow bile, black bile). He identified four personality types (phlegmatic, sanguine, choleric, melancholic) based on these four humors. He tried to establish a composite system of medicine, one that would include formulas/principles that would remove uncertainty from the decisions of practicing physicians. He further developed the theriac, the universal antidote, to include 100 substances, which was to be administered in honey and wine. His advice to physicians (also valid for toxicologists): "If anyone wishes to gain fame through these, and not through clever talk, all that he needs is, without more ado, to accept what I have been able to establish by zealous research."

Paul of Aegina (625–690 AD), celebrated Byzantine physician, authored a seven-volume medical encyclopedia, *Epitome*. It is based on the 70 books by Oribasius and other writings. Book 5 deals with toxicology, specifically bites and wounds of venomous animals. Paul was probably the "last Greek compiler."

The contributions of the Greeks to the advancement of toxicology include comprehensive lists of poisons and antidotes, experimental studies of the biological effects of plants (plant constituents) and metals, and rational methods for the management of poisonings.

Roman

The Romans also had an intense interest in poisons. They derived a great deal of their knowledge of medicine from the Greeks and from other cultures. Aurelius Cornelius Celsus (30 BC–AD 50), the "Cicero of physicians," "Hippocrates of the Romans," the greatest Roman medical writer and an armchair physician, was a Roman nobleman of the Cornelii family, a man of letters, and an encyclopedist who authored the outstanding encyclopedia of his day and a number of books on medical subjects. He provided a systematic survey of medicine, presented sound principles of good surgery, and stressed the application of common sense to medical issues. Only eight volumes of his classic *De Medicina* survived. It was a medical classic and included discussions of many diseases. The importance of dietetics in treatment was stressed. He was the first to identify the four signs of inflammation: calor, rubor, tumor, and dolor.

He also stressed cleanliness, the use of vinegar (currently experiencing a renaissance) and thyme oil to cleanse wounds, the use of ligatures to stop bleeding, and the use of skin from other parts of the body for facial plastic surgery. He believed that "the best medicament is food opportunely given." He also introduced the nutrient enema. *De Medicina* is considered basically Hippocratic with some methodism. Book 5, *Toxicology and Rabies*, included the works of Nicander and Dioscorides and poisons and antidotes. Celsus was not interested in mechanisms or theories of poisoning. He cited others who believed that poisons and animal venoms depressed the vital factor resulting in the loss of innate heat and chilling. Incidentally, *De Medicina* was one of the first medical works to be published after the introduction of the printing press (1478).

Consistent with Hippocratic teaching, Celsus also advocated getting rid of the poison as quickly as possible. He proposed free bleeding, sucking the wound, amputation, promoting evacuation, eliciting heating action (by administering hot, peppery materials or by the application of the warm flesh of a freshly killed fowl or small animal to a wound), and "poisoning the poison" (acrid materials applied to wounds, cupping severe wounds, suction with palms of the hand, and the use of hypertonic salt solutions). In addition, he recommended the use of appropriate antidotes (including the antidote of Mithridates, 37 ingredients in honey). His contributions to toxicology include his list of poisons and antidotes and the management of poisoning.

Pliny the Elder, Gaius Plinius Secundus (23–79 AD), was born in Como. He was a famous Roman naturalist, historian, military tactician, philosopher, and one of the most learned men of his time. He wrote 160 books. Although he was not trained in medicine, he chronicled medical history. His quest for knowledge was insatiable (it is said that he died while trying to observe an eruption of Vesuvius). He collected data about all living things. He was skeptical of the value of mithridatics. He described poisonous plants and animals and the types of injury they cause in his famous *Historia Naturalis* (Natural History), a compendium of information that consisted of 37 books. He advocated the doctrine of signatures, which stated that the therapeutic usefulness of a plant, mineral, or animal was based on its resemblance to the signs of a disease. This doctrine persisted for many centuries and still has a few proponents. He was also interested in adulteration of foods and developed methods for the detection of adulteration (e.g., chalk in flour, herbs, and spices). Like Hippocrates and others, he believed the "the greatest aid to health is moderation in food." His contributions to toxicology include lists of poisons and their biological effects and his questioning of the value of nonspecific antidotes like mithridatics.

Arab

The Arabs made significant contributions to the health professions. For example, their pharmacies are considered to be the forerunners of modern pharmacies. Since Avicenna believed in the importance of keeping patients happy, he instructed pharmacists to make medicines pleasant. To this end, the pharmacists developed sugar-coated pills, mixed rose water or perfumes with medicines, and were the first to wrap medicines (pellets) in silver foil. To make the physician's job easier and to promote more effective healing, Arabian pharmacists are credited with developing or perfecting tinctures, confections, syrups, pomades, plasters, and ointments.

Avicenna (Abu Ali Husain ibn Abdullah ibn Sina, 980–1037), the "Prince of Physicians," was born in Bokhara, Persia. He was a child prodigy who knew the Koran by heart at the age of 10. He studied philosophy, jurisprudence, and mathematics; at the age of 16 he turned to the study of medicine. By 18, his fame as a physician was so great that he was appointed physician to the prince and became physician-in-chief to the hospital in Baghdad. Avicenna was given access to the library of the prince as a token of gratitude and appreciation for healing the prince of a serious ailment. He was also the personal physician to other caliphs. By the age of 21, he had written a 20-volume encyclopedia. He developed a philosophy (avicennism) that was partly Aristotelian and partly new platonic. His most significant medical works were his *Book of Healing* and *Canon of Medicine*, a five-volume treatise that included *The Theory of Medicine, Simpler Drugs, Special Pathology and Therapeutics, General Diseases*, and *Pharmacopoeia*. He also discussed oral and parenteral poisons, bites and stings and their treatment, and classified and discussed poisons as plant, animal, or mineral (cf. Ebers Papyrus). He was also the first to describe the fetid odor exhaled by those poisoned by mercury (Ecobichon, personal communication). In addition, he developed his own psychiatry and believed that psychic alterations were the result of changes in the brain (pathology due to humors [neurotransmitters?]).

His books were logically arranged (an example of "Aristotelian dialectic and Arabian scholasticism"). He was a logical thinker and an astute observer. Some have referred to him as a second Aristotle. Avicenna wanted to develop a system of medicine, to make medicine "a quasi-mathematical discipline." This would remove uncertainty from medical decisions (cf. Galen). His contributions to toxicology include mechanisms of action of poisons including neurotoxicity and metabolic effects. He also recommended the bezoar stone as an antidote for venoms and preventive of disease. Despite his many accomplishments, Avicenna was not "a dryasdust;" he was "a man of the world, he loved wine, women, and song- more ardently, perhaps, than was good for his health. ... But before he reached the age of fifty-eight his bodily powers were exhausted, and he died" (some believe of an overdose of opium). His work was the authoritative text on poisons and antidotes for 500 years.

Note that the Arabs translated most of the important Greek works. The Arabs excelled in chemistry and invented distillation, sublimation, and crystallization. They introduced camphor, benzoin, saffron, laudanum, and naphtha.

> Arabian doctors as a rule watched each other jealously. Disagreements were at times settled by duel-by-poison. In such duels each doctor was expected to take his opponent's poison, then find a quick antidote. Two court physicians once tried it: The first doctor's draught was fierce enough to "melt black stone," but his rival parried with an antidote. Then the second doctor picked a rose, mumbled an incantation, and asked his antagonist to sniff the flower. The first doctor complied, and promptly fell dead. Fright had killed him, for the rose was only a rose.

The Persians also believed in the "Poison Maiden." An attractive young girl was fed poisons (increasing doses of a number of poisons) so she became very "venomous" (double seduction). A kiss or sexual intercourse with her would prove fatal to her lover. Avicenna mentions such a girl; she was so venomous that insects that bit her were poisoned and died.

> "Man should believe nothing that is not attested to (1) by rational proof as in mathematical science, (2) by evidence of the senses or (3) by authority of prophets and saints." (Maimonides)

Rabbi Moses ben Maimon (Moses Maimonides, 1135–1204), was a famous Jewish philosopher and physician, court physician to Saladin, and rabbi of Cairo. His book on poisons, *Poisons and Antidotes/ Upon Poisoning and Its Treatment*, was translated into Latin by Armend and Blasii in 1305, into French in 1865, and into German in 1873 by Steinschneider. He described poisonous insects and animals and noted that the most dangerous bite was that of a fasting human. His treatment of poisons included "ligature of the bite, sucking out the poison by means of cupping glasses or with the oiled lips, again extending Hippocratic teaching to decrease absorption, and the use of external (e.g., salt, onions, asafetida) and internal remedies (e.g., emetics)." It was a much-cited text. His books on health were very advanced and are considered modern. He believed in the importance of preventive medicine and stressed the importance of hygiene; he wrote a four-volume treatise upon hygiene and diet (*Sepher Rephuoth*). His aphorisms are as pertinent today as when they were written.

Others

Pietro de Abano (1250–1316) was born in Abano near Padua. He was a teacher of science and medicine at the University of Padua and one of the most famous teachers and skillful physicians of his time, and the author of *De Venemis*, a book of poisons. Like others before him, he classified poisons as mineral, vegetable, and animal, and he was the first to identify sound as a potential poison. He further noted that poisons can be absorbed from air and through the skin ("poisoning by touch"). The book was very popular and went through 14 editions. He also wrote *Conciliator Differentiarium*, an attempt to reconcile Greek and Arabic medicine. This tradition in toxicology has been maintained even until today, when Marcello Lotti directs an internationally recognized institute of occupational/medicine and toxicology.

The age of observations (recording phenomena) and categorizing and listing poisons gave way to the period of challenge and active investigation—experimental toxicology—through the efforts of one of the most controversial yet influential figures in medicine, Paracelsus. Although others made observations in humans (often after deliberately administering a poison), Paracelsus encouraged the use of animals to study poisons. He also developed and promulgated certain basic principles of the action of chemicals (e.g., dose-response) that still form the scientific underpinnings of modern experimental toxicology.

THE AGE OF EXPERIMENTAL TOXICOLOGY

> "The universities do not teach all things." (Paracelsus)

Philippus Theophrastus Aureolus Bombastus von Hohenheim (Paracelsus, 1492–1541) was born near the village of Einsiedeln near Zurich, Switzerland, on November 10 (or 14), the son of Wilhelm Bombast von Hohenheim, a German physician/alchemist. Following the death of his mother when he was still very young, Paracelsus with his father moved to Villach in southern Austria, where his father taught chemistry, practiced medicine, and became interested in the health problems of the local miners, eventually becoming an expert in occupational medicine. Paracelsus attended the universities of Basel, Tubingen, Wittenberg, Leipzig, Heidelberg, Cologne, and Vienna, from which he received a baccalaureate in medicine in 1510, at the age of 17. He received his doctorate from the University of Ferrara in 1516. Since it was the custom of the humanists at that time to Latinize their names after they received their degree, he began using the name Paracelsus (*para* Celsus, above Celsus), since he considered himself greater than Celsus. Deichmann et al. (1986) claimed that Paracelsus "is a Greco-Roman translation of *Hohenheim* and says 'next to heaven.'" He traveled throughout Europe, England, Scotland, Egypt, the Holy Land, and Constantinople, attempting to learn the most effective means of medical treatment and the latest findings in alchemy.

He wanted to discover "the latent forces of nature" and wrote, "He who is born in imagination discovers the latent forces of Nature ... besides the stars that are established, there is yet another—Imagination—that begets a new star and a new heaven." He returned to Villach in 1524 and became town physician and lecturer in medicine at the University of Basel in 1527. His fame had spread, and students flocked to his lectures.

Paracelsus believed all physicians who preceded him were incompetent, liars, or fakers. "I am to be the monarch, and the monarchy will belong to me." He defied tradition (a young Turk!). Paracelsus drastically and permanently changed the course of medicine. Although a theosophist and an iconoclast, he was a keen student of human behavior, a forerunner of Freud, a chemical anatomist, the founder of medicinal chemistry, and the "godfather of modern chemotherapy," who believed that practicing physicians needed to use common sense, gain experience, travel, and practice humility (good advice that is relevant and sound today). He was a peripatetic physician and was always trying to learn more medicine. His approach to medicine and the body was chemical. For example, he taught that it was more important to learn about the chemical composition of the body than about the muscles. Since God created (caused) diseases, God (Nature) also provided cures. It was the role of the alchemist (chemist) to find these and convert them to effective remedies. Paracelsus began with simple materials, the metals. When the "conservative physicians" warned that metals would poison patients, Paracelsus replied, "This poison, as you call it, has a far better effect than the wagon grease ... with which you are so fond of smearing your patients."

His disdain for established authorities, for everything that had been said by his predecessors, reached its climax on 24 June 1527 when he publicly burned the books of Avicenna and Galen in front of the university. He discarded the old ways, including humoral pathology, but upheld Hippocrates; he attacked medical principles of his time, trusted only his own observations, ideas, and works, and tried to bring chemistry into therapeutics by encouraging the use of mineral salts, acids, and chemically prepared therapeutic agents ("better living through chemistry"), since he believed that the body was a chemical laboratory.

Paracelsus was a free thinker. He developed his own system of medicine and boasted about his contempt for science. One of his methods of learning was theosophical intuition; that is, all knowledge is the result of mystical insight, all wisdom comes directly from God, and one should be in intimate contact with God and God's creation. Submit to the will of God and all knowledge will flow. This intuitive process of learning was also part of gnosticism. He appeared to be contemptuous of the established way of thinking and believed that man was a little world (microcosm) that contained all knowledge. This was based on man's direct descendancy from Adam, who had within himself all sciences since he contained the germs of all creatures. In his book *Paramirum*, Paracelsus described his system of medicine. Health, disease, and human destiny depend upon five entia (cf. Shen Nung); disease is caused by the five entities: ens astrale (influence of the stars), ens venini (influence of nutrition/poisons in food), ens naturale (nature and functions of the body), ens spirituale (spirits, demons), and ens Dei (acts of God directly upon us to restore order and health). His theory of humors included three elementary principles: salt (representing stability), sulfur (representing combustibility), and mercury (representing liquidity). Disease is a separation of one principle from the other two (disequilibrium among humors/principles?). He also believed, according to Cole, that there are five phlegms, five hydropathies, five jaundices, five fevers, five cancers, and so forth. Diseases tend to be localized in a particular "target" organ. Although he tried to bring more chemistry into medicine (e.g., by the use of inorganic salts), he also believed that God will provide cures for us since God is benevolent.

Paracelsus wrote that "nature hints at cures." This is the basis for the doctrine of signatures (cf. Pliny the Elder, "that an agent of nature shows by its external forms its unique qualities"). For example, since turmeric is yellow, use it to treat jaundice, foxglove for heart, figwort for scrofula, and hepatica for liver disease. Cope (1957) described Paracelsus as arrogant and conceited "almost to the point of insanity ... extremely effective in [his] criticisms of the then accepted doctrines ... reveled in the wildest speculations and taught [his] mad conjectures as unassailable truths ... bitter and unscrupulous controversialist ... mystic ... his writings ... so confused and obscure as to be often quite unintelligible ... braggart, scorner of authority ... that Paracelsus scarcely ever lectured except when he was half drunk, or attended a patient until he was wholly drunk." Paracelsus defended himself in his *Seven Arguments, Answering to Several of the Detractions of His Envious Critics*, written in 1537.

But what of Paracelsus's positive contributions? He was an original but eccentric thinker. He is considered by some to be the father (founder) of chemistry and/or medicinal chemistry and the reformer of materia medica. He did not support the humoral basis for disease; he believed that diseases were specific/discrete conditions and are cured by specific/discrete treatments. He taught that observation and experience are essential for success in medicine (and in science?). He is credited with the introduction of the following into the practice of medicine of his day: mineral baths, laudanum, mercury, lead, arsenic, copper sulfate, and iron. He forever destroyed the doctrine of the four humors. His principal works include

Chirurgia magna (1536), *De gradibus* (1568), and *A Treatise on Diseases of Miners* (1567). In one of his books, *Paragranum*, he presents the four pillars upon which medicine should be based: philosophy (knowledge of nature; disease and healing are part of nature); astronomy (heaven paternalistically deals with us); chemistry (provide drugs and insight into biological events; "nature is the ideal chemist"); and virtue (love is the foundation of medicine). In his *Third Defense*, he wrote, "What is there that is not poison? All things are poison and nothing (is) without poison. Solely, the dose determines that a thing is not a poison." (Deichmann et al., 1986). This is often misquoted as "the dose makes the poison." This concept has been expanded to include no-effect level, threshold, extrapolation, and dose-response relationship. His other contributions include target-organ toxicity, animal experimentation to study the effects of chemicals, and the use of inorganic salts in medicine. He was thoroughly seduced by the complexity of chemical–biological interactions and spent his lifetime trying to solve the mysteries of these interactions.

Paracelsus's teachings in psychiatry are often overlooked and may be as significant as his contributions in other medically related areas. For example, he believed that in man there are two antagonistic forces, animal and godly, and that man has to suppress the animal spirit if he is to be successful (yin and yang, id and superego?). He also believed that psychoses are not demonic in origin, the mind (will or spirit) can influence the state of the body (cure or cause some diseases—psychosomatic medicine?) and not the existence of a subconscious, and that women are different from men and must be treated differently ("men are from Mars and women are from Venus").

Paracelsus was a deeply religious man. "He was intensely concerned with the eternity, or soul, in man, and felt that a doctor was neither "pillmaker" nor businessman, but a legate of God, the supreme physician. Medicine was therefore a divine mission, and the doctor must raise his eyes from "excrements and salvepots to the stars." The perfect physician, he felt, was a philosopher, an astrologer, an alchemist and above all, a virtuous man. The character of such a doctor, Paracelsus proclaimed, was far more effective than mere mechanical skill (Amen!) (Bettman, 1959).

Paracelsus died prematurely at age 49. Some say he died in a brawl at the White Horse Tavern in Salzburg on 24 December 1541, presumably exhausted. Despite his early death, he made an indelible mark on medicine and especially on toxicology.

The French physician, poet, and playwright Jacques Grevin (1538–1570), "the father of modern biotoxicology," published his classical work, *Deux Livres des Venins*, in 1568 and further developed the concept of chemical–biological interactions.

Some of the concepts developed by Paracelsus were further developed by others. For example, Felice Abate Fontana (1720–1805), an abbot, physician, physiologist, naturalist, and professor of philosophy at Pisa and director of the Natural History Museum at Florence, advanced the concept of target-organ toxicity; that is, the symptoms of poisoning are the result of poisons acting on a particular organ. He is considered the first modern scientist to study venoms (*Ricerche fisiche sopra il veleno della vipera*, 1767). He is also known for the spaces of Fontana (*Dei moti dell'iride*, 1765). Although Paracelsus drew attention to the plight of miners, little attention was focused on the effects of nondeliberate exposure to chemicals, for example, in the workplace. It was the brilliant Italian physician Bernardino Ramazzini (1633–1714) who effectively and convincingly brought the workplace situation to the attention of the world, especially to the field of medicine. He was the first to describe, in a comprehensive, systematic, and detailed fashion, industrial health problems in his *De Morbis Artificium Diatriba* and his famous *Diseases of Tradesmen/Workers*, which was originally published in 1700; the English edition appeared in 1705. As an astute scientist and physician, he had remarkable powers of observation. He first described "stone mason's consumption [silicosis], potter's sciatica, gilder's ophthalmia and lead poisoning." He is the founder of occupational/industrial medicine. He also advocated the use of cinchona bark to treat malaria, which ran counter to Galen's recommendation that it be treated with purgatives.

The observations of Ramazzini concerning the relationship between workplace exposure and disease were strengthened and extended by the classical studies of Sir Percival Pott (1714–1788), the famed British physician and surgeon to St. Bartholomew's Hospital, who achieved fame in two areas, occupational medicine/toxicology and orthopedics. He sustained an ankle fracture following a fall and described it so well that it became known as Pott's fracture (*Treatise on Fractures*, 1750/1769). Pott's disease (caries of the spine) was first described by Percival Pott. He later described the relationship between scrotal cancer and soot in chimney sweeps (1775). His contributions to toxicology include the identification of chemical carcinogenesis in humans and noting the increased sensitivity of children to chemicals (a concept currently enjoying a resurgence).

Attempts to explain the action of toxins attracted the attention of some of the intellectual giants in the biomedical sciences (intellectual seduction). A few will be mentioned. Ambrose Pare (1510–1590) has been called "the greatest surgeon of the 16th century," the founder of modern surgery, and one of the most famous anatomists of all time. He introduced the use of ligatures of blood vessels as opposed to cauterization and authored many books on medical topics, including anatomy, surgery, malformations, and obstetrics. He investigated CO poisoning and published a report in 1575. On the other side of the channel, Richard Mead (1673–1754), a British physician with a medical degree from Padua who worked at St. Thomas' Hospital and was also physician to the royal family, attempted to explain the action of poisons (venoms) in his book *A Mechanical Account of Poisons* (1702). He described snake poisoning and noted that the venom is only effective parenterally. To prove this, he swallowed the venom and (fortunately) nothing happened. He also authored a book on the influence of the sun and moon on human bodies. The formal beginning of mechanistic toxicology, however, was to await the experiments of Magendie and Bernard, discussed later.

Forensic toxicology, the application of analytical techniques to the detection of poisons, had its beginning with Joseph Jacob Plenck (1738–1807), who noted in his text, *Elementa Medicinae et Chirurgiae Forensis*, that "the only certain sign is the chemical identification of the poison in the organs of the body," which is still a basic principle of forensic toxicology. Unfortunately, his works were not accepted by the medical or scientific communities of his day.

The application of analytical chemistry to matters of food and drug safety formally began with Friedrich Accum (1769–1838), although earlier attempts were made by Theophrastus (370–285 BC), Cato (234–129 BC), Pliny the Elder (23–79), Dioscoridies (40–90), and Galen (131–201). Born in Buckebourg, Germany, Accum moved to London in 1797 as a pharmacist and in 1801 began working with Sir Humphrey Davy. Being entrepreneurial, he also set up his own contract laboratory and supply house. He was the first to use analytical chemistry to detect adulterants in food and published *A Treatise on Adulterations of Food and Culinary Poisons* in 1820, a very successful book that was acclaimed worldwide. He later published *An Attempt to Discover the Genuineness and Purity of Drugs and Medicinal Preparations*. He left England and returned to Germany because of the many (false) charges directed against him.

THE AGE OF MECHANISTIC AND ANALYTICAL TOXICOLOGY

> When you can measure what you are speaking about, and express it in numbers, you know something about it; but when you cannot measure it, when you cannot express it in numbers, your knowledge is of a meager and unsatisfactory kind; it may be the beginning of knowledge, but you have scarcely in your thoughts, advanced to the stage of science. (William Thomson, Lord Kelvin)

The adverse effects of chemicals (including poisons) in humans and extensive lists of poisons and antidotes had been recorded, some poisons had been evaluated in animals, and analytical techniques were being applied to toxicological problems. Toxicology was being recognized as a scientific discipline. But little was being done to answer the basic question, "How do poisons kill?" The era of mechanistic toxicology formally began with the classical studies of the two most famous physiologists in medical history, François Magendie and his pupil Claude Bernard. Contributions had been made by others, but these were limited and not as systematic, fundamental, and far-reaching as those of Magendie and Bernard.

François Magendie (1783–1855), French physician and experimental physiologist, contributed significantly to the advancement of physiology, medicine, and toxicology. For example, he demonstrated the functioning of spinal nerves and he studied blood flow, swallowing, and vomiting. He is credited with the introduction of strychnine, iodine, and bromine compounds into medicine. His interest in the functioning of the nervous system led him to establish the mechanisms of action of emetine and strychnine and the dynamics of movement across body membranes. He was also the first, or one of the first, to observe and describe anaphylactic shock. His most famous pupil, Claude Bernard (1813–1878), the son of a Burgundian vinegrower, studied pharmacy and enjoyed science, but wanted to be a playwright; his critics told him to study medicine and fortunately for humankind, he accepted their advice. He went to Paris and was accepted as an assistant by François Magendie at the Hotel Dieu. He enthusiastically endorsed Magendie's philosophy that physiologists must discover the laws of "vital manifestations" or physiological functions and that observation and experimentation were the only methods of investigation. He received his degree in 1843; his thesis dealt with gastric juice and digestion. He and Magendie did much to advance physiology, especially of the nervous system (autonomic) and the gastrointestinal tract, including the liver. Bernard studied both normal and pathological physiology. His contributions to toxicology include furthering the concept of target organ toxicity, establishing approaches to defining the mechanism of action of drugs and other chemicals (e.g., curare, nicotine, carbon monoxide), demonstrating that the basic principles of pharmacology and toxicology are identical, and showing that drugs and other chemicals can modify the function and structure of tissues. He believed that "the physiological analysis of organic systems ... can be done with the aid of toxic agents" (a new use for poisons!). His works were published in 18 volumes. One of his most famous, *An Introduction to the Study of Experimental Medicine*, was published in

1865 and translated into English in 1949. It is a classic in the field of experimental biology and "must" reading for all students of biology and medicine.

> "One must break the bonds of philosophic and scientific systems as one would break the chains of scientific slavery. Systems tend to enslave the human spirit" (Introduction to *l'Etude de la Medicine experimental*, 1865).

Bernard's work stimulated others to experimentally establish the mechanisms of action of toxic agents and to publish textbooks. For example, Francesco Rognetta (1800–1857), an Italian physician and scientist, significantly advanced our knowledge of the mechanisms of action of toxic agents, especially arsenic. The Florentine physician and scientist R. Bellini (1817–1878) authored the first experimental toxicology text, entitled *Lezioni Sperimentali de Tossicologia*. The discipline of toxicology was also advanced by the outstanding research efforts of such noted pharmacologists as Rudolph Buchheim, Oswald Schmiedeberg, and Lewis Lewin (again noting the closeness of these two disciplines).

The time had come for analytical techniques to be formally incorporated into toxicology. It had been difficult to establish poisons as the cause of death since they could not be identified in tissues, the only scientifically valid proof. Analytical (forensic) toxicology had its formal origins in the outstanding work of Orfila. His investigations were also the forerunner of modern pharmaco- and toxicokinetics and dynamics.

> "Measure what can be measured; make measurable what cannot" (Galileo).

Mathieu Joseph Bonaventure Orfila (1787–1853) was born on the island of Minorca. He was educated in Valencia and Barcelona and studied chemistry and medicine in Paris, receiving his medical degree from the University of Paris in 1811. In 1813–1815, he published his classical and monumental two-volume work, *Traité de Toxicologie: Traité des poisons tirés des regnes mineral, végétal at animal ou toxicologie générale considerée sous les rapports de la physiologie, de la pathologie et de la médecine légale* (Crochard, Paris). This is probably the first book devoted entirely to toxicology and thereby established toxicology as an experimental science different from pharmacology. Orfila classified poisons into six classes including animal, vegetable, and mineral (not unique; cf. Ebers Papyrus and others). He presented the chemical, physical, physiological, and toxic properties of each chemical, methods of treatment and chemical tests for their identification. This classic work, the first of its kind, effectively combined forensic and clinical toxicology with analytical chemistry. It was translated into English in 1817. In 1816, Orfila published *Eléments de chimie médecale* and in 1818, *Secours à donner aux personnes empoisonnées ou asphyxiés*. He provided a rational basis for some antidotes. He demonstrated the toxicity of strychnine in numerous experiments on dogs. At that time, strychnine was widely used in prescriptions and in tonics and was considered by practitioners of medicine to be a safe drug (Magendie later established the mechanism of action of strychnine). He later published *Leçons de médecine légale* (1821), in which he classified poisons as "irritants, narcotics, narcotico-acrids and putrefiants."

Orfila's books were translated into many languages and this helped him to internationalize toxicology (presaging the efforts of Coulston, Doull, Golberg, Zbinden, and others). He was appointed professor of legal medicine at the University of Paris and became dean of the faculty in 1831. He founded the Musée Orfila of Comparative Anatomy. He retired in 1848 and died in 1853. Orfila was an excellent analytical chemist and very capable physician; he was an experimentalist and administered known doses of poisons to animals, carefully observed effects produced, examined organs for evidence of toxicity (target-organ toxicity), and chemically analyzed tissues and body fluids to establish relationships between dose, response, and tissue levels. He was able to demonstrate conclusively and quantitatively that poisons are absorbed from the gastrointestinal tract and accumulate in tissues. His significant contributions to toxicology include the chemical detection of poisons in tissues and fluids, thereby permitting better diagnoses; furthering the concept of target organ toxicity by evaluating tissues grossly and histologically; relating symptoms to specific tissue injury; and extending the concept of dose-response.

His influence on modern toxicology is legendary and probably secondary only to that of Paracelsus and Bernard. His books were published in many languages and used in many countries (including the United States). He spawned other works in toxicology and brought to toxicology the recognition it deserved and needed. For example, Sir Robert Christison (1797–1882), a noted Scottish physician with a medical degree from Edinburgh, studied toxicology with Orfila and became professor of forensic medicine and materia medica at Edinburgh. He published *A Treatise on Poisons* in 1829. The fourth edition, published in 1845, became the first American edition. He also strove to provide a further scientific basis for toxicology. His works helped develop the basis for expert witnessing (and created opportunities for consultants!). Alfred Swaine Taylor (1806–1880), famous British physician and the founder of British forensic medicine, is also the founder of modern medical jurisprudence, a natural sequel to the development of forensic toxicology. He received a diploma from the Apothecaries Society in 1828, his certificate to practice from the Royal College of Surgery in 1830, and presented the first course in medical jurisprudence in England in 1831. He taught chemistry and medical jurisprudence at Guy's Hospital. He was probably the most famous expert witness of his time and published his *Manual of Medical Jurisprudence* in 1842. It became very popular, and the tenth edition was published in 1879.

Other forensic toxicologists of note include the following: Henry Coley, New York City forensic toxicologist, published *Poisons and Asphyxia* in 1832. Included in this book were mineral acids, caustic alkalis, ammonia, nitrates, phosphorus, cyanide, metals, and alkaloids, as well as their chemistry, uses, signs and symptoms of poisoning, cause of death, postmortem findings and treatments. James M. Marsh, developed a test for arsenic (1836). Duflos, developed a test for systematically searching for mineral poisons that involved wet ashing with chlorine (1838). Hugo Reinsch, developed a test for arsenic and mercury (1842). Frensenius and von Bobo reported on a systematic scheme for detection of mineral poisons using wet ashing with chlorine (1844); Jean Servais Stas developed a method for extracting alkaloids from cadavers (1850). T. Graham and A. W. Hofman reported on the adsorbing properties of charcoal (adsorbed strychnine from beer) and proposed utilizing adsorption in toxicological analyses (1853). Theodore George Wormley published *Microchemistry of Poisons*, the first American toxicology textbook (1867). Lieben reported on an iodoform test for alcohol (1870). K. L. Dey developed a test for opium in toxicological analysis. A. W. Blyth published *Poisons: Their Effects and Detection*, an excellent analytical toxicological text (1884). Rudolph A. Witthaus and Tracy C. Becker edited a four-volume text, *Medical Jurisprudence, Forensic Medicine and Toxicology*, which became the standard reference text in the field (1894–1896). Walter S. Haines and Frederick Peterson wrote a toxicology text (1903). Alexander Gettler, who probably influenced the development of forensic toxicology in America more than anyone else, began working in the Office of the Chief Medical Examiner in New York City (1918). Rolla Harger developed the Drunkometer for testing drivers presumed to be under the influence (1937).

Advances in chemistry, physiology, pathology, and clinical medicine in the 18th and 19th centuries resulted in significant advances in toxicology. The discipline of toxicology was recognized in the scientific community as a distinct entity, separate from pharmacology and drawing upon chemical, biological, and physical sciences. Today, toxicology continues to benefit from advances in all the sciences.

The advances in forensic toxicology paralleled advances made in understanding the basic mechanisms of action of chemicals and drugs. The mechanistic studies of Claude Bernard were furthered by many scientists including the brilliant German chemist, microbiologist, and immunologist Paul Ehrlich (1854–1915) who significantly advanced mechanistic toxicology (toxicodynamics) and pharmacology (pharmacodynamics). His keen interest in chemistry and biological structure and function led him to propose the concept of a receptor as the sensitive site for chemical–biological interaction; that "chemical substances in organisms had specific points of attachment" (receptors), and once these were known, specific remedies could be developed. His most famous remedy was the use of arsenic in the management of syphilis (Compound 606, arsphenamine). He subsequently identified several receptors. His successful bout with tuberculosis stimulated his interest in immunity (as did his association with Koch), and he subsequently formulated the concepts of active and passive immunity and the side-chain theory of immunity. His contributions to toxicology and pharmacology include developing the receptor theory (the founder of the receptor theory), underscoring the importance of mechanistic studies and structure–activity relationships. He shared the Nobel prize for physiology and medicine with E. Metchnikoff in 1908.

Rudolph Kobert (1854–1918), a student of Oswald Schmiedeberg (one of the founders of modern pharmacology and toxicology and himself a student of Rudolph Buchheim, the founder of modern pharmacology), published a toxicology textbook (1893). A contemporary, Louis Lewin (1854–1929) reported on the toxicology of alcohols, chloroform, opiates, and plant-derived hallucinogens and also wrote a toxicology text (1929).

Mechanistic studies led to a better understanding of the toxic action of many chemicals and to the development of specific antidotes: for example, the use of BAL (dimercaprol) as an antidote for arsenic (based on the studies of Carl Voegtlin [1923] and Rudolph Peters [1945]), nitrite and thiosulfate for cyanide (K. K. Chen [1934], one of America's most distinguished pharmacologists), and organophosphorus compounds and the use of 2-PAM (Wilson [1951, 1955] and W. Lange and G. Schrader [1952]).

Occupational medicine and industrial toxicology were identified by Paracelsus, systematized and advanced by the pioneering efforts of Bernardo Ramazzini, and further advanced by one of America's foremost physicians, Alice Hamilton (1869–1970). Physician and pathologist, she researched occupational diseases, publicized the hazards of industrial chemicals to workers, and wrote several books on industrial toxicology. She was the foremost woman occupational physician and industrial hygienist, the first woman faculty member of the Harvard Medical School, and the only woman to serve on the Health Committee of the League of Nations. She graphically described the history of industrial toxicology/occupational medicine in the United States in her autobiography, *Exploring the Dangerous Trades* (1943). Others who contributed significantly to this field include Cecil Drinker (1887–1919) of Harvard; R. Bohm (who believed that toxicological information was accumulating very rapidly; mechanisms of toxicity were being elaborated and exposure to chemicals was increasing due to advances [?] in manufacturing); and Ethel Browning (1891–1979), who received her doctorate in medicine in 1927 and wrote the *Toxicity of Industrial Organic Solvents* in 1937. Interestingly, this was the first book on this subject and was written when Browning had no personal occupational medical experience. Her other publications included *Ionizing Radiations* (1959), *Toxicity of Industrial Metals* (1961), and her greatest work, *Toxicity and Metabolism of Industrial Solvents* (1965).

The stage was set for the application of toxicological principles and findings to protection of the public and especially workers from the adverse effects of chemical exposure. Consumers also needed protection from the potentially adverse effects of chemicals found in air, water, foods, and other consumer products.

AGE OF SAFETY EVALUATION, QUANTIFICATION, AND PROGNOSTICATION

> "In no single thing do men approach the gods more readily than in giving of safety to mankind" (Cicero).

In the United States, Harvey Washington Wiley (1844–1930), physician and chemist, served as head of the Bureau of Chemistry of the U.S. Department of Agriculture from 1883 to 1912. His main goal was to provide effective food and drug legislation to protect the unsuspecting public. His efforts culminated in the first U.S. Food and Drug Act (1906), which has been expanded and which formed the basis for food safety legislation worldwide. He issued a number of bulletins summarizing his studies of the effects of food chemicals in human subjects, the "Poison Squad." He wrote, "Injury to public health, in my opinion, is the least important question in the subject of food adulteration, and it is the one which should be considered last of all. The real evil of food adulteration is deception of the consumer." Wiley also served as Director of Foods, Health and Sanitation for Good Housekeeping magazine from 1912 to 1930. He wrote a number of books, including *Principles and Practices of Agricultural Analysis* (three volumes, 1894–1897), *Foods and their Adulteration* (1907), and *History of a Crime Against the Food Law* (1929). Another prominent regulatory pharmacologist/toxicologist was Arnold J. Lehman (1900–1979), who earned his PhD from the University of Washington in Seattle in 1930 and his MD from Stanford in 1936. He taught at a number of universities and joined the U.S. Food and Drug Administration as Director of the Division of Pharmacology in 1946. He and his staff published *Appraisal of the Safety of Chemicals in Foods, Drugs and Cosmetics*, in 1955, the first attempt by the agency to provide guidelines for toxicological studies (this presaged the Redbooks). He and his colleagues, most notably O. Garth Fitzhugh, developed the concept of safety factors (a number applied to the highest dose that did not elicit an adverse effect in a properly designed and executed toxicological study, the no-observed-adverse effect level, NOAEL). He is also renowned for the expression on his office wall: "You too can become a toxicologist in two easy lessons, each ten years long." He was succeeded by Leo Friedman (formerly of MIT), who advocated the use of in utero exposure in lifetime studies. Sandford Miller (also of MIT) served as successor to Friedman. To assist toxicologists concerned with the safety of food and color additives, the U.S. Food and Drug Administration issued a series of guidelines, Redbook I and II. The Organization for Economic Cooperation and Development (OECD) issued similar guidelines. Both of these guidelines are designed to encourage sound science and the conservation of resources while providing adequate data for determining safe exposure limits for consumers. The first comprehensive text to address the principles and practices of toxicology was edited by A. Wallace Hayes.

At the international level, the World Health Organization (WHO), through the enlightened efforts of Frank Lu and Gaston Vettorazzi, applied sound toxicological thinking to establishing safe exposure conditions for food chemicals including pesticides. They developed the concept of an acceptable daily intake (ADI) based on sound toxicological data and the proper use of appropriate safety factors (SF). This concept is recognized and used worldwide and has been found very effective. There have been no significant problems with food chemicals evaluated in this manner. The evaluations are conducted through the auspices of the International Programme on Chemical Safety (IPCS), and implemented by the Joint Expert Committee on Food Additives (JECFA) and the Joint Meeting on Pesticide Residues (JMPR), under the chairmanship of John Herrman.

> "Even while they teach, men [they] learn" (Seneca).

> "Toxicology is the ultimate Renaissance science." (Gillett, 1987)

> "Irrespective of its location and source of identity, toxicology as a field must studiously cross many traditional boundaries. ... The science of toxicology is located somewhere between medicine and the sciences, but drawn toward law by forensic uses and the need to regulate various human activities. Societal values and needs tug the field more into the center of the tetrahedron." (Gillett, 1987).

As toxicology became a recognized scientific discipline and more were seduced by its scientific and public health appeal, training programs began. Although it was very difficult to develop programs that could address the many facets of toxicology including chemistry and biochemistry, physiology and pharmacology, pathology, statistics, and epidemiology, excellent training programs were developed at some of the most prestigious universities. Examples included, in the United States, California, Chicago, Harvard, Iowa, Kansas, Medical College of Virginia, New York University, Rochester, and Vanderbilt; in Germany, Freiburg, Hannover, Tubingen, and Wuurzburg; in Sweden, Karolinska; in Denmark, Copenhagen; in Switzerland, Zurich; in Italy, Bologna, Milan, and Padua; in England, Guy's Hospital, London, and St. Mary's, Surrey; in Ireland, Dublin; and in Australia, Canberra. A list of current training programs in the United States appears in the Appendix following Chapter 37. The continuing (and increasing) popularity of toxicology is due to many factors including its intellectual and emotional appeal. It is multidisciplinary in nature, challenging and demanding, and its experimental findings are relevant and applicable to public health issues, including improving the quality of life and (hopefully) extending it.

> "Knowledge is of two kinds. We know a subject ourselves or we can find information on it." (Samuel Johnson)

The need for a standard textbook became evident. Although several texts were available, none appeared adequate. This issue was addressed and resolved by Louis J. Casarett and John Doull. Dr. Casarett received his PhD in 1958 from the University of Rochester, where he studied respiratory toxicodynamics and morphological changes following exposures to potentially toxic materials, especially to polonium. In 1967 he moved to the University of Hawaii, where he developed a program in toxicology. His research involved drugs of abuse and pesticides. He was considered an excellent researcher and teacher. Dr. Doull received both his PhD in pharmacology and his MD from the University of Chicago. He remained at Chicago for a number of years, then moved to the University of Kansas Medical Center, where he established one of the most outstanding programs in toxicology in the world (and attracted and trained a number of internationally famous toxicologists). Casarett and Doull published *Toxicology, the Science of Poisons* in 1975. It is now in its fifth edition.

Significant contributions to the advancement of toxicology came and continue to come from many sources, academic, governmental/regulatory, and industrial. Government/regulatory toxicologists have made significant contributions especially in the area of safety evaluation, including the quantification of risk. Regulatory agencies demand adequate data of high quality to serve as the basis for establishing safe exposure levels. The extent of testing was and is often determined by the depth of the science, as well as the chemical and physical properties of the agent and the extent of exposure. For example, if absorption, distribution, metabolism, and excretion (ADME) studies were conducted properly, and it was determined that the test material was not absorbed from the gastrointestinal tract, then the need for long-term studies was not compelling. This caused toxicologists who were conducting safety studies to design programs that addressed basic issues early, often resulting in considerable saving of resources. If the agencies had not recommended or required these data, they probably would not have been conducted, or at least not early in the program. The regulators appeared to be driving the science! Academic and industrial and governmental research laboratories continue to advance the frontiers of toxicology by seeking the molecular basis for toxic action. Contract toxicology laboratories have also made a significant contribution to toxicology by providing unique opportunities for those interested in the pragmatic (applied) aspects of toxicology, namely, the conduct of appropriate tests to establish safe conditions of exposure. These studies must consider the latest developments and advances in toxicology and related disciplines and the needs of regulators internationally. This is especially challenging today in this era of increased international trade and harmonization.

As with other recognized, independent scientific disciplines, toxicologists realized a need for a learned society to provide a forum for the exchange of scientific information. Toxicology continued to attract (to seduce) more students and practitioners, and this resulted in more research. The need for an appropriate journal in which to publish, and thus disseminate, the results of investigations was acute. The journal, *Toxicology and Applied Pharmacology* was founded by Fred Coulston; this was followed by *Fundamental and Applied Toxicology* (now *Toxicological Sciences*). Other journals included *Food and Cosmetic* (now *Chemical*) *Toxicology* (founded by Leon Golberg in 1963), *Journal of Applied Toxicology*, *Human and Experimental Toxicology*, and others.

The Society of Toxicology was founded in 1965. This was the first international society for and by toxicologists. Since its founding and as a result of the tremendous growth of toxicology, other societies of toxicology have been established. Almost every developed country has its own society of toxicology, a testimony of the recognition of its importance and its growth.

Toxicology continues to grow. Its uniqueness continues to attract (yes, to seduce by virtue of its attractiveness) some of the brightest students. There is something for everyone: from the molecular to the macro to the modeler, from the gene to the whole animal to the human, from SAR to QSAR. Toxicology's uniqueness and strengths derive from the integration of many chemical and biological sciences and supporting disciplines. This provides a strong base from which to extrapolate data to humans. Toxicology is also one of the few sciences in which academic, industrial, and regulatory scientists can effectively interact to protect the public. The importance of toxicology is recognized by governments worldwide. Toxicology has evolved from listing poisons to protecting the public from the adverse effects of chemicals; from simply identifying effects (qualitative toxicology) to identifying and quantifying human risks from exposure (quantitative toxicology); and from observing phenomena to experimenting and determining mechanisms of action of toxic agents and rational management for intoxication. As Claude Bernard noted:

> Where then, you will ask is the difference between observers and experimenters? It is here: we give the name observer to the man [human] who applies methods of investigation, whether simple or complex, to the study of phenomena which he [she] does not vary and which he [she] therefore gathers as nature offers them. We give the name experimenter to the man [human] who applies methods of investigation, whether simple or complex, so as to make natural phenomena vary, or so as to alter them with some purpose or other, and to make them present themselves in circumstances or conditions in which nature does not show them. In this sense, observation is investigation of a natural phenomenon, and experiment is investigation of a phenomenon altered by the investigator. (Bernard, 1865, p.)

Toxicology has come a long way! As science continues to advance, toxicology will continue to draw from these advances in its constant quest to protect the public from harm. Toxicology has come of age!

It is fitting to close with the daily prayer of Moses Maimonides (appropriate for practicing toxicologists):

> "May there never rise in me the notion that I know enough, but give me strength and leisure to enlarge my knowledge. ... Thou hast chosen me in Thy grace to watch over the life."

> "It is your work in life that is the ultimate seduction." (Pablo Picasso)

QUESTIONS

1. Define poisons and describe several functions for poisons.
2. How has toxicology evolved from an art into a science?
3. How has the receptor concept influenced the development of toxicology?
4. Discuss some of the similarities and differences between toxicology and pharmacology.
5. Should Claude Bernard or Paracelsus be credited with the title, founder of (modern) toxicology? Defend your choice.

SELECTED READINGS

1. Accum, F. (1820): *A Treatise on Adulterations of Food and Culinary Poisons*. ABM Small, Philadelphia, PA (cited in ref. 40).
2. Ackerknecht, E. H. (1982): *A Short History of Medicine*. Johns Hopkins University Press, Baltimore.
3. Albert, A. (1985): *Selective Toxicity*. 1st ed., Methuen, London, 1951; 7th ed., Chapman & Hall, New York, 1985.
4. Baas, J. H. (1889): *Outlines of the History of Medicine*, trans. H. E. Handerson. J. H. Vail, New York.
5. Beeson, B. B. (1930): Orfila: Pioneer toxicologist. *Ann. Med. Hist.*, 2:68–70.
6. Bernard, C. (1865): *An Introduction to the Study of Experimental Medicine*, trans. H. C. Greene. Dover, New York, 1957 edition.
7. Bettmann, O. L. (1979): *A Pictorial History of Medicine*. Charles C. Thomas, Springfield, IL, 5th printing.
8. Breathnach, C. S. (1987): Orfila. *Irish Med. J.* 80:99.
9. Casarett, L. J. (1975): Origin and scope of toxicology. In: *Toxicology: The Basic Science of Poisons*, edited by L. J. Casarett, and J. Doull. Macmillan, New York.
10. Castiglioni, A. (1941): *A History of Medicine*, trans. E. B. Krumbhaar. Alfred A. Knopf, New York.
11. Christison, R. A. (1845): *A Treatise on Poisons*. Barrington & Howell, Philadelphia, PA.
12. Clendening, L. (1942): *Source Book of Medical History*. Paul B. Hober, New York; Dover, New York, 1960.
13. Cope, Z. (1957): *Sidelights on the History of Medicine*. Butterworth, London.
14. Debus, A. G. (1999): *Paracelsus and the Medical Revolution of the Renaissance; A 500th Anniversary Celebration. National Library of Medicine, Paracelsus, Five Hundred Years; Three American Exhibits*.
15. Decker, W. J. (1987): Introduction and history. In: *Handbook of Toxicology*, edited by T. J. Haley and W. O. Berndt. Hemisphere, Washington, DC.
16. Deichmann, W. B., Henschler, D., Holmstedt, B., and Keil, G. (1986): What is there that is not poison? A study of the Third Defense by Paracelsus. *Arch. Toxicol.*, 58:207–213.
17. Doull, J., and Bruce, M. C. (1986): Origin and scope of toxicology. In: *Casarett and Doull's Toxicology: The Basic Science of Poisons*, 3rd ed., edited by C. D. Klaassen, M. O. Amdur, and J. Doull. Macmillan, New York.
18. DuBois, K., and Geiling, E. M. K. (1959): *Textbook of Toxicology*. Oxford University Press, New York.
19. Eckert, W. G. (1980): Historical aspects of poisoning and toxicology. *Am. J. Forens. Med. Pathol.*, 1:261–264.
20. Gallo, M. A., and Doull, J. (1991): History and scope of toxicology. In: *Casarett and Doull's Toxicology*, 4th ed., edited by C. D. Klaassen, M. O. Amdur, and J. Doull. Pergamon Press, New York.
21. Garrison, F. H. (1929): *An Introduction to the History of Medicine*, 4th ed. W. B. Saunders, Philadelphia, PA.
22. Gettler, A. O. (1953): The historical development of toxicology. *J. Forens. Sci.*, 1:1–25.
23. Gillett, J. (1987): *The ICET Newsletter*.
24. Glaister, J. (1954): *The Power of Poison*. William Morrow, New York.
25. Godon, B. L. (1959): *Medieval and Renaissance Medicine*. Philosophical Library, New York.
26. Goulding, R. (1978): Poisoning as a fine art. *SO Med. Leg. J.*, 46:6–17.
27. Goulding, R. (1987): Poisoning as a social phenomenon. *J. R. Coll. Phys. London*, 21:282–286.
28. Gunther, R. T. (1959): *The Greek Herbal of Disocorides*. Hafner, New York.

29. Guthrie, D. A. (1946): *A History of Medicine*. J. B. Lippincott, Philadelphia, PA.
30. Haggard, H. W. (1933): *Mystery, Magic and Medicine*. Doubleday, Doran, Garden City, NY.
31a. Hamilton, A. (1943): *Exploring the Dangerous Trades; The Autobiography of Alice Hamilton, MD*. Little, Brown, Boston.
31b. Hamilton, A. (1925): *Industrial Poisons in the United States*. Macmillan, New York.
31c. Hamilton, A. (1934): *Industrial Toxicology*. Harper & Brothers, New York.
32. Holmstedt, B., and Liljestrand, G. (1981): *Readings in Pharmacology*. Raven Press, New York.
33. Hutt, P. B., and Hutt, P. B. II (1984): A history of governmental regulation of adulteration and misbranding of food. *Food Drug Cosmet. Law J.*, 39:2–73.
34. LaWall, C. H. (1924): *Four Thousand Years of Pharmacy*. J. B. Lippincott, Philadelphia, PA.
35a. Lewin, L. (1920): *Die Gifte in der Weltgeschichte. Toxikologische, allgemeinverstandliche Untersuchungen der historischen Qhellen*. Springer, Berlin.
35b. Lewin, L. (1929): *Gifte und Vergiftungen*. Stilke, Berlin.
36. Loomis, T. A. (1978): *Essentials of Toxicology*. Lea & Febiger, Philadelphia, PA.
37. Macht, D. J. (1931): Louis Lewin: Pharmacologist, toxicologist, medical historian. *Ann. Med. Hist.*, 3:179–194.
38. Massengill, S. E. (1943): *A Sketch of Medicine and Pharmacy*. S. E. Massengill, Bristol, TN.
39. Meek, W. J. (1954): *Medico-Historical Papers: The Gentle Art of Poisoning*. Department of Physiology, University of Wisconsin, Madison.
40. Mettler, C. C., and Mettler, F. A. (1947): *History of Medicine*. Blakiston, Philadelphia, PA.
41. Neuberger, A., and Smith, R. L. (1983): Richard Tecwyn Williams: The man, his work, his impact. *Drug Metab. Rev.*, 14:559–607.
42. Neuburger, M. (1910): *History of Medicine*, trans. Ernest Playfair. Oxford University Press, London.
43. Olmsted, J. M. D. (1938): *Claude Bernard: Physiologist*. Harper & Brothers, New York.
44. Oser, B. L. (1987): Toxicology then and now. *Regul. Toxicol. Pharmacol.*, 7:427–443.
45. Osius, T. G. (1957): The historic art of poisoning. *Univ. Mich. Med. Bull.*, March: 111–116.
46. Pagel, W. (1982): *An Introduction to Philosophical Medicine in the Era of the Renaissance*. Karger, Basel, Switzerland.
47. Peters, R. A., Stocken, L. A., and Thompson, R. H. S. (1945): British anti-lewisite (BAL). *Nature*, 156:616–619.
48. Ramazzini, B. (1713): *Diseases of Workers*, Latin text translated by W. C. Wright.
49. Rhodes, P. (1985): *An Outline History of Medicine*. Buttersworth, London.
50. Rosenfield, L. (1985): Alfred Swaine Taylor (1806–1880), pioneer toxicologist—and a slight case of murder. *Clin. Chem.*, 31:1235–1236.
51. Sigerist, H. E. (1958): *The Great Doctors. A Biographical History of Medicine*. Doubleday, New York.
52. Sonnedecker, G. (1976): *Kremers and Urdang's History of Pharmacy*, 4th ed. J. B. Lippincott, Philadelphia, PA.
53. Talbott, J. H. (1970): *A Biographical History of Medicine. Excerpts and Essays on the Men and Their Work*. Grune & Stratton, New York.
54. Temkin, C. L., Rosen, G., Zilboorg, G., and Sigerist, H. W. (1996): *Four treatises of theophrastus von Hohenheim called Paracelsus*, edited by H. W. Sigerist. Johns Hopkins University Press, Baltimore, MD.
55. Thomas, L. (1979): *The Medusa and the Snail*. Viking Press, New York.
56. Thompson, C. J. S. (1931): *Poisons and Poisoners. With Historical Accounts of Some Famous Mysteries in Ancient and Modern Times*. H. Shaylor, London.
57. Voegtlin, C., Dyer, H. A., and Leonard C. S. (1923): On the mechanism of the action of arsenic upon protoplasm. *Public Health Rep.*, 38:1882–1912.
58. von Oettingen, W. F. (1952): *Poisoning: A Guide to Clinical Diagnosis and Treatment*. Paul B. Hoeber, Harper & Brothers, New York.
59. Williams, R. T. (1959): *Detoxication Mechanisms*. John Wiley, New York.
60. Wooton, A. C. (1910): *Chronicles of Pharmacy*. Macmillan, London.

Principles and Methods of Toxicology,
Fourth Edition, edited by A. Wallace Hayes.
Taylor & Francis, Philadelphia © 2001.

Chapter 2

The Use of Toxicology in the Regulatory Process

Barbara D. Beck, Tracey M. Slayton, Edward J. Calabrese, Linda Baldwin, Ruthann Rudel

BACKGROUND

Regulatory toxicology is that area of toxicology directed at protecting public health by regulating exposure to potentially harmful materials. Historically, regulatory toxicology has developed in a manner that has reflected humankind's ability to relate exposure to certain agents with adverse health effects. Thus, early regulatory attention generally focused on preventing the acute effects of chemical agents, because these effects were observable and could be easily associated with exposure. Once the germ theory of disease was developed and the disease potential of human and animal waste was recognized, the disposal of these materials began to be regulated. Food and drugs were also the focus of early regulation, due, no doubt, to the relative ease in associating acute health effects, such as food poisoning, with exposure to materials in the diet or in medications. Hutt (82) notes that adulteration of the food supply was a serious problem in the ancient world, and quotes Pliny the Elder, writing in the first century AD, as saying, "So many poisons are employed to force wine to suit our taste—and we are surprised that it is not wholesome!"

Occupational exposures were also an early focus of regulation, due again to the fact that the relationship between exposure and effect was often observable. Early industrial hygiene efforts were typically intended to prevent overt or frank effects of materials in the workplace. Some of the first observations of the effects of chronic human exposures to certain chemicals were also made in occupational settings. Hutt (82) notes that during the 16th century, Paracelsus wrote about diseases characteristic of miners. The fact that certain chronic occupational hazards affected the exposed individual at the point of contact also made the connection between agent and effect easier to discern. The first epidemiological study linking human cancer to a specific cause is attributed to Sir Percival Pott, who identified occupational exposure to soot as being responsible for scrotal cancers in young British chimney sweeps (153).

The development of regulatory toxicology during the 20th century has continued to shadow the ability to detect both chemicals and effects; that is, as we have become able to detect chemicals at lower and lower levels and to detect smaller biochemical and physiological changes, we have turned regulatory attention to these "new problems." For example, small increases in airway resistance following exposure to certain air pollutants are currently used as one basis for regulating these air pollutants; historically, no one would have been aware of these subtle effects. The practice of regulatory toxicology has evolved from historical concern about overt effects at high exposure levels to current concern about subtle effects at very low exposure levels, thus paralleling our ability to detect smaller amounts of chemicals and more subtle effects. For example, guidelines for occupational exposures to benzene have decreased by two orders of magnitude from 100 ppm in 1927 to the current Occupational Safety and Health Administration (OSHA) standard of 1 ppm. Ambient criteria for nonoccupational benzene exposures are currently as low as 0.03 ppm in some states (141).

Because of the recent dramatic increase in our ability to detect smaller effects and lower concentrations, programs to regulate chemicals in the environment have increased at an astronomical rate during the last 25 years. Factors contributing to the recent increase in regulatory activity include:

- The realization of the vast number of chemicals that humans have dispersed into the environment and to which humans have been exposed. Approximately 60,000 chemicals that are used commercially have been identified and listed under the Toxic Substances Control Act (TSCA) (214). Advances in analytical chemistry have allowed parts-per-billion levels of chemicals to be detected in "pristine" areas, in wildlife, in food products, and in human body tissues. This message was delivered initially by Rachel Carson in 1962 with the publication of *Silent Spring* (34).
- The realization that historical chemical management practices might not have been protective for the health effects we are concerned with today (effects at low doses), although such practices were consistent with the state of knowledge at the time. For example, during the 1970s, residents of Love Canal realized that they had unknowingly been exposed to chemicals that had migrated from a nearby landfill into their basements. The Comprehensive Emergency Response, Compensation, and Liability Act (CERCLA), also known as Superfund, was enacted shortly after the Love Canal incident.
- The establishment of causal relationships between certain diseases and chronic chemical exposures, such as leukemia and benzene, or mesothelioma and asbestos.
- The reduction in illness and mortality due to microbial diseases and the improved standard of living, which have focused increasing attention on other causes of ill health.

The rapid increase in the number and complexity of regulatory programs to address potential health effects from chemical exposures is also a result of the increased scientific uncertainty about toxicology and risk that has evolved with our increased understanding of these subjects (i.e., the more we learn, the more we realize how much more there is to learn). As we have come to better understand the complexities of toxicology, we have developed more complex procedures for characterizing toxic responses. An example of this is provided in the sixth section of this chapter, which describes probabilistic risk assessment methods.

In 1958, when the Delaney Clause forbidding the addition to food of any substance found to induce cancer in animals or humans was passed (156), the public generally believed that the intent of the law to provide a "zero risk" food supply was achievable. No one foresaw that, 20 years later, scientists would have identified over 500 animal carcinogens, been able to detect chemical concentrations between two and five orders of magnitude lower than they could detect in the 1950s, and found that many naturally occurring chemicals in food could be considered animal carcinogens (213). These developments have forced the recognition that absolute safety is impossible to achieve, even in products regulated to assure safety. Thus, Scheuplein (167) has noted that "the vast improvement in our methods of analytical detection have [sic] exposed carcinogens in the food supply in amounts too minuscule for our carcinogen bioassays and our risk assessment procedures to evaluate with comparable precision. We are capable now, more than before, of asking scientific questions that we cannot answer." (p. 244)

CURRENT REGULATORY FRAMEWORK

At the federal level in the United States, four agencies bear most of the direct responsibility for the regulation of toxic chemicals: the Consumer Product Safety Commission (CPSC), the U.S. Environmental Protection Agency (EPA), the Food and Drug Administration (FDA), and the Occupational Safety and Health Administration (OSHA). Table 2.1 describes the acts that empower these and several other federal agencies.

It is clear from Table 2.1 that there is a broad range of chemical exposures with which federal regulatory auth-

Table 2.1
Federal laws related to exposures to toxic substances

Legislation	Agency	Area of Concern
Food, Drug and Cosmetics Act (1906, 1938, amended 1958, 1960, 1962, 1968, 1976)	FDA	Food, drugs, cosmetics, food additives, color additives, new drugs, animal and food additives, and medical devices
Federal Insecticide, Fungicide and Rodenticide Act (1948, amended 1972, 1975, 1978)	EPA	Pesticides
Dangerous Cargo Act (1952)	DOT, USCG	Water shipment of toxic materials
Atomic Energy Act (1954)	NRC	Radioactive substances
Federal Hazardous Substances Act (1960, amended 1981)	CPSC	Toxic household products
Federal Meat Inspection Act (1967); Poultry Products Inspection Act (1968); Egg Products Inspection Act (1970)	USDA	Food, feed, color additives, and pesticide residues
National Environmental Policy Act (1970; amended 1975, 1985, 1987, 1989, 1996, 1997)	EPA	Ecosystems and natural resources
Occupational Safety and Health Act (1970; amended 1974, 1978, 1982, 1983, 1984, 1986, 1987, 1990, 1992, 1995, 1996, 1997)	OSHA, NIOSH	Workplace toxic chemicals
Poison Prevention Packaging Act (1970, amended 1981)	CPSC	Packaging of hazardous household products
Clean Air Act (1970, amended 1974, 1977, 1990)	EPA	Air pollutants
Hazardous Materials Transportation Act (1972)	DOT	Transport of hazardous materials
Clean Water Act (formerly Federal Water Pollution Control Act; 1972, amended 1977, 1978, 1987)	EPA	Water pollutants
Marine Protection, Research and Sanctuaries Act (1972)	EPA	Ocean dumping
Consumer Product Safety Act (1972, amended 1981)	CPSC	Hazardous consumer products
Lead-based Paint Poison Prevention Act (1973, amended 1976)	CPSC, HEW (HHS), HUD	Use of lead paint in federally assisted housing
Safe Drinking Water Act (1974, amended 1977) and subsequent amendments	EPA	Drinking water, contaminants
Resource Conservation and Recovery Act (1976, amended 1984)	EPA	Solid waste, including hazardous wastes
Toxic Substances Control Act (1976); Asbestos Information Act (1988)	EPA	Hazardous chemicals not covered by other laws, includes premarket review
Federal Mine Safety and Health Act (1977)	DOL, NIOSH	Toxic substances in coal and other mines
Comprehensive Environmental Response, Compensation, and Liability Act (1981); Superfund Amendments and Reauthorization Act (1986); Emergency Planning and Community Right-to-Know Act (1986)	EPA	Hazardous substances, pollutants and contaminants
Radon Gas and Indoor Air Quality Research Act of 1986	EPA	Indoor air
Oil Pollution Act (1990)	DOT	Oil pollution
Pollution Prevention Act (1990)	EPA	Toxics use reduction
Food Quality Protection Act—amendments to FDCA and FIFRA	EPA	Pesticides in food

Note. Adapted from Office of Science and Technology Policy (147).

orities are concerned. Chemicals may be regulated on the basis of environmental medium (e.g., air, water), activity (e.g., food manufacture, chemical transport, ocean dumping), and type of exposure environment (e.g., workplace, residential). While the statutes in Table 2.1 represent almost 100 years of federal legislative history, 17 of the 23 have been written since 1970, illustrating the recent increase in public concern about chemical exposures.

The language of each statute provides the implementing agency with the basis for issuing regulations under the law. Some statutes instruct the agency to limit chemical release or exposure by requiring the use of certain control technologies. Other statutes require the agency to develop and implement risk-based standards, while others require the agency to balance risks with the costs of regulating or the benefits of not regulating. The latter two types of statutes are the most likely to involve regulatory toxicology in their implementation.

Section 307 of the Clean Water Act (CWA) is an example of a statute that requires technology-based standards for pollution control. Under this portion of the CWA, industries discharging to surface water must use the best available control technology to limit their pollutant discharges; installation of the appropriate control technology is required from the discharger to obtain a National Pollutant Discharge Elimination System (NPDES) permit.

Other statutes specify the standard for safety that regulations and standards issued under the law are supposed to provide. A commonly cited example of a law that required health-based, or risk-based, standards for pollution control is Section 112 of the 1970 Clean Air Act (CAA), which required the EPA to set emission standards for hazardous air pollutants (under the National Emissions Standards for Hazardous Air Pollutants [NESHAPS] program) that would "protect public health" with an "ample" margin of safety. Implementation of this standard of safety for carcinogenic air pollutants proved to be so troublesome for the agency that between 1970 and 1990, NESHAPS were set for only seven air pollutants. The difficulty in setting the risk-based standards was that the statute provided no indication of what an "ample margin of safety" was or how such a concept might be applied to carcinogens, given that the agency considered carcinogens to act by a no-threshold mechanism. The 1990 amendments to the CAA replaced the NESHAPS health-based standards with specified technology-based standards for controlling hazardous air pollutants. The statute states that after installation of the control technology, health-based standards must be set to further control emissions where unacceptable risks remain.

The Federal Food, Drug, and Cosmetic Act (FFDCA) is another example of a law requiring health-based standards for limiting the public's exposure to chemicals. Section 409 of the FFDCA requires the sponsor of a food additive to show that no harm to consumers will result when the additive is put to its intended use, and contains the Delaney Clause (discussed earlier), a special provision that forbids the use of any food additives that have been found to induce cancer in humans or animals. The Delaney Clause essentially specifies that the acceptable risks from carcinogens as food additives is zero. This bright line has proven to be very difficult for both the FDA and (until passage of the Food Quality Protection Act in 1996) for the EPA to implement, because the law does not allow the implementing agencies to specify *de minimis*, or acceptable, levels of risk. The EPA regulates pesticides under both the Federal Insecticide, Fungicide, and Rodenticide Act (FIFRA) and the FFDCA. Under the FIFRA, the agency was required to balance the risk from the pesticide with the benefit associated with its use. However, under the FFDCA, the EPA was bound by the Delaney Clause with regard to pesticides that may concentrate in processed foods above the level allowed on the raw agricultural commodity. This dichotomous standard (known as the "Delaney Paradox") forced the EPA to regulate to zero risk for pesticides applied to foods that may concentrate during processing, while regulating using risk-benefit analysis to regulate the same pesticides on raw agricultural commodities (134). In 1992, a Circuit Court ruled that the Delaney Clause does not allow the EPA to permit use of carcinogenic pesticides under the FFDCA, even if their use is associated with negligible risk (1). The Delaney Clause has also been difficult for the FDA to implement as more chemicals (including naturally occurring chemicals in foods) have been determined to be carcinogens, and the FDA has searched for ways to establish acceptable risk levels for food additives. In 1988, the U.S. Court of Appeals for the District of Columbia struck down an effort by the FDA to interpret the Delaney Clause as allowing the agency to set a *de minimis* risk level for two color additives for use in cosmetics and drugs (212).

Other laws require the implementing agency to balance the risks and benefits of alternative regulatory choices. Examples of balancing statutes include Section 408 of the FFDCA, which, until the Food Quality Protection Act (FQPA) of 1996, required tolerances for pesticide residues on raw agricultural commodities to be set at levels necessary to protect the public health, while considering the need for "an adequate, wholesome, and economical food supply" (134). Section 6 of the Toxic Substances Control Act (TSCA) requires the EPA to consider the potential benefits of using a chemical and the economic consequences of restricting its use when determining whether the manufacture, distribution, use, or disposal of a substance presents an unreasonable risk of injury to health or the environment.

Language in the Occupational Safety and Health Act specifies that the Occupational Safety & Health Administration (OSHA) must "adequately assure(s) to the extent feasible ... that no employee will suffer material impairment of health or functional capacity" (145). This statutory language also requires balancing of risks and costs, but is particularly interesting because the dual requirements of "feasibility" and "no employee will suffer" may be impossible to reconcile in certain situations (163).

While the narrative terms *unreasonable risk* and *ample margin of safety* have not been clearly or consistently defined across agencies or across statutes, over the past decade, agencies have generally interpreted this language as requiring a qualitative, and frequently quantitative, estimate of the health risks associated with an exposure and the reduction in risks resulting from regulatory action. A major factor in the increased use of risk analysis by regulatory agencies was the 1980 Supreme Court decision in Industrial Union Department *v.* American Petroleum Institute. In this case, OSHA proposed lowering the occupational standard for benzene from 10 ppm to 1 ppm on the basis that benzene was a carcinogen, that any reduction in exposure would result in a reduction in risk, and that 1 ppm was technologically feasible. The Supreme Court did not find for the Union, stating that "Before he can promulgate any permanent health or safety standard, the Secretary [of Labor] is required to make a threshold finding that a place of employment is unsafe—in the sense that significant risks are present and can be eliminated or lessened by a change in practices" (85). The Court left the decision of what constitutes a "significant risk" to the OSHA. This landmark decision has had a major impact on agencies in addition to OSHA, resulting in an increase in the development and use of tools to quantify risks from exposure to environmental chemicals.

Perhaps one of the most far-reaching (and likely precedent-setting) statutes in recent years is the Food Quality Protection Act (FQPA) of 1996. This statute, which addresses risks from pesticides in food through the setting of tolerance limits, is primarily risk based with limitations on the extent to which EPA can consider benefits. This is in contrast to the risk/benefit balancing requirements of the FFDCA noted earlier. Only in certain narrow circumstances under the FQPA can EPA set pesticide tolerance levels that do not meet health-based criteria. Specifically, the circumstances comprise those situations where the use of the pesticide prevents even greater risks from occurring to consumers (a risk/risk balancing) or where the lack of the pesticide would result in "a significant disruption in domestic production of an adequate, wholesome, and economical food supply." In addition, the FQPA eliminates certain aspects of the "Delaney Paradox" discussed earlier. Tolerance limits for pesticides in both raw agricultural products and processed foods, for both carcinogens and noncarcinogens (the Delaney clause considered carcinogens only), are now to be based on health only. Other important provisions of the FQPA include the requirement that EPA specifically consider exposures and risks to infants and young children in setting pesticide tolerance limits, allowing up to an additional 10-fold safety factor, the need to consider all pathways of exposure (e.g., drinking water, soil/dust ingestion, etc.) to a pesticide in setting tolerance limits for that pesticide in food; the need to consider the cumulative risk for multiple pesticides that act via a common mechanism of action when setting a tolerance limit for any single pesticide of the "common mechanism" class; and the establishment of a very ambitious comprehensive screening program for pesticides that exert estrogenic and possibly other endocrine effects (190). The statute represents a landmark piece of legislation not only in terms of the regulatory implications, but also with respect to the advancement in scientific understanding required to implement the statute.

The combined effect of the increasing use of risk assessment to help make regulatory decisions and the significant uncertainty that accompanies most quantitative estimates of toxicological risk has resulted in considerable debate about the practice of risk assessment. On one side of the debate, the EPA, the FDA, and other agencies have been criticized by the Office of Management and Budget (OMB) and many representatives of the regulated community for being too conservative in their risk assessment procedures (146). On the other side, environmental advocacy groups such as Greenpeace have claimed that "In the real world, quantitative risk assessments are used almost exclusively to justify pollution" (175). Others have noted that "current risk estimates are by no means routinely exaggerated, either for the entire populations they apply to or for highly exposed or highly susceptible individuals within those populations" (58). Much of this difference in opinion is perhaps due to the fact that risk estimates are frequently inadequately defined and presented. Often, risk assessors produce single-value estimates of risk that may apply to some unknown percentage of the population. Because the variability in the exposure and dose-response characteristics of a population are so large, the risk estimates for a small, highly exposed or sensitive subpopulation will generally be very different from the estimates of the most likely risks for the entire population. Although the risk assessment results are supposed to be qualified and uncertainty discussed, the risk number is often used without appropriate explanation of the inherent variability. In a recent effort to address this problem, the EPA prepared guidance to risk assessors on the need to provide fuller, more explicit descriptions of risk when providing such information not only to risk managers but also to the general public (199). For example, the guidance recommends multiple descriptions of risk (e.g., sensitive receptors and general population) as well as clear descriptions of the uncertainties in the risk assessment.

Governmental and nongovernmental agencies other than those already discussed can influence the regulatory process as well. The American Conference of Governmental Industrial Hygienists (ACGIH) sets exposure limits based solely on health protection for approximately 600 workplace chemicals. These exposure limits, known as threshold limit values or TLVs (7), do not carry any regulatory weight, but it is not uncommon for workplaces to adhere to the TLVs for chemicals that OSHA does not regulate or which have an exposure limit that has not been revised since the inception of the OSHA in 1970. The TLVs have also been used by several state environmental agencies to derive acceptable ambient levels for toxic air pollutants.

Agencies in the Department of Health and Human Services that influence the regulatory process include the National Cancer Institute; the National Institute of Environmental Health Sciences, in particular the National Toxicology Program; the National Institute for Occupational Safety and Health (NIOSH) and the Center for Environmental Health (part of the Centers for Disease Control and Prevention, CDC); and the Agency for Toxic Substance and Disease Registry (ATSDR) (183). These agencies affect the regulatory process in several ways, ranging from decisions on which chemicals to test in long-term cancer bioassays, to defining principles for evaluating carcinogens, to conducting site-specific (as with a hazardous waste site) and chemical-specific risk assessments. International organizations such as the World Health Organization (WHO) and the International Agency for Research on Cancer (IARC) also have a significant role in the use of information by regulatory agencies.

The primary focus of this chapter is on the use of regulatory toxicology at the federal level. However, state governments have also been active in regulating exposure to toxins in the environment. For example, in 1986, voters in California overwhelmingly adopted Proposition 65, the Safe Drinking Water and Toxic Enforcement Act of 1986. This act contains two major provisions—one prohibiting the "discharge or release [of] a chemical known to the state to cause cancer or reproductive toxicity into water" and the other, a labeling requirement, mandating that no person expose another individual to any carcinogen or reproductive toxin without providing "clear and reasonable warning." Exemptions for the discharge requirements are provided for carcinogens at discharge levels that will pose lifetime cancer risk to a person drinking the water of less than 1×10^{-5}, or for reproductive toxins for discharges resulting in exposure levels less than 1000 times smaller than the "no-observable-effect level" (NOEL) for reproductive effects.

Some states have also developed their own risk assessment procedures or standards. In the absence of emissions standards for hazardous air pollutants at the federal level, many states developed their own emissions standards for hazardous air pollutants. Under the CWA, states can develop water quality criteria for certain water bodies in the state. Many states also have Superfund-type laws for the cleanup of abandoned hazardous waste sites, and have consequently developed risk assessment procedures for these sites.

RISK ASSESSMENT PARADIGM

In response to a directive from the United States Congress, the FDA contracted with the National Research Council (NRC) of the National Academy of Sciences to evaluate the risk assessment process in the federal government and to make recommendations on how the process could be improved. As a result of this effort, the Committee on the Institutional Means for Assessment of Risks to Public Health published a book in 1983 entitled *Risk Assessment in the Federal Government: Managing the Process* (136). The book summarized past experiences, and although it did not propose new ways to evaluate risks from environmental chemicals, it has nevertheless had an important effect on the use of scientific information by regulatory agencies in its codification of the risk assessment process.

The report has been particularly influential in two areas: (a) the separation of the risk assessment process from the risk management process, and (b) the classification of the risk assessment process into four broad components: *hazard identification, dose-response assessment, exposure assessment*, and *risk characterization*. These concepts are illustrated in Figure 2.1.

More recently, in response to Congressional mandates, both the Committee on Risk Assessment of Hazardous Air Pollutants (established by the NRC under the direction of the EPA) and the Presidential/Congressional Commission on Risk Assessment and Risk Management (CRARM) have reevaluated risk assessment and risk management approaches. The findings of the NRC committee are published in a 1994 book entitled *Science and Judgment in Risk Assessment* (133), and the findings of CRARM are published in a 1997 report entitled *Risk Assessment and Risk Management in Regulatory Decision-Making* (155). While the four components making up the basic risk assessment paradigm and the separation of risk assessment and risk management remain key underlying principles, both committees recommended refinements in risk assessment and risk management

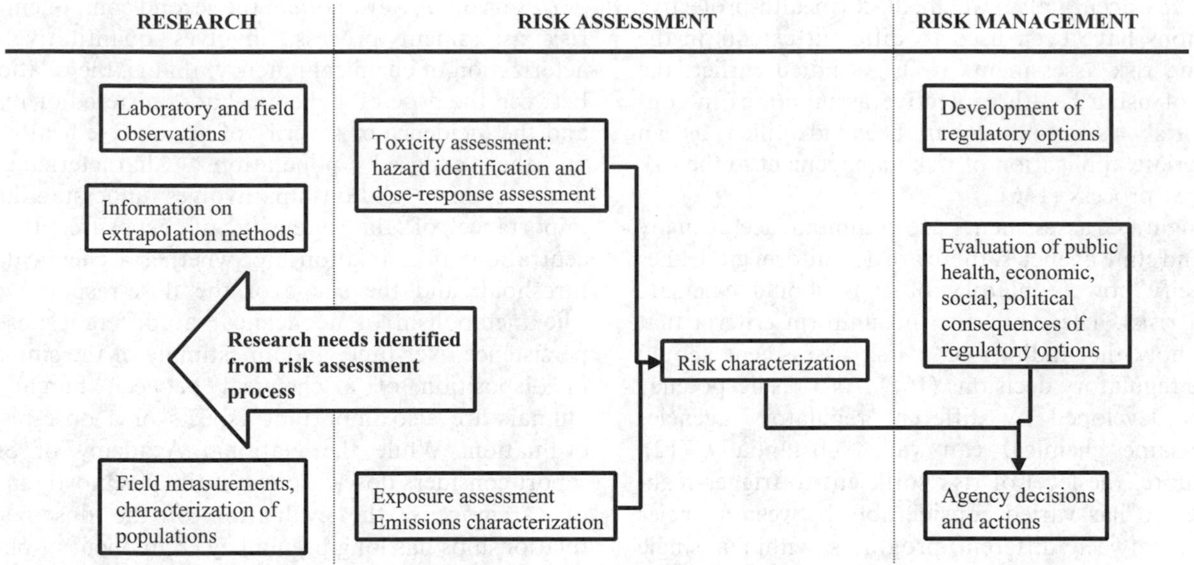

FIG. 2.1. NAS/NRC risk assessment/management paradigm. Adapted from NRC (133).

approaches. For example, the NRC committee highlights the importance of an iterative approach to risk assessment to reduce uncertainties, with each iteration incorporating fewer default assumptions and more specific information, balancing the use of "better science" with the constraints of the available resources (133). CRARM proposes a framework for risk management that encourages early and frequent involvement of all groups affected by the risk management problem, and decision making based on consideration of the risk management problem in the context of the broader, real-world goals of risk reduction and improved health status (155).

Risk assessment is defined as the "systematic, scientific characterization of potential adverse effects of human or ecological exposures to hazardous agents or activities," and involves assessment of the strength of the evidence as well as evaluation of the uncertainties associated with risk estimates (155). In contrast, risk management is "the process of identifying, evaluating, selecting, and implementing actions to reduce risk to human health and ecosystems" (155). Risk managers choose actions that will mitigate risks, considering not only the information derived from risk assessment, but also cultural, ethical, political, social, economic, and engineering information in the decision process.

The distinction between risk assessment and risk management is critical (136). The influence of risk management issues, such as the economic significance of a product, on the risk assessment process can seriously undermine the credibility of the risk assessment. This concern is exemplified in the separation between NIOSH and OSHA. NIOSH, part of the Department of Health and Human Services, is responsible for recommending health-based standards for workplace exposures to OSHA, part of the Department of Labor. As the federal agency actually responsible for setting standards for work place exposures and for implementing them, OSHA is also required to consider feasibility in the choice of exposure limits. It is not uncommon to find that exposure levels permitted by OSHA are different from NIOSH recommended exposure levels (182).

Of course, the distinction between risk assessment and risk management is not nearly so clear in practice. This is because each component of a chemical risk assessment is associated with considerable uncertainty. In the face of this uncertainty, regulatory officials have generally resorted to erring on the side of caution by including health-protective assumptions in their risk assessments. For example, the choice of a low-dose extrapolation model for carcinogens, which leads to a higher estimate of risk than other models, represents a risk management decision as much as a science policy decision. That is, the approach is conservative and provides the regulator with a greater level of confidence that the true risk to the human population is likely to be less than that expressed through the model. This approach has historically been justified as consistent with prudent public health policy when uncertainty is so great that it is difficult to provide a precise estimate of risk (i.e., in the face of uncertainty, it is easier to say the risk is less than *x* than to say the risk equals *y*). However, this practice can lead to inconsistent levels of protection for different chemicals and may direct resources away from the more significant risks (142). For example, the potential cancer risks associated with chemical disinfectants should be compared to the risks of waterborne microbial diseases when making decisions about treating public drinking water supplies, yet such risk/risk trade-offs cannot be accurately weighed if health-protective assumptions have been used to different extents in the underlying risk assessments (67). As noted earlier, the practice of using health-protective assumptions in conducting risk assessments has been identified as an inappropriate application of risk management to the risk assessment process (146).

Although risk assessments are commonplace at many federal and state agencies, there are no uniform guidelines that specify how regulatory officials should calculate chemical risks. There are also no uniform criteria that indicate how the findings of a risk assessment should influence regulatory decisions (165). As a result, potency estimates developed by different regulatory agencies for the same chemical can vary substantially (12). Furthermore, the level of risk sufficient to trigger regulatory action has varied considerably between agencies and even between different programs within a single agency (180). EPA's postregulatory "acceptable" risk levels for arsenic under one statute (the CAA) vary by four orders of magnitude (179).

As discussed earlier, risk assessment is commonly broken down into four components. The first component of risk assessment, *hazard identification*, involves an evaluation of whether a particular chemical can cause an adverse health effect in humans. The hazard identification process can be considered to be a qualitative risk assessment. It involves identifying the potential for exposure as well as the nature of the adverse effect expected. The types of information used in hazard identification include all categories described in the previous section. In hazard identification, the risk assessor must evaluate the quality of the studies (choice of appropriate control groups, sufficient numbers of animals, etc.), the severity of the effect described, the relevance of the toxic mechanisms in animals to those in humans, and many other factors.

The result is a scientific judgment that the chemical can, at some exposure concentrations, cause a particular adverse health effect in humans. The result is not a simple yes-or-no evaluation but a weight-of-evidence estimation of the likelihood that the particular chemical has the potential to cause the particular effect. For example, studies showing that ozone can suppress pulmonary defenses against microbial agents in several species of animals (129), and information on similarities in pulmonary defenses between humans and animals (68), would lead to the conclusion that ozone exposure in humans could, under certain conditions, result in an increased susceptibility to infection (205).

The hazard identification process has been codified mainly for carcinogens, as exemplified in the classification schemes from a variety of agencies including IARC (111), EPA (208), and OSHA (144). These schemes are discussed in more detail later in this chapter.

Dose-response evaluation, the second component of the risk assessment process, involves quantitative characterization of chemical potency, that is, the relationship between the dose of a chemical administered or received and the incidence or severity of an adverse health effect in the exposed population. Characterizing the dose-response relationship involves understanding the importance of the intensity of exposure, the concentration×time relationship, whether a chemical has a threshold, and the shape of the dose-response curve. The metabolism of a chemical at different doses, its persistence over time, and an estimate of the similarities in disposition of a chemical between humans and animals are also important aspects of a dose-response evaluation. While the National Academy of Science report considers dose-response estimates mostly in terms of carcinogens, the evaluation of the dose-response relationships has long been a key component of pharmacology and toxicology for many chemicals (136). Recent advances in dose-response assessment for noncancer risk assessment are described in chapter 8 by Rodericks et al. and in a later section of this chapter.

In *exposure assessment*, the third component of the risk assessment process, a determination is made of the amount of a chemical to which humans are exposed. Data are often very limited for exposure assessment. Measures of chemicals in environmental media, such as air or soil, or in food may be available; however, the extrapolation of those levels to a dose received by humans has many uncertainties. Models exist that can describe the movement of chemicals through a particular medium, and assumptions can be made regarding inhalation, ingestion, or dermal contact rates and the bioavailability of the chemical. This information can then be used to derive an estimate of the dose taken up by humans. Host factors, such as exercise, the use of certain consumer products, or the consumption of particular foodstuffs, will complicate the exposure assessment (see chapter 9, Exposure Assessment).

The use of biological monitoring such as measurement of volatile organic chemicals in exhaled breath for example (219)—and the use of personal sampling devices, such as respirable particulate monitors (178), represent new ways in which the uncertainties of exposure assessment can be reduced. Blood lead testing is another example of biological monitoring that has the ability to reduce the uncertainty in quantifying exposure and in extrapolating from exposure to dose.

The last stage of the risk assessment process, *risk characterization*, involves a prediction of the frequency and severity of effects in the exposed population. That is, the information from the dose-response evaluation (what dose is necessary to cause the effect?) is combined with the information from the exposure assessment (what dose is the population receiving?) to produce an estimate of the likelihood of observing the effect in the population being studied. Most risk assessments, particularly for cancer, performed in the regulatory arena produce a single-number estimate of risk (e.g., lung cancer risk of 1 in a million). These are often designed to represent the risk to the reasonable maximally exposed (RME) individual in a potentially exposed population.

Substantial *variability* exists within any potentially exposed population in exposure rates, intake and uptake rates, and sensitivity to the effect. This variability is such that the risk to the most highly exposed and sensitive portion of the population may be orders of magnitude higher than the risks to the majority of the population. For example, some individuals in a population may never eat locally caught fish, while other individuals may subsist on locally caught fish. The fish intakes of these respective individuals will consequently vary by orders of magnitude. Information should generally be provided on both the risk to individuals and the aggregate risk of the exposed population. Point estimates of risk to a single individual in the population can be misleading when no information is provided to indicate whether that individual's exposure is typical of 50% or 0.001% of the exposed population.

In addition to population variability, there is also significant *uncertainty* present in risk estimates, due to uncertainty in many of the risk assessment components (e.g., model and measurement error). It is critical that the risk characterization step of the risk assessment process describes the biological and statistical uncertainties in the final estimation and identify which component of the risk assessment process (hazard identification, dose-response, or exposure) involved the greatest degree of uncertainty. For example, the dose-response evaluation is generally highly uncertain. This is often due to the model error in extrapolating from animals to humans or short-term to life-time exposures. Information may not be available to characterize the active species, mechanism of effect, the effective dose, or absorption, metabolism, and excretion rates. McKone and Bogen (126) determined that 65% of the variance in the risk assessment results for a case study of tetrachloroethylene in groundwater was due to variance in the estimate of the chemical potency. Because the degree of uncertainty varies greatly among risk assessments for different chemicals, lack of consideration of uncertainty can lead to inappropriate levels of concern for different chemicals.

Monte Carlo uncertainty analysis techniques have been applied to the risk assessment process as one method of attempting to more fully characterize the distribution of potential risks in a population. Rather than using single values to represent input parameters such as contaminant ingestion rates, body weights, and chemical potencies, Monte Carlo analysis uses the range of potential values for each particular input parameter, as well as an estimate of how these values are distributed (termed the probability density function). These individual probability density functions are then used to calculate a probability density function for the risk estimate (47,174,193). Figure 2.2 shows a probability density function, produced by a Monte-Carlo analysis, which was calculated using probability density functions for individual input parameters. Although these techniques provide more information on the distribution of potential risk than a single number risk estimate, they are limited by the availability of information with which to characterize the input probability density functions. Particularly uncertain are estimates of chemical potency, which can vary by orders of magnitude depending upon beliefs regarding carcinogenic mechanisms.

The Committee on Risk Characterization, convened by the NRC, makes recommendations for improving the risk characterization process in its 1996 book entitled *Understanding Risk, Informing Decisions in a Democratic Society* (132). Rather than just a presentation of numerical risk results and associated uncertainties, a risk characterization should also convey the information in a clear and easily understandable way that is useful to risk managers in making informed decisions and that addresses the concerns of interested and affected parties. Therefore, the rigorous scientific analyses involved in risk characterization must be performed in conjunction with frequent deliberations with all interested and affected parties. As explained by the NRC Committee on Risk Characterization, "developing an accurate, balanced, and informative synthesis" involves "getting the science right," "getting the right science," "getting the right participation," and "getting the participation right" (132). The EPA adopted similar values in its 1995 risk characterization guidance (196).

TOXICOLOGY INFORMATION USED IN THE REGULATORY PROCESS

Three main categories of scientific information are employed by agencies in the evaluation and regulation of toxic chemicals in the environment: (a) epidemiology, (b) controlled clinical exposures, and (c) animal toxicology. In vitro studies and structure–activity relationships are typically used by regulatory agencies to support the interpretation of information from the three major categories, and are only occasionally used as a primary source of information.

Epidemiology, studies of clinical exposures, and animal toxicology provide qualitatively different information, with unique advantages and limitations. Environmental epidemiology studies, which attempt to associate disease or other adverse health outcomes with an environmental exposure, have the advantage of measuring an effect in

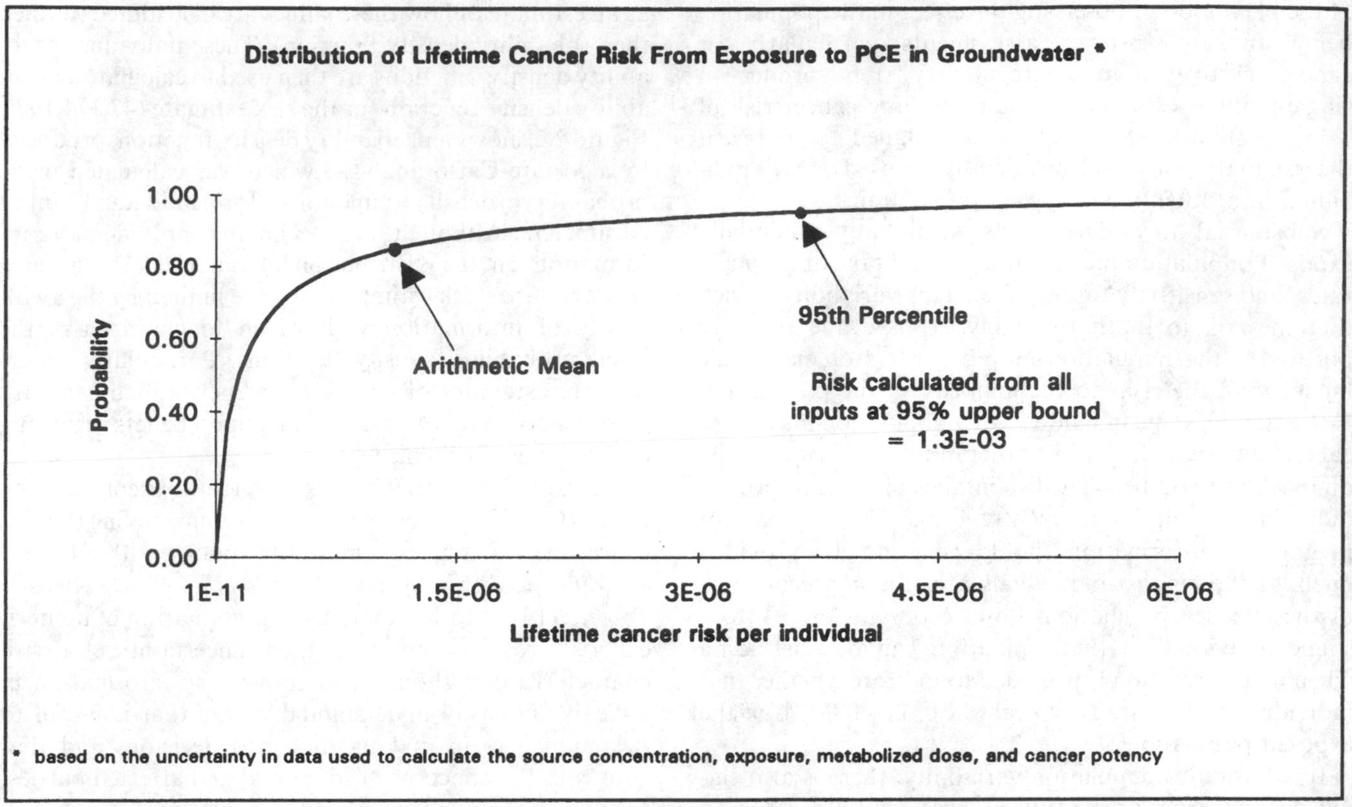

Selected Input Parameters and Distributions

Parameter	Units	Distribution Type	Min	Max	Arithmetic Mean	Arithmetic Std. Dev.	Geometric Std. Dev.
PCE concentration in water	mg/L	empirical			0.0003	0.00035	2.5
Breathing rate per unit body weight	m3/kg-day	lognormal			0.4	0.5	2.7
PCE metabolized cancer potency	kg-day/mg	empirical			0.11	0.14	4.8
Exposure time in house	h/day	uniform	8	20	14		
Skin permeability	m/h	uniform	0.004	0.01	0.007		

FIG. 2.2. Monte Carlo analysis of risk: tetrachloroethylene (PCE) in groundwater. Adapted from McKone and Bogen (126).

humans at exposure conditions that are by definition realistic. The first demonstration that benzene was a carcinogen came from epidemiological studies of rubber workers (86). It wasn't until several years after these studies that benzene was shown to cause cancer in animal studies (124). Studies of the London smog pollution episode in 1952 demonstrated that high levels of pollution from coal combustion could cause mortality, particularly in the very young, the elderly, and those individuals with preexisting cardiopulmonary disease (122). Evaluation of similar effects in animal studies would be difficult, given the complexity of the exposure in London and the lack of good animal models for susceptible populations, such as asthmatics. In general, epidemiology has been particularly helpful in the evaluation of working environments or other environments where exposure concentrations are relatively high.

Several factors limit the use of epidemiological studies by regulatory agencies. One of the major limitations is the lack of well-defined exposure information, both for chemical species and for actual concentrations. For example, the lack of accurate total exposure information limits the ability to quantify the effects of ambient air pollution in the United States. The Harvard University Six City Study showed that outdoor NO_2-monitoring devices are inadequate in accurately assessing total exposure to NO_2, due to the importance of indoor exposure (157). Subsequently, the EPA conducted Total

Exposure Assessment Measurement (TEAM) studies in which personal exposure to VOCs and pesticides were measured and found to be significantly higher than exposures estimated using stationary monitors for indoor or outdoor air (218). In some cases, the use of biological markers of exposure, such as measurements of arsenic levels in urine or lead levels in blood, can provide more accurate information about exposure and help reduce uncertainties in the results of epidemiological studies.

It is also difficult to define the causal element in epidemiological investigations, particularly when complex exposures are involved. For example, several indicators of pollution were measured during the London smog episodes that occurred between 1958 and 1972. Initial evaluations focused on the role of total particulate and SO_2 as causative agents for the elevated mortality levels; however, subsequent analyses of the London studies, as well as studies from other cities, indicate the importance of acid sulfates on mortality (176).

Another limitation is that epidemiological studies are frequently of worker populations, and such studies can be difficult to apply to prediction of health effects in the general population. Occupational studies, in general, focus on healthy adult male workers. The general population is more heterogeneous than the worker population and, for some pollutants, may exhibit a greater range in susceptibility. In general, only more recent epidemiology studies have considered adverse health effects of chemicals specific to women and children, such as developmental, reproductive, or hormonally mediated effects, including cancer. An example of the limitations of occupational epidemiology involves studies of peripheral nerve function in lead-exposed workers, which would underestimate risk of lead exposure in young children, for whom the primary concern is neurobehavioral effects resulting from relatively low-level exposures (217). At the same time, it must be recognized that the young and elderly are not always more susceptible to the effects of chemicals. As noted by Calabrese (25), adults, rather than the young or the elderly, are more susceptible to the renal toxicity of fluorides and mercury. High-risk subgroups are discussed in more detail in a later section of this chapter.

Epidemiology studies are frequently limited by the need for a relatively large increase in disease incidence (twofold or more), given the sample sizes generally available for such investigations. Enterline (55) notes that it would require a large population (1000 deaths, using the Peto model) to detect a 50% excess in deaths from lung cancer at an asbestos level of 2 fibers/cm^3 air.

Controlled clinical studies of humans exposed to pollutants address some of the difficulties of epidemiology studies. The exposures can be controlled and quantified, the effects are observed in humans, and the exposed population can be chosen to consist of susceptible individuals, such as asthmatics or exercising individuals. Thus, changes in airway resistance in asthmatics exposed to SO_2 during exercise (18,164) have been important in the EPA evaluation of the National Ambient Air Quality Standard (NAAQS) for SO_2 (210), because these effects reflect the response of the susceptible population, using an appropriate exposure concentration and a relevant averaging time. Given the subtlety of these changes (nonsymptomatic bronchoconstrictions) and the fact that they occur only in a selected subset of the general population (asthmatics constitute about 4% of the total population), these effects would not have been detectable in the general population.

One of the advantages of controlled clinical exposure studies, that they are performed with humans, is also a major limitation. Since these studies must be limited to short-term effects that are readily reversible, they cannot be used to evaluate the potential of a chemical to cause chronic disease. Furthermore, because of the mildness of the changes observed in these studies, one may question their clinical significance. For example, how does one interpret the change in resistance observed with SO_2 exposure, given that, if not perceptible, the relationship to physical performance may be questionable (72)? Also, although some susceptible populations, such as mild asthmatics, can be tested, individuals with a greater degree of impairment, such as asthmatics who require continual medication, are usually not considered to be appropriate subjects for these studies because of the greater potential for harm during exposure. Later sections in this chapter address the questions of severity of effect on susceptible populations in greater detail.

Animal toxicology studies constitute the third major source of information for assessing the toxicity of chemicals. Animal toxicology studies allow the investigator the greatest degree of control over the exposure conditions, the population exposed, and the effects measured. One can readily evaluate subtle effects of acute and chronic exposure. For example, morphological and numerical changes in the pulmonary type I and type II cell populations, as well as interstitial fibrosis, have been observed in rats exposed to 0.06 to 0.25 ppm O_3 (35,63). It would have been very difficult to describe this effect with other experimental approaches, and yet the effect is clearly of concern for humans who are exposed to comparable concentrations of ozone in certain urban environments.

In animal experiments, the ability to manipulate the experimental conditions permits the evaluation of many variables on the response to toxic chemicals. Thus, Elsayed and Mustafa (53) were able to demonstrate the protective effect of vitamin E on the acute toxicity of NO_2 in mice. In addition, the role of metabolism in susceptibility to polycyclic aromatic hydrocarbon-induced carcinogenesis has been evaluated in studies of genetic variants in mice (120,138). Such studies can be important in predicting modifiers of toxicity in humans and in identifying the susceptible human populations.

The limitations of animal studies fall into two broad categories: (a) those due to uncertainties in extrapolating from animals to humans, and (b) those due to uncertainties in extrapolating from the high exposures in animal studies to the lower exposures typically experienced by humans. Interspecies extrapolation is complicated by the greater homogeneity of laboratory animals than humans, the controlled conditions of housing and diet, innate genetic factors, and other variables. The relevance of trichloroethylene (TCE)-induced hepatocarcinogenesis in the mouse to humans has been questioned on the basis of differences in peroxisomal proliferation in the liver in the two species (52). Similarly, high exposure concentrations typically used in animal studies may result in saturation of detoxification pathways and thus may produce effects that are not relevant to effects produced at ambient exposure concentrations, where detoxification pathways are not saturated. Increased numbers of macrophages and impairment of alveolar clearance are observed in rats exposed to relatively high concentrations of diesel particulates (80). The significance to humans who are exposed to ambient levels of diesel particulates much lower than those employed in the animal studies is uncertain (143).

Historically, in vitro studies and analysis of structure–activity relationships have been used to help set priorities for chemical testing. For example, structure–activity relationships have been used to predict mutagenicity, lethality, and carcinogenicity (54). This type of information can be very useful, for example, in selecting compounds for longer term testing in animals or eliminating chemicals being considered for potential industrial or pharmaceutical applications due to toxicological concerns.

Short-term tests have typically been used indirectly in the regulatory process to support decision making, rather than as a basis per se for decision making. For example, evidence that a chemical is a point mutagen in an in vitro test system might be used to support the classification of a chemical as a possible human carcinogen or the use of a linear dose-response model for carcinogenesis. Metabolism, pharmacokinetic, and mechanistic studies can also provide information to reduce uncertainties in the use of toxicology information. For example, metabolic studies showing that a critical reactive metabolite in rodents is also formed in humans could reduce uncertainties in extrapolating from animals to humans, while mechanistic studies could indicate whether a subtle effect observed in a clinical study is a precursor for later, more serious health endpoints, and therefore of concern as a biomarker of effect.

In some circumstances, short-term tests and structure–activity relationships may be used directly to provide a basis for decision making. For example, Beck and co-workers (16) estimated permissible levels for alkylphenols in water, based on the ability of different alkylphenols to inhibit cyclooxygenase and by comparison with toxic effects of aspirin, a well known cyclooxygenase inhibitor. A critical element in this example is that adequate toxicological data were available for some members of the classes of chemicals being studied and that estimates of risk were applied within a class of chemicals of similar physical/chemical properties.

A summary comparing the differences between epidemiology, controlled clinical exposure, and animal toxicology studies is provided in Tables 2.2 to 2.4.

We can conclude from the preceding discussion that there is no "best" source of information for regulatory agencies. The rational approach is to examine all avail-

Table 2.2
Advantages and disadvantages of epidemiological studies

Advantages	Disadvantages
Exposure conditions realistic	Costly and time-consuming
Occurrence of interactive effects among individual chemicals	Post facto, not protective of public health[a]
Effects measured in humans	Difficulty in defining exposure, problems with confounding exposure
Full range of human susceptibility frequently expressed	Increase in risk must frequently be about twofold to be detected
	Effects measured often relatively crude (morbidity, mortality)

[a] Use of biomarkers in epidemiological studies, rather than disease endpoints, can allow such studies to be public health protective.

Table 2.3
Advantages and disadvantages of controlled clinical studies

Advantages	Disadvantages
Well-defined, controlled exposure conditions	Costly
Responses measured in humans	Relatively low exposure concentrations and short-term exposures
Potential to study subpopulations (e.g., asthmatics)	Limited to relatively small groups (usually <50 individuals)
Ability to measure relatively subtle effects	Limited to short-term, minor, reversible effects
	Usually most susceptible group not appropriate for study

Table 2.4
Advantages and disadvantages of animal toxicology studies

Advantages	Disadvantages
Readily manipulated exposure conditions	Uncertainties in relevance of animal response to human exposure
Ability to measure many types of responses	Controlled housing, diet, etc., of questionable relevance to humans
Ability to assess effect of host characteristics (e.g., gender, age, genetics) and other modifiers (e.g., diet) of response	Exposure concentrations and time frames often very different from those experienced by humans
Potential to evaluate mechanisms	

able sources of information in the evaluation of toxic chemicals. Some kinds of information may be especially useful in hazard identification, the likelihood that a chemical will be toxic to humans, whereas other types of information will be more appropriately applied to the estimation of the dose-response relationship.

EVALUATION OF CARCINOGENS

Background

The public demand for zero risk has made the regulation of carcinogens a formidable challenge. Within the scientific community, there is still no consensus on how to define a potential human carcinogen, much less how to estimate cancer risks under practical conditions of chemical exposure. This uncertainty is due largely to the fact that mechanisms of carcinogenesis for many chemicals are still poorly understood, and different carcinogens act in different ways to induce cancer. The task of regulating carcinogens has been complicated, rather than simplified, by many of the mechanistic discoveries of recent years. The simple picture of the 1950s, when only a very small number of chemicals were thought to be carcinogens, has been replaced by the realization that chemical carcinogenesis takes place in multiple stages, some with reversible steps, which have different dose-response relationships. Essential nutrients and hormones can be carcinogenic in some circumstances. The same chemical can promote or inhibit carcinogenesis, depending on the circumstances of exposure (75,121). Public pressure to regulate carcinogens, even where very little toxicological information exists, has in many circumstances compelled regulatory agencies to treat carcinogens as though they all act by the same mechanisms, even as it has become apparent that they do not. Despite virtual consensus in the scientific and regulatory communities that carcinogens should be regulated in a way that reflects their mechanism of action, sufficient information to allow this to be done does not exist for many chemicals.

From a public health standpoint, the regulatory agencies have generally regulated carcinogens at exposure levels that reflect a very low probability of tumor production (e.g., excess cancer risk of 1 per million exposed). However, for practical reasons, it is impossible to conduct animal studies of a size that would allow observation of effects following treatment at such low doses. The practice has therefore been to conduct animal studies at high dose levels and then extrapolate the results from high to low dose and from animals to humans. Thus, the chronic animal bioassay results, the extrapolation from high to low doses, and the extrapolation across species are used to derive potency factors (i.e., indicators of carcinogenic potency) for carcinogens. These potency factors enable one to relate a dose in humans to a probability of tumor occurring as a result of that dose. It should be noted that even with established human carcinogens, extrapolation procedures are still used to extrapolate carcinogenic response from high to low dose or from one type of exposure condition (e.g., intermittent, subchronic) to another exposure condition (e.g., continuous chronic).

This section on carcinogens first provides some basic information on mechanisms of carcinogenesis. We then describe some of the key issues that agencies address in the interpretation and application of scientific data on carcinogens. These issues fall into the categories of hazard identification and dose-response assessment (136). Hazard identification for carcinogens addresses two questions: (a) What is the evidence that a particular chemical is an animal carcinogen? (b) What is the likelihood that an animal carcinogen is a human carcinogen? Dose-response assessment attempts to determine the probability of tumor production, given a particular exposure or dose level. The dose-response assessment section of this chapter discusses mathematical models used to extrapolate from high to low doses, physiologically based pharmacokinetic (PBPK) modeling to relate administered and effective doses in animals and humans, and issues concerning the relationship between effective dose and response.

Mechanisms of Carcinogenesis

Carcinogenesis is currently understood to be a multistage process that has been described as involving the initiation, promotion, and progression of normal cells into neoplastic cells. Chemicals can act at one or more of these stages, and can act directly (e.g., mutagen) or indirectly (e.g., immune suppression). Initiation is generally understood to be a permanent and irreversible event involving DNA mutation, and the first step in the process of carcinogenesis. Many genotoxic agents are considered to be initiators, thus having the potential to begin the transition from normal to cancer cells. Genotoxic materials have been considered to act via a nonthreshold mechanism, and this belief has formed the basis for linear extrapolation of effects seen at high doses down to low doses. Inferences as to the absence of a threshold for initiating agents comes from the study of mutations that result from these agents. In addition, studies investigating the number of preneoplastic focal lesions induced by an initiating agent did not find a measurable threshold (149). Ionizing radiation is an example of an initiating agent. In addition, certain chemicals (e.g., aflatoxin B_1, diethylnitrosamine, tobacco smoke) are considered to be complete carcinogens, capable of initiation, promotion, and progression. Potential factors modifying the efficiency of initiation include rates of cell division and DNA synthesis as well as the rate of metabolism of a chemical to its active form or rate of metabolic detoxification. (It should therefore be noted that even the no-threshold concept may not be applicable to all genotoxic carcinogens, due to the existence of repair mechanisms and other factors that reduce or eliminate responses at low exposure levels.)

The promotion stage is characterized by clonal expansion of the initiated cells. Promoting agents can act by various mechanisms to increase rates of cell proliferation or decrease rates of cell death. For example, cell proliferation can be induced by cytoxic agents or mitotic agents. Interference with intercellular communication may also be responsible for clonal expansion of initiated cells (181). An important feature of this stage is its reversibility and, in some cases, the existence of a threshold for the effect. In many cancer model systems, withdrawal of the promoting agent halts the development of tumors. The promotion stage is also easily modulated by environmental factors including frequency of dosing, age of test animal, and diet (149,195). Promoting agents are generally thought to exhibit a threshold (or inflection point) in the dose-response curve. Examples of promoting agents include hormones, alcohol, and dietary fat.

Progression is an irreversible stage characterized by the development of malignant neoplasms, and is understood to require a second genetic mutation. Agents that act only during progression, or advance a cell from promotion to progression, have not yet been definitively characterized. It has been hypothesized that malignant neoplasms may all exhibit an abnormal expression of one or more proto- and cellular oncogenes (149). In this scenario, initiation is defined by the first mutation event and progression as the second mutation, resulting in homozygosity at the anti-oncogene locus, and total loss of growth control (130).

Hazard Identification

The question of how to decide whether a particular chemical is a potential human carcinogen is currently the subject of considerable scientific debate. It is an important question because the act of labeling some chemicals "carcinogens" and not labeling others has profound regulatory and societal implications (66). This regulatory paradigm, whereby chemicals are regulated either as carcinogens or as noncarcinogens, requires that the question of whether a particular chemical is a carcinogen or not be answered with a "yes" or "no." In the United States, most regulatory agencies have historically regulated all carcinogens as though they operate via the same no-threshold mechanism. However, different chemicals may act in different ways during the various stages of cancer formation to impact the development of the tumor. These various mechanisms of tumor formation are not all consistent with the mechanistic assumptions that form the basis of the regulatory framework for carcinogens. Thus, the more we learn about carcinogenesis, the less the simple regulatory approach is able to accommodate the new information. A chemical may be carcinogenic via certain routes of exposure and not others, or only above certain dose levels. More flexible classification approaches are being developed (e.g., ref. 195) that allow the incorporation of more science into the classification process.

In the next section, we describe current classification approaches, but the reader is reminded that the current scientific debate on these schemes is continuing to fuel new approaches. Regulatory agencies generally classify potential carcinogens, based on an evaluation of both human and animal studies, as well as supporting information from short-term tests for mutagenicity and structure–activity relationships. Because human evidence exists for so few chemicals, animal studies generally provide most of the available information about the potential carcinogenicity of a chemical to humans.

Animal Studies

The evidence that a chemical is an animal carcinogen frequently derives from long-term animal bioassays. Such studies usually consist of exposing groups of about 50 animals (typically rats or mice) to two concentrations of a chemical over the lifetime of the animals. Sex- and age-matched unexposed animals constitute the control group. At the termination of the bioassay, the animals are killed and the number of tumor-bearing animals and the number and type of tumors per animal are quantified. Interim examinations may be performed, particularly on animals that appear moribund.

The maximum tolerated dose. Dose selection plays a key issue in the design and interpretation of the animal bioassay. Animals are typically exposed at two dose levels: the maximum tolerated dose (MTD) and half the MTD. The MTD is predicted from subchronic toxicity studies as the dose "that causes no more than a 10% weight decrement, as compared to the appropriate control groups, and does not produce mortality, clinical signs of toxicity or pathologic lesions (other than those related to a neoplastic response) that would be predicted [in the long-term bioassay] to shorten an animal's natural lifespan" (171). The MTD is not a nontoxic dose and is expected to produce some level of acceptable toxicity to indicate that the animals were sufficiently challenged by the chemical. The MTD has been justified as a means of increasing the sensitivity of an animal bioassay involving limited numbers of animals so as to be able to predict risks in large numbers of humans (76).

An objection to the use of MTDs has been that metabolic overloading may occur at high dose levels, leading to an abnormal handling of the test compound (131). For example, toxic metabolites could be produced as a consequence of saturation of detoxification pathways. Organ toxicity could occur that might not happen at lower concentrations of the chemical (127), particularly at those concentrations to which humans are typically exposed. Thus, it has been argued that nongenotoxic agents that are determined to be positive in rodent carcinogenicity bioassays, due to target organ toxicity and subsequent cell proliferation, should not be assumed to be carcinogenic at low doses (37).

Ames and co-workers (9,10) have suggested that target-organ toxicity and subsequent mitogenesis is responsible for the fact that over half of all chemicals tested in chronic bioassays at the MTD are determined to be carcinogens in rodents. They observed that both genotoxic and nongenotoxic agents tested at the MTD cause increased rates of mitogenesis, thus increasing the rate of mutation. For several chemicals, induction of tumors was more strongly correlated with cell division than with DNA adducts or mutagenic activity. Others have reported that cancer potency and MTD are inversely correlated and that, consequently, the potency estimate is simply an artifact of the experimental design (161). Goodman and Wilson (65) found that cancer potency and the MTD were more strongly related for nonmutagens than for mutagens in rat bioassays, indicating that the carcinogenic effect and toxicity were more closely associated for nonmutagens than for mutagens. However, they noted that even for most mutagens, their findings suggested that, at high doses, carcinogenicity is induced via mechanisms associated with toxicity.

Haseman and Lockhart (77) compared the sensitivity of the rodent bioassay for detecting carcinogens at the MTD as compared to lower doses. Approximately two-thirds of the chemicals that were positive at the MTD in rodents were also positive at the lower dose, albeit often for fewer tumor sites. One tumor site that was affected disproportionately was the kidney, where a positive response was observed at the lower dose only about one third of the time as compared to the higher dose.

The EPA (195) noted that bioassay results at doses that exceeded the MTD can be rejected if toxic damage to target organs compromises study interpretation. The reason is that dosing above the MTD in a study may result in tumor production secondary to tissue damage rather than a direct carcinogenic influence of the agent tested.

Thus, use of information from testing at fractional doses of the MTD may yield results that are more relevant to human risk. Overall there would be a somewhat modest (except for kidney-only carcinogens) reduction in the total number of carcinogens. It should also be noted that it is still possible that mechanisms may occur at fractional MTD levels that would not occur at the typically lower human exposure levels.

Other issues in hazard identification. Another key issue in the evaluation of animal bioassays is the analysis of the tumors themselves. Considerations include the categorization of benign tumors and whether tumor analysis should be site-specific or based on all sites. The position of the IARC (110) is that "few, if any chemicals exist which produce only benign tumors and no malignant tumors in any species" and that chemicals that cause a marked increase in the number of benign tumors "are now viewed with almost as much suspicion as potential human hazards as they would have been if the induced tumors had been malignant." Thus, it has been the general policy of regulatory agencies to accord almost the same weight to benign tumors as to malignant tumors, especially if there is evidence that the benign tumors could progress to malignancy (208).

It is sometimes stated that one should consider only the overall incidence of tumors, since, from a public health perspective, the concern is with total cancer risk for humans rather than risk at any one site. While this position has an innate appeal, it is difficult to apply in practice for two main reasons:

- This approach greatly decreases the ability of the bioassay to detect a positive effect, given the high background incidence of some tumor types in rodents. For example, the incidence of testicular tumors can be as high as 82% in rats and liver tumors can be as high as 25% in mice (74).
- The grouping of tumor types that do not share a common cellular origin is of questionable biological relevance, since the mechanisms involved in the production of the different tumor types could differ. Furthermore, the metastatic potential of different tumor types is highly variable and would have an important influence on the lethality of a particular type of cancer.

It should also be noted that reductions in tumor incidence are frequently observed in the same cancer bioassays in which tumor increases are observed. A recent analysis by Linkov and co-workers (121) indicates the anticarcinogenic effects observed in rodent bioassays are not explained by random effects. The basis for the reduction is not known and could be a consequence of perturbations in the animal's physiology. These observations lend credence to the concept that animal bioassays must be interpreted with special attention as to whether biological phenomena are induced at high doses that may not occur (or occur with a much lower frequency) at low doses. A similar observation is found in the evaluation of some human carcinogens, in particular those which act through hormonal processes. For example, oral contraceptives are associated with an increased risk of breast cancer, but a decreased risk of ovarian and endometrial cancer (Table 2.5). Anticarcinogenic properties of carcinogens are typically not considered as part of the regulatory process for carcinogens.

In addition, the standard NTP-type 2-year cancer bioassay may not be sensitive to hormonally regulated cancers such as breast cancer. This is because the mouse and rat strains used to perform these bioassays are selected because they are known to be susceptible to liver, kidney, or lung tumors in particular. It has not been demonstrated that these strains are also susceptible to cancers at hormonally sensitive sites. Thus, these bioassays may not detect certain cancer effects that are hormonally regulated (172).

Carcinogen Classification Schemes

The IARC, the European Union (EU), the EPA, the National Toxicology Program (NTP), the German Commission for Investigation of Health Hazards, Health Canada, and the ACGIH have developed classification schemes for carcinogens, based on a weight-of-evidence or strength-of-evidence evaluation of available human and animal studies. These seven classification systems are shown in Table 2.6. The EPA developed guidelines in 1986 (208) and proposed new guidelines in 1996 (195) (Tables 2.7–2.10). Some classification schemes are based on the weight of evidence considering positive and negative evidence (e.g., EPA), whereas others (e.g., IARC) classify chemicals as carcinogens, based on a strength-of-evidence (positive evidence only) basis. The different guidelines use mechanistic information to different degrees.

The EPA (208), IARC (111), and other agencies typically conclude that a chemical demonstrating "sufficient evidence of carcinogenicity" from animal experiments is a potential human carcinogen. To some degree this conclusion is supported by evaluation of known human carcinogens in animal bioassays. For the 67 chemicals, processes or environmental factors associated with cancer indication in humans by IARC (112,177), more than half of those that have been tested have also been positive in animal bioassays (Table 2.5). Recent understanding of carcinogenesis indicates that this assumption is not valid for all animal carcinogens. Species-specific responses or high-dose-only effects indicate that positive animal results are not always evidence of human carcinogenicity.

In 1996, EPA proposed new cancer guidelines (195). These proposed guidelines, in their flexibility and incorporation of new science, represent a significant advance in carcinogen classification schemes. The new guidelines take a weight-of-evidence approach in which human (Table 2.7), animal (Table 2.8), and other relevant

Table 2.5

Chemicals, industrial processes, and environmental factors associated with cancer induction in humans: target organs and main routes of exposure in humans and degree of supporting evidence in animals (IARC)

	Humans		Animals,
Chemical or industrial process	Main type of exposure[a]	Target organ(s)[b]	degree of evidence for carcinogenicity
1-(2-Chloroethyl)-3-(4-methylcyclohexyl)-1-nitrosourea (methyl-CCNU)	Medicinal	Leukemia	Limited
1,4-Butanediol dimethanesulfonate (Myleran)	Medicinal	Leukemia	Limited
2-Naphthylamine	Occupational	Bladder (liver)	Sufficient
4-Aminobiphenyl	Occupational	Bladder	Sufficient
8-Methoxypsoralen (Methoxsalen) plus UV radiation	Medicinal	Skin	Sufficient
Aflatoxins	Environmental	Liver (lung)	Sufficient
Alcoholic beverages	Cultural	Oral cavity, pharynx, larynx, esophagus, liver (breast)	Inadequate
Aluminum production	Occupational	Lung, bladder (lymphoma, esophagus, stomach)	No data
Arsenic compounds[c]	Occupational, medicinal, and environmental	Skin, lung (liver, hematopoietic system, gastrointestinal tract, kidney)	Limited
Asbestos	Occupational	Lung, pleura, peritoneum, gastrointestinal tract, larynx	Sufficient
Auramine manufacture	Occupational	Bladder	No data
Azathioprine	Medicinal	Lymphoma, skin, mesenchymal tumors, hepatobiliary system	Limited
Benzene	Occupational	Leukemia	Sufficient
Benzidine	Occupational	Bladder	Sufficient
Beryllium and beryllium compounds[d]	Occupational	Lung	Sufficient
Betel quid (with tobacco)	Cultural	Oral cavity (pharynx, larynx, esophagus)	Limited
Bis(chloromethyl) ether and chloromethyl methyl ether (technical grade)	Occupational	Lung	Sufficient
Boot and shoe manufacture and repair	Occupational	Leukemia, nasal sinus (bladder, digestive tract)	No data
Cadmium and cadmium compounds[e]	Occupational	Lung	Sufficient
Chlorambucil	Medicinal	Leukemia	Sufficient
Chromium compounds (hexavalent)[c]	Occupational	Lung (gastrointestinal tract)	Sufficient
Ciclosporin[g] (U.S.: cyclosporin)	Medicinal	Lymphoma, Kaposi's sarcoma	Limited
Coal tars and pitches, mineral and shale oils, and soots[f]	Occupational, environmental	Skin, lung, bladder (gastrointestinal tract, leukemia, colon)	Sufficient
Cyclophosphamide	Medicinal	Bladder, leukemia	Sufficient
Diethylstilbestrol	Medicinal	Cervix/vagina, breast, testis (endometrium)	Sufficient
Epstein–Bar–virus[h]	Environmental	Lymphomas, nasopharyngeal carcinoma	Sufficient
Erionite	Environmental, cultural	Pleura, peritoneum	Sufficient
Estrogens (steroidal, nonsteroidal)[c]	Medicinal	Endometrium, breast, cervix/vagina, testis	Sufficient
Estrogen therapy, postmenopausal[i]	Medicinal	Endometrium, breast	No data
Ethylene oxide[c]	Occupational	Lymphatic and hematopoietic systems	Sufficient
Furniture and cabinet making	Occupational	Nasal sinus	Inadequate
Helicobacter pylori[k]	Environmental	Stomach	No data
Hematite mining (with radon exposure)	Occupational	Lung	Inadequate
Hepatitis B virus[l]	Environmental	Liver	Inadequate

Table 2.5 (*continued*)

	Humans		Animals,
Chemical or industrial process	Main type of exposure[a]	Target organ(s)[b]	degree of evidence for carcinogenicity
Hepatitis C virus[m]	Environmental	Liver	Inadequate
Human immunodeficiency virus Type 1[n]	Environmental	Kaposi's sarcoma, non-Hodgkin's lymphoma	Inadequate
Human papilloma virus Types 16 and 18[o]	Environmental	Cervix	None
Human T-cell lymphotropic virus Type 1[p]	Environmental	Adult T-cell leukemia/lymphoma	Inadequate
Ionizing radiation	Environmental	Leukemia, skin, various internal organs	Sufficient
Iron and steel founding	Occupational	Lung (digestive tract, genito-urinary tract, leukemia)	No data
Isopropyl alcohol manufacture (strong acid process)	Occupational	Nasal sinus (larynx)	Inadequate
Magenta manufacture	Occupational	Bladder	Inadequate
Melphalan	Medicinal	Leukemia	Sufficient
MOPP and other combined chemotherapy including alkylating agents	Medicinal	Leukemia	No data
Mustard gas	Occupational	Lung, larynx, pharynx	Limited
Nickel and nickel compounds[c]	Occupational	Nasal sinus, lung (larynx)	Sufficient
N, *N*-Bis(2-chloroethyl)-2-naphthylamine (Chlornaphazine)	Medicinal	Bladder	Limited
Opisthorchis viverrini[a]	Environmental	Liver	Limited
Oral contraceptives, combined[r,s]	Medicinal	Liver (also protective effect against cancers of the ovary and endometrium)	Sufficient
Oral contraceptives, sequential	Medicinal	Endometrium	Sufficient
Painters (occupational exposures as)	Occupational	Lung (esophagus, stomach, bladder)	No data
Phenacetin (in analgesic mixtures)	Medicinal	Renal pelvis/ureter, bladder	Limited
Radon and its decay products	Environmental	Lung	Sufficient
Rubber industry	Occupational	Bladder, leukemia (lymphoma, lung, renal tract, digestive tract, skin, liver, larynx, brain, stomach)	Inadequate
Salted fish[t]	Environmental	Nasopharynx	Limited
Schistosoma haematobium[u]	Environmental	Urinary bladder	Limited
Silica, crystalline[v]	Occupational	Lung	Sufficient
Solar radiation[w]	Environmental	Skin	Sufficient
Talc containing asbestos fibers	Occupational	Lung (pleura)	Inadequate
Tamoxifen[x]	Medicinal	Endometrium (reduces risk for contralateral breast cancer in women with previous diagnosis of breast cancer)	Sufficient
2,3,7,8-Tetrachlorodibenzo-*para*-dioxin[y]	Occupational	Multi-site with no site predominating	Sufficient
Thiotepa[z]	Medicinal	Leukemia	Sufficient
Tobacco products, smokeless	Environmental, cultural	Oral cavity (pharynx, esophagus)	Inadequate
Tobacco smoke	Environmental, cultural	Lung, bladder, oral cavity, larynx, pharynx, esophagus, pancreas, renal pelvis (stomach, liver, cervix)	Sufficient
Treosulphan	Medicinal	Leukemia	No data
Vinyl chloride	Occupational	Liver, lung, brain, lymphatic and hematopoietic system (gastrointestinal tract)	Sufficient
Wood dust[aa]	Occupational	Nasal cavity, paranasalsinus	Inadequate

Note. From IARC (112), Tomatis et al. (177), IARC (115), and references in other footnotes.

[a] The main types of exposure mentioned are those by which the association has been demonstrated; exposures other than those mentioned may also occur.

[b] Suspected target organs in parentheses.

[c] The evaluation of carcinogenicity to humans applies to the group of chemicals as a whole and not necessarily to all individual chemicals within the group.

[d] Source: International Agency for Research on Cancer (87).

[e] Source: International Agency for Research on Cancer (88).

[f] Not all chemicals in this group are associated with all cancers listed.

[g] Source: International Agency for Research on Cancer (89).

[h] Source: International Agency for Research on Cancer (90).

[i] Source: International Agency for Research on Cancer (91).

[j] Source: International Agency for Research on Cancer (92).

[k] Source: International Agency for Research on Cancer (93).

[l] Source: International Agency for Research on Cancer (94).

[m] Source: International Agency for Research on Cancer (95).

[n] Source: International Agency for Research on Cancer (96).

[o] Source: International Agency for Research on Cancer (97).

[p] Source: International Agency for Research on Cancer (98).

[q] Source: International Agency for Research on Cancer (99).

[r] Source: International Agency for Research on Cancer (100).

[s] Source: International Agency for Research on Cancer (101).

[t] Source: International Agency for Research on Cancer (102).

[u] Source: International Agency for Research on Cancer (103).

[v] Source: International Agency for Research on Cancer (104).

[w] Source: International Agency for Research on Cancer (105).

[x] Source: International Agency for Research on Cancer (106).

[y] Source: International Agency for Research on Cancer (107).

[z] Source: International Agency for Research on Cancer (108).

[aa] Source: International Agency for Research on Cancer (109).

toxicological (Table 2.9) evidence are evaluated. As part of this evaluation, the quality of an individual study, as well as the overall consistency across studies, is considered. Demonstration of cancer in humans at the same organ site in multiple studies with well-characterized exposure in the absence of confounding exposures enhances confidence that a chemical is the likely cause of cancer. In contrast to the 1986 guidelines, other evidence relevant to carcinogenicity, such as mechanistic information in animals that attests to the relevance (or lack of relevance) of a particular tumor response, is explicitly considered. Data from human, animal, and other sources are combined to weigh the totality of evidence (Table 2.10) to classify the human carcinogenic potential of a particular chemical. Three descriptors have been proposed:

- Known/likely—Applies to chemicals for which there is convincing human evidence of carcinogenicity or limited (or no) human evidence combined with strong animal evidence that is relevant to the human response.
- Cannot be determined—Applies to chemicals where a conclusion regarding carcinogenicity cannot be drawn for reasons including the presence of conflicting or inadequate data, or suggestive data not sufficiently strong to draw any conclusion.
- Not likely—Applies to chemicals for which there is experimental evidence (in the absence of human data suggesting a carcinogenic potential) that indicates a lack of human hazard potential. Types of evidence include demonstration that a response in animals (e.g., male rat kidney cancer due to $\alpha_{2\mu}$-globulin nephropathy) is not relevant to humans or that well-conducted animal cancer bioassays are negative for carcinogenicity. One noteworthy aspect of the "not likely" category is that, in contrast to the 1986 guidelines, this category allows for conditional classification. For example, a chemical may be classified as likely to be a human carcinogen only with respect to a particular route of exposure, or only above a certain dose level.

Perchloroethylene provides a useful example of how different agencies classify carcinogens. For example, IARC considers perchloroethylene a probable human carcinogen (category 2A), based on limited evidence in humans and sufficient evidence in animals (114). In contrast, Health Canada (123) and ACGIH (6) both consider perchloroethylene as probably not carcinogenic to humans (categories A5 and Group V, respectively). IARC placed greater weight on often times conflicting epidemiological evidence than did ACGIH or Health Canada. For example, IARC considered the positive association between perchloroethylene and certain types of cancer (e.g., non-Hodgkin's lymphoma) as unlikely to be due to chance, while still acknowledging the possible role of confounding factors (e.g., exposure to other solvents). In contrast, Health Canada (123) considered the weaknesses in the epidemiological studies sufficiently large as to make the studies inadequate for drawing any conclusions on perchloroethylene carcinogenicity. With respect to animal studies, both IARC and Health Canada concluded that perchloroethylene causes liver cancer in mice. However, Health Canada concluded that the liver tumors in mice are unlikely to be relevant to humans, based on metabolic differences between humans and mice [humans produce much less trichloroactic acid (TCA) the relevant metabolite in the liver] and species-specific response differences to TCA (humans show little, if any, peroxisomal proliferation, which is likely to play a critical role in hepatic carcinogenesis in response to TCA). Overall, IARC gave greater weight to positive evidence than to negative or conflicting evi-

Table 2.6
Summary of the classification schemes for carcinogens

Agency	Classification	Meaning
DFG/MAK	A1:	Induces malignant tumors in humans.
	A2:	Clearly carcinogenic in animal studies.
	B	Justifiably suspected of having carcinogenic potential.
EU	1	Carcinogenic to humans.
	2	Should be regarded as if carcinogenic to humans.
	3	Cause for concern in humans.
		3A. Substances that are well investigated.
		3B. Substances that are insufficiently investigated.
IARC	1	Carcinogenic to humans.
	2	Reasonably anticipated to be a carcinogen.
		2A. Probably carcinogenic in humans; limited human evidence, sufficient animal evidence.
		2B. Possibly carcinogenic in humans; limited human evidence in the absence of sufficient animal evidence.
	3	Not classified.
	4	Probably not carcinogenic to humans.
ACGIH	A1	Confirmed human carcinogen.
	A2	Suspected human carcinogen, limited human evidence and sufficient relevant animal evidence
	A3	Confirmed animal carcinogen with unknown relevance to human, epidemiologic studies do not confirm risk to humans.
	A4	Not classifiable.
	A5	Not suspected as human carcinogen, based on properly conducted epidemiologic studies or evidence in animal studies.
Health Canada	Group I	Carcinogenic to humans.
	Group II	Probably carcinogenic to humans. Inadequate epidemiologic evidence; sufficient evidence in animal species.
	Group III	Possibly carcinogenic to humans. Inadequate or flawed epidemiologic studies. Limited animal evidence, or adequate animal evidence, but involves epigenetic mechanisms.
	Group IV	Unlikely to be carcinogenic in humans. No evidence in adequate epidemiologic studies; positive animal studies of limited or unlikely relevance to humans.
	Group V	Probably not carcinogenic in humans. No evidence in adequate epidemiologic studies. No evidence or inadequate evidence in animal studies.
U.S. EPA	–A	Human carcinogen. Sufficient epidemiologic evidence.
	–B	Probable human carcinogen.
		B1. Limited epidemiologic evidence, sufficient animal evidence.
		B2. Inadequate or no epidemiologic evidence, sufficient animal evidence.
	–C	Possible human carcinogen. Limited animal evidence, no epidemiologic evidence.
	–D	Not classifiable. Inadequate or no human or animal evidence.
	–E	Evidence of non-carcinogenicity for humans. No evidence for carcinogenicity in at least two adequate animal species in both adequate epidemiologic and animal studies.
NTP	–1	Known to be a carcinogen.
	–2	Reasonably anticipated to be a carcinogen.
		A. Limited evidence in human studies indicating credible causal relationship evidence in human studies.
		B. Sufficient evidence in animal studies.

Note. DFG/MAK, Deutsche Forschungsgemeinschaft/maximale arbeitsplatz-Konzentration (German Commission for the Investigation of Health Hazards of Chemical compounds in the work area) (49, as cited in 140). EU, European Union (56, as cited in 140). IARC, International Agency for Research on Cancer (111,113,115). ACGIH/TLV, American Conference of Governmental Industrial Hygienists, threshold limit values (5). Health Canada (79), Human Health Risk Assessment for Priority Substances, as cited in http://www.terd.org/.tor/methods/cancer.htm. U.S. EPA (208), see Table 7–10 and text for proposed modifications. NTP, National Toxicology Program, as cited in ref. 5.

Table 2.7
Factors for weighing human evidence

Increase Weight	Decrease Weight
Number of independent studies with consistent results	Few studies Equally well designed and conducted studies with null results
Most causal criteria satisfied: • Temporal relationship • Strong association • Reliable exposure data • Dose response relationship • Freedom from bias and confounding or results cannot be explained by bias and confounding • Biological plausibility • High statistical significance	Few causal criteria satisfied

Note. Adapted from U.S. EPA (195).

Table 2.8
Factors for weighing animal evidence

Increase Weight	Decrease Weight
Number of independent studies with consistent results	Single study; inconsistent results
Same site across species, similar response with structural analogues	Single site/species/sex
Multiple positive observations across species, sexes, tumor sites	
Severity and progression of lesions	Benign tumors only
• Early in life tumors/malignancy	
• Lesion progression through malignancy	Hight background of incidence tumors
• Uncommon tumor	
Route of administration like human exposure	Route of administration unlike human exposure

Note. Adapted from U.S. EPA (195).

dence on mechanistic data. In contrast, Health Canada took more of a weight-of-evidence approach, similar to that proposed by EPA in the 1996 guidelines (195).

Dose-Response Assessment

One of the most contentious aspects of the evaluation of animal carcinogens by regulatory agencies is characterizing the dose-response relationship at the exposure levels to which humans are likely to be exposed. Animals are typically exposed to carcinogens at levels that are orders of magnitude greater than those likely to be encountered in the environment by humans. It would be impossible to perform animal experiments with a large enough number of animals to directly estimate the level of risk at low exposure levels. Thus, to obtain a quantitative estimate of the risks that humans are likely to encounter at ambient exposures requires the extrapolation of effects observed at high doses to low doses,

Table 2.9
Factors for weighing other key evidence

Increase Weight	Decrease Weight
A rich set of other key data are available	Few or poor data
Physicochemical data (e.g., electropholicity) support hazard potential	or
Data indicate reactivity with macromolecules	Inadequate data necessitating use of default assumptions
Structure–activity relationships support hazard potential	or
Comparable metabolism and toxicokinetics across species	Mechanistic and other data show that animal findings are not relevant to humans
Toxicological and human clinical data support tumor findings	
Biomarker data support attribution of effects to agent	
Mode-of-action data support causal interpretation of human evidence or relevance of animal evidence	

Note. Adapted from U.S. EPA (195).

Table 2.10
Factors for weighing totality of evidence

Increase weight	Decrease weight
Evidence of human causality	Data not available or do not show causality
Evidence of animal effects relevant to humans	Data not available or not relevant
Consistency across studies	Conflicting data
Comparable metabolism and toxicokinetics between species	Metabolism and toxicokinetics not comparable
Mode of action comparable across species	Mode of action not comparable across species

Note. Adapted from U.S. EPA (195).

and from effects observed in animals to humans. Even the use of carcinogenicity data from human studies (mostly occupational studies) frequently requires the use of extrapolation models to estimate risks to humans exposed at lower ambient levels.

Mechanistic models are being developed to assist in dose-response assessment. Pharmacokinetic models attempt to describe the relationship between exposure and biologically relevant dose to the target tissue. These models characterize absorption, distribution, metabolism, and excretion of chemicals. Pharmacodynamic models attempt to describe the relationship between the dose to target tissue and response. Both of these types of models can assist in extrapolation from high to low doses and across species.

Low-Dose Extrapolation

Extrapolation from high to low dose is done using mathematical models that are hypothesized to characterize the dose-response relationship of carcinogens at both the high dose and response levels observed in animal or human occupational studies and the low dose and response levels of interest for human exposures. The choice of mathematical model depends on two factors: (a) the hypothesis for the mechanism of carcinogenesis for a particular chemical, and (b) the science policy decision to choose, in the absence of data firmly supporting one model or another, the more conservative model (of several biologically plausible models) or to present results from a range of plausible models.

Threshold versus nonthreshold mechanisms. The determination of whether carcinogenesis is a threshold or nonthreshold phenomenon is a key consideration in the choice of the model used to characterize the dose-response relationship. It is considered plausible that carcinogenesis could be a nonthreshold phenomenon for genotoxic agents, particularly those that act directly to cause mutations. For example, the human carcinogen vinyl chloride is an electrophilic agent and is understood to interact with DNA (220). However, there is much debate over whether carcinogenesis is a threshold phenomenon for many chemicals that do not interact directly with DNA (not directly genotoxic) and that may induce cancer through epigenetic mechanisms.

In addition, for many carcinogens, it is unclear whether the dose-response relationship observed at high doses is necessarily the same as the dose-response relationship that might occur at low doses. Because the measure of a chemical's carcinogenic potency is typically determined by fitting a model to the observed data and then extrapolating to low doses, the implicit assumption is that the dose-response relationship is the same at high and low doses. For many chemicals that cause cell damage at high doses, or for chemicals for which detoxification pathways become saturated at high doses, it is likely that a different dose-response relationship will be observed at high and low doses, even for those chemicals where a non-zero slope is plausible at any dose.

Butterworth (22) has noted that there are many different classes of non-DNA-reactive carcinogens, and that the characterization of carcinogens as either genotoxic or nongenotoxic is too simple to adequately reflect the numerous mechanisms by which nongenotoxic carcinogens exert their effects. For example, the potent promoter TCDD, which is characterized as a hormone-type carcinogen, acts by binding to a specific receptor, resulting in enzyme induction via an apparent no-threshold mechanism. Thus, Portier and co-workers have postulated that TCDD may cause cancer by a nonthreshold mechanism despite its characterization as a nongenotoxic carcinogen (152). Other types of nongenotoxic carcinogens include phenobarbital, a non-DNA-reactive carcinogen that is understood to act by altering growth control (increasing mitogenesis), and saccharin, which appears to exhibit initiating/promotional and/or carcinogenic activity as secondary events to the cytotoxicity and increased cell proliferation caused by the high dose levels used in animal bioassays (22). Thus, saccharin would not be anticipated to increase tumor production at doses that do not cause cytotoxicity, and phenobarbital might not be expected to cause cancer at doses that do not affect growth control.

Zeise et al. (222) reviewed the experimental evidence for various shapes of dose-response relationships for carcinogens. They concluded that "reliable high dose data from human studies contains examples of superlinearity (radium injections and bone cancer), linearity (various radiation exposures), and sublinearity (smoking)." (p. 301). Their analysis of animal studies indicated that the "variety of shapes of dose-response curves observed for humans was also seen for animals." Zeise et al. noted that there are no data to indicate the shape of dose-response relationships at doses corresponding to lifetime risks of one in a million; in humans there are some data for incidence rates as low as 1%, and in animals there are two large studies that provide data at lifetime risks of a few tenths of a percent. Because carcinogens act by different mechanisms, it is very likely that different carcinogens, or classes of carcinogens, will exhibit different types of dose-response relationships. Moreover the same carcinogen may cause cancer at different tumor sites via different mechanisms.

A striking example of different dose-response relationships for a single carcinogen is the example of 2-acetylaminofluorene (2-AAF) (40). 2-AAF is a potent mutagenic carcinogen. The dose-response relationship for 2-AAF-induced liver cancer exhibits the expected (for a genotoxic carcinogen) linear dose-response relationship, whereas the dose-response relationship for bladder cancer is highly nonlinear, demonstrating an apparent threshold. The mechanistic basis for the different dose-response relationships appears to involve differences in the relative importance of genetic damage (the likely key event in liver cancer) versus genetic damage *and* hyperplasia of the bladder urothelium (the likely key events in bladder cancer). Thus, selection of the appropriate shape of the dose-response relationship for *any* chemical requires understanding of the mechanism by which tumors are induced.

Mathematical models. The choice of the low-dose extrapolation model can have a major impact on the estimate of risk at low exposure levels. Figure 2.3 shows the estimate of risk from 2-acetylaminofluorene at low exposure levels, using different models. The level of risk varies by many orders of magnitude at the same exposure level, depending on the model chosen to characterize the dose-response curve in the unobservable region. One of the more common models used by regulatory agencies particularly in the United States has been the linearized multistage model (12). The EPA has used the upper 95% confidence limit of this model on the basis of its biological plausibility (it assumes a nonthreshold) and its conservatism (it is unlikely to underestimate risk at low exposure levels) (208) to develop cancer slope factors (CSF), in units of $(mg/kg\text{-}day)^{-1}$. CSFs relate dosage (mg/kg-day) to the probability of an individual developing cancer. Cancer potency estimates for chemicals are highly dependent on model choice. Anderson (12) analyzed cancer potency estimates for TCDD, derived by using different low dose extrapolation

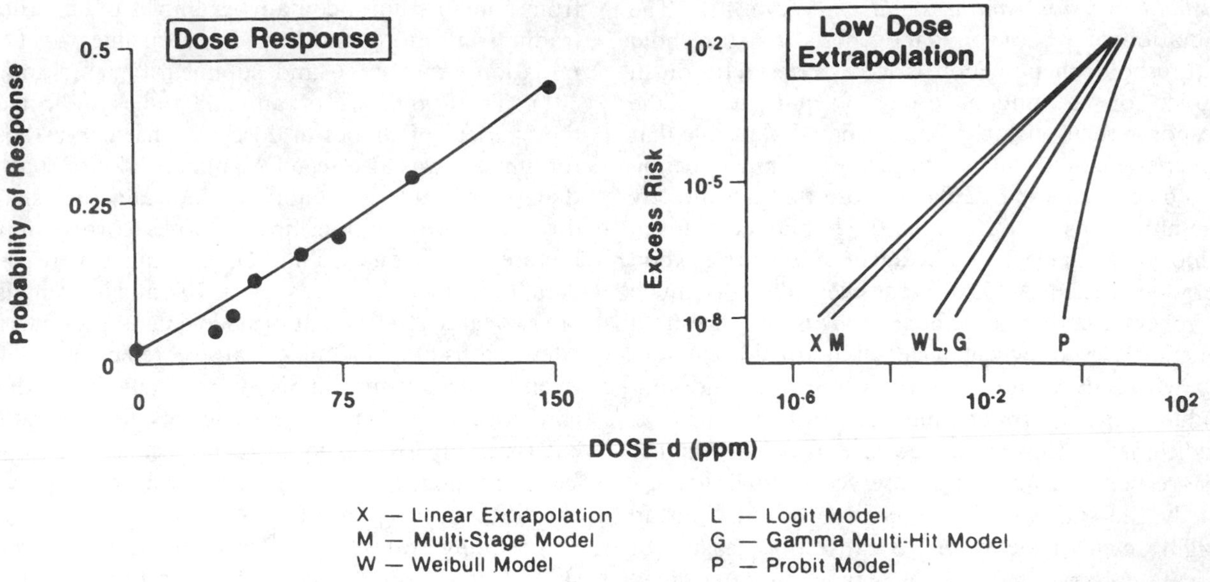

FIG. 2.3. Low-dose extrapolation for 2-acetylaminofluorene under several mathematical models. From Bickis and Krewski (19a).

models and different selection and treatment of bioassay data, and found that model choice alone (Weibull, multistage, log probit) would account for a difference in calculated cancer potency of 13 orders of magnitude.

One difficulty with the use of the upper 95% confidence limit of this model is that this approach basically reduces the model to worst-case curve fitting and does not take basic carcinogenic mechanisms into account. Thus, Cook et al. (43) have stated that if the multistage model as they defined it for carcinogenesis were correct, then the value of k, or the number of stages of cellular transformation, would generally be from four to six. However, the algorithm used in the calculation of cancer risk by the EPA for the multistage model requires k to assume a value not greater than the number of dose levels used in the study. Because three dose levels are usually employed—the MTD, half the MTD, and controls—the value of k is restrained to be, at most, equal to 3. Furthermore, when the MTD dose has been overestimated and excessive mortality occurs, the MTD cannot be used for risk assessment, thereby reducing k from 3 to 2. Allowing the value of k to be determined by the number of dose levels in a study, rather than on an understanding of the process of carcinogenesis, results in risk estimations of the multistage model that have reduced biologic relevance (43).

Because of the uncertainties in dose-response modeling for low dose cancer risk and the growing acceptance of a threshold dose-response relationship for some carcinogens, in the proposed 1996 cancer risk assessment guidelines, the EPA revised the approach to dose-response assessment (195). If sufficient data are available, a biologically based dose-response model represents the most appropriate method for evaluating the observed data and for extrapolating to exposures below the observed dose range. Data are not available for most carcinogens for development of biologically based models. In this case, a "point of departure" approach is recommended. The point of departure represents a dose, within the range of observed data, associated with a 10% extra tumor risk. The point of departure is developed using the linearized multistage model and expressed as the lower 95% confidence limit on the dose associated with 10% extra risk (LED_{10}). Risks below the LED_{10} are characterized either through linear extrapolation (for chemicals believed to act via a linear dose-response relationship (e.g., genotoxic carcinogens), or through a margin-of-exposure analysis (for chemicals whose dose-response relationship is likely to be either threshold or nonlinear). For chemicals where data might support either linear extrapolation or a margin-of-exposure analysis, both analyses are to be presented.

A panel organized by the International Life Sciences Institute (ILSI) recently applied the 1996 EPA guidelines to an assessment of the dose-response relationship for chloroform (64). The ILSI panel evaluated the large database of information relevant to the mode of action by which chloroform induces liver tumors in rodents. The group identified a number of key elements important to chloroform's likely mode of action: lack of evidence of genotoxicity; tumor induction at doses associated with frank toxicity at the tumor sites; and the role of cytotoxicity and compensatory cell proliferation in tumor induction. The group concluded that the evidence did not support a linear dose-response relationship. A margin-of-exposure analysis was considered to represent the most appropriate method for evaluating the potential hazards of chloroform at low doses. The significance of such an approach is potentially quite large with respect to regulatory decision making. In the case of chloroform, use of the margin-of-exposure analysis would yield a permissible level in drinking water in the United States of 300 μg/L, a 60-fold increase beyond the present permissible level of 5 μg/L.

The linearized multistage model is clearly not appropriate for estimating the low-dose carcinogenic potency of some carcinogens. This is largely because experimental evidence indicates that for most chemicals, the dose-response relationship at the high doses used for model fitting is likely to be different than that at low doses. Pharmacokinetic and pharmacodynamic models can and should be used to more accurately characterize the dose-response relationship at low doses. In the absence of information to perform such assessments, alternative approaches, such as those proposed by the U.S. EPA (195), represent a reasonable interim measure.

EVALUATION OF SYSTEMIC TOXICANTS

In its broadest sense, systemic toxicity refers to all adverse effects, but in general it is applied only to chemicals that are postulated to induce an adverse effect through a threshold mechanism. That is, for these chemicals, there is a level of exposure below which there is minimal, if any, chance for an adverse effect. The effects range from skin and eye irritation to subchronic or chronic damage to any organ system, such as pulmonary fibrosis.

The underlying hypothesis for the threshold model for systemic toxicants is that multiple cells must be injured before an adverse effect is experienced, and that the injury must occur at a rate that exceeds the rate of repair. This is in contrast to the commonly used paradigm for carcinogenesis, in which a genotoxic insult to a single cell is theoretically sufficient to allow that cell to grow to a malignant tumor (215). An example of a threshold-type injury can be seen with pulmonary fibrosis due to mineral dust exposure. Fibrotic areas may be present and observed as radiographic or histopathologic changes in the lungs of miners as a consequence of mineral dust exposure in the absence of any physiological impairment such as reduced forced expiratory volume in 1s (FEV_1) or in the absence of changes in lung volume. Physiological impairment will occur as the fibrosis increases and the fibrotic areas begin to coalesce (223).

For effects other than cancer, which still involve genotoxic mechanisms, such as developmental effects, a threshold model may still be the most appropriate choice of dose-response model. This is because multiple cells must still be injured before an effect can be manifested. For example, the prenatal death of a single retinal cell, even through genetic damage, would not result in blindness because of the existence of many retinal cells.

The RfD and Uncertainty Factors

The general approach for setting exposure limits for systemic toxicants differs from that commonly used for carcinogens. Basically, appropriate uncertainty factors are applied to an experimental exposure to yield a level classically defined as the *acceptable daily intake* (ADI). The ADI represents a daily intake level of a chemical in humans that is associated with minimal or no risk of adverse effects. The ADI is expressed in terms of milligrams of chemical per kilogram of body weight per day (135). The EPA refers to such an exposure level as the *risk reference dose* or RfD. The basis for the change in terminology is that the ADI does not represent a magic dividing line between safe and nonsafe, but represents an estimated dose, derived through a consistent methodology, at which the chance of adverse effects is estimated to be negligible. The lack of precision is reflected in EPA's description of the RfD as having an uncertainty perhaps spanning an order of magnitude (200).

An ADI or RfD is typically based on either a no-observed-adverse-effect level (NOAEL) or a lowest-observed-adverse-effect level (LOAEL) from an epidemiology or animal toxicology study. "Uncertainty" factors (UFs), also termed "safety" factors, are then applied to the NOAEL or LOAEL to account for uncertainties in the relationship between exposure to a chemical in an animal study and a particular effect, and the relationship between lifetime daily exposure to the same chemical in the general population of humans and the likelihood of a particular effect.

The history as well as the experimental support for UFs in developing a permissible dose for production against systemic toxicity in humans have been described by Dourson and Stara (51). These authors describe four categories of UFs:

- UF_H: An up to 10-fold uncertainty factor to account for variations in susceptibility in humans. Thus, if a NOAEL was defined from a long-term study in humans, this would be the only UF applied. In a later section of this chapter we discuss in detail the variability in human responsiveness to environmental pollutants and its relevance to the regulatory process.
- UF_A: An up to 10-fold uncertainty factor to extrapolate from animal data to human data. This factor is used for animal studies and is based on the assumption that some humans may be more susceptible than experimental animals to

a particular chemical. The default assumption is that the magnitude of the increased susceptibility is within a factor of 10.

- UF_S: An up to 10-fold uncertainty factor to extrapolate from a subchronic exposure to a chronic exposure. This factor is used for studies that involve less than lifetime exposure and is based on the assumption that if the chemical were given over the lifetime of the animal rather than over a fraction of the lifetime, a smaller amount of chemical would result in the same NOAEL.
- UF_L: An up to 10-fold uncertainty factor to extrapolate from a LOAEL to a NOAEL. This factor is used for studies in which a NOAEL was not identified. The default assumption is that a dose at 1/10 the LOAEL would result in a NOAEL.

More recently, EPA has developed a fifth uncertainty factor, UF_D, which may be applied when the database is incomplete (203). The assumption here is that when the database for a chemical is limited, there is uncertainty as to whether the identified NOAEL might be significantly lower if other studies were performed, or whether a different NOAEL might have been identified if additional health endpoints (such as reproductive toxicity) had been evaluated. A complete database is defined as having two chronic mammalian studies, one mammalian multigeneration study, and two mammalian developmental toxicity studies. If these five studies are available, then there is a high degree of confidence that one has approximated the lowest NOAEL.

Uncertainty factors are used multiplicatively. To derive the RfD, EPA divides the exposure level from the toxicity study by the UFs. Mathematically, this is represented as

$$\text{RfD} = \frac{\text{LOAEL or NOAEL}}{\text{UF}_1 \times \text{UF}_2 \ldots \text{UF}_n}$$

The use of all five UFs (UF_H, UF_A, UF_S, UF_L, UF_D), each representing an order of magnitude, could in theory lead to a total uncertainty factor of 100,000. This would occur if data were from a subchronic animal study that identified only a LOAEL and the database was limited. However, since the multiplication of four or five factors of 10 each is likely to yield unrealistically conservative RfDs, EPA has restricted the total uncertainty factor calculation as follows: when uncertainty exists in four areas, EPA uses a 3000-fold total uncertainty factor, and when uncertainty exists in five areas, EPA uses a 10,000-fold total uncertainty factor (203).

Although 10 represents the default value for a UF, values less than 10 may also be used, depending upon the nature of the available information. For example, in deriving an RfD for chromium(VI), a factor of 3 was applied for the UFs, to account for the fact that the one year exposure duration in the principal study was less than lifetime, but longer than typical subchronic studies in rodents (186). No UFs were used in developing the RfD for fluoride because the NOAEL for the critical effect (dental fluorosis) was observed in the sensitive population (children) for a sufficiently long exposure duration (188).

In addition, a modifying factor (MF) that is greater than 0 and less than or equal to 10 may be used to address uncertainties not addressed in the other factors. For example, the use of a very large number of animals in a study may enhance certainty in the RfD, resulting in the use of a MF less than 1, but greater than 0. Alternatively, when an RfD is based on a very limited number of animals, an MF greater than 1 but less than or equal to 10 may be appropriate (203).

The RfD approach represents a generally accepted (NAS, FDA, and EPA, among others) method for setting lifetime exposure limits for humans, and the use of default 10-fold uncertainty factors has some experimental support, particularly as upper bound estimates (51). For example, the ratio between the subchronic and chronic NOAEL or LOAEL for 52 chemicals was less than 10 in 96% of the cases, as described in the analysis by Dourson and Stara (51). Thus, the uncertainty factor of 10 would be an underestimate for only 4% of these chemicals. A similar analysis regarding subchronic to chronic was performed by Lewis (15), who observed that for 18 chemicals, the ratio of the subchronic to the chronic NOAEL had a ratio of 3.5 or less for 14 chemicals and only 1 had a ratio of greater than 10. If the chemical with a ratio greater than 10 were excluded from the analysis, the mean subchronic to chronic NOAEL ratio was 3.3. Thus, the default UF of 10 for extrapolating from subchronic to chronic exposures would be very protective for most chemicals, and an UF of 3 may be more appropriate than the default value of 10 for many chemicals.

There are several limitations in the RfD approach, the net result of which is that exposures resulting in the same RfD do not imply the same level of risk for all chemicals, and that exposures above the RfD do not represent the same increase in risk for all chemicals. First, the choice of a LOAEL or a NOAEL does not take into consideration the greater experimental confidence associated with, for example, studies using more experimental animals. An exposure concentration defined as a NOAEL in one experiment could turn out to be a LOAEL, had more experimental animals been used (i.e., an effect might have been detected using more animals). As a result, poor experiments may yield anticonservative RfDs, since studies using fewer animals may result in a higher RfD than studies using larger numbers of animals (46).

In addition, the RfD approach does not make use of dose-response information, which is a key determinant in assessing the likelihood of effects. Thus, a chemical with a steep dose-response curve would be associated with a greater likelihood of effects as exposure increased above the RfD and a smaller likelihood of effects with exposures below the RfD than would a chemical with a more shallow dose-response curve (50).

There are also difficulties with the implications of specific UFs. The default value of 10 for the interspecies uncertainty factor (UF*A*) is a reasonable assumption in some cases, but in other cases may not be appropriate. For chemicals for which metabolism is a key determinant of toxicity, interspecies differences may be due mainly to physiological and metabolic differences across species (32). Under this assumption, interspecies differences are believed to scale according to allometric principles, that is, when the dose is expressed on a dose-per-unit surface area, different species are presumed equally sensitive to a chemical (51). According to this interpretation, then, a scaling factor based on surface area (body weight$^{2/3}$) should account for interspecies differences (32,51). For rodent toxicity studies (most commonly used in toxicological risk assessments), such a scaling factor would be about 8 for rats and 13 for mice, similar to the default value of 10 for the UF*A*. However, using this interpretation the default value of 10 would not be adequately protective for much smaller animals, and would be overly protective for much larger animals.

If, however, pharmacokinetic modeling has been used to estimate a biologically effective dose and to extrapolate dose across species, the use of an interspecies UF*A* may be unnecessary. For example, this may apply to chloroform, for which a mechanistically based dose-response model for hepatotoxicity has been developed (42). A similar conclusion has been reached by Jarabek and co-workers, who have developed a methodology for estimating the *reference concentration*, or RfC (116). The RfC is an air concentration of a chemical that is expected to be associated with minimal risk, if any, for adverse effects in humans, including susceptible populations (116,204). As such, the RfC is the functional equivalent of the RfD, except that it is based on an air concentration, rather than an administered dose. Overton and Jarabek (148) noted that when dosimetric adjustments (e.g., through physiologically based pharmacokinetic modeling) are made, use of the value of 10 for the UF*A* for cross-species extrapolation may be inappropriate. This is because the dosimetric adjustment has already addressed some of the basis for interspecies variability. (Additional description of the RfC methodology is provided in chapter 8 by Rodricks et al.)

Differences in metabolism, however, are insufficient to explain all interspecies differences in toxicity. For some chemicals, innate differences in responsiveness are responsible. For example, the difference in susceptibility to the lethal effects of 2,3,7,8-tetrachlorodibenzodioxin is about 10,000-fold greater in guinea pigs than in hamsters and is likely a reflection of differences in Ah receptor activity and other genetic elements (158). Another example is seen in studies involving the fibrogenic mineral dust alpha-quartz. Macrophages of different animal species, when exposed to the fibrogenic mineral dust, alpha-quartz, do not demonstrate the same response in terms of levels or characteristics of fibroblast stimulating factor (73,81). These differences are consistent with differences in the nature and extent of the fibrotic response to intratracheally instilled alpha-quartz (3,21,70).

Alternative Approaches to the RfD

There are alternative approaches to the standard RfD approach. By employing dose-response modeling and statistics, these alternative approaches can address issues of experimental quality, the shape of the dose-response curve, and other limitations of the RfD approach. Examples include the *benchmark dose* method (57,198), probabilistic RfD approaches (13,169), and distributional population approaches. These methods are described next.

The EPA defines a *benchmark dose* (BMD) as "a statistical lower confidence limit on the dose producing a predetermined level of change in adverse response compared with the response in untreated animals" (198). For example, a BMD could represent the 95% lower confidence limit on a dose that produces a 10% increase in a particular adverse health effect. The BMD is then used like a NOAEL or LOAEL, and appropriate UFs are applied to derive an RfD based on a BMD. Calculation of a BMD is illustrated in Figure 2.4.

The BMD approach overcomes many of the weaknesses of the RfD approach (57,198). Because BMDs are determined based on statistical modeling of dose-response data, the approach incorporates information on the sample size and the shape of the dose-response curve, information that is not taken into account using the standard RfD approach. Unlike NOAELs or LOAELs, BMD values are not constrained to be based on one of the experimental doses tested, and are less dependent on the study design. Also, the BMD approach can be used for both threshold and nonthreshold adverse health effects, as well as for both quantal and continuous toxicity data. The BMD approach allows for greater consistency between values derived for different chemicals. A further benefit of the BMD approach is that it allows for possible future harmonization of cancer and noncancer risk assessment methods (45).

For any particular chemical, uncertainty factors applied to NOAELs or LOAELs using the standard RfD approach may not be appropriate to apply to a

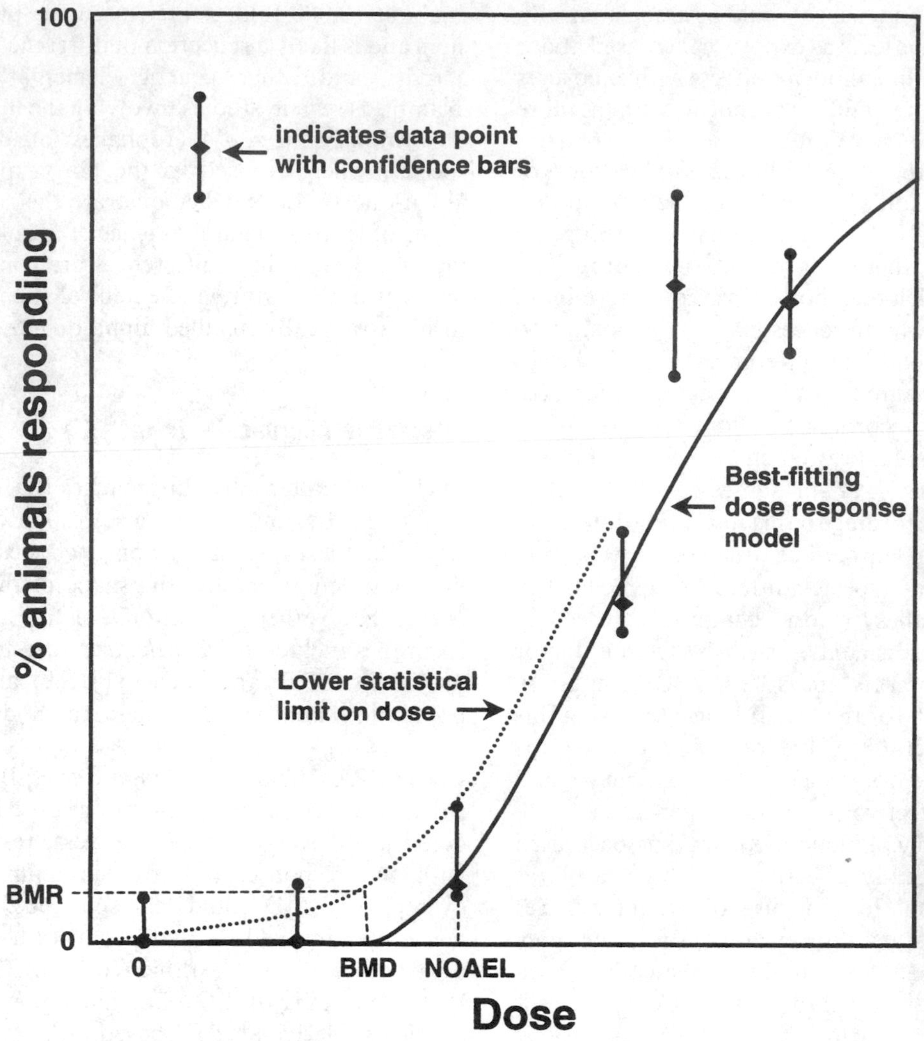

FIG. 2.4. Example of calculation of a BMD. Source: U.S. EPA (198).

BMD. This is because additional dose-response information has already been incorporated into the BMD. For example, when using a BMD, a steeper dose-response curve or a less severe critical effect may warrant a smaller value for UF*L* than would a more shallow dose-response curve or a more severe effect (50).

Recently, the EPA has adopted the BMD approach in developing RfDs for a number of chemicals, including beryllium, methylmercury, and tributyltin oxide (185). Similarly, benchmark concentrations (BMC) have been used to develop RfCs for antimony trioxide, carbon disulfide, methylene diphenyl diisocyanate, methyl methacrylate, phosphoric acid, 1,1,1,2-tetrafluoroethane, and chromium(VI) particulates (185). For all chemicals listed, a 10% relative change was chosen as the benchmark response. Although the EPA has performed a benchmark dose analysis for naphthalene, the resulting RfD (3×10^{-2} mg/kg-day) was very similar to the value derived using a standard NOAEL/RfD approach (2×10^{-2} mg/kg-day), and the EPA decided to use the NOAEL/RfD approach in deriving the final EPA-recommended value (189).

A probabilistic approach for developing RfD or ADI values, combining distributions for each uncertainty factor using a probabilistic approach to generate an overall distribution for the no-adverse-effect level in sensitive human subpopulations, has been recommended by the Netherlands National Institute of Public Health and the Environment (169). This approach allows consideration of all available data on various uncertainties, and minimizes the conservatisms introduced by multiplying numerous UFs. A similar approach has also been recommended by Baird and co-workers (13).

For compounds that have been well studied, particularly in humans (both in terms of exposure and in terms of toxicity), distributional population approaches have been used to evaluate toxicity and to provide input into the decision-making process. Such approaches have been applied mainly to evaluation of the National Ambient Air Quality Standards (NAAQS)—standards for moderately toxic air contaminants that are ubiquitous in the United States. Much of the basis for selection of a NAAQS is based upon human toxicological data, although animal data are used in a supporting role.

An example of a distributional population approach can be seen in the recent evaluation of carbon monoxide (CO) toxicity and exposure by EPA's Ambient Standards Branch (201). As part of this assessment, EPA reviewed several studies that evaluated the relationship between exposure to carbon monoxide, using carboxyhemoglobin (COHb) in blood as an indicator of exposure, and percent decrease in time to angina or pain in the chest, as an indicator of effect. Most of the studies showed an impact of low COHb levels on angina. However, there was no consistent dose-response relationship when studies were analyzed in the aggregate. This may have been due to differences in study design, study populations, and other factors. Because of the lack of a clear dose relationship, EPA evaluated the impact of different concentrations of CO in air upon various "cutoff" points of COHb, from 2.1 to 3.0%. These cutoff points are conceptually similar to the LOAEL used in RfD development. Levels of CO that result in COHb of 2.9 to 3.0% or higher might constitute frank effect levels (FEL). This is because levels of COHb of 2.9 to 3.0% or higher in persons with heart disease are considered as possibly increasing the risk of myocardial ischemia and diminishing blood flow to the heart.

The risk of CO exposure to people with heart disease in Denver, CO (36,345 individuals at the time), was estimated under different carbon monoxide levels (201). The number of person-days where individuals might have at least one hourly COHb level greater than or equal to a defined percent COHb was estimated. Table 2.11 presents some of the results of this analysis. For example, under conditions at the time (considering both indoor and outdoor sources of carbon monoxide), there were approximately 488 person-days in which the Denver population with preexisting heart disease would experience COHb levels greater than 2.1%. If only ambient air is considered, then the person-days drops to 72. If the NAAQS for CO is attained, then the person-days drops to 457 for all sources and 0 for ambient air only. This type of analysis is useful in showing the benefits of CO reduction, as well as identifying the significance of different sources.

Distributional population approaches to evaluating environmental chemicals provide a more comprehensive evaluation of risks than the RfD approach. Rather than focusing on point estimates (e.g., above or below the RfD), this method allows one to more fully characterize variability in responsiveness to chemicals and variability in exposure levels among defined populations. However, this approach is feasible only for a limited number of chemicals and is quite resource intensive.

Endpoints—Developmental Toxicity

Recent refinements in the evaluation of systemic toxicants have focused on specific target-organ systems, such as the nervous system or the developing fetus. In this section, we focus on developmental toxicity as illustrative of the use of a specific endpoint in regulatory toxicology, including, for example, classification schemes and approaches toward setting permissible levels. Evaluation of developmental toxicants presents some unique challenges in risk assessment. This is because standard chronic and subchronic toxicity tests cannot be used to provide information on developmental effects in the offspring of exposed mothers. Rather, animal selection and exposure conditions must be designed specifically to assess developmental effects.

Developmental toxicity has been defined to include "any detrimental effect produced by exposures during embryonic stages of development" (135). These effects may include structural abnormalities, functional abnormalities, growth retardation, or lethality (202).

Table 2.11
Heart person-days with at least one hourly COHb estimate greater than or equal to value for four alternative scenarios

	"As is" air quality		"Just attain" air quality	
Exposure indicators	"Ambient air" plus internal sources	"Ambient air" without internal sources	"Ambient air" plus internal sources	"Ambient air" without internal sources
COHb ≥ 2.1%	488	72	457	0
COHb ≥ 3.0%	37	0	24	0

Note. Adapted from U.S. EPA (201).

The effects may be reversible, such as a temporary reduction in growth rate, or irreversible, such as an overt physical malformation.

We discuss the evaluation of developmental toxicants in the regulatory process by focusing on four main issues:

- Selection of testing protocols.
- Relevance of animal studies to hazard identification in humans, including weight of evidence classifications.
- Use of the RfD approach to assess risk.
- Use of other approaches to assess risk.

Selection of Testing Protocols

The use of animal studies is particularly critical in evaluating developmental toxicants, as compared to chemicals that induce other effects. Reasons for this include the emphasis on adult males in occupational epidemiology studies, the lack of a long-term national registry of birth defects, and the difficulty in identifying certain endpoints, such as resorptions.

Types of studies used to evaluate developmental toxicity include the conventional "segment 2" study, in which the dams are exposed typically during the period of fetal organogenesis, and litters are evaluated for a number of endpoints, including number of viable offspring, types and incidence of skeletal or visceral malformations or variations, and body weight (119,202). Segment 1 tests focus on fertility and reproductive performance of males and females. Segment 3 tests include perinatal and postnatal study after treatment of females only and, as such, may be considered sequential to the segment 2 test. In addition, multigeneration studies are also performed to assess fertility, reproductive performance, and, sometimes, teratology (119).

In the segment 2 tests, maternal toxicity endpoints, such as organ weights and clinical histopathology, are also evaluated. Of particular concern are those compounds that induce toxicity in the offspring in the absence of significant maternal toxicity.

There are significant differences in the protocols for segment 2 tests, particularly between countries. These include differences in animal species, dosing regimen, and specific endpoints evaluated. For example, the Japanese protocol requires that some females be allowed to litter and the pups in the litter are examined for physical, reproductive, and functional development (119), which contrasts with typical U.S. protocols where littering does not occur and only in utero pups are examined.

These differences may be significant, with potential implications for regulatory action. For example, functional deficits in offspring could be observed in the Japanese segment 2 protocol, but not in the standard U.S. segment 2 protocol, where additional testing (segment 3) would be required to detect such effects.

Because of the implication of test differences between countries, an expert panel of scientists has proposed that efforts be made toward "harmonization" of guidelines for reproductive and developmental toxicity testing (119). Harmonization would result in international guidelines for reproductive and developmental toxicity testing to improve the comparability of data from studies. In addition, harmonization of testing schemes would allow for more efficient use of resources and possibly would reduce the need for animal testing, since one country could more readily use the results of studies performed in other countries than is now possible.

In addition to the standard methods, specialized developmental toxicity methods involving, for example, developmental neurotoxicity testing, are available. These can be either an addition to a segment 2 test, or a distinct test. Developmental neurotoxicity testing may be especially critical in evaluating certain chemicals such as lead (217) or polychlorinated biphenyls (PCBs) (216), which have been associated with subtle neurobehavioral changes in offspring from relatively low-level prenatal exposures.

Short-term screening tests and in vitro tests, such as the Chernoff/Kavlock (36), have also been used to evaluate developmental toxicants. In general, these tests are insufficient for performing quantitative risk assessments. However, they may be useful in selecting chemicals for further analysis and in helping to guide the nature of further analyses.

Short-term tests are of particular use when one considers the complexities of animal testing and the relatively high frequency of developmental abnormalities. For example, about 3% of infants are born with major congenital malformations that are recognized in the first year of life (125).

Relevance of Animal Studies to Hazard Identification in Humans, Including Weight-of-Evidence Classifications

Significant species differences have been observed with respect to susceptibility of chemicals to induce developmental toxicity. Perhaps the classic example of species differences is thalidomide. Thalidomide exposure induces comparable target-organ specificity for limb defects in rabbits and various primates, but not in rats. Had initial toxicity tests on thalidomide involved more appropriate animal species, the human tragedy of thalidomide might have been mitigated (125).

Attempts have been made to develop categorical classification schemes and to provide interpretative descriptions of developmental toxicity data. Overall, the aim of such evaluations is to assess the likelihood that a chemical can cause developmental effects in humans. Although not as codified as the cancer classification

Table 2.12
Classification of chemicals based on teratogenic potential

Criteria	Category A	Category B	Category C	Category D
1. Ratio: minimum maternotoxic dose to minimum teratogenic dose	Much greater than 1	Generally greater than 1, teratogenic range starts below the maternotoxic dose range [a] and overlaps it	≤1	No teratogenicity even at maternotoxic doses
2. Incidence of malformations	Dose-related and high	Dose related and high	Dose relatedness of each malformation less obvious, incidence low	—
3. Type of malformation at lower doses	Organ systems involved are specific	Characteristics, possibly specific, generally multiple	Nonspecific involving different organ systems	—
4. Target cell	Specific cells	Specific cells	Nonspecific and generalized	Not known
5. Range of safety factor	1–400	1–300	1–250	1–100

[a] The maternotoxic dose range extends between the dose initiating signs of toxicity and the dose causing 50% mortality (LD_{50}). Source: Khera et al. (119).

schemes described earlier, the use of such schemes for developmental toxicants could be further developed to form a more integral part of the regulatory process. For example, weight-of-evidence schemes could be used for developing regulatory priorities.

A classification scheme for developmental toxicants is shown in Table 2.12. This scheme categorizes chemicals, based on teratogenic potential. Given equal exposure levels, chemicals in category A would present the greatest concern for teratogenic potential. This particular scheme includes several elements: relationship of maternally toxic dose to developmentally toxic dose; shape of the dose-response curve; and the nature of the malformations. The scheme differs from most carcinogen classification schemes in that it takes into consideration elements of the dose-response relationship. For example, the scheme considers the relationship between the maternally toxic and the developmentally toxic dose, and proposes a range of "safety factors" for extrapolating to human risks, depending on category.

An alternative to classification schemes for developmental toxicants is the use of text descriptors of hazard and other risk elements. This approach was recently used by the Institute for Evaluating Health Risk (IEHR) in the report "An Evaluative Process for Determining Human Reproductive and Developmental Toxicity of Agents" (83). This document contains the deliberations of an ad hoc group of industry and government scientists. Using a hypothetical chemical "terminator", the relevance of animal toxicological data for human risk was evaluated, using expert opinion and consensus development, considering factors such as pharmacokinetic differences between humans and animals, absorption potential through different body interfaces, and biological monitoring data. As noted earlier, rather than yield a rigid categorization scheme, the analysis resulted in text descriptors to assist in the interpretation of animal toxicological studies, with respect to potential for hazard in humans.

The use of classification schemes or interpretive text descriptors to evaluate the relevance of animal developmental studies to humans, as described earlier, could significantly improve the use of developmental toxicity data in the regulatory process. In addition, similar approaches are warranted for other endpoints, such as immunotoxicity.

Use of the RfD to Assess Risk

RfDs may be derived for developmental effects, using essentially the same methodology as described earlier for systemic toxicants in which case the value is an RfD_{DT} (202). The RfD_{DT} is derived from a LOAEL or NOAEL from a developmental toxicity study. However, because the relevant exposure period is not chronic, but is the in utero and possibly earlier time period, the RfD_{DT} applies not to a lifetime exposure but only to the study exposure period. At present, RfD_{DT} values are available for only a limited number of chemicals. In general, the use of RfDs for specific endpoints and periods of exposure duration could allow greater comparability of RfDs and better use of toxicological information.

Use of other Methods to Assess Risk

Alternative methods to the RfD_{DT} have been developed to assess risks or to develop protective levels for developmental toxicants. One method described earlier in Table 2.12 involves the use of different safety factors applied to the minimum teratogenic dose depending upon the teratogenic potential category (A–D) to which the chemical belonged. The use of variable "safety" (now termed *uncertainty*) factors for developing permissible levels from a NOAEL or a LOAEL allows better use of information about the specific developmental endpoint and the likelihood of hazard for humans. Nonetheless, this approach still suffers from the basic flaws as the RfD approach, such as the difficulty in evaluating excursions above the RfD level.

The benchmark dose (BMD) approach has also been proposed to improve assessments of developmental toxicants (117). Briefly, the benchmark dose (defined in a previous section) is developed through the use of dose-response modeling and reflects the dose (or the lower confidence limit on the dose) associated with a certain percent response in the population.

Incorporating Information on Severity of Effect

A critical difference in evaluating risks for carcinogenicity versus risks for systemic effects is that, from a regulatory perspective, almost all types of cancer are considered equally severe, while the severity of systemic effects can vary significantly. In general, there is little basis from a regulatory perspective for distinguishing among carcinogens on the basis of malignancy or tumor type. Despite advances in earlier diagnosis and treatment, the fatality rate for cancer is still relatively high. For example, the relative 5-year survival rate for all cancers from 1986 to 1993, excluding nonmelanoma skin cancer, was 60% for whites and 44% for blacks (4). Nonmelanoma skin cancer includes squamous- and basal-cell carcinoma, which can be induced by agents such as ultraviolet light and arsenic and has relatively low (<10%) fatality rates, even when untreated (206).

In contrast, target-organ effects range greatly in severity. For example, using the same target organ and susceptible population—namely, airways in asthmatics—responses may range from imperceptible mild bronchoconstriction induced by low levels of SO_2 to a fatal asthmatic response, as may have been due to acid sulfate pollution in the London smog episode (176,210).

Consideration of severity then becomes important for regulatory development in several ways. For RfD development, is an effect such as a 2% decrease in weight a NOAEL or a LOAEL? Is an effect of sufficient severity to warrant protection of 95% of the population or 99%? Thus, several agencies and groups have developed approaches to incorporate information on severity of effect into the risk assessment or risk management process for environmental chemicals.

In 1985, the American Thoracic Society (ATS) defined an adverse respiratory effect (8). Rather than providing a clear demarcation between nonadverse and adverse, the ATS described a continuum of respiratory effects from mild effects of limited, if any, medical significance (e.g., occasional cough, runny nose) to effects of obvious adverseness and medical significance (e.g., an asthmatic attack). To the extent that the effect caused discomfort and impaired daily function and quality of life, it was viewed as more adverse.

Similarly, EPA has considered severity in its evaluation on the effects of ozone as part of the NAAQS setting process. For example, based on lung function changes, duration of effect, symptoms, and impact on activity level, EPA categorized ozone responses into four categories: mild, moderate, severe, and incapacitating. The mild category includes FEV_1 declines of 5 to 10% and no impact on activity. The EPA (205) recommended that the responses in the mild category *not* be considered an adverse respiratory effect in adults for purposes of defining the NAAQS for ozone.

As noted earlier, the concept of severity of effect is also incorporated into the process for developing the RfD. Specifically, the RfD is based on an effect that, by definition, considers adverseness. The critical effect is adverse, because it may result in functional or structural impairment or is a precursor state to irreversible toxicity (203). For example, fatty infiltration of the liver or a greater than 10% reduction in weight gain versus controls would be considered adverse effects, and the associated dose would be a LOAEL. As the dose increases, the fraction of that population experiencing such effects would increase. Frank effect levels (FELs) are dose levels that result in overt, often clinically apparent toxicity, and are considered "too adverse" to be used in the development of the RfD. Examples of frank effects include liver necrosis or cirrhosis, which are severe and may be irreversible. FELs are not considered appropriate for RfD development because the protection level would be inadequate.

Information on severity has been incorporated into the *reportable quantity* (RQ) definition, under CERCLA. Under this statute, releases of chemicals in amounts greater than some predetermined level, defined as the RQ, require that EPA be notified of the release (48). The amount of release that triggers notification is based on an assessment of the potency of the chemical and the severity of the effect at the dose level where the potency was quantified. The ranking of severity is shown in Table 2.13 (48), where it can be seen that effects range from slight biochemical changes through gross toxicity, including lethality. Unlike the RfD process, this scoring is not restricted to data sets containing information on mildly adverse effects, from subchronic or chronic studies. The RQ process can result in development of scoring indicators from lower quality data sets, involving shorter time periods of exposure and more severe toxicity.

Table 2.13
Rating values for NOAELS, LOAELS, and FELs used to rank chronic toxicity

Rating	Effects
1	Enzyme induction or other biochemical change with no pathologic changes and no change in organ weights.
2	Enzyme induction and subcellular proliferation or other changes in organelles, but no other apparent effects.
3	Hyperplasia, hypertrophy, or atrophy, but no change in organ weights.
4	Hyperplasia, hypertrophy, or atrophy with changes in organ weights.
5	Reversible cellular changes: cloudy swelling, hydropic change, or fatty changes.
6	Necrosis, or metaplasia with no apparent decrement of organ function. Any neuropathy without apparent behavioral, sensory, or physiologic changes.
7	Necrosis, atrophy, hypertrophy, or metaplasia with a detectable decrement of organ functions. Any neuropathy with a measurable change in behavioral, sensory, or physiologic activity.
8	Necrosis, atrophy, hypertrophy, or metaplasia with definitive organ dysfunction. Any neuropathy with gross changes in behavior, sensory or motor performance. Any decrease in reproductive capacity. Any evidence of fetotoxicity.
9	Pronounced pathologic changes with severe organ dysfunction. Any neuropathy with loss of behavioral or motor control or loss of sensory ability. Reproductive dysfunction. Any teratogenic effect with maternal toxicity.
10	Death or pronounced life shortening. Any teratogenic effect without signs of maternal toxicity.

Note. Source: deRosa et al. (48).

The RQ process demonstrates the use of severity information in both risk assessment (developing RQ indicators) and risk management (defining release levels requiring notification as associated with defined RQ values).

Recent efforts involving the use of categorical exposure response modeling demonstrate additional approaches towards consideration of severity. For example Guth and co-workers (as cited in ref. 15) analyzed acute effects resulting from methyl isocyanate exposures of less than 8 h in duration (as seen in Figure 2.5). Effects were separated into three categories: NOAEL (circles), adverse effect level (AEL) (triangles), and lethal (squares). Effect categories were then analyzed on the basis of concentration and time, using logistic regression. Figure 2.5 presents a line above which there is a 90% probability that the true NOAEL lies. This method allows the use of data from a range of severity endpoints and considers various combinations of exposure level and exposure duration. Conceivably, this type of approach could lead to the development of concentration time nomograms for definition of NOAELs for different exposure durations.

PHYSIOLOGICALLY BASED PHARMACOKINETIC MODELS

One of the areas of recent regulatory attention is that of physiologically based pharmacokinetic (PBPK) models and their potential use in risk assessment. This issue is discussed in depth in the chapter 5 by Krishnan and Andersen and chapter 8 by Rodricks et al., we discuss the topic here in terms of regulatory implications.

PBPK models are essentially mechanistic models that describe quantitatively the pharmacokinetic processes affecting the disposition of a chemical and its metabolism from the time it is absorbed to the interaction with different and various body tissues. Once it is determined whether the parent compound or its metabolites are the likely cause of a carcinogenic response, a PBPK model may be developed to quantify the magnitude and the time course of exposure to this agent at the critical target site in the animal model. After the estimates of target tissue dose in the animal model have been made and validated, the information can then be scaled to the human to obtain an estimate of target-organ dose in humans. This estimate may then be used to predict human cancer risk under dif-

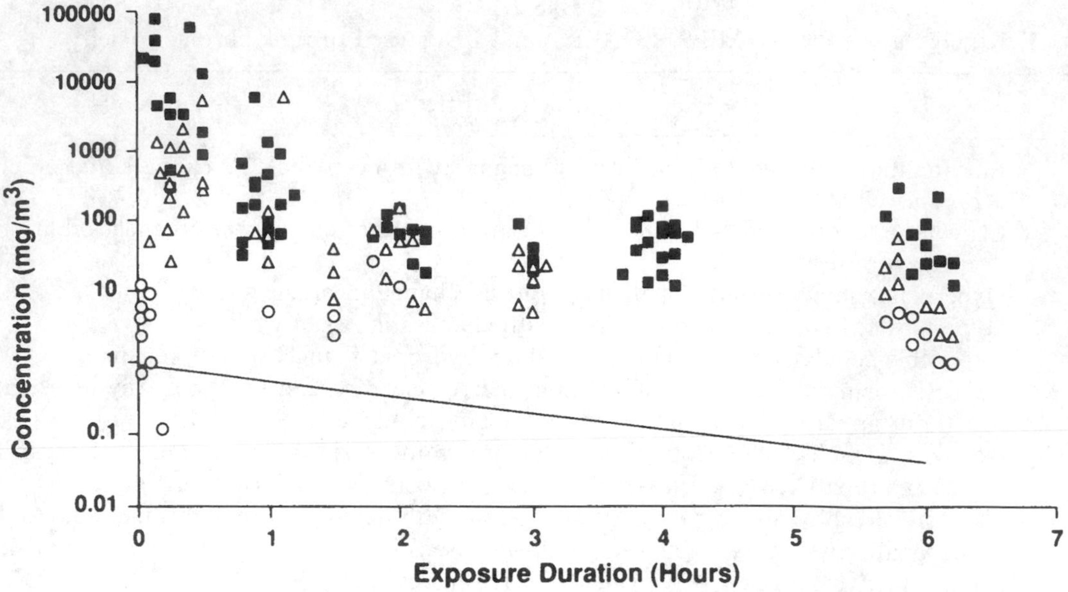

FIG. 2.5. Categorical data from published results on methyl isocyanate for exposures of less than 8 h in duration and shown as NOAEL (circles), AEL (triangles), or lethality (squares). The maximum likelihood model fit is shown by the line representing the model prediction of $p=.1$ that severity is greater than the NOAEL category at the corresponding exposure concentration and duration.

ferent exposure conditions or to develop more precise estimates of the reference dose. It should be emphasized that the PBPK model does not offer an explanation of the most appropriate dose-response relationship, once the dose to target is estimated (11,24). Furthermore, full validation of the model at the relatively low levels of environmental chemicals to which humans are exposed can be difficult.

Despite these limitations, PBPK modeling does offer an important tool for researchers and regulators alike. PBPK models can be used to quantify target organ doses between species and to extrapolate from high to low doses. Of added significance is that new information about the pharmacokinetics of a chemical can be incorporated into the model without affecting the basic structure of the model, thus enhancing its predictive capability.

The use of PBPK models also provides important advantages over conventional pharmacokinetic analyses (11,24). In typical pharmacokinetic modeling, time-course curves are determined for the concentration of the administered agent or its metabolite(s) in blood or some other body compartment. The resulting curves are then described by curve-fitting biostatistical techniques. The approach of conventional pharmacokinetics may be criticized for being more dependent on the mathematical model than on the biological system it purports to represent. However, PBPK models are designed to predict kinetic behavior over a wide range of doses and exposure conditions, and are based on basic physiologic and metabolic parameters. This modeling requires many data on anatomical and physiological parameters, the partitioning of test agents into selected tissues, and the biochemical constants for tissue binding and metabolism in various organs. From these data, a series of mass balance differential equations can be written to describe the interactions between the chemical and the animal model.

PBPK modeling can improve dose-response assessment by accounting for sources of change in the proportions of applied to delivered dose in animals versus humans, and at high versus low doses. Although this approach does not account for the fact that the sensitivity of the target tissue to the delivered dose may differ in humans and animals or between high and low doses, it still addresses some major areas of uncertainty in risk assessment. In fact, many sources of potential nonlinearity in applied dose-response involve saturation or induction of enzymatic processes at high doses, or differences in toxification/detoxification pathways between humans and animals or across doses.

PBPK modeling has been applied to several agents, including methylene chloride and ethylene dichloride (11,24,38). A look at the methylene chloride case illustrates the powerful implications of this approach. Anderson et al. (11) developed a PBPK model based on data indicating two routes of metabolism, one dependent on oxidation by mixed-function oxidase (MFO) and the other dependent on glutathione *S*-transferase (GST) in four species (mouse, rat, hamster, human).

Models were designed to quantify the contributions of the two metabolic pathways in the lung and liver and to allow for extrapolation from rodents to humans. Kinetic constants for the model were obtained from experiments or the literature, with model validation involving a comparison of predicted blood concentration time-course data in rats, mice, and humans, with experimental data from these species.

The capacity of methylene chloride to cause tumors in mice was associated with the target tissue dose and was closely related to the amount of methylene chloride metabolized by the GST but not the MFO pathway. Using the PBPK model, the target tissue doses in humans exposed to low concentrations of methylene chloride were between approximately 50- and 200-fold lower than would have been predicted by the linear extrapolation and body surface area factors used in conventional risk assessment methods. Thus, the PBPK analysis suggested that conventional risk analysis greatly overestimated the risk to humans exposed to low levels of methylene chloride. One of the major uncertainties, however, is the metabolic capacity of the body at low exposure levels where metabolism may not be saturated. Also, the dominant pathway for methylene chloride metabolism at other organ sites has not been determined. Still, the PBPK approach represents an attractive development, since it can increase the biological plausibility of predictive approaches while still incorporating biomathematical approaches for low-dose risk prediction. The EPA has incorporated this pharmacokinetic information into its cancer risk assessment for methylene chloride exposure via inhalation (187).

It is important to note that there are substantial uncertainties in PBPK modeling. For example, Hattis et al. (78) compared PBPK models for perchloroethylene developed by seven different authors and found appreciable differences among the model predictions. Given identical exposure levels in humans, the range of values for metabolized perchloroethylene span a 50-fold range, with 6 of the 7 models having predictions with a 14-fold range. With respect to methylene chloride, Clewell (38) noted the importance of the tissue distribution of GST enzyme activity across species, especially in humans as a source of model uncertainty. Studies to refine estimates of GST enzyme activity across species and within the human population will serve to provide more refined estimates of dose across humans and hence of potential differences in susceptibility.

ROLE OF HIGH-RISK GROUPS

In a previous section, we described the RfD concept as used by regulatory agencies to estimate acceptable levels for noncancer effects. One of the factors in the derivation of this level was to account for variations in population susceptibility. The purpose of this section is to expand upon that issue, to describe the basis for variations in susceptibility and the magnitude of that variation, and to demonstrate the relationship of this issue to the regulatory process. (For more detail the reader is referred to refs. 14, 25, and 139).

There is a high degree of variability in the response of humans to different exposure levels of environmental pollutants (25,44). In fact, the variability in the dose-response relationship in a heterogeneous population makes it difficult to estimate an acceptable level for chemical contaminants that would be protective of the whole population. Perhaps the most critical question is not what is a "safe" numerical standard, but how many individuals are adversely affected at different levels of exposure (33).

Knowing which groups of individuals are at high risk with respect to pollutants is very important in answering this question, since these individuals will be the first to experience morbidity and mortality as pollutant levels increase. If the high risk segments are protected, then the entire population is also protected. Information concerning both the identification and quantification of high-risk groups should play an integral role in the derivation of environmental health standards.

Use of Uncertainty Factors for High-Risk Groups

In trying to assess the role of high-risk groups in the derivation of environmental health standards, it is useful to consider the extent to which the EPA has utilized the concept of high risk groups within the standard setting process. Perhaps the most common approach utilized by the EPA and other regulatory agencies has been the implementation of uncertainty factors for noncancer endpoints. While this approach implicitly recognizes that certain people are more sensitive to pollutants than others, it is inherently imprecise. The precise difference in sensitivity between a statistically "normal" individual and groups at increased risk will vary for the different causes of the high-risk condition and for different pollutants.

The EPA has utilized the uncertainty factor approach in attempting to deal with protection of high risk individuals, as illustrated by the national drinking-water standards for noncarcinogenic chlorinated hydrocarbon insecticides (25). These substances were tested in two animal species, the rat and the dog. Chronic toxicity testing provided an estimate of the lowest level of pollutant (on a milligram of dose per kilogram of body weight) that the animal could ingest with either minimal or no toxic effects. In the absence of data to indicate a basis for an alternative choice, the species that was the most sensitive to the substances was chosen to derive the standard, implying that humans are as sensitive as the most sensitive animal species. In the absence of supporting human exposure data, an uncertainty factor of 500 was applied to the minimally toxic dose in the most sensitive animal species (i.e., the minimally toxic dose was divided by 500). It should be noted that this methodology differs from that of the RfD approach described earlier, in which case a factor of 100 would have been applied. This number was taken to be the total amount of insecticide to which a human could be exposed each day, over an unspecified period of time, without suffering any adverse health effects.

Several questions occur when evaluating such a methodological scheme. For example, on what basis can we assume that the most sensitive humans have the same degree of responsiveness as the most sensitive animals? Why was 500 chosen as a safety factor? What assurances exist that it would provide sufficient protection for the general population as well as high risk groups for these chemicals? Who, in fact, are the groups considered at increased risk?

The main problem with an uncertainty factor approach is its lack of specificity in identifying susceptible subpopulations, the extent of their susceptibility, and, most importantly, what fraction is protected by different standard levels. It should also be realized, however, that when only limited data are available, imprecise safety factors are the only realistic options available. Still, this approach will result in uncertain levels of protection. Alternative approaches must be developed to reduce the magnitude of that uncertainty.

Consideration of Specific High-Risk Groups

A better approach, when data are available to support it, is to consider specific groups at high risk on a chemical-by-chemical basis. There are clear examples of groups more susceptible to particular chemicals and cancer and non-cancer health effects (reviewed in refs. 20, 60, and 69). These include:

- Individuals with genetic variations in metabolism. For example, a slow acetylator phenotype is associated with an increased risk of bladder cancer following exposure to aromatic amine dyes (69).
- Individuals with enzymatic genetic polymorphisms. For example, polymorphisms in cytochrome P450 enzymes can result in differential detoxification or bioactivation of environmental chemicals (60).
- Individuals with inherited genetic defects. For example, xeroderma pigmentosum, an autosomal recessive disease, results in altered DNA repair capacity and increases the risk of skin cancer by more than 1500-fold (60).
- Individuals with preexisting illness. For example, asthmatics may be more susceptible to ozone (20), and those with hepatitis B are more susceptible to liver cancer (69).

Other factors that can affect susceptibility to environmental chemicals include gender, age, and life-style (i.e., cigarettes, alcohol, diet). The role of diet and certain types of cancer is shown in studies demonstrating an inverse relationship between the amount of vitamin A in the diet and susceptibility to hydrocarbon-induced epithelial cancers (41). Also, certain subgroups may be at greater risk, not because of an inherent difference in toxicological susceptibility, but because they are more likely to be exposed. For example, young children are at greater risk from soil contaminants because they tend to accidentally ingest more soil and dust than older children and adults, due to their significant hand-to-mouth activity. Thus, it is likely that, even given the same exposure, individuals are not equally susceptible to the induction of cancer and other adverse health effects, and in many cases the differential susceptibility may be very large.

Recently, there has been increasing attention on the potential for children to be more susceptible to environmental chemicals. In 1996, the EPA emphasized its focus of protecting infants and children in a report entitled "A National Agenda to Protect Children's Health from Environmental Threats" (194). The 1996 FQPA requires use of an additional 10-fold UF for pesticides to account for potential prenatal and postnatal developmental toxicity (191). As noted by Roberts (162), children may be more susceptible because many cells and organs are undergoing growth and development and have not yet matured. A child's diet and physical environment, and therefore his or her exposure potential, may vary significantly from that of an adult. For many routes of exposure (air, food, water, and dermal), chemical intake (on a per kilogram body weight basis) is generally greater for infants and children than adults (150).

However, a subgroup at high risk for one chemical is not necessarily at high risk for other chemical exposures. For example, although children are often assumed to be more sensitive than adults, this is not always the case. Reactions to pharmaceuticals, since they are more widely studied than responses to environmental exposures, can be considered as examples. Acute overdoses of acetaminophen result in less hepatotoxicity in children than in adults with comparable plasma concentrations, possibly due to differences in metabolism (118).

There is currently debate about whether current risk assessment methods adequately account for more highly susceptible groups. In general, setting of levels for carcinogen exposure has not addressed the role of population variability in susceptibility to carcinogens. Consequently, groups at high risk to environmental carcinogens, with the obvious exceptions of smoking as a risk factor for exposure to asbestos, uranium, and coke-oven emission-related cancer, have not generally been addressed. It should be noted, however, that the conservatism of the cancer risk assessment process might result in adequate protection of high-risk groups.

For noncancer effects, there is debate over the appropriate uncertainty factors to account for high-risk subgroups. At a conference organized by the ILSI and the EPA (71), "it was suggested that, in many cases, genetic variation in human susceptibility may be greater than an order of magnitude when comparing differences between children and adults." A coalition of farm food, manufacturing, and pest management organizations concluded that the additional UF of 10 required by the FQPA is not necessary to use "across the board" to protect infants and children (84). They also concluded that the standard default UFs are adequate for a pesticide with a complete and reliable database, and that an additional UF "should only be applied to an endpoint that is relevant to protection of fetuses, infants, and/or children" (84). The EPA is looking into establishing criteria for appropriate use of the 10-fold additional FQPA uncertainty factor (191,192). Overall, the best approach is to consider more susceptible subgroups on a case-by-case basis when data are available, for both carcinogens and noncarcinogens.

Regulatory Applications

The role of population variability should be considered by regulatory agencies in risk assessments for both carcinogens and noncarcinogens. Identification and quantitative characterization of susceptible populations could provide decision makers with a theoretical framework on which to base regulatory action. For example, Tamplin and Gofman (173) have employed knowledge of susceptible populations in predicting the incidence of cancer from radiation pollution in drinking water to help define acceptable levels of exposure. They assumed that the latency period is shorter for in utero exposure than for all radiation exposure beyond birth (i.e., 5 years vs. 15 years). Consideration of the increased susceptibility of the fetus to radiation-induced cancer resulted in greater estimates of cancer risk as compared with traditional methodological approaches, which predict carcinogenic effects at low doses, based on high levels of exposure in adults (160).

The EPA has specifically evaluated the increased sensitivity of specific high-risk groups in setting National Ambient Air Quality Standards for carbon monoxide, lead, nitrogen dioxide, ozone, particulates, and sulfur dioxide, and in establishing drinking-water standards for some environmental chemicals. Examples of the high-risk groups considered are shown in Table 2.14. For instance, the NAAQS for lead considers high-risk populations in a more quantitative way by estimating the fraction of the susceptible subpopulation (children) that would be protected at different air levels of lead (209). Following is a detailed description of the EPA consideration of high-risk groups in the derivation of drinking-water standards for nitrates and cadmium.

Nitrates in Drinking Water

The drinking water standard of 10 mg nitrate (NO_3^2) as milligrams nitrogen per liter is designed to prevent the formation of elevated levels of methemoglobin (MetHb) in infants. In the presence of nitrite (NO_2^-), formed from nitrate in infants, hemoglobin is oxidized to MetHb, which is not able to reversibly combine with oxygen. Levels of 1–2% and 2–5% MetHb are typical in the blood of adults and infants, respectively. When concentrations are less than 5% MetHb, there are no obvious indications of toxicity. However, with levels of MetHb from 5 to 10%, clinical signs of toxicity (e.g., cyanosis) may appear (25).

Infants are at considerable risk for nitrate-related toxicity, as compared to adults. Factors that predispose infants to the development of MetHb formation include:

1. The incompletely developed ability to secrete gastric acid. This permits the gastric pH to be high enough (5–7 pH) to permit the growth of nitrate-reducing bacteria in the gastrointestinal tract, thereby converting nitrate to nitrite before absorption into the circulation (184).
2. The higher levels of fetal hemoglobin in infants. This form of hemoglobin is more susceptible than adult hemoglobin to oxidation to MetHb (19).
3. The diminished enzymatic capability of infants to reduce MetHb to hemoglobin (166).

Research has revealed that levels of nitrate beyond 20 mg/L resulted in a marked upshift in the frequency of methemoglobinemia in infants but not in adults (25). Consequently, a standard of 10 mg/L is principally designed to prevent the occurrence of elevated levels of MetHb in infants. Concentrations twice as great would still protect adults.

Cadmium

Studies with rats show that at a kidney concentration of 200 ppm cadmium (Cd) (211), renal damage is initiated. The EPA calculated that humans would need to ingest 50 g Cd/day for 50 years to reach a level of 200 ppm in their kidneys. In the derivation of the Cd drinking-water standard, the EPA assumed a daily Cd

Table 2.14

High-risk groups in the derivation of standards by the U.S. EPA

A. Drinking-Water Standards

Substance	High-risk condition considered
Arsenic	None
Barium	No specific groups; but a safety factor of 2 incorporated to account for variation (or increased susceptibility) within the human population
Cadmium	None
Fluoride	Children—to prevent mottling of teeth
Lead	Children—to prevent neurological disorders
Mercury	Based on humans who exhibited toxicity at the lowest level of exposure from a group of mercury-poisoned adults
Nitrate	Infants—to protect against methemoglobinemia
Selenium	None
Sodium (no standard)	Individuals with heart and kidney disease
Chlorinated hydrocarbon insecticides (noncarcinogenic)	None
Chlorophenoxy herbicides (noncarcinogenic)	None

B. National Ambient Air Quality Standards

Substance	Original group	Primary groups currently considered
Carbon monoxide	Individuals with neurological or visual impairment	Adults with heart disease (angina, coronary artery disease)
Lead	Children—to protect against neurological and hematological impairment	Same
Nitrogen dioxide	Children—to protect against respiratory infections, also concern for changes in lung structure	Same
Ozone	Asthmatics	Exercisers, individuals with pre existing disease
Particulates	Elderly, individuals with cardiopulmonary disease	Same
Sulfur dioxide	Elderly, individuals with cardiopulmonary disease	Asthmatics

exposure of 75 μg from the diet and 20 μg from water. This 20 μg Cd/day from drinking water would occur at a level of 0.01 mg/L. The total daily Cd exposure is therefore approximately 95 μg Cd/day, and thus a safety factor of 4 was assumed.

In proposing their drinking water standard for cadmium, the EPA requested feedback from the public as to whether the standard should include additional protection for cigarette smokers, since smoking is a source of appreciable cadmium exposure (e.g., approximately 1.5 μg Cd/cigarette) (25). It is interesting to note that of the 52 comments received by the EPA on this issue, only 3 suggested that this standard be modified to include protection for the cigarette smokers. The EPA decided not to incorporate additional safety factors to protect smokers (208). Thus, this example describes a situation in which protection of a high-risk group was not taken into account in derivation of a standard.

HORMESIS

As described in the sections on evaluation of carcinogens and of systemic toxicants, the risk assessment process, as articulated by most regulatory agencies, has generally (but not always) assumed that the shape of the dose-response curve is either, for noncarcinogens, a threshold response below which no toxicity is observed or, for carcinogens, a linear relationship for which there is no exposure without an estimated effect.

Such risk assessment assumptions concerning the nature of the dose-response relationship for different biological endpoints have been challenged in recent years by the recognition that there are many exceptions to the threshold and linearity assumptions. A key exception to the two basic assumptions is that of the U- or inverted U-shaped dose-response relationship (Figure 2.6). Whether a dose-response relationship takes the U or inverted U form is dependent on the endpoint measured. In the case of U-shaped dose-response relationships, the endpoints could be various biological effects or diseases, such as mutation rate, birth defects, and cancer incidence (see ref. 30 for review). In the case of inverted U-shaped dose-response relationships, the types of endpoints include growth rate, fecundity (see ref. 27 for review), and longevity, among others. The phenomenon of stimulatory effects of low-level exposures has been termed *hormesis* and has been applied to both chemicals and radiation. Typical extrapolation processes for both threshold and nonthreshold phenomena ignore such possible U- or inverted U-shaped responses in the low-dose zone. A key implication of U- and the inverted U-shaped dose-response relationships is that, when such phenomena occur, the low-dose response (e.g., disease, incidence, longevity) cannot be readily predicted by responses at higher doses. The rest of this section presents background information on chemical hormesis and discusses some practical implications for both study design and risk-based standards development.

Although the concept of hormesis was seemingly well established by the 1920s at least as far as chemical hormesis is considered, the concept became marginalized within the scientific community in the 1930s and never had any serious impact on the modern concept of the dose-response relationship (26). The principal factors for the demise of the concept are complex, but include the following. One difficulty in differentiating the low-dose stimulatory phenomenon from normal variation was the lack of a study design with an adequate number of appropriately placed doses in the low dose range; this difficulty was further magnified by the fact that

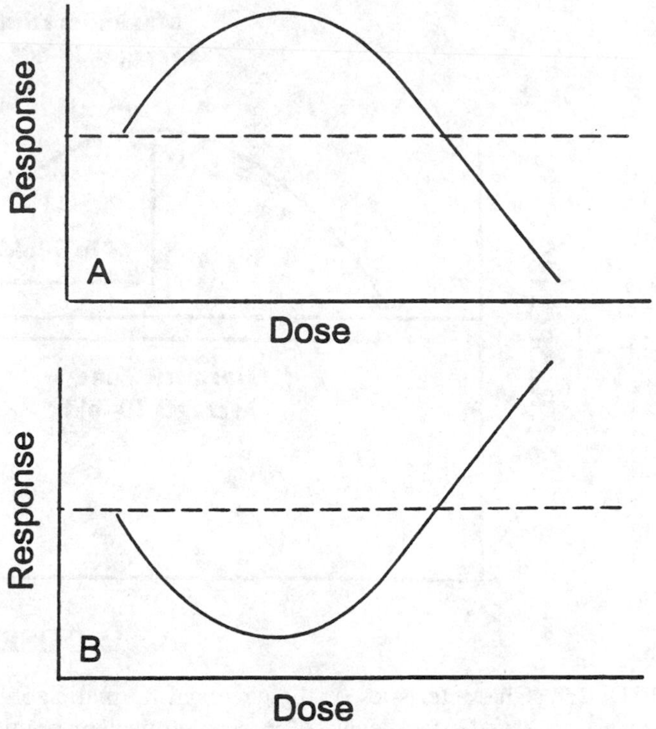

FIG. 2.6. Dose-response curves for hormesis. (A) The most common form of the hormetic dose-response curve depicting low-dosc stimulatory and high-dose inhibitory responses, the β- or inverted U-shaped curve. Examples of endpoints demonstrating the β- or inverted U-shaped dose-response curve include growth, longevity, fecundity, and weight gain. (B) The hormetic dose-response curve depicting low-dose reduction and high-dose enhancement of adverse effects, the J- or U-shaped curve. Examples of endpoints demonstrating the J- or U-shaped dose-response curves include mutations, cancer incidence, and birth-defects incidence. Source: Calabrese and Baldwin (28).

the magnitude of the low-dose stimulatory response has a maximum average of about 30–60% above the control (Figure 2.7). Lack of appreciation for what the hormetic dose-response was coupled with inadequate study design features led to criticism that the phenomenon was simply normal variation.

Over the past several years, Calabrese and Baldwin (30,31) have reinvestigated the hormesis hypothesis and developed rigorous a priori criteria for its evaluation. This investigation has uncovered several thousand examples of well-designed studies published in the peer-reviewed literature that are consistent with the hormesis phenomenon. The hormesis phenomenon has been proposed to result from a modest overcompensation to a disruption in homeostasis. More specifically, the investigation of minor damage induces a generalized repair response. In order to assure that the damage is adequately

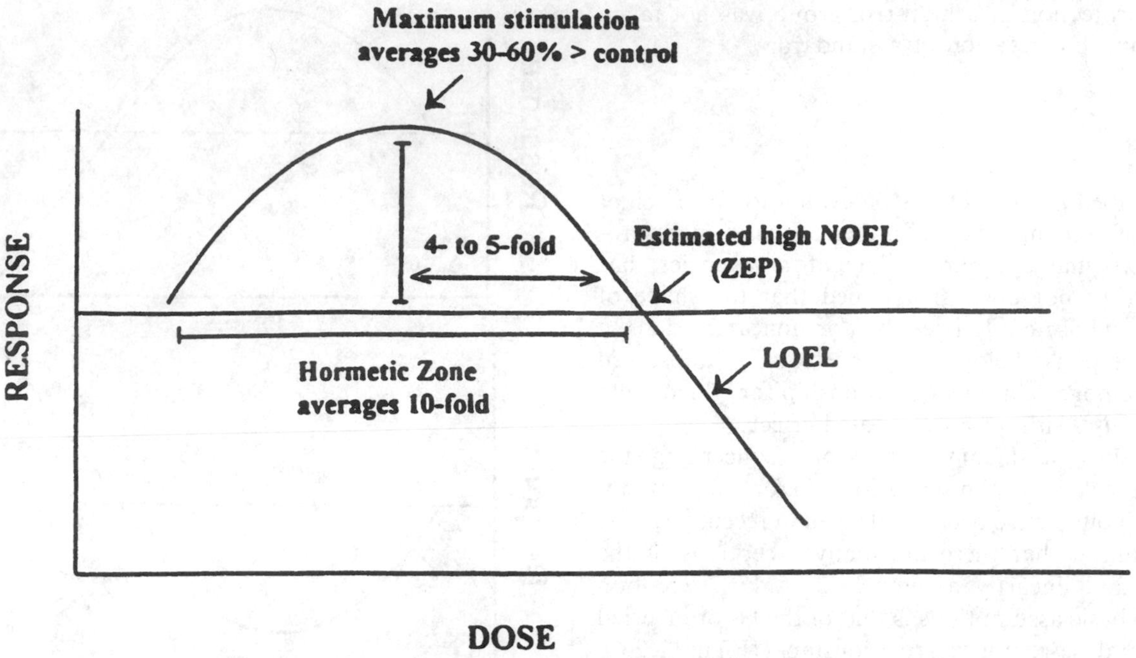

FIG. 2.7. Characteristics of the chemical hormetic zone. Abbreviations: NOEL, no-observed-effect level; LOEL, lowest-observed-effect level; ZEP, zero equivalent point. Source: Calabrese and Baldwin (31).

repaired, there is a slight overcompensation in repair responses. As the dose increases, the capacity to repair the damage decreases and eventually the capacity to repair equals the level of damage when the zero equivalent point (ZEP) is reached [i.e., the no observed adverse effect level (NOAEL)]. At higher doses, frank toxicity occurs. This process provides a framework to understand the basis for the observation that the stimulatory range is modest by up to about 10-fold, that the maximum stimulation averages about 50% above the control, and that the NOAEL/ZEP is only three- to five-fold greater than the maximum stimulatory response. Hormetic responses appear to be generalizable with respect to biological model, chemical class, and toxicological endpoint measured, including critical risk assessment endpoints such as tumor incidence, longevity, and various disease incidences.

Even in the situation where U-shaped dose-response relationships may exist, study design and other factors may reduce the capacity to detect such a relationship (Table 2.15). For example, it is not possible to assess hormesis with the use of certain toxicological parameters such as liver damage as reflected by increased serum enzymes.

To the extent that hormesis exists for a specific chemical, there are several implications for both noncarcinogenic and carcinogenic risk assessment. (a) The dose-response curve would be similar for both the carcinogenic and noncarcinogenic responses. (b) Thresholds would exist for both carcinogens and noncarcinogens. (c) At certain doses below the NOAEL (or ZEP) there would be less damage in the exposed group than observed in the control group. (d) Based on a review of hormetic dose-response relationships, the initial disruption in homeostasis typically occurs approximately 5- to 10-fold below the traditional NOAEL. However, this initial disruption is not only adequately repaired by the induction of adaptive mechanisms, but then background biological damage is also reduced by the induced adaptive mechanisms. (e) Current experimental approaches to assess the dose-response relationship in the hazard assessment process are inadequate since many studies only emphasize the relatively high-dose aspect of the dose-response curve. Thus, the hormetic perspective suggests that new study

Table 2.15

Factors contributing to the inability to detect a hormetic response when one exists

Inappropriate dose range.
Inappropriate spacing of doses.
Inappropriate number of doses.
Inappropriate temporal measurements in relationship to endpoint.
Inappropriate endpoint selection (e.g., serum enzyme levels as bioindicators of liver damage).
Condition of model organism.
Interindividual variability.
Low background in relationship to showing a U- or inverted U-shaped dose-response curve.

design criteria become incorporated into the hazard assessment protocol and that new default parameters become incorporated into the risk assessment framework incorporating the hormetic assumption.

Practical Implications of Hormesis for Quantitative Risk Assessment

Hormesis and Carcinogens

In a recent issue of the BELLE Newsletter, Sielken and Stevenson (168) identified seven ways in which the concept of hormesis should affect quantitative risk assessment (Table 2.16). The seven factors provided by Sielken and Stevenson (168) offer an important and clear blueprint for how the current approaches for both chemical and radiation cancer risk assessment modeling could both include and take advantage of the concept of hormesis and its underlying database. Many of these recommended changes reflect a less biased approach as well. For example, the parameters in the multistage model are typically required for regulatory purposes to be nonnegative values. This restriction determines that the probabilities in the multistage model be increasing as the dose increases. Sielken and Stevenson (168) argue that such nonnegativity restrictions for the parameters in the multistage model should be removed so that the fitted model may reflect the shape of the reported dose-response data. Furthermore, such a change would allow the multistage model enhanced flexibility to explicitly address hormetic effects seen in actual reported data. In addition, when an hormetic effect is present the risk at low dose would be less than for the control group. The lower bound on the "added" risk in the case of hormesis is no longer the zero risk as is now assumed, but would be negative. Clearly, therefore, both upper and lower bounds of uncertainty should be incorporated.

Table 2.16
Implications of hormesis for quantitative risk assessment

Dose-response models need greater flexibility to fit the observed shape of the dose-response data; such models should not be constructed to be forced to always be linearly decreasing at low doses.
Hazard assessment evaluations need to incorporate greater opportunity to identify the hormetic portion of the dose-response relationship.
New dose metrics should be used that incorporate age or time dependence on the dose level rather than a lifetime average daily dose or its analog for a shorter time period.
Low-dose risk characterization should include the likelihood of beneficial effects and the likelihood that a dose level has reasonable certainty of no appreciable adverse health effects.
Exposure assessments should fully characterize the distribution of actual doses from exposure rather than the just upper bounds.
Uncertainty characterizations should include both upper and lower bounds.
Risk should be characterized in terms of the net effect of a dose on health instead of a single dose's effect on a single disease endpoint (i.e., total mortality rather than a specific type of fatal disease).

Note. Adapted from Sielken and Stevenson (168).

Hormesis and Noncarcinogens

The role of hormesis in affecting the risk assessment process for noncarcinogens has also been discussed (28,29,62,197). As discussed in earlier sections, independent of whether hormesis exists or not, the major goal of the hazard assessment process is the derivation of the NOAEL (or in some cases the BMD).

Calabrese and Baldwin (29) have noted that the estimation of the BMD or the NOAEL can be affected by the existence of U-shaped dose-responses in two ways: (a) doses residing in the hormetic zone by affecting the modeling involved in the BMD derivation process, or (b) a dose within the hormetic zone could be selected as the NOAEL. With respect to the former possibility (i.e., BMD derivation), the occurrence of hormetic responses would tend to flatten the model-based dose-response relationship, thereby requiring a higher response to achieve the $BMD_{05/10}$ response. In the latter case (i.e., where the highest dose is not different from the control), a dose with a value lower than the zero equivalent point (ZEP) would be designated the NOAEL. This may be illustrated in Figure 2.8, which shows a typi-

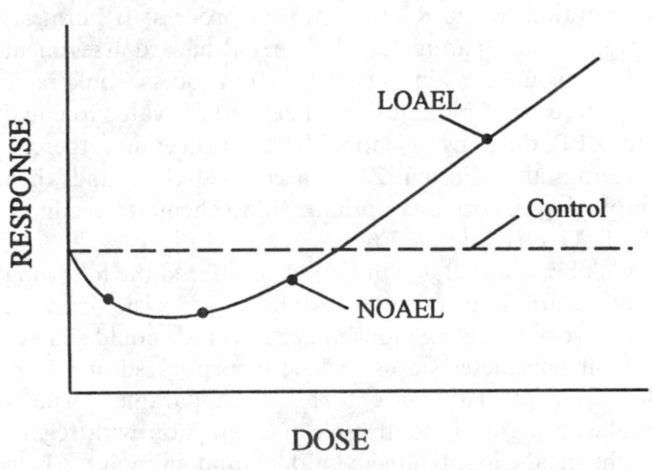

FIG. 2.8. Dose-response relationship presenting NOAEL in the hormetic zone. Source: Calabrese and Baldwin (29).

cal U-shaped dose-response relationship. The highest dose causes a significant toxic effect and is designated the LOAEL. The dose immediately below the highest dose exhibits a response lower than the reference or control group. This hormetic dose would become the NOAEL since it is the highest dose not significantly different with regard to an adverse effect and satisfies the above definitional criteria. Therefore, in these two cases, the concept of the NOAEL is (a) affected by the presence of hormetic doses in the application of the BMD process and (b) being explicitly incorporated into the hormetic portion of the dose-response curve (i.e., traditional NOAEL derivation process).

While the U-shaped dose-response is often seen and appears to be highly generalizable, it is not seen in numerous instances (Table 2.15). For example, it is not possible to assess hormesis if tumor incidence of the background (or control) is very low. This lack of ability to make judgments about hormesis is further seen with respect to other toxicological parameters such as liver damage, which is inferred by increased serum enzymes. Even though the current methods cannot assess hormesis under these conditions, this does not suggest that it does not exist. In fact, hormesis may be predicted to exist independent of the biological incidence of the disease under study.

If hormetic effects were to have an opportunity to affect the RfD derivation process, the hazard assessment process would have to expand the toxicological testing process into the low dose zone by increasing the number of doses from 2–3 to 6–7 doses with an assurance that at least three doses were below the traditional toxicological NOAEL (31). This would help insure that the hormetic phenomenon would have been properly evaluated. Such an expansion of the hazard assessment process would add considerable cost and time to the testing process. An alternative to the expanded testing strategy would be to incorporate hormesis as a default assumption in the RfD derivation process. If hormesis were a default parameter, the current hazard assessment process could remain as is. The RfD process would have to proceed by first adjusting the NOAEL value to equal the ZEP dose by a model-based procedure, thereby deriving an adjusted ZEP-based NOAEL, and then employing a hormesis optimization scheme to facilitate the RfD derivation (23,62).

Calabrese and Baldwin (29) have offered the following considerations in order to establish a decision-making framework for assessing whether hormesis could achieve default parameter status and be incorporated into RfD development. The concept of default parameter status implies a highly generalizable phenomenon with regard to chemical class, biological model, and endpoint, which is linked to the risk assessment process. Consequently, the concept of hormesis would first need to permeate the broad classes of inorganic and organic contaminants, especially those containing agents that are of regulatory concern. Second, the phenomenon of hormesis must be generalizable across species to ensure that hormesis for a particular chemical does not reflect a species- or strain-specific response. The third factor for assessing hormesis as a default parameter in the RfD derivation process concerns biological endpoint. Regulatory actions focus predominantly on adverse endpoints such as organ-specific toxicity, biomarkers of toxic response (e.g., blood lead levels, serum cholinesterase activity), and teratogenic and other reproductive effects, as well as tumor formation. The influence of hormesis is not only in the reduction of already indicated adverse effects and biomarker responses, but also in the enhancement of outcomes such as increased longevity, improved performance, and reduction of disease incidence below background. The ability to incorporate what society considers both beneficial and harmful effects of a chemical into decision making presents a challenge to regulators. Consider, for example, the difficulties in making recommendations on alcohol consumption where moderate levels can reduce risk of heart disease, but excessive drinking clearly takes a toll in terms of morbidity and premature mortality.

The recently developed chemical hormesis database (30) evaluates toxicological investigations for their capacity to demonstrate evidence consistent with the hormesis hypothesis based on study design attributes, response criteria, statistical power, and reproducibility. This database provides evidence that hormesis is likely to be generalizable across the three critical areas listed here and that its relationship to the NOAEL is readily estimated, thus allowing practical incorporation into the risk assessment process. Based on this information, we recommend that regulatory agencies consider the concept of hormesis as a default parameter in the risk assessment process. What would be the practical implication if hormesis were accepted as a default assumption for the RfD derivation process? First, consideration of hormesis would redefine the concept of NOAEL for regulatory purposes. In addition, consideration of hormesis would allow an optimizing process to estimate the dose providing the best balance between preventing the agent-induced adverse effects and enhancing hormetic/adaptive responses within the population.

IMPLICATIONS OF CHEMICAL INTERACTIONS FOR THE REGULATORY PROCESS

One of the major difficulties in current environmental public health practice is that the focus is on a limited number of environmental contaminants, with limited consideration of interactive effects among pollutants. In fact, the number of environmental pollutants in different media is large, making it difficult to estimate the degree of public health protection afforded by our present regulatory apparatus. Still, it is clear that the scientific and regulatory communities must address the issue of multiple chemical exposures. In fact, animal models and human epidemiological studies show that interactions do occur among chemicals and that this can result, under certain circumstances, in greater than additive effects. For example, uranium miners who smoke have a fourfold greater risk of cancer than nonsmokers. However, uranium miners who smoke display a 40-fold greater cancer risk than the general population of nonsmokers (137).

Interactions have been studied for many years by the drug industry, insecticide manufacturers, and forensic/clinical toxicologists. Given the widespread use of multiple drug therapy, the need to anticipate possible interactions has been essential. Thus, much of the basis of our current understanding of toxicological interactions is derived from the pharmaceutical industry. It should be recognized that there is uncertainty in extrapolating from drug exposures where doses are relatively high, that is, by definition at pharmacologically active doses, to environmental exposures, which are typically much lower.

Chemical interactions have been broadly classified by three general terms: *addition* (additivity), when the toxic effect produced by two or more chemicals in combination is equivalent to that expected by simple summation of their individual effects; *antagonism*, when the effect of a combination is less than the sum of the individual effects; and *synergism*, when the effect of the combination is greater than would be predicted by summation of the individual effects. Other terms have been used, such as *indifference* and *potentiation*, which represent specialized aspects of antagonism and synergism, respectively.

In testing for possible interactions, at least two important considerations must be addressed. These include temporal (time) factors and response-endpoint considerations.

Time Factor

While most screening tests for interactions employ simultaneous exposure, this type of exposure approach has the chance of reducing the likelihood of detecting some potential interactions. For example, two agents may affect the same cellular mechanism but may have markedly different times of onset to expression. If a critical threshold of reversible cellular injury is required for the adverse effect, tests of acute toxicity of combinations given simultaneously may show antagonism, whereas an additive action would be observed if the dosing and observation periods were spaced to cause the maximum effect.

Toxic Effect

Since most toxic substances have multiple toxic effects, the nature of any chemical interaction may vary, depending on the measured responses. For example, since chlorinated insecticides and halogenated solvents produce liver injury independently, it is plausible that they could under certain circumstances act in an additive or synergistic manner when combined. However, the insecticide is likely to be a central nervous system stimulant, whereas the solvent may be a central nervous system depressant. Thus, as measured by neurological tests, these chemicals could interact in an antagonistic way.

Predictive Models

Development of predictive models of chemical interaction must rely on an understanding of the basic toxicological principles concerning kinetics of reactions of chemicals with primary sites of action (tissue receptor sites) and with secondary tissue sites of reaction. Four factors have been identified as of central importance:

1. Relative affinities of the individual chemicals for sites of action (e.g., target enzymes, cellular membranes, etc.).
2. Relative affinities for sites of loss of the chemical (e.g., detoxifying enzymes, nonvital tissue binding sites, pathways of excretion, and storage sites).
3. Intrinsic activity of the agents at their sites of action.
4. Sites of bioactivation.

While many of the examples are derived from the pharmacology literature, similar interactions could occur among environmental chemicals.

Pharmacokinetic Drug/Pollutant Interactions

The four factors listed allow us to predict how toxicological interactions may occur. The biological damage caused by a toxic agent is proportional to the amount of the biologically active form of the agents able to react with critical cellular macromolecules. An interaction may occur when the availability of an active chemical is altered by the presence of another agent, or when its reactivity with critical macromolecules is altered by the presence of another agent. The first case involves a site of loss of active chemical, whereas the second involves an interaction at a site of action. Thus, considerable research activity has investigated the capacity of a chemical to affect the absorption, distribution, metabolism, and excretion of another chemical.

Absorption

Absorption of an agent may be affected by a second drug that alters pH or gut motility. For example, aspirin is absorbed more rapidly at low pH because more of the drug is present in the readily diffusible nonionized lipid soluble form. Agents that cause an increase in the pH will slow down the gastric absorption of aspirin when taken simultaneously. Similarly, the absorption of tetracycline is reduced by aluminum hydroxide gels and readily ionized salts of calcium and magnesium. In contrast, the gastrointestinal absorption of acetaminophen is enhanced in the presence of sorbitol.

Protein Binding

Drugs may compete for the same protein binding sites in plasma. When this occurs, the effective biological concentrations of the displaced drug can rise markedly. For example, usually 98% of the anticoagulant drug warfarin is bound to the plasma protein albumin, so that only 2% of the total drug in the plasma is biologically active. If the effect of another drug competing for the same plasma albumin site is to reduce the binding of warfarin from 98 to 96%, the concentration of pharmacologically active warfarin would be doubled. This interaction would have approximately the same effect on clotting time as would doubling the dose of the anticoagulant. This type of interaction with an anticoagulant drug has resulted in a number of clinical incidents, with some resulting in fatal hemorrhagic complications.

Metabolism

Many chemicals, including drugs and environmental contaminants, enhance the metabolic capacity of the liver. Other chemicals may diminish the metabolic capacity of the liver. These interactions could have profound implications. In fact, it is now recognized that several of the insecticide synergists (i.e., agents that, when administered along with insecticides, markedly enhance the insecticide's ability to kill insects) act by blocking the enzymes normally affecting insecticide detoxification (221). For example, the toxicity of the insecticide carbaryl against susceptible female houseflies is enhanced by over 200-fold by certain chemical synergists. Thus, knowledge of synergy has been used to develop more effective insecticide formulations.

Insecticides provide another example of how agencies use information on chemical interactions. In 1957, Frawley et al. (61) reported the first synergistic interaction of two organophosphate insecticides (i.e., malathion and ethyl *p*-nitrophenyl phenyl phosphonothionate or EPN), which led to the development of the FDA requirement that all newly registered organophosphate insecticides be evaluated for possible synergisms with all the already-registered organophosphate insecticides. As more organophosphate insecticides were developed, this regulatory requirement became an extreme testing burden. However, with elucidation of the biochemical mechanism[1] for this interaction, it became possible to assess possible interactions of organophosphate insecticides via biochemical means and thereby circumvent the time-consuming and costly toxicological testing of whole animals. In both examples, that of making a more efficient insecticidal preparation and that of predicting adverse public health effects from multiple agent exposures, chemical interaction predictions were markedly enhanced with a clear understanding of the mechanisms of toxicity.

Implications

The examples just given represent ideal situations, since the mechanisms of toxicity of the insecticides were very well characterized. More frequently, little information is available on toxic mechanisms. Regulatory agencies need to develop approaches in such situations when reasonable mechanistic predictions cannot be made. To this end, Finney (59) developed a theoretical mathematical approach for predicting the degree of toxicity derived from various types of chemical interactions. Pozzani et al. (154) indicated that only 2 of the 36 pairs of mixtures of industrial vapors tested for acute toxicity in rats deviated significantly from the calculations of Finney's theoretical approach for additive joint toxicity. According to Smyth et al. (170), the study by Pozzani et al. (154) supported the hypothesis that the acute toxicity of chemical mixtures randomly chosen has a high likelihood of being accurately predicted by Finney's theoretical formula for additive joint toxicity. In an attempt "to evaluate the overall confidence that can be placed on the prediction of the joint toxicity of many chemical pairs," Smyth et al. (170) studied the toxicity of 27 industrial chemicals in all possible pairs to rats. Their results were consistent with the prediction of Finney (59) that most interactions should be considered as additive until proven otherwise. Smyth et al. (170), in agreement with the general findings of Pozzani et al. (154), concluded that approximately 5% of the various combinations tested exhibited more or less than additive effects.

Most studies have evaluated synergism at only very high or acute levels of exposure. It is important, however, to ask whether synergisms would occur at lower (more realistic) concentrations. Recent investigations using complex mixtures, tested at relatively low levels of

[1] EPN inhibits the nonspecific enzyme carboxyesterase that detoxifies malathion. Thus, in the presence of EPN, malathion is more persistent and causes a greater effect as a cholinesterase inhibitor than would have occurred had enzymatic detoxification mechanisms not been affected.

exposure, indicate that the potential for interactions is likely dose dependent.

Their studies indicated that synergistic interactions, the type of interactions of greatest regulatory concern, may be less likely to occur at environmentally relevant exposure levels than at higher (e.g., pharmaceutical or some occupational) exposure levels.

Approaches Used by Regulatory Agencies to Assess Interactions

Despite the frequent lack of a clear mechanistic understanding of how chemicals may interact, regulatory agencies have developed interim approaches to facilitate the decision-making process. In this section, we highlight some of the typical approaches used by agencies with illustrative examples.

The Hazard Index Approach

Perhaps the simplest approach is the assumption of additivity of hazard. In this approach (applied to noncarcinogens), hazard indices (the ratio between the estimated dose and the reference dose; see section on evaluation of systemic toxicants) are summed across chemicals and across routes of exposure to obtain a total hazard index for a particular exposure setting (207). If the decision criterion of a total hazard index of 1 is exceeded, further review is performed to determine which chemicals act at the same target organ. A subsequent summation is performed for those chemicals only. While this approach is useful as a screening approach, it has several limitations that must be considered when interpreting the results. These include (but are not limited to) the following:

- Reference doses (the denominator in the hazard index) for different chemicals contain different types and magnitudes of uncertainty factors. Thus, differences in the magnitude of a hazard index for a particular chemical or a pathway of exposure may reflect intrinsic differences in hazard as well as differences in the uncertainty of a particular toxicity value.
- Different types of interactive effects are possible, even for chemicals that act at the same target organ. For example, organophosphates that act via the inhibition of acetylcholinesterase at nerve endings would generally be presumed to act in an additive manner (128). In contrast, trichloroethylene (TCE) and alcohol, both of which affect the central nervous system, can when consumed simultaneously, act synergistically (e.g., producing "degreaser's flush"); however, chronic alcohol consumption can, by induction of metabolizing enzymes, diminish the response to TCE (2).

The Toxicity Equivalency Factor Approach

The toxicity equivalency factor (TEF) approach has been applied to a mixture that contains toxicologically and structurally similar chemicals. Perhaps one of the best known examples of the TEF approach is the approach developed by the U.S. EPA (17) for polychlorinated dibenzodioxins (PCDDs) and polychlorinated dibenzofurans (PCDFs). This approach is based on the assumption that PCDDs and PCDFs exert their toxicity through binding to the Ah receptor with subsequent effects on transcription and translational events responsible for toxicity. The most potent PCDD, 2,3,7,8-tetrachlorodibenzodioxin, has the greatest affinity for the Ah receptor and, hence, is the most potent member of this class. TEFs are developed for individual PCDDs and PCDFs, expressed as a fraction (typically in orders of magnitude) of that of TCDD, which is given a TEF of 1.0. Thus, RfDs and cancer slope factors (CSFs) are calculated as a ratio to the RfD and CSF for 2,3,7,8-TCDD. While there is experimental support, based on mixtures of PCDDs and PCDFs, for this approach, there are few, if any, data from long-term studies (17). Other uncertainties in this approach include the assumption of additivity, where competitive interactions may occur at sufficiently high doses, and the choice of a particular TEF value, which can be influenced by selection of endpoint, exposure duration, and dose (151).

The Complex Mixture Approach

There are certain classes of chemicals for which toxicological data exist primary for the complex mixture itself, with limited data for individual constituents. An example of this type of mixture is polychlorinated biphenyls or PCBs. PCBs were manufactured in the United States under the trade name of Aroclors for use in electrical capacitors. Different Aroclor mixtures contained different percentages of chlorine. For example, Aroclor 1242 contained approximately 42% chlorine (159). Much of the toxicity testing of PCBs consists of studies of different Aroclor mixtures (39,159). As a result, toxicity criteria for PCBs are typically expressed as Aroclor-specific values. In the case of Aroclor 1254, for example, the Agency for Toxic Substances and Disease Registry (ATSDR) developed a chronic minimum risk level or MRL, a value conceptually to the RfD, based on immunological effects in monkeys exposed to Aroclor 1254 in feed for 23 months (151). While this approach does not require assumptions on how individual constituents will interact, it does assume that the characteristics of the mixture in the environment are the same as in the laboratory studies. Unfortunately, this assumption is not always correct, since complex mixtures frequently undergo chemical transformations in the environment. Moreover, the individual constituents may partition differently in the environment. In the case of PCBs, for example, the more chlorinated forms bioaccummulate in fish more readily than the less chlorinated forms (39).

Consideration of interactive effects in the regulatory arena is an evolving process. Because data are limited in many cases, simplifying assumptions are often used, such as the assumption of hazard index additivity for chemicals that act via the same target organ. As scientists acquire greater mechanistic understanding of interactive effects in complex mixtures, approaches that better reflect molecular events can be developed, such as the use of TEF approach. Nonetheless, it must be recognized that there is still uncertainty regarding the extent to which such effects occur at environmentally relevant exposure levels and under exposure conditions that do not mimic those tested in the laboratory (e.g., intermittent vs. chronic exposures).

CONCLUSIONS

In this chapter, we have demonstrated the multiple applications of toxicology to the regulatory process. Applications include developing and evaluating chemical testing protocols, such as for developmental toxicants; developing classification schemes (so far mainly for carcinogens) aimed at characterizing the types of toxic effects that might be observed in humans; and developing health-based criteria for chemicals in various media (food, water, air, soil) or notification levels for release of chemicals under accidental circumstances.

In addition, toxicology is used in the regulatory process to help assess potential risk associated with defined exposure levels. The traditional paradigm for assessing such risks is as follows: For carcinogens, potential risk is defined as an upper bound estimate of excess cancer risk based on cancer incidence at high dose levels, and for noncarcinogens, potential risk is defined as the ratio of the estimated exposure to an exposure level associated with negligible, if any, risk. Recent advances in the understanding of toxicological mechanisms indicate that these methodologies are not appropriate in all circumstances. Some carcinogens, such as those that operate by receptor-mediated or cytotoxic mechanisms, may exhibit a threshold or nonlinear dose-response relationship, and thus exposure levels associated with virtually zero risk might be defined. Examples of chemicals with these types of dose-response relationships are saccharin and phenobarbital. The U.S. EPA recent cancer risk assessment guidelines, which consider different dose-response relationships for different carcinogens, represent an important development in this area. Our understanding of certain noncarcinogenic effects, such as angina associated with CO exposure, is reasonably advanced; in this example, risks from CO are more fully described in terms of number of individuals with heart disease who might be expected to exceed defined COHb levels under certain exposure conditions. Benchmark dose and categorical exposure-response modeling represent additional examples of recent advances in noncarcinogenic risk assessment.

Toxicology is frequently applied in the regulatory context of developing permissible exposure levels in different exposure media, such as ambient air, drinking water, or food. As discussed in this chapter, definition of the health-based permissible exposure level is only one part of developing a regulatory standard. Other important factors in the regulatory process include risk management issues such as the definition of acceptable risk, the weighing of the costs and technical feasibility of reducing risk, the availability of alternatives, and the new risks possibly created by reducing the original risk (e.g., use of a less well tested substitute chemical). Issues of equity and whether certain members of the population are unfairly burdened by chemical exposure represent other considerations.

A critical role for toxicologists participating in the regulatory process is to effectively communicate not only the results of a risk assessment, but also the uncertainties associated with risk evaluations, in order to provide risk managers with the full information needed for making sound decisions. In addition, despite pressure to employ older methods for the sake of consistency, toxicologists must work to develop and encourage the use of new methodologies reflecting the advances in our understanding of toxicological mechanisms. We hope this chapter is useful as a guide to the use of better science in the regulatory process.

QUESTIONS

1. How do different approaches used for noncancer risk assessment (e.g., benchmark dose, reference dose, and the distributional population approach) address susceptible populations?
2. Under what circumstances would one use the following approach for assessing risks of complex mixtures: the hazard index approach, the toxicity equivalency factor approach, and the complex mixture?
3. What are some of the advantages and disadvantages of using cancer bioassay results at the maximum tolerated dose (MTD) for interpreting likelihood of carcinogenicity to humans?

REFERENCES

1. Abelson, P. H. (1993): Pesticides and food. *Science*, 259:1235.
2. Agency for Toxic Substances and Disease Registry. (1997): Toxicological profile for trichloroethylene—Update. Prepared by Sciences International, Inc., for U.S. Public Health Services, U.S. EPA. NTIS PB-101165/XAB.
3. Allison, A. C., Harrington, J. S., and Birbeck, M. (1966): An examination of the cytotoxic effects of silica on macrophages. *J. Exp. Med.*, 124:141–154.
4. American Cancer Society. (1998): *Cancer Facts & Figures—1998*. Publication 98-300M-No. 5008.98. American Cancer Society, Inc., Atlanta, GA.
5. American Conference of Governmental Industrial Hygienists. (1998): *Guide to Occupational Exposure Values—1998*. ACGIH, Cincinnati, OH.
6. American Conference of Governmental Industrial Hygienists. (1996): *Documentation of the Threshold Limit Values and Biological Indices*. American Conference of Governmental Industrial Hygienists, Cincinnati, OH. 6th edn. Supplement—Perchloroethylene.
7. American Conference of Governmental Industrial Hygienists. (1992): *Threshold Limit Values for Chemical Substances and Physical Agents*. ACGIH, Cincinnati, OH.
8. American Thoracic Society. (1985): Guidelines as to what constitutes an adverse respiratory health effect with special reference to epidemiologic studies of air pollution. *Am. Rev. Respir. Dis.*, 131:666–669.
9. Ames, B. N., and Gold, L. S. (1990): Too many rodent carcinogens: Mitogenesis increases mutagenesis. *Science*, 249:970–971.
10. Ames, B. N., Swirsky-Gold, L., and Shigenaga, M. K. (1996): Cancer prevention, rodent high-dose cancer tests, and risk assessment. *Risk Anal.*, 16:613–617.
11. Andersen, M. E., Clewell, H. J. III, Gargas, M. L., Smith, F. A., and Reitz, R. H. (1987): Physiologically based pharmacokinetics and the risk assessment process for methylene chloride. *Toxicol. Appl. Pharmacol.*, 87:185–205.
12. Anderson, P. D. (1988): Scientific origins of incompatibility in risk assessment. *Stat. Sci.*, 3(3):320–327.
13. Baird, S. J. S., Cohen, J. T., Graham, J. D., Shlyakhter, A. I., and Evans, J. S. (1996): Noncancer risk assessment: A probabilistic alternative to current practice. *Hum. Ecol. Risk Assess.* 2(1):79–102.
14. Beck, B. D. (1997): The use of information on susceptibility in risk assessment: State of the science and potential for improvement. *Environ. Toxicol. Pharmacol.*, 4:229–234.
15. Beck, B. D., Connolly, R. B., Dourson, M. L., Guth, D., Hattis, D., Kimmel, C., and Lewis, S. C. (1993): Improvements in quantitative noncancer risk assessment. *Fundam. Appl. Toxicol.*, 20:1–14.
16. Beck, B. D., Toole, A. P., Callahan, B. G., and Siddhanti, S. K. (1991): Utilization of quantitative structure activity relationships (QSARs) in risk assessment. *Regul. Toxicol. Pharmacol.*, 14:273–285.
17. Bellin, J. S., Barnes, D. G., Kutz, F. W., and Bottimore, D. P. (1989): Interim procedures for estimating risks associated with exposures to mixtures of chlorinated dibenzo-*p*-dioxins and dibenzofurans (CDDs and CDFs) and 1989 update. Prepared for U.S. EPA, Risk Assessment Forum. EPA-625/3-89-016. NTIS PB90-145756 INZ.
18. Bethel, R. A., Epstein, J., Sheppard, D., Nadel, J. A., and Boushey, H. A. (1983): Sulfur dioxide-induced bronchoconstriction in freely breathing exercising, asthmatic subjects. *Am. Rev. Respir. Dis.*, 128:987–990.
19. Betke, J., Kleihaver, E., and Lipps, M. (1956): Vergleichende Untersucheg uber Sportanozydation von Nabelschnur and Erwachsenenhamoglobin. *Ztschr. Kinderh.* 77:549.

19a. Bickis, M., and Kreski, D. (1985): Statistical design and analysis of the long-term carcinogenicity bioassay. In: *Toxicological Risk Assessment*, Vol. 1, edited by D. B. Clayson, D. Krewski, and I. Munro, pp. 125–147. CRC Press, Boca Raton, FL.

20. Bromberg, P. A. (1998): Risk assessment of the effects of ozone exposure on respiratory health: dealing with variability in human responsiveness to controlled exposures. In: *Human Variability in Response to Chemical Exposure*, edited by D. A. Neumann and C. A. Kimmel, pp. 139–163. ILSI Press, Washington, DC.
21. Burns, C. A., Zarkower, A., and Ferguson, F. G. (1980): Murine immunological and histological changes in response to chronic silica exposure. *Environ. Res.*, 21:298–307.
22. Butterworth, B. E. (1990): Consideration of both genotoxic and nongenotoxic mechanisms in predicting carcinogenic potential. *Mutat. Res.*, 239:117–132.
23. Calabrese, E. J. (1996): Expanding the RfD concept to incorporate and optimize beneficial effects while preventing toxic responses from non-essential toxicants. *BELLE Newslett.*, 4:1–10.
24. Calabrese, E. J. (1987): Animal extrapolation: A look inside the toxicologist's black box. *Environ. Sci. Technol.*, 21:618–623.
25. Calabrese, E. J. (1978): *Pollutants and High Risk Groups*. John Wiley, New York.
26. Calabrese, E. J., and Baldwin, L. A. (1999): The marginalization of hormesis. *Toxicol. Pathol.*, 27:187–194.
27. Calabrese, E. J., and Baldwin, L. A. (1999): Significant biological effects below the NOAEL in reproductive toxicology. In: *Environmental and Human Risk Assessment*, edited by H. Salem, pp. 95–106. Taylor and Francis, Washington, DC.
28. Calabrese, E. J., and Baldwin, L. A. (1998): Can the concept of hormesis be generalized to carcinogenesis? *Regul. Toxicol. Pharmacol.*, 28:230–241.
29. Calabrese, E. J., and Baldwin, L. A. (1998): Hormesis as a default parameter in RfD derivation. *Hum. Exp. Toxicol.*, 17:444–447.
30. Calabrese, E. J., and Baldwin, L. A. (1997): The dose determines the stimulation (and poison): Development of a chemical hormesis database. *Int. J. Toxicol.*, 16:545–559.
31. Calabrese, E. J., and Baldwin, L. A. (1997): A quantitatively-based methodology for the evaluation of chemical hormesis. *Hum. Ecol. Risk Assess.*, 3:545–554.
32. Calabrese, E. J., Beck, B. D., and Chappell, W. R. (1992): Does the animal-to-human uncertainty factor incorporate interspecies differences in surface area? *Regul. Toxicol. Pharmacol.*, 15:172–179.
33. Carnow, B. W. (1976): Panel discussion on TLV's—Lead. In: *Health Effects of Occupational Lead and Arsenic Exposure: A Symposium*, edited by B. W. Carnow, p. 197. U.S. PHS, NIOSH, Washington, DC.
34. Carson, R. L. (1962): *Silent Spring*. Houghton Mifflin, Boston.
35. Chang, L.-Y., Huang, Y., Stockstill, B. L., Graham, J. A., Grose, E. C., Menache, M. G., Miller, F. J., Costa, D. L., and Crapo, J. D. (1992): Epitheliel injury and interstitial fibrosis in the proximal alveolar regions of rats chronically exposed to a simulated pattern of urban ambient ozone. *Toxicol. Appl. Pharmacol.*, 115:241–252.
36. Chernoff, N., and Kavlock, R. J. (1982): An in vivo teratology screen utilizing pregnant mice. *J. Toxicol. Environ. Health*, 10:541–550.
37. Clayson, D. B., and Clegg, D. J. (1991): Classification of carcinogens: Polemics, pedantics, or progress? *Regul. Toxicol. Pharmacol.*, 14:147–166.
38. Clewell, H. J. (1995): The use of physiologically based pharmacokinetic modeling in risk assessment: A case study with methylene chloride. In: *Low-Dose Extrapolation of Cancer Risks*,

edited by S. Olin, W. Farland, C. Park, L. Rhomberg, R. Scheuplein, T. Starr, and J. Wilson, pp. 199–222. ILSI Press, Washington, DC.

39. Cogliano, V. J. (1996): PCBs: Cancer dose-response assessment and application to environmental mixtures. Prepared for U.S. EPA, National Center for Environmental Assessment. NTIS PB96-140603. EPA/600/P-96/001A. NTIS PB96-140603.

40. Cohen, S. M., and Ellwein, L. B. (1995): Biological theory of carcinogenesis: Implications for risk assessment. In: *Low-Dose Extrapolation of Cancer Risks*, edited by S. Olin, W. Farland, C. Park, L. Rhomberg, R. Scheuplein, T. Starr, and J. Wilson, pp. 145–161. ILSI Press, Washington, DC.

41. Colditz, G. A., Stampfer, M. J., and Green, L. C. (1988): Diet. In: *Variations in Susceptibility to Inhaled Pollutants*, edited by B. D. Brain, A. J. Waven, and R. A. Shaiker, pp. 314–331. Johns Hopkins University Press, Baltimore, MD.

42. Conolly, R. B., and Butterworth, B. E. (1995): Biologically based dose response model for hepatic toxicity: a mechanistically based replacement for traditional estimates of noncancer risk. *Toxicol. Lett.*, 82/83:901–906.

43. Cook, P. J., Doll, R., and Fellingham, S. A. (1969): A mathematical model for the age distribution of cancer in man. *Int. J. Cancer*, 4:93–112.

44. Cooper, W. C. (1973): Indicators of susceptibility to industrial chemicals. *J. Occup. Med.*, 15(4):355.

45. Crump, K. S., Clewell, H. J., and Andersen, M. E. (1997): Cancer and non-cancer risk assessment should be harmonized. *Hum. Ecol. Risk Assess.*, 3(4):495–499.

46. Crump, K. S. (1984): A new method for determining allowable daily intake. *Fundam. Appl. Toxicol.*, 4:854–871.

47. Cullen, A. C., and Frey, H. C., eds. (1999): *Probabilistic Techniques in Exposure Assessment. A Handbook for Dealing with Variability and Uncertainty in Models and Inputs*. Plenum Press, New York.

48. deRosa, C. T., Stara, J. F., and Durkin, P. R. (1985): Ranking chemicals based on chronic toxicity data. *Toxicol. Ind. Health*, 1:177–192.

49. Deutsche Forchungsgemeinschaft. (1996): List of Max and BAT values for 1996. VCH Verlagsgeschschaft, Weinheim. As cited in Neumann, H.-G., Thielmann, H. W., Filser, J. G., et al. (1997): Proposed changes in the classification of carcinogenis chemicals in the work area. *Regul. Toxicol. Pharmacol.*, 26:288–295.

50. Dourson, M. L. (1986): New approaches in the derivation of acceptable daily intake (ADI). *Comments Toxicol.*, 1:35–48.

51. Dourson, M. L., and Stara, J. F. (1983): Regulatory history and experimental support of uncertainty (safety) factors. *Regul. Toxicol. Pharmacol.*, 3:224–238.

52. Elcombe, C. R., Rose, M. S., and Pratt, I. S. (1985): Biochemical, histological, and ultrastructural changes in rat and mouse liver following the administration of trichloroethylene: Possible relevance to species differences in hepatocarcinogenicity. *Toxicol. Appl. Pharmacol.*, 79:365–376.

53. Elsayed, N. M., and Mustafa, M. G. (1982): Dietary antioxidants and the biochemical response to oxidant inhalation. I. Influence of dietary vitamin E on the biochemical effects of nitrogen dioxide exposure in rat lung. *Toxicol. Appl. Pharmacol.*, 66:319–328.

54. Enslein, K. (1987): Computer-assisted prediction of toxicity. In: *Toxic Substances and Human Risk. Principals of Data Interpretation*, edited by R. G. Tardiff, and J. V. Rodricks, pp. 317–338. Plenum Press, New York.

55. Enterline, P. E. (1983): Epidemiologic basis for the asbestos standard. *Environ. Health Perspect.*, 52:93–97.

56. European Union. (1993): Annex VI general classification and labeling requirements for dangerous substances and preparation, communication directions 93/21/EEC of April 27, 1993. *Official Journal of the European Communities* L110A 5/4/1993. As cited in Neumann, H.-G., Thielmann, H. W., Filser, J. G., et al. (1997): Proposed changes in the classification of carcinogenis chemicals in the work area. *Regul. Toxicol. Pharmacol.*, 26:288–295.

57. Faustman, E. M. (1996): Review of Noncancer Risk Assessment: Application of Benchmark Dose Methods. Prepared for the Commission on Risk Assessment and Risk Management. Washington, DC. June.

58. Finkel, A. M. (1991): Testimony of Adam M. Finkel, Resources for the Future, before the U.S. House of Representatives Committee on Science, Space, and Technology. Subcommittee on Environment. Hearing on Risk Assessment: Strengths and Limitations of Utilization for Policy Decisions, May 21, 1991. Washington, DC.

59. Finney, D. J. (1952): *Probit Analysis*. Cambridge University Press, London.

60. Frame, L. T., Ambrosone, C. B., Kadlubar, F. F., and Lang, N. P. (1998): Host–environment interactions that affect variability in human cancer susceptibility. In: *Human Variability in Response to Chemical Exposure*, edited by D. A. Neumann and C. A. Kimmel, pp. 165–204. ILSI Press, Washington, DC.

61. Frawley, J. P., Fuyat, H. N., Hagan, E. C., Blake, J. R., and Fitzhugh, O. G. (1957): Marked potentiation in mammalian toxicity from simultaneous administration of two anti-cholinesterase compounds. *J. Pharmacol. Exp. Ther.*, 121:96.

62. Gaylor, D. (1998): Safety assessment with hormetic effects. *Hum. Exp. Toxicol.*, 17:251–253.

63. Germolec, D. R., Yang, R. S., Ackermann, M. F., Rosenthal, G. J., Boorman, G. A., Blair P., and Luster, M. I. (1989): Toxicology studies of a chemical mixture of 25 groundwater contaminants. II. Immunosuppression in B5C3F1 mice. *Fundam. Appl. Toxicol.*, 13:377–387.

64. Golden, R. J., Holms, S. E., Robinson, D. E., Julkunen, P. H., and Reese, E. A. (1997): Chloroform in mode of action: implications for cancer risk assessment. *Regul. Toxicol. Pharmacol.*, 26:142–155.

65. Goodman, G., and Wilson, R. (1992): Comparison of the dependence of the TD_{50} on maximum tolerated dose for mutagens and nonmutagens. *Risk Anal.*, 12(4):525–533.

66. Graham, J. D. (1992): *Recommendations for Improving Cancer Risk Assessment*. Center for Risk Analysis, Harvard School of Public Health, Boston.

67. Graham, J. D., and Wiener, J. B., eds. (1995): *Risk vs. Risk: Tradeoffs in Protecting Health and the Environment*. Harvard University Press, Cambridge, MA.

68. Green, G. M. (1984): Similarities of host defense mechanisms against pulmonary disease in animals and man. *J. Toxicol. Environ. Health*, 13:471–478.

69. Grassman, J. A., Kimmel, C. A., and Neumann, D. A. (1998): Accounting for variability in responsiveness in human health risk assessment. In: *Human Variability in Response to Chemical Exposure*, edited by D. A. Neumann and C. A. Kimmel, pp. 1–26. ILSI Press, Washington, DC.

70. Gross, P., de Villiers, A. J., and de Treveille, R. T. P. (1967): Experimental silicosis: The "atypical reaction" in the Syrian hamster. *Arch. Pathol.*, 84:87–94.

71. Guzelian, P. S., and Henry, C. J. (1992): Conference summary; similarities and differences between children and adults: Implications for risk assessment (November 5–7, 1990, Hunt Valley, Maryland). In: *Similarities and Differences Between Children and Adults: Implications for Risk Assessment*, edited by P. S. Guzelian, C. J. Henry, and S. S. Olin, pp. 1–3. ILSI Press, Washington, DC.

72. Hackey, J. D., and Linn, W. S. (1983): Controlled clinical studies of air pollutant exposure: Evaluating scientific information in relation to air quality standards. *Environ. Health Perspect.*, 52:187–191.

73. Harington, J. S., Ritchie, M., King, P. C., and Miller, K. (1973): The *in-vitro* effects of silica-treated hamster macrophages on collagen production by hamster fibroblasts. *J. Pathol.*, 109:21–37.

74. Hart, R. W., and Fishbein, L. (1985): Interspecies extrapolation of drug and genetic toxicity data. In: *Toxicological Risk Assessment*, Vol. I, edited D. B. Clayson, D. Krewski, and I. Munro, pp. 3–40. CRC Press, Boca Raton, FL.

75. Hart, R. W., and Turturro, A. (1988): Introduction. In: *Banbury Report 31: Carcinogen Risk Assessment: New Directions in the Qualitative and Quantitative Aspects*, edited by R. W. Hart and F. D. Hoerger., pp. 1–14. Cold Spring Harbor Laboratory, Cold Spring Harbor, NY.

76. Haseman, J. K. (1985): Issues in carcinogenicity testing: Dose selection. *Fundam. Appl. Toxicol.*, 5:66–78.

77. Haseman, J. K., and Lockhart, A.-M. (1994): The relationship between use of the maximum tolerated dose and study sensitivity for detecting rodent carcinogenicity. *Fundam. Appl. Toxicol.*, 22:382–391.

78. Hattis, D., White, P., Marmarstein, L., and Koch, P. (1990): Uncertainties in pharmacokinetic modeling for perchloroethylene: I. Comparison of model structure, parameters, and predictions for low-dose metabolism creates for models derived by different authors. *Risk Analysis*, 10(3):449–458.

79. Health Canada (1994): Human Health Risk Assessment for priority substances. As cited in http://www.tera.org/iter/methods/cancer.htm. Downloaded 2/27/99.

80. Heinrich, U., Muhle, H., Takenaka, S., Ernst, H., Fuhst, R., Mohr, U., Pott, F., and Stober, W. (1986): Chronic effects on the respiratory tract of hamsters, mice and rats after long-term inhalation of high concentrations of filtered and unfiltered diesel engine emissions. *J. Appl. Toxicol.*, 6:383–395.

81. Heppleston, A. G. (1984): Pulmonary toxicology of silica, coal and asbestos. *Environ. Health Perspect.*, 55:111–127.

82. Hutt, P. B. (1985): Use of quantitative risk assessment in regulatory decision making under federal health and safety statutes. In: *Risk Quantitation and Regulatory Policy*, edited by D. G. Hoel, R. A. Merrill, and F. P. Perera, pp. 15–29. Banbury Report 19, Cold Spring Harbor Laboratory, Cold Spring Harbor, N.Y.

83. Institute for Evaluating Health Risks. (1992): An evaluative process for determining human reproductive and developmental toxicity of agents, draft version. Institute for Evaluating Health Risks, Washington, DC.

84. Implementation Working Group. (1998): *A science-based, workable framework for implementing the Food Quality Protection Act. Implementation Working Group's "Road Map" Report*. Prepared by Jellinek, Schwartz & Connolly, Inc., McDermott, Will & Emery and Morgan, Lewis & Bockius. (Washington, DC).

85. Industrial Union Department. (1980): AFL-CIO *v.* American Petroleum Institute, 448 U.S. 60165 L. Ed. 2d 1010, 100 S. Ct. 2844.

86. Infante, P. F., Rinsky, R. A., Wagoner, J. K., et al. (1977): Benzene and leukemia. *Lancet*, p. 867–870.

87. International Agency for Research on Cancer. (1999): *IARC Monograph Summary for Beryllium and Beryllium Compounds* (*Group 1*) (*updated 5/4/99*). Downloaded from IARC web site http://193.51.164.11/cgi/iHound/chem/iH_chem_frames.html

88. International Agency for Research on Cancer. (1999): *IARC Monograph Summary for Cadmium and Cadmium Compounds* (*Group 1*) (*updated 5/4/99*). Downloaded from IARC web site http://193.51.164.11/cgi/iHound/chem/iH_chem_frames.html

89. International Agency for Research on Cancer. (1999): *IARC Monograph Summary for Cyclosporin* (*Group 1*) (*updated 5/4/99*). Downloaded from IARC web site http://193.51.164.11/cgi/iHound/chem/iH_chem_frames.html

90. International Agency for Research on Cancer. (1999): *IARC Monograph Summary for Epstein–Barr Virus* (*Group 1*) (*updated 5/4/99*). Downloaded from IARC web site http://193.51.164.11/cgi/iHound/chem/iH_chem_frames.html

91. International Agency for Research on Cancer. (1999): *IARC Monograph Summary for Oestrogen Replacement Therapy* (*Group 1*) (*updated 5/4/99*). Downloaded from IARC web site http://193.51.164.11/cgi/iHound/chem/iH_chem_frames.html

92. International Agency for Research on Cancer. (1999): *IARC Monograph Summary for Ethylene Oxide* (*Group 1*) (*updated 5/4/99*). Downloaded from IARC web site http://193.51.164.11/cgi/iHound/chem/iH_chem_frames.html

93. International Agency for Research on Cancer. (1999): *IARC Monograph Summary for Infection with Helicobacter Pylori* (*Group 1*) (*updated 5/4/99*). Downloaded from IARC web site http://193.51.164.11/cgi/iHound/chem/iH_chem_frames.html

94. International Agency for Research on Cancer. (1999): *IARC Monograph Summary for Hepatitis B Virus* (*Group 1*) (*updated 5/4/99*). Downloaded from IARC web site http://193.51.164.11/cgi/iHound/chem/iH_chem_frames.html

95. International Agency for Research on Cancer. (1999): *IARC Monograph Summary for Hepatitis C Virus* (*Group 1*) (*updated 5/4/99*). Downloaded from IARC web site http://193.51.164.11/cgi/iHound/chem/iH_chem_frames.html

96. International Agency for Research on Cancer. (1999): *IARC Monograph Summary for Human Immunodeficiency Viruses: HIV-1* (*Group 1*); *HIV-2* (*Group 2B*) (*updated 5/4/99*). Downladed from IARC web site http://193.51.164.11/cgi/iHound/chem/iH_chem_frames.html

97. International Agency for Research on Cancer. (1999): *IARC Monograph Summary for Human Papilloma Viruses* (*HPV*): *HPV types 16 and 18* (*Group 1*); *HPV types 31 and 33* (*Group 2A*); *Some HPV types other than 16, 18, 31 and 33* (*Group 2B*) (*updated 5/4/99*). Downloaded from IARC web site http://193.51.164.11/cgi/iHound/chem/iH_chem_frames.html

98. International Agency for Research on Cancer. (1999): *IARC Monograph Summary for Human T-Cell Lymphotropic Viruses: HTLV-I* (*Group 1*); *HTLV-II* (*Group 3*) (*updated 5/4/99*). Downloaded from IARC web site http://193.51.164.11/cgi/iHound/chem/iH_chem_frames.html

99. International Agency for Research on Cancer. (1999): *IARC Monograph Summary for Infection with Liver Flukes* (*Opisthorchis viverrini, Opisthorchis felineus and Clonorchis sinensis*): *Opisthorchis viverrini* (*Group 1*); *Opisthorchis felineus* (*Group 3*); *Clonorchis sinensis* (*Group 2A*) (*updated 5/4/99*). Downloaded from IARC web site http://193.51.164.11/cgi/iHound/chem/iH_chem_frames.html

100. International Agency for Research on Cancer. (1999): *IARC Monograph Summary for Hormonal Contraception and Postmenopausal Hormonal Therapy* (*Vol. 72*) (*2–9 June, 1998*) *In preparation* (*updated 5/4/99*). Downloaded from IARC web site http://193.51.164.11/cgi/iHound/chem/iH_chem_frames.html

101. International Agency for Research on Cancer. (1999): *IARC Monograph Summary for Oral Contraceptives, Combined* (*Group 1*) (*updated 5/4/99*). Downloaded from IARC web site http://193.51.164.11/cgi/iHound/chem/iH_chem_frames.html

102. International Agency for Research on Cancer. (1999): *IARC Monograph Summary for Salted Fish: Chinese-style salter fish* (*Group 1*); *Other salted fish* (*Group 3*) (*updated 5/4/99*). Downloaded from IARC web site http://193.51.164.11/cgi/iHound/chem/iH_chem_frames.html

103. International Agency for Research on Cancer. (1999): *IARC Monograph Summary for Infection with Schistomsomes*

(*Schistosoma haematobium, Schistosoma mansoni and Schistosoma japonicum*): *Schistosoma haematobium* (*Group 1*); *Schistosoma mansoni* (*Group 3*); *Schistosoma japonicum* (*Group 2B*) (*updated 5/4/99*). Downloaded from IARC web site http://193.51.164.11/cgi/iHound/chem/iH_chem_frames.html

104. International Agency for Research on Cancer. (1999): *IARC Monograph Summary for Silica: Crystalline silica-inhaled in the form of quartz or cristobalite from occupational sources* (*Group 1*); *Amorphous silica* (*Group 3*) (*updated 5/4/99*). Downloaded from IARC web site http://193.51.164.11/cgi/iHound/chem/iH_chem_frames.html
105. International Agency for Research on Cancer. (1999): *IARC Monograph Summary for Solar and Ultraviolet Radiation: Solar radiation* (*Group 1*), *Ultraviolet A radiation* (*Group 2A*), *Ultraviolet B radiation* (*Group 2A*), *Ultraviolet C radiation* (*Group 2A*), *Use of sunlamps and sunbeds* (*Group 2A*), *Exposure to fluorescent lighting* (*Group 3*) (*updated 6/2/99*). Downloaded from IARC web site http://193.51.164.11/cgi/iHound/chem/iH_chem_frames.html
106. International Agency for Research on Cancer. (1999): *IARC Monograph Summary for Tamoxifen* (*Group 1*) (*updated 5/4/99*). Downloaded from IARC web site http://193.51.164.11/cgi/iHound/chem/iH_chem_frames.html
107. International Agency for Research on Cancer. (1999): *IARC Monograph Summary for Polychlorinated Dibenzo-para-Dioxins: 2,3,7,8-Tetrachlorodibenzo-para-dioxin* (*Group 1*); *Polychlorinated dibenzo-para-dioxins* (*other than 2,3,7,8-Tetrachlorodibenzo-para-dioxin*): *2,7-DCDD, 1,2,3,6,7,8-/1,2,3,7,8,9-HxCDD, 1,2,3,4,6,7,8-HpCDD* (*Group 3*); *Dibenzo-para-dioxin* (*Group 3*) (*updated 5/4/99*). Downloaded from IARC web site http://193.51.164.11/cgi/iHound/chem/iH_chem_frames.html
108. International Agency for Research on Cancer. (1999): *IARC Monograph Summary for Thiotepa* (*Group 1*) (*updated 5/4/99*). Downloaded from IARC web site http://193.51.164.11/cgi/iHound/chem/iH_chem_frames.html
109. International Agency for Research on Cancer. (1999): *IARC Monograph Summary for Wood Dust* (*Group 1*) (*updated 5/4/99*). Downloaded from IARC web site http://193.51.164.11/cgi/iHound/chem/iH_chem_frames.html
110. International Agency for Research on Cancer. (1980): *Long-term and Short-term Screening Assays for Carcinogens: A Critical Appraisal*. IARC Monographs, Suppl. 2. International Agency for Research on Cancer, Lyons, France.
111. International Agency For Research on Cancer. (1982): *Evaluation of Carcinogenic Risk of Chemicals to Humans*. IARC Monographs, Suppl. 4. International Agency for Research on Cancer, Lyons, France.
112. International Agency For Research on Cancer. (1987): *Overall Evaluations of Carcinogenicity: An Updating of IARC Monographs Volumes 1 to 42*. IARC Monographs, Suppl. 7. International Agency for Research on Cancer, Lyons, France.
113. International Agency for Research on Cancer. (1992): Meeting Report: Working Group on Mechanisms of Carcinogenesis and the Evaluation of Carcinogenic Risks. *Cancer Res.*, 52:2357–2361.
114. International Agency for Research on Cancer. (1997): *IARC Monographs on the Evaluation of Carcinogenic Risks to Humans. Dry Cleaning, Some Chlorinated Solvents and Other Industrial Chemicals*. IARC Monographs, Vol. 63. International Agency for Research on Cancer, Lyons, France.
115. International Agency for Research on Cancer. (1999): *Overall Evaluations of Carcinogenicity to Humans*. Updated by IARC January 20, 1999. http://193.51.164.11/monoeval/crthal.html, downloaded 2/9/99.
116. Jarabek, A. M., Menache, M. G., Overton, J. H., Jr., Douson, M. L., and Miller, F. J. (1990): The U.S. Environmental Protection Agency's inhalation RfD methodology: risk assessment for air toxics. *Toxicol. Ind. Health*, 6:279–301.
117. Kavlock, R. J., Schmid, J. E., and Setzer, R. W. (1996): A simulation study of the influence of study design on the estimation of benchmark doses for developmental toxicity. *Risk Anal.*, 16(3):399–410.
118. Kauffman, R. E. (1992): Acute acetaminophen overdose: An example of reduced toxicity related to developmental differences in drug metabolism. In: *Similarities and Differences Between Children and Adults: Implications for Risk Assessment*, edited by P. S. Guzelian, C. J. Henry, and S. S. Olin, pp. 97–103. ILSI Press, Washington, DC.
119. Khera, K. S., Grice, H. C., and Clegg, D. J. (1989): *Current Issues in Toxicology, Interpretation and Extrapolation of Reproductive Data to Establish Human Safety Standards*. Springer-Verlag, New York.
120. Kouri, R. E., and Nebert, D. W. (1977): Genetic regulation of susceptibility to polycyclic hydrocarbon induced tumors in the mouse. In: *Origins of Human Cancer*, edited by H. H. Hiatt, J. D. Watson, and J. A. Winstyen, pp. 811–835. Cold Spring Harbor Laboratory, Cold Spring Harbor, NY.
121. Linkov, I., Wilson, R., and Gray, G. M. (1998): Anticarcinogenic responses in rodent cancer bioassays are not explained by random effects. *Toxicol. Sci.*, 43:1–9.
122. Lipfert, F. W. (1980): Sulfur oxides, particulates and human mortality: Synopsis of statistical correlations. *J. Air Pollut. Control Assoc.*, 30:366–371.
123. Liteplo, R. G., and Meek, M. E. (1994): Tetrachloroethylene: Evaluation of risks to health from environmental exposure in Canada. *Environ. Carcinogen. & Ecotoxicol. Rev.*, C12(2): 493–506.
124. Maltoni, C., Conti, B., and Cotti, G. (1983): Benzene: A multi-potential carcinogen. Results of long-term bioassays performed at the Bologna Institute of Oncology. *Am. J. Ind. Med.*, 4:589–630.
125. Manson, J. M., and Wise, L. D. (1991): Teratogens. In: *Casarett and Doull's Toxicology*, edited by M. O. Amdur, J. Doull, and C. D. Klaassen, pp. 226–254, Pergamon Press, New York.
126. McKone, T. E., and Bogen, K. T. (1991): Predicting the uncertainties in risk assessment. *Environ. Sci. Technol.*, 25(10): 1674–1681.
127. Melnick, R. L., Boorman, G. H., Haseman, J. K., and Huff, J. (1984): Toxicity and carcinogenicity of melamine in F344 rats and B5C3F1 mice. *Toxicol. Appl. Pharmacol.*, 72:292–303.
128. Mileson, B. E., Chambers, J. E., Chen, W. L., Dettbarn, W., Ehrich, M., Eldefrawi, A. T., Gaylor, D. W., Hamernik, K., Hodgson, E., Karczmar, A. G., Padilla, S., Pope, C. N., Richardson, R. J., Saunders, D. R., Sheets, L. P., Sultatos, L. G., and Wallace, K. B. (1998): Commom mechanism of toxicity: A case study of organophosphorus pesticides. *Toxicol. Sci.*, 41(1):8–20.
129. Miller, F. J., Illing, J. W., and Gardner, D. E. (1978): Effect of urban ozone levels on laboratory-induced respiratory infections. *Toxicol. Lett.*, 2:163–169.
130. Moolgavkar, S. H. (1986): Carcinogenesis modeling: from molecular biology to epidemiology. *Ann. Rev. Public Health*, 7:151–169.
131. Munro, I. C. (1977): Considerations in chronic toxicity testing: The chemical, the dose, the design. *J. Environ. Pathol. Toxicol.*, 1:183–197.
132. National Research Council. (1996): *Understanding Risk: Informing Decisions in a Democratic Society*, edited by P. C. Stern and H. V. Fineberg. National Academy Press, Washington, DC.
133. National Research Council. (1994): *Science and Judgment in Risk Assessment*. National Academy Press, Washington, DC.

134. National Research Council. (1987): *Regulating Pesticides in Food: The Delaney Paradox*. National Academy Press, Washington, DC.
135. National Research Council. (1986): *Drinking Water and Health*, Vol. 6. National Academy Press, Washington, DC.
136. National Research Council. (1983): *Risk Assessment in the Federal Government: Managing the Process*. National Academy Press, Washington, DC.
137. National Research Council. (1980): *Principles of Toxicological Interactions Associated with Multiple Chemical Exposures*. National Academy Press, Washington, D.C.
138. Nebert, D. W. (1989): The Ah locus: Genetic differences in toxicity, cancer, mutation. *Crit. Rev. Toxicol.*, 20:153–174.
139. Neumann D. A., and Kimmel, C. A., eds. (1998): *Human Variability in Response to Chemical Exposure*. ILSI Press, Washington, DC.
140. Neumann, H.-G., Thielmann, H. W., Filser, J. G., Gelbke, H.-P., Greim, H., Kappus, H., Norpoth, K. H., Reuter, U., Vamvakas, S., Wardenbach, P., and Wichmann, H.-E. (1997): Proposed changes in the classification of carcinogenic chemicals in the work area. *Regul. Toxicol. Pharmacol.*, 26:288–295.
141. New York State Department of Environmental Conservation. (1986): *New York State Air Guide–1: Guidelines for the Control of Toxic Ambient Air Contaminants*. Division of Air Resources, Albany.
142. Nichols A. L., and Zeckhauser, R. J. (1986): The perils of prudence; how conservative risk assessments distort regulation. *Regulation*, November/December:13–24.
143. Oberdorster, G., and Yu, C. P. (1990): The carcinogenic potential of inhaled diesel exhaust: a particle effect? *J. Aerosol Sci., Suppl.* 1(21):397–401.
144. Occupational Safety and Health Administration. (1980): Identification, classification, and regulation of potential occupational carcinogens. *Fed. Reg.*, 45:5002–5296.
145. Occupational Safety and Health Act of 1970. 29 U.S.C. 655.
146. Office of Management and Budget. (1990): Current regulatory issues in risk assessment and management. In: *Regulatory Program of the United States Government*. Executive Office of the President, Washington, DC. April 1, 1990–March 31, 1991.
147. Office of Science and Technology Policy. (1986): Chemical carcinogens: A review of the science and its associated principles. U.S. Interagency Staff Group on Carcinogens. *Environ. Health Perspect.*, 67:201–282.
148. Overton, J. H., and Jarabek, A. M. (1989): Estimating equivalent human concentrations of no observed adverse effect levels: A comparison of several methods. *Exp. Pathol.* 37:89–95.
149. Pitot, H. C., and Dragan, Y. P. (1991): Facts and theories concerning the mechanisms of carcinogenesis. *FASEB J.*, 5:2280–2286.
150. Plunkett, L. M., Turnbull, D., and Rodricks, J. V. (1992): Differences between adults and children affecting exposure assessment. In: *Similarities and Differences Between Children and Adults: Implications for Risk Assessment*, edited by P. S. Guzelian, C. J. Henry, and S. S. Olin, pp. 79–94. ILSI Press, Washington, DC.
151. Pohl, H. R., Hansen, H., and Chou, C. H. (1997): Public health guidance values for chemical mixtures: current practice and future directions. *Regul. Toxicol. Pharmacol.*, 26(3):322–329.
152. Portier, C., Tritscher, A., Kohn, M., Sewall, C., Clark, G., Edler, L., Hoel, D., and Lucier, G. (1993): Ligand/receptor binding for 2,3,7,8-TCDD: Implications for risk assessment. *Fundam. Appl. Toxicol*, 20:48–56.
153. Pott, P. (1779): Cancer scroti. In: *Chirurgical Works, A New Edition in Three Volumes*. Vol. I. London.
154. Pozzani, U. S., Weil, C. S., and Carpenter, C. P. (1959): The toxicological basis of TLVs: 5. The experimental inhalation of vapor mixtures by rats, with notes upon the relationship between single dose inhalation and single dose oral data. *Am. Ind. Hyg. Assoc. J.*, 20:364–369.
155. Presidential/Congressional Commission on Risk Assessment and Risk Management. (1997): Risk Assessment and Risk Management in Regulatory Decision-Making (Final Report, Vol. 2). Washington, DC.
156. Public Law 85–929. (1958): Food Additives Amendment of 1958.
157. Quakenboss, J. J., Kanarek, M. S., Spengler, J. D., and Letz, R. (1982): Personal monitoring for nitrogen dioxide exposure: Methodological considerations for a community study. *Environ. Int.*, 8:249–258.
158. Research Triangle Institute. (1998): Toxicological profile for chlorinated dibenzo-*p*-dioxins. National Technical Information Service, Prepared for Agency for Toxic Substances and Disease Registry. NTIS PB99-121998.
159. Research Triangle Institute. (1998): Toxicological profile for polychlorinated biphenyls (PCB) (Update—Draft for public comment). Prepared for U.S. Public Health Service, Agency for Toxic Substances and Disease Registry (*ATSDR*), Atlanta, GA.
160. Riddiough, C. R., Musselmann, R., and Calabrese, E. J. (1977): Is EPA's radium-226 drinking water standard justified? *Med. Hypoth.*, 3(5):171.
161. Rieth, J. P., and Starr, T. B. (1989): Chronic bioassays: Relevance to quantitative risk assessment of carcinogens. *Regul. Toxicol. Pharmacol.* 10:160–173.
162. Roberts, R. J. (1992): Overview of similarities and differences between children and adults: implications for risk assessment. In: *Similarities and Differences Between Children and Adults: Implications for Risk Assessment*, edited by P. S. Guzelian, C. J. Henry, and S. S. Olin, pp. 11–15. ILSI Press, Washington, DC.
163. Rodricks, J. V., and Taylor, M. R. (1989): Comparison of risk management in U.S. regulatory agencies. *J. Haz. Mater.*, 21:239–253.
164. Roger, L. J., Kehrl, H. R., Hazucha, M., and Horstman, D. H. (1985): Bronchoconstriction in asthmatics exposed to sulfur dioxide during repeated exercise. *J. Appl. Physiol.*, 59:784–791.
165. Rosenthal, A., Graf, G. M., and Graham, J. D. (1992): Legislating acceptable cancer risk from exposure to toxic chemicals. *Ecol. Law Q.*, 19:269–362.
166. Ross, J. D., and Des Forges, J. F. (1959): Reduction of methemoglobin by erythrocytes from cord blood. Further evidence of deficient enzyme activity in newborn period. *Pediatrics*, 23:218.
167. Scheuplein, R. J. (1987): Risk assessment and food safety: A scientist and regulator's view. *Food Drug Cosmet. Law J.*, 42:237–250.
168. Sielken, R. L., Jr., and Stevenson, D. E. (1998): Some implications for quantitative risk assessment if hormesis exists. *Hum. Exp. Toxicol.*, 17:259–262.
169. Slob, W., and Pieters, M. N. (1997): A probabilistic approach for deriving acceptable human intake limits and human health risks from toxicological studies: General framework. Report 620110 005. National Institute of Public Health and the Environment, BiHhoven, the Netherlands.
170. Smyth, H. F., Jr., Weil, C. S., West, C. P., and Carpenter, J. S. (1969): An exploration of joint toxic action: 27 Industrial chemicals in rats in all possible pairs. *Toxicol. Appl. Pharmacol.*, 14:340–347.
171. Sontag, J. M., Page, N. P., and Sanotti, U. (1976): Guidelines for carcinogen bioassays in small rodents. DHHS publ. (NIH) 76-801. National Cancer Institute, Bethesda, MD.
172. Strauss, H. S. (1993): Sex biases in the risk assessment of toxic chemicals. Presented at the Annual Meeting of the American Association for the Advancement of Science, Boston, February 12.
173. Tamplin, A. R., and Gofman, J. W. (1970): *Population Control Through Nuclear Pollution*. Nelson-Hill, Chicago.

174. Thompson, K. M., Burmaster, D. E., and Crouch, E. A. C. (1992): Monte-Carlo techniques for quantitative uncertainty analysis in public health risk assessments. *Risk Anal.*, 12(1):53–63.
175. Thorton, J. (1991): Written testimony of J. Thornton, Greenpeace U.S.A., for the U.S. House of Representatives Committee on Science, Space, and Technology, Subcommittee on Environment. Hearing on Risk Assessment: Strengths and Limitations of Utilization for Policy Decisions, May 21.
176. Thurston, G. D., Ito, K., Lippman, M., and Hayes, C. (1989): Reexamination of London, England mortality in relation to exposure to acidic aerosols during 1963–1972 winters. *Environ. Health Perspect.*, 79:73–83.
177. Tomatis, L., Aitio, A., Wilbourn, J., and Shuker, L. (1989): Human carcinogens so far identified. *Jpn. J. Cancer Res.*, 80:795–807.
178. Tosteson, T., Spengler, J. D., and Weber, R. A. (1982): Aluminum, iron, and lead content of respirable particulate samples from a personal monitoring system. *Environ. Int.*, 2:265–268.
179. Travis, C. C., and Hattemer-Fry, H. A. (1988): Determining an acceptable level of risk. *Environ. Sci. Technol.*, 22(8):873–876.
180. Travis, C. C., Richter, S. A., Crouch, E. A. C., Wilson, R., and Klema, E. D. (1987): Cancer risk management. *Environ. Sci. Technol.*, 21(5):415–420.
181. Trosko, J. E., and Chang, C. C. (1988): Nongenotoxic mechanisms in carcinogenesis: Role of inhibited intercellular communication. In: *Banbury Report 31: Carcinogen Risk Assessment: New Directions in the Qualitative and Quantitative Aspects*, edited by R. W. Hart and F. D. Hoerger, pp. 139–170. Cold Spring Harbor Laboratory, Cold Spring Harbor, NY.
182. U.S. Department of Health and Human Services. (1986): NIOSH recommendations for occupational safety and health standards. *Morbid. Mortal. Weekly Rep.*, 35:1S–33S.
183. U.S. Department of Health and Human Services. (1985): Risk assessment and risk management of toxic substances. Report to the Secretary of DHHS from the Executive Committee of the DHHS Committee to Coordinate Environmental and Related Programs. Washington, DC.
184. U.S. Department of Health, Education and Welfare, Public Health Service. (1962): Public Health Drinking Water Standards. Rockville, MD.
185. U.S. Environmental Protection Agency. (1999): Integrated Risk Information System. http://www.epa.gov/iris/
186. U.S. Environmental Protection Agency. (1999): IRIS substance file for chromium(VI); CASRN 18540–29; 9/3/98 (updated 5/21/99). Downloaded from http://www.epa.gov/ngispgm3/iris/subst/0144.htm
187. U.S. Environmental Protection Agency. (1999): IRIS substance file for dichloromethane; CASRN 75-09-2; 1/31/87 (updated 6/14/99). Downloaded from http://www.epa.gov/ngispgm3/iris/subst/0070.htm
188. U.S. Environmental Protection Agency. (1999): IRIS substance file for fluorine (soluble fluoride); CASRN 7782-41-4; 1/31/87 (updated 6/14/99). Downloaded from http://www.epa.gov/ngispgm3/iris/subst/0053.htm
189. U.S. Environmental Protection Agency. (1999): IRIS substance file for naphthalene; CASRN 91-20-3; 9.17/98 (updated 5/21/99). Downloaded from http://www.epa.gov/ngispgm3/iris/subst/0436.htm
190. U.S. Environmental Protection Agency. (1999): Summary of FQPA amendments to FIFRA and FFDCA. Downloaded from http://www.epa.gov/oppfead1/fqpa/fqpa-iss.htm
191. U.S. Environmental Protection Agency. (1998): Framework for addressing key scientific issues presented by the Food Quality Protection Act (FQPA) as developed by the Tolerance Reassessment Advisory Committee (TRAC). *Fed. Reg.*, 63(209):58038-58045.
192. U.S. Environmental Protection Agency. (1998): Presentation for FIFRE Scientific Advisory Panel by Office of Pesticide Programs, Health Effects Division on FQPA Safety Factor for infants and children (draft 3/9/98, updated 3/12/98). Downloaded from http://www.epa.gov/pesticides/SAP/march/10x.htm
193. U.S. Environmental Protection Agency. (1997): Guiding principles for Monte Carlo analysis. EPA/630/R-97/001. USEPA, Risk Assessment Forum (Washington, DC), NTIS PB97-18810 6I.NZ.
194. U.S. Environmental Protection Agency. (1996): A national agenda to protect children's health from environmental threats (ipdated 9/11/96). Downloaded from http://occ-env-med.mc.duke.edu/oem/content/epa.htm
195. U.S. Environmental Protection Agency. (1996): Proposed guidelines for carcinogenic risk assessment; Notice. *Fed. Reg.*, 61(79):17960–18011.
196. U.S. Environmental Protection Agency. (1995): Guidance for risk characterization. Science Policy Council, USEPA, Washington, DC. February 1995.
197. U.S. Environmental Protection Agency. (1995): Proposed guidelines for neurotoxicity risk assessment. *Fed. Reg.*, 60:52032–52056.
198. U.S. Environmental Protection Agency. (1995): The use of the benchmark dose approach in health risk assessment. Risk Assessment Forum, Office of Research and Development, Washington, DC. EPA/630/R-94/007.
199. U.S. Environmental Protection Agency. (1992): Memorandum from F.H. Habicht to assistant administrators and regional administrators, Re: Guidance on risk characterization for risk managers and risk assessors.
200. U.S. Environmental Protection Agency. (1993): Reference dose (RfD): Description and use in health risk assessments (background document 1A), 3/15/93 (updated 5/21/99). Integrated Risk Information System. Downloaded from http://www.epa.gov.ngispgm3/iris/rfd.htm
201. U.S. Environmental Protection Agency. (1992): Review of the National Ambient Air Quality Standards for carbon monoxide 1992 reassessment of scientific and technical information, OAQPS staff paper.
202. U.S. Environmental Protection Agency. (1991): Guidelines for developmental toxicity. *Fed. Reg.*, 56(234):63798–63826.
203. U.S. Environmental Protection Agency. (1990): General quantitative risk assessment guidelines for noncancer health effects. Technical Panel for the Development of Risk Assessment Guidelines for Noncancer Health Effects. ECAO-CIN-538.
204. U.S. Environmental Protection Agency. (1990): Interim methods for development of inhalation reference concentrations (review draft). Environmental Criteria and Assessment Office. EPA/600/8-90/066A.
205. U.S. Environmental Protection Agency. (1989): Review of the National Ambient Air Quality Standard for ozone: Assessment of scientific and technical information. Office of Air Quality Planning and Standards. Research Triangle Park, NC. NTIS PB92-190446. February 26, 1992.
206. U.S. Environmental Protection Agency. (1988): Special report on ingested inorganic arsenic: Skin cancer; nutritional essentiality. Risk Assessment Forum. EPA-625/3-87-013F.
207. U.S. Environmental Protection Agency. (1988): Technical support document on risk assessment of chemical mixtures. National Technical Information Service. EPA/600/8-90/064.
208. U.S. Environmental Protection Agency. (1986): Guidelines for carcinogen risk assessment. *Fed. Reg.*, 51:33992–34003.
209. U.S. Environmental Protection Agency. (1986): *Air Quality Criteria for Lead*, vols. I–IV. EPA-600/8-83/028adf.
210. U.S. Environmental Protection Agency. (1986): Review of the National Ambient Air Quality Standards for sulfur oxides: Updated assessment of scientific and technical information –

addendum to the 1982 OAQPS staff paper. Office of Air Quality, Planning and Standards. EPA-450/5-86-013.

211. U.S. Environmental Protection Agency. (1975): Interim primary drinking water standards. *Fed. Reg.*, 40(51):11990–11998.
212. U.S. Food and Drug Administration. (1988): Color additives: Denial of petition for listing of D&C red no. 19 for use in externally applied drugs and cosmetics. *Fed. Reg.*, 53(136):26831–26883.
213. U.S. Food and Drug Administration. (1986): Listing of D&C orange no. 17 for use in externally applied drugs and cosmectics. Final rule. *Fed. Reg.*, 51(152):28331–28346.
214. U.S. General Accounting Office. (1990): Toxic substances: Effectiveness of unreasonable risk standards unclear. Report to the Chairman, Subcommittee on Health and the Environment, Committee on Energy and Commerce, House of Representatives. GAO/RCED-90-189.
215. U.S. Interagency Staff Group of Carcinogens. (1986): Chemical carcinogens: A review of the science and its associated principals. *Environ. Health Perspect.*, 67:201–282.
216. U.S. Public Health Service, ATSDR. (1989): Toxicological profile for selected PCBs (Arochlor-1260, -1254, -1248, -1242, -1232, -1221, and -1016). Report ATSDR/TP-8821. NTIS PB89-225403.
217. U.S. Public Health Services, Centers for Disease Control. (1991): Preventing lead poisoning in young children: A statement by the Centers for Disease Control. Dept. of Health & Human Services, Public Health Service, Centers for Disease Control, Atlanta, GA.
218. Wallace, L.A. (1991): Comparison of risks from outdoor and indoor exposure to toxic chemicals. *Environ. Health Perspect.*, 95:7–13.
219. Wallace, L.A., Pellizzari, E.D., Hartwell, T.D., Sparacino, C., and Zelon, H. (1983): Personal exposure of volatile organics and other compounds indoors and outdoors: The TEAM study. Proceedings of the 76th Annual Meeting of the Air Pollution Control Association. Air Pollution Control Associatoin, Pittsburgh, PA.
220. Waring, M.J. (1981): DNA modification and cancer. *Annu. Rev. Biochem.*, 50:159–192.
221. Wilkinson, C.F. (1971): Effects of synergists on the metabolism and toxicity of anticholinesterase. *Bull. WHO*, 40:171–190.
222. Zeise, L., Wilson, R., and Crouch, E.A.C. (1987): Dose-response relationships for carcinogens: A review. *Environ. Health Perspect.*, 73:259–308.
223. Ziskind, M., Jones, R.N., and Weil, H. (1976): Silicosis. *Am. Rev. Respir. Dis.*, 113:643–665.

Principles and Methods of Toxicology,
Fourth Edition, edited by A. Wallace Hayes.
Taylor & Francis, Philadelphia © 2001.

Chapter 3

Metabolism: A Determinant of Toxicity

J. Donald deBethizy and Johnnie R. Hayes

As stated in the title of this chapter, the metabolism of *xenobiotics*, compounds foreign to the normal biochemistry of cells, is a major determinant of their toxicity. Most often, toxicologists are interested in the metabolism of potentially toxic compounds to which species may be exposed; however, many of these same enzymes are involved in the detoxication and metabolism of *endobiotics*, which are compounds produced during the normal biochemical reactions that maintain life. For example, some of these enzymes are involved in the detoxication of reactive oxygen species produced during aerobic metabolism that can produce oxidative stress and tissue damage. A toxicologist must have a fundamental knowledge of these detoxication systems to understand, predict, and determine the potential toxicity of a compound. It is our purpose to provide an overview of these various systems that can serve as a foundation for a more comprehensive study of their role in toxicology.

EVOLUTION OF XENOBIOTIC METABOLISM

As the first macromolecules began to organize into complex arrays with the basic attributes of life, environmental factors were present that represented disruptive forces. These forces were physical and chemical. Chemicals present in the early milieu of life could interact with these life forms, disrupting the delicate balance through which they maintained their integrity. Those life forms that developed protective mechanisms, such as the cell membrane, the ability to store energy, and motility, were able to survive. It does not stretch the imagination to hypothesize that these early life forms manufactured molecules capable of reacting with environmental chemicals, including increasing concentrations of oxygen, thereby decreasing their biological activity. An example of such a molecule is glutathione. This nucleophile can react nonenzymatically with many electrophilic chemicals to reduce their toxicity. An early step in the evolution of protective mechanisms may have been the development of macromolecular catalysis to chemically alter disruptive chemicals. These macromolecular catalyses were the first detoxification enzymes. Evidence for such a scenario exists in the occurrence of certain detoxication enzymes in both animal and plant species ranging from simple, single cellular to complex, multicellular organisms.

The cytochrome P450 (P450) monooxygenase system (discussed in detail later) is a large superfamily of hemoproteins whose evolutionary roots have recently been investigated (36,59). This superfamily serves as an example of the evolution of enzymes capable of protecting the organism from toxic chemicals. In fact, its current nomenclature is based on evolutionary and genetic relationships between its isozymes. The P450 superfamily of hemoproteins consists of about 20 gene families, and the functional P450 genes in a mammalian species are estimated to be over 200. The amino acid sequences of more than 100 P450 hemoproteins are known. Phylogenetic trees based on these sequences have been developed to aid in understanding the evolution of these important enzymes (see (58,95) for reviews).

The original ancestral P450 gene may date back 3 billion years or more. The wide distribution of these genes in prokaryotic and eukaryotic organisms emphasizes their importance in maintaining life. About 400 million years ago there appears to have been a major increase in the number of new genes in one of the P450 families (the CYP2 family). It is believed that this evolutionary burst of new genes was associated with animal colonization of land during the Devonian era. In an attempt to protect themselves, plants began to develop toxins to deter their consumption by land animals. This resulted in coevolution of animal cytochromes P450 to detoxify these plant toxins (58). As species began to fill specific ecological niches with unique environmental and dietary chemical challenges, the species diversity in expressed P450 genes that we encounter today developed. The evolution of this single xenobiotic metabolism system illustrates the significance of xenobiotic detoxication systems in the development and maintenance of the diversity of life we encounter on earth today.

An alternative to the hypothesis that the enzymes developed to metabolize foreign compounds is that they represent enzymes of normal anabolic and catabolic metabolism. These enzymes, in addition to functioning in their normal biochemical role, also function in xenobiotic metabolism. Examples of such enzymes certainly exist and include the methyltransferases involved in DNA synthesis and in detoxication, such as the metabolism of nicotine; however, it would appear fortuitous that normal anabolic and catabolic enzymes could have evolved to detoxify the broad array of chemical structures that are foreign to organisms. Another factor that diminishes the confidence in the alternative hypothesis is that many of the xenobiotic metabolizing enzymes can rapidly respond with increased activity to the presence of xenobiotics and environmental change. This would be unlikely if they simply represented enzymes of normal metabolism with the ability to metabolize alternative substrates. Many of the enzymes involved in xenobiotic metabolism are also involved in specific aspects of the metabolism of normal cellular biochemical constituents. Generally these enzymes are isozymes with higher substrate specificity for the endogenous compounds than the isozymes involved in xenobiotic metabolism. This could likely represent a process by which the cell used a preexisting xenobiotic metabolizing enzyme for metabolism of endogenous substrates instead of vice versa. Whatever the evolutionary source of the xenobiotic metabolizing enzymes, it is obvious that they represent a distinct mechanism of metabolizing the thousands of naturally occurring and synthetic chemicals to which cells and tissues are exposed.

GENERAL FEATURES AND BASIC CONCEPTS OF XENOBIOTIC METABOLISM

The majority of organisms studied have *biotransformation* enzymes, although there is diversity in the occurrence, function, and rates of specific enzymes. Certain bacteria contain more primitive or less highly developed systems and may lack certain pathways altogether. Even mammals demonstrate diversity in the activity or rates of specific systems, and, as would be expected of genetically controlled functions, there are species and individual differences. This diversity extends to the organ level in multicellular organisms. Specific organs show different levels of activity, and specific cell types within organs demonstrate variation in biotransformation capability. There is even subcellular diversity in that certain of these enzymes are compartmentalized whereas others are free in the cytoplasm.

The variety of chemicals to which organisms may be exposed requires that the biotransformation enzymes have broad substrate specificity. This characteristic is not shared by the majority of enzymes involved in anabolic and catabolic metabolism. In addition, the types of reactions catalyzed are diverse, as shown in Table 3.1, including oxidation, reduction, epoxidation, deamination, hydroxylation, sulfoxidation, dehalogenation, and conjugation with endogenous compounds, to name a few. Although it is logical to initially focus on one xenobiotic metabolizing system at a time, in many cases, xenobiotic metabolism involves more than a single metabolic route. In addition, the eventual toxicity of a xenobiotic may be modified by a number of factors, including age, gender, physiological status, nutrition, diet, and the presence or absence of disease, among others.

Exposure of an animal to certain xenobiotics can result in the *induction* of specific enzymes associated with xenobiotic metabolism. When induced, their activity can dramatically increase, compared to their basal level. Induction is sometimes coordinated with more than one enzyme induced. Induction results in an increase in the ability of animals to metabolize a xenobiotic, and in most cases this reduces their susceptibility to its toxicity. Induction generally lasts only a few days. When exposure ceases, the enzymes return to their basal levels.

Because xenobiotic metabolism does not always represent detoxication, the term *biotransformation* has come into general use to denote the actions of xenobiotic metabolizing enzymes, although it is still not semantically specific for xenobiotic metabolism. Biotransformation is divided into two distinct phases. *Phase I* reactions result in *functionalization*, the addition or the uncovering of specific functional groups that are required for subsequent metabolism by *phase II* enzymes. Phase II reactions are biosynthetic. These phase I and II reactions are often coordinated, with the product of phase I reactions becoming the substrate for phase II enzymes. A commonality of biotransformation reactions is the conversion of hydrophobic xenobiotics into more polar, more easily excreted compounds. Because the composition of cells is more lipophilic than their environment, nonpolar compounds tend to accumulate. This could lead to bioconcentration of chemicals within the cell to levels higher than that of the environment and increase the likelihood of a cytotoxic event; however, conversion of nonpolar chemicals to more polar metabolites allows them to be more easily excreted by the cell. *Conjugation* of a xenobiotic with an endogenous compound, a phase II reaction, increases water solubility, and, in some cases, the added chemical group is recognized by specific carrier proteins or proteins involved in facilitated diffusion or active transport. This increases the cell's ability to remove the xenobiotic.

Table 3.1
Examples of types of reactions and enzymes that participate in xenobiotic metabolism

Phase I Reactions	
Oxidation	Ester hydrolysis
P450 monooxygenase	Carboxylesterases
Xanthine oxidase	Amidases
Peroxidases	
Amine oxidase	Dehydrogenases
Monoamine oxidase	Alcohol dehydrogenases
Dioxygenases	Aldehyde dehydrogenases
Semicarbizide sensitive amine oxidase	
Reduction	Superoxide dismutase
P450 monooxygenase	
Ketoreductase	
Glutathione peroxidases	
Hydration	
Epoxide hydrolase	
Phase II Reactions	
Glucuronosyltransferase	Methylation
Sulfotransferase	*O*-Methyltransferases
Glutathione *S*-transferase	*N*-Methyltransferases
Glucosyltransferase	*S*-Methyltransferases
Thioltransferase	
Amide synthesis (transacylase)	Acetylation
	N-Acetyltransferase
	Acyltransferases
	Thiosulfate sulfurtransferase (rhodanase)

There are many diverse examples of xenobiotics whose toxicity is directly dependent on the activity of the biotransformation enzymes. For most chemicals, increases in the activity of these enzymes result in decreases in toxicity, whereas decreases in activity result in increased toxicity; however, there are examples in which the product of xenobiotic metabolism is more toxic than the parent compound. Conversion of a foreign compound to a more toxic metabolite is termed *metabolic activation*. For example, the majority of genotoxic and carcinogenic chemicals require metabolic activation to highly reactive species capable of interacting with DNA. The enzymes that protect the animal from the toxicity of certain compounds may be responsible for the toxicity of others. An organism's susceptibility to the toxicity of a particular chemical is dependent, in many cases, on the delicate balance between detoxication and metabolic activation that exist during exposure to the xenobiotic. Due to the sensitivity of the enzymes of xenobiotic biotransformation to both endogenous and exogenous factors, this balance may differ among individuals and at different points in time.

BIOLOGICAL OXIDATION

Cytochrome P450–dependent Monooxygenase System

The P450–dependent monooxygenase system is central to the metabolism of most xenobiotics. Not only is it the primary enzymatic system for metabolism of many xenobiotics, but it is also involved as the initial functionalization step in the further metabolism of many others. Consequently, P450 plays essential roles in several areas of research, including biochemistry, pharmacology, toxicology, physiology, and medicine. Several names for the P450 system exist in the literature. The names most commonly encountered include

1. Mixed function oxidase
2. P450 system
3. P450–dependent monooxygenase system

Generally these names are related either to a specific function or are descriptive of a biochemical mechanism. Currently, it generally is referred to in terms of a monooxygenase system to denote its ability to incorporate one atom of molecule oxygen into its substrates.

Components of the Cytochromes P450 System

The history of the discovery of P450 and the elucidation of its functions and mechanisms of action are intriguing and have recently been reviewed by Estabrook (43). P450 was first described independently in 1958 by Klingenberg (86) and Garfinkel (52) in microsomes isolated from rat liver homogenates and pig liver homogenates, respectively. Klingenberg (86) noted that during 1955 in the laboratory of Britton Chance at the Johnson Foundation G. R. Williams was the first to observe the pigment. The name P450 derived from the occurrence of a pigment that, when reduced and treated with carbon monoxide, yielded a spectrophotometric Soret band at *450* nm. Six years after the publication of the original description of the P450 peak in hepatic microsomes, Omura and Sato (131,132) published their pivotal papers describing P450 as a b-type hemocytochrome. Their work demonstrated that the cytochrome was located in hepatic *microsomes*, which form from the endoplasmic reticulum upon cellular disruption. Upon isolation from the membrane, using proteases, P450 is converted to a form whose reduced carbon monoxide complex produces a spectrophotometric peak at 420 nm. This form was termed *cytochrome P420* (P420) and was found inactive in metabolism. Conversion of P450 to the inactive cytochrome P420 upon isolation from the membrane was one of the major limitations encountered in early attempts to understand the mechanism of this membrane-bound monooxygenase.

Before the discovery of P450, Julius Axelrod and his colleagues (6), in the laboratory of Chemical Pharmacology at the National Heart Institute, were involved with studies on the metabolic disposition of drugs (6). They found that the oxidative metabolism of amphetamine required the co-factor NADPH and the presence of oxygen. An important publication by Estabrook et al. (42) brought together studies of P450 biochemistry and studies of biotransformation. They established that P450 was the terminal oxidase involved with the C-21 hydroxylation of steroids in adrenal cortical microsomes. This was followed by a study from Cooper (32) that demonstrated the involvement of P450 in both steroid and drug metabolism by hepatic microsomes. Many individuals and laboratories have played major roles in the development of the current knowledge concerning P450. Readers who become acquainted with the original literature will no doubt recognize the role of these pioneers in the development of a new field of study: xenobiotic biotransformation.

It soon became obvious that although P450 played a major role in the activity of the monooxygenase, it did not act alone. In 1950, Horecher (70) isolated a flavoprotein from the liver, but no function was identified. This flavoprotein used reducing equivalents from NADPH and was termed *NADPH-cytochrome c reductase* (EC 1.6.2.4). In 1955, La Du et al. (89) showed that cytochrome c could inhibit dealkylation of aminopyrine. This was followed by the studies of Gillette et al. (54) in 1957, which presented additional evidence that cytochrome c reductase was involved in xenobiotic metabolism. Williams and Kamin (188) and Philips and Langdon (136) reported in 1962 that NADPH-cytochrome c reductase occurred in the endoplasmic reticulum of liver cells and might be involved in drug and steroid oxidation. Further proof of the involvement of the flavoprotein came in 1969, when it was shown that antibodies to the reductase inhibited xenobiotic metabolism (88,130), and Lu et al. (100,101) demonstrated its requirement in monooxygenase activity reconstituted from isolated components.

One confusing aspect concerning this flavoprotein is its nomenclature. As previously mentioned, it is sometimes referred to as NADPH-cytochrome c reductase; however, no cytochrome c occurs in the endoplasmic reticulum, and cytochrome c is not its normal substrate. The more appropriate name is NADPH-cytochrome P450 reductase, indicating its natural substrate and function.

Although the major components of the P450–dependent monooxygenase system appear to be P450 and P450 reductase, other components may also be involved with metabolism of specific xenobiotics. Cytochrome b_5 reductase has been proposed to participate in monooxygenase activity through electron transport to cytochrome b_5 and, subsequently, to P450; however, several systems of electron transport in the endoplasmic reticulum and isolated microsomes, as well as other activities, such as peroxidation, have greatly complicated the elucidation of the role of cytochrome b_5. Cytochrome b_5 may affect P450–mediated xenobiotic metabolism by shunting electrons either toward or away from P450 (119). An elucidation of the role of cytochrome b_5 must await further understanding of the complex electron transfer pathways that exist in the endoplasmic reticulum.

Although the catalytic activity of the monooxygenase system appears to require only two proteins—NADPH P450 reductase and P450—it is capable of carrying out a variety of different reactions on a large number of substrates. This ability is based on the occurrence of a variety of P450 isozymes, but it also is based on the basic reaction mechanism of the cytochromes and their apparent overlapping substrate specificity. The nonspecificity of the monooxygenase provides important flexibility to xenobiotic metabolism, but this flexibility comes with a price. Generally, the enzymatic reactions of anabolism and catabolism are both extremely specific in substrate specificity and catalytically efficient, resulting in high activity and high substrate turnover number. The turnover number and efficiency of P450 are considerably lower than most enzymes. This is probably related to the inefficient electron transfer due to the presence of a water molecule at the active site. Some substrates are more efficiently oxidized because they exclude water from the active site (137). Inefficiency of metabolism is more than made up for by the ability to metabolize a variety of chemical structures and the ability to catalyze a variety of reactions. An additional factor that compensates for the relatively low substrate turnover number is the high concentration of the system in organs important in detoxication.

Before a discussion of the various reactions catalyzed by P450, a discussion of the catalytic cycle is appropriate. Knowledge of the catalytic cycle will assist in understanding the various reactions catalyzed by the system and in predicting metabolic pathways for specific xenobiotics.

Catalytic Cycle of the P450–dependent Monooxygenase System

The reaction catalyzed by the cytochrome P450–dependent monooxygenase system and its stoichiometry is illustrated in Figure 3.1. One molecule of substrate reacts with one molecule of molecular oxygen and NADPH to yield oxidized substrate containing one atom from molecular oxygen, water (containing the other oxygen atom), and oxidized NADPH. The incorporation of one oxygen atom from molecular oxygen into the substrate is the source of the term *monooxygenase*. Oxidation of substrate and concomitant reduction of one atom of oxygen to water is the source of the name *mixed function oxidase*. Although the reaction stoichiometry appears simple, obtaining this stoichiometry in the laboratory is difficult (60). The main difficulty is the number of oxidation-reduction reactions that occur simultaneously in the endoplasmic reticulum. These reactions use oxygen and NADPH and may yield water and oxidized NADP. When these diverse reactions have been accounted for, the predicted stoichiometry has been obtained.

It is recommended that the reader carefully follow the reaction sequence illustrated in Figure. 3.2 during this discussion of the catalytic cycle. The initial step of the cycle is binding of the substrate (represented by S in Figure 3.2) to P450. As previously mentioned, P450 exists as a series of closely related isozymes, each of which demonstrates a degree of substrate specificity. This substrate specificity is not absolute, and some overlapping is evident. At any one time, several isozymes of P450 exist in the endoplasmic reticulum. This is dependent on the specific genetic, environmental, and physiological conditions of the organism. Therefore, binding of the substrate to the active site of P450 may represent binding to a single isozyme predominantly but not exclusively. The activity of the catalytic process, as well as the specific metabolites produced, is a function of the particular isozyme profile. Although our understanding of the structure of the active

$$RH + O_2 + NADPH + H^{\oplus} \longrightarrow ROH + H_2O + NADP^{\oplus}$$

FIG. 3.1. Reaction and stoichiometry of P450–dependent monooxygenase.

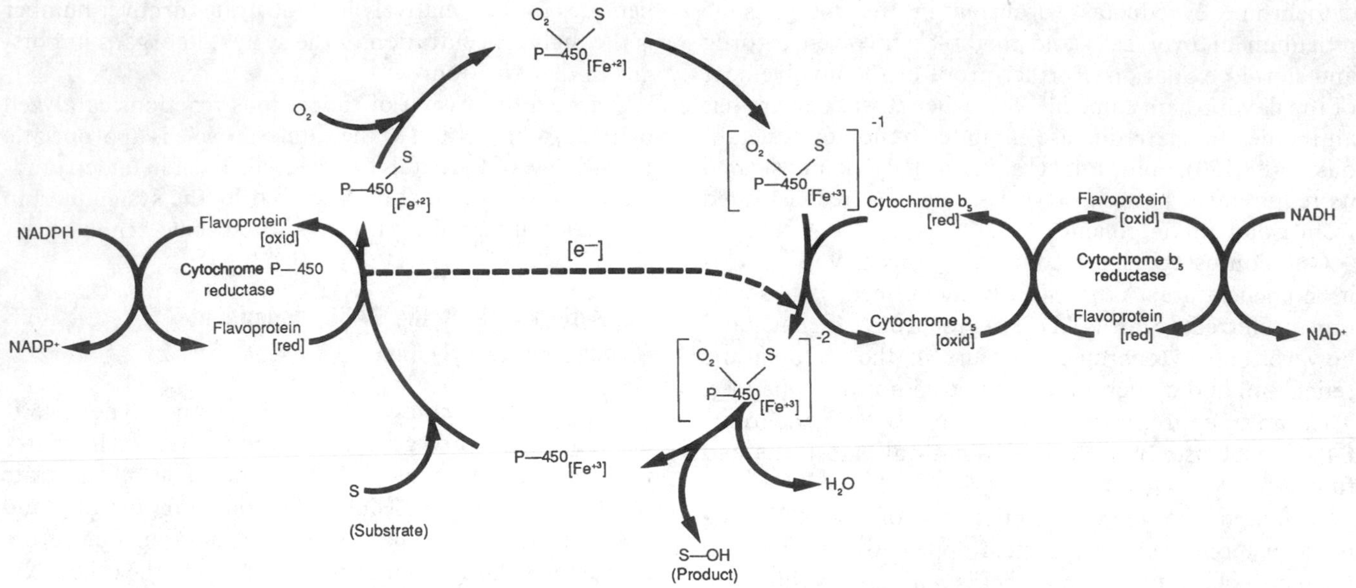

FIG. 3.2. Catalytic cycle of the P450–dependent monooxygenase. The second electron insertion step may be from b_5 (as shown) or from NADPH P450 reductase.

site of P450 is developing (95,96), more needs to be learned. From the nature of the hemoprotein and its substrates, the active site contains the heme and a hydrophobic region. The substrate must have a specific orientation within the active site.

As occurs with many other enzymes, the binding of the substrate to the hemoprotein appears to produce conformational alterations in the enzyme that assist its catalytic activity. For instance, substrate binding results in P450 being more easily reduced by P450 reductase, in part, by lowering its redox potential. Binding of the substrate to the active site changes the absorption spectrum of the cytochrome. Because the oxidized heme iron is paramagnetic, electron paramagnetic resonance (EPR) can be applied to probe the environment of the iron in the heme. These studies have revealed alterations in the EPR signal that correlate with the blue shift in the Soret band from about 419 nm to 390 nm, observed when substrates bind the cytochrome. EPR and visible spectra changes result from the substrate binding in close proximity to the heme iron with a concomitant displacement of a water molecule from the iron. Substrate binding is rapid, the heme is transformed from its low-spin form to the high-spin form, and the substrate is placed in close spatial proximity to the oxygen activation site on the heme. The relationships between the spin state of the cytochrome, interaction with the amino acids at the binding site, and substrate binding is more complex than described here. The reader is referred to discussions of changes in the spin state of P450 in (157,95,140,137).

The next step in the catalytic cycle after substrate binding is the one-electron reduction of the substrate-P450 binary complex. As mentioned, substrate binding and the concomitant alterations in P450 may facilitate this reduction step. The ferric (Fe^{3+}) hemocytochrome P450-substrate complex is reduced by a single electron to the ferrous (Fe^{2+}) hemocytochrome P450-substrate complex. This electron is provided by NADPH through P450 reductase. This flavoprotein contains two flavins: flavin adenine dinucleotide (FAD) and flavin mononucleotide (FMN). The flavoprotein appears to exist in its half-reduced (one-electron reduced) form, and upon reaction with NADPH, is fully reduced (two-electron reduced). The intramolecular electron flow appears to be from FAD to FMN. It is interesting that whereas the flavoprotein is a one-electron donor, its substrate, NADPH, provides two electrons. The mechanism for the two-electron shuttle by the one-electron donor flavoprotein is incompletely understood (7).

The flavoprotein has at least two domains, one of which is imbedded in the endoplasmic reticulum membrane and the other above the plane of the membrane on the cytosolic side. The domain solubilized in the membrane consists mainly of hydrophobic amino acids. The actual interaction with NADPH and oxidation-reduction takes place outside the membrane. Another interesting aspect of P450 reductase is that the quantity of P450 is in large excess to the quantity of reductase (as much as 15-fold to 20-fold or more, dependent upon conditions). This means that each flavoprotein must reduce several P450 molecules, indicating that the interaction between the reductase and P450 is an important consideration, as discussed later.

Upon reduction of the ferric hemocytochrome P450-substrate binary complex to the ferrous state by the reductase, the complex binds oxygen. This results in the ternary complex, ferrous hemocytochrome P450-substrate-oxygen shown in Figure 3.2. The oxygen binds at the free ligand of the heme iron and is believed to be oriented spatially with the substrate binding portion of the active site. Uncoupling (interrupting the flow of electrons) the catalytic cycle at this point can produce the oxidized ferric P450 and a reduced form of oxygen, the superoxide radical. Other reactive oxygen species can be generated by P450 including hydrogen peroxide and the hydroxyl radical. Generation of active oxygen species by P450 has been reviewed in (8).

At this stage of the catalytic cycle, highly critical reactions take place that are still incompletely understood (140). The major event is the activation of the oxygen molecule. The ternary complex accepts a second electron required for reaction. The source of this electron can be either NADH or NADPH, dependent upon the mediator of electron transport. Because the purified, reconstituted system consisting of isolated P450, P450 reductase and phospholipid requires only the presence of NADPH, NADPH P450 reductase can mediate this step; however, as previously mentioned, in some systems it appears that cytochrome b_5 can mediate the electron transfer employing reducing equivalents from NADH through NADH cytochrome b_5 reductase. Whichever the source of the second electron, it results in the production of the peroxy P450-substrate complex, which has a net charge of −2. Determination of the various oxy complexes shown in brackets in Figure 3.2 is critical to understanding the oxygen activation reaction. Of the variety of mechanisms proposed for oxygen activation and insertion into the substrate, two appear to be generally accepted. The first mechanism involves heterolytic cleavage of diatomic oxygen with the abstraction of hydrogen from the substrate and the insertion of oxygen into the substrate. The second mechanism involves homolytic cleavage, whereby two oxygen radicals are generated. Whatever the mechanism, one atom of this reactive oxygen is introduced into the substrate, whereas the other is reduced to water. The oxidized substrate and water are released, regenerating the oxidized ferric P450, which can again initiate the catalytic cycle.

It must be emphasized that other pathways of electron transport in the endoplasmic reticulum can have significant impact on the catalytic activity of the monooxygenase by altering the availability of reducing equivalents. The interested reader is encouraged to consult other sources (7,133) for a more comprehensive discussion of these pathways.

This catalytic cycle is common to cytochromes P450–dependent monooxygenase activity associated with xenobiotic metabolism in a variety of organs and among different species; however, certain of these monooxygenases, especially the more specific forms associated with anabolic and catabolic metabolism, have different mediators of electron transport. For example, the adrenal cortex mitochondria systems use a non-heme iron protein in addition to the P450 reductase in the electron transport chain, as does the monooxygenase in certain microorganisms (137,147).

The P450 system is not totally independent, and its activity is affected by a number of factors. One of these factors is the availability of reducing equivalents. The monooxygenase is primarily dependent on NADPH, as previously discussed, and possibly, to a lesser extent, on NADH. NADPH is generated from the pentose-phosphate shunt, isocitrate dehydrogenase, and the malate enzyme. Under most conditions, these pathways provide saturating levels of NADPH; however, certain conditions can stress the ability of the cell to provide NADPH, and it may become rate limiting. Under conditions of high monooxygenase activity, starvation may reduce the activity toward certain substrates due to reduced levels of NADPH. It is generally believed that the decreased activity due to limiting NADH is an unlikely condition. A discussion of these and other factors that regulate monooxygenase activity can be found in the (171).

An additional factor that influences monooxygenase activity is the endoplasmic reticulum membrane. The asymmetric nature of the protein components of the system in respect to the membrane surface, coupled with the disproportionality of the concentrations of the components (i.e., a 1-to-15–20 ratio between the flavoprotein and P450), indicates an interesting topology and interaction between the components. The membrane topology of the P450 system has been a topic of research for a number of years. The interaction between the protein components of the system and the interaction of these components with the lipid matrix of the membrane are important in the overall reactions of this system. P450 appears to be anchored into the membrane of the endoplasmic reticulum by an anchor peptide at the NH_2-terminal end of the protein with the anchor peptide transversing the membrane. The active site, including the heme, is on the cytoplasmic side of the membrane. The active site portion is rich in alpha helix content, globular in nature, and not associated with membrane lipids. The area around the active site may be associated with the cytosolic surface of the membrane, providing a somewhat rigid character.

P450 appears to exist as multicomponent complexes of six P450 molecules clustered around a single P450 reductase. The NH_2-terminal regions on the opposite side of the membrane may interact to anchor this complex together. This allows for a catalytic advantage because of the close association of the components. This organization implies that each reductase would be capable of sequentially reducing several P450s. P450 may form a transient complex with the reductase that has an extremely short, non-rate-limiting half-life (10,64).

Isozyme Heterogeneity and Substrate Specificity of Cytochrome P450

For many years, P450's apparent lack of substrate specificity intrigued investigators. It appeared that one of the major features of substrate specificity was lipid solubility. There appeared to be few other structural restraints for substrates. Intensive research on the nature of the hemoproteins has revealed that much of this apparent lack of substrate specificity results from the existence of multiple families and multiple subfamilies of P450 isozymes.

As the array of individual isozymes grew in number, nomenclature became a problem. It was sometimes difficult for investigators to know what exact P450 they were working with because of inconsistencies in nomenclature. This led to attempts to develop a systematic nomenclature for the isozymes. P450 nomenclature has evolved from identifications based on spectra peaks to species-dependent nomenclature based on isolated and semi-purified P450s to the current system, which is based on amino acid sequences that result from specific gene sequences (124). P450 are now placed in families, which are further divided into subfamilies. Names are based on the root CYP derived from *cy*tochrome *P*450. The CYP is followed by a number identifying the gene family to which it belongs, such as CYP1, CYP2, CYP3, etc. The number for the gene family is followed by a letter denoting the subfamily to which the P450 belongs, such as CYP1A and CYP2A. The subfamilies are further defined by the addition of a number identifying the gene, such as CYP1A1 and CYP1A2. Thus, P450 nomenclature is based on genetic relationships defined by protein and gene sequences. All P450s within a single family must exhibit a protein sequence similarity greater than 40%. P450s within the same subfamilies have sequence similarities greater than 55% within the same species. Subfamilies have sequence similarity that may be somewhat less than 55% when comparing species that are more distantly related. Members of subfamilies within a species appear to be located on a specific chromosome, and different subfamilies within a gene family may be clustered on the same chromosome. As is generally found in biology, there are exceptions to the classification system resulting from P450s that do not fit the usual patterns. Although this nomenclature provides information on genetic and evolutionary relationships, it provides little information about substrate specificities and the reactions catalyzed by the different P450s. In fact, more is known about the protein and gene sequences of many P450s than about their specific roles in metabolism. With the advent of new methodologies, such as polymerase chain reaction (PCR) techniques, our ability to sequence specific P450s has outgrown our ability to define their specific roles in the metabolism of xenobiotics and endogenous compounds.

Different species may contain a CYP gene or protein that appears to be highly related; these are termed *orthologous genes*, or *orthologs*. Orthologs are believed to have evolved from a single gene that existed before the two species diverged from a single species. Although these genes and their proteins may contain a high degree of sequence homology, it is not necessarily true that they share a catalytic similarity, or vice versa. A small change in an important amino acid sequence can result in a large change in the activity of a P450. Humans and rats have the CYP2 family and the CYP2D subfamily. The rat subfamily contains five genes, one of which is CYP2D1. This P450 has catalytic activity toward debrisoquine metabolism. The human P450 that has the highest catalytic activity toward debrisoquine is CYP2D6, which makes up less than 5% of the complement of P450 in the liver (Figure 3.3). Because these rat and human P450s have similar substrate specificity, it might be assumed they have a high degree of sequence similarity. This was found not to be true. Therefore, even though these two isozymes have similar catalytic activity, they may have been derived from different ancestral genes. Sequence orthologs do not always predict similar catalytic activities. This is important for toxicologists who extrapolate toxicity from animal models to humans, as noted later. It also indicates that such information is important when toxicologists do interspecies extrapolation of toxicity, such as from mice to rats.

The section that follows provides a brief description of the major P450 families involved in xenobiotic metabolism. Those families predominately involved in metabolism of endogenous substrates have been excluded. For a more complete discussion of the P450 families, the reader is referred to the excellent reviews in (73,159).

CYP1 Family

The CYP1 family contains two subfamilies of P450s: CYP1A and CYP1B. CYP1A is much better characterized than the CYP1B subfamily.

CYP1A Subfamily. The CYP1A subfamily contains CYP1A1 and CYP1A2, which appear to occur in all mammals. These two P450s may have been derived from a common ancestor approximately 120 million years ago.

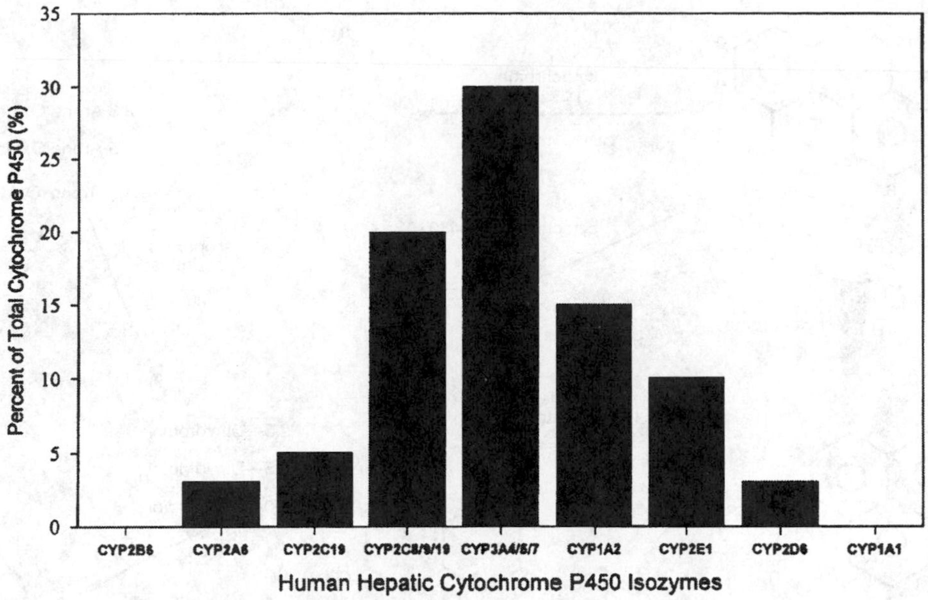

FIG. 3.3. Estimated percentage of distribution of P450 enzymes in human liver. Individual humans may demonstrate significant deviations from this average distribution. CYP2B6 and CYP1A1 may be in very low concentrations and appear only after enzyme induction. Modified from Reference 134.

Both P450s are important in the metabolism of environmental xenobiotics. Although these hemoproteins share a number of physiochemical characteristics, such as similar primary structures, they demonstrate different substrate specificities. For example, CY1A1 is highly active in the metabolism of benzo(a)pyrene (Figure 3.4), whereas CYP1A2 is active in the metabolism of acetanilide. These two P450s were first known as P448, and their classical enzyme inducer is 3-methylcholanthrene. Isosafrole is a specific inducer of CYP1A2. Another characteristic of these P450s is that CYP1A2 is mainly a liver enzyme in humans and animals, whereas CYP1A1 occurs in the liver (Figure 3.3) but also in extrahepatic tissues, such as the lung and kidney. For a number of years there has been an interest in the role of CYP1A1 in the metabolic activation of polycyclic hydrocarbons, such as benzo(a)pyrene. Although many of the investigations on the role of CYP1A1 in activation of polycyclic hydrocarbons have been done in animals with induced CYP1A1, polycyclics may be metabolized by other P450s in uninduced animals. Because its concentration in the liver is low, CYP1A1 may be more important in the metabolic activation of polycyclics in extrahepatic tissues, such as the lung. In humans, CYP1A1 demonstrates genetic polymorphism (discussed later). CYP1A2 has been shown to be associated with the mutagenic activation of heterocyclic amines, such as 4-aminobiphenyl and 2-aminonaphthalene. It also 0-dealkylates phenacetin and 4-hydroxlates acetanilide. Humans can show large differences in the activity of this P450, suggesting it also may be polymorphic. CYP1A2 catalyzes the N3-demethylation of caffeine to paraxanthine. This reaction has been used in vivo as a *substrate probe* for CYP1A2 activity.

CYP2 Family

The CYP2 family contains a number of subfamilies important in xenobiotic metabolism, including CYP2A, CYP2B, CYP2C, CYP2D, and CYP2E.

CYP2A. The CYP2A subfamily contains at least 12 members that differ in their substrate specificity, tissue distribution, and response to inducers and inhibitors, and demonstrate species differences. CYP2A1, CYP2A2, and CYP2A3 are rat P450s, Cyp2a4, Cyp2a5, and Cyp2a12 are found in mice, whereas humans have CYP2A6 and CYP2A7. Rat CYP2A1, along with CYP2A2, hydroxylates testosterone, progesterone, and androsteredione. They can also metabolize aminopyrine, benzphetamine, ethylmorphine, aniline, acetanilide, and N-nitrosodimethylamine. CYP2A1 has low activity toward 3-hydroxylation of benzo(a)pyrene, 7-ethoxycoumarin O-deethylation, and does not metabolize 7-ethoxyresorufin. It occurs in liver and testis, but not kidney and lung. In adult rats it predominates in females and appears to be under endocrine control. CYP2A3 appears to be lung specific, and its substrate specificity has not been well characterized. Human CYP2A6 demonstrates coumarin 7-hydroxylase activity but has

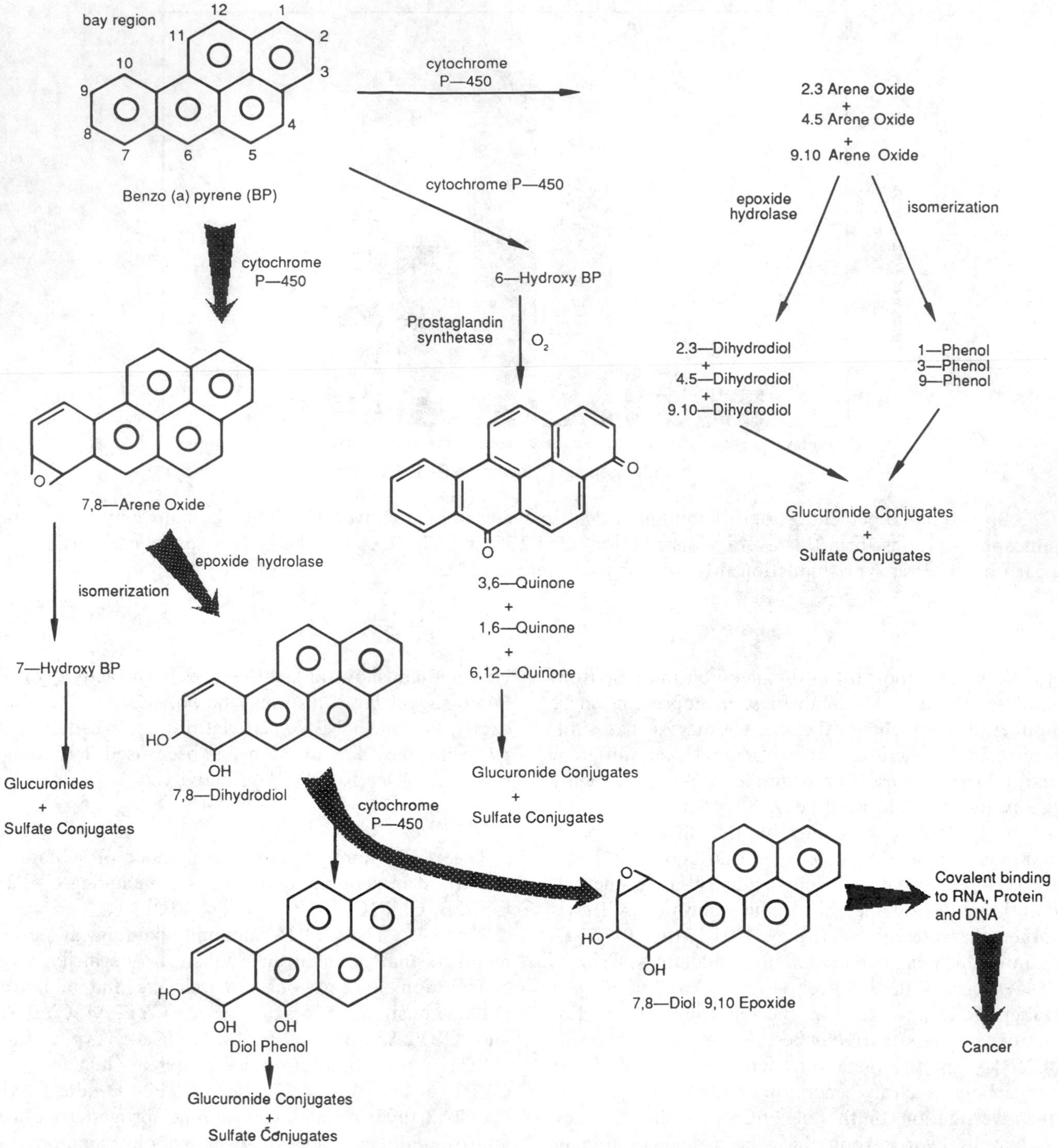

FIG. 3.4. Biotransformation and metabolic activation (*heavy arrows*) of the carcinogen benzo(a)pyrene. (BP).

no activity toward testosterone, in contrast to rat CYP2A1 and CYP2A2. It has no activity toward substrate probes such as 7-ethoxyresorufin, 7-benzyloxyresorufin, ethylmorphine, and testosterone. Although it shows wide variation in activity, there is no evidence that this is a polymorphic P450. Human liver microsomal studies have indicated this P450 may play a role in the metabolic activation of a number of nitrosamines and possibly activation of aflatoxin B_1 to its hepatocarcinogenic epoxide.

CYP2B. This subfamily contains P450s, such as rat CYP2B1 and rat CYP2B2, that are highly induced by phenobarbital. Although the rat P450s in the CYP2B subfamily have been studied for a number of years, the

CYP2B subfamily may have limited importance in humans. The human CYP3A subfamily may be more important in respect to phenobarbital-type induction in humans. Hydroxylation of testosterone at the 16β position is used as a specific substrate probe for this P450 in rats. Other substrates for this subfamily include benzyloxyresorufin, ethoxycoumarin, and pentoxyresorufin. In rats, CYP2B1 has been detected in the lung, adrenal gland, testis, and brain, whereas CYP2B2 occurs in liver and brain. Its role in xenobiotic metabolism has not been thoroughly investigated, although the CYP2B subfamily can metabolically activate xenobiotics, such as bromobenzene, carbon tetrachloride, benzo(a)pyrene, aflatoxin B_1, and some nitrosamines in the rat.

CYP2C. Four CYP2C subfamily members have been identified in humans, CYP2C8, CYP2C9, CYP2C18, and CYP2C19. At least eight members of this subfamily have been identified in rats. Rat CYP2C P450s are gender specific, whereas this is not true for humans. In rats, members of this family are expressed in hepatic and extrahepatic tissues. In humans, CYP2C9 and CYP2C8 are present in the small intestine, and CYP2C8 has been detected in skin. Human CYP2C18 catalyzes the 4-hydroxylation, and CYP2C8 catalyzes the 4- and 7-hydroxylation of warfarin, but at a much lower rate. CYP2C8 also hydroxylates benzo(a)pyrene.

CYP2D. Rats have six members in the CYP2D subfamily, whereas three have been identified in humans: CYP2D6, CYP2D7, and CYP2D8. Mice have five CYP2D members, and this subfamily has been identified in other mammals. Human CYP2D6 was the first human P450 shown to be polymorphic, and is discussed later. Many drugs are metabolized by CYP2D6, and the reactions range from aryl hydroxylation to *N*- and *O*-dealkylation.

CYP2E. The CYP2E subfamily is one of particular interest to toxicologists. Currently, CYP2E1 is the only member of this subfamily in rats, mice, and humans. CYP2E1 appears restricted to mammals, and may have evolved more recently than certain other gene families. It is expressed in liver and kidney and occurs at low levels in a number of other tissues. Although it normally represents less than 10% of total P450 in human liver, it is induced by a broad array of its substrates. Its hepatic concentration can vary up to 50% between different humans. Rat and human forms of CYP2E1 share many similarities, including similar substrate specificities. It is known to metabolize more than 70 different chemicals with diverse structures. Structural requirements for CYP2E1 substrates appear limited to small molecules with hydrophobic character. It does not appear to be active in the metabolism of many drugs but does metabolize a wide array of alcohols, aldehydes, alkanes, aromatic hydrocarbons, ethers, fatty acids, halogenated hydrocarbons (including anesthetics), heterocyclics, and ketones. There are no specific substrate probes for CYP2E1, but aniline hydroxylation, p-nitrophenol hydroxylation, and carbon tetrachloride–dependent lipid peroxidation have been used to follow its activity in vitro.

Interest in the role of CYP2E1 as a mediator of toxicity comes from two of its actions. First, it is known to be important in the metabolic activation/detoxication of a number of carcinogens and heptatoxins. Second, it may have an important role in free-radical production and oxidative stress. For instance, it is believed to be involved in the metabolic activation associated with the carcinogenicity of benzene, nitrosamines, and azoxymethane, and the hepatotoxicity of nitrosamines, acetaminophen, halothane, and enflurane.

In respect to free radical production, it is involved in the formation of a reactive hydroxyethyl radical produced during its metabolism of ethanol to acetaldehyde. This hydroxy radical is believed to play a role in ethanol-related liver damage. It also appears to be involved in the production of a trichloroethyl radical produced by chlorine removal during the metabolism of carbon tetrachloride. This radical may initiate membrane lipid peroxidation associated with carbon tetrachloride–induced hepatotoxicity. An additional mechanism by which CYP2E1 could produce reactive radicals is associated with its potential for futile cycling in the absence of substrate. It appears more loosely coupled than some of the other P450s. Oxygen activation during the catalytic cycle in the absence of substrate results in the production of highly reactive hydroxyl radicals, superoxide anions, and hydrogen peroxide. If these reach concentrations that overcome cellular protection mechanisms, they can initiate oxidative stress leading to tissue damage.

P450s are not evenly expressed in the liver but occur in specific zones. The highest concentration of P450 is generally found in a layer surrounding the terminal hepatic venules. This is especially true for induced CYP2E1. Enhanced CYP2E1 activity in the centrilobular region appears related to the centrilobular necrosis produced by hepatotoxins, such as ethanol, carbon tetrachloride, benzene, nitrosamines, and acetaminophen. It may appear that CYP2E1 is predominately involved with metabolic activation; however, this is not necessarily true. As noted before, P450–mediated xenobiotic metabolism is generally associated with production of less toxic metabolites, but in some cases, more toxic metabolites are produced. CYP2E1 is no exception to this rule and participates in not only metabolic activation, but also detoxication.

CYP3 Family

The CYP3 family of P450s encompasses CYP3A1 and CYP3A2 in rats, Cyp3a-11 and Cyp3a-13 in mice, and

CYP3A3, CYP3A4, CYP3A5, and CYP3A7 in humans, along with others from rabbits, dogs, and other species. The CYP3 family contains P450s that are important in the metabolism of many xenobiotics, especially drugs.

CYP3A. This subfamily contains at least four genes in humans. In many cases, it has been difficult to separate the activities of human CYP3A3 and CYP3A4. CYP3A4 is the major form of P450 expressed in human liver. It is also the major P450 expressed in the human gastrointestinal tract. Small amounts are found in several other organs, such as the kidney and skin. CYP3A4 and other members of the CYP3A subfamily are induced by a number of drugs. These isozymes do not demonstrate a high degree of structural selectivity with respect to their substrates. Generally, their substrates are relatively large, highly lipophilic molecules. Over 150 drugs from 38 classes can be metabolized by CYP3A4. They are also capable of metabolically activating carcinogens, such as aflatoxin B_1 and benzo(a)pyrene. Because of the large number of drugs metabolized by CYP3A4, it may play a role in a number of drug–drug interactions that may result in adverse effects.

An example of how dietary constituents can affect specific isozymes is provided by the interaction between the consumption of grapefruit juice and CYP3A4. Consumption of grapefruit juice can cause an increase in the oral availability of a number of drugs that are CYP3A4 substrates. This affect appears to be associated with intestinal CYP3A4 more so than hepatic CYP3A4. Increased bioavailability is produced by inhibition of intestinal CYP3A4 activity by 6′, 7′-dihydroxybergamottin, which is a component of grapefruit juice. This dietary compound is a mechanism-based inhibitor of CYP3A4 that results in the rapid partial loss of CYP3A4 activity (150). Inhibition of metabolism of the CYP3A4 substrates during their intestinal absorption accounts for the higher-than-anticipated plasma concentration of the drugs.

CYP3A5. This P450 may be polymorphically expressed in humans and has been detected in only 25%–30% of adults. It does not appear to have the broad substrate specificity of CYP3A4 and has lower activity.

Other P450s. There are a large number of P450 families and subfamilies not discussed here. Most of these are involved with the metabolism of endogenous substrates or occur in species that are beyond the scope of the topic of this chapter (see (73) for a more complete discussion).

Reactions Catalyzed by the Cytochromes P450–dependent Monooxygenase System

On first inspection, it appears that P450 can catalyze a bewildering number of reactions (Table 3.2); however, on closer inspection, there is a degree of commonality among these reactions. The first area of commonality is that most of the reactions represent oxidations. Second, the reactions convert lipophilic substrates to more hydrophilic products. Third, many of the reactions can be represented as hydroxylations, as pointed out by Mannering (106). For a review of P450 reactions, see (62).

Table 3.2
Major oxidative reactions catalyzed by the P450 monooxygenase system

Aliphatic hydroxylation
Aromatic hydroxylation
Epoxidation
N-Dealkylation
O-Dealkylation
S-Dealkylation
Deamination
Sulfoxidation
N-Oxidation
Oxidative dehalogenation
Desulfuration

Aliphatic Hydroxylation

Examination of aliphatic hydroxylation reactions is illustrative of several important aspects of monooxygenase activity. The reaction mechanism, which may be common to several other types of monooxygenase metabolism, appears to occur by a hydrogen (or electron) abstraction mechanism. Oxygen activation produces a $[FeO]^{3+}$ at the heme of P450. Hydrogen abstraction from the substrate results in production of the carbon radical. This radical interacts with activated oxygen (through oxygen rebound) to yield hydroxylation. Other reactions, such as *O*-dealkylation of ethers and carboxylic acid esters, may proceed through this mechanism with decomposition of unstable hydroxylation products. Hydrogen abstraction is site selective, resulting in a nonrandom hydroxylation. The specific hydroxylation site is determined by structure and the specific spacial orientation of the substrate at the active site. Different isozymes of P450 show different degrees of site selectivity. For example, n-hexane hydroxylation can occur at C-1, C-2, C-3, C-4. P450 isozymes induced by phenobarbital metabolized n-hexane to yield a four- to fivefold increase in the 2-, 3-, and 4-hydroxylated metabolites and only a slight increase at the 1 position. On the other hand, benzo(a)pyrene-induced isozymes result in decreased yields of the 1- and 2-hydroxylated products but increased yields of the 3- and 4-hydroxylated products (49). Hydroxylation of aliphatic compounds is generally considered detoxication because of the greater water solubility of the products, but one must be cautioned against overgeneralization, as products that are more toxic could be produced by subsequent metabolism.

Aromatic Oxidation

Aromatic oxidation reaction mechanisms are not completely understood but may occur by several mechanisms. The exact mechanism may be based on a number of factors, such as the steric features of the substrate and the configuration of the active site of the specific P450. Potential mechanisms include direct oxygen insertion into the C-H bond to form an epoxide through radicaloid reactions and/or through intermediates bonded to $(FeO)+^3$.

An example of a compound that is hydroxylated by both direct insertion of oxygen at the C-H bond and oxygen addition at the C=C bond is p-chlorobenzene. Both 3- and 4-chlorobenzene oxides are formed by the addition reaction to yield the arene epoxides. These spontaneously rearrange to form the *o*-chlorophenol and *p*-chlorophenol. The occurrence of the *m*-chlorophenol as a metabolite is an example of the direct insertion reaction. The production of arene oxides has been widely studied because of their importance in the formation of epoxide ultimate carcinogens. These epoxides can also be formed in nonaromatic systems, yielding reaction products as illustrated by the metabolism of aflatoxin B_1. This mycotoxin is metabolized to a number of hydroxylated products and to the 8,9-epoxide. It is generally agreed that this epoxide is the ultimate carcinogen of aflatoxin B_1.

Heteroatom Oxidation

P450 not only oxidizes carbon atoms but also nitrogen and sulfur atoms. A number of nitrogen-containing compounds can be oxidized to stable *N*-oxides. Another hepatic enzyme, flavin monooxygenase (FMO), can also catalyze this reaction. P450 and FMO may form *N*-oxides from the same xenobiotic; however, FMO generally prefers substrates with an electron-deficient nitrogen, whereas P450 prefers an electron-rich nitrogen. P450–mediated *N*-oxidation is possible with primary and secondary aromatic amines to produce hydroxylamines. Sulfoxidation can also be catalyzed by P450 and FMO. Sulfoxidation can produce a sulfoxide (SO) that can be further oxidized to a sulfone (SO_2). The mechanism associated with these reactions is believed to be electron abstraction from the heteroatom by $(FeO)^{3+}$.

Heteroatom Dealkylation

P450–dependent heteroatom dealkylation begins like heteroatom oxidation with electron abstraction from N, S, or O. This is followed by abstraction of H^+ from the carbon attached to the heteroatom. This α-carbon is hydroxylated followed by cleavage of the α-carbon and its rearrangement to an aldehyde or ketone. Sulfur atoms generally are not as readily dealkylated as nitrogen and oxygen atoms.

Ether compounds can also be dealkylated. The O-dealkylation is similar to N-dealkylation and is believed to proceed through the initial oxidation of the carbon adjacent to oxygen (i.e., carbon oxidation). The products of this reaction are again an alcohol and aldehyde, analogous to those produced by N-dealkylation.

Oxidative Deamination, Desulfuration, and Dehalogenation

Primary amines can be deaminated by the elimination of ammonia and the formation of an aldehyde or ketone. In a similar manner, P450 can catalyze desulfuration and dehalogenation, with the heteroatom being replaced with oxygen.

Reduction Reactions

An interesting series of reactions in which P450 may participate under special conditions are reductive reactions. These appear to involve transfer of electrons from Fe^{+2} to the substrate. Examples of such reactions are nitro reduction, azo reduction, arene oxide reduction, and reductive dehalogenation. These reactions generally are studied in vitro under anaerobic conditions in the presence of isolated microsomes and NADPH. Because these reactions require low oxygen tension to progress, their in vivo role (if any) is not well understood. Whether or not these reactions represent simply a curious phenomenon associated with P450 or a viable metabolic pathway is not known. It may be possible that under certain cellular conditions of low oxygen tension these reactions could proceed in vivo.

Induction and Inhibition of Cytochromes P450

Induction

When animals are exposed to certain xenobiotics, their ability to metabolize a variety of xenobiotics is increased. This phenomenon is termed *induction*. Induction produces a transitory resistance to the toxicity of many compounds; however, this may not be the case with compounds that require metabolic activation because their toxicity may increase. The exact toxicological outcome of this increased metabolism will be dependent on the specific xenobiotic and its metabolic pathway. Because the toxicological outcome of a xenobiotic exposure can depend on the balance between those reactions that represent detoxication and those that represent activation, increases in metabolic capacity may, at times, produce unpredictable results. Induction of P450 has been reviewed in (17).

One of the initial reports of increased metabolic capacity associated with xenobiotic exposure suggests how induction may provide a survival advantage. In 1954, Brown et al. (19) were studying the metabolism of methylated aminoazo dyes and found that xenobiotics in the animal diets enhanced the P450–dependent demethylation of these compounds. Free-living animals consume a variety of feeds that may contain toxic constituents. If the animal can respond rapidly to these toxic compounds by developing resistance, it can continue to use the feed source and obtain a survival advantage. One mechanism of rapidly developing such resistance is through increased detoxication resulting from stimulation of xenobiotic metabolizing enzyme activity.

Conney (31) published a pivotal review in 1967 that indicated more than 200 chemicals could induce P450–dependent metabolism, and most of these chemicals were monooxygenase substrates. Although the induction of the P450 enzymes has been most intensively investigated, other enzymes of biotransformation can be induced, such as the UDP-glucuronosyltransferases.

The classical definition of enzyme induction requires transcriptional activation at the level of DNA and increased production of mRNA, followed by an increase in the synthesis of the enzyme. The term has taken on a broader definition when used in respect to xenobiotic metabolism. This broader definition includes mechanisms such as mRNA and enzyme stabilization, all of which are associated with xenobiotic "induction." There are a number of "classes" of P450 inducers, which are listed in Table 3.3.

The polycyclic aromatic hydrocarbon class of inducers includes 3-methylcholanthrene, benzo(a)pyrene, and 2, 3, 7, 8 tetrachlorodibenzo-p-dioxin, and their mechanism of induction in animals has been extensively investigated. These inducers induce CYP1A1, which occurs in the liver and extrahepatic tissues of rats and extrahepatic tissues in humans. The low constitutive hepatic concentrations of CYP1A1 result from suppression of transcription by a nuclear repressor protein. Within the cytoplasm of the hepatocyte, there exists a receptor protein termed the *Ah receptor* that is complexed with heat-shock protein (hsp90). When a polycyclic hydrocarbon-type inducer enters the hepatocyte, it binds and activates the Ah receptor, resulting in release of hsp90. The Ah receptor is phosphorylated and subsequently binds to the Ahr nuclear translocator protein (Arnt), which is also activated by phosphorylation. This complex then moves to the nucleus of the hepatocyte. In the nucleus, this complex binds to a DNA regulatory sequence termed the *xenobiotic responsive element* (XRE). A DNA segment similar to rat XRE has been found in mouse and human cells. The XRE has also been found in genes of other xenobiotic metabolism enzymes, such as glutathione *S*-transferase, aldehyde dehydrogenase, and UDP-glucuronosyltransferase, where it may be involved in regulation of their expression. Binding of the ligand-bound-Ah-Arnt complex to XRE enhances transcription of the CYP1A1 gene, resulting in increased quantities of CYP1A1 mRNA followed by an increase in the hepatic concentration of CYP1A1.

In contrast to the polycyclic hydrocarbon class of inducers, no cytoplasmic receptor has been found for the phenobarbital-type inducers. Phenobarbital and other compounds of diverse structure induce expression of CYP2B1 and CYP2B2 and, to a lessor extent, CYP2A1, CYP2C6, CYP3A1, and CYP3A2. It also increases the quantity of endoplasmic reticulum in hepatocytes, increases total microsomal protein, and increases NADPH-cytochrome P450 reductase as well as other xenobiotic metabolizing enzymes, such as UDPG-glucuronosyltransferase and epoxide hydrolase. Its induction of P450s is at the transcription level and is believed to be associated with the removal of a repressor

Table 3.3
Inducers of P450

Class of Inducer	Primary Example	Other Examples	Examples of Induced P450s
Polycyclic hydrocarbon type	3-Methylcholanthrene	Benzo(a)pyrene, β-naphthoflavone, TCDD, chlorpromazine, isosafrole, ketoconazole	CYP1A1, CYP1A2
Phenobarbital type	Phenobarbital	Phenytoin, griseofulvin, chlorpromazine, ketoconazole, dieldrin, butylated hydroxy-toluene	CYP2A1, CYP2B1, CYP2B2, CYP2C6, CYP3A2
Ethanol type	Ethanol	Acetone, heptane	CYP2E1
Glucocorticoid type	Dexamethasone	Pregnenolone-16a-carbonitrile, spironolactone, clotrimazole, prednisolone, methylprenisolone, rifampicin	CYP3A1, CYP3A2, CYP3A4
Clofibrate type	Clofibrate		CYP4

protein from an enhancer region of the DNA, allowing an increase in transcription. Compounds in the phenobarbital inducer class, such as terpenes, organochlorine pesticides, and polychlorinated biphenyls, may act through a common pathway of induction (51).

CYP2E1 induction has been studied in detail in the rat and represents an interesting situation where induction is controlled at the transcription, mRNA stabilization, translation, and enzyme stabilization levels. In addition, diet and pathophysiological conditions can produce induction of this P450. CYP2E1 is induced by the ethanol-type inducers. Although not true for all P450s, the CYP2E1 inducers generally are substrates for the isozyme. In many cases, the regulation of expression of CYP2E1 is controlled by stabilization of CYP2E1 mRNA and stabilization of the enzyme apoprotein, along with possible increased efficiency of translation. Cycloheximide, which blocks translation, blocked the increase in CYP2E1 apoprotein when mRNA was unchanged, indicating the increase in apoprotein was related to increased translation. Actinomycin D, which blocks transcription, did not block the apoprotein increase, indicating it was not transcription related. Many of the CYP2E1 inducers act by post-translational stabilization, including acetone, low ethanol doses, pyridine, and pyrazole. With these inducers, CYP2E1 concentration increases, whereas there is no change in mRNA. This indicates that CYP2E1 degradation decreases while synthesis remains constant, with the net result being increased CYP2E1.

Nutritional factors and disease conditions can also result in increased activity of CYP2E1. High-fat diets and starvation produce an induction of CYP2E1, as does insulin-dependent diabetes and obesity. One common factor in all of these conditions is increased plasma ketone body concentrations. Whether or not this induction is produced by increased ketone bodies, including acetone, or by other factors is currently under investigation.

The glucocorticoid-type inducers, such as dexamethasone and pregnenolone-16α-carbonitrile, induce CYP3A1 and CYP3A2. Induction is associated with transcription activation and mRNA stabilization. The exact mechanism of induction is unknown and its relationship to the glucocorticoid receptor, if any, is uncertain. CYP3A isozymes are involved in the metabolism of a number of drugs, and induction could effect drug–drug interactions.

Clofibrate-type inducers induce the CYP4A subfamily, that is, in most part, associated with metabolism of endogenous compounds. They also cause hepatocyte peroxisome proliferation in rodents. Many compounds that cause peroxisome proliferation in rodent liver are also hepatocarcinogens; however, humans are resistant to peroxisome proliferation, and these compounds do not appear to be a hepatocarcinogenic risk to humans. The low concentrations of CYP4A in human liver and its limited number of xenobiotic substrates, reduce its role in drug–drug interactions in humans. Induction by compounds such as clofibrate appears associated with a peroxisome proliferator-activated receptor (PPAR) involved in activation of transcription and resulting apoprotein synthesis.

Inhibition

Just as induction of xenobiotic metabolism can have important toxicological ramifications, inhibition of the ability to metabolize a xenobiotic can result in profound changes in its toxicity. Inhibition of a compound's metabolism can result in a higher plasma concentration than predicted and unexpected toxicity. During multiple drug treatment, unexpected adverse effects can be produced through drug–drug interactions where one drug inhibits the metabolism of another, resulting in higher than expected plasma concentrations.

Four mechanisms are generally associated with inhibition of P450-mediated detoxication. First, two xenobiotics may be substrates for the same P450 isozyme and will compete for the active site of the enzyme. This is an example of competitive inhibition. A second mechanism of competitive inhibition is the binding of a xenobiotic to the active site of a P450, although it is not a substrate for that P450. The presence of the nonsubstrate at the active site blocks the binding of the true substrate, inhibiting its metabolism. A third mechanism of inhibition involves the metabolism of a xenobiotic to a product that has a higher affinity for the active site than the parent compound. The active site is then occupied and additional substrate cannot bind. This essentially makes the enzyme inactive and is an example of noncompetitive inhibition. The fourth mechanism is another example of noncompetitive inhibition resulting from the production of a highly reactive metabolite that binds (often covalently) to the heme or apoprotein of P450, destroying its activity. This type of inhibitor is termed a *mechanism-based inhibitor* or a *suicide substrate*.

Other, less common mechanisms can result in inhibition of P450-mediated xenobiotic metabolism, including compounds that may modify protein or heme synthesis or degradation, those that may uncouple electron transport to P450, those that may interfere with cofactor availability, and those that may directly inhibit NADPH P450 reductase activity. Just as some substrates may demonstrate a higher affinity for specific P450s and others may not, inhibitors may show a narrow or broad range of affinity for a specific P450. Inhibitors have been useful tools in determining mechanisms associated with xenobiotic metabolism and in attempts to predict specific drug–drug interactions. Induction and inhibition of human cytochromes P450 have been recently reviewed in (135).

Species, Strain, and Gender Differences in Monooxygenase Activity

The activities of cytochromes P450 play a central role in the expression of the toxicity of the majority of xenobiotics. Knowledge of the rates at which a xenobiotic is metabolized and the chemical and biological nature of its metabolites assist not only in understanding its toxicity, but also its mechanism of action. This provides essential information to enable toxicologists to predict its toxicity. One factor that complicates extrapolation of toxicity between species is the quantitative and qualitative differences in how species metabolize xenobiotics. Generally, the basic reactions and major metabolites of a xenobiotic are similar between species; however, subtle differences in metabolism can lead to major differences in susceptibility to the toxicity of a xenobiotic.

A variety of mechanisms can be associated with differences between species in their response to a xenobiotic, including (1) adsorption, (2) distribution, (3) organ differences in metabolic capacity, (4) qualitative and quantitative differences in P450 isozymes and other xenobiotic metabolizing enzymes, (5) excretion, and (6) insensitivity of either the target organ or biochemical target site. Although all of these factors may be more or less important in understanding species differences in the susceptibility to the xenobiotic, it appears that the dominant factor is xenobiotic metabolism.

Mechanisms that may account for species differences include (1) lack of a metabolic pathway or a genetic "defect" in a particular metabolic pathway, (2) differences in the Km and Vmax of specific enzymes, (3) the existence of different isozymes and differences in the ratios of specific isozymes of important enzymes, such as P450, and (4) differences in the ratio of activities of separate enzyme systems that act together to metabolize a specific xenobiotic.

The lack of a specific pathway or a defect in a pathway will make a species or strain susceptible to xenobiotics that are detoxicated via that pathway. Conversely, when the xenobiotic is metabolically activated by that pathway, the species will be resistant. Although there does not appear to be a mammalian example of the lack of the monooxygenase system, examples exist for other enzymes, such as the lack of glucuronidation in cats. A more common explanation of species difference is the variation in the activity (Km, Vmax) and substrate specificity of isozymes associated with xenobiotic metabolism. At low doses or environmental exposures, these differences will be expressed in detoxication and species susceptibility. Caution needs to be used in both the design and interpretation of studies to investigate species differences. As mentioned, doses below enzyme saturation may not reveal species differences. Care must be used when investigating these differences in vitro, as this activity may not mimic in vivo activity.

When one metabolite represents a metabolically activated form and another a detoxicated form, the ratio of these metabolites can dictate a species susceptibility to a xenobiotic. This type of species difference is most commonly encountered when the P450–dependent monooxygenase acts in coordination with another pathway. Species may differ in either the initial monooxygenase functionalization reaction or in the activity of the secondary pathway. This is illustrated by the metabolic activation of benzo(a)pyrene (BP) (see Figure 3.4) in rats and mice. The metabolic activation of BP requires initial epoxidation by the P450–dependent monooxygenase at the 7,8 position, followed by hydration of the epoxide by epoxide hydrolase to yield the 7,8-diol. This diol is then epoxidated by the monooxygenase to yield the ultimate carcinogen of BP, the 7,8-dihydrodiol 9,10-oxide. When mouse hepatic microsomes were used for metabolic activation in the Ames assay for mutagenicity, BP was highly mutagenic, indicating a high degree of metabolic activation; however, when rat hepatic microsomes were employed in the same assay, only slight mutagenicity was evident. This indicates a significantly lower ability for the rats to metabolically activate BP in vitro (127). Although mice do metabolize BP to a greater extent than rats, rats have six- to sevenfold more epoxide hydrolase activity. Further studies (126,127) indicated that both species have adequate monooxygenase to metabolically activate BP and that higher epoxide hydrolase activity in the rat may have been responsible for the lower mutagenicity. Therefore, the species differences in the secondary pathway, epoxide hydrolase, may have controlled the mutagenicity, as opposed to differences in the monooxygenase activity.

Just as species demonstrate differences in metabolism that alters toxicity, different strains of the same species may demonstrate differences in metabolism. For instance, if a different strain of mouse had been used in the studies described above, the data may have been different. It is important to recognize these strain differences when designing toxicological studies. The mechanisms associated with strain differences may be diverse. As with any genetically controlled activity, differences in metabolism are not unusual. Laboratory animals are generally bred in distinct groups, and without extensive outbreeding strain differences can develop quite rapidly. In the wild, such strain differences would be less likely, but individual differences may be greater. Other factors, such as diet, environment, etc., may result in what appears to be strain differences.

Species differences in metabolism and, consequently, susceptibility lead to an important concept in toxicology, that of selective toxicity. Ideally, a pesticide should be toxic only to the organism against which it is directed. This concept of selective toxicity has resulted in efforts to develop selective pesticides. For these activities to be fruitful, it is important that species differences in metabolism are understood and this information is used.

For the toxicologist, the species differences of major importance are those between humans and those species used in toxicological testing. Without an understanding of these species differences, it will be difficult to extrapolate toxicological studies performed with animals to humans. Studies of species differences in animals are difficult to design and interpret, and those involving humans are even more complex. This complexity results from the large differences in xenobiotic biotransformation found in humans. Many factors contribute to these individual differences in metabolism, including the following: (1) humans are free-living and have few restraints to reproductive diversity, diminishing the development of small genetic pools that result in genetically less diverse, more homogeneous control of metabolism; (2) environmental factors, such as diet, nutrition, xenobiotic exposure, etc., are diverse among humans; and (3) humans generally have more control and probably more interest in consumption of varied non-nutritive materials, such as alcohol, drugs, etc. These, as well as other factors, result in a large diversity in susceptibility to xenobiotic exposure. This is, in part, why such large safety factors are employed in risk or hazard assessments of xenobiotics to which humans may be exposed. These safety factors are used to attempt to protect the vast majority of individuals at risk. For further discussions of species differences, the reader is directed to the articles by Walker and Oesch (182) and by Caldwell (22). A discussion of intraindividual and interindividual differences can be found in the monograph by Vesell and Penno (178). For detailed reviews of P450 in a number of species, including plants, see (149).

Gender differences in xenobiotic metabolism may be an important factor in gender-dependent differences in toxicity. The best example of gender differences in xenobiotic metabolism, especially cytochrome P450-mediated metabolism, is the rat. Because the rat is commonly used in toxicological safety assessments, it is important to realize the gender differences in this species and understand how it relates to the extrapolation of rat data to humans.

Generally, male rats have a higher capacity to metabolize xenobiotics than females. This difference is, in most part, related to the cytochromes P450. Although females have 10%–30% less total P450 than males, this difference is not high enough to explain the 2- 20-fold difference seen in metabolism. Much of the differential seen between males and females can be explained by differences in P450 isozymes between the sexes. For instance, males express CYP2C11 whereas females do not. Isozymes that predominate in males are CYP2A1, CYP2A2, and CYP3A2. Adult females also have predominant P450s, such as CYP2C12, which occurs in juvenile and older males but not in young adult males. These differences are under hormonal control and can be altered by procedures such as castration and administration of sex hormones. They also are developmentally controlled, and the stage of life at which these procedures are done can influence their outcome. Neonatal castration of male rats results in different expression of P450 when they become adults. The adult expression of P450s can actually be "imprinted" during the neonatal period. Although sex hormones play an important role in the expression of P450 in rats, other hormones, including growth hormone, thyroxine, insulin, and somatostatin, may play important roles.

These differences between male and female rats also show an age dependency. As male rats age, their P450 isozyme profiles begin to appear more like females. Toxicologists using rats as a model in safety assessments need to be cognizant of these gender- and age-dependent changes. The toxicity data from young rats, generally used in toxicity studies, may not reflect the toxicity seen in old rats. During chronic toxicity and carcinogenicity studies, the response of rats to the toxicity of a test material may change as the study progresses. This is especially true of carcinogenicity studies that begin with in utero exposure. Early developmental changes in P450 in animals and humans may be important in responses to teratogens and embryotoxic compounds (112).

If gender differences in xenobiotic metabolism in rats can complicate toxicity assessments, what about other species, including humans? Rats have been the most intensively investigated species in regard to gender differences; however, studies with other species suggest that they generally do not demonstrate such large gender differences. Mice, another species important in toxicology studies, generally do not show the exaggerated gender differences in xenobiotic metabolism seen in rats. Gender differences in mice seem to be dependent on the specific strain of mouse investigated. Where gender differences do exist in mice, it is generally the female that has the higher metabolic capacity, but the differences are not as great as that seen in rats.

Other species used in toxicological investigations, such as dogs, appear to demonstrate some gender differences in the expression of P450 isozymes, but, again, they are not as exaggerated as in rats. Although there are few reported studies, monkeys have not been reported to demonstrate significant gender differences in xenobiotic metabolism.

Humans have not been shown to demonstrate gender-dependent differences in the expression of P450 isozymes. Although there can be significant differences between human males and females in xenobiotic biodisposition, these appear to be more based on anatomical and physiological differences that affect absorption, distribution, and excretion. There can be large differences between individual humans based on life-style factors and exposure to environmental chemicals, food, and drugs; however, there do not appear to be inherent gender differences in the expression of P450.

This raises the question as to how species, such as rats, can be used to predict toxicity in humans. With care and knowledge of the differences between rats and humans, the rat can serve as a model for human toxicity. This has been shown through decades of use. For instance, rats and humans share similarities between the CYP isozyme subfamilies CYP1A1, CYP1A2, and CYP2E1, and these subfamilies are not expressed in a highly gender-dependent manner in rats. Xenobiotics that are substrates for these isozymes may be metabolized in a similar manner in rats and humans. Gender-dependent differences in xenobiotic metabolism are but one of the reasons toxicologists must use both sexes in the safety assessment of chemicals. Gender differences in xenobiotic metabolism have recently been reviewed (120).

Pharmacogenetics, Human Polymorphism of P450 Isozymes, and Their Toxicological Significance

Pharmacogenetics is the study of the hereditary basis of the observed differences in response (both therapeutic and adverse) to drugs by individuals and populations. The term can be expanded to include not only drugs but also dietary and environmental chemicals. This field has seen a large expansion over the last decade, as the understanding of the genetics, genetic regulation, and interindividual variations in P450 and other xenobiotic metabolism enzymes has increased. New methodologies from molecular biology and refinement of other methodologies to study genetic differences in individuals and populations have spurred interest in the pharmacogenetics of xenobiotic metabolism.

Many studies of the adverse effects of chemicals in animals and humans have indicated there are highly significant differences between animal strains, individual animals, and especially differences in individual humans and different human population groups. These genetic *polymorphisms* can result in unexpected drug and environmental toxicities and complicate safety assessments and the extrapolation of data from animal studies to humans. As discussed later, this has led to recommendations that the specific family and subfamily of P450 that metabolizes a specific drug candidate be determined during early drug discovery efforts. This could avoid unexpected interactions and suggest potential adverse effects before additional developmental efforts with a drug or other chemical product are undertaken.

Several human P450s have been shown to be polymorphically expressed, including CYP1A1, CYP2A6, CYP2C9, CYP2C19, CYP2D6, and CYP2E1. The chromosomal locations of these P450 genes have been identified and the genetic basis for the altered P450 activity is becoming understood. For instance, several alleles in the CYP2D6 family are known to contain specific nucleotide deletions that result in inactive genes and a lack of production of the CYP2D6 protein (34). Individuals homozygous for these gene variations will be "poor metabolizers" of CYP2D6 substrates. In contrast, some individuals have multiple copies of the CYP2D6 gene, possibly due to gene duplication (80). These individuals have enhanced capability to metabolize CYP2D6 substrates and are "ultra-rapid metabolizers" (9). A chemical whose detoxification depends on CYP2D6 would be more toxic than expected in the poor metabolizers, but less toxic than expected in the ultra-rapid metabolizers. In contrast, a chemical that is metabolically activated would be less toxic in poor metabolizers and more toxic in ultra-rapid metabolizers. To predict toxicity, it is obvious that not only must the role of metabolism in the toxicity of a compound be known, but also the potential genotype of exposed individuals.

Major advances have been made in determining the genotypes of individuals in respect to P450 isozymes. These range from the in vivo administration of probe drugs and determination of their metabolites as probes of metabolic capability and P450 genotype to the tools of modern molecular biology. For instance, the CYP2D6 genotype of individuals and populations can be probed using polymerase chain reaction (PCR) technology, followed by restriction endonuclease digestion, as well as other techniques (159). Genotyping studies have shown that the most common CYP2D6 mutations occur in about 7% of Caucasians and less than 1% of Asians.

CYP2D6 represents one of the first P450 polymorphisms discovered and one of the most extensively studied from the aspects of genetics, biochemistry, and clinical significance. It also is an excellent example of how all of these factors come into play to define a P450's role as a determinate of toxicity. Smith and his colleagues were among the first to suggest that the high incidence of side effects associated with debrisoquine, an antihypertensive, might be due to genetic differences in debrisoquine metabolism (103). The early studies led to the knowledge that debrisoquine was metabolized to its 4-hydroxy metabolite by CYP2D6. Investigations of the substrate specificity of this P450 have indicated that its preferred substrates are basic arylalkylamines with an ionized nitrogen at physiological pH. The site of oxidation is generally on or near a planar aromatic system 5–7 A from the basic nitrogen (160). A proposed strong ion pairing between the substrate nitrogen and an aspartic acid in the active site of the P450 suggest it would have a high affinity for its substrates. This is supported by its low K_m and K_i, compared to other P450s.

Although the requirements for a compound to be a substrate for CYP2D6 appear stringent, it has been shown to metabolize over 30 prescribed and over-the-counter drugs, including members of a variety of drug classes such as β-adrenergic blocking agents, antiarrhythmics, and antidepressants, among others. From this listing, it is obvious that CYP2D6 polymorphism is of clinical significance. In addition, it has been linked with increased risk of cancer in several organs, Parkinson's disease, and dopamine neurotransmission.

Regulatory and Product Development Aspects of Xenobiotic Metabolism

International regulatory agencies require some information about the metabolism of drugs and other chemicals that fall under their jurisdiction. The amount of data required will depend on the use of the chemical, its potential exposure to humans, and the potential role of metabolism in its efficacy and toxicity. Early information on the metabolism of drugs is becoming essential for the selection of drug candidates for further development. With the development of combinatorial synthetic chemistry and high-throughput pharmacological screening, the number of potential drug candidates that need to be rapidly screened for their potential metabolism has increased dramatically. This is leading to the development of rapid methods to predict metabolism and potential drug–drug interactions. Data are needed from in vitro and in vivo animal models that will be used in safety assessments to allow the toxicologist to design appropriate studies during the preclinical phase of a safety assessment. Data are also needed concerning the potential human metabolism of the drug candidate to allow the toxicologist to extrapolate animal safety data to humans. In the recent past, it was difficult to obtain in vitro data from human tissues. With the current knowledge of the human P450 isozymes and the commercial availability of human hepatic preparations and cells that express human P450s, it is possible to obtain data concerning human metabolism of drug candidates.

The U.S. Food and Drug Administration (FDA) has recently released a guidance document concerning in vitro drug metabolism and drug–drug interaction studies during the drug development process (173). This document stresses the importance of obtaining information on a drug candidate's metabolism during the early stages of development. This information is important in predicting potential individual differences based on polymorphic expression of xenobiotic metabolism enzymes and in predicting drug–drug interactions. The guidance document is based on the following general observations:

1. The concentrations of a drug or its active metabolite circulating in the body determine the extent of its desirable and/or adverse effects.
2. A major determinant of a drug's concentration is clearance, and metabolism is a major determinant of clearance.
3. Drugs that are not substantially metabolized may impact the metabolism of other drugs.
4. Large differences in blood concentrations can occur because of polymorphic metabolism. Drug–drug interactions can also produce large changes in the blood concentration of a drug.
5. Major advances have been made in availability of human tissue and recombinant enzymes for in vitro studies of drug metabolism.

The guidance document suggests that the goals of in vitro metabolism and interaction studies should be (1) to identify major metabolic pathways and the specific isozymes involved, and (2) to explore and extrapolate the effects of the drug candidate on the metabolism of other drugs and the effect of other drugs on the candidate's metabolism. To accomplish these goals, the FDA suggests starting from human hepatic microsomes, now commercially available, then moving to expression systems that express specific human P450s, which are also commercially available. They note it is possible to move to hepatocytes and precision-cut liver slices but realize there are technical difficulties with these preparations.

Co-incubation of the drug candidate with substrate probes with known metabolic pathways can be used to determine its effects on their metabolism. In addition, assessment of the drug candidates' metabolism by CYP3A4 may provide information on intestinal metabolism that can affect drug bioavailability. Parallel studies using preparations from animal models can aid the toxicologist in choice of species for the toxicological studies. The document points out that in vitro studies currently cannot replace in vivo studies but can give direction for the proper design of in vivo studies. For instance, if the drug candidate is not metabolized by CYP2D6, then it will not be important to study the impact of the slow metabolizer phenotype on potential adverse effects. If the drug candidate is not a substrate for CYP3A4, then there is less concern that inhibition of CYP3A4 by drugs such as ketoconazole and erythromycin or induction by rifampin and anticonvulsants could cause problems.

Role of the Cytochrome P450–dependent Monooxygenase in Toxicity

The toxicity of any agent is dependent on its concentration at its target site. This is a function of many factors, including the route of exposure, the pharmacokinetics of the xenobiotic, the excretion of both the parent compound and its metabolites, and the sensitivity of the target site. The ability of the organism to clear the xenobiotic through excretion will have a profound influence on the concentration at the target site. Directly associated with the ability to clear many xenobiotics is the ability to metabolize the xenobiotic to more water-soluble metabolites.

Without doubt, the P450–dependent monooxygenase plays a pivotal role in the metabolism of xenobiotics. It is the prime metabolic route for the majority of xenobiotics, acting either directly in detoxication or indirectly by priming the xenobiotic for further metabolism through functionalization, as illustrated in other sections of this chapter.

The original interest in the P450 system was associated with its ability to metabolize drugs and decrease both their toxicity and duration of action. It soon became evident that, in certain cases, this enzyme system converted certain drugs from pharmacologically inactive forms to active forms. Examples of the metabolic activation of toxicants, such as the in vivo conversion of the inactive insecticide parathion to its active form, paraoxon, were soon encountered. It was also discovered that this enzyme system could activate stable molecules such as benzo(a)pyrene to highly reactive metabolites capable of damaging cellular macromolecules, as shown in Figure 3.4. Further studies have indicated that metabolic activation plays an important role in the toxicity of a number of xenobiotics.

Studies undertaken to understand the biochemistry of P450 played a large role in the development of the modern fields of biochemical and molecular toxicology. Currently, much effort is placed on the determination of the balance between metabolite activation, detoxication, and detoxication of activated metabolites. This is providing new insight for the toxicologist in understanding the toxicity of xenobiotics. Studies on the active sites of P450 and other xenobiotic metabolism enzymes, and the factors that influence their activity and their expression, are bringing toxicologists closer to being able to predict potential toxicity with more accuracy. These efforts are also aiding toxicologists in the difficult task of predicting human toxicity from studies done with cellular and animal models.

Other Enzymes Associated with Oxidative Metabolism

Microsomal Flavin-containing Monooxygenase

Since 1960, it has been apparent that a microsomal monooxygenase other than P450 could catalyze the oxygenation of nucleophilic nitrogen, sulfur, and phosphorus compounds. Purification to homogeneity indicated it was an NADPH-dependent, flavin-containing monooxygenase that does not contain P450. This monooxygenase (EC 1.14.13.8) has been referred to as amine oxidase, Ziegler enzyme, dimethylaniline monooxygenase, and flavin-containing monooxygenase. This enzyme may be a good example of proteins involved in normal anabolic and catabolic metabolism being recruited for xenobiotic metabolism. The flavin prosthetic group that is characteristic of these enzymes is especially versatile at carrying out redox functions.

The catalytic cycle for the flavin-containing monooxygenase is shown in Figure 3.5. NADPH reduces the FAD of the enzyme, and the oxidized $NADP^+$ remains bound. Oxygen then binds to yield FAD peroxide followed by substrate binding. An oxygen atom from the peroxide is transferred to the substrate leaving the hydroxyflavin. The final and rate-limiting step of the cycle is the dehydration to regenerate FAD, yield water, and release the bound $NADP^+$. NADH can substitute for NADPH, but with lower affinity and activity.

There are at least five isoforms of the flavin-containing monooxygenase, designated as FMO1-FMO5, whose genes are expressed across several species and tissues. These forms have different substrate specificities and are probably related to the species-dependent toxicity

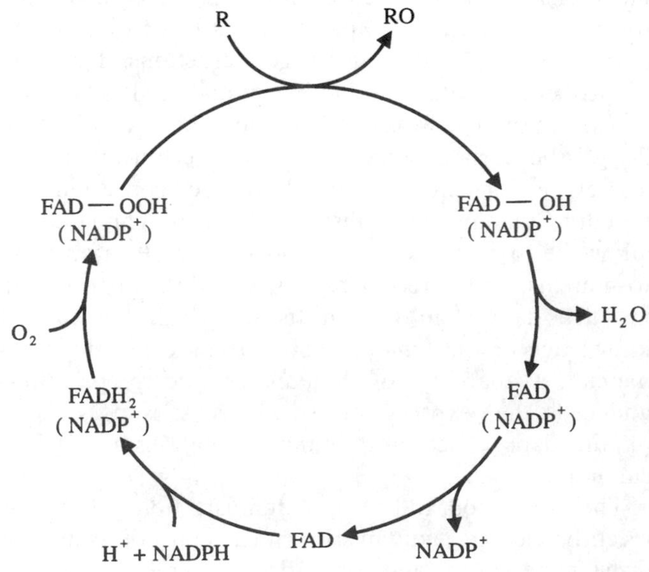

FIG. 3.5. Catalytic cycle of the flavin-containing monooxygenase. Adapted from References 194 and 195.

of certain substrates, such as the pyrrolizidine alkaloids. Humans, rats, and mice have relatively high activity of FMO1 in kidney. Humans and mice have low activity for this form in the liver, whereas the rat has high activity. Humans and mice have high activity of FMO3 in the liver, whereas the rat has low activity. No FMO3 activity has been detected in human kidney but rat and mouse kidney show high activity. In mice, only females express FMO3 and have two- to threefold higher activity of FMO1 compared to males. FMO5 shows no gender differences. Male rats have higher total FMO than females, and two- to threefold more FMO1 than females, but no differences are seen in FMO3 (27). Humans can show considerable individual differences, but no gender differences have been detected. This illustrates the species, gender, and tissue differences that can be encountered with this monooxygenase and emphasizes the importance of choosing an appropriate animal model for toxicological studies of compounds that are potential substrates for this enzyme.

This microsomal enzyme catalyzes the oxidative attack on the nucleophilic nitrogen and sulfur heteroatom of a variety of xenobiotics (195) (See Table 3.4). It was once believed that oxidations of basic aliphatic and tertiary aromatic amines were carried out by the flavin-containing monooxygenase while primary aromatic amines and the acidic nitrogens of amides were catalyzed by P450, whereas secondary amines were oxidized by both enzyme systems. More recent studies with the purified enzymes have demonstrated that there is no clear division between the types of substrates preferred by the two enzymes. Therefore, the metabolism of each nitrogen-containing xenobiotic must be considered on an individual basis. The thermal instability of the flavin monooxygenase in the absence of NADPH (above 35°C) has provided a tool to separate the activity of this enzyme in vitro from that of P450; however, defining the relative contribution of the flavin monooxygenase and P450 to the metabolism of many xenobiotics is difficult because some inhibitors of P450, such as SKF-525A, are substrates for the flavin monooxygenases. More selective inhibitors of P450, such as N-benzylimidazole and aminobentotriazole, are a better choice for distinguishing these two enzymes (195). Antibodies to specific P450 isozymes can be used to inhibit P450 and determine the role of the flavin-containing monooxygenase.

Many nitrogen- and sulfur-containing xenobiotics are metabolized by this phase I enzyme, as seen in Table 3.4. *N*-oxidation of nucleophilic tertiary amines yields *N*-oxides. Primary and secondary amines are oxidized to hydroxylamines. In addition, primary amines can be oxidized to oximes and secondary amines to nitrones. Thiols, thioethers, and other xenobiotics containing sulfur can be oxidized to sulfur oxides. The flavin-containing monooxygenase has a relatively broad substrate specificity, but individual isozymes demonstrate some specificity. Broad substrate specificity and its occurrence in several tissues indicate that it can be a major determinant in oxidative xenobiotic metabolism.

Amine Oxidases

Amine oxidases can play a significant role in the metabolism of specific xenobiotics (167). Monoamine oxidase (MAO) (EC 1.4.3.4) and related amine oxidases catalyze the oxidative deamination of endogenous amines. They can also be involved in the metabolism of primary, secondary, and tertiary xenobiotic amines. Two of the amine oxidases (MAO and semicarbazide-sensitive amine oxidase) will be used as examples of amine oxidases.

Most tissues express two forms of the mitochondrial enzyme MAO, termed MAO-A and MAO-B, each expressed by a separate gene. MAO is a flavoprotein capable of oxidative deamination of primary, secondary, and tertiary amines. Metabolism of primary amines yields an aldehyde and ammonia, whereas secondary amines yield an aldehyde and a primary amine. The aldehyde products may be further metabolized by other enzymes to carboxylic acids or alcohols. Unlike the monooxygenases, the oxygen used in the reaction is derived from water. During the oxidation, the FAD prosthetic group is reduced ($FAD \rightarrow FADH_2$) then reoxidized by oxygen with the production of hydrogen peroxide.

A well-publicized example of an MAO-related toxicity was initiated by individuals attempting to synthesize a narcotic related to demerol. Instead of the intended product, 1-methyl-4-phenyl-1,2,5,6-tetrahydropyridine (MPTP) resulted from the synthesis. Individuals who self-administered MPTP demonstrated Parkinson's disease–like symptoms. This was related to neuro-cytotoxicity in dopaminergic neurons produced by brain MAO-B metabolism of MPTP to 1-methyl-4-phenyl-2,3-dihydropyridine ($MPDP^+$), which oxidizes to the neurotoxic 1-methyl-4-phenylpyridine (MPP^+). The cytotoxicity of MPP^+ results from its inhibition of mitochondrial respiration.

A number of amine drugs have been shown to be substrates for MAO. Some of these act as pro-drugs and require MAO metabolism to produce the active form; others have their activities limited by MAO metabolism. MAO-A and MAO-B have different substrate specificities, but there can be overlap in specificity.

Semicarbazide-sensitive amine oxidases (SSAO) (EC 1.4.3.6), like monoamine oxidase, catalyzes the oxidative deamination of endogenous amines, but also can metabolize xenobiotic amines (102,167). The SSAO do not contain a flavin but do contain copper. They demonstrate a more limited activity than MAO by only catalyzing deamination of primary aliphatic and aro-

Table 3.4
Functional groups oxidized by flavin-containing monooxygenase

Functional group	Compound class	Example
$RSH \rightarrow RSSR$	*Sulfur Oxidation* Thiols	Cystamine → cysteamine
$RSSR \rightarrow RS(=O)SR$	Disulfides	
$RSR \rightarrow RS(=O)R \rightarrow RS(=O)_2R$	Sulfides	Cimetidine, aldicarb
$-N(-)-C(SH)-NH \rightarrow -N(-)-C(=S{=}O)-NH_2 \rightarrow -N(-)-C(SO_2H)=NH$	Thiocarbamides	
$R-C(S)-NH_2 \rightarrow R-C(=S{=}O)-NH_2 \rightarrow R-C(SO_2H)=NH_2$	Thioamides	Thioacetamide, thiobenzamide
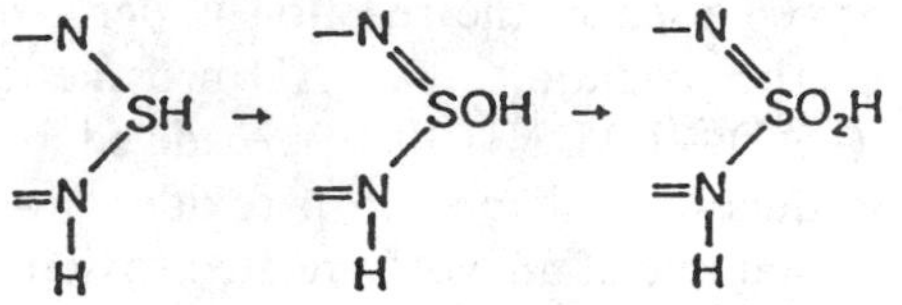	Mercaptopurines and pyrimidines	
	Nitrogen Oxidation	
Acrylic $R-N(R_1)(R_2) \rightarrow R-N(OH)(R_1)-R_2$	Tertiary amines	Chloropromazine, cocaine, fluphenazine, nicotine
Cyclic 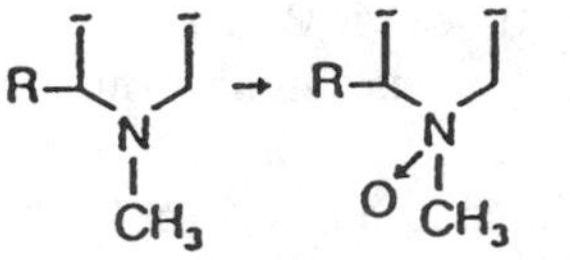		
$R-NH-R_1 \rightarrow R-N(OH)-R_1 \rightarrow R{=}N(\rightarrow O)-R_1$	Secondary amines	Desipramine, *N*-methylaniline
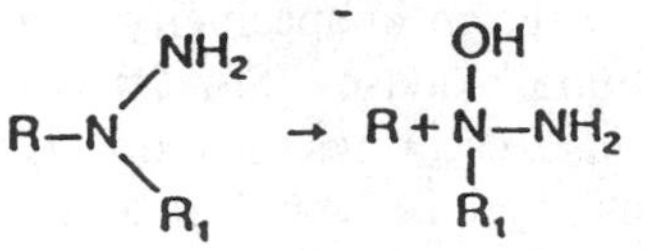	Hydrazines	Dimethylthydrazine, procarbazine, benzylthydrazine
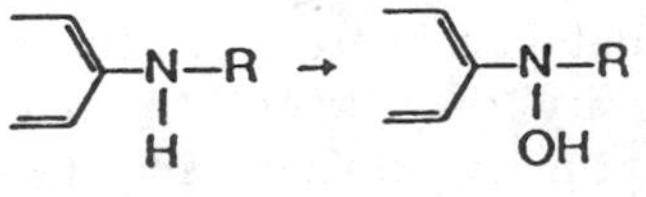	*N*-Alkylarylamines	2-Acetylaminofluorene

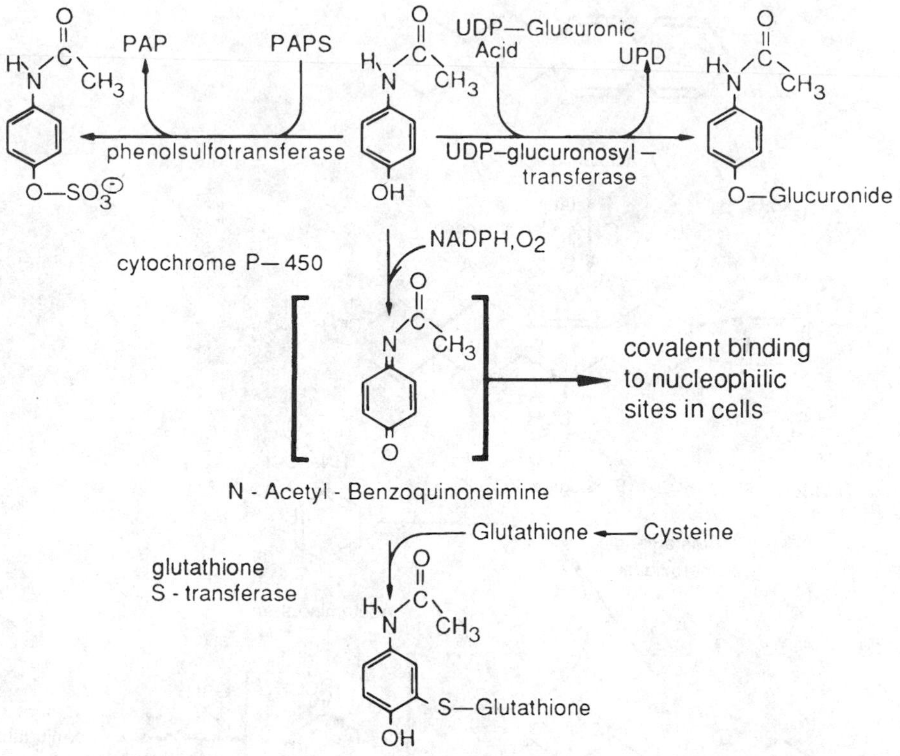

FIG. 3.6. Biotransformation of the analgesic acetaminophen.

matic monoamines. They are sensitive to inhibition by semicarbazide but insensitive to the classic MAO inhibitors. The products of their reaction are an aldehyde, ammonia, and hydrogen peroxide. They occur in most species, including bacteria, fungi, plants, and animals. In animals, they occur in plasma and bound to tissues. Although they can metabolize several endogenous substrates (191), their exact physiological role is currently unknown. There are considerable species differences with SSAO. For instance, rats have relatively low concentrations of plasma SSAO compared to humans. SSAO can metabolize certain xenobiotics to more toxic metabolites. 3-Aminopropene has been used in the manufacture of pharmaceuticals and in rubber vulcanization. Chronic exposure to this compound can produce lesions similar to acute myocardial necrosis and atherosclerosis. SSAO appears to metabolize 3-aminopropene to 2-propenal (acrolein), which alkylates glutathione *S*-transferase and allows excessive peroxidative damage (66). Damage occurs in the heart and aortic tissue, which have high SSAO activity (30).

Co-oxidation of Xenobiotics by Prostaglandin Synthase H

Pathways other than the monooxygenases may be involved in xenobiotic oxidation. Marnett and Reed (107) demonstrated that prostaglandin H synthetase, an enzyme system responsible for prostaglandin biosynthesis, was capable of oxidizing benzo(a)pyrene to quinones. Two catalytic activities co-purify with the synthase: fatty acid cyclooxygenase and prostaglandin hydroperoxidase. The cyclooxygenase catalyzes arachidonic acid oxidation to prostaglandin G_2, and the hydroperoxidase reduces the hydroperoxidase (–OOH) to the corresponding alcohol in prostaglandin H_2, as shown in Figure 3.7. Oxidation of xenobiotics results from a one-electron pathway involving an oxidizing agent produced during the hydroperoxidase-catalyzed reduction of prostaglandin G_2 to the hydroxy endoperoxide, prostaglandin H_2. Prostaglandin synthetase is a major source of alkyl hydroperoxides produced during normal metabolism (108). Most tissues possess prostaglandin synthetase activity and are capable of oxidizing certain xenobiotics, even if the tissue is low in P450 content. In fact, acetaminophen, which is activated to a reactive intermediate by P450 (Figure 3.6), can be activated by prostaglandin synthetase in the medulla of the kidney (Figure 3.7). This tissue is low in P450 activity, but in the presence of arachidonic acid, the medulla activates acetaminophen to a reactive intermediate that covalently binds to tissue macromolecules (14). Other compounds that undergo co-oxidation include aminopyrine, benzphetamine, oxyphenbutazone, benzidine, and benzo(a)pyrene.

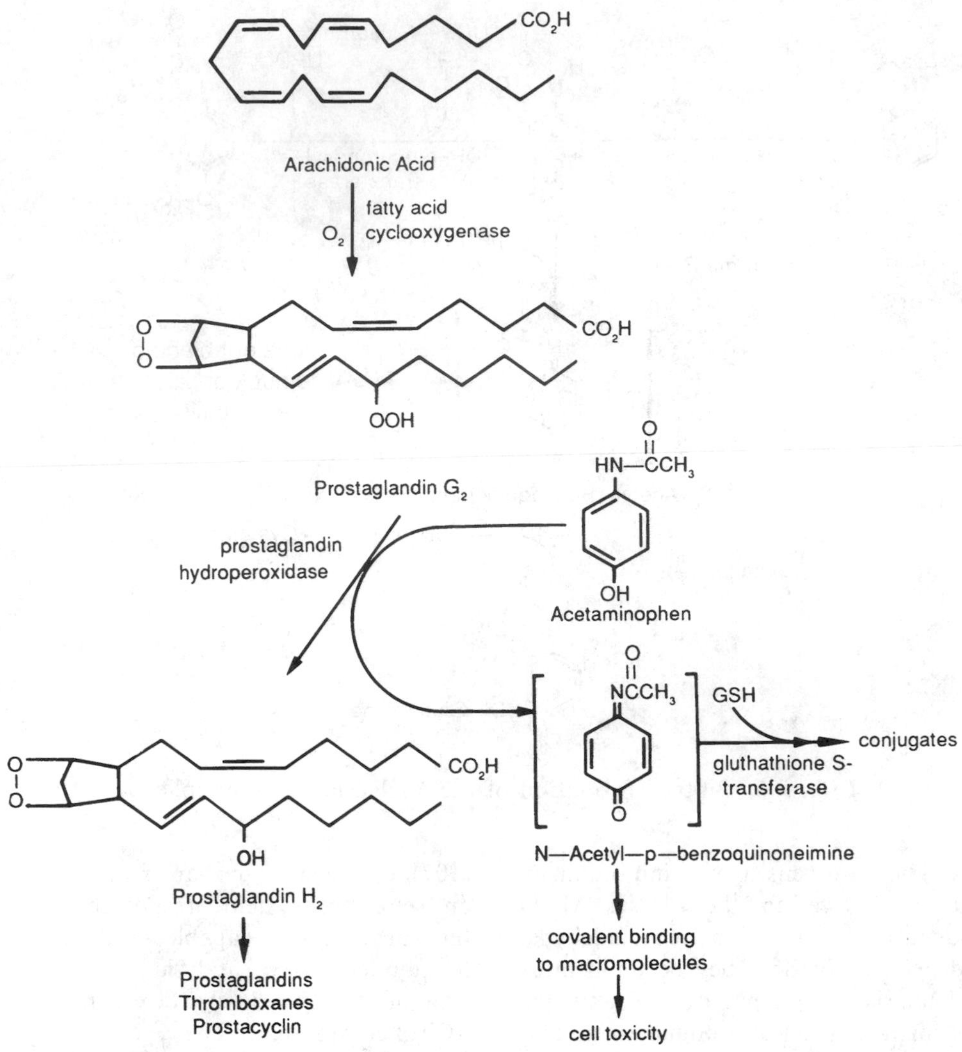

FIG. 3.7. Co-oxidation of acetaminophen by prostaglandin endoperoxide synthetase.

The bladder also possesses high prostaglandin synthetase activity. Mattammal et al. (109) proposed that several structurally diverse renal and bladder carcinogens are metabolically activated by prostaglandin synthetase. For example, the bladder carcinogen 2-amino-4-(5-nitro-2-furyl)thiazole is believed to be activated by prostaglandin synthetase co-oxidation in bladder transitional epithelium to metabolites capable of covalently modifying RNA and DNA. Feeding aspirin to rats can inhibit the bladder lesion induced by 5-nitrofuran, the ultimate carcinogen. This suggests that prostaglandin synthetase is involved in the metabolic activation, as aspirin is a specific inhibitor of prostaglandin synthetase.

Use of the analgesic p-phenetidine has declined because of reports of kidney damage in man following prolonged use of the drug. Andersson et al. (5) proposed a mechanism by which phenetidine is activated by prostaglandin synthetase in the kidney. The primary amine nitrogen of phenetidine undergoes a one-electron oxidation similar to that shown in Figure 3.7 for acetaminophen. This leads to hydrogen abstraction yielding a reactive nitrenium radical. This radical is postulated based on its rate of reaction with reduced glutathione. Benzene can be hydroxylated to phenol in the liver by P450, and the phenol can be further oxidized to hydroquinone. The phenol and hydroquinone can enter the blood stream and be distributed to other tissues. In the bone marrow, the phenol stimulates prostaglandin synthetase peroxidative activation of hydroquinone to reactive metabolites that form adducts with nucleophiles, such as protein and DNA. This is believed to result in the bone marrow suppression seen with chronic exposure to benzene. Phenolic compounds may be converted to reactive phenoxyl radicals by the one-electron oxidative process. Other peroxidases, such as lactoperoxidase and myeloperoxidase, may be involved in xenobiotic metabolism.

BIOCHEMICAL CONJUGATIONS

Mammals can synthesize xenobiotic conjugates that are more polar and readily excreted, compared with the parent compound. Conjugate synthesis is finely controlled through various feedback pathways. Two major reactants are required for conjugate synthesis: a xenobiotic with the appropriate functional group and a cosubstrate that can be conjugated with the xenobiotic. If the xenobiotic does not have a functional group amenable to conjugation, such as a hydroxyl group, it may be oxidized (functionalized) by cytochromes P450. The oxidized product and the cosubstrate must be simultaneously available for conjugation. Both functions must be tightly integrated for rapid excretion of the xenobiotic. Although the forthcoming sections will discuss each conjugating system as a separate entity, it must be emphasized that in vivo metabolism is integrated. Examples showing the integration of the conjugating systems with related pathways will be described.

Glucuronidation: Uridine Diphosphoglucuronosyltransferases

P450s are the principal phase I oxidative enzymes. Similarly, uridine diphospho(UDP)glucuronosyltransferases (also known as UDP-glycosyltransferases) are the principal phase II enzymes. Glucuronosyltranferases can use monooxygenase products to form glucuronides; however, it is not a necessity for substrates of the glucuronosyltransferase to be monooxygenase products. Significant numbers of xenobiotics and certain endobiotics possess the necessary functional groups for glucuronidation and do not require functionalization. These enzymes belong to a superfamily of related genes, and over 30 glucuronosyltransferases have been purified or cloned and expressed.

Whereas the multienzyme complex of the P450 monooxygenase is termed a *system* because the enzymes are closely linked, the multiple enzymes of glucuronidation are not linked, but are interdependent. The general reaction mechanism of the conjugating enzymes involves the activation of an endogenous molecule. Subsequent reaction of this activated form of the endogenous molecule with the xenobiotic produces the conjugate. Activation may occur in a different cellular compartment than conjugation, as is the case with glucuronidation. Activation of glucose occurs in the cytosol, whereas conjugation occurs in the lumen of the endoplasmic reticulum. UDP-glucuronosyltransferases occur in several tissues, but their highest activity is found in the liver. Other tissues containing these enzymes include kidney, intestine, lung, skin, adrenals, and spleen. Extrahepatic glucuronosyltransferases may be differentially expressed and demonstrate different isoforms compared to the liver (123,165).

Although the products of P450 are more water soluble than their parent compounds, some still possess considerable lipophilicity. Subsequent conjugation produces metabolites with higher water solubility. These metabolites can generally be readily excreted in the bile or urine. Transport proteins can recognize the glucuronic acid moiety of the glucuronide and aid in excretion from the liver and kidney. An additional method by which glucuronidation produces less toxic metabolites is via the addition of a bulky moiety to the xenobiotic. This can result in both the shielding of reactive portions of the xenobiotic and in the blocking of reactions between the xenobiotic and the site responsible for the toxicological sequelae. In some cases, the product of glucuronidation has more biological activity than the parent compound, and conjugation can be considered metabolic activation, although examples are far fewer than with P450 oxidation.

Glucuronides are either secreted by the liver into the bile, and consequently found in the feces, or by the kidney into the urine. The excretion route is generally dependent upon the molecular weight of the xenobiotic. The rat excretes glucuronides of xenobiotics with molecular weights greater than about 250–300 in the bile and those with lower molecular weights in the urine. Higher molecular weight xenobiotics, such as morphine, chloramphenicol, and endogenous steroids, are excreted in bile and enter the intestine. Biliary excretion can result in enterohepatic circulation, which can cause prolonged plasma half-lives for some compounds. The intestine contains β-glucuronidase, from the intestinal microflora, that catalyzes the hydrolysis of glucuronides. This releases the xenobiotic in the intestine, where it can be absorbed into the blood. The xenobiotic can then be taken up by the liver, where it is reconjugated and excreted into the bile, where the cycle is again initiated. This can cause prolonged exposure to target organs, such as the liver, and result in unanticipated toxicity.

History of the discovery of glucuronidation and the glucuronosyltransferases is interesting, and the reader is directed to Williams' classic book on detoxication mechanisms (189) and the comprehensive discussions of this enzyme (40,170).

Nomenclature for UDP-Glucuronosyltransferase Gene Superfamily

Nomenclature for the UDP-glucuronosyltransferases has progressed similar to that for the P450 superfamily. It has been proposed that each gene be identified by the root symbol UGT for *U*DP-*g*lucuronosyl*t*ransferase.

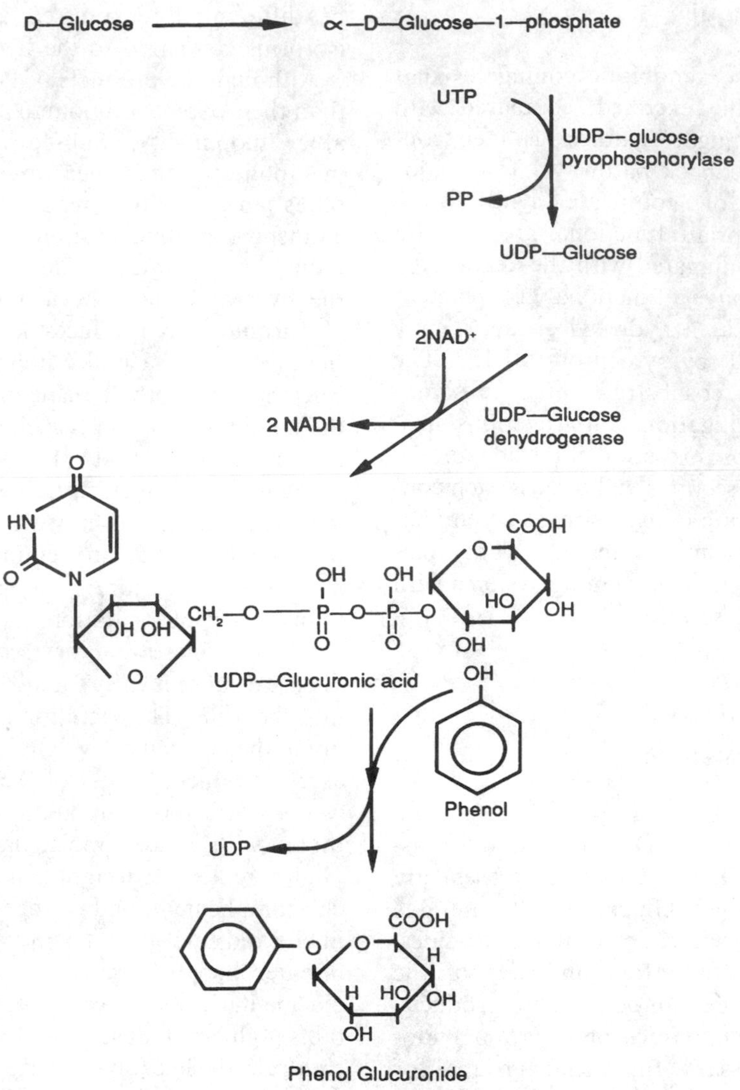

FIG. 3.8. Glucuronidation of phenol. An example of the pathway leading to production of glucuronic acid conjugates.

The gene family is identified by a number and a letter is added to designate the subfamily (UGT2B) followed by a number to identify the gene (UGT2B1). This system, as with the P450 nomenclature, is an attempt to provide isoforms with a name that is not only specific but reflects the evolutionary divergence of the genes. As new discoveries are being made, the nomenclature for these enzymes is evolving.

Biochemistry of Glucuronidation

Glucuronidation (illustrated in Figure 3.8) requires the availability of three reactants:

1. UDP-α-D-glucuronic acid (UDPGA), generated in the cytoplasm.
2. UDP-glucuronosyltransferase (UDPGT, EC 2.4.1.17), bound to the endoplasmic reticulum.
3. Substrate with the requisite functional group and some hydrophobic character.

Maximal enzyme activity is dependent on optimal concentrations of these reactants at the membrane site of catalysis.

As seen in Figure 3.8, D-glucose is the original precursor of UDPGA. During anabolic metabolism, D-glucose is converted to α-D-glucose-1-phosphate. This compound serves as substrate for UDP-glucose pyrophosphorylase (EC 2.7.7.9), which catalyzes its reaction with uridine triphosphate to yield the high-energy phosphate containing UDP-D-glucose and pyrophosphate. UDP-D-glucose then reacts with nicotine adenine dinucleotide (NAD) catalyzed by UDP-glucose dehydrogenase (EC 1.1.1.22) to yield UDP-D-glucuronic acid, which completes glucose activation. This compound is termed the *glycone*, indicating its source. The xenobiotic that is conjugated is termed the *aglycone*. Glucose activation occurs within the cytoplasm, whereas glucuronidation of the aglycone occurs at the endoplasmic reticulum. Because UDP-D-glucose is also used in glycogen synthesis, it generally is available in the cell. This is not true for all conjugation reactions, and may be one of the reasons that glucuronidation is a major conjugation pathway.

The topology of UDP-glucuronosyltransferases is important for understanding substrate specificity and the need to disrupt microsomes with detergents or other means before assaying these enzymes in vitro. It is believed that large interlaboratory variation of in vitro glucuronidation data comes from variation in detergent-released latency. UDP-glucuronosyltransferases are oriented in the endoplasmic reticulum in such a way that the majority of the protein protrudes into the lumen of the endoplasmic reticulum. The intraluminal portion of the protein possesses the UDP-glucuronic acid-binding domain as well as the xenobiotic or endobiotic (endogenous substrates) binding domain. This means that UDP-glucuronic acid must pass through the membrane, possibly by carrier mediation, and that the substrate must also pass through the membrane (63). Molecular biology studies indicate that the C-terminal half of the protein is highly conserved among different UDP-glucuronosyltransferases, whereas the N-terminal region is highly variable. The C-terminal half of the protein contains the transmembrane sequences that anchor the enzyme within the membrane and the short portion of the C terminus that protrudes from the outside surface of the endoplasmic reticulum into the cytoplasm. The C-terminal half of the enzyme may contain a UDP-glucuronic acid binding site. The broad substrate specificity is believed to come from variation in the primary sequence of the N-terminal region where the substrate-binding domain resides (110).

UDP-glucuronic acid and the aglycone (xenobiotic or endobiotic) must be present for the conjugation reaction to be initiated. The number of xenobiotics that have been shown to be substrates for UDPGTs is large and continues to grow (113). The major functional groups forming glucuronides are (a) hydroxyl, (b) carboxyl, (c) amino, and (d) sulfhydryl. The substituents to which these functional groups are attached can be quite variable (see Table 3.5). Similar to the substrate requirements for monooxygenases of the endoplasmic reticulum, the aglycone must be somewhat lipid soluble to be a substrate for the UDPGTs. This requirement reflects the need for the xenobiotic to penetrate the endoplasmic reticulum to gain access to the active site. All of the endobiotics associated with normal metabolism and homeostasis that are substrates for the UDPGTs are lipid soluble and include bilirubin, catechols, such as 3-O-methyladrenaline, serotonin, and 17-hydroxy-containing steroids.

As noted earlier, UDP-glucuronosyltransferases constitute a multigene family, divided into subfamilies, consisting of a number of genes, all but one of which encode for an individual UDPGT isozyme. Evidence accumulated from differential induction and developmental studies, enzyme purification, immunochemical analysis, and the cloning of UDPGT cDNAs suggests the existence of at least 12 different UDPGT isozymes in the rat. Rat isozymes are divided into two gene families. The UGT1 family contains isozymes that appear related to a single gene, and each member of the UGT2 family is related to a unique gene. Some of the UGTI family are inducible by 3-methylcholanthrene and others are inducible by phenobarbital. Two members of the UGT2 family are inducible by phenobarbital.

A similar approach has been applied to human UDPGTs, and the heterogeneity of the enzyme in humans is now recognized. Compared to the rat, the characterization of the isozymes in humans is less complete. The expression of human liver UDPGT cDNAs in tissue culture is providing useful information on the substrate specificity of individual isozymes. Site-directed mutagenesis is proving useful to determine which amino acid sequences are modifying substrate specificity among these isozymes. Human isozymes are also divided into UGT1, which contains at least six isozymes from a single gene, similar to the rat. The human UGT2B family contains at least six isozymes from unique genes.

Reactions Catalyzed by the UDP-glucuronosyltransferases

As with many of the enzymes of detoxication, the glucuronosyltransferases have a low order of substrate specificity. This lack of substrate specificity makes them ideally suitable as detoxication enzymes. Whether or not they evolved as detoxication enzymes or represent enzymes of normal metabolism whose lack of specificity make them suitable for detoxication is open to debate. Of interest in this respect is that they occur only in higher organisms. Glucuronosyltransferases have been found in all mammals, birds, and reptiles that have been investigated, although their specific activities toward specific substrates may vary among different species and strains. Unlike the monooxygenase, they have not been found in bacteria and less developed species. This fact, among others, lends support to Dutton's hypothesis that these transferases evolved to metabolize endogenous compounds, such as bilirubin, catecholamines, and steroids, and not as detoxication enzymes (39).

Table 3.5
Functional groups forming glucuronides

Functional group	Compound class	Example
Hydroxyl → *O*-glucuronide	Alcohols	
–C–OH → –C–O–Glucuronic acid	Aliphatic	Trichlorethanol
	Alicyclic	Hexobarbital
	Benzylic	Methylphenylcarbinol
>N–OH → >N–O–Glucuronic acid	Phenolic	Phenol
	Enols	4-Hydroxycoumarin
Carboxyl → *O*-glucuronide	Hydroxyamines	*N*-hydroxy-2-acetylaminofluorene
	Carboxylic acids	
–C(=O)–OH → –C(=O)–O–Glucuronic acid	Aliphatic	2-Ethylhexanoic acid
	Aromatic	Benzoic acid
Amine → *N*-glucuronide	Arylalkyl	Phenylacetic acid
N-glucuronic acid	Heterocyclic	Nicotinic acid
–O–C(=O)–N(H)–*N*-glucuronic acid	Aromatic	Aniline
(R_3)—N^+—glucuronic acid		
	Carbamate	Meprobamate
R—SO_2—N(H)—glucuronic acid	Aliphatic tertiary Amine	Tripelennamine cotinine
	Sulfonamide	Sulfadimethoxine
Sulfhydryl → *S*-glucuronide		
O–*S*–glucuronic acid	Heterocyclic	Sulfisoxazole
C–*S*–glucuronic acid	Arylthiol	Thiophenol
Carbon → C–glucuronide		
C–glucuronic acid		
	Dithiocarbamic acid	
	1,3-Dicarbonyl system	Phenylbutazone

Modified from Reference 81.

Table 3.5 illustrates the functional groups, generally nucleophilic heteroatoms, that form glucuronides, and examples of the reactions. The glucuronides formed from these functional groups have different properties. Stability is among the most important with respect to detoxication. Breakdown of the glucuronide can lead to reformation of the parent compound, and in certain cases the production of highly reactive electrophilic species. These reactive species may be responsible for the production of acute and chronic toxicity by covalent binding to nucleophilic sites on tissue macromolecules.

Among the most commonly encountered glucuronides are those involving linkage of glucuronic acid and the xenobiotic through an oxygen atom. These *O*-glucuronides may form with a number of chemical classes including, aryl, alkyl, and acyl compounds, as illustrated in Table 3.5.

The alkyl-O-glucuronides are ether-linked glucuronides that can form from a variety of primary, secondary, and tertiary alcohols. Although generally stable at physiological conditions, they can be hydrolyzed under acidic conditions.

The enolic glucuronides are formed from aglycones without a free hydroxyl group. Glucuronides are formed from the enolized keto group. These conjugates lack the stability of the ether glucuronides and are susceptible to both acid and alkaline hydrolysis. They are more stable at neutral and alkaline pH than in acid conditions. Ester glucuronides can be produced from a variety of carboxylic acids, including primary, secondary and tertiary aliphatic acids and both aryl and heterocyclic compounds. They generally are stable in acidic conditions but are susceptible to alkaline hydrolysis.

The chemical properties of *N*-glucuronides are different from those of *O*-glucuronides. One of the most important of these is their lack of stability. They are especially unstable at pH below neutrality. The instability of these compounds may have important biological consequences; examples are discussed in more detail later. Quanternary ammonium *N*-glucuronides are formed by *N*-glucuronidation of cyclic and acyclic tertiary amines. These charged metabolites can be major metabolites of certain xenobiotics in higher primates while not being found in other animal models, such as the rat.

The *S*-glucuronides are not as commonly encountered as the *O*-glucuronides, but they represent important detoxication pathways for thiolic compounds. Their stability is similar to that of the *O*-glucuronides.

The *C*-glucuronides represent recently recognized conjugates, and only a few examples are known, such as phenylbutazone. Generally, they appear to be formed by the transferase, but other possible mechanisms of formation have been suggested.

Role of UDP-glucuronosyltransferases in Detoxication and Metabolic Activation

The foregoing discussion indicates that the UDP-glucuronosyltransferases play a critical role in the metabolism and detoxication of xenobiotics. Some substrates require functionalization by the monooxygenase before metabolism by the transferase, whereas others can be directly conjugated. The conjugates are more water soluble than the parent xenobiotic, and some readily form salts. Addition of the glycone may enable some of the conjugates to be more readily excreted through carrier-mediated mechanisms. Mechanisms other than increased excretion rates may also be important. The addition of the relatively bulky glycone may hide or hinder the biological reactivity of particular functional groups on the xenobiotic. In addition, binding of the toxicant to particular receptors responsible for toxicity may be blocked. Overall, these mechanisms represent an efficient system for detoxication. On the other hand, glucuronidation of certain compounds represents a metabolic activation where the product is more toxic than the parent compound.

Aromatic amines are among the most studied examples of the role glucuronidation plays in metabolic activation of carcinogens. These glucuronides transport the proximate carcinogen to the target site, where it decomposes to the species that react with cellular macromolecules producing the biochemical lesion responsible for generating the pathological lesion.

Several of the arylamines are potent bladder carcinogens, including 4-aminobiphenyl, 1-naphthylamine, and benzidine. Metabolic activation of these carcinogens to the ultimate carcinogen appears similar and requires the action of UDP-glucuronosyltransferase. Metabolic activation begins with P450–dependent activation of the arylamine to the proximate carcinogen, an *N*-hydroxyarylamine. Other specific ring hydroxylated forms may be produced and may represent more stable products. The unstable *N*-hydroxyarylamines are then converted to stable N-glucuronides. These *N*-glucuronides are transported to the bladder. In the bladder, the *N*-glucuronides are subject to β-glucuronidase activity, which splits off the glycone. They are also subject to hydrolysis in acidic urine producing the *N*-hydroxyarylamine. The *N*-hydroxyarylamine spontaneously converts to the electrophilic arylnitrenium ion as illustrated in Figure 3.9.

The electrophilic arylnitrenium ion can then react with nucleophilic centers on macromolecules of the bladder epithelium, especially DNA, to initiate tumor formation. The concentration of the glucuronide in the bladder, in combination with the time the glucuronide remains in

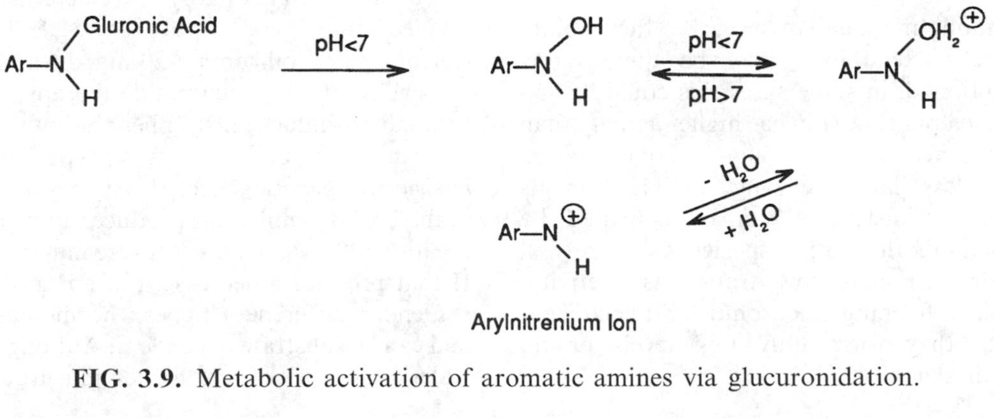

FIG. 3.9. Metabolic activation of aromatic amines via glucuronidation.

the bladder, can modify the potential for tumor formation. Glucuronides may function in this manner with a number of carcinogens and be important in explaining why certain target organs are susceptible to a specific carcinogen and others are not susceptible. In the above example, glucuronidation may protect the liver but make the bladder, the target organ, susceptible.

Glucuronidation has also been implicated in adverse drug reactions of certain carboxylic drugs, which resulted in a toxic immunological response. It is believed that a reactive glucuronide covalently binds to cellular proteins that act as haptens, producing an anaphylactic reaction.

Stable expression of cloned UDP-glucuronosyltransferases in tissue culture cell lines is providing a powerful new tool for understanding their role in the biotransformation of xenobiotics (21).

Species, Gender, and Genetic Differences in UDP-glucuronosyltransferase Activity

Studies of species, strain, and gender differences in glucuronidation are complicated by a number of factors. Activity may be affected by age, hormonal status, environmental exposure to xenobiotics in the diet and other sources, and by nutrition status. Factors associated with the methodology to determine differences in glucuronidation also play a role, including substrate, assay method, method of freeing latent activity, and the method of isolating the preparation employed to measure activity. This has led to a number of reports of differences in activity that could be artifactual. However, the large number of reports concerning differences in glucuronidation among species, strains, and the sexes indicate that certain of these differences are real and may have a genetic basis.

As mentioned previously, lower animals, including prokaryotes and invertebrates, do not produce glucuronides. Fish and reptiles do demonstrate glucuronidation of xenobiotics, but vary dramatically in activity, which is generally 10-fold or more lower than mammalian activity. Birds have glucuronidation ability similar to that of mammals.

Differences among mammalian species in their ability to glucuronidate a xenobiotic may be quite large; however, as mentioned, in some cases this could be artifactual. The guinea pig generally has higher activity than most other laboratory species. This higher activity may be associated with less latent enzyme activity, as its UDPG-glucuronosyltransferases can be activated by much gentler methods than other species. Cats are well known for their extremely low transferase activity. Although capable of forming glucuronides with endogenous compounds, they form only low levels or no glucuronides with xenobiotics.

Glucuronidation of amines is divided into two groups: nonquaternary N-conjugates and quaternary N-conjugates. There does not appear to be major species differences with the nonquaternary N-conjugate group, sulfonamides, arylamines, and cyclic and heterocyclic amines, although quantitative differences do exist. Quaternary glucuronidation occurs in primates, including humans, but not in other species. In humans, quaternary ammonium-linked glucuronides of aliphatic amines appear to be produced by UGT1A3 and UGT1A4 (28,61).

A well-known example of a strain difference is the almost complete lack of bilirubin glucuronidation in the Gunn rat. This rat strain also has low activity toward a number of xenobiotic substrates, but normal activity toward others. There is a genetic component to this, with the low activity being autosomally recessive. The mutation in the Gunn rat responsible for its lack of bilirubin conjugation occurs in the UGT1 family and affects this entire group of isozymes. A frameshift mutation occurs because of a deleted guanine that results in a TGA stop codon occurring sooner than normal. This mutation results in a protein missing 115 amino acids that constitute a hydrophobic region associated with insertion of the protein into the membrane. Lack of insertion negates the activity of this enzyme form and results in degradation of the incomplete protein. The genes in the UGT2 family are normally expressed in the Gunn rat.

Similar defects occur in humans and are known as *unconjugated hyperbilirubinemias*. Gilbert's syndrome is a milder form of the disease that occurs in 2%–5% of the population. This large prevalence in the population makes it an important human genetic deficiency when considering interindividual variation in xenobiotic metabolism. These patients are characterized by mild, chronic, unconjugated hyperbilirubinemia that produces jaundice and an impaired ability to metabolize menthol. Decreased clearance of several drugs, including tolbutamide, rifamycin, josamycin, and paracetamol, has been observed. Crigler–Najjar syndrome is a familial form of severe unconjugated hyperbilirubinemia. Infants often developed severe neurological damage from bilirubin encephalopathy (kernicterus). Patients are divided into two types. Type I is more severe (unconjugated bilirubin >20 mg/dl) and not responsive to barbiturate or glutethimide therapy. Type II patients respond to induction by phenobarbital, which suggests a fundamental difference from type I in the molecular basis of the genetic defect. Type I results from mutations in the UGT1 family that produces a loss of bilirubin conjugation (29), whereas less severe mutations occur in type II that produce a decrease, but not a loss, of activity.

Gender differences appear hormonally related (166) and can be substrate dependent. Although it is sometimes stated that males have higher glucuronidation activity than females, this is substrate dependent, and no general classification should be made. Like monooxygenase activity, activity may be sensitive to imprinting or programming during the neonatal period. As with species and strain differences, care must be taken when extrapolating data obtained with one substrate to other substrates.

Glucuronidation of estradiol and estrone is higher in female rats than male rats (193). Paracetamol, oxazepam, and diflunisal are cleared 30%–50% faster in males, due primarily to enhanced glucuronidation.

Induction of the Glucuronosyltransferases

UDP-glucuronosyltransferases are inducible enzymes, much like cytochrome P450. They are inducible by some of the same inducers. Evidence of a true induction process involving *de novo* protein synthesis and increases in mRNA has been observed for induction of the UDP-glucuronosyltransferases by phenobarbital. Most inducers of CYP1A, CYP2B, CYP3A, and CYP4A can induce these transferases. Rat UGT1A6 and UGT1A7 and human UGT1A6 and UGT1A9 are polycyclic hydrocarbon-inducible transferases. Induction appears mediated by the Ah receptor. Rat UGT1A7 and human UGT1A9 have high activity toward the phenolic and diphenolic metabolites of polycyclics, such as benzo(a)pyrene (11). Few specific inducers of the transferases that do not also induce the monooxygenase are known. For example, trans-stilbene oxide and ethoxyquin appear to only induce the transferases, but more studies are needed to determine if this is a true induction. Induction of the transferases modifies the toxicity of xenobiotics in a manner similar to induction of P450, as previously discussed.

Sulfation: Sulfotransferases

As early as 1815, it was recognized that mammals excrete organic sulfates in their urine (68). The discovery that these organic sulfates were esters produced in the mammalian body by conjugation of endogenous organic compounds with inorganic sulfate came about 50 years later (16). The sulfate conjugates were believed to be ethers formed between the organic aryl group and the inorganic sulfate group. Therefore, they called the urinary fraction containing these metabolites *ethereal sulfates*; however, these metabolites are actually esters of sulfuric acid, and the term ethereal sulfate is only of historical significance (121).

Sulfation, or more appropriately, sulfonation, of xenobiotics and endobiotics is catalyzed by a set of enzymes called *sulfotransferases* (EC 2.8.2). These enzymes belong to a multigene family and occur in prokaryotes, plants, and animals. Some of the enzymes are membrane bound and others occur in the cytosol. The membrane-bound sulfotransferases are found in the Golgi membranes and are involved in the sulfation of endogenous compounds, such as glycosaminoglycans, glycoproteins, and proteins, and peptides secreted by the Golgi apparatus; they are not involved in xenobiotic metabolism. The soluble sulfotransferases can also sulfate endogenous compounds, such as steroids and thyroid hormones, and are involved in the metabolism of xenobiotics. For the most part, sulfation of xenobiotics results in metabolites that are less toxic than the parent compound; however, the sulfotransferases, like many xenobiotic metabolism enzymes, can produce metabolically activated products that have mutagenic and carcinogenic potential.

Until recently, the sulfotransferases have not been as intensely investigated as some of the other xenobiotic metabolism enzymes. Currently there is renewed interest in these enzymes based, in part, on attempts to understand their role in metabolic activation. Utilization of the tools of molecular biology has provided new insight into their roles in metabolism and has revealed the complexity of their gene family (38,139). The ability to sequence the sulfotransferases and identify new isoforms of these enzymes has progressed faster than our understanding of their individual roles in xenobiotic metabolism. The availability of expression systems that express single and multiple sulfotransferases is providing toxicologists a powerful tool to investigate their roles in xenobiotic metabolism.

Biochemistry of Sulfation

A limiting factor in the sulfation of xenobiotics by the sulfotransferases is the availability of 3-phosphoadenosine 5′-phosphosulfate (PAPS) (reviewed in (85)). As illustrated in Figure 3.10, PAPS is synthesized in a two-step process. The first step is formation of adenosine 5′-phosphosulfate (APS) catalyzed by ATP-sulfurylase. Although the synthesis of APS from sulfate and ATP is not energetically favored, the rapid hydrolysis of pyrophosphate and the rapid utilization of APS as a substrate for APS-kinase drives the reaction toward APS synthesis. APS-kinase catalyzes synthesis of PAPS from APS and ATP. This enzyme is tightly coupled with the ATP-sulfurylase, which results in the rapid utilization of APS.

Tissue concentration of PAPS is relatively low (4–80 ng/g tissue), compared to UDPGA, the active form of glucuronic acid used in glucuronidation (200 nmol/g liver). During active sulfation, PAPS becomes rapidly depleted. For example, the sulfotransferase has a high affinity of acetaminophen, which forms a sulfate con-

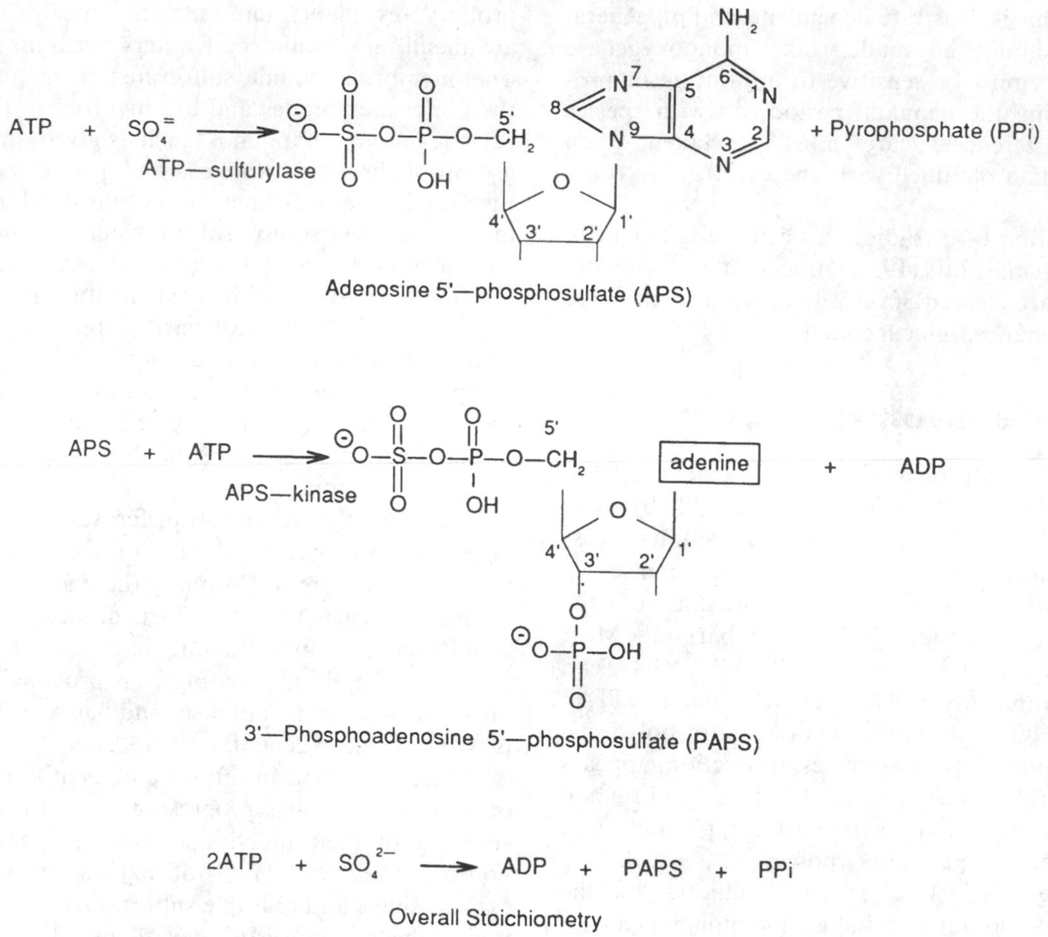

FIG. 3.10. Reactions catalyzing the formation of PAPS from inorganic sulfate and ATP.

jugate. (See Figure 3.6). At low doses, rats excrete the sulfated acetaminophen as a major urinary metabolite. As the dose of acetaminophen is increased, the sulfate metabolite does not increase, whereas the glucuronide of acetaminophen increases dramatically; this is believed to be due to the limited availability of PAPS. The limitation in the synthesis of PAPS is sulfate. The major sources of sulfate include diet and degradation of sulfur amino acids (methionine and cysteine). These sources are inadequate to maintain sulfate concentrations for PAPS synthesis during rapid sulfotransferase activity. In the mouse, sulfation appears more limited by sulfotransferase activity than by PAPS and sulfate.

Reactions Catalyzed by Sulfotransferases

As mentioned, sulfotransferases esterify a variety of endogenous substrates, including steroids, carbohydrates, and proteins. Sulfation also plays a role in the disposition of hormones. Sulfation directs lipophilic compounds, such as the steroidal hormones, to more polar environments, including the active sites of enzymes and to body fluids. For example, sulfation enhances the elimination of steroids from the adrenal gland (116). Sulfation also facilitates deiodination of thyroid hormone and is a rate-limiting step in one of the elimination pathways of thyroid hormone (179).

Xenobiotic conjugation with sulfate (Figure 3.11) is an important route for conversion of lipophilic xenobiotics to more readily excreted polar metabolites (Table 3.6) (79,151). Sulfation of xenobiotics with an aliphatic or aromatic hydroxyl group readily occurs. For example, phenol is excreted as its sulfate conjugate (Figure 3.12). Often it is necessary for phase I metabolism to functionalize a xenobiotic with a hydroxyl group before it can be sulfated. For example, toluene is oxidized to benzyl alcohol before conjugation with sulfate (Figure 3.12).

Role of Sulfotransferases in Detoxication and Metabolic Activation

Alcohols, phenols, aliphatic and aromatic amines, and aromatic hydroxyamines and hydroxyamides can be

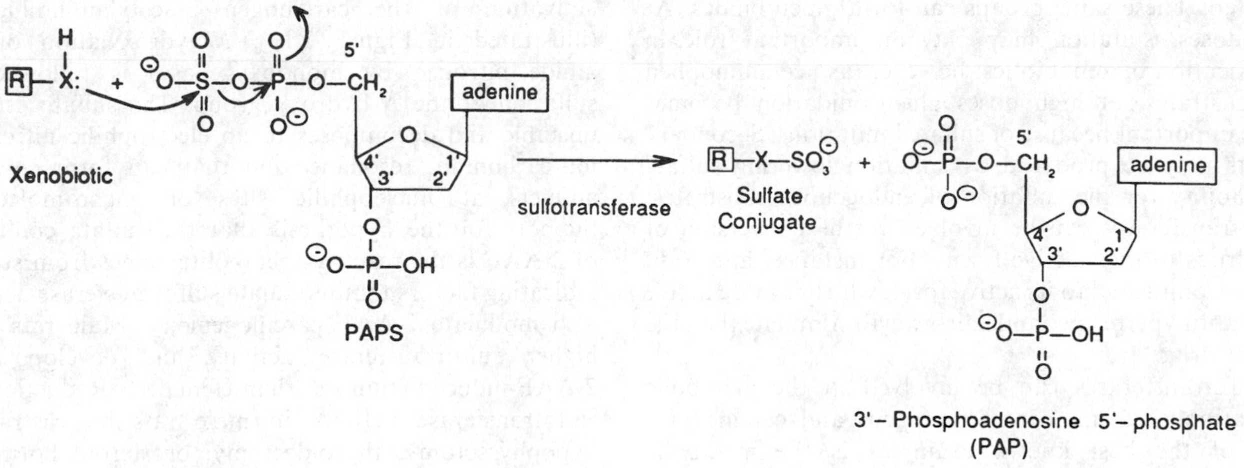

FIG. 3.11. Synthesis of a sulfate conjugate from a model xenobiotic by sulfotransferase.

Table 3.6
Sulfotransferases involved in the metabolism of xenobiotics

EC No.	Name	Example substrates
2.8.2.1	Arylsulfotransferase	2-naphthol, phenol, substituted phenols, serotonin, acetaminophen
2.8.2.2	Alcohol sulfotransferase (also called hydrosteroid sulfotransferase)	Primary and secondary aliphatic alcohols, nonaromatic hydroxysteroids
2.8.2.4	Estrone sulfotransferase	Estrone and other aromatic hydroxysteroids
2.8.2.9	Tyrosine ester sulfotransferase	Tyrosine methyl ester, 2-cyanoethyl-N-hydroxythioacetamide
2.8.2.14	Bile salt sufotransferase	Conjugated and unconjugated bile acids

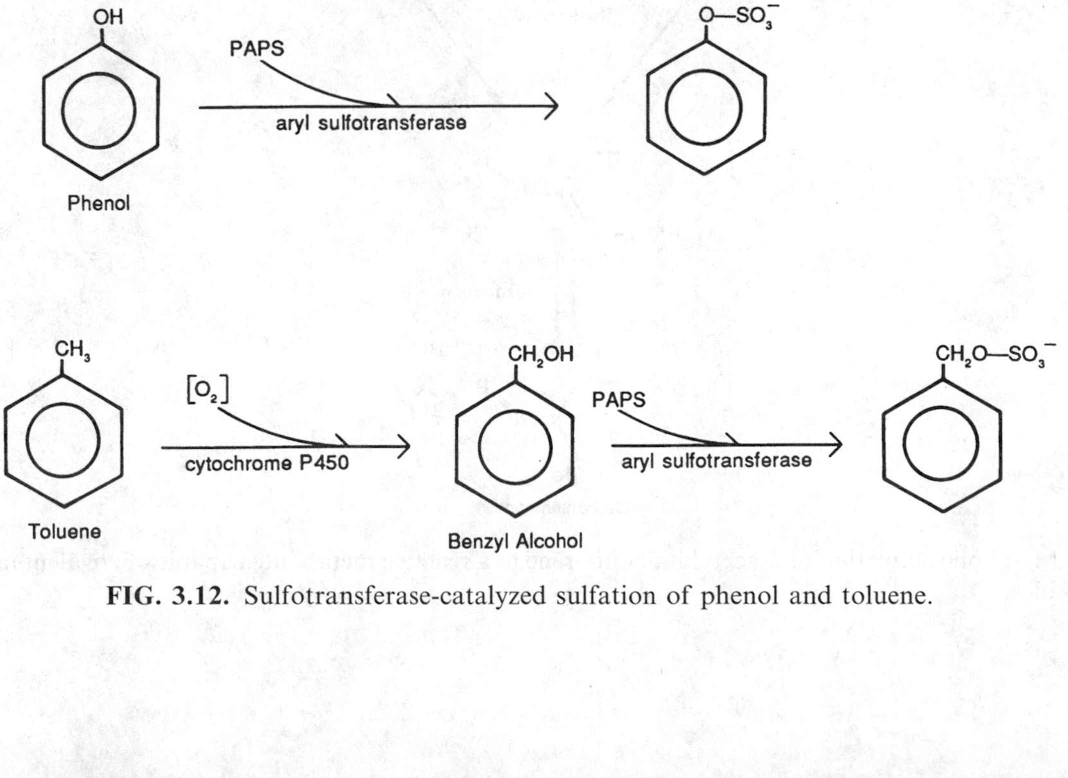

FIG. 3.12. Sulfotransferase-catalyzed sulfation of phenol and toluene.

sulfated. These same groups can form glucuronides. At low doses, sulfation may play an important role in detoxication of xenobiotics; however, as acetaminophen demonstrates, at high doses glucuronidation becomes more important because of sulfate limitations. Secondary effects may be produced by sulfation lowering sulfate availability for the sulfation of endogenous substrates. Sulfotransferases can be involved in the conversion of pro-drugs to their active forms. For instance, minoxidil is sulfoconjugated to its active form, which is more active as an antihypertensive and hair-growth stimulate than the parent drug.

Sulfotransferases can be involved in the metabolic activation of a number of mutagens and carcinogens. One of the best known examples is the metabolic activation of the carcinogen 2-acetylaminofluorene (illustrated in Figure 3.13). *N*-hydroxylation of the amide nitrogen by monooxygenases is followed by sulfation of the *N*-hydroxy group. The sulfate ester is unstable and decomposes to an electrophilic nitrenium ion-carbonium resonance ion that can form covalent adducts at nucleophilic sites on macromolecules. Support for the hypothesis that the sulfate conjugate of 2-AAF is the reactive metabolite comes from studies indicating factors that modulate sulfotransferase activity also modulate 2-AAF carcinogenicity. Male rats have higher sulfotransferase activity and develop more 2-AAF-induced tumors than females. Reduction of sulfotransferase activity in male rats by castration, hypophysectomy, thyroidectomy, or steroid hormones

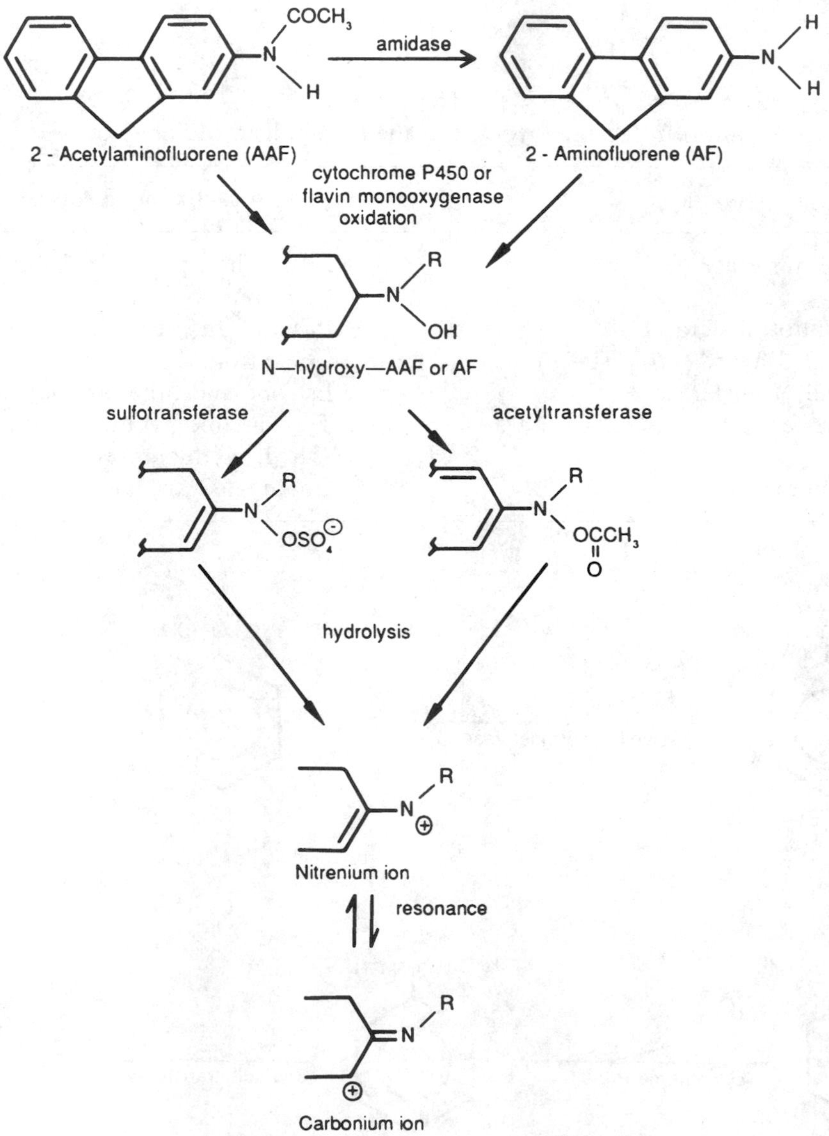

FIG. 3.13. Metabolic activation of 2-acetylaminofluorene to a reactive metabolite capable of covalent modification of macromolecules.

reduces 2-AAF covalent adducts. These results are consistent with the hypothesis that sulfation of 2-AAF is required for covalent modification of DNA. This mechanism is at least partially responsible for the activation of several other xenobiotics, including aromatic amines, mono- and dinitrotoluene, *N*-hydroxyphenacetin, 1′-hydroxysafrole, N_3-hydroxyxanthine, and other *N*-hydroxyarylamides (122). Secondary nitroalkanes, such as 2-nitrobutane and 3-nitropentane, can be metabolically activated by aryl sulfotransferase to mutagens and hepatocarcinogens. Primary nitroalkanes, such as 1-butane and 1-nitropentane, are not activated by aryl sulfotransferase (46).

Sulfotransferases can metabolically activate certain products of CYP1A1 metabolism of polycyclic hydrocarbons. For example, 9-hydroxymethylbenzo(a)pyrene (*see* Figure 3.4) can be sulfated to yield a highly reactive sulfate ester that is heterolytically cleaved to produce an electrophilic cation that damages DNA, RNA, and protein. In addition, 6-hydroxymethylbenzo(a)pyrene can be activated to the carcinogenic 6-sulfooxymethylbenzo(a)pyrene by rat and mouse sulfotransferase (47). Other examples include 5-hydroxymethylchrysene and 7,12-dihydroxymethyl benz(a)anthracene (184). The potential for sulfotransferases to metabolically activate xenobiotics has resulted in the development of new assay systems for genotoxicity. For instance, Glatt's laboratory (55,56) has developed *Salmonella* strains that express rat and human sulfotransferase activity for use in Ames assays. They have also developed Chinese hamster V79-derived cells that express rat sulfotransferase activity.

Sulfotransferase Isoforms, Genetics, and Species Differences

Sulfotransferases belong to a multigene family that produces a number of distinct enzymes that have different, but overlapping, substrate specificities. Some of these enzymes demonstrate species and even tissue specificity in their expression. It is expected that more detailed analysis will identify additional sulfotransferases.

The nomenclature used to describe these enzymes is still evolving, and there is no universal naming system, as yet. Weinshilboum et al. (186) have divided 30 of the known cDNA sequences into three families that have at least a 45% amino acid sequence identity, then into subfamilies with at least 60% homology. Two of the families are expressed in animals and one in plants. The two animal families represent phenol-sulfotransferases and hydroxysteroid sulfotransferases, and the phenol-sulfotransferase are divided into the phenol group and estrogen group. The phenol group contains three human genes, two mouse genes, and one rat gene. The estrogen group contains one human gene, two rat genes, and one mouse gene. The hydroxysteroid family contains one human gene, three rat genes, and three mouse genes. Undoubtedly, more genes will be discovered and the classification system refined; however, this classification demonstrates the diversity of genes in the sulfotransferase family.

Amino acid sequence data indicate that four regions of sulfotransferases have been highly conserved among species. One region, near the carboxy terminus of the proteins, is believed to be the PAPS binding site. A critical lysine may be involved in stabilization of an intermediate form during catalysis.

Humans demonstrate sulfotransferase genetic polymorphisms, which help explain some of the differences between individuals in response to specific xenobiotics. Because sulfotransferases do not appear to be as sensitive to xenobiotic induction of their activity, exposure to xenobiotics may not be as important as with some of the other xenobiotic metabolizing enzymes in producing individual variations in metabolism.

Sulfation occurs in most species, including mammals, birds, reptiles, amphibians, fish, and invertebrates. The most notable exception to this is the low sulfotransferase activity in the pig. Members of the cat family are deficient in glucuronyltransferase activity but have high sulfotransferase activity. This balance of glucuronyltransferase and sulfotransferase must always be kept in mind when evaluating the activity of either enzyme system. A deficiency in one pathway can shift metabolism, as similar functional groups are conjugated by the two enzyme systems. In addition, sulfation appears to have high affinity but low capacity for phenols, whereas glucuronidation has low affinity and high capacity for these substrates.

A large part of our understanding of sulfotransferases comes from study of purified rat enzymes. There are at least six different phenol sulfotransferases and seven different forms of rat liver steroid/bile acid sulfotransferases. By contrast, only three distinct isozymes of cytosolic sulfotransferase have been isolated: two phenol-sulfotransferases and one bile acid sulfotransferase. The two phenol sulfotransferases have been referred to as the monoamine-sulfating form and the phenol-sulfating form. Dopamine, epinephrine, and levodopa are substrates for the monoamine form, and 4-nitrophenol, minoxidil, and acetaminophen are substrates for the phenol form (45).

There is wide species variation in sulfation of two model substrates: isoprenalin and harmol. For example, the activity toward isoprenalin in mouse liver is 10 times that in monkey liver. Sulfation of acetaminophen is limited by PAPS availability in rats. In mice, acetaminophen sulfation is limited by lower sulfotransferase activity. Although mice have lower PAPS synthetic capability than rats, lower sulfotransferase activity is the major limiting factor in mice (98). The activity of acetaminophen sulfotransferase and 17 α-ethinylestradiol sulfotransferase in hepatic preparations from monkeys, dogs, and humans were compared. Rhesus and cynomolgus monkeys and dogs had higher activity acetaminophen sulfotransferase than humans (152).

Four cytosolic sulfotransferases, distinguished by their substrate specificity, have been found in human tissues. Dehydroepiandrosterone or hydroxsteroid sulfotransferases appear to be involved in sulfation of steroids and may be important in regulating their activity and in bile acid sulfation and excretion. Estrogen sulfotransferase is involved in the inactivation of estrogens in target tissue. Other sulfotransferases can also sulfate estrogen, but with lower activity. This transferase does not appear to play an important role in xenobiotic metabolism.

The other two cytosolic sulfotransferases belong to the phenol sulfotransferase group and are involved in xenobiotic metabolism. Phenol-sulfotransferases (PST) are found in a number of tissues, and their discovery in blood platelets has provided an important source for their study. They are divided into two groups: P-PST and M-PST. P-PST sulfates phenols, such as p-nitrophenol and α-naphthol, and aromatic amines, such as 2-naphthylamine. M-PST sulfates monoamine neurotransmitters. Again, substrate specificity overlaps as demonstrated by acetaminophen, which can be sulfated by both sulfotransferases.

As mentioned, nomenclature for the sulfotransferases is currently under development and can cause confusion. Some investigators use the term *aryl sulfotransferase* for a gene family that includes sulfotransferases found in rats, humans, and mice that have a 70% sequence homology and catalyze the sulfation of dopamine, p-nitrophenol, estradiol, and other phenols.

Factors Modifying Metabolism

Sulfotransferases are not induced by the classical inducers, phenobarbital and 3-methylcholanthrene, and these compounds may actually suppress their expression (146). Several inhibitors of sulfotransferase have been discovered and exploited experimentally to study these enzymes. Pentachlorophenol and 2,6-dichloro-4-nitrophenol are potent sulfotransferase inhibitors. Only 0.2 μM pentachlorophenol is required for 50% inhibition of 2-dichloro-4-nitrophenol sulfation by purified arylsulfotransferase (77). Pentachlorophenol and 2,6-dichloro-4-nitrophenol are effective inhibitors because the *ortho-* and *para-*aromatic ring positions are substituted with electron-withdrawing groups. This effect is consistent with the mechanism whereby the sulfotransferases facilitate electrophilic attack of the hydroxyl oxygen by the sulfur (Figure 3.11).

Gender Differences

There are major gender differences in the sulfate conjugation of steroid hormones. For example, female rats have fivefold higher activity for cortisol metabolism than do male rats (154). This gender difference in cortisol metabolism is apparently due more to suppression of sulfotransferase by male hormone levels than to stimulation by the ovaries (153,155). Three steroid sulfotransferases have been isolated from rat liver, and it is the relative amounts of these isozymes that account for the large gender difference. Aryl sulfotransferase concentrations in the livers of male rats were higher than in females. In contrast, hydroxysteroid sulfotransferase concentration was higher in the liver of female rats compared to males (26).

Lower sulfotransferase activity observed in neonatal rats has been attributed to sexual immaturity because as gonads develop, sulfotransferase activity increases. Newborn infants, who characteristically exhibit pronounced immaturity in glucuronidation, have a fully developed phenol sulfotransferase activity. For example, newborns excrete acetaminophen as a sulfate conjugate, whereas adults primarily excrete it as a glucuronide conjugate. Chloramphenicol is extremely toxic in neonates because it is a poor substrate for sulfotransferase and is primarily cleared by glucuronidation in adults.

Glutathione *S*-transferases

A family of cytosolic enzymes known as *glutathione S-transferases* is capable of conjugating relatively hydrophobic electrophilic molecules with the nucleophile-reduced glutathione (Figure 3.14) (24). These enzymes are found in highest concentrations in the liver, kidney, intestines, and lung, but they occur in most tissues. Glutathione conjugates have higher molecular weights and are more water soluble and more likely to be excreted in urine and bile than are the parent compounds. Conjugation with glutathione makes it unlikely the xenobiotic will react with toxicological targets.

Glutathione *S*-transferases involved in xenobiotic metabolism are cytosolic proteins that catalyze the conjugation of glutathione with a substrate bearing an electrophilic atom (74). The transferases facilitate the nucleophilic attack of glutathione thiolate ion (GS^-) on the electron-deficient atom of a relatively hydrophobic electrophilic xenobiotic. There is little specificity in the active site for the xenobiotic other than it must possess hydrophobic character. Substrates for the glutathione *S*-transferases can react with glutathione nonenzymati-

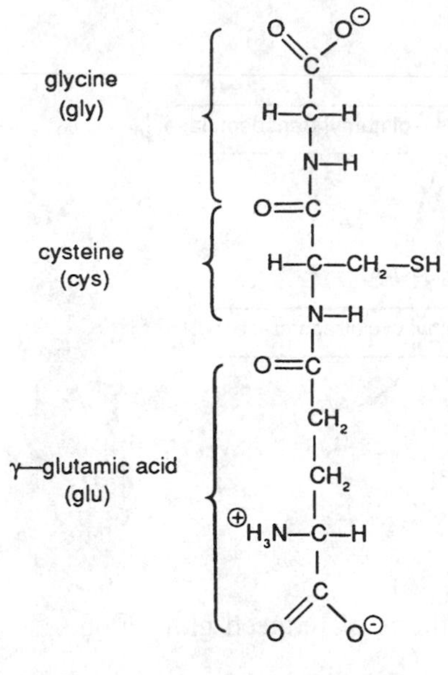

FIG. 3.14. Structure of reduced glutathione (MW 307).

cally but at slower rates than the enzyme-catalyzed reaction.

In addition to catalyzing the conjugation of xenobiotics with glutathione, glutathione *S*-transferases are capable of binding the chemical on the enzyme surface. This binding may or may not inhibit the catalytic activity of the enzyme, but it prevents the xenobiotic from interacting with other critical cellular sites, such as proteins and nucleic acids. A glutathione *S*-transferase possessing this property has been called *ligandin* (161,162). Glutathione *S*-transferases can form covalent bonds between reactive xenobiotics and the enzyme's active site. Binding inactivates the enzyme but also inactivates the reactive xenobiotic and represents an additional detoxication mechanism (76). This process is called *suicide inactivation* and is seen with other detoxication enzymes, such as P450.

Because of these three activities of the glutathione *S*-transferases, the enzymes have been called "a triple threat in detoxification" by Jakoby and Keen (76). Glutathione and the glutathione *S*-transferases can detoxify a broad spectrum of compounds that the organism either may encounter in its environment or generate during normal cellular metabolism. Although not highly efficient in its reactions (operates at relatively high concentrations of the xenobiotic), glutathione *S*-transferases are capable of catalyzing or reacting with a number of reactive chemical functional groups. Any lack of efficiency is made up by the high cellular concentration of glutathione and glutathione *S*-transferase. Liver glutathione concentrations are high (10 mM) and glutathione *S*-transferases can represent as much as 10% of the total hepatocellular proteins (2); however, it is possible for glutathione conjugation to become capacity limited at high doses of xenobiotics. Glutathione utilization can be faster than its synthesis, resulting in decreased conjugation and increased toxicity.

Bromobenzene metabolism is an example of a compound whose glutathione conjugate protects the liver from the toxicity of its P450-generated epoxide. At doses that deplete the cytosolic store of glutathione, the epoxide produces severe hepatotoxicity. Another example is acetaminophen. It is a very safe drug, but at extremely high doses, where glutathione is depleted by reaction with its activated metabolite, *N*-acetyl-benzoquinoneimine (see Figure 3.6), it produces hepatic necrosis.

Glutathione *S*-transferase enzymes are dimers of two protein subunits. They may exist as homodimers, where each subunit is identical, or as heterodimers, where the subunits are expressed by different genes. These transferases are inducible by the classical P450 inducers phenobarbital and 3-methylcholanthrene. The region of the gene that controls the expression of some of these transferases contains the xenobiotic-responsive element (XRE) previously discussed for P450 induction. In the case of the transferases that are heterodimers, the expression of each subunit may be independently regulated.

Different glutathione *S*-transferases have substrate preferences but not a high order of substrate specificity. Substrate selectivity of these enzymes can be based on small changes in the primary structure of the enzymes. For instance, a glutathione *S*-transferase of the P-class contains a tyrosine at a site important for selectivity, whereas a transferase of the A-class contains a valine. When the tyrosine of the P-class enzyme is replaced with a valine, its substrate selectively is changed toward that of the A-class (125).

Biochemistry of Glutathione *S*-transferases

Although the urinary metabolites of glutathione conjugation, mercapturic acids, were first described in the 19th century (16), it was not until the 1950s that glutathione (Figure 3.14) was identified as the source of the cysteine in the mercapturic acid (189). Glutathione is synthesized in the cytosol of most cells by the gamma-glutamyl cycle, a series of six, tightly controlled, enzyme-catalyzed reactions (Figure 3.15). The three amino acids that comprise glutathione—cysteine, glycine, and glutamic acid—can enter the cycle from several biochemical pathways, although the cycle depicts them arising from glutathione.

Some xenobiotics contain sufficiently electrophilic groups to react directly with glutathione, whereas others must first undergo phase I metabolism. Most xenobiotics react with glutathione through the catalytic activity of

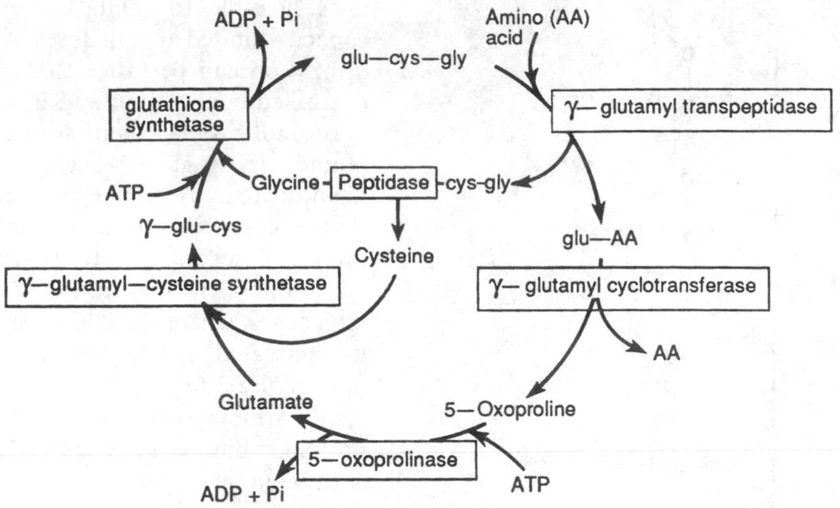

FIG. 3.15. The γ-glutamyl cycle responsible for the biosynthesis of reduced glutathione.

the glutathione *S*-transferases. Glutathione *S*-transferase reactions fall into four broad categories, as depicted in Figure 3.16: reaction with (1) electrophilic carbon, (2) nitrogen, (3) sulfur, and (4) oxygen (50,65,75).

Reaction with Electrophilic Carbon

The reactions of glutathione with electrophilic carbon can be divided into three types, as shown in Figure 3.16: (a) displacement reactions, (b) opening of strained rings, and (c) addition to activated double bonds.

(a) *Displacement of leaving groups such as halides, sulfates, sulfonates, phosphates, and nitro groups from saturated carbon or heteroatoms.* Displacement is facilitated if the saturated carbon atom is allylic or benzylic. Displacement of halide or nitro groups on aromatic rings occurs if there are sufficient electron-withdrawing groups that predispose the ring system toward nucleophilic substitution. The rate of formation of a carbanion intermediate of the aromatic ring governs the overall rate of the reaction. Functional groups that withdraw electrons stabilize the carbanion and

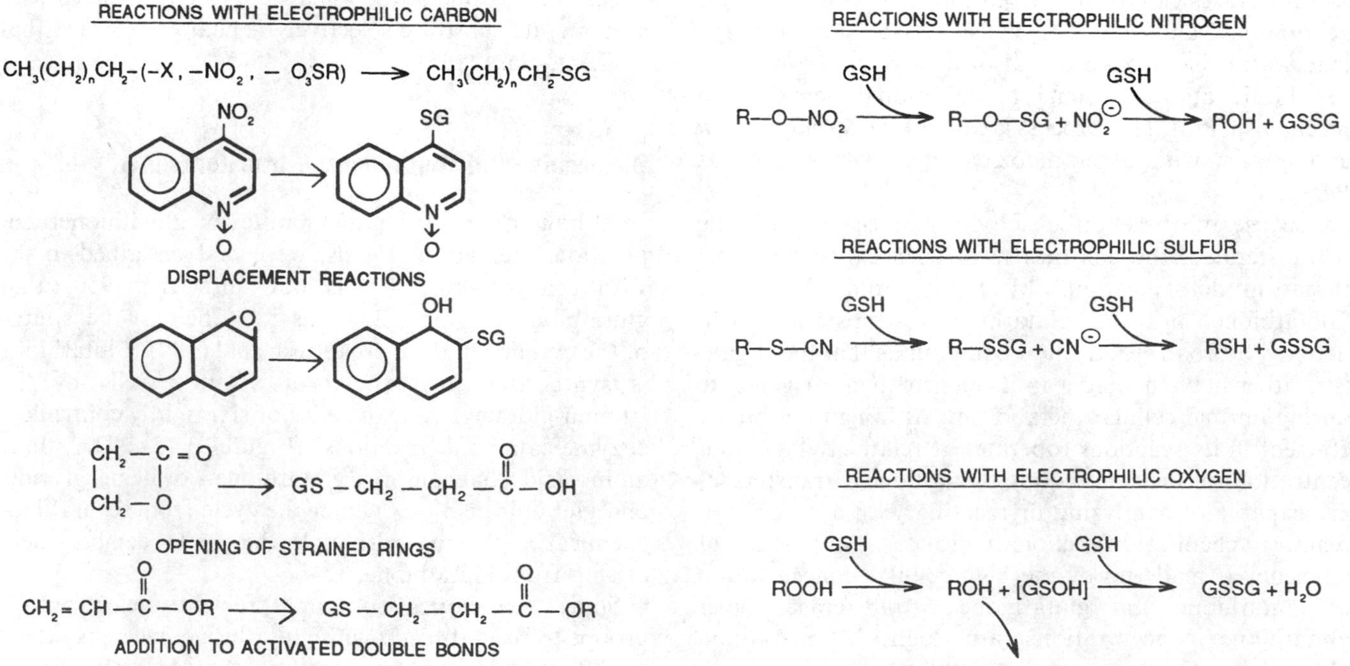

FIG. 3.16. Examples of the reactions catalyzed by the glutathione *S*-transferases.

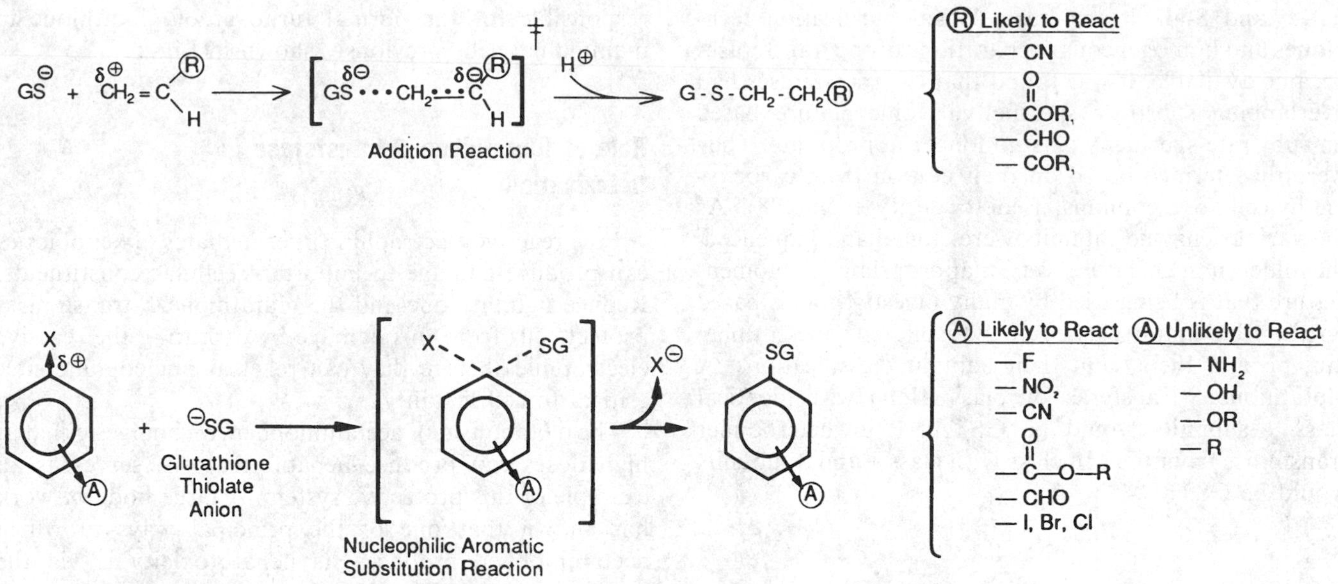

FIG. 3.17. Putative reaction mechanisms for the glutathione *S*-transferase-catalyzed nucleophilic attack of the glutathione thiolate anion on electrophilic xenobiotics where X represents a halogen and R and A represents the listed substituents.

are considered "good leaving groups." Those that donate electrons to the ring deactivate the ring, making displacement of the leaving group by glutathione less likely (Figure 3.16).

(b) *Opening of strained rings, such as epoxides and 4-membered lactones*. As shown in Figure 3.16, the 1,2-epoxide of naphthalene is opened, resulting in a 1-napthol conjugate of glutathione. These reactions can be stereoselective. Epoxide products of P450 are detoxified by this reaction and are an example of a phase II conjugation of a phase I activated metabolite.

(c) *Addition to activated double bonds via Michael addition*. The glutathione thiolate anion will also attack β-unsaturated xenobiotics due to the partial positive charge on the β-carbon, as shown in Figure 3.17 (addition reaction). Figure 3.22 illustrates the addition of glutathione to the β-carbon of an acrylate ester.

Reaction with Electrophilic Nitrogen

The reaction sequence and overall stoichiometry for the reaction of organic nitrate esters with glutathione is shown in Figure 3.16. This reaction was once attributed to a glutathione reductase but is now known to be catalyzed by glutathione *S*-transferases. The transferases catalyze the removal of nitrite from the ester, generating an R-O-S conjugate with glutathione. The vasodilators, nitroglycerin and erythrityl tetranitrate, are two organic nitrate ester substrates for this reaction. As seen in Figure 3.16, the alcohol-glutathione conjugate can react nonenzymatically with another reduced glutathione molecule. This yields an alcohol and oxidized glutathione.

Reaction with Electrophilic Sulfur

Alkyl and aryl thiocyanates are substrates for glutathione *S*-transferase catalyzed conjugations, as shown in Figure 3.16. Products of this nucleophilic attack of the thiolate ion on the sulfur of the xenobiotic result in a mixed disulfide and hydrogen cyanide. The mixed disulfide can react nonenzymatically with another molecule of glutathione to yield a thiol of the xenobiotic (RSH) and oxidized glutathione (GSSG).

Reaction with Electrophilic Oxygen

Figure 3.16 illustrates how glutathione reacts with organic hydroperoxides in a two-step sequence. The first step is catalyzed by glutathione *S*-transferase and forms an alcohol or phenol and a glutathione sulfenic acid intermediate (G-SOH). Another glutathione reacts nonenzymatically with the sulfenic acid to form oxidized glutathione and water. An example of reaction with endogenous hydroperoxides is the conversion of hydroperoxy-$PGF_{2\alpha}$ to PGF*a*. Cumene hydroperoxide is metabolized as rapidly by purified glutathione *S*-transferases as the classical transferase substrate probe 1-chloro-2,4-dinitrobenzene.

Glutathione *S*-transferases Nomenclature

The glutathione *S*-transferases were originally named by their substrate specificity, such as S-epoxide transferase and S-alkyltransferase. When purification techniques and homogeneous preparations of the transferases became available, it was found that the transferases had overlapping substrate specificity. Nomenclature based on substrate specificity was no longer appropriate. They were then termed based on their elution from carboxymethylcellulose columns used to purify them (78). As the various enzyme subunits were cloned and sequenced, the older nomenclature was inappropriate. A nomenclature that is being used by many investigators is based on the four major classes of cytosolic enzymes (alpha, mu, pi, and theta) and their subunit classifications. A *g*lutathione *S-t*ransferase in class *A*lpha with identical class *1* subunits would be GSTA1-1. A heterodimer transferase from the Mu class with class 1 and 2 subunits would be GSTM1-2.

Mercapturic Acid Formation

Mercapturic acids are *N*-acetylated, *S*-substituted, cysteine conjugates that arise from conjugation of a xenobiotic with glutathione (15).

The glutathione conjugates formed in the liver and other tissues as shown in pathway 1 of Figure 3.18 are polar and partition into the aqueous phase of cells and blood. Because 25% of the blood flow passes through the kidney, glutathione conjugates are transported to the kidney via systemic circulation. There, the glutathione conjugate undergoes a series of reactions, shown in pathway 2 of Figure 3.18, which result in mercapturic acid formation.

The initial step in mercapturic acid synthesis is cleavage of glutamic acid from cysteine catalyzed by γ-glutamyltranspeptidase (EC 2.3.2.2). This enzyme is located in the brush border of the proximal tubules in the kidney (187). Evidence that this enzyme is involved in glutathione degradation comes from observations of pronounced glutathionemia and glutathionuria (high levels of glutathione in blood and urine, respectively) in patients who lack detectable γ-glutamyltranspeptidase. This enzyme not only hydrolyzes the glutathione moiety, but also transfers the γ-glutamyl group to a variety of amino acids and dipeptides. These two reactions have been shown to proceed at equivalent rates under physiological conditions (190).

Next, the glycine group is cleaved from the resulting cysteinylglycine conjugate by aminopeptidase M yielding the *S*-substituted cysteine conjugate of the xenobiotic. The cysteine conjugate is a substrate for N-acetyltransferase that acetylates the free amino group of cysteine to yield the mercapturic acid, which is excreted in the urine (pathway 3, Figure 3.18). These two enzymes, γ-glutamyltransferase and aminopeptidase M, are also responsible for the normal turnover of glutathione in mammalian cells previously shown in Figure 3.15.

Role of Glutathione *S*-transferase in Detoxication

Free reactive electrophilic intermediates of xenobiotics can produce damage to important cellular constituents. Reduced glutathione and the glutathione *S*-transferases protect cells from this damage by capturing the reactive electrophiles before they can react at nucleophilic sites critical to cell viability.

The metabolism of acetaminophen, an analgesic that at high doses can produce hepatic necrosis, serves as an example of this protective system. A large body of work has shown that one of the principal ways in which acetaminophen produces its hepatotoxicity is via the reactive intermediate, N-acetyl-p-benzoquinone imine, as shown in Figure 3.6. This intermediate is an electrophile that reacts readily with the nucleophile glutathione. As long as the amount of glutathione present at the site of activation of acetaminophen is sufficient to bind the reactive intermediate, no toxicity ensues; however, as demonstrated in the classic study by Mitchell (115), when glutathione is depleted by pretreatment with diethyl maleate, the benzoquinone imine covalently binds to tissue proteins resulting in tissue necrosis. Mitchell (115) was among the first to propose that glutathione plays a fundamental role in protecting tissues against electrophilic attack by xenobiotics.

Since these early studies demonstrating the protective role of glutathione, many compounds have been shown to form conjugates with glutathione. For a comprehensive review of these reactions, see (25,87).

Factors Affecting Metabolism

Glutathione *S*-transferases have been found in most species, including reptiles, birds, insects, amphibians, and plants. Factors that influence the availability of reduced glutathione drastically alter the effectiveness of glutathione *S*-transferases. As was discussed previously, the toxicity of acetaminophen is modulated by the availability of reduced glutathione. Most xenobiotics that are highly reactive nonenzymatically with glutathione can deplete glutathione. Other mechanisms can also lower glutathione availability. For example, certain individuals have genetic defects in the γ-glutamyl cycle, resulting in low tissue concentrations of glutathione. These individuals generally are anemic due to the lack of glutathione and the resulting loss of protection from oxidative damage to erythrocytes (111).

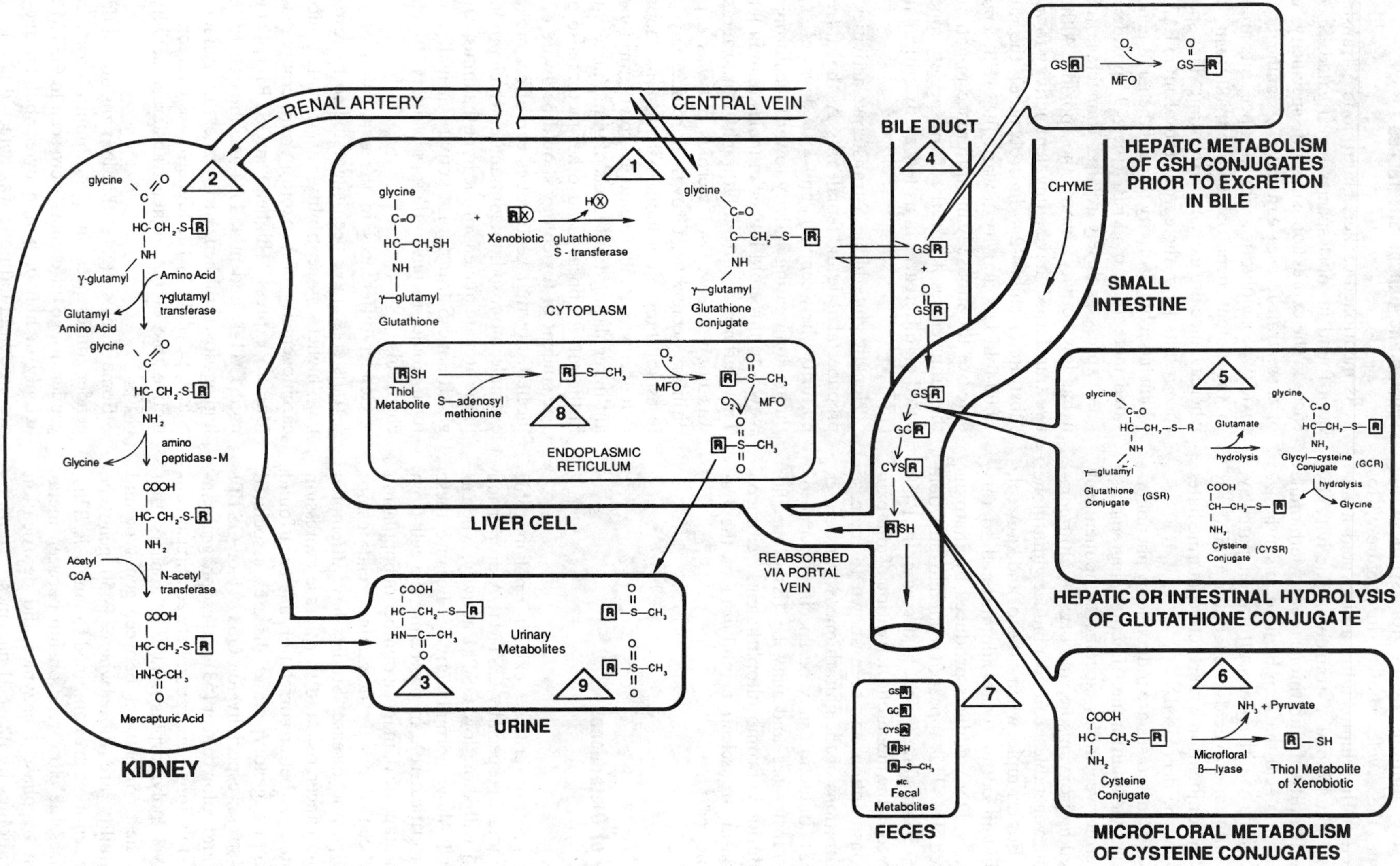

FIG. 3.18. Integration of glutathione conjugate disposition in mammals. Pathway numbers referred to in the text are shown in the triangles.

Cysteine is the limiting factor for synthesis of glutathione via the cycle shown in Figure 3.15. Nutritional factors that limit sulfur amino acid availability decrease glutathione *S*-transferase activity by reducing the availability of glutathione (168). Methionine is an essential amino acid that can be used to synthesize cysteine and cystine via the transsulfuration pathway. If diets low in sulfur amino acids are fed, the availability of glutathione for conjugation with reactive intermediates of xenobiotics can be decreased.

Glutathione *S*-transferases are inducible by phenobarbital and 3-methylcholanthrene. Dietary ingredients, such as cruciferous vegetables, specific components of coffee, butylated hydroxyanisole, and organosulfur compounds of allium vegetables, can also induce glutathione *S*-transferases. For example, when cafestol and kahweol, diterpenes found in coffee, were administered to rats for up to 90 days, DNA adducts produced by aflatoxin B_1 were inhibited 50%. This appeared related to induction of glutathione *S*-transferase and a decrease in P450 isozymes involved in the metabolic activation of aflatoxin (23). Coffee consumption has been shown to increase salivary concentrations of the glutathione *S*-transferases in humans (163). Induction may be specific for one or more of the transferases and may be tissue specific. Triphenyltinchloride, bromosulfophthalein, cibracon blue, and hematin are selective inhibitors of the transferase isozymes (175).

Polymorphisms of Glutathione *S*-transferases

Glutathione *S*-transferases exhibit polymorphic expression in humans, especially GSTM1. A proportion of a population will show low GSTM activity, whereas the majority will show normal activity. Because these enzymes play a critical role in protecting the cell from cytotoxic and mutagenic damage, a number of population studies have been done to determine relationships between genotype and disease. Studies have attempted to correlate lung cancer risk and transferase expression with mixed results. A better correlation has been found between transferase genotype and diseases associated with oxidative stress, especially for GSTM1 or GSTT1 polymorphism and colon cancer (53) and esophageal cancer (97). No correlations were found between breast cancer and GSTM1 polymorphism (1). It appears that some of the highest correlations between genotype and cancer susceptibility are those where P450 genotype and transferase genotype are combined for analysis. This, again, emphasizes the close relationship between metabolic activation by phase I enzymes and detoxication of reactive metabolites by phase II enzymes.

Species and Gender Differences

As mentioned earlier, glutathione *S*-transferases have been found in most species investigated. Species differences in the expression, substrate specificity, and activity of these transferases can have a significant role in the toxicity of xenobiotics. For instance, rats are susceptible to the potent hepatocarcinogen aflatoxin B_1 (AFB_1), whereas mice are extremely resistant. This species difference results from the expression of mGSTA3-3 in mice, which has a high activity toward the P450-generated activated metabolite of AFB_1 (the 8,9 epoxide). Although rats express a closely related transferase (rGSTA3-3), it has low activity toward the epoxide. Although these two transferases have equivalent activity toward a probe substrate (1-chloro-2,4-dinitrobeneze), the rat form has 1,000-fold less activity toward the AFB_1 epoxide compared to the mouse. This difference in activity between the transferases from the two species appears to be based on differences in as few as six critical amino acids (177).

Hepatic glutathione *S*-transferase activities are low in prepubertal male and female rats. As the rats reach sexual maturity between 30 and 50 days of age, glutathione-conjugating activity toward dichloronitrobenzene is two- to threefold higher in males than in females (91). This difference in glutathione *S*-transferase activity was not related to sex steroids but was dependent on pituitary secretions. Growth hormone may play a role in establishing glutathione *S*-transferase activities (90), as it does with P450. Although growth hormone is important in regulating adult levels of glutathione *S*-transferase in the rat, it appears that other factors also play a role. The student of toxicology should be aware of the multifaceted way that xenobiotics can affect organisms. For example, monosodium glutamate, which produces lesions in the arcuate nucleus of the hypothalamus, can lower the glutathione *S*-transferase activity in male rats. This, in turn, could increase their sensitivity to electrophilic chemicals.

Gender differences in the expression of glutathione *S*-transferase have been suggested to be responsible for the higher susceptibility of female mice to the carcinogenicity of benzo(a)pyrene compared to males. Males express higher mGSTP1-1, mGSTA3-3, mGSTM1-1, and mGSTA4-4 compared to females. At higher doses of benzo(a)pyrene this gender difference is lost, possibly by the higher doses overcoming the protective role of the higher transferase activity in males (156).

Some studies suggest that humans do not demonstrate gender differences in glutathione *S*-transferases. No gender or age differences were seen in GSTM and GSTP activity in human lymphocytes, but an age-dependent decrease in glutathione was detected (176).

Role of Glutathione *S*-transferases in Metabolic Activation

Glutathione conjugation does not always produce an innocuous and readily excreted metabolite. For example, Elfarra and Anders (41) compiled a list of 1,2-dihaloalkanes and halogenated alkenes whose glutathione or cysteine conjugates were nephrotoxic (Figure 3.19). Glutathione reacts with these 1,2-dihaloalkanes via a glutathione *S*-transferase–catalyzed reaction that yields sulfur mustards. An electrophilic episulfonium ion can be formed from the mustard when the second halogen atom is displaced by a cellular nucleophile. The episulfonium ion intermediate has been implicated in the toxicity of these chemicals. The major DNA adduct resulting from exposure to the carcinogen, 1,2 dibromoethane, was S-2-*N*-7-guanylethylglutathione (72). A brief review of this bioactivation pathway is included in (4,174).

As shown in Figure 3.18, glutathione and cysteine conjugates (GSR and CySR, respectively) formed in the liver (pathway 1) can be excreted in the bile (pathway 4). Glutathione conjugates can be hydrolyzed to cysteine conjugates by pancreatic peptidases in the small intestine (pathway 5). Cysteine conjugates originating from the bile and those formed by hydrolysis of glutathione conjugates are good substrates for microfloral β-lyase (pathway 6). β-Lyase, an enzyme found in liver, kidney, and in intestinal microflora, cleaves thioether linkages in cysteine conjugates of xenobiotics (169). The resulting thiol compounds are more hydrophobic than the conjugates and can be readily absorbed in the small intestine. These thiol metabolites return to the liver via the portal circulation and act as substrates for thiol *S*-methyltransferase that methylates the thiol group (pathway 8). Enterohepatic circulation (pathways $1 \rightarrow 4 \rightarrow 5 \rightarrow 6 \rightarrow 8$) of glutathione conjugates accounts for some of the unusual sulfur-containing metabolites (pathway 9) that have been found in the urine of animals treated with xenobiotics, such as propachlor (138). A portion of the glutathione-derived sulfur-containing metabolites formed in the small intestine is excreted in the feces (pathway 7 of Figure 3.18).

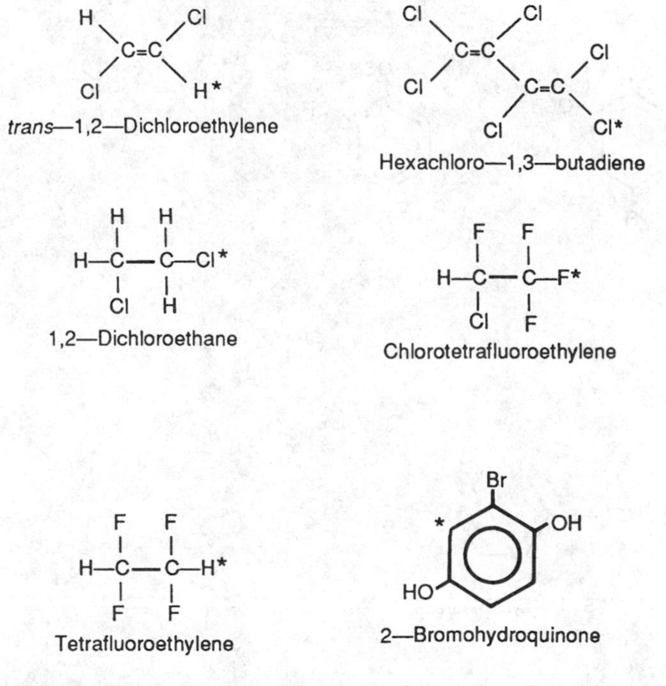

FIG. 3.19. Halogenated hydrocarbons that form glutathione and cysteine S-conjugates that are nephrotoxic. Asterisks indicate the position where the glutathione *S*-transferase–catalyzed displacement (SN_2) occurs.

Reactions of glutathione and cysteinyl conjugates shown in Figure 3.19 are believed to play a role in the nephrotoxicity of several xenobiotics. For example, the cysteinyl conjugate of trichloroethylene, S-(1,2-dichlorovinyl)-L-cysteine (DCVC), is a potent nephrotoxin and a β-lyase substrate. Inhibition of renal β-lyase with aminooxyacetic acid, an inhibitor of pyridoxyl phosphate-dependent enzymes, protected against DCVC-induced nephrotoxicity (41).

In general, glutathione conjugate synthesis results in readily excreted polar metabolites; however, in some cases (depicted in Figure 3.18), the residence time of a glutathione conjugate in the body is prolonged. This can result in formation of metabolites that are more reactive than the original, parent xenobiotic, or the glutathione conjugate. If these reactive metabolites interact with critical cellular sites, toxicity can ensue. For a review, see (3,118).

Glutathione *S*-Transferases as Markers of Liver Damage

Glutathione *S*-transferases may be valuable as an adjunct to serum aminotransferases for detecting acute liver damage. These transferases constitute as much as 3% of cytosolic protein in the hepatocyte and are uniformly distributed across the liver lobule, compared with aminotransferases, which are located periportal. Their plasma half-life is less than 60 minutes, compared to 48 hours for the alanine aminotransferase. Selective use of these different characteristics between aminotransferases and glutathione *S*-transferases have led to more accurate diagnosis of hepatic damage produced by xenobiotics (67). Recently, it has been suggested that determination of glutathione *S*-transferase be included in toxicology studies, and validated methods for rats and dogs have been developed (84).

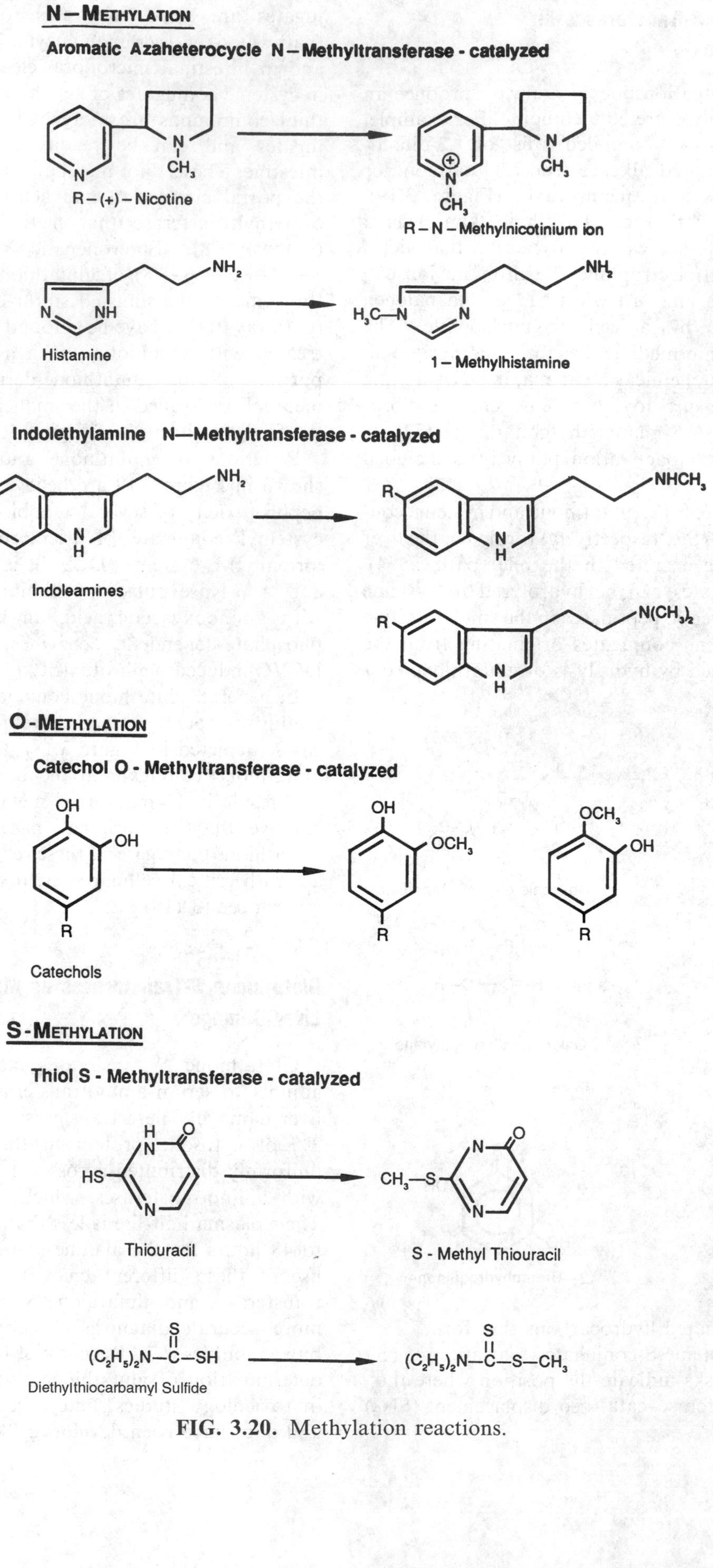
N–METHYLATION
Aromatic Azaheterocycle N–Methyltransferase - catalyzed
R–(+)–Nicotine
R–N–Methylnicotinium ion
Histamine
1–Methylhistamine
Indolethylamine N—Methyltransferase - catalyzed
Indoleamines
O-METHYLATION
Catechol O - Methyltransferase - catalyzed
Catechols
S-METHYLATION
Thiol S - Methyltransferase - catalyzed
Thiouracil
S - Methyl Thiouracil
Diethylthiocarbamyl Sulfide

FIG. 3.20. Methylation reactions.

Methylation

Methyl conjugation is an important pathway in the metabolism of many neurotransmitters, drugs, and xenobiotics. Methylation of endogenous substrates, such as histamine, amino acids, proteins, carbohydrates, and polyamines, is important in the regulation of normal cellular metabolism and accounts for the presence of this activity in mammalian cells. Only when a xenobiotic fits the requirements for the enzymes involved in these normal reactions does methylation become important in the metabolism of foreign compounds.

Methylation can be achieved by two routes. First and foremost is the methyltransferase-catalyzed methylation that requires S-adenosylmethionine (SAM) as a cosubstrate. Most biological methylations require SAM as the methyl donor; however, there are methyl transferases that require SAM as a cosubstrate but vary in other requirements for optimal activity (105). Reactions involving four of these SAM-dependent methyltransferases are shown in Figure 3.20. Two enzymes catalyze nitrogen methylation: aromatic azaheterocycle N-methyltransferase and indolethylamine N-methyltransferase. Oxygen methylation is primarily catalyzed by catechol *O*-methyltransferase and sulfur methylation thiol *S*-methyltransferase. A secondary source of methylation is the N_5-methyltetrahydrofolate (5-CH3-THF)-catalyzed methylation. This methylation is important in the synthesis of nucleic acids; however, 5-CH_3-THF is 1000 times less reactive toward soft nucleophiles (shown in Figure 3.20) than SAM, suggesting that it plays a smaller role in xenobiotic metabolism.

Methylation is a major route for nicotine biodisposition in the guinea pig. The enzyme responsible for nicotine methylation is an aromatic azaheterocycle *N*-methyltransferase that normally methylates histamine (Figure 3.20). Guinea pigs are well known for their ability to methylate histamine. They represent a good animal model for studying xenobiotic methylation. Nicotine is an example of a xenobiotic that can be metabolized by an enzyme of normal cellular metabolism. Because nicotine is a weak base, methylation of the pyridyl nitrogen results in charges at both nitrogens at physiologic pH, increasing water solubility and urinary excretion.

Methylation reactions can be stereoselective. For example, the R(+) enantiomer of nicotine is preferentially methylated over the S(−) enantiomer (33). Stereoselective metabolism of xenobiotics can be important in understanding the metabolic basis of toxicity. Because most biotransformation reactions are catalyzed by enzymes, there is always the possibility that the active site will select one orientation around a chiral center over another.

Individual differences in S-methylation activity have been observed, with activity being trimodal. These data suggested that S-methylation is controlled by a single genetic locus with two alleles, one controlling low activity and one controlling high activity (185). Inherited variations in "methylator" status should be included among those factors responsible for individual variations in the metabolism of thiopurine and catechol xenobiotics.

Amide Synthesis

Amide biosynthesis can take place via two principal routes:

1. Conjugation of a carboxylic acid–containing xenobiotic with the free amino group of an amino acid such as glycine.
2. The acetylation of a xenobiotic containing a primary amine ($-NH_2$).

Amino Acid Conjugation

Xenobiotics that contain a carboxylic acid moiety are susceptible to conjugation with endogenous amino acids. Xenobiotic conjugation occurs in hepatic mitochondria. The free carboxylic acid is activated by reaction with ATP followed by reaction with acetyl coenzyme A (CoA), as shown in reactions 1 and 2 of Figure 3.21. For example, the carboxylic acid of benzoic acid is activated to a thioester CoA intermediate that reacts with the primary amine of glycine to form the amide, hippuric acid.

Glycine has historical significance in xenobiotic conjugation because it is one of the earliest reactions attributed to xenobiotic metabolism. Keller (83), in 1842, administered benzoic acid to himself and then isolated and characterized the major metabolite, hippuric acid, a glycine conjugate. This reaction has been used as a liver function test in humans. The liver is the principal site of glycine conjugation. Amino acids other than glycine can be used for conjugating aromatic and heterocyclic carboxylic acids. For example, arginine is used by arachnids, glutamine by chimpanzees, and ornithine by certain birds.

Acetylation

Acetylation, catalyzed by *N*-acetyltransferases, is the principal pathway of amide formation for primary aromatic amines, endogenous primary aliphatic amines, anutrient amino acids, hydrazines, hydrazides, and sulfonamides. The activated acetyl group is derived from acetyl-CoA. Mercapturic acid formation in the kidney is an example of acetylation that has been presented. In this reaction, the primary amine group of the cysteine conjugate of the xenobiotic is acetylated to form the mercapturic acid. This is an exception to the rule that aliphatic primary amines generally are not good substrates

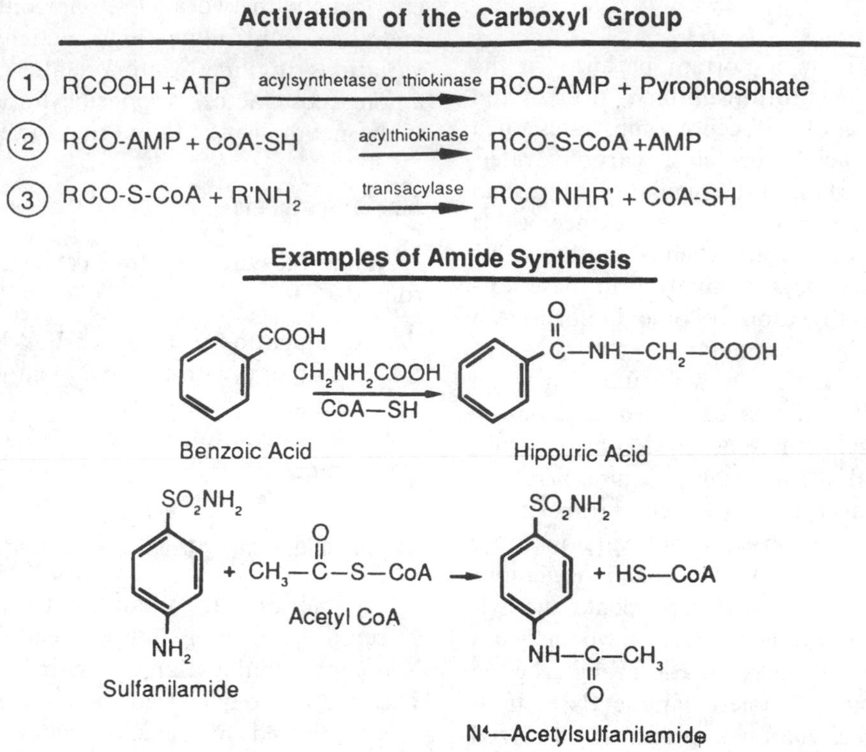

FIG. 3.21. Series of reactions leading to amide formation from either a xenobiotic containing a carboxylic functional group (RCOOH) or a primary amine group ($R'NH_2$).

for the N-acetyltransferases. It is worth noting that the use of the -uric suffix to denote an acidic metabolite was once common. Mercapturic acids, hippuric acid, and salicyluric acid all share this common suffix that is probably derived from the fact that these were acids. Uric acid had similar characteristics and all were isolated from urine.

The N-acetyltransferases are cytosolic enzymes that occur in many tissues. Some species, including humans, express two independently regulated transferases, NAT1 and NAT2, whereas other species express three. NAT1 and NAT2 are similar proteins but have different substrate specificities, although there is some overlap. NAT2 is primarily a liver and intestinal enzyme, whereas NAT1 is expressed in a number of organs. The *N*-acetyltransferases are important in the metabolic disposition of drugs and can also be involved in the metabolic activation of xenobiotics (e.g., aromatic amines).

Human Amide Synthesis Polymorphism

The main route of metabolism of isoniazid (1-isonicotinyl hydrazide) in humans is conjugation with acetyl-CoA to form the amide metabolite (106). Isoniazid is eliminated much faster from the body once it is acetylated. With the widespread use of isoniazid to control tuberculosis, it became obvious that there were major differences in the rates at which individuals eliminated the drug (44). Careful studies of hundreds of patients showed that there were two distinct populations: the fast and the slow acetylators. Slow acetylators inherited the trait as a homozygous recessive allele.

NAT polymorphisms have been reported in several species. Although it is possible that NAT1 may be polymorphic, NAT2 has received the most interest. Slow acetylation is associated with mutations, in the NAT2 gene. Not all slow acetylators show identical mutations, and there is a spectrum of activity in the slow acetylator phenotype. Some mutations affect enzyme activity, whereas others decrease the stability of the enzyme. A number of population studies have been done to determine if the NAT polymorphism alters susceptibility to carcinogens. In some studies, no differences have been reported, whereas in others, associations have been suggested (18). The number of enzymes involved in carcinogen biodisposition and the polymorphisms associated with some of these enzymes makes the task of identifying specific polymorphisms associated with increased cancer risk difficult. As more is learned about the complex interactions of these enzymes, population-based studies will provide valuable information.

HYDROLYSIS

Many xenobiotics and their phase I metabolites contain either a carboxyl ester, an amide bond, or an epoxide that mask hydrophilic functional groups, such as alcohols, carboxylic acids, and amines. The rate at which an organism can hydrolyze these bonds and unmask these function groups can influence their toxicity. In fact, pesticides and therapeutic drugs have been synthesized with intent to modulate the bioavailability of the active species by affecting the rate of hydrolysis of the parent compound.

Hydrolysis normally competes with other detoxication reactions. An example of competition is demonstrated by the metabolism of acrylate esters (Figure 3.22). Most acrylate esters either react with glutathione via a glutathione *S*-transferase–catalyzed pathway or are hydrolyzed by B-esterases to acrylic acid and the corresponding alcohol (Figure 3.22).

Epoxide Hydrolase

Organisms may be exposed to epoxides in the environment, or, they may be produced during the oxidative metabolism of specific xenobiotics from their environment. Epoxides generally are reactive electrophilic compounds due to the highly strained oxirane ring (Figure 3.23). Excess strain energy can be released by ring opening in the presence of nucleophiles. Ring opening may follow either a S_N1-type mechanism with the formation of an intermediate with carbonium ion character or an S_N2 mechanism with bond formation with the attacking nucleophile. The latter case has important toxicological consequences when the nucleophile is on a critical tissue macromolecule, such as DNA, because it results in covalent modification of the macromolecule. Modification of DNA results in a biochemical lesion that may be the precursor to a number of pathological lesions, including cancer. Reaction of the epoxide with cellular nucleophiles, such as proteins, could also lead to other mechanisms producing acute or subchronic toxicity.

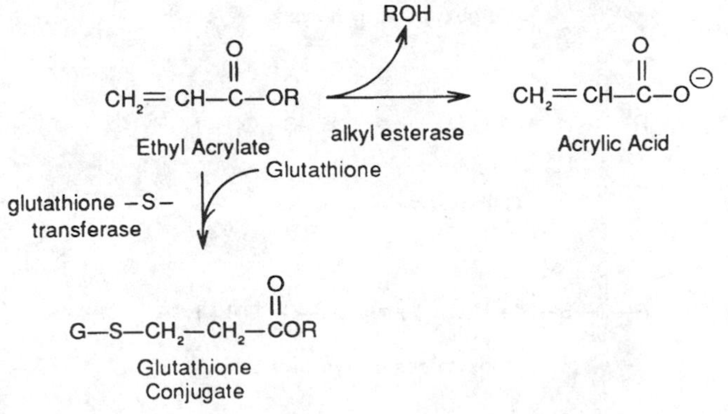

FIG. 3.22. Routes of disposition of ethyl acrylate.

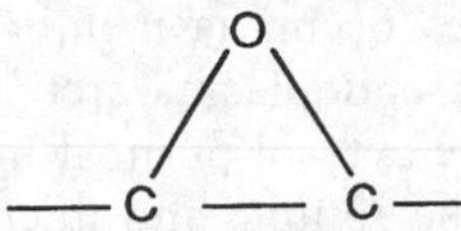

FIG. 3.23. An example of a strained epoxide oxirane ring.

The chemical reactivity and, consequently, the biological activity of epoxides are influenced by the constituents attached to the oxirane ring carbons. Epoxides with asymmetric carbon atoms can exhibit optical activity and exist as enantiomers in a racemic mixture. Reaction of epoxides with nucleophiles with an asymmetrical center will produce diastereoisomers with different spatial orientations around the carbon center. Production of diastereoisomers is important in biological activity in respect to both reaction at critical biochemical sites and subsequent metabolism. For instance, one isomer may react more efficiently at the toxigenic site and be a poor substrate for subsequent metabolism when compared to another isomer.

Although not always the case, the epoxides that are formed in vivo appear to be more toxicologically important than those that occur in the environment. Highly reactive epoxides would most likely interact with nucleophilic sites in the environment, such as proteins in food, and not be absorbed in their active form. Epoxides formed in vivo are produced close to their sites of action and require only diffusion or short transport to their target. Epoxides most frequently formed in vivo represent alkene and arene oxides produced by P450. Their efficient detoxication is important to cellular survival.

Detoxication of epoxides may follow several routes:

(1) Spontaneous decomposition.
(2) Nonenzymatic reaction with glutathione.
(3) Reaction with glutathione catalyzed by glutathione transferase.
(4) Hydration by epoxide hydrolase.
(5) Minor mechanisms such as a P450 hydrolysis.

Nonenzymatic and enzymatic conjugations with glutathione have been previously discussed.

A major route for biodisposition of epoxides is hydration catalyzed by epoxide hydrolase. This enzyme was previously referred to as epoxide hydrase and epoxide hydratase, and readers will sometimes encounter these terms still in use. This microsomal enzyme catalyzes the biotransformation of arene oxides and aliphatic epoxides to vicina (Latin: *vicinalis*, neighboring) dihydrodiols. In most cases, this enzymatic pathway results in less reactive diol metabolites that are more readily excreted from the organism, either as the diol or as a glucuronide or sulfate conjugate of the diol.

Epoxide hydrolases occur as membrane-bound proteins located in the endoplasmic reticulum and as a soluble enzyme in the cytosol of most mammalian cells. The mechanism of the soluble and microsomal epoxide hydrolase-catalyzed reaction appears to be a nucleophilic attack by an amino acid at the active site, possibly asparagine, on the epoxide to form an α-hydroxyacyl-enzyme intermediate. Water hydrolysis of the acyl-enzyme occurs at the carbonyl carbon of the ester bond yielding the active enzyme and diol (12,172). This stereoselective attack usually results in the diols having a transconfiguration. Hydrolysis of the ester is the rate-limiting step in catalysis.

Membrane-bound epoxide hydrolase has a 20 amino acid sequence at the N-terminal end that anchors it to the membrane. The active site of the enzyme occurs outside of the membrane. Unlike P450, if the anchor sequence of the protein is not present, the enzyme retains a portion of its catalytic activity (48).

Epoxide hydrolase has been found in a variety of tissues, including liver, kidney, lung, skin, intestine, colon, testis, ovary, spleen, thymus, heart, and brain. The activity of liver microsomal enzyme is relatively low in newborn rats and increases during neonatal development until adult males have about twice the activity of females. This sexual dimorphism is remarkably similar to that seen in the rat for P450. In contrast, the renal epoxide hydrolase of male and female rats does not demonstrate age-dependent changes or gender differences. Human hepatic microsomal epoxide hydrolase activities increase during gestation, but there does not appear to be a gender difference in humans (129).

Humans demonstrate considerable variation in epoxide hydrolase activity. This, in part, is associated with the inducibility of epoxide hydrolase and environmental exposures and life-style differences among individuals. In addition, there is evidence that there are genetic polymorphisms with the enzymes that result from amino acid sequence differences. These human polymorphisms may not result in significantly altered enzyme activity nor post-transcriptional regulation (93), although more work is needed in this area. Polymorphic expression of epoxide hydrolase has been related to specific human diseases (92,158).

The activity of this enzyme is induced by the classical inducers of cytochromes P450. Although *trans*-stibene oxide has been shown to be an inducer of epoxide hydrolase, no specific inducer of epoxide hydrolase has been reported. Two widely used inhibitors of epoxide hydrolase are trichloropropane oxide and cyclohexene oxide.

Because of its localization in the endoplasmic reticulum, microsomal epoxide hydrolase is ideally situated to catalyze the detoxication of lipophilic epoxides formed by P450; however, it can also be involved in metabolic activation. One example of metabolic activation is the biotransformation of benzo(a)pyrene to the ultimate mutagen benzo(a)pyrene trans-7,8-dihydrodiol-9-10-oxide, which is shown in Figure 3.4 and described under metabolic oxidations. These diol epoxides are poor substrates for further metabolism by epoxide hydrolase and, as shown in Figure 3.4 react with critical cellular macromolecules.

An immunologically distinct epoxide hydrolase has also been identified in the cytosol of some species. This enzyme may play a role in hydrolysis of more water-soluble epoxides that partition out of the endoplasmic reticulum. As discussed earlier, this enzyme completes with glutathione transferases for cytosolic epoxides. The activity of the cytosolic epoxide hydrolase appears to be highest in mice and rabbits and relatively low in rats.

Esterases and Amidases

Hydrolysis of xenobiotics containing ester linkages and amide bonds is catalyzed by a group of enzymes with broad substrate specificity. In general, these enzymes perform endogenous functions and appear to metabolize xenobiotics that have structural similarities to endogenous substrates.

The reactions carried out by this diverse group of enzymes are illustrated in Figure 3.24. Specificity of carboxylesterases depends on the nature of the R groups rather than on the atom (*O*, *N*, or *S*) adjacent to the carbonyl carbon (69). The esterases have been broadly grouped into three categories based on their reactivity with organophosphorous compounds (181). Those esterases preferring carboxylesters with aryl groups in the R position and that can use organophosphate esters as substrates are classified as A-esterases (Table 3.7). Those esterases preferring esters with alkyl groups in

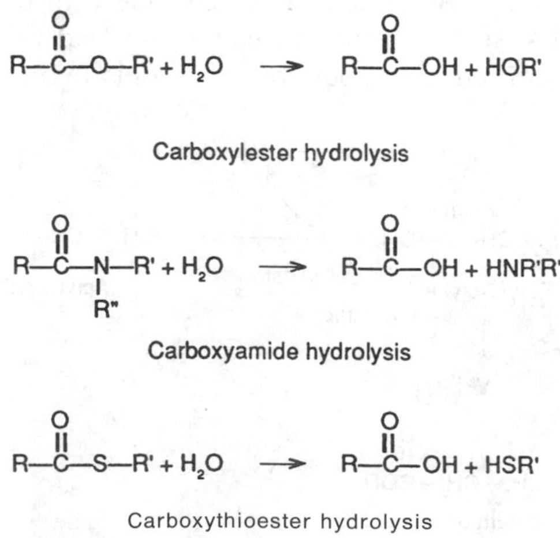

FIG. 3.24. Reactions catalyzed by esterases and amidases.

Table 3.7
Classification of esterases by how they interact with organophosphates and substrate specificity

Esterase	Interaction with organophosphates	Substrates	Examples
A-esterases (arylesterases)	Substrates	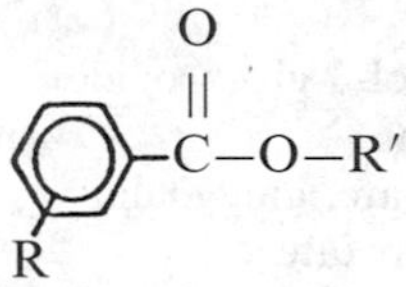 Aromatic Esters	Organophosphate and carbamate insecticides
B-esterases (carboxyltesterases including cholinesterases)	Inhibitors	$R{-}CH_2{-}C({=}O){-}O{-}R'$ Aliphatic Esters	Acetylcholine, acrylate esters, succinylcholine, propanidid
C-esterases (acetylesterases)	No interaction	$CH_3{-}C({=}O){-}O{-}R'$ Acetate Esters	*p*-Nitrophenyl acetate, *n*-propylchloroacetate

the R position and that are inhibited by organophosphate esters are classified as B-esterases. Another group of esterases that prefer acetate esters and do not interact with organophosphates are referred to as C-esterases. This classification has been devised to help organize this multifarious group of enzymes. It also has some practical value in toxicology. The mechanism of organophosphate and carbamate insecticide toxicity is inhibition of acetylcholinesterase, a B-type esterase. Organophosphate insecticides, such as malathion, are detoxified in mammals by A-esterase hydrolysis. Many insects have lower levels of A-esterases than mammals. The selective toxicity of malathion in birds and insects can be explained by the low activity of A-esterases compared to mammals (182).

MICROFLORA METABOLISM

Xenobiotic metabolism by microorganisms can be divided into reactions occurring in the environment and reactions occurring inside the body (141). Metabolism of chemicals by microorganisms in the environment has become familiar through the use of microorganisms to degrade chemical spills (164). The in vivo metabolism of chemicals by microorganisms is not as familiar. Mammals are colonized by microorganisms (only those animals raised in a germ-free environment (gnotobiotic) are microbe-free). The metabolic reactions carried out by these microorganisms are dependent on the substrate and environment in which they are growing. Microbes growing in an aerobic environment are capable of cleavage of aromatic nuclei and can use these xenobiotics as sole carbon sources for biosynthetic reactions and growth. Microbes growing in an anaerobic environment are more likely to carry out reductive metabolism. The hallmark of metabolism by organisms colonizing the intestinal tract of mammals is reduction (Table 3.8).

Because the majority of microbes that colonize various surfaces of the mammalian body reside in the intestinal tract, most of this discussion will center around intestinal microflora metabolism. The intestinal microflora can alter xenobiotic bioavailability by metabolizing the parent compound to a metabolite that may be absorbed to a greater or lesser extent. Intestinal microflora can also metabolize products of xenobiotic biotransformation that are secreted into the intestine either directly from the blood or via the bile, saliva, or by swallowing respiratory tract mucus. Metabolism of secreted metabolites is a common mechanism by which microflora influence xenobiotic toxicity.

Xenobiotic Biotransformation by Microbes Colonizing Mammals

The intestinal tract of mammals contains a variety of microorganisms. The location, total number, and species diversity of microflora vary among mammals. Microflora can range from ruminants that have evolved to be dependent on microflora metabolism for energy needs to monogastric mammals, such as humans, that have great

Table 3.8
Types of metabolic reactions carried out by intestinal bacteria

Reaction	Representative Substrate
Hydrolysis	
Glucuronides	Estradiol-3-glucuronide
Glycosides	Cycasin
Sulfamates	Cyclamate, amygdalin
Amides	Methotrexate
Esters	Acetydigoxin
Nitrates	Pentaerythritol trinitrte
Dehydroxylation	
C-Hydroxy groups	Bile Acids
N-Hydroxy groups	N-Hydroxyfluorenylacetamide
Decarboxylation	Amino acids
N-Demethylation	Biochanin A
Deamination	Amino acids
Dehydrogenase	Cholesterol, bile acids
Dehalogenation	DDT
Reduction	
Nitro groups	*p*-Nitrobenzoic acid
Double bonds	Unsatrated fatty acids
Azo groups	Food dyes
Aldehydes	Benzaldehydes
Alcohols	Benzyl alchols
N-Oxides	4-Nitroquinoline-1-oxide
Other Reactions	
Nitrosamine formation	Dimethylnitrosamine
Aromatization	Quinic acid
Acetylation	Histamine
Esterification	Gallic acid

numbers of bacteria only in the large intestine. Because of this variation in location within the intestinal tract, the types of microorganisms present, and hence the types of microflora metabolism, vary with the mammalian species being studied.

Another factor that relates to the location of the microflora is the disposition of the xenobiotic and its microflora metabolites. Chemicals metabolized by microflora located in the stomach will be distributed differently than chemicals metabolized in the large intestine.

The majority of mammals have a gradient of microflora that increases in numbers and species diversity along the intestinal tract from the foregut to the hindgut. Most research on microflora metabolism has focused on microorganisms that colonize the large intestine of humans, as most of the research in toxicology is directed toward understanding the toxicity of chemicals in humans. In vivo and in vitro models have been developed for studying human colonic flora (145).

Role of Diet and Other Factors in Modulating Microflora Metabolism

The microflora colonizing the digestive tract of mammals play a major role in the digestion of plant cell wall constituents that are indigestible by mammalian enzymes. These dietary fibers provide energy substrates that support the large bacterial populations in the gut. These energy sources also influence the microflora metabolism of xenobiotics. Certain types of dietary fiber, such as the fermentable carbohydrate pectin, can influence the toxicity of xenobiotics that require microflora metabolic activation by increasing the number of anaerobic bacteria colonizing the large intestine (35). This diet-induced elevation in the number of bacteria increases the total metabolic capacity of the large intestine for metabolizing xenobiotics. For reviews of this topic, see (143,144).

Examples of Xenobiotics Whose Toxicity is Dependent on Microflora Metabolism

Nitroaromatics

A body of literature has now accumulated indicating that the toxicity of many nitroaromatic compounds is dependent on microflora metabolism. One of the most studied nitroaromatics is 2,6-dinitrotoluene (DNT), which is hepatocarcinogenic in male rats (94). DNT is metabolized to the 2,6-dinitrobenzylalcohol glucuronide conjugate that is preferentially excreted in the bile of male rats (99) (Figure 3.25). The glucuronide conjugate is hydrolyzed by gut microflora β-glucuronidase, and one or both of the nitro groups are reduced by microflora nitroreductase to a reduced aglycone. The resulting aminobenzyl alcohol is relatively nonpolar and reabsorbed in the intestine, where it returns to the liver via the portal circulation. In the liver, the aglycone is activated to the putative proximate carcinogen by N-hydroxylation of the amine functional group followed by sulfation of the N-hydroxy group (82). Evidence that intestinal microflora were required for the activation of DNT was provided by studies indicating the genotoxicity of DNT in hepatocytes isolated from rats treated with DNT was dependent on the presence of bacteria in the intestinal tract (114). Rats raised in a germ-free environment showed minimal levels of genotoxicity. Additional evidence emphasizing the role of microflora in the metabolic activation of DNT was the observation that DNT was not genotoxic when tested in vitro in isolated hepatocytes (114). These results indicated that liver metabolism was not sufficient to activate the molecule to the ultimate carcinogen. The genotoxicity of DNT to liver cells only occurred when the compound was

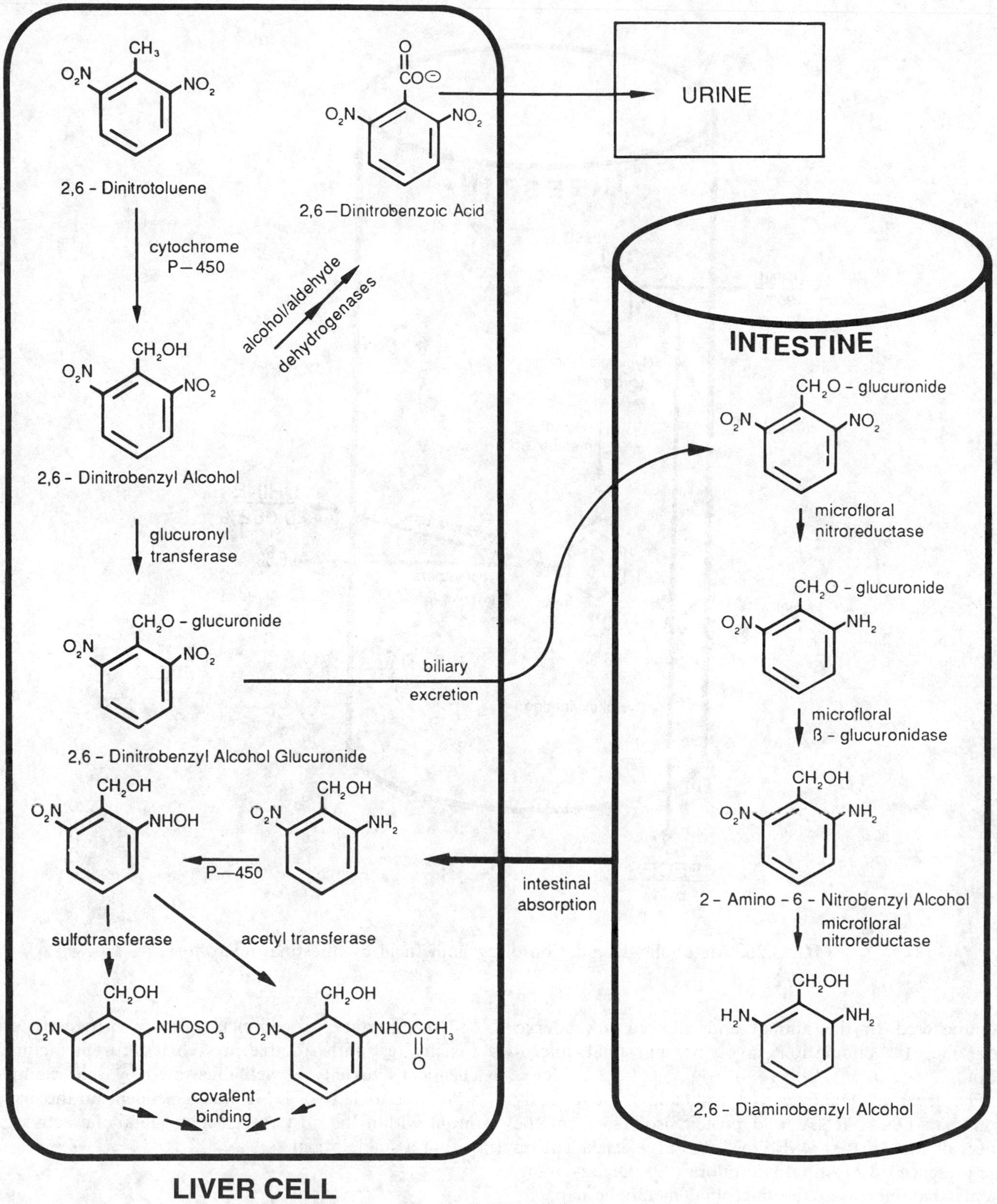

FIG. 3.25. Putative route of disposition of 2,6-dinitrotoluene.

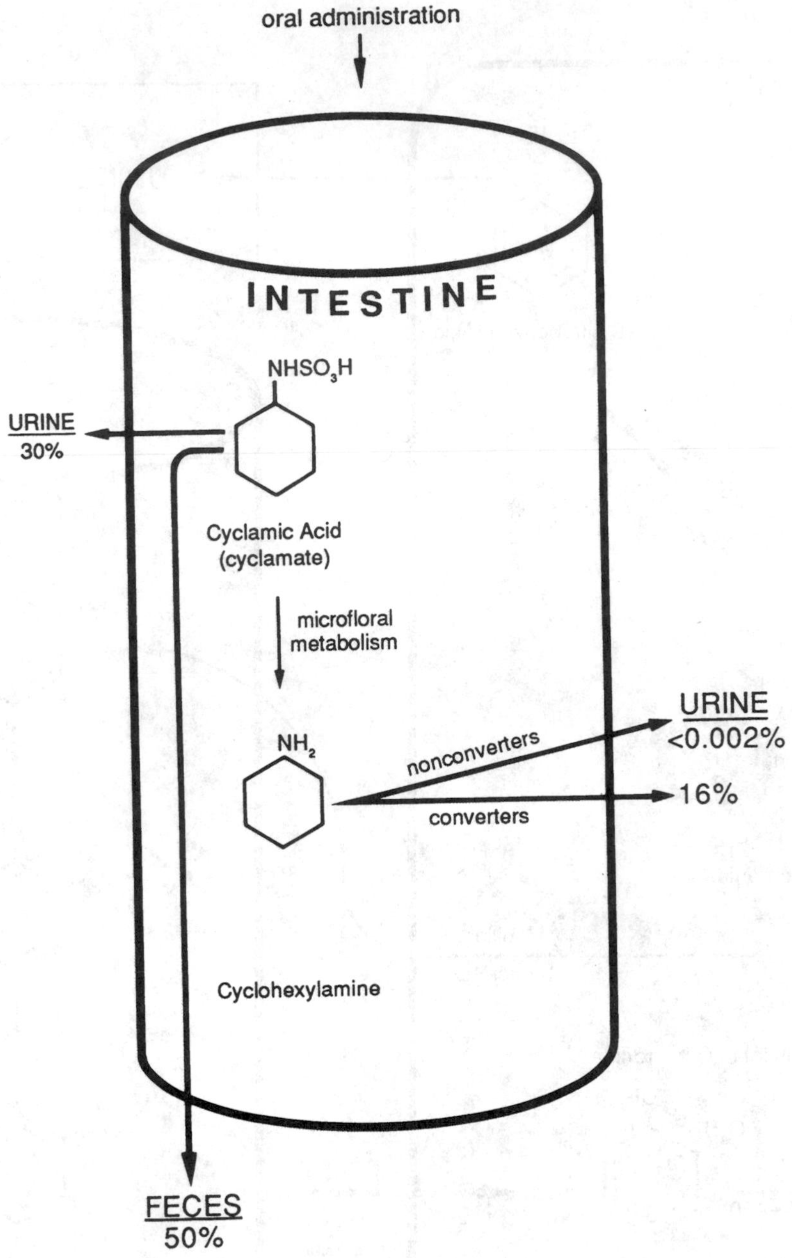

FIG. 3.26. Metabolic degradation of cyclamic acid by intestinal microflora.

administered to the animal and allowed to undergo enterohepatic circulation involving intestinal microflora.

The level of DNT-derived radioactivity covalently bound to DNA, RNA, and protein isolated from the livers of rats treated with DNT was also dependent on the presence of intestinal microflora (99). Dietary treatments that increased the microbial metabolic capacity of the rat's large intestine also increased the covalent binding of DNT-derived radioactivity to hepatic macromolecules (35).

The importance of complementary in vitro short-term toxicity test with suitable in vivo test for predicting a chemical's toxicity is well illustrated by this example, where the toxicity of DNT was dependent on the disposition within the host rather than metabolic activation within a single organ.

Cyclamate

The sodium and calcium salts of cyclamic acid (cyclohexylsulfamic acid) were used as an artificial sweetening agent until 1969 in the United States, when it was removed from the market because a metabolite, cyclohexylamine, was suspected of being a bladder carcinogen.

Most of the hydrolysis of cyclamate to cyclohexylamine takes place in the gut by the microflora, as shown in Figure 3.26 (142). Cyclohexylamine is more lipophilic than the parent acid and is readily absorbed from the intestine and excreted in the urine. Minor urinary metabolites include cyclohexanol and trans-cyclohexane-1, 2-diol.

Although only trace amounts of the cyclohexylamine could be detected in humans administered cyclamate, chronic exposure to the acid increased the capacity to produce this metabolite (104). It was found that certain individuals possessed a greater capacity to metabolize cyclamate to cyclohexylamine; these individuals were called converters. Thus, cyclamate is a good example of how prior exposure to a xenobiotic can alter the disposition of the xenobiotic. For additional reading on intestinal microflora xenobiotic metabolism, see (57,148).

INTEGRATION OF METABOLIC PATHWAYS

To understand a complex system, it is necessary to reduce it to its basic components and study each component separately. After achieving an understanding of the components, it is important to integrate them back into the whole. Xenobiotic metabolism is a complex system. Now that the reader has examined each component of the system in detail, let us examine how they act in concert to protect an organism from toxic injury. Specific examples of integrated biotransformations will be presented.

Bromobenzene

Bromobenzene, an industrial solvent, produces centrilobular necrosis in the rat liver. Bromobenzene's hepatotoxicity results from metabolic activation of the parent compound via epoxidation (Figure 3.27) catalyzed by P450. Bromobenzene-3, 4-epoxide is stable enough to

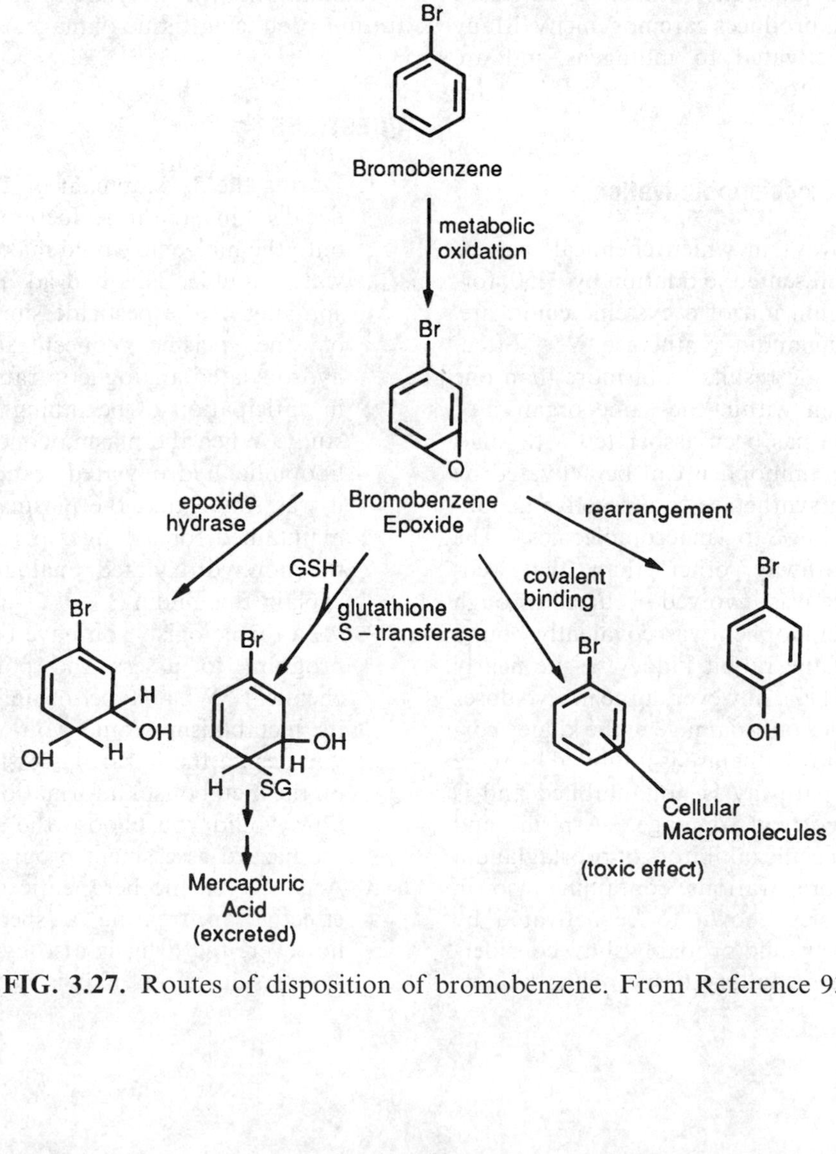

FIG. 3.27. Routes of disposition of bromobenzene. From Reference 93.

diffuse from its site of formation in the endoplasmic reticulum. It can then follow several biodisposition routes, depending on a variety of factors. The epoxide is a substrate for epoxide hydrolase, which would catalyze its hydration to the diol (Figure 3.27). It is also a substrate for glutathione *S*-transferase, which catalyzes thioether formation. The glutathione conjugate is processed by the kidney into its corresponding mercapturic acid, which is excreted in the urine (Figure 3.18). The epoxide can also undergo spontaneous rearrangement to form *p*-bromophenol. This metabolite can cycle through oxidation by P450. If the phase II reactions do not trap the reactive epoxide metabolite formed from the phase I metabolism of bromobenzene, the electrophilic carbon of the epoxide will react nonenzymatically with nucleophilic sites on cellular macromolecules. The ability of electrophilic metabolites to react covalently with critical cellular macromolecules is responsible for many chemical-induced toxicities, including chemical carcinogenicity. The delicate balance between detoxication and metabolic activation determines whether a chemical will be toxic to an organism and in what tissue. Toxic doses of bromobenzene produce centrilobular hepatic necrosis, whereas benzo[a]pyrene, which is activated via a similar mechanism, produces carcinogenicity. Many xenobiotics that are activated to mutagens and are tumorigenic are also cytotoxic.

Multiple Pathways for Xenobiotic Activation

Three different pathways in which chemicals can be nephrotoxic have been presented: oxidation by P450, formation of an episulfonium ion of a cysteine conjugate, and oxidation by prostaglandin synthetase. Very often, the toxicity of a xenobiotic results from more than one route of activation, even within the same organ. For example, acetaminophen has been associated with analgesic nephropathy. Acetaminophen can be activated by P450 and prostaglandin synthetase to a reactive metabolite capable of binding to macromolecules. The realization that a pathway other than the well-characterized P450 route was involved occurred through observations that acetaminophen was covalently bound in the inner medulla of the rabbit kidney, a site nearly devoid of P450 activity (117); however, large in vivo doses of acetaminophen produce only damage in the kidney cortex because prostaglandin synthetase is inhibited by these large doses. The P450 pathway is not inhibited and is responsible for the cortical damage. Aspirin and indomethacin are very specific inhibitors of prostaglandin synthetase. Analgesic preparations containing aspirin and one of the analgesics known to be activated by prostaglandin synthetase would probably show considerably less toxicity to the medullary tissue of the kidney. This gradient of oxidation pathways across the kidney, with the cortex possessing higher P450 activity than prostaglandin synthetase, the outer medulla being intermediate, and the inner medulla possessing far greater prostaglandin synthetase activity, results in certain xenobiotics being more toxic to one region of the kidney than another (192). These examples stress the importance of understanding the metabolic activation of a toxicant in explaining its mechanism of action.

Another example of competing pathways is acrylate ester metabolism. Many acrylate esters are good substrates for both alkyl esterase and glutathione *S*-transferase, and can react with glutathione nonenzymatically. Depending on the dose and route of administration of these compounds, these pathways compete for acrylate metabolism. The alkyl esterase hydrolyzes the acrylate ester to acrylic acid, and the corresponding alcohol (Figure 3.22) and glutathione adds to the β-carbon of the acrylate ester. Both pathways are considered detoxication pathways; however, at high doses glutathione can be depleted faster than it can be resynthesized. Elimination of the glutathione pathway can result in saturation of the esterase pathway and an accumulation of the acrylate ester at the site of administration producing tissue damage.

QUESTIONS

1. During the development of a new pesticide, it was decided that the introduction of a hydroxyl group onto the molecule would make the compound more water soluble. This had advantages in making the spraying of the pesticide simpler. An initial study of the plasma concentrations of the nonhydroxylated analogue in rats had been completed in anticipation of beginning a subchronic toxicity study. When the plasma concentrations of the less lipophilic, hydroxylated pesticide were determined, it was found that the plasma concentrations were maintained for a longer period of time than with the nonhydroxylated analogue. How would you explain this finding?
2. As a toxicologist, you have been asked to design a program to assess the potential hazard of a chemical. What type of information concerning its metabolism would you want to have before you design the hazard assessment program? Based on the metabolism information you have requested, how would you choose the species to be used in the hazard assessment program?
3. A cancer chemotherapeutic drug has been shown effective in treating a specific type of cancer; however, the drug is also cytotoxic and produces severe side effects if it is not rapidly metabolized

by cytochromes P450. Therefore, it is important to not treat a patient with doses of the drug that are too high for the patient's capacity to rapidly metabolize it to the less toxic product. What characteristics of the patient should be considered when attempting to choose a dose that will minimize the side effects?

4. A compound is functionalized by the P450 system and then forms sulfate and glucuronide conjugates and a mercapturic acid before being excreted. How may its metabolism be altered as the dose is increased from a No Observable Effect Level (NOEL) to a dose that produces severe toxicity?
5. Many chemical carcinogens are metabolized by routes that represent detoxication and by other routes that represent metabolic activation. What are the various phenomena that may shift the balance between detoxication and metabolic activation?

REFERENCES

1. Ambrosone, C. B., Coles, B. F., Freudenheim, J. L., and Shields, P. G. (1999): Glutathione S-transferase (GSTM1) genetic polymorphisms do not affect human breast cancer risk regardless of dietary antioxidants. *J. Nutr.*, 129:565–568.
2. Akerboom, T. P. M., and Sies, H. (1981): Assay of glutathione, glutathione disulfide, glutathione mixed disulfides in biological samples. In: *Methods in Enzymology, Vol. 77, Detoxication and Drug Metabolism: Conjugation and Related Systems.*, edited by S. P. Colowick and N. O. Kaplan, p. 376. Academic Press, New York.
3. Anders, M. W. (1988): Glutathione-dependent toxicity: Biosynthesis and bioactivation of cytotoxic S-conjugates. *ISI Atlas Pharmacol.*, 2:99–104.
4. Anders, M. W., Lash, L., Dekant, W., Wlfarra, A. A., and Dohn, D. R. (1988): Biosynthesis and biotransformation of glutathione S-conjugates to toxic metabolites. *CRC Crit. Rev. Toxicol.*, 18:311–341.
5. Andersson, B., Nordenskjold, M., Rahimtula, A., and Moldeus, P. (1982): Prostaglandin synthetase-catalyzed activation of phenacetin metabolites to genotoxic products. *Mol. Pharmacol.*, 22:479–485.
6. Axelrod, J. (1983): The discovery of the microsomal drug-metabolizing enzymes. In: *Drug Metabolism and Distribution: Current Reviews in Biomedicine 3*, edited by J. W. Lamble, pp. 1–6. Elsevier Biomedical Press, New York.
7. Backes, W. L. (1993): NADPH-cytochrome P450 reductase: Function. In: *Cytochrome P450*, edited by J. B. Schenkman and H. Greim, pp. 15–34. Springer-Verlag, Berlin.
8. Bernhardt, R. (1995): Cytochrome P450: Structure, function, and generation of reactive oxygen species. *Rev. Physiol. Biochem. Pharmacol.*, 127:137–221.
9. Bertilsson, L., Dahl, M. L., Sjoqvist, F., Abergwisted, A., Humble, M., Johansson, I., Lundqvist, E., and Ingelman-Sundberg, M. (1993): Molecular basis for rational megaperscribing in ultrarapid hydroxylators of debrisoquine. *Lancet*, 341:63.
10. Blanck, J., and Ruckpaul, K. (1993): Lipid-protein interactions. In: *Cytochrome P450*, edited by J. B. Schenkman and H. Greim, pp. 581–597. Springer-Verlag, Berlin.
11. Bock, K. W., Gschaidmeier, H., Heel, H., Lehmkoster, T., Munzel, P. A., Raschko, F., and Bock-Hennig, B. (1998): Ah receptor-controlled transcriptional regulation and function of rat and human UDP-glucuronosyltransferase isoforms. *Adv. Enzyme Regul.*, 38:207–222.
12. Borhan, B., Jones, A. D., Pinot, F., Grant, D. G., Kurth, M. J., and Hammock, B. D. (1995): Mechanism of soluble epoxide hydrolase: Formation of an α-hydroxy ester-enzyme intermediate through ASP-333. *J. Biol. Chem.*, 270:26923–26930.
13. Boxenbaum, H. G., Bedersky, I., Jack, M. L., and Kaplan, S. A. (1979): Influence of gut microflora on bioavailability. *Drug Metab. Rev.*, 9:259–279.
14. Boyd, J. A., and Eling, T. E. (1981): Prostaglandin endoperoxide synthetase-deficient cooxidation of acetaminophen to intermediates which covalently bind in vitro to rabbit renal medullary microsomes. *J. Pharmacol. Exp. Ther.*, 219:659–664.
15. Boyland, E., and Chasseaud, L. F. (1969): The role of glutathione and glutathione S-transferases in mercapturic acid biosynthesis. *Adv. Enzymol.*, 32:173–219.
16. Braumann and Preusse, (1879): Ueber bromophenylmercaptursaure. *Ber. Dtsch. Chem. Ges.*, 12:806–810.
17. Bresnick, G. (1993): Induction of cytochromes P450 1 and P450 2 by xenobiotics. In: *Cytochrome P450*, edited by J. B. Schenkman and H. Greim, pp 503–524. Springer-Verlag, Berlin.
18. Brockmoller, J., Cascorbi, I., Kerb, R., Sachse, C., and Roots, I. (1998): Polymorphisms in xenobiotic conjugation and disease predisposition. *Toxicol. Lett.*, 102–103: 173–183.
19. Brown, R. R., Miller, J. A., and Miller, E. C. (1954): The metabolism of methylated aminoazo dyes. IV. Dietary factors enhancing demethylation in vitro. *J. Biol. Chem.*, 209:211–217.
20. Burchell, B., and Coughtrie, M. W. H. (1989): UDP-glucuronosyltransferases. *Pharmacol. Ther.*, 43:261–289.
21. Burchell, B., Ebner, T., Baird, S., Bin Senati, S., Clark, D., Brierley, C., and Sutherland, L. (1994): Use of cloned and expressed human liver UDP-glucuronosyltransferases for analysis of drug glucuronide formation and assessment of drug toxicity. *Environ. Health Perspect*, 102 Suppl 9:19–23.
22. Caldwell, J. (1980): Comparative aspects of detoxication in mammals. In: *Enzymatic Basis of Detoxication*, edited by W. B. Jakoby, pp. 85–114. Academic Press, New York.
23. Calvin, C., Holzhauser, D., Constable, A., Huyggett, A.C., and Schilter, B. (1998): The coffee-specific diterpenes cafestol and kahweol protect against aflatoxin B_1 induced genotoxicity through a dual mechanism. *Carcinogenesis*, 19:1369–1375.
24. Chasseaud, L. F. (1973): The nature and distribution of enzymes catalyzing the conjugation of glutathione with foreign compounds. *Drug Metab. Rev.*, 2:185–220.
25. Chasseaud, L. F. (1978): The role of glutathione and glutathione S-transferases in the metabolism of chemical carcinogens and other electrophilic agents. *Adv. Cancer Res.*, 29:175–274.
26. Chen, G., Baron, J., and Duffet, M. W. (1995): Enzyme and sex-specific differences in the interlobular localization and distributions of aryl sulfotransferase IV (tyrosine-ester sulfotransferase) and alcohol (hydroxysteroid) sulfotransferase a in rat liver. *Drug Metab. Dispos.*, 12:1346–1353.
27. Cherrignton, J. J., Cao, Y., Cherrington, J. W., Rose, R. L., and Hodgson, E. (1998): Physiological factors affecting protein expression of flavin-containing monooxygenases 1, 3 and 5. *Xenobiotica*, 28:673–682.
28. Chiu, S. H., and Huskey, S. W. (1998): Species differences in N-glucuronidation. *Drug Metab. Dispos.*, 26:838–847.
29. Ciotti, M., Obaray, R., Martin, M. G., and Owens, I. S. (1997): Genetic defects at the UGT1 locus associated with Crigler-Naffar type I disease, including a prenatal diagnosis. *Am. J. Med. Genet.* 68:173–178.

30. Conklin, D. J., Langford, S. D., and Boor, P. J. (1998): Contribution of serum and cellular semicarbazide-sensitive amine oxidase to amine metabolism and cardiovascular toxicity. *Toxicol. Sci.*, 46:386–392.
31. Conney, A. H. (1967): Pharmacological implications of microsomal enzyme induction. *Pharmacol. Rev.*, 19:317–350.
32. Cooper, D. Y. (1964): Photochemical action spectrum of the terminal oxidase of mixed function oxidase systems. *Science*, 147:400–402.
33. Cundy, K. C., Sato, M., and Crooks, P. A. (1985): Sterospecific in vivo N-demethylation of nicotine in the guinea pig. *Drug Metab.*, 13:175–185.
34. Daly, A. K., Brockmuller, J., Broly, F., Eichelbaum, M., Evans, W. E., Gonzalez, F. J., Huang, J. D., Idle, J. R., Ingelman-Sundberg, M., Ishizaki, T., Jacqzaigrain, E., Meyer, U. A., Nebert, D. W., Steen, V. M., Wolf, C. R., and Zanger, U. M. (1996): Nomenclature for human CYP2D6 alleles. *Pharmacogenetics*, 6:193–201.
35. deBethizy, J. D., Sherrill, J. M., Rickert, D. E., and Hamm, T. E., Jr. (1983): Effects of pectin containing diets on the hepatic macromolecular covalent binding of 2, 6-dinitro[^{3}H]toluene in Fischer-344 rats. *Toxicol. Appl. Pharmacol.*, 69:369–376.
36. Degtyarenko, K. N., and Archakov, A. I. (1993): Molecular evolution of P450 superfamily and P450-containing monooxygenase systems. *Fed. Eur. Biochem. Soc. Let.*, 332:1–8.
37. De Meio, R. H. (1975): Sulfate activation and transfer. In: *Metabolism Pathways, Vol. 7*, Edition 3, edited by D. M. Greenberg, pp. 287–385. Academic Press, New York.
38. Dooley, T. P., and Huang, Z. (1996): Genomic organization and DNA sequences of two human phenol sulfotransferase genes (STP1 and STP2) on the short arm of chromosome 16. *Biochem. Biophys. Res. Commun.*, 228:134–140.
39. Dutton, G. J. (1971): Glucuronide-forming enzymes. In: *Handbook of Experimental Pharmacology. Part 2*, p. 378. Springer-Verlag, New York.
40. Dutton, G. J. (1980): *Glucuronidation of Drugs and Other Compounds*. CRC Press, Boca Raton, Florida.
41. Elfarra, A. A., and Anders, M. W. (1984): Commentary: Renal processing of glutathione conjugates—Role in nephrotoxicity. *Biochem. Pharmacol.*, 33:3729–3732.
42. Estabrook, R. W., Cooper, D. Y., and Rosenthal, O. (1963): The light reversible carbon monoxide inhibition of the steroid C-21-hydroxylase system of adrenal cortex. *Biochem. Z.*, 338:741–755.
43. Estabrook, R. W. (1996): Cytochrome P450: From a single protein to a family of proteins—with some personal reflections. In: *Cytochromes P450: Metabolic and Toxicological Aspects.*, edited by C. Ioannides, pp. 3–28. CRC Press, Boca Raton.
44. Evans, D. A. P. (1989): N-Acetyltransferase. *Pharmacol. Ther.*, 42:157–234.
45. Falany, C. N. (1991): Molecular enzymology of human liver cytosolic sulfotransferases. *Trends Pharmacol. Sci.*, 12:255–259.
46. Fiala, E. S., Sodum, R. S., Hussain, N. S., Rivenson, A., and Dolan, L. (1995): Secondary nitroalkanes: Induction of DNA repair in rat hepatocytes, activation by aryl sulfotransferase and hepatocarcinogenicity of 2-nitrobutane and 3-nitropentane in male F344 rats. *Toxicology*, 99:89–97.
47. Flesher, J. W., Horn, J., and Lehner, A. F. (1997): 6-sulfooxymethylbenzp(a)pyrene is an ultimate electrophilic and carcinogenic form of the intermediary metabolite 6-hydroxymethylbenzo(a)pyrene. *Biochem. Biophys. Res. Commun.*, 234:554–558.
48. Friedberg, T., Lollmann, B., Becker, R., Holler, R., and Oesch, F. (1994): The microsomal epoxide hydrolase has a single membrane signal anchor sequence which is dispensable for the catalytic activity of this protein. *Biochem. J.*, 303:967–972.
49. Frommer, U., Ullrich, V., Staudinger, H., and Orrenius, S. (1972): The monooxygenation of n-heptane by rat liver microsomes. *Biochem Biophys. Acta*, 280:487–494.
50. Fukami, J. I. (1984): Metabolism of several insecticides by glutathione S-transferase. *Int. Encycl. Pharmacol. Ther.*, 113:223–264.
51. Ganem, L. G., Trottier, E., Anderson, A., and Jefcoate, C. R. (1999): Phenobarbital induction of CYP2B1/2 in primary hepatocytes: Endocrine regulation and evidence for a single pathway for multiple inducers. *Tox. Appl. Pharmacol.*, 155:32–42.
52. Garfinkel, D. (1958): Studies on pig liver microsomes. I. Enzymic and pigment composition of different microsomal fractions. *Arch. Biochem. Biophys.*, 77:493–509.
53. Gertig, D. M., Stampfer, M., Haiman, C., Hennekens, X. H., Kelsey, K., and Huner, D. J. (1998): Glutathione S-transferase GSTM1 polymorphisms and colorectal cancer risk: A prospective study. *Cancer Epidemiol. Biomarker Prev.*, 11:1001–1005.
54. Gillette, J. R., Brodie, B. B., and La Du, B. N. (1957): The oxidation of drugs by liver microsomes: On the role of TPNH and oxidase. *J. Pharmacol. Exp. Ther.*, 119–540.
55. Glatt, H. (1997): Bioactivation of mutagens via sulfation. *FASEB J.*, 11:314–321.
56. Glatt, H., Bartsch, I., Coughtrie, M. W., Falany, C. N., Hagen, M., Landsiedels, R., Pabel, U., Phillips, D. H., Seidel, A., and Yamazoe, Y. (1998): Sulfotransferase-mediated activation of mutagens studied using a single membrane signal anchor sequence which is dispensable for the catalytic activity of this protein. *Chem. Biol. Interact.*, 109:195–219.
57. Goldman, P. (1978): Biochemical pharmacology of the intestinal flora. *Annu. Rev. Pharmacol.*, 18:523–539.
58. Gonzalez, F. G., and Nebert, D. W. (1990): Evolution of the P450 gene superfamily: Animal-plant warfare, molecular drive and human genetic differences in drug oxidation. *Trends in Genetics*, 6:182–186.
59. Gonzales, F. (1993): Cytochrome P450: Evolution and nomenclature. In: *Cytochrome P450*, edited by J. B. Schenkman and H. Greim, pp. 211–219. Springer-Verlag, Berlin.
60. Gorsky, L. D., Koop D. R., and Coon, M. J. (1984): On the stoichiometry of the oxidase and monooxidase reaction catalyzed by liver microsomal cytochrome P450. *J. Biol. Chem.*, 259:6812–6817.
61. Green, M. D., and Tephly, T. R. (1998): Glucuronidation of amine substrates by purified and expressed UDP-glucuronosyltransferase proteins. *Drug Metab. Dispos.*, 26:860–867.
62. Guengerich, F. P. (1996): The chemistry of cytochrome P450 reactions. In: *Cytochrome P450: Metabolic and Toxicological Aspects*, edited by C. Ioannides, pp. 55–74. CRC Press, Boca Raton.
63. Gueraud, F., and Paris, A. (1998): Glucuronidation: A dual control. *Gen. Pharmacol.*, 31:683–688.
64. Gut, J. (1982): Rotation of cytochrome P450 II: Specific interactions of cytochrome P450 with NADPH-cytochrome P450 reductase in phospholipid vesicles. *J. Biol. Chem.*, 257:7030–7036.
65. Habig, W. H. (1982): Glutathione S-transferases: Versatile enzymes of detoxification. In: *Radioprotectors and Anticarcinogens*, edited by O. F. Nygaard, pp. 169–190. Academic Press, New York.
66. Haenen, G. R. M., Vermeulen, N. P. E., Tai Tin Tsoni, J. N. L., Regetti, H. M. N., Timmerman, H., and Bast, A. (1988): Activation of the microsomal glutathione S-transferase and reduction of the glutathione dependent protection against lipid peroxidation by acrolein. *Biochem. Pharmacol.*, 37:1933–1938.

67. Hayes, P. C., Bouchier, I. A. D., and Becket, G. J. (1991): Glutathione S-transferases in human health and disease. *Gut*, 32:813–818.
68. Henry, W. (1815): *The Elements of Experimental Chemistry*. Vol. II, Edition 7, p. 352. Baldwin, Cradock and Joy, London.
69. Heyman, E. (1982): Hydrolysis of carboxylic esters and amides. In: *Metabolic Basis of Detoxication*, edited by W. B. Jakoby, J. R. Bend, and J. Caldwell, pp. 229–245. Academic Press, New York.
70. Horecher, B. L. (1950): Triphosphopyridine nucleotide cytochrome c reductase in liver. *J. Biol. Chem.*, 183:593–605.
71. Huttner, W. B. (1982): Sulphation of tyrosine residues: A widespread modification of proteins. *Nature*, 299:273–276.
72. Inskeep, P. B., Koga, N., Cmarik, J. L., and Guengerich, F. P. (1986): Covalent binding of 1,2-dihaloalkanes to DNA and stability of the major DNA adduct, S-[2-(N^7-guanyl)ethyl] glutathione. *Cancer Res.*, 46:2839–2844.
73. Ioannides, C. (1996): *Cytochromes P450: Metabolic and Toxicological Aspects*. CRC Press, Boca Raton.
74. Jakoby, W. B. (1978): The glutathione S-transferases: A group of multifunctional detoxification proteins. *Adv. Enzymol. Relat. Areas Mol. Biol.*, 46:383–414.
75. Jakoby, W. B., and Habig, W. H. (1980): Glutathione transferases. In: *Enzymatic Basis of Detoxification, Vol. II*, edited by W. B. Jakoby, pp. 63–94. Academic Press, New York.
76. Jakoby, W. B., and Keen, J. H. (1977): A triple-threat in detoxification: The glutathione S-transferases. *Trends Biochem. Sci.*, 2:229–231.
77. Jakoby, W. B., Duffel, M. W., Lyon, E. S., and Ramaswamy, S. (1984): Sulfotransferases active with xenobiotics: Comments on mechanism. In: *Progress in Drug Metabolism, Vol. 8*, edited by J. W. Bridges and L. F. Chasseaud, pp. 11–33. Taylor and Francis, London.
78. Jakoby, W. B. (1976): Glutathione S-transferases: Catalytic aspects. In: *Glutathione Metabolism and Function*, edited by I. M. Arias and W. B. Jakoby, pp. 189–211. Raven Press, New York.
79. Jakoby, W. B. (1980): Sulfotransferases. In: *Enzymatic Basis of Detoxification, Vol. II*,, edited by W. B. Jakoby, pp. 199–228. Academic Press, New York.
80. Johansson, I., Lundquist, E., Bertilsson, L., Dahl, M.-L., Sjoqvist, F., and Ingrelman-Sundberg, M. (1993): Inherited amplification of an active gene in the cytochrome P450 CYP2D locus as a cause of ultrarapid metabolism of debrisoquine. *Proc. Nat. Acad, Sci.*, USA, 90:11825–11829.
81. Kasper, C. B., and Henton, D. (1980): Glucuronidation. In: *Enzymatic Basis of Detoxification*, Vol. II, edited by W. B. Jakoby, pp. 3–41. Academic Press, New York.
82. Kedderis, G. L., Dyroff, M. C., and Rickert, D. E. (1984): Hepatic macromolecular covalent binding of the hepatocarcinogen 2,6-dinitrotoluene and its 2,4-isomer in vivo: Modulation by the sulfotransferase inhibitors pentachlorophenol and 2, 6-dichloro-4-nitrophenol. *Carcinogenesis*, 5:1199–1204.
83. Keller, W. (1842): Ueber verwandlung der Benzoesaure in hippursaure. Justus Liebig's *Ann. Chem.*, 43:108–111.
84. Kilty, C., Doyle, S., Hassett, B., and Manning, F. (1998): Glutathione S-transferases as biomarkers of organ damage: Applications of rodent and canine GST enzyme immunoassays. *Chem. Biol. Interact.*, 112:123–135.
85. Klaassen, C. D., and Boles, J. W. (1997): The importance of 3′-phosphoadenosine 5′-phosphosulfate (PAPS) in the regulation of sulfation. *FASEB J.*, 11:404–418.
86. Klingenberg, M. (1958): Pigments of rat liver microsomes. *Arch. Biochem Biophys.*, 75:379–386.
87. Koob, M., and Dekant, W. (1991): Bioactivation of xenobiotics by formation of toxic glutathione conjugates. *Chem. Biol. Interact.*, 77:107–136.
88. Kuriyama, Y., Omura, T., Siekevitz, P, and Palade, G. E. (1969): Effects of phenobarbital on the synthesis and degradation of protein components of rat liver microsomal membranes. *J. Biol. Chem.*, 244:2017–2026.
89. La Du, B. N., Gaudette, L., Trousof, N., and Brodie, B. B. (1955): Enzymatic dealkylation of aminopyrine (Pyramidon) and other alkylamines. *J. Biol. Chem.*, 214:741–752.
90. Lamartiniere, C. A. (1981): The hypothalamic-hypophyseal-gonadal regulation of hepatic glutathione S-transferases in the rat. *Biochem. J.*, 198:211–217.
91. Lamartiniere, C. A., and Lucier, G. W. (1983): Endocrine regulation of xenobiotic conjugation enzymes. *Basic Life Sci.*, (Organ Species Specif. Chem. Carcinog.): 295–312.
92. Lancaster, J. M., Brownlee, H. A., Bell, D. A., Futreahs, R. A., Marks, J. R., Berchuchk, A., Wiseman, R. W., and Taylor, J. A. (1996): Microsomal epoxide hydrolase polymorhphisms as a risk factor for ovarian cancer. *Mol. Carcinog.*, 3:160–162.
93. Laurenzana, E. M., Hassett, C., and Omiecinski, C. J. (1998): Post-transcriptional regulation of human microsomal epoxide hydrolase. *Pharmacogenetics*, 8:157–167.
94. Lenoard, T. B., and Popp, J. A. (1981): Investigation of the carcinogenic initiation potential of dinitrotoluene: Structure-activity study. *Proc. Am. Assoc. Cancer Res.*, 22:82.
95. Lewis, D. F. V. (1996): *Cytochromes P450: Structure, Function and Mechanism*. Taylor and Francis, London.
96. Lewis, D. F. V. (1998): The CYP2 family: Models, mutants and interactions. *Xenobiotica*, 28:617–661.
97. Lin, D. X., Tang, Y. M., Peng, Q., Lu, S.X., Ambrosone, C. B., Kadlubar, F. F. (1998): Susceptibility to esophageal cancer and genetic polymorphisms in glutathione S-transferases T1, P1 and M1 and cytochrome P450 2E1. *Cancer Epidemiol. Biomarkers Prev.*, 11:1013–1018.
98. Lui, L., and Klaassen, C. D. (1996): Different mechanism of saturation of acetaminophen sulfate conjugation in mice and rats. *Toxicol. Appl. Pharmacol.*, 139:128–134.
99. Long, R. M., and Rickert, D. E. (1982): Metabolism and excretion of 2, 6-dinitro-[^{14}C]toluene in vivo and in isolated perfused rat livers. *Drug Metab. Dispos.*, 10:455–458.
100. Lu, A. Y. H, Strobel, H. W., and Coon, M. J. (1969): Hydroxylation of benzphetamine and other drugs by a solubilized form of cytochrome P450 from liver microsomes: Lipid requirement for drug demethylation. *Biochem. Biophys. Res. Commun.*, 36:545–551.
101. Lu, A. Y. H., Strobel, A. H. W., and Coon, M. J. (1970): Properties of a solubilized form of the cytochrome P450-containing mixed-function oxidase of liver microsomes. *Mol. Pharmacol.*, 6:213–220.
102. Lyles, G. A. (1996): Mammalian plasma and tissue-bound semicarbazide sensitive amine oxidase: Biochemical, pharmacological and toxicological aspects. *Int. J. Biochem. Cell Biol.*, 28:259–274.
103. Mahgoub, A., Idles, J. R., Dring, L. G., Lancaster, R., and Smith, R. L. (1977): Polymorphic hydroxylation of debrisoquine in man. *Lancet*, 2:584–586.
104. Mallett, A. K. (1985): Metabolic adaptation of rat faecal microflora to cyclamate in vitro. *Fd. Chem. Toxicol.*, 23:1029–1034.
105. Mandell, H. G. (1981): Pathways of drug biotransformation: Biochemical conjugations. In: *Fundamentals of Drug Metabolism and Drug Disposition*, edited by B. N. La Du, H. G. Mandel, and E. L. Way, pp. 169–171. Robert E. Kreiger, Malabar, Florida.
106. Mannering, G. T. (1971): Microsomal enzyme systems which catalyze drug metabolism. In: *Fundamentals of Drug Metabolism and Drug Disposition*, edited by B. N. La Du, H. G. Mandel, and E. L. Way, pp. 206–252. Robert E. Kreiger, Malabar, Florida.

107. Marnett, L. J., and Reed, G. A. (1979): Peroxidative oxidation of benzo(a)pyrene and prostaglandin biosynthesis. *Biochemistry*, 18:2923–2929.

108. Marnett, L. J., Reed, G. A., and Johnson, J. T. (1977): Prostaglandin synthetase dependent benzo(a)pyrene oxidation: Products of the oxidation and inhibition of their formation by anti-oxidants. *Biochem. Biophys. Res. Commun.*, 79:569–576.

109. Mattammal, M. B., Zenser, T. V., and Davis, B. B. (1981): Prostaglandin hydroperoxidase-mediated 2-amino-4-(5-nitro-2-furyl)[14C]thiazole metabolism and nucleic acid binding. *Cancer Res.*, 41:4961–4966.

110. Meech, R., and Mackenzie, P. I. (1997): Structure and function of uridine diphosphate glucuronosyltransferases. *Clin. Exp. Pharmacol. Physiol.*, 24:907–915.

111. Meister, A., and Tate, S. S. (1976): Glutathione and related gamma-glutamyl compounds: Biosynthesis and utilization. *Annu. Rev. Biochem.*, 45:559–604.

112. Miller, M. S., Juchau, M. R., Guengerich, P., Nebert, D. W., and Raucy, J. L. (1996): Symposium overview: Drug metabolism enzymes in developmental toxicology. *Fund. Appl Toxicol.*, 34:165–175.

113. Miners, J. O., and Mackenzie, P. I. (1991): Drug glucuronidation in humans. *Pharmacol. Ther.*, 51:347–369.

114. Mirsalis, J. C., and Butterworth, B. E. (1982): Induction of unscheduled DNA synthesis in rat hepatocytes following in vivo treatment with dinitrotoluene. *Carcinogenesis*, 3:241–245.

115. Mitchell, J. R. (1973): Acetaminophen-induced hepatic necrosis. IV. Protective role of glutathione. *J. Pharacol. Exp. Ther.*, 187:211–217.

116. Miyazaki, M., Yoshizawa, I. I., and Fishman, J. (1969): Direct methylation of estrogen catechol sulfates. *Biochemistry*, 8:1669–1672.

117. Mohandas, J., Duggin, G. G., Horvath, J. S., and Tiller, D. J. (1981): Metabolic oxidation of acetaminophen (paracetamol) mediated by cytochrome P450 mixed-function oxidase and prostaglandin endoperoxide synthetase in rabbit kidney. *Toxicol. Appl. Pharmacol.*, 61:252–259.

118. Monks, T. J., Anders, M. W., Dekant, W., Stevens, J. L., Lau, S. S., and van Bladeren, P. J. (1990): Glutathione conjugate mediated toxicities. *Toxicol. Appl. Pharmacol.*, 106:1–19.

119. Morgan, E. T., and Coon, M. J. (1984): Effects of cytochrome b_5 on cytochrome P450-catalyzed reactions: Studies with manganese-substituted cytochrome b5. *Drug Metab. Dispos.*, 12:358–364.

120. Mugford, C. A., and Kedderis, G. L. (1998): Sex-dependent metabolism of xenobiotics. *Drug Metab. Rev.*, 30:441–498.

121. Mulder, G. J. (1981): Introduction. In: *Sulfation of Drugs and Related Compounds*, edited by G. J. Mulder, pp. 1–3. CRC Press, Boca Raton, Florida.

122. Mulder, G. J. (1981): Generation of reactive intermediates from xenobiotics by sulfate conjugation: Their potential role in chemical carcinogenesis. In: *Sulfation of Drugs and Related Compounds*, edited by G. J. Mulder, pp. 213–226. CRC Press, Boca Raton, Florida.

123. Munzel, P. A., Bruck, M., and Bock, K. W. (1994): Tissue-specific constitutive and inducible expression of rat phenol UDP-glucuronosyltransferase. *Biochem. Pharmacol.*, 8:1445–1448.

124. Nelson, D. R., Koymang, L., Kamataki, T., Stegeman, J. J., Feyerelsin, R., Waxman, D. J., Waterman, M. R., Gotoh, O., Coon, M. J., Estabrook, R. W., Gunsalus, I. C., and Nebert, D. W. (1996): P450 superfamily: Update on new sequences, gene mapping, accession numbers, and nomenclature. *Pharmacogenetics*, 6:1–42.

125. Nuccetelli, M., Mazzetti, A. P., Rossjohn, J., Parker, M. W., Beard, P., Caccuri, A. M., Federiai, G., Ricci, G., and LoBello, M. (1998): Shifting substrate specificity of human glutathione transferase (from class Pi to class alpha) by a single point mutation. *Biochem. Biophys. Res. Commun.*, 252:184–189.

126. Oesch, F. (1980): Species differences in activating and inactivating enzymes related to in vitro mutagenicity mediated by tissue preparations from these species. *Arch. Toxicol.*, Suppl. 3:179–194.

127. Oesch, F., Bentley, P., and Glatt, H. R. (1970): Prevention of benzp(a)pyrene induced mutagenicity by homogenous epoxide hydratase. *Int. J. Cancer*, 18:448–452.

128. Oesch, F., and Glatt, H. R. (1976): Evaluation of the importance of enzymes involved in the control of mutagenic metabolites. *IARC Sci. Publ.*, 1232:255–274.

129. Omiecinski, C. J., Aicher, L., and Swenson, L. (1994): Developmental expression of human microsomal epoxide hydrolase. *J. Pharmacol. Exp. Ther.*, 269:417–423.

130. Omura, T. (1969): Discussion. In: *Microsomes and Drug Oxidations*, edited by J. R. Gillette, pp. 160–161. Academic Press, New York.

131. Omura, T., and Sato, R. (1964): The carbon monoxide-binding pigment of liver microsomes. I. Evidence for its hemoprotein nature. *J. Biol. Chem.*, 239:2370–2378.

132. Omura, T., and Sato, R. (1964): The carbon monoxide-binding pigment of liver microsomes. II. Solubilization, purification and properties. *J. Biol. Chem.*, 2379–2385.

133. Ortiz de Montellano, P. R. (1986): Oxygen activation and transfer. In: *Cytochrome P450 Structure, Mechanism and Biochemistry*, edited by P.R. Ortiz de Montellano, pp. 217–271. Plenum Press, New York.

134. Ortiz de Montellano, P. R. (1986): *Cytochrome P450 Structure, Mechanism and Biochemistry*. Plenum Press, New York.

135. Pelkonen, O., Maenpan, J., Taavitsainen, P., Rautio, A., and Rautio, H. (1998): Inhibition and induction of human cytochrome P450 (CYP) enzymes. *Xenobiotica*, 28:1203–1253.

136. Phillips, A. H., and Langdon, R. G. (1962): Hepatic triphosphopyridine nucleotide-cytochrome reductase: Isolation, characterization and kinetic studies. *J. Biol. Chem.*, 237A:2652–2660.

137. Poulas, T. L., and Raag, R. (1992): Cytochrome $P450_{cam}$: Crystallography, oxygen activation, and electron transfer. *FASEB J.*, 6:674–679.

138. Rafter, J. J. (1983): Studies on the reestablishment of the intestinal microflora in germ-free rats with special reference to the metabolism of N-isopropyl-alpha-choloracetanilide (Propachlor). *Xenobiotica*, 13:171–178.

139. Raftogianis, R. B., Her, C., and Weinshiboum, R. M. (1996): Human phenol sulfotransferase pharmacogenetics: STP1 gene cloning and structural characterization. *Pharmacogenetics*, 6:473–478.

140. Rein, H., and Jung, C. (1993): Metabolic reactions: Mechanism of substrate oxidation. In: *Cytochrome P450*, edited by J. Schenkman and H. Greim, pp. 106–122. Springer-Verlag, Berlin.

141. Renwick, A. G. (1977): Microbial metabolism of drugs. In: *Drug Metabolism: From Microbe to Man*, edited by D. V. Parke and R. L. Smith, pp. 169–189. Proceeding of the International Symposium, Guilford, England. Taylor and Francis, London.

142. Renwick, A. G., and Williams, R. T. (1972): The fate of cyclamate in man and other species. *Biochem. J.*, 129:869–79.

143. Rowland, I. R., and Wise, A. (1985): The effect of diet on the mammalian gut flora and its metabolic activities. *CRC Crit. Rev. Toxicol.*, 16:31–103.

144. Rowland, I. R. (1988): Factors affecting metabolic activity of the intestinal microflora. *Drug Metab. Rev.*, 19:243–261.

145. Rumney, C. J., and Rowland, I. R. (1992): In vivo and in vitro models of the human colonic flora. *CRC Food Sci. Nutr.*, 31:299–331.
146. Runge-Morris, M. A. (1997): Regulation of expression of the rodent cytosolic sulfotransferases. *FASEB J.*, 11:109–117.
147. Sanglard, D., and Kappeli, O. (1993): Cytochrome P450 in unicellular organisms. In: *Cytochrome P450*, edited by J. Schenkman and H. Greim, pp. 325–349. Springer-Verlag, Berlin.
148. Scheline, R. R. (1973): Metabolism of foreign compounds by gastrointestinal microorganisms. *Pharmacol. Rev.*, 25:451–523.
149. Schenkman, J., and Greim, H. (1993): *Cytochrome P450*. Springer-Verlag, Berlin.
150. Schmiedlin-Ren, P., Edwards, D. J., Fitzsimmons, M. E., He, K., Lown, K. S., Woster, P. M., Rahman, A., Thummel, K. E., Fisher, J. M., Hollenberg, P. F., and Watkins, P. B. (1997): Mechanisms of enhanced oral availability of CYP3A4 substrates by grapefruit constituents: Decreased interocyte CYP3A4 concentration and mechanism-based inactivation by furanocoumarins. *Drug Metab. Disp.*, 25:1228–1233.
151. Sekura, R. D., Marcus, C. J., Lyon, E. S., and Jakoby, W. B. (1979): Assay of sulfotransferases. *Anal. Biochem.*, 95:82–86.
152. Sharer, J. E., Shipley, L. A., Vanderbranden, R. R., Binkley, S. N., and Wrighton, S. A. (1995): Comparisons of phase I and phase II in vitro hepatic enzyme activities of human, dog, rhesus monkey and cynomolgus monkey. *Drug Metab. Dispos.*, 11:1231–1241.
153. Singer, S. S., and Brun, L. (1978): Enzymatic sulfation of steroids—V11. Hepatic cortisol sulfation and glucocorticoid sulfotransferases in old and young male rats. *Exp. Gerontol.*, 13:425–429.
154. Singer, S. S., Giera, D., Johnson, J., and Sylvester, S. (1976): Enzymatic sulfation of steroid. I. The enzymatic basis for the sex difference in cortisol sulfation by rat liver preparations. *Endocrinology*, 98:963–974.
155. Singer, S. S., and Sylvester, S. (1976): Enzymatic sulfation of steroids. II. The control of the hepatic cortisol sulfotransferase activity and of the individual hepatic steroid sulfotransferases of rats by gonads and gonadal hormones. *Endocrinology*, 99:1346–1352.
156. Singh, S. V., Benson, P. J., Hy, X., Pal, A., Srivastava, S. K., Awasthi, S., Zaren, H. A., and Orchard, J. L. (1998): Gender-related differences in susceptibility of A/J mouse to benzo(a)pyrene-induced pulmonary and forestomach tumorigenesis. *Cancer Lett.*, 128:197–204.
157. Sligar, S. G., and Murray, R. I. (1986): Cytochrome P450cam and other bacterial P450 enzymes. In: *Cytochrome P450: Structure, Mechanism, and Biochemistry*, edited by P. R. Ortiz de Montellano, pp. 429–503, Plenum Press, New York.
158. Smith, C. A., and Harrison, D. J. (1997): Association between polymorphism in gene for microsomal epoxide hydrolase and susceptibility to emphysema. *Lancet*, 350: 630–633.
159. Smith, G., Stubbins, M. J., Harries, L. W., and Wolf, C. R. (1998): Molecular genetics of human cytochrome P450 monooxygenase superfamily. *Xenobiotica*, 28:1124–1165.
160. Smith, D. A., and Jones, B. C. (1992): Speculations on the substrate structure activity relationship (SSAR) of cytochrome P450 enzymes. *Biochem. Pharmacol.*, 44:2089–2094.
161. Smith, G. J., and Litwack, G. (1980): Roles of ligandin and the glutathione S-transferases in binding steroid metabolites, carcinogens and other compounds. *Rev. Biochem. Toxicol.*, 2:1–47.
162. Smith, G. J., Ohl, V. S., and Litwack, G. (1977): Ligandin, the glutathione S-transferases, and chemically induced hepatocarcinogenesis: A review. *Cancer Res.*, 37: 8–14.
163. Sreeravan, L., Hedge, M. W., and Sladek, N. E. (1995): Identification of a class 3 aldehyde dehydrogenase in human saliva and increased levels of this enzyme, glutathione *S*-transferases, and DT-diaphorase in the saliva of subjects who continually ingest large quantities of coffee or broccoli. *Clin. Cancer Res.*, 1:1153–1163.
164. Stirling, L. A. (1980): Microorganisms and environmental pollutants. In: *Introduction to Environmental Toxicology*, edited by F. E. Guthrie and J. J. Perry, pp. 329-342. Elsevier North Holland, New York.
165. Strassburg, C. P., Nguyen, N., Manns, M. P., and Tukey, R. H. (1998): Polymorphic expression of the UDP-glucuronosyltransferase UGT1A gene locus in human gastric epithelium. *Mol. Pharmacol.*, 54:647–654.
166. Strasser, S. I., Smid, S. A., Mashford, M. L., Desmond, P. V. (1997): Sex hormones differentially regulate isoforms of UDP-glucuronosyltransferase. *Pharm. Res.*, 14:1115–1121.
167. Strolin Benedetti, M., and Dostert, P. (1994): Contribution of amine oxidases to the metabolism of xenobiotics. *Drug Metab. Rev.*, 26:507–535.
168. Tateishi, N., and Sakamoto, Y. (1983): Nutritional significance of glutathione in rat liver. In: *Glutathione: Storage, Transport and Turnover in Mammals*, edited by S. Y. Sakamoto, T. Higashi, and N. Tateishi, pp. 13–38. Japan Science Society Press, Tokyo/VNH Science Press, Utrecht.
169. Tateishi, M., Suzuki, S., and Shimizu, H. (1978): Cysteine conjugate beta-lyase in rat liver: A novel enzyme catalyzing formation of thiol-containing metabolites of drugs. *J. Biol. Chem.*, 253:8854–8859.
170. Tephly, T. R., and Burchell, B. (1990): UDP-glucuronosyltransferases: A family of detoxifying enzymes. *Trends Pharmacol. Sci.*, 11:276–279.
171. Thurman, R. G. (1987): Regulation of monooxygenation in intact cells. In: *Mammalian Cytochromes P450, Vol. II*, edited by F. P. Guengerich, pp. 131–152. CRC Press, Boca Raton, Florida.
172. Tzeng, H. F., Laughlin, L. T., and Armstrong, R. N. (1998): Semifunctional site-specific mutants affecting the hydrolytic half-reaction of microsomal epoxide hydrolase. *Biochemistry*, 37:2905–2911.
173. U.S. FDA (1997): *Guidance for Industry: Drug metabolism/drug interaction studies in the drug development process: Studies in vitro*. The Drug Information Branch, Center for Drug Evaluation and Research, Rockville, Maryland.
174. Vamvakas, S., and Anders, M. W. (1990): Formation of reactive intermediates by phase II enzymes: Glutathione-dependent bioactivation reactions. In: *Biological Reactive Intermediates IV*, edited by C. M. Witmer, et al., pp. 13–24. Plenum Press, New York.
175. vanBladeren, P. J., and van Ommen, B. (1991): The inhibition of glutathione S-transferases: Mechanisms, toxic consequences and therapeutic effects. *Pharmacol. Ther.*, 51:35–46.
176. van Lieshout, E. M., and Peters, W. H. (1998): Age and gender dependent levels of glutathione and glutathione S-transferases in human lymphocytes. *Carciongenesis*, 19:1873–1875.
177. Van Ness, K. P., McHugh, T. E., Bammler, T. K., and Eaton, D. L. (1998): Identification of amino acid residues essential for high aflatoxin B1-8,9-epoxide conjugation activity in alpha class glutathione S-transferases through site-directed mutagenesis. *Toxicol. Appl. Pharmacol.*, 152:166–174.
178. Vesell, E. S., and Penno, M. B. (1983): Intraindividual and interindividual variations. In: *Biological Basis of Detoxication*, edited by J. Caldwell and W. B. Jakoby, pp. 369–410. Academic Press, New York.
179. Visser, T. J., van Buuren, J. C. J., Rutger, M., Rooda, S. J. E., and deHerder, W. W. (1990): The role of sulfation in thyroid hormone metabolism. *Trends Endocrinol. Metab.*, 1:211–218.

180. Vos, R. A. M. E., and Van Bladeren, P. J. (1990): Glutathione S-transferase in relation to their role in the biotransformation of xenobiotics. *Chem. Biol. Interactions*, 75:241–265.

181. Walker, C. H., and Mackness, M. I. (1983): Esterases: Problems of identification and classification. *Biochem. Pharmacol.*, 32:3265–3269.

182. Walker, C. H., and Oesch, F. (1983): Enzymes in selective toxicology. In: *Biological Basis of Detoxication*, edited by J. Caldwell and W. B. Jakoby, pp. 349–368. Academic Press, New York.

183. Watabe, T., Hiratsuka, A., and Okuda, H. (1985): Sulfate conjugations. *Tok Foramu*, 8:264–277.

184. Watabe, T. (1985): Metabolic activation of 7,12-dimethylbenz(a)anthracene and 7-methylbenz(a)anthracene via hydroxymethyl sulfate esters by P450-sulfotransferase. *Gann Monogr.*, 30:125–139.

185. Weinshilboum, R. (1992): Methylation pharmacogenetics: Thiopurine methyl transferase as a model system. *Xenobiotica*, 22:1055–1071.

186. Weinshilboum, R. M., Otterness, D. M., Aksoy, I. A., Wood, T. C., Her, C., and Raftoginnis, R. B. (1997): Sulfotransferase molecular biology: cDNAs and genes. *FASEB J.* 11:7–14.

187. Wendel, A., Heinle, H., and Silbernagl, S. (1977): The degradation of glutathione derivatives in the rat kidney. *Curr. Probl. Clin. Biochem.*, 8:73–84.

188. Williams, C. H., Jr., and Kamin, H. (1962): Microsomal triphosphopyridine nucleotide-cytochrome c reductase of liver. *J. Biol. Chem.*, 237:587–595.

189. Williams, R. T. (1959): *Detoxication Mechanisms*, Edition 2. Chapman and Hall, London.

190. Wood, J. I. (1970): Biochemistry of mercapturic acid formation. In: *Metabolic Conjugation and Metabolic Hydrolysis, Vol. 2*, edited by W. H. Fishman, pp. 261–299. Academic Press, New York.

191. Yu, P. H., and Zuo, D.-M. (1997): Formation of formaldehyde form adrenaline: A potential risk factor for stress-related antipathy. *Neurochem. Res.*, 22:615–620.

192. Zenser, T. V., Mattammal, M. B., and Davis, B. B. (1979): Demonstration of separate pathways for the metabolism of organic compounds in rabbit kidney. *J. Pharmacol. Exp. Ther.*, 208:418–421.

193. Zhu, B. T., Suchar, L. A., Huang, M. T., and Conney, A. H. (1996): Similarities and differences in the glucuronidation of estradiol and estrone by UDP-glucuronosyltransferase in liver microsomes from male and female rats. *Biochem Parmacol.*, 51:1195–1202.

194. Ziegler, D. M. (1990): Flavin-containing monooxygenases: Enzymes adapted for multisubstrate specificity. *Trends Pharmacol. Sci.*, 11:321–324.

195. Ziegler, D. M. (1993): Recent studies on the structure and function of multisubstrate flavin-containing monooxygenase. *Ann. Rev. Pharmacol. and Toxicol.*, 33:179–199.

Principles and Methods of Toxicology,
Fourth Edition, edited by A. Wallace Hayes.
Taylor & Francis, Philadelphia © 2001.

Chapter 4

Toxicokinetics: Pharmacokinetics in Toxicology

Andrew Gordon Renwick

The term pharmacokinetics is derived from the Greek words *pharmako* (medicine, drug, or poison) and *kinetikos* (motion or movement). Thus, pharmacokinetics is the study of the movement of drugs within the body, that is, the absorption, distribution via the blood, metabolism, and excretion. This term is in contrast to *pharmacodynamics*, which is concerned with the pharmacological actions of the drug within the body, that is, its effects at the site of action/receptor. The word drug is popularly associated with medicines or therapeutic agents, although for certain subjects, for example, drug metabolism, this word has long been applied to any environmental anutrient, that is, drugs, pesticides, environmental contaminants, and plant products. Because the processes concerned with the absorption, distribution, and elimination of therapeutic drugs are nonspecific and shared with other types of anutrients, the principles of pharmacokinetics apply to any environmental anutrient (xenobiotic). It is thus valid to apply the term *pharmacokinetics* to all foreign compounds, although other terms, such as "chemobiokinetics" (32), have been proposed to describe the application of these principles to nontherapeutic substances. *Toxicokinetics* is receiving increasing and even international (122) usage; it has useful connotations with respect to the nonspecific nature of the toxicant and the implicit requirement for kinetic data at toxic doses. However, most of the basic principles were established in relation to therapeutic drugs, and the introductory chapters of many clinical pharmacology textbooks contain much useful basic information. The term *toxicokinetics* is frequently misused and applied to nonspecific data, such as autoradiography, and radiolabeled excretion and metabolism studies. Toxicokinetics, in the present context, is the application of pharmacokinetic principles to animal toxicity studies and to human toxicity data in order to provide information on exposure to the parent compound and its metabolites, and other aspects such as accumulation during chronic exposure. The incorporation of data from animal studies into risk assessment requires data from related studies in humans at appropriate doses.

The understanding and interpretation of toxicological findings requires information on two key areas: (a) delivery of the compound to its site of action (toxicokinetics) and (b) the mechanism of action and potency of the chemical at the site of action (toxicodynamics) (Figure 4.1). Such information may assist in understanding the dose–response relationship in animal toxicity studies and its relevance to humans as well as assisting in the identification of potentially at-risk subgroups of

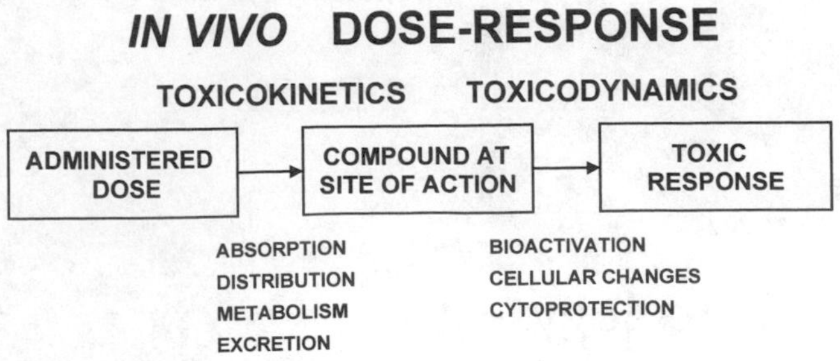

FIG. 4.1. The relationship between in vivo response and toxicokinetics and toxicodynamics.

the exposed human population. Risk assessment has traditionally used different approaches for cancer (and other nonthreshold effects), compared with toxicity believed to show a biological threshold. For cancer, and similar effects, the dose–response relationship in animals is extrapolated down to a very low level of risk, or virtually safe dose; toxicokinetics are frequently incorporated into the process by the use of a physiologically based pharmacokinetic model (PBPK). For threshold toxicity, the approach is to estimate a level of human intake without appreciable health effects; the acceptable daily intake (ADI), or tolerable daily intake (TDI), or reference dose (RfD), for human exposure is derived by dividing the intake of animals treated at the no-observed-adverse-effect level (NOAEL) (on a mg/kg basis) by an appropriate safety or uncertainty factor. A safety factor of 100 is usually applied with a 10-fold factor to allow for extrapolation from animals to humans and a 10-fold factor to allow for interindividual differences in the exposed human population (75,123). A scheme was proposed (76) that would allow appropriate toxicokinetic or mechanistic data to be incorporated into the derivation of a data-derived safety factor by the replacement of part of the relevant 10-fold default factor. The use of such a scheme would produce a more secure basis for the establishment of an ADI/TDI/RfD, while providing a direct return for the investment necessary to produce more than the minimum toxicity database required for regulatory purposes. The greater use of toxicokinetic data in regulatory decisions will provide a more scientific basis for risk assessment, and will encourage the increased generation of such data.

Toxicokinetic studies are important in compound development, and such information is regarded as necessary before proceeding with long-term and carcinogenicity tests (101). If the kinetic evidence indicates tissue accumulation on prolonged dosing, saturation of elimination at subtoxic doses, or the formation of chemically reactive metabolites, chemical analogs without these problems may be selected for development, because these properties mitigate against a high therapeutic index (for drugs) or ADI (for food additives).

Toxicokinetics is concerned with the relationship between the external dose, as usually measured in toxicity studies (e.g., mg/kg body weight per day) and a measure of the internal dose of active compound delivered to the target for toxicity (Figure 4.1), such as the concentration in the general circulation or at the target for toxicity. Frequently the compound administered has to pass many lipid and metabolic barriers prior to reaching the target, as shown in Figure 4.2. An understanding of the extent and nature of these processes may be derived from serial analysis of the concentrations of the chemical in plasma and urine. A knowledge of the concentrations of the parent compound and any metabolites in plasma and tissues, allied to the rate of change on further dosing or cessation of administration, allows logical selection of the animal species most appropriate for toxicity testing, and extrapolation of any toxicity observed in animals to the likely risk for man (2,17,29,65,75,76,122, 123,124).

Therefore, toxicokinetic studies are designed to produce information on the profile of exposure of the site of toxicity to the active moiety, under the conditions which produce the toxicity, and which are the basis for determining the NOAEL. Important toxicokinetic data relate to:

1. Exposure (or internal dose) in animals based on plasma or blood concentrations of the parent compound or its active metabolite
2. Relationship between the dose given to the animals and exposure
3. Relationship between plasma or blood concentrations and those at the site of toxicity
4. Information on appropriate blood/plasma data after the administration of tracer doses to human volunteers in order to allow extrapolation of animal data to humans

The aim of this chapter is to introduce the underlying principles in both biological and mathematical terms, and subsequently to describe methods of obtaining suitable samples from certain animal species, primarily the rat. The final section of the chapter covers the analysis of data, with examples to illustrate the type of information and insights that may be obtained using these techniques. In all cases, the examples and data processing described have been restricted to simple analyses of results, in order to illustrate principles. References are provided for further reading, because the analysis of data using computer programs and more complex mathematical models are not covered in this chapter.

In the past, animal and human disposition studies during drug development utilized slightly different approaches, with absorption, distribution, metabolism, and excretion studies (ADME studies) in animals, which were usually based on the fate of the radiolabeled drug,

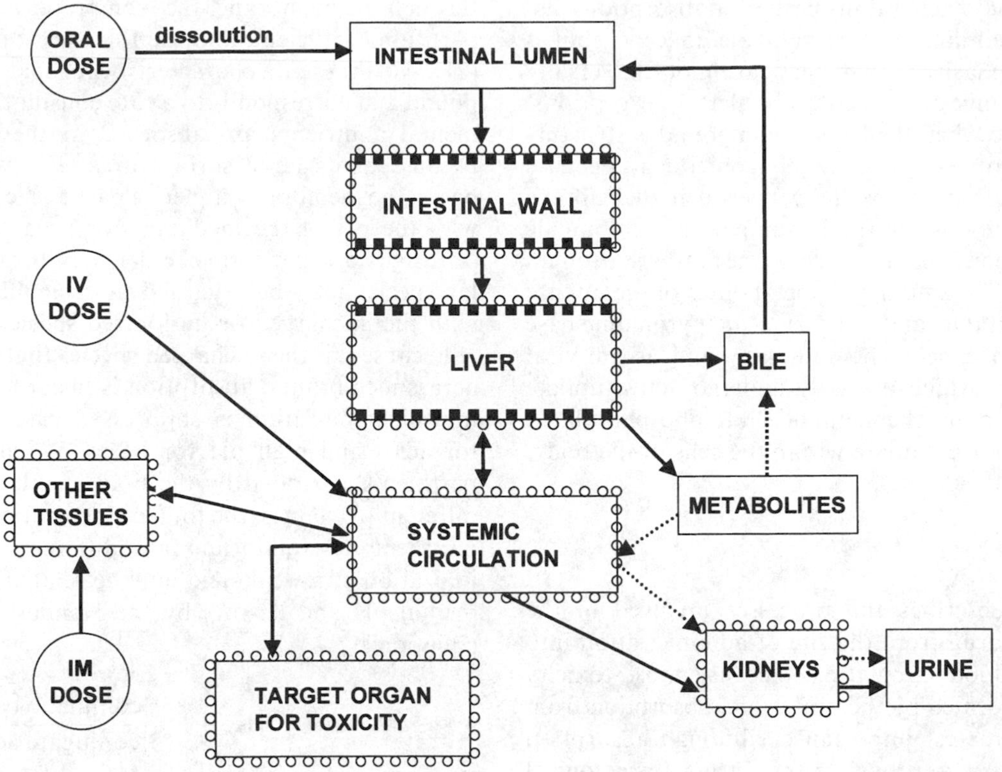

FIG. 4.2. Toxicity in relation to pharmacokinetics. The chemical may be given orally or by injection or inhalation. The concentration at the target organ is in equilibrium with that in the systemic circulation, which is itself in dynamic equilibrium with a large number of other physiological processes tending to increase or decrease that concentration. The transfer from one tissue to another usually involves transfer across a lipid membrane (*open circles*) and frequently entails entering a tissue with high elimination capacity (*solid squares*) such as the liver.

whereas similar radiolabeled studies in humans were frequently supplemented with data on plasma concentration–time curves. The basis for the interpretation of plasma concentration–time curves was the formulation of suitable mathematical models which allowed the derivation of rates of absorption, metabolism, and excretion in humans. It was thus possible, using pharmacokinetic methods, to gain an insight into the rates and extents of processes in humans, which had been shown to occur in animals using serial sacrifice and tissue analysis, and which had been detected in metabolic studies (measurement of urinary metabolites or incubation of the drug with liver microsomes).

However, with the development of automated analytical techniques of high sensitivity and specificity (such as HPLC, LC-MS, and LC-MS-MS), the expansion of laboratories undertaking plasma drug analyses, and the full potential of pharmacokinetics to reveal information on in vivo drug absorption, distribution, and elimination has resulted in these techniques being applied increasingly to toxicology problems in laboratory animals. For therapeutic drugs, the impetus to develop toxicokinetic data in animals has been increased by recent international harmonization initiatives which promote the use of kinetic data in animals and humans to establish maximum dosage levels for toxicity studies. Although there is not acceptance that the top dose for nondrugs can be based on kinetic principles, there is increasing recognition of the value of such data for the interpretation of toxicity studies in which the top dose has been established by tolerability, for example the maximum tolerated dose. Problems of accumulation on repeated dosing and saturation of elimination are particularly pertinent to high-dose animal toxicity studies, and information on these areas can be obtained only from suitably designed in vivo toxicokinetic studies. It must be emphasized at the outset that the key to successful kinetic studies is the development of an assay of high specificity that measures the chemical without interference by its metabolites, and that is of sufficient sensitivity to define the terminal slope accurately (see below).

BIOLOGICAL PRINCIPLES

Certain general principles governing the disposition of therapeutic drugs are applicable to nearly all foreign compounds that are not substrates for normal intermediary metabolism. These general properties of absorption, distribution, and elimination are valuable concepts, but it should be emphasized that they are not universally applicable, and investigators must be alert for exceptions. Exceptions arise when the foreign compound is structurally similar to an endogenous body constituent, because it may then undergo a specific carrier-mediated uptake process or metabolism. Good examples of compounds showing such characteristics include the antiparkinsonian drug levodopa, the amino acid metabolites of the intense sweetener aspartame, and the purine and pyrimidine base analogs used in cancer chemotherapy and as antiviral agents, many of which not only undergo active uptake into cells but also may be metabolized to phosphorylated products, which accumulate within the cells of the body.

Absorption

Absorption describes the processes involved in the transfer of the drug from the site of administration into the systemic blood circulation. Because most toxicity studies are performed by the oral route, absorption from the gut is of greatest importance, although absorption from other sites is appropriate for certain toxicological studies.

Absorption from the Gut

Significant absorption occurs once the compound has dissolved and is present in the gut lumen as a molecular solution. Slow dissolution and release of drugs from oral sustained-release formulations can be useful for therapeutic drugs that are eliminated very rapidly. Dissolution may be slow and be the rate limiting process, especially when high doses have to be administered as a suspension. Slow dissolution of the compound in the gut lumen can affect the rate of absorption, the peak concentrations, and even the magnitude of acute effects.

The extent of absorption is determined largely by the pH of the gut lumen and the pK_a and lipid solubility of the compound. Other biological variables, such as the presence of food, gastric emptying time, intestinal transit time, and the gut microflora, may also play important roles in limiting the rate of absorption and the amount of compound absorbed unchanged. The absorption of chemicals requires passage across lipid membranes (Figure 4.2), which can involve (a) passive diffusion through the membrane, (b) passage through membrane pores, and (c) specialized carrier-mediated processes.

The rate of diffusion of a chemical across a membrane, given by Fick's law, is proportional to the concentration gradient, the membrane surface area, and the permeability coefficient of the compound. The permeability coefficient depends on the diffusivity of the molecule through the membrane, the membrane/aqueous medium partition coefficient, and the thickness of the membrane (21), and thus it is a characteristic for that particular compound and corresponds to a rate constant. Most environmental anutrients are absorbed in the small intestine because of its large surface area. For weak acids and bases, the membrane/aqueous partition coefficient varies with the pH of the medium. For such compounds, the diffusivity and partition coefficient of the ionized molecular species may be regarded as insignificant compared with the uncharged or un-ionized species.

Because it is the uncharged species that readily diffuses across membranes, absorption is faster under conditions in which ionization is suppressed, that is, at low pH for acids and high pH for bases. When the two compartments separated by the lipid membrane are kept at different pH values, the total concentrations in each compartment at equilibrium are different. The extent of ionization of a weak acid may be related to the environmental pH and its pK_a by the Henderson–Hasselbalch equation:

$$\mathrm{pH} = \mathrm{pK_a} + \log\frac{[\text{conjugate base}]}{[\text{conjugate acid}]}$$

At equilibrium, the concentrations of the diffusible form (un-ionized) on each side of the membrane are equal, and the concentration of the ionized form is given by the Henderson–Hasselbalch equation (Figure 4.3).

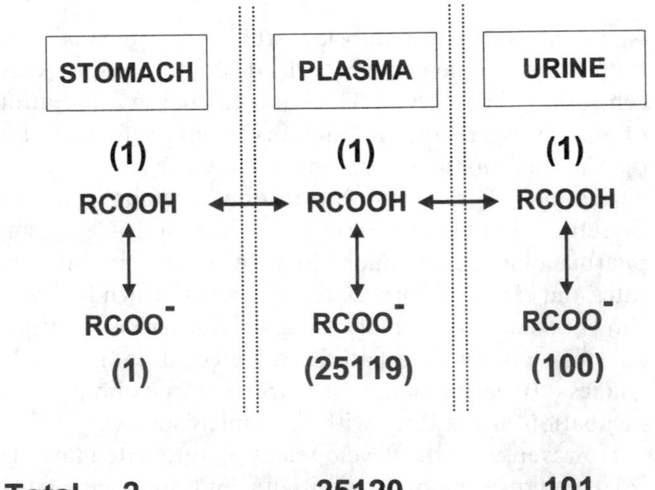

FIG. 4.3. pH partitioning. The numbers give the relative concentration of un-ionized and ionized species in each compartment, as determined by the Henderson–Hasselbalch equation for a weak acid (pK_a 3.0) at the pH of stomach (3.0), plasma (7.4), and urine (5.0). The total concentration is the concentration of compound in each compartment at equilibrium, assuming that the ionized form undergoes negligible diffusion.

It is apparent from Figure 4.3 that weak acids should be absorbed rapidly and extensively in the low pH of the stomach, whereas weak bases should undergo absorption in the intestine and not the stomach. Although this is true for bases, absorption of acids from the stomach is limited, possibly due to the relatively small surface area of the gastric mucosa. Strong organic acids and bases frequently show incomplete absorption from the gut, because they are extensively ionized at all pH values of the gut.

The absorption of foreign compounds by passage through membrane pores, which are about 4 Å in diameter, is largely applicable to small water-soluble molecules (<200 Da) (21). Bulk passage of water across the membrane may act as a driving force and carry small molecules with it (66), and this should be borne in mind when studying the absorption kinetics of large doses of sparingly water-soluble compounds. Under such circumstances, the oral administration of high doses in large volumes of hypotonic solution could result in enhanced absorption. This situation is the opposite of the case for compounds undergoing carrier-mediated absorption, because high concentrations may saturate the carrier, and the rate and extent of absorption may be reduced at high doses. Food can also affect carrier-mediated absorption by competition with the natural substrate for the carrier. Examples of foreign compounds undergoing active absorption are rare and usually apply when the chemical resembles a nutrient (e.g., levodopa).

A number of factors may limit the amount of a compound that reaches the systemic circulation as the original or parent compound after oral administration (bioavailability; see later).

1. Extremes of pH, which may affect the stability of the compound. Species differences can then arise between rats (gastric pH 3.8–5.0) and rabbits (gastric pH 3.9) (98) and humans (gastric pH 1–2).
2. Hydrolytic enzymes. The gut is rich in nonspecific proteases and lipases, which may affect foreign compounds.
3. Gut microflora. The gut flora can perform a wide range of largely degradative metabolic reactions on foreign compounds (91), which may reduce the amount available for absorption or result in the formation of potentially toxic metabolites (72). Species differences in gut flora are seen in both types of organism present and their distribution along the gut (98), with larger numbers in the stomach and upper intestine of rats and mice, compared with rabbits, dogs, and humans, in which the upper intestinal tract is almost sterile because of the low gastric pH.
4. Metabolism by the gut wall. The gut wall has the capacity to inactivate metabolically certain compounds prior to their reaching the hepatic portal vein (first-pass effect) (16). The intestinal wall is rich in enzymes catalyzing general hydrolysis and conjugation reactions (such as glucuronidation and sulfation), monoamine oxidase, and some oxidative enzymes, particularly CYP3A4/5.
5. Metabolism by the liver. Many compounds are effectively removed from the hepatic portal vein by a single passage (first-pass effect) (36). The liver is the main site of foreign compound metabolism in the body, and represents the main metabolic barrier to the parent compound reaching the general circulation.
6. Food present in the gut lumen, which may affect the absorption rate, gastric pH, or gut motility.
7. P-Glycoprotein, which is expressed on the luminal surface of the intestinal epithelium, and can act as an efflux pump for compounds entering the enterocyte.

These barriers to the establishment of effective plasma levels of the compound may be associated with suppression of systemic pharmacological and toxic properties (35) and thus render dietary administration an inappropriate route for the toxicity testing of compounds for which exposure of humans is parenteral.

Absorption from the Nasal Cavity

The nasal cavity has various interesting properties as a route of administration. Although it has relatively small surface area, the mucous membrane is highly permeable, so that after nasal administration even quaternary ammonium compounds, which are poorly absorbed from the gut, show blood levels approaching those present following intravenous administration (103). In addition, the nature of this site and its venous drainage directly into the systemic circulation allow increased absorption of compounds extensively metabolized in the gut lumen (e.g., proteins) or in the liver. Local toxicity may be a problem with this route at high doses (103).

Absorption from the Lung

The lung represents a poor barrier to a chemical entering the blood, as it has a large surface area of thin membrane, a limited capacity to metabolize foreign compounds, and an excellent blood supply. The epithelium acts as a limited permeability barrier, allowing only slow absorption of highly water-soluble compounds (106), although the rate may be greater than that from the gastrointestinal tract. The lung is a major site of inactivation of circulating local hormones such as peptides and prostaglandins; however, for toxicity testing, similar substances would not be likely to be given by this route. Major problems exist with the quantitative analysis of the extent and rate of absorption from the lung, due to poor measurement of the dose given by this route. Particulate matter is largely trapped by the cilia and passed back to be absorbed in the gut. Volatile compounds are absorbed only partially, and the unabsorbed fraction is eliminated in the expired air and not retained for subsequent absorption, as occurs in the gut (37).

Percutaneous Absorption

The extent of percutaneous absorption is highly dependent on the lipophilicity of the compound, because the stratum corneum of the epidermis acts as an effective barrier (37,54). This route is important for the therapeutic administration of potent lipophilic drugs which undergo extensive first-pass metabolism (e.g., organic nitrates in angina) and for workers exposed to environmental aerosols and particulates. Studies in animals and humans suggest that the rate-limiting step is the initial penetration of the stratum corneum (40), which may result in very slow absorption and "flip-flop" kinetics (see following).

Distribution

Foreign compounds are distributed largely via the blood, although the lymphatic system may be important in the initial distribution of some very lipid-soluble chemicals given orally. The rate of uptake of a compound by the tissues may be limited by either diffusion rate or perfusion rate.

1. Diffusion rate. If the diffusion of the chemical across membranes is slow, the rate of entry into tissues is limited by this property of the molecule.
2. Perfusion rate. If the diffusion of the chemical across membranes is rapid, the rate of entry is limited by the rate of delivery to the tissue, that is, the perfusion rate.

As a generalization, diffusion rate limitation applies to highly water-soluble compounds, whereas perfusion rate limitation applies to the entry of lipid-soluble compounds into slowly perfused systems, such as adipose tissue. The perfusion rates of the major organ systems of man (Table 4.1) can be readily divided into well and poorly perfused tissues.

The extent to which chemicals leave the blood and enter tissues depends on their relative affinities for each system. Thus compounds highly bound to plasma protein but not to tissue show a relatively high concentration in the plasma, whereas drugs with a high affinity for tissue components such as proteins or fat have a low plasma concentration. However, it should be remembered that it is the *relative* affinity that determines the extent of distribution to tissues. The dye Evans Blue has a high affinity for plasma protein, and its distribution (Table 4.2) is restricted to the plasma volume (3 L in man); the β-blocker propranolol is highly bound to plasma protein (95%), but it also shows a higher affinity for the tissues,

Table 4.1
Relative organ perfusion rates in man[a]

Organ	Percent Body weight[b]	Blood flow[c] (ml/min)	Percent cardiac output[b,c]	Blood flow[b,c] (ml/min/100 g)
Well perfused				
Lung	1.2	5000	100	1000
Adrenals	0.02	25	1	550
Kidneys	0.4	1260	23	450
Thyroid	0.04	50	2	400
Liver				
Total	2	1350	25	75
Via portal vein		1050	20	60
Heart	0.4	252	5	70
Intestines	2	1050	20	60
Brain	2	750	15	55
Poorly perfused				
Skin	7	462	9	5
Skeletal muscle	40	840	16	3
Connective tissue	7			1
Fat	15	95	2	1

[a] The results are for an adult male under resting conditions and are approximate values only.
[b] Adapted from Reference 14.
[c] Adapted from Reference 5.

Table 4.2
Volumes of body fluids with drugs showing restricted distribution

Fluid	Volume (L)	Percent body weight	Compound[a]
Total body water	41	58	D_2O, antipyrine, ethanol, urea
Extra cellular water	12	17	Na^+, Br^-, tubocurarine, sucrose
Plasma	3	4	Evans Blue, [^{131}]albumin

Adapted from References 14, 33.
[a] Compounds for which the distribution is restricted to a particular body fluid.

so that relatively low concentrations remain in the plasma after distribution.

The volumes of body fluids and chemicals that distribute in them are given in Table 4.2. However, only rarely do compounds distribute to a single physiologically recognizable volume, and usually some degree of tissue selectivity is observed. Thus, a compound may appear to have dissolved in total body water because the apparent volume of distribution (see below) corresponds to about 60% of body weight, but it may actually show a nonuniform tissue distribution.

Many foreign compounds bind reversibly to plasma proteins, with albumin being of the greatest importance, although acid glycoproteins may be important for certain organic bases (68). Foreign compounds bind at specific sites in a reversible, saturable fashion, and the bound material represents an inactive depot of the chemical. Extensive protein binding lowers the concentration of unbound chemical in the blood, which may increase the concentration gradient and thus the rate of diffusion into blood from the gut (during absorption) or reabsorption from the kidney tubules (during elimination) (56). The dissociation of the chemical–protein complex occurs within milliseconds, and by comparison with tissue perfusion times may be regarded as instantaneous. Thus, for tissues in which the free plasma concentration is lowered rapidly by an active uptake process within the tissue (i.e., liver or kidney), the compound can be effectively stripped from plasma proteins in a single passage. The plasma protein binding of foreign compounds has been reviewed and discussed by several authors (19,25,50,56,61).

Elimination

There are two main mechanisms by which the circulating levels of a foreign compound may be reduced: metabolism and excretion. *Metabolism* and its toxicological consequences are discussed in an earlier chapter. Certain mathematical implications are discussed later. The principal routes of excretion are via the urine and feces, and in the case of volatile compounds, the expired air.

Excretion via Urine

There are three major processes affecting elimination in the kidney.

Glomerular filtration. The glomerular membrane has pores of 70–80 Å. Under the positive hydrostatic conditions in the glomerulus, all molecules smaller than about 20,000 Da are filtered. Thus proteins and protein-bound compounds remain in the plasma, and about 20% of the nonbound chemical is carried with 20% of the plasma water into the glomerular filtrate.

Reabsorption. Because the glomerular filtrate contains many important body constituents (e.g., glucose), there are specific active uptake processes to transport them from urine back into blood. Although not normally substrates for these transport processes, lipid-soluble chemicals diffuse back from the tubule into the blood, especially as the urine becomes more concentrated because of water reabsorption. The pH of the urine is generally lower than that of the plasma, and therefore weak acids are more ionized in plasma, so that pH partitioning (see above) tends to increase the reabsorption of weak acids. The pH of the urine can be altered appreciably by treatment with ammonium chloride (decreases pH) or sodium carbonate (increases pH); the buffered plasma shows little change. It is thus relatively easy to affect the pH partitioning of foreign compounds between tubule contents and plasma, and either increase or decrease the elimination rate. This possibility should be considered when preparing dose solutions, because the use of excess acid or alkali to dissolve the test compound could alter its renal elimination.

Tubular secretion. Foreign compounds may be secreted actively into the renal tubule against a concentration gradient by anion and cation carrier processes. These processes are saturable and of relatively low specificity; many basic or acidic compounds and their metabolites (especially the phase II or conjugation products) are removed by them (26). Organic cation transporters are expressed on the luminal membrane of the renal tubule and are important in eliminating charged molecules (125). Because the dissociation rate for the chemical–albumin complex is rapid, it is possible for highly protein-bound compounds to be almost completely cleared at a single passage through the kidney.

Excretion via the Gut

The bile is the most important route allowing foreign compounds to move from the general circulation into the gut. The biological aspects of this mechanism have been reviewed (99), and certain pertinent points have emerged. Organic cation transporters on the sinusoidal membrane transfer large polar cations into the hepatocyte and from the hepatocyte in the bile (125). The bile may be regarded as a complementary pathway to the urine, with small molecules being eliminated by the kidney and large molecules in the bile. Thus the bile becomes the principal excretory route for many xenobiotic conjugates. Species differences exist in the molecular weight requirement for significant biliary excretion, which has been estimated as 325±50 Da in the rat, 440±50 Da in the guinea pig, 475±50 Da in the rabbit (43), and about 500 Da in humans. In the rat, small molecules (<350 Da) are not eliminated in the bile and large molecules (>450 Da) are not excreted in the urine, even if the principal excretory mechanism is blocked by ligation of the renal pedicles or bile duct, respectively. Compounds of intermediate molecular weight (350–450 Da) are excreted by both routes, and ligation of one pathway results in increased use of the other (42).

Foreign compounds may also enter the gut by direct diffusion or secretion across the gut wall, elimination in the saliva, pH partitioning of bases into the low pH of the stomach, and elimination in the pancreatic juice. In most cases, these routes are quantitatively of minor importance, although they may play an important role in toxicity by allowing a foreign compound to undergo metabolism by the gastrointestinal flora (30,72,74). The toxicological implications of the gut microflora have been reviewed by Scheline (91).

MATHEMATICAL PRINCIPLES

In order to adequately describe the changes in blood or plasma concentrations of foreign compounds, it is necessary to assign a suitable mathematical model that accurately predicts the shape of the plasma concentration–time curve. However, certain aspects are model independent and are considered first, because these considerations are usually constituent parts of the various models. In addition, there has been a marked trend away from multicompartmental mathematical analysis, which offers little apart from mathematical predictability, toward physiologically more relevant model-independent concepts such as clearance (17,118). Physiologically related parameters such as clearance and bioavailability represent an intermediate stage between mathematical multicompartment models and PBPK models.

Model-Independent Considerations

Biochemical and physiological processes are usually either zero-order or first-order reactions. In zero-order reactions the rate of change in concentration occurs at a fixed amount per time, that is,

$$\frac{dC}{dt} = k$$

where C is concentration, t is time, and k is a constant with units of amount per time, for example, micrograms per minute. In first-order reactions the rate of change in concentration is proportional to the concentration of the chemical available for the reaction, that is,

$$\frac{dC}{dt} = kC$$

where k is a constant that represents a proportional change with time and has units of time^{-1}, for example, min^{-1}.

Most processes (e.g., diffusion, carrier-mediated uptake, metabolism, excretion) are first-order reactions at low concentrations. *Most of the equations given below make this assumption.* Zero-order reactions are particularly important at high concentrations, when enzymes are working at maximum rate and an increase in C cannot result in an increase in rate. This situation produces nonlinear, or saturation, kinetics, which can assume considerable importance in toxicity studies, and is discussed later.

First-order reactions can be described by equations employing exponential functions. In many cases the entry of a foreign compound into the body or into a tissue follows an exponential increase, which may be described mathematically by

$$\text{Uptake} = 1 - e^{-kt} \quad [1]$$

where the uptake is the concentration present at time t divided by the final concentration when all the compound has entered the body or tissue. This equation assumes that there is no elimination process occurring. The elimination of a compound (by a single mechanism) once it has entered the body or tissue may be described by

$$C = C_0 e^{-kt} \quad [2]$$

where C is the concentration present at time t, and C_0 is the initial concentration. In Eq. (1) and (2), k is the rate constant for that process.

Exponential equations of the type given in Eq. (2) may be solved as

$$\ln C = \ln C_0 - kt$$

or using $\log_{10}$

$$\log C = \log C_0 - \frac{kt}{2.303}$$

which represents an equation of the generalized form

$$y = C + mx$$

where m and C are constants, and x and y are variables. In such cases, a plot of x against y gives a straight line graph with a slope of m and an intercept of C. Thus for toxicokinetics, a graph of ln C against time gives a slope of $-k$ and an intercept of ln C_0 . If such a graph is drawn using log–linear graph paper, the slope must be calculated by taking the $\log_{10}$ of the concentration terms and dividing by the time (see below), and the slope will be $-k/2.303$.

Frequently, the equation necessary to describe the kinetics of a compound in the body requires the use of two exponential rate terms, that is, absorption into a single compartment plus elimination, or elimination from a two-compartment system (see below). In such cases the early time points in the concentration–time curve are influenced by both rates. However, provided the rate constants are sufficiently dissimilar, eventually the influence of the component with the higher rate becomes negligible, whereas the smaller rate constant still affects the concentration. Thus the terminal phase of the concentration–time curve is determined by the process with the smaller rate constant, and the earlier phase by the sum of both processes. This process allows both rate constants to be determined by the procedure known as the method of residuals or stripping (see below).

Tissue Extraction

Removal of a compound from the blood by a tissue is schematized in Figure 4.4. On constant infusion, the rate of entry into the tissue may be regarded as equivalent to a first-order absorption rate (78):

$$\text{Uptake} = 1 - e^{-kt} \qquad [1]$$

where uptake = the fractional uptake = $C_t/C_{\text{equilibrium}}$.

In *perfusion limited uptake*, the value k is related to the flow rate (Q) as follows (Figure 4.4):

$$\text{Fractional uptake} = 1 - e^{-(Q/PV_t)t} \qquad [3]$$

(Q/V_t is the volume-adjusted flow rate and P is the partition ratio). The uptake half-time may be derived as described below for Eq. (19):

$$t_{1/2}(\text{uptake}) = \frac{0.693}{k} = \frac{0.693PV_t}{Q} = \frac{0.693P}{Q/V_t} \qquad [4]$$

For *diffusion-limited uptake*, the value k is related to the diffusion rate constant and thus is not readily measurable.

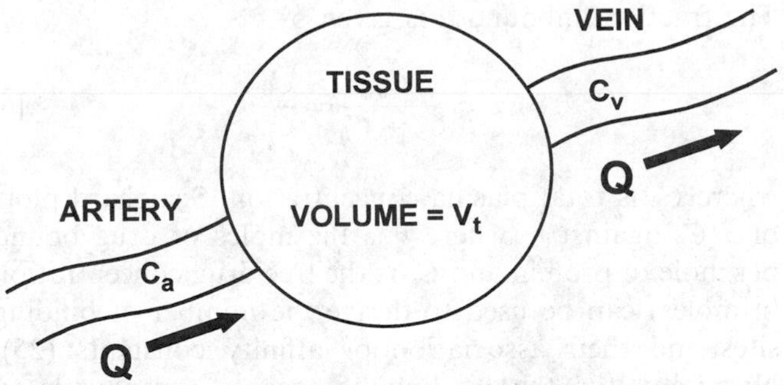

FIG. 4.4. Tissue uptake of foreign compounds. Q is the blood flow, C_a is the arterial concentration, C_v is the venous concentration, C_t is the concentration in tissue, and V_t is the volume of tissue. We define the following parameters: rate of delivery of drug = QC_a, rate of outflow of drug = QC_v, and rate of uptake = $QC_a - QC_v$. The units for these rates are mass time^{-1} (i.e., μg min^{-1}, etc.). Thus

$$\text{Extraction ratio } (E) = \frac{\text{rate of uptake}}{\text{rate of delivery}} = \frac{QC_a - QC_v}{QC_a} = \frac{C_a - C_v}{C_a}$$

$$\text{Partition ratio } (P) = \frac{\text{Concentration in tissue}}{\text{Concentration in blood supply}} = \frac{C_t}{C_a}$$

These relationships are an essential part of PBPK models.

Plasma Protein Binding

The extent of protein binding may be represented by an equilibrium reaction:

$$P^r + C_u \rightleftharpoons C_b$$

where P^r is the free protein, C_u is the unbound compound, and C_b is the compound–protein complex. The equilibrium constant K is given by

$$K = \frac{[C_b]}{[P^r][C_u]} = \frac{[\text{product}]}{[\text{reactants}]} \qquad [5]$$

The fraction unbound α is given by

$$\alpha = \frac{C_u}{C_u + C_b} = \frac{C_u}{C_p} \quad [6]$$

where C_p is total plasma concentration. Scatchard plots of r/C_u against r (where r is the moles of drug bound per mole of protein and C_u is the free drug concentration in moles) can be used to derive the number of binding sites and their association or affinity constants (25). Normally, for the binding of organic compounds to albumin, two or more binding sites are revealed. This approach is valuable for detailed studies on binding to and displacement from albumin, but it could yield multiple binding sites if applied to a complex protein mixture, such as plasma, containing different proteins at different concentrations.

Because it is the unbound compound in plasma that undergoes equilibration with the unbound compound in tissues (Figure 4.5), adequate information may be obtained from a knowledge of α, or of the percentage bound. Detailed knowledge is not required for pharmacokinetic analysis of the plasma data because the plasma concentrations used to calculate kinetic parameters are usually the total concentrations ($C_u + C_b$). (When the nonbound concentration is used this has to be specified in the description of the parameters, e.g. clearance [nonprotein bound]; in the absence of such a description it is assumed that the total plasma concentration has been used). Because plasma protein binding is a saturable process (see later), in vitro binding studies should be performed over a range of concentrations.

Clearance

Clearance (CL) is defined as the ratio:

$$CL = \frac{\text{Rate of elimination}}{\text{Plasma concentration}}$$

and may be regarded as the volume of plasma or blood that is cleared of compound in unit time by the route under consideration. The units are volume time^{-1}, for example, usually ml min^{-1} because if rate is μg min^{-1} and plasma concentration is μg ml^{-1} the plasma clearance will be ml min^{-1}.

Renal Clearance

The renal clearance (CL_R) is given by

$$CL_R = \frac{\text{rate of elimination in urine}}{\text{plasma concentration}} = \frac{C_u \times F_u}{C_p} \quad [7]$$

where C_u is the urine concentration, F_u is the urine flow (volume in unit time), and C_p is the plasma concentration at the midpoint of the urine collection period. The concentration in urine is dependent on a number of variables, which are now described.

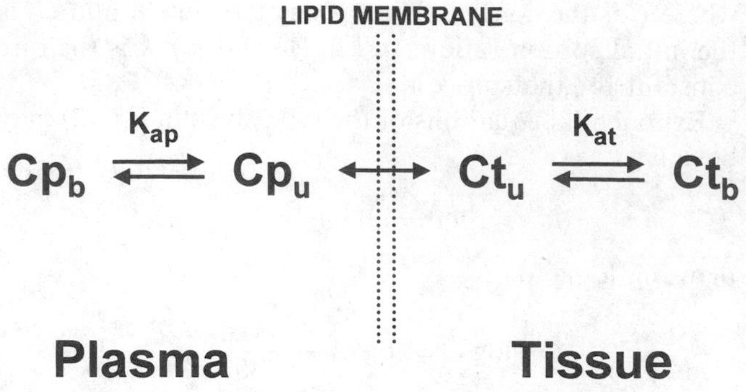

FIG. 4.5. Protein binding and tissue distribution. C_p is the plasma concentration, C_t is the tissue concentration, u=unbound, b=bound, K_{ap} is the association constant for plasma protein binding. At equilibrium, $C_{pu} = C_{tu}$; and the relative distribution between plasma and tissue is determined by the values of K_{ap} and K_{at}.

Glomerular filtration. The rate of filtration is given by

$$\text{GFR} \times C_{\text{pu}} = \text{GFR} \times C_p \times \alpha \quad [8]$$

where GFR is the glomerular filtration rate, C_{pu} is the unbound concentration in plasma, C_p is the total plasma concentration, and α is the fraction unbound.

Thus compounds binding extensively to plasma proteins show limited clearance by glomerular filtration. The protein binding equilibrium is not disturbed in the glomerulus because after loss of 20% free drug and 20% water, C_{pu} is unaltered, whereas the concentrations of both free protein and drug–protein complex increase by 20%, that is,

Before filtration	After filtration
$K_{\text{ap}} = \frac{[\text{complex}]}{[C_{\text{pu}}][P^r]}$	$K_{\text{ap}} = \frac{1.2\,[\text{complex}]}{[C_{\text{pu}}]\,1.2[P^r]}$

where K_{ap} is the protein-binding association constant. Thus, the chemical–protein complex does not dissociate in the glomerulus. The complex dissociates to give more free compound when the plasma is diluted by water reabsorbed in the distal parts of the renal tubule. Under such circumstances, about 99% of the plasma water is reabsorbed, so that the concentrations of the protein and complex return to almost their initial levels, whereas the concentration of unbound compound is diluted to about 80% of its former level, that is, after reabsorption:

$$K_{\text{ap}} \neq \frac{[\text{complex}]}{0.8[C_{\text{pu}}][P^r]}$$

Therefore the complex dissociates to restore the

equilibrium. The glomerular filtration rate is about 130 ml min^{-1} in men and 120 ml min^{-1} in women, or approximately 2 ml $min^{-1}kg^{-1}$, which is lower than that of the Wistar rat (3.4 ml $min^{-1}kg^{-1}$) (100).

Reabsorption. Reabsorption from the renal tubule back into the blood is variable and dependent on the lipid solubility of the compound, the pH of the urine, and the extent of concentration of the urine (i.e., water reabsorption). Mathematical quantitation is impracticable, but an indication of the extent of reabsorption may be obtained (see below). In certain instances the administered foreign compound may be a substrate for carrier mediated reabsorption, in which case the renal elimination is dose dependent and is greater at high doses when this reuptake is saturated. Such a saturable reuptake process is obviously ideal for maintaining a constant low body load of an essential compound, for example, glucose or riboflavin, which might show adverse effects at high body concentrations.

Tubular secretion. Saturable carrier-mediated processes are present in the proximal part of the tubule. They show a relatively low substrate specificity, and the extent of their involvement for a particular compound is dependent on the affinity between the compound and the carrier protein. The extent of clearance by these active processes may be regarded as analogous to hepatic clearance, which is another active, saturable process. The specificities of the carriers have been studied extensively (26,116,125) and structural requirements such as

$$\mathrm{R-\underset{\underset{O}{\|}}{C}-\underset{\underset{H}{|}}{N}-(CHR')_n-COOH}$$

have been proposed. Saturation of secretion causes a decreased elimination at high doses.

All three processes described above can alter, simultaneously and independently, the value of C_u for any given value of C_p. The final renal clearance may be regarded as a composite expression:

$$\text{Renal excretion} = \text{glomerular filtration} - \text{reabsorption} + \text{tubular secretion}$$

$$\text{Rate of excretion} = \text{GFR}\ C_p\alpha - \text{rate of reabsorption} + \text{rate of tubular secretion}$$

The values of GFR, C_p, and α can be determined experimentally. Measurement of inulin clearance (or creatinine clearance in man) determines the GFR, because this compound does not undergo significant reabsorption, tubular secretion, or protein binding; thus for inulin:

$$\text{Rate of renal excretion} = \text{GFR}\ C_p$$

and because

$$\mathrm{CL}_R = \frac{\text{rate of excretion}}{C_p}$$

$$\mathrm{CL}_R = \text{GFR}$$

The extent of reabsorption and secretion of a compound may be inferred from a comparison of its renal clearance with the value of GFR × α.

$\mathrm{CL}_R < \mathrm{GFR} \times \alpha$ Reabsorption must be occurring and is greater than secretion (which may or may not be present).

$\mathrm{CL}_R = \mathrm{GFR} \times \alpha$ Reabsorption, which may or may not be present, is negated by an equal rate of secretion.

$\mathrm{CL}_R > \mathrm{GFR} \times \alpha$ Tubular secretion must be occurring and is greater than reabsorption (which may or may not be present).

The mathematical implications of the renal elimination process have been the subject of a number of reviews (31,115).

Hepatic Clearance

The clearance of a compound by the liver may be regarded as dependent on the rate of delivery to the organ (blood flow) and the efficiency of removal from the blood (extraction ratio; see Figure 4.4). Thus

$$\mathrm{CL}_H = QE \qquad [9]$$

where CL_H is the hepatic (metabolic) clearance, Q is the hepatic blood flow, and E is the extraction ratio.

This simple relationship has been verified experimentally for a number of compounds. However, it is complicated by the finding that the variables Q and E are not independent, because for certain compounds an increase in blood flow decreases the extraction efficiency. This finding led Rowland et al. (87) to propose the following relationship, known as the *perfusion limited model*:

$$\mathrm{CL}_H = Q\left(\frac{\alpha \times \mathrm{CL_{int}}}{Q + \alpha \mathrm{CL_{int}}}\right) \qquad [10]$$

where α is the fraction unbound in plasma, $\mathrm{CL_{int}}$ is the intrinsic metabolic clearance by the hepatocytes from the cell water, and Q is the blood flow (as plasma).

If the metabolic clearance ($\mathrm{CL_{int}}$) is high, the value in parentheses in Eq. (10), which is equivalent to the term E in Eq. (9), approaches unity; under these circumstances the hepatic clearance approximates to the hepatic blood flow and becomes dependent on the blood flow. However, if the metabolic clearance is low, $Q + \alpha\mathrm{CL_{int}}$ approximates to Q, and therefore the extraction ratio (E) decreases with an increase in blood flow and the hepatic clearance remains relatively constant. These equations adequately explain the effects of changes in perfusion rate on the extraction ratio and clearance of compounds that show a range of extraction ratios. In addition, comparison of the hepatic clearance (calculated by measurement of Q and E) with "nonrenal" clearance (calculated as plasma clearance minus renal clearance) can indicate the role of extrahepatic tissues in the elimination of the compound.

Further analysis of this equation (see ref. 117 for discussion) indicates that

$$\mathrm{CL_{int}} = \frac{V_{\max}}{K_m + C_{\mathrm{pu}}} \qquad [11]$$

where $V_{\max}$ and K_m are Michaelis–Menton constants for the enzyme metabolizing the foreign compound, and C_{pu} is the hepatic venous concentration of unbound compound. If C_{pu} is low and is much less than the K_m for the enzyme (i.e., well below saturation levels), this term may be ignored and

$$\mathrm{CL_{int}} = \frac{V_{\max}}{K_m} = \text{constant}$$

When the value of C_{pu} approaches or exceeds K_m, the substrate concentration is sufficient to saturate the enzyme, and the kinetics are grossly altered and become nonlinear. This situation is a distinct possibility in high-dose toxicity testing and is discussed later in more detail. The concepts given above are important for the use of $V_{\max}$ and K_m values in interspecies comparisons. $V_{\max}/K_m$ is taken as a measure of enzyme activity; species differences in clearance will relate to differences in this measure of enzyme activity for low clearance compounds, but will relate to liver blood flow for high clearance compounds (irrespective of differences in $V_{\max}/K_m$). This possible source of error in extrapolation across species is avoided when both the enzyme activity and organ blood flows are part of a PBPK model (see below).

Biliary Clearance

The clearance via the bile CL_B is given, by analogy with renal clearance, as

$$\mathrm{CL}_B = \frac{\text{rate of elimination in bile}}{C_p} = \frac{C_B \times F_B}{C_p} \qquad [12]$$

where C_B is the concentration in bile and F_B is the volume of bile in unit time (bile flow).

Plasma Clearance

Plasma clearance (CL) may be defined as

$$\mathrm{CL} = \frac{\text{rate of elimination from plasma}}{C_p}$$

The plasma clearance is the sum of the various contributory clearance processes:

$$\mathrm{CL} = \mathrm{CL}_R + \mathrm{CL}_H + \mathrm{CL}_B + \text{etc.} \qquad [13]$$

Plasma clearance, which is one of the most valuable toxicokinetic constants, is determined from the plasma concentration–time curve and is discussed in detail later. It may be used to derive other model-independent variables, for example, mean residence time, which are given later under Statistical Moment Analysis.

Physiologically Based Pharmacokinetic Models

In recent years models have been developed which are based on the principles discussed above, that is, organ blood flow, tissue extraction, and rates of metabolism and excretion. These models are derived from the physiology of the test animal and are discussed in detail in Chapter 5. PBPK models have been applied successfully to a number of compounds and have been particularly successful for organic solvents, e.g., benzene (108). This approach represents a powerful method, capable of dealing with saturation of metabolism and valuable for the extrapolation of animal data to humans (69,57,113). However, its ability to predict concentrations is dependent on the precision of the parameter estimates used and the model chosen (9). Therefore, PBPK modeling should be considered as one of three possible approaches to the analysis and interpretation of toxicokinetic data:

1. Simple physiologically related concepts, such as bioavailability and clearance (this chapter)
2. Compartmental analysis, which gives mathematical precision but does not directly reflect organ concentration (this chapter)
3. PBPK modeling, which allows the prediction of target organ concentrations (Chapter 5)

Compartmented Systems: Modeling

In order to describe plasma concentration-time curves mathematically, an appropriate predictive model has to be fitted to the data. The correlation between the actual data and the concentration–time curve generated using the model shows the suitability of the model in describing the experimental results.

Thus considering the data presented in Figure 4.6 and Table 4.3, it is apparent that the same model cannot describe the properties of both compounds, although in both cases the initial and final plasma measurements were the same. The differences in the plasma concentration–time profiles originate in the number of rates at which the compound may leave and enter the plasma.

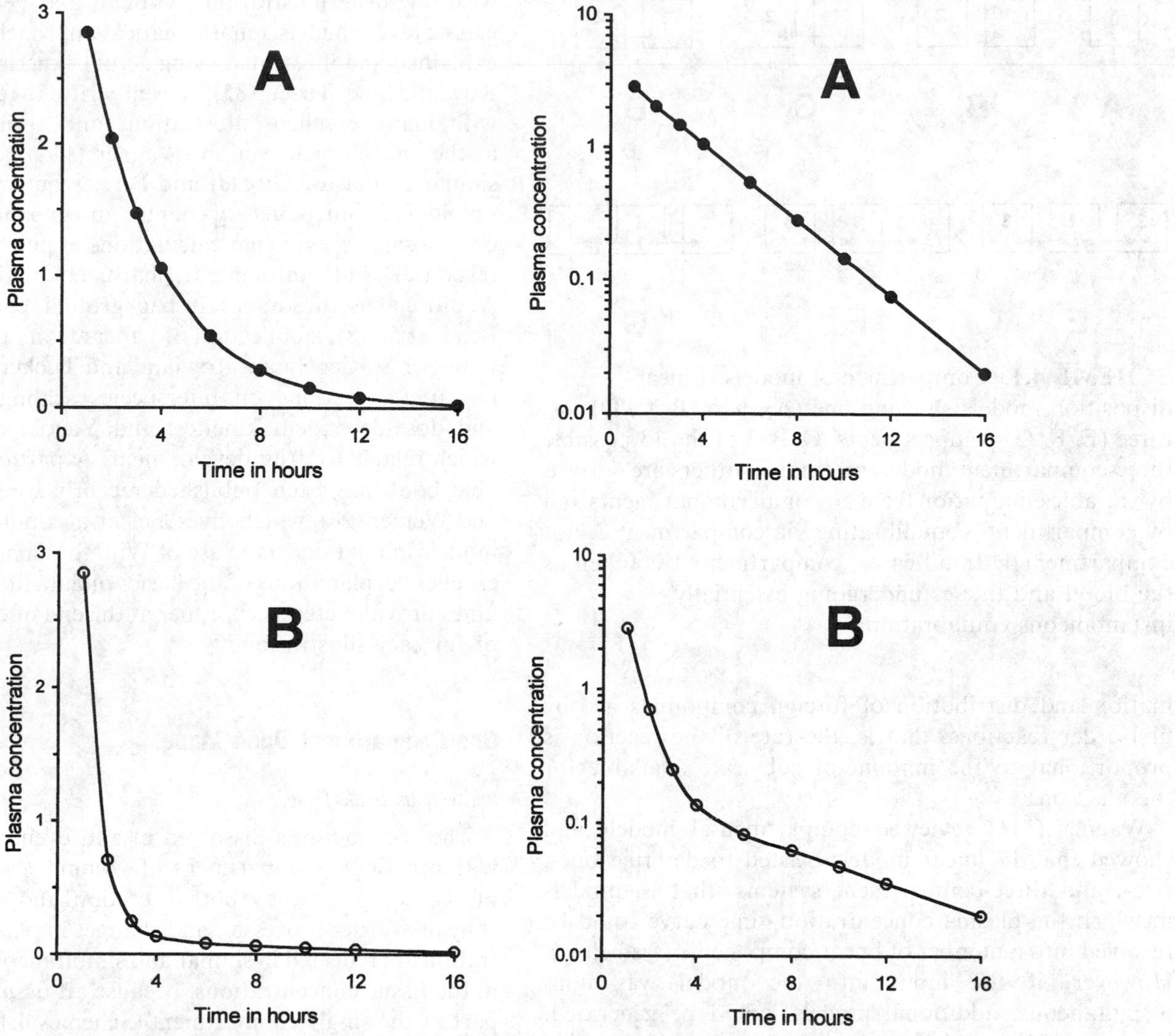

FIG. 4.6. Plasma concentration–time data for two compounds; results are plotted in linear and semilogarithmic forms. The data used to generate the curves are given in Table 4.3.

If the tissues show instantaneous equilibration with plasma, the compound leaves the plasma by a single process (Scheme 4.1A), an elimination process with a simple exponential decrease. Alternatively, the compound may leave the plasma to enter "other tissues" at measurable rates, as well as undergoing elimination from the plasma. Under such circumstances, the "other tissues" may be adequately described mathematically by a second compartment in addition to the plasma (or the central compartment) (Scheme 4.1B). In some cases, two or more additional compartments are required. It is important to realize that these "other tissues" share only one criterion, that is, their associated rate constants, and that biologically diverse tissues may be part of the same compartment. In addition, elimination may occur from compartments other than the central compartment (Schemes 4.1C–G). In most cases the processes of elim-

Table 4.3
Data used for Figure 4.6

Time after IV Dosing (h)	C_p (μg ml^{-1}) Compound A	Compound B
1	2.850	2.850
2	2.040	0.705
3	1.470	0.250
4	1.050	0.136
6	0.540	0.082
8	0.280	0.062
10	0.145	0.047
12	0.075	0.035
16	0.020	0.020

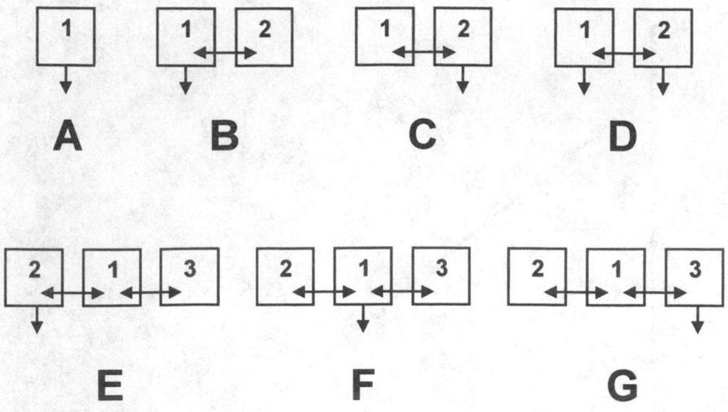

SCHEME 4.1. Compartmental models. Linear disposition models showing one (A), two (B, C, D), or three (E, F, G) compartments. Only 3 of the 13 possible three-compartment models are shown; others are derived by variable elimination from any or all compartments and by compartment 3 equilibrating via compartment 2, not compartment 1. In all cases, compartment 1 is taken as the blood and tissues undergoing essentially instantaneous equilibration.

ination and distribution of foreign compounds are by first-order reactions, that is, the rate of the reaction is proportional to the amount of substrate available for the reaction.

Wagner (111) reviewed compartmental models and showed that 17 linear models existed to describe one-, two-, and three-compartment systems, that is, models in which the plasma concentration–time curve could be resolved into a number of linear components (see below). However, if the input into the model was non-instantaneous, additional models would be generated. Wagner (111) concluded that there were 760 possible pharmacokinetic models comprising up to three distribution compartments and two input compartments, but that in many cases and for many calculations a knowledge of the best-fit model was not necessary. Because the aim of this chapter is to provide an introduction to toxicokinetics (i.e., samples needed, data handling, and the type of information that can be obtained), only simple models are discussed in detail. Readers are referred to standard texts on pharmacokinetics if the plasma data are not fitted by the simple models discussed here. However, the two models selected show widespread applicability, and an understanding of the principles underlying these simple models is essential, if the data generated by computer analysis of more complex models are to have any meaning. In addition, more complex models contain greater numbers of variables, and blood sampling must be increased to define the rate constants accurately.

Texts recommended for further reading include those by Rescigno and Segre (78), a mathematical approach with few drug illustrations; Gibaldi and Perrier (36), a classic text, which is a mathematical approach that is well explained and illustrated using actual experimental data; Rowland and Tozer (85), a well-written, readable text with many excellent illustrations and study problems at the end of each section; Wagner (112), an approach similar to that of Gibaldi and Perrier but with a useful "biological" introductory chapter and expanded sections on dosage regimen calculations, pharmacological response, and automated pharmacokinetic analysis. Additional useful sources for background reading include Benet et al. (8), a collection of papers from a symposium to honor S. Riegelman; Rowland and Tucker (86), which has useful sections on interspecies scaling and time- and dose-dependent kinetics; and Yacobi et al. (124), which relates to drug development. A particularly valuable book has been published recently by Gabrielsson and Weiner (28), which gives a clear account of different models in relation to the use of WinNonlin, and provides excellent explanations of the basics of data fitting. All volumes provide references, either at the end of each chapter or for each illustration.

One-Compartment Open Model

Intravenous Bolus Dose

The compound is dissolved in and evenly distributed within a single compartment of volume V. Elimination of the compound, by both excretion and metabolism, is by first-order processes, and changes in plasma concentration are reflected in similar and simultaneous decreases in the tissue concentrations, because all tissues represent part of the single compartment (Schemes 4.1A and 4.2). In Scheme 4.2, V is the volume of distribution, k_{ex} is the excretion rate constant, and k_m is the metabolism rate constant. The plasma concentration–time curve for a one-compartment system is given in Figure 4.7, the data are presented in Table 4.4. In mathematical terms, such a system may be described adequately by a simple first-order equation, where the rate of removal of a compound from the body (e.g., in milligrams per hour) is proportional to the body load (e.g., in milligrams):

$$\frac{dAb}{dt} = k\text{Ab} \qquad [14]$$

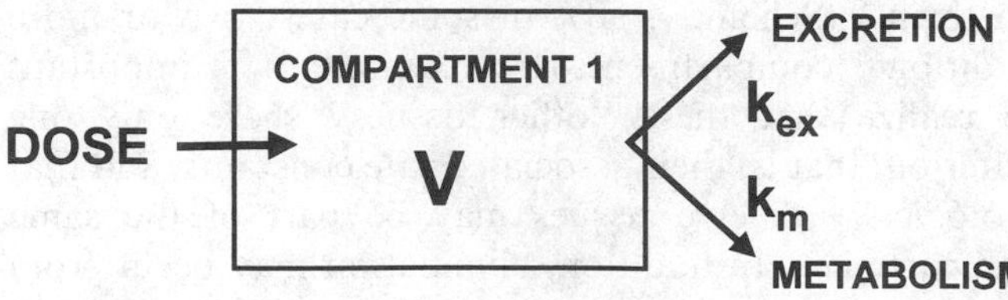

SCHEME 4.2. One-compartment model.

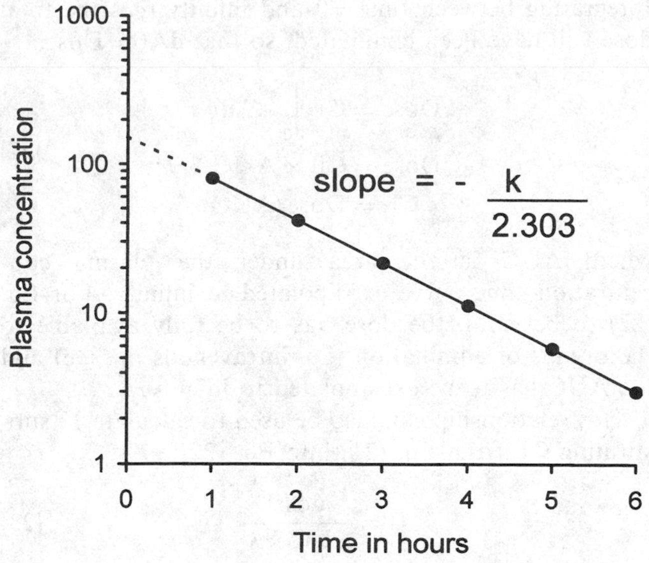

FIG. 4.7. Plasma concentration–time curve after a bolus intravenous dose for a one-compartment system. The data are given in Table 4.4.

Table 4.4
Data used for Figure 4.7[a]

Time (h)	C_p (μg ml^{-1})	ln C_p	
1	80.0	4.382	
2	41.5	3.726	$k = 0.656$ h^{-1}
3	21.5	3.068	$t_{1/2} = 1.06$ h
4	11.2	2.416	
5	5.8	1.758	$C_{p0} = 154.3$ μg ml^{-1}
6	3.0	1.099	$V = 324$ ml kg^{-1}

[a] The plasma concentrations were obtained after an intravenous bolus dose of 50 mg/kg.

where Ab is the amount of compound in the body, and k is the elimination rate constant (k equals $[k_{ex} + k_m]$). A solution to this equation to give the amount remaining in the body at time t after injection is given by

$$\text{Ab}_t = \text{Ab}_0 e^{-kt} \quad [15]$$

where Ab_t is the amount of compound at time t, and Ab_0 is the amount at time zero.

Assuming uniform distribution within a single compartment, the concentration in the plasma (C_p) may be related to Ab by the *apparent volume of distribution* (V). This volume may be regarded as the volume of plasma in which the body burden (body load) would have to be dissolved, in order to give the plasma concentration measured. For a chemical that is lipid soluble or that readily binds to tissue components, the plasma concentration represents a small fraction of the total amount in the body, and thus the compound appears to have been dissolved in a large volume of plasma (see below):

$$C_p = \frac{\text{Ab}}{V} \quad [16]$$

where C_p is the plasma concentration and V is the apparent volume of distribution. Thus Eq. (15) may be rewritten in its more usual form,

$$C_{pt} = C_{p0} e^{-kt} \quad [17]$$

where C_{pt} is the plasma concentration at time t, and C_{p0} is the concentration at time zero. For such a system, we can define the following parameters.

Apparent volume of distribution. The apparent volume of distribution (V) is the apparent volume into which the dose would have been dissolved to give the initial plasma concentration, C_{p0}, that is,

$$V = \frac{\text{Ab}}{C_p} = \frac{\text{dose}}{C_{p0}} \quad [18]$$

The units are in liters, milliliters, liters per kilogram, or milliliters per kilogram.

Elimination rate constant. The elimination rate constant (k) represents the fractional loss of compound from the body per unit time, that is,

$$k = \frac{\text{amount of chemical eliminated in unit time}}{\text{amount of chemical in the body}} = \frac{(d\text{Ab}/dt)}{\text{Ab}}$$

Equation (17) may be rewritten as

$$\text{either} \quad \ln C_{pt} = \ln C_{p0} - kt$$

$$\text{or} \quad \log C_{pt} = \log C_{p0} - \frac{kt}{2.303}$$

Thus a graph of ln C_p against time has a slope of $-k$ and an intercept of ln C_{p0}; a graph of log C_p against time has a slope of $-k/2.303$ and an intercept of log C_{p0} (Figure 4.7). The units of k are h^{-1} or min^{-1}. Thus if the elimination rate constant is determined as 0.4 h^{-1}, it means that 40% of the body load is removed each hour. The value of k is the summation of component elimination rate constants (e.g., k_{ex}, k_m).

Elimination half-life. The elimination half-life ($t_{1/2}$) is the time taken for the amount in the body (Ab) or the plasma concentration (Ab/V) to decrease to one-half. Thus after one half-life, C_p in Eq. (17) equals $C_{p0}/2$, that is,

$$\frac{C_{p0}}{2} = C_{p0} e^{-kt_{1/2}} \quad \text{or} \quad \frac{1}{2} = e^{-kt_{1/2}}$$

Therefore,

$$\ln 0.5 = -kt_{1/2} \quad \text{or} \quad -0.693 = -kt_{1/2}$$

$$t_{1/2} = \frac{0.693}{k} \qquad [19]$$

where the units are hours or minutes.

Plasma clearance. Plasma clearance (CL) is the amount of chemical eliminated in unit time related to the plasma concentration and may be regarded as the volume of blood that is cleared of chemical in unit time. CL is a constant for first-order reactions. In many respects, this measurement is a better reflection of the inherent capacity of the tissues to eliminate the compound than is the half-life or elimination rate constant:

$$\mathrm{CL} = \frac{\text{rate of elimination}}{\text{plasma concentration}}$$

$$\mathrm{CL} = \frac{(\mathrm{dAb}/\mathrm{d}t)}{C_p} \qquad [20]$$

Substituting from Eq. (14),

$$\mathrm{CL} = \frac{k\mathrm{Ab}}{C_p}$$

The amount in the body at any time (Ab) is given by Eq. (16); therefore

$$\mathrm{CL} = \frac{kC_pV}{C_p} = kV \qquad [21]$$

where the units are in $\mathrm{L\,h^{-1}}$, $\mathrm{L\,min^{-1}}$, $\mathrm{ml\,h^{-1}}$, or $\mathrm{ml\,min^{-1}}$. Rearranging Eq. (21),

$$k = \frac{\mathrm{CL}}{V}$$

This equation shows clearly that the elimination rate constant (k) is derived from two independent variables that can be related to physiological processes: the *clearance*, which reflects the capacity of the organs of elimination to remove the compound from the plasma, and the *apparent volume of distribution*, which reflects the proportion of the total body burden that is circulated to the organs of elimination. Plasma clearance may depend on the rate of the active process in the organs of elimination or on the plasma flow to the principal organ(s) of elimination.

Clearance may also be obtained without knowing the value of V. Rearranging Eq. (20),

$$\frac{\mathrm{dAb}}{\mathrm{d}t} = \mathrm{CL} \times C_p$$

or in time dt, the amount lost $\mathrm{dAb} = \mathrm{CL} \times C_p \times \mathrm{d}t$. Integrating between time $= 0$ and infinity (∞) the total dose will have been eliminated, so that dAb = Dose,

$$\mathrm{Dose} = \mathrm{CL}\int_0^\infty C_p\mathrm{d}t$$

$$\mathrm{Dose} = \mathrm{CL} \times \mathrm{AUC} \qquad [22]$$

$$\mathrm{CL} = \mathrm{Dose}/\mathrm{AUC}$$

where AUC is the area under the plasma concentration–time curve extrapolated to infinity. For Eq. (22) to be valid, the dose has to be fully available to the organs of elimination (i.e. intravenous dosage) and the AUC has to be extrapolated to infinity.

This relationship can also be used to calculate V; substituting CL from Eq. (21) into Eq. (22):

$$V = \frac{\text{dose}}{\mathrm{AUC} \times k} \qquad [23]$$

The value of Eqs. (22) and (23) is that both the clearance and the apparent volume of distribution can be derived from infusion or parenteral administration, where the determination of V using Eq. (18) is not possible, because the total dose is not present in the central compartment at $t = 0$. These equations may also be applied to oral administration, providing that allowance is made for incomplete absorption of the dose. This method of calculating CL is also applicable to multicompartment linear systems with elimination from the central compartment.

Information Obtainable from Urinary Data

From Eq. (7), we obtain

$$\text{Rate of urinary excretion} = \mathrm{CL}_R \times C_p$$

where CL_R is the renal clearance. Thus

$$\mathrm{CL}_R \times C_p = k_R \times V \times C_p = k_R \times \mathrm{Ab}$$

from Eqs. (21) and (18), where k_R is the renal excretion rate constant. However, Ab at any time $=$ dose $\times\, e^{-kt}$. Therefore

$$\text{Rate of urinary excretion} = k_R \times \text{dose} \times e^{-kt} \qquad [24]$$

or

$$\log(\text{rate of urinary excretion}) = (\log k_R \times \text{dose}) - \frac{kt}{2.303} \qquad [25]$$

A plot of rate of urinary excretion (amount excreted per time interval) against time gives a straight line on log-linear graph paper, the slope of which is $-k/2.303$, and the intercept is log k_R dose. It is important to note that the slope of this graph gives the overall elimination rate constant, not the specific urinary elimination rate constant. In other words, the decrease in the amount appearing in the urine mirrors the overall decrease in the plasma concentration. It is not possible to obtain information regarding other kinetic parameters (such as CL_R or V) without sampling the central (blood) compartment. The value of k_R may be derived from the values of renal clearance

$$CL_R = \frac{C_u \times F_u}{C_p} \quad [7]$$

and the apparent volume of distribution, V, when $CL_R = k_R \times V$.

The above approach is subject to considerable fluctuation in the excretion rate due to factors such as incomplete bladder emptying. To overcome this problem, the rate constant can be derived more reliably from the amount remaining to be excreted, using the *sigma-minus* method. This method is based on the equation below, which is derived from integration of Eq. 24:

$$A_{ex} = \frac{k_R \times \text{dose}}{k}[1 - e^{-kt}] \quad [26]$$

where A_{ex} is the total amount excreted up to time t. At infinite time, $(1 - e^{-kt})$ equals unity. Therefore

$$A_{ex}^{\infty} = \frac{k_R \times \text{dose}}{k}$$

where A_{ex}^{∞} is the cumulative total amount excreted in urine up to time infinity. Substituting back into Eq. (26)

$$A_{ex} = A_{ex}^{\infty}[1 - e^{-kt}]$$

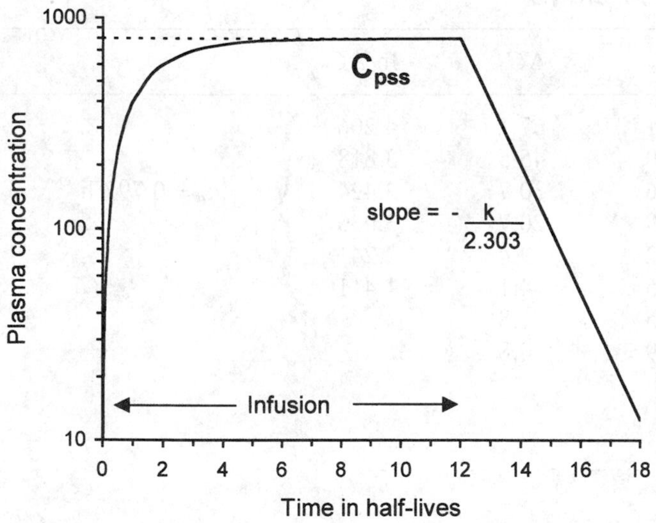

FIG. 4.8. Plasma concentration–time curve for constant intravenous infusion into a single-compartment system. The foreign compound was infused at a constant rate from time =0 to time=12 half-lives when the infusion was stopped.

or

$$A_{ex}^{\infty} - A_{ex} = A_{ex}^{\infty}e^{-kt} \quad [27]$$

The left-hand side of Eq. (27) is equivalent to the amount finally excreted minus the amount excreted up to that time (ΔA_{ex}). Taking logs,

$$\log \Delta A_{ex} = \log A_{ex}^{\infty} - \frac{kt}{2.303} \quad [28]$$

A semilog plot of ΔA_{ex} against time gives a straight line of slope $-k/2.303$. An example of this method is described below under Data Handling.

By analogy with Eq. (22), CL_R may be calculated from the total amount excreted and the plasma AUC

$$CL_R = \frac{A_{ex}}{AUC}$$

where A_{ex} and AUC refer to the same time interval.

Constant Intravenous Infusion

During infusion the plasma concentration (C_p) rises to reach a plateau or steady-state concentration (C_{pss}) at which time the rate of infusion equals the rate of elimination. By analogy with Eq. (1)

$$\frac{C_p}{C_{pss}} = (1 - e^{-kt})$$

or

$$C_p = C_{pss}(1 - e^{-kt}) \quad [29]$$

The various kinetic parameters may be derived from the plasma concentration–time curve for infusion (as given in Figure 4.8).

Decrease at end of infusion. The slope equals $-k$ because on cessation of entry into the single compartment, $C_p = C_{p0}e^{-kt}$. The same slope would be obtained if the infusion was stopped at any stage during the infusion.

Plateau level (C_{pss}). At steady state, the rate of infusion (R) equals the rate of elimination:

$$R = CL \times C_{pss}$$

or

$$CL = \frac{R}{C_{pss}} = V \times k$$

Increase to plateau. Rearranging Eq. (29),

$$C_{pss} - C_p = C_{pss}e^{-kt}$$

Therefore, a plot of ln ($C_{pss} - C_p$) against time gives a straight line with a slope equal to k. The time taken to

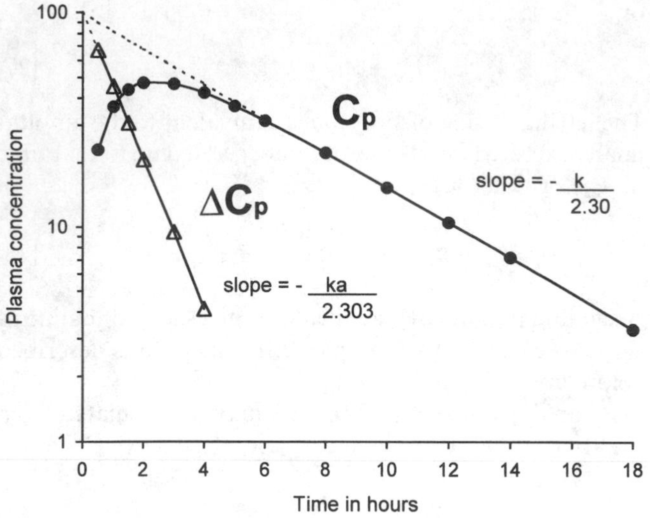

FIG. 4.9. Use of the method of residuals to calculate the absorption rate constant for a one-compartment system. The dose was given at time 0, and plasma levels (C_p) were measured at intervals. The linear terminal phase was extrapolated to yield the values corresponding to the measurement times. The difference values (C_p extrapolated $-C_p$ measured) are plotted (ΔC_p) to yield a line of slope $-k_a/2.303$ or $-k/2.303$; see text. The data are given in Table 4.5.

reach the plateau is therefore similar to the time taken to eliminate the compound after infusion, or about 97% of the final level within five half-lives.

Area under the curve. Both CL and V may be derived using Eqs. (22) and (23).

Oral Administration

Absorption frequently obeys first-order kinetics (80), but may involve a lag time due to delayed gastric emptying. The plasma concentration–time profile may thus resemble Figure 4.9 (see also Table 4.5), and the various pharmacokinetic parameters are related by the equation:

$$C_p = \frac{F \times \text{dose} \times k_a(e^{-kt} - e^{-k_a t})}{V(k_a - k)} \quad [30]$$

where F is the fraction of the dose absorbed and k_a is the absorption rate constant.

Decrease after peak. The decrease after the peak concentration is determined by the slower of the two processes (absorption or elimination), but it is usually elimination, and the slope is equal to $-k$. (Note that for a polar compound showing slow absorption and rapid elimination, this decrease is equivalent to $-k_a$, a situation described by Gibaldi and Perrier (36) as "flip-flop" kinetics [see Figure 4.10]).

Peak plasma concentration. The peak plasma concentration is determined by the relative rates k_a and k. This may be of toxicological importance, especially for acute effects when the extent of toxicity is frequently related to the peak concentration rather than to the area under

Table 4.5
Data used for Figure 4.9

Time (h)	C_p	ln C_p		ln C_{pex}	C_{pex}	ΔC_p	ln ΔC_p	
0.5	23.0			4.501	90.1	67.1	4.206	
1	36.5			4.406	82.0	45.5	3.818	
1.5	43.9			4.312	74.6	30.7	3.424	$k_a = 0.797\ h^{-1}$
2	47.2			4.218	67.9	20.7	3.030	
3	46.8			4.029	56.2	9.4	2.241	
4	42.4			3.840	46.5	4.1	1.411	
5	36.7			3.652	38.5	1.8		
6	31.1			3.463	31.9	0.8		
8	21.8	3.082						
10	15.0	2.708						
12	10.3	2.332	$k = 0.1887\ h^{-1}$					
14	7.1	1.960						
18	3.3	1.194						

Note: The 5- and 6-h points are not included in the residuals analysis, as an error of 3% in the original value of C_p would translate into an error of 61 and 117%, respectively, for the ΔC_p value.
ln C_{pex} = Data generated by linear regression analysis of the terminal phase of ln C_p against time.
C_{pex} = Antilogs.
ΔC_p = The values ($C_{pex} - C_p$) used to draw the residuals line.

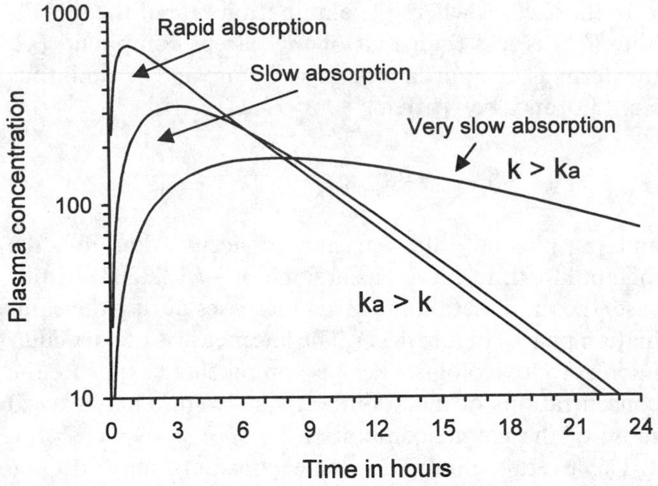

FIG. 4.10. The effect of absorption rate on the shape of the plasma concentration–time curve.

the curve. An increase in the absorption rate may be as important toxicologically therefore as a decrease in elimination rate.

Area under the curve. Both CL and V may be derived using Eqs. (22) and (23), providing that the dose used in the calculation is adjusted for the fraction absorbed (F), that is,

$$\mathrm{CL} = \frac{\mathrm{dose} \times F}{\mathrm{AUC}}$$

It is common to see $\mathrm{CL}_{\mathrm{oral}}$ calculated as (dose/AUC) in the absence of any information on F. Such a term is meaningless physiologically; if the value of F is unknown, oral AUC data should be compared as such. Intravenous data are necessary to relate a nonlinear change in AUC at high oral doses to either altered CL or F.

The value of F may be determined by comparison of oral with intravenous dosing, because CL remains constant.

$$CL = \frac{\mathrm{dose}_o \times F}{\mathrm{AUC}_o} = \frac{\mathrm{dose}_{\mathrm{iv}}}{\mathrm{AUC}_{\mathrm{iv}}}$$
$$F = \frac{\mathrm{dose}_{\mathrm{iv}} \times \mathrm{AUC}_o}{\mathrm{AUC}_{\mathrm{iv}} \times \mathrm{dose}_{\mathrm{o}}} \qquad [31]$$

where o relates to oral and iv relates to intravenous dosing. These relationships are valid only if the AUC/dose ratio is constant: if not, the value of either F or CL must alter with an increase in dose, suggesting saturation of absorption or elimination (see below).

Alternatively, the fraction F may be derived from the cumulative urinary excretion:

$$\mathrm{F} = \frac{A_{\mathrm{exo}}^{\infty}}{A_{\mathrm{exiv}}^{\infty}} \times \frac{\mathrm{dose}_{\mathrm{iv}}}{\mathrm{dose}_o} \qquad [32]$$

Increase to peak. The increase to peak is determined by the more rapid of the two processes, that is, usually absorption. Measurement of the absorption rate constant must make allowance for the excretion occurring throughout the postdosing period; the method of residuals is used (see Gibaldi and Perrier (36) for the mathematical basis of this method). The method is illustrated and explained in Figure 4.9 and Table 4.5. In cases where absorption is slow, the rate of increase may be determined by the elimination rate constant. Thus the value of k_a can be assigned to the increase to peak only after demonstration that the value of k for the decrease is similar to that seen after intravenous dosing.

Metabolite Kinetics

As discussed elsewhere, the biotransformation of xenobiotics usually results in detoxication but is sometimes associated with the formation of a toxic metabolite. Measurement of the rate of metabolism in vivo can provide much useful information on detoxication or bioactivation processes. In most cases, the rate of metabolite formation is governed by in vivo enzyme kinetics, which are first-order only over a limited substrate concentration range. Saturation of metabolism is discussed in more detail below, and the following analysis relates to metabolite formation under first-order reaction conditions, when CL depends on enzyme activity rather than liver blood flow.

The measurements that are available for analysis of metabolite kinetics include plasma levels of unchanged drug (C_p) and metabolite (C_p^m). The simple system given earlier, for the parent compound (Scheme 4.2) can be extended into Scheme 4.3, where V, k_{ex}, and k_m are, respectively, the apparent volume of distribution, excretion rate constant, and metabolism rate constants for the parent compound, and V^m, k_{ex}^m, and k_m^m are the

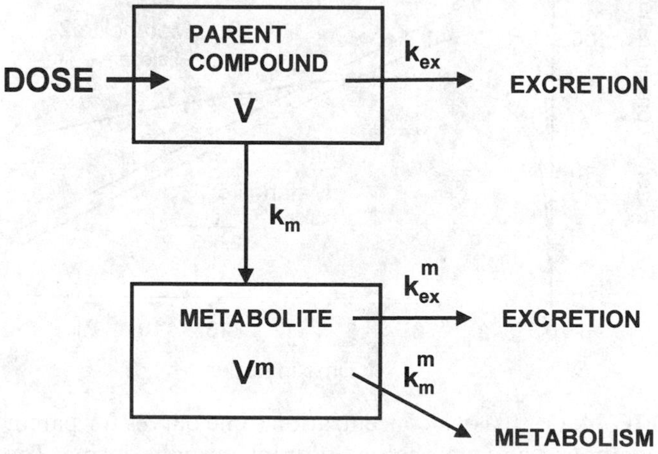

SCHEME 4.3. One-compartment model with metabolite formation.

same parameters for the metabolite. The time course for the metabolite is given by

$$\frac{dM}{dt} = k_m\mathrm{Ab} - k^m M$$

where Ab and M are the amount of parent compound and metabolite in the body, respectively, and k^m is the overall elimination rate constant for the metabolite, that is, $k^m = k^m_{\mathrm{ex}} + k^m_m$. This equation may be solved to yield

$$C^m_p = \frac{k_m \mathrm{dose}(e^{-k_m t} - e^{-kt})}{V^m(k - k^m)} \quad [33]$$

where C^m_p is the plasma concentration of the metabolite at time $= t$.

In many cases the overall elimination rate of the metabolite (k^m) is greater than the overall elimination rate of the parent compound (k) (for example in the case of the formation of a more polar metabolite). In such cases the term $e^{-k^m t}$ approaches zero before e^{-kt}, and thus at late time points Eq. (33) may be rewritten and solved omitting e^{-k^m} when it becomes

$$\log C^m_p = \log \frac{k_m \times \mathrm{dose}}{V^m(k^m - k)} - \frac{kt}{2.303} \quad [34]$$

Thus the log plasma concentration of the metabolite–time curve has a terminal slope similar to that of the parent compound (i.e., $k/2.303$) (Figure 4.11). In this case the rate of elimination of the metabolite is limited by the elimination of the parent drug, and the metabolite/drug ratio remains constant during the elimination phase (Figure 4.11).

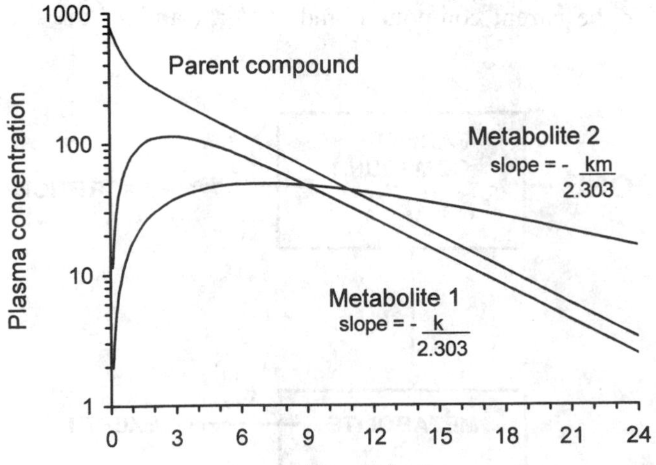

FIG. 4.11. Plasma concentration–time curves for parent compound and metabolites after intravenous dosing. The parent compound was given as an intravenous bolus dose at time=0.

In those cases where the elimination rate of the metabolite (k^m) is less than that of the parent compound (k), the term e^{-kt} approaches zero before $e^{-k^m t}$, and thus Eq. (33) may be written

$$\log C^m_p = \log \frac{k_m \times \mathrm{dose}}{V^m(k - k^m)} - \frac{k^m t}{2.303} \quad [35]$$

and a plot of log plasma concentration of the metabolite–time curve has a slope of $-k^m/2.303$. In this case, the ratio metabolite/drug increases during the elimination phase (Figure 4.11). The latter case is of particular interest to toxicologists because on repeated exposure the concentrations of metabolite at steady state may exceed those of the parent compound.

The overall elimination rate constants may also be derived from urinary metabolite levels as described above for the parent compound, although again the derived rate may be either k or k^m and the identity can be determined only by measuring k and k^m separately after administration of both the parent compound and the metabolite. However, if metabolite kinetics are based solely on urinary excretion data, the formation of more lipid-soluble metabolites may be missed. For example, the active thioether metabolite of sulfinpyrazone is a major circulating metabolite of which negligible amounts are excreted in the urine (102).

Two-Compartment Open Model

Mathematically and physiologically, it is often more appropriate to regard the body as representing a simple two-compartment open system in which the distribution to certain peripheral tissues is not an instantaneous process. In such a system the chemical initially enters a central compartment (the plasma and those tissues for which distribution is instantaneous) and is subsequently distributed to a second, peripheral compartment. Elimination occurs from the central compartment, so that chemical in the peripheral compartment must transfer back to the central compartment in order to be eliminated (Scheme 4.1B or Scheme 4.4). In Scheme 4.4, k_{12} and k_{21} are the rate constants for transfer from compartment 1 to 2 and from 2 to 1, respectively, and k_{10} is the elimination rate from the central compartment.

Intravenous Bolus Dose

After a single intravenous bolus dose into a two-compartment system, the plasma concentration (C_p) at time t may be described by

$$C_p = Ae^{-\alpha t} + Be^{-\beta t} \quad [36]$$

where A and B may be regarded as analogous to C_{p0} for each compartment, and $A + B = C_{p0}$; α and β correspond

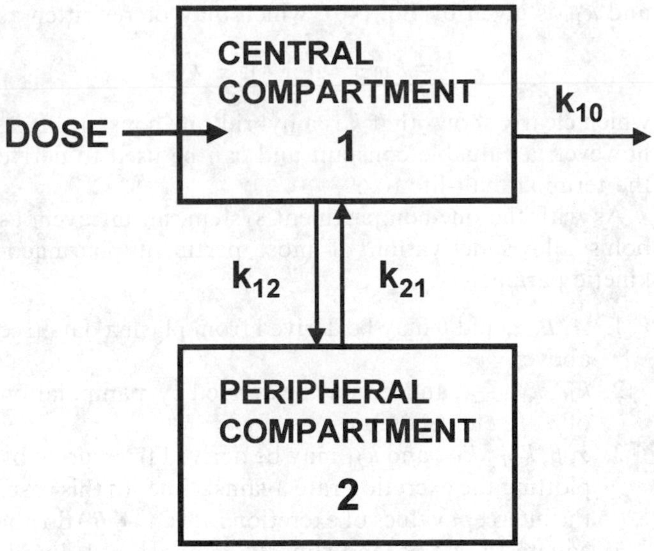

SCHEME 4.4. Two-compartment model.

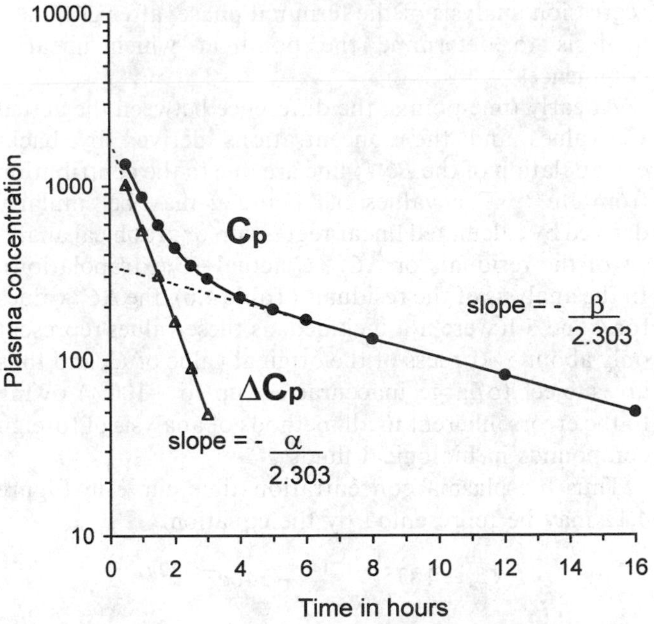

FIG. 4.12. Plasma concentration–time curve for two-compartment system. The data are given in Table 4.6.

to hybrid rate constants, each influenced by all the individual distribution, redistribution, and elimination rate constants, that is, k_{12}, k_{21}, and k_{10} (36). The shape of a typical plasma concentration–time curve following a bolus intravenous dose is given in Figure 4.12 (see also Table 4.6) with the plasma data and the method of derivation of the various constants. As with the determination of absorption rate constants discussed above, the method of residuals or line stripping is used to separate α and β. In the terminal phase, $Ae^{-\alpha t}$ approaches zero, and the data are described by $C_p = Be^{-\beta t}$. For example, using the data in Table 4.6, when $t = 8$ h, $Be^{-\beta t} = 346e^{-0.121\times 8} = 131\ \mu$g/ml, whereas $Ae^{-\alpha t} = 1875e^{-1.214\times 8} = 0.1\ \mu$g/ml; therefore, the contribution of the latter term is negligible. The terminal phase after 8 h is therefore extrapolated back to time 0 when the intercept is equal to B and the slope of log C_p against time is $\beta/2.303$. As described in Table 4.6, the values of B and β may also be derived by least-squares linear

Table 4.6
Data used for Figure 4.12

Time (h)	C_p (μg ml^{-1})	ln C_p	ln C_{pex}	C_{pex}	ΔC_p	ln ΔC_p	
0.5	1345		5.788	326	1,019	6.927	By linear regression
1	864		5.727	307	557	6.323	$\alpha = 1.214$ h^{-1}
1.5	593		5.666	289	304	5.717	ln $C_{p0} = 7.537$
2	438		5.606	272	166	5.112	$\therefore A = 1875\ \mu$g ml^{-1}
2.5	346		5.545	256	90	4.500	
3	290		5.485	241	49	3.892	
4	228		5.364	214	15	2.708	
5	193		5.243	189	4	1.386	
6	168	5.122	Terminal phase; by linear regression				$\beta = 0.1210$ h^{-1}
8	131	4.879					ln $C_{p0} = 5.848$
12	81	4.395					$\therefore B = 346\ \mu$g ml^{-1}
16	50	3.911					

ln C_{pex} = Data generated by linear regression analysis of the terminal phase data for ln C_p against time.
C_{pex} = Antilogs of these extrapolated points; similar values may be obtained from the extrapolated line on the graph.
ΔC_p = The values ($C_p - C_{pex}$); they may be used to derive the $\log_{10}$ residuals line (slope $-\alpha/2.303$) or may be converted to natural logarithms and analyzed by linear regression.

regression analysis of the terminal phase, after graphical analysis to determine the point at which linearity commences.

At early time points, the difference between the actual C_p values and the concentrations derived by back-extrapolation of the $Be^{-\beta t}$ line are due to the contribution from $Ae^{-\alpha t}$. The values of A and α may be similarly derived by calculated linear regression or graphical analysis of the residuals or ΔC_p ($C_p$actual$-C_p$extrapolation). In the analysis of the residuals (Table 4.6), the ΔC_p values for 4 and 5 h were not included, as these values represent only about 5% or less of the original value of C_p and thus are subject to large inaccuracies (up to +100%) owing to the errors inherent in all methods of analysis of foreign compounds in biological fluids.

Thus the plasma concentration–time curve in Figure 4.12 may be represented by the equation:

$$C_p = 1875e^{-1.214t} + 346e^{-0.1210t}$$

The rate constants α and β are composite rate constants, from which it is possible to derive k_{12}, k_{21}, and k_{10} given in Scheme 4.4 using the following equations (see refs. 36 and 112 for derivations):

$$C_{p0} = A + B$$
$$\alpha + \beta = k_{12} + k_{21} + k_{10} \qquad [37]$$
$$V_1 = \frac{\text{dose}}{A + B}$$

where V_1 is the volume of the central compartment, and

$$k_{21} = \frac{A\beta + B\alpha}{A + B} \qquad [38]$$

$$k_{10} = \frac{\alpha\beta}{k_{21}} \qquad [39]$$

$$k_{12} = \alpha + \beta - k_{21} - k_{10} \qquad [40]$$

For the example given in Figure 4.10,

$$k_{21} = \frac{(1875 \times 0.1210) + (346 \times 1.214)}{(1875 + 346)} = 0.291$$

$$k_{10} = \frac{(1.214 \times 0.1210)}{0.291} = 0.505$$

$$k_{12} = 1.214 + 0.1210 - 0.291 - 0.505 = 0.539$$

It is important to note that k_{10} (0.505) and β (0.121) do not relate to the same process, because k_{10} refers to the elimination from the central compartment, whereas β refers to the overall elimination from the body (and is slower due to transfer out of tissues as well as elimination from the central compartment). The relation between β and k_{10} is given by Eq. (40), which may be rewritten as

$$\beta = k_{10} + k_{21} + k_{12} - \alpha$$

which clearly shows that β is a hybrid rate constant. It is, however, a valuable constant and can be used to derive the terminal half-life ($0.693/\beta$).

As with the one-compartment system, an intravenous bolus allows derivation of most pertinent pharmacokinetic parameters:

1. A, B, α, and β may be derived from plasma data (see above).
2. k_{10}, k_{12}, k_{21}, and V_1 may be derived by manipulation of α, β, etc. (see above).
3. α, β, k_{10}, k_{12}, and k_{21} may be derived from urine by plotting the excretion rate against time. In this case, the intercept values of excretion rate ($A' + B'$) do not equate to $A + B$, and thus V_1 cannot be deduced. However, k_{10}, k_{12}, and k_{21} can be obtained from Eqs. (38–40) by substitution of A and B by A' and B'. The renal elimination rate constant (k_R) is given by

$$k_R = \frac{A' + B'}{\text{dose}}$$

4. α, β, k_{10}, k_{12}, and k_{21}, may be derived from urine by the sigma-minus method, where log ($A_{ex}^{\infty} - A_{ex}$) [see Eq. (27)] is plotted against time. Again α and β may be derived by the method of residuals; k_{10}, k_{12}, and k_{21} can be calculated from from α and β and the intercepts (A'' and B'') by substitution in Eqs. (38–40). The renal elimination rate constant (k_R) is given by

$$k_R = \frac{A_{ex}^{\infty}}{\text{dose}} \times k_{10}$$

5. The renal elimination constant, k_R, may be derived also from the renal clearance

$$CL_R = \frac{C_u \times F_u}{C_p}$$

and the value of V_1 as $\text{CL}_R = k_R V_1$.

6. The amount in the peripheral compartment may be calculated from the following equation (which is similar to Eq. (30) for absorption into a single compartment):

$$C_2 = \frac{\text{dose} \times k_{12}(e^{-\beta t} - e^{-\alpha t})}{V_2(\alpha - \beta)} \qquad [41]$$

where C_2 and V_2 are respectively the concentrations in, and volume of, the peripheral or deep compartment.

During the terminal phase of the concentration–time curve, $e^{-\alpha t}$ approaches zero and therefore Eq. (41) may be simplified as

$$C_2 = \frac{\text{dose} \times k_{12} \times e^{-\beta t}}{V_2(\alpha - \beta)}$$

Therefore, a graph of log C_2 against time has a slope of $-\beta/2.303$. Thus the terminal rate of decrease in the peripheral compartment of a two-compartment system is identical to the decrease in the central compartment.

In absolute terms, the calculation of C_2 is not particularly valuable, because the peripheral tissues comprising the deep compartment are not homogeneous, and the compound may not show a uniform concentration. Thus C_2 should not be regarded as the effective drug concentration, even if the target organ lies within the deep compartment. Rather, the concentration in the target organ should be measured, from which subsequent concentrations may be calculated using β defined from the central compartment.

A further useful kinetic parameter (V_β), which relates the total amount of chemical in the body to the plasma concentration, is given by the equation

$$V_\beta \times \beta = V_1 \times k_{10} = \frac{\text{dose}}{\text{AUC}} = \text{CL}$$

Just as β is a hybrid term reflecting overall elimination from the body, so V_β is a composite but valuable function.

$$V_\beta = \frac{\text{dose}}{\text{AUC} \times \beta}$$

Intravenous Infusion

The shape of the plasma concentration–time curve on intravenous infusion into a two-compartment open system is similar to that given in Figure 4.8, but with a biphasic increase at the start of the infusion and a biphasic decrease at the end. The kinetic parameters may be derived from the graph similarly to the one-compartment model, as follows.

Increase to plateau. The increase to plateau follows a complex exponential function with 90 and 99% of the steady-state concentration being reached after four and seven half-lives, respectively.

Plateau level (C_{pss}). At steady state, the rate of infusion (R) equals the rate of elimination. Therefore

$$\frac{R}{C_{pss}} = \text{CL} = V_1 \times k_{10} = V_\beta \times \beta$$

Decrease after plateau. The decrease after plateau follows the equation:

$$C_p = A^* e^{-\alpha t^*} + B^* e^{-\beta t^*}$$

where A^* and B^* are the intercepts by back extrapolation to the end of the infusion of the α and β slopes (determined as described for Figure 4.12) and t^* = time since cessation of infusion.

In many cases, two-compartment characteristics seen after a bolus dose are obscured in postinfusion data, because much of the distribution phase will have occurred during the infusion, so that the duration of the α phase may be reduced.

Area under the curve. The AUC can be used to derive the plasma clearance using Eq. (22).

Oral Administration

Assuming first-order absorption into compartment 1, the plasma concentration at time t is given by

$$C_p = A^{\ddagger} e^{-\alpha t} + B^{\ddagger} e^{-\beta t} + C^{\ddagger} e^{-k_a t}$$

Graphical analysis by a semilogarithmic plot of log C_p against time may reveal three separate phases, from which α, β, and k_a should be measurable using the method of residuals. However, in practice the value of k_a is frequently similar to α, and compounds that require a two-compartment model after intravenous administration appear to fit first-order absorption into a one-compartment model following oral dosing (18). Thus analysis is not possible without reference to intravenous data to determine which rate constant refers to the absorption rate. An example of linear regression analysis to obtain the three rate constants was given by Wagner (112). An alternative method (deconvolution method) may be used that derives the absorption rate constant by a comparison of plasma concentrations for intravenous and oral administration, and does not require fitting the data to a particular one-, two-, or three-compartment model. This method (36,112) does, however, require analysis of the plasma concentrations at the same time points after both oral and intravenous dosing. Various methods of calculating the absorption rate are discussed in Gibaldi and Perrier (36).

The absorption rate is likely to be of greatest importance in acute toxicity studies, whereas the bioavailability (F) may be more significant in chronic studies; the latter may be measured using model-independent equations [Eq. (31) or (32)]. However, absorption from the gastrointestinal tract is complex, as it involves physiologically different membranes at differing luminal pH values. Thus the process may involve more than one first-order rate, or a zero-order component, or both; an alternate approach to compartmental analysis and a valuable measure is the mean absorption time (see below).

Metabolite Kinetics

Frequently, metabolites of foreign compounds fit a two-compartment open model, in which case a second compartment for the metabolite is in equilibrium with the central metabolite compartment, as well as a second compartment for the parent compound (see Scheme 4.3). The equation describing these four compartments requires four exponential terms, but often the concentration–time curve for the metabolite appears as a bi-exponential decrease. The slow terminal phase of the metabolite is given by either β for the parent compound, or the terminal rate for the metabolite (see earlier); the faster rate is a composite of the other three rate constants.

Multiple Dosing: Chronic Administration

On multiple dosing or continuous intake, the plasma levels increase over a period of four to five half-lives to establish a plateau concentration similar to that seen with intravenous infusion (Figure 4.8). The average plateau level is subject to variations around a mean as material is eliminated between "doses." In oral toxicity studies, these "doses" may represent either repeated single-gavage doses or the feeding habits of the animals if the test compound is incorporated into the diet and fed ad libitum. On cessation of chronic intake, the rate of decrease in blood levels is usually but not always similar to that seen after a single dose (22).

One-compartment Open Model

The time taken to reach plateau plasma levels is four to five times the half-time of the terminal phase of the plasma concentration–time curve. The average plateau level is given (by analogy with intravenous infusion) as

$$C_{p\,\mathrm{mean}} = \frac{\mathrm{dose} \times F}{V \times k \times T} \qquad [42]$$

where F is the fraction absorbed, T is the dose interval, and k is the elimination rate constant. However, it is important to realize that this equation is appropriate only if the terminal phase following oral administration is due to elimination. When the compound exhibits slow absorption and rapid elimination, the decrease in plasma levels is determined by the slower absorption rate (k_a). An alternative equation can be derived from the fact that at steady state the rate of input ($F \times \mathrm{dose}/T$) is balanced by the rate of elimination ($C_{p\,\mathrm{mean}} \times \mathrm{CL}$); therefore

$$C_{p\,\mathrm{mean}} = \frac{\mathrm{dose} \times F}{T \times \mathrm{CL}}$$

The fluctuations around the mean plateau level depend on the dosing interval in relation to the terminal elimination rate. Thus compounds with a short half-life show much larger fluctuations, as more of the chemical is eliminated between each dose. In the case of compounds with a short half-life (2–3 h), single daily dosing gives plasma levels approaching zero prior to each dose. Interdose fluctuations may be reduced and blunted by slow absorption. The equations relating to these processes were detailed by Gibaldi and Perrier (36) and Wagner (112). In summary, at steady state after repeated intravenous doses, the minima and maxima are given by

$$C_{p\,\mathrm{minimum}} = \frac{\mathrm{dose}}{V}\left(\frac{e^{-kT}}{1 - e^{-kT}}\right) \qquad [43]$$

$$C_{p\,\mathrm{maximum}} = \frac{\mathrm{dose}}{V}\left(\frac{1}{1 - e^{-kT}}\right) \qquad [44]$$

When absorption from the gut occurs as a first-order process, the fluctuations in the steady-state concentration–time curve can be described by the following equation:

$$C_p = \frac{F \times \mathrm{dose} \times k_a}{V(k_a - k)} \times \left[\left(\frac{1}{1 - e^{-kT}}\right)e^{-kt} - \left(\frac{1}{1 - e^{-k_aT}}\right)e^{-kt}\right] \qquad [45]$$

where C_p is the concentration at time t and T is the dose interval. The similarity between this equation and Eq. (30) for absorption of a single dose is apparent.

The value of the mean plasma concentration at steady state ($C_{p\,\mathrm{mean}}$) may be calculated without knowledge of F, V, k_a, or k by measuring the area under the plasma concentration–time curve for a single oral dose, as

$$\mathrm{AUC_{oral}} = \frac{\mathrm{dose} \times F}{V \times k} = \frac{\mathrm{dose} \times F}{\mathrm{CL}} \qquad [23]$$

where $\mathrm{AUC_{oral}}$ is the area under the plasma concentration–time curve between $t = 0$ and $t = \infty$ for a single oral dose. Substituting into Eq. (42),

$$C_{\mathrm{mean}} = \frac{\mathrm{AUC_{oral}}}{T} \qquad [46]$$

It is important to realize, however, that substitution of Eq. (23) into Eq. (42) assumes that the AUC is directly proportional to the dose, that is, that dose-dependent kinetics are absent and that CL does not alter during chronic administration of the compound. The latter possibility may be assessed by comparison of the $\mathrm{AUC}_{0-\infty}$ for a single dose, with the AUC for a dose interval at steady state, that is, AUC_{0-T} for chronic administration,

$$\mathrm{CL} = \frac{\mathrm{dose\ (single)} \times F}{\mathrm{AUC}_{0-\infty}} = \frac{\mathrm{dose\ (chronic)} \times F}{C_{p\,\mathrm{mean}} \times T} = \frac{\mathrm{dose\ (chronic)} \times F}{\mathrm{AUC}_{0-T}}$$

If $\mathrm{AUC}_{0-T}(\mathrm{chronic}) < \mathrm{AUC}_{0-\infty}(\mathrm{single})$, either induction of metabolism or decreased bioavailability is indicated; conversely if AUC_{0-T}(chronic)>$AUC_{0-\infty}$ (single), then inhibition or saturation of metabolism is suggested.

The extent of accumulation on repeated intake may be measured by the average amount in the body at steady state (Ab_{mean}), divided by the amount in the body after a single dose (Ab), that is,

$$\text{extent of accumulation} = \frac{Ab_{mean}}{Ab} = \frac{Ab_{mean}}{\text{dose} \times F}$$

The amount in the body at the plateau is given by Eq. (42):

$$Ab_{mean} = VC_{p\,mean} = \frac{F \times \text{dose}}{k \times T}$$

Therefore

$$\text{Extent of accumulation} = \frac{1}{k \times T} = \frac{1}{0.693/t_{1/2} \times T} = \frac{1.44 \times t_{1/2}}{T}$$

Two-compartment Open Model

The equations giving the plasma concentration at time t at steady state into a two-compartment system with first-order absorption are considerably more complex than those for the one-compartment system. However, the simplified equation [Eq. (42)] applies in the form

$$C_{p\,mean} = \frac{\text{dose} \times F}{V_1 \times k_{10} \times T} = \frac{\text{dose} \times F}{V_\beta \times \beta \times T}$$

and the value of $C_{p\,mean}$ may still be derived from Eq. (46):

$$C_{p\,mean} = \frac{AUC_{oral}}{T} = \frac{\text{dose} \times F}{CL \times T}$$

In addition, the relationship between the AUC between $t=0$ and $t=\infty$ for a single dose and the AUC for a dose interval at steady state applies on the condition that neither CL or F changes on chronic intake (see above); a difference between these AUC estimates indicates changes in CL or F during chronic treatment.

Statistical Moment Analysis

In recent years both clinical pharmacokinetic and animal toxicokinetic studies have moved away from compartmental analyses, because they involve multiple variables, which require numerous properly timed blood samples to characterize them adequately. Also, curve fitting is dependent on the terminal slope, which is frequently measured using plasma concentrations that approach the limit of detection of the assay method, that is, are the weakest data. In contrast, terms such as clearance are measured from dose and AUC, the latter being determined largely from the highest and most accurately measured concentrations. Such "time-averaged" parameters may be extended to "time-related" parameters by the use of statistical moment theory, which allows assessment of additional useful kinetic parameters such as *mean residence time* (MRT). The plasma concentration–time curve may be regarded as a statistical distribution curve for which the zero and first moments are the AUC and MRT respectively:

$$AUC = \int_0^\infty C_p dt \qquad MRT = \frac{AUMC}{AUC} \quad [48]$$

where AUMC is the area under the first moment of concentration time curve, that is, $\int_0^\infty t \times C_p dt$.

The AUC and AUMC may be calculated using the trapezoid rule, which is illustrated under Data Handling (see Table 4.17). The AUC from the last data point to infinity can be calculated as $C_{p\,last}/\beta$. The AUMC from the last data point to infinity has to be calculated as

$$\frac{t_{last} \times C_{p\,last}}{\beta} + \frac{C_{p\,last}}{\beta^2}$$

Clearly any inaccuracy in the value of β affects the extrapolation of AUMC to infinity more than the extrapolation of AUC. This situation is shown in the data given in Table 4.17, where the extrapolated area is 17% of the AUMC, but only 3% of the AUC.

In the same way that the AUC can be related to CL, k and V, β and V_β, etc., so the AUMC can be used to derive additional useful parameters.

Intravenous Administration

Following an intravenous bolus dose, the MRT can be calculated by Eq. (48) as illustrated in Table 4.17. The *apparent volume of distribution at steady state* (V_{ss}) may be regarded as the volume of plasma in which the compound appears to be dissolved and that has to be "removed" from the body, that is, the product of clearance (ml min^{-1}) and MRT (min):

$$V_{ss} = CL \times MRT = \frac{\text{dose}}{AUC} \times \frac{AUMC}{AUC} = \frac{\text{dose} \times AUMC}{AUC^2} \quad [49]$$

Attempts to separate the MRT, which refers to the whole body, into central and peripheral components (110) may prove to be of value, but are dependent on the data fitting a two-compartment model.

If the compound is too toxic to be given as an instantaneous bolus, the MRT can be calculated from the AUMC determined following an intravenous infusion using the equation:

$$\mathrm{MRT}_{\mathrm{infusion}} = \mathrm{MRT} + \frac{T}{2} \qquad [50]$$

where $\mathrm{MRT}_{\mathrm{infusion}}$ is calculated from the AUMC and AUC by Eq. (48) from the infusion data, and T is the infusion time.

V_{ss} cannot be derived directly from the AUMC and AUC data from infusions, because the AUMC value contains a component due to the infusion time. The following equation therefore applies,

$$V_{ss} = \frac{\text{infused dose} \times \mathrm{AUMC}}{\mathrm{AUC}^2} - \frac{\text{infused dose} \times T}{2 \times \mathrm{AUC}} \qquad [51]$$

In the same way that CL may be related to V by the rate constant k [Eq. (21)], so it may be related to V_{ss} by the first-order rate constant k_{ss} (7,36).

$$\mathrm{CL} = k_{ss} V_{ss} = \frac{V_{ss}}{\mathrm{MRT}}$$

Therefore k_{ss} is equivalent to 1/MRT; for a two-compartment system k_{ss} is intermediate between α and β. The half-life derived from k_{ss} ($0.693/k_{ss}$ or $0.693 \times \mathrm{MRT}$) is therefore a composite half-life, and may be regarded as the "effective" half-life. This is shown in the data analyzed later (Table 4.17) where the half-life derived from MRT ($0.693 \times 25 = 17$ min) is intermediate between that calculated from α ($0.693/0.0705 = 10$ min) and β ($0.693/0.0240 = 34$ min).

Oral Administration

A major strength of the statistical moment theory is its ability to derive meaningful data following oral administration, because it is both more reliable and easier to use than most other methods (18) and does not rely on assumptions about a first-order or zero-order process. The most useful parameter is the *mean absorption time* (MAT), which is the difference between the mean residence times following oral and intravenous dosing:

$$\mathrm{MAT} = \mathrm{MRT}_{\mathrm{oral}} - \mathrm{MRT}_{\mathrm{iv}} \qquad [52]$$

The MAT may be used to derive apparent first-order rate constants and half-lives:

$$k_a = \frac{1}{\mathrm{MAT}}$$

$$\text{Absorption } t_{1/2} = 0.693 \times \mathrm{MAT}$$

Alternatively, if absorption appears to be zero order, by analogy with Eq. (50):

$$\mathrm{MAT} = \frac{T_{\mathrm{abs}}}{2}$$

where T_{abs} is the duration of the absorption process.

The measurement of MAT is generally applied to absorption from a solution. If a sparingly soluble compound is given,

$$\mathrm{MRT}_{\mathrm{oral}} = \mathrm{MRT}_{\mathrm{iv}} + \mathrm{MAT} + \mathrm{MDT}$$

where MDT is the mean dissolution time.

The statistical moment theory is therefore a valuable technique for comparisons on the influence of dosage formulations on absorption (18,79).

Chronic Administration

As discussed previously, the increase to steady state for multicompartment models is complex. AUC data may be used, in the absence of compartmental analysis, to derive the proportion of steady state reached at any time after dosing. The proportion of steady state is equal to the AUC to that time (AUC_{0-t}) calculated as a proportion of the total AUC extrapolated to infinity ($\mathrm{AUC}_{0-\infty}$), that is,

$$\%\ \text{steady state} = 100 \times \frac{\mathrm{AUC}_{0-t}}{\mathrm{AUC}_{0-\infty}}$$

There is, however, a significant complication in the use of statistical moments for the analysis of steady-state data because, unlike AUC data, $\mathrm{AUMC}_{0-\infty}$ for a single dose does not equal AUMC_{0-T} during regular dosing (6). A simple way to overcome this difficulty is to apply a method of residuals to the steady-state plasma concentration prior to the regular dose ($C_{\min}$). Assuming that this level decreases by a single first-order rate (β) determined from the terminal phase of the interdose period (or the terminal phase following a single dose), the contribution of this residue to each subsequent sample can be calculated as $C_{\min}e^{-\beta t}$, where t is the time of that particular sample after $C_{\min}$. The calculated residue is then subtracted from the measured value at each time to derive pseudo-single-dose data ($C - C_{\min}e^{-\beta t}$) that can be used to calculate AUMC.

Dose-Dependent or Nonlinear Kinetics

Whereas simple diffusion obeys first-order kinetics at all concentrations, many of the other processes fundamental to toxicokinetics involve an interaction between the foreign chemical and a specific site on a protein (examples being active transport across the gut, plasma and tissue protein binding, metabolism, and renal tubular secretion). These processes have a finite capacity for interaction between the chemical and the protein; thus at high concentrations of chemical, all the specific sites on the protein may be occupied. Addition of further chemical cannot result in further interaction between the chemical and protein, and the concentration of free compound increases rapidly. Depending on the nature of the protein–chemical interaction, there are a number of possible consequences, which are summarized in Table 4.7. This table represents a considerable simplification because the effect of saturation at one site may affect another protein–chemical interaction. For example, saturation of renal tubular secretion gives increased AUC/dose and elevated plasma concentrations. However, the resultant high concentrations may saturate plasma protein binding, resulting in an increase in free drug and increased glomerular filtration and/or hepatic clearance. Thus the decreased elimination in the renal tubule may be overcome to some extent by increased elimination elsewhere.

Almost all of the processes listed in Table 4.7 may be described by a Michaelis–Menten equation of the type introduced into Eq. (11), that is,

$$-\frac{dC}{dt} = \frac{V_{max} \times C}{K_m + C} \qquad [53]$$

where V_{max} is the theoretical maximum rate of the reaction and K_m is the Michaelis constant (which reflects the concentration giving 50% saturation of the protein).

At low concentrations $C \ll K_m$, and $K_m + C$ approximates to K_m so that

$$-\frac{dC}{dt} = \frac{V_{max} \times C}{K_m}$$

and V_{max}/K_m is equivalent to the first-order rate constant k.

At higher concentrations $C \gg K_m$, and $K_m + C$ approximates to C so that

$$-\frac{dC}{dt} = \frac{V_{max} \times C}{C} = V_{max}$$

and thus the elimination is a zero-order reaction. The shape of the plasma concentration–time curve for a hypothetical compound showing saturation kinetics is given in Figure 4.13, which clearly shows that although low doses are indistinguishable from first-order elimination, the decrease at high plasma concentrations shows zero-order and then first-order reaction components.

It is important to note that the terminal slope and terminal half-life are derived from low plasma concentrations, and do not provide evidence of dose dependence. However, the plasma clearance, which is derived from AUC data and which reflects the capacity of the organs of elimination to remove the chemical from plasma, provides the best evidence of saturation. This is shown clearly by derivation of the appropriate rate constants, etc., for the example given in Figure 4.13 and Table 4.8, which shows a fivefold change in CL; it also illustrates the power of the statistical moment approach, which shows a fourfold increase in MRT. The value of k (0.0485) approximates to V_{max}/K_m (0.050).

Table 4.7
Consequences of saturation of chemical–protein interactions

Site	Interaction	Possible consequences of saturation at high dose
Absorption	Active uptake	Reduced plasma levels and AUC after oral but not IV doses.
	First-pass metabolism	Increased plasma levels and AUC after oral but not IV doses.
Distribution	Plasma protein	Increased volume of distribution; increased glomerular filtration; increased hepatic clearance if extraction ratio is low.
	Tissue protein	Decreased volume of distribution; a graph of C_t/C_p against C_p will be nonlinear.
Metabolism	Metabolizing enzyme (saturation by substrate, depletion of cofactors, product inhibition)	Decreased clearance; AUC/dose ratio increases for parent compound, whereas AUC of metabolite/dose ratio may decrease for both oral and IV doses; enzymes with high K_m values may handle a larger proportion of the dose.
Excretion	Renal tubular secretion	Decreased renal clearance; AUC/dose ratio increases for oral and IV doses; nonrenal routes of elimination become of more importance; total excretion in urine per dose may decrease depending on the availability of other routes of elimination.
	Renal tubular reabsorption (rare)	Opposite of effects for saturation of renal tubular secretion.
	Biliary excretion	Decreased biliary clearance; decreased enterohepatic recirculation; renal route may become more important; AUC/dose ratio increases for oral and IV doses.

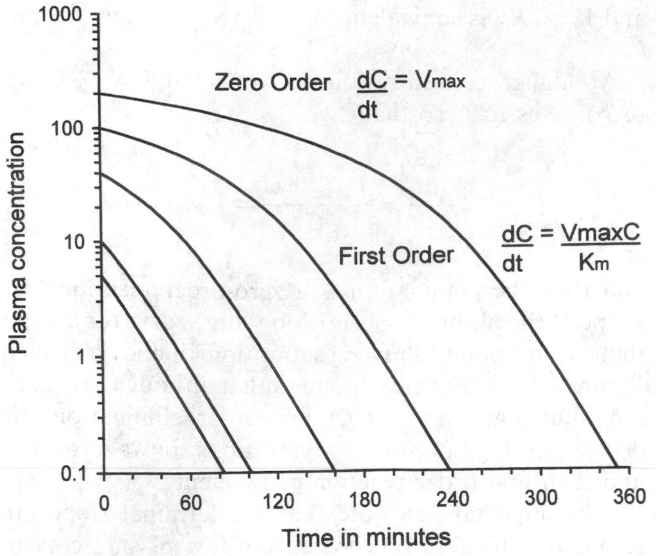

FIG. 4.13. Plasma concentration–time curve for a compound showing saturation kinetics. The data were generated using an apparent V_{max} of 1 μg/min and a K_m of 20 μg/ml for initial concentrations of 5, 10, 40, 100, and 200 μg/ml. Data points were obtained using a derivative of Eq. (53), $V_{max}(t - t_0) = C_{p0} - K_m \ln(C_{p0}/C_p)$.

An increased understanding of saturation kinetics can be obtained by the determination of K_m and V_{max} from in vivo data. The value of K_m which reflects the plasma concentration necessary to give 50% saturation of the active process, is particularly useful for interpreting toxicity dose–response relationships. These constants can be determined following a single intravenous bolus dose using various equations, provided that the elimination is by a single saturable process (see below). The simplest method, applicable to a one-compartment model, is by calculation directly from the plasma concentration–time curve using the equations

$$\ln C_p = \ln C_{p0e} - \frac{V_{max} \times t}{K_m}$$

and

$$K_m = \frac{C_{p0a}}{\ln(C_{p0e}/C_{p0a})}$$

where C_{p0e} is the value of C_p at $t = 0$ derived by back extrapolation of the terminal linear phase, and C_{p0a} is the actual concentration measured at $t = 0$. A plot of $\ln C_p$ against time has a terminal "first-order" slope of V_{max}/K_m.

Applying these equations to the data in Figure 4.13 for the highest dose gives values of 0.0486 for the slope, 200 for C_{p0a}, and 2,701,271 for C_{p0e}. Thus

$$K_m = \frac{200}{\ln(2,701,271/200)} = 21\,\mu g\,ml^{-1}$$

and

$$V_{max} = 0.0486 \times 21 = 1.0\,\mu g\,min^{-1}$$

Alternative equations for the calculation of K_m and V_{max} require calculation of the rate of change of concentration from one sample to the next ($\Delta C_p/\Delta t$) as well as the plasma concentration at the midpoint (C_{pm}).

Table 4.8
Pharmacokinetic parameters derived from data showing saturation kinetics: Figure 4.13

Parameter	Curve 1	Curve 2	Curve 3	Curve 4	Curve 5
Dose (mg/kg)	5	10	40	100	200
C_{p0} ($\mu g\ ml^{-1}$)	5	10	40	100	200
k (min^{-1})[a]	0.0486	0.0486	0.0486	0.0485	0.0486
Half-life (min)[a]	14.3	14.3	14.3	14.3	14.3
AUC ($\mu g\ ml^{-1}\ min$)[b]	115	254	1614	7020	24,027
AUMC ($\mu g\ ml^{-1}\ min^2$)[b]	2437	5702	50,682	355,788	2,002,493
CL ($ml\ min^{-1}\ kg^{-1}$)[c]	43.5	39.4	24.8	14.2	8.3
MRT (min)[d]	21.2	22.4	31.4	50.7	83.3

The parameters were calculated assuming a one-compartment model with a volume of distribution of 1 L/kg, which is not dose-dependent.
[a] Derived from data between 2.0 and 0.1 μg/ml for each dose.
[b] Calculated by the trapezoid rule with extrapolation to infinity. (See Table 4.17 for a worked example.)
[c] CL = dose/AUC [Eq. (22)].
[d] MRT = AUMC/AUC [Eq. (48)].

Lineweaver–Burk plot

$$\frac{1}{\Delta C_p/\Delta t} = \frac{K_m}{V_{max} \times C_{pm}} + \frac{1}{V_{max}}$$

Therefore a plot of $1/(\Delta C_p/\Delta t)$ against $1/C_{pm}$ has a slope of K_m/V_{max} and an intercept of $1/V_{max}$.

Hanes–Woolf plot

$$\frac{C_{pm}}{\Delta C_p/\Delta t} = \frac{K_m}{V_{max}} + \frac{C_{pm}}{V_{max}}$$

Therefore a plot of $C_{pm}/(\Delta C_p/\Delta t)$ against C_{pm} has a slope of $1/V_{max}$ and an intercept of K_m/V_{max}.

Woolf–Augustinsson–Hofstee plot

$$\frac{\Delta C_p}{\Delta t} = V_{max} - \frac{(\Delta C_p/\Delta t)K_m}{C_{pm}}$$

Therefore a plot of $(\Delta C_p/\Delta t)$ against $(\Delta C_p/\Delta t)/C_{pm}$ has a slope of $-K_m$ and an intercept of V_{max}.

When the data for the highest dose in Figure 4.13 are analyzed by these techniques (Table 4.9) the following values are obtained (Figure 4.14):

Lineweaver–Burk plot

$$x\text{-intercept} = -\frac{1}{K_m} = -0.0537; \qquad K_m = 18.6\,\mu\text{g ml}^{-1}$$

$$y\text{-intercept} = \frac{1}{V_{max}} = 1.04; \qquad V_{max} = 0.96\,\mu\text{g min}^{-1}$$

$$\text{Slope} = \frac{V_{max}}{K_m} = 0.0517; \qquad \frac{0.96}{18.6} = 0.0516$$

Hanes–Woolf plot

$$\text{Slope} = \frac{1}{V_{max}} = 0.999; \qquad V_{max} = 1.001\,\mu\text{g min}^{-1}$$

$$\text{Intercept} = \frac{K_m}{V_{max}} = 19.85; \qquad K_m = 19.9\,\mu\text{g ml}^{-1}$$

Woolf–Augustinsson–Hofstee plot

$$\text{Slope} = -K_m = -20.3; \qquad K_m = 20.3\,\mu\text{g ml}^{-1}$$

$$\text{Intercept} = V_{max} = 1.005; \qquad V_{max} = 1.005\,\mu\text{g min}^{-1}$$

The values of V_{max} and K_m may be derived from plateau levels on intravenous infusion, providing that elimination is essentially by a saturable process only, because at

Table 4.9
Calculation of K_m and V_{max} from plasma concentration time data

Time[a]	C_p^a	$\Delta C_p/\Delta t^b$	C_{pm}^c	$1/(\Delta C_p/\Delta t)$	$1/C_{pm}$	$C_{pm}/(\Delta C_p/\Delta t)$	$(\Delta C_p/\Delta t)/C_{pm}$
0	200	0.905	188	1.10	0.0053	207.7	0.0048
22.1	180	0.893	168	1.12	0.0060	188.1	0.0053
44.5	160	0.885	147	1.13	0.0068	166.1	0.0060
67.1	140	0.865	127	1.16	0.0079	146.8	0.0068
90.2	120	0.844	107	1.18	0.0093	126.8	0.0079
113.9	100	0.820	87	1.22	0.0115	106.1	0.0094
138.3	80	0.775	68	1.29	0.0147	87.7	0.0114
164.1	60	0.712	49	1.40	0.0204	68.8	0.0145
192.2	40	0.637	34.2	1.57	0.0292	53.7	0.0186
207.9	30	0.549	24.5	1.82	0.0408	44.6	0.0224
226.1	20	0.467	17.7	2.14	0.0565	37.9	0.0264
236.8	15	0.382	12.5	2.62	0.0800	32.7	0.0306
249.9	10	0.265	7.3	3.77	0.1370	27.5	0.0363
268.8	5	0.141	3.3	7.09	0.3030	23.4	0.0427
290.1	2	0.067	1.4	14.93	0.7140	20.9	0.0479
305.0	1	0.035	0.70	28.57	1.4286	20.0	0.0500
319.3	0.5	0.012	0.225	83.33	4.44	18.8	0.0530
351.9	0.1						

[a] Raw data.
[b] Calculated as 200 − 180/22.1 − 0 = 0.905, etc.
[c] Read off the concentration time curve at midpoint of interval.

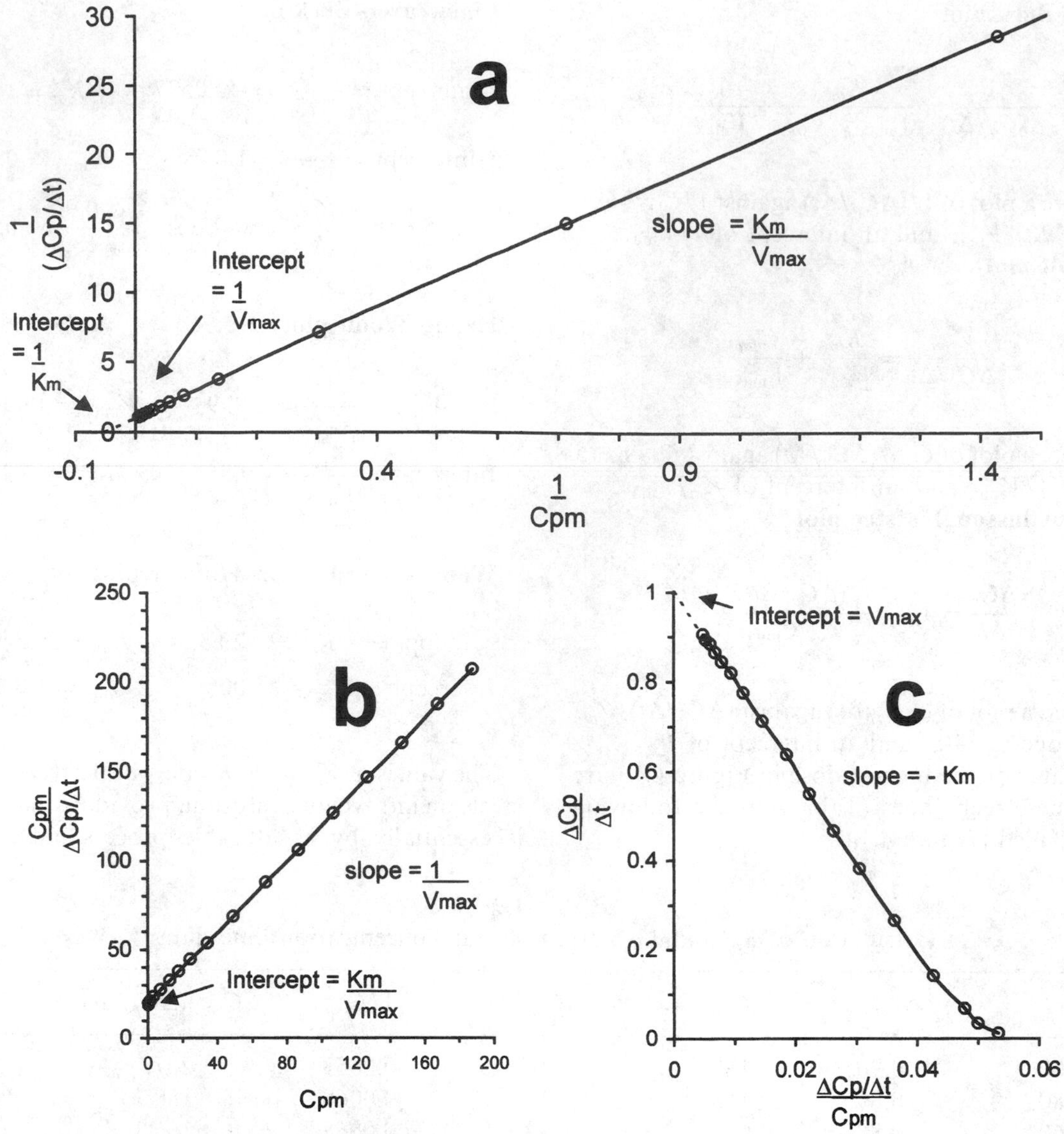

FIG. 4.14. Analysis of the maximum dose given in Figure 4.13 to derive K_m and V_{max} using the data in Table 4.9 and the methods of (a) Lineweaver–Burk, (b) Hanes–Woolf, and (c) Woolf–Augustinssohn–Hofstee.

steady state the rate of input = rate of elimination:

$$R = \frac{V_{\max} \times C_{pss}}{K_m + C_{pss}}$$

where R is the rate of infusion, or

$$R = V_{\max} - \left(K_m \times \frac{R}{C_{pss}} \right)$$

Thus a plot of R for different rates of infusion against R/C_{pss} gives a straight line with a slope of K_m and an intercept of $V_{\max}$ on the R axis.

Frequently, the rate of elimination can be described by a combination of saturable and nonsaturable processes when

$$-\frac{dC}{dt} = \frac{V_{\max} \times C}{(K_m + C)} + k'C$$

where k' is the rate constant for the nonsaturable process: k' may be replaced by CL'/V where CL' is the clearance by the nonsaturable process; for example for glomerular filtration the value $(GFR \times \alpha / V)$ may be substituted for k'.

Of greatest importance for toxicology is the clear demonstration of saturation at high doses, an estimation of the plasma concentration above which first-order kinetics cease to apply, and the plasma concentrations present in animals showing overt toxicity. Wagner (112) proposed five tests for the establishment of saturation or nonlinear kinetics.

1. Graphs of C_p/dose against time should be superimposable for linear kinetics at different doses. Although considerable scatter is seen, an overall trend to increased or decreased levels at higher doses should be apparent for nonlinear systems.
2. Administer different intravenous doses and estimate C_{p0} by fitting only the first two or three early time points to the equation $\ln C_p = \ln C_{p0} - kt$. Graphs of C_p/C_{p0} against time should be superimposable if linear kinetics apply.
3. Fit each set of concentration–time data to a linear model and derive the appropriate kinetic parameters (CL, V, k, k_{12}, k_{21}, V_1, etc.). A dose-dependent change in a parameter indicates nonlinearity or saturation kinetics (which will invalidate some of the derived parameters, e.g., k).
4. If Michaelis–Menten kinetics apply, the percentage metabolized by that pathway decreases with an increase in dose (provided other elimination routes are available), the value of AUC/dose is not constant, and plots of log C_p or ln C_p against time curve downward, as shown in Figure 4.13.
5. Measure the tissue and unbound plasma concentrations over a range of doses. A graph of tissue concentration against unbound concentration in plasma should be a straight line for a linear tissue extraction. Saturation of tissue binding is shown by the tissue concentration having a smaller increase at higher concentrations.

A consequence of nonlinear kinetics is that the time to reach steady state is also dose dependent. In simple terms, this is because the "effective half-life," which can be calculated by 0.693×MRT, increases with an increase in dose (e.g., Table 4.8) so that the time to steady state (four to five half-lives) must also increase. This situation should be borne in mind when planning short term studies. The importance of nonlinear kinetics in toxicology is discussed in greater detail after Data Handling.

PRACTICAL METHODS

General information on techniques may be obtained from the texts by Waynforth (114) and Cocchetto and Bjornsson (20). Waynforth described practical methods ranging from how to hold the animal for injection to such specialist techniques as renal transplantation. The other work, which contains 501 references, is an extensive and invaluable literature review of methods for the collection of body fluids. A number of modifications applicable to other species are given below.

The methods for dosing, blood sampling, urine collection, etc., described below are largely related to the rat, as it is the species most commonly used in toxicological studies.

Administration Techniques

Oral Dosing

Because a number of lipid and metabolic barriers separate the lumen of the gastrointestinal tract from the systemic circulation (Figure 4.2), the plasma levels of test compounds usually increase gradually after oral administration to reach a maximum. Therefore it is possible to give higher doses by this route than by intravenous injection, and this technique is aided by the capacity of the stomach to hold a large volume of liquid. For toxicokinetic studies, the oral route can provide valuable information on elimination and clearance values, provided that the extent of absorption of the parent compound (F) is known. The latter may be determined by measuring either the area under the plasma concentration–time curve or the total amount of the test substance excreted in the urine unchanged after both oral and intravenous administration at low doses. The fraction absorbed is given by Eq. (31), and this value can then be used to calculate the clearance as described in the derivative of Eq. (22). The possibility of saturation of absorption may be determined by plotting the value C_p/dose against time for doses up to and including those producing overt toxicity.

Rats, guinea pigs, and mice may be dosed orally using a syringe fitted with a suitable intubation needle; in rabbits, a polyethylene cannula is passed into the stomach while the jaws are held open by a gag. Certain precautions should be taken to prevent artifacts. For example, it is important that the test chemical is completely dissolved, because if the chemical is given as a suspension, the apparent absorption rate must include a component due to dissolution of the chemical. If this factor is rate limiting, the measured absorption rate reflects the dissolution rate and is not related to the biological availability of the chemical. The ideal vehicle for dissolution is water or a small volume of a water-miscible solvent such as ethanol, propylene glycol (propane-1,2-diol), or dimethylsulfoxide, although for very lipid-soluble compounds, it may be necessary to give the dose in corn oil or as an emulsion. Excess acids or bases should not be used to dissolve the test compound, and the pH of the dose solution should be near pH 7, because pH partitioning in either the gut or the renal tubule could be affected, which could alter the measured absorption or elimination rate constants. If a water-miscible organic solvent is used to dissolve the chemical, water should be added to reduce the dehydrating effect of the solvent within the gut lumen. The volume of water or solvent/water used to dissolve the chemical should be kept low, because excess quantities may distend the stomach and cause rapid gastric emptying. In addition, large volumes of water may carry the chemical through membrane pores and increase the absorption rate. If dose-dependent absorption is suspected, the different doses should be given in the same volume of solution. The maximum volume of aqueous solution that can be administered without the possibility of gross interference with absorption is approximately 5–10 ml/kg. Larger volumes may be given, although nonlinear kinetics seen under such circumstances may be due to solvent-induced alteration of intestinal function.

The use of water-immiscible solvents such as corn oil, which are sometimes used for gavage doses, should be avoided if possible, because mobilization from the vehicle may be rate limiting. However, such a vehicle would obviously be appropriate if it was the method of administration used in toxicity studies, because it would give information on the rate of absorption and bioavailability under the conditions of the toxicity study.

The rate of absorption can have a major effect on the toxicokinetic profile, affecting not only the time to maximum concentration and the maximum concentration but also the total amount entering the systemic circulation by saturating hepatic uptake and first-pass metabolism. The hepatotoxicity of oral carbon tetrachloride is markedly higher after a bolus dose compared with gastric infusion (89).

When toxicity studies are performed by mixing the compound into the animals' diet, it is important to measure the concentration–time curve over a 24-h period at steady state, because both the peak concentration and the AUC may be different from data obtained from bolus gavage studies.

Nasal Administration

Methods have been described for assessing absorption from the nasal cavity based on plasma pharmacokinetics following intranasal and intravenous dosing and by in situ perfusion experiments (45,103). A technique for inhalation with nose-only exposure has been described for studies in guinea pigs (52).

Rectal Administration

Because a number of therapeutic compounds are given in the form of suppositories, an indication of the bioavailability after rectal administration is sometimes required. Normally, toxicity studies and initial drug formulations of such compounds are performed by the oral route, and the rectal formulation comes late in development and marketing. Animal bioavailability studies late in drug development are of limited value because of the differences between laboratory animals and man in intestinal anatomy and microflora of the colon and rectum. However, in cases where an indication of rectal bioavailability is required, the compound may be introduced into the rectum of the rat using an oral dosing needle to prevent tissue damage. To avoid rapid excretion of the unabsorbed dose, anesthetized animals are used and the dose is retained with an inert plug or bung.

Inhalation

As indicated previously, a major problem associated with determining the kinetics of inhalation concerns the measurement of the extent to which the chemical is absorbed across the lung, rather than passed back into the mouth to be swallowed, exhaled in the expired air, or absorbed across the skin. Comparison of the plasma AUC or the total urinary excretion of unchanged compound, after a period of inhalation with the same parameter after a known intravenous dose, can be used to determine the total dose, entering via the lungs plus gut.

A method used successfully by McKenna et al. (59) to obtain kinetic data involved a 6-h exposure to the vapor of [^{14}C]vinylidene chloride in rats, after which the animals were transferred to a metabolism cage. The body load at the time of removal was determined by the total recovery of radioactivity in the expired air, excreta, cage washings, and carcass. This method is appropriate for determining the total dose because the nonspecific measurement of ^{14}C includes parent compound and all metabolites. If the parent compound alone is measured, the inhalation data must be compared to intravenous data in order to measure the extent of exposure after inhalation. The approach of McKenna et al. (59) was capable of revealing differences between fasted and fed animals in their capacity to metabolize vinylidene chloride, which correlated well with the toxicity of this compound. The absorption of most compounds given by inhalation is rapid, although certain compounds, for example the highly polar antiasthmatic drug sodium cromoglycate, may show a measurable first-order absorption across the lungs. It should be remembered that the observed absorption rate after instillation of a micronized powder into the trachea may be that of the formulation, not of the chemical moiety itself.

The metabolism rate constants of inhaled 1,l-dichloroethylene were determined by measurement of the rate of removal of the compound from circulating air in a closed chamber system containing the experimental animal (1). The air was recirculated, with oxygen added to maintain the concentration at 19–21%, and the air was sampled at regular intervals and analyzed for unabsorbed 1,l-dichloroethylene by gas–liquid chromatography. The rate of removal showed two phases: (i) a rapid phase proportional to the mass of the animal and the concentration of chemical, (ii) and a slow phase, which represented metabolism of the compound. The slow phase showed saturation (Michaelis–Menten) kinetics, and rate constants (K_m and V_{max}) were derived in terms of the concentration of chemical in the chamber. This approach is interesting as the data are obtained by a noninvasive method. Also, the kinetic constants are derived in terms of vapor or gas concentrations, which are most appropriate when interpreting inhalation studies in relation to human exposure to volatile agents.

Percutaneous Absorption

The percutaneous route is likely to be of increasing importance in drug formulation in the future. Animals may be used as suitable models; however, there may be major species differences related to the presence of hair follicles and the barrier function of the stratum corneum. An added pharmacokinetic advantage to this route is that the fraction absorbed may be measured as described above for the oral route (i.e., AUC data) and also by analysis of the amount remaining at the site of administration. The dermal absorption of vapors can be assessed in rats using a body-only chamber (58). Shaving the hair from the backs of rats can provide a suitable site for in vivo absorption studies (47), although in vitro data provide a suitable model for extrapolation to humans.

Intravenous Injection

The bolus intravenous dose is the most important single technique for deriving information concerning the kinetics of the distribution and elimination of chemicals. As with oral administration, aqueous or aqueous miscible solvents should be used, although the maximum dosage volume is considerably lower, that is, about 2 ml/kg for aqueous and 1 ml/kg for solvent–aqueous mixtures. Ideally, the solution is made isotonic by the addition of sodium chloride, although in practice dissolution of low doses in isotonic saline is adequate.

There are two important parameters to be considered in such studies. First, the data processing assumes that the material was administered instantaneously at time zero. In practice, a rapid injection may produce considerable toxicity, which a slower injection can prevent. Generally, a "bolus" dose, given over a finite period of up to a few minutes, is regarded as instantaneous provided that the total injection time does not represent more than about 5% of the half-life of the most rapid phase of the plasma concentration–time curve. The other parameter to be considered is the true location of the dose, because in kinetic studies it is important that 100% of the dose is intravenous and none ends up in a perivascular site. The following techniques have proved successful.

Rat. The tail and hind paw veins are convenient for dosing but neither is particularly easy to use or gives 100% intravascular dosing repeatedly and routinely without the necessary expertise. The following technique, although more complex, is preferable because it overcomes the problems experienced with the above routes, and the cannula can be used subsequently for sample collection. The animal is anesthetized with ether, and an incision is made through the skin of the neck to the right of the midline. Blunt dissection is used to separate the thin layer of muscle covering the external jugular vein, which is exposed and cleaned. Thread is passed under the vein at both anterior and posterior ends of the exposed section but is not tied off posteriorly. A small incision is made in the vein, and a length of polyethylene cannula tubing, connected to the dosing syringe, is passed into the vein toward the heart for a distance of about 2 cm. The dose solution is injected and the cannula rinsed with isotonic saline. The tubing may then be removed and the vein tied off, or the cannula tubing can be tied in situ for subsequent sampling, providing that the compound is not adsorbed to the cannula (see below). In anesthetized rats, which will not regain consciousness during the study, an alternative site of injection is the femoral vein, which may be exposed by an incision into the ventral surface of the top of the hind leg.

Guinea pig. A modification of the external jugular method described above may be used for the guinea pig. The external jugular vein of an anesthetized animal is exposed but not cleaned of connective tissue. The dose is injected directly using a fine needle (0.5-mm gauge) bent inward through about 45°, which allows the needle to be positioned without undue stretching or movement of the vein. The vein is clamped, above and below the injection site, as the needle is withdrawn. The vein is subsequently ligated and the incision sutured.

Rabbit. It is relatively easy to administer intravenous doses to rabbits, because the vein running around the periphery of the ear lobe can be readily exposed by shaving with a scalpel blade. This vein is of sufficient size and visibility to give reliable intravenous dosing.

Intravenous Infusion

For intravenous infusion studies, the dose must be given via an indwelling cannula, and the external jugular vein is a suitable site in rats. If the infusion period is prolonged, such that recovery from anesthesia is envisaged, the cannula can be run under the skin from the ventral surface of the neck and exteriorized on the dorsal surface behind the ears. If the cannula is then secured on the dorsal surface, the animal is prevented from damaging it during infusion while being permitted a degree of restricted movement. This method of exteriorization is also valuable as a method of long-term sampling (see below).

The delivery of compound during intravenous infusion must be at a constant but low rate such that the animal is not subjected to excessive hemodilution. To date, the standard method has been to use a high-quality infusion pump. The development of osmotically driven minipumps (Alzet), which can be implanted into the animal and deliver a constant rate as low as 0.5 μl/h for up to 2 weeks, opened up exciting possibilities. Minipumps allow investigations of steady-state plasma and tissue concentrations associated with toxicity, and the pharmacokinetics under similar steady-state conditions. Such devices have been used to study the renal clearance of ^{63}Ni under steady-state conditions; interestingly, these studies revealed diurnal fluctuations in the steady-state levels, probably due to metabolic changes that were not suspected from earlier studies (94).

Sampling Techniques

Blood (Plasma and Serum)

When considering the frequency, timing, and duration of blood sampling, it is important that an adequate number of samples are taken to define each section of the plasma concentration–time curve (Figure 4.6). It has been suggested that plasma samples be collected during the first four to five half-lives, during which time 93–97% of the compound will have been eliminated (119). However, it is possible that such a restriction may mask a quantitatively minor distribution component, for example a third compartment, capable of significant accumulation on continuous ingestion as part of a toxicity test. Such a compartment could be perfusion- or diffusion-limited distribution to a tissue in which the tissue affinity was high. If such a tissue was the site of toxicity on chronic administration, a single-dose kinetic investigation restricted to four half-lives would have failed to throw any light on the process involved. However, autoradiography following a radiolabeled dose may reveal such a selective distribution; but it must be remembered that this method cannot differentiate between parent compound and metabolites. Thus, as a general guideline, the plasma concentrations should be measured until the limit of detection of the analytical method is reached. Obviously, if the limit of detection allows analysis over a large number of half-lives, less frequent sampling is required during the slow terminal phase, which can be defined adequately by about four samples. Thus a three-compartment system can be accurately analyzed by about 12 samples provided that they are correctly timed. The corollary to this situation is that a relatively insensitive analytical method is incapable of yielding full pharmacokinetic data. Considering the data in Figure 4.6, if the limit of detection for compounds A and B were 0.1 μg/ml, both would appear to be represented adequately by a one-compartment model, with different values of k. Indeed, under these circumstances the plasma concentration of both A and B would fall from 2.85 to 0.10, a decrease of 97%, equivalent to about five half-lives.

Using the methods described below, it is possible to withdraw a significant fraction of the total blood volume (64 ml/kg in the rat), thereby modifying the perfusion of the organs of elimination and corrupting the derived pharmacokinetic data. This problem can be avoided by taking the smallest samples consistent with accurate analysis and the minimum number of samples necessary to define adequately the various phases (i.e., smaller samples at early time points). As a general rule, individual blood samples should be restricted to a maximum of about 0.5 ml/kg body weight, providing the total number of samples is small (i.e., less than 10). This general rule takes no account of the duration of the experiment, which may indicate either smaller or larger sample sizes.

Rat. Various methods have been used successfully to obtain small serial blood samples from anesthetized and conscious rats.

Tail vein. Whole-blood samples (approximately 70 μl) are obtained on cutting the tail vein with a scalpel blade and collecting the blood into heparinized capillary tubes. This method is widely used and was employed by Sauerhoff et al. (90) in their study of the dose-dependent kinetics of 2,4,5-trichlorophenoxyacetic acid. Care must be taken to wash the tail to avoid contamination of late blood samples by the much higher concentrations present in urine and feces. Washing the tail vein with warm water will often remove the blood clot and reinstigate blood flow.

Toe vasculature. Blood samples (up to 500 μl) may be collected by clipping the toenail into the vascular bed and allowing the blood to run into heparinized capillary tubes (41), but this would be more stressful for the animal than the use of the tail vein.

Cardiac puncture. Multiple cardiac sampling is possible but involves more trauma than the above methods, and anesthesia (ether) is essential. However, provided that a fine (0.5-mm) needle is used, it is possible, with practice, to obtain a number of samples without evidence of extravascular blood loss, although this technique is also more stressful than a simple incision into the tail vein.

Orbital sinus. The animal is anesthetized with ether and held down by gentle pressure with thumb and forefinger behind the head. A heparinized capillary tube is inserted into the orbit at the anterior apex and moved to rupture the sinus membrane in the anterior dorsal region at the back of the orbit. A considerable blood flow is obtained, which stops on removal of the tube and the pressure at the back of the neck.

External jugular vein. Methods have been described in which silicon medical grade cannula tubing (Silastic; 0.05 cm i.d., 0.09 cm o.d.) implanted in the external jugular vein has remained patent for blood sampling for periods up to 2 months (109). The use of silicon tubing is preferred to polyethylene for such long-term studies because it is more flexible for exteriorization on the dorsal surface and less apt to cause thrombosis.

The tubing is inserted into the vein by either of two methods. First, a suitable size syringe needle shaft is attached, which is passed into the vein and then pushed back out again about 5 mm lower down. The needle shaft is then removed, and the cannula tubing is gently pulled back until it reenters the vein. Alternatively, the end of the cannula is made into a point by a steep diagonal cut and inserted via a small incision in the vein. A shallow diagonal cut (i.e., almost parallel with the longitudinal axis of the tubing) aids insertion but is more prone to obstruction by the vein wall during sampling. Careful positioning of the end of the cannula tubing by gentle maneuvering may be necessary to achieve optimal sampling, which usually involves passing the cannula toward the heart for a distance of about 2 cm. A similar technique has been described (4) in which the cannula is then exteriorized and secured behind the head of the animal. However, under such circumstances a collar may be necessary to prevent the animal damaging the tubing (20).

Common carotid artery. In anesthetized animals in which the external jugular vein is used for infusion, the ipsilateral carotid artery can be used for sampling. The artery lies deep below the sternohyoid muscle and may be reached using blunt dissection. The artery is a robust structure and can be brought to the surface by curved forceps. Cotton ties are placed anterior (×1) and posterior (×2) to the intended site of incision and tied loosely. The artery is then placed under tension by artery forceps attached to the anterior tie and to the posterior tie nearer the heart so as to prevent blood loss during incision. A small incision is made in the artery, and a length of cannula tubing, attached to a saline-filled syringe, is inserted and passed toward the heart, through the first posterior tie. It is tied firmly, and the tension on the second posterior tie is released. The cannula can now be slid through the second posterior tie, which is then tied securely. The anterior tie is now tightened and the artery forceps removed. Blood may be sampled by removing the syringe when the blood pressure is sufficient to expel the saline. The sampling is stopped by clamping the tubing, replacing the syringe, and passing saline back up the tubing. It is important to keep the artery under tension during insertion of the cannula, or significant blood loss may occur. An alternative method of applying tension is to insert a pair of forceps underneath the artery and allow them to open and stretch the artery.

Other species. For experiments performed under anesthesia, a major vein or artery (e.g., jugular, carotid, femoral) can be cannulated. For multiple sampling under temporary ether anesthesia, cardiac puncture has been used successfully for guinea pigs. On the other hand, the orbital sinus is a more appropriate site for the mouse, and the marginal ear vein can be used for the rabbit without anesthesia.

Urine

A knowledge of the urinary excretion rate is necessary for calculating the overall renal clearance of a compound. The bladder causes variable slowing of the output; for compounds with a short half-life, a method of overcoming sporadic urination is necessary. Calculating results by the sigma-minus method, rather than using excretion rate data, reduces the importance of incomplete bladder emptying and the resultant scatter in the data. For compounds with a half-life of many hours, sufficiently frequent samples may be obtained merely by placing the animals in a metabolism cage, which gives adequate separation of urine and feces, and by encouraging reflex urination (20).

Under anesthesia, the effect of the bladder may be overcome by (a) inserting and tying a cannula into the bladder via the urethra or directly across the bladder wall, and emptying and rinsing the bladder with isotonic saline using a syringe; (b) inserting a cannula via the urethra and allowing the urine to be expelled naturally or with the aid of gentle massage (11); or (c) cannulation of both ureters and collection of the urine without it passing through the bladder (77). The third technique was used by the author to analyze the extent of reabsorption of saccharin from the rat urinary bladder, but was found to be technically difficult, because both ureters had to be cannulated with polyethylene tubing stretched to give a suitable taper, and even slight twisting of the ureter effectively blocked the urine flow. This technique is not recommended for routine investigations. However, these studies did reveal that although the intact urinary bladder was relatively impermeable to saccharin (which is highly ionic), manipulation of the bladder with forceps produced a slight increase in permeability, and bladder cannulation (as described above) produced a marked increase in permeability and reabsorption. Thus any damage or irritation caused by the cannula should be kept to a minimum; if a cannula is inserted across the wall into the apex of the bladder, it is essential that the contents be removed and rinsed at frequent intervals, that is, at least every 15 min. Similarly, any palpation used in method (b) above, should not be excessive, or increased reabsorption from the bladder may occur and cause a decreased apparent renal clearance. In addition, cannulae passed via the urethra, which is particularly suitable for female animals, should be positioned carefully such that they do not enter too far into the bladder lumen and damage the epithelium.

Renal clearance studies may be performed either after single doses or during infusion at steady state (when the clearance can be related to total clearance and plasma concentration). Insights into the extent of reabsorption and tubular secretion can be obtained by measuring the renal clearance of inulin given simultaneously (1–20 μCi of [^{14}C]inulin/kg or 50–100 μCi of [^{3}H]inulin/kg).

Bile

Bile may be collected from a cannula inserted into the common bile duct such that the tip is located at the point of bifurcation near the hilar region of the liver. The common bile duct is found by making an incision through the midline into the anterior part of the body cavity. Slight tension on the proximal part of the duodenum reveals the bile duct running through the pancreatic tissue. The bile duct is cleaned, a thread is placed loosely around it, and cannula tubing is inserted via a small incision and tied in place. Bile flow is usually 0.5-1.0 ml/h in the rat. Bile may be collected by either placing the animal in a restraining cage and collecting from the exteriorized cannula or passing the tubing into a suitable container (sealed plastic sachet) placed subcutaneously. The test chemical is usually given soon after establishing the cannula, because changes in bile composition occur if the bile salts are not allowed to recirculate. A modified technique avoiding the use of animals still under the stress of surgery has been demonstrated by Light et al. (55). With this technique, the bile cannula was exteriorized and joined to a second cannula, which passed back into the body cavity and entered the duodenum via the greater curvature of the stomach. The animals were then left for 4 days, after which constant feed intake and body weight were observed. This method could be useful for studies with chronic dietary intake of the chemical; however, chronic intake for more than 4 days might be necessary after surgery in order to reestablish steady-state intake via the diet, which may be different from that of normal animals.

In animal species that possess a gallbladder (i.e., guinea pig and rabbit), it is necessary to prevent this organ from delaying elimination by ligation around its base so that bile has to pass directly down the cannula.

DATA HANDLING

The type of information that can be obtained from kinetic studies, and its derivation from raw plasma, and urine data are illustrated by results obtained by the author and colleagues. Saccharin is a nonnutritive sweetener which causes an increased incidence of tumors of the urinary bladder in male rats when fed at high dietary concentrations (more than 3%) for two generations (88) or from birth (93). The possibility of nonlinear kinetics at such high doses was investigated using the Charles River CD-derived rat, the same strain used in the cancer bioassays. The study, which has been published elsewhere (105), investigated the concentrations of saccharin in the tissues of animals fed saccharin-containing diets and used the techniques outlined above to investigate details of the disposition of this compound. Previous studies using [^{14}C]saccharin had shown that it was incompletely absorbed from the gut, and eliminated in the urine and feces without undergoing detectable metabolism (73).

On feeding rats with saccharin-containing diets ad libitum for a period of 22 days, significant nonlinearity was apparent in the concentrations of saccharin in the plasma and tissues, with elevated concentrations at high dietary levels (Figure 4.15). The following studies were

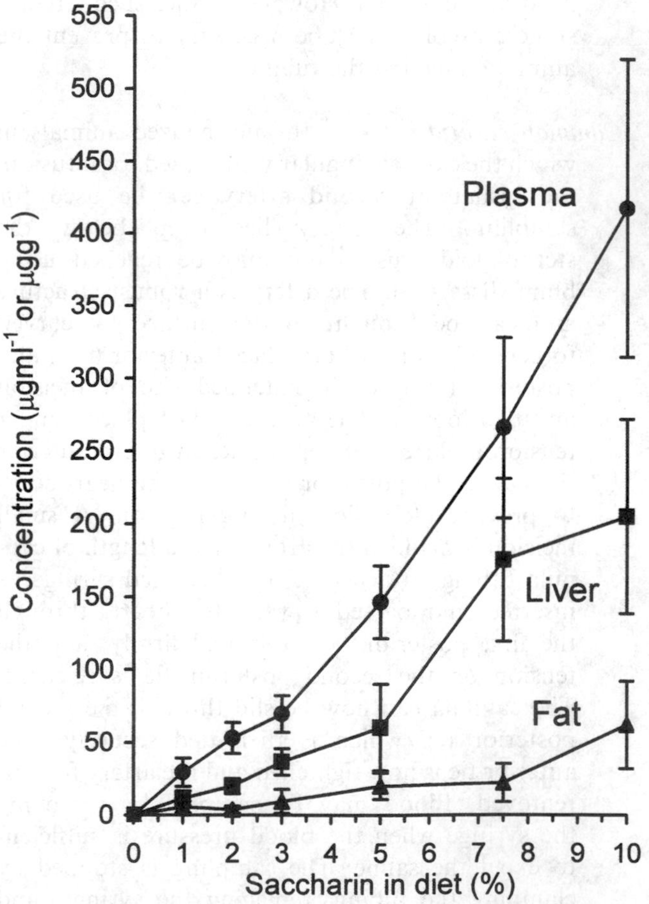

FIG. 4.15. Concentrations of saccharin in the plasma and tissues of rats given saccharin-containing diets. Adult male rats were given saccharin-containing diets ad libitum for 22 days prior to killing at 6 AM. The results are the means with standard deviations represented by vertical bars. From Reference 105.

Table 4.10
Concentrations of saccharin in the plasma and urine of a rat given a single intravenous bolus dose[a]

Plasma		Urine	
Time of sample (min)	Concentration ($\mu g\ ml^{-1}$)	Collection period (min)	Amount excreted (μg)
5	184.3	0–5	7518
15	102.0	5–15	6275
30	50.5	15–30	4989
45	24.9	30–45	2580
60	14.1	45–60	1485
75	8.0	60–75	861
90	5.7	75–90	561
105	4.0	90–105	363
120	2.9	105–120	300

[a] The animal (body weight 570 g) was given a single IV bolus dose of saccharin (50 mg/kg) at time 0.

performed in an attempt to investigate the cause of this phenomenon.

Intravenous Bolus Dose: Plasma Analysis

Saccharin is a strong organic acid (pK_a about 2) that forms a highly water-soluble sodium salt. 5-[^{3}H]Saccharin was used in these studies, and the concentrations in plasma and urine samples were determined by measuring the total radioactivity present (*because saccharin does not undergo metabolism*). A range of doses of saccharin were given (1–1000 mg/kg as a single intravenous bolus over a period of 30 s) to anesthetized male rats via a cannula inserted into the jugular vein. The dead volume in the cannula was displaced with saline. Plasma samples were subsequently withdrawn from the same cannula, because saccharin showed no tendency to adhere to the polyethylene tubing used. The bladder was cannulated, emptied, and rinsed at each plasma collection period. The results for an individual animal given 50 mg/kg are presented in Table 4.10.

A graph of plasma concentration against time (Figure 4.16) clearly shows a biphasic decrease, which may be analyzed graphically using the method of residuals as shown in Table 4.11. Alternatively, the β phase can be analyzed by linear regression analysis to yield the extrapolated values, which can then be analyzed by linear regression to give the values of A, B, α, and β as shown in Table 4.11. The data selected for this discussion were for an individual animal that showed a prolonged $\alpha+\beta$ phase. This choice was necessary, as information on the initial $\alpha+\beta$ phase is decreased when urine data are analyzed. For other animals, the $\alpha+\beta$ phase was apparent only during the first 30 min, and linearity occurred between 30–45 and 120 min, so that the corresponding urine data could not be studied adequately by the methods used in Tables 4.13 and 4.14 (see below). Thus, in the animal selected, the data are actually deficient in that the β phase is dependent on only four

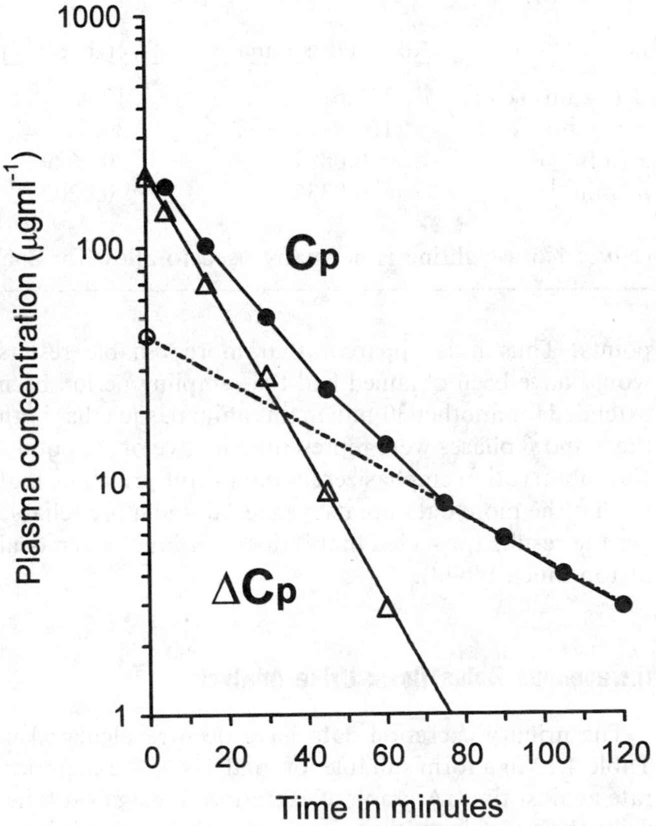

FIG. 4.16. Plasma concentration–time curve after a bolus of saccharin (50 mg/kg IV) into a male rat. The data used are given in Tables 4.10 and 4.11.

Table 4.11
Analysis of plasma data shown in Figure 4.16

Graphical Analysis	Linear regression analysis
75–120 min	
$\beta = \frac{(\log 8.0 - \log 2.9)}{120 - 75} \times 2.303 = 0.0226\ \text{min.}^{-1}$	$\beta = 0.0226\ \text{min}^{-1}$
$B = 42\ \mu g\ ml^{-1}$	$B = 43.7\ \mu g\ ml^{-1}$

Residuals

Time (min)	*Conc. ($\mu g\ ml^{-1}$)*	*Time (min)*	*Conc. ($\mu g\ ml^{-1}$)*
5	184.3 − 37.5 = 146.8	5	184.3 − 39.0 = 145.3
15	102.0 − 30.0 = 72.0	15	102.0 − 31.1 = 70.9
30	50.5 − 21.6 = 28.9	30	50.5 − 22.1 = 28.4
45	24.9 − 15.5 = 9.4	45	24.9 − 15.8 = 9.1
60	14.1 − 11.1 = 3.0	60	14.1 − 11.2 = 2.9

5–45 min (residuals)

Graphical Analysis	Linear regression analysis
$\alpha = \frac{(\log 198 - \log 9.4)}{45 - 0} \times 2.303 = 0.0677\ \text{min}^{-1}$	$\alpha = 0.0683\ \text{min}^{-1}$
$A = 198\ \mu g\ ml^{-1}$	$A = 204.5\ \mu g\ ml^{-1}$

Analysis using WinNonlin

	All weights equal	Weighted $1/y$	Weighted $1/y^2$
A ($\mu g\ ml^{-1}$)	148.6	212.4	218.4
B ($\mu g\ ml^{-1}$)	104.9	30.3	19.2
α (min^{-1})	0.0887	0.0629	0.0585
β (min^{-1})	0.0335	0.0202	0.0162

(*Note*: $1/y$ weighting is normally used to allow for analytical errors of $\pm x\%$.)

points. Thus it is apparent that more reliable results would have been obtained had the sampling period been extended for another 30 min in this animal, such that both the α and β phases were represented by five or six points. This observation emphasizes an important principle, that is, that the more data points measured, the more reliable are the results (provided that it does not involve removal of too much blood).

Intravenous Bolus Dose: Urine Analysis

The urinary excretion data have been recalculated in Table 4.12 in a form suitable for analysis of the excretion rate against time. A graph of excretion rate against time, using the midpoint of the sample collection period (Figure 4.17 and Table 4.13), shows a biphasic decrease similar to that seen in plasma. Because of the scatter in the points of the terminal β phase, it is not clear whether the 52.5-min point should be included in the β or the $\alpha+\beta$ phase. However, from the plasma curve (Figure 4.16), it seems that the β phase started after 60 min, and thus the 52.5-min point was not included in the analysis of β. The residuals line (Figure 4.17) was analyzed with the omission of the 2.5-min point, because this value did not fit the line clearly shown by other points (possibly due to high initial renal elimination prior to mixing of the compound within the central compartment). The constants α and β may be derived from the excretion rate or using the sigma-minus method, which is described by Eq. (28). The total amount finally excreted (Table 4.12) is obtained by extrapolation of the cumulative total (column 5, Table 4.12) to infinity, which may be done either graphically or from the excretion rate data, as shown in Table 4.12. The amount remaining to be excreted (ΔA_{ex}) is calculated by subtracting the running total from the final total for each time point (column 6, Table 4.12). A graph of ΔA_{ex} against time (Figure 4.18)

Table 4.12
Urinary excretion of saccharin after a single bolus dose of 50 mg/kg

Time of collection[a] (min)	Midpoint (min)	Amount excreted (μg)	Excretion rate (μg min^{-1})	Cumulative total (μg)	A_{ex}^{∞} − cumulative total (ΔA_{ex}) (μg)
0–5	2.5	7518	1503.6	7518	18,247
5–15	10.0	6275	627.5	13,793	11,972
15–30	22.5	4989	332.6	18,782	6983
30–45	37.5	2580	172.0	21,362	4403
45–60	52.5	1485	99.0	22,847	2918
60–75	67.5	861	57.4	23,708	2057
75–90	82.5	561	37.4	24,269	1496
90–105	97.5	363	24.2	24,632	1133
105–120	112.5	300	20.0	24,932	833
120–∞	—	833[b]	—	25,765[b]	—

[a] Raw data from Table 4.10.
[b] The additional amount excreted from the last data point to infinity can be calculated as the excretion rate (last) divided by the terminal slope. The graph of rate against time (Figure 4.17; Table 4.13) gives a terminal slope of 0.024 min^{-1}; therefore the amount excreted, 120–∞, equals 20.0 μg min^{-1}/0.024 min^{-1} = 833 μg.

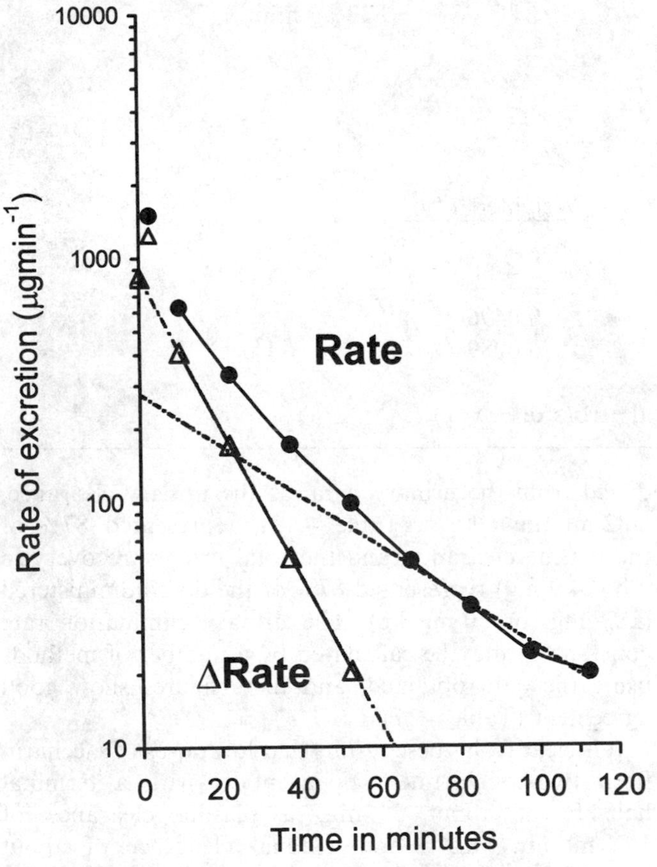

FIG. 4.17. Urinary excretion of saccharin after a single intravenous dose. The results are given as micrograms excreted per minute plotted against the time at the midpoint of the collection period. The data used are given in Table 4.12.

clearly shows a biphasic decrease, although the β phase appears to have started slightly earlier, at 60 min. Analysis of this curve by the method of residuals gave values of α, β, A'', and B'' (Table 4.14).

The renal clearance of the compound can be determined by Eq. (7) using the excretion rate during individual collection periods and the plasma concentrations at the middle of the collection period. These values are given in Table 4.15 and show a clearance of 5.0 ml min^{-1}±10% for seven of the nine time points. The clearance adjusted for body weight was 8.82 ml min^{-1} kg^{-1}. As an alternative to averaging the values derived during the experiment, CL_R may be calculated also from the time-averaged values A_{ex} and AUC (Table 4.15).

Intravenous Bolus Dose: Rate Constants

The values α, β, A, B, A', and so on, derived from plasma and urine, are given in Table 4.16. Using the six values for each constant given in the table, it is interesting that the values of β (0.0222 ± 0.0017 [SD]) and α (0.0691 ± 0.0023 [SD]) show much less variability (±7.5 and ±3.3%, respectively) than the values of k_{21}, k_{10}, and k_{12} derived by Eqs. (38), (39), and (40) (±12, ±16, and ±19%, respectively).

Another important parameter that can be derived from the raw data is the plasma clearance, which is given by Eq. (22). The AUC may be measured by the trapezoid rule, as shown in Table 4.17. With the linear trapezoid method, the concentrations are joined by straight lines; thus after oral dosing, the area during the increase is underestimated and that after the peak is overestimated, as a result

Table 4.13
Analysis of excretion rate data shown in Figure 4.17

Graphical analysis	Linear regression analysis
67.5–112.5 min	
$\beta = \frac{(\log 270 - \log 20)}{110} \times 2.303 = 0.0237\ \text{min}^{-1}$	$\beta = 0.0240\ \text{min}^{-1}$
$B' = 270\ \mu\text{g min}^{-1}$	$B' = 277\ \mu\text{g min}^{-1}$

Residuals

Time (min)	*Rate (μg min^{-1})*	*Time (min)*	*Rate (μg min^{-1})*
2.5	1503.6 − 256 = 1247.6	2.5	1503.6 − 260.5 = 1243.1
10	627.5 − 215 = 412.5	10	627.5 − 217.6 = 409.9
22.5	332.6 − 160 = 172.6	22.5	332.6 − 161.2 = 171.4
37.5	172.0 − 112 = 60.0	37.5	172.0 − 112.5 = 59.5
52.5	99.0 − 79 = 20.0	52.5	99.0 − 78.5 = 20.5

Graphical analysis	Linear regression analysis
10–52.5 min (residuals)	
$\alpha = \frac{(\log 830 - \log 20)}{52.5 - 0} \times 2.303 = 0.0710\ \text{min}^{-1}$	$\alpha = 0.0705\ \text{min}^{-1}$
$A' = 830\ \mu\text{g min}^{-1}$	$A' = 833\ \mu\text{g min}^{-1}$

(Using the 2.5 min point, $\alpha = 0.0784$ and $A' = 1138$)

Analysis using WinNonlin

	All weights equal	Weighted $1/y$	Weighted $1/y^2$
A' (μg min^{-1})	818	898	936
B' (μg min^{-1})	273	161	43.4
α (min^{-1})	0.0680	0.0599	0.0496
β (min^{-1})	0.0248	0.0198	0.0089

(*Note*: $1/y$ weighting is normally used to allow for analytical errors of $\pm x\%$.)

the errors tend to cancel. After intravenous dosing, however, the AUC for each segment is overestimated, the total extent of which depends on the number of time points available. Such errors may be minimized by applying the trapezoid rule to log-transformed data. These points are shown in Table 4.17, which also illustrates the derivation of the model-independent parameters MRT and V_{ss}.

Because the terminal half-life (β phase) from plasma was 30.8 min (0.693/0.0225), the duration of the study was the minimum necessary to adequately define the curve. Ideally, the data collection should have been extended for at least another 30 or 60 min in order to give five half-lives, which was borne out by the fact that the β phase was dependent on only four data points. Because the duration of the experiment was four half-lives, a total of about 94% of the dose should have been eliminated, which is in good agreement with that predicted from the urinary data, as the urinary clearance, 8.82 ml min^{-1} kg^{-1} (Table 4.15), represented 87% of the plasma clearance, and the total urinary recovery in 2 h (24.9 mg) represented 87% of the dose administered (28.5 mg, or 50 mg/kg). The urinary elimination rate constant k_R may be calculated by a number of methods using the data obtained, and these figures show good agreement (Table 4.17).

It is clear from these results that low doses of saccharin fit a two-compartment open model with a terminal half-life of about 30 min, a plasma clearance of 10.1 ml min^{-1} kg^{-1}, and a renal clearance of about 8.8 ml min^{-1} kg^{-1}. The latter value is considerably higher than the glomerular filtration rate in the rat (3.4 ml min^{-1} kg^{-1}). Because glomerular filtration removes only the nonprotein-bound compound and saccharin is about 80% protein-bound (105), the clearance due to filtration would be only about

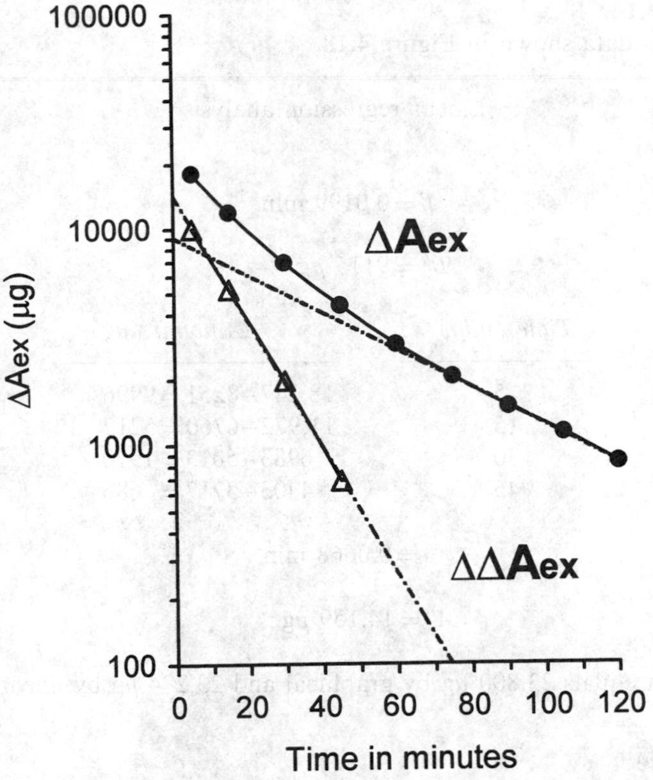

FIG. 4.18. Urinary excretion of saccharin analyzed by the sigma-minus method. The results are the amount remaining to be excreted (ΔA_{ex}) plotted against time. The data used are given in Table 4.12.

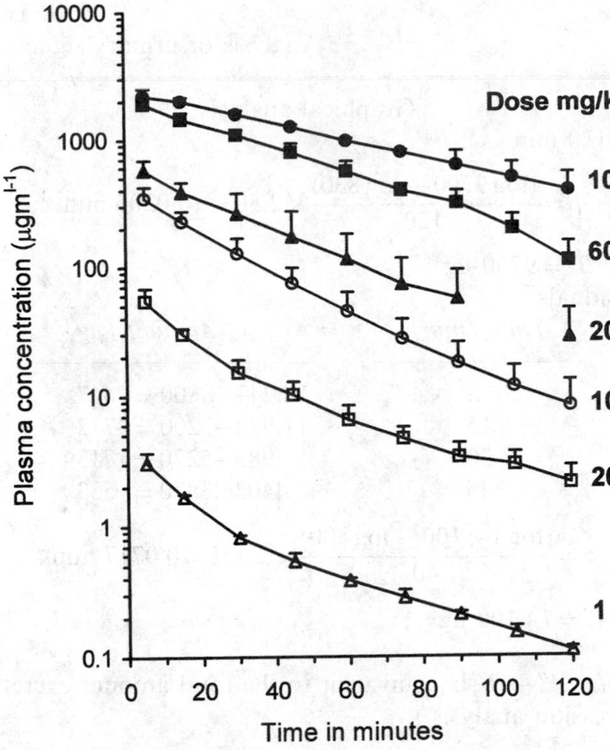

FIG. 4.19. Plasma concentration–time curves for rats given bolus intravenous doses of saccharin. Adult male rats were given [^{3}H]saccharin (1–1000 mg/kg IV) by bolus dose, and plasma levels were measured by liquid scintillation counting. From Reference 105.

0.7 ml min^{-1} kg^{-1}. It is therefore apparent that extensive secretion and negligible reabsorption must be occurring in the renal tubule, and we can conclude that the major route of elimination of saccharin is by renal tubular secretion. Renal tubular secretion is responsible for about 80% $[(8.8-0.7)/10.1 \times 100]$ of total elimination. This finding was confirmed by studies in which the plasma clearance of saccharin was reduced by about 70% by the drug probenecid, which inhibits renal tubular secretion (105).

Because renal tubular secretion is a saturable process, it was possible that the nonlinearity of plasma levels, seen on dietary administration, arose from saturation of this major route of elimination. This possibility was investigated by giving a range of intravenous bolus doses of saccharin (1–1000 mg kg^{-1}) and calculating the plasma clearance. The plasma concentration–time curves for high doses (Figure 4.19) reflected nonlinear kinetics (Figure 4.13) being superimposed on the two-compartment pattern seen at low doses (Figure 4.16). It resulted in high doses appearing to be a simple one-compartment system during the course of the experiment. Obviously, better data would have been obtained if the collection period was extended (105). These data illustrated well that the terminal half-life, which was derived at low plasma levels, did not show a dose-dependent increase and that the best indication of saturation kinetics was given by plasma clearance, which was decreased at doses of 300 mg kg^{-1} or more (Figure 4.20). The increased half-life at the highest dose is probably a reflection of the duration of the study rather than a true value.

Intravenous Infusion

Saturation kinetics apparent after single doses of about 300 mg kg^{-1} (shown by the decreased plasma clearance and altered plasma concentration-time curve) could not be related closely to a particular plasma concentration, because the levels fell from about 500 to 30 μg ml^{-1} during the 2-h study period. Infusion studies were used to relate altered clearance to a particular plasma level, because at steady state the rate of infusion equals the rate of elimination for a *fixed* plasma concentration. CL can be calculated using Eq. (20),

$$CL = \frac{\text{rate of infusion}}{C_{pss}}$$

Table 4.14
Analysis of urinary sigma-minus data shown in Figure 4.18

Graphical analysis		Linear regression analysis	
60–120 min			
$\beta = \frac{(\log 9700 - \log 830)}{120} \times 2.303 = 0.0205\ \text{min}^{-1}$		$\beta = 0.0199\ \text{min}^{-1}$	
$B'' = 9700\ \mu g$		$B'' = 9115\ \mu g$	
Residuals			
Time (min)	*Amount (μg)*	*Time (min)*	*Amount (μg)*
5	18,247−8800 = 9447	5	18,247−8251 = 9996
15	11,972−7200 = 4772	15	11,972−6760 = 5212
30	6983−5270 = 1713	30	6983−5013 = 1970
45	4403−3870 = 533	45	4403−3717 = 686
$\alpha = \frac{(\log 14,100 - \log 800)}{40} \times 2.303 = 0.0717\ \text{min}^{-1}$		$\alpha = 0.0668\ \text{min}^{-1}$	
$A'' = 14,100\ \mu g$		$A'' = 14,159\ \mu g$	

(*Note*: $A'' + B''$ is equivalent to the total amount excreted; it equals 23,800 μg by graphical and 23,274 μg by linear regression analysis.)

Analysis using WinNonlin

	All weights equal	Weighted $1/y$	Weighted $1/y^2$
A'' (μg)	14,669	15,316	15,509
B'' (μg)	8165	7407	7140
α (min^{-1})	0.0608	0.0581	0.0569
β (min^{-1})	0.0193	0.0183	0.0180

(*Note*: $1/y$ weighting is normally used to allow for analytical errors of $\pm x\%$.)

The rats were anesthetized and infused at a rate of 9.6 μl/min with [^{3}H]saccharin solution in isotonic saline via the jugular vein using a Harvard infusion pump. The infusion rate was selected because it approximates 14 ml/day and is therefore not an excessive fluid intake. Each animal was infused at a constant rate, within the range 50–2000 μg min^{-1}, and the plasma was analyzed every 30 min from 90 min onward until three consecutive samples showed the same concentration (C_{pss}). The clearance for each animal was calculated using the equation given above. A graph of clearance against steady-state plasma concentration (Figure 4.21) shows that the clearance was about 8–12 ml min^{-1} kg^{-1} at plasma concentrations below 200 μg ml^{-1}, whereas the clearance decreased to 4–8 ml min^{-1} kg^{-1} at concentrations above 300 μg ml^{-1} (a value similar to that seen after an intravenous bolus dose of 600 mg kg^{-1}).

Thus, based on these studies, the renal tubular secretion of saccharin appears to be saturated by doses giving plasma concentrations of 200–300 μg ml^{-1} or more. This value correlates well with the concentration in the plasma of rats fed a 7.5% saccharin diet, and which was associated with elevated levels in the plasma and most organs (Figure 4.15) (105). [Intravenous infusion in dogs was used to relate serum concentrations of minoxidil at steady state to cardiovascular effects and to cardiac toxicity (60).]

Oral Studies

Because saccharin has a short terminal half-life (30 min), it is possible that there are rapid fluctuations in plasma concentrations during chronic dietary administration. This possibility was investigated by studies on the plasma concentration–time curve for animals maintained on a 5% saccharin diet for an extended period. The diurnal variation showed relatively small changes, with a peak at around 6 AM and a minimum

Table 4.15
Renal clearance of saccharin after an intravenous bolus dose

Time of collection (min)	Midpoint (min)	Excretion rate (μg min^{-1})	Midpoint plasma concentration[a] (μg ml^{-1})	CL_R^b (ml min^{-1})
0–5	2.5	1503.6	225	6.68
5–15	10.0	627.5	138	4.55
15–30	22.5	332.6	71	4.68
30–45	37.5	172.0	35.5	4.84
45–60	52.5	99.0	18.8	5.27
60–75	67.5	57.4	10.6	5.42
75–90	82.5	37.4	6.9	5.42
90–105	97.5	24.2	4.8	5.04
105–120	112.5	20.0	3.4	5.88
			Mean value (5–105 min)	5.03

[a] Data are from Figure 4.16.
[b] Renal clearance, calculated using Eq. (7). Mean renal clearance = 5.03 ml min^{-1} (per 570 g) = 8.82 ml min^{-1} kg^{-1}. CL_R may be calculated also from A_{ex} (Table 4.12) and AUC (Table 4.17) between 0 and 120 min:

$$CL_R = \frac{A_{ex}}{AUC} = \frac{24,932\,\mu g}{4895\,\mu g\,ml^{-1}\,min} = 5.09\,ml\,min^{-1}$$

at 6 PM. (Figure 4.22). The extent of variation was less than might have been expected from the half-life, and the fact that little saccharin-containing feed was consumed between 6 AM and 6 PM. It therefore seemed probable that the rate of absorption from the gut was low and blunted any large change in plasma level. The plasma concentration–time curve after oral administration was studied and showed much lower levels than after similar doses given intravenously (Figure 4.23). The peak concentration was at the time of the first sample, followed by a slow and variable decrease. The decrease in concentration was obviously not related to the value of β, and thus saccharin is a good example of a compound for which the decrease after oral administration is related to k_a, and not to k or β (see Mathematical Principles, above). The decrease was slow and complex, emphasizing that if absorption from the gut is slow, a single rate constant cannot be derived to apply to the many rates occurring simultaneously at different sites within the gastrointestinal tract. The duration of sample collection after oral dosage was inadequate for definition of the $ACU_{0-\infty}$, and thus the bioavailability could not be calculated from these plasma data. The methods for deriving simple absorption rate constants are described above under Mathematical Principles.

In summary, these studies have been used to illustrate the derivation of kinetic data and the insights they can give into the handling of the compound during chronic toxicity studies. The possibility of saturation of one pathway revealing a second pathway of elimination could result in saccharin (which is not metabolized normally) undergoing metabolism in rats fed high-saccharin diets. However, this phenomenon has not been detected for saccharin (104), although Gehring and Young (33) showed that metabolism of 2,4,5-trichlorophenoxyacetic acid was revealed by doses resulting in saturation of renal tubular secretion.

Computation

The use of computer programs to derive kinetic constants from plasma and urinary concentrations can greatly simplify data handling. Because data handling is also optimized, computer usage is the method of choice. There are a number of suitable programs (e.g. BLIN, NONLIN, SIPHAR) available for nonlinear least-squares regression analysis, which is the most appropriate method, and readers are referred to Gibaldi and Perrier (36), Wagner (112), and Gabrielsson and Weiner (28) for further details. The use of such a program would automatically put the best-fit line through the data presented in Figures 4.16–4.18 and would avoid a possibly erroneous decision as to the time at which the α component was exerting an insignificant influence and the line was described by β alone. In the analysis of data by computer program, it is common to apply a suitable weight to each data point to ensure the most appropriate fit. The weights that can be applied to the concentration data include (a) all weights equal, which is applicable if the errors in measurement are a constant amount, for example, ± 2 μg/ml; (b) weighted by $1/y$, which is

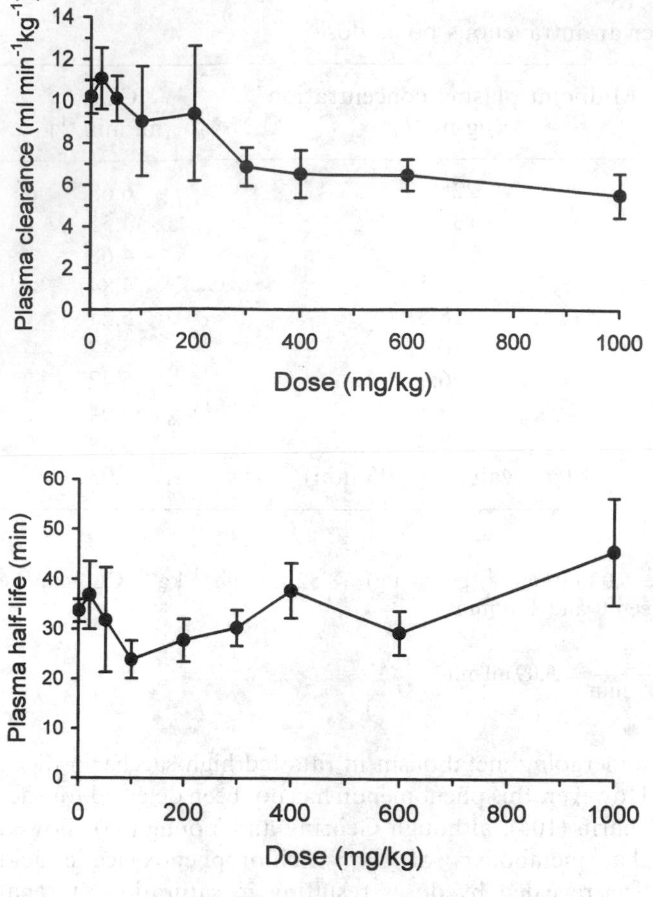

FIG. 4.20. Influence of dose on the plasma clearance and half-life of saccharin in male rats following an intravenous bolus dose. From Reference 105.

applicable if the errors of measurement are a constant proportion, for example ±2%; and (c) weighted by $1/y^2$, which can be used to force the fit through the later time points at the expense of the early higher values. The second option, $1/y$, closely represents the accuracy of most assay procedures and is used most frequently. It is important with computer fitting of data that some indication of appropriateness of fit is obtained by either a graphical representation or analysis of the deviation between observed and calculated concentrations (error analysis). With the latter approach, a consistent positive or negative deviation is more important than wider but randomly distributed deviations, because it indicates an inadequate fit. Reasons for this situation could be the choice of an inappropriate model to fit to the data or incorrect weighting. Another factor to consider is that although adoption of a more complex model may give a closer fit to the data, the sampling times may be inadequate to provide accurate parameter estimates.

It should be realized that although kinetic constants derived from sophisticated computerized line fitting contain the minimum possible errors due to data handling, any errors in the raw data, due to methodological problems, will still be present. Indeed, the adage "rubbish in, rubbish out" is particularly pertinent to the use of sophisticated data handling to analyze inaccurate or badly designed animal toxicokinetic experiments.

Interpretation of Toxicokinetic Data

There are three principle aims of kinetic studies as applied to toxicology. First, toxicokinetics can provide

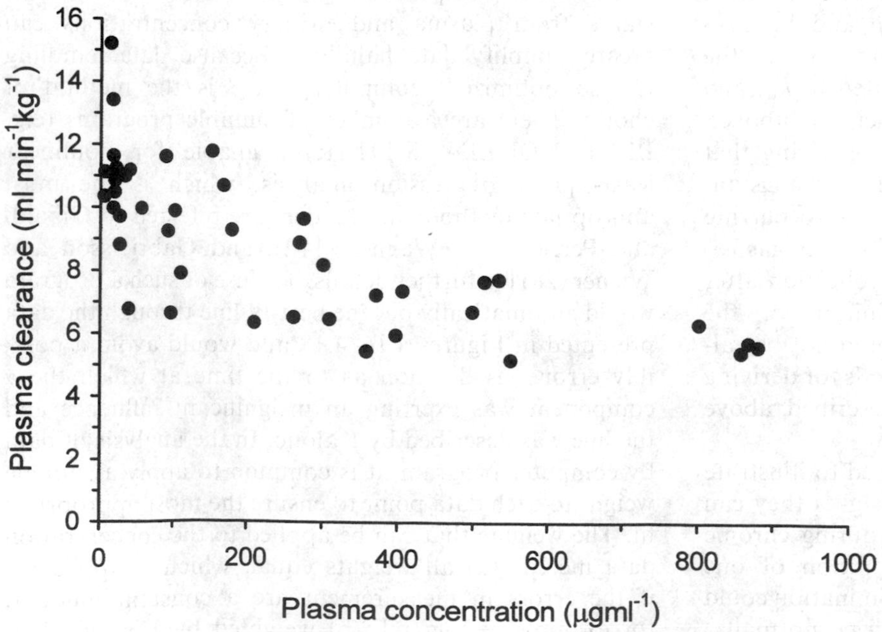

FIG. 4.21. Plasma clearance of saccharin at steady-state plasma concentrations. Adult male rats were given [^{3}H]saccharin in isotonic saline by intravenous infusion (0.0096 ml/min) until a constant plasma ^{3}H concentration was obtained. The plateau saccharin concentration was calculated from the specific activity of the dose solution, and the plasma clearance from the infusion rate and plasma concentration. From Reference 105.

Table 4.16
Summary of kinetic data after intravenous saccharin

Parameter	Plasma		Urine (excretion rate)		Urine (sigmus minus)	
	Graphical	Regression	Graphical	Regression	Graphical	Regression
β (min^{-1})	0.0224	0.0226	0.0237	0.0240	0.0205	0.0199
B or B' or B''	42	43.7	270	277	9700	9115
α (min^{-1})	0.0664	0.0683	0.0710	0.0705	0.0717	0.0668
A or A' or A''	198	204.5	830	833	14,100	14,159
V_1 (ml kg^{-1})	208	201				
k_{21}(min^{-1})	0.0301	0.0307	0.0353	0.0356	0.0414	0.0383
k_{10} (min^{-1})	0.0494	0.0503	0.0477	0.0475	0.0355	0.0347
k_{12} (min^{-1})	0.0093	0.0099	0.0117	0.0113	0.0153	0.0137

$$V_1 = \frac{\text{dose (50 mg/kg)}}{A+B}$$

$$k_{21} = \frac{A\beta + B\alpha}{A+B}; \quad \text{or } A', B'; \quad \text{or } A'', B''$$

$$k_{10} = \frac{\alpha\beta}{k_{21}}$$

$$k_{12} = \alpha + \beta - k_{21} - k_{10}$$

The constants were derived by graphical analysis or by least-squares linear regression analysis applied to β phase and residuals.

$$\text{Renal excretion} = \frac{25,765}{50,000 \times 0.57} \times 100 = 90.4\% \text{ of dose } (0.57 = \text{body weight in kg})$$

Renal elimination rate constant (k_R)

$$k_R = \frac{A' + B'}{\text{dose}} = \frac{277 + 833}{28,500} = 0.039\ \text{min}^{-1}$$

$$k_R = \frac{A_{ex}^{\infty} \times k_{10}}{\text{dose}} = \frac{25,765 \times 0.050}{28,500} = 0.045\ \text{min}^{-1}$$

$$k_R = \frac{CL_R}{V_1} = \frac{8.82}{201} = 0.044\ \text{min}^{-1}$$

$$\text{MRT} = \frac{\text{AUMC}}{\text{AUC}} = \frac{125,072}{5024} = 25\ \text{min}$$

$$V_{ss} = \frac{\text{dose} \times \text{AUMC}}{\text{AUC}^2} = \frac{50,000 \times 125,072}{5024^2} = 248\ \text{ml kg}^{-1}$$

Table 4.17
Plasma clearance and renal elimination of saccharin

Plasma clearance: $CL = \dfrac{\text{dose}}{\text{AUC}}$ Trapezoid rule: AUC = sum of $\dfrac{(t_2 - t_1)}{2}(C_{p1} + C_{p2})$, etc.

time (min) (t)	C_p (μg ml^{-1})	AUC (μg ml^{-1} min)	$t \times C_p$ (μg ml^{-1} min)	AUMC (μg ml^{-1} min^2)
0	242.0[a]	1066	0	2305
5	184.3	1432	922	12,260
15	102.0	1144	1530	22,838
30	50.5	566	1515	19,770
45	24.9	293	1121	14,753
60	14.1	166	846	10,845
75	8.0	103	600	8348
90	5.7	73	513	6998
105	4.0	52	420	5760
120	2.9	129[b]	348	21,195[c]
Total		5024 μg ml^{-1} min		125,072 μg ml^{-1} min^2

Plasma clearance = 50,000 μg kg^{-1}/5024 μg ml^{-1} min = 9.95 ml min^{-1} kg^{-1}
CL = $k_{10}V_1$ = 208 × 0.0494 = 10.27 ml min^{-1} kg^{-1} or 201 × 0.0506 = 10.17 ml min^{-1} kg^{-1} (Table 4.16)
Renal clearance (CL_R) = 8.82 ml min^{-1} kg^{-1} (Table 4.15)

[a]By extrapolation of plasma concentration–time curve.
[b]Calculated by $C_{p\,\text{last}}/\beta = 2.9/0.0225$.
[c]Calculated by $t \times C_{p\,\text{last}}/\beta + C_{p\,\text{last}}/\beta^2 = 348/0.0225 + 2.9/0.000506 = 15.467 + 5728$.

an understanding of the physiological processes that are involved in the fate of the chemical in the body. Second, the relation between dose and toxicokinetics may be the key to either the establishment of appropriate dose levels for chronic studies (101) or the interpretation of such studies. Third, comparative toxicokinetics may be used to assess potential human risks with a more secure basis by reducing the number of unknown variables involved in the extrapolation from animal to humans (see ref. 76).

A good example of the physiological insights that may be obtained is provided by the data on saccharin discussed above. In summary, these data showed that the sweetener is slowly absorbed from the gut. Thus, during chronic feeding of saccharin diets, there are only slight diurnal fluctuations due to the absorption rate producing "flip-flop" kinetics. The absorbed saccharin has a low volume of distribution so that the concentrations in most tissues are similar to or lower than those in plasma. The urinary bladder tissue is part of the central compartment (105). The sweetener is cleared rapidly from plasma, mostly as a result of renal tubular secretion. This process is saturated at the high dietary intakes that are necessary to produce an increase in bladder tumors. Renal tubular secretion is a general mechanism for the elimination of organic acids, and saturation of renal clearance of saccharin at high dietary concentrations is accompanied by decreased renal clearance of indican, a major urinary metabolite of tryptophan (95). Subsequent studies demonstrated that the slow absorption of saccharin from the gut results in altered metabolism of essential nutrients within the gastrointestinal tract (53,95,96). Thus the dietary levels necessary throughout life (≥3%) to increase the incidence of bladder tumors in male rats produce profound perturbations of the physiology and biochemistry of the test animal, although these are not directly related to bladder tumor formation. Neither saturation of renal clearance (73) nor altered excretion of amino acid metabolites (81) has been found in humans following doses equivalent to the highest likely human intake.

The relationship between kinetics, dose, and toxicity is probably the single most important contribution that kinetics can make to the field of toxicity testing. Although a few therapeutic chemicals show nonlinear kinetics at the doses normally given to man (notable examples being salicylates, phenytoin [diphenylhydantoin], and ethanol), the plasma levels of foreign chemicals in humans are usually well below those necessary to saturate any protein-mediated reactions. However, in toxicity testing,

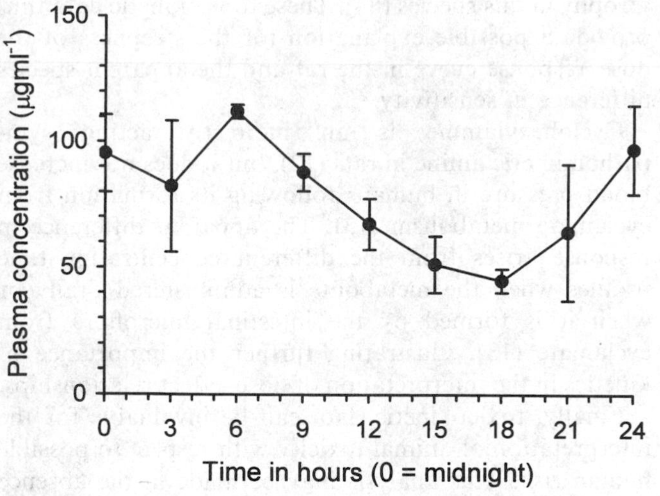

FIG. 4.22. Diurnal variation in the concentration of saccharin in the plasma of rats given a 5% saccharin diet. Adult male rats were given a 5% saccharin (sodium saccharin dihydrate) diet for 66 days ad libitum; plasma samples were collected during a 24-h period and analyzed for saccharin content by HPLC. The results given are the mean concentrations ±*SD* (as sodium saccharin dihydrate) for three animals. From Reference 105.

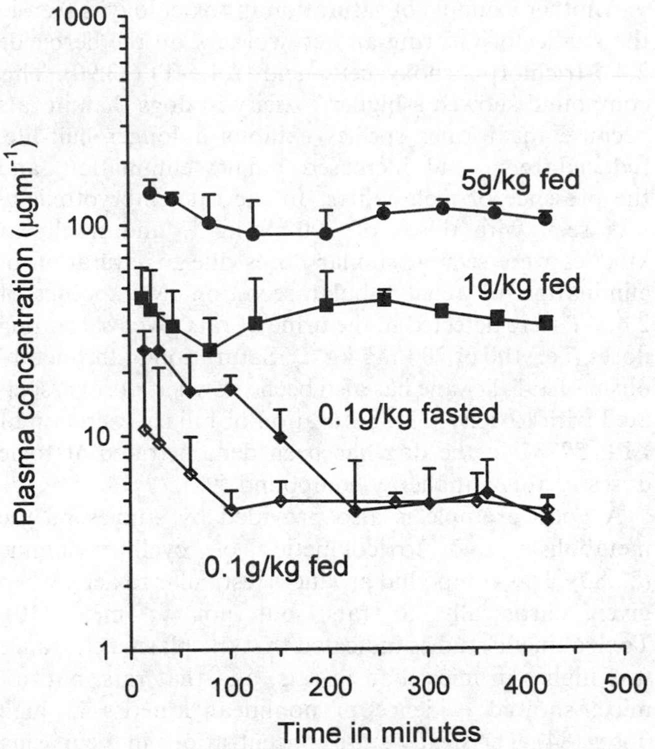

FIG. 4.23. Concentration of saccharin in the plasma of rats given [^{3}H]saccharin orally. Adult male rats were given a single oral dose of [^{3}H]saccharin, and the plasma ^{3}H content was determined by liquid scintillation counting. The saccharin (5, 1, and 0.1 g/kg) was given in aqueous solution (20, 10, and 0.5 ml/kg). The plasma concentration–time curve for 0.1 g/kg was not altered by giving the dose in a large volume (10 ml/kg). The results given are the mean of three animals ±*SD*. From Reference 105.

when the maximum dose tested is designed to show some degree of toxicity, nonlinear kinetics are a distinct possibility and should be fully and carefully investigated. At doses above saturation, the body load of free compound increases steeply with an increase in dose. Under such circumstances, effective tissue concentrations of the chemical will also be considerably higher than predicted by extrapolation from doses showing first-order kinetics. The presence of dose-dependent kinetics may result in an extremely steep dose–response curve for the toxic effect observed. In such circumstances, the nonlinearity in kinetics shown in animal toxicity testing must be taken into account when extrapolating the effects to man.

A possible cause of toxicity associated with large saturating doses of chemicals is that normally minor pathways of metabolism may become of major significance. Thus if a chemical undergoes metabolism by two routes, one with a low K_m (high affinity) and one with a high K_m (low affinity), at low doses most chemical in the cell is eliminated by the former route. However, if the levels increase to saturate the high affinity enzyme, any further input will exceed removal and levels will rise such that the low-affinity enzyme will metabolize the excess. (A useful analogy is that of water pouring into a bucket that has two holes in the side at different heights. Little escapes through the upper hole until the rate of input exceeds the rate of removal by the lower hole.)

There have been some notable examples of toxicity occurring largely at saturating doses of foreign chemicals. In a series of papers by Brodie and co-workers (48,62,63,71), it was shown that the hepatotoxicity of paracetamol (acetaminophen) was related to the metabolism of the compound and occurred only at high doses, which were associated with extensive covalent binding of the compound to tissue components. Little binding occurred at low doses or if the metabolism of toxic doses was inhibited by treatment with piperonyl butoxide. The binding at high doses arose from saturation of the capacity of the hepatocytes to protect themselves from the reactive metabolite produced. The protective mechanism was conjugation with glutathione, and saturation of this system at toxic doses was caused by depletion of the available glutathione.

Another example of saturation in toxicology is seen in the studies of Gehring and co-workers on the herbicide 2,4,5-trichlorophenoxyacetic acid (2,4,5-T) (33,90). This compound showed a higher toxicity in dogs than in rats because the former species exhibits a longer half-life, reduced renal and increased biliary elimination, and the presence of metabolites. In the rat, embryotoxicity was seen with doses of 100 mg kg^{-1}, and nonlinear kinetics were seen at similar doses due to saturation of elimination by renal tubular secretion. Metabolites of 2,4,5-T were detected in the urine of rats given saturating doses (i.e., 100 or 200 mg kg^{-1}). Saturation of the metabolism of 1,4-dioxane has also been shown at doses associated with toxicity (33). Saturation of biliary excretion of FPL 57787 in the dog has been demonstrated at toxic doses of this antiallergy compound (97).

A good example is also provided by studies on the metabolism and toxicokinetics of cyclohexylamine (82,83). This compound produces testicular toxicity when given chronically to rats, but not to mice (10). Toxicokinetic studies indicated that the plasma clearance was higher in mice than in rats, and that rats, but not mice, showed evidence of nonlinear kinetics at high doses (84). The steady-state concentrations in the plasma and testes during chronic administration confirmed dose-dependent kinetics in the rat (Figure 4.24), which coincided with the dose–response curve for testicular

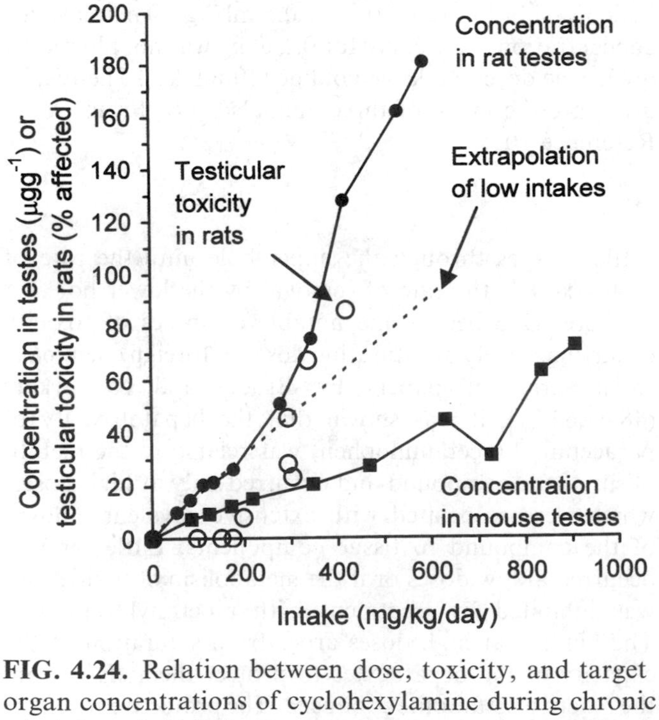

FIG. 4.24. Relation between dose, toxicity, and target organ concentrations of cyclohexylamine during chronic administration; (●) concentration in rat testes; (■) concentration in mouse testes; (○) testicular toxicity in rats. Data from Reference 84.

atrophy in this species (84). These toxicokinetic data thus provide a possible explanation for the steepness of the dose–response curve in the rat and the apparent species difference in sensitivity.

Cyclohexylamine is an indirectly acting sympathomimetic amine in rats (12), but it does not increase blood pressure in humans following its formation from cyclamate metabolism (13). The apparent difference in response arises from the different concentration–time profiles when the metabolite is administered orally or when it is formed by the intestinal microflora from cyclamate (13), illustrating further the importance of kinetics in the interpretation of dose–effect relationships.

Finally, toxicokinetic data can be invaluable for the interpretation of animal toxicity with respect to possible human risk. This analysis may be made in the absence or the presence of human pharmacokinetic data. In the absence of human data, extrapolation may be by either physiological or compartmental modeling methods (3). The physiological approach relies on the scale-up between animals and man of such parameters as tissue volume and blood flow (Figure 4.4) and by their relation to body weight. Assuming that the uptake from blood to tissue (extraction ratio) is a function of the chemical and therefore independent of species, it is possible to derive complex models involving all the major tissues of the body (34). These models may then be scaled up from known animal data to humans based on the known physiological differences. Alternatively and more pragmatically, the plasma kinetics in various species may be fitted by compartmental modeling and then scaled up empirically according to the body mass of the species studied and extrapolated to humans (39,64).

The most secure comparison is when kinetic data are available in animals and humans, allowing direct analysis of the potential risk. In any such analysis the species difference in basic physiological processes such as cardiac output and relative tissue weight usually result in lower clearances and longer half-lives in humans than in animals (75). Thus comparisons of animals and humans on the basis of plasma levels or AUC values, rather than intake or exposure data expressed per kilogram body weight, result in a decreased apparent safety margin compared with intake data. However, by removing important variables from interspecies comparisons, such an approach provides a more secure basis for the safety assessment (76,92).

Toxicokinetic data can also be useful in defining the contributions of parent compound and metabolites to toxicity. Retinol (vitamin A) is an animal and human teratogen, which is metabolized to a number of biologically active species such as all-*trans*-retinoic acid, 13-*cis*-retinoic acid, and 9-*cis*-retinoic acid. The principle sources of exposure to retinol (rather than the precursor carotenoids) are from the consumption of animal livers

Table 4.18
The AUC values for retinol and its metabolites in young women after oral doses of 50 mg and 150 mg of retinol given as retinyl palmitate in a supplement or in cooked calf liver

	AUC values in ng ml^{-1}h					
Dose	Retinyl palmitate	Retinol	All-*trans*-retinoic acid	13-*cis*-retinoic acid	All-*trans*-4-oxo-retinoic acid	13-*cis*-4-oxo-retinoic acid
50 mg S	10,400 (5,300)	2070 (1900)	86 (63)	359 (104)	30 (33)	877 (207)
50 mg L	5900 (3,700)	1530 (2490)	6 (5)	243 (70)	11 (15)	492 (145)
150 mg S	18,900 (20,200)	2300 (1180)	170 (118)	674 (156)	133 (47)	2385 (563)
150 mg L	14,500 (8,800)	2430 (2090)	23 (11)	596 (131)	120 (84)	1820 (294)

S = Supplement given under fasting conditions.
L = Cooked liver as part of a meal.
The results are the mean (with *SD* in parentheses) for 10 subjects dosed at 4-week intervals (data from ref. 14).

and from vitamin supplements. The evidence for teratogenicity in humans is from case reports of excessive consumption of vitamin supplements; there is little evidence of a risk from liver consumption, despite the fact that this source may give similar or even higher intakes than those causing malformations after excessive supplement consumption. The areas under the plasma concentration–time curve of retinol and its metabolites in young women following oral doses of retinyl palmitate as an oral solution (fasting) and as cooked liver (as part of a meal) (14) are given in Table 4.18. The main difference was the 5–10-fold difference in the AUC of all-*trans*-retinoic acid, which is recognized to be the major teratogenic metabolite. However, 13-*cis*-retinoic acid (isotretoin), also a recognized human teratogen, showed no major difference. Therefore, the key issue for the assessment of human risk was the plasma concentration–response relationship for the main metabolites, and whether the teratogenicity of retinol and 13-*cis*-retinoic acid could be explained by their metabolism to all-*trans*-retinoic acid. A subsequent study (107) gave single oral doses of retinol, all-*trans*-retinoic acid and 13-*cis*-retinoic acid to pregnant rats and determined the dose–response relationship (Figure 4.25) and plasma kinetics of the different metabolites for each compound. Both retinol and 13-*cis*-retinoic acid gave measurable levels of all-*trans*-retinoic acid in the plasma. A graph of teratogenic response against the AUC of all-*trans*-retinoic acid for the three compounds (Figure 4.26) shows that whereas the teratogenicity of 13-*cis*-retinoic acid could be explained on the basis of the circulating all-*trans*-retinoic acid, this was not the case for retinol. Retinol was considerably more potent than would be predicted from the plasma AUC of all-*trans*-retinoic acid after retinol administration, possibly due to local bioactivation within the fetus. Consequently, the

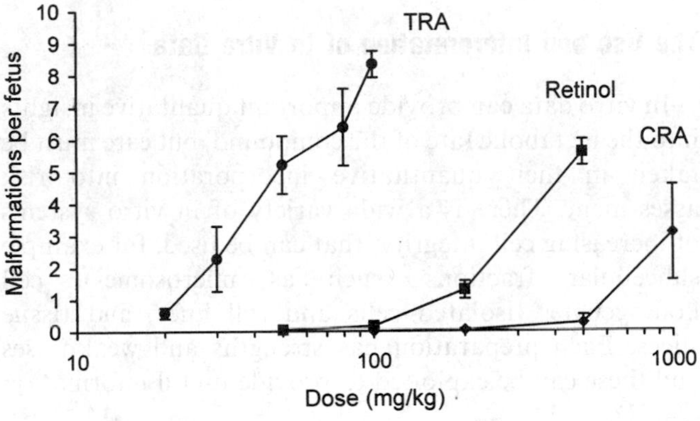

FIG. 4.25. Dose–response relationships for teratogenicity of all-*trans*-retinoic acid (TRA), retinol, and 13-*cis*-retinoic acid (CRA) given as a single oral dose to rats on day 10 of gestation. Data from Reference 107.

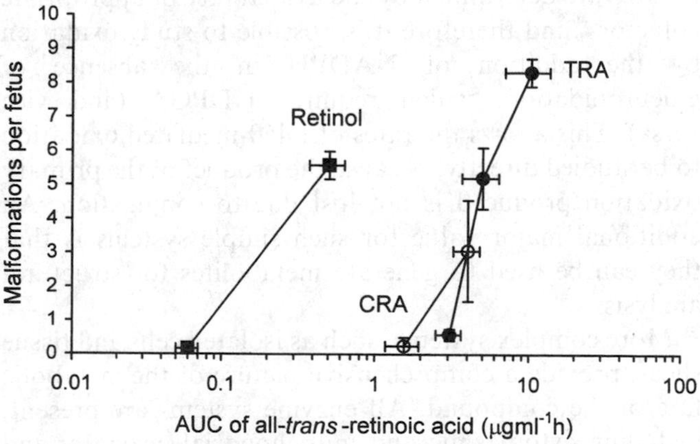

FIG. 4.26. Relationship between AUC of all-*trans*-retinoic acid in maternal plasma and teratogenicity in female rats given all-*trans*-retinoic acid (TRA), retinol, and 13-*cis*-retinoic acid (CRA) on day 10 of gestation. Data from Reference 107.

5–10-fold difference in the AUC of all-*trans*-retinoic acid between liver and supplements (Table 4.18) would not be expected to be translated into a similar difference in teratogenic risk. Using the comparative potency ratios in rats (Figure 4.25) of about 25 : 3 : 1 for all-*trans*-retinoic acid, 13-*cis*-retinoic acid, and retinol, and the AUC data in Table 4.18, the doses of 50 and 150 mg as supplements would be expected to be about 2.2 and 1.8 times, respectively, more active than the equivalent doses given in cooked liver. However, this analysis was heavily biased by the AUC and response data for retinol; also, there could be major species differences in local activation of retinol in the fetus and/or vehicle-dependent differences (liver compared with supplements) in the proportions bound to retinol-binding protein (which could alter this conclusion).

The Use and Interpretation of In Vitro Data

In vitro data can provide important qualitative insights into the metabolic fate of the compound, but care must be taken in their quantitative incorporation into risk assessment. There is a wide variety of in vitro systems of increasing cell integrity, that can be used, for example subcellular fractions (such as microsomes), cell homogenates, isolated cells and cell lines, and tissue slices. Each preparation has strengths and weaknesses and these can be exploited to provide useful information (24,51).

Strengths of In Vitro Systems

Microsomes comprise the smooth endoplasmic reticulum and its associated enzymes, cytochrome P450s and UDP-glucuronyl transferases. The rates of reaction in vitro are determined by the availability of appropriate cofactors, and therefore it is possible to study oxidation by the addition of NADPH in the absence of glucuronidation, which requires UDPGA (and vice versa). This allows the rates of P450-mediated oxidation to be studied directly, because the product of the primary oxidation produced is not lost due to conjugation. An additional major value for such simple systems is that they can be used to generate metabolites for structural analysis.

More complex systems, such as isolated cells and tissue slices, provide a comprehensive picture of the metabolic fate of the compound. All enzyme systems are present, including cytoplasmic and mitochondrial enzymes, and the cell architecture can affect cell uptake and intracellular distribution of the chemical. Perhaps the most integrated in vitro system is the isolated perfused rat liver, which can give excellent correlations with in vivo clearance (23). As a result, these systems can provide information on the relative importance of alternative metabolic pathways.

A major advantage of in vitro systems is that they allow data to be generated on the potential metabolism in humans, without the need for in vivo exposure. This has been particularly valuable for carcinogens, where the generation of in vivo data would be unethical. Identification of the specific isoenzymes of cytochrome P450 involved in metabolism of a compound is important in understanding the potential variability in metabolism within the human population, because of the genetic polymorphism in some of the isoforms, for example CYP2D6. Such information can be generated by in vitro studies in three ways:

1. Comparisons of the rates of metabolism in stored (banked) liver preparations from individuals with characteristic isoenzyme profiles
2. The use of isoenzyme specific inhibitors or inducers (in cell-intact preparations)
3. The use of expression systems in which the DNA for specific isoenzymes is incorporated and expressed by a suitable host, such as a yeast or bacteria (38)

The generation of in vitro data using human tissues allows characterization of species differences both qualitatively and quantitatively by the generation of the appropriate enzyme constants V_{max} and K_m. Such data represent critical components of PBPK models (70) and for the prediction of in vivo clearance (44,46, 120,121).

The outline given above should be sufficient to indicate the huge potential for in vitro studies and explain why these methods have been the basis for much of our understanding of pathways of xenobiotic metabolism.

Precautions with In Vitro Systems

A number of limitations need to be remembered when considering in vitro data.

1. Many studies give data on the extent of metabolism at a single high concentration in vitro and therefore represent V_{max}, which may be of limited relevance to in vivo concentrations. A full analysis of the enzyme kinetics is necessary to give both V_{max} and K_m.
2. The strengths of simple systems, for example microsomes outlined above, will be weaknesses if the data are overinterpreted in relation to the fate in vivo.
3. Changes in enzyme expression occur in vitro, for example isolated cell lines show a different complement of cytochrome P450 activities to those in the same cells at isolation.

4. Many human data are generated from stored liver samples obtained at postmortem. The in vitro enzyme activity could be affected by both in vivo aspects, such as drugs given in attempts at resuscitation, disease, etc., and ex vivo aspects, such as the period between death and freezing and storage (67).
5. In vitro data may still be misleading, even if all of these aspects are optimum. This occurs when the clearance of drug by an organ is blood flow limited rather than enzyme limited (see earlier). Under these conditions, both interspecies differences and inter-individual variability will reflect organ blood flow, rather than $V_{\max}$ and K_m. A good example of this is furan (49) for which the rate of oxidation in vitro would greatly exceed delivery via the liver blood flow.

These problems can be avoided if the in vitro data are incorporated into a PBPK model that will allow for organ blood flow, partitioning between blood and tissue, and enzyme kinetics.

The increasing use of in vitro test systems facilitates a quantitative analysis of the dose–toxicity curve and may provide information on mechanisms of action (24, 27). The logical interpretation of such data with respect to human risk requires information on the steady-state concentrations of the active chemical species in the target organ and plasma of the test animal during chronic toxicity testing, combined with knowledge of the toxicokinetics of the chemical in the test animal at toxic doses and in human at the likely exposure level. It must be emphasized that large safety factors have been introduced to protect us from our own ignorance. The increased use of pharmacokinetic data, especially when combined with knowledge of the mechanism of toxicity, will allow the future use of potentially toxic chemicals to be based on scientific principles and understanding (76,92).

STUDY QUESTIONS

1. A new chemical has been administered to rats and humans by both oral and intravenous routes. Basic toxicokinetic measurements (extrapolated to infinity) are given below.

	Rat	Human
Intravenous		
Dose (mg kg^{-1})	10	1
AUC (μg ml^{-1} min)	2000	500
Terminal slope (min^{-1})	0.0025	0.001
% dose excreted unchanged in urine	1	15
Oral		
Dose (mg kg^{-1})	100	1
AUC (μg ml^{-1} min)	8000	490
Terminal slope (min^{-1})	0.0025	0.001

Calculate appropriate toxicokinetic parameters and suggest biochemical and physiological mechanisms that could explain the species difference.

2. The pharmaceutical company for which you work has synthesized a new antianxiety drug, a basic compound, structurally related to the old drug debrisoquine. The parent drug, the active form, causes enzyme (cytochrome P450) induction and liver enlargement; the hydroxylated metabolite, formed on incubation of the drug with liver microsomes, is inactive. After an oral dose, 40% is excreted in the urine within 24 h as the parent compound, 40% is in urine as an hydroxylated metabolite, and 20% is in feces as the parent drug. After an intravenous dose, 80% is in urine as the parent drug, and 20% is in the urine as the metabolite. What advice would you give the company about the following issues:

a. Is the drug likely to be toxic after oral dosage?
b. Would the oral and intravenous doses associated with toxicity be the same?
c. What are the likely sources of variability in kinetics in young physically healthy adults (20–30 years old)?
d. Would the kinetics be different in the elderly (70–80 years old)?
e. How much would a 50% decrease in liver or kidney function affect the kinetics, and would the toxicity be increased or decreased?
f. How much would a 50% increase in liver or kidney function affect the kinetics, and would the toxicity be increased or decreased?
g. Should the pharmaceutical group develop a slow-release formulation and would this be likely to affect the toxicity?

3. The company you work for has developed a novel opioid for the treatment of intractable pain. The drug is 20 times more potent than morphine in relation to both analgesia and respiratory depression when given to rats by intravenous injection, and binding studies show that it has a high and similar affinity for μ-receptors of rats and humans. Initial kinetic studies in humans after a single intravenous bolus dose of 10 mg gave the following data.

Time after dose (h)	*Plasma concentration (ng/ml)*
0.5	367
1.0	336
2	283
4	200
6	141
10	71
24	6.3

The area under the plasma concentration–time curve (AUC) extrapolated to infinity was 2310 ng ml^{-1} h. Urine was collected over the period 2–4 h after dosing and contained a total of 1.85 mg of the parent drug and 0.1 mg of an hydroxy metabolite. The plasma concentration of parent drug at 3 h was 238 ng/ml.

After a single oral dose of 10 mg the maximum plasma concentration occurred at 8 h and was only 48 ng/ml; the blood concentration reached 6 ng/ml by 36 hours. The AUC to infinity was 1155 ng ml^{-1} h.

Plot the intravenous data on graph paper. Calculate appropriate pharmacokinetic parameters to describe the elimination rate, clearance, distribution, and absorption of the drug. Describe the probable overall fate of the drug in the body (e.g., routes of elimination).

Your research director needs the following advice:

i. What extra studies/data could support your description of the fate of the drug?
ii. What route(s) of administration should the company use for its first trials of clinical effect for pain relief?
iii. How should the drug be administered to provide relief of chronic pain?

Hints and Clues

Question 1

a. Calculate clearance (per kg body weight)—why is it different? (See b).
b. Use urinary excretion data to think about pathways of elimination.
c. Use clearance and "terminal slope" (k or β—we don't know) to calculate the apparent volume of distribution.
d. Use AUC data to calculate bioavailability.
e. Are terminal rates different after oral dosage? What would it mean if they were?
f. What are the likely causes of differences between species? Could clearance and bioavailability be interrelated? If so, how?
g. Would scaling to body surface area affect the calculations and conclusions? If so, how?

Question 2

a. Use urinary excretion data to interpret the potential for exposure (or not) of the liver to the parent compound. (Obviously the dose will affect the response, but is toxicity possible?)
b. Use urinary excretion data to calculate bioavailability. What processes are giving rise to the low bioavailability?
c. Variability in adults: What are the routes of elimination? What is the relevance of debrisoquine?
d. Consider 50% changes in liver in relation to bioavailability and clearance. Then, consider changes in renal function similarly. Will kidney function affect bioavailability?
e. A slow-release formulation is necessary when a drug has a very short half-life (e.g., 3–4 h or less). There is information on the rate of elimination in the question. What can you conclude about half-life? (*Clue*: Could it be 24 h?)

Question 3

a. You can calculate clearance, apparent volume of distribution, and half-life from the intravenous data. But what route is important for elimination? (*Clue*: Use urine data to calculate renal clearance and compare with plasma clearance.)
b. The extra studies should relate to kinetics. (*Clue*: What studies would we normally have before giving the first dose to humans?)
c. What is happening with the oral data? What is the extent of absorption? Why are blood levels at 36 h higher after oral dosage? (*Clue*: You can calculate the concentration at 36 h after IV dosage using the exponential terms derived from the IV data.)
d. Phase 1 studies (initial human studies) are usually by the oral route. Is this likely to produce analgesia or side effects with this compound?
e. Chronic pain relief requires the maintenance of constant concentrations of the analgesic. Which route would be likely to give this profile? If oral dosage could not give effective plasma levels without unacceptable side effects (such as constipation), how could you give the drug parenterally to provide similar constant concentrations?

REFERENCES

1. Andersen, M. E., Gargas, M. L., Jones, R. A., and Jenkins, L. J. (1979): The use of inhalation techniques to assess the kinetic constants of 1,l-dichloroethylene metabolism. *Toxicol. Appl. Pharmacol.*, 47:395–409.
2. Anderson, M. W., Hoel, D. G., and Kaplan, N. L. (1980): A general scheme for the incorporation of pharmacokinetics in low-dose risk estimation for chemical carcinogens: Example—vinyl chloride. *Toxicol. Appl. Pharmacol.*, 55:154–161.
3. Bachmann, K. (1989): Predicting toxicokinetic parameters in humans from kinetic data acquired in three small mammalian species. *J. Appl. Toxicol.*, 9:331—338.
4. Bakar, S. K., and Niazi, S. (1983): Simple reliable method for chronic cannulation of the jugular vein for pharmacokinetic studies in rats. *J. Pharm. Sci.*, 72:1027–1029.
5. Bard, P. (1956): In: *Medical Physiology,*. l0th ed., p. 221. Henry Kimpton, London.
6. Bauer, L. A., and Gibaldi, M. (1983): Computation of model-independent pharmacokinetic parameters during multiple dosing. *J. Pharm. Sci.*, 72:978–979.

7. Benet, L. Z., and Galeazzi, R. L. (1979): Noncompartmental determination of the steady state volume of distribution. *J. Pharm. Sci.*, 68:1071–1074.

8. Benet, L. Z., Levy, G., and Ferraiolo, B. L. (eds.) (1984): *Pharmacokinetics: A Modern View*. Plenum Press, New York.

9. Bois, F. Y., Woodruff, T. J., and Spear, R. C. (1991): Comparison of three physiologically based pharmacokinetic models of benzene disposition. *Toxicol. Appl. Pharmacol.*, 110:79–88.

10. Bopp, B. A., Sonders, R. C., and Kesterson, J. W. (1986): Toxicological aspects of cyclamate and cyclohexylamine. *CRC Crit. Rev. Toxicol.*, 16:213–306.

11. Bourgoignie, J. J., Hwang, K. H., Espinel, C., Klahr, S., and Bricker, N. S. (1972): A natriuretic factor in the serum of patients with chronic uremia. *J. Clin. Invest.*, 51:1514–1527.

12. Buss, N. E., and Renwick, A. G. (1992): Blood pressure changes and sympathetic function in rats given cyclohexylamine by intravenous infusion. *Toxicol. Appl. Pharmacol.*, 115:211–215.

13. Buss, N. E., Renwick, A. G., Donaldson, K. M., and George, C. F. (1992): The metabolism of cylamate to cyclohexylamate and its cardiovascular consequences in human volunteers. *Toxicol. Appl. Pharmacol.*, 115:199–210.

14. Buss, N. E., Tembe, E. A., Prendergast, B. D., Renwick, A. G., and George, C. F. (1994): The teratogenic metabolites of vitamin A in women following supplements and liver. *Human Exp. Toxicol.*, 13:33–43.

15. Butler, T. C. (1971): The distribution of drugs. In: *Fundamentals of Drug Metabolism and Drug Disposition*, edited by B. N. LaDu, H. G. Mandel, and E. L. Way, pp. 44–62. Williams & Wilkins, Baltimore, MD.

16. Caldwell, J., and Varwell Marsh, M. (1982): Metabolism of drugs by the gastrointestinal tract. In: *Presystemic Drug Elimination*, edited by C. F. George, D. G. Shand, and A. G. Renwick, pp. 29–42. Butterworth, Boston.

17. Campbell, D. B., and Ings, R. M. J. (1988): New approaches to the use of pharmacokinetics in toxicology and drug development. *Human Toxicol.*, 7:469–479.

18. Chan, K. K. H., and Gibaldi, M. (1985): Assessment of drug absorption after oral administration. *J. Pharm. Sci.*, 74:388–393.

19. Clinical implications of drug protein binding (1984): (Levy, R. and Shand, D., Eds). *Clin. Pharmacokinet.*, 9 (Suppl. 1):1–104.

20. Cocchetto, D. M., and Bjornsson, T. D. (1983): Methods for vascular access and collection of body fluids from the laboratory rat. *J. Pharm. Sci.*, 72:465–492.

21. Cohn, V. H. (1971): Transmembrane movement of drug molecules. In: *Fundamentals of Drug Metabolism and Drug Disposition*, edited by B. N. LaDu, H. G. Mandel, and E. L. Way, pp. 3–43. Williams & Wilkins, Baltimore, MD.

22. Colburn, W. A., and Matthews, H. B. (1979): Pharmacokinetics in the interpretation of chronic toxicity tests: The last-in, first-out phenomenon. *Toxicol. Appl. Pharmacol.*, 48:387–395.

23. Damian, P., and Raabe, O. G. (1996): Toxicokinetic modeling of dose-dependent formate elimination in rats: *In vivo-in vitro* correlations using the perfused rat liver. *Toxicol. Appl. Pharmacol.*, 139:22–32.

24. Davila, J. C., Rodriguez, R. J., Melchert, R. B., and Acosta, D. (1998): Predictive value of *in vitro* model systems in toxicology. *Annu. Rev. Pharmacol. Toxicol.*, 38:63–96.

25. Davison, C. (1971): Protein binding. In: *Fundamentals of Drug Metabolism and Drug Disposition*, edited by B. N. LaDu, H. G. Mandel, and E. L. Way, pp. 63–75. Williams & Wilkins, Baltimore, MD.

26. Despopoulos, A. (1965): A definition of substrate specificity in renal transport of organic anions. *J. Theor. Biol.*, 8:163–192.

27. Flamm, W. G., and Lorentzen, R. J. (1987): The use of in vitro methods in safety evaluation. *In Vitro Toxicol.*, 1:1–3.

28. Gabrielsson, J., and Weiner, D. (1997): *Pharmacokinetic/Pharmacodynamic Data Analysis: Concepts and Applications*, 2nd ed. Swedish Pharmaceutical Society, Swedish Pharmaceutical Press, Sweden.

29. Garattini, S. (1987): Toxic effects of chemicals: Difficulties in extrapolating data from animals to man. *CRC Crit. Rev. Toxicol.*, 16:1–29.

30. Gardner, D. M., and Renwick, A. G. (1978): The reduction of nitrobenzoic acids in the rat. *Xenobiotica*, 8:679–690.

31. Garrett, E. R. (1978): Pharmacokinetics and clearance related to renal processes. *Int. J. Clin. Pharmacol.*, 16:155–172.

32. Gehring, P. J. (1979): Chemobiokinetics and metabolism. In: *Environmental Health Criteria. 6. Principles and Methods for Evaluating the Toxicity of Chemicals Part 1*, pp. 116–177. WHO, Geneva.

33. Gehring, P. J., and Young, D. J. (1978): Application of pharmacokinetic principles in practice. In: *Proceedings of the First International Congress on Toxicology. Toxicology as a Predictive Science*, edited by G. L. Plaa and W. A. M. Duncan, pp. 119–141. Academic Press, New York.

34. Gerlowski, L. E., and Jain, R. K. (1983): Physiologically based pharmacokinetic modelling: Principles and application. *Pharm. Sci.*, 72:1103–1127.

35. Gibaldi, M., and Perrier, D. (1974): Route of administration and drug disposition. *Drug Metab. Rev.*, 3:185–199.

36. Gibaldi, M., and Perrier, D. (1982): *Pharmacokinetics*, 2nd ed. Marcel Dekker, New York.

37. Goldstein, A., Aranow, L., and Kalman, S. M. (1974): *Principles of Drug Action: The Basis of Pharmacology*. John Wiley, New York.

38. Gonzalez, F. J., and Korzekwa, K. R. (1995): Cytochrome P450 expression systems. *Annu. Rev. Pharmacol. Toxicol.*, 35:369–390.

39. Grene-Lerouge, N. A. M., Bazin-Redureau, M. I., Debray, M., and Scherrmann, J. M. G. (1996): Interspecies scaling of clearance and volume of distribution for digoxin-specific Fab. *Toxicol. Appl. Pharmacol.*, 138:84–89.

40. Guy, R. H., Hadgraft, J., and Maibach, H. I. (1984): Percutaneous absorption in man: A kinetic approach. *Toxicol. Appl. Pharmacol.*, 78:123–129.

41. Hiles, R. A., and Birch, C. G. (1978): Non-linear metabolism and disposition of 3,4,4′-trichlorocarbanilide in the rat. *Toxicol. Appl. Pharmacol.*, 46:323–337.

42. Hirom, P. C., Millburn, P., and Smith, R. L. (1976): Bile and urine as complementary pathways for the excretion of foreign organic compounds. *Xenobiotica*, 6:55–64.

43. Hirom, P. C., Millburn, P., Smith, R. L., and Williams, R. T. (1972): Species variations in the threshold molecular-weight factor for the biliary excretion of organic anions. *Biochem. J.*, 129:1071–1077.

44. Houston, J. B., and Carlile, D. J. (1997): Prediction of hepatic clearance from microsomes, hepatocytes, and liver slices. *Drug Metab. Rev.*, 29:891–922.

45. Huang, C. H., Kimcera, R., Nassar, R. B., and Hussain, A. (1985): Mechanisms of nasal absorption of drugs. I. Physicochemical parameters influencing the rate of in situ nasal absorption of drugs in rats. *J. Pharm. Sci.*, 74:608–611.

46. Ito, K., Iwatsubo, T., Kanamitsu, S., Nakajima, Y., and Sugiyama, Y. (1998): Quantitative prediction of *in vivo* drug clearance and drug interactions from *in vitro* data on metabolism, together with binding and transport. *Annu. Rev. Pharmacol. Toxicol.*, 38:461–499.

47. Jepson, G. W., and McDougal, J. N. (1997): Physiologically based modeling of nonsteady state dermal absorption of halogenated methanes from an aqueous solution. *Toxicol. Appl. Pharmacol.*, 144:315–324.

48. Jollow, D. J., Mitchell, J. R., Potter, W. Z., Davis, D. C., Gillette, J. R., and Brodie, B. B. (1973): Acetaminophen-induced necrosis II. Role of covalent binding in vivo. *J. Pharmacol. Exp. Ther.*, 187:195–202.

49. Kedderis, G. L., and Held, S. D. (1996): Prediction of furan pharmacokinetics from hepatocyte studies: Comparison of bioactivation and hepatic dosimetry in rats, mice and humans. *Toxicol. Appl. Pharmacol.*, 140:124–130.

50. Keen, P. M. (1971): Effect of binding to plasma proteins on the distribution, activity, and elimination of drugs. In: *Handbook of Experimental Pharmacology*, Vol. 28, edited by B. B. Brodie and J. R. Gillette, pp. 213–233. Springer–Verlag, New York.

51. Lake, B. G. (1997): *In vitro* methods. In: *Comprehensive Toxicology, vol. 9, Hepatic and Gastrointestinal Toxicology*, edited by R. S. McCuskey and D. L. Earnest, pp. 233–246. Pergamon Press, New York.

52. Langenberg, J. P., Spruit, H. E. T., van der Wiel, H. J., Trap, H. C., Helmich, R. B., Bergers, W. W. A., van Helden, H. P. M., and Benschop, H. P. (1998): Inhalation toxicokinetics of soman stereoisomers in the atropinized guinea pig with nose-only exposure to soman vapour. *Toxicol. Appl. Pharmacol.*, 151:79–87.

53. Lawrie, C. A., Renwick, A. G., and Sims, J. (1985): The urinary excretion of bacterial amino-acid metabolites by rats fed saccharin in the diet. *Food Chem. Toxicol.*, 23:445–450.

54. Lien, E. J., and Tong, G. L. (1973): Physicochemical properties and percutaneous absorption of drugs. *J. Soc. Cosmet. Chem.*, 24:371–384.

55. Light, H. G., Witmer, C., and Vars, H. M. (1959): Interruption of the enterohepatic circulation and its effects on rat bile. *Am. J. Physiol.*, 197:1330–1332.

56. Lindup, W. E. (1975): Drug-albumin binding. *Biochem. Soc. Trans.*, 3:635–640.

57. Mann, S., Droz, P.-O., and Vahter, M. (1996): A physiologically based pharmacokinetic model for arsenic exposure. *Toxicol. Appl. Pharmacol.*, 140:471–486.

58. McDougal, J. N., Jepson, G. W., Clewell, H. J., and Andersen, M. E. (1985): Dermal absorption of dihalomethane vapours. *Toxicol. Appl. Pharmacol.*, 79:150–158.

59. McKenna, M. J., Zempel, J. A., Madrid, E. O., and Gehring, P. J. (1978): The pharmacokinetics of [^{14}C]vinylidene chloride in rats following inhalation exposure. *Toxicol. Appl. Pharmacol.*, 45:599–610.

60. Mesfin, G. M., Higgins, M. J., Robinson, F. G., and Zhong, W.-Z. (1996): Relationship between serum concentrations, hemodynamic effects, and cardiovascular lesions in dogs, treated with minoxidil. *Toxicol. Appl. Pharmacol.*, 140:337–344.

61. Meyer, M. C., and Guttman, D. E. (1968): The binding of drugs by plasma proteins. *J. Pharm. Sci.*, 57:895–918.

62. Mitchell, J. R., Jollow, D. J., Potter, W. Z., Davis, D. C., Gillette, J. R., and Brodie, B. B. (1973): Acetaminophen-induced hepatic necrosis. I. Role of drug metabolism. *J. Pharmacol. Exp. Ther.*, 187:185–194.

63. Mitchell, J. R., Jollow, D. J., Potter, W. Z., Gillette, J. R., and Brodie, B. B. (1973): Acetaminophen-induced hepatic necrosis. IV. Protective role of glutathione. *J. Pharmacol. Exp. Ther.*, 187:211–217.

64. Mordenti, J. (1985): Pharmacokinetic scale up: Accurate prediction of human pharmacokinetic profiles from animal data. *J. Pharm. Sci.*, 74:1097–1099.

65. Munro, A. M. (1990): Interspecies comparisons in toxicology: The utility and futility of plasma concentrations of the test compound. *Reg. Toxicol. Pharmacol.*, 12:137–160.

66 Ochsenfahrt, H., and Winne, D. (1972): Solvent drag influence on the intestinal absorption of basic drugs. *Life Sci.*, 11:1115–1122.

67. Olinga, P., Merema, M., Hof, I. H., de Jong, K. P., Slooff, M. J. H., Meijer, D. K. F., and Groothuis, G. M. M. (1997): Effect of human liver source on the functionality of isolated hepatocytes and liver slices. *Drug Metab. Disp.*, 26:5–11.

68. Piafsky, K. M., Borga, O., Odar-Cedelof, I., Johansson, C., and Sjoqvist, F. (1978): Increased plasma protein binding of propranolol and chlorpromazine mediated by disease-induced elevations of plasma α_1 acid glycoprotein. *N. Engl. J. Med.*, 299:1435–1439.

69. Pierce, C. H., Dills, R. L., Morgan, M. S., Nothstein, G. L., Shen, D. D., and Kalman, D. A. (1996): Interindividual differences in $^2H_8$-toluene toxicokinetics assessed by a semi-empirical physiologically based model. *Toxicol. Appl. Pharmacol.*, 139:49–61.

70. Ploemen, J.-P. H. T. M., Wormhoudt, L. W., Haenen, G. R. M. M., Oudshoorn, M. J., Commandeur, J. N. M., Vermeulen, N. P. E., de Waziers, I., Beaune, P. H., Watabe, T., and van Bladeren, P. J. (1997): The use of human *in vitro* metabolic parameters to explore the risk assessment of hazardous compounds: The case of ethylene dibromide. *Toxicol. Appl. Pharmacol.*, 143:56–69.

71. Potter, W. Z., Davis, D. C., Mitchell, J. R., Jollow, D. J., Gillette, J. R., and Brodie, B. B. (1973): Acetaminophen-induced hepatic necrosis. III. Cytochrome P450-mediated covalent binding in vitro. *J. Pharmacol. Exp. Ther.*, 187:203–210.

72. Renwick, A. G. (1982): First pass metabolism within the lumen of the gastrointestinal tract. In: *Presystemic Drug Elimination*, edited by C. F. George, D. G. Shand, and A. G. Renwick, pp. 3–28. Butterworth, Boston.

73. Renwick, A. G. (1985): The disposition of saccharin in animals and man—a review. *Food Chem. Toxicol.*, 23:429–435.

74. Renwick, A. G. (1986): Gut bacteria and the enterohepatic circulation of foreign compounds. In: *Microbial Metabolism in the Digestive Tract*, edited by M. J. Hill, pp. 135–153. CRC Press, Boca Raton, FL.

75. Renwick, A. G. (1991): Safety factors and establishment of acceptable daily intakes. *Food Addit. Contamin.*, 8:135–150.

76. Renwick, A. G. (1993): Data derived safety factors for the evaluation of food additives and environmental contaminants. *Food Addit. Contamin.*, 10:275–305.

77. Renwick, A. G., and Sweatman, T. W. (1979): The absorption of saccharin from the rat urinary bladder. *J. Pharm. Pharmacol.*, 31:650–652.

78. Rescigno, A., and Segre, B. (1966): *Drug and Tracer Kinetics*, Blaisdell, London.

79. Riegelman, S., and Collier, P. (1980): The application of statistical moment theory to the evaluation of in vivo dissolution time and absorption time. *J. Pharmacokinet. Biopharm.*, 8:509–534.

80. Riegelman, S., Loo, J. C. K., and Rowland, M. (1968): New method for calculating the intrinsic absorption rate of drugs. *J. Pharm. Sci.*, 57:918–928.

81. Roberts, A., and Renwick, A. G. (1985): The effect of saccharin on the microbial metabolism of tryptophan in man. *Food Chem. Toxicol.*, 23:451–455.

82. Roberts, A., and Renwick, A. G. (1985): The metabolism of ^{14}C-cyclohexylamine in mice and two strains of rat. *Xenobiotica*, 15:477–483.

83. Roberts, A., and Renwick, A. G. (1988): The fate of cyclohexylamine in rat and mouse in relation to testicular toxicity. *Human. Toxicol.*, 7:229.

84. Roberts, A., and Renwick, A. G. (1989): The pharmacokinetics and tissue concentrations of cyclohexylamine in rats and mice. *Toxicol. Appl. Pharmacol.*, 98:230–242.

85. Rowland, M., and Tozer, T. N. (1980): *Clinical Pharmacokinetics: Concepts and Applications*. Lea & Febiger, Philadelphia.

86. Rowland, M., and Tucker, G. (eds.) (1986): *Pharmacokinetics: Theory and Methodology*, Pergamon Press, New York.
87. Rowland, M., Benet, L. Z., and Graham, G. G. (1973): Clearance concepts in pharmacokinetics. *J. Pharmacokinet. Biopharm.*, 1:123–136.
88. *Saccharin: Technical Assessment of Risks and Benefits* (1978): Institute of Medicine, National Research Council–National Academy of Science, Washington, DC.
89. Sanzgiri, U. Y., Kim., H. J., Muralidhara, S., Dallas, C. E., and Bruckner, J. V. (1995): Effect of route and pattern of exposure on the pharmacokinetics and acute hepatoxicity of carbon tetrachloride. *Toxicol. Appl. Pharmacol.*, 134:148–154.
90. Sauerhoff, M. W., Braun, W. H., Blau, G. E., and Gehring, P. J. (1976): The dose-dependent pharmacokinetic profile of 2,4,5-trichlorophenoxyacetic acid following intravenous administration to rats. *Toxicol. Appl. Pharmacol.*, 36:491–501.
91. Scheline, R. R. (1973): Metabolism of foreign compounds by gastrointestinal microorganisms. *Pharmacol. Rev.*, 25:451–523.
92. Scheuplein, R. J., Shoaf, S. E., and Brown, R. N. (1990): Role of pharmacokinetics in safety evaluation and regulatory decisions. *Annu. Rev. Pharmacol. Toxicol.*, 30:197–218.
93. Schoenig, G. P., Goldenthal, E. I., Geil, R. G., Frith, C. H., Richter, W. R., and Carlborg, F. W. (1985): Evaluation of the dose response and in utero exposure to saccharin in the rat. *Food Chem. Toxicol.*, 23:475–490.
94. Shen, S. K., Williams, S., Onkelinx, C., and Sunderman, F. W. (1979): Use of implanted minipumps to study the effects of chelating drugs on renal ^{63}Ni clearance in rats. *Toxicol. Appl. Pharmacol.*, 51:209–217.
95. Sims, J., and Renwick, A. G. (1983): The effects of saccharin on the metabolism of dietary tryptophan to indole, a known cocarcinogen for the urinary bladder of the rat. *Toxicol. Appl. Pharmacol.*, 67:132–151.
96. Sims, J., and Renwick, A. G. (1985): The microbial metabolism of tryptophan in rats fed a diet containing 7.5% saccharin in a two-generation protocol. *Food Chem. Toxicol.*, 23:437–444.
97. Smith, D. A. (1979): Differences in toxicity due to species variation in the metabolism of an oral antiallergy agent. *Br. J. Pharmacol.*, 66:422P–423P.
98. Smith, J. W. (1965): Observations on the flora of the alimentary tract of animals and factors affecting its composition. *J. Pathol. Bacteriol.*, 89:95–122.
99. Smith, R. L. (1973): *The Excretory Function of Bile. The Elimination of Drugs and Toxic Substances in Bile*. Chapman & Hall, London.
100. Solomon, S. (1977): Developmental changes in nephron number, proximal tubular length and superficial glomerular filtration rate of rats. *J. Physiol. (Lond.)*, 272:573–589.
101. Spurling, N. W., and Carey, P. F. (1992): Dose selection for toxicity studies: A protocol for determining the maximum repeatable dose. *Human Exp. Toxicol.*, 11:449–457.
102. Strong, H. A., Renwick, A. G., and George, C. F. (1984): The site of reduction of sulphinpyrazone in the rabbit. *Xenobiotica*, 14:815–826.
103. Su, K. S. E., Campanale, K. M., and Gries, C. L. (1984): Nasal drug delivery system of a quaternary ammonium compound: Clofilium tosylate. *J. Pharm. Sci.*, 73:1251–1254.
104. Sweatman, T. W., and Renwick, A. G. (1979): Saccharin metabolism and tumorigenicity. *Science*, 205:1019–1020.
105. Sweatman, T. W., and Renwick, A. G. (1980): The tissue distribution and pharmacokinetics of saccharin in the rat. *Toxicol. Appl. Pharmacol.*, 55:18–31.
106. Taylor, A. E., and Gaar, K. A. (1970): Estimation of equivalent pore radii of pulmonary capillary and alveolar membranes. *Am. J. Physiol.*, 218:1133.
107. Tembe, E. A., Honeywell, R., Buss, N. E., and Renwick, A. G. (1996): All-*trans*-retinoic acid in maternal plasma and teratogenicity in rats and rabbits. *Toxicol. Appl. Pharmacol.*, 141:456–472.
108. Travis, C. C., Quillen, J. L., and Arms, A. D. (1990): Pharmacokinetics of benzene. *Toxicol. Appl. Pharmacol.*, 102:400–420.
109. Upton, R. A. (1975): Simple and reliable method for serial sampling of blood from rats. *J. Pharm. Sci.*, 61:112–114.
110. Veng-Pedersen, P., and Gillespie, W. (1985): The mean residence time of drugs in the systemic circulation. *J. Pharm. Sci.*, 74:791–792.
111. Wagner, J. G. (1975): Do you need a pharmacokinetic model and, if so, which one? *J. Pharmacokinet Biopharm.*, 3:457–478.
112. Wagner, J. G. (1975): *Fundamentals of Clinical Pharmacokinetics*. Drug Intelligence Publications, Hamilton, Illinois.
113. Wang, X., Santostefano, M. J., Evans, M. V., Richardson, V. M., Diliberto, J. J., and Birnbaum, L. S. (1997): Determination of parameters responsible for pharmacokinetic behavior of TCDD in female Sprague-Dawley rats. *Toxicol. Appl. Pharmacol.*, 147:151–168.
114. Waynforth, H. B. (1980): *Experimental and Surgical Technique in the Rat*. Academic Press, New York.
115. Weiner, I. M. (1967): Mechanisms of drug absorption and excretion: The renal excretion of drugs and related compounds. *Annu. Rev. Pharmacol.*, 7:39–56.
116. Weiner, I. M. (1971): Excretion of drugs by the kidney. In: *Handbook of Experimental Pharmacology*, vol. 28, edited by B. B. Brodie and J. R. Gillette, pp. 329–353. Springer–Verlag, New York.
117. Wilkinson, G. R. (1976): Pharmacokinetics in disease states modifying body perfusion. In: *The Effect of Disease States on Drug Pharmacokinetics*, edited by L. Z. Benet, pp. 13–32. American Pharmaceutical Association, Academy of Pharmaceutical Sciences, Washington, DC.
118. Wilkinson, G. R. (1987): Clearance approaches in pharmacology. *Pharmacol. Rev.*, 39:1–47.
119. Withey, J. R. (1978): Pharmacokinetic principles. In: *Proceedings of the First International Congress on Toxicology. Toxicology as a Predictive Science*, edited by G. L. Plaa and W. A. M. Duncan, pp. 97–117. Academic Press, New York.
120. Worboys, P. D., Bradbury, A., and Houston, J. B. (1994): Kinetics of drug metabolism in rat liver slices. Rates of oxidation of ethoxycoumarin and tolbutamide, examples of high- and low-clearance compounds. *Drug Metab. Disp.*, 23:393–397.
121. Worboys, P. D., Bradbury, A., and Houston, J. B. (1996): Kinetics of drug metabolism in rat liver slices. II. Comparison of clearance by liver slices and freshly isolated hepatocytes. *Drug Metab. Disp.*, 24:676–681.
122. World Health Organization (1986): Principles of toxicokinetic studies. In: *Environmental Health Criteria*, Vol. 57. WHO, Geneva.
123. World Health Organization (1987): Principles for the safety assessment of food additives and contaminants in food. In: *Environmental Health Criteria*, Vol. 70. WHO, Geneva.
124. Yacobi, A., Skelly, J. P., and Batra, V. K. (eds.) (1989): *Toxicokinetics and New Drug Development*. Pergamon Press, New York.
125. Zhang, L., Brett, C. M., and Giacomini, K. M. (1998): Role of organic cation transporters in drug absorption and elimination. *Annu. Rev. Pharmacol. Toxicol.*, 38:431–460.

Principles and Methods of Toxicology,
Fourth Edition, edited by A. Wallace Hayes.
Taylor & Francis, Philadelphia © 2001.

Chapter 5

Physiologically Based Pharmacokinetic Modeling in Toxicology

Kannan Krishnan and Melvin E. Andersen

Pharmacokinetic modeling deals with the development of mathematical descriptions of the time-course of chemical concentration in biota. The temporal change in the concentration of a chemical in blood and tissues of an exposed organism is the net result of its absorption, distribution, metabolism, and excretion. Two commonly used compartmental pharmacokinetic models are:

(a) data-based, and
(b) physiologically based.

The data-based pharmacokinetic models correspond to mathematical equations that describe the available data on the temporal change in the blood or tissue concentration of a chemical in the animal species of interest (see the chapter by Renwick). This procedure considers the organism as a single homogeneous compartment or as a multi-compartmental system with elimination occurring in specific compartments of the model (106,276). The number, behavior, and volume of these hypothetical compartments are estimated by the type of equation chosen to describe the data, and not necessarily by the physiological characteristics of the organism in which the blood/tissue concentration data were acquired.

These data-based pharmacokinetic models can be used for interpolation, but they should not be used for extrapolation outside the range of doses, exposure routes, and species used to generate data for constructing these models. To use the data-based models to describe the pharmacokinetic behavior of a chemical administered at various doses by different routes, extensive animal experimentation would be required to generate similar blood-time course data under respective conditions. Even within the same species of animal, the time-dependent nature of critical biological determinants of disposition (e.g., tissue glutathione depletion and resynthesis) cannot easily be included or evaluated with the data-based pharmacokinetic modeling approach. Further, due to the lack of actual anatomical, physiological, and biochemical realism, these data-based compartmental models cannot easily be used in interspecies extrapolation, particularly to predict pharmacokinetic behavior of chemicals in humans. These various extrapolations, which are essential for the conduct of dose-response assessment of chemicals, can be performed more confidently with a physiologically based pharmacokinetic modeling approach. This chapter presents the basic principles and methods of physiologically based pharmacokinetic (PBPK) modeling as applied to the study of toxicologically important chemicals.

PBPK modeling refers to the development of mathematical descriptions of the uptake and disposition of chemicals based on quantitative interrelations among the critical biological determinants of these processes. These determinants include partition coefficients, rates of biochemical reactions, and physiological characteristics of the animal species. The biological and mechanistic bases of the PBPK models enable them to be used, with limited animal experimentation, for extrapolation of the kinetic behavior of chemicals from high dose to low dose, from one exposure route to another, and from test animal species to people.

The development of PBPK models for volatile and gaseous anesthetics dates back to the research work of Haggard (112) who mathematically described the uptake of inhaled diethyl ether from a physiological perspective. Further developments in PBPK modeling with vapors were contributed by Kety (136) and Riggs (233), who provided mathematical descriptions of the kinetics of chemicals in the body based on parameters such as blood flow rates, tissue volumes, and chemical partitioning into tissues, and by Mapleson (178), who developed PBPK models for inert gases utilizing an electric analog. This electric analog approach was expanded by Fiserova-Bergerova (80) for describing the pharmacokinetic behavior of metabolized vapors and gases relying on numerical integration of mass balance equations. In the pharmaceutics area, PBPK modeling traces back to Teorell's pioneering work in the 1930s (258,259). Beginning in the early 1960s, scientists trained in chemical engineering also developed PBPK models of various drugs, particularly antineoplastic agents such as methotrexate, 5-fluorouracil, and cisplatin (18,42,77). Subsequently, the PBPK modeling approach has found extensive application in toxicology, particularly for conducting various extrapolations essential for the dose-response assessment of chemicals.

The development of PBPK models is initiated in four interconnected steps: model representation, model parameterization, model simulation, and model validation (Figure 5.1). *Model representation* involves the development of conceptual and mathematical descriptions of the relevant compartments of the animal as well as the exposure and metabolic pathways of the chemical. *Model parameterization* involves obtaining independent measures of the mechanistic determinants, such as physiological, physicochemical, and biochemical parameters, which are included in one or more of the PBPK model equations. *Model simulation* involves the prediction of the uptake and disposition of a chemical for defined exposure scenarios, using a numerical integration algorithm, a software program, and a computer. The

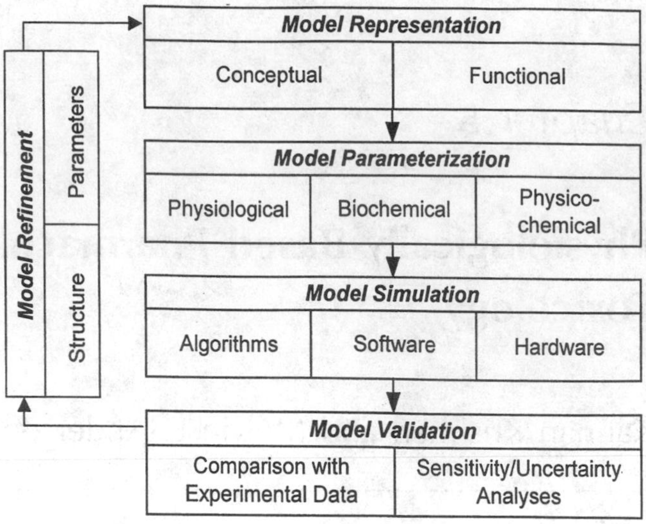

FIG. 5.1. Schematic of the steps involved in the development of physiologically based pharmacokinetic models.

model validation step involves the comparison of the a priori predictions of the PBPK model with experimental data to refute, validate, or refine the model description. PBPK models after appropriate testing or refinement and validation can be used to conduct extrapolations of the pharmacokinetic behavior of chemicals from one exposure route/scenario to another, from high dose to low dose, and from one species to another.

The PBPK model development for a chemical is preceded by the definition of the problem, which, in toxicology, may often be related to the apparently complex nature of toxicity. Examples of such apparently complex toxic responses include non-linearity in dose-response, sex/species differences in tissue response, differential response of tissues to chemical exposure, qualitatively and/or quantitatively different responses for the same cumulative dose administered by different routes/scenarios, and so on. In these instances, PBPK modeling studies can be utilized to evaluate the pharmacokinetic basis of the apparent complex nature of toxicity induced by the chemical. One of the values of PBPK modeling, in fact, is that accurate description of target tissue dose often resolves behavior that appears complex at the administered dose level.

The problem identification step is followed by the specification of the goal(s) of the PBPK modeling effort. At this stage, the integrated model development process begins with the model representation step.

MODEL REPRESENTATION

Model representation refers to the development of conceptual (i.e., diagrammatic) and mathematical descriptions of the relationships among system elements as they relate to system response of interest (e.g., tissue dose).

Conceptual Representation

This step involves the diagrammatic representation of the relevant anatomical and physiological features of the organism, and the uptake and disposition pathways of the chemical. The organism is represented as a network of compartments, each of which is physically, physiologically, and biochemically characterized. The pathways of uptake and disposition of chemicals are indicated by adding arrows to the appropriate compartments in the conceptual representation of the PBPK model. The conceptual representation of the PBPK model for a chemical requires an understanding of the anatomical and physiological characteristics of the test animal species, and the pathways of uptake and disposition of the chemical under study such that both the animal and the chemical can be represented adequately.

Representing the Animal

The diagrammatic representation of the organism (e.g., rat) should correspond to the real system; in other words, it should clearly show how the relevant individual compartments are placed and interconnected in the test organism (Figure 5.2).

In representing the animal system, the organism as a whole in terms of its body weight (e.g., 250 g for a rat) should be accounted for, so the mass balance of chemicals can be accurately maintained. More precisely, maintaining the mass balance in PBPK models requires that the total blood flow (i.e., cardiac output) in the model be equal to the sum of the flows to the tissue compartments of the model. In other words, the tissues that receive the chemical via blood flow need only be represented in the model. Further, it is not necessary to represent these tissues as individual compartments, and they may be lumped together as long as the total flow in the model is accounted for. The simplest conceptual model may consider the organism as a one-compartment system, whereas there is virtually no limit to the number of compartments in larger systems with more detailed representation of events at the cellular/molecular levels.

In addition, the necessity for representing a particular tissue as a separate compartment in a PBPK model is determined by whether its

(a) chemical,
(b) biochemical,
(c) physiological, a1.d/or
(d) anatomical characteristics contribute significantly to the uptake and disposition of the chemical being modeled.

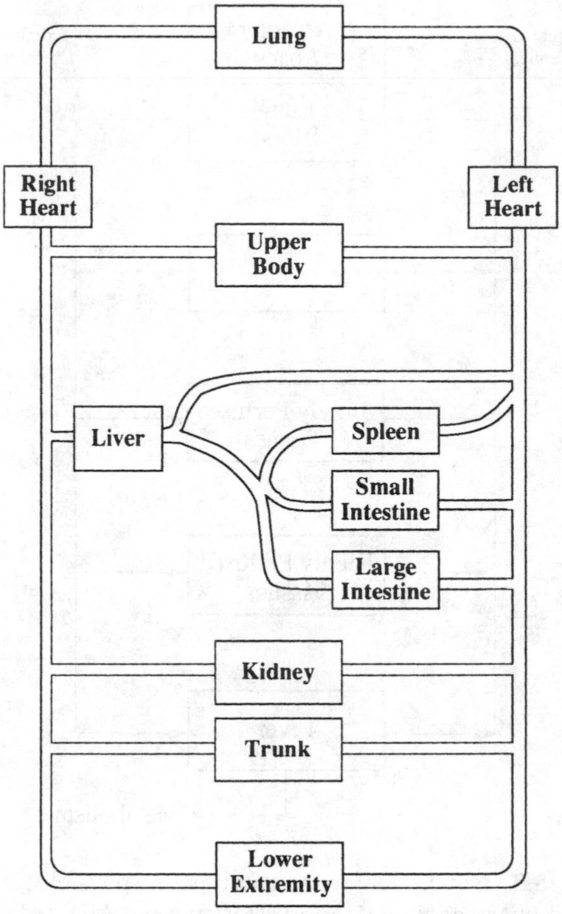

FIG. 5.2. Flow diagram for mammals. Adapted with permission from Reference 17.

The chemical composition of tissues in the present context refers primarily to the water and non-polar lipid contents. These tissue constituents are non-reactive but account for the differential solubility of a chemical among various tissues. In this respect, the adipose tissue is represented as a separate compartment in many PBPK models (Figure 5.3; fat) because of its ability to sequester lipophilic chemicals during exposure and release them after the cessation of exposure. In the case of a hydrophilic chemical, adipose tissue may be combined with the rest of the body since it may not show any particular kinetic behavior that is unique and different from the rest of the body. If other chemical components of the tissue (e.g., chloride levels or pH) are critical determinants of disposition, then individual or groups of tissue compartments defined with this kind of information should be included in the model as necessary.

The biochemical characteristics, in the present context, refer primarily to the binding and metabolizing capacities of the tissues. These properties account primarily for the removal of chemicals from the circulating blood by mechanisms other than chemical partitioning. For

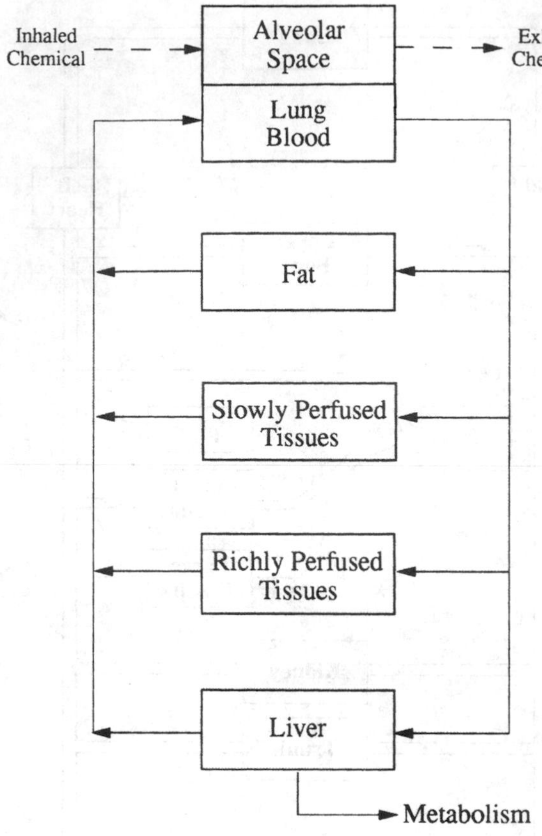

FIG. 5.3. Conceptual representation of a physiologically based pharmacokinetic model for styrene. Adapted with permission from Reference 223.

example, liver is often represented as a compartment in the PBPK models because of its central role in the metabolism of many organic chemicals. Representation of other tissues as separate compartments may be required according to the extent of expression of specific enzyme activities of relevance to the metabolism of the chemical being modeled (e.g., P450 and glutathione S-transferase in lung or kidney, epoxide hydrolase in testis, or myeloperoxidase in bone marrow).

The physiological characteristics refer to breathing rate, cardiac output, glomerular filtration rate, tissue blood flow rates, and so on. These characteristics essentially determine the biodisposition of chemicals. The tissue compartments possessing these properties (i.e., lung, heart, and kidney) or a quantitative description of these physiological processes should be included in the PBPK model. Respiration, urinary excretion, and blood circulation often are represented as quantitative descriptions of the processes themselves. Depending on the proposed use of the model, the tissues involved may be represented individually and characterized for particular aspects. For example, lung is represented as both an uptake and a metabolizing tissue in PBPK models for certain volatile organics (Figure 5.4), whereas it is not characterized separately in the case of nonvolatile organics which are neither eliminated by exhalation nor metabolized significantly by this tissue (Figure 5.5).

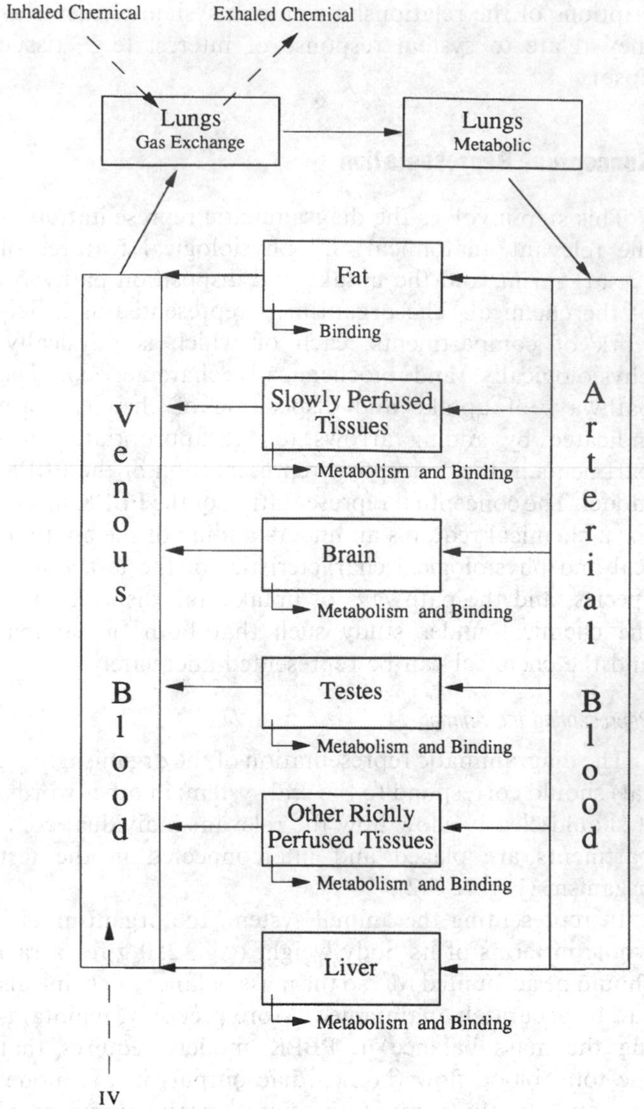

FIG. 5.4. Conceptual representation of a physiologically based pharmacokinetic model for ethylene oxide. Adapted with permission from Reference 151.

The anatomical location of certain tissues makes them particularly important for the uptake and elimination of chemicals. Lung, skin, and gastrointestinal tract serve as portals of entry for chemicals. According to their relevance and relative importance to the pharmacokinetics of a chemical, they should be included in PBPK descriptions. Target organs are included as separate compartments.

In principle, if the characteristic time constants of tissue disposition (i.e., the product of partition coefficient

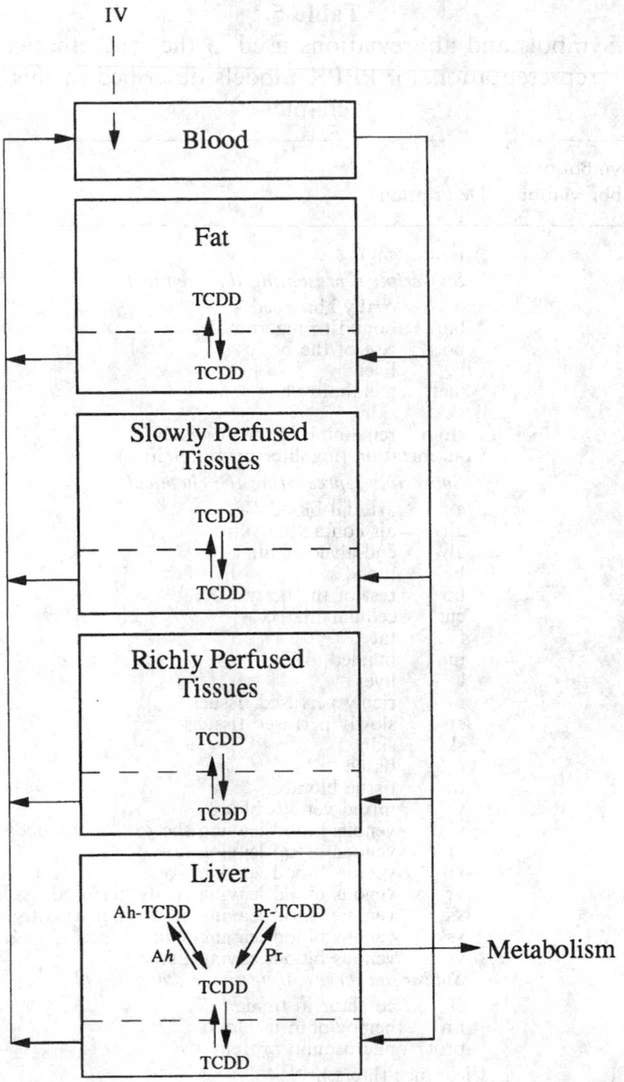

FIG. 5.5. Conceptual representation of a physiologically based pharmacokinetic model for 2,3,7,8-tetrachlorodibenzo-p-dioxin (TCDD). Pr, protein; Ah, Ah receptor. Adapted with permission from Reference 9.

and volume divided by blood flow rate) are similar for various tissues, they can be lumped together to form a single tissue group. In other words, when the critical determinants of pharmacokinetics do not vary quantitatively among several tissues, the time course of the chemical concentration in these tissues will be similar. That is why fat depots such as perirenal, epididymal, and omental fat are frequently grouped and represented as a single "fat" compartment (Figures 5.3–5.5). If necessary, a fat compartment may be subdivided into two or more groups according to the perfusion rates (e.g., inner and subcutaneous adipose tissues). Another example of this kind involves tissues such as adrenal, kidney, thyroid, brain, lung, heart, testis, and hepatoportal system, which often are pooled into one compartment and referred to as "richly perfused tissues" (Figures 5.3 and 5.5). When the contents of relevant metabolizing enzymes quantitatively differ among the richly perfused tissues, the individual organs are represented as separate compartments even though the blood flow rate and solubility characteristics are somewhat similar (Figure 5.4). Tissues with poor blood perfusion characteristics (muscle, skin) are frequently grouped as "slowly perfused tissues." Other groupings of tissues based on perfusion characteristics can also be defined, but this has not been done routinely.

Since the skeletal and structural components of the body have only a negligible perfusion and do not play a significant role in the disposition of many organic chemicals, they have not been included in the PBPK model descriptions for these chemicals. When describing certain metals and metalloids stored in bone, inclusion of this compartment is essential.

In PBPK models for organic and inorganic chemicals that are not stored to a significant extent in the skeletal/structural components of the body, approximately 91% of the body weight is represented by the tissue compartments included in the models (100% body weight minus 9% skeletal/structural component weight). In other words, 91% of the body weight is fractionated into the four, five, or nine compartments included in the models presented in Figures 5.3–5.5. In some models, blood is not described as a separate compartment (Figure 5.3 vs. Figure 5.4) even though blood concentrations are calculated. When blood is not described as a separate compartment, its total volume is apportioned among the tissues implicitly or explicitly.

Although PBPK models are mechanistically based and more detailed than the classical data-based pharmacokinetic models, they still represent a significant simplification of the true complexities of the biological systems. Model complexity and the number of compartments should not be equated with accuracy and usefulness of the model description; oftentimes model complexity yields a multitude of parameters to be estimated and greater uncertainty of the model description. Parsimony in PBPK modeling, on the other hand, refers to the choice of a model structure that has minimal but necessary elements that together adequately describe the pharmacokinetics of a chemical.

Representing the Chemical

The pathways of uptake, distribution, metabolism, and excretion of the chemical should also be conceptually represented in the PBPK model. The pathways of uptake are indicated by adding arrows to appropriate model compartments for representing the port of entry for each exposure route of interest (Figures 5.3–5.5). The interconnections among the individual tissue compartments of the conceptual model serve to represent the working hypothesis of the researcher regarding the distribution of the chemical in the organism. With respect to binding and metabolism, the specific pathways in each of the relevant tissue compartments should be identified/hypothesized so changes in parent chemical concentration and the formation and/or tissue distribution of the metabolite(s) can be followed. Even though there is not much uncertainty regarding the mechanistic basis of the absorption and distribution of chemicals, there are larger uncertainties regarding the importance, basis, and magnitude of specific aspects of binding to tissue macromolecules, metabolic pathways, and extra-hepatic metabolism. In such cases, the extent of metabolism or binding by a particular pathway may be included in the model structure and verified by specific model-directed experiments.

Once the tissue compartments of the animal and the pathways of uptake and disposition of a chemical are identified/hypothesized and conceptually represented, mathematical descriptions of pharmacokinetic processes are developed.

Mathematical Representation

This phase of the PBPK modeling process involves the development of mathematical representations of

(a) the quantitative interrelationships among the mechanistic determinants of the functions of each tissue compartment, and
(b) the interrelationships among the individual tissues.

The functional representation of a PBPK model requires a rudimentary knowledge of calculus. A brief review of basic mathematics and differential calculus required for pharmacokinetic modeling has been provided by O'Flaherty (192).

Prior to the development of mathematical descriptions of the various functions of the tissue compartments, it is essential to characterize them physicochemically, physiologically, and biochemically. The symbols and abbreviations that refer to these characteristics, in the mathematical representations of the PBPK models described in this chapter, are provided in Table 5.1.

In PBPK modeling, each tissue compartment is described with a mass balance differential equation (MBDE) that consists of a series of clearance terms as follows:

$$\frac{dA_t}{dt} = Cl_u C_a - Cl_e C_{vt} - Cl_m C_a - Cl_f C_a \quad (1)$$

Dimensionally, the units for each of the clearance terms is flow per time, that is L/h or ml/min.

Table 5.1
Symbols and abbreviations used in the mathematical representations of PBPK models described in this chapter

Symbol or abbreviation		Description
A		Amount (mg)
		Subscripts representing the chemical
	o	orally absorbed
	bm	bound to macromolecules
	bo	rest of the body
	i	liver
	met	metabolized
	sk	skin
	stom	remaining in the stomach
C		Concentration (mg/liter or mmol/liter)
		Subscripts representing the chemical
	a	arterial blood
	air	air contacting skin
	alv	end-alveolar air
	b	blood
	bo	rest of the body
	cm	cellular matrix
	f	fat
	inh	inhaled air
	l	liver
	r	richly perfused tissues
	s	slowly perfused tissues
	sk	skin
	t	tissue "t"
	tb	tissue blood
	v	mixed venous blood
	vbo	venous blood leaving the rest of the body
	vf	venous blood leaving fat
	vl	venous blood leaving liver
	vr	venous blood leaving richly perfused tissues
	vs	venous blood leaving slowly perfused tissues
	vsk	venous blood leaving skin
	vt	venous blood leaving tissue "t"
		Subscripts representing tissue components
	cf	cofactor in tissue "t"
	hb	hemoglobin in blood
	prot	microsomal protein
Cl		Clearance (liters hr^{-1})
		Subscripts
	e	efflux clearance
	f	functional clearance
	int	intrinsic clearance
	m	metabolic clearance
	u	uptake clearance
D_0		Oral dose of chemical (mg)
E		Hepatic extraction ratio
F		Tissue content (fraction of tissue weight)
		Subscripts
	lb	lipid in blood
	lt	lipid in tissue "t"
	nb	neutral lipid in blood
	nt	neutral lipid in tissue "t"
	nleb	neutral lipid equivalent in blood
	nlet	neutral lipid equivalent in tissue "t"
	pb	phospholipid in blood
	pt	phospholipid in tissue "t"
	wb	water in blood
	wt	water in tissue "t"
	web	water equivalent in blood
	wet	water equivalent in tissue "t"
F_{tiss}		Volume fraction of the tissue (g tissue/g body weight)
k		Transfer constant (liters hr^{-1})
K		Binding affinity constants or metabolic rate constants
		Subscripts representing affinity
	m	Michaelis–Menten affinity constant (mg/liter)

Table 5.1 (*continued*)

Symbol or abbreviation	Description	
	Subscripts representing reaction rates	
	f	first-order metabolism (hr^{-1})
	o	oral absorption (hr^{-1})
	p	skin permeability constant ($cm\ hr^{-1}$)
	s	second-order metabolism ($liters\ mg^{-1}\ hr^{-1}$)
K^0	zero-order infusion constant ($mg\ hr^{-1}$)	
n	Number of binding sites/protein molecule	
P	Partition coefficient	
	Subscripts	
	b	blood : air
	l : a	lipid : air
	o : a	n-octanol : air
	o : w	n-octanol : water
	s : a	skin : air
	s : b	skin : blood
	t	tissue : blood
	t : a	tissue : air
	w : a	water : air
PA_t	Permeation area cross product for tissue "t" ($liters\ hr^{-1}$)	
Q	Flow rate ($liters\ hr^{-1}$)	
	Subscripts	
	bo	blood flow to rest of body
	c	cardiac blood flow
	f	blood flow to fat
	l	blood flow to liver
	p	alveolar ventilation
	r	blood flow to richly perfused tissues
	s	blood flow to slowly perfused tissues
	sk	blood flow to skin
	t	blood flow to tissue "t"
S	Exposed skin surface area (cm^2)	
ss	Steady-state	
t	Elapsed time (hr)	
T_m	Apparent transport maximum of the carrier system ($mg\ hr^{-1}$)	
V	Volume (liters)	
	Subscripts	
	alv	alveolar
	b	blood
	cm	cellular matrix in a tissue
	t	tissue "t"
	tb	tissue blood
V_{max}	Maximal velocity of enzymatic reaction ($mg\ hr^{-1}$)	

Of the various clearance processes described above, the basic process that applies to all PBPK model compartments is chemical uptake, that is, inter- and intra-tissue transfers of chemicals. The uptake of a chemical by a tissue from the blood is described according to Fick's law of simple diffusion, which states that the flux of a chemical is proportional to its concentration gradient:

$$\text{Flux} = \frac{dC_t}{dt} = k\Delta C \tag{2}$$

For high molecular weight compounds, diffusion is often the rate-limiting process; therefore, their uptake through the tissue sub-compartments (Figure 5.6) must be considered. This requires that tissue blood and cellular matrix be described separately.

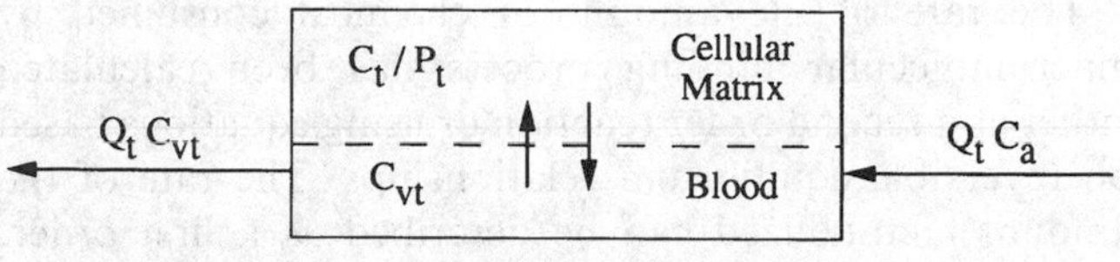

FIG. 5.6. Schematic of a tissue compartment. Q_t is tissue blood flow rate, C_a is arterial blood concentration, C_{vt} is the concentration of the chemical in the venous blood leaving tissue, C_t is the tissue concentration, and P_t is the tissue–blood partition coefficient.

The rate of change in the amount of chemical in cellular matrix is equal to the product of the diffusion rate constant and the net flux from tissue blood:

$$V_{cm}\frac{dC_{cm}}{dt} = PA_t\left(C_{vt} - \frac{C_t}{P_t}\right) \tag{3}$$

The rate of change in the tissue blood sub-compartment equals the sum of the net retention from blood flow plus the net flux from cellular matrix:

$$V_{tb}\frac{dC_{tb}}{dt} = Q_t(C_a - C_{vt}) + PA_t\left(\frac{C_t}{P_t} - C_{vt}\right) \tag{4}$$

If the diffusion of a chemical from tissue blood to cellular matrix is slow with respect to total tissue blood flow, both equations are necessary. On the other hand, if tissue blood flow (i.e., perfusion) is slow with respect to diffusion, tissues are described as homogeneous, well-mixed compartments such that the rate of change in the amount of chemical in the tissue is described with a single equation for the whole tissue mass [cellular matrix plus tissue blood, i.e., Eq. (3) plus Eq. (4)] as follows:

$$V_t\frac{dC_t}{dt} = Q_t(C_a - C_{vt}) \tag{5}$$

In the perfusion-limited tissue descriptions, the transfer constant is the rate of blood flow to the compartment and the effluent venous blood concentration (C_{vt}) is in equilibrium with the tissue concentration (C_t) as specified by the tissue–blood partition coefficient (P_t) such that $C_{vt} = C_t/P_t$.

When a tissue included in a PBPK model contributes to the clearance of the chemical by metabolism and macromolecular binding, the MBDE for that tissue becomes:

$$V_t\frac{dC_t}{dt} = [Q_t(C_a - C_{vt})] - \frac{dA_{met}}{dt} - \frac{dA_{bm}}{dt} \tag{6}$$

Rate of change in the amount of the chemical in the tissue = (blood flow × arteriovenous concentration difference) − rate of loss due to metabolism − rate of loss due to macromolecular binding.

The rate of the amount of chemical consumed by macromolecular binding process has been calculated either as a second order reaction or using equations based on reversible equilibrium relationships. The rate of the amount metabolized can be described as a first order, second order, or a saturable process as follows:

$$\frac{dA_{met}}{dt} = K_f C_{vt} V_t \tag{7}$$

$$\frac{dA_{met}}{dt} = K_s C_{vt} V_t C_{cf} \tag{8}$$

$$\frac{dA_{met}}{dt} = \frac{V_{\max} C_{vt}}{K_m + C_{vt}} \tag{9}$$

Conjugation reactions are traditionally described as a second order process (Equation 5.8) with respect to the concentration of the cofactor and the chemical (70,151). Alternatively, descriptions based on a ping-pong mechanism have also been used successfully (50).

The saturable [Eq. (9)] or first-order [Eq. (7)] metabolism descriptions presented above use the venous blood concentration, and appear to describe metabolism independent of the blood flow limitations. Once this equation becomes a part of Eq. (6), the blood flow limitation is accounted for. Alternatively, metabolism can be described using the following equation:

$$\frac{dA_{met}}{dt} = Q_l \times E \times C_a \tag{10}$$

Since $Q_1 \times E =$ hepatic clearance (L/h), the above equation represents the classical way of calculating the amount of chemical metabolized from knowledge of hepatic clearance and arterial blood concentration. Since $C_{v1} = C_a\ (1 - E)$, and $V_{\max}/K_m$ or $Cl_{int} = Q_l \times E/(1 - E)$, Eqs. (9) and (10) are mathematically equivalent (219).

In several PBPK models, the rate of metabolism has been calculated using Eq. (9) which uses the venous blood concentrations of chemicals (i.e., C_{vl}). This is equivalent to the venous equilibration model for hepatic metabolism. Other types of physiological descriptions of liver metabolism include the parallel tube model and the distributed sinusoidal perfusion model (234,235). The parallel tube model describes the flow of substrate through the sinusoids lined with enzymes, by considering them to be functionally homogeneous. On the contrary, however, the distributed sinusoidal model accounts for the functional heterogeneity among sinusoids by including statistical distributions of enzyme contents and sinusoidal blood flow (234). Although the distributed sinusoidal perfusion model is physiologically more realistic than the venous equilibration model, the latter simpler model may often be sufficient. Even though the predictions of tissue dose might vary in cases where the metabolizing organ alone is considered in isolation (237), the difference in predictions between these models might not be significant when considering the whole-body clearance of chemicals. A recent effort has produced a geometric multicompartmental description for liver, which can be used to simulate regional protein induction (2). The decision to use a multicompartmental liver depends on the objective and intended use of the model.

In perfusion-limited PBPK descriptions, the tissues that exhibit no significant capacity to bind or metabolize chemicals are described with the form of Eq. (5), and those tissues that exhibit significant binding and metabolic capacity are described as per Eq. (6). Thus, the basic form of equation representing chemical flux is the same for all tissues. In the case of metabolizing and eliminating tissues, however, additional terms are included to represent chemical loss due to specific biochemical processes. All tissue compartments receive the chemical via systemic arterial blood and lose the chemical via venous blood (Figures 5.3–5.5). The venous effluents of the various tissue compartments combine to yield a mixed venous concentration.

In PBPK models for volatile chemicals without a specific venous blood compartment, the mixed venous blood concentration has been calculated as follows (223):

$$C_v = \frac{\sum_t^n Q_t C_{vt}}{Q_c} \tag{11}$$

The above equation represents the steady-state solution of the MBDE for venous blood:

$$V_b(dC_b/dt) = \sum_t^n Q_t C_{vt} - C_v Q_c \tag{12}$$

The chemical in venous blood, on reaching the pulmonary compartment, may be exhaled or retained and further introduced into systemic arterial blood along with new chemical that is inhaled during the passage via the lungs. In PBPK models for some volatile chemicals, arterial blood has not been represented as a separate compartment and described with a MBDE, but, instead, described with the steady-state solution of the MBDE for the combined lung tissue-alveolar air compartments (223) as follows:

$$C_a = \frac{Q_p C_{inh} + Q_c C_v}{Q_c + \left(\frac{Q_p}{P_b}\right)} \tag{13}$$

The above algebraic expression is derived from the following mass conservation equation for lung, which specifies that the loss of chemical from the air is balanced by an identical gain of the chemical in the pulmonary blood:

$$Q_p(C_{inh} - C_{alv}) = Q_c(C_a - C_v) \quad (14)$$

Since the lung equilibrates vapor between alveolar air and blood, $C_{alv} = C_a / P_b$. This relationship assumes rapid equilibrium of the chemical across the alveolar walls, no significant metabolism by the lung tissue, and negligible storage capacity in the lungs. Pulmonary metabolism, in addition to uptake, can be included by describing both functions of the lung (151). The concentration of the chemical appearing in the systemic arterial blood is then affected by the pulmonary first-pass effects associated with metabolic processes (6,151). The types of mathematical descriptions used for calculating the rate of uptake following oral, iv, and dermal administrations are presented elsewhere (see below).

It is not essential to have both (arterial and venous) blood compartments or the lung compartment to provide venous-to-arterial interconnections for the tissues. The linkage can be done as well without a lung or a separate blood compartment (223). In these cases, the blood volume is not specified explicitly in the model but distributed implicitly among the tissues (223). However, in such descriptions it is not possible to calculate the amount of chemical in the blood compartment. Therefore, it is important to formulate the questions to be answered with the model during the "problem identification" step so a desirable model structure can be chosen.

PBPK models are based on various assumptions. Some may be reasonable, others might be questionable. Their appropriateness and accuracy should be verified experimentally. The experimentally obtained mechanistic data can then be used to accept, replace, or modify the assumptions/cmpirical descriptions included in the model. Some of the more general assumptions that apply to many PBPK models are (232):

(a) the mixing of the chemical in the effluent blood from the tissues is instantaneous and complete;
(b) blood flow is unidirectional, constant, and non-pulsatile; and
(c) the flow of chemicals through the blood is smaller than the blood flow, with the former not adding appreciably to the total flow.

In basic PBPK models, certain processes are considered together and described in simple mathematical terms; however, simplified terms can later be replaced with specific mechanistic details as relevant information becomes available. The level of mechanistic detail in the model description conforms to the intended use of the model. PBPK models, then, are of varying complexities according to the particular model's intended purpose (2). A list of toxicologically important chemicals for which PBPK models have been developed in one or more species is provided in Table 5.2. The following paragraphs provide examples of prototypical representations employed in PBPK models for diverse groups of chemicals.

Examples of Model Representations

Organic Chemicals

Volatile organics, lipophilic. The tissue uptake of low molecular weight, non-polar, volatile organic chemicals is a perfusion-limited process, whereas the inhalational uptake may either be blood flow- or ventilation-limited (223). The basic mathematical representation that is applicable to many members of this category is provided in Figure 5.7. In this example, the model consists of four tissue compartments—liver, fat, richly perfused tissue group, and slowly perfused tissue group—similar to the conceptual representation shown in Figure 5.3. Here the chemical input to the model results from the inspiration of the chemical in the inhaled air at a flow rate equal to the alveolar ventilation rate. The chemical in alveolar air is assumed to equilibrate very rapidly with arterial blood so that the concentration of chemical in arterial blood and in alveolar air leaving the lungs maintains a constant ratio specified by the blood–air partition coefficient (PC). Arterial blood, flowing at a rate equal to the cardiac output, is apportioned among liver, fat, richly perfused tissue, and slowly perfused tissue. Venous blood leaving each tissue compartment mixes simultaneously to yield the chemical concentration in the mixed venous blood returning to the lungs at a flow rate equal to cardiac output. In this example, tissue uptake of the chemical is assumed to occur rapidly and metabolism is assumed to occur only in the liver by a single saturable process. It is entirely possible that extrahepatic metabolism is important and that there is a need to estimate the total amount of a chemical in the blood (151). In such cases, the metabolic capacity of each tissue included in the model is characterized, and blood is included as a separate compartment and described explicitly (151).

Volatile organics, hydrophilic. In the models presented above, pulmonary uptake is represented by assuming that all the chemicals disappearing from the inspired air appear in the arterial blood and that the chemicals in alveolar air and arterial blood are in instantaneous equilibrium. In these descriptions, the conducting airways (i.e., nasal passages, larynx, trachea, bronchi, and bronchioles) are considered inert tubes that carry the chemical to the pulmonary region, where diffusion occurs. There is mounting evidence that this kind of a simple, continuous ventilation equilibration model is

Table 5.2
Environmental chemicals for which PBPK models have been developed in different mammalian species

Chemicals	Species[a]	References
Organic chemicals		
Acetone	H	154, 126
Acrylic acid	R, H	88
Acrylonitrile & cyanoethylene oxide	R	96, 134
Aldicarb	H	202
Benzene	R, M, H	20, 21, 60, 83, 182, 239, 248, 266
Benzo(a)pyrene	R	237
Benzoic acid	R	175
Bromochloromethane	R	95, 99, 181
Bromodichloromethane	R	166
Bromotrifluoromethane	H	271
Butadiene (1,3-) and metabolites	R, M, H	23, 50, 113, 129, 130, 143, 159, 255
Butanol (2-)	R	66
Butanol (tertiary)	R	24
Butoxyacetic acid (2-)	R, H	44
Butoxyethanol (2-)	R, M, H	44, 46, 125, 160, 247
Carbon tetrachloride	R	95, 98, 201, 245, 264
Chlordecone	R	27
Chlorobenzene	H	153
Chloroethane	R	98
Chloroform	R, M, H	45, 98, 104, 227, 250, 251
Chloromethane	R	98
Chloropentafluorobenzene	R, M, H, Mk	40, 48
Cyclohexane	H	207
Dibromomethane	R	95, 181
Dichloroethane (1,1-)	R	98
Dichloroethane (1,2-)	R, M	98
Dichloroethane (1,2-)	R	70
Dichloroethylene (1,1-)	R	69, 98, 99
Dichloroethylene (*cis* 1,2-)	R	98
Dichloroethylene (*trans* 1,2-)	R	15, 98
Dichlorophenoxyacetic acid (2,4-)	R, Rb	139, 140
Dieldrin	R, H	169
Diethylether	R, H	95, 126
Difluoromethane	R	71, 99
Diisopropylfluorophosphate	R, M	103
Dioxane (1,4-)	R, M, H	161, 229
Dioxin, chlorinated & brominated	R, M, H, Mk	9, 135, 158, 162–164, 238, 240, 277
Ethyl acrylic acid	R	89
Ethylene dibromide	R, H	210
Ethylene dichloride	R	70
Ethylene oxide	R	151
Furans	R, M, H	133, 141
Chlorofluorohydrocarbons	R, M, H, Ha	14, 99, 171–173, 271, 273
Heptafluoropropane	H	271
Hexachlorobenzene	H	90, 282
Hexachloroethane	R	94
Hexanedione (2,5-)	H	205, 206
Isopropene	R, M, H	79

Table 5.2 (*continued*)

Chemicals	Species[a]	References
Lindane	R	61
Methanol	R, M, H, Mk	117, 278
Methoxyacetic acid (2-)	M	36, 261
Methoxyethanol (2-)	M	36
Methyl chloroform	R, M, H	55, 93, 95, 157, 172, 230
Methyl *tertiary*-butyl ether	R	24
Methylene chloride	R, H	6, 8, 12, 98, 99, 181, 251
Methylethylketone	H	165
m-xylene	H, R	132, 156, 257
Naphtalene & naphtalene oxide	R, M	256
n-Hexane	H	205
Nicotine	R	211
Parathion	M	253
PCBs and PBBs	R, M, H, D, Mk	11, 174, 268, 269
p-chlorobenzotrifluoride	R, H	142
Pentachloroethane	R	94
Pentafluoroethane	H	271
Phthalate (diethylhexyl-)	R	137
Polychlorotrifluoroethylene	R	272
Pyrene	R	111
Styrene	R, M, H	8, 209, 223
Tetrachloroethane (1,1,1,2-)	R	94
Tetrachloroethane (1,1,2,2-)	R	94
Tetrachloroethylene	R, M, H, D	28, 29, 52, 53, 98, 144, 225, 229, 279
Tetrahydrofuran	H	68
Toluene	R, H	62, 156, 208, 257
Trichloroacetic acid	R, M, H	1, 82, 86, 87, 108
Trichloroethane (1,1,2-)	R	94, 93
Trichloroethylene and its metabolites	R, M, H	1, 15, 19, 54, 82, 85–87, 98, 108, 144, 157, 252
Trichloropropane (1,2,3-)	R	274
Trifluoroethane	R	172
Trifluoroiodomethane	H	271
Trimethylbenzene (1,2,4-)	H	124
Vinyl acetate	R	212
Vinyl chloride	R	15, 98
Vinyl fluoride	R	31
Inorganic chemicals		
Arsenic	R, H, M, Rb, Ha	176, 177, 283
Carbon dioxide	H	126
Carbon monoxide	R, H	5
Chromium	R	194
Fluoride	R, H	224
Lead	R	56, 193
Mercury, organic & inorganic	R, H, Mk	76, 102, 107
Nickel	R	183
Ozone	R, H, GP	185, 196
Zinc	R	123

[a] Rat (R), mice (M), human (H), monkey (Mk), dog (D), rabbit (Rb), hamster (Ha), guineapig (GP).

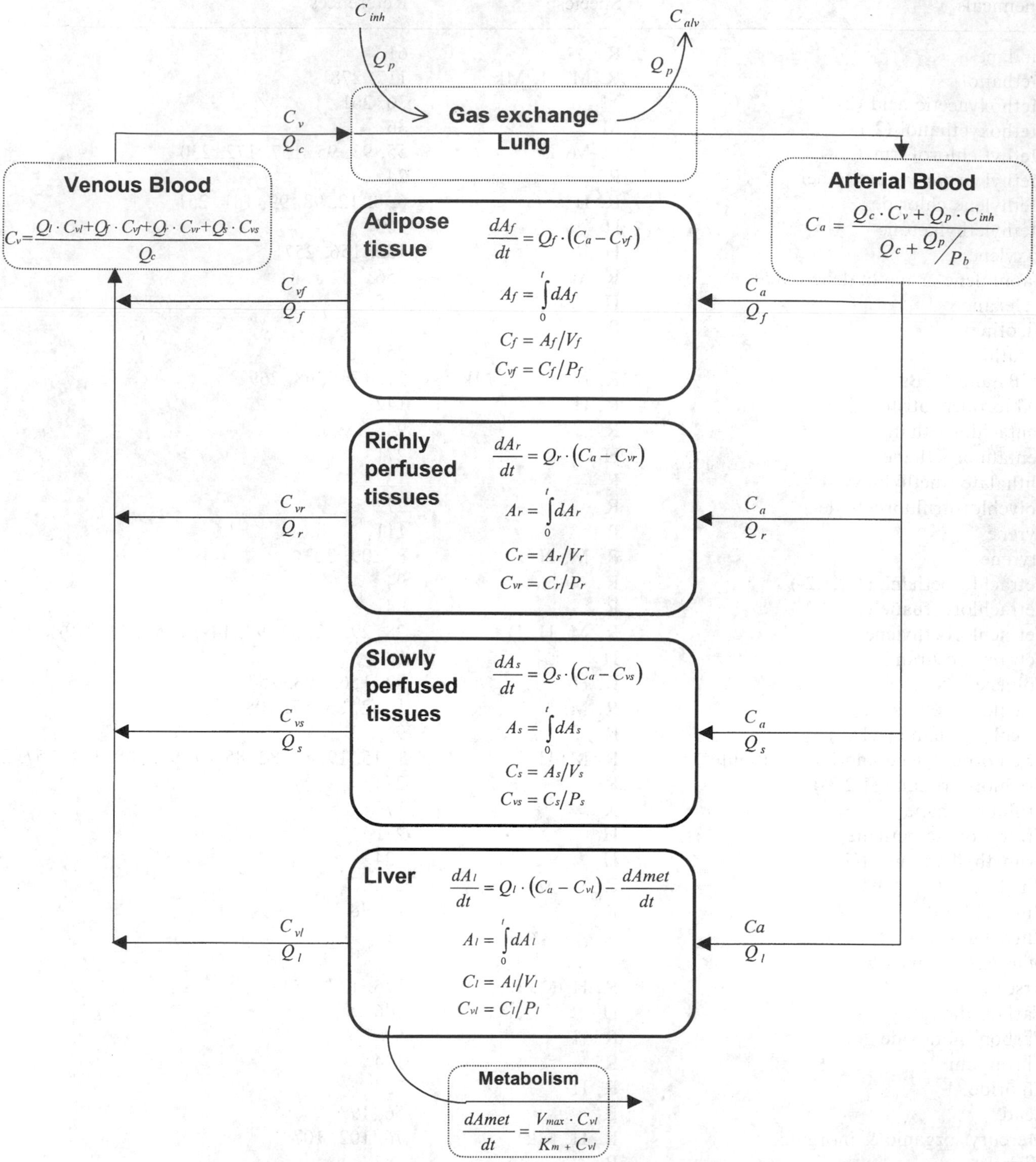

FIG. 5.7. A schematic of the PBPK model for styrene. In this model, the rat is represented as a four-compartment system interconnected by systemic circulation. The input for the system is the product of the inhaled concentration of styrene times the alveolar ventilation rate. The resulting arterial blood concentration is in turn provided as input to the tissue compartments, the effluent venous blood concentrations of which are provided as input for the calculation of mixed venous concentration. All abbreviations are defined in Table 5.1.

not predictive of either total respiratory uptake or regional uptake of highly soluble polar solvents (126). With these chemicals there are complex relationships between uptake and the blood–air partition coefficient. Further, several studies have shown that the total respiratory uptake is less than 100 percent as predicted by the continuous ventilation equilibration model (126). It has been suggested that the reduced pulmonary uptake of polar solvents is due to their adsorption and/or dissolution in the surface of the respiratory epithelium during inhalation, and their desorption during exhalation (126). This adsorption–desorption mechanism is a consequence of both the aqueous solubility of the chemicals and the cyclic nature of respiratory exchange.

PBPK models for polar solvents, then, include a description of the adsorption of vapors during inhalation and desorption during exhalation in addition to accounting for the anatophysiological characteristics of the respiratory tract, blood flow rates, and partition coefficients of the chemical (105,126). The PBPK model for polar solvents developed by Johanson (126) consists of nine serially connected central compartments, each one corresponding to an anatomical level of the respiratory tree. The first central compartment corresponds to the trachea and the last compartment to the alveolar region. Each of the central compartments corresponds to the airway and the outermost layer of mucus lining the airway wall. Radial diffusion of solvent from the outermost layer and deeper portions of the airway wall is accounted for by linking a peripheral compartment with each of the first eight compartments. The central compartment of the ninth and final region corresponds to the pulmonary or gas exchange region of the respiratory tract (respiratory bronchioles, alveolar ducts, and alveoli), the volume of which increases during inhalation and decreases during exhalation. The peripheral compartment of this ninth region represents the rest of the body, where immediate equilibrium between alveolar air and arterial blood is assumed. Either a single compartmental or a multi-compartmental physiological description can be used to account for chemical disposition in the body.

Nonvolatile organic chemicals, uncharged. PBPK models for nonvolatile organics describe chemical uptake as a diffusion-limited or a perfusion-limited process, and accommodate descriptions for chemical input via oral, dermal, intraperitoneal, and intravenous routes. These models typically consist of the following compartments: liver, fat, slowly perfused tissues, richly perfused tissues, and blood. Evidently, lung tissue or a description for pulmonary uptake is not included if its contribution to the overall kinetic behavior of the chemical is negligible (9). When there is evidence to the contrary, and, also, when there is evidence for pulmonary metabolism, lungs should be separated from the richly perfused tissues group and described as a separate compartment. In the case of diffusion-limited uptake description, each tissue compartment has a specified cellular matrix volume and tissue blood volume. The movement of a chemical from tissue blood into cellular matrix is described as being proportional to the permeation coefficient–surface area cross-product (PA_t) for the tissue (t). Tissue uptake is diffusion-limited when $PA_t < Q_t$. Binding to tissue macromolecules and other clearance processes are described as appropriate (9,135,240).

Nonvolatile organic chemicals, charged species. The distribution of water-soluble, charged species, such as weak acids and weak bases, is determined primarily by the pK_a of the compound and pH of the body fluids. The tissue uptake of these chemicals can be defined by the conventional flow-limited exchange between plasma/blood and tissues, with partitioning being determined by the pK_a of the chemical and the pH of the body fluids in accordance with the Henderson–Hasselbach equation (195). The elimination of these chemicals is mainly via urine, and therefore time-course information on this process may be necessary to adequately describe the kinetics of excretion.

Inorganic Chemicals

Gases and vapors. For inorganic gases that do not interact with walls of the conducting airways, simple dosimetry descriptions similar to those discussed in the preceding sections have been employed (5,126). For reactive inorganic gases, however, simulation models should incorporate critical elements of local absorption in the lower respiration tract and reactions with the biological constituents (185,196). Typically, these dosimetry models use quantitative information on the physiology of the lower respiratory tract, i.e., ventilation parameters and varying airway dimensions during breathing cycle. Lung dimensions are taken into account by making use of the airway models, in which airways of the lower respiratory tract are represented by a sequence of sets of right circular cylinders. All cylinders in series corresponding to a particular generation are of the same size. The upper respiratory tract (if used) consists of pre-tracheal generations or sequential segments. For each generation, the simulation model requires the specification of the number of airways or segments and their diameters and lengths. Additionally, for the pulmonary region, the alveolar volume and the surface area for each generation are needed. Similarly, the surface area of each upper respiratory segment is included.

The processes of transport and chemical reactions are described with a series of partial differential equations. In the liquid lining, tissue, and blood compartments, where only the processes of molecular diffusion and chemical reactions are considered, the form of the equation is the same. In the lumen of the airway and in the alveolar air spaces, axial convection, axial dispersion, the loss of chemical to the liquid lining, and lung expansion and contraction are taken into account. With quantitative information on the boundary conditions, initial conditions, and the physical, chemical, and biological parameters, these equations are solved to simulate dose and dose patterns. In this case, computational requirements are greater than those associated with the simpler PBPK models discussed above. More recently, a hybrid computational fluid dynamics and PBPK model has been constructed to estimate the regional tissue dose of organic acids in rodent and human nasal cavity (88).

Metals. The functional description used in PBPK models for metals is basically similar to that for organics; however, the common assumptions of flow-limited tissue uptake and linear partitioning into tissues may not be applicable for some metals (191). Further, the systemic uptake of metals may be mediated by ion channels or carrier-mediated transport mechanisms, and metabolism may be limited to oxidation state transitions and alkylation/dealkylation reactions. In the PBPK models for metals, the uptake has been described as a diffusion-limited process in some tissues and as a flow-limited process in others, to obtain adequate fitting of the model to experimental data (123). Clearance associated with binding to subcellular proteins occurs to a greater extent in the case of metals. Another important phenomenon associated with certain metals is their storage in bone. The metals for which PBPK models have been developed include arsenic, nickel, lead, chromium, zinc, and mercury (Table 5.2).

MODEL PARAMETERIZATION

Model parameterization refers to obtaining independent measures of the mechanistic determinants, namely, physiological parameters, physicochemical parameters, and biochemical rate constants, which are included in one or more of the PBPK model equations.

Physiological Parameters

Physiological parameters included in most PBPK models include alveolar ventilation rate, cardiac output, tissue blood flow rates, and tissue volumes. Additional parameters (e.g., tissue DNA levels, hematocrit) may be required in certain cases. The physiological parameters can generally be measured directly in the animal species of interest (33,67,120,236,244). For example, breathing rates can be measured with the use of a spirometer, plethysmograph, pneumotachograph, hotwire anemometer, or nonbreathing valves (179). Cardiac output has been determined from dye dilution curves using oximeters (65). Representative data from compilations of reference physiological parameters for laboratory animals and humans (13,26,57) are presented in Tables 5.3–5.5.

Physicochemical Parameters

The physicochemical parameters required for PBPK models refer primarily to the partition coefficients (PCs), which represent the relative distribution of a chemical between two phases at equilibrium. Partitioning between

Table 5.3
Reference physiological parameters for mice, rats, and humans[a]

Physiological parameters	Mouse	Rat	Human
Body weight (BW) (kg)	0.025	0.25	70.0
Tissue volume (fraction of BW)			
Liver	0.055	0.04	0.026
Fat	0.10	0.07	0.190
Richly perfused	0.05	0.05	0.05
Slowly perfused	0.70	0.75	0.62
Cardiac output (Qc) (liters/min)	0.017	0.083	6.20
Tissue perfusion (fraction of Qc)			
Liver	0.25	0.25	0.26
Fat	0.09	0.09	0.05
Richly perfused	0.51	0.51	0.44
Slowly perfused	0.15	0.15	0.25
Minute volume (liters/min)	0.037	0.174	7.50
Alveolar ventilation (liters/min)	0.025	0.117	5.00

[a] Reproduced with permission from Reference 265.

Table 5.4
Range of plausible values of the volume and perfusion of selected tissues in mice (26)

Tissue	Volume (% body weight)		Regional blood flow (% cardiac output)	
	Mean	Range	Mean	Range
Adipose	7.0	5–14[a]		
Brain	1.7	1.35–2.03	3.3	3.1–3.5
Heart	0.5	0.4–0.6	6.6	5.9–7.2
Kidneys	1.7	1.35–1.88	9.1	7.0–11.1
Liver	5.5	4.19–7.98	16.1	
Lungs	0.7	0.66–0.86	0.5	
Muscle	38.4	35.8–39.9	15.9	12.2–19.6
Skin	16.5	15.9–20.8	5.8	3.3–8.3

[a] Varies proportionately with body weight.

Table 5.5
Range of plausible values of the volume and perfusion of selected tissues in the rat (26)

Tissue	Volume (% body weight)		Regional blood flow (% cardiac output)	
	Mean	Range	Mean	Range
Adipose	7.0	4.6–12.0[a]	7.0	
Brain	0.6	0.38–0.83	2.0	1.5–2.6
Heart	0.3	0.27–0.40	5.1	4.5–5.1
Kidneys	0.7	0.49–0.91	14.1	9.5–19.0
Liver	3.4	2.14–5.16	18.3	13.1–22.1
Lungs	0.5	0.37–0.61	2.1	1.1–17.8
Muscle	40.4	35.4–45.5	27.8	
Skin	19.0	15.8–23.6	5.8	

[a] Varies proportionately with body weight.

two media (e.g., blood and air) as described by Henry's law for gases is a balance of the solubility of a chemical in the two media. PCs are represented as the ratio of the concentration of a chemical in the two media (e.g., blood : air, tissue : blood) at equilibrium. These physicochemical parameters are necessary to describe the tissue distribution of most uncharged xenobiotics as well as the pulmonary uptake of volatile organic chemicals. Several in vitro, in vivo, and animal replacement methods are available for estimating the PCs of chemicals.

In Vitro Methods

Vial equilibration. This in vitro method involves comparison of the equilibrium concentration of a chemical in the headspace of test vials containing tissues with empty/reference vials (81,97,100,127,242). The experimental procedure for determining the tissue : air and blood : air PCs of volatile organic chemicals by vial equilibration is given below:

1. Prepare a batch of 16 glass vials (volume ~25 ml) stoppered with Teflon septa. Transfer a measured quantity of raw ground tissue (e.g., 200 mg) or blood (e.g., 200 μl) into even-numbered vials. The odd-numbered empty vials are used as reference vials. All vials are placed in a shaker–incubator at 37°C.
2. Aerate the vials after a 5-min initial equilibration at 37°C, and cap them again.
3. Remove a predetermined volume of air (e.g., 0.5 or 1.0 ml) from each vial individually with a gas-tight syringe inserted through the septa, and replace it with an equal volume of air containing a known quantity of the chemical.
4. Draw a sample of headspace atmosphere (e.g., 1.0 ml) from one set of eight individual vials (four reference + four sample) at either of the sampling time points (e.g., 1 h and 2 hr).
5. The tissue : air (or blood : air) PCs is calculated as follows (97):

$$P_{t:a} = \frac{(C_{ref} V_{ref}) - [C_{sam}(V_{ref} - V_{sam})]}{C_{sam} V_{sam}} \tag{15}$$

where C_{ref} = chemical concentration in the headspace of reference vial, C_{sam} = chemical concentration in the headspace of sample vial, V_{ref} = volume of the reference vial, and V_{sam} = volume of sample.

If the $P_{t:a}$ values obtained at both time points are not significantly different from each other, they can be averaged and standard deviations calculated. If the $P_{t:a}$ values obtained at the later time point are significantly different from those obtained at the earlier time point, they are not considered to represent a true measure of solubility. An increase in $P_{t:a}$ values with incubation time indicates chemical reactions in the aqueous phase, and/or the non-attainment of equilibrium during the time points chosen for sampling. In such cases, additional experiments have been conducted to generate a time course of the distribution ratio to estimate $P_{t:a}$ by extrapolating to time 0 (151). Metabolic inhibitors may also be added in excess before introducing the chemical. The latter approach has been shown to eliminate chemical uptake by tissues due to specific and known reactions (e.g., glutathione conjugation) (89,103). On the other hand, if the calculated $P_{t:a}$ value decreases with incubation time, then deterioration of the tissue sample during incubation is likely; in such cases, headspace sampling for the determination of PCs should be conducted at earlier time points.

The tissue and blood samples do not have to be used as raw preparations in these experiments. Especially for chemicals with low solubility, the tissue and blood samples can be prepared as a 1 : 2 or 1 : 3 homogenate in saline (0.9% NaCl). The corresponding reference vials will contain saline alone. The $P_{t:a}$ value in this case is obtained using the following formula (97):

$$P_{t:a} = \frac{[C_{ref}(V_{ref} - V_{liq})] - [C_{sam}(V_{ref} - V_{liq} - V_{sam})] + [(C_{ref} - C_{sam})(V_{liq} P_{liq})]}{C_{sam} V_{sam}} \tag{16}$$

where V_{liq} = volume of the diluent liquid and P_{liq} = diluent liquid-air PC.

PCs for nonvolatile chemicals have been determined in vitro using equilibrium dialysis or ultrafiltration techniques.

Equilibrium dialysis. In this technique, the cell cavities are separated with dialysis membrane of desired molecular weight specifications. The experimental procedure consists of dialyzing the tissue homogenate or whole blood prepared in a buffer (e.g., Tris HCl, 0.1 M, pH 7.4) against the same buffer in a metabolic shaking bath (118,167,254). These experiments are conducted for several different initial concentrations of the chemical (radiolabeled + cold). Preliminary studies using different dialysis durations should be conducted to determine the time needed to attain equilibrium. At the end of the incubation, radioactivity in both the tissue and buffer is determined separately by liquid scintillation counting. The sum of the buffer and tissue radioactivity should account for all the radioactivity initially added to the dialysis cells. The unbound fraction of radioactive chemical in the tissue is determined by dividing the chemical concentration in buffer by the concentration in the tissue homogenate (167,168). The Pt values obtained from these experiments will be accurate only if the ratio of the bound to free form of chemical is constant over a wide range of concentrations.

Ultrafiltration. The ultrafiltration assembly consists of an ultrafiltration device, and a semipermeable membrane. In this approach, the tissue homogenates are spiked with a known amount of a chemical (radiolabeled + cold) and allowed to equilibrate for a predetermined time. Following equilibration, they are transferred into the reservoir portion of the ultracentrifugation device, placed in an angle rotor, and spun in a superspeed centrifuge. The concentrations of the chemical in the tissue homogenate and the buffer are determined and solved for the concentration of the chemical in the tissue (167).

The time and speed of ultracentrifugation should be determined for particular cases so that a desired volume of the ultrafiltrate is collected. Untreated tissues should be used to generate a protein-free ultrafiltrate for measuring the nonspecific binding onto the surface of the ultrafiltration device.

In Vivo Methods

Methods for estimating P_t values based on the analysis of data on blood and tissue concentrations of parent chemical after a single-bolus dose, or at steady-state condition following constant intravenous infusion or administration by other routes, have been published (35,91,92,155). P_t values have also been estimated from the slope of best-fit straight line with a unit slope drawn through the log–log plot of tissue concentration vs. blood concentration of the parent chemical for each tissue (59).

The steady-state approach will work only if the chemical is not removed by active binding/metabolic processes in one or more tissues. In this case where there is active tissue metabolism, the estimated P_t values tend to underestimate the true P_t values. Estimates of P_t for these tissues can be obtained if the amount of chemical consumed by the metabolic process is accounted for. Thus, for metabolizing tissues, the partition coefficients are determined after adjusting for clearance (35).

A potential problem associated with the determination of the PCs relates to the presence of residual blood in the tissues. The contamination of tissues with blood in the tissue vasculature might introduce errors in the estimated PCs. The importance of this problem has been investigated and the means of correcting these errors proposed (138).

Animal Replacement Approaches

Tissue : air partition coefficients. The partitioning of a chemical between two matrices can be predicted if its solubility and binding in each of the matrices can be estimated with reasonable accuracy. Using this basic premise, mechanistic animal replacement approaches for predicting tissue : air, blood : air, and tissue : blood PCs have been developed. Accordingly, the tissue : air PCs of low-molecular-weight VOCs, for which macromolecular binding is negligible, have been calculated as follows (74,200):

$$P_{t:a} = (P_{l:a} \times F_{lt}) + (P_{w:a} \times F_{wt}) \tag{17}$$

In the above equation, $P_{l:a} \times F_{lt}$ represents the partitioning of a chemical between the tissue lipids and air, and $P_{w:a} \times F_{wt}$ represents the partitioning between tissue aqueous phase and air. $P_{o:a}$ has been used as a predictor of $P_{l:a}$, and $P_{w:a}$ as a surrogate of chemical partitioning between tissue water and air (74,200). However, "tissue lipids" is too generic to represent the differential lipophilicity characteristics of neutral lipids (e.g., triglyceride) and polar lipids (e.g., phospholipid). Therefore, the partitioning of a chemical into neutral lipids and polar lipids may have to be considered separately. The physicochemical properties of phospholipids are dependent on the presence of a hydrophobic (e.g., glyceride) and hydrophilic (e.g., phosphomonoester) groups. Therefore, the use of $P_{o:a}$ or $P_{w:a}$ alone cannot adequately predict tissue phospholipid : air PCs. The partitioning of a chemical between tissue polar lipids (i.e., phospholipids) and air can be calculated as a fractional additive function of their partitioning into neutral lipids ($0.3 \times P_{o:a}$) and water ($0.7 \times P_{w:a}$). This approximation of chemical partitioning into tissue phospholipids is based on the assumption that the lipophilicity-hydrophilicity characteristics of tissue phospholipids is similar to that of commercial lecithin (220). Based on this working hypothesis, Poulin and Krishnan (216,217) have proposed the following equation to predict $P_{t:a}$ of volatile organic chemicals, considering separately the partitioning of chemicals into neutral lipid and polar lipid portions:

$$P_{t:a} = (P_{o:a} \times F_{nt}) + (P_{o:a} \times 0.3F_{pt}) + (P_{w:a} \times 0.7F_{pt}) + P_{w:a} \times F_{wt} \quad (18)$$

The above equation can be rewritten as:

$$[P_{t:a} = P_{o:a}(F_{nt} + 0.3F_{pt})] + [P_{w:a}(F_{wt} + 0.7F_{pt})] \quad (19)$$

In Eqs. (18) and (19), the partitioning of a chemical between tissue neutral lipids and air is assumed to correspond directly to $P_{o:a}$, while the partitioning between tissue water and air is assumed to correspond to $P_{w:a}$. Accordingly, $P_{t:a}$ can be calculated with knowledge of tissue composition data (F_{nt}, F_{pt}, F_{wt}), and physicochemical properties of chemicals ($P_{o:a}$ and $P_{w:a}$). Compilations of species-specific tissue composition data (72,216,217,220), $P_{o:a}$ and $P_{w:a}$ values of several VOCs at 37°C are available in the literature (97,200). To facilitate the use of $P_{o:w}$ values instead of $P_{o:a}$ values which are not readily available in the literature, Equation 19 can be rewritten as follows:

$$P_{t:a} = [P_{o:w}P_{w:a}(F_{nt} + 0.3F_{pt})] + [P_{w:a}(F_{wt} + 0.7F_{pt})] \quad (20)$$

Eq. (20) has been used to predict rat and human $P_{t:a}$ (liver, muscle, fat) of several alkanes, haloalkanes, and aromatic hydrocarbons (204,216–219,221). In general, the predicted $P_{t:a}$ values were within a factor of two of the experimentally determined PCs. For chemicals such as alcohols, acetate esters, and ketones, the values of rat and human fat : air calculated using Eq. (20) differed substantially from the experimental data (214,216,217). These results have been explained by the choice of the surrogate of biotic lipid used in Eq. (20). n-Octanol, being an alcohol, would appear to solubilize other alcohols to a greater extent than biotic neutral lipids. Based on its hydrophilicity–lipophilicity characteristics and its fatty acid composition, vegetable oil has been suggested as an acceptable alternative to n-octanol as a surrogate of biotic neutral lipids, especially for hydrophilic organics (214). Then, to predict $P_{t:a}$ of hydrophilic VOCs, especially for fatty tissues, $P_{o:w}$ in Eq. (16) should represent vegetable oil : water PCs. However, in the case of relatively lipophilic VOCs (log $P_{o:w} > 1.25$), there is little difference between the n-octanol : water PCs and vegetable oil : water PCs. Therefore, either one of these PCs can be used as the biotic lipid surrogate for solving Eq. (20) to predict tissue : air PCs of these chemicals (217).

Blood : air partition coefficients. Based on Eq. (20), Poulin and Krishnan (215,217) proposed the following equation for predicting P_b of VOCs that do not bind significantly to blood proteins:

$$P_b = [P_{o:w}P_{w:a}(F_{nlep})] + [P_{w:a}(F_{web})] \quad (21)$$

where F_{nlep} = neutral lipid equivalents, calculated as the sum of neutral lipids plus 0.3 × phospholipid content, and F_{web} = water equivalents, calculated as the sum of tissue water content plus 0.7 × phospholipid content.

Accordingly, P_b of VOCs can be calculated with the knowledge of blood composition data, $P_{o:w}$ and $P_{w:a}$. The data on lipid and water levels in rat and human blood are available in the literature (215) and so are the numerical values of $P_{o:w}$ and $P_{w:a}$ at 37°C for several VOCs (97,127,200) The predictions of rat P_b obtained using Eq. (21) are adequate for relatively hydrophilic organics (e.g., alcohols, ketones, acetate esters), but are not the case for relatively lipophilic organic chemicals (e.g., alkanes, haloalkanes, aromatic hydrocarbons). P_b of a chemical is a composite number that potentially represents two processes occurring in the blood, namely, solubility and binding. While chemical solubility is likely to be determined by the neutral lipid, phospholipid, and water contents in blood, the binding would appear to be associated with plasma proteins and/or hemoglobin. For alcohols, acetate esters, and ketones, rat and human P_b appear to be adequately predicted solubility-based algorithms [i.e., Eq. (21)] (215,217). For more lipophilic VOCs (e.g., alkanes, haloalkanes, aromatic hydrocarbons), however, the rat P_b calculated using Eq. (21) were lower (60–80%) than the experimental data (215,217). The fact that the rat P_b of lipophilic VOCs are under-predicted could be explained by the potential binding of these substances to blood proteins (215), a phenomenon not considered in Eq. (21). At the present time, there does not exist a validated animal replacement algorithm for predicting association constants for blood protein binding of organic chemicals.

Tissue : blood partition coefficients. Tissue : blood PCs of VOCs, for which macromolecular binding in tissue and blood is negligible, can be estimated from n-octanol : water PCs or vegetable : water PCs ($P_{o:w}$) using the following general equation (64,221):

$$P_t = \frac{(P_{o:w} \times F_{nlet}) + F_{wet}}{(P_{o:w} \times F_{nleb}) + F_{web}} \quad (22)$$

The numerator and denominator of Eq. (22) correspond to Eqs. (20) and (21) divided by $P_{w:a}$. In the case of VOCs then, P_t values can be obtained by dividing $P_{t:a}$ by P_b. The predictions of Eq. (22) will therefore be identical to the ratio of the predictions obtained using Eqs. (20) and (21) (214,217,220). In the above equation, the neutral lipid equivalent has in some cases been considered to be equivalent to total lipid content (74). The sum of $F_{nlet} + F_{wet}$ is not equal to 1 in most cases due to the presence of other tissue components such as

Table 5.6
Neutral lipid and water equivalent of major tissues in human and rat blood (221)

	Water equivalent		Neutral lipid equivalent	
Tissues	*Rat*	*Human*	*Rat*	*Human*
Blood	0.8423	0.8217	0.0020	0.0040
Fat	0.1215	0.1514	0.8536	0.7986
Liver	0.7176	0.7400	0.0425	0.0473
Muscle	0.7471	0.7573	0.0117	0.0378

proteins. This aspect should be appropriately considered while using the tissue composition data for calculating PCs of chemicals.

When the tissue : air, blood : air, and tissue : blood PCs of unionized organic chemicals are not known, Eqs. (20), (21), and (22) can be used to provide first-cut estimates. Since the tissue and blood composition data can be estimated experimentally or obtained from literature (Table 5.6), only the numerical values of the physicochemical properties are needed for each new chemical. The $P_{o:w}$ and $P_{w:a}$ of chemicals can be predicted from molecular structure information (217). An example of the prediction of tissue : blood PC from molecular structure information of 1,1,1-trichloroethane is presented in Figure 5.8. Semi-empirical methods relating molecular structure information to tissue : blood and blood : air PCs of chemicals may also be used as appropriate (64,198).

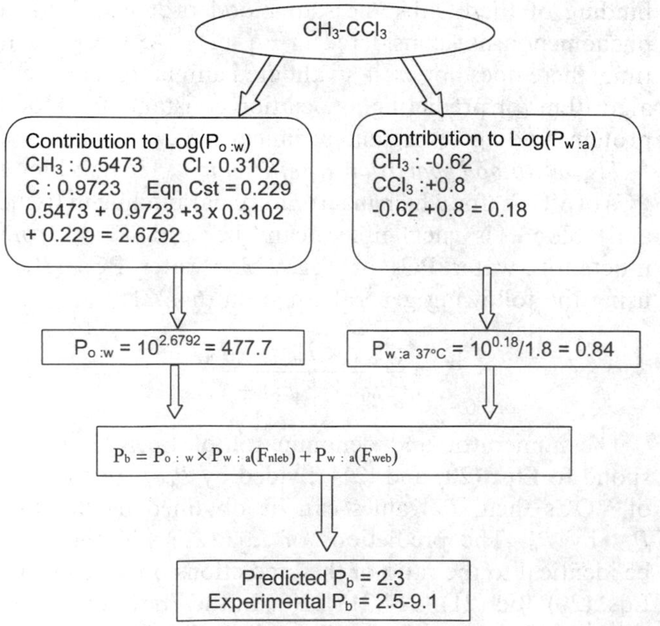

FIG. 5.8. Prediction of the human blood : air partition coefficient (P_b) of 1,1,1-trichloroethane from knowledge of its molecular structure, according to Reference 217.

Biochemical Parameters

Biochemical parameters such as the rates of absorption, biotransformation, macromolecular binding, and excretion can be determined by conducting time-course analysis in vivo or in vitro. One strategy for accurate estimation of specific biochemical parameters in vivo is to conduct experiments under conditions where pharmacokinetic behavior of a chemical is related to one or two dominant factors and thereby derive estimates of these parameters.

Thus, the rate constant for dermal absorption of VOCs has been determined by conducting body-only exposure of animals covered with a latex face mask. The total amount of the chemical absorbed through the skin during exposure is calculated by analyzing the blood-time course data collected during the exposure with a PBPK model that has all parameters except K_p defined. The value of K_p is estimated by fitting PBPK model simulations to the blood-time course concentration data obtained experimentally (180,181).

The skin permeability constant can also be determined in vitro using excised skin tissue. In these experiments, the test material is placed on excised skin in a vehicle and its appearance in the bathing medium determined (3). A plot of concentration in the bath vs. skin has a time lag, a period of increasing slope, and a final phase of constant slope (Figure 5.9). The plot of rate of uptake—the first derivative of this curve—gives the maximum uptake rate. The permeability uptake rate K_p (cm/hr) is calculated by

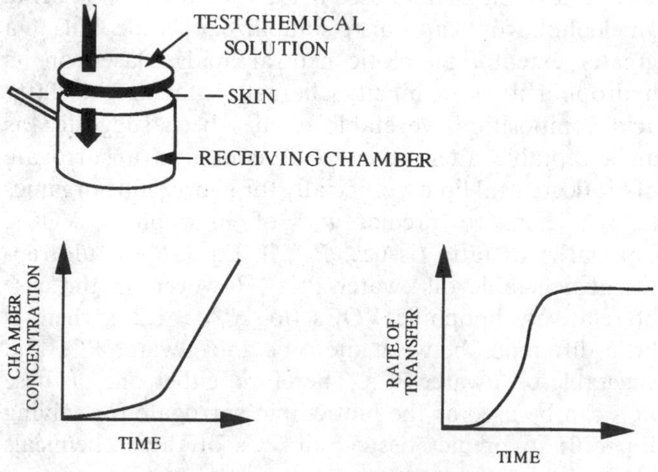

FIG. 5.9. Schematic representation of in vitro approaches to estimate skin permeability constants. Redrawn with permission from Reference 3.

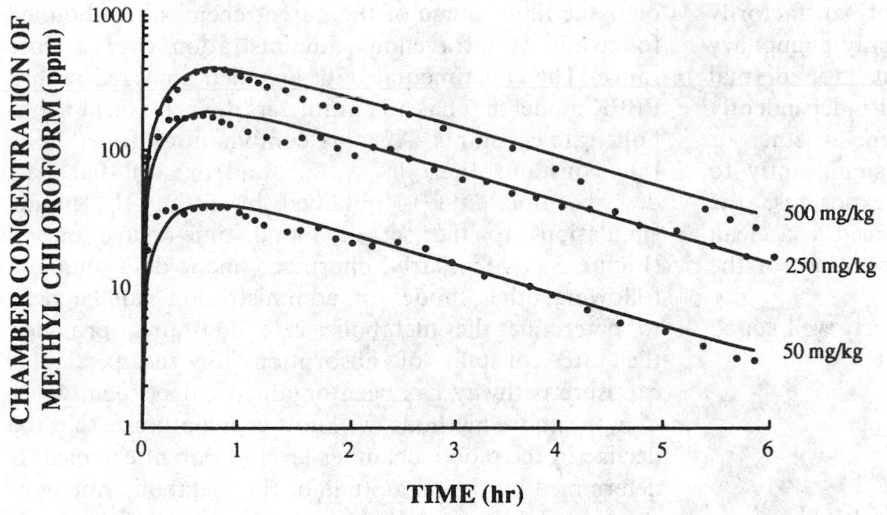

FIG. 5.10. Exhaled breath chamber time course for groups of four mice following oral dose of 50, 250, or 500 mg 1,1,1-trichloroethane/kg body weight. PBPK model simulations (solid lines) obtained using an oral absorption rate constant of 0.72 h^{-1} are compared with the experimental data (closed circles). Redrawn with permission from Reference 93.

dividing the uptake rate ($mg/cm^2/hr$) with applied concentration (mg/cm).

The rate constant for gastrointestinal absorption of volatile organics has been estimated by analyzing the time course of exhalation of the parent chemical after oral administration, with a PBPK model that had all parameters except K_o defined (Figure 5.10) (93). The estimation of the rate of gastrointestinal absorption for hydrophilic chemicals ($P_b > 90$) has been performed by determining the blood concentration following oral dosing and analyzing the data with a PBPK model that defined all parameters except K_o (87).

The rate constants for metabolism can be determined in vivo or in vitro. Two innovative noninvasive methods have been devised for the estimation of the in vivo metabolic rate constants of VOCs. These are

(a) the closed chamber or gas uptake method, and
(b) the exhaled breath chamber method.

The closed chamber or gas uptake method uses a desiccator-type chamber with a recirculating atmosphere for exposing groups of animals to volatile chemicals (7,78). This approach involves periodically monitoring the chamber concentration of a chemical during exposures. The rate of change in the chamber concentration of the chemical both in the absence and in the presence of animals is determined for various starting concentrations. The net difference in the rates determined in these two sets of experiments represents the loss of chemical due to uptake and metabolism by the animals. The rate of spontaneous loss of chemicals in the empty chamber, corresponding to degradation and/or adsorption to chamber surface, should not exceed ~2 percent per hour. Otherwise the decline in the chamber concentration may not be sensitive enough to enable the determination of metabolic rate constants. When animals are placed in the gas uptake chamber, the rate of decline in chamber concentration of the chemical increases, the magnitude being proportional to the rate of metabolism once the chemical has equilibrated within the organism.

The data analysis is conducted with a PBPK model that has all parameters defined except the metabolic rate constants (95). Initially, the PBPK model for closed chamber exposures is run for several starting concentrations with the metabolic rate constants set to 0 (i.e., $V_{max} = 0$, $K_f = 0$). The model simulations obtained at this stage reflect chemical uptake by the organism in the absence of tissue metabolism. Then, by setting the V_{max}, K_m, and K_f to some numerical values, it can be seen that the model simulations correspond to experimentally observed decline in chamber chemical concentrations. By optimization to get the best fit to the set of gas uptake curves, the values of metabolic rate constants are estimated. A single set of K_m and V_{max} obtained in these in vivo experiments has been considered to represent the role of a single isoenzyme, or the average of the sum of the activities of multiple enzymes. This method has been used successfully to obtain metabolic rate constants of VOCs that are biotransformed by a single first-order process, a saturable process, or a combination of both (6,98).

It is important to monitor the oxygen concentration, humidity level, and chamber pressure during gas uptake studies. Any change in the respiratory rate should be investigated so that modeling of gas uptake exposure provides reliable estimates of metabolic rates (51,128). Control gas uptake runs, during which naive animals are placed in the chamber without any added chemical, are necessary to ensure the absence of interfering chromatographic peaks of exhaled endogeneous chemicals.

Since the gas uptake studies involve whole-body exposures, there is a possibility for adsorption to fur and also dermal uptake. If dermal absorption is important, or if the PBPK model cannot satisfactorily simulate the chamber decline data with only pulmonary uptake description, then rate constants for dermal absorption process should be determined independently and included in the model. To determine whether or not adsorption to fur has contributed significantly to chemical uptake during whole-body exposures, the animals, after termination, should be placed in a clean chamber and the time course of the appearance of the chemical determined (94).

The gas uptake method is not particularly well suited for use with those organic chemicals that

(a) have low vapor pressure,
(b) exhibit high chamber loss rates, or
(c) are highly soluble in blood and tissue.

For example, in the case of a chemical with blood–air PC greater than 60, the equilibration phase may become prolonged, thus occupying most of the gas uptake curves. The behavior in these gas uptake curves is restricted largely to tissue uptake. In such cases, the metabolic rate constants have been assessed using an exhaled breath chamber (93,94).

The exhaled breath method involves placing an animal, previously exposed to a chemical, in a flow-through type of chamber and collecting samples of the chamber effluent for chromatographic analysis. Several exhaled breath samples are taken at periodic intervals during the experiment. The time intervals are chosen based on the appearance of the decay phase or whenever transitions in the elimination behavior are expected or observed. These curves are then analyzed with a PBPK model in which all parameters except metabolic rate constants are defined. The metabolic rate constants are estimated by obtaining an optimal fit of the PBPK model simulations to the exhaled breath curves.

Metabolic rate constants also have been determined by measuring the production of a stable metabolite resulting from the conversion of the parent compound in vivo (99). For a particular metabolite to provide a quantitative measure of metabolism of the parent chemical, it is ideal if it is produced in the first step of metabolism and is resistant to further biotransformation. Only very few metabolites exhibit these attributes. An example of this kind is bromide ion resulting from the initial metabolism of dibromomethane. This metabolite is distributed almost exclusively in the extracellular fluid spaces and is excreted slowly in the urine. In this case, the metabolic rate constants were estimated by fitting the simulations of a PBPK model that accounted for the formation, distribution, and excretion of bromide to experimental data on plasma bromide levels (99).

The blood time-course data obtained after intravenous administration also have been used to determine the rate constants of metabolism (229). Accordingly, the blood or tissue time course of the parent chemical is obtained following its intravenous administration over a dose range. The experimental data are then analyzed with a PBPK model that has all parameters defined except metabolic rate constants. A single combination of metabolic rate constants (i.e., V_{max}, K_m, and/or K_f) that best describes the data is obtained by fitting the model simulations to the set of blood time-course curves (Figure 5.11). Similarly, pharmacokinetic data obtained following other modes of administration can be used to determine the metabolic rate constants, provided the rate constant of absorption for the particular exposure pathway has been obtained independently.

In the above methods, we know or hypothesize that the decline in the blood/chamber level of parent chemical is determined by the magnitude of the metabolic rate constants, and that metabolism occurs via a single first-order, second-order, or saturable process, or via a combination of any two processes in a particular tissue. In the case of chemicals that are metabolized by more than two competing metabolic pathways to varying extents in several tissues, the gas uptake, exhaled breath chamber, or intravenous pharmacokinetic studies alone cannot be used to determine the rate constants for each of the multiple pathways occurring in several tissues. The use of these methods in this case will yield one set of rate constants that represent the overall metabolic clearance of the chemical (i.e., the sum total of metabolism via all metabolic pathways). Alternatively, if the rate constants for

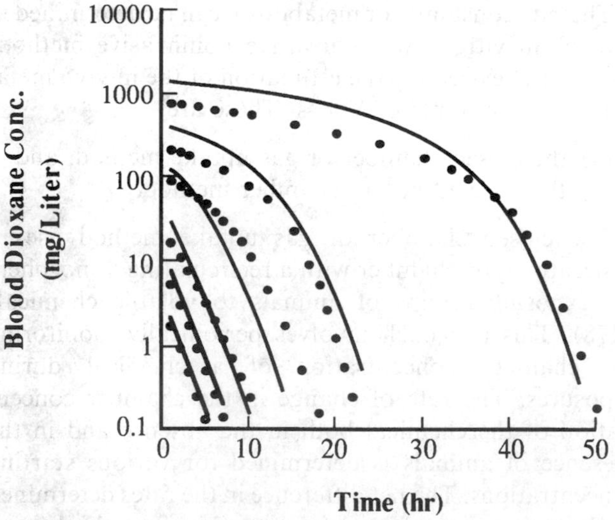

FIG. 5.11. Comparison of PBPK model simulations (solid lines) with the experimental data (symbols) of blood concentrations of 1,4-dioxane following intravenous dosing (3, 10, 30, 100, 300, and 1000 mg/kg). Model simulations were obtained using metabolic rate constants estimated by statistical optimization of the model fit to the experimental data. Redrawn with permission from Reference 229.

all metabolic pathways except one have been determined independently, then an intravenous dosing or a gas uptake study can be conducted to obtain the rate constants for this pathway (151). The rate constants for individual metabolic pathways can potentially be obtained from in vitro studies.

Subcellular fractions, postmitochondrial preparations, isolated cells, tissue slices, and isolated perfused organs are all potentially useful as in vitro systems for the estimation of metabolic rate constants (58,60,62,63,103, 116,121,167,170,186–188,228,231,241). The relevance of rate constants determined in vitro to the intact animal is not clear in all cases. However, several studies using microsomes, post-mitochondrial fractions preparations, or hepatocytes to determine metabolic rate constants for direct incorporation into PBPK models have successfully described the kinetics of volatile and nonvolatile organic chemicals (150). The K_m obtained in in vitro studies has been used directly [or scaled to reflect the in vitro/in vivo ratios in a test species (231)], but the $V_{\max}$ obtained in vitro has been scaled to the whole organism based on the mass recovery of the particular fraction. For example, the $V_{\max}$ for the intact animal has been estimated from the $V_{\max}$ obtained using rat liver microsomes as follows:

$$V_{\max\,(\text{in vivo})} = V_{\max\,(\text{in vitro})} \times 60 \times C_{prot} \times V_t \qquad (23)$$

where $V_{\max\,(\text{in vivo})}$ is expressed in mg/hr/kg, $V_{\max\,(\text{in vitro})}$ is expressed in mg/min/mg protein, 60 is the factor for converting the per-minute rate to per-hour rate, C_{prot} is the concentration of protein in the microsomal sample (mg protein/g tissue), and V_t refers to the volume of tissue (g).

Care must be taken to check the validity of the various in vitro systems to adequately predict the kinetics of chemicals in vivo (50). For example, the clearance of dichloromethane (DCM) by oxidative metabolism estimated in vitro using rat liver microsomes is lower than the actual clearance estimated by in vivo methods. The examination of the in vitro- and in vivo- derived rate constants for oxidative metabolism revealed that the $V_{\max}$ agreed well, but there are differences of up to four orders of magnitude in the K_m values between the two approaches. Use of these in vitro K_m values in a PBPK model would underestimate severely the amount of DCM metabolized via the oxidative pathway at low exposure concentrations (5). Such a description would have the oxidative pathway competing less efficiently with the glutathione (GSH) conjugation pathway, thus over-predicting the metabolite production via the GSH pathway. Products from the GSH pathway have been correlated with tumor outcome and this parameter misspecification would lead to substantial errors in assessing the carcinogenic risk associated with low-level DCM exposures (5).

The identification of in vitro systems for determining metabolic rate constants that give values consistent with those operative in vivo is crucial for eventually predicting human dosimetry. Recent studies indicate that freshly isolated hepatocytes are a better system that provides rate constants comparables to the in vivo estimates (e.g., 133). Other studies have succeeded in conducting extrapolations between in vitro metabolic systems, based on an understanding of biochemical principles at the quantitative level (e.g., Lipscomb et al. (170)). Our ability to predict metabolic rates from one in vitro system to another is a significant step forward in predicting the rate constants for the in vivo system.

Mechanistic animal-replacement approaches for predicting the numerical values of E, $V_{\max}$, K_m, or Cl_{int} of chemicals are not available yet. However, semi-empirical approaches relating the molecular structure information to PBPK model parameters such as PCs and metabolic rate constants have been developed (198,199,281). A major limitation of these approaches is that experimental data need to be collected before developing equations that consistently describe the relationship between molecular structure and PBPK model parameters. Truly predictive approaches can be developed only as our understanding of the biochemical processes improve. At the present, however, the hepatic extraction can be assumed to be complete or negligible in PBPK models in order to generate simulations. Accordingly, the numerical value of E in Eq. (10) should be set to 0 or 1 during the model simulations. The region encompassed by the simulated lines obtained with $E=0$ and $E=1$ will naturally contain the experimental data for that particular exposure scenario (e.g., Figure 5.12).

The rate constants of chemical reaction with hemoglobin and tissue proteins determined in vitro or in vivo, have been incorporated into the PBPK model to make predictions of these phenomena in vivo (89,151). Attempts also have been made to include receptor binding and DNA binding properties of chemicals into a PBPK modeling framework based on in vitro-derived data (77,260).

Some PBPK models, in which perfusion-limited tissue descriptions are used, may predict greater tissue uptake of chemicals than that which actually is observed. In such cases, tissue uptake is described as a diffusion-limited process and the mass transfer coefficient for each tissue is required. PA_t is estimated by fitting model simulations to experimental data on tissue concentration of the parent chemical by varying the numerical value of the PA_t term (9,59) (Figure 5.13).

Once the mathematical representation of a PBPK model is prepared and its parameters estimated, the model can be used to simulate the kinetic behavior of a chemical in the test species.

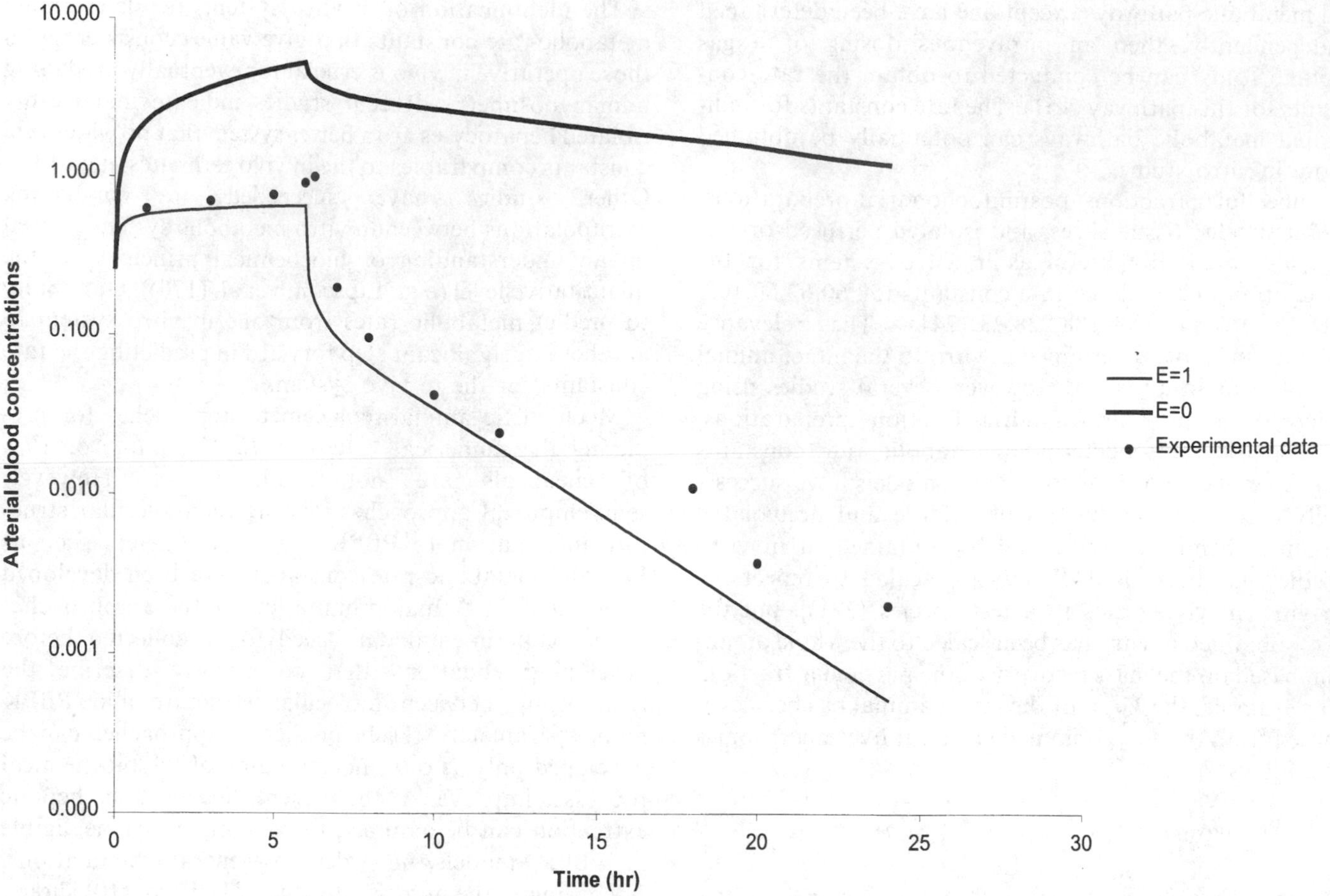

FIG. 5.12. Comparison of experimental data (closed circles) on arterial blood concentration with the envelope simulated by rat PBPK model for a 6-h exposure to 80 ppm styrene (solid lines). The upper line corresponds to the simulation obtained when the hepatic extraction was set to zero, and the lower line represents simulation obtained when the hepatic extraction ratio was set to 1. The experimental data were obtained from Reference 223.

MODEL SIMULATION

Simulation is the system behavior predicted by solving the differential equations representing the quantitative interrelations among the various model parameters. In the context of PBPK modeling, simulation refers to the prediction of the kinetic profiles of chemicals in blood and tissues by solving the set of MBDEs. Typically, simulation is chosen when:

(a) the real system does not exist,
(b) the real system exists but experimentation is expensive,
(c) a forecasting model is required to analyze events occurring over long periods of time in a compressed format, and
(d) the model does not have practical analytical solutions (e.g., stochastic models, nonlinear systems) (232).

Since PBPK models often contain differential equations and describe nonlinear processes, it is usually impractical to obtain analytical solutions and, therefore, a numerical simulation approach is adopted. For conducting computer simulations, the mathematical equations should be written in such a way as to facilitate their solution by a fixed, step-by-step procedure (i.e., algorithm).

Algorithms

Algorithms for simulation are chosen based primarily on the following criteria:

(a) thoroughness of the theoretical basis of the algorithm,
(b) self-starting capability,
(c) automatic control of step size and method order,

(d) ability to deal with both stiff and nonstiff problems and to detect stiffness automatically, and, finally,
(e) proof that the algorithm works for test problems of the same kind as the one(s) under consideration (232).

Some of the commonly used algorithms include those of Euler and Gear, Runge–Kutta routines, and predictor–corrector methods. The general principle underlying these algorithms used for solving first-order ordinary differential equations can be represented in simple terms as follows:

$$\text{New value} = \text{Old value} + (\text{slope} \times dt) \tag{24}$$

For a tissue compartment in PBPK model,

$$A_{t,1} = A_{t,0} + (dA_t/dt \times dt) \tag{25}$$

where dt is the integration interval or the predetermined length of time for which solution is obtained. Using the above algorithm, the numerical solution will approach the reality as long as the dt is prohibitively short. The specific form of the numerical solution represented in Eq. (25) is referred to as the Euler algorithm. In this method, the error arises from the negligence of the second- and other higher-order derivatives of the Taylor expansion series (110). In other words, the error associated with the Euler method is proportional to dt^2. Therefore, with the use of smaller dt values, the error associated with this first-order integration method can be minimized.

Some of the algorithms (e.g., Gear) and not others (e.g., Euler) can deal with stiff systems (101,110). The stiffness in models is reflected by the ratio (generally of several orders of magnitude) of the largest to the smallest time constant in the model. The stiffness requires that variable integration intervals be used as simulation progresses due to the compartments with the smallest time constants attaining steady-state condition gradually. The fact that the integration interval is not changed with the progression of simulation time, in accordance with the

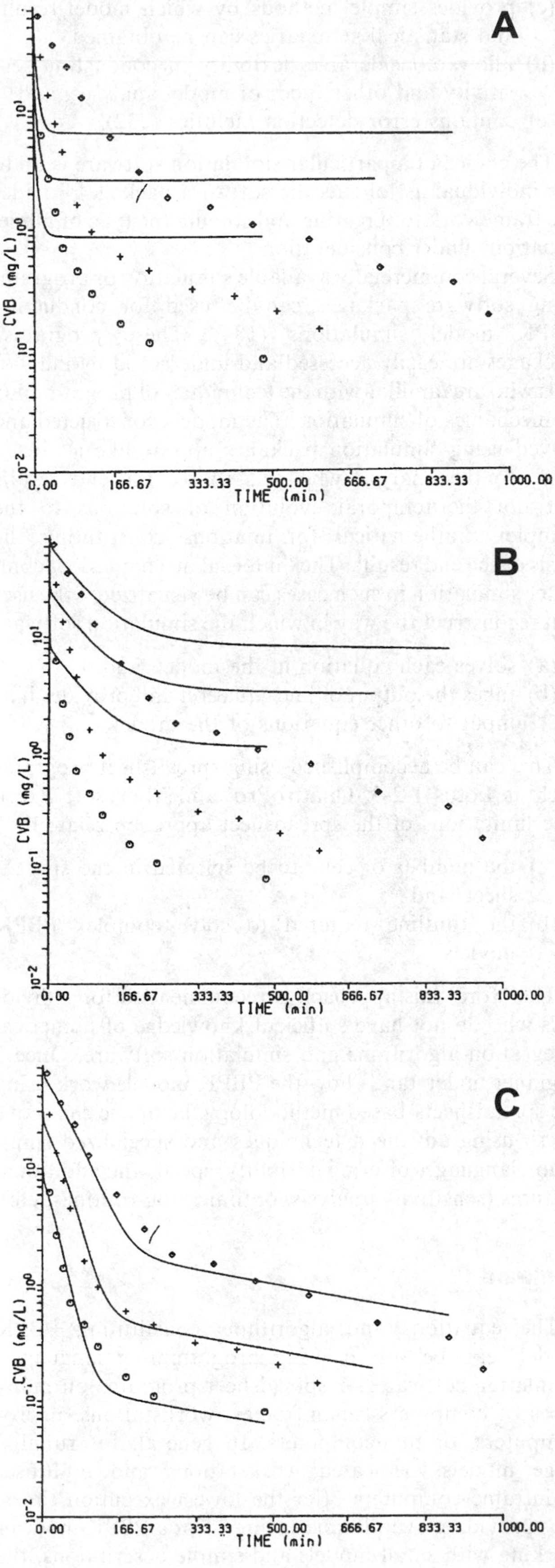

FIG. 5.13. Comparison of the experimental data (symbols) on the venous blood concentration of unchanged pyrene in rats with PBPK model simulations (solid lines). The simulations were obtained with a model that described uptake as a perfusion-limited process in all tissues (A), or as a diffusion-limited process in adipose tissues and slowly perfused tissues (B). With the additional description of metabolism in appropriate tissues, the PBPK model simulations correspond to the experimental data (C). The dose levels were 2,6,15 mg/kg (iv). Reproduced with permission from Reference 111.

existing stiffness state, represents only a disadvantage of the Euler algorithm taking a longer time to complete a given simulation. This is particularly because at steady-state conditions (at which $dAt/dt = 0$) larger integration intervals can be used, thus saving time without losing the accuracy of the simulation. The adequacy of the Euler algorithm for numerical integration of differential equations used in PBPK models has been demonstrated (110,131).

Software

The PBPK model equations, along with the integration algorithms, can be written and solved using programming languages, simulation software, or spreadsheets. In the first two cases, the style of computational representation of a model is determined by the grammatical and precedence rules of the programming language (FORTRAN, BASIC, etc.) or simulation language to be used. Simulation languages are computer programming packages that are general in nature but may have special features for modeling certain types of systems. Examples of simulation languages that possess features particularly useful for PBPK modeling are listed in Table 5.7. When selecting a particular simulation language for modeling, it is important to ensure that it

(a) provides a convenient means for initializing the status of the model (e.g., generating random numbers in case of stochastic models),
(b) permits the introduction of changes in both the status and temporal structure of the model as simulation time evolves (i.e., scheduling the occurrence of events),

Table 5.7
Examples of softwares used in PBPK modeling

Software	Source	Some references
ACSL	Pharsight Corporation, Mountain View, CA	52, 172, 223
	Aegis Research Corporation, Huntsville, AL	
D02EBF	NAG Library	190
Excel	Microsoft	110, 131
Matlab	MATLAB Manual, University of Manchester	222, 275
	Regional Computer Center, NAT 657	
ScoP	Simulation Resources, Inc., Berrien Springs, MI	145, 224
Simusolv	Dow Chemical, Midland, MI	29, 139, 273
	Mitchell and Gauthier Associates, Concord, MA	
STELLA	High Performance Systems, Inc., Hanover, NH	209

(c) provides simple methods by which model results and statistical summaries can be obtained,
(d) allows considerable flexibility in conducting sensitivity and other types of model analyses, and
(e) contains error detection facilities (232).

The choice of a particular simulation software is up to the individual as long as the software package provides the framework for creating and solving the type of model equations under consideration.

Several commercially available simulation or programming software packages can be used for conducting PBPK model simulations (184). These programs/packages are easily accessed and understood by individuals who are familiar with the techniques of programming or mechanics of simulation. The models constructed and solved using simulation packages appear like a "black box" to the analyst, who gets to see the end results but not the temporal evolution of solutions to the complex mathematical formulations constituting the basis of the end results. The "internal mechanics" of computer simulation in such cases can be visualized if the user can reconstruct the way in which the simulation software

(a) solves each equation in the model, and
(b) takes the output of one equation and provides it as input to other equations of the model.

This can be accomplished using spreadsheet programs such as Lotus 1-2-3, QuattroPro, and Microsoft Excel. The limitations of the spreadsheet approach relate to

(a) the number of cells to be selected in the spreadsheet, and
(b) the runtime required to solve complex PBPK models.

Therefore, this approach is recommended for individuals who do not have sufficient knowledge of numerical integration algorithms and simulation software. Once a beginner understands how the PBPK models work using the spreadsheets-based methodology, he or she can move on to using advanced techniques and specialized simulation languages offering flexibility, speed, and additional features (sensitivity analysis, optimization routines, etc).

Hardware

The equations and algorithms constituting PBPK models can be solved using programming languages, simulation software, or spreadsheet programs on many types of computers—mainframes, workstations, microcomputers, or minicomputers. In general, for running large models, dedicated workstations and multiuser mainframe computers offer the lowest execution times, thus providing overall time savings. For a PBPK modeler working with small models and simple descriptions, the

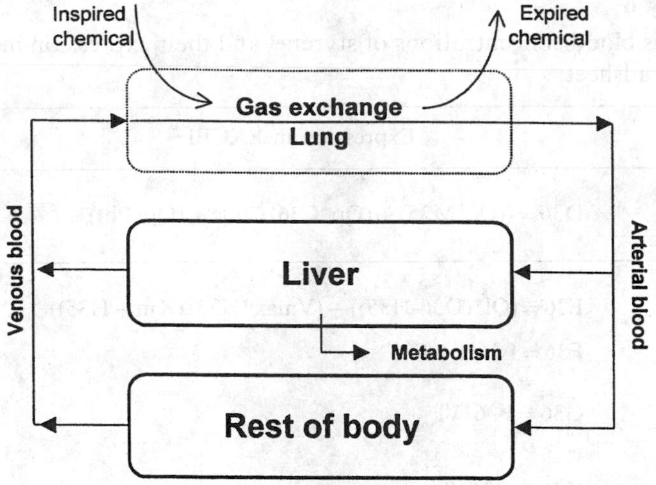

FIG. 5.14. Conceptual representation of a two-compartmental PBPK model for styrene in the rat.

Macintosh or IBM PC-based modeling packages are sufficient (114,131,145,223). The processing speed, hard disk space, and run time memory of computers marketed currently are quite adequate for PBPK modeling. The methodological approach of PBPK modeling using spreadsheets is presented in the following section.

PBPK Modeling Using Spreadsheets

Consider a simple, physiologically based model with compartments interconnected by systemic circulation for simulating the pharmacokinetics of inhaled styrene in the rat (Figure 5.14). The parameters and equations of this hypothetical PBPK model should be entered in spreadsheets to obtain simulations of styrene pharmacokinetics in the rat. The numerical values for each of the PBPK model parameters should be entered into a specific cell in the spreadsheet and identified appropriately. For example, the numerical value contained in cell C5 is referred to as Q_p (Table 5.8). Since the alveolar ventilation is referred to as Q_p in this example, whenever Q_p is typed in any other cell of the spreadsheet, the numerical value found in cell C5 will be imported automatically.

Table 5.9 lists the manner in which the model equations are written in the spreadsheets. In addition to the equations for computing blood concentrations, four equations per compartment are written. These correspond to the tracking of:

(a) the rate of change in the amount of chemical in tissue,
(b) the amount of chemical in tissue,
(c) the concentration of chemical in tissue, and
(d) the concentration of chemical in venous blood leaving tissue.

The calculation of the amount of chemical in tissue is based on the Euler algorithm. If intended, other integration algorithms can be used. In the various equations (Table 5.9), the model parameters are referred to using the appropriate abbreviations (e.g., Q_p, Q_c, V_l) and the variables are referred to with the use of relative reference expressions. The relative reference expression

Table 5.8
List of parameters for the two-compartment PBPK model, their numerical values, and location in Excel spreadsheet.

Parameters	Abbreviation[a]	Numeric values[b]	Place of cell[c]
Cardiac output	Qc	5.64 L/hr	C4
Alveolar ventilation rate	Qp	4.5 L/hr	C5
Hepatic blood flow	Ql	2.11 L/hr	C6
Blood flow in rest of body	Qbo	0.261 L/hr	C8
Liver volume	Vl	0.012 L	D6
Volume of rest of body	Vbo	0.027 L	D8
Liver : blood partition coefficient	Pl	2.7	E6
Rest of body : blood partition coefficient	Pbo	50	E8
Blood : air partition coefficient	Pb	40	F7
Maximal velocity of metabolism	Vmax	3.6 mg/hr	G6
Michaelis–Menten affinity constant	Km	0.36 mg/L	H6

[a] The various model parameters are referred to, with the use of these abbreviations, in the spreadsheet.
[b] All parameters estimates were based on Reference 223.
[c] The cell locations provided here correspond to the column and row coordinates, respectively, that is, the alphabetical letters denote the columns and the Arabic numerals correspond to the rows of the spreadsheet.

Table 5.9

Equations used in the calculation of tissue, arterial and venous blood concentrations of styrene, and their expression in EXCEL spreadsheet.

Compartment	Equations[a]	Expression in EXCEL[b]
Arterial blood	$C_{a,n} = \dfrac{Q_c \times C_{v,n-1} + Q_p \times C_{inh,n}}{Q_c + Q_p/P_b}$	D36 = ((Qc*M35) + (Qp*C36))/(Qc + (Qp/Pb))
Liver	$dA_l/dt_n = Q_l \times (C_{a,n} - C_{vl,n-1}) - \dfrac{V_{\max} \times C_{vl,n-1}}{K_m + C_{vl,n-1}}$	E36 = (Ql*(D36-H35)) – (Vmax*H35/(Km + H35))
	$A_{l,n} = dA_l/dt_{,n} \times t + A_{l,n-1}$	F36 = E36*t + F35
	$C_{l,n} = \dfrac{A_{l,n}}{V_l}$	G36 = F36/Vl
	$C_{vl,n} = \dfrac{C_{l,n}}{P_l}$	H36 = G36/Pl
Rest of body	$dA_{bo}/dt_n = Q_{bo} \times (C_{a,n} - C_{vbo,n-1})$	I36 = Qbo*(D36 – L35)
	$A_{bo,n} = dA_{bo}/dt_n \times t + A_{bo,n-1}$	J36 = I36*t + J35
	$C_{bo,n} = \dfrac{A_{bo,n}}{V_{bo}}$	K36 = J36/Vbo
	$C_{vbo,n} = \dfrac{C_{bo,n}}{P_{bo}}$	L36 = K36/Pbo
Venous blood	$Cv_n = \dfrac{Q_l \times C_{vl,n} + Q_{bo} \times C_{vbo,n}}{Q_c}$	M36 = ((Ql*H36) + (Qbo*L36))/Qc

[a] All abbreviations and symbols used in the equations, except n and n – 1, are defined in Table 5.1. Subscripts n and n – 1 refer to the current and previous simulation times. The difference between n and n – 1 in the styrene example was 0.005 hr.
[b] The components of these equations refer either to absolute references (in the case of constant input parameters, as defined in Table 5.8) or to relative references (in the case of state variables).

involves referring to a cell according to its location relative to another cell where the calculation is being carried out. This option is particularly useful when the output of an equation contained in one cell is to be provided as input for an equation contained in another (e.g., adjacent) cell. Thus, the use of relative reference expressions in spreadsheets may be useful to facilitate loop-type calculations essential for advancing the state of a system during simulations.

Table 5.10 presents a part of the spreadsheet depicting how equations presented in Table 5.9 are actually entered into spreadsheets. Accordingly, in the spreadsheet, the descriptions of the two tissue compartments occupy eight columns (columns E–L, in Table 5.10 and Figure 5.15) and the calculation/representation of the simulation time, exposure concentration, arterial concentration, and venous blood concentration occupy one column each (columns B, C, D, and M, respectively). The mixed venous blood concentration resulting from that of the venous blood exiting the two tissue compartments described in a particular row is calculated in the same row (i.e., cell M35 in Table 5.10 and Figure 5.15). This C_v then is used along with C_{inh} (i.e., cell C36) to calculate C_a in the subsequent row (e.g., cell D36). In this structure then, according to the schematics shown in Figures 5.14 and 5.15, all model equations are interconnected by specifying the proven/hypothetical input–output connections among them.

Once

(a) the numerical values of model parameters are provided,
(b) the equations in the first and subsequent rows of the spreadsheet are entered,
(c) the time interval for integration is specified, and
(d) the required number of cells are chosen, the simulation begins.

One has only to repeat the calculations shown in row 36 of Figure 5.15 for each time interval of integration until the end of the desired duration of simulation. In the present example, the time interval of integration was fixed at 0.005 h. Each line in the Excel spreadsheet then rep-

Table 5.10
A portion of the spreadsheet depicting the entry of model equations

	B	C	D	E	F	G	H	I	J	K	L	M
33				Liver				Body				
34	Time (hr)	Cinh (mg/L)	Ca	dAl/dt	Al	Cl	Cvl	dAbo/dt	Abo	Cbo	Cvbo	Cv
35	=t	=Cinh	=((Qc*0)+ (Qp*C36))/ (Qc+(Qp/Pb))	=(Ql*(D36-0)) − (Vmax*0/ (Km+0))	=E36*t +0	=F36/Vl	=G36/Pl	=Qbo* (D36-0)	=I36*t+ 0	=J36/Vbo	=K36/Pbo	=((Ql*H36)+ (Qbo*L36))/ Qc
36	=t+B35	=Cinh	=((Qc*M35)+ (Qp*C36))/ (Qc+(Qp/Pb))	=(Ql*(D36-H35)) − (Vmax*H35/ (Km+H35))	=E36*t +F35	=F36/Vl	+G36/Pl	=Qbo* (D36-L35)	=I36*t+ J35	=J36/Vbo	=K36/Pbo	=((Ql*H36)+ (Qbo*L36))/ Qc

The row and column coordinates are designated by an Arabic numeral and an alphabetical letter, respectively. The equations found in rows 35 and 36 correspond to calculations at the first and second integration intervals. For continuing the simulation, the set of equations in row 36 should be copied onto desired number of subsequent rows. In this table, column B represents the state of the system which advances during each time interval (t). Column C contains the exposure concentration at any given time during the simulation, and columns D and U represent calculations of arterial and venous blood concentrations of the chemical. In between, four columns per compartment (e.g., liver: columns E–H, rest of the body: columns I–L) are devoted for calculation of

(1) the rate of change in the amount of chemical in tissue,
(2) amount of chemical in tissue,
(3) concentrations of chemical in tissue, and
(4) concentrations of chemical in venous blood leaving tissue. All abbreviations are defined in Table 5.8.

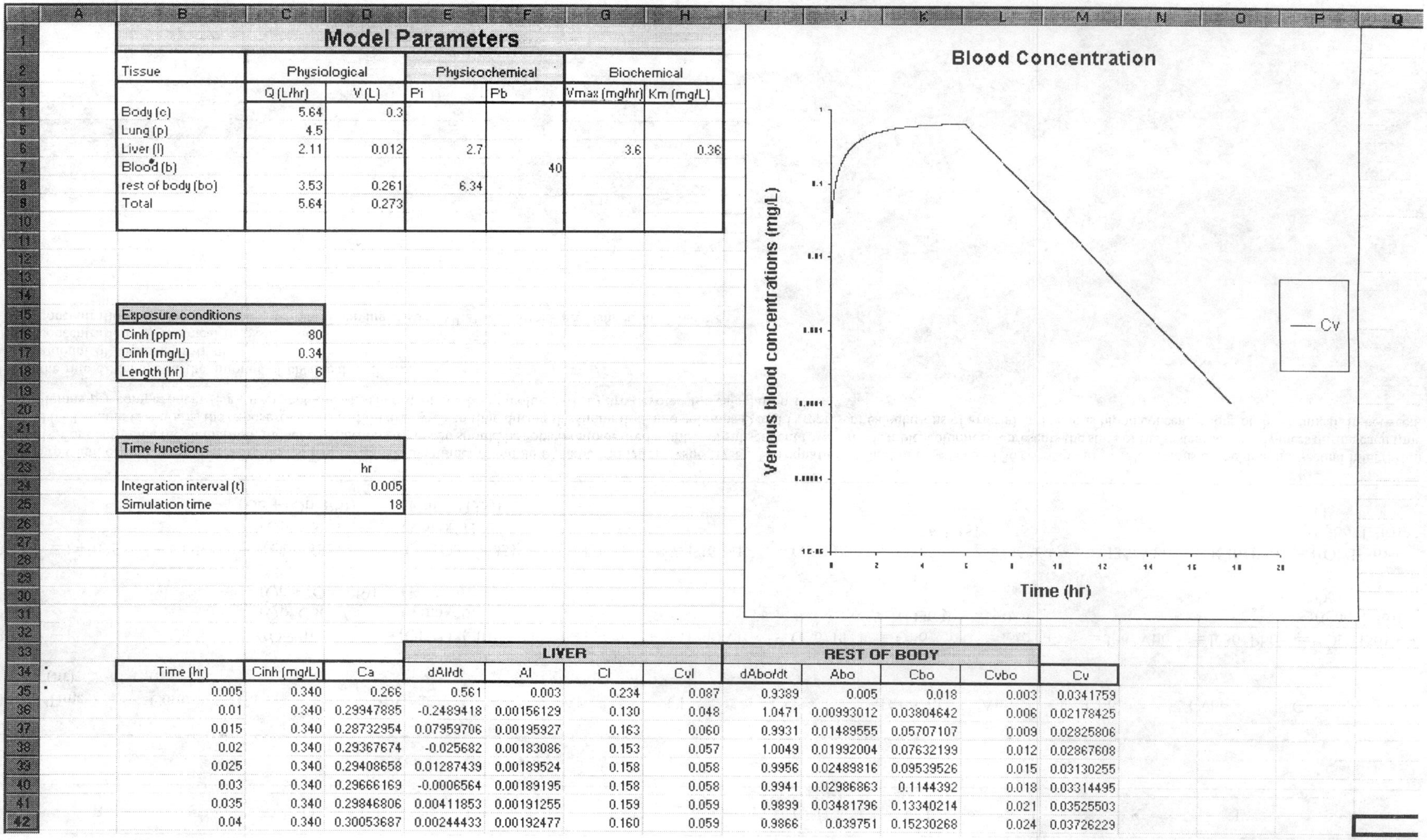

Model Parameters

Tissue	Physiological		Physicochemical		Biochemical	
	Q (L/hr)	V (L)	Pi	Pb	Vmax (mg/hr)	Km (mg/L)
Body (c)	5.64	0.3				
Lung (p)	4.5					
Liver (l)	2.11	0.012	2.7		3.6	0.36
Blood (b)				40		
rest of body (bo)	3.53	0.261	6.34			
Total	5.64	0.273				

Exposure conditions	
Cinh (ppm)	80
Cinh (mg/L)	0.34
Length (hr)	6

Time functions	
	hr
Integration interval (t)	0.005
Simulation time	18

			LIVER				REST OF BODY				
Time (hr)	Cinh (mg/L)	Ca	dAl/dt	Al	Cl	Cvl	dAbo/dt	Abo	Cbo	Cvbo	Cv
0.005	0.340	0.266	0.561	0.003	0.234	0.087	0.9389	0.005	0.018	0.003	0.0341759
0.01	0.340	0.29947885	-0.2489418	0.00156129	0.130	0.048	1.0471	0.00993012	0.03804642	0.006	0.02178425
0.015	0.340	0.28732954	0.07959706	0.00195927	0.163	0.060	0.9931	0.01489555	0.05707107	0.009	0.02825806
0.02	0.340	0.29367674	-0.025682	0.00183086	0.153	0.057	1.0049	0.01992004	0.07632199	0.012	0.02867608
0.025	0.340	0.29408658	0.01287439	0.00189524	0.158	0.058	0.9956	0.02489816	0.09539526	0.015	0.03130255
0.03	0.340	0.29666169	-0.0006564	0.00189195	0.158	0.058	0.9941	0.02986863	0.1144392	0.018	0.03314495
0.035	0.340	0.29846806	0.00411853	0.00191255	0.159	0.059	0.9899	0.03481796	0.13340214	0.021	0.03525503
0.04	0.340	0.30053687	0.00244433	0.00192477	0.160	0.059	0.9866	0.039751	0.15230268	0.024	0.03726229

FIG. 5.15. Printout of a computer screen depicting an EXCEL spreadsheet with

(1) the plot of a two-compartment PBPK model simulation of venous blood concentrations of styrene during and following a 6-h exposure of rats to 80 ppm of this chemical,
(2) the numerical values of the PBPK model parameters, and
(3) a portion of the raw numbers corresponding to the rate of change in the amount of styrene in tissue, amount in tissue, concentration in tissue, and venous blood concentration leaving the tissues, generated during simulations between time 0.005 and 18 h.

resents calculations characterizing the state of the system at every 0.005 h. In the present example, simulations were conducted for 24 h using 0.005 h as the integration interval (Figure 5.15). Therefore, in total, $4800(=24/0.005)$ lines were used up for conducting PBPK simulations. The solution to the set of PBPK model equations is generated every time the numerical values in cells corresponding to model parameters are changed, since these cells are specified in one or more equations appearing in the spreadsheet (Figure 5.15). Figure 5.16 presents simulations of the pharmacokinetics of styrene obtained using the parameters and equations for a four-compartment model developed by Ramsey and Andersen (223).

MODEL VALIDATION

Model validation refers to the evaluation of the adequacy of the conceptual and mathematical representations of the system under study in specific use conditions. Since PBPK models are only simplified representations of the actual systems, only those system variables that the investigator hypothesizes to be critical determinants are described in detail. The purpose of the validation process is then to determine whether all major determinants/processes that are essential for describing the system behavior have been adequately identified and characterized. When model predictions and experimental data agree, there is a higher level of confidence regarding the adequacy of the model and its use in decision-making (i.e., risk assessment). The approaches used for testing the adequacy of PBPK models can be classified into three categories:

(a) inspection approach,
(b) discrepancy measures, and
(c) statistical tests.

Inspection Approach

The testing of the degree of concordance between PBPK model simulations and experimental data to date has been conducted by eye balling or a visual inspection approach. This approach involves visual comparison of the plots of simulated data (usually continuous and represented by solid lines) with experimental values (usually discrete and represented by symbols) against a common independent variable (usually time). The rationale behind this approach is that the greater the commonality between the simulated and experimental data, the greater will be our confidence in the model. Instead of simply visualizing the degree of concordance between experimental data and simulation results, the residuals (i.e., difference between experimental and simulated data) can be examined. The residual analysis can be applied either to the whole model as it is or, in some other cases (as in diagnostic checkup during model building), to some estimated parameters of a tentatively ascertained theoretical model, so as to pinpoint inadequacies (122). The residuals should be random if the model is adequate. Time plots of residuals as well as the plots of residuals with respect to various controllable variables can detect possible model inadequacies, which can shed light on how to improve the model (122).

The inspection approach to model validation continues to be used pending the validation of statistical tests and discrepancy measure tests appropriate for application to PBPK models.

Statistical Tests

Statistical comparison of the model output with experimental observations is not as easy as it might appear. None of the classical tests (t, Mann–Whitney, two-sample X^2, two-sample Kolmogrov, etc.) to determine whether the underlying distributions of the two data sets are similar is applicable, since the output processes of almost all real-world systems and simulations are non-stationary and autocorrelated. Furthermore, there is a question of whether the use of statistical hypothesis tests is even appropriate. Since the model is only an approximation of the actual system, a null hypothesis that the system and model are the same is clearly false. The more appropriate question is to ask whether or not the differences between the system and the model are significant enough to affect conclusions derived from the model. In this regard, Haddad et al. (109) screened various statistical procedures (correlation, regression, confidence interval approach, lack fit F test, univariate analysis of variance, and multivariate analysis of variance) for their potential usefulness in testing the degree of agreement of PBPK model simulations and experimental data obtained in intact animals. According to these authors, the multivariate analysis of variance represents the most appropriate test, with the variance for the simulation data permitting. Alternatively, lack of fit F test represents a useful way of evaluating the adequacy of simulation models. Particularly, this simple procedure permits the consideration of multiple data sets (e.g., data for several endpoints collected at various time intervals) in conducting such an evaluation of model validity.

The F statistic in model fitting may be defined as lack of fit

$$\frac{\text{Mean square}}{\text{Pure error mean square}}$$

This ratio is compared to the critical value of F at the required degree of confidence and the corresponding

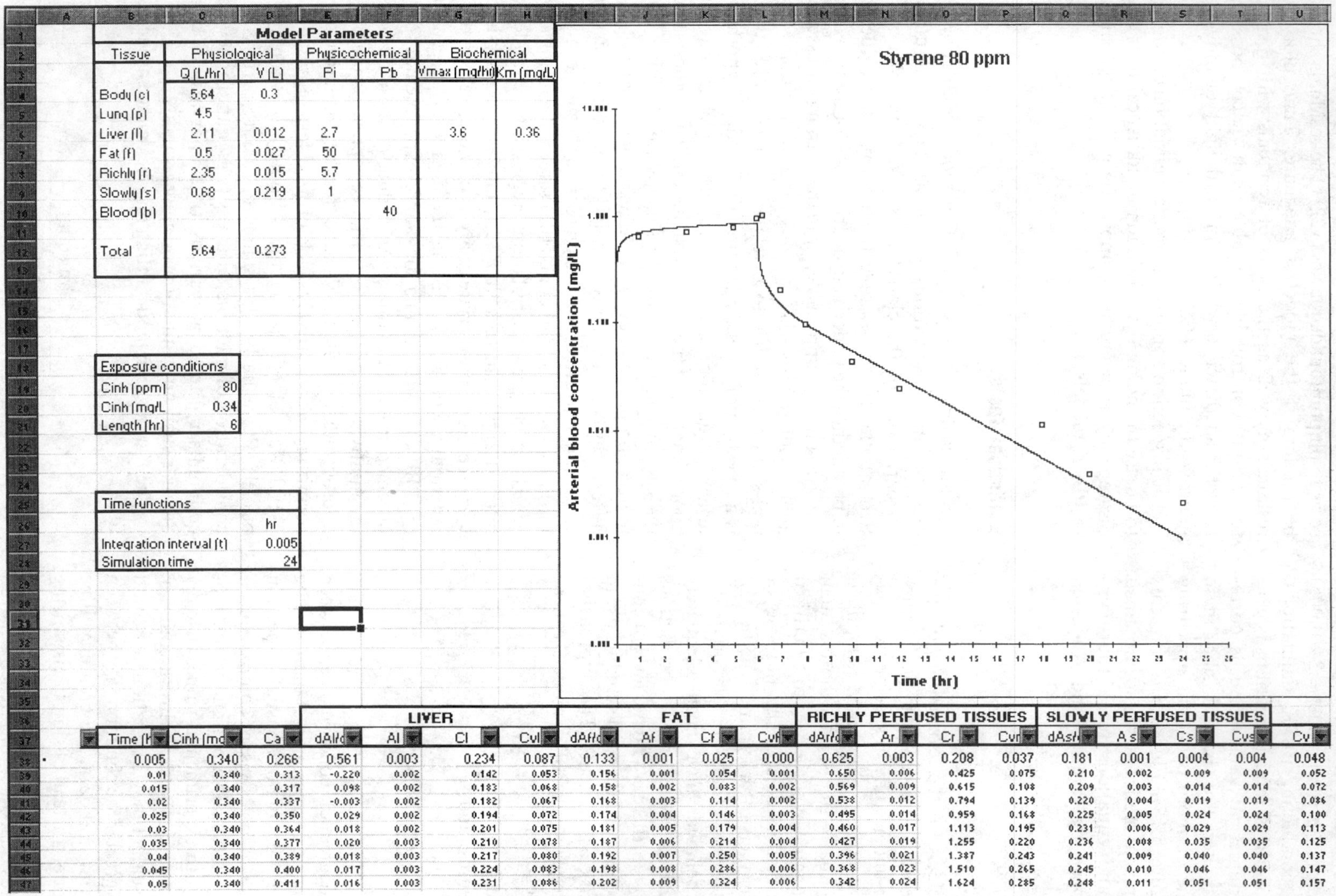

Model Parameters

Tissue	Physiological		Physicochemical		Biochemical	
	Q (L/hr)	V (L)	Pi	Pb	Vmax (mg/hr)	Km (mg/L)
Body (c)	5.64	0.3				
Lung (p)	4.5					
Liver (l)	2.11	0.012	2.7		3.6	0.36
Fat (f)	0.5	0.027	50			
Richly (r)	2.35	0.015	5.7			
Slowly (s)	0.68	0.219	1			
Blood (b)				40		
Total	5.64	0.273				

Exposure conditions	
Cinh (ppm)	80
Cinh (mg/L	0.34
Length (hr)	6

Time functions	
	hr
Integration interval (t)	0.005
Simulation time	24

			LIVER				FAT				RICHLY PERFUSED TISSUES				SLOWLY PERFUSED TISSUES				
Time (h	Cinh (mg	Ca	dAl/d	Al	Cl	Cvl	dAf/d	Af	Cf	Cvf	dAr/d	Ar	Cr	Cvr	dAs/	A s	Cs	Cvs	Cv
0.005	0.340	0.266	0.561	0.003	0.234	0.087	0.133	0.001	0.025	0.000	0.625	0.003	0.208	0.037	0.181	0.001	0.004	0.004	0.048
0.01	0.340	0.313	-0.220	0.002	0.142	0.053	0.156	0.001	0.054	0.001	0.650	0.006	0.425	0.075	0.210	0.002	0.009	0.009	0.052
0.015	0.340	0.317	0.098	0.002	0.183	0.068	0.158	0.002	0.083	0.002	0.569	0.009	0.615	0.108	0.209	0.003	0.014	0.014	0.072
0.02	0.340	0.337	-0.003	0.002	0.182	0.067	0.168	0.003	0.114	0.002	0.538	0.012	0.794	0.139	0.220	0.004	0.019	0.019	0.086
0.025	0.340	0.350	0.029	0.002	0.194	0.072	0.174	0.004	0.146	0.003	0.495	0.014	0.959	0.168	0.225	0.005	0.024	0.024	0.100
0.03	0.340	0.364	0.018	0.002	0.201	0.075	0.181	0.005	0.179	0.004	0.460	0.017	1.113	0.195	0.231	0.006	0.029	0.029	0.113
0.035	0.340	0.377	0.020	0.003	0.210	0.078	0.187	0.006	0.214	0.004	0.427	0.019	1.255	0.220	0.236	0.008	0.035	0.035	0.125
0.04	0.340	0.389	0.018	0.003	0.217	0.080	0.192	0.007	0.250	0.005	0.396	0.021	1.387	0.243	0.241	0.009	0.040	0.040	0.137
0.045	0.340	0.400	0.017	0.003	0.224	0.083	0.198	0.008	0.286	0.006	0.368	0.023	1.510	0.265	0.245	0.010	0.046	0.046	0.147
0.05	0.340	0.411	0.016	0.003	0.231	0.086	0.202	0.009	0.324	0.006	0.342	0.024	1.624	0.285	0.248	0.011	0.051	0.051	0.157

FIG. 5.16. Printout of a computer screen depicting an EXCEL spreadsheet with

(1) the plot of experimental data (symbols) and a four-compartment PBPK model simulations (solid line) of arterial blood concentrations of styrene during and following a 6-h exposure of rats to 80 ppm of this chemical,
(2) the numerical values of the PBPK model parameters, and
(3) a portion of the raw numbers corresponding to the rate of change in the amount of styrene in tissue, amount in tissue, concentration in tissue, and venous blood concentration leaving the tissues, generated during simulations between time 0.005 and 24 h.

Experimental data were obtained with permission from Reference 223.

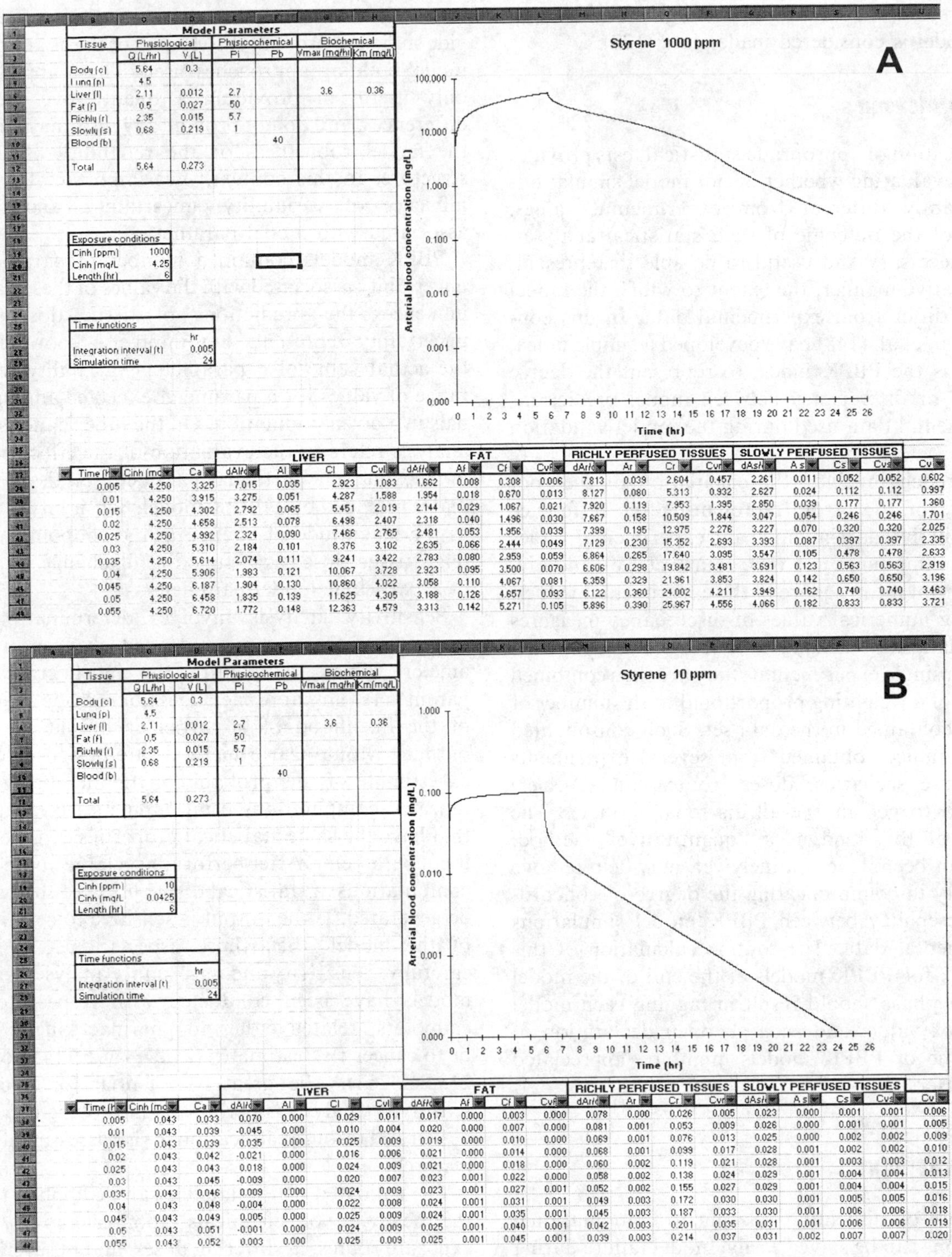

FIG. 5.17. Printout of computer screens depicting EXCEL spreadsheets with the PBPK modeling results obtained in rats exposed to

(A) 1000 ppm and

(B) 10 ppm of styrene.

Each of the two panels contain

(1) a plot of PBPK model simulation of arterial blood concentrations of styrene during and following a 6-h exposure,

(2) the numerical values of the PBPK model parameters, and

(3) a section of the raw numbers corresponding to the rate of change in the amount of styrene in tissue, amount in tissue, concentration in tissue, and venous blood concentration leaving the tissues, generated during simulations between time 0.005 and 24 h.

Note that only the exposure concentration (cell C19), and no other input parameter, differs between the two simulation exercises presented here.

degrees of freedom. If the above ratio is greater than F_{crit}, then the model is considered inadequate (122).

Discrepancy Measures

The application of appropriate statistical tests provides a means of evaluating whether or not model simulations are significantly different from experimental values. Regardless of the outcome of such statistical analyses, it is often necessary and useful to be able to represent, in a quantitative manner, the extent to which the model simulations differ from experimental data. In this context, Krishnan et al. (148) have developed a simple index, referred to as the PBPK index, to represent the degree of closeness or discrepancy between model predictions and experimental data used during the model validation phase.

This approach involved the calculation of the root mean square of the error (representing the difference between the individual simulated and experimental values for each sampling point in a time course curve), and division by the root mean square of the experimental values. The resulting numerical values of discrepancy measures for several data sets (each corresponding to an endpoint) obtained in a single experimental study are then combined on the basis of a weighting proportional to the number of data points contained in the data set. Such consolidated discrepancy indices obtained from several experiments (e.g., exposure scenarios, doses, routes, and species) are averaged to get an overall discrepancy index. The application of this kind of a "quantitative" method, which has not been done routinely yet, may help remove the ambiguity in communicating the degree of concordance or discrepancy between PBPK model simulations and experimental data. The routine calculation of this kind of index for PBPK models at the end of the model development phase should result in tagging each model with an index value, and such an open declaration of the face value of PBPK models might be appreciated by the end users.

MODEL REFINEMENT

Since errors or difficulties relating to computational representations can be solved easily, model failure during the validation stage would primarily reflect incorrect presentation of the system (i.e., conceptual representation), or failure to include specific mechanistic determinants or biochemical processes (i.e., mathematical representation). Further experimentation in such cases has resulted in significant improvement in the biological understanding of the system under study (39,111).

The use of a discrepancy measure test or statistical test to show that a priori predictions of a particular end point are in agreement with the experimental data does not provide sufficient proof of the validity of the assumptions and model-building approaches used. These approaches are only useful in providing a quantitative measure of differences, and do not provide any information on either the model robustness or the reliability of the model structure. In this context, it is important to verify the influence of variability, uncertainty, and sensitivity associated with model parameters.

PBPK models contain a number of parameters; the uncertainty associated with the values of these parameters influences the predictions of tissue dose. Whereas uncertainty represents our imprecise knowledge about the actual value of a parameter, variability reflects the range of values for a parameter expected among individuals in a given population. On the other hand, sensitivity analysis refers to the evaluation of the effect of changes in the value of a particular parameter on tissue dose estimates provided by a PBPK model. Sensitivity is expressed as the magnitude of change in the endpoint of interest (e.g., tissue dose) as a function of change in the value of a particular model parameter.

Sensitivity analysis involves determination of the response of the system to defined changes in the parameter values to identify the most critical model parameters. This approach does not provide an indication of the likelihood of a particular output or range of outputs. Monte Carlo methods are designed to provide an estimate of this probability, the idea being to make repeated computations using inputs selected at random that have the same statistical properties expected of each input parameter. After performing a large number of such computations, a statistical distribution of the output can be generated. If the output is sensitive to certain aspects of the model, then those aspects must be modeled carefully. Sensitivity and uncertainty analyses with PBPK models have been conducted with respect to specific endpoints, related either to pharmacokinetic behavior or to cancer risk estimates (21,22,41,75,114,115,119,146, 213,262,263). The greatest potential for uncertainty/sensitivity analysis is perhaps in improving experimental design and resource allocation in risk assessment-oriented research.

The validated PBPK models can be applied to predict the behavior of chemicals administered by various exposure routes, at differing doses, and in several animal species. This is particularly important because human health risk assessment is based on responses seen in animal toxicity studies in which the test chemical is administered at high doses by routes often different from anticipated human exposures. With advances in mathematical modeling and molecular biology fronts, the tissue dose of chemicals in an individual can be simulated by accounting for the individual-specific information, including data on polymorphism of enzymes (73).

MODEL APPLICATIONS

The principal application of PBPK models is to predict the target tissue dose of the toxic parent chemical or its reactive metabolite. Using the tissue dose of the toxic moiety of a chemical in risk assessment calculations provides a better basis of relating to the observed toxic effects than the external or exposure concentrations of the parent chemical (8,16). Because PBPK models facilitate the prediction of target tissue dose for various exposure scenarios, routes, doses, and species, they can help reduce the uncertainty associated with the conventional extrapolation approaches.

High-Dose to Low-Dose Extrapolation

High-dose–low-dose extrapolation of tissue dose is accomplished with PBPK models by accounting for the nonlinear kinetic behavior of chemicals (39). The description of metabolism in these cases frequently involves the use of a Michaelis–Menten equation. Nonlinearity arising from mechanisms other than saturable metabolism, such as enzyme induction, enzyme inactivation, and depletion of glutathione reserves, also has been described with PBPK models (39,70,151). An example of high-dose–low-dose extrapolation is presented in Figure 5.17. Panel A of this figure shows the blood kinetic profile of styrene in rats exposed for 6 h to 1000 ppm styrene, whereas Panel B depicts the concentration vs. time course profile following a 6-h inhalation exposure to 10 ppm styrene. For conducting high-dose to low-dose simulation, in this particular example, the numerical value of the exposure concentration (indicated in cell C19) alone was changed. With the change in the numerical value of this input parameter, all calculations in the spreadsheet are carried out automatically, thus providing the simulations corresponding to the exposure concentration specified.

Route-to-Route Extrapolation

The extrapolation of the kinetic behavior of a chemical from one exposure route to another can be performed by adding appropriate equations to represent each exposure pathway. For simulating the intravenous administration of a chemical, a single input (K^0) representing the dose administered to the animal can be included in the equation for mixed venous concentration:

$$C_v = (Q_f \times C_{vf} + Q_l \times C_{vl} + Q_r \times C_{vr} + Q_s \times C_{vs} + K^0)/Qc \tag{26}$$

More accurate description of intravenous administration includes the specification of time of infusion to calculate the rate of entry of the chemical. The parameters (iv dose, infusion time, and iv rate) essential for calculating the dose received intravenously should be included and linked to the rest of the equations constituting the PBPK model. Once the equations describing the route-specific entry of chemicals into systemic circulation are included in the model, it is possible to conduct extrapolations of kinetics. This approach is illustrated in Figure 5.18 for inhalation → iv extrapolation of the kinetics of styrene in rats. For simulating the inhalation pharmacokinetics, the iv dose is set to zero, while for simulating styrene kinetics following iv administration C_{inh} is set to 0 (Figure 5.18).

Similarly, for simulating oral absorption of a chemical, appropriate equations should be additionally included to describe process(es) occurring in the stomach compartment. At time zero, there is no chemical in the stomach. Appearance of the chemical in the stomach, and thereafter in the liver, will depend on the rate constant of absorption. For the chemical, whose oral absorption is first order, certain parameters (i.e., oral dose [mg/kg], rate of absorption [h^{-1}]), and equations are added to basic inhalation model depicted in Figure 5.7:

$$\frac{dA_o}{dt} = K_o A_{stom} \tag{27}$$

$$A_{stom} = D_o - \int_0^t \frac{dA_o}{dt} \tag{28}$$

$$\frac{dA_l}{dt} = Q_l(C_a - C_{vl}) - \frac{dA_{met}}{dt} + K_o A_{stom} \tag{29}$$

The above approach requires that parameters to define oral dose in mg/kg, and D_o in mg and rate of oral absorption (K_o) be included along with mass balance equations for the stomach compartment and modifications to the liver reflecting the input from the stomach. More complicated descriptions may be required in certain cases depending on the vehicle of administration, extent of intestinal retention, and other factors (129, 251).

For simulating dermal absorption of chemicals, it is essential to introduce a skin compartment in the model and write the mass balance differential equation (MBDE) for that compartment. The chemical uptake by the skin may be described in the same way as the other tissues. To this MBDE, however, an additional term to account for the absorption of chemical present in the environment should be added as follows (181):

$$\frac{dA_{sk}}{dt} = Q_{sk}(C_a - C_{vsk}) + K_p \times S[C_{air} - (C_{sk}/P_{s:a})] \tag{30}$$

Model Parameters

Tissue	Physiological		Physicochemical		Biochemical	
	Q (L/hr)	V (L)	Pi	Pb	Vmax (mg/hr	Km (mg/L)
Body (c)	5.64	0.3				
Lung (p)	4.5					
Liver (l)	2.11	0.012	2.7		3.6	0.36
Fat (f)	0.5	0.027	50			
Richly (r)	2.35	0.015	5.7			
Slowly (s)	0.68	0.219	1			
Blood (b)				40		
Total	5.64	0.273				

Exposure conditions	
Cinh (ppm)	80
Cinh (mg/L	0.34
Length (hr)	6

IV Administration	
IV Dose (mg/kg)	0
IV Dose (mg)	0
Time of infusion	0.05
IVR (mg/hr)	0

Time functions	
	hr
Integration interval (t)	0.005
Simulation time	24

AUC	3.8042268

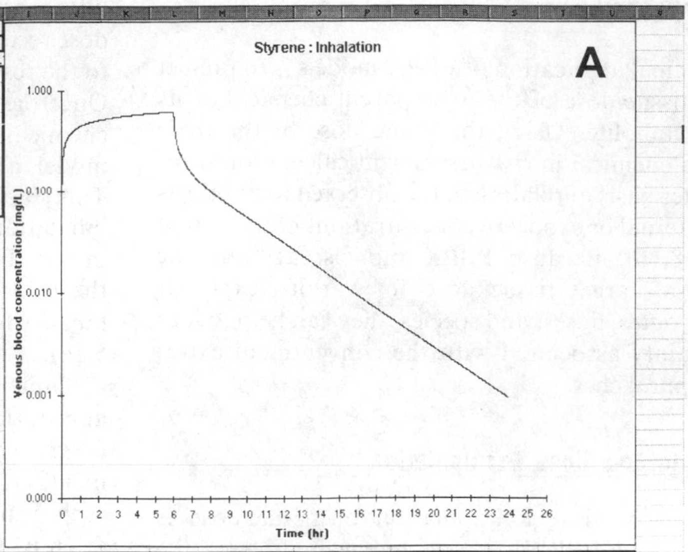

				LIVER				FAT				RICHLY PERFUSED TISSUES				SLOWLY PERFUSED TISSUES				
Time (h	Cinh (mg	IVR	Ca	dAl/d	Al	Cl	Cvl	dAf/d	Af	Cf	Cvf	dAr/d	Ar	Cr	Cvr	dAs/d	A s	Cs	Cvs	Cv
0.005	0.340	0	0.266	0.561	0.003	0.234	0.087	0.133	0.001	0.025	0.000	0.625	0.003	0.208	0.037	0.181	0.001	0.004	0.004	0.048
0.01	0.340	0	0.313	-0.220	0.002	0.142	0.053	0.156	0.001	0.054	0.001	0.650	0.006	0.425	0.075	0.210	0.002	0.009	0.009	0.052
0.015	0.340	0	0.317	0.098	0.002	0.183	0.068	0.158	0.002	0.083	0.002	0.569	0.009	0.615	0.108	0.209	0.003	0.014	0.014	0.072
0.02	0.340	0	0.337	-0.003	0.002	0.182	0.067	0.168	0.003	0.114	0.002	0.538	0.012	0.794	0.139	0.220	0.004	0.019	0.019	0.086
0.025	0.340	0	0.350	0.029	0.002	0.194	0.072	0.174	0.004	0.146	0.003	0.495	0.014	0.959	0.168	0.225	0.005	0.024	0.024	0.100
0.03	0.340	0	0.364	0.018	0.002	0.201	0.075	0.181	0.005	0.179	0.004	0.460	0.017	1.113	0.195	0.231	0.006	0.029	0.029	0.113
0.035	0.340	0	0.377	0.020	0.003	0.210	0.078	0.187	0.006	0.214	0.004	0.427	0.019	1.255	0.220	0.236	0.008	0.035	0.035	0.125
0.04	0.340	0	0.389	0.018	0.003	0.217	0.080	0.192	0.007	0.250	0.005	0.396	0.021	1.387	0.243	0.241	0.009	0.040	0.040	0.137

Model Parameters

Tissue	Physiological		Physicochemical		Biochemical	
	Q (L/hr)	V (L)	Pi	Pb	Vmax (mg/hr	Km (mg/L)
Body (c)	5.64	0.3				
Lung (p)	4.5					
Liver (l)	2.11	0.012	2.7		3.6	0.36
Fat (f)	0.5	0.027	50			
Richly (r)	2.35	0.015	5.7			
Slowly (s)	0.68	0.219	1			
Blood (b)				40		
Total	5.64	0.273				

Exposure conditions	
Cinh (ppm)	0
Cinh (mg/L	0
Length (hr)	6

IV Administration	
IV Dose (mg/kg)	11.767
IV Dose (mg)	3.5301
Time of infusion	0.05
IVR (mg/hr)	70.602

Time functions	
	hr
Integration interval (t)	0.005
Simulation time	24

AUC	3.8043942

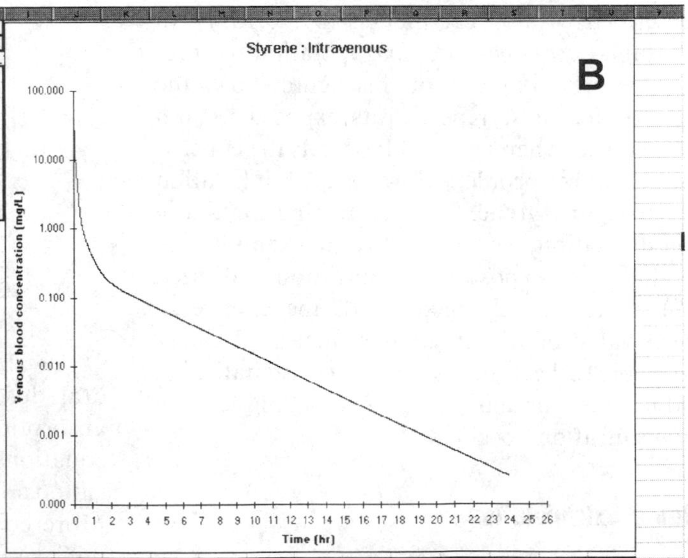

				LIVER				FAT				RICHLY PERFUSED TISSUES				SLOWLY PERFUSED TISSUES				
Time (h	Cinh (mg	IVR	Ca	dAl/d	Al	Cl	Cvl	dAf/d	Af	Cf	Cvf	dAr/d	Ar	Cr	Cvr	dAs/d	A s	Cs	Cvs	Cv
0.005	0.000	70.602	0.000	0.000	0.000	0.000	0.000	0.000	0.000	0.000	0.000	0.000	0.000	0.000	0.000	0.000	0.000	0.000	0.000	12.518
0.01	0.000	70.602	12.273	25.897	0.129	10.790	3.996	6.137	0.031	1.136	0.023	28.842	0.144	9.614	1.687	8.346	0.042	0.191	0.191	14.741
0.015	0.000	70.602	14.453	18.760	0.223	18.607	6.891	7.215	0.067	2.473	0.049	30.000	0.294	19.614	3.441	9.698	0.090	0.412	0.412	16.584
0.02	0.000	70.602	16.260	16.346	0.305	25.418	9.414	8.105	0.107	3.973	0.079	30.124	0.445	29.655	5.203	10.777	0.144	0.658	0.658	18.294
0.025	0.000	70.602	17.936	14.515	0.378	31.466	11.654	8.928	0.152	5.627	0.113	29.924	0.594	39.630	6.953	11.749	0.203	0.926	0.926	19.897
0.03	0.000	70.602	19.507	13.079	0.443	36.915	13.672	9.697	0.200	7.423	0.148	29.504	0.742	49.465	8.678	12.635	0.266	1.215	1.215	21.409
0.035	0.000	70.602	20.990	11.932	0.503	41.887	15.514	10.421	0.253	9.352	0.187	28.933	0.887	59.109	10.370	13.447	0.333	1.522	1.522	22.843
0.04	0.000	70.602	22.396	11.004	0.558	46.472	17.212	11.105	0.308	11.409	0.228	28.261	1.028	68.529	12.023	14.195	0.404	1.846	1.846	24.209

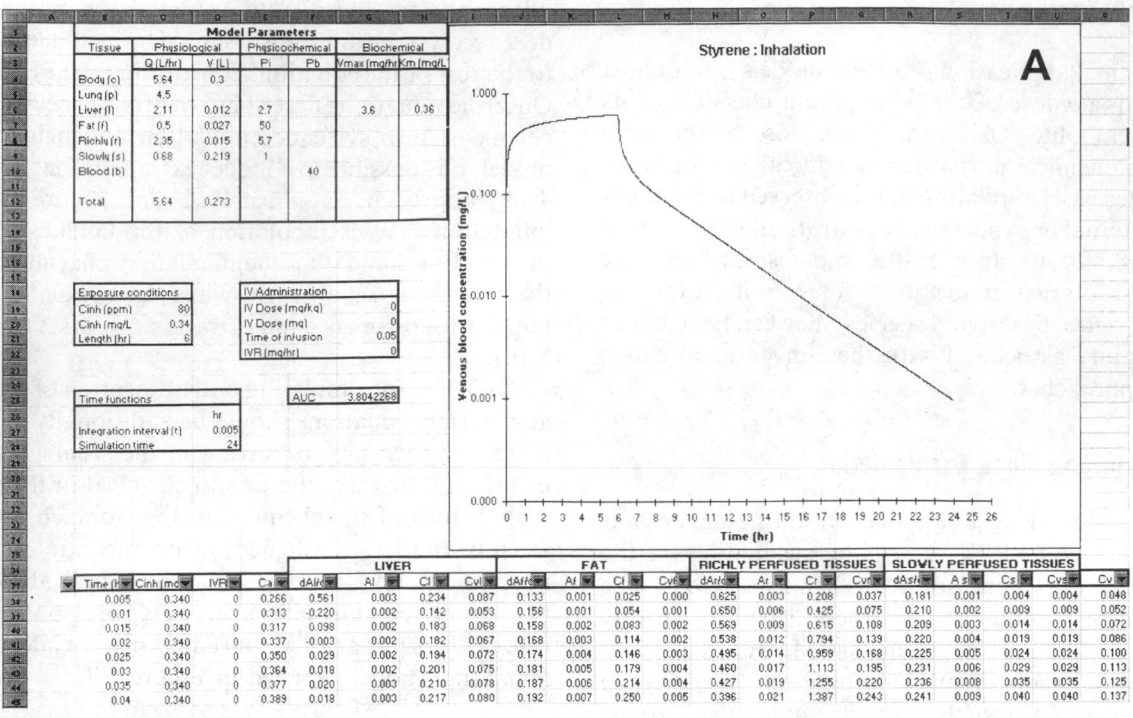

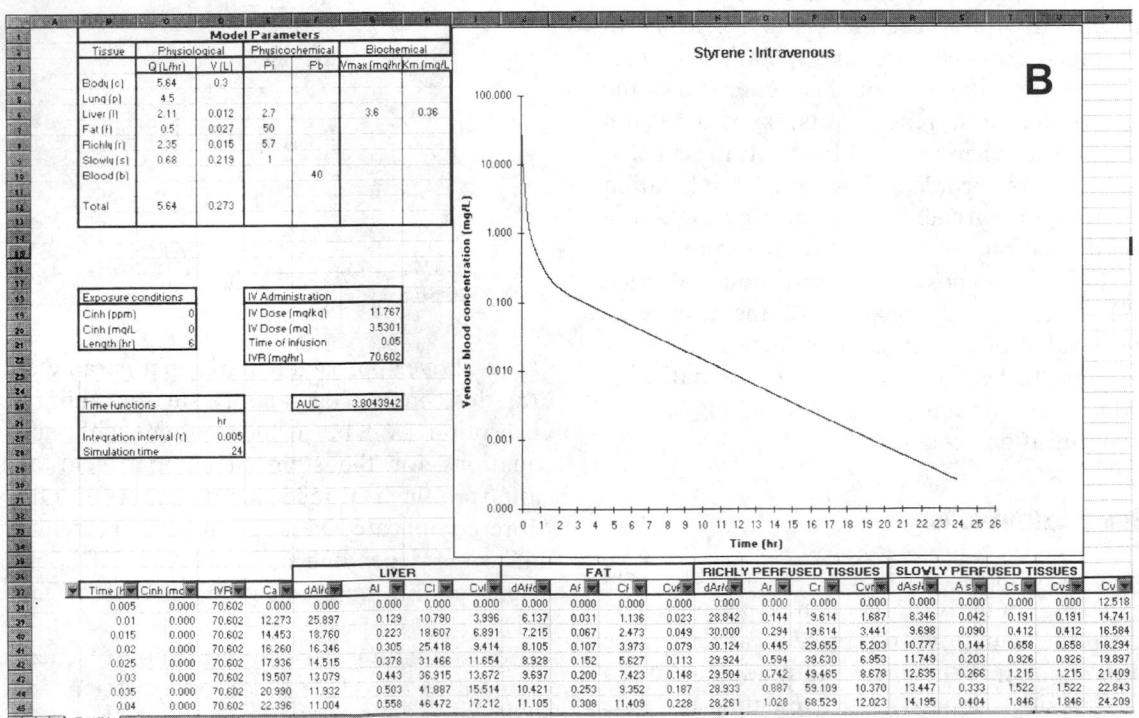

FIG. 5.18. Printout of computer screens depicting EXCEL spreadsheets with the PBPK modeling results obtained in rats exposed to styrene
(A) by inhalation (80 ppm, 6 h) or
(B) by intravenous administration (11.767 mg/kg). Each of the two panels contains
(1) a plot of PBPK model simulation of venous blood concentrations of styrene during and following exposure,
(2) the numerical values of the PBPK model parameters, and
(3) a section of the raw numbers corresponding to the rate of change in the amount of styrene in tissue, amount in tissue, concentration in tissue, and venous blood concentration leaving the tissues, generated during simulations between time 0.005 and 24 h.

Note that only the parameters related to the exposure route (C_{inh}, iv dose) differ between the two simulation exercises presented here.

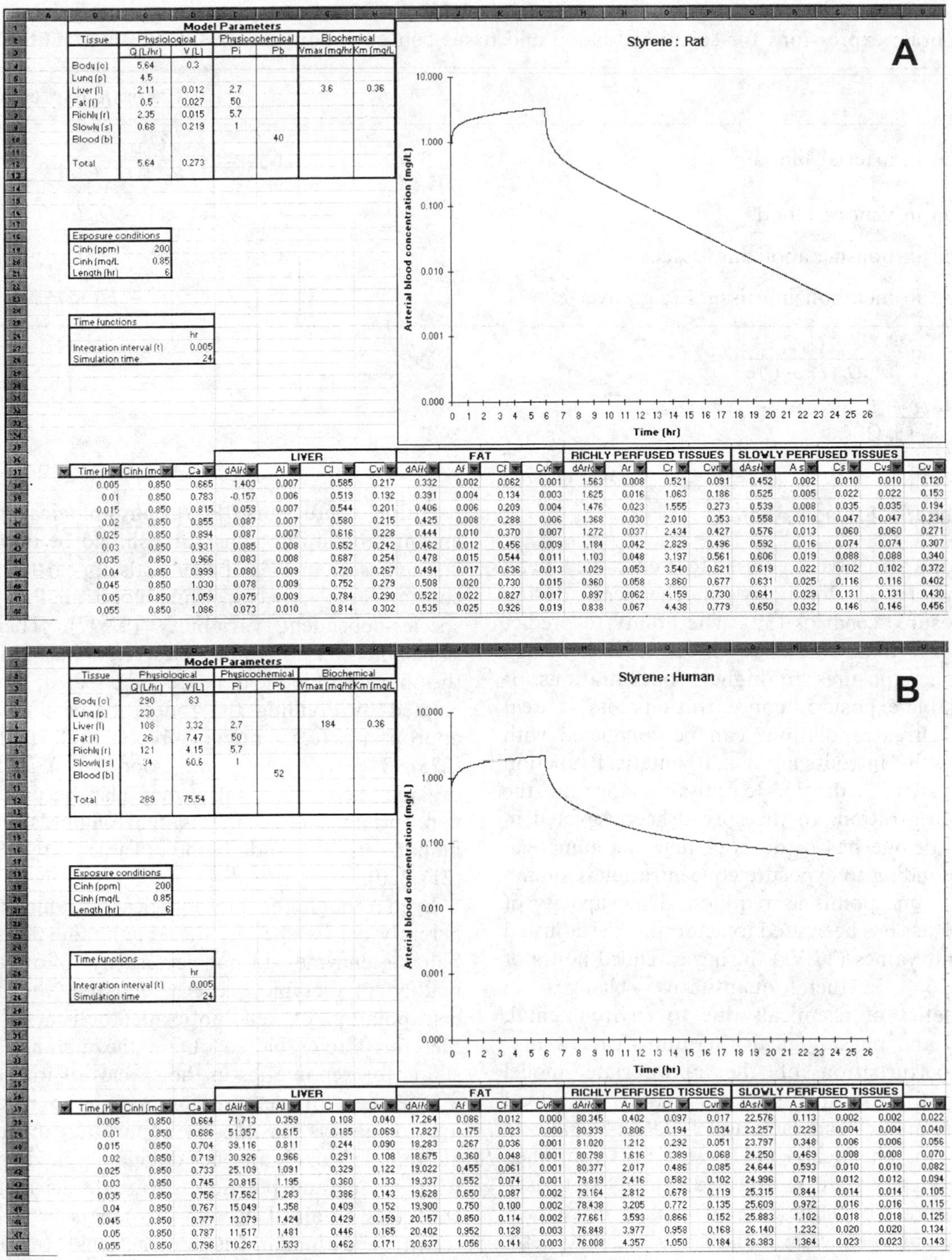

(A) Model Parameters

Tissue	Physiological Q (L/hr)	Physiological V (L)	Physicochemical Pi	Physicochemical Pb	Biochemical Vmax (mg/hr	Biochemical Km (mg/L
Body (c)	5.64	0.3				
Lung (p)	4.5					
Liver (l)	2.11	0.012	2.7		3.6	0.36
Fat (f)	0.5	0.027	50			
Richly (r)	2.35	0.015	5.7			
Slowly (s)	0.68	0.219	1			
Blood (b)				40		
Total	5.64	0.273				

Exposure conditions	
Cinh (ppm)	200
Cinh (mg/L	0.85
Length (hr)	6

Time functions	hr
Integration interval (t)	0.005
Simulation time	24

			LIVER				FAT				RICHLY PERFUSED TISSUES				SLOWLY PERFUSED TISSUES				
Time (h	Cinh (mg	Ca	dAl/d	Al	Cl	Cvl	dAf/d	Af	Cf	Cvf	dAr/d	Ar	Cr	Cvr	dAs/d	A s	Cs	Cvs	Cv
0.005	0.850	0.665	1.403	0.007	0.585	0.217	0.332	0.002	0.062	0.001	1.563	0.008	0.521	0.091	0.452	0.002	0.010	0.010	0.120
0.01	0.850	0.783	-0.157	0.006	0.519	0.192	0.391	0.004	0.134	0.003	1.625	0.016	1.063	0.186	0.525	0.005	0.022	0.022	0.153
0.015	0.850	0.815	0.059	0.007	0.544	0.201	0.406	0.006	0.209	0.004	1.476	0.023	1.555	0.273	0.539	0.008	0.035	0.035	0.194
0.02	0.850	0.855	0.087	0.007	0.580	0.215	0.425	0.008	0.288	0.006	1.368	0.030	2.010	0.353	0.558	0.010	0.047	0.047	0.234
0.025	0.850	0.894	0.087	0.007	0.616	0.228	0.444	0.010	0.370	0.007	1.272	0.037	2.434	0.427	0.576	0.013	0.060	0.060	0.271
0.03	0.850	0.931	0.085	0.008	0.652	0.242	0.462	0.012	0.456	0.009	1.184	0.042	2.829	0.496	0.592	0.016	0.074	0.074	0.307
0.035	0.850	0.966	0.083	0.008	0.687	0.254	0.478	0.015	0.544	0.011	1.103	0.048	3.197	0.561	0.606	0.019	0.088	0.088	0.340
0.04	0.850	0.999	0.080	0.009	0.720	0.267	0.494	0.017	0.636	0.013	1.029	0.053	3.540	0.621	0.619	0.022	0.102	0.102	0.372
0.045	0.850	1.030	0.078	0.009	0.752	0.279	0.508	0.020	0.730	0.015	0.960	0.058	3.860	0.677	0.631	0.025	0.116	0.116	0.402
0.05	0.850	1.059	0.075	0.009	0.784	0.290	0.522	0.022	0.827	0.017	0.897	0.062	4.159	0.730	0.641	0.029	0.131	0.131	0.430
0.055	0.850	1.086	0.073	0.010	0.814	0.302	0.535	0.025	0.926	0.019	0.838	0.067	4.438	0.779	0.650	0.032	0.146	0.146	0.456

(B) Model Parameters

Tissue	Physiological Q (L/hr)	Physiological V (L)	Physicochemical Pi	Physicochemical Pb	Biochemical Vmax (mg/hr	Biochemical Km (mg/L
Body (c)	290	83				
Lung (p)	230					
Liver (l)	108	3.32	2.7		184	0.36
Fat (f)	26	7.47	50			
Richly (r)	121	4.15	5.7			
Slowly (s)	34	60.6	1			
Blood (b)				52		
Total	289	75.54				

Exposure conditions	
Cinh (ppm)	200
Cinh (mg/L	0.85
Length (hr)	6

Time functions	hr
Integration interval (t)	0.005
Simulation time	24

			LIVER				FAT				RICHLY PERFUSED TISSUES				SLOWLY PERFUSED TISSUES				
Time (h	Cinh (mg	Ca	dAl/d	Al	Cl	Cvl	dAf/d	Af	Cf	Cvf	dAr/d	Ar	Cr	Cvr	dAs/d	A s	Cs	Cvs	Cv
0.005	0.850	0.664	71.713	0.359	0.108	0.040	17.264	0.086	0.012	0.000	80.345	0.402	0.097	0.017	22.576	0.113	0.002	0.002	0.022
0.01	0.850	0.686	51.357	0.615	0.185	0.069	17.827	0.175	0.023	0.000	80.939	0.806	0.194	0.034	23.257	0.229	0.004	0.004	0.040
0.015	0.850	0.704	39.116	0.811	0.244	0.090	18.283	0.267	0.036	0.001	81.020	1.212	0.292	0.051	23.797	0.348	0.006	0.006	0.056
0.02	0.850	0.719	30.926	0.966	0.291	0.108	18.675	0.360	0.048	0.001	80.798	1.616	0.389	0.068	24.250	0.469	0.008	0.008	0.070
0.025	0.850	0.733	25.109	1.091	0.329	0.122	19.022	0.455	0.061	0.001	80.377	2.017	0.486	0.085	24.644	0.593	0.010	0.010	0.082
0.03	0.850	0.745	20.815	1.195	0.360	0.133	19.337	0.552	0.074	0.001	79.819	2.416	0.582	0.102	24.996	0.718	0.012	0.012	0.094
0.035	0.850	0.756	17.562	1.283	0.386	0.143	19.628	0.650	0.087	0.002	79.164	2.812	0.678	0.119	25.315	0.844	0.014	0.014	0.105
0.04	0.850	0.767	15.049	1.358	0.409	0.152	19.900	0.750	0.100	0.002	78.438	3.205	0.772	0.135	25.609	0.972	0.016	0.016	0.115
0.045	0.850	0.777	13.079	1.424	0.429	0.159	20.157	0.850	0.114	0.002	77.661	3.593	0.866	0.152	25.883	1.102	0.018	0.018	0.125
0.05	0.850	0.787	11.517	1.481	0.446	0.165	20.402	0.952	0.128	0.003	76.848	3.977	0.958	0.168	26.140	1.232	0.020	0.020	0.134
0.055	0.850	0.796	10.267	1.533	0.462	0.171	20.637	1.056	0.141	0.003	76.008	4.357	1.050	0.184	26.383	1.364	0.023	0.023	0.143

FIG. 5.19. Printout of computer screens depicting EXCEL spreadsheets with the PBPK modeling results obtained in
(A) rats and
(B) humans exposed to 200 ppm of styrene.

Each of the two panels contains

(1) a plot of PBPK model simulation of arterial blood concentrations of styrene during and following a 6-h exposure,
(2) the numerical values of the PBPK model parameters, and
(3) a section of the raw numbers corresponding to the rate of change in the amount of styrene in tissue, amount in tissue, concentration in tissue, and venous blood concentration leaving the tissues, generated during simulations between time 0.005 and 24 h.

Note that the numerical values of all species-specific parameters are different between the two simulation exercises presented here.

Table 5.11
Algebraic expressions for calculated blood and tissue concentrations under steady-state conditions

Parameter	Algebraic expression
Concentration in arterial blood[a,b]	$C_{a,ss} = \dfrac{C_{inh}}{1/P_b + Q_{lc}E}$
Concentration in venous blood[b]	$C_{v,ss} = C_{a,ss}(1 - Q_{lc}E)$
Concentration in non-metabolizing tissues	$C_{t,ss} = C_{a,ss}P_t$
Concentration in metabolizing tissues (e.g., liver)[b]	$C_{l,ss} = C_{a,ss}(1 - E) \times P_l$

[a] If $Q_p \neq Q_c$, $C_{a,ss} = \dfrac{Q_p C_i}{Q_p/P_b + Q_l E}$

[b] $E = \dfrac{V_{\max}/K_m}{(V_{\max}/K_m) + Q_l}$

Exposure Scenario Extrapolation

PBPK models also have been used to predict the kinetic behavior and tissue dosimetry of chemicals during unusual exposure scenarios (39). The ability to predict tissue dose of toxic moieties of chemicals during short-duration exposures to higher concentrations or during variable-exposure concentrations is a real challenge. Such extrapolations can be conducted with PBPK models by introducing a mathematical function that is consistent with the temporal change in the exposure concentration. In the spreadsheet depicted in Figure 5.19, all one has to do is change the numerical value corresponding to exposure concentration (Column C) at specific time points as required. This capacity of the PBPK models has been used to determine the adjusted threshold limit values (TLVs) during extended hours of work (25,156). Further, quantitative changes in pharmacokinetics of chemicals due to environmental, pathological, and physiological alterations can be predicted by perturbation of the appropriate model parameter(s), for example physical activity/workload (156,243), pregnancy and lactation (82,91,149,246), or co-exposure to chemicals (147). During continued exposures, a steady-state is attained. Steady-state is a condition during which the rate of change in concentration of parent chemicals in tissues is equal to zero. The steady-state concentrations predicted using PBPK models can also be obtained using simple algebraic equations (Table 5.11) (203).

Interspecies Extrapolation

For conducting interspecies extrapolation of pharmacokinetic behavior of a chemical, quantitative estimates of species differences in the model parameter values (i.e., partition coefficients [PCs], physiological parameters, and metabolic rate constants) should be obtained.

The tissue–air PCs of chemicals appear to be relatively constant across species, while blood–air PCs show some species-dependent variability (92,97). Therefore, the tissue–blood PCs, for species (e.g., humans) to which the pharmacokinetic data are to be scaled, have been calculated by dividing the rodent tissue–air PCs by the appropriate (e.g., human) blood–air partition values (223). The tissue : air and blood : air PCs for volatile organic chemicals (VOCs) may also be predicted using appropriate data on the content of lipids and water in human tissues and blood (Table 5.6; Figure 5.8) (217,220).

Even though the physiological parameters vary coherently across species, the kinetic constants for metabolizing enzymes do not necessarily follow any type of readily predictable pattern, making the interspecies extrapolation of xenobiotic metabolism difficult. It is therefore preferable to obtain the metabolic rate constants for xenobiotics in the species of interest. In vivo approaches for determining metabolic rate constants are not always feasible for application in humans. The alternative is to obtain such data under in vitro conditions while the default position is to scale the metabolic rate constants obtained in vivo in rodents or in vitro using rodent and human tissue fractions. In the case of chemicals exhibiting high affinity (low K_m) for metabolizing enzymes, $V_{\max}$ has been scaled to approximately the 3/4th power of body weight, keeping the K_m species-invariant. This approach may be useful as a crude approximation but should be used only when other direct measurements of metabolic parameters are not available or feasible. An example of rat–human extrapolation of the kinetics of styrene using a PBPK model is presented in Figure 5.19. In this example, the model was validated using human data for styrene. Whenever the human data

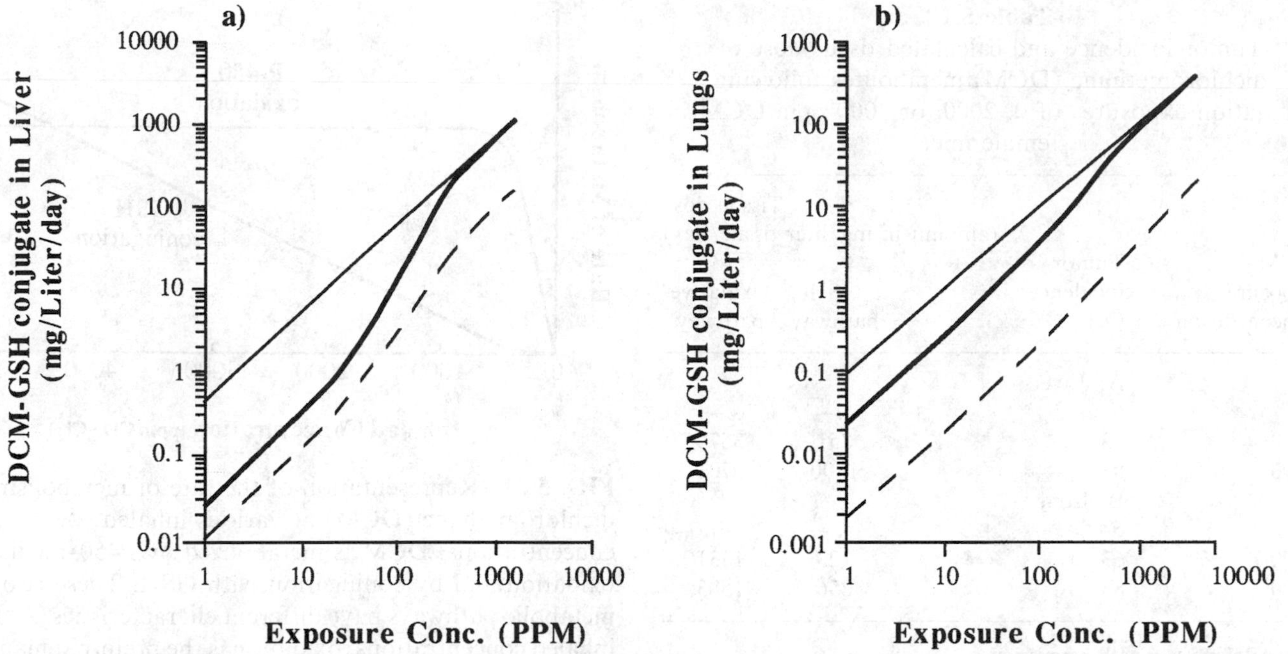

FIG. 5.20. Quantitative relationship between (a) liver or (b) lung dose of DCM-GSH conjugate and external exposure concentration of DCM determined with a PBPK model for B6C3F1 mice (heavy solid line) and humans (dashed line). The lighter solid line depicts linear back-extrapolation to 1 ppm. Redrawn with permission from Reference 10.

for a particular chemical are not available for validation purposes, a corollary approach permitting the use of human data on similar chemicals may be attempted (280).

Example of PBPK Model Application

The usefulness of PBPK models in reducing the uncertainties associated with high-dose–low-dose, route–route, and interspecies extrapolations has been demonstrated during the risk assessment process for a number of chemicals. This aspect was initially demonstrated with dichloromethane (DCM) (5). DCM caused liver and lung tumors in mice exposed to 2000 or 4000 ppm, 6 hr/day, for their lifetimes (189). DCM is metabolized by two processes:

(a) oxidation leading to the production of highly reactive formyl chloride, as well as carbon monoxide and small amounts of carbon dioxide, and
(b) GSH conjugation, yielding chloromethylglutathione (a reactive intermediate) and carbon dioxide (152).

Either of the reactive metabolites resulting from the oxidation or GSH conjugation could be involved in the mutagenic changes leading to cancer. In the PBPK model for DCM, these metabolic pathways were described according to their different kinetic characteristics. DCM metabolism in lung and liver was described with a saturable term for oxidation and with a linear term for reaction with GSH (5).

The PBPK model for DCM developed for the mouse by integrating quantitative information on physiological characteristics, partition coefficients, and metabolic rate constants, described adequately the disposition of DCM. The mouse DCM model then was used to calculate the tissue dose of metabolites and parent chemical arising from exposure scenarios comparable to those of the NTP bioassay studies (Table 5.12). The relationship of tissue dose of metabolic and parent chemical to the observed tumor incidence then was examined. Since the parent chemical is unreactive, it is unlikely to be directly involved in the tumorigenicity. Hence, the relationship between the tissue exposure to its metabolites and tumor incidence was examined (Table 5.12). Although the dose surrogate based on oxidative pathway did not vary between DCM exposure concentrations of 2000 and 4000 ppm, the flux through the GSH pathway did correspond well with the degree of DCM-induced cancer at these exposure concentrations. These observations are consistent with a role for the metabolite(s) arising from the GSH conjugation pathway in DCM-induced lung and liver cancer. The GSH conjugation of DCM, mediated by glutathione *S*-transferase enzymes, yields

Table 5.12
Tumor incidence and calculated tissue dose of dichloromethane (DCM) metabolites following inhalation exposures of 0, 2000, or 4000 ppm DCM in female mice

DCM exposure concentration	Tumor incidence (%)	Tissue dose (amount in mg/liter tissue/day)	
		GSH pathway	Oxidative pathway
	A. Liver		
0	6	—	—
2000	33	851	3575
4000	83	1800	3701
	B. Lung		
0	6	—	—
2000	63	123	1531
4000	85	256	1583

From Reference 6 with permission.

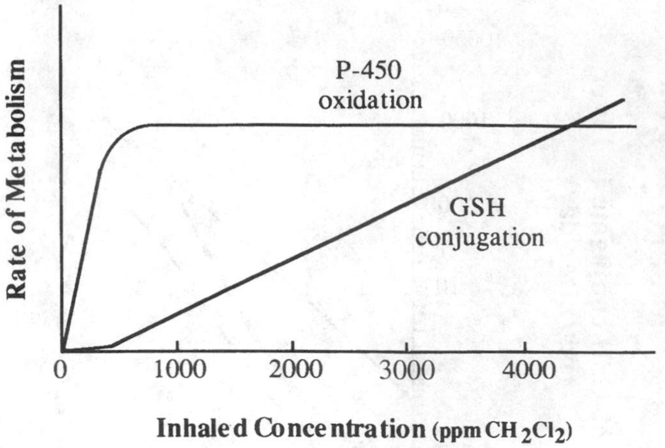

FIG. 5.21. Representation of the rate of metabolism of dichloromethane (DCM) at various inhaled concentrations. DCM is metabolized by P450–mediated oxidation and by conjugation with GSH. These two metabolic pathways have different characteristics. At low inhaled concentrations, oxidation is the preferred manner of metabolism, but at higher concentrations GSH conjugation becomes more favored. From Reference 10, with permission.

formaldehyde as a metabolite. Casanova et al. (32) reported DNA–formaldehyde–protein crosslinks resulting from DCM exposure, further strengthening the case for GSH conjugation as the pathway leading to potentially carcinogenic metabolites. Therefore, high-dose–low-dose extrapolation and interspecies extrapolation of DCM-induced cancer risk were conducted with the tissue dose of the GSH pathway metabolite predicted by the PBPK model.

High-Dose–Low-Dose Extrapolation

The model prediction of the target tissue dose of the DCM-GSH conjugate resulting from 6-h inhalation exposures to 1–4000 ppm of DCM is presented in Figure 5.20. The estimation of target tissue dose of DCM–GSH conjugate by linear back-extrapolation gives rise to a 21-fold higher estimate than that obtained by the PBPK modeling approach. This discrepancy arises from the nonlinear behavior of DCM metabolism at high exposure concentrations (Figure 5.21). At exposure concentrations exceeding 300 ppm, the cytochrome P450–mediated oxidation pathway is saturated, giving rise to a corresponding disproportionate increase in the flux through the GSH conjugation pathway.

Interspecies Extrapolation

The interspecies extrapolation of DCM disposition behavior was possible because the critical biological determinants were first identified in the test species, the mouse. Thus, the physiological parameters in the mouse PBPK model were scaled allometrically, the metabolic parameters were determined experimentally, and the tissue–blood PCs were assumed to be species-invariant. The PBPK model adequately simulated the blood levels of DCM observed in humans after a 6-h inhalation exposure to 100 or 350 ppm DCM. The target tissue–dose for humans was estimated to be some 2.7 times lower than that for the mouse. Considered together, the human tissue dose of DCM-GSH conjugate for a 6-h exposure to 1 ppm DCM is expected to be some 57 times lower than that expected by linear extrapolation of its behavior at high exposure concentrations, such as the ones used in the mouse cancer bioassay.

The cancer risk assessment for DCM, then, was conducted using the linearized multistage (LMS) model to relate tissue dose of DCM-GSH metabolite (rather than DCM exposure concentration) to the tumor incidence rates observed at high exposure concentrations in the mouse. In assessing the tumorigenic risks associated with human exposure to this chemical, it was assumed that humans are as sensitive as the most sensitive test species. Therefore, equal target tissue doses are expected to produce similar tumor incidence regardless of the species. This PBPK model-based DCM risk assessment predicted human low-dose risk about 100- to 200-fold less than that predicted by the U.S. Environmental Protection Agency (EPA) using standard default assumptions (249). With further refinement of the model with the estimation of the metabolic rate constants for humans in vitro (231), the PBPK model-based approach using tissue dose of the DCM-GSH conjugate predicted a cancer risk of 3.7×10^{-8} for a lifetime inhalation exposure of 1 $\mu g/m^3$.

Table 5.13
Examples of chemicals for which risk assessment has been performed using PBPK models

Chemical	References
Benzene	47
Chloroform	227
1,4-Dioxane	161, 229
Methylene chloride	213
Tetrachloroethylene	30, 34, 267
Trichloroethylene	19, 38, 49, 84
Vinyl chloride	38, 226

This risk estimate was still lower, by more than two orders of magnitude, than that calculated by the EPA using the standard default assumptions and exposure concentrations of DCM (270).

Following the DCM example, there have been several reports of the use of PBPK models for enhancing the scientific and mechanistic basis of cancer and non-cancer risk assessments of environmental agents (37,197), (Table 5.13) The use of PBPK models in quantitative risk assessment does not always result in the estimation of risk lower than that derived from the conventional approach adopted by regulatory agencies. For example, if the test chemical is a direct-acting agent, the PBPK approach actually could predict greater risk to humans than conventional methods because enzyme-mediated metabolic clearance (detoxification) is expected to be lower in larger species. Similarly, if the toxicity of a chemical is mediated by reactive intermediates resulting from a saturable metabolic process, then the high-dose–low-dose extrapolation conducted with the PBPK modeling approach would predict a risk greater than that predicted by the linear extrapolation procedure.

CONCLUDING REMARKS

Modeling, in general terms, involves mathematical description of the interrelationships among critical parameters that determine the behavior of the system under study. Mathematical models can be constructed to fit experimental data by adjusting one or more model parameters, or by deriving an equation that describes the data. The latter approach reflects the methodological basis of conventional pharmacokinetic models. This approach might well be sufficient to describe the kinetics of prescription drugs and other pharmaceutical products, since these substances are often tested in humans in the dose range of prescription. Such empirical models are not sufficient in the case of environmental contaminants for which human health risk assessments need to be performed based on data obtained in animal studies conducted by administering high doses of chemicals by routes often different from anticipated human exposures. In this respect, mechanistically based PBPK models are useful for conducting the required extrapolations. So, the kind of modeling approach—physiological or nonphysiological—that is required/sufficient to describe the kinetics of a chemical depends on the intended use. If extrapolation to untested scenarios and design of useful mechanistic toxicology studies is the goal, then the choice will be PBPK modeling. However, the ability to conduct extrapolations with PBPK models will be compromised if the methods employed for developing and validating the models are inappropriate.

For example, PBPK models should not be constructed by assembling sets of equations, in which the parameters are not interpretable in terms of physicochemical, biochemical, or physiological properties. That sort of an approach will compromise the very basis of PBPK modeling, that is, the mechanistic basis. In other words, the mathematical equations employed in PBPK modeling should show clearly the interrelationships among the critical biological determinants. One should be able to dissect each equation into subsections, each of which describes a particular phenomenon (e.g., tissue uptake, metabolism). Further, the dissociation of each term should provide parameters that are biologically meaningful (e.g., breathing rate, tissue volume). If the mathematical descriptions employed in the model do not satisfy this basic criterion (i.e., use biologically relevant parameters), then it should not be considered a "true" physiologically based model, and the appropriateness of the use of such models in conducting extrapolations is questionable. The guiding principles of modeling in toxicology and the characteristics of a good modeling paper are summarized elsewhere (4).

A related problem is circularity in PBPK modeling. This aspect refers to the practice of using sets of experimental data to construct the model and then using the model to simulate the same data. Even though such an approach provides a framework to integrate various data sets, it does not instill confidence in using the model to predict the kinetic behavior of chemicals at untested exposure scenarios. Genuine PBPK modeling efforts should ensure that

(a) the assumptions on which the model is based are appropriate,
(b) the coding of model equations is errorless,
(c) the model parameter values are accurate, and
(d) the model is adequately tested/validated.

The model is as good as the input parameters. Therefore, accurate parameterization is fundamentally important for constructing useful PBPK models.

Methodological aspects of some of the important and widely used techniques for model parameterization were provided in the earlier sections of this chapter. A number of prototypical descriptions have also been provided to serve as examples for developing PBPK models for other chemicals of interest. These prototypical structures and descriptions may not be directly applicable to a chemical of interest to the researcher. The model structure and the phenomena to be represented in a particular model depend on the chemical whose kinetics are being modeled. Each chemical may possess some unique properties, thus presenting some very different problems and requiring the modification of existing model structures and functional representations. This might lead to the development of totally new descriptions. Thus, PBPK modeling is as much an art as a science. The creativity of the researcher is as much implied in the formulation of these models as the experimental techniques to obtain parameter estimates, such that novel model structures and descriptions will evolve continually in this field.

Parameter identifiability and model overspecification are problems inherent in these PBPK models or in any other multiparameter model. Direct measurement of model parameters by experimental methods, independent of analysis of tissue time-course curves, is the preferred approach. Nonetheless, limited numbers of parameters often will still have to be estimated by analysis of time-course data by curve-fitting techniques, under well-defined experimental conditions where the curves are particularly sensitive to the parameter(s) of interest.

The motivation for the use of PBPK models in toxicology research is to uncover the biological determinants of tissue dosimetry. These models are part of a systematic approach to studying how chemicals gain entry into, are distributed within, and are eliminated from the body. A major advantage of PBPK models is their use in designing critical mechanistic toxicological studies. With respect to the design of studies, PBPK and other biologically based models provide an opportunity to evaluate the various plausible hypotheses by computer simulation. We can ask questions of an "if–then" nature. For example, if the model structure is correct and the rate of a reaction or another process is varied, what is the expected impact on tissue dosimetry? The PBPK model can be used to generate quantitative predictions of the expected experimental outcome based on the most attractive hypothesis of the experimentalists, and this then can be verified experimentally. In this case, the model serves as a tool in designing experimental studies to enable efficient resource utilization and maintenance of the focus on human health risk assessment endpoints.

For example, examining the PBPK model-based risk assessment approach for DCM presented in this chapter, the following questions arise: Is GSH conjugation really the key determinant in DCM tumorigenesis? Are all the important biological determinants of uptake, metabolism, and disposition of DCM included in the model description? These are essentially biological, research-oriented questions with answers that rely on the state of knowledge of mechanisms of toxicokinetics and carcinogenicity of this chemical. Further, in the DCM example presented in this chapter, the low-dose extrapolation of the tissue response was conducted with the LMS modeling approach. The improvement over the conventional methodology is that here the independent variable specified in the LMS model—dose—is not administered dose or inhaled concentration; it is the tissue dose of the toxic moiety estimated with the PBPK model. The uncertainties associated with the low-dose extrapolation using the LMS model can be addressed with the use of biologically based response models (43).

Unlike the mandated mathematical models used in conventional risk assessment, the biologically based dosimetry and response models are versatile and, often, but not always, difficult to validate. In contrast to the "mandated" models, which are useful only for generating a risk number, the biologically based models allow integration of various observations, identification of critical data gaps, and estimation of risk numbers, along with attendant appreciation of areas of significant biological uncertainty.

QUESTIONS

1. Calculate the fat : blood partition coefficient for a chemical with a $P_{o:w}$ of 152.
2. Develop a conceptual representation for PBPK modeling of human exposure to airborne n-octane ($P_{o:w} = 151356$, $P_{w:a} = 0.00762$).
3. Calculate the alveolar ventilation rate (Q_p) for a human weighing 64 kg, knowing that the body weight-normalized Q_p for mammals is 15 L/hr/kg.
4. The V_{max} and K_m of pyrene determined in vitro using rat liver post-mitochondrial fractions were 5.935×10^{-4} μmol/min per mg protein and 27.73 μmol/L, respectively. Convert these potentially useful in vitro values for incorporation into in vivo model (protein concentration = 88 mg protein/g liver, and liver weight = 10 g).
5. Using the rat PBPK model for styrene presented in Figure 5.16 of this chapter, determine the external exposure concentration of styrene corresponding to an area under the curve for liver concentration of 150 mg/L/h (for the parent chemical). Set the exposure duration and the length of simulation to 24 hr.

REFERENCES

1. Abbas, R., and Fisher, J. W. (1997): A physiologically based pharmacokinetic model for trichloroethylene and its metabolites, chloral hydrate, trichloroacetate, dichloroacetate, trichloroethanol, and trichloroethanol glucuronide in B6C3F1 mice. *Toxicol. Appl. Pharmacol.*, 147:15–30.
2. Andersen, M. E., Eklund, C. R., Mills, J. J., Barton, H. A., and Birnbaum, L. S. (1997): A multicompartment geometric model of the liver in relation to regional induction of cytochrome P450s. *Toxicol. Appl. Pharmacol.*, 144:135–144.
3. Andersen, M. E., and Keller, W. C. (1984): Toxicokinetic principles in relation to percutaneous absorption and cutaneous toxicity. In: *Cutaneous Toxicity*, edited by V. A. Drill and P. Lazar, pp. 9–27, Raven Press, New York.
4. Andersen, M. E., Clewell, H. J., III, and Frederick, C. B. (1995): Contemporary issues in toxicology. Applying simulation modeling in toxicology and risk assessment—A short perspective. *Toxicol. Appl. Pharmacol.*, 133:181–187.
5. Andersen, M. E., Clewell, H. J., III, and Gargas, M. L. (1991): Physiologically-based pharmacokinetic modeling with dichloromethane, its metabolite carbon monoxide and blood carboxyhemoglobin in rats and humans. *Toxicol. Appl. Pharmacol.*, 108:14–27.
6. Andersen, M. E., Clewell, H. J., III, Gargas, M. L., Smith, F. A., and Reitz, R. H. (1987): Physiologically-based pharmacokinetics and risk assessment process for methylene chloride. *Toxicol. Appl. Pharmacol.*, 87:185–205.
7. Andersen, M. E., Gargas, M. L., Jones, R. A., and Jenkins, L. J. (1980): Determination of the kinetic constants for metabolism of inhaled toxicants in vivo by gas uptake measurements. *Toxicol. Appl. Pharmacol.*, 54:116.
8. Andersen, M. E., MacNaughton, M. G., Clewell, H. J., III, and Paustenbach, D. J. (1987): Adjusting exposure limits for long and short exposure period using a physiological pharmacokinetic model. *Am. Ind. Hyg. Ass. J.*, 48:335–343.
9. Andersen, M. E., Mills, J. J., and Gargas, M. L. (1993): Modeling receptor-mediated processes with dioxin: Implications for pharmacokinetics and risk assessment. *Risk Anal.*, 13:25–36.
10. Andersen, M. E., and Krishnan, K. (1995): Relating in vitro to in vivo exposures with physiologically based tissue dosimetry and tissue response models. In: *Animal Test Alternatives: Refinement, Reduction, Replacement*, edited by H. Salem, pp. 2–25. Marcel Dekker, Inc., New York.
11. Anderson, M. W., Eling, T. E., Lutz, R. L., and Mattews, H. B. (1977): The construction of a pharmacokinetic model for the disposition of PCBs in the rat. *Clin. Pharmacol. Ther.*, 22:765–773.
12. Angelo, M. J., and Pritchard, A. B. (1987): Route to route extrapolation of dichloromethane exposures using a physiological pharmacokinetic model. *Drinking Water and Health*, 8:254–264.
13. Arms, A. D., and Travis, C. C. (1988): *Reference Physiological Parameters in Pharmacokinetic Modeling*. Office of Health and Environmental Assessment, U.S. Environmental Protection Agency (EPA), Washington, D.C. NTIS PB 88–196019.
14. Auton, M. J., and Woollen, B. H. (1991): A physiologically based mathematical model for the human inhalation pharmacokinetics of 1,1,2-trichloro-1,2,2-trifluoroethane. *Int. Arch. Occup. Environ. Health*, 63:133–138.
15. Barton, H. A., Creech, J. R., Godin, S., Randall, G. M., and Seckel, C. S., (1995): Chloroethylene mixtures: Pharmacokinetic modeling and in vitro metabolism of vinyl chloride, trichloroethylene, and trans-1,2-dichloroethylene in rat. *Toxicol. Appl. Pharmacol.*, 130:237–247.
16. Benignus, V. A., Boyes, W. K., and Bushnell, P. J. (1998): A dosimetric analysis of behavioral effects of acute toluene exposure in rats and humans. *Toxicol. Sci.*, 43:186–195.
17. Bischoff, K. B. (1987): Physiogically-based pharmacokinetic modeling. *Drinking Water and Health*, 8:36–64.
18. Bischoff, K. B., Dedrick, R. L., Zakharo, D. S., and Longstreth, J. A. (1971): Methotrexate pharmacokinetics. *J. Pharm. Sci.*, 60:1128–1133.
19. Bogen, K. T., and Gold, L. S. (1997): Trichloroethylene cancer risk: Simplified calculation of PBPK-based MCLs for cytotoxic end points. *Regul. Toxicol. Pharmacol.*, 25:26–43.
20. Bois, F. Y., Smith, M. T., and Spear, R. C. (1991): Mechanism of benzene carcinogenesis. Application of a physiological model of benzene pharmacokinetics and metabolism. *Toxicol. Lett.*, 56:283–298.
21. Bois, F. Y., Woodruff, T. J., and Spear, R. C. (1991): Comparison of three physiologically-based pharmacokinetic models for benzene disposition. *Toxicol. Appl. Pharmacol.*, 110:79–88.
22. Bois, F. Y., Zeise, L., and Tozer, T. N. (1990): Precision and sensitivity of pharmacokinetic models for cancer risk assessment. Tetrachloroethylene in mice, rats and humans. *Toxicol. Appl. Pharmacol.*, 102:300–315.
23. Bond, J. A., Himmelstein, M. W., Seaton, M., Boogaard, P., and Medinsky, M. A. (1996): Metabolism of butadiene by mice, rats, and humans: A comparison of physiologically based toxicokinetic model predictions and experimental data. *Toxicology*, 113:48–54.
24. Borghoff, S. J., Murphy, J. E., and Medinsky, M. A. (1996): Development of a physiologically based pharmacokinetic model for methyl tertiary-butyl ether and tertiary-butanol in male Fischer-344 rats. *Fundam. Appl. Toxicol.*, 30:264–275.
25. Brodeur, J., Laparé, S., Krishnan, K., Tardif, R., and Goyal, R. (1990): Le problème de l'ajustement des valeurs limites d'exposition pour des horaires de travail non-conventionnels: Utilité de la modélisation pharmacocinétique à base physiologique. *Travail et Santé*, 6:S11–16.
26. Brown, R. P., Delp, M. D., Lindstedt, S. L., Rhomberg, L. R., and Belisle, R. P. (1997): Physiological parameter values for physiologically based pharmacokinetic models. *Toxicol. Ind. Health*, 13:407–484.
27. Bungay, P. M., Dedrick, M. L., and Mattews, H. B. (1981): Enteric transport of chlordecone in the rat. *J. Pharmacokin. Biopharm.*, 9:309–341.
28. Byczkowski, J. Z., Kinkead, E. R., Leahy, H. F., Randall, G. M., and Fisher, J. W. (1994): Computer simulation of the lactational transfer of tetrachloroethylene in rats using a physiologically based model. *Toxicol. Appl. Pharmacol.*, 125:228–236.
29. Byczkowski, J. Z., and Fisher, J. W. (1994): Lactational transfer of tetrachloroethylene in rats. *Risk Anal.*, 14:339–349.
30. Byczkowski, J. Z., and Fisher, J. W. (1995): A computer program linking physiologically based pharmacokinetic model with cancer risk assessment for breast-fed infants. *Comput. Methods Programs Biomed.*, 46:155–163.
31. Cantoreggi, S., and Keller, D. A. (1997): Pharmacokinetics and metabolism of vinyl fluoride in vivo and in vitro. *Toxicol. Appl. Pharmacol.*, 143:130–139.
32. Casanova, M., d'Heck, H., and Deyo, D. F. (1992): Dichloromethane (methylene chloride): Metabolism to formaldehyde and formation of DNA-protein crosslinks in B6C3F1 mice and Syrian golden hamsters. *Toxicol. Appl. Pharmacol.*, 114:162–165.
33. Caster, W. O., Poncelet, J., Simon, A. B., and Armstrong, W. B. (1956): Tissue weights of the rat. I. Normal values determined by dissection and chemical methods. *Proc. Soc. Exp. Biol. Med.*, 91:122–126.
34. Chen, C. W., and Blancato, J. N. (1987): Role of pharmacokinetic modeling in risk assessment: Perchloroethylene as an example.

In: *Pharmacokinetics in Risk Assessment. Drinking Water and Health*, 8:369–385.

35. Chen, H. S. G., and Gross, J. F. (1979): Estimation of tissue to plasma partition coefficients used in physiological pharmacokinetic models. *J. Pharmacokin. Biopharm.*, 7:117–125.
36. Clarke, D. O., Elswick, B. A., Welsch, F., and Conolly, R. B. (1993): Pharmacokinetics of 2-methoxyethanol and 2-methoxyacetic acid in the pregnant mouse: A physiologically-based mathematical model. *Toxicol. Appl. Pharmacol.*, 121:239–252.
37. Clewell H. J., Gentry, P. R., and Gearhart, J. M. (1997): Investigation of the potential impact of benchmark dose and pharmacokinetic modeling in noncancer risk assessment. *J. Toxicol. Environ. Health*, 52:475–515.
38. Clewell H. J., Gentry, P. R., Gearhart, J. M., Allen, B. C., and Andersen, M. E. (1995): Considering pharmacokinetic and mechanistic information in cancer risk assessments for environmental contaminants—examples with vinyl chloride and trichloroethylene. *Chemosphere*, 31:2561–2578.
39. Clewell, H. J. III, and Andersen, M. E. (1987): Dose, species and route extrapolation using physiologically-based pharmacokinetic models. *Drinking Water and Health*, 8:159–182.
40. Clewell, H. J. III, and Jarnot, B. M. (1994): Incorporation of pharmacokinetics in noncancer risk assessment: Example with chloropentafluorobenzene. *Risk Anal.*, 14:265–276.
41. Cohn, M. S. (1987): Sensitivity analysis in pharmacokinetic modeling. *Drinking Water and Health*, 8:265–272.
42. Collins, J. M., Dedrick, R. L., Flessner, M. F., and Guarino, A. M. (1982): Concentration dependent disappearance of fluorouracil from peritoneal fluid in the rat: Experimental observations and distributed modeling. *J. Pharm. Sci.*, 71:735–738.
43. Conolly, R. B., and Andersen, M. E. (1991): Biologically based pharmacodynamic models: Tools for toxicological research and risk assessment. *Annu. Rev. Toxicol. Pharmacol.*, 31:503–523.
44. Corley, R. A., Bormett, G. A., and Ghanayem, B. I. (1994): Physiologically based pharmacokinetics of 2-butoxyethanol and its major metabolite, 2-butoxyacetic acid, in rats and humans. *Toxicol. Appl. Pharmacol.*, 129:61–79.
45. Corley, R. A., Mandrela, A. L., and Smith, F. A. (1990): Development of a physiologically-based pharmacokinetic model for chloroform. *Toxicol. Appl. Pharmacol.*, 103:512–527.
46. Corley, R. A., Markham, D. A., Banks, C., Delorme, P., Masterman, A., and Houle, J. M. (1997): Physiologically based pharmacokinetics and the dermal absorption of 2-butoxyethanol vapor by humans. *Fundam. Appl. Pharmacol.*, 39:120–130.
47. Cox. L. A. (1996): Reassessing benzene risks using internal doses and Monte Carlo uncertainty analysis. *Environ. Health Perspect.*, 104 (suppl.6):1413–1429.
48. Crank, W. D., and Vinegar, A. (1992): A physiologically-based pharmacokinetic model for chloropentafluorobenzene in primates to be used in the evaluation of protective equipment against toxic gases. *Toxicol. Ind. Health*, 8:21–35.
49. Cronin, W. J., Oswald, E. J., Shelley, M. L., Fisher, J. W., and Flemming, C. D. (1995): A trichlororthylene risk assessment using a Monte Carlo Analysis of parameter uncertainty in conjunction with physiologically-based pharmacokinetic modeling. *Risk Anal.*, 15:555–565.
50. Csanady, G. A., Kreuzer, P. E., Baur, C., and Filser, J. G. (1996): A physiological toxicokinetic model for 1,3-butadiene in rodents and man: Blood concentrations of 1,3-butadiene, its metabolically formed epoxides, and of haemoglobin adducts-relevance of glutathione depletion. *Toxicology*, 113:300–305.
51. Dallas, C. E., Bruckner, J. V., Megden, J. L., and Weir, F. W. (1986): A method for direct measurement of systemic uptake and elimination of volatile organics in small mammals. *J. Pharmacol. Meth.*, 16:239–250.
52. Dallas, C. E., Chen, X. M., Muralidhara, S., Varkonyl, P., Tackett, L., and Bruckner, J. V. (1995): Physiologically based pharmacokinetic model useful in prediction of the influence of species, dose, and exposure route on perchloroethylene pharmacokinetics. *J. Toxicol. Environ. Health*, 44:301–317.
53. Dallas, C. E., Chen, X. M., O'Barr, K., Muralidhara, S., Varkonyl, P., and Bruckner, J. V. (1994): Development of a physiologically based pharmacokinetic model for perchloroethylene using tissue concentration-time data. *Toxicol. Appl. Pharmacol.*, 128:50–59.
54. Dallas, C. E., Gallo, J. M., Ramanthan, R., Muralidhara, S., and Bruckner, J. V. (1991): Physiological pharmacokinetic modeling of inhaled trichloroethylene in rats. *Toxicol. Appl. Pharmacol.*, 110:303–314.
55. Dallas, C. E., Ramanthan, R., Muralidhara, S., Gallo, G. M., and Bruckner, J. V. (1989): The uptake and elimination of 1,1,1-trichloroethane during the following inhalation exposures in rats. *Toxicol. Appl. Pharmacol.*, 98:385–397.
56. Dalley, J. W., Gupta, P. K., and Hung, C. T. (1990): A physiological pharmacokinetic model describing the disposition of lead in the absence and presence of l-ascorbic acid in rats. *Toxicol. Lett.*, 50:337–348.
57. Davies, B., and Morris, T. (1993): Physiological parameters in laboratory animals and humans. *Pharm. Res.*, 10: 1093–1095.
58. Dedrick, R. L., Forrester, D. D., and Ho, D. H. W. (1972): In vitro–in vivo correlation of drug metabolism: Deamination of 1-β-D-arabinosyl cytosine. *Biochem. Pharmacol.*, 21:1–16.
59. Dedrick, R. L., Zaharko, D. S., and Lutz, R. J. (1973): Transport and binding of methotrexate in vivo. *J. Pharm. Sci.*, 62:882–890.
60. DeJongh, J., and Blaauboer, B. J. (1996): In vitro-based and in vivo-based simulations of benzene uptake and metabolism in rats. *ATLA*, 24:179–190.
61. DeJongh, J., and Blaauboer, B. J. (1997): Simulation of lindane kinetics in rats. *Toxicology*, 122:1–9.
62. DeJongh, J., and Blaauboer, B. J. (1996): Simulation of toluene kinetics in the rat by a physiologically based pharmacokinetic model with application of biotransformation parameters derived independently in vitro and in vivo. *Fundam. Appl. Toxicol.*, 32:260–268.
63. DeJongh, J., and Blaauboer, B. J. (1997): Evaluation of in vitro-based simulations of toluene uptake and metabolism in rats. *Toxicol. in vitro*, 11:485–489.
64. DeJongh, J., Verhaar, H. J. M., and Hermens, J. L. M. (1997): A quantitative property–property relationship (QPPR) approach to estimate in vitro tissue–blood partition coefficients of organic chemical sin rats and humans. *Arch. Toxicol.*, 72:17–25.
65. Delp, M. D., Manning, R. O., Bruckner, J. V., and Armstrong, R. B. (1991): Distribution of cardiac output during diurnal changes of activity in rats. *Am. J. Physiol.*, 261:H1487–1493.
66. Dietz, K. F., Rodriguez-Giaxola, M., Traiger, G. J., Stella, V. J., and Himmelstein, K. J. (1981): Pharmacokinetics of 2-butanol and its metabolites in the rat. *J. Pharmacokin. Biopharm.*, 9:553–573.
67. Domenech, R. J., Hoffman, J. E., Noble, M. M., Saunder, K. B., Hensen, J. R., and Subijanto, S. (1969): Total and regional coronary blood flow measured by radioactive microsphere in conscious and anesthetized dogs. *Circul. Res.*, 25:581–596.
68. Droz, P. O., Berode, M., and Jang, J. Y. (1999): Biological monitoring of tetrahydrofuran: Contribution of a physiologically based pharmacokinetic model. *Am. Ind. Hyg. Ass. J.*, 60:243–248.
69. D'Souza, R. W., and Andersen, M. E. (1988): Physiologically-based pharmacokinetic model for vinylidine chloride. *Toxicol. Appl. Pharmacol.*, 95:230–240.
70. D'Souza, R. W., Francis, W. R., and Andersen, M. W. (1988): Physiological model for tissue glutathione depletion and decreased

resynthesis after ethylene dichloride exposures. *J. Pharmacol. Exp. Ther.*, 245:563–568.

71. Ellis, M. K., Trebilcock, R., Naylor, J. L., Tseung, K., Collins, M. A., Hext, P. M., and Green, T. (1996): The inhalation toxicology, genetic toxicology, and metabolism of difluoromethane in the rat. *Fundam. Appl. Toxicol.*, 31:243–251.
72. El-Masri, H. A., and Portier, C. J. (1998): Physiologically-based pharmacokinetics model of primidone and its metabolites phenobarbital and phenylethylmalonamide in humans, rats and mice. *Drug Metab. Dispos.*, 26:585–594.
73. El-Masri, H. A., Bell, D. A., and Portier, C. J. (1999). Effects of glutathione transferase theta polymorphism on the risk estimates of dichloromethane to humans. *Toxicol. Appl. Pharmacol.*, 158:221–230.
74. Falk, A., Gullstrand, E., Löf, A., and Wigaeus-Hjelm, E. (1990): Liquid/air partition coefficients of four terpenes. *Br. J. Ind. Med.*, 47:62–64.
75. Farrar, D., Allen, B., Crump, K., and Shipp, A. (1989): Evaluation of uncertainty in input parameters to pharmacokinetic models and the resulting uncertainty in output. *Toxicol. Lett.*, 49:371–385.
76. Farris, F. F., Dedrick, R. L., Allen, P. V., and Smith, J. C. (1993): Physiological model for the pharmacokinetics of methylmercury in the growing rat. *Toxicol. Appl. Pharmacol.*, 119:74–90.
77. Farris, F. F., Dedrick, R. L., and King, F. G. (1988): Cisplatin pharmacokinetics: Applications of a physiological model. *Toxicol. Lett.*, 43:117–137.
78. Filser, J. G., and Bolt, H. M. (1979): Pharmacokinetics of halogenated ethylenes in rats. *Arch. Toxicol.*, 42:123–136.
79. Filser, J. G., Csanady, G. A., Denk, B., Hartmann, M., Kauffman, A., Kessler, W., Kreuzer, P. E., Putz, C., Shen, J. H., and Stei, P. (1996): Toxicokinetics of isopropene in rodents and humans. *Toxicology*, 113:278–287.
80. Fiserova-Bergerova, V. (1975): Mathematical modeling of inhalation exposure. *J. Combust. Toxicol.*, 32:201–210.
81. Fiserova-Bergerova, V., and Diaz, M. L. (1986): Determination and prediction of tissue–gas partition coefficients. *Int. Arch. Occup. Environ. Health*, 58:75–87.
82. Fisher, J. W., Whittaker, T. A., Taylor, D. H., Clewell, H. J., and Andersen, M. E. (1990): Physiologically-based pharmacokinetic modeling of the lactating rat and nursing pup: A multiroute exposure model for trichloroethylene and its metabolite, trichloroacetic acid. *Toxicol. Appl. Pharmacol.*, 102:497–513.
83. Fisher, J., Mahle, D., Bankston, L., Greene, R., and Gearhart, J. (1997): Lactational transfer of volatile chemicals in breast milk. *Ind. Hyg. Assoc. J.*, 58:425–431.
84. Fisher, J. W., and Allen, B. C. (1993): Evaluating the risk of liver cancer in humans exposed to trichloroethylene using physiological models. *Risk Anal.*, 13:87–95.
85. Fisher, J. W., Gargas, M. L., Jepson, G. W., Allen, B., and Andersen, M. E. (1991): Physiologically based pharmacokinetic modeling with trichloroethylene and its metabolite, trichloroacetic acid in the rat and mouse. *Toxicol. Appl. Pharmacol.*, 109:183–195.
86. Fisher, J. W., Mahle, D., and Abbas, R. (1998): A human physiologically based pharmacokinetic model for trichloroethylene and its metabolites, trichloroacetic acid and free trichloroethanol. *Toxicol. Appl. Pharmacol.*, 152:339–359.
87. Fisher, J. W., Whittaker, T. A., Taylor, D. H., Clewell, H. J., and Andersen, M. E. (1989): Physiologically-based pharmacokinetic modeling of the pregnant rat: Multiroute exposure model for trichloroethylene and trichloroacetic acid. *Toxicol. Appl. Pharmacol.*, 99:395–414.
88. Frederick, C. B., Bush, M. L., Lomax, L. M., Black, K. A., Finch, L., Kimbell, J. S., Morgan, K. T., Subramaniam, R. P., Morris, J. B., and Ultman, J. S. (1998): Application of a hybrid computational fluid dynamics and physiologically based inhalation model for interspecies dosimetry extrapolation of acidic vapors in the upper airways. *Toxicol. Appl. Pharmacol.*, 152:211–231.
89. Frederick, C. B., Potter, D. W., Chang-Mateu, M. I., and Andersen, M. E. (1992): A physiologically-based pharmacokinetic and pharmacodynamic model to describe the oral dosing of rats with ethyl acrylate and its implications for risk assessment. *Toxicol. Appl. Pharmacol.*, 114:246–260.
90. Freeman, R. A., Rozman, K. K., and Wilson, A. G. E. (1989): Physiological pharmacokinetic model of hexachlorobenzene in the rat. *Health Phys.*, 57:139–147.
91. Gabrielsson, J. L., Paalkow, L. K., and Nordstrom, L. (1987): A physiologically-based pharmacokinetic model for theophylline disposition in the pregnant and nonpregnant rat. *J. Pharmacokin. Biopharm.*, 12:149–165.
92. Gallo, J. M., Lam, F. C., and Perrier, D. G. (1987): Area method for the estimation of partition coefficients for physiological pharmacokinetic models. *J. Pharmacokin. Biopharm.*, 15:271–280.
93. Gargas, M. L. (1990): An exhaled breath chamber system for assessing rates of metabolism and rates of gastrointestinal absorption with volatile chemicals. *J. Am. Coll. Toxicol.*, 9:447–453.
94. Gargas, M. L., and Andersen, M. E. (1989): Determinating the kinetic constants of chlorinated ethane metabolism in the rat from rates of exhalation. *Toxicol. Appl. Pharmacol.*, 99:344–353.
95. Gargas, M. L., Andersen, M. E., and Clewell, H. J. (1986): A physiologically-based simulation approach for determining metabolic rate constants from gas uptake data. *Toxicol. Appl. Pharmacol.*, 86:341–352.
96. Gargas, M. L., Andersen, M. E., Teo, S. K., Batra, R., Fennell, T. R., and Kedderis, G. L. (1995): A physiologically based dosimetry description of acrylonitrile and cyanoethylene oxide in the rat. *Toxicol. Appl. Pharmacol.*, 134:185–194.
97. Gargas, M. L., Burgess, R. J., Voisard, D. E., Cason, G. H., and Andersen, M. E. (1989): Partition coefficients of low molecular weight volatile chemicals in various liquids and tissues. *Toxicol. Appl. Pharmacol.*, 98:87–99.
98. Gargas, M. L., Clewell, H. J., and Andersen, M. E. (1986): Gas uptake inhalation techniques and the rates of metabolism of chloromethanes, chloroethanes and chloroethylenes in the rat. *Inhal. Toxicol.*, 2:319.
99. Gargas, M. L., Clewell, H. J., and Andersen, M. E. (1986): Metabolism of inhaled dihalomethanes in vivo: Differentiation of kinetic constants for two independent pathways. *Toxicol. Appl. Pharmacol.*, 87:211–223.
100. Gargas, M. L., Seybold, P. G., and Andersen, M. E. (1988): Modeling the tissue solubilities and metabolic rate constants of halogenated methanes, ethanes and ethylenes. *Toxicol. Lett.*, 43:235–256.
101. Gear, C. W. (1971): *Numerical Initial Value Problems in Ordinary Differential Equations*. Prentice-Hall, Englewoods Cliffs, New Jersey.
102. Gearhart, J. M., Clewell, H. J. I., Crump, K. S., Shipp, A. M., and Silvers, A. (1995): Pharmacokinetic dose estimates of mercury in children and dose-response curves of perfomance tests in a large epidemiological study. *Water Air Soil Pollut.*, 80:49–58.
103. Gearheart, J. M., Jepson, G. W., Clewell, H. J., Andersen, M. E., and Conolly, R. B. (1990): A physiologically-based model for the in vivo inhibition of acetylcholinesterase by diisopropylfluorophosphate. *Toxicol. Appl. Pharmacol.*, 106:295–310.
104. Georgopoulos, P. G., Roy, A., and Gallo, M. A. (1994): Reconstruction of short-term multi-route exposure to volatile organic compounds using physiologically based pharmacokinetic models. *J. Expos. Anal. Environ. Epidemiol.*, 4:309–328.
105. Gerde, P., and Dahl, A. R. (1991): A model for the uptake of inhaled vapors in the nose of the dog during cyclic breathing. *Toxicol. Appl. Pharmacol.*, 109:276–288.

106. Gibaldi, M., and Perrier, D. (1982): *Pharmacokinetics*. Marcel Dekker, New York.

107. Gray, D. G. (1995): A physiologically based pharmacokinetic model for methyl mercury in the pregnant rat and fetus. *Toxicol. Appl. Pharmacol.*, 132:91–102.

108. Greenberg, M. S., Burton, G. A., and Fisher, J. W. (1999): Physiologically based pharmacokinetic modeling of inhaled trichloroethylene and its oxidative metabolites in B6C3F1 mice. *Toxicol. Appl. Pharmacol.*, 154:264–278.

109. Haddad, S., Gad, S. C., Tardif, R., and Krishnan, K. (1995): Statistical approaches for the validation of physiologically-based pharmacokinetic (PBPK) models. *Toxicologist*, 15 (258).

110. Haddad, S., Pelekis, M., and Krishnan, K. (1996): A methodology for solving physiologically based pharmacokinetic models without the use of simulation softwares. *Toxicol. Lett.*, 85:113–126.

111. Haddad, S., Withey, J., Lapare, S., Law, F., and Krishnan, K. (1998): Physiologically-based pharmacokinetic modeling of pyrene in the rat. *Environ. Toxicol. Pharmacol.*, 5:245–255.

112. Haggard, H. W. (1924): The absorption, distribution and elimination of ethyl ether. Analysis of the mechanism of the absorption and elimination of such a gas or vapor as ethyl ether. *J. Biol. Chem.*, 59:753–770.

113. Hallenbeck, W. H. (1992). Cancer risk assessment for the inhalation 1,3-butadiene using PBPK modeling. *Bull. Environ. Contam. Toxicol.,* 49:66–70.

114. Hattis, D., White, P., Marmorstein, L., and Koch, P. (1990): Uncertainties in pharmacokinetics modeling for perchloroethylene. I. Comparison of model structure, parameters, and predictions for low dose metabolic rates for models by different authors. *Risk Anal.*, 10:449–458.

115. Hetrick, D. M., Jarabek, A. M., and Travis, C. C. (1991): Sensitivity analysis for physiologically-based pharmacokinetic models. *J. Pharmacokin. Biopharm.*, 19:1–20.

116. Hilderbrand, R. L., Andersen, M. E., and Jensen, L. J. (1981): Prediction of in vivo kinetic constants for metabolism of inhaled vapors from kinetic constants measured in vitro. *Fundam. Appl. Toxicol.*, 1:403–409.

117. Horton, V. L., Higuchi, M. A., and Rickert, D. E. (1992): Physiologically based pharmacokinetic model for methanol in rats, monkeys and humans. *Toxicol. Appl. Pharmacol.*, 117:26–36.

118. Igari, Y., Sugiyama, Y., Sawada, Y., Iga, Y., and Hanano, M. (1983): Prediction of diazepam disposition in rat and man by a physiologically-based pharmacokinetic model. *J. Pharmacokin. Biopharm.*, 11:577–593.

119. Iman, R., and Helton, J. (1988): An investigation of uncertainty and sensitivity analysis techniques for computer models. *Risk Anal.*, 8:71–90.

120. International Commission on Radiation Protection (1975): *Report of the task group on reference man*. ICRP Publication No. 23. Pergamon Press, New York.

121. Iwatsubo, T., Suzuki, H., and Sugiyama, Y. (1997). Prediction of species differences (rats, dogs, humans) in the in vivo metabolic clearance of YM796 by the liver from in vitro data. *J. Pharmacol. Exp. Ther.*, 283:462–469.

122. Iyengar, S., and Rao, M. S. (1983): Statistical techniques in modeling of complex systems: Single versus multiresponse models. *IEEE Trans. Syst. Man. Cybernet.*, 13:175–189.

123. Jain, R. K., Gerlowski, L. E., Weissbrod, J. M., Wang, J., and Pierson, R. N. (1982): Kinetics of uptake, distribution and excretion of zinc in rats. *Ann. Biomed. Eng.*, 9:347–361.

124. Järnberg, J., and Johanson, G. (1999): Physiologically based modeling of 1,2,4-trimethylbenzene inhalation toxicokinetics. *Toxicol. Appl. Pharmacol.*, 155:203–214.

125. Johanson, G. (1986): Physiologically-based pharmacokinetic modeling of inhaled 2-butoxyethanol in man. *Toxicol. Lett.*, 34:23–31.

126. Johanson, G. (1991): Modeling of respiratory exchange of polar solvents. *Ann. Occup. Hyg.*, 35:323–339.

127. Johanson, G., and Dynesius, B. (1988): Liquid : air partition coefficients for six commonly used glycol ethers. *Br. J. Ind. Med.*, 45:561–564.

128. Johanson, G., and Filser, J. G. (1992): Experimental data from closed chamber gas uptake studies in rodents suggest lower uptake rate of chemical than calculated from literature values on alveolar ventilation. *Arch. Toxicol.*, 66:291–295.

129. Johanson, G., and Filser, J. G. (1993): A physiologically based pharmacokinetic model for butadiene and its metabolite butadiene monoepoxide in rat and mouse and its significance for risk extrapolation. *Arch. Toxicol.*, 67:151–163.

130. Johanson, G., and Filser, J. G. (1996): PBPK model for butadiene metabolism to epoxides: Quantitative species differences in metabolism. *Toxicology*, 113:40–47.

131. Johanson, G., and Naslund, P. H. (1988): Spreadsheet programming: A new approach in physiologically-based modeling of solvent toxicokinetics. *Toxicol. Lett.*, 41:115–127.

132. Kaneko, T., Endoh, K., and Sato, A. (1991): Biological monitoring of exposure to organic solvent vapors. I. A physiological simulation model of m-xylene pharmacokinetics in man. *Yamanashi Med. J.*, 6:127–135.

133. Kedderis, G. L., and Held, S. D. (1996): Prediction of furan pharmacokinetics from hepatocyte studies: Comparison of bioactivation and hepatic dosimetry in rats, mice, and humans. *Toxicol. Appl. Pharmacol.*, 140:124–130.

134. Kedderis, G. L., Teo, S. K., Batra, R., Held, S. D., and Gargas, M. L. (1996): Refinement and verification of the physiologically based dosimetry description for acrylonitrile in rats. *Toxicol. Appl. Pharmacol.*, 140:422–435.

135. Kedderis, L. B., Mills, J. J., Andersen, M. E., and Birnbaum, L. S. (1993): A physiologically-based pharmacokinetic model of 2,3,7,8-tetrabromo dibenzo-p-dioxin (TBDD) in the rat: Tissue distribution and CYPIA induction. *Toxicol. Appl. Pharmacol.*, 121:87–98.

136. Kety, S. S. (1951): The theory and application of the exchange of inert gas at the lungs. *Pharmacol. Rev.*, 3:1–41.

137. Keys, D. A., Wallance, D. G., Kepler, T. B., and Conolly, R. B. (1999): Quantitative evaluation of alternative mechanisms of blood and testes disposition of di-(2-ethylhexyl)phthalate and mono(2-ethylhexyl)phthalate in rats. *Toxicol. Sci.*, 49:172–185.

138. Khor, S. P., and Mayersohn, M. (1991): Potential error in the measurement of tissue to blood distribution coefficients in physiological pharmacokinetic modeling: Residual tissue blood. I. Theoretical considerations. *Drug Metab. Disp.*, 19:478–485.

139. Kim, C. S., Gargas, M. L., and Andersen, M. E. (1994): Pharmacokinetic modeling of 2,4-dichlorophenoxyacetic acid (2,4-D) in rat and in rabbit brain following single dose administration. *Toxicol. Lett.*, 74:189–201.

140. Kim, C. S., Slikker, W., Ninienda, Z., Gargas, M. L., and Andersen, M. E. (1995): Development of a physiologically based pharmacokinetic model for 2,4-dichlorophenoxyacetic acid dosimetry in discrete areas of the rabbit brain. *Neurotoxicol. Teratol.*, 17:111–120.

141. King, F. G., Dedrick, R. L., Collins, J. M., Mattews, H. B., and Birnbaum, L. G. (1983): Physiological model for the pharmacokinetics of 2,3,7,8-tetra-chloro dibenzofuran in several species. *Toxicol. Appl. Pharmacol.*, 67:390–400.

142. Knaak, J. B., and Smith, L. W. (1998): In vitro hepatic metabolism of PCBTF: Development of V_{max} and K*m* values and partition

coefficients and their use in an inhalation PBPK model. *Inhal. Toxicol.*, 10:65–85.

143. Kohn, M. C., and Melnick, R. L. (1993): Species differences in pharmacokinetics and clearance of 1,3-butadiene metabolites: A mechanistic model indicates predominantly physiological, not biochemical control. *Carcinogenesis*, 14:619–628.

144. Koizumi, A. (1989): Potential of physiological pharmacokinetics to amalgamate kinetic data of trichloroethylene and tetrachloroethylene obtained in rats and man. *Br. J. Ind. Med.*, 46:239–249.

145. Kootsey, J. M., Kohn, M. C., Feezor, M. D., Mitchell, G. R., and Fletcher, P. R. (1986): SCoP: An interactive simulation control program for micro-and minicomputers. *Bull. Math. Biol.*, 48:427–441.

146. Krewski, D., Wang, Y., Bartlett, S., and Krishnan, K. (1995): Uncertainty, variability, and sensitivity analysis in physiological pharmacokinetic models. *J. Biopharm. Statist.*, 5:245–271.

147. Krishnan, K., Andersen, M. E., Clewell, H. J., III, and Yang, R. S. H. (1994): Physiologically-based pharmacokinetic modeling of chemical mixtures. In: *Toxicology of Chemical Mixtures*, edited by R. S. A. Yang, pp. 399–437. Academic Press, New York.

148. Krishnan, K., Pelekis, M. L., and Haddad, S. (1995): A simple index for describing the discrepancy between PBPK model simulations and experimental data. *J. Toxicol. Ind. Health*, 11:413–421.

149. Krishnan, K., and Andersen, M. E. (1998): Physiologically based pharmacokinetic models in risk assessment of developmental neurotoxicants. In: *Handbook Developmental Neurotoxicology*, pp. 709–725.

150. Krishnan, K., Gargas, M. L., and Andersen, M. E. (1993): In vitro toxicology and risk assessment. *Altern. Meth. Toxicol.*, 9:185–203.

151. Krishnan, K., Gargas, M. L., Fennell, T. R., and Andersen, M. E. (1992): A physiologically-based description of ethylene oxide dosimetry in the rat. *Toxicol. Ind. Health*, 8:121–140.

152. Kubic, V. L., Anders, M. W., Engel, R. R., Barlow, C. H., and Caughey, W. S. (1974): Metabolism of dihalomethanes to carbon monoxide. *Drug Metab. Dispos.*, 2:53–57.

153. Kumagai, S., and Matsunaga, I. (1995): Effect of variation of exposure to airborne chlorobenzene on internal exposure and concentrations of urinary metabolite. *Occup. Environ. Med.*, 52:65–70.

154. Kumagai, S., and Matsunaga, I. (1995): Physiologically based pharmacokinetic model for acetone. *Occup. Environ. Med.*, 52:344–352.

155. Lam, G., Chen, M. L., and Chiou, W. L. (1982): Determination of tissue: blood partition coefficients in physiologically-based pharmacokinetic models. *J. Pharm. Sci.*, 71:454–456.

156. Lapare, S., Tardif, R., and Brodeur, J. (1993): Effect of various exposure scenarios on the biological monitoring of organic solvents. I. Toluene and xylene. *Int. Arch. Occup. Environ. Health*, 64:569–580.

157. Lapare, S., Tardif, R., and Brodeur, J. (1995): Effect of various exposure scenarios on the biological monitoring of organic solvents in alveolar air. II. 1,1,1-trichloroethane and trichloroethylene. *Int. Arch. Occup. Environ. Health*, 67:375–394.

158. Lawrence, G. S., and Gobas, F. A. P. C. (1997): A pharmacokinetic analysis of interspecies extrapolation in dioxin risk assessment. *Chemosphere*, 35:427–452.

159. Leavens, T. L., Moss, D. R., and Bond, J. A. (1996): Dynamic inhalation system for individual whole-body exposure of mice to volatile organic chemicals. *Inhal. Toxicol.*, 8:655–677.

160. Lee, K. M., Dill, J. A., Chou, B. J., and Roycroft, J. H. (1998): Physiologically based pharmacokinetic model for chronic inhalation of 2-butoxyethanol. *Toxicol. Appl. Pharmacol.*, 153:211–226.

161. Leung, H. W., and Paustenbach, D. J. (1990): Cancer risk assessment for dioxane based upon a physiologically-based pharmacokinetic modeling approach. *Toxicol. Lett.*, 51:147–162.

162. Leung, H. W., Ku, R. H., Paustenbach, D. J., and Andersen, M. E. (1988): A physiologically-based pharmacokinetic model for 2,3,7,8-tetrachloro dibenzo-p-dioxin in C57BL/6J and DBA/2J mice. *Toxicol. Lett.*, 42:15–28.

163. Leung, H. W., Paustenbach, D. J., Murray, F. J., and Andersen, M. E. (1990): A physiologically-based pharmacokinetic description and enzyme-inducing properties of 2,3,7,8-tetrachlorodibenzo-p-dioxin in the rat. *Toxicol. Appl. Pharmacol.*, 103:399–410.

164. Leung, H. W., Poland, A. P., Paustenbach, D. J., and Andersen, M. E. (1990): Dose-dependent pharmacokinetics of (125-I)-2-iodo-3, 7,8-trichlorodibenzo-p-dioxin in mice: Analysis with a physiological modeling approach. *Toxicol. Appl. Pharmacol.*, 103:411–419.

165. Liira, J., Johanson, G., and Riihimaki, V. (1990): Dose-dependent kinetics of inhaled methylethylketone in man. *Toxicol. Lett.*, 50:195–201.

166. Lilly, P. D., Andersen, M. E., Ross, T. M., and Pegram, R. A. (1998): A physiologically based pharmacokinetic description of the oral uptake, tissue dosimetry, and rates of metabolism of bromodichloromethane in the male rat. *Toxicol. Appl. Pharmacol.*, 150:205–217.

167. Lin, J. H., Sugiyama, Y., Awazu, S., and Hanano, M. (1982): In vitro and in vivo evaluation of the tissue to blood partition coefficients for physiological pharmacokinetic models. *J. Pharmacokin. Biopharm.*, 10:637–647.

168. Lin, J. H., Sugiyama, Y., Awazu, S., and Hanano, M. (1982): Physiological pharmacokinetics of ethoxybenzamine based on biochemical data obtained in vitro as well as on physiological data. *J. Pharmacokin. Biopharm.*, 10:649–661.

169. Lindstrom, F. T., Gillette, J. W., and Rodecap, S. E. (1974): Distribution of HEOD (dieldrin) in mammals. I. Preliminary model. *Arch. Environ. Contam. Toxicol.*, 2:9–42.

170. Lipscomb, J. C., Fisher, J. W., Confer, P. D., and Byczkowski, J. Z. (1998): In vitro to in vivo extrapolation for trichloroethylene metabolism in humans. *Toxicol. Appl. Pharmacol.* 152:376–387.

171. Loizou, G. D., and Anders, M. W. (1995): Gas-uptake pharmacokinetics and metabolism of 2-chloro-1,1,1,2-tetrafluoroethane (HCFC-124) in the rat, mouse, and hamster. *Drug Metab. Dispos.*, 23:875–880.

172. Loizou, G. D., Eldirdiri, N. I., and King, L. J. (1996): Physiologically based pharmacokinetics of uptake by inhalation of a series of 1,1,1-trihaloethanes: Correlation with various physicochemical parameters. *Inhal. Toxicol.*, 8:1-19.

173. Loizou, G. D., Urban, G., Dekant, W., and Anders, M. W. (1994): Gas-uptake pharmacokinetics of 2,2-dichloro-1,1,1-trifluoroethane (HCFC-123). *Drug Metab. Dispos.*, 22:511–517.

174. Lutz, R. J., Dedrick, R. L., Tuey, D., Sipes, I. G., Andersen, M. W., and Mattews, H. B. (1984): Comparison of the pharmacokinetics of several polychlorinated biphenyls in the mouse, rat, dog, and monkey by means of a physiological pharmacokinetic model. *Drug Metab. Dispos.*, 12:527–535.

175. Macpherson, S. E., Barton, C. N., and Bronaugh R. L. (1996): Use of in vitro skin penetration data and a physiologically based model to predict in vivo blood levels of benzoic acid. *Toxicol. Appl. Pharmacol.*, 140:436–443.

176. Mann, S., Droz, P. O., and Vahter, M. (1996): A physiologically based pharmacokinetic model for arsenic exposure. I. Development in hamsters and rabbits. *Toxicol. Appl. Pharmacol.*, 137:8–22.

177. Mann, S., Droz, P. O., and Vahter, M. (1996): A physiologically based pharmacokinetic model for arsenic exposure. II. Validation and application in humans. *Toxicol. Appl. Pharmacol.*, 140:471–486.

178. Mapleson, W. W. (1963): An electric analog for uptake and elimination in man. *J. Appl. Physiol.*, 18:197–204.

179. Mauderly, J. L. (1990): Measurment of respiration and respiratory responses during inhalation exposures. *J. Am. Coll. Toxicol.*, 9:397–406.

180. McDougal, J. N., Jepson, G. W., Clewell, H. J., and Andersen, M. E. (1985): Dermal absorption of dihalomethane vapors. *Toxicol. Appl. Pharmacol.*, 79:150–158.

181. McDougal, J. N., Jepson, G. W., Clewell, H. J., MacNaughton, M. G., and Andersen, M. E. (1986): A physiological pharmacokinetic model for dermal absorption of vapors in the rat. *Toxicol. Appl. Pharmacol.*, 85:286–294.

182. Medinsky, M. A., Sabourin, P. J., Lucier, G., Birnbaum, L. S., and Henderson, R. F. (1989): A physiological model for simulation of benzene by rats and mice. *Toxicol. Appl. Pharmacol.*, 99:193–206.

183. Menzel, D. B. (1988): Planning and using PBPK models: An integrated inhalation and distribution model for nickel. *Toxicol. Lett.*, 43:67–83.

184. Menzel, D. B., Wolpert, R. L., Boger, J. R., and Kootsey, J. M. (1987): Resources available for simulation in toxicology: Specialized computers, generalized software and communication networks. *Drinking Water and Health*, 8:229–254.

185. Miller, F. J., Overton, J. H., Jaskot, R. H., and Menzel, D. B. (1985): A model for the regional uptake of gaseous pollutants in the lung. I. The sensitivity of the uptake of ozone in the human lung to lower respiratory tract secretions and exercise. *Toxicol. Appl. Pharmacol.*, 79:11–27.

186. Mortensen, B., Lokken, T., Zahlsen, K., and Nilsen, O. G. (1997): Comparison and in vivo relevance of two different in vitro headspace metabolic systems: Liver S9 and liver slices. *Pharmacol. Toxicol.*, 81:35–41.

187. Mortensen, B., and Nilsen, O. G. (1988): Allometric species comparison of toluene and n-hexane metabolism: Prediction of hepatic clearance in man from experiments with rodent liver S9 in headspace vial equilibration system. *Pharmacol. Toxicol.*, 82:183–188.

188. Nakajima, T., and Sato, A. (1979): Enhanced activity of liver drug-metabolizing enzymes for aromatic and chlorinated hydrocarbons following food deprivation. *Toxicol. Appl. Pharmacol.*, 50:549–556.

189. National Toxicology Program (1985): NTP Technical Report on the Toxicology and Carcinogenesis Studies of Dichloromethane in Fisher-344 Rats and B6C3F1 Mice (inhalation studies). NTP TR No. 306.

190. Nestorov, I. A., Aarons, L. J., and Rowland, M. (1997): Physiologically based pharmacokinetic modeling of a homologous series of barbiturates in the rat: A sensitivity analysis. *J. Pharmacokin. Biopharm.*, 25:413–447.

191. O'Flaherty, E. (1998): Physiologically based models of metal kinetics. *Crit. Rev. Toxicol.*, pp. 271–317.

192. O'Flaherty, E. J. (1981): *Toxicant and Drugs: Kinetics and Dynamics*. John Wiley, New York.

193. O'Flaherty, E. J. (1991): Physiologically-based models for boneseeking elements. II. Kinetics of lead disposition in rats. *Toxicol. Appl. Pharmacol.*, 111:313-331.

194. O'Flaherty, E. J. (1993): A pharmacokinetic model for chromium. *Toxicol. Lett.*, 68:145–158.

195. O'Flaherty, E. J., Scott, W., Schreiner, C., and Beliles, R. P. (1992): A physiologically-based kinetic model of rat and mouse gestation: Disposition of a weak acid. *Toxicol. Appl. Pharmacol.*, 112:245–256.

196. Overton, J. H., Graham, R. C., and Miller, F. J. (1987): Mathematical modeling of ozone absorption in the lower respiratory tract. *Drinking Water and Health*, 8:302-311.

197. Page, N. P., Singh, D. V., Farland, W., Goodman, J. I., Conolly, R. B., Andersen, M. E., Clewell, H. J., Frederick, C. B., Yamasaki, H., and Lucier, G. (1997): Implementation of EPA revised cancer assessment guidelines: Incorporation of mechanistic and pharmacokinetic data. *Fundam. Appl. Toxicol.*, 37:16-36.

198. Parham, F. M., Kohn, M. C., Matthews, H. B., DeRosa, C., and Portier, C. J. (1997): Using structural information to create physiologically based pharmacokinetic models for all polychlorinated biphenyls. I. Tissue : blood partition coefficients. *Toxicol. Appl. Pharmacol.*, 144:340–347.

199. Parham, F. M., and Portier, C. J. (1998): Using structural information to create physiologically based pharmacokinetic models for all polychlorinated biphenyls. II. Rates of metabolism. *Toxicol. Appl. Pharmacol.*, 151:110–116.

200. Paterson, S., and MacKay, D. (1989): Correlation of tissue, blood, and air partition coefficients of volatile organic chemicals. *Br. J. Ind. Med.*, 46:321–328.

201. Paustenbach, D., Andersen, M. E., Clewell, H. J., and Gargas, M. L. (1988): A physiologically-based pharmacokinetic model for inhaled carbon tetrachloride in the rat. *Toxicol. Appl. Pharmacol.*, 96:191–211.

202. Pelekis, M., and Krishnan, K. (1999): Physiologically based modeling of the pharmacokinetics and pharmacodynamics of aldicarb in humans. In: *Proceeding of the 1999 Medical Science Simulation Conference*, edited by J. G. Anderson, and M. Katzper, pp. 124–128. Society for Computer Simulation International, San Diego, California.

203. Pelekis, M., Krewski, D., and Krishnan, K. (1997): Physiologically based algebraic expressions for predicting steady-state toxicokinetics of inhaled vapors. *Toxicol. Meth.*, 7:205–225.

204. Pelekis, M., Poulin, P., and Krishnan, K. (1995): An approach for incorporating tissue composition data into physiologically based pharmacokinetic models. *Toxicol. Ind. Health*, 11:511–522.

205. Perbellini, L., Mozzo, P., Brugnone, F., and Zedde, A. (1986): Physiologicomathematical model for studying human exposure to organic solvents: Kinetics of blood/tissue n-hexane concentrations and of 2,5-hexanedione in urine. *Br. J. Ind. Med.*, 43:760–768.

206. Perbellini, L., Mozzo, P., Olivata, D., and Brugnone, F. (1990): Dynamic biological exposure indices for n-hexane and 2,5-hexanedione, suggested by a physiologically-based pharmacokinetic model. *Am. Ind. Hyg. Ass. J.*, 51:356–362.

207. Perico, A., Cassinelli, C., Brugnone, F., Bavazzano, P., and Perbellini, L. (1999): Biological monitoring of occupational exposure to cyclohexane by urinary 1,2-and 1,4-cyclohexanediol determination. *Int. Arch. Occup. Environ. Health*, 72:115–120.

208. Pierce, C. H., Dills, R. L., Morgan, M. S., Nothstein, G. L., Shen, D. D., and Kalman, D. A. (1996): Interindividual differences in $^2H_8$-toluene toxicokinetics assessed by a semi-empirical physiologically based model. *Toxicol. Appl. Pharmacol.*, 139:49–61.

209. Pierce, C. H., Becker, C. E., Tozer, T. N., Owen, D. J., and So, Y. (1998): Modeling the acute neurotoxicity of styrene. *J. Occup. Environ. Med.*, 40:230–240.

210. Ploemen, J. P. H. T. M., Wormhoudt, L. W., Haenen, G. R. M. M., Oudhoorn, M. J., Commandeur, J. N. M., Vermeulen, N. P. E., De Wazier, I., Beaune, P. H., Watabe, T., and van Bladeren, P. J. (1997): The use of human in vitro metabolic parameters to explore the risk assessment of hazardous compounds: The case of ethylene dibromide. *Toxicol. Appl. Pharmacol.*, 143:56–69.

211. Plowchalk, D. R., Andersen, M. E., and Bethizy, J. D. (1992): A physiologically-based pharmacokinetic model for nicotine disposition in the Sprague–Dawley rat. *Toxicol. Appl. Pharmacol.*, 116:177–188.

212. Plowchalk, D. R., Andersen, M. E., and Bogdanffy, M. S. (1997): Physiologically based modeling of vinyl acetate uptake, metabolism, and intracellular pH changes in the rat nasal cavity. *Toxicol. Appl. Pharmacol.*, 142:386–400.

213. Portier, C. J., and Kaplan, N. L. (1989): Variability of safe estimated when using complicated models of carcinogenic processes. A dose study: Methylene chloride. *Fundam. Appl. Toxicol.*, 13:533–544.

214. Poulin, P., and Krishnan, K. (1995): An algorithm for predicting tissue blood partition coefficients of organic chemicals from n-octanol : water partition coefficient data. *J. Toxicol. Environ. Health*, 46:117–129.

215. Poulin, P., and Krishnan, K. (1996): A mechanistic algorithm for predicting blood:air partition coefficients of organic chemicals with the consideration of reversible binding in hemoglobin. *Toxicol. Appl. Pharmacol.*, 136:131–137.

216. Poulin, P., and Krishnan, K. (1996): A tissue composition-based algorithm for predicting tissue : air partition coefficients of organic chemicals. *Toxicol. Appl. Pharmacol.*, 136:126–130.

217. Poulin, P., and Krishnan, K. (1996): Molecular structure-based prediction of the partition coefficients of organic chemicals for physiological pharmacokinetic models. *Toxicol. Meth.*, 6:117–137.

218. Poulin, P., and Krishnan, K. (1998): A quantitative structure-toxicokinetic relationship model for highly metabolised chemicals. *ATLA*, 26:45–59.

219. Poulin, P., and Krishnan, K. (1999): Molecular structure-based prediction of the toxicokinetics of inhaled vapors in humans. *Int. J. Toxicol.*, 18:7–18.

220. Poulin, P., and Krishnan, K. (1995): A biologically-based algorithm for predicting human tissue : blood partition coefficients of organic chemicals. *Human Exp. Toxicol.*, 14:273–280.

221. Poulin, P., Beliveau, M., and Krishnan, K. (1999): Mechanistic animal replacement approaches for predicting pharmacokinetics of organic chemicals. In: *Toxicity Assessment Alternatives: Methods, Issues, Opportunities*, edited by H. Salem, and S. A. Katz, pp. 115–139. Humana Press Inc., Totowa, New Jersey.

222. Ramchandani, V. A., Bolane, J., Li, T.-K., and O'Connor, S. (1999): A physiologically-based pharmacokinetic (PBPK) model for alcohol facilitates rapid BrAC clamping. *Alcohol Clin. Exp. Res.*, 23:617–623.

223. Ramsey, J. C., and Andersen, M. E. (1984): A physiologically-based description of the inhalation pharmacokinetics of styrene in rats and humans. *Toxicol. Appl. Pharmacol.*, 73:159–175.

224. Rao, H. V., Beliles, R. P., Whitford, G. M., and Turners, C. H. (1995): A physiologically based pharmacokinetic model for fluoride uptake by bone. *Regul. Toxicol. Pharmacol.*, 22:30–42.

225. Reitz, R. H., Gargas, M. L., Mendrala, A. L., and Schumann, A. M. (1996): In vivo and in vitro studies of perchloroethylene metabolism for physiologically based pharmacokinetic modeling in rats, mice, and humans. *Toxicol. Appl. Pharmacol.*, 136:289–306.

226. Reitz, R. H., Gargas, M. L., Andersen, M. E., Provan, W. M., and Green, T. L. (1996): Predicting cancer risk from vinyl chloride exposure with a physiologically based pharmacokinetic model. *Toxicol. Appl. Pharmacol.*, 137:253–267.

227. Reitz, R. H., Mandrela, A. L., Corley, R. A., Quast, J. F., Gargas, M. L., Andersen, M. E., Staats, D. E., and Conolly, R. B. (1990): Estimating the risk of liver cancer associated with human exposures to chloroform using physiologically-based pharmacokinetic modeling. *Toxicol. Appl. Pharmacol.*, 105:443–459.

228. Reitz, R. H., Mandrela, A. L., and Guengerich, F. P. (1989): In vitro metabolism of methylene chloride in human and animal tissues: Use in physiologically-based pharmacokinetic models. *Toxicol. Appl. Pharmacol.*, 97:230-246.

229. Reitz, R. H., McCroskey, P. S., Park, C. N., Andersen, M. E., and Gargas, M. L. (1990): Development of a physiologically-based pharmacokinetic model for risk assessment with 1,4-dioxane. *Toxicol. Appl. Pharmacol.*, 105:37–54.

230. Reitz, R. H., McDougal, J. N., Himmelstein, M. W., Nolan, R. J., and Schumann, A. M. (1988): Physiologically-based pharmacokinetic modeling with methyl chloroform: Implications for interspecies, high-low dose and dose-route extrapolations. *Toxicol. Appl. Pharmacol.*, 95:185–199.

231. Reitz, R. H., Mendrala, A. L., Park, C. N., Andersen, M. E., and Guengerich, F. P. (1988): Incorporation of in vitro enzyme data into the physiologically-based pharmacokinetic (PBPK) model for methylene chloride: Implications for risk assessment. *Toxicol. Lett.*, 43:97–116.

232. Rideout, V. C. (1991): *Mathematical and Computer Modeling of Physiological Systems*. Prentice-Hall, New York.

233. Riggs, D. S. (1970): *The Mathematical Approach to Physiological Problems: A Critical Treatise*. MIT Press, Cambridge, Massachusetts.

234. Robinson, P. J. (1991): Effect of microcirculatory heterogeneity in the determination of pharmacokinetic parameters: Implications for risk assessment. *Drug Metab. Rev.*, 23:43–64.

235. Robinson, P. J. (1992): Physiologically-based liver modeling and risk assessment. *Risk Anal.*, 12:139–148.

236. Ross, R., Leger, L., Guardo, R., de Guise, J., and Pike, B. G. (1991): Adipose tissue volumes measured by magnetic resonance imaging and computerized tomography in rats. *J. Appl. Physiol.*, 70:2164–2172.

237. Roth, R. A., and Vinegar, A. (1990): Action by the lungs on circulating xenobiotic agents with a case study of physiologically-based pharmacokinetic modeling of benzo(a)pyrene disposition. *Pharmacol. Therap.*, 48:143–155.

238. Roth, W. L., Ernst, S., Weber, L. W. D., Kerecsen, L., and Rozman, K. K. (1994): A pharmacodynamically responsive model for 2,3,7,8-tetrachlorodibenzo-p-dioxin (TCDD) transfer between liver and fat at low and high doses. *Toxicol. Appl. Pharmacol.*, 127:151–162.

239. Roy, A., and Georgopoulos, P. G. (1998): Reconstructing week-long exposures to volatile organic compounds using physiologically based pharmacokinetic models. *J. Expos. Anal. Environ. Epidemiol.*, 8:407–422.

240. Santostefano, M. J., Wang, X., Richardson, V. M., Ross, D. G., DeVito, M. J., and Birnbaum, L. S. (1998): A pharmacodynamic analysis of TCDD-induced cytochrome P450 gene expression in multiple tissues: Dose- and time-dependent effects. *Toxicol. Appl. Pharmacol.*, 151:294–310.

241. Sato, A., and Nakajima, T. (1979): A vial equilibration method to evaluate the drug metabolizing enzyme activity for volatile hydrocarbons. *Toxicol. Appl. Pharmacol.*, 47:41–46.

242. Sato, A., and Nakajima, T. (1979): Partition coefficients of some aromatic hydrocarbons and ketones in water, blood and oil. *Br. J. Ind. Med.*, 36:231–234.

243. Sato, A., Endoh, K., Kaneko, T., and Johanson, G. (1991): A simulation study of physiological factors affecting pharmacokinetic behavior of organic solvent vapors. *Br. J. Ind. Med.*, 48:342–347.

244. Schoeffner, D. J., Warren, D. A., Muralidhara, S., Bruckner, J. V., and Simmons, J. E. (1999): Organ weights and fat volume in rats as a function of strain and age. *J. Toxicol. Environ. Health*, Part A, 56:449–462.

245. Semino, G., Lilly, P., and Andersen, M. E. (1997): A pharmacokinetic model describing pulsatile uptake of orally-administered carbon tetrachloride. *Toxicology*, 117:25–33.

246. Shelley, M. L., Andersen, M. E., and Fisher, J. W. (1989): A risk assessment approach for nursing infants exposed to volatile

organics through the mothers occupational inhalation exposure. *Appl. Ind. Hyg.*, 4:21–26.

247. Shyr, L. J., Sabourin, P. J., Medinsky, M. A., Birnbaum, L. S., and Henderson, R. F. (1993): Physiologically based modeling of 2-butoxyethanol disposition in rats following different routes of exposure. *Environ. Res.*, 63:202–218.
248. Sinclair, G. C., Gray, C. N., and Sherwood R. J. (1999): Structure and validation of a pharmacokinetic model for benzene. *Am. Ind. Hyg. Ass. J.*, 60:249–258.
249. Singh, D. V., Spitzer, H. L., and White, P. D. (1987): *Addendum to the Health Risk Assessment for Dichloromethane. Updated Carcinogenicity Assessment for Dichloromethane*. EPA 600/8-82/004F.
250. Smith, A. E., Gray, G. M., and Evans, J. S. (1995): The ability of predicted internal dose measures to reconcile tumor bioassay data for chloroform. *Regul. Toxicol. Pharmacol.*, 21:339–351.
251. Staats, D. A., Fisher, J. W., and Conolly, R. B. (1991): Gastrointestinal absorption of xenobiotics on physiologically-based pharmacokinetic models. A two-compartmental description. *Drug Metab. Dispos.*, 19:144–149.
252. Stenner, R. D., Merdink, J. L., Fisher, J. W., and Bunge, A. L. (1998): Physiologically-based pharmacokinetic model for trichloroethylene considering enterohepatic recirculation of major metabolites. *Risk Anal.*, 18:261–269.
253. Sultatos, L. G. (1990): A physiologically-based pharmacokinetic model for parathion based on chemical specific parameters determined in vitro. *J. Am. Coll. Toxicol.*, 9:611–617.
254. Sultatos, L. G., Kim, B., and Woods, L. (1990): Evaluation of estimations in vitro of tissue : blood distribution coefficients for organothiophosphate insecticides. *Toxicol. Appl. Pharmacol.*, 103:52–55.
255. Sweeney, L. M., Schlosser, P. M., Medinsky, M. A., and Bond, J. A. (1997): Physiologically based phamacokinetic modeling of 1,3-butadiene, 1,2-epoxy-3-butene, and 1,2:3,4-diepoxybutane toxicokinetics in mice and rats. *Carcinogenesis*, 18:611–625.
256. Sweeney, L. M., Shuler, M. L., Quick, D., and Babish, J. G. (1996): A preliminary physiologically based pharmacokinetic model for naphthalene and naphthalene oxide in mice and rats. *Ann. Biomed. Eng.*, 24:305–320.
257. Tardif, R., Lapare, S., Krishnan, K., and Brodeur, J. (1992): Physiologically-based modeling of the toxicokinetic interaction between m-xylene and toluene in the rat. *Toxicol. Appl. Pharmacol.*, 120:266–273.
258. Teorell, T. (1937): Kinetics of distribution of substances administered to the body. I. The extravascular modes of administration. *Arch. Int. Pharmacodyn.*, 57:205–225.
259. Teorell, T. (1937): Kinetics of distribution of substances administered to the body. II. The intravascular modes of administration. *Arch. Int. Pharmacodyn.*, 57:226–240.
260. Terasaki, T., Iga, T., Sugiyama, Y., Sawada, Y., and Hanano, M. (1984): Nuclear binding as a determinant of tissue distribution of adriomycin, daunomycin, adriamycinol, daunorubicinol and actinomycin D. *J. Pharmacodyn.*, 7:269–277.
261. Terry, K. K., Elswick, B. A., Welsch, F., and Conolly, R. B. (1995): Development of a physiologically based pharmacokinetic model describing 2-methoxyacetic acid disposition in the pregnant mouse. *Toxicol. Appl. Pharmacol.*, 132:103–114.
262. Thomas, R. S., Bigelow, P. L., Keefe, T. J., and Yang, R. S. H. (1996): Variability in biological exposure indices using physiologically based pharmacokinetic modeling and Monte Carlo simulation. *Am. Ind. Hyg. Ass. J.*, 57:23–32.
263. Thomas, R. S., Lytle, W. E., Keefe, T. J., Constan, A. A., and Yang, R. S. H. (1996): Incorporating Monte Carlo simulation into physiologically based pharmacokinetic models using advanced continuous simulation language (ACSL): A computational method. *Fundam. Appl. Pharmacol.*, 31:19–28.
264. Thrall, K. D., and Kenny, D. V. (1996): Evaluation of a carbon tetrachloride physiologically based pharmacokinetic model using real-time breath-analysis monitoring. *Inhal. Toxicol.*, 8:251–261.
265. Travis, C. C., and Hattemer-Frey, H. A. (1991): Physiological pharmacokinetic models. In: *Statistics in Toxicology*, edited by D. Krewski and C. Franklin, p. 170. Gordon and Breach, New York.
266. Travis, C. C., Quillen, J. L., and Arms, A. D. (1990): Pharmacokinetics of benzene. *Toxicol. Appl. Pharmacol.*, 102:400–420.
267. Travis, C. C., White, R. K., and Arms, A. D. (1989): A physiologically based pharmacokinetic approach for assessing the cancer risk of tetrachloroethylene. In: *The Risk Assessment of Environmental and Human Health Hazards. A Textbook of Case studies*, edited by D. J. Paustenbach, pp. 769–796. Wiley-Interscience Publications, New York.
268. Tuey, D. B., and Mattews, D. H. (1980): Distribution and excretion of 2,2′,4′,4′,5,5′-hexabromobiphenyls in rats and man: Pharmacokinetic model predictions. *Toxicol. Appl. Pharmacol.*, 53:420–431.
269. Tuey, D. B., and Mattews, D. H. (1980): Use of a physiological compartmental model for the rat to describe the pharmacokinetics of several chlorinated biphenyls in the mouse. *Drug Metab. Dispos.*, 8:397–403.
270. U.S. EPA (1987): *Update to the Health Risk Assessment Document and Addendum for Dichloromethane: Pharmacokinetics, Mechanism of Action and Epidemiology*. EPA 600/8-87/030A.
271. Vinegar, A., and Jepson, G. W. (1996): Cardiac sensitization thresholds of halon replacement chemicals predicted in humans by physiologically based pharmacokinetic modeling. *Risk Anal.*, 16:571–579.
272. Vinegar, A., Seckel, C. S., Pollard, D. L., Kinkead, E. R., Conolly, R. B., and Andersen, M. E. (1992): Polychlorotrifluoroethylene oligomer pharmacokinetics in F-344 rats: Development of a physiologically-based model. *Fundam. Appl. Toxicol.*, 18:504–514.
273. Vinegar, A., William, R. J., Fisher, J. W., and McDougal, J. N. (1994): Dose-dependent metabolism of 2,2-dichloro-1,1,1-trifluoroethane: A physiologically based pharmacokinetic model in the male Fisher 344 rat. *Toxicol. Appl. Pharmacol.*, 129:103–113.
274. Volp, R. F., Sipes, I. G., Falcoz, C., Carter, D. E., and Gross, J. F. (1984): Disposition of 1,2,3-trichloropropane in the Fischer-344 rats: Conventional and physiological pharmacokinetics. *Toxicol. Appl. Pharmacol.*, 75:8–17.
275. Wada, D. R., Stanski, D. R., and Ebling, W. F. (1995): A PC-based graphical simulator for physiological pharmacokinetic models. *Comput. Methods Programs Biomed.*, 46:245–255.
276. Wagner, J. G. (1975): *Fundamentals of Clinical Pharmacokinetics*. Drug International, Hamilton, Illinois.
277. Wang, X., Santostefano, M. J., Evans, M. V., Richardson, V. M., Diliberto, J. J., and Birnbaum, L. S. (1997): Determination of parameters responsible for pharmacokinetic behavior of TCDD in female Sprague–Dawley rats. *Toxicol. Appl. Pharmacol.*, 147:151–168.
278. Ward, K. W., Blumenthal, G. M., Welsch, F., and Pollack, G. M. (1997): Development of a physiologically based pharmacokinetic model to describe the disposition of methanol in pregnant rats and mice. *Toxicol. Appl. Pharmacol.*, 145:311–322.
279. Ward, R. C., Travis, C. C., Hetrick, D. M., Andersen, M. E., and Gargas, M. L. (1988): Pharmacokinetics of tetrachloroethylene. *Toxicol. Appl. Pharmacol.*, 93:108–117.
280. Williams, R. J., Vinegar, A., McDougal, J. N., Jarabek, A. M., and Fisher, J. W. (1996): Rat to human extrapolation of HCFC-123 kinetics deduced from halothane kinetics—A corollary approach

to physiologically based pharmacokinetic modelling. *Fundam. Appl. Pharmacol.*, 30:55–66.

281. Yamaguchi, T., Yabuki, M., Saito, S., Watanabe, T., Nishimura, H., Isobe, N., Shono, F., and Matsuo, M. (1996): Research to develop a predicting system of mammalian subacute toxicity (3) Construction of a predictive toxicokinetics model. *Chemosphere*, 33:2441–2468.

282. Yesair, D. W., Feder, P. I., and Chin, A. E. (1986): Development, evaluation and use of a pharmacokinetic model for hexachlorobenzene. In: *Hexachlorobenzene: Proceedings of an International Symposium*, edited by C. R. Morris and J. R. P. Cabral, pp. 297-318. Oxford University Press, New York.

283. Yu, D. (1999): A physiologically based pharmacokinetic model of inorganic arsenic. *Regul. Toxicol. Pharmacol.*, 29:128–141.

Principles and Methods of Toxicology,
Fourth Edition, edited by A. Wallace Hayes.
Taylor & Francis, Philadelphia © 2001.

Chapter 6

The Toxicological Assessment of Pharmaceutical and Biotechnology Products

Michael A. Dorato and Mary Jo Vodicnik

GENERAL OVERVIEW OF DRUG DEVELOPMENT

The World Health Organization (WHO) Scientific Group has defined a drug as "... any substance or product that is used or intended to be used to modify or explore physiological systems or pathological states for the benefit of the recipient" (152). The drug discovery process covers a wide range of therapeutic areas and treatment regimens, and is a risky, multifaceted, expensive undertaking. The goal is to develop a new product with therapeutic benefits (efficacy) and few side effects (toxicity) (3). The drug development process for a new chemical entity (NCE) starts at the chemist's bench with its isolation; moves through efficacy pharmacology testing using various in vivo and in vitro models; then proceeds through an abbreviated toxicology profile, including pharmacological profiling (the determination of pharmacological effects other than the desired therapeutic effect), based on the proposed clinical plan for first human dose (FHD).

The principal aim of nonclinical safety testing is to understand the toxicity of the candidate drug well enough to make a judgment that it is safe to initiate clinical trials (89). Provided the efficacy pharmacology and initial toxicology profiles are acceptable, clinical safety, pharmacokinetic, and pharmacodynamic studies are initiated. As the human clinical trials progress, the drug candidate moves through nonclinical subchronic studies, chronic, and developmental toxicology studies, and oncogenic evaluations. Zbinden (209) has provided a summary of the biological parameters that should be evaluated for new drug candidates (Table 6.1).

The technical risks in new drug development programs are enormous. The risk of failure related to one or more of these aspects has been reviewed by Chien (26), where it is reported that <0.02 percent of NCEs result in marketed drug products, and even fewer, 0.002%, return a profit to support continued drug research (Figure 6.1). Very little of what enters the drug development pipeline ever enters the marketplace (58). It has been estimated that the cost of developing a NCE ranges from \$0.5 billion to \$1.2 billion.

By its nature, a drug must modify a biological process, that is, alter or adjust a physiological system in some way (43). Toxicology is a critical part of both early- and late-phase drug development. The role of toxicology in that process has been extensively reviewed (79,55,59). The initial purpose of toxicology testing programs is to identify the circumstances—for example, dose, treatment duration, route—under which a NCE produces potentially harmful effects (44). A general approach to developing a toxicity profile for a pharmaceutical agent is given in Figure 6.2, and will be discussed more extensively below.

During the discovery process, toxicologists employ rapid, quantitative screening methods, focusing on a limited spectrum of toxicity, to help identify potential drug candidates with the best safety profile. These early

Table 6.1
Biological properties of chemicals that should be considered in safety evaluations[a]

Acute Toxicity
Cumulative Toxicity
Absorption from Various Routes
Elimination $t_{1/2}$ and Accumulation in Deep Compartments
Penetration of Barriers
Milk Excretion
Teratogenicity
Mutagenicity
Carcinogenicity
Sensitization
Local Irritation

[a] From Reference 209.

screening procedures, however, are only a prelude to the required comprehensive safety assessments expected from the toxicologist. Regulatory requirements, termed Good Laboratory Practices (GLPs), dictate many aspects of the toxicology study protocol, and must be followed closely for all definitive (those that support human studies) toxicology studies (64). The early toxicology studies, conducted in the discovery phase, are not required to be in full compliance with the GLPs.

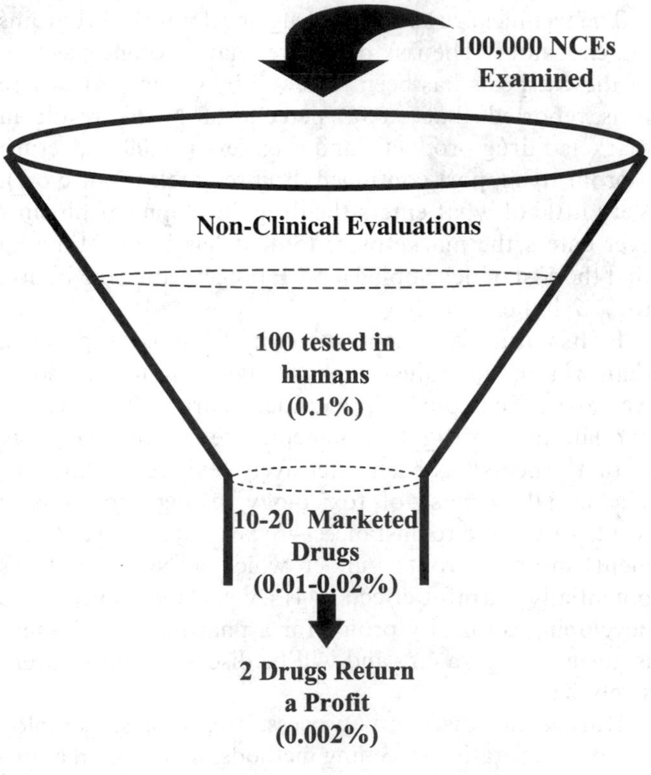

FIG. 6.1. Attrition rate of new drug candidates. Drawn from information presented in Reference 28.

Prior to initiating clinical trials, physicians need an estimate of the extent of toxicity produced by the drug candidate in relevant animal models. Obviously, prior to FHD, the determination of the relevance of animal models, that is, metabolism relative to humans, is limited to in vitro evaluations using human and animal tissue preparations. On the basis of the clinicians' needs, the toxicology profile of a NCE is characterized by a number of questions (124):

- What dose/exposure produces toxic effects in animals?
- What dose/exposure does not produce toxic effects in animals?
- Were the animals relevant models for predicting human toxicity?
- What were the signs and duration of toxic responses?
- Did effects differ following single or multiple dosing?
- Were the toxic responses reversible?
- What were the target organs or systems?
- Was the toxicity expected for this chemical class?
- Are toxic metabolites produced?
- Was accommodation to the toxic effects observed?

The answers to these questions form the basis of the toxicology profile supporting initial and continued clinical trials.

The major objectives of toxicological evaluation change according to the stage of the development process (208). The early stages of development focus on toxicological screening (Table 6.2). Definitive toxicology studies are very time-consuming and costly. Thus, relatively inexpensive, short-term screening procedures are used to eliminate the most toxic compounds (205). Inherent to these initial approaches to evaluate potential drug toxicity are a number of imperfections—the affected systems may not be routinely examined; the assay procedures are inadequate or improperly timed relative to the onset of the toxic response; target organ exposure is insufficient; there is an inability to identify and measure adverse effect (lack of functional evaluations); there is an inability to predict metabolic, anatomical, and physiological differences between species; and, the test animals may not express human-specific responses (212). There is no simple answer to the often asked question: "What toxicity profile would cause a company to stop development of a new drug candidate?" (100). However, the demonstrated toxicity of other compounds in the class, if available, and the gravity of the disease state under study often provide guidance as to what might be an acceptable safety profile for a NCE.

Varied opinions on the occurrence of drug toxicity in the human population have been reported (31,115).

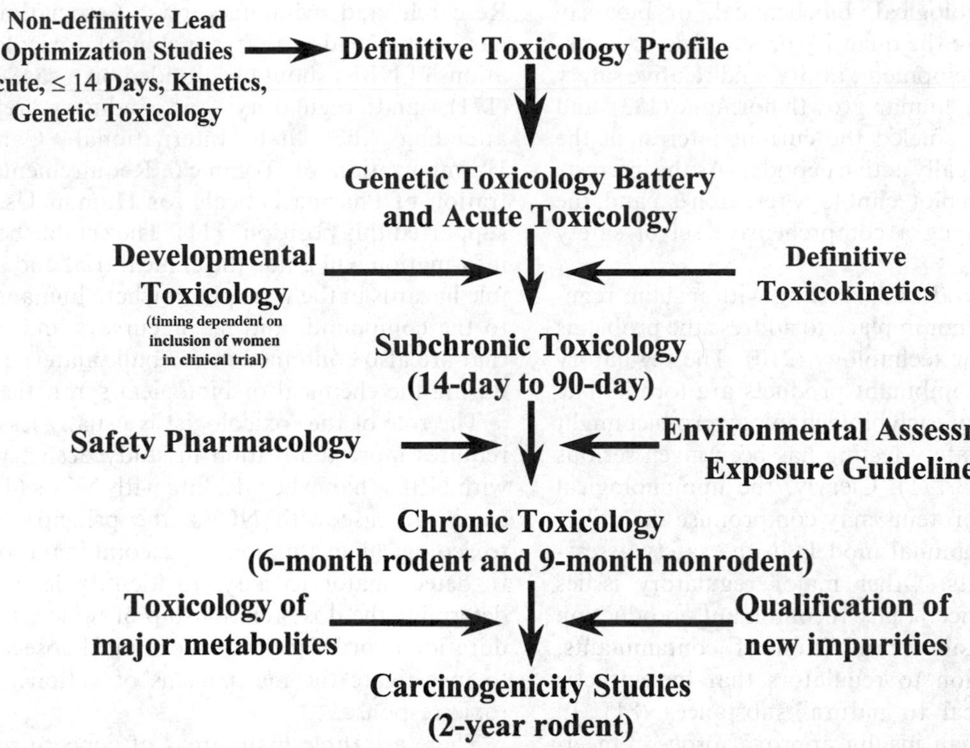

FIG. 6.2. General approach to developing a toxicity profile for pharmaceutical agents.

Although the magnitude of adverse responses seems small—1 per 10,000 patients demonstrates untoward adverse reactions (115)—focus must be placed on identification of all potentially adverse effects (31).

In addition to the drug substance, the delivery system may also require nonclinical evaluation because it may alter pharmacodynamic (action of the drug on the body) and pharmacokinetic (action of the body on the drug) relationships. The regulatory requirements for known and novel drug delivery systems have been reviewed by Weissinger (192).

Commercially advantageous forms of genetic manipulation date back to antiquity, that is, inbreeding, cross fertilization, and so on. The introduction of modern recombinant DNA (rDNA) technology has had a major impact on life science research, and has allowed for the large-scale production of protein pharmacological agents that would have been very difficult to produce by normal chemical synthetic means.

A New Biological Entity (NBE) is defined as a complex, high molecular weight material, which cannot be fully characterized by standard chemical analysis, and which

Table 6.2
Purpose of toxicology evaluations of new drugs[a]

Phase	Principle Activity	Purpose
Discovery	Identification of Candidates	Toxicological Screening
Before FHD	Safety and Principle Target Organs	Regulatory Prerequisites for Human Exposure
During Clinical Trial	Toxicological Spectrum	Cumulative Effects and Mechanisms
Pre-Marketing	Complete Routine Test Program	Regulatory Requirements
Post-Marketing	Identify Special Risks Due to Population or Use Circumstances	Improve Utility and Safety

[a] From Reference 208.

may require immunological, biochemical, or bioassay techniques to measure the quantity present and to assess activity (46). The development, utility, and relative safety of human insulin (83), human growth hormone (133), and interferon (139) have fueled the current interest in the production of biologically active peptides. As the interests of pharmacologists in biotechnology research expand, the difficulties of producing a comprehensive set of safety guidelines increase.

As NBEs were introduced, starting with insulin, regulatory concepts were not in place to address the problems presented by this new technology (210). The regulatory issues relating to recombinant products are formidable, and the possibility that each biotechnology product might require customized safety testing has been given serious consideration (40,163,171). Clearly, the immunological response to foreign proteins may compromise the utility of using traditional animal models in the safety assessment of these agents. Other major regulatory issues include the assurance that recombinant production methods do not result in addition of contaminants, and the demonstration to regulators that biosynthetic products are identical to natural substances (81). In the biosynthetic human insulin approval process, meetings between regulatory agencies and industry scientists to review the manufacturing process, molecular biology, and purification of the hormone, as well as clinical trial programs, were critical in facilitating eventual approvals. Industry and regulatory agency representatives agreed that the chemistry of a NBE should prove its identity (188). The identity and purity of the rDNA insulin, therefore, received much attention (26). Anticipation of problems, and communication of concerns, was the key to the rapid New Drug Application (NDA) approval for biosynthetic human insulin (5.5 months). The U.S. Food and Drug Administration (FDA) has strongly recommended that it be involved early in the nonclinical and clinical development plan to facilitate the approval process for both NCEs and NBEs (87).

The U.S. biotechnology policy states "... the same physical and biological laws govern the response of organisms modified by modern molecular and cellular methods and those produced by classical methods. ... No conceptual distinction exists between genetic modification of plants and microorganisms by classical methods or by molecular techniques that modify DNA and transfer genes" (183). Thus, it would not be expected that NBEs, per se, pose an unusual risk to human health and the environment (183). The toxicologist should be aware, however, that compounds made via rDNA techniques are not necessarily identical to the natural material, as might be assumed (198). Dayan (45) suggested that the toxicology profile for a NBE should be defined in terms of chemical identity of the material, extent of prior knowledge, and intended use. The U.S. Pharmaceutical Research and Manufacturers Association (PhRMA) has recommended that nonclinical toxicological evaluations of NBEs should be decided on a case-by-case basis (171), and regulatory and industry representatives attending the first International Conference on Harmonization of Technical Requirements for Registration of Pharmaceuticals for Human Use (ICH) also supported this position (111). The established toxicology information will guide the clinical trial and address possible hazards in the workplace, where humans are exposed to the compound, and its precursors and contaminants that are also contained in the bulk material to be tested, during the chemical or biological synthetic process.

The role of the toxicologist is usually less routine and requires more innovation in study design when dealing with NBEs than when dealing with NCEs (46). However, as is the case with NCEs, the principal goals of the toxicological evaluation of recombinant products are: to detect major toxicity; to identify lesser toxicity; to determine the dose relationship of toxic effects and their duration in order to guide the clinical dose schedule; and, to investigate the mechanisms of action related to the toxic response.

There are three main areas of concern relative to the toxicity of NBEs: toxicity per se, exaggerated pharmacodynamic effects (anticipated toxicity based on the pharmacological mechanism of action), and allergic reactions (210) (Figure 6.3). Intrinsic toxicity has been defined as undesirable effects having no obvious relationship to the molecule's pharmacodynamic properties. Pharmacodynamic toxicity is defined as an exaggerated pharmacological response, e.g., hypoglycemic shock from insulin. Immunotoxicity has been related to hypersensitivity, cell transformation, and production of neutralizing antibodies. The loss of a recombinant therapeutic agent's biological activity through production of neutralizing antibodies or the development of immune complex disease in experimental animals are factors that must be given individual attention (171). It has been suggested that animal models of immunotoxicity are of limited usefulness because no animal model may be fully suitable for predicting the toxicity of highly species-specific proteins. Friedmann (78) has indicated, however, that the lack of hypersensitivity reactions in response to small peptides in animal experiments may be viewed as an indication of their acceptability in humans. Graham (88) emphasized the use of a case-by-case approach to toxicological evaluations of NBEs based on their similarity to natural human proteins, immune response in animal models, and production of neutralizing antibodies in nonclinical and clinical studies.

The unique regulatory approval of recombinant insulin most likely resulted in unrealistic expectations in the biotechnology industry regarding the rapidity of review

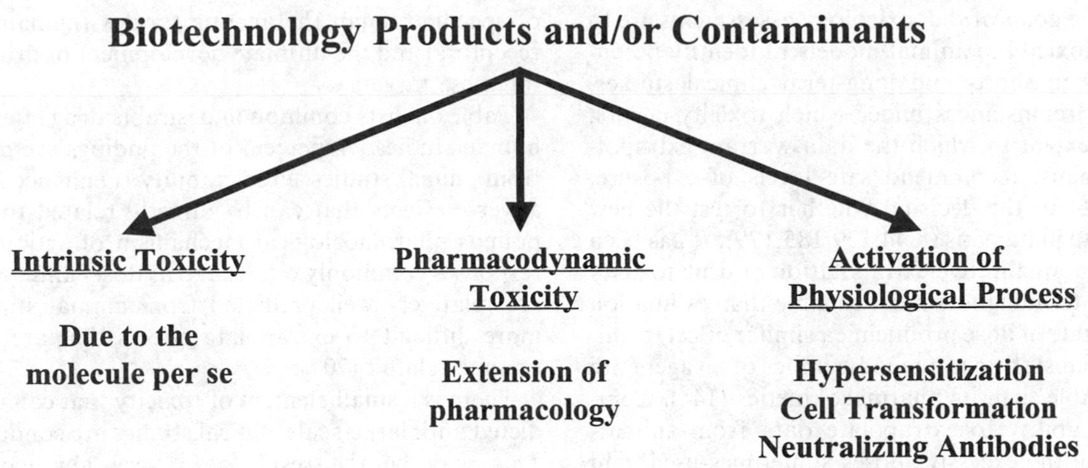

FIG. 6.3. Main areas of concern with response to biotechnology products. Redrawn, with permission, from Reference 210, pp. 143–159.

of NBE applications (121). Two factors facilitate the regulatory approval of NBEs. As is true in the development requirements for all NCEs, the first factor is therapeutic importance, and the FDA has established a "fast-track" rapid approval procedure for NBEs that target unsatisfied indications. The second factor is the relationship of the NBE to an established drug. It appears likely that new therapeutic agents derived from biotechnology will have to satisfy all the usual demands of regulatory agencies (121). The possibility that subtle changes in chemical structure may exist, and may thus influence pharmacokinetics, pharmacodynamics, and/or immunogenicity, is used to support this regulatory position (80).

Questions of safety are not only properly asked about the NBE per se, but about contaminants or residues resulting from the manufacturing and/or purification processes, or antigenic variation or reversion to the wild type of a living organism (46). Worker exposure in the production process may be of concern due to relatively high-level, long-term exposure to various end products of the biotechnology process—live and dead microorganisms and mammalian cells and their derivatives (198). This leads to the area where traditional scientific approaches and techniques do not provide a satisfactory toxicological profile, for example, transfer of an immortalization factor from a mammalian cell; allergic reactions (198).

RELEVANCE OF ANIMAL MODELS IN TOXICOLOGICAL ASSESSMENT

The suitability of experimental animal data for assessing risk to humans is an important contemporary issue in toxicology. Animals and humans have much in common anatomically, physiologically, and biochemically (202). There are two main guiding principles of experimental toxicology: that effects produced in animals, when properly qualified, are applicable to humans; and, that exposure of experimental animals to high doses of a test compound is necessary and valid in determining human hazard (117). Although it is generally agreed that animal assays are not as predictive of human effects as would be desired, they are more predictive than generally thought (93,156). It has been reported that animal assays are predictive of human toxicity in all but 10 percent of comparisons (130). It must be recognized, however, that major differences in response to chemical agents can exist both within and between species (101). The most serious differences between laboratory animal studies and human clinical trials are related to anatomical and physiological "species differences," such as metabolism and genetics (hypersensitivity responses), and experimental design, including quantity, route, and duration of drug administration (122). Humans can be as much as 50 times more sensitive on a mg/kg basis than experimental animals (122).

Regulatory agencies and research-based pharmaceutical companies consider laboratory animal toxicology studies a critical part of the assessment of new drug candidates (74,128). Confidence in the validity of experimental toxicology is based on the large inventory of chemically induced lesions that occur both in animals and humans (215). It may be incorrect to assume that what is demonstrated in animal toxicology studies will occur in human clinical trials, but until it is shown that the toxicity expressed is not relevant to humans, that assumption must be made (8). Also, until our knowledge base expands, animal data must be extrapolated to the human situation using a conservative approach, that is use of relatively high doses, assumption that humans are more sensitive than the most sensitive species, and so on (16).

The ultimate goals of the toxicology assessments are to characterize toxicity in animal models to identify potential problems in short- and long-term clinical studies, identify the circumstances under which toxicity occurs, evaluate the extent to which the data warrant extrapolation to humans, recommend safe levels of exposure, and contribute to the decision whether to test the new drug candidate in humans (8,44,129,185,179). It has been recognized that qualitative extrapolation of drug toxicity from animals to humans is more reliable than estimation of the magnitude of dose producing a similar effect in animals and humans; the pharmacodynamics of an agent are more predictable than its pharmacokinetics (144). Complicating the ability to extrapolate data from animals to humans are the excessive doses sometimes used, and often required, in animal studies. As a result, adverse effects are described that may be the result of frank intoxication of the animal and that are irrelevant in humans. Zbinden (203) has reported that the ability of animal toxicity studies to predict potential human toxicity is related to the mechanism of drug action. Within limitations, animals and humans respond in ways similar enough, from a pharmacodynamic perspective, for animal toxicity evaluations to serve as useful predictors of human toxicity (41,96,125,129,172). However, toxicological evaluations in animals can predict toxic responses in humans only if the response is not unique to humans (74). Those compounds that are toxic to humans but relatively nontoxic to animals—for example thalidomide—are of greatest concern. The extrapolation of animal data to humans is likely to become even more complicated as molecular biology techniques continue to allow the more sophisticated characterization of specific human therapeutic targets (human enzymes, receptors) and the ultimate development of drugs specific for these targets.

Table 6.3 lists common undesirable drug effects seen in human studies; 76 percent of the findings are predictable from animal studies. Predictability is enhanced for those adverse effects that can be directly related to the compounds pharmacological mechanism of action. Adverse responses commonly referred to as dose- and time-related are relatively well predicted from animal studies. It is more difficult to extrapolate effects that are not dose- or time-related (207).

There is a small element of toxicity that cannot be predicted until large-scale clinical studies are conducted (96). This may be the result of a very low incidence of occurrence, or idiosyncratic responses in a small subset of the patient population. However, considering the increased use of pharmaceutical agents and the relative infrequency of major incidence of human toxicity, the initial laboratory studies are clearly serving a valuable function (8). A large majority of human drug exposures are free of toxicity, and in good accordance with the results of animal toxicity studies (207). The use of adequate test systems is critical to the predictive ability of animal toxicity evaluations. Cahn (20) reported that the cardiac effects of calcium antagonists—ectopic beats, ventricular tachycardia, and ventricular fibrillation—were seen in humans, but were not described in long-term animal studies. However, these effects were demonstrable in animals using appropriate functional evaluations not always included in routine toxicological testing. Oftentimes, toxicologically important end points, such as cardiac, pulmonary, or renal function, are not

Table 6.3
Common untoward reactions to drugs[a]

Clinical Side Effect	Predictable from Animal Studies (Y/N)	Clinical Side Effect	Predictable from Animal Studies (Y/N)	Clinical Side Effect	Predictable from Animal Studies (Y/N)
Drowsiness	Y	Hypertension	Y	Anorexia	Y
Nausea	N	Insomnia	Y	Depression	Y
Dizziness	N	Fatigue	N	Increased Appetite	Y
Sedation	Y	Constipation	Y	Tremor	Y
Dry Mouth	Y	Tinnitus	N	Perspiration	Y
Nervousness	Y	Weight Gain	Y	Dermatitis	Y
Epigastric Distress	N	Hypotension	Y	Increased Energy	Y
Headache	N	Dryness of Nasopharynx	Y	Vertigo	N
Vomiting	Y	Heartburn	N	Palpitation	Y
Weakness	Y	Diarrhea	Y	Blurred Vision	Y
Nasal Stuffiness	Y	Skin Rash	Y	Lethargy	Y

[a] From References 145, 204, and 206.

taken into consideration in the design of "routine" toxicology studies. The above example emphasizes the importance of using an adequate test system to evaluate the toxicity of new drug candidates. The toxicologist is challenged to consider potential adverse effects related to the pharmacodynamics of the test compound in the design of appropriate safety studies (172).

As with standard pharmaceuticals, no animal model is fully appropriate to evaluate the toxicity of highly species-specific proteins in humans (88). Animal testing for biotechnology products is limited to the species showing the same pharmacological response as humans, without showing signs of immunity (45,80). This is only feasible when proteins are highly conserved across species. The production of neutralizing antibodies will limit the study duration and, thus, support for clinical trials. Administration of a highly specific human protein to laboratory animals for a sufficient duration to produce immune complex disease will do nothing to reveal effects anticipated in clinical trials. Antigenicity of the test material can be a major complicating factor because the potential allergic etiology of all lesions developing in animals treated with human proteins must be considered (214). Alternatively, nonclinical toxicology studies of biotechnology products may be less predictive of allergic responses that may occur in humans following chronic therapy (198). The appropriate laboratory species for biotechnology product testing should demonstrate similar pharmacodynamics and adverse responses relative to humans. If an animal model demonstrating similar pharmacological response to humans cannot be selected, species selection based on toxicity likely to be representative of effects expected in humans may be acceptable (191). The FDA does not currently require the study of recombinant proteins in primate models, but these animals demonstrate many similarities to humans at the molecular level, and often turn out to be the most appropriate species for toxicity testing (88).

TOXICOKINETICS

Species differences in expression of toxicity (Figure 6.4) due to differences in pharmacokinetics (metabolic processes and physicochemical characteristics of the compound that affect its absorption, disposition, metabolism, and elimination related to the expression of pharmacological endpoints) or toxicokinetics (related to toxicological endpoints), are important factors in toxicology studies (47,152). Toxicokinetic analyses have become common components of nonclinical toxicology profiles of NCEs and NBEs. Toxicokinetic analyses provide information on dose proportionality, potential dose accumulation, and sex and species differences in drug candidate distribution and elimination (42). A major purpose

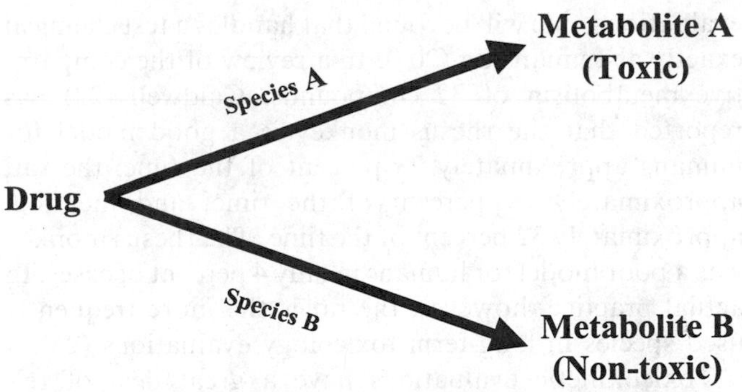

FIG. 6.4. Hypothetical drug metabolism pathways in two species, demonstrating the importance of metabolic data when interpreting toxic responses.

of kinetic studies is to evaluate the level of parent drug or metabolite in various body fluids, tissues, and/or excreta and to use these data to determine suitability of animal data for human hazard assessment (30,43,150,164). Another purpose is to determine the levels of the compound, and its potentially active metabolites, that result in toxicity.

To fully interpret the results and applicability of toxicology studies, the metabolic profile and kinetics of the drug candidate in animal models and in humans must be compared (143). Wherever possible, species that handle the chemical in a manner similar to humans should be used in toxicology studies (190). Rapid detoxification in animals can cause the toxicologist to miss signs of potential human toxicity (207). Alternatively, signs of toxicity in experimental animals may be the result of a metabolic conversion that is only slightly present in humans. For example, the increased liver weights seen with ketotifen (Zaditen, an antianaphylactic agent) in dogs were due to an N-oxide metabolite which is produced in insignificant amounts in humans (172). Toxic responses in humans can be predicted from animal studies more accurately if the absorption, distribution, metabolism, and excretion of the test chemical are compared (10).

The determination of metabolic and pharmacokinetic profiles in animals is of great value in the design of extended clinical trials, once these parameters have also been characterized in initial limited human testing. Specifically, interspecies variation in response that may preclude extrapolation of animal toxicity data to humans could be explained by toxicokinetics (57). Qualitative metabolic profiles are remarkably similar among the four or five laboratory animals commonly used in toxicology studies and humans (23). Quantitative differences in drug metabolism parameters among species, however, are apparently the rule. It may be unreasonable to expect that, from the few animal species used in toxicological evaluations, one will be found that handles a test chemical exactly as humans do (207). In a review of the comparative metabolism of 32 compounds, Caldwell (22) has reported that the rhesus monkey is a good model for humans approximately 73 percent of the time; the rat, approximately 29 percent of the time; and the dog, approximately 32 percent of the time. The rhesus monkey was a poor model for humans in only 4 percent of cases. In actual practice, however, the rat is the more frequently used species in long-term toxicology evaluations (23).

Toxicokinetic evaluations have a great deal of relevance in explaining species differences in toxicology profiles (56). The kinetic parameters that are pertinent to an understanding of toxic responses across species are absorption (extent, rate, and relationship to route of administration); distribution (blood and tissue levels of parent compound and metabolites, accumulation in various body compartments); metabolism (species differences, activation); and elimination (route, rate), better known as ADME (164). These processes are interdependent and occur simultaneously (132). Association of drug toxicity with parent compound or metabolite, or the association of enzyme induction with the late accumulation of a novel metabolite, can be characterized by kinetic evaluations (114).

Toxicokinetic data provide another important contribution to toxicology evaluations, that is, assessment of nonlinear kinetics, which frequently occur at the high dose levels used in toxicity testing (151). In this situation, the relationship of dose to internal concentration is not representative of the relationship at the lower, unsaturated, linear dose levels that occur in humans. It is very important that toxicity be evaluated in conjunction with kinetics over a dose range wide enough to define whether a transition from linear to nonlinear kinetics occurs (151). This kinetic information can be used to establish a more realistic upper dose level for a toxicity study, rather than the maximum tolerated dose (MTD), which may far exceed the metabolic capabilities of the animal, and thus result in irrelevant toxicity. If the kinetic evaluations are not conducted simultaneously with the toxicology study, they should be conducted at doses encompassing those actually used in the toxicity evaluation, as well as those which produce the desired pharmacological effect (185). This assessment of systemic exposure to parent drug and metabolites allows a more realistic expression of the difference between the doses that result in efficacy and toxicity (margin of safety) than comparing the doses administered on a mg/kg basis.

The use of in vitro techniques allows the toxicologist to establish some level of comfort for comparative metabolic similarities between humans and the common species employed in toxicity testing. In vitro techniques have several advantages: rapid assessment of permeability and metabolism; study of molecular mechanisms of toxicity; drug targeting; early studies comparing human and animal systems; and, minimization of animal usage (5). The in vitro models do not provide the entire metabolic picture, but they are useful in illuminating parts of a very complex process. Dedrick and Bischoff (52) have stated that it should be possible to use in vitro comparative metabolic information to provide a basis for predicting drug behavior in any mammalian species, providing anatomy and physiology are known.

Several in vitro methods are available that are applied to human and animal liver samples: liver subcellular fractions (14), that is, postmitochondrial supernatant or microsomes; specific forms of cytochromes P450, that is, species-specific metabolism and effects of enzyme induction/inhibition (62,95); hepatocytes (162); and, liver slices (15,165). Subcellular fractions are easy to prepare and cryopreserve, but may be altered in the preservation process (148). Hepatocytes allow for the study of integrated hepatocellular metabolism, express many of the functional activities of the intact liver, and may provide a good compromise between cell extracts and isolated organs (52,62). Liver slices have the additional advantage of maintaining the structural heterogeneity of the liver, and are not exposed to the potential hepatocyte membrane damaging effects of collagenase used during their preparation. Currently, the most commonly used in vitro preparations are subcellular fractions, hepatocytes, and liver slices (75), and the early assessment of metabolic pathways in cultured human and animal hepatocytes and liver slices is widely practiced (215).

The correlation of the in vitro techniques with in vivo metabolic profiles has been demonstrated with hepatocyte suspensions from rat, rabbit, dog, squirrel monkey, and human livers (90). In general, the metabolic profile from the hepatocytes corresponded to the profile of urinary metabolites previously established for each species (90). As a further positive comparison, the metabolism of caffeine by human liver microsomes, slices, or hepatocyte cultures compared very well with its in vivo metabolism (12). An understanding of the mechanism of species-specific acetaminophen toxicity in rat, rabbit, dog, and cynomolgus monkey was provided by studies in primary hepatocyte cultures (166). The applicability of this in vitro approach has been further demonstrated for diazepam and ketotifen (27,123). Wrighton and Stevens (200) have compared and contrasted specific human P450s, involved in the metabolism of a very large number of endogenous and exogenous lipophilic compounds, with P450s of several experimental animal species. The evaluation of the metabolism of drug candidates by individual P450 isozymes from animals and humans may provide valuable information relative to both species differences and potential idiosyncratic responses in the human population. These in vitro test systems generally provide a more rapid, less expensive means of evaluating toxicity and mechanisms of toxicity, across species during early drug development (165,178).

The use of these in vitro systems may also improve the selection of appropriate species for subsequent in vivo testing. Importantly, how the drug is metabolized relative to other drugs that may be administered simultaneously, may provide critical guidance in the design of subsequent clinical studies to address potential drug–drug interaction issues. Many animal and human subcellular, cellular, and tissue preparations that can aid the toxicologist in selecting species for toxicity testing or extrapolating animal data to humans are now commercially available.

Toxicity studies are designed to produce a higher level of exposure in the experimental animals than anticipated in the human clinical trial. Generally, small animals (rats and mice) have more rapid basal metabolic rates, shorter life spans, and more rapid drug metabolic activity than humans (23). Thus, small animals usually require a higher dose of the drug, administered more frequently, to mimic the human clinical exposure (136). Campbell and Ings (23) have provided an example showing that, all else being equal, rats would have to be dosed at 5 mg/kg/day to achieve similar systemic exposure as humans receiving 1 mg/kg/day. It should be realized, therefore, that a dose multiple comparison based on a mg/kg relationship is often an inappropriate measure of safety. It is now generally accepted that exposure (plasma level) provides a better estimate of safety margin than administered dose. Issues related to tissue accumulation, measures of exposure, and safety margins are discussed below.

The assessment of systemic exposure in toxicity studies has been addressed by the ICH and the objectives of toxicokinetic evaluation and specific recommendations are contained in ICH Topic S3A (107).

TOXICOLOGY GUIDELINES

Drug Development Time Lines

Development time has become an important focus for the pharmaceutical industry. The available data indicate a four fold increase in drug development time between the 1960s and the 1980s. From the early 1980s to 1996, however, mean drug development times have been relatively constant at about 10–12 years, with a very wide variability (177). The pharmaceutical industry has committed to increasing drug discovery/development efficiency leading to a halving of the mean drug development time.

NBEs generally have had a shorter development time than NCEs. The NBEs have a mean development time of approximately 6–9 years. The NBEs registered to date have generally been well-characterized natural molecules and the shorter development time is probably related to a better understanding of their actions in humans. The introduction of analogs of natural proteins, some designed to be used at supra-physiological levels, will probably lead to an increase in development time for NBEs.

Regulatory Guidelines for Toxicity Testing

In this section, the toxicology support packages for the registration of NCEs and NBEs are reviewed from slightly different perspectives. More detailed information on the specific studies conducted, their results, and interpretation are included for the classical agents (omeprazole and zidovudine [AZT]) since the majority of compounds currently in development would fall into this category and thus require similar testing strategies. Omeprazole was selected for discussion because it has a comprehensive toxicology package and represents an example of where additional mechanistic studies were critical in the approval process. Zidovudine is discussed due to its proposed use to treat life-threatening disease where no adequate therapy was available. The rapid approval of AZT, in spite of significant toxicology findings and an abbreviated toxicology support package, demonstrates the inherent flexibility in the approval system even with regard to NCEs.

The discussion of specific human NBEs (gonadotropin-releasing hormone analogs, interferon, human insulin) is presented from a more philosophical perspective. Since these agents are naturally occurring, and since the major limiting toxicity in animal studies (immunogenicity) is not applicable to clinical trials, the design of the toxicology package posed special issues that were considered on a case-by-case basis. Furthermore, the toxicological profile was anticipated based on extensive clinical experience with less specific agents (animal-derived insulins) and/or a broad understanding of the hormones' physiological functions. Thus, the following discussion of the NBEs poses questions, concerns, and general guidelines to be considered in the development of these agents.

Acute, Subchronic, and Chronic Testing

Toxicity testing can be considered to be composed of several major types (44). Acute (single-dose), subchronic (multiple-dose, less than 6 months duration), and chronic (multiple-dose, greater than or equal to 6 months duration), studies are intended to elucidate the target organs for toxicity and demonstrate dose-response relationships. They are useful for determining the mechanism of toxic action and often provide important information for dose selection in other study types. A variety of endpoints are routinely evaluated in subchronic and chronic studies, including body weight, feed consumption, hematology, clinical chemistry, urinalysis, and gross and histological pathology of numerous tissues. A list of common parameters assessed in subchronic/chronic studies is presented in Table 6.4. However, the toxicologist is continually challenged to modify study design to address the anticipated actions of the compound under investigation. This may result in the addition of certain parameters or tissues to be evaluated, or a more comprehensive analysis of tissues (i.e., electron microscopic evaluation, immunohistochemistry). Furthermore, previous studies, or knowledge of the toxicity of other agents in the therapeutic class or those that have a similar structure, may recommend alternative assessments, such as the determination of the propensity of the agent to induce hepatic microsomal enzymes, cause phospholipid accumulation, or result in peroxisome proliferation.

An assessment of bioavailability and pharmacokinetics is often an important endpoint of subchronic and chronic studies. As discussed previously, these data are critical to extrapolate toxicity findings to humans. Often, the kinetic profile of the compound is determined early and late in the study so that the potential for drug accumulation can be revealed. Alternatively, drug levels may be lower toward study termination, or the metabolite profile may differ, due to the induction of drug metabolizing enzymes. Tissues may also be collected for drug analysis, so that levels in affected tissues can be related to the extent of the histopathological findings. Finally, important dose-response relationships can be established, relative to both parent compound and metabolites, that may be critical in the interpretation of toxicity data.

Acute (single dose followed by a 2-week observation period) and subchronic (usually 2-week or 1-month studies) testing is required prior to FHD. One-month studies in one rodent (usually rat or mouse) and one nonrodent (usually dog or primate) species usually will support 1 to 2 weeks of dosing in humans. Where possible, the animal studies should be carried out using the same route of administration anticipated for use in patients. As an aside, it should be acknowledged that clinical studies may initially be conducted by the intravenous route, regardless of the desired ultimate route of administration, particularly for those molecules that are anticipated to show efficacy rapidly, in order to demonstrate the proof of concept of a new pharmacological mechanism. Drug developers might thus avoid the time and expense associated with formulation development and maximization of the desired properties of the chemical if it has been demonstrated that the molecule/mechanism is ineffective. These clinical trials require the support of intravenous toxicology assessments. In these circumstances, it is extremely important to evaluate the risk associated with the potential for demonstrating toxicity in the intravenous study that may be irrelevant to the ultimate route of administration.

Phases II and III, efficacy testing in patients, are supported by longer-term studies. Depending on the proposed duration of human exposure, toxicity studies to support Phases II/III may be of 3, 6, and/or 9/12 months duration. Two or more subchronic/chronic studies may be conducted simultaneously (i.e., 3-month and 6-month studies may be initiated at the same time) so that patients can be placed on the trial earlier (upon completion of the 3-month study), and maintained on the trial longer (supported by the 6-month study) if the human efficacy and safety data support continued therapy. A potential problem with this approach is that dose selection for the more extended study may be found to be inadequate (doses either too low or too high) based on the findings of the shorter test.

There has been much discussion surrounding the utility of 1-year studies. The FDA has been a strong proponent of the 1-year study approach, while Japan and the European Union (EU) have suggested that 1-year studies reveal little new information beyond that gained from 6-month studies. These data have been reviewed by Lumley et al. (127), who suggest that for 154 compounds in which short- ($\leq$6 months) and long- ($>$6 months) term animal data are available, tests lasting longer than 6 months (excluding carcinogenicity studies) have not provided new substantive safety information. They also point out that although new findings became evident after 6 months of treatment in 9 out of 75 cases, the data did not influence the decision whether to continue the development of the compound.

Based on the present ICH position, it is generally accepted that 6-month rodent and 9-month nonrodent multiple-dose studies are acceptable for a tripartite development plan (108). Even so, it is strongly recommended that the sponsor have a written commitment from the appropriate reviewing division of the FDA on the acceptability of the 9-month versus the 1-year nonrodent chronic toxicity study.

Additional Toxicology Studies to Support Clinical Trials

Other tests conducted prior to initial clinical trials include mutagenicity studies and pharmacological assessments. A variety of mutagenicity studies currently are employed that assess various types of DNA damage in vitro and in vivo in an attempt to predict the oncogenic potential of the compound under investigation. In pharmacological screening, the ability of the compound to produce toxicities or "side effects" based on its pharmacological mechanism of action is assessed. For example, an agent that is shown to bind to β-receptors in vitro might be anticipated to influence cardiac function in subsequent toxicity and clinical testing. Both of these study types are often employed as a very early screen in the

Table 6.4
Parameters that might typically be assessed in a subchronic/chronic toxicology study

Live-phase		
Body weight		
Feed consumption		
Efficiency of food utilization (g body weight gained/100 g feed consumed)		
Clinical observations		
Ophthalmology		
Electrocardiogram (large animal)		
Physical examination		
Hematology		
Erythrocyte count	Total leukocyte count	
Hemoglobin	Leukocyte differential	
Packed cell volume	Thrombocyte count	
Mean corpuscular volume	Activated partial thromboplastin time	
Mean corpuscular hemoglobin	Prothrombin time	
Mean corpuscular hemoglobin concentration	M : E ration (bone marrow smears)	
Clinical chemistry		
Glucose	Inorganic phosphorus	
Blood urea nitrogen	Sodium	
Creatinine	Potassium	
Total bilirubin	Chloride	
Alkaline phosphatase	Cholesterol	
Alanine transaminase	Triglycerides	
Aspartate transaminase	Total protein	
Gamma glutamyltransferase	Albumin	
Creatinine phosphokinase	Globulin	
Calcium	Albumin/globulin ratio	
Urinalysis		
Color	Glucose	
Clarity	Occult blood	
Specific gravity	Ketones	
pH	Bilirubin	
Protein	Urobilinogen	
Organ weights		
Kidneys	Prostate	
Liver	Adrenals	
Heart	Thyroids (with parathyroids)	
Ovaries	Brain	
Testes		
Histopathology		
Kidney	Stomach	Skin
Urinary bladder	Duodenum	Skeletal muscle
Liver	Jejunum	Bone
Gallbladder	Ileum	Bone marrow
Heart	Cecum	Adrenal
Aorta	Colon	Thyroid
Trachea	Rectum	Parathyroid
Lung	Ovary	Pituitary
Spleen	Uterus	Cerebrum
Lymph node	Cervix	Cerebellum
Thymus	Vagina	Brain stem
Salivary gland	Testis	Spinal cord
Pancreas	Epididymis	Sciatic nerve
Tongue	Prostate	Eye
Esophagus	Mammary gland	Harderian gland
Other		
Blood levels of parent compound/metabolites		
Hepatic microsomal enzyme activity/cytochromes P450 content		
Hepatic oxidation		
Tissue phospholipid phosphorus concentration		

evaluation of potential drug candidates to select one of a group of structurally related compounds that would be least likely to result in carcinogenicity, and most likely to demonstrate the specific desired pharmacological activity. The types and utility of these studies are further described below.

Finally, special studies might be conducted prior to initial clinical testing to address specific issues, for example, irritation testing of an agent proposed for topical use in the patient population.

Reproductive and Developmental Toxicity Studies

Since the thalidomide incident, there has appropriately been a great deal of concern relative to predictive testing for developmental toxicity, as well as, fertility effects in both males and females. Although regulations have differed substantially among countries, worldwide harmonized guidelines for reproductive toxicity testing have now been established (109,110). The ultimate goal of reproductive and developmental toxicity studies is to assess reproductive risk to adults as well as to the developing individual at all stages from conception to sexual maturity. Traditionally, animal studies have been conducted in three "segments"—in adults, treatment pre-mating through mating in the male, and pre-mating through either implantation or lactation in the female (Segment I); in pregnant animals, treatment during organogenesis (Segment II or teratology studies); and in pregnant/lactating animals, treatment from the completion of organogenesis through lactation (Segment III—perinatal and postnatal study). Although guidelines addressing treatment regimens have been rather similar throughout the world, the required endpoints measured, in both the adult and developing organism, have varied widely, and this is an area where much duplicative testing has occurred to support worldwide registration.

The harmonized ICH guidelines (109,110) stress the need for flexibility in testing for reproductive and developmental toxicity, and challenge the toxicologist to "custom design" a combination of studies that will reveal potential effects on all the parameters considered in the classical Segments I, II, and III studies. For treated adults, these include development and maturation of gametes, mating behavior, fertilization, implantation, parturition, and lactation. In the developing organism, where the maternal animal may be exposed to the drug candidate from prior to mating through lactation, assessments of early embryonic development, major organ formation, fetal development and growth, postnatal development and growth, including behavioral assessments, and attainment of full reproductive function are required. These evaluations might be carried out as one comprehensive study with interim assessments, or they might be segmented into several treatment components. Thus, the new guidelines have not diminished the extent of evaluation, but allow flexibility in study design based on what is already known of the compound under investigation. The harmonized guideline suggests a three-study design that is likely to provide all the developmental toxicity data necessary to support product registration, assuming no untoward toxicity (Figure 6.7). Should toxicity be demonstrated, further mechanistic studies would be conducted to clarify effects and determine whether the responsible mechanism(s) would be applicable to humans. Clearly, the results from previous subchronic/chronic studies (i.e., was there evidence for an effect on spermatogenesis upon histopathological examination of the testes) are critical in the design of an appropriate reproduction package.

Women of child bearing potential are generally first recruited into Phase II trials, and several countries require that efficacy be demonstrated in male patients prior to recruitment of women of child bearing potential into trials, regardless of the outcomes of the nonclinical reproductive studies. However, the FDA has encouraged the inclusion of women of child bearing potential in early clinical trials, especially in the case of drugs intended to treat life-threatening conditions or in the study of disease states that more commonly afflict women. Typically, prior to the inclusion of such women into clinical trials, studies are conducted to evaluate effects on organogenesis (Segment II) in two species (usually the rabbit and the rodent species that has been selected for the subchronic and chronic studies). Female fertility assessments are also usually undertaken prior to longer-term treatment or addition of significant numbers of patients. Early studies in men are supported by histological evaluation of the testes at the conclusion of the subchronic and chronic studies, and specific animal studies to examine drug effects on male fertility are not required until Phase III. Unless there are concerns regarding a specific chemical class or mechanism of action, the more sophisticated analyses of perinatal and postnatal development and behavior (Segment III studies) are often conducted in conjunction with the Phase III clinical trials. Frequently, as is the case with other toxicity evaluations, special studies may be conducted to determine the mechanism(s) of observed reproductive effects in an effort to assess whether these findings are meaningful to humans, and whether use of the compound should be restricted depending on the reproductive status of the patient (i.e., the drug should not be administered to pregnant women). Finally, the inclusion of female patients in clinical trials may be allowed following a more limited assessment of reproductive/developmental parameters if the compound under development is shown to be efficacious, and/or thought to provide distinct advantages over available therapies, in the treatment of life-threatening disease.

Carcinogenicity Studies

Among the final toxicity studies to be conducted to support the registration of chronic-use therapeutics are the carcinogenicity bioassays. These lifetime studies are usually conducted in two rodent species (normally rat and mouse). Selection of the top dose for the carcinogenicity bioassays has been an intensely debated topic of discussion in the international harmonization process. The international consensus has based the selection of the top dose for carcinogenicity bioassay on any one of the following (104):

1. Maximum tolerated dose (MTD) (see discussion below).
2. Area under the plasma concentration : time curve (AUC): ratio of 25-fold (rodent : human): applies when there is no genotoxicity.
3. Saturation of absorption.
4. Dose-limiting pharmacodynamics: that is, hypotension, hypoglycemia, decreased blood clotting time.
5. The use of a limit dose (1500 mg/kg): applies when the maximum recommended human dose is $\leq$500 mg/day, and the AUC (rodent : human) is $\geq$10.

The middle and low doses should also be selected to provide additional information to use in the risk assessment. The consideration of dose linearity, saturation of metabolic pathways, margin of safety, pharmacodynamics, specific animal physiology, threshold effects, and progression of toxic effects should be included in the selection of the middle and low doses for carcinogenicity evaluations.

The use of an MTD as the top dose in a carcinogenicity study is a subject of some controversy. The MTD has been classically defined as the dose that causes no more than a 10 percent decrease in body weight, and does not produce mortality, clinical signs of toxicity, or pathological lesions that would be predicted to shorten the natural life span of an experimental animal for any reason other than the induction of neoplasms (167). The MTD is suggested to produce a level of toxicity indicative of sufficient chemical challenge to define chronic toxic manifestations (99). Many regulatory bodies default to the use of the MTD as the maximum dose in the rodent bioassays. A major concern with the MTD approach is that metabolic saturation, as discussed above, may occur at high doses, leading to abnormal metabolism (138), or in the case of inhaled therapeutics, abnormal clearance (137). Chemicals administered at the MTD in animal bioassays tend to induce mitogenesis as a result of cell death due to frank intoxication, with the target tissues differing among species and sexes (86). This stimulation of cell proliferation, a natural recovery process in response to severe toxicological insult that does not normally occur at reasonable multiples of human exposure levels, can account for the carcinogenic response of nongenotoxic compounds (32). Thus, the fact that a chemical is a carcinogen at MTD levels in rodents may provide little meaningful information relative to low-dose risk assessment in humans (2). MTDs for chronic toxicity studies are usually estimated based on the results of subchronic toxicity studies. However, since compound distribution and disposition may be affected by dose and/or duration of treatment, this may be a very crude estimate (138,140).

The choice of an MTD is a critical aspect of chronic toxicity evaluations (173). Cell proliferation indices in subchronic toxicology studies may provide a useful estimation of an appropriate MTD by determining the highest dose that does not result in the phenomenon (19). The use of kinetic parameters (C_{max}, AUC related to dose), would better predict the dose at which saturation (nonlinearity) might occur, and therefore provide a better estimate of the MTD in a particular species. Also, changes in urinary metabolite profile, in relation to dose, may be a good way of indicating metabolic overload, and aid in more accurately selecting upper dose levels in toxicology studies (199).

The utility of using two rodent species has also been an active area for discussion. The ICH has indicated that the rat would be preferable to the mouse for the conduct of carcinogenicity studies (103). The rat seems to have been given a preference because background mechanistic data are usually available for rats (not mice), studies of metabolic disposition are more often carried out in rats than in mice, and mouse carcinogenicity studies are dominated by liver tumors of questionable relevance to humans. A review of the European Regulatory Database has concluded that studies in the mouse add little to the ability to detect carcinogenic risk from pharmaceuticals (184,34); but it found, however that carcinogenicity studies in two rodent species are necessary to identify transspecies tumorigens. NCEs active across species are considered to pose a relatively greater risk to humans than NCEs positive in only one specie. The conduct of a study using an alternative in vivo carcinogenicity model along with a standard bioassay in one specie was considered to be an acceptable alternative for assessing carcinogenic potential (34).

The use of alternative models for carcinogenicity assessment meet the desire of the FDA to have an assessment in two species, and provides the advantages of using fewer animals, being of shorter duration, and being capable of improving the accuracy of the rodent bioassay (33). A number of transgenic animal models are currently being evaluated as alternatives to the two-year bioassay (84,33,4). It is early, yet, however, to evaluate the contribution of alternative models of carcinogenic potential to the risk assessment process, and it would be advisable to discuss the selection of alternative models with the appropriate regulatory agency prior to study initiation.

Within the FDA, it is highly recommended that protocols, dose justification documents, and supporting data be submitted to the Carcinogenicity Assessment Committee (CAC) for evaluation prior to the initiation of carcinogenicity studies. The CAC provides consultation on study designs, assures consistency and quality in the analysis and interpretation of animal carcinogenicity studies, and monitors scientific developments to ensure that scientific standards of design and interpretation are upheld.

Since 1982, there has been a rise in the number of NBEs presented for registration. Even so, this represents a relatively small number of molecules. Due in part to this lack of practical experience, the safety programs for the NBEs have been designed on a case-by-case basis. The ICH has provided two guidelines that address carcinogenicity studies with products of biotechnology (103,111). There is general acknowledgment that carcinogenicity studies are not appropriate for biotechnology products given essentially as replacement therapy, at physiological levels, especially when clinical experience exists (e.g., insulin, calcitonin, pituitary derived growth hormone) (111, 103,94). Product-specific assessment of carcinogenic potential may be needed depending on clinical dosing regimen, patient population, and/or biological activity of the product. For products that have the potential to induce cell proliferation (e.g., growth factors), an in vitro evaluation of receptor expression, in cells relevant to the patient population, may be conducted. If these data indicate a need for further evaluation of carcinogenic potential, two-year studies in a single rodent species should be considered.

Long-term carcinogenicity evaluations with endogenous peptides and proteins, or their analogs, are generally indicated when (103):

1. there are significant differences in biological effects to the natural substances.
2. modifications lead to significant changes in structure compared to the natural substance.
3. therapeutic exposure levels exceed those that normally occur in the systemic circulation or in tissues.

A specific example of studies recommended for the analog of a naturally occurring decapeptide, gonadotropin-releasing hormone (GnRH), is presented below (149).

Regulatory guidelines exist as to when and why carcinogenicity studies should be conducted with naturally occurring substances and their analogs. There are opinions from industry, academia, and regulatory agencies on the propriety of conducting these studies (94). For each NBE under development, the existing opinions and guidance must be considered, a reasonable plan to establish safety must be developed, and a discussion held with the appropriate regulatory agency to test the plan. Safety evaluation of NBEs is still very much a case-by-case consideration. The pharmaceutical industry must be careful not to over-interpret the position that carcinogenicity studies are not usually appropriate for biotechnology products.

New Chemical Entities

The extent and types of safety testing of synthetic organic pharmaceutical agents in animal models depend on a variety of factors, including the potential duration of treatment of patients (e.g., short-term—antibiotics; chronic—antihypertensives), route of administration, pharmacological mechanism of action, proposed patient population, and clinical experience with other agents in that therapeutic class. Furthermore, the design of animal toxicity studies that occur later in development must carefully consider the results of previous tests in animals and humans relative to bioavailability, unanticipated toxic responses, and relevance of species selected.

Generally, toxicity testing in animals can be considered in three phases—testing to support FHD (single- and multiple-dose, Phase I), testing to support longer-term and broader efficacy studies (weeks to months, Phase II), and testing to support final registration and, if appropriate, chronic treatment (Phase III) (Figure 6.5). Although the great majority of testing is performed prior to registration, special studies may be requested by regulatory agencies during the review and approval processes. Following widespread clinical use of a new agent, further testing may be appropriate to examine potential mechanisms of action for unanticipated side effects that become evident in the increasing patient population or sub-populations. These may occur due to genetic differences, environmental factors, age, patient history, existence of other diseases/pathologies, and drug interactions. Other tests may be considered if new formulations of the drug are developed, if the drug is suggested for new indications, or if it will be used in patient populations that were not anticipated during initial development (e.g., pediatrics).

The primary purposes of initial clinical testing (support for FHD) are to determine the toxicity and pharmacokinetics (and oral bioavailability, if appropriate) of the drug candidate in humans following one or several doses. Usually, the drug is administered to humans at doses below the anticipated efficacious dose, and doses are escalated until a satisfactory multiple over the anticipated efficacious dose is achieved or toxicity becomes evident. Unless the drug candidate has known, serious toxicity, as is the case with many oncolytics, it is usually first tested

	Early Discovery Nonclinical Testing	Phase I	Phase II	Phase III	FDA Review	Phase IV
Years	3.5-6.5	1-1.5	2	3-3.5	2.5-1.5	
Test Population	Nonclinical Laboratory Studies	<100 Healthy Volunteers	< 300 Patients	< 3000 Patients	Data Review	Post-marketing Testing required by FDA (could be related to line extension strategy)
Purpose	Efficacy and Safety	Kinetics Dose Range Safety	Efficacy Safety	Confirm Efficacy Long-term Safety		
Success Rate	100,000 NCEs	100 NCEs Enter Trials (0.1%)			10-20 Approved (0.01-0.02%)	

Short term studies ≤ 2 weeks, 1 or 2 species, in vitro alternatives Detect serious adverse effects

File IND

Genotox., Safety pharmacology, definitive studies ≤ 1 month, 2 species, Safety evaluation in support of FHD

Definitive studies ≤ 6 months (9 months to 1 year nonrodent), support extended clinical trials, Carcinogenicity studies or alternatives

Fertility and teratology studies conducted before inclusion of women of child bearing potential (WCBP) in clinical trials

File NDA

Carcinogenicty studies or other studies dictated by clinical experience

FIG. 6.5. Schematic of the drug development and approval process in the United States. Similar processes are employed for worldwide pharmaceutical testing. From Reference 85.

in a limited male, non-patient population. As indicated above, the FDA supports the early inclusion of women in clinical trials for new therapies, especially those to be used in the treatment of life-threatening diseases (65,66). Because of this interest, studies of developmental toxicity, which usually occur later, may be moved to a much earlier point in the drug development process (142).

When designing animal studies to support FHD, a major consideration in dose selection must be the anticipated "margin of safety" between animals and humans. Ideally, doses in animal studies should provide exposure to the compound well in excess of what is anticipated at the highest doses to be tested in humans. As discussed previously, a comparison of these doses on a mg/kg basis is no longer considered to provide adequate information in this respect due to potential species differences in absorption and rates and routes of metabolism. Thus, a good estimate of the pharmacokinetic behavior of the agent in animals is an important goal of nonclinical testing. There is no firm guideline regarding what should be considered an adequate margin of safety. However, a "smaller" margin between the potentially efficacious dose and a toxic dose is tolerated for those compounds under development for life-threatening diseases, particularly if they are expected to offer a distinct therapeutic advantage over other agents currently marketed in the class.

Based on the activities of the ICH, the designs and goals of clinical trials are similar throughout the world. Figure 6.6 shows the recommendations for the duration of animal tests relative to proposed human exposure to NCEs. It is possible to discuss the nonclinical and clinical programs with regulatory bodies, and, depending on the characteristics and proposed use of the chemical, modify these recommendations.

The duration of animal tests necessary to support a specific duration of clinical trials for NBEs is much more flexible (111). Short-term clinical trials for life-threatening conditions may be supported by 2-week nonclinical toxicology studies. Subchronic clinical trials

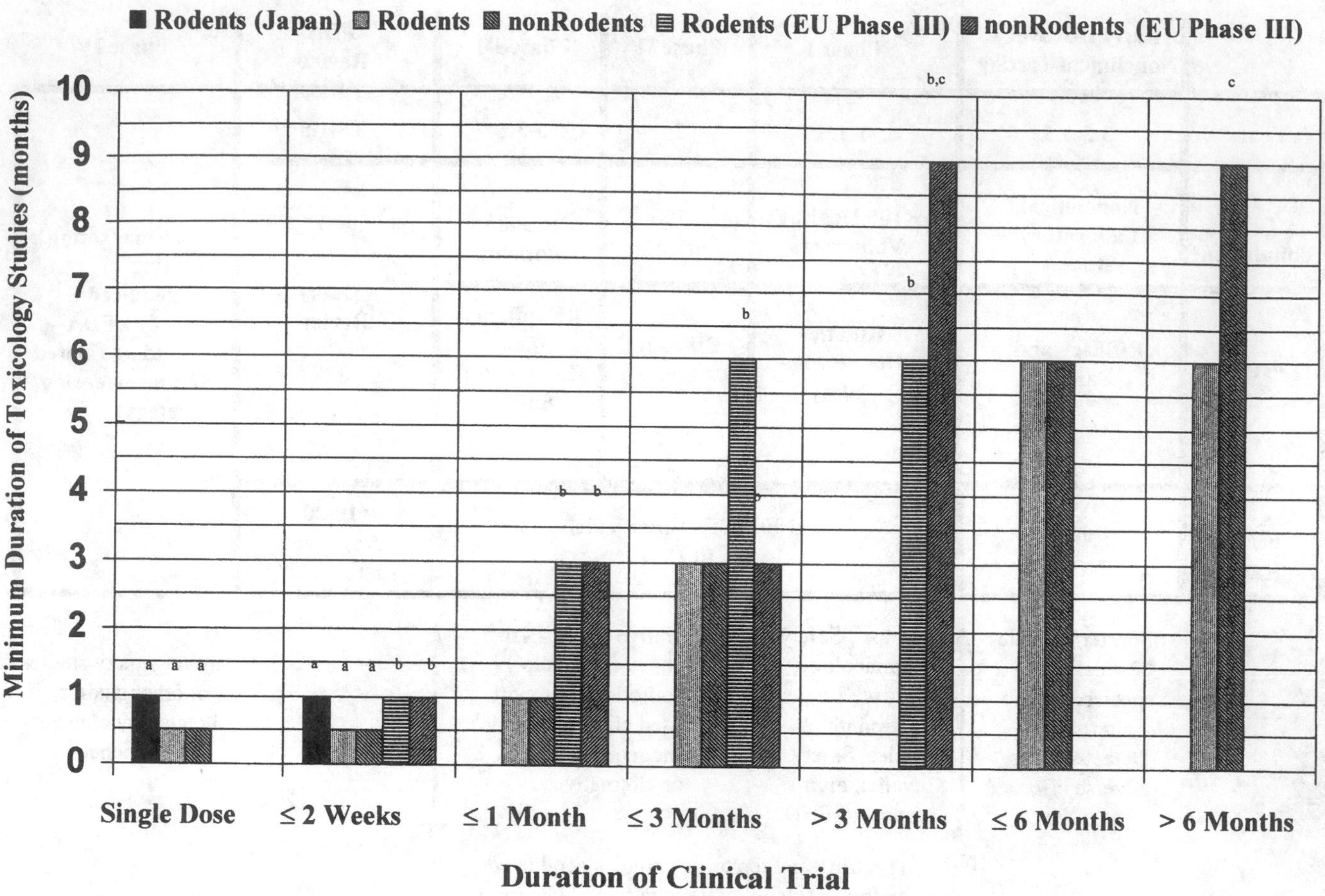

FIG. 6.6. International guidelines for the duration of animal toxicology studies necessary to support clinical trials of various duration. Assessment of reversibility may be necessary in three-month or six-month toxicology studies. Carcinogenicity studies are not needed in advance of clinical trials, unless there is a cause for concern. They may be conducted post-approval for some indications. From Reference 102.

a. In the United States and the European Union (EU), two-week rodent and nonrodent studies are the minimum duration. In: Japan, four-week rodent and two-week nonrodent are needed. In the United States, single-dose toxicity with extended examinations can support single-dose CT.
b. Studies in support of Phase III trials in EU, and marketing in all regions.
c. Nine-month nonrodent study is an international consensus, EU and Japan favor six-month, United States favors 12-month. Check with regulators before initiating study.

can be supported with toxicology studies of 1–3 months. Clinical trials to support long-term, chronic therapy, can be supported with 6-month toxicology studies.

Regulators throughout the world have recognized that resources could be used more efficiently, and efficacious and safe drugs could be made available more rapidly, if guidelines for nonclinical clinical testing and registration were comparable across countries. The ICH has developed a comprehensive set of safety guidelines to harmonize the regulatory requirements of the EU, United States, and Japan. The ICH Expert Working Groups (EWG) have considered appropriate guidelines for all of the various types of toxicity tests, including acute and subchronic testing, chronic and carcinogenicity testing, reproduction and developmental toxicity studies, and mutagenicity testing. The required duration of animal studies to support human exposure has also been addressed. There has been a good deal of collaboration between regulatory agencies and pharmaceutical companies in the development of the safety guidelines.

Dorato and Buckley (59) have provided a more complete discussion of the role of the ICH process in drug development. The ICH guidelines addressing the various nonclinical studies required to support clinical trials and registrations in the three major regions (EU, United States, Japan) are shown in Table 6.5. Selected Internet websites providing information on design of toxicology studies to support clinical trials are shown in Table 6.6.

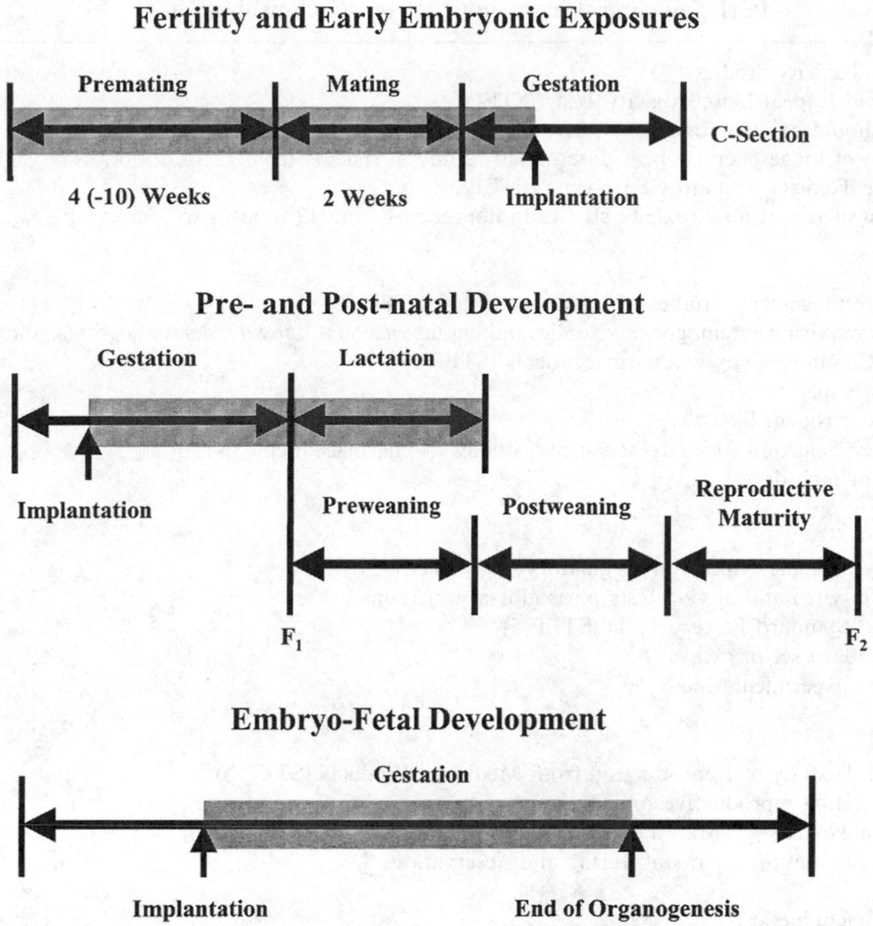

FIG. 6.7. The three-study design proposed for the assessment of reproductive and developmental toxicity for a standard pharmaceutical. From Reference 110.

Specific Agents

Omeprazole (Prilosec)

Omeprazole (Figure 6.8) is a substituted benzimidazole that is a potent inhibitor of H^+/K^+ ATPase ("proton pump") at the secretory surface of the gastric parietal cell, thereby inhibiting gastric acid secretion (155,189). Omeprazole is indicated for the short-term (4- to 12-week) treatment of active duodenal and gastric ulcer, gastroesophageal reflux disease (GERD), severe erosive esophagitis, and the maintenance of healing of erosive esophagitis; and the long-term treatment of pathological hypersecretory conditions such as the Zollinger–Ellison syndrome. It is also approved for use, with clarithromycin, for treatment of *H. pylori* infections. The recommended dosage for the short-term indications is 20–40 mg daily (approximately 0.4–0.8 mg/kg in a 50 kg individual). For the long-term indications, the recommended initial dose is 60 mg daily; however, doses up to 120 mg three times daily have been administered (146). Table 6.7 lists the toxicology studies that were submitted to the FDA (68) to support the U.S. registration of omeprazole. The content of the toxicology package suggests that the intravenous route may have also been a considered route for therapy.

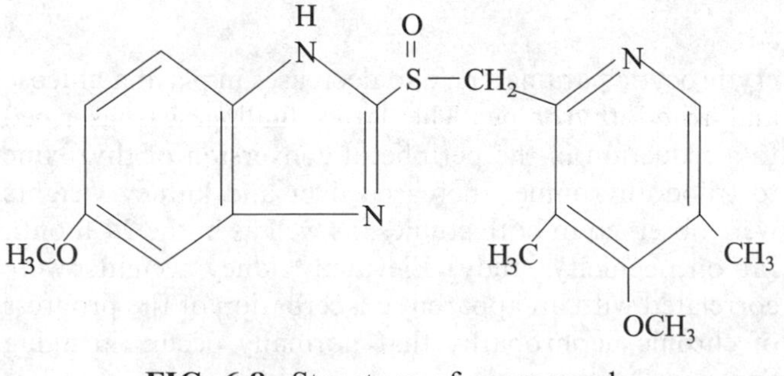

FIG. 6.8. Structure of omeprazole.

The results of acute, subchronic, and chronic studies suggested that the toxicology profile of omeprazole was generally unremarkable (24,61,68,97). The acute

Table 6.5
ICH guidelines for the conduct of nonclinical studies

Single- and Repeat-Dose Toxicity Studies
Topic S4 Single-Dose and Repeat-Dose Toxicity Tests (STEP 5)
- LD_{50} determination should be abandoned
- Reduction in duration of longest-term repeat-dose toxicity study in rodents from 12 to 6 months

Topic S4A Repeat-Dose Toxicity Tests in Nonrodents (STEP 3)
- Reduction of duration of repeat-dose toxicity studies in nonrodents from 12 months to 9 months

Carcinogenicity Studies
Topic S1A Need for Carcinogenicity Studies of Pharmaceuticals (STEP 5)
- Defines circumstances requiring carcinogenicity studies, taking into account known risks, indications, and duration of exposure

Topic S1B Testing for Carcinogenicity in Pharmaceuticals (STEP 5)
- Need for studies in two species
- Alternatives to two-year rodent bioassay

Topic S1C & S1CR Dose Selection for Carcinogenicity Studies in Pharmaceuticals (STEP 5)
- Criteria for selection of high dose

Genotoxicity Studies
Topic S2A Genotoxicity: Specific Aspects of Regulatory Tests (STEP 5)
- Specific guidance for in vitro and in vivo tests pluss glossary of terms

Topic S2B Genotoxicity: Standard Battery Tests (STEP 5)
- Identification of a standard set of assays
- Extent of confirmatory experimentation

Reproductive Toxicology
Topic S5A Detection of Toxicity to Reproduction from Medicinal Products (STEP 5)
- Specific guidance for testing reproductive toxicity

Topic S5B Reproductive Toxicology: Male Fertility Studies (STEP 5)
- Recommendation for pre-mating treatment during and observations

Toxicokinetics and Pharmacokinetics
Topic S3A Toxicokinetics: Guidance on the Assessment of Systemic Exposure in Toxicity studies (STEP 5)
- Integration of kinetic information into toxicity testing

Topic S3B Pharmacokinetics: Guidance for Repeat-Dose Tissue Distribution Studies (STEP 5)
- Need for tissue distribution studies, when appropriate data cannot be derived from other sources

Biotechnology Products
Topic S6 Safety Studies for Biotechnology Products (STEP 5)
- Nonclinical safety studies, use of animal models of disease and other alternative methods, need for genotoxicity and carcinogenicity studies, impact of antibody formation

Multidisciplinary Safety/Efficacy Studies
Topic M3 Timing of Nonclinical Studies in Relation to Clinical Trials (STEP 5)
- Principles for development of nonclinical testing strategies
- Addresses full range of studies to support clinical trials for NCEs

toxicity of the compound in rats and mice was low as demonstrated by oral LD_{50s} (the dose that kills 50% of the animals tested) generally in excess of 4 g/kg. Multiple-dose studies in rats were conducted at doses up to 414 mg/kg/day for 3 months, and up to 138 mg/kg/day for 6 months. There were no consistent effects on body weight or food consumption reported in those studies. Treatment-related findings that occurred at high doses in these studies included decreases in several erythrocytic parameters, and decreases in plasma glucose and triiodothyronine. The latter finding was ascribed to a reduction in the peripheral conversion of thyroxine to triiodothyronine. Increased liver and kidney weights were observed in both studies, as well as in the 24-month rat oncogenicity study. Elevated kidney weights were correlated with an apparent exacerbation of the progress of chronic nephropathy that normally occurs in aging Sprague–Dawley rats.

Table 6.6
Selected internet websites providing information on the design and expectations on nonclinical toxicology studies

1. http://www.fda.gov/cder/guidance

   Access to guidance documents representing the agency's current thinking on a particular subject relating to the drug development process. Includes access to adopted and draft ICH guidelines.

2. http://www.eudra.org/humandocs/humans/swp.htm

   Safety Working Party (SWP) documents covering aspects of safety evaluation in Europe. Includes access to adopted and draft ICH guidelines.

3. http://www.ich.org

   The process and the adopted and draft safety guidelines of the International Conference on Harmonization of Technical Requirements for Registration of Pharmaceuticals for Human Use (ICH).

4. http://www.eudra.org

   The European Agency for the Evaluation of Medicinal Products (EMEA).

5. http://www.cmr.org

   The Centre for Medicines Research International (CMR) is a not-for-profit organization funded by the worldwide research-based pharmaceutical industry to provide unique data and expert analysis to address technical, medical, economic, regulatory, and policy issues in the discovery, development, and safe use of medicines.

Dogs were treated with omeprazole for 3 months at doses up to 138 mg/kg/day or 12 months at doses up to 28 mg/kg/day. Clinical chemistry findings were generally unremarkable, although as observed in the rat, some decreases in hematology parameters and plasma triiodothyronine were noted.

The most significant nonclinical finding in both rats and dogs was a reversible gastric mucosal cell hyperplasia with increases in mucosal thickness and folding. In the 6-month study in rats, omeprazole induced a dose-related eosinophilia of the zymogen granules of the pepsinogen-secreting chief cells, with slight atrophy of these cells occurring at the high dose. Slight chief cell atrophy was also observed in dogs given the high dose of omeprazole for 3 or 12 months. To characterize these gastric changes more rigorously, a rather extensive reversibility study was conducted in rats in which animals were treated with either 0 or 138 mg omeprazole/kg/day for 14 days, and 1, 3, or 6 months. Other groups of animals were treated with that dose of omeprazole for 3 or 6 months, followed by recovery periods of 14 days, and 1, 3, or 6 months. This study demonstrated the time dependency and complete reversibility of the gastric lesions in rats. A 3-month recovery period following 3 months of treatment in dogs showed that the slight chief cell atrophy observed at 3 months was reversible, and a 4-month recovery period following 12 months of treatment in dogs demonstrated the reversibility of mucosal hyperplasia and chief cell atrophy, although increased mucosal folding was still evident.

No teratological findings were observed in the rat at omeprazole doses up to 138 mg/kg/day administered on days 6–15 of pregnancy. The two highest doses tested in rabbits (approximately 70 and 140 mg/kg), administered during days 6–18 of pregnancy, resulted in maternal toxicity as evidenced by anorexia and reduced water intake. Signs were sufficiently severe that treatment of animals at the high dose was discontinued on day 14. Fetal mortality was increased in conjunction with maternal toxicity, but fetal development was unaffected by maternal omeprazole treatment. The major finding of the fertility and perinatal and postnatal studies was a decrease in weight gain of pups of maternal animals given the high dose of 138 mg/kg/day during late pregnancy and lactation. This correlated with a decrease in maternal body weight and food consumption during late lactation. Whether the decrease in pup weight gain was the result of the decrease in maternal feed consumption, or whether it may have been a direct effect on offspring via the breast milk transfer of the compound is not known, and whether nursing or drug therapy ought to be discontinued in the nursing woman, for this and other pharmacological agents, should be considered.

In the mouse oncogenicity study, animals were treated with up to 138 mg omeprazole/kg/day for 18 months. A decrease in survival was noted at the high dose, but no neoplasia was observed in any organ. Different results, however, were obtained in the rat oncogenicity study, in which animals were treated with 13.8, 43, or 138 mg omeprazole/kg/day for 24 months. Enterochromaffin-like (ECL) cell hyperplasia, progressing to ECL cell carcinoids, occurred in dose-related fashion in these animals, with males being affected at doses of 43 and 138 mg/kg/day, and females being affected at all dose levels. These positive findings resulted in the temporary suspension of the clinical trial program. The carcinoids were characterized as "end-of-life" tumors, since the first was discovered at 82 weeks of treatment in an animal that had died prematurely. Carcinoid tumors were not identified as the cause of death in any animals, and no metastases were found. A 2-year study was repeated in females in an attempt to define a dose at which ECL cell carcinoids did not occur. However, carcinoid formation again occurred in a dose-related fashion, including at the lowest dose tested (1.7 mg/kg/day).

A major question that must be addressed following positive results in a carcinogenicity bioassay is whether tumorigenesis was the direct result of chemical insult, or whether it can be related to the pharmacological mechanism of action of the compound. Furthermore, whether the model is appropriate for extrapolation of these findings to humans requires evaluation. For example, at this late stage in the development of a compound, sufficient pharmacokinetic data should be available in both the animal species tested and humans to determine whether a finding might be restricted to a species that metabolizes the compound quite differently from humans. If this is the case, further mechanistic studies can be designed to support or refute the applicability of the findings.

A number of in vivo and in vitro mutagenicity studies were conducted with omeprazole (Table 6.7). An initial mouse micronucleus test with omeprazole administered to animals at a high dose of 5000 mg/kg produced equivocal results, with slight increases in the mean numbers of micronucleated cells compared to controls (approximately 2-fold, compared to 30-fold following a 0.4 mg/kg dose of the positive control, mitomycin C). It was noted that the dose of 5000 mg/kg was not well tolerated. A second mouse micronucleus test was conducted, using a maximum dose of approximately 800 mg/kg, which did not show evidence of mutagenic potential. All other mutagenicity tests conducted produced negative results, suggesting that the tumorigenesis observed in the 2-year rat studies was not the result of a genotoxic action of omeprazole or its metabolites.

Mechanistic studies in dogs and rats, combined with correlative data from clinical trials, ultimately provided the information to support the safe use and registration of omeprazole. At the doses selected for the toxicity studies, the sustained decrease in luminal pH of the stomach resulting from the inhibition of gastric acid secretion by omeprazole caused a substantial increase in the release of gastrin into the blood. In fed rats, gastrin levels in plasma normally range from 150–200 pg/ml. Omeprazole administered at doses of 13.8–138 mg/kg/day increased plasma gastrin concentrations to 1000–3000 pg/ml. Gastrin has a trophic effect on the gastric mucosa and results in the hyperplasia of several cell types, including ECL cells, and consequent mucosal thickening. These data suggest that omeprazole does not inherently cause ECL cell hyperplasia and resulting carcinoid formation. Indeed, in antrectomized dogs, where the major source of gastrin is surgically removed, high doses of omeprazole for 1 year resulted in neither hypergastrinemia nor mucosal hyperplasia (61). Similarly, antrectomy in rats prevents the hypergastrinemia and ECL cell hyperplasia associated with omeprazole treatment (120).

Table 6.7
Summary of toxicology studies conducted to support the registration of omeprazole in the United States

Acute toxicology
Oral study in mice
IV study in mice
Oral study in rats
IV study in rats
Oral study in dogs
Subchronic toxicology
2-Week iv study in rats
1-Month iv study in rats
1-Month iv study in dogs
3-Month oral study in rats
3-Month oral study in mice
3-Month oral study in dogs
3-Month oral study in dogs with 3-month recovery
Chronic toxicology
6-Month oral study in rats
3- and 6-Month oral studies in rats with 2-week to 6-month recovery
2-Year study in female rats to examine gastrin-dependent variables
1-Year oral study in dogs with 4-month recovery
5-Year oral study in dogs (ongoing at time of application)
Genetic toxicology
Ames *Salmonella* test with/without metabolic activation
Mouse lymphoma forward mutation assay
Mouse micronucleus test
Mouse chromosome aberrations
Rat liver DNA damage assay
Reproductive and developmental toxicology
Segment I oral fertility in rats
Segment II oral teratology in rats
Segment II oral teratology in rabbits
Segment III oral perinatal and postnatal in rats
Segment III extended oral perinatal and postnatal in rats
Carcinogenicity studies
78-Week oral study in mice
104-Week oral study in rats
104-Week oral study in female rats

The course of development of omeprazole demonstrates the importance of conducting mechanistic studies to elucidate the significance of findings in animal safety studies, and whether the effects can be meaningfully extrapolated to humans. A close collaboration between the toxicologist and clinician during advancing human trials is critical to resolve questions related to human safety. The extensive clinical experience with omeprazole has confirmed its safe and effective use

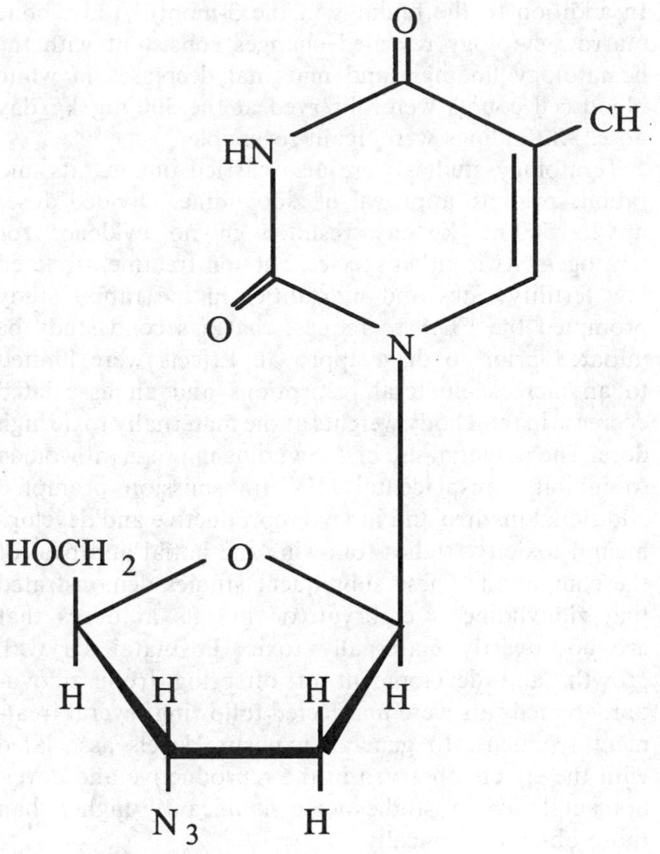

FIG. 6.9. Structure of zidovudine.

for treatment of the described indications (146,11). In a group of patients who required continuous treatment with 40 mg of omeprazole for up to 4 years, there was no evidence for dysplastic or neoplastic changes (39). Over 12,000 endoscopic biopsies further support the clinical safety of omeprazole relative to its potential for causing hyperplastic changes.

Zidovudine (Retrovir/AZT)

Zidovudine (azidothymidine, AZT, Figure 6.9) inhibits viral RNA-dependent DNA polymerase (reverse transcriptase) and, thus, viral replication. Furthermore, as a thymidine analog, zidovudine becomes incorporated into growing strands of DNA by viral reverse transcriptase, and inhibits the further addition of nucleotides. It is intended for use in the management of adult patients with HIV infection when antiretroviral therapy is warranted (147). It is also indicated for the prevention of maternal–fetal HIV transmission during gestation and labor, and in the neonate after birth. The recommended dose for adults is 600 mg/day in divided doses in combination with other antiretroviral agents and 500 mg/day (100 mg every 4 hours while awake) or 600 mg/day in divided doses for monotherapy. Zidovudine is also available for intravenous infusion in

Table 6.8
Summary of toxicology studies submitted for initial FDA review to support the registration of zidovudine in the United States

Acute toxicology	
	IV study in mice
	IV study in rats
Subchronic toxicology	
	2-Week iv study in dogs with 2-week recovery
	2-Week oral study in rats
	2-Week oral study in dogs
	2-Week oral study in monkeys
	1-Month iv study in rats with 2-week recovery
	3-Month oral study in rats with 2-week recovery
	3-Month oral study in monkeys with 6-week recovery
	6-Month oral study in rats with 2-month recovery
Reproductive and developmental toxicology	
	Segment II oral teratology in rats
	Segment II oral teratology in rabbits
Genetic toxicology	
	Mouse lymphoma assay
	Ames *Salmonella* test with/without metabolic activation
	Cell transformation assay
	In vivo cytogenetic study in rats
	In vitro cytogenetic study in human lymphocytes
Summary of toxicology studies planned or in progress at the time of initial FDA review of zidovudine	
	6-Month oral study in monkeys
	Segment I oral reproduction/fertility study in rats
	Segment III oral perinatal and postnatal study in rats
	Segment II oral teratology study in rabbits
	1-Year oral study in rats
	1-Year oral study in monkeys
	Oral carcinogenicity study in rats
	Oral carcinogenicity study in mice

patients with advanced disease and for use in women during labor and delivery. In spite of the intended long-term use of the compound, it was approved with a minimal toxicology package due to the serious nature of the disease and lack of alternative efficacious therapies.

The studies listed in the upper portion of Table 6.8 were either submitted as part of the original NDA in December 1986, or as amendments to the application shortly thereafter (69). At the time of the initial pharmacology–toxicology review, a variety of chronic toxicity studies were still underway or planned. The FDA commentary indicated that

> "nonclinical toxicity data submitted in support of the application include results of studies in rats, dogs and cynomolgus monkeys. FDA guidelines would have prescribed more extensive nonclinical testing than that reported thus far. However, the urgency for developing an anti-AIDS drug has been so great that clinical testing has preceded the usual/customary nonclinical testing. For example, while data from a 6-month *clinical* study are available, results for the supporting 6-month *nonclinical* toxicity studies have not yet been submitted" (emphasis added).

An approvable letter issued by the FDA in March 1987, less than four months following submission of the NDA, stipulated the timing for the conduct of these outstanding studies. Comprehensive reviews of the acute, subchronic, chronic, genetic, carcinogenic, reproductive, and developmental toxicity studies have been published (6,7,91).

Zidovudine demonstrated relatively low acute toxicity with intravenous MLDs (median lethal doses) of greater than 750 mg/kg in rats and mice. The most consistent findings in the subchronic/chronic studies with rats, dogs, and monkeys were effects on hematological parameters. In rats given two divided doses of zidovudine at approximately 50, 150, or 500 mg/kg/day orally for 3 or 6 months, there were reversible decreases in red blood cell counts and hemoglobin concentration primarily in the mid- and high-dose groups. The severity of these effects appeared to progress slightly between 3 and 6 months of treatment. No remarkable histopathology was noted in these studies. A subsequent 1-year study, submitted well following the initial approval of zidovudine, revealed a similar toxicity profile to that observed in the 3- and 6-month studies. The severity of anemia did not progress between 6 and 12 months of exposure, and effects were again reversible following discontinuation of treatment.

Dogs were more sensitive to zidovudine treatment. In a 2-week study in which animals were administered 125–500 mg/kg/day orally in divided doses, decreases in erythroid values, and leukopenia and thrombocytopenia were observed at all dose levels. Cytostatic effects were observed in the small intestine at the high dose, and were also evidenced by slight to moderate non-dose-related lymphoid depletion, and mild to marked dose-related bone marrow hypocellularity at all dose levels. No cytostatic effects were observed at similar or higher doses in either rats or monkeys. Studies revealed that zidovudine was metabolized almost identically in monkeys and humans, and as a result, the continued nonclinical development of the drug was conducted in the monkey, rather than the dog. However, the species differences in metabolism were not of sufficient magnitude to account for the much greater sensitivity of the dog to zidovudine, and the design of subsequent nonclinical and clinical studies continued to respect the significant findings in this species.

Monkeys responded to a 2-week treatment at divided doses of 125–500 mg/kg/day with a slight reduction in hemoglobin concentrations in one animal at the low dose, and in both monkeys given the high dose. In a 3-month monkey study, at divided doses of 35–300 mg/kg/day, dose-related decreases in erythron parameters were noted as early as day 15 of treatment and progressed to live-phase termination. Platelet counts were also increased. Values returned to normal during the 6-week recovery phase of the study. Subsequent (post-approval) 6- and 12-month studies were conducted in the monkey. In addition to the findings in the 3-month study, bone marrow cytology revealed changes consistent with the hematology findings, and marginal decreases in white blood cell counts were observed at the 300 mg/kg/day dose. All findings were again reversible.

Teratology studies were also carried out in rats and rabbits prior to approval of zidovudine. Divided doses up to 500 mg/kg/day resulted in no evidence for teratogenicity in either species, but non-treatment-related low fertility rates and mortalities in the rabbit study prompted the FDA to request that a second study be initiated prior to drug approval. Effects were limited to an increase in fetal resorptions and an associated decrease in fetal body weights at the maternally toxic high dose. The potential use of zidovudine in pregnant women to inhibit transplacental HIV transmission prompted additional in vitro and in vivo reproductive and developmental toxicity studies following the initial approval of the compound. These subsequent studies demonstrated that zidovudine is embryotoxic in rats at doses that are not overtly maternally toxic. Postnatal survival, growth, and development of offspring from zidovudine-treated rats were unaffected following several treatment regimens. In general, exposure levels associated with the effects observed in the reproductive and developmental toxicity studies were significantly higher than those observed clinically.

No evidence for mutagenicity by zidovudine was observed in the Ames Salmonella study either with or without mammalian metabolic activation. The compound was weakly mutagenic in the mouse lymphoma assay without metabolic transformation at concentrations of 4000 and 5000 μg/ml; it was also weakly mutagenic with metabolic activation at concentrations greater than or equal to 1000 μg/ml. A positive response was obtained in the mammalian cell transformation assay at concentrations of 0.5 μg/ml or greater. In an in vitro cytogenetic assay in human lymphocytes, zidovudine caused structural chromosomal abnormalities at concentrations equal to or greater than 3 μg/ml. However, in an in vivo rat assay, no chromosomal abnormalities were noted following the intravenous administration of doses up to 300 mg/kg (plasma levels over 400 μg/ml). Subsequent in vivo micronucleus studies in mice and rats revealed dose-related increases in micronucleated erythrocytes, reflecting chromosome breakage or mitotic spindle damage.

Carcinogenicity studies in mice were initiated using single daily doses of 30, 60, or 120 mg/kg. These doses were reduced to 20, 30, or 40 mg/kg at 3 months of treatment due to treatment-related anemia. Rats were dosed with 80, 220, or 600 mg/kg/day, with the high dose being reduced to 450, then 300 mg/kg. As expected, hematological changes were observed, but there were no deaths or morbidities that were considered treatment-related in either study. In the mouse study, one benign vaginal neoplasm occurred at 30 mg/kg, and five malignant and two benign neoplasms occurred at 40 mg/kg. Two vaginal neoplasms occurred at the high dose of the rat study. In both cases, the tumors were late-occurring and non-metastasizing. An eloquent argument has been put forth suggesting that these vaginal tumors result from high local exposure to zidovudine due to the retrograde flow of urine containing high levels of the excreted compound into the vagina. An additional lifetime mouse study to support this hypothesis was conducted in which animals were administered zidovudine intravaginally. Thirteen vaginal squamous cell carcinomas occurred in animals receiving the highest concentration in that study, supporting the contention that systemic exposure to the drug was unlikely to be responsible for the neoplasia observed in the oral studies.

A variety of adverse reactions have been documented in patients receiving zidovudine. Due to the wide range of symptoms associated with the opportunistic infections seen in AIDS patients, it is difficult to assess which adverse reactions are clearly the result of zidovudine therapy. However, the animal safety studies were highly predictive of the major hematological toxicities of zidovudine described in humans—granulocytopenia and severe anemia.

Similar to what was described previously under the development of omeprazole, additional mechanistic studies were conducted with zidovudine to explain toxicity findings, even though the drug was intended for the treatment of a fatal disease.

Although the toxicology support package for zidovudine ultimately responded to existing guidelines for registration of a chronic-use pharmaceutical in the United States, its development history demonstrates that the approval system allows considerable flexibility in cases where the market for a life-threatening disease is clearly not satisfied (i.e., antivirals, antifungals, oncolytics). This type of development strategy can only occur with close collaboration between the submitter and the regulatory agency, and after careful consideration of the risk–benefit assessments.

New Biological Entities

The development of highly purified species-specific protein pharmaceutical agents, made possible through advances in rDNA technology, presents a significant challenge to toxicologists. The major question presented is, "What nonclinical toxicology evaluations should be conducted to insure safety in human clinical trials?" The major issue is the testing of these specific proteins in nonhomologous animal species, where the possibility of immunogenicity, not applicable to the clinical trial, exists (174). As there are no universally accepted methods/procedures for the nonclinical evaluation of new biological entities (NBEs), decisions of appropriate nonclinical study design are made on a case-by-case basis. The general consensus is that nonclinical toxicity evaluations with species-specific proteins reveal little more than enhanced pharmacodynamic activity rather than predicting the potential for adverse effects. Furthermore, the toxicity observed in animal studies may be the result of an immunological response to the foreign protein. Toxicology studies with NBEs should demonstrate that the product has no adverse effects other than those specifically related to pharmacodynamics, and that safety for the expected clinical dose range, rather than exaggerated toxicity (i.e., MTD), should be demonstrated (9,145,174).

Regulatory agencies have placed great emphasis on chemical characterization of the NBE as a means of establishing that it is identical to the naturally occurring protein (manufacturing contaminant issues aside). Establishing this identity has allowed for appropriate modification of toxicology requirements and abbreviation of the toxicology support package. However, NBEs are being developed that contain amino acid sequences that have been purposefully manipulated to differ from the naturally occurring protein in order, for example, to result in a prolonged duration of action over the naturally occurring agent. These molecules may require a more comprehensive toxicology package, such as established for NCEs (see above).

Safety testing of NBEs can be presented in three categories (Table 6.9). The reasonably clear-cut time sequence of nonclinical and clinical studies established with NCEs often is not feasible with NBEs. The interactions between toxicologists and clinicians are important in addressing suspected adverse reactions in the clinical trials (9). Nonclinical toxicology evaluations of NBEs should be designed according to the risks anticipated from the type of product, the contaminant profile, and the intended clinical use (9). There will continue to be major questions and differences of opinion relative to

Table 6.9
Safety testing of biotechnology products[a]

Category	Requirements
1	Identity, purity, pharmacology, safety pharmacology
2	Category 1 plus: Detailed pharmacological activity (human, animal), relationship of plasma concentration and antibody titer (human, animal, in vitro) tolerance, selected toxicological testing
3	Categories 1 and 2 plus: Studies guided by indication, studies guided by duration of treatment

[a] From Reference 9.

the evolution of nonclinical toxicology testing strategies of NBEs. The major questions will arise concerning appropriate species (174,216), the need to conduct genetic toxicology studies (9,174), and the conduct of reproductive toxicology assessments (174).

As examples of NBEs, we have chosen to discuss toxicology support for the registration of gonadotropin-releasing hormone (GnRH) analogs, interferon, and human insulin. The development of interferon has provided a great deal of guidance for nonclinical toxicity testing of NBEs. The pharmacological effects of insulin are well known from extensive clinical experience. This experience has aided the relatively rapid approval of rDNA insulin products, and has allowed the chemical characterization of test material to play a major role in supporting a more limited toxicology profile. Human insulin, therefore, provides an example of a NBE that was approved rapidly, in approximately five months (121).

Gonadotropin-Releasing Hormone (GnRH) Analogs

GnRH analogs are either agonists or antagonists of the receptor for the naturally occurring hypothalamic decapeptide GnRH. The chemical modifications either increase the biological activity and duration of action or affect the solubility, potency, and kinetics of the molecule. GnRH analogs were first introduced for the treatment of cancer (e.g., prostatic carcinoma) and their toxicological assessment was less complete than usually recommended for new drugs. Since their first introduction, the use of GnRH analogs has expanded into treatment of non-life-threatening conditions, and they now are expected to have to undergo the same rigorous toxicology evaluation as other new drugs (149). In the case of GnRH analogs, the FDA has allowed the multi-dose toxicity studies to be conducted at a multiple of human exposure (30- to 50-fold) rather than at doses that define the toxic limits of the compound. Due to the chronic nature of therapy, and chemical dissimilarity with native GnRH, the FDA has recommended that both rat and mouse carcinogenicity studies be conducted. As is the case with the multiple-dose toxicity studies, the FDA has allowed the MTD not to be used, but required, instead, that some multiple of the human clinical exposure be used to set the top dose in the carcinogenicity studies (e.g., 15- to 50-fold). The full toxicity profile recommended for GnRH analogs includes: single-dose acute toxicity (rodent and nonrodent), repeat-dose toxicity studies through 6 months in rodents and 9 months in nonrodents, genetic toxicology, developmental toxicology, and carcinogenicity (149).

Interferon

Interferons (IFNs) are classified as IFN-α (leukocyte), -β(fibroblast), or γ (immune) (Figure 6.10). IFN-α consists of a family of at least 14 highly homologous species. The amino acid sequence homology of the IFN-α subtypes has been reported to be 52 to 75 percent (168,169,181). The biological activities of IFNs include antiviral, anticellular, and immunomodulatory activities (181). The properties of interferons and their potential uses have been reviewed by Bocci (13).

The adverse clinical experiences reported with the use of IFNs include: fever, chill/rigor, headache, tremor, nausea, vomiting, myalgia, anxiety, fatigue, malaise, anorexia, confusion, local inflammation, cardiovascular toxicity, hepatotoxicity, and abnormal EEGs (71,160,161,169,187). The most commonly reported adverse effects are fever, fatigue, and leukopenia (169). The effects that cause the most distress in clinical subjects are those related to central nervous system (CNS) depression (187). The toxicity seen with very pure and single clone IFN preparations is almost identical to that reported for the less pure, more heterogeneous preparations of IFNs. The responses reported, particularly the influenza-like syndrome, therefore, are likely intrinsically related to IFNs, and not to a contaminant or impurity (169,187).

The species specificity of highly purified human IFNs implies that classical animal (nonhomologous) efficacy and toxicity models are not applicable in evaluation of these materials. Nonclinical safety testing of IFNs has not identified an appropriate animal model (72,98, 153,157,170,213), supporting the recommendation that the routine safety tests applied to NCEs should not be applied haphazardly (174) to NBEs. Yet, given the traditional significance and predictive nature of nonclinical toxicology evaluations, and acknowledging the lack of generally accepted and validated nonclinical animal models for the testing of these entities, drug regulatory agencies have published safety testing guidelines that place NBEs on a level with conventional drugs relative to the comprehensive requirements for animal safety studies (77,112). A representative example of these guidelines/requirements is given in Table 6.10.

Interferon-α_{2a} (Roferon-A,) is a commercially available NBE identical to one of the 15 subtypes of human leukocyte IFN (182). At the time clinical trials were initiated with this drug, considerable clinical data were available from studies with other leukocyte IFNs to indicate the types of adverse reactions, described above, that might be expected (169,187). The species specificity of recombinant IFN-α_{2a} has led to production of neutralizing antibodies in rodent and nonrodent species (182). This has impaired the ability of toxicology studies to detect the expected adverse clinical signs in common toxicology species.

Acute, single-dose toxicology studies (Table 6.11) were conducted in a variety of species in an attempt to disclose any unexpected acute toxicity related to the clinical dos-

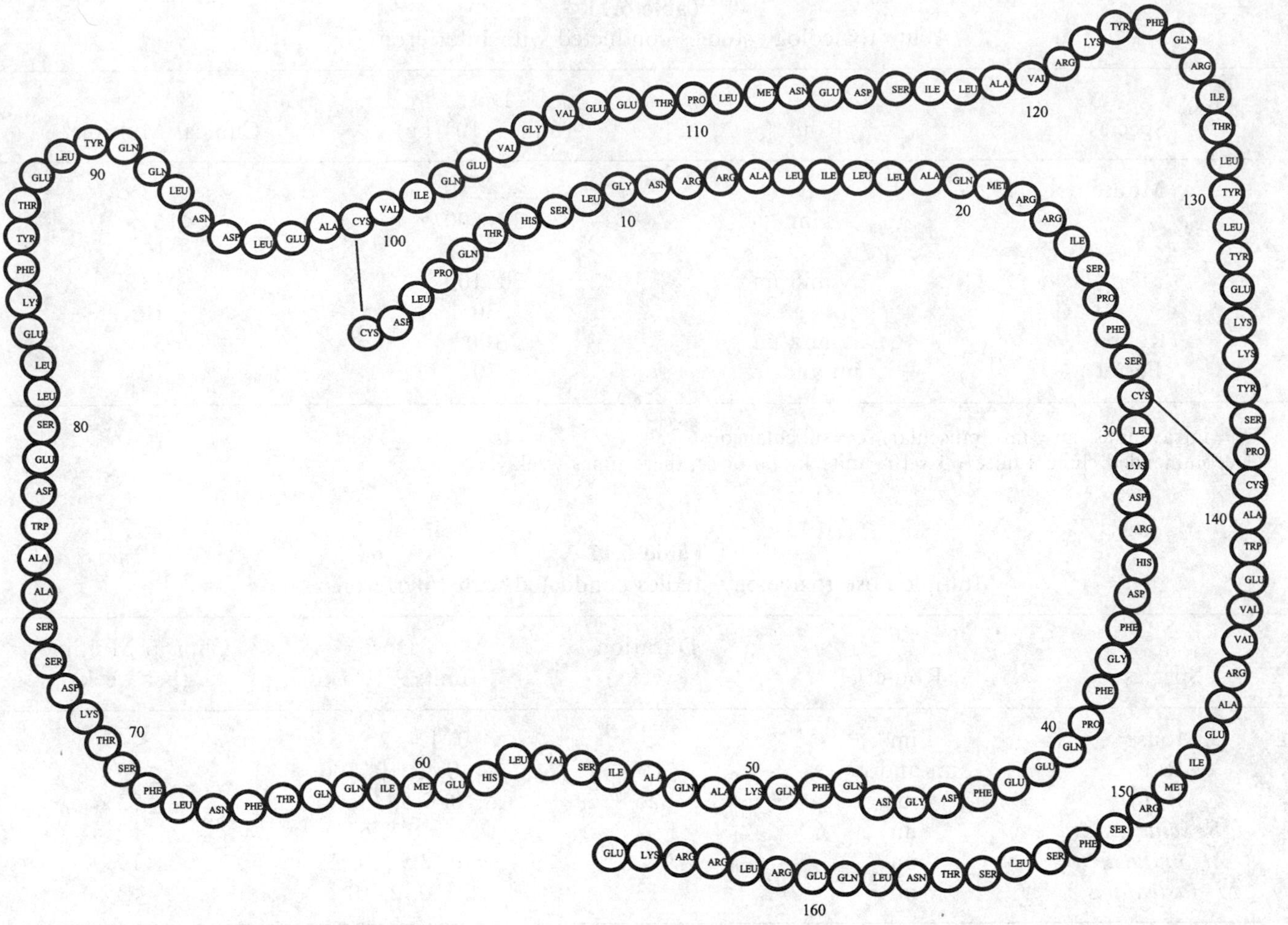

FIG. 6.10. Consensus sequence of human leukocyte interferons. Redrawn with permission from Reference 169.

Table 6.10
Recommendations for Interferon testing by the French Ministry of Social Affairs[a]

Toxicological Test	Recommendation
Acute	2 species, both sexes in 1 species, 2 routes, 2-week observation
Subchronic	2 species, rodent and primate, 3 months daily injection
Reproduction	Segments I, II, III
Mutagenicity	In vivo and in vitro clastogenesis
Carcinogenicity	Not required
Pyrogenicity	Rabbit
Safety Pharmacology	In vivo cardiopulmonary, isolated organs; Neurobehavioral studies
Cell culture	Cytostatic and cytotoxic effects

[a] From Reference 210.

age form (excipients, active ingredients). No mortalities were noted in the species tested. The LD_{50} of IFN-α_{2a} was determined to be $>22.8 \times 10^6$ units/kg iv. These studies were conducted at multiples of a single clinical dose (3×10^6 units/kg), ranging from 10- to 167-fold. Multiple-dose toxicology studies were conducted over a range of 5 to 26 weeks at 3- to 78-fold the weekly clinical dose (9×10^6 units/kg) (Table 6.12). A low frequency of treatment-related adverse findings was reported: slight weight loss in rats; a slight, reversible, increase in platelets and total leukocytes in mice; a slight decrease in hemoglobin and hematocrit in squirrel monkeys; dose-dependent anorexia and weight loss in *M. mulatta*; and transient anorexia in *M. fasicularis*. In studies longer than 2 weeks, neutralizing antibodies developed in rabbits, guinea pigs, and *M. fasicularis* (182). These results were expected, and may have affected the signs of toxicity. Reproductive studies carried out in *M. mulatta* indicated that a dose-dependent increase in abortion was related to the administration of IFN-α_{2a}.

Table 6.11
Acute toxicology studies conducted with Interferon-α_{2a}

Species	Route[a]	Dose (units × 10^6/kg)	Clinical Multiple[b]
Mouse	iv	30, 250	≤83×
	im	30, 500	≤167×
	sc	30	10×
Rat	iv and im	30, 100	≤33×
	sc	30	10×
Rabbit	iv and im	100	33×
Ferret	im and sc	30	10×

[a] iv = intravenous; im = intramuscular; sc = subcutaneous
[b] Recommended clinical dose = 3 × 10^6 units/kg im or sc, there times weekly.

Table 6.12
Multiple dose toxicology studies conducted with Interferon-α_{2a}

Species	Route[a]	Duration (weeks)	Dose (units × 10^6/kg)	Clinical Multiple[b] (per week)
Mouse	im	5	0, 1.4, 2.8, 5.7	≤4×
Rat	im and iv	5	0, 1, 10, 100	≤78×
Rat	im	26	0, 7.5, 15, 30	≤23×
S. sciureus	im	2	0, 2.5	2×
M. mulatta	im	4	0, 2.5, 10, 25	≤19×
M. fasicularis	im	13	0, 2, 10	≤3×

[a] im = intramuscular; iv = intravenous
[b] Recommended clinical dose = 3 × 10^6 units/kg three times weekly (9 × 10^6 units/kg/week)

Insulin

The nonclinical toxicity of biosynthetic human insulin (BHI) (Figure 6.11) was evaluated in an unconventional way. The use of graded increments of dose representing multiples of the projected clinical exposure was not feasible due to the pharmacological effect of hypoglycemia caused by the insulin molecule. Since the pharmacological effects of insulin were well known, a primary goal of the toxicology evaluations was to determine whether BHI contained potentially toxic contaminants/impurities (i.e., *E. coli* proteins, endotoxins, etc.) that are introduced as a result of the synthetic process. Toxicology studies on BHI were conducted simultaneously with purified porcine pancreatic insulin (PPI) as a positive control, at doses previously established to produce hypoglycemia but not mortality. The doses selected for toxicology studies were varied according to species sensitivity, route of administration, and duration of treatment. In acute, single-dose toxicity studies (Table 6.13), the minimal lethal dose of BHI to rats and mice was >10 units/kg sc. Dogs given single doses of two units BHI/kg sc, showed the expected hypoglycemia but no toxicity. No toxic effects were seen in either rats or dogs given BHI sc or iv for one month (Table 6.14). Chronic toxicity, reproductive toxicity, and carcinogenicity studies were not conducted due to the extensive clinical experience with insulin, and the extensive chemical analysis of the NBE, establishing its identical nature with natural human insulin. BHI was negative in a genetic toxicology screen composed of bacterial mutation, DNA repair, and sister chromatid exchange evaluations. BHI was also not pyrogenic. Overall, BHI did not induce any effects different from those induced by PPI, and all effects seen were extensions of known insulin pharmacology. Investigations demonstrating the virtual absence of endogenous *E. coli* proteins, and the absence of antigenic response in rats

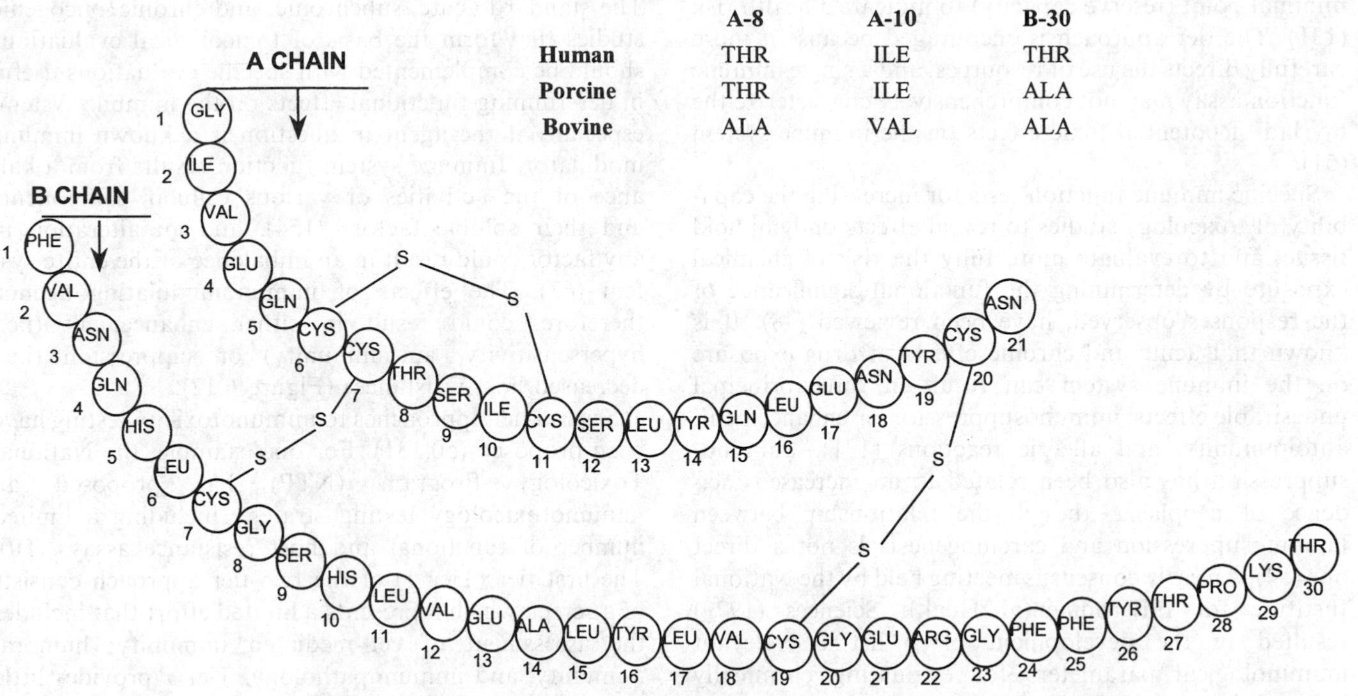

FIG. 6.11. Sequence of biosynthetic human insulin (BHI).

Table 6.13

Acute toxicology studies conducted with biosynthetic human insulin

Species	Route[a]	Dose (units/kg)	Clinical Multiple[b]
Mouse	sc	10	40×
Rat	sc	10	40×
Dog	sc	2	8×
Monkey	iv	0.1	—

[a] sc = subcutaneous; iv = intravenous
[b] Anticipated clinical dose = 0.24 units/kg/day, sc.

Table 6.14

Multiple dose toxicology studies conducted with biosynthetic human insulin

Species	Route[a]	Duration (weeks)	Dose (units/kg)	Clinical Multiple[b]
Rat	sc	4	2.4	10 ×
Dog	sc	4	2.0	8 ×
Dog	iv	4	0.1	—

[a] sc = subcutaneous; iv = intravenous
[b] Anticipated clinical dose = 0.24 units/kg/day, sc.

and guinea pigs sensitized with *E. coli* polypeptides, further addressed the safety of the rDNA-derived human insulin product.

Special Issues

Immunotoxicology

Immunotoxicology can be defined as the discipline concerned with the study of adverse effects on the immune system as a result of exposure to xenobiotics (51). It is not the purpose of this section to review in detail the specific evaluations conducted to define immunotoxicity (48,51,179,201), but, rather, to discuss the use of these evaluations in a hazard assessment tier approach. Adverse responses of the immune system are known to occur secondary to malnutrition, radiation exposure, neonatal thymectomy, and exposure to certain drugs and chemicals (54,186). Historically, few chemicals have been shown to be immunosuppressive in toxicology evaluations, probably because the lymphoid organs and the immune system, in general, have been poorly examined. It would be desirable, therefore, to establish an effective tier approach to detect immunotoxicity in standard subchronic and chronic toxicology studies, and also to evaluate the functional nature of the changes observed as a result of drug exposure. It is presumed that a functional change detected in the immune system is predictive of adverse health effects (201). It must be remembered that a critical function must be depressed beyond a defined, minimal point (reserve capacity) to indicate a health risk (131). The tier approach is encouraged because it more carefully directs the use of resources, and a single immune function assay may not comprehensively characterize the myriad of potential toxic effects on the immune system (51).

Specific immune function tests for increasing the capability of toxicology studies to reveal effects on lymphoid tissue, and to evaluate more fully the risk of chemical exposure by determining the functional significance of the responses observed, have been reviewed (48). It is known that acute and chronic effects of drug exposure on the immune system can result in three principal undesirable effects: immunosuppression or enhancement, autoimmunity, and allergic reactions (131). Immunosuppression has also been related to an increased incidence of neoplasia, though the relationship between immunosuppression and carcinogenesis is not a direct one (54). An early consensus meeting held by the National Institute for Environmental Health Sciences (1979) resulted in the development of a list of relevant immunological parameters for evaluating chemically induced immunotoxicity. This immunology screening panel has been reviewed (48), and includes: pathotoxicology, hematology, host resistance, radiometric delayed hypersensitivity, lymphoproliferation, humoral immunity, and evaluation of bone marrow progenitor cells.

Some of the first guidelines for immunotoxicology testing were those developed by the EU in the late 1970s. The focus of these guidelines was to evaluate the potential risk of chemical exposure by evaluating the functional significance of any histopathological or hematological effects seen on lymphoid organs in routine toxicity studies (141). The intention was to pursue the significance of these effects with specific function tests as necessary. It is known that immunotoxicity following drug exposure may take the form of changes in lymphoid tissue organ weights or histology, or changes in bone marrow or peripheral leukocytes (51). Norbury (141), however, pointed out that the evaluation of drug effects on the immune system is related to immune responsiveness, and is not simply a single point examination of lymphoid tissue using histopathology and hematology. Histopathological changes are generally not believed to be sensitive indicators of drug-induced immunotoxicity, are seen only at fairly high dose levels, and do not necessarily equate with functional immune alterations (51,141,201). The route and time of exposure relative to the maturational development of the immune system are important considerations in designing an immunotoxicity protocol (25,49).

The application of nonspecific immunotherapy for bacterial and viral diseases has led to an increased level of importance in the determination of immunotoxic effects. The standard acute, subchronic, and chronic/oncogenic studies that form the basis of toxicological evaluations should be complemented with specific evaluations useful in determining functional effects on the immune system, especially if the agent in question is a known immune modulator. Immune system function results from a balance of the activities of various cellular components and their soluble factors (154), and an alteration in any factor could result in an imbalance of the entire system (63). The effects of immunomodulating agents, therefore, could result in either enhancement (i.e., hypersensitivity, autoimmunity) or suppression (i.e., decreased host resistance) (Figure 6.12).

Several tier approaches to immunotoxicity testing have been proposed (50,131). For one example, the National Toxicology Program (NTP) has proposed an immunotoxicology testing strategy including a limited number of functional and host resistance assays (50). The first tier (Tier 1) of the two-tier approach consists of a screen which represents a limited effort that includes the assessment of cell-mediated immunity, humoral immunity, and immunopathology. Tier 1 provides little information on the specificity of an observed immune defect, or its relevance to the host; however, it can detect an immune alteration resulting from drug exposure (131). Tier 2 represents an in-depth evaluation, initiated only if functional changes are seen in Tier 1 at otherwise nontoxic doses (131). The in-depth immune function and host resistance evaluations provide information on the mechanism(s) of the immunotoxicity and aid risk assessment. Luster et al. (131) have reported that no compound evaluated to date has been found to produce an effect in Tier 2 without demonstrating some effect in Tier 1. The NTP procedure for detection of immune alterations following chemical or drug exposure in rodents is shown in Table 6.15. The concept of performing func-

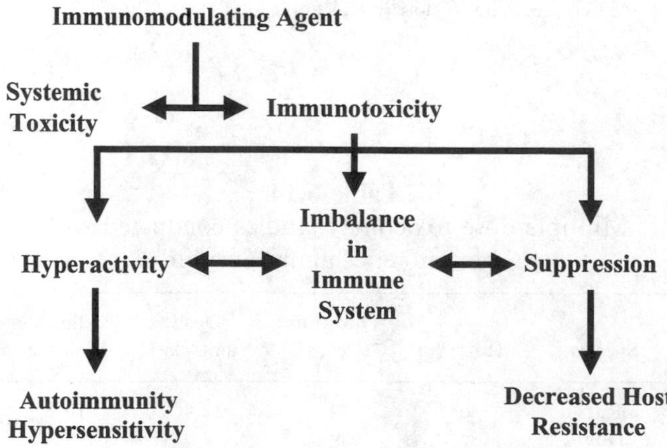

FIG. 6.12. Potential toxic responses of immunomodulating agents. Redrawn, with permission, from Reference 63.

Table 6.15
NTP immunotoxicology procedure[a]

Tier 1		Tier 2	
Immunopathology	Hematology (complete and differential blood count)	Immunopathology	Quantitation of Splenic B and T Cells
	Organ Weights (spleen, thymus, kidney, liver)	Humoral-Mediated Immunity	IgG response to sheep RBCs
	Body Weight	Cell-Mediated Immunity	Delayed Hypersensitivity
	Cellularity (spleen)	Nonspecific Immunity	Macrophage Function
	Histology (spleen, thymus, lymph node)	Host Resistance	Syngenic Tumor Cells (tumor incidence)
Humoral-Mediated Immunity	Plaque-Forming Cells		Listeria monocytogenes (mortality)
Cell-Mediated Immunity	Lymphocyte Blastogenesis to Mitogens		Influenza (mortality)
Nonspecific Immunity	Natural Killer Cell Activity		*Plasmodium yoelii* (parasitemia)

[a] From Reference 131.

tional tests is critical to defining potential mechanisms of the toxic response and their applicability to humans. An international collaborative effort has focused on the evaluation of limited pathology or enhanced pathology evaluations to better understand potential immunotoxicity (176). The enhanced pathology approach—for example, weight determination, examination of additional lymphoid organs, and grading of changes in the principal compartments of lymphoid tissue—was determined to provide an advantage in revealing effects on the immune system.

The direction for pharmaceutical development is to include tests of potential immune system involvement in the traditional toxicological evaluations for subchronic and chronic toxicity. Due to the sensitivity of the immune system to toxicants that could adversely affect the critical balance of the various immune factors, and the adverse health effects that could ensue, it is extremely important to define any potential interaction of a new drug and immune system function (201).

As can be anticipated from the previous discussion, immunogenicity is a major scientific issue relative to the development of biotechnology products. Concern has been raised over the comparison of the recombinant protein and the naturally occurring protein, since animal models are thought to be inadequate to assess the chemically subtle, but potentially immunologically significant, differences in the human response to these molecules. It has been assumed that a recombinant protein, designed for human use, would produce a number of adverse effects, including the production of neutralizing antibodies, in experimental animals. It has now become clear, through chronic exposures in nonclinical studies, that some small molecular weight human proteins are not immunogenic in animals, or are only weakly so. They have also been observed not to produce neutralizing antibodies. In the case where antibodies to human proteins have been detected in nonclinical studies, they do not necessarily cause expected immunopathology or neutralization activity. The rhesus monkey has been shown to predict the relative immunogenicity of several recombinant proteins in humans (216), and may serve as a good model. A further question is, Should all recombinant DNA products be routinely screened in animals prior to their introduction into humans? The major reason for conducting immunotoxicity evaluations in experimental animals is to detect those compounds which could induce anaphylaxis or anaphylactoid reactions in humans (193). New molecules, previously minimally tested in animals, such as enkephalins, would have a greater potential risk than well-known molecules, such as insulin. An approach to testing recombinant proteins, as well as NCEs, for immunogenicity/antigenicity has been suggested based on the extent of the clinical database and the existing regulatory requirements (Figure 6.13). Although studies in animals seem well justified for poorly characterized chemicals, it remains an open question whether or not regulatory agencies will accept an existing extensive clinical database as justification for not performing immunogenicity evaluations. Again, the chemical characterization of the recombinant product relative to

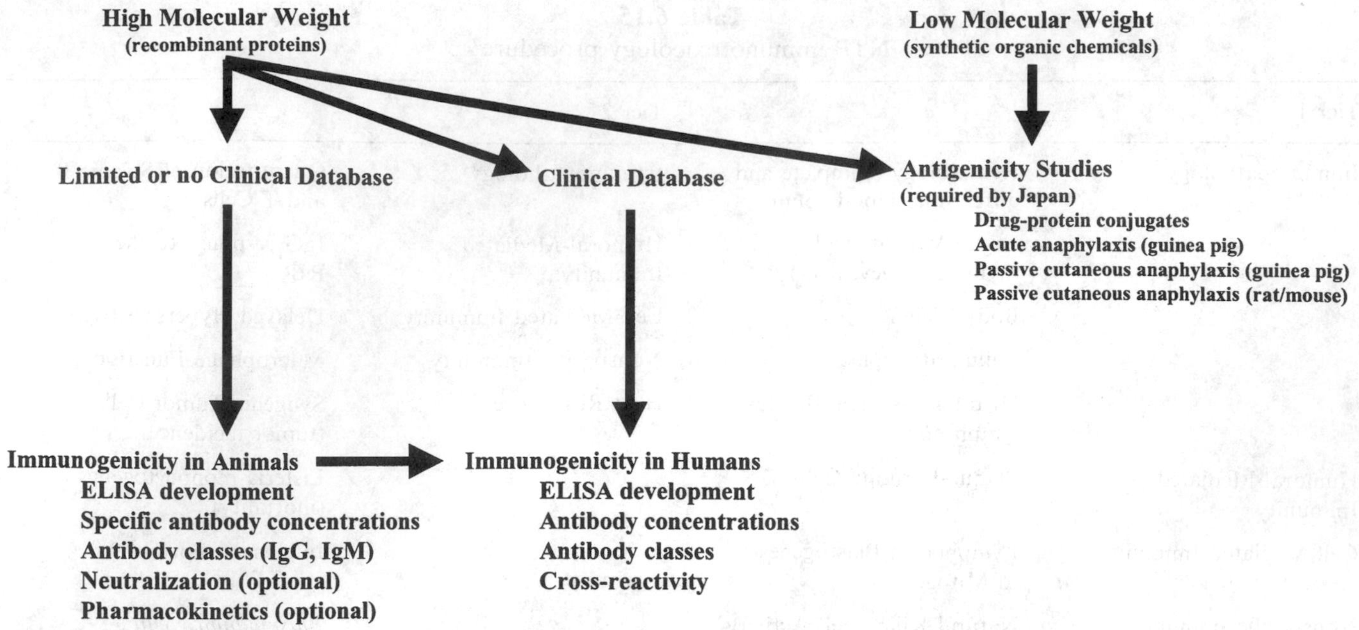

FIG. 6.13. Proposed approach for addressing immunogenicity and antigenicity issues with established and novel biotechnology products and NCEs. From Reference 193.

the natural material will have some bearing on this debate.

Genetic Toxicology

Genotoxicity has been defined as the ability of either a chemical or physical agent to damage DNA, resulting in a mutation (29). An important element of toxicology is the early identification of potentially hazardous substances. Since the actions of toxins are ultimately exerted at the cellular level, isolated cell systems represent an important model for identifying toxic effects. In vitro assays allow a greater control over xenobiotic metabolism (i.e., addition of enzymes or inhibitors), and facilitate mechanistic studies that could not be performed in vivo (113). In vitro tests generally provide a reasonable approximation of the potential for an agent to have an effect on genetic material; in vivo procedures provide a better test for the potential for genetic alterations to occur in the intact organism (119). The short-term in vitro tests for genotoxicity, potentially predictive of in vivo carcinogenicity, are among the most important techniques available for the rapid determination of potential severe undesirable effects of compounds selected for development. They are also useful in the prioritization of compounds to be studied in the more extended and expensive in vivo toxicology studies.

A number of assays are available to evaluate the potential for genotoxicity. The majority opinion is in favor of a battery approach to identify potential genotoxic activity since different assays assess different types of genetic damage (116,158). The ICH has published a guideline on how to conduct genotoxicity tests, and a guideline on the recommended standard genotoxicity testing battery for evaluations of pharmaceuticals (105,106). The ICH test battery includes:

1. gene mutation in bacteria: detect relevant genetic changes and the majority of genotoxic rodent carcinogens.
2. in vitro mammalian cell chromosomal aberration, or in vitro mouse lymphoma tk assay: detect either gross chromosomal damage or detection of gene mutation and clastogenic effects.
3. In vivo chromosomal damage in rodent hematopoietic cells: allows evaluation of additional relevant factors, for example, absorption, distribution, metabolism, and excretion.

This battery may be expanded when appropriate, such as when compounds with structural alerts are negative in the three standard tests (106).

Excellent reviews of methods to study genotoxic potential, and issues concerning nongenotoxic, yet carcinogenic, chemicals are available (17,18,194,195). In vivo exposure assays have the advantage of an intact metabolic system to effectively assay those compounds which must be activated (metabolized to a reactive entity) to achieve an effect. The in vitro assays may be conducted with or without the addition of a postmitochondrial supernatant from livers of rats treated with polychlorinated biphenyls to maximally induce drug metabolizing enzyme activities, and, thus, enhance the detection of indirect-acting agents.

In vitro genotoxicity assays are often used in the early drug discovery process aimed at selecting drug candidates for further development. The definitive in vitro genotoxicity evaluations of mutation and chromosomal damage are generally submitted prior to FHD. The complete battery of recommended tests should be submitted prior to Phase II clinical development.

The conduct of genotoxicity screens on NBEs has been an area of much discussion. The ICH has recognized that the standard genotoxicity testing battery may not be applicable to NBEs (111). Despite this, many pharmaceutical companies conduct genotoxicity evaluations on NBEs primarily to evaluate process impurities, to meet perceived regulatory expectations, or to meet specific regulatory agency requests (94).

Safety Pharmacology

Safety pharmacology involves establishing the pharmacological profile of new drug candidates by evaluating the pharmacodynamics related to the therapeutic indication and by evaluating the pharmacodynamics on other organ systems not related to the therapeutic indication (37). These studies are usually conducted at doses well below those used to establish the toxicology profile. It is not necessary, or even desirable, to produce frank toxicity to establish a valid pharmacological profile.

Pharmacological profiling was initially focused on guiding the synthetic chemist in the discovery of new pharmacologically active chemicals, rather than on the detection of adverse drug effects in humans (204). In reviewing the common adverse drug findings in humans, Zbinden (204) pointed out that some responses are easily detected in both humans and experimental animals, including sedation, anorexia, body weight changes, tremor, and tachycardia; and some responses are only detectable in humans, such as tinnitus, vertigo, nausea, and headache. In any event, when one considers the nature of the functional disturbances encountered in both nonclinical and clinical testing, it becomes evident that pharmacological profiling is critical to the safety evaluation of potential therapeutic agents (196,197). Every chemical that enters the body has the potential for creating effects that may or may not be related to its pharmacological activity. Antihistamines, for example, produce sedation, related to their pharmacological effects, and anticholinergic responses, which are not (196). Pharmacological profiling can help identify the potential incidence of effects unrelated to the known pharmacological activity.

The Japanese Ministry of Health and Welfare (MHW) has published Guidelines for General Pharmacology Studies (60). These studies are designed to characterize effects and potency, and to determine mechanism. The guidelines include studies to determine effects on: general activity and behavior; the CNS; autonomic nervous system and smooth muscle; respiratory and cardiovascular systems; gastrointestinal tract; and, renal excretion.

A proposal has been made to the ICH for establishment of an EWG to harmonize the safety pharmacology requirements for submission in the EU, United States, and Japan. The EU and Japan have completed similar draft guidelines for safety pharmacology (37). The proposed approach is based on a flexible strategy, including a basic evaluation and a complementary evaluation of safety pharmacology parameters. It has been suggested that the basic evaluation include:

1. Central nervous system: behavioral changes, motor activity, reflex responses, and cardiovascular potential.
2. Cardiovascular system: heart rate, ECG, contraction force, resistance, flow rate, and blood pressure.
3. Respiratory system: frequency, tidal volume, resistance, blood gases.

The following have been proposed for the complementary evaluation:

4. Renal system: volume, pH, fluid/electrolyte balance, protein, and glomerular filtration rate.
5. Immune system.
6. Gastrointestinal system: gastric secretion (pH), ulcerogenic potential, and gastrointestinal transit time.

In addition, the EU Committee for Proprietary Medicinal Products (CPMP) has introduced a guideline to address the potential for QT-interval prolongation by non-cardiovascular medicinal products (36).

Measure of Exposure

The relationship of administered dose to toxicological response is not always a simple correlation. Traditionally, the administered dose (mg/kg) has been the most commonly used expression to compare toxicological responses between species. The value of the administered dose term as the most appropriate comparator with toxicological response, however, has been questioned in scientific and regulatory circles. It is becoming increasingly well recognized that both beneficial and toxic effects of therapeutic agents are dependent on the quantity of material reaching the target site (134,211,179).

Knowledge of the magnitude of drug exposure is necessary in substantiating efficacy and drug safety evaluations. Furthermore, exposure data have provided important information relative to the interpretation of unanticipated toxicity (143). Toxicologists, therefore, must make an effort to monitor concentrations of parent compound and/or major active metabolites in the blood and, when possible, the tissues. Measurement of plasma concentrations in toxicology studies provides much

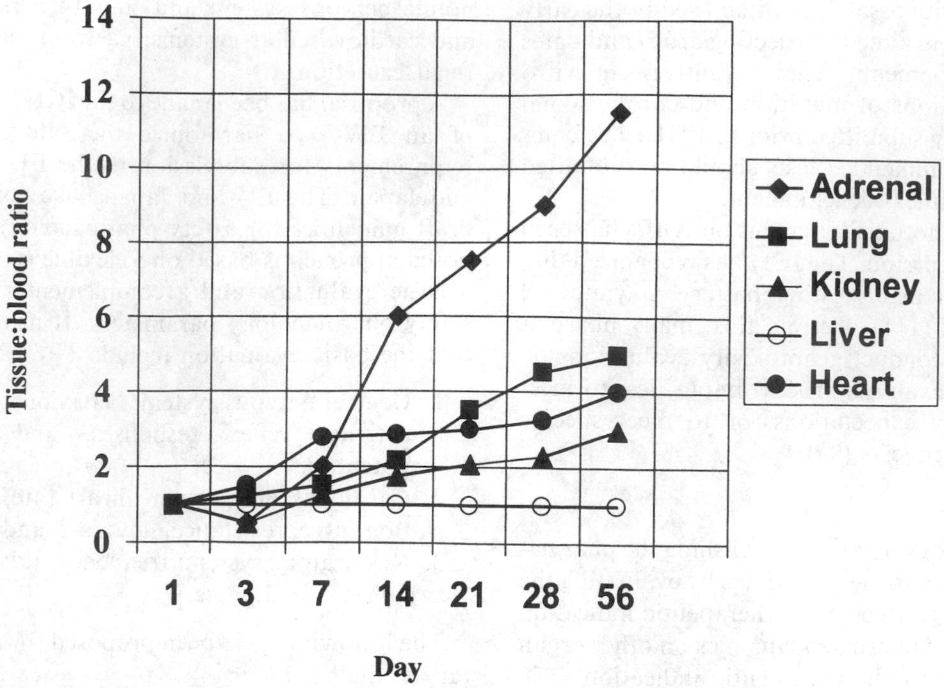

FIG. 6.14. Tissue to blood ratio, over time, in various tissues following single daily doses of chlorphentermine. Redrawn with permission from Reference 126.

needed proof of absorption and exposure. It also, provides a more appropriate dose comparator than administered dose when responses between species are being evaluated. For example, because of differences in metabolism, bioavailability, and so on, rats may have much lower exposure (plasma level) for a given administered (mg/kg) dose than humans receiving the same administered dose. Therefore, the use of multiples of the administered human dose on a mg/kg basis in the experimental animal species may result in an actual exposure that is unpredictable, and differs substantially (either greater or less), from that achieved in patients. The potential of expressing toxicity that is poorly correlated with exposure to a clinical dose, therefore, increases. Setting clinical dose multiples for toxicology studies on the basis of exposure is much more appropriate. Measures of exposure are also useful in establishing nonlinearity in kinetics, which, as described above, is important in explaining toxic responses seen in particular species (134). It seems more rational to establish an upper dose in toxicology studies based on linearity of kinetics rather than at the MTD, since it is often the case that the MTD falls in the range of nonlinear kinetics, saturating normal metabolic processes. Thus, an animal treated at the MTD may be exposed to much higher levels of parent drug, or toxic metabolite(s), than would be observed at meaningful multiples of the clinical dose.

The relationship of administered dose to delivered dose remains a central issue in the interpretation of toxicology data. The measurement of plasma concentrations of parent compound and metabolites represents a partial resolution of this problem. There are limitations, however, in using plasma concentration as a relevant measure of exposure for those compounds that are tissue-sequestered (135). Although many therapeutic agents achieve tissue levels proportional to plasma concentration, some continue to accumulate in tissue with continued dosing (77). In studies of phentermine and chlorphentermine, it was found that the blood to tissue ratios of phentermine remained constant over the entire period of treatment, while those for chlorphentermine significantly increased with time in most of the tissues studied (Figure 6.14) (126). In addition to becoming tightly bound to tissue, chlorphentermine also induced new binding sites during treatment. The difference in behavior between the two closely related chemicals was related to the increased amphiphilic nature of chlorphentermine (126).

Extrapolation of toxicological test results across species is based on the assumption that mammalian species will respond to toxicants in a similar fashion. The convention in toxicology has been to express dose on the basis of mg/kg body weight. Whether body weight is the most appropriate scaling factor for toxicity data has been the subject of much discussion. It had been previously observed that the toxicity of a variety of anticancer drugs was best predicted across species if the dose was expressed on the basis of body surface area rather than body weight (76). Others, however, have

Table 6.16
Dose by weight and surface area (1 mg/kg)[a]

Species	Body Weight (g)	Surface Area (cm^2)	Total Dose (mg/animal)	Administered Dose (mg/cm^2)	Multiple of Human Dose
Mouse	20	45	.02	.00044	0.10
Rat	200	325	.20	.00061	0.16
Monkey	4000	2980	4.00	.00134	0.34
Dog	12000	5770	12.00	.00207	0.53
Human	70000	18000	70.00	.00389	1.00

[a] From References 23, 118.

reported that although heat loss appears to be related to body surface area, basal metabolic rate, an important aspect of toxicity evaluation, is more closely related to body weight (82). The use of surface area for the purpose of dose extrapolation is a more conservative approach than the use of body weight (21,21,82,118) (Table 6.16). Assuming that the average adult mouse (0.02 kg) and the normal adult human (70 kg), are given the same administered dose on a body weight basis, the adult human will receive 3500 times the total dose received by the mouse. The same dose, given on a body surface area basis to mice and men, would represent only a 400-fold difference. Although there is support for using surface area as the most appropriate dose extrapolation factor, there is an increasing body of data that suggest the use of body weight to be the most accurate factor (1). Target organ specificity may be a deciding factor in the selection of the most appropriate allometric relationship (that is, antihypertensives vs. oncolytics). The appropriate scaling factor can probably only be determined on a case-by-case basis using data from a variety of species.

Clinical Trials in Pediatric Populations

The FDA has found that most products indicated for treatment of diseases that occur in both adults and children have little clinical trial support for pediatric use. As a result, a new regulation requiring pediatric studies for certain NCEs and NBEs has been proposed (67). The EU Committee for Proprietary Medicinal Products (CPMP) has also concluded that specific age-dependent differences in pharmacokinetics, pharmacodynamics, growth process and development, and specific pathology require that therapeutic agents be tested in the target age group (35). The ICH has recommended that pediatric clinical trials be supported by repeated dose toxicity studies of an appropriate duration, all developmental toxicity studies, and the full battery of genotoxicity tests. These studies should be concluded before the pediatric clinical trials begin (102). Due to the potentially long duration of treatment, carcinogenicity studies must be considered prior to the initiation of long-term pediatric clinical trials. The performance of nonclinical studies in juvenile animals may also be necessary if previous toxicology evaluations and human safety data are not sufficient or raise a cause for concern.

Nonclinical Evaluation of Anticancer Drugs

The development of drugs for life-threatening diseases, such as cancer and AIDS, requires a modification of the approach established for the safe development of NCEs or NBEs (see above). The treatment of cancer usually includes the use of potent agents designed to halt cell replication. The therapeutic index for these agents is often small. Due to the life-threatening nature of the disease, a greater risk of drug toxicity and a shorter nonclinical testing strategy is generally accepted for therapeutic agents in this class, since serious drug effects are often less threatening than the targeted disease. However, due to the greater intrinsic toxicity of the agents in this class, the early clinical trials are often conducted in patients rather than normal volunteers, as with other therapeutic agents.

The history of anticancer drug development has been extensively reviewed (92,53,180). The basic approach for development of anticancer drugs includes:

1. Establishment of a safe clinical trial entry dose.
2. Determination of potential dose limiting target organ toxicity.
3. Evaluation of reversibility of effects.
4. Determination of MTD in animals.
5. Determination of dose schedule toxicity.

The use of nonclinical studies has been successful in accurate predictions of the MTD in humans and a safe starting dose for clinical trials (92).

The CPMP has provided a specific note for guidance on the nonclinical evaluation of anticancer agents (38). Safety pharmacology is generally required prior to Phase I studies, as are the determination of C_{max} (maximum plasma concentration of the drug) and AUC at the animal MTD. Other kinetic parameters are expected to be determined prior to Phase II/III testing. Determination of the single-dose MTD in rodents and the approximate MTD in nonrodents, using a relevant route of exposure, is also expected prior to Phase I. Repeated-dose toxicity studies in two rodent species are expected prior to Phase I clinical studies. Longer-term repeat-dose studies, in a rodent and nonrodent species, equal in duration to the clinical trial but <6 months, are expected prior to Phase II/III. Genotoxicity testing is not necessary prior to Phase I/II, but the genotoxicity battery is expected to be conducted prior to Phase II/III. Since cytotoxic anticancer agents are known to have an adverse effect on reproduction, developmental toxicity studies are not required but are encouraged.

The development of anticancer drugs and other therapies for life-threatening diseases has unique characteristics based on the life-threatening nature of the disease and the inherent toxicity of the therapeutic agents.

Alternative Methods for Carcinogenicity Determination

The testing for carcinogenic potential has relied primarily on the rodent bioassay. Recently, through the ICH process, the rat has been identified as either the most acceptable or most relevant model for the two-year bioassay. In addition to the rat bioassay, an alternative short-term method of carcinogenicity evaluation is recommended (ICH S1b). These approaches may include studies in transgenic mice—for example, $p53^{+/-}$ heterozygous gene deficient mouse or Tg/AC mouse—or use of a neonatal rodent tumorigenicity model.

To evaluate and verify the available alternative models, the International Life Sciences Institute (ILSI) has initiated a collaborative effort among industry, academic, and government laboratories to study chosen chemicals in the alternative models and evaluate the results in light of the known bioassay data. Currently, there is insufficient information to guide us in the choice of suitable alternative models for carcinogenicity evaluation.

Once validated, the proposed transgenic animal models may be used as follows (33):

1. To confirm results in equivocal 2-year rodent bioassays.
2. To set priorities for 2-year carcinogenicity bioassays.
3. As an alternative to the mouse 2-year bioassay, in conjunction with the rat 2-year bioassay.
4. To assess carcinogenic potential of new genotoxic contaminants/degredants in a drug product after 2-year bioassays are completed.

In addition, the use of transgenic animals may support weight-of-evidence decisions, is relatively short-term, and is generally less expensive than the 2-year rodent bioassay.

Several transgenic mouse models are available to complement the rat 2-year bioassay. The Tg/AC mouse and the $p53^{+/-}$ heterozygous-gene-deficient mouse are taken as examples. It must be remembered that these models are not fully validated.

The Tg/AC mouse model (175) presents an animal model of initiated skin as a target for tumorigenesis. The Tg/AC line may be able to differentiate carcinogens from noncarcinogens, but may not be able to differentiate genotoxic carcinogens from those that cause only tumor promotion activity. This model may only be useful in combination with other transgenic animal models (159).

The $p53^{+/-}$ heterozygous-gene-deficient mouse model is based on rendering mice heterozygous for the p53 tumor suppressor gene (84). These animals are at elevated risk for tumor development. The model has been proposed to best approximate humans at risk for heritable forms of cancer. This model may be able to detect genotoxic carcinogens in a 6-month period.

The neonatal mouse assay has been available longer than the transgenic animal models. The detailed protocol for this 1-year study has been reviewed previously (73). Neonates are treated with the test compound on days 8 and 15 of age, and then observed to 1 year of age. At that time the animals are evaluated for tumor production. This assay is sensitive to direct-acting carcinogens, primarily those that work through formation of covalently bound DNA adducts.

The assessment of carcinogenicity in the drug development process is at a crossroad. The rodent bioassay has been used for over 25 years, and has provided useful data, although it is not a perfect system and is one that has received much criticism. The investigation of alternatives to the standard bioassay in two rodent species has been encouraged by ICH. Conducting a 2-year study in the rat, and an alternative study in the mouse, may provide an acceptable transition. There is, however, much work to be done before the alternative models are validated and fully useful in carcinogenicity risk assessments. The alternative assays are relative newcomers, full of promise but short on experience. There should not be undue enthusiasm about their ability to dramatically improve our carcinogenicity risk assessment process.

Development of Stereoisomeric Drugs

The development of individual enantiomers and racemates requires specific considerations and interactions with regulatory agencies, especially the FDA. In 1992, the FDA, developed a specific policy statement to deal with development of enantiomers and racemates (70). It is recognized that the properties of enantiomers may be similar and desirable. For example, both enantiomers of dobutamine have positive inotropic properties. It may also occur that the isomers may have desirable but different properties, for example, the d-isomer of propoxyphene is an analgesic, the s-isomer is an antitussive. It is also recognized that toxicity may be linked to one member of a stereoisomeric pair, for example, granulocytopenia is ascribed to the d-isomer of the antiparkinsonian drug levodopa.

The FDA position is that the establishment of a relatively benign nonclinical toxicological profile for the racemate should support the clinical development of the enantiomer without a separate toxicological evaluation. Since the FDA policy statement (1992) leaves some room for interpretation of "benign toxicology profile," it is highly advisable to engage in a conversation with the agency before proceeding with development.

The FDA makes specific recommendations for pharmacokinetic and toxicology profiles. The potential for interconversion of the isomers must be monitored in nonclinical studies and compared to the clinical profile. It is sufficient to carry out toxicity studies with the racemate unless toxicity unrelated to the pharmacology of the drug occurs at relatively low multiples of the clinical exposure. In that case, the drug developer should investigate the individual enantiomers to examine whether the pharmacological and toxicological effects can be segregated.

The development of a single stereoisomer after the racemate had been evaluated in nonclinical studies requires abbreviated toxicology studies:

1. 3-month toxicology studies of the single enantiomer in rodent and nonrodent species.
2. Segment II (teratology) developmental toxicology study of the single enantiomer in the most sensitive species.
3. A positive control group consisting of the racemate.

If there are no differences between the toxicological profile of the single enantiomer and the racemate, no further toxicology studies would be needed.

CONCLUSION

The next decade promises to be another exciting one for the industrial toxicologist. The physician and patient continue to demand more efficacious and safer medications more quickly. Basic research efforts in biochemistry, physiology, and pharmacology have allowed the more precise characterization of receptors, and the normal and perturbed sequelae of receptor binding, which continues to stimulate the development of more specific, potent modulators of cellular functions. The etiologies of human diseases are becoming better understood, thanks to the technological ability to elucidate their characteristics at the molecular level. This has resulted in the potential to therapeutically modify the disease process at its origin—the human genome. These molecular approaches have already resulted in the development of agents that are highly species-specific, and the use of these techniques to elucidate normal and pathological cellular function will only continue to escalate. It is unlikely that the classical tools of toxicology will be adequate to ensure the human safety of the highly specific potential therapeutics forthcoming from these sophisticated technologies. The development of NBEs has already challenged the established norms of safety assessment.

Consider the example of an agent that has shown selectivity for modifying the activity of a human-specific enzyme critical to a pathological process. Although traditional animal studies are likely to be predictive of toxicity that is unrelated to the pharmacology of the compound, they will not be useful for the prediction of adverse findings relative to the action of the drug at the enzyme which will occur only in humans. Thus, not only may data generated from classical animal studies be inadequate to predict toxic responses in humans, but the information may be irrelevant or misleading. A major concern is whether modification of this enzyme activity in the only responsive species, humans, might result in unanticipated, severe toxicity. How can this best be predicted prior to the initiation of clinical trials?

The future direction of discovery research suggests that industrial and regulatory toxicologists will need to collaborate more closely in the design of the toxicology studies to support registration, and ultimately, these may have to be considered on a case-by-case basis. Indeed, the current guidelines resulting from global harmonization efforts repeatedly emphasize the need for defending the scientific rationale supporting the design of proposed toxicological assessments. Although these guidelines are viewed as much more flexible than the country-specific regulations of the past, they also place a greater burden on toxicologists relative to defending the relevance of their studies. The era of "checking the tox box" has, thankfully, come to a close.

Another challenge on the horizon concerns the need to improve the efficiency of the drug development process without compromising its quality. Currently, the drug development and approval processes are taking longer, and costing more than ever before. More stringent regulatory requirements have resulted in the conduct of more studies (in both animals and humans), taking more time and costing more money. These costs are passed on to the patient, who ultimately must also compensate for the resultant decreased market life, due to patent length restrictions, of the registered product. Furthermore, the use of large numbers of experimental animals remains a concern from both the ethical and financial points of view. One approach to solving these dilemmas is to ensure that the toxicological studies conducted meet the needs of the regulatory agency, the physician, and, ultimately, the patient. As suggested earlier, this can be most efficiently accomplished by early and routine interactions between the industry and these customers, especially in cases where the agent under development represents a unique therapeutic approach.

Finally, the major role of the toxicologist as a mechanistic scientist will continue to be enhanced. For the reasons discussed above, the interpretation of toxicology data will become increasingly more sophisticated, requiring a broad knowledge base in a variety of other scientific disciplines. Elucidation of the mechanisms responsible for observed toxicities would improve the ability to achieve the traditional, ultimate purpose of the discipline of toxicology—the appropriate extrapolation of these data to humans. Achievement of this goal will surely become more challenging, but also more exciting, in the future.

ACKNOWLEDGMENTS

The authors gratefully acknowledge and appreciate the efforts of Ms. Arlene Adkins in the preparation of this document.

QUESTIONS

1. What are the major objectives of toxicity testing relative to the development of pharmaceuticals?
2. In what major ways would a toxicology submission package differ for a drug intended to be prescribed chronically (e.g., for essential hypertension) as opposed to one that will be used acutely (e.g., an antibiotic)?
3. In what situations would the conduct of oncogenicity studies most likely be encouraged? For NCEs? For NBEs?
4. Why is the use of the maximum tolerated dose (MTD) as the high dose in oncogenicity studies controversial?
5. What are the different phases of clinical testing and what is the purpose of each phase?
6. Why is exposure in animal models considered a better parameter than administered dose when extrapolating toxicity data to humans?
7. Under what conditions might a compound with significant animal toxicity be considered for regulatory approval?
8. What are some of the special considerations necessary in designing the toxicology package for NBEs?

REFERENCES

1. Allen, B. C., Crump, K. S., and Shipp, A. M. (1988): Correlation between carcinogenic potency of chemicals in animals and humans. *Risk Anal.*, 8:531–561.
2. Ames, B. N., and Gold, L. S. (1990): Too many rodent carcinogens: Mitogenesis increases mutagenesis. *Science*, 249:970–971.
3. Ankier, S. I., and Warrington, S. J. (1989): Research and development of new medicines. *J. Internat. Med. Res.*, 17:407–416.
4. Ashby, J. (1996): Alternatives to the 2-species bioassay for the identification of potential human carcinogens. *Human Exper. Toxicol.*, 15(3):183–202.
5. Audus, K. L., Bartel, R. L., Hidalgo, I. J., and Borchardt, R. T. (1990): The use of cultured epithelial and endothelial cells for drug transport and metabolism studies. *Pharm. Res.*, 7(5):435–451.
6. Ayers, K. M., Clive, D., Tucker, W. E., Jr., Hajian, G., and De Miranda, P. (1996): Nonclinical toxicology studies with zidovudine: Genetic toxicity tests and carcinogenicity bioassays in mice and rats. *Fundam. Appl. Toxicol.*, 32:148–158.
7. Ayers, K. M., Tucker, W. E., Jr., Hajian, G., and De Miranda, P. (1996): Nonclinical toxicology studies with zidovudine: Acute, subacute, and chronic toxicity in rodents, dogs, and monkeys. *Fundam. Appl. Toxicol.*, 32:129–139.
8. Baker, S. B. deC., and Davey, D. G. (1970): The predictive value for man of toxicological tests of drugs in laboratory animals. *Br. Med. Bull.*, 26(3):208–211.
9. Bass, R., and Scheibner, E. (1987): Toxicological evaluation of biotechnology products: A regulatory viewpoint. *Arch. Toxicol.*, (Suppl. 11):182–190.
10. Beret, L. Z. (1984): Pharmacokinetics: Basic principles and its use as a tool in drug metabolism. In: *Drug Metabolism and Drug Toxicity*, J. R. Mitchell, and M. G. Horning, pp. 199–211. Raven Press, New York.
11. Berlin, R. G. (1991): Omeprazole: Gastrin and gastric data (August 1991). *Digest. Dis. Sci.*, 36:1501–1502.
12. Berthou, F., Ratanasavanh, D., Riche, C., Picart, D., Voirin, T., and Guillouzo, A. (1989): Comparison of caffeine metabolism by slices, microsomes and hepatocyte cultures from adult human liver. *Xenobiotica*, 19(4):401–417.
13. Bocci, V. (1992): Physicochemical and biological properties of interferons and their potential uses in drug delivery systems. *Crit. Rev. Therapeut. Drug Carrier Syst.*, 9(2):91–133.
14. Boobis, A. R., and Davies, D. S. (1984): Human cytochromes P450. *Xenobiotica*, 14:151–185.
15. Brendel, K., Fisher, R. L., Krumdieck, C. L., and Gandolfi, A. J. (1990): Precision-cut rat liver slices in dynamic organ culture for structure–toxicity studies. *J. Am. Coll. Toxicol.*, 9(6):621–627.
16. Brent, R. L. (1980): The prediction of human diseases from laboratory and animal tests for teratogenicity, carcinogenicity, and mutagenicity. In: *Controversies in Therapeutics*, L. Lasagna, pp. 131–150. W. B. Saunders Co., Philadelphia.
17. Brusick, D. (1989): Genetic toxicology. In: *Principles and Methods of Toxicology*, 2nd ed., edited by A. W. Hayes, pp. 407–434. Raven Press, New York.
18. Butterworth, B. (1989): Nongenotoxic carcinogens in the regulatory environment. *Reg. Toxicol. Pharmacol.*, 9:244–256.
19. Butterworth, B. E., Goldsworthy, T. L., Popp, J. A., and McClellan, R. O. (1991): The rodent cancer test: An assay under siege. *CIIT Activities*, 11(9):1–6.
20. Cahn, J. (1983): Forecasting of cardiac side effects: Vincamine and calcium antagonists, a comparative study in animals and man. In: *Current Problems in Drug Toxicology*, edited by G. Zbinden, J. Y. Detaille, and G. Mazue, pp. 90–94. John Libbey Eurotext, London.
21. Calabrese, E. J., Beck, B. D., and Chappell, W. R. (1992): Does the animal-to-human uncertainty factor incorporate interspecies differences in surface area? *Reg. Toxicol. Pharmacol.*, 15:172–179.
22. Caldwell, J. (1981): The current status of attempts to predict species differences in drug metabolism. *Drug Metab. Rev.*, 12(2):221–237.

23. Campbell, D. B., and Ings, R. M. (1988): New approaches to the use of pharmacokinetics in toxicology and drug development. *Hum. Toxicol.*, 7:469–479.
24. Carlsson, E., Larsson, H., Mattson, H., Ryberg, B., and Sundell, G. (1986): Pharmacology and toxicology of omeprazole—with special reference to the effects on the gastric mucosa. *Scand. J. Gastroent.*, (Suppl. 118):31–38.
25. Chan, P. K., O'Hara, G. P., and Hayes, A. W. (1981): Principles and methods for acute and subchronic toxicity. In: *Principles and Methods of Toxicology*, edited by A. W. Hayes, pp. 1–51. Raven Press, New York.
26. Chance, R. E., Kroeff, E. P., and Hoffman, J. A. (1981): Chemical, physical and biological properties of recombinant human insulin. In: *Insulins, Growth Hormone, and Recombinant DNA Technology*. J. L. Gueriguian, pp. 71–84. Raven Press, New York.
27. Chenery, R. J., Ayrton, A., Oldham, H. G., Standring, P., Norman, S. J., Seddon, T., and Kirby, R. (1987): Diazepam metabolism in cultured hepatocytes from rat, rabbit, dog, guinea pig and man. *Drug Metab. Dispo.*, 15:312–318.
28. Chien, R. E., ed. (1979): *Issues in Pharmaceutical Economics*. Lexington Books, Lexington, Massachusetts.
29. Choy, W. N. (1996): Principles of genetic toxicology. *Drug Chem. Toxicol.*, 19(3):149–160.
30. Clark, B., and Smith, D. A. (1984): Pharmacokinetics and toxicity testing. *Crit. Res. Toxicol.*, 12(4):343–385.
31. Cluff, L. E. (1980): Is drug toxicity a problem of great magnitude? Yes! In: *Controversie in Therapeutics*, edited by L. Lasagna, pp. 44–50. W. B. Saunders Co., Philadelphia.
32. Cohen, S., and Ellwein, L. B. (1990): Cell proliferation in carcinogenesis. *Science*, 249:1007–1011.
33. Contrera, J. F. (1998): Transgenic animals: Refining the two-year rodent carcinogenicity study. *Lab. Animal*, 27(2):30–33.
34. Contrera, J. F., Jacobs, A. C. and DeGeorge, J. J. (1997): Carcinogenicity testing and the evaluation of regulatory requirements for pharmaceuticals. *Reg. Toxicol. Pharmacol.*, 25:130–145.
35. CPMP (1997): Note for guidance on clinical investigation of medicinal products in children. London, 17 March, CPMP/EWP/462/95.
36. CPMP (1997): Points to consider: The assessment of the potential for QT interval prolongation by non-cardiovascular medicinal products. London, 17 December, CPMP/986/96.
37. CPMP (1998): Note for guidance on safety pharmacology studies in medicinal product development (draft of preliminary consultation). CPMP/SWP/872/98.
38. CPMP (1998): Note for guidance on the preclinical evaluation of anticancer medicinal products. CPMP/SWP/997/96. London, 23 July.
39. Creutzfeldt, W., and Lamberts, R. (1991): Is hypergastrinaemia dangerous to man? *Scand. J. Gastroenterol.*, (Suppl. 180): 179–191.
40. D'Agnolo, G. (1983): The control of drugs obtained by recombinant DNA and other biotechnologies. In: *Current Problems in Drug Toxicology*, edited by G. Zbinden, J. Y. Detaille, and G. Mazue, John Libbey Eurotext (London), pp. 241–247.
41. D'Aguanno, W. (1973): Drug toxicity evaluation—Pre-clinical aspects. FDA Introduction to Total Drug Quality. DHEW Publication No. (FDA) 74-3006, pp. 35–40.
42. Dahlem, A. M., Allerheiligen, S. R., and Vodicnik, M. J. (1995). Concomitant toxicokinetics: Techniques for and interpretation of exposure data obtained during the conduct of toxicology studies. *Toxicol. Pathol.*, 23(2):170–178.
43. Davey, D. G. (1964): The study of the toxicity of a potential drug—basic principles. In: *Proceedings of the European Society for the Study of Drug Toxicity*, Vol. III, pp. 2–13. Excerptamedica Foundation, New York.
44. Dayan, A. D. (1981): The troubled toxicologist. *TIPS*, 2(11):1–4.
45. Dayan, A. D. (1986): Preclinical safety studies on genetically engineered medicine for man. *BIBRA J.*, 5(3):12–15.
46. Dayan, A. D. (1988): Risk assessment of biotechnology products. *Hum. Toxicol.*, 7(1):50–52.
47. De Schaepdryver, A. F. (1978): Toxicology: General and special toxicity testing: A situation paper. In: *The Scientific Basis of Official Regulation of Drug Research and Development: Proceedings of a Satellite Symposium of the 7th International Congress of Pharmacology* pp. 25–27. Heymans Foundation, Ghent, Belgium.
48. Dean, J. H., Cornacoff, J. B., Rosenthal, G. J., and Luster, M. I. (1989): Immune System: Evaluation of injury. In: *Principles and Methods of Toxicology*, 2nd ed., edited by A. W. Hayes, pp. 741–760. Raven Press, New York.
49. Dean, J. H., Luster, M. I., and Boorman, G. A. (1982): Methods and approaches for assessing immunotoxicity: An overview. *Environ. Health Perspect.*, 43:27–29.
50. Dean, J. H., Luster, M. I., Boorman, G. A., and Laver, L. D. (1982): Procedures available to examine the immunotoxicity of chemicals and drugs. *Pharmacol. Rev.*, 34:137–148.
51. Dean, J. H., and Vos, J. G. (1986): An introduction to immunotoxicology assessment. In: *Immunotoxicology of Drugs and Chemicals*, edited by J. Descotes, Elsevier Science, New York.
52. Dedrich, R., and Bischoff, K. B. (1980): Species similarities in pharmacokinetics. *Fed. Proc.*, 39:54–59.
53. DeGeorge, J. J., Ahn, C.-H., Andrews, P. A. Brower, M. E., Giorgio, D. W., Goheer, M. A., Lee-Han, D. Y., McGuinn, W. D., Schmidt, W., Sun, C. J., and Tripathi, S. C. (1998). Regulatory considerations for preclinical development of anticancer drugs. *Cancer Chemother. Pharmacol.*, 41:173–185.
54. Descotes, G., Mazue, G., and Richey, P. (1982): Drug immunotoxicological approaches with some selected medical products: Cyclophosphamide, methylprednisolone, betamethasone, cefoxitine, minor tranquillizers. *Toxicol. Lett.*, 13:129–138.
55. Diener, R. M. (1997): Safety assessment of pharmaceuticals. In: *Comprehensive Toxicology, Vol. 2, Toxicology Testing and Evaluation*, edited by I. G. Sipes, C. A. McQueen, and J. Gandolfi, pp. 269–290. Elsevier Science Ltd., New York.
56. Dieterle, W., and Faigle, J. W. (1981): Species differences in the disposition and metabolism of sulfinpyrazone. *Xenobiotica*, 11:559–568.
57. Dietz, F. K., Ramsey, J. C., and Watanabe, P. G. (1983). Relevance of experimental studies to human risk. *Environ. Health Perspect.*, 52:9–14.
58. DiMasi, J. A. (1994): Risks, regulation, rewards in new drug development in the United States. *Reg. Toxicol. Pharmacol.*, 19:228–235.
59. Dorato, M. A., and Buckley, L. A. (1998): Toxicology in the drug development process. In: *Current Protocols in Pharmacology*, edited by S. J. Enna, M. Williams, J. W., Ferkany, T. Kenakin, R. D. Porsolt and J. P. Sullivan, J. Wiley and Sons, New York.
60. Drug Registration Requirements in Japan, 4th ed. (1991). Yakuji Nippo Ltd., Tokyo, pp. 69–73.
61. Ekman, L., Hansson, E., Havu, N., Carlsson, E., and Lundberg, C. (1985): Toxicological studies on omeprazole. *Scand. J. Gastroent.*, (Suppl. 108):53–69.
62. Fabre, G., Combalbert, J., Berger, Y., and Cano, J.-P. (1990): Human hepatocyte as a key in vitro model to improve preclinical drug development. *Eur. J. Drug Metab. Pharmacokinetics*, 15(2):165–171.
63. Falchetti, R., Silvestri, S., Battaglia, A., and Caprino, L. (1983): Toxicological evaluation of immunomodulating drugs. In: *Current Problems in Drug Toxicology*, edited by G. Zbinden, J. Detaille, and G. Mazue, pp. 248–263. John Libbey Eurotext, London.

64. FDA (1987): Good laboratory practice for nonclinical laboratory studies. Final Rule, 21CFR58.
65. FDA (1993): Guideline for the study and evaluation of gender differences in the clinical evaluation of drugs. U.S. DHHS *Federal Register notice*, July 22, 58FR39406.
66. FDA (1997): Investigational new drug applications; proposed amendment to clinical hold regulations for products intended for life-threatening diseases. U.S. DHHS *Federal Register* notice. Sept 24, 62FR499446.
67. FDA (1997): Regulations requiring manufacturers to assess the safety and effectiveness of new drugs and biological products in pediatric patients. U.S. DHHS *Federal Register* notice, July 24, 21CFR201,312,314,601.
68. FDA Summary Basis of Approval for omeprazole. (1990).
69. FDA Summary Basis of Approval for zidovudine. (1989).
70. FDA (1992): FDA's Policy Statement for the Development of New Stereoisomeric Drugs. Corrections made Jan 3, 1997. http://www.fda.gov/cder/guidance/stereo.htm.
71. Fent, K., and Zbinden, G. (1987): Toxicity of interferon and interleukin. *TIPS*, 8:100–105.
72. Finter, N. B., Woodrouffe, J., and Priestman, T. J. (1982): Monkeys are insensitive to pyrogenic effects of human alpha-interferons. *Nature* (London), 298:301.
73. Flammang, J. J., VonTungeln, L. S., Kadlubar, F. F., and Fu, P. P. (1997): Neonatal mouse assay for tumorigenicity: Alternative to the chronic rodent bioassay. *Reg. Toxicol. Pharmacol.*, 26:230–240.
74. Fletcher, A. P. (1978): Drug safety tests and subsequent clinical experience. *J. Royal Soc. Med.*, 71:693–696.
75. Frazier, J. M., Tyson, C. A., McCarthy, C. McCormick, J. J., Meyer, D., Powis, G., and Ducat, L. (1989): Potential use of human tissues for toxicity research and testing. *Toxicol. Appl. Pharmacol.*, 97:387–397.
76. Freireich, E. J., Gehan, E. A., Rall, D. P. Schmidt, L. H., and Skipper, H. E. (1966): Quantitative comparison of toxicity of anticancer agents in mouse, rat, hamster, dog, monkey, and man. *Cancer Chemotherap.*, 50:219–244.
77. French Ministry of Social Affairs (1984): Recommendation concernant le protocole toxicologigue des interferons pour l'obtention d'une autorisation de mise sur le marche: Direction de la Pharmacie et du Medicament, Sous-Direction des Affaires Techniques et Scientifigues, Paris.
78. Friedmann, N. (1985): Thymopentin: Safety overview. *Sur. Immunol. Res.*, 4(Suppl.1):139–148.
79. Gad, S. C., and Chengelis, C. P. (1995): Human health products: Drugs and medicinal devices. In: *Regulatory Toxicology*, edited by C. P. Chengelis, J. F. Holson, and S. C. Gad, pp. 9–49. Raven Press, New York.
80. Galbraith, W. M. (1987): Safety evaluation of biotechnology-derived products. In: *Preclinical Safety of Biotechnology Products Intended for Human Use*, edited by C. Graham, pp. 3–14. Alan R. Liss, Inc., New York.
81. Galloway, J. A., and Chance, R. E. (1984): *Human insulin* rDNA: From rDNA through the FDA. In *Proceedings of the Second World Conference on Clinical Pharmacology and Therapeutics*, edited by L. Lemberger, M. M. Reidenberg, pp. 503–520. ASPET, Bethesda, Maryland.
82. Goddard, M. J., and Krewski, D. (1992): Interspecies extrapolation of toxicity data. *Risk Analysis*, 12(2):315–317.
83. Goeddel, D. V., Kleid, D. G., Boliva, F., Heyneker, M. L., Yansura, D. G., Crea, R., Mirose, T., Kaszewski, A., Itakura, K., and Riggs, A. D. (1979): Expression in *Escherichia coli* of chemically synthesized genes for human insulin. *Proc. Natl Acad. Sci. USA*, 76:106–110.
84. Goldsworthy, T. L., Recio, L., Brown, K., Donehower, L. A., Mirsalis, J. C., Tennant, R. W., and Purchase, I. F. H. (1994): Transgenic animals in toxicology. *Fund. Appl. Toxicol.*, 22:8–19.
85. Gordon, C. V., and Wierenga, D. E. (1992): The drug development and approval process. *New Drug Approvals* (*PMA*), January.
86. Gori, G. B. (1991): Are animal tests relevant in cancer risk assessment? A persistent issue becomes uncomfortable. *Reg. Toxicol. Pharmacol.*, 13:225–227.
87. Goyan, J. (1981): Introduction. In: *Insulins, Growth Hormone and Recombinant DNA Technology*, edited by J. L. Gueriguian, p. xviii. Raven Press, New York.
88. Graham, C. E. (1987): Overview: The industry position. In: *Preclinical Safety of Biotechnology Products Intended for Human Use*, edited by C. E. Graham, pp. 183–187. Alan R. Liss, Inc., New York.
89. Grahame-Smith, D. G. (1982): Preclinical toxicological testing and safeguards in clinical trials. *Eur. J. Clin. Pharmacol.*, 22:1–6.
90. Green, C. E., LeValley, S. E., and Tyson, C. A. (1986): Comparison of amphetamine metabolism using isolated hepatocytes from five species including human. *J. Pharmacol. Exp. Ther.*, 237:931–936.
91. Greene, J. A., Ayers, K. M., Tucker, W. E., Jr., and De Miranda, P. (1996): Nonclinical toxicology studies with zidovudine: Reproductive toxicity studies in rats and rabbits. *Fundam. Appl. Toxicol.*, 32:140–147.
92. Greishaber, C. K. (1991): Prediction of human toxicity of new antineoplastic drugs from studies in animals. In: *The Toxicity of Anticancer Drugs*, edited by G. Powis, and M. P. Hacker, pp. 10–26 Pergamon Press, New York.
93. Griffin, P. J. (1986): Predictive value of animal toxicity studies. In *Long-Term Animal Studies: Their Predictive Value for Man*, edited by S. R. Walker, and A. D. Dayan, pp. 107–116. MTP Press, Lancaster, England.
94. Griffiths, S. A., Ashton, G. A., McAuslane, J. A. N., and Lumley C. E. (1998): Non-clinical safety evaluation of products of biotechnology: Industrial strategies. CMR International report, pp. 5–6.
95. Guengerich, F. P. (1989): Characterization of human microsomal P450 enzymes. *Annu. Rev. Pharmacol. Toxicol.*, 29:241–264.
96. Hanley, T., Udall, V., and Weatherall, M. (1970): An industrial view of current practice in predicting drug toxicity. *Br. Med. Bull.*, 26(3): 203–207.
97. Hansson, E., Havu, N., and Carlsson, E. (1986): Toxicology studies with omeprazole. *Scand. J. Guastroenterol. Suppl.*, 118:89–91.
98. Harada, Y. (1987): Problems presented by animal toxicity studies. In: *Preclinical Safety of Biotechnology Products Intended for Human Use*. edited by C. E., Graham, pp. 127–142. Alan R. Liss, Inc., New York.
99. Haseman, J. K. (1985): Issues in carcinogenicity testing: dose selection. *Fundam. Appl. Toxicol.*, 5:66–78.
100. Hayes, A. H., Jr. (1990): Safety considerations in product development. *Drug Safety*, 5(Suppl. 1):24–26.
101. Homburger, F. (1987): The necessity of animal studies in routine toxicology. *Comments Toxicol.*, 1(5):245–255.
102. ICH Topic M3, STEP 5 (1997): Non-clinical safety studies for the conduct of human clinical trials for pharmaceuticals. ICH Harmonized Tripartite Guideline.
103. ICH Topic S1A, STEP 5 (1995): Need for carcinogenicity studies of pharmaceuticals. ICH Harmonized Tripartite Guideline.
104. ICH Topic S1C(R), STEP 5. (1995): Dose selection for carcinogenicity studies in pharmaceuticals. ICH Harmonized Tripartite Guideline.
105. ICH Topic S2A, STEP 5. (1996): Genotoxicity: Specific aspects of regulatory tests. ICH Harmonised Tripartite Guideline.

106. ICH Topic S2B, STEP 5. (1997): Genotoxicity: Standard battery of tests. ICH Harmonized Tripartite Guideline.
107. ICH Topic S3A, STEP 5. (1995): Toxicokinetics: Guidance on the assessment of systemic exposure in toxicity studies. ICH Harmonized Tripartite Guideline.
108. ICH Topic S4A, STEP 3 (1999): Draft guideline for: Duration of chronic toxicity testing. ICH Harmonized Tripartite Guideline.
109. ICH Topic S5A, STEP 5. (1996): Detection of toxicity to reproduction from medicinal products. ICH Harmonized Tripartite Guideline.
110. ICH Topic S5B, STEP 5 (1996): Reproductive toxicity: Male fertility studies. ICH Harmonized Tripartite Guideline.
111. ICH Topic S6, STEP 5 (1997): Preclinical safety evaluation of biotechnology-derived pharmaceuticals. ICH Harmonized Tripartite Guideline.
112. Japanese Ministry of Health and Welfare (1984): Notification on application data for rDNA drugs. Notification No. 243, Pharmaceutical Affairs Bureau.
113. Jenssen, D., and Romet, L. (1990): Studies of metabolism mediated mutagenicity in vitro. *Altern. Lab. Animals*, 18:243–250.
114. Jollow, D. J., Roberts, S., Price, V., Longacre, S., and Smith, C. (1982): Pharmacokinetic considerations in toxicity testing. *Drug. Metab. Rev.*, 13(6):983–1007.
115. Karch, F. E. (1980): Is drug toxicity a problem of great magnitude? Probably not. In: *Controversy in Therapeutics*, edited by L. Lasagna, pp. 51–57. W. B. Saunders Co., Philadelphia.
116. Kier, L. D. (1985): Use of the Ames Test in toxicology. *Reg. Toxicol. Pharmacol.*, 5:59–64.
117. Klaassen, C. D., and Doull, J. (1980): Evaluation of safety: Toxicologic evaluation. In: *Toxicology: The Basic Science of Poisons*, 2nd ed., edited by J. Doull, C. D. Klaassen, and M. O. Amdur, pp. 11–27. Macmillan, New York.
118. Klaassen, C. D., and Eaton, D. L. (1991): Principles of Toxicology. In: *Toxicology: The Basic Science of Poisons*, 4th ed., edited by M. O. Amdur, J. Doull, and C. D. Klaassen, pp. 12–49. Pergamon Press, New York.
119. Kluwe, W. M. (1995): The complementary roles of in vitro and in vivo tests in genetic toxicology assessment. *Reg. Toxicol. Pharmacol.*, 22:268–272.
120 Larsson, H., Carlsson, E., Mattsson, H., Lundell, L., Sundler, F., Sundell, G., Wallmark, B., Watanabe, T., and Hakanson, R. (1986): Plasma gastrin and gastric enterochromaffin-like cell activation and proliferation: Studies with omeprazole and ranitidine in intact and antrectomized rats. *Gastroenterology*, 90:391–399.
121. Lasagna, L. (1986): Clinical testing of products prepared by biotechnology. *Reg. Toxicol. Pharmacol.*, 6:385–390.
122. Lasagna, L. (1987): Predicting human drug safety from animal studies: Current issues. *J. Toxicol. Sci.*, 12:439–450.
123. Le Bigot, J. F., Begue, J. M., Kiechel, J. R., and Guillouzo, A. (1987): Species differences in metabolism of ketotifen in rat, rabbit and man: Demonstration of similar pathways in vivo and in cultured hepatocytes. *Life Sci.*, 40:883–891.
124. Lemberger, L. (1987): Early clinical evaluation in man: The buck stops here. *Xenobiotica*, 17(3):267–273.
125. Litchfield, J. T. (1961): Forecasting drug effects in man from studies in laboratory animals. *J. Am. Med. Assoc.*, 177:104–108.
126. Lullman, H., Rossen, E., and Seiler, K.-V. (1973): The pharmacokinetics of phentermine and chlorphentermine in chronically treated rats. *J. Pharm. Pharmacol.*, 25:239–243.
127. Lumley, C. E., Parkinson, C., and Walker, S. R. (1992): An international appraisal of the minimum duration of chronic animal toxicity studies. *Hum. Exptl. Toxicol.*, 11:155–162.
128. Lumley, C. E., and Walker, S. R. (1985): A toxicology databank based on animal safety evaluation studies of pharmaceutical compounds. *Hum. Toxicol.*, 4:447–460.
129. Lumley, C. E., and Walker, S. R. (1985): The value of chronic animal toxicology studies of pharmaceutical compounds: A retrospective analysis. *Fundam. Appl. Toxicol.*, 5:1007–1024.
130. Lumley, C. E., and Walker, S. R. (1988): Investigation of the relationship between animal and clinical data. Abstr. 29th Congress *Eur. Soc. Toxicol.* p. 188.
131. Luster, M. I., Munson, A. E., Thomas, P. T., Holsapple, M. P., Fenters, J. D., White, Jr., K. L., Laver, L. D., Germolee, D. R., Rosenthal, G. J., and Dean, J. H. (1988): Development of a testing battery to assess chemical-induced immunotoxicity: National Toxicology Program's Guidelines for immunotoxicity evaluation in mice. *Fundam. Appl. Toxicol.*, 10:2–19.
132. Malmfors, T. (1981): Toxicology as science. *TIPS*, 2(1):1.
133. Martial, J. A., Hallewell, R. A., Baxter, J. D., and Goddman, H. M. (1979): Human growth hormone: Complementary DNA cloning and expression in bacteria. *Science*, 205:602–607.
134. Monro, A. (1992): What is an appropriate measure of exposure when testing drugs for carcinogenicity in rodents? *Toxicol. Appl. Pharmacol.*, 112:171–181.
135. Monro, A. M. (1990): Interspecies comparisons in toxicology: The utility and futility of plasma concentrations of the test substance. *Regul. Toxicol. Pharmacol.*, 12(2): 137–160.
136. Mordenti, J. (1986): Man versus beast: Pharmacokinetic ceiling in mammals. *J. Pharm. Sci.*, 75(11):1028–1038.
137. Morrow, P. E. (1992): Dust overloading of the lungs: Update and appraisal. *Toxicol. Appl. Pharmacol.*, 113:1–12.
138. Munro, I. C. (1977): Considerations in chronic toxicity testing: The chemical, the dose, the design. *J. Environ. Pathol. Toxicol.*, 1:183–197.
139. Nagata, S., Taira, M., Mall, A., Johnsrud, L., Streuli, M., Ecsodi, J., Bell, W., Cantell, K., and Weissman, C. (1980): Synthesis in *E. coli* of a polypeptide with human leukocyte interferon activity. *Nature* (London), 284:316–320.
140. National Toxicology Program (NTP). (1984): Report of the NTP Ad Hoc Panel on Chemical Carcinogenesis Testing and Evaluation, USDHHS publication.
141. Norbury, K. C. (1982): Immunotoxicology in the pharmaceutical industry. *Environ. Health Perspect.*, 43:53–59.
142. Parkinson, C., Thomas, K. E., and Lumley, C. E. (1997): Reproductive toxicity testing of pharmaceutical compounds to support the inclusion of women in clinical trials. *Human Exper. Toxicol.*, 16:239–246.
143. Peck, C. C., Barr, W. H., Benet, L. Z., Collins, J., Desjardins, R. E., Furst, D. E., Harter, J. G., Levy, G., Ludden, T., Rodman, J. H., Sonathanan, L., Schentag, J. J., Shah, V. P., Sheiner, L. B., Skelly, J. P., Stanski, D. R., Temple, R. J., Viswanathan, C. T., Weissinger, J., and Yacobi, A. (1992): Opportunities for integration of pharmacokinetics, pharmacodynamics, and toxicokinetics in rational drug development. *J. Pharm. Sci.*, 81(6):605–610.
144. Peck, H. M. (1968): An appraisal of drug safety evaluation in animals and the extrapolation of results to man. In: *Importance of Fundamental Principles in Drug Evaluation.* edited by D. E., Tedeschi, and R. E., Tedeschi, pp. 450–471, Raven Press, New York.
145. Petricciani, J. C. (1983): An overview of safety and regulatory aspects on new biotechnology. *Reg. Toxicol. Pharmacol.*, 3:428–433.
146. *Physicians' Desk Reference* (1999): Medical Economics Data, Montvale, New Jersey, pp. 584–587.
147. *Physicians' Desk Reference* (1999): Medical Economics Data, Montvale, New Jersey, pp. 1202–1210.
148. Powis, G., Jardine, I., Van Dyke, R., Weinshilbaum, R., Moore, D., Wilke, T., Rhodes, W., Nelson, R., Benson, L., and Szumlanski, C. (1988): Foreign compound metabolism studies with

human liver obtained as surgical waste: Relation to donor characteristics and effects of tissue storage. *Drug Metab. Dispo.*, 16:582–589.

149. Raheja, K. L., and Jordan, A. (1994): FDA recommendations for preclinical testing of gonadotropin-releasing hormone (GnRH) analogues. *Reg. Toxicol. Pharmacol.*, 19:168–175.
150. Rahmani, R., Richard, B., Fabre, G., and Cano, J.-P. (1988): Extrapolation of preclinical pharmacokinetic data to therapeutic drug use. *Xenobiotica*, 18(Suppl. 1):71–88.
151. Ramsey, J. C. (1982): Nonlinear pharmacokinetics relative to toxicity and use of toxicological data. *Drug Metab. Rev.*, 13(15):779–797.
152. Report of a WHO Scientific Group (1966): Principles for pre-clinical testing of drug safety. *Wld. Hlth. Org. Techn. Rep. Ser.*, 341:3–22.
153. Ronneberger, H., and Hilfenhaus, J. (1983): Toxicity studies with human fibroblast interferon. *Arch. Toxicol.*, (Suppl. 6):391–394.
154. Rumjanek, V. M., Hanson, J. M., and Morley, J. (1982): Lymphokines and monokines. In: *Immunopharmacology*, edited by P. Sirois, and M. Pleszczymski, pp. 267–285. Elsevier Press, Amsterdam.
155. Sachs, G., Carlsson, E., Lindberg, P., and Wallmark, B. (1988): Gastric H,K-ATPase as therapeutic target. *Ann. Rev. Pharmacol. Toxicol.*, 28:269–284.
156. Schein, P. S., Davis, R. D., Carter, S., Newman, R. R., and Rall, D. P. (1970): The evaluation of anti-cancer drugs in dogs and monkeys for the prediction of qualitative toxicities in man. *Clin. Pharmacol. Ther.*, 11:3–40.
157. Schellebens, H., de Reus, A., and von den Meide, P. H. (1984): The chimpanzee as a model to test side effects of human interferons. *J. Med. Primatol.*, 13:235–245.
158. Schreiner, C. A. (1983): Application of short-term tests to safety testing of industrial chemicals. *Ann. NY Acad. Sci.*, 407:367–373.
159. Schwetz, B., and Gaylor, D. (1997): New directions for predicting carcinogenesis. *Mol. Carc.*, 20:275–279.
160. Scott, G. M. (1982): Interferon: Pharmacokinetics and toxicity. *Phil. Trans. R. Soc. Lond.* B299:91–107.
161. Scott, G. M. (1983): The toxic effects of interferon in man. *J. Interferon Res.*, 5:85–114.
162. Seddon, T., Michele, I., and Chenery, R. J. (1989): Comparative drug metabolism of diazepam in hepatocytes isolated from man, rat, monkey and dog. *Biochem. Pharmacol.*, 38:1657–1665.
163. Segre, G. (1983): New toxicological problems and proposed solutions: An introduction. In: *Current Problems in Drug Toxicology*, edited by G. Zbinden, J. Y. Detaille, and G. Mazue, pp. 239–240. John Libbey Eurotext, London.
164. Singhvi, S. M., Keim, G. R., and Migdalaf, B. H. (1985): Application of pharmacokinetics in drug safety evaluation. *Reg. Toxicol. Pharmacol.*, 5:3–17.
165. Sipes, I. G., Fisher, R. L., Smith, P. F., Stine, E. R., Gandolfi, A. J., and Brendel, K. (1987): A dynamic liver culture system: A tool for studying chemical biotransformation and toxicity. *Arch. Toxicol.*, 11:20–23.
166. Smolarek, T. A., Higgins, C. V., and Amacher, D. E. (1990): Metabolism and cytotoxicity of acetaminophen in hepatocyte cultures from rat, rabbit, dog and monkey. *Drug Metab. Disp.*, 18(5):659–663.
167. Sontag, J. M., Page, N. P., and Safiotti, V. (1976): Guidelines for carcinogen bioassays in small rodents. DHHS pub. (NIH) 76-801. National Cancer Institute, Bethesda, Maryland.
168. Stebbing, N. (1984): Pharmacological assessment of interferons for clinical use. In: *Proceedings of the Second World Conference on Clinical Pharmacology and Therapeutics*, edited by L. Lemberger, and M. M. Reidenberg, pp. 521–534. *Am. Soc. Pharmacol. Exp. Therp.*, Bethesda, Maryland.
169. Stebbing, N., and Weck, P. K. (1984): Preclinical assessment of biological properties of recombinant DNA derived human interferons. In: *Recombinant DNA Products: Insulin, Interferon and Growth Hormone*, edited by A. P. Bollon, pp. 75–114. CRC Press, Inc., Boca Raton, Florida.
170. Stebbing, N., Weck, P. K., Fenno, J. T., Estell, D. A., and Rinderknecht, E. (1983): Antiviral effects of bacteria derived human leukocyte interferons against encephalomyocarditis virus infection of squirrel monkeys. *Arch. Virol.*, 76:365–372.
171. Stoll, R. E. (1987): The preclinical development of biotechnology-derived pharmaceuticals: The PMA perspective. In: *Preclinical Safety of Biotechnology Products Intended for Human Use*. edited by C. E. Graham, pp. 169–171. Alan R. Liss, Inc., New York.
172. Suter, K. E. (1983): Relevance of standard toxicological tests. Comparison of the experimental and clinical data of six pharmaceutical preparations. In: *Current Problems in Drug Toxicology*, edited by G. Zbinden, J. Y. Detaille, and G. Mazue, pp. 77–89. John Libbey Eurotext, London.
173. Swenberg, J. A. (1995): Bioassay design and MTD setting: Old methods and new approaches. *Reg. Toxicol. Pharmacol.*, 21:44–51.
174. Teelmann, K., Hohbach, C., Lehmann, H., and the International Working Group (1986): Preclinical safety testing of species-specific proteins produced with recombinant DNA techniques. *Arch. Toxicol.*, 59:195–200.
175. Tennant, R. W., Spalding, J., and French, J. F. (1996): Evaulation of transgenic mouse bioassays for identifying carcinogens and noncarcinogens. *Mutation Res.*, 365:119–127.
176. The ICICIS Group Investigators. (1998): Report of validation study of assessment of direct immunotoxicity in the rat. *Toxicol.*, 125:183–201.
177. Spence, C., ed. (1997): The Pharmaceutical R&D Compendium: CMR International/SCRIP's Complete Guide to Trends in R&D. CMR International and PJB Publishers Ltd., Surrey, United Kingdom.
178. Thenot, J. P., Durand, A., and Morselli, P. L. (1990): In vitro techniques for metabolism studies during drug development. *Acta Pharm. Jugosl.*, 40:395–408.
179. Thomas, P. T. (1990): Approaches used to assess chemically induced impairment of host resistance and immune function. *Toxic Substan. J.*, 10:241–278.
180. Tomaszewski, J. E., and Smith, A. C. (1997): Safety testing of antitumor agents. In: *Comprehensive Toxicology, Vol. 2, Toxicity Testing and Evaluation*, edited by P. D. Williams and G. H. Hottendorf, pp. 299–309. Elsevier Science Ltd., New York.
181. Trotta, P. P. (1986): Preclinical biology of alpha interferons. *Seminars in Oncol.*, 13(3):3–12.
182. Trown, P. W., Wills, R. J., and Kamm, J. J. (1986): The preclinical development of Roferon-A. *Cancer*, 57(8):1648-1656.
183. U. S. Biotechnology Policy. (1992): *Nature*, 356:1–2.
184. Van Oosterhoot, J. P. J., Vanderhann, J. W., DeWaal, E. J., Olejiniczak, K., Hilgenfeld, M., Schmidt, V., and Bass, R. (1997): The utility of two rodent species in carcinogenic risk assessment of pharmaceuticals in Europe. *Reg. Toxicol. Pharmacol.*, 25:6–17.
185. Voisin, E. M., Ruthsatz, M., Collins, J., and Hoyle, P. C. (1990): Extrapolation of animal toxicity to humans: Interspecies comparisons in drug development. *Reg. Toxicol. Pharmacol.*, 12:107–116.
186. Vos, J. G. (1977): Immune suppression as related to toxicology. *CRC Crit. Rev. Toxicol.*, 5:67–101.
187. Wagstaff, J., Chadwick, G. Howell, A., Thatcher, N., Scarffe, J. H., and Crowther, D. (1984): A phase I toxicity study of human rDNA interferon in patients with solid tumors. *Cancer Chemother. Pharmacol.*, 13:100–105.

188. Waife, S. O., and Lasagna, L. (1985): From DNA to NDA—The impact of recombinant DNA technology on new drug development. *Reg. Toxicol. Pharmacol.*, 5:212–224.
189. Wallmark, B. (1986): Mechanism of action of omeprazole. *Scand. J. Gastroent.*, (Suppl. 118):11–16.
190. Weil, C. S. (1972): Guidelines for experiments to predict the degree of safety of a material for man. *Toxicol. Appl. Pharmacol.*, 21:194–199.
191. Weissinger, J. (1989): Nonclinical pharmacologic and toxicologic considerations for evaluating biologic products. *Reg. Toxicol. Pharmacol.*, 10:255–263.
192. Weissinger, J. (1990): Pharmacology and toxicology of novel drug delivery systems: Regulatory issues. *Drug Safety*, 5(Suppl 1):107–113.
193. Wierda, D. (1992): Personal communication. Biochemical Toxicology, Eli Lilly and Company, Greenfield, Indiana.
194. Williams, G. M., Dunkel, V. C., Ray, V. A., eds. (1983): Cellular systems for toxicity testing. *Ann. NY Acad. Sci.*, V. 407.
195. Williams, G. M., and Weisburger, J. H. (1991): Chemical carcinogenesis. In: *Toxicology: The Basic Science of Poisons*, 4th ed., edited by M. O. Amdur, J. Doull, and C. D. Klaassen, pp. 127–200. Pergamon Press, New York.
196. Williams, P. (1990): The role of pharmacological profiling in safety assessment. *Reg. Toxicol. Pharmacol.*, 12(3):238–252.
197. Williams, P. D., Calligaro, D. O., Colbert, W. E., Helton, D. R., Shetler, T., Turk, J. A., and Jordan, W. H. (1991): General pharmacology of a new potent 5-hydroxytryptamine antagonist. *Arzneim. Forsch.*, 41(1):189–195.
198. Wilson, A. B. (1987): The toxicology of the end products from biotechnology processes. *Arch. Toxicol.*, (Suppl. II):194–199.
199. Wolf, F. J. (1980): Effect of overloading pathways on toxicity. *J. Environ. Pathol. Toxicol.*, 3:113–134.
200. Wrighton, S. A., and Stevens, J. C. (1992): The human hepatic cytochromes P450 involved in drug metabolism. *CRC Crit. Rev. Toxicol.*, 22(1):1–21.
201. Yoshida, S., Golub, M. S., and Gershwin, M. E. (1989): Immunological aspects of toxicology: Premises not promises. *Reg. Toxicol. Pharmacol.*, 9:56–80.
202. Zapp, J. A., Jr. (1977): Extrapolation of animal studies to the human situation. *J. Toxicol. Environ. Health*, 2:1425–1433.
203. Zbinden, G. (1964): The problem of the toxicologic examination of drugs in animals and their safety in man. *Clin. Pharmacol. Ther.*, 5:537–545.
204. Zbinden, G. (1966): The significance of pharmacologic screening tests in the preclinical safety evaluation of new drugs. *J. New Drugs*, 6:1–7.
205. Zbinden, G. (1976): A look at the world from inside the toxicologist's cage. *Eur. J. Clin. Pharmacol.*, 9:333–338.
206. Zbinden, G. (1978): Application of basic concepts to research in toxicology. *Pharmacol. Rev.*, 30(4):605–616.
207. Zbinden, G. (1980): Predictive value of pre-clinical drug safety evaluation. In: *Proceedings of the First World Conference on Clinical Pharmacology and Therapeutics* (London), edited by P. Turner, C. Padghan, and A. Hedges, p. 9–14. Macmillan, London.
208. Zbinden, G. (1982): Current trends in safety testing and toxicological research. *Naturwissenschaften*, 69:255–259.
209. Zbinden, G. (1986): Acute toxicity testing, public responsibility and scientific challenges. *Cell Biol. Toxicol.*, 2(3):325–335.
210. Zbinden, G. (1987): Biotechnology products intended for human use, toxicological targets and research strategies. In: *Preclinical Safety of Biotechnology Products Intended for Human Use*, edited by C. E. Graham, pp. 143–159. Alan R. Liss, Inc., New York.
211. Zbinden, G. (1988): Biopharmaceutical studies, a key to better toxicology. *Xenobiotica*, 18(1):9–14.
212. Zbinden, G. (1989): Improvement of predictability of subchronic and chronic toxicity studies. *J. Toxicol. Sci.*, 14(Suppl. 3):3–21.
213. Zbinden, G. (1990): Effects of recombinant human alpha-interferon in a rodent cardiotoxicity model. *Toxicol. Lett.*, 50:25–35.
214. Zbinden, G. (1990): Safety evaluation of biotechnology products. *Drug Safety*, 5(Suppl. 1):58–64.
215. Zbinden, G. (1991): Predictive value of animal studies in toxicology. *Reg. Toxicol. Pharmacol.*, 14:167–177.
216. Zwickl, C. M., Cocke, K. S., Tamura, R. N., Holzhausen, L. M., Brophy, G. T., Bick, P. H., and Wierda, D. (1991): Comparison of the immunogenicity of recombinant and pituitary human growth hormone in rhesus monkeys. *Fundam. Appl. Toxicol.*, 16:275–287.

Principles and Methods of Toxicology, Fourth Edition, edited by A. Wallace Hayes.
Taylor & Francis, Philadelphia © 2001.

Chapter 7

Statistics For Toxicologists

Shayne C. Gad

Over the years that have passed since the writing of the third edition of this chapter, the rate of change in toxicology, statistics, and in the interface between these two disciplines has continued to accelerate. The author is hopeful that this complete revision adequately reflects these changes.

PHILOSOPHY AND GENERAL PRINCIPLES

This chapter has been written for both practicing and student toxicologists as both a basic text and a practical guide to the common statistical problems encountered in toxicology and the methodologies that are available to solve them. The chapter has been enriched by the inclusion of discussions of why a particular procedure or interpretation is recommended, by the clear enumeration of the assumptions that are necessary for a procedure to be valid, and by worked-through examples and problems drawn from the actual practice of toxicology.

Since 1960, the field of toxicology has become increasingly complex and controversial in both its theory and practice. Much of this change is due to the evolution of the field. As in all other sciences, toxicology started as a descriptive science. Living organisms, be they human or otherwise, were dosed with or exposed to chemical or physical agents, and the adverse effects which followed were observed, but as a sufficient body of descriptive data was accumulated, it became possible to infer and study underlying mechanisms of action to determine in a broader sense why adverse effects occurred. Toxicology has thus entered a later state of development, the mechanistic stage, where active contributions to the field encompass both descriptive and mechanistic studies.

Studies continue to be designed and executed to generate increased amounts of data. The resulting problems of data analysis have then become more complex and toxicology has drawn more deeply from the well of available statistical techniques. Statistics have also been very active and growing during the last 35 years, to some extent, at least, because of the parallel growth of toxicology. These simultaneous changes have led to an increasing complexity of data and, unfortunately, to the introduction of numerous confounding factors that severely limit the utility of the resulting data in all too many cases.

A major difficulty is that there is a very real need to understand the biological realities and implications of a problem, as well as to understand the peculiarities of toxicological data before procedures are selected and employed for analysis. These characteristics include the following:

(1) The need to work with a relatively small sample set of data collected from the members of a population (laboratory animals, cultured cells, bacterial cultures) that are not actually the population of interest (i.e., humans or a target animal population).

(2) Dealing frequently with data resulting from a sample that was censored on a basis other than by the investigator's design. By censoring, of course, we mean that not all data points were collected as might be desired. This censoring could be the result of either a biological factor (the test animal being dead or too debilitated to manipulate) or a logistic factor (equipment being inoperative or a tissue being missed in necropsy).

(3) The conditions under which our experiments are conducted are extremely varied. In pharmacology (the closest cousin to at least classical toxicology), the possible conditions of interaction of a chemical or physical agent with a person are limited to a small range of doses via a single route over a short course of treatment to a defined patient population. In toxicology, however, all of these variables (dose, route, time span, subject population) are determined by the investigator.

(4) The time frames available to solve our problems are limited by practical and economic factors. This frequently means that there is not time to repeat a critical study if the first attempt fails, so a true iterative approach is not possible.

The training of most toxicologists in statistics remains limited to a single introductory course that concentrates on some theoretical basics. As a result, the armamentarium of statistical techniques of most toxicologists is limited and the tools that usually are used (t-tests, chi-square, analysis of variance, linear regression) are neither fully developed nor well understood. It is hoped that this chapter will help change this situation.

As a point of departure, it is essential that any analysis of study results be interpreted by a professional who firmly understands three concepts: the difference between biological significance and statistical significance, the nature and value of different types of data, and causality.

For the first concept, we should consider the four possible combinations of these two different types of significance for which we find the relationship shown below.

		STATISTICAL SIGNIFICANCE	
		NO	YES
BIOLOGICAL SIGNIFICANCE	NO	CASE I	CASE II
	YES	CASE III	CASE IV

Cases I and IV give us no problems, as the answers are the same statistically and biologically, but cases II and III present problems. In case II (the false-positive) we have a circumstance where there is a statistical significance in the measured difference between treated and control groups, but there is no true biological significance to the finding. This is not an uncommon happening (e.g., in the case of clinical chemistry parameters). This is called type I error by statisticians, and the probability

Table 7.1
Approximate total sample sizes for comparisons using the t-test and equal group sizes

	$\beta=0.1$		$\beta=0.2$	
Δ/σ	$\alpha=0.05$	$\alpha=0.10$	$\alpha=0.05$	$\alpha=0.10$
0.25	672	548	502	396
0.50	168	138	126	98
0.75	75	62	56	44
1.00	42	34	32	24
1.25	28	22	20	16
1.50	18	16	14	12

Δ is the difference in the treatment group means and σ is the standard deviation.

of this occurring is called the α (alpha) level. In case III (the false-negative) we have no statistical significance, but the differences between groups are biologically/toxicologically significant. This is called type II error by statisticians, and the probability of such an error happening by random chance is called the β (beta) level. An example of a type II error is when a few of a very rare tumor type are seen in treated animals. For both type I and II errors, numerical analysis, no matter how well done, is no substitute for professional judgment. One must have a feeling for the different types of data and for the value or relative merit of each. Note that the two error types interact, and in determining sample size we need to specify both α and β levels. Table 7.1 demonstrates this interaction in the case of the t-test.

There are many reasons that biological and statistical significance are not identical and often are multiple, but certainly a central reason is causality. Through our consideration of statistics, we should keep in mind that just because a treatment and a change in an observed organism are seemingly or actually associated with each other does not "prove" that the former caused the latter. Though this fact is now widely appreciated for correlation (e.g., the fact that the number of storks' nests found each year in England is correlated with the number of human births that year does not mean that storks bring babies), it is just as true in the general case of significance. Timely establishment and proof that treatment causes an effect requires an understanding of the underlying mechanism and proof of its validity. At the same time, it is important that we realize that not finding a good correlation or suitable significance associated with a treatment and an effect likewise does not prove that the two are not associated (that a treatment does not cause an effect). At best, it gives us a certain level of confidence that under the conditions of the current test, these items are not associated.

These points, along with other common pitfalls and shortcomings associated with the method, will be discussed in greater detail in the Assumptions section for each method. To help in better understanding the sections to come, terms frequently used in discussion throughout this chapter should first be considered. These are presented in Table 7.2.

Each measurement we make—each individual piece of experimental information we gather—is called a datum; however, we gather and analyze multiple pieces at one time, with the resulting collection being called data. Data are collected on the basis of their association with a treatment (intended or otherwise) as an effect (a property) that is measured in the experimental subjects of a study, such as body weights. These identifiers (i.e., treatment and effect) are termed *variables*. Treatment variables (those that the researcher or nature control and that can be directly controlled) are termed *independent*, whereas effect variables (such as weight, life span, and number of neoplasms) are termed dependent variables (their outcome is believed to dependent on the "treatment" being studied).

All of the possible measures of a given set of variables in all of the possible subjects that exist are termed the population for those variables. Such a population of variables cannot be truly measured (e.g., one would have to obtain, treat, and measure the weights of all the Fischer-344 rats that were, are, or ever will be). Instead, we deal with a representative group—a sample. If our sample of data is appropriately collected and of sufficient size, it serves to provide good estimates of the characteristics of the parent population from which it was drawn.

Two terms refer to the quality and reproducibility of our measurements of variables. The first, accuracy, is an expression of the closeness of a measured or computed value to its actual or "true" value in nature. The second, precision, reflects the closeness or reproducibility of a series of repeated measurements of the same quantity.

If we arrange all of our measurements of a particular variable in order as a point on an axis marked as to the values of that variable, and if our sample were large enough, the pattern of distribution of the data in the sample would begin to become apparent. This pattern is a representation of the frequency distribution of a given population of data (i.e., of the incidence of different measurements, their central tendency, and dispersion).

The most common frequency distribution—and one we will talk about throughout this chapter—is the normal (or Gaussian) distribution. The normal distribution is such that two thirds of all values are within one standard deviation of the mean (or average value for the entire population), and 95% are within 1.96 standard

Table 7.2
Some frequently used terms and their general meanings (171)

Term	Meaning
95% confidence interval	A range of values above, below, or above and below the sample mean, median, mode, etc., has a 95% chance of containing the true value of the population (mean, median, mode). Also called the fiducial limit equivalent to the Pc 0.05.
Bias	Systemic error as opposed to a sampling error. For example, selection bias may occur when each member of the population does not have an equal chance of being selected for the sample.
Degrees of freedom	The number of independent deviations, usually abbreviated *df*.
Independent variables	Also known as predictors or explanatory variables.
P-value	Another name for significance level; usually 0.05 or 0.01
Power	The effect of the experimental conditions on the dependent variable relative to sampling fluctuation. When the effect is maximized, the experiment is more powerful. Power can also be defined as the probability that there will not be a type II error (1-Beta). Conventionally, power should be at least .07.
Random	Each individual member of the population has the same chance of being selected for the sample.
Robust	Having inferences or conclusions little effected by departure from assumptions.
Sensitivity	The number of subjects experiencing each experimental condition divided by the variance of scores in the sample.
Significance level	The probability that a difference has been erroneously declared to be significant, typically 0.05 and 0.01 corresponding to 5% and 1% chance of error, respectively.
Type I error (false-positives)	Concluding that there is an effect when there really is not an effect. Its probability is the alpha level.
Type II error (false-negatives)	Concluding there is not an effect when there really is an effect. Its probability is the beta level.

deviations of the mean. The mathematical equation describing the normal distribution is

$$y = \frac{1}{\sigma\sqrt{2\pi}} e^{-(x-\mu)^2/2\sigma^2}$$

where μ is the mean and σ is the standard deviation. Other common frequency distributions include the Poisson and chi square.

In all areas of biological research, optimal design and appropriate interpretation of experiments require that the researcher understand both the biological and technological underpinnings of the system being studied and of the data being generated. From the point of view of the statistician, it is vitally important that the experimenter both knows and is able to communicate the nature of the data and understands its limitations. One classification of data types is presented in Table 7.3.

The nature of the data collected is determined by three considerations. These are the biological source of the data (the system being studied), the instrumentation and techniques being used to make measurements, and the design of the experiment. The researcher has some degree of control over each of these, with least control over the biological system (he/she normally has a choice of only one of several models to study) and most control over the design of the experiment or study. Such choices, in fact, dictate the type of data generated by a study.

Statistical methods are based on specific assumptions. Parametric statistics—those that are most familiar to the majority of scientists—have more stringent underlying assumptions than do nonparametric statistics. Among the underlying assumptions for many parametric

Table 7.3
Types of variables (data) and examples of each type

Classified by		Type	Example
Scale	Continuous	Scalar	Body weight
		Ranked	Severity of a lesion
	Discontinuous	Scalar	Weeks until the first observation of a tumor in a carcinogenicity study
		Ranked	Clinical observations in animals
		Attribute	Eye colors in fruit flies
		Quantal	Dead/alive or present/absent
Frequency distribution		Normal	Body weights
		Bimodal	Some clinical chemistry parameters
		Others	Measures of time to incapacitation

statistical methods (such as the analysis of variance) is that the data are continuous. The nature of the data associated with a variable (as described previously) imparts a "value" to that data, the value being the power of the statistical tests that can be employed.

Continuous variables are those that can at least theoretically assume any of an infinite number of values between any two fixed points (such as measurements of body weight between 2.0 and 3.0 kg).

Limitations on our ability to measure a specific parameter constrain the extent to which the real-world situation approaches the theoretical, but many of the variables studied in toxicology are, in fact, continuous. Examples of these are lengths, weights, concentrations, temperatures, periods of time, and percentages. For these continuous variables, we may describe the character of a sample with measures of central tendency and dispersion that we are most familiar with—the mean, denoted by the symbol μ and also called the arithmetic average, and the standard deviation SD, which is denoted by the symbol σ and is calculated as being equal to

$$\sqrt{\frac{\sum X^2 - \frac{(\sum X)^2}{N}}{N-1}},$$

where X is the individual datum and N is the total number of data in the group.

Contrasted with these continuous data, however, we have discontinuous (or discrete) data that can only assume certain fixed numerical values with no possible intermediate values (such as counts of 5 and 6 dead animals respectively). In these cases our choice of statistical tools or tests is, as we will find later, more limited.

Probability

Probability is simply the frequency with which, in a sufficiently large sample, a particular event will occur or a particular value will be found. Hypothesis testing, for example, generally is structured so that the likelihood of a treatment group being the same as a control (the so called "null hypothesis") can be assessed as being less than a selected low level (very frequently 5%), which implies that we are 1.0-α (i.e., 1.0–0.05, or 95%) sure that the groups are *not* equivalent.

Functions of Statistics

Statistical methods may serve to do any combination of three possible tasks. The one we are most familiar with is hypothesis testing (i.e., determining if two [or more] groups of data differ from each other at a predetermined level of confidence). A second function is the construction and use of models that may be used to predict future outcomes of chemical–biological interactions. This is most commonly seen in linear regression or in the derivation of some form of correlation coefficient. Model fitting allows us to relate one variable (typically a treatment or "independent" variable) to another. The third function, reduction of dimensionality, continues to be less commonly used than the first two. This final category includes methods for reducing the number of variables in a system while only minimally reducing the amount of information, therefore making a problem easier to visualize and to understand. Examples of such techniques are factor analysis and cluster analysis. A subset of this last function, discussed later under descriptive statistics, is the reduction of raw data to single expressions of central tendency and variability (such as the mean and standard deviation). There also is a special subset of statistical techniques that is part of both the second and third functions of statistics. This is data transformation, which includes such things as the conversion of numbers to log or probit values.

This chapter is primarily designed to address the first of the three functions of statistical methods that we presented (hypothesis testing). The second function, modeling (especially in the form of risk assessment), is becoming increasingly important as the science continues to evolve from the descriptive phase to a mechanistic phase. Likewise, because the interrelation of multiple factors is becoming a real concern, a discussion of reduction of dimensionality has been included.

Descriptive Statistics

Descriptive statistics are used to summarize the general nature of a data set. As such, the parameters describing any single group of data have two components. One of these describes the location of the data, whereas the other gives a measure of the dispersion of the data in and about this location. Often overlooked is the fact that the choice of which parameters are used to give these pieces of information implies a particular type of distribution for the data.

Most commonly, location is described by giveing the (arithmetic) mean and dispersion by giving the standard deviation (SD) or the standard error of the mean (SEM). The calculation of the first two of these has already been described. If we again denote the total number of data in a group as N, then the SEM would be calculated as

$$\mathrm{SEM} = \frac{\mathrm{SD}}{\sqrt{N}}.$$

The SD and the SEM are related to each other but yet are quite different. To compare these two, let us first demonstrate their calculation from the same set of 15 observations:

Data Points (X_i): 1,2,3,4,4,5,5,5,6,6,6,7,7,8,9

$\mathrm{Sum}\left(\sum\right) = 78.$

Squares (X_i^2): 1,4,9,16,16,25,25,25,36,36,36,49,49,64,81

Sum = 472

The standard deviation can then be calculated as

$$\mathrm{SD} = \frac{\sqrt{472 - \dfrac{(78)^2}{15}}}{15-1} = \frac{\sqrt{472 - \dfrac{(6084)}{15}}}{14}$$

$$= \frac{\sqrt{472 - 405.6}}{14} = \sqrt{4.7428571} = 2.1778$$

with a mean ($\bar{x}$) of $\frac{78}{15} = 5.2$ for the data group. The SEM for the same set of data, however, is

$$\mathrm{SEM} = \frac{2.1778}{\sqrt{15}} = \frac{2.1778}{3.8730} = 0.562303.$$

The SEM is quite a bit smaller than the SD, making it very attractive to use in reporting data. This size difference is because the SEM actually is an estimate of the error (or variability) involved in measuring the means of samples and not an estimate of the error (or variability) involved in measuring the data from which means are calculated. This is implied by the *Central Limited Theorem*, which tells us three major things:

- The distribution of sample means will be approximately normal regardless of the distribution of values in the original population from which the samples were drawn.
- The mean value of the collection.
- The standard deviation of the collection of all possible means of samples of a given size, called the SEM, depends on both the standard deviation of the original population and the size of the sample.

The SEM should be used only when the uncertainty of the estimate of the mean is of concern, which is almost never the case in toxicology. Rather, we are concerned with an estimate of the variability of the population, for which the standard deviation is appropriate.

The use of the mean with either the SD or SEM implies, however, that we have reason to believe that the sample of data being summarized are from a population that is at least approximately normally distributed. If this is not the case, then we should rather use a set of statistical descriptions that do not require a normal distribution. These are the median, for location, and semiquartile distance, for a measure of dispersion. These somewhat less familiar parameters are characterized as follows.

Median

When all of the numbers in a group are arranged in a ranked order (i.e., from smallest to largest), the median is the middle value. If there is an odd number of values in a group, then the middle value is obvious (in the case of 13 values, for example, the seventh largest is the median). When the number of values in the samples is even, the median is calculated as the midpoint between the (N/2)th and the ([N/2] + 1)th number. For example, in the series of numbers 7, 12, 13,19, the median value would be the midpoint between 12 and 13, which is 12.5.

Semiquartile Distance

When all the data in a group are ranked, a quartile of the data contains one ordered quarter of the values. Typically, we are most interested in the borders of the middle two quartiles Q_1 and Q_3, which together represent the semiquartile distance and which contain the median as their center. Given that there are N values in an ordered group of data, the upper limit of the jth quartile (Q_j)

may be computed as being equal to the [(jN÷1)/4th] value. Once we have used this formula to calculate the upper limits of Q_1 and Q_3, we can then compute the semiquartile distance (which is also called the quartile deviation, and as such is abbreviated as the QD) with the formula $QD = (Q_3 - Q_1)/2$.

For example, for the 15 value data set 1, 2, 3, 4, 4, 5, 5, 5, 6, 6, 6, 7, 7, 8, 9, we can calculate the upper limits of Q_1 and Q_3 as

$$Q_1 = \frac{1(15+1)}{4} = \frac{16}{4} = 4,$$

$$Q_3 = \frac{3(15=1)}{4} = \frac{48}{4} = 12.$$

The 4th and 12th values in this data set are 4 and 7, respectively. The semiquartile distance can then be calculated as

$$QD = \frac{7-4}{2} = 1.5.$$

One final sample parameter that sees some use in toxicology (primarily in inhalation studies) is the geometric mean, denoted by the term $\bar{X}_g$. This is calculated as

$$\overline{X}_g = (X_1.X_2 \ldots X_N)^{1/N}$$

and has the attractive feature that it does not give excessive weight to extreme values (or "outliers"), such as the mass of a single very large particle in a dust sample. In effect, it "folds" extreme values in toward the center of the distribution, decreasing the sensitivity of the parameter to the undue influence of the outlier. This is particularly important in the case of aerosol samples, where a few very large particles would cause the arithmetic mean of particle diameters to present a misleading picture of the nature of the "average" particle.

There are times when it is desired to describe the relative variability of one or more sets of data. The most common way of doing this is to compute the coefficient of variation (CV), which is calculated simply as the ratio of the SD to the mean, or

$$CV = \frac{SD}{\overline{X}}$$

A CV of 0.2 or 20% thus means that the standard deviation is 20% of the mean. In toxicology the CV is frequently between 20% and 50% and may at times exceed 100%.

Outliers and Rounding of Numbers

These two considerations in the handling of numerical data can be, on occasion, of major concern to the toxicologist because of their pivotal nature in cases of borderline significance. Outliers should also be of concern for other reasons, however. On the principle that one should always have a plan to deal with all reasonably likely contingencies in advance of their happening, early decisions should be made to select a policy for handling both outliers and the rounding of numbers.

Outliers

Outliers are extreme (high or low) values that are widely divergent from the main body of a group of data and from what is our common experience. They may arise from an instrument (such as a balance) being faulty, the apparently natural urge of some animals to frustrate research, or they may be indicative of a "real" value. Outlying values can be detected by visual inspection of a data, use of a scattergram (described later), or (if the data set is small enough, which is usually the case in toxicology) by a large increase in the parameter estimating the dispersion of data, such as the SD.

When we can solidly tie one of the above error-producing processes (such as a balance being faulty) to an outlier, we can safely delete it from consideration, but if we cannot solidly tie such a cause to an outlier (even if we have strong suspicions), we have a much more complicated problem, for then such a value may be one of several other things. It could be the result of a particular parameter that is the grounds for the entire study (i.e., the very "effect" that we are looking for) or it could be because of the collection of legitimate effects which constitute sample error. As will be discussed later (under exploratory data analysis), and is now more widely appreciated, outliers can be an indication of a biologically significant effect that is not yet statistically significant. Variance inflation can be the result of such outliers and can be used to detect them. Outliers, in fact, by increasing the variability within a small sample set, decrease the sensitivity of our statistical tests and actually preclude our having a statistically significant result (12).

Alternatively, the outlier may be the result of, for example, an unobserved technician error and may change the decisions made from a set of data. In this case we want to reject the data point—to exclude it from consideration with the rest of the data, but how can one identify these legitimate statistical rejection cases?

There are a wide variety of techniques for data rejection. Their proper use depends on one's having an understanding of the nature of the distribution of the data. For normally distributed data with a single extreme value, a simple method such as Chauvenet's criterion (107) may legitimately be employed. This states that if the probability of a value deviating from the mean is greater than 1/2 N, one should consider that there are adequate grounds for its rejections. This approach is demonstrated below.

USE OF CHAUVENET'S CRITERION

Having collected 20 values as a data set, we find they include the following values: 1, 6, 7, 8, 8, 9, 9, 9, 10, 10, 10, 10, 10, 11, 11, 11, 12, 12, 13 and 14. Was the lowest value (1) erroneous and should it be rejected as a outlier? Some simple calculations are performed, as

Mean (X) = 9.55,

Standard deviation (SD) = 2.80,

Chauvenet's Criterion Value $= \frac{1}{2}N = \frac{20}{2} = 10$.

So we would reject the value of "1" if its probability of occurrence were less than 10%. Going to a table of Z scores, we see that 10% of the values in a normal distribution are beyond ±1.645 SDs of the mean. Multiplying this by the SD for the sample, we get (1.645)(2.80) = 4.606. This means we would reject values beyond this range from the mean—that is, less than (9.55–4.606) = 4.944 or greater than (9.55 + 4.606) = 14.156. We therefore reject the value of "1."

One should note that as the sample size gets bigger, the rejection zone for Chauvenet's Criterion will also increase, as N of 20 is about as large as this method is useful for.

A second relatively straightforward approach, for use when the data are normally distributed but contain several extreme values is to winsorize the data. Though there are a number of variations to this approach, the simplest (called the *G-1 method*) calls for replacing the highest and lowest values in a set of data. In a group of data consisting of the values 54, 22, 18, 15, 14, 13, 11, and 4, we would replace 54 with a second 22, and 4 with a replicate 11. This would give us a group consisting of 22, 22, 18, 15, 14, 13, 11, and 11, which we would then treat as our original data. Winsorizing should not be performed, however, if the extreme values constitute more than a small minority of the entire data set.

Another approach is to use Dixon's Test (42) to determine if extreme values should be rejected. In Dixon's test, the set of observations is first ordered according to their magnitude (as we did earlier for the data set used to demonstrate Chauvenet's Criterion, though there this step was simply to make the case clearer). The ratio of the difference of an extreme value from one of its nearest neighbor values in the range of values in the sample is then calculated using a formula that varies with sample size. This ratio is then compared to a table value, and if found to be equal or greater, is considered to be an outlier at the $p \leq 0.05$ level. The formula for the ratio varies with sample size and according to whether it is the smallest or largest value that is suspect.

If we have more information as to the nature of the data or the type of analysis to be performed, there are even better techniques to handle outliers. Extensive discussions of these may be found elsewhere (10,12, 76,137).

Rounding Off

When the number of digits in a number is to be reduced (due to limitations of space or to reflect the extent of significance of a number), we must carry out the process of rounding off a number. Failure to have a rule for performing this operation can lead to both confusion and embarrassment for a facility (during such times as study audits). One common rule follows.

A digit to be rounded is not changed if it is followed by a digit less than 5; the digits following it are simply dropped off ("truncated"). If the number is followed by a digit greater than 5 or by a 5 followed by other nonzero digits, it is increased to the next highest number. When the digit to be rounded is followed by 5 alone or by 5 followed by zeros, it is unchanged if it is even but increased by one if it is odd. Examples of this rule, in effect, are (in a case where we must reduce to 3 digits)

137.4 becomes 137
137.6 becomes 138
138.52 becomes 139
137.5 becomes 138
and 138.5 becomes 138

The rationale behind this procedure is that over a period of time the results should even out—as many digits that increased are also decreased.

Sampling

Sampling—the selection of which individual data points will be collected, whether in the form of selecting which animals to collect blood from or to remove a portion of a diet mix from for analysis—is an essential step upon which all other efforts toward a good experiment or study are based. There are three assumptions about sampling that are common to most of the statistical analysis techniques that are used in toxicology. These are that the sample is collected without bias, that each member of a sample is collected independently of the others, and that members of a sample are collected with replacements. Precluding bias, both intentional and unintentional, means that at the time of selection of a sample to measure, each portion of the population from which that selection is to be made has an equal chance of being selected. Ways of precluding bias are discussed in detail in the section on experimental design.

Independence means that the selection of any portion of the sample is not affected by and does not affect the selection or measurement of any other portion.

Finally, sampling with replacement means that, in theory, after each portion is selected and measured, it is returned to the total sample pool and thus has the opportunity to be selected again. This is a corollary of the assumption of independence. Violation of this assumption (which is almost always the case in toxicology and all of the life sciences) does not have serious consequences if the total pool from which samples are taken is sufficiently large (say 20 or greater) so that the chance of reselecting that portion is small anyway.

There are four major types of sampling methods—random, stratified, systematic, and cluster. Random is by far the most commonly employed method in toxicology. It stresses the fulfillment of the assumption of avoiding bias. When the entire pool of possibilities is mixed or randomized (procedures for randomization are presented in a later section), then the members of the group are selected in the order that they are drawn from the pool.

Stratified sampling is performed by first dividing the entire pool into subsets or strata and then random sampling from each strata. This method is employed when the total pool contains subsets that are distinctly different but the data within each subset are similar. An example is a large batch of a powdered pesticide in which it is desired to determine the nature of the particle size distribution. Larger pieces or particles are on the top, whereas progressively smaller particles have settled lower in the container; at the very bottom, the material has been packed and compressed into aggregates. To determine a timely representative answer, proportionally sized subsets from each layer or strata should be selected, mixed, and randomly sampled. This method is used more commonly in diet studies.

In systematic sampling, a sample is taken at set intervals (such as every fifth container of reagent or taking a sample of water from a fixed sample point in a flowing stream every hour). This is most commonly employed in quality assurance or (in the clinical chemistry lab) in quality control.

In cluster sampling, the pool is already divided into numerous separate groups (such as bottles of tablets), and we select small sets of groups (such as several bottles of tablets) and then select a few members from each set. This results in a cluster of measures. Again, this is a method most commonly used in quality control or in environmental studies when the effort and expense of physically collecting even a small number of data points is significant.

In classical toxicology studies, sampling arises in a practical sense in a limited number of situations. The most common of these are as follows:

(1) Selecting a subset of animals or test systems from a study to make some measurement (which either destroys or stresses the measured system or is expensive) at an interval during a study. This may include such cases as doing interim necropsies in a chronic study or collecting and analyzing blood samples from some animals during a subchronic study.
(2) Analyzing inhalation chamber atmospheres to characterize aerosol distributions with a new generation system.
(3) Analyzing diet in which test material has been incorporated.
(4) Performing quality control on an analytical chemistry operation by having duplicate analyses performed on some materials.
(5) Selecting data to audit for quality assurance purposes.

EXPERIMENTAL DESIGN

Toxicological experiments generally have two purposes. The first is to determine whether or not an agent results in an effect on a biological system. The second, never far behind, is to find how much of an effect is present. It has become increasingly desirable that the results and conclusions of studies aimed at assessing the effects of environmental agents be as clear and unequivocal as possible. It is essential that every experiment and study yield as much information as possible and that the results of each study have the greatest possible chance of answering the questions it was conducted to address. The statistical aspects of such efforts, so far as they are aimed at structuring experiments to maximize the possibilities of success, are called *experimental design*.

We have now become accustomed to developing exhaustively detailed protocols for an experiment or study prior to its conduct. A priori selection of statistical methodology (as opposed to the post hoc approach) is as significant a portion of the process of protocol development and experimental design as any other and can measurably enhance the value of the experiment or study. Prior selection of statistical methodologies is essential for proper design of other portions of a protocol such as the number of animals per group or the sampling intervals for body weight. Implied in such a selection is the notion that the toxicologist has both an in-depth knowledge of the area of investigation and an understanding of the general principles of experimental design, as the analysis of any set of data is dictated to a large extent by the manner in which the data are obtained.

The four basic statistical principles of experimental design are replication, randomization, concurrent ("local") control, and balance. In abbreviated form, these may be summarized as follows.

Replication: Any treatment must be applied to more than one experimental unit (animal, plate of cells, litter of offspring, etc.). This provides more accuracy in the measurement of a response than can be obtained from a single observation, as underlying experimental errors tend to cancel each other out. It also supplies an estimate of the experimental error derived from the variability among each of the measurements taken (or "replicates"). In practice, this means that an experiment should have enough experimental units in each treatment group (i.e., large enough "N") so that reasonably sensitive statistical analysis of data can be performed. The estimation of sample size is addressed in detail later in this chapter.

Randomization: This is practiced to ensure that every treatment has its fair share of extreme high and extreme low values. It also serves to allow the toxicologist to proceed as if the assumption of "independence" is valid (i.e., there is not avoidable [known] systematic bias in how one obtains data).

Concurrent Control: Comparisons between treatments should be made to the maximum extent possible between experimental units from the same closely defined population. Therefore, animals used as a "control" group should come from the same source, lot, age, etc. as test group animals. Except for the treatment being evaluated, test and control animals should be maintained and handled in exactly the same manner.

Balance: If the effect of several different factors is being evaluated simultaneously, the experiment should be laid out in such a way that the contributions of the different factors can be separately distinguished and estimated. There are several ways of accomplishing this using one of several different forms of design, as will be discussed later.

Types of Experimental Design

There are four basic experimental design types used in toxicology: the randomized block, latin square, factorial design, and nested design. Other designs that are used are really combinations of these and are rarely employed in toxicology. Before examining these four basic types, however, we must first examine the basic concept of blocking.

Blocking is, simply put, the arrangement or sorting of the members of a population (such as all of an available group of test animals) into groups based on certain characteristics that may (but are not sure to) alter an experimental outcome. Such characteristics, which may cause a treatment to give a differential effect, include genetic background, age, sex, overall activity levels, and so on. The process of blocking then acts (or attempts to act) so that each experimental group (or block) is assigned its fair share of the members of each of these subgroups.

We should now recall that randomization is aimed at spreading out the effect of undetectable or unsuspected characteristics in a population of animals or some portion of this population. The merging of the two concepts or randomization and blocking leads to the first basic experimental design, the randomized block. This type of design requires that each treatment group have at least one member of each recognized group (such as age), with the exact members of each block being assigned in an unbiased (or random) fashion.

The second type of experimental design assumes that we can characterize treatments (whether intended or otherwise) as belonging clearly to separate sets. In the simplest case, these categories are arranged into two sets that may be thought of as rows (for, say, source litter of test animal, with the first litter as row 1, the next as row 2, etc.), and the secondary set of categories may be thought of as columns (for, say, our ages of test animals, with 6–8 weeks as column 1, 8–10 weeks as column 2, and so on). Experimental units are then assigned so that each major treatment (control, low dose, intermediate dose, etc.) appears once and only once in each row and each column. If we denote our test groups as A (control), B (low), C (intermediate), and D (high), such an assignment would appear as below:

		Age			
Source Litter		6–8 Weeks	8–10 Weeks	10–12 Weeks	12–14 Weeks
1	:	A	B	C	D
2	:	B	C	D	A
3	:	C	D	A	B
4	:	D	A	B	C

The third type of experimental design is the factorial design in which there are two or more clearly understood treatments, such as exposure level to test chemical, animal age, or temperature. The classical approach to this situation (and to that described under the latin square) is to hold all but one of the treatments constant and at any one time to vary just that one factor. Instead, in the factorial design, all levels of a given factor are combined with all levels of every other factor in the experiment. When a change in one factor produces a different change in the response variable at one level of a factor than at other levels of this factor, there is an interaction between these two factors that can then be analyzed as an interaction effect.

The last of the major varieties of experimental design are the nested designs, where the levels of one factor are nested within (or are subsamples of) another factor. That is, each subfactor is evaluated only within the limits of its single larger factor.

Censoring

A second concept and its understanding are essential to the design of experiments in toxicology, that of censoring.

Censoring is the exclusion of measurements from certain experimental units, or indeed of the experimental units themselves, from consideration in data analysis or inclusion in the experiment at all. Censoring may occur either prior to initiation of an experiment (where, in modern toxicology, this is almost always a planned procedure), during the course of an experiment (when they are almost universally unplanned, resulting from events such as the death of animals being tested), or after the conclusion of an experiment (when data usually are excluded because of being identified as some form of outlier).

In practice, a priori censoring in toxicology studies occurs in the assignment of experimental units (such as animals) to test groups. The most familiar example is in the practice of assignment of test animals to acute, subchronic, and chronic studies, where the results of otherwise random assignments are evaluated for body weights of the assigned members. If the mean weights are found not to be comparable by some preestablished criterion (such as a 90% probability of difference by analysis of variance), then members are reassigned (censored) to achieve comparability in terms of starting body weights. Such a procedure of animal assignment to groups is known as a *censored randomization*.

Sample Size

The first precise or calculable aspect of experimental design encountered is determining sufficient test and control group sizes to allow one to have an adequate level of confidence in the results of a study (i.e., in the ability of the study design with the statistical tests used to detect a true difference—or effect—when it is present). The statistical test contributes a level of power to such a detection. Remember that the power of a statistical test is the probability that a test results in rejection of a hypothesis, say H_0 (the null hypothesis) when some other hypothesis, say H, is valid. This is termed the power of the test "with respect to the (alternative) hypothesis H."

If there is a set of possible alternative hypotheses, the power, regarded as a function of H, is termed the *power function* of the test. When the alternatives are indexed by a single parameter θ, simple graphical presentation is possible. If the parameter is a vector θ, one can visualize a *power surface*.

If the power function is denoted by $\beta(\theta)$ and H_0 specifies $\theta = \theta_0$, then the value of β (Π)—the probability of rejecting H_0 when it is in fact valid—is the significance level. A test's power is greatest when the probability of a type II error is the least. Specified powers can be calculated for tests in any specific or general situation.

Some general rules to keep in mind are

- The more stringent the significance level, the greater the necessary sample size. More subjects are needed for a 1% level test than for a 5% level test.
- Two-tailed tests require larger sample sizes than one-tailed tests. Assessing two directions at the same time requires a greater investment.
- The smaller the critical effect being measured, the larger the necessary sample size. Subtle effects require greater efforts.
- Any difference can be significant if the sample size is large enough.
- The larger the power required, the larger the necessary sample size. Greater protection from failure requires greater effort. The smaller the sample size, the smaller the power (i.e., the greater the chance of failure).
- The requirements and means of calculating necessary sample size depends on the desired (or practical) comparative sizes of test and control groups.

The necessary sample size (N) can be calculated, for example, for equalised test and control groups using the formula

$$N = \frac{(t_1 + t_2)^2}{d^2} S,$$

where t_1 is the one-tailed t value with N-1 degrees of freedom corresponding to the desired level of confidence, t_2 is the one-tailed t value with N-1 degrees of freedom corresponding to the probability that the sample size will be adequate to achieve the desired precision, d is the population standard deviation and S is the sample standard deviation, derived typically from historical data and calculated as

$$S = \sqrt{\frac{1}{N-1} \sum (V_1 - V_2)^2}.$$

Determination of the necessary sample size is demonstrated in Example 1.

Example 1

In a subchronic dermal study in rabbits, the principal point of concern is the extent to which the compound causes oxidative damage to erythrocytes. To quantitate this, the laboratory will be measuring the numbers of reticulocytes in the blood. What then would be an adequate sample size to allow the question at hand to be addressed with reasonable certitude?

To do this, we use the one-tailed t value for an infinite number of degrees of freedom at the 95% confidence level (i.e., $p \leq 0.05$). Going to a set of t tables, we find this number to be 1.645. From prior experience, we know that the usual values for reticulocytes in rabbit blood are from 0.5 to 1.9×10^6/ml. The acceptable range of variation, 0, is therefore equal to the span of this range, or 1.4. Likewise, examining the control data from previous rabbit studies, we find our sample standard deviation to be 0.825. When we insert all of these numbers into the equation (presented above) for sample size, we can calculate the required sample size (N) to be

$$= \frac{(1.645 + 1.645)^2}{(1.4)^2}$$

$$= \frac{10.824}{1.96}(0.825)$$

$$= 4.556.$$

In other words, in this case where there is little natural variability, measuring the reticulocyte counts of groups of only five animals each should be sufficient. There are many formulas for calculating sample sizes. Readers are referred to Gad (62) for a more detailed presentation.

Toxicology Experimental Design

There are a number of aspects of experimental design that are specific to the practice of toxicology. Before we look at a suggestion for step-by-step development of experimental designs, these aspects should first be considered as follows:

1. Frequently, the data gathered from specific measurements of animal characteristics are such that there is wide variability in the data. Often, such wide variability is not present in a control or low-dose group, but in an intermediate dosage group, variance inflation may occur (i.e., there may be a large SD associated with the measurements from this intermediate group). In the face of such a set of data, the conclusion that there is no biological effect based on a finding of no statistically significant effect might well be erroneous.
2. In designing experiments, a toxicologist should keep in mind the potential effect of involuntary censoring on sample size. In other words, though the study described in Example 1 might start with five rabbits per group, this provides no margin should any die before the study is ended and blood samples are collected and analyzed. Including just enough experimental units per group frequently leaves too few at the end of a study to allow meaningful statistical analysis, and allowances should be made accordingly in establishing group sizes.
3. It is certainly possible to pool the data from several identical toxicological studies. For example, after first having performed an acute inhalation study where only three treatment group animals survived to the point at which a critical measure (such as analysis of blood samples) was performed, we would not have enough data to perform a meaningful statistical analysis. We could then repeat the protocol with new control and treatment group animals from the same source. At the end, after assuring ourselves that the two sets of data are comparable, we could combine (or pool) the data from survivors of the second study with those from the first. The costs of this approach, however, would then be both a greater degree of effort expended (than if we had performed a single study with larger groups) and increased variability in the pooled samples (decreasing the power of our statistical methods).
4. Another frequently overlooked design option in toxicology is the use of an unbalanced design (i.e., of different group sizes for differential levels of treatment). There is no requirement that each group in a study (control, low dose, intermediate dose, high dose) have an equal number of experimental units assigned to it. Indeed, there frequently are good reasons to assign more experimental units to one group than to others, and, as we shall see later in this chapter, all of the major statistical methodologies have provisions to adjust for such inequalities, within certain limits. The two most common uses of the unbalanced design have larger groups assigned to either the highest dose to compensate for losses due to possible deaths during the study, or to the lowest dose to give more sensitivity in detecting effects at levels close to an effect threshold (or more confidence to the assertion that no effect exists).
5. We frequently are confronted with the situation where an undesired variable is influencing our experimental results in a nonrandom fashion. Such a variable is called a confounding variable. Its presence, as discussed earlier, makes the clear attribution and analysis of effects at best difficult and at worst impossible. Sometimes such confounding variables are the result of conscious design or management decisions, such as the use of different instruments, personnel, facilities, or procedures for different test groups within the same study. Occasionally, however, such confounding variables are the result of unintentional factors or actions, called a *lurking variable*. Examples of such variables almost always are the result of standard operating procedures being violated—water not being connected to a rack of animals over a

weekend, a set of racks not being cleaned as frequently as others, or a contaminated batch of feed being used.

6. Finally, some thought must be given to the clear definition of what is meant by experimental unit and concurrent control. The experimental unit in toxicology encompasses a wide variety of possibilities. It may be cells, plates of microorganisms, individual animals, litters of animals, etc. The importance of clearly defining the experiment unit is that the number of such units per group is the "N," which is used in statistical calculations or analyses and critically affects such calculations.

The experimental unit is the unit that receives treatments and yields a response that is measured and becomes a datum. What this means in practice is that, for example, in reproduction or teratology studies, where we treat the parental generation females and then determine results by counting or evaluating offspring, the experimental unit is still the parent. Therefore, the number of litters, not the number of offspring, is the N (162).

A true concurrent control is one that is identical in every manner with the treatment groups except for the treatment being evaluated. This means that all manipulations, including gavaging with equivalent volumes of vehicle or exposing to equivalent rates of air exchanges in an inhalation chamber, should be duplicated in control groups just as they occur in treatment groups.

The goal of the four principles of experimental design is statistical efficiency and the economizing of resources. The single most important initial step in achieving such an outcome is to clearly define the objective of the study—get a clear statement of what questions are being asked. For the reader who would like to further explore experimental design, there are a number of more detailed texts available that include more extensive treatments of the statistical aspects of experimental design (28,39,54,85,99,108).

GENERALIZED METHODOLOGY SELECTION

One approach for the selection of appropriate techniques to employ in a particular situation is to use a decision-tree method. Figure 7.1 is a decision tree that leads to the choice of one of three other trees to assist in technique selection, with each of the subsequent trees addressing one of the three functions of statistics that was defined earlier in this chapter. Figure 7.2 is for the selection of hypothesis-testing procedures, Figure 7.3 for modeling procedures, and Figure 7.4 for reduction of dimensionality procedures. For the vast majority of situations, these trees will guide the user into the choice of the proper technique. The tests and terms in these trees will be explained subsequently.

Computational Devices

The range, scope, and availability of aids for the calculation of mathematical techniques in general and for statistical techniques in particular have increased at an almost geometric rate since the mid-1970s. There is no longer any reason to use paper and pencil to perform such calculations; the capabilities of electronic systems are sufficiently developed at each level (as discussed later), and the cost, compared to labor savings, are minimal.

There are now three tiers of computational support available for statistical analysis (though it may be argued that the middle two tiers are becoming indistinguishable), and this chapter will attempt an overview of the major systems available within these tiers and the general

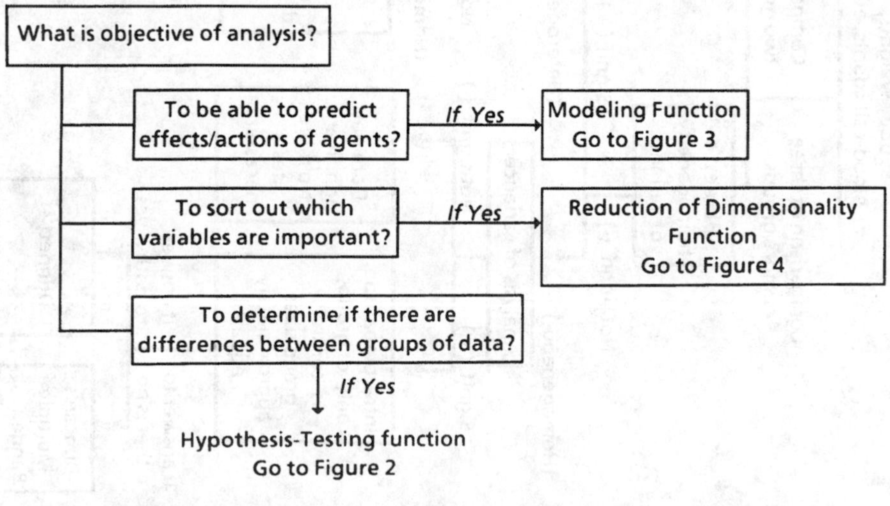

FIG. 7.1. Overall decision tree for selecting statistical procedures.

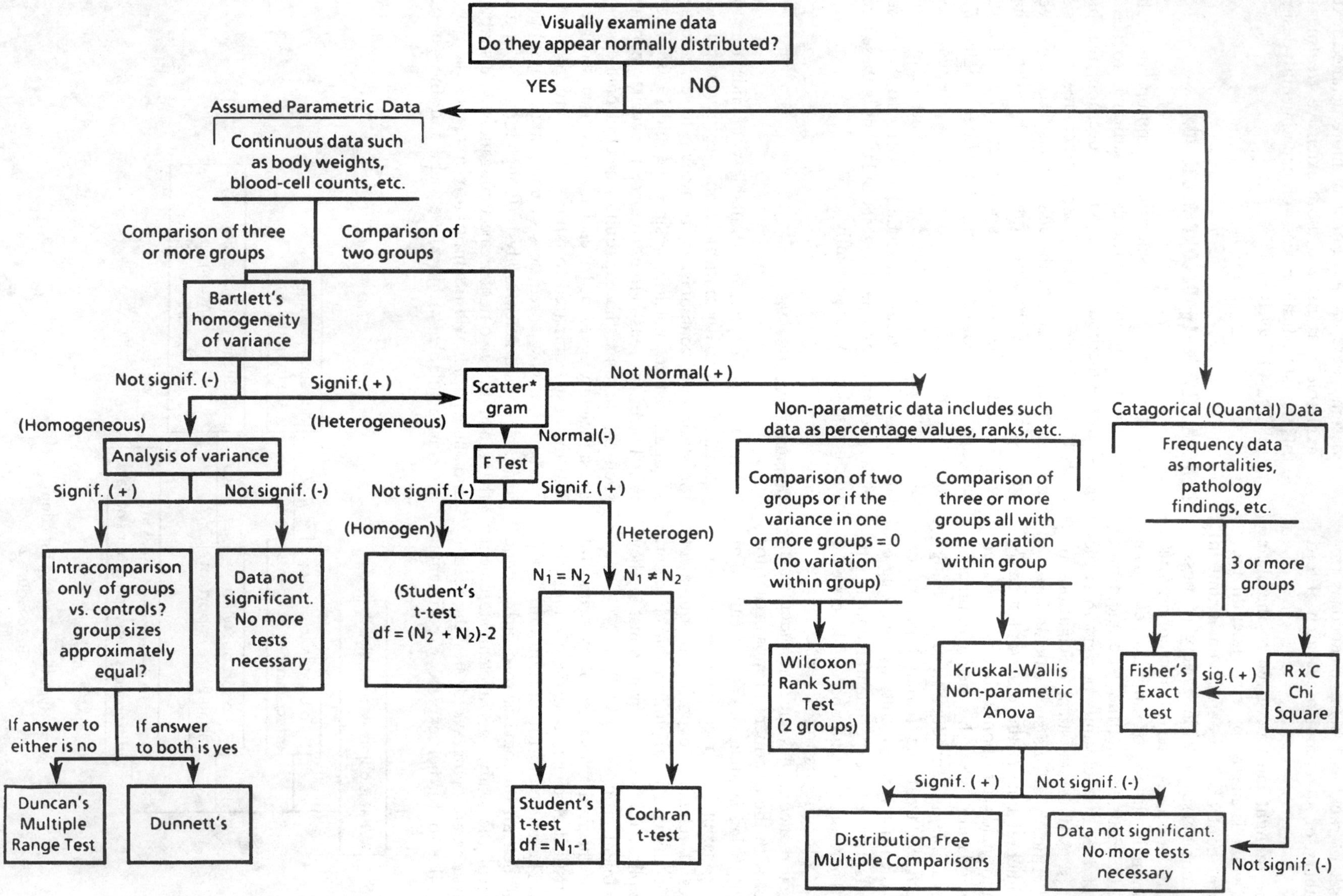

*If plot does not clearly demonstrate lack of normality exact tests may be employed.
– If continuous data, Kalmogorov–Smirnov test.
– If disconyinuous data, Chi-Square Goodness of Fit test may be used.

FIG. 7.2. Decision tree for selecting hypothesis-testing procedures.

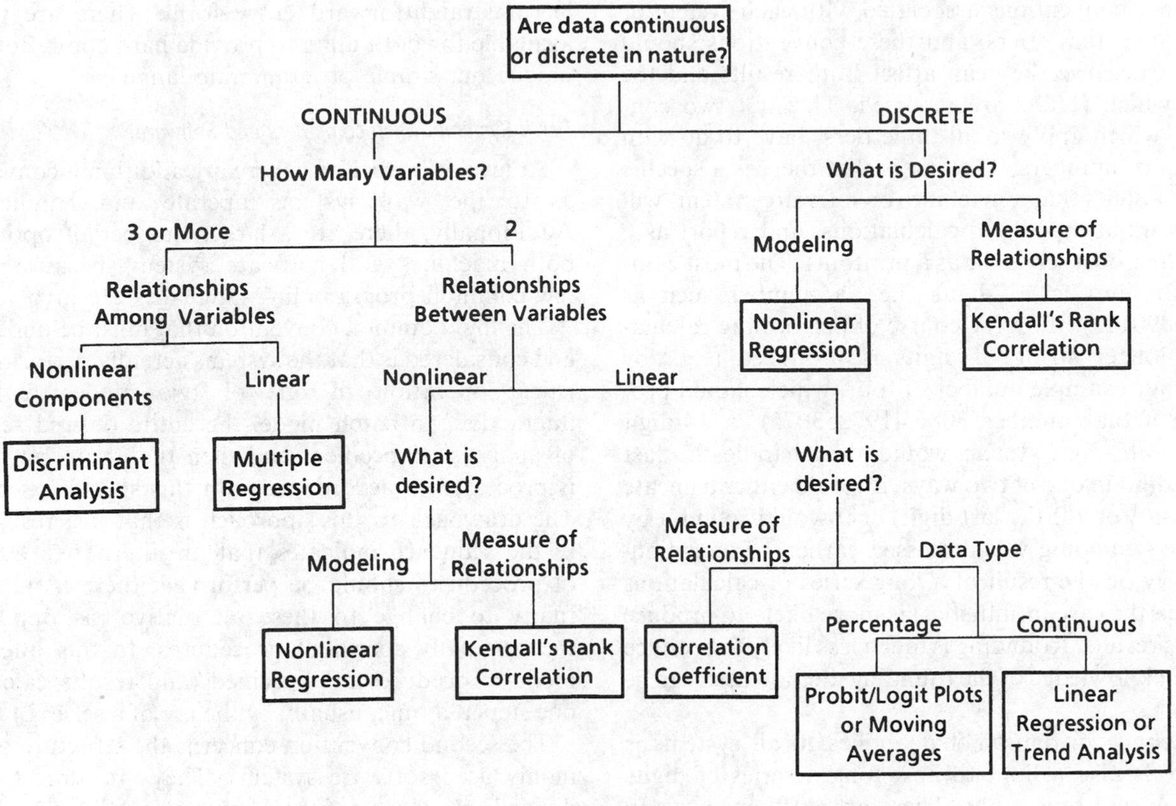

FIG. 7.3. Decision tree for selecting modeling procedures.

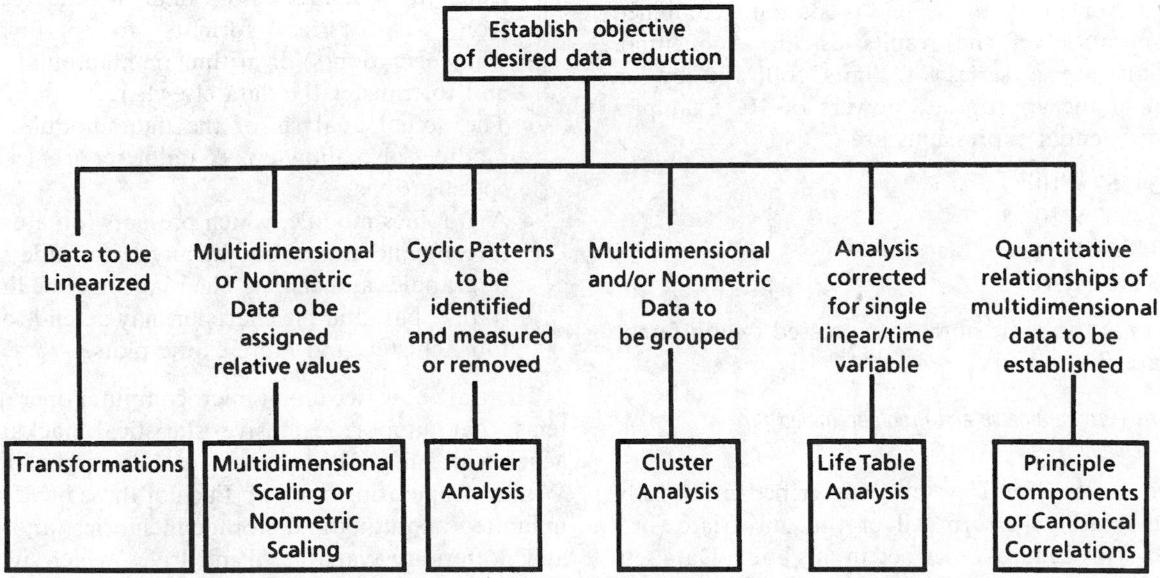

FIG. 7.4. Decision tree for selection of reduction of dimensionality procedures.

characteristics and limitations of each. The three tiers range from programmable calculators (which represent Tier I and include such devices as the Texas Instruments TI-83 and the Hewlett-Packard HP-41) to complete statistical packages available on mainframe computers (the Tier III systems, which include such packages as Statistical Analysis System [SAS], Statistical Package for Social Sciences [SPSS], and Minitab). As a general rule, as one goes from the systems in Tier 1 to those in Tier II, the cost, power, and capabilities of the systems increase, whereas ease of use ("user friendliness") and flexibility decrease.

There are conventions associated with each system or instrument in these tiers, and these conventions should be known because they can affect both results and the ways in which results are reported. The first two conventions, which apply to all three tiers, have to do with the length of numbers. The first is that there is a specific number of digits that a machine (or software system) will accept as input, handle in calculations, and report as a result (either on a screen or as a printout). The most common such limit is 13 digits (i.e., a number such as 12325.67890123). If, in the course of performing calculations, a longer string of digits is produced (e.g., by dividing our example number of four, which should produce the actual number 3086.4197253075), a 14-digit number, a 13-digit system would then handle the last ('extra") digit in one of two ways: it would either truncate it (i.e., just drop off the last digit) or it would round it by some rule (rounding was discussed earlier). Truncation, particularly on the result of a long series of calculations (as is often the case in statistics) is more likely to produce erroneous results. Rounding is much less likely to produce errors, but knowledge of the rounding method used can be helpful.

The second convention that applies to all systems is that there is also a limit to how long a series of digits any system will report out. There are different ways in which systems report out, and there are different ways in which systems report longer digit series. The first, less common, is truncation; the second is rounding combined with presentation of the results as an exponential. Exponentials are a series of digits followed by an expression of the appropriate powers of 10. Examples of such exponential expressions are

(a) 1.234567×10^{16}
(b) 1.234567×10^{-16}
(c) 1.234567 E 16
(d) 1.234567 E-16

(a) and (c) are the same number expressed two different ways, as are (b) and (d).

Tier I Systems (Programmable and Preprogrammed Statistical Calculators)

The two major Tier I systems (described more fully below) can readily perform all of the univariate (i.e., two variable) procedures described in this book. Data sets may also be stored, and by the clever coding of programs and data sets of extreme length may be processed, but longer programs or longer data sets run extremely slowly. Accordingly, use of these instruments is limited, in practice, to univariate procedures and small data sets.

The two Tier I systems are the Texas Instruments TI-83 and the Hewlett-Packard HP-41. These differ mainly in that the HP programs and data entry systems are in reverse Polish notation (RPN) form, whereas the TI has a straightforward entry form. There are printers available for both units to provide hard copy. Both have unique but simple programming languages.

Tier II Systems (Microcomputers and Software)

At levels above Tier I there are additional conventions as to the way systems operate and handle data. Additionally, there are a larger number of options for both machines and software systems because only a few common programming languages are involved.

The first common convention that must be understood and considered is that the systems actually perform a statistical operation in one of two modes: batch or interactive. In batch mode, the entire desired sequence of analysis is specified, and then the entire set of data is processed in accordance with this specified sequence. The drawback to this approach is that if a result early in the sequence indicates that an alternative latter set of procedures should be performed, there is no opportunity to change to these alternative (as opposed to the originally specified) procedures. In this interactive mode, procedures are specified (and results calculated) one step at a time, usually by the use of a series of menus.

The second convention concerns the structure of commonly used software systems. They are almost always divided into three separate parts or modules:

- A database manager, which allows the person using the system to store data in (and recall it from) a desired format, to perform a transformation(s) or arithmetic manipulation(s), and to transfer the data elsewhere.
- The actual analysis of the data module. Such modules also allow one to tailor reports to one's specifications.
- A graphics module, which presents (on a display screen) and prints out in any of a wide range of graphics and charts. The range may be limited to line, bar, and pie charts or may extend to contour, cluster, and more exotic plots.

There are now two major microcomputer operating systems that support extensive statistical packages: the Macintosh and IBM/clone (usually some form of Windows operating system). Each of these have virtually unlimited operating and storage memories, and printers and plotters are available. "Zip" drives, which significantly expand working memory, are also available for both.

Before reviewing software packages, several considerations should be presented. First, systems perform in one of two modes, either as libraries of programs, each of which can be selected to perform an individual procedure, or as an integrated system, where a single loading of the file allows access to each and every procedure. In the first mode, each step in an analysis (such as Bartlett's test, analysis of variance, and Duncan's multiple range test) requires loading a separate file and then executing the procedure. Second, software may load from CD-ROMs or Zip drive media. Third, the available range of transformations should be carefully considered. At least a small number (log, reciprocal, probit, addition, subtraction, multiplication, division, and absolute value) is essential. If unusual data sets are to be handled or exploratory data analysis (discussed later) performed regularly, a more extensive set is required. Fourth, all of the packages listed in Table 7.4 have at least a basic set of capabilities. They can each perform, besides database management and basic transformation and graphic functions, the following simple tests:

- Analysis of Variance (ANOVA)
- 2 × 2 Chi Square
- Linear Regressions
- Student's t-Test

Table 7.4 presents an overview of 12 widely available commercially statistical packages for microcomputers that the author is familiar with; there are at least 120 additional packages available. Woodward et al. (168) presents an overview of many of these. For each package, the following information is presented:

TITLE—the name of the package.
OPERATING SYSTEMS—which systems the package will operate on
EDA—does the system perform exploratory data analysis?
GRAPHICS—how extensive are the graphic functions that the package performs?
SPREADSHEET IMPORT/EXPORT—can the system accept data-give output to popular spreadsheets such as EXCEL and LOTUS?
MENU (M) OR COMMAND (C) DRIVEN—how does the user primarily interface with the system?

Tier III Systems (Main Frame Programs)

The Tier III system programs are all large commercial software packages that run on large computer systems on a time-sharing basis. By definition, this means that these programs operate in a batch mode and use a unique (for each package) code language. Four of these libraries are briefly described below.

PACKAGE	REFERENCE	DESCRIPTION
SPSS	113	With manipulation, SPSS will perform all the procedures described in this book and the full range of graphics.
BMD	41	Has generally wider capabilities than SPSS (which are constantly being added to) and easily manipulated.
SAS	127	Widely available. Easier to format and very strong on data summarization. Has its own higher-level programming language.
MINITAB	125	Easiest to use and least expensive of these six, but does not have the full range of capabilities.

The difficulty with the recently achieved, wide availability of automated analysis systems is that it has become increasingly easy to perform the wrong tests on the wrong data and from there to proceed to the wrong conclusions. This serves to make at least a basic understanding of the procedures and discipline of statistics a vital necessity for the research toxicologist.

Methods for Data Examination and Preparation

The data from toxicology studies should always be examined before any formal analysis. Such examinations should be directed to determining if the data are suitable for analysis, and if so, what form the analysis should take (see Figure 7.2). If the data as collected are not suitable for analysis or if they are only suitable for low-powered analytical techniques, one may wish to use one of many forms of data transformation to change the data characteristics so that they are more amenable to analysis.

The above two objectives, data examination and preparation, are the primary focus of this chapter. For data examination, two major techniques are presented—the scattergram and Bartlett's test. Likewise, for data preparation (with the issues of rounding and outliers having been addressed in a previous chapter), two techniques are presented—randomization (including a test for randomness in a sample of data) and transformation. Exploratory data analysis (EDA) is presented and briefly reviewed later. This is a broad collection of techniques and approaches to "probe" data (i.e., to both examine and to perform some initial, flexible analysis of the data).

Scattergram

Two of the major points to be made throughout this chapter are (a) the use of the appropriate statistical tests and (b) the effects of small sample sizes (as is often the case in toxicology) on our selection of statistical techniques. Frequently, simple examination of the nature and distribution of data collected from a study can also suggest patterns and results that were unanticipated

Table 7.4
Popular microcomputer statistical packages

Title	Operating Systems	EDA Performed	Graphics	Spreadsheet Import/Export	Menu(M) or Command(C) Driven
BMD8	Windows	No	Largely	Limited	C
DATA DESK	Mac Windows	Yes	Complete	Full	M
E CHIP	Windows	No	Largely	Limited	M
JMP	Windows Mac	Yes	Largely	Largely	M
NCSS	Windows	Yes	Complete	Full	M
SAS/STAT	MSDOS Windows	Yes	Complete	Full	C
SPSS/PC	MSDOS Windows	No	Complete	Full	C
STAT/MOST	Windows	Yes	Complete	Full	M
STATISTICA	Windows Mac	Yes	Complete	Full	M
STATVIEW	Mac Windows	Yes	Complete	Full	M
STATXALT	Windows	Yes	Complete	Full	M
SYSTAT	Windows	No	Complete	Full	C

and for which the use of additional or alternative statistical methodology is warranted. It was these three points that caused the author to consider a section on scattergrams and their use essential for toxicologists.

Bartlett's test may be used to determine if the values in groups of data are homogeneous. If they are, this (along with the knowledge that they are from a continuous distribution) demonstrates that parametric methods are applicable, but, if the values in the (continuous data) groups fail Bartlett's tests (i.e., are heterogeneous), we cannot be secure in our belief that parametric methods are appropriate until we gain some confidence that the values are normally distributed. With large groups of data, we can compute parameters of the population (kurtosis and skewness, in particular), and from these parameters determine if the population is normal (with a certain level of confidence). If our concern is especially marked, we can use a chi-square goodness-of-fit test for normality, but when each group of data consists of 25 or fewer values, these measures or tests (kurtosis, skewness, chi-square goodness-of-fit) are not accurate indicators of normality. Instead, in these cases we should prepare a scattergram of the data and then evaluate the scattergram to estimate if the data are normally distributed. This procedure consists of developing a histogram of the data and then examining the histogram to get a visual appreciation of the location and distribution of the data.

The abscissa (or horizontal scale) should be in the same scale as the values and should be divided so that the entire range of observed values is covered by the scale of the abscissa. Across such a scale we then simply enter symbols of each of our values. Example 2 shows such a plot.

Example 2

Suppose we have the two data sets below:

Group 1: 4.5, 5.4, 5.9, 6.0, 6.4, 6.5, 6.9, 7.0, 7.1, 7.0, 7.4, 7.5, 7.5, 7.5, 7.6., 8.0, 8.1, 8.4, 8.5, 8.6, 9.0, 9.4, 9.5, and 10.4.

Group 2: 4.0, 4.5, 5.0, 5.1, 5.4, 5.5, 5.6, 6.5, 6.5, 7.0, 7.4, 7.5, 7.5, 8.0, 8.1, 8.5, 8.5, 9.0, 9.1, 9.5, 9.5, 10.1, 10.0, and 10.4.

Both of these groups contain 24 values and cover the same range. From them we can prepare the following scattergrams.

Group 1

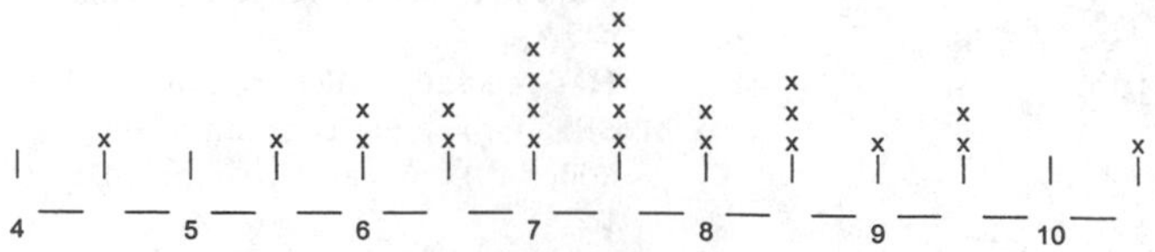

Group 2

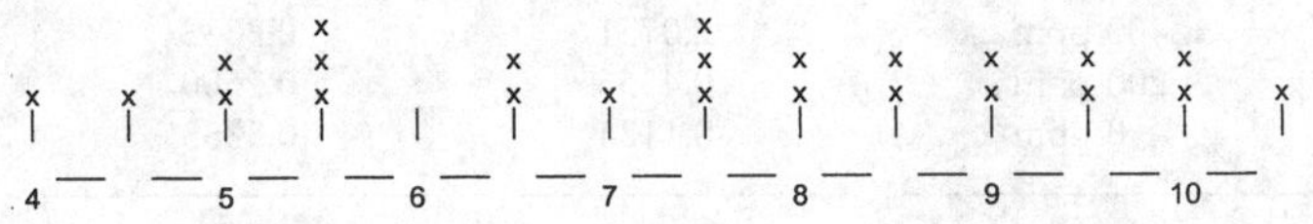

Group 1 can be seen to approximate a normal distribution (bell-shaped curve); we can proceed to perform the appropriate parametric tests with such data, but group 2 clearly does not appear to be normally distributed. In this case, the appropriate nonparametric technique must be used.

Example 2 is a traditional and rather limited form of scatterplot, but such plots can reveal significant information about the amount and types of association between the two variables, the existence and nature of outliers, the clustering of data, and a number of other two-dimensional factors (7,23).

Current technology allows us to add significantly more graphical information to scatterplots by means of graphic symbols (letters, faces, or different shapes, such as squares, colors, etc.) for the plotted data points. One relatively simple example of this approach is shown in Figure 7.5, where the simple case of dose (in a dermal study), dermal irritation, and white blood cell count are presented. This graph quite clearly suggests that as dose (variable x) is increased, dermal irritation (variable y) also increases, and as irritation becomes more severe, white blood cell count (variable z), an indicator of immune system involvement suggesting infection or persistent inflammation, also increases. There is no direct association of variables x and z, however.

Cleveland and McGill (25) presented an excellent, detailed overview of the expanded capabilities of the scatterplot, and the interested reader should refer to that article. Cleveland expanded this to a book (26). Tufte (145) has also expanded on this.

Bartlett's Test for Homogeneity of Variance

Bartlett's test (138) is used to compare the variances (values reflecting the degree of variability in data sets) among three or more groups of data, where the data in the groups are continuous sets (such as body weights, organ weights, red blood cells counts, or diet consumption measurements). It is expected that such data will be suitable for parametric methods (normality of data is assumed), and Bartlett's is frequently used as a test for the assumption of equivalent variances.

Bartlett's is based on the calculation of the corrected χ^2 (chi-square) value by the formula

$$\chi^2_{corr} = 2.3026 \frac{\sum df\left(\log_{10}\left[\frac{\sum[df(S^2)]}{\sum df}\right]\right) - \sum[df(\log_{10} S^2)]}{1 + \frac{1}{3(K-1)}\left[\sum \frac{1}{df} - \frac{1}{\sum df}\right]},$$

where $S^2 = \text{variance} = \frac{{}^{n}\sum x^2 - \frac{(\sum x)^2}{n}}{n-1}$,

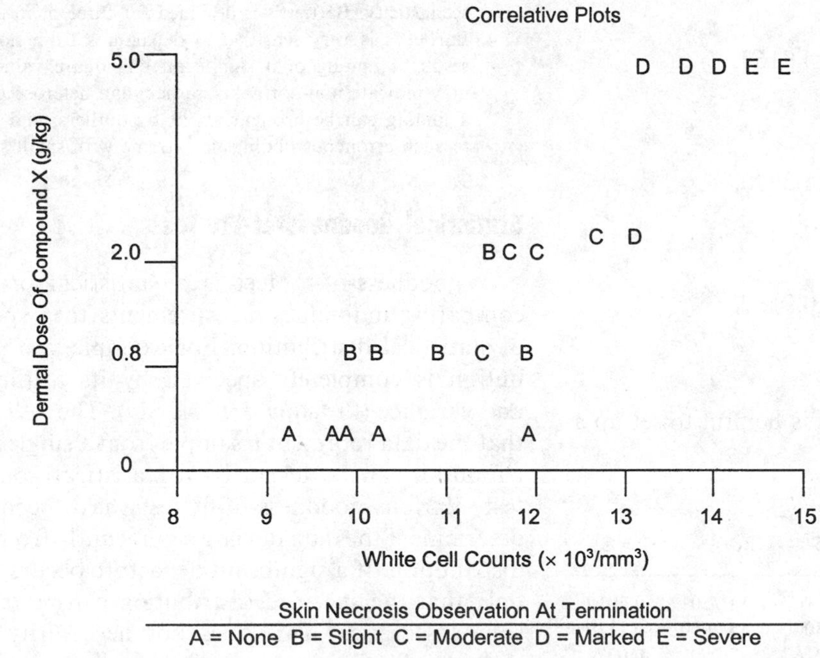

FIG. 7.5. Exploratory data analysis.

X = individual datum within each group;
n = number of data within each group;
K = number of groups being compared;
df = degrees of freedom for each group = (N − 1).

The corrected χ^2 value yielded by the above calculations is compared to the values listed in the chi square table according to the numbers of degrees of freedom (such as found in ref. 137, pp. 470–471).

If the calculated value is smaller than the table value at the selected p level (traditionally 0.05), the groups are accepted to be homogeneous and the use of ANOVA is assumed proper. If the calculated χ^2 is greater than the table value, the groups are heterogeneous and other tests (as indicated in Figure 7.2, the decision tree) are necessary. This is demonstrated in Example 3.

Example 3

If the monocytes in a sample of rat blood taken in the course of an inhalation study were counted, the results might appear as follows:

400 ppm		200 ppm		0 ppm	
(X_1)	$(X_1)^2$	(X_2)	$(X_2)^2$	(X_3)	$(X_3)^2$
9	81	5	25	7	49
5	25	5	25	6	36
5	25	4	16	5	25
4	16	6	36	7	49
		7	49		
$\Sigma X_1 = 23$	$\Sigma X_1^2 = 147$	$\Sigma X_2 = 27$	$\Sigma X_2^2 = 151$	$\Sigma X_3 = 25$	$\Sigma X_3^2 = 159$

$$ {}^2_1 = \frac{\dfrac{4(147) - (23)^2}{4}}{4 - 1} = 4.9167, $$

$$ {}^2_2 = \frac{\dfrac{5(157) - (27)^2}{5}}{5 - 1} = 1.3000, $$

$$ {}^2_3 = \frac{\dfrac{4(159) - (25)^2}{4}}{4 - 1} = 0.9167. $$

In continuing the calculations, it is helpful to set up a table as follows:

Concentration	n	*df* = (N − 1)	S^2	(*df*)(S^2)	log S^2
400 ppm	4	3	4.9167	14.7501	0.6917
200 ppm	5	4	1.3000	5.2000	0.1139
0 ppm	4	3	0.9167	2.7501	−0.0378
Sums (Σ)	13	10		22.7002	

Concentration	(*df*)(log S^2)	$\frac{1}{\text{df}}$
400 ppm	2.0751	0.3333
200 ppm	0.4556	0.2500
0 ppm	−0.1134	0.3333
Sums (Σ)	2.4173	0.9166

Now we substitute into our original formula for corrected χ^2

$$ \chi^2 = 2.3026 \frac{10\left[\log_{10}\left(\dfrac{22.7002}{10}\right)\right] - 2.4173}{\dfrac{1}{3(3-1)}\left(0.9166 - \dfrac{1}{10}\right)} $$

$$ = 2.3026 \frac{10(0.3560) - 2.4173}{1 + 0.1667(0.8166)} $$

$$ = 2.32. $$

The table value for two degrees of freedom at the 0.05 level is 5.99. As our calculated value is less than this, the corrected χ^2 is not significant and the variances are accepted as homogeneous. We may thus use parametric methods (such as ANOVA) for further comparisons.

ASSUMPTIONS AND LIMITATIONS

1. Bartlett's test does not test for normality, but rather homogeneity of variance (also called equality of variances or homoscedasticity).
2. Homoscedasticity is an important assumption for Student's t-test, analysis of variance, and analysis of covariance.
3. The F-test (covered in the next chapter) is actually a test for the two-sample (i.e., control and one test group) case of homoscedasticity. Bartlett's is designed for three or more samples.
4. Bartlett's is very sensitive to departures from normality. As a result, a finding of a significant chi-square value in Bartlett's may indicate non-normality rather than heteroscedasticity. Such a finding can be brought about by outliers, and the sensitivity to such erroneous findings is extreme with small sample sizes.

Statistical Goodness-of-Fit Tests

A goodness-of-fit test is a statistical procedure for comparing individual measurements to a specified type of statistical distribution. For example, a normal distribution is completely specified by its arithmetic mean and variance (the square of the SD). The null hypothesis, that the data represent a sample from a single normal distribution, can be tested by a statistical goodness-of-fit test. Various goodness-of-fit tests have been devised to determine if the data deviate significantly from a specified distribution. If a significant departure occurs, it indicates only that the specified distribution can be rejected with some assurance. This does not necessarily mean that the true distribution contains two or more subpopulations. The true distribution may be a single distribution based on a different mathematical relationship (e.g., log-normal). In the latter case, logarithms of the measurement would not be expected to exhibit by a goodness-of-fit test a statistically significant departure from a log-normal distribution.

Everitt and Hand (51) recommended using a sample of 200 or more to conduct a valid analysis of mixtures of populations. Even the maximum likelihood method, the best available method, should be used with extreme caution, or not at all, when separation between the means of the subpopulations is less than 3 SD and sample sizes are less than 300. None of the available methods conclusively establish bimodality, which may occur when separation between the two means (modes) exceeds 2 SD. Conversely, inflections in probits or separations in histograms *less than* 2 SD apart may arise from genetic differences in test subjects.

Mendal et al. (106) compared eight tests of normality to detect a mixture consisting of two normally distributed components with different means but equal variances. Fisher's skewness statistic was preferable when one component comprised less than 15% of the total distribution. When the two components comprised more nearly equal proportions (35%–65%) of the total distribution, the Engelman and Hartigan test (50) was preferable. For other mixing proportions, the maximum likelihood ratio test was best. Thus, the maximum likelihood ratio test appears to perform very well, with only small loss from optimality, even when it is not the best procedure.

The method of *maximum likelihood* provides estimators that usually are quite satisfactory. They have the desirable properties of being consistent, asymptotically normal, and asymptotically efficient for large samples under quite general conditions. Often they are biased, but the bias is frequently removable by a simple adjustment (Examples 4 and 5). Other methods of obtaining estimators are also available, but the maximum likelihood method is the most frequently used.

Maximum likelihood estimators also have another desirable property: *invariance*. Let us denote the maximum likelihood estimator of the parameter θ by $\hat{\sigma}$. Then, if $f(\theta)$ is a single-valued function of θ, the maximum likelihood estimator of $f(\theta)$ is $f(\hat{\sigma})$. Thus, for example, $\hat{\sigma} = (\hat{\sigma}^2)^{1/2}$.

The principle of maximum likelihood tells us that we should use as our estimate that value which maximizes the likelihood of the observed event. The following examples demonstrate the technique.

Example 4

Derive the maximum likelihood estimator p of the binomial probability p for a coin-tossing experiment in which a coin is tossed n times and r heads are obtained.

We know that the likelihood of the observed event is

$$L = \binom{n}{r} p^r (1-p)^{n-r}.$$

According to the principle of maximum likelihood, we choose the value of p which maximizes L. This value also maximizes

$$\text{In}\, L = \ln\binom{n}{r} + r\ln p + (n-r)\ln(1-p).$$

At the maximum, the derivative with respect to p must be zero; that is,

$$\frac{\partial}{\partial \rho}\text{In}\, L = r/p - (n-r)/\ln(1-p) = 0$$

and

$$\hat{p} = r/n.$$

Example 5

A sample of n observations $x_1, \ldots, x_n$ is drawn from a normal population. Derive the maximum likelihood estimators $\hat{\mu}$ and $\hat{\sigma}_2$ for the mean and variance of the population. The likelihood of the observed event is

$$L = \left[\frac{1}{\sigma(2\pi)\frac{1}{2}}\exp\left\{-\frac{1}{2}\left(\frac{x_1-\mu}{\sigma}\right)^2\right\}\right]$$

$$\times \Lambda\left[\frac{1}{\sigma(2\pi)\frac{1}{2}}\exp\left\{-\frac{1}{2}\left(\frac{x_n-\mu}{\sigma}\right)^2\right\}\right].$$

According to the principle of maximum likelihood, we choose those values of μ and σ^2 which maximize L. The same values maximize $\ln L$. So we equate the partial derivatives of $\ln L$ with respect to $\hat{\mu}$ and $\hat{\sigma}^2$ to zero and find that

$$\hat{\mu} = \bar{x}-$$

and

$$\hat{\sigma}^2 = \frac{1}{n}\sum_{i=1}^{n}(x_i - \bar{x})^2.$$

The latter estimator is slightly biased, but the bias can be removed by multiplying by $n/(n-1)$ and using the estimator

$$\hat{\sigma}^2 \frac{1}{n-1}\sum_{i=1}^{n}(x_i - \bar{x})^2.$$

These maximum likelihood methods can be used to obtain *point estimates* of a parameter, but we must remember that a point estimator is a random variable distributed in some way around the true value of the parameter. The true parameter value may be higher or lower than our estimate. It is often useful, therefore, to obtain an interval within which we are reasonably confident the true value will lie, and the generally accepted method is to construct what are known as *confidence limits*.

The following procedure will yield upper and lower 95% confidence limits with the property that when we say that these limits include the true value of the parameter, 95% of all such statements will be true and 5% will be incorrect:

1. Choose a (test) statistic involving the unknown parameter and no other unknown parameter.
2. Place the appropriate sample values in the statistic.
3. Obtain an equation for the unknown parameter by equating the test statistic to the upper 2.5% point of the relevant distribution.
4. The solution of the equation gives one limit.
5. Repeat the process with the lower 2.5% point to obtain the other limit.

One can also construct 95% confidence intervals using unequal tails (e.g., using the upper 2% point and the lower 3% point). We usually want our confidence interval to be as short as possible, however, and with a symmetric distribution such as the normal or t, this is achieved using equal tails. The same procedure very nearly minimizes the confidence interval with other nonsymmetric distributions (e.g., chi-square) and has the advantage of avoiding rather tedious computation.

When the appropriate statistic involves the square of the unknown parameter, both limits are obtained by equating the statistic to the upper 5% point of the relevant distribution. The use of two tails in this situation would result in a pair of nonintersecting intervals. When two or more parameters are involved, it is possible to construct a region within which we are reasonably confident the true parameter values will lie. Such regions are referred to as confidence regions. The implied interval for p_1 does not form a 95% confidence interval, however, nor is it true than an 85.7375% confidence region for p_1, p_2, and p_3 can be obtained by considering the intersection of the three separate 95% confidence intervals because the statistics used to obtain the individual confidence intervals are not independent. This problem is obvious with a multiparameter distribution, such as the multinomial, but it even occurs with the normal distribution because the statistic that we use to obtain a confidence interval for the mean and the statistic that we use to obtain a confidence interval for the variance are not independent. The problem is not likely to be of great concern unless a large number of parameters is involved, as illustrated in Example 6.

Example 6

A sample of nine is drawn from a normal population with unknown mean and variance. The sample mean is 4.2 and the sample variance is 1.69. Obtain a 95% confidence interval for the mean μ. The confidence limits are obtained from the equations

$$\sqrt{9}(4.2 - \mu)/(1.69)^{1/2} = 2.306;$$

$$\sqrt{9}(4.2 - \mu)/(1.69)^{1/2} = -2.306.$$

From these we determine that the 95% confidence interval is from 3.2 to 5.2.

Randomization

Randomization is the act of assigning a number of items (plates of bacteria or test animals, for example) to groups in such a manner that there is an equal chance for any one item to end up in any one group. This is a control against any possible bias in assignment of subjects to test groups. A variation on this is censored randomization, which ensures that the groups are equivalent in some aspect after the assignment process is complete. The most common example of a censored randomization is one in which it is ensured that the body weights of test animals in each group are not significantly different from those in the other groups. This is done by analyzing group weights both for homogeneity of variance and by analysis of variance after animal assignment, then re-randomizing if there is a significant difference at some nominal level, such as $p \leq 0.10$. The process is repeated until there is no significant difference.

There are several methods for actually performing the randomization process. The three most commonly used are card assignment, use of a random number table, and use of a computerized algorithm.

For the card-based method, individual identification numbers for items (plates or animals, for example) are placed on separate index cards. These cards are then shuffled, placed one at a time in succession into piles corresponding to the required test groups. The results are a random group assignment.

The random number table method requires only that one have unique numbers assigned to test subjects and access to a random number table. One simply sets up a table with a column for each group to which subjects are to be assigned. We start from the head of any one column of numbers in the random table (each time the table is used, a new starting point should be used). If our test subjects number less than 100, we use only the last two digits in each random number in the table. If they number more than 99 but less than 1000, we use only the last three digits. To generate group assignments, we read down a column one number at a time. As we come across digits that correspond to a subject number, we assign that subject to a group (enter its identifying number in a column), proceeding to assign subjects to groups from left to right filling one row at a time. After a number is assigned to an animal, any duplication of its unique number is ignored. We use as many successive columns of random numbers as we may need to complete the process.

The third (and now most common) method is to use a random number generator that is built into a calculator or computer program. Procedures for generating these are generally documented in user manuals.

One is also occasionally required to evaluate whether a series of numbers (such as an assignment of animals to test groups) is random. This requires the use of a randomization test, of which there are a large variety. The chi-square test, described later, can be used to evaluate the goodness-of-fit to a random assignment. If the result is not critical, a simple sign test will work. For the sign test, we first determine the middle value in the numbers being checked for randomness. We then go through a list of the numbers assigned to each group, scoring each as a "+" (greater than our middle number) or "–" (less than our middle number). The number of pluses and minuses in each group should be approximately equal. This is demonstrated in Example 7.

Example 7

In auditing a study performed at a contract lab, we wish to ensure that their assignment of animals to test groups was random. Thirty-three animals numbered 1 to 33 were assigned to groups of 11 animals each. Using the middle value in this series (17) as our check point, we assign signs as below.

Control		Test Group A		Test Group B	
Animal Number	Sign	Animal Number	Sign	Animal Number	Sign
17	0	18	+	11	–
14	–	1	–	2	–
7	–	12	–	22	+
26	+	9	–	28	+
21	+	5	–	19	+
15	–	20	+	3	–
16	–	33	+	29	+
6	–	27	+	10	–
25	+	8	–	23	+
32	+	24	+	30	+
4	–	31	+	13	–
Sum of signs	–2		+1		+1

Note that 17 is scored as zero, ensuring (as a check on results) that the sum of the sums of the three columns would be zero. The results in this case clearly demonstrate that there is no systematic bias in animal number assignments.

Transformations

If our initial inspection of a data set reveals it to have an unusual or undesired set of characteristics (or to lack a desired set of characteristics), we have a choice of three courses of action. We may proceed to select a method or test appropriate to this new set of conditions, or abandon the entire exercise, or transform the variable(s) under consideration in such a manner that the resulting transformed variates (X′ and Y′, for example, as opposed to the original variates X and Y) meet the assumptions or have the characteristics that are desired.

The key to all this is that scale of measurement of most (if not all) variables is arbitrary. Although we are most familiar with a linear scale of measurement, there is nothing that makes this the "correct" scale on its own, as opposed to a logarithmic scale (familiar logarithmic measurements are that of pH values, or earthquake intensity (Richter scale)). Transforming a set of data (converting X to X′) is really as simple as changing a scale of measurement.

There are at least four good reasons to transform data:

(1) To normalize the data, making them suitable for analysis by our most common parametric techniques, such as analysis of variance (ANOVA). A simple test of whether a selected transformation will yield a distribution of data which satisfies the underlying assumptions for ANOVA is to plot the cumulative distribution of samples on probability paper (i.e., a commercially available paper that has the probability function scale as one axis). One can then alter the scale of the second axis (i.e., the axis other than the one that is on a probability scale) from linear to any other (logarithmic, reciprocal, square root, etc.) and see if a previously curved line indicating a skewed distribution becomes linear to indicate normality. The slope of the transformed line gives us an estimate of the SD, and if the slopes of the lines of several samples or groups of data are similar, we accordingly know that the variance of the different groups are homogeneous.

(2) To linearize the relationship between a paired set of data, such as dose and response. This is the most common use in toxicology for transformations and is demonstrated in the section under probit/logit plots.

Table 7.5
Common Data Transformations

Transformation	How Calculated[a]	Example of Use
Arithmetic	$x' = \frac{x}{y}$ or $x' = x + c$	Organ weight/body weight
Reciprocals	$x' = \frac{1}{x}$	Linearizing data, particularly rate phenomena
Arcsine (also called Angular)	$x' = \text{arcsine } \sqrt{x}$	Normalizing dominant lethal and mutation rate data
Logarithmic	$x' = \log x$	pH values
Probability (Probit)	$x' = \text{probability } X$	Percentage responding
Square roots	$x' = \sqrt{x}$	Surface area of animal from body weights
Box cox	$x' = (x^v - 1)v$: for $v \neq 0$; $x' = \ln x$: for $v = 0$	A family of transforms for use when one has no prior knowledge of the appropriate transformation to use
Rank transformations	Depends on nature of samples	As a bridge between parametric and nonparametric statistics (174)

[a] x and y are original variables, x′ and y′ transformed values. "C" stands for a constant.
Note: Plotting a double reciprocal (that is, $\frac{1}{x}$ versus $\frac{1}{y}$) will linearize almost any data set. So will plotting the log transforms of a set of variables.

(3) To adjust data for the influence of another variable. This is an alternative in some situations to the more complicated process of analysis of covariance. A ready example of this usage is the calculation of organ weight to body weight ratios in in vivo toxicity studies, with the resulting ratios serving as the raw data for an analysis of variance performed to identify possible target organs. This use is discussed in detail later in this chapter.

(4) Finally, to make the relationships between variables clearer by removing or adjusting for interactions with third, fourth, etc. Uncontrolled variables that influence the pair of variables of interest. This case is discussed in detail under time series analysis.

Common transformations are presented in Table 7.5.

Exploratory Data Analysis

Over the past 20 years, an entirely new approach has been developed to get the most information out of the increasingly larger and more complex data sets that scientists are faced with. This approach involves the use of a very diverse set of fairly simple techniques that comprise exploratory data analysis (EDA). As expounded by Tukey (148), there are four major ingredients to EDA:

Displays: These visually reveal the behavior of the data and suggest a framework for analysis. The scatterplot (presented earlier) is an example of this approach.

Residuals: These are what remain of a set of data after a fitted model (such as a linear regression) or some similar level of analysis has been removed.

Re-expressions: These involved questions of what scale would serve to best simplify and improve the analysis of the data. Simple transformations, such as those presented earlier in this chapter, are used to simplify data behavior (e.g., linearizing or normalizing) and clarify analysis.

Resistance: This is a matter of decreasing the sensitivity of analysis and summary of data to misbehavior so that the occurrence of a few outliers, for example, will not complicate or invalidate the methods used to analyze the data. For example, in summarizing the location of a set of data, the median (but not the arithmetic means) is highly resistant.

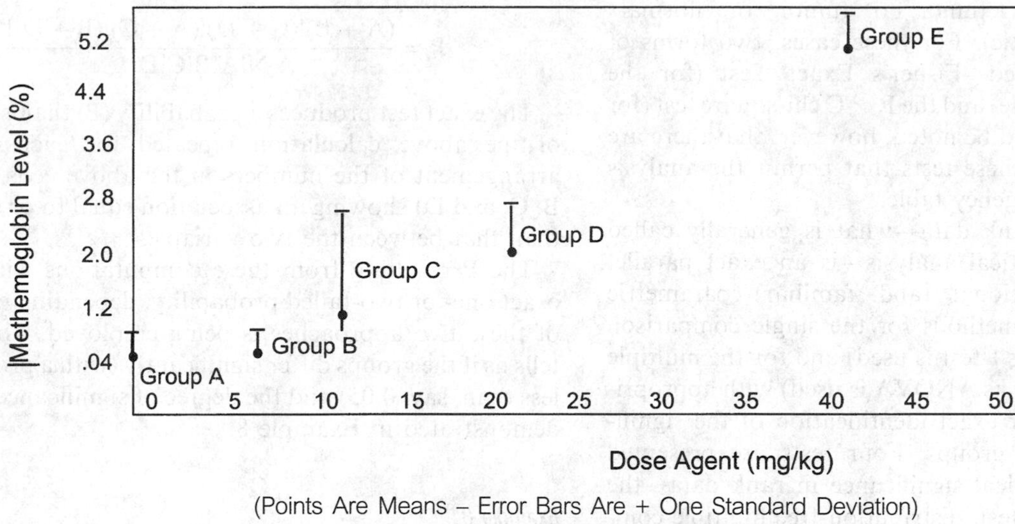

FIG. 7.6. Variance inflation.

These four ingredients are used in a process falling into two broad phases: an exploratory phase and a confirmatory phase. The exploratory phase isolates patterns in and features of the data and reveals them, allowing an inspection of the data before any firm choice of actual hypothesis testing or modeling methods has been made.

Confirmatory analysis allows evaluation of the reproducibility of the patterns or effects. Its role is close to that of classical hypothesis testing, but also often includes steps such as (a) incorporating information from an analysis of another closely related set of data, and (b) validating a result by assembling and analyzing additional data. These techniques are, in general, beyond the scope of this text; however, Velleman and Hoaglin (149) and Hoaglin et al. (86) present a clear overview of the more important methods, along with codes for their execution on a microcomputer (they have also now been incorporated into Minitab). A short examination of a single case of the use of these methods, however, is in order.

In the field of toxicology it has long been recognized that no population—animal or human—is completely uniform in its response to any particular toxicant. Rather, a population is composed of a (presumably normal) distribution of individuals, some resistant to intoxication (hyporesponders), the bulk that respond close to a central value (such as an LD_{50}), and some that are very sensitive to intoxication (hyperresponders). Taking advantage of this population distribution can, in fact, result in additional statistical techniques. The sensitivity of techniques such as ANOVA is reduced markedly by the occurrence of outliers (extreme high or low values, including hyper- and hyporesponders), which, in fact, serve to markedly inflate the variance (standard deviation) associated with a sample. Such variance inflation is particularly common in small groups that are exposed or dosed at just over or under a threshold level, causing a small number of individuals in the sample (who are more sensitive than the other members) to respond markedly. Such a situation is displayed in Figure 7.6, which plots the mean and standard deviations of methaemoglobin levels in a series of groups of animals exposed to successively higher levels of a hemolytic agent.

Though the mean level of methaemoglobin in group C is more than double that of the control group (A), no hypothesis test will show this difference to be significant because it has such a large SD associated with it. Yet this "inflated" variance exists because a single individual has such a marked response. The occurrence of the inflation is certainly an indicator that the data need to be examined closely. Indeed, all tabular data in toxicology should be visually inspected for both trend and variance inflation.

A concept related (but not identical) to resistance and exploratory data analysis is that of robustness. Robustness generally implies insensitivity to departures from assumptions surrounding an underlying model, such as normality.

In summarizing the location of data, the median, though highly resistant, is not extremely robust, but the mean is both nonresistant and nonrobust.

HYPOTHESIS TESTING OF CATEGORICAL AND RANKED DATA

Categorical (or contingency table) presentations of data can contain any single type of data, but generally the contents are collected and arranged so that they can be classified as belonging to treatment and control groups, with the members of each of these groups then classified as belonging to one of two or more response categories (such as tumor/no tumor or normal/hyperplastic/neoplastic). For these cases, two forms of analysis are presented—Fisher's Exact Test (for the 2 × 2 contingency table) and the R × C chi-square test (for large tables). It should be noted, however, that there are versions of both of these tests that permit the analysis of any size of contingency table.

The analysis of rank data—what is generally called nonparametric statistical analysis—is an exact parallel of the more traditional (and familiar) parametric methods. There are methods for the single comparison case (just as Student's t-test is used) and for the multiple comparison case (just as ANOVA is used) with appropriate post hoc tests for exact identification of the significance with a set of groups. Four tests are presented for evaluating statistical significance in rank data—the Wilcoxon rank–sum test, distribution-free multiple comparisons, Mann-Witney U Test, and the Kruskal–Wallis nonparametric analysis of variance. For each of these tests, tables of distribution values for the evaluations of results can be found in any of a number of reference volumes (62).

It should be clearly understood that for data that do not fulfill the necessary assumptions for parametric analysis, these nonparametric methods are either as powerful, or, in fact, more powerful than the equivalent parametric test.

Fisher's Exact Test

Fisher's exact test should be used to compare two sets of discontinuous, quantal (all or none) data. Small sets of such data can be checked by contingency data tables, such as those of Finney et al. (56). Larger sets, however, require computation, including frequency data, such as incidences of mortality or certain histopathological findings, etc. Thus, the data can be expressed as ratios. These data do not fit on a continuous scale of measurement but usually involve numbers of responses classified as either negative or positive (i.e., a contingency table situation) (138).

The analysis is started by setting up a 2 × 2 contingency table to summarize the numbers of "positive" and "negative" responses as well as the totals of these responses as follows:

	"Positive"	"Negative"	Total
Group I	A	B	A + B
Group II	C	D	C + D
Totals	A + C	B + D	$A+B+C+D=N_{total}$

Using the above set of symbols, the formula for P appears as follows:

$$P = \frac{(A+B)!(C+D)!(A+C)!(B+D)!^{*}}{N!A!B!C!D!}$$

The exact test produces a probability (P) that is the sum of the above calculation repeated for each possible arrangement of the numbers in the above cells (i.e., A, B, C, and D) showing an association equal to or stronger than that between the two variables.

The P resulting from these computations will be the exact one- or two-tailed probability, depending on which of these two approaches is being employed. This value tells us if the groups differ significantly (with a probability less than, say, 0.05) and the degree of significance. This is demonstrated in Example 8.

Example 8

The pathology reports from 35 control and 20 treated rats show that 2 control and 5 treated animals have tumors of the spleen. Setting this up as a contingency table, we see:

	Tumor-bearing	No tumors	Total
Control	2	33	35
Treated	5	15	20
Total	7	48	55

The probability for the worst case on this calculates as

$$prob_1 = \frac{(35)! \bullet (20)! \bullet (7)! \bullet (48)!}{(55)! \bullet (2)! \bullet (5)! \bullet (33)! \bullet (15)!} = 0.046.$$

Similarly, the probabilities for the secondary may be computed as $prob_2 = 0.007$ and the tertiary as $prob_3 = 0.000$, respectively. The exact one-tailed p-value is $p = 0.046 + 0.007 + 0.000 = 0.053$. Because this is greater than 0.05, we would not reject the hypothesis of equal proportions at a significance level of 0.05 (this is close to 0.05, however, and may give the researcher encouragement to conduct a larger study).

ASSUMPTIONS AND LIMITATIONS

1. Tables are available that provide individual exact probabilities for small sample size contingency tables (see ref. 171, pp. 518–542).
2. Fisher's exact must be used in preference to the chi-square test when there are small cell sizes.
3. The probability resulting from a two-tailed test is exactly double that of a one-tailed test from the same data.
4. Ghent (69) has developed and proposed a good (though, if performed by hand, laborious) method extending the calculation of exact probabilities to 2 × 3, 3 × 3, and R × C contingency tables.
5. Fisher's probabilities are not necessary symmetric. Although some analysts will double the one-tailed p-value to obtain the two-tailed result, this method usually is overly conservative.

* A! is A factorial. For 4!, as an example, this would be (4) (3) (2) (1) = 24.

2 × 2 Chi Square

Though Fisher's Exact Test is preferable for analysis of most 2 × 2 contingency tables in toxicology, the chi-square test is still widely used and is preferable in a few unusual situations (particularly if cell sizes are large yet only limited computational support is available). The formula is simply:

$$\chi^2 = \frac{(0_1 - E_1)^2}{E_1} + \frac{(0_2 - E_2)^2}{E_2}$$
$$= \sum \frac{(0_i - E_i)^2}{E_i},$$

where 0 are observed numbers (or counts) and E are expected numbers. The common practice in toxicology is for the observed figures to be test or treatment group counts. The expected figure is calculated as

$$E = \frac{\text{(column total)(row total)}}{\text{grand total}}$$

for each box or cell in a contingency table. Example 9 illustrates this.

Example 9

In an subacute toxicity study, there were 25 animals in the control group and 25 animals in the treatment group. Seven days after dosing, control and 13 treatment animals were observed to be exhibiting fine muscle tremors; all other animals had no tremors. Do significantly more treatment animals have tremors?

	Tremors		No tremors		Σ
	Observed	(Expected)	Observed	(Expected)	
Control	5	(8.5)	20	(16.5)	25
Treated	12	(8.5)	13	(16.5)	25
Σ	17		33		50

$$\chi^2 = \frac{(5-8.5)^2}{8.5} + \frac{(12-8.5)^2}{8.5} + \frac{(20-16.5)^2}{16.5} + \frac{(13-16.5)^2}{16.5}$$

$$= \frac{12.25}{8.5} + \frac{12.25}{8.5} + \frac{12.25}{16.5} + \frac{12.25}{16.5}$$

$$= 1.441 + 1.441 + 0.762 + 0.742$$

$$= 4.366.$$

Our degrees of freedom are (R − 1)(C − 1) = (2 − 1)(2 − 1) = 1. Looking at a chi-square table for one degree of freedom we see that this is greater than the test statistic at 0.05 (3.84) but less than that of 0.01 (6.64) so that $0.05 > p > 0.01$.

ASSUMPTIONS AND LIMITATIONS

Assumptions:

(1) Data are univariate and categorical.
(2) Data are from a multinomial population.
(3) Data are collected by random, independent sampling.
(4) Groups being compared are of approximately same size, particularly for small group sizes.

When to use:

(1) When the data are of a categorical (or frequency) nature.
(2) When the data fit the assumptions above.
(3) To test goodness-to-fit to a known form of distribution.
(4) When cell sizes are large.

When not to use:

(1) When the data are continuous rather than categorical.
(2) When sample sizes are small and very unequal.
(3) When sample sizes are too small (e.g., when total N is less than 50 or if any expected value is less than 5).
(4) For any 2 × 2 comparison (user Fisher's Exact test instead).

R × C Chi Square

The R × C chi-square test can be used to analyze discontinuous (frequency) data as in the Fisher's exact or 2 × 2 chi-square tests; however, in the R × C test (R = row, C = column) we wish to compare three or more sets of data. An example would be comparison of the incidence of tumors among mice on three or more oral dosage levels. We can consider the data as "positive" (tumors) or "negative" (no tumors). Thc expected frequency for any box is equal to (row total)(column total)/(N_{total}).

As in the Fisher's exact test, the initial step is setting up a table (this time an R × C contingency table). This table would appear as follows:

	Positive	Negative	Total
Group I	A_1	B_1	$A_1 + B_1 = N_1$
Group II	A_2	B_2	$A_2 + B_2 = N_2$
	↓	↓	
Group R	A_R	B_R	$A_R + B_R = N_R$
Totals	N_A	N_B	N_{total}

Using these symbols, the formula for chi-square (χ^2) is

$$\chi^2 = \frac{N_{tot}^2}{N_A N_B N_K}\left(\frac{A_1^2}{N_1} + \frac{A_2^2}{N_2} + \ldots \frac{A_K^2}{N_K} - \frac{N_A^2}{N_{tot}}\right).$$

The resulting χ^2 value is compared to table values (138, pp. 470–471) according to the number of degrees of freedom, which is equal to (R − 1)(C − 1). If χ^2 is smaller than the table value at the 0.05 probability level, the groups are not significantly different. If the calculated χ^2 is larger, there is some difference among the groups, and 2 × R chi square or Fisher's exact tests will have to be compared to determine which group(s) differ from which other group(s). Example 10 demonstrates this.

Example 10

The R × C square can be used to analyze tumor incidence data gathered during a mouse-feeding study as follows:

Dosage (mg/kg)	No. of mice with tumors	No. of mice without tumors	Total no. of mice
2.00	19	16	35
1.00	13	24	37
0.50	17	20	37
0.25	22	12	34
0.00	20	23	43
Totals	91	95	186

$$\chi^2 = \frac{(186)^2}{91(95)}\left[\frac{19^2}{35}+\frac{13^2}{37}+\frac{17^2}{37}+\frac{22^2}{34}+\frac{20^2}{43}-\frac{91^2}{186}\right]$$
$$= (4.00)(1.71)$$
$$= 6.84$$

The smallest expected frequency would be (91)(34)/186 + 16.6, well above 5.0. The number of degrees of freedom is (5 – 1)(2 – 1) = 4. The chi-square table value for four degrees of freedom is 9.49 at the 0.05 probability level. Therefore, there is no significant association between tumor incidence and dose or concentration.

ASSUMPTIONS AND LIMITATIONS

(1) Based on data being organized in a table (such as below) so that there are *cells* (below, A, B, C, and D are cells):

		Columns (C)		
		Control	Treated	Total
Rows (R)	No Effect	A	B	A + B
	Effect	C	D	C + D
Total		A + C	B + D	A + B + C + D

(2) None of the "expected" frequency values should be less than 5.0.
(3) Chi-square test is always one tailed.
(4) Without the use of some form of correction, the test becomes less accurate as the differences between group sizes increases.
(5) The results from each additional column (group) is approximately additive. Due to this characteristic, chi-square can be readily used for evaluating any R × C combination.
(6) The results of the chi-square calculation must be a positive number.
(7) Test is weak with either small sample sizes or when the expected frequency in any cell is less than 5 (this latter limitation can be overcome by "pooling"—combining cells.).
(8) Test results are independent of order of cells, unlike Kolmogorov–Smirnov.
(9) Can be used to test the probability of validity of any distribution.

$$\frac{(N)(N+1)}{2},$$

where N is the total number of data in both groups. The result should be equal to the sum of the sum of ranks for both groups.

The sum of rank values are compared to table values (14, pp. 409–413) to determine the degree of significant differences, if any. These tables include two limits (an upper and a lower) that are dependent on the probability level. If the amount of data is the same in both groups ($N_1 = N_2$), then the lesser sum of ranks (smaller N) is compared to the table limits to find the degree of significance. Normally the comparison of the two groups ends here and the degree of significant difference can be reported. This is demonstrated in Example 11.

Example 11

If we recorded the approximate times of death (in hours) of rats dosed with 5.0 g/kg (Group B) or 2.5 g/kg (Group A) or a given material, we might obtain the following results:

Hours to Death (Group A)		Hours to Death (Group B)	
4	3	7	4
6	6	3	3
7	1	6	1
7	7	7	2
2	7	2	5
5	4	5	4
7	6		
7	3		

With $n_1 = 16$, $n_2 = 12$ and $n = 28$, the ranked value of the responses are as shown in parenthesis below:

(Group A)				(Group B)			
4	(11.5)	3	(7.5)	7	(24.5)	4	(11.5)
6	(18.5)	6	(18.5)	3	7.5	3	(7.5)
7	(24.5)	1	(1.5)	6	(18.5)	1	(1.5)
7	(24.5)	7	(24.5)	7	(24.5)	2	(4)
2	(4)	7	(24.5)	2	(4)	5	(15)
5	(15)	4	(11.4)	5	(15)	4	(11.5)
7	(24.5)	6	(18.5)				
7	(24.5)	3	(7.5)				

Sums $R_1 = (261)$, $R_2 = (145)$.

As a check, $R_1 + R_2 = 406$, $\frac{(28)(29)}{2} = 406 = R_1 + R_2$. The test's statistic, based on a significance level of $\mu = 0.05$ in a normal approximation, becomes

Null hypothesis: $H_0 : \theta_1 = \theta_2$.

Alt. hypothesis: $H_A : \theta_1 \neq \theta_2$.

Test statistic: $Z = \frac{|R_1 - \mu_{R_1}| - 0.5}{\sigma_{R_1}}$.

$$\frac{(261 - 232) - 0.5}{\sqrt{448.38}} = 1.346.$$

Decision rule: reject H_0 if $|Z| > 1.96$.

Conclusion: Because 1.346 is not >1.96, we do not reject H_0, concluding that there is insufficient evidence of a difference between the two doses in terms of time of death.

Distribution-Free Multiple Comparison

The distribution-free multiple comparison test should be used to compare three or more groups of nonparametric data. These groups are then analyzed two at a time for any significant differences (87, pp. 124–129). The test can be used for data similar to those compared by the rank-sum test. We often employ this test for reproduction and mutagenicity studies (such as comparing survival rates of offspring of rats fed various amounts of test materials in the diet).

As shown in Example 12, two values must be calculated for each pair of groups: the difference in mean ranks and the probability level value against which the difference will be compared. To determine the difference in mean ranks we must first arrange the data within each of the groups in order of increasing values. Then we must assign rank values, beginning with the smallest overall figure. Note that this ranking is similar to that in the Wilcoxon test except that it applies to more than two groups.

The ranks are then added for each of the groups. As a check, the sum of these should equal

$$\frac{N_{tot}(N_{tot} + 1)}{2},$$

where N_{tot} is the total number of figures from all groups. Next we can find the mean rank (R) for each group by dividing the sum of ranks by the numbers in the data (N) in the group. These mean ranks are then taken in those pairs that we want to compare (usually each test group versus the control) and the differences are found ($|R_1 - R_2|$). This value is expressed as an absolute figure (i.e., it is always a positive number).

The second value for each pair of groups (the probability value) is calculated from the expression

$$z[a/K(K-1)]\sqrt{\frac{N_{total}(N_{total}+1)}{12}}\sqrt{\frac{1}{N_1}\frac{1}{N_2}},$$

where a is the level of significance for the comparison (usually 0.05, 0.01, 0.001, etc.), K is the total number of groups, and Z is a figure obtained from a normal probability table and determining the corresponding "Z-score".

The result of the probability value calculation for each pair of groups is compared to the corresponding mean difference $|R_1 - R_2|$. If $|R_1 - R_2|$ is smaller, there is no significant difference between the groups; if it is larger, the groups are different and $|R_1 - R_2|$ must be compared to the calculated probability values for $a = 0.01$ and $a = 0.001$ to find the degree of significance.

Example 12

Consider the following set of data (ranked in increasing order), which could represent the proportion of rats surviving given periods of time during diet inclusion of a test chemical at four dosage levels (survival index):

I 5.0 mg/kg		II 2.5 mg/kg		III 1.25 mg/kg		IV 0.0 mg/kg	
% Value	Rank	% Value	Rank	% Value	Rank	% Value	Rank
40	2.0	40	2.0	50	5.5	60	9.0
40	2.0	50	5.5	50	5.5	60	9.0
50	5.5	80	12.0	60	9.0	80	12.0
100	17.5	80	12.0	100	17.5	90	14.0
		100	17.5	100	17.5	100	17.5
						100	17.5
Sum of ranks	27.0		49.0		55.0		79.0

$N_I = 4, \quad N_{II} = 5, \quad N_{III} = 5, \quad N_{IV} = 6.$

$N_{tot} = 20$

Check sums of $= 210$, $\frac{20(21)}{2} = 210$.

Mean ranks (R): $R_1 = \frac{27.0}{4} = 6.75$, $R_2 = \frac{49.0}{5} = 9.80$,

$R_3 = \frac{55.0}{5} = 11.00$, $R_4 = \frac{79.0}{6} = 13.17$.

Comparison Groups	$\|R1–R2\|$	Probability test values
5.0 versus 0.0	6.42	$(0.05/4(3)) = Z_{0.00417} = 2.637$ $\sqrt{\frac{(20)(21)}{12}}\sqrt{\frac{1}{4}+\frac{1}{6}} = 10.07$
2.5 versus 0.0	3.37	$(0.05/4(3)) = Z_{0.00417} = 2.637$ $\sqrt{\frac{(20)(21)}{12}}\sqrt{\frac{1}{5}+\frac{1}{6}} = 9.45$
1.25 versus 0.0	2.17	$(0.05/4(3)) = Z_{0.00417} = 2.637$ $\sqrt{\frac{(20)(21)}{12}}\sqrt{\frac{1}{5}+\frac{1}{6}} = 9.45$

Because each of the $|R_1 - R_2|$ values is smaller than the corresponding probability calculation, the pairs of groups compared are not different at the 0.05 level of significance.

ASSUMPTIONS AND LIMITATIONS

1. As with the Wilcoxon Rank–Sum, too many tied ranks inflate the false-positive.
2. Generally, this test should be used as a post hoc comparison after Kruskal–Wallis.

Mann–Whitney U Test

This is a nonparametric test in which the data in each group are first ordered from lowest to highest values, and then the entire set (both control and treated values) is ranked, with the average rank being assigned to tied values (i.e., if two values tie for 12th rank—and therefore would be ranked 12th and 13th—both would be assigned the average rank of 12.5). The ranks are then summed for each group and U is determined according to

$$U_t = n_c n_t + \frac{n_t(n_t + 1)}{2} - R_t,$$

$$U_c = n_c n_t + \frac{n_c(n_c + 1)}{2} - R_c,$$

where n_c, n_t = sample size for control and treated groups and R_c, R_t = sum of ranks for the control and treated groups. For the level of significance for a comparison of the two groups, the larger value of U_c or U_t is used. This is compared to critical values as found in tables in Reference 137.

As demonstrated in Example 13, the Mann–Whitney U test is employed for the count data, but which test should be employed for the percentage variables should be decided on the same grounds as described later in a discussion of statistical requirements for reproduction studies.

Example 13

In a 2-week study, the levels of serum cholesterol in treatment and control animals are successfully measured and assigned ranks as follows:

	Treatment		Control	
	Value	Rank	Value	Rank
	10	1	19	4
	18	3	28	13
	26	10.5	29	14.5
	31	16	26	10.5
	15	2	35	19
	24	8	23	7
	22	6	29	14.5
	33	17	34	18
	21	5	38	20
	25	9	27	12
SUM OF RANKS		77.5		132.5

The critical value for one tailed $p \leq 0.05$ is $U \geq 73$. We then calculate

$$U_t = (10)(10) + \frac{10(10 + 1)}{2} - 77.5$$

$$= 100 + \frac{110}{2} - 77.5 = 77.5$$

$$U_c = (10)(10) + \frac{10(10 + 1)}{2} - 132.5 = 22.5.$$

As 77.5 is greater than 73, these groups are significantly different at the 0.05 level.

ASSUMPTIONS AND LIMITATIONS

1. It does not matter whether the observations are ranked from smallest to largest, or vice versa.
2. This test should not be used for paired observations.
3. The test statistics from a Mann–Whitney are linearly related to those of Wilcoxon. The two tests will always yield the same result. The Mann–Whitney is presented here for historical completeness, as it has been much favored in reproductive and developmental toxicology studies; however, it should be noted that the authors do not include it in the decision tree for method selection (Figure 7.2).

Kruskal–Wallis Nonparametric ANOVA

The Kruskal–Wallis nonparametric one-way analysis of variance should be the initial analysis performed when we have three or more groups of data that are by nature nonparametric (either not a normally distributed population, or of a discontinuous nature, or all the groups being analyzed are not from the same population) but not a categorical (or quantal) nature. Commonly these will be either rank-type evaluation data (such as behavioral toxicity observation scores) or reproduction study data. The analysis is initiated (119, pp. 170–173) by ranking all the observations from the combined groups to be analyzed. Ties are given the average rank of the tied values.

The sum of ranks of each group ($r_1, r_2, \ldots r_k$) is computed by adding all the rank values for each group. The test value H is then computed as

$$H = \frac{12}{n(n+1)} \sum r_1^2/n_1 + r_2^2/n_2 + \cdots + r_k^2/n_k) - 3(n+1),$$

where $n_1, n_2, \ldots n_k$ are the number of observations in each group. The test statistic is then compared with a table of H values. If the calculated value of H is greater than the table value for the appropriate number of observations in each group, there is significant difference between the groups, but further testing (using the distribution-free multiple comparisons method) is necessary to determine where the difference lies (as demonstrated in Example 14).

Example 14

As part of a neurobehavioral toxicology study, righting reflex values (whole numbers ranging from 0 to 10) were determined for each of five rats in each of three groups. The values observed, and their ranks, are as follows:

Control group		5 mg/kg group		10 mg/kg group	
Reflex Score	Rank	Reflex Score	Rank	Reflex Score	Rank
0	2	1	5	4	11
0	2	2	7.5	4	11
0	2	2	7.5	5	13
1	5	3	9	8	14.5
1	5	4	11	8	14.5
Sums of ranks (r)	16		40		64

From these the H value is calculated as

$$H = \frac{12}{15(15+1)}\left[\frac{16^2}{5} + \frac{40^2}{5} + \frac{64^2}{5}\right] - 3(15+1)$$

$$= \frac{12}{240}\left[\frac{(256 + 1600 + 4096)}{5}\right] - 48$$

$$= \frac{1}{20}(1190.4) - 48$$

$$= 59.52 - 48$$

$$= 11.52$$

Consulting a table of values for H, we find that for the case where we have three groups of five observations each, the test values are 4.56 (for $p = 0.10$), 5.78 (for $p = 0.05$), and 7.98 (for $p = 0.01$). As our calculated H is greater than the $p = 0.01$ test value, we have determined that there is a significant difference between the groups at the level of $p < 0.01$ and would now have to continue to a multiple comparisons test to determine where the difference is.

ASSUMPTIONS AND LIMITATIONS

1. The test statistic H is used for both small and large samples.
2. When we find a significant difference, we do not know which groups are different. It is not correct to then perform a Mann–Whitney U test on all possible combinations. Rather, a multiple comparison method must be used, such as the distribution-free multiple comparisons.
3. Data must be independent for the test to be valid.
4. Too many tied ranks will decrease the power of this test and also lead to increased false-positive levels.
5. When $k = 2$, the Kruskal–Wallis chi-square value has 1 d.f. This test is identical to the normal approximation used for the Wilcoxon Rank–Sum Test. As noted in previous sections, a chi-square with 1 d.f. can be represented by the square of a standardized normal random variable. In the case of $k = 2$, the h-statistic is the square of the Wilcoxon Rank–Sum Z-test (without the continuity correction).
6. The effect of adjusting for tied ranks is to slightly increase the value of the test statistic, h. Therefore, omission of this adjustment results in a more conservative test.

Log–Rank Test

The log-rank test is a statistical methodology for comparing the distribution of time until the occurrence of the event in independent groups. In toxicology, the most common event of interest is death or occurrence of a tumor, but it could just as well be liver failure, neurotoxicity, or any other event that occurs only once in an individual. The elapsed time from initial treatment or observation until the *event* is the *event time*, often referred to as "survival time," even when the event is not "death."

The log–rank test provides a method for comparing "risk-adjusted" event rates, useful when test subjects in a study are subject to varying degrees of opportunity to experience the event. Such situations arise frequently in toxicology studies due to the finite duration of the study, early termination of the animal, or interruption of treatment before the event occurs.

Examples where use of the log–rank test might be appropriate include comparing survival times in carcinogenity bioassay animals that are given a new treatment with those in the control group or comparing times to liver failure for several dose levels of a new nonsteroidal anti-inflammatory drug (NSAID) where the animals are treated for 10 weeks or until cured, whichever comes first.

If every animal were followed until the event occurrence, the event times could be compared between two groups using the Wilcoxon Rank–Sum Test, however, some animals may die or complete the study before the event occurs. In such cases, the actual time of the event is unknown since the event does not occur while under study observation. The event times for these animals are based on the last known time of study observation and are called "censored" observations because they represent the lower-bound of the true, unknown event times. The Wilcoxon Rank–Sum Test can be highly biased in the presence of the censored data.

The null hypothesis tested by the Log–Rank Test is that of equal event time distributions among groups. Equality of the distributions of event times implies similar event rates among groups not only for the clinical trial as a whole, but also for any arbitrary time point during the trial. Rejection of the null hypothesis indicates that the event rates differ among groups at one or more time points during the study.

The idea behind the log–rank test for comparison of two life tables is simple. If there were no difference between the groups, the total deaths occurring at any time should split between the two groups at that time. So if the numbers at risk in the first and second groups in (say) the sixth month were 70 and 30, respectively, and 10 deaths occurred in that month, we would expect

$$10 \times \frac{70}{70+30} = 7$$

of these deaths to have occurred in the first group, and

$$10 \times \frac{30}{70+30} = 3$$

of the deaths to have occurred in the second group.

A similar calculation can be made at each time of death (in either group). By adding together for the first group the results of all such calculations, we obtain a single number, called the extent of exposure (E_1), which represents the "expected" number of deaths in that group if the two groups had the distribution of survival time. An extent of exposure (E_2) can be obtained for the second group in the same way. Let O_1 and O_2 denote the actual total numbers of deaths in the two groups. A useful arithmetic check is that the total number of deaths $O_1 + O_2$ must equal the sum $E_1 + E_2$ of the extents of exposure.

The discrepancy between the O's and E's can be measured by the quantity

$$\chi^2 = \frac{(|O_1 - E_1| - 1/2)^2}{E_1} + \frac{(|O_2 - E_2| - 1/2)^2}{E_2}.$$

For rather obscure reasons, X^2 is known as the *Log–Rank statistic*. An approximate significance test of the null hypothesis of identical distributions of survival time in the two groups is obtained by referring X^2 to a chi-square distribution on 1 degree of freedom. This is demonstrated in Example 15.

Example 15

In a study of the effectiveness of a new monoclonal antibody to treat a specific cancer, the times to reoccurrence of the cancer in treated animals in weeks were as follows:

Control Group			Treatment Group		
1	5	11	6	10	22
1	5	12	6	11	23
2	8	12	6	13	25
2	8	15	6	16	32
3	8	17	7	17	32
4	8	22	9	19	34
4	11	23	10	20	35

The table opposite presents the calculations for the log–rank test applied to these times. A chi-square value of 13.6 is significant at the $p<0.001$ level.

Illustration:

$$t = 23, 2 \times \frac{6}{7} = 1.7143, 2 \times \frac{1}{7} = 0.2857.$$

Test of significance:

$$x^2 = \frac{\left(|O_1 - E_1| - \frac{1}{2}\right)^2}{E_1} + \frac{\left(|O_2 - E_2| - \frac{1}{2}\right)^2}{E_2}$$

$$= \frac{\left(|9 - 19.2| - \frac{1}{2}\right)^2}{19.2} + \frac{\left(|21 - 10.8| - \frac{1}{2}\right)^2}{10.8} = 13.6.$$

Estimate of relative risk:

$$\theta = \frac{(O_1/E_1)}{(O_2/E_2)}$$

$$\hat{\theta} = \frac{9/19.2}{21/10.8} = 0.24.$$

The log–rank test as presented by Peto et al. (118) uses the product-limit life-table calculations rather than the actuarial estimators shown above. The distinction is unlikely to be of practical importance unless the grouping intervals are very coarse.

Peto and Pike (118) suggest that the approximation in treating the null distribution of χ^2 as a chi-square is conservative, so it will tend to understate the degree of statistical significance. In the formula for χ^2 we have used the continuity correction of subtracting $1/2$ from $|O_1 - E_1|$ and $|O_2 - E_2|$ before squaring. This is recommended by Peto et al. (118) when, as in nonrandomized studies, the permutational argument does not apply. Peto et al. (118) gives further details of the log–rank test and its extension to comparisons of more than two treatment groups and to tests that control for categorical confounding factors.

Log-Rank Calculation for Tumor Data

Time,	At Risk			Relapses			Extent of Exposure		
t	T	C	Total	T	C	Total	T	C	Total
1	21	21	42	0	2	2	1.0000	1.0000	2
2	21	19	40	0	2	2	1.0500	0.9500	2
3	21	17	38	0	1	1	0.5526	0.4474	1
4	21	16	37	0	2	2	1.1351	0.8649	2
5	21	14	35	0	2	2	1.2000	0.8000	2
6	20.5	12	32.5	3	0	3	1.8923	1.1077	3
7	17	12	29	1	0	1	0.5862	0.4138	1
8	16	12	28	0	4	4	2.2857	1.7143	4
10	14.5	8	22.5	1	0	1	0.6444	0.3556	1
11	12.5	8	20.5	0	2	2	1.2295	0.7705	2
12	12	6	18	0	2	2	1.3333	0.6667	2
13	12	4	16	1	0	1	0.7500	0.2500	1
15	11	4	15	0	1	1	0.7333	0.2667	1
16	11	3	14	1	0	1	0.7857	0.2143	1
17	9.5	3	12.5	0	1	1	0.7600	0.2400	1
22	7	2	9	1	1	2	1.5556	0.4444	2
23	6	1	7	1	1	2	1.7143	0.2857	2
Total				9	21 (O_1)	30 (O_2)	19.2080 (E_1)	10.7920 (E_2)	30

ASSUMPTIONS AND LIMITATIONS

(1) The endpoint of concern is or is defined so that it is "right censored"—once it happens, it does not reoccur. Examples are death or a minimum or maximum value of an enzyme or physiologic function (such as respiration rate).

(2) The method makes no assumptions on distribution.

(3) Many variations of the Log–Rank Test for comparing survival distributions exist. The most common variant has the form

$$\chi^2 = \frac{(O_1 - E_1)^2}{E_1} + \frac{(O_2 - E_2)^2}{E_2},$$

where O_i and E_i are computed for each group, as in the formulas given previously. This statistic also has an approximate chi-square distribution with 1 degree of freedom under H_0.

A continuity correction can also be used to reduce the numerators by one half before squaring. Use of such a correction leads to even further conservatism and may be omitted when sample sizes are moderate or large.

(4) The Wilcoxon Rank–Sum Test could be used to analyze the event times in the absence of censoring. A "Generalized Wilcoxon" Test, sometimes called the Gehan Test, based on an approximate chi-square distribution, has been developed for use in the presence of censored observations. Both the Log–Rank and the Generalized Wilcoxon Tests are nonparametric tests and require no assumptions regarding the distribution of event times. When the event rate is greater early in the trial than toward the end, the Generalized Wilcoxon Test is the more appropriate test because it gives greater weight to the earlier differences.

(5) Survival and failure times often follow the exponential distribution. If such a model can be assumed, a more powerful alternative to the Log–Rank Test is the Likelihood Ratio Test. This parametric test assumes that event probabilities are constant over time. That is, the chance that a patient becomes event-positive at time t given that he is event-negative up to time t does not depend on t. A plot of the negative log of the event times' distribution showing a linear trend through the origin is consistent with exponential event times.

(6) Life tables can be constructed to provide estimates of the event time distributions. Estimates commonly used are known as the Kaplan–Meier estimates.

HYPOTHESIS TESTING: UNIVARIATE PARAMETRIC TESTS

Univariate case* data from normally distributed populations generally have a higher information value associated with them, but the traditional hypothesis testing techniques generally are neither resistant nor robust. All the data analyzed by these methods are also, effectively, continuous (i.e., at least for practical purposes, the data may be represented by any number and each such data number has a measurable relationship to other data numbers).

Student's t-Test (Unpaired t-Test)

Pairs of groups of continuous, randomly distributed data are compared via this test. We can use this test

*That is, where each datum is defined by one treatment and one effect variable.

to compare three or more groups of data, but they must be intercompared by examination of two groups taken at a time and are preferentially compared by analysis of variance (ANOVA). Usually this means comparison of a test group versus a control group, although two test groups may be compared as well. To determine which of the three types of t-tests described in this chapter should be employed, the F-test usually is performed first. This will tell us if the variances of the data are approximately equal, which is a requirement for the use of the parametric methods. If the F-test indicates homogeneous variances and the numbers of data within the groups (N) are equal, then the Student's t-test is the appropriate procedure (138). If the F is significant (the data are heterogeneous) and the two groups have equal numbers of data, the modified Student's t-test is applicable (42).

The value of t for Student's t-test is calculated using the formula

$$t = \frac{\bar{X}_1 - \bar{X}_2}{\sum D_1^2 + \sum D_2^2} \sqrt{\frac{N_1 N_2}{N_1 + N_2}(N_1 + N_2 - 2)},$$

where the value of $\Sigma D^2 = [N \sum X^2 - (\sum X)^2]/N$.

The value of t obtained from the above calculations is compared to the values in a t-distribution table according to the appropriate number of degrees of freedom (df). If the F value is not significant (i.e., variances are homogeneous), the df $= N_1 + N_2 - 2$. If the F was significant and $N_1 = N_2$, then the df $= N - 1$. Although this case indicates a nonrandom distribution, the modified t-test is still valid. If the calculated value is larger than the table value at $p = 0.05$, it may then be compared to the appropriate other table values in order of decreasing probability to determine the degree of significance between the two groups. Example 16 demonstrates this methodology.

Example 16

Suppose we wish to compare two groups (a test and control group) of dog weights following inhalation of a vapor. First, we would test for homogeneity of variance using the F-test. Assuming that this test gave negative (homogeneous) results, we would perform the t-test as follows:

	Test weight		Control weight	
Dog	(X_1 in kg)	X_1^2	(X_2 in kg)	X_2^2
1	8.3	68.89	8.4	70.56
2	8.8	77.44	10.2	104.04
3	9.3	86.49	9.6	92.16
4	9.3	86.49	9.4	88.36
Sums	$\Sigma X_1 = 35.7$	ΣX_1^2 319.31	$\Sigma X_2 = 37.6$	ΣX_2^2 355.12
Means	8.92		9.40	

The difference in means $= 9.40 - 8.92 = 0.48$.

$$\sum D_1^2 = \frac{4(319.31) - (35.7)^2}{4} = \frac{2.75}{4} = 0.6875,$$

$$\sum D_2^2 = \frac{4(355.12) - (37.6)^2}{4} = \frac{6.72}{4} = 1.6800,$$

$$t = \frac{0.48}{\sqrt{0.6875 + 1.6800}} \sqrt{\frac{4(4)}{4+4}(4+4-2)} = 1.08.$$

The table value for t at the 0.05 probability level for $(4+4-2)$, or six degrees of freedom, is 2.447. Therefore, the dog weights are not significantly different at $p = 0.05$.

ASSUMPTIONS AND LIMITATIONS

1. The test assumes that the data are univariate, continuous, and normally distributed.
2. Data are collected by randomly sampling.
3. The test should be used when the assumptions in 1 and 2 are met and there are only two groups to be compared.
4. Do not use when the data are ranked, when the data are not approximately normally distributed, or when there are more than two groups to be compared. Do not use for paired observations.
5. This is the most commonly misused test method, except in those few cases where one is truly only comparing two groups of data and the group sizes are roughly equivalent. Not valid for multiple comparisons (because of resulting additive errors) or where group sizes are very unequal.
6. Test is robust for moderate departures from normality and, when N_1 and N_2 are approximately equal, robust for moderate departures from homogeneity of variances.
7. The main difference between the Z-test and the t-test is that the Z-statistic is based on a known standard deviation, σ, whereas the t-statistic uses the sample standard deviation, s, as an estimate of σ. With the assumption of normally distributed data, the variance σ^2 is more closely estimated by the sample variance s^2 as n gets large. It can be shown that the t-test is equivalent to the Z-test for infinite degrees of freedom. In practice, a "large" sample usually is considered $n \geq 30$.

Cochran t-test

The Cochran test should be used to compare two groups of continuous data when the variances (as indicated by the F-test) are heterogeneous and the numbers of data within the groups are not equal ($N_1 \neq N_2$). This is the situation, for example, when the data, though expected to be randomly distributed, were found not to be (28, pp. 100–102).

Two t values are calculated for this test, the "observed" t (t_{obs}) and the "expected" t (t′). The observed t is obtained by

$$t_{obs} = \frac{\bar{X}_1 - \bar{X}_2}{\sqrt{W_1 + W_2}}$$

where $W = \text{SEM}^2$ (standard error of the mean squared),

$$= S^2/N,$$

where S (variance) can be calculated from

$$S = \frac{\dfrac{N\sum X^2 - (\sum X)^2}{N}}{N-1}$$

The value for t' is obtained from

$$t' = \frac{t_1' W_1 + t_2' W_2}{W_1 + W_2}$$

where t_1' and t_2' are values for the two groups taken from the t-distribution table corresponding to N–1 degrees of freedom (for each group) at the 0.05 probability level (or such level as one may select).

The calculated t_{obs} is compared to the calculated t′ value (or values, if t′ values were prepared for more than one probability level). If t_{obs} is smaller than a t′, the groups are not considered to be significantly different at that probability level. This procedure is shown in Example 17.

Example 17

If we wished to compare the red blood cell count (RBC) of rats receiving a test material in their diet with the RBCs of control rats, we might obtain the following results:

Test RBC (X_1)	X_1^2	Control RBC (X_2)	X_2^2
8.23	67.73	7.22	52.13
8.59	73.79	7.55	57.00
7.51	56.40	7.53	56.70
6.60	46.56	7.32	53.58
6.67	44.49		
$\sum X_1 = 37.60$	$\sum X_1^2$ 285.97	$\sum X_2 = 29.62$	$\sum X_2^2$ 219.41

$$\bar{X}_1 = \frac{37.60}{5} = 7.52, \quad W_1 = \frac{0.804}{5} = 0.1608,$$

$$\bar{X}_2 = \frac{29.62}{4} = 7.40, \quad W_2 = \frac{0.025}{4} = 0.0062,$$

(note that S^2 values of 0.804 and 0.025 are calculated in Example 17)

$$t_{obs} = \frac{7.52 - 7.40}{\sqrt{0.1608 + 0.0062}} = 0.29.$$

From the t-distribution table we use $t_1 = 2.776$ ($df = 4$) and $t_2 = 3.182$ ($df = 3$) for the 0.05 level of significance; there is no statistical difference at $p = 0.05$ between the two groups.

ASSUMPTIONS AND LIMITATIONS

1. The test assumes that the data are univariate, continuous, normally distributed, and that group sizes are unequal.
2. The test is robust for moderate departures from normality and very robust for departures from equality of variances.

F-Test

This is a test of the homogeneity of variances between two groups of data (138). It is used in two separate cases. The first is when Bartlett's indicates heterogeneity of variances among three or more groups (i.e., it is used to determine which pairs of groups are heterogeneous). Second, the F-test is the initial step in comparing two groups of continuous data that we would expect to be parametric (two groups not usually being compared using ANOVA), the results indicating whether the data are from the same population and whether subsequent parametric comparisons would be valid.

The F is calculated by dividing the larger variance (S_1^2) by the smaller one (S_2^2). S^2 is calculated as

$$S^2 = \frac{\dfrac{N\sum X^2 - (\sum X)^2}{N}}{N-1},$$

where N is the number of data in the group and X represents the individual values within the group. Frequently, S^2 values may be obtained from ANOVA calculations. Use of this is demonstrated in Example 18.

The calculated F value is compared to the appropriate number in an F value table for the appropriate degrees of freedom (N–1) in the numerator (along the top of the table) and in the denominator (along the side of the table). If the calculated value is smaller, it is not significant and the variances are considered homogeneous (and the Student's t-test would be appropriate for further comparison). If the calculated F value is greater, F is significant and the variances are heterogeneous (and the next test would be modified Student's t-test if $N_1 = N_2$ or the Cochran t-test if $N_1 \neq N_2$; see Figure 7.2 to review the decision tree).

Example 18

Using the RBC comparison from Example 17 (with $N_1 = 5$, $N_2 = 4$), the following results were determined:

$$\text{Variance for } X_1 = S_1^2 = \frac{\dfrac{5(285.97) - (37.60)^2}{5}}{5-1} = 0.804,$$

$$\text{Variance for } X_2 = S_3^2 = \frac{\frac{4(219.41) - (29.62)^2}{4}}{4-1} = 0.025,$$

$$F = \frac{0.804}{0.025} = 32.16.$$

From a table for F values, for 4 (numerator) versus 3 (denominator) df, we read the limit of 9.12 at the 0.05 level. As our calculated value is larger (and, therefore, significant), the variances are heterogeneous and the Cochran t-test would be appropriate for comparison of the two groups of data.

ASSUMPTIONS AND LIMITATIONS

1. This test could be considered as a two-group equivalent of the Bartlett's test.
2. If the test statistic is close to 1.0, the results are (of course) not significant.
3. The test assumes normality and independence of data.

Analysis of Variance

ANOVA is used for comparison of three or more groups of continuous data when the variances are homogeneous and the data are independent and normally distributed. A series of calculations are required for ANOVA, starting with the values within each group being added ($\sum X$) and then these sums being added ($\sum\sum X$). Each figure within the groups is squared, and these squares are then summed ($\sum X^2$) and these sums added ($\sum\sum X^2$). Next the "correction factor" (CF) can be calculated from the following formula:

$$CF = \frac{\left(\sum_1^K \sum_1^N X\right)^2}{N_1 + N_2 + \ldots N_k},$$

where N is the number of values in each group and K is the number of groups. The total sum of squares (SS) is then determined as follows:

$$SS_{total} = \sum_1^K \sum_1^N X^2 - CF.$$

In turn, the sum of squares between groups (bg) is found from

$$SS_{bg} = \frac{(\sum X_1)^2}{N_1} + \frac{(\sum X_2)^2}{N_2} + \cdots \frac{(\sum X_k)^2}{N_k} - CF.$$

The sum of squares within group (wg) is then the difference between the last two figures, or

$$SS_{wg} = SS_{total} - SS_{bg}.$$

Now there are three types of degrees of freedom to determine. The first, total df, is the total number of data within all groups under analysis minus one ($N_1 + N_2 + \cdots N_k - 1$). The second figure (the df between groups) is the number of groups minus one (K–1). The last figure (the df within groups or "error df") is the difference between the first two figures (df_{total}—df_{bg}).

The next set of calculations requires determination of the two mean squares (MD_{bg} and MS_{wg}). These are the respective sum of square values divided by the corresponding df figures (MS = SS/df). The final calculation is that of the F ratio. For this, the MS between groups is divided by the MS within groups ($F = MS_{bg}/MS_{wg}$).

A table of the results of these calculations (using data from Example 19 at the end of this section) would appear as follows:

	df	SS	MS	F
Bg	3	0.04075	0.01358	4.94
Wg	12	0.03305	0.00275	
Total	15	0.07380		

For interpretation, the F ratio value obtained in the ANOVA is compared to a table of F values. If $F \leq 1.0$, the results are not significant and comparison with the table values is not necessary. The degrees of freedom (df) for the greater mean square (MS_{bg}) are indicated along the top of the table. Then read down the side of the table to the line corresponding to the df for the lesser mean square (MS_{wg}). The figure shown at the desired significance level (traditionally 0.05) is compared to the calculated F value. If the calculated number is smaller, there is no significant differences among the groups being compared. If the calculated value is larger, there is some difference, but further (post hoc) testing will be required before we know which groups differ significantly.

Example 19

Suppose we want to compare four groups of dog kidney weights, expressed as percentage of body weights, following an inhalation study. Assuming homogeneity of variance (from Barlett's test), we could complete the following calculations:

	400 ppm	200 ppm	100 ppm	0 ppm
	0.43	0.49	0.34	0.34
	0.52	0.48	0.40	0.32
	0.43	0.40	0.42	0.33
	0.55	0.34	0.40	0.39
$\sum X$	1.93	1.71	1.56	1.38

$$\sum\sum X = 1.93 + 1.71 + 1.56 + 1.38 = 6.58.$$

Next, the preceding figures are squared:

	400 ppm	200 ppm	100 ppm	0 ppm
	0.1849	0.2401	0.1156	0.1156
	0.2704	0.2304	0.1600	0.1024
	0.1849	0.1600	0.1764	0.1089
	0.3025	0.1156	0.1600	0.1521
$\sum X^2$	0.9427	0.7461	0.6120	0.4790

$$\sum\sum X^2 = 0.9427 + 0.7461 + 0.6120 + 0.4790 = 2.7798.$$

$$\text{CF} = \frac{(6.58)^2}{4+4+4+4} = 2.7060,$$

$$\text{SS}_{\text{total}} = 2.7798 - 2.7060 = 0.0738,$$

$$\text{SS}_{\text{bg}} = \frac{(1.93)^2}{4} + \frac{(1.71)^2}{4} + \frac{(1.56)^2}{4} + \frac{(1.38)^2}{4} - 2.7060$$
$$= 0.04075,$$

$$\text{SS}_{\text{wg}} = 0.07380 - 0.04075 = 0.03305.$$

The total degrees of freedom (df) $= 4+4+4+4-1 = 15$,

$$\text{df}_{\text{bg}} = 4 - 1 = 3 \quad \text{df}_{\text{wg}} = 15 - 3 = 12,$$

$$\text{MS}_{\text{bg}} = \frac{0.4075}{3} = 0.01358,$$

$$\text{MS}_{\text{wg}} = \frac{0.03305}{12} = 0.00275,$$

$$\text{F} = \frac{0.01358}{0.00275} = 4.94.$$

Going to a table of F values, we find that for 3 df_{bg} (greater mean square) and 12 df_{wg} (lesser mean square), the 0.05 value of F is 3.49. As our calculated value is greater, there is a difference among groups at the 0.05 probability level. To determine where the difference is, further comparisons by a post hoc test will be necessary.

ASSUMPTIONS AND LIMITATIONS

1. What is presented here is the workhorse of toxicology—the one-way analysis of variance. Many other forms exist for more complicated experimental designs.
2. The test is robust for moderate departures from normality if the sample sizes are large enough. Unfortunately, this is rarely the case in toxicology.
3. ANOVA is robust for moderate departures from equality of variances (as determined by Bartlett's test) if the sample sizes are approximately equal.
4. It is not appropriate to use a t-test (or a 2-groups-at-a-time version of ANOVA) to identify where significant differences are within the design group. A multiple-comparison post hoc method must be used.

Post Hoc Tests

There is a wide variety of post hoc tests available to analyze data after finding significant result in an ANOVA. Each of these tests has advantages and disadvantages, proponents, and critics. Four of the tests are commonly used in toxicology and are presented here. These are Duncan's, Scheffe's, and Dunnett's t-test and Williams' t-test. Two other tests that are available in many statistical packages are Tukey's method and the Student–Newman–Keuls method (171, pp. 151–161).

If ANOVA reveals no significance, it is not appropriate to proceed to perform a post hoc test in hope of finding differences. To do so would only be another form of multiple comparisons, increasing the type I error rate beyond the desired level.

Duncan's Multiple Range Test

Duncan's (44) is used to compare groups of continuous and randomly distributed data (such as body weights, organ weights, etc.). The test normally involves three or more groups taken one pair at a time. It should only follow observation of a significant F value in the ANOVA and can serve to determine which group (or groups) differs significantly from which other group (or groups).

There are two alternative methods of calculation. The selection of the proper one is based on whether the number of data (N) are equal or unequal in the groups.

Groups with Equal Number of Data ($N_1 = N_2$)

Two sets of calculations must be carried out. First, the determination of the difference between the means of pairs of groups; second, the preparation of a probability rate against which each difference in means is compared (as shown in the first of the two examples in this section).

The means (averages) are determined (or taken from the ANOVA calculation) and ranked in either decreasing or increasing order. If two means are the same, they take up two equal positions (thus, for four means we could have ranks of 1, 2, 2, and 4 rather than 1, 2, 3, and 4). The groups are then taken in pairs and the differences between the means ($\bar{X}_1 - \bar{X}_2$), expressed as positive numbers, are calculated. Usually, each pair consists of a test group and the control group, though multiple test groups may be intracompared if so desired. The relative rank of the two groups being compared must be considered. If a test group is ranked "2" and the control group is ranked "1," then we say that there are two places between them, whereas if the test group were ranked "3," then there would be three places between it and the control.

To establish the probability table, the standard error of the mean (SEM) must be calculated as presented earlier, or as

$$\sqrt{\frac{\text{error mean square}}{\text{N}}} = \sqrt{\frac{\text{mean square within group}}{\text{N}}},$$

where N is the number of animals or replications per dose level. The mean square within groups (MS_{wg}) can be calculated from the information given in the ANOVA procedure (refer to the earlier section on ANOVA). The SEM is then multiplied by a series of table values (14,80) to set up a probability table. The table values used for the calculations are chosen according to the probability levels (note that the tables have sections for 0.05, 0.01, and 0.001 levels) and the number of means apart for the groups being compared and the number of "error" degrees of freedom (df). The "error" df is the number of df within the groups. This last figure is determined from the ANOVA calculation and can be taken from ANOVA output. For some values of df, the table values are not given and should thus be interpolated. Example 20 demonstrates this case.

Example 20

Using the data given in Example 19 (4 groups of dogs, with 4 dogs in each group), we can make the following calculations:

Ranks	1	2	3	4
Concentration	0 ppm	100 ppm	200 ppm	400 ppm
Mean kidney weight ($\bar{X}$)	0.345	0.390	0.428	0.482

Groups compared	$\bar{X}_1 - \bar{X}_2$	No of means apart	Probability
2 vs. 1 (100 vs 0 ppm)	0.045	2	p>0.05
3 vs. 1 (200 vs 0 ppm)	0.083	3	p>0.05
4 vs. 1 (400 vs 0 ppm)	0.137	4	0.01>p>0.001
4 vs. 2 (400 vs 100 ppm)	0.092	3	0.05>p>0.01

The mean square within groups from the ANOVA example was 0.00275. Therefore, the SEM = $\sqrt{0.00275/4} = 0.02622$. The "error" $df(df_{wg})$ was 12, so the following table values are used.

	Probability levels		
No. of means apart	0.05	0.01	0.001
2	3.082	4.320	6.106
3	3.225	4.504	6.340
4	3.313	4.662	6.494

When these are multiped by the SEM we get the following probability table:

	Probability levels		
No. of means apart	0.05	0.01	0.001
2	0.0808	0.1133	0.1601
3	0.0846	0.1161	0.1662
4	0.0869	0.1212	0.1703

Groups with Unequal Numbers of Data ($N_1 \neq N_2$)

This procedure is very similar to that discussed above. As before, the means are ranked and the differences between the means are determined ($\bar{X}_1 - \bar{X}_2$). Next, weighing values ("a_{ij}" values) are calculated for the pairs of groups being compared in accordance with

$$a_u = \sqrt{\frac{2N_iN_j}{(N_i + N_j)}} = \sqrt{\frac{2N_1N_2}{(N_1 + N_2)}}$$

This weighting value for each pair of groups is multiplied by ($\bar{X}_1 - \bar{X}_2$) for each value to arrive at a "t" value. It is the "t" that will later be compared to a probability table.

The probability table is set up as above except that instead of multiplying the appropriate table values by SEM, SEM^2 is used. This is equal to $\sqrt{MS_{wg}}$.

For the desired comparison of two groups at a time, the ($\bar{X}_1 - \bar{X}_2$) value (if $N_1 = N_2$) is compared to the appropriate probability table. Each comparison must be made according to the number of places between the means. If the table value is larger at the 0.05 level, the two groups are not considered to be statistically different. If the table value is smaller, the groups are different and the comparison is repeated at lower levels of significance. Thus, the degree of significance may be determined. We might have significant differences at 0.05 but not at 0.01, in which case the probability would be represented at $0.05 > p > 0.01$. Example 21 demonstrates this case.

Example 21

Suppose that the 400 ppm level from the above example had only 3 dogs, but that the mean for the group and the mean square within groups were the same. To continue Duncan's we would calculate the weighing factors as follows:

100 ppm vs. 0 ppm,

200 ppm vs. 0 ppm $N_1 = 4$; $N_2 = 4$ $a_{ij} = \sqrt{\frac{2(4)(4)}{4+4}} = 2.00$,

400 ppm vs. 0 ppm $N_2 = 3$; $N_4 = 4 a_{ij} = \sqrt{\frac{2(3)(4)}{3+4}} = 1.852$, 400 ppm vs. 100 ppm.

Using the $\bar{X}_1 - \bar{X}_2$ from the above example we can set up the following tables:

Concentrations ppm	No. of means apart	$\bar{X}_1 - \bar{X}_2$	a_{ij}	$(\bar{X}_1 - \bar{X}_2)a_{ij}$
100 versus 0	2	0.045	2.000	2.000(.045) = .090
200 versus 0	3	0.083	2.000	2.000(.083) = .166
400 versus 0	4	0.137	1.852	1.852(.137) = .254
400 versus 100	3	0.092	1.852	1.852(.092) = .170

Next we calculate SEM[2] as being $\sqrt{0.00275} = 0.05244$. This is multiplied by the appropriate table values chosen for 11 $df(df_{wg}$ for this example). This gives the following probability table.

No. of means apart	Probability levels 0.05	0.01	0.001
2	0.1632	0.2303	0.3291
3	0.1707	0.2401	0.3417
4	0.1753	0.2463	0.3501

Comparing the "t" values with the probability table values we get the following:

Comparison	Probability
100 ppm vs. 0 ppm	$p > 0.05$
200 ppm vs. 0 ppm	$p > 0.05$
400 ppm vs. 0 ppm	$0.01 > p > 0.001$
400 ppm vs. 100 ppm	$0.05 > p > 0.01$

ASSUMPTIONS AND LIMITATIONS

1. Duncan's assures a set alpha level or type I error rate for all tests when means are separated by no more than ordered step increases. Preserving this alpha level means that the test is less sensitive than some others, such as the Student–Newman–Keuls. The test is inherently conservative and not resistant or robust.

Scheffe's Multiple Comparisons

Scheffe's is another post hoc comparison method for groups of continuous and randomly distributed data. It also normally involved three or more groups (79, 131). It is widely considered a more powerful significance test than Duncan's.

Each post hoc comparison is tested by comparing an obtained test value (F_{contr}) with the appropriate critical F value at the selected level of significance (the table F value multiplied by K–1 for an F with K–1 and N–K degrees of freedom[2]). F_{contr} is computed as follows:

(a) Compute the mean for each sample (group);
(b) Denote the residual mean square by MS_{wg};
(c) Compute the test statistic as

$$F_{contr} = \frac{C_1\bar{X}_1 + C_2\bar{X}_2 + \ldots + C_k\bar{X}_k^2)}{(K-1)MS_{wg}(C_1^2/n_1 + \ldots + C_K^2/n_k},$$

where C_k is the comparison number such that the sum $C_1, C_2 \cdots C_k = 0$ (see Example 22) and

[2]Where K = the number of groups and N = the total number of data.

Example 22

At the end of a short-term feeding study, the following body weight changes were recorded:

	Group 1	Group 2	Group 3
	10.2	12.2	9.2
	8.2	10.6	10.5
	8.9	9.9	9.2
	8.0	13.0	8.7
	8.3	8.1	9.0
	8.0	10.8	
		11.5	
Totals	51.6	76.1	46.6
Means	8.60	10.87	9.32

$MS_{wg} = 1.395$

To avoid logical inconsistencies with pairwise comparisons, we compare the group having the largest sample mean (group 2) with that having the smallest sample mean (group 1), then with the group having the next smallest sample mean, and so on. As soon as we find a non-significant comparison in this process (or no group with a smaller sample mean remains), we replace the group having the largest sample mean with that having the second largest sample mean and repeat the comparison process.

Accordingly, our first comparison is between groups 2 and 1. We set $C_1 = -1$, $C_2 = 1$, and $C_3 = 0$ and calculate our test statistic

$$F_{contr} = \frac{(10.87 - 8.60)^2}{(3-1)1.395(1/6 + 1/7)} = 5.97.$$

The critical region for F at $p \leq 0.05$ for 2 and 11 degrees of freedom is 3.98. Therefore, these groups are significantly different at this level. We next compare groups

2 and 3, using $C_1 = 0$, $C_2 = 1$, and $C_3 = -1$:

$$F_{contr} = \frac{(10.87 - 9.32)^2}{(3-1)1.395(1/7 + 1/5)} = 2.51.$$

This is less than the critical region value, so these groups are not significantly different.

ASSUMPTIONS AND LIMITATIONS

1. The Scheffe procedure is robust to moderate violations of the normality and homogeneity of variance assumptions.
2. It is not formulated on the basis of groups with equal numbers (as one of Duncan's procedures is), and if $N_1 \neq N_2$, there is no separate weighing procedure.
3. It tests all linear contrasts among the population means (the other three methods confine themselves to pairwise comparison, except they use a Bonferroni type correlation procedure).
4. The Scheffe procedure is powerful because of its robustness, yet it is very conservative. Type I error (the false-positive rate) is held constant at the selected test level for each comparison.

Dunnett's t-Test

Dunnett's t-test (45,46) has as its starting point the assumption that what is desired is a comparison of each of several means with one other mean and only one other mean; in other words, that one wishes to compare each and every treatment group with the control group, but not compare treatment groups with each other. The problem here is that, in toxicology, one is frequently interested in comparing treatment groups with other treatment groups; however, if one does want only to compare treatment groups versus a control group, Dunnett's is a useful approach. In a study with K groups (one of them being the control), we will wish to make K-1 comparisons. In such a situation, we want to have a P level for the entire set of K-1 decisions (not for each individual decision). The Dunnett's distribution is predicated on this assumption. The parameters for using a Dunnett's table, such as found in his original article, are K (as above) and the number of degrees of freedom for mean square with groups (MS_{wg}). The test value is calculated as

$$t = \frac{|T_j - T_i|}{\sqrt{2MS_{wg}/n}}$$

where n is the number of observations in each of the groups. The mean square within group (MS_{wg}) is as we have defined it previously; T_j is the control group mean and T_i is the mean of, in order, each successive test group observation. Note that one uses the absolute value of the positive number resulting from subtracting T_i from T_j. This is to ensure a positive number for our final t.

Example 23 demonstrates this test, again with the data from Example 19.

Example 23

The means, N's, and sums for the groups previously presented in Example 19 are

	Control	100 ppm	200 ppm	400 ppm
Sum ($\sum X$)	1.38	1.56	1.71	1.93
N	4	4	4	4
Mean	0.345	0.39	0.4275	0.4825

The MS_{wg} was 0.00275, and our test t for 4 groups and 12 df is 2.41. Substituting in the equation, we calculate our t for the control versus the 400 ppm to be

$$= \frac{|0.345 - 0.4825|}{\sqrt{2(0.00275)/4}}$$

$$= \frac{0.1375}{\sqrt{0.001375}}$$

$$= \frac{0.1375}{0.037081} = 3.708.$$

which exceeds our test value of 2.41, showing that these two groups are significantly different at $p \leq 0.05$. The values for the comparisons of the control versus the 200 and 100 ppm groups are then found to be, respectively, 2.225 and 1.214. Both of these are less than our test value, and therefore the groups are not significantly different.

ASSUMPTIONS AND LIMITATIONS

1. Dunnett's seeks to ensure that the type 1 error rate will be fixed at the desired level by incorporating correction factors into the design of the test value table.
2. Treated group sizes must be approximately equal.

Williams' t-Test

Williams' t-test (164, 165) is also popular, although its use is quite limited in toxicology. It is designed to detect the highest level (in a set of dose/exposure levels) at which there is no significant effect. It assumes that the response of interest (such as change in body weights) occurs at higher levels but not at lower levels and that the responses are monotonically ordered so that $X_0 \leq X_1 \ldots \leq X_k$. This frequently is not the case, however. The Williams' technique handles the occurrence of such discontinuities in a response series by replacing the offending value and the value immediately preceding it with weighted average values. The test also is adversely affected by any mortality at high dose levels. Such moralities "impose a severe penalty, reducing the power of detecting an effect not only at level K but also at all lower doses" (165, p. 529). Accordingly, it is not generally applicable in toxicology studies.

Analysis of Covariance

ANCOVA is a method for comparing sets of data that consist of two variables (treatment and effect, with our effect variable being called the "variate") when a third variable (called the "covariate") exists that can be measured but not controlled and that has a definite affect on the variable of interest. In other words, it provides an indirect type of statistical control, allowing us to increase the precision of a study and to remove a potential source of bias. One common example of this is in the analysis of organ weights in toxicity studies. Our true interest here is the effect of our dose or exposure level on the specific organ weights, but most organ weights also increase (in the young, growing animals most commonly used in such studies) in proportion to increases in animal body weight. As we are not interested in the effect of this covariate (body weight), we measure it to allow for adjustment. We must be careful before using ANCOVA, however, to ensure that the underlying nature of the correspondence between the variate and covariate is such that we can rely on it as a tool for adjustments (3,97).

Calculation is performed in two steps. The first is a type of linear regression between the variate Y and the covariate X. This regression, performed as described under the linear regression section, gives us the model

$$Y = a_1 + BX + e,$$

which in turn allows us to define adjusted means ($\bar{Y}$ and $\bar{X}$) such that $\bar{Y}_{1a} = \bar{Y}_1 - (\bar{X}_1 - X^*)$.

If we consider the case where K treatments are being compared such that $K = 1, 2, \ldots K$, and we let X_{ik} and Y_{ik} represent the predictor and predicted values for each individual i in group k, we can let X_k and Y_k be the means. Then, we define the between-group (for treatment) sum of squares and cross products as

$$T_{xx} = \sum_{k-1}^{K} n_k(\bar{X}_K - \bar{X})^2,$$

$$T_{yy} = \sum_{k-1}^{K} n_k(\bar{Y}_K - \bar{Y})^2,$$

$$Txy = \sum_{k-1}^{K} n_k(\bar{X}_k - \bar{X})(\bar{Y}_k - \bar{Y}_k - \bar{Y}).$$

In a like manner, within-group sums of squares and cross products are calculated as

$$\sum xx = \sum_{k=1}^{k} \sum_{i} (X_{ik} - X_k)^2,$$

$$\sum yy = \sum_{k=1}^{k} \sum_{i} (Y_{ik} - Y_k)^2,$$

$$\sum xy = \sum_{k=1}^{k} \sum_{i} (X_{ik} - X_k)(Y_{ik} - Y_k),$$

where i indicates the sum from all the individuals within each group; $f' =$ total number of subjects minus the number of groups

$$S_{xx} = T_{xx} + \sum\nolimits_{xx},$$
$$S_{yy} = T_{yy} + \sum\nolimits_{xx},$$
$$S_{xy} = T_{xy} + \sum\nolimits_{xy}.$$

With these in hand, we can then calculate the residual mean squares of treatments (St^2) and error (Se^2):

$$St^2 = \frac{T_{yy} - \dfrac{S_{xy}^2}{S_{xx}} + \dfrac{\sum_{xy}^2}{\sum_{xx}}}{k-1},$$

$$Se^2 = \frac{\left(\sum_{yy} - \dfrac{\sum_{y}^2}{\sum_{xx}}\right)}{f-1}.$$

These can be used to calculate an F statistic to test the null hypothesis that all treatment effects are equal:

$$F = \frac{St^2}{Se^2}.$$

The estimated regression coefficient of Y or X is

$$B = \frac{\sum_{xy}}{\sum_{xx}}.$$

The estimated standard error for the adjusted difference between two groups is given by

$$Sd = Se\frac{1}{n_i} + \frac{1}{n_j} + \frac{(X_i - X_j)^2}{\sum_{xx}},$$

where n_i and n_j are the sample sizes of the two groups. A test of the null hypothesis that the adjusted differences between the groups is zero is provided by

$$t = \frac{Y_i - Y_j - B(X_i - X_j)}{Sd}.$$

The test value for the t is then looked up in the t-table with f–1 degrees of freedom. Computation is markedly simplified if all the groups are of equal size, as demonstrated in Example 24.

Example 24

An ionophere was evaluated as a potential blood-pressure-reducing agent. Early studies indicated that there was an adverse effect on blood cholesterol and hemoglobin levels, so a special study was performed to evaluate this specific effect. The hemoglobin (Hgb) level covariate was measured at study start along with the percentage changes in serum triglycerides between study start and at the end of the 13-week study. Was there a difference in effects of the two ionopheres?

Ionophere A		Ionophere B	
Hgb (X)	Serum Triglyceride, %—Change (Y)	Hgb (X)	Serum Triglyceride, %—Change (Y)
7.0	5	5.1	10
6.0	10	6.0	15
7.1	–5	7.2	–15
8.6	–20	6.4	5
6.3	0	5.5	10
7.5	–15	6.0	–15
6.6	10	5.6	–5
7.4	–10	5.5	–10
5.3	20	6.7	–20
6.5	–15	8.6	–40
6.2	5	6.4	–5
7.8	0	6.0	–10
8.5	–40	9.3	–40
9.2	–25	8.5	–20
5.0	25	7.9	–35
		5.0	0
		6.5	–10

To apply ANCOVA using Hgb as a covariate, we first obtain some summary results from the data as follows:

	Ionophere A (Group 1)	Ionophere B (Group 2)	Combined
$\sum x$	112.00	119.60	231.60
$\sum x^2$	804.14	821.64	1625.78
$\sum y$	–65.00	–185.00	–250.00
$\sum y^2$	4575.00	6475.00	11050.00
$\sum xy$	–708.50	–1506.50	–2215.00
$\bar{x}$	7.000	6.6444	6.8118
$\bar{y}$	–4.625	–10.2778	–7.3529
n	16	18	34

We compute for the ionophere group (i = 1):

$$S_{xx(1)} = 804.14 - (112)^2/16 = 20.140,$$
$$S_{yy(1)} = 4575.00 - (-65)^2/16 = 4310.938,$$
$$S_{xy(1)} = -708.50 - (112)(-65)/16 = -253.500.$$

Similarly, for the ionophere B group (i = 2), we obtain

$$S_{xx(2)} = 26.964,$$
$$S_{yy(2)} = 4573.611,$$
$$S_{xy(2)} = -277.278.$$

Finally, for the combined data (ignoring groups), we compute

$$S_{xx} = 48.175,$$
$$S_{yy} = 9211.765,$$
$$S_{xy} = -512.059.$$

The sums-of-squares can now be obtained as

$$TOT(SS) = 9211.8,$$

$$SSE = (20.140 + 26.964)(4310.938 + 4573.611) \frac{-[-253.500 - 277.28]^2}{(20.140 + 26.964)} = 2903.6,$$

$$SSG = \frac{(48.175)(9211.765) - (-512.059)^2}{48.175} - 2903.6 = 865.4,$$

$$SSX = (4310.938 + 473.611) - 2903.6 = 5980.9,$$

and the ANCOVA summary table can be completed as follows:

SOURCE	*df*	*SS*	*MS*	*F*
TREATMENT	1	865.4	865.4	9.2*
X (Hgb)	1	5980.9	5980.9	63.8
Error	31	2903.7	93.7	
Total	33	9211.8		

* Significant ($p<0.05$); critical F-value = 4.16.

The F-statistics are formed as the ratios of effect mean-squares (MS) to the MSE (93.7). Each F-statistic is compared with the critical F value with 1 upper and 31 lower degrees of freedom. The critical F-value for $\alpha = 0.05$ is 4.16.

The significant covariate effect ($F = 63.8$) indicates that the triglyceride response has a significant linear relationship with HbA_{1c}. The significant F-value for TREATMENT indicates that the mean triglyceride response adjusted for hemoglobin effect differs between treatment groups.

ASSUMPTIONS AND LIMITATIONS

1. The underlying assumptions for ANCOVA are fairly rigid and restrictive. The assumptions include the following:

a. The slopes of the regression lines of a Y and X are equal from group to group. This can be examined visually or formally (i.e., by a test). If this condition is not met, ANCOVA cannot be used.
b. The relationship between X and y is linear.
c. The covariate X is measured without error. Power of the test declines as error increases.
d. There are no unmeasured confounding variables.
e. The errors inherent in each variable are independent of each other. Lack of independence effectively (but to an immeasurable degree) reduces sample size.
f. The variances of the errors in groups are equivalent between groups.
g. The measured data which form the groups are normally distributed. ANCOVA is generally robust to departures from normality.

2. Of the seven assumptions above, the least robust are the first four.

Modeling

The mathematical modeling of biological systems, restricted even to the field of toxicology, is an extremely large and vigorously growing area. Broadly speaking, modeling is the principal conceptual tool by which toxicology seeks to develop as a mechanistic science. In an iterative process, models are developed or proposed, tested by experiment, reformulated, and so on in a continuous cycle. Such a cycle could also be described as two related types of modeling—explanatory (where the concept is formed) and correlative (where data are organized and relationships derived). An excellent introduction to the broader field of modeling of biological systems can be found in Gold (72).

In toxicology, modeling is of prime interest in seeking to relate a treatment variable with an effect variable and, from the resulting model, predict effects at exact points where no experiment has been done (but in the range where we have performed experiments, such as "determining" LD_{50}s) to estimate how good our prediction is, and occasionally, simply to determine if a pattern of effects is related to a pattern of treatment.

For use in prediction, the techniques of linear regression, probit/logit analysis (a special case of linear regression), moving averages (an efficient approximation method), and nonlinear regression (for doses where data cannot be made to fit a linear pattern) are presented. For evaluating the predictive value of these models, both the correlation coefficient (for parametric data) and Kendall's rank correlation (for nonparametric data) are given. Finally, the concept of trend analysis is introduced and a method presented.

When we are trying to establish a pattern between several data points (whether this pattern is in the form of a line or a curve), what we are doing is interpolating. It is possible for any given set of points to produce an infinite set of lines or curves that pass near (for lines) or through (for curves) the data points. In most cases we cannot actually know the "real" pattern, so we apply a basic principle of science—Occam's razor. We use the simplest explanation (or, in this case, model) that fits the facts (or data). A line is, of course, the simplest pattern to deal with and describe, so fitting the best line (linear regression) is the most common form of model in toxicology.

Linear Regression

Foremost among the methods for interpolating within a known data relationship is regression—the fitting of a line or curve to a set of known data points on a graph and the interpolation ("estimation") of this line or curve in areas where we have no data points. The simplest of these regression models is that of linear regression (valid when increasing the value of one variable changes the value of the related variable in a linear fashion, either positively or negatively). This is the case we will explore here, using the method of least squares.

Given that we have two sets of variables, x (say, mg/kg of test material administered) and y (say, percentage of animals so dosed that die), what is required is solving for a and b in the equation $Y_i = a + bx_i$ (where the uppercase Y_i is the fitted value of y_i at x_i, and we wish to minimize $(y_i - Y_i)^2$). So we solve the equations

$$b = \frac{\sum x_1 y_1 - n\bar{x}\bar{y}}{\sum x_1^2 - n\bar{x}^2}$$

and

$$a = \bar{y} - b\bar{x},$$

where a is the y intercept, b is the slope of the time, and n is the number of data points. Use of this is demonstrated in Example 25.

Note that in actuality, dose-response relationships often are not linear and instead we must use either a transform (to linearize the data) or a nonlinear regression method (65).

Note also that we can use the correlation test statistic (to be described in the correlation coefficient section) to determine if the regression is significant (and, therefore, valid) at a defined level of certainty. A more specific test for significance would be the linear regression analysis of variance (119). We start by developing the appropriate ANOVA table, as demonstrated in Example 25, then proceed to perform the linear regression portion of the ANOVA, as shown in Example 26.

Example 25

From a short-term toxicity study we have the following results:

Dose Administered (mg/kg)	% Animals dead		
x_i	x_i^2	y_i	$x_i y_i$
1	1	10	10
3	9	20	60
4	16	18	72
5	25	20	100
Sums $x_l = 13$	$x_i^2 = 51$	$y_i = 68$	$x_i y_i - 242$

$$\bar{x} = 3.25, \quad \bar{y} = 17,$$

$$b = \frac{242 - (4)(3.25)(17)}{51 - (4)(10.5625)} = \frac{21}{8.75} = 2.40,$$

$$a = 17 - (2.4)(3.25) = 9.20.$$

We therefore see that our fitted line is $Y = 9.2 + 2.4X$.

These ANOVA table data are then used as shown in Example 26.

Linear regression analysis of variance

Source of variation (1)	Sum of squares (2)	Degrees of freedom (3)	Mean square (4)
			equal to $\left(\frac{2}{3}\right)$
Regression	$b_1^2(\sum x_1^2 - n\bar{x}^2)$	1	By division
Residual	By difference	n–2	By division
Total	$\sum y_1^2 - n\bar{y}^2$	n–1	

We then calculate

$$F_{1,n-2} = \frac{\text{regression mean square}}{\text{residual mean square}}.$$

Example 26

We desire to test the significance of the regression line in Example 25:

$$\sum y_i^2 = 10^2 + 20^2 + 18^2 + 20^2,$$

$$\text{Regression } SS = (2.4)^2[51 - 4(3.25)^2] = 50.4,$$

$$\text{Total } SS = 1224 - 4(17^2) = 68.0,$$

$$\text{Residual } SS = 68.0 - 50.4 = 17.6,$$

$$F_{1,2} = 50.4/8.8 = 5.73.$$

This value is not significant at the 0.05 level; therefore, the regression is not significant. A significant F value (as found in an F distribution table for the appropriate degrees of freedom) indicates that the regression line is an accurate prediction of observed values at that confidence level. Note that the portion of the total sum of squares explained by the regression is called the coefficient of correlation, which in the above example is equal to 0.86^2 (or 0.74). Calculation of the correlation coefficient is described later in this chapter.

Finally, we might wish to determine the confidence intervals for our regression line (i.e., given a regression line with calculated values for Y_i given x_i, within what limits may we be certain [with say a 95% probability] what the real value of Y_i is)?

If we denote the residual mean square in the ANOVA by s^2, the 95% confidence limits for *a* (denoted by A, the notation for the true—as opposed to the estimated—value for this parameter) are calculated as

$$t_{n-2} = \frac{a - A}{\sqrt{\dfrac{s^2(\sum x^2)}{n\sum x_1^2 - n^2\bar{x}^2}}},$$

$$\frac{9.2 - A}{\sqrt{\dfrac{8.8(51)}{4(51) - (16)(10.562)}}} = \frac{9.2 - A}{\sqrt{\dfrac{448}{35.008}}}$$

$$= \frac{9.2 - A}{3.58} = \pm 4.303,$$

$$9.2 - A = \pm 15.405,$$

$$A = 9.2 \pm 15.405.$$

ASSUMPTIONS AND LIMITATIONS

1. All the regression methods are for interpolation, not extrapolation. That is, they are valid only in the range that we have data—the experimental region—not beyond.
2. The method assumes that the data are independent and normally distributed and it is sensitive to outliers. The x-axis (or horizontal) component plays an extremely important part in developing the least square fit. All points have equal weight in determining the height of a regression line, but extreme x-axis values unduly influence the slope of the line.
3. A good fit between a line and a set of data (i.e., a strong correlation between treatment and response variables) does not imply any casual relationship.
4. It is assumed that the treatment variable can be measured without error, that each data point is independent, that variances are equivalent, and that a linear relationship does not exist between the variables.
5. There are many excellent texts on regression, which is a powerful technique, including (53,54), which are not overly rigorous mathematically.

Probit/Log Transforms and Regression

As we noted in the preceding section, dose-response problems (among the most common interpolation problems encountered in toxicology) rarely are straightforward enough to make a valid linear regression directly from the raw data. The most common valid interpolation methods are based on probability ("probit") and logarithmic ("log") value scales, with percentage responses (death, tumor incidence, etc.) being expressed on the probit scale whereas doses (Y_i) are expressed on the log scale. There are two strategies for such an approach. The first is based on transforming the data to these scales, then doing a weighted linear regression on the transformed data (if one does not have access to a computer or a high-powered programmable calculator, the only practical strategy is not to assign weights). The second requires the use of algorithms (approximate calculation techniques) for the probit value and regression process and is extremely burdensome to perform manually.

Our approach to the first strategy requires that we construct a table with the pairs of values of x_i and y_i listed in order of increasing values of Y_i (percentage response). Beside each of these columns a set of blank columns should be left so that the transformed values may be listed. We then simply add the columns described in the linear regression procedure. Log and probit values may be taken from any of a number of sets of tables and the rest of the table is then developed from these transformed x_i' and y_i' values (denoted as x_i' and y_i'). A standard linear regression is then performed (see Example 27).

The second strategy we discussed has been broached by a number of authors (16, 32, 103, 12). All of these methods, however, are computationally cumbersome. It is possible to approximate the necessary iterative process using the algorithms developed by Abramowitz and Stegun (1), but even this merely reduces the complexity to a point where the procedure may be readily programmed on a small computer or programmable calculator.

Example 27

Our interpolated log of the LD_{50} (calculated by using $Y = -0.200591 - 0.240226\ x$, where x equals 5.000—the probit of 50%—in the regression equation) is 1.000539. When we convert this log value to its linear equivalent, we get an LD_{50} of 10.0 mg/kg.

Finally, our calculated correlation coefficient is $r = 0.997$. A goodness-of-fit of the data using chi-square may also be calculated.

Percentage of animals killed x_i	Probit of $x_i = x_i$	Dose of chemical (mg/kg) y_i	Log of $y_1 = y_i'$	$(x_i')^2$	$x_i'y_i'$
2	2.9463	3	0.4771	8.6806	1.40568
10	3.7184	5	0.6990	13.8264	2.59916
42	4.7981	10	1.0000	23.0217	4.79810
90	6.2816	20	1.3010	39.4585	8.17223
98	7.2537	30	1.4771	52.6162	10.4190
	$\sum x_i = 24.9981$		$\sum y_i' = 4.9542$	$\sum x_i'^2 = 137.6034$	$\sum x_i'y_i' = 27.68974$

ASSUMPTIONS AND LIMITATIONS

1. The probit distribution is derived from a common error function, with the midpoint (50% point) moved to a score of 5.00.
2. The underlying frequency distribution becomes asymptotic as it approaches the extremes of the range. That is, in the range of 16%–84%, the corresponding probit values change gradually—the curve is relatively linear, but beyond this range they change ever more rapidly as they approach either 0% or 100%. In fact, there are no values for either of these numbers.
3. A normally distributed population is assumed, and the results are sensitive to outliers.

Moving Averages

An obvious drawback to the interpolation procedures we have examined to date is that they do take a significant amount of time (though they are simple enough to be done manually), especially if the only result we desire is an LD_{50}, LC_{50}, or LT_{50}.

The method of moving averages (144,161) gives a rapid and reasonable accurate estimate of this "median-effective-dose" (m) and the estimated SD of its logarithm.

Such methodology requires that the same number of animals be used per dosage level and that the spacing between successive dosage exposure levels be geometrically constant (i.e., levels of 1, 2, 4, and 8 mg/kg or 1, 3, 9, and 27 ppm). Given this and access to a table for the computation of moving averages, one can readily calculate the median effective dose with the formula (illustrated for dose):

$\log m = \log D + d(K - 1)/2 + df$, where m = median effective dose or exposure.
D = the lowest dose tested.

d = the log of the ratio of successivedoses/exposures.

f = a table value taken from Gad (62) for the proper K (the total number of levels tested minus 1).

Example 28 demonstrates the use of this method.

Example 28

As part of an inhalation study, we exposed groups of 5 rats each to levels of 20, 40, 80 and 160 ppm of a chemical vapor. These exposures killed 0, 1, 3, and 5 animals, respectively. From the N = 5, K = 3 tables on the r value 0, 1, 3, 5 line, we get an f of 0.7 and an α_f^4 of 0.31623. We can then calculate the LC_{50} to be

$$\begin{aligned} \text{Log}LC_{50} &= 1.30130 + 0.30103(2)/2 + 0.30103(0.7) \\ &= 1.30103 + 0.51175 \\ &= 1.81278, \\ \therefore LC_{50} &= 65.0 \text{ ppm with 95\% confidence intervals of} \\ &\pm 2.179\, d\sigma_f \text{ or } \pm 2.179(0.30103)(0.31623) \\ &= \pm 0.20743. \end{aligned}$$

Therefore, the log confidence limits are 1.81278 $\pm$ 0.20743 = 1.60535 to 2.02021; on the linear scale = 40.3 to 104.8 ppm

ASSUMPTIONS AND LIMITATIONS

1. A common misconception is that the moving average method cannot be used to determine the slope of the response curve. This is not true. Weil has published a straightforward method for determining slope in conjunction with a moving average determination of the LD_{50} (161).
2. The method also provides confidence intervals.

Nonlinear Regression

More often than not in toxicology we find that our data demonstrate a relationship between two variables (such as age and body weight) that are not linear. That is, a change in one variable (say age) does not produce a directly proportional change in the other (e.g., body weight), but some form of relationship between the variables is apparent. If understanding such a relationship and being able to predict unknown points is of value, we have a pair of options available to us. The first, which was discussed and reviewed earlier, is to use one or more transformations to linearize our data and then to make use of linear regression. This approach, though most commonly used, has a number of drawbacks. Not all data can be suitably transformed; sometimes the transformations necessary to linearize the data require a cumbersome series of calculations, and the resulting linear regression is not always sufficient to account for the differences among sample values—there are significant deviations around the linear regression line (i.e., a line may still not give us a good fit to the data or do an adequate job of representing the relationship between the data). In such cases we have available a second option—the fitting of data to some nonlinear function such as some form of the curve. This is, in general form, nonlinear regression and may involve fitting data to an infinite number of possible functions, but most often we are interested in fitting curves to a polynomial function of the general form

$$Y = a + bx + cx^2 + dx^2 + \cdots,$$

where x is the independent variable. As the number of powers of x increases, the curve becomes increasingly complex and will be able to fit a given set of data increasingly well. Generally in toxicology, however, if we plot the log of a response (such as body weight) versus a linear scale of our dose or stimulus, we get one of four types of nonlinear curves. These are (137)

(1) Exponential growth, where

$\log Y = A(B^x)$, such as the growth curve for the log phase of a bacterial culture.

(2) Exponential decay, where

$\log Y = A(B^{-x})$, such as a radioactive decay curve.

(3) Asymptotic regression, where

$\log Y = A - B(p^x)$, such as a first-order reaction curve.

(4) Logistic growth curve, where

$\log Y = A/(1 + Bp^x)$, such as a population growth curve.

In all these cases, A and B are constant whereas p is a log transform. These curves are illustrated in Figure 7.7.

All four types of curves are fit by iterative processes (i.e., best guess numbers are initially chosen for each of the constants and, after a fit is attempted, the constants are modified to improve the fit). This process is repeated until an acceptable fit has been generated. Analysis of variance or covariance can be used to objectively evaluate the acceptability of it. Needless to say, the use of a computer generally accelerates such a curve-fitting process.

ASSUMPTIONS AND LIMITATIONS

1. The principle of using least squares may still be applicable in fitting the best curve if the assumptions of normality, independence, and reasonably error-free measurement of response are valid.
2. Growth curves are best modeled using a nonlinear method.

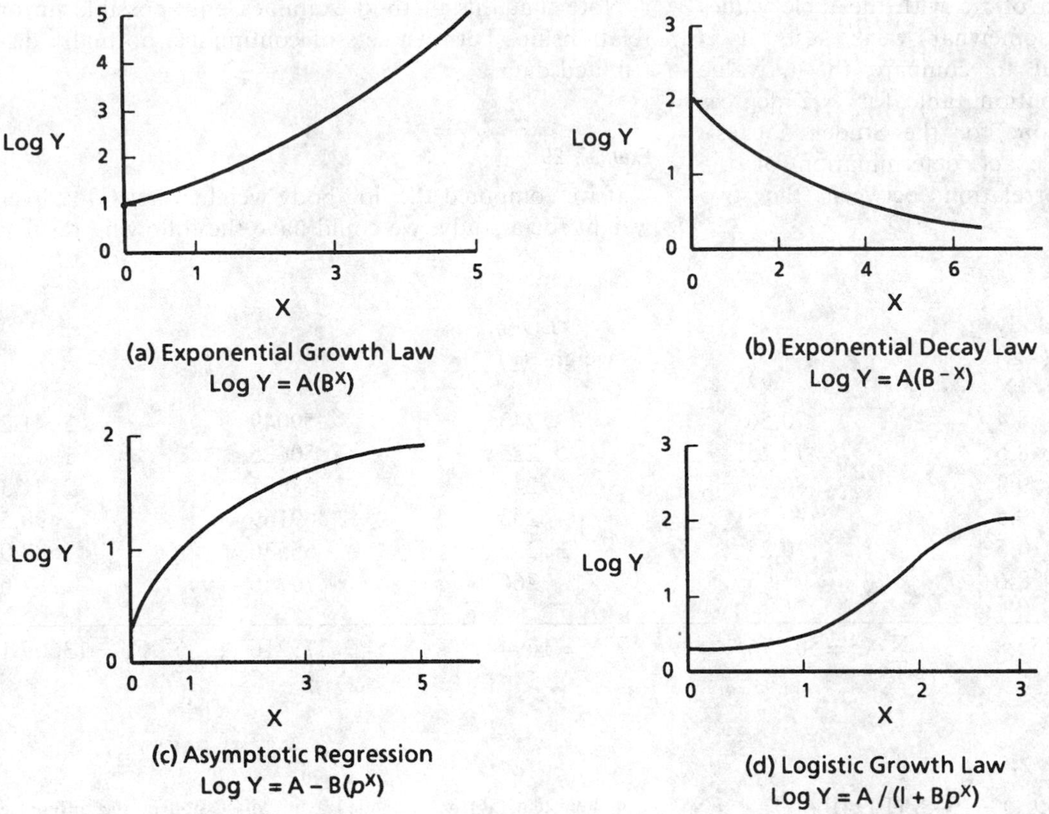

FIG. 7.7. Common curvilinear curves.

Correlation Coefficient

The correlation procedure is used to determine the degree of linear correlation (direct relationship) between two groups of continuous (and normally distributed) variables. It will indicate whether there is any statistical relationship between the variables in the two groups. For example, we may wish to determine if the liver weights of dogs on a feeding study are correlated with their body weights. Thus, we will record the body and liver weights at the time of sacrifice and then calculate the correlation coefficient between these pairs of values to determine if there is some relationship.

A formula for calculating the linear correlation coefficient (r_{xy}) is as follows:

$$r_{xy} = \frac{N\sum XY - (\sum X)(\sum Y)}{\sqrt{N\sum X^2 - (\sum X)^2}\sqrt{N\sum Y^2 - (\sum Y)^2}},$$

where X is each value for one variable (such as the dog body weights in the above example), Y is the matching value for the second variable (the liver weights), and N is the number of pairs of X and Y. Once we have obtained r_{xy}, it is possible to calculate t_r, which can be used for more precise examination of the degree of significant linear relationship between the two groups. This value is calculated as follows:

$$t_r = \frac{r_{zy}\sqrt{N-2}}{\sqrt{1 - r_{zy}^2}}.$$

This calculation is also equivalent to r = sample covariance/$(S_x S_y)$, as was seen earlier under ANCOVA.

The value obtained for r_{xy} can be compared to table values (137) for the number of pairs of data involved minus two. If the r_{xy} is smaller (at the selected test probability level, such as 0.05), the correlation is not significantly different from zero (no correlation). If r_{xy} is larger than the table value, there is a positive statistical relationship between the groups. Comparisons are then made at lower levels of probability to determine the degree of relationship (note that if r_{xy} = either 1.0 or –1.0, there is complete correlation between the groups). If r_{xy} is a negative number and the absolute is greater than the table value, there is an inverse relationship between the groups (i.e., a change in one group is associated with a change in the opposite direction in the second group of variables). Both computations are demonstrated in Example 29.

Because the comparison of r_{xy} with the table values may be considered a somewhat weak test, it is perhaps more meaningful to compare the t_r value with values in a t-distribution table for N-2 degrees of freedom (df), as is done for the Student's t-test. This will give a more exact determination of the degree of statistical correlation between the two groups.

Note that this method examines only possible linear relationships between sets of continuous, normally distributed data.

Example 29

If we computed the dog body weight versus dog liver weight for a study, we could have the following results:

Dog#	Body weight (kgj) X	X^2	Liver weight (g) Y	Y^2	XY
1	8.4	70.56	243	59049	2041.2
2	8.5	72.25	225	50625	1912.5
3	9.3	86.49	241	58081	2241.3
4	9.5	90.25	263	69169	2498.5
5	10.5	110.25	256	65536	2688.0
6	8.6	73.96	266	70756	2287.6
Sums	$\sum X = 54.8$	$\sum X^2 = 503.76$	$\sum Y = 1494$	$\sum Y^2 = 373216$	$\sum XY = 13669.1$

$$r_{xy} = \frac{6(13669.1) - (54.8)(1494)}{\left(\sqrt{6(503.76) - (54.8)^2}\right)\left(\sqrt{6(373216) - (1494)^2}\right)}$$

$$= 0.381.$$

The table value for six pairs of data (read beside the N–2 value, or 6–2 = 4) is 0.811 at a 0.05 probability level. Thus, there is a lack of statistical correlation (at $p = 0.05$) between the body weights and liver weights for this group of dogs.

The t_r value for these data would be calculated as follows:

$$t_r = \frac{0.381\sqrt{6-2}}{\sqrt{1-(0.381)^2}} = 0.824.$$

The value for the t-distribution table for four df at the 0.05 level is 2.776; therefore, this again suggests a lack of significant correlation at $p = 0.05$.

ASSUMPTIONS AND LIMITATIONS

1. A strong correlation does not imply that a treatment causes an effect.
2. The distances of data points from the regression line are the portions of the data not "explained" by the model. These are called residuals. Poor correlation coefficients imply high residuals, which may be due to many small contributions (variations of data from the regression line) or a few large ones. Extreme values (outliers) greatly reduce correlation.
3. X and Y are assumed to be independent.
4. Feinstein (55) has provided a fine discussion of the difference between correlation (or association of variables) and causation.

Kendall's Coefficient of Rank Correlation

Kendall's rank correlation, represented by τ(tau), should be used to evaluate the degree of association between two sets of data when the nature of the data is such that the relationship may not be linear. Most commonly, this is when the data are not continuous and/or normally distributed. An example of such a case is when we are trying to determine if there is a relationship between the length of hydra and their survival time in a test medium in hours, as is presented in Example 30. Both of our variables here are discontinuous, yet we suspect a relationship exists. Another common use is in comparing the subjective scoring done by two different observers.

Tau is calculated at $\tau = N/n(n-1)$, where n is the sample size and N is the count of ranks, calculated as $N = 4(^nC_i) - n(n-1)$, with the computing of ^nC_i being demonstrated in the example.

If a second variable Y_2 is exactly correlated with the first variable Y_1, then the variates Y_2 should be in the same order as the Y_1 variates; however, if the correlation is less than exact, the order of the variates Y_2 will not correspond entirely to that of Y. The quantity N measures how well the second variable corresponds to the order of the first. It has maximum value of $n(n-1)$ and a minimum value of $-n(n-1)$.

A table of data is set up with each of the two variables being ranked separately. Tied ranks are assigned as demonstrated earlier under the Kruskal–Wallis test. From this point, disregard the original variates and deal only with the ranks. Place the ranks of one of the two variables in rank order (from lowest to highest), paired with the rank values assigned for the other variable. If one (but not the other) variable has tied ranks, order the pairs by the variables without ties (138).

The most common way to compute a sum of the counts is also demonstrated in Example 30. The resulting value of tau will range from –1 to +1, as does the familiar parametric correlation coefficient, *r*.

Example 30

During the validation of an in vitro method, it was noticed that larger hydra seem to survive longer in test media than do small individuals. To evaluate this, 15 hydra of random size were measured (mm) and then placed in test media. How many hours each individual survived was recorded over a 24-hour period. These data are presented below, along with ranks for each variable:

Length	Rank(R_1)	Survival	Rank(R_2)
3	6.5	19	9
4	10	17	7
6	15	11	1
1	1.5	25	15
3	6.5	18	8
3	6.5	22	12
1	1.5	24	14
4	10	16	6
4	10	15	5
2	3.5	21	11
5	13	13	3
5	13	14	4
3	6.5	20	10
2	3.5	23	13
5	13	12	2

We then arrange this based on the order of the rank of survival time (there are no ties here). We then calculate our counts of ranks. The conventional method is to obtain a sum of the counts, C_i, as follows: examine the first value in the column of ranks paired with the ordered column. In the following case this is rank 15. Count all ranks subsequent to it that ranks greater than 15. There are 14 ranks following the 2 and all of them are less than 15. Therefore, we count a score of $C_1 = 0$. We repeat this process for each subsequent rank of R_1, giving us a final score of 1 (by this point it is obvious that our original hypothesis—that larger hydrae live longer in test media than do small individual—was in error).

R_2	R_1	Following (R_2) ranks greater than (R_1)	Counts (C_i)
1	15		$C_1 = 0$
2	13		$C_2 = 0$
3	13		$C_3 = 0$
4	13		$C_4 = 0$
5	10		$C_5 = 0$
6	6.5	10	$C_6 = 0$
7	10	—	$C_7 = 0$
8	6.5		$C_8 = 0$
9	6.5		$C_9 = 0$
10	6.5		$C_{10} = 0$
11	3.5	6.5	$C_{11} = 0$
12	6.5	—	$C_{12} = 0$
13	3.5	—	$C_{13} = 0$
14	1.5	—	$C_{14} = 0$
15	1.5	—	$C_{15} = 0$
			$C_i = 1$

Our count of ranks, N, is then calculated as

$$N = 4(1) - 15(15 - 1)$$
$$= 4 - 15(14)$$
$$= -206.$$

We can then calculate tau as

$$= \frac{-206}{15(15-1)}$$
$$= \frac{-206}{210}$$
$$= -0.9810.$$

In other words, there is a strong negative correlation between our variables.

ASSUMPTIONS AND LIMITATIONS

1. A very robust estimator that does not assume normality, linearity, or minimal error of measurement.

Trend Analysis

Trend analysis is a collection of techniques that have been "discovered" by toxicology since the mid-1970s (141). The actual methodology dates back to the mid-1950s (29).

Trend analysis methods are a variation on the theme of regression testing. In the broadcast sense, the methods are used to determine whether a sequence of observations taken over an ordered range of a variable (most commonly time) exhibit some form of pattern of change (either an increase-upward trend) associated with another variable of interest (in toxicology, some form or measure of dosage or exposure).

Trend corresponds to sustained and systematic variations over a long period of time. It is associated with the structural causes of the phenomenon in question (e.g., population growth, technological progress, new ways of organization, or capital accumulation).

The identification of trend has always posed a serious statistical problem. The problem is not one of mathematical or analytical complexity but of conceptual complexity. This problem exists because the trend, as well as the remaining components of a time series, are latent (nonobservable) variables, and therefore, assumptions must be made on their behavioral pattern. The trend is generally thought of as a smooth and slow movement over a long term. The concept of "long" in this connection is relative, and what is identified as trend for a given series span might well be part of a long cycle once the series is considerably augmented. Often, a portion of a long cycle is treated as a trend because the length of the observed time series is shorter than one complete cycle.

The ways in which data are collected in toxicology studies frequently serve to complicate trend analysis, as the length of time for the phenomena underlying a trend to express themselves is frequently artificially censored. To avoid the complexity of the problem posed by a statistically vague definition, statisticians have resorted to two simple solutions. One consists of estimating trend and cyclical fluctuations together, calling this combined movement *trend-cycle*; the other consists of defining the trend in terms of the series length, denoting it as the longest nonperiodic movement.

Trend Models

Within the large class of models identified for trend, we can distinguish two main categories: deterministic trends and stochastic trends. Deterministic trend models are based on the assumption that the trend of a time series can be approximated closely by simple mathematical functions of time over the entire span of the series. The most common representation of a deterministic trend is by means of polynomials or of transcendental functions. The time series from which the trend is to be identified is assumed to be generated by a nonstationary process where the nonstationarity results from a deterministic trend. A classical model is the regression or error model (4), where the observed series is treated as the sum of a systematic part or trend and a random part or irregular part. This model can be written as

$$Z_t = Y_t + U_{t'},$$

where U_1 is a purely random process; that is, $U_t \sim$ i.i.d. (O_u^2) (independent and identically distributed with expected value 0 and variance σ_u^2).

Trend tests generally are described as "k-sample tests of the null hypothesis of identical distribution against an alternative of linear order"; i.e., if sample I has distribution function F_1, i = 1, then the null hypothesis

$$H-: F_1 = F_2 - \ldots = F_k$$

is tested against the alternative

$$H1: F_1 \geq F_2 \geq \ldots = F_k$$

(or its reverse); there, at least one of the inequalities is strict. These tests can be thought of as special cases of tests of regression or correlation in which association is sought between the observations and its ordered sample index. They are also related to analysis of variance except that the tests are tailored to be powerful against the subset of alternatives H_1, instead of the more general set $\{F_1 \neq F_j$, some $i \neq j\}$.

Different tests arise from requiring power against specific elements or subsets of this rather extensive set of alternatives. The most popular trend test in toxicology is currently that presented by Tarone (141) in 1975 because it is that used by the National Cancer Institute in the analysis of carcinogenicity data. The Armitage and Doll method also is recommended by UIS and Canadian regulatory agencies. A simple but efficient alternative is the Cox and Stuart test (29) which is a modification of the sign test. For each point at which we have a measure (such as the incidence of animals observed with tumors), we form a pair of observations—one from each of the groups we wish to compare. In a traditional National Cancer Institute (NCI) bioassay this would mean pairing control with low dose and low dose with high dose (to explore a dose-related trend) or each time period observation in a dose group (except the first) with its predecessor (to evaluate time-related trend). When the second observation in a pair exceeds the earlier observation, we record a plus sign for that pair. When the first observation is greater than the second, we record a minus sign for that pair. A preponderance of plus signs suggests a downward trend whereas an excess of minus signs suggests an upward trend. A formal test at a preselected confidence level can then be performed.

More formally put, after having defined what trend we want to test for, we first match pairs as $(X_1 - X_{1+c})$, (X_2, X_{2+c}), ... $(X_{n'-c}, X_{n'})$, where $c = n'/2$ when n' is even and $c = (n' + 1)/2$ when n' is odd (where n' is the number of observations in a set). The hypothesis is then tested by comparing the resulting number of excess positive or negative signs against a sign test table such as are found in Beyer.

	Control		Low Doses					
Month of Study	Total X Animal with Tumors	Change (X_{A-B})	Total Y Animals with Tumors	Change (Y_{A-B})	Compared to Control (Y-X)	Total Z Animals with Tumors	Change (Z_{a-b})	Compared to Control (Z-X)
12(A)	1	NA	0	NA	NA	5	NA	NA
13(B)	1	0	0	0	0	7	2	(+)2
14(C)	3	2	1	1	(−)1	11	4	(+)2
15(D)	3	0	1	0	0	11	0	0
16(E)	4	1	1	0	(−)1	13	2	(+)1
17(F)	5	1	3	2	(+)1	14	1	0
18(G)	5	0	3	0	0	15	1	(+)1
19(H)	5	0	5	2	(+)2	18	3	(+)3
20(I)	6	1	6	1	0	19	1	0
21(J)	8	2	7	1	(−)1	22	3	(+)1
22(K)	12	4	9	2	(−)2	26	4	0
23(L)	14	2	12	3	(+)1	28	2	0
24(M)	18	4	17	5	(+)1	31	3	(−)1
				Sum of signs	4+ 4−		Sum of signs	6+ 1−
				Y-X	=0 (No trend)		Z-X	=5

Reference to a sign table is not necessary for the low-dose comparison (where there is no trend), but clearly shows the high dose to be significant at the $p \leq 0.5$ level.

We can, of course, combine a number of observations to allow ourselves to actively test for a set of trends, such as the existence of a trend of increasing difference between two groups of animals over a period of time. This is demonstrated in Example 31.

Example 31

In a chronic feeding study in rats, we tested the hypothesis that in the second year of the study there as a dose-responsive increase in tumor incidence associated with the test compound. We utilize below a Cox–Stuart test for trend to address this question. All groups start the second year with an equal number of animals.

ASSUMPTIONS AND LIMITATIONS

1. Trend tests seek to evaluate whether there is monotonic tendency in response to a change in treatment. That is, the dose response direction is absolute—as dose goes up, the incidence of tumors increases. Thus, the test loses power rapidly in response to the occurrences of "reversals"—for example, a low-dose group with a decreased tumor incidence. There are methods (47) that "smooth the bumps" of reversals in long data series. In toxicology, however, most data series are short (i.e., there are only a few dose levels).

Tarone's trend test is most powerful at detecting dose-related trends when tumor onset hazard functions are proportional to each other. For more power against other dose-related group differences, weighted versions of the statistic are also available (19,32).

In 1985, the United States *Federal Register* (53) recommended that the analysis of tumor incidence data is carried out with a Cochran–Armitage (8,27) trend test.

The test statistic of the Cochran–Armitage test is defined as this term:

$$T_{CA} = \sqrt{\frac{N}{((N-r))r}}, \frac{\sum_{i=0}^{k}\left(R_1 - \frac{n_1}{N}r\right)d_1}{\sqrt{\sum_{i=0}^{k}\frac{n_i}{N}d_i^2 - \left(\sum_{i=0}^{k}\frac{n_i}{N}d_1\right)^2}}$$

with dose scores d_i. Armitage's test statistic is the square of this term (T^2_{CA}). As one-sided tests are carried out for an increase of tumor rates, the square is not considered. Instead, the above-mentioned test statistic, which is presented by Portier and Hoel (120), is used. This test statistic is asymptotically standard normal distributed. The Cochran–Armitage test is asymptotically efficient for all monotone alternatives (141) but this result only holds asymptotically. Tumors are rare events, so the binominal proportions are small. In this situation approximations may become unreliable. Therefore, exact tests can be performed using two different approaches: conditional and unconditional are considered. In the first case, the total number of tumors r is regarded as fixed. As a result, the null distribution of the test statistic is independent of the common probability p. The exact conditional null distribution is a multivariate hypergeometric distribution.

The unconditional model treats the sum of all tumors as a random variable. Then the exact unconditional null distribution is a multivariate binomial distribution. The distribution depends on the unknown probability.

METHODS FOR THE REDUCTION OF DIMENSIONALITY

Techniques for the reduction of dimensionality are those that simplify the understanding of data, either visually or numerically, while causing only minimal reductions in the amount of information present. These techniques operate primarily by pooling or combining groups of variables into single variables, but may also entail the identification and elimination of low-information-content (or irrelevant) variables.

Descriptive statistics (calculations of means, SDs, etc.) are the simplest and most familiar form of reduction of dimensionality. Here we first need to address classification, which provides the general conceptual tools for identifying and quantifying similarities and differences between groups of things that have more than a single linear scale of measurement in common (e.g., which have both been determined to have or lack a number of enzyme activities). Then we will consider two collections of methodologies that combine graphic and computational methods, multidimensional/nonmetric scaling, and cluster analysis. Multidimensional scaling (MDS) is a set of techniques for quantitatively analyzing similarities, dissimilarities, and distances between data in a display-like manner. Nonmetric scaling is an analogous set of methods for displaying and relating data when measurements are nonquantitative (the data are described by attributes or ranks). Cluster analysis is a collection of graphic and numerical methodologies for classifying things based on the relationships between the values of the variables that they share.

The final pair of methods for reduction of dimensionality that will be tackled in this chapter are Fourier analysis and the life table analysis. Fourier analysis seeks to identify cyclic patterns in data and then either analyze the patterns or the residuals after the patterns are taken out. Life table analysis techniques are directed to identifying and quantitating the time course of risks (such as death or the occurrence of tumors).

Classification

Classification is both a basic concept and a collection of techniques that are necessary prerequisites for further analysis of data when the members of a set of data are (or can be) each described by several variables. At least some degree of classification (which is broadly defined as the dividing of the members of a group into smaller groups in accordance with a set of decision rules) is necessary prior to any data collection. Whether formally or informally, an investigator has to decide which things are similar enough to be counted as the same and develop rules for governing collection procedures. Such rules can be simple as "measure and record body weights only of live animals on study," or as complex as that demonstrated by the expanded weighting classification presented in Example 32. Such a classification also demonstrates that the selection of which variables to measure will determine the final classification of data.

Example 32

I.	Is animal of desired species?	Yes/No
II.	Is animal member of study group?	Yes/No
III.	Is animal alive?	Yes/No
IV.	Which group does animal belong to? A. Control B. Low dose C. Intermediate dose D. High dose	
V.	What sex is animal?	Male/Female
VI.	Is the measured weight in acceptable range?	Yes/No

Classifications of data have two purposes (73,81): data simplification (also called a descriptive function) and prediction. Simplification is necessary because there is a limit to both the volume and complexity of data that the human mind can comprehend and deal with conceptually. Classification allows us to attach a label (or name) to each group of data, to summarize the data (i.e., assign individual elements of data to groups and to characterize the population of the group), and to define the relationships between groups (i.e., develop a taxonomy).

Prediction, meanwhile, is the use of summaries of data and knowledge of the relationships between groups to develop hypotheses as to what will happen when further data are collected (as when more animals or people are exposed to an agent under defined conditions) and as to the mechanisms which cause such relationships to develop. Indeed, classification is the prime device for the discovery of mechanisms in all of science. A classic example of this was Darwin's realization that there were reasons (the mechanisms of evolution) behind the differences and similarities in species that had caused Linaeus to earlier develop his initial modern classification scheme (or taxonomy) for animals.

To develop a classification, one first sets bounds wide enough to encompass the entire range of data to be considered but not unnecessarily wide. This is typically done by selecting some global variables (variables every piece of data has in common) and limiting the range of each so that it just encompasses all of the cases on hand. Then one selects a set of local variables (characteristics which only some of the cases have, say, the occurrence of certain tumor types, enzyme activity levels, or dietary preferences) which thus serve to differentiate between groups. Data are then collected, and a system for measuring differences and similarities is developed. Such measurements are based on some form of measurement of distance between two cases (x and y) in terms of each single variable scale. If the variable is a continuous one, then the simplest measure of distance between two pieces of data is the Euclidean distance, (d[x, y]), defined as

$$= \frac{0.1375}{0.037081} = 3.708.$$

For categorical or discontinuous data, the simplest distance measure is the matching distance, defined as:

$$d(x, y) = \text{number of times } x_i \neq y_i.$$

After we have developed a table of such distance measurements for each of the local variables, some weighting factor is assigned to each variable. A weighting factor seeks to give greater importance to those variables that are believed to have more relevance or predictive value. The weighted variables are then used to assign each piece of data to a group. The actual act of developing numerically based classifications and assigning data members to them is the realm of cluster analysis and will be discussed later in this chapter. Classification of biological data based on qualitative factors has been well discussed (70,73) and does an excellent job of introducing the entire field and mathematical concepts.

Relevant examples of the use of classification techniques range from the simple to the complex. Schaper et al. (130) developed and used a very simple classification of response methodology to identify those airborne chemicals which alter the normal respiratory response induced by CO_2. At the other end of the spectrum, Kowalski and Bender (98) developed a more mathematically based system to classify chemical data (a methodology they termed *pattern recognition*).

Statistical Graphics

The use of graphics in one form or another in statistics is the single most effective and robust statistical tool, and at the same time, one of the most poorly understood and improperly used. Graphs are used in statistics (and in toxicology) for one of four major purposes. Each of the four is a variation on the central theme of making complex data easier to understand and use. These four major functions are exploration, analysis, communication and display of data, and graphical aids. Exploration (which may be simply summarizing data or trying to expose relationships between variables) is determining the characteristics of data sets and deciding on one or more appropriate forms of further analysis, such as the scatter plot. Analysis is the use of graphs to formally evaluate some aspect of the data, such as whether there are outliers present or if an underlying assumption of a population distribution is fulfilled. As long ago as 1960 (5), some 18 graphical methods for analyzing multivariate data relationships were developed and proposed.

Communication and display of data are the most commonly used function of statistical graphics in toxicology, whether used for internal reports, presentations at meetings, or formal publications in the literature. In communicating data, graphs should not be used to duplicate data that are presented in tables, but rather to show important trends and/or relationships in the data. Though such communication is most commonly of a quantitative compilation of actual data, it can also be used to summarize and present the results of statistical analysis. The fourth and final function of graphics is one that is largely becoming outdated as microcomputers become more widely available. Graphical aids to calculation include nomograms (the classic example in toxicology of a nomogram is that presented by Litchfield and Wilcoxon for determining median effective doses) and extrapolating and interpolating data graphically based on plotted data.

There are many forms of statistical graphics (a partial list, classified by function, is presented in Table 7.6), and a number of these (such as scatter plots and histograms) can be used for each of a number of possible functions. Most of these plots are based on a Cartesian system (i.e., they use a set of rectangular coordinates), and our review of construction and use will focus on these forms of graphs.

Construction of a rectangular graph of any form starts with the selection of the appropriate form of graph followed by the laying out of the coordinates (or axes). Even graphs that are going to encompass multivariate data (i.e., more than two variables) generally have as their starting point two major coordinates. The vertical axis, or ordinate (also called the Y axis), is used to present an independent variable. Each of these axes is scaled in the units of measure that will most clearly present the trends of interest in the data. The range covered by the scale of each axis is selected to cover the entire region for which data is presented. The actual demarking of

Table 7.6
Forms of statistical graphics (by function)

EXPLORATION		
Data Summary	**Two Variables**	**Three or More Variables**
Box and whisker plot	Autocorrelation plot	Biplot
Histogram	Cross-correlation plot	Cluster trees
Dot-array diagram	Scatter plot	Labeled scatter plot
Frequency polygon	Sequence plot	Glyphs and metroglyphs
Ogive		Face plots
Stem and leaf diagram		Fourier plots
		Similarity and preference maps
		Multidimensional scaling displays
		Weathervane plot
ANALYSIS		
Distribution Assessment	**Model Evaluation and Assumption Verification**	**Decision Making**
Probability plot	Average versus standard deviation	Control chart
Q-Q plot	Component-plus-residual plot	Cusum chart
P-P plot	Partial-residual plot	Half-normal plot
Hanging histogram	Residual plots	Ridge trace
Rootagram		Youden plot
Poissonness plot		
COMMUNICATION AND DISPLAY OF DATA		
Quantitative Graphics	**Summary of Statistical Analyses**	**Graphical Aids**
Line chart	Means plot	Confidence limits
Pictogram	Sliding reference distribution	Graph paper
Pie chart	Notched box plot	Power curves
Contour plot	Factor space/response	Nomographs
Stereogram	Interaction plot	Sample-size curves
Color Map	Contour plot	Trilinear coordinates
Histogram	Predicted response plot	
	Confidence region plot	

the measurement scale along an axis should allow for easy and accurate assessment of the coordinates of any data point, yet should not be cluttered.

Actual data points should be presented by symbols that present the appropriate indicators of location, and if they represent summaries of data from a normal data population, it would be appropriate to present a symbol for the mean and some indication of the variability (or error) associated with that population, commonly by using "error bars" which present the SD (or standard error) from the mean. If, however, the data are not normal or continuous, it would be more appropriate to indicate location by the median and present the range or semiquartile distance for variability estimates. The symbols that are used to present data points can also be used to present a significant amount of additional information. At the simplest level a set of clearly distinct symbols (circles, triangles, squares, etc.) are very commonly used to provide a third dimension of data (most commonly, treatment group), but by clever use of symbols, all sorts of additional information can be presented. Using a method such as Chernoff's faces (79), in which faces are used as symbols of the data points (and various aspects of the faces present additional data, such as the presence or absence of eyes denoting presence or absence of a secondary pathological condition), it is

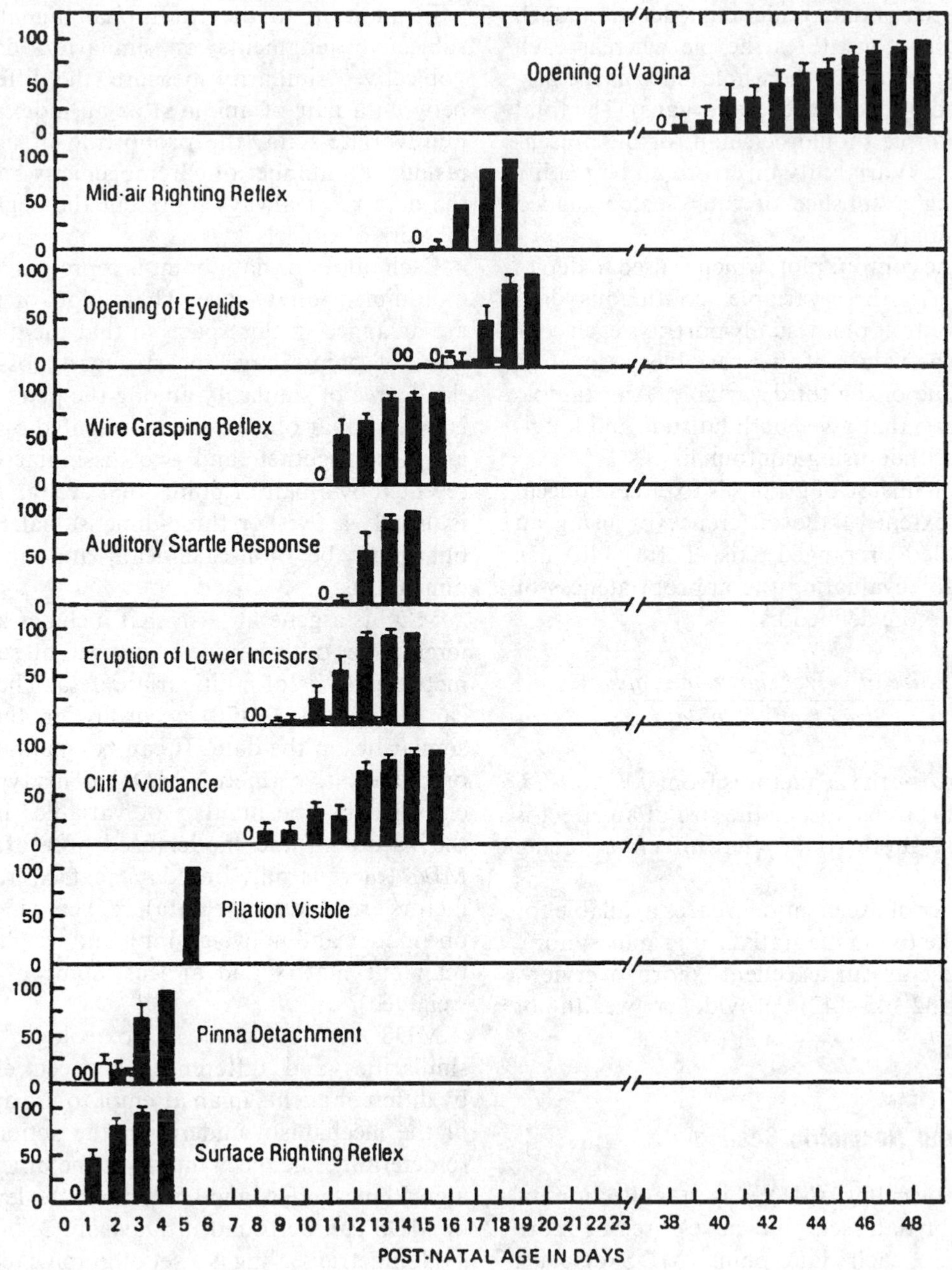

FIG. 7.8. Acquisitions of postnatal development landmarks in rats.

possible to present a large number of different variables on a single graph.

The three other forms of graphs that are commonly used in toxicology are histograms, pie charts, and contour plots. Histograms are graphs of simple frequency distribution. Commonly, the abscissa is the variable of interest (such as lifespan or litter size) and generally is shown as classes or intervals or measurements (such as age ranges of 0 to 10 weeks, 10 to 20 weeks, etc.). The ordinate, meanwhile, is the incidence or frequency of observations. The result is a set of vertical bars, each of which represents the incidence of a particular set of observations. Measures of error or variability about each incidence are reflected by some form of error bar on top of or in the frequency bars, as shown in Figure 7.8. The size of class intervals may be unequal (in effect, one can combine or pool several small class intervals), but it is proper in such cases to vary the width of the bars to indicate differences in interval size.

Pie charts are the only common form of quantitative graphic technique that is not rectangular. Rather, the figure is presented as a circle out of which several "slices" are delimited. The only major use of the pie chart is in presenting a breakdown of the components of a group.

Typically the entire set of data under consideration (such as total body weight) constitutes the pie whereas each slice represents a percentage of the whole (such as the percentages represented by each of several organs). The total number of slices in a pie should be small for the presentation to be effective. Variability or error can be readily presented by having a subslice of each sector shaded and labeled accordingly.

Finally, there is the contour plot, which is used to depict the relationships in a three-variable, continuous data system. That is, a contour plot visually portrays each contour as a locus of the values of two variables associated with a constant value of the third variable. An example would be a relief map that gives both latitude and longitude of constant altitude using contour lines.

The most common misuse of graphs is to either conceal or exaggerate the extent of the difference by using an inappropriately scaled or ranged axis. Tufte (146) has termed a statistic for evaluating the appropriateness of scale size, the lie factor, defined as

$$\text{Lie factor} = \frac{\textit{Size of effect shown in graph}}{\textit{Size of effect in data}}.$$

An acceptable range for the lie factor is from 0.95 to 1.05. A value less than this range means the size of an effect is being understated, more than the effect is being exaggerated.

There are a number of excellent references available for those who would like to pursue statistical graphics more. Anscombe (7) presents an excellent short overview, whereas others (132,145–147) provide a wealth of information.

Multidimensional and Nonmetric Scaling

Multidimensional scaling (MDS) is a collection of analysis methods for data sets that have three or more variables making up each data point. MDS displays the relationships of three or more dimensional extensions of the methods of statistical graphics.

MDS presents the structure of a set of objects from data that approximate the distances between pairs of the objects. The data, called similarities, dissimilarities, distances, or proximities, must be in such a form that the degree of similarities and differences between the pairs of the objects (each of which represents a real-life data point) can be measured and handled as a distance (remember the discussion of measures of distances under classifications). Similarity is a matter of degree, small differences between objects cause them to be "similar" (a high degree of similarity) whereas large differences cause them to be considered dissimilar (a small degree of similarity).

In addition to the traditional human conceptual or subjective judgments of similarity, data can be an "objective" similarity measure (the difference in weight between a pair of animals) or an index calculated from multivariate data (the proportion of agreement in the results of a number of carcinogenicity studies); however, the data must always represent the degree of similarity of pairs of objects.

Each object or data point is represented by a point in a multidimensional space. These plots or projected points are arranged in this space so that the distances between pairs of points have the strongest possible relation to the degree of similarity among the pairs of objects. That is, two similar objects are represented by two points that are close together, and two dissimilar objects are represented by a pair of points that are far apart. The space is usually a two- or three-dimensional Euclidean space, but may be non-Euclidean and may have more dimensions.

MDS is a general term that includes a number of different types of techniques; however, all seek to allow geometric analysis of multivariate data. The forms of MDS can be classified (170) according to the nature of the similarities in the data. It can be qualitative (nonmetric) or quantitative (metric MDS). The types can also be classified by the number of variables involved and by the nature of the model used—for example, classical MDS (there is only one data matrix, and no weighting factors are used on the data), replicated MDS (more than one matrix and no weighting), and weighted MDS (more than one matrix and at least some of the data being weighted).

MDS can be used in toxicology to analyze the similarities and differences between effects produced by different agents in an attempt to use an understanding of the mechanism underlying the actions of one agent to determine the mechanisms of the other agents. Actual algorithms and a good intermediate level presentation of MDS can be found in Davison (35).

Nonmetric scaling is a set of graphic techniques closely related to MDS, and is definitely useful for the reduction of dimensionality. Its major objective is to arrange a set of objects (each object, for our purposes, consisting of a number of related observations) graphically in a few dimensions while retaining the maximum possible fidelity to the original relationships between members (i.e., values that are most different are portrayed as most distant). It is not a linear technique and it does not preserve linear relationships (i.e., A is not shown as twice as far from C as B, even though its "value difference" may be twice as much). The spacings (interpoint distances) are kept such that if the distance of the original scale between members A and B is greater than that between C and D, the distances on the model scale shall likewise be greater between A and B than between C and D. Figure 7.5 uses a form of this technique in adding a third dimension by using letters to present degrees of effect on the skin.

This technique functions by taking observed measures of similarity or dissimilarity between every pair of M objects and then finding a representation of the objects as points in Euclidean space that the interpoint distances in some sense "match" the observed similarities or dissimilarities by means of weighting constants.

Cluster Analysis

Cluster analysis is a quantitative form of classification. It serves to help develop decision rules and then use these rules to assign a heterogeneous collection of objects to a series of sets. This is almost entirely an applied methodology (as opposed to theoretical). The final result of cluster analysis is one of several forms of graphic displays and a methodology (set of decision-classifying rules) for the assignment of new members into the classifications.

The classification procedures used are based on either density of population or distance between members. These methods can serve to generate a basis for the classification of large numbers of dissimilar variables, such as behavioral observations and compounds with distinct but related structures and mechanisms (63,64), or to separate tumor patterns caused by treatment from those caused by old age (14).

There are five types of clustering techniques (52):

a. Hierarchical techniques: Classes are subclassified into groups, with the process being repeated at several levels to produce a tree that gives sufficient definition to groups.
b. Optimizing techniques: Clusters are formed by optimization of a clustering criterion. The resulting classes are mutually exclusive; the objects are partitioned clearly into sets.
c. Density- or mode-seeking techniques: Clusters are identified and formed by locating regions in a graphic representation that contains concentrations of data points.
d. Clumping techniques: A variation of density-seeking techniques in which assignment to a cluster is weighted on some variables so that clusters may overlap in graphic projections.
e. Others: Methods that do not clearly fall into classes a–d.

Romesburg (124) provides an excellent step-by-step guide to cluster analysis.

Fourier or Time Analysis

Fourier analysis (16) is most frequently a univariate method used for either simplifying data (which is the basis for its inclusion in this chapter) or for modeling. It can, however, also be a multivariate technique for data analysis. In a sense it is like trend analysis; it looks at the relationship of sets of data from a different perspective. In the case of Fourier analysis, the approach is by resolving the time dimension variable in the data set. At the most simple level it assumes that many events are periodic in nature, and if we can remove the variation in other variables because of this periodicity (by using Fourier transforms), we can better analyze the remaining variation from other variables. The complications to this are (a) there may be several overlying cyclic time-based periodicities, and (b) we may be interested in the time cycle events for their own sake.

Fourier analysis allows one to identify, quantitate, and (if we wish) remove the time-based cycles in data (with their amplitudes, phases, and frequencies) by use of the Fourier transform:

$$nJ_i = x_i \exp(-iw_i t),$$

where

n = length
J = The discrete Fourier transform for that case,
x = actual data,
i = increment in the series,
w = frequency,
t = time.

A graphic example of the use of Fourier analysis in toxicology is provided in Figure 7.9.

Life Tables

Chronic in vivo toxicity studies generally are the most complex and expensive studies conducted by a toxicologist. Answers to a number of questions are sought in such a study—notably if a material results in a significant increase in mortality or in the incidence of tumors in those animals exposed to it, but we are also interested in the time course of these adverse effects (or risks). The classic approach to assessing these age-specific hazard rates is by the use of life tables (also called survivorship tables).

It may readily be seen that during any selected period of time (t_i) we have a number of risks competing to affect an animal. There are risks of (a) "natural death," (b) death induced by a direct or indirect action of the test compound, and (c) death due to such occurrences of interest as tumors (77). We are indeed interested in determining if (and when) the last two of these risks become significantly different than the "natural" risks (defined as what is seen to happen in the control group). Life table methods enable us to make such determinations as the duration of survival (or time until tumors develop) and the probabil-

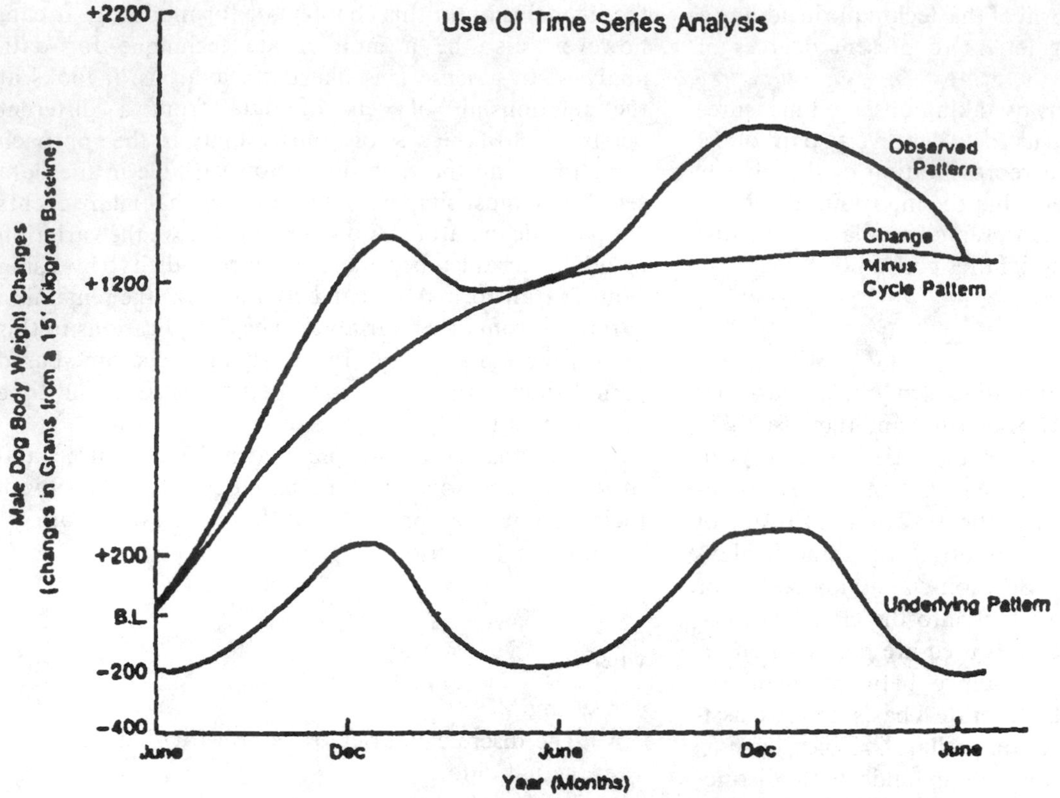

FIG. 7.9. Use of time series analysis.

ity of survival (or of developing a tumor) during any period of time.

We start by deciding the interval length (t_i) we wish to examine within the study. The information we gain becomes more exact as the interval is shortened, but as interval length is decreased, the number of intervals increases and calculations become more cumbersome and less indicative of time-related trends because random fluctuations become more apparent. For a 2-year or lifetime rodent study, an interval length of a month is commonly employed. Some life table methods, such as the Kaplan–Meyer, have each new event (such as a death) define the start of a new interval.

Having established the interval length, we can tabulate our data (33). We start by establishing the following columns in each table (a separate table being established for each group of animals—i.e., by sex and dose level):

(a) The interval of time selected (t_i).
(b) The number of animals in the group that entered that interval of the study alive (l_i).
(c) The number of animals withdrawn from study during the interval (such as those taken for an interim sacrifice or that may have been killed by a technician error) (ω_i).
(d) The number of animals that died during the interval (d_i).
(e) The number of animals at risk during the interval, $l_i = l_i - 1/2\omega_I$, or the number on study at the start of the interval minus one half of the number withdrawn during the interval.
(f) The proportion of animals that died $= D_i = d_i/l_i$.
(g) The cumulative probability of an animal surviving until the end of that interval of study, $P_i = 1 – D_i$, or one minus the number of animals that died during that interval divided by the number of animals at risk.
(h) The number of animals dying until that interval (M_i).
(i) Animals found to have died during the interval (m_i).
(j) The probability of dying during the interval of the study $c_i = 1–(M_i + m_i/l_i)$, or the total number of animals dead until that interval plus the animals discovered to have died during that interval divided by the number of animals at risk through the end of that interval.
(k) The cumulative proportion surviving, p_i, is equivalent to the cumulative product of the interval probabilities of survival (i.e., $p_i = p_1 \cdot p_2 \cdot p_3 \cdots p_x$).
(l) The cumulative probability of dying, C_i, equal to the cumulative product of the interval probabilities to that point (i.e., $C_i = c_1 \cdot c_2 \cdot c_3 \cdots c_x$).

With such tables established for each group in a study (as shown in Example 33), we may now proceed to test the hypotheses that each of the treated groups has a significantly shorter duration of survival or that the treated groups died more quickly (note that plots of total animals dead and total animals surviving will give one an appreciation of the data, but can lead to no statistical conclusions).

Now, for these two groups, we wish to determine effective sample size and to compare survival probabilities in the interval months 14 to 15.

For the exposure group we compute sample size as

$$\ell_{E14-15} = \frac{0.8400(1 - 0.8400)}{(0.0367)^2} = 99.7854$$

Likewise, we get a sample size of 98.1720 for the control group.

The standard error of difference for the two groups here is

$$SD = \sqrt{0.0367^2 + 0.0173^2} = 0.040573$$

The probability of survival differences is $P_D = 0.9697 - 0.8400 = 0.1297$. Our test statistic is then $0.1297/0.040573 = 3.196$. From our z value table we see that the critical values are

$$p \leq 0.05 = 1.960$$
$$p \leq 0.01 = 2.575$$
$$p \leq 0.001 = 3.270$$

As our calculated value is larger than all but the last of these, we find our groups to be significantly different at the 0.01 level ($0.01 > p > 0.001$).

There are a multiplicity of methods for testing significance in life tables, with (as is often the case) the power of the tests increasing as does the difficulty of computation (30,83,126,141).

We begin our method of statistical comparison of survival at any point in the study by determining the standard error of the K interval survival rate as (66)

$$S_K = P_k \sqrt{\sum_{1}^{k}\left(\frac{D_i}{1'_x - d_x}\right)}.$$

We may also determine the effective sample size (l_1) in accordance with

$$l_1 = \frac{P(1 - P)}{S^2}.$$

Example 33

Test level 1

Interval (months) I_i	Alive at Beginning of interval I_i	Animals withdrawn w_i	Died during interval d_i	Animals at risk I_i	Proportion of animals dead D_i	Probability of survival P_i	Cumulative proportion surviving P_i	Standard error of survival S_i
8–9	109	0	0	109	0	1.0000	1.0000	0.0000
9–10	109	0	2	109	0.0184	0.9816	0.9816	0.0129
10–11	107	0	0	107	0	1.0000	0.9816	0.0128
11–12	107	10	0	102	0	1.0000	0.9816	0.0128
12–13	97	0	1	97	0.0103	0.9897	0.9713	0.0162
13–14	96	0	1	96	0.0104	0.9896	0.9614	0.0190
14–15	95	0	12	95	0.1263	0.8737	0.8400	0.0367
15–16	83	0	2	83	0.0241	0.9759	0.8198	0.0385
16–17	81	0	3	81	0.0370	0.9630	0.7894	0.0409
17–18	78	20	1	68	0.0147	0.9853	0.7778	0.0419
18–19	57	0	2	57	0.0351	0.6949	0.7505	0.0446
Control Level								
11–12	99	0	1	99	0.0101	0.9899	0.9899	0.0100
12–13	98	0	0	98	0	1.0000	0.9899	0.0100
13–14	98	0	0	98	0	1.0000	0.9899	0.0100
14–15	98	0	2	98	0.0204	0.9796	0.9697	0.0172
15–16	96	0	1	96	0.0104	0.9896	0.9596	0.0198
16–17	95	0	0	95	0	1.0000	0.9596	0.0198
17–18	95	20	2	85	0.0235	0.8765	0.9370	0.0249
18–19	73	0	2	73	0.0274	0.9726	0.9113	0.0302

We may now compute the standard error of difference for any two groups (1 and 2) as

$$S_D = \sqrt{S_1^2 + S_2^2}.$$

The difference in survival probabilities for the two groups is then calculated as

$$P_D = P_1 - P_2.$$

We can then calculate a test statistic as

$$t' = \frac{P_D}{S_D}.$$

This is then compared to a z distribution table. If $t' > z$ at the desired probability level, it is significant at that level. Example 33 illustrates the life table technique for mortality data. With increasing recognition of the effects of time (both as age and length of exposure to unmeasured background risks), life table analysis has become a mainstay in chronic toxicology. An example is the reassessment of the ED_{01} study (139), which radically changed interpretation of the results and understanding of underlying methods when adjustment for time on study was made.

Now, for these two groups, we wish to determine effective sample size and to compare survival probabilities in the interval months 14–15.

For the exposure group we compute sample size as

$$S_{xx} = T_{xx} + \sum\nolimits_{xx}.$$

Likewise, we get a sample size of 98.1720 for the control group.

The standard error of difference for the two groups here is

$$SD = \sqrt{0.0367^2 + 0.0173^2} = 0.040573.$$

The probability of survival differences is $P_D = 0.9697 - 0.8400 = 0.1297$. Our test statistic is then $0.1297/0.040573 = 3.196$. From our z value table we see that the critical values are

$$p \leq 0.05 = 1.960,$$
$$p \leq 0.01 = 2.575,$$
$$p \leq 0.001 = 3.270.$$

As our calculated value is larger than all but the last of these, we find our groups to be significantly different at the 0.01 level ($0.01 > p > 0.001$).

The increased importance and interest in the analysis of survival data has not been restricted to toxicology, but rather has encompassed all of the life sciences. Those with further interest should consult Lee (101) or Elandt-Johnson and Johnson (49), both general in their approach to the subject.

Multivariate Methods

In a chapter of this kind, an in-depth explanation of the available multivariate statistical techniques is an impossibility; however, as the complexity of problems in toxicology increases, we can expect to confront more frequently data that are not univariate but rather multivariate (or multidimensional). For example, a multidimensional study might be one in which the animals are being dosed with two materials that interact. Suppose we measure body weight, tumor incidence, and two clinical chemistry values for test material effects and interaction. Our dimensions, or variables, are now A = dose "x," B = dose "y," W = body weight, C = tumor incidence, D and E = levels of clinical chemistry parameters, and possibly also t (length of dosing).

These situations are particularly common in chronic studies (129). Though we can continue to use multiple sets of univariate techniques as we have in the past, there are significant losses of power, efficiency, and information when this is done, as well as an increased possibility of error (34).

Here we will also look briefly at the workings and uses of each of the most commonly employed multivariate techniques, together with several examples from the literature of their employment in toxicology and the other biological sciences. We shall group the methods according to their primary function: hypothesis testing (are these significant or not?), model fitting (what is the relationship between these variables, or what would happen if a population would be exposed to x?), and reduction of dimensionality (which variables are most meaningful?). It should be noted (and will soon be obvious), however, that most multivariate techniques actually combine several of these functions.

The most fundamental concept in multivariate analysis is that of a multivariate population distribution. By this point it is assumed that the reader is familiar with the univariate random variable and with such standard distributions as the normal distribution. Here we extend these to the multivariate normal distribution.

Multivariate data are virtually never processed and analyzed other than by computer. One must first set up an appropriate database file and then enter the data, coding some of them to meet the requirements of the software being used (e.g., if only numerical data are analyzed, sex may have to be coded as 1 for male and 2 for females).

Having recorded the data, it is then essential to review for suspect values and errors of various kinds. There are many different types of suspect values, and it is helpful to distinguish among them:

(a) Outliers: These are defined to be observations that appear to be inconsistent with the rest of the data. They may be caused by gross recording or entering errors, but it is important to realize that an apparent outlier may occasionally be genuine and indicate a non-normal distribution or valuable data point.
(b) Inversions: A common type of error occurs when two consecutive digits are interchanged at the recording, coding, or entering stage. The error may be trivial if, for example, 56.74 appears as 56.47, but it may generate an outlier if 56.74 appears as 65.74.
(c) Repetitions: At the coding or entering stage, it is quite easy to repeat an entire number in two successive rows or columns of a table, thereby omitting one number completely.
(d) Values in the wrong column: It is easy to get numbers into the wrong columns.
(e) Other errors and suspect values: There are many other types of error, including possible misrecording of data of a minor nature.

The general term used to denote procedures for detecting and correcting errors is *data editing*. This includes checks for completeness, consistency, and credibility. Some editing can be done at the end of the data entry stage. In addition, many routine checks can be made by the computer itself, particularly those for gross outliers. An important class of such checks are range tests. For each variable an allowable range of possible values is specified and the computer checks that all observed values lie within the given range. Bivariate and multivariate checks are also possible. For example, one may specify an allowable range for some functions of two or more variables. A set of checks called "if-then" checks are also possible. For example, if both age and date of birth are recorded for each animal, then one can check that the answers are consistent. If the date of birth is given, then one can deduce the corresponding age. In fact, in this example the age observation is redundant. It is sometimes a good idea to include one or two redundant variables as a check on accuracy. Various other general procedures for detecting outliers are described by Barnett and Lewis (10).

When a questionable value or error is detected, the toxicologist must decide what to do about it. One may be able to go back to the original data source and check the observation. Inversions, repetitions, and values in the wrong column can often be corrected in this way. Outliers are more difficult to handle, particularly when they are impossible to check or have been misrecorded in the first place. It may be sensible to treat them as missing values and try to insert a value "guessed" in an appropriate way (e.g., by interpolation or by prediction from other variables). Alternatively, the value may have to be left as unrecorded and then either all observations for the given individual will have to be discarded or one will have to accept unequal numbers of observations for the different variables. With a univariate set of observations, the analysis usually begins with the calculation of two summary statistics, namely the mean and standard deviation. In the multivariate case, the analysis usually begins with the calculation of the mean and standard deviation for each variable, and, in addition, the correlation coefficient for each pair of variables is usually calculated. Their summary statistics are vital in having a preliminary look at the data.

The sample mean of the jth variable is given by

$$\bar{x}_j = \sum_{r=1}^{n} x_{rj}/n,$$

and the sample mean vector, x, is given by $x^T = [x_1, x_2, x_n, \ldots, xn]$. If the observations are a random sample from a population with mean $\bar{x}$, then the sample mean vector x is usually the point estimate of x, and this estimate can easily be shown to be unbiased.

The SD of the jth variable is given by

$$Sj = \sqrt{\left[\sum_{r=1}^{n} (x_{rj} - \bar{x}_j^2)/(n-1)\right]}.$$

The correlation coefficient of variables i and j is given by

$$r_{ij} = \sum_{r=1}^{n} (x_{ri} - \bar{x}_j)(x_{rj} - \bar{x}_j)/(n-1)S_i s_j.$$

These coefficients can be conveniently assembled in the sample correlation matrix, R, which is given by

$$R = \begin{bmatrix} 1 & r_{12} & \cdots & r_{1n} \\ r_{21} & 1 & \cdots & r_{2n} \\ \vdots & & & \\ r_n^1 & r_n^2 & \cdots & 1 \end{bmatrix}.$$

Note that the diagonal terms are all unity.

The interpretation of mean and standard deviations is straightforward. It is worth looking to see if, for example, some variables have much higher scatter than others. It is also worth looking at the form of the distribution of each variable and considering whether any of the variables need to be transformed. For example, the logarithmic transformation is often used to reduce positive skewness and produce a distribution that is closer to normal.

One may also consider the removal of outliers at this stage.

There are three significant multivariate techniques that have hypothesis testing as their primary function: MANOVA, MANCOVA, and factor analysis.

MANOVA (multivariate analysis of variance) is the multidimensional extension of the ANOVA process we explored before. It can be shown to have grown out of Hotelling's T^2 (88), which provides a means of testing the overall null hypothesis that two groups do not differ in their means on any of p measures. MANOVA accomplishes its comparison of two (or more) groups by reducing the set of p measures on each group to a simple number applying the linear combining rule $W_i = w_j X_{ij}$ (where w_j is a weighting factor) and then computing a univariate F-ratio on the combined variables. New sets of weights (w_j) are selected in turn until that set which maximizes the F-ratio is found. The final resulting maximum F-ratio (based on the multiple discriminant functions) is then the basis of the significance test. As with ANOVA, MANOVA can be one way or higher order, and MANOVA has as a basic assumption a multivariate normal distribution.

Gray and Laskey (75) used MANOVA to analyze the reproductive effects of manganese in the mouse, allowing identification of significant effects at multiple sites. Witten et al. (167) utilized MANOVA to determine the significance of the effects of dose, time, and cell division in the action of abrin on the lymphocytes.

Multivariate analysis of covariance (MANCOVA) is the multivariate analog of analysis of covariance. As with MANOVA, it is based on the assumption that the data being analyzed are from a multivariate normal population. The MANCOVA test uses the two residual matrices using the statistic and is an extension of ANCOVA with two or more uncontrolled variables (or covariables). A detailed discussion can be found in Tatsuoka (142).

Factor analysis is not just a technique for hypothesis testing; it can also serve a reduction of dimensionality function. It seeks to separate the variance unique to particular sets of values from that common to all members in that variable system and is based on the assumption that the intercorrelations among the n original variables are the result of there being some smaller number of variables ("factors") that explain the bulk of variation seen in the variables. There are several approaches to achieving the end results, but they all seek a determination of what percentage of the variance of each variable is explained by each factor (a factor being one variable or a combination of variables). The model in factor analysis is $y = Af + xz$, where

y = n dimensional vector of observable responses;
A = factor loading an $n \times q$ matrix of unknown parameters;
f = q dimensional vector of common factor;
z = n dimensional vector of unique factor.

Used for the reduction of dimensionality, factor analysis is said to be a linear technique because it does not change the linear relationships between the variables being examined.

Joung et al. (92) used factor analysis to develop a generalized water quality index that promises suitability across the United States, with appropriate weightings for 10 parameters. Factor analysis promises great utility as a tool for developing models in risk analysis, where a number of parameters act and interact.

Now we move on to two multivariate modeling techniques: multiple regression and discriminant analysis.

Multiple regression and correlation seeks to predict one (or a few) variable from several others. It assumes that the available variables can be logically divided into two (or more) sets and serves to establish maximal linear (or some other scale) relationships among the sets;

The linear model for the regression is simply

$$Y = b_0 + b_1X_1 + b_2X_2 + \cdots + b_pX_p,$$

where Y = the predicted value, b = values set to maximize correlations between X and Y, and X and Y = the actual observations (with X's being independent of predictor variables and Y's being dependent variables or outcome measures). One of the outputs from the process will be the coefficient of multiple correlation, which is simply the multivariate equivalent of the correlation coefficient (r).

Schaeffer et al. (128) have neatly demonstrated the utilization of multiple regression in studying the contribution of two components of a mixture to its toxicologic action, using quantitative results from an Ames test as an end point. Paintz et al. (116) similarly used multiple regression to model the quantitative structure-activity relationships of a series of 14 1-benzoyl-3-methyl-pyrazole derivatives.

Discriminant analysis has for its main purpose finding linear combinations of variables that maximize the differences between the populations being studied, with the objective of establishing a model to sort objects into their appropriate populations with minimal error. At least four major questions are, in a sense, being asked of the data:

1. Are there significant differences among the K groups?
2. If the groups do exhibit statistical differences, how do the central masses (or centroids, the multivariate equivalent of means) of the populations differ?
3. What are the relative distances among the K groups?

4. How are known (or at this point unknown) members allocated to *establish* groups? How do you predict the set of responses of characteristics of an as yet untried exposure case?

The discriminant functions used to produce the linear combinations are of the form

$$D_i = d_{i1}X_i + d_{i2}Z_2 \cdots + d_{ip}Z_p,$$

where

D1 = the score on the discriminant function I,
d's = weighing coefficients,
Z's = standardized values of the discriminating variables used in the analysis.

It should be noted that discriminant analysis can also be used for the hypothesis testing function by the expedient of evaluating how well it correctly classifies members into proper groups (say, control, treatment 1, treatment 2, etc.) Taketomo et al. (140) used discriminant analysis in a retrospective study of gentamycin nephrotoxicity to identify patient risk factors (i.e., variables which contributed to a prediction of a patient being at risk).

Finally, we introduce four techniques whose primary function is the reduction of dimensionality: canonical correlation analysis, principal components analysis, biplot analysis, and correspondence analysis.

Canonical correlation analysis provides the canonical R, an overall measure of the relationship between two sets of variables (one set consisting of several outcome measures, the other of several predictor variables). The canonical R is calculated on two numbers for each subject:

$$W_i = \sum w_j X_{ij} \text{ and } V_i = \sum v_i Y_{ij},$$

where

X's = predictor variables,
Y's = outcome measures,
W_j and V_j = canonical coefficients.

MANOVA can be considered a special case of canonical correlation analysis. Canonical correlation can be used in hypothesis testing also for testing the association of pairs of sets of weights, each with a corresponding coefficient of canonical correlation, each uncorrelated with any of the preceding sets of weights, and each accounting for successively less of the variation shared by the two sets of variables. For example, Young and Matthews (169) used canonical correlation analysis to evaluate the relationship between plant growth and environmental factors at 12 different sites.

The main purpose of principal components analysis is to describe as economically as possible the total variance in a sample in a few dimensions: one wishes to reduce the dimensionality of the original data while minimizing the loss of information. It seeks to resolve the total variation of a set of variables into linearly independent composite variables that successively account for the maximum possible variability in the data. The fundamental equation is Y = AZ, where

A = matrix of scales eigenvectors,
Z = original data matrice,
Y = principal components.

The concentration here, as in factor analysis, is on relationships within a single set of variables. Note that the results of principal components analysis are affected by linear transformations.

Cremer and Seville (31) used principal components to compare the difference in blood parameters resulting from each of two separate pyrethroids. Henry and Hidy (84), meanwhile, used principal components to identify the most significant contributors to air quality problems.

The biplot display (58) of multivariate data is a relatively new technique but promises wide applicability to problems in toxicology. It is, in a sense, a form of exploratory data analysis, used for data summarization and description.

The biplot is a graphical display of a matrix Y_{nmx} of N rows and M columns by means of row and column marker. The display carries one marker for each row and each column. The "bi" in biplot refers to the joint display of rows and columns. Such plots are used primarily for inspection of data and for data diagnostics when such data are in the form of matrices.

Shy-Modjeska et al. (135) illustrated this usage in the analysis of aminoglycoside renal data from beagle dogs, allowing the simultaneous display of relationships among different observed variables and presentation of the relationship of both individuals and treatment groups to these variables.

Correspondence analysis is a technique for displaying the rows and columns of a two-way contingency table as points in a corresponding low-dimensional vector space. As such, it is equivalent to simultaneous linear regression (for contingency table data, such as tumor incidences, which is a very common data form in toxicology). As such, it can be considered a special case of canonical correlation analysis. The data are defined, described, and analyzed in a geometric framework. This is particularly attractive to such sets of observations in toxicology as multiple end point behavioral scores and scored multiple tissue lesions.

There are a number of good surveys of multivariate techniques available (9,21,133) that are not excessively mathematical. More rigorous mathematical treatments on an introductory level are also available (71). Most of the techniques we have described are available in the better computer statistical packages.

Table 7.7
Classification of Data Commonly Encountered in Toxicology, by Type

Continuous normal:	Body weights Food consumption Organ weights: Absolute and relative Mouse Ear Swelling Test (MEST) measurements Pregnancy rates Survival rates Crown–Rump lengths Hematology (some) Clinical chemistry (some)
Continuous but not normal:	Hematology (some—WBC) Clinical chemistry (some) Urinalysis
Scalar data:	Neurobehavioral signs (some) PDI scores Histopathology (some)
Count data:	Resorption sites Implantation sites Stillborns Hematology (some—reticulocyte counts//Howel–Jolly//WBC differentials)
Categorical data	Clinical signs Neurobehavioral signs (some) Ocular scores GP sensitization scores Mouse ear swelling tests (MEST) sensitization Counts Fetal abnormalities Dose/mortality data Sex ratios Histopathology data (most)

DATA ANALYSIS APPLICATIONS IN TOXICOLOGY

Having reviewed basic principles and provided a set of methods for statistical handling of data, the remainder of this book will address the practical aspects and difficulties encountered in day-to-day toxicological work. As a starting point, we present in Table 7.7 an overview of data types actually encountered in toxicology, classified by type (as presented at the beginning of this book). It should be stressed, however, that this classification is of the most frequent measure of each sort of observation (such as body weight) and will not always be an accurate classification.

There are now common practices in the analysis of toxicology data, though they are not necessarily the best. These are discussed in the remainder of this chapter, which seeks to review statistical methods on a use-by-use basis and to provide a foundation for the selection of alternatives in specific situations.

Median Lethal and Effective Doses

For many years, the starting point for evaluating the toxicity of an agent was to determine its LD_{50} or LC_{50}, which are the dose or concentration of a material at which half of a population of animals would be expected to die. These figures are analogous to the ED_{50} (effective dose for half a population) used in pharmacologic activities, and are derived by the same means. It is important to keep in mind the three dimensions of dose response.

As the dose increases,

Incidence of responders in an exposed population increases.
Severity of response in effected individuals increases.
Time to occurrence of response or of progressive stage of response decreases.

To calculate either the LD_{50} or LC_{50}, we need, at each of several dosage (or exposure) levels, the number of animals dosed and the number that died. If we seek only to establish the median effective dose in a range-finding test, then 4 or 5 animals per dose level, using Thompson's method of moving averages, is the most efficient methodology and will give a sufficiently accurate solution. With two dose levels, if the ratio between the high and low dose is two or less, even total or no mortality at these two dose levels will yield an acceptably accurate medial lethal dose, although a partial mortality is desirable. If, however, we wish to estimate a number of toxicity levels (LD_{10}, LD_{90}) and are interested in more precisely establishing the slope of the dose/lethality curve, the use of at least 10 animals per dosage level with the log/probit regression technique is the most common approach. Note that in the equation $Y_i = a + bx_1$, b is the slope of the regression line and that our method already allows us to calculate 95% confidence intervals about any point on this line. Note that the confidence interval at any one point will be different from the interval at other points and must be calculated separately. Additionally, the nature of the probit transform is such that toward the extremes—LD_{10} and LD_{90}, for example—the confidence intervals will "balloon" (i.e., they become very wide). Because the slope of the fitted line in these assays has a very large uncertainty, in relation to the uncertainty of the LD_{50} itself (the midpoint of the distribution), much caution must be used with calculated Ld_xs other than LD_{50}s. The imprecision of the LD_{35}, a value close to the LD_{50}, is discussed by Weil (153), as is that of the slope of the log dose-probit line (152). Debanne and Haller (37) recently reviewed the statistical aspects of different methodologies for estimating a median effective dose.

There have been questions for years as to the value of LD_{50} and the efficiency of the current study design (which uses large numbers of animals) in determining it. As long ago as 1953, Weil et al. (154) presented forceful arguments that an estimate having only minimally reduced precision could be made using significantly fewer animals. More recently, the last few years have seen an increased level of concern over the numbers and uses of animals in research and testing and have produced additional arguments against existing methodologies for determining the LD_{50} or even the need to make the determination at all (172). In response, a number of suggestions for alternative methodologies have been advanced (20,38,59).

Body and Organ Weights

Among the sets of data commonly collected in studies where animals are dosed with (or exposed to) a chemical are body weight and the weights of selected organs. In fact, body weight is frequently the most sensitive indication of an adverse effect. How to best analyze this and in what form to analyze the organ weight data (as absolute weights, weight changes, or percentages of body weight) have been the subject of a number of articles (90,155,156,162).

Both absolute body weights and rates of body weight change (calculated as changes from a baseline measurement value that is traditionally the animal's weight immediately prior to the first dosing with or exposure to test material) are almost universally best analyzed by ANOVA followed by a post hoc test, if called for. Even if the groups were randomized properly at the beginning of a study (no group being significantly different in mean body weight from any other group, and all animals in all groups within two SDs of the overall mean body weight), there is an advantage to performing the computationally, slightly more cumbersome (compared to absolute body weights) analysis of changes in body weight. The advantage is an increase in sensitivity because the adjustment of starting points (the setting of initial weights as a "zero" value) acts to reduce the amount of initial variability. In this case, Bartlett's test is performed first to ensure homogeneity of variance, and the appropriate sequence of analysis follows.

With smaller sample sizes, the normality of the data becomes increasingly uncertain, and nonparametric methods, such as Kruskal–Wallis, may be more appropriate (171).

The analysis of relative (to body weight) organ weights is a valuable tool for identifying possible target organs (59). How to perform this analysis is still a matter of some disagreement, however.

Weil (155) presented evidence that organ weight data expressed as percentages of body weight should be analyzed separately for each sex. Furthermore, because the conclusions from organ weight data of males differed so often from those of females, data from animals of each sex should be used in this measurement. Others (17,18,157,162) have discussed in detail other factors that influence organ weights and must be taken into account.

The two competing approaches to analyzing relative organ weights call for either

(1) calculating organ weights as a percentage of total body weight (at the time of necropsy) and analyzing the results by ANOVA, or
(2) analyzing results by ANCOVA, with body weights as the covariates, as discussed previously by the author (156).

A number of considerations should be kept in mind when these questions are addressed. First, one must keep a firm grasp on the difference between biological significance and statistical significance. In this particular case, we are especially interested in examining organ weights when an organ weight change is not proportional to changes in whole body weights. Second, we are now required to detect smaller and smaller changes while still retaining a similar sensitivity (i.e., the $p<0.05$ level).

There are several devices to attain the desired increase in power. One is to use larger and larger sample sizes (number of animals) and the other is to use the most powerful test we can; however, the use of even currently employed numbers of animals is being vigorously questioned and the power of statistical tests must, therefore, now assume an increased importance in our considerations.

The biological rationale behind analyzing both absolute body weight and the organ weight to body weight ratio (this latter as opposed to a covariance analysis of organ weights) is that in the majority of cases, except for the brain, the organs of interest in the body change weight (except in extreme cases of obesity or starvation) in proportion to total body weight. We are particularly interested in detecting cases where this is not so. Analysis of actual data from several hundred studies (unpublished data) has shown no significant difference in rates of weight change of target organs (other than the brain), compared to total body weight for healthy animals in those species commonly used for repeated dose studies (rats, mice, rabbits, dogs). Furthermore, it should be noted that analysis of covariance is of questionable validity in analyzing body weight and related organ weight changes, as a primary assumption is the independence of treatment—that the relationship of the two variables is the same for all treatments (123). Plainly, in toxicology this is not true.

In cases where the differences between the error mean squares are much greater, the ratio of F-ratios will diverge in precision from the result of the efficiency of covariance adjustment. These cases are where either sample sizes are much larger or where the differences between means themselves are much larger. This latter case is one that does not occur in the designs under discussion in any manner that would leave analysis of covariance as a valid approach because group means start out being very similar and cannot diverge markedly unless there is a treatment effect. As we have discussed earlier, a treatment effect invalidates a prime underpinning assumption of analysis of covariance.

Shirley and Newnham (134) have argued the case for ANCOVA but without providing answers to arguments presented above.

Clinical Chemistry

A number of clinical chemistry parameters are commonly determined on the blood and urine collected from animals in chronic, subchronic, and, occasionally, acute toxicity studies. In the past, and still in some places, the accepted practice has been to evaluate these data using univariate-parametric methods (primarily t-tests and/or ANOVA); however, this can be shown to be not the best approach on a number of grounds.

First, such biochemical parameters are rarely independent of each other. Neither is our interest often focused on just one of the parameters. Rather, there are batteries of the parameters associated with toxic actions at particular target organs. For example, increases in creatinine phosphokinase (CPK), γ-hydroxybutyrate dehydrogenase (γ-HBDH), and lactate dehydrogenase (LDH), occurring together, are strongly indicative of myocardial damage. In such cases we are not just interested in a significant increase in one of these, but in all three. Table 7.8 gives a brief overview of the association of various parameters with actions at particular target organs. A more detailed coverage of the interpretation of such clinical laboratory tests can be found in other references (65,78,103,105).

Similarly, the serum electrolytes (sodium, potassium, calcium) interact with each other; a decrease in one is frequently tied, for instance, to an increase in one of the others. Furthermore, the nature of the data (in the case of some parameters), either because of the biological nature of the parameter or the way in which it is measured, is frequently either not normally distributed (particularly because of being markedly skewed) or not continuous in nature. This can be seen in some of the reference data for experimental animals in Mitruka and Rawnsley (109) or Weil (158) in, for example, creatinine, sodium, potassium, chloride, calcium, and blood.

Hematology

Much of what we said about clinical chemistry parameters is also true for the hematologic measurements made in toxicology studies. Which test to perform should be evaluated by use of a decision tree until one becomes confident as to the most appropriate methods. Keep in mind that sets of values and (in some cases) population distribution vary not only between species, but also between the commonly used strains of species, and that "control" or "standard" values will "drift" over the course of only a few years.

Again, the majority of these parameters are interrelated and highly dependent on the method used to determine them. RBC, platelet counts, and mean corpuscular volume (MCV) may be determined using a device such as a Coulter counter to take direct measurements, and the resulting data are usually stable for parametric methods. The hematocrit, however, may actually be a value calculated from the RBC and MCV values, and if so, is dependent on them. If the hematocrit is measured directly, instead of being calculated from the RBC and MCV, it may be compared by parametric methods.

Hemoglobin is directly measured and is an independent and continuous variable; however, and probably because at any one time a number of forms and conformations (oxyhemoglobin, deoxyhemoglobin, methemoglobin, etc.) of hemoglobin are actually present, the distribution seen is not typically a normal one, but rather may be a multimodal one. Here a nonparametric technique such as the Wilcoxon or multiple Rank–Sum is called for.

Consideration of the white blood cell (WBC) and differential counts leads to another problem. The total WBC is, typically, a normal population amenable to parametric analysis, but differential counts are normally determined by counting, manually, one or more sets of 100 cells each. The resulting relative percentages of neutrophils are then reported as either percentages or are multiplied by the total WBC count with the resulting "count" being reported as the "absolute" differential WBC. Such data, particularly in the case of eosinophils (where the distribution does not approach normality) should usually be analyzed by nonparametric methods. It is widely believed that "relative" (percentage) differential data should not be reported because they are likely to be misleading.

Lastly, it should always be kept in mind that it is rare for a change in any single hematologic parameter to be meaningful. Rather, because these parameters are so interrelated, patterns of changes in parameters should be expected if a real effect is present, and analysis and interpretation of results should focus on such patterns of changes. Classification analysis techniques often provide the basis for a useful approach to such problems.

Histopathologic Lesion Incidence

The last 30 years have seen increasing emphasis placed on histopathological examination of tissues collected

Table 7.8

Association of changes in biochemical parameters with actions at particular target organs

	ORGAN SYSTEM								
PARAMETER	BLOOD	HEART	LUNG	KIDNEY	LIVER	BONE	INTESTINE	PANCREAS	NOTES
Albumin				↓	↓				Produced by the liver. Very significant reductions indicate extensive liver damage.
ALP (alkaline phosphatase)					↑	↑	↑		Elevations usually are associated with cholestasis. Bone alkaline phosphatase tends to be higher in young animals.
Bilirubin (total)	↑				↑				Usually elevated due to cholestasis—either due to obstruction or hepatopathy.
BUN (blood urea nitrogen)				↑	↓				Estimates blood filtering capacity of the kidneys. Doesn't become significantly elevated until kidney function is reduced 60%–75%.
Calcium				↑					Can be life threatening and result in acute death.
Cholinesterase				↑	↓				Found in plasma, brain and RBC.
CPK (creatinine phosphokinase)		↑							Most often elevated due to skeletal muscle damage but can also be produced by cardiac muscle damage. Can be more sensitive than histopathology.
Creatinine				↑					Also estimates blood filtering

Table 7.8 (*continued*)

				ORGAN SYSTEM					
PARAMETER	BLOOD	HEART	LUNG	KIDNEY	LIVER	BONE	INTESTINE	PANCREAS	NOTES
									capacity of kidney as BUN does More specific than BUN.
Glucose								↑	Alterations other than those associated with stress are uncommon and reflect an effect on the pancreatic islets or anorexia.
GGT (gamma glutamyl transferase)					↑				Elevated in cholestasis. This is a microsomal enzyme and levels often increase in response to microsomal enzyme induction.
HBDH (hydroxybutyric dehydrogenase)		↑			↑				
LDH (lactic dehydrogenase		↑	↑	↑	↑				Increase usually due to skeletal muscle, cardiac muscle and liver damage. Not very specific.
Protein (total)				↓	↓				Absolute alterations are usually associated with decreased production (liver) or increased loss (kidney). Can see increase in case of muscle "wasting" (catabolism).

Table 7.8 (*continued*)

PARAMETER	BLOOD	HEART	LUNG	KIDNEY (ORGAN SYSTEM)	LIVER (ORGAN SYSTEM)	BONE	INTESTINE	PANCREAS	NOTES
SGOT (serum glutamic-oxaloacetic transaminase); also called AST (aspartate amino transferase)		↑		↑	↑			↑	Present in skeletal muscle and heart and most commonly associated with damage to these.
SGPT (serum glutamic-pyruvic transaminase); also called ALT (alanine amino transferase)					↑				Elevations usually associated with hepatic damage or disease.
SDH (sorbitol dehydrogenase)					↑ or ↓				Liver enzyme that can be quite sensitive but is fairly unstable. Samples should be processed as soon as possible.

Arrow indicates increase (↑) or decrease (↓).

from animals in subchronic and chronic toxicity studies. Whereas it is not true that only those lesions that occur at a statistically significant increased rate in treated/exposed animals are of concern (for there are the cases where a lesion may be of such a rare type that the occurrence of only one or a few such in treated animals "raises a flag"), it is true that, in most cases, a statistical evaluation is the only way to determine if what we see in treated animals is significantly worse than what has been seen in control animals. Although cancer is not our only concern, this category of lesions is of greatest interest.

Typically, comparison of incidences of any one type of lesion between controls and treated animals are made using the multiple 2 × 2 chi-square test or Fisher's exact test with a modification of the numbers of animals as the denominators. Too often, experimenters exclude from consideration all those animals (in both groups) that died prior to the first animals being found with a lesion at that site. The special case of carcinogenicity bioassays will be discussed in detail later in this chapter.

An option that should be kept in mind is that frequently a pathologist cannot only identify a lesion as present, but also grade those present as to severity. This represents a significant increase in the information content of the data that should not be given up by performing an analysis based only on the perceived quantal nature (present/absent) of the data. Quantal data, analyzed by chi-square or Fisher's exact tests, are a subset (the 2 × 2 case) of categorical or contingency table data. In this case it also becomes ranked (or "ordinal") data—the categories are naturally ordered (e.g., no effect<mild lesion<moderate lesion<severe lesion). This gives a 2 × R table if there are only one treatment and one control group, or an N × R ("multiway") table if there are three or more groups of animals.

The traditional method of analyzing multiple, cross-classified data has been to collapse the N × R contingency table over all but two of the variables and to follow this with the computation of some measure of association between these variables. For an N-dimensional table, this results in N (N–1)/2 separate analyses. The result is crude, "giving away" information and even (by inappropriate pooling of data) yielding a faulty understanding of the meaning of data. Though computationally more laborious, a multiway (N × R table) analysis should be used.

Reproduction

The reproductive implications of the toxic effects of chemicals are becoming increasingly important. Because of this, reproduction studies, together with other closely related types of studies (such as teratogenesis, dominant lethal, and mutagenesis studies, which are discussed later in this chapter), are now a common companion to chronic toxicity studies.

One point that must be kept in mind with all reproduction-related studies is the nature of the appropriate sampling unit. What is the appropriate N in such a study? The number of individual pups, the number of litters, pregnant females? Fortunately, it is now fairly well accepted that the first case (using the number of offspring as the N) is inappropriate (162). The real effects in such studies actually occur in the female that was exposed to the chemical or that is mated to a male that was exposed. What happens to her and to the development of the litter she is carrying is biologically independent of what happens to every other female/litter in the stud. This cannot be said for each offspring in each litter (e.g., the death of one member of a litter can and will be related to what happens to every other member). The effect on all of the offspring might be similar for all of those from one female and different or lacking for those from another.

As defined by Oser and Oser (115), there are four primary variables of interest in a reproduction study. First, there is the fertility index (FI), which may be defined as the percentage of attempted matings (i.e., each female housed with a male) that resulted in pregnancy, with pregnancy being determined by a method such as the presence of implantation sites in the female. Second, there is the gestation index (GI), which is defined as the percentage of mated females, as evidenced by a vaginal plug being dropped or a positive vaginal smear, which deliver viable litters (i.e., litters with at least one live pup). Two related variables that may also be studied are the mean number of pups born per litter and the percentage of total pups per litter that are stillborn. Third, there is the viability index (VI), which is defined as the percentage of offspring born that survive at least 4 days after birth. Finally (in this four-variable system) there is the lactation index (LI), which is the percentage of animals per litter that survive 4 days and also survive to weaning. In rats and mice, this is classically taken to be 21 days after birth. An additional variable that may reasonably be included in such a study is the mean weight gain per pup per litter.

Given that our N is at least 10 pregnant animals, we may test each of these variables for significance using a method such as the Wilcoxon–Mann–Whitney U test, or the Kruskal–Wallis nonparametric ANOVA. If N is less than 10, we cannot expect the central limit theorem to be operative and should use the Wilcoxon sum of ranks (for two groups) or the Kruskal–Wallis nonparametric ANOVA (for three or more groups) to compare groups.

Developmental Toxicology

When the primary concern of a reproductive/developmental study is the occurrence of birth defects or deformations (terata, either structural or functional) in the offspring of exposed animals, the study is one of developmental toxicology (teratology). In the analysis of the data from such a study, we must consider several points.

First is sample size. Earlier a method to estimate sufficient sample size was presented previously. The difficulties with applying these methods here revolve around two points: (1) selecting a sufficient level of sensitivity for detecting an effect, and (2) factoring in how many animals will be removed from study (without contributing a datum) by either not becoming pregnant or not surviving to a sufficiently late stage of pregnancy. Experience generally dictates that one should attempt to have 20 pregnant animals per study group if a pilot study has provided some confidence that the pregnant test animals will survive the dose levels selected. Again, it is essential to recognize that the litter, not the fetus, is the basic independent unit for each variable.

A more fundamental consideration, alluded to in the section on reproduction, is that as we use more animals, the mean of means (each variable will be such in a mathematical sense) will approach normality in its distribution. This is one of the implications of the Central Limit Theorem: even when the individual data are not normally distributed, their means will approach normality in their distribution. At a sample size of 10 or greater, the approximation of normality is such that we may use a parametric test (such as a t-test or ANOVA) to evaluate results. At sample sizes less than 10, a nonparametric test (Wilcoxon rank–sum or Kruskal–Wallis nonparametric ANOVA) is more appropriate. Other methodologies have been suggested (100,112) but do not offer any prospect of widespread usage. One nonparametric method that is widely used is the Mann–Whitney U test, which was described earlier. Williams and Buschbom (163) further discuss some of the available statistical options and their consequences, and Rai and Ryzin (22) have recommended a dose-responsive model.

Dominant Lethal Assay

The dominant lethal study is essentially a reproduction study that seeks to study the end point of lethality to the fetuses after implantation and before delivery. The proper identification of the sampling unit (the pregnant female) and the design of an experiment so that a sufficiently large sample is available for analysis are the prime statistical considerations. The question of sampling unit has been adequately addressed in earlier sections. Sample size is of concern here because the hypothesis-testing techniques that are appropriate with small samples are of relatively low power, as the variability about the mean in such cases is relatively large. With sufficient sample size (e.g., from 30–50 pregnant females per dose level per week (11)), variability about the mean and the nature of the distribution allow sensitive statistical techniques to be employed.

The variables that are typically recorded and included in analysis (for each level/week) are as follows: (a) the number of pregnant females, (b) live fetuses/pregnancy, (c) total implants/pregnancy, (d) early fetal deaths (early resorptions)/pregnancy, and (e) late fetal deaths/pregnancy.

A wide variety of techniques for analysis of these data have been (and are) used. Most common is the use of ANOVA after the data have been transformed by the arc sine transform (111).

Beta binomial (2,151) and Poisson distributions (36) have also been attributed to these data, and transforms and appropriate tests have been proposed for use in each of these cases (in each case with the note that the transforms serve to "stabilize the variance" of the data). With sufficient sample size, as defined earlier in this section, the Mann–Whitney U test is recommended for use here. Smaller sample sizes necessitate the use of the Wilcoxon rank–sum test.

Diet and Chamber Analysis

Earlier we presented the basic principles and methods for sampling. Sampling is important in many aspects of toxicology, and here we address its application to diet preparation and the analysis of atmospheres from inhalation chambers.

In feeding studies we seek to deliver doses of a material to animals by mixing the material with their diet. Similarly, in an inhalation study we mix a material with the air the test animals breathe. In both cases we must then sample the medium (food or atmosphere) and analyze these samples to determine what levels or concentrations of material were actually present and to assure ourselves that the test material is homogeneously distributed. Having an accurate picture of these delivered concentrations and how they varied over the course of time is essential on a number of grounds:

1. The regulatory agencies and sound scientific practice require that analyzed diet and mean daily inhalation atmosphere levels be ±10% of the target level.
2. Excessive peak concentrations, because of the overloading of metabolic repair systems, could result in extreme acute effects that would lead to results in a chronic study that are not truly indicative of the chronic low-level effects of the compound, but rather of periods of metabolic and physiologic overload. Such results could be misinterpreted if true exposure or diet levels were not maintained at a relatively constant level.

Sampling strategies are not just a matter of numbers (for statistical aspects), but of geometry, so that the contents of a container or the entire atmosphere in a chamber is truly sampled, and of time, in accordance with the stability of the test compound. The samples must be both randomly collected and representative of the entire mass of what one is trying to characterize. In the special case of sampling and characterizing the physical properties of aerosols in an inhalation study, some special considerations and terminology apply. Because of the physiologic characteristics of the respiration of humans and of test animals, our concern is very largely limited to those particles or droplets that are of a respirable size. Unfortunately, "respirable size" is a complex characteristic based on aerodynamic diameter, density, and physiological characteristics. Unfortunately, while those particles with an aerodynamic diameter of less than 10 μm are generally agreed to be respirable in humans (i.e., they can be drawn down to the deep portions of the lungs), 3 μm in aerodynamic diameter is a more realistical value. Typically, it then becomes a matter of the calculation of measures of central tendency and dispersion statistics, with the identification of those values that are beyond acceptable limits (15).

Genotoxicity

Over the last 25 years a wide variety of tests (see ref. 96 for an overview of those available) for genotoxicity have been developed and brought into use. These tests give us a quicker and cheaper (though not as conclusive) way of predicting whether a material of interest is a mutagen, and possibly a carcinogen, than do longer-term, whole-animal studies.

How to analyze the results of the multitude of tests (Ames, DNA repair, micronucleus, chromosome abberation, cell transformation, and sister chromatid exchange, to name a few) is an extremely important question. Some workers in the field hold that it is not possible (or necessary) to perform statistical analysis and that the tests can simply be judged to be positive or not positive on the basis of whether or not they achieve a particular increase in the incidence of mutations in the test organism. Quantitations of potency are complicated by the fact that we are dealing with a nonlinear phenomenon, and although low dose of most genotoxins produce a linear response curve with increasing dose, the curve will flatten out (and even turn into a declining curve) as the higher doses provoke an acute response.

Several concepts different from those we have previously discussed need to be examined, for our concern has now shifted from how a multicellular organism acts in response to one of a number of complex actions to how a mutational event is expressed, most frequently by a single cell. Given that we can handle much larger numbers of experimental units in systems that use smaller test organisms, we can seek to detect both weak and strong mutagens.

Conducting the appropriate statistical analysis and using the results of such an analysis properly must start with an understanding of the biological system involved and, from this understanding, developing the correct model and hypothesis. We start such a process by considering each of five interacting factors (74,150):

1. α, which is the probability of our committing a type I error (saying an agent is mutagenic when it is not, equivalent to our p in such earlier considered designs as the Fisher's exact test); false-positive.
2. β, which is the probability of our committing a type II error (saying an agent is not mutagenic when it is); false-negative.
3. Δ, our desired sensitivity in an assay system (such as being able to detect an increase of 10% in mutations in a population).
4. σ, the variability of the biological system and the effects of chance errors.
5. n, the single necessary sample size to achieve each of these (we can, by our actions, change only this portion of the equation) as n is proportional to

$$\frac{\sigma}{\alpha, \beta, \text{and } \Delta}$$

The implications of this are, therefore, that (a) the greater σ is, the larger n must be to achieve the desired levels of α, β, and Δ; (b) the smaller the desired levels of α, β, and/or Δ, if n is constant, the larger our σ is.

What is the background mutation level and the variability in our technique? As any good genetic or general toxicologist will acknowledge, matched concurrent control groups are essential. Fortunately, with these test systems, large n's are readily attainable, though there are other complications to this problem, which we shall consider later. An example of the confusion that would otherwise result is illustrated in the intralaboratory comparisons on some of these methods done to date, such as that reviewed by Weil (159).

New statistical tests based on these assumptions and on the underlying population distributions have been proposed, along with the necessary computational background, to allow one to alter one of the input variables (α, β, or Δ). A set that shows particular promise is that proposed by Katz (94,95) in his two articles. He described two separate test statistics: Φ for when we can accurately estimate the number of individuals in both the experimental and control groups, and θ for when we do not actually estimate the number of surviving individuals in each group, we can assume that the test material is only mildly toxic in terms of killing the test organisms. Each of these two test statistics is also formulated on the basis of only a single exposure of the organisms to the test chemicals. Given this, then we may compute

$$\phi = \frac{a(M_E - 0.5) - Kb(M_C + 0.5)}{\sqrt{Kab(M_E + M_C)}},$$

where a and b are the number of groups of control (c) and experimental (e) organisms, respectively.

N_C and N_E are the numbers of surviving microorganisms:

$$[K = N_E/N_C].$$

M_E and M_C are the numbers of mutations in experimental and control groups; μ_e and μ_c are the true (but unknown) mutation rates (as μ_c gets smaller, N's must increase).

We may compute the second case as

$$\theta = \frac{a(M_E - 0.5) + (M_C + 0.5)}{ab(M_E + M_C)}$$

with the same constituents.

In both cases, at a confidence level for I of 0.05, we accept that $\mu_c = \mu_e$ if the test statistic (either Φ or θ) is less than 1.64. If it is equal to or greater than 1.64, we may conclude that we have a mutagenic effect (at $\alpha = 0.05$).

In the second case (θ, where we do not have separate estimates of population sizes for the control and experimental groups), if K deviates widely from 1.0 (if the material is markedly toxic), we should use more containers of control organisms (tables for the proportions of each to use given different survival frequencies may be found in ref. 96). If different levels are desired, tables for θ and Φ may be found in Kastenbaum and Bowman (94).

An outgrowth of this is that the mutation rate per surviving cells (μ_c and μ_e) can be determined. It must be remembered that if the control mutation rate is so high that a reduction in mutation rates can be achieved by the test compound, these test statistics must be adjusted to allow for a two-sided hypothesis (48). The α levels may likewise be adjusted in each case, or tested for, if we want to assure ourselves that a mutagenic effect exists at a certain level of confidence (note that this is different from disproving the null hypothesis).

It should be noted that there are numerous specific recommendations for statistical methods designed for individual mutagenicity techniques, such as that of Bernstein et al. (13) for the Ames test.

Behavioral Toxicity

A brief review of the types of studies/experiments conducted in the area of behavioral toxicology and a classification of these into groups is in order. Although there are a small number of studies that do not fit into the following classification, the great majority may be fitted into one of the following four groups. Many of these points were first covered in earlier articles (61,63).

The first type of study is observational. Observational score-type studies are based on observing and grading the response of an animal to its normal environment or to a stimulus that is imprecisely controlled. This type of result is generated by one of two major sorts of studies. Open-field studies involve placing an animal in the center of a flat, open area and counting each occurrence of several types of activities (grooming, moving outside a designated central area, rearing, etc.) or timing until the first occurrence of each type of activity. The data generated are scalar of either a continuous or discontinuous nature but frequently are not of a normal distribution. Tilson et al. (144) presented some examples of this sort.

Observational screen studies involve a combination of observing behavior and evoking a response to a simple stimulus, the resulting observation being graded as normal or as deviating from normal on a graded scale. Most of the data so generated are rank in nature, with some portions being quantal or interval. Irwin (89) and Gad (61) have presented schemes for the conduct of such studies, which became the basis of the commonly used functional observational battery. Table 7.9 gives an example of the nature (and of one form of statistical analysis) of such data generated after exposure to one material.

The second type of study is one that generates rates of response as data. The studies are based on the number of responses to a discrete controlled stimulus or are free of direct connection to a stimulus. The three most frequently measured parameters are licking of a liquid (milk, sugar water, ethanol, or a psychoactive agent in water), gross locomotor activity (measured by a photocell or electromagnetic device), or level pulling. Examples of such studies have been published by Annau (6) and Norton (114). The data generated are most often of a discontinuous or continuous scalar nature and are often complicated by underlying patterns of biological rhythm.

The third type of study generates a variety of data that are classified as error rate. These are studies based on animals learning a response to a stimulus or memorizing a simple task (such as running a maze or a Skinner box–type shock avoidance system). These tests or trials are structured so that animals can pass or fail on each of a number of successive trials. The resulting data are quantal, though frequently expressed as a percentage.

The final major type of study is that which results in data that are measures of the time to an endpoint. They are based on animals being exposed to or dosed with a toxicant and the time taken for an effect to be observed is measured. Usually the endpoint is failure to continue to be able to perform a task and can, therefore, be death, incapacitation, or the learning of a response to a discrete stimulus. Burt (22) and Johnson et al. (91) present data of this form. The data are always of a censored nature (i.e., the period of observation is always artificially limited, as in measuring time-to-incapacitation in combustion toxicology data, where animals are exposed to the thermal decomposition gases to test materials for a period of 30 minutes). If incapacitation is not observed during these 30 minutes, it is judged not to occur. The data generated by these studies are continuous, discontinuous, or rank in nature. They are discontinuous because the researcher may check, or may be restricted to checking for the occurrence of the endpoint only at certain discrete points in time. On the other hand, they are rank if the periods to check for occurrence of the endpoint are far enough apart, in which case one may actually only know that the endpoint occurred during a broad period of time, but not where in that period.

Table 7.9
Functional Observational Battery parameters showing significant differences between treated and control groups

Parameter	Rats (18-crown-6 animals given 40 mg/kg i.p.) Control sum of ranks	N_c	18-crown-6 treated sum or ranks	N_T	Observed difference in treated animals (as compared to controls)
Twitches	55.0	10	270.0	15	Involuntary muscle twitches
Visual placing	55.0	10	270.0	15	Less aware of visual stimuli
Grip strength	120.0	10	205.0	15	Considerable loss of strength, especially in hind limbs
Respiration	55.0	10	270.0	15	Increased rate of respiration
Tremors	55.0	10	270.0	15	Marked tremors

All parameters above are significant at $p < 0.05$.

There is a special class of test that should also be considered at this point—the behavioral teratology or reproduction study. These studies are based on dosing or exposing either parental animals during selected periods in the mating and gestation process or pregnant females at selected periods during gestation. The resulting offspring are then tested for developmental defects of a neurological and behavioral nature. Analysis is complicated by a number of facts:

(1) The parental animals are the actual targets for toxic effects, but observations are made on offspring.
(2) The toxic effects in the parental generation may alter the performance of the mother in rearing its offspring, which in turn can lead to a confusion of prenatal and postnatal effects.
(3) Different capabilities and behaviors develop at different times (discussed further later).

A researcher can, by varying the selection of the animal model (species, strain, sex), modify the nature of the data generated and the degree of dispersion of these data. In behavioral studies particularly, limiting the within-group variability of data is a significant problem and generally should be a highly desirable goal.

Most, if not all, behavioral toxicology studies depend on at least some instrumentation. Very frequently overlooked here (and, indeed, in most research) is that instrumentation, by its operating characteristics and limitations, goes a long way toward determining the nature of the data generated by it. An activity monitor measures motor activity in discrete segments. If it is a "jiggle cage"-type monitor, these segments are restricted so that only a distinctly limited number of counts can be achieved in a given period of time and then only if they are of the appropriate magnitude. Likewise, technique can also readily determine the nature of the data. In measuring response to pain, for example, one could record it as a quantal measure (present or absent), a rank score (on a scale of 1–5 for decreased to increased responsiveness, with 3 being "normal"), or as scalar data (by using an analgesia meter, which determines either how much pressure or heat is required to evoke a response).

Study design factors are probably the most widely recognized of the factors that influence the type of data resulting from a study. Number of animals used, frequency of measures, and length of period of observation are three obvious design factors that are readily under the control of the researcher and which directly help to determine the nature of the data.

Finally, it is appropriate to review each of the types of studies presently seen in behavioral toxicology, according to the classification presented at the beginning of this section, in terms of which statistical methods are used now and what procedures are recommended for use. The recommendations, of course, should be viewed with a critical eye. They are intended with current experimental design and technique in mind and can only claim to be the best when one is limited to addressing the most common problems from a library of readily and commonly available and understood tests.

Table 7.10 summarizes this review and recommendation process.

Carcinogenesis

The experimental evaluation of potentially carcinogenic substances is generally based on the exposure of nonhuman species to some relatively high dose and an attempt is made to predict the occurrence and level of

Table 7.10
Overview of statistical testing in behavioral toxicology: Those tests commonly used[a] as opposed to those recommended

Type of observation	Most commonly used procedures	Suggested procedures
Observational scores	Either Student's t-test or one-way ANOVA	Kruskal–Wallis nonparametric ANOVA or Wilcoxon Rank sum
Response rates	Either Student's t-test or one-way ANOVA	Kruskal–Wallis ANOVA or one way ANOVA
Error rates	ANOVA followed by a post-hoc test	Fisher's exact, or RxC chi-square, or Mann–Whitney U-test
Times to endpoint	Either Student's t-test or one-way ANOVA	ANOVA then a post-hoc test or Kruskal–Wallis ANOVA
Teratology and reproduction	ANOVA followed by a post-hoc test	Fisher's exact test, Kruskal–Wallis ANOVA, or Mann–Whitney U-test

[a] These are the most commonly used procedures. The reader need only look at the example articles cited in this chapter to verify this fact.

Table 7.11
Sample size required to obtain a specified sensitivity at $p<0.05$

Background tumor incidence	P[a]	Treatment Group Incidence 0.95	0.90	0.80	0.70	0.60	0.50	0.40	0.30	0.20	0.10
0.30	0.90	10	12	18	31	46	102	389			
	0.50	6	6	9	12	22	32	123			
0.20	0.90	8	10	12	18	30	42	88	320		
	0.50	5	5	6	9	12	19	28	101		
0.10	0.90	6	8	10	12	17	25	33	65	214	
	0.50	3	3	5	6	9	11	17	31	68	
0.05	0.90	5	6	8	10	13	18	25	35	76	464
	0.50	3	3	5	6	7	9	12	19	24	147
0.01	0.90	5	5	7	8	10	13	19	27	46	114
	0.50	3	3	5	5	6	8	10	13	25	56

[a] P = Power for each comparison of treatment group with background tumor incidence.

tumorogenesis in humans at much lower levels. This topic is addressed in Chapter 8 as well as in Gad (62).

The single most important statistical consideration in the design of carcinogenicity bioassays in the past was based on the point of view that what was being observed and evaluated was a simple quantal response (cancer occurred or it didn't) and that a sufficient number of animals needed to be used to have reasonable expectations of detecting such an effect. Though the single fact of whether or not the simple incidence of neoplastic tumors is increased due to an agent of concern is of interest, a much more complex model must now be considered. The time to tumor, patterns of tumor incidence, effects on survival rate, and age at first tumor all must now be included in a model.

Bioassay Design

As presented earlier in the section on experimental design, the first step that must be taken is to clearly state the objective of the study to be undertaken. Carcinogenicity bioassays have two possible objectives.

The first objective is to detect possible carcinogens. Compounds are evaluated to determine if they can or cannot induce a statistically detectable increase in tumor rates over background levels, and only by happenstance is information generated that is useful in risk assessment. Most older studies have such detection as their objective. Current belief is that at least two species must be used for detection, though the necessity of a second species (the mouse) is increasingly questioned.

The second objective for a bioassay is to provide a range of dose response information (with tumor incidence being the response) so that a risk assessment may be performed. Unlike detection, which requires only one treatment group with adequate survival times (to allow expression of tumors), dose response requires at least three treatment groups with adequate survival. We will shortly look at the selection of dose levels for this case; however, given that the species is known to be responsive, only one species of animal need be used for this objective.

To address either or both of these objectives, three major types of study designs have evolved. First is the classical skin painting study, usually performed in mice. A single, easily detected endpoint (the formation of skin tumors) is evaluated during the course of the study. Though dose response can be evaluated in such a study (dose usually being varied by using different concentrations of test material in volatile solvent), most often detection is the objective of such a study. Though others have used different frequencies of application of test material to vary dose, there are data to suggest that this only serves to introduce an additional variable (166). Traditionally, both test and control groups in such a test consist of 50 to 100 mice of one sex (males being preferred because of their very low spontaneous tumor rate). This design is also used in tumor initiation/promotion studies.

The second common type of design is the original National Cancer Institute (NCI) bioassay. The announced objective of these studies was detection of moderate to strong carcinogens, though the results have also been used in attempts at risk assessment. Both mice and rats were used in parallel studies. Each study used 50 males and 50 females at each of two dose levels (high and low) plus an equal-sized control group. The National Toxicology Program (NTP) has subsequently moved away from this design because of a recognition of its inherent limitations. More animals per group and more dose groups are now used.

Table 7.12

Average number of animals needed to detect a significant increase in the incidence of an event (tumors, anomalies, etc.) over the background incidence (control) at several expected incidence levels using the Fisher exact probability test ($p = 0.05$)

Background incidence, %	Expected Increase in Incidence, % 0.01	0.1	1	3	5	10
0	46,000,000[a]	460,000	4,600	511	164	46
0.01	46,000,000	460,000	4,600	511	164	46
0.1	47,000,000	470,000	4,700	520	168	47
1	51,000,000	510,000	5,100	570	204	51
5	77,000,000	770,000	7,700	856	304	77
10	100,000,000	1,000,000	10,000	1,100	400	100
20	148,000,000	1,480,000	14,800	1,644	592	148
25	160,000,000	1,600,000	16,000	1,840	664	166

[a] Number of animals needed in each group, controls as well as treated.

Finally, there is the standard industrial toxicology design, which uses at least two species (usually rats and mice) in groups of no fewer that 100 males and females each. Each study has three dose groups and at least one control. Frequently, additional numbers of animals are included to allow for interim terminations and histopathological evaluations. In both this and the NCI design, a long list of organs and tissues are collected, processed, and examined microscopically. This design seeks to address both the detection and dose response objectives with a moderate degree of success.

Selecting the number of animals to use for dose groups in a study requires consideration of both biological (expected survival rates, background tumor rates, etc.) and statistical factors. The prime statistical consideration is reflected in Table 7.11. It can be seen in this table that if, for example, we were studying a compound that caused liver tumors and were using mice (with a background or control incidence of 30%), we would have to use 389 animals per sex per group to be able to demonstrate that an incidence rate of 40% in treatment animals was significant compared to the controls at the $p = 0.05$ level.

Perhaps the most difficult aspect of designing a good carcinogenicity study is the selection of the dose levels to be used. At the start it is necessary to consider the first underlying assumption in the design and use of animal cancer bioassays—the need to test at the highest possible dose for the longest practical period.

The rationale behind this assumption is that though humans may be exposed at very low levels, detecting the resulting small increase (over background) in the incidence of tumors would require the use of an impractically large number of test animals per group. This point is illustrated by Table 7.11, where, for instance, while only 46 animals (per group) are needed to show a 10% increase over a zero background (i.e., a rarely occurring tumor type), 770,000 animals (per group) would be needed to detect a tenth of a percent increase above a 5% background. As we increase dose, however, the incidence of tumors (the response) will also increase until it reaches the point where a modest increase (say, 10% over a reasonably small background level (say, 1%)) could be detected using an acceptably small-sized group of test animals (in Table 7.12 we see that 51 animals would be needed for this example case). There are, however, at least two real limitations to the highest dose level. First, the test rodent population must have a sufficient survival rate after receiving a lifetime (or two years) of regular doses to allow for meaningful statistical analysis. Second, we really want the metabolism and mechanism of action of the chemical at the highest level tested to be the same as at the low levels, where human exposure would occur. Unfortunately, toxicologists usually must select the high dose level based only on the information provided by a subchronic or range-finding study (usually 90 days in length), but selection of either too low or too high a dose will make the study invalid for detection of carcinogenicity and may seriously impair the use of the results for risk assessment.

There are several solutions to this problem. One of these solutions has been the rather simplistic approach of the NTP Bioassay Program, which is to conduct a 3-month range-finding study with sufficient dose levels to establish a level that significantly (10%) decreases the rate of body weight gain. This dose is defined as the maximum tolerated dose (MTD) and is selected as the highest dose. Two other levels, generally one half MTD and one quarter MTD, are selected for testing as the intermediate and low-dose levels. In many earlier NCI studies, only one other level was used.

The dose range–finding study is necessary in most cases, but the suppression of body weight gain is a scientifically questionable bench mark when dealing with establishment of safety factors. Physiologic, pharmacologic, or metabolic markers generally serve as better indicators of systemic response than body weight. A series of well-defined acute and subchronic studies designed to determine the "chronicity factor" and to study onset of pathology can be more predictive for dose setting than body weight suppression.

Also, the NTP's MTD may well be at a level where the metabolic mechanisms for handling a compound at real-life exposure levels have been saturated or overwhelmed, bringing into play entirely artifactual metabolic and physiologic mechanisms (68). The regulatory response to questioning the appropriateness of the MTD as a high-dose level (82) has been to acknowledge that occasionally an excessively high dose is selected, but to counter by saying that using lower doses would seriously decrease the sensitivity of detection.

QUESTIONS

1. If the results of an analysis of variance establish that differences between groups is significant at the $p \leq 0.05$ level, what are the chances that the two groups are not different?
   a) 5% or less. That is, one in twenty or less.
2. If a set of 17 measured values are ranked in ascending order, the median value is which value in order?
   a) The 9th value.
3. Analysis of variance assumes that the data it is evaluating is from a normally distributed population. The test is robust for deviation from this assumption if what?
   a) The sample size is large enough.
4. In what manner does a lag profit transformation of a dose response curve alter its shape?
   a) It linearizes it.
5. Does the occurrence of outliers in a sample increase or decrease the sensitivity of any hypothesis testing (such as ANOVA)?
   a) Decreases Sensitivity.

Groups of incidence data are usually compared by contingency table tests (such as Fishers Extract Test) of ANOVA?

a) Contingency table analysis.

REFERENCES

1. Abramowitz, M., and Stegun, I. A. (1964): *Handbook of Mathematical Functions*, pp. 925–964. National Bureau of Standards, Washington.
2. Aeschbacher, H. U., Vautaz, L., Sotek, J., and Stalder, R. (1977): Use of the beta binomial distribution in dominant-lethal testing for "weak mutagenic activity," Part 1. *Mutat. Res.*, 44:369–390.
3. Anderson, S., Auquier, A., Hauck, W. W., Oakes, D., Vandaele, W., and Weisburg, H. I. (1980): *Statistical Methods for Comparative Studies*. John Wiley & Sons, New York.
4. Anderson, T. W. (1971): *The Statistical Analysis of Time Series*. Wiley, New York.
5. Anderson, E. (1960): A semigraphical method for the analysis of complex problems. *Technomet.*, 2:387–391.
6. Annau, Z. (1972): The comparative effects of hypoxia and carbon monoxide hypoxia on behavior. In: *Behavioral Toxicology*, edited by B. Weiss and V. G. Laties, pp. 105–127. Plenum Press, New York.
7. Anscombe, F. J. (1973): Graphics in statistical analysis, *The American Statistician*, 27:17–21.
8. Armitage, P. (1955) Tests for linear trends in proportions and frequencies. *Biometrics.*, 11:375–386.
9. Atchely, W. R., and Bryant, E. H. (1975): *Multivariate Statistical Methods: Among Groups Covariation*. Dowden, Hutchinson and Ross, Stroudsburg.
10. Barnett, V., and Lewis, T. (1984): *Outliers in Statistical Data*, Edition 2. John Wiley, New York.
11. Bateman, A. T. (1977): The dominant lethal assay in the male mouse. In: *Handbook of Mutagenicity Test Procedures*, edited by B. J. Kilbey, M. Legator, W. Nichols, and C. Ramel, pp. 325–334. Elsevier, New York.
12. Beckman, R. J., and Cook, R. D. (1983): Outliers. *Technometrics*, 25:119–163.
13. Bernstein, L., Kaldor, J., McCann, J., and Pike, M. C. (1982): An empirical approach to the statistical analysis of mutagenesis data from the Salmonella test. *Mutation Res.*, 97:267–281.
14. Beyer, W. H. (1976): *Handbook of Tables for Probability and Statistics*. CRC Press, Boca Raton, FL.
15. Bliss, C. I. (1935): The calculation of the dosage-mortality curve. *Ann. Appl. Biol.*, 22:134–167.
16. Bloomfield, P. (1976): *Fourier Analysis of Time Series: An Introduction*. John Wiley, New York.
17. Boyd, E. M., and Knight, L. M. (1963): Postmortem shifts in the weight and water levels of body organs. *Tox. Appl. Pharm.*, 5:119–128.
18. Boyd, E. M. (1972): *Predictive Toxicometrics*. Williams & Wilkins, Baltimore.
19. Breslow, N. (1984): Comparison of survival curves. In: *Cancer Clinical Trials: Methods and Practice*, edited by M. F. Buse, M. J. Staguet, and R. F. Sylvester, pp. 381–406. Oxford University Press, Oxford.
20. Bruce, R. D. (1985): An up-and-down procedure for acute toxicity testing. *Fund. Appl. Toxicol.*, 5:151–157.
21. Bryant, E. H., and Atchely, W. R. (1975): *Multivariate Statistical Methods: Within-Groups Covariation*. Dowden, Hutchinson and Ross, Stroudsburg.
22. Burt, G. S. (1972): Use of behavioral techniques in the assessment of environmental contaminants. In: *Behavioral Toxicology*, edited by B. Weiss and V. G. Laties, pp. 241–263. Plenum Press, New York.
23. Chambers, J. M., Cleveland, W. S., Kleiner, B., and Tukey, P. A. (1983): *Graphical Methods for Data Analysis*. Wadsworth, Belmont.
24. Chernoff, H. (1973): The use of faces to represent points in K-dimensional space graphically. *J. Amer. Stat. Assoc.*, 68:361–368.
25. Cleveland, W. S., and McGill, R. (1984): Graphical perception: Theory, experimentation, and application to the development of graphical methods, *Journal of the American Statistical Association*, 79:531–554.
26. Cleveland, W. S. (1985): *The Elements of Graphing Data*. Wadsworth Advanced Books, Monterey, CA.

27. Cochran, W. F. (1954): Some models for strengthening the common x^2 tests. *Biometrics.*, 10:417–451.
28. Cochran, W. G., and Cox, G. M. (1975): *Experimental Designs.* John Wiley, New York.
29. Cox, D. R., and Stuart, A. (1955): Some quick tests for trend in location and dispersion. *Biomet.*, 42:80–95.
30. Cox, D. R. (1972): Regression models and life-tables. *J. Roy. Stat. Soc.*, 34B:187–220.
31. Cremer, J. E., and Seville, M. P. (1982): Comparative effects of two pyrethroids dietamethrin and cismethrin, on plasma catecholamines and on blood glucose and lactate. *Toxicol. Appl. Pharmacol.*, 66:124–133.
32. Crowley, J., and Breslow, N. (1984): Statistical analysis of survival data. *Annual Review of Public Health*, 5:385–411.
33. Cutler, S. J., and Ederer, F. (1958): Maximum utilization of the life table method in analyzing survival. *J. Chron. Dis.*, 8:699–712.
34. Davidson, M. L. (1972): Univariate versus multivariate tests in repeated-measures experiments. *Psych. Bull.*, 77:446–452.
35. Davison, M. L. (1983): *Multidimensional Scaling.* John Wiley, New York.
36. Dean, B. J., and Johnston, A. (1977): Dominant lethal assays in the male mice: Evaluation of experimental design, statistical methods and the sensitivity of Charles River (CD1) mice. *Mutat. Res.*, 42:269–278.
37. Debanne, S. M., and Haller, H. S. (1985): Evaluation of statistical methodologies for estimation of median effective dose. *Tox. Appl. Pharm.*, 79:274–282.
38. DePass, L. R., Myers, R. C., Weaver, E. V., and Weil, C. S. (1984): An assessment of the importance of number of dosage levels, number of animals per dosage level, sex and method of LD_{50} and slope calculations in acute toxicity studies. In: *Alternate Methods in Toxicology, Vol. 2: Acute Toxicity Testing: Alternate Approaches*, edited by A. M. Goldberg. Mary Ann Liebert, Inc., New York.
39. Diamond, W. J. (1981): *Practical Experimental Designs.* Lifetime Learning Publications, Belmont, CA.
40. Diem, K., and Lentner, C. (1975): *Documenta Geigy Scientific Tables*, pp. 158–159. Geigy, New York.
41. Dixon, W. J. (1994): *BMD-Biomedical Computer Programs.* University of California Press, Berkeley.
42. Dixon, W. J., and Massey, F. J., Jr. (1969): *Introduction to Statistical Analysis*, Edition 3. McGraw-Hill, New York.
43. Draper, N. R., and Smith, H. (1998): *Applied Regression Analysis*, Edition 3. John Wiley, New York.
44. Duncan, D. B. (1955): Multiple range and multiple F tests. *Biomet.*, 11:1–42.
45. Dunnett, C. W. (1955): A multiple comparison procedure for comparing several treatments with a control. *J. Am. Stat. Assoc.*, 50:1096–1121.
46. Dunnett, C. W. (1964): New tables for multiple comparison with a control. *Biomet.*, 16:671–685.
47. Dykstra, R. L., and Robertson, T. (1983): On testing monotone tendencies. *J. Amer. Stat. Associ.*, 78:342–350.
48. Ehrenberg, L. (1977): Aspects of statistical inference in testing genetic toxicity. In: *Handbook of Mutagenicity Test Procedures*, edited by B. J. Kilbey, M. Legator, W. Nichols, and C. Ramel, pp. 419–459. Elsevier, New York.
49. Elandt-Johnson, R. C., and Johnson, N. L. (1980): *Survival Models and Data Analysis.* John Wiley, New York.
50. Engelman, L., and Hartigan, J. A. (1969): Percentage points of a test for clusters. *Journal of the American Statistical Association*, 64:1647–1648.
51. Everitt, B. S., and Hand, D. J. (1981): Finite mixture distributions. Chapman and Hall, New York.
52. Everitt, B. (1980): *Cluster Analysis.* Halsted Press, New York.
53. *Federal Register* (1985): No. 50, Vol. 50. Washington.
54. Federer, W. T. (1955): *Experimental Design.* Macmillan, New York.
55. Feinstein, A. R. (1979): Scientific standards versus statistical associations and biological logic in the analysis of causation. *Clin. Pharmacol. Therapeu.*, 25:481–492.
56. Finney, D. J., Latscha, R., Bennet, B. M., and Hsu, P. (1963): *Tables for Testing Significance in a 2 × 2 Contingency Table.* Cambridge University Press, Cambridge.
57. Finney, D. K. (1977): *Probit Analysis*, Edition 3. Cambridge University Press, Cambridge.
58. Gabriel, K. R. (1981): Biplot display of multivariate matrices for inspection of data and diagnosis. In: *Interpreting Multivariate Data*, edited by V. Barnett, pp. 147–173. John Wiley, New York.
59. Gad, S. C., Smith, A. C., Cramp, A. L., Gavigan, F. A., and Derelanko, M. J. (1984): Innovative designs and practices for acute systemic toxicity studies. *Drug Chem. Toxicol.*, 7:423–434.
60. Gad, S. C., and Chengelis, C. P. (1992): *Animal Models in Toxicology.* Marcel Dekker, New York.
61. Gad, S. C. (1982): A neuromuscular screen for use in industrial toxicology. *J. Toxicol. Env. Health*, 9:691–704.
62. Gad, S. C. (1998): *Statistics and Experimental Design for Toxicologists.* CRC Press, Boca Raton, FL.
63. Gad, S. C. (1984): Statistical analysis of behavioral toxicology data and studies. *Arch. Toxicol. Suppl.*, 5:256–266.
64. Gad, S. C., Reilly, C., Siino, K. M., and Gavigan, F. A. (1985): Thirteen cationic ionophores: Neurobehavioral and membrane effects. *Drug and Chemical Toxicology*, 8:451–468.
65. Gallant, A. R. (1975): Nonlinear regression. *Am. Stat.*, 29:73–81.
66. Garrett, H. E. (1947): *Statistics in Psychology and Education*, pp. 215–218. Longmans, Green, New York.
67. Gaylor, D. W. (1978): Methods and concepts of biometrics applied to teratology. In: *Handbook of Teratology, Vol. 4*, edited by J. G. Wilson and F. C. Fraser, pp. 429–444. Plenum Press, New York.
68. Gehring, P. J., and Blau, G. E. (1977): Mechanisms of carcinogenicity: Dose response. *J. Environ. Path. Toxicol.*, 1:163–179.
69. Ghent, A. W. (1972): A method for exact testing of 2 × 2, 2 × 3, 3 × 3 and other contingency tables, employing binomiate coefficients. *American Midland Naturalist*, 88:15–27.
70. Glass, L. (1975): Classification of biological networks by their qualitative dynamics. *J. Theor. Bio.*, 54:85–107.
71. Gnanadesikan, R. (1977): *Methods for Statistical Data Analysis of Multivariate Observations.* John Wiley, New York.
72. Gold, H. J. (1977): *Mathematical Modeling of Biological System: An Introductory Guidebook.* John Wiley, New York.
73. Gordon, A. D. (1981): *Classification.* Chapman and Hall, New York.
74. Grafe, A., and Vollmar, J. (1977): Small numbers in mutagenicity tests. *Arch. Toxicol.*, 38:27–34.
75. Gray, L. E., and Laskey, J. W. (1980): Multivariate analysis of the effects of manganese on the reproductive physiology and behavior of the male house mouse. *J. Toxicol. Environ. Health*, 6:861–868.
76. Grubbs, F. E. (1969): Procedure for detecting outlying observations in samples. *Technometrics*, 11:1–21.
77. Hammond, E. C., Garfinkel, L., and Lew, E. A. (1978): Longevity, selective mortality, and competitive risks in relation to chemical carcinogenesis. *Environ. Res.*, 16:153–173.
78. Harris, E. K. (1978): Review of statistical methods of analysis of series of biochemical test results. *Ann. Biol. Clin.*, 36:194–197.
79. Harris, R. J. (1975): *A Primer of Multivariate Statistics*, pp. 96–101. Academic Press, New York.
80. Harter, A. L. (1960): Critical values for Duncan's new multiple range test. *Biomet.*, 16:671–685.

81. Hartigan, J. A. (1983): Classification. *Encyclopedia of Statistical Sciences*, Vol. 2, edited by S. Katz and N. L. Johnson. John Wiley, New York.
82. Haseman, J. K. (1985): Issues in carcinogenicity testing: Dose selection. *Fund. App. Toxicol.*, 5:66–78.
83. Haseman, J. K. (1977): Response to use of statistics when examining life time studies in rodents to detect carcinogenicity. *J. Toxicol. Environ. Health*, 3:633–636.
84. Henry, R. D., and Hidy, G. M. (1979): Multivariate analysis of particulate sulfate and other air quality variables by principle components. *Atmos. Environ.*, 13:1581–1596.
85. Hicks, C. R. (1982): *Fundamental Concepts in the Design of Experiments*. Holt, Rinehart, and Winston, New York.
86. Hoaglin, D. C., Mosteller, F., and Tukey, J. W. (1983): *Understanding Robust and Explanatory Data Analysis*. John Wiley, New York.
87. Hollander, M., and Wolfe, D. A. (1999): *Nonparametric Statistical Methods*, Edition 2. John Wiley, New York.
88. Hotelling, H. (1931): The generalization of Student's ratio. *Ann. Math. Stat.*, 2:360–378.
89. Irwin, S. (1968): Comprehensive observational assessment. Systematic, quantitative procedure for assessing the behavioral and physiologic state of the mouse. *Psychopharmacologia.*, 13:222–257.
90. Jackson, B. (1962): Statistical analysis of body weight data. *Toxicol. Appl. Pharmacol.*, 4:432–443.
91. Johnson, B. L., Anger, W. K., Setzer, J. V., and Xinytaras, C. (1972): The application of a computer controlled time discrimination performance to problems. In: *Behavioral Toxicology*, edited by B. Weiss and V. G. Laties, pp. 129–153. Plenum Press, New York.
92. Joung, H. M., Miller, W. M., Mahannah, C. N., and Guitjens, J. C. (1979): A generalized water quality index based on multivariate factor analysis. *J. Environ. Qual.*, 8:95–100.
93. Kastenbaum, M. A., and Bowman, K. O. (1970): Tables for determining the statistical significance of mutation frequencies. *Mutat. Res.*, 9:527–549.
94. Katz, A. J. (1978): Design and analysis of experiments on mutagenicity. I: Minimal sample sizes. *Mutat. Res.*, 50:301–307.
95. Katz, A. J. (1979): Design and analysis of experiments on mutagenicity. II: Assays involving micro-organisms. *Mutat. Res.*, 64:61–77.
96. Kilbey, B. J., Legator, M., Nicholas, W., and Ramel, C. (1977): *Handbook of Mutagenicity Test Procedures*, pp. 425–433. Elsevier, New York.
97. Kotz, S., and Johnson, N. L. (1982): *Encyclopedia of Statistical Sciences, Vol. 1*, pp. 61–69. John Wiley & Sons, New York.
98. Kowalski, B. R., and Bender, C. F. (1972): Pattern recognition: A powerful approach to interpreting chemical data. *J. Amer. Chem. Soc.*, 94:5632–5639.
99. Kraemer, H. C., and Thiemann, G. (1987): *How Many Subjects? Statistical Power Analysis in Research*. Sage Publications, Newbury Park, California.
100. Kupper, L. L., and Haseman, J. K. (1978): The use of a correlated binomial model for the analysis of certain toxicological experiments. *Biomet.*, 34:69–76.
101. Lee, E. T. (1980): *Statistical Methods for Survival Data Analysis*. Lifetime Learning Publications, Belmont.
102. Litchfield, J. T., and Wilcoxon, F. (1949): A simplified method of evaluating dose effect experiments. *J. Pharmacol. Exp. Ther.*, 96:99–113.
103. Loeb, W. F., and Quimby, F. W. (1989): *The Clinical Chemistry of Laboratory Animals*. Pergamon Press, New York.
104. Marriott, F. H. C. (1991): *The Dictionary of Statistical Terms*. Longman Scientific & Technical, Essex, England.
105. Martin, H. F., Gudzinowicz, B. J., and Fanger, H. (1975): *Normal Values in Clinical Chemistry*. Marcel Dekker, New York.
106. Mendal, N. R., Finch, S. J., and Thode, H. C., Jr. (1993): Where is the likelihood ratio test powerful for detecting two component normal mixtures? *Biometrics*, 49:907–915.
107. Meyer, S. L. (1975): *Data Analysis for Scientists and Engineers*, pp. 17–18. John Wiley, New York.
108. Myers, J. L. (1972): *Fundamentals of Experimental Designs*. Allyn and Bacon, Boston.
109. Mitruka, B. M., and Rawnsley, H. M. (1977): *Clinical Biochemical and Hematological Reference Values in Normal Animals*. Masson, New York.
110. Montgomery, D. C., and Smith, E. A. (1983): *Introduction to Linear Regression Analysis*. John Wiley, New York.
111. Mosteller, F., and Youtz, C. (1961): Tables of the Freeman-Tukey transformations for the binomial and Poisson distributions. *Biometrika*, 48:433–440.
112. Nelson, C. J., and Holson, J. F. (1978): Statistical analysis of teratologic data: Problems and advancements. *J. Environ. Pathol. Toxicol.*, 2:187–199.
113. Nie, N. H., Hall, C. H., Jenkins, J. G., Steinbrenner, K., and Bent, D. H. (1995): *Statistical Package for the Social Sciences*. McGraw-Hill, New York.
114. Norton, S. (1973): Amphetamine as a model for hyperactivity in the rat. *Physiol. Behav.*, 11:181–186.
115. Oser, B. L., and Oser, M. (1956): Nutritional studies in rats on diets containing high levels of partial ester emulsifiers. II: Reproduction and lactation. *J. Nutr.*, 60:429.
116. Paintz, M., Bekemeier, H., Metzner, J., and Wenzel, U. (1982): Pharmacological activities of a homologous series of pyrazole derivatives including quantitative structure: Activity relationships (QSAR). *Agents Actions* (Suppl.), 10:47–58.
117. Peto, R., Pike, M. C., Armitage, P., Breslow, N. E., Cox., D. R., Howard, S. V., Kantel, N., McPherson, K., Peto, J., and Smith, P. G. (1977): Design and analysis of randomized clinical trials requiring prolonged observations of each patient, II, Analyses and examples, *British Journal of Cancer*, 35:1–39.
118. Peto, R., and Pike, M. C. (1973): Conservatism of approximation; $(0\text{—}E)^2$ E in the Log Rank Test for survival data on tumour incidence data, *Biometrics*, 29:579–584.
119. Pollard, J. H. (1977): *Numerical and Statistical Techniques*. Cambridge University Press, New York.
120. Portier, C., and Hoel, D. (1984): Type I error of trend tests in proportions and the design of cancer screens. *Comm. Stat. Theory Meth.*, A13:1–14.
121. Prentice, R. L. (1976): A generalization of the probit and logit methods for dose response curves. *Biomet.*, 32:761–768.
122. Rai, K., and Ryzin, J. V. (1985): A dose-response model for teratological experiments involving quantal responses. *Biomet.*, 41:1–9.
123. Ridgemen, W. J. (1975): *Experimentation in Biology*, pp. 214–215. Wiley, New York.
124. Romesburg, H. C. (1984): *Cluster Analysis for Researchers*. Lifetime Learning Publications, Belmont. 43:45–58.
125. Ryan, T. A., Joyner, B. L., and Ryan, B. F. (1996): *Minitab Reference Manual*. Duxbury Press, Boston.
126. Salsburg, D. (1980): The effects of life-time feeding studies on patterns of senile lesions in mice and rats. *Drug Chem. Tox.*, 3:1–33.
127. SAS Institute (1996): *SAS Users Guide 1996 Edition*. SAS Institute, Cary, NC.
128. Schaeffer, D. J., Glave, W. R., and Janardan, K. G. (1982): Multivariate statistical methods in toxicology, III: Specifying joint toxic interaction using multiple regression analysis. *J. Toxicol. Env. Health*, 9:705–718.

129. Schaffer, J. W., Forbes, J. A., and Defelice, E. A. (1967): Some suggested approaches to the analysis of chronic toxicity and chronic drug administration data. *Toxicol. Appl. Pharmacol.*, 10:514–522.
130. Schaper, M., Thompson, R. D., and Alarie, Y. (1985): A method to classify airborne chemicals which alter the normal ventilatory response induced by CO_2. *Toxicol. Appl. Pharmacol.*, 79:332–341.
131. Scheffe, H. (1959): *The Analysis of Variance*. Wiley, New York.
132. Schmid, C. F. (1983): *Statistical Graphics*. John Wiley, New York.
133. Seal, H. L. (1964): *Multivariate Statistical Analysis for Biologists*. Methuen, London.
134. Shirley and Newman (1954).
135. Shy-Modjeska, J. S., Riviere, J. E., and Rawldings, J. O. (1984): Application of biplot methods to the multivariate analysis of toxicological and pharmacokinetic data. *Toxicol. Appl. Pharmacol.*, 72:91–101.
136. Siegel, S. (1956): *Nonparametric Statistics for the Behavioral Sciences*. McGraw-Hill, New York.
137. Snedecor, G. W., and Cochran, W. G. (1980): *Statistical Methods*, Edition 7. Iowa State University Press, Ames.
138. Sokal, R. R., and Rohlf, F. J. (1994): *Biometry*, Edition 3. W.H. Freeman, San Francisco.
139. SOT ED_{01} Task Force (1981): Reexamination of the ED_{01} study–adjusting for time on study. *Fundam. Appl. Toxicol.*, 1:8–123.
140. Taketomo, R. T., McGhan, W. F., Fushiki, M. R., Shimada, A., and Gumpert, N. F. (1982): Gentamycin nephrotoxicity application of multivariate analysis. *Clin. Pharm.*, 1:554–549.
141. Tarone, R. E. (1975): Tests for trend in life table analysis. *Biometrika*, 62:679–682.
142. Tatsuoka, M. M. (1971): *Multivariate Analysis*. John Wiley, New York.
143. Thompson, W. R., and Weil, C. S. (1952): On the construction of tables for moving average interpolation. *Biomet.*, 8:51–54.
144. Tilson, H. A., Cabe, P. A., and Burne, T. A. (1980): Behavioral procedures for the assessment of neurotoxicity. In: *Experimental and Clinical Neurotoxicology*, edited by P. S. Spencer and N. H. Schaumburg, pp. 758–766. Williams & Wilkins, Baltimore.
145. Tufte, E. R. (1990): *Envisioning Information*. Graphics Press, Cheshire, CT.
146. Tufte, E. R. (1983): *The Visual Display of Quantitative Information*. Graphics Press, Cheshire, CT.
147. Tufte, E. R. (1997): *Visual Explanations*. Graphics Press, Cheshire, CT.
148. Tukey, J. W. (1977): *Exploratory Data Analysis*. Addison-Wesley Publishing Co., Reading, PA.
149. Velleman, P. F., and Hoaglin, D. C. (1981): *Applications, Basics and Computing of Exploratory Data Analysis*. Duxbury Press, Boston.
150. Vollmar, J. (1977): Statistical problems in mutagenicity tests. *Arch. Toxicol.*, 38:13–25.
151. Vuataz, L., and Sotek, J. (1978): Use of the beta-binomial distribution in dominant-lethal testing for "weak mutagenic activity," Part 2. *Mutat. Res.*, 52:211–230.
152. Weil, C. S. (1975): Toxicology experimental design and conduct as measured by inter-laboratory collaboration studies. *J. Assoc. Off. Anal. Chem.*, 58:687–688.
153. Weil, C. S. (1972): Statistics versus safety factors and scientific judgment in the evaluation of safety for man. *Toxicol. Appl. Pharmacol.*, 21:459–472.
154. Weil, C. S., Carpenter, C. P., and Smith, H. I. (1953): Specifications for calculating the median effective dose. *Amer. Indust. Hyg. Assoc. Quart.*, 14:200–206.
155. Weil, C. S. (1962): Applications of methods of statistical analysis to efficient repeated-dose toxicological tests. I: General considerations and problems involved: Sex differences in rat liver and kidney weights. *Toxicol. Appl. Pharmacol.*, 4:561–571.
156. Weil, C. S., and Gad, S. C. (1980): Applications of methods of statistical analysis to efficient repeated-dose toxicologic tests. 2: Methods for analysis of body, liver and kidney weight data. *Toxicol. Appl. Pharmacol.*, 52:214–226.
157. Weil, C. S. (1973): Experimental design and interpretation of data from prolonged toxicity studies. In: *Proc. 5th Int. Congr. Pharmacol.*, Vol. 2, pp. 4–12. Beacon Press, San Francisco.
158. Weil, C. S. (1982): Statistical analysis and normality of selected hematologic and clinical chemistry measurements used in toxicologic studies. *Arch. Toxicol.*, (Suppl.) 5:237–253.
159. Weil, C. S. (1978): A critique of the collaborative cytogenetics study to measure and minimize interlaboratory variation. *Mutat. Res.*, 50:285–291.
160. Weil, C. S. (1952): Tables for convenient calculation of median-effective dose (LD_{50} or ED_{50}) and instructions in their use. *Biomet.*, 8:249–263.
161. Weil, C. S. (1983): Economical LD_{50} and slope determinations. *Drug Chem. Toxicol.*, 6:595–603.
162. Weil, C. S. (1970): Selection of the valid number of sampling units and a consideration of their combination in toxicological studies involving reproduction, teratogenesis or carcinogenesis. *Food Cosmet. Toxicol.*, 8:177–182.
163. Williams, R., and Buschbom, R. L. (1982): Statistical Analysis of Litter Experiments in Teratology. *Battelle PNL-4425*.
164. Williams, D. A. (1971): A test for differences between treatment means when several dose levels are compared with a zero dose control. *Biomet.*, 27:103:117.
165. Williams, D. A. (1972): The comparison of several dose levels with a zero dose control. *Biomet.*, 28:519–531.
166. Wilson, J. S., and Holland, L. M. (1982): The effect of application frequency on epidermal carcinogenesis assays. *Toxicol.*, 24:45–53.
167. Witten, M., Bennet, C. E., and Glassman, A. (1981): Studies on the toxicity and binding kinetics of abrin in normal and Epstein Barr virus-transformed lymphocyte culture-I: Experimental results. *Exp. Cell. Biol.*, 49:306–318.
168. Woodward, W. A., Elliott, A. C., and Gray, H. L. (1985): *Directory of Statistical Microcomputer Software*. Marcel Dekker, New York.
169. Young, J. E., and Matthews, P. (1981): Pollution injury in Southeast Northumberland, England UK: The analysis of field data using economical correlation analysis. *Environ. Pollut. Sen. B. Chem. Phys.*, 2:353–366.
170. Young, F. W. (1985): Multidimensional scaling. In: *Encyclopedia of Statistical Sciences*, Vol. 5, edited by S. Katz and N. L. Johnson, pp. 649–659. John Wiley, New York.
171. Zar, J. H. (1974): *Biostatistical Analysis,* p. 50. Prentice-Hall, Englewood.
172. Zbinden, G., and Flury-Roversi, M. (1981): Significance of the LD_{50} test for the toxicological evaluation of chemical substances. *Arch. Toxicol.*, 47:77–99.
173. Conover, J. W., and Inman, R. L. (1981): Rank transformation as a bridge between parametric and nonparametric statistics, *The American Statistician*, 35:124–129.

Principles and Methods of Toxicology,
Fourth Edition, edited by A. Wallace Hayes.
Taylor & Francis, Philadelphia © 2001.

Chapter 8

Quantitative Extrapolations in Toxicology

Joseph V. Rodricks, David W. Gaylor, and Duncan Turnbull

The purpose of this chapter is to describe the scientific basis for extrapolation of toxicity findings in laboratory animals to predict outcomes in human populations. Such extrapolation is often said to comprise two components, one qualitative in nature, the second quantitative. Qualitative extrapolations generally concern the nature of the toxic response (are the specific toxicity endpoints observed in test animals also expected in similarly exposed human beings?), while quantitative extrapolations concern issues such as the magnitude and duration of the dose at which human beings and test animals are expected to be at equal risk of toxicity. Although both types of extrapolation are important, scientific understanding of the basis for quantitative extrapolations across species is more limited than is the basis for qualitative extrapolations. At the same time, because results from animal toxicity studies have become such important determinants of regulatory and other public health protection activities, and because the latter typically require the establishment of quantitative limits on human exposure, questions regarding quantitative extrapolations have come to be seen as ultimately of greater significance than those that are purely qualitative in character. Thus, as in many other areas in which science plays a significant role in the development of social policies, the questions that are of most importance tend to be those about which science has the least clear answers. It is therefore no surprise that there is so much public skepticism about the predictions of toxicologists and risk assessors.

The scientific basis for quantitative extrapolations across species is not, however, as feeble as it is sometimes made out to be by those who would minimize the importance of toxicology, and science in general, in regulatory and public health decisions. The principal purpose of this chapter is to describe that basis as it is understood today, and to point to the many active areas of research that are devoted to furthering that understanding. As has been the case in the evolution of other areas of science, the greatest understanding comes with the ability to provide quantitatively accurate, empirical descriptions of physical and biological phenomena, and to build from these generally applicable, predictive models of those phenomena. It is true, of course, that quantitative understanding never provides a complete description of these phenomena—the qualitative aspects will always be necessary to complete the picture.

Following brief discussions of the historical context of and need for interspecies extrapolation, and a description of the problem, the chapter continues with five sections on different aspects of the problem of extrapolation (these are outlined in the section on the need for extrapolation), and concludes with a discussion of the overall strategy for scientifically based, interspecies extrapolation.

HISTORICAL CONTEXT

The use of experimental animals to study biological phenomena arose in the mid 19th century, but their modern use in toxicology had its origin during the third decade of the 20th century, when several investigators began to study the effects of vitamins, minerals, and other food constituents. At about the same time, efforts were initiated to identify and breed species and strains of laboratory animals whose genetic and physiological characteristics, and nutritional requirements, could be sufficiently well defined that they could be reliably used in controlled experiments. By the mid-1930s a number of government and industrial laboratories in the United States, Europe, and Japan had begun the fairly routine use of laboratory animals to study occupational chemicals, and soon thereafter, reports of studies of food additives, pesticides, and pharmaceutical agents began to appear in the literature. These early efforts to use laboratory animals to investigate chemical toxicity were no doubt motivated by the belief that responses in animals were useful indicators of potential human responses, but there was little explicit discussion of how data from these studies should be used for that purpose.

Two FDA scientists, Arnold Lehman and O. Garth Fitzhugh, were perhaps the first toxicologists to deal explicitly with the issue. In a short but famous paper published in 1954 (39), the two scientists described the basis for the belief that results from animal studies could be used qualitatively to predict responses in humans, but that quantitative predictions were more problematic. To deal with this problem, Lehmann and Fitzhugh postulated that "average" humans would likely respond to a chemical exposure at a lower dose than would a group of experimental animals, and that within the human population, some individuals would respond at lower doses than would the "average" person. In modern parlance, these authors recognized that the *variability* in response at a given dose was likely to be much greater in a highly diverse human population than it is in a group of inbred, and otherwise homogeneous and healthy, experimental animals. They further recognized that if toxicology data from experimental animals were to be used to establish protective limits[1] (what Lehman and Fitzhugh called "safe levels") for humans, it would be necessary to "adjust" the experimental results. From their discussion and review arose the concept of "safety factors": a factor of 10 was proposed to adjust (downward) the animal dose (specifically the no-observed-adverse-effect level, NOAEL) to estimate the NOAEL for the "average" human, and another factor of 10 to estimate the NOAEL for the "most sensitive" members of the human population. They offered the term *acceptable daily intake* (ADI) as their notion of a "safe level" of chronic chemical exposure for the general population, and the ADI was to be obtained by dividing experimental NOAELs from chronic animal toxicology studies by a factor of 100 (10 × 10). This system, though modified in several significant ways, remains in place today. It is used to establish various protective limits for chemical exposures in the general population. It is interesting that in the 1954 Lehman–Fitzhugh paper, an attempt is made to find an empirical basis for the two factors of 10, but the authors recognized that the database available for such an analysis was extremely limited (39).

Although the Lehman–Fitzhugh approach to quantitative extrapolation recognized the phenomena of inter- and intraspecies variability, it assumed implicitly that no toxic response was likely to occur in any individual unless exposures exceeded some threshold dose. The problem was to define that threshold for a large and diverse human population when the only significant data available arose from experimental studies. During the 1940s and 1950s an influential body of scientists working in the area of experimental carcinogenesis espoused the view that this particular class of toxic agents behaved biologically in ways that called into question the viability of the threshold concept (45). Government policies incorporated this view, which was until the 1970s captured by the phrase *no safe level*. By that time regulators saw that such a policy provided little useful guidance for decision making, and turned to the scientific literature to identify specific methodologies that could be applied to animal carcinogenicity data to estimate low-dose risks to humans for substances that might act by "no-threshold" mechanisms (45). The concept of safety also took a turn at this time, as scientists and decision makers recognized

[1] *Protective limits* is our term, used through the chapter as a description of any quantitative measure that is derived from toxicology or epidemiology data and that is intended to establish the upper limit on exposure that is thought to be without significant risk of toxicity to humans. It is recognized that it is not possible to provide absolute assurance that such limits will protect every person in a population; moreover, exposures greater than these limits may pose no risk to many persons. The term is used here as a simple, one-phrase description of a concept that has in practice unfortunately attracted many different names (described later).

that safety could be defined only in relative terms. In an influential 1983 study issued by the National Research Council, the notion arose that decisions regarding levels of risk that were sufficiently small to ensure protection of the public health properly fell within the domain of *risk management*: Scientists have the task of assessing toxic risks and describing how their magnitudes change with exposure, but policymakers have the task of deciding how much risk reduction is needed to protect public health, and of how any needed risk reduction is to be achieved (45,48).

As these developments regarding the uses of toxicology data in decision making evolved, so did the work of experimental toxicologists. Since the 1950s, animal studies have provided increasingly complete data on the effects of chemical exposures. Thus, increasing amounts of information have developed on the influences of dose, duration, and routes of exposure, on the roles of chemical kinetics and metabolism, and on the biological and molecular mechanisms underlying the production of toxicity. Experimentalists continue to find useful ways to examine the influences of exogenous compounds on a greater variety of targets, including complex systems of the body. Alongside the work of toxicologists must now be placed developments in the field of epidemiology, because these offer increased possibilities for testing hypotheses generated in the toxicology laboratory.

These various developments, which emerge more completely in the discussions to follow, place greater demands on the risk managers who must use the results of risk assessments in the formulation of health protection policies. At the same time, they provide better tools for risk assessment—of which interspecies extrapolation is a highly important component—and are proving to be of value in improving the scientific basis for risk-based decision making. This is, after all, what toxicology is about.

THE NEED FOR EXTRAPOLATION

Experimental and Epidemiological Methods and Their Limits

In the best of all possible worlds there would be no need for any form of extrapolation. Second best would be a world in which well-founded predictive models were available to extrapolate from one set of conditions to another. In the area of predictive toxicology, we now live in a third-best world, and perhaps our goal is to achieve the second best. The "best" world is probably not within our reach.

Why is extrapolation necessary? The answer to this question may seem so obvious that it is unnecessary to offer an explicit discussion. But because so many observers see science as a purely empirical subject in which all forms of extrapolation are merely speculative (a highly naive view of science), or as a subject in which extrapolation is justified only when well-supported predictive models have come to be available (a more credible and, indeed, a proper view of science), the question of "why engage in extrapolation?" is not as easy to answer as it might appear to be.

Given that there is a social need, expressed in many federal and state laws, to protect people from the toxic properties of chemicals in the environment, in foods, consumer products, medicines, and so on, it is necessary to rely upon one or both of the two basic methods available for acquiring toxicological data—the epidemiological and the experimental. Both have strengths and limits (Table 8.1), but neither method is capable of providing direct measurements of toxic risks that are applicable in all situations of potential interest. Animal studies allow us to understand toxicity characteristics of a chemical before human exposure is allowed to occur, whereas the epidemiological method generally does not. They also allow much more thorough examination of the effects of chemical exposure, under a much wider variety of conditions, than do the methods of epidemiology. They usually provide better information on dose-response characteristics, and also allow causal relations to be more readily established. They suffer, of course, one large disadvantage, in that they do not reveal responses directly in the species of interest. Thus, extrapolation from animal data is necessary in many if not most cases if anything at all is to be said about potential human risk and protection of human populations.

Both methods, experimental and epidemiological, suffer from additional limitations. Most importantly, the information they yield, even under the best conditions, is restricted to that portion of the dose-response curve that is within the detection power of the method used; in both cases the size of the population that can be studied, along with some other aspects of that population, is the principal determinant of detection power. Thus, empirical dose-response data will be limited to the relatively "high dose–high risk" portion of the dose-response curve. Most conditions about which toxicity dose-response data are sought concern exposures and doses that fall outside of (well below) the observable range, and therefore outside of the area of direct measurement.

It is also important to emphasize that although epidemiological data derive from studies in humans, there always remains the question of the representativeness of the studied population for the population whose risk is being assessed. The typical problem concerns the use of information obtained in occupational cohorts for assessing toxic risk in the general population.

Other extrapolation issues arise and cannot be avoided, because it is often necessary to reach decisions in the absence of complete data. The most common problems

Table 8.1
Comparison of epidemiology and animal studies for identifying toxic properties

	Epidemiology studies	Animal studies
Opportunity to conduct study	Often not possible	Generally possible
Opportunity to obtain information prior to human exposure	No	Yes
Time requirements	Years to decades	Weeks to years
Species of interest	Yes[a]	No
Cause–effect determination	Difficult	Not as difficult
Opportunity to obtain quantitative dose-response data	Not frequently	Always

[a] Note that epidemiology studies may not provide data on both sexes or on all relevant subgroups of the human population.

arise when it is necessary to assess risk for a given route of exposure when data are available only for another route, and when the assessment concerns risks associated with chronic exposures when only relatively short-term data on toxicity are available.

Thus, if toxicity and epidemiology data are to be used at all to assess human risk and to establish protective limits, extrapolations will be necessary, sometimes several types.

Using Epidemiological and Experimental Data: Distinguishing "Prudence" From "Science"

When engaging in any form of extrapolation for which a reliable, well-established model or empirical basis is not available, judgments must be made that, strictly speaking, go beyond the realm of pure science (45). If such judgments are not introduced, then, as described earlier, no useful conclusions can be reached. Because of the social need to provide conclusions, however tentative and uncertain, judgments must be introduced, whether they concern qualitative or quantitative issues. The National Research Council (NRC), in its 1983 report on risk assessment in the federal government (45) and also in its 1994 report on the same subject (48) recommended that regulatory agencies use the best available science, but that the agencies also adopt guidelines that would specify what judgements they would make (these have come to be loosely called "defaults") to fill knowledge and data gaps. The NRC notion was that these defaults would be specified in advance, in the form of guidelines, and that they would be applied consistently, in specific risk assessments, to avoid case-by-case "manipulations" and to ensure explicitness in the assessment. The NRC also recommended flexibility in the use of defaults, so that chemical-specific data, if reliable, could be used in specific cases to replace one or more generic defaults.

The choice of defaults is a difficult topic, having both scientific and policy components. The U.S. Environmental Protection Agency (EPA) guidelines for carcinogen risk assessment can be consulted for information on the choice of defaults (73). The emphasis in this chapter is on the scientific basis for extrapolation and its limits, and the regulatory defaults are discussed only in passing. It is important, however, to attempt to distinguish what is in the area of well-established science from what is a "science-policy" choice. The truth is that all science is accompanied by uncertainty, and that there is no sharp distinction between what is known with such high certainty that little or no judgment is called for, and that which is insufficiently certain to stand on its own. (It would be interesting to poll the community of toxicologists on how much of any decision to extrapolate from experimental animals to humans they may think is based upon "science," and what part is based on "prudence"—"I'm not sure of its relevance to people but I'll use it anyway, because I want to be careful.")

DESCRIPTION OF THE PROBLEM

The several types of extrapolations necessary to assess risks of toxicity in human populations from data obtained in experimental animals are described in the next five sections of this chapter, along with what are called the empirical and biological bases for each. Both qualitative and quantitative aspects are described, with emphasis on the latter.

Cross-species extrapolations are those pertaining to the attempt to describe expected toxic responses and their relationship to dose in human populations based on responses and their relationship to dose observed experimentally in animals.

Within-species extrapolations are those pertaining to the attempt to describe the expected variability in response within human populations, based either on observations in limited segments of that population, or on responses predicted for limited segments of that population from observations in experimental animals.

Cross-dose extrapolations are those pertaining to the attempt to describe toxic responses and their relationship to dose for the range of the dose-response relationship that falls below the range that is subject to direct measurement, and within the range expected to be experienced by the population that is the subject of the risk assessment.

Cross-route extrapolations are those pertaining to the attempt to describe expected toxic responses and their relationships to dose in populations exposed by one route, based on responses and their relations to dose observed when exposure occurs by another route.

Cross-time extrapolations are those pertaining to the attempt to describe toxic responses and their relationships to dose for various exposure durations, based on responses and their relationships to dose observed over more limited exposure durations.

In each case the empirical and biological bases for such extrapolations are summarized. By *empirical* is meant an analysis based upon comparisons made in more limited circumstances of actual observations relevant to the extrapolation being considered. Thus, for example, compilations and comparisons of human and animal dose-response data for several carcinogens are available, and these comparisons allow at least limited generalizations to be made regarding cross-species extrapolations. By *biological* bases is meant the use of basic knowledge in biology to provide support for particular forms of extrapolation. Both the empirical and biological bases are limited, but often inferences drawn from them converge and thus may provide support for some aspects of extrapolation.

The emphasis in this chapter is on quantitative extrapolations and on the types of scientific data and theories that are regarded as the basis for such extrapolations. As noted in the concluding sections, practical applications of many of the issues discussed in the following are not yet generally available; the thrust of the discussion thus concerns the directions necessary to improve the scientific basis for human risk assessment.

CROSS-SPECIES EXTRAPOLATION

Defining the Problem

When extrapolating toxicological data from one species to another, it is necessary to consider the various factors that may differentially affect the response of different species to the exposure of interest. As a first approximation, of course, for both cross-species and within-species extrapolation, it is common to normalize the toxicant dose to the body weight, and express it as milligrams per kilogram body weight per day. This approach assumes that it is the concentration of the toxicant in the body or at the target site (or some measure directly proportional to it) that determines the magnitude of the toxic effect. Although this appears to address at least one of the differences between species (body size), there are many examples in the literature showing that direct extrapolation simply on the basis of body weight is not accurate. Other aspects of differences among species need to be considered.

Two broad, overlapping classes of factors may affect differential responses: those related to the "effective dose" of the toxicant (determined in part by its pharmacokinetic and metabolic behavior), and those related to the inherent sensitivity of different species. In the absence of differences in inherent sensitivity (often called pharmacodynamic[2] differences), it is generally assumed that different species will show similar responses when exposed to the same effective dose of the toxicant. The effective dose may in turn be influenced by species differences in body size, life span, anatomy and physiology, and pharmacokinetics and metabolism. For a direct-acting toxicant that follows first-order kinetics, the effective dose may be simply proportional to the administered dose. For a chemical with a more complex pattern of kinetics and metabolism to generate a reactive metabolite, pharmacokinetic modeling may be needed to accurately predict the effective dose.

Two general approaches have been used to evaluate methods for interspecies extrapolation: empirical, and biologically based. Empirical approaches rely on collection of data from multiple species exposed to the same substances under comparable conditions, and evaluation of the data to identify consistent relationships among species that permit the prediction of the magnitude of the response in one species (typically humans) based on data from another species. This approach has the advantage of simplicity, but does not readily allow consideration of chemical-specific factors that may affect interspecies scaling. Biologically based approaches make use of scientific knowledge of factors that may influence interspecies scaling, such as anatomical and physiological parameters and especially pharmacokinetics, metabolism, and mechanism of action.

[2] The terms *pharmacokinetic* and *pharmacodynamic* derive from the pharmacological sciences. They have been retained by many toxicologists to describe the behavior of substances having toxic effects. Some have advocated the terms *toxicokinetics* and *toxicodynamics*, but, though those terms seem more descriptive, they have not become widespread in use.

Empirical Approaches

Empirical approaches to cross-species scaling have been studied since the end of the nineteenth century, when Rubner (62) noted that oxygen utilization and caloric expenditure scaled among dogs of different sizes approximately on the basis of body surface area more closely than simply on body mass. Subsequently, this work was extended to other species and other parameters, including the development of criteria for selecting doses for cancer chemotherapeutic drugs (26,53). These authors noted that, for a number of chemotherapeutic drugs, the repeat-dose LD_{10} in mice, rats, and hamsters (treated daily for 5 days), the maximum tolerated dose in dogs and monkeys (the highest daily dose that killed no animals), and the maximum tolerated dose used clinically in humans were more closely comparable when the doses were expressed on a milligrams per square meter body surface area basis than when expressed on the basis of body weight. Because of the difficulty in accurately measuring body surface area, as an approximation based on the relationship between the mass and surface area of a sphere, this surface-area scaling is generally approximated as (body weight)$^{2/3}$.

A more recent reevaluation of these and other repeat toxicity data by Travis and White (69), however, suggested that (body weight)$^{3/4}$ scaling gave a better correlation. Travis and White (69) reanalyzed the repeat toxicity data in mouse, rat, dog, rhesus monkey, and human with 14 chemotherapeutic drugs described by Freireich et al. (26), and similar data in mouse, hamster, rat, dog, monkey, and human for an additional 13 chemotherapeutic drugs. Based on all of these data sets, and the use of a multiple linear regression model, the exponent of body weight giving the best correlation ($r^2 = .96$) among species was 0.73, with 95% confidence bounds of .69 to 0.77.

Recently, Rhomberg and Wolff (59) reported an analysis of cross-species scaling for acute oral LD_{50} values covering ten mammalian species and a wide range of chemical types. They used data from the NIOSH Registry of Toxic Effects of Chemical Substances (RTECS) database, which contains information on over 135,000 substances. Several thousand of these had oral LD_{50} data from at least two species to permit comparisons. Overall, based on the log–log scatter plots of LD_{50} values in pairs of species (e.g., rat vs. mouse; mouse vs. rabbit), and log–log plots of mean ratio of LD_{50} values versus body weight for all species-pair comparisons, body-weight scaling appeared to give a better correlation among species than did body surface area, (body weight)$^{2/3}$ or (body weight)$^{3/4}$. The authors suggested that the difference between the apparent optimal scaling procedure for acute lethality (mg/kg) and that for repeat-dose lethality [(mg/kg$^{2/3}$) or (mg/kg$^{3/4}$)] may be related to differences in the mechanism of lethality. With single acute doses, the lethal dose may depend upon the level of defense capacities or reserves, proportional to body mass; with repeated exposure, survival may, to a larger extent, be a function of repair or replacement rate, which may show scaling patterns more like those for basal metabolic rate or other rates. As discussed later, these rates tend to scale across species as a function of body surface area or (body weight)$^{3/4}$.

Empirical approaches have also been used extensively in attempts to identify the most appropriate approach for scaling of cancer data between species (2,15,28). In one of the most extensive of these studies, Allen et al. (2) evaluated 23 chemicals for which data permitted quantitative estimation of cancer potency in humans and animals. As their measure of "potency," Allen et al. (2) calculated "risk-related doses" (RRDs), defined as the average daily dose per kilogram body weight that would be expected to result in an extra cancer risk of 25% over a lifetime. Allen et al. examined several different ways of expressing the dose, different scaling procedures, different subsets of animal data (restricted by experimental design, route of exposure, species, sex, tumor types), different statistical measures (maximum likelihood estimates and lower confidence limits on RRD), and different ways of considering results from multiple studies of the same chemicals (median response, most sensitive species/sex combination). When the logarithms of the RRDs derived from epidemiological studies were plotted against the logarithms of the predicted RRDs from animal studies, the scaling procedure giving the strongest correlation (by a slight margin) between humans and animals was scaling on the basis of body weight. However, there were wide variations in the apparent relative potency for individual chemicals, and given the uncertainties in the experimental and epidemiological data, it was not possible to rule out surface-area scaling [(body weight)$^{2/3}$], or some intermediate procedure, such as (body weight)$^{3/4}$, as being appropriate. Wide variations in apparent relative potency were also reported in the other comparisons (14,15,28). These studies considered mostly potency comparisons between rats and mice. On average in these studies, rats appeared to be slightly more sensitive than mice when compared on a body-weight basis, as would be expected if the "correct" scaling was on the basis of (body weight)$^{2/3}$ or (body weight)$^{3/4}$. Because of the small sample sizes and wide variation for individual chemicals, however, these comparisons are of limited predictive value.

The U.S. Environmental Protection Agency (72) published an extensive discussion on the selection of a default scaling procedure for cancer risk assessment based on these and other considerations. Its conclusion was that, although there was considerable uncertainty in the

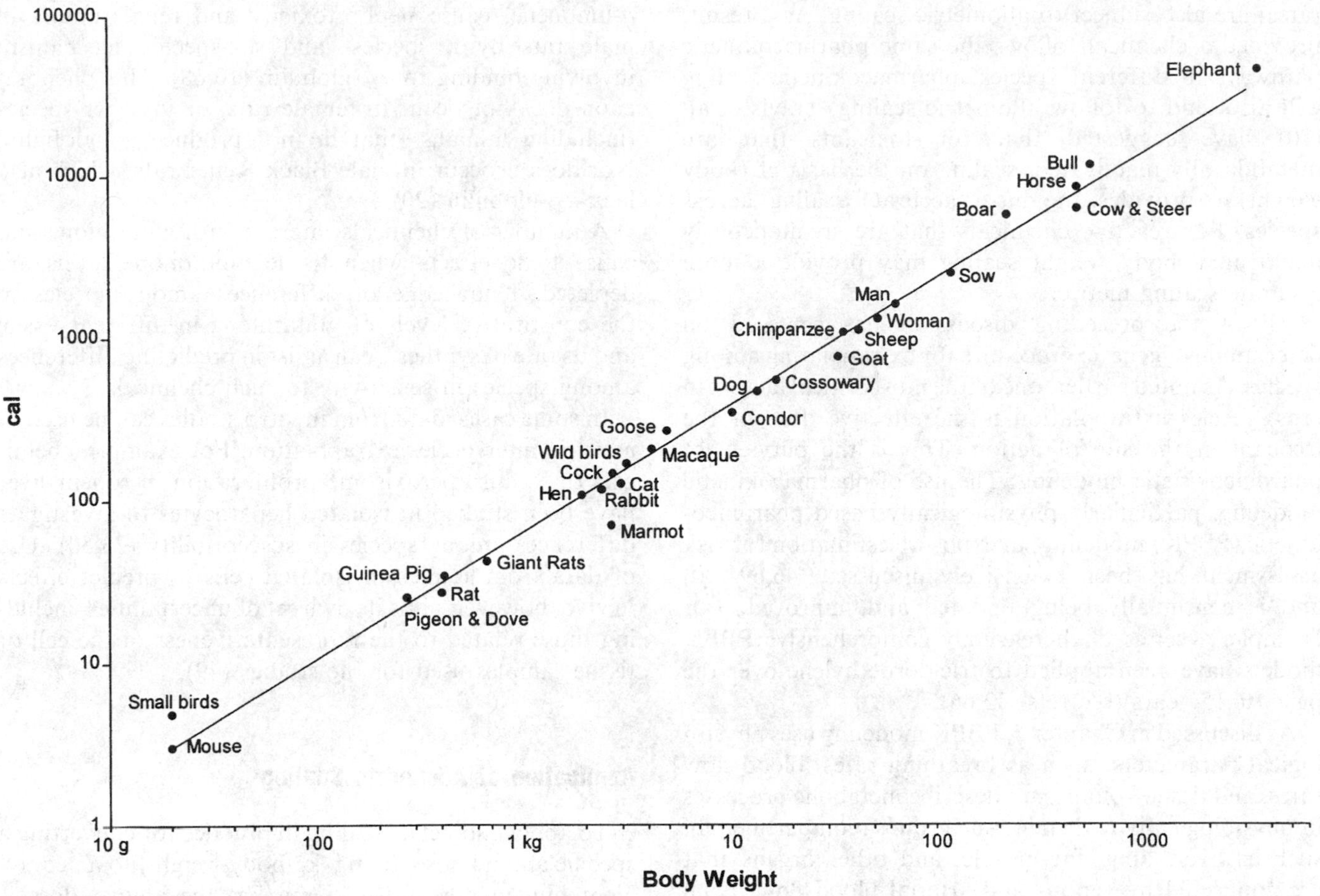

FIG. 8.1. Benedict's (7) mouse-to-elephant graph showing the relationship between species body weight and basal metabolic rate.

selection of any generic scaling procedure, the balance of evidence supported the use of (body weight)$^{3/4}$ as a general procedure when no chemical-specific data provided support for an alternative procedure.

Biologically Based Approaches

Allometry

The work of Rubner (62) and others (e.g., refs. 1, 34, 35) on the relationship between body size and metabolism, mentioned previously, led to the study of allometry, the relationships between body weight and various biological and physiological parameters. A large number of biological and physiological parameters have been found to show a relation to body weight of the form:

$$Y = aW^b$$

where Y is the biological parameter of interest (organ size, blood flow rate, basal metabolic rate, etc.), and a and b are constants relating Y to body weight (W).

When the exponent b in the allometric equation is 1.0, cross-species scaling is based on relative body-weights. When it is 0.67, the biological or physiological measure is said to scale on the basis of relative surface areas.

In examining a wide number of measurements, measures of size (organ weights, blood volumes, etc.) tended to show an exponent (b) of approximately 1.0, while measures of rates (ventilation rate, basal metabolic rate, drug clearance rate, etc.) typically showed values closer to 0.67 (1). There was considerable variation in the best estimate of the exponent, b, for different parameters, and other authors have suggested that the value of b for metabolic and other rates falls closer to 0.75 (11,54,64). Figure 8.1, for example, shows a plot of basal metabolic rate versus body weight for warm blooded animals, ranging from mouse to elephant (7). The slope of this line corresponds to a b value of 0.76 (see ref. 19a).

Pharmacokinetics

Parameters affecting pharmacokinetic differences across species (organ sizes, physiological and metabolic rates) are also subject to allometric scaling. As a result, provided a chemical follows the same pharmacokinetic pathways in different species, pharmacokinetic scaling will also tend to follow allometric scaling. Travis et al. (70) have suggested that for toxicants that are metabolically inactivated, scaling on the basis of (body weight)$^{3/4}$ provides the most accurate scaling across species. For reactive chemicals that are spontaneously inactivated, body weight scaling may provide a more accurate scaling metric.

All of the preceding discussion has centered on determining a generic procedure for extrapolating among species. As noted earlier, one of the most critical factors in cross-species extrapolation is the effective dose of the toxicant at the site of action. This is the purview of pharmacokinetic modeling. The use of pharmacokinetic modeling, particularly physiologically based pharmacokinetic (PBPK) modeling, in exposure estimation for risk assessment has been extensively discussed (46,69a,70) and is continually being updated and improved. For example, a series of increasingly comprehensive PBPK models have been applied to trichloroethylene over the past 10–15 years (see refs. 32,66).

As discussed in Chapter 5, PBPK modeling uses physiological parameters, such as breathing rates, blood flow rates, and tissue volumes, to describe metabolic processes in physiologically realistic tissue groups (compartments), such as liver, lung, fat muscle, and other organs that are connected by venous and arterial blood flow. Each compartment is described mathematically by a set of differential equations. Such models can be used to relate exposure concentrations—for example, in air, water, or food—to concentrations of the parent compound or its metabolites in different tissues, including the target tissue. A major strength of PBPK models is that one can use the same model developed for a chemical in one species to predict chemical transport and metabolism in other species (including humans) by substituting species- specific physiological, biochemical, and metabolic parameters in the model.

Pharmacodynamics

Pharmacokinetics deals with the movement of chemicals in the body. Pharmacodynamics examines the interactions of chemicals and their metabolites with tissue constituents, their biological and physiological effects, and mechanisms of action. Even if one uses allometric scaling or pharmacokinetic modeling to identify an "equivalent" dose of a chemical at a target site, there may be differences in response in different species because of differences in pharmacodynamics or susceptibility. Thus, for example, a diverse group of chemicals, including unleaded gasoline, decalin, and *d*-limonene, cause nephrotoxicity and renal tumors in male rats by a species- and sex-specific mechanism involving binding to α_{2u}-globulin (10,68). This phenomenon does not occur in female rats, or in other species (including humans) that do not produce α_{2u}-globulin. Nor does it occur in male Black Reiter rats, which also lack α_{2u}-globulin (20).

A number of chemicals interact with glutathione and cause toxic effects when tissue glutathione levels are depleted. Knowledge of differences among species in the constitutive levels of glutathione in different tissue and its rate of synthesis can assist in predicting differences among species in sensitivity to such chemicals.

In some cases, data from in vitro studies can be used to assist in interspecies extrapolation. For example, chemicals that cause peroxisome proliferation in rodent liver have been studied in isolated hepatocytes to investigate differences among species in susceptibility (23,50). Use of data from studies in isolated cells to predict effects in vivo, however, adds its own set of uncertainties, including those related to the representativeness of the cell or tissue samples used for the studies (49).

Application of Allometric Scaling

To apply allometric scaling in practice for converting a specific animal dose (in mg/kg body weight) to an equivalent human dose (also in mg/kg) the animal dose is multiplied by the ratio of animal to human body weight to the $(1-b)$ power. Thus, for scaling on the basis of (body weight)$^{3/4}$, the equivalent human dose is calculated as:

$$\text{Human dose (mg/kg)} = \text{animal dose (mg/kg)} \times \left(\frac{\text{animal body weight}}{\text{human body weight}}\right)^{1/4}$$

This scaling factor is derived as follows. For (body weight)^b scaling:

$$\frac{D_\mathrm{h}}{(W_\mathrm{h})^b} = \frac{D_\mathrm{a}}{(W_\mathrm{a})^b}$$

where D_h is the human dose (mg), D_a is the animal dose (mg), W_h is the human body weight (kg), and W_a is the animal body weight. Rearranging this equation and dividing both sides by the human body weight gives:

$$\frac{D_\mathrm{h}}{W_\mathrm{h}} = \frac{D_\mathrm{a}}{W_\mathrm{h}} \times \left(\frac{W_\mathrm{h}}{W_\mathrm{a}}\right)^b$$

Table 8.2
Cross-species scaling factors based on allometric scaling (based on equations described in text)

Allometric scaling	Mouse–human scaling factor	Rat–human scaling factor
$W^{1.0}$	$(0.035/70)^0 = 1.0$	$(0.3/70)^0 = 1.0$
$W^{0.75}$	$(0.035/70)^{0.25} = 0.150$	$(0.3/70)^{0.25} = 0.256$
$W^{0.67}$	$(0.035/70)^{0.33} = 0.0794$	$(0.3/70)^{0.33} = 0.162$

Note. Assumes human body weight of 70 kg, mouse body weight of 35 g, and rat body weight of 300 g. The scaling factor indicates the dose for a human (mg/kg/day) that is equivalent to 1 mg/kg/day for a mouse or rat. For example with $W^{0.75}$ scaling, a dose of 1 mg/kg/day in a mouse is equivalent to 0.150 mg/kg/day for a 70-kg human.

Multiplying the top and bottom of the right side by the animal body weight W_a gives:

$$\frac{D_h}{W_h} = \frac{D_a}{W_a} \times \frac{(W_h)^b \times W_a}{(W_a)^b \times W_h}$$

$$= \frac{D_a}{W_a} \times \frac{(W_a)^{1-b}}{(W_h)^{1-b}}$$

$$= \frac{D_a}{W_a} \times \left(\frac{W_a}{W_h}\right)^{1-b}$$

Examples of the application of these relationships are illustrated in Table 8.2.

Current Trends

At the present time there is extensive work under way aimed at improving our ability to perform cross-species extrapolation, particularly in the areas of pharmacokinetic and pharmacodynamic modeling. As with other types of extrapolation, cross-species extrapolation is aided by an understanding of the mechanism of action of the toxicant under consideration. Because of the limitations of studying toxicants in humans, efforts are also underway to use isolated human cells to address some pharmacodynamic questions and, hence, improve the accuracy of extrapolation.

WITHIN-SPECIES EXTRAPOLATION—VARIABILITY IN HUMAN RESPONSE

Defining the Problem

The term *extrapolation* is, in this context, used somewhat differently than it is in the four other areas discussed in this chapter. The human population is without question highly *heterogeneous* with respect to all of the many differences that affect response to a given dose of a given chemical. If the distribution of toxic responses at a specified dose were known with accuracy, it would be possible to specify a dose at which a specified fraction of the population would be at a given risk of toxicity. Moreover, if the distribution of threshold doses for the population were known, it would be possible to specify the dose at which, for example, the vast majority of individuals would not be at risk; the specific fraction at the tail of the distribution that might remain at risk would be selected as a matter of policy (such a selection would be necessary on the assumption that any plausible distribution of population thresholds would not include an identifiable dose at which there were absolutely zero responders).

In practice such population distributions are not available, and the traditional "default" approach has been, first, to estimate a threshold dose for some hypothetical person described as "average" with respect to responsiveness, and, second, to divide this threshold estimate by a factor, usually 10, that is thought to lead to an estimate of the threshold dose somewhere near the tail of the underlying, but unknown, distribution at which the "most sensitive" members of the population are expected to be found. This estimate is usually considered protective for the "most sensitive" individuals and, necessarily, for all less sensitive individuals. Factors other than 10 have been used if there is some reason to believe that the data supporting a threshold represent individuals more or less sensitive than the hypothetical "average." This relatively crude procedure thus involves extrapolation from so-called "average" to "sensitive" individuals. Interestingly, there is no methodological tradition within the realm of carcinogen risk assessment that is specifically designed to account for population variability (48).

The traditional approach to deriving protective doses offers no insight into the degree of population protection provided. Whether it is underprotective or extraordinarily overprotective depends upon where on the true (but unknowable) distribution of threshold doses the protective dose happens to lie.

Movement away from the "default" approach toward a more scientifically rigorous one that provides some insight into the degree of protection from toxic risk provided at various doses depends upon the development and incorporation of scientific information relevant to the question of population variability. The factors known to influence variability are described in the next subsection, and this is followed by a review of some empirical data on this question.

Biological Bases for Interindividual Variability

Three major sources of interindividual variability in response to a chemical exposure can be described. First,

Table 8.3
Major sources of interindividual variability in responses to chemical exposures

Source	Cause of variability	Some major influences
Uptake	Differences in contact with and absorption of chemical from its environmental sources	Age Diet Smoking Health status of skin, respiratory tract, and gastrointestinal tract
Pharmacokinetics and metabolism	Differences in distribution, metabolism, and elimination, leading to different target site concentrations	Age Gender Health status Other exposures (dietary, drug, chemicals) Genetic polymorphisms Pregnancy
Response at target site(s) (pharmacodynamics)	Differences in biological response at a given target site concentration	Age Gender Health status Nutritional status Hormonal status Pregnancy Immune status Genetic polymorphisms

individuals vary in uptake of a chemical from the environment. Second, pharmacokinetic and metabolic behaviors of chemicals vary among individuals; and third, interindividual variability exists with respect to the response at the target site to a given dose (concentration × time) of a toxicologically active compound (pharmacodynamic differences). These three influences lead to variability in the size of the dose (concentration × time) of active compound (administered compound or, more often, a metabolite thereof) that reaches the target site, and the magnitude of the response to that dose, even when all individuals are exposed to identical concentrations of a chemical in their environment. In addition, variability exists with respect to the intake of a chemical because of differences in the nature and extent of human contacts with the environmental media in which the chemical is present. In Table 8.3 are listed some of the major contributors to interindividual variability in toxic response.

Although there is substantial empirical support for the fact of human variability, there is large uncertainty regarding its magnitude. In any given exposure situation, some factors may serve to increase the relative responsiveness of some individuals, while in other exposure situations these same individuals may be at less relative risk. Thus, for example, infants lacking metabolic capacity, which does not fully develop until about 1 year of age, may be less susceptible to substances requiring metabolic activation, yet be more sensitive to other substances because of their less than fully functional immune systems. The number of factors influencing responsiveness is so large and variable within the human population, and the cumulative direction of their effects (to increase or decrease sensitivity) so unpredictable in any given exposure situation, that no attempt to derive a generally applicable model of variability based on biological understanding of each of the factors known to influence it has proved successful. Instead, empirical evidence that captures the cumulative effects of all important influences has been generally regarded as of more value (48).

Empirical Approaches to Understanding Interindividual Variability

Little empirical data supported Lehmann and Fitzhugh's original 1954 proposal to extrapolate from "average" to "sensitive" individuals by the incorporation of the assumption of a 10-fold difference in sensitivity, and this assumption has become the standard "default" uncertainty factor, typically used by regulators when there is no known basis for another factor. Although it has never been explicitly described, the adoption of the 10-fold factor suggests that the total variability in response in the human population ranges over about 100-fold, assuming a symmetrical distribution of responses about the average. Of course, the location of the "least" and "most" sensitive individuals on the actual distribution is unknown, so it is not possible to describe the actual range.

By the early 1980s, sufficient empirical information had accumulated to allow limited analysis of variability (21). Dourson and Stara's 1983 review of a number of data sets (21) concluded that a 10-fold factor was likely to reflect a wider range of interindividual variability than could be documented for the vast majority of chemicals. This analysis suggested that the 10-fold factor was adequately protective. Review of differences in human metabolism of chemicals (12) has found that a 10-fold factor covered the total range of variability for 80–95% of the population; this finding suggests that the range from "average" to "sensitive" is significantly less than 10-fold. LD_{50} ratios of adults to newborns for 238 chemicals have been evaluated (65) as a measure of intraspecies variability. Although it was found that the median ratio reflected only a 2.6-fold variability, and that 86% of the ratios were less than 10, the fact that most of the data derived from experimental animal studies casts some doubt on its applicability to humans.

In a review published in 1996, Dourson et al. (22) concluded, based on evaluations of the type just described, that:

> In general, the default value of 10 for interhuman variability appears to be protective when starting from a median response, or by inference, from a NOAEL assumed to be from an average group of humans. However, when NOAEL's are available in a known sensitive human subpopulation, or if human toxicokinetics or toxicodynamics are known with some certainty, this default value should be adjusted or replaced accordingly. (p. 111)

Some authors have proposed to examine variability separately for factors influencing delivery of target site dose (uptake, pharmacokinetics, metabolism) and those affecting response. One reviewer suggested that variability in the former factor was generally larger than it was for the latter, and he proposed that the 10-fold factor be subdivided into factors of 4 (pharmacokinetics) and 2.5 (pharmacodynamics) (58).

The limited empirical analysis supporting the factor of 10, or its subfactors, is perhaps reassuring. Little effort has been devoted to developing more complete descriptions of variability distributions. Heterogeneity in response might be derived by treating human data, where available, as animal data are often treated (56). Probit plots have, for example, been developed using data derived from studies in Iraq of neurobehavioral outcomes in humans exposed in utero to methylmercury. A probit plot is one useful way of describing the variability in thresholds among individuals in a population. If it is assumed that the distribution is lognormal in character, then a plot of probit against log dose yields a straight line, the slope of which reflects variability; steep slopes reveal less variability than do shallower ones. (Lognormal distributions arise when the factors contributing to variability act multiplicatively—addition of the logarithms of variables is identical to multiplying the variables themselves.) It has been suggested that some responses to methylmercury show a probit slope as low as 1, corresponding to a geometric standard deviation of 10 (56). It is inferred from this that 95% of the population would have thresholds spread over a range of 10,000-fold in dosage—from 100-fold lower to 100-fold higher than the threshold dose for individuals at the median. Such estimates provide the type of description of variability that could increase the level of risk information provided to decision makers, because they allow more explicit analysis of the areas of the distribution that might be selected as the focus of regulation. At the same time, numerous difficulties attend the use of such statistical methods, not the least of which is its failure to incorporate data on biological mechanisms. It nevertheless suggests the possibility of a more quantitative direction for this aspect of risk assessment.

QUANTITATIVE STRATEGIES FOR HIGH- TO LOW-DOSE EXTRAPOLATION

In the production and use of chemicals, it is necessary to consider the health risks and benefits. Both the degree of risks and benefits depend upon the amount of chemical present. For some chemicals, such as genotoxic carcinogens, trace amounts may pose a small risk. For other relatively nontoxic chemicals, large doses may be required before adverse health effects result. In either case, the goal is to eliminate or at least minimize the occurrence of adverse health effects. This generally entails establishing a dose-response curve that relates the incidence of disease, that is, the proportion of individuals that develop a disease, to the dose of a chemical. This provides a method for estimating doses associated with low probability of disease.

In the case of cancer, regulatory decisions regarding exposures to carcinogens are generally made to limit the estimated lifetime probability of cancer (risk) to less than 1 in 10,000 and often to less than 1 in 1,000,000 (60). This creates a difficult problem. For studies conducted in laboratory animals, it would require tens of thousands of animals to estimate the incidence of cancer with precision at doses producing cancer risks below 1 in 10,000. Resources simply are not available to conduct such studies. Instead, experiments are conducted in animals at doses high enough to elicit potential toxic effects that can be observed in a moderate number, generally 50 or less, of animals per dose group. Such studies generally must produce incidence rates in excess of 10% in order to achieve statistical significance; this limit is 1,000 to

100,000 times greater than the risks that are the subject of regulation. Often, these studies require doses that are tens, hundreds, or even thousands of times higher than human doses. In cancer studies, the highest dose generally is selected that is anticipated not to cause death, other than due to tumors, and does not cause average body weight losses greater than 10% compared to control animals. The use of high doses necessitates extrapolation to estimate the incidence of adverse health effects at human dose levels.

Occasionally, human data are available to access risk. Often these studies are based on occupational exposures that are higher than those experienced by the general public. Hence, extrapolation to lower doses is required, albeit much less than from animal studies.

Toxicity studies for drugs often are conducted from near human dose levels up to perhaps 100 times higher. In such studies, some extrapolation to lower dose levels may be required.

A question almost always arises from toxicological studies about extrapolating the results from high doses to lower doses experienced by humans. In the following sections the biological and empirical basis for low-dose extrapolation is summarized. Finally, the uncertainties and future directions for low-dose extrapolation are discussed.

Biologically Based Models for Low-Dose Extrapolation

Very few biological processes are understood well enough to make quantitative predictions of outcomes based on toxic insults. When we speak of biologically based dose-response models, it usually only means that some general principles are accepted that dictate to some extent the shape of the dose-response model. For example, it may be reasonable to assume that a threshold dose exists below which adverse health effects do not occur. Or, arguments may be presented that suggest no threshold dose exists. Arguments may be presented that support the saturation of toxic or detoxification pathways leading to asymptotic curves that flatten at high or low doses, respectively. Even if the general shape of a dose-response model can be established from knowledge of the biological mode of action or mechanisms, considerable variation may exist in available experimental data, resulting in imprecise estimates of risk particularly at doses below the experimental dose range. However, such estimates are generally considered more reliable than estimates based solely on empirical fits to data from an array of plausible dose-response models.

Threshold Doses

For noncancer endpoints, it generally is assumed that small doses of chemicals can be tolerated without any adverse health effects. Experimental data often are compatible with the existence of a threshold dose. However, experimental data can only demonstrate that an effect is likely to be within certain limits. For example, with no adverse effect in 100 animals, it can be stated with 95% confidence that the true incidence is likely to be less than 3%. Threshold doses generally cannot be estimated with precision even in animal studies with homogeneous animals. Estimation of threshold doses for a heterogeneous human population is even more problematic.

The general approach to safety assessment for noncancer effects is to establish an acceptable daily intake (reference dose) based on dividing an experimental no-observed-adverse-effect level (NOAEL) by a series of safety (uncertainty) factors up to 10 for each to allow for extrapolation from animals to humans, when necessary, and to allow for sensitive individuals in a population (6). Hopefully, this results in a reference dose (RfD) that is below the threshold dose for most individuals, resulting in negligible risks. Since the RfD based on animal data is generally a factor of 100 or more below doses that produce adverse effects in bioassays, it is presumed that risks are negligible at these lower doses. There generally is no dose-response modeling attempted to estimate the risk at or below the reference dose.

There is no explicit use of a dose-response curve in the safety assessment process described earlier. There is no estimate of the risk at the NOAEL and no extrapolation to lower risks at lower doses. Gaylor (27) demonstrated that estimated risks of embryo/fetal death and malformations at the NOAEL varied from 0 to 4.5% for typical bioassays. Leisenring and Ryan (40) show that risks at the NOAEL could be as high as 20% for quantal (incidence) data from typical bioassays. Recognizing the wide variation in risks at the NOAEL and the fact that smaller sample sizes result in larger NOAELs, Crump (16) suggested that rather than the NOAEL, the point of departure for RfDs should be a benchmark dose (BD) corresponding to a specified low level (1 to 10%) of risk. A lower confidence limit for the BD is used to allow for experimental variation, and an additional uncertainty factor is introduced to account for the point of departure being associated with a low level of risk.

The whole concept of threshold doses is challenged by the additivity-to-background argument. Obviously, all adverse health effects of concern occur in the human population. For those health effects that may be the result of chemical exposure, either endogenous and/or exogenous, threshold doses have been surpassed for some individuals. Hence, the addition of any chemical dose, no matter how small, will have an additional effect if it augments an existing toxic chemical pathway (19). At low doses, the relationship between added health risk and dose is approximately linear (19). For this to be true, the added chemical dose must not be a toxic effect that has a mechanism of action independent of existing mechanisms.

U-Shaped Dose-Response

For some essential vitamins and minerals, a U-shaped dose-response curve may occur. At deficient levels health risks increase, but health risks may also occur at excessive levels, such as for vitamin A and iron. Hence, there is an optimum dose or range that minimizes risk with risk increasing below and above the optimum level. If the dose-response can be modeled for both the deficient and excessive dose risks, assuming these two processes are independent, the overall risk can be estimated by adding the risk from the two components.

There is some evidence for hormetic effects. For example, low doses of a chemical may induce a detoxification process that actually lower risks, but becomes overwhelmed at higher doses. Such a process also may produce a U-shaped dose-response for risk.

Clearly, U-shaped dose-response curves require special attention. Risk assessment procedures that only consider high-dose risk may result in recommended doses that produce risks at low doses, particularly for essential or beneficial nutrients.

Noncancer Effects

The Michaelis–Menten equation is used widely in enzyme kinetics to relate the velocity (V) of an enzyme-mediated reaction to the substrate dose (d), where V increases rapidly for small doses and then levels off, approaching a maximum rate ($V_{\max}$) at high doses:

$$V = \frac{V_{\max} d}{K + d}$$

where K is the dose at which V equals one-half of the maximum value ($V_{\max}$). $V_{\max}$ and K are generally estimated by a double-reciprocal plot of $1/V$ versus $1/d$ that gives a linear relationship with an intercept of $1/V_{\max}$ and slope of K times the intercept:

$$\frac{1}{V} = \frac{1}{V_{\max}} + \frac{K}{V_{\max}}\left(\frac{1}{d}\right)$$

In the event that an endogenous dose is present that is equivalent to d_e, then

$$V = \frac{V_{\max}(d + d_e)}{K + (d + d_e)}$$

Now nonlinear regression procedures are required to estimate the parameters.

The Hill equation is a generalization where

$$V = \frac{V_{\max}(d + d_e)^n}{K + (d + d_e)^n}$$

If $n > 1$, the relationship between V and d is sigmoidal.

If risk is proportional to the amount of V present, then

$$\text{Risk} = \frac{B(d + d_e)^n}{K + (d + d_e)^n}$$

where $B \leq 1$ when risk is expressed as a probability on the scale of 0 to 1. Even though there may be a biological basis for this dose-response curve, estimates of B, K, d_e, and n may be quite imprecise unless there are adequate numbers of animals over a wide range of doses. Also, the relationship between risk and V is crucial.

For developmental effects, Gaylor and Chen (29) proposed that birth defects may be related to decreased fetal weight. It was assumed that fetal growth was exponential and that the growth rate constant was effected by chemical exposure during gestation. Gaylor and Chen (29) suggested two models that fit a number of dose-response data about equally well for predicting the incidence (P) of a variety of structural malformations.

$$P = 1 - \exp[-(b_0 + b_1 d^k)]$$

and

$$P = 1 - \exp[-(b_0 + b_1 d + b_2 d^2 + \cdots + b_k d^k)]$$

where the d is the daily dose and the b terms and k are estimated from the data.

Leroux et al. (41) developed a mathematical model to describe aspects of the dynamic process of organogenesis, based on branching models of cell kinetics. The biological information incorporated in the model includes timing and rates of dynamic cell processes such as differentiation, migration, growth, and replication. The dose-response models produced can explain patterns of malformation rates as a function of both dose and time of exposure.

Cancer

More attention has been devoted to dose-response modeling for cancer than to noncancer effects for risk assessment. For a genotoxic carcinogen, theoretically one molecule interacting with DNA at the right place and time could result in a mutation that initiates a carcinogenic process. Even though the probability that this event occurs is infinitesimally small, it argues against absolute threshold doses for genotoxic carcinogens. Further, the probability of an initiated cell is a stochastic process that is proportional to the number of molecules available to interact with DNA. This argues for low-dose linearity at the target site. As discussed earlier, additivity of doses to background processes also argues for linear, nonthreshold dose-response for risk. The question is not, does low-dose linearity exist for genotoxic carcinogens; rather, the question is, over what dose range does linearity hold? High-dose studies may alter metabolic pathways and saturate detoxification processes. Nonlinear kinetics will result in nonlinear dose-response curves for risk, at least at high doses.

The most widely used model for estimating tumor risk is the multistage model of carcinogenesis. This model assumes that cancer is a progression of mutagenic or mutageniclike events that transform a normal cell into a malignant cell. These events may be the formation of DNA adducts, activation of oncogenes, deactivation of tumor suppressor genes, or mutations. The probability (p) of a tumor appearing within a specified period of time (t) is expressed in a simplified form as:

$$P = 1 - \exp[-(q_0 + q_1 d + q_2 d^2 + \cdots + q_k d^k)]t^k$$

where the q terms generally are restricted to be nonnegative and are estimated from tumor incidence data, and d is the active dose at the target tissue site. In practice, the term t^k is dropped and absorbed into the estimates of the q terms. In the absence of information to the contrary, it often is assumed that the target tissue dose is proportional to the administered dose. This model does not explicitly take into account pharmacokinetics, or the rates of cell proliferation, apoptosis, or DNA repair. Clearly, these factors may influence tumor incidence. However, the polynomial form of the model is flexible enough to provide an adequate fit to most data.

The value of k is the number of stages affected by the chemical. It is generally believed from the examination of data that k often ranges from 3 to 6. If only one stage is effected, a one-hit supralinear model is obtained:

$$P = 1 - \exp[-(q_0 + q_1 d)]$$

This produces a concave dose-response that rises approximately linearly at low doses and then levels off.

At low doses the multistage model is approximately linear up to doses that double the background tumor incidence (19). The extra risk is approximately linear versus dose:

$$(P - P_0)/(1 - P_0) \approx q_1 d$$

where P_0 is the background tumor incidence. The upper confidence limit on the estimate of q_1 is denoted as q_1^*. When the dose-response has a sigmoid shape, $k \geq 2$, at low doses the dose-response curves upward. Linear extrapolation tends to overestimate the risk in this range. The upper bound estimate of extra risk at low doses is given by

$$\text{Risk} \leq q_1^* \times d$$

which is the so-called linearized multistage estimate.

Crude tumor incidence rates (number of animals with tumors divided by the number of animals examined for a dose group) may provide poor fits for dose-response models. Animals may die at some doses before late occurring tumors appear, often resulting in lower crude incidence rates at higher doses than lower doses. To account for different noncancer mortality across dose groups, Peto et al. (51) proposed a dose-response trend test consisting of two parts: nonfatal tumors that are incidentally discovered when an animal dies from a cause other than the tumor type of concern or is sacrificed, and fatal tumors that cause the death of the animal. Bailer and Portier (4) and Bieler and Williams (9) provided a dose-response trend test that does not require knowledge of the cause of death but does utilize the age of death of the animal.

Moolgavkar and Venzon (44) and Moolgavkar and Knudson (43) introduced a two-stage model that included initiated cell cloning. This model considers the rate that normal cells are initiated, the birth and death rates of initiated cells, and the mutation rate of initiated cells to malignant cells. The exact solution that provides the probability of tumor by age t is given in a NRC report (47) as

$$P(t) = 1 - \left[\frac{2Ce^{-(\beta-\delta-\mu+C)t/2}}{(\beta - \delta - \mu + C)e^{-Ct} - (\beta - \delta - \mu - C)}\right]^{v/\beta}$$

where $C = [(\beta + \delta + \mu)^2 - 4\beta\delta]^{1/2}$ and the parameters v, β, δ, and μ are defined as follows. It is assumed that the number of normal cells that are dividing per day remains relatively constant resulting in an average number, v of new initiated cells per day, β is the probability that an initiated cell undergoes division in a day, δ is the daily probability that an initiated cell is removed, and μ is the daily probability that an initiated cell divides into another initiated cell and a mutated cancer cell. In general, the values of these parameters as a function of dose are not known. However, changes in the tumor incidence can be calculated for changes in the parameters. For example, Gaylor and Zheng (30) showed that a sustained increase of 20% in the net cell proliferation rate $(\beta - \delta)$ can double the lifetime tumor incidence. Zheng et al. (74) extended the model to describe a sequence of mutational changes that constitute the G : C–A : T base substitution.

Empirical Models for Low-Dose Extrapolation

All empirical models must be biologically plausible if they are to fit bioassay data. The models described next do not arise from specific biologically based mechanisms, but generally accommodate saturation of detoxification and toxic processes. Unfortunately, several different models may fit bioassay data about equally well in the experimental dose range but unfortunately may result in widely different estimates of risk at low doses of interest (25). For this reason, linear extrapolation often is used to provide an upper bound on the risk for low doses of convex dose-responses that curve upward. Linear extrapolation does not mean that a linear model is fit to curvilinear dose-response data. A curvilinear model is still fit to the data and linear extrapolation is only used from the low end of the experimental dose range to an excess risk of zero at zero dose.

Statistical Models

The simplest model is linear where y is a response and d is dose:

$$y = b_0 + b_1 d$$

The intercept (b_0) representing the background response and b_1, the slope, are estimated from the data. A linear model often is used to approximate a dose-response curve over a limited range of doses. The response may be the incidence of risk of an adverse effect. A linear approximation may be adequate at low doses, but obviously must level off as the incidence (probability of risk) approaches 1.

The linear-quadratic model allows for some curvature, either up or down, in the dose-response curve:

$$y = b_0 + b_1 d + b_2 d^2$$

This model often will fit data adequately up to the inflection point where the response curvature changes from convex to concave or concave to convex.

The probit model has a long history in biology (24). It belongs to a class of tolerance distributions. The probit model is based on the Gaussian (normal) bell-shaped distribution. The tolerance distribution describes the relative probability that an individual will respond—suffer an adverse health effect—at a dose d. If there is a large number of factors that act in an additive manner to determine the dose at which an individual responds, then by the Central Limit Theorem a normal distribution is obtained. Integrating (summing the relative probabilities) up to a dose d gives the proportion (probability) of individuals that develop an adverse effect at or below the dose d. The normal distribution is defined by the mean (μ) and standard deviation (σ). At the mean dose, 50% of the individuals are affected. Special probability (probit) graph paper is available such that plotting the proportion of effected individuals versus dose gives a straight line. The slope of the line is the reciprocal of the standard deviation.

Often, a probit model describes experimental data better when the logarithm of dose is used. This distribution could arise when a number of factors multiplicatively determine the dose at which an individual responds. The log-probit model has been used extensively for the analysis of dichotomous bioassay data (24). This model assumes that the distribution of log-dose thresholds is normal. For the log-probit model, the probability of a tumor induced by an exposure to a dose d of a chemical is given by

$$P(d) = \phi(b_0 + b_1 \log d)$$

where ϕ denotes the standard cumulative normal distribution.

Another model that has been used extensively in the analysis of dichotomous bioassay data is the log-logistic model (8):

$$P(d) = [1 + \exp(b_0 + b_1 \log d)]^{-1}$$

where $P(d)$ is the probability (incidence) of an adverse effect by a specified time at a dose d, and b_0 and b_1 are estimated from the data.

Data from reproductive/developmental studies pose special problems where pregnant animals are dosed and the results are measured in the offspring/fetuses. Correlation of results among offspring/fetuses within a litter must be considered. Kodell et al. (37) assumed that the incidence of adverse effects for the offspring/fetuses of a litter behaves according to a binomial distribution and that the probability of adverse effects varies among litters according to a beta distribution. Further, it is assumed that the probability of an adverse effect may be a function of the size s (number of offspring/fetuses in a litter). The expected probability of an adverse effect for an offspring/fetus in a litter of size s at dose d is

$$P(d, s) = 1 - \exp\{-[b_0 + b_1(s - \bar{s})]\}$$

for d less than or equal to a threshold dose of d_0 and $\bar{s}$ is the average litter size across all dose groups in a bioassay. For doses above the threshold dose of d_0,

$$P(d, s) = 1 - \exp(-\{b_0 + b_1(s - \bar{s}) + [b_3 + b_4(s - \bar{s})](d - d_0)^k\})$$

where the $b \geq 0$ and $k \geq 1$ are estimated from the data, and where

$$[b_0 + b_1(s - \bar{s})] \geq 0 \quad \text{and} \quad [b_3 + b_4(s - \bar{s})] \geq 0 \quad \text{for all } s$$

Kupper et al. (38) proposed a model for reproductive/developmental data of the form

$$P(d, s) = b_0 + b_1 s + [1 - b_0 - b_1 s] / \{1 + \exp[b_3 + b_4 s - b_5 \log(d - d_0)]\}$$

Ryan (63) discussed multivariate models that simultaneously consider two or more biological effects, such

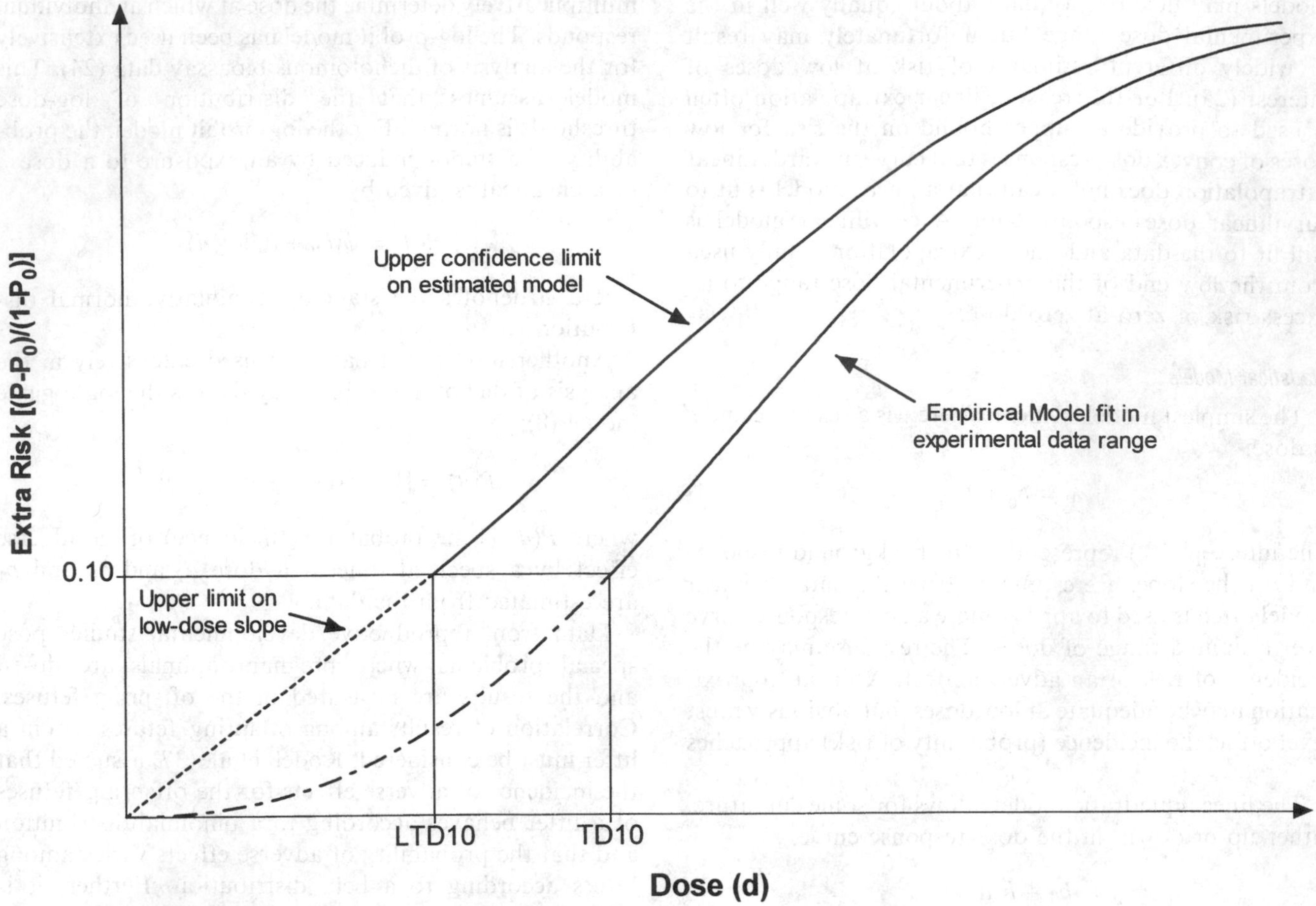

FIG. 8.2. Illustration of the low-dose extrapolation of the empirical model and likely overestimation of low-dose risk.

as the proportion of malformed fetuses in a litter and the proportion of dead/resorbed fetuses in a litter.

Microbial risk assessment is an area currently receiving more attention than in the past. Haas (33) proposed that the probability of infection could be described as a function of the number N of colony-forming-units by

$$P = 1 - [1 + (N/\beta)]^{-\alpha}$$

where α and β are estimated from dose-response data.

Low-dose extrapolation using empirical models is suspect. The model may fit adequately in the experimental dose range, but there is little assurance of accuracy below the experimental dose range. However, linear extrapolation can serve as an upper bound estimate of risk for dose-responses that are convex (curve upward).

Recognizing that current methodology generally does not permit precise estimates of cancer risks below 10%, the proposed U.S. Environmental Protection Agency (73) carcinogen cancer risk assessment guidelines suggest estimating the dose associated with a 10% tumor risk (TD_{10}) as a point of departure for low-dose extrapolation. In order to account for experimental variation, a lower confidence limit (LTD_{10}) is calculated for this benchmark dose. If a nonlinear (thresholdlike) dose-response is likely below this benchmark dose, the LTD_{10} is divided by appropriate uncertainty (safety) factors to arrive at a reference dose that is not likely to cause an appreciable cancer risk. If a nonlinear dose-response below the benchmark dose cannot be justified, the regulatory default is linear extrapolation from the LTD_{10} to zero (Figure 8.2). This gives a low-dose cancer potency slope factor of $0.10/LTD_{10}$. This often is similar to the value of q_1^*, discussed earlier, which is estimated from the multistage model of carcinogenesis. If data are adequate, a benchmark dose below a 10% level of estimated cancer risk may be used as a point of departure for low-dose cancer risk assessment (73).

Uncertainties and Future Directions

There is a tremendous amount of research being conducted to examine the mechanisms of toxicity. Presumably this will provide better information to develop biologically based dose-response models that can facilitate low-dose extrapolation. In order to employ the

Moolgavkar–Venzon–Knudson two-stage clonal model of carcinogenesis to estimate cancer risk, for example, it is necessary to identify directly or indirectly initiated cells and to obtain a measure of the rate at which initiated cells arise from normal cells, divide, and are removed, all as a function of dose of the carcinogen. Further, the mutation rate of an initiated cell to a malignant state is needed as a function of dose. Seldom will all of this information be available. Hence, assumptions regarding some of these rates generally will be needed in order to use this model. Currently, there are relatively large uncertainties, up to a factor of 100, for cancer risk estimates based on animal data (31). Many scientists have questioned the validity of long-term bioassays conducted at the maximum tolerated dose. Several authors (17,55) have suggested that in the absence of extrapolatable data which can be extrapolated to low doses the same approach to safety assessment should be used for carcinogens as for noncancer effects. That is, establish a relatively safe dose and divide by a series of uncertainty factors to account for extrapolation from animals to humans, sensitive individuals, and other uncertainties to arrive at a relatively safe dose without any numerical estimates of risk. Several publications in recent years have addressed the size of uncertainty factors needed to provide adequate safety. Baird et al. (5) have shown that the products of current default values of 10 appear to provide adequate coverage for these uncertainties. Doubtless, research will continue to explore mechanisms of toxicity that will lead to better predictive models. Hopefully, the development of biomarkers of exposure will expand the use of human data for dose-response modeling.

CROSS-ROUTE EXTRAPOLATION

It is often necessary, particularly in the regulatory setting, to make some estimate of the likely toxic effect associated with exposure to a chemical by one route of exposure (e.g., inhalation) when toxicity data only from studies of exposure by a different route (e.g., oral) are available. Such extrapolation is subject to considerable uncertainty, and often is not attempted. In particular, chemicals quite frequently show route-specific toxic effects, especially at or near the site of administration (in the respiratory tract by inhalation, in the upper gastrointestinal tract by oral administration, or on the skin by dermal exposure). Such local effects may be indicative of a potential effect at a local site by another route of administration (e.g., a chemical that causes local dermal irritation when applied to the skin will very likely also cause local irritation when inhaled or ingested). However, quantitative extrapolation of such effects is generally not possible because of difficulties in identifying the effective dose of the toxicant at the target site and particularly because of differences in sensitivity of different tissues.

For systemic effects at distant sites, a crude cross-route adjustment can be performed (if absorption data are available) by simply normalizing the dose to a body-weight basis, and adjusting for relative absorption by the different routes of exposure. This procedure can be quite misleading, however. For example, if the chemical is subject to a significant first-pass effect in the liver (either activating a protoxicant, or inactivating a direct-acting toxicant), the ingestion and inhalation routes may show substantially different responses even with the same total absorbed dose. Clearly, if relevant metabolic and pharmacokinetic data are available, a preferred approach would be the development of a pharmacokinetic model that would take these factors into consideration (see Chapter 4).

CROSS-TIME EXTRAPOLATION: QUANTITATIVE STRATEGIES FOR ADJUSTING FOR DIFFERENCES IN EXPOSURE DURATIONS

Dosing animals with chemicals in toxicological studies may vary from a single administration to continuous exposure over the lifetime of the animal. Likewise, human exposure may vary from a single episode to continuous lifetime exposure. Often, a 2-year rodent lifetime is considered equivalent to a 70-year human lifetime. Hence, an exposure of an animal for 1 year is assumed to be equivalent to a 35-year exposure in humans. Generally, the durations of animal studies are chosen to mimic likely human exposure conditions. However, resources are not available to test chemicals at all of the possible human exposure conditions. Hence, statistical techniques have been devised to estimate the effects of short-term exposures from studies conducted with long-term exposures and vice versa.

Biological Models

Generally, estimates of cancer risk are based on the average daily lifetime exposure. That is, the total dose is divided by the number of days in a lifetime. This is a plausible approach for a genotoxic carcinogen where it is assumed that carcinogenesis is a stochastic process. In such a case, the probability of a biological event is proportional to the number of molecules of the chemical available to interact with biological matter. In order to predict biological effects for different durations of exposures, it is necessary that dose-response models contain a time or age element.

As discussed earlier, the multistage model of carcinogenesis does contain an element of time. Crump and Howe (18) provided estimates of risk as a function of age and duration of exposure. Kodell et al. (36) showed that the use of the average daily lifetime dose may overestimate risk but never underestimates the cancer risk by more than a factor of k (generally 3 to 6) for a k-stage model. For example, based on the average daily lifetime dose, the estimated risk for exposure for one-tenth of a lifetime would be one-tenth of the risk for continuous lifetime exposure at that daily dose. According to Kodell et al. (36), this estimated risk should be multiplied by a factor of 3 to 6 to allow for exposure during a sensitive age.

For the Moolgavkar–Venson–Knudson two-stage clonal expansion model of carcinogenesis, Chen et al. (13) showed that the use of the average daily lifetime dose generally does not underestimate risk by more than a factor of ten. For exposures longer than one-tenth of a lifetime, the estimated risk would be the same as for a continuous lifetime exposure. For exposures for a fraction (f) less than one-tenth of a lifetime, the estimated risk is taken to be less than 10 times the upper limit on the estimated lifetime risk with continuous exposure. For the extreme case of only a single exposure to N milligrams of a carcinogen, the average daily lifetime (75-year) dose for a 70-kg person is $N/(70 \times 75 \times 365) = 5 \times 10^{-7} \times N$ mg/kg. If $q_1{}^*$ is the estimated upper bound of the cancer risk per milligram per kilogram body weight per lifetime daily exposure, the estimated risk from a single exposure is $5 \times 10^{-6} \times q_1{}^*$ where a factor of 10 is included to allow for exposure at a sensitive age.

Empirical Models

For noncancer effects, extrapolation of subchronic to chronic exposures is generally accompanied by an uncertainty factor of 10 (6). That is, it is assumed that an effect observed with a subchronic exposure is not likely to occur at less than one-tenth that dose for a chronic exposure. Swartout (67) compared NOAELs and LOAELs for subchronic and chronic exposures for about 100 cases. The median ratio of subchronic to chronic doses producing equivalent effects was 2 with a 95th percentile of 17. On the average, a chronic exposure to one-half of the dose for a subchronic exposure produced the same biological effect. For 5% of the cases, the chronic dose was less than 1/17th of the subchronic dose for the same biological effect. The convention default factor of 10 for subchronic to chronic extrapolation covered about 89% of the cases. Pieters et al. (52) conducted a similar study for 149 cases and obtained median ratio of subchronic to chronic doses for similar effects of 1.7 with a 95th percentile of 29.

Haber's Rule has been used extensively to make small extrapolations between durations of exposure. Haber's Rule states that equal biological effects are expected for equal exposures of concentration (c) times duration (t). That is, equal values of $c \times t$ are expected to produce equal biological effects. For example, if the exposure duration is doubled, the concentration would need to be halved to obtain the same biological effect. A generalization of Haber's Rule is given by tenBerge et al. (71) where values of $c^n \times t$ are expected to produce equal biological effects. Estimation of the exponent n requires dose-response data collected for different durations of exposure. For several data sets, tenBerge et al. (71) observed that n varied from about 1 to 3 and tended to center around $n=2$. In the absence of duration–dose-response data, the recommended extrapolation to different durations of exposure is calculated on the basis of $c^2 \times t$. For example, if the exposure time is increased by a factor of 4, the concentration needs to be halved to obtain an equivalent biological effect. In order to be conservative, it is recommended that $c^3 \times t$ be used when extrapolating from long to shorter exposure times and $c \times t$ be used when extrapolating from short to longer exposure durations.

AN OVERALL STRATEGY FOR SCIENTIFICALLY BASED INTERSPECIES EXTRAPOLATION

Assessing risks to human populations from exposures to potentially toxic substances, based upon data from experimental studies, always requires cross-species and within-species extrapolations, almost always requires cross-dose extrapolations, and often requires cross-route and cross-time extrapolations. The need for specific types of extrapolation depends upon (a) the specific risk situation under assessment and (b) the nature of the data available for that assessment. Embarking upon a risk assessment thus requires, at the outset, a careful delineation of the problem to be evaluated. Once this is accomplished, efforts are made to collect all data that might be relevant to the risk question at hand. A matching of the data available with the problem to be assessed allows identification of the types of extrapolation that will have to be undertaken.

At the present stage of development of the toxicological sciences, most extrapolations are undertaken using the so-called "default" approaches discussed earlier. Increasingly, however, attempts are being made to search for the types of information needed to avoid resorting to such defaults, and to use approaches with more fully developed scientific bases.

Table 8.4 describes the types of inquiries that might be made to move toward a more purely science-based approach. It is assumed that the risk assessment problem to be addressed requires the use of animal toxicology data (there is no significant epidemiology data available), and that all five forms of extrapolation will be required. Thus, for example, the assessment might involve chronic, gen-

Table 8.4
Overall strategy for science-based interspecies extrapolation: The search for information necessary to improve the scientific basis for human risk assessment based upon experimental data

Type of extrapolation	Type of inquiry
Cross-species	Can data be found for quantitative cross-species comparisons of target site doses and their relationships to administered doses?
	Can PBPK models be developed to accomplish above?
	Can mechanistic data be developed to estimate differences in target-site responsiveness across species?
Within species	Can quantitative estimates be developed, on a chemical-specific basis, of the ranges of human variability in uptake, pharmacokinetic and metabolic handing, and target-site responsiveness?
	Can methods be developed to integrate these sources of variability?
Cross-dose	Can the data necessary to apply biologically based models for low-dose extrapolation be identified or developed?
Cross-route	Can pharmacokinetic data be developed to permit accurate assessment of interroute differences?
Cross-time	Can empirical data be found to support extrapolations from one exposure duration to another? Are there biologically based mechanistic considerations to guide such extrapolations?

eral population exposure to a drinking-water or food contaminant for which the only available toxicity data involves gavage or even inhalation exposure over 90 days in one or more species of experimental animals. Before resorting to the usual defaults for each of these types of required extrapolation, and assuming that they are simply scientific uncertainties that cannot be overcome, it is now expected that toxicologists will inquire more fully, along the lines outlined in Table 8.4, into the possibility that alternative, data-based approaches can be developed. At the same time, it must be recognized that development of the data necesary for science-based extrapolations will necessarily introduce new uncertainties that have to be accommodated. Thus, while most would agree that reliable pharmacokinetic data can provide useful information on interspecies differences, it is likely that scientists will disagree on just how complete such data need to be before they can be used in risk assessment. Regulators typically display a high degree of skepticism about the incorporation of such data, and tend to remain close to the usual defaults, not because they dispute their relevance, but because they question their completeness. Thus, risk assessors must work to reach consensus not only on the types of data needed to improve risk assessments, but also on the difficult question of how complete they must be before they can be used for important public health decisions.

QUESTIONS

1. Why is it necessary to extrapolate?
2. How is a dose-response curve selected?
3. Does a threshold dose always exist? Ever exist?
4. Is the risk zero at the no-observed-adverse-effect level? Explain.
5. When does linear extrapolation to lower doses overestimate risk?
6. Describe the basis for a probit model.
7. Construct a numerical example that illustrates Haber's Rule.
8. When is a safety factor not an uncertainty factor?
9. What factors affect interspecies differences in response?
10. What factors account for variability in response within species?
11. What is the difference between variability and uncertainty?
12. What is the difference between a biologically based extrapolation and an empirically based extrapolation? Is one more reliable than the other?
13. How does science develop *general* explanations for phenomena such as interspecies differences in response?
14. Under what circumstances would cross-route extrapolation not be appropriate?

REFERENCES

1. Adolph, E. F. (1949): Quantitative relations in the physiological constitutions of mammals. *Science*, 109:579.
2. Allen, B. C., Shipp, A. M., Crump, K. S., Kilian, B., Hogg, M. L., Tudor, J., and Keller, B. (1987): Investigation of cancer risk assessment methods: Summary. EPA/600/6-87/007a. NTIS PB88-127105. September.
3. Armitage, P., and Doll, R. (1961): Stochastic models for carcinogenesis. In: *Proc 4th Berkeley Symposium on Mathematical Statistics and Probability*. Vol. 4, pp. 19–38. University of California Press Berkeley, CA.
4. Bailer, A. J., and Portier, C. J. (1988): Effects of treatment-induced mortality and tumor-induced mortality on tests for carcinogenicity in small samples. *Biometrics*, 44:417–431.
5. Baird, S. J. S., Cohen, J. T., Graham, J. D., Shlyakhter, A. I., and Evans, J. S. (1996): Noncancer risk assessment: A probabilistic alternative to current practice. *Hum. Ecol. Risk Assess.*, 2:79–102.
6. Barnes, D. G., and Dourson, M. (1988): Reference dose (RfD): Description and use in health risk assessments. *Regul. Toxicol. Pharmacol.*, 8:471–486.
7. Benedict, F. G. (1938): *Vital Energetics: A Study in Comparative Basal Metabolism*. Carnegie Institute of Washington, Washington, DC.
8. Berkson, J. (1944): Application of the logistic function to bio-assay. *J. Am. Stat. Assoc.*, 39:357–365.
9. Bieler, G. S., and Williams, R. L. (1993): Ratio estimates, the delta method, and quantal response tests for increased carcinogenicity. *Biometrics*, 49:793–801.
10. Borghoff, S. J., Short, B. G., and Swenberg, J. A. (1990): Biochemical mechanisms and pathobiology of alpha 2μ-globulin nephropathy. *Annu. Rev. Pharmacol. Toxicol.*, 30:349–367.
11. Boxenbaum, H., and Ronfeld, R. (1983): Interspecies pharmacokinetic scaling and the Dedrick plots. *Am. J. Physiol.*, 245: R768–R775.
12. Calabrese, E. J. (1985): Uncertainty factors and interindividual variation. *Regul. Toxicol. Pharmacol.*, 5:190–196.
13. Chen, J. J., Kodell, R. L., and Gaylor, D. W. (1988): Using the biological two-stage model to assess risk from short-term exposures. *Risk Anal.*, 8:223–230.
14. Crouch, E. (1983): Uncertainties in interspecies extrapolations of carcinogenicity. *Environ. Health Perspect.*, 50:321–327.
15. Crouch, E., and Wilson, R. (1979): Interspecies comparison of carcinogenic potency. *J. Toxicol. Environ. Health*, 5:1095–1118.
16. Crump, K. S. (1984): A new method for determining allowable daily intakes. *Fundam. Appl. Toxicol.*, 4:854–871.
17. Crump, K. S. (1996): The linearized multistage model and the future of quantitative risk assessment. *Hum. Exp. Toxicol.*, 15:787–798.
18. Crump, K. S., and Howe, R. B. (1984): The multistage model with a time-dependent dose pattern: Applications to carcinogen risk assessment. *Risk Anal.*, 4:163–179.
19. Crump, K. S., Hoel, D. G., Langley, C. H., and Peto, R. (1976): Fundamental carcinogenic processes and their implications for low dose risk assessment. *Cancer Res.*, 36:2973–2979.

19a. Davidson, I. W. F., Parker, J. C., and Beliles, R. P. (1986): Biological basis for extrapolation across mammalian species. *Regul. Toxicol. Pharmacol. 6:* 211–237.

20. Dietrich, D. R., and Swenberg, J. A. (1991): NCI-Black-Reiter (NBR) male rats fail to develop renal disease following exposure to agents that induce α-2u-globulin (α_{2u}) nephropathy. *Fundam. Appl. Toxicol.*, 16:749–762.
21. Dourson, M. L., and Stara, J. F. (1983): Regulatory history and experimental support of uncertainty (safety) factors. *Regul. Toxicol. Pharmacol.*, 3:224–238.
22. Dourson, M. L., Felter, S. P., and Robinson, D. (1996): Evolution of science-based uncertainty factors. *Regul. Toxicol. Pharmacol.*, 24:108–120.
23. Elcombe, C. R., Bell, D. R., Elias, E., Hasmall, S. C., and Plant, N. J. (1996): Peroxisome proliferators: Species differences in response of primary hepatocyte cultures. *Ann. NY Acad. Sci.*, 804:628–635.
24. Finney, D. J. (1964): *Probit Analysis*. 2nd ed. Cambridge University Press, Cambridge.
25. Food and Drug Administration (1971): Advisory Committee on Protocols for Safety Evaluation. Panel on Carcinogenesis Report on Cancer Testing in the Safety Evaluation of Food Additives and Pesticides. *Toxicol. Appl. Pharmacol.*, 20:419–438.
26. Freireich, E. J., Gehan, E. A., Rall, D. P., Schmidt, L. H., and Skipper, H. E. (1966): Quantitative comparison of toxicity of anticancer agents in mouse, rat, hamster, dog, monkey, and man. *Cancer Chemother. Rep.*, 50:219–244.
27. Gaylor, D. W. (1992): Incidence of developmental defects at the no observed adverse effect level (NOAEL). *Regul. Toxicol. Pharmacol.*, 15:151–160.
28. Gaylor, D. W., and Chen, J. J. (1986): Relative potency of chemical carcinogens in rodents. *Risk Anal.*, 6:283–290.
29. Gaylor, D. W., and Chen, J. J. (1993): Dose-response models for developmental malformations. *Teratology*, 47:291–297.
30. Gaylor, D. W., and Zheng, Q. (1996): Risk assessment of nongenotoxic carcinogens based upon cell proliferation/death rates in rodents. *Risk Anal.*, 16:221–225.
31. Gaylor, D. W., Chen, J. J., and Sheehan, D. M. (1993): Uncertainty in cancer risk estimates. *Risk Anal.*, 13:149–154.
32. Greenberg, M. S., Burton, G. A., Jr., and Fisher, J. W. (1999). Physiologically based pharmacokinetic modeling of inhaled trichloroethylene and its oxidative metabolites in $B6C3F_1$ mice. *Toxicol. Appl. Pharmacol.*, 154:264–278.
33. Haas, C. N. (1983): Estimation of risk due to low doses of microorganisms: A comparison of alternative methodologies. *Am. J. Epidemiol.*, 118:573–582.
34. Kleiber, M. (1932): Body size and metabolism. *Hilgardia*, 6:315–353.
35. Kleiber, M. (1947): Body size and metabolic rate. *Physiol. Rev.*, 27:511–541.
36. Kodell, R. L., Gaylor, D. W., and Chen, J. J. (1987): Using average lifetime dose rate for intermittent exposures to carcinogens. *Risk Anal.*, 7:339–345.
37. Kodell, R. L., Howe, R. B., Chen, J. J., and Gaylor, D. W. (1991): Mathematical modeling of reproductive and developmental toxic effects for quantitative risk assessment. *Risk Anal.*, 11:583–590.
38. Kupper, L., Portier, C., Hogan, M., and Yamamoto, E. (1986): The impact of litter effects on dose-response modeling in teratology. *Biometrics*, 42:85–98.
39. Lehman, A. J., and Fitzhugh, O. G. (1954): 100-fold margin of safety. *Assoc. Food Drug Off. U.S. Q. Bull.*, 18:33–35.
40. Leisenring, W., and Ryan, L. (1992): Statistical properties of the NOAEL. *Regul. Toxicol. Pharmacol.*, 15:161–171.
41. Leroux, B. G., Leisenring, W., Moolgavkar, S. H., and Faustman, E. M. (1996): A biologically-based dose-response model for development toxicology. *Risk Anal.*, 16:449–458.
42. Lewis, S. C. (1993): Reducing uncertainty with adjustment factors. Improvements in non-cancer risk assessment. *Fundam. Appl. Toxicol.*, 20:2–4.
43. Moolgavkar, S. H., and Knudson, A. G. (1981): Mutation and cancer: A model for human carcinogenesis. *JNCI*, 66:1037–1052.
44. Moolgavkar, S. H., and Venzon, D. J. (1979): Two-event models for carcinogenesis: Incidence curves for childhood and adult tumors. *Math Biosci.*, 47:55–77.

45. National Research Council. (1983): *Risk Assessment in the Federal Government: Managing the Process*. National Academy Press, Washington, DC.
46. National Research Council. (1987): *Drinking Water and Health Volume 8: Pharmacokinetics in Risk Assessment*. National Academy Press, Washington, DC.
47. National Research Council. (1993): *Issues in Risk Assessment*. National Academy Press, Washington, DC.
48. National Research Council. (1994): *Science and Judgement in Risk Assessment*. National Academy Press, Washington, DC.
49. Paine, A. J. (1996): Validity and reliability of in vitro systems in safety evaluation. *Environ. Toxicol. Pharmacol.*, 2:207–212.
50. Perrone, C. E., Shao, L., and Williams, G. M. (1998): Effect of rodent hepatocarcinogenic peroxisome proliferators on fatty acyl-CoA oxidase, DNA synthesis and apoptosis in cultured human and rat hepatocytes. *Toxicol. Appl. Pharmacol.*, 150:277–286.
51. Peto, R., Pike, M. C., Day, N. E., Gray, R. G., Lee, P. N., Parish, S., Peto, J., Richards, S., and Wahrendorf, J. (1980): Guidelines for simple, sensitive significance tests for carcinogenic effects in long-term animal experiments. *IARC Monogr. Suppl. 2* IARC, Lyon, France.
52. Pieters, M. N., Kramer, H. J., and Slob, W. (1998): Evaluation of the uncertainty factor for subchronic-to-chronic extrapolation: Statistical analysis of toxicity data. *Regul. Toxicol. Pharmacol.*, 27:108–111.
53. Pinkel, D. (1958): The use of body surface area as a criterion of drug dosage in cancer chemotherapy. *Cancer Res.*, 18:853–856.
54. Prothero, J. W. (1980): Scaling of blood parameters in mammals. *Comp. Biochem. Physiol. A.*, 67:649–657.
55. Purchase, I. F. H., and Auton, T. R. (1995): Thresholds in chemical carcinogenesis. *Regul. Toxicol. Pharmacol.*, 22:199–205.
56. Rees, D. C., and Hattis, D. (1994): Developing quantitative strategies for animal to human extrapolation. In: *Principles and Methods of Toxicology*, 3rd ed., edited by A. W. Hayes, pp. 275–315. Raven Press, New York.
57. Renwick, A. G. (1991): Safety factors and establishment of acceptable daily intake. *Food Addit. Contam.*, 8(2):135–150.
58. Renwick, A. G. (1993): Data-derived safety factors for the evaluation of food additives and environmental contaminants. *Food Addit. Contam.*, 10(3):275–305.
59. Rhomberg, L. R., and Wolff, S. K. (1998): Empirical scaling of single oral lethal doses across mammalian species based on a large database. *Risk Anal.*, 18:741–753.
60. Rodricks, J. V., Brett, S., and Wrenn, G. (1987): Significant risk decisions in federal regulatory agencies. *Regul. Toxicol. Pharmacol.*, 7:307–320.
61. Rodricks, J. V., Rudenko, L., Starr, T. B., and Turnbull, D. (1997): Risk assessment. In: *Comprehensive Toxicology. Vol. I. General Principles*, edited by J. Bond. Pergamon, Elsevier Science, New York.
62. Rubner, M. (1883): Ueber den einfluss der köpergrösse auf stoff und kraft wechsel. *Z. Biol*, 1919:535–562.
63. Ryan, L. (1992): Quantitative risk assessment for developmental toxicity. *Biometrics*, 48:163–174.
64. Schmidt-Nielson, K. (1984): *Scaling: Why Is Animal Size So Important*? Cambridge University Press, Cambridge.
65. Sheehan, D., and Gaylor, D. W. (1990): Analyses of the adequacy of safety factors. *Teratology*, 41:590–591.
66. Stenner, R. D., Merdink, J. L., Fisher, J. W., and Bull, R. J. (1998): Physiologically-based pharmacokinetic model for trichloroethylene considering enterohepatic recirculation of major metabolites. *Risk Anal.*, 18:261–269.
67. Swartout, J. (1996): Subchronic-to-chronic uncertainty factor for the reference dose. Abstr. F2.03. Society for Risk Analysis Annual Meeting, New Orleans, LA.
68. Swenberg, J. A., Short, B., Borghoff, S., Strasser, J., and Charbonneau, M. (1989): The comparative pathobiology of alpha 2μ-globulin nephropathy. *Toxicol. Appl. Pharmacol.*, 97:35–46.
69. Travis, C. C., and White, R. K. (1988): Interspecific scaling of toxicity data. *Risk Anal.*, 8:119–125.
69a Travis, C. C., White, R. K., and Arms, A. D. (1989): A physiologically based pharmacokinetic approach for assessing the cancer risk of tetrachloroethylene. In: *The Risk Assessment of Environmental Hazards*, edited by D. J. Paustenbach, Wiley Interscience, New York.
70. Travis, C. C., White, R. K., and Ward, R. C. (1990): Interspecies extrapolation of pharmacokinetics. *J. Theoret. Biol.*, 142:285–304.
71. tenBerge, W. F., Zwart, A., and Appelman, L. M. (1986): Concentration–time mortality response relationship of irritant and systemically acting vapours and gases. *J. Hazard. Mater.* 3:301–309.
72. U.S. Environmental Protection Agency. (1992): Draft report: A cross-species scaling factor for carcinogen risk assessment based on equivalence of $mg/kg^{3/4}/day$. *Fed. Reg.*, 57:24152–24173.
73. U.S. Environmental Protection Agency. (1996): Proposed guidelines for carcinogen risk assessment. *Fed. Reg.*, 61:17960–18011.
74. Zheng, Q., Lutz, W. K., and Gaylor, D. W. (1997): A carcinogenesis model describing mutational events at the DNA adduct level. *Math. Biosci.*, 144:23–44.

Principles and Methods of Toxicology,
Fourth Edition, edited by A. Wallace Hayes.
Taylor & Francis, Philadelphia © 2001.

Chapter 9

The Practice of Exposure Assessment

Dennis J. Paustenbach

INTRODUCTION

Health risk assessment is the process wherein toxicology data from animal studies and human epidemiology are evaluated, a mathematical formula is applied to predict the response at low doses, and then information about the degree of exposure is used to predict quantitatively the likelihood that a particular adverse response will be seen in a specific human population (229,257). More simply, risk assessment is a process by which scientists evaluate the potential for adverse health effects from exposure to naturally occurring or synthetic agents (335). Regulatory agencies have used the risk assessment process for nearly 50 years, most notably the U.S. Food and Drug Administration (U.S. FDA) (189). However, the difference between assessments performed in the 1950s and 1960s and those performed in the 1980s and 1990s is that dose-extrapolation models, quantitative exposure assessments, and quantitative descriptions of uncertainty have been added to the process (63). Because of increased understanding of many relevant issues, the availability of desktop computers, and better quantitative methods for predicting the low-dose response (such as physiologically based pharmacokinetic ([PBPK] models), risk assessments conducted today provide more accurate risk estimates than in the past (257).

Since 1980, most environmental regulations and some occupational health standards have, at least in part, been based on health risk assessments (61,390). They include standards for pesticide residues in crops, drinking water, ambient air, and food additives, as well as exposure limits for chemicals found in indoor air, consumer products, and other media. Risk managers increasingly rely on risk assessment to decide whether a broad array of risks are significant or trivial: an important task since, for example, more than 400 of the about 2000 chemicals routinely used in industry have been labeled carcinogens in various animal studies (234). In theory, the results of risk assessments in the United States should influence virtually all regulatory decisions involving so-called "toxic agents" (238,278,279).

The risk assessment process has four parts: hazard identification, dose-response assessment, exposure assessment, and risk characterization (234). Although progress has been made over the past 20 years in how to conduct and interpret toxicology and epidemiology studies (e.g., hazard identification), and scientists believe that they are doing a better job of dose-response extrapolation than in the past, most significant advances in the risk assessment process have occurred in the field of exposure assessment (405).

In recent years, an increasing number of environmental scientists have embraced the view that "toxicology data are important, but they do not mean much without quantitative information about human exposure." For this reason, each year since about 1990, the toxicology community has shown increasing interest in understanding the exposure assessment field (246,247). Fortunately, a significant amount of research has been conducted to identify better values for many exposure parameters, and major improvements have been made in applying these exposure factors to various scenarios. This chapter is intended to familiarize toxicologists, risk assessors, and others with this evolving field.

BASIC CONCEPTS

Description of Exposure Assessment

Exposure assessment is the step in the risk assessment process that quantifies the uptake of an agent resulting from contact with various environmental media (e.g., air, water, soil, food) (1,257,375). Exposure assessments can address past, current, or future anticipated exposures, although uncertainties can become significant when attempting to anticipate what might happen or estimate what happened long ago (98,130,262,263,294,345).

Exposure assessment in various forms dates back at least to the early twentieth century, and perhaps earlier, particularly in the fields of epidemiology (106,204), industrial hygiene (212,256), and health physics (360). Epidemiology is the study of disease occurrence and the causes of disease. Exposure assessment combines elements of industrial hygiene, radiological health, and air pollution and relies upon aspects of statistics, biochemical toxicology, large-animal toxicology, atmospheric sciences, analytical chemistry, food sciences, physiology, environmental modeling, and others (377).

Fundamentally, an exposure assessment describes the nature and size of the various populations exposed to a chemical agent and the magnitude and duration of their exposures (371,382). It determines the degree of contact a person has with a chemical and estimates the magnitude of the absorbed dose (69). Several factors need to be considered when estimating the absorbed dose, including exposure duration, exposure route, chemical bioavailability from the contaminated media (e.g., soil), and, sometimes, the unique characteristics of the exposed population (e.g., hairless mice absorb a greater percent of chemical than other mice). By definition, "duration" is the period of time over which the person is exposed.

Knowledge of the chemical concentration in an environmental medium is essential to determine the magnitude of the absorbed dose. This information is usually obtained by analytical measurements of samples of the contaminated medium (air, water, soil, sediment, food, or dust). Estimates can also be made using mathematical models, such as models relating air concentrations at various distances from a point of release (e.g., a smoke stack) to factors including release rate, weather conditions, distance, and stability of the agent (312,430). Needless to say, a significant number of factors need to be considered to quantitatively evaluate a typical contaminated site (Figure 9.1).

In general, since about 1995, our ability to perform exposure assessments has matured to a degree that they will usually possess less uncertainty than other steps in the risk assessment. Admittedly, many factors should be considered when estimating exposure; for example, it is a complicated procedure to understand the transport and distribution of a chemical that has been released into the environment. Nonetheless, available data indicate that scientists can now do an adequate job of quantifying chemical concentrations in various media, and the resulting uptake by exposed persons, if they account for the majority of factors that should be considered (268).

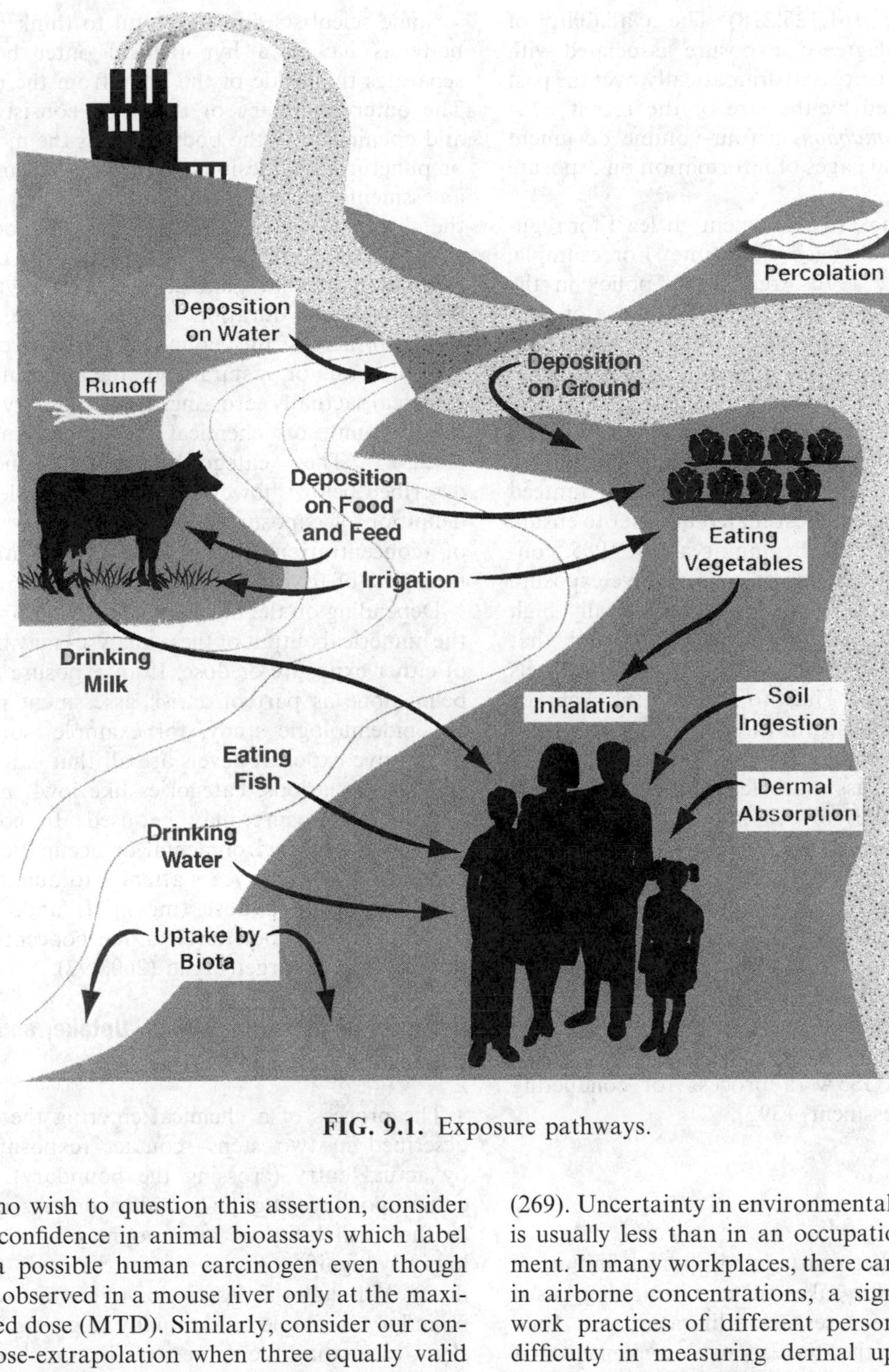

FIG. 9.1. Exposure pathways.

For those who wish to question this assertion, consider our level of confidence in animal bioassays which label a chemical a possible human carcinogen even though tumors were observed in a mouse liver only at the maximum tolerated dose (MTD). Similarly, consider our confidence in dose-extrapolation when three equally valid models yield risk estimates that are 1000-fold different at a typical environmental dose.

The primary routes of human exposure to chemicals in the ambient environment are dust and vapor inhalation, dermal contact with contaminated soils or dusts, and ingestion of contaminated food, water, dust, or soil. In the workplace, the predominant exposure route usually is inhalation, followed by dermal uptake and, to a lesser extent, dust ingestion due to hand-to-mouth contact (269). Uncertainty in environmental exposure assessment is usually less than in an occupational exposure assessment. In many workplaces, there can be large fluctuations in airborne concentrations, a significant difference in work practices of different persons, and there is real difficulty in measuring dermal uptake and incidental ingestion (166,256,259).

Scientists in the field of radiological health were the first to quantitatively estimate human uptake of environmental contaminants (301); health physics publications can be a source of valuable information when conducting assessments of chemical contaminants (20). This work, which was conducted after World War II, provided numerous methodologies for estimating human uptake of environmental contaminants. These have been refined over the past decade (161,125,218). The availability of information on the degree of exposure associated with various scenarios has increased dramatically over the past 15 years, as evidenced by the size of the recent *EPA Exposure Factors Handbook,* a four-volume document containing nearly 1000 pages of information on exposure assessment (382–384,386).

The practice of exposure assessment, at least for regulatory purposes, has changed over time. For example, beginning in the late 1970s, regulatory policy in the United States encouraged or mandated the use of conservative approaches when conducting exposure assessments. This was codified in the U.S. EPA original document entitled *Risk Assessment Guidance for Superfund,* called RAGS (372). At that time, standardization of exposure assessments used to satisfy regulatory agencies was considered prudent because it guaranteed that risks would not be underestimated in order to ensure protection of public health. Beginning about 1985, concern evolved that repeated use of conservative exposure factor assumptions was producing unrealistically high estimates of exposure (81,209,242,254,259) and that the cost of achieving the recommended cleanup levels was becoming enormous. Thus, to improve the accuracy of many of the factors used in these assessments, a significant amount of new research was initiated.

Around 1990, risk assessors learned how to apply Monte Carlo techniques to evaluate both typical and highly exposed persons. Application of Monte Carlo techniques to exposure assessment has dramatically improved our understanding of the certainty of our estimates, and has decreased the problems associated with the repeated use of conservative assumptions, thereby altering the field permanently (44,117,353,354). The U.S. EPA and other agencies have now embraced this approach, which is well described in the recent document called RAGS3A (a process for conducting probabilistic risk assessment) (392).

What Is Exposure?

Because there has been no agreed-upon definition of where or when exposure takes place, terminology used in published exposure assessment literature has been inconsistent. Although there is reasonable agreement that human exposure means contact with the chemical or the agent (4,372,375), there has not yet been widespread agreement as to whether this means contact with (1) the visible exterior of the person (e.g., an aluminum strip touches the skin but can't be absorbed), or (2) the so-called exchange boundaries where absorption takes place (skin, lungs, gastrointestinal tract) (377). The differing definitions have led to some ambiguity in the use of terms and units for quantifying exposure.

Some scientists find it helpful to think of the human body as having a hypothetical outer boundary that separates the inside of the body from the outside (377). The outer boundary of the body consists of the skin and openings into the body, such as the mouth, nostrils, or punctures and lesions in the skin. In most exposure assessments, chemical exposure is defined as contact of the chemical with some part of this boundary. An exposure assessment is the quantitative or qualitative evaluation of that contact. It describes the intensity, frequency, and duration of contact, the route of the chemical across the boundary (exposure route, e.g., dermal, oral, or respiratory), the resulting amount of chemical actually crossing the boundary (dose), and the amount of chemical absorbed (internal dose) (192,375). These categories can be further refined as described below; however, a very workable quantitative definition of exposure is to think of it as "the product of (concentration), (time), and (duration), or rate of transport of toxicant (mg/cm^2-min)" (166).

Depending on the purpose of the exposure assessment, the numerical output of these analyses may be an estimate of either exposure or dose. If an exposure assessment is being done as part of a risk assessment in support of an epidemiologic study, for example, sometimes only qualitative exposure levels are all that can be provided. In these situations, categories like low-, medium-, and high-level exposure may be used. In contrast, most assessments of environmental or occupational exposure conducted in recent years attempt to quantitatively predict the absorbed dose (mg/kg-d) and, occasionally, the circulating blood level or the concentration of the toxicant in the target organ (260,292).

Concepts of Exposure, Intake, Uptake, and Dose

The process of a chemical entering the body can be described in two steps—contact (exposure), followed by actual entry (crossing the boundary). Absorption, either upon crossing the boundary or subsequently, leads to the availability of an amount of chemical to biologically significant sites within the body (target tissue dose). Although the description of contact with the outer boundary is simple conceptually (e.g., mg benzene/cm^2 skin), estimating the degree to which a chemical crosses this boundary is somewhat more complex.

In the early 1990s, some scientists described the transport of chemicals into the body as involving two separate steps: intake and uptake. Intake involved physically moving the chemical in question through an opening in the outer boundary (usually the mouth or nose), typically via inhalation, eating, or drinking. Normally, the chemical was contained in a medium such as air, food, water, or dust/soil. Here, the key question was the mass inhaled or ingested. Uptake, in contrast to intake, involved absorption of the chemical through the skin or across other barriers.

Today, most persons tend to lump intake and uptake together, simply calling the amount of chemical entering the body "uptake." In some cases, chemicals are absorbed completely, so systemic absorption (uptake) is the same as that eaten or in contact with the skin (intake). In other cases, the chemical is often contained in a carrier medium, and the medium itself typically is not absorbed at the same rate as the "contaminant of interest," so estimates of the amount of chemical crossing the boundary cannot be made directly. For example, benzene on the surface of a contaminated soil particle will move quickly through the skin, but benzene in the center of the soil particle may never completely reach the surface, and therefore it is not bioavailable and will not enter the bloodstream. Of course, for many inorganic chemicals like arsenic or lead in soil, oral and dermal bioavailability can be very low since the chemical is bound to the interstices of the soil particle and, therefore, uptake is very low. In short, if a chemical cannot be released from a media, it has no bioavailability and, consequently, since there is no uptake the chemical does not pose a risk.

Dermal absorption is an example of direct uptake across the outer boundary of the body. A chemical uptake rate is the amount of chemical absorbed per unit of time. In this process, mass transfer occurs by diffusion, so uptake will depend on the concentration gradient across the boundary, permeability of the barrier, and other factors (192,214,215). Chemical uptake rates can be expressed as a function of the exposure concentration, permeability coefficient, and surface area exposed, or as flux (269).

Bioavailability

The study of the bioavailability of chemicals in various media began around 1980 and continues to be an important topic (305).

Most studies are of oral bioavailability, although the dermal and inhalation bioavailability of chemicals have also been evaluated. This area of research has been a bit confusing due to a lack of standard terminology (159). A recent review paper by Ruby et al. (305) is probably the most authoritative one on this topic. The following definitions should be used in future assessments:

Bioavailability: Oral bioavailability is defined as the fraction of an administered dose that reaches the central (blood) compartment from the gastrointestinal tract. Bioavailability defined in this manner is commonly referred to as *absolute bioavailability,* and is equal to the oral absorption fraction.

Relative bioavailability: Relative bioavailability refers to comparative bioavailabilities of different forms of a substance or for different exposure media containing the substance (e.g., bioavailability of a metal from soil relative to its bioavailability from water), expressed in this document as a relative absorption factor (RAF).

Relative absorption factor: The RAF describes the ratio of the absorbed fraction of a substance from a particular exposure medium relative to the fraction absorbed from the dosing vehicle used in the toxicity study for that substance (the term *relative bioavailability adjustment,* RBA, is also used to describe this factor).

Bioaccessibility: The oral bioaccessibility of a substance is the fraction that is soluble in the gastrointestinal environment and is available for absorption. It is imortant to note that the bioaccessible fraction is not necessarily equal to the RAF (or RBA) but depends on the relation between results from a particular in vitro test system and an appropriate in vivo model.

There are both in vitro and in vivo tests for evaluating bioavailability, and many different approaches have been suggested over the past 20 years (159,165,321,358).

As noted by Ruby et al. (305), a number of in vitro tests are available. Simple extraction tests have been used for several years to assess the degree of metals dissolution in a simulated gastrointestinal-tract environment. The predecessor of these systems was developed originally to assess the bioavailability of iron from food, for studies of nutrition. In these systems, various metal salts or soils containing metals are incubated in low-pH solution for a period intended to mimic residence time in the stomach. The pH is then increased to near neutral, and incubation continues for a period intended to mimic residence time in the small intestine. Enzymes and organic acids are added to simulate gastric and small-intestinal fluids. The fraction of lead, arsenic, or other metals that dissolves during the stomach and small-intestinal incubations represents the fraction that is bioaccessible (i.e., is soluble and available for absorption).

A number of in vivo tests have also been used with varying success. For example, gastrointestinal absorption of lead in humans varies with the age, diet, and nutritional status of the subject as well as with the chemical species and the particle size of lead that is administered. For example, age is a well-established determinant of lead absorption; adults typically absorb 5–7% of lead ingested from dietary sources, while estimates of lead absorption from dietary sources in infants and children range from 40 to 53%. For the purpose of modeling exposure to lead in soil, the U.S. EPA currently assumes that the absolute bioavailability of lead in diet and water is 50% and that the absolute bioavailability of lead in soil is 30% for children. This corresponds to a soil RAF of 0.60 (60%) for the bioavailability of soil lead relative to lead in water (i.e., RAF = 0.3/0.5) (305).

The results of bioavailability studies need to be considered in virtually all assessments involving human exposure. Often the effects in uptake will be minor, while in other cases one may find that insignificant quantities of a chemical are absorbed even though the applied dose or exposure is quite high (358,396).

Applied Dose or Potential Dose

Applied dose has been defined as the amount of chemical available at the absorption barrier (skin, lung, gastrointestinal tract) (377). It is useful to know the applied dose if a relationship can be established between the applied dose and the internal dose, a relationship that can sometimes be established experimentally. This relationship can be estimated either through modeling or by direct measurement. For example, some researchers have analyzed phenol concentrations in the blood of volunteers over time after placing their hands in a bucket of nitrobenzene in an attempt to quantify the flux rate (273,275). Usually it is difficult to measure the applied dose directly, as many of the absorption barriers are internal to the human, and not localized in such a way to make measurement easy. An approximation of applied dose can be made, however, using the concept of potential dose (377).

Potential dose is simply the amount of chemical that is ingested or inhaled, or the amount of chemical contained in material applied to the skin. It is a useful term or concept in those instances when there is a measurable amount of chemical or transport medium. The potential dose for ingestion and inhalation is analogous to the administered dose in a dose-response experiment.

For the dermal route, potential dose is the amount of chemical applied, or the amount of chemical in the medium applied (for example, as a small amount of soil deposited on the skin). Note that because all of the chemical in the soil particulate is not contacting the skin, this differs from exposure (the concentration in the particulate times the duration of contact) and applied dose (the amount in the layer actually touching the skin) (377).

As previously noted, the amount of chemical that reaches the exchange boundaries of the skin, lungs, or gastrointestinal tract may often be less than the potential dose if the material is only partly bioavailable. For example, only about 0.001% to 1.0% of dioxins or polycyclic aromatic hydrocarbons (PAHs) on fly ash in contact with the skin are likely to penetrate (321). When bioavailability data are known, adjustments to the potential dose should be made to convert it to the absorbed or internal dose (159,321).

Internal Dose

The amount of chemical that has been absorbed and is available for interaction with biologically significant receptors (e.g., target organs) is called the *internal dose.* Estimating internal dose is the first objective of a good exposure assessment (288,381).

Transport models are available to assist in this process (219). Once absorbed, the chemical can be metabolized, stored, excreted, or transported within the body. The amount transported to an individual organ, tissue, or fluid of interest is termed the *delivered dose* (68). The delivered dose may be only a small part of the total internal dose. For example, although 1 mg of PCB may be absorbed into the body, at any given time the amount in the liver (the target organ) may only be 0.001 mg. Work to refine the techniques used to estimate delivered dose has been among the most exciting areas of exposure assessment research over the past 15 years. Currently, the best approach to estimate delivered dose is to directly measure blood or to use physiologically based pharmacokinetic (PBPK) models (12,194).

The *biologically effective dose* (BED), or the amount that actually reaches cells, sites, or membranes where adverse effects occur (235), may represent only a fraction of the delivered dose, but it is obviously the best one for predicting adverse effects. To understand BED is the ultimate goal of exposure assessment. Thus far, toxicologists have rarely been able to estimate BED or measure it for most chemicals (377), but models allow us to estimate it.

Currently, most risk assessments dealing with environmental chemicals (as opposed to pharmaceutical assessments) rely upon dose-response relationships based on the potential (administered) dose or the internal dose, because our understanding of how to estimate the delivered dose or the biologically effective dose is insufficient for most chemicals. In general, the best method currently available for estimating the dose to the target organ is to use PBPK models. These have been developed for about 60 high-volume industrial chemicals (193) (Table 9.1).

Often it is more convenient in risk assessment to refer to dose rates, or the amount of a chemical dose (applied or internal) per unit time (e.g., mg/d), or as dose rates on a per unit body weight basis (e.g., mg/kg-d). Most exposure data found in the various editions of the U.S. EPA *Exposure Factors Handbook* and other guidance documents are presented as dose rates (e.g., grams of fish consumed each day) rather than as dose (8,382–384).

Exposure and Dose Relationships

Depending on the purpose of the exposure assessment, different estimates of exposure and dose may require

Table 9.1
Examples of PBPK models for toxic substances

Benzene	Lead
Benzo[a]pyrene	Methanol
Butoxyethanol	Methoxyethanol (2-ME)
Carbon tetrachloride	Methyl ethyl ketone (MEK)
Chlorfenvinphos	Nickel
Chloralkanes	Nicotine
Chloroform	Parathion
Chloropentafluorobenzene	Physostigmine
cis-Dichlorodiammine platinum	PBB
Dichloroethane	PCBs
Dichloroethylene	Styrene
Dichloromethane	Toluene
Dieldrin	TCDF
Diisopropylfluorophosphate	TCDD (Dioxin)
Dimethyloxazolidine dione	Tetrachloroethylene
Dioxane	Trichloroethane
Ethylene oxide	Trichloroethylene
Ethyoxy ethanol (2-EE)	Trichlorotribluoroethane
Formaldehyde	Vinyl chloride
Hexane	Vinylidene fluoride
Hexavalent chromium	Xylene
Kepone	

Note. This table is an expansion of one presented in a paper by Leung and Paustenbach (193).

calculation. Often, estimates of uptake will be presented in units used in the toxicology study which may not be useful for exposure calculations.

When risk is a function of time of exposure, exposure or dose profiles can be very useful. In these profiles, the exposure concentration or dose is plotted as a function of time (19). Concentration and time are used to depict exposure, while amount and time characterize dose.

Such profiles are important for use in risk assessment where the severity of the effect depends on the pattern by which the exposure occurs, rather than on the total (integrated) exposure. For example, a developmental toxicant may only produce effects if exposure occurs during a particular stage of development. As shown in Figure 9.2, during the time above a certain dose rate (the shaded portion), there was an increased risk to the fetus of certain birth defects. Similarly, a single acute exposure to very high dose may induce adverse effects, even if the average is much lower than apparent no-effect levels. To understand the probability of an adverse effect, one must generally consider the pharmacokinetics of the specific chemical. For example, for a chemical that has a long biologic half-life, internal exposure continues long after the chemical is ingested because blood levels remain high until the substance is completely released from poorly perfused tissues like adipose, and then is metabolized and/or eliminated.

In general, there is a need to consider the time elements of exposure assessment. Specifically, it is useful to understand the relationship between the biological half-lives of toxicants and the subsequent critical time element of their exposure. Indeed, the appropriate consideration of these elements should drive the specified averaging times for both toxicant exposure limits and exposure assessment (258,295).

If a chemical or agent causes its biological damage quickly and is gone from the body in a short time, then how we test its toxicity is critical. For example, consider

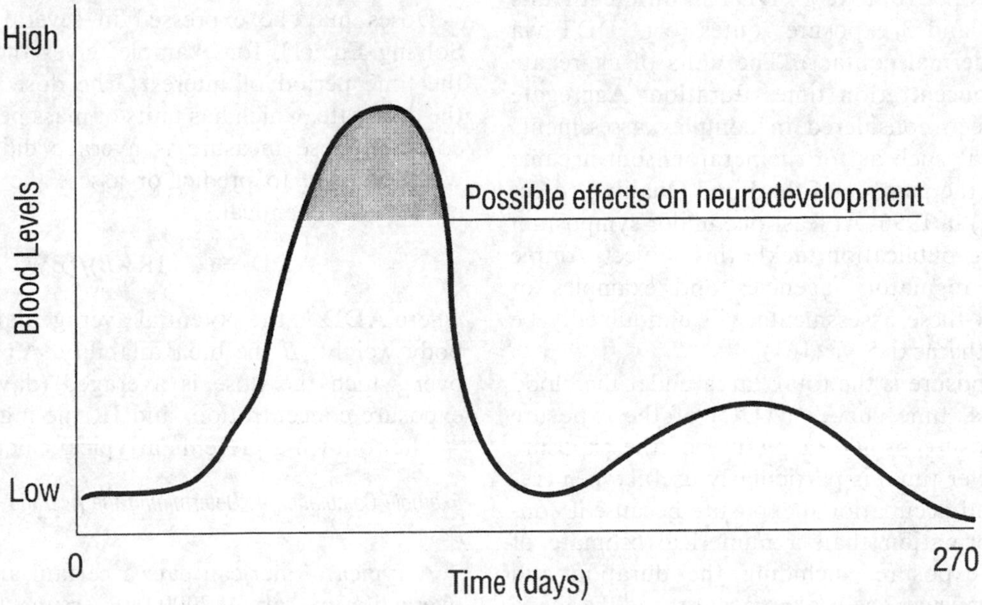

FIG. 9.2. Time course of exposure to a developmental toxicant. Note that the shaded portion represents the blood concentration of toxicant which is necessary to offer some probability that an inverse effect might occur.

a material with a half-life of a few minutes in the body. If we were to test it by spreading or apportioning the daily dose of this material over 24 h via inhalation, it will produce a different toxicity than if the animal got the same amount in a couple of 1-h inhalation exposures. The same dose of this quick-acting material would do much more damage amassed in a bolus dose of a few minutes or even an hour or two than spread over 24 h.

Thus, dosing times in toxicological studies should be commensurate with the biological half-life for the relatively quick-acting chemicals. We often need to measure the exposure over an appropriately short period of time where the worst-case exposure may occur. The same logic also holds for the dermal (topically applied) and oral (normally ingested) exposures in that they should occur in time frames that are comparable to what we would expect in use. Bolus dosing by gavage or injection would, of course, be worst case.

On the other hand, if the biological half-life of the compound is longer than a few days, then relatively high spikes of exposure over a day or two are not particularly significant from a health impact perspective. What is important from a chronic toxicity perspective for these types of compounds is, of course, the weighted average over a significantly longer time period.

As such, it would only seem appropriate to use an annual average exposure when you are dealing with a compound with a very long (greater than 90 d) half-life in the body and no evidence of acute toxicity at high short-term dose rates (289,291,295).

Aggregate exposure is the sum total of exposure to a chemical via all routes of exposure (and all media). It is now commonplace to add as many as 6 to 10 different exposure sources per route (e.g., DDT in different fruits and vegetables) and 3 exposure routes (e.g., DDT via food, air, and dermal contact). The units of aggregate exposure are concentration times duration. Aggregate exposure has been considered in complex assessments of the past 10 yr, such as for incinerators, but it came to the fore with the passage of the Food Quality Protection Act (FQPA) in 1996. At least one major symposium and the resulting publication tackle this subject. Ample guidance from regulatory agencies and examples of how to perform these assessments will undoubtedly be published over the next 5 yr (161).

Integrated exposure is the total "area under the blood concentration vs. time curve" (AUC) of the exposure profile. An exposure profile (a picture of the exposure concentration over time) is particularly useful when trying to understand occupational exposure because it contains more information than a numerical estimate of the integrated exposure, including the duration and periodicity of exposure, the peak exposure, and the shape of the area under the time-concentration curve (Figure 9.2). The risk posed by most systemic toxicants with chronic effects are often best understood by evaluating the blood concentration versus time relationship.

The last way to characterize exposure is the time-weighted average (TWA). This is particularly relevant when conducting a carcinogen risk assessment. In cancer risk assessments, the time over which exposure is integrated is usually 70 yr (377). A TWA dose rate is the total dose divided by the time period of dosing, usually expressed in units of mass per unit time, or mass/time normalized to body weight (e.g., mg/kg-d). TWA dose rates such as the lifetime average daily dose (LADD) are used in dose-response equations to estimate lifetime risk.

Measures of Dose

For risk assessment purposes, dose estimates should be expressed in a manner that can be compared with available dose-response data from animal or human studies. For example, if data on human exposure are in milligrams of lead per deciliter of blood (mg/dl), it would be best to use the blood concentrations in an animal or human study to predict the risk. Frequently, dose-response relationships are based on potential dose (called administered dose in animal studies), although dose-response relationships are sometimes based on internal dose. These differences need to be accounted for. The measure of dose selected should be based on the mode of action of the adverse effect (10,13,19,375,381). For example, to assess a nasal irritant, the airborne concentration of the chemical is a relevant dose, and an even better dose metric would be mg of chemical contacting a square centimeter of nasal mucosa.

Doses may be expressed in several different ways. Solving Eq. (1), for example, gives the dose rate over the time period of interest. The dose per unit time is the dose rate, which has units of mass per time. The most common dose measure is average daily dose (ADD), which is used to predict or assess the noncarcinogenic effects of a chemical.

$$\mathrm{ADD} = (C \cdot \mathrm{IR} \cdot B)/(\mathrm{BW} \cdot \mathrm{AT}) \qquad (1)$$

where ADD is the potential average daily dose, BW the body weight, B the bioavailability, AT the time period over which the dose is averaged (days), C the mean exposure concentration, and IR the ingestion rate.

The following presents a typical calculation.

Example Calculation 1: Determining the Average Daily Dose

A typical American eats a certain amount of lettuce over a lifetime (about 2000 kg). Assume that on any given week, the maximum quantity ingested is 0.5 kg, and the maximum on any one day is 0.04 kg/d. Assume that the typical aldrin residue is 4 mg/kg on all lettuce ingested over the person's lifetime. What is the ADD of aldrin for the maximum week? Assume the oral bioavailability of aldrin in lettuce is 90%.

Given:

$$C = 4\ \text{mg/kg (aldrin)}$$
$$\text{BW} = 70\ \text{kg}$$
$$\text{AT} = 7\ \text{d}$$
$$\text{IR} = 0.5\ \text{kg}$$
$$B = 0.9$$

Therefore:

$$\text{ADD} = (C \cdot \text{IR} \cdot B)/(\text{BW} \cdot \text{AT})$$
$$\text{ADD} = (4\ \text{mg/kg})(0.5\ \text{kg})(0.9)/(70\ \text{kg})(7\ \text{d})$$
$$\text{ADD} = 0.004\ \text{mg/kg-d}$$

When the primary health risk posed by a chemical is cancer or another chronic effect, then the biological response is usually described in terms of lifetime probabilities (e.g., the increased risk of developing cancer during a 70-yr lifetime is 2 in 100,000). In these circumstances, even though exposure may not occur over the entire lifetime, doses are usually presented as LADDs (377). The LADD takes the form of Eq. (2), with lifetime (LT) replacing the averaging time (AT):

$$\text{LADD} = (C \cdot \text{IR} \cdot B)/(\text{BW} \cdot \text{LT}) \qquad (2)$$

Example Calculation 2: Determining the Lifetime Average Daily Dose

Assume that the reasonable maximum ingestion lifetime uptake of lettuce over a 70-yr lifetime (99% person) is 14,000 kg and that it contains 4 mg/kg of aldrin. What is the LADD?

Given:

$$C = 4\ \text{mg/kg (aldrin in lettuce)}$$
$$\text{IR} = 14,000\ \text{kg}$$
$$B = 0.9$$
$$\text{BW} = 70\ \text{kg}$$
$$\text{LT} = 70\ \text{yr} = 25,550\ \text{d}$$

where

$$\text{LADD} = (\text{C} \cdot \text{IR} \cdot \text{B})/(\text{BW} \cdot \text{LT})$$

Then

$$\text{LADD} = (4)(14,000)(0.9)/(70)(25,550)$$
$$\text{LADD} = 0.028\ \text{mg/kg-d}$$

Although other measures of chronic dose may be more appropriate for predicting the hazard posed by specific chronic toxicants, such as an area under the blood concentration (AUC) curve or the peak target tissue concentration, the LADD is the most common dose metric used in carcinogen risk assessment (Figure 9.3).

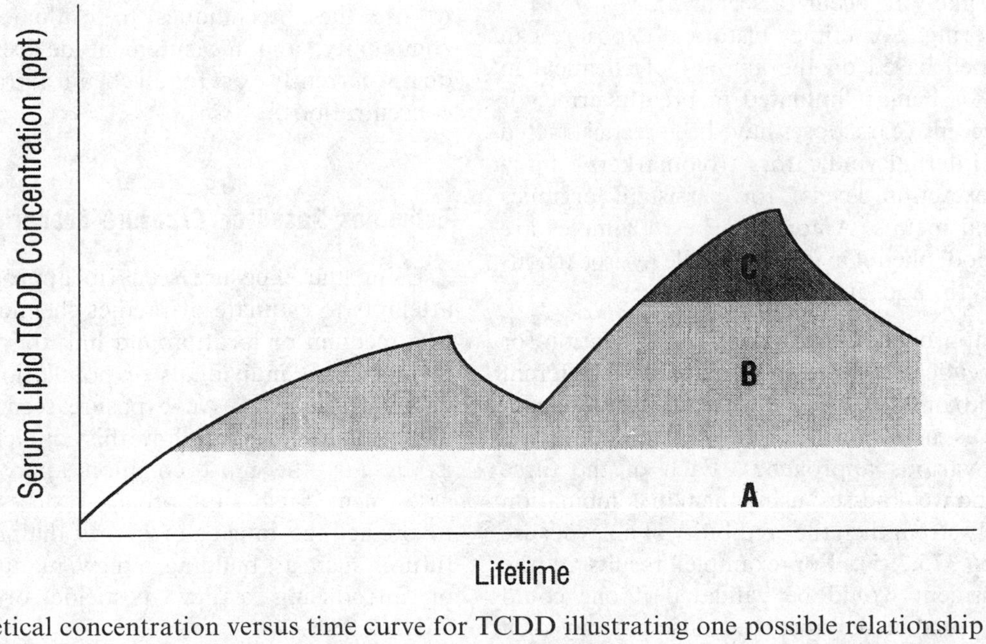

FIG. 9.3. Theoretical concentration versus time curve for TCDD illustrating one possible relationship between AUC and response. This figure illustrates the possible combination of AUC and thresholds for production of various responses: area A, no effect; area B, enzyme induction occurs; area C, significant increased cell proliferation. From Reference 19.

CONCEPTUAL APPROACHES TO EXPOSURE ASSESSMENT

Quantifying Exposure

Although exposure assessments are conducted for a variety of reasons, the process of estimating exposure can be approached using one of the following three methods (377):

1. Direct measurement: The exposure can be measured at the point of contact (the outer boundary of the body) while it is taking place, measuring the exposure concentration and time of contact and integrating them (point-of-contact measurement). An example is the measurement of the amount of contaminated soil on an exposed hand of someone digging a hole to plant a tree. The relevant exposure information would be contaminant concentration in soil (μg/g), surface area of the hand in contact with the soil (100 m^2), and time of exposure (2 h).
2. Exposure scenario: Sometimes one is concerned about an exposure that may or may not occur, so a hypothetical exposure scenario is developed. In these assessments, specific data cannot actually be collected, but relevant information can be found. For example, if an incinerator were built, it would not be known today how much of each chemical in the airborne emissions would reach the various compartments in the environment (food, soil, sediment, surface water), but one can describe what would be likely to occur (a scenario).
3. Biomonitoring: Sometimes historical exposure can be estimated based on the amount of chemical in the body or being eliminated in breath, urine, or feces. In recent years, doses have been reconstructed through internal indicators (biomarkers, body burden, excretion levels) for persistent organics and several metals. Among the best examples are lead in blood, phenol in urine, volatile hydrocarbons in the breath, and dioxins in blood fat.

These three approaches to exposure quantification (or dose) are independent because each is based on different assumptions and/or data. The fact that they are independent measures is useful in verifying or validating the results of the various approaches. Each of the three has strengths and weaknesses; using them in combination can considerably strengthen the credibility of an exposure assessment (236,375,395). For example, results of the exposure assessment would be validated if one could mathematically predict the absorbed dose per day of a chemical, estimate the resulting blood concentrations, and confirm these estimates by sampling the blood of the exposed population (268).

Estimates Based on Direct Measurement

Point-of-contact or direct exposure assessment evaluates the exposure as it occurs. Measuring chemical concentrations at the interface between the person and the environment as a function of time yields an exposure profile. The best known example of point-of-contact measurement is the output of a radiation dosimeter. This small badgelike device measures radiation exposure as it occurs and provides an integrated exposure estimate for the period of time over which the measurement has been taken (377). The Total Exposure Assessment Methodology (TEAM) studies (369) conducted by the U.S. EPA made use of direct measurements. In the TEAM studies, a small pump with a collector and an absorbent was attached to a person's clothing to measure his or her exposure to airborne solvents or other pollutants as it occurred, just as has been done in industrial hygiene studies of the past 60 yr (7). In both of these examples, the measurements are taken at the interface between the person and the environment while exposure is occurring.

The area of exposure assessment known as agricultural hygiene has developed very sophisticated techniques for estimating the uptake (absorption) of chemicals during the mixing and application of pesticides. These have been described in numerous articles (179,180). A recent paper by Kissel and Fenske (175) is also useful.

Providing that the measurement devices are accurate, the direct measurement method likely gives the best exposure value for the period of time over which the measurement was taken. It is often expensive, however, to use these techniques to evaluate persons in the community, and measurement devices and techniques do not currently exist for all chemicals (at least at ambient concentrations).

Estimates Based on Exposure Scenarios

Using the exposure scenario approach, the assessor attempts to estimate or predict chemical concentrations in a medium or location and link this information with the time that individuals or populations are in contact with the chemical. An exposure scenario is the set of assumptions describing how this contact takes place. This is, by far, the most common approach to exposure assessment. Such an approach is necessary when trying to predict the impact of events that may occur in the future, such as building a new manufacturing facility or introducing a new pesticide or herbicide (239, 261,262,284).

The first step to building a scenario is to determine the concentration of the contaminated media. This is typically accomplished indirectly by measuring, modeling, or using existing data on concentrations in the media of concern, rather than at the point of contact (for example, pesticide residues on food or metal emissions on residential soils). Often, we assume that the concentration in the bulk medium is the same as the concentration at the point of exposure. This can be a source of potential error and should be discussed in the uncertainty analysis. For example, over the past 20 yr, most assessments of the hazard posed by contaminated soil were based on soil samples collected in the top 6 in of soil, even though most persons were exposed routinely to the surface soil (usually the top 2½ in). Arguments can be made in either direction about the appropriateness of this assumption.

The next step in conducting an exposure scenario is to estimate the contact time, identify who is likely to be exposed, and then develop estimates of the exposure frequency and duration. Like chemical concentration characterization, this is usually done indirectly using demographic data, survey statistics, behavior observation, activity diaries, activity models, or, in the absence of more substantive information, assumptions about behavior (386,387).

Chemical concentration and population characterizations are ultimately combined in an exposure scenario. One of the major problems in evaluating dose equations is that the limiting assumptions used to derive them (e.g., steady-state assumptions) do not always hold true. Two approaches to this problem are available: (1) to evaluate the exposure or dose equation under conditions when the limiting assumptions do hold true, or (2) to build a dynamic model that accounts for both accumulation and degradation. The microenvironment method, which is usually used to evaluate air exposures, is an example of the first approach. This method evaluates segments of time and location when the assumption of constant concentration is approximately true, and then sums the time segments to determine the total exposure for the respiratory route, effectively removing some of the uncertainty (282). In occupational hygiene, this is done by combining time–motion data with short-term air concentration data. While exposure concentration and time of contact may be estimated in some situations, the concentration and time of contact can be measured for each microenvironment. This avoids much of the error due to summing average values in cases where concentration and time of contact vary widely.

In the second approach, a computer model can efficiently predict dose if enough data are available (51,204,430). When conducting modeling, there are various tools used to describe parameter variation, such as Monte Carlo analysis, and these may be necessary in some assessments.

Estimating Exposure Using Biological Monitoring

Exposure can often be estimated after it has taken place. The key factor is whether the biological half-life of the chemical is sufficiently long to allow for accurate measurement. If a total dose is known or can be reconstructed, and information about intake and uptake rates is available, an average past exposure rate can be estimated (19,276,309,333,346). Dose reconstruction relies on measuring biological fluids (blood, urine), hair, nails, or feces after exposure, intake, and uptake have already occurred, and using these measurements to back-calculate dose (19). However, data on body burden levels or biomarkers cannot be used directly unless a relationship can be established between these levels (or biomarker indications) and internal dose.

Biological monitoring can be used to evaluate the amount of a chemical in the body by measuring one or more parameters (Table 9.2). In general, if these measurements can be made and the biologic half-life is acceptable, then past exposure estimates can be reasonably accurate. Not all of these can be measured for every chemical (377). Following is a list of possible measurements:

- The concentration of the chemical itself in biological tissues or sera (blood, urine, breath, hair, adipose tissue, etc.).
- The concentration of the chemical's metabolite(s).
- The biological effect that occurs as a result of human exposure to the chemical (e.g., alkylated hemoglobin or changes in enzyme induction).
- The amount of a chemical or its metabolites bound to target molecules.

The results of biomonitoring can be used to estimate chemical uptake during a specific interval, if background levels do not mask the marker and the relationship between uptake and the selected marker is known (89). The sampling time for biomarkers is often critical. Establishing a correlation between exposure and measurement of the marker, including pharmacokinetics, is necessary to properly back-calculate historical exposure (377).

The strengths of this method are that it demonstrates that exposure and absorption of the chemical has actually taken place, and theoretically it can give a good indication of past exposure. The drawbacks are that (1) it will not work for every chemical because of interferences or the reactive nature of the chemical, or because the biological half-life of the agent is too short; (2) that the approach has been applied to only a few chemicals; (3) that data relating internal dose to exposure are needed; and (4) that it may be expensive.

Table 9.2
Examples of types of measurements to characterize exposure-related media and parameters

Type of measurement (sample)	Usually attempts to characterize (whole)	Examples	Typical information needed to characterize exposure
Breath	Total internal dose for individuals or population (usually indicative of relatively recent exposures).	Measurement of volatile organic compounds (VOCs), alcohol. (Usually limited to volatile compounds.)	1. Relationship between individuals and population; exposure history (i.e., steady-state or not) pharmacokinetics (chemical half-life), possible storage reservoirs within the body. 2. Relationship between breath content and body burden.
Blood	Total internal dose for individuals or population (may be indicative of either relatively recent exposures to fat-soluble organics or long-term body burden for metals).	Lead studies, pesticides, heavy metals (usually best for soluble compounds, although blood lipid analysis may reveal lipophilic compounds).	1. Same as for breath. 2. Relationship between blood content and body burden.
Adipose	Total internal dose for individuals or population (usually indicative of long-term averages for fat-soluble organics).	NHATS, dioxin studies, PCBs (usually limited to lipophilic compounds).	1. Same as for breath. 2. Relationship between adipose content and body burden.
Nails, hair	Total internal dose for individuals or population (usually indicative of past exposure in weeks to months range; can sometimes be used to evaluate exposure patterns).	Heavy metal studies (usually limited to metals).	1. Same as for breath. 2. Relationship between nails, hair content and body burden.
Urine	Total internal dose for individuals or population (usually indicative of elimination rates); time from exposure to appearance in urine may vary, depending on chemical.	Studies of tetrachloroethylene and trichloroethylene.	1. Same as for breath. 2. Relationship between urine content and body burden.

Note. From Reference 385.

For those chemicals where biological monitoring can be used to estimate past exposure, the information obtained can be invaluable for conducting retrospective exposure assessments that can be used in epidemiology studies. Some examples of chemicals for which past exposure can reliably be estimated include several metals, as well as numerous large organic chemicals (e.g., DDT, chlordane, dioxin, polybrominated biphenyl [PBB], PCB) (19).

INFORMATION UPON WHICH EXPOSURE ASSESSMENTS ARE BASED

Comprehensive exposure assessment of a complex scenario may require several hundred exposure factors to estimate the various chemical concentrations in one of several dozen different media. Among the most complex exposure assessments are those that address the risks posed by airborne emissions from combustors (125,281,388) (Figure 9.4). To estimate the concentration, numerous dispersion models, as well as fate and transport models, may be required. In addition, the assessor may need to search the literature to identify relevant studies from as many as 10 related fields of research. Sometimes, hundreds of published papers and government guidance documents need to be evaluated, used, and cited. In short, the exercise can be formidable, especially for assessments involving food chain contamination. Equally difficult and highly complex exposure assessments are those that attempt to estimate the uptake of fish by various members of the angling public (428).

Obtaining Data on Intake and Uptake

The numerous editions of the *Exposure Factors Handbook* (382–384, 386) present statistical data on many of the factors used to assess exposure, including intake rates, and these provide citations for primary references. Today, this series of publications represents the most comprehensive, single source of exposure assessment information. Some of the many intake factors in the various volumes include:

- Drinking water consumption rates.
- Breast milk ingestion rates for infants.
- Consumption rates for homegrown fruits, vegetables, beef, and dairy products.

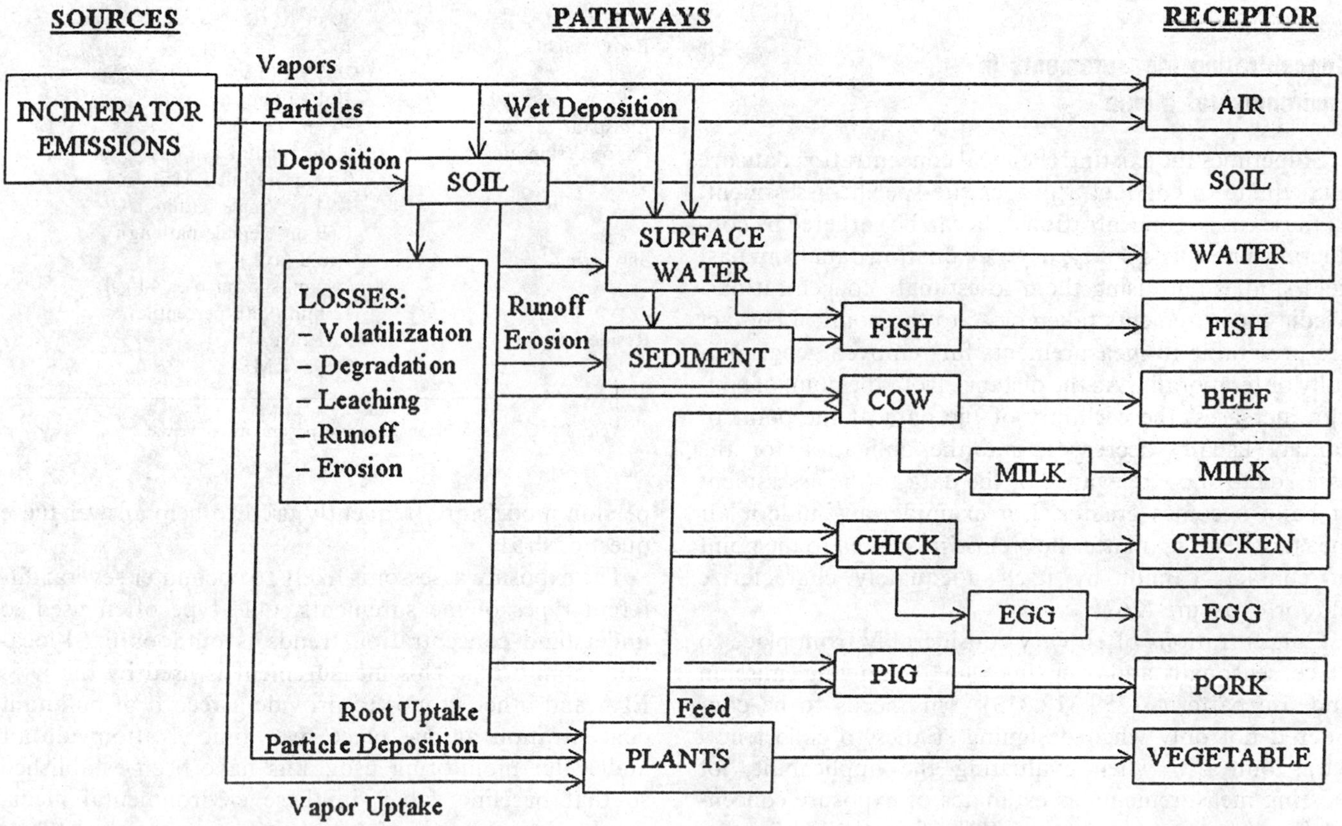

FIG. 9.4. EPA's conceptual approach to dealing with direct and indirect exposure pathways as illustrated by assessments of incinerator emissions.

- Consumption rates for recreationally caught fish and shellfish.
- Incidental soil ingestion rates.
- Pulmonary ventilation rates.
- Surface area of various parts of the human body.
- Body weight for various age groups.

Table 9.3 presents examples of some of the standard or default exposure factors used in risk assessment.

The *Exposure Factors Handbook* is updated routinely to include additional factors and to include new research data on previously discussed factors. It also provides default parameter values, which can be used when site-specific data are not available. Obviously, general default values should not be used in place of known, valid data that are more relevant to the assessment being conducted. The U.S. EPA handbook, though substantial, may not contain all available information on exposure factors or relevant studies, so a supplemental literature search should be conducted to ensure that pertinent literature has been identified. As discussed later, if a probabilistic or Monte Carlo assessment is to be conducted, the document titled *Risk Assessment Guidance for Superfund: Process for Conducting Probabilistic Risk Assessment* (392) and other publications should be consulted.

Table 9.3
Some standard regulatory default assumptions used in exposure assessment

Variable	Assumption
Drinking water	2 L/d (RME adult)
	1.4 L/d (adult ave.)
	1.0 L/d (child)
	0.1 L/d (incidental ingestion during swimming)
Soil (ingestion)	200 mg/d (child ave.)
	800 mg/d (child 90th percentile)
	100 mg/d (adult)
Food	2000 g/d (adult total)
Beef (home-grown)	44 g/d (ave.)
	75 g/d (RME)
	100 g/d (all sources)
Dairy (home-grown)	160 g/d (ave.)
	300 g/d (RME)
	400 g/d (all sources)
Fruit (home-grown)	28 g/d (ave.)
	42 g/d (RME)
	140 g/d (all sources)
Vegetables (home-grown)	50 g/d (ave.)
	80 g/d (RME)
	200 g/d (all sources)
Sport fish	30 g/d (ave.)
	140 g/d (RME)
Inhalation	10 m^3/d (ave. 8-h shift.)
	20 m^3/d (adult ave.)
	30 m^3/d (RME)
Body weight	13.2 kg (2–5 yr)
	20.8 kg (6 yr)
	70 kg (adult ave.)
Lifespan	70 yr
Exposed skin area	0.2 m^2 (adult ave.)
	0.53 m^2 (adult RME)
	1.94 m^2 (male bathing)
	1.69 m^2 (female bathing)
Showering	7 min (ave.)
	(5-min. shower uses 40 gal)
	12 min (90th percentile)
Residence time	9 yr (ave.)
	30 yr (RME)

Note. RME, reasonable maximum exposure; ave., average.

Concentration Measurements in Environmental Media

Sometimes the existing chemical concentration data are inadequate to conduct a proper site-specific assessment. In these cases, concentration data can be gathered by conducting a new field study, or by evaluating data from past field studies and using them to estimate concentrations. Media measurements taken close to the point of contact are preferable to measurements far removed geographically or temporally. As the distance from the point of contact increases, the certainty of the data at the point of contact usually decreases, and the obligation for the assessor to show relevance of the data to the assessment at hand becomes greater. For example, an outdoor air measurement, no matter how close it is taken to the point of contact, cannot by itself adequately characterize indoor exposure (267).

Concentrations often vary considerably from place to place, seasonally and over time due to changing emission and use patterns (259,312,313). This needs to be considered not only when designing studies to collect new data, but also when evaluating the applicability of existing measurements as estimates of exposure concentrations in a new assessment. It is of particular concern when the measurement data will be used to extrapolate to long time periods, such as lifetimes. Transport and dispersion models are frequently used to help answer these questions (51).

The exposure assessor is likely to encounter several different types of measurements. One type often used to understand concentration trends is outdoor fixed-location monitoring. This measurement is used by the U.S. EPA and other groups to provide a record of pollutant concentration at one place over time. Nationwide air and water monitoring programs have been established so that baseline values in these environmental media can be documented. Although it is not practical to set up a national monitoring network to gather data for a particular exposure assessment, data from existing networks can be evaluated for relevance to an exposure assessment. These data are often far removed from the point of contact. Adapting data from previous studies usually presents specific challenges.

Indoor air contaminant concentrations can vary as much as or more than those in outdoor air (298,410–413). Consequently, indoor exposure is best represented by measurements taken at the point of contact. However, because pollutants such as carbon monoxide can exhibit substantial outdoor penetration, indoor exposure estimates should consider potential outdoor, as well as indoor, sources of the contaminant(s) under evaluation (247,377).

Contaminant concentrations in food and drinking-water measurements can also be measured. General characterization of these media, such as market basket studies (where representative diets are characterized), shelf studies (where foodstuffs are taken from store shelves and analyzed), or drinking-water quality surveys, are usually far removed from the point of contact for an individual, but may be useful in evaluating exposure concentrations for a large population. Measurements of tap water or foodstuffs in a home and how they are used are closer to the point of contact. In evaluating the relevance of data from previous studies, variation in the distribution systems must be considered, as well as the space–time proximity (377).

Consumer or industrial product analysis is sometimes done to characterize the chemical concentrations in products. Product formulations can change substantially over time, similar products do not necessarily have similar formulations, and regional differences in product formulation can also occur. These should be considered when determining the relevance of existing data and when setting up sampling plans to gather new data (377).

Another type of concentration measurement is the microenvironmental measurement. Rather than using measurements to characterize the entire medium, this approach defines specific zones in which the concentration in the medium of interest is thought to be relatively homogeneous, and then characterizes the concentration in that zone (283,375). Typical microenvironments include the home or parts of the home, office, automobile, or other indoor settings. Microenvironments can also be divided into time segments (e.g., kitchen during the day, kitchen during the night). This approach can produce measurements that are closely linked with the point of contact, both in location and time, especially when new data are generated for a particular exposure assessment. The more specific the microenvironment, however, the greater is the burden on the exposure assessor to establish that the measurements are representative of the population of interest.

The concentration measurement that provides the closest link to the actual point of contact is personal monitoring. In virtually all cases, if available, this information should be the basis of exposure assessments of individuals. An obvious exception is the work environment where lapel sampling is conducted while the person is wearing a respirator; in this case, personal sampling would not reflect genuine exposure.

Models and Their Role

Often the most critical element in an exposure assessment is estimating pollutant concentrations at exposure points. This is usually carried out by combining field data and modeling results. In the absence of field data, this process often relies on the results of mathematical models of aerial dispersion, such as ISCLT, or of water movement, such as MODFLOW (107,364,366–368). The U.S. EPA Science Advisory Board and others have recommended that modeling ideally should be linked with monitoring data in regulatory assessments, although this is not always possible.

A modeling strategy has several aspects, including setting objectives, model selection, obtaining and installing the code, calibrating and running the computer model, and validation and verification. Many of these aspects are analogous to the quality assurance and quality control measures applied to measurements.

Regardless of whether models are extensively used in an assessment or whether a formal modeling strategy is documented in the exposure assessment plan, when computer simulation models such as fate and transport models and exposure models are used in exposure assessments, the assessor must be aware of the performance characteristics of the model and state how the exposure assessment requirements are satisfied by the model (51).

The site must be characterized if models are to be used to simulate pollutant behavior at a specific site. Site characterization for any modeling study includes examining all data on the site, such as source characterization, dimensions and topography of the site, location of receptor populations, meteorology, soils, geohydrology, and ranges and distributions of chemical concentrations. For exposure models that simulate both chemical concentration and time of exposure (through behavior patterns), data on these two parameters must be evaluated (262,264,375).

Criteria are provided by the U.S. EPA (368) for selecting surface water models and groundwater models, respectively; the reader is referred to this document for details. Similar selection criteria exist for air dispersion models.

A primary consideration in selecting a model is whether to perform a screening study or a detailed evaluation. A screening study makes a preliminary evaluation of a site or a general comparison between several sites. It may be generic to a type of site (i.e., an industrial segment or a climatic region) or may pertain to a specific site for which sufficient data are not available to properly characterize the site. Screening studies can help direct data collection at the site by, for example, providing an indication of the level of detection and quantification that would be required and the distances and directions from a point of release where chemical concentrations might be expected to be highest.

An example of a screening-level modeling effort would be to estimate the amount of lead deposited by an incinerator onto local crops using a basic air dispersion model, without considering local geographical or weather conditions. The next level of complexity would consider the presence of mountains, their proximity to the stack, the local weather patterns, and the number of atmospheric inversions per year. A higher level of analysis could incorporate yet other, more subtle factors.

The value of the screening-level analysis is that it is simple to perform and may indicate that no significant contamination exists. Screening-level models are frequently used to get a first approximation of the concentrations that may be present. Often these models use very conservative assumptions; that is, they tend to overpredict concentrations or exposures. If the results of the conservative screening procedure predict concentrations or exposures at less than a predetermined no-concern level, then more detailed analysis is probably not necessary. If the screening estimates are above that level, refinement of the assumptions or a more sophisticated model are necessary to generate a more realistic estimate (377).

Screening-level models also help the user conceptualize the physical system, identify important processes, and locate available data. The assumptions used in the preliminary analysis should represent conservative conditions, such that the predicted results overestimate potential conditions, limiting false negatives. If the limited field measurements or screening analyses indicate that a contamination problem may exist, then a detailed modeling study may be useful.

In contrast, the purpose of the detailed evaluation is to use the best data available to make the best estimate of spatial and temporal chemical distributions of a specific site. Detailed studies typically require higher quality data and more sophisticated models.

Accounting for Background Concentrations

Background exposure to so-called "toxic" or industrial chemicals, especially environmentally persistent ones, can occur due to natural or anthropogenic sources (355). In most exposure assessments, background soil concentrations are the focus of attention, but the same issue can be relevant when evaluating sediments, ambient air, groundwater, and vegetation (foodstuffs). At some sites, it is important that these so-called "background" concentrations be accounted for because removing the quantity of toxicant due to humans may, in fact, not appreciably change the concentrations or be sufficient to reduce the risk to acceptable levels. For example, naturally occurring concentrations of lead, arsenic, and cadmium, in some locations, may be higher than cleanup levels established by various regulatory agencies (94,95). The exposure assessor should try to determine local background concentrations by gathering data from nearby locations clearly unaffected by the site under investigation, or by referring to published works that have assessed this issue. Statistical approaches are applicable to address this issue (245).

Description of Background Levels

When assessing soils, background levels can be viewed in at least four different ways (107):

- "Pristine" levels—Some would like to equate background levels with those associated with the "pristine" state, that is, soils or landscapes unaffected by human activity. This rather idealistic situation probably no longer exists; even in Antarctica, mercury and dioxin concentrations can be detected in some media. Toxic elements mainly associated with the solid phase of some natural material (such as soil dust, plant or volcanic ash, vegetable matter) are relatively mobile in a global sense. For example, Nriagu (243) has suggested that about 40 million tons of heavy metals have been dispersed atmospherically over the many centuries of human activity.

  Increases in pollutant metal concentrations have been measured up to 60 km from smelters, and automotive lead (fine particles) has been measured in soils and rainfall up to about 50 km downwind from major cities. Soil contamination up to 50–100 m from highways by automotive lead (coarser particles) is an example of short-range transport, and contrasts with transport of toxic metals on a continental or global scale (e.g., contamination of the Greenland ice sheets from the northern United States, mercury in the Florida Everglades due to aerial releases in South America, the snows of the New Zealand Alps by soil dust from inland Australia) (107).
- "Normal" levels—The question could be asked: Are soils contaminated at farms in the higher rainfall areas of the Appalachians, which used to receive automotive exhaust particulates from

the New York metropolitan area 200 km away? These soils are not pristine, but the chemical concentrations are perfectly safe for growing food, raising farm animals, and residential living. Soils from such areas would have a range of what is often called "normal" background values. To most exposure assessors, this mosaic of normal soils, which is only affected by the minor pollution of everyday activities associated with modern rural and urban life, should be the basis for defining background values. Statistically, this range of normal background values would constitute a single lognormally distributed population. Obviously, one needs to exclude the outliers or "hot" spots due to a geochemical anomaly, or localized pollution arising from either industrial emissions, disposal of waste products, or intensive (excessive) use of farm chemicals (107).

- Historically polluted regions—Local community and regulatory policies often affect what are defined as background levels. A community with highly developed environmental consciousness may insist on very low, possibly unreasonable, reference values. Some densely populated areas with historically derived pollution, perhaps from former mining activities, may sustain apparently healthy populations who pragmatically must accept higher "background" level values. The cities of Philadelphia, Baltimore, and New York, and parts of Japan, for example, may fit in this category.
- Geochemical variation—Background levels of some potentially toxic elements may vary among geographical regions because of differences in soil type. The resulting concentrations are often called naturally occurring levels.

An important factor is the composition of rocks and sediments that weather from soils. Some extreme examples are high concentrations of nickel, cobalt, and chromium in igneous rocks such as basalts that cover extensive areas in western Victoria and Tasmania, Australia; and high concentrations of boron in soils on marine sediments in the Riverina, Mallee, and Wimmera districts of South Australia, and in Victoria, Eyre Peninsula and parts of western Australia.

Some regulatory agencies have provided written guidance describing how to select soil or sediment cleanup values that account for background chemical concentrations. In past years, these have varied significantly, but within the past 5 yr, there appears to be some convergence regarding the definition of background, how to measure it, and how it should affect exposure assessment calculations.

ESTIMATING UPTAKE VIA THE SKIN

When attempting to predict chemical risks in the environmental or occupational setting, the dermal exposure route can vary in its importance from negligible to significant. In most evaluations of hazardous waste sites and ambient air or water contaminants, this is not a major route of exposure. Although the uptake of chemicals via the skin has generally been overlooked in most workplace exposure assessments, it probably represents a substantial portion of the exposure for many occupations. Even though gloves are more frequently used than in years past and training has increased on the possible hazards of dermal exposure, there is still ample evidence to indicate that, in order to conduct a complete exposure assessment, this route deserves attention (192,253,265).

In addition to the risks associated with systemic toxicity due to uptake via the skin, it is sometimes necessary to evaluate the allergic contact dermatitis hazard (ACD). In recent years, techniques have been developed to quantitatively predict the likelihood of elicitation and induction of ACD (164,240). Some regulatory agencies are concerned with ACD and have developed cleanup standards based on this health endpoint.

In the workplace, a worker's skin frequently comes into contact with solvents or chemicals mixed in water (aqueous materials). In most environmental settings where persons can be exposed to contaminated soil or contaminated water, dermal uptake must be assessed. Fortunately, a good deal of research has been conducted to understand the rate at which chemicals pass through the skin. Percutaneous absorption of neat chemicals (i.e., the pure liquid) was often studied in humans until the late 1970s (100,101,113,184,225,274,275,347). Because of the potential toxicity of many chemicals and improved laboratory techniques, in vivo human studies have been largely supplanted by experiments with laboratory animals, in vitro studies, or athymic rodents grafted with human skin (178). Historical research has shown that, in general, chemical penetration of the human skin is similar to that of a pig or monkey, and much slower than that of the rat and rabbit (26). Thus, for many chemicals, there is some level of confidence that the rate of dermal uptake of a chemical by humans can be inferred from animal data.

Starting in the 1980s, in vitro studies using human skin began to be conducted on a more routine basis. In these studies, a piece of excised skin is attached to a diffusion apparatus with a top chamber to hold the applied chemical and a temperature-controlled bottom chamber containing saline or other fluids (plus a sampling port to withdraw fractions for analysis) (123). Although human forearm skin is optimal, it is difficult to obtain, so abdominal or breast skin is commonly used. Generally, a properly conducted in vitro test can be a reasonably good predictor of the absorption rate in vivo (34). However, due to the fragile nature of the technique, these studies must be carefully interpreted (22). Often, depending on the conditions of the test, the results are not applicable to humans.

Aside from neat liquids and exposure to contaminated water, dermal exposures can also occur through contact with dust or dirt on surfaces, and by way of contact with soil or dust-bound contaminants (267). Few studies (96,119,156,169,177,191,286,300,317) have directly estimated soil loading on human skin, and only one of them attempted to measure dermal contact of contaminated equipment by workers (206). The available studies probably provide sufficient data to generate point estimates of soil adherence and perhaps can provide a reasonable probability density function (PDF) for most persons exposed to contaminated soils. The degree of representativeness of the data to the general population is difficult to assess (48).

Recently, a few studies measured the adherence of soil to multiple skin surfaces (hands, forearms, lower legs, faces, and feet) under ambient and recreational conditions (156,177). Dermal loading on the hands was found to vary over five orders of magnitude and to be dependent on the type of activity. Differences between pre- and postactivity adherence demonstrated the episodic nature of dermal contact with soil. However, due to the activity-dependent nature of soil exposure, data from these studies must be interpreted for their relevance to the type of activity, frequency, duration, and otherwise site-specific nature of exposure. The various studies involving contaminated soil are informative for providing an estimate of exposure; however, they are probably a couple orders of magnitude greater than what might be expected in an occupational setting. Nonetheless, this work is a "starting point" for bracketing potential exposure to dusts in the workplace.

Recently, there has been a reasonable level of research investigating exposure to house dust. The basis for this concern has been increasing evidence that controlling exposure to house dust, especially in homes located near sites with considerable surface soil contamination, is more important for reducing the health hazard than remediating the soil (267). Numerous papers in recent years have shown that in-house exposure to toxics is much greater than that encountered due to ambient (so-called environmental) contamination (247,405).

Along these lines, and of particular interest to those who study indoor exposure, is the recent work to develop standardized approaches for collecting wipe samples and estimating the amount of dust loading on the palm of the hand (197,198). Although dermal absorption of toxicants in house dust will almost always pose a relatively low dermal uptake hazard, the uptake of toxicants due to hand-to-mouth contact can be substantial (267).

Quantitative Description of Dermal Absorption

For the purposes of risk assessment, percutaneous absorption is defined as transport of externally applied chemicals through cutaneous structures and the extracellular medium to the bloodstream (375,391). In many settings, such as for agricultural workers, platers, mechanics, and others, dermal uptake is the primary route of exposure. The simplest way to describe the rate of skin absorption is to apply Fick's first law of diffusion at steady state (349,418):

$$J = dQ/dt = DK\nabla C/e \approx K_p C \qquad (3)$$

where J ($= dQ/dt$) is the chemical flux or rate of chemical absorbed (mg/cm^2-h), D is the diffusivity in the stratum corneum (cm^2/h), K the stratum corneum/vehicle partition coefficient of the chemical (unitless), ∇C the concentration gradient (mg/cm^3), e the thickness of the stratum corneum (cm), K_p the permeability coefficient (cm/h), and C the applied chemical concentration (mg/cm^3). The concentration gradient is equal to the difference between the concentration above and below the stratum corneum. Because the concentration below is small compared to the concentration above, ∇C can be approximated as equal to the applied chemical concentration. From the preceding equation, it can be seen that the rate of absorption is directly proportional to the applied concentration. The diffusivity represents the rate of migration of the chemical through the stratum corneum. Since the stratum corneum has a nonnegligible thickness, there is a period of transient diffusion (lag time), during which the transfer rate rises to reach a steady state. In these studies, the steady state is maintained indefinitely, provided the system remains constant. Depending on the type of chemical, the lag time can range from minutes to days (192). From an exposure assessment standpoint, if the exposure duration is shorter than the lag time, it is unlikely that there will be any significant systemic absorption (142,349).

The partition coefficient (K_p) is one of the key parameters that influences the degree to which a chemical penetrates the skin (14,122,128,142,349). Fatty chemicals tend to accumulate in the stratum corneum. Conversely, the stratum corneum is an effective barrier for hydrophilic substances, which tend to have low skin absorption rates. Because stratum corneum/vehicle partition coefficients are difficult to measure, the three parameters (D, k, and e) are combined to give an overall permeability coefficient (K_p). It is noteworthy that Eq. (3) only approximates most in vivo exposure situations in which true steady-state conditions are rarely attained. In spite of its limitations, this equation has yielded satisfactory estimations of the actual absorption rates of chemicals for many situations (Table 9.4).

Pharmacokinetic Models for Estimating the Uptake of Chemicals in Aqueous Solution

Pharmacokinetic models predict the uptake of a chemical through the skin based on fundamental thermodynamics. Several different models have been proposed. For example, a four-compartment pharmacokinetic model was developed in 1982 (128). This model, which uses first-order rate constants, describes chemical movement through the compartments representing the various skin structures. It has been used successfully to predict the chemical disposition in the skin and plasma as a function of their physicochemical properties, and when an input rate constant to the skin surface is added to the model, it can be used to assess vehicle effects. A similar model that treats the barrier membrane as a series of spaces filled with immiscible liquids has also been developed (14); its advantage is that it allows examination of non-steady-state conditions where Fick's law does not apply.

Under an infinite-dose situation where the amount of a chemical lost by penetration is too small to alter the applied concentration (e.g., where one is swimming), the rate of absorption is essentially linear once steady-state has been reached. In the finite-dose system, however, the chemical solution is applied as a thin film and the concentration decreases as penetration proceeds (e.g., a splash). All other model parameters being the same, penetration is reduced under finite-dose conditions. This is because the chemical concentration is continuously reduced over time, resulting in a decrease in the gradient across the stratum corneum. These modeling results indicate that the mechanism by which fluxes are affected must be considered when extrapolating to non-steady-state conditions.

Although classic pharmacokinetic modeling like that described by Guy et al. (42) can provide a good mathematical description of the disposition of chemicals, it does not depict exactly the biological processes in the intact animal. Fortunately, due to recent improvements in available computer hardware and software, pharmacokinetic methods based on physiological principles are now feasible alternatives for analysis of in vivo skin penetration studies. These so-called PBPK models realistically describe the disposition of the chemical in the intact animal in terms of rates of blood flow, permeability of membranes, and partitioning of chemicals into tissues (12,14). Characterizing dermal absorption in terms of actual anatomical, physiological, and biochemical parameters facilitates extrapolations to the real species of interest, humans.

In 1991, a PBPK model was developed to describe percutaneous absorption of volatile organic contaminants in dilute aqueous solutions (316). The exposure scenario modeled was either hand or full-body immersion into a vessel of solute-contaminated water. Modeling results suggested that chemical uptake in aqueous solutions is most markedly influenced by epidermal blood flow rates, followed by epidermal thickness and lipid content of the stratum corneum. In general, thicker and fattier skin provides a better barrier to dermal penetration of chemicals. These are precisely the principles under which barrier creams offer their protection for increasing the effective thickness and lipophilicity of the skin. This model also predicted that the dose of some volatile organic chemicals in water absorbed through the skin during a 20-min bath may be equivalent to the amount inhaled (316).

Among the most complex and best validated of the various models for dermal uptake of liquids is that developed by McDougal (213). This team has successfully predicted dermal uptake rates for humans for more than a dozen chemicals based on animal data. One advantage of dermal PBPK models over traditional in vivo methods is their ability to accurately describe nonlinear biochemical and physical processes. For example, describing skin penetration based on blood concentrations or excretion rates as "percent absorbed" assumes that all processes have a simple linear relationship with the exposure concentration. This is often not the case. The kinetics become nonlinear when the absorption, distribution, metabolism, or elimination of a chemical is saturated at high exposure concentrations. This model and models developed since then address this phenomenon in a reasonable manner.

Factors Used to Estimate Dermal Uptake

Many factors need to be quantitatively accounted for in order to estimate the likely systemic uptake of a chemical that comes into contact with the skin, either as a liquid or when present in soil or dust (269,376).

Dermal Bioavailability

The typical media of concern for assessing cutaneous contact to environmental chemicals, in contrast with occupational exposure, are house dust, soil, fly ash, and sediment. In the workplace, dermal uptake is due to direct contact with liquids and contact with surfaces contaminated with dirt or liquids. A number of parameters can influence the degree of cutaneous bioavailability of chemicals in complex matrices. These may include aging (time following contamination), soil type (e.g., silt, clay, and sand), type and concentration

Table 9.4
Human cutaneous permeability coefficient values for some industrial chemicals in aqueous medium

	MW	K_{ow}	Observed	Calculated[a]
Organic chemicals				
2-Amino-4-nitrophenol	154.13	21.38	0.00066	0.019
4-Amino-2-nitrophenol	154.13	9.12	0.0028	0.0081
Aniline	93.12	7.94	0.041[b]	0.091
Benzene	78.11	134.90	0.11	0.39
p-Bromophenol	173.02	389.05	0.036	0.25
Butane-2,3-diol	90.12	0.12	<0.00005	0.0009
n-Butanol	74.12	7.59	0.0025	0.024
2-Butanone	72.10	1.94	0.0045	0.007
Carbon disulfide	76.14	100.00	0.54[b]	0.3
Chlorocresol	142.58	1258.93	0.055	1.31
S-Chlorophenal	128.56	147.91	0.033	0.19
p-Chlorophenal	128.56	257.04	0.036	0.34
Chloroxylenal	156.61	1621.81	0.059	1.35
m-Cresol	108.13	100.00	0.015	0.18
o-Cresol	108.13	100.00	0.016	0.18
p-Cresol	108.13	85.11	0.018	0.15
Decanol	158.28	37153.52	0.08	30.11
2,4-Dichlorophenol	163.01	1995.26	0.06	1.5
1,4-Dioxane	88.10	0.38	0.00043	0.0016
Ethanol	46.07	0.49	0.0008	0.0036
2-Ethoxyethanol	90.12	0.29	0.0003	0.0013
Ethylbenzene	106.16	1412.54	1.215[b]	2.65
Ethylether	74.12	6.76	0.016	0.022
p-Ethylphenol	122.17	549.54	0.035	0.79
Heptanol	116.20	257.04	0.038	0.41
Hexanol	102.17	107.15	0.028	0.21
Methanol	32.04	0.17	0.0016	0.0026
Methyl hydroxybenzoate	152.15	91.20	0.0091	0.082
β-Naphthol	144.16	691.83	0.028	0.7
3-Nitrophenol	139.11	100.00	0.0056	0.11
4-Nitrophenol	139.11	81.28	0.0056	0.09
Nitrosodiethanolamine	134.13	0.13	0.0000055	0.0005
Nonanol	144.26	2951.21	0.06	2.99
Octanol	130.22	933.25	0.061	1.19
Pentanol	88.15	36.31	0.006	0.091
Phenol	94.11	32.36	0.0082	0.074
Propanol	60.09	2.00	0.0017	0.0088
Resorcinol	110.11	6.03	0.00024	0.011
Styrene	104.14	891.25	0.635[b]	1.72
Thymol	150.21	1995.26	0.053	1.84
Toluene	92.13	489.78	1.01	1.15
2,4,6-Trichlorophenol	197.46	2344.23	0.059	1.02
3,4-Xylenol	122.16	169.82	0.036	0.25
Inorganic chemicals				
Cobalt chloride	129.84		0.0004	
Lead acetate	325.29		0.0000042[b]	
Mercuric chloride	271.50		0.00093	
Nickel chloride	129.60		0.001	
Nickel sulfate	154.75		<0.000009	
Silver nitrate	169.87		<0.00035[b]	
Sodium chromate	161.97		0.0021[b]	

Note. From Reference 192.
[a] Permeability coefficients calculated using equation presented in Leung and Paustenbach (192).
[b] All the observed permeability coefficients were obtained by using in vitro techniques except those denoted with superscript *b*, which were determined in vivo.

of cocontaminants (e.g., oil and other organics), and the concentration of the chemical contaminant in the media (321). The bioavailability of a chemical in soil will usually be affected by its physicochemical properties. High-molecular-weight chemicals tend to bind to soil/dust and be less water soluble, while smaller molecules will frequently be water soluble, less tightly bound, and relatively bioavailable (159,215). The cutaneous bioavailability of perhaps 20 to 30 chemicals in soils has been determined in animals (159,321,326,358,359,420). These studies show that different media and different chemicals can yield dramatically different cutaneous bioavailabilities. The results of these studies, for example, produce values of bioavailability for different chemicals that range from 0.001 to 3% for chemicals in soil.

Skin Surface Area

There is an abundance of information about the surface area of different portions of the body. One simple approach is to use the "rule of nines" for estimating the surface area of the human body (334): the head and neck are 9%, upper limbs are each 9%, lower limbs are each 18%, and the front or back of the trunk is 18% (254). The U.S. EPA has estimated an exposed surface area (arms, hands, legs, and feet) of 2900 cm^2 for children 0 to 2 yr old; 3400 cm^2 for children 2 to 6 yr old; and 2940 cm^2 for adults (an adult is assumed to wear pants, an open-neck short-sleeve shirt, shoes, and no hat or gloves) (377). When assessing chemical exposure in the ambient environment, most of the necessary surface area information can be found in the U.S. EPA *Exposure Factors Handbook* (386). Table 9.5 presents the skin surface areas commonly used when conducting exposure assessments (334). A distribution plot of skin area versus body weight has been developed (42).

Soil Loading on the Skin

A key factor to consider when estimating dermal uptake via soil is the soil-to-skin adherence rate. Values of 0.5 to 0.6 mg/cm^2 and 0.2 to 2.8 mg/cm^2 have been reported for adults and children, respectively (59, 96,259,286). Recent works by Finley et al. (119), Kissel et al. (177), and Holmes et al. (156) have built on prior studies to show that dermal loading can vary significantly among different activities and different people. Based on data collected in past studies, in 1992 the U.S. EPA suggested a default soil-to-skin adherence rate of 0.2 mg/cm^2 (median) and 1.0 mg/cm^2 (95th percentile) for an adult. The recent edition of the *Exposure Factors Handbook* gives considerable attention to this topic (382,384). One approach to improving dermal uptake calculations is to use area-weighted adherence factors as recently suggested by the U.S. EPA.

Table 9.5
Representative surface areas of the human body (Adult male)

Body portion	Area (cm^2)
Whole body	18,000
Head and neck	1,620
Head	1,260
Back of head	320
Neck	360
Back of neck	90
Torso	6,480
Back	2,520
Chest	2,520
Sides	1,440
Upper limbs	3,240
Upper arms (elbow–shoulder)	1,440
Lower arms (elbow–wrist)	1,080
Hands	720
Palms	360
Upper arms (back of)	360
Lower arms (back of)	270
Lower limbs	6,480
Thighs	3,240
Lower legs (knee–ankle)	2,160
Feet	1,080
Soles of feet	540
Thighs (back of)	810
Lower legs (back of)	540
Perineum	180

Note. Data adapted from Reference 334.

Interpreting Wipe Samples

In some workplaces, wipe sampling has been conducted historically to assess the degree of surface contamination. Hospitals were among the first occupational settings, as long ago as 1940, to rely on this method to determine microbial levels in operating rooms. In pharmaceutical manufacturing, wipe sampling has been used as an indicator of hygienic conditions since the 1960s. The health physics profession has utilized wipe samples extensively as an indicator of the need for better housekeeping and decontamination; this group performed most of the early work in quantifying the relationship of wipe sample concentrations to dermal and oral uptake.

Over the years, few papers have discussed how to collect and interpret wipe samples (60,109,110,114,176,210). When the primary effect of a chemical is skin discoloration, allergic contact dermatitis (ACD), or chloracne, wipe sampling was nearly always the preferred approach for assessing the acceptability of the workplace (rather than relying on air samples). Beginning in the 1980s, a substantial number of wipe samples were collected in office buildings contaminated with dioxins and furans after electrical transformer fires to estimate the potential human exposure (222). The interpretation of these data was often mishandled and, as a result, a number of decisions by risk managers were less than optimal, resulting in significant unnecessary expenses. Today, better approaches are available.

Although wipe sampling data have generally been used as an indicator of cleanliness (60), these data can also be used to estimate systemic uptake of a contaminant if the degree of skin contact with the contaminated surfaces is known. While historical wipe sampling methods were rather imprecise, they were useful for obtaining a rough estimate of the possible exposure, which could be refined later by other means, such as biological monitoring.

If one knows that wipe sampling results are representative of what comes into contact with the hands (i.e., actually able to be absorbed), then the procedures for converting wipe sample data to estimates of systemic uptake are straightforward (35). For example, if one knows the number of times a surface (e.g., valve handle, instrument controller, or drum) is touched, the surface area of the hand touching these items (usually the palm), and the percutaneous chemical absorption rate, then the uptake can be estimated using wipe sample information. The best wipe sampling data were those collected in a reliable and consistent manner, with a focus on the mass per unit area. Hand wash sampling is often more representative than wipe samples (115).

Until recently, no standardized approaches existed for conducting wipe sampling. Differences in the use of wetting agent (acetone, methylene chloride, water, saline, isopropanol, and ethanol) and sampling media (paper, cotton, and synthetic fibers) produced drastically different results. In some procedures, especially those that used methylene chloride (in which the paint was concurrently stripped by the solvent), the chemical in the paint matrix was assumed to be bioavailable (a completely unreasonable assumption). Clearly, much of the previous work, which measured the amount of chemical released following aggressive scrubbing of the contaminated surfaces with detergent or solvent, did not reflect a realistic exposure scenario. Thus, there has been a need for standard techniques that attempt to mimic the conditions in which a hand comes into contact with a contaminated surface (210). Some of the techniques have been developed by hygienists involved in agricultural exposure assessment (179,187,188,277).

In an attempt to fill this need, fairly sophisticated work to standardize these procedures has been conducted by researchers at Rutgers University. In fact, some of their wipe sampling procedures and devices have been patented (197). They have also developed a dry contact sampling device (198) that offers promise for understanding the hazard from surface dusts. The implications from recent wipe sampling research are that: (1) a minimum number of samples is needed to have statistical confidence; (2) the pressure applied to the cloth during sample collection should be standardized; (3) neat solvent should not be used as a collection media; (4) the size of the sample area needs to be sufficient to collect enough contaminant for quantification; and (5) the technique should be validated by using glove analyses.

Estimating the Dermal Uptake of Chemicals in Soil

One of the most frequently occurring exposure scenarios involving environmental exposures is that of contaminated soil (259). Unfortunately, dermal uptake of chemicals found on soil has rarely been evaluated experimentally (192). A model to estimate the amount of an organic chemical in soil that crosses the stratum corneum into the underlying tissue layer has been developed (215). To differentiate this absorptive process from bioavailability, which also includes transport into blood, McKone refers to the percentage of available chemical as an uptake fraction. The approach is based on the fugacity concept, which measures the tendency of a chemical to move from one phase to another. Because the skin has a fat content of about 10% and soil has an organic carbon content on the order of 1 to 4%, an organic chemical in soil placed on the skin will move from the soil to the underlying adipose layers of the skin. However, this transfer depends on the period of time between deposition on the skin and removal by evaporative processes. The mass-transfer coefficients of the soil-to-skin layer and the soil-to-air layer define the rate at which these competing processes occur.

Results of this model suggest that the chemical uptake fraction in soil varies with the exposure duration, soil deposition rate, and physical properties of the chemical, and is particularly sensitive to the values of K_{ow}, as well as the mass or depth of soil deposited on the skin. When the amount of soil on the skin is low ($<1\ mg/cm^2$), a high uptake fraction, approaching unity in some cases, is predicted. With higher soil loading ($20\ mg/cm^2$), an uptake of only 0.5% is predicted. Because of the diverse variations of the uptake fraction with soil loading, results obtained from experiments with a single soil loading should be applied with caution to human soil-exposure scenarios.

The dermal uptake of chemicals in soil is a complex process, but its behavior is predictable if the controlling factors are accounted for and quantified (192,215). In situations involving a relatively thin layer of a chemical on the skin for purposes of screening assessments, a few generalizations can be made. First, for chemicals with a high K_{ow} and a low air:water partition coefficient, it is reasonable to assume 100% uptake in 12 h. Second, for chemicals with an air:water partition coefficient greater than 0.01, the uptake fraction is unlikely to exceed 40% in 12 h. Third, for chemicals with an air:water partition coefficient greater than 0.1, one can expect less than 3% uptake in 12 h. In most occupational settings, contaminated soil will rarely be in contact with the skin for greater than 4 h before it is washed off. Consequently, this should be accounted for when attempting to predict systemic uptake.

Dermal Uptake of Contaminants in Soil

To estimate chemical uptake, one needs to know the percutaneous absorption rate, the exposed skin area, the chemical concentration, and the exposure duration. One scenario would be a thin film of chemical on the skin. For this finite-dose scenario, Eq. (5) is useful:

$$\text{Uptake (mg)} = (C)(A)(x)(f)(t) \qquad (5)$$

where C is the concentration of the chemical (mg/cm^2), A the skin surface area (cm^2), x the thickness of the film layer (cm), f the absorption rate (percent per hour), and t the duration of exposure (h).

Another scenario would be an excess amount of a chemical on the skin (i.e., infinite dose). In this case, the thickness of the chemical layer is not calculated and steady-state kinetics are assumed. For a chemical in an aqueous or gaseous media:

$$\text{Uptake (mg)} = (C)(A)(K_p)(t)(d) \qquad (6)$$

where K_p is the permeability coefficient (cm/h) and d is the distribution factor.

For a neat liquid chemical,

$$\text{Uptake (mg)} = (A)(J)(t) \qquad (7)$$

where J is the flux of chemical (mg/cm^2-h).

The U.S. EPA has suggested using the following equation for estimating percutaneous absorption of chemicals in soil (376):

$$\text{Uptake (mg)} = (C)(A)(r)(B) \qquad (8)$$

where C is the concentration of the chemical in soil (mg/g), A the skin surface area (cm^2), r the soil-to-skin adherence rate (g/cm^2), and B the cutaneous bioavailability (unitless).

Example Calculation 3: Skin Uptake of a Chemical in Soil

A person gardens with soil contaminated on average with 250 ng dioxin/soil (250 ppb). Assuming that the person's hands and lower arms are in contact with the soil, the soil loading is equal to 0.2 mg/cm^2, and the cutaneous bioavailability of dioxin in soil is 1% (321), what is the plausible uptake of dioxin by this person [using Eq. (8)]? Assume that the person washes his or her hands every 4 h and the exposed area of skin is 1800 cm^2.

$$\text{Uptake (ng)} = (C)(A)(r)(B)$$

where:

$$C = 250\ \text{ng/g}$$
$$A = 1800\ \text{cm}^2$$
$$r = 0.2\ \text{mg/cm}^2$$
$$B = 0.01$$

By substitution:

$$\text{Uptake} = \left(\frac{250\ \text{ng TCDD}}{1\ \text{g soil}}\right)\left(\frac{0.2\ \text{mg soil}}{\text{cm}^2\ \text{skin}}\right)\left(\frac{1\ \text{g}}{10^3\ \text{mg}}\right) \times (1800\ \text{cm}^2\ \text{skin})(0.01) = 0.9\ \text{ng TCDD}$$

Note: A preferred method for performing this calculation, if data are available, is to use a flux rate (ng/cm^2-h) for the chemical. Assume that rate is 500 ng/cm^2-h:

$$\text{Uptake (ng)} = (C)(J)(A)(t)$$

where

$$J = 500\ \text{ng/cm}^2\text{-h}$$
$$t = 4\ \text{h}$$

By substitution:

$$\text{Update} = \left(\frac{250\ \text{ng TCDD}}{1\ \text{g soil}}\right)\left(\frac{1\ \text{g}}{10^9\ \text{ng}}\right)(1800\ \text{cm}^2\ \text{skin})(4\text{h}) \times \left(\frac{500\ \text{ng}}{\text{cm}^2 - \text{h}}\right) = 0.9\ \text{ng TCDD}$$

Uptake of Chemicals in an Aqueous Matrix

Published estimates of dermal uptake of chemicals in water have generally focused on evaluating workplace or environmental exposure. A number of different scenarios have been evaluated (50,117a,168,173,314). If interested in the possible uptake of a chemical present in water, the amount of chlordane absorbed through the skin by a man swimming for 4 h in water containing 1 ppb chloroform has been estimated (168). This is useful to compare various approaches. For example, the amount of chloroform absorbed by a boy swimming for 3 h in water has been calculated (277). Some have compared the amounts absorbed through the skin during a 10-min shower versus a 20-min bath with water containing 1 ppb 1,1,1-trichlorethane (171).

About 10 yr ago, it was recognized that in the indoor environment, oral exposure to volatile chemicals present in drinking water may not necessarily represent the vast majority of the risk. Specifically, it was found that inhalation exposure due to the release of vapors from liquids to which people were in close contact could be relatively high. For example, comparisons have been made of the chloroform concentration in exhaled breath after a shower to that after an inhalation-only exposure (168). The concentration after showering was about twice that after the inhalation-only exposure, indicating that the absorbed dose from the skin is approximately equivalent to that from inhalation absorption.

Example Calculation 4: Skin Uptake of a Chemical From Water

A person has filled his swimming pool with shallow well water contaminated with 0.002 mg/ml (2 ppb) toluene. What is the plausible dermal uptake of toluene while swimming in the contaminated water for half an hour? Assume that 18,000 cm^2 of skin is exposed and the K_p is 1.01 cm/h. From Eq. (6):

$$\text{Uptake} = (C)(A)(K_p)(t)(d)$$

where

$$C = 0.002\,\text{mg/ml}$$
$$A = 18,000\,\text{cm}^2$$
$$K_p = 1.01\,\text{cm/h}$$
$$t = 0.5\,\text{h}$$
$$d = \text{distribution factor (1 ml of water covers 1 cm}^3\text{)}$$

By substitution:

$$\text{Uptake} = (0.002\,\text{mg/ml})(18{,}000\,\text{cm}^2)(1.01\,\text{cm/h})(0.5\,\text{h}) \times (1\,\text{ml water}/1\,\text{cm}^3) = 18\,\text{mg}$$

Percutaneous Absorption of Liquid Solvents

While the percutaneous absorption of chemical solutes generally proceeds by simple diffusion, the skin uptake of neat chemical liquids is not necessarily exclusively governed by Fick's law. Consequently, the uptake of neat liquid through the skin needs to be estimated using direct in vivo skin contact techniques. Table 9.6 presents the percutaneous absorption rates of some neat industrial liquid solvents that have been determined in human volunteer studies.

Table 9.6
Absorption rates of some neat industrial liquid chemicals in human skin in vivo

Chemical	Absorption rate (mg/cm^2-h)
Aniline	0.2–0.7
Benzene	0.24–0.4
2-Butoxyethanol	0.05–0.68
2-(2-Butoxyethoxy)ethanol	0.035
Carbon disulfide	9.7
Dimethylformamide	9.4
Ethylbenzene	22–23
2-Ethoxyethanol	0.796
2-(2-Ethyoxyethoxy)ethanol	0.125
Methanol	11.5
2-Methoxyethanol	2.82
2-(2-Methoxyethoxy)ethanol	0.206
Methyl butyl ketone	0.25–0.48
Nitrobenzene	2
Styrene	9–15
Toluene	14–23
Xylene (mixed)	4.5–9.6
m-Xylene	0.12–0.15

Note. From Reference 192.

Example Calculation 5: Skin Uptake of a Neat Liquid Chemical

Due to carelessness or a leak, the inside of a glove becomes contaminated with 2-methoxyethanol. How much can be absorbed if a worker wears the contaminated glove on one hand for half an hour? Assume the surface area of exposed skin is 360 cm^2 and the flux rate is 2.82 mg/cm^2-h. From Eq. (7),

$$\text{Uptake} = (A)(J)(t)$$

where

$$A = 360\,\text{cm}^2$$
$$J = 2.82\,\text{mg/cm}^2\text{-h}$$
$$t = 0.5\,\text{h}$$

By substitution,

$$\text{Uptake} = (360\,\text{cm}^2)(2.82\,\text{mg/cm}^2\text{-h})(0.5\,\text{h}) = 508\,\text{mg}$$

To understand the relative hazard from skin exposure versus inhalation exposure, the dose of 2-methoxyethanol absorbed by the same worker via inhalation for 8 h (10 m^3

Table 9.7
Percutaneous absorption rates for chemical vapors in vivo

Chemical	Skin update in combined exposure (%)[a]	Permeability coefficient K_p (cm/h)	
		Rat	Human
Styrene	9.4	1.75	0.35–1.42
m-Xylene	3.9	0.72	0.24–0.26
Toluene	3.7	0.72	0.18
Perchloroethylene	3.5	0.67	0.17
Benzene	0.8	0.15	0.08
Halothane	0.2	0.05	
Hexane	0.1	0.03	
Isoflurane	0.1	0.03	
Methylene chloride		0.28	
Dibromomethane		1.32	
Bromochloromethane		0.79	
Phenol			15.74–17.59
Nitrobenzene			11.1
1,1,1-Trichloroethane			0.01

Note. Rat data from Reference 214.
[a]In combined exposure, rats are simultaneously absorbing chemical vapors by inhalation and by whole-body absorption through the skin.

of air inhaled), assuming a threshold limit value (TLV) of $16\,mg/cm^3$, can be estimated and compared to the dose due to inhalation exposure. Assume an 80% inhalation uptake efficiency.

$$\text{Inhalation uptake} = (16\,mg/m^3)(10\,m^3)(0.8) = 128\,mg$$

Thus, the uptake of 2-methoxyethanol following 30 min of skin exposure of a single hand can be as much as 4 times that from inhalation for 8 h at the TLV concentration, a presumably safe level of exposure. From this example, it is clear that the cutaneous route of entry can, in some situations, significantly contribute to the total absorbed dose, especially in the occupational setting.

Percutaneous Absorption of Chemicals in the Vapor Phase

Until the 1990s, it was generally assumed that the plausible dose resulting from vapors absorbed through the skin was too low to pose a hazard. Only a few studies have examined this issue (173,184,391). A few clinical reports have encouraged some limited in vivo research to evaluate the absorption of several chemicals in the gaseous phase through the human skin (Table 9.7). A chamber system to measure the whole-body percutaneous absorption of chemical vapors in rats has been described by McDougal et al. (214), and this approach has produced some interesting results (208). In this system, chemical flux across the skin is determined from the chemical concentration in blood during exposure by using a PBPK model. In most cases, vapor absorption through the skin amounts to less than 10% of the total dose received from a combined skin and inhalation exposure. While there is good agreement between the rat and human in the relative ranking of the permeability coefficients among the chemicals studied, for an individual chemical the rat skin appears to be two to four times more permeable than the human skin. These observations are consistent with previously reported data (22,34,274,275,321).

It is generally not necessary to account for the contribution from percutaneous uptake of vapors when the occupational exposure limit (OEL) is used as a guideline for acceptable exposure, because uptake of vapors through the skin is usually inherent in the data; that is, the studies of animals or humans from which data were collected were usually exposed via inhalation (whole body) so dermal uptake of the vapor occurred. However, although good work practices and the law require that situations where persons are placed in atmospheres that are life-threatening, sometimes in emergency situations, airline (supplied air) respirators or self-contained breathing apparatus (SCBA) are worn in environments containing chemical concentrations 10-fold to 1000-fold greater than the TLV. In these cases, it is important to account for vapor uptake through either exposed or covered skin.

Although nearly all data on vapor absorption involve bare skin, the role of clothing in preventing skin uptake has occasionally been evaluated. For example, a study of workers wearing denim clothing indicated no decreased uptake of phenol vapors (274), but found a 20% and 40% reduction in uptake of nitrobenzene (273) and aniline vapors, respectively (100). Although standard clothing may slightly decrease the amount of a chemical transferred from air through the skin, it can be a significant source of continuous exposure if the clothing has been contaminated.

Example Calculation 6: Skin Uptake of a Chemical Vapor

Assume that a person needs to repair a leaking pump, so he enters a room wearing an airline respirator. Assume the room contains 500 mg/m^3 nitrobenzene (100 times the current TLV) and it takes 30 min to repair the pump. How much nitrobenzene might be absorbed through the skin?

The head, neck, and upper limbs are assumed to be exposed (surface area = 4860 cm^2), and the rest of the body (surface area = 13,140 cm^2) is covered with clothing. Assume the percutaneous K_p of nitrobenzene is 11.1 cm/h, and that the clothing has reduced the skin uptake rate of vapors by about 20% (273). From Example 5.

$$\text{Uptake} = (C)(A)(K_p)(t)$$

$$\begin{aligned}\text{Uptake through exposed skin} &= (500\,\text{mg/m}^3)(4860\,\text{cm}^2)\\ &\times (11.1\,\text{cm/h})(0.5\,\text{h})\\ &\times (1\,\text{m}^3/10^6\,\text{cm}^3)\\ &= 13.5\,\text{mg}\end{aligned}$$

$$\begin{aligned}\text{Uptake through clothing} &= (500\,\text{mg/m}^3)(13{,}140\,\text{cm}^2)\\ &\times (11.1\,\text{cm/h})(0.8)(0.5\,\text{h})\\ &\times (1\,\text{m}^3/10^6\,\text{cm}^3)\\ &= 29\,\text{mg}\end{aligned}$$

$$\text{Total uptake} = 13.5 + 29 = 42.5\,\text{mg}$$

From this example, it is clear that if one enters an environment containing a high concentration of an airborne contaminant, even if a supplied-air respirator is worn, the degree of skin uptake of the vapor may be worthy of evaluation to ensure that the worker is protected. These kinds of calculations sometimes have to be conducted in difficult work environments that are in a state of alert (e.g., submarines, chemical plants during emergency situations, etc.).

ESTIMATING INTAKE VIA INGESTION

If the appropriate information is available, estimating the intake of various chemicals due to ingestion is a relatively straightforward exercise. In general, one is concerned with the ingestion of the following media: drinking water, other liquids, food, soil, and house dust. Drinking-water contamination may occur because of soil contamination from leaking underground storage tanks, landfills, or hazardous waste sites, as well as discharges from contaminated streams or water transport systems. Nearly all foods in Western society contain a number of intentional and unintentional chemicals, including pesticide residues, naturally occurring chemicals, and food additives that serve as preservatives or enhancers of taste or visual appeal. Soils are ingested as a result of eating incompletely washed vegetables, hand-to-mouth contact, and through direct ingestion by children. Soils are also ingested when particles too large to reach the lower respiratory tract are inhaled (and then are swallowed). House dust contaminated with a number of chemicals can be ingested due to contact with foods and hand-to-mouth activities (267).

Estimating Intake of Chemicals in Drinking Water

Estimating the magnitude of the potential dose of toxics from drinking water requires knowledge of the amount of water ingested, the chemical concentrations in the water, and the chemical bioavailability in the gastrointestinal tract. The amount of water ingested per day varies with each person and is usually related to the amount of physical activity. A good deal of literature has addressed the amount of water ingested by persons engaged in different kinds of activities (364,366,386).

Currently, the U.S. EPA suggests that when little is known about the specifics of exposure, a value of 2 L/d for adults and 1 L/d for infants (body weight of less than 10 kg) should be used as the default value. These rates include drinking water consumed in the form of juices and other beverages.

Numerous studies cited in the U.S. EPA *Exposure Factors Handbook* (383,384) have generated data on drinking-water intake rates. In general, these sources support the U.S. EPA use of 2 L/d for adults and 1 L/d for children as upper percentile tap-water intake rates. Many of the studies have reported fluid intake rates for both total fluids and tap water. Total fluid intake is defined as consumption of all types of fluids including tap water, milk, soft drinks, alcoholic beverages, and water intrinsic to purchased foods. Total tap water is defined as water consumed directly from the tap as a bev-

Table 9.8
Summary of tap-water intake by age

Age group	Intake (ml/d) Mean	Intake (ml/d) 10th–90th Percentiles	Intake (ml/kg-d) Mean	Intake (ml/kg-d) 10th–90th Percentiles
Infants (<1 yr)	302	0–649	43.5	0–100
Children (1–10 yr)	736	286–1,294	35.5	12.5–64.4
Teens (11–19 yr)	965	353–1,701	18.2	6.5–32.3
Adults (20–64 yr)	1,366	559–2,268	19.9	8.0–33.7
Adults (65+ yr)	1,459	751–2,287	21.8	10.9–34.7
All ages	1,193	423–2,092	22.6	8.2–39.8

Note. From Reference 108.

erage or used to prepare foods and beverages (i.e., coffee, tea, frozen juices, soups, etc.). Data for both consumption categories are presented in numerous publications. Table 9.8 presents typical information reported from these studies (377).

All currently available studies on drinking water intake are based on short-term survey data. Although short-term data may be suitable for obtaining mean intake values that are representative of both short- and long-term consumption patterns, upper percentile values may be different for short-term and long-term data because there is generally more variability in short-term surveys. It should also be noted that most of the currently available drinking water surveys are based on recall. This may be a source of uncertainty in the estimated intake rates because of the subjective nature of this type of survey technique (377).

To estimate the intake of toxics via direct ingestion of drinking water, the calculation is straightforward:

$$\text{Intake} = (V)(C)(B)$$

where V is the volume of water (L/d), C the concentration of chemical in water (μg/L), and B the bioavailability (unitless).

One of the more interesting observations of the past 15 yr is that ingestion of contaminated drinking water is sometimes not the primary route of exposure to the toxicant in drinking water. Uptake of volatile chemicals via inhalation can be nearly as great in some homes as ingestion, which is the result of the presence of these chemicals in air due to showering, off-gases from the dishwasher, and other opportunities for volatilization of the chemical (168,171,173,208,391).

The Importance of Soil Ingestion When Estimating Human Exposure

Between 1980 and 1995, predicted risks associated with the ingestion of contaminated soil were the primary drivers for remediating many (if not most) hazardous waste sites. As discussed by Paustenbach et al. (259), there was no better example than the site in Times Beach, MO. Hundreds of millions of dollars can be needed to clean up these kinds of sites to levels that would not pose a significant risk if children actually ate significant quantities of contaminated soil. Because of the expense of remediation, a good deal of research has been conducted over the past 15 yr to attempt to quantitatively understand this route of exposure.

Clearly, the ingestion of soil and house dust is a potential source of human exposure to toxicants (296–298). The potential for contaminant exposure via this source is greater for children because they are more likely to ingest greater quantities of soil than adults. Inadvertent soil ingestion among children may occur through the mouthing of objects or hands. Mouthing behavior is considered to be a normal phase of childhood development. Adults may also ingest soil or dust particles that adhere to food, cigarettes, or their hands. Deliberate soil ingestion is defined as pica and is considered to be relatively uncommon. Because normal, inadvertent soil ingestion is more prevalent and data for individuals with pica behavior are limited, the focus of most exposure assessments is on normal levels of soil ingestion that occur as a result of mouthing or unintentional hand-to-mouth activity (73,174,259,377).

Mouthing activities by children, which are generally accepted as normal and commonplace [e.g., Barltrop (23) estimated that almost 80% of all children at age

1 yr exhibited mouthing tendencies], are potential exposure routes to trace amounts of soil and/or dust adhering to fingers, hands, and objects placed in the mouth. The available data indicate that soil exposure occurs through several indirect routes:

1. Soil contributes to house dust (e.g., by local dust deposition, and mud and dirt carried in by shoes and pets, etc.).
2. House dust (fine particles) adheres to objects and to children's hands.
3. Children ingest dust particles when sucking and mouthing objects and fingers.

Obviously, in some situations, exposure may be direct (a child playing outdoors may eat dirt directly). In other situations, oral exposure to chemicals in soil may occur via contamination of domestic water supplies or contamination of fruit and vegetable produce grown onsite. However, the content and concentration of dusts in the indoor environment, which may represent the most important source of indirect exposure to soil, need to be better understood (107,267).

Many studies have been conducted to estimate the amount of soil ingested by children. Most of the early studies attempted to quantify the amount of soil ingested by measuring the amount of dirt present on children's hands and making generalizations based on behavior. More recently, soil intake studies have been conducted using a methodology that measures trace elements in feces and soil that are believed to be poorly absorbed in the gut. These measurements are used to estimate the amount of soil ingested over a specified period of time.

Studies of Soil Ingestion

In light of the importance of soil ingestion for estimating human exposure to contaminated soil, several literature surveys have been undertaken to identify the typical amount of soil consumed by children and adults (107,174,259,377,382). Research evaluating lead uptake by children from ingestion of contaminated soil, paint chips, dust, and plaster provides the best source of information. Walter et al. (417) estimated that a normal child typically ingests very small quantities of dust or dirt between the ages of 0 to 2 yr, the largest quantities between 2 to 7 yr, and nearly insignificant amounts thereafter. In the classic text by Cooper (71), it was noted that the desire of children to eat dirt or place inedible objects in their mouths becomes established in the second year of life and disappears more or less spontaneously by the age of 4 to 5 yr. A study by Charney et al. (65) also indicated that mouthing tends to begin at about 18 mo and continues through 72 mo, depending on several factors such as nutritional and economic status, as well as race. Work by Sayre et al. (310) indicated that ages 2 to 6 yr are the important years, but that "intensive mouthing diminishes after 2 to 3 years of age."

An important distinction that is often blurred is the difference between the ingestion of very small quantities of dirt due to mouthing tendencies and the disease known as pica. Children who intentionally eat large quantities of dirt, plaster, or paint chips (1 to 10 g/d), and consequently are at greater risk of developing health problems, can be said to suffer from the disease known as pica. This disease is known as geophagia if the craving is for dirt alone. Geophagia, rather than pica, is generally of greatest concern in areas with contaminated soil.

Duggan and Williams (99) have summarized the literature on the amount of lead ingested through dust and dirt. In their opinion, a quantity of 50 mg lead was the best estimate for daily ingestion of dust by children. Lepow et al. (191) estimated an ingestion rate equal to 100 to 250 mg/d (specifically, 10 mg ingested 10 to 25 times a day). Barltrop (23) and Barltrop et al. (25) also estimated that the potential uptake of soils and dusts by a toddler is about 100 mg/d. In a Dutch study, the amount of lead on hands ranged from 4 to 12 ng. By assuming maximum lead concentrations of 500 ng/g (concentrations were typically lower) and complete ingestion of the contents adsorbed to a child's hand on 10 separate occasions, the amount of ingested dirt would equal 240 mg. Thus, in order to eat 10,000 mg soil/d, the rate once suggested by the Centers for Disease Control (174), children would have to place their hands into their mouths 410 times a day, a rate that seems improbable (232,252).

A report by the National Research Council (232) addressing the hazards of lead suggested a rate of 40 mg/d. Day et al. (88) measured the amount of dirt transferred from children's hands (age range from 1 to 3 yr) to a sticky sweet, and estimated a daily intake of 2 to 20 sweets would lead to dirt intake of 10 to 1000 mg/d. Bryce-Smith (36) estimated 33 mg/d. In its document addressing lead in air, the U.S. EPA assumed that children ate 50 mg/d of household dust, 40 mg/d of street dust, and 10 mg/d of dust derived from their parents' clothing (i.e., a total of 100 mg/d).

Kimbrough et al. (174) used a series of assumptions about soil exposure when estimating the possible risks of contaminated soil at Times Beach, MO, based upon unpublished observations about children's behavior and hand–mouth activity. A few years later, Kimbrough noted that their estimate of up to 10,000 mg/d was clearly an exaggeration and her personal estimate would be nearer 50 mg/d (107).

La Goy (186) based his soil ingestion estimates upon a review of the literature, in particular using empirical data derived by Binder et al. (28) and Van Wijnen et al. (397). Similarly, Paustenbach et al. (264) based their estimates upon a review of the literature, including the mass-balance quantitative study conducted by Calabrese et al. (55).

De Silva (90,91) adopted a different approach that may overcome some of the uncertainties inherent in the assumptions of the above indirect studies. She applied a "slope factor" increase of 0.6 mg/dl in children's blood lead levels for each 1000 ppm increase in soil lead [this factor was developed by Barltrop et al. (25) following his work on blood lead levels in children from villages on old mining sites]. De Silva then deduced that an increase of 0.6 mg/dl in blood indicates an extra oral intake of 3.75 mg lead/d, based upon a U.S. EPA (367) calculation that an increase of 1.0 mg lead/d in children's diets produces an increase of 0.16 in the blood lead level. With a soil lead value of 1000 ppm, 3.75 mg soil would contain 3.75 mg lead, suggesting that 3.75 mg/d (say 4 mg) of soil was ingested by the children. However, the slope factor used here may not be the most appropriate, since mining soil wastes typically have larger sized particles, which tends to decrease lead bioavailability compared with soil contaminated by lead smelter activity, and therefore reduces the slope factor.

A major step forward beyond estimating soil ingestion using indirect measurements has been the attempt to study tracer elements found in soil with elements measured in the urine and feces of children. Several studies have been conducted thus far that have used this approach (28,53,55–57,90,91,336–339). One early tracer study evaluated the amount of soil eaten by 24 hospitalized and nursery-school children. They analyzed the amount of aluminum, titanium, and acid-soluble residue in the feces of children aged 2 to 4 yr. The data were normally distributed. They found an average of 105 mg/d of soil in the feces of nursery children, and 49 mg/d in hospitalized children. Even with the limited number of children in the study, the difference between the two groups was significant ($p < .01$). If the value for the hospitalized children is assumed to be the background level because these substances are taken in from nonsoil sources (e.g., diet and toothpastes), the estimated average amount of soil ingested by the nursery school children would be 56 mg/d. This value is in the lower range of estimates in the literature and supports the use of 100 mg/d as a conservative uptake of soil by toddlers (ages 2 to 4 yr).

There have been two major studies completed by Calabrese et al. (53,55–57; 52,58,336,341). In the first, they quantitatively evaluated 6 different tracer elements in the stools of 65 school children aged 2 to 4 yr. They attempted to evaluate children from diverse socioeconomic backgrounds. This study, conducted in Massachusetts, was more definitive than prior investigations because they analyzed the children's diets, assayed for the presence of tracers in the diapers, assayed house dust and surrounding soil, and corrected for the pharmacokinetics of the tracer materials.

In the second study, soil ingestion estimates were obtained from a stratified, simple random sample of 64 children aged 1–4 years residing on a superfund site in Montana. The study was conducted during the month of September for 7 consecutive days (58). Soil ingestion was estimated by each soil tracer via traditional methods as well as by an improved approach using five trace elements (Al, Si, Ti, Y, and Zr), called the Best Tracer Method (BTM), which substantially corrects for error due to misalignment of tracer input and output as well as error occurring from ingestion of tracers from nonfood, nonsoil sources, while being insensitive to the particle size of the soil/dust ingested. According to the BTM, the median soil ingestion was less than 1 mg/day while the upper 95% was 160 mg/day. No significant age (1 year vs. 2, vs. 3) or sex-related differences in soil ingestion were observed. These estimates are lower than estimates observed in the first study, which was conducted in New England during September and October.

Based on the series of papers by the researchers at the University of Massachusetts (53,55–57; 52,336), a few generalizations can be made. These studies were difficult to conduct and interpret. Second, only children from a single climate were studied, and it can be expected that rates vary with the amount of time spent indoors and outdoors. Third, only a handful of children have been studied (less than 500), so it is not possible to characterize the percentage of children who might tend to ingest large quantities of soil or house dust. Fourth, the relevant amount of soil or house dust ingested indoors versus outdoors is not known yet. In most cases, the contaminant concentrations in dust can be quite different when found in a carpet versus the yard (267). Fifth, although there is some degree of uncertainty in the results of the various studies, it appears that a best estimate of soil intake for most children resides in the area of 10 to 25 mg/d. It appears that perhaps 1 to 5% of the children may ingest much larger amounts during certain days or weeks (e.g., 2000 mg/d), but these tendencies do not occur on a chronic basis.

It has been proposed that one can estimate uptake over the period of one year and they have proposed lifetime values (337). Recent work by Calabrese and Stanek (52) suggests that prior work yielded reasonable results for purposes of risk assessment. Most of the values discussed here are presented in Table 9.9. As mentioned previously, another area of research impacting exposure assessments of contaminated soil, which has been and continues to be actively pursued, is the bioavailability of the contaminant in the soil matrix (159).

Table 9.9
Values for childhood and adult soil ingestion rates that have been used in health risk assessments conducted between 1984 and 2000

Author	Age	Soil and dust (mg/d)
Barltrop (24)	2–6 yr	100
Lepow et al. (190)	2–6 yr	100–250
Day et al. (88)	2–6 yr	10–1000
Kimbrough et al. (174) (CDC)	0–9 mo	0
	9–18 mo	1000
	1.5–3.5 yr	10,000
	3.5–5 yr	1000
	5+ yr	100
Hawley (149)	0–2 yr	Negligible
	2–6 yr	90
	6–18 yr	21
	18–70 yr	57
La Goy (186)	1–6 yr	500 (max.)
	1–6 yr	100 (ave.)
Calabrese et al. (55)	1–4 yr	27–85 (mean)
		9–16 (median)
Paustenbach (262)	2–4 yr	25–50
	Adults	2–5
De Silva (91)	Children	~4
U.S. EPA (386)	Children	200
Calabrese & Stanek (52)	Children	30–60 (best estimate)

What is the Significance of Pica?

There appears to be some confusion in the literature over what constitutes "pica." Pica can be defined as "the habitual ingestion of substances not normally regarded as edible," but some authors have included mouthing and sucking activities in their definitions (201). Others appear to assume that all children with pica necessarily must be habitual soil eaters. In fact, pica behavior may be generalized to the ingestion of many different (nonfood) substances, or may be specific to one substance such as paper, soap, or earth. It is likely that repetitive pica behavior specifically for dirt, or habitual "geophagia," rarely occurs in the general population in most industrialized countries (84,350).

Pica should, therefore, be considered a "normal" temporary phenomenon in some children. In the general population, the prevalence of both mouthing and pica, and the range of articles ingested, has been shown to decrease with age (23). In the 1-yr-old age group, 78% of children mouthed objects and 35% ingested them; this behavior decreased at the age of 4 yr, when 33% were mouthing and only 6% had pica.

It is also relevant to note that in certain circumstances, pica for soil may be culturally determined (such as eating clay, high in silicon and aluminum, for its medicinal properties in the relief of stomach discomfort and diarrhea by some Aborigines; or the custom of eating earth during pregnancy in certain cultures) (107). For example, some women in the southern portions of the United States report a craving for and eat certain clays during pregnancy.

Pica may be associated with physical disorders, including iron deficiency. However, it has been debated whether pica represents a cause or an effect of these deficiencies. Pica can also be associated with mental illness. It has also been reported that 25% of institutionalized mentally handicapped adults indulged in pica of one kind or another (including bizarre objects ranging from rags and string to rocks, insects, and feces) (84).

Calabrese and Stanek (52) have indicated that in their studies, they have observed great variability in soil ingestion by children. They have noted, for example, that some children are highly variable in their soil ingestion activities, displaying little propensity for soil ingestion on one day while ingesting copious amounts the next day. While there has not been any concerted focus on the soil pica child, the available data indicate that some children ingest over 50 g of soil on particular days. They note that while it is true that some children will ingest large amounts of soil, it is far from certain whether soil pica is behavior that only a small subgroup displays over a limited number of years (e.g., one to six) or whether most children, on occasion, display this behavior or some combination of both behavioral patterns. Clearly, additional work is needed to understand this topic.

Soil Ingestion by Adults

For most persons beyond the ages of 5 to 6 yr, the daily uptake of dirt due to intentional ingestion is generally thought to be quite low. With the exception of some lower income persons who eat clays due to tradition or mineral deficiency, adults will not usually intentionally ingest dirt or soil. However, there are two other important ways in which adults eat dirt—incidental hand-to-mouth contact and through dust on vegetables. It has been shown that most soil ingested from crops comes from leafy vegetables. Interestingly, investigations at nuclear weapons trials have shown that particles exceeding 45 μm are seldom retained on leaves. Further, superficial contamination by smaller particles is readily lost from leaves, usually by mechanical processes or rain, and certainly by washing (308). As a result, unless the soil contaminant is absorbed into the plant, superficial contamination of plants by dirt will rarely present a health hazard (207,259).

The estimated deposition rate of dust from ambient air in rural environments is about 0.012 mg/cm^2-d, assuming that rural dust contains about 300 mg/g of lead (the substance for which these data were obtained). The U.S. EPA has estimated that even at very high air concentrations (0.45 mg/m^3 total dust), it is unlikely that surface deposition alone can account for more than 0.6 to 1.5 mg lead/g dust (2 to 5 μg/g lettuce) on the surface of lettuce during a 21-d growing period (252). These data suggest that daily ingestion of dirt and dust by adults due to eating vegetables is unlikely to exceed about 0 to 5 mg/d even if all of the 137 g of leafy and root vegetables, sweet corn, and potatoes consumed by adult males each day were replaced by family garden products.

In its document on lead, the U.S. EPA used worst-case assumptions to estimate that persons could ingest up to 100 mg of lead each day due to unwashed vegetables. The actual uptake by adults from vegetables should actually be much less, and is probably negligible, because the U.S. EPA estimate assumed that all of the suspended dust is contaminated; persons do not wash the vegetables; garden vegetables are eaten throughout the year, rather than only during the growing season; and persons actually replace most vegetables with their own garden products.

With respect to the second route—incidental ingestion—only a very limited amount of work has been conducted which addresses dust ingestion via this route. It has been suggested that the primary route of uptake will be through accidental ingestion of dirt on the hands, which may be of special concern to smokers, who tend to have more frequent hand-to-mouth contact. It is true that before the importance of this route of entry was recognized, persons who worked in lead factories between 1890 and 1920 probably received a large portion of their body burden of lead due to poor hygiene and ingestion of dust; however, such conditions are now rare in the United States and most developed countries.

Some persons have evaluated the exposure experience of agricultural workers who apply or work with pesticide dusts. Due to the frequency and degree of pesticide exposure during its manufacture or application, these data do not appear to be appropriate surrogates for estimating soil uptake from the hands of persons who live on or near sites having contaminated soil. In addition, most of the published studies on pesticides involve liquids such as the organophosphates, rather than "soil-like" particles. Exposure studies of persons who apply granular pesticides might be more useful for defining upper bound estimates of dermal exposure than estimates based on dusty workplaces (181).

At least one study has been conducted to specifically address soil uptake by adults involved in remediating waste sites (52,284,339: also see ref. 431). The results suggest that the amount of soil eaten by these workers is much less than the default value of 100 mg/d suggested by the U.S. EPA in a number of guidance documents and risk assessments. Based on all the available data, it appears that a value of 5–25 mg/day for soil ingestion by most adults is a reasonable one.

Estimating the Intake of Chemicals Via Food

Without question, the information necessary to accurately estimate the ingestion of xenobiotics via foods is one the most complex of all exposure calculations. The hundreds of different possible foods and dozens of different chemicals that can be present as a pesticide residue, coupled with the background concentrations of various chemicals in soil, make this a formidable task.

The methodology for estimating uptake via ingestion must account for the quantity of food ingested each day, the concentration of contaminant in the ingested material, and the bioavailability of the contaminant in the media. Over the past 20 yr, a significant amount of work has been directed at understanding these exposure factors. Specifically, an entire volume of the U.S. EPA *Exposure Factors Handbook* (Volume II) is devoted to this topic (386).

The approach to estimating uptake via foods was first applied in the late 1940s by the Food and Drug Administration (361) and had not changed appreciably through 2000. However, because of the passage of the Food Quality Protection Act of 1996 (FQPA), the methodology for estimating uptake of chemicals from foods will be changing dramatically over the next 5–10 yr. Specifically, the FQPA requires that all pesticide residues from foods be added together, in a prescribed manner based on target organ, with the goal of understanding the total daily dose of all residual pesticides in the diet. Then, if necessary, the pesticide manufacturers are expected to calculate the necessary residue level that their chemical may have in a particular food so that the total dose does not exceed a fraction of the acceptable daily intake (ADI). Since there are hundreds of foods and dozens of residues, this presents a formidable challenge.

Ingestion of contaminated fruits and vegetables is a potential pathway of human exposure to chemicals. Fruits and vegetables may become contaminated by several different pathways. Ambient air pollutants may be deposited on or absorbed by plants, or dissolved in rainfall or irrigation waters that contact the plants. Plant roots may also absorb pollutants from contaminated soil and groundwater. The addition of pesticides, soil additives, and fertilizers may also result in food contamination (386). Formulas are available to predict the concentration of chemicals from the soil, which have deposited from the air, and remain after treatment with a pesticide.

The primary information source on consumption rates of fruits and vegetables among the U.S. population is the U.S. Department of Agriculture (USDA) Nationwide Food Consumption Survey (NFCS) and the USDA Continuing Survey of Food Intakes by Individuals (CSFII). Data from the NFCS have been used in various studies to generate consumer-only and per-capita intake rates for individual fruits and vegetables, as well as total fruits and total vegetables. CSFII data from the 1989–1991 survey have been analyzed by the U.S. EPA to generate per-capita intake rates for various food items and food groups (362,365,386).

Consumer-only intake is defined as the quantity of fruits and vegetables consumed by individuals who ate these food items during the survey period. Per-capita intake rates are generated by averaging consumer-only intakes over the entire population of users and nonusers. In general, per-capita intake rates are appropriate for use in exposure assessment for which average dose estimates for the general population are of interest, because they represent both individuals who ate the foods during the survey period and individuals who may eat the food items at some time but did not consume them during the survey period. Total fruit intake refers to the sum of all fruits consumed in a day, including canned, dried, frozen, and fresh fruits. Likewise, total vegetable intake refers to the sum of all vegetables consumed in a day, including canned, dried, frozen, and fresh vegetables.

Intake rates may be presented on either an as-consumed or a dry-weight basis. As-consumed intake rates (g/d) are based on the weight of food in the form in which it is consumed. In contrast, dry-weight intake rates are based on the weight of food consumed after the moisture content has been removed. In calculating exposures based on ingestion, the unit of weight used to measure the contaminant concentration in the produce will vary. Intake data from the individual NFCS and CSFII components are based on "as eaten" (i.e., cooked or prepared) forms of the food items or groups. Thus, no corrections are required to account for changes in portion sizes from cooking losses (249,363).

Estimating source-specific exposures to chemicals in fruits and vegetables may also require information on the amount of fruits and vegetables exposed to or protected from contamination as a result of cultivation practices, the physical nature of the food product itself (i.e., those having protective coverings that are removed before eating would be considered protected), or the amount grown beneath the soil (i.e., most root crops such as potatoes). The percentages of foods grown above and below ground will be useful when the contaminant concentrations in foods are estimated from concentrations in soil, water, and air. For example, vegetables grown below ground would more likely be contaminated by soil pollutants, but leafy above-ground vegetables would more likely be contaminated by deposition of air pollutants on plant surfaces. Some examples of various exposure factors and confidence ratings for liquids and food are presented in Table 9.10 (386).

Individual average daily intake rates calculated from NFCS and CSFII data are based on averages of reported individual intakes over 1 d or 3 consecutive days. Such short-term data are marginally suitable for estimating mean average daily intake rates representative of both short-term and long-term consumption. However, the distribution of average daily intake rates generated using short-term data (e.g., 3 day) does not necessarily reflect the long-term distribution of average daily intake rates. The distributions generated from short-term and long-term data will differ to the extent that each individual's intake varies from day to day; the distributions will be similar to the extent that individuals' intakes are constant from day to day (386).

Day-to-day intake variation among individuals will be greatest for food items or groups that are highly seasonal, and for items or groups that are eaten year-round but are not typically eaten every day. For these foods, the intake distribution generated from short-term data will not reflect long-term distribution. On the other hand, for broad categories of foods (e.g., vegetables), which are eaten on a daily basis throughout the year with minimal seasonality, the short-term distribution may be a reasonable approximation of the true long-term distribution, although it will show somewhat more variability.

Other relevant fruits and vegetables intake studies include the U.S. EPA Dietary Risk Evaluation System (DRES), Office of Pesticide Programs (OPP). The OPP uses the DRES (formerly the Tolerance Assessment System) to assess the dietary risk of pesticide use as part of the pesticide registration process (249,363). The OPP sets tolerances for specific pesticides on raw agricultural commodities based on estimates of dietary risk. These estimates are calculated using pesticide residue data for the food item of concern and relevant consumption data. Intake rates are based primarily on the USDA 1977–1978 NFCS, although intake rates for some food items are based on estimations from production volumes or other data (i.e., some items were assigned an arbitrary value of 0.000001 g/kg-d) (386). The OPP has calculated per-capita intake rates of individual fruits and vegetables for 22 subgroups of the population (age, regional, and seasonal) by determining the composition of NFCS food items and disaggregating complex food dishes into their component raw agricultural commodities (RACs) (386,422).

The advantage of using these data is that complex food dishes have been disaggregated to provide intake rates for a very large number of fruits and vegetables. These data are also based on the individual body weights of the respondents. Therefore, using these data to calculate

Table 9.10
Summary of default exposure factor recommendations and confidence ratings for citizens of United States

Exposure factor	Recommendation	Confidence rating
Drinking-water intake rate	21 ml/kg-d or 1.4 L/d (average)	Medium
	34 ml/kg-d or 2.3 L/d (90th percentile)	Medium
	Percentiles and distribution also included	
	Means and percentiles also included for pregnant and lactating women	
Total fruit intake rate	3.4 g/kg-d (per capita average)	Medium
	12.4 g/kg-d (per capita 95th percentile)	Low
	Percentiles also included	
	Means presented for individual fruits	
Total vegetable intake rate	4.3 g/kg-d (per capita average)	Medium
	10 g/kg-d (per capita 95th percentile)	Low
	Percentiles also included	
	Means presented for individual vegetables	
Total meat intake rate	2.1 g/kg-d (per capita average)	Medium
	5.1 g/kg-d (per capita 95th percentile)	Low
	Percentiles also included	
	Percentiles also presented for individual meats	
Total dairy intake rate	8.0 kg-d (per capita average)	Medium
	29.7 g/kg-d (per capita 95th percentile)	Low
	Percentiles also included	
	Means presented for individual dairy products	
Grain intake	4.1 g/kg-d (per capita average)	High
	10.8 g/kg-d (per capita 95th percentile)	Low in long-term upper percentiles
	Percentiles also included	
Breast-milk intake rate	742 ml/d (average)	Medium
	1,033 ml/d (upper percentile)	Medium
Fish intake rate	General population	
	20.1 g/d (total fish) average	High
	14.1 g/d (marine) average	High
	6.0 g/d (freshwater/estuarine) average	High
	63 g/d (total fish) 95th percentile long-term	Medium
	Percentiles also included	
	Serving size	
	129 g (average)	High
	326 g (95th percentile)	High
	Recreational marine anglers	
	27 g/d (finfish only)	Medium
	Recreational freshwater	
	8 g/d (average)	Medium
	25 g/d (95th percentile)	Medium
	Native American subsistence population	
	70 g/d (average)	Medium
	170 g/d (95th percentile)	Low

Note. From Reference 385.

chemical exposure may provide more representative estimates of potential dose per unit body weight. However, because the data are based on the NFCS short-term dietary recall, the same limitations discussed previously for other NFCS data sets also apply here. In addition, consumption patterns may have changed since the data were collected in 1977–1978. The OPP is in the process of translating consumption information from the USDA CSFII 1989–1991 survey to be used in DRES (386).

The USDA has also conducted a study entitled *Food and Nutrient Intakes of Individuals in One Day in the U.S.* (362,386). The USDA calculated mean intake rates for total fruits and total vegetables using NFCS data from 1977–1978 and 1987–1988, and CSFII data from 1994–1995 (362,386). Mean per-capita total intake rates are based on intake data for 1 d from the 1977–1978 and 1987–1988 USDA and NFCS, respectively. Data from both surveys are presented in the *Exposure Factors Handbook* to demonstrate that although the 1987–1988 survey had fewer respondents, the mean per-capita intake rates for all individuals agree with the earlier survey. Also, slightly different age classifications were used in the two surveys, providing a wider range of age categories from which exposure assessors may select appropriate intake rates. The age groups used in this data set are the same as those used in the 1987–1988 NFCS. Information for per-capita intake rates and consumer-only intake rates for various ages of individuals is also available. Intake rates for consumers-only were calculated by dividing the per-capita consumption rate by the fraction of the population using vegetables or fruits in a day (386).

The advantages of using these data are that they provide intake estimates for all fruits, all vegetables, or all fats combined. Again, these estimates are based on 1-d dietary data which may not reflect usual consumption patterns (386).

Intake of Fish and Shellfish

Contaminated finfish and shellfish are potential sources of human exposure to persistent chemicals and metals. Pollutants are carried in surface waters, but also may be stored and accumulated in sediments as a result of complex physical and chemical processes. Consequently, various aquatic species can be exposed to pollutants and may become sources of contaminated food (386).

Accurately estimating exposure to various chemicals in a population that consumes fish from a polluted water body requires an estimation of caught-fish intake rates by fishermen and their families. Commercially caught fish are marketed widely, making the prediction of an individual's consumption from a particular commercial source difficult. Because the catch of recreational and subsistence fishermen is generally not diluted in this way, these individuals and their families represent the population that is most vulnerable to exposure by intake of contaminated fish from a specific location (386).

Over the years, fish consumption survey data have been collected using a number of different approaches, which need to be considered when interpreting the survey results. Generally, surveys are either "creel" studies in which fishermen are interviewed while fishing, or broader population surveys (using mailed questionnaires or phone interviews). Both data types can be useful for exposure assessment purposes, but somewhat different applications and interpretations are needed. In fact, creel study results have often been misinterpreted because of inadequate knowledge of survey principles (280,285,386).

The typical survey seeks to draw inferences about a larger population from a smaller sample of that population. The larger population from which the survey sample is taken and to which the survey results are generalized describes the target population of the survey. In order to generalize from the sample to the target population, the probability of being sampled must be known for each member of the target population. This probability is reflected in weights assigned to each survey respondent, with weights being inversely proportional to sampling probability. When all members of the target population have the same probability of being sampled, all weights can be set to 1 and essentially ignored (102,306).

In a mail or phone study of licensed anglers, the target population generally involves all licensed anglers in a particular area, and in these studies, the sampling probability is essentially equal for all target population members. In a creel study, the target population is anyone who fishes at the locations being studied; generally in a creel study, the probability of being sampled is not the same for all members of the target population. For instance, if the survey is conducted for 1 d at a site, then it will include all persons who fish there daily, but only about 1/7 of the people who fish there weekly, 1/30 of the people who fish there monthly, etc. In this example, the probability of being sampled (or inverse weight) is seen to be proportional to the frequency of fishing. However, if the survey involves interviewers who revisit the same site on multiple days, and persons who are only interviewed once for the survey, then the probability of being in the survey is not proportional to frequency; in fact, it increases less proportionally with greater frequency of fishing. If the same site is surveyed every day of the survey period with no reinterviewing, all members of the target population would have the same probability of being sampled, regardless of fishing frequency, implying that the survey weights should all equal 1 (102,302).

On the other hand, if the survey protocol calls for individuals to be interviewed each time an interviewer encounters them (i.e., without regard to whether they were previously interviewed), then the inverse weights will again be proportional to fishing frequency, no matter how many times interviewers revisit the same site. Note that when individuals can be interviewed multiple times, the results of each interview are included as separate records in the database, and the survey weights should be inversely proportional to the expected number of times that an individual's interviews are included in the database (102,302,386).

Fish and shellfish exposure assessments are among the most complicated of all assessments (227). A significant portion of the *Exposure Factors Handbook* addresses this topic (386). Recently, fairly complex Monte Carlo methods have been applied to resolve many of the difficulties estimating exposure of anglers and their families (428).

Aggregate Exposure and FQPA

Pesticides are regulated under both the Federal Insecticide, Fungicide, and Rodenticide Act (FIFRA) and the Federal Food, Drug, and Cosmetics Act (FFDCA). In 1996, Congress passed the Food Quality Protection Act (FQPA) that amended both FIFRA and FFDCA. These laws mandated the U.S. EPA to register pesticides and set tolerances based on a safety determination, a reasonable certainty that use of a given pesticide or consumption of raw agricultural commodity of processed foods that contain the pesticide and its residues will cause no harm to human health or the environment. The U.S. EPA evaluates risks posed by the use and usage of each pesticide to make a determination of safety. Based upon this determination, the agency regulates pesticides to ensure that use of the chemical is not unsafe.

In the past, the U.S. EPA evaluated the safety of pesticides based on a single-chemical, single-exposure-pathway scenario. However, FQPA requires that the agency consider aggregate exposure in its decision-making process. Section 408(a)(4)(b)(2)(ii) of FFDCA specifies with respect to a tolerance that there must be a determination "that there is a reasonable certainty that no harm will result from aggregate exposure to the pesticide chemical residue, including all anticipated dietary exposures and all other exposures for which there is reliable information." Section (b)(2)(C)(ii)(I) states that "there is a reasonable certainty that no harm will result to infants and children from aggregate exposure to the pesticide chemical residues" *Aggregate dose* is defined as the amount of a single substance available for interaction with metabolic processes or biologically significant receptors from multiple routes of exposure. *Aggregate risk* is defined as the likelihood of the occurrence of an adverse health effect resulting from all routes of exposure to a single substance. Conversely, *cumulative risk* is defined as the likelihood of the occurrence of an adverse health effect resulting from all routes of exposure to a group of substances sharing a common mechanism of toxicity.

As shown in Figure 9.5, the most basic concept underlying all aggregate exposure assessments is that exposure occurs to an individual. The integrity of the data concerning this exposed individual must be maintained throughout the aggregate exposure assessment. In other words, each of the individual "subassessments" must be linked back to the same person (394). Because exposures are based on that received by a single individual, aggregate exposure assessments must agree in time, place, and demographic characteristics. Each of these parameters have imbedded attributes that must be matched to create a reasonable assessment. Some of these imbedded attributes include:

- Time (duration, daily, seasonally).
- Place (location and type of home, urbanization, watersheds, region).
- Demographics (age, gender, reproductive status, ethnicity, personal preference).

To develop realistic aggregate exposure and risk assessments requires that the appropriate temporal, spatial, and demographic exposure factors be correctly assigned. Examples of some of these factors include sex- and age-specific body weights, regional specific drinking-water concentrations of the pesticide being considered, seasonally based pesticide residues in food, and frequency of residential pest control representative of housing type. Once an aggregate exposure and risk assessment is completed for one individual, population and subpopulation distributions of exposures and risk may be constructed by probabilistic techniques (161).

An aggregate exposure and risk assessment is distinct from a cumulative risk assessment. Cumulative risk is defined as "the measure or estimate of distributions of exposures (doses) for a set of chemicals that act by a common mechanism of toxicity" (390). Cumulative risk assessment evaluates risks from multiple chemicals via all routes and pathways of exposure. The cumulative risk assessment considers the combined toxicological effect of a group of chemicals with a common mechanism of toxicity. The definition of a common mechanism of toxicity is "two or more pesticide chemicals that produce an adverse effect(s) to human health by the same, or essentially the same, sequence of major biochemical events. The underlying basis of the toxicity is the same, or essentially the same, for each chemical" (390). Specific guidance concerning conducting a cumulative risk assessment is currently being developed (161).

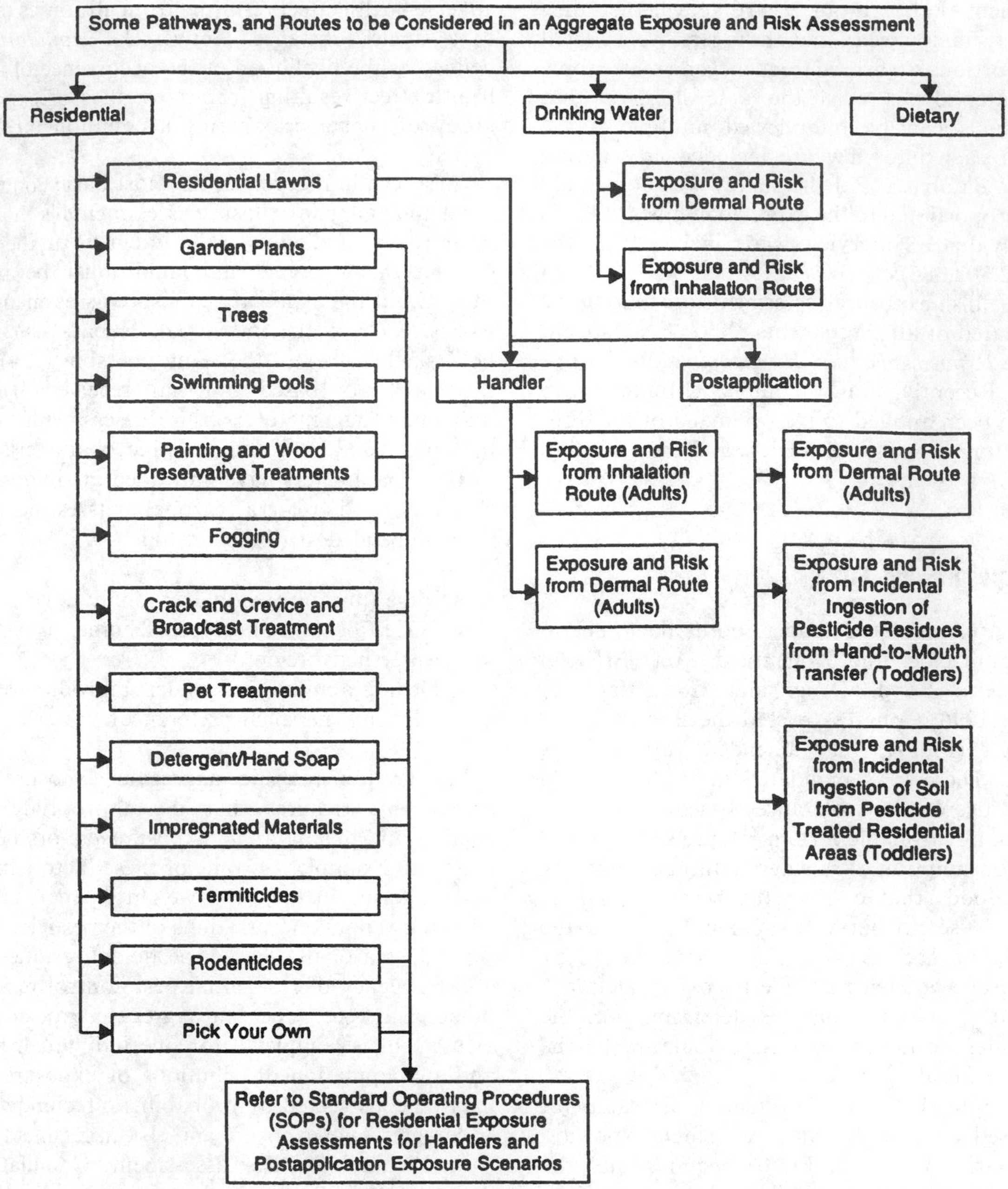

FIG. 9.5. Factors to consider in an aggregate exposure assessment of a pesticide. From Reference 394.

Breast Milk

Breast milk is a potential source of exposure to toxic substances for nursing infants. Lipid-soluble chemical compounds accumulate in body fat and may be transferred to breastfed infants in the lipid portion of breast milk. Because nursing infants obtain most (if not all) of their dietary intake from breast milk, they are especially vulnerable to exposures to these compounds. In fact, some models predict that the peak body burdens of certain chemicals (like dioxin) can reach their lifetime peak (μg/kg) on the last day of nursing at age 12–24 mo. Estimating the magnitude of the potential dose to infants from breast milk and the resulting body burdens of blood levels is quite complicated. It requires information on the quantity of breast milk consumed per day and the duration (months) over which breastfeeding occurs. Information on the fat content of breast milk is also needed for estimating dose from breast-milk residue concentrations that have been indexed to lipid con-

Table 9.11
Default values for daily intakes of breast milk

Age	Number of infants surveyed at each time period	Mean intake (ml/d)	Range of daily intake (ml/d)
Completely breast-fed			
1 mo	11	600 ± 159	426–989
3 mo	2	833	645–1000
6 mo	1	682	616–786
Partially breast-fed			
1 mo	4	485 ± 79	398–655
3 mo	11	467 ± 100	242–698
6 mo	6	395 ± 175	147–684
9 mo	3	<554	451–732

Note. From Reference 249. Data expressed as mean ± standard deviation.

tent (331,386). Until recently, these were considered the key parameters but it is now clear that one must account for the quickly increasing body weight of the infant, the differences in the blood perfusion of the fat compartments in the infant versus the mother, and other factors (172,185).

Several studies have generated data on breast-milk intake (182,230,241,332). Typically, breast-milk intake has been measured over a 24-h period by weighing the infant before and after each feeding without changing its clothing (test weighing). The sum of the difference between the measured weights over the 24-h period is assumed to be equivalent to the amount of breast milk consumed daily. Intakes measured using this procedure are often corrected for evaporative water losses (insensible water losses) between infant weighings (230). Neville et al. (241) evaluated the validity of the test-weight approach among bottle-fed infants by comparing the weight of milk taken from bottles with the difference between the before and after feeding weights of infants. Once corrected for insensible water loss, test-weight data were not significantly different from bottle weights. Conversions between weight and volume of breast milk consumed are made using the density of human milk (approximately 1.03 g/ml) (230). Recently, techniques for measuring breast-milk intake using stable isotopes have been developed; however, few data based on this new technique have been published (230).

Studies among nursing mothers in industrialized countries have shown that infant intake averages approximately 750 to 800 g/d (728 to 777 ml/d) during the first 4 to 5 mo of life, with a range of 450 to 1200 g/d (437 to 1165 ml/d) (230,386). Similar intakes have also been reported for developing countries (230,386). Infant birth weight and nursing frequency have been shown to influence the rate of intake (230,386). Infants who are larger at birth and/or nurse more frequently have been shown to have higher intake rates. Also, breast-milk production among nursing mothers has been reported to be somewhat higher than the amount actually consumed by the infant (102,386).

Like exposure assessments of fishes, techniques for estimating chemical uptake by children of breast milk continue to evolve. One of the more interesting papers on this topic was recently presented by Kerger et al. (172), which put into question most of the prior calculation approaches for estimating dose to nursing infants based, in part, on work conducted by Kreuzer et al. (185). A portion of the U.S. EPA *Exposure Factors Handbook* addresses this topic, and a few published papers have offered some novel approaches (331,386,387). Some examples of breast-milk intake rates are presented in Table 9.11. A distribution for breast-milk consumption has been suggested by Kerger et al. (1999).

ESTIMATING UPTAKE VIA INHALATION

Estimating intake via inhalation depends on only a few exposure factors, such as inhalation rate; airborne chemical concentration; bioavailability; and, if it is a particle, particle size. In general, uncertainty in estimates of intake via inhalation is among the smallest for all exposure calculations.

Inhalation rates are known to vary directly with the amount of physical activity of the persons being evaluated. The default value used by the U.S. EPA and others is 20 m^3/d. When conducting occupational exposure assessments, it is common to assume that workers inhale about 10 m^3 in an 8-h workday (377).

Airborne chemical concentrations are obtained through either direct measurement or modeling. The form of the chemicals in the air will be a gas (includes vapors) or particles (dusts or fumes). Generally, it is assumed that virtually all of the vapors or gases will be absorbed if inhaled (9,184,377). This may not be the case for volatile chemicals, if the concentration in the blood is approaching steady state. In those cases, a significant fraction of the inhaled vapors will be present in the exhaled breath and, therefore, not absorbed (275).

It is usually assumed that if particles enter the lower respiratory tract, they will eventually be absorbed unless the chemical is highly insoluble. Generally, it is assumed that particles less than 150 μm in diameter are inhalable, but virtually all particles greater than 10 μm will be captured in the upper respiratory tract (nose and throat) and then ingested. It has often been assumed that particles less than 10 μm in diameter will be captured in the lower respiratory tract and the majority of these (by mass rather than particle number) will eventually be absorbed. Notably, for some chemicals, the adverse effect is related to the particle size, so this must be taken into account. For example, it is thought that beryllium particles should be collected in several different size fractions and that the severity of the adverse effect varies according to particle size.

Various Inhalation Rates

A significant amount of research has been done to correlate various inhalation rates with different tasks and body weights. Most studies on this subject have been summarized in the most recent U.S. EPA *Exposure Factors Handbook* (382). Data are available for dozens of different levels of physical activity and the distributions for several populations are presented.

A number of equations have been proposed for predicting the inhalation rate based on body weight (386). The *Exposure Factors Handbook* and other sources provide a number of tables that relate physical activity with inhalation rate (see Table 9.12).

Bioavailability of Airborne Chemicals

Because the mass of particles inhaled is usually quite small, and because most particles less than 10 μm in diameter are thought to be fairly easily absorbed, it is generally assumed that particles are 100% bioavailable after they are trapped in the lower lung. Likewise, it is generally assumed that most vapors and gases are completely absorbed (100% bioavailable) if they reach the lower respiratory tract. Both are conservative assumptions that should be reassessed on a case-by-case basis.

Table 9.12
Daily inhalation rates estimated from daily activities

	Inhalation rate (IR)		Daily inhalation
Subject	Resting (m^3/h)	Light activity (m^3/h)	rate (DIR)[a] (m^3/d)
Adult man	0.45	1.2	22.8
Adult woman	0.36	1.14	21.1
Child (10 yr)	0.29	0.78	14.8
Infant (1 yr)	0.09	0.25	3.76
Newborn	0.03	0.09	0.78

Note. From Reference 334. Assumptions made were based on 8 h resting and 16 h light activity for adults and children (10 yr); 14 h resting and 10 h light activity for infants (1 yr); 23 h resting and 1 h light activity for newborns.

$$^a\mathrm{DIR} = \frac{1}{T}\sum_{i=1}^{k} \mathrm{IR}_i t_i$$

where IR_i is corresponding inhalation rate at ith activity, t_i is hours spent during the ith activity, k is number of activity periods, and T is total time of the exposure period (i.e., a day).

ROLE OF UNCERTAINTY ANALYSIS

Exposure assessment uses a wide array of information sources and techniques. Even when actual exposure-related measurements exist, assumptions or inferences will still be required. Most likely, data will not be available for all aspects of the exposure assessment and these data may be of questionable or unknown quality. In these situations, the exposure assessor will have to rely on a combination of professional judgment, inferences based on analogy with similar chemicals and conditions, estimation techniques, and the like. The net result is that the exposure assessment will be based on a number assumptions with varying degrees of uncertainty (377).

The decision analysis literature has focused on the importance of explicitly incorporating and quantifying scientific uncertainty in risk assessments (227,302). Reasons for addressing uncertainties in exposure assessments include (377):

- Uncertainty information from different sources and of different quality must be combined.
- A decision must be made about whether and how to expend resources to acquire additional information (e.g., production, use, and emissions data; environmental fate information; monitoring data; population data) to reduce the uncertainty.

- So much empirical evidence exists that biases may occur, resulting in so-called best estimates that are not very accurate. Even when all that is needed is a best-estimate answer, the quality of the answer may be improved by incorporating a frank discussion of uncertainty into the analysis.
- Exposure assessment is an iterative process. The search for an adequate and robust methodology to handle the problem at hand may proceed more effectively, and to a more certain conclusion, if the associated uncertainty is explicitly included and it can be used as a guide in the process of refinement.
- A decision is rarely made on the basis of a single piece of analysis. Further, it is rare for there to be one discrete decision; a process of multiple decisions spread over time is the more common occurrence. Chemicals of concern may go through several levels of risk assessment before a final decision is made. During this process, decisions may be made based on exposure considerations. An exposure analysis that attempts to characterize the associated uncertainty allows the user or decision maker to conduct a better evaluation in the context of the other factors being considered.
- Exposure assessors have a responsibility to present not just numbers, but also a clear and explicit explanation of the implications and limitations of their analyses. Uncertainty characterization helps to achieve this.

Essentially, constructing scientifically sound exposure assessments and analyzing uncertainty go hand-in-hand. The reward for analyzing uncertainties is knowing that the results have integrity or that significant gaps exist in available information that can make decision making a tenuous process.

Variability Versus Uncertainty

While some authors treat variability as a specific component of uncertainty, the U.S. EPA (62) and others advise risk assessors (and, by analogy, the exposure assessor) to distinguish between variability and uncertainty (236). Specifically, uncertainty represents a lack of knowledge about factors affecting exposure or risk, whereas variability arises from true heterogeneity across people, places, or time. In other words, uncertainty can lead to inaccurate or biased estimates, whereas variability can affect the precision of the estimates and the degree to which they can be generalized.

Variability and uncertainty can complement or confound one another. The National Research Council (236) has drawn an instructive analogy based on estimating the distance between the earth and the moon. Prior to fairly recent technological developments, it was difficult to accurately measure this distance, resulting in measurement uncertainty. Because the moon's orbit is elliptical, the distance is a variable quantity. If only a few measurements were taken without knowledge of the elliptical pattern, then either of the following incorrect conclusions might be reached:

- The measurements were faulty, thereby ascribing to uncertainty what was actually caused by variability; or
- The moon's orbit was random, thereby not allowing uncertainty to shed light on seemingly unexplainable differences that are in fact variable and predictable.

A more fundamental error in this situation might be to incorrectly estimate the true distance and assume that a few observations were sufficient. This latter pitfall—treating a highly variable quantity as if it were invariant or only uncertain—is most relevant to the exposure or risk assessor (377).

Now consider a situation that relates to exposure, such as estimating the average daily dose by one exposure route—ingestion of contaminated drinking water. Suppose that it is possible to measure an individual's daily water consumption (and concentration of the contaminant) exactly, thereby eliminating uncertainty in the measured daily dose. The daily dose still has an inherent day-to-day variability, however, because of changes in the individual's daily water intake or concentration of the contaminant in the water (377).

Clearly, it is impractical to measure the individual's dose every day. For this reason, the exposure assessor may estimate the average daily dose (ADD) based on a finite number of measurements, in an attempt to "average out" the day-to-day variability. The individual has a true (but unknown) ADD, which has now been estimated based on a sample of measurements. Because the individual's true average is unknown, it is uncertain how close the estimate is to the true value. Thus, the variability across daily doses has been translated into uncertainty in the ADD. Although the individual's true ADD has no variability, the estimate of the ADD has some uncertainty (377).

The preceding discussion pertains to the ADD for one person. Now consider a distribution of ADDs across individuals in a defined population (e.g., the general U.S. population). In this case, variability refers to the range and distribution of ADDs across individuals in the population. By comparison, uncertainty refers to the exposure assessor's state of knowledge about that distribution, or about parameters describing the distribution (e.g., mean, standard deviation, general shape, various percentiles) (377).

As noted by the National Research Council (1994), the realms of variability and uncertainty have fundamentally different ramifications for science and judgment. For example, uncertainty may force decision makers to judge how probable it is that exposures have been overestimated or underestimated for every member of the exposed population, whereas variability forces them to cope with the certainty that different individuals are subject to exposures both above and below any of the exposure levels chosen as a reference point (377).

Types of Variability

Variability in exposure is related to an individual's location, activity, and behavior or preferences at a particular point in time, as well as pollutant emission rates and physical/chemical processes that affect concentrations in various media (e.g., air, soil, food, and water). The variations in pollutant-specific emissions or processes, and in individual locations, activities, or behaviors are not necessarily independent of one another. For example, both personal activities and pollutant concentrations at a specific location might vary in response to weather conditions, or between weekdays and weekends (377).

At a more fundamental level, three types of variability can be distinguished:

- Variability across locations (spatial variability).
- Variability over time (temporal variability).
- Variability among individuals (inter-individual variability).

Spatial variability can occur both at regional (macroscale) and local (microscale) levels. For example, fish intake rates can vary depending on the region of the country. Higher consumption may occur among populations located near large bodies of water such as the Great Lakes or coastal areas. As another example, outdoor pollutant levels can be affected at the regional level by industrial activities and at the local level by activities of individuals. In general, higher exposures tend to be associated with closer proximity to the pollutant source, whether it be an industrial plant or related to a personal activity such as showering or gardening. In the context of exposure to airborne pollutants, the concept of a "microenvironment" has been introduced to denote a specific locality (e.g., a residential lot or a room in a specific building) where the airborne concentration can be treated as homogeneous (i.e., invariant) at a particular point in time.

Temporal variability refers to variations over time, whether long or short term. Seasonal fluctuations in weather, pesticide applications, use of woodburning appliances, and fraction of time spent outdoors are examples of longer term variability. Examples of shorter term variability are differences in industrial or personal activities on weekdays versus weekends or at different times of the day.

Interindividual variability can be either of two types: (1) human characteristics such as age or body weight, and (2) human behaviors such as location and activity patterns. Each of these variabilities, in turn, may be related to several underlying phenomena that vary. For example, the natural variability in human weight is due to a combination of genetic, nutritional, and other lifestyle or environmental factors. Variability arising from independent factors that combine multiplicatively generally will lead to an approximately lognormal distribution across the population, or across spatial/temporal dimensions (377; 153,154).

Monte Carlo Analysis

Among the most promising and exciting techniques to emerge in the area of exposure assessment in recent years is the application of Monte Carlo or other probabilistic analyses to environmental health issues (98,223,379). Monte Carlo analysis has existed as an engineering analytical tool for many years, but the development of the personal computer and software [e.g., Crystal Ball (Decisioneering, Boulder, CO), @RISK (Palisades Corp., Newfield, NY)] has allowed its application to new areas. As discussed previously, one criticism of many exposure assessments has been a reliance on overly conservative assumptions about exposure, as well as the problem of how to properly account for the highly exposed (but usually small) populations that do exist (44,242). The Monte Carlo technique offers an approach to addressing this issue.

The probabilistic or Monte Carlo model accounts for the uncertainty in select parameters evaluating the range and probability of plausible exposure levels. Instead of specifying input parameters as single values, this model allows for consideration of the probability distributions. The Monte Carlo statistical simulation is a statistical model in which the input parameters to an equation are varied simultaneously. The values are chosen from the parameter distributions, with the frequency of a particular value being equal to the relative frequency of the parameter in the distribution. The simulation involves the following three steps:

1. The probability distribution of each equation parameter (input parameter) is characterized, and the distribution is specified for the Monte Carlo simulation. If the data cannot be fit to a distribution, the data are "bootstrapped" into the simulation,

meaning that the input values are randomly selected from the actual data set without a specified distribution.

2. For each iteration of the simulation, one value is randomly selected from each parameter distribution, and the equation is run. Many iterations are performed, such that the random selections for each parameter approximate the distribution of the parameter. Five thousand iterations are typically performed for each dose equation.
3. Each iteration of the equation is evaluated and saved; hence a probability distribution of the equation output (possible doses) is generated.

This technique generates distributions that describe the uncertainty associated with the risk estimate (resultant doses). The predicted dose for every 50th percentile to the 95th percentile of the exposed population and the true mean are calculated. Using these models, the assessor is not forced to rely solely on a single exposure parameter or the repeated use of conservative assumptions to identify the plausible dose and risk estimates. Instead, the full range of possible values and their likelihood of occurrence is incorporated into the analysis to produce the range and probability of expected exposure levels (15,43,49,98, 120,332).

The methodology is illustrated in the following examples. The first example characterizes the time needed to go shopping. Time spent shopping each month (minutes) is estimated by the product of two parameters: the number of trips per month and the total time spent in the store (minutes). Total time spent in the store is the sum of time spent shopping and time spent waiting in line. Using Monte Carlo techniques, a distribution of likely values is associated with each of these parameters. These distributions depend upon the detail of information available to characterize each parameter. For example, the distribution compares all of the information, such as those days when the line at the check-out counter is short, as well as those when the line is long. It is noteworthy that each parameter has a different distribution: lognormal, gaussian, and square. Total time spent shopping is then calculated repeatedly by combining parameter values that are randomly selected from these distributions. The result is a distribution of likely time spent shopping each month. Using this technique, information concerning each parameter is carried along to the final estimate.

The second example, which directly applies to toxicologists, is to build a distribution that describes the various soil ingestion rates for children. As shown in Figure 9.6, the three pertinent distributions are the basis for constructing the overall exposure distribution.

Most of the variables used in an exposure assessment actually exist as ranges, rather than single point values and this is captured in Monte Carlo analysis. For instance, the common assumption that adult body weight is 70 kg will be replaced by the appropriate distribution (i.e., normal) of body weights (including maximum, minimum, mean, and standard deviation). Using this approach, virtually every exposure variable, whether physiological, behavioral, environmental, or chronological, can be replaced with a probability distribution (15,43,45–47,49,119,120,133,162,226,282,306,332,351,353, 354,357). Since no population (or individual) is exposed to a single concentration; breathes, eats, or drinks at a single rate; or is exposed for the same length of time, it is not appropriate to assess them as such. To be protective, high values are employed, resulting in the problems of compounding conservatisms mentioned previously (5,44,81,124,209).

The probabilistic analysis addresses the main deficiencies of the point estimate approach because it imparts more information to risk managers and the public, and uses all of the available data (27,221). The range of values (i.e., the distribution) for all the variables used in an exposure assessment is determined (e.g., normal, lognormal, uniform, triangular, etc.) and combined into a "distribution of distributions." Because of the extrapolations involved and the assumptions made, the area of single greatest uncertainty in risk assessment is associated with the dose-response evaluations.

It should also be clear that, in addition to exposure variables, data forming the basis of the toxicological criteria (carcinogenic potency factors [CPFs] and reference doses [RfDs]) are also amenable to Monte Carlo–style analysis where a robust database exists (21,33,76, 78,79,111,112,152,319,322–324,398). As with exposure variables, the advantage to this approach is that it allows all data to be used (and weighted appropriately, where necessary), thus avoiding reliance on a single experiment or endpoint.

Probabilistic analyses have in recent years been recognized in regulatory guidance (376), and the U.S. EPA Risk Assessment Forum has published a document of principles for conducting Monte Carlo analyses (76) (Table 9.13). Recently, the U.S. EPA (392) published a comprehensive guidance document on how to conduct Monte Carlo assessments.

Like traditional exposure analysis, one challenge to performing a Monte Carlo analysis properly is having appropriate distributions for use in the analysis. Numerous studies on individual variables have been published in the risk assessment literature (27,41,42,73,74,117,129, 315,330,337,338,387), and the impact on the distributions employed on the outcome has also been discussed (40,72,143,146,148,154). It should be pointed out that these techniques can be combined with other advanced risk assessment methods (i.e., PBPK modeling) to further reduce uncertainty in risk estimates (77,325). Recently,

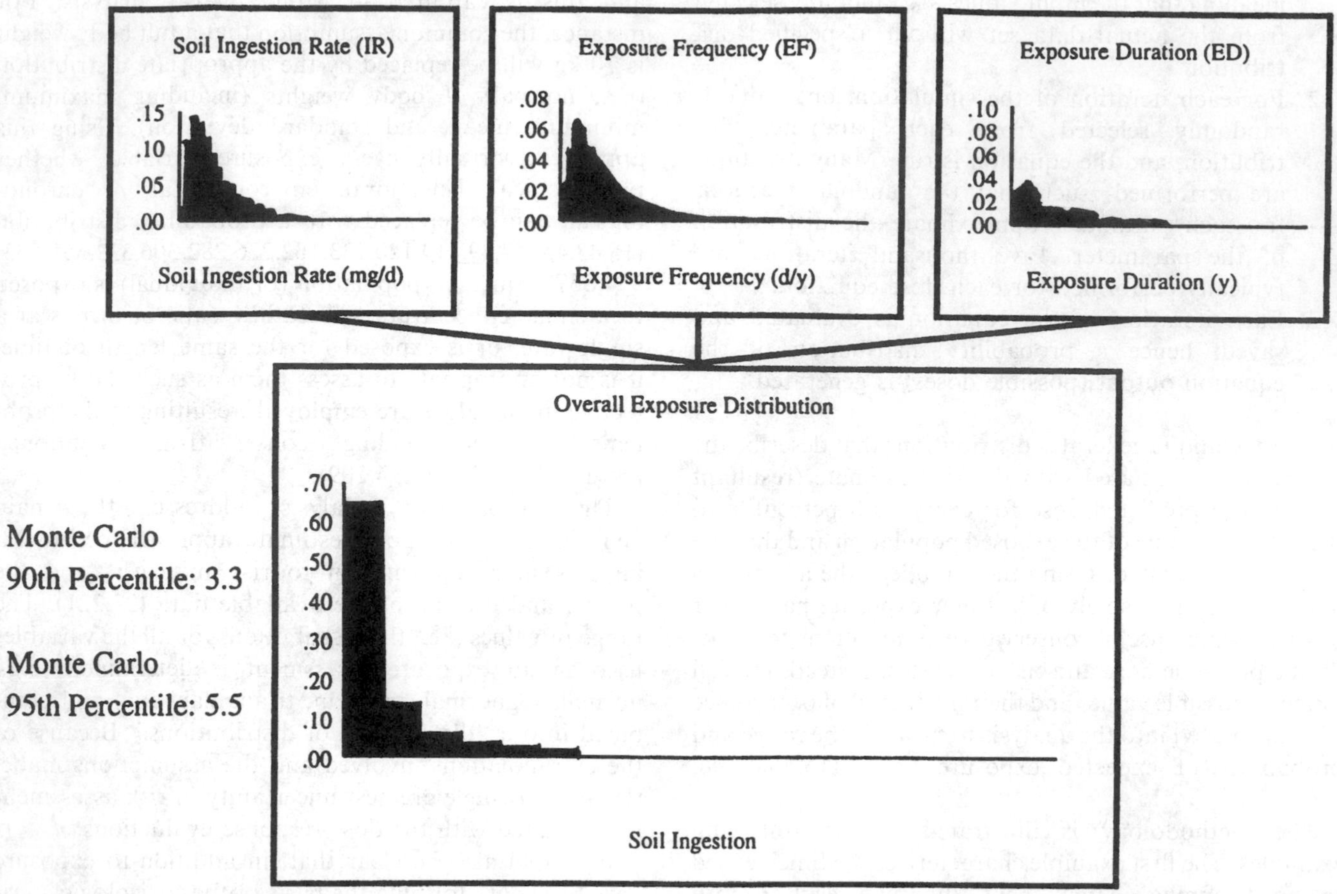

FIG. 9.6. Example of how probability density functions (distributions) for three different related exposure factors are combined to form a distribution for the amount of soil ingested by a population of children. The Monte Carlo technique allows the risk assessor to account for the variability in many exposure parameters within a population and then produce a distribution that characterizes the entire population.

two-dimensional Monte Carlo analyses have been developed that take into account both variability and uncertainty (82,399). Information appropriate to probabilistic analyses can often be found in published papers in fields quite distant from the environmental sciences.

Case Study Using Monte Carlo Technique

An example might be useful (129). Assume that persons are likely to be exposed to contaminated drinking water at the maximum contaminant limit (MCL). Concern has been raised that these regulatory limits are not sufficiently protective, and that certain federal and state regulatory programs (i.e., Resource Conservation and Recovery Act) are justified in requiring groundwater remediation to levels below that of drinking water standards. To test this supposition, it is necessary to evaluate the possible incremental cancer risk of exposure via tap-water ingestion, dermal contact with water while showering, inhalation of indoor vapors, and ingestion of produce irrigated with groundwater, using a probabilistic approach. Probability density functions for each exposure variable (e.g., water ingestion, skin surface area, fraction of exposed skin, showering time, inhalation rate, air exchange and water use rates, exposure time, etc.) are then identified and used in the appropriate exposure equation to calculate dose and risk. A commercially available software package (i.e., @RISK) could be used to conduct the Monte Carlo analysis (357).

Some have suggested that the Latin hypercube (LHC) approach offers some advantages to traditional approaches for identifying the correct number of iterations. Often, one can reach convergence sooner with LHC than the Monte Carlo option in @RISK/Crystal Ball. In addition, LHC is more reproducible (to the hundredth decimal place). The Monte Carlo option needs more iterations to reach convergence.

The results of such an analysis are presented in Table 9.14 (129). The risk associated with exposure to water at the current maximum contaminant level (MCL) level for four different contaminants, as well as the 50th

Table 9.13
U.S. EPA guiding principles for Monte Carlo analysis

1. Conduct preliminary sensitivity analyses to identify important contributors to the assessment endpoint and its variability and uncertainty.
2. Based on the results of the sensitivity analyses, include probabilistic assessments only for the important pathways and parameters.
3. Use the entire database of information when selecting input distributions.
4. When using surrogate data, identify sources of uncertainty, and whenever possible, validate the use of these data by collecting site/case specific data.
5. If empirical data are collected for use in the assessment, use collection methods that improve the representativeness and quality of these data (especially at the tails of the distribution.)
6. Identify when expert judgment, rather than hard data, is used in the assessment.
7. Separate uncertainty and variability during the analysis.
8. Use appropriate methods to address uncertainty and variability, e.g., two-dimensional Monte Carlo.
9. Discuss the numerical stability of estimates at the tails of the distribution.
10. Identify which sources of uncertainty are addressed by the assessment, and which are not.
11. Provide a detailed description of all models used.
12. Provide a detailed description of the input distributions, including a distinction between variability and uncertainty in these distributions, and a graphical representation of the probability density and cumulative distribution functions.
13. Provide a graphical representation of the probability density and cumulative distribution functions of each output distribution.
14. Consider the potential covariance between important parameters. If the covariance cannot be determined, evaluate the impact of a range of potential covariances on the output distributions.
15. Present point estimates and identify where they fall on the exposure distribution. If there are large differences between point estimates and Monte Carlo estimates, explain if the differences are due to changes in the data or models used.
16. Present results in a tiered approach.

Note. From Reference 161.

Table 9.14
Risks calculated for exposure to four halogenated solvents in water using probabilistic analysis at the MCL level and for the 50th and 95th percentile exposure

Chemical	50th Percentile risk	95th Percentile risk	MCL risk
Tetrachloroethylene	0	0.000005	0.000007
Chloroform	0.000009	0.00014	0.000017
Bromoform	0.000002	0.000016	0.000023
Vinyl chloride	0.000005	0.000029	0.000054

Note. Adapted from Reference 117.

and 95th percentile of exposure as determined by the probabilistic analysis, are shown. At the 50th percentile level ("the best estimate"), the risk ranges from 6×10^{-7} (tetrachloroethylene) to 9×10^{-6} (chloroform), while at the 95th percentile ("the upper-bound risk"), these risks range from 4×10^{-6} (tetrachloroethylene) to 1.5×10^{-4} (chloroform). These values can be compared to the point estimate risks calculated for the MCLs, which range from 7×10^{-6} (tetrachloroethylene) to 5.4×10^{-5} (vinyl chloride). For the 50th percentile (average) person, all calculated risks are within the range of "acceptable" risks adopted by regulatory authorities for Superfund sites (1×10^{-4} to 1×10^{-7}). For the 95th percentile person (upper bound), the risks are still mostly below the 1×10^{-4} benchmark risk level generally used to separate acceptable from unacceptable risks. For tetrachloroethylene, these results are 30 (50th percentile) to 3 (risk at the MCL) times below the reasonable maximum exposure (RME) risk of 2×10^{-5} developed by combining the 95th percentile values for each exposure variable using standard U.S. EPA risk assessment methodologies. This point estimate is greater than the 99th percentile of risk and is consistent with statements regarding the conservatism of the RME approach. These results suggest that chemical residues in drinking water at the MCL levels will be health protective and that remedial goals based on de minimis requirements (1×10^{-6}) might be unnecessarily low (129).

In terms of estimates for the reasonably maximally exposed (RME) individual, which often serve as the basis for regulatory decisions, several observations on the utility of probabilistic assessment can be made. First, exposure assessments that incorporate two to three direct exposure pathways usually show that the 95th percentile probabilistic estimates are three to five times below the traditional RME estimates. Second, for multipathway assessments that contain several indirect exposure pathways, the 95th percentile probabilistic estimates can be as much as an order of magnitude below the RME estimates. Third, when the number of distributions used in the exposure assessment is 10 or more, the difference between the 50th and 95th percentile estimates may be between 5 and 10. Finally, in such assessments, the difference between the RME estimates and the 95th percentile probabilistic estimates can be as high as 100 (117). In the probabilistic approach to estimating exposure and risk, the complete range of potential risks can be illustrated along with the likelihood estimates and estimates of uncertainty associated with such risks. While the availability and confidence of distributions for exposure variables differ, risk assessors ought to take advantage of this and similar approaches in their risk assessments to advance and improve the process. Additionally, since the highest degree of uncertainty in risk assessment tends to be the CPFs, attention ought to be directed to applying probabilistic analysis to the development of toxicity criteria in a similar manner (111,116,398).

Sensitivity Analysis

In addition to establishing exposure and risk distributions, probabilistic analysis can also identify variables with the greatest impact on the estimates and illuminate uncertainties associated with exposure variables through sensitivity analysis (30,160,287,299,319). This provides some insight into the confidence that resides in exposure and risk estimates, and has two important results. First, it identifies the inputs that would benefit most from additional research to reduce uncertainty and improve risk estimates. Second, assuming that a thorough assessment has been conducted, it is possible to phrase the results in more accessible terms, such as "the risk assessment of PCBs in smallmouth bass is based on a large amount of high-quality reliable data, and we have high confidence in the risk estimates derived. The analysis has determined that 90 percent of the increased cancer risk could be eliminated through a ban on carp and catfish, but there is no appreciable reduction in risk from extending such a ban to bass and trout." Such a description provides all stakeholders with considerably more information than a simple point estimate of risk based on a traditional exposure and risk assessment (257).

If the most "sensitive" exposure variables are based on limited or uncertain data, confidence in these estimates will be poor. Robust data sets, on the other hand, lead to increased confidence in the resulting estimates. In the preceding example involving smallmouth bass, sensitivity is defined as the ratio of the relative change in risk produced by a unit relative to change in the exposure variables used. A Gaussian approximation (the product of the normalized sensitivity and the standard deviation of the distribution) of intake was used to allow both sensitivity and uncertainty to be gauged. In this case, the true mean of each distribution was chosen as the baseline point value, and the differential value for each variable was calculated by increasing this value by 10%. For each variable, the differential value was substituted, the risks recalculated, and the baseline value replaced (129). Sensitivity was calculated using the following formula:

$$\text{Sensitivity} = \frac{|\text{Risk}_{\text{baseline}} - \text{Risk}_{10\%}|}{|X_{\text{baseline}} - X_{10\%}|} \cdot [\sigma]$$

where X_{baseline} and $X_{10\%}$ are baseline and differential values for the variable X, and σ is the standard deviation for the distribution of variable X. The sensitivity of each variable relative to one another is assessed by summing the unitless sensitivity values and determining the relative percent that each variable contributes to the total.

Table 9.15 indicates which are the most important variables in a probabilistic analysis of tetrachloroethylene in household tap water. In this case, the most sensitive exposure variables in household exposure to tap water are exposure time in shower and exposure duration. Relatively small changes in these variables will result in relatively large changes in the risk estimates. Since these estimates are based on actual time–use studies and census information, this suggests a high level of confidence can be placed on this estimate, particularly if site-specific data are being used. If the critical variables (in terms of sensitivity) were not based on robust data, this would suggest that the risk assessment could be improved by additional research on these exposure variables. It is interesting that the form of the distribution chosen for

Table 9.15
Results of sensitivity analysis for tetrachloroethylene exposure in household water

Exposure variable	Sensitivity (unitless)	Percentage rank
Shower exposure time	0.000004	55.0%
Exposure duration	0.000001	20.0%
Plant–soil partition factor	0	8.4%
Water ingestion rate	0	4.6%
Surface area of exposed skin	0	4.4%
Body weight	0	3.8%
Dermal permeability constant	0	1.8%
Skin fraction contacting water	0	1.5%

Note. Adapted from Reference 117.

Table 9.16
Effect of matrix and aging on the bioavailability of lead from soil

Treatment			
Lead acetate (ppm diet)	Soil lead (ppm)	Tibial lead (standard deviation)	Relative lead absorption
—	—	0.3 (0.3)	—
—	11.3	0	—
50	—	247 (10)	100
50	11.3	130 (30)	53
—	706	40 (6)	16
—	995	108 (26)	44
—	1080	37 (7.3)	15
—	1260	53.6 (7)	22
—	10420	173 (22)	70

Note. Lead acetate in the diet results in an increase in tibial lead, while lead acetate mixed with soil is only 50% as well absorbed. Aged lead from garden soil must reach high levels before significant absorption occurs. Adapted from Reference 64.

the variables is less important than the validity of the data (118). When the empirical distribution of the tapwater ingestion rate from Ershow and Cantor (108) was substituted with a lognormal distribution developed by Roseberry and Burmaster (303), the resultant change in the risk estimates was less than 1% (357).

In this case, the value of the sensitivity analysis is that it allows input variables to be ranked in order of importance and confidence in the output to be established to a higher degree than previously possible. As pointed out by the U.S. EPA, where possible, exposure assessors should report variability in exposures as numerical distributions and should characterize uncertainty as probability distributions. They need to identify clearly where they are using point estimates for 'bounding' potential exposure variables or estimates; these point estimates should not be misconstrued to represent, for example, the upper 95th percentile when information on the actual distribution is lacking (324). As noted by the U.S. EPA, such explicit presentation of the data reduces the temptation to use the exposure assessment process for veiling policy judgments (141).

ISSUES IN EXPOSURE ASSESSMENT

The field of exposure assessment will continue to benefit from ongoing research efforts. The following are some fruitful areas of ongoing research.

Bioavailability

Applied research that will improve the practice of exposure assessment include bioavailability, speciation, chemical fate, and the role of biological monitoring. Bioavailability has become an increasingly important issue in the exposure assessment process (159,202,266,305, 311). Alexander (3) has shown that a variety of organic chemicals in soil lose the ability to interact with biological receptors over time, despite the fact that the chemical concentration in soil remains largely the same. The alteration in bioavailability extends across the various routes of exposure as well (307,321,326,358,359,420,421). Inorganic compounds, even those posing a potentially significant degrees of hazard (i.e., cyanide) react similarly (85–87,318). These losses in hazard potential are presumably due to irreversible chemical interactions with soil constituents. Table 9.16 indicates that the bioavailability of lead added to soil is immediately halved and that it is further reduced over time (64). This would suggest that an assumption of 100% bioavailability of this compound (and many others) from soil is erroneous. It is also clear that the environmental media in which the compound occurs will influence its uptake into the body (307). The U.S. EPA recognized this fact when it developed two reference doses (RfDs) for manganese depending on whether it occurred in solid matrices (e.g., food, soil, etc.) or water (390). One simple method to improve bioavailability estimates is to conduct extractions under more biologically relevant conditions.

Bench-scale extraction experiments in simulated gastric fluids or sweat can be used to inexpensively and accurately measure how readily environmental residues can be released from the media in which they occur (157,304,305). As with inhalation or ingestion of vapors or solutions, both the release and absorption rates of agents from an environmental matrix (i.e., soil) across biological membranes need to be incorporated into the risk assessment when such data are available, and generated when absent. This need is particularly great when assessing dermal exposure. The problem for materials in aqueous solutions is less problematic than from solid matrices (192). For liquids, permeability constants expressed in terms of agent weight per unit area per time (mg/cm^2-min) have been developed for a number of agents, and in vivo and in vitro techniques or mathematical models exist to develop similar flux rates if needed (22,26,29,31,123,142,217,316,349,419,420). From soil, however, the typical approach in many risk assessments has been to assume a constant percent absorbed from soil adhered to skin as a default. For volatiles, an absorption rate of 25% has sometimes been used. For semivolatiles and inorganics, absorption rates of 10% and 1% have been used, respectively.

Some experimental data for absorption are available for a few agents (e.g., PCBs, DDT, dioxin, benzo[a]pyrene, etc.), suggesting that the simple assumption of a constant percentage absorbed may overestimate or underestimate the dose depending on the agent, cocontaminants, soil type, exposure duration, and similar considerations (321,326,420,421). The impact of using this default approach results in an instantaneous dermal dose being assumed, regardless of whether the soil remains in contact with the skin for 1 min or 1 day. This assumption, together with the questionable route-to-route adjustment of toxicity criteria from oral to dermal, results in a predicted dermal absorption of agents from soil, which arguably should present a minor risk in most cases, being a major driver in the risk assessment of soilbound contaminants.

Chemical Fate

Risk assessors ought to incorporate information on the fate of chemicals in the environment in their exposure estimates, whenever possible (86). Many organic compounds tend to degrade over time, and may disappear from exposed surfaces relatively quickly or otherwise change (6,255). As already suggested, inorganic compounds may also undergo changes in the environment over time that affect their fates (64,318). Influencing factors include degradation by sunlight, soil and water microbes, evaporation, and chemical interactions. The resultant changes can dramatically alter the outcome of exposure assessments (87,266). For instance, much of the criticism of incinerators has focused on the inhalation risk of dioxin emitted from the stacks. As it turns out, the environmental half-life of dioxin (as a vapor) is only 90 min because of photolytic degradation. In contrast, the half-life for dioxin in soil or fly-ash is 50 to 500 yr. The focus of concern is often not the main risk issue when environmental fate is considered because levels and availability change over time (269). Incorporation of half-life data into risk assessments can have substantial benefits for improving understanding of the potential exposures and risks associated with a specific situation (32).

In a similar manner, the risk from persistent contaminants (i.e., DDT) in fish has usually been assessed using results from the analysis of raw fish fillets in combination with assumptions about the size and number of fish meals. The effects of cleaning and cooking on these residues are not typically considered, but have been shown to be reduced substantially in many cases (i.e., 50% or greater) when cooked or processed (224,427). Since many of these risk assessments form the basis of fish advisories or bans with potentially significant economic repercussions, there is obviously an important reason to make these exposure estimates as accurate as possible. Additionally, since there are known health benefits to fish consumption, making recommendations against eating fish based on theoretical risk deserves careful evaluation (352).

Biomarkers and Molecular Epidemiology

The past decade has witnessed a dramatic increase in the level of research activity, derivation of theoretical constructs, and development of practical applications for the direct measurement of biological events or responses that result from human exposure to xenobiotics (89,147). These measurements, conveniently grouped under the descriptor "biological markers" or "biomarkers," reflect molecular and/or cellular alterations that occur along the temporal and mechanistic pathways connecting ambient exposure to a toxicant and eventual disease. As such, an almost limitless array of biomarkers is theoretically available for assessment, and only a minute fraction of these has been recognized and investigated to date (147,155,220). Some events that can technically be classified as biomarkers of chemical exposure (e.g., hematological changes following high levels of exposure to lead or benzene, acetylcholinesterase inhibition by organophosphates) have been measured for decades. However, the recent surge of interest in this field has been driven by technical advances in analytical chemistry and molecular genetic techniques and by the recognition that "classical" toxicology and epidemiology may not be able to alone resolve critical questions regarding causation of environmentally induced disease (89).

Biomarkers are an important component of the emerging discipline of molecular epidemiology, which seeks to expand the capabilities and overcome the limitations of classical epidemiology by incorporating biological measurements collected in exposed humans (89,429). Early efforts at utilizing biomarkers to make quantitative estimates of exposure and to predict human cancer risk were made by Ehrenberg and Osterman-Golkar (105). Using ethylene oxide as a model xenobiotic, these investigators explored the use of macromolecular reaction products (i.e., hemoglobin adducts) as internal dosimeters. By employing hemoglobin adduction data, they predicted the level of ambient ethylene oxide that would correspond to a tumorigenic dose of g-radiation, which they termed the "rad-equivalent dose." Seminal work in the area of biomarkers as applied to the molecular epidemiology of cancer was performed by Perera and Weinstein (271), who proposed the use of such techniques to identify environmental contributors to human cancer incidence. Important early applications of biomarkers to characterize environmental and occupational exposure have also been explored by several other groups in the United States and abroad.

As presented in the original NRC report, biomarkers of internal dose reflect the absorbed fraction of a xenobiotic, that is, the amount of material that has successfully crossed physiological barriers to enter the organism. Consequently, the magnitude of the biomarker accounts for bioavailability and is influenced by numerous parameters such as route of exposure, physiological characteristics of the receptor, and chemical characteristics of the xenobiotic. Generally, simple measurement of xenobiotic levels in biological media (blood, tissue, urine) can provide data on internal dose, and this is called biomonitoring (17,18,203). Biomarkers, on the other hand, reflect internal dose (in terms of proximity to downstream events in the sequence) and could include the measurement of a metabolite in selected biological media, particularly if such metabolite is active or critical to the toxic effects seen (89).

Very useful exposure biomarkers for reactive xenobiotics or their activated (i.e., electrophilic) metabolites are macromolecular reaction products. Substantial research effort has been devoted to the use of protein and DNA adducts as molecular dosimeters. Ehrenberg and co-workers first proposed using hemoglobin (Hb) adducts to monitor the internal dose of alkenes and epoxides such as ethylene oxide over two decades ago (105). This methodology has since evolved into a widely-used and highly sensitive technique for quantitating N-terminal Hb adducts of a variety of xenobiotic metabolites in human blood. Hb adducts have been employed as internal exposure biomarkers for aromatic amines, nitrosamines, polycyclic aromatic hydrocarbons (PAHs), and other compounds (89).

Protein and DNA adducts can be considered as biomarkers of either internal or biologically effective dose (BED), depending upon how close their relationship is to actual disease occurrence. The NRC report defined BED as dose at the site of action, dose at the receptor site, or dose to target macromolecules (233). This definition is troublesome since, strictly speaking, complete characterization of molecular site and mechanism of action for a given xenobiotic would be necessary in order to assign a particular measured end point as a marker of biologically effective dose. For example, protein adducts cannot be considered as effective dose biomarkers for carcinogens, since they do not satisfy these criteria. Ambiguity exists even for DNA adducts, since in no reported instance has xenobiotic-induced adduction of a specific base within a particular DNA sequence in a target cell type been unequivocally linked to a specific clinical outcome in people (89). Despite these uncertainties, adducts in total lymphocyte DNA are considered as appropriate BED biomarkers for carcinogens, based upon the postulated mechanism of chemical carcinogenesis and limited experimental data indicating correlations between DNA adducts in lymphocytes and target tissues (89).

Ideally, a biomarker should be biologically relevant, sensitive, and specific (i.e., valid). In addition, it should be readily accessible, inexpensive, and technically feasible. This combination of requirements is rarely achieved, and some trade-off is inevitable in order to obtain useful biomarker data in a timely manner. A few promising examples are presented in Table 9.17. The validation process for a biomarker involves determining the relationship between the biological parameter measured and both upstream and downstream events in the continuum, that is, the dose-response curve must be characterized (89). For example, an Hb adduct considered for use as an exposure biomarker for a xenobiotic should exhibit a predictable relationship to ambient exposure level. In addition, if used as a surrogate for DNA adduction, then a reproducible correlation between Hb and DNA adducts must be demonstrated. Biological relevance refers to the nature of the phenomenon being measured and its mechanistic involvement in the pathway from exposure to disease. For biomarkers of exposure, disease relevance is not as critical a requirement as is a predictable exposure–response relationship; the opposite is true for biomarkers of effect (89).

There are a few terms that are used when discussing biomarkers that help define their usefulness. *Sensitivity,* for example, reflects the ambient exposure level that can be detected by means of the biomarker. Highly sensitive markers are necessary to quantitate the low ambient levels typical of environmental exposures in industrialized Western nations. *Specificity* is the probability that the biomarker is indicative of actual exposure to the specific xenobiotic that it is designed to detect. For example, certain macromolecular adducts can be derived from exposure to a number of chemical species and are thus less specific than one unique to a single compound. Biomarkers must also be reasonably accessible. Thus, with the exception of occasional tissue biopsies, samples for use in exposure biomarker studies generally consist of blood, urine, milk, or other readily obtainable biological media. Since these are rarely target tissues for toxicological or carcinogenic effects, how the concen-

Table 9.17
Biomarkers examined for selected occupational and environmental chemicals

Chemical	Biomarker: Exposure	Biomarker: Effect	Biomarker: Susceptibility
PAH	DNA adducts[a] Hb adducts SA adducts Urinary 1-HP[a] Sister chromatid exchange (SCE) SCE (high-frequency cells)	*hprt* mutation *gpa* mutation *fes* oncogene activation *ras* p21 level DNA single-strand breaks Chromosomal aberrations Micronuclei	GST-M1 NAT-2 CYP1A1 CYP1A2
1,3-Butadiene	Hb adducts[a] Sister chromatid exchange (SCE) Urinary metabolites	*hprt* mutation Chromosomal aberrations Micronuclei *ras* oncogene activation	
Acrylamide	Hb adducts[a] Urinary metabolites		

Note. From Reference 89.
[a]Biomarkers for which cumulative data indicate best correlation with ambient exposure.

tration relates to the incidence of disease must be inferred. Finally, cost and technical feasibility are important considerations in selection of appropriate biomarkers for applied studies (89).

Statistical and Analytical Issues

Despite the use of precise and reproducible analytical methods, we often do not have enough data of chemical concentrations to estimate exposure with great certainty. Due to resource availability, over the past 15–20 yr it has often been the case that a single round of analytical results or samples collected for other purposes (140) serves as input and the surrogate for long-term or lifetime exposure. As noted previously, chemical concentrations vary over both time and space, which makes the task of dose estimation all the more difficult (224). For instance, to use the (estimated) average dose to predict the typical lifetime dose may seriously overestimate or underestimate the actual dose. Additionally, the average dose may be less important in the biological scheme of things than peak exposures or exposures at specific times (i.e., developmental effects), and ought to be considered as such in the evaluation of exposure (11). Techniques do exist for estimating long-term exposure from short-term data (37,38,328), but the reliability of these estimates is uncertain. Similarly, various mathematical or bench-scale models exist that have been used to estimate exposure in the absence of measurements or long-term monitoring data (342). As has been noted on several occasions, "all models are wrong, but some are useful," and risk assessors should carefully evaluate mesoscale and microscale models, as well as model outputs, for relevance and accuracy. Often, field measurements can serve as useful and relatively inexpensive "reality checks" on model results.

Equally important in exposure assessment are the statistics used to analyze field data. Environmental data are most often lognormally distributed. Under such conditions, a geometric average is generally assumed to be a better measure of the central tendency of data than the arithmetic mean (80). Despite this, the arithmetic mean (and the 95% upper confidence limit of the arithmetic mean) is typically used to identify environmental concentrations for use in exposure assessment. Since the advances in analytical chemistry have improved our ability to measure trace amounts of chemicals in different media and identify potential sources in some situations, less reliance should be placed on the use of mathematical models to predict the distribution of chemical and physical agents in the environment, and actual field data should be collected.

Another important issue in exposure assessment is how the analytical limit of detection (LOD) is handled in calculations. An agent reported as a nondetect may be treated as a numerical zero, or occurring at the LOD or some fraction of the LOD, typically one-half, for purposes of calculating statistics. The manner in which censured data are assessed may affect the outcome of the risk assessment process (132,144,150,158,251,272, 290,356). For instance, analysis of highly contaminated samples or samples containing interfering substances may result in high LODs. Under such conditions and in the absence of additional analysis, assuming that nondetects are present at one-half the LOD could result in the exposure assessment and subsequent risk assessment being driven by compounds that are not truly present in the environmental media. When such an approach is used on a site that may be only 2 to 10% contaminated (based on surface area), the predicted severity of the level of contamination will be much higher than what actually occurs (80).

The practical result of these decisions can be illustrated by considering the following 11 data points resulting from analysis of field samples: Nondetect (ND), ND, ND, ND, ND, 5, 6, 6, 8, 55, and 500 ppm. The results are lognormally distributed as expected. The detection limit is 0.05 ppm, and nondetects are assumed to be present at one-half the detection limit (0.025 ppm). Using these assumptions, the arithmetic mean of the data set is 52.7 ppm, while the geometric mean is 1.3 ppm. The practical consequence of choosing one descriptor over the other may be to mischaracterize the dose and ultimately the risk, and this could influence regulatory decisions involving remediation or regulation.

CLOSING THOUGHTS

The field of exposure assessment has evolved significantly over the past 20 yr. We have learned a great deal about where people are exposed to xenobiotics and the relative degree of exposure. Not that long ago, most of our concerns were about industrial chemicals in our water, ambient air, and the soil. Today, we know that indoor exposure to particles, vapors, and gases (influenced by smoking) often represents the predominant source of exposure for most persons. A greater portion of our work in the future will undoubtedly focus on better understanding of both occupational and indoor exposure, rather than environmental exposures.

It is my personal view that of the four portions of a risk assessment, exposure assessment has made the biggest improvement in quality over the 20-yr history of health risk assessment. Usually, exposure assessments will contain less uncertainty than other steps in a risk assessment, especially the dose-response portion. Admittedly, there are a large number of factors to consider when estimating exposure, and it is a complicated procedure to understand the transport and distribution of a chemical that has been released into the environment. Nonetheless, the available data indicate that scientists can do an adequate job of quantifying the concentration of the chemicals in the various media and the resulting uptake by exposed persons if they account for all the factors that should be considered.

There are at least 11 significant lessons we have learned about conducting exposure assessments in recent years. Had we not had to learn through experience, avoiding these lessons could potentially have saved the United States hundreds of millions of dollars and thousands of person-years of work. First, experience has shown that in our attempts to be prudent, we placed too much emphasis on the "so-called" maximally exposed individual (MEI) (117,242). Often, the results of those analyses were misinterpreted by the public and/or misrepresented by some scientists or lawyers. Often, as a result, poor decisions were made by risk decision makers.

Second, as we have learned how to accurately characterize the risks of exposure for about 95% of the population, more emphasis has been placed on evaluating the various special groups (e.g., Eskimos, subsistence fishermen, dairy farmers). Although the risk for these populations, who can be exposed to particularly high doses (the 95–99.99% group) needs to be understood, the typical levels of exposure for the majority of the population should be the initial focus of the assessment. Perhaps the most significant change in exposure asessment of the past three years has been the national interest in characterizing the risks to children.

The third lesson is a variation of the second: Do not allow the repeated use of conservative assumptions to dictate the results of the assessment. In recent years, many investigators have addressed this issue and have demonstrated its importance. Monte Carlo techniques can generally be successful in addressing this problem.

Fourth, we have learned that risk managers and the public want to understand the statistical confidence in our estimates of risk. Sensitivity analyses can yield important information about the critical exposure variables (132,144,290,356). Further, most risk assessments can benefit from analyses of both variability and uncertainty. Without these, risk managers are not fully informed.

Fifth, we have improved our techniques for statistically handling data; and particularly for samples that have no detectable amount of a contaminant. In the past, regulatory agencies have used the limit of detection (LOD) of the analysis or one-half the LOD in the exposure calculations relying on the premise that the contaminant might be present at that level. We learned that when such an approach is used (without reflection) on a site that may only be 2–10% contaminated (based on surface area), the impact of a few samples on the results could lead us to improper conclusions about the actual level of risk to persons who live there or nearby.

Sixth, we have gained a significant degree of confidence in our ability to estimate historical exposures; so-called dose-reconstruction or retrospective risk assessments, a term that this author coined in 1983. Over the past ten years, for use in epidemiology studies, the likely exposure of workers and/or those in the community nearly forty to fifty years ago have been estimated using chemical usage and emission data, measured data, and models (145,265,294,333,345,424).

Seventh, we now understand the need to quantitatively account for indirect pathways of exposure. For example, the uptake of a contaminant in water by humans due to ingestion is obvious (and direct), but the uptake of the same contaminant by garden vegetables due to watering and the uptake via the inhalation of volatile contaminants from the water while showering are indirect pathways that had not always been evaluated in assessments. Perhaps the most important indirect route of exposure, which had not been considered before 1986 when regulating airborne nonvolatile chemicals, was the ingestion of particulate emissions that have deposited onto soil and plants and were subsequently eaten by grazing animals (125,388). Much additional research in this area will be conducted, and the results will probably change our views about the hazards posed by numerous chemicals.

Eighth, we have learned that children and their exposure patterns are unlike those of adults. As some have said, in more ways than one, children are not miniature adults! Their intake of certain foods, percentage of time spent outdoors, proximity to carpets, and inhalation rates per body weight are all different than adults.

The ninth lesson learned is to use biological monitoring to validate or confirm the predicted degree of human exposure. Over the past 5 to 10 yr, analytical chemists have increased their ability to detect very small quantities of dozens of chemicals in blood, urine, hair, feces, breath, and fat. For many chemicals, these data represent a direct indicator of recent exposure, and in some cases (like PCBs and dioxins), chronic exposure. Validation of our exposure assessments should be one of the major areas of study during the next decade (through both biomonitoring and molecular epidemiology).

Tenth, it has become clear that in most cases, the most significant risks due to exposure to chemicals occur in the workplace. Even though great strides have been made in industrial hygiene over the past 50 yr, the doses to which persons can legally be exposed are much greater (often by a factor of 100) than those to which most persons not in the community will ever be exposed.

Eleventh, and perhaps most important, we have learned that (for most persons) exposures to chemicals and bacteria in the home pose a greater risk than to those in the ambient air or through the ingestion of water. Many fine studies conducted in the 1970s through the current day continue to show that in-home exposures to most chemicals are often about 2–20 times greater than that present in the ambient environment (83,131,167,183,195, 196,247,407). Recently, more than 200 scientists in the fields of epidemiology, exposure assessment, and medicine signed a document called a "consensus statement," which states that future research should focus on personal monitoring; especially of the indoor environment (104).

We have come a long way in a short time. Several professional societies, including the International Society of Exposure Analysis (ISEA), Society for Risk Analysis (SRA), American Industrial Hygiene Association (AIHA), Air and Waste Management Association (AWMA), American Chemical Society (ACS), Society of Toxicology (SOT), International Society for Regulatory Toxicology and Pharmacology (ISRTP), and others, have placed an emphasis on improving the practice of exposure assessment. All indications are that the information we have gained has significantly improved the quality of recent risk assessments, and it can be expected that due to better exposure assessments, future decisions by risk managers will be much better informed.

QUESTIONS

1. What are the routes of exposure normally considered in an exposure assessment?
   Answer: Dermal, inhalation, and ingestion
2. What is the definition of exposure assessment?
   Answer: Exposure assessment is the step in the risk assessment that quantifies the uptake of an agent resulting from contact with various media (e.g., air, water, soil and food). These assessments can address past, current or future anticipated exposures.
3. When estimating uptake through the skin, what are the factors to be considered?
   Answer: Percutaneous absorption rate, surface area of exposed skin, the chemical concentration, exposure duration, and interspecies scaling factor (if data were not collected using human skin).
4. What is a PB-PK model and why are they considered an important improvement over traditional toxicological methods?
   Answer: A physiologically-based pharmacokinetic (PB-PK) model is a quantitative description of the absorption, distribution, metabolism and excretion (ADME) of a chemical in living organism (fish, laboratory animal or human). These models are usually capable of scaling-up animal data to predict the behavior of the toxicologically important substance (parent or metabolite) in humans, thus representing a major improvement over traditional qualitative or semi-quantitative approaches.

5. Uncertainty analyses are an important component of exposure assessments. In these analyses, uncertainty is contrasted with variability. What is the difference between these two terms and give an example?

   Answer: Uncertainty represents a lack of knowledge about factors affecting exposure. For example, if one can precisely measure a particular value, such as the amount of chicken eaten by a specific person on a particular day, then there would be no uncertainty in the measurement. On the other hand, if one wanted to understand the ingestion of chicken during adulthood, this would vary from day to day and week to week; thus this would represent variability. To understand the degree of variability, which could be measured, then a large number of measurements would be necessary. The three most common forms of variability are the variability across locations, variability over time, and variability among individuals.

6. Over the past ten years, monte carlo or probabilistic techniques have become an important and useful component of exposure assessment. Describe the technique and discuss what is learned from their application.

   Answer: Monte carlo techniques attempt to describe the uncertainty in select exposure parameters without having to make a particular measurement during every event over a lifetime. For example, these techniques allow one to estimate with confidence the daily ingestion of water by a typical adult male without having to collect every glass of water drunk by a person (or group of persons) over their lifetimes. The technique generates distributions that describe the uncertainty associated with the risk estimate. By using this approach, the assessor is not forced to rely solely on a single exposure parameter or the repeated use of conservative assumptions to identify the possible dose and risk estimates for a population of persons.

REFERENCES

1. Agency for Toxic Substances and Disease Registry. (1995): *Public health assessment guidance manual.* Lewis, Ann Arbor, MI.
2. Aggazzotti, G., Fantuzzi, G., Righi, E., Tartoni, P., Cassinadri, T., and Predieri, G. (1993): Chloroform in alveolar air of individuals attending indoor swimming pools. *Arch. Environ. Health*, 48:250–254.
3. Alexander, M. (1995): How toxic are chemicals in soil? *Environ. Sci. Technol.*, 29:2713–2717.
4. Allaby, M. (1983): *A dictionary of the environment*, 2nd ed., p. 195. New York University Press, New York.
5. Allen, B., Gentry, R., Shipp, A., and Van Landingham, C. (1998): Calculation of benchmark doses for reproductive and developmental toxicity observed after exposure to isopropanol. *Regul. Toxicol. Pharmacol.*, 28:38–44.
6. American Chemical Society. (1983): *Fate of chemicals in the environment*, edited by R. L. Swann and A. Eschenroeder. ACS Symp. Ser. 225. American Chemical Society, Washington, DC.
7. American Conference of Governmental Industrial Hygienists (ACGIH). (1998): *Industrial hygiene instruments handbook.* American Conference of Governmental Industrial Hygienists, Cincinnati, OH.
8. American Industrial Health Council. (1994): *Exposure factors sourcebook.* American Industrial Health Council, Washington, DC.
9. Andelman, J. B. (1985): Human exposures to volatile halogenated organic chemicals in indoor and outdoor air. *Environ. Health Perspect.*, 62:313–318.
10. Andersen, M. E., and Conolly, R. B. (1998): Mechanistic modeling of rodent liver tumor promotion at low levels of exposure: An example related to dose-response relationships for 2,3,7,8-tetrachlorodibenzo-*p*-dioxin. *Hum. Exp. Toxicol.*, 17(12):683–690.
11. Andersen, M. E., MacNaughton, M. G., Clewell, H. J., and Paustenbach, D. J. (1987): Adjusting exposure limits for long and short exposure periods using a physiological pharmacokinetic model. *Am. Ind. Hyg. Assoc. J.*, 48(4):335–343.
12. Andersen, M. E., Clewell, H. J. III, Gargas, M. L., MacNaughton, M. G., Reitz, R. H., Nolan, R. J., and McKenna, M. J. (1991): Physiologically based pharmacokinetic modeling with dichloromethane, its metabolite, carbon monoxide, and blood carboxyhemoglobin in rats and humans. *Toxicol. Appl. Pharmacol.*, 108:14–27.
13. Andersen, M. E., Clewell, H. J., and Krishnan, K. (1995): Tissue dosimetry, pharmacokinetics modeling and interspecies scaling factors. *Risk Anal.*, 15:533–537.
14. Anderson, B. D., Higuchi, W. I., and Raykar, P. V. (1988): Heterogeneity effects on permeability: Partition coefficient relationships in human stratum corneum. *Pharmacol. Res.*, 5:566–573.
15. Anderson, P. D., and Yuhas, A. L. (1996): Improving risk management by characterizing reality: A benefit of probabilistic risk assessment. *Hum. Ecol. Risk Assess.*, 2:55–58.
16. Antoine, S. R., DeLeon, I. R., and O'Dell-Smith, R. M. (1986): Environmentally significant volatile organic pollutants in human blood. *Bull. Environ. Contam. Toxicol.*, 36:364–371.
17. Ashley, D. L., Bonin, M. A., Cardinali, L., McCraw, J. M., and Wooten, J. V. (1994): Blood concentrations of volatile organic compounds in a nonoccupationally exposed US population and in groups with suspected exposure. *Clin. Chem.*, 40:1401–1404.
18. Ashley, D. L., Bonin, M. A., Cardinali, F. L., McCraw, J. M., and Wooten, J. V. (1996): Measurement of volatile organic compounds in human blood. *Environ. Health Perspect.*, 104(suppl. 5):871–877.
19. Aylward, L. L., Hays, S. M., Karch, N. J., and Paustenbach, D. J. (1996): Relative susceptibility of animals and humans to the cancer hazard posed by 2,3,7,8-tetrachlorodibenzo-*p*-dioxin using internal measures of dose. *Environ. Sci. Technol.*, 30(12):3534–3543.
20. Baes, C. F. III, Sharp, R. D., Sjoreen, A., and Shor, W. R. (1984): *A review and analysis of parameters for assessing transport of environmental released radionuclides through agriculture.* ORNL-5786. U.S. Department of Energy, Oak Ridge National Laboratory, Oak Ridge, TN.
21. Baird, S. J. S, Cohen, J. T., Graham, J. D., Shlyakhter, A. I., and Evans, J. S. (1996): Noncancer risk assessment: a probabilistic alternative to current practice. *Hum. Ecol. Risk Assess.*, 2:79–102.
22. Barber, E. D., Teetsel, N. M., Kolberg, K. F., and Guest, D. (1992): A comparative study of the rates of in vitro percutaneous absorption of eight chemicals using rat and human skin. *Fundam. Appl. Toxicol.*, 19:493–497.
23. Barltrop, D. (1966): The prevalence of pica. *Am. J. Dis. Child.*, 112(2):116–123.

24. Barltrop, D. (1973): Sources and significance of environmental lead for children. *Proc. Int. Symp. Environmental Health Aspects of Lead.*, Commission of European Communities, Center for Information and Documentation, Luxembourg.
25. Barltrop, D., Stehlow, C. D., Thornton, I., and Webb, J. S. (1975): Absorption of lead from dust and soil. *Postgrad. Med. J.*, 5:801–804.
26. Bartek, M. J., LaBudde, J. A., and Maibach, H. I. (1972): Skin permeability *in vivo*: Comparison in rat, rabbit, pig and man. *J. Invest. Dermatol.*, 58:114–123.
27. Beck, B. D., and Cohen, J. T. (1997): Risk assessment for criteria pollutants versus other noncarcinogens: The difference between implicit and explicit conservatism. *Hum. Ecol. Risk Assess.*, 3:617–626.
28. Binder, S., Sokal, D., and Maughan, D. (1986): Estimating soil ingestion: The use of tracer elements in estimating the amount of soil ingested by young children. *Arch. Environ. Health*, 41:341–345.
29. Bogen, K. T. (1994): A note on compounded conservatisms. *Risk Anal.*, 14:379–382.
30. Bogen, K. T., and Spear, R. C. (1987): Integrating uncertainty and interindividual variability in environmental risk assessment. *Risk Anal.*, 7:427–435.
31. Bogen, K. T., Keating, G. A., Meissner, S., and Vogel, J. S. (1998): Initial uptake kinetics in human skin exposed to dilute aqueous trichloroethylene. *J. Expos. Anal. Environ. Epidemiol.*, 8:253271.
32. Borgert, S. J., Roberts, S. M., Harbison, R. D., and James, R. C. (1995): Influence of soil half-life on risk assessment of carcinogens. *Regul. Toxicol. Pharmacol.*, 22:143–151.
33. Boyce, C. P. (1998): Comparison of approaches for developing distributions for carcinogenic potency factors. *Hum. Ecol. Risk Assess.*, 4:527–578.
34. Bronaugh, R. L., Stewart, R. F., Congdon, E. R., and Giles, A. L., Jr. (1982): Methods for *in vitro* percutaneous absorption studies: I. Comparison with *in vitro* results. *Toxicol. Appl. Pharmacol.*, 62:474–480.
35. Brouwer, D. H., and Van Hemmen, J. J. (1992): Elements of a sampling strategy for dermal exposure assessment (abstr.). *Proc. Int. Occup. Hyg. Assoc.,* First International Scientific Conference, 710 December. Brussels, Belgium.
36. Bryce-Smith, D. (1974): Lead absorption in children. *Phys. Bull.*, 25:178–181.
37. Buck, R. J., Hammerstrom, K. A., and Ryan, P. B. (1995): Estimating long-term exposures from short-term measurements. *J. Expos. Anal. Environ. Epidemiol.*, 5:359–374.
38. Buck, R. J., Hammerstrom, K. A., and Ryan, P. B. (1997): Bias in population estimates of long-term exposure from short-term measurements of individual exposure. *Risk Anal.*, 17:455–465.
39. Buckley, T. J., Prah, J. D., Ashley, D., Wallace, L. A., and Zweidinger, R. A. (1997): Body burden measurements and models to assess inhalation exposure to methyl tertiary butyl ether (MTBE). *J. Air Waste Manage. Assoc.*, 47(7).
40. Bukowski, J., Korn, L., and Wartenberg, D. (1995): Correlated inputs in quantitative risk assessment: The effects of distributional shape. *Risk Anal.*, 15:215–219.
41. Burmaster, D. E. (1998): A lognormal distribution for time spent showering. *Risk Anal.* 18:33–36.
42. Burmaster, D. E. (1998): Lognormal distributions for skin area as a function of body weight. *Risk Anal.*, 18:27–32.
43. Burmaster, D. E., and Anderson, P. D. (1994): Principles of good practice for the use of Monte Carlo techniques in human health and ecological risk assessment. *Risk Anal.*, 14:477–491.
44. Burmaster, D. E., and Harris, R. H. (1993): The magnitude of compounding conservatisms in Superfund risk assessments. *Risk Anal.*, 13:131–134.
45. Burmaster, D. E., and Huff, D. A. (1997): Using lognormal distributions and lognormal probability plots in probabilistic risk assessments. *Hum. Ecol. Risk Assess.*, 3:223–234.
46. Burmaster, D. E., and Maxwell, N. I. (1991): Time and loading-dependence in the McKone model for dermal uptake of organic chemicals from a soil matrix. *Risk Anal.*, 11:491–497.
47. Burmaster, D. E., and Thompson, K. M. (1995): Back calculating cleanup targets in probabilistic risk assessments when the acceptability of cancer risk is defined under different risk management policies. *Hum. Ecol. Risk Assess.*, 1:101–120.
48. Burmaster, D. E., and Thompson, K. M. (1997): Estimating exposure point concentrations for surface soils for use in deterministic and probabilistic risk assessments. *Hum. Ecol. Risk Assess.*, 3:363–384.
49. Burmaster, D. E., and von Stackelberg, K. (1991): Using Monte Carlo simulations in public health risk assessments: Estimating and presenting full distributions of risk. *J. Expos. Anal. Environ. Epidemiol.*, 1:491–521.
50. Byard, J. (1989): Hazard assessment of 1,1,1-trichloroethane in groundwater. In *The risk assessment of environmental and human health hazards: A textbook of case studies,* edited by D. J. Paustenbach, pp. 331–334. John Wiley & Sons, New York.
51. Calabrese, E. J., and Kostecki, P. T. (1992): *Risk assessment and environmental fate methodologies.* Lewis, Ann Arbor, MI.
52. Calabrese, E. J., and Stanek, E. J. III. (1998): Soil ingestion in children and adult: A dominant influence in site-specific risk assessment. *Environ. Law Reporter*, 28:10,660–10,671.
53. Calabrese, E. J., and Stanek, E. J. III. (1991): A guide to interpreting soil ingestion studies, II: Qualitative and quantitative evidence of soil ingestion. *Regul. Toxicol. Pharmacol.*, 13:278–292.
54. Calabrese, E. J., and Stanek, E. J. III. (1991): Evidence of soil pica behavior and quantification of soil ingestion. *Human Exp. Toxicology*, 10:245–249.
55. Calabrese, E. J., Barnes, R., Stanek, E. J. III, Pastides, H., Gilbert, C. E., Veneman, P., Wang, X. R., Lasztity, A., and Kostecki, P. T. (1989): How much soil do young children ingest: An epidemiologic study. *Regul. Toxicol. Pharmacol.*, 10:123–137.
56. Calabrese, E. J., Stanek, E. J., Gilbert, C. E., and Barnes, R. M. (1990): Preliminary adult soil ingestion estimates: Results of a pilot study. *Regul. Toxicol. Pharmacol.*, 12:88–95.
57. Calabrese, E. J., Stanek, E. J., and Barnes, R. (1996): Methodology to estimate the amount and particle size of soil ingested by children: implications for exposure assessment at waste sites. *Regul. Toxicol. Pharmacol.*, 24:264–268.
58. Calabrese, E. J., Stanek, E. J. III, Pekow, P., and Barnes, R. M. (1997): Soil ingestion estimates for children residing on a Superfund site. *Ecotoxicol. Environ. Safety*, 36:258–268.
59. California Department of Health Services. (1986): *Development of applied action levels for soil contact: A scenario for the exposure of humans to soil in a residential setting.* California Department of Health Services, Sacramento, CA.
60. Caplan, K. (1993): The significance of wipe samples. *Am. Ind. Hyg. Assoc. J.*, 53(2):70–75.
61. Carnegie Commission on Science, Technology, and Government. (1993): *Risk and the environment. Improving regulatory decision-making.* Carnegie Commission on Science, Technology, and Government, New York.
62. Carrington, C. D., and Bolger, P. M. (1998): Uncertainty and risk assessment. *Hum. Ecol. Risk Assess.*, 4:253–258.
63. Center for Risk Analysis. (1994): *Historical roots of health risk assessment.* Harvard University, School of Public Health, Cambridge, MA.
64. Chaney, R. L., Sterrett, S. B., and Mielke, H. W. (1984): The potential for heavy metal exposure from urban gardens and soils. *Proc. Symp. Heavy Metals in Urban Gardens,* edited by J. R. Preer,

pp. 37–44. Agricultural Experiment Station, University of District of Columbia, Washington, DC.

65. Charney, E., Sayre, J., and Coulter, M. (1980): Increased lead absorption in inner city children: Where does the lead come from? *Pediatrics*, 65:226–231.
66. Clayton, C. A., Perritt, R. R., Pellizzari, E. D., Thomas, K. W., Whitmore, R. W., Özkaynak, H., Spengler, J. D., and Wallace, L. A. (1993): Particle Total Exposure Assessment Methodology (PTEAM) study: Distributions of aerosol and elemental concentrations in personal, indoor, and outdoor air samples in a Southern California community. *J. Expos. Anal. Environ. Epidemiol.*, 3:227–250.
67. Cleek, R. L., and Bunge, A. L. (1993): A new method for estimating dermal absorption from chemical exposure. 1. General approach. *Pharm. Res.*, 10(4):497–506.
68. Clewell, H. J. (1995): The application of physiologically based pharmacokinetics modeling in human health risk assessment of hazardous substances. *Toxicol. Lett.*, 79:207–217.
69. Committee on Advances in Assessing Human Exposure to Airborne Pollutants. (1991): *Human exposure assessment for airborne pollutants.* National Research Council Board of Environmental Studies and Toxicology, National Academy of Science. National Academy Press, Washington, DC.
70. Conner, J. M., Oldaker, G. B. III, and Murphy, J. J. (1990): Method for assessing the contribution of environmental tobacco smoke to respirable particles in indoor microenvironments. *Environ. Technol.*, 11:189–196.
71. Cooper, M. (1957): *Pica,* pp. 60–74. Charles C. Thomas, Springfield, IL.
72. Cooper, J. A., Ferson, S., and Ginzburg, L. (1996): Hybrid processing of stochastic and subjective uncertainty data. *Risk Anal.*, 16:785–792.
73. Copeland, T. L., Paustenbach, D. J., Harris, M. A., and Otani, J. (1993): Comparing the results of a Monte Carlo analysis with EPA's reasonable maximum exposed individual (RMEI): A case study of a former wood treatment site. *Regul. Toxicol. Pharmacol.*, 18:275–312.
74. Copeland, T. L., Holbrow, A. H., Otani, J. M., Connor, K. T., and Paustenbach, D. J. (1994): Use of probabilistic methods to understand the conservatism in California's approach to assessing health risks posed by air contaminants. *J. Air Waste Manage. Assoc.*, 44:1399–1413.
75. Costa, M., Zhitkovich, A., Harris, M., Paustenbach, D., and Gargas, M. (1997): DNA–protein crosslinks produced by various chemicals in cultured human lymphoma cells. *J. Toxicol. Environ. Health*, 30:101–116.
76. Cox, L. A., Jr. (1996): More accurate dose-response estimation using Monte Carlo uncertainty analysis: The data cube approach. *Hum. Ecol. Risk Assess.*, 2:150–174.
77. Cronin, W. J., Oswald, E. J., Shelley, M. L., Fisher, J. W., and Fleming, C. D. (1995): A trichloroethylene risk assessment using a Monte Carlo analysis of parameter uncertainty in conjunction with physiologically-based pharmacokinetic modeling. *Risk Anal.*, 15:555–566.
78. Crouch, E. A. C. (1996): Uncertainty distributions for cancer potency factors: Combining epidemiological studies with laboratory bioassays—The example of acrylonitrile. *Hum. Ecol. Risk Assess.*, 2:130–149.
79. Crouch, E. A. C. (1996): Uncertainty distributions for cancer potency factors: Laboratory animal carcinogenicity and interspecies extrapolation. *Hum. Ecol. Risk Assess.*, 2:103–129.
80. Crump, K. S. (1998): On summarizing group exposures in risk assessment: Is an arithmetic mean or a geometric mean more appropriate? *Risk Anal.*, 18:293–297.
81. Cullen, A. C. (1994): Measures of compounding conservatism in probabilistic risk assessment. *Risk Anal.*, 14(4):389–393.
82. Cullen, A. C., and Frey, H. C. (1999): *Probabilistic techniques in exposure assessment.* Plenum Press, New York.
83. Daisey, J. M., Hodgson, A. T., Fish, W. J., Mendell, M. J., and Ten Brinke, J. (1994): Volatile organic compounds in 12 California office buildings: Classes, concentrations, and sources. *Atmos. Environ.*, 28(22):3557–3562.
84. Danford, D. C. (1982): Pica and nutrition. *Annu. Rev. Nutr.*, 2:303–322.
85. Davis, A., Ruby, M. V., and Bergstrom, P. D. (1992): Bioavailability of arsenic and lead from the Butte, Montana, mining district. *Environ. Sci. Technol.*, 26:461–468.
86. Davis, A., Drexter, J. W., Ruby, M. V., and Nicholson, A. (1993): Micromineralogy of mine waste in relation to lead bioavailability, Butte, Montana. *Environ. Sci. Technol.*, 27:1415–1425.
87. Davis, A., Bloom, N. S., and Que Hee, S. S. (1997): The environmental geochemistry and bioaccessability of mercury in soils and sediments: A review. *Risk Anal.*, 17:557–569.
88. Day, J. P., Hart, M., and Robinson, M. S. (1975): Lead in urban street dust. *Nature* (*Lond.*), 253:343–345.
89. DeCaprio, A. P. (1997): Biomarkers: Coming of age for environmental health and risk assessment. *Environ. Sci. Technol.*, 31(7):1837–1848.
90. de Silva, P.E. (1991): Assessment of Health Risk to Residents of Contaminated Sites. AMCOSH, Occupational Health Services Report to Gas and Fuel Corporation, Melbourne, Australia.
91. de Silva, P. E. (1994): How much soil do children ingest—A new approach. *Appl. Occup. Environ. Hyg.*, 9:40–43.
92. Delzell, E., Sathiakumar, N., Hovinga, M., Macaluso, M., Julian, J., Larson, R., Cole, P., and Muir, D. C. (1996): A follow-up study of synthetic rubber workers. *Toxicology*, 113(13):182–189.
93. Dockery, D. W., Schwartz, J., and Spengler, J. D. (1992): Air pollution and daily mortality: Associations with particulates and acid aerosols. *Environ. Res.*, 59:362–73.
94. Dragun, J. (1998): *The soil chemistry of hazardous materials,* 2nd ed. Amherst Scientific, Amherst, MA.
95. Dragun, J., and Chiasson, A. (1991): *Elements in North American soil.* Hazardous Materials Control Resources Institue, Greenbelt, MD.
96. Driver, J. H., Konz, J. J., and Whitmyre, G. K. (1989): Soil adherence to human skin. *Bull. Environ. Contam. Toxicol.*, 17(9):1831–1850.
97. Duan, N. (1991): Stochastic microenvironmental models for air pollution exposure. *J. Exp. Anal. Environ. Epidemiol.*, 1(2):235–257.
98. Duan, N., and Mage, D. T. (1997): Combination of direct and indirect approaches for exposure assessment. *J. Exp. Anal. Environ. Epidemiol.*, 7(4):439–470.
99. Duggan, M. J., and Williams, S. (1977): Lead-in-dust in city streets. *Sci. Total Environ.*, 7:91–97.
100. Dutkiewicz, T., and Piotrowski, J. (1961): Experimental investigations on the quantitative estimation of aniline absorption in man. *Pure Appl. Chem.*, 3:319–323.
101. Dutkiewicz, T., and Tyras, H. (1967): A study of the skin absorption of ethylbenzene in man. *Br. J. Ind. Med.*, 24:330–332.
102. Ebert, E., Harrington, N., Boyle, K., Knight, J., and Keenan, R. (1993): Estimating consumption of freshwater fish among Maine anglers. *North Am. J. Fisheries Manage.*, 13:737–745.
103. Ebert, E. S., Price, P. S., and Keenan, R. E. (1994): Selection of fish consumption estimates for use in the regulatory process. *J. Expos. Anal. Environ. Epidemiol.*, 4:373–394.
104. Editor. (2000): Pollution monitoring should get personal, scientists say. *Environment. Sci. Tech.*, February 1, pp. 64–65.

105. Ehrenberg, L., and Osterman-Golkar, S. (1980): Alkylation of macromolecules for detecting mutagenic agents. *Teratogen. Carcinogen. Mutagen.* 1(1):105–127.
106. Eisenbud, M. (1978): *Environment, technology, and health: Human ecology in historial perspective.* New York University Press, New York.
107. El Saadi, O., and Langley, A. (1994): The health risk assessment and management of contaminated sites. *Proc. National Workshop on the Health Risk Assessment and Management of Contaminated Sites.* South Australian Health Commission, Adelaide.
108. Ershow, A. G., and Cantor, K. P. (1989): *Total tapwater intake in the United States: Population-based estimates of quantities and sources.* Life Sciences Research Office, Federation of American Societies for Experimental Biology, Bethesda, MD.
109. European Center for Ecotoxicology and Toxicology of Chemicals (ECETOC). (1993): Percutaneous absorption. Monograph 20. Brussels: European Center for Ecotoxicology and Toxicology of Chemicals.
110. European Center for Ecotoxicology and Toxicology of Chemicals (ECETOC). (1993): *Strategy for assigning a "skin notation."* Revised ECETOC Document 31. European Center for Ecotoxicology and Toxicology of Chemicals, Brussels.
111. Evans, J. S., Graham, J. D., Gray, G. M., and Sielken, R. L., Jr. (1994): A distributional approach to characterizing low-dose cancer risks. *Risk Anal.*, 14:25–33.
112. Evans, J. S., Gray, G. M., Sielken, R. L., Jr., Smith, A. E., Valdez-Flores, C., and Graham, J. D. (1994): Use of probabilistic expert judgment in uncertainty analysis of carcinogenic potency. *Regul. Toxicol. Pharmacol.*, 20:15–36.
113. Feldmann, R. J., and Maibach, H. I. (1974): Percutaneous penetration of some pesticides and herbicides in man. *Toxicol. Appl. Pharmacol.* 28:126–132.
114. Fenske, R. A. (1993): Dermal exposure assessment techniques. *Ann. Occup. Hyg.*, 37:687–706.
115. Fenske, R., and Lu, C. (1994): Determination of handwash removal efficiency: Incomplete removal of chloropyrifos from skin by standard handwash techniques. *Am. Ind. Hyg. Assoc. J.*, 55:425–432.
116. Finley, B., Kirman, C., Scott, P., Spivack, A., Bernhardt, T., Warmerdam, J., and Pittignano, A. (2000): A probabilistic risk assessment of a PCB-contaminated waterway: A case study. *J. Soil Contam.*, in press.
117. Finley, B. L., and Paustenbach, D. J. (1994): The benefits of probabilistic exposure assessment: Three case studies involving contaminated air, water, and soil. *Risk Anal.*, 14(1):53–73.
118. Finley, B. L., Scott, P., and Paustenbach, D. J. (1993): Evaluating the adequacy of maximum contaminant levels as health protective cleanup goals: An analysis based on Monte Carlo techniques. *Regul. Toxicol. Pharmacol.*, 18:438–455.
119. Finley, B. L., Scott, P. K., and Mayhall, D. A. (1994): Development of a standard soil-to-skin adherence probability density function for use in Monte Carlo analyses of dermal exposure. *Risk Anal.*, 14:555–569.
120. Finley, B. L., Proctor, D., Scott, P., Harrington, N., Paustenbach, D., and Price, P. (1994): Recommended distributions for exposure factors frequently used in health risk assessment. *Risk Anal.*, 14(4):533–553.
121. Fitzgerald, E. F., Hwang, S.-A., Brix, K. A., Bush, B., Cook, K., and Worswick, P. (1995): Fish PCB concentrations and consumption patterns among Mohawk women at Akwesasne. *J. Expos. Anal. Environ. Epidemiol.*, 5:1–20.
122. Flynn, G. L. (1990): Physicochemical determinants of skin absorption. In *Principles of route-to-route extrapolation for risk assessment,* edited by T. R. Gerrity and C. J. Henry, pp. 93–127. New York: Elsevier.
123. Frantz, S. W. (1990): Instrumentation and methodology for *in vitro* skin diffusion cells. In *Methods for skin absorption,* edited by B. W. Kemppainen and W. G. Reifenrath, pp. 35–59. CRC Press, Boca Raton, FL.
124. Frey, H. C., and Rhodes, D. S. (1998): Characterization and simulation of uncertainty frequency distributions: Effects of distribution choice, variability, uncertainty, and parameter dependence. *Hum. Ecol. Risk Assess.*, 4:423–469.
125. Fries, G. F., and Paustenbach, D. J. (1990) Evaluation of potential transmission of 2,3,7,8-tetrachlorodibenzo-*p*-dioxin-contaminated incinerator emissions to humans via foods. *J. Toxicol. Environ. Health*, 29:1–43.
126. Fries, G. F., Paustenbach, D. J., Mathur, D. B., and Luksemburg, W. J. (1999): A congener specific evaluation of transfer of chlorinated dibenzo-*p*-dioxins and dibenzofurans to milk cows following ingestion of pentachlorophenol-treated wood. *Environ. Sci. Technol.*, 33(8):1165–1170.
127. Gallacher, J. E., Elwood, P. C., Phillips, K. M., Davies, B. E., and Jones, D. T. (1984): Relation between pica and blood lead in areas of differing lead exposure. *Arch. Dis. Child.*, 59:40–44.
128. Gargas, M. L., Burgess, R. J., Voisard, D. E., Cason, G. H., and Andersen, M. E. (1989): Partition coefficients of low molecular weight volatile chemicals in various liquids and tissues. *Toxicol. Appl. Pharmacol.*, 98:87–99.
129. Gargas, M. L., Finley, B. L., Paustenbach, D. J., and Long, T. F. (1999): Environmental health risk assessment: Theory and practice. In *General and applied toxicology,* vol. 3, eds. B. Ballantyne, T. Marrs, and T. Syversen, 2nd ed., pp. 1749–1809. Macmilllan, London.
130. Georgopoulos, P. G., and Lioy, P. J. (1994): Conceptual and theoretical aspects of human exposure and dose assessment. *J. Exp. Anal. Environ. Epidemiol.*, 4:253–285.
131. Gesell, T. F., and Prichard, H. M. (1980): The contribution of radon in tap water to indoor radon concentrations. In *Natural radiation environment III,* vol. 2, edited by T. F. Gesell and W. M. Lowder, pp. 1347–1363. Department of Energy, Washington, DC. CPMF-780422.
132. Gilbert, R. O. (1987): *Statistical methods for environmental pollution monitoring.* Van Nostrand Reinhold, New York.
133. Glickman, T. S. (1986): A methodology for estimating time-of-day variations in the size of a population exposed to risk. *Risk Anal.*, 6:317–323.
134. Goldstein, B. (1995): Risk management will not be improved by mandating numerical uncertainty analysis for risk assessment. *University of Cincinnati Law Review*, 63:1599–1610.
135. Gómez, M. R. (1997): Factors associated with exposure in occupational safety and health administration data. *Am. Ind. Hyg. Assoc. J.*, 58(3):186–195.
136. Gómez, M. R. (1997): Recommendations for optimizing the usefulness of existing exposure databases for public health applications. *Am. Ind. Hyg. Assoc. J.*, 58(3):181–182.
137. Gómez, M. R. (2000): Exposure assessment must stop being local. *Appl. Occup. Environ. Hyg.*, 15(1):15–20.
138. Gómez, M. R., and Rawls, G. R. (1995): Conference on occupational exposure databases: A report and look at the future. *Appl. Occup. Environ. Hyg.*, 10(4):238–243.
139. Goodman, M., Paustenbach, D., Sipe, K., Malloy, C. D., Chapman, P., Figueroa, R., Zhao, K., and Exuzides, K. A. (2000): Epidemiologic study of pulmonary obstruction in workers occupationally exposed to ethyl and methyl cyanoacrylate. *J. Toxicol. Environ. Health A*, 59:135–163.
140. Graham, J. D., Green, L., and Roberts, M. J. (1988): *In search of safety: Chemicals and cancer risks,* pp. 80–114. Harvard University Press, Cambridge, MA.

141. Graham, J., Berry, M., Bryan, E. F., Callahan, M. A., Fan, A., Finley, B., Lynch, J., McKone, T., Ozkaynak, H., Sexton, K., and Walker, K. (1992): The role of exposure databases in risk assessment. *Arch. Environ. Health*, 47:408–420.
142. Guy, R. H., Hadgraft, J., and Maibach, H. I. (1982): A pharmacokinetic model for percutaneous absorption. *Int. J. Pharmacol.*, 11:119–129.
143. Haas, C. N. (1997): Importance of the distributional form in characterizing inputs to Monte Carlo risk assessments. *Risk Anal.*, 17:107–113.
144. Haas, C. N., and Scheff, P. A. (1990): Estimation of averages in truncated samples. *Environ. Sci. Technol.*, 24:912–919.
145. Hallock, M. F., Smith, T. J., Woskie, S. R., and Hammond, S. K. (1994): Estimation of historical exposures to machining fluids in the automotive industry. *Am. J. Ind. Med.*, 26:621–634.
146. Hamed, M. M., and Bedient, P. B. (1997): On the effect of probability distributions of input variables in public health risk assessment. *Risk Anal.*, 17:97–105.
147. Hattis, D. B. (1986): The promise of molecular epidemiology for quantitative risk assessment. *Risk Anal.*, 6(2):181–194.
148. Hattis, D., and Burmaster, D. (1994): Assessment of variability and uncertainty distributions for practical risk analyses. *Risk Anal.*, 14:713–729.
149. Hawley, J. K. (1985): Assessment of health risk from exposure to contaminated soil. *Risk Anal.*, 5(4):289–302.
150. Helsel, D. R. (1990): Less than obvious: statistical treatment of data below the detection limit. *Environ. Sci. Technol.*, 24:1766–1774.
151. Hewitt, D. J., Millner, G. C., Nye, A. C., Webb, M., and Huss, R. G. (1995): Evaluation of residential exposure to arsenic in soil near a Superfund site. *Hum. Ecol. Risk Assess.*, 1:323–335.
152. Hill, R.A., and Hoover, S. M. (1997): Importance of the dose-response model form in probabilistic risk assessment: A case study of health effects from methylmercury in fish. *Hum. Ecol. Risk Assess.*, 3:465–481.
153. Hoffman, F. O., and Hammonds, J. S. (1992): *An introductory guide to uncertainty analysis in environmental and health risk assessment.* Martin Marietta. ES/ER/TM-35.
154. Hoffman, F. O., and Hammonds, J. S. (1994): Propagation of uncertainty in risk assessments: The need to distinguish between uncertainty due to lack of knowledge and uncertainty due to variability. *Risk Anal.*, 14:707–711.
155. Holdway, D. A. (1996): The role of biomarkers in risk assessment. *Hum. Ecol. Risk Assess.*, 2:263–267.
156. Holmes, K. K., Kissel, J. C., and Richter, K. Y. (1996): Investigation of the influence of oil on soil adherence to skin. *J. Soil Contam.*, 5(4):301–308.
157. Horowitz, S. B., and Finley, B. L. (1993): Using human sweat to extract chromium from chromite ore processing residue: Applications to setting health-based cleanup levels. *J. Toxicol. Environ. Health*, 40:585–599.
158. Horwitz, W. (1984): Effects of scientific advances on the decision-making process: Analytical chemistry. *Fundam. Appl. Toxicol.*, 4:S309–S317.
159. Hrudey, S. E., Chen, W., and Rousseaux, C. (1996): *Bioavailability.* CRC–Lewis Publishers, New York.
160. Iman, R. L., and Helton, J. C. (1991): The repeatability of uncertainty and sensitivity analyses for complex probabilistic risk assessments. *Risk Anal.*, 11:591–606.
161. International Life Science Institute (ILSI). (1998): *Aggregate exposure assessment.* Washington, DC.
162. Israeli, M., and Nelson, C. B. (1992): Distribution and expected time of residence for U.S. households. *Risk Anal.*, 12:65–72.
163. Jayjock, M. A. (1997): Uncertainty analysis in the evaluation of exposure. *Am. Ind. Hyg. Assoc. J.*, 58(5):380–382.
164. Jayjock, M. A. (1998): Risk assessment of contact allergens. *Am. J. Contact Dermatitis*, 9(3):155161.
165. Jayjock, M. A., Hazelton, G. A., Lewis, P. G., and Wooder, M. F. (1996): Formulation effect on the dermal bioavailability of isothiazolone biocide. *Food Chem. Toxicol.*, 34(3):277–282.
166. Jayjock, M. A., Lynch, J. R., and Nelson, D. I. (2000): *Risk assessment: Principles for the industrial hygienist.* ACGIH Press, Cincinnati, OH.
167. Jenkins, P. L., Phillips, T. J., Mulberg, E. J., and Hui, S. P. (1992): Activity patterns of Californians: Use of and proximity to indoor pollutant sources. *Atmos. Environ.*, 26A(12):2141–2148.
168. Jo, W. K., Weisel, C. P., and Lioy, P. J. (1988): Routes of chloroform exposure and body burden from showering with chlorinated tap water. *Risk Anal.*, 10:575–580.
169. Johnson, J. E., and Kissel, J. C. (1996): Prevalence of dermal pathway dominance in risk assessment of contaminated soils: A survey of Superfund risk assessments, 1989–1992. *Hum. Ecol. Risk Assess.*, 2:356–365.
170. Johnson, T. R. (1995): Recent advances in the estimation of population exposure to mobile source pollutants. *J. Expos. Anal. Environ. Epidemiol.*, 5(4):551–571.
171. Kerger, B., and Paustenbach, D. (2000): Exposure to 1,1,1 TCE vapors in a home due to contaminated groundwater. *Risk Anal.*, in press.
172. Kerger, B. D., Stabile, I., and Copeland, T. L. (1999): *Mass balance problems with the USEPA model for estimating dioxin dose via breast milk.* Society for Risk Analysis Annual Meeting, Atlanta, GA, 3–7 December.
173. Kezic, S., Mahieu, K., Monster, A. C., and de Wolff, F. A. (1997): Dermal absorption of vaporous and liquid 2-methoxyethanol and 2-ethoxyethanol in volunteers. *Occup. Environ. Med.*, 54:38–43.
174. Kimbrough, R. D., Falk, H., Stehr, P., and Fries, G. F. (1984): Health implications of 2,3,7,8-tetrachlorodibenzo-*p*-dioxin (TCDD) contamination of residential soil. *J. Toxicol. Environ. Health*, 14:47–93.
175. Kissel, J., and Fenske, R. (2000): Improved estimation of dermal pesticide dose to agricultural workers upon reentry. *Appl. Occup. Environ. Hyg.* 15(3):284–290.
176. Kissel, J. C., Richter, K. Y., and Fenske, R. A. (1996): Factors affecting soil adherence to skin in hand-press trails. *Bull. Environ. Contam. Toxicol.* 56:722–728.
177. Kissel, J. C., Richter, K. Y., and Fenske, R. A. (1996): Field measurement of dermal soil loading attributable to various activities: Implications for exposure assessment. *Risk Anal.*, 16(1):115–125.
178. Klain, G. J., and Black, K. E. (1990): Specialized techniques: Congenitally athymic (nude) animal models. In *Methods for skin absorption,* edited by B. W. Kemppainen and W. G. Reifenrath, pp. 165–174. CRC Press, Boca Raton, FL.
179. Knaak, J. B., Iwata, Y., and Maddy, K. T. (1989): The worker hazard posed by reentry into pesticide-treated foliage: Development of safe reentry times, with emphasis on chlorhiophos and carbosulfan. In *The risk assessment of environmental hazards; a textbook of case studies,* edited by D. J. Paustenbach, pp. 797–842. John Wiley and Sons, New York.
180. Knaak, J. B., Dary, C. C., Patterson, G., and Blancato, J. N. (2001): The worker hazard posed by reentry into pesticide-treated foliage: Reassessment of reentry intervals using foliar residue transfer-percutaneous absorption PB-PK/PD models, with emphasis on isofenphos and parathion. In *Human and ecological risk assessment: Theory and practice,* edited by D. J. Paustenbach. J. Wiley and Sons, New York.
181. Knarr, R. D., Cooper, G. L., Brian, E. A., Kleinschmidt, M. G., and Graham, D. G. (1985): Worker exposure during aerial application of a liquid and a granular formulation of ordram selective herbicide to rice. *Arch. Environ. Contam. Toxicol.*, 14:523–527.

182. Kohler, L., Meeuwisse, G., and Mortensson, W. (1984): Food intake and growth of infants between six and twenty-six weeks of age on breast milk, cow's milk formula, and soy formula. *Acta Paediatr. Scand.*, 73:40–48.
183. Krieger, R. I., Ross, J. H., and Thongsinthusak, T. (1992): Assessing human exposures to pesticides. *Rev. Environ. Contam. Toxicol.*, 128:1–15.
184. Krivanek, N. D., McLaughlin, M., and Fayweather, W. E. (1978): Monomethylformide levels in human urine after repetitive exposure to dimethylformamide. *J. Occup. Med.*, 20:179–187.
185. Kreuzer, P. E., Csanady, G. Y., Baur, C., Kessler, W., Papke, O., Greim, H., and Filser, J. Y. (1997): 2,3,7,8 Tetrachlorodibenzo-p-dioxin (TCDD) and congeners in infants:A toxicokinetic model of human lifetime body burdens. *Arch. Toxicol.*, 71:383–400.
186. La Goy, P. K. (1987): Estimated soil ingestion rates for use in risk assessment. *Risk Anal.*, 7(3):355–359.
187. Lavy, T., Shepard, J., and Bouchard, D. (1980): Field worker exposure and helicopter spray pattern of 2,4,5-T. *Bull. Environ. Contam. Toxicol.*, 24(1):90–96.
188. Lavy, T., Walstad, J., Flynn, R., and Mattice, J. (1982): (2,4-Dichlorophenoxy)acetic acid exposure received by aerial application crews during forest spray operations. *J. Agric. Food Chem.*, 30:375–361.
189. Lehmann, A. J., and Fitzhugh, O. G. (1954): 100-fold margin of safety. *Q. Bull. Assoc. U.S. Food & Drug Administration*, 18:33.
190. Lepow, M. L., Bruckman, L., Robino, R. A., Markowitz, S., Gillette, M., and Kapish, J. (1974): Role of airborne lead in increased body burden of lead in Hartford children. *Environ. Health Perspect.*, 6:99–101.
191. Lepow, M. L., Bruckman, L., Gillette, M., Markowitz, S., Robino, R., and Kapish, J. (1975): Investigations into sources of lead in the environment of urban children. *Environ. Res.*, 10:415–426.
192. Leung, H. W., and Paustenbach, D. J. (1994): Techniques for estimating the percutaneous absorption of chemicals due to environmental and occupational exposure. *Appl. Environ. Occup. Hyg.*, 9(3):187–197.
193. Leung, H. W., and Paustenbach, D. J. (1995): Physiologically based pharmacokinetic and pharmacodynamic modeling in health risk assessment and characterization of hazardous substances. *Toxicol. Lett.*, 79:55–65.
194. Lilly, P. D., Andersen, M. E., Ross, T. M., and Pegram, R. A. (1998): A physiologically based pharmacokinetic description of the oral uptake, tissue dosimetry, and rates of metabolism of bromodichloromethane in the male rat. *Toxicol. Appl. Pharmacol.*, 150(2):205–217.
195. Lioy, P., Waldman, J. M., Greenberg, A., Harkov, R., and Pietarinen, C. (1988): The Total Human Environmental Exposure Study (THEES) to Benzo(a)pyrene: Comparison of the inhalation and food pathways. *Arch. Environ. Health*, 43(4):304–312.
196. Lioy, P., Waldman, J. M., Buckley, T., Butler, J., and Pietarinen, C. (1990): The personal, indoor, and outdoor concentrations of PM-10 measured in an industrial community during the winter. *Atmos. Environ.*, 24B(1):57–60.
197. Lioy, P. J., Wainman, T., and Weisel, C. (1993): A wipe sampler for the quantitative measurement of dust on smooth surfaces: Laboratory performance studies. *J. Exp. Anal. Environ. Epidemiol.*, 3:315–320.
198. Lioy, P. J., Yiin, L. M., Adgate, J., Weisel, C., and Rhoads, G. G. (1998): The effectiveness of a home cleaning intervention strategy in reducing potential dust and lead exposures. *J. Exp. Anal. Environ. Epidemiol.*, 8(1):17–35.
199. Lipton, J., Shaw, W. D., Holmes, J., and Patterson, A. (1995): Short communication: Selecting input distributions for use in Monte Carlo analysis. *Regul. Toxicol. Pharmacol.*, 21:192–198.
200. Lotens, W. A., and Wammes, L. J. A. (1993): Vapour transfer in two-layer clothing due to diffusion and ventilation. *Ergonomics*, 36(10):1223–1240.
201. Lourie, R. S., and Cayman, E. M. (1963): Why children eat things that are not food. *Children*, 10:143–146.
202. Lucier, G. W., and Schecter, A. (1998): Human exposure assessment and the national toxicology program. *Environ. Health Perspect.*, 106:623–626.
203. Lynch, A. L. (1994): *Biological monitoring.* Wiley, New York.
204. Lynch, J. R. (1985): Measurement of worker exposure. In *Patty's industrial hygiene and toxicology,* vol. 3a, *The work environment,* eds. L. J. Cralley and L. V. Cralley, 2nd ed., pp. 569–615. Wiley-Interscience, New York.
205. Mage, D., Wilson, W., Hasselblad, V., and Grant, L. (1999): Assessment of human exposure to ambient particulate matter. *J. Air Waste Manage.*, 49:174–183.
206. Marlow, D., Sweeney, M. H., and Fingerhut, M. (1990): *Estimating the amount of TCDD absorbed by workers who manufactured 2,4,5-T.* Tenth Annual International Dioxin Meeting, Bayreuth, Germany.
207. Martin, W. E. (1964): Loss of Sr-90, Sr-89 and I-131 from fallout of contaminated plants. *Radiat. Bot.*, 4:275–281.
208. Mattie, D. R., Bates, G. D., Jr., Jepson, G. W., Fisher, J. W., and McDougal, J. N. (1994): Determination of skin: Air partition coefficients for volatile chemicals: Experimental method and applications. *Fundam. Appl. Toxicol.*, 22:51.
209. Maxim, D. (1989): Problems associated with the use of conservative assumptions in exposure and risk analysis. Chapter 14. In *The risk assessment of environmental and human health hazards: A textbook of case studies,* edited by D. J. Paustenbach, pp. 526–560. J. Wiley and Sons, New York.
210. McArthur, B. (1992): Dermal measurement and wipe sampling methods: A review. *Appl. Occup. Environ. Hyg.*, 7:599–606.
211. McBride, S. G., Ferro, A., Ott, W., Switzer, P., and Hildemann, L. (1999): Investigation of the proximity effect for pollutants in the indoor environment. *J. Exp. Anal. Environ. Epidemiol.*, 9(6):602–621.
212. McCord, C. P. (1943): *Industrial hygiene for engineers.*, Chicago: Martin Press.
213. McDougal, J. N. (1996): Physiologically-based pharmacokinetic modeling. In *Dermatoxicology,* edited by F. N. Marzulli and H. I. Maibach. Taylor and Francis, Washington, DC.
214. McDougal, J. N., Jepson, G. W., Clewell H. J. III, Gargas, M. L., and Andersen, M. E. (1990): Dermal absorption of organic chemical vapors in rats and humans. *Fundam. Appl. Toxicol.*, 14:299–308.
215. McKone, T. E. (1990): Dermal uptake of organic chemicals from a soil matrix. *Risk Anal.*, 10:407–419.
216. McKone, T. E. (1991): Human exposure to chemicals from multiple media and through multiple pathways: Research overview and comments. *Risk Anal.*, 11(1):5–10.
217. McKone, T. E. (1993): Linking a PB-PK model for chloroform with measured breath concentrations in showers: Implications for dermal exposure models. *J. Exp. Anal. Environ. Epidemiol.*, 3:339–365.
218. McKone, T. E., and Bogen, K. T. (1991): Predicting the uncertainties in risk assessment. *Environ. Sci. Technol.*, 25:16–74.
219. McKone, T. E., and Bogen, K. T. (1992): Uncertainties in health-risk assessment: An integrated case study based on tetrachloroethylene in California groundwater. *Regul. Toxicol. Pharmacol.*, 15:86–103.
220. McMillan, A., Whittemore, A. S., Silvers, A., and DiCiccio, Y. (1994): Use of biological markers in risk assessment. *Risk Anal.*, 14(5):807–813.

221. Mertz, C. K., Slovic, P., and Purchase, L. F. H. (1998): Judgments of chemical risks: Comparisons among senior managers, toxicologists, and the public. *Risk Anal.*, 18:391–403.
222. Michaud, J. M., Huntley, S. L., Sherer, R. A., Gray, M. N., and Paustenbach, D. J. (1994): PCB and dioxin re-entry criteria for building surfaces and air. *J. Exp. Anal. Environ. Epidemiol.*, 4(2):197–227.
223. Morgan, M. D., and Henrion, M. (1990): *Uncertainty: A guide to dealing with uncertainty in quantitative risk and policy analysis.* Cambridge University Press, Cambridge.
224. Morgan, J. N., Berry, M. R., and Graves, R. L. (1997): Effects of commonly used cooking practices on total mercury concentration in fish and their impact on exposure assessments. *J. Exp. Anal. Environ. Epidemiol.*, 7:119–133.
225. Mraz, J., and Nohova, M. (1992): Percutaneous absorption of *N,N*-dimethylformamide in humans. *Int. Arch. Occup. Environ. Health*, 64:79–83.
226. Murray, D. M., and Burmaster, D. E. (1992): Estimated distributions for total body surface area of men and women in the United States. *J. Exp. Anal. Environ. Epidemiol.*, 2:451–462.
227. Murray, D. M., and Burmaster, D. E. (1994): Estimated distributions for average daily consumption of total and self-caught fish for adults in Michigan angler households. *Risk Anal.*, 14:513–520.
228. National Academy of Public Administration (NAPA). (1995): Setting Priorities, Getting Results: A New Direction for EPA. Washington, DC.
229. National Academy of Sciences. (1983): *Risk assessment in the federal government: Managing the process.* National Academy Press, Washington, DC.
230. National Academy of Sciences. (1991): *Nutrition during lactation.* National Academy Press, Washington, DC.
231. National Committee on Radiation Programs. (1996): *A guide for uncertainty analysis in dose and risk assessments related to environmental contamination.* Commentary No. 14. National Committee on Radiation Programs, Scientific Committee, Washington, DC.
232. National Research Council. (1974): *Lead in the environment.* National Academy Press, Washington, DC.
233. National Research Council. (1987): Biological markers in environmental health research. Committee on Biological Markers of the National Research Council. *Environ. Health Perspect.*, 74:39.
234. National Research Council. (1989): *Improving risk communication.* National Academy Press, Washington, DC.
235. National Research Council. (1990): *Human exposure assessment for airborne pollutants: Advances and applications.* Committee on Advances in Assessing Human Exposure to Airborne Pollutants, Committee on Geosciences, Environment, and Resources, NRC. National Academy Press, Washington, DC.
236. National Research Council. (1994): *Science and judgment in risk assessment.* National Academy Press, Washington, DC.
237. National Research Council. (1994): *Building consensus through risk assessment.* National Academy Press, Washington, DC.
238. National Research Council. (1996): *Understanding risk: Informing decisions in a democratic society.* National Academy Press, Washington, DC.
239. Nessel, C. S., Butler, J. P., Post, G. B., Held, J. I., Gochfeld, M., and Gallo, M. A. (1991): Evaluation of the relative contribution of exposure routes in a health risk assessment of dioxin emissions from a municipal waste incinerator. *J. Expos. Anal. Environ. Epidemiol.*, 1:283–308.
240. Nethercott, J., Paustenbach, D. J., Adams, R., Horowitz, S., Finley, B. E., Fowler, J., Marks, J., Morton, C., and Taylor, J. (1994): A study of chromium induced allergic contact dermatitis with 54 volunteers: Implications for environmental risk assessment. *Occup. Environ. Med.*, 51(6):371–380.
241. Neville, M. C., Keller, R., Seacat, J., Lutes, V., Neifert, M., Casey, C., Allen, J., and Archer, P. (1988): Studies in human lactation: Milk volumes in lactating women during the onset of lactation and full lactation. *Am. J. Clin. Nutr.*, 48:1375–1386.
242. Nichols, A. L., and Zeckhauser, R. J. (1988): The perils of prudence: How conventional risk assessments distort regulations. *Regul. Toxicol. Pharmacol.*, 8:61–75.
243. Nriagu, J. (1979): *Heavy metals in the environment.* John Wiley and Sons, New York.
244. Ott, W., Thomas, J., Mage, D., and Wallace, L. (1988): Validation of the Simulation of Human Activity and Pollutant Exposure (SHAPE) model using paired days from the Denver, CO, carbon monoxide field study. *Atmos. Environ.*, 22:249–267.
245. Ott, W. R. (1995): *Environmental statistics and data analysis.* CRC Lewis, Boca Raton, FL.
246. Ott, W. R. (1995): Human exposure assessment: the birth of a new science. *J. Expos. Anal. Environ. Epidemiol.*, 5(4):449–472.
247. Ott, W. R., and Roberts, J. W. (1998): Everyday exposure to toxic pollutants. *Sci. Am.*, 278:86–91.
248. Özkaynak, H., Xue, J., Spengler, J., Wallace, L., Pellizzari, E., and Jenkins, P. (1996): Personal exposure to particles and metals: Results from the particle TEAM study in Riverside, CA. *J. Expos. Anal. Environ. Epidemiol.*, 26(1):57–78.
249. Pao, E. M., Fleming, K. H., Guenther, P. M., and Mickle, S. J. (1982): *Foods Commonly Eaten by Individuals: Amount per Day and per Eating Occasion.* Home Economics Report No. 44. U.S. Department of Agriculture, Beltsville, MD.
250. Park, C. N., and Snee, R. D. (1983): Quantitative risk assessment: State-of-the-art for carcinogenesis. *Fundam. Appl. Toxicol.*, 3:320–333.
251. Parkin, T. B., Melsinger, J. J., Chester, S. T., Starr, J. L., and Robinson, J. A. (1988): Evaluation of statistical estimation methods for lognormally distributed variables. *Soil Sci. J.*, 52:323–329.
252. Paustenbach, D. J. (1987): Assessing the potential environmental and human health risks of contaminated soil. *Comments Toxicol.*, 1:185–220.
253. Paustenbach, D. J. (1988): Assessment of the developmental risks resulting from occupational exposure to select glycol ethers within the semiconductor industry. *J. Toxicol Environ. Health*, 23:29–75.
254. Paustenbach, D. J. (1989): A survey of environmental risk assessment. In *The risk assessment of environmental and human health hazards: A textbook of case studies,* edited by D. J. Paustenbach, pp. 139. J. Wiley and Sons, New York.
255. Paustenbach, D. J. (1989): *The risk assessment of environmental hazards: A textbook of case studies.* John Wiley & Sons, New York.
256. Paustenbach, D. J. (1990): Health risk assessment and the practice of industrial hygiene. *Am. Ind. Hyg. Assoc. J.*, 51(7):339–351.
257. Paustenbach, D. J. (1995): The practice of health risk assessment in the United States (1975–1995): How the U.S. and other countries can benefit from that experience. *Hum. Ecol. Risk Assess.*, 1(1):29–79.
258. Paustenbach, D. J. (2000): Pharmacokinetics and unusual work schedules. In *Patty's industrial hygiene and toxicology*, Chapter 40, pp. 1787–1901. John Wiley and Sons, New York.
259. Paustenbach, D. J., Shu, H. P., and Murray, F. J. (1986): A critical examination of assumptions used in risk assessment of dioxin contaminated soil. *Regul. Toxicol. Pharmacol.*, 6:284–307.
260. Paustenbach, D. J., Clewell, H. J. III, Gargas, M. L., and Andersen, M. E. (1988): A physiologically-based pharmacokinetic model for carbon tetrachloride. *Toxicol. Appl. Pharmacol.*, 96:191–211.
261. Paustenbach, D. J., Rinehart, W. E., and Sheehan, P. J. (1991): The health hazards posed by chromium-contaminated soils in residen-

tial and industrial areas: Conclusions of an expert panel. *Regul. Toxicol. Pharmacol.*, 13:195–222.

262. Paustenbach, D. J., Meyer, D. M., Sheehan, P. J., and Lau, V. (1991): An assessment and quantitative uncertainty analysis of the health risks to workers exposed to chromium contaminated soils. *Toxicol. Ind. Health*, 7:159–196.
263. Paustenbach, D. J., Jernigan, J., Bass, R., Kalmes, R., and Scott, P. (1992): A proposed approach to regulating contaminated soil: Identify safe concentrations for seven of the most frequently encountered exposure scenarios. *Regul. Toxicol. Pharmacol.*, 16:21–56.
264. Paustenbach, D. J., Wenning, R. J., Lau, V., Harrington, N. W., Rennix, D. K., and Parsons, A. H. (1992): Recent developments on the hazards posed by 2,3,7,8-tetrachlorodibenzo-*p*-dioxin in soil: Implications for setting risk-based cleanup levels at residual and industrial sites. *J. Toxicol. Environ. Health*, 36:103–148.
265. Paustenbach, D. J., Price, P. E., Bradshaw, R. D., Ollison, W., Peterson, D., and Blank, C. (1992): Re-evaluation of benzene exposure for the pliofilm workers (1939–1976). *J. Toxicol. Environ. Health*, 36:177–232.
266. Paustenbach, D. J., Bruce, G. M., and Chrostowski, P. (1997): Current views on the oral bioavailability of inorganic mercury in soil: The impact on health risk assessments. *Risk Anal.*, 17:533–545.
267. Paustenbach, D. J., Finley, B. L., and Long, T. F. (1997): The critical role of house dust in understanding the hazards posed by contaminated soils. *Int. J. Toxicol.*, 16:339–362.
268. Paustenbach, D. J., Hays, S., Sururi, S., and Underwood, P. (1997): Comparing the estimated uptake of TCDD using exposure calculations with the actual uptake: A case study of residents of Times Beach, Missouri. *Proc. Int. Dioxin Conf.*, Indianapolis, IN.
269. Paustenbach, D. J., Leung, H. W., and Rothrock, J. (1999): Health risk assessment. In *Occupational skin disease*, edited by R. Adams, 3rd ed., pp. 291–323. W. B. Saunders, Philadelphia, PA.
270. Pellizzari, E. D., Perritt, R. L., and Clayton, C. A. (1999): National human exposure assessment survey (NHEXAS): Exploratory survey of exposure among population subgroups in EPA Region V. *J. Expos. Anal. Environ. Epidemiol.*, 9:4955.
271. Perera, F. P., and Weinstein, I. B. (1982): Molecular epidemiology and carcinogen–DNA adduct detection: New approaches to studies of human cancer causation. *J. Chron. Dis.*, 35(7):581–600.
272. Perkins, J. L., Cutter, G. N., and Cleveland, M. S. (1990): Estimating the mean, variance, and confidence limits from censored (‹limit of detection), lognormally-distributed exposure data. *Am. Ind. Hyg. Assoc. J.*, 51:416–419.
273. Piotrowski, J. K. (1967): Further investigations on the evaluation of exposure to nitrobenzene. *Br. J. Ind. Med.*, 24:60–65.
274. Piotrowski, J. (1971): Evaluation of exposure to phenol: Absorption of phenol vapor in the lungs and through the skin and excretion of phenol in urine. *Br. J. Ind. Med.*, 28:172–178.
275. Piotrowski, J. (1977): *Exposure tests for organic compounds in industrial toxicology.* National Institute for Occupational Safety and Health, Cincinnati, OH.
276. Plato, N., Krantz, S., Gustavsson, P., Smith, T. J., and Westerholm, P. (1995): A cohort study of Swedish man-made mineral fiber (MMMF) production workers. Part I: Fiber exposure assessment in the rock/slag wool production industry 1938–1990. *Scand. J. Work Environ. Health*, 21:345–352.
277. Popendorf, W. J., and Leffingwell, J. T. (1982): Regulating OP pesticide residues for farmworker protection. In *Residue review 82,* pp. 125–201. Springer-Verlag, New York.
278. Presidential/Congressional Commission on Risk Assessment and Risk Management (CRAM). (1997): *Framework for environmental health risk management, Final report,* Vol. 1, U.S. Government Printing Office, Washington, DC.
279. Presidential/Congressional Commission on Risk Assessment and Risk Management (CRAM). (1997): *Risk assessment and risk management in regulatory decision-making, Final report,* Vol. 1, U.S. Government Printing Office, Washington, DC.
280. Price, P. S., Su, S. H., and Gray, M. N. (1994): The effect of sampling bias on estimates of angler consumption rates in creel surveys. *J. Expos. Anal. Environ. Epidemiol.*, 4:355–372.
281. Price, P. S., Su, S. H., Harrington, J. R., and Keenan, R. E. (1996): Uncertainty and variation in indirect exposure assessments: An analysis of exposure to tetrachlorodibenzo-*p*-dioxin from a beef consumption pathway. *Risk Anal.*, 16:263–277.
282. Price, P. S., Curry, C. L., Goodrum, P. E., Gray, M. N., McCrodden, J. I., Harrington, N. W., Carlson-Lynch, H., and Keenan, R. E. (1996): Monte Carlo modeling of time-dependent exposures using a microexposure event approach. *Risk Anal.*, 16:339–348.
283. Price, P. S., Scott, P. K., Wilson, N. D., and Paustenbach, D. J. (1998): An empirical approach for deriving information on total duration of exposure from information on historical exposure. *Risk Anal.*, 18:611–619.
284. Proctor, D. M., Zak, M. A., and Finley, B. L. 1997. Resolving uncertainties associated with the construction worker soil ingestion rate: A proposal for risk-based remediation goals. *Hum. Ecol. Risk Assess.*, 3:299–304.
285. Puffer, H. W., Azen, S. P., Duda, M. J., and Young, D. R. (1981): Consumption Rates of Potentially Hazardous Marine Fish Caught in the Metropolitan Los Angeles Area. EPA Grant R807 120010.
286. Que Hee, S. S., Peace, B., Clark, C. S., Boyle, J. R., Bornschein, R. L., and Hammond, P. B. (1985): Evolution of efficient methods to sample lead sources, such as house dust and hand dust, in the homes of children. *Environ. Res.*, 38:77–95.
287. Rai, S. N., and Krewski, D. (1998): Uncertainty and variability analysis in multiplicative risk models. *Risk Anal.*, 18:37–45.
288. Ramsey, J., and Andersen, M. (1984): A physiologically based description of the inhalation pharmacokinetics of styrene in rats and humans. *Toxicol. Appl. Pharmacol.*, 73:159–175.
289. Rappaport, S. M. (1985): Smoothing of exposure variability at the receptor—Implications for health standards. *Ann. Occup. Hyg.*, 29:201–214.
290. Rappaport, S. M., and Selvin, J. (1987): A method for evaluating the mean exposure from a lognormal distribution. *Am. Ind. Hyg. Assoc. J.*, 48:374–379.
291. Rappaport, S. M., and Spear, R. C. (1988): Physiological damping of exposure variability during brief periods. *Ann. Occup. Hyg.*, 32:21–33.
292. Reitz, R. H., Gargas, M. L., Andersen, M. E., Provan, W. M., and Green, T. L. (1996): Predicting cancer risk from vinyl chloride exposure with a physiologically based pharmacokinetic model. *Toxicol. Appl. Pharmacol.*, 137:253–267.
293. Rhomberg, L. R. (1997): A survey of methods for chemical risk assessment among federal regulatory agencies. *Hum. Ecol. Risk Assess.*, 3:1029–1196.
294. Ripple, S. R. (1992): Looking back: The use of retrospective health risk assessment. *Environ. Sci. Tech.*, 26:1270–1277.
295. Roach, S. A. (1966): A more rational basis for air-sampling programs. *Am. Ind. Hyg. Assoc. J.*, 27:1–12.
296. Roberts, J. W., and Dickey, P. (1995): Exposure of children to pollutants in house dust and indoor air. *Rev. Environ. Contam. Toxicol.*, 143:59–78.
297. Roberts, J. W., Budd, W. T., Ruby, M. G., Camann, D. E., Fortmann, R. C., Lewis, R. G., Wallace, L. A., and Spittler, T. M. (1992): Human exposure to pollutants in the floor dust of homes and offices. *J. Expos. Anal. Environ. Epidemiol. Suppl.*, 1:127–146.
298. Roberts, J. W., Budd, W. T., Chuang, J., and Lewis, R. G. (1993): Chemical Contaminants in House Dust: Occurrences and Sources.

EPA/600/A-93/215. U.S. Environmental Protection Agency, Washington, DC.

299. Robinson, R. B., and Hurst, B. T. (1997): Statistical quantification of the sources of variance in uncertainty analysis. *Risk Anal.*, 17:447–454.
300. Roels, H. A., Buchet, J. P., Lauwenys, R. R., Claeys-Thoreau, F., Lafontaine, A., and Verduyn, G. (1980): Exposure to lead by oral and pulmonary routes of children living in the vicinity of a primary lead smelter. *Environ. Res.*, 22:81–94.
301. Romney, E. M., Lindberg, N. G., Hawthorne, H. A., Bystrom, B. B., and Larson, K. H. (1963): Contamination of plant foliage with radioactive nuclides. *Annu. Rev. Plant Physiol.*, 14:271–279.
302. Roseberry, A. M., and Burmaster, D. E. (1991): A note: Estimating exposure concentrations of lipophilic organic chemicals to humans via finfish. *J. Expos. Anal. Environ. Epidemiol.*, 1:513–521.
303. Roseberry, A. M., and Burmaster, D. E. (1992): Lognormal distributions for water intake by children and adults. *Risk Anal.*, 12:99–104.
304. Ruby, M. V., Davis. A., Kempton, J. H., Drexter, J. W., and Bergstrom, P. D. (1992): Lead bioavailability under simulated gastric conditions. *Environ. Sci. Technol.*, 26:1242–1248.
305. Ruby, M. V., Schoof, R., Brattin, W., Goldade, M., Post, G., Harnois, M., Mosby, D. E., Casteel, S. W., Berti, W., Carpenter, M., Edwards, D., Cragin, D., and Chappell, W. (1999): Advances in evaluating the oral bioavailability of inorganics in soil for use in human health risk assessment. *Environ. Sci. Technol.*, 33(21):3697–3705.
306. Ruffle, B., Burmaster, D. E., Anderson, P. D., and Gordon, H. D. (1994): Lognormal distributions for fish consumption by the general U.S. population. *Risk Anal.*, 14(4):395–404.
307. Ruoff, W. L., Diamond, G. L., Velazquez, S. F., Stiteler, W. M., and Gefell, D. J. (1994): Bioavailability of cadmium in food and water: A case study on the derivation of relative bioavailability factors for inorganics and their relevance to the reference dose. *Regul. Toxicol. Pharmacol.*, 20:139–160.
308. Russell, R. S. (1966): Entry of radioactive materials into plants. In *Radioactivity and human diet,* edited by R. S. Russell, chap. 5. Pergamon Press, New York.
309. Sathiakumar, N., Delzell, E., Hovinga, M., Macaluso, M., Julian, J. A., Larson, R., Cole, P., and Muir, D. C. (1998): Mortality from cancer and other causes of death among synthetic rubber workers. *Occup. Environ. Med.*, 55(4):230–235.
310. Sayre, J. W., Charney, E., Vostal, J., and Pless, B. (1974): House and hand dust as a potential source of childhood lead exposure. *Am. J. Dis. Child.*, 127:167–170.
311. Schoof, R. A., and Nielsen, J. B. (1997): Evaluation of methods for assessing the oral bioavailability of inorganic mercury in soil. *Risk Anal.*, 17:545–555.
312. Scott, P. K., Sung, H., Finley, B. L., Schulze, R. H., and Turner, D. B. (1997): Identification of an accurate soil suspension/dispersion modeling method for use in estimating health-based soil cleanup levels of hexavalent chromium in chromit-ore processing residues. *J. Air Waste Manage.*, 47(7):753–765.
313. Scott, P. K., Harris, M. A., Rabbe, D. E., and Finley, B. L. (1997): Background air concentrations of Cr(VI) in Hudson County, New Jersey: Implications for setting health-based standards for Cr(VI) in soil. *J. Air Waste Manage.* 47:592–600.
314. Scow, K., Wechsler, A. E., Stevens, J., Wood, M., and Callahan, M. A. (1979): Identification and Evaluation of Waterborne Routes of Exposure From Other Than Food and Drinking Water. U.S. Environmental Protection Agency, Washington, DC. EPA/440/4-79/016.
315. Sedman, R., Funk, L. M., and Fountain, R. (1998): Distribution of residence duration in owner occupied housing. *J. Exp. Anal. Environ. Epidemiol.*, 8:51–57.
316. Shatkin, J. A., and Brown, H. S. (1991): Pharmacokinetics of the dermal route of exposure to volatile organic chemicals in water. A computer simulation model. *Environ. Res.*, 56:90–108.
317. Sheppard, S. C., and Evenden, W. G. (1994): Contaminant enrichment and properties of soil adhering to skin. *J. Environ. Qual.*, 23:604–613.
318. Shifrin, N. S., Beck, B. D., Gauthier, T. D., Chapnick, S. D., and Goodman, G. (1996): Chemistry, toxicology, and human health risks of cyanide compounds in soils at former manufactured gas plant sites. *Regul. Toxicol. Pharmacol.*, 23:106–116.
319. Shlyakhter, A. I. (1994): An improved framework for uncertainty analysis: Accounting for unsuspected errors. *Risk Anal.*, 14:441–447.
320. Shlyakhter, A., Goodman, G., and Wilson, R. (1992): Monte Carlo simulation of rodent carcinogenicity bioassays. *Risk Anal.*, 12:73–82.
321. Shu, H., Paustenbach, D., Murray, F. J., Marple, L., Brunck, B., Dei Rossi, D., and Teitelbaum, P. (1988): Bioavailability of soil-bound TCDD: Dermal bioavailability in the rat. *Fundam. Appl. Toxicol.*, 10:648–654.
322. Sielken, R. L., Jr. (1989): Useful tools for evaluating and presenting more science in quantitative cancer risk assessments. *Tox. Subst. J.*, 9:353–404.
323. Sielken, R. L., Jr., and Stevenson, D. E. (1997): Opportunities to improve quantitative risk assessment. *Hum. Ecol. Risk Assess.*, 3:479–490.
324. Sielken, R. L., Jr., and Valdez-Flores, C. (1996): Comprehensive realism's weight-of-evidence based distributional dose-response characterization. *Hum. Ecol. Risk Assess.*, 2:175–193.
325. Simon, T. (1997): Combining physiologically based pharmacokinetic modeling with Monte Carlo simulation to derive an acute inhalation guidance value for trichloroethylene. *Regul. Toxicol. Pharmacol.*, 26:257–270.
326. Skrowronski, G. A., Turkall, R. M., and Abdel-Rahman, M. S. (1988): Soil absorption alters bioavailability of benzene in dermally exposed male rats. *Am. Ind. Hyg. Assoc. J.*, 49:506–511.
327. Slob, W. (1994): Uncertainty analysis in multiplicative models. *Risk Anal.*, 14(4):571–576.
328. Slob, W. (1996): A comparison of two statistical approaches to estimate long-term exposure distributions from short-term measurements. *Risk Anal.*, 16:195–200.
329. Smith, A. (1994): Risk evaluation of breast milk. *J. Toxicol. Environ. Health,*
330. Smith, A. E., Ryan, P. B., and Evans, J. S. (1992): The effect of neglecting correlations when propagating uncertainty and estimating population distribution of risk. *Risk Anal.*, 12:467–474.
331. Smith, A. H. (1987): Infant exposure assessment for breast milk dioxins and furans derived from waste incineration emissions. *Risk Anal.*, 7(3):347–353.
332. Smith, R. L. (1994): Use of Monte Carlo simulation for human exposure assessment at a Superfund site. *Risk Anal.*, 14(4):433–439.
333. Smith, T. J., Hammond, S. K., and Wong, O. (1993): Health effects of gasoline exposure: I: Exposure assessment for U.S. distribution workers. *Environ. Health Perspect.*, 101(6):13–21.
334. Snyder, W. S. (1975): *Report of the task group on reference man.* International Commission on Radiological Protection Pub. 23. Pergamon Press, New York.
335. Society of Toxicology. (2000): Risk assessment: What's it all about? *Communique,* special issue, pp. 4. Society of Toxicology, Reston, VA.
336. Stanek, E. J. III, and Calabrese, E. J. (1991): A guide to interpreting soil ingestion studies, I: Development of a model to estimate the soil ingestion detection level of soil ingestion studies. *Regul. Toxicol. Pharmacol.*, 13:263–277.

337. Stanek, E. J. III, and Calabrese, E. J. (1995): Daily estimates of soil ingestion in children. *Environ. Health Perspect.*, 103:276–285.

338. Stanek, E. J. III, and Calabrese, E. J. (1995): Improved soil ingestion estimates for use in site evaluations using the best tracer method. *Hum. Ecol. Risk Assess.*, 1:133–157.

339. Stanek, E. J. III, and Calabrese, E. J. (1995): Soil ingestion estimates for use in site evaluation based on the best tracer method. *Hum. Ecol. Risk Assess.*, 1:133–156.

340. Stanek, E. J. III, and Calabrese, E. J. (1998): Prevalence of soil mouthing/ingestion among healthy children aged 1 to 6. *Soil Contam.*, 2:27–42.

341. Stanek, E. J. III, Calabrese, E. J., and Xu, L. (1997): Soil ingestion in adults: Results of a second pilot study. *Ecotoxicol. Environ. Safety*, 36:249–257.

342. Stanek, E. J. III, Calabrese, E. J., and Xu, L. (1998): A caution for Monte Carlo risk assessment of long term exposures based on short term exposure data. *Hum. Ecol. Risk Assess.*, 4:409–422.

343. Stern, A. H., Korn, L. R., and Ruppel, B. E. (1996): Estimation of fish consumption and methylmercury intake in the New Jersey population. *J. Expos. Anal. Environ. Epidemiol.*, 6:503–525.

344. Stewart, P., and Stenzel, M. (2000): Exposure assessment in the occupational setting. *Appl. Occup. Environ. Hygiene*, 15:435–444.

345. Stewart, P. A., and Herrick, R. F. (1991): Issues in performing retrospective exposure assessment. *Appl. Occup. Environ. Hyg.*, ???

346. Stewart, P. A., Lees, P. S. J., and Francis, M. (1996): Quantification of historical exposures in occupational cohort studies. *Scand. J. Work Environ. Health*, 22:405–414.

347. Stewart, R. D., and Dodd, H. C. (1964): Absorption of carbon tetrachloride, trichloroethylene, tetrachloroethylene, methylene chloride, and 1,1,1-trichloroethane through the human skin. *Am. Ind. Hyg. Assoc.*, J. 25:439–446.

348. Stone, R. A., Marsh, G. M., Youk, A. O., Smith, T. J., and Quinn, M. M. (1996): Statistical estimation of exposure to fibres in jobs for which no direct measurements are available. *Occup. Hyg.*, 3:91–101.

349. Surber, C., Wilhelm, K. P., Maibach, H. I., Hall, L. L., and Guy, R. H. (1990): Partitioning of chemicals into human stratum corneum: Implications for risk assessment following dermal exposure. *Fundam. Appl. Toxicol.*, 15:99–107.

350. Taylor, E. R. (1983): How much soil do children eat? In *The health risk assessment and management of contaminated sites,* edited by O. El Saadi and A. Langley, pp. 7277. South Australian Health Commission, Adelaide.

351. Taylor, A. C., Evans, J. S., and McKone, T. E. (1993: The value of animal test information in environmental control decisions. *Risk Anal.*, 13:403–412.

352. Thomas, K. W., Sheldon, L. S., Pellizzari, E. D., Handy, R. W., Roberds, J. M., and Berry, M. R. (1997): Testing duplicate diet sample collection methods for measuring personal dietary exposures to chemical contaminants. *J. Expos. Anal. Environ. Epidemiol.*, 7:17–36.

353. Thompson, K. M., and Burmaster, D. E. (1991): Parametric distributions for soil ingestion by children. *Risk Anal.*, 11:339–342.

354. Thompson, K. M., Burmaster, D. E., and Crouch, E. A. C. (1992): Monte Carlo techniques for quantitative uncertainty analysis in public health risk assessments. *Risk Anal.*, 12(1):53–63.

355. Travis, C. C., and Hester, S. T. (1990): Background exposure to chemicals: What is the risk? *Risk Anal.*, 10:463–466.

356. Travis, C. C., and Land, M. L. (1990): Estimating the mean of data sets with nondetectable values. *Environ. Sci. Technol.*, 24:961–962.

357. Trowbridge, P. R., and Burmaster, D. E. (1997): A parametric distribution for the fraction of outdoor soil in indoor dust. *J. Soil Contam.*, 6:161–168.

358. Umbreit, T. H., Hesse, E. J., and Gallo, M. A. (1986): Acute toxicity of TCDD contaminated soil from an industrial site. *Science*, 232:497–499.

359. Umbreit, T. H., Hesse, E. J., and Gallo, M. A. (1986): Comparative toxicity of TCDD contaminated soil from Times Beach, Missouri and Newark, New Jersey. *Chemosphere*, 15:121–2124.

360. Upton, A. C. (1988): Evolving perspectives on the concept of dose in radiobiology and radiation protection. *Health Phys.*, 55(4):605–614.

361. U.S. Department of Agriculture. (1972): *Food consumption: Households in the United States, seasons and year 1965–1966.* U.S. Department of Agriculture, Washington, DC.

362. U.S. Department of Agriculture. (1980): Food and Nutrient Intakes of Individuals in One Day in the United States, Spring 1977. Nationwide Food Consumption Survey 1977–1978. U.S. Department of Agriculture, Washington, DC. Preliminary Report 2.

363. U.S. Department of Agriculture. (1992): Food and Nutrient Intakes by Individuals in the United States, 1 Day, 1987–88. Nationwide Food Consumption Survey 1987–1988. U.S. Department of Agriculture, Washington, DC. Human Nutrition Information Service, NFCS Report 87-1-1.

364. U.S. Environmental Protection Agency. (1983–1989): *Methods for assessing exposure to chemical substances, Vol. 113.* U.S. Environmental Protection Agency, Washington, DC. Office of Toxic Substances, Exposure Evaluation Division, EPA/560/5-85/002, NTIS PB86-107067.

365. U.S. Environmental Protection Agency. (1984) *An estimation of the daily food intake based on data from the 1977–1978 USDA nationwide food consumption survey.* U.S. Environmental Protection Agency, Washington, DC. Office of Radiation Programs, EPA/520/1-84/015.

366. U.S. Environmental Protection Agency. (1985): *Development of statistical distributions or ranges of standard factors used in exposure assessments.* U.S. Environmental Protection Agency, Washington, DC. Office of Health and Environmental Assessment, EPA/600/8-85/010.

367. U.S. Environmental Protection Agency. (1986): *Guidelines on air quality models* (rev.). U.S. Environmental Protection Agency, Research Triangle Park, NC. Office of Air Quality Planning and Standards, EPA/450/2-78/027R.

368. U.S. Environmental Protection Agency. (1987): *Selection criteria for mathematical models used in exposure assessments: Surface water models.* U.S. Environmental Protection Agency, Washington, DC. Office of Health and Environmental Assessment, Office of Research and Development, EPA/600/8-87/042, NTIS PB88-139928/AS.

369. U.S. Environmental Protection Agency. (1987): *The Total Exposure Assessment Methodology (TEAM) study. Volume 1: Summary and analysis.* U.S. Environmental Protection Agency, Office of Acid Deposition, Environmental Monitoring and Quality Assurance, Research and Development, EPA/600/6-87/002a.

370. U.S. Enviornmental Protection Agency. (1987): *Methods for assessing exposure to chemical substances, Vol. 7, Methods for assessing consumer exposure to chemical substances.* U.S. Environmenmental Protection Agency, Washington, DC. Office of Toxic Substances, EPA/560/5-85/007.

371. U.S. Environmental Protection Agency. (1988): Proposed guidelines for exposure-related measurements. *Fed. Reg.*, 53(232):48830–48853.

372. U.S. Environmental Protection Agency. (1989) *Risk assessment guidance for Superfund. Volume I. Human health evaluation manual (Part A).* Interim final. U.S. Environmental Protection Agency, Washington, DC. Office of Emergency and Remedial Response, EPA/540/1-89/002.

373. U.S. Environmental Protection Agency. (1991): *Risk assessment guidance for Superfund (RAGS). Volume I: Human health evaluation manual (HHEM) (Part B). Development of risk-based preliminary remediation goals.* U.S. Environmental Protection Agency, Washington, DC. Office of Emergency and Remedial Response, EPA/540/R-92/003, NTIS PB92-963333.
374. U.S. Environmental Protection Agency. (1991): *Time spent in activities, locations, and microenvironments: A California-national comparison.* Office of Research and Development, Las Vegas, NV. Environmental Monitoring Systems Laboratory, EPA/600/4-91/006.
375. U.S. Environmental Protection Agency. (1992): *Supplemental guidance to RAGS: Calculating the concentration term.* U.S. Environmental Protection Agency, Washington, DC. Office of Solid Waste and Emergency Response, OSWER Directive 9285.7-081.
376. U.S. Environmental Protection Agency. (1992): *Dermal exposure assessment: Principles and applications.* U.S. Environmental Protection Agency, Washington, DC. Office of Health and Environmental Assessment, Office of Research and Development, EPA/600/8-91/011.
377. U.S. Environmental Protection Agency. (1992): Guidelines for exposure assessment; Notice. *Fed. Reg.*, 57(104):22888–22938.
378. U.S. Environmental Protection Agency. (1992): Safeguarding the future: Credible science, credible decisions. Report of the Expert Panel on the Role of Science at EPA. Washington, DC, EPA/600/9-91/050.
379. U.S. Environmental Protection Agency. (1995): *Guidance for risk characterization.* U.S. Environmental Protection Agency, Washington, DC. Science Policy Council.
380. U.S. Environmental Protection Agency. (1996): *Summary report for the workshop on Monte Carlo analysis.* U.S. Environmental Protection Agency, Washington, DC. Office of Research and Development, EPA/630/R-96/010.
381. U.S. Environmental Protection Agency (EPA). (1996): Draft guidelines for carcinogen risk assessment. *Fed. Reg.*, 61(79):17960–18011.
382. U.S. Environmental Protection Agency. (1996): *Exposure factors handbook. Volume I of III: General factors—SAB Review Draft.* U.S. Environmental Protection Agency, Washington, DC. Office of Research and Development, EPA/600/P-95/002Ba.
383. U.S. Environmental Protection Agency. 1996d. *Exposure factors handbook. Volume II of III: Food ingestion factors—SAB Review Draft.* Washington, DC: U.S. Environmental Protection Agency, Office of Research and Development, EPA/600/P-95/002Bb.
384. U.S. Environmental Protection Agency. 1996e. *Exposure factors handbook. Volume III of III: Activity factors—SAB Review Draft.* U.S. Environmental Protection Agency, Washington, DC. Office of Research and Development, EPA/600/P-95/002P.
385. U.S. Environmental Protection Agency. (1997): *Lognormal distribution in environmental applications.* U.S. Environmental Protection Agency, Washington, DC. Office of Solid Waste and Emergency Response, EPA/600/R-97/006.
386. U.S. Environmental Protection Agency. (1997): *Exposure factors handbook* (update to the May 1989 edition). U.S. Environmental Protection Agency, Washington, DC. EPA/600/P-95/002Fa.
387. U.S. Environmental Protection Agency. (1997): *Guiding principles for Monte Carlo analysis.* U.S. Environmental Protection Agency, Washington, DC. Office of Research and Development, Risk Assessment Forum, EPA/630/R-97/001.
388. U.S. Environmental Protection Agency. (1997): *Methodology for assessing health risks associated with multiple exposure pathways to combustor emissions.* U.S. Environmental Protection Agency, Washington, DC. National Center for Environmental Assessment, NCEA-C-0238.
389. U.S. Environmental Protection Agency. (1997): *The parameter guidance document.* U.S. Environmental Protection Agency, Cincinnati, OH.
390. U.S. Environmental Protection Agency. (1998): *Integrated risk information system (IRIS).* U.S. Environmental Protection Agency, Washington, DC.
391. U.S. Environmental Protection Agency. (1999): *Risk assessment guidelines for dermal assessment.* U.S. Environmental Protection Agency, Washington, DC.
392. U.S. Environmental Protection Agency. (1999): *Risk assessment guidance (RAGS3A) for conducting probabilistic risk assessment.* U.S. Environmental Protection Agency, Washington, DC.
393. U.S. Environmental Protection Agency. (1999): *Sociodemographic data used for identifying potentially highly exposed populations.* U.S. Environmental Protection Agency, Washington, DC. EPA/600/R-99/060.
394. U.S. Environmental Protection Agency. (1999): *Guidance for performing aggregate exposure and risk assessments under the Food Quality Protection Act.* (Draft). U.S. Environmental Protection Agency, Washington, DC. Office Periodicals Program.
395. U.S. Office of Science and Technology Policy. (1993): *Researching health* risks. Office of Technology Assessment, Washington, DC.
396. Van Den Berg, M., Olie, K., & Hutzinger, O. (1984): Uptake and selective retention in rats of orally administered chlorinated dioxins and PCDF from fly ash. *Chemosphere,* pp. 531–544.
397. Van Wijnen, J. H., Clausing, P., and Brunekreef, B. (1990: Estimated soil ingestion by children. *Environ. Res.*, 51:147–162.
398. Velazquez, S. F., McGinnis, P. M., Vater, S. T., Stiteler, W. S., Knauf, L. A., and Schoeny, R. S. (1994): Combination of cancer data in quantitative risk assessments: Case study using bromodichloromethane. *Risk Anal.*, 14:285–292.
399. Vose, D. (1996): *Quantitative risk analysis: A guide to Monte Carlo simulation modelling.* Wiley, New York.
400. Wallace, L. A. (1986): The Total Exposure Assessment Methodology (TEAM) study: Direct measurement of personal exposures through air and water for 600 residents of several U.S. cities. In *Pollutants in a multimedia environment,* edited by Y. Cohen, pp. 289–315. Plenum Press, New York.
401. Wallace, L. A. (1987) *The TEAM study: Summary and analysis: Volume I.* U.S. Environmental Protection Agency, Washington, DC, EPA 600/6-87/002a, NTIS PB 88-100060.
402. Wallace, L. A. (1989): The Total Exposure Assessment Methodology (TEAM) study: An analysis of exposures, sources, and risks associated with four chemicals. *J. Am. Coll. Toxicol.*, 8:883–895.
403. Wallace, L. A. (1993): A decade of studies of human exposure: What have we learned? *Risk Anal.*, 13(2):135–143.
404. Wallace, L. A. (1996): Environmental exposure to benzene: An update. *Environ. Health Perspect.*, 104(suppl. 6):1129–1136.
405. Wallace, L. A. (1998): The Weslowski Lecture. Personal correspondence.
406. Wallace, L. (2000): Correlations of personal exposure to particles with outdoor air measurements: A review of recent studies. *Appl. Occup. Environ.*, in press.
407. Wallace, L. A. (2000): Real-time monitoring of particles, PAH, and CO in an occupied townhouse. *Appl. Occup. Environ. Hyg.*, 15:19.
408. Wallace, L. A., and Pellizzari, E. D. (1995): Recent advances in measuring exhaled breath and estimating exposure and body burden for volatile organic compounds (VOCs). *Environ. Health Perspect.*, 103:95–98.
409. Wallace, L. A., and Slonecker, T. (1997): Ambient air concentrations of fine manganese ($PM_{2.5}$) in U.S. national parks and in California and Canadian cities: The possible impact of adding MMT to unleaded gasoline. *J. Air Waste Manage. Assoc.*, 47:(6)642–652.

410. Wallace, L. A., Pellizzari, E., Hartwell, T., Sparacino, C., Sheldon, L., and Zelon, H. (1985): Personal exposures, indoor-outdoor relationships and breath levels of toxic air pollutants measured for 355 persons in New Jersey. *Atmos. Environ.*, 19:1651–1661.
411. Wallace, L. A., Pellizzari, E. D., Hartwell, T. D., Whitmore, R., Sparacino, C., and Zelon, H. (1986): Total Exposure Assessment Methodology (TEAM) study: Personal exposures, indoor–outdoor relationships, and breath levels of volatile organic compounds in New Jersey. *Environ. Int.*, 12:369–387.
412. Wallace, L. A., Pellizzari, E. D., Hartwell, T. D., Sparacino, C., Whitmore, R., Sheldon, L., Zelon, H., and Perritt, R. (1987): The "TEAM" study: Personal exposures to toxic substances in air, drinking water, and breath of 400 residents of New Jersey, North Carolina, and North Dakota. *Environ. Res.*, 43:290–307.
413. Wallace, L. A., Pellizzari, E., Leaderer, B., Hartwell, T., Perritt, R., Zelon, H., and Sheldon, L. (1987): Emissions of volatile organic compounds from building materials and consumer products. *Atmos. Environ.*, 21:385–393.
414. Wallace, L. A., Pellizzari, E., and Wendel, C. (1991): Total volatile organic concentrations in 2700 personal, indoor, and outdoor air samples collected in the US EPA TEAM studies. *Indoor Air* 4:465–477.
415. Wallace, L. A., Duan, N., and Ziegenfus, R. (1994): Can long-term exposure distributions be predicted from short-term measurements? *Risk Anal.*, 14:75–85.
416. Wallace, L. A., Buckley, T., Pellizzari, E. D., and Gordon, S. (1996): Breath measurements as VOC biomarkers: EPA's experience in field and chamber studies. *Environ. Health Perspect.*, 104(suppl. 5):861–869.
417. Walter, S. D., Yankel, A. J., and von Lindern, I. H. (1980): Age-specific risk factors for lead absorption in children. *Arch. Environ. Health*, 35:53–58.
418. Wepierre, J., and Marty, J. P. (1979): Percutaneous absorption of drugs. *Trends Pharmacol. Sci.*, 1:23–26.
419. Wester, R. C., and Noonan, P. K. (1980): Relevance of animal models for percutaneous absorption. *Int. J. Pharmacol.*, 7:99–110.
420. Wester, R. C., Bucks, D. A. W., and Maibach, H. I. (1993): Percutaneous absorption of contaminants from soil. In *Health risk assessment: Dermal and inhalation exposure and absorption of toxicants,* edited by R. G. M. Wang, J. B. Knaak, and H. I. Maibach. CRC Press, Boca Raton, FL.
421. Wester, R. C., Maibach, H. I., Sedik, L., Melendres, J., Wade, M., and DiZio, S. (1993): Percutaneous absorption of pentachlorphenol from soil. *Fundam. Appl. Toxicol.*, 20:68–71.
422. White, S. B., Peterson, B., Clayton, C. A., and Duncan, D. P. (1983): The Construction of a Raw Agricultural Commodity Consumption Database. Interim Report 1. Prepared by Research Triangle Institute for U.S. Environmental Protection Agency. Office of Pesticide Programs.
423. Whitmore, R. W., Immerman, F. W., Camann, D. E., Bond, A. E., Lewis, R. G., and Schuam, J. L. 1994. Non-occupational exposures to pesticides for residents of two U.S. cities. *Arch. Environ. Contam. Toxicol.* 26:47–59.
424. Widner, T. (2000): Dose-reconstruction for radionuclides and chemicals released from the federal nuclear facility in Oak Ridge, Tennessee. In *Human and ecological risk assessment: Theory and practice,* edited by D. J. Paustenbach. John Wiley and Sons, New York.
425. Wilschut, A., and ten Berge, W. F. (1995): Two mathematical skin permeation models for vapours. Abstracts of presentations at the Fourth International Prediction of Percutaneous Penetration Conference, La Grande Motte, April 1995. *Prediction of Percutaneous Penetration,* vol. 4a. 3M Medica.
426. Wilschut, A., ten Berge, W. F., Robinson, P. J., and McKone, T. E. (1995): Estimating skin permeation. The validation of five mathematical skin permeation models. *Chemosphere*, 30:1275–1296.
427. Wilson, N. D., Shear, N. D., Paustenbach, D. J., and Price, P. S. (1998): The effect of cooking practices on the concentration of DDT and PCB compounds in the edible tissue of fish. *J. Expos. Anal. Environ. Epidemiol.*, 8:423–440.
428. Wilson, N. D., Price, P., and Paustenbach, D. J. (2000): An assessment of the risk of DDT and PCB in fish from the Palos Verdes shelf. In *Human and ecological risk assessment: Theory and practice,* edited by D. J. Paustenbach. John Wiley & Sons, New York.
429. Wolfe, D. A. (1996): Insights on the utility of biomarkers for environmental impact assessment and monitoring. *Hum. Ecol. Risk Assess.*, 2:245–250.
430. Zannetti, P. (1992): Particle modeling and its application for simulating air pollution phenomena. In *Environmental modeling,* edited by P. Melli, chap. 11. Macmillan, UK.
431. Zartarian, V. G., Ferguson, A. C., and Leckie, J. O. (1998): Quantified mouthing activity data from a four-child pilot field study. *J. Expos. Anal. Environ. Epidemiol.*, 8(4):543–553.
432. Zweig, G., Leffingwell, J. T., and Popendorf, W. J. (1985): The relationship between dermal pesticide exposure by fruit harvesters and dislodgeable foliar residues. *J. Environ. Sci. Health B*, 20:27–60.

Principles and Methods of Toxicology,
Fourth Edition, edited by A. Wallace Hayes.
Taylor & Francis, Philadelphia © 2001.

Chapter 10

Epidemiology for Toxicologists

Ralph R. Cook

The search for scientific "truth" regarding the causes of human disease is a laborious multistep process, a winnowing of a large number of postulated hypotheses down to the few that can be supported with data derived from testing and observation. It depends upon the replication of results, coherence of evidence from many different fields and, ultimately, an understanding of the underlying biological mechanisms of action. In evaluating the potential human health effects of chemical exposures, there are three major sources of scientific information used by the courts, various government agencies, and the larger scientific community: experimental laboratory research, controlled clinical investigations, and observational epidemiology studies. These three are not mutually exclusive in method or thought; each makes a unique contribution toward understanding the etiologies of human disease; but each has certain inherent limitations. Ultimately, the determination of causation depends upon the demonstration of a meaningful elevated risk for the disease among those with the "exposure" and a biological explanation for the excess. The former can only be obtained via epidemiology studies; the latter usually comes from an interplay of information derived from experimental laboratory research and controlled clinical investigations.

Toxicology is one of the key experimental disciplines. In toxicology, investigators are able to carefully control the exposures of genetically homogeneous groups of animals, some purposefully bred so that they exhibit a marked predilection for specific diseases. The latter can provide toxicologists and pharmacologists with important clues about the biological mechanisms which predispose, aggravate, or cause disease. Toxicologists also have the opportunity of evaluating each and every subject to the same exquisite detail. Therefore, at least in theory, the experimental method can provide comprehensive results unperturbed by extraneous variables; but it is increasingly being recognized that this approach does not automatically eliminate, or reduce to a level of insignificance, all forms of technical bias (97). Nor does it protect against personal bias, a problem that can plague all types of research irrespective of the affiliations of the investigators (70,74,118). Toxicology also has become stylized to the extent that the format of research results is both predictable and quantitative. This has made it very convenient for information derived from toxicology experiments to be used in quantitative risk assessments and related regulations. Paradoxically, this convenience facilitates a major violation of scientific principles: an extrapolation beyond the data to make inferences about health effects not only for levels of exposure that were not administered but also for species who were not studied.

Clinical investigators also administer measured doses according to a predetermined schedule, but do so to the species of major interest, humans. Although this type of work is "controlled," it is at best quasi-experimental because humans are not passive participants in health research. At the very least, they must consent to be studied. Some do not and key characteristics of those who do and do not may be markedly different. In other words, most study groups used in clinical trials are not random samples of the general population. This means that care must be exercised in extrapolating the findings too broadly.

On the plus side, clinical research can collect data both on objective signs of pathology and also on more subjective symptoms, data that animal research cannot provide. On the negative side, an equivalent and comprehensive data set for each study subject may not be obtainable. For example, histopathology of all the organs is only available on those few of the deceased whose next-of-kin allow an autopsy to be performed. Any study of humans also means that the research subjects are not homogeneous with regard to either genetic makeup or alternative exposures such as diet, personal habits, or medications. To address this problem, randomization of subjects to different treatment groups is utilized during study design, the assumption being that key alternative variables are randomly distributed across groups and confounding thereby controlled. Sometimes it doesn't work.

There are two major strengths of observational epidemiology research. One, it studies humans. Two, it deals with the effects of real exposures—actual levels, durations and patterns of exposure to individual agents and to mixtures. If epidemiology studies are well done, they furnish results that reasonably can be extended to larger populations. Unfortunately, epidemiologists are often forced to handle exposure as a qualitative variable (either as a yes/no or some variation of high, medium and low). This can limit the utility of the research results for those who require quantitative information. In addition, because the research is observational in the sense that the investigators simply observe natural experiments and do not exercise control over the key variables, epidemiologists routinely must grapple with a number of technical biases that are largely transparent to those in the other two fields. If these biases—in particular, selection, misclassification, and confounding—are not adequately addressed during study design or data analysis, the study results may be unduly imprecise and important associations missed. Alternatively, the results may be relatively precise but precisely inaccurate, thereby leading to interpretations that are incorrect. Some of these problems can be exacerbated if the epidemiologist utilizes secondary sources of data (data originally gathered for purposes other than the specific research project, possibly even for reasons unrelated to research), especially if the methods for the original data collection process were poorly documented.

There is one other point that differentiates epidemiology from the other two fields. Although acceptance into the American College of Epidemiology provides an imprimatur of professional competence, in practice epidemiology requires no graduate degree, certification, or licensure. Some enter the field with strong statistical skills; others have extensive training in human biology. The formal graduate degree programs require a proficiency in both; but anyone with any level of education can gather a data set, analyze it, report the results, and call their efforts epidemiology research. There is no law against it and no professional body condemns the practice. Epidemiologists can be very egalitarian. The rule of thumb for the consumer of epidemiology results, therefore, especially if a report appears in other than the peer reviewed literature, is *caveat emptor*.

Epidemiology has been defined as the study of the distribution and determinants of disease in humans (75). Although commonly used, this definition is incomplete. Although epidemiologists certainly search for the factors associated with human disease, they also attempt to identify both interventions that likely will benefit those who are at risk for getting the condition (perhaps because of unique patterns of exposure to combinations of putative agents or a genetic predisposition for reacting adversely to such exposures) and treatments that will help control or cure any significant pathology once it occurs. They also, implicitly or explicitly, try to determine which agents do not cause a specific disease, which interventions will not be successful, and which treatments are not effective.

As with toxicology and clinical research, good epidemiology is an amalgam of subject-specific knowledge and methods. And just as there are clinical specialties and areas of expertise in toxicology that have evolved with the growing complexities of each of those two fields, epidemiology is divided into a number of overlapping subgroups: occupational, environmental, reproductive, cardiovascular, cancer, infectious disease, molecular, genetic, nutritional, medical device, clinical, etc. Some of these are subdivided still further, for example, AIDS is a subcategory of viral which, in turn, is a subset of infectious disease. Although certain knowledge and techniques may be unique to a subgroup, many concepts are common across the discipline.

The primary objective of this chapter is to introduce those concepts that span the field so that toxicologists might become better consumers of the epidemiology literature. Table 10.1 provides an outline of the major topics: data, measures of disease frequency, measures of risk and association, methods, and issues. All of these are interrelated so the order of presentation is somewhat arbitrary; but the first three set the stage for the last one,

Table 10.1
Major topics

Data
Prevalence
Incidence
Measures of disease frequency
Prevalence rate
Incidence rate
Measures of risk and association
Absolute risk
Relative risk
Standardized mortality ratio (SMR)
Proportional mortality ratio (PMR)
Rate difference
Attributable risk
Methods
Cohort
Case control
Cross-sectional
Case studies or case series
Issues
Selection
Misclassification
Confounding
Chance
Causation

in particular the key issues impacting validity—selection, misclassification, and confounding. Each of these in turn is presented to show how it can bias the measures of association. The intent is to make the readers more sensitive to possible flaws so that they might determine for themselves how well the investigators recognized a potential problem and addressed it during study design, data collection or data analysis, and during data interpretation.

Most of the major points are illustrated with recent examples from the epidemiology literature or, to a lesser extent, with toxicology or clinical references. In part, this was done to emphasize the point that all science—experimental, quasi-experimental, and observational—is based upon assumptions that may not be correct. Some of these assumptions are relatively innocuous. Conversely, some are so important that, if violated, the science is severely flawed and any policies based upon that science likely also are flawed. Those are the two poles of a continuum; but validity is not a dichotomous variable like pregnancy. The challenge for the consumer of scientific reports is to determine which provide useful information, which do not, and which lie somewhere in between—intriguing enough to warrant additional research, but not strong enough to merit intervention. This winnowing equates to first, identifying potential problems that may have compromised the validity of the research; second, determining the probability to which the problems occurred; and third, estimating the impact, if any, they had upon the results.

This chapter is by design a limited overview. For those who wish to have a more detailed presentation of the field, the list of references includes a number of recently published textbooks (19,48,62,98,101). Note, throughout this chapter key ''terms of art'' are emphasized with italics. A small number of these are defined in the book's glossary; but most can be found in Last's *Dictionary of Epidemiology* (72), an invaluable resource to any technical library. Additionally, at the end of the chapter there is an appendix: the *Guidelines for Good Epidemiology Practices for Occupational and Environmental Epidemiologic Research* (GEPs), an analog of *Good Laboratory Practices* (GLPs).

DATA AND MEASURES OF DISEASE FREQUENCY

Data, information, and knowledge are related but not equivalent terms. Data are the raw materials gathered by the investigator during the course of an investigation, information is analyzed data, and knowledge is meaningful information that can be used to predict or solve problems. By way of analogy, data are bricks, information the wall, and knowledge the building. Just as good bricks can be put together poorly to build an unstable wall, so can data be valid, but aggregated in a fashion that produces useless information. Pseudoknowledge may be a function of either bad data or useless information, just as a structurally unsound building may result from poor quality bricks or an unstable wall.

Prevalence and Incidence

For the epidemiologist, there are two general types of data: *prevalence* and *incidence*. Prevalence is what is observed at a single point; a snapshot of what is prevalent, what exists, at a specific point in chronological or biological time. For example, the number of toxicologists currently employed by federal regulatory agencies is prevalence data.

Incidence is the number of incidents, of new events, that develop over time. Because it represents a delta, a change, incidence data have to be gathered at two or more points in time. In a sense, if prevalence is a snap-shot, incidence is a movie. The number of toxicologists hired by federal agencies in any given year is an example of incidence data. They didn't work for the agencies at the start of the year (observation point one); but they did work for the government later in the year (observation points two or more).

Parenthetically, when epidemiologists speak of prevalence data they are usually referring to *point prevalence* but they may mean *period prevalence*. Period prevalence is a combination of what exists at the beginning as well as what occurs during a specified period. The number of toxicologists who were employed by federal agencies at any time during a given year is period prevalence data. It includes those who were working at the beginning of the year (point prevalence data) and those who were hired during the year (incidence data). Period prevalence may or may not be the same as the number of those who were employed at the end of the year (more point prevalence data) because some toxicologists may have left government employment during the period of observation.

Whether data are period prevalence or incidence can sometimes be difficult to discern, because both refer to events occurring during a span of time. The key is whether the data represent a combination of existing and new events (period prevalence) or just new events (incidence). Unless otherwise noted, the term prevalence is used in this chapter as a synonym for point prevalence.

The difference between prevalence and incidence data is important for at least three reasons. One, incidence data can be used to evaluate cause and effect; prevalence data usually cannot, at least not without additional assumptions. Two, because prevalence data can be gathered at a single point in time, it is much easier to obtain and therefore many reports in the medical literature are based upon prevalence data. Three, the medical literature often incorrectly uses the two terms interchangeably. As a consequence, reports that use valid prevalence data to develop nonsense information about cause and effect appear in even the most prestigious journals.

Although the two are different, they are related. Prevalence (P) is a function of both the incidence (I) and the duration (D) of the disease ($P = I \times D$). What that means is a chemical may not cause a disease, may not increase the incidence of the disease, but it may still be associated with a higher prevalence of the condition. Whether that is good news or bad depends upon the circumstances. For example, the incidence of diabetes may be quite stable in a population; but if that population is given access to a chemical called insulin, the prevalence of the condition likely will increase dramatically. It will increase because the insulin extends the duration of the disease by allowing more of the afflicted to live longer.

Conversely, the prevalence of minor birth defects (prevalence because the events are measured at a single point in biological time, birth) may be lower among live children born to women exposed to some agent, not because the agent prevents the development of minor defects in utero, but because the agent and causes major malformations that lead to early spontaneous abortions.

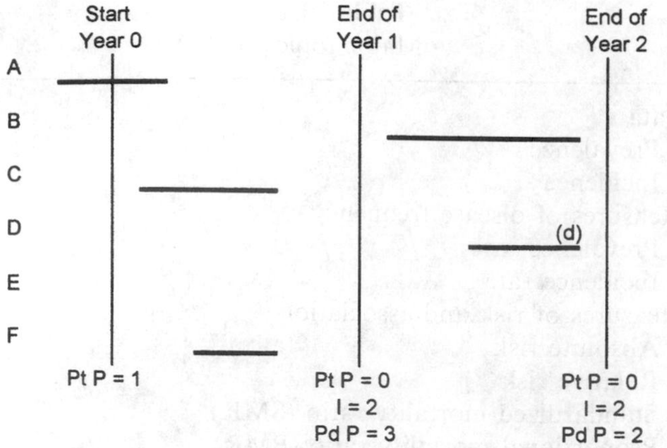

Pt P is point prevalance; I is incidence; and Pd P is period prevalence.

FIG. 10.1. Prevalence versus incidence (time-limited condition).

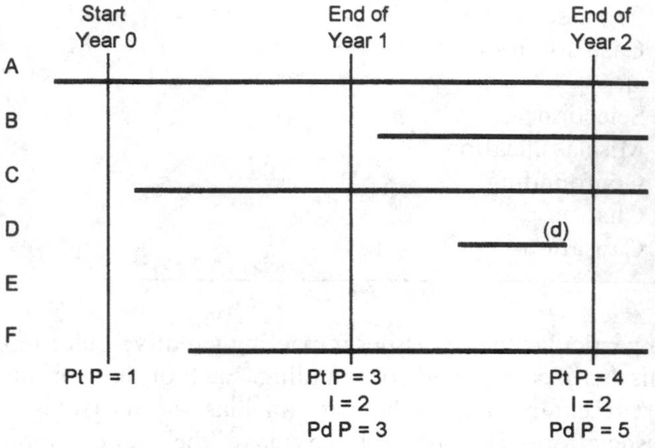

Pt P is point prevalance; I is incidence; and Pd P is period prevalence.

FIG. 10.2. Prevalence versus incidence (condition chronic).

The incidence of minor defects is quite stable in this example, but their duration has been shortened and therefore fewer malformations observed among live births.

Figures 10.1 and 10.2 illustrate these points. In both, a group of six patients (A through F) is observed for 2 years. In Figure 10.1, the condition is time limited. It either spontaneously resolves, is cured through some treatment, or the patient dies. The point prevalence at the initial baseline observation (year 0) is one. Two additional cases subsequently occur and all three resolve before year's end. At the end of year 1, the point prevalence is zero, the incidence is two, and the period prevalence is three. During the following year, two more cases develop and one patient dies (patient D) of an unrelated cause before the end of the year. Therefore, at year's end, the point prevalence is zero, the incidence two, and the period prevalence also two.

In Figure 10.2, the condition is chronic, perhaps because, like diabetes, it has been extended through treatment. Note the incidence is exactly the same as in the previous example. It is two in each year. However, the extended duration has impacted both measures of prevalence. The point prevalence at the time of the three observations is respectively one, three, and four. The period prevalence for the first year is three. For the second, it is five even though patient D died before year's end. Each of these three measures of disease provides valuable information, but using either type of prevalence data for interpretations about cause and effect depends upon assumptions about *incidence time* (i.e., when the health event actually occurred) and disease duration that are often untestable or incorrect.

Rates

Technically, the terms incidence and prevalence refer to numerator data; however, in both the epidemiology and medical literature, these terms often are used interchangeably with, respectively, *incidence rate* and *prevalence rate*. An incidence rate is the number of new events of a disease in a defined population that occur during some specified period of time. A prevalence rate is the number of cases of disease observed in a defined population at a point in time. In both, the numerator is a subset of the denominator. Obviously, errors of count in either the numerator or the denominator can impact the accuracy of a rate. Nonetheless, in some technical reports the former may not be a subset of the latter and the description as to how either was compiled may be less than clear.

Rather than presenting a rate as the actual numerator (the exact number of new events observed) in comparison to the actual denominator (the precise count of the group under study) at or during the period of observation, for convenience a rate is usually given as the number of cases per 100 or per 1000 or per 10,000. For example, if there were 486 persons in the study group and 5 new events occurred during a 12-month period of observation, the incidence rate might be presented as 1.0 per 100 per year (5 divided by 486 times 100) or, alternatively, as 10.3 per 1000 per year.

As opposed to toxicology, in epidemiology the study groups can be either *fixed* or *open* (sometimes called *dynamic*). In a fixed study group, those included are defined at the start and followed over time. If no losses occur during the period of study, the group may be called a *closed population*. In an open study group, individuals may be added or lost during the time of study. Just the events that occur and just that time that passes during the period each individual was under observation are counted. This so-called *person–time experience* assumes that observing 10 people for 1 year is the same as observing 1 person for 10 years. In some situations, the assumption is appropriate. In others, it may not be. Determining which is which depends upon the underlying biological model.

MEASURES OF RISK AND ASSOCIATION

Absolute Risk

It is an immutable fact of life that we are all going to get ill at sometime and ultimately we are all going to die. On a personal level, the questions for each of us are by what disease and when? Epidemiologists are also interested in those questions, but they are particularly interested in whether the disease occurs more frequently or more severely in association with some type of exposure. In other words when it comes to identifying the causes of disease, what is at issue is whether the *absolute risk* for a specific disease among the exposed is greater than the absolute risk of that same disease in the unexposed.

Relative Risk

An incidence rate provides a measure of absolute risk. The ratio of the incidence rates in two different groups is a *rate ratio*, *risk ratio*, or *relative risk*, a key measure of association between exposure and disease. If the relative risk (*RR*) is appreciably greater than 1 among those with a particular exposure, it is evidence that the agent may be causing the disease. May be. Conversely, if the relative risk is below 1, the agent may be protecting against the disease. May be. And if the relative risk approximates 1, there may be no meaningful association between the two variables. Once again, may be. May be is an important caveat in all three situations because how well the *apparent relative risk* (the number derived as the result of a particular investigation) corresponds to the *true relative risk* (the actual underlying biological truth) depends not only on the statistical stability of the estimate of relative risk, but also on how well the potential technical biases of selection, misclassification, and confounding were controlled in study design, during data collection, and by data analyses.

Standardized Mortality Ratio (SMR)

In cohort mortality studies, the measure of association may be provided as a *standardized mortality ratio* or SMR. Because this is simply the ratio of the number of deaths observed in the study group to the number that would have been expected if the study group had the same death rate as a reference (i.e., standard) population, it is sometimes presented as *observed to expected* deaths or

O/E. By convention, this measure of association is given as a percentage, but the interpretations parallel those of the relative risk. A SMR of 150 is analogous to a RR of 1.5; a SMR of 75 to a RR of 0.75; and a SMR of 100 to a RR of 1.0. Because the observed number of deaths occurs in discrete increments and the number of expected deaths is for all intents and purposes a continuous variable (i.e., the expected deaths might be a biologically impossible number such as 1.27365...), by convention many epidemiologists will not calculate a SMR if the number of observed deaths is less than 2 (19). They may simply provide the two numbers, the observed and the expected, or just give a confidence interval. Sometimes, they'll do neither and merely indicate that the numbers were too small to be meaningful

Note, the "controls," the comparison group, in a SMR analysis are essentially those in a hypothetical group statistically constructed from the reference population to have approximately the same age, race, and gender characteristics as the exposed group. For many occupational studies, the mortality experience of United States white males is used as a reference even if a small number of those in the occupational cohort are of a different race or ethnic group, the assumption being that the calculations of expected deaths will be adequate. Using a SMR approach also means the investigator is assuming that no one in the reference population was exposed to the agent of interest. If the exposure is relatively rare among those in the reference population, the assumption is probably reasonable because the mortality experience of those few who were exposed would have had very little impact on the population statistics. On the other hand, if the exposure is relatively common—for example, something like chlorinated drinking water—the assumption may be unreasonable and another type of study would have to be done to obtain valid information.

An interpretation of a "crude" measure of association assumes that both the exposed group and the reference population had similar habits regarding smoking, dietary preferences, medical care, etc. This assumption may be incorrect. For example, a number of years ago a study was done in California of men who lived in communities adjacent to petrochemical facilities along the Sacramento river (8). The comparison population was composed of those who lived in the same county, but remote from the industrial sector. An apparent elevated risk for lung cancer was discovered and the finding was initially presumed, at least by the news media, to be due to emissions from the petrochemical plants. However, during this first stage of the investigation, no attempt had been made to control for the effects of cigarette smoking. For efficiency, that activity had been deferred to subsequent stages of the research. It was later found that those who lived near the plants were largely blue collar workers and those who lived elsewhere tended to be white collar professionals who commuted to work in San Francisco. Why was this important? Blue collar workers on average smoke more than white collar workers (at least that has been past experience) and therefore blue collar workers have higher rates of lung cancer. When the subsequent research gathered the necessary data and adjusted for these differences, the elevated risk disappeared (20). As a result, the proposed intervention strategies changed from targeting industrial emissions to implementing smoking cessation programs.

The SMR can also be an acronym for a *standardized morbidity ratio*. Instead of death being the outcome of interest, it is illness; but the calculations and the resultant interpretations are basically the same. So too are the underlying assumptions. If the assumptions were violated to the degree that the study results were affected, the reader should look for confirmation elsewhere.

Proportional Mortality Ratio (PMR)

Neither the RR or the SMR should be confused with a *PMR*, a *proportional mortality* (*or morbidity*) *ratio*. The PMR is a measure of the relative importance of an individual category of disease among those with disease. As such, both numbers in the ratio are "numerator data." Although it is a convenient measure to obtain, it must be used with caution in etiologic research because it compares proportions and not rates. It makes the assumption that a higher proportion of a particular disease is the same as an increased frequency of that disease. Because a PMR calculation works like a teeter-totter, that assumption may be invalid. Although a higher proportion of disease A may be due to an increased incidence of disease A, it also simply may be a function of a lower frequency (and therefore a lower proportion) of some other condition, disease B. For example, a higher PMR for cancer among an occupational group with a certain exposure may mean that more of those with the exposure were developing (and dying) from cancer than those in the standard population; but it is also consistent with the interpretation that those with the exposure were not dying more often from cancer, they were just dying less often from noncancer events. In other words, in a PMR analysis an apparently "adverse" finding may be spurious, for example, solely a function of the *healthy worker effect* (79).

Rate Difference and Attributable Risk

With two incidence rates it is possible to calculate not only a rate ratio, but also a *rate difference*. If the association between the exposure and the disease is truly causal, the rate difference provides a measure of the excess burden of disease an exposed population might expect to experience as a result of the exposure. Stated another way, it represents the amount of the disease that would never have occurred if the exposure had been prevented. In such situations, it may be called an *attributable risk*, *attributable risk percent*, *attributable fraction*, or a number of other related terms as derived for just the exposed group or for the general population as a whole. Unfortunately, some will calculate a risk difference and use the term "attributable" even when causation has not been established.

Note the two measures, the rate ratio and the rate difference, provide very different information. The higher a RR is above one, the greater the likelihood that there is a true cause-and-effect relationship; but a high RR for a very rare disease among a few individuals with a unique exposure may be of *de minimis* concern from a public health perspective, whereas a lower RR for a relatively common condition might equate to an enormous number of cases. By way of example, it is generally accepted that excess exposures to vinyl chloride monomer cause angiosarcoma of the liver. The RR for this association is quite high; but the total number of excess cases, worldwide, approximates 100. By way of contrast, the RR for heart disease among cigarette smokers is only about 1.5; but the rate difference equates to a large number of cases—many, many orders of magnitude more than 100. This is because both the disease and the exposure are relatively common. From a public health perspective, it is much more important to control the excess risk of disease related to smoking than it is the risk associated with vinyl chloride monomer. Yet for the purpose of establishing a cause for the disease, it took many fewer epidemiology studies to establish an etiologic association between vinyl chloride monomer and liver angiosarcomas than it did for cigarettes and cardiovascular problems.

Rate ratios and rate differences are derived from research in which two groups are defined based upon exposure status and the disease patterns of each are followed forward in time. On occasion, it is easier to get groups based upon whether they do or do not have a specific disease and then collect data on previous exposures. For example, it may be more convenient to identify all those who developed lung cancer during some period, possibly via the use of data from a tumor registry, and identify a comparable group of healthy individuals from the general population, perhaps by means of random digit dialing within the same area codes as the cases. Gathering data on previous exposures from those in each group (or from their next of kin) would allow the calculation of an *odds ratio* or *OR*, that is, the odds of having been exposed to a particular agent given one had the disease versus the odds of having been exposed to that same agent among the healthy controls. If a study is done properly, the OR will approximate the RR. For example, if the RR for getting lung cancer among cigarette smokers is 10, the OR of having been a cigarette smoker among those with lung cancer also will be about 10. For simplicity, the rest of the text will focus predominately on two measures of association, the relative risk and the odds ratio.

METHODS

Cohort

Over the years, epidemiologists have developed a variety of methods to evaluate cause and effect. The most intuitively obvious, and the most analogous to the approach used in toxicology, is the *cohort* study. A cohort is simply a group with some common characteristic, for example, gender, ethnic background, health behavior, or exposure to a particular chemical or medicine. In a cohort study, the health experiences of at least two cohorts are compared, one with an exposure to the agent of interest and one without. Ideally, multiple cohorts, each with a different level of exposure, are identified so that the effects of low, medium, and higher levels of exposure can be assessed. Irrespective of the number of groups, conceptually exposure status is determined first and health data—on subsequent mortality, morbidity, blood cholesterol levels, etc.—are then gathered forward in time. If the exposure status is determined in the present and the health data then gathered into the future, the term *prospective cohort study* is used.

Prospective cohort studies, for all of their advantages, may not be the method of choice in preliminary investigations of the causes of disease, especially if the disease has a long latency. As opposed to toxicologists who dose animals of species with relatively short life spans (a standard chronic feeding study of mice takes 2 years), epidemiologists examine a long-lived species, humans; therefore if they only did prospective cohort studies of chronic disease, they likely would complete very few projects during their professional careers. To overcome this problem, epidemiologists often times will use historical records—personnel files, medical archives, industrial hygiene reports, etc.—to define their exposed and unexposed study groups at some arbitrary date in the past. They will then gather health data on each individual in the study groups from that point up to the present. These are sometimes called *retrospective cohort studies* or, to differentiate them from the case control method that also gathers data on former events, they may be labeled *nonconcurrent prospective studies* or *historical prospective studies* or even *retrospective prospective studies*. Irrespective of whether the starting point for a cohort study is at the present or in the past, the results

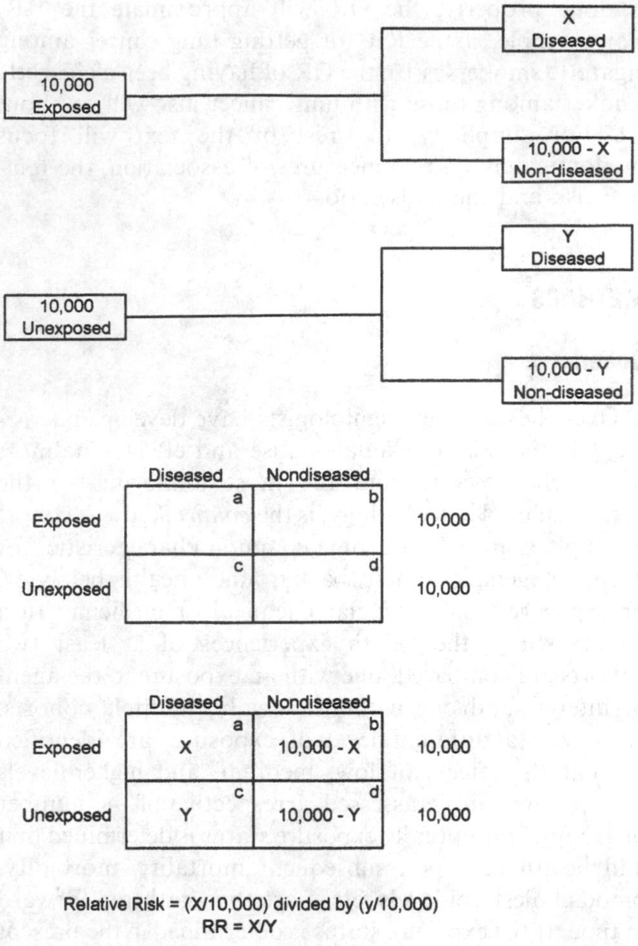

FIG. 10.3. Illustration of the cohort method.

are based on incidence data presented as relative risks (and, if appropriate, risk differences).

Figure 10.3 illustrates how this is done. Two groups of healthy individuals are identified at a point in time. One group is selected because they have (or had) a known or presumptive exposure to a specific agent; the second, because they don't have (and ideally never had) the exposure. The health experience of those in each group is then compiled in an equivalent fashion over some defined period of time. This health experience is converted into incidence rates and the rates compared by means of a relative risk. It is possible to calculate relative risks for all health events combined (e.g., total causes of mortality) or for any number of distinct outcomes (e.g., just deaths due to angiosarcoma of the liver). When the cohort approach is used in exploratory data analysis, it can be considered "an exposure in search of a disease," a hypothesis generating exercise. If it targets just one or a limited number of specific associations of a priori concern, it is akin to hypothesis testing. Many epidemiology studies are a combination of both and it may be difficult for the reader to discern which associations were of concern at the beginning of the research and which were simply serendipitous findings (3). At times, it is possible to make this determination only by reviewing the original study protocol—if there was one.

In the example shown in Figures 10.3, there were 10,000 individuals in each group at the start of the study. Therefore, the marginals for the 2 by 2 table are both 10,000. During the period of study, *X* individuals in the exposed group were observed to have developed the disease (cell a) whereas the remainder, 10,000 minus *X*, did not (cell b). Therefore, the incidence rate for the exposed is *X* divided by 10,000 (10,000 being the totals of those in cells a and b). Among the unexposed, *Y* developed the same disease (cell c) and 10,000 minus *Y* did not (cell d). The incidence rate among the unexposed is therefore *Y* divided by 10,000. Dividing *X* over 10,000 by *Y* over 10,000 gives the relative risk. Because both groups had the same denominator, this particular RR simplifies to *X*/ *Y*. In real life that seldom happens.

Hypothetically, the investigators might have found that 50 individuals among the exposed developed the disease and only 10 among the unexposed (Figure 10.4). After plugging these numbers into the table, the resultant calculations would produce a RR of 5. The exposed had five times the risk of developing the disease as did the unexposed—assuming there was no selection, misclassification, or confounding bias, and the finding was not a chance occurrence.

Note, in a cohort study those in both groups must be free of the condition at the start of the investigation. This implies that no one in either the exposed or the unexposed group is eligible until they are first examined and determined to be disease free. In other words, the first step of any prospective incidence study is, conceptually, a *cross-sectional* or *prevalence study*. The data from this cross-sectional study, even though they are collected on two or more "cohorts," cannot be used to make interpretations concerning etiology. They are prevalence data.

In actual practice, it may be impossible to determine baseline health status. For example, in a nonconcurrent cohort morbidity study, an investigator cannot go back in time to examine the study participants in any of the groups. Moreover, even when the study has a prospective orientation, it may not be feasible to examine those in the control group if a SMR-type approach is used, because that would mean everyone in the standard group (e.g., the U.S. white male population) would have to be examined, a logistical impossibility. Nevertheless, if the natural history of the health condition is well understood, adjustments can be made to overcome this problem. With diseases of long latency, the investigators might simply ignore the health data from the first couple of years. For mortality research, a person might be pre-

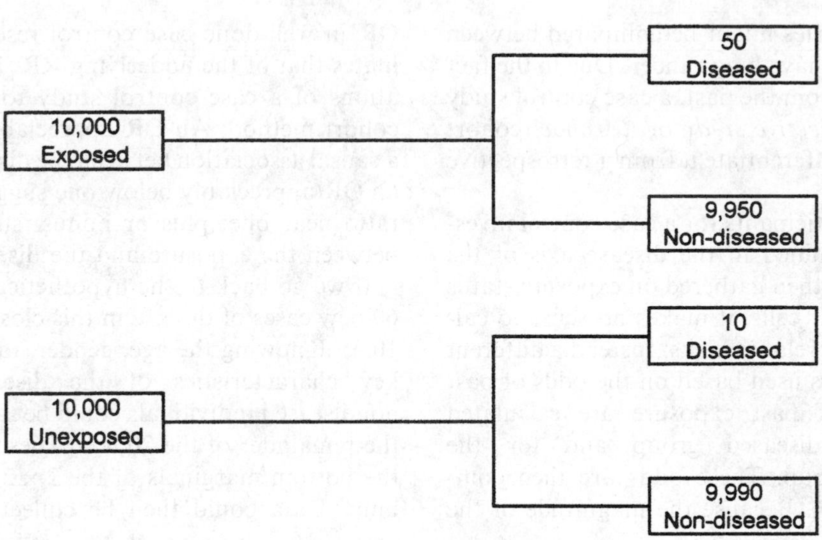

	Diseased	Nondiseased	
Exposed	a 50	b 9,950	10,000
Unexposed	c 10	d 9,990	10,000

Relative Risk = (50/10,000) divided by (10/10,000)
RR = 50/10
RR = 5

FIG. 10.4. Illustration of the cohort method, $RR = 5$.

sumed living at the start of the study if he or she was then employed, paying taxes, or receiving retirement benefits.

A cohort study can be a very labor-intensive process. Exposure histories have to be compiled and validated. Study subjects (or their next of kin) may have to be traced and contacted and data obtained on personal habits, hobbies, and a host of other variables. Medical records then must be collected and coded. Many things can complicate the process.

The first major obstacle is simply finding the study subjects. In our society, it is not unusual for someone to change their residence multiple times during his or her lifetime. Women may leave the workforce, get married, and, in the process, assume a new last name. Conversely, someone may have a name so common that it is very difficult to determine which "John Miller" is the right study subject and which is not.

A second major obstacle is finding comparable health data on each individual. The amount of medical information can vary from person to person simply because of differences in health care–seeking behavior. The study subjects may have many different physicians, each providing a different level of care, possessing diverse diagnostic skills, and having office records with unique formats. Many states and municipalities have disparate rules governing access to government records such as death certificates. In addition, litigation and regulations may obstruct the process of data collection (5,7,29).

Case Control

Even if all of these obstacles can be satisfactorily addressed, it means that a great deal of effort may be needed to gather a lot of data that produce relatively little useful information. In the hypothetical example, 20,000 individuals were tracked to identify the 60 who actually got the disease. To overcome the inefficiencies of cohort studies, epidemiologists developed the *case control* method. With case control studies, the past exposures of those with some disease are compared to the past exposures of those who don't have the disease. For example, smoking histories might be compared between men who do and do not have lung cancer. Due to the fact that data are gathered from the past, a case control study may be called a *retrospective study* or a *trohoc* (cohort spelled backwards) to differentiate it from a retrospective cohort study.

Because the study participants for a case control investigation are first determined in the disease axis of the 2 × 2 table and data are then gathered on exposure status to fill in each of the four cells, it makes no sense to calculate incidence rates or relative risks. Instead a different measure of association is used based on the odds of past exposure. The odds of past exposure are calculated respectively for the diseased group and for the nondiseased control group. These odds are then compared to develop an OR. Because the magnitude of the OR in well-done case control research closely approximates that of the underlying RR, it allows the interpretations of a case control study to parallel those of the cohort method: An OR appreciably above one suggests a causal association between the disease and the exposure; an OR appreciably below one suggests protection; and a ratio near one, plus or minus, suggests no association between the exposure and the disease.

If we go back to the hypothetical example, there were 60 new cases of disease in this closed population (Figure 10.5). Knowing the age, gender, race, and perhaps other key characteristics of the diseased, 60 "matched" nondiseased individuals could be randomly selected from the remainder of the 20,000. These 120 would constitute the bottom marginals of the 2 × 2 table, 60 in each column. Data could then be collected on past exposure.

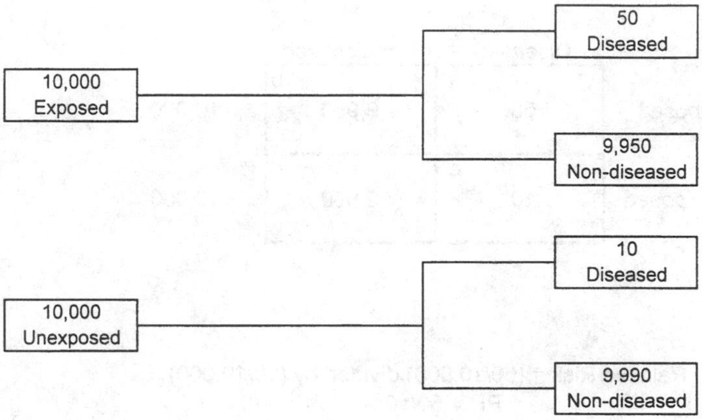

	Diseased	Nondiseased	
Exposed	a	b	
Unexposed	c	d	
	60	60	20,000

	Diseased	Nondiseased	
Exposed	a 50	b 30	
Unexposed	c 10	d 30	
	60	60	20,000

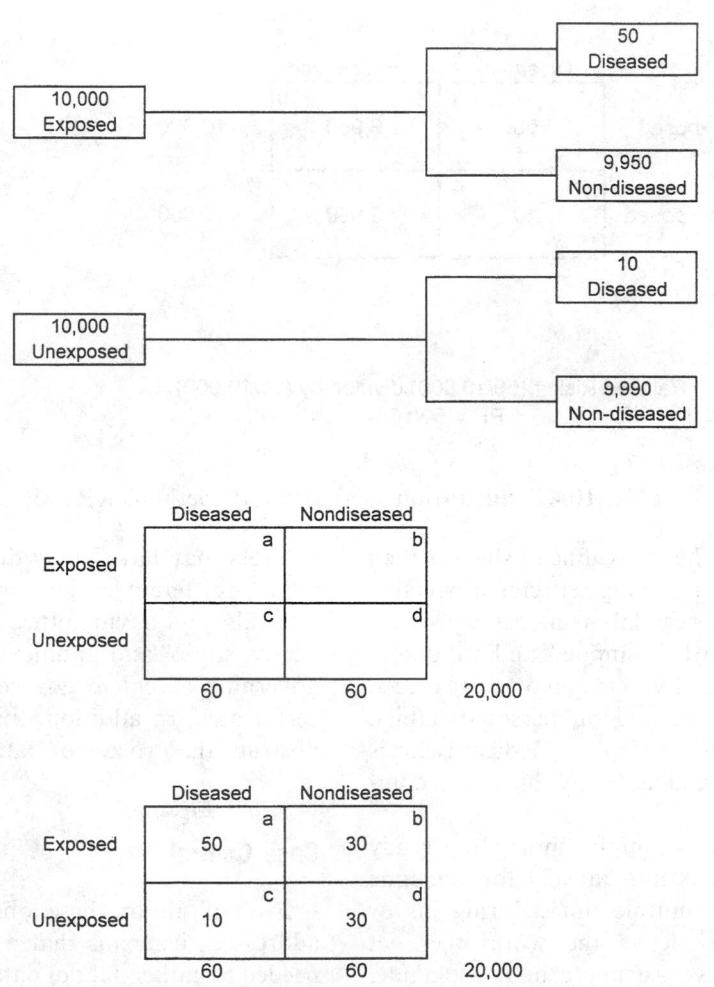

Odds Ratio = odds of exposure among the diseased versus the odds of exposure among the nondisease
Odds Ratio = 50/10 divided by 30/30
OR = 5
the cross-product ratio is *ad* divided by *bc*
OR = 50 x 30 divided by 30 x 10
OR = 5

FIG. 10.5. Illustration of the case control method, OR = 5.

In this particular example, 50 of the diseased group would end up in cell a and 10 in cell c. Among the nondiseased, approximately 30 would end up in cell b and another 30 in cell d. Parenthetically, the nondiseased in each exposure category were approximately the same, 9950 and 9990. Therefore, random sampling of 60 from the aggregate 19,940 should select equal numbers from each group: 30 and 30. With data in all four cells, the odds of exposure among the patients would be 50 to 10 (5 to 1) and the odds of exposure among the controls would be 30 to 30 (1 to 1), giving an odds ratio or OR of 5. Conveniently, the calculations for case control studies often simplify to a *cross-product ratio*, ad divided by bc. In the example, 50 times 30 divided by 30 times 10 simplifies to 5.

For this case control study, an evaluation of just 120 individuals provided the same information as a study of 20,000. In the context of the time, effort, and cost, the need to gather data on such a limited number of study subjects can be a tremendous advantage. Paradoxically, the small size of the study can also be a problem because seemingly minor amounts of bias can have a dramatic impact on the OR.

Unfortunately, avoiding inadvertent bias can be more difficult in case control studies because the health outcome has already occurred. If the investigators or the study subjects are not properly "blinded," this knowledge can impact both the participants in the research and the data they provide. Social forces still may influence the results even if "blinding" is incorporated. For example, those with disease may be more inclined to participate in the research because they have a greater need to understand why they became ill. Furthermore, the cases who selectively participate may expend greater effort toward trying to remember their past exposures and thereby may provide more comprehensive or more valid data than the controls. This is called *recall* or *rumination bias*. It is a type of *information bias* that very often leads to overestimates of risk.

There is one other problem. A case control study may utilize a combination of prevalence and incidence data instead of just incidence data and thereby limit its utility for etiologic interpretations. For all of these reasons, results from case control studies are considered "lesser evidence" than those derived from cohort research.

Even with its limitations, a case control approach can be very attractive. Because the two groups are initially defined based on disease status, data on any number of exposures can be collected. As a consequence, a large number of different associations can be evaluated simultaneously and rapidly reduced to just a few that deserve further study. For that reason, an exploratory case control study can be considered "a disease in search of an exposure," the mirror image of the hypothesis-generating exercise done in a cohort mode.

A case control study also can focus in depth on just one disease-exposure association, testing a hypothesis derived from case reports or other types of research with much greater sophistication than might be feasible in a cohort study. In certain situations, it can be advantageous to use the cohort and the case control approaches in series to generate a relatively small and well-defined number of hypotheses. Such a *nested case control study* can combine the strengths of both methods. For example, the cohort approach could be used to identify a cluster of disease within a broadly defined group, perhaps all those ever employed at a multiple chemical manufacturing facility, and a case control study could then be implemented within the larger cohort not only to narrow the focus to those few agents that appear to be most important for that particular disease but also to do so with proper adjustments for confounding. This integrated approach, therefore, can achieve both efficiency and rigor.

Cohort and case control studies are sometimes called *analytic* research—in contrast to other types of epidemiology investigations that are simply *descriptive* of time, place, and person. In theory, the term "analytic" should be restricted to those studies that are designed to test a priori hypotheses; but in practice, it is often used more broadly to refer to any cohort or case control research, irrespective of whether it generates or tests hypotheses. That is unfortunate because it blurs the distinction between these two important concepts and the role each plays in the search for the causes of human disease.

As illustrated by the cartoon strip Sally Forth (Figure 10.6), determining disease etiology is basically a four-step process. Step 1 is formulating a theory. Step 2 is testing that theory. To be tested, it must be constructed in a form that is refutable. Although the theory may be stated as "exposure X is associated with an increased risk to disease Y," conceptually it has to be tested in the null (i.e., exposure X *is not* associated with an increased risk to disease Y) and the null disproved (4). If the null is rejected, that is, if an epidemiology study detects an apparent increased risk for disease among those with a particular exposure and the reasons for this excess are not otherwise obvious, step 3 is research to understand the underlying biological mechanisms of the association. Finally, step 4 is to be confident that the key results derived in the second and third steps were not statistical flukes or the consequence of one or more technical biases, each has to be replicated. As a rule of thumb, the more important the association, the more important is the need to replicate the findings.

Case Studies or Case Series

Hypotheses for analytic epidemiology may originate from toxicology studies or from epidemiology investiga-

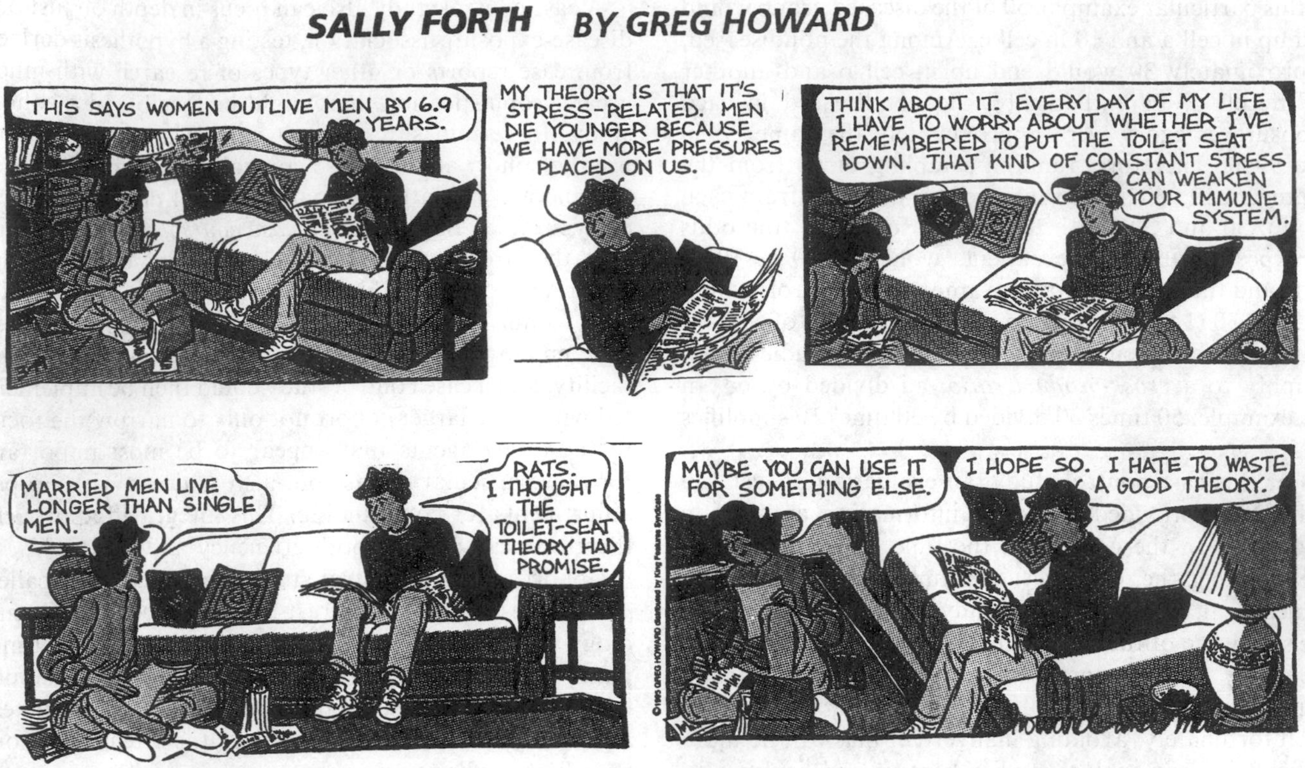
SALLY FORTH BY GREG HOWARD
THIS SAYS WOMEN OUTLIVE MEN BY 6.9 YEARS.
MY THEORY IS THAT IT'S STRESS-RELATED. MEN DIE YOUNGER BECAUSE WE HAVE MORE PRESSURES PLACED ON US.
THINK ABOUT IT. EVERY DAY OF MY LIFE I HAVE TO WORRY ABOUT WHETHER I'VE REMEMBERED TO PUT THE TOILET SEAT DOWN. THAT KIND OF CONSTANT STRESS CAN WEAKEN YOUR IMMUNE SYSTEM.
MARRIED MEN LIVE LONGER THAN SINGLE MEN.
RATS. I THOUGHT THE TOILET-SEAT THEORY HAD PROMISE.
MAYBE YOU CAN USE IT FOR SOMETHING ELSE.
I HOPE SO. I HATE TO WASTE A GOOD THEORY.

FIG. 10.6. Determining the etiology of human disease. Copyright 1996. Reprinted with permission of King Features Syndicate.

tions; but many evolve from clinical observations and are published in the form of *case studies* or *case series*. Although based a great deal on intuition, a case study is a time-honored way for a physician to develop new theories about the causes of human disease. It has been said, with some justification, that every human carcinogen was first identified by an astute clinician who published his findings in the form of a case study or case series. Nonetheless, that does not mean case studies can be used to unerringly identify new etiologic associations. Although the theories derived from case studies are not always wrong, history teaches that they are seldom right (9,31,95). Determining which is which depends upon data developed by others using experimental, quasi-experimental, and observational research. If we go back to the 2 × 2 table, we can see why.

To test a hypothesis about a new cause for human disease (to identify an elevated risk in analytic epidemiology research), data are needed in all four cells of the 2 × 2 table—data that are properly defined on both variables. Case studies tend to focus just on those in one of the four cells, cell a, the exposed with disease. Very little, if any, data are gathered by the clinician on those in the other three cells. Furthermore, those from whom data are gathered are a *convenience sample*. They are not a representative sample of any well-defined group, especially not a representative sample of the healthy—irrespective of their exposure history. They are not because physicians tend to direct their efforts toward diagnosing and treating those with medical problems.

In Figure 10.7, examples a through c, the three 2 × 2 tables represent the three possible types of association. In the first, the 50 in cell a translates to a RR of 5; in the second, the 30 to a RR of 1; and in the third, the 20 to a RR of 0.5. The three relative risks have very different meanings. Although it is conceivable that any clinician practicing in a community might become suspicious if a cluster of three or so patients came to him with the same rare disease and all had a similar exposure history, based upon the information available he would not be able to determine whether the cluster was a subset of those in cell a from example 10.7a, or from 10.7b, or from 10.7c. Most clusters, however provocative, are meaningless (96). Furthermore, additional case reports do not satisfy the need for replication and confirmation. Once a testable hypothesis has been formulated, additional case reports proposing the same hypothesis contribute nothing.

By way of example, in the silicone breast implant controversy, it was originally hypothesized that women who received this medical device were at increased risk for breast cancer. The theory was based on clinical observations and concern was increased because of an animal toxicology study that demonstrated an Oppenheimer

Example a. Relative Risk is 5

	Diseased	Nondiseased	
Exposed	50	9,950	10,000
Unexposed	10	9,990	10,000
	60	19,940	20,000

Example b. Relative Risk is 1

	Diseased	Nondiseased	
Exposed	30	9,950	10,000
Unexposed	30	9,990	10,000
	60	19,940	20,000

Example c. Relative Risk is 0.5

	Diseased	Nondiseased	
Exposed	20	9,950	10,000
Unexposed	40	9,990	10,000
	60	19,940	20,000

A physician sees three patients with the condition and all three were exposed to the same chemical leading him to conclude that the disease in all three was caused by the chemical exposure. Is he correct?

FIG. 10.7. Case studies and case series.

effect, the tumorigenic properties of foreign bodies as observed in rodents (12,45,83). As a result of subsequent research, both experimental and observational, something between examples 10.7b and 10.7c is now thought to most closely approximate the association between silicone breast implants and human breast cancer. It is being theorized that these medical devices or the materials from which they were constructed offer some type of protective effect against breast cancer (15,120). The current data-based theory is in exact opposition to the hypothesis originally derived from the case reports. Interestingly, no action has been taken on this information. Why? Probably because even though the epidemiology study results have been reasonably consistent and demonstrate coherence with the findings of the experimental animal research, and the public health implications of such an association could be profound considering both the frequency and the life-threatening characteristics of the cancer, the underlying biological mechanisms of protection have not been identified.

ISSUES

Peer review is an imperfect process. Even the most prestigious journals publish findings that are wrong. As a consequence, everything must be read with a degree of healthy skepticism (90). This can be difficult enough within a single field; but it is truly a daunting task when a scientist tries to evaluate the merit of work from a different discipline. If a toxicologist understands the basics of data, measures of disease frequency, measures of association and methods, the epidemiology literature can be screened fairly rapidly using the "mantra" of *selection, misclassification, confounding, chance,* and *causation*. Consultation with an epidemiologist or biostatistician might still prove necessary; but only for the smaller number of studies.

The order of this mantra is important. If there are obvious technical biases related to selection, misclassification or confounding, it may make very little sense to spend time trying to evaluate the merit of the investigators statistical machinations, much less to assume the findings of statistical significance have biological meaning. It is no accident that the scientific literature has a highly stylized format: some variation of abstract, introduction, methods and materials, results, discussion, and conclusion. This format allows the reader to rapidly focus on the key components of the work. If the authors provide a one-sided presentation of the topic in the introduction, supply insufficient detail regarding their methods and materials, or do not critique their own work in the discussion—pointing out the potential biases of selection, misclassification, and confounding and how they were addressed—the reader should exercise extreme caution before accepting either the results or the conclusions, even as provisional truth.

Selection

In epidemiology, the term *bias* is used to denote a deviation from the truth; but not necessarily to imply that the deviation occurred intentionally (3,125). *Selection bias* refers to errors that are related to systematic differences between those who are and are not selected into a study. Therefore, even if the data gathered are valid for the examined, it may be inappropriate to use any information derived from these data for purposes of extrapolation to a larger population. For example, the results of a study of hormone replacement therapy among women cannot logically be extended to men. In epidemiology research, various types of selection bias can be introduced by the study subjects, by the investigators, or even by traditional medical practice and other social forces.

Self-selection occurs in both clinical research and some epidemiology studies. It is well recognized that those who participate in controlled clinical investigations, those who actually sign informed consents, may not be representative of the general population. Therefore, even with subsequent randomization of treatment, care must be taken before extending the study results too broadly. A similar problem occurs in observational studies in which some type of active participation, some type of action on the part of the study subjects, is required. For example, informed consent is needed for any epidemiology study in which biological samples are collected. Usually the more invasive the procedure, the more disinclined are the potential subjects to participate, and the greater the potential for bias. However in other situations, this bias may be less obvious or, paradoxically, so obvious that it is largely overlooked. For example, how many times have you received a questionnaire in the mail and, rather than filling it out, tossed it away? By doing so, you introduced a potential *participation bias* into that investigator's work.

In certain types of observational research, self-selection is not a problem. Projects that can be conducted without the active cooperation of the subjects often are able to achieve close to 100% follow-up. For example, occupational cohort mortality studies that utilize personnel records and industrial hygiene reports to identify the exposed, and death certificates to document the cause of death, can be conducted with little or no self-selection (84).

The same arguably holds for some studies that utilize medical records, but only if the medical records relate to the total health experience of a well-defined population. Such is the case in certain countries with socialized medicine in which all the hospital and clinic records are available for the entire citizenry. In the United States, such opportunities are rare and even those few are disappearing rapidly. For example, Mayo Clinic is a world renowned referral center, providing both state-of-the-art medical treatment and highly sophisticated research on the underlying mechanisms of disease. In addition, it serves most of the primary medical needs for those who live in the relatively isolated community of Rochester, Minnesota, and shares medical records by agreement with the few other primary care facilities that operate in that area (49,50). Having access to the total health experience on those in the community has allowed the Mayo epidemiologists to focus some of their research just on the residents and thereby to conduct high quality population-based epidemiology research that had minimal self-selection or referral bias. Recently, ostensibly for reasons of privacy and confidentiality, the state legislature passed a law requiring study-specific informed consent from all study subjects before any of their data may be utilized for research purposes, even if the patients had previously expressed a willingness to have their medical records used for any such activities

WANTED

Kansas farmers suffering from non-Hodgkins lymphoma especially those exposed to herbicdes such as 2,4-D. Needed to interview for research article. Please send name, address, and phone number to Box P7629 Classified Dept. The Star, 1729 Grand, K.C., MO 64108

FIG. 10.8. Recruitment of study subjects.

(69). This action by the Minnesota legislature, although undoubtedly politically expedient, will not only complicate the logistics of future research at Mayo Clinic, it unfortunately may also compromise the validity of the work.

Either intentionally or not, investigators can introduce selection bias when they decide who to study, especially if they make a greater effort to get participation among the exposed than the unexposed, or the diseased rather than the healthy. Figure 10.8 is an advertisement that appeared in a Kansas paper in the late 1980s. It apparently was placed by investigators who wished to identify more subjects for a research project and thereby improve its statistical power. What they presumptively did not recognize was that by recruiting simultaneously on both health outcome (non-Hodgkin's lymphoma) and exposure (2,4-dichlorophenoxyacetic acid), they would introduce a significant selection bias into their work, one potentially so severe as to invalidate any of their findings.

More recently, a study was published in the *Journal of the American Medical Association* of children with esophageal dysfunction who had been born to mothers with silicone breast implants (73). Once again, the key study subjects had been selected on the dual characteristics of health outcome and exposure. The investigators characterized their work as a case control study and indicated they had findings that were supportive of a cause and effect association. The fact that their report was little more than a case series was missed during the peer review process and corrected later in the form of an obscure errata, and apparently only then because of ad hoc peer review, that is, a series of highly critical letters to the editor (25,36,39,87).

Figure 10.9 illustrates the dynamic which leads to *Berkson's bias*, a particular type of selection bias that occurs as a result of the patterns of referral, either self-referral or physician-referral (51). Although there is some merit in asserting that the 250 individuals who

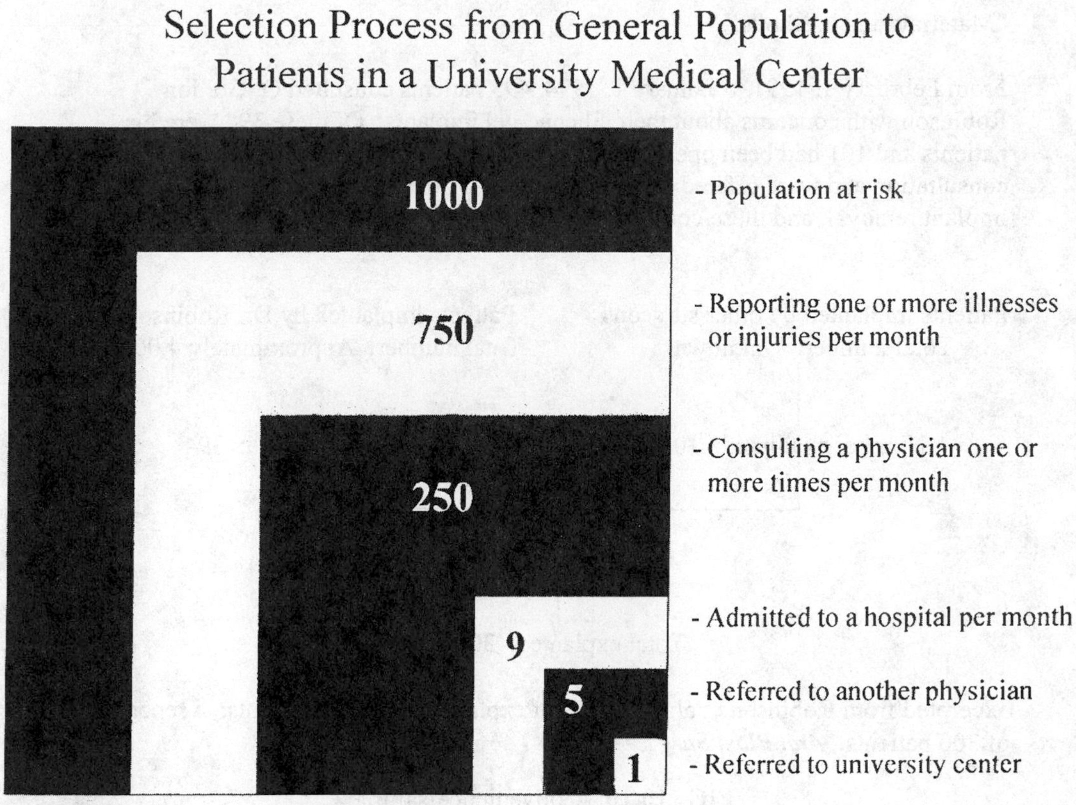

Source: Gehlbach SH. Interpreting the Medical Literature. New York: McGraw-Hill, Inc., 1993. (Ref. 51).

FIG. 10.9. Berkson's bias: potential selection bias by referral.

initially consulted a physician represent those with the more definitive illness among the 1000 in the population at risk and thus were legitimate subjects for etiologic research, it is less likely that the same thing can be said about the 5 referred to a specialist or the 1 who finally ended up at a university center. Patients seen by specialists or at tertiary referral centers include a disproportionate number whose disease is complicated, obscure, or atypical. In our chemophobic society, these patients also may be referred because of a suspicion that the condition is related to what Peter Huber has called the latest *terror du jour* (64). A spuriously elevated relative risk will predictably be found in any research in which the study subjects are selected on the joint characteristics of the condition of interest and the putative agent of concern.

Even if no formal study is conducted, the specialist may develop a marked suspicion concerning the presumptive cause for the condition—and then act upon that presumption. Once it becomes known in the community that a physician or a referral center is interested in patients with a particular condition, especially when it occurs in conjunction with exposure to a specific agent, additional referrals or self-referrals further compromise the value of the sample for etiologic research (115). Ironically, the more caring the physician in the sense of being more willing to provide therapy to those who have been unsuccessfully treated or refused treatment by others, the more that physician becomes a magnet for these patients.

The 1995 publication by Robinson and colleagues entitled "Analysis of explanted silicone implants: A report of 300 patients" illustrates a number of different types of selection bias (93). Among the 300 women who Dr. Robinson explanted over the course of 3 years, 214 (71.3%) reportedly had "disruption" (defined as frank rupture of an implant or severe silicone bleed). Interestingly, these authors noted that there was "virtually no difference in the disruption rates between those patients relating symptoms to their implants and those who did not (71.8% versus 70.9%)," suggesting health complaints were not a consequence of implant status. Nonetheless, they extrapolated from this sample to predict that most implants will lose their integrity somewhere between 8 and 14 years and recommended that all gel-filled implants be removed "preferably before 8 years from implantation."

Robinson et al. based their "rates," their interpretations, and formulated a policy of explantation on

"Materials and Methods

From February 1, 1991 to January 1, 1994, 495 patients consulted O. Gordon Robinson with concerns about their silicone-gel implants. Of these 394 were his patients and 101 had been operated on elsewhere. All 495 had the same consultation and were offered implant removal. Of the 495 patients, 300 elected implant removal, and these constitute our study group."

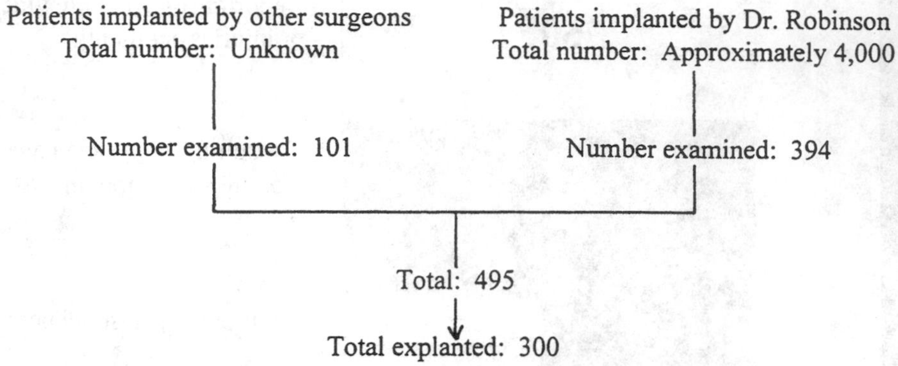

Excerpted from Robinson et al. Analysis of explanted silicone implants: a report of 300 patients. *Ann Plast Surg* 1995;34:1-7

FIG. 10.10. Convenience sample.

data from a denominator of 300; but that was not the group they actually studied (Figure 10.10). According to the paper, Dr. Robinson saw 495 women who would have been eligible for this investigation, 101 who had been implanted by other surgeons, and 394 of his own patients. The 300 were drawn from the 495, but note, even if he had studied all 495, he still would not have been able to develop rates that were free of potential selection bias. Even with 100% participation of his sample, he would not have been able to develop rates that meaningfully could be extrapolated back to a larger group. That is because the 495 were a convenience sample, an ill-defined and likely highly biased sample of the larger population from whence they came. The larger population included all of Dr. Robinson's implant patients and, by implication, all the breast implant patients of the other 15 to 20 plastic surgeons who practiced concurrently in the same community (2). Court records indicate that Dr. Robinson implanted approximately 4000 women and it is quite possible that at least some of the surgeons in his community implanted comparable numbers (92).

So what can we make of the Robinson information? The data collected for this report were prevalence data. Although gathered over a 3-year period, for the individual study subjects they were obtained at a single point in biological time, time of surgical explantation. Because they had prevalence data, the researchers could not differentiate between events that occurred at the time of surgical implantation, during the period the implant was within the body, or at explantation. Therefore, their interpretation that implant failure was a function of the aging of the device, presumptively related to biological degradation of the silicone elastomer shell, required assumptions (e.g., the incidence time of rupture was just before explantation) that were not adequately addressed in this research.

Based on the work of others, at least some of those assumptions appear to be incorrect. Rapaport et al. have found an appreciable number of implant ruptures occur secondary to micropunctures caused by needles or other medical devices used during the implant procedure (88). Others have done work that expands on this observation (13). Brandon and colleagues, using lot-matched controls, reported that the material properties of the silicone shell were not affected by implantation for time periods up to 21 years, and concluded "that the silicone elastomer undergoes little or no change during implantation" (14). Also, Slavin and Goldwyn noted that approximately 25% of the implant ruptures they observed occurred during the explant procedure (110). At least two other mechanisms contribute to implant ruptures in vivo: closed capsulotomies (manual compression of the breast to rupture the tissue capsule surrounding the medical device) and so-called "fold flaws" (disruption of the elastomer by excessive flexing at the site of folds in the shell). Both involve mechanical trauma. Obviously, different approaches might better be used to prevent, control, or otherwise address implant ruptures caused by different mechanisms.

Setting aside the questions of the validity of the data and the causes of implant rupture, if the 300 who were explanted were a representative sample of the ever-implanted, then it is quite possible that a high proportion of implanted women have "disrupted" implants. Further, if "disruption" equates to implant rupture, either overt or occult, it suggests there may be a high rupture rate for these medical devices, at least for those brands and models favored by Dr. Robinson and his colleagues (22). On the other hand, if the 214 with disrupted implants are the majority of those in the numerator of a true rate, especially if disruption does not equate to rupture, then it is likely that the actual rupture rate is quite low, quite possibly a single-digit phenomenon. Of course if neither scenario is correct, then the information is invalid and has no utility at all. Furthermore—and in spite of the question about rupture rates—if these authors are correct in their observation that there is a lack of association between implant integrity and health outcome, a conclusion reached independently by others, is it good public health policy to expose all implanted women to the predictable risks of explant surgery (17,131)? Probably not.

There are a number of lessons to be learned from this report. One, not understanding the difference between prevalence and incidence data can lead to flawed interpretations (26–28,53–55). Two, selection bias can occur even when 100% of those selected for the study participate because the selection process itself may be flawed. Three, anytime there is less than 100% participation among those originally selected, even in a descriptive study of just the exposed group, the results are susceptible to an additional selection bias. Particularly troublesome are those situations in which the participation rates differ between the groups in analytic research—that is, among the exposed and the unexposed for a cohort study or the diseased and the healthy in a case control study—because this suggests the reasons for participation may not have been equivalent and therefore there may have been a spurious correlation between health outcome and exposure among one group or the other. The consequence of selection bias is an incorrect measure of association, possibly an underestimate of risk but often an overestimate. Complicating the situation still further, the dynamics of selection bias can change over time as a result of a well-publicized environmental controversy, a lawsuit, a provocative news program, or any number of other things. Thus, different types of selection bias can wax and wane. Four, flawed studies can lead to flawed policies, policies that ironically may put those whom they are designed to protect at greater risk.

In evaluating the literature, the reader needs to ask two questions related to selection bias. One, was the sample that the investigators were attempting to study truly representative of some larger group? Two, were the researchers successful in getting participation from all or a large majority of those they sought to study? An individual epidemiology report probably will have little or no value if the answer to either question is "no."

The operative term in the last sentence is "probably." It is important to note that not every potential selection bias is real and therefore not every study in which there is less than 100% participation need be dismissed as meaningless. The question is how one determines whether a study with less than optimal participation provides relatively unbiased results. Usually one cannot make that determination from the single study. The question can only be addressed in the context of the larger body of literature. If the results of the potentially flawed study are comparable with those of other work in which selection bias is a lesser concern, the consistency suggests a cross-validation of findings. On the other hand, if the results of multiple studies are markedly different, it raises concern that the findings of one or more of the reports are biased.

Misclassification

Measurement or *misclassification bias*, also called *information bias*, is systematic error arising from the inaccurate measurement or inappropriate classification of subjects on the study variables—either exposure (to the putative agent or confounder) or health outcome. At some level, all measurement or classification is inaccurate. The errors may be large or small and, in turn depending upon the use to which the data are put, these errors may be important or meaningless. For example, in measuring blood pressure some physicians routinely round up to the next increment of 5 (e.g., 140 mm Hg systolic and 90 diastolic, or 145 and 95, etc.), others round down, and still others record to the closest unit of 2. The experienced clinician tends to make these measurements consistently on the same two of the five Korotkoff sounds; but which two may vary from physician to physician (47). These variations from the true blood pressure probably have very little importance in the clinical setting if the patient is consistently measured and treated by the same physician; but they could be very important if treatment is provided by multiple physicians. They also could be important if the clinical data were used to judge the relative efficacy of a variety of treatments as administered by different physicians.

Misclassification can be introduced into an epidemiology study by the study subjects, the measurement tool, the observer, or even, after the fact, by the consumer of the research findings. For example, Edwards and associates conducted interviews to gather data on alcohol consumption (37). They observed that men reported significantly lower age-adjusted mean levels of alcohol use when a third party was present during the interview (probably the spouse in most instances). Conversely, study subjects may over-report specific conditions. Cautioning against placing too much reliance on self reported data, Star et al. noted that the self-reported diagnosis of rheumatoid arthritis could be confirmed in only about 20% of elderly women, a finding replicated more broadly across age strata by Sanchez-Guerrero and colleagues in a larger study of nurses (102,116).

Overreporting or underreporting by study subjects may be a function of a number of factors unrelated to the biology of the disease (59). For example, medical students tend to develop the symptoms of the latest disease they are studying even to the extent that some male students reportedly have complained of sympathetic labor pains during their obstetrics training! To address such *reporting bias*, Turner and associates emphasized the importance of "double blinding" in clinical trials of pain medications, positing that even inadvertent clues of voice inflection or facial expression by an "unblinded" investigator could influence how a patient might report his or her symptoms (124).

There are various techniques that an epidemiologist might use to avoid or reduce the potential for either purposeful or unintentional misreporting. Concealing the intent of the research from the study subjects is one; but such "blinding" of subjects is increasingly difficult to use in a climate of mandated informed consent and almost instantaneous dissemination of news about the latest health controversy. Another approach is to add a dummy health variable whose association with the exposure is biologically implausible. For example, a query about dental caries could be incorporated into a study evaluating the effects of exercise on angina. If there is a strong correlation between the frequency with which the study subjects reported the dummy variable and the health outcome of concern, one should suspect a misreporting problem. In such a situation, it may be necessary to validate the reports—perhaps, if feasible, by examining a subset of the respondents or via review of medical records that predate the controversy or by use of a biological marker such as salivary cotinine for cigarette smoking (71,94,128).

At a minimum, the processes by which the data were collected should be well defined. Even then, there could be problems. It is well recognized by the seasoned researcher that mechanical or electronic instruments of assessment periodically must be calibrated to assure a consistency of measurement over time. To achieve validity, they need to be calibrated to an external standard. Yet the application of other data collection tools like questionnaires may be less than rigorous. With survey instruments, the order in which the questions were posed can be important. Even if the questionnaire is not open-ended, the words themselves may have alternative connotations for different ethnic or racial groups. To the extent possible, epidemiology research should use tools whose strengths and limitations are well recognized, or should incorporate a validation pilot into the research project.

Diagnostic bias, a type of observer bias, occurs when a physician's diagnosis is influenced by his or her knowledge of certain exposures or surrogates of such exposures. In a study of eosinophilia-myalgia syndrome, Wagner et al. found up to a sixfold increase in diagnosing the condition when physicians were told the patients had ingested L-tryptophan, even though use of this dietary supplement was not part of the definition for the condition (129). In unpublished work, Cook submitted a series of chest x-rays to a board-certified radiologist and resubmitted the same x-rays about 1 month later. As is customary, a short description of each patient accompanied his respective radiograph. During one submission the patients were identified as office workers, during the other as pipe-fitters. When presented as pipe-fitters, they were more frequently diagnosed as having asbestosis.

Even laboratory tests that logically should be free of this bias may not be. In attempting to satisfy himself of the utility of a new laboratory test that purported to distinguish between those who did and did not have a particular environmental exposure, Young found a stronger correlation between test positivity and a history of exposure than the correlation with actual exposure, even when some of the histories had been fabricated. He concluded that "since the test costs at least $350, it is probably wise for surgeons to advise their patients to find a better way to spend their money" (130).

Conflict of interest is another form of observer bias. It occurs when special interests of the investigators unintentionally or intentionally compromise observer objectivity. Journal requirements for disclosure of the authors affiliations and financial interests are an attempt to control this bias, or at least make the readers aware of its potential; but this implies that affiliation and money are the only threats to objectivity (41,56,77,97). There are others that are much more insidious: power, prestige, position, promotion, social philosophy, and a need to publish being just a few. The best protection against observer bias, whatever the cause, is for the investigators to be aware that it might exist and design it out at the project's inception. This equates to a well–thought out protocol, review and approval of the protocol by an appropriate third party, slavish adherence to the approved procedures, and possibly even independent oversight of the conduct of the research. In other words, it requires good epidemiology practices.

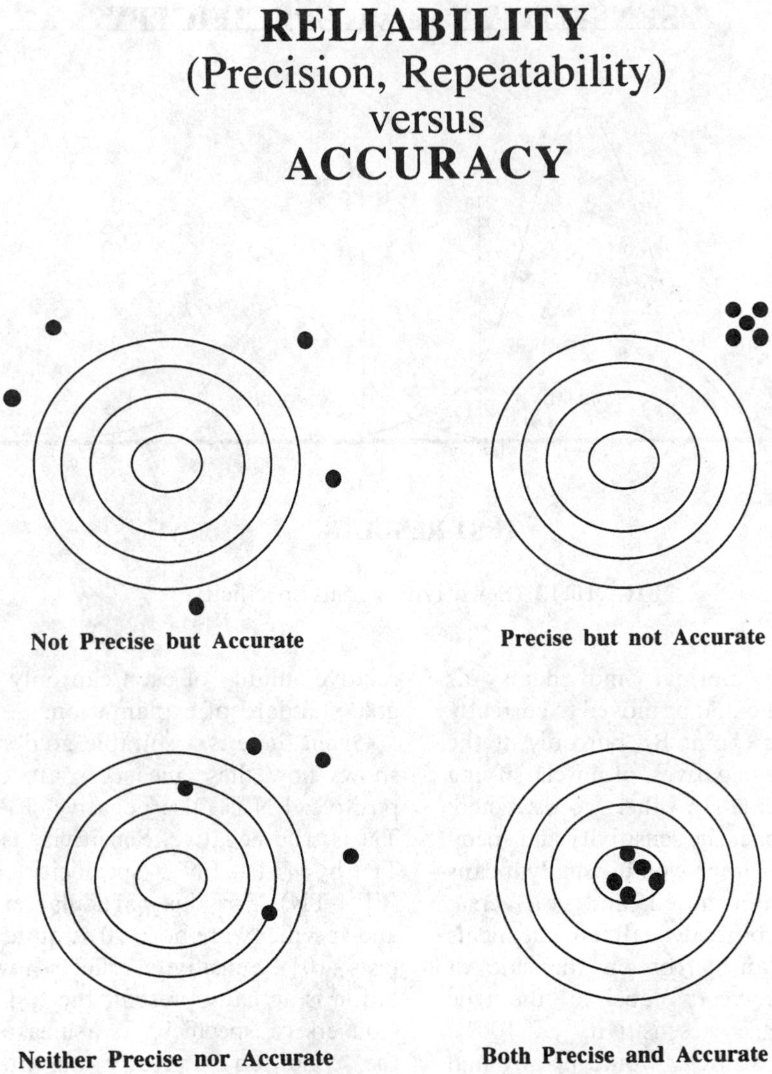

FIG. 10.11. Precision and accuracy.

Misclassification can even occur after a study has been published! In the Robinson et al. article, silicone breast implants were classified as "disrupted" if, at time of explantation, the device shell was broken or it was simply judged subjectively that there was an excess of what appeared to be silicone gel surrounding the intact implant (93). Others, referencing the published paper, erroneously have implied that all the "disrupted" implants were ruptured (17,53). Familiarity with the literature is the best protection against this form of misclassification bias. For those new to a field or an issue, it may be necessary to go back to the original sources before accepting the conclusions of a literature review or a meta-analysis.

Sensitivity and Specificity

Consistency or precision of measurement, although important, does not assure the absence of measurement bias, whatever its underlying cause. As illustrated in Figure 10.11, it is possible to be precise and precisely inaccurate. What is more important is accuracy, that is the validity of the data. The key measures of validity are *sensitivity* and *specificity*. Sensitivity is a measure of how well the test identifies a true condition (disease or exposure). Specificity is a measure of how well it documents a true noncondition (the absence of disease or exposure).

It is actually more complicated than that. A number of tests that are used in medicine, like blood cholesterol or antinuclear antibody status, do not clearly separate the normal individuals from those who are abnormal (62,121). The distribution of values in each group overlap (Figure 10.12). In such situations, the operational diagnostic break point between the two can be somewhat arbitrary. It can be set to identify all the true abnormals (point A), all the true positives, but only at the expense of accepting a certain number of false positives, of

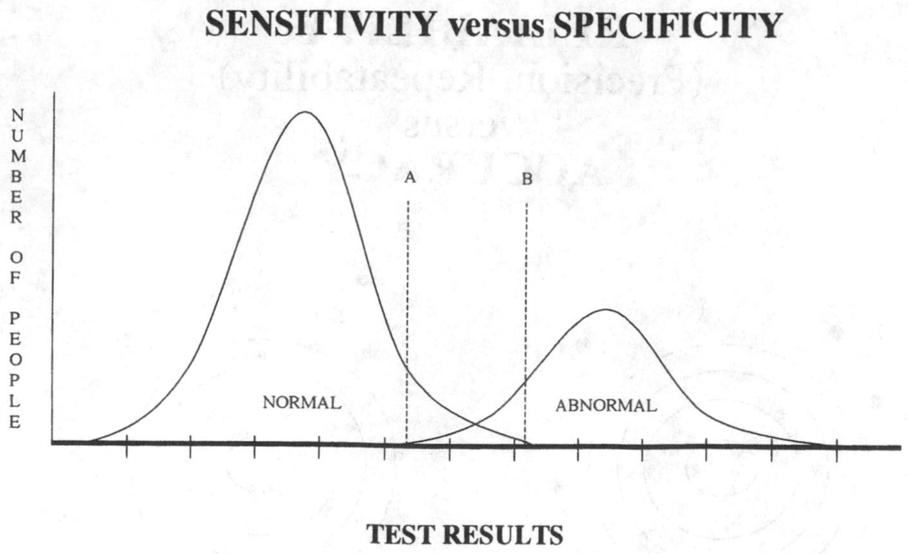

FIG. 10.12. Sensitivity versus specificity.

incorrectly labeling some normal individuals as abnormal. Or the break point could be moved to correctly identify all the true normals (point B), but only at the expense of getting more false negatives, of misclassifying some of the abnormal patients. In other words, where the break point is set can impact the sensitivity and specificity of a test; if sensitivity is improved it usually means the specificity has been compromised, and visa versa. For example, one could arbitrarily call all chemicals human carcinogens. Such an "error on the side of caution" would certainly correctly label all the true carcinogens, would guarantee a sensitivity of 100%; but the specificity of such a strategy would be abysmal because the number of false positives would be huge.

Note, to determine the sensitivity and specificity of a test, its results must be compared to those of a *gold standard*, an accepted test or procedure that reliably determines the presence or absence of the condition. Why then is it necessary to have the new test? Why not just use the gold standard? The new test may be needed because the gold standard is not as useful a tool in the clinical setting. It might be more expensive, inconvenient, invasive, or dangerous.

Paradoxically, data gathered by means of a gold standard actually might have little utility for etiologic research in and by itself, but still may be important for the development of tools that can be used in such investigations. Explantation, for example, is the gold standard for determination of implant rupture (17). However, for both technical and ethical reasons, it can only be used to collect prevalence data. There are other noninvasive techniques like mammography, ultrasound, and magnetic resonance imaging (MRI) that can collect incidence data and at lesser risk to the patient; but the relative validity of each can only be established via the gold standard of explantation.

Given there is a suitable gold standard, Figure 10.13 shows how these measures are calculated. TP is true positive, FN is false negative, FP is false positive, and TN is true negative. Sensitivity is obtained by dividing TP by (TP + FN), specificity by dividing TN by (FP + TN). For this particular example, the sensitivity and specificity are both 90%, quite good for most clinical tests (101). Sensitivity reflects how well, given the condition is actually present, the test detects the condition. Conversely, specificity is a measure of how well, given the condition is really absent, the test does not erroneously document its presence.

Predictive Value Positive and Predictive Value Negative

In real life, whether the condition is actually present or not is unknown before the test is performed. That's the reason for doing the test! For most investigations, what is of greatest interest is the predictive capabilities of a test: how well, given the test result is positive or negative, it respectively predicts the presence or absence of the condition. These measures, *predictive value positive* (PV+) and *predictive value negative* (PV−), can be obtained by making calculations in the vertical axis of the 2×2 table (Figure 10.14). In this example, the PV+ is 50% and the PV− is 98.8%. What this indicates is that among those who are diagnosed as having an illness on the basis of an "abnormal" test result, only 50% of them are truly diseased; and among those whose test result was in the "normal" range, 98.8% are actually healthy.

The two sets of measures are related but not equivalent. Although the sensitivity and specificity are relatively

	Test: positive	Test: negative	
Disease present	TP	FN	TP + FN
Disease absent	FP	TN	FP + TN
			TOTAL

Sensitivity = TP/(TP+FN)

Specificity = TN/(FP+TN)

	Test: positive	Test: negative	
Disease present	90	10	100
Disease absent	90	810	900
			1,000

Sensitivity = 90/100 or 90%

Specificity = 810/900 or 90%

FIG. 10.13. Sensitivity and specificity.

	Test: positive	Test: negative	
Disease present	TP	FN	
Disease absent	FP	TN	
	TP + FP	FN + TN	TOTAL

Predictive Value Positive = TP/(TP+FP)

Predictive Value Negative = TN/(FN+TN)

	Test: positive	Test: negative	
Disease present	90	10	
Disease absent	90	810	
	180	820	1,000

Predictive Value Positive = 90/180 or 50%

Predictive Value Negative = 810/820 or 98.8%

FIG. 10.14. Predictive value positive and predictive value negative.

stable attributes of a test, the predictive values vary widely as a function of the background frequency of the condition being studied. Figure 10.15 illustrates this point. For a given test, the less frequent the condition, the lower the PV+ and the higher the PV−. When the disease frequency drops to 1 in a 1000, the PV+ is less than 1%. In other words, if used as a screening tool, the test would label patients as "abnormal" incorrectly more than 99 times out of a hundred. This interplay between the underlying validity of a test and the relative frequency of the condition being studied impacts not only epidemiology, it also has important implications for medical surveillance (and the government regulations that mandate, fund, or otherwise support such procedures) as well as toxicology, in particular as it impacts risk assessment.

For example, a blue ribbon panel of experts recently recommended that routine mammography screening be restricted to women over 50 or those in high risk groups. In both, the frequency of breast cancer is orders of magnitude higher than it is in the general population of younger aged women. This recommendation ignited a fire storm of controversy and the panel, in part apparently due to pressure from Congress, subsequently modified its recommendation to include younger women (40). This probably will prove to be a mistake. Predictably what will happen is that the medical system will be flooded with false positives (38).

There are a number of downsides to a false-positive breast cancer screening test among younger women. One, a false-positive test can severely frighten patients. Even among those subsequently told the test was incorrect, many will retain a lingering anxiety at the very least. Two, an abnormal mammogram is often checked by means of a biopsy. This surgical procedure is associated with a cer-

Given:

Sensitivity = 90%

Specificity = 90%

Disease Frequency	PV+	PV-
1 in 10	50%	98.8%
1 in 100	8.3%	99.9%
1 in 1,000	0.9%	99.99%

FIG. 10.15. Predictive values as a function of disease frequency.

tain small but predictable risk of infection, bleeding, loss of sensation, and adverse reactions to anesthesia. For women without breast cancer, it is an unnecessary risk. Three, false positives put a strain on our medical care delivery system and misdirect limited resources. Four, even procedures that produce false results cost money, a financial burden that must be borne by the individual patient in the form of direct payments and by society at large in the form of increased insurance premiums and higher taxes. Five, arguably of greatest importance, some young women after one, two, or more false positive reports may lose confidence in the procedure. A certain number of these will drop out of the mammography program and never re-enroll. This means that they will not get the screening test later when they would benefit from it most.

The results of toxicology studies are not immune to this problem, in part because their results are routinely extrapolated to humans. If a high dose of an agent is found to cause tumors among rodents, it is current policy to assume it will cause some form of cancer in humans at lower levels of exposure. Unfortunately, although the sensitivity of toxicology research is quite high (but not perfect), its PV+ for extrapolations between different species of rodents is low, in the order of 50% in a study of various chemicals purposefully selected because of their presumed carcinogenicity (67). Arguably its PV+ is even lower for humans, especially for chemicals being tested simply to satisfy a mandated protocol (see questions).

Nondifferential and Differential Misclassification

Descriptive epidemiology research such as that done by Robinson and colleagues focuses on a single group (93). Nonetheless, misclassification obviously can produce erroneous information. In analytic epidemiology, the problem is compounded because data are gathered on and compared between two or more groups. This can lead to errors which are either *nondifferential* or *differential*.

With the *nondifferential mismeasurement* or *misclassification*, error is equivalent across all study groups. For example, an investigator may wish to compare the effects of growth between two groups with different dietary habits. As the health outcome, height might be assessed and recorded to the nearest inch. Even if the measurements were made carefully, two individuals with identical recorded values could easily vary in height by a half inch or more. In spite of the mislabeling, if the measurements were conducted consistently, the rank order of the various study subjects by height, short to tall, would be reasonably accurate. Furthermore, this would be the situation irrespective of the exposure group to which a particular individual might belong. As a consequence, meaningful comparisons could be made between the two groups. What the nondifferential misclassification might do is add a degree of statistical variability to the data and thereby bias the measure of association, the RR or OR, towards the null—to a greater or lesser extent depending upon the magnitude of the bias.

With *differential misclassification bias*, the relative invalidity of the data varies by study group. This may give rise to unpredictable shifts of the RR or OR either toward or away from the null and may generate marked under- or overestimates of RR depending on the size and direction of the differential error. It can even generate large measures of apparent excess risk where none really exists. In addition, this error is magnified as a function of the underlying frequency of the condition. Figure 10.16 illustrates these points. In this example, the respective sensitivities and specificities were quite high; but a slightly better job of identifying problems was done among the employees exposed: there was a better sensitivity, but also a concomitant decrement in the measure of specificity. Although the *true relative risk* was 1, that is, there was no excess risk in either group, the *apparent relative risks* among the exposed employees in plant A were quite high.

Does this happen in real life? Yes. Dr. Irving Selikoff justifiably has been recognized as one of the icons of modern occupational medicine. In 1968, he and his associates published a paper in the *Journal of the American Medical Association* entitled "Asbestos exposure, smoking and neoplasia" in which they reported an excess risk of lung cancer among insulation workers (104). Quoting from the article, "A copy of the death certificate was obtained for each of the 94 deaths. In addition we examined hospital records, postmortem findings (41 cases), as well as the surgical and pathological reports when surgery was performed (39 cases). We also re-examined histologic

Givens:
True relative risk = 1, i.e., background incidence rate equivalent in the exposed and the unexposed
Differential misclassification fixed
Sensitivity and specificity among the exposed: 95% and 90%, respectively
Sensitivity and specificity among the unexposed: 90% and 99%, respectively

Background Incidence Rate	Apparent Relative Risk
10 per 100 per year	1.9
1 per 100 per year	5.5
1 per 1,000 per year	9.2

FIG. 10.16. Risk estimates in presence of differential misclassification.

specimens. It was found that the death certificate was inaccurate in 14 instances." For comparison numbers, that is, expected deaths by cause, they used "United States 1964 life tables for white males." In their well-meaning attempts to be thorough, they introduced a significant bias into their study because, by using multiple sources to diagnose the exposed and only one source (life tables based on death certificates) to determine cause of death among the unexposed, they compromised their study results with differential misclassification. As a consequence, they overestimated the true relative risk.

Differential misclassification continues to contaminate research and clinical practice. Propelled by a series of case reports in the late 1980s and early 1990s, a cascade of systemic diseases were alleged to have been caused by silicone breast implants (105,108,114). Many of these theories have been evaluated in case control and cohort studies and found wanting (33,119). An unresolved question is whether women with implants are at higher risk to something called atypical connective tissue disease (ACTD) or, by some, siliconosis and, more recently, systemic silicone related disease (SSRD) (107,111). One of the problems with this alleged condition is that no one can define it well enough so that it can be rigorously studied to determine whether it occurs uniquely or more frequently among women with breast implants. Investigators who have tried have reported that the condition is essentially the same as fibromyalgia or chronic fatigue syndrome and the risks appear to be equivalent in women who both do and do not have breast implants (21). However, those who allege a unique disease does exist and waits to be discovered criticize this work as "studying the wrong disease" (112,132).

To address this presumptive shortcoming, one physician proposed epidemiologists utilize a set of criteria that he developed to diagnose SSRD in his medical practice (113). It is based on a series of inclusionary, exclusionary, and relatively nonspecific clinical criteria. By definition, one of the two inclusionary criteria are needed to make a diagnosis, either "current or past silicone gel-filled breast implants" or a "local disease" such as capsular contracture or implant rupture. Parenthetically, neither of the latter could occur unless a woman had an implant. They are, therefore, surrogates for the exposure of interest, silicone breast implants.

Restricting a diagnosis of SSRD to those with the joint characteristics of exposure and health outcome means that two women with exactly the same signs and symptoms, one with silicone breast implants and the other without, could never be classified as having the same condition. By means of the inclusionary criteria, Dr. Solomon assured, however inadvertently, that any epidemiology study that used his definition would be biased by essentially a 100% differential misclassification (113). In theory, any etiologic research based on his definition would produce a spurious elevated relative risk that approached infinity.

Similar biases occur in toxicology research, both nondifferential and differential. The traditional acceptance of tumors, benign and malignant, as a surrogate for cancer is one form of misclassification. In well-conducted studies, it probably is nondifferential; but any time the methods for disease determination differ between the exposed animals and the controls, it could be differential. For example, if more histopathological slides are made or read for the exposed animals than the controls, it is more likely that small occult tumors will be found among the exposed. This is differential misclassification, one that would introduce an overestimate of risk.

The reader of scientific reports can garner clues regarding the potential for misclassification bias, both nondifferential and differential, from the Methods and Materials section of these articles. The variables, both exposure and disease, should be well defined and equivalent throughout. If they are not, the reasons for the differences should be discussed. The techniques for data collection should be reasonable and applied consistently across all groups. It is important to be particularly vigilant if a study report did not discuss the potential for misclassification bias and how it was addressed. This suggests the authors were either naïve regarding the problem or chose to ignore it. In either situation, the potential for bias could be high.

Confounding

A potential *confounder* is a determinant for the disease in question, an alternative "cause" whose effects may confound or confuse the results of an epidemiology study. It can either be an agent itself or a surrogate for that agent. For instance, age is a surrogate for a constellation of biological, environmental, and social factors that individually and in aggregate are associated with increased risks to certain diseases. The same can be said for race and ethnic background. One of the two major characteristics of a confounder is that it is a "cause" for the disease under study. Different agents have different effects. None are universal confounders.

A confounder is not the same as an *effect modifier,* although an agent, depending on the study, can be one, both, or neither. With effect modification, there is a nonuniformity of effect across various levels of the effect modifier (98). For example, the consequences of exposure to pathogenic organisms varies by immunization status.

In addition to being an alternate cause, the other major attribute of a confounder is that it must be unequally distributed across study groups. That is, *confounding* only occurs when a determinant of the outcome of interest (a confounder) is unequally distributed among the exposed and the unexposed in a cohort study or among the diseased and the nondiseased in a case control study. As with the biases related to selection and misclassification, the degree of differential distribution determines the direction and magnitude of the error. In addition, the relative "potency" of the confounder can also, to a greater or lesser extent, influence the apparent relative risk or odds ratio.

For example, cigarette smoking is one of the major determinants of lung cancer. Any epidemiology study investigating the carcinogenic potential of a particular agent vis-à-vis lung cancer has to take this into consideration, has to "control for smoking." If not, the greater the proportion of the exposed who are or were smokers, the greater will be the overestimate of actual risk. On the other hand, if more controls smoked, the true risk to the putative agent will be underestimated.

Smoking is also associated with mortality due to cardiovascular disease; but not to the degree to which it causes lung cancer. In other words, equivalent amounts of unequal distribution between the two study groups may not have the same impact on the measures of risk for different conditions because the potency, the biological activity of a confounder, varies from disease to disease. With lung cancer, smoking equates to a relative risk of perhaps 10, whereas for cardiovascular mortality the relative risk lies closer to 1.5, and for still other diseases it has a RR which approximates 1 (no effect).

Very few, if any, diseases have only one etiology. Even a rare malignancy like angiosarcoma of the liver has a number of alternative causes aside from vinyl chloride monomer (42). Agents with high potency are relatively easy to discern. It is those with lesser biological activity that are more difficult to identify. An indeterminate number of the latter undoubtedly have not yet been discovered. Theoretically, because all the causes for the various diseases are unknown, some level of confounding may occur in any epidemiology study (and any toxicology study for that matter). In addition, it is highly likely that there are synergistic and antagonistic actions between various agents, both exogenous and endogenous, further complicating the picture. Evidence is also growing that suggests that effects seen at high dose may actually be reversed at low dose, a phenomenon that makes the interpretation of the dose response curve more challenging (18).

In experimental studies, the number of variables are purposefully kept to a minimum and ostensibly all of them are under the control of the investigators. Those who conduct observational studies of humans do not have the same advantages. The number of variables are only limited by life itself. Each participant in an epidemiology study has his or her own unique genetic makeup and own unique pattern of extraneous exposures (diet, medications, personal habits, etc.). Although either or both may be only weak confounders for a particular health outcome under investigation, they may be one reason why epidemiology research, especially any single study, has difficulty in reliably identifying putative agents with lesser biological potency, with true relative risks less than 3 or so (123). That is because even in the absence of selection and misclassification biases, the signal may be swamped by the noise of uncontrolled confounding. In epidemiology, the signal-to-noise ratio is improved via more research, especially more targeted research. As the exposure–disease associations become more focused, the relative risks should increase in size. If they don't, be suspicious of claims of causation. Also be suspicious of etiologic interpretations based on one study unless there is supporting evidence.

Control of Confounding

Confounding can be addressed through study design, data analysis, or a combination of both. For example, if smoking is a confounder for a particular disease (i.e., those who smoke get the disease more frequently than those who don't smoke, but those who don't smoke still get the disease), confounding by smoking can be dealt with via a technique called *subject category restriction*; that is, by restricting the study subjects (both those exposed to the putative agent and the controls) to just those who never smoke. This design strategy simplifies the analysis and interpretation of the data; but it also restricts how broadly the results can be extrapolated. If only nonsmokers are studied, the results derived from the sample usually only apply to the larger population of nonsmokers. Comparable information about smokers must come from another study restricted to exposed and unexposed individuals, all of whom smoked.

Alternatively, if a certain number of subjects are being evaluated and it is known that a proportion of those in the exposed and unexposed groups were smokers, controlling for confounding could be attempted at the analysis stage of the research, possibly by means of a *stratified data analysis* whereby different strata of smokers are analyzed and the results combined across strata. With the advent of high speed computers, ever more sophisticated statistical techniques have been developed to control confounding; but most of these incorporate assumptions that may or may not be valid depending upon the circumstances and, because they involve complex calculations within a "black box," it is often impossible for the reader (and perhaps even the investigators) to assess the relative impact of the various assumptions on the results.

Matching on potential confounders—age, race, gender, smoking, etc.—is an intuitively attractive way of addressing confounding that combines elements of both study design and data analysis. However, it is not a panacea (98). Not only may it be difficult to do properly, it also places certain constraints on the types of information that can be developed. And it may lead to *overmatching*, that is, to matching on surrogates of exposure or health outcome (54).

No matter what method is used to prevent or control confounding, decisions about which specific potential confounders might be important need to be made at the stage of protocol development, if for no other reason than to assure that adequate data are collected. Obviously, it would be impossible to control for smoking during the analysis stage of the research if no data had been collected concerning cigarette smoking.

Confounding is not restricted to epidemiology research. It also occurs in toxicology. For example, Hart and associates have explored the impact of food intake in laboratory animals (61). They noted that animals fed *ad libitum* have poorer health and longevity than those whose diet has been restricted. The total caloric load appears to play a role, but trace contaminants may also be important. As reported recently by Paolini and colleagues, most standardized diet formulations used by cancer research laboratories worldwide, "contain the well-known mutagenic carcinogenic element manganese at the same level and, in some cases, at an even higher level (up to ninefold) compared to that used to study the carcinogenicity of manganese itself" (85). Obviously, the more animals eat, the higher their caloric load and the higher their dose of this carcinogen. However, the amount ingested could be an unintended consequence of the experiment, for example, ever larger amounts of the test chemical mixed with the food may make the food less and less palatable. For those experiments in which ingestion varied by dose level of the experimental agent, it is quite possible that the results reflect a measure of confounding, and perhaps effect modification. Paolini et al. also summarized a number of problems with using historical controls. For example, "B6C3F$_1$ mice have a higher natural incidence of tumors than humans, and this incidence has also changed over time, increasing in excess of 50% over a period of just 10 years."

Although it is impossible to control for all possible confounders in any single study, the reader of epidemiology reports should determine whether attempts were made to control those factors which likely would have had the greatest impact on the results. As with other types of potential bias, a paper can offer a number of clues as to how well this issue was or was not properly managed. If confounding was ignored or obviously inadequately addressed, be skeptical of the information. Look for confirmation in other work which did try to minimize confounding.

Chance

Within the mantra of selection, misclassification, confounding, chance, and causation, the rubric "*chance*" covers all things mathematical and statistical and some that are methodological. For example, did the investigators add, subtract, multiply, and divide properly? Were the number of subjects consistently the same in the abstract, results, discussion, and tables? With more complex statistical procedures, especially those conducted in the mode of exploratory data analysis, it is possible for even the most seasoned epidemiologist to inadvertently lose part of a data set or to ignore a key assumption and thereby produce erroneous results. If numbers are inconsistent within a report, do the authors explain why? If they do, does the explanation seem appropriate or does it smack of gerrymandering or numerology? If either of the latter, look for confirmation of the results elsewhere. Or look for a correction published as an errata in a subsequent issue of the journal.

The term "statistical significance" is used by both epidemiologists and toxicologists. It means that within some acceptable measure of statistical "wobble" two findings were not equivalent, a measure of association such as the relative risk was different than 1, a trend was found, two variables were highly correlated, etc. It is not the same as biological significance because it does not speak to the underlying validity of the data. As a consequence, if it is apparent that the data set in a research study is likely biased by selection, misclassification, or confounding, it may make very little sense to analyze the data or to accept any information resulting from a data analysis.

Nor does statistical significance equate to cause and effect even in situations where the underlying data may be valid. For example, Vojandi, Campbell, and Brautbar published a study in 1992 that compared the results of a large number of tests of immune function among women who had breast implants for more than 10 years with those of a sex- and age-matched control group composed of women who did not have these medical devices (127). In this study, they identified a number of differences ($p < .001$) between the exposed and the unexposed and concluded that "these immunological abnormalities in individuals who underwent silicone breast augmentation indicate a mechanism of tissue injury to these patients causing autoimmune diseases or syndromes . . ."

Their data may have been valid; but their inference regarding breast implants was not. In the study, all of the implanted women had "symptomatology in relation to the musculoskeletal and nervous system" and all the unimplanted women did not. In the context of the 2×2 table, they only collected data for two of the four cells, a and d: the exposed/diseased and the unexposed/healthy. As a consequence, they could not disentangle the two variables and determine whether the implants "caused" the disease. They could not calculate a relative risk or odds ratio and therefore could not determine whether women with breast implants were more likely to get disease. At best, what their study could do was to appraise the efficacy of their test battery for differentiating between those who did and did not have disease, irrespective of exposure (24). But even for that, the exercise was of little utility because the "disease" was so poorly defined and the battery of tests so broad.

p Values and Confidence Intervals

Increasingly, epidemiologists are moving away from the use of *p values* and toward *confidence intervals* (*CI*) (43). *p* values, although useful, can obscure important characteristics of the underlying data set. By itself, a *p* value less than .05 or .01 suggests a finding that deviates from the null (e.g., a RR that differs from 1), but not whether the result is higher or lower. Nor does it necessarily provide insight regarding statistical power. With confidence intervals, one set of numbers representing the range of values which are consistent with the data observed, for example, the 95% confidence interval, provides not only an indication of where the point estimate of risk lies relative to the null, but also gives the reader a sense of the underlying variability of the data and, therefore, the *statistical power* of the study to detect a problem given one exists. If 1 lies within a 95% CI, it indicates the finding is not statistically significantly different from 1. If the lower value of a 95% CI is greater than 1, the estimate of risk is statistically significantly elevated. If the upper value is less than 1, it is statistically significantly decreased. Furthermore, the width of a confidence interval is an indication of the power of that study, at least for that particular outcome. If narrow, the power of the study was large. Conversely, if wide, the power was low.

It is important to note that a study result may have a wide confidence interval and still be valid. Statistical power and study validity are not equivalent concepts. One addresses precision, the other accuracy. In fact, a result from a small study relatively unbiased by selection, misclassification, and confounding may be more valid than the result from a larger study that has a narrower confidence interval. Although the former may have limited utility in and by itself to support or refute causation as a consequence of its low power, when combined with the results of other studies of comparable quality, it may prove to be very valuable. This is the rationale underlying *meta-analysis*.

Meta-Analysis

Meta-analysis refers to the use of statistical tools to combine the results of different studies. Originally, it was confined to randomized controlled clinical trials, to combining results of multiple small studies of the equivalent design, that is, those with identical dosing regimens and comparable, well-defined outcomes. It is increasingly being used to aggregate the findings of multiple epidemiology studies, even when their results were derived by means of disparate methods (e.g., cohort and case control studies), the sample sizes varied by orders of magnitude, the categories of exposure differed, and the disease outcomes were similar but not equivalent (11). Although some decry the use of meta-analysis for this purpose, others view it as an important adjunct to the traditional, more subjective literature review. Done properly, meta-analysis promises not only an aggregate quantitative measure of risk that has a narrower confidence interval than each individual study, but it also facilitates the identification of any studies that may be outliers, perhaps because of various types of technical bias or differences in study design.

Meta-analysis is not the same as *data pooling*. Whereas meta-analysis depends upon the research results as obtained from epidemiology reports, pooling refers to the aggregation of the actual raw data from many different studies and the subsequent analysis of this larger, single data set. Conceptually, pooling has some advantages over meta-analysis; but in practice it also has a number of disadvantages, a major one being access to the data. Unlike meta-analysis where the results have been distributed publicly via the scientific journals, data are not as readily available. In part, this is because of concerns related to protecting the privacy of individual study subjects and the confidentiality of their data (6).

The validity of a meta-analysis is dependent upon the validity of the studies included in the exercise. To address this problem, some have suggested that a priori rules must be established with respect to which studies to include or exclude. Unfortunately, these rules may reflect the personal biases of the person doing the meta-analysis. For that reason, a type of sensitivity analysis is arguably a better approach (86). In this type of analysis, the results of all available studies are first evaluated together and then various combinations are used to better understand how the different methods, number of study subjects, classifications of exposure, or definitions of health outcome may have influenced the calculations. It can even be used to compare and contrast the results of different studies that may have different types of bias and to explore whether potential bias is a likely explanation for why one or just a few of the studies seem to be outliers. If a comprehensive sensitivity analysis is conducted and the results published, readers also have the opportunity to make their own interpretations, something that can be difficult to do with the traditional literature review or even with pooling.

There is one particular type of bias to which meta-analyses are particularly prone: *publication bias.* Publication bias is a type of selection bias. It refers to the tendency of authors to submit and editors preferentially to accept studies with provocative findings (3,34,68). This has also been called *positive results bias* and can be exacerbated by a *hot stuff bias* (100). The publication of "I had a patient like that too" case reports is an example of the latter. Such a flurry of case reports following the initial announcement of an interesting finding in either a medical journal or the popular press can give undue credibility to hypothesized associations, even if they are not real. There are a number of different approaches that can be used to assess the possibility of publication bias, but the best way to avoid it is to aggressively search for pertinent research reports, including those in the form of dissertations, abstracts, and publications in obscure journals (90).

Exploratory Data Analysis and Multiple Comparisons Bias

To the general public, all findings of statistical significance have basically the same merit. They either accept them as exact and correct or, when faced with apparent contradictions, become frustrated with science. The late Senator Edmund Muskie, following an exhaustive series of federal hearings in which various experts testified about a complex environmental issue, epitomized that frustration when he reportedly said that he wanted to meet a one-armed scientist, someone who did not always say, "On the one hand this, but on the other hand that."

Scientific discovery is not a destination. It is a journey with many side trips along the way. It starts with a hypothesis, a theory whose genesis may be any number of things ranging from the subjective (clinical observations that seem unusual for intuitive reasons) to the super quantitative (statistically significant findings derived during *exploratory data analysis* of a large medical data set, e.g., the health claim files of a private insurance company or of Medicare/Medicaid). Before these findings can be accepted as even provisional truth, they have to be confirmed by additional research, preferably well-focused hypothesis-testing research.

In both hypothesis-generating and hypothesis-testing exercises, the same statistical tools and the same levels of statistical significance may be used. Yet the findings of the former do not carry the same interpretive weight as those from the latter (109). That's because the former, in addition to uncontrolled confounding, are subject to a *multiple comparisons bias* (122).

The statistical tests used in health research factor in both a type I and a type II error. A type I is the error of rejecting a null hypothesis, of concluding that a difference exists when, in truth, it does not. By convention, the alpha level (the probability of a type I error) is usually set at .05 (that equates to a 95% CI). This means that a certain predictable number of statistically significant findings are incorrect, about 1 in 20. The greater the number of comparisons, the greater is the number of spurious associations that may be found, that is, the larger is the multiple comparisons bias. Various techniques have been developed to address this bias, the simplest perhaps being the *Bonferroni correction* in which the putative alpha is divided by the total number of comparisons and the "corrected alpha" used to determine the presence or absence of statistical significance (78). For example, if the study alpha level was preset at .05 and 10 comparisons were made, a Bonferroni-corrected 95% CI would, in essence, be a 99.5% CI.

In many studies in which a large number of comparisons are made, the authors will do a Bonferroni correction or some analogous procedure and report the confidence intervals with and without the adjustment. In others, they will not; but they will indicate the total number of comparisons and thus allow the reader to develop his or her own opinions about the merit of the findings. In still others, it may be difficult for the reader to recognize the potential for a multiple comparisons bias, especially if investigators practice surreptitious data dredging—engage in exploratory statistical analyses of large and diverse data sets, but selectively report only those results which support their own pet theories (82,103,122). Because few comparisons are presented, the reader is given the erroneous impression that only those few were considered and therefore they must have been of some a priori concern. This approach can be particularly attractive to quasi-scientific advocacy groups who recognize the publicity value of a statistically significant cluster.

Post Hoc Reasoning

The latter is but one of a number of variations on the theme of purposefully biased science (66,81). In another, the investigator simply scans a data set and determines which hypotheses he wishes to test. Or he may gerrymander the data set and thereby construct an artificial cluster. In either case, by having foreknowledge of what the cluster is and where it is located in the data set, he can reduce the total number of actual statistical procedures and therefore, even with "overly conservative" corrections for multiple comparisons, claim to have refuted the null hypothesis. The nefarious may even point to a hypothesis in a protocol that predated the formal statistical analysis. Although the work seems to fit the scientific method, giving the results an aura of biological credibility, the findings are a product of *post hoc reasoning.* They are worthless. Using this approach, statistically significant clusters even can be generated from a table of random numbers.

Investigators who are guilty of post hoc reasoning are sometimes derisively called *Texas sharpshooters* (58).

In most target shooting, one shoots at a bull's eye. The Texas sharpshooter first shoots at the side of the barn (perhaps from very close to the building) and then draws the bull's eye around the holes. By doing so, he claims his marksmanship is both precise and accurate.

If clusters of disease are the catalyst for an epidemiology study, they can introduce another form of self-fulfilling reasoning into the research. It occurs when an investigator stumbles upon a cluster of disease, perhaps in an occupational group, and then uses the cluster both to develop a hypothesis about one or more of the chemicals to which the group was exposed and also to test this hypothesis, that is, the cluster is incorporated into any subsequent analytic research. If the disease is rare, it is quite possible that an elevated relative risk will be found in the formal epidemiology study even if no new cases are discovered in the expanded cohort. Although the additional research in this situation may be designed, initiated, and conducted after the theory was developed, it will not be an independent test of hypothesis (3,23,44).

In summary, even the most precise results may be wrong, a consequence of simple mathematical errors, technical bias, or less innocent intent. Although exploratory data analysis is a valuable tool, more is not always better. This maxim applies equally well to epidemiology, toxicology, and clinical medicine (Figure 10.17). To be interpreted properly, the results of tests must be put in the context of the size of the data set, the number of tests that were performed, the body of information that is already available, and even, if possible, the mind-set of the investigators at the inception of the research. The latter may be obvious from the introduction of the paper or from the protocol; but sometimes it can only be surmised.

Causation

Even when selection, misclassification, and confounding are minimal, the identification of the causes of human disease is not simply an exercise of calculating which exposure–disease associations are statistically significant. It is a thoughtful process based upon the preponderance of evidence and a logical ordering of that information. Sir Bradford Hill, a British statistician/epidemiologist, presented his criteria for determining causation in the mid-1960s and subsequently refined them for his textbook (63). These criteria are still in wide use. In interpreting data, he noted that an investigator must deal with two basic problems: *significance* (the statistical reliability of a finding) and *inference* (the deductions one might make from such a finding). With the former, he cautioned against overinterpreting statistical significance and also noted that, if absent, "chance is a not unlikely reason" for an apparent difference, for an apparent association, and for an apparent elevated relative risk. As for inference, he offered nine criteria for differentiating between "causation or merely association" when faced "with a clear and significant association

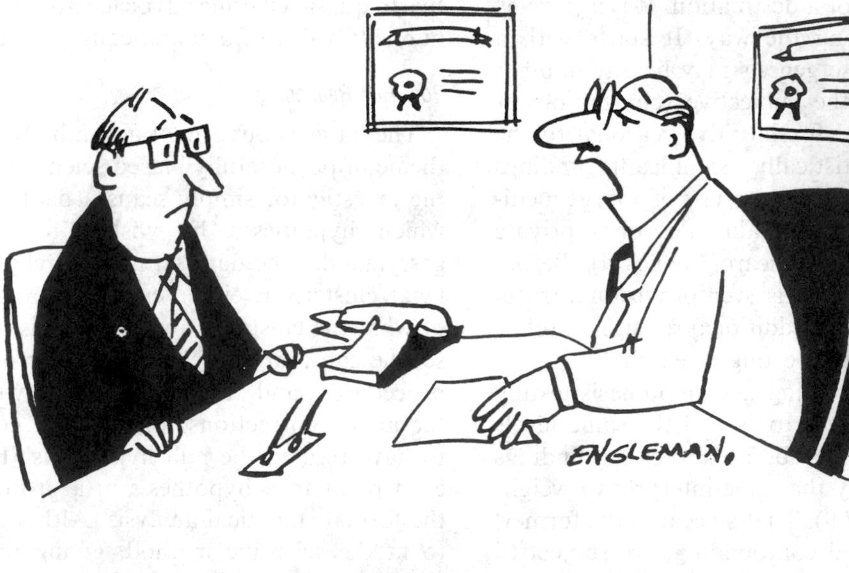

You seem to be in fine health
but let's run a few tests.
I'm sure we can find something wrong with you.

FIG. 10.17. Multiple comparisons bias in clinical medicine.

Table 10.2
Hill criteria for causation

Strength of the association
Consistency
Specificity
Temporal relationship
Biological gradient
Biological plausibility
Coherence of the evidence
Experiment
Reasoning by analogy

Adapted from Reference 63.

between some form of sickness and some feature of the environment" (Table 10.2).

His first criterion was *strength of the association;* in other words, the size of the relative risk or odds ratio. Obviously not every statistically significant relative risk is meaningful; but the larger the number, the less likely any observed association is simply the result of random error or the consequence of selection, misclassification, and confounding. The question is, "How large is large enough?" For isolated findings, seasoned epidemiologists are reluctant to accept relative risks of less than 3 or 4 (123).

Sir Bradford's second criterion was *consistency,* the finding of similar relative risks for the same condition and exposure in different epidemiology studies conducted by different investigators on different groups of participants. In part, this is important because it is unlikely that the equivalent errors would be replicated in all the studies. Therefore, a finding that is consistent across many studies is more likely true. It logically follows that a summary measure of risk as derived from consistent findings will more likely reflect the underlying biological truth than the results of any single study. As mentioned earlier, meta-analysis provides such a summary measure. It is a way of teasing out a signal from the cacophony of noise that is inherent to epidemiology. If statistically significant, the findings of multiple small studies may be biologically important; but also meaningful can be the absence of elevated risks in study after study or as de Grasse Tyson has emphasized, "Null results matter, too" (31). Although it is theoretically impossible to prove the negative, when multiple studies fail to identify an association between disease and a particular exposure, pragmatic scientists conclude proof of causation is lacking and move on.

As his third criterion, Sir Bradford offered *specificity,* elevated risks to a single or small number of well defined health problems. When many disparate conditions are attributed to an agent, at some point it becomes questionable whether any of them are a likely consequence of exposure. The need for specificity also applies to the disease itself. No meaningful body of etiologic research can be conducted to determine if a condition occurs more frequently among the exposed if the "disease" cannot be defined because, perforce, each individual study would be evaluating a different outcome. The same holds for exposure. Although the initial stages of investigation may incorporate broader categories of disease such as "pulmonary disease" and mixtures of chemicals, knowledge comes with focus.

Sir Bradford's fourth criterion dealt with the *temporal relationship* of the exposure and the disease or, as he put it, "which is the cart and which is the horse?" In cross-sectional or prevalence research, it is often impossible to make this determination. Conditions with long latency or those whose signs and symptoms wax and wane over time can further complicate the picture (124). Nonetheless, if the condition occurs before the exposure, it cannot have been caused by the exposure.

His fifth criterion was *biological gradient*, that is, if small doses cause harm, do larger doses cause greater harm? Parenthetically, this is not a variation of the assumption inherent to quantitative risk assessment, that is, that if large doses are associated with health problems, lesser doses cause lesser problems (18). Something akin to linear extrapolation back through zero exposure must be assumed for the latter. Such an assumption is not required for the former.

Biological plausibility was presented as a sixth criterion. This he implicitly categorized one of the lesser tier of criteria because "what is biologically plausible depends on the biological knowledge of the day." Some consider this necessary to prove causation, that is, that the underlying mechanisms of action must be understood before cause and effect can be accepted. For many, it is too stringent a requirement. They are satisfied if a meaningful association is found for a risk factor even if the exact causal agent and the process by which it works is unknown. In a sense, biological plausibility also is a lesser criterion because it is subordinate to other criteria. For example, a biologically plausible explanation for a disease excess is meaningless if there is no disease excess.

The seventh criteria addressed the *coherence of the evidence,* the amalgamation of what is known concerning the natural history and biology of the disease, the presumptive actions of the etiologic agent, the results of experimental research on animals, and the contributions of other types of information. The evidence can come from within a single study or across studies from many different disciplines. Cigarette smoking, for example, is associated with both an increase in lung cancer and an excess risk for a constellation of other diseases, in part because smoke is a mixture of noxious agents. Although lung cancer may be the outcome of interest in a particular study, say one evaluating the impact of low levels of smoking, an increase in both lung cancer and the other pertinent diseases would add coherence to any evidence of harm. As for multidisciplinary evidence, the decrease of mammary tumors among methylnitroso urea–exposed animals implanted with silicone gel–filled devices adds credibility to the epidemiology findings of lower breast cancer risk among women with silicone breast implants (120).

The next attribute was *experiment;* but not necessarily in the context of a laboratory experiment. He also considered the removal of the presumptive etiologic agent a type of experiment. If a problem resolves following such removal, it may provide support for cause and effect; but even this is not absolute proof. Diseases wax and wane. If the putative exposure is removed at the apex of disease severity, resolution may take place coincidentally and the condition, in the absence of exposure, may return at a later date. If that were the case, it would suggest the original "experiment" was incomplete and therefore lent fallacious support to conclusions about cause and effect. To eliminate this possibility, there must be adequate follow-up of the patients following removal of the putative agent. Even then, there are a number of other things that can confound such experiments. Humans react to subliminal clues, exhibiting both placebo and nocebo effects, and these can present as either subjective symptoms or more objective signs of disease (117). Resolution of a condition may be related to concomitant treatment. Alternatively, its original presentation and subsequent resolution can be due to malingering (106).

Sir Bradford's ninth and final criterion was *reasoning by analogy*, that is, if agent *X* can cause disease *Y*, then perhaps a material similar to X can cause a disease comparable to Y. Some have argued that because new environmental immunologically mediated diseases such as eosinophilia myalgia secondary to L-tryptophan exposure are still being identified, it is possible (they imply probable) that silicone is also associated with a new disease. However, eosinophilia myalgia has a relatively short latency. It also has a characteristic clinical presentation. Both of these attributes are missing with silicone. If there is an epidemic of a unique autoimmune disease caused by silicone, it has not yet been discovered. If this is because it is a disease of long latency and therefore the epidemic has not yet occurred, one has to ask the question, "What then is the basis for the legal controversy?"

Legal Causation

At one time, courts tended to disregard epidemiology as simply a statistical exercise that provided information of little probative value; however, within the last 10 to 15 years, it has become key to the legal theory of causation as used in a particular type of litigation, that dealing with tort or product liability (10). Epidemiology research not only helps establish whether an agent is causally associated with a particular disease, but also whether the association supports a finding of "more likely than not." This equates to an attributable risk percent of greater than 50% and, with knowledge of the relative risk, can be calculated with the following formula: $AR\% = (RR - 1)/RR$. For example, a relative risk of 3 would equate to an attributable risk percent of 67%.

As mentioned earlier, the various calculations regarding attributable risk have no meaning until causation for human disease is established, until an acceptable number of the Hill Criteria have been satisfied. Therefore, in theory, there are four characteristics of an exposure–disease association that are needed before a claim of causation logically can be accepted in legal deliberations. One, the putative agent must be a known cause of the disease. Two, the causal relationship must be more likely than not. Three, the plaintiff must have been exposed to the agent in adequate quantity and for sufficient duration. Four, the plaintiff must have developed the appropriate disease after the exposure. The first two deal with *general causation*. The last two pertain to *specific causation*. In tort liability cases, the plaintiff has the burden to prove all four, at least in theory. Trials are emotional events and jury deliberations can sometimes be more influenced by the subjective rather than the objective.

Prior to the 1993 Daubert decision, juries were the triers of fact and judges basically functioned as the umpires of the proceedings (30,46,89). They made rulings regarding process but few about content. The Daubert case changed that. After a series of appeals that went all the way to the Supreme Court, judges were given the additional responsibility of "gate-keepers." Juries retained the role of triers of fact; but judges were charged with determining which body of "facts" were relevant and reliable versus which were simply "junk science"—which testimony would "assist" the jury in their deliberations and "whether the 'probative value' of the testimony substantially outweighed the risks of prejudice, confusion or wasted time" (65). In practice, this means federal judges now must decide which "expert witnesses" can and cannot testify and what opinions they will be permitted to convey to the jury. Many state courts are also moving toward a process based upon the Daubert principles.

Some courts have done an impressive job in rendering judgments that included sophisticated legal arguments well infused with scientific principles (80). Others have accomplished the same result with the help of outside experts employed directly by the court, an option acknowledged in the Daubert decision (60). Still others at the state level have yet to apply the Daubert principles, in part because some judges feel uncomfortable with their new role and in part because the new rules technically pertain to just the Federal judiciary (35).

Lawyers and judges, even at the federal level, are still exploring the limits of the gatekeeper function and how certain statistical and epidemiologic thought might be translated into legal concepts. For example, statistical significance means a finding has a lower confidence limit above 1, that is, there is some assurance that the estimate of risk is different than 1. The legal notion of "more likely than not" requires a relative risk above 2; but it is unclear whether the key finding, to be admissible, has to be statistically significantly different than 1 or statistically significantly different than 2. When there is just one or a limited number of epidemiology studies, the latter makes more sense. However, the former is not inconsistent with epidemiology opinion when there are a large number of studies which have similar results.

Clinical Causation

Neither epidemiology causation (what Sir Bradford Hill called "medical causation") nor legal causation should be confused with *clinical causation*. The primary goal of clinical medicine is diagnosis and treatment. In a sense, the major reason for a diagnosis is to predict which treatment will most successfully reverse, eliminate, or control a patient's troublesome symptoms or signs of pathology. If the diagnosis is correct, the resulting treatment works and the patient is well served. If not, the patient likely gets no better, possible may get worse, or even may develop additional adverse outcomes as a result of the inappropriate therapy.

Experienced clinicians are adept at the technique of *differential diagnosis*. Through the use of various signs, symptoms, and test results, and factoring in the risks inherent to alternative treatments, they identify the most probable diagnoses, weigh the merits of each, and use the resultant information to help select a treatment that likely will be most successful. If that particular treatment does not work, they move on to the next most likely diagnosis and a different treatment—and if that doesn't work to still another, continually balancing benefit and risk.

When clinicians speak of searching for the "cause" of a patient's problems, they usually are referring to identifying the most likely diagnosis, quite possibly one whose underlying mechanisms of action are unknown. Arguably, knowledge regarding the underlying cause of a particular disease is only important in the clinical setting if it materially impacts treatment decisions; for example, if a specific type of bacterial pneumonia is more efficaciously treated by a particular antibiotic. Also, the underlying causes are not initially discovered by the process of differential diagnosis. Such knowledge is derived from experimental animal research, controlled clinical investigations, and observational epidemiology studies. Contrary to what some physicians have asserted, differential diagnosis, no matter how sophisticated, does not obviate the need for etiologic research (1,52,57,91). As the many programs of the National Institutes of Health demonstrate, research regarding cause and effect and that related to diagnosis and treatment are complementary but not equivalent.

Parenthetically, proper diagnoses are made by means of pattern recognition; by what Margolis has called "habits of the mind" (76). Within the context of clinical causation, this has a number of implications. One, the more extensive a physician's training and experience, the larger the number of mental templates he acquires against which he can compare the next patient's combination of signs, symptoms, and test results. Thus, even if the underlying etiology for a condition is unknown (i.e., the condition is "idiopathic"), a physician may develop successful strategies for treating the syndrome. Two, this knowledge, no matter how prodigious, is always finite. Physicians recognize this. They specialize so that they might concentrate their energy on developing in-depth knowledge within one sector of medical practice; and even within that specialty, they refer patients to their peers, a tacit acknowledgment that another physician may be better suited to diagnose and treat a particular individual. Three, because the number of templates increases as a direct result of experience, the more seasoned the clinician, the greater his ability to diagnose and paradoxically, the greater the potential for a multiple comparisons bias. The latter is reflected in case reports.

CONCLUSION

As de Grasse Tyson noted in his recent essay, entitled "Certain Uncertainties," "the frontier of science is a messy place" (32). As a consequence, to the uninitiated, science appears to provide contradictory and therefore unreliable findings, irrespective of whether the research is experimental, quasi-experimental, or observational; but perhaps more so for the latter (Figure 10.18). Part of the reason for the apparent inconsistencies is related to technical bias: selection, misclassification, and confounding; but part is due to overinterpretation of the findings of any single study, either by the study investigators or by the consumers of research reports.

One of the primary goals of any scientist should be the elimination of bias from his or her research. The first step is to acknowledge that various types of bias exist. The second is to understand how they occur. The third is to develop methods and procedures to avoid, minimize, or control bias. Over the years, well-trained epidemiologists have found ways to address potential error and improve the validity of their research. The same can be said for toxicologists and clinical investigators. The scientific method has been core to all of these endeavors.

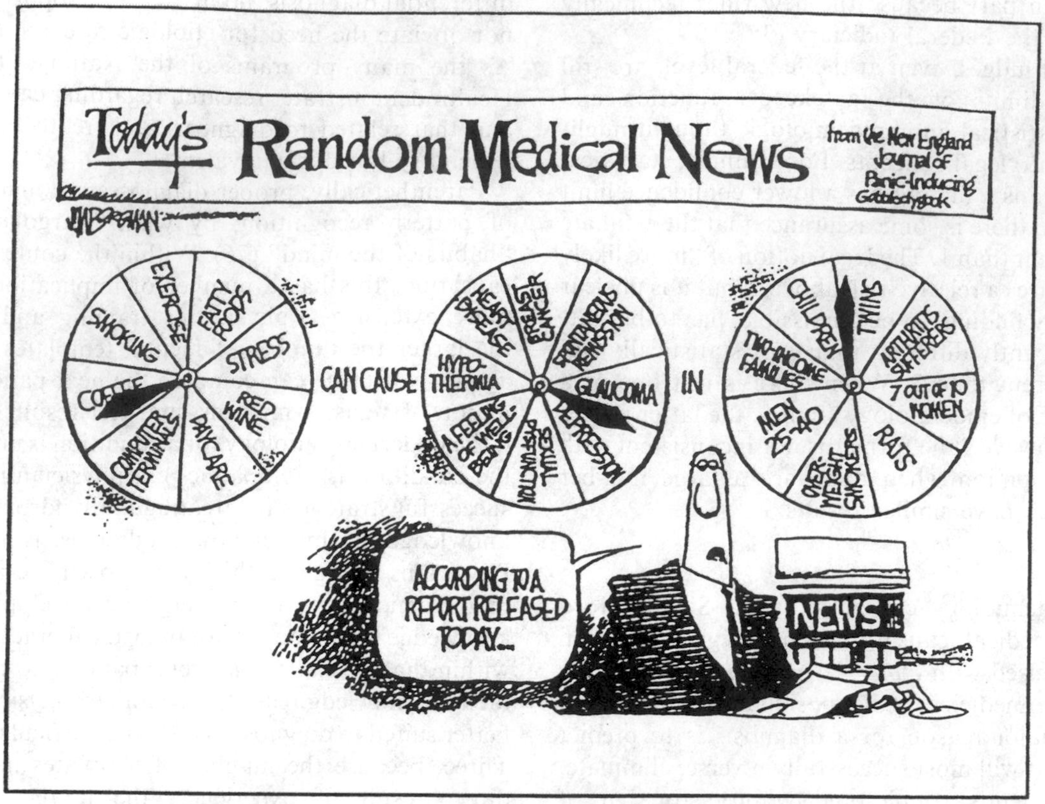

BY JIM BORGMAN

FIG. 10.18. Today's random medical news. Copyright 1997, *The Cincinnati Enquirer*. Reprinted with special permission of King Features Syndicate.

The scientific method is one of the major discoveries in human history (16,126). It has allowed mankind to gain a more objective view of the universe; to better understand the workings of the atom; and to successfully identify the causes of disease and with that understanding to treat, control, and even eliminate some of the major scourges that once were endemic worldwide. Unfortunately, the scientific method can be laborious, inconvenient, time consuming, and expensive. The temptation to take shortcuts can be great; but history teaches that shortcuts often just lead to further confusion (99). Identifying the truth can be difficult enough even in the best of circumstances; but it is impossible with biased data, inappropriate methods, or muddled logic.

One of the responsibilities of the technical journals is to screen research papers and determine which have sufficient rigor in data, methods, and interpretation to warrant publication. However, scientific investigation is a human endeavor and peer review an imperfect process, therefore flawed studies still get published, even in the best of journals. For that reason, the ultimate judgment regarding the value of any single report or group of reports may have to be made by the consumer: the epidemiologist, toxicologist, physician, lawyer, judge, newspaper reporter, or other member of the general public less well versed in the scientific method. This chapter provides a conceptual framework whereby such winnowing of fact from fancy might be accomplished. Within a basic understanding of epidemiology data, measures of association, and methods, it is based on the mantra of selection, misclassification, confounding, chance, and causation.

QUESTIONS

Exercise One

Among 50 employees of a chemical company producing ethylmethyl chicken wire, the company physician identified 2 last year with lung cancer. In the general population, the incidence rate of lung cancer is 5 per 1000 per year. What is the relative risk for lung cancer among the chemical company employees? Does this finding support the legal concept of "general causation"? What about "medical causation" as defined by Sir Bradford Hill?

Answer

Based upon the information provided, the presumptive incidence rate for lung cancer among the employees was 2 per 50 per year, which is the same as 4 per 100 or 40 per 1000 per year. Because the incidence rate in the general population is 5 per 1000 per year, the apparent relative risk is 40 divided by 5 or 8.0.

To support the legal concept of "general causation," two conditions must be satisfied. One, the putative agent must be a known cause of the condition. Two, the association must be "more likely than not." In other words, the relative risk must be above 2 and statistically significant. In this situation, we don't know whether ethylmethyl chicken wire is generally accepted as a known cause for lung cancer, in part because we have no knowledge of the results of any other experimental or observational research on this chemical. Furthermore, we don't know whether the finding in this particular study is statistically significantly greater than 2 or even whether it is significantly above 1. Calculating the 95% confidence interval could be done; but, with due consideration for the small number of cases that were observed, it is quite possible that this was a chance occurrence.

General causation aside, even if this had been the first report of lung cancer associated with the chemical, the data provided are insufficient to conclude that ethylmethyl chicken wire should be considered a potential risk factor for this type of malignancy. For example, we don't know how the two diagnoses of lung cancer were made. Were they based on x-ray or confirmed by biopsy? The former is much less likely to be correct than the latter. We also don't know whether the two lung cancers developed before or after first exposure. Although the determination of the exact incident time of a malignancy is usually impossible to determine, if the company had been producing the chemical for just a short time or the two employees had just recently been hired, the known latency of lung cancer would suggest that the condition predated any possible putative exposure. Moreover, who made the original diagnosis and when? If the diagnoses had been made earlier by the employees' personal health providers and only "identified" later by the company physician during the course of a routine clinic visit, the cancers could have been *prevalence* and not *incidence* cases.

In addition to more information about those in the numerator, what about the denominator? Did this company only have 50 employees? If there were considerably more and only 50 had been seen at the company's medical clinic, it is quite possible that a *selection bias* could have artificially inflated the incidence rate for lung cancer. If such was the case, the relative risk was seriously elevated.

Furthermore, to calculate the incidence rate for the plant population, we had to assume the two who developed the condition, given they were diagnosed accurately, actually were exposed. If they worked in a part of the company remote from the production facilities, for example, in accounting or sales, an incorrect assumption that they were exposed could have introduced a *misclassification bias* into the calculations, one that resulted in another spurious elevation in relative risk.

Finally, the comparison incidence rate, the absolute risk among the unexposed, 5 per 1000 per year, was that of the general population. That means there were other causes for lung cancer, like smoking. Furthermore, the term "general population" suggests the rate was based upon the experience of both men and women. The two genders have distinctly different incidence rates of lung cancer. If the distribution of either the attribute of gender or smoking was not the similar in both the exposed and controls, then *confounding* could have biased the results.

Exercise Two

There are two hospitals in the same city, a smaller one with 30 births a month and a larger one with 300 births a month. At the end of the year, which hospital is likely to have experienced more months with more than 60% male births?

Answer

The sample size is smaller for the smaller hospital. As a consequence, the variability of the data is greater. Thus there is a greater chance that the smaller hospital will have more months with more than 60% male births.

Exercise Three

In a study of chemicals associated with site-specific neoplasia in rodents, Huff and colleagues reported that "25 chemicals were carcinogenic to the liver in both rats and mice, 9 chemicals caused liver cancer only in rats; 53 caused liver cancer only in mice; and in 226/313 studies, no chemically related liver tumors were observed in either rats or mice" (67). They also stated that "the overall interspecies concordance in liver carcinogenicity is 80% (251/313)." That means if the mouse bioassay were used as a screening test of the carcinogenic potential of chemicals for rats, it would have a sensitivity of 73.5% and a specificity of 81.0%. In this example, what was the predictive value positive and the predictive value negative of the mouse bioassay?

Answer

The easiest way to solve this problem is to set up a 2 × 2 table similar to that found in Figure 10.14. If the outcomes in rats is the "truth" that we wish to predict, there were 25 true positives (TP), 9 false negatives (FN), 53 false positives (FP), and 226 true negatives (TN).

Predictive value positive was TP/(TP + FP) or 25/78. In other words, less than a third (32.1%) of the chemicals that were positive in the mouse bioassay were actually carcinogenic to rats.

Predictive value negative was TN/(TN + FN) or 226/235. The mouse bioassay correctly predicted which chemicals would not cause liver tumors in rats 96.2% of the time.

Exercise Four

In Exercise Three, 34 of the 313 chemicals tested caused liver tumors in rats, about 1 in 10. If among additional chemicals to be tested randomly, only one in a hundred would actually cause liver tumors in humans, how predictive would be the results of the mouse bioassay? Calculate the predictive value positive, the predictive value negative, and the concordance. Assume the same level of sensitivity and specificity for the mouse bioassay as found with rats. For convenience, assume also that 3400 chemicals were tested.

Answer

Among the 3400 chemicals tested, 34 are actually human carcinogens. With a sensitivity of 73.5%, that would mean 25 would be true positives (TP) and 9 would be false negatives (FN). With a specificity of 81%, among the remaining 3366 chemicals, approximately 2726 would be true negatives (TN) and 640 would be false positives. Using these numbers, a 2 × 2 table can be set up, and the predictive values and the concordance calculated.

Predictive value positive would be TP/(TP + FP) or 25/665 or 3.8%. Of the 665 positive tests in mice, less than 4% of them would correctly predict what would happen in humans.

Predictive value negative would be TN/(TN + FN) or 2726/2735 or 99.7%. In other words, of the 2735 negative mouse bioassay studies, 99.7% would correctly predict that the chemicals would not produce cancer in humans.

Concordance would be (TP + TN)/(TP + FN + TN + FP) or 2751/3400 or 80.9%, basically the same as that found by Huff for his interspecies study.

REFERENCES

1. *Allison v. McGhan Medical Corp.*, #1:93-CV-2051-RLV (N.D.Ga. November 3, 1998).
2. *American Society of Plastic and Reconstructive Surgery and the Plastic Surgery Education 1996 Combined Roster*. ASPRS/PSEF, Arlington Heights, IL.
3. Anderson, B. (1990): *Methodological Errors in Medical Research—An Incomplete Catalog*. Blackwell Scientific Publications, Oxford.
4. Angell, M. (1997): *Science on Trial: The Clash of Medical Evidence and the Law in the Breast Implant Case*. W. W. Norton & Company, New York.
5. Anon. (1997): Informed consent litigation could severely hamper epidemiologic research. In: *The Epidemiology Monitor*, edited by R. H. Bernier and V. M. Mason, pp. 18(8):1–3.
6. Anon. (1999): OMB explains how it intends to implement new requirements for release of research data collected under federal grant dollars. In *The Epidemiology Monitor*, edited by R. H. Bernier and V. M. Mason, pp. 20(3):7–10.
7. Anon. (1997): Pharmacoepidemiologists moving to protect access to medical record information. In: *The Epidemiology Monitor*, edited by R. H. Bernier and V. M. Mason, pp. 18(6):1–3.
8. Austin, D. F. (1979): *Preliminary Report, Cancer Incidence Rates, Industrial and Non-Industrial Areas of Contra Costa County*. California Department of Health Services (unpublished). Emeryville, CA.
9. Bender, A. P., Williams, A. N., Johnson, R. A., and Jagger, H. G. (1990): Appropriate publish health responses to clusters: The art of being responsibly responsive. *Am. J. Epidemiol.*, 132:S48–S52.
10. Black, B. (1990): Matching evidence about clustered health events with tort law requirements. *Am. J. Epidemiol.*, 132:S79–S86.
11. Blair, A., Burg, J., Foran, J., Gibb, H., Greenland, S., Morris, Raabe, G., Savitz, D., Teta, J., Wartenberg, D., Wong, O., and Zimmerman, R. (1995): Guidelines for application of meta-analysis in environmental epidemiology. *Regul. Toxicol. Pharmacol.*, 22:189–197.
12. Brand, K. G., Johnson, K. H., and Buoen, L. C. (1976): Foreign body tumorigenesis. *CRC Crit. Rev. Toxicol.*, 4:353–94.
13. Brandon, H. J., Young, V. L., Jerina, K. L., Wolf, C., and Schorr, M. W. (1997): Diagnosis of breast implant failure mechanisms. *Presented at the 13th European Conference on Biomaterials*, Goteborg, Sweden. (4–7 September, 1997).
14. Brandon, H. J., Young, V. L., Wolf, C., and Jerina, K. L. (1997): Long-term material stability of explanted breast implants. *Plast. Surg. Forum*, XX:215–216.
15. Brinton, L. A., Malone, K. E., Coates, R. J., Schoenberg, J. B., Swanson, C. A., Daling, J. R., and Stanford, J. L. (1996): Breast enlargement and reduction: Results from a breast cancer case-control study. *Plast. Reconstr. Surg.*, 97:269–75.
16. Bronowski, J. (1956): *Science and Human Values*. Harper & Row, New York.
17. Brown, S. L., Silverman, B. G., and Berg, W. A. (1997): Rupture of silicone-gel breast implants: Causes, sequelae and diagnosis. *Lancet*, 350:1531–1537.
18. Calabrese, E. J., and Baldwin, L. A. (1997): A quantitatively-based methodology for the evaluation of chemical hormesis. *Hum. Ecol. Risk Assess.*, 3:545–554.

19. Checkoway, H., Pearce, N., and Crawford-Brown, D. (1989): *Research Methods in Occupational Epidemiology*. Oxford University Press, New York.
20. Cheevers, J. (1981): CC industry may not be cancer culprit. *Contra Costa Times*. Walnut Creek, California.
21. Chow, H. Y., Cash, J. M., Calabrese, H. H., and Wilke, W. S. (1996): Patients with chronic fatique syndrome (CFS) and silicone-associated disease (SAI) are similarly disabled. *Arthritis Rheum.*, 38 (Suppl. 9):S52.
22. Collis, N., and Sharpe, D. T. (1998): Rupture of silicone-gel breast implants. *Lancet*, 351:520.
23. Cook, R. R. (1981): Dioxin, chloracne and soft tissue sarcoma. *Lancet*, 1:618–619.
24. Cook, R. R. (1993): But is it significant? *Ann. Plast. Surg.*, 31:94–5.
25. Cook, R. R. (1994): Sclerodermalike esophageal disease in children breast-fed by mothers with silicone breast implants. *J. A. M. A.*, 272:767–768.
26. Cook, R. R., Curtis, J. M., Perkins, L. L., and Hoshaw, S. J. (1998): Rupture of silicone-gel breast implants. *Lancet*, 351:520–521.
27. Cook, R. R., Hoshaw, S. J., and Perkins, L. L. (1998): Failure of silicone gel breast implants: Analysis of literature data for 1652 explanted protheses. *Plast. Reconstr. Surg.*, 101:1162.
28. Cook, R. R., Hoshaw, S. J., and Perkins, L. L. (1999): Failure of silicone gel breast implants. *Plast. Reconstr. Surg.*, 103:1091–1092.
29. Cook, R. R., Tirey, S. L., Spadacene, N. W., and Woodbury, M. (1994): Access to data for epidemiological studies. In: *Environmental Epidemiology: Effects of Environmental Chemicals on Human Health*, pp. 231–244, edited by W. M. Draper. American Chemical Society, Washington, DC.
30. *Daubert v. Merrell Dow Pharmaceuticals, Inc.*, 509 U.S. 579 (1993).
31. de Grasse Tyson, N. (1998): Belly up to the error bar. *Natural History*, 11:70–74.
32. de Grasse Tyson, N. (1998): Certain uncertainties. *Natural History*, 10:86–88.
33. Diamond, B. A., Hulka, B. S., Kerkvliet, N. I., and Tugwell, P. (1998): Silicone breast implants in relation to connective tissue diseases and immunologic dysfunction: A report by a national science panel to the Honorable Sam C. Pointer, Jr., coordinating judge for the Federal Breast Implant Multi-District Litigation in *In re Silicone Breast Implants Products Liability Litigation (MDL 926)*, #CV 92-10000-S (N.D. AL November 17, 1998).
34. Dickersin, K. (1990): The existence of publication bias and risk factors for its occurrence. *J. A. M. A.*, 263:1385–1389.
35. *Dow Chemical Company v. Mahlum*, 970 P.2d 98 (Nev. Supreme Court 1998).
36. Editors of the JAMA. (1994): Correction: Incorrect study design in abstract. *J. A. M. A.*, 272:770.
37. Edwards, S. L., Slattery, M. L., and Ma, K. (1998): Measurement errors stemming from nonrespondents present at in-person interviews. *Ann. Epidemiol.*, 8:272–877.
38. Elmore, J. G., Barton, M. B., Moceri, V. M., Polk, S., Arena, P. J., and Fletcher, S. W. (1998): Ten-year risk of false positive screening mammograms and clinical breast examinations. *N. Engl. J. Med.*, 338:1089–1096.
39. Epstein, W. A. (1994): Sclerodermalike esophageal disease in children breast-fed by mothers with silicone breast implants. *J. A. M. A.*, 272:768–769.
40. Ernster, V. L. (1997): Mammography screening for women 40 through 49: A guidelines saga and a clarion call for informed decision making. *Am. J. Public Health*, 87:1103–1106.
41. Fairweather, W. E., Higginson, J., and Beauchamp, T. L., eds. (1991): *Ethics in Epidemiology*. Pergamon Press, New York.
42. Falk, H., Herbert, J., Crowley, S., Ishak, K. G., Thomas, L. B., Popper, H., and Caldwell, G. (1981): Epidemiology of hepatic angiosarcoma in the United States: 1964-1974. *Environ. Health Perspect.*, 40:107–113.
43. Feinstein, A. R. (1998): P-values and confidence intervals: Two sides of the same unsatisfactory coin. *J. Clin. Epidemiol.*, 51:355–360.
44. Fingerhut, M. A., Halperin, W. E., Marlow, D. A., Piactelli, D. A., Honchar, P. A., Sweeney, M. A., Griefe, A. L., Dill, P. A., Steenland, K., and Suruda, A. J. (1991): Cancer mortality in workers exposed to 2,3,7,8-tetrachlorodibenzo-p-dioxin. *N. Engl. J. Med.*, 324:212–218.
45. Food and Drug Administration. (1991): *Background Information on the Possible Health Risks of Silicone Breast Implants* (Revised February 8, 1991). FDA, Rockville, MD.
46. Foster, K. R., and Huber, P. W. (1997): *Judging Science: Scientific Knowledge and the Federal Courts*. MIT Press, Cambridge, MA.
47. Fraser, G. E. (1986): *Preventive Cardiology*. Oxford University Press, New York.
48. Friedman, G. D. (1994): *Primer in Epidemiology*, 4th ed. McGraw-Hill, New York.
49. Gabriel, S. E., O'Flalon, W. M., Kurland, L. T., Beard, C. M., Woods, J. E., and Melton, L. J., III. (1994): Risk of connective-tissue diseases and other disorders after breast implantation. *N. Engl. J. Med.*, 330:1697–1702.
50. Gabriel, S. E., Woods, J. E., O'Fallon, W. M., Beard, C. M., Kurland, L. T., and Melton, L. J., III. (1997): Complications leading to surgery after breast implantation. *N. Engl. J. Med.*, 336:677–682.
51. Gehlbach, S. H. (1993): *Interpreting the Medical Literature*. McGraw-Hill, New York.
52. Gershwin, E. (1997): Testimony in *Spitzfaden v. Dow Corning Corporation*, #CV 92-2589 (La. Civ. Dist. Ct. April 22, 1997).
53. Goldberg, E. P., Widenhouse, C., Marotta, J., and Martin, P. (1997): Failure of silicone gel breast implants: Analysis of literature data for 1652 explanted protheses. *Plast. Reconstr. Surg.*, 100:281–284.
54. Goldberg, E. P., Widenhouse, C., Marotta, J., and Martin, P. (1998): Failure of silicone gel breast implants: Analysis of literature data for 1652 explanted protheses. *Plast. Reconstr. Surg.*, 101:1163–1164.
55. Goldberg, E. P., Widenhouse, C., Marotta, J., and Martin, P. (1999): Failure of silicone gel breast implants. *Plast. Reconstr. Surg.*, 103:1092.
56. Goldwyn, R. M. (1997): Financial disclosure is not full disclosure. *Plast. Reconstr. Surg.*, 99:2034–2035.
57. Gorman C. (1999): The web of deceit. *Time*, 153(5):76.
58. Grufferman, S. (1982): Hodgkin's disease. In: *Cancer Epidemiology and Prevention*, p. 744, edited by D. Schottenfeld and J. F. Fraumeni. W. B. Saunders Company, Philadelphia.
59. Hahn, R. A. (1997): The nocebo phenomenon: Concept, evidence and implications for public health. *Prevent. Med.*, 26:607–611.
60. *Hall v. Baxter Healthcare Corporation*, 947 F. Supp. 1387 (D. OR 1996).
61. Hart, R. W., Neumann, D. A., and Robertson, M. (1995): *Dietary Restriction: Implications for the Design and Interpretation of Toxicity and Carcinogenicity Studies*. ILSI Press, Washington, DC.
62. Hennekens, C. H., and Buring, J. E. (1987): *Epidemiology in Medicine*, edited by S. L. Mayrent. Little, Brown and Company, Boston.
63. Hill, A. B. (1971): *Principles of Medical Statistics*, 9th ed. Oxford University Press, New York.
64. Huber, P. (1997): The health scare industry. *Forbes*, October 6, 1997:15.
65. Huber, P. (1998): Joiner, Scheffer and Kumbo: Refining the standards of evidence. *Civil Justice Memo*, 35:1–5.

66. Huff, D. (1954): *How to Lie with Statistics*. W. W. Norton & Company, New York.
67. Huff, J., Cirvello, J., Haseman, J., and Bucher, J. (1991): Chemicals associated with site-specific neoplasia in 1394 long-term carcinogenesis experiments in laboratory rodents. *Environ. Health Perspect.*, 93:247–270.
68. Ioannidis, J. P. A. (1998): Effect of the statistical significance of results on the time to completion and publication of randomized efficacy trials. *J. A. M. A.*, 279:281–286.
69. Jacobsen, S. J., Xia, Z., Campion, M. E., Darby, C. H., Plevak, M. F., and Melton, L. J. (1997): Authorization for research use of medical records: Who declines. In: *Proceedings of The American College of Epidemiology Annual Scientific Sessions*, (abstract A-3). September 21–23, 1997, Cambridge, MA.
70. Kohn, A. (1986): *False Prophets: Fraud and Error in Science and Medicine*. Basil Blackwell, Oxford.
71. Kvien, T. K., Glennas, A., Knudsrod, O. G., and Smedstad, L. M. (1996): The validity of self-reported diagnosis of rheumatoid arthritis: Results from a population survey followed by clinical examinations. *J. Rheumatol.*, 23:1866–1871.
72. Last, J. M. (1995): *A Dictionary of Epidemiology*, 3rd ed. Oxford University Press, New York.
73. Levine, J. J., and Ilowite, N. T. (1994): Sclerodermalike esophageal disease in children breast-fed by women with silicone breast implants. *J. A. M. A.*, 271:213–216.
74. Lock, S. (1988): Misconduct in medical research: Does it exist in Britain? *B. M. J.*, 297:1531–1535.
75. MacMahon, B., and Pugh, T. F. (1970): *Epidemiology: Principles and Methods*. Little, Brown and Company, Boston.
76. Margolis, H. (1993): *Paradigms and Barriers: How Habits of the Mind Govern Scientific Beliefs*. University of Chicago Press, Chicago.
77. Marshall, E. (1997): Journals joust over conflict-of-interest. *Science*, 276:524.
78. Matthews, D. E., and Farewell, V. (1985): *Using and Understanding Medical Statistics*. Karger, Basel.
79. McMichael, A. J. (1976): Standardized mortality ratios and the "healthy worker effect"—scratching beneath the surface. *J. Occup. Med.*, 18:165–168.
80. *Merrell Dow Pharmaceuticals, Inc. v. Havner*, 953 S.W.2d 706 (Tex. 1997).
81. Michael, M., III, Boyce, W. T., and Wilcox, A. J. (1984): *Biomedical Bestiary: An Epidemiologic Guide to Flaws and Fallacies in the Medical Literature*. Little, Brown and Company, Boston.
82. Mills, J. L. (1993): Data torturing. *N. Engl. J. Med.*, 329:1196–1199.
83. Moore, G. E., and Palmer, W. N. (1977): Money causes cancer: Ban it! *J. A. M. A.*, 238:397.
84. Olsen, G. W., Lacy, S. E., Bodner, K. M., Chau, M., Arceneaux, T. G., Cartmill, J. B., Ramlow, J. M., and Boswell, J. M. (1997): Mortality from pancreatic and lymphopoietic cancer among workers in ethylene and propylene chlorohydrin production. *Occup. Environ. Med.*, 54:592–598.
85. Paolini, M., Biagi, G. L., and Cantelli-Forti, G. (1997): A hidden paradox in carcinogenesis bioassays. *J. Natl. Cancer Inst.*, 89:736.
86. Perkins, L. L., Clark, B. D., Klein, P. J., and Cook, R. R. (1995): A meta-analysis of breast implants and connective tissue diseases. *Ann. Plast. Surg.*, 35:561–570.
87. Placik, O. J. (1994): Sclerodermalike esophageal disease in children breast- fed by mothers with silicone breast implants. *J. A. M. A.*, 272:768–769.
88. Rapaport, D. P., Stadelmann, W. K., and Greenwald, D. P. (1997): Incidence and natural history of saline-filled implant deflations: Comparison of blunt-tipped versus curring and tapered needles. *Plast. Reconstr. Surg.*, 100:1028–1032.
89. Reed, M. E. (1997): *Daubert* and the breast implant litigation: how is the judiciary addressing the science. *Plast. Reconst. Surg.*, 100:1322–1326.
90. Riegleman, R. K., and Hirsch, R. P. (1996): *Studying a Study and Testing a Test: How to Read the Health Science Literature*, 3rd ed. Little, Brown and Company, Boston.
91. Roberts, H. J. (1988): Reactions attributed to aspartame-containing products: 551 cases. *J. Appl. Nutr.*, 40:85–94.
92. Robinson, O. G. (1994): Deposition testimony in *In re Silicone Breast Implants Product Liability Litigation (MDL 926)*, #CV 92-P-10000-S (N.D. AL March 12, 1994).
93. Robinson, O. G., Bradley, E. L., and Wilson, D. S. (1995): Analysis of explanted silicone implants: A report of 300 patients. *Ann. Plast. Surg.*, 34:1–7.
94. Roht, L. H., Vernon, S. W., Weir, F. W., Pier, S. M., Sullivan, P., and Reed, L. J. (1985): Community exposure to hazardous waste disposal sites: Assessing reporting bias. *Am. J. Epidemiol.*, 122:418–433.
95. Rothman, K. J. (1987): Clustering of disease. *Am. J. Public Health*, 77:13–15.
96. Rothman, K. J. (1990): A sobering start for the cluster busters' conference. *Am. J. Epidemiol.*, 132:S6–S13.
97. Rothman, K. J. (1993): Conflict of interest: The new McCarthyism in science. *J. A. M. A.*, 269:2782–2784.
98. Rothman, K. J., and Greenland, S. (1998): *Modern Epidemiology*, 2nd ed. Lippincott-Raven Publishers, Philadelphia.
99. Rousseau, D. L. (1992): Case studies in pathological science. *Am. Sci.*, 80:54–62.
100. Sackett, D. L. (1979): Bias in analytic research. *J. Chronic Dis.*, 32:51–63.
101. Sackett, D. L., Haynes, R. B., Guyatt, G. H., and Tugwell, P. (1991): *Clinical Epidemiology*: A Basic Science for Clinical Medicine, 2nd ed. Little, Brown and Company, Boston.
102. Sanchez-Guerrero J., Colditz, G. A., and Karlson, E. W. (1995): Silicone breast implants and the risk of connective tissue diseases and symptoms. *N. Engl. J. Med.*, 332:1666–1670.
103. Schneiderman, M. A. (1994): More on torturing data. *N. Engl. J. Med.*, 330:861–862.
104. Selikoff, I. J., Hammond, E. C., and Churg, J. (1968): Asbestos exposure, smoking and neoplasia. *J. A. M. A.*, 204:106–112.
105. Shoaib, B. O., Patten, B. M., and Calkins, D. S. (1994): Adjuvant breast disease: An evaluation of 100 symptomatic women with breast implants for silicone fluid injections. *Keio J. Med.*, 43:79–87.
106. Shorter, E. (1992): *From Paralysis to Fatigue: A History of Psychosomatic Illness in the Modern Era*. The Free Press, New York.
107. Silverman, S., Borenstein, D., Solomon, G., Espinoza, L., and Colin, M. (1996): Preliminary operational criteria for systemic silicone related disease (SSRD). *Arthritis Rheum.*, 39 (Suppl. 9):S51.
108. Silverstein, M. J., Handel, N., Gamagami, P., Waisman, J. R., Gierson, E. D., Rosser, R. J., Steyskal, R., and Colburn, W. (1988): Breast cancer in women after augmentation mammaplasty. *Arch. Surg.*, 123:681–685.
109. Skrabanek, P. (1994): The emptiness of the black box. *Epidemiology*, 5:553–555.
110. Slavin, S. A., and Goldwyn, R. M. (1995): Silicone gel implant explantation: Reasons, results and admonitions. *Plast. Reconstr. Surg.*, 95:63–69.
111. Solomon, G. (1993): Clinical and serologic features of 176 women with silicone implants: Evidence for a novel disease siliconosis. *Arthritis Rheum.*, 36 (Suppl. 9):S117.

112. Solomon, G., Espinoza, L., and Silverman, S. (1994): Breast implants and connective-tissue disease. *N. Engl. J. Med.*, 331:1231.
113. Solomon, G. E. (1996): Operational criteria for systemic silicone related disease (SSRD). Declaration submitted in *In re Breast Implant Litigation*, #92-182-JO-LEAD (E.D.NY August 2, 1996).
114. Spiera, H. (1988): Scleroderma after silcone augmentation mammoplasty. *J. A. M. A.*, 260:236–238.
115. Spiera, H., and Kerr, L. D. (1993): Scleroderma following silicone implantation: A cumulative experience of 11 cases. *J. Rheumatol.*, 20:958–961.
116. Star, V. L., Scott, J. C., Sherwin, R., Lane, N., Nevitt, M. C., and Hochberg, M. C. (1996): Validity of self-reported rheumatoid arthritis in elderly women. *J. Rheumatol.*, 23:1862–1865.
117. Staudenmayer, H. (1999): *Environmental Illness: Myth and Reality*. Lewis Publishers, London.
118. Steimle, S. (1998): Will Germany's Good Scientific Practice Guidelines prevent fraud? *J. Nat. Cancer Inst.*, 90:1694–1695.
119. Sturrock, R. D., Batchelor, J. R., Harpwood, V., Long, D. R., Milward, T. M., Silman, A. J., and Sloane, J. P. (1998): *Silicone Gel Breast Implants: The Report of the Independent Review Group*. Medical Device Agency of the British Department of Health, London.
120. Su, C. W., Dreyfuss, D. A., Krizek, T. J., and Leoni, K. J. (1995): Silicone breast implants and the inhibition of cancer. *Plast. Reconstr. Surg.*, 96:513–520.
121. Tan, E. M., Feltkamp, T. E. W., Smolen, J. S., Butcher, B., Dawkins, R., Fritzler, M. J., Gordon, T., Hardin, J. A., Kalden, J. R., Lahita, R. G., Maini, R. N., McDougal, J. S., Rothfield, N. F., Smeenk, R. J., Takasaki, Y., Wiik, A., Wilson, M. R., and Koziol, J. A. (1997): Range of antinuclear antibodies in "healthy" individuals. *Arthritis Rheum.*, 40:1601–1611.
122. Tannock, I. F. (1996): False-positive results in clinical trials: Multiple significance tests and the problem of unreported comparisons. *J. Nat. Cancer Inst.*, 88:206–207.
123. Taubes, G. (1995): Epidemiology faces its limits. *Science*, 269:164–169.
124. Turner, J. A., Deyo, R. A., Loeser, J. D., Von Korff, M., and Fordyce, W. E. (1994): The importance of placebo effects in pain treatment and research. *J. A. M. A.*, 271:1609–1614.
125. Ungar, W. (1998): Bias—it's everywhere! *Pharmacoepidemiol. Drug Safety*, 7:425–427.
126. Van Doren, C. (1991): The invention of the scientific method. In: *A History of Knowledge*, pp. 184–212. Ballantine Books, New York.
127. Vojandi, A., Campbell, A., and Brautbar, N. (1992): Immune functional impairment in patients with clinical abnormalities and silicone breast implants. *Toxicol. Ind. Health*, 8:415–29.
128. Wagenknecht, L. E., Burke, G. L., Perkins, L. L., Haley, N. J., and Friedman, G. D. (1982): Misclassification of smoking status in the CARDIA study: A comparison of self-report with serum cotinine levels. *Am. J. Public Health*, 82:33–36.
129. Wagner, K. R., Elmore, J. G., and Horwitz, R. I. (1996): Diagnostic bias in clinical decision making: An example of L-tryptophan and the diagnosis of eosinophilia-myalgia syndrome. *J. Rheum.*, 23:2079–2085.
130. Young, V. L. (1996): Testing the test: An analysis of the reliability of the silicone sensitivity test (SILS) in detecting immune-mediated responses to silcone breast implants. *Plast. Reconstr. Surg.*, 97:681–683.
131. Young, V. L., Elliott, L. F., Peters, W. J., and Lassus, C. (1997): Panel discussion: Management of displaced breast implants. *Aesthetic Surg. J.*, 17:247–253.
132. Zuckerman, D. (1999): Uncertainty about breast implants' safety won't stop thousands from trying them. *San Jose Mercury News*, C2, pp. 1–2, February 21, 1999.

APPENDIX *Guidelines for good epidemiology practices for occupational and environmental epidemiologic research*

The *Guidelines for Good Epidemiology for Occupational and Environmental Epidemiologic Research* are included in this text by courtesy of the Chemical Manufacturers Association (CMA). They were developed by the CMA Epidemiology Task Group as part of the Epidemiology Resource and Information Center (ERIC) Pilot Project and, prior to publication in 1991, were modified following review and comment by an ad hoc panel of epidemiologists from academia, various government agencies, and the private sector. Although they do not have the force of law, they have been recognized by a number of groups and are analogous to the toxicology *Good Laboratory Practice Standards* or GLPs. The *Guidelines for Good Epidemiology Practices* (GEPs) were developed in part to provide an alternative to the GLPs, one that would appropriately address the issues confronted by epidemiologists conducting nonexperimental research.

The *Guidelines for Good Epidemiology Practices* address the conduct of studies generally undertaken to answer questions about human health in relation to the work place or the environment. The GEPs propose minimum practices and procedures that should be considered in order to help ensure the quality and integrity of data used in epidemiologic research and to provide adequate documentation of the research methods. Epidemiologic studies often evolve through a number of stages that precede the development of a protocol, for example, proposals, feasibility studies, and measurement instrument validation. Although the GEPs are intended to address all activities that begin with protocol development, it was the opinion of the Task Group that adherence to the spirit of the guidelines would prove beneficial for those activities preceding protocol development as well as more informal investigations such as health hazard assessments/evaluations or small cluster investigations.

A copy of the original guidelines as published by ERIC can be obtained from the CMA. The complete document includes an introduction, eight sections, and three appendices. Only the eight sections are presented here, and in a slightly abridged form. A more detailed discussion of these GEPs can be found in the proceedings of a conference published in December 1991 issue of the *Journal of Occupational Medicine*.

I. Organization and Personnel

A. Organizational Structure

The organization or individual conducting the research shall be fully responsible for the operation and performance of the research. The organization shall be a legal entity with a governing body that sets policy and that is fully responsible for the administrative aspects of the organization and its related research activities. The relationship, roles, and responsibilities of the organizations and/or individuals sponsoring or conducting the study should be carefully defined in writing.

B. *Personnel*

Personnel engaged in epidemiologic research and related activities shall have the education, training, and/or experience necessary to competently perform the assigned functions. The organization shall maintain a current summary of training and experience of these personnel. A job description for each individual engaged in or supervising activities shall be maintained and updated periodically.

II. Facilities, Resource Commitment, and Contractors

A. *Facilities*

Adequate physical facilities shall be provided to all those engaged in epidemiologic research and related activities. Sufficient resources, for example, office space, relevant equipment, and office/professional supplies, shall be available to ensure timely completion of all studies. Suitable storage facilities shall be available to maintain research materials in a safe and secure environment.

B. *Resource commitment*

Sufficient commitment shall be made at the beginning of each study to ensure its timely and proper completion.

C. *Contractors*

For the purposes of ensuring and documenting the contractor's conformance with the *Guidelines for Good Epidemiology Practices*, it is recommended that the study sponsor have the right during the course of the study, and for a reasonable period following completion of the study, to inspect the contractor's facilities, including equipment, technical records, and records relating to the work conducted under the sponsor's contract.

III. Protocol

Each study shall have a written protocol. This protocol must be approved before the study begins. The protocol should include the following:

A. A descriptive title.

B. The names, titles, degrees, addresses, and affiliations of the study director, principal investigator, and all coinvestigators.

C. The name and address of the sponsor.

D. An abstract of the protocol.

E. The proposed study tasks and milestones, including study approval date (date protocol signed by all signatories), study start date (first date that the protocol is implemented), periodic progress review dates, and estimated completion date.

F. A statement of the research objectives, specific aims, and rationale. The statement should identify the immediate purpose of the investigation. For example, it might indicate whether the study will be exploratory data analysis, hypothesis testing, or a combination of both.

G. A critical review of the relevant literature to evaluate applicable findings. This should include pertinent animal and human experiments, clinical studies, vital statistics, and previous epidemiologic studies. The literature review should be in sufficient depth to identify potential confounders and effect modifiers and to determine areas where new knowledge is needed.

H. A description of the research methods, including:
   1. The overall research design and the reasons for choosing the proposed study design.
   2. The data sources for exposure, health status, and risk factors.
   3. Clear definitions of health outcomes, exposure, and other measured risk factors as well as selection criteria, as appropriate, for exposed and nonexposed persons, morbidity and mortality cases, and referent groups.
   4. The project's study size and, if appropriate, statistical power.
   5. The methods to be used in assembling the study data, including a description of, or reference to, methods used to control, measure, or reduce various forms of error—for example, bias due to selection, misclassification, interviewer, or confounding—and their impact on the study. Pretesting procedures for research instruments and any manuals and formal training to be provided to interviewers, abstractors, coders, or data entry personnel also should be described or referenced.
   6. The procedures for handling the data in the analysis.
   7. The methods for data analysis.
   8. The major limitations of the study design, data sources, and analytic methods.
   9. The criteria for interpreting the results.

I. A description of plans for protecting human subjects.

J. The quality assurance and quality control procedures for all phases of the study. As appropriate, a certification and/or qualifications of any supporting laboratory or research groups.
K. A description of plans for disseminating and communicating study results.
L. The resources required to conduct the study.
M. The bibliographic references.
N. Addenda, as appropriate; for example informed consent forms, questionnaires, and representative samples of other documents to be used in the study.
O. A data protocol review and approval sign-off sheet for the study director, principal investigator, coinvestigators, and all reviewers.
P. The dated amendments to the protocol.

IV. Review and Approval

A. *Scientific Review*

The study protocol shall receive appropriate scientific review by qualified persons who are not part of the investigative team to ensure that the study is designed to address the objectives of the research and that the protocol is written according to the *Guidelines for Good Epidemiology Practices*. The nature and the circumstances of this review shall be documented.

B. *Ethical Review*

The ethical aspects of each study protocol shall be reviewed by an institutional review board or other comparable review procedure. This review should consider:

1. Obligations to research subjects.
2. Obligations to society.
3. Obligations to funders and employers.
4. Obligations to colleagues.

C. *Administrative Review*

The administrative aspects of the study protocol shall receive appropriate review and written approval by sponsors, contractors, and associated third parties to ensure that sufficient resources are available to complete the study in a timely and proper fashion.

V. Study Conduct

While the study director shall be responsible for the overall research program, the principal investigator shall be responsible for the individual research project, including the day-to-day conduct of the study, interpretation of the study data, and preparation of a final report. These responsibilities extend to all aspects of the study including periodic reporting of study progress as well as quality assurance. In some situations, the study director and the principal investigator may be the same person. To ensure the proper conduct of the study, personnel shall adhere to sound research principles and practices established according to the protocol. A protocol must be approved before the study begins. The study shall be conducted in accordance with the protocol; all deviations from the protocol shall be properly documented and authorized by the principal investigator. If a decision is made not to complete a research project, the reasons for that decision shall be put in writing, dated, and signed by the responsible party, that is, the individual who makes the decision to terminate the study.

A. *Protection of Human Subjects*

Procedures for protecting human subjects shall be followed. Confidential information about study subjects shall be protected using established procedures. If stipulated by the study protocol and/or required by an institutional review board, each study subject shall be informed about the purpose of the study and any risks associated with participating in the study. Written consent, if required, shall be obtained from each study subject before he/she participates in the study. Written consent shall include at a minimum:

1. The purpose of the research or study.
2. The names, addresses, and phone numbers of personnel available to answer questions about the research and the rights of study subjects.
3. The expected duration of a subject's participation
4. The eligibility requirements for study participation.
5. The possible benefits of the study results to the study subject or others.
6. A statement on the voluntary nature of participation in the study and the right of the study subject to discontinue participation at any time.
7. A statement of confidentiality of records identifying the study subject, including reasonable exceptions to absolute confidentiality, for example, sharing of information with the study subject's personal physician or as required by court order.
8. A description of any foreseeable risks or discomforts to the study subject.
9. A statement of the availability of the results.

B. *Data Collection and Verification*

All data collected for the study should be recorded directly, accurately, promptly, and legibly. The individuals responsible for the integrity of the data, computerized and hard copy, shall be identified. All procedures used to verify and promote the quality and integrity of the data shall be outlined in writing. A historical file of these procedures shall be maintained, including all revisions and the dates of such revisions. Any changes in data entries shall be documented.

C. *Analysis*

All data management and statistical analysis programs and packages used in the analyses should be documented. All dated versions used in research shall be kept with accompanying documentation.

D. *Study Report*

Completed studies shall be summarized in a final report that accurately and completely presents the study objectives, methods, results, and the principal investigator's interpretation of the findings. Although the content and length of any technical publication based on the research may be subject to requirements of the particular journal, if a more comprehensive report is written, it should include:

1. A descriptive title.
2. An abstract.
3. The purpose (objectives) of the research as stated in the protocol.
4. The names, titles, degrees, addresses, and affiliations of the study director, principal investigator, and all the coinvestigators.
5. The name and address of the sponsor.
6. The dates on which the study was initiated and completed.
7. An introduction with background, purpose, and specific aims of the study.
8. A description of the research methods, including:
   a. The selection of study subjects and controls.
   b. The data collection methods.
   c. The transformations, calculations, or operations on the data.
   d. The statistical methods used in data analyses.
9. A description of circumstances that may have affected the quality or integrity of the data.
10. A summary of the data analyses, including sufficient tables, graphs, and illustrations to present the pertinent data and to reflect the analyses performed.
11. A statement of the conclusions drawn from the analyses of the data.
12. A discussion of the implications of the study results.
13. A list of references.
14. A statement describing the location where all source data and the final report are stored.
15. A dated study report review sign-off sheet for the study director, principal investigator, coinvestigators, and reviewers and/or auditors.

VI. Communication

Each organization shall predetermine procedures under which communications of the intent, conduct, results, and interpretations of an epidemiologic study will occur, including what function individuals associated with the research will fulfill. These individuals should include the principal investigator, study director, and/or the sponsor. This procedure may be documented in the form of a standard operating procedure, in the study protocol, or through contractual agreement. Government agencies shall be informed of study results in a manner that complies with applicable regulatory requirements. To the extent possible, scientific peers shall be informed of study results by publication in the scientific literature or via presentations at scientific conferences, workshops, or symposia. As feasible, all study subjects shall be informed of the study results and any interpretations of the study findings and conclusions. Information about the study results should be presented in language appropriate to the audience.

VII. Archiving

Physically secure archives must be designated for the orderly storage and expedient retrieval of all study-related material. An index shall be prepared to identify the archived contents and their location, and to identify by name and location any material that by their general nature are not retained in a specific study archive. Access to the archives shall be controlled and limited to authorized personnel only. Special procedures may be necessary to ensure that confidential information about study subjects is protected. Individual study archives should contain, or refer to, the following:

A. The original signed and dated study protocol and all approved modifications.
B. The original signed and dated final report of the study.
C. All source data and, where feasible, biological specimens. A printed sample of the master computer data files with reference to the location of the machine readable master.
D. Documentation adequate to identify and locate all computer programs and statistical procedures used, including version numbers where appropriate.
E. Copies of computer printouts, including relevant execution code, that form the basis of any tables, graphs, discussions, or interpretations in the final report. Any manually developed calculations shall be documented on a work sheet and similarly retained.
F. Correspondence pertaining to the study, standard operating procedures, informed consent releases, copies of all relevant representative material, copies of signed institutional review board and other external reviewer reports, and copies of all quality assurance reports and audits. As appropriate, this would

include questionnaires, the name, make and model numbers of relevant measurement instruments and calibration information and procedures.

G. Original documents for the certain research materials that may be unique to the study such as laboratory notebooks and coder modification records.

VIII. Quality Assurance

Written procedures shall be established to ensure the quality of the data used in a study. These procedures shall address data collection and completeness, coding and computer input, storage and retrieval, and data validation and analysis. Any deviations from the GEPs shall be explained and documented in the final report. An individual who is not part of the investigative team should be assigned as a study quality assurance auditor. This individual shall, no less than annually, review study compliance with the written quality-assurance procedures. The study quality-assurance auditor shall prepare a written summary of the audit. The principal investigator should respond in writing to the audit report, including any remedial actions taken. Quality-assurance activities shall address the preceding sections of these guidelines as well as monitor conformance with established standard operating procedures.

Principles and Methods of Toxicology,
Fourth Edition, edited by A. Wallace Hayes.
Taylor & Francis, Philadelphia © 2001.

Chapter 11

Food-Borne Toxicants

Chada S. Reddy and A. Wallace Hayes

Chemicals capable of causing adverse effects in humans are present in food as naturally occurring components, contaminants, intentional additives, or as components formed in the course of food processing. The simultaneous presence of dietary components capable of enhancing or protecting against the adverse effects of food toxicants has, without a doubt, contributed to the lack of correlation between experimental animal and epidemiological data. An understanding of such agents and direction and magnitude of their effects on specific toxicants in the complex dietary milieu is presently lacking. This together with a lack of good methods for risk extrapolation of mixtures of toxicants/anti-toxicants from animals to humans hampers our effort toward realistic human risk estimations related to food toxicants.

NATURAL TOXICANTS

Natural toxicants are derived from food and feed components of plants and animals. Acute intoxications from chemicals naturally occurring in the human diet are limited to individuals and to selected classes of compounds, for example, favism in individuals deficient in RBC glucose-6-phosphate dehydrogenase (123). Food derived from animal sources can also contain toxic components/contaminants that causes acute intoxications. However, long-term or delayed effects resulting from plant and animal toxins are more widespread and are likely to be more important.

Toxicants in Foods of Plant Origin

Foods of plant origin account for most (>70%) of the world's supply of protein. Although plants with obvious toxic effects have been excluded from human diet by trial and error, deleterious (toxic as well as antinutritive) effects from the following groups of compounds are deemed significant for human health.

Alkaloids

Nitrogenous heterocyclic organic compounds have protective roles against herbivorous consumption and attack by insects, parasites, and competitors. Major alkaloid groups of concern from the standpoint of human consumption include pyrrolizidines, xanthines, and solanines. Others including piperidines from *Conium* and tobacco; quinolizidines from *Lupinus*; and indolizidines from *Astragalus*, *Swainsona*, and red clover are mainly consumed by grazing animals and potentially can be transferred to humans through milk. For a review of toxic effects of alkaloids in humans and animals see Cheeke (38).

Pyrrolizidine alkaloids (PAs) are a group of more than 250 geographically ubiquitous plant metabolites posing a major threat to animal health by their presence in plants including *Senecio, Crotalaria*, and *Heliotropium*, among others. Human exposure and possible health effects result from the wide use of coltsfoot (*Tussilago*), comfrey (*Symphytum*) and petasites (*Petasites*), as herbal remedies, foods (salads, etc.), and tea; contamination of food grains with seeds from PA-containing plants; honey derived from pansy ragwort (*Senecio sp.*) and Patterson's Curse (*Echium sp*); and/or through milk from animals grazing on these alkaloid-containing plants (44).

Among the several structural groups of PAs, the acyclic diesters and macrocyclic diesters such as retronecine, senecionine, and petasitenine are more toxic (77). Highly reactive pyrrole derivatives of PAs and/or their hydrolysis products formed by the action of mixed function oxidases are considered responsible for the toxic effects of PA (130). Huxtable (83) reviewed human intoxications with PA. Typically, liver involvement with venoocclusive disease is characterized by occlusion of small branches of the hepatic vein thus leading to ascites, edema, reduced urinary output, and high mortality which occur mostly in children. Survivors often manifest cirrhosis. Histologically, endothelial proliferation and medial hypertrophy lead to occlusion of small hepatic veins which then advances to centrilobular congestion resulting in sinusoidal widening and blood pooling. Necrosis and fibrosis ultimately result. Certain dehydro PAs, monocrotaline in particular, are known to induce similar occlusive changes in pulmonary arterioles, developing into pulmonary hypertension and right ventricular hypertrophy and, ultimately, to cor pulmonale (right heart congestive failure). Impairment of serotonin and norepinephrine clearance by endothelial cells appears to contribute to pulmonary hypertension (83).

Many PAs and their pyrrole metabolites are bifunctional alkylating agents crosslinking to macromolecules, including DNA (77,83), thus accounting for their mutagenicity and carcinogenicity in experimental animals (77). At least six species of plants (*Senecio longilobus, Petasites japonicus, Tussilago farfara, Symphytum officinale, Farfugium japonicum*, and *Senecio cannabifolis*) and eight PAs have been shown to induce one or more of the following types of cancer: hepatic carcinoma, hepangioendothelial sarcoma in the liver, liver cell adenoma, cholangiosarcoma, astrocytoma, squamous cell carcinoma of the skin, pulmonary adenoma, adenocarcinoma of the small intestines, adenomyoma of the ileum, and rhabdomyosarcoma (77). One of the PAs, heliotrine, was shown to be teratogenic in rats. Oberved malformations included lower jaw hypoplasia, musculoskeletal defects involving ribs, and general growth retardation (77).

Solanum alkaloids, predominantly, solamine, chaconine, and tomatine are found in potato, eggplant, and tomato (species of *Solanum genus*) among others. Reviews on the biosynthesis, occurrence, and toxicology of solanum alkaloids include those by Sharma and Salunkhe (183) and Keeler et al. (94).

Potatoes, especially the sprouted, greened, blighted, injured, or spoiled, have raised the most concern relating to alkaloid intoxication with over 200 cases of human poisonings documented (141). Signs of human intoxication, some of which may be related to the irritant and cholinesterase-inhibiting activity of the alkaloids, appear at >20 mg alkaloid/100 g of tuber and include headache, vomiting, diarrhea, neurological signs, debilitation, and death. Association of consumption of blighted potatoes to the incidence of anencephaly-spina bifida (ASB) in humans has been questioned by subsequent studies which failed to produce defects in animals consistent with ASB in humans (177). Although normal levels of glycoalkaloids in potato conform to the U.S. Department of Agriculture (USDA) guideline of 20 mg/100 g of tuber, exposure to light, immature tubers, wounding of potatoes, and stresses such as fungal attack can increase its content severalfold (25). Baking, boiling, or microwaving do not destroy solanine or chaconine in potatoes. Some simple methods to prevent glycoalkaloid formation during storage appear to be protection of tubers from sunlight, γ-irradiation, soaking in water under controlled conditions, dipping damaged potatoes in emulsified water, treating potatoes with sprout inhibitors during storage, waxing, and heating, dipping in oils (corn, olive, or mineral), spraying tubers with lecithin (such as PAM), or simply spray rinsing tubers with an aqueous solution of an edible surfactant (Tween 85) (183).

Xanthine alkaloids. Three major related alkaloids, caffeine, theobromine, and theophylline, are found as major components of coffee (*Coffea arabica*), cocoa (*Theobroma cocas*), and tea (*Thea sinenis*), respectively. Caffeine, in addition, is added to many beverages, foods, and medications (56). Caffeine-related adverse effects begin when 0.5–1.0 g of caffeine (10 cups of coffee) is ingested by an adult, leading to fatalities at 5 g in children and 5 to 10 g in adults (45,56). Caffeine and other methylxanthines inhibit phosphodiesterase, leading to intracellular accumulation of cyclic AMP, blockage of adenosine receptors, and increased release of Ca^{2+} from the terminal cisternae of the sarcoplasmic reticulum (45). Major effects of xanthines involve the central nervous system (CNS) stimulation (hyperesthesia to convulsions), emesis, cardiovascular effects (cardiac stimulation to arrhythmias), diuresis, and smooth muscle effects leading to decreased vascular resistance and bronchodilation (45). In addition, caffeine enhances gastric secretion of acid and pepsin. Caffeine and theobromine are mutagenic in bacterial systems and can potentiate DNA damage caused by other genotoxins but are neither directly carcinogenic in animals nor are they associated with human cancer (10,45). Caffeine is teratogenic in experimental animals, causing mostly limb and facial defects (177). Although high caffeine consumption during pregnancy may increase the risk of low birth-weight babies, no correlation exists between caffeine consumption and birth defects in humans (190). In 1980, the U.S. Food and Drug Administration (FDA) however, issued a warning to pregnant women to limit coffee consumption (45).

Allergens

Food allergies are a group of disorders characterized by an exaggerated immunological response to a component of food. All foods are capable of eliciting an allergic reaction. Most allergens in foods are heat-stable proteins, glycoproteins, or peptides with a MW between 5000 and 70,000. Prevalence of food allergies appears to be age-dependent, with up to 8 percent of children under 3 years and 1.5 percent of adults (155,174) affected. Milk (casein, β-lactoglobulin) and eggs (ovomucoid, ovalbumin) are the most commonly incriminated agents (13), followed by peanuts (Aha I & II, aglutinin), wheat (globulins, glutenine), soy proteins (in formulae), fish, crustaceans, tomatoes, strawberries, chocolate, and certain beverages (15,26,213). Although multiple tissues of the body are often affected, the skin (eczema and urticaria) and the respiratory tract (rhinitis, pneumonitis, asthma, etc.) account for 90 percent of food allergies (156). Abdominal distress, vomiting and diarrhea, hypotens in and shock secondary to hypovolemia, and nervous system involvement as indicated by headaches, convulsions, and behavioral problems (156) are also suggestive of allergic reaction to food. Rapid-onset allergies are dependent on reaction of the antigens with circulating antibodies of the IgE class (reagin) and the eventual release of vasoactive substances such as serotonin and histamine, sometimes leading to life-threatening anaphylaxis. Non-IgE-type food allergies are dependent on specifically sensitized lymphocytes that are attracted to the site of antigen exposure by lymphokines released by already existing T-lymphocytes and require several hours or days to fully manifest. Recent evidence suggests a role for food allergies in autoimmune disorders (celiac disease), juvenile or insulin-dependent diabetes mellitus, migraine, and arthritis in children (26,97). Idiosyncratic reactions such as lactose intolerance, a result of genetic deficiency of lactase leading to luminal accumulation of lactic acid and osmotic diarrhea, must be differentiated from immunologically mediated allergic reactions.

Cyanogens

Cyanogenic glycosides which release highly toxic hydrocyanic acid on hydrolysis are derived not only from plants (more than 2000 species) but, also, from fungi, bacteria, and even members of the animal kingdom (140). Although cassava, sweet potatoes, yam, maize, millets, bamboo, sugarcane, peas, beans, almond kernel, lemon, lime, apple, pear, cherry, apricot, prune, and plum constitute sources for humans, poisonings are mainly associated with the consumption of improperly processed cassava in Africa, Asia, and Latin America (140,158). Among more than 20 glycosides identified, only four (i.e., amygdalin, dhurrin, linamarin, and lotaustralin) appear to be of toxicological importance. Cyanogenic lipids, although of unknown toxicological significance, are also present in plants and yield carbonyl compounds and HCN upon hydrolysis (50).

The hydrolysis of the glycoside is triggered by physical disruption (mastication, trampling, etc.) or stress (drought, cooking, frost, etc.) and is catalyzed by β-glucosidase and hydroxynitrile lyase, which are present within the plant or in bacteria found in the gastrointestinal tract of humans and animals (158). The scheme of breakdown leading to the formation of glucose and hydrosynitrile from the glycoside, followed by breakdown of hydroxynitrile into carbonyl compounds and HCN, is presented in Figure 11.1. Rhodanese catalyzes the conversion of HCN to thiocyanate in the presence of thiosulfate (158).

Animals have often been acutely poisoned by young sorghum and arrow grass. Young bamboo shoots and tea made from peach leaves are examples of dietary sources of HCN poisoning in children. The minimal lethal dose of HCN in humans and animals is 0.5–3.5 mg/kg and 2–10 mg/kg, respectively. The acute effects of HCN result from its affinity toward metalloporphyrin-containing enzymes, more specifically, cytochrome oxidase. Cyanide concentration of only 33 μM can completely block electron transfer through the mitochondrial electron transport chain and thus prevent O_2 utilization (158). Death results from generalized cytotoxic anoxia. Signs of acute cyanide poisoning in humans are hyperventilation, headache, nausea and vomiting, generalized weakness, coma, and death due to respiratory depression and failure. Treatment of acute cyanide intoxication involves, in addition to artificial respiration, the conversion of hemoglobin in the blood to methemoglobin with nitrites (sodium or amyl). Methemoglobin competes with cytochrome oxidase for HCN and forms cyanmethemoglobin. Co-administration of sodium thiosulfate will convert free cyanide present in the blood to thiocyanate, which is eliminated. As free cyanide in the blood decreases, additional cyanide dissociates from the cyanmethemoglobin and is subsequently eliminated (36).

Tropical ataxic neuropathy (TAN), characterized by myelopathy, bilateral optical atrophy, deafness, and polyneuropathy; konzo, an irreversible upper moto-

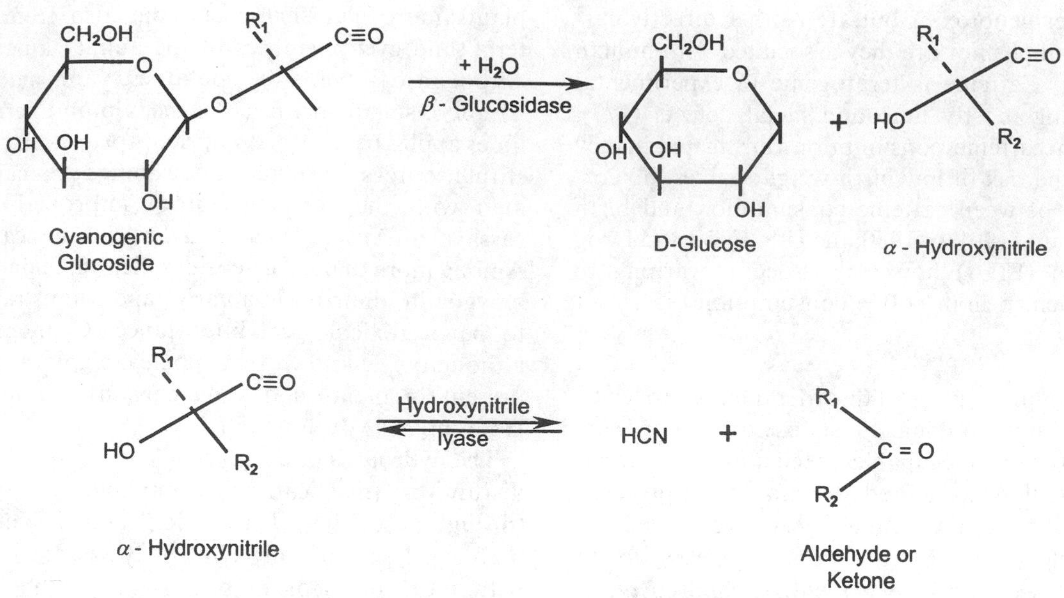

FIG. 11.1. Enzymatic hydrolysis of cyanogenic glycosides. Initially, the glycoside is hydrolyzed by a β-glucosidase releasing glucose and α-hydroxynitrile. The hydroxynitrile dissociates either enzymatically or nonenzymatically to yield HCN and the corresponding aldehyde or ketone.

neuron paralytic disease (20) of women and children; goiter; epigastric burning pain; dizziness; abdominal distension and vomiting (2)—all have been linked to longer-term consumption of cassava diets in Africa and other tropical countries (150). These diets were also poor in protein and sulfur-containing amino acids which can detoxify HCN to thiocyanoalanine and subsequently to the inert 2-amino-4-thiazolidine carboxylic acid (158). Although it is generally assumed that chronic effects of cyanogen exposure are due to thiocyanates, recent evidence suggests that the glycoside, linamarin, itself may be responsible for konzo in cassava-consuming populations (20).

Enzyme Inhibitors

Although plant and animal foods contain inhibitors of proteases, amylases, and lipases, only the inhibitors of proteases pose some hazard to human health, if any.

Kunitz inhibitor, the major protease inhibitor of soybeans, is a heat labile protease capable of inhibiting trypsin and, to a lesser degree, other proteases (93). The cationic form, which accounts for a majority of human trypsin activity, is only weakly inhibited, whereas the anionic form is fully inhibited (114). In addition, there appear to be a heat stable, lower molecular weight Bowman–Birk inhibitor, an insect protease inhibitor, and a papain inhibitor associated with raw soybeans. Egg white, milk, a number of varieties of beans, peas, cereal grains, alfalfa, and potatoes also have been shown to contain one or more protease inhibitors (86).

The major effects of protease inhibitors in animal diets include pancreatic hypertrophy, adenomas, and nodular hyperplasia associated with growth depression (115). Pancreatic hypertrophy is postulated to result from constant pancreatic hypersecretion necessitated by release of a humoral agent (possibly cholecystokinin pancreozymin) in the upper small intestine in response to the lack of free trypsin and chymotrypsin following their binding with the inhibitor (66). Although any single food source such as soybean is likely to be consumed by humans in quantities of toxicological significance, consumption of multiple sources of protease inhibitors may increase the risk of pancreatic hypertrophy and cancer. Ironically, soybean trypsin inhibitors are gaining attention for their inhibition of initiation and promotion, as well as dissemination of transformed cells during the carcinogenic process (46).

Estrogens

There are more than 220 species of plants containing estrogenic isoflavonoids (e.g., genistein, glycetein, daidzein) and/or their glycosides (genistin, glyectin, daidzin). Coumestans (e.g., coumestrol, 4-O-methylcoumestrol) and lignans represent other important groups of plant estrogens (3,191). Phytoestrogens, although capable of causing infertility in animals heavily grazing on estrogen(coumestan)-containing forages (subterranean clover, alfalfa), have not been proven to cause human problems. Genistein (soybeans) appears to be the plant estrogen of most (if any) significance in human health (6). Zearalenone and zearalenol, two major resorcylic acid lactone estrogens, are produced in corn in response to infection by toxigenic strains of the fungus *Fusarium roseum* and are discussed later. Human infants can be exposed to 4 mg/kg body weight or more of isoflavones from soy-based formula (6). Phytoestrogens bind to the same intracellular receptors as those that bind estradiol but at 20–200 times lower affinity, resulting in 500–10,000 times lower potency in vivo, compared to estradiol. Recently, Safe (173) estimated that human adults are exposed to 102 μg estrogenic equivalents (reflecting both potency and exposure) daily compared to 3.35 mg/day for estrogen replacement and 16.7 mg/day for oral contraceptives. Due to inefficient binding, phytoestrogens can actually impede the action of endogenous mammalian steroidal estrogen and at higher doses also induce antigonadotropic effects at the hypothalarnic, pituitary, and gonadal levels in both sexes (6). In addition to the above effects, genistein inhibits protein tyrosine kinases associated with a number of growth factors and other enzymes with roles in cell proliferation and differentiation (6).

The only reported animal effects of phytoestrogens include infertility in sheep fed subterranean clover and cattle consuming alfalfa (6), and feminization of males following exposure during development (40). In humans, however, although reversible changes in menstrual cycle and FSH and LH surges in premenopausal women appear to result from soy consumption, no developmental or infertility problems were noted in populations consuming large quantities of phytoestrogen (6). Phytoestrogens, on the contrary, may protect humans against coronary heart disease, cancer of the breast, prostate, and colon, and postmenopausal osteoporosis (4), possibly due to their antiestrogenic effects. Phytoestrogens are not mutagenic in the Ames assay (22) and appear to be noncarcinogenic when given orally (206). Whether exposure to relatively high levels of isoflavones in soy-based formulae in human infants leads to longer-term effects needs to be investigated.

Glucosinolates

Glucosinolates (GS) are a group of more than 100 flavor-imparting thioglucoside compounds found at up to 60 mg/g in crucifers such as broccoli, cabbage, brussels sprouts, cauliflower, calabrese, turnip, radish, horseradish, mustard, rapeseed, and related plants. Common names of some important GS include sinigrin, progoitrin, epi-progoitrin, glucobrassicin, and neoglucobrassicin. Not only the parent GS but, also, their products of plant and human digestive tract bacterial myrosinase (thioglucosidase) hydrolyze—isothiocyanates, nitriles, oxazolidinethione (OZT), and thiocyanate ions—contribute to their biological activity (208).

Although evidence is lacking in humans, in animals the thiocyanate ion inhibits the uptake of iodine by the thyroid, leading to iodine-reversible hyperplasia and hypertrophy of the thyroid (cabbage and legume goiter) and growth suppression. OZT also inhibits thyroxine synthesis and induces goiter (brassica seed goiter) in rats by inhibiting the incorporation of iodine into precursors of thyroxine (129). This condition is not reversible by iodine supplementation. In addition to goiter, epiprogoitrin and progoitrin also induce liver and kidney enlargement and death at 2.6 percent in the diet via their nitrile metabolites (203). Bile duct hyperplasia, hepatocyte necrosis, and megalocytosis of renal tubular epithelium were also seen in these animals (200).

Isothiocyanates are embryocidal and cause fetal weight reduction (25). Isothiocyanates and certain GS (e.g., sinigrin) are mutagenic in the Ames assay, whereas thiocyanates are not (25). Higher intake of cruciferous vegetables in humans and animals, however, may exert an anticarcinogenic effect attributable to the formation of isothiocyanates (at least seven), indoles, indole-3-carbinol, 3-indoleacetonitrile, and 3,3′-diindolylmethane (208). Anticarcinogenic effects of glucosinolates may result from their induction of phase II enzymes (quinone reductase) in the gastrointestinal (GI) tract and liver (197) and stimulation of apoptosis (188).

Lectins (Phytohemagglutinins)

Lectins are high MW (100,000 to 150,000), heat labile proteins, lipoproteins, or glycoproteins (up to >10% of total seed protein) detected in over 800 edible plant species, including 600 that belong to the leguminosae (beans, peas, etc.). In addition, lectins are also present in animals including sponges, crustaceans, mollusks, fish (blood), amphibian (eggs), and even mammals (tissue) (50). Their interactions with membrane glycoproteins (e.g., red blood cells causing hemolysis) made them suitable in the study of blood typing, tumor cell recognition, cell adhesion, signal transduction, mitogenesis, immune function, and cell death (139).

Binding of lectins from edible sources to cells in the crypts and villi of the intestines followed by nonspecific inhibition of active and passive absorption of many nutrients (amino acids, fats, vitamins, minerals, thyroxin, etc.) across the intestinal mucosa and necrosis of intestinal epithelial cells (96) appears to account for growth reduction and possibly goiter after long-term oral exposure to high levels (86). Mortality following acute systemic lectin exposure is associated with damage to the liver (84) and other organs. The most toxic lectin, ricin from castor bean, can cause severe intestinal epithelial cell necrosis and death from multi-organ damage (204). Recent evidence has suggested that lipid peroxidation mediated by reactive oxygen species may be involved in ricin-induced thyroid damage (175). Epithelial-bound ricin is taken up by cells via clathrin-dependent as well as clathrin-independent endocytosis and then subjected to lysosomal degradation. A portion of ricin enters golgi and ER, inhibits protein synthesis, and causes cell death (176,204). Less toxic lectins may act by the same mechanism to stimulate protein synthesis, mitogen activation, and immune stimulation.

Lipids

Adverse effects can result from naturally occurring plant lipids when factors such as the departure from established food use patterns, the use of new lipids in human diets, or inborn errors of metabolism are introduced. Erucic acid (cis-13-docosanoic acid) is a predominant component of rape (*Brassica napus* and *B. campestris*) and mustard (*B. hirta* and *B. juncea*) seeds. Canada, Argentina, Mexico, China, India, Pakistan, Japan, and several European countries are the major producers and users of these oils. Growth suppression, myocardial fatty infiltration, mononuclear cell infiltration, and fibrosis were observed in weanling rats fed erucic acid at levels supplying greater than 20 percent of the dietary calories. In addition, ducklings showed hydropericardium and cirrhosis, and guinea pigs developed splenomegaly and hemolytic anemia (131). Organ-specific inhibition of glutamate oxidation and adenosine triphosphate (ATP) synthesis in cardiac mitochondria (79) could be mechanistically involved in the pathogenesis of these lesions. In humans, however, although the long-term use of Lorenzo's oil (oleic acid and erucic acid) in the treatment of adrenoleukodystrophy or adrenomyeloneuropathy leads to thrombocytopenia and lymphopenia (202), adverse effects from dietary consumption of erucic acid have not been reported.

Refsum is disease is a genetic peroxisomal fatty acid oxidase and catalase deficiency resulting in an inability of the affected individuals to convert phytanic acid (3,7,11,15-tetramethylhexadecanoic acid, a product of chlorophyll metabolism in the rumen) from dairy products and ruminant fats to α-hydroxyphytanic acid in preparation for further oxidation. This results in accumulation of lipids containing phytanic acid in many tissues and a disorder characterized by poor physical and mental growth, blindness, deafness, and other neurological signs (38). Elimination of dairy and ruminant fats from the diet of these individuals results in partial remission.

Cyclopropene fatty acids such as sterculic acid (C19) and malvalic acid (C18) are natural components of oils from plants of the order *Malvales*, most important of which are cotton and kapok seeds. Cyclopropene fatty acids have been incriminated in the pink discoloration of egg whites and reduced egg production in cottonseed-fed laying hens, growth suppression and impaired female reproduction in rats, and increased saturated fatty acids (possibly causing atherosclerosis) in the tissues of pigs and other animals (131). Cyclopropene fatty acids are carcinogens and markedly increase the carcinogenicity of aflatoxin in trout (10).

Increased consumption of dietary polyunsaturated fatty acids to lower blood cholesterol, although beneficial in decreasing the incidence of coronary disease, has raised concern about adverse effects such as induction of Vitamin E deficiency (131). Carrol (32) reported a strong correlation between dietary fat and age-adjusted mortality rates for breast and intestinal cancer. Pancreatic cancer was found to be enhanced by a diet containing 20 percent corn oil but not by one containing 18 percent hydrogenated coconut oil and 2 percent corn oil (167). Unsaturated fatty acids are easily oxidized during cooking to a variety of mutagens, enols and other aldehydes, and alkoxy and hydroperoxy radicals (10). Lipid oxidation products alter signal transduction pathways (196) and thus enhance cell proliferation and promote carcinogenesis. Lipid-induced inhibition of immune responses and enhanced formation of some of the known tumor promotors such as prostaglandins and bile acids also have been reported (32). Interestingly, Hayasu et al. (74) showed that oleic and linoleic acids may, in fact, be antimutagenic. The overall effect of dietary fats may depend on the ratio of beneficial fatty acids to causative fatty acids for each effect.

Oxalates and Phytates

Certain plants including spinach, rhubarb, beet leaves, tea, and cocoa contain high (0.2–2.0% on a fresh weight basis) levels of oxalic acid. Although dietary oxalates present little problem in humans, cattle and sheep have been poisoned following ingestion of the toxic plants *Halogeton* and *Sarcobatus* (grease wood). Toxic signs result from binding of the oxalic acid to serum calcium leading to hypocalcemia, coagulation defects, and tetany. Degeneration and necrosis of kidneys and vasculature from Ca^{++} oxalate deposition may result in severe cases. Oxalates also interfere with absorption of calcium, iron, magnesium, and copper and inhibit succinate dehydrogenase and carbohydrate metabolism (151). Approximately 2.5 kg of tomato or 0.5 kg of spinach leaves need to be consumed to approach a lethal dose (5 g or more) of oxalates.

Phytic acid, the hexaphosphoric ester of myo-inositol, is present at high levels (up to 1.5 g%) in the bran and germ of wheat followed by other cereals, nuts, seeds, spices, and legumes (87). Phytates bind di- and tri-valent metals in the order: $Cu^{++} > Zn^{++} > Co^{++} > Mn^{++} > Fe^{+++} > Ca^{++}$, causing mineral deficiencies (especially of Ca^{++} and Fe^{+++}) in developing countries that are heavily reliant on cereals as the exclusive source of protein. Inclusion of phytase, an enzyme that releases phosphate from plant phytic acid, in animal feeds ensures phosphate utilization and reduces environmental phosphate pollution from animal production. Supplementation with minerals and Vitamin D can antagonize most effects of oxalates and phytates (87).

Plant Phenolics

Plant phenolics comprise a group of several thousand substituted phenolic compounds occurring in trace amounts as esters or glycoconjugates. Acute human and animal poisonings are mostly caused by phenolics uncommon in human food and include coumarius, aflatoxins, and gossypol. Phenolics common in human foods belong to three general classes, that is, non-flavonoids (gallic, syringic, caffeic, and other acids); flavonoids (flavones such as tangeritin, flavonols such as kaempferol and quercetin, isoflavones such as coumestrol, aurones, chalcones, and anthocyanin pigments); and polyphenols (tannins and lignin). Polyphenols are widely distributed and present in relatively large amounts in cereals, millets, legumes, and fruits. Deleterious effects of long-term exposure of both hydrolyzable (polyphenolic acid) and condensed (polyflavonoid) tannins include reductions in the digestibility of foods and feeds, protein utilization, and body weight gain, damage to and sloughing of the mucosal lining of the gastrointestinal tract, and cancer of the mouth and esophagus (77,164). In contrast to mild acute effects in humans, livestock losses can exceed $10 million annually, attributable to the toxic effects of hydrolyzable oak tannins consumed when other forages are unavailable (186).

Epidemiological correlation exists between high consumption of condensed tannins (sorghum and dark beer prepared from sorghum, tea, red wines, and areca nuts) and high rates of oral and esophageal cancer (50). Parenteral exposure to tannins reportedly has led to high incidence of liver and other tumors in rodents (77). On the other hand, a negative association between tea drinking and stomach cancer (192) and coffee consumption and kidney cancer (85) also exists.

Polyphenols, however, are not directly damaging to DNA (35) and experimental evidence of anticarcinogenic effects of penta-O-gallyl-beta-D-glucose and epigallocatechin gallate, two green tea tannins (64), exists. Flavonoids and non-flavonoids exert no less than 40 different physiological and pharmacological actions accounting for their therapeutic and health food use. These include anticoagulant, antihistaminic, antihypercholesterolemic, anti-inflammatory, antioxidant, antiproliferative, antipruritic, antipyretic, antirheumatic, antiseptic, antithrombogenic, antitumor, apoptotic, estrogenic, and vasoactive effects. Many if not all of these actions are based on their UV-absorbing, chelating, oxidative phosphorylation uncoupling and antioxidant properties. In addition, their sparing effect on vitamins C and E; induction of P450-mediated enzymes; and alteration of enzymes (phospholipases, ATPases, cycloxygenases, lipoxygenases, protein kinases), oncogenes, and other signaling components critical for cell survival and proliferation (35,61) contribute to an array of opposing effects in many systems.

Although human consumption of flavonoids alone can be greater than 1 g/day (87), the toxicological implications of exposure to flavonoids and other simple phenolics arise from lifetime exposure to them. Recently, high intake of flavonoid supplements was suggested to have caused acute renal failure due to hemolysis (116). More than 30 flavonoids, including the most abundant quercetin, kaempferol, myricetin, hesperetin, naringenin, wogonin, and norwogonin, as well as their glycosides have been shown to be mutagenic in bacterial and/or mammalian systems (77,122). Quercetin induced hyperplasia and benign renal tubular epithelial tumors and appeared to enhance pancreatic pre-tumorous lesions induced by nitrosomethylurea in rats fed a 5% dietary level for 2 years (21,54). The proponderance of evidence (77), however, points to the antagonistic effects of flavonoids against mutagenic and carcinogenic effects of a number of genotoxicants and promotors in many organs (18,35,77,117). These conflicting results are likely due to differences in test systems and the dose levels used because phenolics exert antioxidant effects at low doses and prooxidant effects at higher doses (219).

On balance, however, both polyphenols and simple phenolics may play a protective role against the carcinogenic and oxidative influences (e.g., those causing coronary heart disease) in humans. Anticarcinogenic effects of phenolics are likely due to the inhibition of metabolic enzymes leading to reduced levels of reactive intermediates, induction of detoxifying enzymes such as glutathione-*S*-transferase, reduced formation of oxidation products, and/or inhibition of enzymes such as protein kinases and oncogenes that stimulate cell proliferation, among other mechanisms (117,215). Cardiovascular protection appears to result from reduced low-density lipoprotein oxidation (antiatherogenic effect), reduced platelet aggregation (antithrombotic), vasodilation, relaxation of cardiovascular smooth muscle, and antihypercholesterolemic effects of flavonoids (61,80).

Gossypol (1,1,6,6,7,7-hexahydroxy-5,5-diisopropyl-3, 3-dimethyl [2,2-binaphthalene]-8,8-dicarboxaldehyde), a yellow phenolic pigment in cottonseed, can bind to proteins and minerals and reduce the biological availability of iron and lysine (86). Similar to other phenolics, free gossypol (>60 ppm) inhibits oxidative phosphorylation and causes myriad other effects leading to acute toxicity in animals on a high cottonseed diet. In general, higher acute doses cause cardiac failure associated with liver and lung (pulmonary edema) damage whereas chronic exposure leads to general malnutrition and reproductive effects (35). Signs of gossypol toxicity include loss of appetite and body weight; rough hair coat; edematous fluid in body cavities, lungs, and pericardium giving rise to gasping; hemorrhagic degenerative changes in liver, and necrosis of cardiac myocytes (223). Changes in plasma K^+ (increase in calves and decrease in humans) may be responsible for gossypol toxicity. Olive discoloration of yolk and decreased egg hatchability occur in poultry (35). Male antifertility effects of gossypol in mammals are only partially reversible and include reduced sperm production as well as motility during the late stages of spermatogenesis, likely caused by mitochondial damage (160) or inhibition of protein kinases (199). Gossypol is not mutagenic in the Ames test (35) but appears to induce genetic damage (dominant lethal mutations) in rats and may be both an initiator and promotor of carcinogenesis (10).

Gossypol and polyphenol (tannin) toxicity can be prevented by the addition of iron, supplemental protein, vitamin K, and alkalinizing agents such as sodium hydroxide. In addition, non-ionic detergents such as Tween 80, methyl donors such as choline and methionine, and dehulling and peeling of grains and fruits have also been shown to counteract the toxic effects of tannins (49,186). A glandless (gossypol-free) variety of cottonseed, although it is expected to eliminate gossypol toxicity in animals, appears to be more susceptible to insect attack and has yet to gain popularity.

Proteins and Peptides

In the average American diet protein supplies 15 percent of total calories. Long-term consumption of higher amounts of protein, especially animal-derived, may contribute to diabetes, renal glomerular sclerosis, Crohn's disease, and osteoporosis (by increased Ca^{++} loss from bones in response to acidosis) (23,185,217).

Protein toxicants such as allergens, hemagglutinins (lectins) and enzyme inhibitors have been discussed. Certain microbial protein toxins are discussed in subsequent sections. Toxic peptides from mushrooms are discussed below.

Mushroom peptides. Among several thousand species of mushrooms only about 100 may be toxic and 12 are known to contain lethal toxins (57,108,214).

Emesis and profuse diarrhea followed by rapidly developing hepatic and renal insufficiency (similar to acute hepatitis) and death are characteristic of poisoning by mushrooms related to *Amanita verna* (destroying angel) in the United States and *A. phalloides* (green death cap) in Europe (209). Approximately one-half of a mature cap of *A. phalloides* can be lethal in an adult (132). Among the three classes of thermostable peptide toxins (amatoxins, phallotoxins, and virotoxins) in the deadly Amanitas, the cyclic octapeptides, amatoxins (Figure 11.2), appear to be responsible for the observed clinical effects which begin to appear after a 12-hour latency period. Evidence of hepatotoxicity includes an increase in serum transaminases, decrease in blood glucose and clotting factors, and, occasionally, jaundice. Hepatogenous encephalopathy and renal failure may be present terminally.

Fatalities are common even following intensive symptomatic care, which includes fluid replacement, activated charcoal hemoperfusion, and forced diuresis, etc. In countries other than France and the United States, use of silibinin (from *Silybum marianum*), which prevents hepatocyte uptake of amatoxins, has produced beneficial effects in direct relationship with the speed of onset of therapy (132,209). A return toward normal glucose, factor V, and fibrinogen is prognostic of recovery (132). Amatoxins inhibit RNA polymerase II by binding to the enzyme directly, and subsequently inhibit mRNA synthesis by blocking the formation of phosphodiester bonds at the elongation step, due to stabilization of the ternary complex of template, enzyme, and the nascent ribonucleotide chain (209).

The other two groups of polypeptide toxins, the phallotoxins and virotoxins, are capable of causing toxic effects only at relatively higher doses. The effects of phallotoxins include swelling of the liver due to engorgement of hepatic sinusoids with blood, and depletion of blood in the peripheral circulation, leading to shock. Reduction of cellular G-actin concentration by a combined effect of stimulated G-actin polymerization into F-actin, and inhibition of F-actin depolymerization leading to a loss of membrane elasticity and thus cell surface vesiculation may explain subsequent hepatocyte damage (209).

The toxic effects of several mushroom species that are rarely lethal are summarized in Table 11.1. Treatment in most cases is supportive. Other identified human conditions associated with mushroom production, commerce, and consumption are: hypersensitivity to edible mushrooms in certain populations; hypersensitive allergic alveolitis and other pulmonary allergic changes in mushroom workers from spores of certain edible mushrooms (mushroom worker's lung); hemolytic reactions following consumption of mushrooms belonging to the genera *Gyromitra, Boletus*, and *Paxillus*; and dermatitis (allergic) from contact with one or more species of the genera *Boletus, Lactarius, Calvaria*, and *Agaricus*.

Saponins

The saponins are bitter-tasting, steroidal (C27) or mono-, di-, tri-, and sesqui-terpenoid (C30) glycosides from plants, fish, and sponges, and are capable of reducing surface tension, hemolyzing red blood cells, and causing toxic effects in cold-blooded animals. Their occurrence, biological effects, and relevance to food,

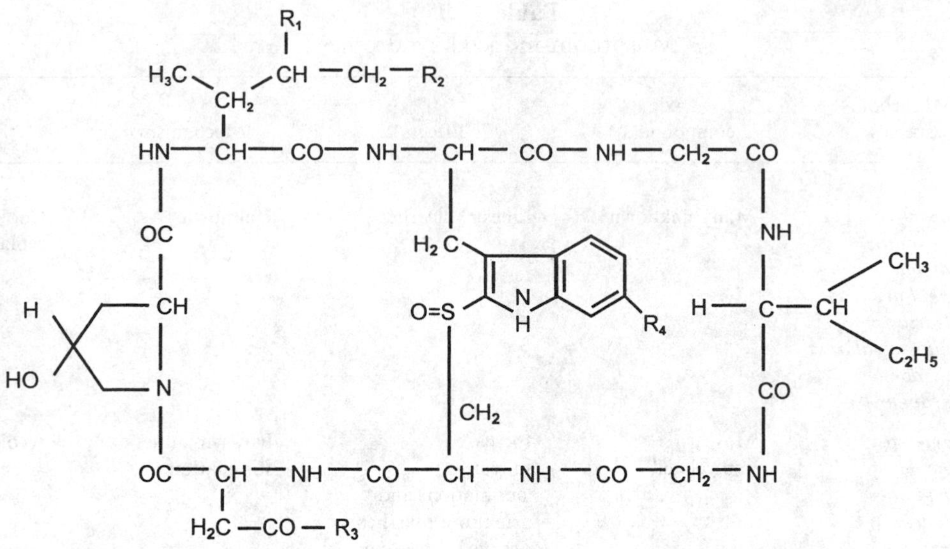

	R_1	R_2	R_3	R_4
α-Amanitin	• OH	• OH	• NH_2	• OH
β-Amanitin	• OH	• OH	• OH	• OH
γ-Amanitin	• CH	• H	• NH_2	• OH
ε-Amanitin	• OH	• H	• OH	• OH
Amanin	• OH	• OH	• OH	• H
Amanullin	• H	• H	• NH_2	• OH
Amaninamide	• OH	• OH	• NH_2	• H

FIG. 11.2. The structures of amatoxins.

agriculture, and medicine are reviewed by Walker and Yamazaki (211,212).

So far, d-limonene from citrus oils, ginseng saponins, and medicagenic acid and hederosides in alfalfa and *Hedera helix*, respectively, and oleanolic and ursolic acid in a variety of food, medicinal, and other plants, as well as their aglycones (sapogenins), have been studied to some extent. Their analgesic, anti-atherosclerotic, anticarcinogenic, anticholinergic, antihypercholesteremic, antihyperglycemic, anti-inflammatory, antitubercular, cardioprotective, diuretic, and hepatoprotective effects are likely to encourage increased dietary, supplemental, and medicinal utilization of saponin-containing plants such as ginseng (119,124,161,218). Mechanisms of protection involve Ca^{++}-antagonistic and vasodilatory/venoconstrictive; immune-modulatory, bile acid-binding, anti-proliferative, and membrane permeabilizing; and antioxidant and anti-cytochrome P450 effects (119,161). Feeding high levels of saponin from a variety of sources, however, resulted in lower growth rate; increased serum LDH and GOT associated with hepatocellular necrosis; and increased BUN, hematuria, and proteinuria associated with renal tubular necrosis (99,143) in animals. Several steroidal and nonsteroidal saponins from pasture weeds such as *Hypericum perforatum* and *Narthecium ossifragum*, vines such as *Tribulus terrestris*, and tropical grasses such as *Brachiaria* and *Panicum* sp. cause primary or hepatogenic photosensitization in animals (34). Alpha-hederin, a saponin that induces metallothionein in maternal tissues, appears to induce visceral and skeletal defects in offspring born to exposed rat dams by possibly reducing zinc availability to the fetus (52). Similar to phenolics, the beneficial effects of saponins can be derived from daily doses present in a balanced diet.

Toxic Amino Acids

In general, foodstuffs do not contain individual amino acids of nutritional importance in amounts that cause adverse reactions. Therapeutic use of greater than ten times the required dose of amino acids, on the other hand, when given on an empty stomach, can lead to adverse effects, including gastric distress (essential amino acids), nausea, febrile reaction and/or headaches (methionine, isoleucine, and threonine), and disorientation (methionine and tryptophan) in psychiatric patients treated with monoamine oxidase inhibitors (73).

Monosodium glutamate (MSG) had long been used as a flavor enhancer in commercially processed foods. MSG, as well as other acidic amino acids, but not basic or neutral amino acids, produced lesions in rats and mice

Table 11.1
Mushroom-induced syndromes

	Mushroom species	Toxic compound(s)	Effects	Mechanism	Prevention/ Treatment
Rapid onset: Syndrome	*Chlorophyllum molybditis* *Entoloma lividum* *Omphalotus olearius* *Paxillus involutus* *Trichodoma pardinum*	Many unknown	Emesis, diarrhea	Unknown	Cooking/Fluid replacement
Parasympathetic	*Inocyte* sp. *Clitocybe* sp. *Omphalotus illudens* *Amanita* sp.	Muscarine and related	Increased salivation, lacrimation, and urination; diarrhea; dyspnea; sweating; bradycardia; tremors, etc.	Parasympathetic stimulation	Avoid/Atropine
CNS Syndrome	*Psilocybe* sp. *Panaeolus* sp. *Copelandia* sp. *Gymnopilus* sp.	Psilocybin Psilocin	Hallucinations involving all sensations; hyperthermia, convulsions, coma, and death.	Serotonin agonist	Avoid/Diazepam and cooling
	Amanita pantheria *A. muscaria*	Ibotenic acid, muscinol, stizolobic and stizolobinic acid	Alternating depression and neuromuscular stimulation	Stimulation of bicuculin-reactive post-synaptic receptors	Avoid/Diazepam and respiration
Alcohol sensitization	*Coprinus* sp. *Clitocybe claviceps* *Boletus luridus* *Verpa bohemica*	Coprine and others	Nausea, vomiting, headache, hypotension, tingling, palpitations, tachycardia; testicular damage, etc.	Inhibit acetaldehyde dehydrogenase	Avoid mushroom and Alcohol/ supportive
Delayed onset: Headache	*Gyromitra; esculenta* (false morel) *Gyromitra* sp.	Gyromitrin, Monomethyl hydrazine, etc.	Fatigue, head and body ache, vomiting, liver damage, death, carcinogenic	Interfere with pyridoxine?	Cook or dry, don't inhale vapors
Nephropathy	*Cortinarius* sp.	Orellanine Cortinarin	Polydypsia, oliguria, nausea, head and body aches, chills, etc., Renal tubular and liver necrosis, death	Membrane damage from oxygen-derived free radicals (similar to paraquat)	Hemodialysis
Carcinogenic	*Agaricus bisporus* (edible)	Agaritine, hydrazines	Lung tumors	Genotoxic	Cooking
Hepatotoxic	*Amanita phalloides* (Europe) *A. Virosa* (United States) *Galerina* sp. *Lepiota* sp.	Amatoxins, phallotoxins, and virotoxins	Emesis and diarrhea, increase in serum enzymes, decrease in glucose and clotting factors, hepatic and renal damage, jaundice, coma, and death	1. Inhibit RNA polymerase 2. Enhance G-actin polymerization into F-actin 3. Inhibit F-actin depolymerization	1. Correct glucose and clotting effects 2. Decontaminate 3. Penicillin and silobinin 4. Supportive 5. Transplant liver

in the arcuate nucleus of the hypothalamus, retina, and lateral geniculate nucleus, and in other brain areas devoid of the blood–brain barrier (148). Numbness of the neck and back, weakness, and palpitations, typical signs of the so-called Chinese restaurant syndrome, were later found not to be associated with dietary MSG (198).

Hypoglycin A (β-methylene cyclopropyl alanine) and its γ-glutamyl conjugate, hypoglycin B, are components of the fruit of the plant, *Blighia sapida* (ackee in Jamaica and isin in Nigeria). Consumption of this fruit in the unripened stage has been associated with hypoglycemia, resulting from inhibition of gluconeogenesis involving inhibition of fatty acyl-CoA dehydrogenases and thus β-oxidation of fatty acids by cyclopropylacetyl CoA (a metabolite of hypoglycin A). Signs of intoxication include vomiting, convulsions, hypothermia, coma, and even death. Pretreatment with clofibrate (stimulator of peroxismal fatty acid oxidases) prevented many but not all signs, lesions, and biochemical effects (205).

Koa haoli (*Leucaena leucocephala*), a legume found in Hawaii, and other legume species belonging to the Mimosidae family, have potentially high nutritive value for animals and humans (144). However, use of these legumes is precluded in ruminants by the goitrogenic effect of the metabolite (3,4-dihydroxypyridine) of an unusual amino acid, mimosine [3-N-(3-hydroxypyridone-4)-2-aminopropionic acid], present in this plant. Mimosine also causes reversible destruction of the hair follicle matrix (loss of hair), reduced bone strength and mineral composition in poultry, and growth depression in both ruminants and nonruminants. The ability of mimosine to chelate Zn and Mg, reduce plasma thyroid and other hormone levels (159), inhibit a large number of enzymes leading to DNA synthesis inhibition and cell-cycle arrest (88,113) explains many of the effects.

Djenkolic acid, which is an amino acid that is structurally similar to cystine, is present in the djenkol bean (*Pithocolobium lobatum*), found in Sumatra and Java. It can neither substitute for cystine nor can it be totally metabolized, but it can crystallize in the kidney, causing hematuria and crystalluria (113).

Favism, a hemolytic disease (accompanied by jaundice and hemoglobiuuria) in persons genetically deficient in glucose-6-phosphate dehydrogenase (G6PD) and, thus, in NADPH and reduced glutathione content, results from the consumption of the amino acid, 3,4-dihydroxyphenylalanine, and the pyrimidine aglycones (divicine and isouramil) of the glycosides vicine and convicine in broad beans (*Vicia faba*), mainly in the Mediterranean region and in the Middle East (37). Ohga et al. (147) observed beneficial effects of human heptaglobin administration in managing this crisis.

The etiology of the neurological disease characterized by posterior sensory ataxia in cattle consuming cycads may be an amino acid, β-N-methylamino-L-alanine. Certain seleno-amino acids such as methylselenocysteine, selenocystathionine, selenocysteine, and selenomethionine in plants that grow on high Se soils (113), when incorporated into structural animal proteins, may, during longer-term exposure in livestock, produce defective hair and hooves that are eventually lost. In human beings, a syndrome characterized by abdominal distress, nausea, vomiting, diarrhea, and loss of scalp and body hair had been reported following consumption of coco de momo (*Lecythis ollaria*) nuts containing high levels of selenocystathionine (16).

The amino acids L-2,4-diaminobutyric acid (DABA), 3-N-oxalyl-L-2,3-diaminopropionic acid (ODAP) 3-cyanoalanine, 4-glutamylcyanoalanine, and related homologues, present in seeds of several species of *Lathyrus* and *Vicia sativa* in the Indian subcontinent, have been implicated in the pathogenesis of neurolathyrism, a syndrome characterized by muscular rigidity, weakness, paralysis of leg muscles, and death following long-term, high-level consumption of *L. sativus* seeds (204). The mechanism of action appears to involve irreversible binding of ODAP to the glutamate receptor, and enhanced release/reduced re-uptake of glutamine at relevant nerve terminals, leading to vascular degeneration and necrosis of neurons (152). In certain individuals, amino acids such as β-aminopropionitrile and the dipeptide (N-γ-glutamyl) aminopropionitrile as well as certain urides, hydrazides, and hydrazines from the green parts of *Lathyrus* and other plants, lead to osteolathyrism characterized by bone deformities and reduction in the tensile strength of the aorta (72) resulting from the irreversible inhibition of lysyl oxidase and interference with crosslinking of collagen (216).

Creeping indigo (*Indigofera endecapylla*), a tropical forage, contains a nitric oxide synthase inhibitor, indospicine, which causes liver damage in sheep, rats, and mice by inhibiting the incorporation of arginine, the amino acid it resembles, into protein (113,154). 3-Nitropropionic acid, a neurotoxin capable of inhibiting mitochondrial succinate dehydrogenase and, thus, cellular respiration, is also present (7).

Vaso- and Psychoactive Substances

High levels of amines such as tyramine and its methyl derivatives octopamine, dopamine, epinephrine, norepinephrine, histamine, serotonin, and others are present in cheese, yeast products, fermented foods, beer, wine, pickled herring, snails, chicken liver, coffee, broad beans, chocolate, and certain cream products, and in plants such as pineapple, banana, plantain, and avocado (121). Moderate amounts of cheese and yeast products often contain sufficient tyramine (10 mg) to cause severe hypertensive crisis in individuals treated with non-selective monoamine oxidase (MAO) inhibitors for mood disorders (19). Inhibition of MAO leads to a combined vasopressor effect of unmetabolized biogenic as well as dietary amines. In addition, tyramine enhances release of catecholamines that are present in supranormal amounts in the adrenal medulla (19). Palpitations, migraine headaches, and, in some instances, intracranial bleeding and death may ensue. Use of selective (MAO-A or B) inhibitors for therapy appears not to sensitize individuals to dietary tyramine (101).

Psychoactive substances include CNS stimulants such as xanthines (caffeine, theophylline, and theobromine present in coffee, tea, and cocoa); depressants such as alcohol and high doses of atropine (from jimsonweed and henbane); and hallucinogens such as myristicin from nutmeg, psilocybin and psilocin from mushrooms, and nondietary sources of cocaine and lysergic acid derivatives (130). Chronic overindulgence in xanthine beverages may lead to restlessness, disturbed sleep, myocardial stimulation reflected as premature systoles and tachycardia (palpitations), and tremors. Herbs containing psychoactive agents include California poppy, catnip, cinnamon, hops, hydrangea, juniper, kola nut, nutmeg, periwinkle, thornapple, and wild lettuce (25). The essential oils of coffee and the tannins in tea may cause diarrhea and constipation, respectively (45). Caffeine is neither mutagenic by itself nor enhances the mutagenic effects of other compounds in mammalian cells and may actually be anticarcinogenic (39).

Vitamins and Antivitamins

Vitamins A (retinol), D, and pyridoxine have a lower safety margin (ten times the RDA) and should be used on a longer-term basis only under medical supervision (126). Other vitamins with a safety ratio of 50–100 relative to the RDA are generally safe. Therapeutic uses of vitamin A for night blindness, steatorrhea, hyperkeratosis, acne vulgaris, certain immune disorders, and cancer, along with daily consumption of carotenoids and vitamin A in plant and animal tissues (especially the liver), account for the total vitamin A exposure in humans (149). Oral doses of 18,000–60,000 IU/day and 100,000 IU/day can cause hypervitaminosis A in infants and adults, respectively, with premature epiphyseal closure and retardation of long bone growth in children; and headaches, blurred vision, fatigue, hair loss, drying and flaking of skin, pruritus, nose bleeds, anemia, and liver and spleen enlargement in adults (149). Therapy of acute promyelocytic leukemia with tretinoin (all-trans-retinoic acid) as an adjunct to antineoplastic therapy induces retinoic acid syndrome (fatal leukocytosis, body weight gain, respiratory distress, cardiac and renal failure) in 25 percent of cases (60). Excess vitamin A (retinoids) is teratogenic, causing craniofacial, thymic, heart, and CNS malformations subsequent to interaction with cellular retinoic acid/retinol binding proteins (47). The oral doses of vitamin A not exceeding 6000 IU/day are considered safe during pregnancy in human beings.

Vitamin D, following hydroxylation at C_{25} and C_1 in the liver and kidney, respectively, functions to facilitate the action of parathyroid hormone to release Ca^{++} from bone and to promote intestinal absorption of Ca^{++} and inhibit its renal loss. Ergosterol (a plant steroid) converted to ergocalciferol (Vit-D_2) by ultraviolet light, endogenous dehydrocholesterol (in skin) converted to cholecalciferol (Vit D_3) by sunlight, and vitamin D-fortified milk are predominant sources of vitamin D for humans (149). While the recommended dose is 400 IU/day, excessive exposure to vitamin D from 1000–3000 IU/day in infants and 10,000–500,000 IU/day in adults has resulted in toxicosis. Poisonings in dogs and cats have resulted from accidental consumption of insecticidal vitamin D packages. Toxic signs of vitamin D in humans, which are similar to those seen in laboratory animals, are a result of hypercalcemia leading to extraskeletal calcifications, especially blood vessel walls and kidneys, leading to hypertension, renal failure, and cardiac insufficiency (149). Recent evidence suggests that supplementation with vitamin D_3 may lead to an increase in LDL and may negate putative cardioprotection by hormone replacement therapy in post-menopausal women (76), and may exacerbate intimal hyperplasia in balloon-damaged rat arteries (106).

Long-term supplemental use of vitamin E can result in coagulopathy (by reduced iron utilization and increased vitamin K requirement) as well as tumor promotion (both stage I and II); such use of pyridoxine can result in photoallergic reaction and sensory neuropathy (126,137, 149). Table 11.2 lists examples of anti-vitamin factors in foods, the effects of which, in general, only manifest in individuals with already low levels of the vitamin in question.

Miscellaneous Plant Toxicants

A common human intoxication called milk sickness was one of the most dreaded diseases from colonial times to the early 19th century in an area extending from North Carolina to Virginia and to the midwestern United States (112). The disease manifested as weakness, nausea and vomiting, constipation, tremors, prostration, delirium, and even death, resulted from consumption of dairy products made from milk derived from cows (even healthy ones) grazing on white snakeroot (*Eupatorium rugosum*) or rayless goldenrod (*Haplopappus heterophillus*). The causative agent appears to be trematol, an unsaturated alcohol, in combination with a resin acid (112). Other plant toxins excreted through milk that pose toxic hazards for children and nursing animals include pyrrolizidine, piperidine, and quinolizidine alkaloids; sesquiterpene lactones of bitterweed and rubberweed; and glucosinolates (153). Animals grazing high Se forages

Table 11.2
Examples of anti-vitamin factors in foods

Vitamin	Antagonist(s)	Mechanism	Effect(s)	Source(s)
A	Lipoxidase	oxidize β-carotene	Lower blood Vit A level	Soybeans
	Citral	inhibit retinoic acid (P=450) dehydrogenase	Endothelial damage cardiovascular disease?	Oranges
B Thiamine	Thiaminase, tannins, and ortho-catechols	inactivate thiamine	Neurological syndrome	Bracken fern other plants and seafood
Riboflavin			Vomiting, sickness	
Niacin	Hypoglycin A		Pellagra	Ackee plum
Biotin	Leucine?	Irreversible binding		Cereal crops
Pyridoxine	Avidin,	Hydrazine metabolites		Egg white
	Linatine, Agaritine	condense with the vitamin		Flaxseed, Shiitake mushroom
Pantothenic acid				Pea seedlings
	Unknown			Soybeans
B12	Unknown	Unknown		
C	Ascorbic acid oxidase	Oxidizes Vit C	Normally none	Fruits and vegetables
D	β-carotene, plant steroids (some)	Reduce absorption	Rickets and osteomalacia	Green leafy vegetables
	Unknown	Unknown		Soybeans
E	α-tocoferol oxidase	Oxidizes Vit E	Muscular dystrophy	Kidney beans and others
	Polyunsaturated fatty acids	Increases Vit E demand	Liver necrosis	Vegetable oils Beans
K	Diconmarol	Inhibit epoxide reductase	Hemorrhages	Sweet clover

may excrete high levels of Se in milk and contribute to chronic Se toxicosis in the offspring (153). Current processing methods have kept these conditions in check for the most part. In cattle, consumption of 5–10 pounds of snakeroot causes weakness and trembling of various groups of muscles, labored respiration, and death.

Fool's parsley (*Aethusa cynapium*) and other members of the *Umbelliferae* family contain highly toxic acetylene derivatives (e.g., aethusin) that are responsible for many human poisonings (114). Carotatoxin and other acetylene compounds in carrots are neurotoxic (25) but are not likely to cause problems in humans.

Purple mint (*Perilla frustescens*), widely distributed in the United States and Japan, is used as a flavoring agent, for medicinal purposes, and as animal feed. The presence, in mint, of a ketone-substituted furan capable of causing acute pulmonary emphysema and other lung lesions in cattle and other animals (181) raises questions about the safety of these uses in humans and animals.

Cycads, the palm-like plants adapted for adverse climatic conditions of the tropical and subtropical areas of the world, are still used (seeds and stem) as a source of starch in Guam, Kenya, Amami Oshima, Miyako Island, and southern Japan by small groups of people (128). Adverse effects result from incomplete extraction of toxicants, including cycasin and β-N-methylamino-L-alanine (BMAA), during preparation of the flour. Several neurological conditions, including a paralytic disease (amyotrophic lateral sclerosis, ALS) and Parkinsonism–dementia (PD) were observed among the native Chamorro in Guam who consume cycad, gait disturbances, motor weakness, and paralysis in cattle grazing on cycads, and Parkinsonian features and degenerative changes in CNS motor neurons in monkeys—all appear to be related to either or both of these cycad toxicants (128,190). Attenuation of the cycad-induced neurotoxic syndrome by AP7 and MK801, two selective antagonists of N-methyl-D-aspartate receptor and its associated ion channel, suggests a role of the excitatory neurotransmitters in the causation of ALS–PD, other motor-system diseases (Huntington's chorea, Parkinson's disease, and olivopontocerebellar atrophy), and Alzheimer's disease (190). Other effects of cycasin, its aglycone, or cycad flour include hepatic necrosis, subserosal hemorrhages, accumulation of yellow fluid in serosal cavities, benign and malignant tumors in the liver, kidney, lungs, and gastrointestinal tract (mainly colon), neuroteratological effects in offspring, death in experimental animals, and mutagenic effects in a variety of in vitro and in vivo systems. Interestingly, cycasin is neither toxic nor carcinogenic when given parenterally to conventional rats or when given either orally or parenterally to germ-free rats, suggesting that the intestinal flora mediate cycasin toxicity. Bacterial β-glucosidase hydrolyzes cycasin to the active carcinogen, methylazoxymethanol (MAM), which produces hepatomas in rats. MAM spontaneously breaks down to methyldiazonium hydroxide which methylates hepatic DNA, RNA, and proteins (128). Certain cycad glycosides inhibit aromatase and may be useful in the treatment of estrogen-dependent cancer (102).

Toxicants in Foods of Animal Origin

The discussion on plant toxicants has included certain agents from this category (e.g., vasoactive agents in cheese, plant-derived toxicants in milk). Others such as bacterial toxins in meats are discussed in a subsequent section. Residues, in meats and milk, from pesticides, antibiotics, and growth promotants (including hormones such as estrogenic substances) are addressed briefly in the section on food additives and in the chapter dealing with pesticides. Natural toxicant hazards in foods of animal origin are mostly limited to those derived from marine sources.

Marine Toxins in Food

Of the many marine organisms containing toxins (up to 1200 species), only a few are involved in food poisoning. Problems of seafood poisoning have spread to inland areas from coastal fishing sites as a result of modern transportation and shipping. Toxicants may be produced by the fish itself, and/or by the marine plankton or algae consumed by the fish, with or without the aid of certain marine bacteria. Leftley and Hannah (111) and Russell and Dart (172) have presented a detailed discussion of the toxicological information relating to fish-borne toxins.

Shellfish poisoning is one of several (amnesic, digestive, neurotoxic–paralytic) disease entities resulting from the consumption of shellfish (clams, crustaceans, lobsters, mussels, oysters, scallops, etc.) that have ingested toxic marine algae, especially certain dinoflagellates. The shellfish are toxic during seasons of heavy algal bloom (such as red tide) containing 200 organisms/ml or more. Toxicity increases in proportion to the concentration of algae and disappears within two weeks after the toxic plankton has disappeared from the waters (171). Saxitoxin, neosaxitoxin, and gonyautoxins are the most potent of the more than 20 toxins present in the group of paralytic shellfish poison, produced by dinoflagollates belonging to *Alexandrium, Gymnodinium, Guanyalax*, and *Pyrodinium* sp.

Saxitoxin blocks the action potential in nerves and muscles by preferential blockade of inward flow of sodium ions with no effect on the flow of potassium or chloride ions (90). Consumption of 1 mg of the toxin (in 1 to 5 mussels or clams weighing 150 g each) can be mildly toxic whereas 4 mg can be fatal if not treated vigorously. Toxic symptoms begin as numbness of the lips, tongue, and fingertips within minutes after eating. Numbness then extends to the legs, arms, and neck and is followed by general muscular incoordination, which progresses to respiratory paralysis and death. Decreased heart rate and contractile force, headache, dizziness, increased sweating, and thirst may also be noted. Boiling in bicarbonate-treated water and discarding the broth is suggested as a means of preventing shellfish poisoning (71).

Diarrhetic shellfish poisoning results from consumption of shellfish contaminated by one of several species of *Dinophysis* that containing okadaic acid (OA) and/or dinophysistoxins (DPT). Both OA and DPT are powerful inhibitors of protein phosphatases and potent tumor promoters (101). Whether protein phosphatase inhibition by OA leads to the observed increase in the permeability of intestinal epithelial cells OA and the diarrhetic effect is unknown.

Neurotoxic shellfish poisoning is characterized by nausea, vomiting, diarrhea, chills, headache, muscle weakness and pain, eye and nasal irritation, and, in severe cases, paresthesia, difficulty in breathing, double vision, dysphonea, and dysphagia. It has been reported along the Gulf of Mexico, the eastern coast of Florida, and New Zealand following consumption of shellfish with a heavy load of *Gymnodinium breve* and/or similar organisms (111). The lipophilic polyether toxin, the brevitoxin, promotes Na^+ influx and thus depolarization by its action on site-5 of the voltage-dependent Na^+ channels (111).

Amnetic shellfish poisoning, characterized by short-term and sometimes permanent memory loss associated with gastrointestinal signs and hallucinatory state, has been reported mostly from coastal areas in North America. Damage to the hippocampus, coma, and death result in severe cases. A water-soluble acidic non-protein amino acid, domoic acid (and its isomers), produced by the diatom *Pseudonitzschia* sp. and acting as a competitive glutamate antagonist at various sites, has been ascribed the etiological agent (111).

Between 300 and 400 tropical reef and semipelagic species of edible marine animals, including barracudas, groupers, sea basses, snappers, surgeon fishes, parrot fishes, jacks, wrasses, eels, and certain gastropods, accumulate in their liver and other viscera toxins capable of causing ciguatera poisoning, with an estimated 20,000 cases/year worldwide (118). The intoxication, common in the South Pacific and the Caribbean, appears to follow the spacial and temporal pattern of the distribution of a photosynthetic dinoflagellate *Gamblerdiscus toxicus*, which is consumed by the smaller herbivorous fish and, in turn, by the ciguatoxic fish (171).

Ciguatoxins, the colorless and heat stable lipophilic polyethers (MW of 1100), appear to play a major role in intoxication with some contribution from the water-soluble maitotoxin (111). Ciguatoxins increase membrane permeability to sodium ions causing depolarization of nerves. In addition, ciguatoxin inhibits subsequent inactivation of open Na^+ channels and possesses anticholinesterase activity in experimental animals (111,171). Maitotoxin, on the other hand, inactivates voltage-dependent and receptor-mediated Ca^{++} channels leading to high intracellular Ca^{++} and cell death (111). In humans, tingling of the lips, tongue, and throat, followed by numbness, nausea, vomiting, abdominal pain, diarrhea, pruritus, bradycardia, dizziness, and muscle and joint pain occurs. Severe cases exhibit paresis of the legs and, infrequently, death due to cardiovascular and/or respiratory failure (111,171). Prevention of ciguatera poisoning is difficult, although extensive evisceration of fish may help.

Pufferfish (fugu fish) poisoning, known to occur as far back as 2000–3000 B.C. in China and Japan, results from consumption of tetrodotoxin present in the liver and ovaries of puffer fish, ocean sunfishes, porcupine fishes, blue-ringed octopus, and certain amphibians of the family *Salamandridae* (91,171). Toxin accumulation is greatest just prior to spawning in the spring. Tetrodotoxin (TTx), with a cyclic hemilactal structure, is highly lethal (LD_{50}, 10 mg/kg) to all vertebrates and is active after boiling for one hour but is inactivated under alkaline conditions (63). Tetrodotoxin prevents the increase in the early Na^+ permeability in both motor and sensory neuronal membranes similar to that of saxitoxin (171). In humans, numbness of the lips, tongue, fingers, and arms, muscular paralysis and ataxia, hypotension, and respiratory paralysis leading to death progress rapidly beginning 30–60 minutes after consumption of 1 to 2 mg of tetrodotoxin (1–10 g of roe or liver). Although current treatment is only symptomatic, experimental evidence (33,166) indicates that anti-TTx antibodies or 4-aminopyridine may be effective in antagonizing the cardiorespiratory effects of tetrodotoxin. Training of personnel in proper evisceration techniques and licensing of fugu restaurants is a must.

Scombroid poisoning is the most widespread fish-borne intoxication. It results from the consumption of inadequately preserved abalone, amberjack, bluefish, tuna, mackerel, mahi-mahi, and sardines in which histamine and saurine are produced by bacterial scombrotoxic action (118). Scombroid fish apparently has a sharp or peppery taste. Signs of intoxication include nausea, vomiting, diarrhea, epigastric distress, flushing of the face, throbbing headache, and burning of the throat followed by numbness and urticaria. Severe cases may lead to cyanosis and respiratory distress but, rarely, death. These signs appear within 2 hours of the meal and disappear in 16 hours (171). The disease readily responds to antihistamine treatment.

FOOD CONTAMINANTS

Although some naturally occurring toxicants and food additives impart resistance against pests to plants and help preserve and/or enhance the nutritional quality of the diet, respectively, the biological and synthetic industrial chemical contaminants sometimes increase the risk of food-borne illness and deserve a much broader margin of safety in their control than food additives. The FDA, in consultation with other federal agencies, establishes legal action levels, that is, the maximal level of a contaminant allowed in foods and feeds based on economic considerations and technological feasibility (75).

Bacterial Toxins

Foods contaminated with microbial agents are a major source of human disease estimated to afflict up to 80 million people and to cost $22 billion annually in the United States (8). With a few exceptions, these can be prevented by adequate cooking and proper cooling, storage, and reheating of cooked foods in clean containers (127). Bacterial food-borne disease may result from the consumption, in food, either of bacteria (e.g., *Salmonella* sp. and *Clostridium perfringens*) that can cause disease by multiplying in the intestinal mucosa where they may elaborate toxins (enterotoxins), or of a sufficient amount of preformed microbial toxins (staphylococcal enterotoxins and botulinum toxin). In addition to the above well-known etiologies, genetic changes in bacteria that increase virulence, changes in eating habits, altered food production and distribution systems, the increased number of immunocompromised consumers, and improved detection systems have led to identification of other pathogens such as *Escherichia coli, Listeria* sp., and *Yersinia* sp. as causing food-borne illness.

C. perfringens frequently causes food-borne infections which subsequently lead to sporulation of the organism in the large intestine. The enterotoxin, released during sporulation of the bacteria, is capable of causing fluid accumulation in the intestines. The α-toxin, possessing lethal, necrotizing, and hemolytic activities, is also produced by certain types. Among the five distinct types of *C. perfringens* (type A through E), type A is almost always involved in food-borne gastroenteritis and associated signs in human beings in the United States. Only meat and fish products are capable of providing all the amino acids and growth factors required for the growth of *C. perfringens*. Roast beef, beef stew, gravy, and meat pies for type A, and pork, other meats, and fish for type C, are frequently involved (27). Typically, foods involved are cooked at 100°C for less than an hour and are subsequently kept warm or slowly cooled. Spores that survive the heat shock multiply faster in the food than those not subjected to heat treatment, and elaborate the enterotoxin in the gut. The enterotoxin appears to form ion-permeable channels in the cell membrane, leading to movement of extracellular calcium and water into the cells, leading to cell death (194). Entry of the toxin into the blood stream leads to release of potassium from hepatocytes, hyperkalemic cardiac failure, and death (194). Due to the ubiquitous distribution of the organism in soil, and in the gastrointestinal tract of humans and animals, prevention of contamination is difficult. Multiplication and toxin production can be inhibited by heating food to the proper temperature (165–212°F), prompt and effective cooling, and avoiding prolonged reheating before consumption.

Staphylococcus aureus is probably the leading cause of food-borne disease worldwide. The organisms are gram-positive, non-motile, and non-spore-forming cocci that occur ubiquitously in the environment. Although humans are the leading source of food contamination by way of nasal discharge and infected cuts and wounds, the organism can be present in milk derived from mastitic cows and meat derived from arthritic poultry (136). Baked ham, poultry, fish and shellfish, meat and potato salads, cream-filled bakery goods, and high-protein leftover foods are frequently involved in such intoxication (27). Multiplication of *S. aureus* in raw food products is inhibited by other spoilage organisms present. As a result, mostly cooked products subsequently contaminated by infected handlers and stored at warm temperature for several hours before consumption cause intoxication. The causative agent is one of more than six immunologically distinct heat stable enterotoxic proteins (MW 26,000–34,000) whose secretion is genetically regulated during growth (A, D, and E by chromosomes or by plasmids B and C). In addition, *S. aureus* also produces many other substances such as coagulase, DNase, hemolysins, lipases, fibrinolysin, and hyaluronidase, that are toxic to one or more animal species. Although all strains of *S. aureus* are potentially pathogenic, the enterotoxin production is closely related to the presence of coagulase and DNase. Signs and symptoms begin one to six hours after consumption of contaminated food, and include nausea, salivation, vomiting, retching, occasional diarrhea, abdominal cramps, sweating, dehydration, and weakness followed by recovery in one to three days. Severe cases may show fever, chills, a drop in blood pressure, and prostration (136). Preventive measures effective against *S. aureus* food intoxication include education of food handlers regarding hygienic practices to reduce post-cooking contamination of high-protein foods and eliminating prolonged storage of cooked foods at room temperature before consumption.

Botulism is a neurotoxic syndrome caused by consumption of improperly cooked and stored foods containing one of seven (A through G) heat labile neurotoxins produced by *Clostridium botulinum*. It is an ubiquitous, anaerobic, gram-positive, and motile rod capable of forming heat-resistant spores. High moisture, a pH above 4.6, and prolonged anaerobic storage are required for sufficient toxin production (136). Common foods involved are home canned fruits and vegetables such as beans, corn, leafy vegetables, and, especially, peppers, all of which contain toxins A and B. Non-poultry meats contain toxin B, and cheese and other dairy products contain toxin A. Type E is isolated mostly from fish products (136). Types C and D, which cause botulism in animals and birds, do not affect humans.

Botulinum toxin is stable in the acid pH of the stomach where it is protected from the gastric juice and pepsin by a nontoxic component of the toxin molecule. Once in the duodenum, it is activated by trypsin, with no change in molecular size, and subsequently absorbed into the lymphatics. The toxin irreversibly binds to the myoneural junction and, acting as a Zn endopeptidase, degrades peptides involved in the release of acetylcholine (ACh), thus inhibiting its release at the peripheral cholinergic nerve endings (136). Signs and symptoms of botulism usually appear 12–24 hours (range: 2 hours to 6 days) following consumption of the toxin-containing food. Initial signs of nausea, vomiting, and diarrhea are followed later by predominantly neurological symptoms including headache, dizziness, blurred and/or double vision, loss of light reflex, weakness of facial muscles, and pharyngeal paralysis (difficulty in speech and swallowing). Fever is absent. Sensory reflexes and mental alertness are intact. Paralysis of the respiratory muscles leads to failure of respiration and death, usually in 3–10 days (187). Food-borne botulism can be prevented by proper canning technique, boiling vegetables for at least 3 minutes before serving, and discarding all swollen and damaged canned products. Treatment of botulism involves the use of monovalent (E), bivalent (A and B), or polyvalent (A, B, and E) antitoxin, recall of all involved commercial products, proper reporting, and epidemiological investigation. Boiling for 3 minutes or heating at 80°C for 30 minutes destroys the preformed toxin, and the use of salt, the antimicrobial compound nisin, polyphosphates, smoke, spices, lactic acid, and nitrite can inhibit the growth of *C. botulinum* and, thus, toxin formation (136). If the nitrite content of cured meats and fish as well as fermented sausages is reduced from current levels as a means of decreasing the carcinogenic dietary nitrosamines, it is conceivable that the incidence of botulism from the consumption of such foods could increase unless suitable replacements are found.

Food-borne disease outbreaks involving *Bacillus cereus* have occurred in Northern and Eastern Europe. A diarrheal illness involving a wide variety of meats and vegetables, various desserts, fish, pasta, milk, and ice cream (similar to that of *C. perfringens*), and a vomiting illness involving flour-based foods such as cereals and fried rice served in Chinese restaurants (similar to that of *S. aureus*) are both apparently caused by this organism (136). At least seven toxins including a heat stable (121°C for 90 minutes) emetic toxin and a heat labile (56°C for 5 minutes) enterotoxin contribute to the syndrome (136). The enterotoxin appears to disrupt cell membranes, leading to increased permeability, whereas the mechanism of emetic toxin is unknown.

Salmonella sp. consists of over 2200 serotypes possessing somatic O, flagellar H, and capsular Vi antigens, of which 50 serotypes commonly occur. *S. typhi, S. paratyphi*, and *S. sendai* are adapted to human hosts which serve as the sole carrier for those organisms. Feces of infected humans, domestic and wild animals, and birds serve as sources of contamination in a variety of meat and milk products, causing severe gastrointestinal signs along with fever, septicemia, shock, and the sequelae of embolism including pneumonia, meningitis, and abortion. Mortality is rare and occurs in very young, very old, and immunocompromised patients. Enteritis can result from bacterial multiplication within the mucosa or from enterotoxins secreted by some serotypes. Salmonella-free birds can be raised in salmonella-free environments using salmonella-free pelleted feed or by vaccination. Thorough cooking of meats; pasteurization of milk and dairy and egg products; prevention of cross-contamination between cooked and raw products; and, finally, testing, isolation, and treatment of carrier animals and food handling personnel are all extremely important in controlling the incidence of this most common food-borne disease (58).

Campylobacter jejuni and other species in this genus (*C. sputorum* etc.) are associated with up to 4 million cases of diarrheal illness similar in many respects to salmonellosis (9). Reactive arthritis, inflammation of the urethra and conjunctiva, and Guillain-Barré syndrome have been described as sequalae in occasional cases (9).

Escherichia coli, a close relative of the genus *Shigella*, has recently raised concern as a fatal, food-borne disease agent. There are more than 160 serotypes (based on O, H, or capsular K antigen), of which 43 have been associated with bloody diarrhea and hemolytic uremic syndrome (HUS) in humans (165). Pneumonia, meningitis, thrombotic and thrombocytopenric purpura, bladder and kidney infections, and septicemia may also result from *E. coli* infections. Based on virulence factors (which bestow the organism with the ability to attack, invade, and produce toxin in the host cells) located in the plasmids, five virotypes have been identified as pathogenic. These are: enterotoxigenic *E. coli* (ETEC), enteroaggregative *E. coli* (Eagg EC), enteropathogenic *E. coli* (EPEC), enterohemorrhagic *E. coli* (EHEC), and enteroinvasive *E. coli* (EIEC). Serogroup O 157 : H7, belonging to the EHEC group and producing a shiga-like toxin, may be the most common serotype causing bloody diarrhea and HUS mainly traceable to consumption of contaminated beef products (165). Less frequently, unpasteurized milk and juices; ham, turkey, and cheese sandwiches; dry fermented sausage; salad; and non-chlorinated water have been involved. Once in the intestines, *E. coli* produce shiga-like toxins SL1 and SL2 which similar to vicin, act by inactivating ribosomes to cause intestinal cell death (165).

Listeriosis, in addition to being transmitted by other routes, is an emerging food-borne disease resulting from the consumption of *Listeria monocytogenes*-contaminated soft cheeses, milk and other milk products, poultry, meat (especially delicatessen meats and frankfurters), and coleslaw and other products (salads, etc.) derived from contaminated vegetables. Food products are contaminated by contact with soil, feces, discharges, and urine from infected animals and humans. The clinical food-borne disease, occurring mostly in pregnant women, neonates, older, and immunocompromised adults, is characterized by gastrointestinal or flu-like symptoms within 12 hours of exposure followed by bacteremia leading to abortions, stillbirths, or premature births in pregnant women; meningitis, respiratory distress, and skin nodules in neonates; and meningitis-related signs in adults (41). The disease can be treated with antibiotics and other supportive measures. Prevention involves improvement of sanitation of the environment and equipment, and education to identify and avoid contaminated food products.

Another recent controversy involves food-borne transmission of *spongiform encephalopathies* (SE) of animals (bovine SE [BSE] and scrapie of sheep and goats) to humans that may manifest as Creutzfeldt–Jakob (CJ) disease, characterized by fatal neuronal vacuolization and cell death (70). Although experimental evidence suggests that these diseases can sometimes be orally transmitted, no definitive proof exists that human disease results from consumption of edible animal products or that toxins play a role in its pathogenesis (70). Nevertheless, the fact that BSE may be transmitted to other species should increase the vigilance of the veterinarians responsible to ensure that products from animals with progressive degenerative neurological disease do not enter the human food chain.

Yersiniosis resulting from consumption of improperly cooked chitterlings (porcine large intestines), cryptosporidiosis from contaminated water and unpasteurized apple cider, *Cyclospora* infection from contaminated water and fresh berries, and brucellosis from unpasteurized milk and meats from infected cattle, sheep, goats, and their products are other examples of potential food-borne outbreaks.

Prevention and Control of Microbial Food Hazards The National Animal Health Monitoring System (USDA) has stepped up efforts to monitor food animal and poultry health on the farm and thus develop strategies to deal with potential increases in existing as well as emerging food-borne disease threats. The USDA's Food Safety Inspection Service (FSIS) began implementing a hazard analysis and critical control point system (HACCP) for pathogen reduction in 1996 for all slaughter and processing operations. The HACCP directs each processing unit to: conduct a hazard analysis; identify critical control points at which a safety hazard can be prevented; establish limits at each point; develop monitoring procedures and corrective action when limits are exceeded; and implement record keeping that will allow subsequent verification for compliance by FSIS (78). Data for the *E. coli* and salmonella burden of carcasses are used as evidence of fecal and enteric pathogen reduction. Together, these two programs are aimed at minimizing overall food-borne disease from animal foods in the U.S. population. The approval, by FDA, of low-dose irradiation of red meats to control pathogens, coupled with previously approved irradiation of poultry for pathogen reduction, pork for control of trichinae, fruits, vegetables, and grains for insect control, and spices, seasonings, and dry enzymes used in food processing for microbial reduction (14), should not only contribute to the prevention of food-borne disease caused by microbial pathogens but also help in increasing the shelf life of such products without undesirable organoleptic, toxicological, or nutritional changes. Irradiation is yet to be approved for pathogen control of seafood products and is unsuitable for dairy products because of development of off-flavors and discoloration. In the final analysis, however, the key to minimizing the microbial food-borne illness is at the food preparer/consumer level in the form of proper canning, cooking at the correct temperature, hygienic service, and/or prompt and appropriate storage and reheating.

Mycotoxins

From the standpoint of human and animal health, toxigenic molds belonging to the genera *Aspergillus, Fusarium*, and *Penicillium* have received the most attention, owing to their frequent occurrence in food and feed commodities. Unfavorable conditions such as drought and damage to seeds by insects or mechanical harvesting can enhance fungal toxin (mycotoxin) production during both growth and storage thus making mycotoxicoses a problem of both developing and developed countries. Although more than a hundred mycotoxins have been identified, the public health significance of most remains unknown.

Aflatoxins

The aflatoxins are a group of highly substituted coumarins containing a fused dihydrofuran moiety (Figure 11.3) and produced by the molds *Aspergillus flavus* and *A. parasiticus*. Four major aflatoxins designated B1, B2, G1, and G2 (based on blue or green fluorescence under ultraviolet light) are produced in varying quantities in a variety of products that has not been adequately dried at harvest and has been stored at relatively high temperatures (30). Commodities most often shown to contain aflatoxins are peanuts, various other nuts, cottonseed, corn, and figs. Human exposure can occur from consumption of aflatoxins from these sources and the products derived from them, as well as from tissues and the milk (AFM_1, a hydroxylated metabolite) of food animals consuming contaminated feeds.

Aflatoxin B_1 (AFB_1), the most potent and the most commonly occurring aflatoxin, is acutely toxic (LD_{50}, 0.3–0/9.0 mg/kg) to all species of animals, birds, and fishes (42). Acute effects of AFB_1 in animals include death without signs, or signs of anorexia, depression, ataxia, dyspnea, anemia, and hemorrhages from body orifices. In subchronic cases icterus, hypoprothrombinemia, hematomas, and gastroenteritis are common. Chronic aflatoxicosis, characterized by bile duct proliferation, periportal fibrosis, icterus, and cirrhosis of the liver, and associated with loss of weight and reduced resistance to disease, is more prevalent in domestic animals and is also likely to occur in humans (151). Prolonged exposure to low levels of AFB_1 in animals also leads to hepatoma, cholangiocarcinoma, or hepatocellular carcinoma and other tumors (30).

The National Research Council (146) reviewed epidemiological studies to conclude that the risk of primary hepatocellular carcinoma from AFB_1 exposure may be

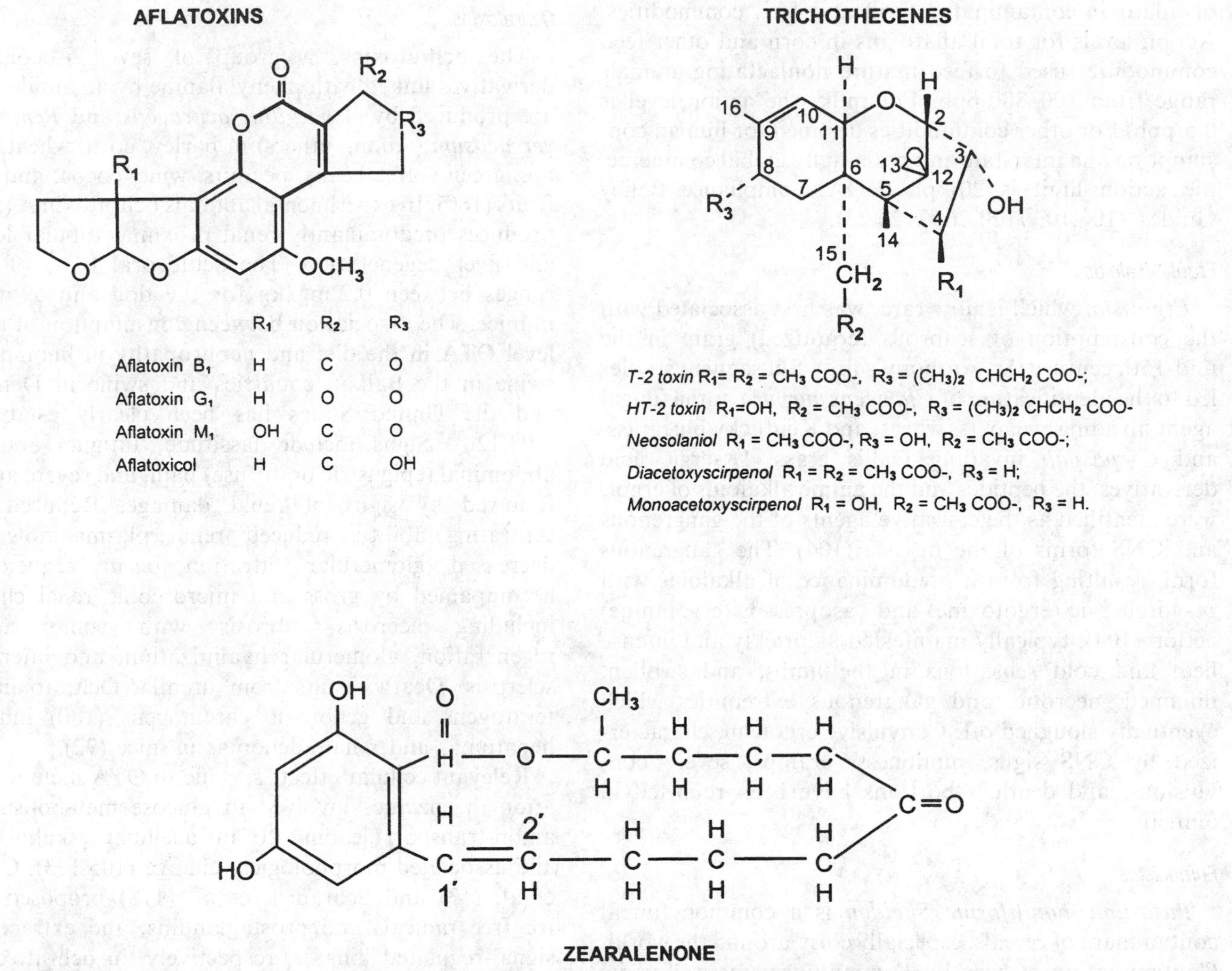

FIG. 11.3. The structure of the mycotoxins, aflatoxins, trichothecenes, ochratoxin A, and zearalenone.

one in 10,000 in the United States. However, in populations infected with hepatitis B, the risk may be 10 to 100 times higher. AFB_1 is mutagenic following metabolic activation in many systems including HeLa cells, *Bacillus subtilis*, *Neurospora crossa*, and *Salmonella typhimurium* (30). A portion of AFB_1 is metabolized by microsomal mixed-function oxidase system in the liver into a variety of reactive products (AFB_1 2,3-epoxide, or e.g.) that from adducts with DNA. Hsieh (82) suggested that subsequent formation of repair-resistant adduct, apurination, or error-prone DNA repair may lead to single strand breaks, base-pair substitution, transversion, or frame shift mutations. Recent evidence has suggested that a higher proportion of liver cancer in high aflatoxin-exposure areas had mutations of the *ρ*53 gene involving $G > T$ transversions of codon 249 (109) and that such effect-biomarkers as well as exposure biomarkers such as AFB_1-DNA or AFB_1-albumin adducts can be used to assess the effectiveness of preventive agents and strategies in public and animal health (95). In addition, AFB_1 inhibits DNA synthesis, DNA-dependent RNA polymerase activity, and messenger RNA synthesis and protein synthesis (81) which may be related to several lesions and signs of aflatoxicosis including fatty liver (failure to mobilize fats from the liver), coagulopathy (inhibition of prothrombin synthesis), and reduced immune function.

Other less widespread human clinical syndromes in which aflatoxins have been implicated include childhood cirrhosis in India; possibly Reye's syndrome in many parts of the world, and, rarely, acute hepatitis (aflatoxicosis) in India, Taiwan, and certain countries in Africa (182).

Widespread concern regarding the toxic effects of aflatoxins in humans and animals and the possible transfer of residues from animal tissues and milk to humans has led to regulatory actions governing the interstate as well as global transport and consumption of aflatoxin-contaminated food and feed commodities. Action levels for total aflatoxins in corn and other feed commodities used to feed mature nonlactating animals range from 100–300 ppb. For milk, the action level is 0.5 ppb. For other commodities destined for human consumption and interstate and potentially global commerce, the action limit is 20 ppb (FDA Compliance Policy Guides 7106.10, 7120.26, 7126.23).

Ergot Alkaloids

Ergotism, which is now rare, was first associated with the consumption of scabrous (ergotized) grain in the mid-16th century (St. Anthony's fire). Subsequent studies led to the identification of *Claviceps purpura* as the fungal agent invading rye, oats, wheat, and Kentucky bluegrass, and *C. paspali* invading Dallis grass. Lysergic acid derivatives, the peptides and the anime alkaloids of ergot, were identified as the causative agents of the gangrenous and CNS forms of the disease (104). The gangrenous form, resulting from a predominance of alkaloids with $\propto$-adrenergic (ergotoxine) and vasopressor (ergotanine) action (104), typically manifested as prickly and intense heat and cold sensations in the limbs, and swollen, inflamed, necrotic, and gangrenous extremities which eventually sloughed off. Convulsive ergotism, characterized by CNS signs, numbness, cramps, severe convulsions, and death. Abortions have been reported in animals.

Fumonisins

Fusarium moniliforme Sheldon is a common fungal contaminant of cereals, especially corn, around the world. Contamination of corn by *F. moniliforme* as well as its major metabolites, fumonisins B_1 and B_2, can induce one of several human and animal diseases including leukoencephalomalacia (LEM) in horses, pulmonary edema in swine, renal and hepatotoxicosis in horses, swine, and rats, and hepatocarcinogenic effect in rats (55). Recent evidence has suggested that FB_1 increases chromosomal aberrations in primary rat hypatocytes (98) and developmental effects in the offspring of pregnant mice (163). Consumption of high levels of fumonisins in home-grown corn has been associated with an higher incidence of human esophageal cancer in certain regions of South Africa and China (125). Although the mechanisms of the toxic and carcinogenic effects are not understood, inhibition of spingolipid biosynthesis (210), enhancement of lipid peroxidation (1), elevated secretion of tumor necrosis factor-alpha (53), depletion of glutathione levels (89), elevated nitric oxide synthesis (169), induction of protein kinase C translocation via its action on phorbolester binding site (222), and inhibition of protein serine/threonine phosphotases (65) are among the changes that can explain some of the effects of FB_1.

Ochratoxins

The ochratoxins, a group of seven isocoumarin derivatives linked with phenylalanine by an amide bond, are produced by *Aspergillus ochraceus* and *Penicillium verrucosum* (among others) in barley, corn, wheat, oats, rye, green coffee beans, peanuts, wine, cocoa, and dried fruits (180). In experimental animals ochratoxin A (OTA) produces predominantly renal proximal tubular lesions and liver degeneration. The acute oral LD_{50} of OTA ranges between 0.2 mg/kg for the dog and 59 mg/kg in mice. The association between consumption of a high level OTA in the diet and nephropathy in humans and swine in the Balkan countries and swine in Denmark and the United States has been clearly established (103,120). Signs include lassitude, fatigue, anorexia, abdominal (epigastric or diffuse) pain, and severe anemia followed by signs of renal damage. Reduced concentrating ability, reduced renal plasma flow, and decreased glomerular filtration occur sequentially, accompanied by gross and microscopic renal changes including necrosis, fibrosis with some tubular regeneration, glomerular hyalinization, and interstitial sclerosis. Death results from uremia. Ochratoxins are teratogens and genotoxic carcinogens (180) inducing hepatomas and renal adenomas in mice (92).

Relevant cellular effects specific to OTA include alteration in enzymes involved in glucose metabolism and anion-transport leading to intracellular alkalinization and associated morphological change (105,133). Creppy et al. (43) and Schramek et al. (178) proposed roles for free radicals and prostaglandins, and extracellular signal-regulated kinases, respectively, in ochratoxin-induced renal damage.

Psoralens

Psoralens are furocoumarin compounds that have been used in repigmenting achromatic skin lesions in an acquired disease called vitiligo, in some suntan lotions, and in drugs used to treat psoriasis (31). Abuse of such compounds can result in dermatitis following exposure to the sun along with nausea, vomiting, vertigo, and mental excitation. A phototoxic dermatitis in celery pickers has been linked to the presence of psoralens (8-methoxypsoralen, 5-methoxypsoralen, and trimethylpsoralen) in stalks infected with *Sclerotinia sclerotiorum* (pink rot), *S. rolfsii*, *Rhizoctonia solani*, or *Erwinia aroideae*, or in celery stalks soaked in 5 percent NaCl (182). Fig, parsley, parsnip, lime, and clove also contain psoralens. 8-Methoxypsoralen appears to undergo epoxidation of the furan ring similar to aflatoxins and may react with DNA in a similar fashion. Treatment with 8-methoxypsoralen and ultraviolet light led to squamous cell carcinomas of the ear in mice (31).

Unlike other photosensitizing agents, psoralens seem to act by photoreacting with DNA, and to a lesser extent, with RNA. The mechanism of psoralen photosensitivity appears to involve intercalation and crosslinking of psoralen in the DNA which occurs in three steps:

(a) reversible intercalation of psoralen between two pyrimidines on opposing sides of the helix;
(b) formation of a monoadduct with the 5,6 double bond of the pyrimidine following absorption of 1 quantum of ultraviolet light; and
(c) crosslink formation by absorption of a second quantum of ultraviolet light and linking of the monoadduct to the 5,6 double bond of thymidine (179). In general, there is an excellent correlation between photoadduct formation and photosensitization of psoralens.

Trichothecenes

Trichothecenes are a group of 12,13-epoxy trichothecenes produced by *Fusarium poae, F. tricinctum, F. graminearum, F. nivale, F. solani, Myrothecium roridum*, and *Stachybatrys atra*, among others, in cereal grains, including wheat. The group of macrocyclic trichothecenes including satratoxins, verrucarins, and roridins is produced mainly by *Stachybotrys* sp. in hay. Although more toxic, this group does not pose significant human health threat due to lack of prevalence. Group A trichothecenes (T-2 toxin, diacetoxyscirpenol) contain a side chain and are relatively less polar compared to group B (nivalenol, deoxynivalenol, fusarenon). A two-volume treatise about trichothecene toxins and their role in human and animal health is available (24).

Most trichothecenes of health significance are produced by *Fusarium* sp. Characteristic signs of alimentary toxic aleukia (ATA), caused by T-2 toxin and related trichothecenes, including radiometric damage such as irritation and necrosis of skin and mucous membranes, hemorrhage, destruction of the thymus and bone marrow, hematological changes, and nervous disturbances; necrotic angina and shock are common to all toxic syndromes (24). Feed refusal, vomiting, and immune suppression are common problems in farm animals, especially swine, in the midwestern United States and are associated predominantly with the presence of the trichothecene, deoxynevalenol (vomitoxin) in wheat and corn (151). Paradoxically, nivalenol and deoxynivalenol exposure of a prolonged duration induced autoimmune-like effects similar to human IgA nephropathy (170). Trichothecenes (T-2 toxin) can cause fetal death, abortions, and teratogenic effects (24). Although several trichothecenes are genotoxic in bacterial, yeast, and cell culture systems (98,201), they exhibit no initiator or promoter effect in whole animal systems (107).

Metabolism of trichothecenes occurs rapidly through deacetylation and hydroxylation and subsequent glucuronidation in the liver and kidneys (24,170), thus posing little problem of residues in meats from contaminated animals. Trichothecenes inhibit protein synthesis which either by itself or together with their ability to induce apoptosis (138) can explain many of their toxic effects. In addition, deoxynivalenol and possibly other trichothecenes affect serotonergic pathways in the brain and also induce expression of a number of cytokines (170). The significance of these effects in trichothecene intoxication in humans and animals is unknown.

Zearalenone

Zearalenone and zearalenol are nonsteroidal estrogenic contaminants (produced by *Fusarium roseum*) in grains such as corn, wheat, sorghum, barley, and oats. Zearalenone induces effects consistent with those produced by excessive steroidal estrogens, that is, anabolic and uterotropic activities and regulation of serum gonadotropins. Although swine appear to be the most sensitive species and exhibit signs of hyperestrogneic syndrome—that is, changes in serum leutinizing hormone, swollen and edematous vulva, hypertrophic myometrium, vaginal cornification and prolapse (in extreme cases), and infertility (151)—human exposure to zearalenone and its metabolites by way of cereal products can also be significant.

The mode of action of zearalenone involves interaction with estrogen receptors, translocation of the receptor–zearalenone complex to the nucleus, combination with chromatin receptors, selective RNA transcription leading to biochemical effects including increased water and lowered lipid content in muscle, and increased permeability of the uterus to glucose, RNA, and protein precursors (67). Available evidence indicates that rapid conversion of zearalenone and zearalanol to conjugated metabolites to be excreted in urine and feces makes consumption of meat and milk from animals receiving Ralgro an insignificant risk to humans.

Zearalenone is genotoxic in bacterial systems (68), forms DNA adducts in female mouse tissues, and induces hepatocellular adenomas in female mice (157). Unknown presently is the carcinogenic risk to humans and whether potentiative interaction exists between the adverse effects of zearalenone and those of dietary or endogenous estrogens as well as the xenoestrogens in the environment.

Other Mycotoxins

A number of other mycotoxins (Table 11.3) have been identified either as contaminants in foods destined for human consumption, or as metabolites of fungi isolated from human foods (29). Although some of these have been associated with outbreaks of domestic animal diseases, no link between human consumption and disease

Table 11.3
Miscellaneous Mycotoxins

Mycotoxin	Major producing organisms	Source of fungi	Principal toxic effects
Alternariol and alternariol methyl ether	*Alternaria* sp.	sorghum, peanuts, wheat	highly teratogenic to mice; cytotoxic to HeLa cells; lethal to mice
Altenuene, altenuisol	*Alternaria* sp.	peanuts	cytotoxic to HeLa cells
Altertoxin 1	*Alternaria* sp.	sorghum, peanuts, wheat	cytotoxic to HeLa cells; lethal to mice
Ascladiol	*Aspergillus clavatus*	wheat flour	lethal to mice
Austamide and congeners	*Aspergillus ustus*	stored foodstuffs	toxic to ducklings
Austadiol	*Aspergillus ustus*	stored foodstuffs	toxic to ducklings
Austin	*Aspergillus ustus*	peas	lethal to chicks
Austocystins	*Aspergillus ustus*	stored foodstuffs	toxic to ducklings; cytotoxic to monkey kidney epithelial cells
Chaetoglobosins	*Penicillium aurantio-virens Chaetomium globosum*	pecans	toxic to chicks; cytotoxic to HeLa cells
Citreoviridin	*Penicillium citreoviride*	rice	neurotoxic, producing convulsions in mice
Citrinin	*Penicillium viridicatum, Penicillium citrinum*	corn, barley	nephrotoxic, swine
Cyclopiazonic acid	*Penicillum cyclopium*	ground nuts, meat products	nephrotoxic, enterotoxic
Cytochalasins	*Aspergillus clavatus* *Phoma* sp. *Phomopsis* sp. *Hormiscium* sp. *Helminthosporium dematioideum* *Metarrhizium anisopliae*	rice, potatoes millet, pecans, tomatoes	Cytotoxic to HeLa cells, teratogenic to mice and chickens
Diplodiatoxin	*Diplodia maydis*	corn	nephrotoxic and enterotoxic to cattle and sheep
Emodin	*Aspergillus wentii*	chestnuts	lethal to chicks
Fumigaclavines	*Aspergillus fumigatus*	silage	enterotoxic to chicks
Kojic acid	*Aspergillus flavus*	squash, spices	lethal to mice
Malformins	*Aspergillus niger*	onions, rice	lethal to rats
Maltoryzine	*Aspergillus oryzae*	malted barley	hepatotoxic and causes paralysis
Moniliformin	*Fusarium moniliforme*	corn	cardiotoxic in rodents
Oosporein (chaetomidin)	*Chaetomium trilaterale*	peanuts	lethal to chicks
Paspalamines	*Claviceps paspali*	Dallisgrass	neurotoxic to cattle and horses; causes paspalum staggers
Patulin	*Penicillium urticae*	apple juice	lethal to mice; mutagenic; teratogenic to chicks; pulmonary effects in dogs; carcinogenic to rats

Table 11.3 (*continued*)

Mycotoxin	Major producing organisms	Source of fungi	Principal toxic effects
Penicillic acid	*Penicillium* sp.	corn, dried beans	lethal to mice; mutagenic; carcinogenic to rats
PR toxin	*Penicillium roqueforti*	mixed grains	hepatotoxic and nephrotoxic to rats; abortion in cattle
Roseotoxin B	*Trichothecium roseum*	corn	toxic to mice and ducklings
Rubratoxins	*Penicillium rubrum*	corn	causes hemorrhage in animals; hepatoxic to cattle
Secalonic acids	*Aspergillus aculeatus* *Penicillium oxalicum*	rice, corn	lethal, cardiotoxic, lung-irritant, and teratogenic to mice
Slaframine	*Rhizoctonia leguminicola*	red clover	salivation and lacrymation in horses and cattle
Sporidesmins	*Pithomyces chartarum*	pasture grasses	hepatotoxic, causes photosensitization in ruminants
Sterigmatocystin	*Aspergillus flavus*	mammals	mutagen, carcinogen, and hepatotoxic to mammals
Tenuazonic acid	*Alternaria* sp.	grains, nuts	lethal to mice
Terphenyllins	*Aspergillus candidus*	wheat flour	hepatoxic to mice; cytotoxic to HeLa cells
Tremorgenic Mycotoxins			
Fumitremorgens A and B	*Aspergillus fumigatus*	rice	neurotoxic (prolonged tremors and convulsions)
Paxilline	*Penicillium paxilli*	pecans	neurotoxic (prolonged tremors and convulsions)
Penitrems A, B, and C	*Penicillium cyclopium*	peanuts, meat products, cheese	neurotoxic (prolonged tremors and convulsions) to cattle, sheep, dogs, and horses
Tryptoquivalines	*Aspergillus clavatus*	rice	neurotoxic (prolonged tremors and convulsions)
Verruculogen (TR-1)	*Penicillium verru culosum*	peanuts	neurotoxic (prolonged tremors and convulsions)
Unidentified Toxin(s)	*Aspergillus terrus* *Balansia epichloe* *Epichloe typhina* *Fusarium tricinctum* and others	fescue grass	gangrene (Fescue foot); summer slump syndrome; fat necrosis and agalactia in cattle
Xanthoascin	*Aspergillus candidus*	wheat flour	hepatotoxic and cardiotoxic to mice

Condensed and modified from Reference 29.

has been established. Others have been shown to induce toxic and lethal effects in laboratory animals with no association between consumption of these toxins by animals or humans and a disease syndrome. Several of these, for example, cytochalasins and secalonic acid D (162), have been used to expand our understanding of normal as well as abnormal cellular responses to xenobiotics.

Although it is difficult to assess the total significance of the consumption of mycotoxins in human foods, it is easy to conceive that such a task requires extensive research into hundreds of known and a potentially large number of as yet unknown mycotoxins. In spite of the vast number of toxic metabolites, reduction in mycotoxin levels in foods and feeds and the prevention of mycotoxicoses in humans and animals can be achieved for the most part by avoiding stress in crops and damage to seeds by pests and by mechanical harvesting. Rapid postharvest drying and avoiding conditions that promote mold growth during storage are equally important.

Pesticides

Pesticides are essential in agriculture. The National Monitoring Program for Food and Feed, comprised of three federal surveillance programs (i.e., the Total Diet Study of market foods by the FDA, nationwide monitoring of unprocessed food and feed by the FDA, and analysis of meat and poultry by the USDA), monitors residues of chlorinated hydrocarbon insecticides, organophosphates and carbamates, and, very infrequently, herbicides and inorganic pesticides such as Arsenic and bromide in various agricultural products. Despite the ban on DDT in 1972 and aldrin and dieldrin in 1975, a partial ban on heptachlor and chlordane in 1978, and a complete ban on heptachlor in 1983 and others later, residues of these and other chlorinated pesticides and their metabolites continue to appear, especially in dairy products, meat, fish, and poultry. In most cases, however, the daily intake of a pesticide did not exceed the ADI established by a Joint Food and Agriculture Organization (FAO)/World Health Organization (WHO) Expert Committee on Pesticide Residues. Intoxication with a pesticide usually results from accidental or suicidal ingestion, careless storage, or improper use. The toxic effects of individual pesticides are discussed in Chapter 13.

Toxic Metals

A high proportion of the general population's total daily exposure to metals occurs from their natural presence in foods. Beverages, water, air, and contact with metal-containing consumer products contribute to the rest. Children consume more calories per unit body weight and have a higher absorption rate than adults, placing them at a higher risk for metal toxicity than adults.

Industrial and agricultural uses of metal products pose the hazard of food-contamination associated with their use, storage, accidental spillage, and improper disposal. The recent decline in the use of heavy metal-based pesticides, including herbicides, makes acute poisonings from dietary toxic metals less likely. A decline in the use of containers with metal coatings that dissolve during food manufacture, cooking, and storage has also contributed to the decline in acute toxicities associated with metals. Food-borne intoxications from metals are mostly limited to long-term consumption of water and food products from environments that contain naturally high levels of metals (e.g., selenium and fluoride) or that are contaminated by mining, smelting, and industrial discharge (e.g., methylmercury and Minamata disease). The reader is referred to Chapter 14 for information on the toxic effects of metals.

FOOD ADDITIVES

The increasing demand for food by an ever-increasing world population, and for ready-to-eat foods because of changes in lifestyles in developed societies, has necessitated the use of chemical additives to help preserve, nutritionally fortify, and process foods. Concerns about adulteration (masking of low-quality food by chemical additives) and of toxic effects from chronic dietary chemical exposure have led to the passage of the Food and Drug Act of 1906; the Food, Drug, and Cosmetic Act of 1938; the Miller Pesticide Amendment of 1954; the Food Additive Amendment of 1958; the Color Additive Amendment of 1960; the Animal Drug Amendment of 1968; the Federal Food, Drug, and Cosmetic Act (FFDCA) of 1976; and the Federal Food Quality Protection Act (FFQPA) of 1996. The term, *food additive*, is defined in these acts as

> "...any substance the intended use of which results or may reasonably be expected to result, directly or indirectly, in its becoming a component or otherwise affecting the characteristic of any food (including any substance intended for use in producing, manufacturing, packing, processing, preparing, treating, packaging, transporting, or holding food; and including any source of radiation intended for any such use), if such substance is not generally recognized, among experts qualified by scientific training and experience to evaluate its safety, as having been adequately shown through scientific procedures (or, in the case of substances used in food prior to January 1, 1958, through either scientific procedures or experience based on common use in food) to be safe under the conditions of its intended use..."

Food additives fall into two broad categories, direct and indirect. Direct additives are those intentionally added to foods to preserve or improve the quality of the product or to aid in the processing. Some examples of 32 functional classes of direct additives are antioxidants, inhibitors of bacterial and mold growth, vitamins and minerals, color, and antifoaming agents. Among the approximately 3000 direct additives, more than 500 are "generally recognized as safe" (GRAS), and about 150 are sanctioned as safe prior to September 6, 1958, with their number likely to increase. They are exempt from regulation as food additives unless the scientific review of these substances currently underway warrants reclassification in the future. Sucrose, corn syrup, dextrose, and salt (all on GRAS list) account for 93 percent, by weight, of all the food additives used. Indirect additives are chemicals that gain their way into foods unintentionally or unavoidably during some phase of production, processing, storage, or packaging. Components of packaging containers and materials that migrate into foods fall under this category. In addition, the presence of pesticide residues in crops and processed foods and residues from animal drugs in milk, meat, and eggs is allowed based on their potential health risk as balanced against the benefits of their use.

Safety Assessment of Food Additives

Foods in their natural forms are assumed safe unless they are "ordinarily injurious." The presence of avoidable contaminant(s) posing a risk of injury to health renders the food unsafe and subject to recall, while the presence of unavoidable contaminant(s) posing such risk is considered unsafe if it exceeds tolerance levels set by FDA (or EPA) or action levels (informal and not subject to law) set by FDA. Intentional additives other than those GRAS or those that are prior sanctioned (e.g., colors) are subject to regulations described above and can only be used at levels posing a risk at or below the level considered acceptable.

Safety evaluation of direct food additives involves establishment of a no observable adverse effect level (NOAEL) in experimental animals followed by establishment of acceptable daily intake (ADI) in the total diet for human beings using a suitable safety factor (usually 100). For unavoidable contaminants, tolerance levels are set to limit the quantity of the agent in each commodity based on risk–benefit–cost analysis.

The FDA-recommended safety testing approach is based on the concept of "level of concern" (28). Level of concern is based on the level of exposure, structural correlation with known toxic compounds (if no toxicity data are available), and existing toxicological data. Subjective categorization of additives into concern levels I, II, or III (level III being of highest concern) is done for compounds contributing <0.05 pmm, 0.05–1.0 ppm, and >1.0 ppm, respectively, to the total diet. Also, low, medium, or high toxicity or a structural similarity to compounds with low, medium, or high toxicity places a compound in concern levels I, II, or III, respectively. Furthermore, formation of active metabolites would place the compound in level III.

Table 11.4 lists recommended toxicological tests for each level of concern. This testing scheme allows compounds producing effects only at high levels and those with lower levels of human exposure to be tested less extensively. Protocols for testing color additives and indirect food additives are similar to direct food additive testing. Safety testing of animal drugs and feed additives, however, is more complex not only because an additional animal species (target animal) is involved but also because of the necessity of understanding the impact of target animal metabolism on the diversity and toxic potential of the metabolites to humans, the need for the development of residue detection methods and elimination strategies in the target animal species, and to set maximum allowable residues (tolerance) of the parent compound and metabolites in tissues of the target animal.

Food and color additive use is regulated by a special anti-cancer clause, the Delaney Clause, in the Food Additive Amendment. The Delaney Clause prohibits the use of these additives "if they are found to induce cancer when ingested by man or animal, or if found, after tests which are appropriate to the evaluation of safety of such substances, to induce cancer in man or animal" (59). Although the addition of the Delaney Clause reflected the then-prevailing concern for cancer, subsequent scrutiny and recent developments in the understanding of the mechanisms of carcinogenesis required changes as reflected in the FQPA of 1996. Currently, the regulation of pesticide residues has become the responsibility of EPA and, thus, is not an issue for the FDA as a food additive. EPA can approve pesticide applications if it concludes that there is "a reasonable certainty that no harm will result from its aggregate exposure." This would translate to no greater than a risk of 1 in 1 million lifetime risk for carcinogens and levels with a 100-fold safety margin to NOAEL for threshold-limited effects. For already approved carcinogenic pesticides, EPA is allowed to retain tolerance posing greater than negligible risk (1 in 1 million) if the pesticide either protects consumers from a greater health risk or is necessary to avoid disruption of an adequate, wholesome, and economical food supply (134). In addition, the FQPA directs EPA to take higher intakes for certain pesticides in children into consideration in setting tolerances and to apply an additional safety factor of 10 for threshold effects in calculating ADI.

Animal Drugs

All new animal drugs and feeds containing them must receive premarket clearance from the Bureau of Veterin-

Table 11.4
Test schedule recommended by FDA for additives at various concern levels

Concern Level I	Concern Level II	Concern Level III
1. Short-term (at least 28 days) feeding study in a rodent species 2. Short-term test for carcinogenic potential	1. Subchronic feeding study in a rodent species 2. Subchronic feeding study in a non-rodent species 3. Multi- (at least two) generation reproduction study with teratology, in a rodent species 4. Short-term test for carcinogenic potential	1. Chronic (at least 1 yr) feeding study in a rodent species 2. Chronic (at least 1 yr) feeding study in a non-rodent species 3. Multi- (at least two) generation reproduction study with teratology, in a rodent species 4. Short-term test for carcinogenic potential 5. Carcinogenicity studies in two rodent species (test 1 can be a part of this)

ary Medicine of the FDA. Antibiotics and steroidal as well as nonsteroidal growth promotants are used in feeds for the prevention of disease or for growth promotion in raising 60 to 100 percent of food-producing animals. Two major concerns with the use of antibiotics in animal feeds are: the development of resistance in enteric bacteria in animals that could be transferred via plasmids to pathogenic bacteria in the gut of animals and, thus, to humans through meat or milk, making antibiotics currently used in human medicine ineffective; and, the presence of carcinogenic residues in meat or residues that form carcinogenic nitrosamines following reaction with nitrite in the meat. Increasing pressure on the FDA has already resulted in the exclusion of many antibiotics (kanamycin, gentamicin, semisynthetic penicillins, chloramphenicol etc.) as feed additives with exclusion of all likely in the future.

Similarly, concerns about the use of hormonal and other growth promotants in feeds are related to possible chronic toxic effects, mainly carcinogenicity. The synthetic estrogen, diethylstilbestrol (DES), was banned as a feed additive due to its carcinogenic effects and the lack of a method sensitive enough to detect residues of health significance (causing >1 life time cancer in 1 million population). Steroids approved for feed additive use in one or more animal species include estradiol, progesterone, testosterone, melengestrol acetate, and zearalanol. Other additives commonly used in animal production include monensin, iodides (EDDI), phenothiazine, and thiabendazole. Carcinogenic animal drugs can be approved for use by the FDA if an adequate withdrawal period is recommended between the last dose of the additive and slaughter to allow residues to fall below those judged capable of inducing greater than negligible (1 lifetime cancer in 1 million) incidence of cancer.

Toxic reactions associated with the use of selected additives that have been restricted, banned, or are currently being critically reviewed are presented below.

Direct Food Additives

Aspartame (Nutrasweet)

The use of aspartame (L-aspartyl-L-phenylalanine methyl ester) as a sweetener in a large variety of food products increases the likelihood that acceptable daily intake is exceeded. Previously suspected association between aspartame consumption and the anecdotal reports of headache, dizziness, and seizures in adults and hyperkinesia in children appears to be unsupported. Although nitrosation products of aspartame are moderately mutagenic (184), the question of the role of aspartame in the recent increase of lymphoma of the brain remains unresolved. The metabolism of aspartame to phenyl alanine led to the suggestion that patients with phenylketonuria should avoid aspartame-containing products.

Butylated Hydroxy Anisole (BHA)

Synthetic phenolic antioxidant BHA has been GRAS and used for decades as an antioxidant to retard the autoxidation of lipids and prevent rancidity in foods. Together with ascorbic acid, α-tocopherol, gallate esters, and BHT, it fulfills almost 100 percent of the antioxidant needs of foods. BHA may be a rodent carcinogen involving squamous cells in the forestomach but these cells are not the human equivalent of glandular or other cells. The carcinogenicity of BHA appears to involve O-demethylation of BHA to tertiarybutyl hydroquinone (TBHQ), oxidation of TBHQ to tertiary butyl semiquinone and tertiary butylquinone (TBQ), conjugation of TBQ with glutathione (GSH), and formation of DNA-reactive oxygen species including the hydroxyl radical (207). However, genotoxicity of BHA has not been demonstrated. Since humans lack a forestomach, evidence for direct genotoxic effect is lacking, and since human exposure is well below inducing nongenotoxic effects it is highly unlikely that BHA carcinogenicity in rodents is relevant to the safety of BHA in human foods.

Cyclamates

Sodium and calcium cyclamate were introduced as non-nutritive sweeteners in 1950 and were included in the 1959 GRAS list. Significant consumption of cyclamates in low-calorie foods and drinks followed. Subsequent demonstration of cancer-promoting or co-carcinogenic activity in animals led to the removal of cyclamates from the GRAS list and, thus, from food additive use in the United States, despite a lack of evidence in human beings (5). Cyclamates, however, are still used in many other countries.

Monosodium Glutamate (MSG)

MSG has been on the GRAS list since 1958, used as both a seasoning agent and a flavor enhancer with an ADI of 120 mg/kg. The demonstration of lesions in the retina and the lateral geniculate nucleus in MSG-exposed neonatal rats and mice led to a voluntary discontinuation of its use in infant foods in the United States. This appears justified since neonatal effects of MSG may last through adulthood (193). In adults, the MSG symptom complex (headache, muscle tightness, numbness/tingling, general weakness, and flushing, among others) occurs in a third of the population with a threshold dose of 2.5 g of MSG (220).

Nitrates, Nitrites, and Nitrosamines

Of the total daily dietary intake of nitrates of 10—150 mg/day (48), leafy vegetables contribute 99 percent. Nitrate use to cure meats (to give characteristic flavor and pink color, to prevent rancidity, and to prevent growth of the spores of *Clostridium botulinum*) contributes <0.1 mg/day (48). Nitrates can be reduced endogenously by microbial systems to nitrites which then oxidize the hemoglobin to methemoglobin (heme iron from ferrous to ferric state). Methemoglobin, being unable to combine with oxygen, following accumulation in sufficient quantities, can lead to anoxia. The use of water with high (>30 mg/l) nitrate content (from soils, fertilizers, etc.) in making baby formula and foods, spinach with high nitrate content, and occasionally meats with high levels of added nitrates and nitrites have resulted in life-threatening methemoglobinemia in humans, especially children. The consumption of plants high in nitrates by animals has caused significant economic loss for owners. In adult humans, however, the daily intake of nitrate and nitrite amount to less than 69 percent and 0.7 percent of the ADI of 3.64 and 0.135 mg/kg/day (48).

Nitrite reacts with secondary amines to form a variety of N-nitrosamines which are present in foods, pharmaceuticals, cosmetics, agricultural chemicals, tobacco, and tea. In vivo, nitrosamines are converted to unstable hydroxyalkyl compounds which subsequently form reactive alkyl carbonium ions capable of alkylating DNA (207). Nitrosamines are mutagens and rodent carcinogens, producing cancer in a variety of organs, including the liver, respiratory tract, kidney, urinary bladder, esophagus, stomach, lower gastrointestinal tract, and pancreas (207). Nitrite itself may promote carcinogenesis. Because they are not added to foods, however, nitrosamines are not subject to the restrictions of the Delaney Amendment. Inhibition of nitrosamine formation in foods by ascorbate, cysteine, gallic acid, tannins, sodium sulfite, and sodium erythorbate prompted the FDA to suggest that one of these compounds be concurrently added to meats during curing to reduce nitrite added from 200 to 120 ppm. Such a practice, however, is ill-advised until a suitable additive is found to deal with the threat of *C. botulinum* growth at reduced nitrate levels and while consumers accept the ensuing changes in the appearance and organoleptics properties of meat cured with this combination. Perhaps a change to lower nitrate-containing vegetables to reduce nitrate intake is a less dangerous option.

Saccharin

After having been in use since the beginning of the 20th century and surviving a ban and an attempted ban of its use due to suspected weak bladder cancer-promoting activity (142) at high doses, saccharin continues to be used as a sweetener in soft drinks and in table top uses. The average intake is 7.1 mg/day in the United States and 15.0 mg/day in Europe per capita, reaching as high as 25 mg/day in certain subpopulations (86). In 2000,

Saccharin was delisted as a human carcinogen by the National Toxicology Program.

Safrole

Safrole and other alkenylbenzene compounds (β-asarone, methyleugenol, estragole, and isosafrole) are active components of many spice flavors. Sassafras, which contains high levels of safrole, has been used as a flavoring agent in sarsaparilla root beer. Safrole also is consumed in the form of sassafras oil and sassafras tea, the latter still occurring to a limited extent in the United States. A total dose of only 0.5–1.5 mg of safrole orally or intraperitoneally to infant male mice caused high liver tumor incidence. Dihydrosafrole, a synthetic safrole, caused esophageal tumors in rats, and some of the other natural alkenylbenzenes also are carcinogenic (135). These findings resulted in the FDA ban on the use of safrole, sassafras, and sassafras oil from commercial use in foods, including root beer, in 1960. Safrole continues to be used in the European Community, however. A metabolite, 1-hydroxy sulfate ester, is apparently the ultimate carcinogen, forming adducts with guanine and adenine (135).

Other chemical additives initially approved as safe by a regulatory body but now prohibited from use due to a potential risk or to lack of demonstration of safety include calamus and its derivatives in 1968 (containing aklenylbenzene flavoring agents); coumarin flavoring compounds in 1953; chlorofluorocarbon propellants in self-pressurized containers in 1978 (due to their role in the dissolution of the earth's ozone layer, which results in increased skin cancer risk from ultraviolet radiation); diethyl pyrocarbonate (DEPC), an antimicrobial agent in beers and juices (cold pasteurization) and a ferment inhibitor, in 1972, due to the presence of the carcinogen urethan in DEPC-treated products; and dulcin, a sweetener, in 1950, due to liver and bladder cancer in rats. On the other hand, the ultimate determination of the safety of recently approved additives such as the fat substitute, Olestra (long-chain fatty acid esters with sugar), must await longer-term consumer use.

Food Colors

Color is a quality of foods that makes them visually acceptable and aids in their recognition. Foods containing added colors include candy and confections, bakery goods, soft drinks, cereals, and dairy products such as butter, ice cream, and sherbet, margarine, snack foods, jams and jellies, and dessert powders. Following the passage of the Color Additive Amendment of 1960, 20 natural colors (compromising preparations such as dried algae meal, beet powder, grape skin extract, fruit juice, paprika, caramel, carrot oil, cochineal extract, ferrous gluconate, and iron oxide) were exempted from certification, whereas all the synthetic colors, including the ones approved prior to the amendment, were required to be retested if questions arose regarding their safety. A provisional certification was given to those in use that required further testing. Currently, there are seven certified synthetic colors (FD&C colors Blue No. 1, Red No. 3, Red No. 40, and Yellow No. 5 are permanently listed whereas FDB Blue No. 2, Green No. 3, and Yellow No. 6 are provisionally listed) with unlimited uses (according to good manufacturing practices) and one permanently listed color (Citrus Red No. 2) used only for coloring skins of oranges at 2 ppm. Several colors including Green No. 1, Green No. 2, Orange No. B, Red No. 2, Red No. 4, and Violet No. 1 were delisted due to concerns about their carcinogenicity and other chronic toxic effects. A controversy linking food colors to allergies and hyperkinesis in children failed to draw supportive evidence.

Packaging Materials

Packaging is an essential part of food processing that aids in the preservation of the wholesomeness of foods by preventing

(a) contamination or destruction by dirt, microorganisms, insects, and rodents,
(b) loss or gain of moisture, odors, flavors, or aroma, and
(c) deterioration from air, light, heat, and contaminating gases (69).

Other functions served by packaging include assembling a variety of items, convenient handling, labeling, and, finally, sales promotion. A variety of materials, ranging from metal foils to complex plastic substances, are in use. Examples of package modifications employing chemical additives are oleoresinous coating with or without suspended ZnO, which is used in the preservation of acid foods that do (e.g., seafood) or do not (e.g., cherries) produce sulfides; stabilizers to prevent degradation of plastic when exposed to heat and light; and hot-melt adhesives used to glue multilayered packages (tea, hydrated soups, potato chips, etc.). A complete list of additives approved for use in packaging is given by Gilchrist (69).

To approve new packaging material, FDA requires extraction studies involving one or more of aqueous (8% alcohol), alcoholic (50% alcohol), or lipid solvents (corn oil or triglycerides), followed by toxicity testing depending upon the extent of extraction, >1 ppm requiring extensive testing including chronic toxicity. The National Science Foundation (NSF) estimated that as many as 3000 chemicals may enter foods indirectly from the process of packaging itself (75). A safety review by the FDA has resulted in banning the adhesive Flectol

H, polyurethane resins and curing agents food packaging adhesives containing 4, 4-methylenebis (2-chloroanaline), and the synthetic chemicals, mercaptoimidazoline and 2-mercaptoimidazoline, used in the production of rubber articles (75). The use of polyvinylchloride for packaging liquors has been banned in the United States. Among the packaging-derived contaminants likely to be encountered in U.S. diets, benzene and vinyl chloride are known carcinogens; acrylonitrile, 1,3-butadiene, epidilorohydrin, formaldehyde, propylene oxide, and styrene oxide, are probable carcinogens; and 2,4-diaminololuene, dibutyl and diethylhexylphthalates, dimethylformamide, 1,4-dioxane, ethylacrylate, phenyl glycidil ether, styrene, and toluene diisocyanate are possible carcinogens (86,146).

Toxic Factors Produced During Processing

Food processing is aimed at improving the quality of foodstuffs, ensuring safety, and enhancing the ease of preparation. This requires various chemical and physical treatments of food which may result in

(a) partial or complete destruction or removal of nutrients,
(b) inferior digestibility or utilization of nutrients, and
(c) generation of new, potentially harmful chemicals.

The first two effects can be overcome by nutritional supplementation. The latter represents a need for appropriate toxicological investigation. In addition, similar products can be formed during storage due to the continuous effects of heat, humidity, light, oxygen, and catalysts present in foods.

Formation of crosslinked amino acid side chains such as lysinoalanine, ornithinoalanine, and lanthionine, as well as racemization of amino acids to D-analog appear to take place during alkali treatment, for example, of soybean protein for preparing imitation meat (62). These products, especially lysinoalanine, have been shown to cause nephrocytomegaly (enlarged nuclei and cytoplasm) of the pars recta cells. Nonenzymatic browning reactions (Maillard reactions) occurring during heating of foods (drying, frying, roasting, baking, and broiling) involve chemical interactions between amino acids and reducing sugars (aldoses and ketoses), forming mutagenic reductones, furans, amino-carbonyls, pyrazines, and other premelanoid secondary amine derivatives (Amadori and Heyns' products) which are hypothesized to inhibit growth, impair reproduction, damage the liver, cause allergies, play a role in aging, and induce lens lesions (86).

In general, high-protein foods appear to possess more mutagenic activity compared with foods rich in carbohydrates and/or fats. Pyrolysis of proteins and amino acids at high temperatures (300°C or more) yields a series of heterocyclic compounds which can be metabolized to mutagenic products were positive in one or more rodent species for carcinogenicity (86,195). Using estimates of various heterocyclic amines ingested and cancer potencies in animal studies, Layton et al. (110) estimated that only 0.25 percent of human colorectal cancer may be due to these compounds. Certain cooking practices such as frying of high nitrite foods such as cured bacon results in the formation of nitrosamines whose carcinogenic effects have already been discussed.

A variety of polycyclic aromatic hydrocarbons (PAH) are formed in foods by pyrolysis during cooking or by their prior contact with petroleum and/or coal tar products. Although the carcinogenic effects of PAH are known, the contribution of dietary PAH to cancer in humans is likely to be insignificant.

Fats (polyunsaturated) undergo three basic changes during storage and/or heat treatments, that is, autoxidation, thermal oxidation, and thermal polymerization. Autoxidation occurs at below 100°C in the presence of enzymes (lipoxygenases) or upon exposure to light and results in the generation of hydroperoxides via a free-radical or singlet oxygen mechanism leading to rancidity (86). Hydroperoxides can be degraded into alkanes, aldehydes, and ketones, among others. Termination of peroxidative reactions generally involves scavenging of the radicals or their polymerization into nonreactive products. Lipid hydroperoxides, at subtoxic levels, can stimulate signal transduction mediated by Ca^{++} and protein phosphorylation by acting as second messengers in pathways involved in cell proliferation, chemotaxis, apoptosis, and other cellular mechanisms (196). High levels of rancid fats (5% or more of the diet) can cause decreased food consumption, diarrhea, weight loss, leukopenia, and hair loss. Hydroperoxides and/or their products (hydroxynonenal, melon-dialdehyde, etc.) can disrupt gap-junctional communication and form DNA adducts, and are mutagenic and carcinogenic, increasing the incidence of tumors and atherosclerosis (86,221). Components of heated oils that fail to form adducts with urea, especially the cyclic monomeric fatty acids followed by polymers of fatty acids, appear to be toxic. Toxic effects include, in addition to those described above, hepatomegaly and carcinogenicity.

Yeast-fermented foods and beverages such as yogurt, cider, malt beverages, bread, soy sauce, wine, and sake, in addition to psychoactive and vasoactive amines discussed earlier, contain mutagenic and carcinogenic ethyl carbamate (urethane) derived, in the presence of heat and light, from arginine, asparagine, cyanogenic glycosides, or ethanol in the fermented commodity. Levels of <10 ppb or less for soft drinks and <30–400 ppb for various alcoholic beverages have been recommended as acceptable by the FAO/WHO and the Canadian government, respectively (87).

The major fermentation product consumed by humans is ethanol which, in addition to death from toxic effects, contributes to human deaths from occupational as well as automobile accidents. The toxic effects of ethanol, although they can manifest themselves in many organ systems, display major CNS involvement (dependence and depression), and impact the developing fetus (fetal alcohol syndrome of mental deficiency and microcephaly) and the liver (hepatomegaly followed by cirrhosis). Mechanisms of ethanol toxicosis may involve the direct effects of alcohol, effects of its metabolite acetaldehyde, ethanol-induced malnutrition, ethanol-induced endotoxin release by intestinal bacteria that stimulate release of reactive chemicals by Kupfer's cells, ethanol-induced potentiation of other hepatotoxic agents, or a combination. An International Agency for Research on Cancer (IARC) expert panel considered ethanol a human carcinogen causing tumors of the oral cavity, pharynx, esophagus, and liver (189).

Toxic effects of processed food as a whole, however, cannot be estimated by simply adding up the toxic, mutagenic, and/or carcinogenic potential of the products present in it. This is due to the fact that chemical derivatives which both enhance as well as antagonize the myriad toxic effects of other dietary components are formed during processing (146). At present, these chemicals and their interactions with each other, for the most part, are unknown. As a result, the overall adverse effects of cooked foods can only be determined reliably based on the assessment of risk from the complex milieus of the product in question.

CARCINOGENS AND MUTAGENS IN FOODS

Cancer, a disease of most public concern for the past half a century, is, experimentally, a multistage process involving initiation (induction of DNA damage, thus resulting in a transformed cell), promotion (a nongenotoxic effect leading to a rapid multiplication of the transformed cell and, thus, establishment of a cancerous lesion), and progression. Multistage models involving a sequence of multiple genetic events with the incidence increasing in proportion to the exponent of time, however, seem to fit most human cancers (146). Naturally occurring food toxicants provide examples of both initiators and promoters, with up to 70 percent of cancer deaths being attributed to dietary factors (51). Examples of likely dietary carcinogens as reviewed by the National Research Council (NRC) (146) are provided in Table 11.5. This list includes carcinogens derived from natural products both by commercial processing (e.g., alcohol) as well as biotransformation in the body (e.g., allylisothiocyanate and nitrosamines); and initiators (e.g., aflatoxins, furocoumarins, pyrrolizidine alkaloids) as well as promoters (e.g., phorbol esters, fat, caffeine). In addition, residues of synthetic chemicals can be present in foods subsequent to their accidental contact or intentional use to increase production. An added dimension to diet is the formation of animal and possibly human carcinogens during cooking, including nitrosamines, aromatic hydrocarbons, amino acid pyrrolysates, carbolines, imidazoquinolines, quinoxalines, and fat oxidation products inducing cancer of the liver, stomach, intestines, zymbal and clitoral glands, skin, and oral cavity and others (146). Coffee, in addition to caffeine, is known to yield several animal carcinogens including caffeic acid, catechol, furfural, hydrogen peroxide, and hydroquinone during roasting and/or brewing (11). Carcinogenic natural pesticides are present in all classes of plant foods including fruits, vegetables, and spices (11).

Balancing this bewildering array of toxins and carcinogens, in almost every food item, is another group of chemicals capable of antagonizing these effects. The dietary antimutagens and anticarcinogens, whose mechanisms of action are not always understood, belong to a wide variety of chemical structures (Table 11.6). As with mutagens, multiple species of antimutagens/anticarcinogens appear to be present in each dietary component (at least five are known in soybeans and three or more in broccoli). Interactions between carcinogens and anticarcinogens are complicated as indicated by the study of indole-3-carbinol, a component of cruciferous vegetables, known to inhibit mammary and forestomach neoplasia in rodents. When given as a pretreatment, indole carbinol reduced the carcinogenicity of aflatoxin B_1, while exposure to indole carbinol after the carcinogen exposure resulted in an increase in aflatoxin carcinogenicity (17).

Natural versus Synthetic Chemicals

The widely held belief that naturally (free of synthetic chemicals) grown foods are inherently safer than those grown with the aid of synthetic chemicals is flawed. Certain natural chemicals in the human diet (such as indole carbinol in cruciferous vegetables) interact with the same receptor (Ah) as dioxin (TCDD), one of the most feared synthetic toxicants, interacts (12). An EPA reference dose, a dose estimated to produce one cancer in one million individuals (6 fg/kg/day), of TCDD is comparable to 5 mg of indole carbinol per 100 g of broccoli or cabbage, a level of exposure not unrealistic. The EPA ban on alar—using a worst-case scenario risk estimation in response to public outcry resulting from less-than-objective reporting by the media and a passive attitude by knowledgeable academicians and researchers (168)—suggests that regulatory agencies also may subscribe to this misconception.

The NRC (146), however, considers natural carcinogens at least as potent and, considering the extent of exposure, more potent than synthetic carcinogens. The fact that disproportionately fewer natural chemicals have been tested suggests a greater need to test natural chemicals, a daunting task considering that all toxicants in all classes of foods are not known and that exposures to those that are known are wide-ranging and not well documented.

Table 11.5
Naturally occurring carcinogens and potential carcinogens in the diet

Carcinogen/Mutagen	Major Foods Containing the Chemical
Alcohol	grains and fruits (derived from . . .)
Allylisothiocyanate	cabbage, collard greens, brussels sprouts, mustard (brown)
Caffeic acid, Caffeine, and Theobromine	coffee, cocoa, fruits, and vegetables
Cyclopropene fatty acids	cotton seed oil, kapok, and okra
Fat (unsaturated and cholesterol-containing)	vegetable and animal fats
Flavonoids (Quercetin, etc.)	vegetables, tea, coffee
Furocoumarins (psoralen)	celery, figs, parsley, parsnips
Gossypol	cottonseed oil
Hormones (estrogen, testosterone, progestins, and related)	meats as residues, supplements
Hydrazines (agaritine, gyromitrin)	mushrooms
d-Limonine	citrus juices
Methylazoxymethanol, cycasin	cycads
Mycotoxins (aflatoxins, fumonisins, ochratoxin A, sterigmatocystin)	corn, cottonseed, peanuts, wheat, and other grains
Nitrosamines	beets, celery, spinach, meat preserved in nitrite
Phorbol esters	croton oil, other Euphorbaceae (herbal teas)
Polyphenols (tannic acid)	beverages (tea, cider, cocoa, red wine), fruits
Ptaquiliside	bracken fern
Pyrrolizidine alkaloids	herbs, herbal teas, honey
Safrole, estragole, methyleugenol, piperine, etc.	nutmeg, other spices, black pepper
Cooked food carcinogens/mutagens	all cooked foods
Polyaromatic hydrocarbons (mono and dibenzo derivatives)	
Maillard reaction products	
Amino acid pyrrolysates (Trp-P-1-, Trp-P-2; Glu-P-1, Glu-P-2)	
Carbolines	
Imidazoquinolines and quinoxalines (IQ, MeIQ, MeIQx)	
Fat oxidation products	
Coffee-derived mutagens/carcinogens	

Table 11.6
Important antimutagens and anticarcinogens naturally occurring in foods

Class/subclass	Examples	Foods containing them
Alkaloids	indole-3-carbinol, caffeine	broccoli, cabbage, cauliflower, coffee
Amino acids	cysteine and tryptophan, curcumin	many plants and animals
Arylheptanoids		tumeric
Benzenoids	gingerol, paradol	ginger root and related plants
Cyclitols	myoinostol, phytic acid	wheat, other cereals, nuts, and meats?
Estrogens	sitosterol	soybeans, alfalfa, etc.
Fatty acid derivatives	conjugated linoleic and arachidonic acid	vegetable oils
Fiber	acid-soluble, neutral, etc.	fruits and vegetables, cereal bran
Minerals	Se, Ca^{++}	crops grown on Se-containing soils, milk, meat
Phenolics		
Phenolic acids	gallic and protocatechuic acids,	many fruits and vegetables
Phenyl propanoids	caffeic, cinnamic, chlorogenic and ferrulic acids, enginol, myristicin	broccoli, other vegetables
Flavones	apigenin, myricetin, quercetin, robinetin, rutin	fruits, herbs, and vegetables
Isoflavones	biochanin A, genistein, daidzein, etc.	soybeans and others
Polyphenols		
Lignans	sesamin	sesame seed
Tannins	ellagic and tannic acids, epigallo-catechin-gallate	Chinese green tea, other teas, cereals, legumes, and fruits
Protease Inhibitors	antipain, elastatinal	
Porphyrins	chlorophyll, chlorophyllin, cytochrome C, hemin, hemoglobin, myoglobin	green leafy vegetables, meats
Sulfur-containing compounds	benzyl isothiocyanate, cysteanine, diallyl sulfide and disulfide, glutathione, isothiocyanate, phenethyl, sinigrin, sulforaphane	broccoli, cabbage, cauliflower, and others
Terpenoids		
Monoterpenes	carveol, limonene, menthols	citrus fruits, grapes, mint, other plants, wine
Diterpenes	cafestol, kahweol	coffee, variety of plants, sponges, corals, etc.
Triterpenes	glycerrhetinic acid, its glycoside, limonin, oleanolic acid, and ursolic acid	citrus fruits and a variety of medicinal plants
Sesquiterpenes	nerolidol	medicinal plants and herbs
Unidentified	unknown	in beef, cabbage, germinating wheat, mushrooms, etc.
Vitamins		
Carotenoids	canthaxanthin, $\propto$ and β-carotene, fucoxanthin	fresh green, leafy vegetables
Others	vitamins A, C, E, and riboflavin	fruits and vegetables (fresh), meats, fish

Adding to this complexity is the fact that simultaneous exposure to two initiators, an initiator and a promotor, or to two promotors can lead to additive, multiplicative, and supramultiplicative carcinogenic responses in experimental settings (100). However, at exposure levels as low as those occurring in natural foods, the differences are lost so that the overall risk of a mixture becomes only additive (145). Furthermore, making the safety assessment of human dietary ingredients an almost impossible task is the presence of protective (anticarcinogens, etc.) agents in the same mixture, with interactive effects among themselves and their combined antagonistic effect against the effects of mixture of carcinogens and other toxicants present.

Testing various crude solvent extracts of each dietary ingredient or even selected total diets (composed of average daily per capita amounts of each of the common dietary ingredients in the United States, for example) may reduce the amount of testing. Interactions between components of various extracts and between extractable and non-extractable components will still need to be estimated or tested further. The best but not a perfect approach to a more realistic risk appraisal, however, may involve testing pelleted dehydrated edible whole product such as meat, fruit, or vegetable individually or in combination in animals at doses reflecting human intake. Such an approach not only reduces the cost of testing compared to an individual chemical testing strategy but, also, provides data more relevant to natural exposure to a complex diet.

At the same time, transgenic plants—with improved nutritional quality, capabilities to withstand processing, resistance to spoilage, lower levels of toxic compounds (using anti-sense or other recombinant DNA technology to inactivate gene[s] regulating biosynthesis and/or metabolism), and reduced susceptibility to fungal infestation—should be developed and the lower risk associated with consumption of such plants must be confirmed prior to extensive consumer use. Reduction in fungal susceptibility can be achieved by lowering the micro- and/or macronutrients in the plant needed for fungal growth, or other appropriate techniques (146). Success in risk reduction is also likely if preservation, processing, and storage methods to reduce the levels and/or the effects of natural toxicants in foods are developed and put in practice. Methods to process cassava root to extract/neutralize cyanide; evisceration of fugu fish to eliminate tetrodotoxicosis; waxing, heating, dipping in corn oil, spraying with lecithin, and/or immersion in dilute detergents of potatoes to reduce their glycoalkaloid content; and prudent addition of antioxidants to reduce formation of harmful agents such as lipid oxidation products and nitrosamines—all are examples of such processes. Last, but not the least, of the strategies in dealing successfully with natural dietary chemicals involves public education in avoiding/reducing exposure to natural dietary hazards.

CONCLUSION

Although there has been much progress in our understanding of identification and management of food-borne hazards, large gaps in knowledge exist in the areas of mechanisms of pathogenesis of known human intoxications associated with foods; interactions between multiple toxicants present simultaneously, between toxicants and nutritional components, and between toxicants and antitoxicants (including antimutagens and anticarcinogens) in foods; methods of realistic human health risk extrapolation from animal data; and the development of safer plant varieties and processing and cooking methodologies that minimize toxic hazards to consumers.

Considering the facts that natural dietary toxicants are, at least, as toxic as the synthetic ones and that human exposure to them is greater in quantity and consistency than to synthetic toxicants, U.S and worldwide research resources should be shifted to achieve a realistic balance, in the study of health hazards, more toward the natural dietary components. Present testing of purified individual food toxicants in animals is inadequate and must be succeeded by feeding realistic levels of such compounds in the complex milieus of the product in which the toxicant is naturally present (smoked meats, for example) or even, perhaps, in the total human diet. Realistically speaking, although this task is impossible because of the vastly variable composition of individual food ingredients as well as of the total human diet, we can edge closer to this goal by designing a diet containing various dietary ingredients (vegetables, fruits, grain, dairy products, and meats) at a level equal to percentages of their average per capita human consumption.

Education of the consumers to minimize dietary risks using practicable methods similar to those cited above and to shatter the myths that "natural is healthy" and "man made or synthetic is toxic" needs to be vigorously pursued. An educated populace is less likely to be unduly alarmed and is more likely to accept prudent regulatory actions resulting from realistic scenarios of risk estimation. Finally, application of newer molecular methodologies (such as PCR) to confirm intoxication from bacterial and other biotoxins and intensified activities by national animal health monitoring systems combined with more rigorous application of HACCP will lead to a significant reduction in the currently widespread incidence of microbial diseases from food sources.

ACKNOWLEDGMENT

The authors acknowledge Kathy Craighead and Sarah Young for their excellent word processing skills and timely completion of this manuscript.

QUESTIONS: FOOD FOR THOUGHT

1. Design a Hazard Analysis Critical Control Point System for a food-borne microbial agent of your choice. Can this system, in principle, be used to control other toxic (both natural and synthetic) hazards? If not, is it possible to modify the HACCP system or to develop a similar system to suit such needs?
2. Using the information provided in this chapter (start with #2 of the recommended reading list) and other chapters of this book as well as other available resources (including your imagination), propose a strategy to test natural dietary toxicants in a way that allows more realistic extrapolation to humans than is currently used.
3. Do synthetic chemicals pose a greater hazard than food-borne chemicals in your informed opinion (use #3 of the recommended reading list and others)? If so, are we doing all we can to keep them out of our food supply? Is there more that can be done to achieve this goal? If not, how can we use our resources in the right context of food safety?

REFERENCES

1. Abado-Becognee, K., Mobio, T. A., Ennamany, R., Fleurat-Lessard, F., Shier, W. T., Badria, F., and Creppy, E. E. (1998): Cytotoxicity of fumonisin B1: Implication of lipid peroxidation and inhibition of protein and DNA syntheses. *Arch. Toxicol.*, 72(4):233–236.
2. Abuye, C., Kelbassa, U., and Wolde-Gebriel, S. (1998): Health effects of cassava consumption in South Ethiopia. *East African Med. J.*, 75:166–170.
3. Adams, H. R. (1989): Phytoestrogens. In: *Toxicants of Plant Origin*, Vol. IV, Phenolics, edited by P. R., Cheeke, pp. 23–51. CRC Press, Boca Raton, Florida.
4. Adlercreutz, H. (1995): Phytoestrogens: Epidemiology and a possible role in cancer protection. *Environ. Hlth. Perspect.*, 103 (supp 7):103–112.
5. Ahmed, F. E., and Thomas, D. B. (1992): Assessment of the carcinogenicity of the non-nutritive sweetener cyclamate. *Crit. Rev. Toxicol.*, 22:81–118.
6. Aldridge, D., and Tahourdin, C. (1998): Natural oestrogenic compounds. In *Natural Toxicants in Foods*, edited by D. H. Watson, pp. 54–83. CRC Press, Boca Raton, Florida.
7. Alston, T. A., Mela, L., and Bright, H. G. (1977): 3-Nitropropionate, the toxic substance of Indigofera, is a suicide activator of succinate dehydrogenase. *Proc. Natl. Acad. Sci. (USA)*, 74:3767-3771.
8. Altekruse, S. F., Swerdlow, D. L., and Wells, S. J. (1998): Factors in the emergence of food borne diseases. In: *Microbial Food Borne Pathogens*, edited by L. Tollefson, *Vet. Clin. N. Amer. (Food Anim. Pract.)* 14:1–15.
9. Altekruse, S. F., Swerdlow, D. L., and Stern, N. J. (1998): *Campylobacter jejuni*. In: *Microbial Food-Borne Pathogens*, edited by L. Tollefson, *Vet. Clin. N. Amer. (Food Anim. Pract.)*, 14:31–40.
10. Ames, B. N. (1983): Dietary carcinogens and anticarcinogens: Oxygen radicals and degenerative diseases. *Science*, 221: 1256–1264.
11. Ames, B. N., and Gold, L. S. (1990): Too many rodent carcinogens: Mitogenesis increases mutagenesis. *Perspect. Science*, 249: 970–971.
12. Ames, B. N., Profet, M., and Gold, L. S. (1990): Nature's chemicals and synthetic chemicals: Comparative toxicology. *Proc. Natl. Acad. Sci. (USA)*, 87:7782–7786.
13. Anderson, J. A. (1997): Milk, eggs, and peanuts: Food allergies in children. *Amer. Fam. Phys.*, 56:1365–1374.
14. Andrews, L. S., Ahmedna, M., Grodner, R. M., Liuzzo, J. A., Murano, P. S., Murano, E. A., Rao, R. M., Shane, S., and Wilson, P. M. (1998): Food preservation using ionizing radiation. *Rev. Environ. Contam. Toxicol.*, 154:1–53.
15. Angus, F. (1998): Nut allergens. In: *Natural Toxicants in Food*, edited by D. H. Watson, pp. 84–104. CRC Press, Boca Raton, Florida.
16. Aronow, L., and Kerdel-Vegas, F. (1965): Selino-cystathionine, a pharmacologically active factor in the seeds of Lecythis ollaria: Cytotoxic and depilatory effects. *Nature*, (London) 205: 1185–1186.
17. Bailey, G., Goeger, D., Hendricks, J., Nixon, J., and Pawlowski, N. (1985): Indole-3-carbinol promotion and inhibition of aflatoxin B_1 carcinogenesis in rainbow trout. *Proc. Am. Assoc. Cancer Res.*, 26:115: (abst).
18. Balasubramanian, S., and Govindaswamy, S. (1996): Inhibitory effect of dietary flavonol, quercetin, on 7,12-cimethylbenzanthracine-induced hamster baccal pouch carcinogenesis. *Carcinogenesis*, 17:877–879.
19. Baldessarini, R. J. (1985): Drugs and the treatment of psychiatric disorders. In: *Goodman and Gilman's The Pharmacological Basis of Therapeutics*, 7th ed., edited by A. G. Gilman, L. S. Goodman, T. W. Rall, and F. Murad, pp. 387–445. Macmillan Publishing Co. Inc., New York.
20. Banea-Muyambu, J. P., Tylleskar, T., Gitebo, N., Mtadi, N., Gebre-Medhim, M., and Rosling, A. (1997): Geographical and seasonal association between linamarin and cyanide exposure from cassava and the upper motor neuron disease Konzo in former Zaire. *Trop. Medi. Int. Health*, 2:1143–1151.
21. Barotto, N. N., Lopez, C. B., Eynard, A. R., Fernandez-Zapico, M. D., and Valentich, M. A. (1998): Quercetin enhances pre-tumorous lesions in the NMU model of rat pancreatic carcinogenesis. *Cancer Lett.*, 129:1–6.
22. Bartholomew, R. M., and Ryan, D. A. (1980): Lack of mutagenicity of some phytoestrogens in the Salmonella/mammalian microsome assay. *Mut. Res.*, 78:317–321.
23. Barzel, U. S., and Massey, L. K. (1998): Excess dietary protein can adversely affect bones. *J. Nutr.*, 128:1051–1053.
24. Beasley, V. R. (1989): *Trichothecene Mycotoxicosis: Pathophysiologic Effects*, Vols. 1–2, CRC Press, Boca Raton, Florida.
25. Beier, R. C. (1990): Natural pesticides and bioactive components in foods. *Rev. Environ. Contam. Toxicol.*, 113:47–137.
26. Bruggink, T. (1997): Food allergy and food intolerance. In: *Food Safety and Toxicity*, edited by J. DeVries, pp. 183–194. CRC Press, Boca Raton, Florida.
27. Bryan, F. L. (1979): Infections and intoxications caused by other bacteria. In: *Foodborne Infections and Intoxications*, 2nd ed.,

edited by H. Riemann, and F. L. Bryan, pp. 212–298. Academic Press, New York.

28. Bureau of Foods (1982): *Toxicological Principles for the Safety Assessment of Direct Food Additives and Color Additives Used in Food*. U. S. Food and Drug Administration, Washington, D.C.
29. Busby, W. F., Jr., and Wogan, G. N. (1979): Foodborne mycotoxins and alimentary mycotoxicoses. In: *Foodborne Infections and Intoxications*, 2nd ed., edited by H. Riemann, and F. L. Bryan, pp. 519–610. Academic Press, New York.
30. Busby, W. F., Jr., and Wogan, G. N. (1981): Aflatoxins. In: *Mycotoxins and Nitroso Compounds: Environmental Risks*, Vol. 2, edited by R. C. Shank, pp. 3–28. CRC Press, Boca Raton, Florida.
31. Busby, W. F., Jr., and Wogan, G. N. (1981): Psoralens. *Mycotoxins and Nitroso Compounds: Environmental Risks*, Vol. 2, edited by R. C. Shank, pp. 105–119. CRC Press, Boca Raton, Florida.
32. Carrol, K. K. (1982): Dietary fat and its relationship to human cancer. In: *Carcinogens and Mutagens in the Environment*, Vol. 1, edited by H. F. Stich, pp. 31–38. CRC Press, Boca Raton, Florida.
33. Chang, F. C. T., Spriggs, D. L., Benton, B. J., Ketter, S. J., and Capucio, B. R. (1997): 4-aminopyridine reverses saxitoxin and tetrodotoxin-induced cardiorespiratory depression in chronically instrumented guinea pigs. *Fundam. Appl. Toxicol.*, 38:75–88.
34. Cheeke, P. R. (1996): Biological effects of feed and forage saponins and their impacts on animal production. *Adv. Exper. Med. Biol.*, 405:377–385.
35. Cheeke, P. R. (1989): Toxicants of plant origin. In: *Phenolics*, Vol. 1–4, CRC Press, Boca Raton, Florida.
36. Chen, K. K., and Rose, C. L. (1952): Nitrite and thiosulfate therapy in cyanide poisoning. *J. A. M. A.*, 149:113–119.
37. Chevion, M., Mager, J., and Claser, G. (1983): Favism producing agents. In: *Handbook of Naturally Occurring Food Toxicants*, edited by M. Rechcigl, Jr., pp. 63–79. CRC Press, Boca Raton, Florida.
38. Chow, C. W., Poulos, A., Fellenberg, A. J., Christodoulon, J., and Danks, D. M. (1992): Autopsy findings in two siblings with infantile Refsum's disease. *Acta Neuropath.*, 83:190–195.
39. Chung, F. L., Wang, M., Rivenson, A., Iatropoulous, M. J., Reinhardt, J. C., Pittman, B., Ho, C. T., and Amin, S. G. (1998): Inhibition of lung carcinogenesis by black tea in Fischer rats treated with a tobacco-specific carcinogen: Caffeine as an important constituent. *Cancer Res.*, 58(18):4096–4101.
40. Clarkson, T. B. (1995): Estrogenic soybean isoflavones and chronic disease. *Trends Endocrin. Metab.*, 6:11–16.
41. Cooper, J., and Walker, R. D. (1998): Listeriosis. *Vet. Clin. N. Amer.* (*Food Anim. Pract.*), 14(1):113–125.
42 Coulombe, R. A., Jr. (1991): Aflatoxins. In: *Mycotoxins and Phytoalexins*, edited by R. P. Sharma, and D. K. Salunkhe, pp. 103–143. CRC Press, Boca Raton, Florida.
43. Creppy, E. E., Baudrimont, I., and Betbeder, A. M. (1995): Prevention of nephrotoxicity of ochratoxin A, a food contaminant. *Toxicol. Lett.*, 82–83:869–877.
44. Crews, C. (1998): Pyrrolizidine alkaloids. In: *Natural Toxicants in Food*, edited by D. H. Watson, pp. 11–28. CRC Press, Boca Raton, Florida.
45. Daly, J. W. (1993): Mechanism of action of caffeine. In: *Coffee, Caffeine, and Health*, edited by S. Garattini, pp. 97–150. Raven Press. New York.
46. DeClerk, Y. A., and Inven, S. (1994): Protease inhibitors: Role and potential therapeutic use in human cancer. *Eur. J. Cancer*, 30A:2170–2180.
47. Dencker, L., Gustafson, A. L., Annerwall, E., Busch, C., and Eriksson, U. (1991): Retinoid-binding proteins in craniofacial development. *J. Craniofac. Gen. Dev. Biol.*, 11(4):303–314.
48. Derks, H. J. G. M., Groen, C., Olling, M., and Zeilmaker, M. J. (1997): Extrapolation of toxicity data in risk assessment. In: *Food Safety and Toxicity*, edited by J. DeVries, pp. 241–254. CRC Press, Boca Raton, Florida.
49. Deshpande, S. S., Sathe, S. K., and Salunkhe, D. K. (1984): Chemistry and safety of plant polyphenols. In: *Nutritional and Toxicological Aspects of Food Safety*, edited by M. Friedman, pp. 457–495. Plenum Press, New York.
50. Deshpande, S. S., and Sathe, S. K. (1991): Toxicants in plants. In: *Mycotoxins and Phytoalexins*, edited by R. P. Sharma, and D. K. Salunkhe, pp. 671–730. CRC Press, Boca Raton, Florida.
51. Doll, R., and Peto, R. (1981): The causes of cancer: Quantitative estimates of avoidable risks of cancer in the United States today. *J. Nat. Cancer Inst.*, 66:1193–1308.
52. Duffy, J. Y., Baines, D., Overmann, G. J., Keen, C. L., and Daston, G. P. (1997): Repeated administration of alpha-hederin results in alterations in maternal zinc status and adverse developmental outcome in the rat. *Teratol.*, 56(5):327–334.
53. Dugyala, R. R., Sharma, R. P., Tsunoda, M., and Riley, R. T. (1998): Tumor necrosis factor-alpha as a contributor in fumonisin B1 toxicity. *J. Pharm. Exper. Ther.*, 285(1):317–324.
54. Dunnick, J. K., and Hailey, J. R. (1992): Toxicity and carcinogeniality studies of quercetin, a natural component of foods. *Fnd. Appl. Toxicol.*, 19:423–431.
55. Dutton, M. F. (1996): Fumonisins, mycotoxins of increasing importance: Their nature and their effects. *Pharmacol. Ther.*, 70:137–161.
56. Ellenhorn, M. J., and Barceloux, D. G. (1988): *Medical Toxicology: Diagnosis and Treatment of Human Poisoning*, pp. 508–514, 606–613, Elsevier, New York.
57. Ellenhorn, M. J., Schonwald, S., Ordog, G., and Wesserberger, J. (1997): Natural toxins: Plants, mycotoxins, mushrooms. In: *Ellenhorn's Medical Toxicology*, pp. 1880–1896. Williams & Wilkins, Philadelphia.
58. Ekperigen, H. E., and Nagaraja, K. V. (1998): Salmonella. In: *Microbial Food-Borne Pathogens*, edited by L. Tollefson, *Vet. Clin. N. Amer.* (*Food Anim. Pract.*), 14:17–29.
59. *Federal Food, Drug, and Cosmetic Act, as Amended.* (1976): U.S. Government Printing Office, Washington, D.C.
60. Fenaux, P., and DeBotton, S. (1998): Retinoic acid syndrome. Recognition, prevention, and management. *Drug Safety*, 18(4):273–279.
61. Formica, J. V., and Regelson, W. (1995): Review of the biology of quercetin and related bioflavonoids. *Food & Chem. Toxicol.*, 33(12):1061–1080.
62. Friedman, M., Gumbmann, M. R., and Masters, P. M. (1984): Protein–alkali reactions: Chemistry, toxicology, and nutritional consequences. In: *Nutritional and Toxicological Aspects of Food Safety*, edited by M. Friedman, pp. 367–412. Plenum Press, New York.
63. Fuhrman, F. A. (1983): Toxic constituents of animal foodstuffs: Eggs of fishes and amphibians. In: *Handbook of Naturally Occurring Food Toxicants*, edited by M. Rechcigl, Jr., pp. 301–311. CRC Press, Boca Raton, Florida.
64. Fujiki, H., Yoshizawa, S., Horiuchi, T., Sugamura, M., Yatsunami, J., Nishiwaki, S., Okabe, S., Nishiwaki-Matsushima, R., Okuda, T., and Sugimura, T. (1992): Anticarcinogenic effects of penta-O-gallyl-beta-D-glucose and epigallocatedmin gallate. *Prev. Med.*, 21:503–509.
65. Fukuda, H., Shima, H., Vesonder, R. F., Tokuda, H., Nishino, H., Katoh, S., Tamura, S., Sugimura, T., and Nagao, M. (1996): Inhibition of protein serine/threonine phosphatases by fumonisin

B1, a mycotoxin. *Biochem. Biophys. Res. Commun.*, 220(1):160–165.

66. Gallaher, D., and Schneeman, B. O. (1984): Nutritional and meolic response to plant inhibitors of digestive enzymes. *Adv. Exp. Med. Biol.*, 177:299–320.
67. Gentry, P. A. (1986): Comparative biochemical changes associated with mycotoxicosis other than aflatoxicosis and trichothecene toxicosis. In: *Diagnosis of Mycotoxicoses*, edited by J. R. Richard, and J. R. Thurston, pp. 125–139. Martinus Nijhoff Publishers, Dordrecht, Netherlands.
68. Ghedira-Chekir, L., Maaroufi, K., Zakhama, A., Ellouz, F., Dhouib, S., Creppy, E. E., and Bacha, H. (1998): Induction of a SOS repair system in lysogenic bacteria by zearalenone and its prevention by vitamin E. *Chemico-biol. Interact.*, 113(1):15–25.
69. Gilchrist, A. (1981): *Foodborne Disease and Food Safety*. American Medical Association, Monroe, Wisconsin.
70. Godon, K. A. H., and Houstead, J. (1998): Transmissible spongiform encephalopathies in food animals, *Vet. Clin. N. Amer. (Food Anim. Prac.)*, 14(1):49–70.
71. Halstead, B. W. (1978): *Poisonous and Venomous Marine Animals of the World.*. Darwin Press, Inc., Princeton, New Jersey.
72. Haque, A., Hossain, M., Lambein, F., and Bell, E. A. (1997): Evidence of osteolathyrism among patients suffering from neurolathyrism in Bangladesh. *Nat. Tox.*, 5(1):43–46.
73. Harper, A. E. (1973): Amino acids of nutritional importances. In: *Toxicants Occurring Naturally in Foods*, 2nd ed., edited by the Committee on Food Protection, NRC, pp. 130–152. National Academy of Sciences Press, Washington, D.C.
74. Hayatsu, S., Arimoto, K., Togawa, K., and Mokita, M. (1981): Inhibitory effects of the ether extract of human feces on activities of mutagens: Inhibition of oleic and linoleic acids. *Mutat. Res.*, 81:287–293.
75. Hayes, J. R., and Campbell, T. C. (1986): Food additives and contaminants. In: *Casarett and Doull's Toxicology, the Basic Science of Poisons*, 3rd ed., edited by C. D. Klaassen, M. O. Amdur, and J. Doull, pp. 771–800. Macmillan Publishing Co., New York.
76. Heikkinen, A. M., Tuppurainen, M. T., Niskanen, L., Komulainen, M., Penttila, I., and Saarikoski, S. (1997): Long-term vitamin D_3 supplementation may have adverse effects on serum lipids during postmenopausal hormone replacement therapy. *Eur. J. Endocrin.*, 137(5):495–502.
77. Hirono, I. (1987): *Naturally occurring carcinogens of plant origin: Toxicology, Pathology, and Biochemistry*, pp. 1–227. Kodansha/Elsevier, New York.
78. Hogue, A. T., White, P. L., and Heninover, J. A. (1998): Pathogen reduction and hazard analysis and critical control point (NACCP) systems for meat and poultry. *Vet. Clin. N. Amer.* (*Food Anim. Pract.*), 14(1):151–164.
79. Houtsmuller, U. M. T., Struijk, C. B., and Van Der Beek, A. (1970): Decrease in rate of ATP synthesis of isolated rat heart mitochondria induced by dietary erucic acid. *Biochime. Biophys. Acta*, 218:564–566.
80. Howard, B. V., and Kritchevsky, D. (1996): Phytochemicals and cardiovascular disease: A statement for health care professionals from the American Heart Association. *Circulation*, 95(11):2591–2593.
81. Hsieh, D. P. H. (1979): Basic meolic effects of mycotoxins. In: *Interactions of Mycotoxins in Animal Production*, pp. 43–55. National Academy of Science, Washington, D.C.
82. Hsieh, D. P. H. (1986): Genotoxicity of mycotoxins. In: *New Concepts and Developments in Toxicology*, edited by P. L. Chambers, P. Gebring, and F. Sakai, pp. 251–259. Elsevier Science Publishers, New York.
83. Huxtable, R. J. (1989): Human health implications of pyrrolizidine alkaloids and herbs containing them. In: *Toxicants of Plant Origin*, Vol. I, Alkaloids, edited by P. R. Cheeke, pp. 41–86. CRC Press, Boca Raton, Florida.
84. Ikeguonu, F. I., and Bassir, O. (1977): Effects of phytohemagglutinins from immature legume seeds on the function and enzyme activities of the liver and on the organs of the rat. *Toxicol. Appl. Pharmacol.*, 40:217–226.
85. Jacobsen, B. K., and Bjelke, E. (1982): Coffee consumption and cancer: A prospective study. In: Proceedings of the 13th International Cancer Congress, Seattle, Washington (abstr).
86. Janssen, M. M. T. (1997): Antinutritives; Food contaminants; Food additives; Nutrients. In: *Food Safety and Toxicity*, edited by J. De Vries, pp. 39–52; 53–62; 63–74; 75–98. CRC Press, Boca Raton, Florida.
87. Janssen, M. M. T., Put, H. M. T., and Nout, M. J. R. (1997): Natural toxins. In: *Food Safety and Toxicity*, edited by J. De Vries, pp. 7–38. CRC Press, Boca Raton, Florida.
88. Kalejta, R. F., and Hamlin, J. L. (1997): The dual effect of mimosine on DNA replication. *Exper. Cell Res.*, 231(1):173–183.
89. Kang, Y. J., and Alexander, J. M. (1996): Alterations of the glutathione redox cycle status in fumonisin B1-treated pig kidney cells. *J. Biochem. Toxicol.*, 11(3):121–126.
90. Kao, C. Y. (1967): Comparison of the biological actions of tetrodotoxin and saxitoxin. In: *Animal Toxins*, edited by F. E. Russell, and P. R. Saunders, pp. 109–114. Pergamon Press, Oxford.
91. Kao, C. Y. (1966): Tetrodotoxin, saxitoxin, and their significance in the study of excitation phenomena. *Pharmacol. Rev.*, 18:997–1049.
92. Kanisawa, M., and Suzuki, S. (1978): Induction of renal and hepatic tumors in mice by ochratoxin A, a mycotoxin. *Gann*, 69:599–600.
93. Kassell, B. (1970): Inhibitors of proteolytic enzymes. *Methods Enzymol.*, 19:839–906.
94. Keeler, R. F., Baker, D. C., and Gaffield, W. (1991): Solanum alkaloids. In: *Mycotoxins and Phytoalexins*, edited by R. P. Sharma, and D. K. Salunkhe, pp. 607–636. CRC Press, Boca Raton, Florida.
95. Kensler, T. W., Groopman, J. D., and Roebuck, B. D. (1998): Use of aflatoxin adducts as intermediate endpoints to assess the efficacy of chemopreventive interventions in animals and man. *Mut. Res.*, 402(1–2):165–172.
96. King, T. P., Pusztai, A., and Clarke, E. M. W. (1980): Kidney bean lectin-induced lesions in rat small intestine, I. Light microscopic studies. *J. Comp. Pathol.*, 90:585–593.
97. Kitts, D., Yuan, Y., Joneja, J., Scott, F., Szilagyi, A., Amiot J., and Zarkadas, M. (1997): Adverse reactions to food constituents: Allergy, intolerance, and autoimmunity. *Can. J. Physiol. Pharm.*, 75(4):241–254.
98. Knasmuller, S., Bresgen, N., Kassie, F., Mersch-Sundermann, V., Gelderblom, W., Zohrer, E., and Eckl, P. M. (1997): Genotoxic effects of three fusarium mycotoxins, fumonisin B1, moniliformin and vomitoxin in bacteria and in primary cultures of rat hepatocytes. *Mut. Res.*, 391(1–2):39–48.
99. Kobayashi, M., Suzuki, K., Nagasawa, S., and Mimaki, Y. (1993): Purification of toxic saponins from narthecium asiaticum maxim. *J. Vet. Med. Sci.*, 55(3):401–407.
100. Kodell, R. L., Krewski, D., and Zielinski, J. M. (1991): Additive and multiplicative risks in the two-stage clonal expansion model of carcinogenesis. *Risk Anal.*, 11:483–490.
101. Korn, A., Wagner, B., Moritz E., and Dingemanse, J. (1996): Tyramine pressor sensitivity in healthy subjects during combined treatment with moclobemide and selegiline. *Eur. J. Clin. Pharm.*, 49(4):273–278.
102. Kowalska, M. T., Itzhak, Y., and Puett, D. (1995): Presence of aromatase inhibitors in cycads. *J. Ethnopharm.*, 47(3):113–116.

103. Krogh, P., Hald, B., Plestina, R., and Ceovic, S. (1977): Balkan nephropathy and food-borne ochratoxin A: Preliminary results of a survey of foodstuffs. *Acta Pathol. Microbiol. Scand. Sect. B*, 85:238–240.
104. Kunkel, D. B., and Jallo, D. S. (1990): Ergot. In: *Clinical Management of Poisoning and Drug Overdose*, 2nd ed., edited by L. M. Haddad, and J. F. Winchester, pp. 1401–1406. W.B. Saunders Co., Philadelphia.
105. Kuramochi, G., Gekle, M., and Silbernagle, S. (1997): Derangement of pH homeostasis in the renal papilla: Ochratoxin A increases pH in vasa recta blood. *Nephron.*, 76(4):472–476.
106. Lamawansa, M. D., Wysocki, S. J., House, A. K., and Norman, P. E. (1996): Vitamin D3 exacerbates intimal hyperplasia in balloon-injured arteries. *Br. J. Surg.*, 83(8):1101–1103.
107. Lambert, L. A., Hines, F. A., and Eppleyl, R. M. (1995): Lack of initiation and promotion potential of deoxynivalenol for skin. *Food & Chem. Toxicol.*, 33(3):217–222.
108. Lampe, K. F. (1983): Mushroom poisoning. In: *Handbook of Naturally Occurring Food Toxicants*, edited by M. Rechcigl, Jr., pp. 193–212. CRC Press, Boca Raton, Florida.
109. Lasky, T., and Magder, L. (1997): Hepatocellular carcinoma p53 G > T transversions at codon 249: The fingerprint of aflatoxin exposure? *Environ. Health Perspect.*, 105(4):392–397.
110. Layton, D. W., Bogen, K. T., Knize, M. G., Hatch, F. T., Johnson, V. M., and Felton, J. S. (1995): Cancer risk of heterocyclic amines in cooked foods: An analysis and implications for research. *Carcinogenesis*, 16:39–52.
111. Leftley, J. W., and Hannah, F. (1998): Phycotoxins in seafood. In: *Natural Toxicants in Food*, edited by D. H. Watson, pp. 182–224. CRC Press, Boca Raton, Florida.
112. Lewis, W. H., and Elvin-Lewis, M. P. F. (1977): *Medical Botany: Plants Affecting Human Health*, p. 57. John Wiley & Sons, New York.
113. Liener, I. E. (1980): Miscellaneous toxic factors. In: *Toxic Constituents of Plant Foodstuffs*, 2nd ed., edited by I. E. Liener, pp. 429–467. Academic Press, New York.
114. Liener, I. E., and Kakade, M. L. (1980): Protease inhibitors. In: *Toxic Constituents of Plant Foodstuffs*, 2nd ed., edited by I. E. Liener, pp. 7–71. Academic Press, New York.
115. Liener, I. E. (1995): Possible adverse effects of soybean anti--carcinogens. *J. Nut.* 125(3 Suppl):744–750.
116. Lin, J. K., Chen, Y. C., Huang, Y. T., and Lin-Shiau, S. Y. (1997): Suppression of protein kinase C and nuclear oncogene expression as possible molecular mechanisms of cancer chemoprevention by apigenin and curcumin. *J. Cell. Biochem.*, Suppl 28–29:39–48.
117. Lin, J. L., and Ho, Y. S. (1994): Flavonoid-induced acute nephropathy. *Am. J. Kidney Dis.*, 3(3):433–440.
118. Lipp, E. K., and Rose, J. B. (1997): The role of seafood in food borne diseases in the United States of America. *Revue Scientifique et Technique*, 16:620–640.
119. Liu, J., Liu, Y., Bullock, P., and Klaassen, C. D. (1995): Suppression of liver cytochrome P450 by alpha-hederin: Relevance to hepatoprotection. *Toxicol. Appl. Pharm.*, 134(1):124–131.
120. Lloyd, W. E., Daniels, G. N., and Stahr, H. M. (1985): Cases of nephrotoxic mycotoxicoses in cattle and swine in the United States. In: *Trichothecenes and Other Mycotoxins*, edited by J. Lacey, pp. 545–548. John Wiley & Sons, New York.
121. Lovenberg, W. (1973): Some vaso- and psychoactive substances in food. In: *Toxicants Occurring Naturally in Foods*, 2nd ed., edited by the Committee on Food Protection, NRC, pp. 170–188. National Academy of Sciences Press, Washington, D.C.
122. MacGregor, J. T. (1984): Genetic and carcinogenic effects of plant flavonoids: An overview. In: *Nutritional and Toxicological Aspects of Food Safety*, edited by M. Friedman, pp. 497–526. Plenum Press, New York.
123. Mager, J., Chevion, M., and Claser, G. (1980): Favism. In: Toxic Constituents of Plant Foodstuffs, 2nd ed., edited by I. E. Liener, pp. 266–294. Academic Press, New York.
124. Malinow, M. R., Bardana, E. J. Jr., Pirofsky, B., Craig, S., and McCluagblin, P. (1982): Systemic lupus erythematosus-like syndrome in monkeys fed alfalfa sprouts: Role of a non-protein amino acid. *Science*, 216:415–417.
125. Marasas, W. F. (1995): Fumonisins and their implications for human and animal health. *Nat. Toxins*, 3:193–198.
126. Marks, J. (1989): The safety of the vitamins: An overview. *Int. J. Vit. Nut. Res. Suppl*, 30:12–20.
127. Marth, E. H. (1981): Food-borne hazards of microbial origin. In: *Food Safety*, edited by H. R. Roberts, pp. 15–65. John Wiley & Sons, New York.
128. Matsumoto, H. (1983): Cycasin. In: *Handbook of Naturally Occurring Food Toxicants*, edited by M. Rechcigl, Jr., pp. 43–61. CRC Press, Boca Raton, Florida.
129. Matsumoto, T., Itoh, H., and Akiba, Y. (1968): Goitrogenic effects of 5-vinyl-2-oxazolidinethione, a goitrogen in rapeseed, in growing chicks. *Poultry Sci.*, 47:1323–1330.
130. Mattocks, A. R. (1986): *Chemistry and Toxicology of Pyrrolizidine Alkaloids*. Academic Press, New York.
131. Mattson, F. H. (1973): Potential toxicity of food lipids. In: *Toxicants Occurring Naturally in Foods*, 2nd ed., edited by the Committee on Food Protection, NRC, pp. 189–209. National Academy of Sciences Press, Washington, D.C.
132. McPartland, J. M., Vigaly, R. J., and Cubeta, M. A. (1997): Mushroom poisoning. *Am. Fam. Phys.*, 55:1797–1811.
133. Meisner, H., and Cimbala, M. (1985): Effect of ochratoxin A on gene expression in rat kidneys. In: *New Concepts and Developments in Toxicology*, edited by P. L. Chambers, P. Gehring, and F. Sakai, pp. 261–271. Elsevier Science Publishers, New York.
134. Merril, R. A. (1997): Food safety regulation: Reforming the Delaney clause. *Ann. Rev. Pub. Health*, 18:313–340.
135. Miller, J. A., Miller, E. C., and Phillips, D. H. (1982): The metabolic activation and carcinogenicity of alkenylbenzenes that occur naturally in many spices. In: *Carcinogens and Mutagens in the Environment*, Vol. 1, edited by H. F. Stich, pp. 93–96. CRC Press, Boca Raton, Florida.
136. Miller, I., Gray, D., and Kay, H. (1998): Bacterial toxins found in foods. In: *Natural Toxicants in Food*, edited by D. H. Watson, pp. 105–146. CRC Press, Boca Raton, Florida.
137. Mitchel, R. E., and McCann, R. (1993): Vitamin E is a complete tumor promoter in mouse skin. *Carcinogenesis*, 14(4):659–662.
138. Miura, K., Nakajima, Y., Yamanaka, N., Terao, K., Shibato, T., and Ishino, S. (1998): Induction of apoptosis with fusarenon-X in mouse thymocytes. *Toxicol.*, 127(1-3):195–206.
139. Mody, R., Joshi, S., and Chaney, W. (1995): Use of lectins as diagnostic and therapeutic tools for cancer. *J. Pharmacol. Toxicol. Meth.*, 33:1–10.
140. Montgomery, R. D. (1980): Cyanogens. In: *Toxic Constituents of Plant Foodstuffs*, 2nd ed., edited by I. E. Liener, pp. 143–160. Academic Press, New York.
141. Morris, S. C., and Lee, T. H. (1984): The toxicity and teratogenicity of Solanaceae glycoalkaloids, particularly those of the potato (*Solanum tuberosum*): A review. *Food Technol. Aust.*, 36:118–124.
142. Nakanishi, K., Hagiwara, A., Shibata, M., Imaida, K., Tetematsu, M., and Ito, N. (1980): Dose response of saccharin induction of urinary bladder hyperplasia in Fisher 344 rats pretreated with N-butyl N- (4-hydroxybutyl) nitrosamine. *J. Natl. Cancer Inst.*, 65:1005–1010.
143. Nakhla, H. B., Mohamed O. S., Abu, I. M., Fatuh, A. L., and Adam, S. E. (1991): The effect of *Trigonella foenum graecum*

(fenugreek) crude saponins on Hisex-type chicks. *Vet. Hum. Toxicol.*, 33(6):561–564.
144. National Academy of Sciences. (1977): *Leucaena, Promising Forage, and Tree Crop for the Tropics*. NAS Press, Washington, D.C.
145. National Research Council (NRC). (1988): Complex mixtures: Methods for in vivo toxicity testing. National Academy Press, Washington, D.C.
146. NRC. (1996): *Carcinogens and anticarcinogens in the human diet*, pp. 1–417. National Academy Press, Washington, D.C.
147. Ohga, S., Higashi, E., Nomura, A., Matsuzaki, A., Hirono, A., Miwa, S., Fujii, H., and Ueda, K. (1995): Haptoglobin therapy for acute favism: A Japanese boy with glucose-6-phosphate dehydrogenase Guadalajara. *Br. J. Haematol.*, 89(2):421–423.
148. Olny, J. W. (1982): The toxic effects of glutamate and related compounds in the retina and the brain. *Retina*, 2:341–359.
149. Omaye, S. T. (1984): Safety of megavitamin therapy. In: *Nutritional and Toxicological Aspects of Food Safety*, edited by M. Friedman, pp. 169–203. Plenum Press, New York.
150. Osuntokun, B. O. (1973): Ataxic neuropathy associated with high cassava diets in West Africa. In: *Chronic Cassava Toxicity*, edited by B. Nestel, and R. MacIntyre, pp. 127–138. International Development Research Center, Ottawa.
151. Osweiler, G. D., Carson, T. L., Buck, W. B., and Van Gelder, G. A. (1985): *Clinical and Diagnostic Veterinary Toxicology*, Kendall-Hunt Publishing Co., Dubuque, Iowa.
152. Padmanaban, G. (1980): Lathyrogens. In: *Toxic Constituents of Plant Foodstuffs*, 2nd ed., edited by I. E. Liener, pp. 239–263. Academic Press, New York.
153. Panter, K. E., and James, L. F. (1990): Natural plant toxicants in milk: A review. *J. Anim. Sci.*, 68:892–904.
154. Pass, M. A., Arab, H., Pollitt, S., and Hegarty, M. P. (1996): Effects of the naturally occurring arginine analogues indospicine and canavanine on nitric oxide mediated functions in aortic endothelium and peritoneal macrophages. *Nat. Toxins*, 4(3):135–140.
155. Pearl, E. R. (1997): Food allergy. *Lippincott's Primary Care Practice* 1:154–167.
156. Perlman, F. (1980): Allergens. In: *Toxic Constituents of Plant Foodstuffs*, 2nd ed., edited by I. E. Liener, pp. 295–327. Academic Press, New York.
157. Pfohl-Leszkowicz, A., Chekir-Ghedira, L., and Bacha H. (1995): Genotoxicity of zearalenone, and estrogenic mycotoxin: DNA adduct formation in female mouse tissues. *Carcinogenesis*, 16(10):2315–2320.
158. Poulton, J. E. (1983): Cyanogenic compounds in higher plants and their toxic effects. In: *Handbook of Natural Toxins, Vol 1, Plant and Fungal Toxins*, edited by R. F. Keeler, and A. T. Tu, pp. 117–160. Marcel Dekker, Inc., New York.
159. Puchala, R., Pierzynowski, S. G., Sahlu, T., and Hart, S. P. (1996): Effects of mimosine administered to a perfused area of skin in Angora goats. *Br. J. Nutr.*, 75(1):69–79.
160. Randel, R. D., Chase, C. C., and Wyse, S. J. (1992): Effect of gossypol and cottonseed products on reproduction in mammals. *J. Anim. Sci.*, 70:1628–1638.
161. Rao, A. V., and Sung, M. K. (1995): Saponins as anticarcinogens. *J. Nutr.*, 125(3 suppl):717S-724S.
162. Reddy, C. S., Hanumaiah, B., Hayes, T. G., and Ehrlich, K. (1986): Developmental stage specificity and dose response of secalonic acid D-induced cleft palate and the absence of cytotoxicity in the developing mouse palate. *Toxicol. Appl. Pharmaco.*, 84:346–354.
163. Reddy, R. V., Johnson, G., Rottinghaus, G. E., Casteel, S. W., and Reddy, C. S. (1996): Developmental effects of fumonisin B in mice. *Mycopathologia*, 134:161–166.
164. Reed, J. D. (1995). Nutritional toxicology of tannins and related polyphenols in forage legumes. *J. Anim. Sci.*, 43:1516–1528.
165. Riemann, H. P., and Oliver, D. O. (1998): Escherichia coli O157 : H7. *Vet. Clin. N. Amer. (Food Anim. Pract.)*, 14(1):41–48.
166. Rivera, V. R., Pol, M. A., and Bignami, G. S. (1995): Prophylaxis and treatment with a monoclonal antibody of tetrodotoxin poisoning in mice. *Toxicon*, 33:1231–1237.
167. Roebuck, B. D., Yeager, J. D. Jr., Longnecker, D. S., and Wilpone, S. A. (1981): Promotion by unsaturated fat of azaserine-induced pancreatic carcinogenesis in the rat. *Cancer Res.*, 41:3961–3966.
168. Rosen, J. D. (1990): Much ado about alar. *Iss. Sci. Technol.*, VIII:85–90.
169. Rotter, B. A., and Oh, Y. N. (1996): Mycotoxin fumonisin B1 stimulates nitric oxide production in a murine macrophage cell line. *Nat. Toxins*, 4(6):291–294.
170. Rotter, B. A., Prelusky, D. B., and Pestka, J. J. (1996): Toxicology of deosynivalenol (vomitoxin). *J. Toxicol. Environ. Health*, 48(1):1–34.
171. Russell, F. E. (1986): Toxic effects of animal toxins. In: *Casarett and Doull's Toxicology, the Basic Science of Poisons*, 3rd ed., edited by C. D. Klaassen, M. O. Amdur, and J. Doull, pp. 706–756. Macmillan Publishing Co., New York.
172. Russell, F. E., and Dart, R. C. (1991): Toxic effects of animal toxins. In: *Casarett and Doull's Toxicology, the Basic Science of Poisons*, 4th ed., edited by M. O. Amdur, J. Doull, and C. D. Klaassen, pp. 753–803. Pergamon Press, New York.
173. Safe, S. H. (1995): Environmental and dietary estrogens and human health: Is there a problem? *Environ. Health Perspect.*, 103:346–351.
174. Sampson, H. A. (1997): Food allergy. *JAMA*, 278:1888–1894.
175. Sandani, G. R., Soman, C. S., Deodhar, K. K., and Nadharni, G. D. (1997): Reactive oxygen species involvement in ricin-induced thyroid toxicity in the rat. *Hum. Exper. Toxicol.*, 16:254–256.
176. Sandvig, K., and Van Deurs, B. (1997): Endocytosis, intracellular transport and cytotoxic action of shiga toxin and ricin. *Physiol. Rev.*, 76:949–966.
177. Schardein, J. L. (1985): *Chemically Induced Birth Defects*, pp. 709–716. Marcel Dekker Inc., New York.
178. Schramek, H., Wilflingseder D., Pollack, V., Freudinger, R., Mildenberger, S., and Gekle, M. (1997): Ochratoxin A-induced stimulation of extracellular signal-regulated kinases 1/2 is associated with Madin–Darby canine kidney–C7 cell dedifferentiation. *J. Pharm. Exper. Ther.*, 283(3):1460–1468.
179. Scott, B. R., Pathak, M. A., and Mohn, G. R. (1976): Molecular and genetic basis of furocoumarin reactions. *Mutat. Res.*, 39:29–74.
180. Scudamore, K. A. (1998): Mycotoxins. In: *Natural Toxins in Foods*, edited by D. H. Watson, pp. 147–181. CRC Press, Boca Raton, Florida.
181. Selman, I. E., Wiseman, A., Breeze, R. G., and Pirie, H. M. (1976): Fog fever in cattle: Various theories on its etiology. *Vet. Rec.*, 99:181–184.
182. Shank, R. C. (1981): Environmental toxicoses in humans. In: *Mycotoxins and Nitroso Compounds: Environmental Risks*, Vol. 1, edited by R. C. Shank, pp. 107–140. CRC Press, Boca Raton, Florida.
183. Sharma, R. P., and Salunkhe, D. K. (1989): Solanum glycoalkaloids. In: *Toxicants of Plant Origin*. Vol. I, Alkaloids, edited by P. R. Cheeke, pp. 179–236. CRC Press, Boca Raton, Florida.
184. Shephard, S. E. (1993): Mutagenic activity of peptides and artificial sweetener aspartame after nitrosation. *Food Chem. Toxicol.*, 31:323–329.
185. Shoda, R., Matsueda, K., Yamamoto, S., and Umeda, N. (1996): Epidemiologic analysis of Crohn's disease in Japan: Increased diet-

ary intake of n-6-polyunsaturated fatty acids and animal protein relates to increased incidence of Crohn's disease. *Am. J. Clin. Nutr.*, 63:741–745.

186. Singleton, V. L., and Kratzer, F. H. (1973): Plant phenolics. In: *Toxicants Occurring Naturally in Foods*, 2nd ed., edited by the Committee on Food Protection, NRC, pp. 309–345. National Academy of Sciences Press, Washington, D.C.
187. Smith, L. D. (1977): *Botulism: The Organism, Its Toxins, the Disease*. Charles C. Thomas Publishers, Springfield, Illinois.
188. Smith, T. K., Lund, E. K., and Johnson, I. K. (1998): Inhibition of dimethyl-hydrazine induced aberrant crypt foci and induction of apoptosis in rat colon following oral administration of the glucosinolate, sinigrain. *Carcinogens*, 19:267–273.
189. Snyder, R., and Andrews, L. S. (1996): The effects of solvents and vapors. In: *Casarett and Doull's Toxicology: The Basic Science of Poisons*, 5th ed., edited by C. D. Klaassen, pp. 737–771. McGraw-Hill Co., New York.
190. Spencer, P. D., Nunn, P. B., Hugon, J., Ludolph, A. C., Ross, S. M., Roy, D. N., and Robertson, R. C. (1987): Guam amyotrophic lateral sclerosis-parkinsonism-dementia linked to a plant-excitant neurotoxin. *Science*, 237:517–522.
191. Stob, M. (1983): Estrogens. In: *Handbook of Naturally Occurring Food Toxicants*, edited by M. Rechcigl, Jr., pp. 81–100. CRC Press, Boca Raton, Florida.
192. Stocks, P. (1970): Cancer mortality in relation to national consumption of cigarettes, solid fuel, tea, and coffee. *Br. J. Cancer*, 24:215–225.
193. Stricker-Krongrad, A., Burlet, C., and Beck, B. (1998): Behavioral deficits in monosodium glutamate rats: Specific changes in structure and behavior. *Life Sci.*, 62:2127–2132.
194. Sugimoto, N., Horiguchi, Y., and Matsuda, M. (1996): Mechanism of action of *Clostridium perfringens* enterotoxin. In: *Natural Toxins II*, edited by B. R. Singh, and A. Tu, pp. 257–269. Plenum Press, New York.
195. Sugimura, T. (1986): Past, present, and future of mutagens in cooked foods. *Environ. Health Perspect.*, 67:5–10.
196. Suzuki, Y. J., Forman, H. J., and Sevanian, A. (1997): Oxidants as stimulators of signal transduction. *Free Radical Biol. Med.*, 22:269–285.
197. Talaley, P., and Zhang, Y. (1996): Chemoprotection against cancer by isothiocyanates and glucosinolates. *Biochem. Soc. Transact.*, 24:806–810.
198. Tarasoff, L., and Kelly, M. F. (1993): Monosodium L-glutamate: A double-blind study and review. *Food Chem. Toxicol.*, 31(2):1019–1035.
199. Teng, C. S. (1995): Gossypol-induced apoptotic DNA fragmentation correlates with inhibited protein kinase C activity in speratocytes. *Contraception*, 52:389–395.
200. Tookey, H. L., Van Etten, C. H., and Daxenbichler, M. E. (1980): Glucosinolates. In: *Toxic Constituents of Plant Foodstuffs*, 2nd ed., edited by I. E. Liener, pp. 103–142. Academic Press, New York.
201. Tsuda, S., Kosaka, Y., Murakami, M., Matsuo, H., Matsusaka, N., Taniguchi, K., and Sasaki, Y. F. (1998): Detection of nivalenol genotoxicity in cultured cells and multiple mouse organs by the alkaline single-cell gel electrophoresis assay. *Mut. Res.*, 415(3):191–200.
202. Unkrig, C. J., Schroeder, R., Scharf, R. E., and Aubourg, P. (1994): Lorenzo's oil and lymphocytopemia (letter) *New Engl. J. Med.*, 330:577.
203. Van Etten, C. H., and Tookey, H. L. (1983): Glucosinolates. In: *Handbook of Naturally Occurring Food Toxicants*, edited by M. Rechcigl, Jr., pp. 15–30. CRC Press, Boca Raton, Florida.
204. Van Genderen, H. (1997): Adverse effects of naturally occurring non-nutritive substances. In: *Food Safety and Toxicity*, edited by J. DeVries, pp. 147–162. CRC Press, Boca Raton, Florida.
205. Van Hoff, F., Hue, L., Vamecq, J., and Sherratt, H. S. (1985): Protection of rats by clofibrate against the hypoglycaemic and toxic efects of hypoglycin and pent-4-enoate. An ultrastructural and biochemical study. *Biochem. J.*, 229(2):387–397.
206. Verdeal, K., Brown, R. R., Richardson, T., and Ryan, D. S. (1980): Affinity of phytoestrogens for the estradiol-binding proteins and effect of coumestrol on growth of 7,12-dimethylbenz (A) anthracene-induced rat mammary tumors. *J. Natl. Cancer Inst.*, 64:285–290.
207. Verhagen, H. (1997): Adverse effects of food additives. In: *Food Safety and Toxicity*, edited by J. DeVries, pp. 121–132. CRC Press, Boca Raton, Florida.
208. Verkerk, R., Dekker, M., and Jongen, W. M. F. (1998): Glucosinolates. In: *Natural Toxicants in Foods*, edited by D. H. Watson, pp. 29–53. CRC Press, Boca Raton, Florida.
209. Vetter, J. (1998): Toxins of *Amanita phalloides*. *Toxicon*, 36:13–24.
210. Voss, K. A., Chamberlain, W. J., Bacon, C. W., Riley, R. T., and Norred, W. P. (1995): Subchronic toxicity of fumonisin B1 to male and female rats. *Food Addit. Contam.*, 12(3):473–478.
211. Walker, G. R., and Yamazaki, K. (1996): Saponins in food and agriculture. *Adv. Exp. Med. Biol.*, 404: pp. 1–422.
212. Walker, G. R., and Yamazaki, K. (1996): Saponins in traditional and modern medicine. *Adv. Exp. Med. Biol.*, 405: pp. 1–576.
213. Whitley, B. D., Holmes, A. R., Shepherd, M. G., and Ferguson, M. M. (1991): Peanut sensitivity as a cause of burning mouth. *Oral. Surg., Oral Med., Oral Path.*, 72:671–674.
214. Wieland, T., and Faulstich, H. (1983): Peptide toxins from *Amanita*. In: *Handbook of Natural Toxins*, Vol. 1., Plant and Fungal Toxins, edited by R. F. Keeler, and A. T. Tu, pp. 117–160. Marcel Dekker, Inc., New York.
215. Williamson, G., Faulkner, K., and Plumb, G. W. (1998): Glucosinolates and phenolics and antioxidants from plant foods. *Eur. J. Cancer Prev.*, 7(1):17–21.
216. Wilmarth, K. R., and Froines, J. R. (1992): In vitro and in vivo inhibition of lysyl oxidase by aminopropionitriles. *J. Toxicol. Environ. Health*, 37:411–423.
217. Wolever, T. M., Hamad, S., Gittelsohn, J., Gao, J., Hanley, A. J., Harris, S. B., and Zinman, B. (1997): Low dietary fiber and high protein intake associated with newly diagnosed diabetes in a remote aboriginal community. *Am. J. Clin. Nutr.*, 66: 1470–1474.
218. Xu, R., Zhao, W., Xu, J., Shao, B., and Qin, G. (1996): Studies on bioactive saponins from Chinese medicinal plants. *Adv. Exper. Med. Biol.*, 404:371–382.
219. Yamanaka, N., Oda, O., and Nagao, S. (1997): Prooxidant activity of caffeic acid, dietary non-flabonoid phenotic acid, on Cu^{24}-induced low density lipoprotein oxidation, *FEBS Lett.*, 405:186–190.
220. Yang, W. H., Drouin, M. A., Herbert, M., Mao, Y., and Karsh, J. (1997): The monosodium glutamate symptom complex: Assessment in double-blind placebo-controlled, randomized study. *J. Aller. Clin. Immun.*, 99:757–762.
221. Esterbauer, H. (1993): Cytotoxicity and genotoxicity of lipid peroxidation products. *Amer. J. Clin. Nutr.*, 57:779–786.
222. Yeung, J. M., Wang, H. Y., and Prelusky, D. B. (1996): Fumonisin B1 induces protein kinase C translocation via direct interaction with diacylglycerol binding site. *Toxicol. Appl. Pharmacol.*, 141(1): 178–184.
223. Zelski, R. Z., Rothwell, J. T., Moore, R. E., and Kennedy, D. J. (1995): Gossypol toxicity in preruminant calves. *Aust. Vet. J.*, 72:394–398.

FURTHER READINGS

ICMSF (International Commission on Microbiological Specifications for Foods). (1988): *Microorganisms in Foods: 4. Application of the Hazard Analysis Critical Control Point (HACCP) System to Ensure Microbiological Safety and Quality*. Blackwell Scientific Publications, Oxford.

National Research Council (NRC) (1988): Complex mixtures: methods for in vivo toxicity testing. National Academy Press, Washington, D.C.

NRC (1996): *Carcinogens and Anticarcinogens in the Human Diet*. National Academy Press, Washington, D.C.

Principles and Methods of Toxicology,
Fourth Edition, edited by A. Wallace Hayes.
Taylor & Francis, Philadelphia © 2001.

Chapter 12

Solvents and Industrial Hygiene

Robert C. Spiker, Jr. and Gary B. Morris

Solvent use by industry and the general public is widespread, encompassing numerous products and applications. As Table 12.1 illustrates, billions of pounds of organic solvents are produced annually (11,12). Solvents may be utilized individually (e.g., acetone or toluene) or as mixtures containing several ingredients (e.g., paint thinners, cleaning agents). Alternative, nontraditional solvents, as described later, are also finding widespread applicability.

To better understand the hazards that these materials may present, we must first learn something about their basic physical, chemical, and toxicological properties. Table 12.2 contains a list of physical properties of commonly encountered organic solvents (4,101). This is followed by a brief explanation of the properties. For ease of comparison, inhalation, dermal, and oral toxicological data for solvents are often discussed in relation to the chemical groups to which they belong (aromatics, alcohols, halogenated hydrocarbons, etc.). Much of the text is devoted to a review of the basic toxicology of some widely used solvents as well as several alternative compounds.

Modern industrial hygiene practices have done much to characterize and minimize workplace solvent exposures. A number of these practices, such as workplace monitoring, local exhaust ventilation, and personal protective equipment are discussed in this chapter. Because solvent use in small businesses and the home is often not as well controlled as in major industrial settings, large populations may be at risk. A challenge to the health and

Table 12.1
Ten-year trends in production volumes for some common solvents[a]

Name	Production (millions of pounds) 1997	1996	1995	1994	1993	1992	1991	1990	1989	1988
Acetone	NA[b]	NA	2761	2664	2430	2435	2347	2329	2524	2303
Aniline	1339	1079	1391	1263	991	1009	961	989	1016	1029
Benzene[c]	2342	2116	2168	2074	1677	1636	1569	1699	1631	1608
Cumene	6119	5879	5625	5217	4393	4666	4168	4311	4426	4455
Ethanol (Synthetic)	NA	NA	626	648	678	698	526	546	549	562
Ethylbenzene	12691	10359	13656	10758	9336	11108	8871	8369	9235	9929
Ethylene dichloride	26294	11336	17263	16762	17947	15150	13713	13849	13383	13028
Ethylene glycol	NA	NA	5230	6090	5200	5128	4809	5070	5461	5517
2-Ethylhexanol	768	760	743	732	695	692	657	650	612	743
Formaldehyde (37%)	NA	NA	8110	8165	8189	8278	6612	6720	5893	6280
Isopropyl alcohol	1478	1384	1424	1451	1272	1463	1342	1456	1474	1389
Methanol (Synthetic)	NA	NA	11292	12176	10506	8082	8704	8344	8167	8142
Methylene chloride	NA	NA	NA	403	354	362	389	461	482	504
Styrene	11366	11874	11386	11294	9594	9000	8114	8017	8337	8984
Toluene[c]	NA	NA	927	931	880	833	873	861	806	892
Xylenes[d]	8880	7054	7356	7170	6622	6574	6117	6143	6327	6572

[a] Data from References 11 and 12.
[b] NA = data not available
[c] Millions of gallons
[d] ortho- and para-isomers

safety community is to help educate these groups about the safe use of solvents.

PROPERTIES OF SOLVENTS

Vapor Pressure

Vapor pressure is the amount of pressure exerted by a saturated vapor above its own liquid in a closed container. Vapor pressure increases with increasing temperature of the solvent, slowly at lower temperatures and then more rapidly at higher temperatures (85). The higher the vapor pressure, the greater the tendency for the substance to evaporate into the atmosphere. Units of vapor pressure are usually expressed as millimeters of mercury (mm Hg) at 20°C (68°F).

The vapor pressure of a mixture of two miscible solvents differs from that of the individual constituents (85). If the mixture is left open to the environment, the more volatile component evaporates first, leaving the remaining mixture rich in the less volatile solvent. This process will continue until either the more volatile solvent is gone or an azeotropic (constant boiling) mixture is formed. If the azeotrope is formed, then both vapor constituents escape simultaneously. Examples of solvents that form azeotropic mixtures are water/ethanol (95.57% by weight ethanol, boiling at 78.15°C) and chloroform/acetone (20.0% by weight acetone, boiling at 64.7°C) (85). Vapor pressure and evaporation rate (see below) can be used to estimate how quickly a substance becomes airborne and, thus, how soon an individual may be exposed to it.

Boiling Point

The boiling point of a liquid is the temperature at which the liquid's vapor pressure equals the surrounding atmospheric pressure. This is characterized by formation of bubbles of vapor within the liquid which escape into the vapor phase. The normal boiling point is measured in degrees centigrade (°C) or degrees Fahrenheit (°F), usually at one atmosphere pressure (760 mm Hg or 14.7 psi). Generally, the solvent with the lower boiling point will have the higher vapor pressure.

Evaporation Rate

The rate of evaporation of a solvent is also an important property to consider when selecting a material for a particular process or when evaluating its fire and health hazard potential. Since evaporation rates depend on a number of intrinsic properties as well as external conditions, evaporation rates cannot be stated in absolute numbers (120). One common way of expressing evaporation rate, however, is to compare the rate for the solvent in question to a reference material under identical conditions. Such a reference is normal butyl acetate (n-BuAc), which is given an evaporation rate of 1.0, by definition. Solvents evaporating more quickly have a value greater than 1.0 (e.g., ethyl ether and hexane) and those evaporating more slowly have a value less than 1.0 (e.g., xylene and mineral spirits).

Specific Gravity

Specific gravity is the ratio of the density of a substance to the density of a reference material at a specified temperature. Water is the reference standard for liquids and solids (density 1 g/ml at 4°C). A chemical with a specific gravity greater than 1.0 (e.g., perchloroethylene), if insoluble in water, will sink. A material having a specific gravity of less than 1.0 (e.g., toluene) is lighter than water and, if not soluble, will float on it. As can be seen, specific gravity takes on special significance in fire fighting and chemical spill cleanup operations, since many flammable liquids have a specific gravity of less than 1.0 and if insoluble, will remain on top of a pool of water.

Vapor Density

Vapor density is expressed by the ratio of the mass of a vapor or gas to the mass of an equal volume of air at the same temperature (average mass for gases in air, 29 grams per mole). The density of dry air is 0.075 lb/ft^3 or 1.2 kg/m^3 at 70°F and 1 atmosphere (3). Materials heavier than air (e.g., carbon disulfide, perchloroethylene, and chlorine) tend to settle in low places such as sumps, manholes, and trenches. If there is little or no air movement or temperature variability that could promote mixing, then a potentially hazardous situation exists.

Flash Point

The flash point of a solvent is the lowest temperature at which vapor is given off in sufficient quantity so that the air–vapor mixture above the surface of the solvent will ignite momentarily in a flame. The flash point is determined by heating or cooling the solvent in a closed or open cup apparatus (e.g., Setaflash, Pensky–Martens, Tag, or Cleveland) and measuring the temperature at which the flash will be obtained when a small flame is introduced into the vapor above the surface of the solvent. The Occupational Safety and Health Administration (OSHA) and the NFPA (National Fire Protection Association) define a flammable liquid as a liquid having a flash point below 100°F (37.8°C).

When vapors of a flammable solvent are mixed with air in the proper proportions, ignition is possible. This proportion, called the flammable range, is also known as the explosive range. Concentrations of vapor too lean or too rich cannot be ignited. Figure 12.1 depicts the flammability characteristics of a vapor-air mixture as concentration and temperature vary (134).

Partition Coefficient

The partition coefficient (sometimes called distribution coefficient) is the ratio of the distribution at equilibrium of a solute between two insoluble solvents. This ratio is constant at a given temperature and is valid as long as the solute does not undergo a change in solution such as dissociation. For example, the partition coefficient for iodine in water and chloroform at 25°C is 0.0117 (85). In biological systems, the partition coefficient can describe the partitioning of a toxicant between other media such as air and blood or blood and fat, and so on. Lists of partition coefficients for solvents into biological media or other compounds such as olive oil have been published (44,51,106,119).

CHEMICAL CLASSIFICATION FOR SOLVENTS

Most solvents fall into one of 11 chemical groups, which are characterized by a specific chemical radical that gives the individual members the properties typical of the group. Figure 12.2 presents the chemical configurations for these classifications along with examples of common solvents belonging to each group (92). Additionally, current American Conference of Governmental Industrial Hygienists (ACGIH) eight-hour time-weighted average (TWA) threshold limit values (TLVs) are given with these examples.

OCCUPATIONAL EXPOSURE LIMITS

Various organizations and governmental agencies in the U.S. and throughout the world have issued occupational exposure limits (OELs) to help protect the health and well being of the workforce. Exposure limits com-

Table 12.2
Solvent properties[a,b]

Compound	Boiling point	Freezing point	Flash point	Vapor pressure
Acetaldehyde	20°C	−123°C	−36°F	740 mm
Acetone	56°C	−95°C	0°F	180 mm
n-Amyl acetate	149°C	−71°C	77°F	4 mm
Benzene	80°C	5.5°C	12°F	75 mm
Bromoform	149°C	8°C	None	5 mm
2-Butanone	79°C	−86°C	16°F	78 mm
n-Butyl acetate	125°C	−77°C	72°F	10 mm
n-Butyl alcohol	118°C	−90°C	84°F	6 mm
Carbon disulfide	47°C	−112°C	−22°F	297 mm
Carbon tetrachloride	77°C	−23°C	None	91 mm
Chlorobenzene	132°C	−46°C	82°F	9 mm
Chloroform	61°C	−63°C	None	160 mm
m-Cresol	203°C	12°C	187°F	0.14 mm @25°C
Crotonaldehyde	104°C	−74°C	45°F	19 mm
Cumene	152°C	−96°C	96°F	8 mm
Cyclohexane	81°C	7°C	0°F	78 mm
Cyclohexanol	161°C	25°C	154°F	1 mm
Cyclohexanone	156°C	−45°C	146°F	5 mm
Cyclohexylamine	134°C	−18°C	88°F	11 mm
1,2-Dichlorobenzene	181°C	−17°C	151°F	1 mm
Diethylamine	56°C	−50°C	−15°F	192 mm
Dimethylphthalate	284°C	6°C	295°F	0.01 mm
Dimethyl sulfate	188°C	−32°C	182°F	0.1 mm
Ethanol	78°C	−114°C	55°F	44 mm
Ethyl acetate	77°C	−83°C	24°F	73 mm
Ethylene glycol	198°C	−13°C	232°F	0.06 mm
Ethylene glycol n-butyl ether	171°C	−77°C	143°F	0.8 mm
Ethylene glycol monoethyl ether	135°C	−90°C	110°F	4 mm
Ethylene glycol monethyl ether acetate	156°C	−62°C	124°F	2 mm
Ethylene glycol monomethyl ether	124°C	−85°C	102°F	6 mm
Ethylene glycol monomethyl ether acetate	145°C	−65°C	120°F	2 mm
Ethyl ether	34°C	−116°C	−49°F	440 mm
Formaldehyde (37% in water)	101°C	NA	185°F	1 mm
Formamide	211°C	2.8°C	310°F	0.1 mm @30°C
Furfural	162°C	−37°C	140°F	2 mm
Furfuryl alcohol	170°C	−14°C	149°F	0.6 mm @25°C
Heptane	98°C	−91°C	25°F	40 mm @22°C
n-Hexane	69°C	−95°C	−7°F	124 mm
Hexone	117°C	−84°C	64°F	16 mm
Isopropyl acetate	90°C	−69°C	36°F	42 mm
Isopropyl alcohol	83°C	−88°C	53°F	33 mm
Isopropyl ether	68°C	−60°C	−18°F	119 mm
Methanol	64°C	−98°C	52°F	96 mm
Methylcyclohexane	101°C	−127°C	25°F	37 mm
Methylene chloride	40°C	−95°C	None	350 mm
Nitroethane	114°C	−90°C	82°F	21 mm @25°C
Nitromethane	101°C	−29°C	95°F	28 mm
1-Nitropropane	132°C	−93°C	96°F	8 mm
n-Pentane	36°C	−130°C	−57°F	420 mm
Perchloroethylene	121°C	−19°C	None	14 mm
Propylene glycol monomethyl ether	120°C	−95°C	97°F	12 mm @25°C
Pyridine	116°C	−42°C	68°F	16 mm
Stoddard solvent	154–202°C	NA	102–110°C	NA
Styrene	145°C	−31°C	88°F	5 mm
Tetrahydrofuran	66°C	−108°C	6°F	132 mm
Toluene	111°C	−95°C	40°F	21 mm
1,1,1-Trichloroethane	74°C	−31°C	None	100 mm
Trichloroethylene	87°C	−73°C	None	58 mm
Turpentine	154–170°C	−50–−60°C	95°F	4 mm
Vinyl acetate	72°C	−93°C	18°F	83 mm
VM&P naphtha	95–160°C	NA	20–55°F	2–20 mm
o-Xylene	144°C	−25°C	63°F	7 mm

[a] Data from References 4 and 101.
[b] C, degrees centigrade; Ceiling, concentration that should not be exceeded during any part of the working exposure; F, degrees Fahrenheit; LEL, lower explosive limit; mm, mm Hg; ppm, parts per million; NA, noT available or not applicable; Specific gravity, at 20°C referenced to water at 4°C; TLV, threshold limit value; skin, potential exposure contribution due to cutaneous absorption; UEL, upper explosive limit; Vapor pressure at 20°C unless otherwise indicated.

Table 12.2
Solvent properties (*continued*)

Specific Gravity	LEL	UEL	TLV
0.79	4.0%	60%	25 ppm (ceiling)
0.79	2.5%	12.8%	500 ppm
0.88	1.1%	7.5%	50 ppm
0.88	1.2%	7.8%	0.5 ppm (skin)
2.89	NA	NA	0.5 ppm (skin)
0.81	1.4% @93°C	11.4% @93°C	200 ppm
0.88	1.7%	7.6%	150 ppm
0.81	1.4%	11.2%	50 ppm (ceiling, skin)
1.26	1.3%	50%	10 ppm (skin)
1.59	NA	NA	5 ppm (skin)
1.11	1.3%	9.6%	10 ppm
1.48	NA	NA	10 ppm
1.03	1.1% @150°C	NA	5 ppm (skin)
0.87	2.1%	15.5%	0.3 ppm (ceiling, skin)
0.86	0.9%	6.5%	50 ppm
0.78	1.3%	8%	300 ppm
0.96	NA	NA	50 ppm (skin)
0.95	1.1% @100°C	9.4%	25 ppm (skin)
0.87	1.5%	9.4%	10 ppm
1.30	2.2%	9.2%	25 ppm
0.71	1.8%	10.1%	5 ppm (skin)
1.19	0.9%	NA	5 mg/m^3
1.33	NA	NA	0.1 ppm (skin)
0.79	3.3%	19%	1000 ppm
0.90	2.0%	11.5%	400 ppm
1.11	3.2%	15.3%	100 mg/m^3(ceiling)
0.90	1.1% @93°C	12.7% @135°C	20 ppm (skin)
0.93	1.7% @93°C	15.6% @93°C	5 ppm (skin)
0.98	1.7%	NA	5 ppm (skin)
0.96	1.8%	14%	5 ppm (skin)
1.01	1.7%	8.2%	5 ppm (skin)
0.71	1.9%	36%	400 ppm
1.00	7%	73%	0.3 ppm (ceiling)
1.13	NA	NA	10 ppm (skin)
1.16	2.1%	19.3%	2 ppm (skin)
1.13	1.8%	16.3%	10 ppm (skin)
0.68	1.05%	6.7%	400 ppm
0.66	1.1%	7.5%	50 ppm
0.80	1.2% @93°C	8.0% @93°C	50 ppm
0.87	1.8% @38°C	8%	250 ppm
0.79	2.0%	12.7% @93°C	400 ppm
0.73	1.4%	7.9%	250 ppm
0.79	6.0%	36%	200 ppm (skin)
0.77	1.2%	6.7%	400 ppm
1.33	13%	23%	50 ppm
1.05	3.4%	NA	100 ppm
1.14	7.3%	NA	20 ppm
1.00	2.2%	NA	25 ppm
0.63	1.5%	7.8%	600 ppm
1.62	NA	NA	25 ppm
0.96	1.6 (calc.)	13.8% (calc.)	100 ppm
0.98	1.8%	12.4%	5 ppm
0.78	NA	NA	100 ppm
0.91	0.9%	6.8%	20 ppm
0.89	2%	11.8%	200 ppm
0.87	1.1%	7.1%	50 ppm (skin)
1.34	7.5%	12.5%	350 ppm
1.46	8% @25°C	10.5% @25°C	50 ppm
0.86	0.8%	NA	100 ppm
0.93	2.6%	13.4%	10 ppm
0.73–0.76	1.2%	6.0%	300 ppm
0.88	0.9%	6.7%	100 ppm

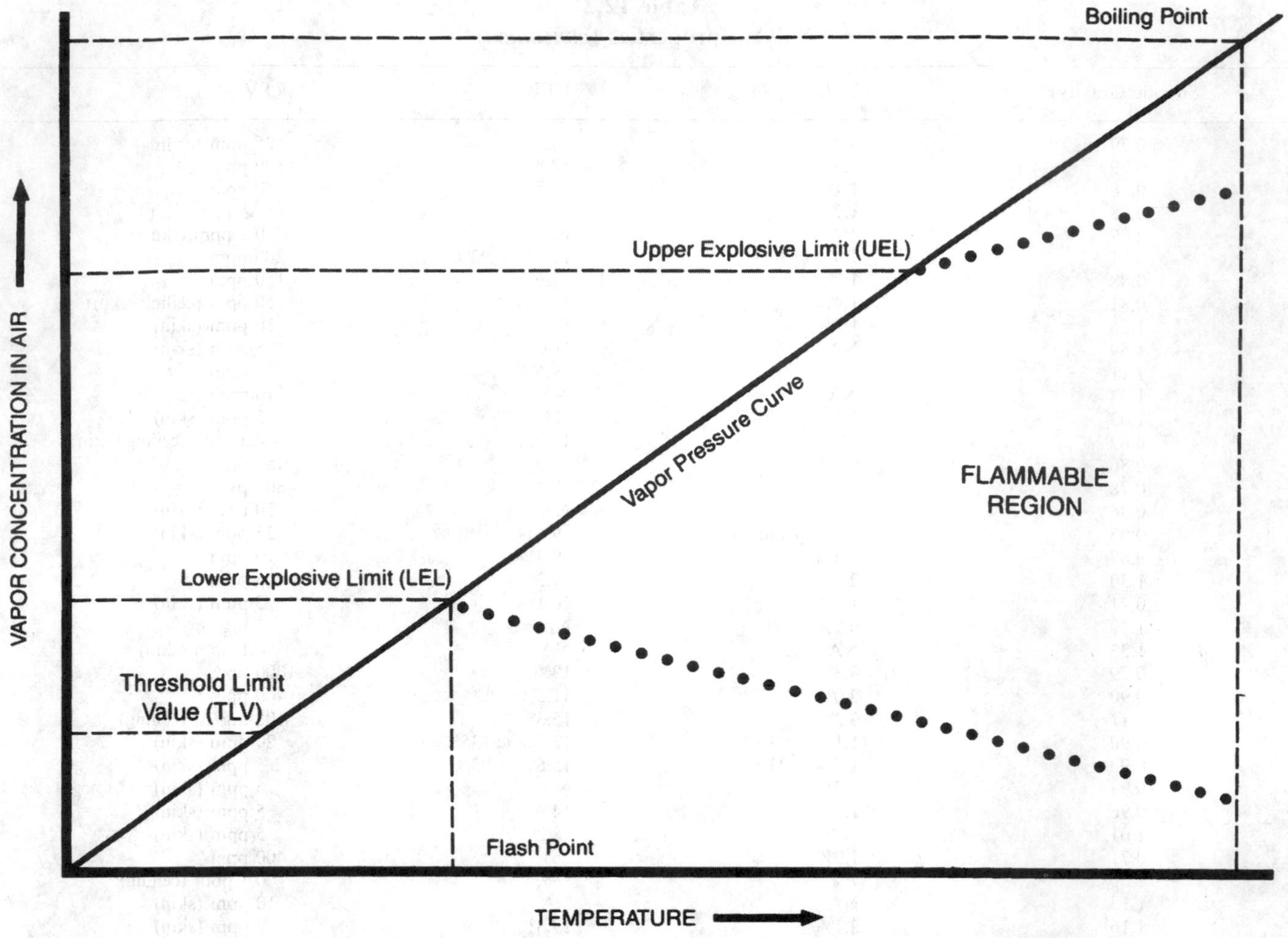

FIG. 12.1. Diagram of vapor pressure versus temperature showing relation between upper and lower flammable (explosive) limits, flammable and nonflammable regions, threshold limit value, boiling point, flash point, and vapor pressure curve. This diagram shows what happens to a vapor/air mixture as concentration and temperature vary.

monly accepted in the United States and in many parts of the world are the TLVs and the biological exposure indices (BEIs), which are updated yearly by the ACGIH. Other limits in the United States include the workplace environmental exposure level guides (WEEL) of the American Industrial Hygiene Association (AIHA), the recommended exposure limits (REL) of the National Institute for Occupational Safety and Health (NIOSH), and the permissible exposure limits (PEL) promulgated by OSHA. Exposure limits in Germany are the DFG (Deutsche Forschungsgemeinschaft) Maximum Concen- ıtion Values in the Workplace (MAKs) (2). In the ted Kingdom, the COSHH (Control of Substances rdous to Health) Regulations mandate adherence imum Exposure Limits (MEL) and Occupational Standards (OES) for protection of workers litional regulations may apply for extremely ubstances such as carcinogens. The processes by which various occupational exposure standards are developed have been reviewed for the United States, Russia, Australia, Britain, and Norway (139). OELs are intended solely for the protection of the workforce and should not be applied to exposures unrelated to the occupational environment.

Threshold limit values are airborne concentrations of substances to which most workers may be exposed during an 8-h workday and a 40-h work week without suffering detrimental health effects (4). Most are presented as TWAs. TWAs permit excursions above the limit, provided there are compensating equivalent exposures below the limit during the workday. Importantly, TLVs are not to be considered as absolute values differentiating between hazardous and nonhazardous concentrations, nor should they be used as a relative index of toxicity. Table 12.3 presents data used by ACGIH in developing TLVs.

Table 12.3
Data used in developing threshold limit values

Physical properties
Lipid solubility
Water solubility
Vapor pressure
Odor threshold
Acute toxicity data
Oral toxicity, LD_{50}
Dermal toxicity, LD_{50}
Dermal and eye irritation
Inhalation toxicity, LC_{50}
Subchronic data (oral, dermal, or inhalation)
14 day, NOEL[a]
90 day, NOEL
6 month, NOEL
Other data
Developmental (teratology and embryotoxicity)
Mutagenicity (Ames test, *Drosophila*, etc.)
Fertility
Reproductive (3-generation)
Reversibility study
Dermal absorption tests
Pharmacokinetics
Cancer bioassay (2-year)
Epidemiological data
Morbidity
Mortality
Case reports
Industrial hygiene exposure data
Area samples
Personal samples

[a] NOEL, no observed effect level.

To illustrate the TWA concept, consider a worker who is degreasing metal parts at two different workstations using trichloroethylene (50 ppm TLV). The employee spends 240 minutes at Station 1 with an average exposure of 30 ppm, followed by 45 minutes with no exposure (lunch), then 195 minutes at Station 2 with an exposure of 60 ppm. Calculating the 8-h TWA:

$$[(30\text{ ppm} \times 240\text{ min}) + (0\text{ ppm} \times 45\text{ min}) + (60\text{ ppm} \times 195\text{ min})]/480\text{ min} = 39\text{ ppm} \quad (1)$$

The TLV–TWA has not been exceeded. However, one may want to evaluate the employee's work practices and other aspects of the operation to reduce the exposure as much as possible (refer to sections on Exposure Controls and Personal Protective Equipment).

The TLV of a mixture is given by:

$$C_1/T_1 + C_2/T_2 \ldots + C_n/T_n = 1 \quad (2)$$

provided the components have similar toxicological effects and the air is analyzed for each component. The letters C and T represent the concentration and TLV of each chemical, respectively. If the calculation gives a value greater than 1, then the TLV has been exceeded.

As an example, suppose a worker was exposed to a mixture of 25 ppm trichloroethylene and 20 ppm perchloroethylene (25 ppm TLV) during the shift. The calculated TLV is:

$$25\text{ ppm}/50\text{ ppm} + 20\text{ ppm}/25\text{ ppm} = 0.5 + 0.8 = 1.3 \quad (3)$$

The threshold limit has been exceeded and action should be taken to reduce this exposure. For other examples of TLVs for mixtures, refer to the most current ACGIH TLV handbook (4).

Other categories of TLVs are short-term exposure limits (STEL) and ceilings. A STEL is a 15-minute time-weighted average exposure (above the 8-h TWA) that should not be exceeded during the workday. Allowances are made for up to four STEL excursions per day as long as there are at least 60 min between exposure periods and the 8-h TLV–TWA has not been exceeded. The STEL is supplementary to the TWA limit and should not be used exclusively as an exposure limit. Methanol is an example of a solvent having both an 8-h TLV–TWA (200 ppm) and a STEL (250 ppm). A ceiling limit is an airborne concentration that should not be exceeded, even instantaneously. Hexylene glycol is a solvent having such a limit (25 ppm).

For certain compounds a *skin* notation has been added to indicate a possible significant contribution to overall exposure from absorption through the skin, mucous membranes, or the eyes. Both methanol and propanol have skin notations.

BEIs denote levels of determinants (primarily from exhaled air, blood, and urine) likely to be found in workers exposed to the same degree as a worker with inhalation exposure to the TLV. The determinants are primarily the chemical itself or its metabolites. BEIs are a measure of the amount of chemical in the body and may be useful when evaluating the possibility of skin absorption, effectiveness of personal protective equipment, or nonoccupational exposure. BEIs are strictly related to 8-h exposures (5 days a week) and to the specified timing for the collection of the sample. A determinant for n-hexane is 2,5-hexanedione in urine (5 mg/g creatinine), measured at the end of the shift. In the case of altered work schedules, BEIs may be

Aliphatic Hydrocarbons

Straight or branched chains of carbon and hydrogen.

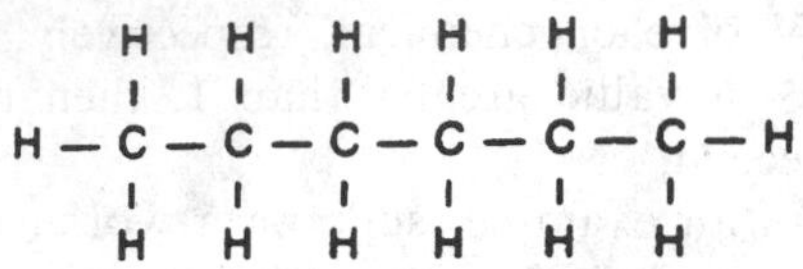

*Hexane	—	50 ppm
Heptane	—	400 ppm
VM&P Naphtha	—	300 ppm

Aromatic Hydrocarbons

Contain a 6-carbon ring structure with one hydrogen per carbon bound by energy from several resonant forms.

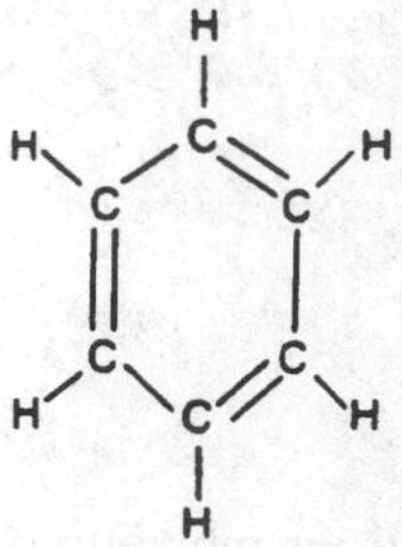

Benzene	—	0.5 ppm
Toluene	—	50 ppm
Xylene	—	100 ppm

Cyclic Hydrocarbons

Ring structure saturated and unsaturated with hydrogen.

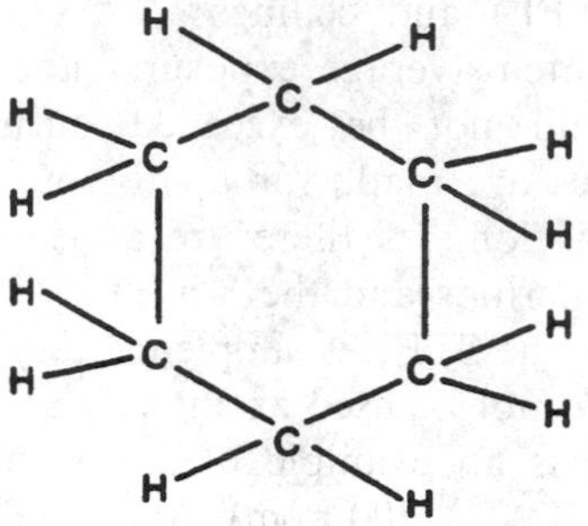

Cyclohexane	—	300 ppm
Turpentine	—	100 ppm

Alcohols

Contain a single hydroxyl group.

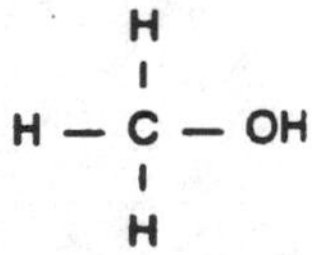

Methanol	—	200 ppm
Ethanol	—	1000 ppm
Isopropanol	—	400 ppm

Esters

Formed by interaction of an organic acid with an alcohol.

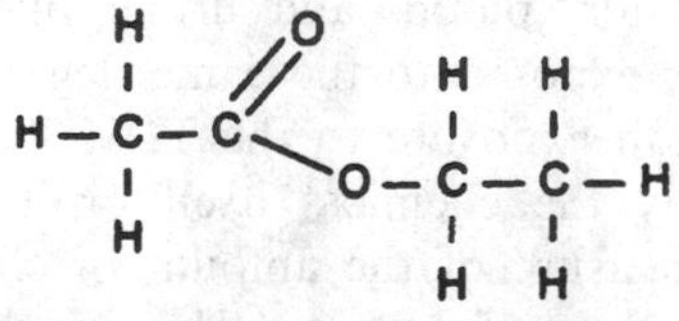

Ethyl Acetate	—	400 ppm
Isopropyl Acetate	—	250 ppm

Ketones

Contain a double bonded carbonyl group, C=O, with two hydrocarbon groups on the carbon.

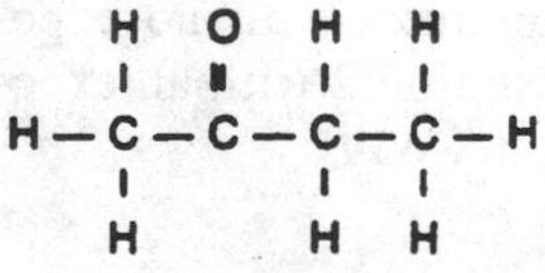

Methyl Ethyl Ketone	—	200 ppm
Acetone	—	500 ppm
Methyl Isobutyl Ketone	—	50 ppm

*TLV - American Conference of Governmental Industrial Hygienists (ACGIH) Threshold Limit Value (TLV-TWA), 1998.

FIG. 12.2. Classes of organic solvents.

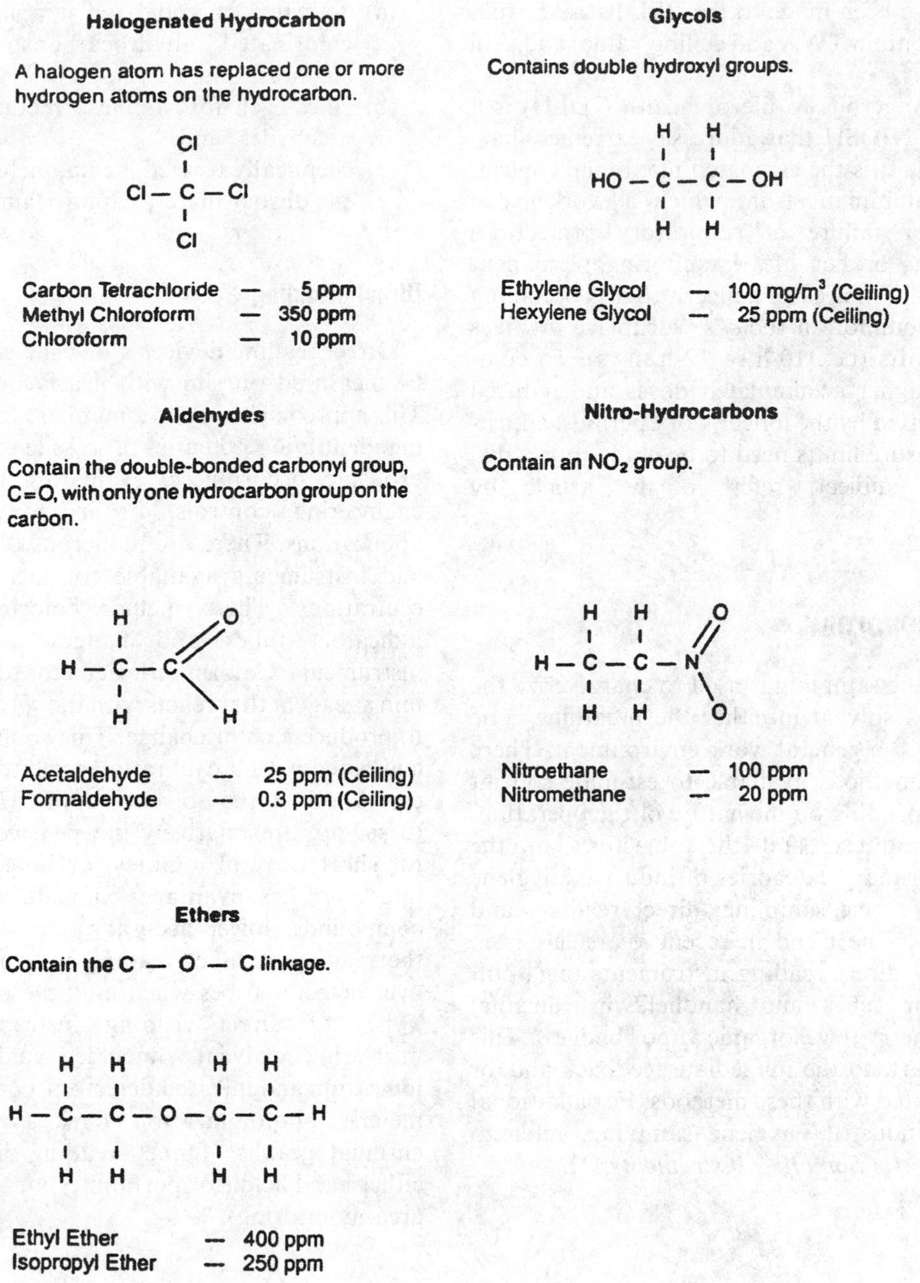

Halogenated Hydrocarbon
A halogen atom has replaced one or more hydrogen atoms on the hydrocarbon.
Carbon Tetrachloride — 5 ppm
Methyl Chloroform — 350 ppm
Chloroform — 10 ppm
Glycols
Contains double hydroxyl groups.
Ethylene Glycol — 100 mg/m3 (Ceiling)
Hexylene Glycol — 25 ppm (Ceiling)
Aldehydes
Contain the double-bonded carbonyl group, C=O, with only one hydrocarbon group on the carbon.
Acetaldehyde — 25 ppm (Ceiling)
Formaldehyde — 0.3 ppm (Ceiling)
Nitro-Hydrocarbons
Contain an NO2 group.
Nitroethane — 100 ppm
Nitromethane — 20 ppm
Ethers
Contain the C — O — C linkage.
Ethyl Ether — 400 ppm
Isopropyl Ether — 250 ppm

FIG. 12.2. (*continued*)

extrapolated based on pharmacokinetic and pharmacodynamic considerations (4).

The AIHA WEEL Committee develops WEELs for agents that have no current exposure guidelines established by other organizations. WEELs are expressed as TWAs; however, different time periods are specified depending on the properties of the agent. A skin notation is used in the same manner as the ACGIH TLV.

NIOSH RELs are expressed as either a TWA or a ceiling or both. These recommended limits are published as criteria documents and are periodically revised. They are established for up to a 10-h workday and are intended to provide the maximum possible protection for all workers against acute and chronic effects of exposure. Skin notations are applied.

OSHA PELs are the legal allowable concentrations of airborne contaminants. They were derived from existing standards during the enactment of the Occupational Safety and Health Act of 1970. Although the ACGIH revises some TLVs each year, the PELs remain as created unless changes are made in the law. A number of revisions and additions have been made to the PEL list since that time. The PELs contain TWA and ceiling values and skin notations.

Immediately dangerous to life or health (IDLH) is a limit specified by NIOSH that addresses extremely hazardous conditions. It is the estimated maximum concentration of a contaminant from which a worker can escape (i.e., after failure of respiratory protection) without losing his or her life or suffering permanent health impairment. An area of concern that is becoming more and more common in today's workplace involves extended work shifts (i.e., 10-h or 12-h days). To compensate for the higher accumulated doses and reduced recovery times caused by the longer work periods, adjustments to the exposure limits need to be made. For a discussion of this subject, refer to the article by Paustenbach (104).

SAMPLING METHODOLOGY

Industrial hygiene sampling is used to characterize the concentration of a solvent in either the breathing zone of a worker or in the general work environment. There are a number of methods available to estimate solvent concentration, depending on the nature of the operation, the solvent of interest, and the objectives of the evaluation. The primary categories of industrial hygiene sampling include active sampling, direct reading, and passive dosimetry. The trend in recent years has been toward the use of direct reading instruments (e.g., colorimetric detector tubes and handheld instruments) and passive dosimetry (e.g., organic vapor badges). This is due, in large part, to the immediate feedback and/or ease of use associated with these methods. For additional information on industrial hygiene sampling, refer to the ACGIH text, *Air Sampling Instruments* (1).

Active Sampling

Active sampling involves the use of a battery-powered sampling pump to draw contaminated air onto suitable collection medium, which is then analyzed in the laboratory to determine the amount of material collected. The sampling pump requires field and/or laboratory calibration to ensure that it is pulling air at the desired flow rate. The collection medium is connected to the sampling pump via tubing and is attached to the worker in his or her breathing zone (typically the shirt collar). When completed, the medium is returned to the laboratory where the chemical of interest is extracted and analyzed. Various types of collection media are available for solvents, depending on the material being evaluated. Examples include:

(a) activated charcoal for sampling solvents such as chlorinated hydrocarbons, gasoline, many alcohols, and ketones;
(b) silica gel for amines, methanol, phenols, and aldehydes; and,
(c) chemically treated media, including filters for toluene diisocyanates, naphthylamines, and toluidines.

Direct Reading

Direct reading devices allow solvent concentrations to be measured on site with nearly instantaneous results. This approach is used in a number of applications, including identifying potential process leaks, determining peak exposure occurrences, evaluating the effectiveness of engineering controls, or in continuous monitoring applications. There are numerous direct reading devices and instruments available for measuring solvent concentrations. These include colorimetric detector (or indicator) tubes and badges, and direct reading instruments. Colorimetric detector tubes and badges contain a reagent that reacts with the solvent vapor of interest to produce a color change. This color change, or stain, is compared with a calibration scale to determine the concentration of the solvent vapor. These tubes are easy to set up, are relatively inexpensive, and may be used for short (several minutes) or longer (hours) sampling intervals. Disadvantages include possible interfering compounds, lower accuracy, and some subjectivity in the readings. Direct reading instruments are preferred over detector tubes when multiple readings are desired. Types of direct reading instruments suitable for measuring solvents include analyzers with flame ionization and infrared detectors, combustible gas/vapor meters, photoionization devices, and portable gas chromatographs. Direct reading instruments can be either hand held (for portability) or fixed (for continuous area monitoring).

Passive Dosimetry

Passive samplers (e.g., organic vapor monitors) utilize the principles of molecular diffusion rather than a sampling pump to direct samples onto a collection medium (charcoal for organic vapor monitors). This technology is particularly well suited for personal monitoring because these devices

(a) are lightweight,
(b) are unobtrusive,
(c) require no external power source,
(d) require no calibration, and
(e) can be used to obtain short-term or full-shift exposures (19).

Organic vapor monitors are accurate and can be used to sample for many industrial solvents. Analysis is similar to charcoal tubes mentioned above.

EXPOSURE CONTROLS

Solvent overexposure may be avoided through proper planning, equipment design, and the use of process controls, where necessary. The approach to exposure control will depend on which route(s) of exposure are expected, primarily inhalation, skin contact, or a combination of both. Specific controls may be mandated by federal health and safety regulations (as in the case of benzene and vinyl chloride) or when exposure levels exceed established limits (such as permissible exposure limits or threshold limit values). The types of controls employed include engineering and administrative controls and the use of personal protective equipment. Control of solvent exposure is often achieved with a combination of these methods.

The preferred approach in controlling solvent exposure is through the use of engineering controls. Types of engineering controls (in order of preference) include change in a process to eliminate or reduce solvent usage; substitution with a less hazardous solvent; isolation of the process to minimize worker involvement; and ventilation to reduce the concentration of solvent vapor in the work environment. A discussion of each type of control follows.

Process Change/Solvent Elimination

Organic solvent-based processes can often be changed to eliminate or reduce solvent exposure. Eliminating the solvent is considered the best approach to controlling exposure and should be employed during the initial design of the process. Elimination has been used extensively in various organic solvent-based processes such as degreasing, cleaning, printing, painting, and metal treatment. These initiatives are the result of a combination of health and safety concerns, good business practices, and government regulations. In addition to minimizing worker exposure, elimination of organic solvents may have additional benefits as well, including the reduction of emissions into the environment and the cost savings associated with decreased waste disposal and personal protective equipment purchases. Two examples of process changes are replacing spray painting with paint dipping and replacing compressed air spray painting with electrostatic methods (less paint overspray). Examples of organic solvent elimination include: replacing chlorinated solvent degreasers with water-based detergent or subcritical carbon dioxide systems (discussed later); replacing solvent-based paints with water-based paints; improving flux application systems in circuit board manufacturing to eliminate the need for cleaning with chlorinated compounds; and using water-based or vegetable oil-based inks to eliminate solvent-based inks.

Substitution

In addition to directly eliminating solvents or using water-based materials, substitution of one organic solvent for another with lower toxicity or higher flash point is often employed. Substitutions may be made within a chemical series by retaining the active group. For example, substitution of butyl cellosolve for methyl cellosolve may be advantageous. The general group also can be retained such as in the substitution of aromatic naphtha for toluene, or toluene for benzene. Substituting a solvent with similar polar characteristics, but different toxicity, such as ethanol for methanol, may also be possible. Other examples include replacing perchloroethylene with citrus-based products in metal degreasing; substituting iosocyanate-containing coatings with toluene-based materials; and replacing formaldehyde used in preserving laboratory specimens with glycol-based compounds. Common solvents according to a group classification are shown in Table 12.4.

Isolation

A process can sometimes be enclosed and/or automated, to isolate the worker from the hazards of operation. When total enclosure of a solvent-based process is not possible, the operation can be separated from adjacent areas to minimize the number of workers exposed to the vapor. The isolation by enclosure of a solvent-based process usually requires the introduction of local exhaust ventilation (see below) to prevent the accumulation of vapors within the enclosure (fire/explosion hazard). Examples of isolation are found in most manufacturing environments. For instance, manual painting in automotive assembly plants and manual metal plating operations have been replaced with robotic systems. These automated processes often can be operated and monitored from remote locations.

Ventilation

When the methods discussed above are not feasible or available, introducing mechanical ventilation to the process can control solvent exposure. For industrial situations, this involves the delivery of uncontaminated air into the work area (dilution ventilation) and/or direct removal of contaminated air (local exhaust ventilation).

Typical applications for dilution ventilation are heat control (as in foundries), or regulation of humidity

Table 12.4
Common solvents classified by group

Aliphatic Hydrocarbons	
Gasoline	Hexane
Pentane	Octane
Mineral spirits	Heptane
Aromatic Hydrocarbons	
Benzene	Ethylbenzene
Styrene	Toluene
Cumene	Xylene
Halogenated Hydrocarbons	
1,1,1,-Trichloroethane	Chlorobenzene
Ethylene dichloride	Perchloroethylene
Methylene chloride	Trichloroethylene
Alcohols	
Amyl alcohol	Methyl alcohol
Benzyl alcohol	Butyl alcohol
Ethyl alcohol	Isopropyl alcohol
Ketones	
Methyl ethyl ketone	Diacetone alcohol
Cyclohexanone	Acetone
Esters	
Acetates	Lactates
Alkyl formates	Propionates
Ethers	
Butyl ether	Isopropyl ether
Ethyl ether	Ethylene glycol monoethyl ether

and odor. If dilution ventilation is to be used to reduce the concentration of solvent vapors in the ambient air, at least four conditions must be met:

1. The quantity of solvent vapor generated must not be too great because the air volume necessary for dilution will become impractical.
2. The worker must be far enough away from the source of solvent vapor generation so that the TLV is not exceeded.
3. The solvent must have low toxicity.
4. The solvent vapor must be released into the work environment at a uniform rate (3).

In contrast to dilution ventilation, which dilutes vapors to acceptable levels by adding fresh air, local exhaust ventilation (LEV) removes the solvent vapors at the source. It is generally more effective than dilution ventilation and cheaper to operate since lower air volumes and smaller fans are required. LEV systems consist of a hood, ductwork, and fan, and an optional cleaner for contaminant removal prior to discharge to the outside environment. Figure 12.3 shows a typical local exhaust ventilation system (6).

The decision of whether or not to install LEV for solvent exposure control is based on a number of factors, including: the lack of more cost-effective controls, amount and toxicity of the solvent vapor generated by the process, governmental requirements, or simply good management practice (6).

In LEV systems, the air is exhausted to the outside environment either directly or by passing the airstream through a cleaner. There are three types of LEV hoods

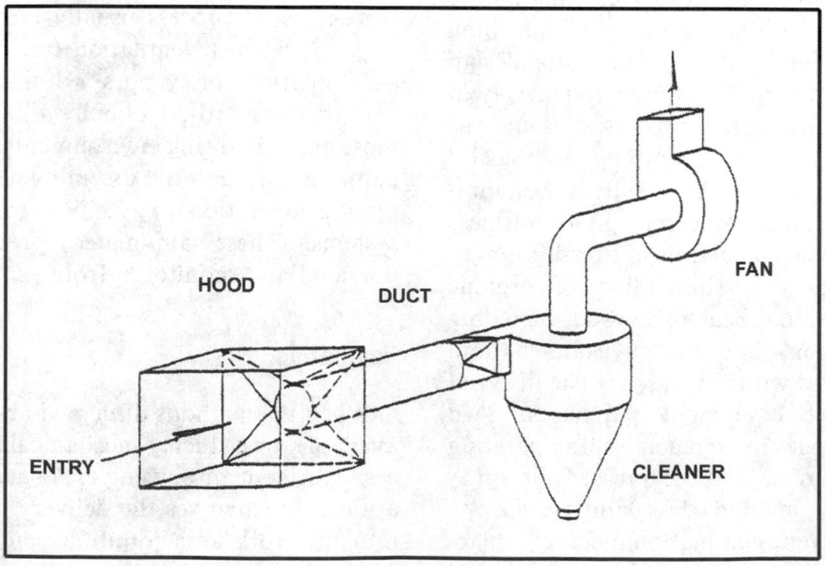

FIG. 12.3. Typical local exhaust system components. Reprinted with permission of the American Industrial Hygiene Association.

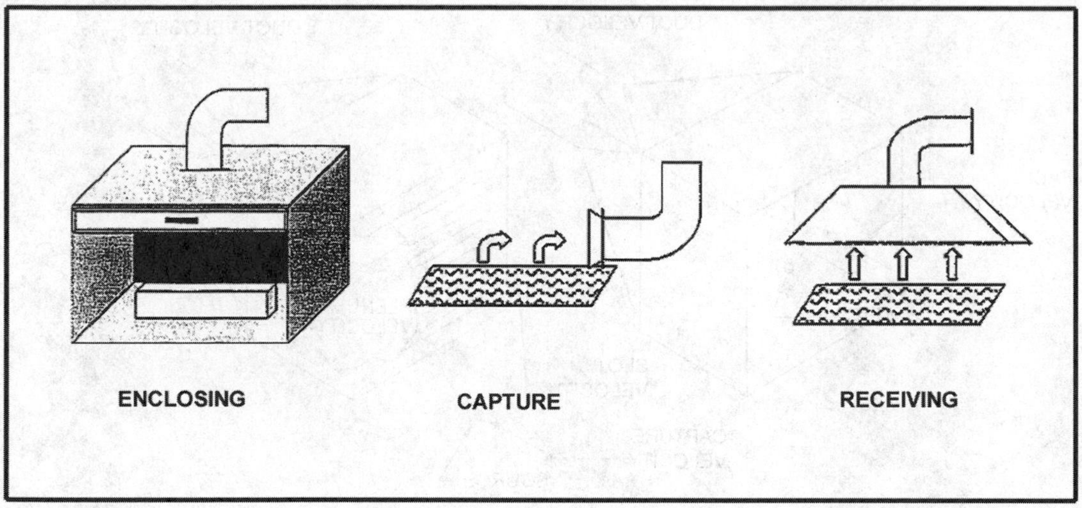

FIG. 12.4. Three types of local exhaust ventilation hoods.

used for solvent vapor control: enclosing, exterior (or capture), and receiving hoods. Figure 12.4 provides an illustration of each. Enclosing hoods are those which partially or completely enclose the process so that the point of contaminant generation is located within the hood. Enclosing the process as much as possible increases the effectiveness of LEV systems. Examples of enclosing systems include laboratory chemical fume hoods and spray paint hoods. Exterior hoods are those that are located near the point of contaminant generation, but that do not enclose it. Examples of exterior hoods are slot-type hoods used on vapor degreasing processes and flexible hoods used to exhaust solvent-based mixing processes. Receiving hoods are typically canopy-type hoods used for exhausting hot processes, for example, ovens and detergent baths. They are generally less suitable for solvent operations such as metal cleaning and degreasing.

Careful evaluation of the process should be carried out prior to selecting and designing a LEV system. Input should be provided from various disciplines, including engineering, planning, industrial hygiene, and labor. In addition to choosing the correct flow rates, designers must ensure that the arrangement of the hood and ductwork does not interfere with the work or other aspects of the facility's operation. In general, designers of LEV systems should take into account the flammability (e.g., use of approved wiring and motors) and toxicity of the solvent and the concentration generated, possible interfering air currents in the room, whether access to the work area is needed, and the amount of airflow or capture velocity required to adequately exhaust the contaminant (6).

As defined, capture velocity is the air velocity, at any point in front of the hood or at the hood opening, necessary to overcome air currents and to capture the contaminated air at that point by causing it to flow into the hood. Recommended capture velocities for solvents vary between 50 and 500 feet per minute depending on the conditions of solvent dispersion into the air (3).

Figures 12.5–12.7 detail principles of local exhaust ventilation, including hood nomenclature and design considerations. For further reading on local exhaust ventilation systems, refer to the fundamental text, *Industrial Ventilation: A Manual of Recommended Practice*, published by the American Conference of Governmental Industrial Hygienists (3).

Administrative Controls

Although generally not the preferred approach, administrative controls may be the only feasible method to control worker exposure in certain instances or while engineering controls are being implemented. Administrative controls may include job rotation or reduction in time permitted in the area of concern. One disadvantage of limiting individual solvent exposures through job rotation is that exposures may be spread over a greater number of workers. Furthermore, administrative controls often require the continual observance of employees and additional training.

Personal Protective Equipment

If engineering or administrative controls discussed above are not feasible and/or do not provide adequate protection, personal protective equipment (PPE) must be used to minimize exposures. PPE should always be considered a last resort and managed carefully by qualified individuals. This is due to a number of limiting factors associated with PPE, which include the following:

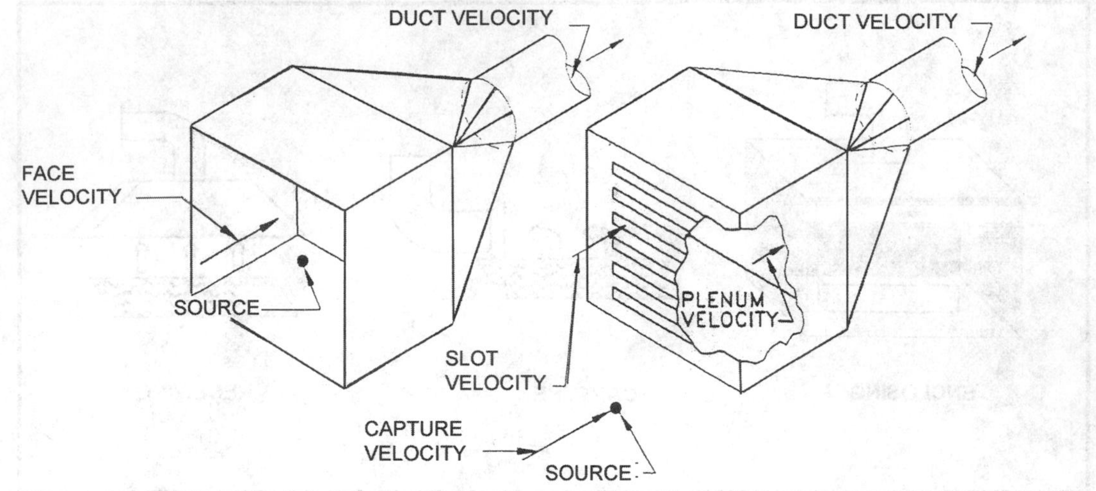

CAPTURE VELOCITY—AIR VELOCITY AT ANY POINT IN FRONT OF THE HOOD OR AT THE HOOD OPENING NECESSARY TO OVERCOME OPPOSING AIR CURRENTS AND TO CAPTURE THE CONTAMINATED AIR AT THAT POINT BY CAUSING IT TO FLOW INTO THE HOOD.

FACE VELOCITY— AIR VELOCITY AT THE HOOD OPENING.

SLOT VELOCITY— AIR VELOCITY THROUGH THE OPENINGS IN A SLOT-TYPE HOOD. IT IS USED PRIMARILY AS A MEANS OF OBTAINING UNIFORM AIR DISTRIBUTION ACROSS THE FACE OF THE HOOD.

PLENUM VELOCITY—AIR VELOCITY IN THE PLENUM. FOR GOOD AIR DISTRIBUTION WITH SLOT-TYPES OF HOODS, THE MAXIMUM PLENUM VELOCITY SHOULD BE 1/2 OF THE SLOT VELOCITY OR LESS.

DUCT VELOCITY— AIR VELOCITY THROUGH THE DUCT CROSS SECTION. WHEN SOLID MATERIAL IS PRESENT IN THE AIR STREAM, THE DUCT VELOCITY MUST BE EQUAL TO OR GREATER THAN THE MINIMUM AIR VELOCITY REQUIRED TO MOVE THE PARTICLES IN THE AIR STREAM.

AMERICAN CONFERENCE OF GOVERNMENTAL INDUSTRIAL HYGIENISTS	*HOOD NOMENCLATURE LOCAL EXHAUST*			
	DATE	*4–91*	FIGURE	*3–1*

FIG. 12.5. Principles of exhaust hoods. From American Conference of Governmental Industrial Hygienists (ACGIH) (1992) (3). Reprinted with permission.

1. PPE does not eliminate the hazard. When PPE is used to control solvent exposure, the hazard continues to exist since protection is achieved by creating a barrier between the hazard and the worker. Thus, if the protection fails (such as a tear in a glove or a leak in a respirator), the worker is directly exposed to the hazard.
2. PPE requires continual worker and supervisor involvement. The effectiveness of the PPE depends not only on matching the protective device against the hazard, but, also, on the worker using the equipment properly and using it when needed. This is especially important for chemical-resistant gloves and respirator cartridges since no single glove or cartridge provides protection against every solvent.
3. Appropriate training is required. Federal regulations require that potential users be trained in the correct use and care of PPE.
4. PPE may provide a false sense of security. Some workers may believe that PPE provides complete protection, leading them to take chances when handling solvents. This is particularly true in emergency

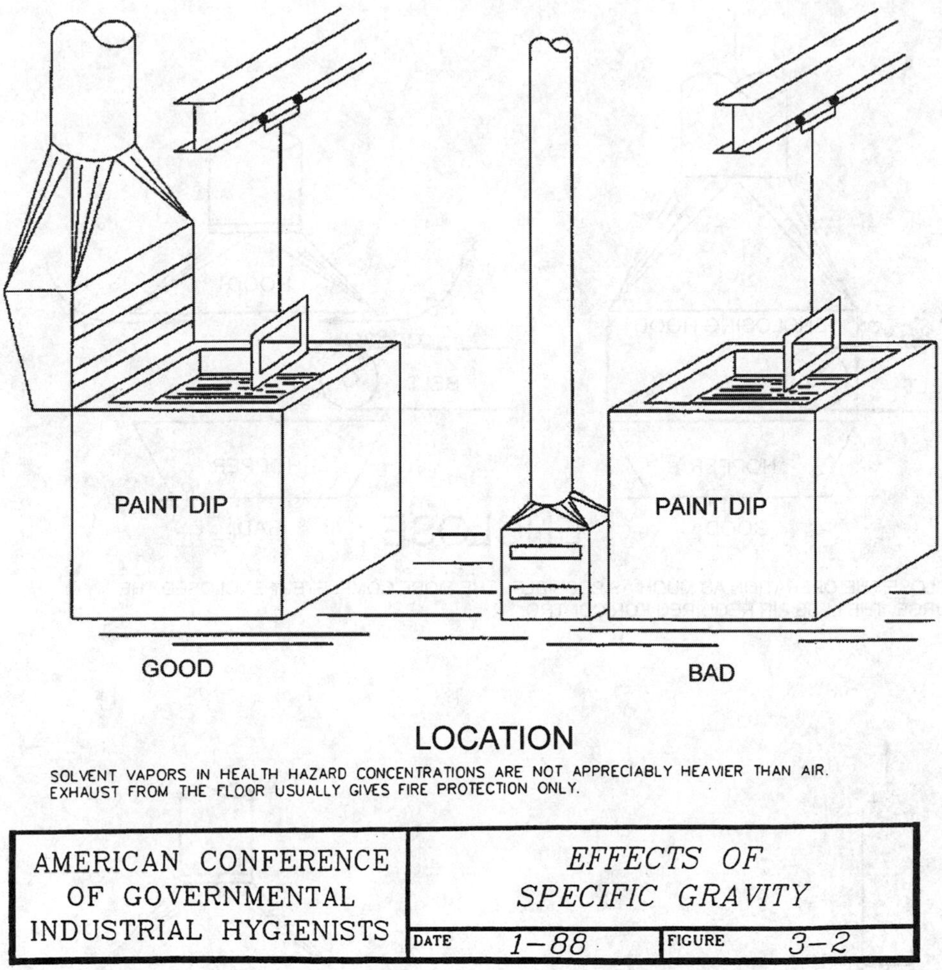

FIG. 12.6. Principles of exhaust hoods. From American Conference of Governmental Industrial Hygienists (ACGIH) (1992) (3). Reprinted with permission.

incidents where a worker may attempt to address a spill with PPE that might not be designed for the type of chemical or concentration involved.

There are various types of PPE used in the workplace, but the primary categories associated with solvent hazards are respiratory protection, protective clothing (including chemical-resistant gloves), and eye and face protection. The specific type of PPE must be carefully matched against the hazard. Often, a combination or mixture of chemicals exists, which can make PPE selection a challenge. As a general recommendation, it is always best to consult with manufacturers prior to purchasing PPE. Following is a discussion of PPE used to control solvent exposure.

Respirators

Respiratory protection is used to prevent or reduce the level of worker exposure to airborne hazards. It is often employed to control intermittent exposures that can occur during entry into contaminated areas or during emergency repair and maintenance. However, respirators also may be the only feasible method of protection for exposures that may occur during normal work operations.

When LEV or other control methods are not feasible, the employer should provide workers with respiratory protection and implement an effective respiratory protection program. The goal is to ensure that the appropriate type of respiratory protection is selected and used correctly. OSHA has established requirements for a respiratory protection program in 29 CFR (*Code of Federal Regulations*) 1910.134. The standard instructs employers to develop written standard operating procedures to direct the respiratory protection program. Elements of the program include respirator selection, user training and fit testing, medical approval, and specific instructions for cleaning and maintenance. (See 1998 update).

The two major categories of respiratory protection are air-purifying and atmosphere-supplying respirators.

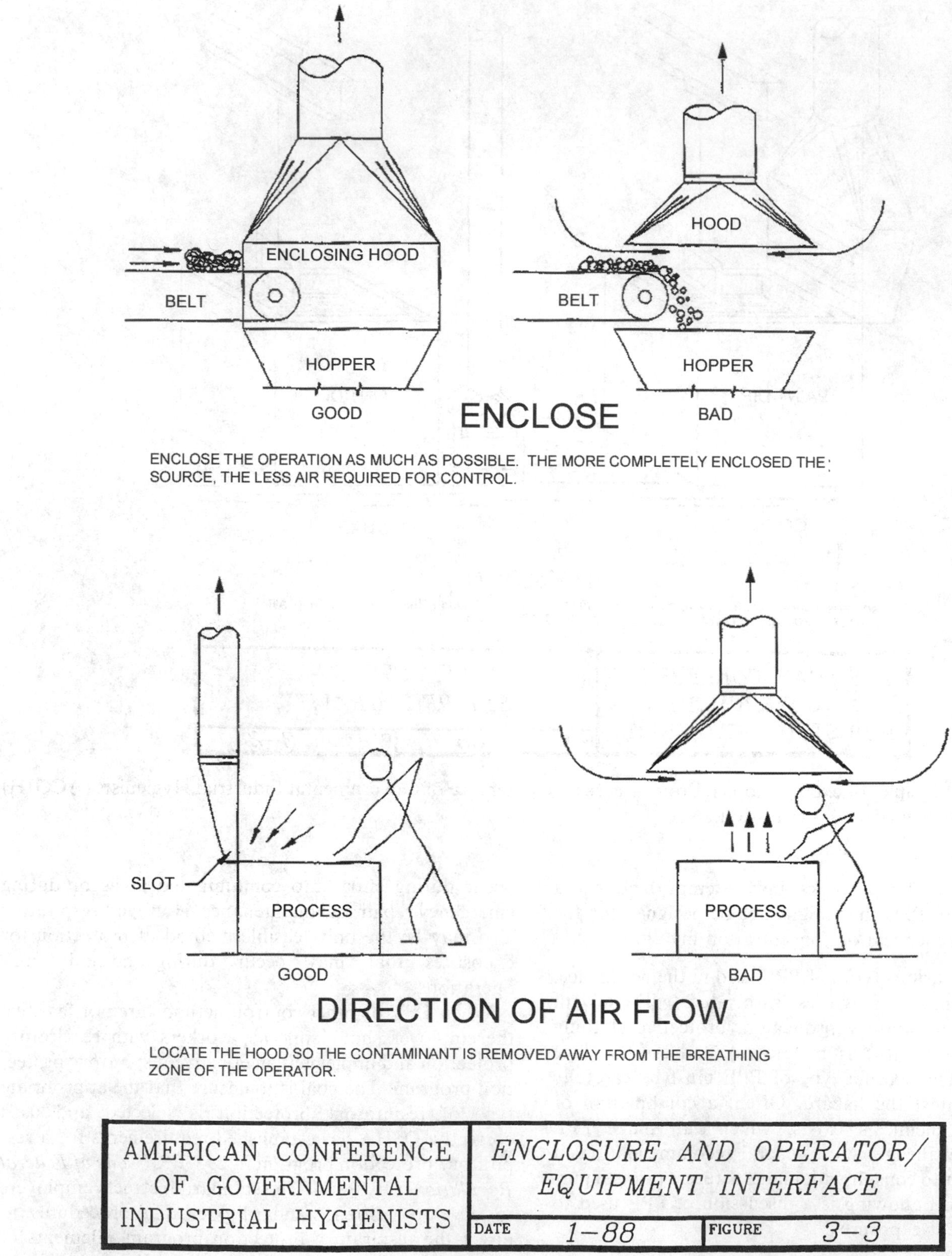

FIG. 12.7. Principles of exhaust hoods. From American Conference of Governmental Industrial Hygienists (ACGIH) (1992) (3). Reprinted with permission.

Air-purifying devices for solvent exposure protect the worker by removing the contaminant from the airstream prior to its reaching the worker's respiratory system. This is accomplished by passing the contaminated air through a cartridge containing a sorbent such as charcoal. Air-purifying respirators come in various models, including half-mask, full-face, and powered air-purifying devices. Atmosphere-supplying respirators provide the user with a source of clean air separate from the local environment. Examples of atmosphere-supplying respirators include air-line devices and self-contained breathing apparatus (SCBA). Only approved respirators (i.e., by the National Institute for Occupational Safety and Health) should be worn.

Other factors that must be considered when selecting respiratory protection are the type of hazard, including oxygen deficiency, concentration of the contaminant, and adequacy of warning properties. For situations involving very high solvent concentrations and/or oxygen-deficient atmospheres, air-purifying respirators do not provide adequate protection. Thus, assessment of the hazard through industrial hygiene sampling is a key component in the selection process. Warning properties, such as odor, taste, and respiratory irritation provide an indication to the user that the device is not functioning properly (e.g., the service life of the sorbent has been reached) or the device is being worn incorrectly (e.g., leak around the face seal). Air-purifying respirators should not be worn for chemicals with poor warning properties (6). Since people vary greatly in their ability to detect odors, other methods such as cartridge replacement schedules or end-of-service-life indicators are being developed by various groups to ensure greater safety when using air-purifying equipment.

Protective Clothing

Protective clothing protects against dermal exposure by forming a barrier between the skin and the solvent. Protective clothing includes gloves, laboratory coats, rubber aprons, chemical resistant suits, and boots. Various types of chemical-resistant clothing are available, depending on the solvent of concern, the work involved, and the level of protection desired. Classifications include neoprene, nitrile, natural or butyl rubber, polyvinyl chloride, and viton. Some operations may require only partial protection (such as a rubber apron) while others may need full-body enclosures (such as those used by emergency response workers). The type of material and degree of protection chosen could affect the mobility, vision, and manual dexterity of the worker. Encapsulating suits can also present potential heat stress hazards for work conducted outdoors in the summer or work conducted indoors around heat-generating operations.

The amount of protection afforded by a given type of chemical-protective clothing is related to three primary performance factors: permeation, degradation, and penetration. Permeation is the ability of a chemical to pass through the molecules of a protective film (e.g., the clothing or glove). Degradation is a reduction in one or more of the physical properties of protective clothing or gloves due to contact with a chemical. Penetration is the flow of a chemical through physical aspects of the clothing or glove, such as zippers, seams, pores, or imperfections in the material.

Manufacturers of protective clothing determine product-specific performance data via laboratory tests conducted in accordance with methods established by the American Society for Testing and Materials (ASTM). All three factors should be considered when choosing protective clothing since data for two or three of the factors may not correlate for a given type of clothing and target chemical. For example, a glove may have acceptable degradation ratings for a chemical, but the chemical may readily permeate the material. No single glove or type of protective clothing provides adequate protection against every hazard. Furthermore, a glove type from one manufacturer often has different performance data from the same glove type produced by another manufacturer. Another general source of information is *Chemical Protective Clothing*, published by the American Industrial Hygiene Association (5). This two-volume set provides data needed to select and use chemical protective clothing. Included in the document is a discussion of permeation theory, testing methods, and available vendors.

Eye and Face Protection

Eye and face protection is used to prevent injuries that may occur while handling or transporting solvents. Two types of protective eyewear typically used to prevent exposure are chemical splash goggles and face shields. Chemical splash goggles are designed to completely enclose the eyes (as opposed to safety glasses, which are designed to prevent physical injuries that may result from an object striking the eye). Some goggles may also prevent vapor exposure to the eye in addition to contact with the liquid. Face shields are often worn in conjunction with goggles to protect the face and neck. Face shields and goggles that meet recognized safety standards bear the engraving of ANSI Z-87, which indicates that the device has passed safety performance tests conducted by the American National Standards Institute.

ABSORPTION OF SOLVENTS AND INHALATION EXPOSURE

A key factor in the absorption of solvents, whether by ingestion, dermal exposure, or inhalation, is the partitioning (solubility) of the chemical into blood and tissues.

When considering solvent exposure by inhalation, the rate of solvent uptake and subsequent equilibrium concentration in tissues are also dependent on pulmonary ventilation and the minute volume of blood flow through the lung and other organs.

Solvents that are highly soluble in blood and tissues are absorbed very readily by inhalation, and blood concentrations can rise rapidly. The driving force is the difference in concentration between inspired air and blood. The amount diffusing through the alveolar capillary membrane is dependent on the air–blood partition coefficient. Tissue equilibrium concentrations with solvents such as xylene, styrene, and acetone, which are highly soluble in blood and tissues, are not limited by pulmonary ventilation because the tissues act as a sink for the inhaled solvent. As pulmonary ventilation is increased, the blood and tissue concentrations continue to rise. The limiting factor in attaining the tissue equilibrium concentration is the blood flow through the tissues and the blood–tissue partition coefficient.

Solvents such as methyl chloroform, methylene chloride, trichloroethylene, and toluene, which have lower solubilities in blood and tissues, reach equilibrium rapidly because of low solubility or low blood–air partition coefficients. Tissue concentrations also will reach equilibrium rapidly because of low tissue–blood partition coefficients. Tissue concentration is limited, then, by tissue solubility and pulmonary ventilation. To achieve a higher concentration in tissues and blood, pulmonary ventilation must increase, allowing more solvent to enter the blood and a new blood–tissue equilibrium to be obtained (13,14).

DERMAL UPTAKE OF SOLVENTS

The opportunity for solvents to enter the body through dermal contact is enhanced, in part, due to the large surface area of the skin (18 ft^2). Fortunately, the barrier properties of the skin, which are associated with filamentous proteins and lipids of the stratum corneum, naturally inhibit penetration by harmful substances. Disruption of this barrier, however, by injury, illness, or removal of lipids, can facilitate passage of these materials. For example, treatment of the skin with polar organic solvents, detergents, and some surfactants can remove the lipids, thereby increasing the skin's permeability.

Penetration of the skin also depends on a number of factors such as the thickness and integrity of the skin layer, the difference in concentration of solvent on both sides of the epithelium, and a number of physical constants. In addition, hydration can increase absorption by affecting the permeability of the skin. Movement of water-soluble compounds may be impeded, however, when the stratum corneum is highly hydrated. Although hair follicles and sweat glands comprise only a small proportion of the skin's surface area, they, too, provide pathways for solvent penetration.

Solvents can damage the skin by removing lipids, resulting in irritation, cellular hyperplasia, and swelling. For example, the careless use of solvents without proper hand and arm protection frequently leads to cases of dermatitis in the workplace. In a study of skin lipid removal by solvents, it was found that the ability of a solvent to penetrate the skin depends on the polarity of the solvent and the surface charge of the skin. Results comparing penetration or removal of lipids by several solvents showed that ethanol, the solvent with the greatest polarity, extracted the most lipids, followed by acetone and then ether (17).

Treatment of the skin with solvents can also increase the penetration rate of other compounds. In a study using excised human skin, the effect of several solvents including DMSO, dimethylacetamide, formamide, and dimethylformamide on the penetration rate of sarin was examined (86). Results showed that solvent pretreatment increased the rate of sarin transport by a factor of 10–100 over that of sarin on control skin.

Penetration of solvents by the dermal route in humans was studied for toluene, xylene, and styrene vapors. Volunteers were exposed to 300 or 600 ppm for 3.5 h in a dynamic exposure situation in which the subjects wore full-face respirators to prevent pulmonary absorption of the solvents. A 10-min exercise period was sufficient to make the subjects perspire and to raise the skin temperature about 0.5°C. Perspiration and warm skin temperature enhance the hydration of the skin and subsequent percutaneous absorption. After termination of exposure, these solvents displayed biphasic elimination from the blood into exhaled air with a short half-life of about 1 h and a much longer half-life of approximately 10 hr. Xylene and styrene had slightly delayed excretion in exhaled air after percutaneous exposure when compared with inhalation exposure. Delayed excretion after dermal exposure may be accounted for by a slow release from the skin after termination of exposure.

Overall percutaneous absorption of the compounds above corresponded to only about 0.1 percent of the amount estimated to be absorbed by the pulmonary route, thus indicating a very small absorption potential by the percutaneous route. When the percutaneous absorption of xylene vapor was compared to earlier work with xylene liquid, the vapor displayed an approximately 10-fold greater efficiency in penetrating the skin than did the liquid. According to the authors, it was not uncommon to observe greater penetration with vapor exposure because liquid solvents removed the lipids from the stratum corneum and thus interfered with absorption. Additionally, exercise promoted the absorption of solvents because of the warm hydrated skin. In general, under reasonable exposure conditions in the workplace, percutaneous absorption of solvent vapors would not contribute significantly to the total blood concentrations of these solvents (116).

TOXICOLOGY OF SELECTED SOLVENTS

This section deals with solvents of occupational concern that have had neurotoxic, reproductive, or carcinogenic effects in humans. Examples are provided for these as well as less toxic, alternative solvents. Generally speaking, acute exposure to high levels of solvents (i.e., greater than the TLV) results in alterations of central nervous system (CNS) function. Repeated solvent exposures give rise to the organ-specific pathology described below for individual chemicals.

Effects of Acute Solvent Exposure on the Central Nervous System

Although varying widely in chemical structure and physical properties, solvents produce a rather stereotypical set of toxicological manifestations upon acute exposure (10). Most commonly these include evidence of dysfunction of the CNS and, if exposure is sufficiently severe, narcosis. Exposure to certain solvents has been associated with alterations of cognitive and psychomotor function following short-term exposures at or near the TLV. For example, controlled studies of volunteers exposed to toluene (100 ppm for about 6 h) revealed decreased manual dexterity, visual perception, and color discrimination (15). Exposure to greater concentrations may provoke symptoms including, for instance, headache, dizziness, ataxia, a sense of euphoria, drowsiness, lightheadedness, disorientation and confusion, tremulousness, and nausea. These symptoms are readily reversible under single exposure conditions upon removal of the individual to a solvent-free environment. Exposure to potentially lethal levels of solvents can result in stupor, loss of consciousness, coma, respiratory depression, and abnormal cardiac function. Information on neurotoxic symptoms associated with acute exposure to specific solvents is found in the latter portion of this chapter.

Other Toxic Effects of Solvent Exposure

Exposure to solvents at concentrations too low to induce many of the acute symptoms cited above is of special concern with regard to neurotoxicity, because the capacity of nervous tissues for post-toxicity regeneration is limited and repeated insults may lead to cumulative damage. The subtlest symptoms of chronic solvent exposure include relatively mild alterations of mood and behavior not accompanied by quantifiable evidence of dysfunction on neurobehavioral tests (18,57). Although dose-response and causal relationships have been difficult to study in the absence of animal models, symptoms of chronic solvent exposure may include increased irritability, decreased span of attention, and loss of interest in daily activities. More severe damage to the nervous system, both central and peripheral, occurs upon repeated exposure to certain solvents such as carbon disulfide and n-hexane (discussed later).

Numerous neurobehavioral and functional tests have been used to detect such changes in both clinical and experimental settings (69,112). Whether the acute effects of solvents play a role in determining the pathogenesis of toxic lesions observed after chronic exposure to the same solvents is uncertain. However, current thought is that the acute effects on the nervous system are mediated through nonspecific interactions of solvents with the cell membrane, that is, increases in membrane fluidity or functional alteration of cell surface receptors, while the effects of chronic exposure are mediated by specific biochemical actions of solvents.

Organs that receive a high percentage of the cardiac output are exposed to greater doses of absorbed toxicants than poorly perfused tissues. A major determinant of target organ selectivity for the toxicity of solvents is xenobiotic metabolism. While pharmacokinetics defines the quantity of solvent reaching a particular organ or tissue after absorption, metabolism may yield products with increased toxic potential relative to the parent chemical. Thus, well-perfused organs with high capacities for specific types of biotransformation reactions, mainly those catalyzed by the cytochrome P450, are common targets for solvent-induced toxicity. In particular, the liver is vulnerable to the toxicity of many solvents, owing to its high capacity for xenobiotic metabolism. Many common hepatotoxic solvents yield toxic intermediates or end products upon biotransformation, for example, carbon tetrachloride (113), chloroform (109), and trichloroethylene (16). However, some solvents, such as ethanol, may exert their hepatotoxic effects indirectly by altering cellular redox balance during metabolism and thereby deranging normal liver function and structure (117).

The kidney, as a filtering and concentrating organ of excretion, receives not only untransformed solvents but also the products of hepatic metabolism of solvents. These biotransformation products—for example, conjugates of trichloroethylene—may be more toxic than the parent chemical and produce renal-specific toxicity (81). The ion transport and solute concentrating functions of renal tubules also contribute to the vulnerability of the kidney to certain chemical toxicants (82). In addition, biochemical peculiarities of certain species and genders may play a major role in bringing about solvent-induced renal toxicity. A notable example is the susceptibility of the male rat to renal toxicity caused by 1,4-dichlorobenzene, Stoddard solvent, VM&P naphtha, and other hydrocarbon solvents. This has been attributed to the male rat–specific abundance of the low molecular weight protein α_{2u}-globulin, which acts as a carrier for lipophilic molecules (128). α_{2u}-Globulin is normally degraded in renal tubule lysosomes and binding to a solvent ligand slows degradation of the protein so that the α_{2u}-globulin-hydrocarbon complex is sequestered by lysosomes (77). The sequestered protein apparently disrupts lysosomal function and cytotoxicity results when large amounts of α_{2u}-globulin accumulate (121). There is apparently no counterpart to this type of nephrotoxicity in species other than the rat (7).

Organs that catalyze relatively few types of chemical biotransformation reactions or have low rates of xenobiotic metabolism, such as lung, nasal mucosa, and testes, may also be target organs for the toxicity of some solvents. For example, ethylene glycol monomethyl ether and related glycol ethers are testicular toxicants (58,95) as are hexane and the hexane metabolite 2,5-hexanedione (22). Recently, special attention has been paid to the potential susceptibility of the tissues lining the upper airways—the nasal mucosa—to solvent-induced toxicity. These tissues have high levels of certain xenobiotic-metabolizing enzymes and, in addition, are exposed to high solvent concentrations relative to the lung and other organs. In particular, esters such as propylene glycol monomethyl ether acetate, dimethylphthalate, and dimethylsuccinate are enzymatically transformed by nasal carboxylesterase to yield acidic products that may accumulate to toxic levels in the nasal mucosa (95,126,133). Certain solvents need no metabolism to adversely affect the tissues of the upper respiratory tract; vapors or aerosols of aldehydes cause local tissue damage to the nasal epithelium (97), presumably due to the activity of these solvents in forming protein–protein and protein–DNA crosslinks (61).

It is well known that neurotoxic chemicals can have a negative impact on the sensory function. Often, the first symptoms reported following chemical exposure are those related to the senses (48). Toluene, xylene, styrene, trichloroethylene, and carbon disulfide are examples of solvents associated with adverse affects on the auditory system (98). In the industrial environment, workers are often exposed to solvents as well as high levels of noise, which is known to damage the inner ear and cause hearing loss. In recent years, evidence has emerged from workplace studies and animal experimentation that the combined effects of noise and ototoxic solvents may increase the susceptibility to hearing loss (68,98). In one animal study, rats were exposed to toluene or noise or toluene followed by noise and then had their auditory functions tested. Results showed that rats exposed to toluene followed by noise exhibited a decrease in auditory sensitivity greater than the sum of the effects of toluene and noise alone (98). The risk for hearing loss may be increased by factors other than noise, such as drugs or other chemicals, and can also be influenced by heredity and aging (98). It is important to take all of these factors into account when addressing hearing loss in the workplace.

Solvent Mixtures

Humans are often exposed to multiple chemicals at work or in the home. An example, as reported by Worksafe Australia (the Australian National Occupational Health and Safety Commission), involved solvent exposure and health effects in spray-painter apprentices (143). Their study identified 32 different solvents contained in 20 thinner products used by the painters. The solvents represented six classes of compounds: alcohols, aromatic hydrocarbons, esters, glycol ethers, ketones, and mixtures. Of significance was the fact that the workers commonly perceived the thinners to be equivalent and safe to use. This underscores the need for chemical communication programs to inform workers about the potential hazards of working with mixtures of chemicals.

Exposure to multiple chemicals, either simultaneously or sequentially, may alter the toxicological interactions of the individual chemicals, leading to a change in the toxicity as predicted by summing their individual effects. Thus, one chemical may alter the absorption, distribution, metabolism, and/or excretion of other chemicals in a mixture (74). The study of chemical interactions has been developed most extensively for therapeutic drugs. Although some information exists on interactions of industrial chemicals, most toxicological research to date has dealt with single, pure chemicals. These single chemical studies are important because they allow researchers to gather fundamental knowledge about the mechanisms of toxicity under conditions that are well controlled. Additional research is required to examine the potential health effects associated with exposures to multiple compounds (148).

Glycol Ethers

Glycol ethers represent an important category of solvents that are widely used in mixtures for industrial and consumer applications. They are grouped as ethylene glycol, propylene glycol, or butylene glycol ethers, with the ether portion of the molecule containing methyl, ethyl, propyl, butyl, or higher molecular weight moieties (52). Additional members of this class of compounds are the corresponding acetate esters. The miscibility of glycol ethers with water and many organic compounds make them ideally suited as solvents in oil–water compositions. Production capacity of the ethylene-based ethers in 1992 exceeded one billion pounds, with the coatings (paint) industry being the major consumer (52). In addition to coatings, glycol ethers are found in many household goods such as brake fluids, waxes, cleaners, dyes, detergents, degreasers, and inks. 2-Butoxyethanol has been formulated into hundreds of consumer products (27).

The current ACGIH TLV–TWAs and German MAKs for three widely used glycol ethers, 2-methoxyethanol (ME), 2-ethoxyethanol (EE), and 2-butoxyethanol (BE), are 5 ppm, 5 ppm and 20 ppm, respectively. The NIOSH RELs and proposed OSHA PELs for ME and EE are significantly lower at 0.1 ppm and 0.5 ppm, respectively. All have skin notations. ACGIH based their limit for ME on possible blood, reproductive, and CNS effects. For EE and BE, effects on reproduction and the blood were considered, respectively. The TLV and REL for propylene glycol monomethyl ether (PGME) are both 100 ppm and are based on potential irritation and CNS effects (2,4,101).

The commonly encountered glycol ethers are colorless liquids with mild odors. The primary routes of exposure in the industrial environment are inhalation and skin absorption (52). Some cases of accidental or intentional ingestion of products containing glycol ethers by children and adults have been reported (27). In general, the ethylene glycol ethers exhibit low acute oral toxicity (52). Experiments in rats have shown that the methyl, ethyl, and butyl ethers are readily absorbed through the skin (118). As the molecular weights of the glycol ethers increase, the potential for inhalation exposure and skin absorption decreases. Because the methyl and ethyl ethers of ethylene glycol and their acetates have demonstrated adverse reproductive, embryotoxic, teratogenic, and developmental effects in animal studies (58–60,99,100), their use in consumer products has declined (52).

Monoalkyl ethers of ethylene glycol are converted to their respective alkoxyacetic acids via the actions of alcohol dehydrogenase (27). Many of the observed adverse effects caused by ethylene glycol ethers in animals, such as hemotoxicity (e.g., 2-butoxyethanol) and testicular toxicity, are attributed to these toxic metabolites. Whereas rat erythrocytes have demonstrated vulnerability to the hemolytic effects of 2-butoxyacetic acid (from BE), human erythrocytes have been shown to be much less susceptible to these effects (27).

PGME and its acetate (PGMEA) are relatively innocuous compounds when compared to the ethylene glycol ethers discussed above. Overexposure to PGME has been associated only with increased liver weight and CNS depression. Studies have shown that EE and PGME are metabolized by different routes and the types of metabolites produced are responsible for the marked differences in toxicity. For example, methoxyacetic acid is the primary metabolite of EE, while propylene glycol is the main biotransformation product of PGME and PGMEA (94,96).

Investigators have studied the potential interaction of ethanol and EE because of similar metabolic pathways and the likelihood of concomitant exposure to ethanol in some individuals (100). EE, when presented to rats alone or in combination with ethanol, seemed to increase the duration of pregnancy. Exposure to EE during gestational days 7–13 caused a decrease in certain behavioral tests such as rotorod performance. However, when EE was exposed to animals that also consumed ethanol the behavioral deficit was diminished. When EE was administered alone during late gestation, motor activity of pups was depressed and performance at avoidance conditioning trials was retarded. Combined administration of EE and ethanol seemed to exaggerate the behavioral deficits induced by EE and to depress both activity and learning.

Examination of neurotransmitters in 21-day-old pups that had been whelped by dams exposed to EE alone on gestational days 7–13 revealed an increase in several neurotransmitters such as acetylcholine, dopamine, and norepinephrine. Pups that were whelped by dams that had the combined treatment displayed a decrease in acetylcholine, dopamine, and 5-hydroxytryptamine. Thus, it was observed that ethanol during late gestation altered the neurochemical effects of EE.

In summary, concomitant exposure to ethanol can have differential effects depending on the stage of gestation. Ethanol administration during the early period of gestation ameliorated both the behavioral and neurochemical effects of EE to approximately 50 percent of the response produced by EE alone. In the late stage of gestation the combination of ethanol with EE exaggerated the effects of EE alone. This indicates that the possibility exists for ethanol-induced exaggeration of the potential toxic effects of EE exposure in pregnant workers.

Retrospective epidemiological studies of workers exposed to ME and EE have reported evidence of adverse effects on the male reproductive system, with increased frequency of reduced sperm counts (145). Evaluation of sperm production in several species has shown that the output of human sperm is about one-fourth that of other mammals when compared on a per-gram tissue basis. This finding suggests that humans may be more susceptible to occupational toxicants than predicted by laboratory animals (130). As is the case with many widely used chemicals with potentially harmful effects, substitutes are being considered. PGMEA and ethyl-3-propionate have been identified as useful and less toxic alternatives to ethylene glycol ether solvents (23).

Benzene

Benzene has been used extensively over the years as a raw material in the manufacturing of polymers, detergents, pesticides, dyes, plastics, and resins, and as a solvent for waxes, oils, natural rubber, and other compounds (93,123). In addition, benzene is a component of gasoline and is generally present at low levels throughout the environment (64).

Exposure to benzene in the workplace is primarily through inhalation, but skin absorption may also contribute to the overall body burden. OSHA regulates benzene as a potential occupational carcinogen with a PEL of 1 ppm and a STEL of 5 ppm (102). The ACGIH TLV–TWA and STEL for benzene are 0.5 ppm and 2.5 ppm (skin notation), respectively, and ACGIH has designated benzene as a confirmed human carcinogen (4). The NIOSH REL and STEL for benzene are 0.1 and 1 ppm, respectively. NIOSH additionally lists benzene as a potential occupational carcinogen (2). The ACGIH BEI for benzene is 25 μg of the metabolite S-phenylmercapturic acid per gram of creatinine in urine, measured at the end of the work shift (4).

Because of its high lipid solubility, acute exposure to benzene can cause depression of the CNS to the point of narcosis. Headache, dizziness, nausea, and vomiting are all features of benzene overexposure. Exposure to benzene at high concentrations can lead to blurring of vision, unconsciousness, convulsions, ventricular irregularities, and respiratory failure. Death as a result of exposure to extremely high concentrations of benzene may occur because of respiratory failure or cardiac arrhythmias (123,144). Concomitant exposure to benzene and high concentrations of catecholamines can sensitize the heart and lead to ventricular fibrillation.

Benzene is hematotoxic and carcinogenic following repeated exposure to high concentrations (90). There are numerous rodent studies that also show that benzene can cause cytogenetic damage in vivo (64). In addition, examination of the chromosomes of humans exposed to high levels of benzene revealed an elevated rate of chromosomal aberrations that persisted after cessation of exposure (47). Chronic exposure to benzene leads to a progressive depression of bone marrow function (83). Epidemiological studies have demonstrated that blood dyscrasias such as pancytopenia, aplastic anemia, and acute myelogenous leukemia can develop in humans as a result of this exposure (90,123). Furthermore, clinical investigations have shown that it may take several years after the termination of exposure for benzene-induced leukemia to appear (138).

Enzymes linked to the metabolic activation of benzene and its metabolites are the cytochrome P450 monooxygenases and myeloperoxidase (90). The major metabolic pathway for benzene appears to be oxidation to a phenol, which is then converted to a sulfate conjugate and excreted in urine. Other hydroxylated metabolites include hydroquinone and catechol. Benzene metabolism can be effected by interactions of benzene with its metabolites or other compounds. For example, experiments in mice suggest that benzene can inhibit the oxidation of phenol. Furthermore, animal and human studies have demonstrated that coexposure to toluene may significantly alter the formation of benzene metabolites. Finally, treatment with ethanol induces benzene and phenol metabolism in the liver, resulting in higher levels of active metabolites (90).

The mechanism of benzene-induced leukemia is not known. Potential mechanisms for benzene-induced bone marrow disease include metabolism of the parent compound to phenols and other metabolites, in particular, quinone-type metabolites such as catechol, quinol, and pyrogallol which could react with chromosomes and interfere with mitosis. Another possibility could be the depletion of sulfur available for glutathione detoxification, thereby leading to interaction of toxic intermediates with critical elements of the bone marrow. Another suggested mechanism involves transfer of benzene metabolites from the liver to the bone marrow (123). Researchers have investigated the metabolism and binding of radiolabeled benzene in the isolated hind limb of rats in which benzene was administered directly into the bone marrow space. Metabolites of benzene were found covalently bound to macromolecules in the bone marrow, indicating that the bone marrow has the potential of metabolizing benzene to reactive intermediates (67). The fact that benzene or benzene metabolites have been shown to inhibit the multiplication of erythrocyte precursor cells in the bone marrow may imply an additional mode of action (76).

The potential for benzene to induce leukemia in experimental animals has been difficult to demonstrate. In an inhalation study involving Sprague–Dawley rats and AKR mice, benzene vapor (300 ppm) was administered for 6 h a day, 5 days a week, for the lifetime of the animals. The rats showed signs of lymphocytopenia, mild anemia, and slightly decreased survival. The mice displayed severe lymphocytopenia and anemia with significantly decreased weight gain and survival. However, no evidence of a leukemic or pre-leukemic response was observed in either species (122). In a 2-year carcinogenicity study, rats and mice fed benzene in corn oil developed dose-related leukopenia and tumors in multiple organs, but the study failed to show benzene-associated leukemia (64).

Toluene

Toluene is a flammable solvent that has been used extensively in the chemical, rubber, paint, and drug industries. It is also useful as a solvent for paints, inks, lacquers, dyes, and other compounds, and as an additive for gasoline. Sources of toluene in the environment include manufacturing plants, automobile emissions, gasoline evaporation, and cigarette smoke (31,93).

Various exposure limits and biological indicators of exposure apply to toluene. The ACGIH TLV–TWA, German MAK, and NIOSH REL for toluene are 50 ppm (skin notation), 50 ppm, and 100 ppm, respectively. NIOSH adds a 150 ppm STEL and has established an IDLH of 500 ppm. The current OSHA PEL is 200 ppm with a 300 ppm ceiling limit. The ACGIH BEIs are 0.05 mg toluene per liter of venous blood, collected before the last shift of the work week, 1.6 grams of hippuric acid per gram of creatinine in the urine, collected at the end of the shift, and 0.5 mg of o-cresol per liter of urine, collected at the end of the shift (2,4,101). Toluene in expired air has also been evaluated to determine its usefulness as an indicator of exposure. Analysis of expired air in toluene-exposed workers revealed that the toluene concentration was correlated to the exposure environment, representing approximately 15–20 percent of the environmental concentration (28).

The principal toxic effect of toluene is injury to the nervous system. Toluene is most rapidly absorbed by inhalation, followed by ingestion and skin contact. A substantial amount of inhaled toluene is retained in the body. The toxicity of toluene is similar to that of benzene except that it does not exhibit the hematopoietic effects characteristic of benzene. Toluene is an eye and skin irritant and animal studies indicate that its acute oral toxicity is less than that of other alkylbenzenes (31). In humans, acute effects of toluene exposure can resemble alcoholic intoxication by first stimulating and later depressing the central nervous system. Groups of volunteers exposed to 100 ppm of toluene vapor for 6 hr, complained of fatigue, sleepiness, and the feeling of intoxication. Irritation of the eyes, nose, and throat was reported as well as decreased manual dexterity and accuracy in visual perception (15).

Exposure to high concentrations of toluene, as seen in cases of solvent abuse (e.g., glue sniffing), may cause death by sensitizing the myocardium (115,144). In chronic abusers of toluene, irreversible neurological toxicity and reversible renal damage have also been reported (129,142). Symptoms associated with intentional inhalation of high concentrations of toluene include euphoria, mild tremors, unsteady gait, and changes in behavior. Encephalographic examination of these individuals has shown abnormalities indicative of cerebellar atrophy (71). Toluene is a lipid soluble compound that readily crosses the placenta and, as such, may pose a teratogenic risk in cases of high exposure, as with intentional abuse. A pattern of teratogenicity like that of the fetal alcohol syndrome (described in the section on ethanol) is prevalent in human studies relating to excessive in utero exposure to toluene. Coabuse of alcohol and toluene may heighten the risks (142).

Toluene is metabolized to benzoic acid, which is subsequently conjugated with glycine or glucuronic acid to form hippuric acid or benzoylglucuronates, respectively. These conjugates, as well as another metabolite, o-cresol, are excreted in the urine (75). In human studies ethanol was shown to inhibit the metabolism of toluene at blood ethanol concentrations of 21 mmol/liter (42). Results indicated that the concentration of toluene in alveolar air of the toluene/ethanol-exposed group was significantly higher than that of the toluene control group. Additionally, hippuric acid and o-cresol excretion was significantly reduced as compared to controls. During the 24 hours following the last exposure, excretion of both hippuric acid and o-cresol was about 40–50 percent of that excreted by subjects who received toluene alone. These results suggest that ethanol may alter the metabolism of inhaled toluene and prolong its elimination from the body. Therefore, the possibility of ethanol consumption should be considered during biological monitoring since ethanol intake could lead to an underestimation of the actual toluene exposure (42).

In contrast to the above, pretreatment of rats with phenobarbital (PB) showed that the metabolism of toluene could be enhanced to form benzoic acid. The pretreatment did not, however, appear to effect the rate of conjugation of benzoic acid with glycine to form hippuric acid. The hippuric acid concentration in the urine of PB pretreated rats was about three times that of rats receiving toluene only. In addition, the toluene concentration in the blood of the PB pretreated group was only about one-half that in the toluene-exposed rats. Not only did the phenobarbital pretreatment enhance metabolism of toluene to benzoic acid (with subsequent conversion to hippuric acid), it also reduced the blood concentration of toluene and thus shortened the sleeping time induced by the narcotic effect of toluene (66).

The mechanism of the neurotoxic effect of toluene is not well understood. Some experimental work with rats found that exposure to 30,000 ppm toluene for a few minutes reduced the concentration of tryptophan and tyrosine in plasma by about 50 percent and 20 percent, respectively, compared to controls. Tryptophan and tyrosine are known to be precursors of the neurotransmitters noradrenaline, dopamine, and 5-hydroxytryptamine. The reason for the decrease in the precursors was unknown, but it was speculated to be an alteration in the hepatic uptake or utilization of these amino acids (141).

A potential factor in toluene-induced neurotoxicity is production of reactive oxygen species that can cause cell damage. Experiments using rats suggested that benzaldehyde, a metabolite of toluene, accelerates the production of these reactive oxygen species within the nervous system, and may also contribute to the overall neurotoxicity (87).

n-Hexane

n-Hexane is a flammable liquid and one of the most toxic of the alkanes. It is an excellent organic solvent that has been used in industrial applications such as printing, low-temperature thermometers, adhesives, extractions, and cleaning processes (30,62).

The primary routes of exposure in the industrial setting are by inhalation and skin contact. The ACGIH TLV–TWA, NIOSH REL, and German MAK are all 50 ppm. ACGIH added a skin notation and NIOSH established an IDLH value of 1100 ppm (10% of the lower explosive limit). ACGIH set the TLV based on possible neuropathy, CNS effects, and irritation (2,4,101).

Acute toxic responses after accidental ingestion include nausea, gastrointestinal irritation, and CNS effects. Inhalation overexposure leads to dizziness, a sense of euphoria, and numbness of the extremities. Exposure to high concentrations causes vertigo and a marked anesthetic effect. Hexane is also an irritant to the skin upon dermal exposure (30).

Many cases of polyneuropathy in workers exposed to n-hexane have been noted, with the earliest occurring in Japan (147). The severity of symptoms in the Japanese workers varied directly with degree and duration of exposure and in some cases there was incomplete recovery (62). Polyneuropathy has also been reported in cases of solvent abuse (30). The neurotoxic effect of n-hexane has characteristically been a progressive motor or sensorimotor neuropathy with symptoms usually reported after several months of exposure (62). In cases from occupational exposure, symptoms have often been sensory, with numbness and paresthesia in the distal extremities, most notably the feet or hands. Improvement of symptoms is noted after cessation of exposure, and mild cases can recover completely.

Hexane is readily absorbed in laboratory animals and has an affinity for tissues high in lipid content (24). It is rapidly metabolized to hydroxylated compounds prior to being converted to a keto form (72,84). 2,5-Hexanedione and methyl n-butyl ketone are the metabolites suspected of being responsible for the production of neurotoxicity.

The mechanism of 2,5-hexanedione-induced neuropathy is not known but several hypotheses have been presented (39). These include reduction in energy production in the axon resulting in disruption of axonal transport, alteration of protein structure, and inadequate proteolysis of neurofilaments in the nerve terminal. 2,5-Hexanedione has been shown to interact with glyceraldehyde-3,5-dehydrogenase and phosphofructokinase, inhibiting their glycolytic properties and resulting in decreased energy production and possible disruption of axonal flow. Reaction of 2,5-hexanedione with lysine amine moieties to form pyrrole adducts and modification of neurofilament or axonal skeletal proteins is also an attractive hypothesis (40). Modification of the proteins may lead to crosslinking of the neurofilaments, which could cause difficulty in neurofilament passage through narrow regions of the axon such as the node of Ranvier, and therefore an accumulation of proteins at the site of constriction. Possible biophysical membrane changes as a result of 2,5-hexanedione may influence the degeneration of the axon. 2,5-Hexanedione binding and inactivation of calcium-dependent proteases that are important for degradation of neurofilament proteins is the last mechanism mentioned that might lead to accumulation of neurofilaments. Although none of the mechanisms mentioned fully answers all of the questions concerning n-hexane-induced neurotoxicity, these hypotheses offer some contributions to the understanding of the toxic response. It may be that several mechanisms act in parallel to produce the neurotoxic effects.

Repeated exposure of rats to n-hexane not only produces the characteristic pattern of neurotoxicity but results in testicular lesions as well (146). The testicular effects are linked to disruption of the cytoskeleton of Sertoli cells. Secondary effects, caused by a loss in functional spermatogonial cells, are seen in affected tubules. Acute exposure led to reversible effects but inhalation or oral exposures of two to five weeks led to irreversible effects. Although the neurotoxic effect of n-hexane is observed in humans, the testicular effect seen in rats has not been well documented in humans.

Methyl n-Butyl Ketone

Methyl n-butyl ketone (2-hexanone, MBK) has been used as a solvent or cosolvent (e.g., with methyl ethyl ketone) for adhesives, lacquers, vinyl coatings, printing inks, oils, varnish removers, and other materials (25,73).

Occupationally, the principal routes of exposure to MBK are via inhalation and skin contact with the liquid. The ACGIH lowered the TLV–TWA for MBK in 1998 to 5 ppm (skin notation) to protect against possible neuropathy. The German MAK is also 5 ppm. The NIOSH REL and IDLH for MBK are 1 ppm and 1600 ppm, respectively (2,4,101).

Methyl n-butyl ketone has low acute oral toxicity. Inhalation of high vapor concentrations causes eye and respiratory tract irritation followed by CNS depression and narcosis (131). MBK easily penetrates the skin, and inhalation exposure yields approximately 80–85 percent pulmonary retention. In addition, MBK is widely distributed in the tissues, the highest concentrations being found in the blood and the liver (25). Chronic exposure to low doses may produce degenerative axonal changes, primarily in the peripheral nerves and long spinal cord tracts (124,125,131).

Depending on the route of administration, a number of metabolites in varying amounts can be detected in the blood. The primary neurotoxic metabolite, as with n-hexane, is 2,5-hexanedione. Other metabolites identified following oral, intraperitoneal, or respiratory exposures include 2-hexanol and 5-hydroxy-2-hexanediol (25).

MBK was implicated as a neurotoxic agent in the 1970s after instances of neurotoxicity were reported in the printing and painting industries (9,91). Inhalation was the primary route of exposure, with the severity of the developed neurotoxicity proportional to the extent of exposure. The characteristic disorder caused by methyl n-butyl ketone begins several months after chronic exposure commences. Symptoms include weight loss and distal sensory neuropathy marked by a tingling sensation in the hands or feet. The muscular weakness that develops usually involves the hands and feet, but in severe cases may extend to the legs and thighs. The sensory loss is symmetrical and may progress to the legs and thighs in severe cases. There is also a moderate reduction of nerve conduction velocity in affected peripheral nerves (8,9).

When volunteers were given MBK by inhalation, orally, or by dermal application, 2,5-hexanedione was detected in the serum. Radioactivity associated with the radiolabeled MBK was found to be excreted slowly, indicating that repeated exposures to high concentrations of methyl n-butyl ketone may lead to prolonged exposure to its neurotoxic metabolites (41).

The relative neurotoxicity of methyl n-butyl ketone, n-hexane, and their metabolites was investigated in rats. Potency was estimated by the time required to produce evidence of severe hind limb weakness or paralysis. Results showed 2,5-hexanedione to be most toxic followed by 5-hydroxy-2-hexanone, 2,5-hexanediol, methyl n-butyl ketone, 2-hexanol, and n-hexane. An examination of the data showed that the neurotoxic potency was related to the amount of 2,5-hexanedione metabolically produced (73).

Carbon Disulfide

Carbon disulfide (CS_2) is a toxic and highly flammable solvent that has found extensive use in the manufacturing of rayon, soil disinfectants, carbon tetrachloride, and electronic vacuum tubes. It is commonly used as a solvent in industrial hygiene analyses. Other applications include its use as a fumigant for grain and a corrosion inhibitor (21,93).

Inhalation and skin contact are the main routes of occupational exposure. Because adaptation to carbon disulfide's characteristic rotten egg odor occurs rapidly, the sense of smell is not useful in judging exposure. The current ACGIH, OSHA, and NIOSH exposure limits are 10 ppm, 20 ppm, and 1 ppm, respectively, all with skin notations (2,4). The ACGIH TLV–TWA was set to protect against cardiovascular, central nervous system, and neuropathic effects. NIOSH has established an IDLH value of 500 ppm (101). In addition to these levels, there have been proposals in the literature to lower the occupational exposure limit to 4 ppm to prevent neurological sequelae (63). The Biological Exposure Index recommended by ACGIH is 5 mg of the metabolite 2-thiothiazolidine-4-carboxylic acid (TTCA) per gram of creatinine in urine, measured at the end of the work shift (4).

Acute exposure to high concentrations of carbon disulfide can result in restlessness, euphoria, nausea, vomiting, headache, mucous membrane irritation, unconsciousness, and fatal convulsions. Chronic exposure can lead to abnormalities such as irritability, hallucinations, auditory and visual disturbances, and weight loss (21,55,78,93,137). Distal sensorimotor neuropathy is the most common chronic effect associated with CS_2 exposure. This has been confirmed in experimental animals as a neurofilamentous axonopathy that effects long axons in the CNS and peripheral nervous system (36,54). Peripheral neuropathy takes place only after frequent and prolonged exposures to CS_2 and is characterized by a loss of distal sensory and motor function. The condition can progress more proximally with continued exposure. Chronic exposure to CS_2, as well as hexane, 2-hexanone, and their metabolite 2,5 hexanedione, results in large swellings of the distal axons which are filled with neurofilaments. Continued exposure causes axonal degeneration distal to the axonal swellings. (34,54). In addition to these effects, encephalopathy, detected by neurological examination and neuropsychological testing, has been reported.

There is evidence that exposure to CS_2 accelerates the rate of atherosclerosis (54). In addition, an investigation to determine a possible association between CS_2 exposure and ischemic heart disease mortality found that the relationship is meaningful only for workers exposed to high levels for many years. Price has suggested a safe level of between 15 and 20 ppm (111).

Approximately 70–90 percent of absorbed CS_2 is metabolized and excreted in the urine. The remaining 10–30 percent is exhaled in the breath unchanged. In addition to TTCA mentioned above, other metabolites found in workers' urine include 2-mercapto-2-thiazolin-5-one and thiocarbamide (63,107,108,135,136).

In a study of rayon production workers with long-term exposure to carbon disulfide at concentrations well above the TLV, evidence of neuropathy was observed in a significant number of workers and consisted of distal sensory loss, altered tendon reflexes, reduced muscle power, and reduction in nerve conduction velocity. These abnormalities persisted for up to 10 years after removal from exposure and were considered to be permanent impairments in nervous system physiology (35).

Methanol

As Table 12.1 shows, synthetic methanol (or methyl alcohol, wood alcohol) production exceeded one billion pounds in 1995. Methanol's largest use is in the production of MTBE (methyl t-butyl ether), an additive in gasoline. It is also utilized as a denaturant for ethanol, a raw material in the production of numerous other chemicals such as formaldehyde and acetic acid, and as a solvent or antifreeze in paints and strippers, cleaners, and windshield washer compounds (43).

The major routes of exposure to methanol in the industrial environment are through inhalation and dermal contact. The ACGIH TLV–TWA of 200 ppm (250 ppm STEL) is based on potential ocular toxicity and CNS effects. The OSHA PEL and NIOSH REL have also been set at 200 ppm. NIOSH has further established an IDLH value of 6000 ppm for methanol, and ACGIH and NIOSH have added skin notations as indications that skin absorption can be a contributor to the overall body burden. The ACGIH BEI is 15 mg methanol per liter of urine, collected at the end of the work shift (2,4,101).

Most information regarding methanol toxicity in humans is gathered from acute exposures, primarily from ingestion, but there are reports of adverse health effects from inhalation and dermal exposures (80). In one NIOSH study, teachers' aides reported headaches, blurred vision, and other symptoms following inhalation exposure to methanol used in duplicating machines. Concentrations at the site were about 2–15 times the current REL. Adverse effects have also been reported following skin applications of methanol for various purposes, although inhalation may have also contributed to these exposures (80).

Methanol is readily absorbed following oral, inhalation, or dermal exposure and is distributed throughout the body according to water content of the tissues (80). Ingestion of as little as 2 teaspoonfuls may cause toxicity, whereas the fatal dose in humans is between 2 and 8 oz (53). In the absence of medical treatment, a dose of between 4 and 10 mL can lead to blindness (114), and depending on the amount of methanol ingested, mild to severe CNS depression can occur. A latent period, commonly 12 to 24 hr, usually ensues followed by severe abdominal pain, difficult breathing, blurred vision, and pain in the eyes, among other symptoms. Visual impairment or total blindness may occur within days depending on individual susceptibility and the time when treatment began (80). Metabolic acidosis due to formic acid production is thought to be the cause of the delayed symptoms and the ocular toxicity (114).

Metabolism of methanol in the liver accounts for a high percentage of absorbed methanol in both nonhuman primates and rats. Lesser amounts are excreted unchanged in the urine and breath. Metabolism is important not only because of its primary role in clearance, but because of the connection between its metabolites and the acute toxic effects mentioned above. Methanol is oxidized by a catalase-peroxidative system in rats, rabbits, and guinea pigs and an alcohol dehydrogenase system in humans and primates. The metabolic sequence proceeds from methanol to formaldehyde to formic acid (formate) and finally to carbon dioxide and water. Formic acid is metabolized in both rats and primates via a folate-dependent pathway. Rats are able to utilize this pathway more efficiently than primates, allowing for a more rapid conversion to carbon dioxide. Because the process is slower in humans and primates, high doses of methanol cause a buildup of formate in tissues, including the eye, resulting in the observed toxicity (114).

Administration of ethanol has been used in treating methanol poisoning because ethanol inhibits the oxidation of methanol by competing for the same metabolic pathway. Prompt hemodialysis (able to remove both methanol and formate), coupled with concurrent administration of ethanol and bicarbonate, has been successful in many poisoning cases (53).

Ethanol

Ethanol (ethyl alcohol, grain alcohol) is produced in large quantities (see Table 12.1) and is utilized extensively as a solvent in industry, in numerous consumer preparations, and as an additive to gasoline (gasohol). It is used industrially as a raw material in the production of drugs, plastics, perfumes, cosmetics, and other compounds. Other applications include products such as hairsprays, mouthwashes, cleaning products, and drug formulations (53,80). Denaturants are added to the alcohol in a number of these products to discourage ingestion. Synthesis from ethylene represents the largest source of ethanol; smaller amounts are made from fermentation of natural materials (80).

Human exposure to ethanol is primarily through ingestion of alcoholic beverages and inhalation of ethanol vapors from industrial processes and consumer products. Percutaneous absorption appears to be much less important (80). OSHA, ACGIH, and many countries have established an exposure limit of 1000 ppm for ethanol (2,4). The NIOSH IDLH of 3300 ppm was set because of safety concerns (10% of the lower explosive limit) rather than toxicological considerations (101).

Although there is no clear evidence that ethanol is carcinogenic in animals, it has been shown to be a tumor promoter. Additionally, the International Agency for Cancer Research (IARC) has classified alcoholic beverages as a Group 1 carcinogen based on the occurrence of a variety of tumors in humans that have been causally related to ingestion of these beverages (80).

An unfortunate occurrence associated with chronic maternal consumption of large amounts of alcohol is a pattern of congenital abnormalities commonly called fetal alcohol syndrome. Effects may include growth retardation, microcephaly, mental deficiency, facial abnormalities, and poor coordination. Children who have been effected may display a few or many of the features characteristic of the syndrome (33,80, 110).

Ethanol is a CNS depressant that is capable of inducing all stages of anesthesia. It is readily absorbed by the GI tract and the lungs and is distributed throughout the body water (53). Absorption can be delayed, however, by food in the stomach. Subjects exposed to 5000–10,000 ppm of ethanol vapor experienced eyc irritation and coughing (114). Individuals with tolerance to alcohol experienced headache, drowsiness, and stupor when exposed to concentrations of 9400–13,200 mg/m^3 (5000–7000 ppm) for a period of 110 minutes (114). Ingestion of approximately one liter of an alcoholic beverage (40–55% ethanol) within several minutes can result in death (53). Individuals with blood alcohol levels of approximately 0.05–0.15 percent (50–150 mg/dl) may exhibit decreased inhibitions, poor coordination, blurred vision, and slowed reaction time. Increasing blood levels to 0.15–0.30 percent can result in slurred speech, visual impairment, hypoglycemia, and staggering. At 0.3–0.5 percent blood alcohol content (severe intoxication), symptoms can include muscular incoordination, hypothermia, vomiting and nausea, and convulsions. In adults, coma and death are typically associated with levels exceeding 0.5 percent (80,114). The wide ranges reported above reflect the differences in tolerance and susceptibility of individuals to the effects of alcohol.

Like methanol, ethanol is metabolized primarily (about 90%) by the liver. Elimination from the body by urinary excretion and pulmonary exhalation is minimal (80). Oxidation of ethanol to acetaldehyde occurs via alcohol dehydrogenase within the cytosol. Acetaldehyde is then converted to acetic acid by action of aldehyde dehydrogenase. Both enzymes utilize oxidized nicotinamide adenine dicucleotide (NAD) as a cofactor (53). Following release to the blood, acetic acid is metabolized to carbon dioxide and water in the peripheral tissues (80). Alternative, but less active, metabolic pathways have been demonstrated in humans and other species. These include catalase and microsomal ethanol-oxidizing systems (26,79). Adults metabolize ethanol at a rate of about 7–10 g/hr. This rate remains essentially constant for each individual within a wide range of exposure. Metabolic rates are higher for chronic alcoholics and children (80,114).

The interaction of ethanol with other hepatotoxins is well known. Ethanol pretreatment has been shown to increase the toxicity of carbon tetrachloride, chloroform, trichloroethylene, dimethylnitrosamine, chlorpromazine, and other compounds (127). The induction of cytochrome P450 isozymes may be responsible for their metabolic effects (80).

Methylene Chloride

Methylene chloride (dichloromethane) is widely used in a number of diverse applications including manufacturing of polyurethane foams, production of pharmaceuticals, boat building, paint stripping, vapor degreasing, extraction of caffeine from coffee and tea, and various consumer products. Its high volatility, good solvent properties for fats, oils, and other compounds, and relatively good water solubility compared to other chlorinated compounds have made it quite valuable (103,132).

Because of methylene chloride's high vapor pressure, the primary route of human exposure is through inhalation; however, dermal contact can be significant, depending on the application. The ACGIH TLV–TWA of 50 ppm was set to protect against CNS effects and anoxia. In addition, ACGIH has designated methlyene chloride as a confirmed animal carcinogen, but they also state that available epidemiological studies do not confirm an increased risk of cancer in exposed humans (4). NIOSH recommends that methylene chloride be regarded as a potential occupational carcinogen (101). OSHA considers methylene chloride a potential human carcinogen and has reduced the PEL for methylene chloride from 500 ppm to 25 ppm, with a STEL of 125 ppm (15 min) and an action level of 12.5 ppm that triggers certain requirements (103). The current German MAK is 100 ppm (2).

The primary acute hazards associated with exposure to methylene chloride are CNS depression and eye, skin, and respiratory tract irritation. In addition, one of the products of methylene chloride metabolism is carbon monoxide, which can impair health in a manner similar to direct exposure to carbon monoxide. The resulting carboxyhemoglobin levels reduce the supply of oxygen to the heart and may aggravate preexisting heart disease (103).

Metabolism of methylene chloride can proceed via two pathways, one by a route involving cytochrome P450 mixed-function oxidase (MFO) and the other by a route utilizing glutathione *S*-transferase (GST). Carbon dioxide is an end product in both systems, but carbon monoxide is only produced via the MFO route. At low concentrations the MFO system appears to dominate, but at higher concentrations (above 300–500 ppm) the glutathione pathway increases in a disproportionate manner (132).

Methylene chloride was shown in a 1986 National Toxicology Program inhalation study to produce lung and liver tumors in male and female mice and benign mammary tumors in male and female rats (56). Recent research has suggested that mice may be uniquely sensitive at high exposures to methylene chloride-induced lung and liver cancer (56). The tumors appear to be caused by a genotoxic mechanism involving metabolites of the GST pathway. The particular metabolites responsible are not found in high concentrations in lung or liver tissue in humans or rats.

In a study to determine the effects of alcohols and toluene upon methylene chloride-induced carboxyhemoglobin in the rat and monkey, it was shown that ethanol, methanol, isopropanol, and toluene inhibited the formation of carboxyhemoglobin. In addition, neither the rat nor the monkey demonstrated the methanol potentiation of carboxyhemoglobin that has been reported to occur in humans (32).

A study of the pharmacokinetics of [^{14}C]methylene chloride in rats at 50, 500, and 1500 ppm for 6 h showed that metabolic processes were saturated above the 50 ppm exposure concentration. At 48 h postexposure, approximately 95 percent of the body burden attributable to the 50 ppm exposure was metabolized, in contrast to 69 percent and 45 percent at 500 and 1500 ppm, respectively (89). In addition, the production of carboxyhemoglobin reached a steady-state range of 10–13 percent regardless of the exposure concentration, suggesting that the CO metabolic pathway was saturated. Tetrachloroethylene (perchloroethylene) is another solvent in which patterns of elimination are altered when metabolic pathways become saturated (105). In a study comparing oral and inhalation exposure of rats to [^{14}C]tetrachloroethylene, it was found that with increasing dose, metabolism was saturated resulting in more of the parent compound being eliminated unchanged at 72 h after exposure (105). These results with methylene chloride and tetrachloroethylene indicate that just increasing the exposure concentration does not always increase the body burden in a linear manner. Such information may be useful for safety evaluations to avoid overestimation of body burden.

NONTRADITIONAL SOLVENTS

Given the negative health and environmental impacts created by some of the more widely used solvents, a great deal of effort has gone into finding suitable replacements. The following compounds are examples of nontraditional materials that show promise as replacement solvents.

d-Limonene

d-Limonene is a naturally occurring monocyclic terpene found in citrus peel oils, spices, evergreens, and human milk (140). It is considered to have low acute toxicity and is listed as GRAS (generally recognized as safe) as a food additive by the Food and Drug Administration (FDA) (21 CFR 182.60). It has found wide application as a solvent in numerous cleaning and degreasing applications, replacing more toxic and environmentally undesirable chlorinated solvents, glycol ethers, xylene, and chlorofluorocarbons (CFCs) (46). Skin contact with d-limonene may cause irritation and sensitization (attributed to the oxidation product d-limonene oxide) (140). d-Limonene has been shown to produce hyaline droplet nephropathy and renal tubular tumors in male rats. However, these effects are attributed to the unique presence of α_{2u}-globulin in the male rat and are not deemed relevant to other species, including humans (45). Among the attributes of d-limonene are its antimicrobial, antiviral, antifungal, and antilarval properties (29). d-Limonene and related monoterpenes have also demonstrated chemopreventive and chemotherapeutic efficacy in experimental cancer-therapy models (37).

Based on similar metabolic pathways in rats and humans and the therapeutic successes in rodents, it has been suggested that d-limonene may be an efficacious chemotherapeutic agent for human malignancies (37).

Carbon Dioxide

Carbon dioxide is a gas under standard temperature and pressure conditions. It can be converted, however, to the liquid and supercritical phases by increasing pressure and temperature. The critical point of carbon dioxide is 31°C and 73 atm. Below this point, CO_2 can be maintained in a liquid state (e.g., 65 atm and 25°C), whereas above 31°C no amount of pressure can be applied to liquify it (supercritical phase) (65). In either of these dense phases, CO_2 exhibits good solvent properties. Beneficial characteristics include liquidlike density, gaslike diffusivity, and low surface tension. In particular, liquid CO_2 acts like a hydrocarbon solvent, it has good homogenizing properties (i.e., immiscible liquids form a single phase when mixed with CO_2), and it is a good solvent for many aliphatic hydrocarbons and most small aromatic hydrocarbons. Other chemical groups such as halocarbons, esters, ketones, and low molecular weight alcohols also exhibit good solvency in CO_2 (65). Since the mid-1970s, supercritical CO_2 technology has been employed in the food, beverage, pharmaceutical, and perfume industries. Applications include production of spice extracts, natural dyes, decaffeinated coffee and tea, plant extracts, active substances from drugs, and volatile oils (20,38,88). It has also been used in wastewater treatment, chemical analysis, and at times as an aerosol propellant. More recently, liquid CO_2 has found favor as an alternative for metal parts degreasing and as a solvent for dry-cleaning clothes (38,70).

One such CO_2 degreasing system is being used in a pen manufacturing operation to replace perchloroethylene. It consists primarily of two separate systems, a hot oil pretreatment process, and an automated system that employs liquid carbon dioxide in a pressure vessel. The application is to degrease and remove chips from ball points after machining. The hot oil unit is used to displace fatty esters contained in machining oil and to remove chips in the point cavity. The automated unit then removes oil from the points using liquid carbon dioxide. The carbon dioxide and oil are separated in a recycling system and the carbon dioxide is used again during the next cleaning cycle.

Advantages of CO_2 usage over conventional solvents are numerous. Carbon dioxide is nonflammable, noncorrosive, nonreactive, nontoxic, inexpensive, and plentiful. Products obtained are solvent-free. Selective separations are possible. Finally, there are no environmental problems, since the gas is recovered for future use. One of the disadvantages of CO_2 systems involves the relatively high start-up costs for equipment. However, these may be recouped through improved productivity and reduced costs for waste disposal, for example.

Ionic Liquids

Ionic systems, which are made up of salts that are liquid at room temperature, are finding applications in a number of chemical processes. Ionic liquids have good solvent properties for many inorganic, organic, and, polymeric materials and, in some cases, these compounds can serve as both catalyst and solvent (49). Research has indicated that partitioning of organic solvents between an ionic liquid and water corresponds closely with that found for molecular organic solvents and water. Thus, ionic liquids have the potential to replace the toxic, flammable, and volatile organic compounds currently used in liquid–liquid separations (50). The room-temperature ionic compounds, such as 1-butyl-3-methylimidazolium hexafluorophosphate and 1-butylpyridinium nitrate, consist of nitrogen-containing organic cations and inorganic anions. Their physical and chemical properties can be altered according to the choice of ions. Advantages compared to conventional organic solvents include low volatility and relative ease of recycling (50). Other potential uses include removal of organic contaminants from wastewater, soil cleanup, replacement of corrosive mineral acids in refinery processes, and spent nuclear fuel treatment (49). The safety and toxicological profiles of these compounds has yet to be thoroughly developed; therefore caution must be exercised before they are put into general use.

OPPORTUNITIES IN THE TOXICOLOGICAL EVALUATION OF SOLVENTS

Human exposure to solvents is quite common in today's society. These exposures frequently involve multiple chemicals that are found in numerous products such as cleaning agents, paint thinners, and fuels. Although most toxicological research to date has dealt with single chemicals, questions remain about the long-term health effects associated with low-level exposures to multiple chemicals and the sensitivity of the toxicological endpoints that are currently being relied upon. Development of innovative experimental protocols and new quantitative mechanistic approaches to the study of chemical interactions may be beneficial in this regard (74,148).

Economic concerns and the desire for less toxic and more environmentally friendly chemicals have resulted in the introduction of numerous alternative compounds into the marketplace. In some cases, little may be known about the health and environmental impacts of these materials; examples include the ionic liquids discussed above. It is therefore essential that sufficient toxicological and environmental data be gathered before replacements are introduced on a wide scale.

Research has shown that many neurotoxic chemicals are capable of adversely affecting the sensory function. Minor changes in vision or hearing, for example, can dramatically alter job performance and the overall quality of life. While most reports to date have dealt with changes in the visual system, additional investigations into the effects of solvents on hearing, taste, and smell would provide important new information on this subject (48).

ACKNOWLEDGMENTS

The authors wish to thank Dr. Henry Ciuchta, Dr. Joseph Morton, and Mark Savell for reviewing portions of the manuscript and also Peter Kahla for his help with one of the figures. The authors also gratefully acknowledge the significant contributions of the previous writers Paul H. Ayres, W. David Taylor, and Michael J. Olson.

QUESTIONS

1. You are a toxicologist with industrial hygiene responsibilities in a large manufacturing company. Your boss has just told you that the solvent the factory is using to degrease metal parts will be banned by the EPA within the next six months. Your job is to lead a team of employees, who have a vested interest in the current solvent, in coming up with a suitable alternative material. What are your considerations in recommending a replacement? Explain.
2. Assume that the solvent chosen above will be used in six locations in the factory. You surmise that some sort of ventilation will be required to protect the employees. What factors must you take into account in recommending the proper system?
3. One of your employees has begun using a solvent mixture containing xylene and toluene. To ensure the safety of the worker, you have conducted personal air monitoring throughout the day and have come up with the following sampling times and monitoring results: 0800–1000: 60 ppm xylene and 25 ppm toluene; 1000–1200: 92 ppm xylene and 45 ppm toluene; 1200–1300: no exposure because employee left for lunch; 1300–1600: 110 ppm xylene and 47 ppm toluene. Calculate the TWA exposure for each chemical. Assume that there is no dermal exposure and that the toxic effects contributed by each solvent are additive. Has the TLV–TWA been exceeded?
4. Match each solvent or metabolite with the appropriate fact listed below.

Solvent/Metabolite	*Fact*
1. d-Limonene	a. Antidotal in methanol poisonings
2. Carbon Disulfide	b. Associated with bone marrow disease in humans
3. 2,5-Hexanedione	c. Potentially useful in cancer therapy
4. Toluene	d. Teratogen and embryotoxin
5. Methanol	e. Metabolism produces carboxyhemoglobin
6. 2-Butoxyacetic Acid	f. Frequently "sniffed" to obtain euphoric effect
7. Ethylene Glycol Monomethyl Ether	g. Used in rayon production
8. Benzene	h. A few ml can lead to blindness
9. Ethanol	i. Primary causative agent in polyneuropathy
10. Methylene Chloride	j. Produces hemolytic effects in rats

REFERENCES

1. American Conference of Governmental Industrial Hygienists, Inc. (ACGIH). (1995): *Air Sampling Instruments for Evaluation of Atmospheric Contaminants* 8th ed., ACGIH, Cincinnati, OH.
2. ACGIH. (1998): *Guide to Occupational Exposure Values—1998*. ACGIH, Cincinnati, OH.
3. ACGIH. (1998): *Industrial Ventilation: A Manual of Recommended Practice*, 23rd ed., ACGIH, Inc., Cincinnati, OH.
4. ACGIH. (2000): *2000 TLVs® and BEIs®, Threshold Limit Values for Chemical Substances and Physical Agents, and Biological Exposure Indices*. ACGIH, Cincinnati, OH.
5. American Industrial Hygiene Association (AIHA). (1990): *Chemical Protective Clothing*, edited by J. S. Johnson and K. J. Anderson. AIHA, Akron, OH.
6. AIHA. (1997): *The Occupational Environment—Its Evaluation and Control*, edited by S. R. DiNardi. AIHA Press, Fairfax, VA.
7. Alden, C. L. (1986): A review of unique male rat hydrocarbon nephropathy. *Toxicol. Pathol.*, 14:109–111.
8. Allen, N. (1979): Solvents and other industrial organic compounds. In: *Handbook of Clinical Neurology Intoxications of the Nervous System*, Part 1(36), edited by P. J. Vinken and G. W. Bruyn, pp. 361–389. Elsevier/North-Holland, New York.
9. Allen, N., Mendell, J. R., Billmaier, D. J., Fontaine, R. E., and O'Neill, J. (1975): Toxic polyneuropathy due to methyl n-butyl ketone. *Arch. Neurol.*, 32:209–218.
10. Anger, W. K. (1986): Workplace exposures. In: *Neurobehavioral Toxicology*, edited by Z. Annau, pp. 331–347. Johns Hopkins University Press, Baltimore.
11. Anon. (1997): Facts and figures for the chemical industry. *Chem. Eng. News*, 75(25):38–79.
12. Anon. (1998): Facts and figures for the chemical industry. *Chem. Eng. News*, 76(26):40–81.
13. Astrand, I. (1975): Uptake of solvents in the blood and tissues of man. *Scand. J. Work Environ. Health*, 1:199–218.
14. Astrand, I. (1985): Uptake of solvents from the lungs. *Br. J. Ind. Med.*, 42:217–218.
15. Baelum, J., Anderson, I., Lundqvist, G. R., Molhave, L., Pedersen, O. F., Vaeth, M., and Wyon, D. P. (1985): Response of solvent-exposed printers and unexposed controls to six-hour toluene exposure. *Scand. J. Work Environ. Health*, 11:271–280.
16. Baerg, R. D., and Kimberg, D. V. (1970). Centrilobular hepatic necrosis and acute renal failure in "solvent sniffers." *Ann. Intern. Med.*, 73:713–720.
17. Bahl, M. K. (1985): ESCA studies on skin lipid removal by solvents and surfactants. *J. Soc. Cosmet. Chem.*, 36:287–296.

18. Baker, E. L. (1988): Organic solvent neurotoxicity. *Annu. Rev. Public Health*, 9:223–232.

19. Bamberger, R. L., Esposito, G. G., Jacobs, B. W., Podolak, G. E., and Mazur, J. F. (1978): A new personal sampler for organic vapors. *Am. Ind. Hyg. Assoc. J.*, 39:701–708.

20. Basta, N., and McQueen, S. (1985): Supercritical fluids: Still seeking acceptance. *Chem. Eng.*, 92:14–17.

21. Beliles, R. P., and Beliles, E. M. (1993): Phosphorus, selenium, tellurium, and sulfur. In: *Patty's Industrial Hygiene and Toxicology*, Vol. IIA, 4th ed., edited by G. D. Clayton and F. E. Clayton, pp. 818-822. John Wiley, New York.

22. Boekelheide, K. (1987): 2,5-Hexanedione alters microtubule assembly. 1. Testicular atrophy, not nervous system toxicity, correlates with enhanced tubulin polymerization. *Toxicol. Appl. Pharmacol.*, 88:370–382.

23. Boggs, A. (1989): Comparative risk assessment of casting solvents for positive photo resist. *Appl. Ind. Hyg.*, 4:81–87.

24. Bohlen, P., Schlunegger, U. P., and Lauppi, E. (1973): Uptake and distribution of hexane in rat tissues. *Toxicol. Appl. Pharmacol.*, 25:242–249.

25. Bos, P. M., deMik, G., and Bragt, P. C. (1991): Critical review of the toxicity of methyl n-butyl ketone: Risk from occupational exposure. *Am. J. Ind. Med.*, 20:175–194.

26. Bradford, B. U., Seed, C. B., Handler, J. A., Forman, D. T., and Thurman, R. G. (1993): Evidence that catalase is a major pathway of ethanol oxidation in vivo: Dose-response studies in deer mice using methanol as a selective substrate. *Arch. Biochem. Biophys.*, 303:172–176.

27. Browning, R. G., and Curry, S. C. (1994): Clinical toxicology of ethylene glycol monoalkyl ethers. *Human and Exper. Toxicol.*, 13:325–335.

28. Brugnone, F., Perbellini, L., Gaffuri, E., and Apostoli, P. (1980): Biomonitoring of industrial solvent exposures in workers' alveolar air. *Int. Arch. Occup. Environ. Health*, 47:245–261.

29. Cavender, F. (1994): Alicyclic hydrocarbons: Limonene. In: *Patty's Industrial Hygiene and Toxicology*, Vol. IIB, 4th ed., edited by G. D. Clayton and F. E. Clayton, pp. 1282–1283. John Wiley, New York.

30. Cavender, F. (1994): Aliphatic hydrocarbons: Hexanes. In: *Patty's Industrial Hygiene and Toxicology*, Vol. IIB, 4th ed., edited by G. D. Clayton and F. E. Clayton, pp. 1233–1234. John Wiley, New York.

31. Cavender, F. (1994): Aromatic hydrocarbons: Toluene. In: *Patty's Industrial Hygiene and Toxicology*, Vol. IIB, 4th ed., edited by G. D. Clayton and F. E. Clayton, pp. 1326–1332. John Wiley, New York.

32. Ciuchta, H. P., Savell, G. M., and Spiker, R. C. (1979): The effects of alcohols and toluene upon methylene chloride-induced carboxyhemoglobin in the rat and monkey. *Toxicol. Appl. Pharmacol.*, 49:347–354.

33. Clarren, S. K., and Smith, D. W. (1978): The fetal alcohol syndrome. *N. Engl. J. Med.*, 198:1063–1067.

34. Colombi, A., Maroni, M., Picchi, O., Rota, E., Castano, P., and Foa, V. (1981): Carbon disulfide neuropathy in rats. A morphological and ultrastructural study of degeneration and regeneration. *Clin. Toxicol.*, 18:1463–1474.

35. Corsi, G., Maestrelli, P., Picotti, G., Manzoni, S., and Negrin, P. (1983): Chronic peripheral neuropathy in workers with previous exposure to carbon disulphide. *Br. J. Ind. Med.*, 40:209–211.

36. Costa, L. G., and Manzo, L. (1998): Biological monitoring of occupational neurotoxicants. In: *Occupational Neurotoxicology*, edited by L. G. Costa and L. Manzo, p. 90. CRC Press, Boca Raton, FL.

37. Crowell, P. L., Elson, C. E., Bailey, H. H., Elegbede, A., Haag, J. D., and Gould, M. N. (1994): Human metabolism of the experimental cancer therapeutic agent d-limonene. *Cancer Chemother. Pharmacol.*, 35:31–37.

38. Darvin, C. H., and Hill, E. A. (1996): Demonstration of liquid CO_2 as an alternative for metal parts cleaning. *Precision Cleaning*, 4(9):25–32.

39. DeCaprio, A. P. (1985): Molecular mechanisms of diketone neurotoxicity. *Chem. Biol. Interact.*, 54:257–270.

40. DeCaprio, A. P., and O'Neill, E. A. (1985): Alterations in rat axonal cytoskeletal proteins induced by in vitro and in vivo 2,5-hexanedione exposure. *Toxicol. Appl. Pharmacol.*, 78:235–247.

41. DiVincenzo, G. D., Hamilton, M. L., Kaplan, C. J., Krasavage, W. J., and O'Donoghue, J. L. (1978): Studies on the respiratory uptake and excretion and the skin absorption of methyl n-butyl ketone in humans and dogs. *Toxicol. Appl. Pharmacol.*, 44:593–604.

42. Dossing, M., Baelum, J., Hansen, S. H., and Lundqvist, G. R. (1984): Effect of ethanol, cimetidine and propranolol on toluene metabolism in man. *Int. Arch. Occup. Environ. Health*, 54:309–315.

43. Environmental Protection Agency (EPA), Office of Pollution Prevention and Toxics. (1994): Chemical summary for methanol. *EPA 749-F-94-013a*, pp. 1–9.

44. Fiserova-Bergerova, V., and Diaz, M. L. (1986): Determination and prediction of tissue–gas partition coefficients. *Int. Arch. Occup. Environ. Health*, 58:75–87.

45. Flamm, W. G., and Lehman-McKeeman, L. D. (1991): The human relevance of the renal tumor-inducing potential of d-limonene in male rats: Implications for risk assessment. *Reg. Toxicol. Pharm.*, 13:70–86.

46. Florida Chemical Co. Inc. (1997): *d-Limonene Product Data Sheet*. Winter Haven, FL.

47. Forni, A. M., Cappellini, A., Pacifico, E., and Vigliani, E. C. (1971): Chromosome changes and their evolution in subjects with past exposure to benzene. *Arch. Environ. Health*, 23:385–391.

48. Fox, D. S. (1998): Sensory system alterations following occupational exposure to chemicals. In: *Occupational Neurotoxicology*, edited by L. G. Costa and L. Manzo, pp. 169–184. CRC Press, Boca Raton, FL.

49. Freemantle, M. (1998): Designer solvents. *Chem. Eng. News*, 13:32–37.

50. Freemantle, M. (1998): Ionic liquids show promise for clean separation technology. *Chem. Eng. News*, 34:12.

51. Gargas, M. L., Burgess, R. J., Voisard, D. J., Cason, G. H., and Andersen, M. E. (1989): Partition coefficients of low molecular weight volatile chemicals in various liquids and tissues. *Toxicol. Appl. Pharmacol.*, 98:87–99.

52. Gingell, R., Boatman, R. J., Bus, J. S., Cawley, R. J., Knaak, J. B., Krasavage, W. J., Skoulis, N. P., Stack, C. R., and Tyler, T. R. (1994): Glycol ethers and other selected glycol derivatives. In: *Patty's Industrial Hygiene and Toxicology*, Vol. IID, 4th ed., edited by G. D. Clayton and F. E. Clayton, pp. 2761–2966. John Wiley, New York.

53. Gosselin, R. E., Smith, R. P., and Hodge, H. C. (1984): Ethyl alcohol and methyl alcohol. In: *Clinical Toxicology of Commercial Products*, Section III, 5th ed., pp. 166–171, 275–279. Williams & Wilkins, Baltimore/London.

54. Graham, D. G., Amarnath, V., Valentine, W. M., Pyle, S. J., and Anthony, D. C. (1995): Pathogenic studies of hexane and carbon disulfide neurotoxicity. *Crit. Rev. Toxicol.*, 25(2):91–112.

55. Grasso, P., Sharratt, M., Davies, D. M., and Irvine, D. (1984): Neurophysiological and psychological disorders and occupational exposure to organic solvents. *Food Chem. Toxicol.*, 22:819–852.

56. Halogenated Solvents Industry Alliance (1998): Methylene chloride white paper. *HSIA*, pp. 1–6, Washington, DC.

57. Hanninen, H. (1985): Twenty-five years of behavioral toxicology within occupational medicine: A personal account. *Am. J. Ind. Med.*, 7:19–30.
58. Hardin, B. D. (1983): Reproductive toxicity of the glycol ethers. *Toxicology*, 27:91–102.
59. Hardin, B. D., Bond, G. P., Sikov, M. R., Andrew, F. D., Beliles, R. P., and Niemeier, R. W. (1981): Testing of selected workplace chemicals for teratogenic potential. *Scand. J. Work Environ. Health*, 7:66–75.
60. Hardin, B. D., Niemeier, R. W., Smith, R. J., Kuczuk, M. H., Mathinos, P. R., and Weaver, T. F. (1982): Teratogenicity of 2-ethoxyethanol by dermal application. *Drug Chem. Toxicol.*, 5:277–294.
61. Heck, H. d'A., Casanova, M., and Starr, T. B. (1990): Formaldehyde toxicity: New understanding. *CRC Crit. Rev. Toxicol.*, 20:397–426.
62. Herskowitz, A., Ishii, N., and Schaumburg, H. (1971): n-Hexane neuropathy. *N. Engl. J. Med.*, 285:82–85.
63. Hoet, P., and Lauwerys, R. (1998): Biological monitoring of occupational neurotoxicants. In: *Occupational Neurotoxicology*, edited by L. G. Costa and L. Manzo, pp. 57–58. CRC Press, Boca Raton, FL.
64. Huff, J. E., Haseman, J. K., DeMarini, D. M., Eustis, S., Maronpot, R. R., Peters, A. C., Persing, R. L., Chrisp, C. E., and Jacobs, A. C. (1989): Multiple-site carcinogenicity of benzene in Fischer 344 rats and B6C3F mice. *Environ. Health Perspect.*, 82:125–163.
65. Hyatt, J. A. (1984): Liquid and supercritical carbon dioxide as organic solvents. *J. Org. Chem.*, 49:5097–5101.
66. Ikeda, M., and Ohtsuji, H. (1971): Phenobarbital-induced protection against toxicity of toluene and benzene in the rat. *Toxicol. Appl. Pharmacol.*, 20:30–43.
67. Irons, R. D., Dent, J. G., Baker, T. S., and Rickert, D. E. (1980): Benzene is metabolized and covalently bound in bone marrow in situ. *Chem. Biol. Interact.*, 30:241–245.
68. Johnson, A., and Nylen, P. (1995): Effects of industrial solvents on hearing. *Occup. Med.*, 10(3):623–640.
69. Johnson, B. L., ed. (1990): *Advances in Neurobehavioral Toxicology: Applications in Environmental and Occupational Health.* Lewis, Chelsea, MI.
70. Kaplan, K. (1997): A new spin on dry cleaning. *Los Angeles Times*, September 8, 1997.
71. Knox, J. W., and Nelson, J. R. (1966): Permanent encephalopathy from toluene inhalation. *N. Engl. J. Med.*, 273:1494–1496.
72. Kramer, A., Staudinger, H., and Ullrich, V. (1974): Effect of n-hexane inhalation on the monooxygenase system in mice liver microsomes. *Chem. Biol. Interact.*, 8:11–18.
73. Krasavage, W. J., O'Donoghue, J. L., DiVincenzo, G. D., and Terhaar, C. J. (1980): The relative neurotoxicity of methyl n-butyl ketone, n-hexane and their metabolites. *Toxicol. Appl. Pharmacol.*, 52:433–441.
74. Krishnan, K., Andersen, M. E., Clewell III, H .J., and Yang, R. S. H. (1994): Physiologically based pharmacokinetic modeling of chemical mixtures. In: *Toxicology of Chemical Mixtures*, edited by R. S. H. Yang, pp. 399–433. Academic Press, San Diego.
75. Laham, S. (1970): Metabolism of industrial solvents. *Ind. Med.*, 39:61–64.
76. Lee, E. W., Kocsis, J. J., and Snyder, R. (1974): Acute effects of benzene on 59-Fe incorporation into circulating erythrocytes. *Toxicol. Appl. Pharmacol.*, 27:431–436.
77. Lehman-McKeeman, L. D., Rivera-Torres, M. I., and Caudill, D. (1990): Lysosomal degradation of α_{2u}-globulin and α_{2u}-globulin-xenobiotic conjugates. *Toxicol. Appl. Pharmacol.*, 103: 539–548.
78. Lewey, F. H. (1941): Neurological, medical, and biochemical signs and symptoms indicating chronic industrial carbon disulphide absorption. *Ann. Intern. Med.*, 15:869–883.
79. Lieber, C. S., and DeCarli, L. M. (1970): Hepatic microsomal ethanol-oxidizing system. *J. Biol. Chem.*, 245:2505–2512.
80. Lington, A. W., and Bevan, C. (1994): Alcohols. In: *Patty's Industrial Hygiene and Toxicology*, Vol. IID, 4th ed., edited by G. D. Clayton and F. E. Clayton, pp. 2585–2622. John Wiley, New York.
81. Lock, E. A. (1988): Studies on the mechanism of nephrotoxicity and nephrocarcinogenicity of halogenated alkenes. *CRC Crit. Rev. Toxicol.*, 19:23–42.
82. Lock, E. A., and Ishmael, J. (1985): Effect of the organic acid transport inhibitor probenicid on renal cortical uptake and proximal tubular toxicity of hexachloro-1,3-butadiene and its conjugates. *Toxicol. Appl. Pharmacol.*, 81:32–42.
83. Longacre, S. L., Kocsis, J. J., and Snyder, R. (1981): Influence of strain differences in mice on the metabolism and toxicity of benzene. *Toxicol. Appl. Pharmacol.*, 60:398–409.
84. Lu, A. Y. H., Strobel, H. W., and Coon, M. J. (1970): Properties of a solubilized form of the cytochrome P450-containing mixed-function oxidase of liver microsomes. *Mal. Pharmacol.*, 6:213–220.
85. Maron, S. H., and Prutton, C. F. (1965): *Principles of Physical Chemistry*, 4th ed., pp. 215–216, 285. Macmillan Company, New York.
86. Matheson, L. E., Jr., Wurster, D. E., and Ostrenga, J. A. (1979): Sarin transport across excised human skin. II: Effect of solvent pretreatment on permeability. *J. Pharm. Sci.*, 11:1410–1413.
87. Mattia, C. J., LeBel, C. P., and Bondy, S. C. (1991): Effects of toluene and its metabolite on cerebral reactive oxygen species generation. *Biochem. Pharmacol.*, 42:879–882.
88. McHugh, M. A. (1986): Extraction with supercritical fluids. In: *Recent Developments in Separation Science*, Vol. 9, edited by N. Li and J. Calo, pp. 75-105. CRC Press, Boca Raton, FL.
89. McKenna, M. J., Zempel, J. A., and Braun, W. H. (1982): The pharmacokinetics of inhaled methylene chloride in rats. *Toxicol. Appl. Pharmacol.*, 65:1–10.
90. Medinsky, M. A., Schlosser, P. M., and Bond, J. A. (1994): Critical issues in benzene toxicity and metabolism: The effect of interactions with other organic chemicals on risk assessment. *Environ. Health Perspect.*, 102(9):119–124.
91. Mendell, J. R., Saida, K., Ganansia, M. F., Jackson, D. B., Weiss, H., Gardier, R. W., Chrisman, C., Allen, N., Couri, D., O'Neill, J. J., Marks, B. H., and Hetland, L. B. (1974): Toxic polyneuropathy produced by methyl n-butyl ketone. *Science*, 185:787–789.
92. Menger, F. M., Goldsmith, D. J., and Mandell, L. (1972): *Organic Chemistry—A Concise Approach*, p. 450. W. A. Benjamin, Menlo Park, CA.
93. Merck Index. (1996): 12th ed., edited by S. Budavari. Merck & Co., Inc., Whitehouse Station, NJ.
94. Miller, R. R., Hermann, E. A., Langvardt, P. W., McKenna, M. J., and Schwetz, B. A. (1983): Comparative metabolism and disposition of ethylene glycol monomethyl ether and propylene glycol monomethyl ether in male rats. *Tox. Appl. Pharmacol.*, 67:229–237.
95. Miller, R. R., Hermann, E. A., Young, J. T., Calhoun, L. L., and Kastl, P. E. (1984): Propylene glycol monomethyl ether acetate (PGMEA) metabolism, disposition, and short-term vapor inhalation toxicity studies. *Toxicol. Appl. Pharmacol.*, 75:521–530.
96. Miller, R. R., Hermann, E. A., Young, J. T., Landry, T. D., and Calhoun, L. L. (1984): Ethylene glycol monomethyl ether and propylene glycol monomethyl ether: Metabolism, disposition, and subchronic inhalation toxicity studies. *Environ. Health Persp.*, 57:233–239.

97. Monteiro-Riviere, N. A., and Popp, J. A. (1986): Ultrastructural evaluation of acute nasal toxicity in the rat respiratory epithelium in response to formaldehyde gas. *Fund. Appl. Toxicol.*, 6:251–262.
98. Morata, T. C., and Dunn, D. E. (1994): Occupational exposure to noise and ototoxic organic solvents. *Arch. Environ. Health*, 49: 359–365.
99. Nelson, B. K., Setzer, J. V., Brightwell, W. S., Mathinos, P. R., Kuczuk, M. H., Weaver, T. E., and Goad, P. T. (1984): Comparative inhalation teratogenicity of four glycol ether solvents and an amino derivative in rats. *Environ. Health Persp.*, 57:261–271.
100. Nelson, B. K., Brightwell, W. S., Setzer, J. V., and O'Donohue, T. L. (1984): Reproductive toxicity of the industrial solvent 2-ethoxyethanol in rats and interactive effects of ethanol. *Environ. Health Persp.*, 57:255–259.
101. NIOSH (1997): *Pocket Guide to Chemical Hazards*. pp. 1–341. NIOSH Publications, Cincinnati, OH.
102. Occupational Safety and Health Administration (OSHA). (1998): Benzene. *29 CFR 1910.1028*, pp. 235–253.
103. OSHA. (1997): Methylene Chloride. *29 CFR 1910.1052*, pp. 479–496.
104. Paustenbach, D. J. (1994): Occupational exposure limits, pharmacokinetics, and unusual work schedules: In: *Patty's Industrial Hygiene and Toxicology*, Vol. IIIA, 4th ed., edited by G. D. Clayton and F. E. Clayton, pp. 191–348. John Wiley, New York.
105. Pegg, D. G., Zempel, J. A., Braun, W. H., and Watanabe, P. G. (1979): Disposition of tetrachloro(14C)ethylene following oral and inhalation exposure in rats. *Toxicol. Appl. Pharmacol.*, 51:465–474.
106. Perbellini, L., Brugnone, F., Caretta, D., and Maranelli, G. (1985): Partition coefficients of some industrial aliphatic hydrocarbons (C5–C7) in blood and human tissues. *Br. J. Ind. Med.*, 42:162–167.
107. Pergal, M., Vukojevic, N., and Djuric, D. (1972): Isolation and identification of thiocarbamide. *Arch. Environ. Health*, 25:42–44.
108. Pergal, M., Vukojevic, N., Cirin-Popov, N., Djuric, D., and Bojovic, T. (1972): Carbon disulfide metabolites excreted in the urine of exposed workers. *Arch. Environ. Health*, 25:38–41.
109. Pohl, L. R. (1979): Biochemical toxicology of chloroform. In: *Reviews in Biochemical Toxicology*, Vol. 1, edited by E. Hodgson, J. R. Bend, and R. M. Philpot, pp. 79–107. Elsevier/North Holland, New York.
110. Pratt, G. E. (1982): Alcohol and the developing fetus. *Br. Med. Bull.*, 38:48–53.
111. Price, B., Bergman, T. S., Rodriquez, M., Henrich, R. T., and Moran, E. J. (1997): A review of carbon disulfide exposure data and the association between carbon disulfide exposure and ischemic heart disease mortality. *Reg. Toxicol. Pharmacol.*, pp. 119–128.
112. Rafales, L. S. (1986): Assessment of locomotor activity. In: *Neurobehavioral Toxicology*, edited by Z. Annau, pp. 54–68. Johns Hopkins University Press, Baltimore.
113. Recknagel, R. O. (1967): Carbon tetrachloride hepatotoxicity. *Pharmacol. Rev.*, 19:145–208.
114. Reese, E., and Kimbrough, R. D. (1993): Acute toxicity of gasoline and some additives. *Environ. Health Prospect. Suppl.*, 101 (Suppl. 6):115–131.
115. Reinhardt, C. F., Mullin, L. S., and Maxfield, M. E. (1973): Epinephrine-induced cardiac arrhythmia potential of some common industrial solvents. *J. Occup. Med.*, 15:953–955.
116. Riihimaki, V., and Pfaffli, P. (1978): Percutaneous absorption of solvent vapors in man. *Scand. J. Work Environ. Health*, 4:73–85.
117. Rubin, E., and Lieber, C. S. (1972): The effects of ethanol on the liver. In: *International Review of Experimental Pathology*, edited by G. W. Richter and M. A. Epstein, pp. 177–232. Academic Press, New York.
118. Sabourin, P. J., Medinsky, M. A., Thurmond, F., Birnbaum, L. S., and Henderson, R. F. (1992): Effect of dose on the disposition of methoxyethanol, ethoxyethanol, and butoxyethanol administered dermally to male F344/N rats. *Fund. Appl. Toxicol.*, 19:124–132.
119. Sato, A., and Nakajima, T. (1979): Partition coefficients of some aromatic hydrocarbons and ketones in water, blood, and oil. *Br. J. Ind. Med.*, 36:231–234.
120. Scheflan, L., and Jacobs, M. B. (1953): *The Handbook of Solvents*, p. 728. Van Nostrand Reinhold, New York.
121. Short, B. G., Burnett, V. L., Cox, M. G., Bus, J. S., and Swenberg, J. A. (1987): Site-specific renal cytotoxicity and cell proliferation in male rats exposed to petroleum hydrocarbons. *Lab. Invest.*, 57:564–577.
122. Snyder, C. A., Goldstein, B. D., Sellakumar, A., Wolman, S. R., Bromberg, L., Erlichman, M. N., and Laskin, S. (1978): Hematotoxicity of inhaled benzene to Sprague–Dawley rats and AKR mice at 300 ppm. *J. Toxicol. Environ. Health*, 4:605–618.
123. Snyder, R., and Kocsis, J. J. (1975): Current concepts of chronic benzene toxicity. *CRC Crit. Rev. Toxicol.*, 3:265–288.
124. Spencer, P. S., and Schaumburg, H. H. (1977): Ultrastructural studies of the dying-back process. IV. Differential vulnerability of PNS and CNS fibers in experimental central–peripheral distal axonopathies. *J. Neuropathol. Exp. Neurol.*, 36:300–320.
125. Spencer, P. S., Schaumburg, H. H., Raleigh, R. L., and Terhaar, C. J. (1975): Nervous system degeneration produced by the industrial solvent methyl n-butyl ketone. *Arch. Neurol.*, 32:219–222.
126. Stott, W. T., and McKenna, M. J. (1985): Hydrolysis of several glycol ether acetates and acrylate esters by nasal mucosal carboxylesterase in vitro. *Fund. Appl. Toxicol.*, 5:399–404.
127. Strubelt, O. (1980): Interaction between ethanol and other hepatotoxic agents. *Biochem. Pharmacol.*, 29:1445–1449.
128. Swenberg, J. A., Short, B., Borghoff, S., Strasser, J., and Charbormeau, M. (1989): The comparative pathobiology of α_{2u}-globulin nephropathy. *Toxicol. Appl. Pharmacol.*, 97:35–46.
129. Taher, S. M., Anderson, R. J., McCartney, R., Popovtzer, M. M., and Schrier, R. W. (1974): Renal tubular acidosis associated with toluene "sniffing." *N. Engl. J. Med.*, 290:765–768.
130. Thomas, J. A., and Ballantyne, B. (1990): Occupational reproductive risk: Sources, surveillance, and testing. *J. Occup. Med.*, 32:547–554.
131. Topping, D. C., Morgott, D. A., David, R. M., and O'Donoghue, J. L. (1994): Ketones. In: *Patty's Industrial Hygiene and Toxicology*, Vol. IIC, 4th ed., edited by G. D. Clayton and F. E. Clayton, pp. 1739–1787. John Wiley, New York.
132. Torkelson, T. R. (1994): Halogenated aliphatic hydrocarbons containing chlorine, bromine, and iodine. In: *Patty's Industrial Hygiene and Toxicology*, Vol. IIE, 4th ed., edited by G. D. Clayton and F. E. Clayton, pp. 4034–4045. John Wiley, New York.
133. Trela, B. A., and Bogdanffy, M. S. (1991): Carboxylesterase-dependent cytotoxicity of dibasic esters (DBE) in rat nasal explants. *Toxicol. Appl. Pharmacol.*, 107:285–301.
134. Van Dolah, R. W. (1965): Flame propagation, extinguishment, and environmental effects on combustion. *Fire Technol.*, 2:138– 145.
135. van Doorn, R., Delbressine, L. P. C., Leijdekkers, C. M., Vertin, P. G., and Henderson, P. H. (1981): Identification and determination of 2-thiothiazolidine-4-carboxylic acid in urine of workers exposed to carbon disulfide. *Arch. Toxicol.*, 47:51–58.
136. van Doorn, R., Leijdekkers, C. P. M. J. M., Henderson, P. T., Vanhoome, M., and Vertin, P. G. (1981): Determination of thio compounds in urine of workers exposed to carbon disulfide. *Arch. Environ. Health*, 36:289–297.
137. Vigliani, E. C. (1950): Clinical observations on carbon disulfide intoxication in Italy. *Ind. Med. Surg.*, 19:240–242.
138. Vigliani, E. C., and Fomi, A. (1976): Benzene and leukemia. *Environ. Res.*, 11:122–127.

139. Vincent, J. H. (1998): International occupational exposure standards: A review and commentary. *Am. Ind. Hyg. Assoc. J.*, 59:729–742.

140. Von Burg, R. (1995): Toxicology update: Limonene. *J. Appl. Toxicol.*, 15(6):495–499.

141. Voog, L., and Eriksson, T. (1984): Toluene-induced decrease in rat plasma concentrations of tyrosine and tryptophan. *Acta Pharmacol. Toxicol.*, 54:151–153.

142. Wilkins-Haug, L. (1997): Teratogen update: Toluene. *Teratology*, 55:145–151.

143. Winder, C., and Ng, S. K. (1995): The problem of variable ingredients and concentration in solvent thinners. *Am. Ind. Hyg. Assoc. J.*, 56:1225–1228.

144. Winek, C. L., and Collom, W. D. (1971): Benzene and toluene fatalities. *J. Occup. Med.*, 13:259–261.

145. World Health Organization (WHO). (1990): 2-methoxyethanol, 2-ethoxyethanol, and their acetates. *Environ. Health Crit.*, 115.

146. WHO (1991): n-Hexane. *Environ. Health Crit.*, 122.

147. Yamada, S. (1964): An occurrence of polyneuritis by n-hexane in the polyethylene laminating plants. *Jpn. J. Ind. Health*, 6:192–194.

148. Yang, R. S. H. (1994): Introduction to the toxicology of chemical mixtures. In: *Toxicology of Chemical Mixtures*, edited by R. S. H. Yang, pp. 1-10. Academic Press, San Diego.

Principles and Methods of Toxicology,
Fourth Edition, edited by A. Wallace Hayes.

Chapter 13

Crop Protection Chemicals

James T. Stevens and Charles B. Breckenridge

The control of pests using chemicals dates back to more than 1000 BC by the Chinese (93). Sulfur, the first documented material, was found somewhat effective as a fumigant. However, for nearly 2500 years no additional pest control products were found. In the 16th century, the Chinese discovered arsenic could be used as an insecticide (159). Tobacco leaf (nicotine) and the seed of *Strychnos nux vomica* (strychnine) were established as possessing rodenticidal properties in 1700 (102). It was not until the mid-1800s that the insecticidally active botanicals, rotenone from the root of *Derris eliptica* and pyrethrum from the flowers of chrysanthemums, were added as insecticides. In 1880, Bordeaux mixture (copper sulfate, lime, calcium hydroxide, and water) was introduced for mildew control (93,159). Paris green (copper arsenite) and later calcium arsenite were used extensively at the turn of the century for Colorado potato beetle (102). The inorganic arsenicals and nature's botanicals were used for insecticides, and inorganic sulfur products for herbicides and fungicides. It was with this limited level of achievement that mankind entered the 20th century (160).

The Age of Synthetic Chemistry was ushered in with the synthetic organochlorine chemical called dichlorodiphenyltrichloroethylene or DDT (Figure 13.1). A German chemist named Zeidler (148) synthesized DDT in 1874. However, it was not until 1939 that its insecticidal properties were fully realized. DDT was developed as part of the carefully planned and targeted research of an industrial chemist, Dr. Paul Mueller (158). Despite its persistence and bioaccumulating properties, DDT has probably been responsible for saving more human lives than any other synthetic chemical in history (157).

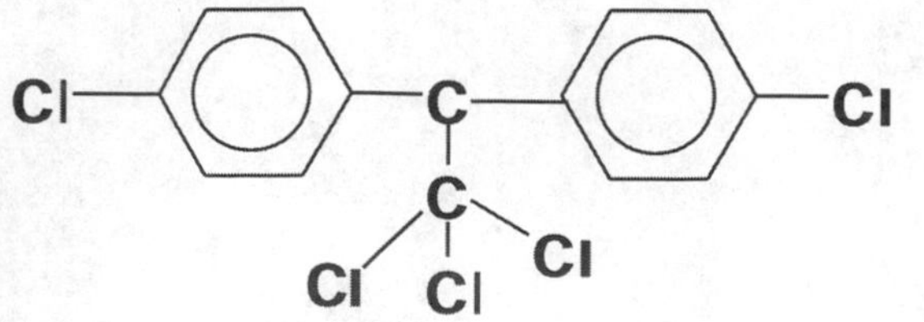

FIG. 13.1. The structure of dichlorodiphenyltrichloroethylene (DDT).

Of all the communicable diseases, malaria has had the greatest impact on society living in tropical and subtropical areas (157). During the first half of the 20th century, every year more than 300 million people suffered from malaria. The mortality rate was estimated at 1%; 3 million people dying annually. By 1965, or less than a quarter of century after its introduction, DDT had effectively eradicated malaria as a threat to 953 million people (319). In addition to malaria, DDT controlled the outbreak of louse-borne typhus, the plague, and yellow fever, the three other most significant diseases in human history. DDT also has been credited as offering some level of control for 20 other human diseases including viral encephalitis, shigellosis, cholera, and tularemia (157).

The development and growth of the agricultural chemistry industry was rapid, particularly in regard to synthetic insect control and weed control agents, following World War II (90). Clearly, there was an intense focus on a diverse number of structures arising from the targeted application of principles of chemistry to the mechanism(s) of action toward specific and selective pest control. The use of synthetic organic crop protection chemicals grew in the United States until 1980 and then has gradually declined thereafter (98). The figures for 1992 sales were essentially the same as the 1985 number or 1.1 billion lb; 1993 sales were estimated as 1.3 billion lb (160), and 1.2 billion lb in 1995 (1).

In the United States during the last 50 years, the use of synthetic organic pesticides has enabled agriculturalists to increase crop yields as much as 50% while affording a reduction in the farm population involved by 69% (2). Despite the reduction in the number of farmers from approximately 7% to 2% of the population, the individual farmer produces enough food to feed an average of 129 people. Control of crop pests leads to healthier plants and thus reduction of mycotoxins and endotoxins, which can present significant human health risk.

Even with the extensive use of pesticides, the U.S. Food and Drug Administration (FDA) estimates that pests destroy approximately one-third of the world's food crops every year (3). The loss in the United States alone is nearly $20 billion per year. Despite the clear benefits from pesticide use, the potential hazard from their application has long been recognized and their uses are tightly regulated and monitored.

The risks associated with pesticides are evaluated by assessing the toxicity of each chemical, and estimating the magnitude of exposure from sources in the workplace, in the environment, in food, and in water. The need to balance the risk of damage to the environment and man against benefits associated with using pesticides is clear (87).

In the United States, the regulation of pesticides is covered by several legislative acts and enforced by several federal and state agencies. A brief historical review of pesticide legislation is provided as a background for current provisions for federal regulation of pesticides by the U.S. Environmental Protection Agency (EPA). Further details for the toxicology study requirements ascribed by the U.S. EPA in its guidelines (171) will be considered. In addition, guidelines, which have been generally harmonized with the U.S. EPA guidelines, are put forth by the Japanese Ministry of Agriculture, Forestry and Fisheries (MAFF), and the Organization for Economic Cooperation and Development or OECD (149,155). Further, the U.S. EPA guidelines have been generally harmonized with those of the European Economic Community (96). This is only logical, as the United States is a member nation of the EEC and Japan belongs to the OECD. The OECD nations include Australia, Austria, Belgium, Canada, Denmark, Finland, France, Germany, Italy, Japan, the Netherlands, Norway, Spain, Sweden, Switzerland, Turkey, the United Kingdom, and the United States.

HAZARD CHARACTERIZATION OF PESTICIDES

Federal Insecticide, Fungicide, and Rodenticide Act

Several years after the introduction of DDT and other synthetic insecticides, the Federal Insecticide, Fungicide, and Rodenticide Act (FIFRA) was passed in 1947 (169). The legislation was administered by the U.S. Department of Agriculture (USDA) and remained primarily a labeling requirement. FIFRA has been amended several times since that time and its registration provisions strengthened. Conner et al. (89) provided a detailed review of FIFRA, with its history and regulations.

Pesticides are also regulated under the Federal Food, Drug, and Cosmetic Act (FFDCA). FFDCA was amended with Section 408 (the Miller Amendment), establishing pesticide tolerances on foodstuffs, in 1954, and Section 409, which established tolerances for food additives in processed foods, was added in 1958 (170).

Section 409 of FFDCA contains the Delaney Clause, which forbids use of carcinogens as food additives. Although Section 409 directly addresses food additives only, interpretations of this section by the U.S. EPA have determined that pesticides, which concentrate during food processing, require food additive tolerances. Thus, the Delaney Clause applies only to pesticides, which concentrate during the processing of food. In the absence of concentration, only Section 408 applies.

Public concern for environmental and health issues as well as an interest in greater efficiency in regulations led to the formation of the U.S. EPA in 1970 (89). This new creation (162,163) did not significantly alter the process of pesticide registration, but it did centralize it in a single agency instead of the previous two (USDA and FDA).

To protect human health and the environment, it is necessary to thoroughly evaluate health and environmental effects of all new products before manufacture and distribution. Specific toxicology study requirements for registration of pesticides around the world have been harmonized (95,96,149,155,171). As testing procedures are enhanced or new guidelines developed, these are added to the specific requirements shown in Table 13.1 (243).

Acute toxicity studies are conducted by administering the chemical orally, dermally, or by inhalation to determine the dose that causes mortality in 50% of the animals tested (LD_{50} or LC_{50}). Acute studies are conducted to evaluate the irritation potential of the chemical after application to skin and eyes. Finally, the potential of the chemical to cause an allergic reaction (i.e., sensitization) is determined. Because this reaction is an all-or-nothing response, chemicals are classified as either sensitizers or nonsensitizers. Acute oral and inhalation studies are usually conducted in rats, dermal and irritation studies are conducted in rabbits or rats, and the sensitization study is carried out in guinea pigs. These tests are used to establish the product labels for all crop protection chemicals (163). The criteria used are presented in Table 13.2.

Dermal toxicity is evaluated by applying the chemical to the skin for 6 h/day for 21 days (rats) to 28 days (rabbits). Feeding studies are used to evaluate the toxicological effects of the chemical when a known dose is administered orally.

The oral feeding studies involve feeding rats, mice, or dogs diets containing the chemical for various lengths of time. Rat and mouse feeding studies are conducted for 28 days, 90 days, 1 year, and for the lifetime of the animals (24 months for rats, 18 months for mice). In dogs, the studies are usually conducted for 28 days, 90 days, 1 year, or 2 years. In all cases, animals are divided into test groups, 10 to 50 rats or mice and 4 to 6 dogs. At least four test groups are used in each study, one receiving no chemical (controls) and three groups receiving low, medium, or high concentrations of chemical in their diets. In these studies, urinalysis, hematology, and clinical chemistry parameters are evaluated, and gross and microscopic pathology examinations are performed on up to 50 tissues. Maximum tolerated doses are tested in order to demonstrate toxicity (up to 1000 mg/kg/day in the diets). In this fashion, it is possible to determine whether a chemical damages or alters any organ or tissue, and to establish levels of the chemical that produce no observable effects (no-observed effect level, NOEL) and the lowest level at which effects are noted (the lowest-observed effect level, LOEL).

Hazard testing also includes the examination of the potential of a chemical to affect the development of offspring, and to identify whether it induces birth defects in either the rat or rabbit. These tests have been described as teratology studies, but are now usually referred to as developmental toxicity studies. In addition to developmental toxicity studies, a reproduction study is conducted in rats. This study involves feeding diets containing the chemical to young adult male and female rats for approximately 3 months prior to mating. The females are allowed to produce a litter of offspring that are then reared to adulthood. The animals are fed diets containing the chemical during this entire period. After reaching sexual maturity, the second-generation animals are allowed to mate.

It was noted by Weisburger (316) that certain chemical carcinogens are capable of interacting directly with genetic material such as DNA. Based upon this association, several short-term tests to identify the alteration of genetic material or mutation were introduced into hazard testing for crop protection chemicals. These include tests to examine the possible interaction with (a) genes (gene mutation tests), (b) the chromosome (clastogenic tests), and (c) directly with DNA (classified as other tests).

Since individuals may be exposed to low levels of crop protection chemicals in their diet or water over a portion of their life span, studies to evaluate lifetime exposure are conducted in animal bioassays. An important aspect of these studies is an assessment of the potential of the chemical to cause cancer. An increase in the number of tumors or the earlier onset of tumors as a result of treatment will identify a chemical as a potential carcinogen. For laboratory studies, mice and rats are divided into at least 3 treatment groups and a control group with a minimum of 50 animals/sex/group. These groups of mice and rats are fed selected concentrations of the test chemical in their diet for 18 months and 24 months, respectively. The levels of the test chemical administered in the diet are generally selected from repeated-dose feeding studies at least 90 days in duration, and are normally used to establish the NOEL, LOEL, and the maximum tolerated dose (MTD) (97). The MTD is defined as the highest concentration of test chemical that can be administrated that can be tolerated without causing the death of the animal; often a 10% reduction in body weight gain has been used as the criterion for establishing the MTD.

Table 13.1
Series 870—Health effects test guidelines (242)

OPPTS Number	Name	Existing Numbers		
		OPPT	OPP	OECD
	Group A—Acute Toxicity Test Guideline.			
870.1000	Acute toxicity testing—background	none	none	none
870.1100	Acute oral toxicity	798.1175	81-1	401
870.1200	Acute dermal toxicity	798.1100	81-2	402
870.1300	Acute inhalation toxicity	798.1150	81-3	403
870.2400	Acute eye irritation	798.4500	81-4	405
870.2500	Acute dermal irritation	798.4470	81-5	404
870.2600	Skin sensitization	798.4100	81-6	406
	Group B—Subchronic Toxicity Test Guidelines.			
870.3100	90-Day oral toxicity in rodents	798.2650	82-1	408
870.3150	90-Day oral toxicity in nonrodents	none	82-1	409
870.3200	21/28-Day dermal toxicity	none	82-2	410
870.3250	90-Day dermal toxicity	798.2250	82-3	411
870.3465	90-Day inhalation toxicity	798.2450	82-4	413
870.3700	Prenatal developmental toxicity study	798.4900	83-3	414
870.3800	Reproduction and fertility affects	798.4700	83-4	416
	Group C—Chronic Toxicity Test Guidelines.			
870.4100	Chronic toxicity	798.3260	83-1	452
870.4200	Carcinogenicity	798.3300	83-2	451
870.4300	Combined chronic toxicity/carcinogenicity	798.3320	83-5	453
	Group D—Genetic Toxicity Test Guidelines.			
870.5100	Bacterial reverse mutation test	798.5100, 798.5265	84-2	471, 472
870.5140	Gene mutation in Aspergillus nidulans	798.5140	84-2	none
870.5195	Mouse biochemical specific locus test	798.5195	84-2	none
870.5200	Mouse visible specific locus test	798.5200	84-2	none
870.5250	Gene mutation in Neurospora crassa	798.5250	84-2	none
870.5275	Sex-linked recessive lethal test in Drosophila	798.5275	84-2	477
870.5300	In vitro mammalian cell gene mutation test	798.5300	84-2	476
870.5375	In vitro mammalian chromosome aberration test	798.5375	84-2	473
870.5380	Mammalian spermatogonial chromosomal aberration	798.5380	84-2	483
870.5385	Mammalian bone marrow chromosomal aberration test	798.5385	84-2	475
870.5395	Mammalian erythrocyte micronucleus test	798.5395	84-2	474
870.5450	Rodent dominant lethal assay	798.5450	84-2	478
870.5460	Rodent heritable translocation assays	798.5460	84-2	none
870.5500	Bacterial DNA damage or repair tests	798.5500	84-2	none
870.5550	Unscheduled DNA synthesis in mammalian cells	798.5550	84-2	482
870.5575	Mitotic gene conversion in Saccharomyces cerevisiae	798.5575	84-2	481
870.5900	In vitro sister chromatid exchange assay	798.5900	84-2	479
870.5915	In vivo sister chromatid exchange assay	798.5915	84-2	none
	Group E—Neurotoxicity Test Guidelines.			
870.6100	Acute and 28-day delayed neurotoxicity of Organophosphorus substances	798.6450, 798.6540 798.6560	81-7, 82-5, 82-6	418, 419
870.6200	Neurotoxicity screening battery	798.6050, 798.6200, 798.6400	81-8, 82-7, 83-1	424
870.6300	Developmental neurotoxicity study	none	83-6	none
870.6500	Schedule-controlled operant behavior	798.6500	85-5	none
870.6850	Peripheral nerve function	798.6850	85-6	none
870.6855	Neurophysiology: Sensory evoked potentials	798.6855	none	none
	Group F—Special Studies Test Guidelines.			
870.7200	Companion animal safety	none	none	none
870.7485	Metabolism and pharmacokinetics	798.7485	85-1	417
870.7600	Dermal penetration	none	85-3	none
870.7800	Immunotoxicity	none	85-7	none

Table 13.2
U.S. EPA acute toxicity classification scheme (163)

Toxicology Category	Signal Word	Oral LD_{50} (mg/kg)	Dermal LD_{50} (mg/kg)	Inhalation LC_{50}(mg/L)	Eye Irritation	Skin Irritation
I	Danger[1]	Up To 50	Up To 200	Up To 0.2	Corrosive. Corneal Opacity Not Reversed In 7 Days	Corrosive
II	Warning	From 50 Through 500	From 200 Through 2000	From 0.2 Through 2.0	Corneal Opacity Reversed In 7 Days; Irritation Persisting 7 Days	Severe Irritation At 72 Hours
III	Caution	From 500 Through 5000	From 2000 Through 5000	From 2.0 Through 20	No Corneal Opacity; Irritation Reversed Within 7 Days	Moderate Irritation At 72 Hours
IV	Caution	Greater Than 5000	Greater Than 5000	Greater Than 20	No Irritation	Mild Or Slight Irritation At 72 Hours

[1] The word "Poison" is used on the label if the "Danger" category is based on oral, dermal or inhalation toxicity.

Following lifetime feeding studies at the prescribed treatment levels, veterinary pathologists examine approximately 50 tissues from each animal for the presence of tumors or other evidence of tissue damage. If a statistically significant increase in the incidence of any tumor in any tissue above the incidence in the control animals is observed, then it is considered in a weight-of-evidence approach as described in the EPA cancer classification scheme (146). In a weight-of-evidence analysis, the evidence of oncogenicity in humans comes from long-term animal studies, and from epidemiology (studies of humans in exposed populations). Results from these studies are supplemented with available information from other sources that include mutagenicity and other short-term tests (for genetic effects), metabolic or kinetic studies, and other relevant toxicological studies. Using this approach, the oncogenic response is classified into one of several categories as indicated in Table 13.3.

The U.S EPA has essentially taken the approach that animal tumorigens are human carcinogens (146). This approach has been taken as a default assumption almost without regard to quality of the study, the level of test material administered, or the mechanism by which the tumor response is manifest (166). In this regard, all animal carcinogens are treated as though they have no threshold or there is a real risk at all exposure levels. The U.S. EPA has published a list identifying crop protection chemicals as known, probable, or possible human carcinogens without appropriate consideration of the mechanism by which the tumors occur or their relevance to humans (150).

However, most of the other OECD and EEC countries have long recognized that genotoxic agents exist (96,168). For genotoxic agents, there is evidence of mutagenic and/or clastogenic responses in standard laboratory tests, and nongenotoxic chemicals are devoid of any mutagenic and/or clastogenic behavior (150). It is considered that genotoxic agents will most likely be carcinogenic in animal tests and most probably will be human carcinogens (168). These genotoxic carcinogens would be regulated as if they are devoid of a threshold, and it would be assumed that there would be a risk at all doses. On the other hand, nongenotoxic agents would be charac-

Table 13.3
U.S. Environmental Protection Agency's classification of carcinogens

Carcinogen Category	Criteria for Classification		Evaluation: Uncertainty Factor	Evaluation: Mathematical Modeling
A – Human	Sufficient evidence in man			X
B – Probable Human	B1	· Limited evidence in man · Sufficient evidence in animal (two species with tumors)		X
	B2	· Inadequate human evidence · Sufficient animal evidence		X
C – Possible Human		· No evidence in man · Limited evidence in animals	X or	X
D – Not Classifiable		· Inadequate animal or human evidence	X	
E – Not a Human Carcinogen		· Sufficient animal testing with no evidence of carcinogenicity and human experience	X	

terized as having thresholds and a safety factor would be used.

Although new U.S. EPA guidelines for cancer classification based on animal data are in development (192), they have not been finalized.

Food Quality Protection Act of 1996

The Food Quality Protection Act (FQPA) amendments to the Food Drug and Cosmetic Act (170) and FIFRA (169), direct the U.S. EPA to consider a number of factors in assessing risk as part of the tolerance setting procedure (5). FQPA 1996 provides for a single, health-based standard, eliminates long-standing problems posed by multiple standards for pesticides in raw and processed foods, and requires the U.S. EPA to consider all nonoccupational sources of exposure, including drinking water, and exposure to other pesticides with a common mechanism of toxicity when setting tolerances. Most of these provisions *originally reflected* concerns that children may be especially susceptible to pesticide exposure and embodied key recommendations of a National Academy of Sciences report, "Pesticides in the Diets of Infants and Children" (153). The FQPA directs the U.S. EPA to set a tolerance for pesticide residues in food. In order to accomplish this task, the U.S. EPA uses an extra 10-fold safety factor to account for susceptibility of children including effects of in utero exposure and to evaluate the cumulative effects of exposure to the pesticide. Further, the agency is directed to consider substances having a common mode of action and to consider aggregate exposure for all consumers (i.e., other routes, such as drinking water). Finally, the agency must define techniques for evaluating potential for endocrine-disrupting effects.

Unlike previous law, which contained an open-ended provision for the consideration of pesticide benefits when setting tolerances, the new law places specific limits on benefit considerations. Benefits cannot be considered for pesticides that result in reproductive or other threshold effects.

In addition, FQPA 1996 reauthorizes Federal Insecticide, Fungicide, and Rodenticide Act provisions (FIFRA) and requires tolerances to be reassessed as part of the reregistration program (5). Further, it expedites review of safer pesticides to help them reach the market sooner and replace older and potentially more risky chemicals. Minor-use pesticides and antimicrobial pesticides are given greater attention under this new law.

FUNGICIDES

The world market for agricultural and noncrop fungicides amounted to nearly $6 billion in 1995 (139). The

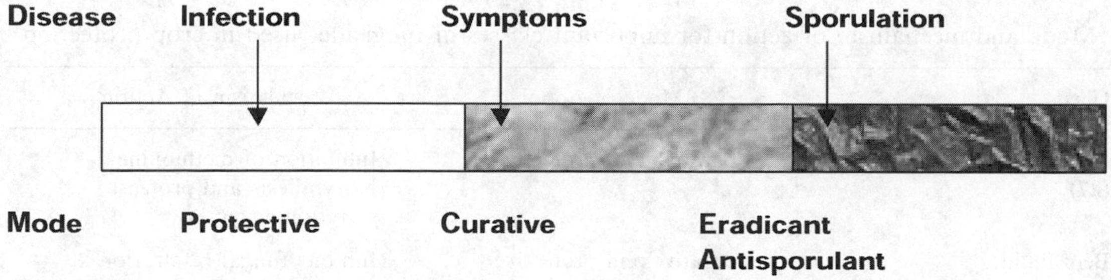

FIG. 13.2. Representation of the disease process and efficacy by mode of action.

United States, western Europe, and Japan accounted for 75% of the total world market. Tree fruits and nuts, citrus, and grapes constitute the largest market for fungicides worldwide. This sector was 28.5% of the total world market, followed by cereals, rice, vegetables, and potatoes. In western Europe, half of the $2 billion spent for fungicides was used on wheat and barley, followed by vines, tree fruits, and other crop and noncrop markets. For the Japanese market of over $1 billion, about 40% of the fungicides were applied to rice, with vegetables and tree fruits the next most important market. The U.S. market for fungicides amounted to about $800 million, with tree and vine crops accounting for 30%, followed by turf ornamentals, then vegetable crops, and finally peanuts and potatoes.

Fungicides have been classified in several different manners. Mode of action in affecting the development of fungal diseases is one of the systems used. Schematically, the disease process along with the mode of action for fungicides is presented in Figure 13.2 (91).

A *protective* or *preventative* mode of action is ascribed to fungicidal activity when the disease is prevented. *Curative* relates to activity that interrupts the development of established infection. An *eradicant*, as the name implies, stops the development of the disease after symptoms are visible in the plant, and an *antisporulant* stops or decreases spore production. Mode of action and mechanism of action determine the major classes of fungicides used in crop protection, presented in Table 13.4.

Individual fungicides representing each mode of action are discussed here. It is not feasible to discuss all fungicides within the scope of this chapter. Therefore, no attempt to consider every fungicide within a group has been made. Instead, an attempt was made to consider only those fungicides with current significant economic importance or use. Therefore, discussions focus on selected agents.

Anilinopyrimidines

The spectrum of activity for anilinopyrimidines is limited to *Ascomycetes* and *Deuteromycetes* (27). Their unique mode of action of inhibiting methionine biosynthesis as well as protease secretion necessary for infection affords both protective and curative action. The anilinopyrimidines are used to control gray mold on vines, fruits, vegetables, and ornamentals, and leaf scab on pome fruit. The anilinopyrimidines are a new class of fungicides currently represented by two commerically available products. The structures, uses, and hazard profiles of cyprodinil and pyrimethanil are presented in Table 13.5.

The profiles for the mammalian toxicity studies conducted with these fungicides suggest minimal hazard to humans from their use (224,231).

Benzanilides

Benzanilides, which inhibit the succinate dehydrate complex in the electron transport chain and thus stop the synthesis of aspartate and glutamate, are represented by flutolanil (43). Flutolanil is a systemic fungicide with protective and curative action. It is used for control of sheath blight, white mold, and snow blight in rice, cereals, sugar beet, and other crops. The structure, uses, and hazard profile of flutolanil are given in Table 13.6.

It exhibits minimal acute toxicity and possesses a good hazard profile (186).

Benzimidazoles

The benzimidazoles have broad-spectrum activity in the inhibition of mitosis by preventing polymerization of beta-tubulin (15). Important members of this class are benomyl, thiabendazole, and thiophanate-methyl. Their structures, uses, and hazard profiles are presented in Table 13.7.

The hazards for benomyl, thiabendazole, and thiophanate-methyl have been carefully reviewed by either the U.S. EPA or WHO (106,132,216). Benomyl has been classified as Category C (possible human carcinogen) based on mouse liver tumors (100).

Table 13.4
Mode and mechanism of action for important classes of fungicides used in crop protection

Class	Mode of Action	Mechanism of Action
Anilinopyrimidines (27)	Curative and protective	Inhibition of methionine biosynthesis and protease secretion enzymes
Benzanilides (16)	Curative and protective	Inhibits fungal respiration at succinate dehydrogenase complex
Benzimidazoles (15)	Curative and protective	Inhibition of mitosis by preventing polymerization of tubulin in a broad spectrum of fungi
Phenylamides (54)	Curative and protective	Inhibition of RNA synthesis
Sterol Biosynthesis sterol Inhibitors (26)	Curative, protective, and eradicants	Interferes with biosynthesis essential for cell wall formation
Strobilurins (12)	Curative, protective, and antisporulants	Disruption of electron transport in cytochrome bc_1 complex
Dicarboximides (53)	Protective, and antisporulants	Inhibition of spore germination
Dithiocarbamates (39)	Protective	Interferes with oxygen uptake and inhibits sulfur-containing enzymes
Ethylenediothio-carbamates (54)	Protective	Breaks down to cyanide which reacts with thiol compounds in the cells and interferes with sulfhydryl groups
Inorganic (23–25,74)	Protective	Blocks enzymes and stops respiration
Organometallics (37)	Protective, some curative and antisporulant	Destroys cell membranes, and inhibits metabolism and respiration
Phenylpyrroles (35)	Protective	Interferes with membrane transport
Phthalimides (16)	Protective and curative	Inhibits enzymes by thiophosgene production
Substituted Benzenes (20)	Protective	Inhibits sulfur-containing enzymes

Phenylamides

This class of fungicides includes two products, metalaxyl and mefenoxam (55). Metalaxyl is a mixture of *R* and *S* enantiomers. Mefenoxam is the *R* enantiomer of metalaxyl. The spectrum of activity for mefenoxam is quite narrow controlling downy mildew and late blight; it is used in maize, peas, sorghum, sunflowers, and tobacco (55).

Mefenoxam is efficacious at approximately half the rate of metalaxyl; therefore, the registration of metalaxyl has been voluntarily canceled (180,218). The structure, uses, and hazard profile for mefenoxam are presented in Table 13.8.

Table 13.5
Structures, uses, and hazard profiles for major anilinopyrimidine fungicides

Fungicide	Structure	Crops/uses	Use Rates gm (a.i.)/ha
Cyprodinil Vangard® (27)	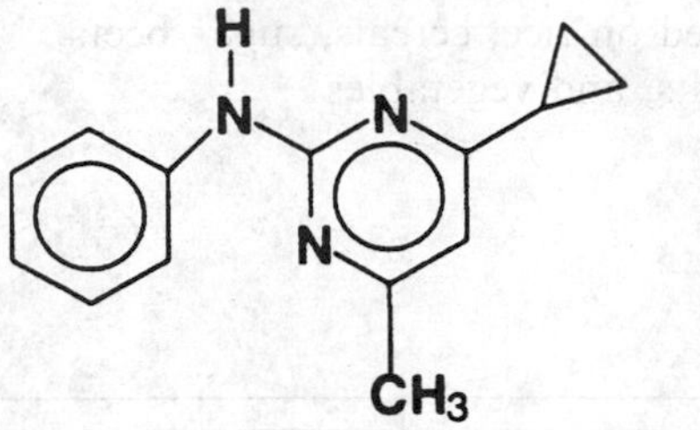	Used on cereals, grapes, pome fruit, stone fruit, almonds, strawberries, vegetables, field crop and as a seed dressing	95–160
Pyrimethanil Mythos®, Scala® (68,224)	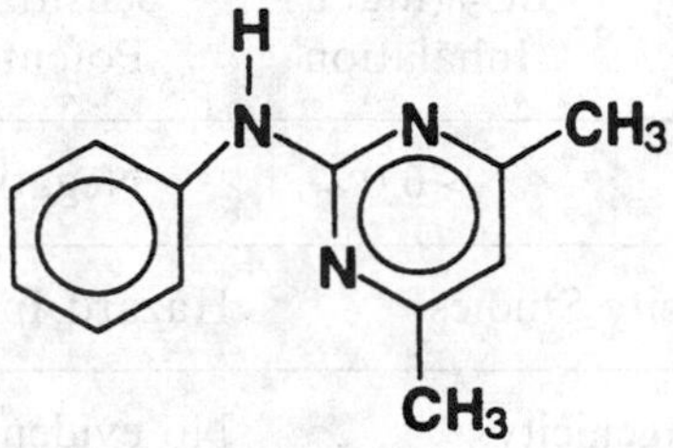	Used on pome fruit, vine crops, vegetables and ornamentals.	1000–3000

	Irritation		LD_{50} (mg/kg)		LC_{50} (mg/L)		
Fungicide	Eye	Skin	Oral	Dermal	Inhalation	Sensitizing Potential	Signal Word
Cyprodinil (27)	Minimal Irritant	Slight Irritant	2796	> 2000	> 1.2	Positive	Caution
Pyrimethanil (68)	Slight Irritant	Non-irritant	> 4149	> 5000	> 1.98	No positive	Caution

Fungicide	Species/study	NOEL[1] (mg/kg/day)	Toxicity Studies	Hazard Indicator
Cyprodinil (231)	Rat/2-year	3.75	Mutagenicity	No evidence
	Dog/52-week	65.6	Developmental	Not teratogenic
	Mouse/18-month	16.1 ♂	Reproductive	No evidence
	RfD[2]	0.038	Oncogenicity	E(No evidence)[3]
Pyrimethanil (224)	Rat/2-year	20	Mutagenicity	No evidence
	Dog/52-week	30	Developmental	Not teratogenic
	Mouse/18-month	211 ♂	Reproductive	No evidence
	RfD[2]	0.2	Oncogenicity	C with RfD[3] (thyroid tumors in rats)

[1] No observable effect level
[2] RfD = reference dose
[3] See Table 13.3 for US EPA classification scheme

Mefenoxam is without any significant hazard to humans.

Sterol Biosynthesis Inhibitors

The sterol biosynthesis inhibitors or sterol demethylase inhibitors (DMIs) group are comprised of imidazoles, piperazines, pyridines, pyrimidines, and triazoles that produce their effect on fungi by inhibition of the synthesis of ergosterol (26). Ergosterol is essential for cell-wall integrity in fungi. The structures and crop uses for the most prominent DMIs are given in Table 13.9.

The ability of these fungicides to inhibit cytochrome P450 demethylase required for the synthesis of ergosterol

Table 13.6
Structure, uses and hazard profile for flutolanil (Folistar®) (187)

Structure	Crops/uses	Use Rates gm (a.i.)/ha
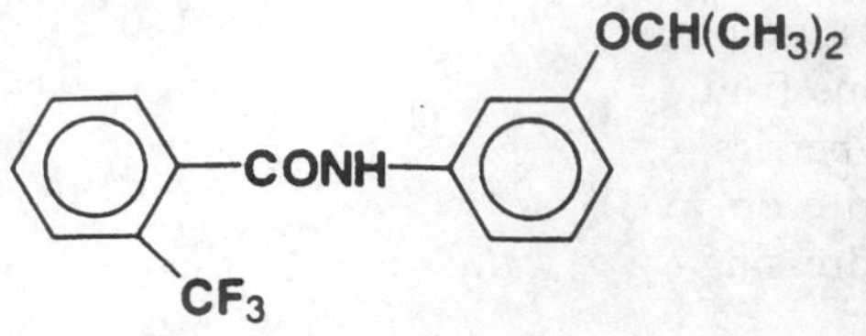	Used on rice, cereals, sugar beets, fruits, and vegetables	NA

Irritation Eye	Irritation Skin	LD_{50}(mg/kg) Oral	LD_{50}(mg/kg) Dermal	LC_{50}(mg/L) Inhalation	Sensitizing Potential	Signal Word
Slight Irritant	Non-irritant	> 10000	> 5000	> 6.0	Negative	Caution

Species/study	NOEL[1] (mg/kg/day)	Toxicity Studies	Hazard Indicator
Rat/2-year	87	Mutagenicity	No evidence
Dog/2-Year Oral	50	Developmental	Not teratogenic
Mouse/18-month	735	Reproductive	No evidence
RfD[2]	0.2 (based rat reproduction; UF[3] = 300	Oncogenicity	E (No evidence)[4]

[1] No observable effect level
[2] RfD = reference dose
[3] UF = Uncertainty factor
[4] See Table 13.3 for US EPA classification scheme
NA = Not Available

in fungi also occurs in mammalian systems and often manifests itself as an induction of liver cytochrome P450 as well as inhibiting these enzymes (31). Inherent in the chemical structure of these compounds is specificity to alter the activity of cytochrome P450 isozymes responsible for the metabolism of steroids, or xenobiotics. In some instances, these liver effects are seen following chronic feeding as liver tumors in the mouse. The hazard profiles for the selected sterol biosynthesis inhibitors are presented in Table 13.10 and 13.11.

Several fungicides produce liver tumors in mice, but all are not genotoxic. Cyproconazole (177) and triadimenol (112) elicit some evidence of developmental toxicity.

Strobilurins

The strobilurins inhibit mitochondrial respiration by blocking electron transfer between cytochrome *b* and cytochrome c_1 (12). These materials have their origins as a natural substance derived from mushrooms and are modified synthetically. Numerous chemicals in this class are under development, but only one strobilurin is available commercially, azoxystrobin. Azoxystrobin has a broad mode of action that includes protective, eradicant, and antisporant activity. The structure, uses, and hazard profile for azoxystrobin are presented in Table 13.12.

Azoxystrobin presents a rather innocuous hazard profile (196).

Inorganic Fungicides

Inorganics, such as sulfur, were used before 1000 BC as previously discussed (102). Yet elemental sulfur and forms of copper (hydroxide, oxychloride, and sulfate) are the only commercially significant fungicides in this class remaining in use. The mode of action of the inorganic fungicides is protective or preventative; they exert their effects by blockage of enzymes and inhibiting respiration (74). These materials are cheap and are applied at high use rates, from thousands to ten thousand of grams per hectare. Severe eye irritation is seen with copper hydroxide (23); copper oxychloride and copper sulfate do not exhibit this inherent hazard (24,25).

Table 13.7
Structures, uses, and hazard profiles for important benzimidazoles

Compound	Structure	Crops/uses	Use Rates gm (a.i.)/ha
Benomyl Benlate® (15)	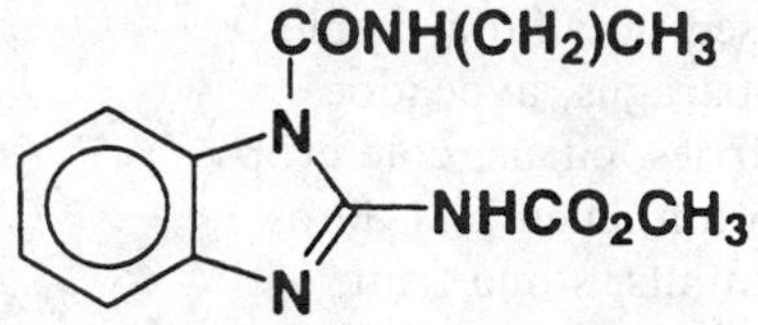	Used against *Ascomycetes* and *Basidomycetes* in cereals, grapes, pome and stone fruit, rice and vegetables.	Field: 140–550 Tree: 550–1100 Storage; 25–200
Thiabenazole Mertech® (77)	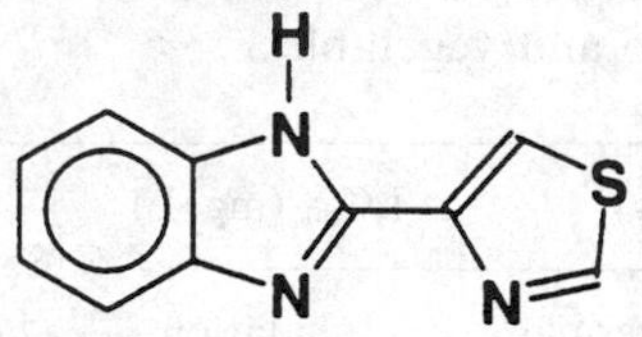	Used for the control of *Aspergillus, Botrytis*, and others in vegetables, bananas, cereals, cabbage, stone fruit, citrus fruit, and hops.	~250
Thiophanate-methyl Topsin-M® (78)	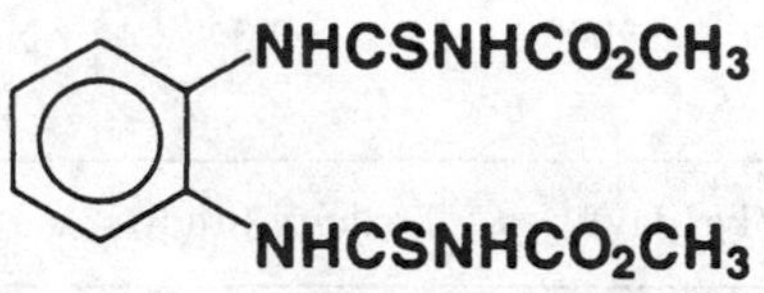	Used for eyespot on cereals, scab and rot on apples and pears, powdery mildew on pome fruit, stone fruit, vegetables, strawberries, and vines	30–50

Fungicide	Irritation		LD_{50} (mg/kg)		LC_{50} (mg/L)	Sensitizing Potential	Signal Word
	Eye	Skin	Oral	Dermal	Inhalation		
Benomyl (15)	Moderate Irritant	Slight Irritant	>10000	>5000	>2.0	Negative	Caution
Thiabendazole (51)	Non-irritant	Non-irritant	3100	>2000	>0.4	Negative	Caution
Thiophanate-methyl (78)	Moderate Irritant	Mild Irritant	6640 ♀	>10000	>5.0	Negative	Caution

Fungicide	Species/study	NOEL[1] (mg/kg/day)	Toxicity Studies	Hazard Indicator
Benomyl (132,173)	Rat/2-year	125	Mutagenicity	No evidence
	Dog/52-week	12.5	Developmental	Inconclusive evidence
	Mouse/18-month	40	Reproductive	Decreased fertility
	RfD (based on reproduction study)[2]	0.05	Oncogenicity	C with RfD (liver tumors in mice)[3]
Thiabendazole (106)	Rat/2-year	20	Mutagenicity	No evidence
	Dog/2-Year Oral	20	Developmental	Effects only at maternally toxic doses
	Mouse/18-month	6	Reproductive	No evidence
	ADI (human study)[2]	0.035	Oncogenicity	Thyroid tumors in rats
Thiophanate-Methyl (135)	Rat/2-year	8.0	Mutagenicity	No evidence
	Dog/52-week	50	Developmental	Minimal evidence
	Mouse/18-month	23	Reproductive	↓spermatogenesis
	RfD[2]	0.08	Oncogenicity	No evidence

[1] No observable effect level
[2] RfD = reference dose and ADI = acceptable daily intake
[3] See Table 13.3 for US EPA classification scheme

Table 13.8
Structure, uses, and hazard profile for the phenylamide fungicide mefenoxam

Fungicide	Structure	Principle Uses/Crops	Application Rate gm(a.i.)/ha
Mefenoxam (Metalaxyl-M) Ridomil Gold® (55)	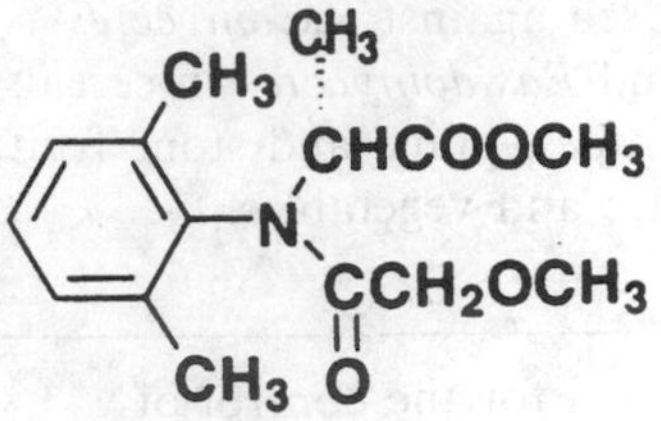	Used on alfalfa, apples, asparagus, avocadoes, berries, citrus, cole crops, cotton, cucurbits, hops, peanuts, stone fruit, soybeans, sugar beets, tobacco and vegetables.	70–1680

Fungicide	Irritation		LD_{50} (mg/kg)		LC_{50} (mg/L)	Sensitizing Potential	Signal Word
	Eye	Skin	Oral	Dermal	Inhalation		
Mefenoxam (55)	Severe Irritant	Slight Irritant	490	>2000	>2.3	Negative	Warning

Fungicide	Species/study	NOEL[1] (mg/kg/day)	Toxicity Studies	Hazard Indicator
Mefenoxam (199,218)	Rat/2-year	13	Mutagenicity	No evidence
	Dog/52-week	8	Developmental	Not teratogenic
	Mouse/18-month	38	Reproductive	No evidence
	RfD(based on 6-Month Dog)[2]	0.08	Oncogenicity	No evidence

[1] No observable effect level
[2] RfD = reference dose

Elemental sulfur is considered practically nontoxic to humans and animals (74).

Dicarboximides

The dicarboximides have a narrow spectrum of activity with strengths on *Botrytis, Sclerotinia, Monifinia*, and *Altemaria*. These fungicides appear to inhibit spore germination (51). The dicarboximides are used to treat infections in turf, strawberries, stone fruit, peanuts, and vines. Iprodione and vinclozolin represent the dicarboximide fungicides; the structures, uses, and mammalian toxicology for these agents are presented in Table 13.13.

Iprodione interferes with androgen synthesis (134); this effect results in testicular effects including interstitial-cell tumors in male rats at feeding levels of 1600 ppm and above. Vinclozolin has been shown to be metabolized to antiandrogenic metabolites, 2-1[(3,5-dichlorophenyl) carbamoyl] oxyl-2-methyl-3-butenoic acid and 3,5′-dichloro-2-hydroxy-2-methylbut-3-enanilide, that appear to lead to infertility in male rats (140). This response is thought to be due to feminization of the outer genital organs of males exposed during development to a dietary concentration of 1000 ppm or more of vinclozolin (227).

Dithiocarbamates

The dithiocarbamates are broad-spectrum protective fungicides with multiple sites of action (39). They are use to control scab on pome fruit, blue mold on tobacco, rust on ornamentals, and diseases on vegetables. These agents interfere with oxygen uptake and inhibit sulfur-containing enzymes. The dithiocarbamates are applied at rates of 500 to over 10,000 g/hectare. Ferbam, thiram, and ziram are the commercially important chemicals in this group. Their structures, uses, and hazard profiles are given in Table 13.14.

Ferbam, thiram, and ziram have significant acute toxicity by the inhalation route. Both ferbam and ziram have been shown to alter spermatazoa in mice and thus would be placed under the endocrine disruptor category as suggested in the FQPA 1996 (5).

Table 13.9
Selected sterol synthesis inhibitors

Fungicide	Structure	Crops/uses
Cyproconazole Alto® (26)	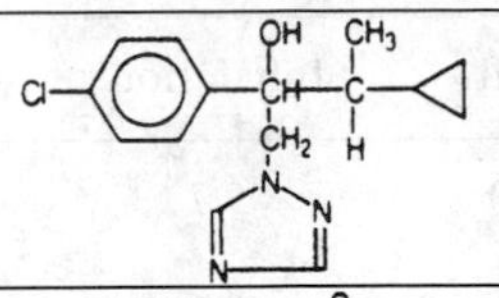	Cereal, sugar beets, fruit trees, vines, coffee, turf, bananas, and vegetables for treatment of rust, powdery mildew, *Septoria*, *Venturia*, and others.
Difenoconazole Dividend® (31)	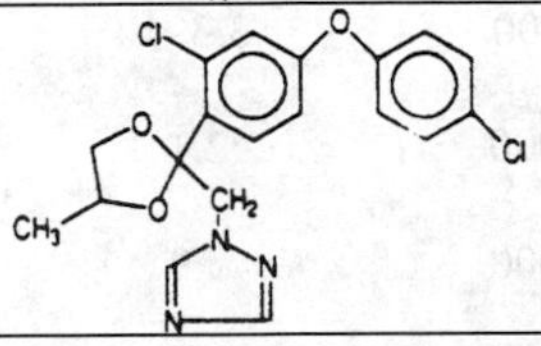	Seed treatment, grapes, fruit trees, potatoes, sugar beets, oilseed rape, banana, ornamentals and vegetables for treating a variety of fungal diseases.
Fenbuconazole Indar® (34)	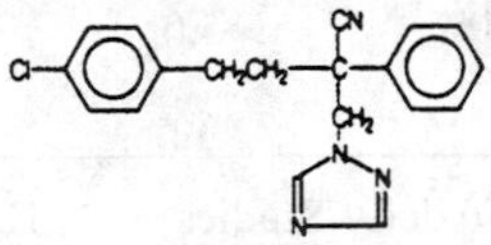	Cereals, fruit trees, vines, beans, sugar beets, rice, bananas, ornamentals, tree nuts and vegetables
Hexaconazole Amizol® (46)	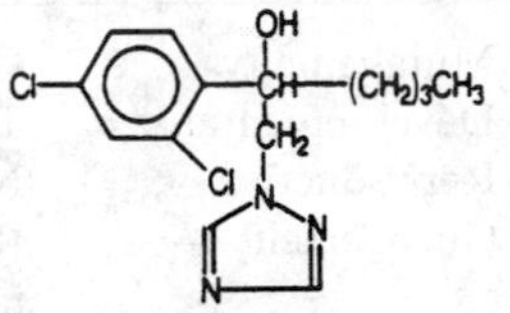	Vine, coffee, bananas, peanuts, and vegetables for treating a variety of fungal diseases.
Myclobutanil Rally®, Nova® (58)	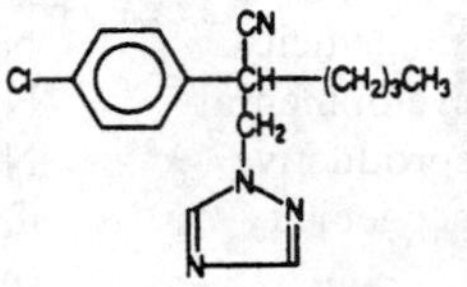	Seed treatment, grapes, fruit trees, rice, cotton, barley, wheat, maize, grass seed, ornamentals and vegetables for treating a variety of fungal diseases
Propiconazole Tilt® (64)	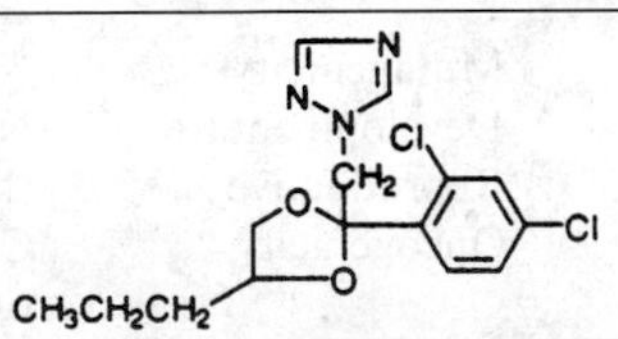	Wheat, rice, coffee, bananas, peanuts, stone fruit, maize and turf for treating a variety of fungal diseases. Rates: 24 to 110 gm (a.i.)/ha
Tebuconazole Folicur® (75)	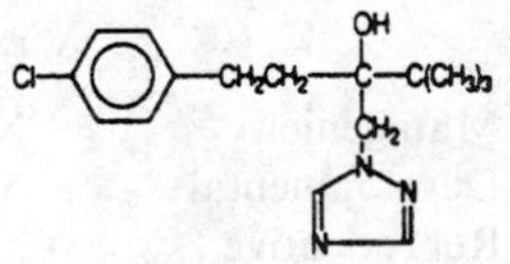	Seed treatment, cereals, coffee, fruit trees, grapes, grass seed, oilseed rape, soybeans, sugar beets, bananas, ornamentals, turf and vegetables for treating a variety of fungal diseases
Triadimefon Bayleton® (80)	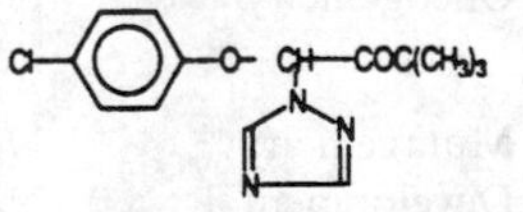	Cereals, corn, fruit trees, vines, berries, sugar cane, tobacco and vegetables for treating a variety of fungal diseases
Triadimenol Baytan® (82)	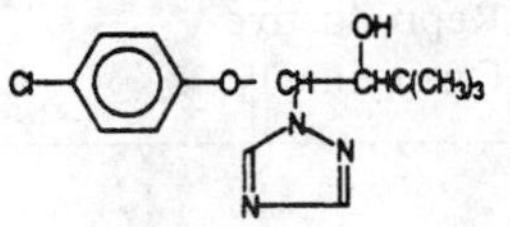	Seed treatment, cereals, fruit trees, hops, vines and vegetables for treating a variety of fungal diseases
Imazalil Fungaflor® (48)	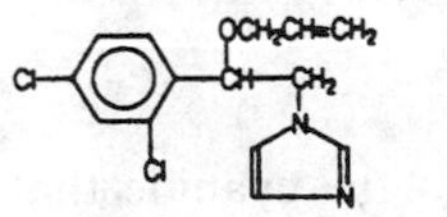	Seed, fruit trees, potatoes, bananas, vegetables, ornamentals and cereals for treating a variety of fungal diseases. Rates of 4–5 (a.i.) 100 kg seed
Prochloraz Sportak® (62)	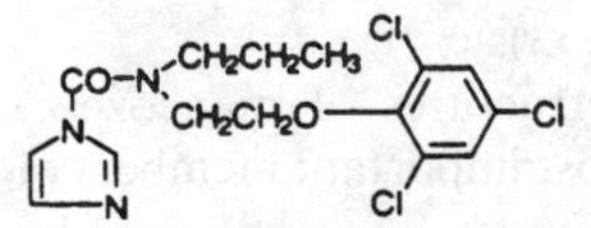	Citrus, tropical fruit (dip), beets, oilseed rape, mushrooms, ornamentals and cereals (seed treatment). Rates: 400–600 gm (a.i.)/ha

Table 13.10
Hazard profile for sterol synthesis-inhibiting fungicides

Fungicide	Irritation		LD_{50} (mg/kg)		LC_{50} (mg/L)	Sensitizing Potential	Signal Word
	Eye	Skin	Oral	Dermal	Inhalation		
Cyproconazole (26)	Non-irritant	Non-irritant	> 1020	> 2000	5.7	Negative	Caution
Difenoconazole (31)	Moderate Irritant	Slight Irritant	1453	>2000	3.3	Negative	Caution
Fenbuconazole (34)	Non-irritant	Non-irritant	> 2000	> 5000	> 2.1	Negative	Caution
Hexaconazole (46)	Mild Irritant	Non-irritant	2189	> 2000	> 5.9	Positive	Caution
Myclobutanil (58)	Irritant	Non-irritant	> 1600	> 5000	> 5.0	Positive	Danger

Fungicide	Species/study	NOEL[1] (mg/kg/day)	Toxicity Studies	Hazard Indicator
Cyproconazole (177)	Rat/2-year	2.2	Mutagenicity	Clastogenic (CHO)
	Dog/52-week	1.0	Developmental	Teratogenic in rabbit
	Mouse/18-month	1.8	Reproductive	No evidence
	RfD[2]	0.01	Oncogenicity	B2 (Mouse liver tumors in both sexes)[3]
Difenoconazole (204)	Rat/2-year	1.0	Mutagenicity	No evidence
	Dog/52-week	3.4 ♂	Developmental	Not Teratogenic
	Mouse/18-month	4.7 ♂	Reproductive	No evidence
	RfD[2]	0.01	Oncogenicity	C with RfD (Mouse liver tumors in both sexes)[3]
Fenbuconazole (178)	Rat/2-year	3.0	Mutagenicity	No evidence
	Dog/52-week	3.8 ♂	Developmental	Not teratogenic
	Mouse/18-month	1.4 ♂	Reproductive	(No evidence)[3]
	RfD[2]	0.03	Oncogenicity	C with RfD (Mouse liver tumors—both sexes/ thyroid tumors—male rats)[3]
Hexaconazole (187a)	Rat/2-year	0.5	Mutagenicity	No evidence
	Dog/52-week	2.0	Developmental	Not teratogenic
	Mouse/18-month	4.7 ♂	Reproductive	No evidence
	RfD[2]	0.005	Oncogenicity	C with CSF (Male rat Leydig cell tumor)[3]
Myclobutanil (219)	Rat/2-year	2.5	Mutagenicity	No evidence
	Dog/52-week	3.1 ♂	Developmental	Not teratogenic
	Mouse/18-month	13.7 ♂	Reproductive	Testicular atrophy
	RfD[2]	0.025	Oncogenicity	E (No evidence)[3]

[1] No observable effect level
[2] RfD = reference dose, ADI = acceptable daily intake, and CSF = cancer slope factor
[3] See Table 13.3 for US EPA classification scheme

Ethylenebisdithiocarbamates

The ethylenebisdithiocarbamates (EBDCs) have a broad spectrum of activity, although their mode of action is primarily protective. Their mechanism of action is to break down to the cyanide that reacts with thiol compounds in the cell and thus interferes with sulfhydryl groups (53).

The structures of mancozeb, maneb, and zineb, the three most important members of this class, are presented

Table 13.11
Hazard profile for more sterol synthesis inhibitor fungicides

Fungicide	Irritation: Eye	Irritation: Skin	LD_{50} (mg/kg): Oral	LD_{50} (mg/kg): Dermal	LC_{50} (mg/L): Inhalation	Sensitizing Potential	Signal Word
Propiconazole (64,191)	Mild Irritant	Slight Irritant	1517	> 6000	> 5.8	Negative	Caution
Tebuconazole (225)	Mild Irritant	Non-irritant	> 3933 ♂	> 5000	> 0.37	Negative	Caution
Triadimefon (80)	Non-irritant	Non-irritant	> 363	> 2000	> 3.6	Positive	Warning
Triadimenol (81)	Non-irritant	Non-irritant	> 1100	> 5000	> 0.9	NA	Caution
Imazalil (48)	Non-irritant	Mild Irritant	> 227	4200	16	Negative	Warning
Prochloraz (62)	Irritant	Mild Irritant	1600	3000	0.42	Negative	Caution

Fungicide	Species/study	NOEL[1] (mg/kg/day)	Toxicity Studies	Hazard Indicator
Propiconazole (64,191)	Rat/2-year	3.6	Mutagenicity	No evidence
	Dog/26-Week Oral	1.3	Developmental	Not teratogenic
	Mouse/18-month	15	Reproductive	No evidence
	RfD[2]	0.013	Oncogenicity	C with RfD (Mouse liver tumors in males)[3]
Tebuconazole (225)	Rat/2-year	7.4	Mutagenicity	No evidence
	Dog/52-week	3.0	Developmental	Teratogenic in rat
	Mouse/18-month	2.9	Reproductive	No evidence
	RfD[2]	0.03	Oncogenicity	C with RfD (Mouse liver tumors in both sexes)[3]
Triadimefon (111,194)	Rat/2-year	16.4 ♂	Mutagenicity	No evidence
	Dog/2-Year Oral	11.4	Developmental	Not teratogenic
	Mouse/18-month	40	Reproductive	No evidence
	RfD (52-wk dog study with 300 × UF[4])[2]	0.04	Oncogenicity	C with RfD (Mouse liver tumors in both sexes)[3]
Triadimenol (112)	Rat/2-year	7.0	Mutagenicity	No evidence
	Dog/52-week	3.75	Developmental	Teratogenic in rat
	Mouse/18-month	30	Reproductive	No evidence
	ADI[2]	0.038	Oncogenicity	C with RfD (liver tumors in female mice)[3]
Imazalil (119)	Rat/2-year	5.0	Mutagenicity	No evidence
	Dog/52-week	2.5	Developmental	Not teratogenic
	Mouse/18-month	40	Reproductive	No evidence
	ADI[2]	0.025	Oncogenicity	C with CSF (Mouse liver)[3]
Prochloraz (110)	Rat/2-year	1.9	Mutagenicity	No evidence
	Dog/52-week	0.9	Developmental	Not teratogenic
	Mouse/18-month	11.7	Reproductive	Decreased litter size
	ADI[2]	0.009	Oncogenicity	C with CSF (Mouse liver tumors in both sexes)[3]

[1] No observable effect level
[2] RfD = reference dose, ADI = acceptable daily intake, and CSF = cancer slope factor
[3] See Table 13.3 for US EPA classification scheme
[4] UF = Uncertainty factor
NA = Not Available

Table 13.12
Structure, uses, and hazard profile for azoxystrobin (Heritage®) (112,196)

Structure	Principle Uses/Crops	Application Rate gm (a.i.)/ha
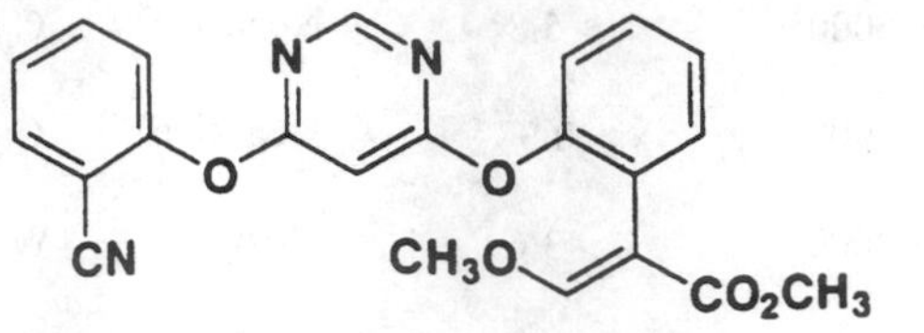	Used on vine crops, apples, cereals, cucurbits, tomatoes, pecans, coffee, potatoes, peanuts, peaches, citrus, rice and turf	100–375

Irritation		LD_{50} (mg/kg)		LC_{50} (mg/L)	Sensitizing Potential	Signal Word
Eye	Skin	Oral	Dermal	Inhalation		
Slight Irritant	Slight Irritant	> 5000	> 2000	> 0.7	Not positive	Caution

Species/study	NOEL[1] (mg/kg/day)	Toxicity Studies	Hazard Indicator
Rat/2-year	18	Mutagenicity	No evidence
Dog/1-Year Oral	25	Developmental	Not teratogenic
Mouse/18-month	38 ♂	Reproductive	No evidence
RfD[2]	0.18	Oncogenicity	E(No evidence)[3]

[1] No observable effect level
[2] RfD = reference dose
[3] See Table 13.3 for US EPA classification scheme

with their toxicologically significant metabolite, ethylenethiourea, in Figure 13.3.

The hazard profiles for mancozeb, maneb, and zineb are presented in Table 13.15.

Both mancozeb and maneb are classified as B2, probable human carcinogens (100), based on the formation of mouse liver tumors and/or thyroid follicular cell tumors in rats. Although zineb was not found to be oncogenic in the rat or mouse, it was observed to produce nonneoplasic hyperplasia of the follicular cells of the thyroid in rats (217). All three fungicides are metabolized to ethylenethiourea. This is known to inhibit thyroid peroxidase and to cause progressive lesions in the thyroid follicular cells, often leading to tumor formation (126,127,129). The U.S. EPA has regulated the risk associated with the EBDCs using a cancer slope factor of 0.06 $(mg/kg/day)^{-1}$ (216).

Organometallic Fungicides

The organometallic fungicides are limited in spectrum of disease control, but are effective as protective, curative, and antisporulants in early and late blight, scab, leaf blotch, and powdery mildew (37). Triphenyltin, whose structure, uses, and hazard profile are presented in Table 13.16, works through destruction of cell membranes and inhibition of respiration (37).

Triphenyltin hydroxide has been classified by the U.S. EPA as category B2, probable human carcinogen, based on mouse liver and pituitary and testicular tumors in rats (100).

Phenylpyrroles

The phenylpyrrole fungicides are a recent entry into the marketplace. They represent a new mechanism of action through interference with membrane transport (35). The structures, uses, and hazard profiles of these two new fungicides, fenpiclonil and fludioxonil, are presented in Table 13.17.

Both of these products are not acutely toxic, and do not exhibit remarkable toxicity profiles. Fludioxonil represents an exception as it has been classified as a category D or nonclassifiable in regard to carcinogenicity. This conclusion is based on the statistically significant increase in liver tumors in female rats for combined adenoma/carcinoma only. Despite the lack of a tumorigenic response in male rats or in either sex of the mouse, additional mutagenicity studies have been required (202).

Table 13.13
Structures, uses, and hazard profiles for dicarboximide fungicides

Fungicide	Structure	Principle Uses/Crops	Application Rate gm (a.i)/ha
Iprodione Rovral® (51)	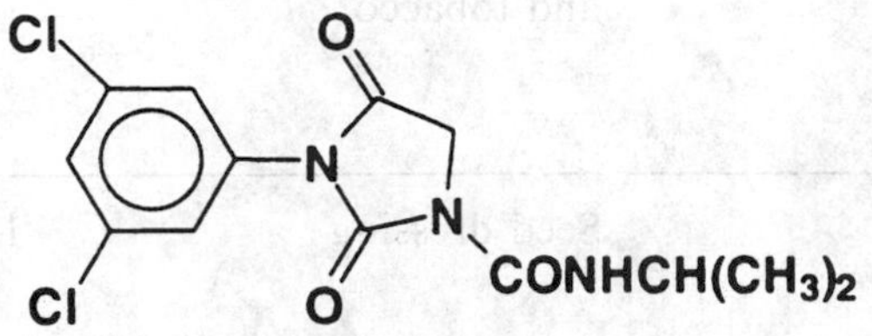	Sunflowers, cereals, fruit trees, berries, oilseed rape, rice, cotton, vegetables, vines, turf and seed treatment.	500–12000
Vinclozolin Roilan® (83)	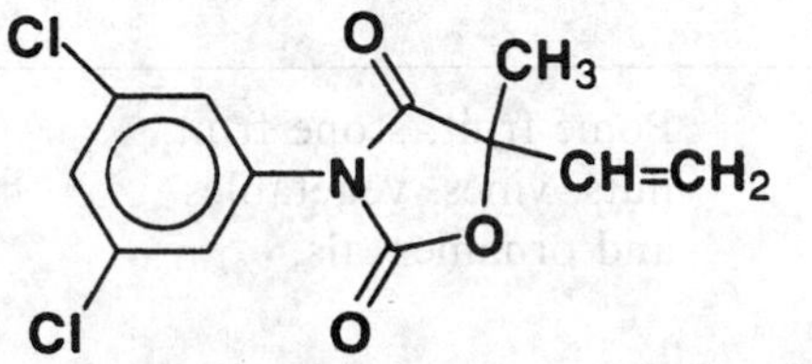	Pome and stone fruit, oilseed rape, vegetables, vines, turf and ornamentals	300–430

Fungicide	Irritation Eye	Irritation Skin	LD_{50} (mg/kg) Oral	LD_{50} (mg/kg) Dermal	LC_{50}(mg/L) Inhalation	Sensitizing Potential	Signal Word
Iprodione (174)	Mild Irritant	Non-irritant	4468	> 2000	> 5.2	Negative	Caution
Vinclozolin (83)	Minimal Irritant	Minimal Irritant	> 15000	> 5000	29.1	Positive	Caution

Fungicide	Species/study	NOEL[1] (mg/kg/day)	Toxicity Studies	Hazard Indicator
Iprodione (134,174)	Rat/2-year	6.0	Mutagenicity	No evidence
	Dog/52-week	4.2	Developmental	Not teratogenic
	Mouse/18-month	1870	Reproductive	No evidence
	RfD[2](300 × UF)	0.04	Oncogenicity	B2 (liver, testes)[3]
Vinclozolin (136,227)	Rat/2-year	1.2	Mutagenicity	No evidence
	Dog/52-week	2.4	Developmental	Not teratogenic
	Mouse/18-month	21	Reproductive	Anti-androgenic metabolite
	RfD[2]	0.012	Oncogenicity	B2 with RfD (multiple benign tumors in rats)[3]

[1] No observable effect level
[2] RfD = reference dose
[3] See Table 13.3 for US EPA classification scheme

Phthalimides

The phthalimide fungicides represent a relatively old group of synthetic chemicals. Of this group of fungicides, only captan remains significant in regard to use. Captan has a broad spectrum of activity that owes its action to degradation to thiophosgene (16). The structure, uses, and hazard profile of captan are given in Table 13.18.

Captan has been shown to bind to DNA in vitro but not in vivo. Further, captan is classified by the U.S. EPA as category B2, probable human carcinogen, based on gastrointestinal-tract tumors in the mouse (100).

Table 13.14
Structures, uses, and hazard profiles for dithiocarbamate fungicides

Fungicide	Structure	Principles Uses/Crops	Application Rate gm (a.i.)/ha
Ferbam (39)	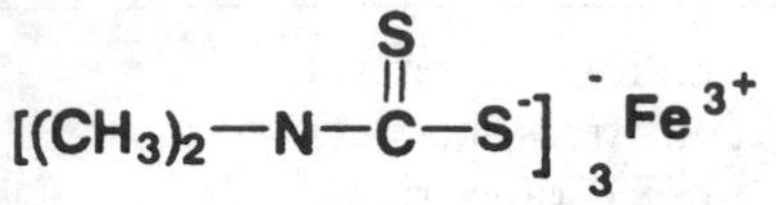	Pome fruit, peaches, and tobacco.	300–500
Thiram Vitavax® (79)	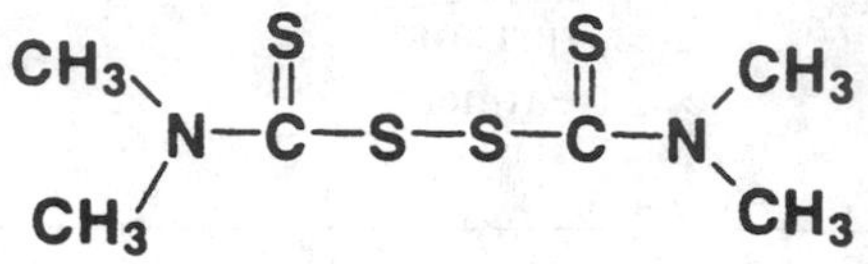	Seed dressing	13–18 gm/100 lbs seed
Ziram (86)	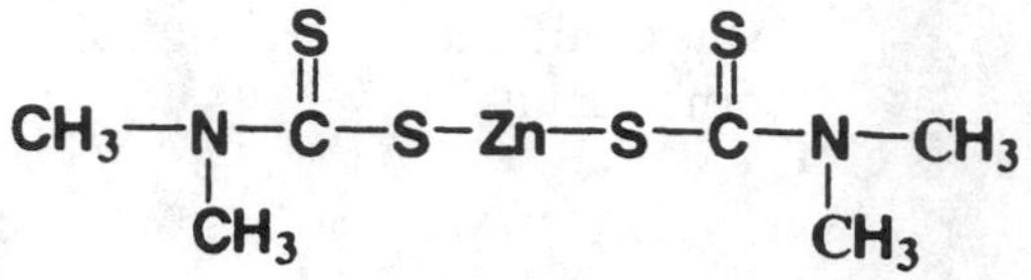	Pome fruit, stone fruit, nuts, vines, vegetables and ornamentals.	1550–2760

Fungicide	Irritation Eye	Irritation Skin	LD_{50} (mg/kg) Oral	LD_{50} (mg/kg) Dermal	LC_{50} (mg/L) Inhalation	Sensitizing Potential	Signal Word
Ferbam (39)	Mild Irritant	Slight Irritant	> 4000	> 4000	0.4	Weak Positive	Warning
Thiram (79)	Slight Irritant	Irritant	> 1800	> 2000	> 0.1	Positive	Warning
Ziram (86)	Severe Irritant	Non-irritant	270	> 2000	0.06	Positive	Danger

Fungicide	Species/study	NOEL[1] (mg/kg/day)	Toxicity Studies	Hazard Indicator
Ferbam (137)	Rat/2-year	12.0	Mutagenicity	No evidence
	Dog/52-week	5.0	Developmental	Not teratogenic
	Mouse/18-month	NA	Reproductive	Effects on sperm in mice
	ADI[2]	0.003 (interim)	Oncogenicity	No evidence
Thiram (121)	Rat/2-year	1.2	Mutagenicity	Positive Ames and SCE
	Dog/2-Year Oral	0.84	Developmental	Teratogenic in mice and hamster at high doses
	Mouse/18-month	3.0	Reproductive	No evidence
	ADI[2]	0.008	Oncogenicity	No evidence
Ziram (138)	Rat/2-year	<2.5	Mutagenicity	Clastogenic
	Dog/52-week	1.6	Developmental	Not teratogenic
	Mouse/18-month	3.0	Reproductive	Effects on sperm in mice
	ADI[2] (1000 × UF)	0.003	Oncogenicity	No evidence

[1] No observable effect level
[2] ADI = acceptable daily intake
[3] See Table 13.3 for US EPA classification scheme
NA = Not Available

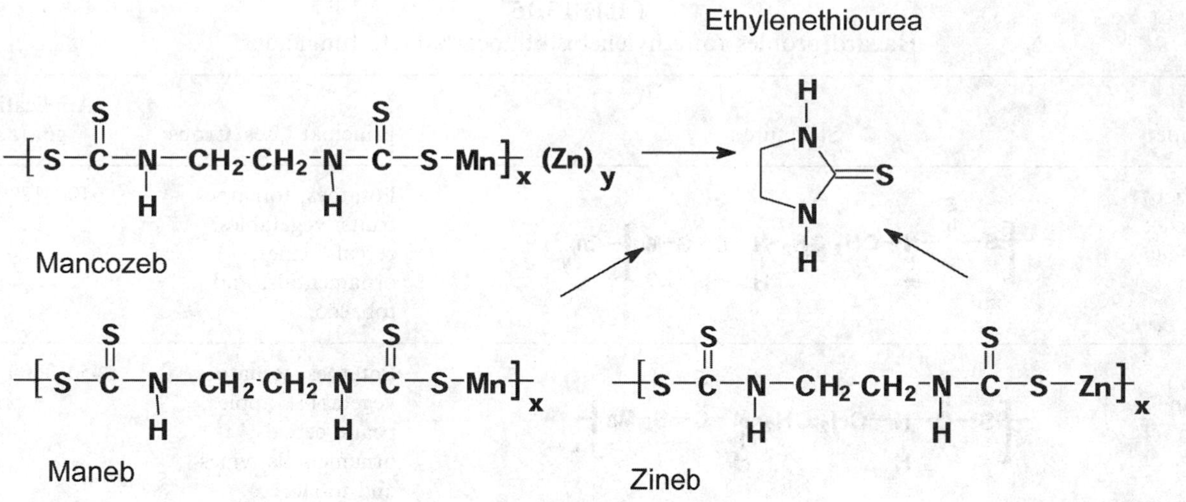

FIG. 13.3. Structures for ethylenedithiocarbamate fungicides.

Substituted Benzenes

The substituted benzene fungicides have a broad spectrum of activity and are considered protective. Chlorothalonil, in this class, controls fungal infection by inhibiting sulfur-containing enzymes (20). The structure, uses, and hazard profile of chlorothalonil are given in Table 13.19.

The U.S. EPA has classified chlorothalonil as B2, probable human carcinogen, based on kidney and forestomach tumors in both rats and mice (100,201).

INSECTICIDES

In 1995, insecticide worldwide sales represented \$3.5 billion and 13.7 million lb of product (1). Discussion of insecticides here emphasizes the major classes of commercial compounds by mode of action. Discussion of insecticide mode of action focuses on their interactions with cell-membrane proteins and the resulting expression of toxicity in the insect (8). No attempt is made to include all the important compounds within a group.

The modes and mechanisms of actions for these major groups of insecticides are included in Table 13.20.

Many of these classes are newly discovered and often originate from nature (8).

Acetylcholine Mimics

Nicotine has been used as an insecticide since the middle of the 18th century (102). Nicotine exhibits contact activity in insects and across phyla including humans (264). Nicotine mimics the action of acetylcholine, which is a major excitatory neurotransmitter in the insect central nervous system (CNS). After the presynaptic cell releases acetylcholine, it binds to the postsynaptic nicotinic acetylcholine receptor and activates an intrinsic cation channel. This results in depolarization of the postsynaptic cell due to an influx of sodium and calcium ions. The synaptic action of acetylcholine is terminated by the enzyme acetylcholinesterase, which rapidly hydrolyzes the ester linkage in acetylcholine. This activity is depicted in Figure 13.4.

A newer compound in this class is the nitroguanidine, imidacloprid. Imidacloprid generally works best as a stomach poison, and has plant systemic activity (50). Nicotine and imidacloprid activate the nicotinic acetylcholine receptors. This persistent activation leads to an overstimulation of cholinergic synapses, and results in hyperexcitation, convulsions, paralysis, and death of the insect (152). The structures, uses, and hazard profiles of these products are presented in Table 13.21.

Imidacloprid is much less toxic to mammals than nicotine (214).

Carbamates

In contrast to the nicothinoids, the carbamate insecticides inhibit acetylcholinesterase (AChE) so that acetylcholine is not destroyed, resulting in continued stimulation of cholinergic receptors. Carbamates behave in biological systems almost identically to the organophosphate insecticides. Carbamate insecticides exist as esters of carbamic acid, typically having an aryl (ring) substituent as the leaving group. The interaction of the carbamate insecticide with acetylcholinestherase (AChE) is depicted in Figure 13.5.

Carbamates react with the serine group on acetylcholinesterase to yield a carbamylation of the serine hydroxyl group. A hydoxylated leaving group is also

Table 13.15
Hazard profiles for ethylenebisdithiocarbamate fungicides

Fungicide	Structure	Principal Uses/Crops	Application Rate gm (a.i.)/ha
Mancozeb Dithane®; Manzate® (52)	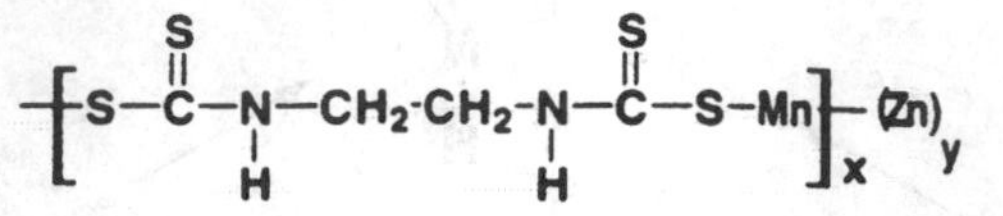	Potatoes, tomatoes, fruits, vegetables, cereals, vines, ornamentals, and tobacco.	6400–12700
Maneb Kypman® (53)	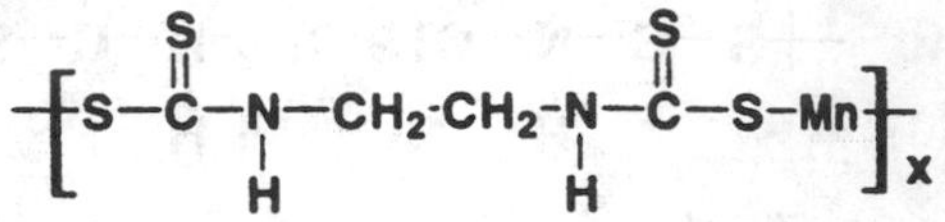	Potatoes, tomatoes, vegetables, apples, pears, cereals, ornamentals, vines and tobacco.	450–3600
Zineb Kypzin® (85)	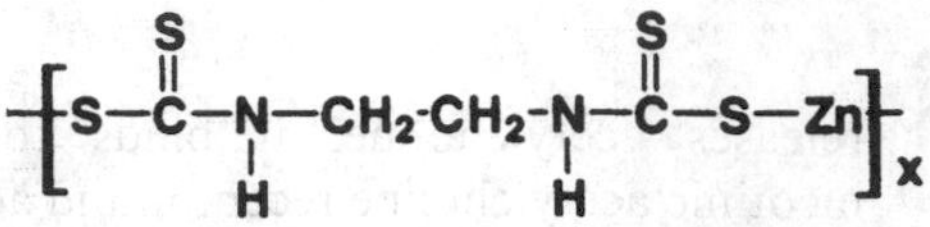	Brassicas, lettuce, onions, oilseed rape, vegetables, berries, apples, pears, stone and citrus fruit, bananas, currants, olives, celery, potatoes, tomatoes, hops, and vines.	NA

Fungicide	Irritation Eye	Irritation Skin	LD_{50} (mg/kg) Oral	LD_{50} (mg/kg) Dermal	LC_{50} (mg/L) Inhalation	Sensitizing Potential	Signal Word
Mancozeb	Severe Irritant	Slight Irritant	> 5000	> 5000	5.14	Positive	Danger
Maneb	Moderate Irritant	Slight Irritant	6750	> 5000	7.38	Positive	Warning
Zineb	Mild Irritant	Slight Irritant	> 5200	> 6000	NA	Negative	Caution

Fungicide	Species/study	NOEL[1] (mg/kg/day)	Toxicity Studies	Hazard Indicator
Mancozeb	Rat/2-year	4.8	Mutagenicity	Equivocal evidence
(216)	Dog/52-week	7.0	Developmental	Teratogenic at high doses
	Mouse/18-month	17	Reproductive	No evidence
	ADI[2]	0.03[4]	Oncogenicity	B2 (Thyroid tumors in rats of both sexes)[3]
Maneb	Rat/2-year	5.0	Mutagenicity	No evidence
(127,216, 217)	Dog/52-week	6.4	Developmental	Not teratogenic
	Mouse/18-month	11	Reproductive	No evidence
	ADI[2]	0.03[4]	Oncogenicity	B2 (Liver tumors in mice of both sexes; thyroid tumors in rats)[3]
Zineb	Rat/2-year	<25	Mutagenicity	No evidence
(129)	Dog/52-week	50	Developmental	Not teratogenic
	Mouse/18-month	No adequate study	Reproductive	No evidence
	ADI[2]	0.03[4]	Oncogenicity	No evidence

[1] No observable effect level
[2] ADI = acceptable daily intake
[3] See Table 13.3 for US EPA classification scheme
[4] Based in a group ADI for mancozeb, alone or in combination with maneb, metiram, and/or zineb, because of similarity in structure to ethylenethiourea (216)
NA = Not Available

Table 13.16
Hazard profile for triphenyltin (Fentin®) acetate and hydroxide (37)

Structure	Principles Uses/Crops	Application Rate gm (a.i.)/ha
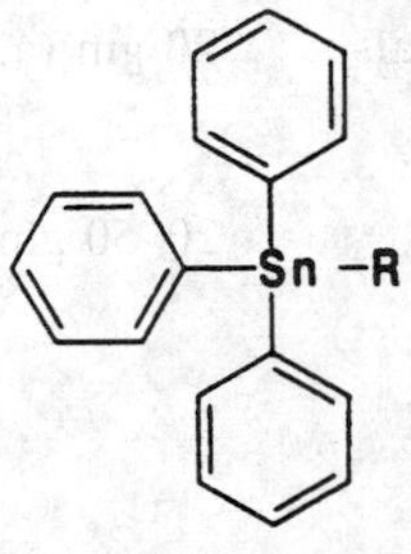 R = acetate or hydroxide	Used on potatoes, celery, onions, sugar beets, peanuts, beans, wheat, coffee and pecans.	160–240

Fungicide	Irritation		LD_{50} (mg/kg)		LC_{50} (mg/L)	Sensitizing Potential	Signal Word
	Eye	Skin	Oral	Dermal	Inhalation		
Triphenyltin Acetate	Severe Irritant	Non-irritant	140	450	0.044	Positive	Danger
Triphenyltin Hydroxide	Severe Irritant	Slight Irritant	110	1600	0.060	Negative	Danger

Fungicide	Species/study	NOEL[1] (mg/kg/day)	Toxicity Studies	Hazard Indicator
Triphenyltin Hydroxide[3] (37)	Rat/2-year	< 0.3	Mutagenicity	No evidence
	Dog/52-week	0.2	Developmental	Not teratogenic
	Mouse/18-month	1.4 ♀	Reproductive	No evidence
	ADI[2]	0.0005	Oncogenicity	B2 (mouse liver and pituitary and testicular tumors in rats)[4]

[1] No observable effect level
[2] ADI = acceptable daily intake
[3] Repeat dose studies conducted with triphenyltin hydroxide and not the acetate form.
[4] See Table 13.3 for US EPA classification scheme (100)

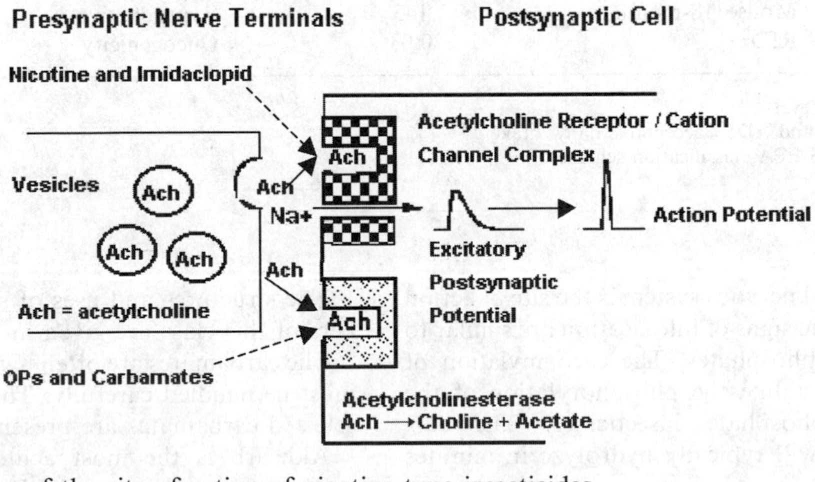

FIG. 13.4. Representation of the site of action of nicotine-type insecticides.

Table 13.17
Structures, uses, and hazard profiles for phenylpyrrole fungicides

Fungicide	Structure	Principle Uses/Crops	Application Rate Gm (a.i.)/ha
Fenpiclonil Beret®, Gambit® (35)	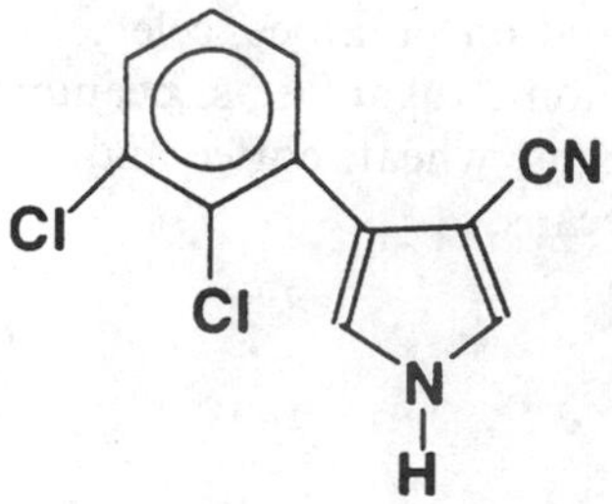	Seed treatment on cereals and peas	20 gm (a.i.)/100 kg
		Potato seed dressing	20–50 gm (a.i.)/ton
Fludioxonil Maxim® (42)	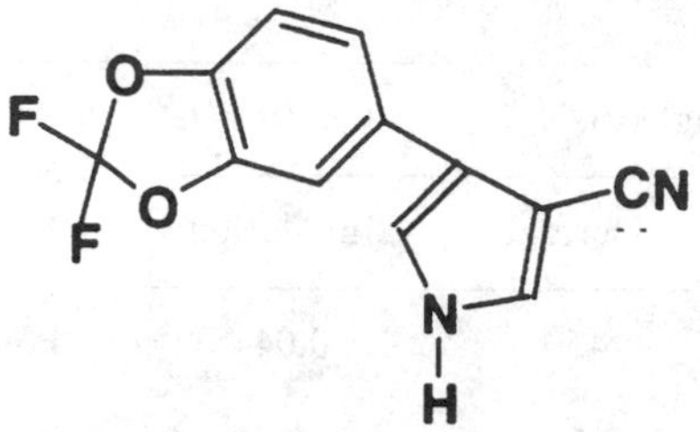	Used for seed treatment on rice, and on grapes, stone fruit, vegetables, field crops, turf and ornamentals	2.5 gm (a.i.)/100 kg

Fungicide	Irritation Eye	Irritation Skin	LD_{50} (mg/kg) Oral	LD_{50} (mg/kg) Dermal	LC_{50} (mg/L) Inhalation	Sensitizing Potential	Signal Word
Fenpiclonil (35)	Non-irritant	Non-irritant	> 5000	> 2000	> 1.5	Negative	Caution
Fludioxonil (42)	Slight Irritant	Non-irritant	> 5000	> 2000	> 2.6	Negative	Caution

Fungicide	Species/study	NOEL[1] (mg/kg/day)	Toxicity Studies	Hazard Indicator
Fenpiclonil (35)	Rat/2-year	1.25	Mutagenicity	No evidence
	Dog/52-week	100	Developmental	Not teratogenic
	Mouse/18-month	20	Reproductive	No evidence
	ADI[2]	0.013	Oncogenicity	No evidence
Fludioxonil (210,257)	Rat/2-year	50	Mutagenicity	Clastogenic (in vitro)
	Dog/52-week	3.3	Developmental	Not teratogenic
	Mouse/18-month	143	Reproductive	No evidence
	RfD[2]	0.03	Oncogenicity	D with RfD[3]

[1] No observable effect level
[2] RfD = reference dose and ADI = acceptable daily intake
[3] See Table 13.3 for US EPA classification scheme

generated. The central nervous system is the site of action of carbamates, and the signs of intoxication are similar to those of the organophosphates. The carbamylation of AChE is reversible, unlike the phosphorylation of the AChE by organophosphate insecticides. The carbamylated complex will typically hydrolyze in minutes (8).

The structures and uses of some representative members of this class are given in Table 13.22.

The carbamates are often highly toxic to mammals and must be handled carefully. The hazard profiles of these selected carbamates are presented in Table 13.23.

Aldicarb is the most acutely toxic of the selected carbamates, with an oral LD_{50} below 1 mg/kg as well

Table 13.18
Hazard profile for captan (16,133)

Structure	Principle Uses/Crops	Application Rate gm (a.i.)/ha
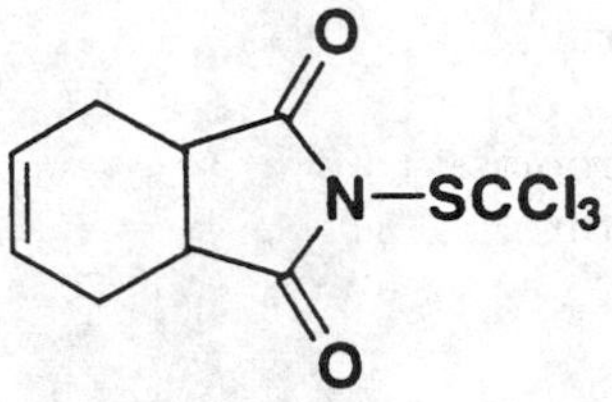	Used on stone fruit, citrus, almonds, vegetables, potatoes, tomatoes, oilseed rape, berries, and ornamentals	340–5050

Irritation		LD_{50} (mg/kg)		LC_{50} (mg/L)		
Eye	Skin	Oral	Dermal	Inhalation	Sensitizing Potential	Signal Word
Corrosive	Mild Irritant	9000	> 4500	5.8	Positive	Danger

Species/study	NOEL[1] (mg/kg/day)	Toxicity Studies	Hazard Indicator
Rat/2-year	25	Mutagenicity	Positive in vitro
Dog/66-Week Oral	60	Developmental	Positive in monkey and hamster
Mouse/18-month	NA	Reproductive	No evidence
RfD[2](based on rat reproduction)	0.13	Oncogenicity	B2 (G.I. tract tumors—mouse; kidney—rat)[3]

[1] No observable effect level
[2] ADI = acceptable daily intake
[3] See Table 13.3 for US EPA classification scheme
NA = Not Available

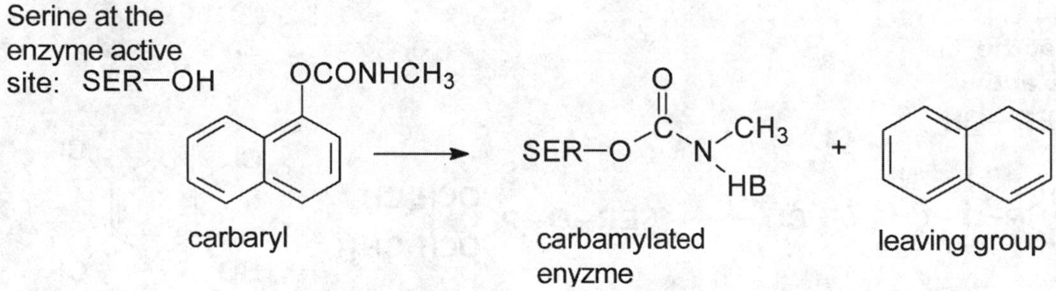

FIG. 13.5. Representation of the interaction of carbamate insecticides with acetylcholinesterase.

as a dermal LD_{50} of 20 mg/kg. Aldicarb, carbofuran, methomyl, and propoxur have been classified as category C (possible human carcinogens) or D(aldicarb) by the U.S. EPA (100). These four materials elicited liver tumors in mice in the 18-month studies.

Organophosphorus Insecticides

Organophosphorus insecticides (OPs) vary tremendously in chemical structure and chemical properties (8). These chemicals are classified into groups depending on the positioning of the central phosphorus—hence their classification as phosphates, phosphonates, phosphorothionates, phosphorodithioates, and phosphoroamidothioates. Selected examples representing these different groups are presented in Table 13.24.

The OPs react with acetylcholinesterase at the serine hydroxyl group within the enzyme active site. In this reaction, this hydroxyl group is phosphorylated, yielding a leaving group (Figure 13.6).

Table 13.19
Hazard profile for chlorothalonil (Bravo®) (20,120,201)

Structure	Principle Uses/Crops	Application Rate gm (a.i.)/ha
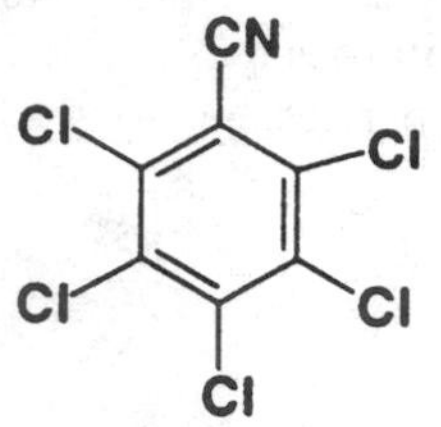	Used on pome fruit, stone fruit, citrus, cane fruit, vegetables, corn, ornamentals, mushrooms, tobacco, soya and turf.	1050–2190

Irritation		LD_{50} (mg/kg)		LC_{50} (mg/L)		
Eye	Skin	Oral	Dermal	Inhalation	Sensitizing Potential	Signal Word
Severe Irritant	Mild Irritant	> 10000	> 10000	0.093 ♀	Negative	Danger

Species/study	NOEL[1] (mg/kg/day)	Toxicity Studies	Hazard Indicator
Rat/2-year	2.0	Mutagenicity	No evidence
Dog/52-Week	150	Developmental	Not teratogenic
Mouse/18-month	5.35	Reproductive	No evidence
ADI[2]	0.03 (JMPR)	Oncogenicity	B2 with CSF of 0.0076 $(mg/kg/day)^{-1}$ (Forestomach tumors in mice and kidney tumors in rats)[3]
RfD (Non-cancer)	0.02		
RfD (Cancer)	0.015		

[1] No observable effect level
[2] RfD = reference dose and ADI = acceptable daily intake
[3] See Table 13.3 for US EPA classification scheme; CSF = cancer slope factor

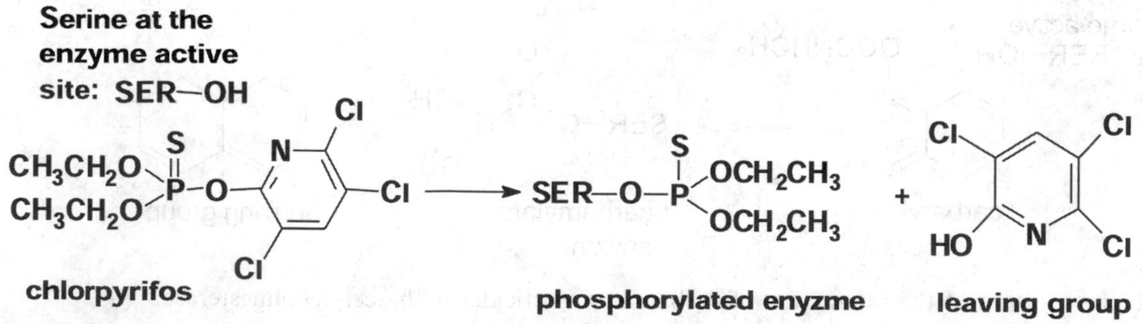

FIG. 13.6. Representation of the interaction of organophosphate insecticides with acetylcholinesterase.

The phosphorylated acetylcholinesterase is inactivated, blocking acetacholine degradation in the synapse. This results in a buildup of this neurotransmitter and central nervous system hyperstimulation. The signs of intoxication include restlessness, hyperexcitability, tremors, convulsions, and paralysis. Reactivation of the enzyme can take many hours or even days. The toxicologic profiles for selected OPs are presented in Table 13.25.

GABA Agonists (Avermectins)

The avermectins are a group of closely related macrocyclic lactones isolated from the fungus *Streptomyces avermitilis* (Turner and Schaeffer, 1989). The structures of abamectin and emamectin-benzoate, the commercially available insecticides in this class, are shown in Figure 13.7. In addition to the avermectins,

Table 13.20
Mode and mechanism of action for important classes of insecticides used in crop protection

Class	Mode of Action	Mechanism of Action
Acetylcholine Mimics (50,59)	Systemic acting as a contact and stomach poison	Bind to acetylcholine receptor
Cholinesterase Inhibitors (10,11)	Systemic acting as a contact and stomach poison	React with a serine hydroxyl group within the enzyme active site and inactivates the enzyme blocking the degradation of the neurotransmitter acetylcholine.
GABA (γ-amino-butyric acid) Agonists (9)	Systemic acting as contact and stomach poison	Act by stimulating the release of GABA, an inhibitory neurotransmitter, by increasing chloride ion flux at the neuromuscular junction.
GABA Antagonists [Channel Blockers] (33)	Non-systemic acting as contact, stomach, and respiratory poison	Act antagonistically at the GABA receptor-chloride channel complex
Compounds Affecting Voltage-Dependent Sodium Channels (36)	Non-systemic acting as contact and stomach poison	Prolong the current flowing through sodium channels by slowing or preventing the shutting of the channels
Juvenile Hormone Mimics (32)	Insect growth regulator preventing metamorphosis to viable adults	Mimic the action of the juvenile hormones and disrupts molting and reproduction
Molt Inhibitors (76)	Systemic acting to inhibit molting and feeding	Inhibit chitin synthesis
Ecdysone Agonists (249)	Lethally accelerates the molting process	Act by binding to the receptor site for ecdysone
Larvicides (28)	Insect growth regulator with contact action	Inhibit embryo development interfering with molting and pupation
Pheromones (147)	Modifies the behavior of other individuals of the same species	Volatile chemicals, natural or synthetic, act for signaling and homing
Respiratory Inhibitors and Uncouplers (19)	Non-systemic acting against all stages of insect development	Inhibit mitochondrial electron transport

spinosad is derived from the fungus *Saccharopolyspora spinasa* (Figure 13.7).

The mode on action of these three products in insects is paralysis. The avermectins stimulate the release of the inhibitory neurotransmitter gamma-aminobutyric acid (GABA) at the neuromuscular junction (88,167). The agonistic release of GABA evokes an electrical activity in vertebrate and invertebrate nerve and muscle by increasing the membrane conductance to chloride ions. The ionic concentration within the neuron increases continuously until a trigger level is reached and the action potential is produced. This activity is depicted in Figure 13.8.

Table 13.21
The hazard profile for the acetylcholine mimic insecticides

Fungicide	Structure	Principle Uses	Application Rate gm (a.i.)/ha
Imidacloprid Admire® Provado® (50)	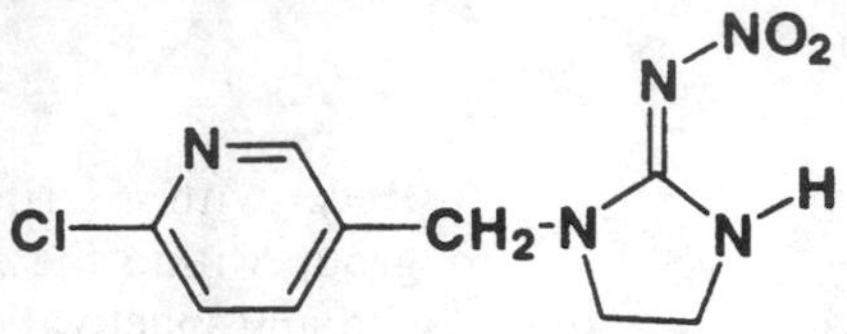	Used to control sucking insects including asphids, thrips, and whiteflies.	290
Nicotine Nico® Soap (59)	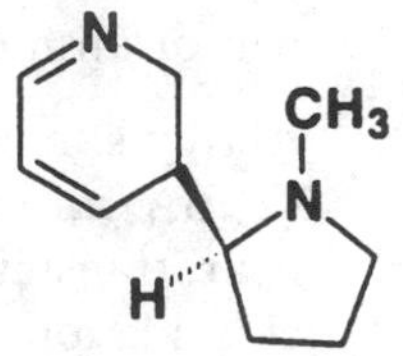	Used to control sucking insects including ricehoppers, asphids, thrips, and whiteflies	Limited Use

	Irritation		LD_{50} (mg/kg)		LC_{50} (mg/L)		
Insecticide	Eye	Skin	Oral	Dermal	Inhalation	Sensitizing Potential	Signal Word
Imidacloprid (50)	Non-irritant	Non-irritant	424	>5000	0.07	Negative	Warning
Nicotine (59)	Irritant	Mild Irritant	50	50	NA	Negative	Danger

Insecticide	Species/study	NOEL[1] (mg/kg/day)	Toxicity Studies	Hazard Indicator
Imidacloprid (214)	Rat/2-year	5.7	Mutagenicity	No evidence
	Dog/2-Year Oral	41	Developmental	Not teratogenic
	Mouse/18-month	208	Reproductive	No evidence
	RfD[2]	0.057	Oncogenicity	E (No evidence)[3]
Nicotine (59)	Rat/2-year	NA	Mutagenicity	No evidence
	Dog/52-week	NA	Developmental	Not teratogenic
	Mouse/18-month	NA	Reproductive	NA
	RfD[2]	NA	Oncogenicity	NA

[1] No observable effect level
[2] RfD = reference dose and ADI = acceptable daily intake
[3] See Table 13.3 for US EPA classification scheme
NA = Not Available

Avermectin intoxication in mammals begins with hyperexcitability, tremors, and incoordination, and later develops into ataxia and coma-like sedation (141). The toxicity profiles of abamectin, emamectin-benzoate, and spinosad are given in Table 13.26.

Both abamectin and emamectin benzoate have the propensity to produce neurotoxicity. This toxicity is reduced or prevented in test animals having a fully intact P-glycoprotein blood–brain barrier. Much of the early testing of the hazards of these avermectins was performed in the CF-1 mouse. The CF-1 mouse has been found to be heterozygous for P-glycoprotein and has been ruled out as an experimental model for human risk assessment (122,142,143,251).

Channel Blockers

Organochlorines

The channel-blocking convulsants represent one of the oldest groups of synthetic organic insecticides, dating back to the early 1940s (148). These lipophilic compounds were found to be environmentally stable and persistent, and many, like dieldrin, endrin, and DDT, have been

Table 13.22
Structures and uses of selected carbamate insecticides

Insecticide	Structure	Principle Uses/Crops	Treatment Rate gm (a.i.)/ha
Aldicarb Temik® (11)	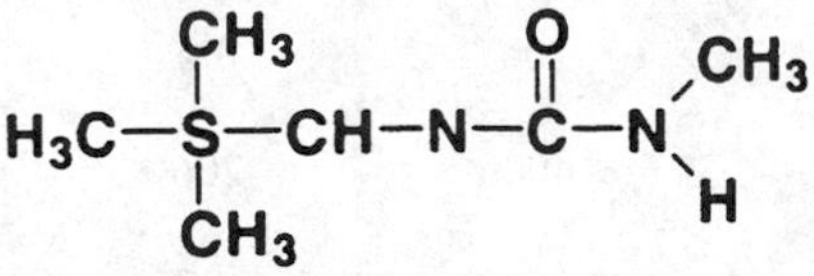	Controls chewing and sucking insects in vegetables and crops.	350–5600
Carbaryl Sevin® (17)	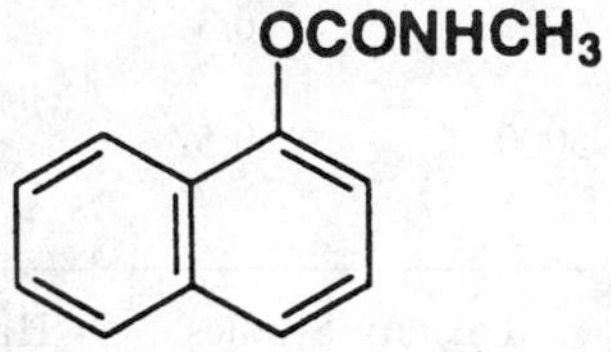	Controls chewing and sucking insects in vegetables and various crops	250–2000
Carbofuran Furadan® (18)	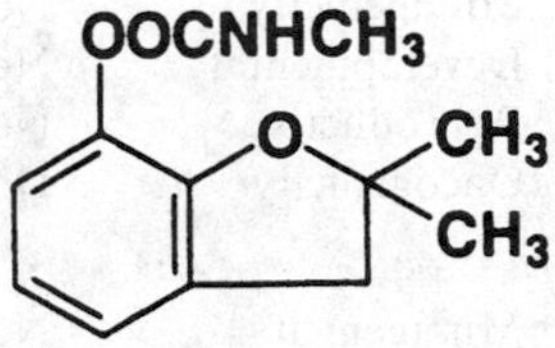	Controls soil dwelling and foliar feeding insects in food crops	260–2050
Methomyl LanoxC® (56)	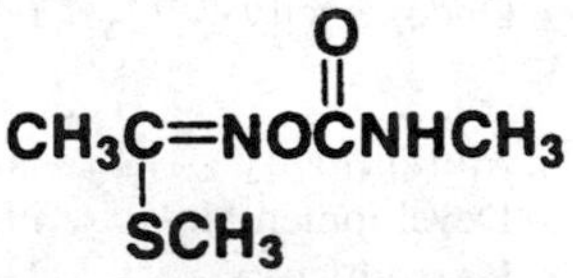	Controls chewing and sucking insects in vegetables, food crops and turf.	120–2000
Propoxur Aprocarb® (65)	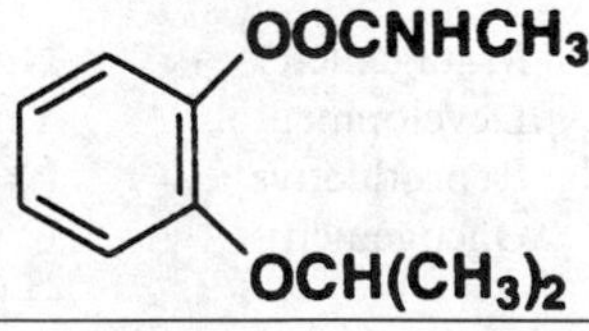	Controls cockroaches, flies, fleas, ants, and mosquitoes.	NA

banned in the United States. However, some of the more biodegradable materials like lindane and endosulfan still find use today. Fipronil is an aryl heterocycle with a similar mode of action, but improved selective toxicity toward insects.

In both insects and mammals, chloride channel-blocking insecticides cause hyperexcitability and convulsions (7). These effects occur via poisoning of the CNS through antagonism of the inhibitory neurotransmitter γ-aminobutyric acid (GABA). Normally, when GABA is released from the presynaptic nerve terminal, it binds to a postsynaptic receptor protein containing an intrinsic chloride ion channel. When GABA binds to the receptor, the channel is opened, and Cl ions flow into the postsynaptic neuron (see Figure 13.8). This chloride permeability can significantly hyperpolarize the membrane potential and has a dampening effect on nerve impulse firing. The structures, uses, and toxicology profiles for selected channel blockers are given in Table 13.27.

The organochlorine channel-blocking insecticides are generally not mutagenic, developmental, or reproductive toxins or oncogenic.

Pyrethroids

The pyrethroid insecticides, typically esters of chrysanthemic acid, were isolated from the flowers of

Table 13.23
Hazard profile for the carbamate insecticides

Insecticide	Irritation: Eye	Irritation: Skin	LD_{50} (mg/kg): Oral	LD_{50} (mg/kg): Dermal	LC_{50} (mg/L): Inhalation	Sensitizing Potential	Signal Word
Aldicarb (11)	Non-irritant	Non-irritant	0.93	20	0.2	Negative	Danger
Carbaryl (20)	Non-irritant	Non-irritant	500 ♀	> 4000	206	Negative	Caution
Carbofuran (18)	Mild irritant	Mild irritant	8	> 3000	0.075	Negative	Danger
Methomyl (56)	Irritant	Non-irritant	17	> 5000	0.3	NA	Danger
Propoxur (65)	Slight Irritant	Non-irritant	50	> 5000	0.5	Negative	Warning

Insecticide	Species/study	NOEL[1] (mg/kg/day)	Toxicity Studies	Hazard Indicator
Aldicarb (131,172)	Rat/2-year	0.3	Mutagenicity	No evidence
	Dog/104-week	0.1	Developmental	Not teratogenic
	Mouse/18-month	0.3	Reproductive	No evidence
	ADI[2]	0.003	Oncogenicity	D[3]
	RfD[2]	0.001		
Carbaryl (107)	Rat/2-year	200	Mutagenicity	No evidence
	Dog/52-week	1.43	Developmental	Not Teratogenic
	Mouse/18-month	NA	Reproductive	No evidence
	Human	0.01	Oncogenicity	E (No evidence)[3]
	RfD[2]	0.01		
Carbofuran (108)	Rat/2-year	20	Mutagenicity	No evidence
	Dog/2-Year Oral	10	Developmental	Not teratogenic
	Mouse/18-month	20	Reproductive	No evidence
	RfD[2]	0.002	Oncogenicity	C with RfD (Mouse liver tumors in both sexes)[3]
Methomyl (116)	Rat/2-year	200	Mutagenicity	No evidence
	Dog/52-week	200	Developmental	Teratogenic in mice
	Mouse/18-month	500	Reproductive	No evidence
	ADI[2]	0.02	Oncogenicity	C with RfD (liver tumors —female mice)[3]
Propoxur (117)	Rat/2-year	5.0	Mutagenicity	No evidence
	Dog/52-week	1.25	Developmental	Not teratogenic
	Mouse/18-month	40	Reproductive	No evidence
	ADI[2]	0.01	Oncogenicity	C with RfD[3]

[1] No observable effect level
[2] RfD = reference dose and ADI = acceptable daily intake
[3] See Table 13.3 for US EPA classification scheme
NA = Not Available

chrysanthemums (160). Synthetic pyrethroid chemistry and action are classified as Type 1 or Type 2, depending on the alcohol substituent (6). The members of the Type 1 group are generally unstable in the environment, which has prevented their use in row crops. The Type 2 pyrethroids are more narrowly defined in terms of their chemical structure. They specifically contain an α-cyano-3-phenoxybenzyl alcohol, which increases insecticidal activity about 10-fold.

The signs of intoxication by pyrethroids develop rapidly, and there exist different poisoning syndromes for the two types of compounds (6). Type 1 pyrethroids

Table 13.24
Structures and uses of selected organophosphate insecticides

Insecticide	Structure	Principle Uses/Crops	Treatment Rate gm (a.i.)/ha
Monocrotophos Monocron® (57)	phosphate 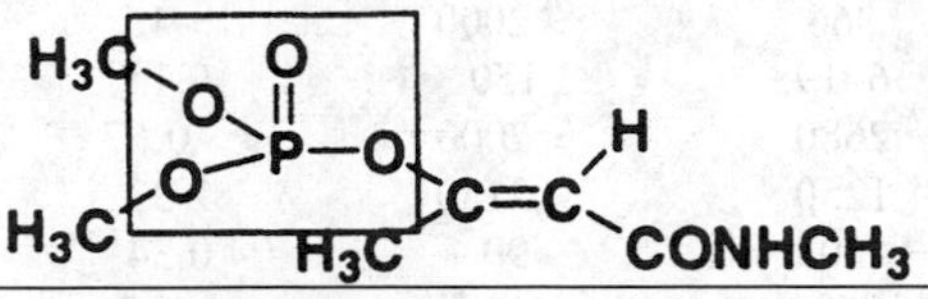	Control of sucking, chewing, and boring insects and spider mites.	NA
Dichlorvos Vapona® (30)	phosphonate 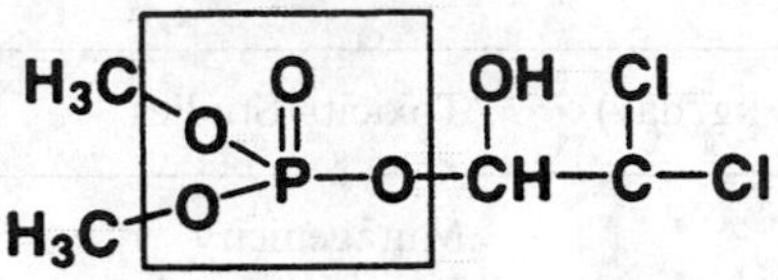	Control of sucking, and chewing insects and spider mites in household sprays, etc.	100
Acephate Amithene® (10)	phosphoramidothiate 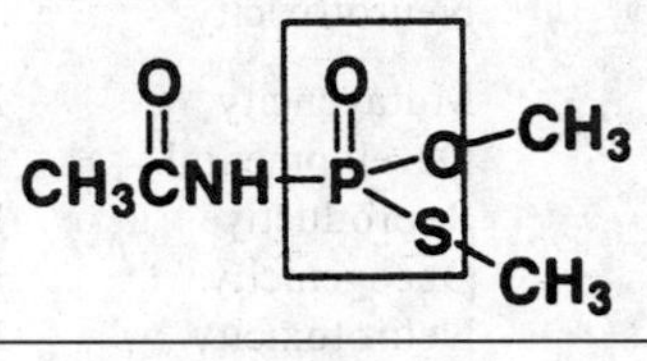	Control sucking, and chewing insects.	500
Diazinon Spectracide® (29,123)	phosphorothionate 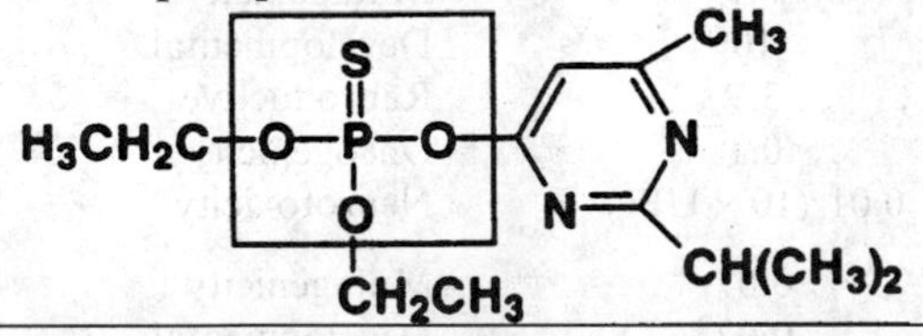	Control of sucking, and chewing insects and mites.	400–800
Chlorpyrifos Lorsban® (21)	phosphorothionate 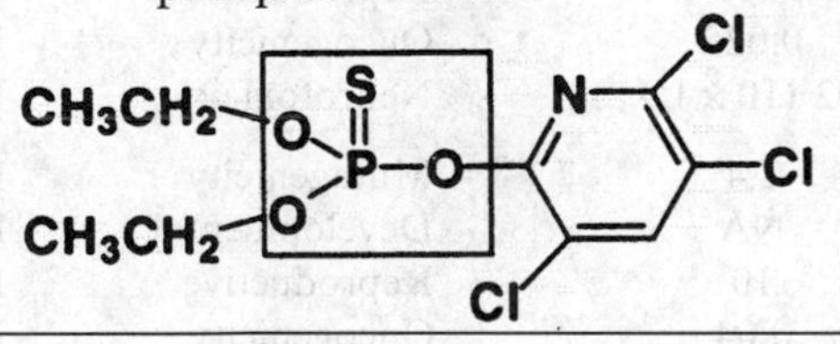	Control of sucking, chewing, and boring insects	470–950
Azinphos-methyl Guthion® (118)	phosphorodithionate 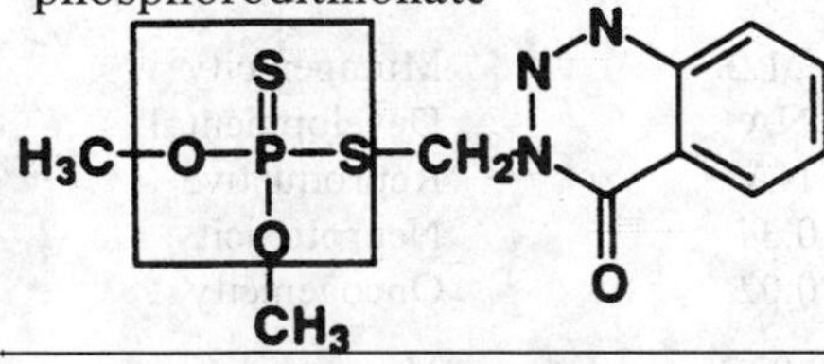	Control of sucking, and chewing insects.	NA
Malathion Acimal® (320)	phosphorodithionate 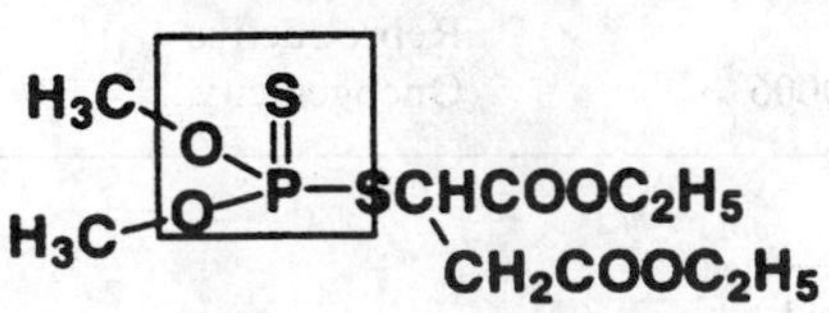	Control of sucking, and chewing insects.	570

Table 13.25
Hazard profiles for selected organophosphate insecticides

Insecticide	Irritation: Eye	Irritation: Skin	LD$_{50}$ (mg/kg): Oral	LD$_{50}$ (mg/kg): Dermal	LC$_{50}$ (mg/L): Inhalation	Sensitizing Potential	Signal Word
Acephate	NA	Non-irritant	866	> 2000	> 15	Negative	Caution
Azinphos-methyl	Mild irritant	Non-irritant	6–19	150	0.15	Positive	Danger
Chlorpyrifos	Non-irritant	Non-irritant	2680	> 2000	> 0.67	Negative	Caution
Diazinon	Non-irritant	Non-irritant	1250	> 2150	2.33	Negative	Caution
Dichlorvos	Irritant	Irritant	50	90	0.34	Negative	Danger
Malathion	NA	NA	1000 ♀	4100	> 5.2	NA	Caution
Monocrotophos	Non-irritant	Non-irritant	18	130	0.08	NA	Danger

Insecticide	Species/study	NOEL[1] (mg/kg/day)	Toxicity Studies	Hazard Indicator
Acephate (113)	Rat/2-year	0.5	Mutagenicity	No evidence
	Dog/26-Week Oral	0.75	Developmental	Not teratogenic
	Mouse/18-month	NA	Reproductive	No evidence
	Human	0.3	Oncogenicity	C (Mouse liver tumor)[4]
	ADI[2]	0.03 (10 × UF[3])	Neurotoxicity	Not delayed neurotoxin
Azinphos-methyl (118)	Rat/2-year	0.86	Mutagencity	Effects in vitro; no in vivo
	Dog/52-Week Oral	0.74	Developmental	No evidence
	Mouse/18-month	0.88	Reproductive	Effects on fertility
	Human	0.005	Oncogenicity	E (No evidence)[4]
	ADI[2]	0.005	Neurotoxicity	Not delayed neurotoxin
Chlorpyrifos (109)	Rat/2-year	0.1	Mutagenicity	No evidence
	Dog/13-Week Oral	10	Developmental	Not Teratogenic
	Mouse/18-month	3.9	Reproductive	No evidence
	Human	0.1	Oncogenicity	No evidence
	ADI[2]	0.01 (10 × UF[3])	Neurotoxicity	Not delayed neurotoxin
Diazinon (123)	Rat/2-year	0.07	Mutagenicity	No evidence
	Dog/2-Year Oral	0.02	Developmental	Not teratogenic
	Mouse/18-month	NA	Reproductive	No evidence
	Human	0.025	Oncogenicity	No evidence
	ADI[2]	0.002 (10 × UF[3])	Neurotoxicity	Not delayed neurotoxin
Dichlorvos (124)	Rat/2-year	2.4	Mutagenicity	May be mutagenic
	Dog/52-week	NA	Developmental	Not Teratogenic
	Mouse/18-month	10	Reproductive	No evidence
	Human/21-day	0.04	Oncogenicity	No evidence
	ADI[2]	0.004 (10 × UF[3])	Neurotoxicity	Delayed neuropathy
Malathion (320)	Rat/2-year	< 1.2	Mutagenicity	No evidence
	Dog/52-week	NA	Developmental	Not teratogenic
	Mouse/18-month	NA	Reproductive	Effects on litter size
	Human/56-day	0.34	Neurotoxicity	Not delayed neurotoxin
	ADI[2]	0.02	Oncogenicity	No evidence
Monocrotophos (130)	Rat/2-year	0.025	Mutagenicity	No evidence
	Dog/52-week	0.0125	Developmental	Not teratogenic
	Mouse/18-month	–	Reproductive	No evidence
	ADI[2]	0.0006	Oncogenicity	No evidence

[1] No observable effect level
[2] ADI = acceptable daily intake
[3] Uncertainty factor of 10 used based on human cholinesterase used
[4] See Table 13.3 for US EPA classification scheme
NA = Not Available

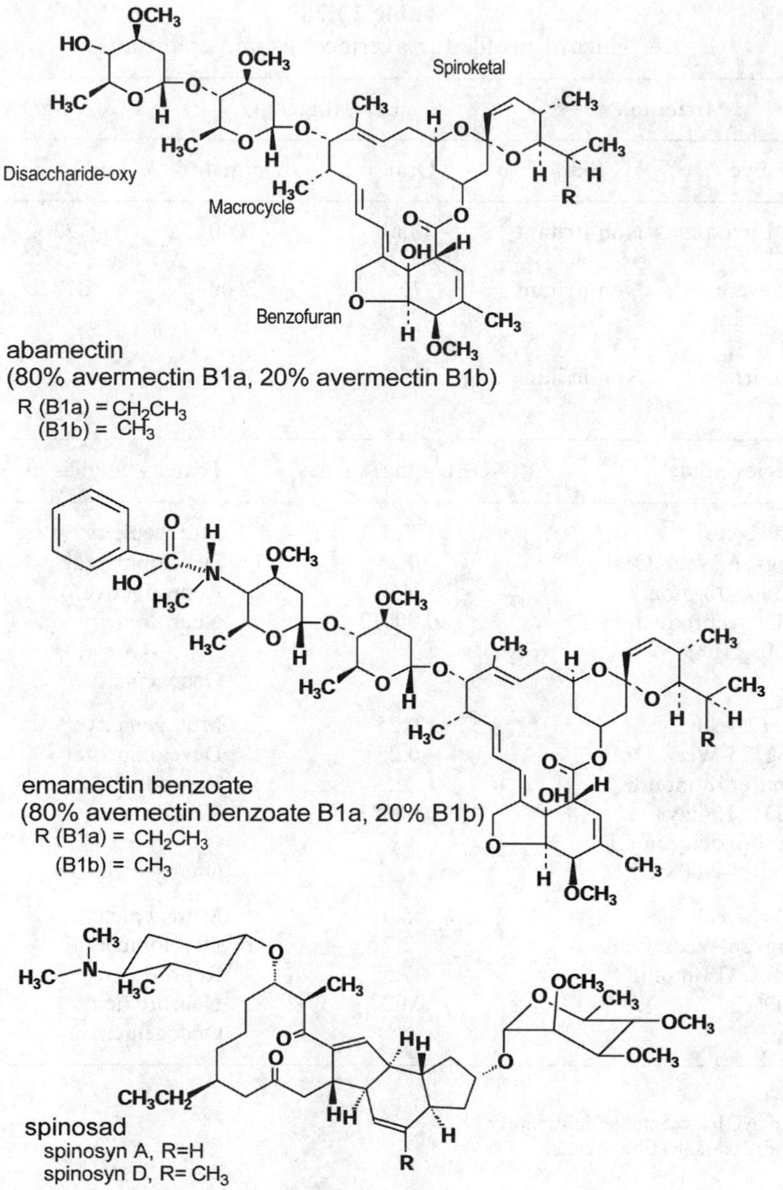

FIG. 13.7. The structures of avermectins and spinosad.

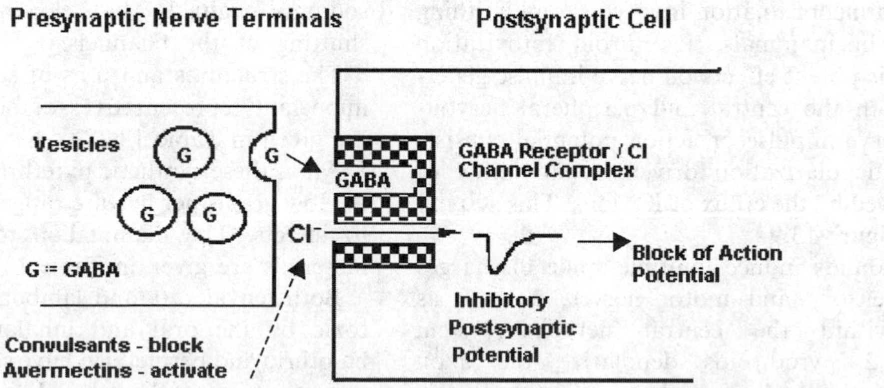

FIG. 13.8. Representation of the action of the avermectins at the presynaptic inhibitory terminal.

Table 13.26
Hazard profile for avermectins and spinosad

Insecticide	Irritation: Eye	Irritation: Skin	LD_{50} (mg/kg): Oral	LD_{50} (mg/kg): Dermal	LC_{50} (mg/L): Inhalation	Sensitizing Potential	Signal Word
Abamectin (9)	Mild irritant	Non-irritant	13.6	> 2000	5.73	Negative	Danger
Emamectin benzoate (256)	Severe Irritant	Non-irritant	76	> 2000	2.12	Negative	Danger
Spinosad (84,193)	Non-irritant	Non-irritant	3738	> 5000	> 5.18	Negative	Caution

Insecticide	Species/study	NOEL[1] (mg/kg/day)	Toxicity Studies	Hazard Indicator
Abamectin (122,136,251)	Rat/2-year	1.5	Mutagenicity	No evidence
	Dog/26-Week Oral	0.25	Developmental	Not teratogenic
	Mouse/18-month	4.0	Reproductive	No evidence
	RfD[2] (reproduction—1000×UF[4])	0.00012	Neurotoxicity	Neurotoxicity exhibited in rodents, and dogs
			Oncogenicity	E (No evidence)[3]
Emamectin Benzoate (256)	Rat/2-year	0.25	Mutagenicity	No evidence
	Dog/25-Week Oral	0.25	Developmental	Not teratogenic
	Mouse/18-month	2.5	Reproductive	No evidence
	RfD[2] (15-day neurotoxicity in CF-1 Mouse—900×UF[4])	0.00083	Neurotoxicity	Neurotoxicity exhibited in rodents, and dogs
			Oncogenicity	E (No evidence)[3]
Spinosad (193)	Rat/2-year	5.0	Mutagenicity	No evidence
	Dog/26-Week Oral	2.7	Developmental	Not teratogenic
	Mouse/18-month	7.5	Reproductive	No evidence
	RfD[2]	0.027	Neurotoxicity	Not Neurotoxic
			Oncogenicity	E (No evidence)[3]

[1] No observable effect level
[2] RfD = reference dose and ADI=acceptable daily intake
[3] See Table 13.3 for US EPA classification scheme
[4] Uncertainty factor

cause hyperexcitability and convulsions in insects and a whole-body tremor in mammals. Type 2 pyrethroids cause ataxia and incoordination in insects, and writhing and salivation in mammals. Pyrethroid intoxication results from their potent effects on nerve impulse generation within both the central and peripheral nervous systems. The nerve impulse or action potential consists of a transient depolarization driven by an influx of Na^+ ions, followed by the efflux of K^+ ions. This activity is depicted in Figure 13.9.

Type 1 compounds induce multiple spike discharges in peripheral sensory and motor nerves, as well as interneurons within the central nervous system (CNS). Type 2 pyrethroids depolarize the axon membrane potential, which reduces the amplitude of the action potential and eventually leads to a loss of electrical excitability. These effects occur because pyrethroids prolong the current flowing through sodium channels by slowing or preventing the shutting of the channels.

The structures and uses of some of the economically important representatives of both types of pyrethroids are given in Table 13.28.

All of these synthetic pyrethroids are generally used in the low grams per hectare range because of their toxicity to insects. The mammalian toxicity profiles of these materials are given in Table 13.29.

Both fenvalerate and lambda-cyhalothrin are acutely toxic by the oral and inhalation route. Lambda-cyhalothrin and permethrin have some potential to produce neurotoxicity, and both exhibit some weak oncogenic potential in animal models.

Table 13.27
Hazard profiles for the organochlorine chloride channel blockers

Insecticide	Structure	Principle Uses	Application Rates gm (a.i./ha)
Endosulfan (33)	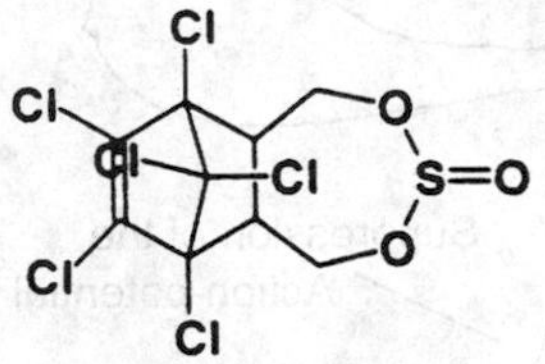	Used to control sucking, chewing and boring insects in a variety of crops including fruit, vines, vegetables, cotton and cereal	1120
Fipronil (40)	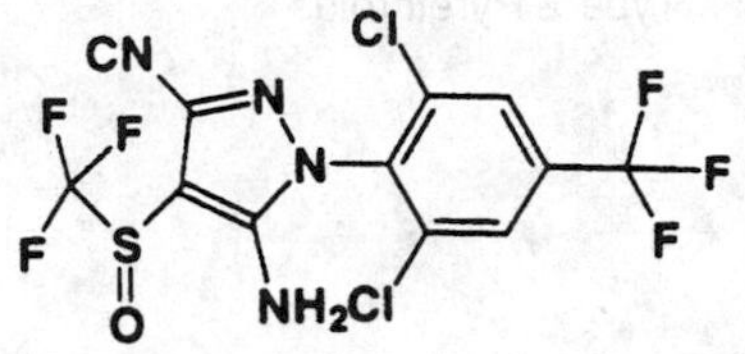	Used to control thrips, corn root worms, and termites	100–200
Gamma-HCH (44)	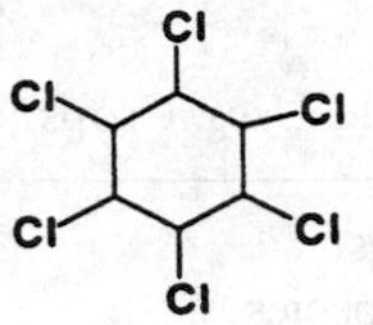	Used to control soil-inhabiting insects, public-health pests, and animal ectoparasites	250–750

Insecticide	Irritation		LD_{50} (mg/kg)		LC_{50} (mg/L)	Sensitizing Potential	Signal Word
	Eye	Skin	Oral	Dermal	Inhalation		
Endosulfan	Non-irritant	Non-irritant	70	359	> 0.034	Negative	Danger
Fipronil	Non-irritant	Non-irritant	97	> 2000	0.68	Negative	Warning
Gamma-HCH	Irritant	Irritant	> 88	> 900	1.6	Negative	Warning

Insecticide	Species/study	NOEL[1] (mg/kg/day)	Toxicity Studies	Hazard Indicator
Endosulfan (114)	Rat/2-year	0.60	Mutagenicity	No evidence
	Dog/52-week	0.57	Developmental	Not teratogenic
	Mouse/18-month	0.84	Reproductive	No evidence
	ADI[2]	0.006	Oncogenicity	No evidence[3]
Fipronil (209)	Rat/2-year	0.20	Mutagenicity	No evidence
	Dog/52-week	0.30	Developmental	Not teratogenic
	Mouse/18-month	0.50	Reproductive	No evidence
	RfD[2]	0.0002	Oncogenicity	No evidence[3]
			Neurotoxicity	Not neurotoxic
Lindane (Gamma-HCH) (115)	Rat/2-year	0.75	Mutagenicity	No evidence
	Dog/52-week	1.6	Developmental	Not teratogenic
	Mouse/18-month	NA	Reproductive	No evidence
	ADI[2]	0.008	Neurotoxicity	Not neurotoxic
			Oncogenicity	No evidence[3]

[1] No observable effect level
[2] RfD = reference dose and ADI = acceptable daily intake
[3] See Table 13.3 for US EPA classification scheme
NA = Not Available

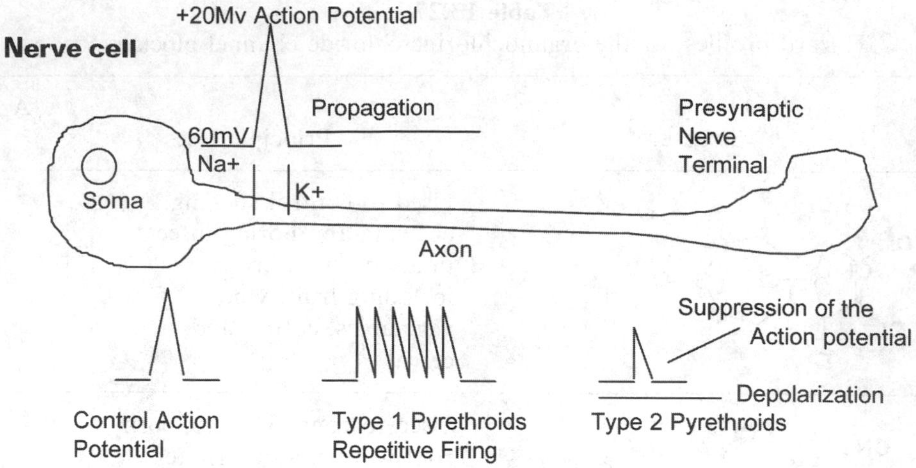

FIG. 13.9. Sites of action of the pyrethroids on nerve impulses.

Table 13.28
Structures and uses of selected pyrethroid insecticides

Insecticide	Structure	Principle Uses/Crops	Treatment Rate gm (a.i.)/ha
Fenpropathrin Danitol® (36)	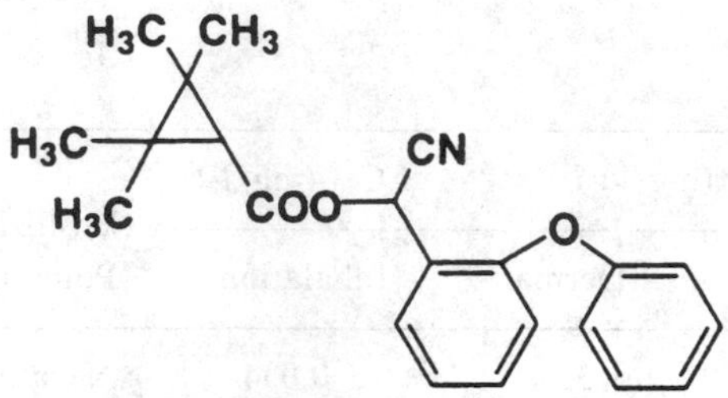	Controls many species of mites and insects.	20–30
Fenvalerate Fenbaz® (38)	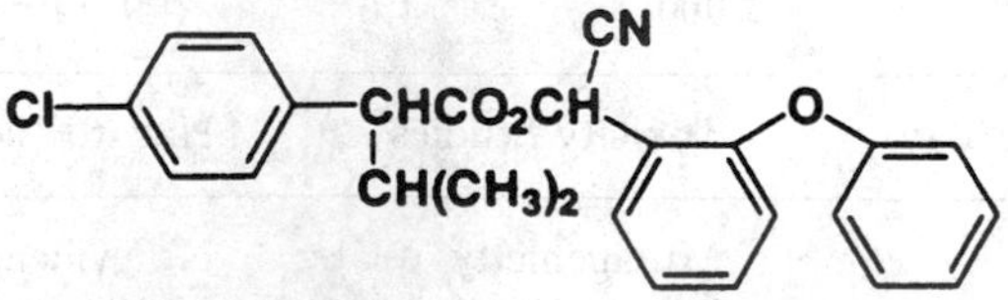	Controls chewing, sucking and boring insects.	20–25
Lambda-cyhalothrin Karate® (51)	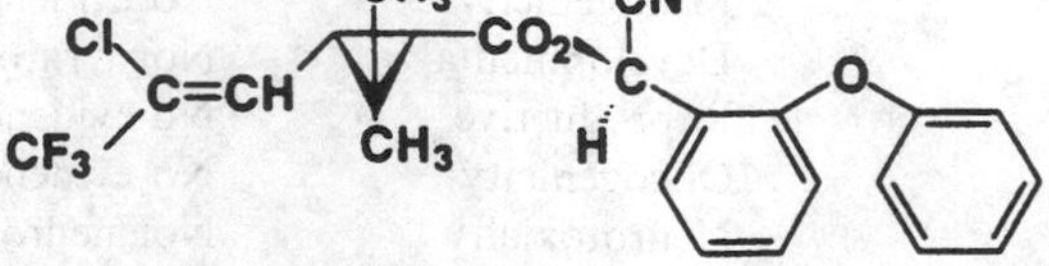	Controls a broad spectrum of chewing and piercing insects.	10–450
Permethrin (Type 1) Ambush® (61)	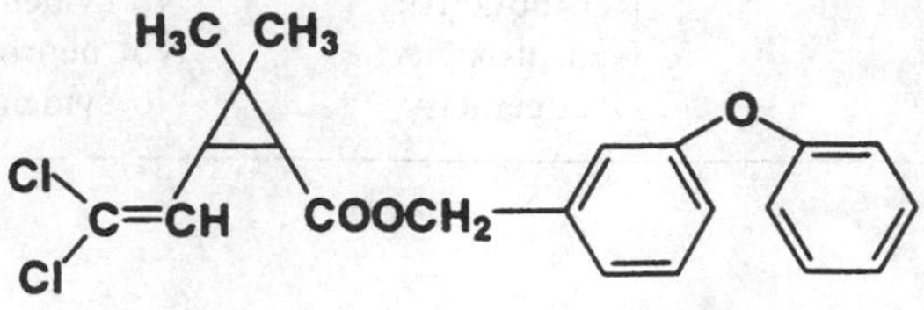	Controls leaf and fruit-eating *Lepidoptera* and *Coleoptera* in cotton.	45–65

Table 13.29
Hazard profiles for the selected synthetic pyrethroids

Insecticide	Irritation: Eye	Irritation: Skin	LD_{50} (mg/kg): Oral	LD_{50} (mg/kg): Dermal	LC_{50} (mg/L): Inhalation	Sensitizing Potential	Signal Word
Fenpropathrin (36)	Not irritant	Not irritant	> 870	> 2000	0.096	Negative	Danger
Fenvalerate (38)	Slight irritant	Irritant	87	> 2000	0.40	Negative	Warning
Lambda-cyhalothrin (52)	Not irritant	Mild irritant	56	632	0.60	Negative	Danger
Permethrin (61)	Not irritant	Not irritant	430	> 2000	> 0.68	Moderate positive	Warning

Insecticide	Species/study	NOEL[1] (mg/kg/day)	Toxicity Studies	Hazard Indicator
Fenpropathrin (125,207)	Rat/2-year	7.0	Mutagenicity	No evidence
	Dog/52-week	3.0	Developmental	Not teratogenic
	Mouse/18-month	56	Reproductive	No evidence
	ADI[2]	0.03	Oncogenicity	E(No evidence)[3]
			Neurotoxicity	Not neurotoxic
Fenvalerate (208)	Rat/2-year	12.5	Mutagenicity	No evidence
	Dog/52-week	2.25	Developmental	Not Teratogenic
	Mouse/18-month	1.5	Reproductive	No evidence
	RfD[2]	0.02	Oncogenicity	E(No evidence)[3]
			Neurotoxicity	Neurotoxic
Lambda-Cyhalothrin (241)	Rat/2-year	2.5	Mutagenicity	No evidence
	Dog/2-Year Oral	0.1	Developmental	Not teratogenic
	Mouse/18-month	14.2	Reproductive	No evidence
	RfD[2]	0.001	Oncogenicity	D (not classifiable)[3]
			Neurotoxicity	Neurotoxic
Permethrin (128)	Rat/2-year	5.0	Mutagenicity	No evidence
	Dog/52-week	5.0	Developmental	Not teratogenic
	Mouse/18-month	7.1	Reproductive	No evidence
	ADI[2]	0.05	Oncogenicity	C/RfD (lung and liver tumors in female mice)[3]
			Neurotoxicity	Neurotoxic

[1] No observable effect level
[2] RfD = reference dose and ADI = acceptable daily intake
[3] See Table 13.3 for US EPA classification scheme

Endotoxins

Bacillus Thuringiensis

Bacillus thuringiensis (Bt) is an aerobic spore-forming gram-positive, rod-shaped bacterium. At sporulation, Bt forms a crystalline inclusion body that contains a number of insecticidal protein toxins (13). When consumed by the insect, the inclusion is dissolved in the midgut and releases δ-endotoxins. The toxin proteins contain a few hundred to over 1000 amino acids. After they are ingested, the δ-endotoxins are cleaved to an active form by proteases within the midgut. The active toxins bind specifically to the membranes of the midgut epithelia and alter their ion permeability properties by forming a cation channel or pore. Ion movements through this pore disrupt potassium and pH gradients and lead to lysis of the epithelium, gut paralysis, and death (99).

Bt has been used directly as a preparation created from grinding up insects infected with Bt or genetically engineered into plants. In regulating this insecticide, the U.S. EPA considered that microbial preparations of Bt have been commercially available for the last 30 years. As these bacterial strains are found in nature, the mammalian hazard test requirements are not as extensive as for synthetic pesticides (197,229). Generally, the hazard tests performed are acute oral toxicity, in vitro digestibility under gastric conditions, and amino acid homology evaluations and comparisons.

Insect Growth Regulators

Juvenile Hormone Mimics

The juvenile hormone mimics (JHMs) are compounds bearing a structural resemblance to the juvenile hormones of insects. Juvenile hormones are lipophilic sesquiterpenoids containing epoxide and methyl ester groups. The JHMs mimic the action of the juvenile hormones on a number of physiological processes, such as molting and reproduction. Exposure to these compounds at molting results in the production of insects containing mixed larval/pupal or larval/adult morphologies. The efficacy of these compounds is greatest when normal juvenile hormone titers are low, namely, in the last larval or early pupal stages (8,263). Thus, timing of application is important for successful control. Another useful property of these compounds is that, in adults, they disrupt normal reproductive physiology.

The structures, uses, and hazard profiles of three of these compounds are presented in Table 13.30.

All three of these compounds have excellent acute and repeated-dose hazard profiles.

Molt Inhibitors

These compounds are classified as benzoylphenylureas and possess a number of halogen substituents. Insects exposed to these compounds are unable to form normal cuticle because the ability to synthesize chitin is lost. Fifty percent of the cuticle is comprised of chitin, which is a polysaccharide of *N*-acetylglucosamine. In the absence of chitin, the cuticle is unable to support the insect.

The compounds are generally not very toxic to mammals but exhibit a high degree of lipophilicity and are stored in the fat. The structures, uses, and hazard profiles of diflubenzuron and teflubenzuron are presented in Table 13.31.

Diflubenzuron and teflubenzuron have excellent hazard profiles with no evidence of significant developmental or reproductive toxicity; neither is carcinogenic.

Molt Accelerators or Ecdysone Agonists

The ecdysone agonist tebufenozide acts upon ingestion, causing the larvae to cease feeding and successfully molt. This compound is also selective, bringing a quick kill to lepidoptera pests (263). The structure, uses, and hazard profile of tebufenozide are presented in Table 13.32.

Tebufenozide is not acutely toxic and does not produce a hazard in regard to repeated-dose toxicity or developmental, reproductive, and oncogenic potential.

Other Modes of Action

Larvicides

The larvicidal agents do not all belong to the same class of chemistry as characterizes some of the previously described mode of action groups. Clofentezine is used as an acaricide/ovicide for deciduous fruits, citrus, cotton, cucurbits, vines, and ornamentals. Cyromazine, an insect growth inhibitor with contact poison features interfering with molting and pupation, is used as a foliar spray, for fly control on treated surfaces, and as a feed premix. Hexythiazox acts as an acaricide, larvicide, and nymphicide. It is used to control eggs and larvae on fruits, vines, vegetables, and cotton. The exact mechanism of action of these three chemicals is not well understood. The structures, principle uses, and hazard profiles for these novel insecticides are given in Table 13.33.

The larvicides possess limited mammalian toxicity. Although cyromazine has not been shown to have any carcinogenic potential in animal studies, both clofentezine and hexythiazox have been classified as category C carcinogens. Clofentezine is to be managed using a reference dose (RfD), whereas, hexythiazox's is regulated using a cancer slope factor value.

Pheromones

Pheromones are common chemical sex attractants secreted by special glands of one or both sexes in insects. These chemicals work to identify and/or locate insects of the opposite gender (147). A pheromone (including an identical synthetic compound) is defined by the U.S. EPA as a compound produced by an arthropod (insect, arachnid, or crustacean) that modifies the behavior of other individuals of the same species (179).

Lepidopteran pheromones, produced by a member of the order Lepidoptera, including butterflies and moths, share a physicohemical feature common to all pheromones: their volatility, which is the basis for the signaling and homing mechanism. The U.S. EPA has registered 17 arthropod pheromones active ingredients, 11 of which are lepidopteran pheromones (179). The information submitted covered compounds that were from 6- to 16-carbon unbranched alcohols, acetates, and aldehydes. The structure for the major lepidopteran pheromone, tetradecenyl acetate, is shown in Figure 13.10.

The U.S. EPA has assumed that pheromones and other similar natural chemicals are different from conventional

Table 13.30
Hazard profile for juvenile hormone mimics

Fungicide	Structure	Principle uses	Application rates gm (a.i.)/ha
Diofenolan (32)	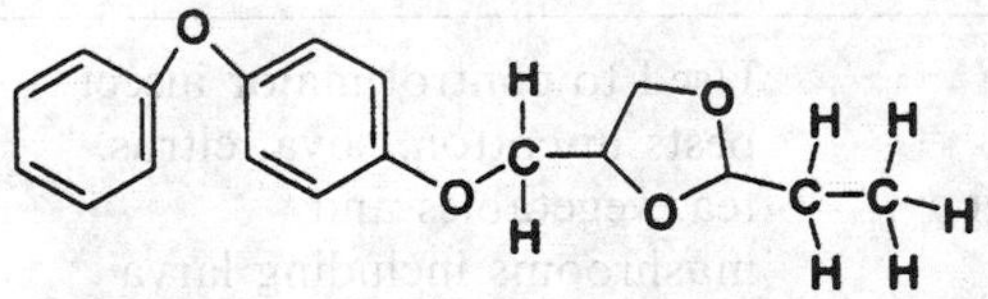	Used to control most scale insects and eggs in fruits and ornamentals	25–50
Pymetrozine Sterling® (67)	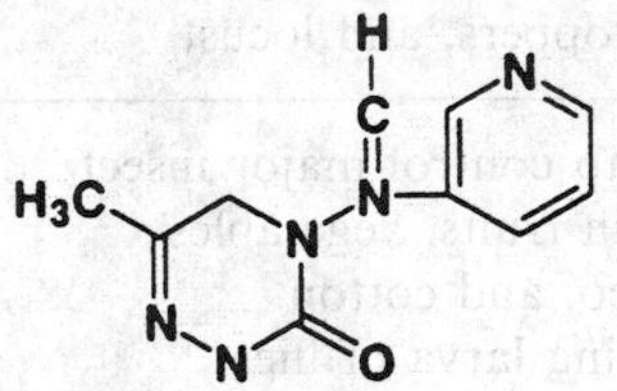	Used to control asphids and whiteflies in vegetables, ornamentals, cotton and field crops	25–50
Pyriproxifen Knack® (70,260)	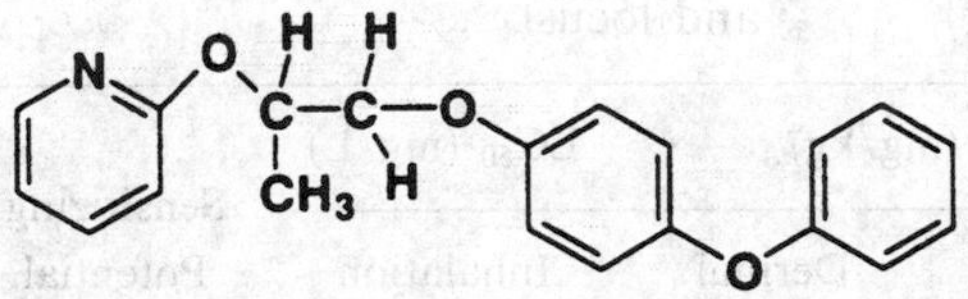	Used to control public health insect pests	25–50

Insecticide	Irritation: Eye	Irritation: Skin	LD_{50} (mg/kg): Oral	LD_{50} (mg/kg): Dermal	LC_{50} (mg/L): Inhalation	Sensitizing Potential	Signal Word
Diofenolan (32)	Not irritant	Not irritant	> 5000	> 2000	> 3.1	Negative	Caution
Pymetrozine (67)	Not irritant	Not irritant	> 5820	> 2000	> 1.8	Negative	Caution
Pyriproxifen (70,260)	Not irritant	Not irritant	> 5000	> 2000	> 3.1	Negative	Caution

Insecticide	Species/study	NOEL[1] (mg/kg/day)	Toxicity Studies	Hazard Indicator
Diofenolan (32)	Rat/13-Week Oral	12	Mutagenicity	No evidence
	Dog/13-Week Oral	12	Developmental	Not teratogenic
	Mouse/18-month	–	Reproductive	No evidence
	ADI (provisional)[2]	0.006(Based on 13-wk. rat with 500 UF[4])	Oncogenicity	NA
Pymetrozine (245,246)	Rat/2-year	3.7	Mutagenicity	No evidence
	Dog/52-week	0.57	Developmental	Not teratogenic
	Mouse/18-month	12	Reproductive	No evidence
	RfD[2]	0.0057	Oncogenicity	No evidence
Pyriproxifen (248)	Rat/2-year	35	Mutagenicity	No evidence
	Dog/52-week	100	Developmental	Not teratogenic
	Mouse/18-month	85	Reproductive	No evidence
	RfD[2]	0.35	Oncogenicity	E(No evidence)[3]

[1] No observable effect level
[2] RfD = reference dose and ADI = acceptable daily intake
[3] See Table 13.3 for US EPA classification scheme
[4] UF = Uncertainty factor
NA = Not Available

Table 13.31
Structures, uses, and hazard profiles for the molt inhibitors (chitin synthesis inhibitors)

Insecticide	Structure	Principle uses	Application Rates gm (a.i.)/ha
Diflubenzuron Amilin® (233,234)	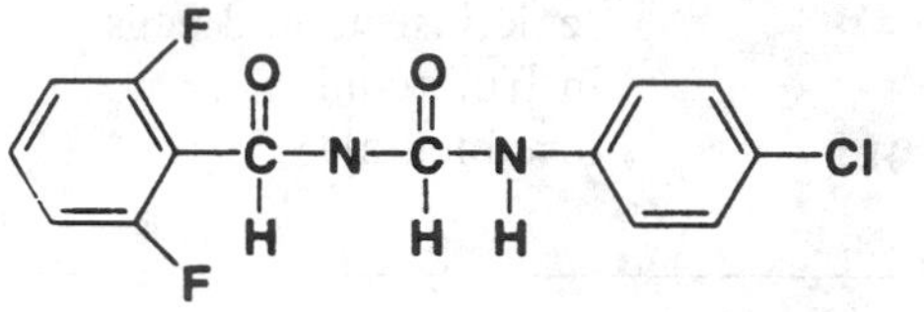	Used to control major insect pests in cotton, soya, citrus, tea, vegetables and mushrooms including larva of flies, mosquitoes, grasshoppers, and locust.	25–75
Teflubenzuron Nomolt® (76)	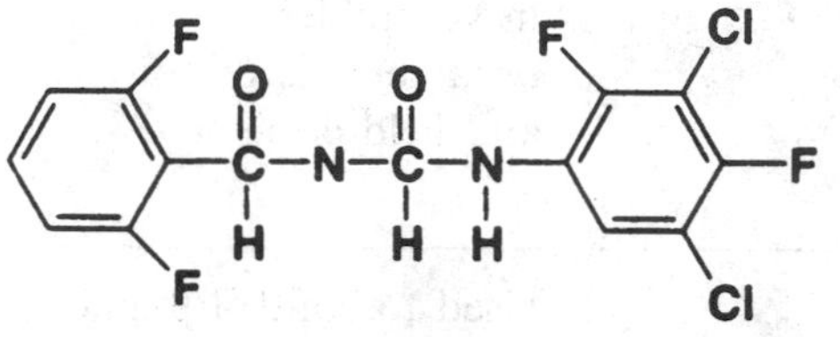	Used to control major insect pests in fruits, vegetables tobacco, and cotton including larva of flies, mosquitoes, grasshoppers, and locust	NA

Insecticide	Irritation: Eye	Irritation: Skin	LD_{50} (mg/kg): Oral	LD_{50} (mg/kg): Dermal	LC_{50} (mg/L): Inhalation	Sensitizing Potential	Signal Word
Diflubenzuron (234)	Not irritant	Not irritant	> 4640	> 10000	> 35	Negative	Caution
Teflubenzuron (76)	Not irritant	Not irritant	> 5000	> 2000	> 3.1	Negative	Caution

Insecticide	Species/study	NOEL[1] (mg/kg/day)	Toxicity Studies	Hazard Indicator
Diflubenzuron (233,234)	Rat/2-year	2.0	Mutagenicity	No evidence
	Dog/52-week	2.0	Developmental	Not teratogenic
	Mouse/18-month	2.0	Reproductive	No evidence
	RfD[2]	0.02	Oncogenicity	E(No evidence)[3]
Teflubenzuron (76)	Rat/2-year	4.8	Mutagenicity	No evidence
	Dog/52-week	3.2	Developmental	Not teratogenic
	Mouse/18-month	2.1	Reproductive	No evidence
	ADI[2]	0.01 (based on the 18-month mouse with a 200×UF[4])	Oncogenicity	No evidence

[1] No observable effect level
[2] RfD = reference dose and ADI = acceptable daily intake
[3] See Table 13.3 for US EPA classification scheme
[4] UF = Uncertainty factor
NA = Not Available

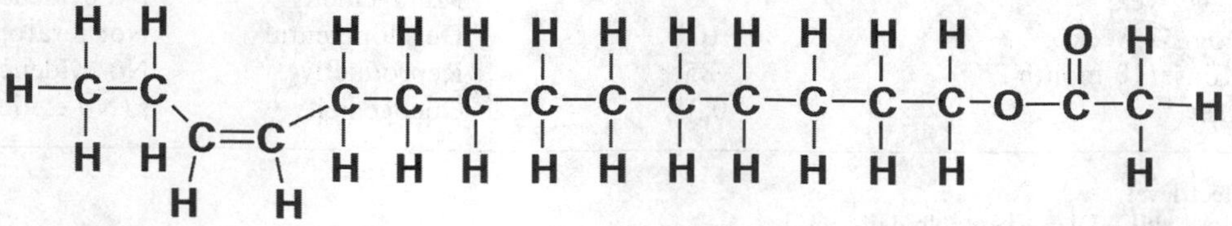

FIG. 13.10. The structure of the lepidopteran pheromone tetradecenyl acetate.

Table 13.32
Structure, uses, and hazard profile for the ecdysone agonist tebufenozide (Confirm®) (249)

Structure	Primary Uses	Application Rates gm (a.i.)/ha
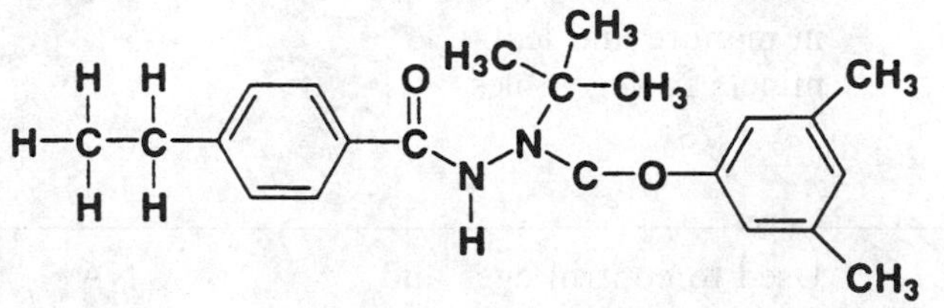	Used for control lepidopteran larvae on rice, fruit, row crop, nut crops, vegetables, and vines.	NA

Insecticide	Irritation Eye	Skin	LD_{50} (mg/kg) Oral	Dermal	LC_{50} (mg/L) Inhalation	Sensitizing Potential	Signal Word
Tebufenozide	Not irritant	Not irritant	> 5000	> 5000	4.5	Negative	Caution

Insecticide	Species/study	NOEL[1] (mg/kg/day)	Toxicity Studies	Hazard Indicator
Tebufenozide	Rat/2-year	4.8	Mutagenicity	No evidence
	Dog/52-week	1.8	Developmental	Not teratogenic
	Mouse/18-month	143	Reproductive	No evidence
	RfD[2]	0.018	Oncogenicity	E(No evidence)[3]

[1] No observable effect level
[2] RfD = reference dose
[3] See Table 13.3 for US EPA classification scheme
NA = Not Available

synthetic pesticides. Therefore, there are fewer data requirements for registering pheromones.

In fact, most of the hazard data for these pheromones are anecdotal. The data available on both lepidopteran and other arthropod pheromones, including several aromatic pheromones, have indicated no acute mammalian toxicity at the limit dose levels tested. The acute toxicity profile generally reveals oral and dermal LD_{50} values of greater than 5000 mg/kg and 2000 mg/kg, respectively (226). The acute inhalation LC_{50} value is generally >5 mg/L. Eye and skin irritation potential fall in the mild or not irritating range, with no evidence of sensitization potential. Since a miniscule amount of the pheromone will be adsorbed to the inside of the bait station, there is practically no human contact with the pheromone. Therefore, the full data package required for conventional pesticides is waived by the U.S. EPA (226).

Respiratory Inhibitors and Uncouplers

Compounds that disrupt energy metabolism have been identified from both natural and synthetic sources. An important natural product is rotenone, which is derived from cube or derris root (160). The synthetic compounds in this group include a number of nitrogen-containing heterocycles, such as pyridaben (144). Disruption of energy metabolism occurs in the mitochondria and usually takes the form of either an inhibition of the electron transport system or an uncoupling of the transport system from ATP production. Inhibition of the electron transport system blocks the production of ATP and causes a decrease in oxygen consumption by the mitochondria. These uncouplers act on coenzyme Q oxidoreductase in the electron transport chain or the cytochrome b–c_1 complex (103). The electron transport system functions normally, but the production of ATP is uncoupled from the electron transport process due to a dissipation of the proton gradient across the inner mitochondrial membrane. In the presence of uncouplers, oxygen consumption increases, but no ATP is produced (104). The disruption of energy metabolism and the subsequent loss of ATP results in a slowly developing toxicity, and the effects of all these compounds include inactivity, paralysis, and death.

The structures, uses, and hazard profiles of three compounds in this group registered in the United States are given in Table 13.34.

Table 13.33
Hazard profiles for selected larvicides

Insecticide	Structure	Principle uses	Application Rates gm (a.i.)/ha
Cyromazine Trigard® (28)	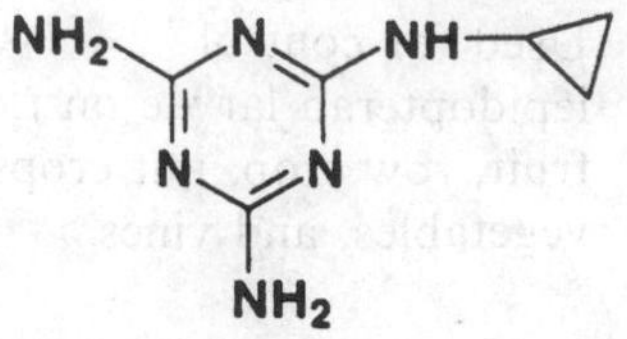	Used to control fly larvae in manure and leaf miners in vegetables.	140
Clofentezine Apollo® (252,253)	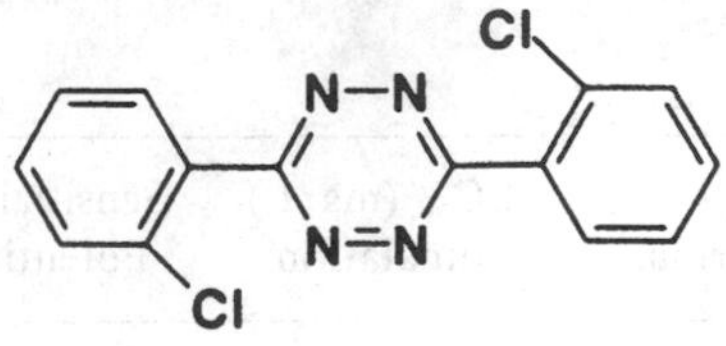	Used to control eggs and young mobile stages of mites in vegetables and fruit.	NA
Hexythiazox Nissorun® (237)	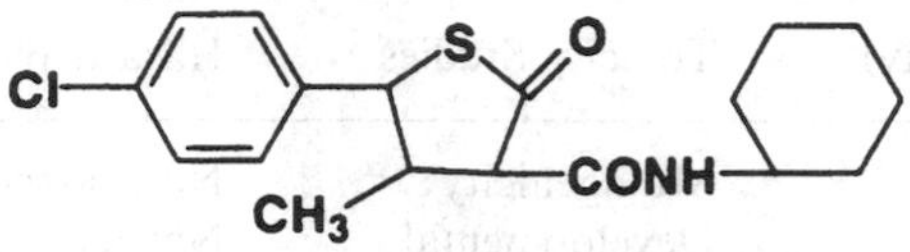	Used to control larvae and eggs phygophagous mites in fruit, vines, cotton and vegetables.	NA

	Irritation		LD_{50} (mg/kg)		LC_{50} (mg/L)		
Insecticide	Eye	Skin	Oral	Dermal	Inhalation	Sensitizing Potential	Signal Word
Cyromazine	Not irritant	Mild Irritant	2029	> 1370	> 2.7	Negative	Caution
Clofentezine	Not irritant	Not irritant	> 5200	> 2100	> 2.0	Weak positive	Caution
Hexythiazox	Mild irritant	Not irritant	> 5000	> 5000	> 2.0	Negative	Caution

Insecticide	Species/study	NOEL[1] (mg/kg/day)	Toxicity Studies	Hazard Indicator
Cyromazine (28,255)	Rat/2-year	1.8	Mutagenicity	No evidence
	Dog/26-Week Oral	0.75	Developmental	Not teratogenic
	Mouse/18-month	6.5	Reproductive	No evidence
	RfD[2]	0.008	Oncogenicity	E(No evidence)[3]
Clofentezine (252,253)	Rat/2-year	2.0	Mutagenicity	No evidence
	Dog/26-Week Oral	1.25	Developmental	Not teratogenic
	Mouse/18-month	7.1	Reproductive	No evidence
	RfD[2]	0.012	Oncogenicity	C with Q* (thyroid tumors in male rats)[3]
Hexythiazox (237,238)	Rat/2-year	21.5	Mutagenicity	No evidence
	Dog/26-Week Oral	2.5	Developmental	Not teratogenic
	Mouse/18-month	37.5	Reproductive	No evidence
	RfD[2]		Oncogenicity	C with CSF (based on liver tumors)[3]

[1] No observable effect level
[2] RfD = reference dose, CSF = cancer slope factor
[3] See Table 13.3 for US EPA classification scheme
NA = Not Available

Table 13.34
Hazard profile for the respiration-inhibiting insecticides

Insecticide	Structure	Principle uses	Application Rates gm (a.i.)/ha
Chlorfenapyr Pirate® (19)	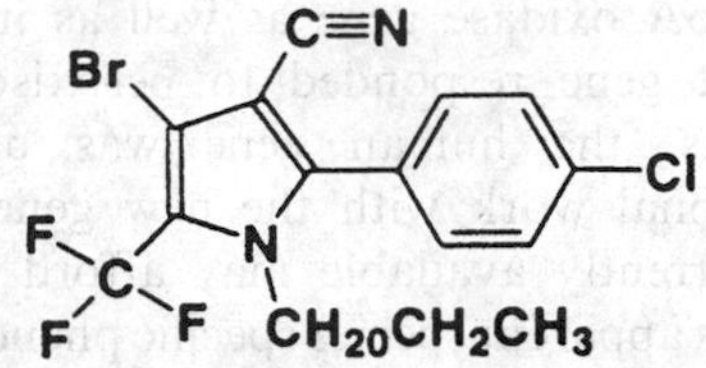	Used to control many insects and mites in cotton, vegetables, citrus, vines and soya beans.	NA
Hydramethylnon Amdro® (47)	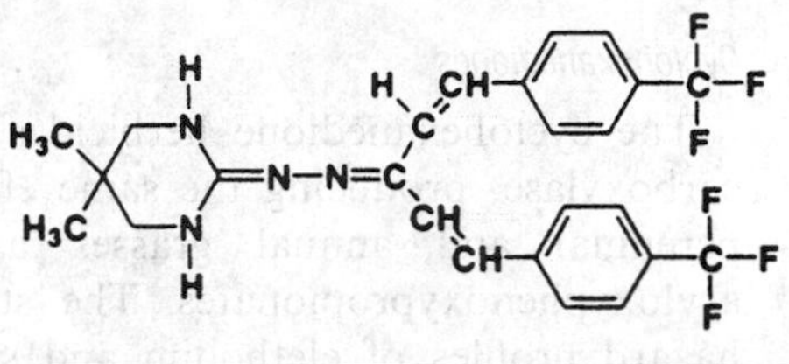	Used to control agricultural and household *Formicidae*	NA
Pyridaben Poseidon® (223)	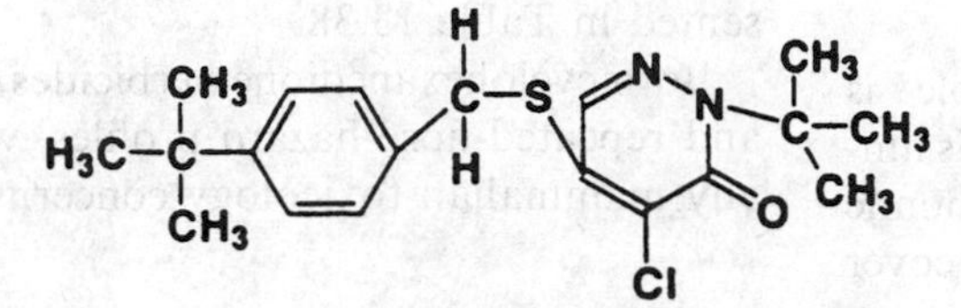	Used to control acarids on field crops, fruits, vegetables and ornamentals	100–300

Insecticide	Irritation: Eye	Irritation: Skin	LD_{50} (mg/kg): Oral	LD_{50} (mg/kg): Dermal	LC_{50} (mg/L): Inhalation	Sensitizing Potential	Signal Word
Chlorfenapyr	Moderate irritant	Not irritant	441	> 2000	1.9	Negative	Warning
Hydramethylnon	Mild irritant	Not irritant	817	> 2000	2.9	Negative	Caution
Pyridaben	Slight irritant	Not irritant	820	> 2000	0.66	Negative	Caution

Insecticide	Species/study	NOEL[1] (mg/kg/day)	Toxicity Studies	Hazard Indicator
Chlorfenapyr (200)	Rat/2-year	2.9	Mutagenicity	No evidence
	Dog/52-week	4.0	Developmental	Not teratogenic
	Mouse/18-month	2.8	Reproductive	No evidence
	RfD[2]	0.03	Oncogenicity	E(No evidence)[3]
			Neurotoxicity	Not neurotoxic
Hydramethylnon (47,237)	Rat/2-year	50	Mutagenicity	No evidence
	Dog/52-week	1.0	Developmental	Not teratogenic
	Mouse/18-month	25	Reproductive	No evidence
	ADI[2]	0.01	Oncogenicity	C-RfD (based on lung/liver tumors in mice)[3]
			Neurotoxicity	Not neurotoxic
Pyridaben (223)	Rat/2-year	1.13	Mutagenicity	No evidence
	Dog/52-week	< 0.5	Developmental	Not teratogenic
	Mouse/18-month	2.78	Reproductive	No evidence
	ADI[2]	0.005	Oncogenicity	E (No evidence)[3]
			Neurotoxicity	Not neurotoxic

[1] No observable effect level
[2] RfD = reference dose and ADI = acceptable daily intake
[3] See Table 13.3 for US EPA classification scheme
NA = Not Available

All of these materials possess low to moderate toxicity to mammals. The U.S. EPA has classified hydramethylnon as category C (possible human carcinogen) based on lung tumors in mice.

HERBICIDES

Herbicides are the leading type of pesticides, in terms of both user expenditures and amount used (1). In 1995, approximately \$6.25 billion (United States) and \$16.25 billion (worldwide) were spent by users on herbicides; this constitutes 55% and 45% of the U.S. and worldwide markets, respectively. Quantity-wise, 556 (46%) and 2210 (39%) million lb of active ingredient were purchased in the U.S. and worldwide markets, respectively. This market has been significantly impacted with the introduction of new chemistry, such as, the sulfonylureas (active in the grams per acre range), and new technology such as corn bioengineered against the phytotoxicity of the nonspecific herbicide glyphosate (198).

As the sheer number of herbicides available is significant, the number of herbicides presented here is limited with a focus on those considered to have economic and high agronomic value. There is an attempt to cover all the different mechanisms of actions in this process. The modes and mechanisms of action for important classes of herbicides used in crop protection are presented in Table 13.35.

Acetyl-CoA Carboxylase Inhibitors

Herbicides that act via inhibition of acetyl coenzyme A (acetyl-CoA) carboxylase alter lipid biosynthesis in weeds. The lipid inhibitors include the aryloxyphenoxypropionate and cyclohexanedione herbicides. These herbicides prevent the formation of fatty acids, components essential for the production of plant lipids. Lipids are vital to the integrity of cell membranes and to new plant growth. The lipid inhibitor herbicides inhibit a single key enzyme involved in fatty acid synthesis (154). Broadleaf plants are tolerant to these herbicide families, but many of the perennial and annual grasses are susceptible. Injury symptoms are slow to develop (7 to 10 days) and appear first on new leaves emerging from the whorl of the grass plant. These herbicides are taken up by the foliage and move in the phloem to areas of new growth (92).

Aryloxyphenoxypropionates

The structures, uses, and hazard profiles for six acetyl-CoA carboxylase-inhibiting aryloxyphenoxypropionate herbicides are presented in Tables 13.36 and 13.37.

These materials are generally not acutely toxic. Clodinafop-propargyl and haloxyfop have been identified as peroxisomal proliferators (pp) in the rodent. The relevance of peroxisomal proliferation to humans is still unresolved. However, studies involving the peroxisomal proliferator response element upstream of the human acyl-CoA oxidase gene as well as in rats showed that the rat gene responded to peroxisomal proliferators; whereas, the human gene was unresponsive (318). Additional work with the new gene technologies that are currently available may afford an opportunity to put this apparent species specific phenomenon into proper perspective.

Cyclohexanediones

The cyclohexanedione herbicides inhibit acetyl-CoA carboxylase, producing the same effects on susceptible perennial and annual grasses as noted with the aryloxyphenoxypropionates. The structures, uses, and hazard profiles of clethodim and sethoxydim are presented in Table 13.38.

Both cyclohexanedione herbicides have excellent acute and repeated-dose hazard profiles, which do not trigger any mammalian toxicology concerns.

Acetolactate Synthase Inhibitors

The sulfonyureas, imidazolinones, triazolopyridimidines, and pyriidinyl thiobenzoates constitute acetolactate synthase (ALS) inhibitors. The ALS inhibitors interact with the acetolactate synthase enzyme, inhibiting biosynthesis of an essential amino acid (297).

Sulfonylureas

Sulfonylurea herbicides belong to a class of compounds comprised of three distinct components. These are an aryl group linked to a nitrogen-containing hetrocycle via a sulfonylurea bridge. Sulfonylurea herbicides inhibit root and shoot growth in rapidly growing plants by suppressing cell division (4). Initial research conducted on *Escherichia coli* and *Salmonella typhimurium* and latter confirmed in plants and yeasts indicate that the herbicidal activity is due to the inhibition of acetolactate synthase (ALS), an enzyme necessary for the biosynthesis of branched chain amino acids in bacteria, fungi, and higher plants.

A large number of sulfonylurea herbicides have been developed for commercial use in North America and Europe (Tables 13.39 and 13.40).

Sulfonylurea herbicides generally are not acutely toxic or irritating to the skin and eye, nor are they mutagenic, developmentally toxic, or oncogenic (203). Their hazard profiles are given in Tables 13.41 through 13.43.

Table 13.35
Mode and mechanism of action for important classes of herbicides used in crop protection

Class	Mode of Action	Mechanism of Action
Acetyl CoA Carboxylase (ACCase) Inhibitors (41)	Systemic grass herbicides	Inhibit ACCase lipid biosynthesis.
Acetolactate Synthase (ALS) Inhibitors (297)	Selective systemic herbicides	Normal function of the ALS enzyme is blocked, inhibiting biosynthesis of essential amino acids.
Photosynthesis Inhibitors (268)	Selective systemic herbicides	Block the photosynthetic reaction, and disrupt cellular membranes so that captured light cannot be converted to chemical energy.
Protoporphyrin Inhibitors (265)	Selective contact herbicides	Inhibits the enzyme protoporphyrinogen oxidase.
Bleaching Herbicides (301)	Selective systemic herbicides	Disrupt synthesis of carotenoid pigments which protect chlorophyll pigments in light. Lack of carotenoids lead to chlorophyll destruction and white, bleached appearance.
EPSP Synthase Inhibitors (287)	Non-selective systemic herbicides	Inhibit 5-enolpyruvlshikimate-3-phosphate synthase preventing the biosynthesis of essential amino acids.
Glutamine Synthase Inhibitors (286)	Non-selective contact herbicides	Inhibit glutamine synthase leading to accumulation of ammonium ions, and inhibition of photosynthesis.
Dihydropteroate (DHP) Synthase Inhibitors (267)	Selective systemic herbicides	Inhibit DHP synthase involved in folic acid synthesis needed for the formation of purine nucleotides required for cell division.
Microtubule Assembly Inhibitors (14)	Selective systemic herbicides	Affect seed germination and prevents weed growth.
Mitosis Inhibitors (303)	Selective systemic herbicides	Affect cell growth and cell elongation.
Inhibitors of Cellulose Synthesis (294)	Selective systemic herbicides	Inhibit cell wall biosynthesis through inhibiting the formation of cellulose.
Membrane Disruptors (302)	Non-selective contact herbicides	Disrupt internal cell membranes by formation of a superoxide preventing the cell from manufacturing energy.
Inhibitors of Lipid Synthesis (308)	Selective systemic herbicides	Block formation of lipids in the shoot (meristem) and roots of grass plants.
Synthetic Auxins (Mimic or Inhibit Indoleacetic Acid) (82)	Selective systemic herbicides	Affect growth in the meristems and leaves by affecting protein synthesis and normal cell division.

Table 13.36
Structures, uses, and hazard profiles of acetyl-CoA carboxylase-inhibiting aryloxyphenoxypropionate herbicides

Chemical/ Common Names	Structure	Principle Uses/Crops	Application rates gm (a.i.)/ha
Clodinafop-propargyl/ Discover® (22)	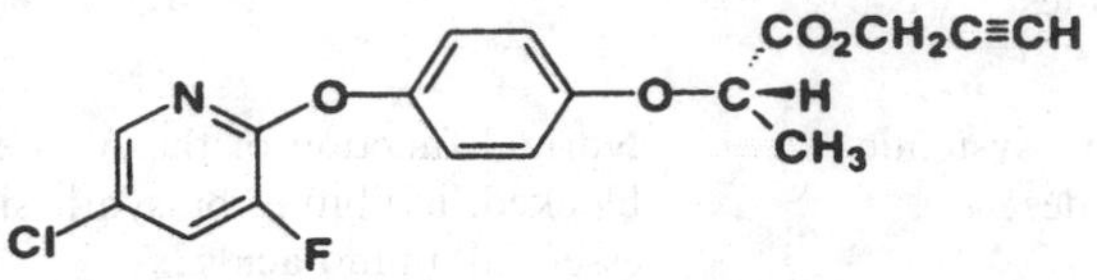	Cereals	20–80
Diclofop-methyl Hoelon® (278)	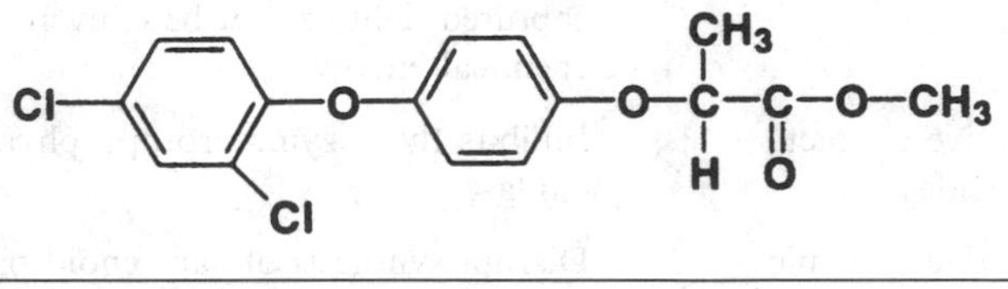	Cereals	840–1680
Fenoxaprop-ethyl (206)	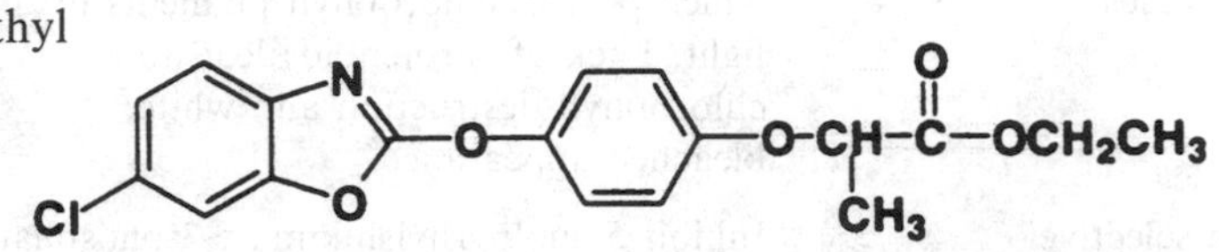	Cereals, soybeans, and turf	37.5–111

Herbicide	Irritation: Eye	Irritation: Skin	LD_{50} (mg/kg): Oral	LD_{50} (mg/kg): Dermal	LC_{50} (mg/L): Inhalation	Sensitizing Potential	Signal Word
Clodinafop-propargyl	Non-irritant	Non-irritant	1829	> 2000	2.325	Positive	Caution
Diclofop-methyl	Non-irritant	Non-irritant	2020	> 5000	> 3.83	NA	Caution
Fenoxaprop-ethyl	Slight irritant	Slight irritant	2565	> 2000	> 0.511	Negative	Caution

Herbicide	Species/study	NOEL[1] (mg/kg/day)	Toxicity Studies	Hazard Indicator
Clodinofop-Propargyl	Rat/2-year	0.35	Mutagenicity	Not a mutagen
	Dog/52-week	3.3	Developmental	Not a developmental toxin
	Mouse/18-month	1.2	Reproductive	Not a reproductive toxin
	ADI (2-yr. rat)[2]	0.004	Oncogenicity	Rodent peroxisomal proliferator (Mouse liver tumors)
Diclofop-Methyl	Rat/2-year	20	Mutagenicity	Not a mutagen
	Dog/15-Mo. Oral	8.0	Developmental	Not a developmental toxin
	Mouse/18-month	NA	Reproductive	Not a reproductive toxin
	ADI[2]	0.001 (proposed)	Oncogenicity	NA
Fenoxaprop-Ethyl	Rat/2-year	1.5	Mutagenicity	Not a mutagen
	Dog/15-Mo. Oral	0.375	Developmental	Not a developmental toxin
	Mouse/18-month	5.7	Reproductive	Not a reproductive toxin
	RfD (rat reproduction)[2]	0.0025	Oncogenicity	C(pending)[3]-adrenal tumors

[1] No observable effect level
[2] RfD = reference dose and ADI = acceptable daily intake
[3] See Table 13.3 for US EPA classification scheme
[4] UF = Uncertainty factor
NA = Not Available

Table 13.37
More structures, uses, and hazard profiles of acetyl-CoA carboxylase-inhibiting aryloxyphenoxypropionate herbicides

Herbicide	Structure	Principle Uses/Crops	Application rates gm (a.i.)/ha
Fluazifop-P-Butyl Fusilade® (41)	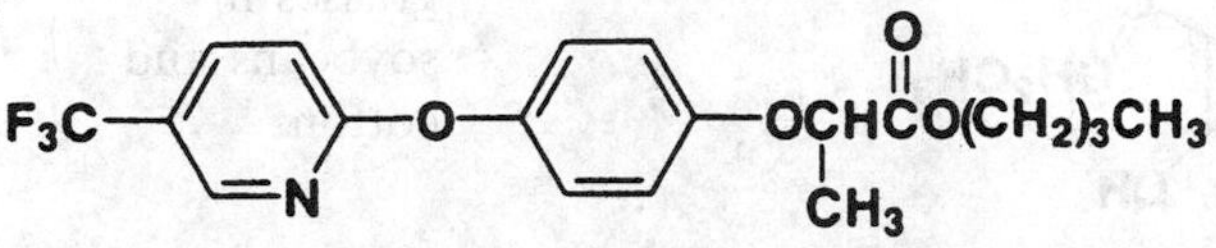	Cotton, fruit, and soybeans	53–210
Haloxyfop Galant™ (288)	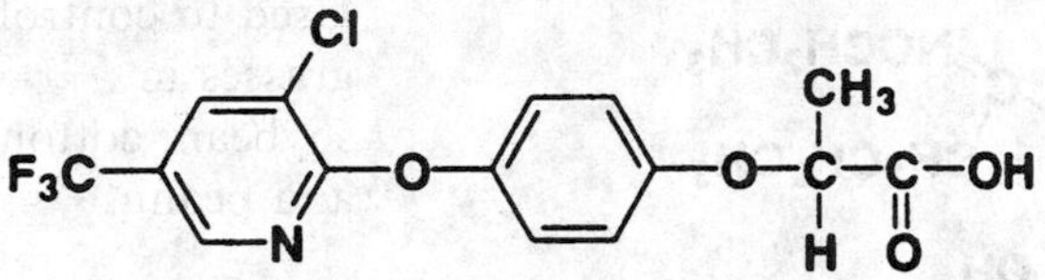	Cotton, soybeans, sunflowers, oilseed rape	140–600
Propaquizafop AGIL® (63)	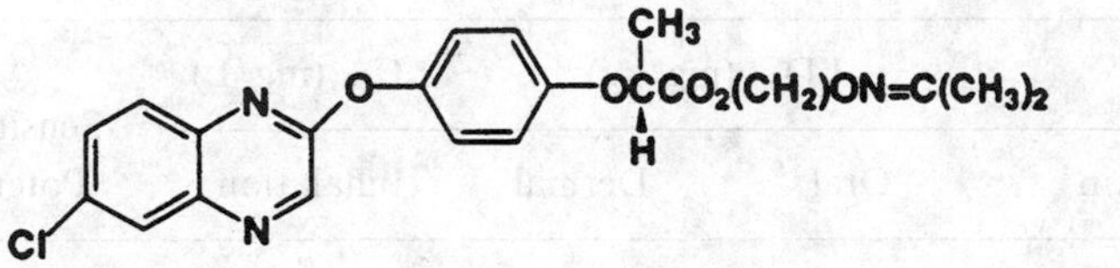	Soybeans, cotton, sunflower, sugar beets, potatoes, oilseed rape, vegetables, peanuts, tobacco	NA

Herbicide	Irritation		LD50 (mg/kg)		LC50 (mg/L)	Sensitizing	Signal
	Eye	Skin	Oral	Dermal	Inhalation	Potential	Word
Fluazifop-P-Butyl	Mild Irritant	Slight Irritant	4096	> 2420	> 5.24	Negative	Caution
Haloxyfop	Moderate Irritant	Non-irritant	518	> 5000	NA	Negative	Caution
Propaquizafop	Moderate Irritant	Non-irritant	> 5000	> 2000	2.5	Possibly positive	Caution

Herbicide	Species/study	NOEL[1] (mg/kg/day)	Toxicity Studies	Hazard Indicator
Fluazifop-P-Butyl	Rat/2-year	NA	Mutagenicity	NA
	Dog/52-week	NA	Developmental	NA
	Mouse/18-month	NA	Reproductive	NA
	RfD[2]	0.01	Oncogenicity	NA
Haloxyfop	Rat/2-year	0.065	Mutagenicity	No evidence
	Dog/52-week	0.5	Developmental	Not a developmental toxin
	Mouse/18-month	0.6	Reproductive	No evidence
	ADI[2]	0.0003	Oncogenicity	Rodent peroxisomal proliferator
Propaquizafop	Rat/2-year	1.5	Mutagenicity	NA
	Dog/52-week	20	Developmental	NA
	Mouse/18-month	1.5	Reproductive	NA
	ADI[2]	0.015	Oncogenicity	NA

[1] No observable effect level
[2] RfD = reference dose and ADI = acceptable daily intake
[3] See Table 13.3 for US EPA classification scheme
NA = Not Available

Table 13.38
Structures, uses, and hazard profiles of acetyl-CoA carboxylase-inhibiting cyclohexanedione herbicides

Herbicide	Structure	Principle Uses/Crops	Application Rate gm (a.i.)/ha
Clethodim Select® (275)	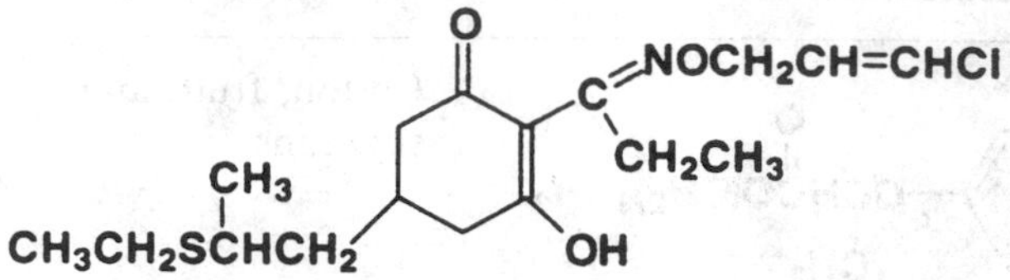	Used to control grasses in soybeans and cotton.	105–280
Sethoxydim Nabu® (308)	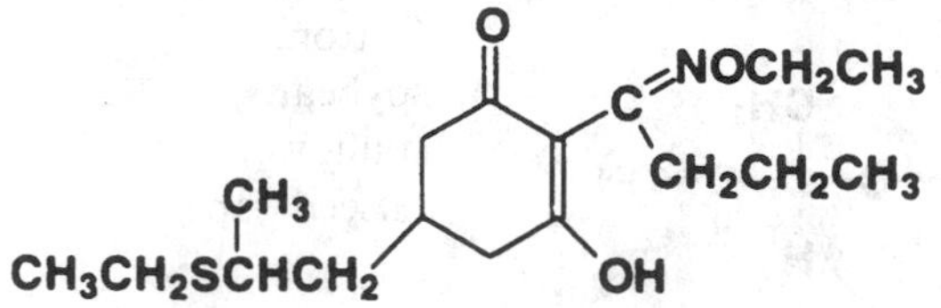	Used to control grasses in soybean, cotton and peanut	112–560

Herbicide	Irritation: Eye	Irritation: Skin	LD_{50} (mg/kg): Oral	LD_{50} (mg/kg): Dermal	LC_{50} (mg/L): Inhalation	Sensitizing Potential	Signal Word
Clethodim	NA	Non-irritant	1360	> 2000	> 3.9	NA	Caution
Sethoxydim	Non-irritant	Non-irritant	2676	> 5000	6.1	Negative	Caution

Herbicide	Species/study	NOEL[1] (mg/kg/day)	Toxicity Studies	Hazard Indicator
Clethodim	Rat/2-year	19	Mutagenicity	Not a mutagen
	Dog/52-week	1	Developmental	Not a developmental toxin
	Mouse/18-month	28	Reproductive	Not a reproductive toxin
	ADI[2]	0.01	Oncogenicity	No evidence
Sethoxydim	Rat/2-year	17.2	Mutagenicity	Not a mutagen
	Dog/52-week	8.9	Developmental	Not a developmental toxin
	Mouse/18-month	14	Reproductive	Not a reproductive toxin
	ADI[2]	0.14	Oncogenicity	No evidence

[1] No observable effect level
[2] RfD = reference dose and ADI = acceptable daily intake
[3] See Table 13.3 for US EPA classification scheme
NA = Not Available

Various target organs have been identified at high doses in chronic studies in rodents and dogs, including bone marrow, liver, kidney, testes, and the peripheral and central nervous systems. Tumor incidence was elevated above control levels in the liver (primisulfuron) and heart (oxasulfuron) at doses that exceed the maximum tolerated dose. An earlier appearance of mammary tumors has also been observed in female Sprague-Dawley rats (prosulfuron, tribenuron).

A unitary mode of action underlying effects of this class of chemical on mammalian systems is not discernable. The diversity of the effects observed in various target organs is attributed to specific functional groups and not to the defining characteristic of the class, the sulfonylurea bridge.

Imidazolinones

There are a restricted number of registered chemicals in this class of ALS-inhibiting herbicides. They include imazameth and imazamethabenzmethyl. The hazard profiles for these chemicals (Table 13.44) indicate that this class of herbicide is relatively nontoxic, even at high doses, with no evidence of mutagenic, developmental, or oncogenic effects.

Table 13.39
Structures and uses of the ALS sulfonylurea herbicides

Chemical/ Common Names	Structure	Principle Uses/Crops	Application Rate gm (a.i.)/ha/yr.
Bensulfuron-methyl Londax® (269)	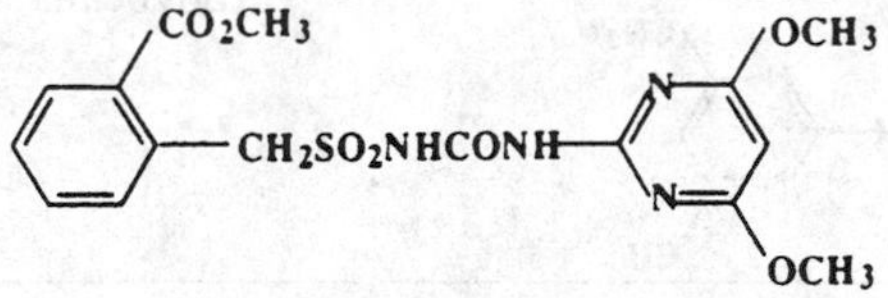	Rice	30–100
Chlorimuron-ethyl Classic® (275)	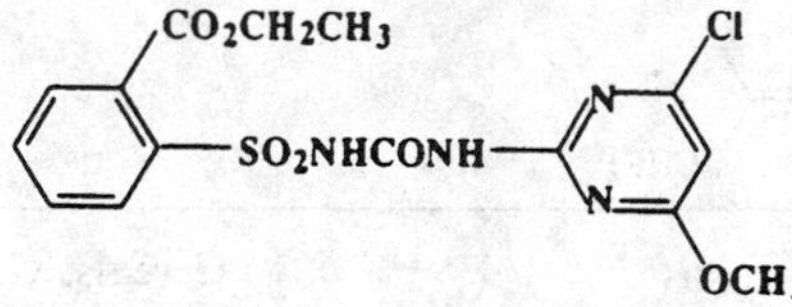	Soybeans, Peanuts	9–13
Chlorsulfuron Glean® (274)	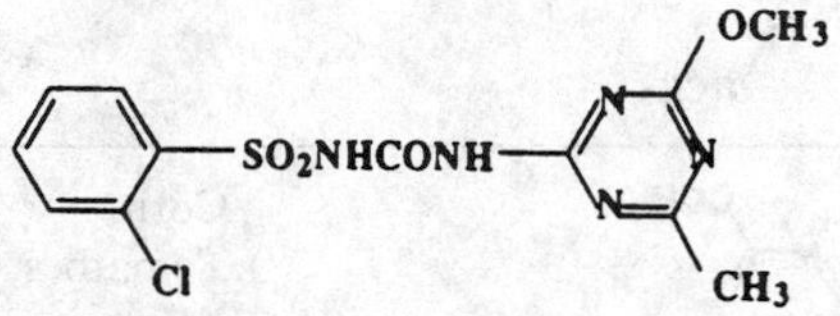	Cereals, IWC	5–25
Halosulfuron-methyl Permit® (45)	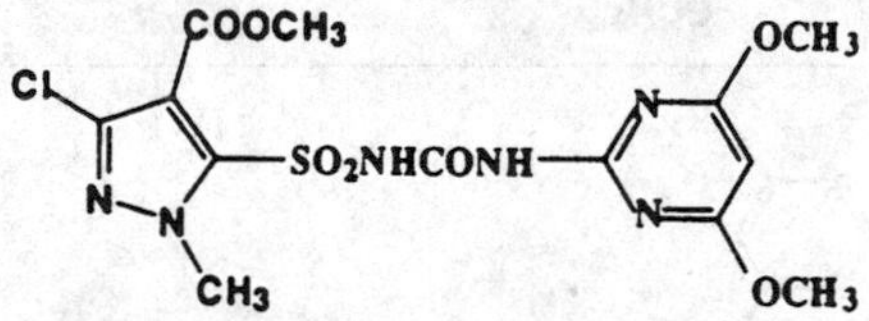	Cereals, Corn Sorghum, Turf	NA
Imazosulfuron Sibatito®, Takeoff® (49)	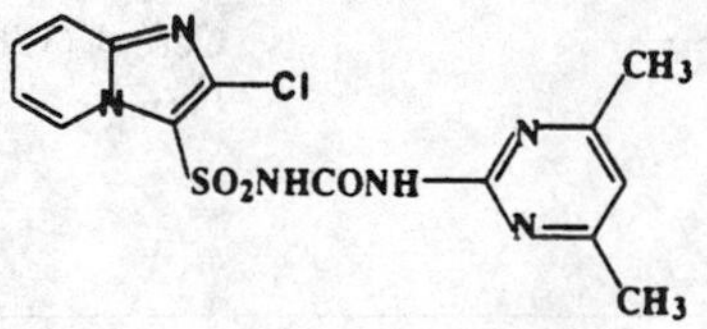	Cereals, Rice, Turf	75–95
Metsulfuron-methyl Ally®, Escort® (297)	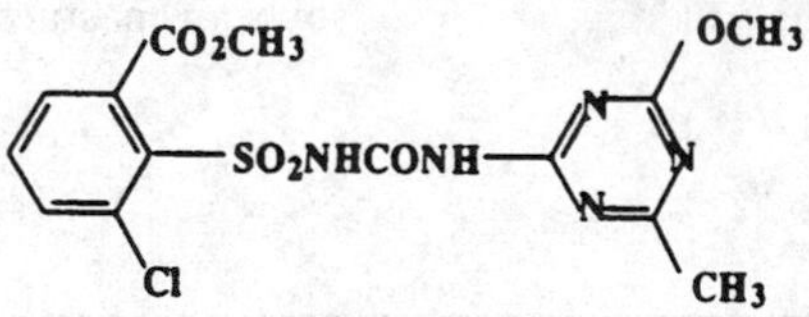	Cereals	4–7.5
Nicosulfuron Accent® (300)	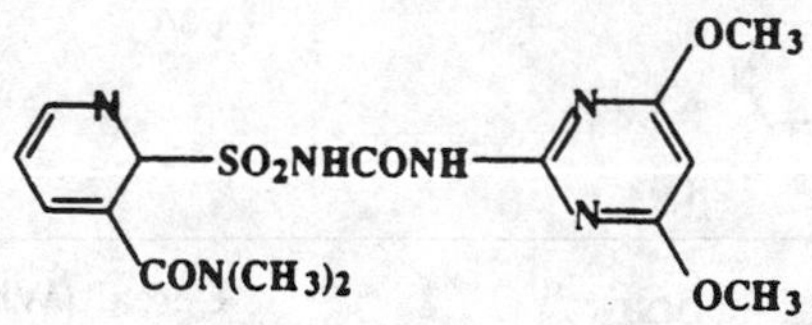	Corn	35–70

Table 13.40
More structures and uses of the ALS sulfonylurea herbicides

Chemical/ Common Names	Structure	Principle Uses/Crops	Application Rate (grams a.i./ha/yr.)
Oxasulfuron Expert® (60)	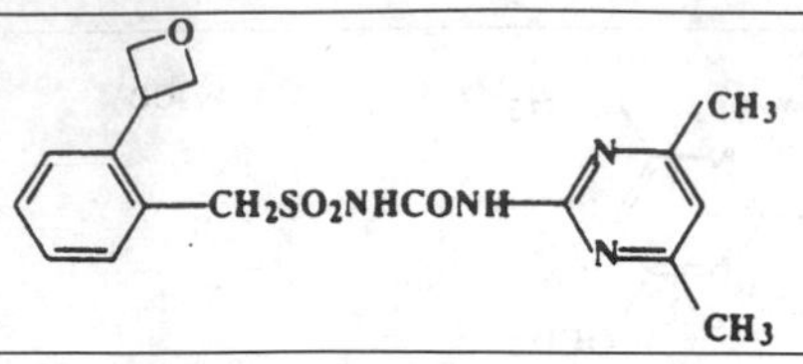	Soybeans	32
Primisulfuron-methyl Beacon® (304)	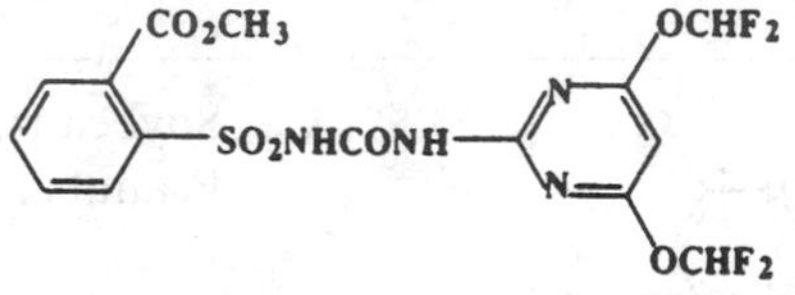	Corn	20–40
Prosulfuron Peak® (66)	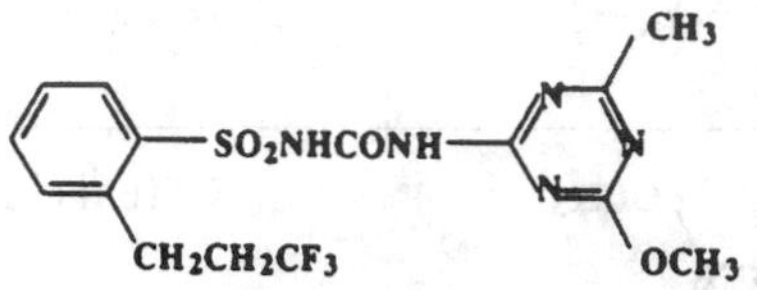	Cereals, Corn, Sorghum, Pasture	10–40
Rimsulfuron Matrix® (71)	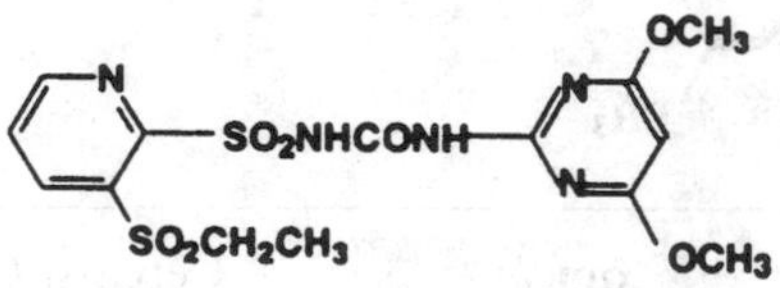	Corn, Tomatoes, and potatoes	15000
Sulfometuron-methyl Oust® (310)	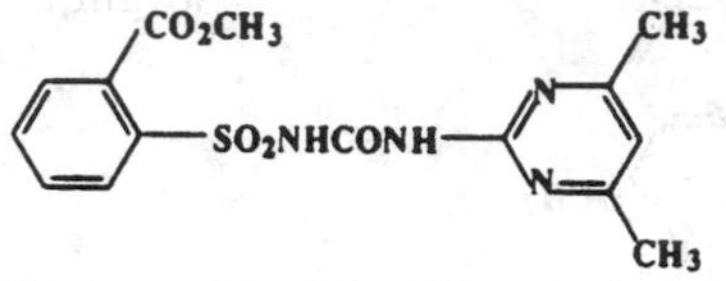	IWC	NA
Sulfosulfuron (Under Development) (73)	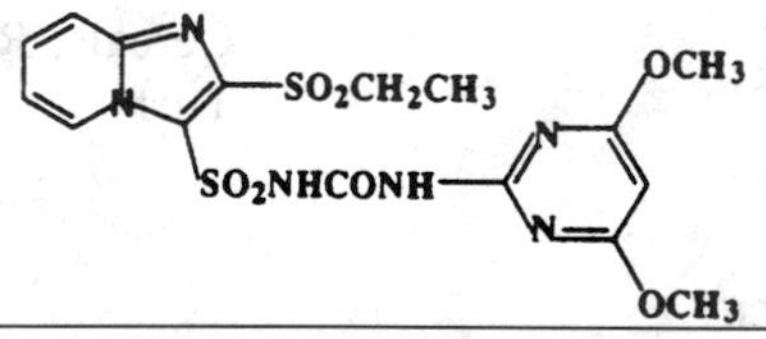	Cereal (Wheat) IWC	10–35
Thifensulfuron-methyl Pinnacle®, Harmony® (312)	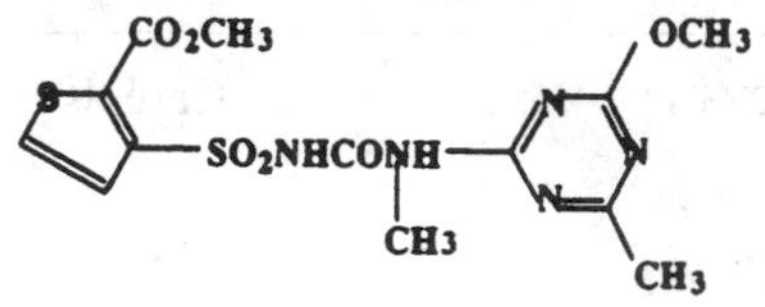	Cereals, corn, soybean, pastures	9–60
Triasulfuron Amber®, Logran® (313)	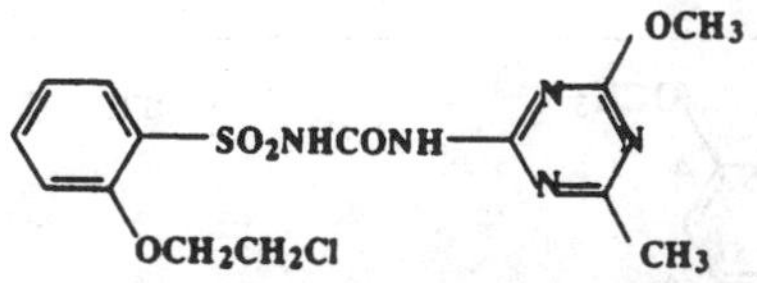	Cereal (Wheat), IWC	10
Tribenuron-methyl Express® (314)	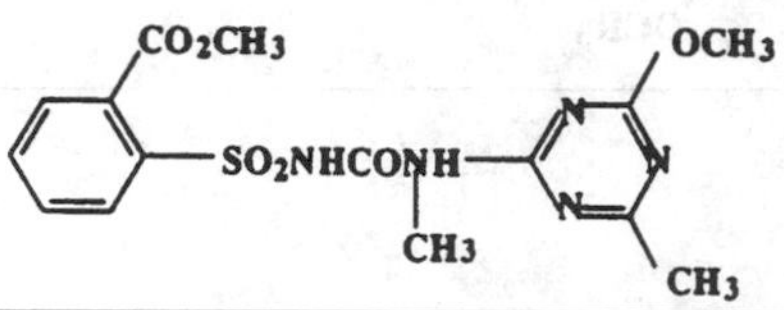	Cereal (Wheat)	9–30

NA = Not Available

Table 13.41
Hazard profile for ALS sulfonylurea herbicides

	Irritation		LD_{50} (mg/kg)		LC_{50} (mg/L)		
Herbicide	Eye	Skin	Oral	Dermal	Inhalation	Sensitizing Potential	Signal Word
Bensulfuron (269)	Non-Irritant	Non-Irritant	> 5000	> 2000	> 7.5	NA	Caution
Chlorimuron (276)	Non-Irritant	Non-Irritant	4102	> 2000	> 5.0	Negative	Caution
Chlorsulfuron (274)	Slight Irritant	Non-Irritant	5545(♂)	2500	> 5.9	Negative	Caution
Halosulfuron (236)	NA	NA	8866	> 2000	NA	NA	Caution
Imazosulfuron (49)	Non-Irritant	Non-Irritant	> 5000	> 2000	> 2.4	Negative	Caution
Metsulfuron (297)	Mod. Irritant	Mild Irritant	> 5000	> 2000	> 5.0	Negative	Caution

Herbicide	Species/study	NOEL[1] (mg/kg/day)	Toxicity Studies	Hazard Indicator
Bensulfuron	Rat/2-year	37.5	Mutagenicity	No evidence
	Dog/52-week	227	Developmental	Not teratogenic
	Mouse/18-month	455	Reproductive	Not reproductive toxin
	ADI[2]	0.2	Oncogenicity	No evidence
Chlorimuron	Rat/2-year	12.5	Mutagenicity	No evidence
	Dog/52-week	6.25	Developmental	Not Teratogenic
	Mouse/18-month	180	Reproductive	No evidence
	ADI[2]	0.02	Oncogenicity	No evidence
Chlorsulfuron	Rat/2-year	5	Mutagenicity	No evidence
	Dog/52-week	50	Developmental	Not teratogenic
	Mouse/18-month	71	Reproductive	No evidence
	RfD[2]	0.05	Oncogenicity	No evidence
Halosulfuron	Rat/2-year	50	Mutagenicity	No evidence
	Dog/52-week	10	Developmental	Not Teratogenic
	Mouse/18-month	430	Reproductive	No evidence
	ADI[2]	0.1	Oncogenicity	No evidence
Imazosulfuron	Rat/2-year	106(♂)	Mutagenicity	No evidence
	Dog/52-week	75	Developmental	Teratogenic in mice
	Mouse/18-month	NA	Reproductive	No evidence
	RfD or ADI[2]	NA	Oncogenicity	No evidence
Metsulfuron	Rat/2-year	25	Mutagenicity	No evidence
	Dog/52-week	12.5(♀)	Developmental	Not teratogenic
	Mouse/18-month	710	Reproductive	No evidence
	ADI (Germany)[2]	0.0125	Oncogenicity	No evidence

[1] No observable effect level; Dietary concentration (ppm) was converted to daily dose (mg/kg/day) by dividing by 20, 7, or 40 for the rat, mouse and dog, respectively.
[2] RfD = reference dose and ADI = acceptable daily intake
[3] See Table 13.3 for US EPA classification scheme
NA = Not Available

Table 13.42
Hazard profile for more ALS sulfonylurea herbicides

Herbicide	Irritation: Eye	Irritation: Skin	LD_{50} (mg/kg): Oral	LD_{50} (mg/kg): Dermal	LC_{50} (mg/L): Inhalation	Sensitizing Potential	Signal Word
Nicosulfuron (300)	Mod. Irritant	NA	> 5000	> 2000	5.47	Negative	Caution
Oxasulfuron (60)	Non-Irritant	Non-Irritant	> 5000	> 2000	5.08	Negative	Caution
Primisulfuron (304)	Slight Irritant	Non-Irritant	> 5050	> 2010	> 4.8	Negative	Caution
Prosulfuron (66)	Non-Irritant	Non-Irritant	986	> 2000	> 5.0	Negative	Caution
Rimsulfuron (71,262)	Mod. irritant	Non-Irritant	> 5000	> 2000	> 5.4	Negative	Caution
Sulfometuron (310)	Slight irritant	Slight irritant	> 5000	> 2000	> 11	Negative	Caution

Herbicide	Species/study	NOEL[1] (mg/kg/day)	Toxicity Studies	Hazard Indicator
Nicosulfuron	Rat/2-year	1000	Mutagenicity	No evidence
	Dog/52-week	125	Developmental	Not teratogenic
	Mouse/18-month	1070	Reproductive	No evidence
	ADI[2]	1.25	Oncogenicity	No evidence
Oxasulfuron	Rat/2-year	8.3	Mutagenicity	No evidence
	Dog/52-week	1.3	Developmental	Not teratogenic
	Mouse/18-month	1.5	Reproductive	No evidence
	ADI[2]	0.0026	Oncogenicity	No evidence
Primisulfuron	Rat/2-year	13	Mutagenicity	No evidence
	Dog/52-week	25	Developmental	Not teratogenic
	Mouse/18-month	45	Reproductive	Testicular degeneration
	ADI[2]	0.13	Oncogenicity	D (Liver tumor in ♂ mice doses>MTD)[3]
Prosulfuron	Rat/2-year	8.6	Mutagenicity	No evidence
	Dog/52-week	1.9	Developmental	Not teratogenic
	Mouse/18-month	80	Reproductive	No evidence
	ADI[2]	0.019	Oncogenicity	D (mammary tumors in ♀ rats—early onset)[3]
Rimsulfuron	Rat/2-year	11.8	Mutagenicity	No evidence
	Dog/52-week	1.6	Developmental	Not teratogenic
	Mouse/18-month	351	Reproductive	No evidence
	RfD[2]	0.016	Oncogenicity	No evidence
Sulfometuron	Rat/2-year	2.5	Mutagenicity	No evidence
	Dog/52-week	5.0	Developmental	Teratogenic: 2 species
	Mouse/18-month	140	Reproductive	No evidence
	ADI[2]	0.025	Oncogenicity	No evidence

[1] No observable effect level; Dietary concentration (ppm) was converted to daily dose (mg/kg/day) by dividing by 20, 7, or 40 for the rat, mouse and dog, respectively.
[2] RfD = reference dose and ADI = acceptable daily intake
[3] See Table 13.3 for US EPA classification scheme
NA = Not Available

Table 13.43
Hazard profile for other ALS sulfonylurea herbicides

Herbicide	Irritation		LD_{50} (mg/kg)		LC_{50} (mg/L)	Sensitizing	Signal
	Eye	Skin	Oral	Dermal	Inhalation	Potential	Word
Sulfosulfuron (73)	Non-Irritant	Slight irritant	> 5000	> 5000	NA	Negative	Caution
Thifensulfuron (312)	Slight Irritant	Non-Irritant	> 5000	> 2000	> 7.9	Negative	Caution
Trisulfuron (313)	Slight Irritant	Non-irritant	> 5000	> 2000	> 5.1	Negative	Caution
Tribenuron (314)	Slight Irritant	Non-irritant	> 5000	> 2000	> 5.0	Positive	Caution

Herbicide	Species/study	NOEL[1] (mg/kg/day)	Toxicity Studies	Hazard Indicator
Sulfosulfuron	Rat/2-year	NA	Mutagenicity	NA
	Dog/52-week	NA	Developmental	NA
	Mouse/18-month	NA	Reproductive	NA
	ADI[2]	NA	Oncogenicity	NA
Thifensulfuron	Rat/2-year	2.6	Mutagenicity	No evidence
	Dog/52-week	19	Developmental	Not teratogenic
	Mouse/18-month	1070	Reproductive	No evidence
	ADI[2]	0.026	Oncogenicity	No evidence
Triasulfuron	Rat/2-year	32.1	Mutagenicity	No evidence
	Dog/52-week	33	Developmental	Not teratogenic
	Mouse/18-month	1.2	Reproductive	No evidence
	ADI[2]	0.012	Oncogenicity	No evidence
Tribenuron	Rat/2-year	1.25	Mutagenicity	No evidence
	Dog/52-week	8.2	Developmental	Not teratogenic
	Mouse/18-month	30	Reproductive	No evidence
	ADI[2]	0.011	Oncogenicity	C (Mammary tumors in ♀ rats—early onset)[3]

[1] No observable effect level; Dietary concentration (ppm) was converted to daily dose (mg/kg/day) by dividing by 20, 7, or 40 for the rat, mouse and dog, respectively.
[2] RfD = reference dose and ADI = acceptable daily intake
[3] See Table 13.3 for US EPA classification scheme
NA = Not Available

Triazolopyrimidines

The triazolopyrimidine class of ALS inhibitors registered for herbicidal use includes imazamox, imazapyr, imazaquin, and imazethapyr. As with the imidazolinones, these chemicals also have excellent hazard profiles (Table 13.45). No evidence of significant target organ toxicity or mutagenic, developmental, or oncogenic potential has been realized even at doses that approximate the limit dose of 1000 mg/kg.

Pyrimidinylthiobenzoates

The members of this class of ALS-inhibiting herbicides, flumetsulam and pyriminobac-methyl (Table 13.46), are less well tolerated in mammalian systems than for other ALS inhibitors as evidence by lower no observed effect levels. However, the hazard profile for these chemicals is still favorable since no mutagenic, developmental, or oncogenic effects have been reported.

Photosynthesis Inhibitors

The photosynthesis inhibitors include triazines, phenylureas, uracils, benzothiadiazoles, nitriles, carbamate, and dicarboxylic acid. Photosynthesis inhibitors shut down the photosynthetic (food-producing) process in susceptible plants by binding to specific sites within

Table 13.44
Structures, uses, and hazard profiles of the ALS imidazolinone herbicides

Chemical/ Common Names	Structure	Principle Uses/Crops	Application Rate (grams a.i./ha/yr.)
Imazameth Cadre® (188)	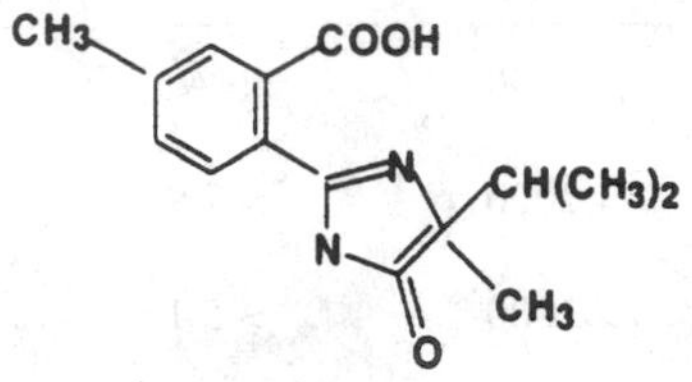	Soybeans, peanuts, sugarcane	NA
Imazamethabenz -methyl Assert® (289)	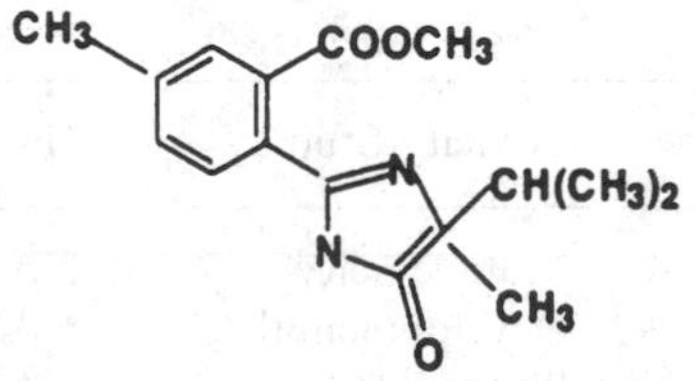	Wheat, barley Sunflower	350–530 Post 200–430 Post

Herbicide	Irritation		LD_{50} (mg/kg)		LC_{50} (mg/L)	Sensitizing Potential	Signal Word
	Eye	Skin	Oral	Dermal	Inhalation		
Imazameth	NA	Non-irritant	> 5000	> 5000	2.38	NA	Caution
Imazamethabenz -methyl	Slight Irritant	Non-irritant	> 5000	> 2000	> 5.8	Negative	Caution

Herbicide	Species/study	NOEL[1](mg/kg/day)	Toxicity Studies	Hazard Indicator
Imazameth	Rat/2-year	1029 ♂	Mutagenicity	No evidence
	Dog/52-week	>137	Developmental	Not teratogenic
	Mouse/18-month	1134 ♂	Reproductive	No evidence
	RfD[2](300×UF[4])	0.5	Oncogenicity	No evidence
Imazamethabenz-methyl	Rat/2-year	12.5	Mutagenicity	No evidence
	Dog/52-week	6.25	Developmental	Not teratogenic
	Mouse/18-month	19.5	Reproductive	No evidence
	ADI[2]	0.06	Oncogenicity	No evidence

[1] No observable effect level; Dietary concentration (ppm) was converted to daily dose (mg/kg/day) by dividing by 20, 7, or 40 for the rat, mouse and dog, respectively.
[2] RfD = reference dose and ADI = acceptable daily intake
[3] See Table 13.3 for US EPA classification scheme
[4] Uncertainty factor
NA = Not Available

the plant chloroplast. Inhibition of photosynthesis could result in a slow starvation of the plant; however, in many situations rapid death occurs, perhaps from the production of secondary toxic substances (101). The triazines, uracils, substituted ureas, benzothiadiazoles, and phenylpyridazines inhibit electron flow in Photosystem II, leading to destruction of cellular membranes and plant death. The bipyridyliums inhibit Photosystem I electron flow.

Injury signs include yellowing (chlorosis) of leaf tissue followed by death (necrosis) of the tissue. Three of the herbicide families (triazines, phenylureas, and uracils) are taken up into the plant via the roots or foliage and move in the xylem to plant leaves. As a result, injury signs will first appear on the older leaves, along the leaf margin. Foliar-applied photosynthetic inhibitors generally remain in the foliar portions of the treated plant, and movement from foliage to roots is negligible.

Table 13.45
Structures, uses, and hazard profiles of the ALS triazolopyrimidines

Chemical/ Common Names	Structure	Principle Uses/Crops	Application Rate gm (a.i)/ha
Imazamox Raptor®: Pending (213)	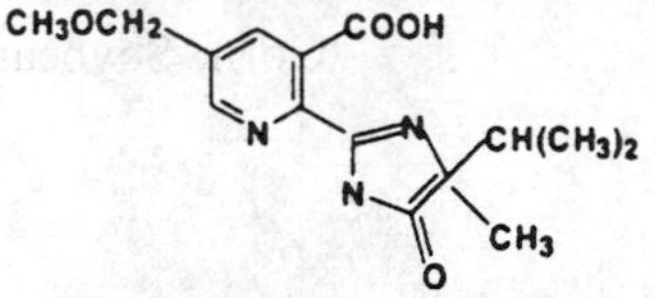	Soybeans, legumes	0.032–0.04 lbs./acre
Imazapyr Arsenal® (290)	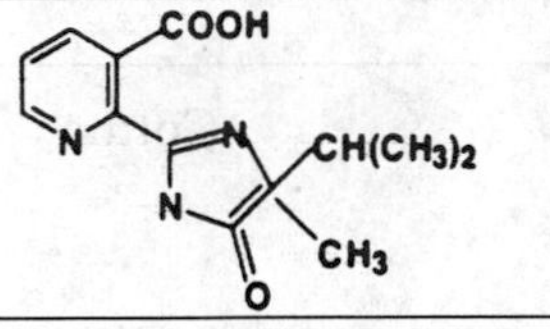	IWC	560–1700 POST
Imazaquin Scepter® (291)	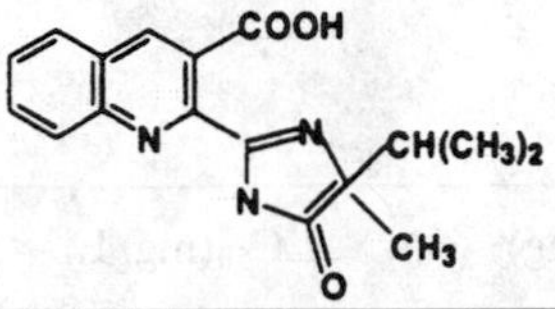	Soybeans	70–140 Pre-Plant, PPI, PRE POST
Imazethapyr Pursuit® (292)	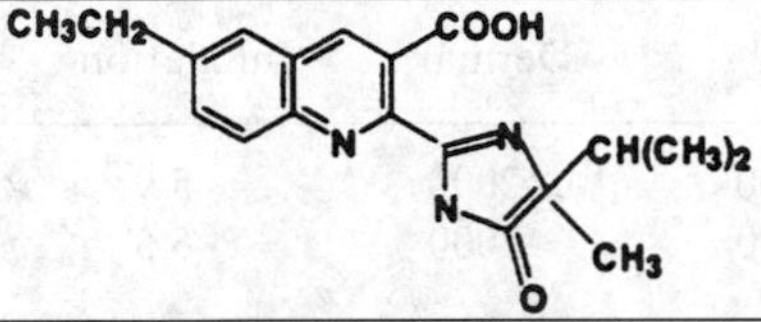	Soybeans, Corn Legume, Peanuts	35–70 Early Pre-Plant, PPI, PRE, POST

Herbicide	Irritation: Eye	Irritation: Skin	LD_{50} (mg/kg): Oral	LD_{50} (mg/kg): Dermal	LC_{50} (mg/L): Inhalation	Sensitizing Potential	Signal Word
Imazamox	Mild irritant	Non-irritant	> 5000	> 4000	> 6.3	Negative	Caution
Imazapyr	Irreversible	Non-irritant	> 5000	> 2000	> 1.3	Negative	Danger
Imazaquin	Non-irritant	Slight irritant	> 5000	> 2000	> 5.7	Negative	Caution
Imazethapyr	Slight Irritant	Slight Irritant	> 5000	> 2000	> 2.6	Negative	Caution

Herbicide	Species/study	NOEL[1] (mg/kg/day)	Toxicity Studies	Hazard Indicator
Imazamox	Rat/2-year	1068	Mutagenicity	No evidence
	Dog/52-week	1165	Developmental	Not teratogenic
	Mouse/18-month	NA	Reproductive	No evidence
	RfD[2]	3.0	Oncogenicity	E (No evidence)[1]
Imazapyr	Rat/2-year	500	Mutagenicity	No evidence
	Dog/52-week	250	Developmental	Not teratogenic
	Mouse/18-month	1500	Reproductive	No evidence
	ADI[2]	2.5	Oncogenicity	No evidence
Imazaquin	Rat/2-year	500	Mutagenicity	No evidence
	Dog/52-week	25	Developmental	Not teratogenic
	Mouse/18-month	150	Reproductive	No evidence
	ADI[2]	0.25	Oncogenicity	No evidence
Imazethapyr	Rat/2-year	500	Mutagenicity	No evidence
	Dog/52-week	25	Developmental	Not teratogenic
	Mouse/18-month	750	Reproductive	No evidence
	ADI[2]	0.25	Oncogenicity	No evidence

[1] See Table 13.3 for US EPA classification scheme
NA = Not Available

Table 13.46
Structures, uses, and hazard profiles of the ALS pyrimidinylthiobenzoates

Chemical/ Common Names	Structure	Principle Uses/Crops	Application Rate gm (a.i.)/ha
Flumetsulam Broadstrike® (282)	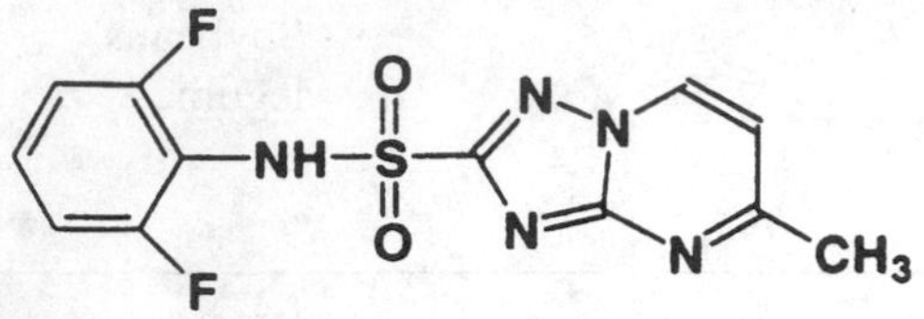	Corn, Soybeans	52.5–78
Pyriminobac-methyl Prosper® (69)	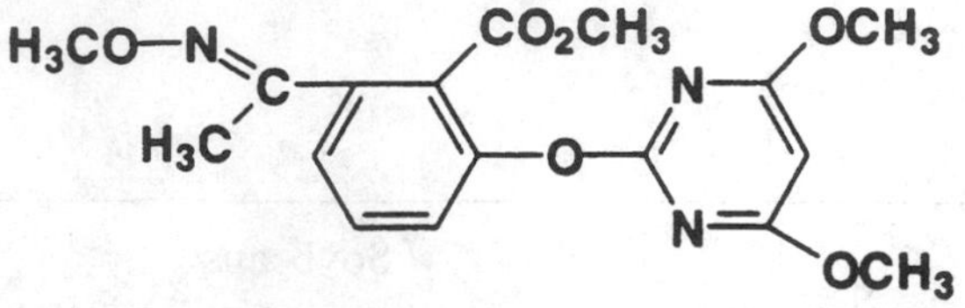	Cotton	70–105

Herbicide	Irritation		LD_{50} (mg/kg)		LC_{50}(mg/L)	Sensitizing Potential	Signal Word
	Eye	Skin	Oral	Dermal	Inhalation		
Flumetsulam	Slight irritant	Non-irritant	> 5000	> 2000	> 5.9	Negative	Caution
Pyriminobac-methyl	Slight irritant	Slight irritant	> 5000	> 2000	> 5.5	NA	Caution

Herbicide	Species/study	NOEL[1] (mg/kg/day)	Toxicity Studies	Hazard Indicator
Flumetsulum	Rat/2-year	35	Mutagenicity	No evidence
	Dog/52-week	100	Developmental	Not teratogenic
	Mouse/18-month	32	Reproductive	No evidence
	ADI[2]	0.32	Oncogenicity	No evidence
Pyriminobac-methyl	Rat/2-year	0.9	Mutagenicity	No evidence
	Dog/52-week	NA	Developmental	Not teratogenic
	Mouse/18-month	8.1	Reproductive	No evidence
	ADI[2]	0.009	Oncogenicity	No evidence

[1] No observable effect level; Dietary concentration (ppm) was converted to daily dose (mg/kg/day) by dividing by 20, 7, or 40 for the rat, mouse and dog, respectively.
[2] RfD = reference dose and ADI = acceptable daily intake
[3] See Table 13.3 for US EPA classification scheme
NA = Not Available

Triazines and Triazinone

The triazine herbicides inhibit the Hill reaction in the process of photosynthesis (161). This unique mechanism of action is specific to photosynthesizing plants. Therefore, the triazines do not exhibit significant mammalian toxicity but rather target-species selectivity. The structures and uses of the symmetrical triazines and an asymmetrical triazine or triazinone, metribuzin, are presented in Table 13.47.

The hazard profiles of these agents are presented in Tables 13.48 and 13.49.

These triazines are generally not acutely toxic, nor do they cause a significant repeated dose toxicity. The one exception appears to be the symmetrical chlorotriazines, atrazine, cyanazine, propazine, and simazine, which in lifetime feeding studies in Sprague-Dawley female rats induce an earlier onset and/or an increase in the incidence of mammary tumors (161,176). The relevance of these tumors to humans has been the subject of intense research and evaluation (94,164,317).

Recently, the International Agency for Research on Cancer reexamined atrazine and simazine (105). Both were classified as "not classifiable as to carcinogenicity

Table 13.47
Structures and uses of selected photosynthesis-inhibiting herbicides: Triazines and triazinones

Herbicide	Structure	Principle Crops/uses	Use rates
Atrazine Aatrex® (268)	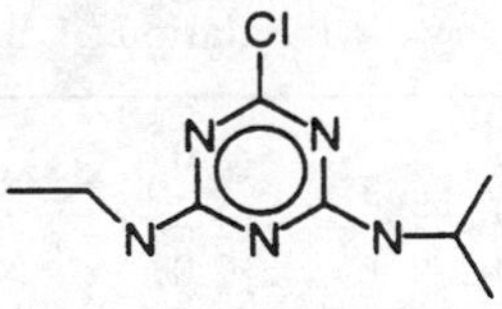	Pre- and post-emergence control of annual broad-leaved and annual grasses in corn, sorghum, sugar cane, and pineapple	1.5 to 2.5 kilograms (a.i.)/hectare
Cyanazine Bladex® (276)	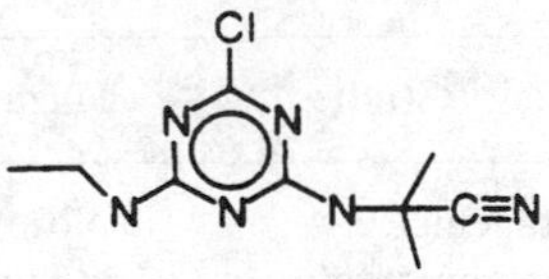	Pre-emergence in broad beans, corn and peas; and post-emergence in barley and wheat	1 to 3 kilograms (a.i.)/hectare 0.26 to 0.33 kilograms (a.i.)/hectare
Propazine Milo-Pro® (222)	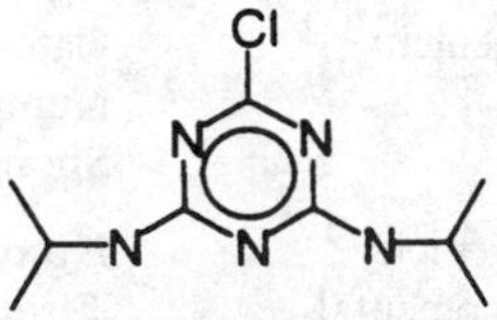	Pre- and post-emergence control of annual broad-leaved and annual grasses in sorghum, carrots, chervil, and parsley	0.5 to 3 kilograms (a.i.)/hectare
Simazine Princep® (309)	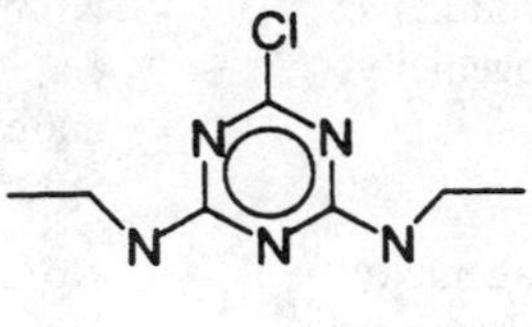	Pre- and post-emergence control of annual broad-leaved and annual grasses in pome fruit, stone fruit, citrus, vines, corn, sorghum, sugar cane, and pineapple	1.5 to 3 kilograms (a.i.)/hectare
Ametryn Evik® (266)	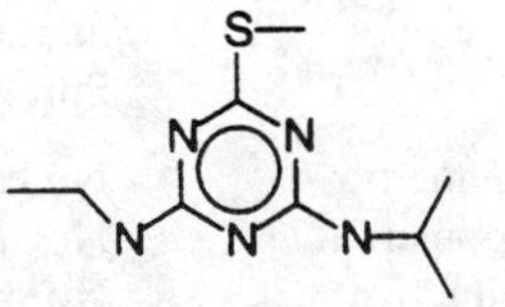	Pre- and post-emergence control of annual broad-leaved and annual grasses in bananas, citrus fruit, corn, coffee, sugar cane, and pineapple	2 to 4 kilograms (a.i.)/hectare
Prometryn Caparol® (244,306)	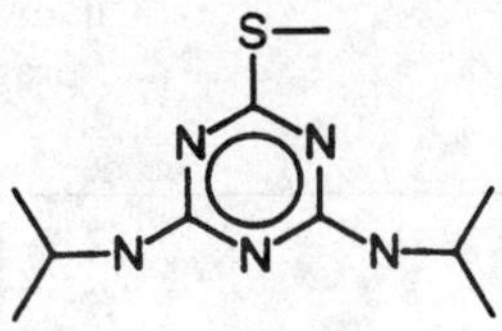	Pre-emergence in vegetables, cotton, sunflower, and peanuts and post-emergence in cotton and vegetables	0.8 to 2.5 kilograms (a.i.)/hectare 0.8 to 1.5 kilograms (a.i.)/hectare
Prometon Pramitol® (305)	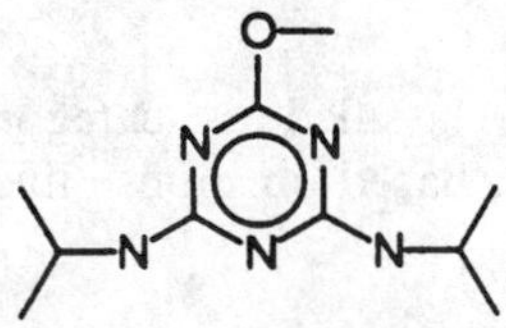	Control of most annual and many perennial broad-leaved weeds, grasses and brush weeds in non-crop areas	10 to 20 kilograms (a.i.)/hectare
Metribuzin Sencor® (296)	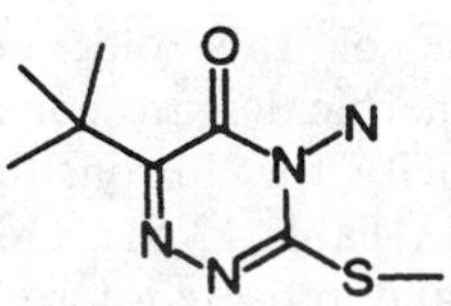	Pre- and post-emergence control of annual broad-leaved and annual grasses in soya beans, potatoes, corn, cereals, sugar cane, alfalfa, and asparagus	0.35 to 0.7 kilograms (a.i.)/hectare

Table 13.48
Hazard profiles for selected photosynthesis-inhibiting herbicides: Triazines (165)

Herbicide	Irritation: Eye	Irritation: Skin	LD_{50} (mg/kg): Oral	LD_{50} (mg/kg): Dermal	LC_{50} (mg/L): Inhalation	Sensitizing Potential	Signal Word
Atrazine	Not irritant	Not irritant	3090	> 3100	> 5.0	Positive	Caution
Cyanazine	Not irritant	Not irritant	182	> 2000	> 5.3	Negative	Warning
Propazine	Mild irritant	Not irritant	> 7000	> 3100	> 2.0	Negative	Caution
Simazine	Not irritant	Mild irritant	> 5000	> 3100	> 5.5	Negative	Caution

Herbicide	Species/study	NOEL[1] (mg/kg/day)	Toxicity Studies	Hazard Indicator
Atrazine	Rat/2-year	0.5	Mutagenicity	No evidence
	Dog/52-week	3.75	Developmental	Not teratogenic
	Mouse/18-month	1.2	Reproductive	No evidence
	ADI[2]	0.005	Oncogenicity	Category C with CSF (based mammary tumors in female Sprague-Dawley rats)[3]
Cyanazine	Rat/2-year	12	Mutagenicity	No evidence
	Dog/52-week	25	Developmental	Teratogenic in rats and rabbits
	Mouse/18-month	1.4	Reproductive	No evidence
	ADI[2]	NA	Oncogenicity	Category C with CSF (based mammary tumors in female Sprague-Dawley rats)[3]
Propazine	Rat/2-year	5.8	Mutagenicity	No evidence
	Dog/52-week	1.3	Developmental	Not teratogenic
	Mouse/18-month	15	Reproductive	No evidence
	RfD[2]	0.02 (based on the 2-yr. rat study with 300×UF[4])	Oncogenicity	Category C with CSF (based mammary tumors in female Sprague-Dawley rats)[3]
Simazine	Rat/2-year	0.5	Mutagenicity	No evidence
	Dog/52-week	7.5	Developmental	Not teratogenic
	Mouse/18-month	5.7	Reproductive	No evidence
	ADI[2]	0.005	Oncogenicity	Category C with CSF (based mammary tumors in female Sprague-Dawley rats[3]

[1] No observable effect level
[2] RfD = reference dose and ADI = acceptable daily intake
[3] See Table 13.3 for US EPA classification scheme, CSF = cancer slope factor
[4] UF = Uncertainty factor

to humans" when mechanistic data were taken into account in making the overall evaluation.

Uracils and Pyridazinones

The structures, uses, and toxicity profiles for two uracils and a pyridazinone herbicide are given in Table 13.50.

The acute hazard associated with bromacil, terbacil, and norflurazon is unremarkable. None of these products have been found to represent a mutagenic, teratogenic, or reproductive hazard. However, bromacil and norflurazon have been classified as category C (possible human carcinogen), based on mouse liver tumors.

Ureas

Three ureas of this older class of photosynthesis-inhibiting herbicides are considered. The structures, uses, and toxicity for diuron, flumeturon, and linuron are provided in Table 13.51.

The acute and repeated-dose toxicity of these three ureas is nonproblematic until the oncogenic potential of these compounds is examined. Both diuron and linuron

Table 13.49

Hazard profiles for more selected photosynthesis-inhibiting herbicides: More triazines and triazinone (165)

Herbicide	Irritation		LD_{50} (mg/kg)		LC_{50} (mg/L)	Sensitizing Potential	Signal Word
	Eye	Skin	Oral	Dermal	Inhalation		
Ametryn	Not irritant	Not irritant	1160	> 2020	> 5.1	Positive	Caution
Prometryn	Slight irritant	Not irritant	4550	> 2020	> 5.1	Negative	Caution
Prometon	Irritant	Mild irritant	1518	> 2020	> 3.2	Negative	Warning
Metribuzin	Not irritant	Not irritant	1090	> 20000	> 0.65	Negative	Caution

Herbicide	Species/study	NOEL[1] (mg/kg/day)	Toxicity Studies	Hazard Indicator
Ametryn	Rat/2-year	2.5	Mutagenicity	No evidence
	Dog/52-week	10	Developmental	Not teratogenic
	Mouse/18-month	1.5	Reproductive	No evidence
	RfD[2]	0.025	Oncogenicity	E (No evidence)[3]
Prometryn	Rat/2-year	37	Mutagenicity	No evidence
	Dog/106-Week Oral	3.7	Developmental	Not teratogenic
	Mouse/102-Week Oral	1.0	Reproductive	No evidence
	RfD[2]	0.037 (based on the 2-yr. dog study with 100 × UF[4])	Oncogenicity	E (No evidence)[3]
Prometon	Rat/2-year	1.0	Mutagenicity	No evidence
	Dog/52-week	5.0	Developmental	Not teratogenic
	Mouse/18-month	70	Reproductive	No evidence
	RfD[2]	0.01	Oncogenicity	No evidence
Metribuzin	Rat/2-year	5.0	Mutagenicity	No evidence
	Dog/104-Week Oral	2.5	Developmental	Not teratogenic
	Mouse/18-month	120	Reproductive	No evidence
	RfD[2]	0.025 (based on 2-yr. dog—100×UF[4])	Oncogenicity	No evidence

[1] No observable effect level
[2] RfD = reference dose and ADI = acceptable daily intake
[3] See Table 13.3 for US EPA classification scheme
[4] UF = Uncertainty factor

have been classified by the U.S. EPA with the known or likely designation as defined in the EPA 1996 classification scheme (192) or as category C (possible human carcinogen) based on the earlier scheme (146). The classification of flumeturon is still pending.

Amides and Nitriles

The structures of two nitriles, dichlobenil and ioxynil, and one amide, isoxaben, are presented along with their uses and toxicology profiles in Table 13.52.

Ioxynil's profile suggests minimal hazard. Dichlobenil is flagged for its oncogenic potential and received a category C designation based on mouse liver tumors. Isoxaben represents a bit more concern as it has been found to be weakly mutagenic and elicits liver tumors in the mouse and adrenal tumors in the rat.

Benzothiadiazoles and Phenylpyridazine

One example of a benzothiazole and a phenylpyridazine photosynthesis inhibitor are presented in Table 13.53.

Bentazon and pyridate have been found to have acute and repeated-dose profiles that suggest minimal hazard to humans.

Bipyridyliums

Diquat and paraquat, bipyridylium photosynthesis inhibitors, are unlike the triazines, uracils, substituted ureas, benzothiadiazoles, and phenylpyridazines in that they inhibit electron flow in Photosystem I. The structures, uses, and hazard profiles for diquat and paraquat are provided in Table 13.54.

Table 13.50
Structures, uses, and hazard profiles for selected photosynthesis-inhibiting herbicides: Uracils and pyridazinone

Herbicide	Structure	Principle Uses/Crops	Application Rate gm (a.i.)/ha
Bromacil Hyvar® (271)	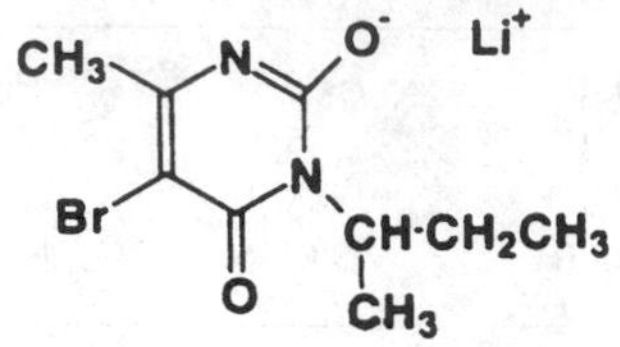	Used to control grasses, broadleaf weeds, and brush in non-cropland area	900–7180
Terbacil Sinbar® (301)	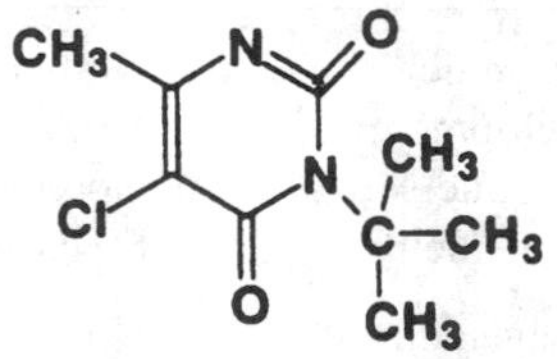	Used to control grasses, and broadleaf weeds in nut trees, mint, alfalfa, and fruits.	450–3580
Norflurazon Predict® (311)	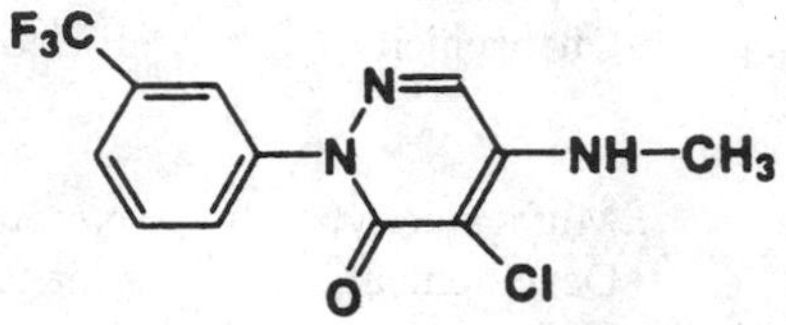	Used to control broadleaf weeds and sedges in fruits, nuts and berries.	560–4500
		Also used on right of ways	9000

Herbicide	Irritation		LD_{50} (mg/kg)		LC_{50} (mg/L)	Sensitizing Potential	Signal Word
	Eye	Skin	Oral	Dermal	Inhalation		
Bromacil	Mild irritant	Mild irritant	5175	> 5000	> 4.8	Positive	Caution
Terbacil	Mild irritant	Not irritant	1255	> 5000	> 4.4	Negative	Caution
Norflurazon	Not irritant	Not irritant	9000	> 20000	NA	Negative	Caution

Herbicide	Species/study	NOEL[1] (mg/kg/day)	Toxicity Studies	Hazard Indicator
Bromacil	Rat/2-year	2.5	Mutagenicity	No evidence
	Dog/52-week	15.6	Developmental	Not teratogenic
	Mouse/18-month	NA	Reproductive	No evidence
	RfD[2]	0.1	Oncogenicity	C (liver tumors in male mice)[3]
Terbacil	Rat/2-year	2.5	Mutagenicity	No evidence
	Dog/104-week	1.25	Developmental	Not teratogenic
	Mouse/18-month	7.1	Reproductive	No evidence
	ADI[2]	0.013	Oncogenicity	E(No evidence)[3]
Norflurazon	Rat/2-year	19	Mutagenicity	No evidence
	Dog/26-week	1.6	Developmental	Not teratogenic
	Mouse/18-month	41	Reproductive	No evidence
	RfD[2]	0.02	Oncogenicity	C (Liver tumors in mice)[3]

[1] No observable effect level
[2] RfD = reference dose
[3] See Table 13.3 for US EPA classification scheme
NA = Not Available

Table 13.51
Structures, uses, and hazard profiles for selected photosynthesis-inhibiting herbicides: Ureas

Herbicide	Structure	Principle Uses/Crops	Application Rate gm (a.i.)/ha
Diuron Diumate® (205,281)	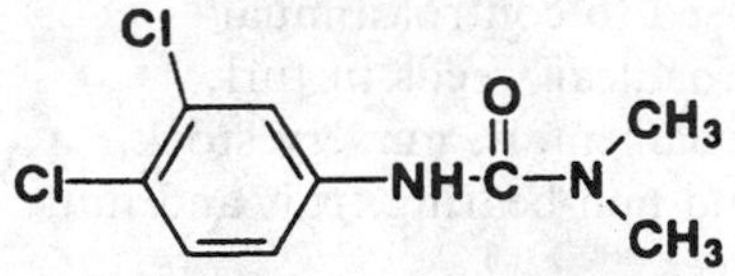	Used to control many annual weeds at lower rates and perennials at higher rates in nuts, berries, spices, and cereals.	200–6400
Fluometuron Cotoran® (284)	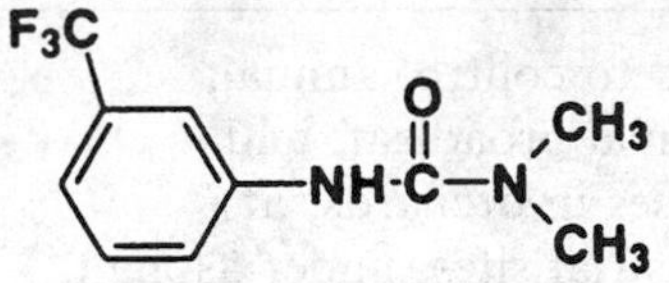	Used to control broadleaf weeds and grasses.	1120–2240
Linuron Lorox® (295)	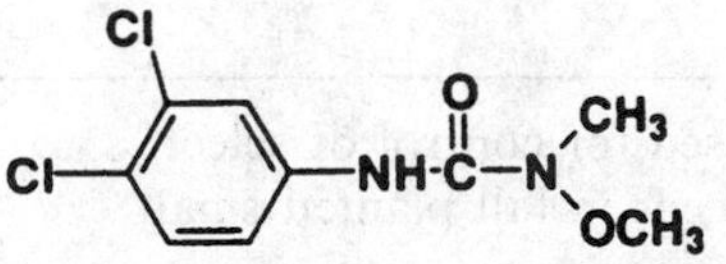	Used to control broadleaf weeds in vegetable and cereals.	250–2240

Herbicide	Irritation: Eye	Irritation: Skin	LD_{50} (mg/kg): Oral	LD_{50} (mg/kg): Dermal	LC_{50} (mg/L): Inhalation	Sensitizing Potential	Signal Word
Diuron	Mild irritant	Not irritant	3400	2000	>2.5	Negative	Caution
Fluometuron	Slight irritant	Not irritant	6416	> 10000	> 2.0	Negative	Caution
Linuron	Not irritant	Not irritant	1090	> 20000	> 0.65	Negative	Caution

Herbicide	Species/study	NOEL[1] (mg/kg/day)	Toxicity Studies	Hazard Indicator
Diuron (205)	Rat/2-year	<1.02	Mutagenicity	No evidence
	Dog/104-week	0.625	Developmental	Not teratogenic
	Mouse/18-month	>50 (LDT)	Reproductive	No evidence
	RfD[2] (300×UF[5])	0.002	Oncogenicity	"Known/Likely" (liver/mice; bladder/rats)[4]
Fluometuron	Rat/2-year	0.55	Mutagenicity	No evidence
	Dog/52-week	10	Developmental	Not teratogenic
	Mouse/18-month	1.3	Reproductive	No evidence
	ADI[2]	0.0055	Oncogenicity	Classification pending[3]
Linuron	Rat/2-year	2.5	Mutagenicity	No evidence
	Dog/104-Week Oral	0.77	Developmental	Not teratogenic
	Mouse/18-month	21	Reproductive	No evidence
	RfD[2]	0.008	Oncogenicity	C (Interstitial cell tumors in male rats)[3]

[1] No observable effect level
[2] RfD = reference dose
[3] See Table 13.3 for US EPA classification scheme
[4] 1996 US EPA carcinogen classification system
[5] UF = Uncertainty factor

Table 13.52
Structures, uses, and hazard profile for selected photosynthesis-inhibiting herbicides: Amides and nitriles

Herbicide	Structure	Principle Uses/Crops	Application Rate gm (a.i.)/ha
Isoxaben Gallery™ (294)	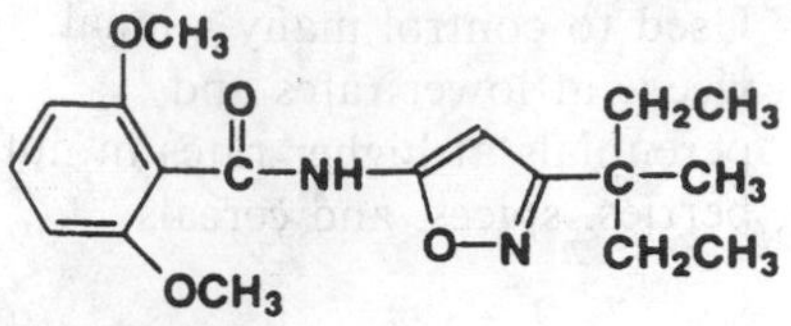	Used to control annual broadleaf weeds in turf, ornamentals, nursery stock, and non-bearing fruit and nut trees.	560–1120
Dichlobenil Acme® (277)	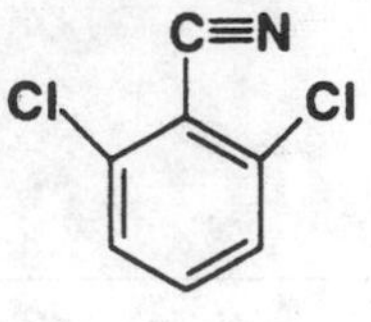	Used to control annual, biennial broadleaf, and grasses in orchards, at industrial sites, under asphalt, and in non-crop areas.	2700–22400
Ioxynil Totril® (293)	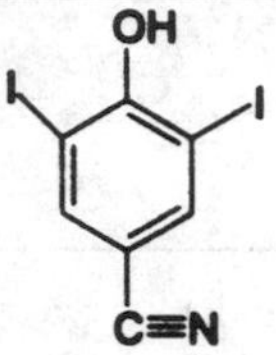	Used for control of select weeds in fall planted small grains.	200–400

Herbicide	Irritation		LD_{50} (mg/kg)		LC_{50} (mg/L)	Sensitizing Potential	Signal Word
	Eye	Skin	Oral	Dermal	Inhalation		
Isoxaben	Moderate Irritant	Slight irritant	> 10000	> 5000	> 2.7	Negative	Caution
Dichlobenil	Non-irritant	Non-irritant	> 1000	> 2000	> 0.25	Negative	Warning
Ioxynil	Non-irritant	Mild irritant	110	1050	> 0.40	Negative	Warning

Herbicide	Species/study	NOEL[1] (mg/kg/day)	Toxicity Studies	Hazard Indicator
Isoxaben	Rat/2-year	5.0	Mutagenicity	Weakly mutagenic
	Dog/52-week	10	Developmental	Not teratogenic
	Mouse/18-month	< 118	Reproductive	No evidence
	RfD[2]	0.05	Oncogenicity	C (liver tumors in mice; adrenal in rats)[3]
Dichlobenil	Rat/2-year	2.5	Mutagenicity	No evidence
	Dog/52-week	1.25	Developmental	Not teratogenic
	Hamster/18-Month Oral	10	Reproductive	No evidence
	RfD[2]	0.013	Oncogenicity	C (liver tumors in female rats)[3]
Ioxynil	Rat/2-year	0.5	Mutagenicity	No evidence
	Dog/30-Week Oral	1.0	Developmental	Not teratogenic
	Mouse/18-month	< 1.5	Reproductive	No evidence
	ADI	0.005	Oncogenicity	No evidence

[1] No observable effect level
[2] RfD = reference dose and ADI = acceptable daily intake
[3] See Table 13.3 for US EPA classification scheme

Table 13.53

Structures, uses, and hazard profiles for selected photosynthesis-inhibiting herbicides: Benzothiadiazole and phenylpyridazine

Herbicide	Structure	Principle Uses/Crops	Application Rate gm (a.i.)/ha
Bentazon Basagran® (270)	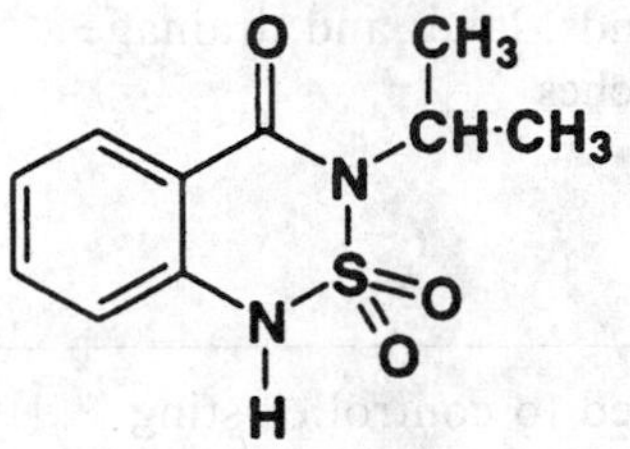	Used to control annual broadleaf weeds in soybeans, peas, peanuts and cereals.	560–2240
Pyridate (247,307)	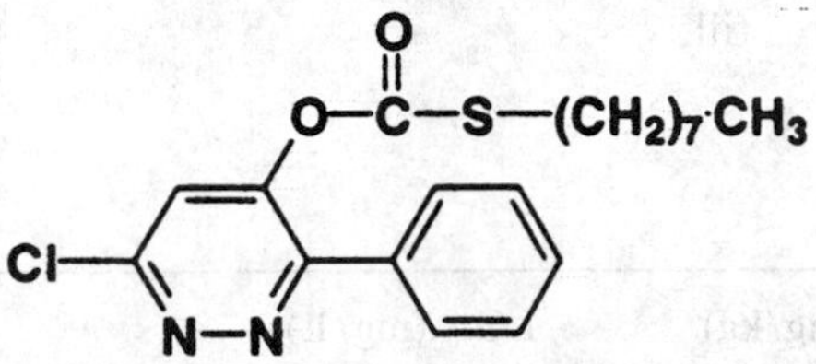	Used to control annual broadleaf weeds in cereals, turf and vegetables.	530–1050

Herbicide	Irritation: Eye	Irritation: Skin	LD_{50} (mg/kg): Oral	LD_{50} (mg/kg): Dermal	LC_{50} (mg/L): Inhalation	Sensitizing Potential	Signal Word
Bentazon	Moderate Irritant	Moderate Irritant	1100	> 2500	5.1	NA	Caution
Pyridate	Non-irritant	Moderate Irritant	4690	> 2000	> 4.7	Positive	Caution

Herbicide	Species/study	NOEL[1] (mg/kg/day)	Toxicity Studies	Hazard Indicator
Bentazon	Rat/2-year	17.5	Mutagenicity	No evidence
	Dog/52-week	3.2	Developmental	Not teratogenic
	Mouse/18-month	50	Reproductive	No evidence
	RfD[2]	0.03	Oncogenicity	E (No evidence)[3]
Pyridate	Rat/2-year	10.8	Mutagenicity	No evidence
	Dog/104-Week Oral	20	Developmental	Not teratogenic
	Mouse/18-month	<48	Reproductive	No evidence
	RfD[2]	0.11	Oncogenicity	E (No evidence)[3]

[1] No observable effect level
[2] RfD = reference dose
[3] See Table 13.3 for US EPA classification scheme
[4] UF = Uncertainty factor
NA = Not Available

Diquat is less acutely toxic than paraquat. Neither bipyridylium is mutagenic, teratogenic, or carcinogenic, nor have they been demonstrated to be reproductive toxicants.

Protoporphyrinogen Inhibitors

The mode of action for this class of herbicides is to interfere with critical enzymes needed in the biosynthesis of chlorophyll in plants. Unfortunately, mammalian systems possess a similar chromophore, namely, heme, that relies on a similar set of enzymes that are also affected by these chemicals. Therefore, it is not uncommon to find evidence of anemia in mammals exposed to protoporphyrinogen-inhibiting chemicals and other photobleaching herbicides (145,151,321). In addition to effects on heme synthesis, it is theorized that light-(phorryhia) and oxygen-dependent peroxidation of cell membrane lipids may lead to cell lysis and death, particu-

Table 13.54
Structures, uses, and hazard profiles for selected photosynthesis-inhibiting herbicides: Bipyridyliums

Herbicide	Structure	Principle Uses/Crops	Application Rate gm (a.i)/ha
Diquat WEEDTRINE® (185,280)	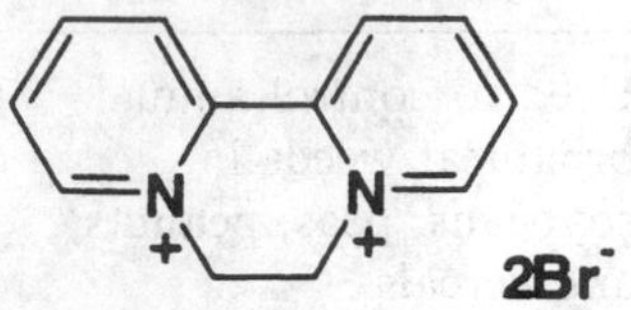	Used to control algae in ponds, lakes and drainage ditches	240 gm/liter of water
Paraquat Cyclone® (183,302)	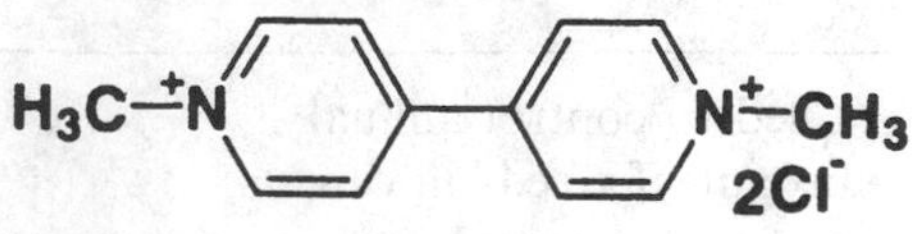	Used to control existing vegetation at planting or no till.	280–1050

Herbicide	Irritation		LD_{50} (mg/kg)		LC_{50} (mg/L)	Sensitizing Potential	Signal Word
	Eye	Skin	Oral	Dermal	Inhalation		
Diquat	Non-irritant	Slight irritant	> 5000	> 5000	> 6	Negative	Caution
Paraquat	NA	Irritant	112	240	NA	Negative	Warning

Herbicide	Species/study	NOEL[1] (mg/kg/day)	Toxicity Studies	Hazard Indicator
Diquat	Rat/2-year	0.6	Mutagenicity	No evidence
	Dog/52-week	0.5	Developmental	Not teratogenic
	Mouse/18-month	3.5	Reproductive	No evidence
	RfD[2]	0.005	Oncogenicity	E (No evidence)[3]
Paraquat	Rat/2-year	1.25	Mutagenicity	No evidence
	Dog/52-week	0.45	Developmental	Not teratogenic
	Mouse/18-month	1.87	Reproductive	No evidence
	RfD[2]	0.0045	Oncogenicity	E (No evidence)[3]

[1] No observable effect level
[2] RfD = reference dose and ADI = acceptable daily intake
[3] See Table 13.3 for US EPA classification scheme
NA = Not Available

larly in organs where these metabolites form or bioconcentrate. Such a theory is consistent with the experimental observation that liver damage and liver tumor formation, particularly in mice, are often a consequence of exposure to these chemicals. An alternate viewpoint is that liver damage and subsequent tumor response may result from peroxosome proliferative effects of chemicals in this class.

Diphenyl Ethers

Acifluorfen, formesafen, lactofen, and oxyfluorfen represent the diphenyl ether protoporphyrin inhibitors. The structures, uses, and toxicity profiles for the products are presented in Table 13.55.

Lactofen is a severe eye irritant; otherwise, the acute hazards associated with these protoporphyrin inhibitors are not remarkable. These diphenyl ethers are classified as B2 (probable human carcinogens) in the case of acifluorfen and lactofen (liver and stomach tumors), or C (possible human carcinogens) in the case of oxyfluorfen and formesafen (liver tumors).

N-Phenylphthalimides, Thiadiazoles, and Triazolinones

Only one representative for each of these chemical groups is featured in Table 13.56.

Table 13.55
Structures, uses, and hazard profiles for selected protoporphyrin inhibitors: Diphenylethers

Herbicide	Structure	Principle Uses/Crops	Application Rate gm (a.i.)/ha
Acifluorfen Scepter® (195, 265)	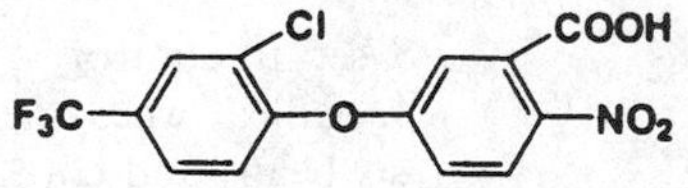	Used to control annual broadleaf weeds in peanuts, beans, and rice.	140–420
Fomesafen Flosil® (212)	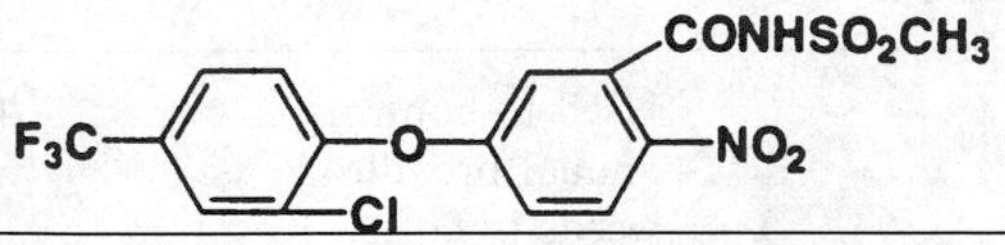	Used to control annual broadleaf weeds in soybeans.	280–420
Lactofen Cobra® (189)	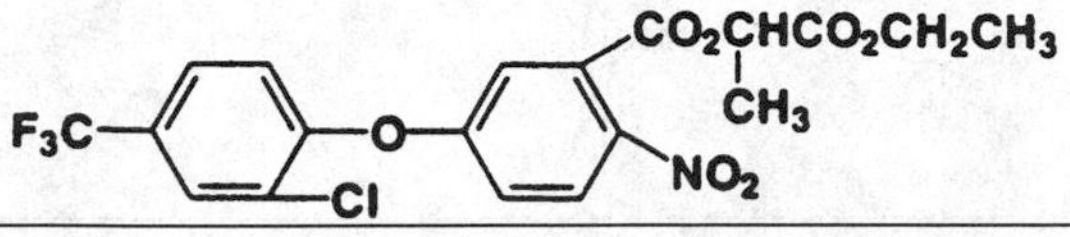	Used to control annual broadleaf weeds in cereals, potatoes, soya, and rice.	70–220
Oxyfluorfen Goal® (182)	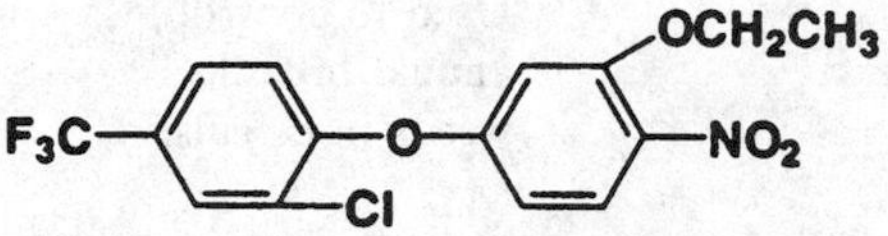	Used to control annual broadleaf weeds in conifers, vegetables, nuts and vine crops.	250–2240

	Irritation		LD_{50} (mg/kg)		LC_{50} (mg/L)		
Herbicide	Eye	Skin	Oral	Dermal	Inhalation	Sensitizing Potential	Signal Word
Acifluorfen	Non-irritant	Moderate irritant	1450	> 2000	> 6.9	Negative	Caution
Fomesafen	Moderate irritant	Mild irritant	1250	> 1000	4.97	Negative	Caution
Lactofen	Severe irritant	Non-irritant	> 5000	2000	NA	NA	Danger
Oxyfluorfen	Moderate irritant	Non-irritant	> 5000	> 5000	NA	Negative	Caution

Herbicide	Species/study	NOEL[1] (mg/kg/day)	Toxicity Studies	Hazard Indicator
Acifluorfen	Rat/2-year	25	Mutagenicity	No evidence
	Dog/52-week	NA	Developmental	Not teratogenic
	Mouse/18-month	38	Reproductive	No evidence
	RfD (rat reproduction)[2]	0.013	Oncogenicity	B2 (liver/stomach tumors)[3]
Fomesafen	Rat/2-year	0.25	Mutagenicity	No evidence
	Dog/52-week	1.0	Developmental	Not teratogenic
	Mouse/18-month	1.0	Reproductive	No evidence
	RfD[2]	0.0025	Oncogenicity	C with CSF (liver tumors in mice)[3]
Lactofen	Rat/2-year	25	Mutagenicity	No evidence
	Dog/52-week	5.0	Developmental	Not teratogenic
	Mouse/18-month	1.5	Reproductive	No evidence
	RfD[2] (mouse—1000×UF[4])	0.002	Oncogenicity	B2 (liver/stomach tumors)[3]
Oxyfluorfen	Rat/2-year	2.0	Mutagenicity	No evidence
	Dog/2-Year Oral	2.5	Developmental	Not teratogenic
	Mouse/18-month	0.3	Reproductive	No evidence
	RfD[2]	0.003	Oncogenicity	C (liver tumors in mice)[3]

[1] No observable effect level
[2] RfD = reference dose, CSF = cancer slope factor
[3] See Table 13.3 for US EPA classification scheme
NA = Not Available

Table 13.56
Structures, uses, and hazard profiles for selected protoporphyrin Inhibitors: *N*-Phenylphthalimide, thiadiazole, and triazolinone

Chemical/ Common Name	Structure	Principle Uses/Crops	Application Rate gm (a.i.)/ha
Flumiclorac-pentyl Resource® (283)	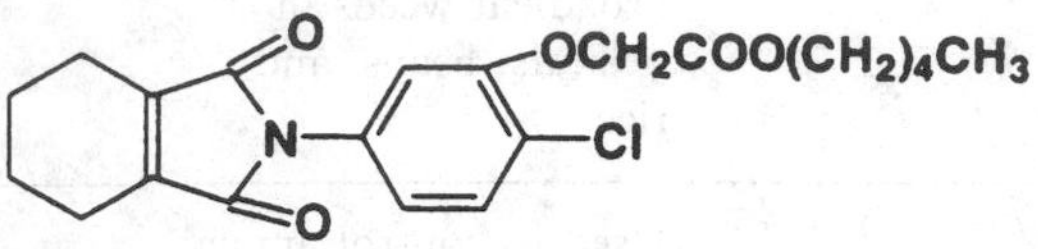	Used to control broadleaf weeds in soybeans and corn.	30–90
Fluthiacet-methyl Action® (211,258)	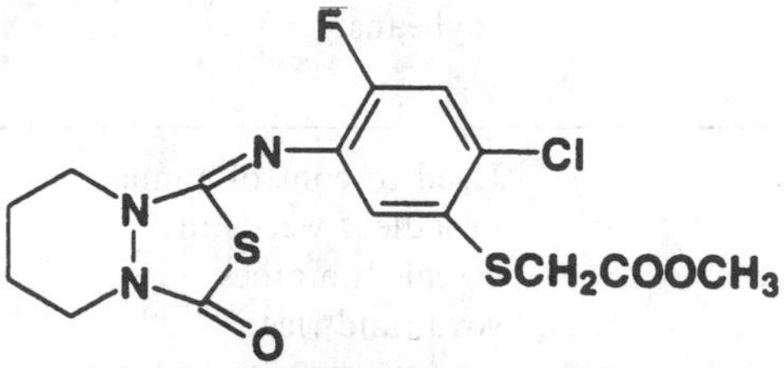	Used to control annual broadleaf weeds in corn, soybeans, and cereals.	4–15
Carfentrazone-ethyl Affinity®, Aurora® (230)	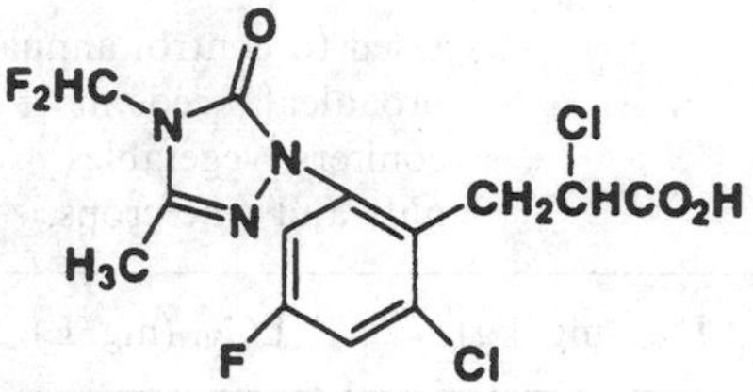	Used to control annual broadleaf weeds in cereals.	9–35

Herbicide	Irritation: Eye	Irritation: Skin	LD_{50} (mg/kg): Oral	LD_{50} (mg/kg): Dermal	LC_{50} (mg/L): Inhalation	Sensitizing Potential	Signal Word
Flumiclorac-pentyl	Slight Irritant	Non-irritant	> 5000	> 2000	> 5.9	Negative	Caution
Fluthiacet-methyl	Slight Irritant	Non-irritant	> 5000	> 2000	> 5.0	NA	Caution
Carfentrazone-ethyl	Minimal Irritant	Non-irritant	5143	> 4000	> 5.0	Negative	Caution

Herbicide	Species/study	NOEL[1] (mg/kg/day)	Toxicity Studies	Hazard Indicator
Flumiclorac-Pentyl	Rat/2-year	35	Mutagenicity	No evidence
	Dog/52-week	100	Developmental	Not teratogenic
	Mouse/18-month	32	Reproductive	No evidence
	RfD[2]	0.32	Oncogenicity	E (No evidence)[3]
Fluthiacet-Methyl	Rat/2-year	2.1	Mutagenicity	No evidence
	Dog/52-week	30	Developmental	Not teratogenic
	Mouse/18-month	0.1	Reproductive	No evidence
	RfD[2]	0.001	Oncogenicity	Likely carcinogen (liver in mice/pancreas in rats)[4]
Carfentrazone-Ethyl	Rat/2-year	3.0	Mutagenicity	No evidence
	Dog/52-week	50	Developmental	Not teratogenic
	Mouse/18-month	10	Reproductive	No evidence
	RfD[2]	0.03	Oncogenicity	Not likely a carcinogen[4]

[1] No observable effect level
[2] RfD = reference dose
[3] See Table 13.3 for US EPA classification scheme
[4] Proposed 1996 US EPA classification scheme
NA = Not Available

Flumiclorac-pentyl is applied in the 30 to 90 g/hectare range and has an acute and repeated-dose hazard profile that should not evoke concern in regard to human health. The thiadiazole, fluthiacet-methyl, which is applied at a remarkable low rate of 4–15 g/hectare, exhibits an unremarkable acute hazard, but has been found to produce liver tumors in mice and pancreatic tumors in the rat. Carfentrazone-ethyl, which is applied at the very low rate of 9–35 g/hectare, incurs little concern based on the acute or repeated-dose hazard evaluation.

Bleaching Herbicides

The bleaching herbicides disrupt the synthesis of carotenoid pigments, which protect chlorophyll pigments in light. In the absence of carotenoids, chlorophyll is destroyed and turns white, thus having a bleached appearance. The pyridazinones, triketones, and isoxazoles bleaching herbicides are considered here. The pyridazinones, triazoles, and isoxazolidinones inhibit carotenoid biosynthesis at the phytoene desaturase step, whereas, the triketones and isoxazoles inhibit the 4-hydroxyphenylpyruvate dioxygenase enzyme (156).

Pyridazinones

The structures, uses, and hazard profiles for norflurazon and fluridone are given in Table 13.57.

Neither norflurazon nor fluridone is acutely toxic; the repeated-dose profile for fluridone is unremarkable. Norflurazon is classified as category C (possible human carcinogen) based on mouse liver tumors.

Triazoles and Isoxazolidinones

Amitrole (triazole) and clomazine (isoxazolidinone) are presented with regard to their structures, uses, and toxicity profiles in Table 13.58.

These compounds are not acutely toxic. Clomazone has an unremarkable repeated-dose hazard profile. Amitrole has been classified as category B2 (probable human carcinogen) based on thyroid tumors in rats and liver tumors in mice.

Triketones and Isoxazoles

The structures, uses, and hazard profile for sulcotrione (triketone) and isoxaflutole (isoxazole) are presented in Table 13.59.

Although the acute toxicity information for sulcotrione does not suggest that it represents a hazard, the available data for its repeated-dose profile are inadequate for full hazard assessment. Isoxaflutole does not represent an acute hazard but has been shown to be a potential developmental toxin, a neurotoxin, and potential carcinogen.

EPSP Synthase, Glutamine Synthase, and Dihydropteroate (DHP) Synthase Inhibitors

A single member of each of these classes of synthase inhibitors was selected for this review. The inhibition of 5-enolpyruvlshikimate-3-phosphate (EPSP) synthase prevents the biosynthesis of essential amino acids (287). The inhibition of glutamine synthase leads to an accumulation of ammonium ions, and inhibition of photosynthesis (286). Inhibition of DHP synthase inhibits folic acid synthesis, which is needed for the formation of purine nucleotides required for cell division (267).

The structures, uses, and hazard profiles for representative ESSP synthase, glutamine synthase, and dihydropteroate synthase inhibitors are given in Table 13.60.

It can be seen that glyphosate, glufosinate-ammonium, and asulam are not acutely toxic. Both glyphosate and glufosinate-ammonium have excellent repeated-dose toxicity profiles. Asulum is also not mutagenic, teratogenic, or a reproductive toxin, but does produce tumors in male rat.

Microtubule Assembly Inhibitors

The structures, uses, and hazard profiles of three commercially important dinitroaniline microtubule assembly inhibitors are given in Table 13.61.

Benfluralin, pendimethalin, and trifluralin are not acutely toxic. There are inadequate data to access the repeated-dose hazards for benfluralin. Both pendimethalin and trifluralin were classified as category C (possible human carcinogens) by the U.S. EPA (100).

Cell Division Inhibitors

The structures, uses, and toxicology profiles for four chloracetamide inhibitors of cell division are provided in Table 13.62.

All four chloracetamide herbicides are potential sensitizers. Alachlor and acetochlor both exhibit mutagenic potential and significant oncogenic potential in both rats and mice. Dimethenamid also has exhibited weak genotoxiciy and a tumor response in the female rat. Metolachlor showed a weak oncogenic response in the liver of the female rat.

Cellulose and Lipid Synthesis Inhibitors

The structures, uses, and hazard profiles of the cellulose synthesis inhibitor isoxaben and of the lipid synthesis inhibitors butylate and molinate are given in Table 13.63.

Isoxaben exhibits a low acute toxicity hazard. Butylate is a potential sensitizing agent, and molinate has signifi-

Table 13.57
Structures, uses, and hazard profile for selected bleaching herbicides: Pyridazinones

Chemical/ Common Names	Structure	Principle Uses/Crops	Application Rate gm (a.i.)/ha
Norflurazon Evital® (220)	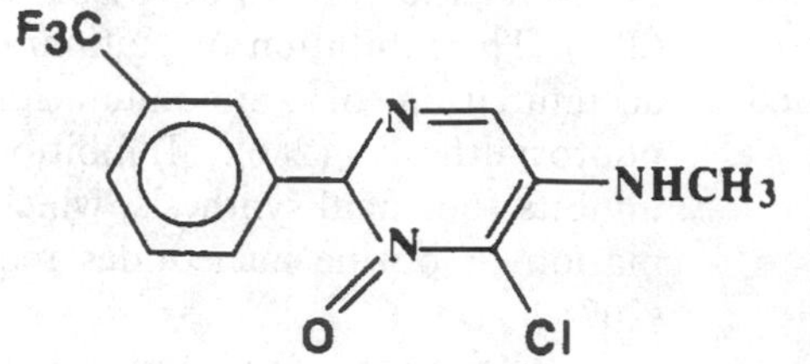	Fruit Tree, Nut, & Vine crops, Soybean, Peanut, Ornamentals, Cotton, and IWC,	500–3360
Fluridone Sonar® (285)	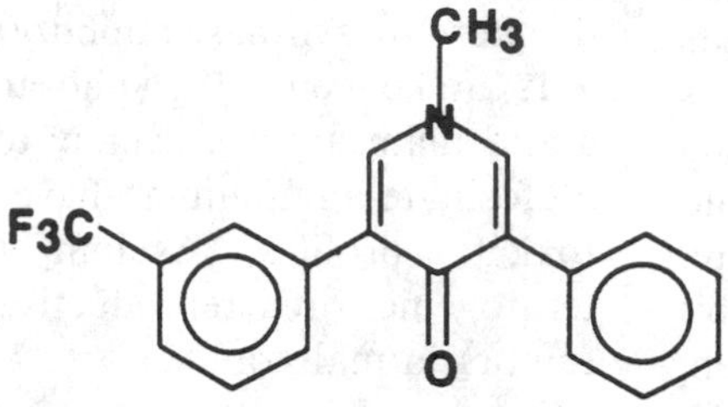	Aquatic herbicide	2240 (0.075–0.15 mg/L)

Herbicide	Irritation: Eye	Irritation: Skin	LD_{50} (mg/kg): Oral	LD_{50} (mg/kg): Dermal	LC_{50} (mg/L): Inhalation	Sensitizing Potential	Signal Word
Pyridazinone	Non-Irritant	Non-irritant	> 9000	> 20000	> 0.2	Negative	Caution
Fluridone	Slight	Non-irritant	> 10000	> 5000	> 4.12	Negative	Caution

Herbicide	Species/study	NOEL[1] (mg/kg/day)	Toxicity Studies	Hazard Indicator
Pyridazinone	Rat/2-year	19	Mutagenicity	No evidence
	Dog/52-week	1.5	Developmental	Not teratogenic
	Mouse/18-month	41	Reproductive	No evidence
	RfD[2]	0.02	Oncogenicity	C (mouse liver tumors)[3]
Fluridone	Rat/2-year	8.0	Mutagenicity	No evidence
	Dog/52-week	11.4	Developmental	Not teratogenic
	Mouse/18-month	11.6	Reproductive	No evidence
	RfD[2]	0.08	Oncogenicity	E (No evidence)[3]

[1] No observable effect level
[2] RfD = reference dose
[3] See Table 13.3 for US EPA classification scheme
NA = Not Available

cant acute inhalation toxicity. Isoxaben has some mutagenic, developmental, and oncogenic potential. The lipid synthesis inhibitor butylate appears not to exhibit significant repeated-dose toxicity. Much of the critical assessment data for molinate is not available, making full evaluation impossible; however, from the available data, molinate appears to have reproductive toxicity and oncogenic potential.

Synthetic Auxin Mimics (Phenoxy, Benzoic, and Pyridine Acids)

The synthetic auxins alter growth in the meristems and leaves by affecting protein synthesis and normal cell division. 2,4-D (phenoxy), dicamba (benzoic), and clopyralid and picloram (pyridine acids) represent this

Table 13.58
Structures, uses, and hazard profiles for selected bleaching herbicides: Triazole and isoxazolidinone

Herbicide	Structure	Principle Uses/Crops	Application Rate gm (a.i.)/ha
Amitrole Amizol® (261)	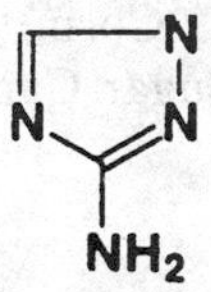	Fruit trees, grapes, olives Ornamentals, cereal, IWC, Aquatic plants	2000–9000
Clomazone Command® (254)	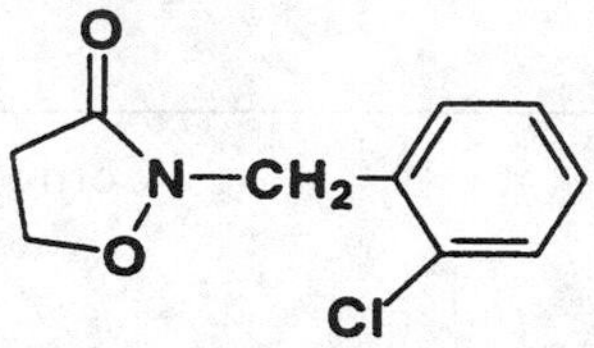	Soybeans, peas, peppers,	560–1700

Herbicide	Irritation: Eye	Irritation: Skin	LD_{50} (mg/kg): Oral	LD_{50} (mg/kg): Dermal	LC_{50} (mg/L): Inhalation	Sensitizing Potential	Signal Word
Amitrole	Slight irritant	Slight irritant	> 5000	> 2000	NA	NA	Caution
Clomazone	Non-irritant	Minimal	2077	> 2000	4.23 (female)	Negative	Caution

Herbicide	Species/study	NOEL[1] (mg/kg/day)	Toxicity Studies	Hazard Indicator
Amitrole	Rat/2-year	0.5	Mutagenicity	No evidence
	Dog/52-week	NA	Developmental	Not teratogenic
	Mouse/18-month	1.4	Reproductive	No evidence
		CSF = 1.13 $(mg, kg, day)^{-1}$	Oncogenicity	B2 (thyroid tumor rats; liver tumor mice)[3]
Clomazone	Rat/2-year	4.3	Mutagenicity	No evidence
	Dog/52-week	12.5	Developmental	Not teratogenic
	Mouse/18-month	143	Reproductive	No evidence
	RfD[2]	0.043	Oncogenicity	E (No evidence)[3]

[1] No observable effect level
[2] See Table 13.3 for US EPA classification scheme
NA = Not Available

class. The structures, uses, and hazard profiles of these synthetic auxins are provided in Table 13.64.

Dicamba and clopyralid were found to exhibit sensitization potential. Dicamba was shown also to have some mutagenic and weak, questionable carcinogenic potential.

Herbicides with Unknown Mechanism of Action

The structures, uses, and hazard profiles of two of these products are presented in Table 13.65.

Monosodium methanearsonic acid (MSMA), an organic arsenical, has a rather unremarkable acute toxicity profile; it has, however, been shown to decrease fertility in rats and is classified as category B2 (probable human carcinogen) based on bladder tumors in the rat. Difenzoquat is labeled as a danger because of its corrosive effects on the eyes; however, it possesses a non-problematical repeated-dose hazard profile.

CONCLUSION

Although older products, like the practically irreplaceable DDT and chlordane, have been banned because of their persistence in the environment, their replacements, the organophosphate insecticides, currently are under fire by the U.S. EPA. Therefore, this

Table 13.59
Structures, uses, and hazard profiles for selected bleaching herbicides: Triketone and isoxazole

Chemical/ Common Names	Structure	Principle Uses/Crops	Application Rate gm (a.i.)/ha
Sulcotrione Mikito® (72)	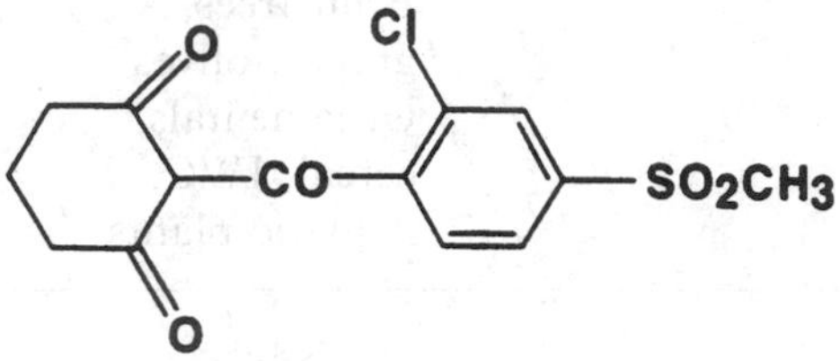	Corn, Sugar Cane	200–300
Isoxaflutole (215,240)	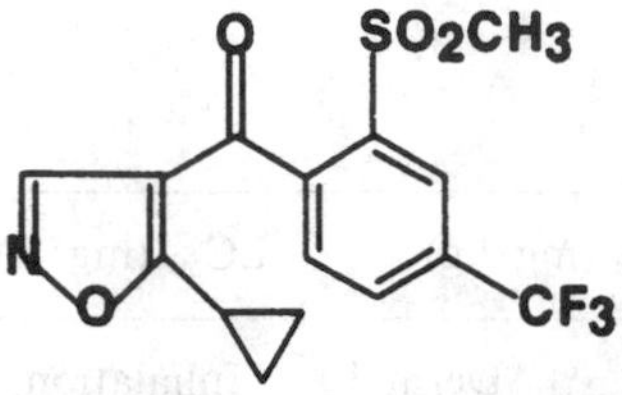	Corn	75–140

Herbicide	Irritation: Eye	Irritation: Skin	LD_{50} (mg/kg): Oral	LD_{50} (mg/kg): Dermal	LC_{50} (mg/L): Inhalation	Sensitizing Potential	Signal Word
Sulcotrione	Mild irritant	Non-irritant	> 5000	> 4000	> 1.6	Positive	Caution
Isoxaflutole	Mild irritant	Minimal	> 5000	> 2000	> 5.3	Negative	Caution

Herbicide	Species/study	NOEL[1] (mg/kg/day)	Toxicity Studies	Hazard Indicator
Sulcotrione	Rat/2-year	NA	Mutagenicity	No evidence
	Dog/52-week	NA	Developmental	Not teratogenic
	Mouse/18-month	NA	Reproductive	NA
	RfD or ADI[2]	NA	Oncogenicity	NA
Isoxaflutole	Rat/2-year	2.0	Mutagenicity	No evidence
	Dog/52-week	45	Developmental	Evidence of developmental toxicity
	Mouse/18-month	3.2	Reproductive	No evidence
	RfD[2]	0.002	Neurotoxicity	Evidence of neurotoxicity
			Oncogenicity	Likely to be a carcinogen[4] (liver tumors in both sexes of rats and mice).

[1] No observable effect level
[2] RfD = reference dose, and ADI = acceptable daily intake
[3] See Table 13.3 for US EPA classification scheme
[4] Proposed 1996 US EPA carcinogen classification system
NA = Not Available

overview of crop protection chemicals and modalities has focused primarily on the newer products used for disease control, insect control, and weed control.

Besides the movement toward more natural chemistry, such as with the avermectins, the chemicals of the late 1980s and 1990s are efficacious at a low grams per acre rate with pest-specific toxicity and limited mammalian toxicity, such as for the ALS sulfonylurea herbicides. In order to reduce the area of exposure due to application, applying materials directly to the seed to be planted is

Table 13.60

Structures, uses, and hazard profiles for selected inhibitors of EPSP: Glutamine and DHP synthase

Common Name Trade Name	Structure	Principle Uses/Crops	Application Rate gm (a.i.)/ha
Glyphosate Roundup® EPSP synthase Inhibitor (235,287)	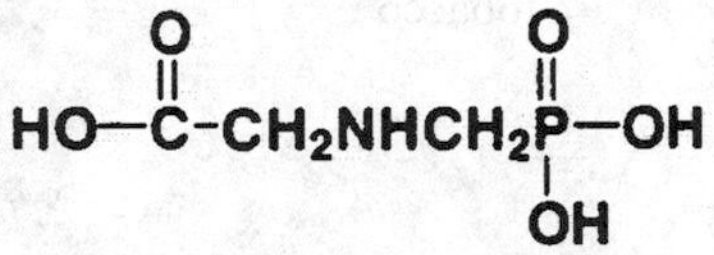	Corn, Soybeans IWC	210–4200
Glufosinate-ammonium Finale® Glutamine synthase inhibitor (287)	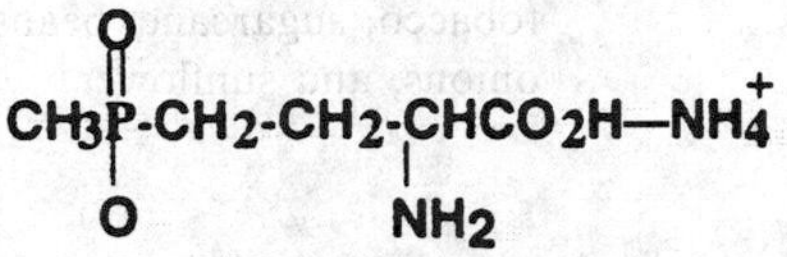	Fruit trees, grapes, rubber, palm ornamentals, vegetables, IWC	280–1700
Asulam Asulux® DHP synthase Inhibitor (267)	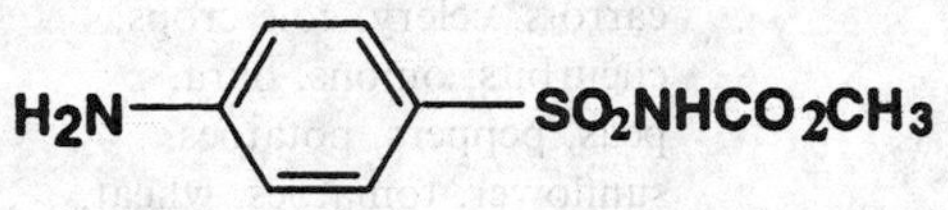	Sugar cane, alfalfa, banana, coffee, tea, cocoa, pasture forestry	1120–4000

Herbicide	Irritation: Eye	Irritation: Skin	LD_{50} (mg/kg): Oral	LD_{50} (mg/kg): Dermal	LD_{50} (mg/L): Inhalation	Sensitizing Potential	Signal Word
Glyphosate	Slight	Non-irritant	5600	> 5000	NA	Negative	Caution
Glufosinate-ammonium	Non-irritant	Non-irritant	1620 ♀	4000	1.26 ♂	NA	Caution
Asulam	Irritant	Slight Irritant	> 5000	> 2000	> 1.8	Negative	Caution

Herbicide	Species/study	NOEL[1] (mg/kg/day)	Toxicity Studies	Hazard Indicator
Glyphosate	Rat/2-year	400	Mutagenicity	No evidence
	Dog/52-week	500	Developmental	Not teratogenic
	Mouse/18-month	4500	Reproductive	No evidence
	RfD[2]	0.1	Oncogenicity	E (No evidence)[3]
Glufosinate-ammonium	Rat/2-year	2.1	Mutagenicity	No evidence
	Dog/52-week	NA	Developmental	Not teratogenic
	Mouse/18-month	NA	Reproductive	No evidence
	RfD[2]	0.02	Oncogenicity	Not oncogenic
Asulam	Rat/2-year	36	Mutagenicity	No evidence
	Dog/52-week	60	Developmental	Not teratogenic
	Mouse/18-month	713	Reproductive	No evidence
	RfD or ADI[2]	0.36	Oncogenicity	C (adrenal tumors in male rats)[3]

[1] No observable effect level
[2] RfD = reference dose, and ADI = acceptable daily intake
[3] See Table 13.3 for US EPA classification scheme
NA = Not Available

Table 13.61

Structures, uses, and hazard profiles for selected dinitroaniline inhibitors of microtuble assembly

Common Name Trade Name	Structure	Principle Uses/Crops	Application Rate gm (a.i.)/ha
Benfluralin Balan®, Benefin® (14)	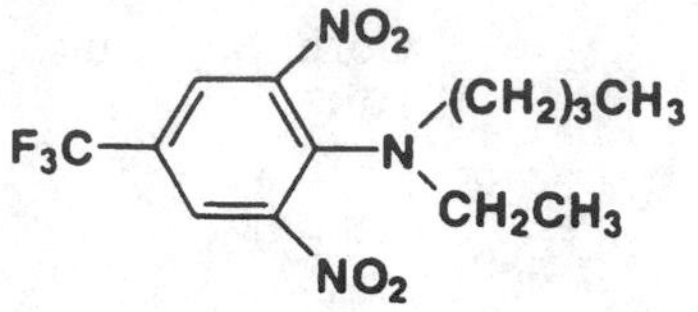	Alfalfa, clover, lettuce and tobacco	1260–1680
Pendimethalin Prowl® (221,303)	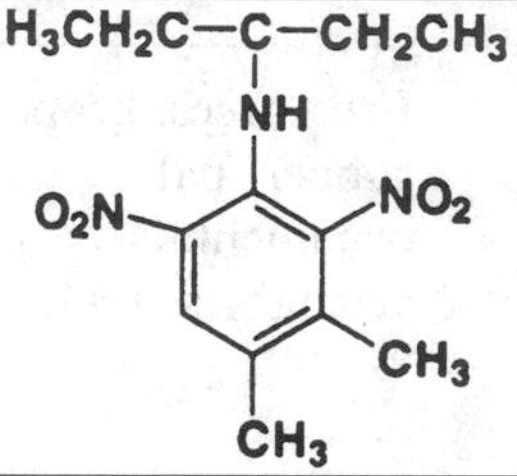	Corn, sorghum, rice, soybeans, cotton, potatoes, tobacco, sugarcane, beans, onions, and sunflower	560–3360
Trifluralin Treflan® (315)	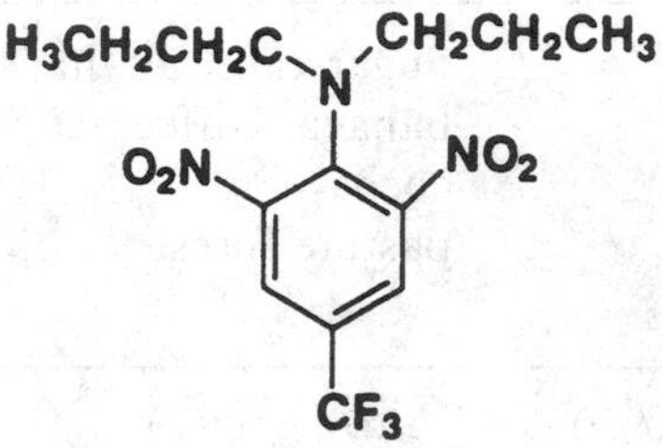	Alfalfa, asparagus, beans, carrots, celery, cole crops, cucurbits, onions, okra, peas, peppers, potatoes, sunflower, tomatoes, wheat, barley, flax, soybeans, corn, sorghum, and ornamentals	340–2240

Herbicide	Irritation		LD_{50} (mg/kg)		LD_{50} (mg/L)	Sensitizing Potential	Signal Word
	Eye	Skin	Oral	Dermal	Inhalation		
Benfluralin	Slight irritant	Slight irritant	> 5000	> 2000	NA	Positive	Caution
Pendimethalin	Slight irritant	Non-irritant	1050♀	> 5000	320 (nominal)	Negative	Caution
Trifluralin	Slight Irritant	Non-irritant	> 5000	> 5000	> 4.8	Positive	Caution

Herbicide	Species/study	NOEL[1] (mg/kg/day)	Toxicity Studies	Hazard Indicator
Benfluralin	Rat/2-year	1000	Mutagenicity	NA
	Dog/52-week	25	Developmental	NA
	Mouse/18-month	6.5	Reproductive	NA
	RfD[2]	0.3	Oncogenicity	NA
Pendimethalin	Rat/2-year	10.0	Mutagenicity	No evidence
	Dog/104-week	12.5	Developmental	Not teratogenic
	Mouse/18-month	75	Reproductive	No evidence
	RfD or ADI[2]	0.13	Oncogenicity	C with RfD (thyroid follicular cell adenomas)[3]
Trifluralin	Rat/2-year	2.5	Mutagenicity	No evidence
	Dog/52-week	2.4	Developmental	Not teratogenic
	Mouse/18-month	7.5	Reproductive	No evidence
	RfD or ADI[2]	0.024	Oncogenicity	C with CSF (bladder, kidney, thyroid tumors)[3]

[1] No observable effect level
[2] RfD = reference dose, ADI = acceptable daily intake, and CSF = cancer slope factor
[3] See Table 13.3 for US EPA classification scheme
NA = Not Available

Table 13.62
Structures, uses, and hazard profiles for selected chloroacetamide inhibitors of cell division

Common Name Trade Name	Structure	Principle Uses/Crops	Application Rate gm (a.i.)/ha
Alachlor Lassco® (228)	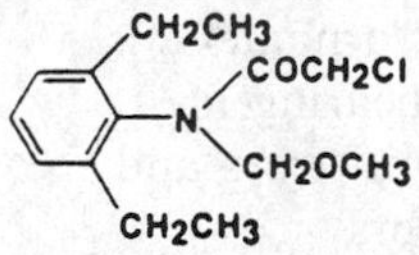	Corn, beans, peanuts, sorghum, soybeans, sunflowers and ornamentals	1.5–4.5 1500–4500
Acetochlor Surpass® (175)	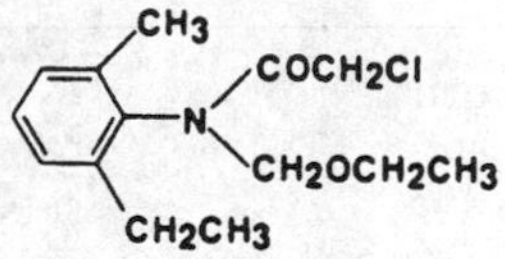	Corn, soybeans, sorghum, and wheat	0.9–3.36 900–3360
Metolachlor Dual® (242)	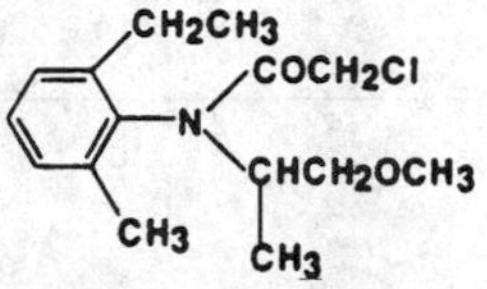	Corn, soybeans, and sorghum, cucurbits, onions, peas, pecans, peppers, potatoes, sugar beets	1.25–6.2 1250–6200
Dimethenamid Frontier® (184)	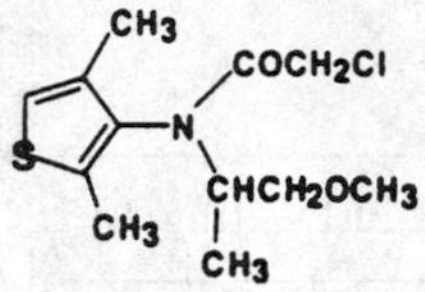	Corn and soybeans	590

Herbicide	Irritation: Eye	Irritation: Skin	LD_{50} (mg/kg): Oral	LD_{50} (mg/kg): Dermal	LD_{50} (mg/L): Inhalation	Sensitizing Potential	Signal Word
Alachlor	Non-irritant	Non-irritant	930	13,300	> 1.04	Positive	Caution
Acetochlor	Slight Irritant	Non-irritant	2148	4166	> 3.0	Positive	Caution
Metolachlor	Non-irritant	Minimal Irritant	> 2780	> 10000	> 1.75	Positive	Caution
Dimethenamid	Slight Irritant	Non-irritant	1570	> 2000	> 5.0	Positive	Caution

Herbicide	Species/study	NOEL[1] (mg/kg/day)	Toxicity Studies	Hazard Indicator
Alachlor	Rat/2-year	2.5	Mutagenicity	Positive (UDS)
	Dog/52-week	1.0	Developmental	Not teratogenic
	Mouse/18-month	16.6♂	Reproductive	No evidence
	RfD[2]	0.01	Oncogenicity	C/RfD(nasal; rats; lung; mice)[3]
Acetochlor	Rat/2-year	8.0	Mutagenicity	Positive (CHO, UDS, mouse lymphoma)
	Dog/52-week	2.0	Developmental	Not teratogenic
	Mouse/18-month	13	Reproductive	No evidence
	RfD[2]	0.02	Oncogenicity	B2 (liver, thyroid, nasal, rats; lung tumors in mice)[3]
Metolachlor	Rat/2-year	15	Mutagenicity	No evidence
	Dog/52-week	10	Developmental	Not teratogenic
	Mouse/18-month	120	Reproductive	No evidence
	RfD[2]	0.1	Oncogenicity	C/RfD (liver tumors; ♀ rats)[3]
Dimethenamid	Rat/2-year	5.0	Mutagenicity	Weak positive (CHO: UDS)
	Dog/52-week	9.6	Developmental	Not teratogenic
	Mouse/18-month	40♀	Reproductive	No evidence
	RfD[2]	0.05	Oncogenicity	C/RfD (liver, ovary; ♀ rats)[3]

[1]No observable effect level
[2]RfD = reference dose and ADI = acceptable daily intake
[3]See Table 13.3 for US EPA classification scheme

Table 13.63

Structures, uses, and hazard profiles for selected benzamide and thiocarbamate inhibitors of cellulose or lipid synthesis

Herbicide	Structure	Principle Uses/Crops	Application Rate gm (a.i.)/ha
Isoxaben Gallery® (294)	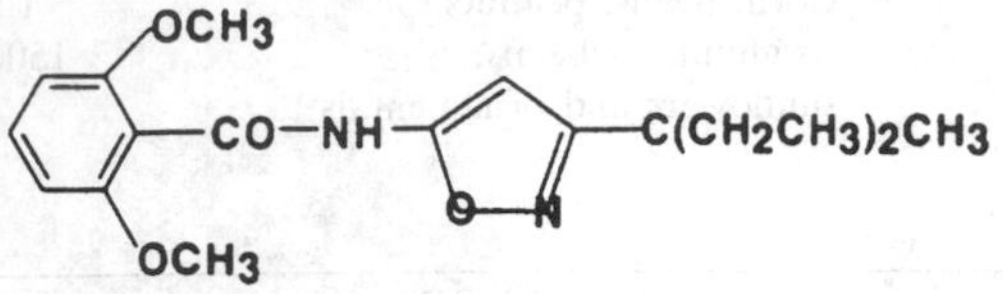	Turf, ornamentals, non-bearing fruit and nut trees and conifers	560–1120
Butylate Sutan® (272)	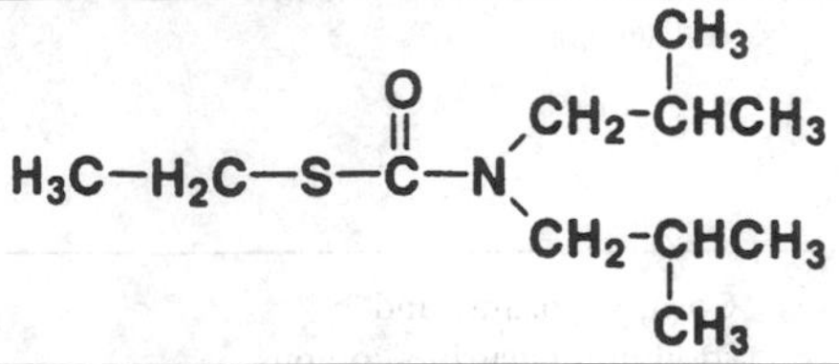	Corn	3500–6900
Molinate Ordram® (298)	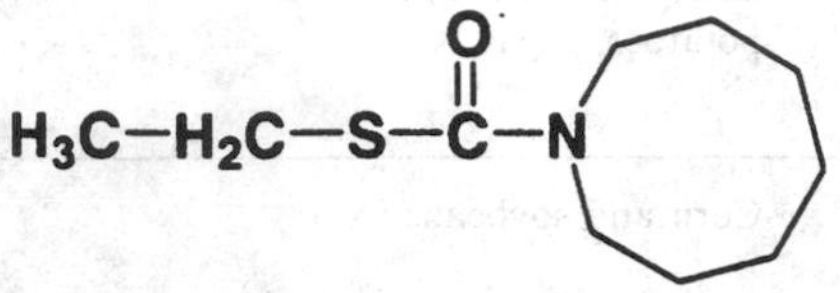	Rice	2240–5600

Herbicide	Irritation		LD_{50} (mg/kg)		LD_{50} (mg/L)	Sensitizing Potential	Signal Word
	Eye	Skin	Oral	Dermal	Inhalation		
Isoxaben	Moderate Irritant	Slight Irritant	> 10000	> 2000	> 2.68	Negative	Caution
Butylate	Non-irritant	Mild Irritant	4659 ♂	1659	4.64	Positive	Caution
Molinate	Moderate Irritant	Mild Irritant	720	~4000	0.003	Negative	Danger

Herbicide	Species/study	NOEL[1] (mg/kg/day)	Toxicity Studies	Hazard Indicator
Isoxaben	Rat/2-year	5.0	Mutagenicity	Positive micronucleus test
	Dog/52-week	10.0	Developmental	Positive only at maternal toxic doses
	Mouse/18-month	NA	Reproductive	No evidence
	RfD or ADI[2]	0.05	Oncogenicity	C (adrenal and liver tumors)[3]
Butylate	Rat/2-year	50	Mutagenicity	No evidence
	Dog/52-week	5.0	Developmental	Not teratogenic
	Mouse/18-month	NA	Reproductive	NA
	RfD or ADI[2]	0.05	Oncogenicity	E (No evidence)[3]
Molinate	Rat/2-year	NA	Mutagenicity	NA
	Dog/52-week	NA	Developmental	NA
	Mouse/18-month	NA	Reproductive	Effect on sperm
	RfD or ADI[2]	0.002	Oncogenicity	C with CSF (kidney tumors in rats)[3]

[1] No observable effect level
[2] RfD = reference dose and CSF = cancer slope factor
[3] See Table 13.3 for US EPA classification scheme
NA = Not Available

Table 13.64
Structures, uses, and hazard profiles for selected synthetic auxin mimics (phenoxy, benzoic, and pyridine acids)

Chemical Class Common Name	Structure	Principle Uses/Crops	Application Rate gm (a.i.)/ha
2,4-D Wedare® (250)	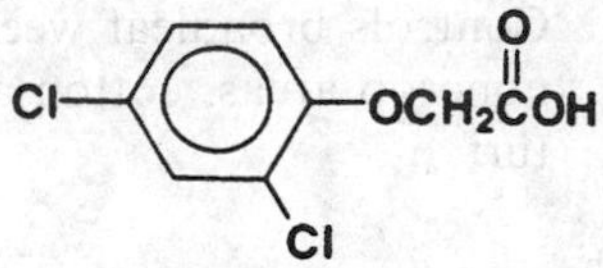	Turf, cereals, sorghum, corn, soybeans, asparagus, and fruit trees	280–2240
Dicamba Banvel® (232)	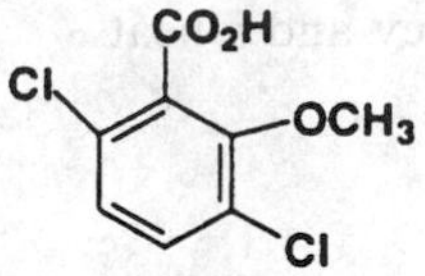	Corn, turf, sorghum, cereals, pastures, and asparagus	70–2240
Clopyralid Reclam® (202)	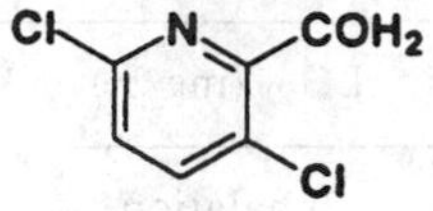	Sugar beets, corn, grass seed, conifers, and pasture	105–560
Picloram Tordon® (259)	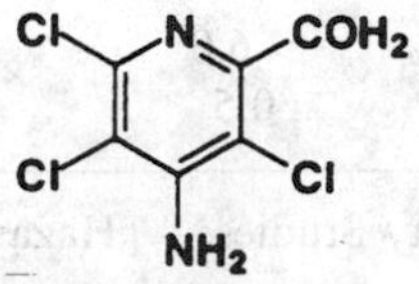	Industrial Weed Control, forestry, pasture, and range land.	35–1120

Herbicide	Irritation: Eye	Irritation: Skin	LD_{50} (mg/kg): Oral	LD_{50} (mg/kg): Dermal	LD_{50} (mg/L): Inhalation	Sensitizing Potential	Signal Word
2,4-D	Severe Irritant	Moderate Irritant	639♂	> 2000	1.8	Negative	Warning
Dicamba	Corrosive	Non-irritant	1851♀	> 2000	> 9.6	Positive	Danger
Clopyralid	Severe Irritant	Slight Irritant	4300	> 2000	1.3	Negative	Warning
Picloram	Moderate Irritant	Non-irritant	4012♀	> 2000	> 0.035	Positive	Danger

Herbicide	Species/study	NOEL[1] (mg/kg/day)	Toxicity Studies	Hazard Indicator
2,4-D	Rat/2-year	5.0	Mutagenicity	No evidence
	Dog/52-week	1.0	Developmental	Not teratogenic
	Mouse/18-month	1.0	Reproductive	No evidence
	RfD or ADI[2]	0.01	Oncogenicity	D (Not classifiable)[3]
Dicamba	Rat/2-year	125	Mutagenicity	Positive (*B. subtilis*; UDS)
	Dog/52-week	60	Developmental	Not teratogenic
	Mouse/18-month	108♂	Reproductive	No evidence
	RfD or ADI[2]	0.6	Oncogenicity	D (Not classifiable)[3]
Clopyralid	Rat/2-year	50	Mutagenicity	No evidence
	Dog/52-week	100	Developmental	Not teratogenic
	Mouse/18-month	500	Reproductive	No evidence
	RfD or ADI[2]	0.5	Oncogenicity	E (No evidence)[3]
Picloram	Rat/2-year	20	Mutagenicity	No evidence
	Dog/52-week	35	Developmental	Not teratogenic
	Mouse/18-month	500	Reproductive	No evidence
	RfD or ADI[2]	0.2	Oncogenicity	E (No evidence)[3]

[1] No observable effect level
[2] RfD = reference dose
[3] See Table 13.3 for US EPA classification scheme

Table 13.65

Structures, uses, and hazard profiles for selected herbicides whose mode of action is unknown

Chemicals Class Common Name	Structure	Principle Uses/Crops	Application Rate gm (a.i.)/ha
MSMA Drexar® (181,299)	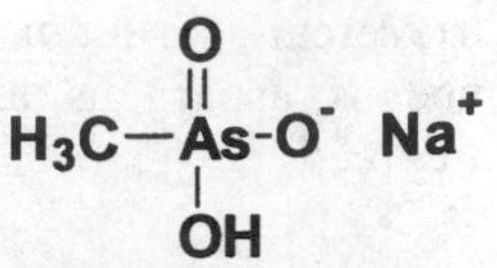	Controls broadleaf weeds in noncrop areas, cotton and turf.	2220–2770
Difenzoquat Avenge® (279)	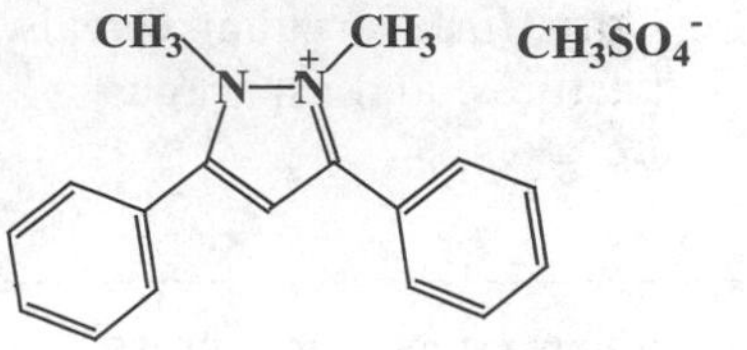	Barley and wheat	700–1120

Herbicide	Irritation: Eye	Irritation: Skin	LD_{50} (mg/kg): Oral	LD_{50} (mg/kg): Dermal	LC_{50} (mg/L): Inhalation	Sensitizing Potential	Signal Word
MSMA	Mild Irritant	Mild Irritant	1059E	> 2000	> 6.0	NA	Caution
Difenzoquat	Corrosive	Moderate Irritant	373E	> 2000	0.5	Negative	Danger

Herbicide	Species/study	NOEL[1] (mg/kg/day)	Toxicity Studies	Hazard Indicator
MSMA	Rat/2-year	3.2	Mutagenicity	NA
	Dog/52-week	NA	Developmental	Not teratogenic
	Mouse/18-month	NA	Reproductive	Decreased fertility
	RfD[2]	0.01	Oncogenicity	B2 (Bladder fibrosarcomas)[3]
Difenzoquat	Rat/2-year	25	Mutagenicity	NA
	Dog/52-week	20	Developmental	Not teratogenic
	Mouse/18-month	75	Reproductive	No evidence
	RfD[2]	0.20	Oncogenicity	E (No evidence)[3]

[1] No observable effect level
[2] RfD = reference dose (190)
[3] See Table 13.3 for US EPA classification scheme
NA = Not Available

being used extensively. More recently, seeds have been genetically engineered to incorporate the natural insecticide control stock of *Bacillus thuringiensis*. Most recently, a gene has been installed in crop seed to protect the crop from a nonspecific herbicide. It can be seen that crop protection chemicals are evolving to superefficacious agents. In most cases, this enhanced efficacy for the target pest did not come at the expense of human or environmental safety.

The crop protection industry has become a significant business during the last 50 years. However, with the harvest reaped by this industry, there have been substantial benefits provided to society. Looking beyond the lives saved by DDT from its use in disease control, the agriculturist's ability to produce food and fiber have significantly increased and labor costs have significantly decreased. Despite a 69% decrease in the number of U.S. farmers from the 1930s to the 1990s, the individual farmer can now feed an average of 129 people; this is up from 19 in the 1930s. Currently less than 2% of our population now grows enough food to feed the entire U.S. population, with surplus.

The average life expectancy has increased from 60 years in 1930 to in excess of 75 years today, primarily due to the availability of an adequate and healthy supply of food. It has been less than 60 years since DDT was first used as an insecticide, and we have learned a lot about the need to develop chemicals that do not disturb our environment.

We are also learning that nature itself may provide us with better ways of achieving that objective. The challenge is ours. In the next 60 years, world agriculture must be able to provide food for more than 11 billion people. This means that we must triple our output over the next six decades while eliminating any impact on the environment.

QUESTIONS

1. Farmers must contend with some 80,000 plant diseases, 30,000 species of weeds, and 1000 species of nematodes and more than 10,000 species of insects. Today, national and international agricultural organizations estimate that as much as 45% of the world's crops continue to be lost to these types of hazards. In the United States alone, about $20 billion worth of crops (one-tenth of production) is lost each year. What do you think would be the status of our national food production capacity without the use of pesticides?
2. Who assures that pesticides can be used without unacceptable hazard to the consumer to protect food crops and maximize yields?
3. How stringent are the testing requirements for the registration of a pesticide when compared to those for products used in the household and yard, industrial chemicals, or even pharmaceuticals?
4. Has the introduction of pesticides into your food supply had a positive or negative impact on the quality of your life?

REFERENCES

1. Aspelin, A. L. (1996): *Pesticide Industry Sales and Useage 1994 and 1995 Market Estimates Reports*. Economic Analysis Branch, Biological and Economic Analysis Division. http://www.epa.gov/oppbead1/95pestsales/Intro.html (accessed 5/99).
2. Avery, D. (1993): Environmental agriculture. 60 Years of inspiration. *National Agricultural Chemicals Association and Farm Chemicals Magazine*, 1:1–13.
3. Ballantine, L. G. (1992): An overview of the U.S. pesticide registration guidelines. *Agric. Newsletter*, 3(2):1–6.
4. Beyer, E. M., Jr., Duffy, M. J., Hay, J. V., and Schlueter, D. D. (1988): Sulfonylureas. In: *Herbicides; Chemistry, Degradation and Mode of Action*, edited by P. C. Kearney and D. D. Kaufman, pp. 117–189. Marcel Dekker, New York.
5. Bliley, R. (1996): *Food Quality Protection Act of 1996*. 104 Congress, 2nd Session. Report 104–669, part 2, pp. 1–89. Government Printing Office, Washington, DC.
6. Bloomquist, J. R. (1993a): Neuroreceptor mechanisms in pyrethroid mode of action and resistance. *Rev. Pestic. Toxicol.*, 2:185–226.
7. Bloomquist, J. R. (1993b): Toxicology, mode of action, and target site-mediated resistance to insecticides acting on chloride channels. *Mini Rev. Comp. Biochem. Physiol.*, 106C:301–314
8. Bloomquist, J. R. (1999): Insecticides: Chemistries and characteristics. At *Radcliffe's IPM World Textbook Home Page*. http://ipmworld.umn.edu/chapters/bloomq.htm (Accessed 4/99).
9. British Crop Protection Council (BCPC). (1997): Abamectin. In: *A World Compendium: The Pesticide Manual*, 11th ed., edited by C. D. S. Tomlin, pp. 3–5. British Crop Protection Council, Farnham, Surrey.
10. British Crop Protection Council (BCPC). (1997): Acephate. In: *A World Compendium: The Pesticide Manual*, 11th ed., edited by C. D. S. Tomlin, pp. 7–9. British Crop Protection Council, Farnham, Surrey.
11. British Crop Protection Council (BCPC). (1997): Aldicarb. In: *A World Compendium: The Pesticide Manual*, 11th ed., edited by C. D. S. Tomlin, pp. 26–28. British Crop Protection Council, Farnham, Surrey.
12. British Crop Protection Council (BCPC). (1997): Azoxystrobin. In: *A World Compendium: The Pesticide Manual*, 11th ed., edited by C. D. S. Tomlin, pp. 70–72. British Crop Protection Council, Farnham, Surrey.
13. British Crop Protection Council (BCPC). (1997): *Bacillus thuringiensis*. In: *A World Compendium: The Pesticide Manual*, 11th ed., edited by C. D. S. Tomlin, pp. 73–78. British Crop Protection Council, Farnham, Surrey.
14. British Crop Protection Council (BCPC). (1997): Benfluralin. In: *A World Compendium: The Pesticide Manual*, 11th ed., edited by C. D. S. Tomlin, pp. 94–95. British Crop Protection Council, Farnham, Surrey.
15. British Crop Protection Council (BCPC). (1997): Benomyl. In: *A World Compendium: The Pesticide Manual*, 11th ed., edited by C. D. S. Tomlin, pp. 100–102. British Crop Protection Council, Farnham, Surrey.
16. British Crop Protection Council (BCPC). (1997): Captan. In: *A World Compendium: The Pesticide Manual*, 11th ed., edited by C. D. S. Tomlin, pp. 177–179. British Crop Protection Council, Farnham, Surrey.
17. British Crop Protection Council (BCPC). (1997): Carbaryl. In: *A World Compendium: The Pesticide Manual*, 11th ed., edited by C. D. S. Tomlin, pp. 180–182. British Crop Protection Council, Farnham, Surrey.
18. British Crop Protection Council (BCPC). (1997): Carbofuran. In: *A World Compendium: The Pesticide Manual*, 11th ed., edited by C. D. S. Tomlin, pp. 186–188. British Crop Protection Council, Farnham, Surrey.
19. British Crop Protection Council (BCPC). (1997): Chlorfenapyr. In: *A World Compendium: The Pesticide Manual*, 11th ed., edited by C. D. S. Tomlin, pp. 209–211. British Crop Protection Council, Farnham, Surrey.
20. British Crop Protection Council (BCPC). (1997): Chlorothalonil. In: *A World Compendium: The Pesticide Manual*, 11th ed., edited by C. D. S. Tomlin, pp. 227–229. British Crop Protection Council, Farnham, Surrey.
21. British Crop Protection Council (BCPC). (1997): Chlorpyrifos. In: *A World Compendium: The Pesticide Manual*, 11th ed., edited by C. D. S. Tomlin, pp. 235–237. British Crop Protection Council, Farnham, Surrey.
22. British Crop Protection Council (BCPC). (1997): Clodinafop-propargyl. In: *A World Compendium: The Pesticide Manual*, 11th ed., edited by C. D. S. Tomlin, pp. 251–253. British Crop Protection Council, Farnham, Surrey.
23. British Crop Protection Council (BCPC). (1997): Copper Hydroxide. In: *A World Compendium: The Pesticide Manual*, 11th ed., edited by C. D. S. Tomlin, p. 268. British Crop Protection Council, Farnham, Surrey.
24. British Crop Protection Council (BCPC). (1997): Copper oxychloride. In: *A World Compendium: The Pesticide Manual*,

11th ed., edited by C. D. S. Tomlin, pp. 269–270. British Crop Protection Council, Farnham, Surrey.

25. British Crop Protection Council (BCPC). (1997): Copper sulfate. In: *A World Compendium: The Pesticide Manual*, 11th ed., edited by C. D. S. Tomlin, pp. 270–272. British Crop Protection Council, Farnham, Surrey.
26. British Crop Protection Council (BCPC). (1997): Cyproconazole. In: *A World Compendium: The Pesticide Manual*, 11th ed., edited by C. D. S. Tomlin, pp. 317–318. British Crop Protection Council, Farnham, Surrey.
27. British Crop Protection Council (BCPC). (1997): Cyprodinil. In: *A World Compendium: The Pesticide Manual*, 11th ed., edited by C. D. S. Tomlin, pp. 319–321. British Crop Protection Council, Farnham, Surrey.
28. British Crop Protection Council (BCPC). (1997): Cyromazine. In: *A World Compendium: The Pesticide Manual*, 11th ed., edited by C. D. S. Tomlin, pp. 321–322. British Crop Protection Council, Farnham, Surrey.
29. British Crop Protection Council (BCPC). (1997): Diazinon. In: *A World Compendium: The Pesticide Manual*, 11th ed., edited by C. D. S. Tomlin, pp. 354–356. British Crop Protection Council, Farnham, Surrey.
30. British Crop Protection Council (BCPC). (1997): Dichlorvos. In: *A World Compendium: The Pesticide Manual*, 11th ed., edited by C. D. S. Tomlin, pp. 849–852. British Crop Protection Council, Farnham, Surrey.
31. British Crop Protection Council (BCPC). (1997): Difenoconazole. In: *A World Compendium: The Pesticide Manual*, 11th ed., edited by C. D. S. Tomlin, pp. 389–390. British Crop Protection Council, Farnham, Surrey.
32. British Crop Protection Council (BCPC). (1997): Diofenolan. In: *A World Compendium: The Pesticide Manual*, 11th ed., edited by C. D. S. Tomlin, pp. 430–431. British Crop Protection Council, Farnham, Surrey.
33. British Crop Protection Council (BCPC). (1997): Endosulfan. In: *A World Compendium: The Pesticide Manual*, 11th ed., edited by C. D. S. Tomlin, pp. 459–461. British Crop Protection Council, Farnham, Surrey.
34. British Crop Protection Council (BCPC). (1997): Fenbuconazole. In: *A World Compendium: The Pesticide Manual*, 11th ed., edited by C. D. S. Tomlin, pp. 508–509. British Crop Protection Council, Farnham, Surrey.
35. British Crop Protection Council (BCPC). (1997): Fenpiclonil. In: *A World Compendium: The Pesticide Manual*, 11th ed., edited by C. D. S. Tomlin, pp. 522–523. British Crop Protection Council, Farnham, Surrey.
36. British Crop Protection Council (BCPC). (1997): Fenpropathrin. In: *A World Compendium: The Pesticide Manual*, 11th ed., edited by C. D. S. Tomlin, pp. 524–525. British Crop Protection Council, Farnham, Surrey.
37. British Crop Protection Council (BCPC). (1997): Fentin. In: *A World Compendium: The Pesticide Manual*, 11th ed., edited by C. D. S. Tomlin, pp. 533–537. British Crop Protection Council, Farnham, Surrey.
38. British Crop Protection Council (BCPC). (1997): Fenvalerate. In: *A World Compendium: The Pesticide Manual*, 11th ed., edited by C. D. S. Tomlin, pp. 539–541. British Crop Protection Council, Farnham, Surrey.
39. British Crop Protection Council (BCPC). (1997): Ferbam. In: *A World Compendium: The Pesticide Manual*, 11th ed., edited by C. D. S. Tomlin, pp. 541–543. British Crop Protection Council, Farnham, Surrey.
40. British Crop Protection Council (BCPC). (1997): Fipronil. In: *A World Compendium: The Pesticide Manual*, 11th ed., edited by C. D. S. Tomlin, pp. 545–547. British Crop Protection Council, Farnham, Surrey.
41. British Crop Protection Council (BCPC). (1997): Fluazifop-P-butyl. In: *A World Compendium: The Pesticide Manual*, 11th ed., edited by C. D. S. Tomlin, pp. 547–549. British Crop Protection Council, Farnham, Surrey.
42. British Crop Protection Council (BCPC). (1997): Fludioxonil. In: *A World Compendium: The Pesticide Manual*, 11th ed., edited by C. D. S. Tomlin, pp. 566–568. British Crop Protection Council, Farnham, Surrey.
43. British Crop Protection Council (BCPC). (1997): Flutolanil. In: *A World Compendium: The Pesticide Manual*, 11th ed., edited by C. D. S. Tomlin, pp. 608–609. British Crop Protection Council, Farnham, Surrey.
44. British Crop Protection Council (BCPC). (1997): Gamma-HCH. In: *A World Compendium: The Pesticide Manual*, 11th ed., edited by C. D. S. Tomlin, pp. 664–666. British Crop Protection Council, Farnham, Surrey.
45. British Crop Protection Council (BCPC). (1997): Halosulfuron-methyl. In: *A World Compendium: The Pesticide Manual*, 11th ed., edited by C. D. S. Tomlin, pp. 657–659. British Crop Protection Council, Farnham, Surrey.
46. British Crop Protection Council (BCPC). (1997): Hexaconazole. In: *A World Compendium: The Pesticide Manual*, 11th ed., edited by C. D. S. Tomlin, pp. 674–675. British Crop Protection Council, Farnham, Surrey.
47. British Crop Protection Council (BCPC). (1997): Hydramethylnon. In: *A World Compendium: The Pesticide Manual*, 11th ed., edited by C. D. S. Tomlin, pp. 681–683. British Crop Protection Council, Farnham, Surrey.
48. British Crop Protection Council (BCPC). (1997): Imazalil. In: *A World Compendium: The Pesticide Manual*, 11th ed., edited by C. D. S. Tomlin, pp. 691–694. British Crop Protection Council, Farnham, Surrey.
49. British Crop Protection Council (BCPC). (1997): Imazosulfuron. In: *A World Compendium: The Pesticide Manual*, 11th ed., edited by C. D. S. Tomlin, pp. 703–706. British Crop Protection Council, Farnham, Surrey.
50. British Crop Protection Council (BCPC). (1997): Imidacloprid. In: *A World Compendium: The Pesticide Manual*, 11th ed., edited by C. D. S. Tomlin, pp. 706–708. British Crop Protection Council, Farnham, Surrey.
51. British Crop Protection Council (BCPC). (1997): Iprodione. In: *A World Compendium: The Pesticide Manual*, 11th ed., edited by C. D. S. Tomlin, pp. 724–726. British Crop Protection Council, Farnham, Surrey.
52. British Crop Protection Council (BCPC). (1997): Lambda-cyhalothrin. In: *A World Compendium: The Pesticide Manual*, 11th ed., edited by C. D. S. Tomlin, pp. 300–302. British Crop Protection Council, Farnham, Surrey.
53. British Crop Protection Council. (1997): Mancozeb. In: *A World Compendium: The Pesticide Manual*, 11th ed., edited by C. D. S. Tomlin, pp. 761–763. British Crop Protection Council, Farnham, Surrey.
54. British Crop Protection Council. (1997): Maneb. In: *A World Compendium: The Pesticide Manual*, 11th ed., edited by C. D. S. Tomlin, pp. 764–766. British Crop Protection Council, Farnham, Surrey.
55. British Crop Protection Council (BCPC). (1997): Metalaxyl-M. In: *A World Compendium: The Pesticide Manual*, 11th ed., edited by C. D. S. Tomlin, pp. 794–795. British Crop Protection Council, Farnham, Surrey.
56. British Crop Protection Council (BCPC). (1997): Methomyl. In: *A World Compendium: The Pesticide Manual*, 11th ed., edited by

C. D. S. Tomlin, pp. 815–817. British Crop Protection Council, Farnham, Surrey.

57. British Crop Protection Council (BCPC). (1997): Monocrotophos. In: *A World Compendium: The Pesticide Manual*. 11th ed., edited by C. D. S. Tomlin, pp. 849–852. British Crop Protection Council, Farnham, Surrey.
58. British Crop Protection Council (BCPC). (1997): Myclobutanil. In: *A World Compendium: The Pesticide Manual*., 11th Ed., edited by C. D. S. Tomlin, pp. 854–855. British Crop Protection Council, Farnham, Surrey.
59. British Crop Protection Council (BCPC). (1997): Nicotine. *A World Compendium: The Pesticide Manual*., 11th ed., edited by C. D. S. Tomlin, pp. 879–880. British Crop Protection Council, Farnham, Surrey.
60. British Crop Protection Council (BCPC). (1997): Oxasulfuron. In: *A World Compendium: The Pesticide Manual*, 11th ed., edited by C. D. S. Tomlin, pp. 911–914. British Crop Protection Council, Farnham, Surrey.
61. British Crop Protection Council (BCPC). (1997): Permethrin. In: *A World Compendium: The Pesticide Manual*, 11th ed., edited by C. D. S. Tomlin, pp. 944–946. British Crop Protection Council, Farnham, Surrey.
62. British Crop Protection Council (BCPC). (1997): Prochloraz. In: *A World Compendium: The Pesticide Manual*. 11th ed., edited by C. D. S. Tomlin, pp. 1000–1002. British Crop Protection Council, Farnham, Surrey.
63. British Crop Protection Council (BCPC). (1997). Propaquizafop. In: *A World Compendium: The Pesticide Manual*, 11th ed., edited by C. D. S. Tomlin, pp. 1021–1024. British Crop Protection Council, Farnham, Surrey.
64. British Crop Protection Council (BCPC). (1997): Propiconazole. In: *A World Compendium: The Pesticide Manual*, 11th ed., edited by C. D. S. Tomlin, pp. 1030–1032. British Crop Protection Council, Farnham, Surrey.
65. British Crop Protection Council (BCPC). (1997): Propoxur. In: *A World Compendium: The Pesticide Manual*, 11th ed., edited by C. D. S. Tomlin, pp. 1036–1039. British Crop Protection Council, Farnham, Surrey.
66. British Crop Protection Council (BCPC). (1997): Prosulfuron. In: *A World Compendium: The Pesticide Manual*, 11th ed., edited by C. D. S. Tomlin, pp. 1041–1043. British Crop Protection Council, Farnham, Surrey.
67. British Crop Protection Council (BCPC). (1997): Pymetrozine. In: *A World Compendium: The Pesticide Manual*, 11th ed., edited by C. D. S. Tomlin, pp. 1045–1046. British Crop Protection Council, Farnham, Surrey.
68. British Crop Protection Council (BCPC). (1997): Pyrimethanil. In: *A World Compendium: The Pesticide Manual*, 11th ed., edited by C. D. S. Tomlin, pp. 1068–1069. British Crop Protection Council, Farnham, Surrey.
69. British Crop Protection Council (BCPC). (1997): Pyriminobac-methyl. In: *A World Compendium: The Pesticide Manual*, 11th ed., edited by C. D. S. Tomlin, pp. 1071–1072. British Crop Protection Council, Farnham, Surrey.
70. British Crop Protection Council (BCPC). (1997): Pyriproxyfen. In: *A World Compendium: The Pesticide Manual*, 11th ed., C. D. S. Tomlin, pp. 1072–1073. British Crop Protection Council, Farnham, Surrey.
71. British Crop Protection Council (BCPC). (1997): Rimsulfuron. In: *A World Compendium: The Pesticide Manual*, 11th ed., edited by C. D. S. Tomlin, pp. 1095–1097. British Crop Protection Council, Farnham, Surrey.
72. British Crop Protection Council (BCPC). (1997): Sulcotrione. In: *A World Compendium: The Pesticide Manual*, 11th ed., edited by C. D. S. Tomlin, pp. 1124–1125. British Crop Protection Council, Farnham, Surrey.
73. British Crop Protection Council (BCPC). (1997): Sulfosulfuron. In: *A World Compendium: The Pesticide Manual*, 11th ed., edited by C. D. S. Tomlin, pp. 1130–1131. British Crop Protection Council, Farnham, Surrey.
74. British Crop Protection Council (BCPC). (1997): Sulfur. In: *A World Compendium: The Pesticide Manual*, 11th ed., edited by C. D. S. Tomlin, pp. 1133–1134. British Crop Protection Council, Farnham, Surrey.
75. British Crop Protection Council (BCPC). (1997): Tebuconazole. In: *A World Compendium: The Pesticide Manual*, 11th ed., edited by C. D. S. Tomlin, pp. 1144–1146. British Crop Protection Council, Farnham, Surrey.
76. British Crop Protection Council (BCPC). (1997): Teflubenzuron. In: *A World Compendium: The Pesticide Manual* 11th ed., edited by C. D. S. Tomlin, pp. 1158–1159. British Crop Protection Council, Farnham, Surrey.
77. British Crop Protection Council (BCPC). (1997): Thiabendazole. In: *A World Compendium: The Pesticide Manual*, 11th ed., edited by C. D. S. Tomlin, pp. 1183–1185. British Crop Protection Council, Farnham, Surrey.
78. British Crop Protection Council (BCPC). (1997): Thiophanate-methyl. In: *A World Compendium: The Pesticide Manual*, 11th ed., edited by C. D. S. Tomlin, pp. 1201–1203. British Crop Protection Council, Farnham, Surrey.
79. British Crop Protection Council (BCPC). (1997): Thiram. In: *A World Compendium: The Pesticide Manual*, 11th ed., edited by C. D. S. Tomlin, pp. 1203–1205. British Crop Protection Council, Farnham, Surrey.
80. British Crop Protection Council (BCPC). (1997): Triadimefon. In: *A World Compendium: The Pesticide Manual*, 11th ed., edited by C. D. S. Tomlin, pp. 1216–1218. British Crop Protection Council, Farnham, Surrey.
81. British Crop Protection Council (BCPC). (1997): Triadimenol. In: *A World Compendium: The Pesticide Manual*, 11th ed., edited by C. D. S. Tomlin, pp. 1218–1220. British Crop Protection Council, Farnham, Surrey.
82. British Crop Protection Council (BCPC). (1997): Trichlopyr. In: *A World Compendium: The Pesticide Manual*, 11th ed., edited by C. D. S. Tomlin, pp. 1237–1239. British Crop Protection Council, Farnham, Surrey.
83. British Crop Protection Council (BCPC). (1997): Vinclozolin. In: *A World Compendium: The Pesticide Manual*, 11th ed., edited by C. D. S. Tomlin, pp. 1267–1268. British Crop Protection Council, Farnham, Surrey.
84. British Crop Protection Council (BCPC). (1997): XDE-105 (Spinosad). In: *A World Compendium: The Pesticide Manual*, 11th ed., edited by C. D. S. Tomlin, pp. 1272–1273. British Crop Protection Council, Farnham, Surrey.
85. British Crop Protection Council (BCPC). (1997): Zineb. In: *A World Compendium: The Pesticide Manual*, 11th ed., edited by C. D. S. Tomlin, pp. 1276–1277. British Crop Protection Council, Farnham, Surrey.
86. British Crop Protection Council (BCPC). (1997): Ziram. In: *A World Compendium: The Pesticide Manual*, 11th ed., edited by C. D. S. Tomlin, pp. 1277–1279. British Crop Protection Council, Farnham, Surrey.
87. British Industrial Biological Research Association (BIBRA). (1988): *Screening for Safety: Pesticides*, p. 3. Liebling Stewart Design Associates, London.
88. Clark, J. M., Scott, J. G., Campos, F., and Bloomquist, J. R. (1995): Resistance to avermectins: Extent, mechanisms, and management implications. *Annu. Rev. Entomol.*, 40:1–30.

89. Conner, J. D., Jr., Ebner, L. S., Landfair, S. W., O'Connor, C. III, Weinstein, K. W., and Jovanovich, A. P. (1991): *Pesticide Regulations Handbook*, 3rd ed., p. 1. Executive Enterprises, New York.
90. Cremlyn, R. (1978): *Pesticides. Preparation and Mode of Action*. John Wiley and Sons, New York.
91. Delp, C. P. (1985): *Fungicide Resistance in North America*, edited by C. P. Delp, pp. 1–20. American Phytopathology Society Press, St. Paul, MN.
92. Duke, S. O., and Kenyon, W. H. (1988): Polycyclic alkanoic acids. In: *Herbicides; Chemistry, Degradation and Mode of Action*, edited by P. C. Kearney and D. D. Kaufman, pp. 71–116. Marcel Dekker, New York.
93. Ecobichon, D. J. (1993): Toxic effects of pesticides. In: *Casarett and Doull's Toxicology: The Basic Science of Poisons*, 4th ed., edited by J. Doull, C. D. Klaassen, and M. O. Amdur, pp. 565–621. Macmillan, New York.
94. Eldridge, J. C., Stevens, J. T., Wetzel, L. T., Tisdel, M. O., Breckenridge, C. B., McConnell, R. F., and Simpkins, J. W. (1996): Atrazine: Mechanisms of hormonal imbalance in female SD rats. *Fundam. Appl. Toxicol.* 24(12):2–5.
95. European Economic Community (ECC). (1993): Commission Directive 93/67/EEC: 1993. Laying Down the Principles for Assessment of Risks to Man and the Environment of Substances Notified in accordance with Council Directive 67/548/EEC. July 20, 1993.
96. European Economic Community (EEC). (1994): Commission Directive 94/79/EC of December 1994 amending Council Directive 91/414/ EEC concerning the placing of plant protection products on the market. *Off. J. Euro. Communities*, December 31:L354/16.
97. Farber, T. M. (1987): Pesticide assessment guidelines, Subdivision F. Position Document: Selection of a Maximum Tolerated Dose (MTD) in oncogenicity studies. Toxicology Branch, Hazard Evaluation Division, Office of Pesticides Programs, U.S. Environmental Protection Agency, Washington, DC. NTIS PB88-116736.
98. Gianessi, L. P. (1986): *A National Pesticide Useage Data Base*, pp. 1–14. Resources for the Future, Washington, DC.
99. Gill, S. S., Cowles, E. A., and Pietrantonio, P. V. (1992): The mode of action of *Bacillus thuringiensis* endotoxins. *Ann. Rev. Entomol.*, 37:615–36.
100. Goldman, L. R. (1998): Chemicals and children's environment: What we don't know about risk. *Environ. Health Perspect.*, 106(suppl. 3):875–880.
101. Gunsolus, G. L., and Curran, W. S. (1999): Herbicide Mode of Action and Injury Symptoms. http://www.mes.umn.edu/Documents/D/C/DC3832.htm (Accessed 6/99).
102. Hayes, W. J., Jr. (1991): Introduction. In *Handbook of Pesticide Toxicology. Volume 1. General Principles*, pp. 1–37. Academic Press, San Diego.
103. Hollingshaus, J. (1987): Inhibition of mitochondrial electron transport by hydramethylnon: A new amidinohyrazone insecticide. *Pestic. Biochem. Physiol.*, 27:61–70.
104. Hollingworth, R. Ahmmadsahib, K. Gedelhak, G., and McLaughlin, J. (1994): New inhibitors of complex I of the mitochondrial electron transport chain with activity as pesticides. *Biochem. Soc. Trans.* (*Lond.*), 22:230–233.
105. International Agency for Research on Cancer (IARC). (1998): Monographs working group—Volume 73: Evaluation or re-evaluation of some agents which target specific organs in rodent bioassays (in preparation). http://193.51.164.11/past&future/OCT98.html (Accessed 11/98).
106. Joint Expert Committee on Food Additives (JECFA). (1997): Tiabendazole (Thiabendazole). *JECFA Monograph Series 31*. World Health Organization, WHO/JECMONO.31.4, pp. 1–23.
107. Joint Meeting of the FAO/WHO Panel of Experts on Pesticide Residues in Food (JMPR). (1974): Carbaryl. FAO Agricultural Studies., No. 92: WHO Technical Report Series, No. 545, 1974. 1973 Evaluation of Some Pesticide Residues in Food. FAO/AGP/1974/M/11.
108. Joint Meeting of the FAO/WHO Panel of Experts on Pesticide Residues (JMPR). (1983): Carbofuran. FAO Plant Production and Protection Paper 46. 1982. FAO Plant Production and Protection Paper 46.
109. Joint Meeting of the FAO/WHO Panel of Experts on Pesticide Residues (JMPR). (1983): Chlorpyrifos. Pesticide Residues in Food—1982 Evaluations. FAO Plant Production and Protection Paper 46.
110. Joint Meeting of the FAO/WHO Panel of Experts on Pesticide Residues (JMPR). (1985): Prochloraz. FAO Plant Production and Protection Paper 56. 1984. Pesticide residues in food—1984 Evaluations. FAO Plant Production and Protection Paper 61.
111. Joint Meeting of the FAO/WHO Panel of Experts on Pesticide Residues (JMPR). (1985): Triadimefon. FAO Plant Production and Protection Paper 68, Pesticide Residues in Food—1985 evaluations; Part II—Toxicology. FAO Plant Production and Protection Paper 72/2.
112. Joint Meeting of the FAO/WHO Panel of Experts on Pesticide Residues (JMPR). (1989): Triadimenol. FAO Plant Production and Protection Paper 99. Pesticide Residues in Food—1989 Evaluations; Part II—Toxicology. FAO Plant Production and Protection Paper 100/2.
113. Joint Meeting of the FAO/WHO Panel of Experts on Pesticide Residues in Food (JMPR). (1990): Acephate. FAO Plant Production and Protection Paper 103. Pesticide Residues in Food—1990 Evaluations; Part II—Toxicology. World Health Organisation, WHO/PCS/92.47.
114. Joint Meeting of the FAO/WHO Panel of Experts on Pesticide Residues (JMPR). (1990): Endosulfan. FAO Plant Production and Protection Paper 99. Pesticide Residues in Food—1989 Evaluations; Part II—Toxicology. FAO Plant Production and Protection Paper 100/2.
115. Joint Meeting of the FAO/WHO Panel of Experts on Pesticide Residues (JMPR). (1990): Lindane. FAO Plant Production and Protection Paper 99. Pesticide Residues in Food—1989 Evaluations; Part II—Toxicology. FAO Plant Production and Protection Paper 100/2.
116. Joint Meeting of the FAO/WHO Panel of Experts on Pesticide Residues (JMPR). (1990): Methomyl. FAO Plant Production and Protection Paper 99. Pesticide Residues in Food—1989 Evaluations; Part II—Toxicology. FAO Plant Production and Protection Paper 100/2.
117. Joint Meeting of the FAO/WHO Panel of Experts on Pesticide Residues (JMPR). (1990): Propoxur. FAO Plant Production and Protection Paper 99. Pesticide Residues in Food—1989 Evaluations; Part II—Toxicology. FAO Plant Production and Protection Paper 100/2.
118. Joint Meeting of the FAO/WHO Panel of Experts on Pesticide Residues in Food (JMPR). (1991): Azinphos-methyl. FAO Plant Production and Protection Paper 111. Pesticide Residues in Food—1991 Evaluations; Part II—Toxicology. http://www.inchem.org/documents/jmpr/jmpmono/v91pr02.htm (Accessed 6/99).
119. Joint Meeting of the FAO/WHO Panel of Experts on Pesticide Residues (JMPR): (1992) Imazalil. FAO Plant Production and Protection Paper 111. Pesticide Residues in Food—1991 Evaluations; Part II—Toxicology & Environment. World Health Organization, WHO/PCS/92.52.
120. Joint Meeting of the FAO/WHO Panel of Experts on Pesticide Residues in Food (JMPR). (1993): Chlorothalonil. FAO Plant Pro-

duction and Protection Paper 116. Pesticide Residues in Food—1992 Evaluations; Part II—Toxicology. World Health Organization, WHO/PCS/93.34.

121. Joint Meeting of the FAO/WHO Panel of Experts on Pesticide Residues in Food (JMPR). (1993): Thiram. FAO Plant Production and Protection Paper 116. Pesticide Residues in Food—1992 Evaluations; Part II—Toxicology. World Health Organization, WHO/PCS/93.34.
122. Joint Meeting of the FAO/WHO Panel of Experts on Pesticide Residues (JMPR). (1994): Abamectin. Pesticide Residues in Food—1993. Report of the Joint Meeting of the FAO Panel of Experts on Pesticide Residues in Food and the Environment and the WHO Expert Group on Pesticide Residues. FAO Plant Production and Protection Paper 127, pp. 15–17.
123. Joint Meeting of the FAO/WHO Panel of Experts on Pesticide Residues in Food (JMPR). (1994): Diazinon. Pesticide Residues in Food—1993 Evaluations; Part II—Toxicology. FAO Plant Production and Protection Paper 122. World Health Organization, WHO/PCS/94.4.
124. Joint Meeting of the FAO/WHO Panel of Experts on Pesticide Residues in Food (JMPR). (1994): Dichlorvos. FAO Plant Production and Protection Paper 122. Pesticide Residues in Food—1993 Evaluations; Part II—Toxicology. World Health Organization, WHO/PCS/94.4.
125. Joint Meeting of the FAO/WHO Panel of Experts on Pesticide Residues (JMPR). (1994): Fenpropathrin. FAO Plant Production and Protection Paper 122. Pesticide Residues in Food—1993 Evaluations; Part II—Toxicology. WHO/PCS/94.4.
126. Joint Meeting of the FAO/WHO Panel of Experts on Pesticide Residues in Food (JMPR). (1994): Mancozeb. FAO Plant Production and Protection Paper 122. Pesticide Residues in Food—1993 Evaluations; Part II—Toxicology. World Health Organization, WHO/PCS/94.4.
127. Joint Meeting of the FAO/WHO Panel of Experts on Pesticide Residues in Food (JMPR). (1994): Maneb. FAO Plant Production and Protection Paper 122. Pesticide Residues in Food—1993 Evaluations; Part II—Toxicology. World Health Organization, WHO/PCS/94.4.
128. Joint Meeting of the FAO/WHO Panel of Experts on Pesticide Residues (JMPR). (1994): Permethrin. FAO Plant Production and Protection Paper 122. Pesticide Residues in Food—1993 Evaluations; Part II—Toxicology. WHO/PCS/94.4.
129. Joint Meeting of the FAO/WHO Panel of Experts on Pesticide Residues in Food (JMPR). (1994) Zineb. FAO Plant Production and Protection Paper 122. Pesticide Residues in Food—1993 Evaluations; Part II—Toxicology. World Health Organization, WHO/PCS/94.4.
130. Joint Meeting of the FAO/WHO Panel of Experts on Pesticide Residues in Food (JMPR). (1995): Monocrotophos. FAO Plant Production and Protection Paper 133. Pesticide Residues in Food—1994 Evaluations; Part II—Toxicology & Environment. World Health Organization, WHO/PCS/96.48.
131. Joint Meeting of the FAO/WHO Panel of Experts on Pesticide Residues in Food (JMPR). (1996): Aldicarb. FAO Plant Production and Protection Paper 133. Pesticide Residues in Food—1995 Evaluations; Part II—Toxicology & Environment. World Health Organization, WHO/PCS/96.48.
132. Joint Meeting of the FAO/WHO Panel of Experts on Pesticide Residues in Food (JMPR). (1996): Benomyl. FAO Plant Production and Protection Paper 133. Pesticide Residues in Food—1995 Evaluations; Part II—Toxicology & Environment. World Health Organization, WHO/PCS/96.48, pp. 3–32.
133. Joint Meeting of the FAO/WHO Panel of Experts on Pesticide Residues in Food (JMPR). (1996): Captan. FAO Plant Production and Protection Paper 133. Pesticide Residues in Food—1995 Evaluations; Part II—Toxicology & Environment. World Health Organization, WHO/PCS/96.48.
134. Joint Meeting of the FAO/WHO Panel of Experts on Pesticide Residues in Food (JMPR). (1996): Iprodione (addendum). FAO Plant Production and Protection Paper 133. Pesticide Residues in Food—1995 Evaluations; Part II—Toxicology & Environment. World Health Organization, WHO/PCS/96.48, pp. 231–237.
135. Joint Meeting of the FAO Panel of Experts on Pesticide Residues in Food (JMPR). (1996): Thiophanate-methyl. FAO Plant Production and Protection Paper 133. Pesticide Residues in Food—1995 Evaluations; Part II—Toxicology & Environment. World Health Organization, WHO/PCS/96.48, pp. 351–374.
136. Joint Meeting of the FAO/WHO Panel of Experts on Pesticide Residues (JMPR). (1996): Vinclozolin. FAO Plant Production and Protection Paper 133. Pesticide Residues in Food—1995 Evaluations; Part II—Toxicology & Environment. World Health Organization, WHO/PCS/96.48, pp. 375–404.
137. Joint Meeting of the FAO/WHO Panel of Experts on Pesticide Residues in Food (JMPR). (1997): Ferbam. FAO Plant Production and Protection Paper 140. Pesticide Residues in Food—1996 Evaluations; Part II—Toxicology & Environment. World Health Organization, WHO/PCS/97.06.
138. Joint Meeting of the FAO/WHO Panel of Experts on Pesticide Residues in Food (JMPR). (1997): Ziram. FAO Plant Production and Protection Paper 140. Pesticide Residues in Food—1995 Evaluations; Part II—Toxicology & Environment. World Health Organization, WHO/PCS/97.12.
139. Kaufman, S. (1997): Fungicides. In: *SRI International's Chemical Economics Handbook*, pp. 1–144. SRI Press, Menlo Park, CA.
140. Kelce, W. R., Monosson, E., Gamcsik, M. P., Laws, S. C., and Gray, L. E., Jr. (1994): Environmental hormone disruptors: Evidence that vinclozolin developmental toxicity is mediated by antiandrogenic metabolites. *Toxicol. Appl. Pharmacol.*, 126:276–285.
141. Lankas, G. R., and Gordon, L. R. (1989): Toxicology. In: *Ivermectin and Abamectin*, edited by W. R. Campbell, pp. 89–112. Springer-Verlag, New York.
142. Lankas, G. R., Minsker, D. H., and Robertson, R. T. (1989): Effects of ivermectin on reproduction and neonatal toxicity in rats. *Food Chem. Toxicol.*, 27:523–529.
143. Lankas, G. R., Cartwright, M. E., and Umbenhauer, D. (1997): P-glycoprotein deficiency in a subpopulation of CF-1 mice enhances avermectin-induced neurotoxicity. *Toxicol. Appl. Pharmacol.*, 143:357–365.
144. Larson, L. L. (1999): Novel organic and natural product insect management tools. *National IPM Network*. hppt://ipmworld.umn.edu/chapters/larson.htm (Accessed 1/99).
145. Matringe, M., Clair, D., and Scala, R. (1990): Effects of peroxidizing herbicides on protoporphyrin IX levels in non-chlorophyllous soybean cell culture. *Pestic. Biochem. Physiol.*, 36:300–307.
146. McGaughy, R. (1986): Guidelines for carcinogen risk assessment. *Fed. Reg.*, 51(185):33992–34003.
147. Meister, R. T. (1997): Pheromone. In: *Farm Chemical Handbook '97*, p. C286. Meister, Willoughby, OH.
148. Mellanby, K. (1992): *The DDT Story*, pp. 6–7. British Crop Protection Council, Farnham, Surrey.
149. Ministry of Agriculture, Forestry and Fisheries (MAFF). (1985): Notification of the Director-General. Requirements for Safety Evaluation of Agricultural Chemicals, Agricultural Production Bureau, Ministry of Agriculture, Forestry and Fisheries, Japan, 59 NohSan No. 4200, January 28.
150. Moolenaar, R. J. (1994): Default assumptions in carcinogenic risk assessment used by regulatory agencies. *Regul. Toxicol. Pharmacol.*, 20:S135–S141.

151. Morishima, Y., Osabe, H., and Goto, Y. (1990): Action mechanism of DLH-1777, a novel 4-pyridone-3-carboxamide herbicide: Peroxidizing activity and accumulation of porphyrins. *J. Pestic. Sci.*, 15:553–559.

152. Mullins, J. W. (1993): Imidacloprid: A new nitroguanidine insecticide. ACS Symp. Ser. 524: Newer Pest Control Agents and Technology with Reduced Environmental Impact. ACS, Washington, DC.

153. National Research Council (NRC). (1993): *Pesticides in the Diets of Infants and Children*, National Academy Press, Washington, DC.

154. Nikolau, B. J., Wurtele, E. S., Caffrey, J., Chen, Y., Crane, V., Diez, T., Huang, J.-Y., Mc Dowell, M. T., Shang, X.-M., Song, J., Wang, X. and Weaver, L. M. (1993): The biochemistry and molecular biology of acetyl-CoA carboxylase and other biotin enzymes. In: *Biochemistry and Molecular Biology of Membrane and Storage Lipids of Plants*, edited by N. Murata and C. Somerville, pp. 138–149. American Society of Plant Physiologists Press. Brentwood, TN.

155. Organization for Economic Cooperation and Development. (1981): OECD Guideline for Testing of Chemicals, Section 4, Health Effects, adopted May 12, 1981. OECD. Paris, France.

156. Retzinger, J. E., Jr., and Mallory-Smith, C. (1999): Classification of Herbicides by Site of Action for Weed Resistance Management Strategies.
http://www.css.orst. edu/weeds/Publications/site_action.htm (Accessed 5/99).

157. Simmons, S. W. (1959): The use of DDT insecticides in human medicine. In: *DDT: The Insecticide Dichlorodiphenyl-Trichloroethane and Its Significance*, edited by P. Miller, Vol. 2, pp. 251–502. Birkhaeriger, Basel.

158. Spindler, M. (1990): DDT: Health aspects in relation to man and risk/benefit assessment based thereupon. *Residue Rev.*, 90:1–34.

159. Stetter, J. (1993): Trends in the future development of pest and weed control—An industrial point of view. *Regul. Toxicol. Pharmacol.*, 17:346–370.

160. Stevens, J. T. (1994): Aspects related to uses of organic and inorganic chlorine compounds: Pesticides. In: *Toxicology Forum. Chlorinated Organic Chemicals. Their Effects on Human Health and the Environment*, pp. 567–580. Berlin.

161. Stevens, J. T., Wetzel, L. T., Breckenridge, C. B., Gillis, J. H., Luempert, L. G. III and Eldridge, J. C. (1994): Hypothesis for mammary tumorigenesis in female Sprague-Dawley rats exposed to chloro-*s*-triazine herbicides. *J. Toxicol. Environ. Health*, 43(2):139–154.

162. Stevens, J. T. (1997): Risk assessment of pesticides. In: *Comprehensive Toxicology. Vol. 2. Toxicological Testing and Evaluation*, edited by I. G. Sipes, C. A. McQueen, and A. J. Gandolfi, pp. 17–26. Elsevier Science, Oxford.

163. Stevens, J. T., Sumner, D. D., and Luempert, L. (1995): Agricultural chemicals: The impact of regulations under FIFRA on science and economics. In: *Primer on Regulatory Toxicology*, edited by C. Chenzelis, J. Holson, and S. Gad, pp. 133–163. Raven Press, New York.

164. Stevens, J. T., Breckenridge, C. B., Wetzel, L. T., Thakur, A. K., Liu, C., Werner, C., Luempert, L. C. III, and Eldridge, J. C. (1999). A risk characterization for atrazine: Oncogenicity profile. *J. Toxicol. Environ. Health, A*, 56:69–109.

165. Stevens, J. T., Werner, C., Breckenridge, C. B., and Sumner, D. D. (1999): Hazard assessment for selected symmetrical and asymmetrical triazine herbicide. In: *The Triazine Herbicides*, edited by H. M. LeBaron, J. McFarland, O. Burnside, and R. Clark. In press.

166. Sumner, D. D., and Stevens, J. T. (1994): Pharmacokinetic factors influencing risk assessment: Saturation of biochemical processes and co-factor depletion. In: *Pharmacokinetics: Defining Dosimetry for Risk Assessment. Environ. Health Perspect.*, 102(suppl. 11):13–22.

167. Turner, M. J., and Schaeffer, J. M. (1989): Chapter 5: Mode of Action of Ivermectin. In: *Ivermectin and Abamectin*, edited by W. R. Campbell, pp. 73–88. Springer-Verlag, New York.

168. U.K. Department of Health. (1991): Guidelines for the Evaluation of Chemicals for Carcinogenicity, p. 1. Committee on Carcinogenicity of Chemicals in Food, Consumer Products and the Environment, UK Department of Health, London.

169. U.S. Congress. (1947): Federal Insecticide, Fungicide and Rodenticide Act (FIFRA). Pub. L. No. 80-104, 61 Stat. 163, 1947, p. 1.

170. U.S. Congress. (1958): Food additive amendments to the Federal Food, Drug, and Cosmetic Act (FFDCA) 409. Pub. L. No. 85-929, 72 Stat., 1785, 1958, p. 1.

171. U.S. Environmental Protection Agency (EPA). (1982): Pesticide Assessment Guidelines, Subdivision F. Hazard Evaluation: Human and Domestic Animals. Environmental Protection Agency, 540/9-82-025. Available from NTIS, Springfield, VA.

172. U.S. Environmental Protection Agency (EPA). (1983): Aldicarb. CASRN 116-06-3. Integrated Risk Information System. http://www.epa.gov/iris/subst/0003.htm (Accessed 3/99).

173. U.S. Environmental Protection Agency (EPA). (1987): Benomyl. CASRN 17804-35-2. Integrated Risk Information System. http://www.epa.gov.ngispgm3/Iris/subst/0011.htm (Accessed 3/99).

174. U.S. Environmental Protection Agency (EPA). (1988): Iprodione. CASRN 36734-19-7. Integrated Risk Information System. http://www.epa.gov.ngispgm3/Iris/subst./0291.htm (Accessed 3/99).

175. U.S. Environmental Protection Agency (EPA). (1994): Acetochlor; Pesticide tolerance. *Fed. Reg.*, 59(56):13654–13558.

176. U.S. Environmental Protection Agency (EPA). (1994): Atrazine, simazine and cyanazine; Notice of initiation of special review. http://www.epa.gov/fedrgstr/ EPA-PEST/1994/November/ Day-23/pr-54.html (accessed 3/99).

177. U.S. Environmental Protection Agency (EPA). (1995): Cyproconazole; Pesticide tolerance. *Fed. Reg.*, 60(153):40545–40548.

178. U.S. Environmental Protection Agency (EPA). (1995): Fenbuconazole: Pesticide tolerances. *Fed. Reg.*, 60(100):27419–27421.

179. U.S. Environmental Protection Agency (EPA). (1995): Lepidopteran pheromones: Tolerance exemption. Final rule. *Fed. Reg.*, 60(168):45060–45062.

180. U.S. Environmental Protection Agency (EPA). (1995): Metalaxyl: Pesticide tolerance. *Fed. Reg.*, 60(244):65579–65581.

181. U.S. Environmental Protection Agency (EPA). (1995): Monosodium methanearsonate and disodium methanearsonate; Toxic chemical release reporting; Community right to know. *Fed. Reg.* http://www.epa.gov?fedrgstr/EPA-TRI/April/Day-20/pr-13.html (Accessed 6/99).

182. U.S. Environmental Protection Agency (EPA). (1995): Oxyfluorfen: Pesticide tolerance. *Fed. Reg.*, 60(187):49816–49818.

183. U.S. Environmental Protection Agency (EPA). (1995): Paraquat: Pesticide tolerance. *Fed. Reg.* http://www.epa.gov/fedrgstr/EPA-Pest/1995/March/Day-15/pr-178.html (Accessed 6/99).

184. U.S. Environmental Protection Agency (EPA). (1996): Dimethenamid. Pesticide tolerance petition: Notice of filing. *Fed. Reg.*, 61(62):10681–10684.

185. U.S. Environmental Protection Agency (EPA). (1996): Diquat. Pesticide tolerance. *Fed. Reg.*, 61(60):13474–13476.

186. U.S. Environmental Protection Agency (EPA). (1996): Flutolanil. Pesticide tolerance. *Fed. Reg.*, 61(124):33041–33044.

187. U.S. Environmental Protection Agency (EPA). (1996): Glufosinate-ammonium. Pesticide tolerance petition: Notice of filing. *Fed. Reg.*, 61(223):58684–58688.

187a. U.S. Environmental Protection Agency (EPA). (1996): Hexaconazole: Pesticide tolerance. *Fed. Reg.*, 61(70):15895–15896.

188. U.S. Environmental Protection Agency (EPA). (1996): Imazameth. Pesticide tolerance for cadre. *Fed. Reg.*, 61(55):11311–11313.

189. U.S. Environmental Protection Agency (EPA). (1996): Lactofen: Pesticide tolerance. *Fed. Reg.*, 61(47):9399–9401.

190. U.S. Environmental Protection Agency (EPA). (1996): Office of Pesticide Programs Reference Dose Tracking Report, pp. 1–77. Office of Prevention, Pesticides, and Toxic Substances.

191. U.S. Environmental Protection Agency (EPA). (1996): Propiconazole: Pesticide tolerances for emergency exemptions. *Fed. Reg.*, 61(220):58135–58140.

192. U.S. Environmental Protection Agency (EPA). (1996): Proposed Guidelines for Carcinogen Risk Assessment. Office of Research and Development. Washington, DC. EPA/600/p-92/003c.

193. U.S. Environmental Protection Agency (EPA). (1996): Spinosad; Pesticide tolerance petition. Notice of filing. *Fed. Reg.*, 61(227): 59437–59440.

194. U.S. Environmental Protection Agency (EPA). (1996): Triadimefon: Pesticide tolerances for emergency exemptions. *Fed. Reg.*, 61(232):63726–63726.

195. U.S. Environmental Protection Agency (EPA). (1997): Acifluorfen. Notice of filing of pesticide petitions. *Fed. Reg.*, 62(143):39967–39974.

196. U.S. Environmental Protection Agency (EPA). (1997): Azoxystrobin. Notice of filing of pesticide petitions. *Fed. Reg.*, 62(48):11441–11447.

197. U.S. Environmental Protection Agency (EPA). (1997): *Bacillus thuringiensis* subspecies tolworthi Cry9C. Notice of filing of pesticide petitions. *Fed. Reg.*, 62(182):49224–49226.

198. U.S. Environmental Protection Agency (EPA). (1997): BASF Monsanto and Dekalb Genetics Corporation; Receipt of petition for determination of nonregulated status for genetically engineered corn. *Fed. Reg.*, 62(156):43311–43312.

199. U.S. Environmental Protection Agency (EPA). (1997): CGA329351. Notice of filing of pesticide petitions. *Fed. Reg.*, 62(143):40080–40086.

200. U.S. Environmental Protection Agency (EPA). (1997): Chlorfenapyr. American Cyanamid Company. Pesticide tolerance petition filing. *Fed. Reg.*, 62(24):5399–5403.

201. U.S. Environmental Protection Agency (EPA). (1997): Chorothalonil; ISK Biosciences Corporation; Pesticide tolerance petition filing. *Fed. Reg.*, 62(63):15700–15704.

202. U.S. Environmental Protection Agency (EPA). (1997): Clopyralid. Pesticide tolerance for emergency exemption. *Fed. Reg.*, 62(48): 11360–11364.

203. U.S. Environmental Protection Agency (EPA). (1997): Cloransulam-methyl. Pesticide tolerance for emergency exemption. *Fed. Reg.*, 62(48):11360–11364.

204. U.S. Environmental Protection Agency (EPA). (1997): Difenoconazole. Notice of filing of pesticide petitions. *Fed. Reg.*, 62(143):40075–40080.

205. U.S. Environmental Protection Agency (EPA). (1997): Diuron. Drexel Chemical Company; Pesticide tolerance petition filing. *Fed. Reg.*, 62(16):3685–3688.

206. U.S. Environmental Protection Agency (EPA). (1997): Fenoxaprop-ethyl; Notice of filing of pesticide petitions. *Fed. Reg.*, 62(180):48837–48842.

207. U.S. Environmental Protection Agency (EPA). (1997): Fenpropathrin. Pesticide tolerances for emergency exemptions. *Fed. Reg.*, 62(134):37516–37522.

208. U.S. Environmental Protection Agency (EPA). (1997): Fenvalerate; Pesticide tolerances. *Fed. Reg.*, 62(228):63019–63037.

209. U.S. Environmental Protection Agency (EPA). (1997): Fipronil. Notice of filing of pesticide petitions. *Fed. Reg.*, 62(119): 33641–33647.

210. U.S. Environmental Protection Agency (EPA). (1997): Fludioxonil: Pesticide tolerance petition filing. *Fed. Reg.*, 62(24): 5403–5406.

211. U.S. Environmental Protection Agency (EPA). (1997): Fluthiacet-methyl: Pesticide tolerance petition filing. *Fed. Reg.*, 63(193):53660–53662.

212. U.S. Environmental Protection Agency (EPA). (1997): Fomesafen. Pesticide tolerance for emergency exemption. Final Rule. *Fed. Reg.*, 62(223):61639–61645.

213. U.S. Environmental Protection Agency (EPA). (1997): Imazamox. Pesticide tolerance. Final rule. *Fed. Reg.*, 62(105):29669–29673.

214. U.S. Environmental Protection Agency (EPA). (1997): Imidacloprid. Bayer Corporation: Pesticide tolerance petition filing. *Fed. Reg.*, 62(38):8734–8734 .

215. U.S. Environmental Protection Agency (EPA). (1997): Isoxaflutole; Pesticide tolerance petition filing. *Fed. Reg.*, 62(38):8737–8740.

216. U.S. Environmental Protection Agency (EPA). (1997): Mancozeb, maneb, and ethylenethiourea tolerances. Notice of filing of pesticide petitions. *Fed. Reg.*, 62(148):41383–41386.

217. U.S. Environmental Protection Agency (EPA). (1997): Maneb: Pesticide tolerances for emergency exemptions. *Fed. Reg.*, 62(185):49918–49925.

218. U.S. Environmental Protection Agency (EPA). (1997): Mefenoxam: Pesticide tolerance for emergency exemptions. *Fed. Reg.*, 62(149):42019–42030.

219. U.S. Environmental Protection Agency (EPA). (1997): Myclobutanil: Pesticide tolerance for emergency exemptions. *Fed. Reg.*, 62(6):1284–1288.

220. U.S. Environmental Protection Agency (EPA). (1997): Norflurazon. BASF Corporation. Pesticide tolerance petition filing. *Fed. Reg.*, 62(58):14423–14426.

221. U.S. Environmental Protection Agency (EPA). (1997): Pendimethalin: Pesticide tolerance for emergency exemptions. *Fed. Reg.*, 62(100):28355–28361.

222. U.S. Environmental Protection Agency (EPA). (1997): Propazine. Pesticide tolerance petition filing. *Fed. Reg.*, 63(193):53657–53660.

223. U.S. Environmental Protection Agency (EPA). (1997): Pyridaben. BASF Corporation. Pesticide tolerance petition filing. *Fed. Reg.*, 62(48):11450–11453.

224. U.S. Environmental Protection Agency (EPA). (1997): Pyrimethanil. Pesticide tolerance. *Fed. Reg.*, 62(231):63662–63669.

225. U.S. Environmental Protection Agency (EPA). (1997): Tebuconazole: Pesticide tolerance petition filing. *Fed. Reg.*, 62(43):10047–10050.

226. U.S. Environmental Protection Agency (EPA). (1997): *trans*-11-Tetradecenyl Acetate Technical Pheromone Pesticide Fact sheet. Unconditional Registration. February 1997. http://www.epa.gov/fedrgstr/EPA-PEST/1997/rJune/Day-13/f-p15562.htm (Accessed 6/99).

227. U.S. Environmental Protection Agency (EPA). (1997): Vinclozolin: Pesticide tolerance petition filing. *Fed. Reg.*, 62(53):13000–13005.

228. U.S. Environmental Protection Agency (EPA). (1998): Alachlor. Registration Eligibility Decision for Alachlor. http://www.epa.gov/docs/oppsrrd1/REDs/index.html (Accessed 6/99)

229. U.S. Environmental Protection Agency (EPA). (1998): *Bacillus thuringiensis* variety kurstaki. Notice of filing of pesticide petitions. *Fed. Reg.*, 63(67):17174–17176.

230. U.S. Environmental Protection Agency (EPA). (1998): Carfentrazone-ethyl; Pesticide tolerances. *Fed. Reg.*, 63(189):52174–52180.
231. U.S. Environmental Protection Agency (EPA). (1998): Cyprodinil. Novartis Crop Protection Inc., Approval of a pesticide product. *Fed. Reg.*, 63(108):30749–3070.
232. U.S. Environmental Protection Agency (EPA). (1998): Dicamba. Notice of filing of pesticide petitions. *Fed. Reg.*, 63(2240): 64481–64484.
233. U.S. Environmental Protection Agency (EPA). (1998): Diflubenzuron. Notice of filing of pesticide petitions. *Fed. Reg.*, 63(37):9528–9532.
234. U.S. Environmental Protection Agency (EPA). (1998): Diflubenzuron. Temporary pesticide tolerance. *Fed. Reg.*, 63(92): 26481–26488.
235. U.S. Environmental Protection Agency (EPA). (1998): Glyphosate; Pesticide tolerance. Final rule. *Fed. Reg.*, 63(195): 54058–54066
236. U.S. Environmental Protection Agency (EPA). (1998): Halosulfuron-methyl; Pesticide tolerance petition filing. *Fed. Reg.*, 63(103):29401–29409.
237. U.S. Environmental Protection Agency (EPA). (1998): Hexythiazox. Notice of filing of pesticide tolerance. Notice. *Fed. Reg.*, 63(18):4252–4255.
238. U.S. Environmental Protection Agency (EPA). (1998): Hexythiazox. BASF Corporation. Pesticide tolerance petition filing. *Fed. Reg.*, 63(137):38644–38646.
239. U.S. Environmental Protection Agency (EPA). (1998): Hydramethylnon. American Cyanamid Company. Pesticide tolerance petition filing. *Fed. Reg.*, 63(157):43702–43705.
240. U.S. Environmental Protection Agency (EPA). (1998): Isoxaflutole; Pesticide tolerances. *Fed. Reg.*, 63(184):50773–50784.
241. U.S. Environmental Protection Agency (EPA). (1998): Lambda-cyhalothrin; Pesticide tolerances. *Fed. Reg.*, 63(30): 7291–7299.
242. U.S. Environmental Protection Agency (EPA). (1998): Metolachor; Pesticide tolerances for emergency exemptions. *Fed. Reg.*, 63(176):48586–48594.
243. U.S. Environmental Protection Agency (EPA). (1998): Pesticide Assessment Guidelines. http://www.epa.gov/docs/OPPTS_Harmonized/870_Health_Effects_Test_Guidelines/Series (Accessed 3/99).
244. U.S. Environmental Protection Agency (EPA). (1998): Prometryn; Pesticide tolerances. *Fed. Reg.*, 63(37):9494–9499.
245. U.S. Environmental Protection Agency (EPA). (1998): Pymetrozine. Notice of filing of pesticide petitions. *Fed. Reg.*, 63(97):27723–27727.
246. U.S. Environmental Protection Agency (EPA). (1998): Pymetrozine. Notice of filing of pesticide petitions. *Fed. Reg.*, 63(194):53906–53909.
247. U.S. Environmental Protection Agency (EPA). (1998): Pyridate; Pesticide tolerances. Final rule. *Fed. Reg.*, 63(194):53837–53844.
248. U.S. Environmental Protection Agency (EPA). (1998): Pyriproxyfen; Pesticide tolerances. Final rule. *Fed. Reg.*, 63(128):33366–36373.
249. U.S. Environmental Protection Agency (EPA). (1998): Tebufenozide. Rohm and Haas Company; Notice of filing of pesticide tolerance. Notice. *Fed. Reg.*, 63(160):44439–44456.
250. U.S. Environmental Protection Agency (EPA). (1999): 2,4-D; Time-limited pesticide tolerances. Final rule. *Fed. Reg.*, 64(46):11792–11799.
251. U.S. Environmental Protection Agency (EPA) (1999): Avermectin; Pesticide tolerances for emergency exemptions; Final rule. *Fed. Reg.*, 64(66):16843–16850 (Appendix 3).
252. U.S. Environmental Protection Agency (EPA). (1999): Clofentezine. Pesticide tolerance. Petition filing. *Fed. Reg.*, 64(18):4414–4418.
253. U.S. Environmental Protection Agency (EPA). (1999): Clofentezine. Pesticide tolerance. Petition filing. *Fed. Reg.*, 64(74):19042–19050.
254. U.S. Environmental Protection Agency (EPA). (1999): Clomazone. Pesticide tolerance. Petition filing. *Fed. Reg.*, 64(32):8087–8090.
255. U.S. Environmental Protection Agency (EPA). (1999): Cyromazine; Pesticide tolerances for emergency exemptions. Final rule. *Fed. Reg.*, 62(168):45735–45741.
256. U.S. Environmental Protection Agency (EPA). (1999): Emamectin benzoate; Pesticide tolerance: Final rule. *Fed. Reg.*, 64(96):27192–27200.
257. U.S. Environmental Protection Agency (EPA). (1999): Fludioxonil; Pesticide tolerance for emergency exemptions: Final rule. *Fed. Reg.*, 64(76):19484–19489.
258. U.S. Environmental Protection Agency (EPA). (1999): Fluthiacet-methyl; Pesticide tolerance: Final rule. *Fed. Reg.*, 64(7):18351–18357.
259. U.S. Environmental Protection Agency (EPA). (1999): Picloram. Time-limited pesticide tolerances. Final rule. *Fed. Reg.*, 64(2):418–425.
260. U.S. Environmental Protection Agency (EPA). (1999): Pyriproxyfen; Notice of filing of pesticide petitions. *Fed. Reg.*, 64(34):8638–8641.
261. U.S. Environmental Protection Agency (EPA) (1999): Reregistration Eligibility Document. Amitrole. http://www.epa.gov/docs/oppsrrd1/REDs/0095/html (Accessed June 1999).
262. U.S. Environmental Protection Agency (EPA). (1999): Rimsulfuron; Pesticide tolerances for emergency exemptions. Final rule. *Fed. Reg.*, 64(41):10227–10233.
263. Valentine, B. J., Gurr, G. M. and Thwaite, W. G. (1996): Efficacy of the insect growth regulators tebufenozide and fenoxycarb on lepidopteran pest control in apples, and their compatibility with biological control for integrated pest management. *Austr. J. Exp. Agric.*, 36:501–506.
264. Ware, G. W. (1999): An introduction to insecticides. Radcliffe's IPM World Textbook Home Page. http://ipmworld.umn.edu/chapters/bloomq.htm (Accessed 4/99).
265. Weed Science Society of America (WSSA). (1994): Acifluorfen. In: *Herbicide Handbook*, 7th ed., edited by W. H. Ahrens, pp. 5–7. Weed Science Society of America, Champaign, IL.
266. Weed Science Society of America (WSSA). (1994): Ametryn. In: *Herbicide Handbook*, 7th ed., edited by W. H. Ahrens, pp. 12–14. Weed Science Society of America, Champaign, IL.
267. Weed Science Society of America (WSSA). (1994): Asulum. In: *Herbicide Handbook*, 7th ed., edited by W. H. Ahrens, pp. 18–19. Weed Science Society of America, Champaign, IL.
268. Weed Science Society of America (WSSA). (1994): Atrazine. In: *Herbicide Handbook*, 7th ed., edited by W. H. Ahrens, pp. 20–23. Weed Science Society of America, Champaign, IL.
269. Weed Science Society of America (WSSA). (1994): Bensulfuron. In: *Herbicide Handbook*, 7th ed., edited by W. H. Ahrens, pp. 28–30. Weed Science Society of America, Champaign, IL.
270. Weed Science Society of America (WSSA). (1994): Bentazon. In: *Herbicide Handbook*, 7th ed., edited by W. H. Ahrens, pp. 32–34. Weed Science Society of America, Champaign, IL.
271. Weed Science Society of America (WSSA). (1994): Bromacil. In: *Herbicide Handbook*, 7th ed., edited by W. H. Ahrens, pp. 37–39. Weed Science Society of America, Champaign, IL.
272. Weed Science Society of America (WSSA). (1994): Butylate. In: *Herbicide Handbook*, 7th ed., edited by W. H. Ahrens, pp. 43–45. Weed Science Society of America, Champaign, IL.

273. Weed Science Society of America (WSSA). (1994): Chlorimuron. In: *Herbicide Handbook*, 7th ed., edited by W. H. Ahrens, pp. 56–58. Weed Science Society of America, Champaign, IL.
274. Weed Science Society of America (WSSA). (1994): Chlorsulfuron. In: *Herbicide Handbook*, 7th ed., edited by W. H. Ahrens, pp. 58–60. Weed Science Society of America, Champaign, IL.
275. Weed Science Society of America (WSSA). (1994): Clethodim. In: *Herbicide Handbook*, 7th ed., edited by W. H. Ahrens, pp. 62–64. Weed Science Society of America, Champaign, IL.
276. Weed Science Society of America (WSSA). (1994): Cyanazine. In: *Herbicide Handbook*, 7th ed., edited by W. H. Ahrens, pp. 72–74. Weed Science Society of America, Champaign, IL.
277. Weed Science Society of America (WSSA). (1994): Dichlobenil. In: *Herbicide Handbook*, 7th ed., edited by W. H. Ahrens, pp. 94–96. Weed Science Society of America, Champaign, IL.
278. Weed Science Society of America (WSSA). (1994): Diclofop. In: *Herbicide Handbook*, 7th ed., edited by W. H. Ahrens, pp. 101–103. Weed Science Society of America, Champaign, IL.
279. Weed Science Society of America (WSSA). (1994): Difenzoquat. In: *Herbicide Handbook*, 7th ed., edited by W. H. Ahrens, pp. 106–108. Weed Science Society of America, Champaign, IL.
280. Weed Science Society of America (WSSA). (1994): Diquat. In: *Herbicide Handbook*, 7th ed., edited by W. H. Ahrens, pp. 108–110. Weed Science Society of America, Champaign, IL.
281. Weed Science Society of America (WSSA). (1994): Diuron. In: *Herbicide Handbook*, 7th ed., edited by W. H. Ahrens, pp. 113–115. Weed Science Society of America, Champaign, IL.
282. Weed Science Society of America (WSSA). (1994): Flumetsulam. In: *Herbicide Handbook*, 7th ed., edited by W. H. Ahrens, pp. 131–133. Weed Science Society of America, Champaign, IL.
283. Weed Science Society of America (WSSA). (1994): Flumiclorac-pentyl. In: *Herbicide Handbook*, 7th ed., edited by W. H. Ahrens, pp. 133–135. Weed Science Society of America, Champaign, IL.
284. Weed Science Society of America (WSSA). (1994): Fluometuron. In: *Herbicide Handbook*, 7th ed., edited by W. H. Ahrens, pp. 135–137. Weed Science Society of America, Champaign, IL.
285. Weed Science Society of America (WSSA). (1994): Fluridone. In: *Herbicide Handbook*, 7th ed., edited by W. H. Ahrens, pp. 141–143. Weed Science Society of America, Champaign, IL.
286. Weed Science Society of America (WSSA). (1994): Glufosinate-ammonium. In: *Herbicide Handbook*, 7th ed., edited by W. H. Ahrens, pp. 147–149. Weed Science Society of America, Champaign, IL.
287. Weed Science Society of America (WSSA). (1994): Glyphosate. In: *Herbicide Handbook*, 7th ed., edited by W. H. Ahrens, pp. 149–152. Weed Science Society of America, Champaign, IL.
288. Weed Science Society of America (WSSA). (1994): Haloxyfop. In: *Herbicide Handbook*, 7th ed., edited by W. H. Ahrens, pp. 153–156. Weed Science Society of America, Champaign, IL.
289. Weed Science Society of America (WSSA). (1994): Imazamethabenz. In: *Herbicide Handbook*, 7th ed., edited by W. H. Ahrens, pp. 159–161. Weed Science Society of America, Champaign, IL.
290. Weed Science Society of America (WSSA). (1994): Imazapyr. In: *Herbicide Handbook*, 7th ed., edited by W. H. Ahrens, pp. 161–163. Weed Science Society of America, Champaign, IL.
291. Weed Science Society of America (WSSA). (1994): Imazaquin. In: *Herbicide Handbook*, 7th ed., edited by W. H. Ahrens, pp. 163–166. Weed Science Society of America, Champaign, IL.
292. Weed Science Society of America (WSSA). (1994): Imazethapyr. In: *Herbicide Handbook*, 7th ed., edited by W. H. Ahrens, pp. 166–168. Weed Science Society of America, Champaign, IL.
293. Weed Science Society of America (WSSA). (1994): Ioxynil. In: *Herbicide Handbook*, 7th ed., edited by W. H. Ahrens, pp. 168–171. Weed Science Society of America, Champaign, IL.
294. Weed Science Society of America (WSSA). (1994): Isoxaben. In: *Herbicide Handbook*, 7th ed., edited by W. H. Ahrens, pp. 173–175. Weed Science Society of America, Champaign, IL.
295. Weed Science Society of America (WSSA). (1994): Linuron. In: *Herbicide Handbook*, 7th ed., edited by W. H. Ahrens, pp. 177–179. Weed Science Society of America, Champaign, IL.
296. Weed Science Society of America (WSSA). (1994): Metribuzin. In: *Herbicide Handbook*, 7th ed., edited by W. H. Ahrens, pp. 200–203. Weed Science Society of America, Champaign, IL.
297. Weed Science Society of America (WSSA). (1994): Metsulfuron. In: *Herbicide Handbook*, 7th ed., edited by W. H. Ahrens, pp. 203–205. Weed Science Society of America, Champaign, IL.
298. Weed Science Society of America (WSSA). (1994): Molinate. In: *Herbicide Handbook*, 7th ed., edited by W. H. Ahrens, pp. 205–206. Weed Science Society of America, Champaign, IL.
299. Weed Science Society of America (WSSA). (1994): MSMA. In: *Herbicide Handbook*, 7th ed., edited by W. H. Ahrens, pp. 209–211. Weed Science Society of America, Champaign, IL.
300. Weed Science Society of America (WSSA). (1994): Nicosulfuron. In: *Herbicide Handbook*, 7th ed., edited by W. H. Ahrens, pp. 216–217. Weed Science Society of America, Champaign, IL.
301. Weed Science Society of America (WSSA). (1994): Norflurazon. In: *Herbicide Handbook*, 7th ed., edited by W. H. Ahrens, pp. 218–220. Weed Science Society of America, Champaign, IL.
302. Weed Science Society of America (WSSA). (1994): Paraquat. In: *Herbicide Handbook*, 7th ed., edited by W. H. Ahrens, pp. 226–228. Weed Science Society of America, Champaign, IL.
303. Weed Science Society of America (WSSA). (1994): Pendimethalin. In: *Herbicide Handbook*, 7th ed., edited by W. H. Ahrens, pp. 230–233. Weed Science Society of America, Champaign, IL.
304. Weed Science Society of America (WSSA). (1994): Primisulfuron. In: *Herbicide Handbook*, 7th ed., edited by W. H. Ahrens, pp. 238–240. Weed Science Society of America, Champaign, IL.
305. Weed Science Society of America (WSSA). (1994): Prometon. In: *Herbicide Handbook*, 7th ed., edited by W. H. Ahrens, pp. 243–244. Weed Science Society of America, Champaign, IL.
306. Weed Science Society of America (WSSA). (1994): Prometryn. In: *Herbicide Handbook*, 7th ed., edited by W. H. Ahrens, pp. 245–247. Weed Science Society of America, Champaign, IL.
307. Weed Science Society of America (WSSA). (1994): Pyridate. In: *Herbicide Handbook*, 7th ed., edited by W. H. Ahrens, pp. 256–258. Weed Science Society of America, Champaign, IL.
308. Weed Science Society of America (WSSA). (1994): Sethoxydim. In: *Herbicide Handbook*, 7th ed., edited by W. H. Ahrens, pp. 266–267. Weed Science Society of America, Champaign, IL.
309. Weed Science Society of America (WSSA). (1994): Simazine. In: *Herbicide Handbook*, 7th ed., edited by W. H. Ahrens, pp. 270–272. Weed Science Society of America, Champaign, IL.
310. Weed Science Society of America (WSSA). (1994): Sulfometuron. In: *Herbicide Handbook*, 7th ed., edited by W. H. Ahrens, pp. 274–276. Weed Science Society of America, Champaign, IL.
311. Weed Science Society of America (WSSA). (1994): Terbacil. In: *Herbicide Handbook*, 7th ed., edited by W. H. Ahrens, pp. 278–280. Weed Science Society of America, Champaign, IL.
312. Weed Science Society of America (WSSA). (1994): Thifensulfuron. In: *Herbicide Handbook*, 7th ed., edited by W. H. Ahrens, pp. 282–283. Weed Science Society of America, Champaign, IL.
313. Weed Science Society of America (WSSA). (1994): Triasulfuron. In: *Herbicide Handbook*, 7th ed., edited by W. H. Ahrens, pp. 287–289. Weed Science Society of America, Champaign, IL.

314. Weed Science Society of America (WSSA). (1994): Tribenuron. In: *Herbicide Handbook*, 7th ed., edited by W. H. Ahrens, pp. 290–291. Weed Science Society of America, Champaign, IL.
315. Weed Science Society of America (WSSA). (1994): Trifluralin. In: *Herbicide Handbook*, 7th ed., edited by W. H. Ahrens, pp. 296–299. Weed Science Society of America, Champaign, IL.
315a. WSSA (1994).
315b. WSSA (1994).
316. Weisburger, J. H. (1975): In: *Toxicology, The Basic Science of Poisons*, edited by L. J. Casarett and J. Doull, pp. 333–378. Macmillan, New York.
317. Wetzel, L. T., Luempert, L. C. III, Breckenridge, C. B., Tisdel, M. O., Stevens, J. T., Thakur, A. K., Extrom, P. J. and Eldridge, J. C. (1994): Chronic effects of atrazine on estrus and mammary tumor formation in female Sprague-Dawley and Fischer 344 rats. *J. Toxicol. Environ. Health*, 43(2):182–196.
318. Woodyatt, N. J., Lambe, K. G., Myers, K. A., Tugwood, J. D., and Roberts, R. A. (1999): The peroxisome proliferator (PP) response element upstream of the human acyl CoA oxidase gene is inactive among a sample human population: Significance for species differences in response to PPs. *Carcinogenesis*, 20(3):369–372.
319. World Health Organization (WHO). (1967): WHO Expert Committee on Malaria. Thirteenth Report. WHO Tech. Rep. Serv. No. 357. World Health Organization, Geneva.
320. World Health Organization (WHO). (1977): Malathion. Data Sheets on Pesticides No. 29. http://www.inchem.org/documents/jmpr/jmpmono/v91pr02.htm (Accessed 5/99).
321. Yanase, D., and Andoh, A. (1989): Porphyrin synthesis involvement in diphenyl ether-like mode of action of TNPP-ethyl, a novel phenylpyrazole herbicide. *Pestic. Biochem. Physiol.* 35:70–80.

Principles and Methods of Toxicology, Fourth Edition, edited by A. Wallace Hayes.
Taylor & Francis, Philadelphia © 2001.

Chapter 14

Metals

Jill C. Merrill, Joseph J. P. Morton, Stephen D. Soileau

Metals are elements generally characterized by ductility, luster, being electropositive with a tendency to lose electrons, and having the property of conducting heat and electricity. However, a number of the elements individually discussed in the body of the chapter are not true metals (e.g., arsenic, fluorine). The attempt was made to include elements that have physiological actions (both beneficial and toxic) by virtue of their chemical ionic form. Elements such as oxygen and sulfur, which are essential to life in some forms (e.g., water, amino acids) but which also exist in forms that are chemically reactive and hence toxic (e.g., hydroperoxide, sulfuric acid), are not covered in this chapter.

Metals can have a variety of physiological effects, and it is often possible to demonstrate the toxicity of any given metal in any given organ, provided that the dose is both high and prolonged (but not so high and prolonged that the primary target organ receives a fatal dose). Essential elements may be toxic at a dose that overwhelms homeostatic controls on absorption and excretion, and the mechanism of toxicity is commonly related to an essential physiological role of the metal (e.g., control of osmolarity for sodium consumption in excess of water intake, neurotransmission for potassium consumption in excess of water intake; redox reactions for iron intake in excess of protein binding capacity). Physiological actions of nonessential elements include substituting for essential elements in enzymatic reactions, energy metabolism, neurotransmission, structural components (bone), reacting covalently or noncovalently with enzymes, membranes, DNA, and stimulating the production of active oxygen species (223). The variety of physiological effects makes it difficult to determine which action is responsible for toxicity in the most sensitive target organ. In some cases, organs are most sensitive for a biochemical reason (e.g., thallium interferes with energy metabolism, and target organs are those with the highest energy requirement); in other cases, the most sensitive organ is simply the organ in which the accumulation is greatest (e.g., cadmium and uranium accumulate in the kidneys, which are the target organs). Metals can interact with each other either to enhance toxicity (e.g., by affecting the same target organ) or to reduce toxicity (e.g., by stimulating defense mechanisms); this must be particularly kept in mind for the interpretation of animal experiments (e.g., levels of calcium, iron, and zinc should be controlled in investigations of cadmium toxicity) and epidemiological studies (e.g., fluoride reduces the incidence of dental caries: therefore, a population with the lowest fluoride exposure is likely to have the highest exposure to mercury and other metals used in dental restorations). The number of combinations of metals that could potentially be investigated is huge, and such studies are most useful either when a sensitive subpopulation is identified (e.g., individuals with insufficient intake of specific nutrients) or when a specific mechanism is revealed. Few treatments for metal toxicity are based on interfering with the mechanism of action; rather, measures are designed to reduce gastrointestinal absorption (from acute poisoning) by removing or binding the metal or are designed to speed elimination from the body (e.g., chelation therapy) (172). Prevention of excessive exposure is generally the best way to reduce the potential for metal toxicity.

The variety of physiological effects that metals can have is also the reason that adverse effects can often be demonstrated in most organ systems. Reproductive, developmental, immunological, and neurological toxicity, which are often not investigated in routine bioassays, are endpoints of increasing concern. For metals in particular, which on general principles would be expected to at least have the potential for these types of toxicity, toxicological understanding should not be considered complete without some information on whether these systems might be the most sensitive.

QUANTIFICATION OF TOXICOLOGICAL EFFECTS OF METALS

Consideration of the toxicity of metals must be quantitative because of the need to identify the most sensitive organ among all the systems that can be affected by the metal, and also because metals are naturally occurring and ubiquitous. Exposure to any metal cannot be banned the way exposure to, for example, an organic pesticide or food additive can be banned; some elements are essential to life, and even for those that are not, with sufficiently sensitive analytic techniques their presence can be demonstrated in any given sample of food, water, soil, or air. The quantification of the toxic effects of metals must attempt to precisely identify the highest level that is not expected to cause undue adverse effects because in many cases the traditional approach of using a safety/uncertainty factor of 10 would quickly lead to calculated levels that are below those essential for health (e.g., zinc, molybdenum) or levels that are below background exposures from food or water and hence extremely costly to achieve (e.g., cadmium, arsenic).

An example of the need to quantify toxicity is in the U.S. Environmental Protection Agency (U.S. EPA) program to address abandoned hazardous waste sites. For each site, a quantitative risk assessment is performed to determine the need for and extent of remediation (583). Essentially this risk assessment calculates doses of contaminants based on the concentration in a medium (air, soil, food, water) and the intake of that medium (e.g., adults are assumed to ingest 100 mg of soil per day). This dose to the maximally exposed person is then compared to two quantitative toxicological values. The first is the reference dose (RfD) or reference concentration (RfC), which is the highest dose or concentration not thought to be associated with adverse noncancer health effects (the "threshold"). The derivation of RfDs and RfCs is described in the chapter by Beck et al. (chapter 2) in this volume. RfDs quantify oral (and potentially dermal) toxicity, and RfCs quantify inhalation toxicity; separate values may be derived for acute, intermediate, and chronic exposure duration. The second toxicological value is the slope factor, which quantifies the cancer risk corresponding to a given lifetime dose (see Chapter 2). There are commonly separate slope factors for the inhalation and oral routes; risks from less-than-lifetime exposure are evaluated by dividing the duration of exposure by an (assumed) 70-year lifetime. Cleanup standards for a site are commonly set as the concentrations that would deliver a dose to the most exposed individual that is less than the RfD for each chemical, and that results in an "acceptable" cancer risk (e.g., 10^{-4} to 10^{-6} incremental lifetime cancer risk). For metals, one important issue is whether they are present at the hazardous-waste site at levels exceeding the natural background level (which are not necessarily below what would pose an unacceptable risk to the most exposed individual). Another issue that arises is incorporation of uncertainty into derivation of cleanup standards. One example is chromium, commonly measured as total chromium, which leads to uncertainty because only the rarer hexavalent form, not the more common trivalent form, is considered a carcinogen (589); considering all chromium detected at a hazardous to be hexavalent will lead to an overestimate of the risk and the need for cleanup, by an unknown amount. Another example is antimony, which has an oral RfD derived with a safety factor of 1000 (589); it is likely that this safety factor is too conservative and that cleanup standards will be more stringent, and therefore more expensive, than needed. For both chromium and antimony, additional information (speciation at the site for chromium; better toxicology data for antimony) would allow risk assessments to determine more precisely acceptable levels, which would prevent the setting of potentially unnecessarily strict standards.

On the other hand, there may be situations where current standards of exposure are not strict enough. Human activities such as mining and smelting, fossil fuel burning and incineration, fertilizer-intensive agriculture, and other industrial processes have increased human exposure to many elements to levels far above those of the preindustrial environment. Lead and cadmium are two examples of metals for which the level of exposure deemed acceptable has dropped many times over the years, as concern about frank toxicity among workers was replaced by concern about more subtle signs of toxicity in workers, which was in turn replaced by concern about even more subtle adverse effects in the general population exposed through environmental (including dietary) routes (94,108). There are numerous examples of metals for which our knowledge of toxicology primarily consists of information on frank toxicity in exposed workers and a few animals studies, very similar to the extent of information that was used to derive standards for lead and cadmium that we now know could cause substantial toxicity in the general population. One of the major reasons for the advances in knowledge about lead, cadmium, and a few other metals was the development of biomarkers of exposure (blood lead levels and urinary cadmium levels) that provide a way to quantify environmental exposure and thus allow studies linking exposure to health effects in the general population. Biomarkers of exposure commonly provide much more precise quantification of exposure than is possible by traditional means, particularly for the general population that may be exposed by several routes (food, air, water), all of which are variable in time and location. One important future direction for investigation of metals toxicology is developing and validating biomarkers of exposure, and using these biomarkers to investigate potential adverse effects in the general population.

For most metals, quantification of toxicological effects has not been done using human studies with validated biomarkers. Instead, the traditional methods are used (discussed in more detail in Chapter 2): assembling the entire data set, surveying the data to determine the most sensitive target organ (the organ exhibiting an adverse effect at the lowest dose), identifying the no-observed-adverse-effect level (NOAEL) or the lowest-observed-adverse-effect level (LOAEL), and applying safety or uncertainty factors to derive a threshold below which no noncancer effects are expected to occur. For cancer risk assessment, the process involves determining a weight-of-evidence judgment as to whether the element has the potential to cause cancers in humans (the U.S. EPA uses classifications of group A, known human carcinogen; group B, probable human carcinogen; group C, possible human carcinogen; and group D, not classifiable as to human carcinogenicity); a separate step is to quantify the cancer risk associated with a given dose, on the no-threshold assumption that any exposure carries some cancer risk, with a safety margin built in by using the most sensitive sex/species/organ carcinogenic response and by using the upper 95th percentile confidence limit of the slope (583).

Several issues for the qualitative and quantitative evaluation of toxicity pertain particularly to metals.

Essentiality

Recommended dietary allowances (RDA) are defined as "the levels of intake of essential nutrients that, on the basis of scientific knowledge, are judged by the National Research Council's (NRC) Food and Nutrition Board to be adequate to meet the known nutrient needs of practically all healthy persons" (420). They are revised and published periodically by the NRC, which convenes expert committees to estimate the mean dietary requirement for the population based on deficiency studies, balance studies, nutritional intakes, bioavailability, interactions, and homeostatic regulatory mechanisms

(446). A normal Gaussian distribution for the range of requirements within the population and a coefficient of variation of 15% are generally assumed. The RDA is then set at two standard deviations above the mean. Statistically, the RDA represents the 97.5th percentile of the nutrient requirement in the healthy population (86). The first RDAs were set during World War II, when food was rationed, and it was important to set minimum requirements to prevent frank deficiency diseases. Today, although preventing nutrient-deficient diseases is still important, public health concerns are directed toward defining the amounts of nutrients needed to ensure optimum health, provide excellent physiological and mental function, and prevent degenerative diseases (291). For example, the 1989 recommendation for selenium is based on the amount needed to support maximal activity of the selenium-dependent enzyme glutathione peroxidase and prevent cardiomyopathy (420); however, recent epidemiological studies suggest selenium has cancer preventive activity at levels significantly higher than that needed to support maximal activity of glutathione peroxidase (125,126,627). A higher recommendation for selenium might be set if a reduction in cancer risk were chosen instead of preventing the disease process associated with frank selenium deficiency, cardiomyopathy (135). This will require a "reconstructed," trilevel RDA, tentatively named the dietary reference intake (DRI) (397), which will address (a) the amount needed to prevent the deficiency disease, (b) the amount needed to provide specific health benefits, and (c) the amount associated with health hazards. The Food and Nutrition Board of the Institute of Medicine, National Academy of Sciences, has formed the Committee on the Scientific Evaluation of Dietary Reference Intakes to address these issues.

Route of Exposure

Two major routes of exposure to metals are by inhalation and oral exposure. Inhalation of metals, particularly as fumes or dusts, commonly causes systematic effects on the lung, ranging from mild, self-limiting metal fume fever from acute exposure and benign pneumoconiosis from chronic exposure for some metals to severe chronic obstructive lung disease for others (254,430). Standards for inhalation exposure to metals are developed by the American Conference of Governmental Industrial Hygienists (ACGIH), based primarily on occupational data; the highest allowable standard, 10 mg/m^3, pertains to dusts that are not chemically reactive but present a cumulative, physical burden on the lung that can be harmful from long-term exposure (31). Oral exposure to many metals with known lung toxicity often has no adverse effects (although at high enough oral doses, most metals cause acute gastrointestinal irritation and distress) (172), possibly due in part to the faster turnover of gastrointestinal versus lung cells. Another important route distinction has to do with carcinogenicity. Several metals are considered to be carcinogenic by the inhalation route, but not by the oral route (e.g., cadmium, chromium, nickel). This classification is based on the observation of an increased rate of lung but not other forms of cancer among workers and experimental animals exposed by inhalation, and on no observed increased rate among experimental animals exposed orally. However, these metals could have weak rather than no oral carcinogenicity; on theoretical grounds, it could be argued that most mechanisms by which an element is carcinogenic to lung tissue could operate in other tissues as well, and certain metals such as arsenic are known to be both lung carcinogens and systemic carcinogens. The potential human oral carcinogenicity of metals, particularly those known to be inhalation carcinogens, is an area deserving further study, and again, valid biomarkers of exposure would be very valuable for such studies.

Another point concerning route of exposure is that some metals, such as cadmium, are known to have very different toxicokinetic and toxicological properties by parenteral routes than by oral or inhalation routes. For cadmium at least, this is most likely due to the binding to metallothionein as a required step in oral or inhalation absorption, which is bypassed by parenteral exposure (16). Cancers can be induced in experimental animals by implantation of solids (metals as well as other solids); this "solid-state" carcinogenicity is typically considered to be only marginally relevant to human exposures. However, solid-state carcinogenesis may be relevant in humans with implanted metal-containing prosthetic devices (605). In general, studies using parenteral routes of exposure are often of limited use, unless the goal is to evaluate human parenteral exposure from medical procedures. A final point with respect to route of exposure is that most metals are considered not to be absorbed through the skin (with certain exceptions such as mercury and thallium); however, few data actually exist to substantiate this assumption, and further studies would be useful to quantify the dermal absorption of metals.

Form

Some metals, such as mercury, exist in elemental, ionic, and organic forms, and each of these forms has a unique toxicity. Other metals, such as chromium, may exist in two or more valence states with different effects. Still others, such as nickel, may be primarily protein bound in food sources but primarily free ions in water, which may affect absorption. Finally, there are some metals, such as cadmium, that appear to have similar toxicological effects regardless of their form. Ideally, information would be available to do a separate quantification for each toxicologically distinct form; this would only be useful, of course, in situations where the form to which humans are to be exposed is actually known. Failing this ideal, the attempt is made to derive a standard for the most toxic form of a given metal; however, in many cases this leads to overly stringent standards, and in some cases lack of information on the most toxic form of a metal may lead to standards that are too lax.

Duration of Exposure

The influence of duration of exposure on the quantitative, and even qualitative, toxicology of a metal depends on its toxicokinetics. Cadmium is an example of a cumulative toxin. To a relatively good approximation, the same total dose given over a week, a month, or a year will accumulate in the kidneys to the same extent and have the same physiological effect (16). Other metals, particularly essential elements, are excreted so efficiently that any dose that can be tolerated for a day can also be tolerated for a lifetime (420). For well-studied metals, information is generally available to account for duration of exposure. One example is that ACGIH commonly derives threshold limit values (TLVs) as time-weighted averages (TWAs), but may also derive a short-term exposure limit (STEL) or a TLV ceiling (TLV-C) for substances that have acute as well as chronic effects (31). For less studied metals, many standards are derived based on animal data with very little information on toxicokinetics, which means that extrapolation to durations of exposure other than those used in the study at hand are quite uncertain.

Age at Exposure

Infants and young children may be particularly sensitive to toxic effects of metals both because they often absorb a greater fraction of ingested metals than older children or adults and because some developing systems (particularly the nervous system) are more sensitive to toxic effects than mature systems. Lead is an example of a metal that is known to be most deleterious to fetuses, infants, and toddlers (108,109). The elderly are another group that may be more sensitive than healthy adults to the toxic effects of metals due to diminution of homeostatic and adaptive mechanisms. Definition of a safe level of exposure has an inherent uncertainty for metals lacking data on effects on infants and the elderly.

Animal Versus Human Data

For well-studied metals, animal and human toxicity appear to be in general qualitative agreement, although there are some exceptions, such as the difficulty in demonstrating that arsenic is carcinogenic to experimental animals. However, quantitative differences do occur; for example, gastrointestinal absorption of cadmium is about two to three times lower in experimental animals than humans (16). Use of a 10-fold safety factor for animal-to-human extrapolation in this case would yield a toxicological value about 3 times more stringent than necessary. This emphasizes the importance of using human data whenever possible for quantification of toxicity.

Toxicokinetic Modeling

Toxicokinetic modeling is very useful for evaluating the toxicity of well-studied metals. Good models can integrate information on the effects of routes of exposure, chemical forms, age at exposure, duration of exposure, and interindividual variation on absorption, distribution, excretion, and target-organ sensitivity. The toxicokinetic model developed for quantifying the systemic toxicity of cadmium is discussed later in this chapter. In addition, toxicological modeling is used in the quantification of the cancer risk from exposure to radioactive elements. Principles of radiological toxicity are covered in detail in the chapter on radioactivity (Chapter 15); the following is a brief description highlighting the use of toxicokinetic modeling for radioactive elements. Radioactive elements can cause damage at levels of exposure many orders of magnitude below those at which their nonradioactive forms cause chemical damage because radioactive decay involves the release of a large amount of energy in the form of alpha particles, beta particles, and/or gamma rays. A single radioactive decay can initiate a cascade of events that creates a huge number of active oxygen species, which are thought to be the ultimate cause of radioactive damage. This damage can cause cell death at high levels of exposure; of greater concern is the possibility of mutations that can initiate or promote cancer or result in hereditary defects (582).

Quantification issues are addressed for individual metals in the remainder of this chapter. The reader should recognize that the U.S. EPA continually reviews and revises toxicity values, and that the numbers presented here are simply the values that were specified in December 2000.

Sources of Information

There are numerous sources of information on toxicity of metals, many of which are updated on a regular basis. The U.S. EPA maintains the Integrated Risk Information System (IRIS), which has a summary of information (including RfD and RfC values) on numerous toxic chemicals, including a number of metals (589). This database is regularly updated, and is available on the EPA web site (http://www.epa.gov). The American Conference of Governmental Industrial Hygienists (ACGIH) publishes annually a listing of all chemicals for which threshold limit values (TLV) and biological exposure indices (BEI) exists (32). The documentation for the development of these values is also available, with the latest update of this publication occurring in 1996 (31). The U.S. Agency of Toxic Substances Disease Registry has published many documents that summarize the toxicological effects of elements and chemicals; documents exist for many of the elements discussed in this chapter. Finally, the series *Patty's Industrial Hygiene and Toxicology* contains a vast amount of information on the toxicity of metals and other elements and compounds, with the major emphasis being on industrial exposures and effects (63,64,142,460). Treatments for exposures to metals and other compounds are described in detail in *Clinical Toxicology of Commercial Products* (222) and in *Diagnosis and Treatment of Human Poisoning* (172).

ESSENTIAL ELEMENTS

Calcium

Calcium is essential both for the physical structure of bone and for normal physiological function (e.g., nerve conduction, muscle contraction, blood clotting, membrane permeability, enzyme activation, acetylcholine synthesis) (27). The average healthy adult body contains about 1200 g of calcium, 99% of which is found in bone and teeth, with the remaining 1% in extracellular fluids, intracellular structures, and cell membranes. The average calcium content of the blood ranges from 9.0 to 10.5 mg/dl with tight physiological controls. Decreased body calcium leads to loss of bone mineral, reduction of bone strength, increased susceptibility to fractures (479), and may increase blood pressure (382), particularly among pregnant women (65). Calcium deficiency is also associated with convulsions and tetany. The RDA for calcium is derived from the need to maintain skeletal calcium, using an estimated 200–250 mg/day obligatory loss and an oral absorption fraction of 30–40%, leading to a recommendation of 1200 mg/day for ages 11–24 years and 800 mg/day for older age groups, except that 1200 mg/day is recommended throughout pregnancy and lactation (420). In 1994 a National Institutes of Health Consensus Conference on Optimal Calcium Intakes recommended all Americans over 5 years of age consume levels of calcium higher than the current RDA, with the greatest change in calcium intake being for elderly persons, who should consume 1500 mg/day (419).

Calcium is not a very toxic metal, but adverse effects may occur at intakes greater than 2000 mg/day (419). Intestinal absorption of calcium decreases as intake increases; however, very large intakes of calcium can increase the calcium body burden (420) as well as interfere with the absorption of magnesium (515), zinc (195), and iron (240). Very large chronic intakes are associated with hypercalcemia and/or hypercalciuria. Other symptoms of calcium excess include renal failure and soft tissue calcification. High-calcium diets could increase the risk of kidney stones in susceptible individuals and reduce the biovailability of zinc and iron. Although excessive calcium intake from food and municipal water was previously seen mainly in individuals with conditions predisposing them to increased calcium absorption, such as parathyroidectomy (379), the consumption of calcium-fortified foodstuffs (e.g., sparkling water, breakfast cereal, orange juice) in addition to a diet containing generous amounts of dairy products could theoretically reach levels of concern (615). Education of health-care professionals and the general public is needed to prevent both overconsumption of calcium in one population and the risk of calcium deficiency in another. A potential adverse effect associated with habitual intake of calcium supplements is ingestion of heavy metals, such as arsenic, cadmium, and lead, which have been found to contaminate some calcium supplements (84,614). With the increased interest in daily calcium supplementation as a preventive measure for colon cancer, osteoporosis, and hypertension, the possible contaminants of these supplements warrant further investigation. The Food and Drug Administration (FDA) does not regulate nutritional supplements; the amount of trace metal contaminants is variable.

Chlorine

Chloride is the principal extracellular inorganic ion. It is required for maintenance of fluid and electrolyte balance and for the production of gastric acid (420). Dietary chloride deficiency is rare, but prolonged loss of electrolytes from vomiting, diarrhea, heavy sweating, and so forth can lead to hypochloremic metabolic alkalosis. The minimum requirement of chloride, based on its close association with sodium in both dietary sources and physiological losses, is 750 mg/day (420).

Reactive chlorine compounds (chlorine gas, hydrochloric acid, hypochlorite, chlorine dioxide, etc.) are irritating to the tissues they contact, but neutral chloride solutions are nontoxic (179). Habitual excess intake of table salt may contribute to hypertension in susceptible individuals, and animal data suggest that the chloride ion may play a role as well as the sodium ion (410). This question has more than theoretical implications because potassium chloride is widely used as a salt substitute by individuals seeking to restrict their sodium intake. However, the sparse human data on the association between chloride intake and blood pressure are generally negative, and more studies are needed before restriction of chloride intake, independent of sodium intake, could be suggested to have a beneficial effect in the general population. The U.S. EPA has not derived any toxicity values for chloride (589).

Chromium

Chromium is a first series transition metal, with its name derived from the Greek word for color, because most chromium compounds are brightly colored. The only important chromium ore is chromite. Chromium is used as an alloy with other metals, and is also used for plating of metals (63). Although chromium can have valences from −2 to +6, the most important valences are +3 and +6 (31).

Trivalent chromium is the most abundant form of chromium in the environment. Chromium(III) is an essential nutrient that plays a role in glucose metabolism (35,63). Although Cr^{3+} is poorly absorbed orally (158), absorption is greatly enhanced by the presence of the "glucose tolerance factor," which forms a complex with Cr^{3+} (513). Chromium(III) is considered to be relatively nontoxic in vivo (63). Micc exposed to chromium(III) acetate in drinking water for over 2 years did not show an increased incidence of tumors (502).

Hexavalent chromium is the most important valence from a toxicity standpoint. Unlike chromium(III), chromium(VI) is readily absorbed by all tissues. Because chromate (CrO_4^{2-}) is structurally similar to phosphate and sulfate (139), it readily enters all cells via the general anion channel protein. Chromium(VI) is acutely toxic, with most reports of human toxicity occurring as a result of accidental or intentional ingestion. The lethal oral dose of soluble chromates in humans is estimated to be in the range of 50–70 mg/kg. Symptoms of acute toxicity include vomiting and generalized gastrointestinal tract damage, with gastrointestinal bleeding leading to cardiovascular shock. If the victim survives the initial toxic effects, liver necrosis, tubular necrosis of the kidney, and damage to the blood-forming tissues can occur (63). Long-term occupational exposure to chromium has been associated either with low-molecular-weight proteinuria, or with elevated levels of proteins normally found in the urine (63, 139). Although animal studies have shown that parenteral administration of 15 mg/kg potassium chromate (+6) is nephrotoxic, chronic renal disease due to occupational or environmental exposure has not yet been reported (63).

Dermal exposure to potassium dichromate and other chromium compounds can lead to the development of a sensitization reaction. The resulting hypersensitivity results from chromium binding to proteins and becoming a hapten (151). Prior to the implementation of appropriate industrial hygiene precautions, occupational inhalation exposure to Cr^{6+} was associated with changes in the septal mucosa, ranging from irritation to septal perforation (63). However, inhalation exposure rarely causes asthma (430).

The carcinogenicity of chromium in the respiratory tract has been well established, beginning when the first nasal tumors were described among Scottish chrome pigment workers in the late 19th century (432), and has been reviewed in the recent literature (63,130,139). The mechanism of action believed to be from a direct modification of DNA (444). After hexavalent chromate enters a cell, it is rapidly reduced to Cr^{3+}. During the reduction process, unstable and reactive intermediates, including Cr(IV), Cr(V), hydroxide, thiyl and organic (RS and R) radicals, and active oxygen radicals are formed, and it is believed that these moieties are responsible for chromium carcinogenicity (130). Because Cr^{6+} is readily absorbed by all tissues, one could postulate that chromium-induced cancers should be noted in other organs. Although the evidence is not as strong, exposure to hexavalent chromium is associated with an increased incidence of may types of cancers (139).

The U.S. EPA has established an oral RfD for chromium(III) of 1.5 mg/kg/day, an oral RfD for chromium(VI) of 5 μg/kg/day, an inhalation RfC for chromic acid mists and dissolved Cr(VI) aerosols of 8.6×10^{-3} $\mu g/m^3$, and an inhalation RfC for Cr(VI) particulates of $1 \times 10^{-1} \mu g/m^3$. The U.S. EPA has classified chromium(III) as a group D (not classifiable) carcinogen and chromium(VI) as a group A (human) carcinogen.

Cobalt

Cobalt is an essential component of vitamin B_{12}, which is involved in intermediary metabolism, nucleic acid synthesis, and single-carbon metabolism, and is required to prevent macrocytic megaloblastic anemia, atrophic gastritis, achlorhydria, neurologic degeneration, and dementia (27). Vitamin B_{12} is synthesized by bacteria, fungi, and algae, but not by yeasts, plants, or animals (420). Cobalt deficiency may develop in animals dependent on gut microflora for their vitamin B_{12}, such as ruminants, and in strict vegetarians consuming no animal products. The RDA for vitamin B_{12} is 2 μg/day, and although cobalt is known to activate the enzyme arginase (554), the only recognized requirement for cobalt is as a component of vitamin B_{12}. Cobalt is a hard, silvery metal widely distributed in rocks and soils and always occurs with nickel and usually with arsenic (13). It is primarily used in the production of superalloys, as a drier in paints, and in magnets, and in the production of prosthetic devices. Occupational exposure occurs in the hard metal industry, among cobalt blue dye plate painters, and in coal miners, and this exposure is reflected in elevated levels of cobalt in tissues and body fluids.

Cobalt can be toxic. For the general population, ingestion is the primary route of exposure (13). Oral exposure to cobalt caused cardiomyopathy among individuals who drank excessive amounts of beer (8–25 pints/day) containing cobalt as a foam stabilizer (405). This effect may have been potentiated by a combination of alcohol, preexisting heart damage, and/or poor diets associated with heavy alcohol consumption, because anemic individuals have been exposed to higher levels of cobalt without a similar effect (405,516). Cobalt can cause allergic dermatitis (eczema and urticaria, mainly of the hands) (28,598), and cross-reaction with nickel is frequent (595,493). Inhalation exposure to cobalt alloyed to tungsten carbide (hard metal) is associated with hard metal disease, which is characterized by interstitial fibrosis and restrictive respiratory impairment (352). The toxic mechanism of hard metal particles is thought to involve both cobalt sensitivity and the generation of oxygen radicals by the carbide particles (352,431). Cobalt by itself has caused occupational asthma in diamond polishers, and the effect has been attributed to an immunologic mechanism with cobalt acting as a hapten (207).

The carcinogenicity of cobalt is uncertain. Animal studies are positive only for subcutaneous, intramuscular, or intratracheal administration, but not for inhalation, and the excess rates of lung cancer observed in men occupationally exposed to cobalt dust could be explained by simultaneous exposure to nickel, arsenic, and/or tobacco (338,439).

The U.S. EPA has not derived toxicity values for cobalt. The ACGIH has adopted TLV-TWA values for cobalt carbonyl and cobalt hydrocarbonyl of 0.1 mg Co/m^3 (32).

Copper

Copper occurs naturally as the free metal and occurs in compounds in +1 or +2 valence state. Copper is incorporated into several enzymes involved in hemoglobin formation, carbohydrate metabolism, catecholamine biosynthesis, and cross-linking of collagen, elastin, and hair keratin (6). These enzymes include cytochrome *c* oxidase, dopamine β-hydroxylase, ascorbic acid oxidase, and superoxide dismutase, as well as interaction with ceruloplasmin and metallothionein. Copper deficiency causes anemia, neutropenia, and impaired growth, particularly in children (420). The ingestion of copper in foods is the primary source for copper intake. The intake from copper plumbing and unpolluted fresh water is not significant. The estimated safe and adequate daily dietary adult intake is 1.5 to 3.0 mg/day (420). The U.S. EPA action level for copper in tap water is 1.3 mg/L (129).

Copper is readily absorbed following oral ingestion, but homeostatic mechanisms limit further intake once requirements are met. Copper overload is normally further controlled by binding to metallothionein. Copper is either active or in transit, with little or no excess copper being normally stored (350). Following absorption, copper is bound to albumin and transcuprein, and is mainly deposited in liver hepatocytes with lesser amounts in the kidney. Biliary excretion is the major route with small amounts secreted in the urine. Considering these homeostatic mechanisms following oral intake, absorption through the inhalation or dermal routes may allow toxic levels to pass unimpeded into the blood.

The consumption of water containing high levels of copper or suicide attempts with copper sulfate can result in vomiting, diarrhea, nausea, abdominal pain, hemolytic anemia, hepatic and renal neurosis, and death. Industrial exposure may occur to copper fumes resulting in metal fume fever with dyspnea, chills, headache, and nausea (63). The ACGIH has adopted TLV-TWA values for copper of 1 mg Cu/m^3 for dusts and mists and 0.2 mg Cu/m^3 for fumes (32). The OSHA PEL differs with 0.1 mg/m^3 for copper fume. Copper can be dermally absorbed from copper-containing topical products (335,465,466). Dermal irritation and contact allergic dermatitis have been associated with copper jewelry, intrauterine contraceptive devices, and through occupational exposure to electroplating and copper containing agricultural products (335).

Wilson's disease is one of several examples of toxicity involving copper in humans. This disease is due to an autosomal recessive disorder that affects normal copper homeostasis. There is an excessive retention of hepatic copper, decreased concentration of plasma ceruloplasmin, impaired biliary copper excretion, and hypercupremia, resulting in hepatic and renal lesions and hemolytic anemia (6). Menkes's disease is a multisystemic lethal disorder characterized by neurodegenerative symptoms and connective tissue manifestations. The disease is attributable to a deficiency of one or more copper-dependent enzymes (571).

Fluorine

Fluorine, the most reactive of the elements, is a pale yellow gas with a pungent odor. The chief fluoride sources are fluorspar (CaF_2) and cryolite (Na_3AlF_6). Fluorine, hydrogen fluoride, and other fluorine compounds are used in a wide number of applications in the nuclear (in the synthesis of uranium hexafluoride), agrochemical (pesticides), drug (anticaries agents), and other industries (31,63). Fluorine gas is a severe eye, mucosal, and skin irritant (31).

Hydrogen fluoride (HF) is a weak acid that causes severe burns on the skin and in the eye, either in aqueous solution or as the anhydrous acid (63). In addition to causing dermal and ocular damage, hydrogen fluoride is readily absorbed through the skin. Once absorbed, fluoride complexes with calcium and causes hypocalcemia. If the hypocalcemia is severe, death can occur via cardiac arrhythmia. Hydrogen fluoride burns over as little as 2.5% of the body surface have caused fatalities, depending on the concentration of HF (113,118,318).

Fluoride is incorporated into bones and tooth enamel, making teeth more resistant to caries, but fluoride deficiency has never been conclusively demonstrated in humans or animals, although goats fed <1 mg F/kg dry ration had reduced growth and survival (40). The NRC classifies fluoride as a beneficial but not an essential element (420). Fluoride replaces hydroxyl ions in enamel, yielding an apatite crystal that is more resistant to acid. Some studies suggest that fluoride supplements may also increase bone strength (452). Fluoride in aqueous solutions is virtually 100% absorbed, while absorption of fluoride in bone meal may be as low as 40% (420). The estimated safe and adequate daily dietary intake for fluoride from both food and water is set equal at 1.5–4 mg/day, based on the range of fluoride composition of diets in the United States (420). Although serious complications are rare (because of limitations set by the U.S. Food and Drug Administration on the total amount of fluoride in an over-the-counter anticaries drug product), acute fluoride toxicity can occur from accidental ingestion of fluoride containing products. In his review of reported accidental fluoride poisoning cases, Whitford (612,613) proposed a "probably toxic dose" of 5 mg/kg, although toxicity has been reported at doses as low as 0.1 mg/kg (23).

Doses of fluoride above 2 mg/day can cause mottled teeth in children, doses over 8 mg/day can cause osteosclerosis, and doses of 20 mg/day for 10–20 years can cause hypermineralization of bone leading to crippling skeletal fluorosis and renal toxicity (378,420). Fluoride increases bone mass but decreases its tensile strength, and is apparently not a treatment for osteoporosis (55). Case reports indicate that administration of sodium fluoride for treatment of osteoporosis can exacerbate rheumatoid arthritis, possibly by stimulating leukocytes and other mediators of the acute inflammatory response (163). Human epidemiological studies have found no evidence that fluoride causes gastrointestinal, respiratory, reproductive, or developmental toxicity (92). Skeletal and dental changes can be seen in rodents exposed to fluoride, as well as chronic stomach inflammation and ulcers (92,378). The U.S. EPA has derived an oral RfD for fluorine based on a no-observed-effect level (NOEL) for objectionable mottling of the teeth (dental fluorosis), which may occur in children drinking water with more than 1 ppm fluoride, leading to a NOEL of 0.06 mg/kg/day in a 20-kg child drinking 1 L/day and ingesting 0.1 mg/kg/day of dietary fluoride (589). The endpoint of dental fluorosis is not considered toxic or adverse. The ACGIH has adopted a TLV-TWA value for fluorides of 2.5 mg F/m^3, with carcinogenicity classification A4 (not classifiable as a human carcinogen) (32).

The potential carcinogenicity of fluoride is debatable. No increase in tumors was found among mice exposed to 1.75 mg/kg/day of sodium fluoride in water for 30 months (297). Sprague-Dawley rats had no statistically significant increase in tumors following 2 years of exposure to doses up to 25 mg/kg/day (378). The National Toxicology Program 2-year drinking water study of sodium fluoride at doses up to 10 mg/kg/day found no evidence for carcinogenicity in female rats, male mice, or female mice, and equivocal evidence of carcinogenicity in male rats (92). The evidence in male rats consisted of an increase in bone osteosarcomas with a dose-response trend that was statistically significant but an incidence in the highest dose group that was not significantly elevated compared to controls (92). Also, no osteosarcomas were found in female rats even though they accumulated fluoride in bones to the same extent as the male rats and they exhibited fluoride-induced osteosclerosis (92). The U.S. EPA has not yet evaluated fluoride for potential human carcinogenicity (589). While human epidemiology studies have generally been negative, the question of whether fluoride is a potential human carcinogen is still open, and more studies are needed to resolve this question of some public health importance (55,92,378).

Iodine

Iodine is the heaviest of the halogens that are of industrial interest. In solid form, iodine takes the form of gray-black plates or granules. It volatilizes at room temperature, yielding a violet vapor (460). The major sources of iodine are oil and natural gas brines, with Japan's natural gas-well brines being credited with as much as four-fifths of the world's iodine reserve (460). Topical iodine solutions (2% iodine and 2% NaI in 50% alcohol, USP) have been used for decades as germicides and antiseptics (31). When inhaled, iodine vapor can be intensely irritating to mucous membranes and affects the upper and lower portions of the pulmonary tract (30). Flury and Zernik (194) reported that humans could work undisturbed at 0.1 ppm, work with difficulty at 0.2 ppm, and could not work at 0.3 ppm. Topical application of iodine solutions can cause irritation, and strong solutions can cause burns (31).

Iodide is required for the synthesis of the thyroid hormones thyroxine and triiodothyronine. Iodide is efficiently absorbed, and excess iodide is excreted in the urine (420). Deficiency of iodide causes hypothyroidism and goiter, and severe deficiency in the newborn may cause cretinism and mental retardation (183). The RDA for iodine is 150 μg/day for adults, with an extra 25 μg/day during pregnancy and 50 μg/day during lactation (420). Chronic absorption of high levels of iodide can lead to a condition known as iodism. This condition is characterized by sleeplessness, tremor, rapid heart rate, diarrhea, weight loss, conjunctivitis, rhinitis, and bronchitis. This syndrome is usually associated with long-term ingestion of iodide containing medications (31). The U.S. EPA and ACGIH have not derived toxicity values for iodide (32,589).

Iron

Iron is a silver-white solid metal found mainly in combination with other elements as oxides, carbonates, sulfides, and silicates (63). It exists in two stable oxidation states, oxidized ferric (Fe^{3+}) and reduced ferrous (Fe^{2+}), which accounts for its essentiality as a trace element and its crucial role in the oxygen and electron transport reactions of all living cells. Dietary iron is available as either heme or nonheme (27). Heme iron is found in meats and is relatively well absorbed compared with nonheme iron, which is also found in meats, grains, and vegetables. Intestinal absorption of iron depends on iron status, with 10% of the total (heme plus nonheme) being absorbed when iron status is normal, but up to 20% in deficiency states. Adequate intakes of vitamin C increase the intestinal absorption of nonheme iron by two- to fourfold (138), which may be of significance to the iron status of vegetarians. Iron is lost through the shedding of cells, sweat, nails, hair, blood loss, menstruation, and in the urine. Early symptoms of iron deficiency are nonspecific and include fatigue and weakness. This progresses to iron-deficiency anemia, which is characterized by small red blood cells with low hemoglobin content (microcytic hypochromic anemia). These symptoms resolve after administration of iron. The RDA for iron is derived using an adequate body store of 300 mg, estimated losses of 1 mg/day in men and 1.5 mg/day in women, and an oral absorption fraction of 10–15%, leading to a recommendation of 10 mg/day for adults males and 15 mg/day for adults females, with an additional 15 mg/day recommended during pregnancy (420).

Free iron is an oxygen-reactive substance, highly toxic to cells, and will enhance the formation of free radicals and peroxidation of membrane lipids (49,50,491). Humans are unable to eliminate excess iron and regulate body iron stores by limiting absorption (381). Divalent iron is taken up by intestinal mucosa and converted to the trivalent form. The trivalent form is bound to transferrin (63,247), a glycoprotein with two iron-binding sites (363). Iron is transported as transferrin to the liver or spleen, where it is stored as ferritin, which has a high iron storage capacity and prevents iron from participating in the Fenton reaction (59, 389). Of the typical 4-g body iron stores found in adults, 66% is bound as hemoglobin, 10% as the protein myoglobin, with a minute amount in iron-containing enzymes, and the rest as intracellular storage proteins. The physiological controls on this essential but potentially toxic metal can be overwhelmed, either by an acute large intake (accidental ingestion of dietary supplements by children) or by chronic excessive intake (endogenous sub-Saharan African populations with a probable genetic defect who consume beverages brewed in steel drums may develop pancreatic, hepatic, and/or renal toxicity from their accumulation of excessive iron) (221). Inhalation exposure to iron dust or fumes has resulted in pulmonary siderosis; fibrosis does not develop and the clinical course is benign (430). Hepatotoxicity is typically seen in patients with iron overload and can progress from portal fibrosis to cirrhosis (541). A gray-bronze hyperpigmentation of the skin caused by increased melanin and iron deposition usually resolves after iron removal. Free radical stress and lipid peroxidation have both been suggested as factors in the etiology of diabetes (443), and increased iron stores have been reported to contribute to the development of non-insulin-dependent diabetes (495). An increased risk of infection by a number of microorganisms, including *Vibrio vulnificus, Listeria monocytogenes, Yersinia enterocoloitica, Eschericia coli*, and *Candida* species, may result from excessive iron intake, due to direct effects on the immune system and/or enhanced bacterial growth due to the increased availability of iron (220,249). Epidemiologic evidence suggests excess dietary iron is a coronary risk factor (494,573,574) and regular blood donation in middle-aged males is associated with a reduced risk of myocardial infarction (496).

Iron poisoning is the most common fatal poisoning in children reported to poison control centers in the United States (354,610). Despite supplements being packaged in child-resistant packages and carrying warning labels, the public perception of their potential danger is low (274) and fatalities in children have recently increased (34,68,610). Iron poisoning is characterized by four distinct clinical stages, but individual patients do not always demonstrate each stage (172,228,385): Stage I (initial period) occurs 0.5–2 h postingestion and is characterized by the onset of acute gastrointestinal symptoms (vomiting and diarrhea), but central nervous system (CNS) symptoms (lethargy and coma) may be present in severe cases;

stage II (quiescent period) occurs 6–24 h postingestion and the victim may be asymptomatic or appear to have improved; stage III (recurrent period) occurs 12–48 h postingestion and is characterized by gastrointestinal perforation, coma, convulsions, cardiovascular collapse, hepatic and renal failure, and metabolic acidosis; and stage IV (late period) occurs 3 to 4 weeks postingestion with the appearance of gastrointestinal scarring. The failure to recognize a patient in stage II iron poisoning has been noted as a "pitfall" in the medical management of iron poisoning (396) and has resulted in premature discharge (172). Gastrointestinal symptoms typically occur following the ingestion of 20 mg elemental iron/kg body weight, and doses greater than 60 mg/kg are often lethal. Treatment involves stabilizing vital functions, removing unabsorbed iron from the gastrointestinal tract, and intravenous administration of deferoxamine if symptoms are severe (34,385,396). Deferoxamine is an iron chelator produced by *Streptomyces pilosus* and removes iron from transferrin and ferritin, but not hemoglobin (359,555). Current research is directed toward the design of an orally active, nontoxic, selective iron chelator (258,320). The FDA recently issued regulations requiring all iron-containing products to carry a label stating the dangers of iron overdosage and unit-dose packaging for products containing 30 mg or more per dosage unit (591). The U.S. EPA has not derived any toxicity values for iron (589); the ACGIH has adopted TLV-TWA values for iron of 5 mg Fe/m^3 for iron oxide dust and fume and 1 mg Fe/m^3 for soluble iron salts (32).

Magnesium

Magnesium is essential to a large number of biochemical and physiological processes including neuromuscular conduction in skeletal and cardiac muscle (63). It is also an important structural component of bone (420). Plasma concentrations of magnesium are regulated within a narrow range (0.65–1.0 m*M*), primarily by adjustments in the reabsorption of filterable magnesium in the loop of Henle, and also by the passive buffering by bone magnesium (420). Magnesium deficiency can occur secondarily to general malnutrition, alcoholism (480), or other disease states that affect gastrointestinal electrolyte absorption or excretion or renal cation reabsorption. Magnesium deficiency results in reduced levels of potassium and calcium, as well as symptoms of nausea, muscle weakness, irritability, and mental derangement (525). The RDA for magnesium is derived from balance studies indicating that magnesium balance can be maintained in healthy men at intakes of 3.0–4.5 mg/kg/day, leading to a recommendation of 350 mg/day for men and 280 mg/day for women, with an extra 20 mg/day during pregnancy and 75 mg/day during lactation (420). Average intakes of U.S. adults are not much above the RDAs; however, there is no definitive evidence of effects attributable to magnesium deficiency (420). Vitamin D facilitates the absorption of magnesium (398).

Oral exposure to magnesium is not toxic except in individuals with impaired renal function, who may experience nausea, vomiting, and hypotension, followed by CNS depression accompanied by a sharp drop in blood pressure and respiratory paralysis (63,420). Magnesium salts are poorly absorbed orally and are commonly used as antacids or cathartics. Inhalation exposure to magnesium oxide can cause metal fume fever (19,63,430). The U.S. EPA has not derived toxicity values for magnesium; the ACGIH has adopted a TLV-TWA value for magnesium oxide fumes of 10 mg/m^3 (nuisance dust) (32).

Manganese

Manganese is a silver-gray soft metal and occurs in ores mainly as oxides (63). Manganese and its compounds are used in numerous products and applications including iron and steel alloys, dry cell batteries, paints, inks, fertilizers, and fungicides (208). Manganese is an essential trace metal that is a component of several mitochondrial enzymes, pyruvate carboxylase and superoxide dismutase, and activates a wide variety of enzymes (decarboxylases, transferases, hydrolases). It occurs in meats, poultry, nuts, grains, green leafy vegetables, and tea. Although outright manganese deficiency has not been observed in the human population, suboptimal manganese intake may be a concern (589). In animals, manganese deficiency can cause impaired growth, skeletal abnormalities, and altered metabolism of carbohydrates and lipids (22). The estimated safe and adequate daily dietary intake for manganese is set equal to current U.S. dietary intakes, based on a lack of evidence for human manganese deficiency, yielding a range of 2–5 mg/day (420). The U.S. EPA has reviewed numerous human and animal studies and related information and concluded that an appropriate chronic oral reference dose for manganese is 10 mg/day (0.14 mg/kg/day) (589). Only between 3 and 10% of dietary manganese is absorbed in normal adults, and total body stores are controlled by a complex homeostatic mechanism regulating absorption and excretion. Calcium, iron deficiencies, age, and other factors may increase manganese absorption (22,589).

Occupational inhalation exposure is the primary route for manganese toxicity. The primary toxic effect of occupational inhalation exposure is neurological damage (483); however, inhalation exposure to manganese can also affect the lung directly, causing metal fume fever, pneumonitis, chronic obstructive lung disease, and pneumonia (22,430). Occupational exposure to manganese at levels of about 1 mg/m^3 may decrease male fertility (205,337). The neurological effects of inhalation of manganese dusts, termed manganism, typically begin with weakness and lethargy, and may progress to disturbances in speech and gait, a mask-like face, tremor, and possibly hallucinations and psychosis (483). Symptoms may resemble Parkinson's disease, but there is only minimal response to L-dopa therapy. The pathobiochemical aspects of manganism involve the striatum and globus pallidus. Cell damage may be due to the auto-oxidation of dopamine with the formation of free radicals (596). Manganese applied to the nasal cavity in rats is taken up in the olfactory receptor cells and transported along the primary neurons to the olfactory bulbs, with subsequent migration into most parts of the brain. This route circumvents the blood–brain barrier (559). More subtle nonclinical neurological damage can be identified by neurobehavioral tests (reaction time, finger tapping, hand steadiness, etc.) in men chronically exposed to levels as low as 0.14 mg/m^3 for 1–35 years (283). Impairment of speed and coordination of motor function are noted.

The U.S. EPA has derived a recent inhalation RfC of 0.05 $\mu g/m^3$ based on studies of Roels et al. (483,589). The previous RfC was 0.4 $\mu g/m^3$. The ACGIH has also lowered the TLV-TWA value to 0.2 mg Mn/m^3 for elemental and inorganic compounds (32). Manganese cyclopentadienyl tricarbonyl (MMT) is a gasoline octane enhancer in use since 1970. The major combustion products of MMT are manganese particulates of manganese phosphate with some sulfates and a small amount of oxides. The TWA-TLV for MMT is 0.1 mg Mn/m^3, with a notation noting the potential for dermal absorption (32). Little evidence exists to suggest that manganese has carcinogenic potential. A 2-year bioassay of manganese sulfate monohydrate in the diet found no evidence of carcinogenicity to rats and equivocal evidence of carcinogenicity to mice (22). The U.S. EPA has classified manganese as a group D carcinogen (not classifiable as to human carcinogenicity), based on inadequate evidence in humans and animals (589).

Molybdenum

Molybdenum is a silver-white metal of the second transition series. The primary molybdenum-containing ore is molybdenite (MoS_2), with minor ores being powellite ($CaMoO_4$) and wulfenite ($PbMoO_4$). Metallic molybdenum is used in a number of important applications, such as in high temperature and tool steel alloys, and in missile and aircraft parts. Molybdenum disulfide is used as a dry lubricant or as a component in lubricants (31).

Molybdenum is a constituent of several enzymes, including aldehyde oxidase, xanthine oxidase, and sulfide oxidase (420). Deficiency is extremely rare; one patient on total parenteral nutrition had disturbed sulfur and uric acid metabolism that resolved after molybdenum supplementation (420). The estimated safe and adequate daily dietary intake for molybdenum is set equal to the current U.S. dietary intake for molybdenum, based on the lack of evidence for human molybdenum deficiency, yielding a range of 75–250 $\mu g/day$ (420). High levels of molybdenum in herbage eaten by cattle caused diarrhea in cattle (186), which could be alleviated by the administration of copper salts (429). Further study has shown an inverse relationship between molybdenum and copper. When molybdenum intake in cattle is increased, the concentration of utilizable copper in the liver decreases (63).

The acute oral toxicity of molybdenum compounds is related to their solubility. Molybdenum trioxide, calcium molybdate, and ammonium molybdate caused fatalities in rats when administered at doses from 1.2 to 6.0 g Mo/kg. Conversely, administration of insoluble molybdenum disulfide to rats at concentrations as great as 6.0 g Mo/kg did not cause any fatalities (182). The U.S. EPA derived an oral RfD for molybdenum of 5 $\mu g/kg/day$ (250 $\mu g/day$ for a 70-kg adult) based on an increase in urinary uric acid levels in humans exposed to 10 mg Mo/day in the diet with an uncertainty factor of 30 (589). Rodent bioassays of molybdenum trioxide indicate that this compound is carcinogenic in rats and mice, causing an increased incidence of alveolar/bronchiolar adenoma or carcinoma (combined). Male rats and mice appear to be more sensitive to the carcinogenic effects of molybdenum trioxide (114).

Dental technicians exposed to dust of vitallium alloy, which contains chromium, cobalt, and molybdenum, can develop pneumoconiosis that is clearly different from hard-metal lung disease associated with cobalt exposure (430), and there are some data to suggest that molybdenum inhalation can cause pneumoconoiosis (31). The ACGIH has adopted TLV-TWA values of 10 mg Mo/m^3 for insoluble compounds and 5 mg Mo/m^3 for soluble compounds (32).

Phosphorus

Phosphorus is an essential component of bone and also participates in many important biochemical reactions (420). Approximately 85% of the body store of phosphorus is in bone, with the rest as soluble phosphate ion and a component of a variety of biomolecules. Absorption of phosphate ranges from 50–70% when intake is adequate, to 90% when intake is low (420). Dietary phosphorus deficiency is rare but can occur following prolonged use of the antacid aluminium hydroxide, which binds phosphorus into an unavailable form. Symptoms of phosphorus deficiency include bone loss, weakness, anorexia, and pain. The RDA for phosphorus is set equal to the RDA for calcium, based on a lack of evidence for either phosphorus deficiency or toxicity at usual U.S. intakes, yielding 1200 mg/day for ages 11–24 years, 800 mg/day for older age groups, with an extra 400 mg/day throughout pregnancy and lactation (420).

High-level phosphate intake in the forms of phosphate-fortified infant formulas, phosphoric acid in carbonated beverages, or purified amino acids may cause calcium loss, which can be adverse in situations of inadequate calcium intake; however, phosphorous in the form of complex proteins does not seem to have this effect (420,537). Certain reactive forms of phosphate may be chemically irritating, but neutral phosphate solutions are essentially nontoxic (304). Phosphorus as the free element does not occur in nature. It exists either as relatively nontoxic red phosphorus or toxic yellow (or white) phosphorus (150). Toxic exposure to yellow phosphorus can occur through the oral, dermal, or respiratory routes. Rodenticides and insecticides containing yellow phosphorus have accounted for poisonings characterized initially by gastrointestinal burning and severe abdominal pain, vomiting, and diarrhea. Acute cardiovascular collapse may occur (276,463). If survived, a second stage of symptoms may occur up to several weeks later, resulting in systemic toxic effects on the liver, heart, kidneys, or central nervous system. Phosphorus can cause necrotic skin burns. The fumes are irritating to the respiratory tract, eyes, and skin. Phosphorous is converted to phosphates and excreted in the urine. The U.S. EPA has derived a chronic oral RfD for elemental phosphorus based on studies of Condray (137), which found increased mortality in pregnant rats near the end of gestation at a dose of 0.075 mg/kg/day for 80 days prior to mating and during gestation. A NOAEL of 0.015 mg/kg/day was converted to an RfD of 0.02 μg/kg/day (1.4 μg/day for a 70 kg adult) with low confidence, using an uncertainty factor of 1000 (a factor of 10 for interspecies variation, 10 for intraspecies variation, and 10 for incomplete reproductive/developmental data and a less-than-adequate lifetime study), and a modifying factor of 1 (589). The ACGIH has adopted TLV-TWA values for phosphorus of 0.2 ppm for phosphorus trichloride, 1 mg/m^3 for phosphorus pentasulfide, 0.1 ppm for phosphorus pentachloride, 0.1 ppm for phosphorus oxychloride, and 0.02 ppm for yellow phosphorus (32). No data exist to suggest that phosphorus may have carcinogenic potential.

Potassium

Elemental potassium is a highly reactive soft metal with a silver-colored appearance and is not found in nature. Potassium compounds are common. Elemental potassium is even more reactive than sodium and must be stored under airtight anhydrous conditions, such as under xylene. Oxidation on the surface of the metal may form highly reactive superoxides, which can detonate the bulk, causing spattering and skin and eye penetration (326). Autoignition can occur at room temperature. Dermal and ocular thermal burns and liquefaction necrosis due to the formation of potassium hydroxide are the primary effects following exposure. Imbedded particles require surgical debridement. Water irrigation is contraindicated. Potassium is the principal cation of intracellular fluid, accumulating to a concentration about 30 times higher than in plasma. Potassium in plasma is involved in nerve transmission, muscle contraction, and blood-pressure homeostasis. The gastrointestinal absorption of potassium is nearly complete; plasma concentrations are kept within a narrow range by regulation of urinary excretion, and by depletion of body stores in cases of low potassium intake (420). Dietary potassium deficiency is rare, but prolonged vomiting, diarrhea, or diuretic use may deplete potassium enough to cause weakness, anorexia, nausea, drowsiness, irrational behavior, and, in severe cases, potentially fatal cardiac arrhythmias (420). Potassium appears to moderate the effect of increased sodium intake on elevating blood pressure, probably by affecting renal sodium excretion (410). The minimum requirement for potassium is based on the need for 1600 mg/day to maintain normal body stores and plasma levels (420). Dietary potassium is not toxic if sufficient water is ingested and renal function is adequate to maintain homeostasis; symptoms of hyperkalemia from dehydration or acute renal failure are similar to those of hypokalemia, including muscle weakness, fatigue, and paralysis (74). The U.S. EPA has not derived any toxicity values for potassium.

Selenium

Selenium is widely distributed in nature and found in combination with sulfides and other minerals (20,64). It has semiconducting properties and is used in photocopying machines, light meters, and rectifiers; cadmium selenide is a pigment used for car taillights; and it is used in agriculture and personal care as a component of fertilizers, pesticides, animal feeds, and antidandruff shampoo (20,31,196). Although selenium has long been known to protect vitamin E-deficient rats from liver necrosis (512) a specific biochemical role was not elucidated until Rotruck et al. (487) demonstrated it to be an essential constituent of glutathione peroxidase. This enzyme protects polyunsaturated fatty acids in the cell membrane from oxidative damage caused by free radicals. Its identification in human erythrocytes established selenium as an essential trace element in human nutrition (46). Selenium deficiency has been identified as the major causal factor in the potentially fatal cardiomyopathy affecting young children and women of child-bearing age in the Keshan region of the People's Republic of China (303). A diet based primarily on local produce grown in the selenium-poor soil resulted in a selenium deficiency, alleviated by supplementing the diet with selenium-fortified table salt (123). Additional evidence for essentiality in humans is provided by the observed cardiomyopathy seen in patients maintained on long-term total parenteral nutrition (292,355,594). Selenium also plays an important role in the control of thyroid hormone (70), which is essential for normal growth, development, and metabolism. The selenoenzymes, iodothyronine deiodinases, are responsible for the activation of thyroxine (T4) to triiodothyronine (T3), and a selenium deficiency may cause reduced growth rates. The RDA for selenium was derived from the intake associated with a plateauing of plasma glutathione peroxidase activity in Chinese adult males (40 μg/day) (625), adjusted for differences in body weight between the reference Chinese and North American male, with an additional safety factor of 1.3 to account for individual variation (346,420). The RDA for selenium is 70 and 55 μg/day in males and females, respectively with additional recommendations of 10 μg/day during pregnancy and 20 μg/day during lactation. Selenium is readily absorbed from the gastrointestinal tract, and the average U.S. diet typically provides 60–150 μg/day (539), which should be adequate to prevent cardiomyopathy in the general population.

Selenium toxicity has long been observed in cattle grazing on milk vetch (legumes of *Astragalus* species) grown in the seleniferous soils of Wyoming and South Dakota (246,299,374,408). Acute intoxication in livestock is known as "blind staggers" and is characterized by signs of CNS impairment (ataxia, impaired vision, disorientation), and respiratory distress. Chronic exposure to moderately toxic selenium levels is known as "alkali disease" and results in skin lesions with alopecia, hoof necrosis and loss, growth retardation, anemia, and cardiac atrophy. In humans, chronic sublethal selenium toxicity has been observed in individuals living in seleniferous areas and is characterized by hair or nail loss, thickened or brittle nails, garlicky breath, tooth decay (235,236), skin lesions, gastrointestinal disorders, and CNS abnormalities including peripheral anesthesia, acroparesthesia, and pain in the extremities (503,534,625). It has also been reported following the ingestion of superpotent selenium dietary supplements, and consumers need to be aware of its potential for toxicity (253,289). The deterioration of keratinized tissue is thought to result from the replacement of sulfur with selenium in methionine, cystine, and other sulfur-containing amino acids. Acute selenium intoxication resulting from ingestion is rare in humans (204), but has been reported following suicidal, accidental, and homicidal exposure (102,323,364,490). Symptoms include gastrointestinal disturbances due to the irritative properties of selenium, a characteristic garlicky breath from the exhalation of dimethyl selenide (384), formication of the nose, signs of rhinitis, neurological symptoms ranging from mild tremors to myoclonic jerks, and cardiovascular shock. Acute inhalation of hydrogen selenide has been reported to cause severe dyspnea with abnormal pulmonary function tests (501), and chronic inhalation of the gas leads to garlicky breath, gastrointestinal disturbances, dental caries, nail deformities, and conjunctivitis (24). Chronic overexposure to selenium has been associated with the motor neuron disease amyotrophic lateral sclerosis (329,599). Although selenium is known to be an avian teratogen (198,264,408) there is inconclusive evidence linking it to mammalian teratogenesis (287,521); Yang et al. (624,625) did not observe teratogenesis in babies during epidemiological studies in seleniferous regions where malformed chicks hatched from local eggs.

The U.S. EPA has established a chronic oral RfD for selenium using the study of Yang et al. (624) and corroborated by Longnecker et al. (357). The NOAEL of 0.85 mg Se/day was converted to a dose of 0.015 mg/kg/day (based on an average adult body weight of 55 kg), and an RfD of 5 μg/kg/day was derived using an uncertainty factor of 3 (less than a full factor of 10 was used to account for sensitive individuals because of the availability of epidemiological data from two independent studies of moderate size) (589). Confidence in this RfD is considered high (589). The U.S. EPA has not derived RfCs for selenium. The ACGIH has adopted a TLV-TWA value for selenium of 0.2 mg Se/m^3 (32).

Various animal models report a protective effect of pharmacologic levels of selenium against chemical carcinogenesis (127,282,473,557). In 1969, Shamberger and Frost (520) reported an inverse relationship between cancer mortality rates in the United States and plant selenium levels as mapped by Kubota et al. (328). Subsequent epidemiological studies have reported promising but inconclusive findings (136,273,319). A recent randomized cancer prevention trial reports that 200 μg selenium daily did not protect against the development of recurrent skin cancers, but was inversely associated with mortality from total prostrate, lung, and colorectal cancers (125,126). Another study reports an inverse relationship between advanced prostrate cancer and toenail selenium concentration (627), an indicator of past selenium intake. One of the authors, Gerald Combs, pointed out that "the greatest value of epidemiology is in generating hypotheses, not testing them" (184), and stressed the requirement for further research before a beneficial effect of increased selenium intake can be established.

Selenium sulfide has been shown to be a rodent carcinogen by the oral (417) but not dermal (416,418) route. A 2-year gavage bioassay of selenium sulfide by the National Toxicology Program produced evidence of carcinogenicity in male rats (liver), female rats (liver), and female mice (liver and lung), but not in male mice (417). The U.S. EPA classifies selenium sulfide as a group B2 carcinogen (probable human carcinogen), based on inadequate data from human studies and sufficient evidence from rodent studies; no quantitative risk assessment was performed (589). Other selenium compounds are classified as group D carcinogens (not classifiable as to carcinogenicity in humans) based on inadequate evidence in both humans and animals (589). The suggested beneficial antioxidant effects of selenium and the potential widespread use of selenium supplements make it important to gain a fuller understanding of selenium toxicology.

Sodium

Sodium is a highly reactive soft metal with a silver appearance that is not found in the elemental form in nature (326). Sodium compounds are ubiquitous in nature. Elemental sodium must be stored under airtight anhydrous conditions, such as under oil, to prevent oxidation, which can produce autoignition at room temperature. Superoxides may form resulting in a violent explosion. Dermal and ocular thermal burns and liquefaction necrosis due to the formation of sodium hydroxide are the primary effects following sodium exposure. Explosion may cause particles to imbed in the skin and eye requiring surgical debridement. Water irrigation is contraindicated.

Sodium is the principal cation of extracellular fluid and the primary regulator of extracellular fluid volume. Sodium also regulates osmolarity, acid–base balance, and membrane potential, and participates in active transport across cell membranes. Renal excretion of sodium maintains homeostasis over a wide range of intakes and losses, via aldosterone control of tubular excretion. Sodium deficiency is very uncommon but may occur after heavy and prolonged sweating, chronic diarrhea, or renal disease, and constitutes a medical emergency. Dietary sodium is not toxic if sufficient water is ingested and renal function is adequate to maintain homeostasis (420). Lifelong excess intake of sodium may predispose sensitive individuals to hypertension, and individuals diagnosed with high blood pressure are commonly advised to limit sodium intake to 1–2 g/day or less (410). At present, the public health benefit of restricting sodium intake in the general population is not firmly established (420). The U.S. EPA has not derived any toxicity values for sodium.

Zinc

Zinc is a bluish-white, soft metal extracted from ore and is used in alloys, for galvanizing iron to prevent corrosion and oxidation, and in numerous compounds including use in cosmetics, pharmaceuticals, and dry-cell batteries (190). At temperatures approaching its boiling point, zinc volatilizes and oxidizes to the white fume of zinc oxide (31). Zinc is an essential trace element and is a required component of many enzymes (420). Zinc is stored in bone and muscle, but is not readily released from these stores during deficiency. Gastrointestinal absorption of zinc is higher when body stores are lower, and is also higher from more refined diets. Zinc deficiency causes loss of appetite, growth retardation, and slow wound healing; no single enzyme function has been identified as associated with these signs of zinc deficiency. Severe zinc deficiency causes hypogonadism and dwarfism, which are alleviated with zinc supplementation. The RDA for zinc is derived from an estimated 2.2–2.8 mg daily loss and an oral absorption fraction of 20%, plus a 20% safety factor, leading to a recommendation of 15 mg/day for adult men and 12 mg/day for adult women, with an additional 3 mg/day during pregnancy and 7 mg/day during lactation (420).

Inhalation exposure to zinc oxide fume can cause metal fume fever (31). Zinc chloride fume is a corrosive material that has caused chemical pneumonitis, alveolar and bronchial obliteration, and death (21). Zinc compounds are absorbed orally and excreted primarily in the feces. Zinc has low human toxicity by the oral route, but high levels can cause gastrointestinal (GI) distress (21). Long term oral intakes of zinc at levels of 18.5–25 mg/day can interfere with copper absorption, and intakes 10–30 times the RDA can impair immune responses and decrease serum high-density lipoprotein (420). The U.S. EPA has derived an oral RfD for zinc of 0.3 mg/kg/day (589). No inhalation RfC has been derived for zinc. The U.S. EPA has classified zinc as a group D carcinogen (not classifiable as to human carcinogenicity) based on inadequate evidence in humans and animals. The ACGIH has adopted TLV-TWA values for zinc of 10 mg/m^3 for zinc dust, 5 mg/m^3 for zinc oxide fume, and 1 mg/m^3 for zinc chloride fume (32).

A summary of quantitative values for essential elements is given in Table 14.1. Elements are listed in the order of highest to lowest dietary requirement.

MAJOR TOXIC METALS

Arsenic

Arsenic is a Group VA element of the periodic table, the 52nd most abundant element in the earth's crust.

Table 14.1
Essential elements

Element	Recommended intake (mg/kg/day)[a]	Chronic oral toxicity: RfD[b] (mg/kg/day)	Chronic oral toxicity: Confidence	Chronic inhalation toxicity: RfC[c] (μg/m^3)	Chronic inhalation toxicity: Confidence	Carcinogenicity: Inhalation slope factor [risk/(μg/m^3)]	Carcinogenicity: Classification[d]
Potassium	30	—	—	—	—	—	—
Calcium	20	—	—	—	—	—	—
Phosphate	20	—	—	—	—	—	—
Chloride	10	—	—	—	—	—	—
Sodium	7	—	—	—	—	—	—
Magnesium	5	—	—	—	—	—	—
Iron	2×10^{-1}	—	—	—	—	—	—
Zinc	2×10^{-1}	3×10^{-1}	Medium	—	—	—	D
Manganese	$3–7 \times 10^{-2}$	1.4×10^{-1}	Medium	5×10^{-2}	Medium	—	D
Fluoride	$2–6 \times 10^{-2}$	6×10^{-2} (Cosmetic)	High	—	—	—	—
	—	12×10^{-2} (Adverse)	High	—	—	—	—
Copper	$2–4 \times 10^{-2}$	—	—	—	—	—	D
Iodide	2×10^{-3}	—	—	—	—	—	—
Molybdenum	$1–4 \times 10^{-3}$	5×10^{-3}	Medium	—	—	—	—
Chromium	$0.7–3 \times 10^{-3}$	1.5 (Cr^{3+})	Low	—	—	(Cr^{3+}	D(Cr^{3+}
	—	3×10^{-3} (Cr^{6+})	Low	8×10^{-3}[e]	Low	1.2×10^{-2} (Cr^{6+})	A(Cr^{6+})
	—	—	—	1×10^{-1}[f]	Medium	—	—
Selenium	1×10^{-3}	5×10^{-3}	High	—	—	—	B2 (SeS_2) D (all)
Cobalt	1×10^{-6}[g]	—	—	—	—	—	—

[a] For a 70-kg adult; see text for actual values.
[b] RfD, reference dose.
[c] RfC, reference concentration.
[d] Group A, known human carcinogen; group B2, probable human carcinogen; group D, not classification as to human carcinogenicity.
[e] Chromic acid mists and soluble Cr(VI) aerosols
[f] Chromium(VI) particulates
[g] Based on cobalt content of vitamin B_{12}.

Arsenic is refined from the minerals arsenopyrite and loellingite, or it can be prepared from the reduction of arsenic trioxide. The main use of arsenic in the United States is in the production of herbicides and other agricultural chemicals. Arsenic is also used in the semiconductor industry (32). Although arsenic can exist in several valence states, the +3 and +5 states are the most prevalent, with arsenic (+3) being more toxic than arsenate (+5) (172). Dietary consumption of arsenic is generally low; the typical daily American intake is 145 μg/day from both food and water (60). However, consumption of seafood can increase the amount of arsenic ingested (278,570).

Arsenic is readily absorbed via the gut (63), and excretion occurs primarily in the urine (93,141,369,549). Two processes are involved in the metabolism of arsenate and arsenite; the interconversion of arsenate and arsenite, and the conversion of these moieties to monomethyl arsenic acid and dimethyl arsenic acid. Because the methylated forms of arsenic are less toxic and because methylation results in lower tissue retention of inorganic arsenic, the methylation process is viewed as a detoxification mechanism (15).

Arsenic is believed to exert its toxic effects through at least two mechanisms, depending on its valence state. Arsenate inhibits ATP synthesis by uncoupling oxidative phosphorylation, whereas arsenite reacts with thiol groups on the active sites of many enzymes and tissue proteins, such as keratin (i.e., skin, nails, and hair) (550). Because of this reactivity with thiol groups, arsenic concentrates in the skin, hair, and nails. Mee's lines (horizontal white lines on the fingernails) appear in exposed individuals after the exposed nail bed grows to the exterior (390). At one time, inorganic arsenic was widely used as a "criminal poison" because it was odorless and nearly tasteless. The lethal dose of arsenic trioxide can be as low as 0.2 g (222). Acute toxicity is characterized by severe gastrointestinal symptoms, which occur from 30 min to several hours after ingestion. Eventually, severe gastrointestinal hemorrhaging occurs, leading to profound losses of fluid and electrolytes, resulting in collapse, shock, and death (222). If the victim survives the initial toxic sequelae, jaundice, renal failure, and peripheral neuropathology can develop (172,222).

In cases of acute intoxication, chelation therapy can be very effective in reducing or preventing symptoms. The agent of choice is British anti-lewisite (BAL), which is dimercaptopropanol (620). D-Penicillamine is also effective as a chelating agent, but nephrotoxicity and optic neuritis can result from long-term use (172). Therefore, BAL remains the treatment of choice in arsenic poisoning (222).

Chronic ingestion of arsenic can be difficult to diagnose. Diarrhea and abdominal pain can occur, as well as hyperpigmentation, hyperkeratosis, and numerous other skin- and hair-related disorders (48,101,172,267, 553). Peripheral vascular occlusive disease has also been linked to chronic exposure to high levels of arsenic in drinking water in Chile (Raynaud's phenomenon) (83) and in Taiwan (blackfoot disease) (566). Neurological changes have been associated with occupational inhalation exposure to inorganic arsenic by smelter workers (81,185,257). Neurologic changes included peripheral neuropathy of sensory and motor neurons, as measured by motor and sensory deficits (406) and encephalopathy, as evidenced by hallucinations and other psychological disturbances (61).

Chronic exposure to arsenic in drinking water is associated with an increased incidence of cancer. Numerous studies have been conducted in Taiwan, comparing residents in the blackfoot disease endemic area with residents in areas with low levels of arsenic in drinking water. These studies have consistently shown an increase in the incidence of skin cancer and several internal cancers in areas with high arsenic consumption (119–122,566,567,621). A similar study was conducted in Japan, which showed an association between high levels of ingested arsenic and lung and urinary-tract cancer (569).

Chronic exposure to arsenic via the inhalation route is also associated with the development of tumors. Studies of smelter worker populations have shown strong associations between exposure and an increased incidence of lung cancer (47,175,341,476,560), as have studies of pesticide manufacturing workers (362,451) case reports of lung cancer in arsenical pesticide applicators (486). Although the carcinogenicity of arsenic is well established in humans, carcinogenicity in animal models has been more difficult to establish. Of the many animal carcinogenicity studies reviewed by the IARC in 1980 (570), only two gave positive results: one with subcutaneous/intravenous administration of sodium arsenite in mice in a multigenerational study (450), and one with intratracheal installation of copper and calcium arsenate in rats (285). Later studies showed that both calcium arsenate and arsenic trioxide are carcinogenic when administered intratracheally to Syrian golden hamsters (284,461,462). The mechanism of carcinogenicity is postulated to be related to the multistep metabolism of pentavalent arsenic to dimethyl arsenic acid, during which free radicals are produced (63,550).

Arsine, AsH_3, is a gaseous form to arsenic that is formed whenever arsenic is in the presence of hydrogen (222) and as such can be generated in metal tanks storing acids that contain arsenic impurities (63). The toxicity profile of arsine is different from all other arsenic compounds. The hallmark of arsine toxicity is hemolysis, sometimes followed by acute renal failure (222). BAL and D-penicillamine are not effective treatments for arsine poisoning (222).

The U.S. EPA has established the following RfDs for arsenic compounds: inorganic arsenic, 0.3 μg/kg/day (group A (human) carcinogen); arsine 0.05 $\mu g/m^3$ (589). The ACGIH has adopted the following TLVs for arsenic compounds: arsenic, elemental arsenic, and inorganic compounds, as As, 0.01 mg/m^3 (A1 carcinogenicity notation; confirmed human carcinogen); arsine, 0.05 ppm (32).

Cadmium

Cadmium is a soft silver-white metal, often found in association with zinc and obtained primarily as a by-product of zinc preparation (63). It is used primarily in the production of nickel–cadmium batteries (35%), but also for metal plating (30%), pigments (15%), plastics and synthetics (10%), and miscellaneous uses (10%) (16). The toxicity of cadmium has been widely investigated, and cadmium has been shown to affect nearly every organ system if the dose is high enough (71). Acute effects of cadmium depend on the route of exposure. Symptoms of acute inhalation exposure to cadmium develop 4–10 h postexposure and initially simulate metal fume fever (fever, nausea, vomiting, headache, cough, dyspnea, nasopharyngeal irritation), but with progression to chemical pneumonitis and a potentially fatal pulmonary edema (71,76,79,164). A fatal dose can be inhaled by exposed individuals who are unaware of either the presence of cadmium or its inhalation hazard (71,360). Cadmium absorption following inhalation exposure is dependent on particle size and solubility and ranges from 20 to 50% of the amount inhaled (200). Fatal doses have been estimated at 50 mg/m^3 for 1 h (57,96) and 9 mg/m^3 for 5 h (71). Recovery following acute high-level exposure or chronic exposure at lower levels may be accompanied by pulmonary fibrosis (56,144,562). Oral exposure to cadmium is rarely fatal because the gastrointestinal irritation leads to vomiting, eliminating most of the dose before absorption (52,95,361,440,526). Gastrointestinal absorption is about 5%, but can reach 20% with concurrent calcium or iron deficiency (192,200). Rats exposed by intravenous injection to 4 mg Cd/kg developed a potentially lethal hepatic necrosis (162,213).

Chronic inhalation or ingestion of cadmium results in kidney damage, characterized by tubular and/or glomerular dysfunction with proteinuria, low concentration capacity, and decreased inulin clearance (200). Increased urinary excretion of β_2-microglobulin, a low-molecular-weight protein normally reabsorbed in the proximal tubule, is an early indicator of renal dysfunction and should be regarded as an adverse effect because it is predictive of an increase in the age-related decline in the glomerular filtration rate (484). Absorbed cadmium is first transported to the liver, where it stimulates the synthesis of metallothionein and is sequestered as cadmium–metallothionien. Small amounts of liver cadmium–metallothionein are released into the plasma following normal cell turnover, filtered with the primary urine, and reabsorbed into the proximal tubular cells, where lysosomes degrade the metallothionein portion, with the release of cadmium, which then induces renal metallothionein synthesis. Renal damage results when the kidneys can no longer produce sufficient metallothionein to sequester the cadmium ion and prevent its interaction with critical macromolecules (224). Free cadmium may inactivate metalloenzymes, activate calmodulin, and/or damage cell membranes through activation of oxygen (602). This threshold level is commonly called the *critical concentration*. Kjellström et al. (314) proposed the term *population critical concentration* (PCC), where a PCC-10 indicates the cadmium concentration in the renal cortex that is likely to result in renal dysfunction in 10% of an exposed population—that is, 10% of the exposed population will have exceeded their individual critical concentrations. They estimated the PCC-10 to be 180–220 μg/g and the PCC-50 to be 25% higher. Excess inhalation or ingestion exposure to cadmium leads to abnormalities of calcium metabolism, and susceptible individuals may develop a painful bone disease as first discovered in a cadmium-contaminated area in Japan (Toyama Prefecture) and termed itai-itai (ouch-ouch) disease (412,568). The disease is characterized by osteomalacia and osteoporosis with an increased tendency to spontaneous fracture and is associated with bone pain and renal tubular dysfunction. Cadmium has been shown to increase bone resorption and inhibit bone formation in both in vivo and in vitro systems (73). Current knowledge suggests that bone changes associated with pregnancy, lactation, and menopause may enhance cadmium's effect on bone. There is conflicting evidence concerning cadmium exposure and the risk of developing hypertension, with human studies reporting either positive, negative, or no effect (16,413). This suggests that a cadmium effect on blood pressure is small to nonexistent compared to other established risk factors. Cadmium-exposed populations are not reported to have elevated death rates associated with cardiovascular disease. Maternal and fetal toxicity of cadmium is well documented in rodents (16,453). Elevated levels of cadmium in neonates are associated with a decreased birth weight (271), but further research is required to determine if developmental effects of cadmium are of concern at environmental levels. Tobacco plants are known to concentrate soil cadmium, and it is estimated 1-pack/day smokers can absorb 1–3 μg cadmium/day (347). Pregnant smokers have an increased cadmium concentration in both maternal and cord blood (117), and cadmium–metallothionein mobilized into the serum has been suggested to be the toxic serum factor associated with preeclampsia (124). High doses of parenteral cadmium will induce testicular necrosis in male rodents, and this effect is thought to be related to cadmium inhibition of a testes-specific enzyme (16). Pretreatment or concurrent treatment with various substances, including zinc and selenium, will inhibit the acute toxic effect of cadmium, but the precise protective mechanism is unknown (527).

The U.S. EPA has derived a chronic oral RfD for cadmium based on an early version of the toxicokinetic model for cadmium (201). Separate values were derived for food and water exposure, assuming 2.5% absorption of cadmium from food and 5% from water with a 0.01% per day excretion, and a kidney concentration of 200 μg Cd/g wet human renal cortex is considered the NOAEL (589). An uncertainty factor of 10 was used for intrahuman variability, and the resulting RfD values are 0.001 mg Cd/kg/day (food) and 0.0005 mg Cd/kg/day (water); confidence in these values is considered high. No reference concentration values for chronic cadmium inhalation exposure were calculated. The Agency for Toxic Substances and Disease Registry (ATSDR) has calculated chronic minimal risk levels (MRLs) for cadmium based on human studies with measured exposures (16). The inhalation MRL was calculated from a NOAEL for renal effects in workers exposed to 0.0016 mg/m^3 (288); adjusting for continuous lifetime exposure and using an uncertainty factor of 10 to account for sensitive members of the population, the chronic inhalation MRL is 0.0002 mg/m^3. A chronic oral MRL of 0.0007 mg/kg/day was calculated from a study in a Japanese population exposed to cadmium in rice (438). The average nonsmoking American absorbs approximately 1–3 μg Cd/day from the diet (16), which is only 2 to 4 times lower than the oral MRL, indicating that there is not a large margin of safety with respect to cadmium toxicity, particularly given evidence that postmenopausal women and diabetics may be more sensitive to cadmium toxicity than members of the general population (94).

The carcinogenicity of cadmium is the subject of much discussion. In animals, inhalation exposure causes lung cancer in rats but not in mice or hamsters (211,252,547). In humans, increases in lung cancer rates were associated with cadmium exposure in one cohort (558), but not in three others (4,170,535); in these same cohorts, early indications of an increase in prostate tumors were not borne out by longer term follow-up. The role of arsenic and/or smoking in the cohort with the increased rate of lung cancer is controversial (156,331,542). Studies investigating environmental cadmium and its role in prostate cancer have been hampered by a lack of dose quantification (2,53,611), and results from studies with occupational exposure have been mixed (315,536). In animals, older studies found no significant increase in tumors following lifetime oral exposure to cadmium, but the doses in these studies were relatively low and histological examination was limited compared to present standards (133,358,502). A more recent study reports prostate tumors in male rats after oral cadmium exposure (603). Further research is required to establish the role of cadmium in human prostate cancer (604). Cadmium is genotoxic (248); it has been reported to induce apoptosis, which may serve to remove critically damaged cells (234,241). The International Agency for Research on Cancer (IARC) accepts cadmium as a category 1 (human) carcinogen (281) based primarily on its role in lung cancer (542). The U.S. EPA classifies cadmium as a group B1 carcinogen (probable human carcinogen) (589) based on evidence in humans and animals (547,558). An inhalation unit risk of 1.8×10^{-3} per ($\mu g/m^3$) was calculated from the study of Thun et al. (558).

If future research were to establish that present levels of exposure to cadmium carry an unacceptable risk of either noncancer or cancer effects, difficult questions would arise. The primary difficulty would be how to reduce exposure; the main source of cadmium exposure is the diet, but reducing this exposure, by removing cadmium from fertilizer, would be costly and difficult. Another policy issue is whether cigarette smokers should be considered a sensitive subpopulation deserving extra protection, so that exposure must be controlled to levels that would be safe for smokers, or whether smokers should be considered individuals with a demonstrated lack of concern for, and need for protection from, adverse health effects.

Lead

Lead is a heavy, bluish-gray metal and, although it serves no biological purpose, is the most widely used nonferrous metal (17,187). Lead and/or lead compounds have been used in many industrial applications, including batteries, ammunition, paints and varnishes, gasoline, pigments, radiation shields, medical equipment, solder, glass, and ceramic glazes (17). Inhalation and ingestion are the main routes of exposure for inorganic lead (261). Adults are primarily exposed occupationally (17), and this occurs by inhalation with 35–40% of inhaled lead dust or fumes deposited in the lungs with extensive (95%) blood absorption (342). Children are primarily exposed by ingestion and absorb 50% of an ingested dose through the gastrointestinal tract. In contrast, adults absorb 10% of an ingested dose, but gastrointestinal absorption will vary with particle size (inverse proportion), solubility, nutritional status, and fasting. Excretion is mainly in the urine, with lesser amounts in the feces, sweat, hair, and nails.

In adults, early symptoms are often nonspecific (fatigue, depression, sleep disturbance, anorexia, intermittent abdominal pain, nausea, constipation, diarrhea, and myalgia) (261). Blood lead level (PbB) is the single best diagnostic test for lead exposure (261). Epidemiologic studies and animal experimentation suggest PbB levels as low as 14 $\mu g/dl$ may elevate blood pressure (245,510), but the results are not definitive (256). A recent study (269) suggests that long-term lead accumulation—measured as bone lead, as opposed to PbB, which reflects recent exposure—is associated with developing hypertension. However, other researchers report no consistent effect (540), and the subject remains controversial. Reversible slowing of nerve conduction velocity has been observed at PbB as low as 30 $\mu g/dl$ (519), and adverse effects on reaction time, mood, and visual–motor coordination at 30–50 $\mu g/dl$ (51,544). Anemia is not seen until PbB are in excess of 50 $\mu g/dl$ (270). Overt neurotoxicity (wrist drop) is reported at levels in excess of 80 $\mu g/dl$ (219). Chronic irreversible nephropathy requires high and sustained PbB exposure (225), but recent evidence suggests low-level lead exposure (PbB$<$10 $\mu g/dl$) is associated with renal impairment, as measured by an increase in serum creatinine (308).

Morphological alterations and decreases in sperm count, density, and motility have all been reported in heavily exposed males (PbB$>$40 $\mu g/dl$) (42,45,345,572). Paternal occupational lead exposure has been reported to increase the risk of low birth weight and prematurity (349). Lead readily crosses the placenta to the fetus (305,482), and maternal PbBs in excess of 15 $\mu g/dl$ are associated with low birth weights and preterm delivery, and PbB in excess of 30 $\mu g/dl$ with spontaneous abortions (176,180,485).

Lead poisoning in children caused by ingestion of lead paint was first noted in Australia and became recognized as a public health problem in the United States in the 1920s (351). Early symptoms of chronic poisoning in children are often nonspecific, including headaches, anorexia, vomiting, and constipation, progressing to anemia with

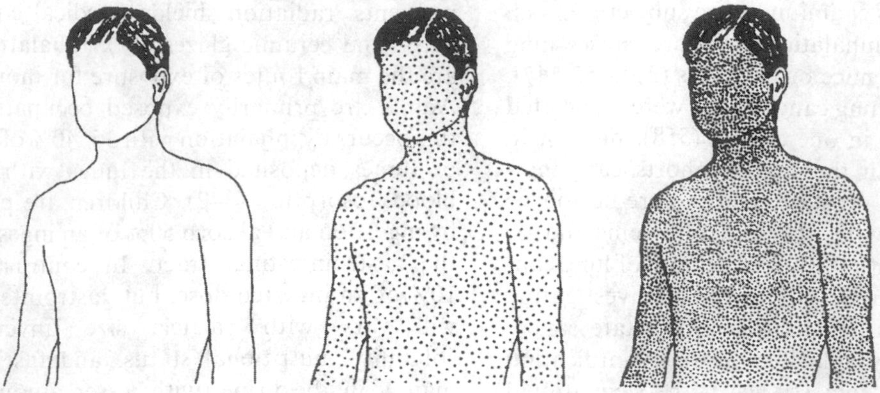

FIG. 14.1. Comparison of lead body burden (from left to right): ancient people uncontaminated by industrial lead (1 dot); typical American (1000 dots); level associated with clinical lead poisoning (4000 dots). Each dot represents 40 μg Pb/70 kg person. Reprinted from Patterson et al. (455), *Sci. Total Environ.*, copyright 1991, pp. 205–236, with permission from Elsevier Science.

basophilic stippling of red cells, Burton's line, chronic nephritis, peripheral neuropathy (manifested as wrist and/or foot drop), and radiographs of long bones revealing lead deposits (442,459). Frank encephalopathy (PbB>80 μg/dl) is characterized by ataxia, coma, convulsions, cerebral edema, and even death. The long-term neurologic consequences of childhood lead poisoning were recognized in 1943 when Byers and Lord follow up 20 "cured" cases and found poor academic performance in all but 1 (98). In 1975, de la Burde and Choate (147) reported school failure due to learning and behavioral problems in asymptomatic lead-exposed children. Asymptomatic children with elevated dentine lead levels in first and second grade scored lower on standardized tests, especially in areas measuring verbal performance and auditory processing, and were more likely to exhibit disruptive behavior relative to controls (152,427). Reexamined 11 years later as adolescents, those with greater lead exposure were more at risk for dropping out of school, reading disability, absenteeism, poor hand–eye coordination, and low scholastic class standing (66,428,511,561).

Since 1970, the CDC has repeatedly lowered the level of concern for PbB from 70 to 10 μg/dl, and the following federal laws have been enacted to reduce lead exposure: the 1971 Lead-Based Paint Poisoning Prevention Act (575); the U.S. EPA phaseout of lead in gasoline, starting in 1973 (581) with completion in 1995 (587); the U.S. EPA ban on lead in plumbing, fixtures, fittings, and solder (576); the Consumer Product Safety Commission (CPSC) 1978 ban on the use of paint containing more than 0.06% lead by weight for interior/exterior residential surfaces, toys, and furniture (579); the FDA ruling to eliminate lead-solder in food cans by December 1995 (590); and the Residential Lead-Based Paint Hazard Reduction Act of 1992 (577). Results of two National Health and Nutrition Examination Surveys, NHANES II (1976 to 1980) and NHANES III (phase I, 1988 to 1991; phase II, 1991 to 1994), indicate a substantial decline in PbB (111,216,464). Since the late 1970s, the average PbB in children 1–5 years of age has declined from 15 μg/dl to 2.7 μg/dl, and the reduction of lead in gasoline and dietary sources (primarily through the former use of lead-soldered cans for food and beverages) is believed responsible for this effect (88,464). Although this decline is substantial, Patterson et al. (455) estimate today's average American has a mean body burden of 40 mg industrial Pb/70 kg, whereas analysis of pre-Columbian American Indian skeletons indicates their mean body burden was 40 μg Pb/70 kg (Figure 14.1). Based on bone : blood lead ratios, this equates with a PbB of 0.016 μg/dl, which is 600-fold lower than the current level considered acceptable for children (i.e., 10 μg/dl) (193) and places current guidelines much closer to lethal Pb levels than natural (529). It is estimated that 890,000 (4.4%) U.S. preschool children have a PbB of 10 μg/dl or higher (111). Further reductions in PbB will require primary prevention efforts to reduce exposure to lead remaining in housing and soil (334,464,530). The Centers for Disease Control and Prevention (CDC) 1997 lead poisoning prevention program recommends targeted screening and follow-up care for high-risk children (i.e., children who live in older-homes, children from low-income families) (111). Although controversial (367), it reserves universal screening of young children to those meeting at least one of the following criteria: (a) child resides in ZIP code where at least 27% of the housing predates 1950; (b) child receives public assistance for the poor; or (c) caretaker's response to a risk assessment questionnaire suggests child is at risk.

The use of car radiators containing lead solder for the illegal distillation of alcohol (moonshine) has long been associated with lead poisoning (178), and recent reports suggest middle-aged men in rural settings continue to be at risk (173,456). Excessive PbB (>40 μg/dl) have been reported in automobile radiator repair mechanics, and "take-home" lead is a potential source of elevated PbB in their children (217), as has been reported in other lead-related industries (300). Apart from congenital intoxication, lead poisoning in infants has been reported from the use of traditional folk remedies, which are often known by their common names of azarcon, greta, and ghasard (104–107); the use of lead-contaminated water to prepare formula (523); use of a lead-soldered samovar (urn) for formula preparation (522); and household renovation (110). Lead as galena (PbS) was the main constituent of eye cosmetics (kohls) in Oman (243) and may contribute to lead poisoning in households with children practicing pica. Lead poisoning in children with pica has been reported following the ingestion of foreign objects including an imported clothing accessory (177), fishing sinkers (407), and curtain weights (77). The dissolution of retained lead gunshot has resulted in lead poisoning (306,368), with rapid onset when the bullet lodges in contact with synovial fluid (392). Lead in crystal leaches into alcoholic beverages, and lead contents as high as 21.5 mg/L have been reported in beverages stored in crystal decanters (227). The lead content of various calcium supplements (bonemeal, dolomite, calcium carbonate) has been tested, and levels of supplementation providing 800 mg calcium would also contain over 6 μg lead in over one-quarter of the 70 different brands tested (85, 614). Although cases of lead intoxication by this route have not been reported, pregnant women and children are the populations most at risk from this source. Lead-contaminated heroin has been reported as a source of lead intoxication, and physicians need to be aware of this possibility (454).

The primary treatment for lead poisoning is to identify and eliminate exposure. For children with venous PbB >45 μg/dl the CDC (108) currently recommends chelation therapy. In 1991 the U.S. FDA approved the use of *meso*-2,3-dimercaptosuccinic acid (DMSA, Succimer), which is an effective oral chelating agent and is more specific for lead than $CaNa_2EDTA$, the use of which is associated with urinary loss of essential trace elements. PbB ranging from 20 to 44 μg/dl is treated with chelation therapy if a provocative test indicates substantial lead can be mobilized. Pharmacological treatments are not currently available for PbBs<20 μg/dl. Iron deficiency is associated with increased lead absorption (365) and should be treated in all cases (36).

The adverse health effects associated with lead occur at PbBs so low as to be without a threshold, and the U.S. EPA considers it inappropriate to derive RfD values for lead (589). The U.S. EPA classifies lead as a group B2 carcinogen (probable human carcinogen) based on sufficient evidence in animals with dietary and subcutaneous exposure and inadequate evidence in humans. The U.S. EPA considers it inappropriate to quantify the carcinogenic risk from oral exposure because toxicokinetic differences between humans and animals cannot be taken into account using the standard procedures.

Mercury

Mercury is a silver-white fluid trace metal found in igneous and sedimentary rocks and in the form of the ore cinnabar (mercury sulfide) (63). It is biologically nonessential and toxic to all organisms. Mercury may occur in the elemental form, or as inorganic and organic compounds. Mercury and its compounds are used in electrical meters, chloralkali production, thermometers, and as antimicorbial preservatives in paints, cosmetics, and pharmaceuticals. Use in dry-cell batteries is now restricted due to environmental toxicity concerns following disposal (578,588). Use in interior latex paints is prohibited (584). Toxicity is related to the covalent binding of mercury to sulfhydryl groups, as well as to carboxy, amide, amine, and phosphoryl groups, thereby inactivating cellular functions (100).

Acute elemental mercury ingestion is usually of no significance due to poor absorption from the GI tract. Acute exposure to high concentrations of elemental mercury vapors are irritating to the respiratory tract. Chronic exposure to the vapors produces CNS toxicity, which includes muscle weakness and tremors, nervousness, memory loss, and anorexia. Inorganic mercury compounds generally demonstrate local irritant or corrosive activity. Acute ingestion may result in necrosis to the GI tract and renal tubular necrosis. Chronic effects produce CNS toxicity similar to that noted for elemental mercury. Organic mercury compounds have been used for treatment of syphillis and as diuretics, but have been replaced by less toxic drugs. Organic mercury compounds, such as phenylmercuric acetate, thimerosal, and mercurochrome, are primarily used as antimicrobial preservatives in ophthalmic preparations, vaccines, and nasal sprays (100). Contact dermatitis may occur to both inorganic and organic mercurials, with cross-sensitivity to each being reported (18,188). Elemental mercury and its compounds are excreted in urine, feces, and through respiration.

Dietary intake, from agricultural products treated with mercurial fungicides and fish from mercury-polluted water, is the major route for toxicity of organic mercury compounds. Metallic and inorganic mercury can enter the air and water from rock and ore deposits, burning of fossil fuels, industrial and agricultural emissions,

Table 14.2
Major toxic metals

Metal	Chronic oral toxicity: RfD[a] (mg/kg/day)	Chronic oral toxicity: Confidence	Chronic inhalation toxicity: RfC[b] ($\mu g/m^3$)	Chronic inhalation toxicity: Confidence	Carcinogenicity: Oral slope factor [risk/(mg/kg/day)]	Carcinogenicity: Inhalation slope factor [risk/($\mu g/m^3$)]	Classification[c]
Lead	—[d]	—	—	—	—[e]	—	B2
Cadmium	1×10^{-3} (food) 5×10^{-4} (water)	High	—	—	—	1.8×10^{-3}	B1
Mercury	—	—	3×10^{-1}	Medium	—	—	D
Arsenic	3×10^{-4}	Medium	—	—	1.5	4.3×10^{-3}	A

[a] RfD, reference dose.
[b] RfC, reference concentration.
[c] Group A, known human carcinogen; group B1, B2, probable human carcinogen; group D, not classifiable as to human carcinogenicity.
[d] U.S. EPA quantifies lead toxicity using a biokinetic model; threshold is equivalent to intake of about 5×10^{-3} mg/kg/day.
[e] U.S. EPA has not quantified lead carcinogenicity; slope factor would be in the range of $1\text{–}4 \times 10^{-3}$/(mg/kg/day).

and trash disposal and incineration. Atmospheric fallout adds to water pollution. Inorganic mercury compounds may be methylated by the microflora of soil and water to form methylmercury. Through the food chain, edible fish can concentrate methylmercury to levels a thousands times greater than in the environment (100). Methylmercury is neurotoxic, and the effects are both dose and time dependent (63). Ataxia is an early symptom, followed by slurred speech, weakness, vision and hearing loss, tremors, coma, and death. Well-documented poisonings from contaminated fish and grains occurred in Japan and Iraq (63,100). Additionally, methylmercury is a well-known neuroteratogen (18).

Recently, the use of dental amalgam fillings has generated concern, both because exposure of dental workers may exceed occupational standards and because a variety of illnesses (multiple sclerosis, rheumatoid arthritis, leukemia, etc.) have been attributed to dental mercury exposure in the general population (41,203,330,601). Contact dermatitis is experienced by some dental patients, and for those in which symptoms do not quickly subside with antihistamine treatment, replacement of fillings with nonmercury materials may alleviate immunological and dermatological symptoms (203,330). However, other diseases have not been firmly linked to mercury exposure, and at present replacement of mercury-containing fillings cannot be justified in nonallergic individuals, while the issue of whether mercury should continue to be used for new dental fillings is more controversial (41,203,330). Additional research is needed before the potential for dental amalgams to cause harm, and the benefit of substituting more costly or less durable materials, can be reasonably evaluated. Concern must include the potential risk of effects on the fetus (18).

The U.S. EPA has derived a chronic inhalation exposure RfC for elemental mercury (vapor) of 0.3 $\mu g/m^3$ based on critical effects of hand tremor, memory disturbances, and autonomic dysfunction (acrodynia) with a medium level of confidence (589). There is no current chronic oral exposure RfD pending further review (589). The ACGIH has adopted TLV-TWA values for inorganic forms and metallic mercury of 0.025 mg/m^3, for aryl mercury compounds of 0.1 mg/m^3, and 0.01 mg/m^3 for alkyl compounds (32). These TLV-TWA values carry a skin notation that points out the potential for dermal absorption. The ACGIH and EPA consider mercury as not classifiable as to human carcinogenicity, based on no evidence of carcinogenicity in humans and inadequate evidence in animals (32,589).

A summary of some quantitative toxicity values for these four major toxic metals is given in Table 14.2. Metals are listed in approximate reverse order of toxicity (least toxic first).

MINOR TOXIC METALS WITH RfDs

Antimony

Antimony is a brittle silver-colored metal extracted from ores (63). Compounds of antimony cover the full range of toxicity. Less toxic compounds have found use in cosmetic pigments (antimony sulfide) and medicinals (antimony potassium tartrate; tartar emetic). Stibine, the metal hydride of antimony, is a colorless highly toxic gas used in the manufacture of semiconductors (63). Ingestion of antimony compounds can cause gastrointestinal, cardiac, dermatological, hepatic, and neurological toxicity in humans and animals (9). Mechanisms for these effects include binding to sulfhydryl groups and inhibiting protein and carbohydrate metabolism (380). Acute inhalation exposure to antimony trichloride or antimony pentachloride may cause pneumonitis, but the injury may be caused by the chloride rather than by the antimony itself; acute exposure to antimony hydride can cause hemolysis, but, again, the antimony itself may not be responsible (430). Long-term inhalation exposure to antimony can cause benign pneumoconiosis (430) and may raise blood pressure (9). Dermatological reactions to antimony (eczema, pustules) exhibit signs of an acute inflammatory response but do not appear to be an allergic reaction (380). The U.S. EPA has derived a chronic oral RfD for antimony based on the study of Schroeder et al. (508), which found changes in blood glucose and cholesterol levels in rats exposed to antimony in drinking water at a dose of 0.35 mg/kg/day. This LOAEL was converted to an RfD of 0.4 μg/kg/day using an uncertainty factor of 1000 (10 for interindividual variation, 10 for interspecies variation, and 10 for use of a LOAEL rather than a NOAEL). Confidence in the RfD was considered low (589). However, a recent study of potassium antimony tartrate in rats following 90-day exposure via drinking water gave a NOAEL level of 0.06 mg/kg/day (467). Using a 100-fold safety factor, as just described, 0.6 μg/kg/day approximates the RfD. The U.S. EPA has not derived an inhalation RfC for antimony (589). The ACGIH has adopted a TLV-TWA value for antimony of 0.5 mg Sb/m^3 (32).

The carcinogenicity of antimony is uncertain. Mice given antimony potassium tartrate in drinking water at a dose of 0.88 mg/kg/day for 33 months had no increased incidence of lung, liver, or total tumors (297). Workers exposed to antimony concentrations well over 5 mg Sb/m^3 had an increased risk of lung cancer (155); however, exposure to arsenic may have caused the excess (380). Female rats exposed to >30 mg Sb/m^3 had an increased incidence of lung tumors (433). A chronic inhalation oncogenicity study in rats of antimony trioxide dust at doses less than 30 mg Sb/m^3 did not show carcinogenicity (233). Antimony has not been evaluated for human carcinogenic potential by the U.S. EPA (589). The ACGIH has classified antimony trioxide production as a suspect human carcinogen for which exposure levels should be as low as reasonably achievable (31,32).

Barium

Barium is a silvery-white alkaline earth metal and is found in nature in combination with other elements (10). The barium ion is highly reactive and its toxicity is dependent on the solubility of the specific compound, with water-soluble forms (i.e., chloride, hydroxide, nitrate) being more toxic than insoluble forms (i.e., sulfate, carbonate). Barium compounds are used primarily as lubricating agents in drilling muds, but also in the manufacture of paints, bricks, tiles, glass, rubber, and pesticides. Barium sulfate is used medically as a contrast agent in x-ray diagnosis. Hospital staff familiar with this use may fail to recognize barium as a potential toxic agent, and this has contributed to at least one fatality (159). The general population is exposed by ingestion (i.e., food, drinking water) and inhalation. Some plants bioconcentrate barium from the soil, with brazil nuts having very high concentrations (3000–4000 ppm) (62).

Occupational exposure to inhaled barium sulfate can cause a benign pneumoconiosis (baritosis) (154), which resolves with cessation of exposure. Acute ingestion of soluble Ba^{2+} salts acts as a muscle poison characterized by stimulation followed by paralysis (475). Symptoms of poisoning start with the gastrointestinal muscles (gastric pain, vomiting, diarrhea) and progress to skeletal and cardiac muscle with ventricular fibrillation followed by death due to respiratory muscle paralysis (5,153,475,488). The barium ion is thought to act as a potassium antagonist, producing an extracellular hypokalemia (488) relieved by intravenous infusion of potassium salts (5,153,475). However, potassium infusion does not relieve the hypertension (153,488,589). Prompt oral administration of sodium sulfate to form the highly insoluble barium sulfate (1 g dissolves in 400,000 parts water) has been used to prevent absorption (5,475). The U.S. EPA has derived an oral RfD for barium based on two studies involving humans, one experimental (618) and one epidemiological (87), and the subchronic and chronic rodent studies performed by the National Toxicology Program (NTP) (423). Wones et al. (618) found a NOAEL of 0.21 mg Ba/kg/day (the highest dose tested) in healthy male volunteers exposed to barium in drinking water. Brenniman and Levy (87) found no convincing evidence of a difference in hypertension or other effects between 2 communities, one exposed to <0.2 mg Ba/L and the other to a mean of 7.3 mg Ba/L (0.20 mg Ba/kg/day). These very similar NOAELs were converted to an RfD of 0.07 mg/kg/day using an uncertainty factor of 3 (to account for database deficiencies and to protect sensitive individuals; a factor lower than 10 was considered appropriate because the supporting studies considered adult males, those likely to be most sensitive to barium's hypertensive effects) (589). Confidence in the RfD was considered medium. The ACGIH has adopted a TLV-TWA value of 0.5 mg Ba/m^3 for soluble barium compounds and 10 mg Ba/m^3 for barium sulfate (32).

The National Toxicology Program (NTP) performed a 2-year rodent bioassay with barium chloride dihydrate in drinking water and found no carcinogenic effects in either rats or mice (423). The U.S. EPA classifies barium as group D (not classifiable as to human carcinogenicity) (589). The carcinogenic potential of inhaled barium cannot be determined due to the lack of adequate animal inhalation studies.

Beryllium

Beryllium is an alkaline earth metal that is the lightest of the structural metals. Beryllium is a rare metal, and is extracted primarily from bertrandite (beryllium–silicate ore) and beryl (beryllium–aluminum oxide–silicate ore). The primary uses of beryllium are as a structural metal in lightweight applications, in metal alloys, and in nuclear reactor technology, as beryllium is an excellent neutron reflector and moderator (31,63).

As beryllium is a rare metal, its toxic effects were not completely recognized until it became widely used in the 1940s. Although beryllium and its compounds can cause contact dermatitis, the primary target organ is the lung. Two types of beryllium-induced lung injury can occur, acute and chronic. The acute and frequently fatal syndrome resembles chemical pneumonitis and is associated with exposure to soluble forms of beryllium (e.g., beryllium sulfate and beryllium fluoride), where the concentration of airborne beryllium is greater than 0.1 mg/m^3 (168). First reported in the early 1930s (63,593), this syndrome has been virtually eliminated in the workplace after 1950, because of controls limiting the concentration of these beryllium compounds in the air (11,169).

Chronic beryllium disease was first reported in 1946 as a delayed pneumonitis (244). The disease (also known as berylliosis) is characterized by granuloma formation, fibrosis, emphysema, and reduction in vital capacity of the lung, and total lung capacity (11). The chronic disease has two forms, one that occurs during exposure, and a second where the disease becomes evident 10 or more years after the cessation of exposure (63). The mechanism of the delayed onset of the condition is not known. The disease has a strong immunological component; chelation treatment has little effect on the course of the disease, whereas corticosteroid treatment has been effective in disease suppression (63).

Beryllium dermatitis is a hypersensitivity reaction that is usually noted 1 to 2 weeks after exposure to soluble beryllium salts. Patch tests of individuals with soluble beryllium salts provoke a positive response. Beryllium can also induce dermal ulceration if particles of beryllium salts become imbedded in the skin (63). The ulceration can be long-lasting, and surgical intervention can be required to resolve the condition (556).

Beryllium compounds are also carcinogenic. The IARC reviewed the available literature and in 1993 published its findings that there was sufficient evidence in humans and animals for the carcinogenicity of beryllium (281). In several retrospective epidemiologic studies conducted in the 1970s and 1980s, a consistent (but small) increase has been noted in the incidence of lung cancer in workers exposed to beryllium. The decade of hire was one of the strongest correlates of lung cancer mortality.

The U.S. EPA has established the following toxicity values for beryllium: oral, RfD, 2 μg/kg/day; inhalation, RfC, 0.02 μg/m^3 and has classified it as a group B1, probable human carcinogen (589). The ACGIH has adopted TLV values for beryllium of 0.002 mg Be/m^3 as an 8-h TWA and 0.01 mg Be/m^3 as a STEL/C. An A1 carcinogenicity notation (confirmed human carcinogen) is present (32).

Boron

Boron is a metalloid. It is a solid element and, because of its high affinity for oxygen, always occurs in nature bound to oxygen in the form of inorganic borates (12,167,400). Boron and associated compounds have many industrial applications, including the production of borosilicate glass, laundry bleaches (sodium perborate), wood preservatives, fire retardants, pesticides (cockroach control), cosmetics, and pharmaceuticals (12). In 1875, Lister used boric acid as an antiseptic (353), but its effectiveness has since been discredited. The world's two largest borate deposits occur in the Mojave Desert (near Boron, California) and in Western Turkey (167). Borates have long been known to be essential for plants, but a specific biochemical role remains to be determined (80). Although boron deficiency has been reported in rats, chickens, and humans, as yet no requirement has been established in humans (420). Nielsen in 1996 (436,437) classified it as an ultratrace element, and the World Health Organization (WHO) Expert Committee on Trace Elements in Human Nutrition came to the conclusion that it is "probably essential" in human nutrition (140). Biochemical and physiological consequences of boron deprivation in humans suggest it affects calcium and magnesium metabolism (435). Inadequate dietary boron (<0.2 mg B/day) has been suggested as a factor contributing to osteoporotic bone loss (434).

Inorganic borates exhibit a low order of acute toxicity in mammals, with the oral LD_{50} for boric acid in male rats being 4.5 g/kg body weight (142). However, inadvertent use of a 2.5% boric acid solution in preparation of infant formula has resulted in toxicity and death (619). The oral lethal dose in adults has been reported as 15–20 g (528), but 80–297 g has been tolerated in a single ingestion (600). Nausea with vomiting and diarrhea, both a characteristic blue-green color, are common. Frequently the skin shows signs of erythema, desquamation (boiled lobster appearance), and exfoliation. Death generally occurs several days after ingestion and results from renal injury, circulatory collapse, and shock. Although the use of boric acid solutions as an antiseptic is now obsolete, concentrated boric acid is still readily available as a household pesticide, and householders, particularly those with young children, need to be familiar with symptoms of poisoning (528,532). Borates are not absorbed through intact skin (166), including that of newborns (202), unless the skin is damaged, abraded, or otherwise compromised (161). The use of boric acid as a dusting power during diapering has resulted in fatalities (215). The Cosmetic Ingredient Review Expert Panel (72) reviewed the use of borates in cosmetics and concluded that "cosmetic formulations containing free sodium borate or boric acid at this concentration (5%) should not be used on infant or injured skin". Animal experiments indicate that chronic oral exposure to boric acid or borax is toxic to the male reproductive system, with testicular lesions being observed in rats, dogs, and mice (181,422,609), and boric acid is a developmental toxicant in all three mammalian species tested (rat, mouse, rabbit) (251,469,470). The rat was the most sensitive species for developmental effects, with a NOAEL of 9.6 mg B/kg/day (469). The effect of boron on male fertility has been investigated indirectly in an occupationally exposed population using a questionnaire to determine the standardized birth ratio (SBR; ratio of the observed number of births to the expected); no adverse reproductive effects were reported (617).

The U.S. EPA has derived a chronic oral RfD for boron (589) using the study of Weir and Fisher where dogs were exposed to boric acid in the diet for 2 years (609) as the pivotal study. Testicular atrophy occurred at a dose of 29 mg/kg/day, whereas no effects were noted at 8.8 mg/kg/day. This NOAEL was converted to an RfD of 90 μg/kg/day using an uncertainty factor of 100 (a factor of 10 each for both inter- and intraspecies variation); confidence in this RfD was considered medium. Other risk assessments of boron (411,616) considered the 1972 Weir and Fisher dog study (609), which predated Good Laboratory Practices, to be of insufficient power and design for use as a pivotal study, using instead the rat developmental study of Price et al. (469), where decreased fetal body weight occurred in a dose-dependent manner. No inhalation RfC has been derived for boron. The ACGIH has adopted several TLV values for boron compounds: TWA values of 10 mg/m^3 for boron oxide, 5 mg/m^3 for sodium tetraborate decahydrate, and 1 mg/m^3 for sodium tetraborate pentahydrate and anhydrous, and ceiling values of 1 ppm for boron tribromide and boron trifluoride (32). NTP conducted a 2-year carcinogenesis biosassay in male and female $B6C3F_1$ mice and reported testicular atrophy and interstitial-cell hyperplasia in males receiving 201 mg B/kg/day, but found no evidence of carcinogenicity (422). The U.S. EPA has not evaluated the potential human carcinogenicity of boron, but classifies it as group D (not classifiable as to human carcinogenicity) (589) based on lifetime studies conducted in mice (422) and rats (609).

Nickel

Nickel is member of the Group VIIB series of transition metals. There are three principal classes of nickel ores: sulfide, silicate, and arsenide. Nickel is used in a wide variety of applications, with 80% of the nickel in the United States being used in the production of nickel metal and alloys (63). The essentiality of nickel in humans is debatable. Nickel deficiency can be experimentally induced in rats and larger mammals (38,420). There is some evidence that nickel is essential for methyl metabolism and iron, calcium, and zinc absorption (38,457), but that if essential, the amount of nickel required would be amply met by the amount of nickel in a typical American diet (457).

Animal experiments have indicated that nickel compounds can be nephrotoxic, hepatotoxic, immunotoxic, and teratogenic (546). In humans, nickel can cause allergic contact dermatitis, particularly in young women using nickel-containing earrings in pierced ears (97), and is the most frequent disease among nickel workers. Statistical evaluations showed that up to 17% of all occupational allergies may be related to nickel occupational exposure (63). Allergic asthma is rare (430), but case reports have been published (63). Acute inhalation exposure to metallic nickel can cause metal fume fever (430). Nickel carbonyl is a colorless, volatile liquid that is particularly hazardous. It has been estimated that exposure to 30 ppm nickel carbonyl for 30 min may be lethal in humans (33). Acute inhalation exposure to this material can cause immediate and delayed toxic effects. Headache, dizziness, and nausea are the immediate manifestations. Ten to 36 h after exposure, substernal pain, coughing, and dyspnea, consistent with chemical pneumonitis, are observed (31,63). Sodium diethyldithiocarbamate (dithiocarb—a chelating agent) has been employed in the therapy of nickel carbonyl-exposed workers (33). Recovery is protracted and is characterized by fatigue upon slight exertion (63). Short-term exposure to 150 ppb $Ni(CO)_4$ can cause immediate but not delayed symptoms, whereas short-term exposure to concentrations on the order of a few parts per million can cause the more severe, delayed-type reactions (63). The U.S. EPA has derived a chronic oral RfD for soluble salts of nickel of 20 μg/kg/day. Neither oral nor inhalation

RfDs have been established for nickel subsulfide, nickel refinery dust, nor nickel carbonyl (589).

Inhalation of nickel compounds can cause lung cancer. The initial observation of excessive lung cancer and nasal tumors among nickel refinery workers was made as early as 1932 (63,404). Since the initial observation, numerous epidemiologic studies have been conducted that show conclusively the association between occupational exposure to nickel refinery dust and nickel subsulfide and lung and nasal cancer (63). The latency period for nickel-induced lung cancer was 13 to 14 years and that for nasal cancer was 15 to 24 years after first employment (31). Nickel exposure has not been clearly associated with respiratory cancer in any of the industries using nickel (31). The U.S. EPA has classified nickel subsulfide and nickel refinery dust as group A carcinogens (human carcinogen) on the basis of animal and epidemiologic carcinogenicity data; nickel carbonyl has been classified as a group B2 carcinogen (probable human carcinogen) (589). IARC has classified nickel compounds as carcinogenic to humans (280). The National Toxicology Program published results on the carcinogenicity of inhaled nickel oxide (424), nickel subsulfide (425), and nickel sulfate hexahydrate (426) in rats and mice. There was no evidence of carcinogenicity of nickel sulfate hexahydrate in either species, clear evidence of carcinogenicity of nickel subsulfide in both species, and either no, equivocal, or some evidence of carcinogenicity of nickel oxide, depending on species and sex. The ACGIH has adopted the following TLVs for nickel compounds: elemental/metal, 1.5 mg/m^3; soluble compounds, 0.1 mg/m^3; insoluble compounds, 0.2 mg/m^3; nickel carbonyl, 0.05 ppm; nickel subsulfide, 0.1 mg/m^3 (32).

Silver

Alloys of silver are used in jewelry, tableware, photographic materials, electronics, dental products, and as topical antibacterial agents for the treatment of burn wounds (63,266). Silver is generally low in toxicity. It is absorbed following inhalation, ingestion, or topical application (31). Accumulation of silver results in argyria, a blue-gray discoloration of the skin, mucous membranes, and eyes. Silver sulfadiazine used in the management of burn wound sepsis has resulted in argyria, ocular injury, leukopenia, and toxicity in kidney, liver, and neurological tissues. Silver may affect the immune system, and contact dermatitis has been observed following exposure to various silver compounds (7). Toxicity has been attributed to the free silver ion released into solution and interaction with sulfhydryl, amino, carboxyl, and other groups on membrane or enzyme proteins (266). Excretion from oral, respiratory, or topical exposure is primarily through the GI tract (7). Mucociliary escalator activity accounts for removal of silver following respiratory exposure. Silver is not considered to be a carcinogen or a reproductive or developmental toxicant (7,589). The U.S. EPA has derived a chronic oral RfD for silver of 5 μg/kg/day (589). No inhalation RfC has been derived for silver. The ACGIH has adopted TLV-TWA values for silver of 0.1 mg Ag/m^3 for the metal and 0.01 mg Ag/m^3 for soluble compounds (32). The ionic form is highly toxic to fish, but is found at extremely low concentrations in the aquatic environment, and other more common forms of silver show only low to moderate toxicity (265).

Strontium

Radiotoxicity is beyond the scope of this chapter and the following discussion pertains to stable strontium. Strontium is a soft silvery metal that turns yellow upon formation of the oxide (63). Its salts are used in the manufacture of color television screens, pyrotechnics (metal and salts impart a characteristic red color to flames), and electrical materials (586). Over 99% of the typical body burden of 320 mg is found in bone, and there is no conclusive evidence it is an essential trace element in mammals (63). Epidemiologic data suggest drinking water containing strontium in the presence of fluoride (5–6 mg Sr2+ and 1 mg F^-/L) decreases the incidence of dental caries in children (143). The gastrointestinal absorption of the strontium ion is poor (586) and acute strontium toxicity is low, with an oral LD_{50} of 2250 mg/kg body weight reported for strontium chloride in rats (99). Acute lethality is due to respiratory failure (132). In contrast, bone is the target organ following chronic strontium exposure. High doses inhibit calcification of the epiphyseal cartilage and cause deformities of long bones (533). Strontium causes these effects by substituting for calcium in the hydroxyapatite crystal during calcification or displacing calcium from existing calcified bone. The metabolic basis of strontium's effect on calcium metabolism is thought to be inhibition of the renal synthesis of 1,25-dihydroxyvitamin D_3 (447). Young animals (still growing) are more susceptible to the toxic effects of strontium than adults, with widening of the epiphyseal cartilage being observed at lower levels of dietary strontium (545). Dietary calcium plays a protective role in strontium toxicity. Weanling rats maintained on diets containing 950 mg Sr/kg and 0.69% calcium for 4 weeks exhibited rachitic changes that were not seen in rats supplemented with 1.6% calcium (174). In contrast to these toxic effects, pharmacologic treatment with low doses of strontium suppresses bone resorption (372), and low-dose strontium lactate has been used to treat osteoporosis (383). The U.S. EPA has derived an oral RfD for strontium of 0.6 mg/kg/day, and confidence in this value is medium (589). Stable strontium has not been adequately evaluated for carcinogenic potential.

Thallium

Thallium is a soft bluish-white metal, widely but sparingly distributed in the earth (63). Historically it has been used to treat gout, venereal disease, dysentery, ringworm, and tuberculosis (115). Thallium sulfate was widely used as a rodenticide, but its use was banned in the United States in 1972 (63). It is still used as a rodenticide in other parts of the world, and rodent resistance to warfarin may cause this use to increase (301). Thallium intoxication from contaminated heroin, presumably imported from areas where thallium is still used as a rodenticide, has been reported (472). It is currently used in the electronics industry and in the manufacture of prisms, imitation jewelry, low-temperature thermometers, and infrared spectrometers. Thallium is well absorbed following oral ingestion and causes severe gastrointestinal symptoms followed by painful paresthesia of the extremities, motor paralysis, and death from respiratory failure (255,316,366,393,409). Individuals surviving the acute phase suffer characteristic scalp alopecia about 10 days postingestion (255,409,592). For an adult the LD_{50} has been calculated to be 8 to 12 mg Tl/kg (409). Treatment involves the use of activated charcoal and oral Prussian blue (ferric ferrocyanide, C.I. 77510), which prevents enterohepatic recirculation and enhances fecal elimination, hemodialysis, and forced diuresis (316,391,409,592). The FDA has yet to approve the human use of Prussian blue (391,409), making suitably pure material difficult to obtain, although it is used as a diagnostic agent in pathology laboratories. The effectiveness of Prussian blue in thallotoxicosis is dependent on the size of the crystal lattice (325). Chelating agents (dithiocarb) have caused a redistribution of thallium to target organs, with an increase in toxicity (172,295). The precise mechanism of toxicity is unknown, but likely involves the substitution of the thallous ion for potassium in the sodium/potassium ATPase pump and/or interference with sulfhydryl enzymes (409). Interference with tissue riboflavin with subsequent effects on metabolic pathways has also been suggested (103). The U.S. EPA has derived a chronic oral RfD for thallium based on its own 90-day study of rats exposed to aqueous thallium sulfate by gavage at doses up to 0.20 mg Tl/kg/day (589). Treatment-related effects of serum chemistry changes, alopecia, and lacrimation without histopathological changes were not considered adverse, and 0.2 mg/kg/day was considered the NOAEL (589). This NOAEL was converted to an RfD of 0.09 μg/kg/day using an uncertainty factor of 3000 (10 for intraspecies extrapolation, 10 for interspecies variation, 10 for less than chronic exposure duration, and 3 for lack of reproductive and chronic toxicity data). Confidence in the RfD was considered low. No inhalation RfC has been derived for thallium. The ACGIH has adopted a TLV-TWA of 0.1 mg Tl/m^3 for elemental and soluble thallium compounds (32). Thallium is classified as group D (not classifiable as to human carcinogenicity), based on two inadequate negative studies in humans and a lack of animal studies designed to examine carcinogenic endpoints (589). Existing data do not indicate thallium is mutagenic (343).

Uranium

Uranium is a soft, malleable metal of the actinide series in the periodic table. The primary uranium ores are pitchblende (uranium oxide) and carnotite (uranium/vanadium-containing mineral). Uranium is primarily used as nuclear fuel, but there are some minor uses, such as a colorant in ceramics or glass, or in armor-piercing projectiles (31). Occupational exposure occurs in mining operations and in uranium enrichment (uranium hexafluoride).

Acute inhalation exposure to uranium hexafluoride can cause pneumonitis, but the injury may be caused by the fluoride rather than the uranium itself (430). Chronic inhalation exposure of uranium dioxide dust at concentration of 5 mg U/m^3 produced no observable adverse effects in rats, dogs, or monkeys (339). The kidney is the main target of uranium's chemical toxicity, with the targets being the pars recta of the proximal tubules, the ascending limb of the loop of Henle, and collecting tubules (31). Attempts have been made to define a "critical concentration" of uranium in the kidney that constitutes a threshold for renal damage (197). Experimental evidence clearly indicates that the "consensus value" of 3 μg/g is above the level shown to produce toxic effects by a factor of 5–10; however, studies of workers exposed to uranium at levels derived from this consensus value have shown no evidence of chemical toxicity (197). This may reflect differences between animal and human metabolism (e.g., binding of uranium to metallothionein or other detoxifying proteins) or differences between the route and duration of the animal and human exposures. The U.S. EPA developed a chronic RfD of soluble salts of uranium of 3 μg U/kg/day; no inhalation RfC has been derived for uranium (589).

Uranium isotopes are radioactive, but only weakly due to their extremely long half-lives. Natural uranium has a radioactivity of about 0.7 pCi/μg (585). No direct evidence exists that uranium is carcinogenic to humans or animals. However, based on the fact that uranium does emit ionizing radiation as it decays, the U.S. EPA has classified uranium as a group A carcinogen (known human carcinogen) and has proposed to quantify the cancer risk of uranium in drinking water using toxicokinetic modeling (585).

Vanadium

Vanadium is a white to gray common trace metal that does not occur in nature but occurs in combination with oxygen, sodium, sulfur, and chloride. Vanadium deficiency can occur in laboratory animals on a very strict diet (39,420), and there is evidence that vanadium helps regulate some phosphoryl transfer enzymes (457). A requirement for vanadium extrapolated from animal experiments is 10–25 μg/day, whereas typical intake is 8–18 μg/day (457); however, the National Research Council believes that there is only weak evidence that vanadium is essential and that any vanadium requirement would be met by naturally occurring levels (420).

Inhalation exposure to vanadium pentoxide can cause tracheobronchitis with persistent bronchial hyperreactivity and inflammation (14,31,430). A greenish-black discoloration of the tongue, gastrointestinal symptoms, neurotoxicity, and renal toxicity have also been reported in workers exposed to vanadium pentoxide. The short term repeated inhalation in rats of vanadium metavanadate (8 h/day for 4 days) at a concentration encountered by humans over a typical work week altered pulmonary immune cell function and produced significant changes in the lungs themselves (131). Oral exposure to vanadium can be toxic to the gastrointestinal, renal, and neurological systems. Vanadium is rapidly excreted in feces and urine following termination of exposure. The U.S. EPA has derived a chronic oral RfD for vanadium pentoxide of 5 μg V/kg/day (9 μg VO_5/kg/day), which was derived using an uncertainty factor of 100 (10 for interindividual variation and 10 for interspecies variation); confidence in this RfD was considered low (589). The U.S. EPA has not derived an inhalation RfC for vanadium compounds. The ACGIH has adopted TLV-TWA values for vanadium of 1 mg/m^3 for ferrovanadium dust and 0.05 mg/m^3 for vanadium pentoxide (32).

The results of behavior testing show that oral sodium metavanadate in rats resulted in significant reductions in both general activity and learning (498). Mice given vanadyl sulfate in drinking water at doses up to 1 mg/kg/day for up to 33 months had no significant increase in tumor incidence (296,505). The U.S. EPA has not evaluated the potential human carcinogenicity of vanadium (589).

Table 14.3 presents the quantitative toxicity values derived by the U.S. EPA for the metals listed in this

Table 14.3
Minor toxic metals with RfDs

	Chronic oral toxicity		Chronic inhalation toxicity		Carcinogenicity		
Metal	RfD[a] (mg/kg/day)	Confidence	RfC[b] (μg/m^3)	Confidence	Oral slope factor [risk/(mg/kg/day)]	Inhalation slope factor [risk/(μg/m^3)]	Classification
Boron	9×10^{-2}	Medium	—	—	—	—	—
Barium	7×10^{-2}	Medium	—	—	—	—	D
Nickel	2×10^{-2}	Medium	—	—	—	2.4×10^{-4}	A
Ni refinery dust					—	4.8×10^{-4}	A
Ni_3S_2					—		B2
$Ni(CO)_4$					—	—	—
Soluble Ni							
Vanadium	9×10^{-3}	Low	—	—	—	—	—
Silver	5×10^{-3}	Low	—	—	—	—	D
Beryllium	2×10^{-3}	Low–medium	2×10^{-2}	Medium	—	2.4×10^{-3}	B1
Uranium	3×10^{-3}	Medium	—	—	—	—	A
Antimony	4×10^{-4}	Low	—	—	—	—	—
Thallium	9×10^{-5}	Low	—	—	—	—	D

[a] RfD, reference dose.
[b] RfC, reference concentration.
[c] Group A, known human carcinogen; group B1, probable human carcinogen; group D, not classifiable as to human carcinogenicity.

section, with metals listed in reverse order of toxicity (least to most toxic).

MINOR TOXIC METALS WITHOUT RfDs

Aluminum

Aluminum is the third most abundant element in the earth's crust, and is extracted from bauxite ore. Although aluminum is not an essential element, humans consume a substantial amount in the diet and are exposed to aluminum from a number of nondietary sources. On average, American adults consume 2 to 25 mg Al daily from food and beverages (230), with average amounts being 8.2 mg/day for males and 7.1 mg/day for females (458). Aluminum is naturally present at low levels in most foods, but the primary source of dietary aluminum is from food additives. Over-the-counter antacids contain large amounts of aluminum hydroxide, and millions of consumers are dermally exposed to aluminum salts from the use of antiperspirants and deodorants (230).

Aluminum is generally considered to have a low order of toxicity, but it can cause reproductive toxicity when administered in high doses to experimental animals (218). The potential role of aluminum in either causing Alzheimer's disease or speeding its progression is highly controversial. Aluminum is certainly neurotoxic. In renal dialysis patients, excessive parenteral exposure to aluminum can cause a progressive, fatal neurological syndrome known as dialysis dementia (26). In addition, injection of aluminum salts into the brain of rabbits leads to the development of neurofibrillary tangles, but not β-amyloid plaques, which are also indicators of Alzheimer's disease (317). Some studies have found elevated levels of aluminum in some regions of the brain (327,564,606,622,626), whereas others have found no difference in aluminum levels between Alzheimer's and control brain tissue (286,373,565).

Epidemiologic studies do not show an association between aluminum exposure and the incidence of Alzheimer's disease. Canadian miners, between 1944 and 1979, were exposed to high concentrations of aluminum and aluminum oxide powder (McIntyre Powder) preceeding each shift as a prophylactic treatment against silicotic lung disease. In an initial study of this population, there was no increased incidence of neurological disorders in exposed miners, but there was an increase in neurological impairment as measured by cognitive testing (478). A follow-up study was conducted to address several methodological weaknesses in the initial study. No statistically significant differences were noted between exposed and nonexposed miners in either neurological disease or cognitive impairment incidence (477). Similarly, an association was noted with aluminum in drinking water and the incidence of Alzhemier's disease (376). A follow-up study (with methodological improvements) found no evidence of such an association (375). Another recent study has shown no association between occupational exposure to aluminium and the incidence of Alzheimer's disease (226).

The ACGIH has adopted TLV-TWA values for aluminum of 10 mg Al/m^3 for metal dust and aluminium oxide, 5 mg Al/m^3 for pyro powders and welding fumes, and 2 mg Al/m^3 for soluble salts and alkyls (32).

Bismuth

Elemental bismuth is a soft lustrous metal and can occur naturally or in combined forms in ores. Bismuth is used in low-melting alloys. Insoluble bismuth salts are poorly absorbed orally or dermally. Excretion is primarily through the GI tract. Bismuth compounds demonstrate a low order of toxicity (63). They are used as coloring agents in cosmetics, and in pharmaceuticals, including use for diarrhea, gastroesophageal reflux, and in ulcer therapy. Bismuth subsalicylate used in ulcer therapy has no substantial capacity to neutralize gastric acid, but rather provides cytoprotection involving enhanced secretion of mucous and HCO_3^-, inhibition of pepsin activity, and the formation of bismuth protein complexes that may afford a protective barrier against peptic digestion. Primary activity may be due to the antibacterial effect of bismuth compounds against the bacteria *H. pylori* in the gastrointestinal mucosa (90). Toxic bismuth levels are not reached with normal use, although salicylism has been reported following use of bismuth subsalicylate (597). Rats exposed to bismuth oxychloride in the diet for 2 years at doses up to 2.0 mg/kg/day were found to have no increased incidence of tumors (468). The ACGIH has adopted a TLV-TWA value for bismuth telluride of 10 mg/m^3 (32).

Bromine

Bromine is a reddish-brown, noncombustible liquid. Although the earth's crust contains a vast amount of bromine, the most readily recoverable sources of bromine are in salt lakes and brines. The largest use of bromine is in the production of fire retardants, gasoline antiknock agents, and in the agricultural chemical industry (460). Bromine vapors are highly toxic; exposure to 1000 ppm bromine is rapidly fatal in humans, and exposure to 40–60 ppm is dangerous for brief exposures (460). The symptoms of inhalation exposure include coughing, nosebleed, dizziness and headache, and abdominal pain and diarrhea; sometimes a measles-like eruption on the trunk and extremities can occur (460). Bromine vapor is extremely irritating to the eyes, skin, and mucous membranes and produces inflammatory lesions in the upper respiratory tract (25). Prolonged contact with the skin causes ulceration (460).

Bromine may be an essential element. A bromine-deficient diet impaired the growth and reproductive success of goats; however, the evidence for the essentiality of bromine is weak, and no cases of human deficiency are likely to occur, due to the widespread distribution of bromine in foods (37).

Excessive oral intake of bromide can cause neurological symptoms in humans (headache, lethargy, ataxia, disorientation, etc.), and high levels of bromine in the diet (400–1200 mg/kg) can cause CNS depression in mice (543). Potassium bromate is a widely used form of bromine. Its primary use is as a conditioner for flour and dough (460). Potassium bromate has been investigated for possible carcinogenic activity. Renal and other tumors were induced in male and female Fischer 344 rats exposed to potassium bromate in drinking water in a 2-year bioassay; tumor formation was dose dependent (279). The IARC has classified potassium bromate as a group 2B (possibly carcinogenic to humans) carcinogen. Conversely, mice and rats fed diets high in bread containing up to 75 mg/kg potassium bromate showed no increase in tumor incidence (191,210). The lack of a carcinogenic effect could be attributable to the degradation of potassium bromate during the baking process (279).

The ACGIH has adopted TLV values for bromine gas of 0.1 ppm as an 8-h TWA and 0.2 ppm as a STEL/C (32). Although the U.S. EPA has established a number of toxicity values for bromine-containing compounds, the U.S. EPA has not derived any toxicity values for bromine (589).

Cerium

Cerium is a lanthanous rare earth metal and is used in fireworks and cigarette lighter flints, self-cleaning ovens, and as an abrasive for polishing glass (63). Occupational inhalation exposure has been reported to cause a pneumoconiosis without pulmonary functional impairment (275). Intravenous administration of cerium chloride produces severe hepatotoxicity in rats (414). The U.S. EPA has not derived toxicity values for cerium (589).

Gallium

Gallium is a relatively rare metal that has found uses in diagnostic radiology (63), as an antineoplastic agent (82), and for the control of cancer-related hypercalcemia (157,607). It is used in the manufacture of alloys and semiconductor electronic devices. There are limited indications of occupationally related toxicity. Occupational exposure to GaF_3 fumes resulted in a rash with subsequent reversible neurological effects consisting of muscular weakness (63). Gallium is excreted in urine. Renal toxicity is noted in rats with the formation of precipitates of gallium complexed with calcium and phosphate (63). No adverse effects were noted in a reproduction study conducted in male mice (134). There are no occupational health standards for gallium or its compounds (63). The U.S. EPA has not derived toxicity values for gallium.

Germanium

Germanium is a Group IVA semiconducting metal. The pure metal has a metallic appearance, but is very brittle, much like glass. Germanium is not found in the free state, but always in combination with other elements, such as silver, copper, and arsenic. Germanium is used in the semiconductor industry (germanium was used in the first transistor), and it is often used in combination with other materials, such as arsenic and antimony, and alloyed with aluminum, gallium, and indium. It is also used in certain optic applications, as the pure metal is transparent to infrared radiation. Industrial exposures are to the dusts and fumes of germanium metal during extraction from ore and metal fumes from welding operations (63). Germanium oxide and germanium sesquioxide have been used in "elixirs" for the treatment of cancer and AIDS (552).

In longer term oral animal studies, germanium and germanium oxide have been shown to be nephrotoxic (497), neurotoxic (309,377), and myotoxic (377). The potential for germanium to induce lung injury is unclear; in one 4-week inhalation toxicity study of germanium powder in rats, histopathologic changes consistent with pulmonary toxicity were present (43), but a follow-up study using germanium dioxide showed no treatment-related histopathologic effects (44). Germanium does not appear to be carcinogenic; in fact, certain germanium compounds appear to have antineoplastic activity (206). In a lifetime feeding study in rats, animals receiving 5 ppm sodium germanate in water had a significantly lower incident of tumors than the control animals (297).

Because of this anticancer activity, germanium-containing elixirs have been sold, first in Japan, and then in other countries as a treatment for cancer and other diseases. To date, there have been at least 31 reported cases of toxicity associated with oral intake of germanium compounds, of which 9 were fatal (552). Nephrotoxicity is the primary manifestation of germanium intoxication, although neurotoxicity and myotoxicity have been reported (548,552).

No TLV has been set for germanium or germanium oxide, but a TLV-TWA of 0.2 ppm has been set for germanium tetrahydride (32).

Gold

Gold is a soft yellowish metal and belongs to Group IB of the periodic table. Its excellent heat and electrical conductivity and malleability have made it important in industrial applications (62). Medically, it is used either orally or by intramuscular injection to slow the progression of rheumatoid arthritis, but treatment is associated with a high incidence of toxicity (277). Adverse skin and mucous membrane effects (dermatitis, stomatitis, pruritus) are most frequent, with incidence and severity less for oral as opposed to parenteral treatment (563). A mild proteinuria is the most common renal effect, but gold-induced nephrosis may occur. Aplastic anemia is relatively rare and has been associated with poor prognosis (623), which may improve with bone marrow transplantation (293). Although traditionally regarded as inert, gold is being recognized as a common contact allergen (268). In Sweden it is second only to nickel (91), and results from the North American Contact Dermatitis Group rank it among the 10 most common allergens in the United States (386). Gold hypersensitivity is characterized by late reactions, and failure to monitor the test site for a minimum of 3 weeks may result in false negatives. The U.S. EPA has not derived toxicity values for gold (589).

Hafnium

Hafnium is a gray metallic element having a silverlike luster and is found in association with zirconium ores (31,171). It has outstanding corrosion resistance and is used for this characteristic in atomic reactors, in electronic components, and in alloys. Hafnium compounds show moderate toxicity in acute animal tests by several routes of administration (239). Studies indicate concentration in the liver and skeleton. Hafnium is poorly absorbed orally (313) and the dust is considered to have relatively low toxicity. Workers exposed to 150 mg/m^3 of hafnium- and zirconium-containing dusts showed no adverse effects after 2–6 years (165). The ACGIH has adopted a TLV-TWA value for hafnium of 0.5 mg/m^3 (32).

Indium

Indium is a Group IIIA metal that is widely distributed in the earth's crust. It is not found in the free state, but most commonly in association with copper, zinc, and sulfur. Indium is used in surface protection of metals, and in many alloys because of its ability to increase hardness. Indium compounds are also used in the photovoltaic and semiconductor industry. Industrial exposures to indium occur during extraction and purification, and in plating and the manufacture of certain electronic instruments (63). Absorption of indium compounds is highly dependent on form; insoluble indium compounds are poorly absorbed and distributed, whereas soluble compounds, such as $InCl_3$ and $In_2(SO_4)_3$, are rapidly absorbed and distributed (63,628). Consistent with these findings, soluble indium compounds are also more toxic than their insoluble counterparts. The acute lethal dose range for the soluble compound indium chloride in rabbits, rats, and dogs was 0.33 to 3.6 mg/kg (160), whereas the minimum lethal dose for insoluble indium oxide in rats was 955 mg/kg (3), and the oral and intraperitoneal LD_{50} for insoluble indium phosphide was greater than 5 g/kg (294).

Indium compounds are toxic when inhaled. Copper indium diselenide and indium trichloride, when acutely administered intratracheally to rats at high doses (higher than would be expected in an industrial exposure), induced a persistent inflammatory response (78,402). Copper indium diselenide was only slightly fibrogenic to the lung, and this corresponds with the limited solubility of this compound (403). Subchronic inhalation of indium sesquioxide in rats induced a persistent inflammatory response; no fibrosis was noted (31). Hamsters were treated once per week for 15 weeks with either indium arsenide or indium phosphide (dose = 7.5 mg arsenic or phosphorus) by intratracheal installation and were examined at the end of their lifespan. Adverse histopathologic findings were significantly higher in the treated groups (551).

Several studies have investigated the reproductive and developmental toxicity of indium compounds. Indium arsenide, administered intratracheally, reduced epididymal sperm counts in rats (449) but not hamsters (448); intratracheal instillation of indium chloride in mice did not affect reproductive performance of either males or females, but it was fetotoxic (116).

The ACGIH TLV-TWA for indium and its compounds is 0.1 mg In/m^3 (32).

Lithium

Lithium is a silvery-white metal and the lightest solid element. Although it is used in batteries, organic synthesis (Grignard reagent), the space industry, as a swimming pool sanitizer, and in air conditioners, industrial intoxication has not been reported (344). Lithium hydride in contact with water releases hydrogen gas (flammable), and it must be stored under air-tight anhydrous conditions (63). Inhalation exposure to lithium hydride can cause pulmonary edema, but the hydride rather than the lithium is likely responsible (430). The ACGIH has adopted a TLV-TWA value for lithium hydride of 0.025 mg/m^3 (32). Oral lithium salts are widely used in the treatment of manic-depressive disorders, but frequent individual monitoring of serum concentrations is required because of the narrow therapeutic index (232,371). The same levels of lithium are devoid of psychotropic effects in individuals not suffering manic-depressive disorders (371). Effective treatment generally requires levels between 0.8 and 1.2 mEq/L, and toxic effects have been seen at serum levels above 1.5 mEq/L. Signs of lithium toxicity are primarily neurologic and range from fine tremors and muscle weakness in mild cases, to dysarthria, hyperreflexia, coma, and collapse. Lithium therapy may produce lasting neurologic consequences (231). Lithium has properties similar to sodium, and substitution for body cations (sodium, potassium) may account for these effects (592). There is no specific antidote. Renal symptoms of intoxication include polyuria, polydipsia, and renal failure (445). Lithium therapy during pregnancy has been associated with an increase risk of cardiac anomalies, and there are sufficient animal and human data to indicate lithium can cause developmental toxicity (399). The U.S. EPA has not derived toxicity values for lithium (589).

Niobium

Niobium is a white, soft metal found in ores in combination with tantalum and other elements (63). Niobium is used in alloys and may find use in surgical implants and dental applications (63,69,518). Organometallic niobium compounds have shown antitumor and anti-HIV activity in vitro and in mice (321,322,507). Acute and chronic animal tests have been conducted on several niobium compounds (238,307,508). Niobium is poorly absorbed from the GI tract. Parenteral administration of niobium pentachloride results in decreased respiration, lethargy, and death. The compound is a moderate to severe skin irritant, with less irritation noted in rabbit eyes. Life-term studies of sodium niobate in mice and rats did not show carcinogenicity (297). Occupational or general health standards have not been established for niobium in the United States. No reports of occupational health hazards from dust or fumes associated with forging or other fabrication techniques of niobium metal and alloys have been reported (63).

Osmium

Osmium is a platinum-group metal. Osmium tetroxide is a noncombustible, colorless to pale yellow solid, with a disagreeable chlorine-like odor. Osmium tetroxide is apparently formed quite readily from finely divided osmium metal by heating in air, or even at room temperature (242). Osmium is found in combination with platinum and nickel-bearing ores. The major use of osmium is as osmium tetroxide, which is used as a biological stain for adipose tissues (31).

Metallic osmium and most of its other compounds are not considered highly toxic (31); however, osmium tetroxide has been shown to be toxic in animals and in man. The oral LD_{50} for osmium tetroxide has been reported to be 14 mg/kg in the rat and 162 mg/kg in the mouse; the intraperitoneal LD_{50} for the mouse was 14 mg/kg (63). The reported LC_{50} for the rat and mouse is 400 mg/m^3 (31). Additionally, rabbits exposed for 30 minutes to osmium tetroxide at a concentration of 130 mg/m^3 died after 4 days from pulmonary edema (89). Application of a drop of a 1% solution of osmium tetroxide to the rabbit eye caused severe corneal damage, permanent opacity, and superficial vascularization (89). Toxic effects have also been reported on guinea pig bone marrow, although the route of administration, dose, and duration were not reported (242).

Osmium tetroxide-induced toxicity in humans has been reported in the early toxicology literature. Inhalation exposure to OsO_4 can cause irritation of the nose and throat, which can persist for at least 12 h (242). Industrial exposure to osmium tetroxide concentrations ranging from 0.1 to 0.6 mg/m^3 induced lacrimation and disturbances in vision (i.e., the appearance of rings around lights). Other complaints included conjunctivitis, cough, and headache. Recovery usually occurred within a few days (387). One human fatality has been reported, resulting from inhalation of osmium tetroxide (387). The exposure concentration was not reported; death was attributed to capillary bronchitis and pulmonary edema.

The ACGIH has adopted a TLV-TWA of 0.0002 ppm and a STEL/C of 0.0006 ppm for osmium tetroxide, both measured as osmium (32).

Platinum

Although platinum is relatively rare, it is found both as the pure metal and in combination with nickel, copper, and gold (63). Platinum is used as a catalyst in the automotive, chemical, and pharmaceutical industries, and its nobility (resistance to oxidation) makes it important in the manufacture of laboratory equipment (481). Metallic platinum is relatively inert, but the complex salts are frequent sensitizers, producing conjunctivitis, urticaria, dermatitis, and eczema following inhalation and/or dermal exposure (212). A syndrome formerly known by the misnomer "platinosis" is characterized by lacrimation, sneezing, rhinorrhea, cough, dyspnea, bronchial asthma (from chloroplatinates), and cyanosis (212). This term suggests a pneumoconiosis and fibrosis, which are not a part of platinum allergy syndrome, and the condition is more accurately known as "allergy to platinum compounds containing reactive halogen ligands" (272). The mentioned symptoms are elicited by either an immediate (type I) or delayed (type II, within 24 h) hypersensitivity reaction (212). The platinum analogue cisplatin has been used as a chemotherapeutic agent against various cancers, especially testicular and ovarian tumors, despite nephrotoxicity at therapeutic doses (212). More recently, carboplatin has been used with comparable efficacy (for many types of cancer) and less toxicity, with thrombocytopenia being the major side effect (212,356). The ACGIH has adopted TLV-TWA values of 1 mg/m^3 for platinum metal and 0.002 mg/m^3 for soluble salts (32). The TLV for platinum salts protects against sensitization, but does not offer protection to a previously sensitized individual. No increased risk of cancer has been reported from occupational exposure to platinum (212). The U.S. EPA has not evaluated the toxicity of platinum (589).

Rhodium

Rhodium is a silver-white, hard metal that can form highly corrosive resistant alloys and coatings used in electrical contacts, reflectors, and jewelry (31,212). Unlike the related platinum compounds, rhodium compounds have not been found to be clinically active in cancer therapy. Antimalarial activity is reported for a rhodium–chloroquine complex (499). Only a limited toxicity profile has been developed for rhodium and its compounds. Intravenously administered rhodium trichloride was moderately low in acute toxicity in rats and rabbits (~200 mg/kg), with death possibly due to central nervous system depression (333). Oral rhodium trichloride was low in toxicity (LD_{50}>500 mg/kg) (212). A chronic feeding study showed slight carcinogenic activity in mice (504). Rhodium has been reported to cause allergic contact urticaria (189). The ACGIH has adopted a TLV-TWA of 1 mg Rh/m^3 for elemental and insoluble compounds, and 0.01 mg Rh/m^3 for soluble rhodium compounds, concurrent with the determination that elemental and rhodium compounds are not classifiable as human carcinogens (31,32). The OSHA PEL values for elemental, insoluble, and soluble rhodium compounds are one-tenth these levels (31).

Tantalum

Tantalum is a gray, hard metal found in ores in combination with niobium and other metals. It is used in electric capacitors, as the carbide for tools, and has found a wide range of use in medical diagnostic and surgical implant applications (31,63,75). Elemental tantalum and its principal oxide are essentially nontoxic in vitro and in vivo. Occupational exposure to tantalum and its oxide has shown no overt adverse health effects (31). Medical uses include tantalum gauze in the repair of hernias, implant plates and screws, and radiographic lung and bone markers (75). The TLV-TWA for tantalum metal and oxide as dust is 5 mg Ta/m^3 (32).

Tellurium

Tellurium is placed in Group IVA of the periodic table. Tellurium has a number of industrial uses and is also found in a variety of food products (e.g., condiments, dairy products, nuts, fish) in high concentration. Pneumonitis and hemolytic anemia are prominent features of acute tellurium intoxication (29). Tellurium hydride has been shown to be highly toxic, causing pulmonary irritation and intravascular hemolysis (608). Acute oral or parenteral tellurium intoxication resulted in numerous symptoms, with hematuria noted in all animals treated (29,388). Weanling rats fed 1% tellurium in the diet developed a peripheral neuropathy characterized by a transient demyelinating/remyelinating event (67,332).

There have been no reports of serious illness or death in workers exposed to tellurium and its compounds. However, absorbed tellurium is slowly metabolized to dimethyl telluride and is excreted in urine, sweat, and breath (149). It is dimethyl telluride that is responsible for the "garlic breath" that is associated with tellurium exposure (336). Two fatalities occurred after unintentional treatment with 2 g sodium tellurite by ureteral catheter (302). Autopsy revealed acute fatty degeneration and edema of the liver. The ACGIH has adopted a TLV-TWA value of 0.1 mg Te/m^3 for tellurium and compounds (32).

Tin

Tin is a soft, white metal that occurs in combination with other chemicals (e.g., chlorine, oxygen) (8). It is alloyed with other metals to make pewter, solder, bronze, and a special cast bronze termed bell metal (up to 24% tin), which is noted for its tonal quality (63). Most of the tin used in the United States is for plating steel cans. The fluoride is used in toothpaste, and the chloride is used to make frost-free windshields (500). Organotins function as antimicrobials in agriculture and industry, as stabilizers in polyvinyl chloride (PVC) plastics, and as marine antifouling agents (63). Although Schwarz et al. (514) in 1970 reported a significant growth effect of dietary tin in weanling rats maintained on purified diets, this has not since been independently confirmed and tin is not considered to be essential. Inorganic tin compounds are poorly absorbed from the gastrointestinal tract [i.e., rats dosed orally absorbed 2.8% of Sn(II) and less than 1% of Sn(IV) (260)] and are therefore relatively nontoxic; acute oral LD_{50} for $SnCl^2$ in rats is

700 mg/kg (99), but after intravenous administration it is reported as 100 mg Sn/kg (517). Soluble salts of inorganic tin are gastric irritants producing nonspecific signs of nausea, vomiting, and diarrhea. Rats maintained on diets containing 0.3% or more as soluble inorganic tin salts (i.e., stannous chloride) experienced growth retardation and anemia (146). Injected stannous chloride is a potent inducer of rat renal microsomal heme oxygenase, enhancing heme breakdown (298). Diets supplemented with high levels of iron and copper protected rats from the anemia, but did not alleviate growth depression (145). Tin has adverse effects on the absorption and metabolism of the essential elements iron, copper, and zinc (145,146,229). In contrast, organotins, especially the trialkyl derivatives, are highly toxic [i.e., rat acute oral LD_{50} of 10 mg/kg (310)]. Triethyltin compounds are skin irritants and potent neurotoxins, producing a decrease in myelin content of the CNS and edema of the white matter (492). Uncoupling of oxidative phosphorylation has been proposed as the mechanism of action (401). Acute inhalation exposure to tin can cause metal fume fever and chronic exposure can cause a benign pneumoconiosis, stannosis (430). The ACGIH has adopted TLV-TWA values of 2 mg/m^3 for the inorganic compounds (except tin hydride, SnH^4) and a TLV-TWA of 0.1 mg/m^3 for organic tin compounds (32). Although the U.S. EPA has not evaluated tin and tin-containing compounds for carcinogenicity, the NTP has performed a 2-year bioassay for stannous chloride in rats and mice with negative results in all but male rats, where the results were equivocal for thyroid C-cell tumors (421).

Titanium

Titanium is a silver-gray metal that can occur naturally in several forms including titanium dioxide. Titanium is a component of several alloys, and is used in surgical implants where it is considered nontoxic (250). Titanium dioxide, the most common oxide of titanium, is extensively used as a white pigment in paints, plastics, inks, and cosmetics (63,209). Titanium dioxide is generally considered to be essentially nontoxic by the oral, dermal, and inhalation routes. A 2-year feeding study of titanium dioxide at maximum doses of 2.5 g/kg/day in rats and 6.4 g/kg/day in mice found no evidence of carcinogenicity (415), although the dose-response relationship was statistically significant for thyroid tumors in female rats and keratoacanthomas in male rats (214). Toxicity from the more prevalent respiratory exposure to titanium dioxide has been investigated. A 2-year inhalation study was conducted in rats with acceptable results at a level of 10 mg/m^3; high levels produced squamous-cell carcinomas, which are postulated to be the result of saturation of normal pulmonary clearance mechanisms (31,340). Epidemiological findings and related information do not conclusively support a relationship between occupational exposure to titanium dioxide and pulmonary fibrosis, cancer, or other adverse health effects (31). The ACGIH has adopted a TLV-TWA value of 10 mg/m^3 for titanium dioxide (32).

Tungsten

Tungsten is a member of the third series of transition metals and occurs in nature in combination with iron, manganese, and calcium. The major use of tungsten is in cutting and wear resistant materials (63). The bulk of inhaled tungsten oxide is rapidly excreted in dogs (1). Although exposure to soluble tungsten compounds can be toxic in experimental animals (311,531), insoluble tungsten compounds have a low order of toxicity (148,199,312,395). Male and female rats given sodium tungstenate in water for $2\frac{1}{2}$ years at doses of 0.25 and 0.29 mg/kg/day had no significant increase in tumor incidence (506).

Pulmonary fibrosis observed in men with inhalation exposure to cobalt-cemented tungsten carbide (394) has been attributed to cobalt (63). Evaluation of workers with long-term exposure to tungsten or its insoluble compounds showed no development of pneumoconioses (31).

The tungsten ion antagonized the normal metabolic action of the molybdate ion, and therefore can inhibit molybdate-dependent enzymes (259,290,441). The ACGIH has adopted TLV-TWA values of 5 mg W/m^3 for insoluble compounds and 1 mg W/m^3 for soluble compounds (32).

Yttrium

Yttrium has a silvery luster and is used primarily as the matrix producing the red color in television tubes (63). Yttrium chloride has been reported to cause granulomatous changes in the rat lung following intratracheal instillation (262), and the liver and spleen are reported to be the primary target organs following intravenous injection (263). Despite a long history of industrial use, there are no definitive reports of adverse effects in workers (63). The LD_{50} for yttrium chloride following intraperitoneal injection in rats is 132 mg Y/kg body weight (128). The U.S. EPA has not derived toxicity values for yttrium. The ACGIH had adopted a TLV-TWA value of 5 mg Y/m^3 but reduced this to 1 mg Y/m^3 (31,32) based on a report that yttrium inhalation caused severe lung damage (63).

Zirconium

Zirconium is a grayish-white element of the second series of transition metals. The metal is produced from two main sources of ore, zircon ($ZrO\ SiO_2$), and baddeleyite (ZrO_2); hafnium is always associated with zirconium (32). Zirconium is used for the cladding in nuclear fuel rods, and zirconium compounds are also used in foundry and sandblasting applications. Industrial exposure occurs during mining and purification operations, and in foundry and other industries. A significant percentage of the general population is exposed (dermally) to aluminum zirconium chlorohydrate complexes in commercially marketed antiperspirant products.

Zirconium oxide has a low order of toxicity via the inhalation route in animals (538); slight toxicity was noted in dogs when exposed to an airborne mist of zirconium chloride at 6 mg Zr/m^3 for 2 months. Zirconium oxide and zirconium chloride exposure at 3.5 mg Zr/m^3 for 1 year had no measurable adverse effect on the animals exposed (63). Similarly, in most studies of industrially exposed workers, no adverse effects have been associated with inhalation exposure to zirconium fumes or other zirconium compounds (237,370,474). However, several cases of either fibrotic (58) or granulomatous (324,348) changes in the lung associated with inhalation exposure to zirconium compounds have been reported. Long-term exposure of mice to zirconium sulfate was not associated with increased tumor incidence (297).

Certain zirconium compounds, such as zirconium lactate, when applied to human skin (54,63,489,524) or the skin of experimental animals (471), can produce dermal granulomas of allergic origin. Aluminum zirconium chlorohydrate complexes, used as active ingredients in antiperspirants, do not appear to cause these granulomatous reactions, but because of risk/benefit considerations, the U.S. Food and Drug Administration banned the use of these materials in aerosolized drug and cosmetic products (580). The ACGIH has adopted a TLV-TWA value of 5 mg Zr/m^3 and a STEL/C value of 10 mg Zr/m^3 for zirconium compounds (32).

ACKNOWLEDGMENTS

The authors gratefully acknowledge the significant contributions of the previous author, Fanny K. Ennever.

QUESTIONS

1. Margins of safety are normally calculated by determining a no-observable-adverse-effect level (NOAEL) in an animal species and modifying the value by factors to account for inter- and intraspecies variability. U.S. EPA reference doses (RfD) are calculated using a similar approach. How does the oral RfD for the essential metal molybdenum show the limitations of this approach for calculating margins of safety?

   Answer: The estimated safe and adequate daily dietary intake for molybdenum is set at the current U.S. dietary intake of 75–250 μg/day, whereas the oral RfD for molybdenum is 350 μg/day, a value very close to the current dietary intake. In fact, the U.S. EPA had initially derived an RfD of 280 μg/day, essentially the same as current U.S. dietary intake levels. These calculations show that the indiscriminate use of safety factors (without consideration of other relevant information) can lead to overestimation of the toxicity of a substance.

2. Your 15-kg patient has ingested 10 tablets, each containing 324 mg ferrous sulfate. How much elemental iron did the child ingest? (Ferrous sulfate contains 20% elemental iron.)

   Answer: $10 \times 324 \times 0.20 = 648$ mg elemental iron. Then $648/15 = 43.2$ mg Fe/kg body weight. Inaccurate calculation of the dose of elemental iron ingested is a known pitfall in the management of iron poisoning.

3. Why is toenail selenium used instead of blood or hair selenium concentrations for estimating past selenium intake?

   Answer: Hair selenium content is difficult to accurately measure because of the common use of selenium-containing antidandruff shampoos. Blood selenium is not a good indicator of past selenium intake because the life of an erythrocyte is only 120 days.

4. Some metals elicit clinical neurotoxicity at certain workplace exposure levels. For example, manganism is often characterized by Parkinson-like symptoms. Describe tests useful in determining neurotoxicity prior to clinical symptoms in order that safe exposure levels may be established and corrective action taken.

   Answer: Nonclinical neurological injury can be evaluated by controlled neurobehavioral tests that evaluate reaction time, eye–hand coordination, and hand steadiness.

REFERENCES

1. Aamodt, R. L. (1975): Inhalation of ^{181}W labeled tungstic oxide by six beagle dogs. *Health Phys.*, 28:733–742.
2. Abd Elghany, A., Schumacher, M. C., Slattery, M. L., et al. (1990): Occuaption, cadmium exposure, and prostate cancer. *Epidemiology*, 1:107–115.
3. Adamson, R. H., Canellos, G. P., and Sieber, S. M. (1975): Studies on the antitumor activity of gallium nitrate and other group IIIa metal salts. *Cancer Chemother. Rep.*, 59:599–610.
4. Ades, A. E., and Kazantis, G. (1988): Lung cancer in a nonferrous smelter: The role of cadmium. *Br. J. Ind. Med.*, 45:435–442.

5. Agarwal, A. K., Ahlawat, S. K., Gupta, S., et al. (1995): Hypokalemic paralysis secondary to acute barium carbonate poisoning. *Tropical Doctor*, 25:101–103.
6. Agency for Toxic Substances and Disease Registry (ATSDR). (1990): *Toxicological Profile for Copper*. Atlanta, GA.
7. Agency for Toxic Substances and Disease Registry (ATSDR). (1990): *Toxicological Profile for Silver*. Atlanta, GA.
8. Agency for Toxic Substances and Disease Registry (ATSDR). (1990): *Toxicological Profile for Tin*. Atlanta, GA.
9. Agency for Toxic Substances and Disease Registry (ATSDR). (1991): *Toxicological Profile for Antimony*. Atlanta, GA.
10. Agency for Toxic Substances and Disease Registry (ATSDR). (1992): *Toxicological Profile for Barium*. Atlanta, GA.
11. Agency for Toxic Substances and Disease Registry (ATSDR). (1992): *Toxicological Profile for Beryllium*. Atlanta, GA.
12. Agency for Toxic Substances and Disease Registry (ATSDR). (1992): *Toxicological Profile for Boron*. Atlanta, GA.
13. Agency for Toxic Substances and Disease Registry (ATSDR). (1992): *Toxicological Profile for Cobalt*. Atlanta, GA.
14. Agency for Toxic Substances and Disease Registry (ATSDR). (1992): *Toxicological Profile for Vanadium*. Atlanta, GA.
15. Agency for Toxic Substances and Disease Registry (ATSDR). (1993): *Toxicological Profile for Arsenic*. Atlanta, GA.
16. Agency for Toxic Substances and Disease Registry (ATSDR). (1993): *Toxicological Profile for Cadmium*. Atlanta, GA.
17. Agency for Toxic Substances and Disease Registry (ATSDR). (1993): *Toxicological Profile for Lead*. Atlanta, GA.
18. Agency for Toxic Substances and Disease Registry (ATSDR). (1993): *Toxicological Profile for Mercury*. Atlanta, GA.
19. Agency for Toxic Substances and Disease Registry (ATSDR). (1994): *Toxicological Profile for Magnesium*. Atlanta, GA.
20. Agency for Toxic Substances and Disease Registry (ATSDR). (1994): *Toxicological Profile for Selenium*. Atlanta, GA.
21. Agency for Toxic Substances and Disease Registry (ATSDR). (1994): *Toxicological Profile for Zinc*. Atlanta, GA.
22. Agency for Toxic Substances and Disease Registry (ATSDR). (1998): *Toxicological Profile for Manganese*. Draft for Public Comment (Update). Atlanta, GA.
23. Akiniwa, K. (1997): Re-examination of acute toxicity of fluoride. *Fluoride*, 30:89–104.
24. Alderman, L. C., and Bergin, J. J. (1986): Hydrogen selenide poisoning: An illustrative case with review of the literature. *Arch. Environ. Health*, 41:354–358.
25. Alexandrov, D. D. (1983): Bromine and Compounds. In: *Encylopaedia of Occupational Health and Safety*, 3rd ed., Volume 1, edited by L. Parmeggiani, pp. 326–329. International Labour Organization, Geneva.
26. Alfrey, A. C. (1993): Aluminum toxicity in patients with chronic renal disease. *Ther. Drug Metab.*, 15:593–597.
27. Allen, L. A. (1996): Nutritional products. In: *Handbook of Nonprescription Drugs*, pp. 361–392. American Pharmaceutical Association, Washington, DC.
28. Alomar, A., Conde-Salazar, L., and Romaguera, C. (1985): Occupational dermatoses from cutting oils. *Contact Dermatitis*, 12:129–138.
29. Amdur, M. L. (1958): Tellurium oxide, An animal study in acute toxicity. *AMA Arch. Ind. Health*, 17:665–667.
30. Amdur, M. O. (1978): Respiratory response to iodine vapor alone and with sodium chloride aerosol. *J. Toxicol. Environ. Health*, 4:619–630.
31. American Conference of Governmental and Industrial Hygienists (ACGIH). (1996): *Documentation of the threshold limit values and biological exposure indicies*, 6th ed. and suppl. ACGIH, Cincinnati, OH.
32. American Conference of Governmental Industrial Hygienists (ACGIH). (2000): *2000 TLV's and BEI's*. ACGIH, Cincinnati, OH.
33. American Industrial Hygiene Association (AIHA). (1968): *Hygienic Guide Series—Nickel Carbonyl* (rev. 1968), pp. 304–307. AIHA, Fairfax, VA.
34. Anderson, A. C. (1994): Iron poisoning in children. *Curr. Opin. Pediatr.*, 6:289–294.
35. Anderson, R. A. (1997): Chromium as an essential nutrient for humans. *Regul. Toxicol. Pharmacol.*, 26:S35–S41.
36. Angle, C. R. (1993): Childhood lead poisoning and its treatment. *Annu. Rev. Pharmacol. Toxicol.*, 32:409–434.
37. Anke, M., Groppel, G., and Arnhold, W. (1990): Essentiality of the trace element bromine. *Acta Agronom. Hung.*, 39:297–303.
38. Anke, M., Groppel, G., and Krause, U. (1991): Essentiallity of the toxic elements cadmium, arsenic, and nickel. In: *Trace Elements in Man and Animals*, Vol. 7. edited by B. Momcilovic, pp. 11–6 to 11–8. IMI, Zagreb, Croatia.
39. Anke, M., Groppel, G., and Krause, U. (1991): Essentiality of the toxic elements aluminum and vanadium. In: *Trace Elements in Man and Animals*, Vol. 7, edited by B. Momcilovic, pp. 11–9 to 11–11. IMI, Zagreb, Croatia.
40. Anke, M., Groppel. G., and Krause, U. (1991): Fluorine deficiency in goats. In: *Trace Elements in Man and Animals*, Vol. 7, edited by B. Momcilovic, pp. 26–28 to 26–27. IMI, Zagreb, Croatia.
41. Anneroth, G., Ericson, T., Johansson, I., et al. (1992): Comprehensive medical examination of a group of patients with alleged adverse effects from dental amalgams. *Acta Odontolog. Scand.*, 50:101–111.
42. Apostoli, P., Kiss, P., Porru, S., Bonde, J. P., Vanhoorne, M., and ASCLEPIOS. (1998): Male reproductive toxicity of lead in animals and humans. *Occup. Environ. Med.*, 55:364–374.
43. Arts, J. H. E., Reuzel, P. G. J., Falke, H. E., and Beems, R. B. (1990): Acute and sub-acute inhalation toxicity of germanium metal powder in rats. *Food Chem. Toxicol.*, 28:571–579.
44. Arts, J. H. E., Til, H. P., Kuper, R., and Swennen, B. (1994): Acute and subacute inhalation toxicity of germanium dioxide in rats. *Food Chem. Toxicol.*, 32:1037–1046.
45. Assennato, G., Paci, C., Baser, M. E., Molinini, R., Candela, R. G., Altamura, B. M., and Giorgino, R. (1987): Sperm count suppression without endocrine dysfunction in lead-exposed men. *Arch. Environ. Health*, 42:123–127.
46. Awasthi, Y. C., Beutler, E., and Srivastava, S. K. (1975): Purification and properties of human erythrocyte glutathione peroxidase. *J. Biol. Chem.*, 250:5144–5149.
47. Axelson, O., Dahlgren, E., Jansson, C.-D., and Rehnlund, S. O. (1978): Arsenic exposure and mortality: A case referent study from a Swedish copper smelter. *Br. J. Ind. Med.*, 35:8–15.
48. Ayres, S., Jr., and Anderson, N. P. (1934): Cutaneous manifestations of arsenic poisoning. *Arch. Dermatol. Syphil.*, 30:33–43.
49. Bacon, B. R., and Britton, R. S. (1990): The pathology of hepatic iron overload: A free radical mediated process? *Hepatology*, 11:127–137.
50. Bacon, B. R., Tavill, A. S., Brittenham, G. M., et al. (1983): Hepatic lipid peroxidation in vivo in rats with chronic iron overload. *J. Clin. Invest.*, 71:429–439.
51. Baker, E. L., White, R. F., Pothier, L. J., et al. (1985): Occupational lead neurotoxicity: Improvement in behavioral effects after reduction of exposure. *Br. J. Ind. Med.*, 42:507–516.
52. Baker, T. D., and Hafner, W. G. (1961): Cadmium poisoning from a refrigerator shelf used as an improvised barbecue grill. *Public Health Rep.*, 76:543–544.
53. Bako, G., Smith, E. S., Hanson, J., et al. (1982): The geographical distribution of high cadmium concentrations in the environment and prostate cancer in Alberta. *Can. J. Pub. Health*, 73:92–94.

54. Baler, G. R. (1965): Granulomas from topical zirconium in poison ivy dermatitis. *Arch. Dermatol.*, 91:145–148.
55. Banting, D. W. (1991): The future of fluoride. An update one year after the National Toxicology Program study. *J. Am. Dental Assoc.*, 123:86–91.
56. Barnhart, S., and Rosenstock, L. (1984): Cadmium chemical pneumonitis. *Chest*, 86:789–791.
57. Barret, H. M., and Card, B. Y. (1947): Studies on the toxicity of inhaled cadmium. II. The acute lethal dose cadmium oxide for man. *J. Ind. Hyg. Toxicol.*, 29:286–293.
58. Bartter, T., Irwin, R. S., Abraham, J. L., Dascal, A., Nash, G., Himmelstein, J. S., and Jederlinic, P. J. (1991): Zirconium compound-induced pulmonary fibrosis. *Arch. Intern. Med.*, 151:1197–1201.
59. Bast, A., Haenen, G. R., and Doelman, C. J. (1991): Oxidants and antioxidants: State of the art. *Am. J. Med.*, 91(suppl. 3C):2–13.
60. Bates, M. N., Smith, A. H., and Hopenhayn-Rich, C. (1992): Arsenic ingestion and internal cancers: A review. *Am. J. Epidemiol.*, 135:462–476.
61. Beckett, W. S., Moore, J. L., Keogh, J. P., and Bleecker, M. L. (1986): Acute encephalopathy due to occupational exposure to arsenic. *Br. J. Ind. Med.*, 43:66–67.
62. Beliles, R. P. (1979): The lesser metals. In: *Toxicity of Heavy Metals in the Environment*, edited by F. W. Oehme, pp. 547–615. Marcel Dekker, New York.
63. Beliles, R. P. (1994): The metals. In: *Patty's Industrial Hygiene and Toxicology*, edited by G. D. Clayton and F. E. Clayton, pp. 1879–2352. John Wiley & Sons, New York.
64. Beliles, R. P., and Beliles, E. M. (1994): Phosphorus, selenium, tellurium, and sulfur. In: *Patty's Industrial Hygiene and Toxicology*, edited by G. D. Clayton and F. E. Clayton, pp. 783–829. John Wiley & Sons, New York.
65. Belizan, J. M., Villar, J., Zalazar, A., et al. (1983): Preliminary evidence of the effect of calcium supplementation on blood pressure in normal pregnant women. *Am. J. Obstet. Gynecol.*, 146:175–180.
66. Bellinger, D., Leviton, A., Waternaux, C., Needleman, H., and Rabinowitz, M. (1987): Longitudinal analyses of prenatal and postnatal lead exposure and early cognitive development. *N. Engl. J. Med.*, 316:1037–1043.
67. Berciano, M. T., Calle, E., Fernández, R., and Lafarga, M. (1998): Regulation of Schwann cell numbers in tellurium-induced neuropathy: Apoptosis, supernumerary cells and internodal shortening. *Acta Neuropathol.*, 95:269–279.
68. Berkovitch, M., Matsui, D., Lamm, S. H., et al. (1994): Recent increases in numbers and risk of fatalities in young children ingesting iron preparations. *Vet. Hum. Toxicol.*, 36:53–55.
69. Berry, J. P., Bertrand, F., and Galle, P. (1993): Selective intra-lysosomal concentration of niobium in kidney and bone marrow cells: A microanalytical study. *BioMetals*, 6:17–23.
70. Berry, M. J., and Larsen, P. R. (1992): The role of selenium in thyroid hormone action. *Endocr. Rev.*, 13:207–219.
71. Beton, D. C., Andrews, G. S., Davies, H. J., et al. (1966): Acute cadmium fume poisoning: Five cases with one death from renal necrosis. *Br. J. Ind. Med.*, 23:292–301.
72. Beyer, K. H., Bergfeld, W. F., and Berndt, W. O. (1983): Final report on the safety assessment of sodium borate and boric acid. *J. Am. Coll. Toxicol.*, 2:87–125.
73. Bhattacharyya, M. H., Jeffery, E., and Silbergeld, E. K. (1996): Bone metabolism: Effects of essential and toxic trace metals. In: *Toxicology of Metals*, edited by L. W. Chang, pp. 959–971. CRC Press, New York.
74. Birch, N. J., and Karim, A. R., (1988): Potassium. In: *Handbook on Toxicology of Inorganic Compounds*, edited by N. G. Sieler and H. Sigel, pp. 543–553. Marcel Dekker, New York.
75. Black, J. (1994): Biological performance of tantalum. *Clin. Materials*, 16:167–173.
76. Blanc, P., and Boushey, H. A. (1993): The lung in metal fume fever. *Semin. Resp. Med.*, 14:212–225.
77. Blank, E., and Howieson, J. (1983): Lead poisoning from a curtain weight. *J. Am. Med. Assoc., 249:2176–2177.*
78. Blazka, M. E., Dixon, D., Haskins, E., and Rosenthal, G. J. (1994): Pulmonary toxicity to intratracheally administered indium trichloride in Fischer 344 rats. *Fundam. Appl. Toxicol.*, 22:231–239.
79. Blejer, H. P. (1966): Death due to cadmium oxide fumes. *Ind. Med. Surg.*, 35:363–364.
80. Blevins, D. G. and Lukaszewski, K. M. (1994): Proposed physiologic functions of boron in plants pertinent to animal and human metabolism. *Environ. Health Persp.*, 102(suppl. 7):31–33.
81. Blom, S., Lagerkvist, B., and Linderholm, H. (1985): Arsenic exposure to smelter workers: Clinical and neurophysiological studies. *Scand. J. Work Environ. Health*, 11:265–269.
82. Bockman, R. S., Wilhelm, F., Siris, E., Singer, F., Chausmer, A., Britton, R., Kotler, J., Bosco, J., Eyre, D. R., and Levenson, D. (1995): A multicenter trial of low dose gallium nitrate in patients with advanced Paget's disease of bone. *J. Clin. Endocrinol. Metab.* 80:595–602.
83. Borgoño, J. M., Vicent, P., Venturino, H., and Infante, A. (1977): Arsenic in the drinking water of the city of Antofagasta: Epidemiological and clinical study before and after the installation of a treatment plant. *Environ. Health Perspect.*, 19:103–105.
84. Boulos, B. M., and von Smolinski, A. (1988): Alert to users of calcium supplements as antihypertensive agents due to trace metal contaminants. *Am. J. Hypertens.*, 1:137S–142S.
85. Bourgoin, B. P., Evans, D. R., Cornett, J. R., et al. (1993): Lead content in 70 brands of dietary calcium supplements. *Am. J. Public Health*, 83:1155–1160.
86. Bowman B. A., and Rishert, J. F. (1994): Comparison of the methodological approaches used in the derivation of recommended dietary allowances and oral reference doses for nutritionally essential elements. In: *Risk Assessment of Essential Elements*, edited by W. Mertz, C. O. Abernathy, S. S. Olin, pp. 63–73. ILSI Press, Washington, DC.
87. Brenniman, G. R., and Levy, P. S. (1984): Epidemiological study of barium in Illinois drinking water supplies. In: *Advances in Modern Toxicology*, Vol. 9, edited by E. J. Calabrese, pp. 231–249. Princeton Scientific, Princeton, NJ.
88. Brody, D. J., Pirkle, J. L., Kramer, R. A., et al. (1994): Blood lead levels in the US population. Phase 1 of the 3rd National health and Nutrition Examination Survey. *J. Am. Med. Assoc.*, 272:277–283.
89. Brunot, F. R. (1933): The toxicity of osmium tetroxide (osmic acid). *J. Ind. Hyg.*, 15:136–143.
90. Brunton, L. L. (1996): Bismuth Compounds. In: *Agents for Control of Gastric Acidity and Treatment of Peptic Ulcers*, edited by J. G. Hardman, L. E. Limberd, P. B. Molinoff, and R. W. Ruddon, pp. 901–915. McGraw-Hill, New York.
91. Bruze, M., Hedman, H., Bjorkner, B., and Moller, H. (1995): The development and course of test reactions to gold sodium thiosulfate. *Contact Dermatitis*, 33:386–391.
92. Bucher, J. R., Hejtmanick, M. R., Toft, J. D., et al. (1991): Results and conclusions of the National Toxicology Program's rodent carcinogenicity studies with sodium fluoride. *Int. J. Cancer*, 48:733–737.
93. Buchet, J. P., Lauwerys, R., and Roels, H. (1981): Urinary excretion of inorganic arsenic and its metabolites after repeated ingestion of sodium metaarsenite by volunteers. *Int. Arch. Occup. Environ. Health*, 48:111–118.

94. Buchet, J. P., Lauwerys, R., Roels, H., et al. (1990): Renal effects of cadmium body burden of the general population. *Lancet*, 336:699–702.

95. Buckler, H. M., Smith, W. D., and Rees, W. D. (1986): Self poisoning with oral cadmium chloride. *Br. Med. J.*, 292:1559–1560.

96. Bulmer, F. M. R., Rothwell, N. F., and Frankish, E. R. (1938): Industrial cadmium poisoning, a report of fifteen cases, including two deaths. *Can. Public Health J.*, 29:19–26.

97. Burrows, D. (1988): Mischievous metals—Chromate, cobalt, nickel and mercury. *Clin. Exp. Dermatol.*, 14:266–272.

98. Byers, R. K., and Lord, E. E. (1943): Late effects of lead poisoning on mental development. *Am. J. Dis. Child.*, 66:471–494.

99. Calvery, H. O. (1942): Trace elements in food. *Food Res.*, 7:313–331.

100. Campbell, D., Gonzales, M., and Sullivan, J. B., Jr. (1992): Mercury. In: *Hazardous Materials Toxicology*, edited by J. B. Sullivan, Jr., and G. R. Krieger, pp. 824-833. Williams & Wilkins, Baltimore, MD.

101. Carleton, A. B., Peters, R. A., and Thompson, R. H. S. (1948): The treatment of arsenical dermatitis with dimercaptopropanol (BAL). *Q. J. Med.*, 17:49–79.

102. Carter, R. F. (1966): Acute selenium poisoning. *Med. J. Aust.*, 1:525–528.

103. Cavanagh, J. B. (1991): What have we learnt from Graham Frederick Young? Reflections on the mechanism of thallium neurotoxicity. *Neuropathol. Appl. Neurobiol.*, 17:3–9.

104. Centers for Disease Control (CDC). (1981): Use of lead tetroxide as a folk remedy for gastrointestinal illness. *Morbid. Mortal. Weekly Rep.*, 30:546–547.

105. Centers for Disease Control (CDC). (1983): Folk remedy-associated lead poisoning in Hmong children—Minnesota. *Morbid. Mortal. Weekly Rep.*, 32:555–556

106. Centers for Disease Control (CDC). (1983): Lead poisoning from Mexican folk remedies—California. *Morbid. Mortal. Weekly. Rep.*, 32:554–555.

107. Centers for Disease Control (CDC). (1984): Lead poisoning-associated death from Asian Indian folk remedies—Florida. *Morbid. Mortal. Weekly Rep.*, 33:638, 643–645.

108. Centers for Disease Control (CDC). (1991): *Preventing lead poisoning in young children: A statement by the Centers for Disease Control—October 1991*. Centers for Disease Control, U.S. Department of Health and Human Services, Atlanta, GA.

109. Centers for Disease Control (CDC). (1991): *Strategic plan for the elimination of childhood lead poisoning*. Centers for Disease Control, U.S. Department of Health and Human Services, Atlanta, GA.

110. Centers for Disease Control (CDC). (1996): Children with elevated blood lead levels attributed to home renovation and remodeling activities—New York, 1993–1994. *Morbid. Mortal. Weekly Rep.*, 45:1120–1123.

111. Centers for Disease Control (CDC). (1997): *Screening young children for lead poisoning: Guidance for state and local public health officials*. Centers for Disease Control, U.S. Department of Health and Human Services, Atlanta, GA.

112. Centers for Disease Control (CDC). (1997): Update: Blood lead levels—United States, 1991–1994. *Morbid. Mortal. Weekly Rep.*, 46:141–146.

113. Chan, K.-M., Svancarek, W. P., and Creer, M. (1987): Fatality due to acute hydrofluoric acid exposure. *J. Toxicol. Clin. Toxicol.*, 25:333–339.

114. Chan, P. C., Herbert, R. A., Roycroft, J. H., Haseman, J. K., Grumbein, S. L., Miller, R. A., and Chou, B. J. (1998): Lung tumor induction by inhalation exposure to molybdenum trioxide in rats and mice. *Toxicol. Sci.*, 45:58–65.

115. Chandler, H. A., and Scott, M. (1986): A review of thallium toxicology. *J. Roy. Nav. Med. Serv.*, 72:75–79

116. Chapin, R. E., Harris, M. W., Hunter, S., Davis, B. J., Collins, B. J., and Lockhart, A. C. (1995): The reproductive and developmental toxicity of indium in the Swiss mouse. *Fundam. Appl. Toxicol.*, 27:140–148.

117. Chatterjee, M. S., Abdel-Rahman, M., Bhandal, A., et al. (1988): Amniotic fluid cadmium and thiocyanate in pregnant women who smoke. *J. Reprod. Med.*, 33:417–420.

118. Chela, A., Reig, R., Sanz, P., Huguet, E., and Corbella, J. (1989): Death due to hydrofluoric acid. *Am. J. Forens. Med. Pathol.*, 10:47–48.

119. Chen, C.-J., Chuang, Y.-C., Lin, T.-M., and Wu, H.-Y. (1985): Malignant neoplasms among residents of a blackfoot disease-endemic area in Taiwan: High-arsenic artesian well water and cancers. *Cancer Res.*, 45:5895–5899.

120. Chen, C.-J., Chuang, Y.-C., You, S.-L., Lin, T.-M., and Wu, H.-Y. (1986): A retrospective study on malignant neoplasms of bladder, lung and liver in blackfoot disease endemic area in Taiwan. *Br. J. Cancer*, 53:399–405.

121. Chen, C.-J., and Wang, C.-J. (1990): Ecological correlation between arsenic level in well water and age-adjusted mortality from malignant neoplasms. *Cancer Res.*, 50:5470–5474.

122. Chen, C.-J., Wu, M.-M., Lee, S.-S., Wang, J.-D., Cheng, S.-H., and Wu, H.-Y. (1988): Atherogenicity and carcinogenicity of high-arsenic artesian well water. Multiple risk factors and related malignant neoplasms of blackfoot disease. *Arteriosclerosis*, 8:452–460.

123. Cheng, Y.-Y., and Qian, P.-C. (1990): The effect of selenium-fortified table salt in the prevention of Keshan disease on a population of 1.05 million. *Biomed. Environ. Sci.*, 3:422–428.

124. Chisolm, J. C., and Handorf, C. R. (1996): Further observations on the etiology of pre-eclampsia: Mobilization of toxic cadmium-metallothionein into the serum during pregnancy. *Med. Hypoth.*, 47:123–128.

125. Clark, L. C., Combs, G. F., Jr., Turnbull, B. W., et al. (1996): Effects of selenium supplementation for cancer prevention in patients with carcinoma of the skin. *J. Am. Med. Assoc.*, 276:1957–1963. [Published erratum appears in *J. Am. Med. Assoc.*, 1997, 277:1520].

126. Clark, L. C., Dalkin, B., Krongrad, A., et al. (1998): Decreased incidence of prostate cancer with selenium supplementation: Results of a double-blind cancer prevention trial. *Br. J. Urol.*, 81:730–734.

127. Clayton, C. C., and Bauman, C. A. (1949): Diet and azo dye tumors: Effect of diet during a period when the dye is not fed. *Cancer Res.*, 9:575–582.

128. Cochran, K. W., Doull, J., Mazur, M., and DuBois, K. P. (1950): Acute toxicity of zirconium, columbium, strontium, lanthanum, cesium, tantalum and yttrium. *Arch. Ind. Health*, 1:637–650.

129. *Code of Federal Regulations*. Protection of the Environment. (1997): National primary drinking water standards. Volume 40: Part 141.80. U.S. Government Printing Office, Washington, DC.

130. Cohen, M. D., Kargacin, B., Klein, C. B., and Costa M. (1993): Mechanisms of chromium carcinogenicity and toxicity. *Crit. Rev. Toxicol.*, 23:255–281.

131. Cohen, M. D., Yang, Z., Zelikoff, J. T., and Schlesinger, R. B. (1996): Pulmonary immunotoxicity of inhaled ammonium metavanadate in Fisher 344 rats. *Fundam. Appl. Toxicol.*, 33:254–263.

132. Cole, V. V., Harned, B. K., and Hafkesbring, R. (1941): The toxicity of strontium and calcium. *J. Pharmacol. Exp. Ther.*, 71:1–5.

133. Collins, J. F., Brown, J. P., Painter, P. R., et al. (1996): On the oral carcinogenicity of cadmium. *Regul. Toxicol. Pharmacol.*, 23:298–299.
134. Colomina, J. M., Llobtet, J. M., Sirvent, J. J., Domingo, J. L., and Corbella, J. (1993): Evaluation of the reproductive toxicity of gallium nitrate in mice. *Food Chem. Toxicol.*, 31:847–851.
135. Combs, G. F. (1996): Should intakes with beneficial actions, often requiring supplementation, be considered for RDAs? *J. Nutr.*, 126:2373S–2376S.
136. Comstock, G. W., Bush, T. L., and Helzlsouer, K. (1992): Serum retinol, beta-carotene, vitamin E, and selenium as related to subsequent cancer of specific sites. *Am. J. Epidemiol.*, 135:115–121.
137. Condray, J. R. (1985): *Elemental yellow phosphorus one-generation reproduction study in rats.* IR-82-215, IRD No. 401-189. Monsanto Company, St. Louis, MO.
138. Cook, J. D., and Monsen, E. R. (1977): Vitamin C, the common cold, and iron absorption. *Am. J. Clin. Nutr.*, 30:235–241.
139. Costa, M. (1997): Toxicity and carcinogenicity of Cr(VI) in animal models and humans. *Crit. Rev. Toxicol.*, 27:431–442.
140. Coughlin, J. R. (1996): Inorganic borates: Chemistry, human exposure, and health and regulatory guidelines. *J. Trace Elem. Exp. Med.*, 9:137–151.
141. Crecelius, E. A. (1977): Changes in the chemical speciation of arsenic following ingestion by man. *Environ. Health Perspect.*, 19:147–150.
142. Culver, B. D., Smith, R. G., Brotherton, R. J., et al. (1994): Boron. In: *Patty's Industrial Hygiene and Toxicology*, edited by G. D. Clayton and F. E. Clayton, pp. 4411–4448. John Wiley & Sons, New York.
143. Curzon, M. E. J., Spector, P. C., and Iker, H. P. (1978): An association between strontium in drinking water supplies and low caries prevalence in man. *Arch. Oral Biol.*, 23:317–321.
144. Davison, A. G., Fayers, P. M., Taylor, A. J., et al. (1988): Cadmium fume inhalation and emphysema. *Lancet*, 1(8587):663–667.
145. De Groot, A. P. (1973): Subacute toxicity of inorganic tin as influenced by dietary levels of iron and copper. *Food Cosmetic. Toxicol.*, 11:955–962.
146. De Groot, A. P., Feron, V. J., and Til, H. P. (1973): Short-term toxicity studies on some salts and oxides of tin in rats. *Food Cosmetic. Toxicol.*, 11:19–30.
147. de la Burde, B., and Choate, M. S. (1975): Early asymptomatic lead exposure and development at school age. *J. Pediatr.*, 87:638–642.
148. Delahant, A. B. (1955): An experimental study of the effects of rare metals on animal lungs. *AMA Arch. Ind. Health*, 12:116–120.
149. DeMeio, R. H. (1947): Tellurium. II. Effect of ascorbic acid on the tellurium breath. *J. Ind. Hyg. Toxicol.*, 29:393–395.
150. Desai, H. (1992): Phosphorus and phosphorus compounds. In: *Hazardous Materials Toxicology*, edited by J. B. Sullivan, Jr., and G. R. Krieger, pp. 937–939. Williams & Wilkins, Baltimore, MD.
151. Descotes, J. (1989): *Immunotoxicology of Drugs and Chemicals.* Elsevier, Amsterdam.
152. Dietrich, K. N. (1991): Human fetal lead exposure: Intrauterine growth, maturation and postnatal neurobehavioral development. *Fundam. Appl. Toxicol.*, 16:17–19.
153. Digenott, D., Rozsa, O., Levy, N., and Muammar, S. (1964): Hypokalemia in barium poisoning. *Lancet*, 2:343–344.
154. Doig, A. T. (1976): Baritosis: A benign pneumoconiosis. *Thorax*, 31:30–39.
155. Doll, R. (1985): Relevance of epidemiology to policies for the prevention of cancer. *Hum. Toxicol.*, 4:81–96.
156. Doll, R. (1992): Is cadmium a human carcinogen? *Ann. Epidemiol.*, 2:335–337.
157. Domingo, J. L., and Corbella, J. (1991): A review of the health hazards from gallium exposure. *Trace Elem. Med.*, 8:56–64.
158. Donaldson, R. M., and Barreras, R. F. (1966): Intestinal absorption of trace quantities of chromium. *J. Lab. Clin. Med.*, 68:484–493.
159. Downs, J. C., Milling, D., and Nichols, C. A. (1995): Suicidal ingestion of barium-sulfide-containing shaving powder. *Am. J. Forens. Med. Pathol.*, 16:56–61.
160. Downs, W. L., Scott, J. K., Steadman, L. T., and Maynard, E. A. (1959): *The toxicity of indium.* Univ. Rochester At. Energy Rep. UR-588.
161. Draize, J. H., and Kelley, E. A. (1959): The urinary excretion of boric acid preparations following oral administration and topical applications to intact and damaged skin of rabbits. *Toxicol. Appl. Pharmacol.*, 1:267–276.
162. Dudley, R. E., Svoboda, D. J., and Klaassen, C. D. (1982): Acute exposure to cadmium causes severe liver injury in rats. *Toxicol. Appl. Pharmacol.*, 65:302–313.
163. Duell, P. B., and Chesnut, C. H. III. (1991): Exacerbation of rheumatoid arthritis by sodium fluoride treatment of osteoporosis. *Arch. Intern. Med.*, 151:783–784.
164. Dunphy, B. (1967): Acute occupational cadmium poisoning: A critical review of the literature. *J. Occup. Med.*, 9:22–26.
165. Duverger-van Bogaert, and Lambotte-Vandepaer M. (1988): Hafnium. In: *Handbook on Toxicity of Inorganic Compounds*, edited by H. G. Sieler and H. Sigel, pp. 313–318. Marcel Dekker, New York.
166. ECETOC. (1995): Reproductive and general toxicology of some inorganic borates and risks assessment for human beings. *Tech. Rep.* No. 63, Brussels, Belgium.
167. ECETOC. (1997): *Ecotoxicology of some inorganic borates.* Special Rep. No. 11, Brussels, Belgium.
168. Eisenbud, M., Berghout, C. F., and Steadman, L. T. (1948): Environmental studies in plants and laboratories using beryllium: The acute disease. *J. Ind. Hyg. Toxicol.*, 30:282–285.
169. Eisenbud, M., and Lisson, J. (1983): Epidemiological aspects of beryllium-induced nonmalignant lung disease: A 30-year update. *J. Occup. Med.*, 25:196–202.
170. Elinder, C. G., Kjellström, T., Hogstedt, C., et al. (1985): Cancer mortality of cadmium workers. *Br. J. Ind. Med.*, 42:651–655.
171. Elinder, C. G., and Zenz, C. (1994): Other metals and their compounds: Hafnium and its compounds. In: *Occupational Medicine*, edited by C. Zenz, O. B. Dickerson, and E. P. Horvath, Jr., pp. 595–616. Mosby-YearBook, St. Louis, MO.
172. Ellenhorn, M. J., and Barceloux, D. G. (1988). *Medical Toxicology: Diagnosis and Treatment of Human Poisoning*, Elsevier, New York.
173. Ellis, T., and Lacy, R. (1998): Illicit alcohol (moonshine) consumption in West Alabama revisited. *S. Med. J.*, 91:858–860.
174. Engfeldt, B., and Hjertquist, S. O. (1969): Effect of strontium administration on bones and teeth of rats maintained on diets with different calcium contents. *Virchows Arch. Abt. A Pathol. Anat.*, 346:330–344.
175. Enterline, P. E., and Marsh, G. M. (1982): Cancer among workers exposed to arsenic and other substances in a copper smelter. *Am. J. Epidemiol.*, 116:895–911.
176. Ernhart, C. B. (1992): A critical review of low-level prenatal lead exposure in the human: Effects on the fetus and newborn. *Reprod. Toxicol.*, 6:9–19.
177. Esernio-Jenssen, D., Donatelli-Guagenti, A., and Mofenson, H. C. (1996): Severe lead poisoning from an imported clothing accessory: "Watch" out for lead. *Clin. Toxicol.*, 34:329–333.
178. Eskew, A. E., Crutcher, J. C., Zimmerman, S. L., et al. (1961): Lead poisoning resulting from illicit alcohol consumption. *J. Forens. Sci.*, 6:337–350.
179. Ewers, U., Manojilovic, N., Hadnagy, W., and Grover, Y. P. (1988): Chlorine. In: *Handbook on Toxicity of Inorganic Compo-*

unds, edited by H. G. Sieler and H. Sigel, pp. 223–237. Marcel Dekker, New York.

180. Fahim, M. S., Fahim, Z., and Hall, D. G. (1976): Effects of subtoxic lead levels on pregnant women in the State of Missouri. *Res. Commun. Chem. Pathol. Pharmacol.*, 13:309–331.
181. Fail, P. A., George, J. D., Seely, J. C., Grizzle, T. B., and Heindel, J. J. (1991): Reproductive toxicity of boric acid in Swiss (CD-1) mice: Assessment using the continuous breeding protocol. *Fundam. Appl. Toxicol.*, 17:225–239.
182. Fairhall, L. T., Dunn, R. C., Sharpless, N. E., and Pritchard, E. A. (1945): *The toxicity of molybdenum*. Public Health Bull. No. 293, U.S. Government Printing Office, Washington, D.C.
183. Farwell, A. P. and Braverman, L. E. (1996): Thyroid and antithyroid drugs. In: *Goodman and Gilman's The Pharmacological Basis of Therapeutics*, edited by J. G. Hardman, L. E. Limbird, and A. G. Gilman, p. 1392. McGraw-Hill, New York.
184. FDC Reports. (1997): Selenium cancer reduction health claim needs further clinical evidence. *Tan Sheet*, 5(39):8–10.
185. Feldman, R. G., Niles, C. A., Kelly-Hayes, M., Sax, D. S., Dixon, W. J., Thompson, D. J., and Landau, E. (1979): Peripheral neuropathy in arsenic smelter workers. *Neurology*, 29:939–944.
186. Ferguson, W. S., Lewis, A. H., and Watson, S. J. (1938): Action of molybdenum in nutrition of milking cows. *Nature*, 141:553.
187. Fischbein, A. (1992): Occupational and environmental lead exposure. In: *Environmental and Occupational Medicine*, edited by W. N. Rom, pp. 735–758. Little, Brown, Boston.
188. Fisher, A. A. (1986): Antiseptics and disinfectants. In: *Contact Dermatitis*, pp. 178–194. Lea and Febiger, Philadelphia.
189. Fisher, A. A. (1986): Contact urticaria. In: *Contact Dermatitis*, p. 698. Lea and Febiger, Philadelphia.
190. Fisher, D. (1992): Zinc. In: *Hazardous Materials Toxicology*, edited by J. B. Sullivan, Jr., and G. R. Krieger, pp. 865–868. Williams & Wilkins, Baltimore, MD.
191. Fisher, N., Hutchinson, J. B., Berry, R., Hardy, J., Ginocchio, A. V., and Waite, V. (1979): Long-term toxicity and carcinogenicity studies of the bread improver potassium bromate. I. Studies in rats. *Food Cosmet. Toxicol.*, 17:33–39.
192. Flanagan, P. R., McLellan, J. S., Haist, J., et al. (1978): Increased dietary cadmium absorption in mice and human subjects with iron deficiency. *Gastroenterology*, 74:841–846.
193. Flegal, A. R., and Smith, D. R. (1992): Lead levels in preindustrial humans. *N. Engl. J. Med.*, 326:1293–1294.
194. Flury, F., and Zernik, F. (1931): *Schädliche gase däpfe, nebel, rauch- und staubarten*, p. 309. Verlag von Julius Springer, Berlin.
195. Forbes, R. M. (1960): Nutritional interactions of zinc and calcium. *Fed. Proc. FASEB*, 19:643–647.
196. Foster, L. H., and Sumar, S. (1997): Selenium in health and disease: A review. *Crit. Rev. Food Sci. Nutr.*, 37:211–228.
197. Foulkes, E. C. (1990): The concept of critical levels of toxic heavy metals in target tissues. *CRC Crit. Rev. Toxicol.*, 20:327–339.
198. Franke, K. W., Moxon, A. L., Poley, W. E., and Tully, W. C. (1936): Monstrosities produced by the injection of selenium salts into hens' eggs. *Anat. Rec.*, 65:15–22.
199. Fredrick, W. G., and Bradley, W. R. (1946): Toxicity of some materials used in the manufacture of cemented tungsten carbide tools. *Ind. Med.*, 15:482–483.
200. Friberg, L. (1984): Cadmium and the kidney. *Environ. Health Perspect.*, 54:1–11.
201. Friberg, L., Piscator, M., Nordberg, G. F., et al. (1974): *Cadmium in the Environment*. CRC Press, Boca Raton, FL.
202. Friis-Hansen, B., Aggerbeck, B., and Jansen, J. A. (1982): Unaffected blood boron levels in newborn infants treated with a boric acid ointment. *Food Chem. Toxicol.*, 20:451–454.
203. Fung, Y. K., and Molvar, M. P. (1992): Toxicity of mercury from dental environment and from amalgam restorations. *Clin. Toxicol.*, 30:49–61.
204. Gasmi, A., Garnier, R., Galliot-Guilley, M., et al. (1997): Acute selenium poisoning. *Vet Hum. Toxicol.*, 39:304–308.
205. Gennart, J.-P., Buchet, J.-P., Roels, H., Ghyselen, P., Ceulemans, E., and Lauwerys, R. (1992): Fertility of male workers exposed to cadmium, lead, or manganese. *Am. J. Epidemiol.*, 135:1208–1219.
206. Gerber, G. B., and Léonard, A. (1997): Mutagenicity, carcinogenicity and teratogenicity of germanium compounds. *Mutat. Res.*, 387:141–146.
207. Gheysens, B., Auwerx, J., Van den Eeckhout, A., and Demedts, M. (1985): Cobalt-induced bronchial asthma in diamond polishers. *Chest*, 88:740–744.
208. Gilmore, D. A., Jr., and Bronstein, A. C. (1992): Manganese and magnesium. In: *Hazardous Materials Toxicology*, edited by J. B. Sullivan, Jr., and G. R. Krieger, pp. 896–901. Williams & Wilkins, Baltimore, MD.
209. Gilmore, D. A., Jr., and Bronstein, A. C. (1992): Titanium. In: *Hazardous Materials Toxicology*, edited by J. B. Sullivan, Jr., and G. R. Krieger, pp. 904–905. Williams & Wilkins, Baltimore, MD.
210. Ginocchio, A. V., Waite, V., Hardy, J., Fisher N., Hutchinson, J. B., and Berry, R. (1979): Long-term toxicity and carcinogenicity studies of the bread improver potassium bromate. 2. Studies in mice. *Food Cosmet. Toxicol.*, 17:41–47.
211. Glaser, U., Hochrainer, D., Otto, F. J., and Oldiges, H. (1989): Carcinogenicity and toxicity of four cadmium compounds inhaled by rats. *Toxicol. Environ. Chem.*, 27:153–162.
212. Goering, P. L. (1992): Platinum and related metals: Palladium, indium, osmium, rhodium, and ruthenium. In: *Hazardous Materials Toxicology*, edited by J. B. Sullivan, Jr., and G. R. Krieger, pp. 874–881. Williams & Wilkins, Baltimore, MD.
213. Goering, P. L., and Klaassen, C. D. (1984): Zinc-induced tolerance to cadmium hepatotoxicity. *Toxicol. Appl. Pharmacol.*, 74:299–307.
214 Gold, L. S., Sawyer, C. B., Magaw, R., et al. (1984): A carcinogenic potency database of the standardized results of animal bioassays. *Environ. Health Perspect.*, 58:9–319.
215. Goldbloom, R. B., and Goldbloom, A. (1953): Boric acid poisoning: Report of four cases and a review of 109 cases from the world literature. *J. Pediatr.*, 43:631–643.
216. Goldman, L. R. (1998): Linking research and policy to ensure children's environmental health. *Environ. Health Perspect.*, 106:S857–S862.
217. Goldman, R. H., Baker, E. L., Hannan, M., and Kamerow, D. B. (1987): Lead poisoning in automobile radiator repair mechanics. *N. Engl. J. Med.*, 317:214–218.
218. Golub, M. S., and Domingo, J. L. (1996): What we know and what we need to know about developmental aluminum toxicity. *J. Toxicol. Environ. Health*, 48:585–597.
219. Gompertz, D. (1981): Assessment of risk by biological monitoring. *Br. J. Ind. Med.*, 38:198–201.
220. Gordeuk, V. R., McLaren, G. D., and Samowitz, W. (1994): Etiologies, consequences, and treatment of iron overload. *Crit. Rev. Clin. Lab. Sci.*, 31:89–133.
221. Gordeuk, V. R., Mukiibi, J., Hasstedt, S. J., et al. (1992): Iron overload in Africa. Interaction between a gene and dietary iron content. *N. Engl. J. Med.*, 326:95–100.
222. Gosselin, R. E., Smith, R. P., and Hodge, H. C. (1984): Arsenic. In: *Clinical Toxicology of Commercial Products*, edited by R. E. Gosselin, R. P. Smith, and H. C. Hodge, pp. III-42 to III-47. Williams & Wilkins, Baltimore, MD.

223. Goyer, R. A. (1986): Toxic effects of metals. In: *Casarett and Doull's Toxicology: The Basic Science of Poisons*, 3rd ed., edited by C. D. Klaassen, M. O. Amdur, and J. Doull, pp. 582–635. Macmillan, New York.

224. Goyer, R. A., Miller, C. R., Zhu, S.-Y., and Victery, W. (1989): Non-metallothionein-bound cadmium in the pathogenesis of cadmium nephrotoxicity in the rat. *Toxicol. Appl. Pharmacol.*, 101:232–244.

225. Goyer, R. A., and Rhyne, B. C. (1973): Pathological effects of lead. *Int. Rev. Exp. Pathol.*, 12:1–77.

226. Graves, A. B., Rosner, D., Echeverria, D., Mortimer, J. A., and Larson, E. B. (1998): Occupational exposures to solvents and aluminum and estimated risk of Alzheimer's disease. *Occup. Environ. Med.*, 55:627–633.

227. Graziano, J. H., and Blum, C. (1991): Lead exposure from lead crystal. *Lancet*, 337:141–142.

228. Greengard, J. (1975): Iron poisoning in children. *Clin. Toxicol.*, 8:575–597.

229. Greger, J. L., and Johnson, M. A. (1981): Effect of dietary tin on zinc, copper, and iron utilization by rats. *Food Cosmet. Toxicol.*, 19:163–166.

230. Greger, J. L., and Sutherland, J. E. (1997): Aluminum exposure and metabolism. *Crit. Rev. Clin. Lab. Sci.*, 34:439–474.

231. Grignon, S., and Bruguerolle, B. (1996): Cerebellar lithium toxicity: A review of recent literature and tentative pathophysiology. *Therapie*, 51:101–106.

232. Groleau, G. (1994): Lithium toxicity. *Conc. Controv. Toxicol.*, 12:511–531.

233. Groth, D. H., Stettler, L. E., and Burg, J. R. (1986): Carcinogenic effects of antimony trioxide and antimony ore concentrate in rats. *J. Toxicol. Environ. Health*, 18:607–626.

234. Habeebu, S. S. M., Liu, J., and Klaassen, C. D. (1998): Cadmium-induced apoptosis in mouse liver. *Toxicol. Appl. Pharmacol.*, 149:203–209.

235. Hadjimarkos, D. M. (1965): Effect of selenium on dental caries. *Arch. Environ. Health*, 10:893–899.

236. Hadjimarkos, D. M., Storvick, C. A., and Remmert, L. F. (1952): Selenium and dental caries. *J. Pediatr.*, 40:451–455.

237. Hadjimichael, O. C., and Brubaker, R. E. (1981): Evaluation of an occupational respiratory exposure to a zirconium-containing dust. *J. Occup. Med.*, 23:543–547.

238. Haley, T. J., Komesu, N., and Raymond, K. (1962): Pharmacology and toxicology of niobium chloride. *Toxicol. Appl. Pharmacol.*, 4:385–392.

239. Haley, T. J., Raymond, K., Komesu, N., and Upham, H. C. (1962): The toxicologic and pharmacologic effects of hafnium salts. *Toxicol. Appl. Pharmacol.*, 4:238–246.

240. Hallberg, L., Brune, M., Erlandsson, M., et al. (1991): Calcium: Effect of different amounts of nonheme- and heme-iron absorption in humans. *Am. J. Clin. Nutr.*, 53:112–119.

241 Hamada, T., Tanimoto, A., and Sasguri, Y. (1997): Apoptosis induced by cadmium. *Apoptosis*, 2:359–367.

242. Hamilton, A., and Hardy, H. (1974): Osmium. In: *Industrial Toxicology*, pp. 155–156. Publishing Sciences Group, Acton, MA.

243. Hardy, A. D., Vaishnav, R., Al-Kharusi, S. S. Z., Sutherland, H. H., and Worthing, M. A. (1998): Composition of eye cosmetics (kohls) used in Oman. *J. Ethnopharmacol.*, 60:223–234.

244. Hardy, H. L., and Tabershaw, I. R. (1946): Delayed chemical pneumonitis occurring in workers exposed to beryllium compounds. *J. Ind. Hyg. Toxicol.*, 28:197–211.

245. Harlan, W. R. (1988): The relationship of blood lead levels to blood pressure in the U.S. population. *Environ. Health Perspect.*, 78:9–13.

246. Harr, J. R., and Muth, O. H. (1972): Selenium poisoning in domestic animals and its relationship to man. *Clin. Toxicol.*, 5:175–186.

247. Hartman, R. S., Conrad, M. E., Hartman, R. E., et al. (1963): Ferritin-containing bodies in human small intestinal epithelium. *Blood*, 22:397–405.

248. Hartwig, A. (1994): Role of DNA repair inhibition in lead- and cadmium-induced genotoxicity: A review. *Environ. Health Perspect.*, 102(suppl. 3):45–50.

249. Hatchcock, J. N., and Rader, J. I. (1990): Macronutrient safety. *Ann. NY Acad. Sci.*, 587:257–266.

250. Haug, R. H. (1996): Retention of asymptomatic bone plates used for orthognathic surgery and facial fractures. *J. Oral Maxillofac. Surg.*, 54:611–617.

251. Heindel, J. J., Price, C. J., Field, E. A., et al. (1992): Developmental toxicity of boric acid in mice and rats. *Fundam. Appl. Toxicol.*, 18:266–277.

252. Heinrich, U., Peters, L., Ernst, H., et al. (1989): Investigation on the carcinogenic effects of various cadmium compounds after inhalation exposure in hamsters and mice. *Exp. Pathol.*, 37:253-258.

253. Helzlsouer, K., Jacobs, R., and Morris, S. (1985): Acute selenium poisoning in the United States. *Fed. Proc. FASEB*, 44:1670.

254. .Henderson, Y., and Haggard, H. W. (1943): *Noxious Gases*, p. 133. Reinhold, New York.

255. Herrero, F., Fernandez, E., Gomez, J., et al. (1995): Thallium poisoning presenting with abdominal colic, paresthesia, and irritability. *Clin. Toxicol.*, 33:261–264.

256. Hertz-Picciotto, I., and Croft, J. (1993): Review of the relation between blood lead and blood pressure. *Epidemiol. Rev.*, 15:352–373.

257. Heyman, A., Pfeifer, J. B., Willett, R. W., and Taylor, H. M. (1956): Peripheral neuropathy caused by arsenical intoxication. *N. Engl. J. Med.*, 254:401–408.

258. Hider, R. C., Choudhury, R., Rai, B. J., et al. (1996): Design of orally active iron chelators. *Acta Haematol.*, 95:6–12.

259. Higgins, E. S., Richert, D. A., and Westerfeld, W. W. (1956): Molybdenum deficiency and tungstate inhibition studies. *J. Nutr.*, 59:539–559.

260. Hiles, R. A. (1974): Absorption, distribution, and excretion of inorganic tin in rats. *Toxicol. Appl. Pharmacol.*, 27:366–379.

261. Hipkins, K. L., Materna, B. L., Kosnett, M. J., et al. (1998): Medical surveillance of the lead exposed worker. *AAOHN J.*, 46:330–339.

262. Hirano, S., Kodama, N., Shibata, K., and Suzuki, K. T. (1990): Distribution, localization, and pulmonary effects of yttrium chloride following intratracheal instillation into the rat. *Toxicol. Appl. Pharmacol.*, 104:301–311.

263. Hirano, S., Kodama, N., Shibata, K., and Suzuki, K. T. (1993): Metabolism and toxicity of intravenously injected yttrium chloride in rats. *Toxicol. Appl. Pharmacol.*, 121:224–232.

264. Hoffman, D. J., Ohlendorf, H. M., and Aldrich, T. W. (1988): Selenium teratogenesis in natural populations of aquatic birds in central California. *Arch. Environ. Contam. Toxicol.*, 17:519–525.

265. Hogstrand, C., and Wood, C. M. (1998). Toward a better understanding of the bioavailability, physiology, and toxicity of silver in fish: Implications for water quality criteria. *Environ. Toxicol. Chem.*, 17:547–561.

266. Hollinger, M. A. (1996): Toxicological aspects of topical silver Pharmaceuticals. *Crit. Rev. Toxicol.*, 26:255–260.

267. Holmquist, I. (1951): Occupational arsenical dermatitis. A study among employees at a copper ore smelting work including investigations of skin reactions to contact with arsenic compounds. *Acta Dermatol. Venereol.*, 31(suppl. 26).

268. Hostynek, J. J. (1997): Gold: An allergen of growing significance. *Food Chem. Toxicol.*, 35:839–844.

269. Hu, H., Aro, A., Payton, M., Korrick, S., Sparrow, D., Weiss, S. T., and Rotnitzky, A. (1996): The relationship of bone and blood lead to hypertension. *J. Am. Med. Assoc.*, 275:1171–1176.
270. Hu, H., Watanabe, H., Payton, M., Korrick, S., and Rotnitzky, A. (1994): The relationship between bone lead and hemoglobin. *J. Am. Med. Assoc.*, 272:1512–1517.
271. Huel, G., Boudene, C., and Ibrahim, M. A. (1981): Cadmium and lead content of maternal and newborn hair: Relationship to parity, birth weight and hypertension. *Arch. Environ. Health*, 36:221–227.
272. Hughes, E. G. (1980): Medical surveillance of platinum refinery workers. *J. Soc. Occup. Med.*, 30:27–30.
273. Hunter, D. J., Morris, J. S., Stampfer, M. J., et al. (1990): A prospective study of selenium status and breast cancer risk. *J. Am. Med. Assoc.*, 264:1128–1131.
274. Huott, M. A., and Storrow, A. B. (1997): A survey of adolescents' knowledge regarding toxicity of over-the-counter medications. *Acad. Emerg. Med.*, 4:214–218.
275. Husain, M. H., Dick, J. A., and Kaplan, Y. S. (1980): Rare earth pneumoconiosis. *J. Soc. Occup. Med.*, 30:15–19.
276. Hussey, H. H. (1976): Phosphorus poisoning in children. *J. Am. Med. Assoc.*, 235:1366.
277. Insel, P. A., (1995): Analgesic-antipyretic and antiinflammatory agents and drugs employed in the treatment of gout. In: *Goodman & Gilman's The Pharmacological Basis of Therapeutics*, edited by J. G. Hardman, L. E. Limbird, and A. G. Gilman, pp. 617–657. McGraw-Hill, New York.
278. International Agency for Research on Cancer. (1980): Some metals and metallic compounds, *IARC Monogr. Eval. of the Carcinogen. Risk of Chem. Hum.*, 23:39–141.
279. International Agency for Research on Cancer. (1986): Potassium bromate. *IARC Monogr. Eval. Carcinogen. Risks Hum.*, 40.
280. International Agency for Research on Cancer. (1990): Chromium, nickel and welding. *IARC Monogr. Eval. Carcinogen. Risks Hum.*, 49:257–445.
281. International Agency for Research on Cancer. (1993): Beryllium, cadmium, mercury, and exposures in the glass manufacturing industry. *IARC Monogr. Eval. Carcinogen. Risks Hum.*, 58:41–237.
282. Ip, C. (1985): Selenium inhibition of chemical carcinogenesis. *Fed. Proc. FASEB*, 44:2573–2578.
283. Iregren, A. (1990): Psychological test performance in foundry workers exposed to low levels of manganese. *Neurotoxicol. Teratol.*, 12:673–675.
284. Ishinishi, N., Yamamoto, A., Hisanaga, A., and Inamasu, T. (1983): Tumorigenicity of arsenic trioxide to the lung in Syrian golden hamsters by intermittent instillations. *Cancer Lett.*, 21:141–147.
285. Ivankovic, S., Eisenbrand, G., and Preussmann, R. (1979): Lung carcinoma induction in BD rats after a single intratracheal instillation of an arsenic-containing pesticide mixture formerly used in vineyards. *Int. J. Cancer*, 24:786–788.
286. Jacobs, R. W., Duong, T., Jones, R. E., Trapp, G. A., and Scheibel, A. B. (1989): A reexamination of aluminum in Alzheimer's disease: Analysis by energy dispersive x-ray microprobe and flameless atomic absorption spectrophotometry. *Can J. Neurol. Sci.*, 16:498–503.
287. Jaffe, W. G., and Velez, F. B. (1973): Selenium intake and congenital malformations in humans. *Arch. Latinoam. Nutr.*, 23:515–517.
288. Jarup, L., Elinder, C. G., and Spang, G. (1988): Cumulative blood-cadmium and tubular proteinuria: A dose-response relationship. *Int. Arch. Occup. Environ. Health*, 60:223–229.
289. Jensen, R., Closson, W., and Rothenberg, R. (1984): Selenium intoxication—New York. *Morbid. Mortal. Weekly Rep.*, 33:157–158.
290. Johnson, J. L., and Rajagopalan, K. V. (1974): Molecular basis of the biological function of molybdenum. *J. Biol. Chem.*, 249:859–866.
291. Johnson, P. E. (1996): New approaches to establish mineral element requirements and recommendations: An introduction. *J. Nutr.*, 126:2309S–2311S.
292. Johnson, R. A., Baker, S. S., Fallon, J. T., et al. (1981): An occidental case of cardiomyopathy and selenium deficiency. *N. Engl. J. Med.*, 304:1210–1212.
293. Jones, G., and Brooks, P. M. (1996): Injectable gold compounds: An overview. *Br. J. Rheumatol.*, 35:1154–1158.
294. Kabe, I., Omae, K., Nakashima, H., Nomiyama, T., Uemura, T., Hosoda, K., Ishizuka, C., Yamazaki, K., and Sakurai, H. (1996): In vitro solubility and in vivo toxicity of indium phosphide. *J. Occup. Health*, 38:6–12.
295. Kamerbeek, H. H., Rauws, A. G., Ham, M. T., et al. (1971): Redistribution of thallium by treatment with sodium diethyldithiocarbamate. *Acta Med. Scand.*, 189:149–154.
296. Kanisawa, M., and Schroeder, H. A. (1967): Life term studies on the effect of arsenic, germanium, tin and vanadium on spontaneous tumors in mice. *Cancer Res.*, 27:1192–1195.
297. Kanisawa, M., and Schroeder, H. A. (1969): Life term studies on the effect of trace elements on spontaneous tumors in mice and rats. *Cancer Res.*, 29:892–895.
298. Kappas, A., and Maines, M. D. (1976): Tin: A potent inducer of heme oxygenase in kidney. *Science*, 192:60–62.
299. Katz, S. A. (1995): The toxicity/essentiality of dietary minerals: A review on some micronutrients prepared in honor of the award for life achievement to Doctor Krist Kostial. *Arh. Hig. Rada. Toksikol.*, 46:333–345.
300. Kaye, W. E., Novotny, T. E., and Tucker, M. (1987): New ceramics-related industry implicated in elevated blood lead levels in children. *Arch. Environ. Health*, 42:161–164.
301. Kazantzis, G. (1979): Thallium. In: *Handbook on the Toxicology of Metals*, edited by L. Friberg, G. F. Nordberg, and V. B. Vouk, pp. 599–612. Elsevier/North Holland, New York.
302. Keall, J. H. H., Martin, N. H., and Tunbridge, R. E. (1946): A report of three cases of accidental poisoning by sodium tellurite. *Br. J. Ind. Med.*, 3:175–176.
303. Keshan Disease Research Group. (1979): Epidemiologic studies on the etiologic relationship of selenium and Keshan isease. *Chin. Med. J.*, 92:477–482.
304. Kettrup, A., and Hüppe, U. (1988): Phosphorus. In: *Handbook on Toxicity of Inorganic Compounds*, edited by H. G. Sieler and H. Siegel, pp. 521–532. Marcel Dekker, New York.
305. Khera, A. K., Wibberley, D. G., and Dathan, J. G. (1980): Placental and stillbirth tissue lead concentrations in occupationally exposed women. *Br. J. Ind. Med.*, 37:394–396.
306. Kikano, G. E., and Stange, K. C. (1992): Lead poisoning in a child after a gunshot injury. *J. Fam. Pract.*, 34:498–504.
307. Kim, G.-S., Judd, D. A., Hill, C. L., and Schinazi, R. F. (1994): Synthesis, characterization, and biological activity of a new potent class of anti-HIV agents, the peroxoniobium-substituted heteropolytungstates. *J. Med. Chem.*, 37:816-820.
308. Kim, R., Rotnitzky, A., Sparrow, D., Weiss, S. T., Wager, C., and Hu, H. (1996): A longitudinal study of low-level lead exposure and impairment of renal function. *J. Am. Med. Assoc.*, 275:1177–1181.
309. Kim, T. S., and Yim, S. Y. (1997): Peripheral nerve and muscle diseases I. *Brain Pathol.*, 7:1117–1121.
310. Kimbrough, R. D. (1976): Toxicity and health effects of selected organotin compounds: A review. *Environ. Health Perspect.*, 14:51–56.
311. Kinard, F. W., and van de Erve, J. (1940): Rat mortality following sodium tungstate injection. *Am. J. Med. Sci.*, 199:668–670.

312. Kinard, F. W., and van de Erve, J. (1943): Effect of tungsten metal diets in the rat. *J. Lab. Clin. Med.*, 28:1541–1543.
313. Kittle, C. F., King, E. R., and Brucer, M. (1951): The tissue distribution and excretion of radioactive hafnium mandelate in the rat. *J. Pharmacol. Exp. Ther.*, 101:21.
314. Kjellström, T., Elinder, C.-G., and Friberg, L. (1984): Conceptual problems in establishing the critical concentration of cadmium in human kidney cortex. *Environ. Res.*, 33:284–295.
315. Kjellström, T., Friberg, L., and Rahnster, B. (1979): Mortality and cancer morbidity among cadmium-exposed workers. *Environ. Health Perspect.*, 28:199–204.
316. Klaassen, C. D. (1995): Nonmetallic environmental toxicants, In: *Goodman & Gilman's The pharmacological basis of therapeutics*, 9th ed., edited by J. G. Hardman, L. E. Limbird, and A. G. Gilman, pp. 1673–1696. McGraw-Hill, New York.
317. Klatzo, I., Wesniewski, H., and Streicher, E. (1965): Experimental production of neurofibrillary degeneration. *J. Neuropathol. Exp. Neurol.*, 24:187–199.
318. Kleinfeld, M. (1965): Acute pulmonary edema of chemical origin. *Arch. Environ. Health*, 10:942–946.
319. Kok, F. J., de Bruijn, A. M., Hofman, A., et al. (1987): Is serum selenium a risk factor for cancer in men only? *Am. J. Epidemiol.*, 125:12–16.
320. Kontoghiorghes, G. J. (1995): Comparative efficacy and toxicity of desferrioxamine, deferiprone and other iron and aluminum chelating agents. *Toxicol. Lett.*, 80:1–18.
321. Köpf-Maier, P., and Klapötke, T. (1992): Antitumor activity of ionic mobecene and molybdenocene complexes in high oxidation states. *J. Cancer Res. Clin. Oncol.*, 118:216–221.
322. Köpf-Maier, P., and Köpf, H. (1994): Organometallic titanium, vandadium, niobium, molybdenum and rhenium complexes-early transition metal antitumour drugs. In: *Metal Compounds in Cancer Therapy*, edited by S. P. Fricker, pp. 109–146. Chapman and Hall, London.
323. Koppel, C., Baudisch, H., Beyer, K.-H., et al. (1986): Fatal poisoning with selenium dioxide. *Clin. Toxicol.*, 24:21–35.
324. Kotter, J. M., and Zieger, G. (1992): Sarkoidale Granulomatose nach mehrjähriger zircokoniumexposition, eine "zirkoniumlunge." *Pathologe*, 13:104–109.
325. Kravzov, J., Rios, C., Altagracia, M., Monroy-Noyola, A., and Lopez, F. (1993): Relationship between physiochemical properties of Prussian blue and its efficacy as antidote against thallium poisoning. *J. Appl. Toxicol.*, 13:213–216.
326. Krenzelok, E. P. (1992): Sodium and potassium. In: *Hazardous Materials Toxicology*, edited by J. B. Sullivan, Jr., and G. R. Krieger, pp. 797–799. Williams & Wilkins, Baltimore, MD.
327. Krishnan, S. S., Harrison, J. E., and Crapper McLachlan, D. R. (1987): Origin and resolution of the aluminum controversy concerning Alzheimer's neurofibrillary degeneration. *Biol. Trace Element Res.*, 13:35–42.
328. Kubota, J., Allaway, W. H., Carter, D. L., et al. (1967): Selenium in crops in the United States in relation to selenium-responsive diseases of animals. *J. Agric. Food Chem.*, 15:448–453.
329. Kurtzke, J. F. (1991): Risk factors in amyotrophic lateral sclerosis. *Adv. Neurol.*, 56:245–270.
330. Laine, J., Kalimo, K., Forssell, H., and Happonen, R. P. (1992): Resolution of oral lichenoid lesions after replacement of amalgam restorations in patients allergic to mercury compounds. *Br. J. Dermatol.*, 126:10–15.
331. Lamm, S. H., Parkinson, M., Anderson, M., et al. (1992): Determinants of lung cancer risk among cadmium-exposed workers. *Ann. Epidemiol.*, 2:195–211.
332. Lampert, P. W., and Garret, R. S. (1971): Mechanism of demyelination in tellurium neuropathy. Electron microscope observations. *Lab. Invest.*, 25:380–388.
333. Landolt, R. R., Berk, H. W., and Russell, H. T. (1972): Studies on the toxicity of rhodium trichloride in rats and rabbits. *Toxicol. Appl. Pharmacol.*, 21:589–590.
334. Lanphear, B. P. (1998): The paradox of lead poisoning prevention. *Science*, 281:1617–1618.
335. Lansdown, A. B. G. (1995): Physiological and toxicological changes in the skin resulting from the action and interaction of metal ions. *Crit. Rev. Toxicol.*, 25:397–462.
336. Larner, A. J. (1995): Biological effects of tellurium: A review. *Trace Elem. Electrol.*, 12:26–31.
337. Lauwerys, R., Roels, H., Benet, P., et al. (1985): Fertility of male workers exposed to mercury vapor or to manganese dust: A questionnaire study. *Am. J. Ind. Med.*, 7:171–176.
338. Lauwerys, R. R. (1989): Metals—Epidemiological and experimental evidence for carcinogenicity. *Arch. Toxicol.* (*Suppl*), 13:21–27.
339. Leach, L. J., Maynard, E. A., Hodge, H. C., Scott, J. K., Yuile, C. L., Sylvester, G. E., and Wilson, H. B. (1970): A five year inhalation study with uranium dioxide (UO_2) dust. I. Retention and biologic effect in the monkey, dog and rat. *Health Phys.*, 18:599–612.
340. Lee, K. P., Henry, N. W., III, Trochimowicz, H. J., and Reinhardt, C. F. (1986): Pulmonary response to impaired lung clearance in rats following excessive TiO_2 dust deposition. *Environ. Res.*, 44:144–167.
341. Lee-Feldstein, A. (1983): Arsenic and respiratory cancer in man: Follow-up of an occupational study, In: *Arsenic: Industrial, Biomedical, and Environmental Perspectives*, edited by W. H. Lederer and R. J. Fensterheim, pp. 245–265. Van Nostrand Reinhold, New York.
342. Leggett, R. W. (1993): An age-specific kinetic model of lead metabolism in humans. *Environ. Health Perspect.*, 101:598–616.
343. Leonard, A., and Gerber, G. B. (1997): Mutagenicity, carcinogenicity and teratogenicity of thallium compounds. *Mutat. Res.*, 387:47–53.
344. Leonard, A., Hantson, P., and Gerber, G. B. (1995): Mutagenicity, carcinogenicity and teratogenicity of lithium compounds. *Mutat. Res.*, 339:131–137.
345. Lerda, D. (1992): Study of sperm characteristics in persons occupationally exposed to lead. *Am. J. Ind. Med.*, 22:567–571.
346. Levander, O. A. (1991): Scientific rationale for the 1989 Recommended Dietary Allowance for selenium. *Perspect. Pract.*, 91:1572–1576.
347. Lewis, G. P., Coughlin, L., Jusko, W., et al. (1972): Contribution of cigarette smoking to cadmium accumulation in man. *Lancet*, 1:291–292.
348. Liipo, K. K., Anttila, S. L., Taikina-aho, O., Ruodonen, E.-L., Toivonen, S. T., and Tuomi, T. (1993): Hypersensitivity pneumonitis and exposure to zirconium silicate in a young ceramic tile worker. *Am. Rev. Respir. Dis.*, 148:1089–1092.
349. Lin, S., Hwang, S. A., Marshall, E. G., and Marion, D. (1998): Does paternal occupational lead exposure increase the risks of low birth weight or prematurity? *Am. J. Epidemiol.*, 148:173–181.
350. Linder, M. C., and Hazegh, M. (1996): Copper biochemistry and molecular biology. *Am. J. Clin. Nutr.*, 63:797S–811S.
351. Lin-Fu, J. S. (1980): Lead poisoning and undue lead exposure in children: History and current status. In: *Low Level Lead Exposure: The Clinical Implications of Current Research*, edited by H. L. Needleman, pp. 5–16. Raven Press, New York.
352. Lison, D. (1996): Human toxicity of cobalt-containing dust and experimental studies on the mechanism of interstitial lung disease (hard metal disease). *Crit. Rev. Toxicol.*, 26:585–616.
353. Lister, J. (1875): Recent improvements in the details of antiseptic surgery. *Lancet*, 603–605.

354. Litovitz, T. L., Holm, K. C., Bailey, K. M., and Schmitz, B. F. (1992): 1991 Annual report of the American Association of Poison Control Centers National Data Collection System. *Am. J. Emerg. Med.*, 10:452–505.
355. Lockitch, G., Taylor, G. P., Wong, L. T. K., et al. (1990): Cardiomyopathy associated with nonendemic selenium deficiency in a caucasian adolescent. *Am. J. Clin. Nutr.*, 52:572–577.
356. Lokich, J., and Anderson, N. (1998): Carboplatin versus cisplatin in solid tumors: An analysis of the literature. *Ann. Oncol.*, 9:13–21.
357. Longnecker, M. P., Taylor, P. R., Levander, O. A., et al. (1991): Selenium in diet, blood, and toenails in relation to human health in a seleniferous area. *Am. J. Clin. Nutr.*, 53:1288–1294.
358. Loser, E., (1980): A two year oral carcinogenicity study with cadmium on rats. *Cancer Lett.*, 9:191–198.
359. Lovejoy, F. H. (1982): Chelation therapy in iron poisoning. *J. Toxicol. Clin. Toxicol.*, 19:871–874.
360. Lucas, P. A., Jariwalla, A. G., Jones, J. H., Gough, J., and Vale, P. T. (1980): Fatal cadmium fume poisoning. *Lancet*, 2(8187):205.
361. Lufkin, N. H., and Hodges, F. T. (1944): Cadmium poisoning, report of outbreak. *U.S. Nav. Med. Bull.*, 43:1273–1276.
362. Mabuchi, K., Lilienfeld, A. M., and Snell, L. M. (1979): Lung cancer among pesticide workers exposed to inorganic arsenicals. *Arch. Environ. Health*, 34:312–320.
363. MacGillivray, R. T., Mendez, E., Sinha, S. K., et al. (1982): The complete amino acid sequence of human serum transferrin. *Proc. Natl. Acad. Sci. USA*, 79:2504–2508.
364. Mack, R. B. (1990): The fat lady enters stage left. *N. Carol. Med. J.*, 51:636–638.
365. Mahaffey-Six, K., and Goyer, R. A. (1972): The influence of iron deficiency on tissue content and toxicity of ingested lead in the rat. *J. Lab. Clin. Med.*, 79:128–136.
366. Malbrain, M. L., Lambrecht, G. L., Zandijk, E., et al. (1997): Treatment of severe thallium intoxication. *Clin. Toxicol.*, 35:97–100.
367. Manheimer, E. W., and Silbergeld, E. K. (1998): Critique of CDC's retreat from recommending universal lead screening for children. *Public Health Rep.*, 113:38–46.
368. Manton, W. I. (1994): Lead poisoning from gunshots—A five century heritage. *Clin. Toxicol.*, 32:387–389.
369. Mappes, R. (1977): Versuche zur ausscheidung von arsen im urin. *Int. Arch. Occup. Environ. Health*, 40:267–272.
370. Marcus, R. L., Turner, S., and Cherry, N. M. (1996): A study of lung function and chest radiograms in men exposed to zirconium compounds. *Occup. Med.*, 46:109–113.
371. Marcus, W. L. (1994): Lithium: A review of its pharmacokinetics, health effects, and toxicology. *J. Environ. Path. Toxicol. Oncol.*, 13:73–79.
372. Marie, P. J., Gabra, M.-T., Hott, M., and Miravet, L. (1985): Effect of low doses of stable strontium on bone metabolism in rats. *Miner. Electrolyte Metab.*, 11:5–13.
373. Markesbery, W. R., Ehmann, W. D., Hossain, T. I. M., Aluaddin, M., and Goodin, D. T. (1981): Instrumental neutron activation analysis of brain aluminum in Alzheimer disease and aging. *Ann. Neurol.*, 10:511–516.
374. Martin, J. L., and Gerlach, M. L. (1972): Selenium metabolism in animals. *Ann. NY Acad. Sci.*, 192:193–199.
375. Martyn, C. N., Coggon, D. N., Inskip, H., Lacey, R. F., and Young, W. F. (1997): Aluminum concentrations in drinking water and risk of Alzheimer's disease. *Epidemiology*, 8:281–286.
376. Martyn, C. N., Osmond, C., Edwardson, J. A., Barker, D. J. P., Harris, E. C., and Lacey, R. F. (1989): Geographical relation between Alzheimer's disease and aluminum in drinking water. *Lancet*, 1:59–62.
377. Matsumuro, K., Izumo, S., Higuchi, I., Ronquillo, A. T., Takahashi, K., and Osame, M. (1993): Experimental germanium dioxide-induced neuropathy in rats. *Acta Neuropathol.*, 86:547–553.
378. Maurer, J. K., Cheng, M. C., Boysen, B. G., and Anderson, R. L. (1990): Two-year carcinogenicity study of sodium fluoride in rats. *JNCI*, 82:1118–1126.
379. McAlister, N. H., Abrams, H. B., Schlosser, R., and Sturtridge, W. (1990): Unintentional self-intoxication with inorganic calcium. *J. Intern. Med.*, 228:193–195.
380. McCallum, R. I. (1989): The industrial toxicology of antimony. The Ernestine Henry Lecture 1987. *J. R. Coll. Physicians Lond.*, 23:28–32.
381. McCance R. A., and Widdowson, E. M. (1937): Absorption and excretion of iron. *Lancet*, 2:680.
382. McCarron, D. A., Morris, C. D., and Cole, C. (1982): Dietary calcium in human hypertension. *Science*, 217:267–269.
383. McCaslin, F. E., and Janes, J. M. (1959): The effect of strontium lactate in the treatment of osteoporosis. *Mayo Clin. Proc.*, 34:329–334.
384. McConnell, K. P., and Portman, O. W. (1952): Excretion of dimethyl selenide by the rat. *J. Biol. Chem.*, 195:277–282.
385. McGuigan, M. A. (1996): Acute iron poisoning. *Pediatr. Ann.*, 25:33–38.
386. McKenna, K. E., Dolan, O., Walsh, M. Y., et al. (1995): Contact allergy to gold sodium thiosulfate. *Contact Dermatitis*, 32:143–146.
387. McLaughlin, A. I. G., Milton, R., and Perry, K. M. A. (1946): Toxic manifestations of osmium tetroxide. *Br. J. Ind. Med.*, 3:183–186.
388. Mead, L. D., and Geis, W. J. (1901): Physiological and toxicological effects of tellurium compounds, with a special study of their influence on nutrition. *Am. J. Physiol.*, 5:104–149.
389. Medeiros, D. M., Wildman, R., and Liebes, R. (1997): Metal metabolism and toxicities. In: *Handbook of Human Toxicology*, edited by E. J. Massaro, pp. 149–188. CRC Press, New York.
390. Mees, R. A. (1919): The nails with arsenical polyneuritis. *J. Am. Med. Assoc.*, 72:1337.
391. Meggs, W. J., Cahill-Morasco, R., Shih, R. D., et al. (1997): Effects of Prussian blue and *N*-acetylcysteine on thallium toxicity in mice. *Clin. Toxicol.*, 35:163–166.
392. Meggs, W. J., Gerr, F., Aly, M. H., et al. (1994): The treatment of lead poisoning from gunshot wounds with succimer (DMSA). *Clin. Toxicol.*, 32:377–385.
393. Meggs, W. J., Hoffman, R. S., Shih, R. D., et al. (1994): Thallium poisoning from maliciously contaminated food. *Clin. Toxicol.*, 32:723–730.
394. Miller, C. W., Davis, M. W., Goldman, A., and Wyatt, J. P. (1953): Pneumoconiosis in the tungsten-carbide tool industry. *AMA Arch. Ind. Hyg. Occup. Med.*, 8:453–465.
395. Miller, J. W., and Sayers, R. R. (1941): The response of peritoneal tissue to industrial dusts. *U.S. Public Health Serv. Rep.*, 56(1):264–272.
396. Mills, K. C., and Curry, S. C. (1994): Acute iron poisoning. *Conc. Controv. Toxicol.*, 12:397–413.
397. Monsen, E. R. (1996): New Dietary Reference Intakes proposed to replace the Recommended Dietary Allowances. *J. Am. Diet. Assoc.*, 96:754–755.
398. Moon, J. (1994): The role of vitamin D in toxic metal absorption: A review. *J. Am. Coll. Nutr.*, 13:559–569.
399. Moore, J. A. (1995): An assessment of lithium using the IEHR evaluative process for assessing human developmental and reproductive toxicity of agents. *Reprod. Toxicol.*, 9:175–210.
400. Moore, J. A. (1997): An assessment of boric acid and borax using the IEHR Evaluative process for assessing human developmental and reproductive toxicity of agents. *Reprod. Toxicol.*, 11:123–160.

401. Moore, K. E., and Brody, T. M. (1961): Effect of triethyl tin on mitochondrial swelling. *Biochem. Pharmacol.*, 6:134–142.
402. Morgan, D. L., Shines, C. J., Jeter, S. P., et al. (1997): Comparative pulmonary absorption, distribution, and toxicity of copper gallium diselenide, copper indium diselenide, and cadmium telluride in sprague-dawley rats. *Toxicol. Appl. Pharmacol.*, 147:399–410.
403. Morgan, D. L., Shines, C. J., Jeter, S. P., Wilson, R. E., Elwell, M. P., Price, H. C., and Moskowitz, P. D. (1995): Acute plumonary toxicity of copper gallium diselenide, copper indium diselenide, and cadmium telluride intratracheally instilled into rats. *Environ. Res.*, 71:16–24.
404. Morgan, J. G. (1958): Some observations on the incidence of respiratory cancer in nickel workers. *Br. J. Ind. Med.*, 15:224–234.
405. Morin, Y., and Daniel, P. (1967): Quebec beer-drinkers' cardiomyopathy: Etiological considerations. *Can. Med. Ass. J.*, 97:926–928.
406. Morton, W. E., and Caron, G. A. (1989): Encephalopathy: An uncommon manifestation of workplace arsenic poisoning? *Am. J. Ind. Med.*, 15:1–5.
407. Mowad, E., Haddad, I., and Gemmel, D. J. (1998): Management of lead poisoning from ingested fishing sinkers. *Arch. Pediatr. Adolesc. Med.*, 152:485–488.
408. Moxon, A. L., and Rhian, M. (1943): Selenium poisoning. *Physiol. Rev.*, 23:305–337.
409. Mulkey, J. P., and Oehme, F. W. (1993): A review of thallium toxicity. *Vet. Hum. Toxicol.*, 35:445–453.
410. Muntzel, M., and Drüeke, T. (1992): A comprehensive review of the salt and blood pressure relationship. *Am. J. Hypertens.*, 5:1S–42S.
411. Murray, F. J. (1995): A human health risk assessment of boron (boric acid and borax) in drinking water. *Regul. Toxicol. Pharmacol.*, 22:221–230.
412. Nakada, T., Furuta, H., Koike, H., et al. (1989): Impaired urine concentrating ability in itai–itai (ouch–ouch) disease. *Int. J. Urol. Nephrol.*, 21:201–209.
413. Nakagawa, H., and Nishijo, M. (1996): Environmental cadmium exposure, hypertension and cardiovascular risk. *J. Cardiovasc. Risk*, 3:11–17.
414. Nakamura, Y., Tsumura, Y., Tonogai, Y., et al. (1997): Differences in behavior among the chlorides of seven rare earth elements administered intravenously to rats. *Fundam. Appl. Toxicol.*, 37:106–116.
415. National Cancer Institute. (1978): *Bioassay of titanium dioxide for possible carcinogenicity*. Techn. Rep. No. 97. NCI, Bethesda, MD.
416. National Cancer Institute. (1980): *Bioassay of selenium sulfide (dermal study) for possible carcinogenicity*. NCI Tech. Rep. Ser. No. 197, NTP No. 80-18.
417. National Cancer Institute. (1980): *Bioassay of selenium sulfide (gavage) for possible carcinogenicity*. NCI Tech. Rep. Ser. No. 194, NTP No. 80-17.
418. National Cancer Institute. (1980): *Bioassay of Selsun (trade name) for possible carcinogenicity*. NCI Tech. Rep. Ser. No. 199, NTP No. 80-19.
419. National Institutes of Health. (1994): Optimal calcium intake. *NIH Consens. Stat.*, 12:1–31.
420. National Research Council. (1989): *Recommended Dietary Allowances*, 10th ed. National Academy Press, Washington, DC.
421. National Toxicology Program. (1982): *Bioassay of stannous chloride for possible carcinogenicity*. Tech. Rep. No. 231. NTP, Research Triangle Park, NC.
422. National Toxicology Program. (1987): *Toxicology and carcinogenesis studies of boric acid (CAS No. 10043-35-3) in B6C3F$_1$ mice*. U.S. Department of health and Human Services, National Institute of Health, Techn. Rep. Ser. 324, October.
423. National Toxicology Program. (1994): Toxicology and carcinogenesis studies of barium chloride dihydrate (CAS no. 10326-27-9) in F344/N rats and B6C3F$_1$ mice (drinking water studies). Tech. Rep. No. 432. NTP, Research Triangle Park, NC.
424. National Toxicology Program. (1996): Tech. Rep. Ser. No. 451: *Toxicology and carcinogenesis studies of nickel oxide in F344/N rats and B6C3F$_1$ Mice*. NIH Publication No. 96-3367. National Institute of Environmental Health Sciences, Research Triangle Park, NC.
425. National Toxicology Program. (1996): Tech. Rep. Ser. No. 453: *Toxicology and carcinogenesis studies of nickel subsulfide in F344/N rats and B6C3F$_1$ Mice*. NIH Publication No. 96-3369. National Institute of Environmental Health Sciences, Research Triangle Park, NC.
426. National Toxicology Program. (1996): Tech. Rep. Ser. No. 454: *Toxicology and carcinogenesis studies of nickel sulfate hexahydrate in F344/N rats and B6C3F$_1$ Mice*. NIH Publication No. 96-3370. National Institute of Environmental Health Sciences, Research Triangle Park, NC.
427. Needleman, H. L., Gunnoe, C., Leviton, A., et al. (1979): Deficits of psychologic and classroom performance of children with elevated dentine lead levels. *N. Engl. J. Med.*, 300:689–695.
428. Needleman, H. L., Schell, A., Bellinger, D., et al. (1990): The long-term effects of exposure to low doses of lead in childhood. An 11-year follow-up report. *N. Engl. J. Med.*, 322:83–88.
429. Neilands, J. B., Strong, F. M., and Elvehjem, C. A. (1948): Molybdenum in the nutrition of the rat. *J. Biol. Chem.*, 172:431–439.
430. Nemery, B. (1990): Metal toxicity and the respiratory tract. *Eur. Respir. J.*, 3:202–219.
431. Nemery, B., Lewis, C. P. L., and Demerts, M. (1994): Cobalt and possible oxidant-mediated toxicity. *Sci. Total Environ.*, 150:57–64.
432. Newman, D. (1890): A case of adeno-carcinoma of the left inferior turbinated body, and perforation of the nasal septum, in the person of a worker in chrome pigments. *Glasgow Med. J.*, 33:469.
433. Newton, P. E., Bolte, H. F., Daly, I. W., Pillsbury, B. D., Terrill, J. B., Drew, R. T., Ben-Dyke, R., Sheldon, A. W., and Rubin, L. F. (1994): Subchronic and chronic inhalation toxicity of antimony trioxide in the rat. *Fundam. Appl. Toxicol.*, 22:561—576.
434. Nielsen, F. H. (1992): Facts and fallacies about boron. *Nutr. Today*, 27:6–12.
435. Nielsen, F. H. (1994): Biochemical and physiologic consequences of boron deprivation in humans. *Environ. Health Perspect.*, 102(suppl. 7):59–63.
436. Nielsen, F. H. (1996): Evidence for the nutritional essentiality of boron. *Trace Elem. Exp. Med.*, 9:215–229.
437. Nielsen, F. H. (1996): How should dietary guidance be given for mineral elements with beneficial actions suspected of being essential? *J. Nutr.*, 126:2377S–2385S.
438. Nogawa, K., Honda, R., Kido, T., et al. (1989): A dose-response analysis of cadmium in the general environment with special reference to total cadmium intake limit. *Environ. Res.*, 48:7–16.
439. Nordberg, G. (1994): Assessment of risks in occupational cobalt exposures. *Sci. Total Environ.*, 150:201–207.
440. Nordberg, G., Stenstrom, T., and Slorach, S. (1973): [Cadmium poisoning caused by a cooled-soft-drink machine.] *Lakartidningen*, 70:601–604. [Swedish, English translation]
441. Notton, B. A., and Hewitt, E. J. (1971): The role of tungsten in the inhibition of nitrate reductase in spinach (*Spinacea oleracea* L.) leaves. *Biochem. Biophys. Res. Comm.*, 44:702–710.
442. Nye, L. J. J. (1929): An investigation of the extraordinary incidence of chronic nephritis in young people in Queensland. *Med. J. Austr.*, 2:145–169.
443. Oberley, L. (1988): Free radicals and diabetes. *Free Radical Biol. Med.*, 5:113–124.

444. O'Brien, P., and Kortenkamp, A. (1995): The chemistry underlying chromate toxicity. *Transition Met. Chem.*, 20:636–642.

445. Okusa, M. D., and Crystal, L. J. T. (1994): Clinical manifestations and management of acute lithium intoxication. *Am. J. Med.*, 97:383–389.

446. Olin, S. S. (1998): Between a rock and a hard place: Methods for setting dietary allowances and exposure limits for essential metals. *J. Nutr.*, 128:364S–367S.

447. Omdahl, J. L., and DeLuca, H. F. (1971): Strontium induced rickets: Metabolic basis. *Science*, 174:949–951.

448. Omura, M., Hirata, M., Tanaka, A., Zhao, M., Makita, Y., Inoue, N., Gotoh, K., and Ishinishi, N. (1996): Testicular toxicity evaluation of arsenic-containing binary compound semi-conductors, gallium arsenide and indium arsenide, in hamsters. *Toxicol. Lett.*, 89:123–129.

449. Omura, M., Tanaka, A., Hirata, M., Zhao, M., Marita, Y., Gotoh, K., and Ishinishi, N. (1996): Testicular toxicity of gallium arsenide, indium arsenide, and arsenic oxide in rats by repetitive intratracheal instillation. *Fundam. Appl. Toxicol.*, 32:72–78.

450. Osswald, H., and Goerttler, K. (1971): Arsenic-induced leucoses in mice after diaplacental and postnatal application. *Verh. Dtsch. Ges. Pathol.*, 55:289–293.

451. Ott, M. G., Holder, B. B., and Gordon, H. L. (1974): Respiratory cancer and occupational exposure to arsenicals. *Arch. Environ. Health*, 29:250–255.

452. Pak, C. Y. C., Sakhafe, K., Zerwekh, J. E., Parcel, C., Peterson, R., and Johnson, K. (1989): Safe and effective treatment of osteoporosis with intermittent slow release sodium fluoride: augmentation of vertebral bone. *J. Clin. Endocrinol. Metab.*, 68:150–159.

453. Parizek, J. (1965): The peculiar toxicity of cadmium during pregnancy. An experimental "toxaemia of pregnancy" induced by cadmium salts. *J. Reprod. Fertil.*, 9:111–112.

454. Parras, F., Patier, J. L., and Ezpeleta, C. (1987): Lead-contaminated heroin as a source of inorganic-lead intoxication. *N. Engl. J. Med.*, 316:755.

455. Patterson, C., Ericson, J., Manea-Krichten, M., and Shirahata, H. (1991): Natural skeletal levels of lead in *Homo sapiens sapiens* uncontaminated by technological lead. *Sci. Total Environ.*, 107:205–236.

456. Pegues, D. A., Hughes, B. J., and Woernle, C. H. (1993): Elevated blood lead levels associated with illegally distilled alcohol. *Arch. Intern. Med.*, 153:1501–1504.

457. Pennington, J. A., and Jones, J. W. (1987): Molybdenum, nickel, cobalt, vanadium, and strontium in total diets. *J. Am. Diet. Assoc.*, 87:1644–1650.

458. Pennington, J. A., and Shoen, S. A. (1995): Estimates of dietary exposure to aluminum. *Food Addit. Contam.*, 12:119–128.

459. Perlstein, M. A., and Attala, R. (1966): Neurologic sequelae of plumbism in children. *Clin. Pediatr.*, 5:292–298.

460. Perry, W. G., Smith, F. A., and Kent, M. B. (1994): The halogens. In: *Patty's Industrial Hygiene and Toxicology*, edited by G. D. Clayton and F. E. Clayton, pp. 4449–4521. John Wiley & Sons, New York.

461. Pershagen, G., and Bjorklund, N.-E. (1985): On the pulmonary tumorigenicity of arsenic trisulfide and calcium arsenate in hamsters. *Cancer Lett.*, 27:99–104.

462. Pershagen, G., Nordberg, G., and Björklund, N.-E. (1984): Carcinomas of the respiratory tract in hamsters given arsenic trioxide and/or benzo[a]pyrene by the pulmonary route. *Environ. Res.*, 34:227–241.

463. Pietras, R., Stavrakos, C., Gunnar, R. M., Tobin, J. R., Jr., (1968): Phosphorus poisoning simulating acute myocardial infarction. *Arch. Intern. Med.*, 122:430–434.

464. Pirkle, J. L., Brody, D. J., Gunter, E. W., et al. (1994): The decline in blood lead levels in the United States. The National Health and Nutrition Examination Surveys (NHANES). *J. Am. Med. Assoc.*, 272:284–291.

465. Pirot, F., Millet, J., Kalia, Y. N., and Humbert, P. (1996): In vitro study of percutaneous absorption, cutaneous bioavailability and bioequivalence of zinc and copper from five topical formulations. *Skin Pharmacol.*, 9:259–269.

466. Pirot, F., Panisset, F., Agache, P., and Humbert, P. (1996): Simultaneous absorption of copper and zinc through human skin in vitro. *Skin Pharmacol.*, 9:43–52.

467. Poon, R., Chu, I., Lecavalier, P., Valli, V. E., Foster, W., Gupta, S., and Thomas, B. (1998). Effects of antimony on rats following 90-day exposure via drinking water. *Food Chem. Toxicol.*, 36:21–35.

468. Preussmann, R., and Ivankovic, S. (1975): Absence of carcinogenic activity in BD rats after oral administration of high doses of bismuth oxychloride. *Food Cosmet. Toxicol.*, 13:503–508.

469. Price, C. J., Marr, M. C., and Myers, C. B. (1994): Determination of the no-observable-adverse-effect-level (NOAEL) for developmental toxicity in Sprague-Dawley (CD) rats exposed to boric acid in feed on gestational days 0 to 20, and evaluation of postnatal recovery through postnatal day 21. Report 65C-5657-200. Research Triangle Institute, Research Triangle Park, NC.

470. Price, C. J., Marr, M. C., Myers, C. B., et al. (1991): Final report on the developmental toxicity of boric acid (CAS No. 10043-35-3) in New Zealand white rabbits. NIEHS/NTP Order PB92-129550.

471. Prior, J. T., Rustad, H., and Cronk, G. A. (1957): Pathological changes associated with deodorant preparations containing sodium zirconium lactate: An experimental study. *J. Invest. Dermatol.*, 29:449–463.

472. Questel, F., Dugarin, J., and Dally, S. (1996): Thallium-contaminated heroin. *Ann. Intern. Med.*, 124:616.

473. Reddy, B. S., Rivenson, A., El-Bayoumy, K., et al. (1997): Chemoprevention of colon cancer by organoselenium compounds and impact of high- or low-fat diets. *JNCI*, 89:506–512.

474. Reed, C. E. (1956): A study of the effects on the lung of industrial exposure to zirconium dusts. *AMA Arch. Ind. Health*, 13:578–580.

475. Reeves, A. L. (1979): Barium. In: *Handbook on the Toxicology of Metals*, edited by L. Friberg, G. F. Nordberg, and V. B.Vouk, pp. 321–328. Elsevier, New York.

476. Rencher, A. C., Carter, M. W., and McKee, D. W. (1977). A retrospective epidemiological study of mortality at a large western copper smelter. *J. Occup. Med.*, 19:754–758.

477. Rifat, S. L., Corey, P. N., and McLachlan, D. R. C. (1997): Neuropsychiatric disorders in a follow-up study of northern Ontario miners. *Am. J. Epidemiol.*, 145:S16.

478. Rifat, S. L., Eastwood, M. R., Crapper McLachlan, D. R., and Corey, P. N. (1990): Effect of exposure of miners to aluminum powder. *Lancet*, 336:1162–1165.

479. Riggs, B. L., and Melton, L .J. (1983): Evidence for two distinct syndromes of involutional osteoporosis. *Am. J. Med.*, 75:899–901.

480. Rivlin, R. S. (1994): Magnesium deficiency and alcohol intake: Mechanisms, clinical significance and possible relation to cancer development (a review). *J. Am. Coll. Nutr.*, 13:416–423.

481. Rodgers, K. (1998): Platinum. In: *Immunotoxicology of Environmental and Occupational Metals*, edited by J. T. Zelikoff and P. T. Thomas, pp. 195–206. Taylor & Francis, Bristol, PA.

482. Roels, H. A., Hubermont, G., Buchet, J. P., and Lauwerys, R. (1978): Placental transfer of lead, mercury, cadmium, and carbon monoxide in women. *Environ. Res.*, 16:236–247.

483. Roels, H. A., Lauwerys, R., Buchet, J. P., et al. (1987): Epidemiological survey among workers exposed to manganese: Effects on lung, central nervous system, and some biological indices. *Am. J. Ind. Med.*, 11:307–327.

484. Roels, H. A., Lauwerys, R. R., Buchet, J. P., et al. (1989): Health significance of cadmium induced renal dysfunction: A five year follow up. *Br. J. Ind. Med.*, 46:755–764.
485. Rom, W. N. (1976): Effects of lead on female reproduction: A review. *Mt. Sinai J. Med.*, 43:542–552.
486. Roth, F. (1958): Über den Brochialkrebs Arsengeschädigter Winzer. *Virchows Arch.*, 331:119–137.
487. Rotruck, J. T., Pope, A. L., Ganther, H. E., et al. (1973): Selenium: Biochemical role as a component of glutathione peroxidase. *Science*, 179:588–590.
488. Roza, O., and Berman, L. B. (1971): The pathophysiology of barium: Hypokalemic and cardiovascular effects. *J. Pharmacol. Exp. Ther.*, 177:433–439.
489. Rubin, L. Slepyan, A. H., Weber, L. F., and Neuhauser, I. (1956): Granulomas of the axillas caused by deodorants. *J. Am. Med. Assoc.*, 162:953–955.
490. Ruta, D. A., and Haider, S. (1989): Attempted murder by selenium poisoning. *Br. Med. J.*, 299:316–317.
491. Ryan, T. P., and Aust, S. D. (1992): The role of iron in oxygen-mediated toxicities. *CRC Crit. Rev. Toxicol.*, 22:119–141.
492. Rybak, L. P. (1992): Hearing: The effects of chemicals. *Otolaryngol. Head Neck Surg.*, 106:677–686.
493. Rystedt, I., and Fischer, T. (1983): Relationship between nickel and cobalt sensitization in hard metal workers. *Contact Dermatitis.*, 9:195–200.
494. Salonen, J. T., Nyyssonen, K., Korpela, H., et al. (1992): High stored iron levels are associated with excess risk of myocardial infarction in eastern Finnish men. *Circulation*, 86:803–811.
495. Salonen, J. T., Tuomainen, T. P., Nyyssonen, K., et al. (1998): Relation between iron stores and non-insulin dependent diabetes in men: Case-control study. *Br. Med. J.*, 317:727.
496. Salonen, J. T., Tuomainen, T. P., Salonen, R., et al. (1998): Donation of blood is associated with reduced risk of myocardial infarction. The Kuopio Ischaemic Heart Disease Risk Factor Study. *Am. J. Epidemiol.*, 148:445–451.
497. Sanai, T., Okuda, S., Onoyama, K., Oochi, N., Takaichi, S., Mizuhira, V., and Fujishima, M. (1991): Chronic tubulointerstitial changes induced by germanium dioxide in comparison with carboxyethylgermainum sesquioxide. *Kidney Int.*, 40:882–890.
498. Sanchez, D. J., Colomina, M. T., and Domingo, J. L. (1998): Effects of vanadium on activity and learning in rats. *Phys. Behav.*, 63:345–350.
499. Sanchez-Delgado, R. A., Navarro, M., Perez, H., and Urbina, J. A. (1996): Toward a novel metal-based chemotherapy against tropical diseases. 2. Synthesis and antimalarial activity in vitro and in vivo of new ruthenium and rhodium-chloroquine complexes. *J. Med. Chem.*, 39:1095–1099.
500. Schafer, S. G., and Femfert, U. (1984): Tin—A toxic heavy metal? A review of the literature. *Regul. Toxicol. Pharmacol.*, 4:57–69.
501. Schecter, A., Shanske, W., Stenzler, A., et al. (1980): Acute hydrogen selenide inhalation. *Chest*, 77:554–555.
502. Schroeder, H. A., Balassa, J. J., and Vinton, W. H., Jr. (1964): Chromium, lead, cadmium, nickel and titanium in mice: Effect on mortality, tumors and tissue levels. *J. Nutr.*, 83:239–250.
503. Schroeder, H. A., Frost, D. V., and Balassa, J. J. (1970): Essential trace elements in man: Selenium. *J. Chron. Dis.*, 23:227–243.
504. Schroeder, H. A., and Mitchener, M. (1971): Scandium, chromium(VI), gallium, yttrium, rhodium, palladium, indium in mice: Effects on growth and life span. *J. Nutr.*, 101:1431–1437.
505. Schroeder, H. A., and Mitchener, M. (1975): Life-term effects of mercury, methyl mercury, and nine other trace metals on mice. *J. Nutr.*, 105:452–458.
506. Schroeder, H. A., and Mitchener, M. (1975): Life-term studies in rats: Effects of aluminum, barium, beryllium, and tungsten. *J. Nutr.*, 105:421–427.
507. Schroeder, H. A., Mitchener, M., Balassa, J. J., Kanisawa, M., and Naron, A. P. (1968): Zirconium, niobium, antimony and fluorine in mice: Effects on growth, survival and tissue levels. *J. Nutr.*, 95:95–101.
508. Schroeder, H. A., Mitchener, M., and Nason, A. P. (1970): Zirconium, niobium, antimony, vanadium and lead in rats: Life term studies. *J. Nutr.*, 100:59–68.
509. Schroeder, H. A., Mitchner, M., and Nason, A. P. (1970): Zirconium, niobium, indium, antimony, vanadium and lead in rats: Life term studies. *J. Nutr.*, 100:59–68.
510. Schwartz, J. (1988): The relationship between blood lead and blood pressure in NHANES II survey. *Environ. Health Perspect.*, 78:15–22.
511. Schwartz, J. (1994): Societal benefits of reducing lead exposure. *Environ. Res.*, 66:105–124.
512. Schwarz, K., and Foltz, C. M. (1957): Selenium as an integral part of factor 3 against dietary necrotic liver degeneration. *J. Am. Chem. Soc.*, 79:3292–3293.
513. Schwarz, K., and Mertz, W. (1959): Chromium(III) and the glucose tolerance factor. *Arch. Biochem. Biophys.*, 85:292–295.
514. Schwarz, K., Milne, D. B., and Vinyard, E. (1970): Growth effects of tin compounds in rats maintained in a trace element-controlled environment. *Biochem. Biophys. Res. Comm.*, 40:22–29.
515. Seelig, M. S., and Master, A. C. N. (1994): Consequences of magnesium deficiency on the enhancement of stress reactions: Preventive and therapeutic implications (a review). *J. Am. Coll. Nutr.*, 13:429–446.
516. Seghizzi, P., D'Adda, F., Borleri, D., Barbic, F., and Mosconi., G. (1994): Cobalt cardiomyopathy. A critical review of literature. *Sci. Total Environ.*, 150:105–109.
517. Seifert, J. (1943): Intravenous injections of soluble tin compounds. *J. Lab. Clin. Med.*, 28:1344–1348.
518. Semlitsch, M., Staub, F., and Weber, H. (1985): Titanium–aluminum–niobium alloy, development for biocompatible, high strength surgical implants. *Biomed. Tech.*, 30:334–339.
519. Seppalainen, A. M., Hernberg, S., Vesanto, R., and Kock, B. (1983): Early neurotoxic effects of occupational lead exposure: A prospective study. *Neurotoxicology*, 4:181–192.
520. Shamberger, R. J., and Frost, D. V. (1969): Possible protective effect of selenium against human cancer. *Can. Med. Assoc. J.*, 100:682.
521. Shamberger, R. J. (1971): Is selenium a teratogen? *Lancet*, 1316.
522. Shannon, M. (1998): Lead poisoning from an unexpected source in a 4-month old infant. *Environ. Health Perspect.*, 106:313–316.
523. Shannon, M., and Graef, J. W. (1989): Lead intoxication from lead-contaminated water used to reconstitute infant formula. *Clin. Pediatr.*, 28:380–382.
524. Shelley, W. B., and Hurley, H. (1958): The allergic origin of zirconium deodorant granulomas. *Br. J. Dermatol.*, 70:75–101.
525. Shils, M. E. (1988): Magnesium in health and disease. *Annu. Rev. Nutr.*, 8:429–460.
526. Shipman, D. L. (1986): Cadmium food poisoning in a Missouri school. *J. Environ. Health*, 49:89.
527. Shiraishi, N., and Waalkes, M. P. (1996): Acquired tolerance to cadmium-induced toxicity in rodent testes. *Toxic Subst. Mechan.*, 15:27–42.
528. Siegel, E., and Wason, S. (1986): Boric acid toxicity. *Pediatr. Clin. North Am.*, 33:363–367.
529. Silbergeld, E. K. (1996): Lead poisoning: the implications of current biomedical knowledge for public policy. *Maryland Med. J.*, 45:209–217.
530. Silbergeld, E. K. (1997): Preventing lead poisoning in children. *Ann. Rev. Public Health*, 18:187–210.

531. Sivjakov, K. I., and Braun, H. A. (1959): The treatment of acute selenium, cadmium, and tungsten intoxication in rats with calcium disodium ethylenediaminetetraacetate. *Toxicol. Appl. Pharmacol.*, 1:602–608.

532. Skipworth, G. B., Goldstein, N., and McBride, W. P. (1967): Boric acid intoxication from "medicated talcum powder." *Arch. Dermatol.*, 95:83–86.

533. Skoryna, S. C. (1984): Metabolic aspects of the pharmacologic use of trace elements in human subjects with specific reference to stable strontium. In: *Trace Substances in Environmental Health*, edited by D. D. Hemphill, pp. 3–20. University of Misssouri, Columbia.

534. Smith, M. I., Franke, K. W., and Westfall, B. B. (1936): The selenium problem in relation to public health. *Public Health Rep.*, 51:1496–1505.

535. Sorahan, T. (1987): Mortality from lung cancer among a cohort of nickel cadmium battery workers: 1946–1984. *Br. J. Ind. Med.*, 44:803–809.

536. Sorahan, T., and Waterhouse, J .A. H. (1983): Mortality study of nickel–cadmium battery workers by the method of regression models in life tables. *Br. J. Ind. Med.*, 40:293–300.

537. Spencer, H., Kramer, L., and Osis, D. (1988): Do protein and phosphorus cause calcium loss? *J. Nutr.*, 118:657–660.

538. Spiegl, C. J., Calkins, M. C., DeVoidre, J. J., et al. (1956): Inhalation toxicity of zirconium compounds. I. Short-term studies. Atomic Energy Commission Project, Report No. UR-460. University of Rochester, Rochester, NY.

539. Stadtman, T. C. (1977): Biological function of selenium. *Nutr. Rev.*, 35:161–166.

540. Staessen, J. A., Roels, H., and Fagard, R. (1996): Lead exposure and conventional and ambulatory blood pressure. *J. Am. Med. Assoc.*, 275:1563–1570.

541. Stal, P. (1995): Iron as a hepatotoxin. *Dig. Dis.*, 13:205–222.

542. Stayner, L., Smith, R., Thun, M., et al. (1992): A dose-response analysis and quantitative assessment of lung cancer risk and occupational cadmium exposure. *Ann. Epidemiol.*, 2:177–194.

543. Sticht, G., and Käferstein, H. (1988): Bromine. In: *Handbook on Toxicity of Inorganic Compounds*, edited by H. G. Sieler and H. Siegel, pp. 143–154. Marcel Dekker, New York.

544. Stollery, B. T. (1996): Reaction time changes in workers exposed to lead. *Neurotoxicol. Teratol.*, 18:477–483.

545. Storey, E. (1961): Strontium "rickets": Bone, calcium and strontium changes. *Aust. Ann. Med.*, 10:213–222.

546. Sunderman, F. W., Jr. (1988): Nickel. In: *Handbook on Toxicity of Inorganic Compounds*, edited by H. G. Sieler and H. Sigel, pp. 454–468. Marcel Dekker, New York.

547. Takenaka, S., Oldiges, H., Konig, H., et al. (1983): Carcinogenicity of cadmium chloride aerosols in W rats. *J. Natl. Cancer Inst.*, 70:367–373.

548. Takeuchi, A., Yoshizawa, N., Oshima, S., Kubota, T., Oshikawa, Y., Akashi, Y., Oda., T., Niwa, H., Imazeki, N., Seno, A., and Fuse, Y. (1992): Nephrotoxicity of germanium compounds: Report of a case and review of the literature. *Nephron*, 60:436–442.

549. Tam, G. K., Charbonneau, S. M., Bryce, F., Pomroy, C., and Sandi, E. (1979): Metabolism of inorganic arsenic (^{74}As) in humans following oral ingestion. *Toxicol. Appl. Pharmacol.*, 50:319–322.

550. Tamaki, S., and Frankenberger, W. T., Jr. (1992): Environmental biochemistry of arsenic. *Rev. Environ. Contam. Toxicol.*, 124:79–110.

551. Tanaka, A., Hisanaga, A., Hirata, M., Omura, M., Makita, Y., Inoue, N., and Ishinishi, N. (1996): Chronic toxicity of indium arsenide and indium phosphide to the lungs of hamsters. *Fukuoka Acta Med.*, 87:108–115.

552. Tao, S.-H., and Bolger, P. M. (1997): Hazard assessment of germanium supplements. *Regul. Toxicol. Pharmacol.*, 25:211–219.

553. Tay, C.-H., and Seah, C.-S. (1975): Arsenic poisoning from anti-asthmatic herbal preparations. *Med. J. Aust.*, 2:424–428.

554. Taylor, A., and Marks, V. (1978): Cobalt: A review. *J. Hum. Nutr.*, 32:165–177.

555. Tenenbein, M. (1996): Benefits of parenteral deferoxamine for acute iron poisoning. *Clin. Toxicol.*, 34:485–489.

556. Tepper, L. B., Hardy, H. L., and Chamberlin, R. I. (1961): *Toxicity of Beryllium Compounds* Elsevier, New York.

557. Thompson, H. J., and Becci, P. J. (1980): Selenium inhibition of *N*-methyl-*N*-nitrosourea-induced mammary carcinogenesis in the rat. *J. Natl. Cancer Inst.*, 1299–1301.

558. Thun, M. J., Schnorr, T. M., Smith., A. B., et al. (1985): Mortality among a cohort of U.S. cadmium production workers—An update. *J. Natl. Cancer Inst.*, 74:325–333.

559. Tjalve, H., and Henriksson, J. (1997): Manganese uptake in the brain via olfactory pathways. Abstract. Fifteenth International Neurotoxicology Conference, Little Rock, AR.

560. Tokudome, S., and Kuratsune, M. (1976): A cohort study on mortality from cancer and other causes among workers at a metal refinery. *Int. J. Cancer*, 17:310–317.

561. Tong, S., Baghurst, P., McMichael, A., et al. (1996): Lifetime exposure to environmental lead and children's intelligence at 11–13 years: The Port Pirie cohort study. *Br. Med. J.*, 312:1569–1575.

562. Townshend, R. H. (1982): Acute cadmium pneumonitis: A 17-year follow-up. *Br. J. Ind. Med.*, 39:411–412.

563. Tozman, E. C. S., and Gottlieb, N. L. (1987): Adverse reactions with oral and parenteral gold preparations. *Med. Toxicol.*, 2:177–189.

564. Trapp, G. A., Miner, G. D., Zimmerman, R. L., Mastri, A. R., and Heston, L. L. (1978): Aluminum levels in brain in Alzheimer's disease. *Biol. Psychiatry*, 13:709–718.

565. Traub, R. D., Rains, T. C., Garruto, R. M., Gadjusek, D. C, and Gibbs, C. J. (1981): Brain destruction alone does not elevate brain aluminum. *Neurology*, 31:986–990.

566. Tseng, W. P. (1977): Effects and dose-response relationships of skin cancer and blackfoot disease with arsenic. *Environ. Health Perspect.*, 19:109–119.

567. Tseng, W. P., Chu, H. M., How, S. W., Fong, J. M., Lin, C. S., and Yeh, S. (1968): Prevalence of skin cancer in an endemic area of chronic arsenicism in Taiwan. *J. Natl. Cancer Inst.*, 40:453–463.

568. Tsuchiya, K. (1969): Causation of ouch-ouch disease (itai-itai byo): An introductory review. Part 1. Nature of the disease. *Keio J. Med.*, 18:181–194.

569. Tsuda, T., Babazono, A., Yamamoto, E., et al. (1995): Ingested arsenic and internal cancer: A historical cohort study followed for 33 years. *Am. J. Epidemiol.*, 141:198–209.

570. Tsuda, T., Inoue, I., Kojima, M., and Aoki, S. (1995): Market basket and duplicate portion estimation of dietary intakes of cadmium, mercury, arsenic, copper, manganese, and zinc by Japanese adults. *J. Assoc. Off. Anal. Chem. Intl.*, 78:1363–1368.

571. Tümer, Z., and Horn, N. (1996): Menkes disease: Recent advances and new insights into copper metabolism. *Ann. Med.*, 28:121–129.

572. Tuohimaa, P., and Wickmann, L. (1985): Sperm production of men working under heavy-metal or organic solvent exposure. In: *Occupational Hazards and Reproduction*, edited by K. Hemminki, M. Sorsa, and H. Vanio, pp. 73–80. Hemisphere, New York.

573. Tuomainen, T. P., Punnonen, K., Nyyssonen, K., and Salonen, J. T. (1998): Association between body iron stores and the risk of acute myocardial infarction in men. *Circulation*, 97:1461–1466.

574. Tzonou, A., Lagiou, P., Trichopoulou, A., et al. (1998): Dietary iron and coronary heart disease risk: A study from Greece. *Am. J. Epidemiol.*, 147:161–166.

575. U.S. Congress. (1971): Lead-Based Paint Poisoning Prevention Act. Public Law 91-695. U.S. Government Printing Office, Washington, DC.

576. U.S. Congress. (1986): Amendments to the Safe Drinking Water Act. Public Law 99-339. U.S. Government Printing Office, Washington, DC.

577. U.S. Congress. (1992): Residential Lead-Based Paint Hazard Reduction Act of 1992. Public Law 102-550, Title X. U.S. Government Printing Office, Washington, DC.

578. U.S. Congress. (1996): Mercury-Containing and Rechargeable Battery Management Act. Public Law 104-142. U.S. Government Printing Office, Washington, DC.

579. U.S. Consumer Product Safety Commission. (1977): Lead-containing paint and certain consumer products bearing lead-containing paint. *Fed. Reg.*, 42:44199–44201.

580. U.S. Department of Health, Education, and Welfare, Food and Drug Administration. (1977): 21 CFR Parts 310.510 and 700.16, Final Rule. *Fed. Reg.*, 42:41374–41376.

581. U.S. Environmental Protection Agency. (1973): Control of lead additives in gasoline. *Fed. Reg.*, 38:33734–33741.

582. U.S. Environmental Protection Agency. (1989): *Office of Radiation Programs. Risk Assessment Methodology, Environmental Impact Statement for NESHAPS Radionuclides. Vol. I. Background Information Document*. U.S. Environmental Protection Agency, Washington, DC. EPA 520/1-89-005.

583. U.S. Environmental Protection Agency. (1990): *Office of Emergency and Remedial Response. Risk Assessment Guidance for Superfund, Vol. I. Human Health Evaluation Manual* (*Part A*). Interim final. U.S. Environmental Protection Agency, Washington, DC. EPA/540/1-89/002.

584. U.S. Environmental Protection Agency. (1990): Pesticide products containing phenylmercury and other mercury compounds; Receipt of requests for voluntary cancellation and amendments to delete uses. *Fed. Reg.*, 55:26754–26756.

585. U. S. Environmental Protection Agency. (1991): National primary drinking water regulations: Radionuclides; proposed rule. *Fed. Reg.*, 56:33050–33127.

586. U.S.Environmental Protection Agency. (1992): Health and environmental effects document for stable strontium. Office of Solid Waste and Emergency Response, Washington, DC (ECAO-CIN-G111).

587. U.S. Environmental Protection Agency. (1996): Prohibition on gasoline containing lead or lead additives for highway use. *Fed. Reg.*, 61:3832–3838.

588. U.S. Environmental Protection Agency. (1997): Implementation of the Mercury-Containing and Rechargeable Battery Management Act. Washington, DC.

589. U. S. Environmental Protection Agency. (1998): Integrated Risk Information System (IRIS). http://www.epa.gov/ngispgm3/iris/subst-fl.htm (As of July, 2000).

590. U.S. Food and Drug Administration. (1995): Lead-soldered food cans. *Fed. Reg.*, 60:33106–33109.

591. U.S. Food and Drug Administration. (1997): Iron-containing supplements and drugs: Label warning statements and unit-dose packaging requirements; Final rule. *Fed. Reg.*, 62:2217–2250.

592. van der Voet, G. B., and de Wolff, F. A. (1996): Human exposure to lithium, thallium, antimony, gold, and platinum. In: *Toxicology of Metals*, edited by L. Magos and T. Suzuki, pp. 455–460. CRC Press, New York.

593. Van Ordstrand, H. S., Hughes, R., and Carmody, M. G. (1943): Chemical pneumonia in workers extracting beryllium oxide. *Cleve. Clin. Q.*, 10:10–18.

594. Van Rij, A. M., Thomson, C. D., McKenzie, J. M., and Robinson, M. F. (1979): Selenium deficiency in total parenteral nutrition. *Am. J. Clin. Nutr.*, 32:2076–2085.

595. Veien, N. K., Hattel, T., Justesen., O., and Norholm, A. (1987): Oral challenge with nickel and cobalt in patients with positive patch tests to nickel and/or cobalt. *Acta Dermato-Venereol.*, 67:321–325.

596. Verity, M. A. (1997): Manganese neurotoxicity: Pathobiochemical aspects. Abstract. Fifteenth International Neurotoxicology Conference, Little Rock, AR.

597. Vernace, M. A., Bellucci, A. G., and Wilkes, B. M. (1994): Chronic salicylate toxicity due to consumption of over-the-counter bismuth subsalicylate. *Am. J. Med.*, 97:308–309.

598. Vilaplana, J., Grimalt, F., Romaguera, C., and Mascaro, J. M. (1987): Cobalt content of household cleaning products. *Contact Dermatitis*, 16:139–141.

599. Vinceti, M., Guidetti, D., Pinotti, M., et al. (1996): Amyotrophic lateral sclerosis after long-term exposure to drinking water with high selenium content. *Epidemiology*, 7:529–532.

600. Von Burg, R. (1992): Boron, boric acid, borates and boron oxide. *J. Appl. Toxicol.*, 12:149–152.

601. Votaw, A. L., and Zey, J. (1991): Vacuuming a mercury-contaminated dental office may be hazardous to your health. *Dent. Assist.*, 60:27–29.

602. Waalkes, M. P., and Goering, P. L. (1990): Metallothionein and other cadmium-binding proteins: Recent developments. *Chem. Res. Toxicol.*, 3:281–288.

603. Waalkes, M. P., and Rehm, S. (1992): Carcinogenicity of oral cadmium in the male Wistar (WF/NCr) rat: Effect of chronic dietary zinc deficiency. *Fundam. Appl. Toxicol.*, 19:512–520.

604. Waalkes, M. P., and Rehm, S. (1994): Cadmium and prostate cancer. *J. Toxicol. Environ. Health*, 43:251–169.

605. Ward, J. J., Thronbury, D. D., Lemons, J. E., and Dunham, W. K. (1990): Metal-induced sarcoma: A case report and literature review. *Clin. Orthopaed. Related Res.*, 252:299–306.

606. Ward, N. I., and Mason, J. A. (1987): Neutron activation analysis techniques for identifying elemental status in Alzheimer's disease. *J. Radioanal. Nuclear Chem.*, 113:515–526.

607. Warrell, R. P. (1997): Gallium nitrate for the treatment of bone metastases. *Cancer* (*Suppl.*), 80:1680–1685.

608. Webster, S. H. (1946): Volatile hydrides of toxicological importance. *J. Ind. Hyg. Toxicol.*, 28:167–182.

609. Weir, R. J., and Fisher, R. S. (1972): Toxicologic studies on borax and boric acid. *Toxicol. Appl. Pharmacol.* 23:351–364.

610. Weiss, B., Alkon, E., Weindlar, F., et al. (1993): Toddler deaths resulting from ingestion of iron supplements-Los Angeles. *Morbid. Mortal. Weekly Ref.*, 42:111–113.

611. West, D. W., Slattery, M. L., Robison, L. M., et al. (1991): Adult dietary intake and prostate cancer risk in Utah: A case-control study with special emphasis on aggressive tumors. *Cancer Causes Control*, 2:85–94.

612. Whitford, G. M. (1987): Fluorides in dental products: Safety considerations. *J. Dent. Res.*, 66:1056–1060.

613. Whitford, G. M. (1992): Acute and chronic fluoride toxicity. *J. Dent. Res.*, 71:1249–1254.

614. Whiting, S. J. (1994): Safety of some calcium supplements questioned. *Nutr. Rev.*, 52:95–97.

615. Whiting, S. J., and Wood, R. J. (1997): Adverse effects of high-calcium diets in humans. *Nutr. Rev.*, 55:1–9.

616. WHO (1998): Boron, Environmental Health Criteria 204, World Health Organization, Geneva.

617. Whorton, M. D., Haas, J. L., Trent, L., and Wong, O. (1994): Reproductive effects of sodium borates on male employees: Birth rate assessment. *Occup. Environ. Med.*, 51:761–767.

618. Wones, R. G., Stadler, B. L., and Frohman, L. A. (1990): Lack of effect of drinking water barium on cardiovascular risk factors. *Environ. Health Perspect.*, 85:355–359.

619. Wong, L. C., Heimbach, M. D., Truscott, D. R., and Duncan, B. D. (1964): Boric acid poisoning: Report of 11 cases. *Can. Med. Assoc. J.*, 90:1018–1023.

620. Woody, N. C., and Kometani, J. T. (1948): BAL in the treatment of arsenic ingestion of children. *Pediatrics*, 1:372–378.

621. Wu, M.-M., Kuo, T.-L., Hwang, Y.-H., and Chen, C.-J. (1989): Dose-response relation between arsenic concentration in well water and mortality from cancers and vascular diseases. *Am. J. Epidemiol.*, 130:1123–1132.

622. Xu, N., Majidi, V., Markesbery, W. R., and Ehmann, W. D. (1992): Brain aluminum in Alzheimer's disease using an improved GFAAS method. *Neurotoxicology*, 13:735–744.

623. Yan, A., and Davis, P. (1990): Gold induced marrow suppression: A review of 10 cases. *J. Rheumatol.*, 17:47–51.

624. Yang, G., Yin, S., Zhou, R., et al. (1989): Studies of safe maximal daily dietary Se-intake in a seleniferous area in China. II. Relation between Se-intake and the manifestation of clinical signs and certain biochemical alterations in blood and urine. *J. Trace Elem. Electrolytes Health Dis.*, 3:123–130.

625. Yang, G.-Q., Wang, S. Z., Zhou, R. H., and Sun, S. Z. (1983): Endemic selenium intoxication of humans in China. *Am. J. Clin. Nutr.*, 37:872–881.

626. Yoshimasu, F., Yasui, M., Yoshiro, Y., Iwata, S., Gajdusek, C., Gibbs, C. J., and Chen, K.-M. (1980): Studies on amyotrophic lateral sclerosis by neutron activiation analysis—2. Comparative study of analytical results on Guam PD, Japanese ALS and Alzheimer disease cases. *Folia Psychiat. Neurolog. Jpn.*, 34:75–82.

627. Yoshizawa, K., Willett, W. C., Morris, S. J., et al. (1998): Study of prediagnostic selenium level in toenails and the risk of advanced prostate cancer. *J. Natl. Cancer. Inst.*, 90:1219–1224.

628. Zheng, W., Winter, S. M., Kattnig, M. J., Carter, D. E., and Sipes, I. G. (1994): Tissue distribution and elimination of indium in male Fisher 344 rats following oral and intratracheal administration of indium phosphide. *J. Toxicol. Environ. Health*, 43:483–494.

Principles and Methods of Toxicology, Fourth Edition, edited by A. Wallace Hayes.
Taylor & Francis, Philadelphia © 2001.

Chapter 15

Ionizing Radiation

Lorris G. Cockerham, Thomas L. Walden, Jr., Cham E. Dallas, Michael R. Landauer, and G. Andrew Mickley, Jr.

The increasing use of radiation in the modern world and recent incidents of massive radiation exposure dictate that certain basic elements of radiation toxicity be addressed.

Radiation toxicology is the study of the adverse effects of radiation on living organisms. It is a multidisciplinary science, borrowing freely from several of the basic sciences. The cytopathological consequences of radiation exposure are similar to those induced in other types of cellular injury. Radiation-induced cell changes may result in death of the organism, death of the cells, modulation of physiological activity, or cancers that have no features distinguishing them from those induced by other types of cell injury.

Electromagnetic radiation is divided into nonionizing and ionizing radiation according to the energy required to eject electrons from molecules (575). Ionizing radiation, which may exhibit the properties of both waves and particles, has sufficient energy to produce ionization in matter. The ionizing radiations that exhibit corpuscular properties include alpha and beta particles whereas those that behave more like waves of energy include x-rays and gamma rays.

Radiation exposure comes from many sources and may be *directly ionizing* or *indirectly ionizing*. Directly ionizing radiation carries an electric charge that directly interacts, by electrostatic attraction or repulsion, with atoms in the tissue or medium exposed. Indirectly ionizing radiation is not electrically charged, but results in production of charged particles by which its energy is absorbed. A characteristic of charged particles produced directly or indirectly is *linear energy transfer* (LET), the energy loss per unit of distance traveled, usually expressed in kiloelectron volts (keV) per micrometer (μm). The LET, depending on the velocity and charge of the particle, may vary from about 0.2 to more than 1000 keV/μm.

DOSIMETRY AND EXPOSURE

Système Internationale

The International Commission on Radiological Units and Measurement (ICRU) introduced the "Système Internationale" or SI units in 1980 to express radiation dose (268). The gray (Gy), the SI unit for absorbed dose, corresponds to an energy absorption of 1 joule/kg or 100 rads. This concept of energy absorption is useful for determining absorbed doses of x-rays and gamma rays. However, determination of the absorbed dose in tissues exposed to fast neutron radiation involves more elaborate calculations. The absorbed dose of neutron radiation depends on the transfer of energy from neutrons to directly ionizing particles in the tissue and is described by the kinetic energy released in the material.

For general use, a quantity different from the rad or gray has been introduced, the dose equivalent. The dose equivalent allows for the relative effectiveness of a particular type of radiation. Gamma rays and x-rays are regarded as the standard and a quality factor of 1 is multiplied by the dose to compute the dose equivalent. Therefore, the dose equivalent (Seiverts, Sv) for x-rays and gamma rays is equal to the dose (grays). However, neutrons are thought to be roughly 10 times more effective in producing tissue damage than x-rays and therefore are assigned a quality factor of 10.

Exposure Factors

Before discussing the effects of ionizing radiation, some of the factors that influence the toxicity of radiation should be reviewed. One of the major factors related to the exposure is the dose or total amount of radiation received (Table 15.1). The absorbed dose of radiation is the quotient dE/dm where dE is the differential energy deposited into a differential mass, dm (268). The unit of absorbed dose, in the CGS (centimeter-gram-second) system, is the rad (radiation-absorbed dose) and 1 rad = 100 ergs/g (a dose of 1 rad of ionizing radiation has been absorbed when 100 ergs of energy have been deposited in each gram of material) (555). Another term commonly used, particularly in the field of radiation protection, is the rem (roentgen equivalent man). This unit was developed to enable radiation protection personnel to set standards of exposure (rem = rad × quality factor × distribution factor). The quality factor is a unit to equate the relative biological effectiveness (RBE) of one radiation to another and the distribution factor

Table 15.1
Radiation quantities and units used in radiobiology[a]

Unit or quantity	Symbol	Application
Becquerel	Bq	SI quantity of radioactivity Bq = 1 disintegration/s Bq = 2.7×10^{-11} Ci
Curie	Ci	Quantity of radioactivity 1 Ci = 3.7×10^{10} dps 1 Ci = 3.7×10^{10} Bq
Gray	Gy	SI unit of absorbed dose 1 Gy = 100 rad = 1 J/kg
Rad	rad	Unit of absorbed dose 1 rad = 0.01 Gy = 100 erg/g
Rem	rem	Unit of dose equivalent rad × Q × other modifying factor 1 rem = 0.01 Sv
Sievert	Sv	SI unit of dose equivalent rad × Q × other modifying factor 1 Sv = 100 rem
Linear energy transfer	LET	Energy deposition per unit of path length Usually in eV/micron
Relative biological effectiveness	RBE	Same effect from same dose of reference radiation Used in radiobiology
Quality factor	Q	Biological effectiveness of radiations
Working level	WL	1.3×10^{-5} MeV α-energy/L air
Working level month	WLM	1 WL × 170 h
Electron volt	eV	Unit of energy; 1 eV = 1.6×10^{-12} ergs 1 eV = 1.6×10^{-19} J

[a] From References 50 and 437.

attempts to compensate for the varying sensitivity of the different parts of the body. The roentgen, the amount of radiation required to produce one electrostatic unit of charge per cubic centimeter of air, is an older radiation exposure term that may still be seen in literature. This is a measure of only the actual ionizations produced by x-ray or gamma ray irradiation in air.

A second factor influencing the toxicity of radiation is the dose rate, $D = dD/dt$, the differential dose with respect to time; when there is no variability in dose dE/dm, $D = D/t$. When reviewing experiments in radiation toxicology, the variables, total dose, dose rate, type of radiation, and variability of the model, must be considered.

The exposure to radon (^{222}Rn) and radon daughters may be expressed, by convention, as the concentration of radon daughters measured in working levels (WL), and cumulative exposures over time are measured in working level months (WLM) (49). The WL is defined as any combination of radon daughters in 1 liter of air that results in the ultimate release of 1.3×10^5 MeV of potential alpha energy. This is approximately the alpha

Table 15.2
Average annual effective dose equivalent of ionizing radiations[a]

	Dose equivalent		Effective dose equivalent	
Source	mSv	mrem	mSv	%
Natural				
Radon	24.0	2400	2.0	55.0
Cosmic	0.27	27	0.27	8.0
Terrestrial	0.28	28	0.28	8.0
Internal	0.39	39	0.39	11.0
Total natural	—	—	3.0	82.0
Artificial				
Medical				
X-ray diagnosis	0.39	39	0.39	11
Nuclear medicine	0.14	14	0.14	4.0
Consumer products	0.10	10	0.10	3.0
Occupational	0.009	0.9	<0.01	<0.3
Nuclear fuel cycle	<0.01	<1.0	<0.01	<0.03
Fallout	<0.01	<1.0	<0.01	<0.03
Miscellaneous	<0.01	<1.0	<0.01	<0.03
Total artificial	—	—	0.63	18
Total natural and artificial	—	—	3.6	100

[a] From Reference 50. Reprinted with permission from *Health Effects of Exposure to Low Levels of Ionizing Radiation(BEIR V)*. Copyright 1990 by the National Academy of Sciences. Courtesy of the National Academy Press, Washington, DC.

energy emitted by the radon daughters in equilibrium with 100 pCi of radon. The WLM is defined as exposure to this concentration for a working month of 170 h.

SOURCES

The quantity of radiation present could range from the irreducible natural background levels to large scale releases such as occurred at Chernobyl and Chelyabinsk in Eastern Europe. Biological damage may be detected at levels only slightly above the former, whereas the latter would result in extreme biological toxicity of unknown proportions. The sources of radiation may be broken into two major components: technologically induced or man-made radiation and natural radiation (Table 15.2).

Technologic or Man-Made Radiation

Health Sciences

The use of man-made radiation in the health sciences is normally divided into three areas: (i) diagnostic x-ray examinations, (ii) nuclear medicine, and (iii) therapeutic radiation. In the more highly developed countries, exposure from medical sources may equal or exceed natural background radiation, but in undeveloped countries, the relative contribution of medical irradiation may be only about 5% of the total exposure (437).

The use of x-rays in diagnostic examinations, including dental, represents the single largest man-made source of radiation exposure in the U.S. population. The Bureau of Radiological Health, Food and Drug Administration (FDA), estimated that approximately 65% of the people in the United States were exposed to x-rays for medical and dental diagnostic examinations in 1970. The mean active bone marrow dose to adults was 103 mrads with the 65 and older age group receiving the highest per capita dose (48). Dental x-ray examinations are the most common of the diagnostic examinations and approximately 30% of the total diagnostic examinations are received on an outpatient basis (437).

The use of radiopharmaceuticals in nuclear medicine has almost doubled over a 10-year period. It is estimated that up to 12 million doses of radiopharmaceuticals are given each year in the U.S. for diagnostic purposes (48). However, the per capita effective dose equivalent from these procedures in the United States is only about 140 μSv (437).

Radiation therapy has been used almost exclusively for the treatment of malignant neoplasms. The high absorbed dose, 50–70 Gy, required in most malignant conditions, leads to *nonstochastic* or direct effects such as cell death.

Therefore, some of the normal tissue surrounding the neoplasm may be exposed and incur some long-range risk. The risk, however, is usually eclipsed by the immediate benefits normally associated with increased life expectancy.

Nuclear Weapons

The first atomic weapon was detonated in 1945 on a New Mexico desert north of Alamagordo. Since that day hundreds of test explosions have been conducted by the United States, the Soviet Union, the United Kingdom, India, France, and the People's Republic of China. Between 1945 and 1984, the total estimated yield of all atmospheric nuclear explosions was approximately 546 megatons (437). A one-megaton (MT) explosion equals the explosive force of 1 million tons of 2,4, 6-trinitrotoluene (TNT).

The radioactive fallout from nuclear explosions may be divided into three portions depending on the yield and height of the burst. The larger, intensively radioactive particles fall out close to the site within hours. Slightly smaller particles behave somewhat like aerosols and are dispersed into the troposphere where they will stay for a matter of months. The fallout from this portion remains in bands around the earth at the latitude of the detonation. The third portion penetrates the stratosphere and its particles are deposited worldwide over a period of months to years (196). Most of the radioactive fallout is downwind from the explosion and up to 70% is in the larger particle portion, returning to the earth close to the detonation site within hours. The intensity of the radioactivity varies inversely with distance from the site of explosion. With a steady wind, the pattern of accumulated dose of radioactivity assumes nested cigar-shaped contours, each contour denoting a particular dose.

A one-MT thermonuclear weapon detonating at ground level with a steady wind of approximately 15 miles per hour would produce a fallout radioactivity dose rate of 400 rem in 24 h in an area of approximately 400 square miles. At a dose rate of 2 rem per year, more than 20 times the maximum recommended by the U.S. Environmental Protection Agency (EPA), an area of 1200 square miles would remain unfit for use for a year and more than 20,000 square miles would be uninhabitable for a month (201).

In a nuclear explosion over 400 radioactive isotopes are released into the biosphere. Among these, about 40 radionuclides are considered potentially hazardous. Of particular interest are those isotopes whose organ specificity and long half-lives present a danger of irreversible damage or induction of malignant alterations. Both early and delayed fallout result in the deposition of radioactive material in the environment (102). The annual average whole-body fallout rate in the United States is now approximately 45 μSv (4.5 mrem) and is projected to stay at this level through the year 2000 (48,437).

Nuclear Power Production

When radiation exposure from nuclear power production is mentioned, most persons immediately think of nuclear power reactors and the environmental dispersion of radionuclides, particularly krypton 85, tritium, carbon 14, and iodine 129. However, exposure from nuclear power production should also include mining, uranium fuel fabrication, and waste storage and disposal (437).

Although uranium mines increase the amount of uranium and its decay products, along with radon and its daughters, the environmental risks from the radioactive emissions from uranium mines is insignificant (196,290). However, mill tailings may represent a significant source of environmental radiation due to the emanation of ^{222}Rn, dispersion of the tailings by wind and water, and by the use of mill tailings in building construction.

About 1000 land-based nuclear reactors have been constructed and operated at some time throughout the world. Some of the reactors were built for research, or the production of radioisotopes and plutonium. Approximately 200 naval vessels throughout the world are powered by nuclear reactors. Yet, the environmental release from nuclear operations in the United States results in a dose rate for the average person of less than 1 mrem/year (48).

Accidents

Although the environmental release of radionuclides from nuclear reactor operations is approximately 1 mrem/year per person, malfunctions can develop and accidents can happen (48). The contents of the reactor at the time of an accident, the amount of contaminant, including its physical and chemical properties, depend on the reactor type, its application, and the duration of operation (596). Not all of the nearly 800 nuclides produced in reactors are radioactive and of these only 54 are considered significant in risk assessment (196). With core damage, the severity of the accident and therefore the risk, depends on the radioactivity, mainly as ^{131}I and ^{137}Cs, being released to the environment.

Since 1952, there have been 14 reactor accidents that involved core damage. One, the Windscale, U.K. Atomic Energy Works accident, was the first time radioactive material was released from a reactor accident. In October 1957, a plutonium production reactor located on the coast of Cumbria in northwest England released approximately 740 TBq ^{131}I, 22 TBq ^{137}Cs, 8.8 TBq ^{210}Po, and 3 TBq ^{89}Sr (122,196). The core in the No. 1 Pile of the two air-cooled, graphite-moderated, natural uranium reactors was partially consumed by fire, releasing the fission products onto the seashore and foothills southwest of the Cumbrian Mountains, over much of England, and parts of northern Europe. As an aftermath of this accident, the village of Seascale has had four fatal leukemia cases in children who were under 20 years of age between 1950 and 1980. Based on statistics, only 0.5 cases would have been expected (617).

On March 28, 1979, the worst accident in the history of U.S. commercial nuclear power generation occurred on Three Mile Island (TMI) in Pennsylvania (290). Even though the accident at TMI-2 released the radionuclides ^{131}I, ^{133}Xe, and ^{135}Xe into the environment, the collective dose equivalent to the population from the release was less than 1% of the dose accrued from natural background radiation in a year (596). As with the Windscale accident, the radionuclide identified as principal concern was ^{131}I, but in this case, only 1 TBq ^{131}I was released and the fission products at TMI were retained within the vessel (121,122). Although radiation exposure to the plant workers and the public was insignificant, the nuclear power industry was set back almost a decade. Even orders for the construction of new nuclear plants were canceled (196).

The largest airborne dispersion of radionuclides thus far occurred from the explosion and ensuing 10-day fire of the graphite-moderated reactor of Unit No. 4 of the Chernobyl nuclear power station in the former Soviet Union (now Ukraine) on April 26, 1986. It has been estimated that this has been the single most costly industrial accident in history (122,196,310,596). One revealing evaluation of the economic loss from this accident has been the estimate that from 8 to 10 annual budgets for the Republic of Belarus will be consumed in order to appropriately address the effects of this disaster, just for the needs generated in that country alone (91). Another more conservative estimate puts the costs of modestly dealing with the Chernobyl nuclear accident at 45 billion dollars, not including, of course, the human and ecological toll (594). The health care needs, for instance, are only now becoming apparent (154).

Fallout from the Chernobyl nuclear disaster was very widespread, with a large amount of a variety of radionuclides distributed throughout the northern hemisphere (20,214,355,661). In Eastern Europe and Scandinavia, it has been estimated that approximately 4×10^{18} Becquerels (Bq) were dispersed by the accident (315,534,608). The radioactive cloud moved outside of the area of the Soviet Union in the first few days after the accident, and the event only became publicized when radioactive levels in Sweden became elevated, reaching 14 times background levels (121). The importance of meteorological conditions at the time and place of nuclear accidents or thermonuclear detonations was clearly evidenced in the dispersion patterns of the fallout. The majority of the ensuing environmental radioactivity now resides in the newly created nation of Belarus (immediately north of the Chernobyl nuclear complex), which now has the distinction of having approximately 30% of its territory with a significant contamination from the accident, including 20% of the forests and 18% of the farmland (315). Ukraine and Russia have most of the remainder of the inventory that was released. The most prominent radionuclides released, in terms of quantity and widespread geographic dispersion, were ^{137}Cs, ^{90}Sr, and ^{131}I. Although less widespread, significant levels of ^{239}Pu and various transuranics were also distributed in the areas around the reactor complex.

The International Atomic Energy Agency (IAEA) report published by the Soviet Union in 1987 determined a radiation dose for the two most highly contaminated areas as (i) a 106,340-man-Sv collective 50 year dose for a population of 10.1 million in Belarus, and (ii) a 80,660-man-Sv collective 50 year dose for a population of 29.8 million in Ukraine (664). Although many east European scientists in post-Soviet scientific circles challenge these estimates as too low, they do indicate a significant radiation dose to a large number of people in the contaminated areas of these two countries. Indeed, newer estimates are that the one million people in the most contaminated areas of Belarus and Ukraine will accumulate between 150,000 and 200,000 Sv (as much as the total dose for both countries in the 1987 report), with the total population dose approaching 1,000,000 Sv (429). Many villages surrounding the Chernobyl reactor area had to be abandoned, along with the entire city of Pripyat, formerly housing over 50,000 people. This made Pripyat the first sizable city in history to be abandoned solely on the basis of radioactive fallout. Some of the inhabitants of the abandoned villages were calculated to have been expected to accumulate at least 35 rem per person (429). In Belarus alone, approximately 2.2 million people live in the areas significantly contaminated by the accident, including 800,000 children (154). At least 135,000 people were evacuated just from the Chernobyl exclusion zone, now established in the areas immediately around the reactor complex (613,699).

One result of the Chernobyl accident has been that the people and the ecosystem of the contaminated areas of Belarus, Ukraine, and Russia have become a living laboratory of the consequences of widespread radioactive contamination. In the ecosystem, deposition of the radionuclides from the reactor fire and dispersion tended to be very "patchy," with variation of over 100% in soil and sediment samples even taken only meters apart (318). Uptake of radionuclides into wildlife around the reactor was very high, with radiocesium concentrations averaging 18,000 Bq/g in one rodent species (363) and up to 200 Bq/g in fish (318). Food contamination from environmental radioactivity resulted in leafy vegetables reaching 10 μCi/kg and iodine levels in milk commonly measured at 1 μCi/L (196).

The ecotoxicological effects from the Chernobyl accident have also provided an unprecedented observation recently of the widespread dispersion of radionuclides in the environment. Evaluations of the blood cell DNA of fish from the radioactively contaminated aquatic habitats near the reactor revealed abnormal DNA distributions, hyperdiploidy, and cell cycle perturbations, though there were no gross physical malformations (155,156,386,628). An even more extensive evaluation of rodents in Chernobyl-contaminated areas has been published in the last few years. A reduction in fertility and various other physiological disorders were reported in some mammalian species in the years immediately following the accident (223,365). Cytogenetic and other mutagenic effects were observed in rodents from sites ranging from the Chernobyl power plant vicinity to Sweden (142,143,250,603). At least some of the variation in response observed can be attributed to a species difference in sensitivity, such as the high radioresistance reported for *Clezhrionomys glareolus* from Chernobyl-contaminated areas (308,363). Species differences in oxidative stress enzyme response were also found in rodents from these areas, with *C. glareolus* showing radioresistance relative to another species (298), despite a much higher deposition of radionuclides measured internally (114). There was sufficient radioactivity released in the accident to kill about 400 hectares of pine forest, and more than one million square meters of ground was bulldozed and buried (430).

The human health effects of the Chernobyl nuclear accident are only now becoming evident, with additional reports appearing each year. A relatively high incidence of thyroid cancer has been documented in Belarus, Ukraine, and Russia (66,232,517). The incidence of leukemia is still under investigation, but a statistically relevant increase related to the accident has not yet been substantiated (249,334,604,703,712). An increased frequency of chromosomal aberrations have been detected in the blood cells of people living in the contaminated areas, or those who worked as liquidators in the cleanup after the accident (582,618). An increased mutation rate at human minisatellites was found in children born in a contaminated region of Belarus relative to a control population (187,188). These minisatellites provided perhaps the only currently available system for the efficient monitoring of germline mutation in humans, and it was concluded that the damage was probably not due to DNA damage induced directly at the minisatellites, but from radiation-induced damage at other sites in the genome (188). Somatic minisatellite mutation events were present in a subset of radiation-induced, but not sporadic, thyroid cancers, suggesting that this type of genomic instability may play a role in radiation-induced tumorigenesis in the thyroid gland (496). There was an increased frequency in both lymphocyte micronuclei (an assay of chromosomal integrity) and somatic mutations in erythrocytes at the glycophorin A locus of residents of Chernobyl-contaminated cities in Belarus, and these effects were significantly correlated with radiocesium content (391,537). Somatic mutation responses were also found in the glycophorin A locus of erythrocytes from Chernobyl workers from the Baltic countries (61,62) and in immigrants to Israel (707). There has been some indication that children exposed to low LET radiation due to Chernobyl may have an increase in cataract formation (166). Among children in Belarus, it was also reported that after the accident there were increases in endocrine and dermatologic diseases, digestive organ diseases, autoimmune thyroiditis, and chronic tonsillitis and adenoiditis (393).

Another serious radiation accident occurred in the central Brazilian plateau state of Goias and went virtually unnoticed by most of the world (144). The Instituto Goiano de Radioterapia, a private radiotherapy clinic in Goiânia, Brazil, ceased operation in 1985, leaving a ^{137}Cs radiotherapy unit in an insecure situation in an abandoned treatment room. In September 1987, the 50.9-TBq ^{137}Cs source was removed from the protective housing of the therapy unit. With the later rupture of the container, the ^{137}Cs became widely dispersed throughout the city's one million population. Exposure to the ^{137}CsCl resulted in 4 deaths, 28 other cases of acute radiation sickness, and 3500 m^3 of radioactive waste. The four persons who died received estimated doses ranging from 4.5 to 6.0 Gy. Other than massive accidents with widespread contamination such as occurred at Chernobyl, this is one of the most serious radiation accidents that has ever occurred.

Nuclear Waste Management

The disposal of radioactive waste is part of a dilemma facing a technologically advanced society. One of the basic demands of such a growing society is availability of convenient and inexpensive sources of energy. As the demand for energy increases, the reliance on nuclear power will increase, as will the production of radioactive waste.

Radioactive waste is classified by its physical and chemical properties as well as its source (196,236). Three general categories of radioactive waste are: (i) low level, (ii) transuranic, and (iii) high level. Low-level radioactive waste (LLRW) includes residues from laboratory research, medical institutions, uranium mill tailings, and waste generated in the cleanup of uranium, radium, and thorium processing plants. LLRW is further subdivided into classes A, B, and C, depending on the concentration, energy levels, half-life and the sources of the radionuclides in the waste. Radionuclides found in LLRW include ^{241}Am, ^{14}C, ^{242}Cm, ^{60}Co, ^{137}Cs, ^{129}I, ^{241}Pu, ^{226}Ra ^{90}Sr, ^{99}Tc, ^{230}Th, and ^{235}U. Because the national inventory of LLRW waste is growing at 10^5 m^3/year (30% from medical institutions), management of the waste is facing a crisis in storage and disposal.

Transuranic (TRU) wastes are materials containing radionuclides with atomic numbers greater than uranium, such as americium, curium, and plutonium. These wastes originate mainly as by-products in the production and fabrication of plutonium for military purposes. Resulting from an industrial process involving transuranic materials, the TRU wastes are predominantly contaminated with ^{238}Pu and ^{239}Pu. These wastes tend to be water-soluble and pose a distinct health hazard because they can contaminate a variety of physical forms ranging from absorbent papers and rubber to discarded tools.

The most radioactivity and the highest concentration of radionuclides associated with nuclear wastes is found in spent fuel from civilian nuclear power reactors, and the reprocessing of civilian and military spent fuel. Typical radionuclides found in this high-level radioactive waste (HLRW) are: ^{60}Co, ^{137}Cs, $^{239-242}$Pu, ^{106}Ru, and ^{90}Sr. Because of the high hazard duration ($>10^5$ years) associated with these nuclides, large quantities (80 million gallons in 1982) (196,236) of highly toxic liquid and solid HLRW must be isolated from the environment for thousands of years.

At present much of the HLRW is stored at temporary sites in concrete-encased steel tanks a few meters below the surface of the ground. Considering the finite lifetime of the steel tanks (15–40 years), it becomes clear that these wastes must be transferred to other containers or sites in the future. Several options for the permanent repository of radioactive waste have been considered (196,251) and the method currently in favor is in deep underground mined cavities.

The worst example of nuclear waste management has been the experience of the Soviet nuclear weapons production complex, MAYAK, which started in 1948 on the Techa River in the Ural mountains of the Soviet Union (about 60 miles from the city of Chelyabinsk). The city constructed nearby to support the facility was originally called Chelyabinsk-65 (it is now called Ozersk), and this nuclear contamination area is now usually referred to simply as Chelyabinsk. Over 2×10^7 Ci were released over time into the surrounding area, making this the largest release of radionuclides at a single site in history (428,652). Most of this inventory was released in 1957 in an explosion in a fuel reprocessing plant, referred to afterwards as the Kyshtym accident. The workers in the MAYAK facility were reported to have had high levels of radioactive exposure, exceeding 1 Gy annually for 25% of the radiochemical workers in the first 5 years of operation, with 11% of the workers overall receiving 6.3 Gy over the first decade (249). This resulted in some deaths from chronic radiation lung injury (359) and elevated lung cancer deaths and leukemia in the workers (360). In the people living in the villages along the Techa River and in the areas contaminated by the Kyshtym accident, there were also reports of high internal radionuclide doses (249) and an increased incidence of leukemia (361).

Natural Environmental Radiation

Natural background radiation is the greatest contributor to radiation exposure in the world. In most countries natural background radiation contributes slightly more than half of the absorbed radiation dose (437). Relative contributions to the total absorbed dose may range from 42% in highly developed countries to 94% in most developing countries. Exposure to natural sources of irradiation is unavoidable and life has evolved under a continuous exposure of ionizing radiation. This background radiation has three components: (a) cosmic radiation (external), (b) terrestrial radiation (external), and (c) naturally occurring radionuclides (internal).

Cosmic and Solar Radiation

Cosmic and solar radiation originate predominately from galactic sources and consist mostly of high-energy protons and alpha particles (48,437,555). Cosmic radiation at the earth's surface varies with altitude, geomagnetic latitude, and solar modulation (214,290). For instance, in the United States, 48% of the population lives at sea level to 152.5 m and receives a dose rate of approximately 27 mrem/year (0.27 μSv/year), whereas in Leadville, Colorado (altitude 3200 m), the residents receive about 125 mrem/year. This effect of altitude becomes increasingly important to passengers and crews of high-flying aircraft. It is estimated that cabin attendants and crew members receive approximately 160 mrem/year above that received at sea level (196). The cosmic rays are reduced by the earth's atmosphere, resulting in a shielding effect. This shielding effect decreases with altitude, with cosmic ray exposure doubling every 1500 m above the earth's surface (437).

Above the earth's atmosphere the radiation consists of two main components. One is the dose from highly energetic cosmic radiation geomagnetically trapped in the earth's magnetic field. The second component is received beyond the earth's magnetic field and is due to background cosmic radiation of about 85% protons and 14% alpha particles. Astronauts traveling into outer space must traverse two belts of geomagnetically trapped radiation, the primary cosmic radiation, radiation from solar flares, and directed beams of gamma rays emitted by certain quasars and pointed directly at Earth (206).

Within the United States the effect of latitude on cosmic radiation dose rate is less than 10%, with an average dose rate at sea level of about 270 μSv/year (437).

However, in the United Kingdom the annual dose rate varies from about 280 μSv a year in the south of England to 310 μSv a year in the north of Scotland (214). The dose rate variation with latitude depends primarily upon the variations in the earth's magnetic field, with which cosmic radiation interacts (48).

Terrestrial Radiation

Terrestrial radiation levels and rates from natural background sources are functions of geographic location and living habits. In most areas on earth the terrestrial radiation level varies within relatively narrow limits, but in certain regions of Brazil, China, France, Italy, Madagascar, and Nigeria, the terrestrial radiation substantially exceeds the normal range (196,398,437). For instance, a person suntanning on some beaches along the Atlantic coast of Brazil may receive as much as 17.5 cGy/year from the sand alone (437). Meanwhile, the exposure from the fine monazite particles of the soil in the Donganling and Tongyou regions of China would run between 18 cGy and 20 cGy per year (398).

The conterminous United States may be divided into three general radiation regions (48). The Atlantic and gulf costal plains receive an average of 23 mrems/year whereas the range in the Colorado plateau area may be as high as 140 mrems/year. The average terrestrial level for the remainder of the United States is only 46 mrems/year, with an estimated national average of 40 mrems/year.

The terrestrial radiation rate varies with the type of soil in the area and the naturally occurring radionuclide content of the soil. Approximately 70 of the 340 nuclides found in nature are radioactive (196). These radionuclides have existed on the earth's crust since its formation and are known as *primordial radionuclides*. These primordial radionuclides have half-lives comparable to the age of the universe and are the source of terrestrial radiation (437).

Three distinct chains of primordial radioactive elements are found in the earth's crust and account for much of the terrestrial radiation exposure (437). These are: (i) the uranium series, (ii) the thorium series, and (iii) the actinium series. Uranium, the origin of the actinium series, is found in various quantities in rocks and soils. The uranium isotopes are alpha emitters and therefore do not contribute to the gamma background radiation. The presence of uranium in soils and in fertilizers leads to its presence, via the food chain, in plant and animal tissues. At equilibrium, an adult human male may be expected to have a uranium content of 100–125 μg. The thorium (^{232}Th) decay series may also move through the food chain, but, due to its relative insolubility and low specific gravity, it is present in biological materials only in insignificant amounts (196). Thorium may be found in silty clay and peaty soils, and in such vegetables as potatoes, corn, carrots, beans, and squash. However, the principal source of human exposure is inhalation of soil particles. Thorium is removed very slowly from bone and its concentration increases with age.

Radium 226 (^{226}Ra), an alpha emitter originating in the uranium decay series, is present in varying amounts in all rocks, soils, and water, and is of special importance, along with its daughter products (437). ^{226}Ra, with a half-life of 1622 years, decays to radon (^{222}Rn), a noble gas radionuclide with a half-life of 3.8 days. Radon, to be discussed later, also emits alpha particles but adds to the gamma radiation level of the environment through its gamma-emitting descendants.

Radium is very similar to calcium and is absorbed by plants from the soil like calcium. It then passes through the food chain to humans, where 70–90% is concentrated in bone. The amount of ^{226}Ra moving through the food chain depends upon its content in the soils and its rate of absorption by plants. This rate of absorption by plants is related to the amount of exchangeable calcium in the soil. Brazil nuts, because of their tendency to concentrate barium, another chemical very similar to radium, may have a ^{226}Ra content approximately 1000 times greater than the average diet.

Radionuclides

Internal radiation results from naturally occurring radionuclides contained within the body, and contributes approximately 11–17% of the average radiation exposure of the population (50,614). Although some of the radioactive emitters may be freely dispersed throughout the body, others are concentrated in specific organs and all of the emitted decay energy is absorbed locally (555,716). The deposition of naturally occurring radionuclides such as bismuth, carbon, hydrogen, lead, polonium, potassium, radium, radon, thorium, and uranium results primarily from the inhalation and ingestion of these materials in air, food, and water (48).

In a terrestrial ecosystem, radionuclides such as ^{210}Ra, ^{226}Ra, and ^{222}Rn that occur in the soil, or are deposited in the soil, are incorporated metabolically into plants (196). In addition to root absorption, plants are contaminated by direct foliar deposition. Foliar deposition is potentially a major source of food chain radionuclide contamination because the radionuclide may be absorbed metabolically by the plant or transferred directly to animals consuming or coming in direct contact with the foliage. Individual radionuclides pass from the roots or the leaves to the remainder of the plant. Mean ^{232}Th concentrations of 0.018±0.022 Pci/kg have been found in the edible portions of 25 vegetables, including beans, carrots, corn, potatoes, and squash. Flora near the summit of the Morro do Ferro, a hill in the state of Minas Gerais, Brazil, have absorbed so much ^{228}Ra that they can easily be autoradiographed (196).

Atmospheric radionuclides are eventually deposited on surface waters as well as on the soil. Therefore, the atmosphere is coupled to soils, surface waters, and subsurface aquifers. Radionuclides are eventually transported into streams or subsurface aquifers. Those that appear in deep underground aquifers may eventually reach surface waters and become incorporated into the biosphere again.

Rivers, estuaries, and coastal waters are major receptors of effluent radionuclides from industrial plants and cities. These waters are of special importance because of their high biological activity and productivity. Phytoplankton in these relatively shallow waters convert mineral resources in the aquatic environment into food for higher organisms. Zooplankton, the basic food of several higher trophic levels, use phytoplankton as their source of nourishment. Certain bottom-dwelling fish and animals also use phytoplankton as a source of nourishment.

Once the radionuclides have settled in an aquatic system over time, they tend to accumulate in the bottom sediments. In a collection pond built to contain a significant radioactive spill, 85% of the primary radionuclide present (radiocesium) was irreversibly bound up in the sediments, with some of the rest of the radionuclides available for remobilization from the sediment and subsequent exchange with the water column (700,701). This accumulation in the sediments is an important factor in determining uptake and deposition in various aquatic species, with bottom-dwellers tending to accumulate more radionuclides than some other organisms in the water column.

The importance of radionuclides in marine and fresh water foods depends, in part, on where the radionuclide is located in the organism. A radionuclide is a higher risk if it concentrates in an organ consumed by higher organisms, such as humans, than if it is deposited in a portion that is not eaten. The radionuclides of cobalt (^{60}Co) and zinc (^{65}Zn) concentrate in edible tissues whereas those of radium (^{226}Ra) and strontium (^{90}Sr), although concentrated by clams, oysters, scallops, and certain crabs, are stored in the shell, which is not ordinarily consumed (196).

Uptake and retention of radionuclides is influenced by the portal of entry, chemistry and solubility, metabolism, and particle size. Internal contamination normally occurs via three principal routes of entry: inhalation, ingestion, and skin absorption. Of the three, inhalation is the biggest problem.

Direct ingestion from contaminated food is also a problem. Gastrointestinal exposure depends upon transit time through the gut, whereas absorption depends upon the solubility of the radionuclide. Contamination of skin with radionuclides is of less consequence because the skin forms a formidable barrier. However, contamination of an open wound may result not only in continuous radiation of the surrounding tissue, but in the introduction of the radionuclide into the rest of the body.

Regardless of the portal of entry, the radionuclide passes throughout the body of the animal and into the milk, flesh, internal organs, and eggs. When the radioactive material enters the body it becomes an internal emitter. It will continue to radiate the body until it is excreted by some physiological process, mainly through urine and feces, or until its radioactivity decays (102). The time it takes an organism to eliminate half of the radionuclide is known as the *biologic half-life* and the time necessary for a radionuclide to decay to half of its activity is the *physical half-life* (Table 15.3). If the biologic and physical half-lives are known for a particular radionuclide, the *effective half-life* may be calculated (437).

Radon

Radon (^{222}Rn), the short-lived radionuclide decay product of ^{226}Ra, accounts for approximately 60% of the effective dose equivalent from internal emitters (437). As seen in Table 15.2, radon and its decay products or progeny (^{222}Rn, ^{214}Bi, ^{214}Pb, ^{214}Po, ^{218}Po) contribute 55% of the total average annual effective dose equivalent of 3.6 mSv.

Since 1974, international concern has centered upon radon, with radon progeny as indoor air pollutants that concentrate in nearly airtight homes and office buildings, resulting from efforts directed toward energy conservation. These energy-efficient homes cause exposure to all segments of the population in which much lower air concentrations of radon progeny may be inhaled during life-span exposures (that is, at much lower dose

Table 15.3
Half-lives of some biologically significant radionuclides[a]

	Half-life		
Nuclide	Physical	Biological[b]	Effective
^{241}Am	458 y	100 y	100 y
^{14}C	5730 y	40 d	40 d
^{137}Cs	30 y	70 d	70 d
^{131}I	8 d	138 d	8 d
^{55}Fe	657 d	2000 d	494 d
^{32}P	14 d	260 d	14 d
^{239}Pu	24,000 y	180 y	180 y
^{24}Na	15 h	11 d	14 h
^{90}Sr	28 y	36 y	16 y
^{3}H	12 y	12 d	12 d
^{235}U	7.1×10^8 y	20 d	15 d
^{65}Zn	245 d	400 d	152 d

[a] From References 102, 196, 437, and 575.
[b] Whole body.

rates than those that have occurred in uranium mining populations). In addition, the low dust concentrations in such buildings with very low air changeover rates result in greatly increased fractions of radon progeny that are unattached to air carrier aerosols, causing proportionately higher radiological doses in the basal-cell epithelium of the conducting airways of the lungs. Measurements of air concentrations in Colorado Plateau uranium miners showed less than 2% unattached radon progeny, but in regions of quiet air such as in private homes, levels became an order of magnitude higher; 81% of the attached RaA may become unattached upon decay (275). During the years 1940 to 1988, many models were developed to calculate the radiation dose to the lungs as a whole or to selected regions of the respiratory tract. Dose conversion factors of rad/WLM show considerable increases above unity as the unattached fraction of radon progeny increases.

In order to define the role of attachment of radon progeny to aerosols and the incidence and site of radon progeny–induced respiratory carcinoma, a series of experimental studies used specific pathogen–free Wistar rats (627). Groups of 32 rats received inhalation exposure during 84 hours per week to 900 WL radon progeny attached to 15 mg/m^3 carnotite uranium ore dust. Exposures lasted for 150 days and the animals were then held for life-span carcinogenesis studies. These animals showed 60% incidence of squamous carcinoma or adenocarcinoma in the periphery of the respiratory tract following these prolonged inhalation exposures to radon progeny that were 98–99% attached to uranium ore dust aerosol, but the animals showed no tumors of the nasal pharynx. In marked contrast, matched groups of rodents that received exposure to radon progeny with only room-air aerosol (from 10–25% unattached, as likely to occur in private homes) displayed less than 6% squamous carcinoma in the peripheral lung but 100% nasal squamous metaplasia and several cases of squamous carcinoma in the nasal pharynx, plus 22% squamous metaplasia in the major conducting airways such as the bronchi and first generations of secondary bronchi (627). Additional studies in the same laboratory involved rats exposed to several concentrations of radon progeny attached to uranium ore dust, designed to determine the effect of exposure rate and unattached fraction of radon progeny on the nature and incidence of pulmonary carcinoma (147). Groups of 32 or 48 male specific pathogen-free Wistar rats received inhalation exposures to radon progeny in groups having unattached percentages of 1.6 and 10, the latter representing exposure conditions that might occur in minimally ventilated dwellings. Pulmonary neoplasms included epidermoid carcinoma, adenocarcinoma, adenosquamous carcinoma, mesothelioma, and adenoma. Exposure regimes included background level, 250, 500, and 1000 WL, with total exposures of 640 or 2560 WLM. Percentages of lung tumors resulting from these exposures ranged from none in the case of animals receiving background exposures to laboratory air to 47% in those animals at the 500 WL dose rate, with the total received exposure of 2560 WLM. Pathological evaluation resulting from the dose rate exposure study indicated an increase in the risk of pulmonary lung tumors as the exposure rate *decreased*.

Epidemiological studies of the incidence of bronchiogenic carcinoma among uranium miners in the Colorado Plateau, as well as in several European uranium mining studies, show considerable consistency in the relationship of the risk of bronchial carcinoma *per* WLM (275). Studies using human volunteers that inhaled significant concentrations of radon progeny attached to uranium mine aerosols in the Colorado Plateau underground mines showed 90–100% attached radon progeny that were deposited in the regions of bronchi and subsegmental bronchi (146). Because of the efficient deposition of unattached RaA in the brachia and major bronchi, the dose to bronchial epithelium from unattached RaA can be greater than three times that of unattached progeny per unit concentration in the atmosphere. Values for the dose conversion factor of rad/WLM in this region of the respiratory tract are 0.5 for underground miners. Analyses of exposures of individuals in the general population indicate values of 0.7 rad/WLM for men, 0.6 for women, 1.2 for children, and 0.6 for infants (275). The unit WLM is defined only in terms of potential alpha energy from radon progeny per liter of air. There can be very significant changes in the magnitude of this dose, with factors of up to twofold higher, due to differing characteristics of inhaled atmospheres. These significant differences are not accounted for when using WLM alone as a unit or exposure.

In 1984, the focus of attention of carcinogenesis resulting from radon progeny inhalation by humans shifted from the miners of the Colorado Plateau to the discovery of unusually high radon levels in a home built upon a geological formation called the Reading Prong in Pennsylvania. It soon became evident that each state had different problems associated with radon exposure to the general population. Whereas Pennsylvania had about 22,000 homes on its section of the Reading Prong, more than 250,000 homes were located on the New Jersey Reading Prong (495).

In order to explain the current concern concerning radon/radon progeny levels in the home, a further definition of the working levels is necessary. Because it is far simpler to measure radon, the parent, rather than the individual radon progeny, even though the latter contribute 95–98% of the dose to the respiratory epithelium, the "working level" can be defined according to its original estimate, that is, 100 pCi of radon per liter of air, which at 100% equilibrium with its progeny will give, by definition, 1.0 working level. In 1984, the National Council on Radiation Protection and Measurement Report No. 74 recommended an action level of 8 pCi per liter environmental exposures, that is, exposures to the general population. Because only 50% of equilibrium is generally assumed for radon progeny ^{218}Po, ^{214}Pb, ^{214}Bi, and ^{214}Po (i.e., one-half the concentration of the parent ^{222}Rn), this corresponds to an equivalent of 0.04 working level.

In 1986, in order to provide a more conservative position, the EPA issued a citizen's guide to radon recommending 4 pCi/L as an action level (663). The recommended caution level by the EPA is based upon linear extrapolations of high-dose level exposure over 5–30 years of a small mining population on the Colorado Plateau (663); the equating of lung cancer risk from a specified level of radon progeny to a given level of cigarette smoking is particularly difficult in that there is a close synergism between incidence of bronchogenic carcinoma in the uranium miner population and high levels of cigarette smoking by these men. The wide limits of uncertainty found in the lung cancer risk estimate associated with a given total exposure level and the importance of dose rate factors, demonstrated by recent animal and epidemiological studies, have resulted in risk estimate calculations by agencies within the United States as well as in Canada and Europe, that suggest possible lower risk per WLM or pCi/L exposure level. The action level for homes recommended by the EPA of 4 pCi/L is low when compared with that recommended by Canada and Finland (110). It is likely that countries of the European Union will follow the example of these two countries with action levels at 8 or 20 pCi/L.

RADIATION BIOCHEMISTRY

Radiation toxicity represents a dynamic interaction between radiation physical constraints and molecular damage, which are further amplified by biological processes resulting in injury (Figure 15.1). Biochemistry provides this important link through which a quantity of energy sufficient to raise the temperature of a liter of water by 0.1°C, an amount less than the caloric energy of a candy bar, can elicit toxicity resulting in death, or the beneficial therapy of a malignant tumor, diverse extremes, and yet mechanistically similar at the molecular level, the initial injurious events that occur in 10^{-17}–10^{-5} s, may be irreversible and may require seconds to years for expression. The expression of injury for some cancers is so slow that it may not be observed over the individual's lifetime. The four processes mediating and amplifying radiation toxicity, ionization and excitation, molecular injury, biochemical damage, and amplification and expression of injury, are illustrated in Figure 15.1. The first three will be discussed in this section, followed by amplification and expression of biological injury in the remaining sections. The latter sections emphasize the important roles of biological mediators and hormones in this process, as well as delineating specific risk concerns such as cancer.

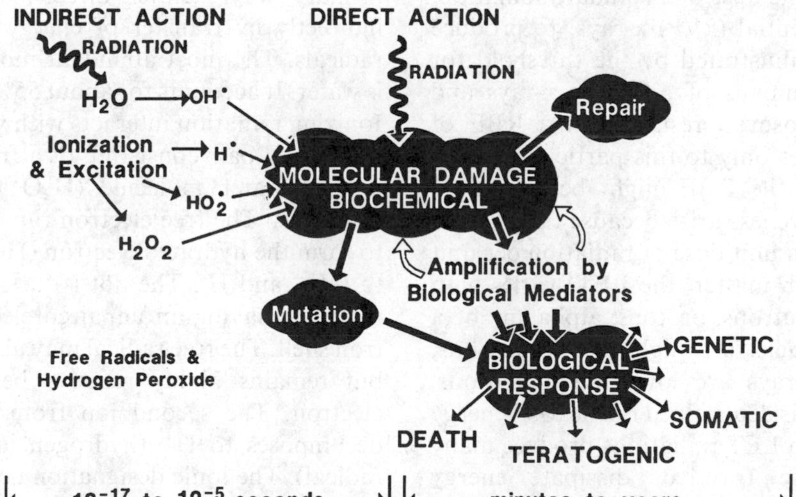

FIG. 15.1. Schematic for radiation injury to biological systems. The small quantity of radiation interacts with matter by ionization and excitation, producing both direct and indirect damage; the latter occurs primarily through free-radical attack. Because free radicals induce chain reaction of free-radical injury, the initial event is magnified. The molecular and biochemical damages in turn stimulate further amplification through the release of biological mediators and hormones. At each of these points, actions can be taken (i.e., radioprotection, radiosensitization) that will enhance or suppress the biological expression of injury. (From References 296 and 685. Used with permission.)

There are four basic possibilities for the interaction of ionizing radiation with an atom: direct and indirect ionization, excitation, and pair production. Ionization occurs through the impartation of sufficient energy to eject an electron out of its orbit, resulting in formation of an ion pair, the positively charge atom and the negatively charged electron. If the ejected electron is also imparted with additional energy, then it too may interact with other atoms to produce additional ion pairs, and this is an indirect ionization process. With excitation, the energy imparted to the electron is sufficient to raise it to a higher electron orbital, but not to escape. Ionization does not occur, but the energy may be sufficient to break chemical bonds. Between 20 to 35 electron volts (eV) are required to produce an ion pair, whereas hydrogen bonds can be broken by 5 eV (686,692). Lastly, photon radiation with energies greater than 1.02 MeV are capable of interacting with the electromagnetic field of the nucleus to convert the energy into the formation of positron and an electron, *pair production*. Neutrons, alpha particles, and other particulate radiations also produce ionization and excitation. Further, in the process of nuclear activation, the neutron is absorbed by the nucleus, forming a radioactive isotope.

Although differing types of radiation may be equal in their initial energy, they differ in the pattern in which the radiation is imparted to matter and, as a result, differ in their biological responsiveness. These differences are quantified for their *relative biological effectiveness* (RBE), determined as the dose of a given type of radiation (neutron, gamma, x-ray, etc.) to produce a reference biological effect divided by the dose of a standard radiation, usually 250 kilovolt potential (kVP) x-rays, to produce the same effect. This is illustrated by the threshold for cataract formation in humans of 2 Gy for x-rays and 0.2 Gy for neutron exposures, resulting in a RBE of 10 (48). This RBE applies only to this particular effect; for a different response the RBE might be 1 or even 50. Differences in effectiveness arise because the amount of energy transferred by a unit dose of radiation per unit pathway traveled through matter, the LET, varies with the type of radiation. Neutrons, protons, alpha and beta particles, and atomic nuclei are high LET radiations, whereas gamma and x-rays are low LET radiations. The depth of penetration is determined by the total energy and the LET factor. High LET radiations produce many ionizations per distance traveled, dissipate energy quickly, and have low depths of penetration. In fact, alpha particles dissipate all of their energy before they can transverse through a sheet of paper, a layer of paint, or the stratum corneum of the skin. The consequence of such a concentrated delivery to a biological system is that more ionizations and therefore more damage is concentrated in a smaller area, making it more difficult to repair the damage (49,686,687,692). Higher RBEs for neutrons (up to 46 for life shorting and 80 for cancer transformation) are elicited when lower doses and dose rates are used because of the better ability of cells to repair injury due to low LET radiation (115,269,493). Low dose neutron exposure is more carcinogenic for mammary tissue than x-rays, and a low environmental or accidental exposure to neutron could therefore be more damaging than the total exposure dose alone might indicate (50). In general, the LET increases from electrons to neutrons to alpha particles. The RBE increases with increasing LET up to 100–125 keV/μ (50,269). Of particular concern, low dose and dose rate exposures to high LET neutron radiation may be more effective at causing cancers than similar exposures to low LET radiation.

Radiation interacts with matter by direct and indirect processes to form ion pairs, some of which may be free radicals. These ion pairs rapidly interact with themselves and other surrounding molecules to produce free radicals. Both the indirect and direct activities of ionizing radiation lead to molecular damage which is then translated to biochemical damage. Biochemical damage may then be amplified and expressed as biological injury in one of three basic processes, including damage to the DNA which may become expressed, stimulation and release of biological mediators, and alteration of nutritional vascular support.

Radiolysis of Water

Radiation may impart energy to matter in one of two primary ways, either directly through ionizations or indirectly by transfer of energy and formation of free radicals. The most abundant molecule in living systems is water. It accounts for about 55% of the mass in humans. Ionizing radiation interacts with water molecules to form an ionized pair consisting of a free electron (e^-) and an ionized water molecule (H_2O^+) in a process termed radiolysis. The free electron rapidly interacts with water to form the hydrated electron (H_2O^-) which decomposes to OH^- and $H^\cdot$. The dot ($\cdot$) designates a free radical, a molecule having an unpaired electron in the outer electron shell. The free radical may also be electrically neutral but remains highly reactive because of the unpaired electron. The second ion from the ion pair, (H_2O^+), decomposes to H^+ (hydrogen ion) and $OH^\cdot$ (hydroxyl radical). The ionic designation depends on the molecular charge, so it is possible for a molecule to be a free radical and an ion. The hydroxyl radical contains nine protons and nine electrons, and is electrically neutral.

The end products of the radiolysis of water without oxygen are $H^\cdot$, $OH^\cdot$, H^+, and OH^-. Of these, $H^\cdot$ and $OH^\cdot$ are the most important, and comprise 55% of the initial relative yield (49). Both are highly reactive and have half-lives of 10^{-11} s. This allows for the initial impact of the radiation ionization event, which may have missed the biological target, membrane or DNA, etc., to diffuse away from the initial site and produce damage by free-radical attack of a nearby molecule. The two primary factors influencing the formation of free radicals are the presence of oxygen and the LET. Radiolysis in the presence of oxygen produces the hydroperoxy radical ($HO_2^{\cdot}$), the hydroperoxy ion (HO_2^-), and hydrogen peroxide (H_2O_2). These chemical entities are powerful oxidizing agents with longer half-lives on the order of 10^{-10} and may diffuse even farther from the initial site of ionization (49,296,692). The type of radical species formed is also governed by how closely or how rapidly radicals are formed, because they may interact to form H_2, H_2O, and H_2O_2, neutralizing the radical attack before reaching the biological target. For example, $H^{\cdot}$ reacts with $OH^{\cdot}$ to form H_2O. High LET radiations produce more ionizing events closer together, with a greater chance of free-radical neutralization. Hence, direct effects tend to predominate with high LET. The net effect of the above processes is that biological material irradiated in a dry state and in the presence of oxygen, is more resistant to injury than when the reverse conditions are present. Interaction of a free radical with a biological molecule (RH) results in the formation of an organic free radical and stabilization of the initial radical:

$$OH \cdot + RH \rightarrow H_2O + R \cdot$$

The Oxygen Effect

The most effective sensitizer of biological tissues is oxygen (269). Biological material and living systems irradiated in the presence of oxygen are more susceptible to injury than when irradiation occurs without oxygen. This response, known as the *oxygen effect* was first observed in 1909 by Gottwald Schwartz who noted that pressure applied to the forearm during irradiation reduced the resulting erythema (686). He was not aware that lack of oxygen per se was responsible. The effectiveness of oxygen in modifying the response to radiation is expressed as the *oxygen enhancement ratio* (OER), the radiation dose in the absence of oxygen to observe a given response divided by the radiation dose required to observe the response in the presence of oxygen. OERs for low LET radiations are generally 2.8 to 3, and tend to decrease as the RBE increases, up to a point, between 100 to 200 keV/μ. The radiosensitizing effects of oxygen are particularly important in radiotherapy because tumors may have hypoxic centers either because of poor vascular supply, tumor compression from the outer cells, or altered metabolism. Therapeutic attempts to address this issue have tried to increase tumor oxygenation (through increased vascularization, vasodilation, hyperbaric oxygen, or increased oxygen delivery to tissues using intravascular perfluorocarbons) or to use electronegative compounds that mimic oxygen (269). Hypoxia decreases the radiosensitivity of tissues, but increases the sensitivity to hyperthermic treatments. The oxygen concentration must be reduced below 2.0% to see any appreciable protection, which increases rapidly with decreasing oxygen concentrations below 0.5% (3 mm partial pressure of oxygen, compared to 40 mm in venous blood and 60–80 mm in oxygenated arterial blood), at which point the OER is about 2 (269). Oxygen results in the formation of hydroperoxy and hydrogen peroxide radicals that are more damaging because of their longer half-life. Free radical damage is "fixed" through reaction of oxygen leading to formation of peroxy and hydroperoxy organic products that are more resistant to biochemical repair processes (263,269). The presence of oxygen can also enhance the therapeutic efficacy of some chemotherapeutic agents, whereas some agents including misonidazole, mitomycin C, doxorubicin, and tirapazamine are more effective in hypoxic environments (269,640,641). Ethanol, narcotics, leukotrienes, and some thiols are radioprotective in part through their ability to induce hypoxia (238,686). Ethanol and narcotics suppress the respiratory center in the central nervous system, resulting in hypoxia.

Effects of Radiation on Macromolecules

Radiation-induced modification of biomolecules can be divided into structural degradation and decomposition, cross-linking of molecules, and breakage of chemical bonds (12,263,296,680,685,686,692). The individual responses for the different classes of macromolecules are presented in Table 15.4. Bond breakage occurs through energy transfer, ionization transfer, or electron transfer. Cross-linking can occur between similar and also different classes of molecules: protein–protein, lipid–lipid, protein–DNA, etc. Structural and conformational changes may alter or eliminate biochemical activity directly and expose internal sites to radical attack (117,233,692). The DNA bases are protected from free-radical attack because of their position in the center of the helix, but are exposed by strand breaks, breakage of hydrogen bonds, and unwinding processes. Conformation is also critical for enzyme activity and structural proteins. The response of macromolecules in vitro may vary from the effects in vivo due to molecular interaction and biological repair processes.

Lipid Peroxidation

Radiation injury of lipids in vitro and in vivo occurs primarily through peroxidation by free radical attack at the double bonds and carbonyls (543,685,686). Lipid

Table 15.4
Effects of ionizing radiation on macromolecules

Amino acids	Liberation of ammonia, hydrogen sulfide, pyruvic acid, carbon dioxide, and hydrogen.
Carbohydrates	Cleaveage of glycosidic bonds, depolymerization of individual monomers, oxidation of terminal alcohols to aldehydes.
DNA	Degradation with base loss or modification; breakage of hydrogen bonds or sugar-phosphate bonds; cross-linking of DNA–DNA or DNA–protein; strand breakage; formation of guanyl, thymidyl, and sugar radicals.
Lipids	Peroxidation; bond rearrangement—conjugated diene formation, aldehyde formation, β-scission, cross-linking; increased microviscosity.
Proteins	Degradation and modification of amino acids, chain scission, and cross-linkage. Denaturation and changes in molecular weight, and solubility.
Thiols	Oxidation, reduction, radical formation, cross-linkage.

Table 15.5
Steps in lipid peroxidation[a]

Initiation	
	Enzymatic
	$LH + \text{Ionizing Radiation} \rightarrow LH^{\cdot} + H^{\cdot}$
	$LH + OH^{\cdot} \rightarrow L^{\cdot} + H_2O$
	$LH + R^{\cdot} \rightarrow L^{\cdot} + RH$
Propagation	
	$L^{\cdot} + O_2 \rightarrow LOO^{\cdot}$
	$LOO^{\cdot} + LH \text{ (or RH)} \rightarrow\rightarrow L^{\cdot} \text{ (or } R^{\cdot}) + LO_2H$
Termination	
	$LOO^{\cdot} + LOO^{\cdot}$ (or $ROO^{\cdot}$)
	$L^{\cdot} + LOO^{\cdot}$
	$LO^{\cdot} + LO^{\cdot}$
	$L^{\cdot} + L^{\cdot}$
	$L^{\cdot} + R^{\cdot}$
	$L^{\cdot} + H^{\cdot}$
	$L^{\cdot}$ + free radical scavenger
	(L = lipid and R = other organic molecules)

[a] From References 357 and 543.

peroxidation, as illustrated in Table 15.5, consists of three phases: initiation, propagation, and termination. Lipid peroxidation is important to homeostasis and is associated with the formation of lipid mediators, including the prostaglandins and leukotrienes, as well as lipid degradation (Figure 15.2). Peroxidation may be mediated by three possible initial events (543,686) (Table 15.5). Initiation may occur enzymatically, as with cyclooxygenase and lipoxygenase enzymes, and requires molecular oxygen and ferric cofactors. Radiation-induced lipid peroxidation is initiated by direct or indirect ionization, or by free-radical attack. The primary radical species involved are the hydroxyl radical and superoxide (193,543).

Lipid peroxidation is affected by the lipid structure and composition, the presence of oxygen and antioxidants, pH, temperature, and the conditions of irradiation (193,543,686). Increasing the number of double bonds in the lipid carbon backbone enhances its susceptibility to free-radical oxidation in solution. For example, arachidonic acid possesses four double bonds and is more sensitive than linoleic acid which has three double bonds (477). The greater the lipid concentration, the greater the likelihood that the free radicals propagate the chain reaction by attacking another lipid molecule. On the other hand, with increased rate of radical formation, the risk of radical interaction and neutralization increases. Therefore, unlike other radiation-induced molecular injury processes, greater lipid peroxidation product yield is obtained with lower radiation doses and exposure rates.

Lipid peroxidation is a chain reaction in which interaction of the lipid radical with another organic molecule results in conversion of that organic molecule to the free-radical state and propagation of damage. Alternatively, the lipid radical may terminate the reaction by one of several different processes as outlined in Table 15.5. It may react with another free radical or with a free-radical scavenger. The primary free-radical scavengers in biological systems are vitamins A and E and the thiols, and their membrane concentrations influence cellular radiosensitivity (357,686,687). In addition, at least eight enzyme systems are associated with detoxification and repair of free-radical injury, not including DNA-specific repair enzymes (368,686). These include glutathione transferase, NADPH-dependent glutathione reductase, selenium-dependent glutathione peroxidase, selenium independent glutathione peroxi-

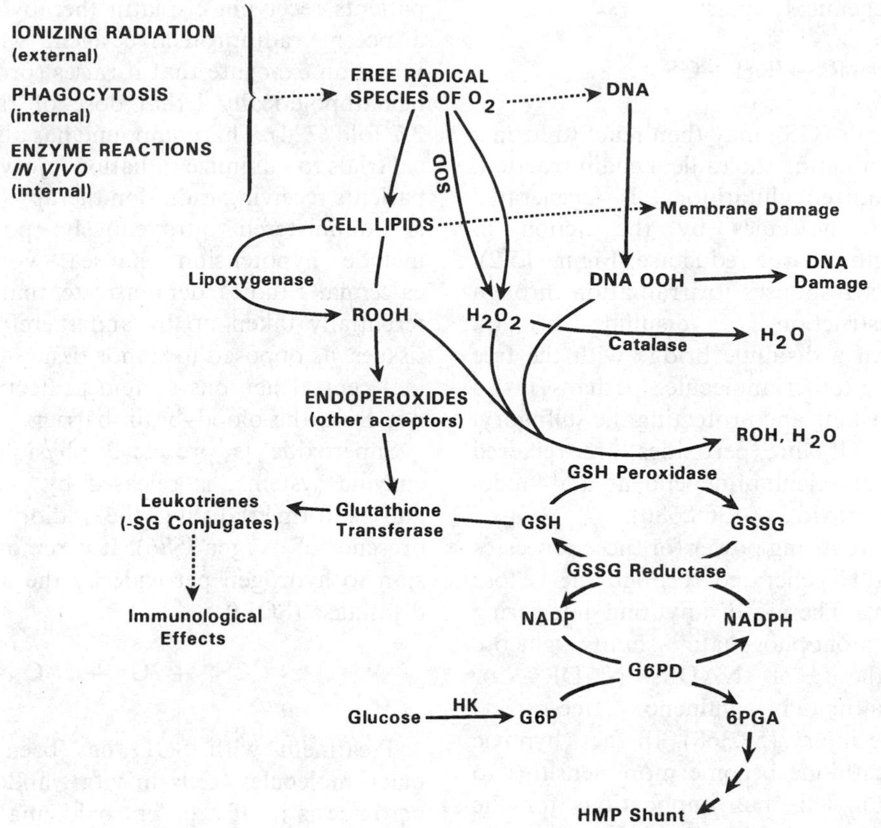

FIG. 15.2. Enzymatic repair of peroxide damage. Reactive oxygen species formed by enzymatic and nonenzymatic processes may induce oxidative attack of DNA, lipids, and other biomolecules. Repair of this damage can be mediated by glutathione (GSH-reduced glutathione) or glutathione dependent peroxidases. As shown, oxidized glutathione (GSSH-glutathione disulfide) can be reduced/renewed, and most of the system can be maintained as long as a sufficient supply of reducing power (NADPH-nicotinamide adenosine diphosphate) generated by the metabolism of glucose is available. DNA-deoxyribonucleic acid; G6PD-glucose 6-phosphate dehydrogenase; HK-Hexokinase; HMP-hexose monophosphate shunt; ROOH-organic peroxide; SOD-superoxide dismutase. (From Reference 368. Used with permission.)

dase, ferric superoxide dismutase, manganese superoxide dismutase, copper-zinc superoxide dismutase, and catalase. Metallothionein is another protein with free-radical scavenging ability, because one third of its amino acids are cysteine residues. Synthesis of this protein is enhanced under stress situations, including lipid peroxidation and radiation injury (686), and can be induced by zinc supplementation. Another thiol-containing protein, thioredoxin, participates in the reduction of a number of important DNA enzymes and transcription factors, including ribonucleotide reductase (225), and is a radioprotectant. It is itself reduced by NADPH-dependent thioredoxin reductase, a selenoprotein. Vitamin E is an important free-radical scavenger that is located primarily in the cell membrane. Once modified or activated by free-radical attack, it is detoxified and renewed by specific enzymatic pathways. Vitamin E interacts with organic radicals to form a stable organic alcohol (357). In this process, vitamin E is converted to an excited state that is restored by interaction with vitamin C. Vitamin C, in turn, is renewed through the action of an NADH-dependent enzyme. Interestingly, melatonin, the pineal gland hormone, has been demonstrated to scavenge free radicals (546), and pretreatment of human lymphocytes irradiated in vitro reduced subsequent micronuclei damage (678).

Thiols are molecules containing free or potential sulfhydryl groups (SH^-) in their structure. Examples include the amino acids methionine and cysteine, and the complex lipid thiol ether, leukotriene C_4. The most abundant nonprotein thiol, the tripeptide glutathione (GSH), is present intracellularly at 1–3 mM. Thiols act as cofactors for some enzymatic processes and participate in radical scavenging and detoxification processes. Their activities are dependent on cellular concentration, location, synthesis, and catabolism. During the reaction of a thiol with a free radical, donation of hydrogen by the reduced sulfhydryl of the thiol to the organic radical results in a form of chemical repair:

$$GSH + R^{\cdot} \rightarrow RH + GS^{\cdot}$$

Two glutathione radicals ($GS^{\cdot}$) may then react to form a disulfide (GSSG), terminating the radical chain reaction. This disulfide, or oxidized glutathione, is regenerated to yield two GSH molecules by the action of NAPDH-dependent glutathione reductase (Figure 15.2). Thiols may also affect responses to irradiation through formation and destruction of disulfide bridges. Glutathione may form a disulfide bridge with the free sulfhydryl group of another molecule, perhaps in an enzyme active site, masking and protecting the sulfhydryl from radical injury. Organic peroxides are repaired through the actions of selenium-dependent and -independent glutathione peroxidases (368,686).

Hydrogen donation reducing power for these processes is provided by NADPH generated through the hexose monophosphate shunt. Therefore, anything interfering with the hexose monophosphate shunt, glucose utilization, or synthesis of NAD^+, $NADP^+$, or glutathione may ultimately influence free-radical scavenging and tissue injury (59,368). In fact, hypoxic cells depleted of glutathione become more sensitive to radiation (59,463,686). This has implications for the radiotherapy of tumor cells, although sensitization has not been consistently observed for aerobic cells (686). The difficulty arises in that glutathione concentrations must be reduced below 5% for sensitization to be observed (463,686). Yet, even at these low levels, glutathione-dependent enzymes usually maintain activity because they retain glutathione. The depletion of glutathione levels by use of specific glutathione synthetase inhibitors, such as buthionine sulfoximine, may have a greater effect on DNA damage, because glutathione synthesis does not take place in the nucleus (29). Glutathione must diffuse into the nucleus. As a result, glutathione depletion in the nucleus would subject the DNA to greater free-radical damage. The participation of other non-glutathione-dependent enzyme systems for modification of oxidative damage also limits the significance of glutathione during irradiation under aerobic conditions. Under aerobic conditions, the electron transport chain ensures a steady supply of NADPH to drive the glutathione-dependent repair enzymes. Because of their roles in free-radical scavenging, chemical repair, and, in some instances, the induction of hypoxia, thiol compounds have been studied extensively as potential agents for radioprotection.

Amifostine (WR-2721) is an organothiophosphate initially developed through the Antioxidation Drug Development Program of the Walter Reed Army Institute of Research, and is approved by the Food and Drug Administration for chemoprotection of the kidneys in patients receiving cisplatin therapy. Amifostine is such a potent radioprotective agent when given prior to radiation exposure that it raises (protects) the necessary hematopoietically lethal dose of radiation by 2.5- to 2.7-fold (724). This compound has also been used in clinical trials to minimize radiation injury to normal tissues of patients receiving radiation therapy (115,178,269,353). It is administered intravenously; potential side effects include hypotension, nausea, vomiting, and hypocalcemia. Studies demonstrate that amifostine is preferentially taken up by and therefore protects normal tissues, as opposed to tumor tissues (725). There is minimal central nervous system protection, because it does not cross the blood–brain barrier.

Superoxide is produced physiologically by several enzyme systems, is released by activated neutrophils, and is formed during the radiolysis of water in the presence of oxygen (686). It is removed through conversion to hydrogen peroxide by the action of superoxide dismutase (SOD):

$$2H^+ + 2O_2 \rightarrow H_2O_2 + O_2$$

Treatment with SOD has been shown to protect macromolecules, cells in vitro, and animals. Hydrogen peroxide is itself a potent oxidizing agent that can also be converted, in the presence of ferric compounds, to yield hydroxyl radicals. Hydrogen peroxide is decomposed by catalase:

$$2H_2O_2 \rightarrow 2H_2O + O_2$$

Nitric oxide, NO, is a neurotransmitter and also acts as endothelial cell relaxation factor, a vasodilator. Superoxide interacts with nitric oxide to form NO_2 and NO_3, processes that are inhibited by SOD. As such, SOD potentiates the response to nitric oxide. Peroxynitrite ($ONOO^-$) is a toxic oxidant product from superoxide and nitric oxide interaction that can breakdown to hydroxyl and nitrous oxide radicals that participate in lipid peroxidation (203). There is much interest in the biological roles of nitric oxide, with as yet little information on modification by ionizing radiation. There are three isozymes of nitrite synthetase, one of which is an inducible form, which has been shown to stimulated in the rate colon and ileum (401). The increase in nitric oxide is thought to be associated with radiation-induced ileal dysfunction (401). Exposure of mice to 7 Gy of gamma irradiation has been shown to stimulate the L-arginine–dependent production of nitric oxide from the terminal guanidine group in mouse liver, lung, brain, and spleen (679). Treatment of mice with a specific inhibitor of nitric oxide synthetase, or with DEA/NO, a nitric oxide–releasing agent, results in increased animal survival of the irradiated mice. Interestingly, both agents have been shown to increase the hypoxic fraction of the mouse bone marrow, and this may be related to alterations in regional blood flow (induction of acute hypoxia). Protection is most effective when these compounds are given close to and before irradiation.

Because of its similarities to oxygen, nitric oxide has also been evaluated as a radiosensitizing agent to hypoxic cells in vitro, with a sensitization enhancement ratio of 2.4 (464). It is thought that under hypoxic conditions, the free radical, nitric oxide, interacts with carbon-based free radicals to "fix" radiation-induced free-radical injury in a manner similar to oxygen.

Effects on Amino Acids, Peptides, and Proteins

The primary effects of radiation on amino acids and proteins in solution are provided in Table 15.4 (12,384,686). Radiation-induced breakage of hydrogen bonds and disulfide bridges, or cross-linkage formation, can affect conformation and therefore activity/function. The radiation dose to inactivate proteins in the dried state is proportional to the molecular weight, that is, a larger target requires more radiation. This relationship has established radiation-inactivation of proteins as an accepted method of determining molecular weights. Further alterations may occur from moderation of radiation synthesis, although, in general, protein synthesis is not affected by radiation doses within the lethal range for humans (12,507). RNA synthesis usually decreases following irradiation of radiosensitive tissues (12,686). Radiation effects on inducible enzyme systems depend on the particular system and vary between species and sexes. Some drug detoxification enzymes are reduced in males in association with decreased testosterone synthesis. Chronic radiation exposure has been shown to induce the hsp 70 heat shock protein (hsp) in mouse lung (436), whereas 0.25 Gy to cells in vitro induces PBP74/mortalin/Grp75, another member of the heat shock protein family (571). Induction of heat shock proteins have been related to increased radioresistance.

Effects on Carbohydrates

The basic effects of carbohydrates in solution are shown in Table 15.4. Radiation may cause depolymerization of glycogen, because the α-glycosidic linkages found in glycogen and cellulose are more radiosensitive than β-glycosidic linkages that might be found in bacterial cell walls (686). In vivo, the effects of radiation on carbohydrates are dominated by alterations in metabolic processes. Radiation promotes glycogenesis and gluconeogenesis during the first several days post-irradiation primarily as a result of hormonal influences and alterations in metabolic enzymes (12,113,686). Insulin and adrenocorticoid release stimulates an increase in blood glucose, providing a source for the glycogen synthesis which is further supplemented by shunting of amino acids released by tissue injury. Decreases in hexokinase, aldolase, and pyruvate kinase and an increase in transketolase are observed (113,686). Additional NAPDH reducing power is obtained by shunting of carbohydrates through the pentose phosphate pathway.

Effects on Nucleic Acids and DNA

Ionizing radiation exposure of DNA may cause degradation of bases and sugars, breakage of hydrogen or sugar phosphate bonds or cross-linking (Table 15.4, Figure 15.3) (117,233,263,296,680,692). The incidences for the individual types of damage is base damage>single-strand breaks>DNA–protein cross-links>double-strand breaks (692). In base damage, sensitivity is thymine>cytosine>adenine>guanine (263). At radiation doses of 200 kGy, it is proposed that the two primary radicals formed in DNA are the thymine anion and the guanine cation (295,680,681). Radicals may be of a charged anion,

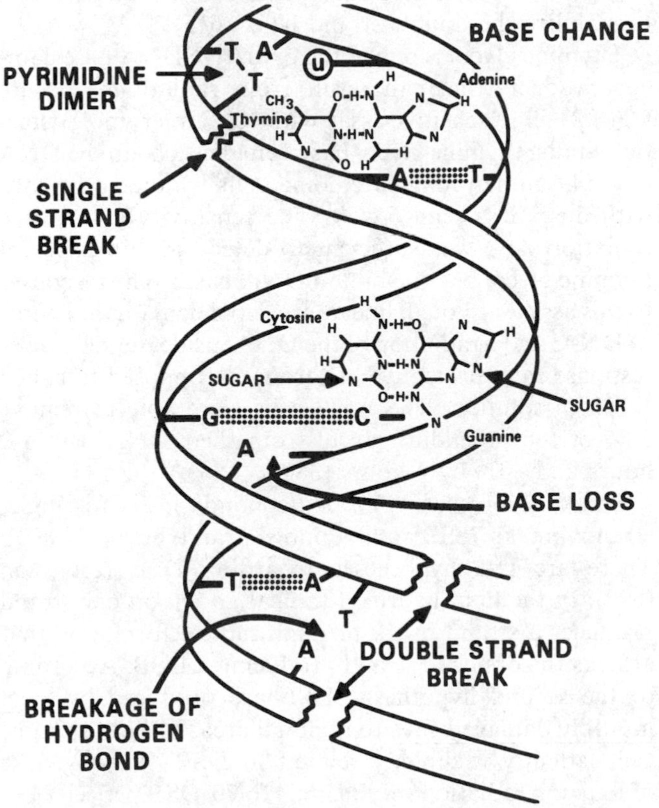

FIG. 15.3. Radiation damage to deoxyribonucleic acid. The basic categories of molecular damage, degradation, bond breakage, and cross-linking that occur in biomolecules following radiation exposure are illustrated for this double-stranded segment of DNA. The dotted lines represent hydrogen bonding between the bases, three between cytosine (C) and guanine (G), and two between adenine (A) and thymine (T). (From Reference 685. Used with permission.)

deprotonated cation, H-addition radicals, H-abstraction radical, and opened sugar ring nature (295). DNA damage to the carbohydrate produces strand breakage, glycosylic bond breakage, and formation of precursors to malonaldehyde (263,681,692). DNA cross-linkages occur between DNA and DNA, DNA and proteins, or DNA and lipids. DNA to DNA cross-links may form between adjacent bases on the same strand or between different strands. The most common DNA–protein adducts would be between DNA and the associated histones and are more likely to involve tyrosine or lysine residues (508). DNA–protein cross-links formation is more common in expanded chromatin than in compressed chromatin (117). Intracellularly, DNA–protein cross-links are enhanced by glutathione depletion but are reduced in the presence of oxygen. Important factors controlling injury are the medium composition, DNA conformation, and presence of repair enzymes (686,692). For example, metal ions are thought to induce structural changes inhibiting free radical access to key sites and to stabilize the double-strand helix (615).

Thymine glycol is one of the oxidative DNA base damage products that can result from radiation exposure (380). Using a sensitive assay with 10^{-15} micromole detection limits, thymine glycol has been identified in the DNA of A549 human lung carcinoma cells irradiated in vitro with doses less than 5 cGy. The sensitivity at this low radiation dose was sufficient to detect 4.3 molecules of thymine glycol per one billion DNA bases. The responses to this assay, although linear, are dependent on the source of DNA, and irradiation of the DNA inside the cell (lower response rate, protective of DNA), as opposed to naked DNA in solution. The A549 cells were able to remove 50% of the thymidine glycol from their DNA within 2 hours and 80% by 4 hours (380).

Breakage of sugar phosphate bonds leads to single-strand breaks (SSB) and double-strand breaks (DSB). There are two hypotheses regarding DSB formation (692). In the first, hydroxyl radical attack on one strand produces a strand break through radical formation that attacks the opposite strand producing a DSB. According to the second hypothesis, DSB are produced by local multiply damaged sites to regional areas of both strands. Cell lethality is directly related to DSB. A 1-Gy dose of ionizing radiation results in 63 to 70 DSB per cell (49). The importance of DSB over SSB in relation to radiation-induced lethality is illustrated by the fact that a radiation dose that kills 63% of the exposed cells, produced 1000 SSB, but only 40 DSB (692). There would also be an estimated 440 locally multiply damaged sites. Exposure to hydrogen peroxide, by comparison, would require production of over 2.5 million SSB per cell to kill 63% of the cells. SSBs are chemical assay phenomena that do not lead to mutational events or expression of injury because the remaining strand is intact, holding the two ends together for repair by DNA ligase. With DSBs, there is no stable end point for repair, and the chromosomal material may be lost during the subsequent cell division or rejoined to a different chromosome, forming a chromosomal aberration.

Several types of chromosomal aberrations are observed following irradiation. These include rejoining to the original chromosome—normal, inversions, and translocations; terminal or interstitial deletions; and ring and dicentric formation. Irradiation of the chromosomes in G1 results in chromosomal aberrations, whereas exposure after DNA synthesis in G2 results in chromatid aberrations. Chromosomal exchanges occurring during G1 irradiation may either be reciprocal (two chromosomes) or nonreciprocal (three chromosomes). In human fibroblasts irradiated in vitro, 50% of the chromosomal exchanges were nonreciprocal (80). The rate of chromosomal aberrations is directly related to the radiation dose and is higher for higher LET irradiation and higher dose rates (49,685,686). Chromosomal aberrations were still evident in the lymphocyte chromosomes of the Japanese atomic bomb survivors 35 years after the bombing (544), and elevations have been identified in radiotherapy patients and in persons receiving occupational radiation exposures such as the uranium miners (49,50,685). Chromosomal aberrations have also been demonstrated to be elevated in the lymphocytes of astronauts who completed long-term space flights on the Russian MIR space station (502). They represent a reasonable means of biological dosimetry and can be detected by several methods including phytohemagglutinin-stimulated peripheral blood lymphocytes, premature chromosomal condensation, micronuclei technique, and fluorescent in situ hybridization (FISH; "chromosome painting"), and the comet assay (192,339,395,685,686). The results are influenced by the scoring criteria, type of irradiation, percent of body irradiated, degree of time following radiation exposure, culture time, and age of the individual, as well as exposure to other environmental toxins or agents that might also produce aberrations. Assays also exist for detection of somatic cell mutations including the hypoxenthine-guanine phosphoribosyltransferase (HPRT) locus and the glycophorin A locus. The latter codes for a glycoprotein found on the surface of red blood cells (similar to and in conjunction with the ABO blood grouping) and expressed by alleles M and N (can also have "null," O). Increases in glycophorin A variants are dose dependent and have been elevated in the atomic bomb survivors, and in patients from the radiation accidents in Goiana, Brazil, and Chernobyl (377). The assay required 0.1 ml of blood and can be completed in less than 1 day. An example of a variant of somatic mutation would be the detection of an MO allele expression in a person who was genetically MN (or MM).

The final expression of DNA damage is modified by repair processes. Repair may occur at several levels: nonspecific suicide enzymatic repair, excision/ligation repair, SOS repair (mismatch repair), single base repair as with DNA glycosylases and methylation. Depending on the process, more than one enzyme may be required. Excision/ligation repair involves several enzymes, one to make a nick on the DNA strand containing the damaged site, presuming radiation has not already provided that nick, an excinuclease that excises damaged bases, synthesis of the new sequences based on the complimentary strand by the action of a DNA polymerase, and, finally, rejoining of the two loose ends by a DNA ligase (263,381,685,686,692). The main repair enzyme in bacteria is DNA polymerase I and, in mammals, DNA polymerase II. In addition, bacteria have a second category of repair enzymes called SOS-repair, or error-prone repair. As the name implies, they play a major role in repair of DSBs and are associated with a high error rate (263). Similar mismatch-repair genes have been identified in humans, and are designated hMSH1, hMSH2, hMLH1, and PMS2 (213). Cells with functional mismatch repair genes are more sensitive to ionizing radiation (cell survival) than mutants lacking active forms of these repair genes (213). The hardest break to repair without errors is the DSB; the repair depends on whether the two breaks are coincident, with possible loss of intervening information, or if the two breaks are separated with overlapping sequences to ensure proper rejoining and repair (49,692). The closer the approximation of the two breaks, the greater the chance of loss.

Mechanisms

The biochemical response of a biological system to ionizing radiation is influenced by eight major groups of factors as outlined in Table 15.6. Repair, reoxygenation, redistribution, and regeneration have been called the "four Rs of radiotherapy" (708). It is appropriate to continue the "R" series. The first group of factors relates to the radiation itself (49,686). Most biochemical responses are dose dependent or at least may have a damage threshold (12,686). In addition, the rate at which the radiation dose is delivered and whether the dose is delivered in fractions or in a single exposure affect the biological response, and depend on the process and cell type in question. In general, increasing the dose rate over the range of 1 to 100 cGy/min results in an enhancement of the effectiveness of the radiation in producing injury secondary to overcoming compensating mechanisms of repair of sublethal damage and cellular proliferation (46,269). Cells have specific repair processes for DNA and the ability to repair small amounts of damage to cell membranes. Therefore, damage that occurs at rates below the cellular capacity will not be as cumulatively injurious. LET is another factor influencing damage. High LET radiation produces more ionizations per unit of matter and more localized damage, making repair difficult. Larger radiation doses given in single treatments tend to cause more injury than the same dose given in fractions or over a more prolonged period. Injury to early responding tissues (hematopoietic stem cells, intestinal crypt stem cells, and many tumors) is reduced by prolonging the duration of the exposure (or in the case of cancer therapy, by extending the treatment over days or weeks), whereas the total dose and fraction size are important to the degree of an effect on late responding tissues (muscle, connective tissue, and nerve tissue) (269). Internal exposure is also a consequence for alpha and beta emitters; for example, ^{214}Po, ^{218}Po, ^{222}Rn, or ^{236}U cause alpha exposure to lung alveoli (49,50). Transmutation produces both radiation exposure and chemical instability. The transmutation of carbon 14 in a key structural position to nitrogen causes mutations in *Drosophila* and in mice (48). Transmutation of tritium also causes mutations. However, the major effect of a transmutation is the radiation exposure (48,50). The ability of beta-emitters to produce localized irradiation has been successfully applied to the use of ^{89}Sr and samarium 153 to treat painful bone metastases in patients with breast cancer, prostate cancer, and multiple myeloma. These compounds are incorporated into bone similar

Table 15.6
Eight "Rs" influencing biochemical reactions to ionizing radiation exposure[a]

Radiation factors
Dose
Dose rate
Dose fractionation
Radiation quality (LET)
Internal versus external irradiation
Radioprotectors/radiosensitizers
Reoxygenation
Resilience
Age/health/individual
Vascular integrity
Response
Nutritional/homeostasis
Biological mediators
Mutational
Circadian
Repopulation
Recovery
Repair

[a] From References 12, 48, 49, 269, 686, 687, and 708.

to calcium, and concentrated at sites of increased bone remodeling/growth activity, such as a fracture, or in a medical use, a cancerous lesion in bone. The localized radionuclide then releases radiation to the surrounding area and tumor as it radioactively decays. Similar therapies are under development to bring radioactive nuclides in contact with soft tissue tumors by attaching the radionuclide to a monoclonal antibody directed to the tumor. The incorporation of ^{90}Sr and ^{131}I through the food chain represents a concern for human exposure from nuclear weapon fallout and nuclear power plant accidents, like Chernobyl.

Biochemical responses may be modified by the presence of radioprotective or radiosensitizing agents (238,686, 688). Substances may induce radioprotection by several mechanisms, including hypoxia, free-radical scavenging, immunomodulation, hematopoietic and intestinal stem cell recovery, and modulation of the cell cycle (239). Reversal of these same processes is radiosensitizing. Cells exposed to ultraviolet radiation or hyperthermia are more sensitive to ionizing radiation, whereas animals exposed to hypothermia are more resistant to ionizing radiation. Radiation may affect core body temperature through prostaglandin synthesis and histamine release (332). Many biological processes, enzymatic rates, and fidelity are temperature dependent. Even the normal spontaneous depurination of DNA can be accelerated by elevations in temperature and this could affect mutations. Irradiated tissues remain sensitive to extreme temperature variations. Cold temperatures can accelerate the degeneration of irradiated skin (624).

An interesting observation that may ultimately prove useful in the development of a radioprotective agent for the medical/civil defense/space environments is the paradoxical nature of many of the biological mediators, such as the cytokines, prostaglandins, leukotrienes, histamines, and serotonin (494,685,687,688). Their release following radiation exposure plays a key role in the biological amplification of injury, yet when administered before radiation, they are the most potent of the naturally occurring biological substances. The degree of protection afforded by a radioprotective agent is described by its dose reduction factor (DRF) or dose modifying factor (DMF). Both values are ratios greater than 1 for protection, and represent the radiation exposure in the presence of a radioprotective agent to produce a given biological response divided by the radiation dose required without the agent. Radiosensitizing substances are described by the sensitizer enhancement ratio (SER). It is a positive value representing the dose of radiation required to produce a given biological endpoint without a protective agent divided by the radiation dose in the presence of the radioprotective agent. Many of the chemotherapeutic drugs (e.g., Adriamycin, bischloroethylnitrosourea (BCNU), bleomycin, cisplatin, fludarabine, gemcitabine, hydroxyurea, cyclophosphamide, cytosine arabinoside, doxorubicin, 5-fluorouracil, interferon, taxol, and topotecan) have additive or synergistic responses when given with radiation exposures (112,267,269). These may be beneficial for tumor therapy but may also adversely affect normal tissues such as heart (Adraimycin), lung (bleomycin), bone marrow, and mucosal tissue (such as the inner lining of the mouth and rectum). Significant advances in oncology have been made using combined modality therapy (chemotherapy and radiotherapy) to improve local control, disease-free survival, and even overall survival. Some patients with laryngeal, bladder, or rectal cancer are able to receive organ preservation therapies involving chemo- and radiation therapy without compromising survival. Patients with nasopharyngeal carcinomas who are treated by concomitant cisplatin/5-fluorouracil chemotherapy with radiation therapy have a greater overall survival than patients who receive an identical course of radiotherapy alone, 78% versus 47% 3-year overall survival, respectively (9). The chemotherapy is thought to reduce the tumor volume, radiosensitize the tumor, and to provide systemic treatment to prevent distant metastases.

For some drugs, because the mode of injury is similar, there may be a memory response equivalent to, or resembling a fractionated radiation exposure, rather than drug injury at one time and radiation injury at another. Caffeine and the cardiac glycosides, digoxin and ouabain, as well as metoclopramide, an antiemetic agent, are also radiosensitizers. Drugs that produce free-radical damage and/or alkylation of DNA, or produce biological responses similar to ionizing radiation, are described as *radiomimetic* (30,269). Examples include azaserine, benzene, bleomycin, BCNU, cyclophosphamide, diethylthiocarbamate, furazolidone, hydrogen peroxide, mitomycin C, neocarzinostatin, nitrofurantoin, nitrosoureas, nitrosoguanidine, ozone, superoxide, streptonigrin, sulfur mustard, tetranodecanoylphorbor acetate, thiotepa, and the trichothecene mycotoxin T-2 (30,269).

Alterations in cell populations influence biochemical responses by several mechanisms. Radiation may alter the population of the cell type responsible for producing a particular product, as in the reduction of estrogen which may occur following ovarian irradiation, or it may alter the population of a controlling or modifying cell. These processes may have dire consequences such as decrease in prostaglandin (PG) production by the bone marrow stromal support cells responsible for maintaining a microenvironment suitable for hematopoietic stem cell development. Studies of bone marrow populations in culture demonstrate that radiation doses that do not kill the hematopoietic stem cells may still halt stem cell progression by injuring the stromal support cells. When stromal synthesis of prostaglandins was inhibited by ionizing radiation treatment, the hematopoietic stem cell development stopped (239). It resumed when the marrow stromal cells were treated with a 100-Gy dose killing the stromal cells, but stimulating endogenous prostaglandin release. Repopulation kinetics and cell–cell influences play important roles in some forms of radiation-induced congenital anomalies where loss, reduction, or inhibition of one cell or tissue type influences the development of surrounding tissues and organs.

Hormonal control of homeostasis is affected by ionizing radiation and at the same time may affect biochemical responses and even survival to ionizing radiation. Physiological processes may be influenced by electrolyte imbalances, polydipsia, and polyuria following irradiation (686,722). As mentioned later in the chapter, levels of the stress hormone adrenocorticotropin hormone (ACTH), glucagon, cortisol, insulin, and growth hormone are altered by ionizing radiation exposure. Radiation acts as a general stressing agent on the body (12,685,686). Estrogen and testosterone both induce radioprotection when administered to animals, and radiosensitivity has been shown to vary throughout the estrous cycle (685,686). Correspondingly, testosterone acts as a growth stimulus for prostate cancer cells. The use of lutenizing hormone–releasing hormone agonists that reduce testosterone levels, in combination with radiation therapy can improve the success of therapy in some stages of prostate cancer (531). Circadian rhythm and season variations also modify responses. The spontaneous induction rate for congenital anomalies and the ability of radiation to induce anomalies are both enhanced during the winter months (685). The sensitivity of the individual to ionizing radiation is modified by the state of health, individual genetic and physiological variations, and the presence of combined injuries. Patients with medical histories of scleroderma and xeroderma pigmentosum have worse skin reactions to ionizing radiation. Although the lethal radiation dose for humans is approximately 4.5 Gy, a 5% lethality is estimated for a 2-Gy dose (722). In large radiation exposures, the presence of combined injuries such as infections or pathophysiological injuries, including burns, wounds, or other trauma, plays an important factor in survival (139,197). Other factors are more difficult to describe. For example, a study on the ability of ^{210}Po to induce lung cancers in hamsters found a 0% incidence of lung cancers when 40 nCi of ^{210}Po was introduced by intratracheal administration, but a 5% incidence of lung tumors if the same administration was followed by an injection of saline (387).

Radiation induces a block in the G2 phase of the cell cycle and a prolongation of S phase (12,269,270,566,686). Cells are more sensitive when irradiated during the mitosis and G2 phases of the cell cycle and progressively less sensitive during early and late S phases, where preparation for and synthesis of DNA occurs. The G2 delay is probably related to repair processes. Studies with inhibitors of protein synthesis indicate that radiation inhibits the synthesis of a protein or key proteins necessary to proceed through the cell cycle (686). Decreased synthesis and phosphorylation of histones is observed after irradiation (511). When mitosis resumes, there is usually an increase in the percentage of cells undergoing mitosis compared to the unirradiated population due to a partial synchronization and abortive mitoses. There may also be an overcompensation from stimulation of cells normally in the G0 stage back into active cycling. Increasing the radiation dose proportionally increases the mitotic delay time up to a point at which the possibility of radiation-induced cell death becomes a more likely outcome. This delay in resumption of mitosis has significant consequences for repopulation kinetics and potential lethality. There are four major acute radiation lethality syndromes: instantaneous, hematopoietic, intestinal, and central nervous system death (722). Of these, the hematopoietic and intestinal cell deaths are governed by repopulation of the respective stem cell compartments. Hematopoietic death results in humans from doses between 2 and 7 Gy, with lethality occurring between 2 weeks to 2 months postirradiation. Death is directly attributable to the mitotic inhibition/death of two stem cell populations, one responsible for hematopoiesis and one for marrow support. The formed components of blood, red and white blood cells, and platelets have finite lifetimes, 4.5 days for platelets to 120 days for red blood cells. They are continually replaced by the bone marrow; but, if marrow production is halted, maturation depletion occurs with hematopoietic progenitor cells in various stages of development. An acute aplastic anemia develops without the continued formation of new progenitors. The duration of mitotic delay is crucial in the recovery process because a point might be reached at which the pathological consequences of the loss of platelets and white blood cells cannot be reversed by the onset of new hematopoiesis in time to avert death. In theory, survival or transplantation of a single hematopoietic stem cell (with proper stromal support) can repopulate the entire hematopoietic system, resulting in survival. Bone marrow transplantation has been used to treat victims of radiation accidents. It is not necessary for the entire marrow to be mitotically inhibited for the acute hematopoietic syndrome to be initiated. Production can be suppressed below a threshold. With a loss of platelets and white blood cells, hemorrhaging and infectious processes lead to death. A similar inhibition of the intestinal crypts of Lieberkuhn by radiation doses greater than 12 Gy progresses to acute intestinal syndrome death between 3 to 7 days postirradiation. Intestinal villi cells continue to be sloughed off or die without replacement. This produces a decrease in villi height, with an associated decrease in absorptive area, followed by eventual denuding of the villi surface, loss of electrolytes, and loss of the protective barrier permitting infection and hemorrhaging. Attempts to transplant intestinal crypt cells have not been successful. A person may survive a hematopoietically lethal dose of radiation only to die instead, and at an earlier period, from the acute intestinal syndrome. Agents that are radioprotective for the hematopoietic system may not necessarily affect the intestinal crypt cells in the same manner.

Radiation is unique among environmental mutagens in that it may affect any of the three stages of tumor development: initiation, promotion, and latency (48,49,269,685,686). There are several chromosomal breakage syndromes, such as xeroderma pigmentosum and ataxia telangiectasia, that are associated with deficiencies in DNA repair and are, therefore, more susceptible to radiation-induced mutational injury. Cancer induction has been related to the activation of proto-oncogenes to oncogenic status. Oncogenes may influence the development of cancer by direct stimulatory effects through altered or amplified gene products or by suppressive activity. In the latter case, the normal function of the gene acts to suppress cancer, and inactivation or loss leads to expression of transformation of cells and carcinogenesis. The most studied human suppressor oncogene, p53, is associated with the induction of retinoblastoma, colon cancer, and lung cancers in humans. Deletions and point mutations in the p53 gene have been observed in some radiation-induced cancers, including, in one study, 7 of 19 radon-associated lung cancers from uranium miners (666), and 16 of 52 in another study (639). Interestingly, 31% of the miners with lung cancer in the second study had a specific transversion of A<u>G</u>G to A<u>T</u>G (arginine to methionine) at codon 249 (639). This codon was not mutated in miners from the first study.

Radiation-induced genetic injury may arise from chromosomal loss of a gene or an entire chromosome, deletions resulting in codon loss, or frameshifts and point mutations involving base substitutions that produce amino acid substitutions or stop codons. Radiation-induced mutations have been observed in the p53, c-*myc*, c-*abl*, β 2M, c-*fms*, K-*ras*, and H-*ras* oncogenes. Analyses of radiation induced gene inactivation in vitro suggest that induced mutations are more likely to be expressed through DNA deletions or rearrangements than as point mutations (643). Interestingly, the types of activated K-*ras* point mutations observed in neutron radiation-induced murine thymic lymphomas were lower in yield and differed from the spectrum of *ras* point mutations induced by gamma irradiation (612). They also lacked a characteristic point mutation of adenine for guanine in codon 12 that was present in 87% of the gamma-radiation induced *ras* mutations. Characteristic deletions have been observed for other radiation-induced cancers, such as the deletions on chromosome 2 in low LET radiation-induced murine myeloid leukemias (653).

Radiation exposure may alter both enzyme levels and the availability of substrates and cofactors. For example, the increase of PGs in mouse spleens following exposure to 2 Gy was shown to be related to a decrease in the activity of the enzyme associated with PG degradation, 15-hydroxy-PG dehydrogenase (689). This effect was not observed in irradiated human colon tissues (224). Prostaglandin synthesis has also been studied in the pig skin following X-irradiation (731). There was an increase in PGE_2 levels within 12 hours after 10-Gy irradiation followed by decreases 24 to 48 hours postirradiation (731). Interestingly, during this same period $PGF_{2\alpha}$ increased. Both changes were related to an increase in NADPH-dependent PGE_2 9-keto reductase, an enzyme that converts PGE_2 to $PGF_{2\alpha}$. In general, PGE_2 antagonizes the actions of $PGF_{2\alpha}$, much like prostacyclin (PGI_2) antagonizes the actions of platelet-clotting activity of thromboxane.

Exposure to ionizing radiation results in induction of a number of "immediate early genes" and early response genes (47, 60, 195, 207, 270, 490, 509, 535, 566, 571, 573). There are more than 100 stress-inducible genes, or "immediate early genes" induced by ionizing radiation (535). Several of these genes have been detected within 15 min postirradiation and have been elicited with doses as low as 10–50 cGy of ionizing radiation. Many of these can also be induced by oxidative stress and free-radical production (270,619), and are associated with transcription (including *c-fos*, *c-jun*, and NF-κB), translation, cell cycle regulation, carcinogenesis, and immunosuppression (270). Several are proto-oncogenes, including c-*fos*, c-Ha-*ras*, c-*jun* and c-*myc* (270,535). In addition, radiation exposure produces biological mediators and second messengers, such as the cytokines (α-interferon, interleukin [IL]-1, interleukin-6, tumor necrosis factor [TNF]-α, and transforming growth factor-β) (18,39,270,565), which in turn can induce specific gene transduction (270). Some genes are down-regulated producing postirradiation consequences. The decreased production of cyclin B following radiation exposure is an underlying factor in radiation-induced mitotic delay (173,270,305). Cyclin A and topoisomerase II-alpha also decrease following radiation exposure (173).

There are a number of important biological mediators that amplify and/or elicit inflammation, fibrosis, or biological end points. Among these mediators are hormones, histamine, serotonin, leukotrienes, PGs, phospholipids, cyclic nucleotides, and cytokines. Each of these may have unique or cooperative interactions resulting in injury, death, or may even be necessary for recovery processes. Histamines and prostaglandins are mediators of radiation-induced skin erythema (85,686). The cytokines are a diverse class of proteins produced by lymphoid cells and other tissues that mediate cell–cell interactions in a hormonal manner. These proteins include IL-1 and IL-12, TNF, granulocyte/macrophage colony stimulating factor (GM-CSF), stem cell factor (SCF), transforming growth factor-β, and the interferons to name a few. These molecules act through specific receptors, and have important physiological and pathological functions/responses. Lung pneumonitis and fibrosis postirradiation are in part related to elevation of transforming growth factor-β and to interleukin-1α, both of which are capable of stimulating collagen gene expression and fibrosis. Prolonged plasma elevation of transforming growth factor-β in patients receiving radiotherapy has been associated with increased risk of developing pulmonary toxicity (18,88,494). Depending on the situation and the cytokine interactions, many of these compounds are able to elicit radioprotective properties or radiosensitization (494). TNF, SCF, and IL-1 and IL-12 are radioprotective in mice when administered individually 18–24 hours prior to irradiation, whereas IL-6 interferons α and β and transforming growth factor-β act as radiosensitizers (494). The end point of study is important, because administration of IL-12 to mice results in radioprotection of hematopoietic tissue, but gastrointestinal radiosensitization. Other cytokines including granulocyte colony-stimulating factor, keratinocyte growth factor, and transforming growth factor-β, are being examined in terms of their wound-healing effects and are undergoing clinical trial tests in patients receiving radiotherapy in order to minimize the injury to normal tissues, while not affecting the tumor tissues (657). Other agents that modify cytokine activity, such as lisofylline reduction of inflammatory cytokines, are also under evaluation to minimize radiation toxicity (657). Granulocyte colony-stimulating factor has been used to increase white blood cell production in patients who have become neutropenic to combinations of ionizing radiotherapy and chemotherapy. Thrombopoietin has been isolated, and is being investigated in clinical trials. It too should have advantages in those patients with radiation-induced bone marrow suppression (but not ablation), but its use will have to await appropriate clinical trials and FDA approval.

Biological processes may also be altered through changes in receptor expression (686). PG, leukotriene, β-adrenergic, histamine, serotonin, alpha IIb β 3 integrin, and 3H-corticosterone receptors have been studied in irradiated cells or animals. Radiation exposure had no effect on the specific binding of leukotriene C_4 at doses up to 20 Gy (688). Adrenergic receptors play important roles in homeostasis by the autonomic nervous system. Radiation induces a decrease in adrenergic receptors in both the rat and rabbit during the first week postirradiation (378,647). In rats, this is followed by an increase in β-adrenergic receptors apparently associated with a late developing radiation-induced congestive heart failure (378). Changes in receptor expression can be related to increased production or to increased use and destruction. An exposure of 2 Gy (a common daily fraction size in clinical radiation oncology) has been shown to increase the mRNA synthesis of the epidermal growth factor receptor in cells irradiated in vitro within the first 24 hours (584). The serotonin$_3$, or 5HT$_3$, receptor is active in radiation-induced emesis, and specific receptor antagonists (ondansetron or granisetron) have been successful in reducing emesis in radiotherapy patients. Administration of 5-HT$_3$ antagonists to ferrets reportedly stopped radiation-induced emesis within 30 s of administration (58). Some radiation-induced receptor changes may have dire consequences because the increased expression of integrin receptors by B16 murine melanoma cells following irradiation is associated with increased lung colony forming ability, or metastasis (510). Expression of the integrin receptor was detected within 15 min postirradiation with downregulation occurring by 4 hours postirradiation.

There are several important signal transduction pathways and cascades that are variously activated by ionizing radiation with important resultant modifications of cellular physiology (329,341,583,619). Among these are the stress-activated protein kinase pathway (SAPK), mitotic-activated protein kinase pathway (MAPK), protein kinase C, modifications of intracellular calcium with corresponding activation of calcium-dependent enzymes, bioactive lipids synthesized or released by phospholipases, and the nuclear transcription factor NF-κB (341,583). Activation of the MAPK pathway, with corresponding stimulation of mitogenic proliferation is thought to account for the accelerated repopulation of irradiated cells that affects the sensitivity and response of cells (including tumor cells) to chronic low doses as might occur environmentally or accidentally (e.g., Chernobyl), or fractionated doses of ionizing radiation (that are routinely used clinically) (583). The steps involved in the activation of this pathway by ionizing radiation are illustrated in Figure 15.4. This pathway can be activated by binding of the receptors on the membrane cell surface to their ligands (including TNF and other cytokines released or elevated by ionizing radiation) (341), or intracellularly through reactive oxygen intermediates (341,619), changes in intracellular calcium, and phosphorylated activation of the epidermal growth factor receptor (583). Inhibition of epidermal growth factor receptor phosphorylation in vitro has been shown to block ionizing radiation-induced cellular proliferation (583). In addition, use of specific inhibitors of MAPK in vitro, resulted in an enhancement of double-stranded DNA breaks and reproductive cell death (95). NF-κB, a nuclear transcription factor, is one of the

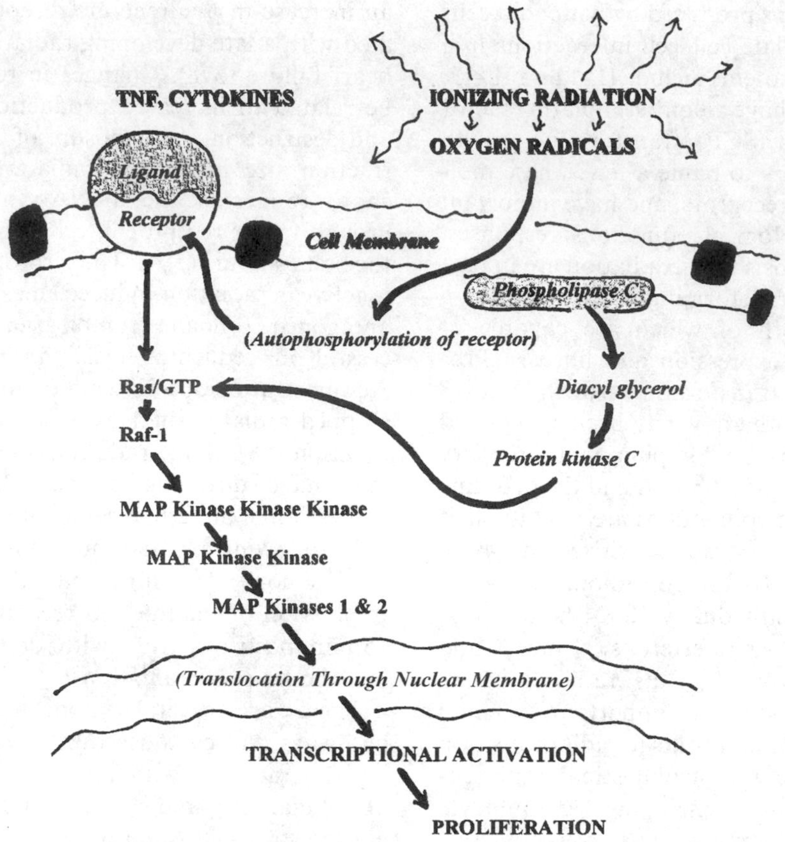

FIG. 15.4. Mitogen-activated protein (MAP) kinase signal transduction pathways can be stimulated in response to ionizing radiation. Radiation exposure results in signal transduction activation of the MAP kinase pathway. The MAP kinase pathway can normally be elicited by cytokines including tumor necrosis factor (TNF). The best characterized receptor-mediated initiation has been the radiation-induced activation through the epidermal growth factor (EGF) receptor by autophosphorylation. The exact mechanism is under investigation, and may involve reactive oxygen intermediates, intracellular calcium mobilization, or indirectly through other biological mediators (diacyl glycerol is released from the phospholipid membrane through the action of phospholipase C). The pathway involves activation of several kinases (phosphorylation activation), and can also be inhibited by phosphatase activities. The resultant pathway action is cell proliferation and differentiation. (Based on References 329,583,619.)

early response genes induced by ionizing radiation exposure (270,341). Its regulation is dysfunctional in people with the genetic disease, ataxia telangiectasia, and is thought to account for their increased sensitivity to ionizing radiation (341). There is also an ataxia telangiectasia-mutated gene (ATM) that participates in DNA repair and recombination, suppression of apoptosis, and induction of p53 (566). The mutated gene is deficient in these functions.

MOLECULAR AND CELLULAR EFFECTS

Effects on Energy Systems

Radiation exposure affects biological energy processes by specific and nonspecific interactions. Nonspecifically, absorptive functions in the stomach and colon may be altered and lead to prolonged gastric emptying times (185), induction of nausea and vomiting, increased stool frequency, loose stools or diarrhea, fatigue, and/or loss of appetite. Radiation affects carbohydrate metabolism by the release of stress-related hormones and by reducing the levels of the thyroid hormones triiodothyronine and thyroxine (686). The reduced thyroid activity is also reflected by an increase in thyroid-stimulating hormone (TSH). In humans receiving radiotherapy, a single dose of 7.5 Gy results in a 35% incidence of elevated TSH (610). Subclinical hypothyroidism is more common (normal thyroid hormone level, elevated TSH), and like clinical hypothyroidism, responds to thyroid hormone (levothyroxine) supplementation.

Specifically, radiation exposure causes an uncoupling of nuclear and oxidative phosphorylation with corresponding decreases in oxygen-dependent ATP synthesis

(12,686). It has been suggested as a mechanism for radiation-induced interphase death (354). This effect has been observed in the rat spleen with doses as low as 1 Gy (668) and as early as 15 min postirradiation (37). It is observed in the spleen, liver, and thymus but is not present in all tissues. The decrease in oxidative phosphorylation is preceded by a decrease in NAD^+ levels, and the decreases in ATP are preceded by reductions in AMP and ADP. The losses are attributable to decreased synthesis, use of remaining stores, and increased leakage through the cell membrane. In nuclei, macrophages, and neutrophils, a specific membrane NADPH oxidase consumes molecular oxygen to produce superoxide but depletes NADPH in the process. The depletion of NADPH, coupled with radiation-induced inhibition of glucose-6-phosphate dehydrogenase, results in the uncoupling of oxidative phosphorylation.

NAD concentrations also decrease following irradiation. Decreases are observed within 15 min postirradiation and have been elicited with doses as low as 0.25 Gy, although doses of 9 Gy or higher are usually required to observe changes (686). This decrease is related to the activation of adenosine 5′-diphospho-5-β-D-ribosyl transferase (ADPRT) by double-stranded DNA breaks. ADPRT uses the ADP contained in NAD to form a poly (ADP-ribosyl) chain that attaches to histones and to several DNA-repair enzymes, including DNA ligase II, Ca^{2+}- and Mg^{2+}-dependent endonucleases, and to protein elongation factor 2. Although its specific function is not known, poly (ADP-ribosyl) affects many biological processes, including DNA repair and cell growth and differentiation. It is also important in some infectious processes because cholera and diphtheria toxins have ADPRT activity. The Poly (ADP-ribosyl) binds to the histones initiating a relaxation of chromatin, facilitating DNA repair. As long as double-stranded DNA damage is present, ADPRT will remain activated and the poly (ADP-ribosyl) chain will remain attached to the histones, preventing condensation of DNA necessary for metaphase. A suicide model of cell death has been proposed in which extensive DNA damage leads to activation of ADPRT, with the subsequent use and depletion of NAD (56). The decrease in NAD for electron transport results in decrease in ATP synthesis, leading to a decrease in other biosynthetic and active transport processes, with a consequential interphase cell death. Most cells can maintain sufficient NAD concentrations to avoid this complication with radiation doses under 20 Gy. Because poly (ADP-ribosyl) participates in both DNA repair, where inhibition would be radiosensitive, and in this cell death model, where inhibition would be protective, the use of ADPRT inhibitors such as caffeine, nicotinamide, and 3-aminobenzamine have produced mixed results (686).

Human immunodeficiency virus (HIV) activation is not a major response to ionizing radiation exposure; however, both ultraviolet (UV) radiation (732) and X-irradiation can stimulate the in vitro replication of the HIV responsible for the acquired immunodeficiency syndrome (AIDS) in humans (497). A 200% increase in viral replication was observed following a 1.5-Gy X-irradiation dose. The increase was thought to be mediated by a cAMP-dependent process. Much larger doses of either UV- or X-irradiation are required for inactivation (282). The LD_{37} dose was 4.5 kGy. In another study, transcription of the HIV promoter could be activated in cells in vivo by doses as low as 25 cGy (198). Radiotherapy remains an effective means of treating Kaposi's sarcomas, lymphomas, and other radiosensitive tumors in AIDS patients (140). Radiation can also cause activation of the herpes zoster virus responsible for chicken pox and shingles (zoster) in humans. Reactivation of the virus (shingles) has been reported in 16% (up to 50% in some studies) of patients receiving radiation therapy for Hodgkin's Disease (257). Most cases occurred within 18 months following completion of radiation therapy and was most common in patients receiving chemotherapy and radiotherapy, and in children.

The Target

The "target" for radiation-induced cellular injury depends on the end point examined. The membrane appears to be the target for some of the behavioral alterations following ionizing radiation, while the chromosome material is thought to be the target for cell lethality. This is supported by the results of microsurgical techniques on irradiated amoeba to transfer the nucleus to unirradiated amoeba and to transfer an unirradiated nucleus to the irradiated cytoplasm. Significantly greater lethality followed the irradiated nucleus. The unirradiated amoeba that contained the irradiated nucleus behaved as if the entire nucleus had been irradiated, whereas the amoeba with the irradiated cytoplasm containing the unirradiated nucleus required much higher doses to the cytoplasm for lethality (255).

In a classic set of experiments, Munro (486) irradiated either the cytoplasm or the nucleus of Chinese hamster fibroblast cells using a needle made of ^{210}Po, an alpha emitter. When the needle remained in the cytoplasm, away from the nucleus, the alpha radiation doses of 250 Gy were dissipated in the cytoplasm with no effect. However, when the needle was placed close to the nucleus, cell lethality resulted from much smaller doses. Finally, cell lethality is directly proportional to the number of chromosomal aberrations observed after irradiation. They may be detected by several methods including phytohemagglutinin (PHG)-stimulated peripheral blood lymphocytes, premature chromosomal condensation, micronuclei technique, and FISH (686). The result is influenced by radiation factors, the degree of time following exposure to ionizing radiation, culture time, and age of the individual. The premature chromosomal condensation technique can be assayed in 2 h, whereas the other assays require 48–52 h to allow the stimulated lymphocytes to grow sufficiently for assay. The basic technique permits growth of the blood lymphocytes to permit sufficient numbers of cells to conduct the assay. The complete assay time including culturing the blood lymphocytes takes 3–5 days.

Other experiments that indicate that the DNA is the main target for radiation injury are those conducted with the halogenated pyrimidines, 5-iododeoxyuridine and 5-bromodeoxyuridine (269,309). These compounds are incorporated into the DNA and increase cellular radiosensitivity by increasing susceptibility to free-radical attack (including the hydrated electron) and damage and by modification of DNA repair (269,309,325). Cells in exponential growth are more sensitive than cells in plateau growth containing equivalent amounts of base substitution. Experiments incorporating ^{125}I-iododeoxyuridine into cellular DNA, or iodinated proteins into cell membranes, further demonstrated that the nucleus, rather than the plasma membrane, is the target for radiation-induced chromosomal instability that occurs after several cell divisions as well as later after radiation exposure (333).

Cellular Responses

There are three basic categories of cellular damage and eight basic responses of cells to ionizing radiation. The basic categories of damage are sublethal damage, potentially lethal damage, and lethal damage. Potentially lethal damage is radiation-induced damage that would result in cell death if not repaired (63), and is affected by postradiation therapy or environment (269). The basic responses of cells to ionizing radiation include no visible response, mitotic delay, transformation, hyperplasia without accompanying cell division leading to giant cells, instant cell death, interphase cell death, reproductive cell death, and apoptosis.

The cell cycle describes the process of cells preparing for and undergoing cell division. Some cells are in a resting phase, termed G_0, and are not actively dividing or preparing for division. Cells go through a G1 (Gap 1) phase incurring growth prior to initiating the S phase (synthesis), during which the chromosomes are replicated. This is followed by a second gap (G2), in between DNA synthesis and cell division (mitosis). Classical radiobiology studies of synchronized cells in culture have shown that cells tend to be most sensitive to ionizing radiation when irradiated in G2 and mitosis, and to be less sensitive when irradiated in S phase. Because cells in mitosis and G2 are more sensitive than the other stages of the cell cycle, cells that are rapidly cycling have more likelihood to be in a radiosensitive phase of the cell cycle than cells that are slowly dividing or cells that are removed from the cell cycle (G_0, or resting phase). This can be particularly important in radiation therapy where differences in radiosensitivity are exploited to maximize tumor kill and patient cure. In fact, agents that affect cell cycle progression, or synchronize cells (for example hydroxyurea), can be used for radiosensitization.

Molecular and cellular biology studies are providing insight both on cell cycle regulation and how radiation is able to affect the cell cycle (270,487,566). There are two key check points in the cell cycle which can be inhibited by ionizing radiation, the first is at G1/S, and the second is at G2/M. Several sets of key proteins are involved. The first set of proteins, called cyclins, are specific for particular phases of the cell cycle. They bind to and activate phosphorylating enzymes called cyclin-dependent kinases (566). There may be several cyclins within a particular class, and there are specific inhibitors for the activated cyclin/cyclin-dependent kinase complexes. Seven different cyclins, A–E, G, and H, have been identified (Table 15.7).

Radiation results in stimulation/accumulation of p53 (Figure 15.5), a tumor suppressor protein with DNA transcriptional and other regulatory roles, which in turn induces transcription of the protein, p21 (Cip1/waf1). Increased levels of p21 inhibits both cyclin E cyclin-dependent kinase 2 (cdk2) and cyclin A-cdk2 kinase with a resultant arrest in G1 (189,270,566). The cdk4/cyclin D kinase activity is also inhibited. In the presence of p21, the cyclin E-cdk2 complex remains in the unphosphorylated and inactivated form. Cells with normal expression of the p53 protein are called "wild type" (normal). Cells with p53 deficiencies or mutations are unable to elicit the inhibition of cyclin E-cdk2 activation, or cell cycle inhibition at G1 (269,270,566). Irradiated mice with deficiencies in p21 (p21 −/−) are still able to elicit G1 cell cycle inhibition, but to a lesser degree (169). This indicates that dual pathways can result

Table 15.7
Role of cyclins in radiation-induced cell cycle response

Cyclin	*Dependent kinase*	*Cell cycle phase*	*Radiation Effect*
Cyclin A	cdk2	S	G1/S Block
Cyclin B	cdk1	G2/M	*G2/M Block*
Cyclin C	cdk, cdk9	G1/2, G2/M	?
Cyclin D	cdk4, cdk6	G0, G1	G1 Block
Cyclin E	cdk2	G1/S	*G1 Block*
Cyclin G	cdk5	G1/S, G2/M	G2/M Block
Cyclin H	cdk7	G2/M	?

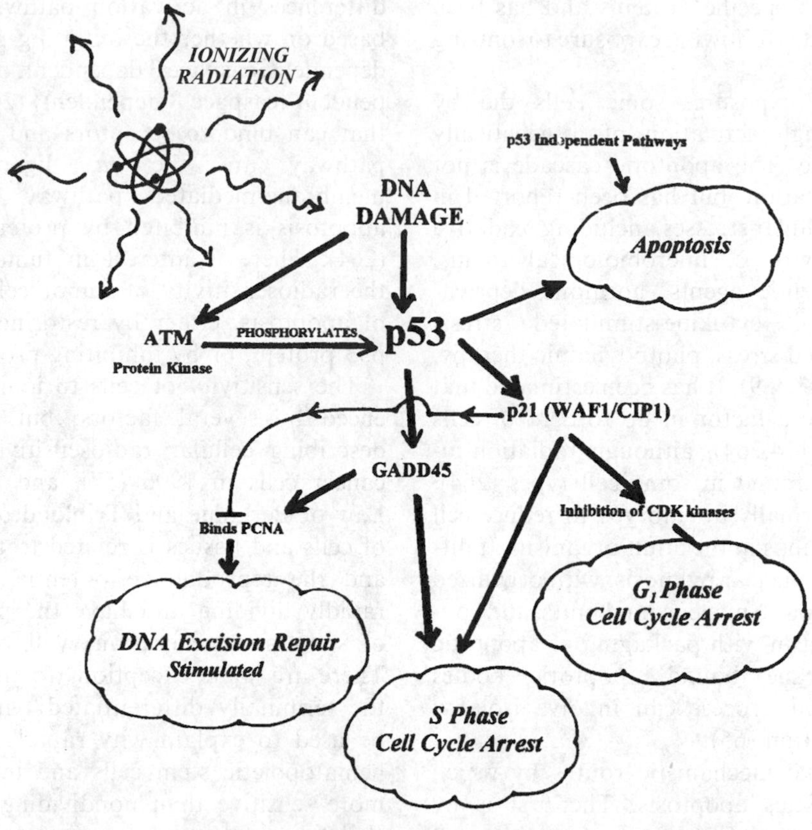

FIG. 15.5. Roles of p53 in response to ionizing radiation. Radiation or DNA damage results in activation of the ataxia telangectasia gene (ATM), a protein kinase that phosphorylates and activates the tumor suppressor/transcriptional activator protein, p53. The actions controlled by p53 are shown. p53 induces transcription of p21, a protein that subsequently inhibits kinases, regulating cell cycle control. p53 increases GADD45 protein levels, which can interact with PCNA (proliferating cell nuclear antigen) to stimulate DNA repair (as shown, p21 can inhibit PCNA binding and activity). p53, in turn, is important in mediating apoptosis, but there are also p53-independent pathways (ceramide signalling) that result in apoptosis.

in G1 inhibition, but that the major pathway is through p53 induction of p21. In general, cells with deficient p53 genes do not get blocked at the G1 check point after exposure to ionizing radiation.

Radiation also produces a delay in the cell cycle by blocking the G2 check point. Combination of the cyclin B with cdk1 forms a phosphorylated complex called the *mitotic proliferating factor*. Ionizing radiation results in a decrease in the cdc25 protein that normally dephosphorylates the threonine 14 and tyrosine 15 position of the mitotic proliferating factor, resulting in its activation, and allowing the cell to proceed through mitosis (270,305,566). The radiation-induced decrease in cdc25 results in an unactivated/phosphorylated mitotic proliferating factor and, in turn, inhibition at the G2 check point. Reduction in cyclin B transcription, decreased stability of the cyclin B mRNA, and increases in elongation factor 1-delta following irradiation have also been implicated in cell cycle blockage at G2 (270,305,487,566). This a simplified description of a more complicated interaction involving over- and under-expression of cyclin-dependent kinase inhibitors, upstream regulators, and other integrated pathways. Interestingly, overexpression of cyclins have been identified in several cancers (566).

If the reproductive potential of a cell has been eliminated but other functional components of a cell remain intact, the cell may continue to grow without dividing, forming a giant cell. In interphase, death occurs after an individual/organism receives a dose of radiation with so much resulting damage that the cell dies before it can undergo mitosis and potentially gets "stuck" in mitosis. The lymphocyte is considered a very radiosensitive cell in humans where doses of 0.05 Gy have been shown to kill lymphocytes (722). Reproductive death refers to the cellular processes by which a cell dies by inhibition in metaphase within several cell divisions after radiation exposure. Apoptosis, characterized by nuclear pyknosis, cytoplasmic condensation, and cellular phagocytosis with appearance of apoptotic bodies, requires the synthesis of specific proteins and has been observed in rat thymocytes following exposure to ionizing radiation (715).

Following radiation exposure, some cells die by apoptotic death, through activation of a genetically preprogrammed cascade. The apoptotic cascade is not specific to ionizing radiation, but has been reported in cells exposed to other cellular stresses, including oxidative stress, hyperthermia, viruses, microbiological toxins, cytotoxic chemotherapeutic agents, hormone deprivation, steroid therapy, cytokine-stimulated stress, antibody/immune-related stress, photodynamic therapy, and UV light (65,264,342,489). It has been estimated that apoptotic death may be a factor in up to 25% of cells dying from radiation (174,264), although radiation-induced apoptosis is not found in some cell types (264). Apoptosis functions normally in embryos to reduce cell numbers, and also functions in the adult organism. It differs from necrosis in the nuclear pyknosis, with organized degradation of the DNA into nucleosomal units, and condensation of the cytoplasm with packaging of apoptotic products into membrane bound apoptotic bodies (65,340). This organized process can involve isolated cells, without inflammation (65).

There are at least two mechanistic routes by which ionizing radiation initiates apoptosis. The first is by initiation of DNA damage (65,264,342) and the second is mediated through the cell membrane action of sphingomyelinase, releasing the second messenger ceramide (118,264). The pathway mediated through DNA damage requires nonmutated/functional (wild type) expression of the p53 protein, which controls production of bax, an apoptotic inducing protein. Cells that have a mutated p53 protein (as many cancer cells have) do not undergo apoptotic death in response to radiation-induced DNA damage and p53 activation, but may still be induced to undergo apoptosis through the membrane-induced (ceramide) pathway (118,264). Bcl-2 and bcl-x_l are suppressor proteins of apoptosis that are thought to bind to each other and to bax (65,264), forming either homodimers or heterodimers. The key events in apoptosis are speculated to occur either from homodimerization of bax, and/or from decreased availability of the bcl-2 and bcl-x_L suppressors (65). Membrane receptor mediated events can inactivate bad, another apoptotic promoter that would otherwise bind to and inactivate bcl-x_L. Bcl-2 and bcl-x_L prevent the translocation of cytochrome c from the mitochondria (209). In the cytoplasm, cytochrome c acts as an apoptotic protease-activating factor, leading to the activation of cysteinyl-containing aspartate-specific proteases (caspaces, there are at least nine types) that mediate the apoptotic cascade, including a caspace activated DNase (209). Activation of caspaces 3, 8, and 9 are considered important in the apoptotic cascade, and further differences in activation pathways can be delineated based on whether the initiating processes are caspace 9 dependent, caspace 3 dependent, or caspaces 3 and 9 independent (caspace 8 dependent) (265). Among the ligands that can bind to receptors and activate the apoptosis pathway are the *fas* ligand and TNF. The membrane-mediated pathway for radiation-induced apoptosis is inhibited by protein kinase C activation (264). There is interest in tumor therapy to enhance the radiosensitivity of tumor cells through stimulation of apoptosis, either by restoring a normal (wild type) p53 protein, or by inhibiting protein kinase C.

The sensitivity of cells to ionizing radiation is influenced by several factors, but the general principles describing cellular radiosensitivity were described for cancer cells in 1906 (57), and are referred to as the Law of Bergonie and Triblondeau. The radiosensitivity of cells and tissues is related to the rate of cell division and the reproductive potential. Cells that are more rapidly dividing and have the potential for a number of successive generations will be more radiosensitive. There are some exceptions to these principles, such as the terminally differentiated lymphocytes, but it may be used to explain why rapidly dividing cells such as hematopoietic stem cells and intestinal crypt cells are more sensitive than nondividing tissues such as heart, skeletal muscle, and nerve cells. The law is usually presented as an explanation for the radiosensitivity of cancer tissues that are rapidly dividing and have unstable chromosome compositions. There may not be sufficient time to repair the chromosomal damage before the next cell division. The expression of injury in some biological systems may require long periods simply because the rate of cell division in a particular tissue is very slow. Even if radiation exposure produced so great a damage as to modify or prevent cell division, it would take years for the cell to reach the point where the division would occur and injury is expressed. The cell cycle time of some ocular cells is 3 years, explaining in part the long latency period for expression of radiation-induced cataract formation (48).

Prokaryotes and insects also represent contradictions to the Law of Bergonie and Triblondeau. Mammals are much more sensitive, with the LD_{50}s for pigs, mice, and men being 2.5 Gy, 6–8 Gy and 4.5 Gy, respectively (23). The LD_{50} for *Escherichia coli* is between 20–50 Gy, compared to 100–1000 Gy for insects and 1000 Gy for amoeba (23). Plant sensitivities range from 4–400 Gy, with 75–90 Gy being lethal for the common chrysanthemum (36). These differences are explained in part by application of the target theory, in that cells with large chromosome numbers and large nuclear to cytoplasmic ratios tend to be more radiosensitive in part because they have larger critical target sizes (36). The chrysanthemum has a polyploidy of 22. Some plant species such as pine

Table 15.8
Radiation dose ranges and associated pathophysiological events[a]

Dose range (cGy)	Pathophysiological events: Prodromal effects	Manifest–illness effects	Survival
75–150	Mild	Slight decrease in blood cell count	Virtually certain
150–300	Mild to moderate	Beginning symptoms of bone marrow damage	Probable (>90%)
300–530	Moderate	Moderate to severe bone marrow damage	Possible bottom third of range: $LD_{5/60}$ Middle third: $LD_{10/60}$ Top third: $LD_{50/60}$
530–830	Severe	Severe bone marrow damage	Death within $3\frac{1}{2}$–6 weeks Bottom half: $LD_{90/60}$ Top half: $LD_{99/60}$
830–1100	Severe	Bone marrow pancytopenia and moderate intestinal damage	Death within 2–3 weeks
1100–1500	Severe	Combined gastrointestinal and bone marrow damage; hypotension	Death within 1–$2\frac{1}{2}$ weeks
1500–3000	Severe	Severe gastrointestinal damage with upper half of range: early transient incapacitation (ETI); gastrointestinal death	Death within 5–12 days
3000–4500		Gastrointestinal and cardiovascular damage	Death within 2–5 days

[a] From Reference 42.

trees have radiosensitivities similar to humans, making them ideal biological dosimeters surrounding nuclear facilities (255).

One last interesting aspect of radiobiology is that radiation exposure does not always result in harm. Hormesis describes the beneficial responses to biologically harmful agents such as poison and even radiation. Radiation has been used to improve the growth of seeds, separate from production of genetic mutations. It has even been reported to extend the life span of female mice, although it did so by sterilization, which eliminated the repeated stress of pregnancy.

SOMATIC EFFECTS OF RADIATION

In higher animals there is no simple, direct relationship between nuclear chromosome volume and sensitivity to ionizing radiation. Rather, the effects of irradiation on specific organ systems are more critical (504).

Acute Radiation Syndrome

There have been less than 25 documented fatalities worldwide, between 1946 and 1985, that may be attributed to radiation accidents (437). Although exposure of the whole body to lethal amounts of ionizing radiation is very rare, any discussion of the biological effects of ionizing radiation would be incomplete without mentioning acute radiation sickness and the acute radiation syndrome (ARS).

Acute radiation sickness is manifest in characteristic clinical sequelae known as the ARS, a combination of syndromes determined primarily by the total radiation dose received, the rate the radiation is delivered, and how the radiation is distributed in the body (722). Signs and symptoms of the ARS result from injury to bone marrow, gastrointestinal system, cardiovascular system, central nervous system, gonads, and skin. The variation in radiation sensitivity of these tissues causes the signs and symptoms of the ARS to occur in three successive phases: an initial prodromal phase, a later latent period, and the manifest illness phase. The length of each phase may vary directly with the radiation dose and the time between each phase may vary indirectly with the dose, so at an extremely high dose of radiation, the phases will blend, with the latent period disappearing completely (Table 15.8).

The prodromal phase may begin about 2–4 h after doses of 3–5 Gy or within minutes after exposure to

45 Gy or higher. The initial prodromal phase is characterized by a combination of gastrointestinal and neuromuscular symptoms such as anorexia, nausea, vomiting, diarrhea, apathy, tachycardia, fever, headaches, insomnia, dizziness, and vertigo. The pathogenesis of the prodromal phase is not known, but several causal factors have been suggested, including direct radiation effects on the central and autonomic nervous systems, disturbance of the endocrine balance, and the production and release of various chemical mediators (176, 687). The latent period, which follows the prodromal phase, is relatively asymptomatic and is believed to be the time between initial cell damage and the interference of radiation with cell renewal in the affected organs (722).

The manifest illness phase of the ARS is classically divided into three major syndromes, traditionally known as the hemopoietic, gastrointestinal, and central nervous system (CNS) syndromes (410). However, the current view replaces the CNS syndrome with the neurovascular syndrome (722).

The hemopoietic syndrome may be encountered after exposure to 2–7 Gy, and 1 Gy or more can significantly damage the blood-forming capability of the body. Radiation kills the mitotically active hemopoietic precursors of red cells, white cells, and platelets. Pathophysiological consequences include increased susceptibility to infection, bleeding, anemia, and lowered immunity. Death usually results from hemorrhage and infection (410,437,722).

Radiation exposure above 7 Gy contributes to the gastrointestinal syndrome by inhibiting the renewal of the cells lining the digestive tract. At doses of 3–8 Gy, tight junctions between the epithelial cells are disrupted, allowing increased fluid and electrolyte loss and permitting the movement of bacterial endotoxins into the blood. At higher doses (10–15 Gy), denudation of the mucosa occurs and death results from dehydration, electrolyte imbalance, and septicemia (437,722).

The neurovascular syndrome is the least understood of the radiation-induced deaths. The syndrome is unique in that death occurs very quickly before damage to the gastrointestinal and hemopoietic systems becomes apparent. Readily obvious CNS signs and symptoms include disorientation, loss of muscular coordination, respiratory distress, apathy, prostration, convulsive seizures, and coma associated with death. Some researchers believe that 50 Gy is necessary for the neurovascular syndrome and doses above 100 Gy are required for direct damage of the nervous system. However, ionizing radiation exposure modified electroencephalographic activity (649) and in vivo exposure decreased hippocampal synaptic transmission and spike generation (297) at lower doses than anticipated. Details of nervous system effects are given later.

Radiation-Induced Developmental Effects

Preimplantation in utero is never succeeded directly by postimplantation, the two being separated by the time it takes the placenta to develop into a functioning organ (472). This interval of development takes 1–2 days in rodents and 10–14 days in humans. Therefore, the traditional categories of prenatal development known as preimplantation, postimplantation, and fetal are replaced by conceptus, embryo, and fetus. The term conceptus is used for the stage of development lasting from ovulation until the placenta becomes a functioning organ. Even though there is some controversy about the maturation of an embryo to a fetus, most classifications of human developmental stages agree that this metamorphosis occurs in the last portion of the first trimester of gestation (289).

The developing conceptus and early embryo have a variety of rapidly dividing progenitor cells. These proliferating cells are much more sensitive to irradiation than differentiated, nondividing cells, making an organism more radiosensitive during its early stages of development than at any other stage of its life. The conceptus exhibits the lowest LD_{50} of any stage of development and is easily killed by doses of ionizing radiation that would cause abnormalities at later stages of development (77,555). Rather than a malformed organism developing to term, it dies in the conceptus stage due to irradiation-induced chromosomal damage (77). Thus, it is believed by some that the highest risk of irradiation during this stage is the death of the developing organism rather than teratogenesis (472).

In some animals, exposure to ionizing radiation in utero can result in anomalies in every organ system and the concept has been formulated that irradiation, however small, can inflict damage to the embryo or fetus (555,558). Irradiation-induced anomalies occurring during the middle stages of development may result in death of the organism or abnormal development of one or more organ systems. However, instead of lethality, morphological abnormalities are associated with irradiation during this time. Exposure during this period may result in gross malformations, growth retardation at term or as an adult, and structural pathology (437,726). In the human, most major organogenesis occurs during the first trimester of pregnancy with embryonic death and congenital abnormalities resulting from irradiation exposure during this period (555).

During late organogenesis and in the perinatal period, just before and just after birth, radiation damage tends to be functional rather than structural. Perinatal irradiation with x-rays and gamma rays (140–180 cGy) induces changes in tissue enzyme activity (14), hormone production (190,311), and hemopoiesis (247,471). The major effects of perinatal in utero exposure in humans is seen in the developing CNS with neurological damage and behavioral changes not always obvious in histological examination (77,133,458,470,499,555).

Susceptibility to radiation carcinogenesis is relatively high during prenatal development (440,556,684). During the last four decades, a major concern has been the risk of childhood leukemia and other neoplasms following irradiation in utero (50,55,77,247,437,527,685). Studies of the effects of ionizing radiation on the fetus are extremely important because there seems to be no biological reason to expect the fetus to be resistant (160). The embryo may be 50 times more vulnerable than the adult to irradiation-induced leukemia (77) and the risk of a child dying of cancer before the 10th birthday may be increased 40–60% by in utero irradiation (476).

The developing conceptus, embryo, and fetus show high susceptibility to ionizing radiation and the extent of injuries depends on the stage of development as well as the dose of radiation. Developmental anomalies are induced with doses much lower than previously used to demonstrate anomalies in adults (317,440,458,471).

The risk of leukemia in children with Down syndrome (trisomy 21) is estimated to be about 20 times higher than in the normal population and there has been some evidence that preconceptional ionizing radiation is linked to the nondisjunction of chromosome 21 (638). Clusters of cases of Down syndrome have been observed in Germany following the passage of the radioactive cloud from Chernobyl and experimental results have demonstrated that ionizing radiation may induce nondisjunction in oogenesis and spermatogenesis (674).

Even though there is a long latency period of radiation-induced cancer, a dramatic increase of up to 100-fold in the number of childhood thyroid cancers have been observed in the heavy radiation contaminated areas of Belarus and Ukraine and the Bryansk regions of Russia following the Chernobyl accident (28,569). A strong relationship is indicated between the thyroid cancer and radiation from the Chernobyl cloud.

The in utero developing nervous system is particularly vulnerable to ionizing radiation with defects of the eye and of spinal development among some of the more common malformations encountered following early gestational exposure (83,84,243). Later prenatal radiation exposure may result in dose related abnormalities of the hippocampus with disorganized and loosely scattered neurons in the CA-1 and CA-3 regions and agenesis of the corpus callosum (455). Perinatal irradiation, during neuronal migration and differentiation, resulted in delay of migration and severe reduction of neuronal tissue in the cerebral and cerebellar cortex and in the hippocampus (220,221,321). Postnatal cephalic irradiation of newborn rat pups produced an increase (122%) in noradrenaline activity and a marked decrease (38%) in monoamine oxidase activity in the cerebellum (177). The irradiation-induced 60% reduction in cerebellar weight may account for some of the marked increase (223%) in noradrenaline concentration and increase (206%) in tyrosine hydroxylase activity.

Direct Effects of Radiation on Reproductive Organs

During a period of approximately 20 years in the early part of this century, radiation was used in an attempt to increase fertility. Exposure normally was to 1.5–2.5 Gy over a period of 3 weeks. These levels apparently had little effect on fertility or on any later conceived children (437). However, neonatal irradiation of rats (211,212) and hamsters (637) demonstrated impaired fertility in mature male and female animals. In utero irradiation of male rat pups resulted in atrophy of the testes, ventral prostates, and seminal vesicles with a complete disappearance of germinal cells from the testes (629). Irradiation treatment of children 15 years of age and younger with Hodgkin's disease resulted in azoospermia in many of the mature males and ovarian injury in some of the mature females (512).

The safety of radiation levels is often questioned because the threshold for the effects of ionizing radiation on male reproduction is difficult to predict (588). Although fully developed sperm cells and primary spermatocytes are relatively radioresistant, the quiescent and proliferating spermatogonial cells of the testis are highly sensitive to ionizing radiation (437,555,670,671). Germ cell dysfunction is common following testicular irradiation and a dose-dependent impairment of spermatogenesis with gradual recovery may be seen following doses of up to 6 Gy (274,351,611). The effects of ionizing radiation on spermatogenesis are normally reversible with the recovery of fertility predictable. Although an acute irradiation dose of 6 Gy to the testis is likely to produce permanent sterility, conception has occurred for males after years of either aspermic or hypospermic conditions following absorbed doses between 2.3 and 3.7 Gy (437,555). However, following the Chernobyl nuclear reactor disaster there has been a widespread fear of damage to the reproductive system, with implications for fertility problems and adverse effects on offspring. A pilot study of 18 salvage workers (liquidators) revealed incomplete genesis of sperm characterized by certain ultramorphological parameters of the sperm head (205). The frequency of amorphous sperm head shape in the study group was significantly higher than in the local Ukrainian control group of 18 men.

Although the human testis is considered relatively resistant to the carcinogenic effects of radiation (50), occupational radiation exposure of the testis produces significant changes in serum gonadotropins and semen parameters. Testicular irradiation may be associated with elevated plasma levels of follicle-stimulating hormone (FSH) and luteinizing hormone (LH), reduced levels of androgen-binding protein (ABP) and testosterone, and reduced prostate and seminal vesicle weights (246,330,351,432,529,686). The decreased ABP levels and increased FSH levels are associated with Sertoli cell dysfunction, although the FSH increase may be a secondary result of germ cell depletion rather than a direct effect of irradiation. The changes in LH and testosterone levels and the decrease in prostate and seminal vesicle weights are indicative of Leydig cell function impairment.

As a direct effect of ionizing radiation, the human prostate epithelial cells may also display malignant transformation after multiple exposure (366). After a cumulative x-ray dose of 30 Gy, tumors characterized as poorly differentiated adenocarcinomas developed from prostate epithelial cells. This report may provide the first evidence of malignant transformation of human prostate epithelial cells resulting from direct exposure to ionizing radiation.

Although there are no proliferating stem cells in the mature female reproductive system, the oocytes are in follicles in various stages of development. Animal experiments indicate that radiosensitivity of the ova depends on the maturity of the follicle (555). Irradiation depletion of the radiosensitive mature and intermediate follicles will result in periods of temporary sterility followed by fertility due to maturation of surviving immature follicles. Sensitivity varies among species and temporary sterility can be produced in humans with doses as low as 1.5 Gy (686). Cases have been reported of irradiated women receiving as much as 6.4 Gy becoming pregnant as long as 2 years later and delivering normal children (437). However, the estimated dose required to produce permanent sterility in the female ranges between 6.25 and 30 Gy, depending on age of the subject (555), sensitivity increasing with the approach of menopause (686).

Ovarian failure is associated with whole body irradiation (149), abdominal irradiation (690,691), or radiation therapy for cervical carcinoma (425). Pubertal failure or premature menopause was common in females irradiated in childhood (690,691). Premenopausal women receiving radiation therapy may produce sign and symptoms associated with menopause, such as amenorrhea, dyspareunia, hot flashes, irritability, and loss of libido (199).

Breast cancer, the most frequent spontaneous malignancy diagnosed in women in the western world is increasing in incidence (568). Exposure of the breast to ionizing radiation is now known to increase the risk of breast cancer, especially for younger women (420,421). The risk of developing breast cancer is very high in women exposed to ionizing radiation before or during puberty, when the differentiation of terminal mammary end buds and alveolar structures is occurring (605). In fact, the carcinogenic effects of ionizing radiation on the vestigial male breast may be quite similar to that seen in the prepubertal female breast (644). The male breast displays an increase in risk for breast cancer with three or more radiographic examinations.

The Lymphohematopoietic System and Immune Competency

One of the systems most sensitive to irradiation is the hematopoietic system. Because of the rapidly proliferating hematopoietic elements of the bone marrow, the hemopoietic syndrome may be encountered following irradiation of 100 cGy or more (475,555). Approximately 50% of individuals exposed to 300 cGy ($LD_{50/60}$) will die within 2 months. The signs and symptoms result from radiation damage to the bone marrow, lymphatic organs, and immune system. The hematopoietic syndrome is characterized by a depression in the peripheral blood levels of mature erythrocytes, granulocytes, lymphocytes, monocytes, and platelets. Except for lymphocytes, the mature blood cells are relatively radioresistant and function normally in the peripheral blood after irradiation levels that will produce bone marrow damage.

Mature cells in peripheral blood have limited life spans and the replacement of their functional cell types is dependent on the proliferation of the hematopoietic elements of the bone marrow. One type of stem cell, a pluripotent stem cell (PPSC), has the dual capability of self-perpetuation and differentiation, and can meet the demands of the lymphohematopoietic and reticuloendothelial systems.

The progeny of the PPSC have specific functions in the body. Granulocytes are involved in activities against invasive bacteria and are related to the nonspecific immune response, whereas the cell-mediated and humoral responses of the lymphocytes are related to the specific immune response. The monocyte migrates into specific tissues and differentiates into a macrophage of the reticuloendothelial system. The platelet is a critical element of hemostasis and thrombocytopenia may result in hemorrhage and purpura. Thus, radiation damage to the PPSC may seriously compromise all of these systems, resulting in hemorrhage, infection, and death.

Depression of the mature cells in circulating blood is dose dependent (437,475). At radiation doses near the LD_{50} changes in the small lymphocytes can be seen in 1 h and lymphocytes may totally disappear from peripheral blood in 2–3 days (245,409,418,437,555). Although lymphocyte depletion may be measured in hours, granulocytes and platelets are depleted over days, and depletion of erythrocytes may be measured in weeks.

The small lymphocytes in lymphoid tissue are some of the most radiosensitive cells in the body and the small lymphocyte is the earliest to decrease in the peripheral blood following irradiation of man or animals. The lymphocyte not only shows the most rapid reduction in number, but it is the slowest to return to normal (418). The reduction in lymphocytes leads to impaired specific immune responses and immunosuppression. Regeneration of both the T- and B-lymphocyte levels depends on the lymphoid stem cells, which in turn depend on the PPSC of the bone marrow. Radiation-induced alterations in the nuclear material of lymphocytes might also have a significant impact on the function of this cell type. Chromosomal aberrations have been found in individuals exposed to radiation from both the Chernobyl accident-related cleanup activities (618) and to the subsequent fallout afterward (582).

Radiation depresses nonspecific immune responses by reducing the levels of circulating monocytes and granulocytes (475). Granulocytes serve as the first line of bactericidal defense at wounds whereas the macrophage, a progeny of the monocyte, can phagocytize and catabolize foreign substances such as microorganisms and toxins. The macrophage is also involved in the humoral specific immune response by processing foreign substances and presenting them as antigens for recognition. Radiation-induced depression of both specific and nonspecific immune responses through the reduction of monocytes, granulocytes, and lymphocytes is potentially life-threatening because of the enhanced susceptibility to opportunistic infections (197,521).

Ionizing radiation induces functional and quantitative abnormalities in the lymphoid cells of both man and experimental animals (6,252). Although ionizing radiation was found to deplete both T and B murine cells in equal proportions in the spleen (252), studies of late effects of atomic-bomb radiation on the immune system showed alteration of the balance and interaction between T and B cells, with a decrease in the T-cell population and an increase in the B-cell population in the periphery (6). Autoimmune deviations, both humoral and cellular, were observed in residents of areas contaminated from the Chernobyl accident and subjects participating in the clean-up of the accident (27,159,473,607). Structural and functional changes seen in the kidney, thyroid, and crystalline lens of the eye well may be associated with significant changes in the humoral immunity systems related to ionizing radiation exposure.

Irradiation usually does not depress the platelet (thrombocyte) count significantly in a healthy individual (437,475). The platelet's life span is 9–12 days and depression in circulating levels reach an initial nadir 10 days after irradiation. The individual will face problems similar to those of a patient with aplastic anemia: thrombocytopenia, capillary fragility, abnormal bleeding, and purpura. When the platelets reach a critical level, hemorrhage is likely to occur and may result in death of the individual. Therefore, platelet transfusion becomes critical for the irradiated individual.

Because of the relative radioresistance and long life span of erythrocytes (120 days), circulating blood levels fall slowly without complicating hemorrhage or infection (475). In the presence of thrombocytopenia and hemorrhage, transfusions may be required. Erythrocyte recovery after irradiation normally follows granulocyte and platelet recovery.

Radiation at the $LD_{50/30}$ dose level (350–400 cGy in humans) may kill more than 99% of the critical cells in the hematopoietic tissue (437,475). At this dose level cytological restoration of the bone marrow begins about the 25th day postirradiation in man. The PPSC will self-replicate and differentiate to produce hematopoietic progenitor cells. The risk of death from hematopoietic radiation injury depends on the regeneration rate of bone marrow stem cells (306), and the level of medical treatment provided (593). With bone marrow transplantation and heroic supportive therapy, survival is possible following whole-body irradiation as high as 1200 cGy (105,293,437). Although bone marrow transplantation certainly may be indicated, other clinical support regimens will stimulate hematopoietic regeneration, accelerate recovery, increase the $LD_{50/30}$, and enhance survival (405,406,518–520,592).

The most common neoplastic disorder of the hematopoietic system are the leukemias and several different types of leukemia have been observed in a variety of experimental animals following exposure to ionizing radiation (550,713). Leukemias account for about 32% of all cancer diagnosed in children, with about 85% of leukemias classified as acute (728). The acute leukemias in children may be related to parental occupational exposures to a number of carcinogenic substances or with prenatal and postnatal exposures to ionizing radiation.

Clinical evidence leads to the concept that ionizing radiation can cause leukemia by inducing DNA damage. Two hematopoietic cell lines were subjected to gamma irradiation to investigate the susceptibility of human cells to irradiation at the genetic recombination stage of leukemogenesis (168). The irradiation induced the formation of fusion genes characteristic of leukemia in both cell lines. The cell lines studied showed differences in susceptibility and frequency at which the different fusion genes were formed. These differences in selectivity may help to explain the differences in risk development of some types of leukemia that have been observed following high doses of irradiation.

Digestive Tract Dysfunction

The digestive tract includes the esophagus, small and large intestine, and rectum. The mucosa of the digestive tract undergoes continuous stress and in order for its functions to remain unimpaired, it must renew itself rapidly to replace lost cells. This fast turnover supported by a marked mitotic activity makes the digestive tract mucosa extremely radiosensitive. The duodenum is the most radiosensitive region of the digestive tract, followed by jejunum, ileum, esophagus, stomach, colon, and rectum, in order of decreasing radiosensitivity (45).

Surprisingly little has been written about radiation damage to the esophagus (665). The mucosal cells are characterized by a rapid proliferation rate and a relatively high degree of radiosensitivity. Acute radiation injuries are quite symptomatic with submucosal congestion and leukocytic infiltration, followed by mucosal necrosis and sloughing. Healing occurs rapidly and in animals with esophageal irradiation, the mucosa appeared completely normal 1 year following 2.5 Gy exposure. Humans who received 7.3–7.6-Gy irradiation exhibited narrowing of the esophageal lumen, partial loss of the mucosa and muscularis, and widening of the submucosa for 2–8 months following exposure. In spite of the initial radiation injury, radiation therapy for esophageal carcinoma results in very low mortality.

At radiation doses of 7–50 Gy, injury to the gastrointestinal tract inhibits the renewal of the cell lining. The intestinal epithelial stem cell is the target of radiation damage, and the resulting decrease in mitotic activity leads to denudation of the intestinal mucosa, fluid and electrolyte imbalance, and bacteremia (258). The symptoms of the gastrointestinal syndrome include lethargy, emesis, diarrhea, dehydration, and sepsis. At doses of 3–8 Gy, temporary injury to the tight junctions between epithelial cells of the mucosal lining permit the escape of bacterial endotoxins into the bloodstream. As dose increases, the epithelial lining is more extensively depleted. With doses of 10–15 Gy, denudation of the mucosa exacerbates the loss of fluid and electrolytes. Beginning at about 12.5 Gy, early mortality occurs due to dehydration and electrolyte imbalance, with death occurring 4–5 days postexposure.

At doses of 1 Gy or more irradiation of many mammals produces nausea and vomiting, signifying the prodromal phase of the acute radiation syndrome (45,186,258,349). Radiation-induced emesis, often accompanied by delayed gastric emptying, may be associated with areas of the brain known as the area postrema and the vomiting center, both located in the medulla (258). Ablation of the area postrema has been observed to abolish radiation-induced emesis in some mammals (258) and zacopride, an antiemetic, inhibited radiation-induced emesis and suppression of gastric emptying in the monkey (186) and abolished radiation-induced emesis in ferrets (350). Inhibition of radiation-induced emesis has been achieved also through the use of the selective 5-hydroxytryptamine (5-HT_3) receptor antagonists granisetron (58,305), ondansetron (284,536), and Y-25130 (216).

Functional alteration of the stomach by radiation included a decrease in the production and secretion of HCl, pepsinogen, and mucus (45), and an increase is serum levels of pepsinogen and gastrin (696). Histopathological alterations included vasodilation and edema indicative of increased microvascular permeability (86), and marked degenerative features including atrophic mucosa and ulceration (45,75).

Intestinal mucosa cells originate from a single stem cell type located at the base of the intestinal crypts. As the cells proliferate and differentiate they move to the tips of the villi, a journey of 3–5 days. The differentiated cells are shed continuously from the tips of the villi. Radiation damage to the cells of the crypt leads to the death of some cells and an arrest of mitotic activity of others (15,45,491). The severely damaged crypt stem cells do not divide and replace the cells lost from the tips of the villi. This results in decreased absorption and allows a ready entry for intestinal flora into the systemic circulation (103,259,515). Electrolyte transport is also altered in the jejunum and ilium following exposure to ionizing radiation and this functional change may be related to the decreased mast cells and histamine (402,403).

Intestinal absorption may also be decreased due to vascular concrescence. In examinations of irradiated animals the villous capillaries showed initial marked vasodilation followed by constriction, with many capillaries becoming totally nonpatent while the endothelial cells showed changes consistent with vascular damage (2,3,402). These findings were consistent with functional changes seen in several studies reviewed by Cockerham and Hawkins (131).

The colon has a relatively high radiotolerance, possibly due to the long turnover of its cells, and the rectum may tolerate more than 50 Gy irradiation (45). Postirradiation pathological events are essentially the same as in the small intestine with inhibition of mitosis, changes in cell morphology, and edema and vascular changes in the submucosal and serosal layers. An inflammatory response occurs within 24 h and a progressive degeneration leading to ulcerations occurs after high doses (86). A late development of colorectal irradiation seen in murine studies was a dose-dependent decrease in compliance (417), possibly due to altered ratios of collagen isotypes, especially in the circular muscle layer and villi (416). As with the other portions of the gastrointestinal tract, the loss of water and electrolyte imbalance due to diarrhea and the development of bacteremia are considered the most important factors in the gastrointestinal syndrome (258). The rat colon also becomes unresponsive to neurally evoked electrolyte transport following exposure to ionizing radiation of 10 Gy (208). This response also correlates with decreased mast cells and histamine.

Cardiovascular Dysfunction

Cardiovascular dysfunction (CVD) has been defined as the inability of any element of the cardiovascular system to perform adequately upon demand. The maintenance of cardiovascular integrity is determined by the changes in (i) the pumping action of the heart, (ii) compliance of the vascular beds, (iii) resistance of the peripheral circulation, (iv) quantity of blood in the vascular system, and (v) viscosity of the blood. Failure of any of the mechanisms to respond properly may compromise the integrity of the entire cardiovascular system (131, 272,280). Exposure to supralethal doses of radiation has been shown to induce alterations in cardiovascular function in many species, including human. The extent of the radiation-induced CVD and its etiology may vary with the species, level of exposure, and dose rate.

Radiation-induced CVD is surprisingly common (26) and may be manifest as circulatory shock. Although postirradiation hypotension does not occur with equal frequency in all species, it has been reported in rats, monkeys, and dogs (124,130,242,441). However, evidence indicates than even if sublethal doses of radiation induce a functional cardiovascular deficiency that manifests itself as early hypotension, the lesion may be masked during a period of circulatory deterioration because of cardiovascular reserve (230,488). When the cardiovascular reserve is no longer capable of maintaining homeostasis the damage may then be recognized as radiation-induced shock (278).

Irradiated rats displayed compromised myocardial function with a decline in cardiac output and an increased left ventricular end-diastolic volume (591,719), which correlated with a decline in capillary density and focal degeneration of the myocardium. Cardiac performance after irradiation using an isolated working rat heart preparation showed a dose-dependent decrease in cardiac function and Frank–Starling curves, suggesting a loss of contractile function of the myocardium (712). Ultrastructural findings in the irradiated rat heart included intercalated disc damage and mitochondrial damage of the myocytes and swelling of the capillary endothelial cells and collapse of the capillaries (120). Mediastinal irradiation of human patients damages endothelial cells with loss of capillaries and ischemia, leading to increase in collagen and fibrous tissue throughout the heart (26). Long-term side effects of mediastinal irradiation include pericarditis, accelerated coronary artery disease, myocardial fibrosis, and valvular injury (26,93).

The response of the gastrointestinal microcirculation to radiation has received little attention, although this may be an important factor in the development of both the cardiovascular and gastrointestinal subsyndromes. Here, as in other parts of the vascular system, the endothelial cell is one of the most radiosensitive cells (545). The initial expression of radiation injury to the endothelial cells is an increased vascular permeability leading to changes in extracellular environment (24). Following a single irradiation of 10–20 Gy, acute damage to endothelial cells may be detected in 1–5 days. Although not identical, radiation-induced endothelial damage in the lungs, kidney, myocardium, and intestine are similar and characterized by the plasma membrane becoming irregular with projections into the vascular lumen, followed by focal or generalized cytoplasmic swelling that narrows the lumen and may obstruct it completely. Damaged endothelial cells may retract from the basement membrane, causing exposure of the membrane. This results in platelet adhesion, followed by aggregation and the development of thrombosis and vascular occlusion. Damaged capillaries may be manifest by telangiectasia or be replaced by a collagen scar formation (38,545). When reviewing the response of any microcirculation to irradiation, the variables of total dose, dose rate, type of radiation, variability of the animal model, and postirradiation time of observation must be considered. Irradiation damage to the microcirculation may cause dilation or constriction and either an increase or decrease in blood flow, depending on the above factors (131).

A complication involving the endothelium of intracerebral vessels is the impaired integrity of the blood–brain barrier (BBB) following irradiation (279). Functional alterations of the BBB are manifest in the endothelium by the activation of pinocytotic vesicular transport (162,655) and in astrocytes by glycogen deposition. The changes in BBB permeability seem to be the result of the intense vesicular response of the endothelium rather than opening of endothelial tight junctions or altered regional blood flow (162,656). The opening of the BBB has been associated with cerebral vasogenic edema and ischemia (352,630). However, Gobbel et al. (248) suggest that postirradiation edema-induced vascular compression was not responsible for changes in regional cerebral blood flow observed in dogs.

A reduction in systemic blood pressure can reduce the driving force required to maintain cerebral blood flow and result in cerebral ischemia. The acute irradiation-induced hypotension in the monkey has a temporal, if not causal, relationship with observed postirradiation reduction in regional cerebral blood flow (134). However, the reduced cerebral blood flow seen in hippocampi and cortices of rat brains and the hypothalamus of humans 10–24 weeks postirradiation was probably due to the telangiectatic vessels, spreading edema, focal regions of necrosis, and hemorrhage observed in the brains (31,115,358,392).

Several biochemical mediators have been implicated in postirradiation CVD and reduced cerebral blood flow, including histamine, serotonin, opiate peptides, platelet-activating factor, eicosanoids, cyclic nucleotides, and catecholamines (176,279,686). Evidence that further implicates histamine includes the finding that plasma histamine increases precipitously in dogs and monkeys after exposure to radiation (126,132). Infusing histamine into humans resulted in decreased blood pressure and altered cerebral blood flow (8,602). Pretreatment with antihistamines diminished the cardiovascular effects of irradiation in dogs and monkeys (125,132), further implicating histamine in postirradiation CVD. However, in another study infusing histamine into humans, Krabbe and Olesen (362) were unable to alter either blood pressure or cerebral blood flow. Likewise, the "histamine hypothesis" does not explain the postirradiation response of the rat (279). Considering that the etiology of postirradiation CVD may vary with the species, perhaps the radiation-induced production or release of other intermediates such as serotonin (129) or free radicals (123) may account for the CVD.

Radiation Effects on Bone, Cartilage, and Muscle

Mature bone is relatively radioresistant and radionecrosis of bone is very rare (437,585). Many of the effects from irradiation seen in bone may be attributed to a reduction in the number of blood vessels supplying the bone and a decreased blood flow. Radiation damage to bone may be apparent only after months or years following irradiation because of impaired progenitor cell proliferation (161,702). If the vascular support of the bone can recover, mitotic activity may reappear within 2 weeks after a dose of less than 17.5 Gy. However, osteoradionecrosis, the characteristic late bone injury, often accompanied by osteomyelitis, occurs at a minimum dose of 50 Gy (585).

Radiation-damaged adult bone characteristically displays a decreased ability to resist infection, increased susceptibility to fractures, and poor healing after damage (148,437). The most common site for osteoradionecrosis and postirradiation complications is the mandible, probably due to its less than abundant blood supply. Clavicles and ribs have an increased incidence of fractures after radiation therapy for breast cancer and tumor-induced fractures of long bones do not heal following radiotherapy of approximately 30 Gy (585). Following surgical trauma of rat femur, a dose-dependent radiation-induced delay is seen in new bone formation (25).

Radiation effects on bone are age dependent, with developing bone more sensitive to irradiation than adult bone, with the most pronounced effects seen during organogenesis (437,585). However, a reduction in number of blood vessels and decreased blood flow are not thought to be the primary causes of reduction in growth. Impaired progenitor cell proliferation may be the reason, because a single dose of 6 Gy has been demonstrated to produce a decrease in mitotic activity.

Internal irradiation of bone by radionuclides may occur through occupational exposure or therapeutic administration (437). A famous case of iatrogenic poisoning was the use of Radithor, a patent medicine used as a metabolic stimulant and aphrodisiac (400). Unfortunately, the victim died of radium poisoning after his skeleton accumulated a dose that may have been greater than 350 Sv.

Probably a more famous case of radioisotope poisoning involved the manufacture of watch dials painted with luminous compounds containing radium (437,564). The radioisotopes ^{226}Ra and ^{228}Ra were ingested by the women workers when they tipped the brushes with their lips. Isotopes of radium, strontium, and calcium are considered *volume seekers* and ultimately are included in the matrix of bone, whereas plutonium and thorium isotopes are considered *surface seekers* and accumulate on the periosteum and endosteal surfaces of the bone. The accumulation of radium in the bones of the female dial painters correlated with fractures of long bones, coarsening of the trabecular pattern, bone infarcts, and aseptic osteonecrosis. Bone sarcomas and head carcinomas have occurred at a higher than normal rate.

More than 3000 children of the 1495 women dial painters in the basic group were exposed continuously to an alpha and gamma-enhanced radiation environment during their entire period of gestation (564), but no evidence exists to suggest that any effects have occurred.

Growing cartilage is more radiosensitive than growing bone (585). Radiation doses exceeding 18 Gy cause permanent cessation of growth but chondrocytes recover from irradiation less than 10 Gy. Children aged 6 years and under and during puberty are the most vulnerable to irradiation-induced growth depression. Uneven irradiation of the spine results in scoliosis and doses up to 20 Gy result in major deformities. Pronounced growth retardation occurs above 35 Gy.

Mature cartilage, like adult bone, is fairly radioresistant (437,585). Doses of 60–70 Gy may be tolerated by mature cartilage if the irradiation is applied over 6–7 weeks. However, if the same dose is given in less than 6 weeks, radionecrosis of the cartilage is to be expected.

Although atrophy of muscle fibers may be seen following fractionated irradiation of 22–54 Gy, doses more than 500 Gy are required to produce acute radionecrosis of skeletal muscle (437). Recently, destructive alterations in muscle proteins were observed after ^{60}Co gamma irradiation as low as 1.0 kGy, with a three-fold decrease in elasticity with doses of 15 kGy (356). Ischemia from a radiation-damaged vascular supply may result in fibrosis, but the extent of muscle damage depends, in part, on whether the entire muscle was exposed, or only a portion.

Radiation Dermatosis

The effects of ionizing radiation on the skin range from erythema to necrosis. The regular sequence of change progresses, as the dose is increased, over two periods, one occurring within 70–120 days and the other from 4 months to years later (22). The first period is characterized by erythema, pigmentation, epilation, dry desquamation, and moist desquamation, whereas the second period is characterized by atrophy, telangiectasia, fibrosis, and necrosis. Erythema, associated with an increased vascular permeability, appears after a single dose of 500 cGy or more and after multiple-dose fractions when the total dose is 1200 cGy or more (22). The first phase of erythema, presumably due to release of vasoactive amines, usually occurs within the first 1–2 days and lasts for a week. The second phase begins at about 10–12 days, reaches a maximum at about 20 days, and lasts for 30–40 days. This second phase is due to vascular damage and increased blood flow (437). The fading of erythema merges with increased pigmentation that may be permanent or fade for days or weeks as dry desquamation proceeds (22,437). This pigmentation is associated with an increased melanin content of the basal layer.

Some epilation may be noted at 10 days following irradiation with a single dose of 300–600 cGy (22,437). The evolution and time course of epilation are not dose dependent but epilation may be complete at 4 weeks with hair beginning to return in the second month and continuing for up to a year. However, a single dose of 700 cGy may cause permanent epilation (437). Radiation epilation sensitivity varies with body area; the scalp and beard are the most sensitive, followed by chest, axillary, abdominal, eyebrow, eyelash, and pubic hair.

Dry desquamation, preceded by decreasing erythema and an increasing pigmentation, is characterized by a loss of epidermal cells accompanied by replacement. The cells may scale off or peel off in a sheet, leaving an intact, erythematous epidermal surface. The regenerative capacity usually exceeds the destructive capacity as long as the single dose does not exceed 2000 cGy, or the multiple fraction total does not exceed 4500 cGy (22,437). The reduced proliferative potential and regenerative capacity of irradiated skin cells may be manifest also in an interference with wound healing at doses of 400 cGy or greater (141).

If the dose exceeds the levels allowing regeneration to occur, 2400 cGy for single dose and 5000 cGy for multiple fraction total, the epidermal cell population becomes depleted and the loss of epidermis allows serum leakage and a moist desquamation (22). A bullous-type, moist desquamation may occur with the small blisters tending to coalesce and rupture (437). Blisters may even form beneath the basal layer and the lesion may appear, similar to a second- or third-degree thermal burn. The ruptured blisters may become infected and ulceration may occur. The ulceration is usually associated with a reduction in circulation due to obliterative arteriolar and small artery changes.

Late skin damage may follow the early reactions by week to years or not at all. Alternatively, late skin damage may be manifest without an earlier reaction. The late reaction is, in part, dose dependent and may progress or remain static (22).

In the weeks or months following irradiation at a single dose level of 1700–2400 cGy or a multiple fraction total of 4500–5000 cGy, telangiectasia manifest as superficial, elongated, and dilated blood vessels (22). Radiation-damaged endothelial cells are lost and the microvessels shorten, uncoil, and dilate. A loss of total microvasculature occurs as well as a decrease in functional vessels. The formation of telangiectatic vessels is dose dependent and if the epidermal response is severe, focal keratosis and dysplasia may be present.

Skin changes occurring months to years following irradiation may include increased induration, stiffening, and thickening of the dermis associated with increasing fibrosis (22,437). Although the onset and formation of fibrosis are dose dependent, once started, fibrosis is progressive with a characteristic proliferation of the small arteries and arterioles. As the degree of fibrosis increases, so does the probability that necrosis will be the result.

Following a single dose of radiation that exceeds 2700 cGy or a multiple fraction total dose greater than 6000 cGy, the end stage of radiation dermatosis is a nonhealing necrosis (22). Radiation-induced necrosis is associated with the progressive loss of the dermal microvasculature and is the end stage to progressive fibrosis.

Chronic exposure to low-dose (0.015 cGy/s) x-ray for 9–18 months (total doses equal 2.025 and 4.05 cGy) will produce a hyperkeratinization in the rat, along with a decrease in skin concentration of zinc and an increased concentration of iron (111). The chronic sequelae following cutaneous radiation may include telangiectases, radiation keratoses, radiation ulcers, hemangiomas, splinter hemorrhages in the distal nail bed, lentiginous hyperpigmentation, and severe subcutaneous fibrosis (525). This predominant involvement of the skin is sometimes described as the cutaneous radiation syndrome and can become the characteristic feature of chronic cutaneous irradiation.

The Urinary System

The kidney is relatively radiosensitive compared to other abdominal organs and has a definite but low sensitivity to radiation carcinogenesis (48,50,437,714). The time course for pathophysiological and histopathological changes are dose dependent with a fractionated tolerance dose (TD) of 20–23 Gy for the human kidney (437,714). The kidneys are considered to be late-reacting organs with the effects of radiation nephropathy appearing months to years after exposure. However, pathological changes in the endothelial cells of the renal microvasculature seen soon after exposure may have long-lasting effects and later tubule and glomeruli degeneration may be secondary to renal ischemia (714). Functional changes seen in mice following fractionated irradiation with x-rays include decreased EDTA clearance, increased urine output, and reduced hematocrit (623).

Reports of patients dying of renal failure and hypertension following therapeutic radiation include subacute changes of intimal necrosis, subendothelial thickening, fibrinoid thrombosis, atrophy of tubules, and replacement with collagen (437). In some instances myointimal proliferation with "foamy cells" and sclerosis of the glomeruli may be seen as well.

There are no human data on acute radiation effects following exposure to single doses (437). However, acute pathological changes seen in animals are hyperemia, increased capillary permeability, interstitial edema, and microvascular endothelial degeneration. These changes are usually followed by occlusive changes in the interlobular arteries and afferent arterioles, reducing blood flow to the nephron. Although in many cases the changes are transient, they may progress to severe diffuse endarteritis and necrotizing vasculitis, which may result in malignant hypertension (714).

Irradiation of pigs with a single ^{60}Co gamma ray dose of 7.8 Gy or higher resulted in a dose-dependent reduction in effective renal plasma flow (ERPF) and glomerular filtration rate (GFR) (553,554). A normochromic normocytic anemia, with a significant reduction in erythrocyte count, hematocrit, and hemoglobin levels, developed within 6–8 weeks following irradiation. Studies in pigs (552) and mice (620) indicate that the kidney fails to exhibit complete recovery in function following irradiation and that irradiation of a previously irradiated kidney is likely to lead to severe renal damage.

Chronic renal dysfunction develops 1–5 years after irradiation and involves a slow evolution of anemia, hypertension, and impairment of renal function (437). The changes are progressive and irreversible, with the treatment usually symptomatic. The pathology is an extension of that seen in short term radiation-induced renal dysfunction. Chronic glomerulonephritis has been reported in subjects participating in the clean-up after the Chernobyl accident (159). The renal pathology was associated with significant changes in the humoral immunity system manifested by increased serum levels of immunoglobulin M, immunoglobulin G, and circulating immune complexes. However, chronic ingestion of drinking water containing uranium (0.004–9 $\mu g/kg$ body weight) indicated that the proximal tubule, rather than the glomerulus, was the site of injury (727).

The urinary bladder is relatively more radioresistant than the kidney and can usually tolerate 55–60 Gy if the dose is fractionated (437). Bladder complications are seen most often in humans following radiotherapy for cancer of the cervix, prostrate, or bladder (626). The symptoms of acute radiation cystitis appear 4–6 weeks following treatment and include dysuria, nocturia, and increased frequency. Edema, hyperemia, and partial desquamation of the mucosa may be seen. Acute pathological changes in humans are less well documented than those in animals.

Acute changes in the bladders of dogs following irradiation are more pronounced than those seen in rodents (626). Acute and short term pathophysiological changes in the rodent bladder include an increase in urination frequency, reduced bladder volume, decreased compliance of the bladder wall, and diminished pressure during micturition (179,396,439,620). Reirradiation tolerance for late bladder damage was inversely related to the first dose and independent of the interval between treatments (622).

Late-occurring or chronic pathological alterations seen in the urinary bladders of dogs following irradiation are similar to those observed in humans. These include a small, shrunken, and contracted bladder with thick and fibrotic walls (437,626). There may be multiple areas of edema and telangiectasia and collagen may replace muscular tissue. Squamous metaplasia is common and extensive mucosal ulceration may extend into and beyond the muscle layers. In women treated for cervical carcinoma, this ulceration can lead to vesicovaginal fistulas.

The most radioresistant portion of the urinary system is said to be the ureter (437). However, others classify the ureter as radiosensitive, with ureteral fibrosis, stenosis, and obstruction following doses of 12.5 Gy (292,600).

Dogs have been shown to tolerate 17.5-Gy irradiation of the ureter with early injury due to ulceration of the epithelium seen at 25 Gy or above (241). However, histological evidence suggested that chronic injury of the canine ureter seen after 5 years was of vascular etiology.

Radiation-Induced Hepatic Dysfunction

Early literature describing hepatic irradiation contained many contradictory reports concerning the radiosensitivity of the liver (322,437). The hepatic cells are relatively radioresistant and there is a marked capacity for regeneration following destruction of a large portion of the liver. The liver is able to tolerate fractionated doses of 30–35 Gy over 3–4 weeks, but 35 Gy should not be exceeded (322). Following liver damage the regenerating portion is more radiosensitive (437).

Radiation-induced hepatic injury represents a continuum of clinical, pathological, and radiographic findings, ranging from asymptomatic biochemical changes to fulminant, fatal hepatic failure (322). Radiolesions in the liver are dose dependent in animals (74,260,261) and are primarily due to damage to the fine vasculature and connective tissue (234,235,322). Characteristic changes following liver irradiation portray a nonspecific form of venous occlusive disease (VOD) resembling pathologically the Budd–Chiari syndrome (322,437).

Pathological changes that occur following irradiation of the liver to doses greater than 35 Gy may be divided into two stages. The acute phase may begin 2–6 weeks postirradiation and continue for 3–6 months. Clinical signs include hepatomegaly, ascites, jaundice, and elevated serum alkaline phosphatase and serum transaminases (SGOT and SGPT) (74,234,322,437). A distinct decrease in hepatic biotransformation and tolerance to a wide variety of drugs may be seen within a few days postirradiation (480,711). These clinical manifestations are usually associated with pathological changes that include sinusoidal congestion, occlusion of the central vein, disrupted intrahepatic blood flow, and parenchymal cell damage, atrophy, and necrosis (235,322,437).

The late phase of pathological changes and hepatic dysfunction manifests itself more than 6 months postirradiation (322,437). There is less hepatic congestion, but the signs and symptoms of portal hypertension and right-sided congestive heart failure are manifest. Pathological findings are those of a veno-occlusive process leading to obstruction of hepatic outflow. The centrilobular veins may be obliterated with dense collagen and periportal fibrosis is extensive. The liver appears shrunken and pale, and atrophy due to cell loss is evident. Serum phosphatase and transaminase levels may be slightly elevated or normal but the serum albumin levels are decreased (322,480). The postirradiation VOD seen in the liver is unique but is similar to conditions caused by various drugs (437).

Radiation Pneumonitis and Pulmonary Fibrosis

The lung is relatively radiosensitive and lesions in the lung are common after any irradiation. Involvement of even a small portion of the thorax results in some degree of pulmonary damage (437,654).

The lung's response to irradiation is biphasic (231). The first phase, *radiation pneumonitis*, may vary in postirradiation time of onset depending on species, type of radiation, and dose (231,379,526,646). A clinical threshold of 6–7 Gy and a maximum of 8 Gy in a single dose has been suggested for the development of radiation pneumonitis (437).

During the pneumonitis phase functional changes are prominent, including respiratory distress, hypoxemia, increased bronchoalveolar lavage protein, impaired surfactant function, decrease in pulmonary blood flow, and pulmonary hypertension (231,526,646). Alveolar epithelium and endothelial damage (379,526) may be associated with a radiation-induced production of free radicals, release of histamine, leukotriene, and prostaglandin, and the acceleration of lipid peroxidation (78,253,501). Pulmonary blood flow problems are indicative of loss of fine vasculature, pulmonary hypertension, right ventricular hypertrophy, and radiation-induced heart failure (54, 599).

The second phase of pulmonary injury, *pulmonary fibrosis*, is seen with or without the presence of pneumonitis (654). Although many patients are asymptomatic during the fibrosis phase, functional changes include arterial hypoxia, a decreased lung volume, decreased compliance, and a reduced maximum breathing capacity. Endothelial and epithelial cell damage may contribute to the development of postirradiation pulmonary fibrosis (526), but the final picture includes replacement of septa by collagen, decreased total alveolar volume, reduced functional microvasculature, and atelectasis (437,654).

Radiation Effects on Endocrine Function

Many discussions of radiation effects of the endocrine system are limited to the pituitary, thyroid, parathyroid, and adrenal glands (437). Other endocrine glands less often considered are the pineal, pancreas, ovary, and testis. Although most endocrine glands are relatively radioresistant with direct effects of radiation resulting from injury to the fine vasculature, endocrine abnormalities are relatively common following irradiation of the head and neck (437).

Pineal Gland (Epiphysis)

Melatonin, a hormone that inhibits ovarian and testicular function, is synthesized and secreted by the pineal gland (148,686). In several species, including human, melatonin synthesis and secretion increase during the dark period of the day and is at a lower level during the daylight hours (228). Pineal synthesis of melatonin in response to the light cycle is altered by radiation, with a decreased synthesis seen in rats following 3.5-Gy exposure (686). However, melatonin has been shown to be radioprotective, with cellular destruction occurring postirradiation in other glands without melatonin (369,686). Even so, the function of melatonin and the pineal in the radiation response of human remains relatively obscure.

Pituitary Gland (Hypophysis)

Physiologically, the pituitary gland is divisible into two distinct portions: the *anterior pituitary* or the *adenohypophysis*, and the *posterior pituitary* or the *neurohypophysis*. Most control of secretion by the pituitary comes from the *hypothalamus* by either nervous or hormonal signals. Secretion by the anterior pituitary is controlled by hormones secreted within the hypothalamus and transported to the anterior pituitary through the *hypothalamic–hypophysial portal system* of blood vessels. Secretion from the posterior pituitary is controlled by nerve fibers originating in the hypothalamus and terminating in the posterior pituitary. The hypothalamus receives signals from sources throughout the nervous system and uses this information to control secretion of the pituitary hormones (228,262).

Six important hormones are secreted by the anterior pituitary and play major roles in the control of metabolic functions throughout the body. These six hormones are (i) *growth hormone* (GH), (ii) *adrenocorticotropic hormone* (ACTH, corticotropin), (iii) *thyroid-stimulating hormone* (TSH, thyrotropin), (iv) *prolactin* (luteotropic hormone, LTH), (v) *follicle-stimulating hormone* (FSH), and (vi) *luteinizing hormone* (LH). The two hormones secreted in the posterior pituitary are, (i) *antidiuretic hormone* (vasopressin, ADH), which controls water excretion, and (ii) *oxytocin*, which helps deliver milk from the glands to the nipple and may help in delivery at the end of gestation. ADH and oxytocin are formed in the supraoptic and paraventricular nuclei of the hypothalamus and released from nerve endings in the posterior pituitary (228,262).

Hypothalamic–pituitary failure is a common complication of cranial and neck irradiation and signs of endocrine deficiency may appear from 1–15 years postirradiation. Some researchers propose that radiation-induced alterations in pituitary function can be attributed to effects of radiation on the hypothalamus (574). There is good evidence that the earliest irradiation damage to the hypothalamic–pituitary axis is at the level of the hypothalamus and that any subject receiving a total irradiation dose of 20 Gy or more to the axis is at risk of hypopituitarism (302,370,388). In general, the direct effects of radiation on the hypothalamic–pituitary axis result in hypopituitarism manifested through alterations of the direct actions of the pituitary hormones or through their influence on other endocrine glands (389,437). Radiation-induced pituitary dysfunction may result in loss of weight, loss of body hair, dry skin, slow pulse, low body temperature, dwarfism in children, genital atrophy, primary amenorrhea in females, failure of sexual development in males, and other dysfunctions associated with the endocrine system (437,574).

Thyroid

Thyrotropin-releasing hormone (TRH) is secreted by the hypothalamus, and stimulates the release of TSH by pituitary thyrotrophs and the release of *calcitonin* from the C cells of the thyroid. TSH stimulates all thyroidal functions associated with the production and release of *triiodothyronine* (T_3) and *tetraiodothyronine* (thyroxine, T_4). Through a classic feedback loop, excessive amounts of T_3 and T_4 suppress the release of TSH by the pituitary (343). Calcitonin, from the C cells or parafollicular cells in the thyroid gland, serves to lower the serum calcium and phosphate levels (228).

Radiation-induced injury of the hypothalamic–pituitary axis may be manifest in the development of hypothyroidism (370,388). However, direct irradiation of the thyroid gland results in decreased production of T_3 and T_4 (686). Estimates of irradiation doses required to produce hypothyroidism vary from 2–50 Gy, with thyroid ablation a possible result of the larger doses. Data confirm the high incidence of thyroid dysfunction when the gland is included in the radiation field (19,202,273,505,718).

Radiation hypothyroidism, through the feedback loop, will result in an increase in TSH secretion by the pituitary. This increase in TSH has been associated with increases in radiation-induced thyroid cancer (686). TSH has also been studied in relation to radiation exposure in children, particularly after the Chernobyl nuclear disaster (249,538).

The latent period for radiation-induced thyroid cancer was in excess of 15 years following the exposure of the Japanese to the atomic bomb explosions at Hiroshima and Nagasaki. Increased numbers of thyroid cancer cases became evident within just 4 or 5 years following the Chernobyl nuclear accident, however, and continued to increase substantially over the next decade (66,232). Another interesting aspect of the dynamics of thyroid cancer incidence in that accident was that geographic correlation of thyroid cancers was more closely related to the transportation corridors than to the isopleths of ^{131}I distribution or to population density (517).

Hypothyroidism following 10-Gy irradiation has been associated with a shift in the ratio of the alpha-myosin heavy chain to the beta-myosin heavy chain in the rat heart, a shift usually associated with overload of the heart or aging (686). This change may correspond with a low resting ejection fraction and decreased response to exercise seen in cardiac scans following therapy for Hodgkin's disease (431).

Therapy for hyperthyroidism using ^{131}I decreases basal calcitonin levels and may cause C cell deficiency (43). However, this may not be of extreme consequence because total thyroidectomy does not reduce the circulating level of the hormone to zero (228).

The thyroid gland of children is especially vulnerable to the carcinogenic action of ionizing radiation, with one of the highest risk coefficients of any organ and may be the only tissue with convincing evidence for risk at about 0.10 Gy (559). This vulnerability is dramatically illustrated in the 100-fold increase in the number of childhood thyroid cancers observed in heavily contaminated areas of Belarus, Ukraine, and the Bryansk regions of Russia following the accident at the Chernobyl nuclear power plant in 1986 (28,569).

Parathyroid

In humans there are usually four parathyroid glands embedded in the poles of the thyroid gland. Chief cells in the parathyroid are sensitive to circulating levels of ionized calcium and act to secrete parathyroid hormone (PTH) in response to decreased Ca^{2+} levels. The PTH acts directly on bone to increase bone resorption and mobilize Ca^{2+}. PTH also acts to depress plasma phosphate by increasing phosphate excretion (228).

Although parathyroid cells are relatively resistant to radiation, data confirm an association between hyperparathyroidism and radiation exposure (44,215, 437). The hyperparathyroidism may be secondary to a depletion of calcium that occurs in mammals following exposure to greater than 3 Gy radiation (686,687). Other biological responses occurring as a result of irradiation-induced calcium loss include increased blood clotting, bone damage, and convulsions (686).

Adrenal Glands

The endocrine functions of the adrenal glands are associated with the adrenal cortex that produces over 30 different steroids. Only two of these corticosteroids are of exceptional importance to the endocrine function of the adrenal cortex: *aldosterone*, the principal mineralocorticoid and *cortisol*, the principal glucocorticoid. The mineralocorticoids affect the levels of the electrolytes of the extracellular fluids and the glucocorticoids serve to increase blood glucose concentration and affect protein and fat metabolism. Aldosterone secretion is regulated by: (i) potassium ion concentration in extracellular fluid, (ii) renin–angiotensin system, (iii) quantity of sodium in the body, and (iv) ACTH. Secretion of cortisol is controlled almost entirely by ACTH (262).

Radiation-induced changes in the endocrine functions of the adrenal glands are difficult to document because stress factors, including radiation, result in increased release of ACTH from the pituitary (437,686). ACTH acts on the adrenal cortex stimulating the synthesis and release of aldosterone and cortisol. Even though irradiation of the hypothalamic–pituitary axis produces a defect in ACTH release, adrenal corticosterone levels may be normal or elevated following irradiation, indicating a possible hypersensitivity to the ACTH present or the presence of some other controlling factor (686).

The direct effects of radiation on the adrenal glands are manifest in three phases of activity, each associated with increases in plasma and adrenal corticosterone levels (686). The first phase occurs early postirradiation and the second peak of activity is associated with gastrointestinal damage. The third phase of activity is associated with hematopoietic injury. The increase in activity may be seen following absorbed doses of 15–35 Gy (437,686). However, if the dose exceeds 35 Gy, normal steroidogenesis may occur under nonstress conditions, but the ability to respond to stress is impaired. Hypertrophy of the adrenal cortex has been demonstrated following irradiation with 15 Gy and higher (172,686).

Pancreas

The pancreas has both endocrine and exocrine functions. The islets of Langerhans in the pancreas are associated with its endocrine function and act to secrete *insulin* and *glucagon*. Insulin is produced by the beta cells of the islets and glucagon by the alpha cells. The secretion of insulin and glucagon is controlled by the blood glucose concentration. An increase in blood glucose concentration stimulates insulin secretion and inhibits glucagon secretion. A decrease in blood glucose concentration has the opposite effect on both hormones. Insulin acts to increase glucose uptake by most tissues of the body and to stimulate glycogen synthesis. Glucagon stimulates breakdown of hepatic glycogen and adipose tissue, and also stimulates gluconeogenesis from amino acids. All its actions increase blood glucose concentration (228).

The pancreas is relatively radioresistant compared to the surrounding structures such as the liver and small intestine (437). The islet cells show more postirradiation changes than do the acinous cells, with the beta cells of the islets being more radioresistant than the alpha cells (172,477). Decreases in insulin and glucagon have been observed following radiotherapy and impaired insulin secretion and hypoglycemia were seen in rats 4 days after 10-Gy irradiation (576,686). One month postirradiation the insulin secretion impairment persisted and was accompanied by a reduced number of beta cells.

Ovaries

The two types of ovarian hormones are the *estrogens* and *progestins* and are secreted by the ovaries in response to FSH and LH from the anterior pituitary. FSH and LH, in turn, are secreted by the anterior pituitary in response to luteinizing hormone-releasing hormone (LHRH) from the hypothalamus. By far the most important of the estrogens is *estradiol*, secreted by the theca interna and granulosa cells of the ovarian follicles and by the corpus luteum. The most important progestin is *progesterone*, secreted by the corpus luteum (228,262).

Ovarian radiation severely reduces the formation of ovarian steroid hormones, even to the point of gonadal failure (389,691). Estrogen decreases have been seen in humans following radiation doses of 6–100 Gy (389,686,691), with large doses producing premature menopause (686). Persistently elevated gonadotrophin levels (FSH and LH) and amenorrhea were associated with the reduced ovarian hormones (389,691). Abdominal radiation of females in childhood resulted in pubertal failure or premature menopause (690). Neonatal irradiation of rats with 15 cGy produced a decrease in progesterone levels, but not estradiol levels, in adult animals (211).

Testes

The testes secrete several hormones that are called *androgens* because of their masculinizing effects. *Testosterone*, considered to be the most significant testicular androgen, is formed by the interstitial cells of Leydig. As in the female, LHRH from the hypothalamus stimulates secretion of LH by the anterior pituitary. LH in turn stimulates hyperplasia of the Leydig cells and the production of testosterone by these cells (228,262).

The most dramatic endocrine effect of irradiation of the testis is the increase in FSH and LH secretion from the anterior pituitary (432). FSH levels have been used as an indication of damage to the germinal epithelium. Elevated LH levels associated with normal testosterone levels are indicative of Leydig cell damage (97,351, 390,432,530). This condition may occur at irradiation doses of 2–12 Gy, because damage to the Leydig cells may be compensated by an increase in the number of cells (hyperplasia) in response to the elevated LH (686). Higher doses of irradiation (20–30 Gy) have been shown to produce Leydig cell damage, decrease testosterone production, and increase secretion of LH (246,432,597). Of course, sperm cells and the less differentiated cells giving rise to sperm cells are also known to be affected by radiation exposure. For example, ultramorphological sperm characteristics have been altered in workers cleaning up materials containing relatively high levels of radioactivity following the Chernobyl nuclear accident (205).

Nervous System

Radiogenic Effects on Sensory Functioning

Ionizing radiation can be sensed at extremely low levels (698). For instance, the olfactory response threshold to radiation is less than 1.0×10^{-4} Gy and the visual system is sensitive to levels below 5.0×10^{-6} Gy. Ionizing radiation has been shown to be as efficient as light in producing retinal activity (as assessed by the electroretinogram), and the visibility of ionizing radiation is now firmly established (344).

Whereas visual system pathomorphology occurs only at high doses (219), this is not true of visual function disruption. Rats trained to a brightness discrimination task were unable to differentiate shades of gray after 3.6 Gy or to make sensitivity changes after 6 Gy of whole-body x-rays (for review, see 344). Chimpanzees showed impaired accuracy and visual acuity on visual discrimination tests after about 4 Gy of gamma irradiation (551). Kekcheyev (337) reported that 1 day after exposure to 0.3–1.0 Gy of x-rays, temporary decrements in scotopic visual sensitivity were observed in humans. Further, Lenoir (383) found long-term delays (20–36 days) in dark adaptation in patients exposed to 4–62 Gy of x-rays.

Most of the literature suggests that significant hearing changes, unlike vision changes, require massive doses (e.g., 10–70 Gy) of radiation (for review, see 217). Heinz (285), using fractionated head-only exposures of baboons to x-rays, found that 10, 12, and 15 Gy caused a long-term hearing deficit. The highest exposure produced a hearing loss of >90 dB that was not frequency specific. Lower doses of x-rays caused slowly developing, transient elevations in auditory reaction times. Vestibular function may be more radiosensitive than audition. Depression in vestibular function may exist at doses close to the LD_{50}, with higher doses producing longer lasting disruptions than low doses (21).

Although not much literature is available, several reports exist of olfactory, gustatory, and cutaneous sensory changes in patients exposed to therapeutic irradiation (217). Altered taste perception was found in patients exposed to 36 Gy of x-rays, with a metallic taste being the most common report. Transient changes in taste and olfactory sensitivity were also reported in radiotherapy patients and rats (see review in 344). There is empirical evidence of radiogenic changes in pain perception. While gamma photons produce a dose-dependent analgesia in mice (642), data also suggest that X- or gamma rays do not alter the analgesic effects of morphine or the anesthetic effects of halothane in rats, except under a narrow set of experimental conditions (89,181). Miyachi and colleagues reported that the olfactory system of mice is important in detecting radiation (467) as well as modulating radiation-induced analgesia (465).

Radiogenic Pathology of the Adult Nervous System

A review of standard radiobiology textbooks revealed the common belief that the adult CNS is relatively resistant to damage from ionizing radiation exposure (96). This conclusion was derived, in part, from early clinical reports suggesting that radiation exposures, given to produce some degree of tumor control, produced no immediate morphological effects on the CNS (299). However, this view was changed when it was later shown that the latency period for the appearance of radiation damage in the CNS is simply longer than it is in other organ systems (399). Later interest in the pathogenesis of delayed radiation necrosis in clinical medicine has produced a significant body of literature. Studies of radiation-induced brain damage in patients used computed axial tomography (CAT) technology to confirm CNS abnormalities that are not associated with tumor treatment but that occur because of the radiotherapy (294).

General, although not universal, agreement exists that there is a threshold dose below which no late radiation-induced morphological sequelae in the CNS occur. In laboratory animals, single doses of radiation up to 10 Gy produced no late morphological changes in the brain or spinal cord (281,385). Necrotic lesions were observed in the forebrain white matter from doses of 15 Gy (92,100,338). In human, the "safe" dose has been a topic of considerable debate. Depending on the radiation field size, the threshold for CNS damage was estimated to be 30–40 Gy if the radiation was given in fractions (516); spinal cord damage occurred with fractionated doses as low as 25 Gy (191). The difference between a safe and a pathogenic radiation dose to the brain may be as small as 4.3 Gy (414).

Different topographical regions of the brain may vary in susceptibility to ionizing radiation (667). The most sensitive area is the brain stem (24). The cerebral cortex may be less sensitive than the subcortical structures (385), such as the hypothalamus (720), the optic chiasm, and the dorsal medulla (562). Although radiation lesions occur more frequently in brain white matter (307,557,669), the radiosensitivity of white matter also appears to vary from region to region (385). It may be that selective necrosis of white matter is due to the slow reproductive loss of glia or their precursors. The radiosensitivity of certain types of glial cells (beta astrocyte) is well recognized (547,548). The earliest sign of their damage is widening of the nodes of Ranvier and segmental demyelination as early as 2 weeks after a dose of 5–60 Gy (419).

The technique and end points selected to assess neuropathology can profoundly influence its detection. In proton-irradiated brain tissue stained with silver to detect degenerating neural elements, punctate brain lesions were found within 3 days after as little as 2 Gy (631). The lesions were not detectable with standard hematoxylin and eosin stain. These effects are similar to a multi-infarction syndrome in which the effects of small infarctions accumulate and may become symptomatic. Similarly, Philpott and his associates (528) found that both the synaptic density and the spine length in area CA1 of the hippocampus were lower in mice irradiated with 0.005 or 0.5 Gy of ^{40}Ar. Because this pathology was observed at doses of radiation previously believed to be completely safe, confirmation of these data may profoundly influence our view of the radiosensitivity of brain tissue.

The phenomenon of latent CNS radiation damage with doses above threshold has been well documented (55,96,567). The long latent period has led to considerable speculation on the likely pathogenesis of late radiation lesions: (a) radiation may act primarily on the vascular system, with necrosis secondary to edema and ischemia; and (b) radiation may have a primary effect on cells of the neural parenchyma, with vascular lesions exerting a minor influence (299).

The first evidence in support of a vascular hypothesis was obtained when canine brains that had been exposed to x-rays were examined (399). It was suggested that delayed damage of capillary endothelial cells may occur, leading to a breakdown of the blood–brain barrier. This would result in vasogenic edema (163), the elevated pressure-impaired circulation of cerebral spinal fluid, and eventually neuronal and myelin degeneration (100,101). The finding that hypertension accelerated the appearance of vascular lesions in the brain after irradiation with 10–30 Gy also supports a hypothesis of vascular pathogenesis (300). The occlusive effects of radiation on arterial walls may cause a transient cerebral ischemia (288). Sequential monkey-brain CAT scans revealed brain edema and hydrocephalus that accompanied hypoactivity and the animal's loss of alertness following 20 Gy of radiation (271). Head-only exposure of rabbits to 4, 6, or 8 Gy of x-rays disturbed the blood–brain barrier permeability, which returned to normal after only 6 days (704). The transient nature of the vascular phenomena may partially explain some of the behavioral deficits observed after exposure to intermediate or large doses of ionizing radiation (426,601).

Evidence of the direct action of radiation on the parenchymal cells of the nervous system, rather than the indirect effect through the vascular bed, was first provided when brain tissue in irradiated human patients was examined (503). None of the brain lesions could be attributed to vascular damage because they were (a) predominantly in white matter and not codistributed with blood vessels, (b) not morphologically typical of ischemic necrosis, and (c) often found without any vascular effects (146,301,312,533,729). Thus, it appears that direct neuronal or glial mechanisms caused at least some of the observed radiogenic brain lesions.

Alterations in Nervous System Physiology and Functioning

In addition to radiogenic changes in CNS morphology, a variety of changes in parameters of brain function were reported. For example, changes in brain metabolism were reported after very low (0.11–0.24 Gy) doses of ionizing radiation (194). In a more detailed analysis with the ^{14}C-2-deoxyglucose method of measuring local cerebral glucose utilization, a dose of 15 Gy of x-rays was administered to the rat brain (313). Significantly lower rates of glucose use were found in 16 different rat brain structures at 4 days after irradiation and in 25 structures at 4 weeks. Although large radiogenic changes existed in the metabolism of particular brain nuclei, a weighted average rate for the irradiated brains was approximately 15% below that for the controls.

Researchers measured the functional sensitivity of some brain areas and the insensitivity of others (4,444). The activation of behaviors through electrical stimulation of the lateral hypothalamus (but not of the sepal nucleus or substantia nigra) is still possible after 100 Gy (119,452). However, years after clinical irradiations, dysfunctions of the hypothalamus are prominent even without evidence of hypothalamic necrosis (427). Local subcortical changes may exist in the reticular formation and account for radiation-induced convulsability of the brain (560,561). Similarly, postirradiation spike discharges are more likely to be observed in the hippocampal electroencephalograph (EEG) than in the cortical EEG (226). This idea of selective neurosensitivity is further supported by experiments in which electrical recordings were made from individual nerve fibers after irradiation (237). These data reveal a hierarchy of radiosensitivity in which gamma nerve fibers are more sensitive than beta fibers, and alpha nerve fibers are the least sensitive.

Electrophysiology

Measures of electrophysiology illustrate changes in brain function after exposure to ionizing radiation. Several studies were reported in which cortical EEG changes were observed in humans and in animals following doses as low as 0.05 Gy (382). Typically, an initial temporary increase in bioelectric amplitude was followed, within minutes, by a depression. Other investigations frequently needed higher doses of radiation to observe changes in EEG. For example, changes were not seen in EEGs after 0.03–0.04 Gy x-rays, but significant alterations were observed after 2 Gy (266). At a higher dose (15 Gy), monkey cortical EEG abnormalities consisted of the slowing of activity, with an increase in amplitude (562). Spiking and patterns of *grand mal* seizure also occurred. A rapid onset of high-amplitude slow waves (delta waves) seemed to relate to periods of behavioral incapacitation (424). Exposures to 4–6 Gy ^{60}Co gamma radiation appeared to stimulate spontaneous activity in the neocortex, whereas exposures of higher than 9 Gy inhibited all brain activities (474). Many of the liquidators involved in the cleanup of the Chernobyl nuclear accident were reported to have abnormal EEGs (682,730).

The hippocampus shows significant changes in physiological activities after gamma irradiation with even less than half of the 18-Gy threshold dose needed to produce changes in cortical activities (24,227). Hippocampal spike discharges were first identified in cats (226) and later confirmed in rabbits (227). This spiking developed soon after irradiation (2–4 Gy x-rays) when no other clinical signs of neurological damage or radiation sickness were present.

The apparent radiosensitivity of the hippocampus and its importance in critical functions, such as learning, memory, and motor performance, have led others to investigate the electrophysiology of this brain area. The firing of hippocampal neurons was found to be altered by exposure to 4 Gy of ^{60}Co gamma radiation in rabbits (40). In guinea pigs exposed to 5 or 10 Gy x-rays, significant changes in hippocampal neuronal function were observed to be time, dose, and dose-rate dependent (523). Higher doses (40–65 Gy x-rays) decreased the ability of hippocampal neurons to generate an action potential (524). In addition, in vitro experiments suggested that spontaneous discharges of hippocampal pacemaker-like neurons were induced by X- and gamma rays at a dose of only 0.08 Gy (522). If confirmed, these data suggest that hippocampal electrophysiology may be the most sensitive measure of functional brain changes after irradiation.

Alterations in the thresholds and patterns for audiogenic and electroconvulsive seizures have been produced by exposing animals to ionizing radiations. Such effects are interpreted as reflecting gross changes in CNS reactivity. Early work with dogs showed that spontaneous seizures sometimes occurred following very large doses of radiation (399). Later experiments confirmed that seizures can be induced by whole-body or head-only exposures to 30–250 Gy in a variety of species. For example, rats were exposed to 5 Gy of X-radiation and the electroconvulsive shock (ECS) threshold was determined for 180 days after irradiation (560). ECS thresholds were reduced in irradiated rats over the entire test period. Later studies (561) reported that considerably lower doses (perhaps as little as 0.01 Gy) also reduced the thresholds for ECS seizures and audiogenic seizures (457,532).

Unlike the CNS, peripheral nerves are quite resistant to the functional alterations produced by ionizing radiation. Most data indicate that peripheral nerves do not show any changes in electrophysiology with x-ray exposures below 100 Gy (577). After higher doses, the action-potential amplitude and the conduction velocity temporarily increase but then gradually decrease (32–35,577). Also, alpha and beta particles are more destructive to peripheral nerves than gamma or x-rays, and usually cause a monophasic depression of function without the initial enhancement of activity (222,229,717). Perhaps the lowest dose of ionizing radiation ever found to produce an alteration in the function of peripheral nerves was reported in a study in which T-shaped preparations of isolated frog sciatic nerves were produced when the nerves were partially divided longitudinally (364). Electrical stimulation was applied to the intact stem of the T, and electrical recordings were made from the ends of the two branches. A small segment of one of the branches was irradiated with 0.04–0.06 Gy of alpha particles, producing a definite decrease in action-potential amplitude and an increase in chronaxy. These results were remarkable because of the much higher doses required to affect these peripheral nerve functions in most other studies.

Paralysis of the hind limbs of animals can result from localized irradiation of the spinal cord. Rabbits developed this paralysis at 4–33 weeks after exposure of the upper thoracic region to 30–110 Gy of X-radiation at 2.5 Gy/day (586). The minimum single exposure found to produce paralysis at 5 months was 20 Gy (587). As in other model systems, the interval between irradiation and the appearance of neurological symptoms decreased as dose increased. For example, 50 Gy of x-rays to the monkey midthoracic spinal cord produced immediate paraplegia, whereas 40 Gy was effective only after a latent period of about 5.5 months (164).

Radiation effects on the electrophysiology of the synapse were first studied using the cat spinal reflex (394,578–581). These studies showed that excitatory synaptic transmission was significantly increased by x-ray exposures of 4–6 Gy. Synaptic transmission at the upper cervical ganglion of the cat was also facilitated 15–20 min after exposure to 8 Gy of x-rays (481). Both monosynaptic and polysynaptic spinal reflexes were significantly augmented immediately after exposure to 5 Gy of X-radiation. Interestingly, significant augmentation of monosynaptic excitatory postsynaptic potentials (EPSPs) was found immediately after exposure to 6–12 Gy of x-rays, whereas inhibitory postsynaptic potentials (IPSPs) recorded from the same cell were not significantly affected by a 12-Gy exposure (578,581). Similarly, polysynaptic EPSPs were significantly augmented as the dose increased, whereas the polysynaptic IPSPs were little influenced even by an exposure of 158 Gy. At higher doses (50–200 Gy), ionizing radiation may damage both synaptic and postsynaptic functioning, probably through different molecular mechanisms (649). These radiogenic changes in synaptic transmission may be important factors underlying the complicated functional changes that occur in the CNS following radiation exposures.

Neurochemistry

Ion flow across the neuronal semipermeable membrane is one of the most important mechanisms of postirradiation nervous transmission to be studied. In particular, the flow of sodium ions is believed to be involved in the control of neuronal excitability (99) and apparently can be disrupted after either a very high or very low dose of radiation. A study using the radioactive isotope ^{24}Na compared the sodium intake across the membrane of the squid giant axon before and after exposure to x-rays (563). A significant increase in sodium intake was found to occur during the initial hyperactive period induced by a dose of 500 Gy. These observations were confirmed, although a simultaneous decrease in the rate of sodium extrusion also occurred in a study of frog sciatic nerves that had been irradiated with 1500–2000 Gy of alpha particles (222). As was described earlier, peripheral nerves may be less radiosensitive than CNS neurons and perhaps differ in their radiation response. In a study that used a different technique, the artificially stimulated uptake of sodium into brain synaptosomes was significantly reduced by an ionizing radiation exposure (high-energy electrons or gamma radiation) of 0.1–1000.0 Gy (485,709).

The brain has been described as a radiosensitive biochemical system (194); in fact, many significant changes in brain neurochemistry have been observed after irradiation. An early study revealed that 1–2 days after an exposure to 3 Gy of X-radiation, neurosecretory granules in the hypophysial–hypothalamic system showed a transient increase in number over the controls (634). A leaking of brain monoamines from the neuronal terminals of rats irradiated with 40 Gy of x-rays was also observed (153). These changes in neuronal structure may correlate with radiogenic alterations of neurotransmitter systems.

Normal catecholamine functioning appears to be damaged following exposure to intermediate or high doses of ionizing radiation. After 100 Gy ^{60}Co gamma radiation, a transient disruption in dopamine functioning (similar in some ways to dopamine-receptor blockade) was demonstrated (303). This radiogenic change in dopaminergic systems is further supported by the finding that a 30-Gy ^{60}Co radiation exposure increased the ability of haloperidol (a dopamine-receptor-blocking drug) to produce cataleptic behavior (328). Relatively low doses of ^{56}Fe (0.1–1.0 Gy) also caused a profound reduction in K^+-stimulated dopamine release from perfused striatal slices of rat brain (326,327). This decrement lasted as long as 180 days postexposure. Radiation-induced effects on dopamine have been correlated in time with behavioral deficits. However, other neuromodulators (such as prostaglandins) also seemed to influence dopaminergic systems to help produce some radiation-induced behavioral changes (328). A transient reduction in the norepinephrine content of a monkey hypothalamus was observed on the day of exposure to 6.6 Gy of gamma radiation. Levels of this neurotransmitter returned to normal 3 days later (367). Similar effects were reported elsewhere (673), but another study found no change in noradrenaline after 8.5 Gy of x-rays (323). An increase in the catecholamine enzyme monoamine oxidase (MAO) was reported within 4 min of exposure and lasted for at least 3 h (98).

A variety of functions involving the neurotransmitter acetylcholine (ACH) are significantly altered by exposure to ionizing radiation. ACH synthesis rapidly increased in the hypothalamus of the rat after as little as 0.02 Gy of beta radiation, but it was inhibited at only slightly higher radiation doses (194). A dose of 4 Gy of ^{60}Co gamma radiation produced a long-term increase in the rate of ACH synthesis in dogs (165). Also, high-affinity choline uptake (a correlate of ACH turnover and release) slowly increased to 24% above control levels 15 min after irradiation with 100 Gy (303). Choline uptake returned to normal by 30 min after exposure. Massive doses of gamma or x-rays (up to 600 Gy) were required to alter brain acetylcholinesterase activity (570), whereas much smaller doses depressed plasma acetylcholinesterase by 30% (397).

Exposure to large doses of ionizing radiation resulted in postirradiation hypotension in monkeys (82,133,279), with arterial blood pressure decreasing to less than 50% of normal (184). Postirradiation hypotension also produced a decrease in cerebral blood flow immediately after a single dose of either 25 or 100 Gy of ^{60}Co gamma radiation (106,107,128,130). This hypotension may be responsible for the early transient incapacitation (ETI; see later description) observed after a supralethal dose of ionizing radiation (82,108,658). A study with untrained monkeys, whose postirradiation blood pressures were maintained by norepinephrine or other pressor drugs, showed that as long as arterial pressure was above a critical level, the monkeys remained attentive and alert (456). However, in a follow-up study on monkeys trained to perform a task, norepinephrine maintained blood pressure but did not consistently improve performance during the first 30 min after irradiation (660). Other authors observed no close association between blood pressure and behavioral changes (424). Further contrary evidence was obtained from experiments with the spontaneously hypertensive rat (SHR), in which exposure to ionizing radiation reduced the blood pressure of most rats to near-normal levels. However, the irradiated SHRs still showed a significant behavioral deficit after exposure to 100 Gy of high-energy electrons (453). Finally, a significant association was found between the degree of hypotension and the frequency of early performance deficits (EPDs) (82). Still, half the monkeys with a 50% drop in blood pressure did not show behavioral decrements. Thus, even though the relationship between decreased blood pressure and impaired performance is intriguing, simple changes in blood pressure may not be sufficient to explain transient behavioral changes.

The massive release of histamine observed after exposure to a large dose of ionizing radiation was proposed as a mediator of radiogenic hypotension and EPDs (183). Histamine was found to be a very active biogenic amine and putative neurotransmitter located in neurons and mast cells throughout the body, especially around blood vessels (180). Attempts to alter the development of behavioral deficits by treating animals with antihistamines before exposure have been encouraging (73,182,184). Monkeys pretreated with chlorpheniramine (H_1-receptor blocker) performed better and survived longer after irradiation than did controls (184). Similar benefits were observed in irradiated rats (442). Further, the use of diphenhydramine (a histamine H_1-receptor antagonist) inhibited radiation-induced cardiovascular dysfunction (11). Because these antagonists produced only partial relief from radiation effects, it appeared that the histamine hypothesis explained just a portion of the behavioral and physiological deficits observed after radiation exposure (94).

When most animal species were exposed to a sufficiently large dose of ionizing radiation, they exhibited lethargy, hypokinesia, and deficits in performance (109,344,452). Because these behaviors seemed similar to those observed after a large dose of morphine, a role was proposed for endogenous opioids (endorphins) in the production of radiation-induced behavioral changes (171,314). Endogenous morphine-like substances were thought to be released as a reaction to some (5,254,283), but not all (413), stressful situations. Like a sufficiently large injection of morphine, endogenous opioids produced lethargy, somnolence, and reduction in behavioral responsiveness (335,413). Cross-tolerance between endorphins and morphine was demonstrated for a variety of behavioral and physiological measures (81,632). Because of the similarity of radiation- and opiate-induced symptoms, it is not surprising that endorphins are involved in some aspects of radiogenic behavioral change. Ionizing radiation produced dose-dependent analgesia in mice, and this radiogenic analgesia was reversed by the opiate antagonist naloxone (642). In another experiment, morphine-induced analgesia of the rat was significantly enhanced 24 h after neutron (but not gamma) irradiation, suggesting some combined delayed effects of endogenous and exogenous analgesics that may be radiation specific (89). Ionizing radiation exposure also attenuated the naloxone-precipitated abstinence syndrome in morphine-dependent rats (152).

Further supporting the hypothesis that endorphins are involved in radiation-induced behavioral change, C57Bl/6J mice exhibited a stereotypic locomotor hyperactivity similar to that observed after morphine injection, after receiving 10–15 Gy of ^{60}Co gamma radiation (451). This radiogenic behavior was reversed by administering naloxone or by pre-exposing the mice to chronically stressful situations, a procedure that produces endorphin tolerance (447). In addition, opiate-experienced mice reduced the self-administration of morphine after irradiation, suggesting that the internal production of an endorphin reduced the requirement for an exogenous opioid compound (450). Biochemical assays also revealed changes in mouse brain beta-endorphin after exposure to ionizing radiation (449). Rats and monkeys had enhanced blood levels of beta-endorphin after irradiation (10,158), and morphine-tolerant rats showed less performance decrement after irradiation than nontolerant subjects (448). Further, naloxone (1 mg/kg) given immediately before exposure to 100 Gy of high-energy electrons significantly attenuated the early behavioral deficits observed in rats (10). Conversely, rats either underwent no change or were made more sensitive to radiation effects after chronic treatment with naloxone on a schedule that increased the number of endorphin receptors (479). However, the manipulation of opioid systems did not produce total control over postirradiation performance deficits. Thus, these data do not suggest an exclusive role for endorphins in radiogenic behavioral change.

BEHAVIORAL EFFECTS OF IONIZING RADIATION

Behavioral and Neurophysiological Effects of Prenatal or Neonatal Radiation Exposure

The developing nervous system is significantly more radiosensitive than the adult nervous system, because ionizing radiation, like other teratogenic agents, is apt to affect embryonic cells with high proliferative and metabolic activity (for reviews, see refs. 347,645). Thus, prenatal exposure to ionizing radiation can cause either organogenic malformations (abnormal closure of the neural tube) or histogenic abnormalities (abnormal proliferation or migration of neurons) (331,542). Because postnatal neurogenesis may be protracted (256), radiosensitivity of selected brain areas (e.g., the dentate gyrus) may well extend into the neonatal period and even young adulthood in some species. For example, 4 Gy of ^{60}Co gamma radiation caused a significant reduction in synaptic contacts made by hippocampal neurons from 7-day-old rats (272). Early postnatal exposure to ^{137}Cs (5–25 Gy) produced a dose-dependent reduction in myelin synthesis (316).

Other cells important to the functioning of the CNS (e.g., glia) develop early in gestation and continue to divide in the mature organism. Glia guide neuronal migration in the fetal brain and subserve neuronal activity in the adult. The present limit for detection of morphological changes in glia was determined to be as low as 0.2 Gy x-rays (549).

Corresponding behavioral alteration may also be observed after relatively low doses of ionizing radiation if exposure occurs prenatally or soon after birth when many cells are actively dividing or migrating (104). In fact, behavioral indicators were shown to be more sensitive indicators of radiogenic damage than were morphological assessments of brain development (331,513). Schull and Otake (590) estimated that survivors exposed in utero to the atomic bombings in Hiroshima and Nagasaki exhibited a diminution in intelligence score of 21–27 points/Gy. The highest risk of severe mental retardation occurred during the 8th–15th week of gestation when radiation exposure coincided with the most rapid period of proliferation of neuronal elements and the migration of immature neurons to the cerebral cortex (514,589).

The behavioral results of prenatal irradiation are discussed in several in-depth reviews (76,344,347). Most of the work focuses on motor performance. Prenatal irradiation can cause significant alterations in gait. For example, D'Amato and Hicks (157) observed a hopping locomotion in rats exposed to 1.5 Gy on gestation days 14 and 15. After some initial difficulty, these animals learned to traverse horizontal ladders by adapting their hopping gait to navigate the rungs. Norton and Kimler (498) also found that rats exposed to 1 Gy from ^{137}Cs source on gestation day 15 showed deficits in muscular endurance as measured by their ability to sustain their own weight by hanging from a rod. This behavioral deficit (and others) were correlated with reduced thickness of the cerebral cortex. Fractionation of the radiation dose resulted in less damage to the developing rat cerebral cortex, as measured by postnatal growth, behavioral tests, and morphological assessment (348,675). Motor deficits were also observed in rats exposed to a low dose (0.6 Gy) on gestation day 16 (73). These animals had difficulty obtaining a reward if they were required to make motor responses in rapid succession (pressing a lever four times in 2 s).

Locomotor hyperactivity was reported after prenatal or perinatal radiation exposure (445). In particular, locomotor activity was enhanced in mice irradiated with 1 Gy ^{137}Cs on gestation day 14 (461), and in rats exposed to 1.25 Gy x-rays on gestation days 14 or 15 (500) as well as 2 Gy x-rays on gestation day 17 (321). Mice exposed to 1.0 Gy ^{137}Cs on day 14 of gestation exhibited higher levels of open-field activity at 19–20 months, but not at 6–7 or 12–13 months of age. Thus, it was concluded that later behavioral changes of prenatally irradiated animals may depend on the age of testing (460).

Other behaviors were also affected by prenatal irradiation. Male mice irradiated with 2 Gy ^{137}Cs on gestation day 14 and tested at 100–135 days of age exhibited increased aggressiveness compared to controls (459). When rats were exposed to 2 Gy X-irradiation on gestation day 17 and tested as adults, they showed enhanced performance on an active avoidance task (requiring movement in a shuttle box) (321,633), whereas passive avoidance (requiring a freezing response) was impaired (633). Rats exposed to 1.5 Gy ^{60}Co gamma radiation on gestation day 15 exhibited a hyperresponse and delayed habituation on an acoustic startle test (462). Mice receiving 0.1–0.5 Gy x-rays (609) or 0.5 Gy mixed neutron/gamma radiation (175) on gestation day 18 and tested in adulthood showed impairment on a spatial memory task (609). Administration of *d*-amphetamine 10 min before testing as adults, however, alleviated neonatally induced X-irradiation-related deficits in short-term memory of rats (286). Radiogenic deficits were also observed when animals (previously irradiated in utero) performed tasks with substantial cognitive components (79). In 90-day-old squirrel monkeys exposed to gamma radiation (0.5 or 1 Gy) on gestation days 89–90, the correct responses in visual orientation, discrimination, and reversal learning tasks were significantly lower than that of controls. Decrements in reversal learning persisted undiminished in the irradiated subjects at 2 years of age.

Cognitive dysfunction is a common sequela of cranial radiation therapy (16), particularly in young children treated for acute lymphoblastic leukemia (1,13,287,672). A dose of 24 Gy or more of radiation to the CNS of children under 5 years of age resulted in neurocognitive deficits that, it was reported, may not become apparent until 2–5 years after treatment (478). Young children are most vulnerable due to toxicity to the developing brain. Mullenix and her colleagues, at this writing, are using a neonatal rat model to investigate the use of drugs to mitigate the effects of cranial radiation-induced behavioral deficits (483,484).

Significant changes in neurotransmitter levels can be measured in brains of rats exposed prenatally (e.g., 0.95 Gy on day 10, 12, or 15 of pregnancy). Marked changes in serotonin and serotonin receptors were found in several brain structures (e.g., hippocampus) and dopamine increased significantly in striatum. There were also significant increases in glutamate, glutamine, and γ-aminobutyric acid (GABA) in cortex, hippocampus, striatum, and thalamus (170). Interestingly, these radiogenic changes in concentrations of neurotransmitters did not correspond with changes in receptor binding (648). Administration of the N-methyl-D-aspartate (NMDA) receptor antagonist, dizocilpine (MK-801), a glutamate blocker, before neonatal X-irradiation produced a dose-dependent behavioral protection in adult rats with radiation-induced hippocampal damage (446). In a related study, dizocilpine administered 20 min after neonatal ^{60}Co irradiation significantly reduced neuronal damage in rats 6 h after exposure (7).

Behavioral Effects of Adult Radiation Exposure

Naturalistic Behaviors

Naturalistic behaviors (normal parts of an animal's response repertoire) may be altered by radiation exposure. In particular, spontaneous locomotor activity is of interest because this behavior is an important component of many other responses. Jones et al. (324) reported an immediate depression in rat volitional activity-wheel performance following an acute, whole-body dose of 2–7 Gy x-rays. Exposure of rats to 10 Gy high-energy electrons (200) or mice to 10 Gy ^{60}Co gamma radiation (408) resulted in reductions in both horizontal and vertical activity within 1 h of exposure. Radiation-induced hypoactivity has also been reported for a variety of species (for review, see ref. 444). A biphasic locomotor response to radiation exposure (initial decrease, followed by partial recovery and then secondary hypoactivity) was reported for mice (371), and is consistent with the phasic postirradiation clinical symptomatology observed in humans (219).

Exposure to ionizing radiation also produces a dose-dependant reduction in food and water consumption, as well as nausea and vomiting (emesis) in a variety of species (217,218,344,350,422,650). Taste-aversion learning (an association between a distinctive taste and radiation-induced malaise) appears to be an especially sensitive indicator of radiation's effects on consummatory behaviors (539,541). The ED_{50} for the formation of a taste aversion following ^{56}Fe exposure was only 0.21 Gy (540). Diltiazem, a calcium channel blocker, prevented the onset of radiation-induced taste aversions in rats (482).

Another indicator of gastrointestinal malaise, vomiting, is more likely observed after irradiation with neutrons than gamma rays (185). Increasing doses of radiation up to 10 Gy (neutron : gamma = 0.4), corresponded with the enhanced likelihood of vomiting in the monkey (454). Above 10 Gy, however, the number of monkeys that vomited decreased with increasing dose. The ED_{50} was approximately 4.5 Gy. Eighty percent of monkeys exposed to mixed neutron/gamma radiation (6 Gy), with a high neutron : gamma ratio of 0.85, vomited in about 45 min (415).

The relationship between vomiting and performance decrement was shown to be complex (721), with irradiated animals rarely vomiting during early behavioral incapacitations (see later discussions). For example, Franz (210), found no relationship between vomiting and early performance deficits in monkeys performing in a physical activity wheel and exposed to less than 50 Gy of mixed neutron/gamma radiation. Animals that were not incapacitated but received the same dose as the incapacitated animals vomited as expected (721,723). Although these data are revealing, the relationship between radiation-induced vomiting and behavioral deficits remains to be fully elucidated. Serotonin receptor blocking agents were shown to be effective against radiation-induced vomiting (51,186,211,415), and to have relatively few behavioral side effects (53,54, 68).

Social behaviors have not received much attention from radiobiologists. Miyachi and colleagues reported a paradoxical effect when both sexual (468) and aggressive (466,469) behavior of mice were reduced following exposure to doses of 0.05–0.15 Gy x-rays but not after higher doses of 0.25–0.35 Gy. Maier and Landauer (407,408) found that aggressive behaviors were surprisingly robust after 10 Gy (electron or ^{60}Co gamma radiation) and persisted until radiogenic moribund behavior was evident.

Motor Performance

Several studies revealed chronic deterioration of motor performance after doses of radiation at or below the LD_{50}. For example, Stapleton and Curtis (616) reported a long-term (42-week) progressive deterioration of forced wheel running behavior in mice exposed to a LD_{50} dose of neutron radiation. Kimeldorf et al. (346) also found significant reductions in motor capacity of rats swimming daily to exhaustion before and after exposure to 3–10 Gy of x-rays. Rats performing a task where they had to press a bar 20 times rapidly to avoid footshock showed significant performance decrements following 7.5 Gy ^{60}Co gamma radiation. This decrement persisted for the first 4 weeks after exposure (434).

Performance of a physically demanding motor task can alter survival after irradiation. Kimeldorf and Jones (345) reported that swimming to exhaustion before and after X-irradiation significantly reduced rat performance and lowered the LD_{50} by about 2 Gy. Bogo and colleagues (67,71) observed a similar phenomenon in rats performing a strenuous, shock-motivated motor task after irradiation.

Learning, Memory, and Cognition

A number of studies suggest learning can be altered by ionizing radiation exposure. Meyerson (438) conditioned rabbits to associate a light and tone stimulus with the respiratory reflex of apnea (cessation of breathing) produced by inhalation of ammonia vapor. A 15-Gy exposure to ^{60}Co gamma radiation produced an absent, or considerably reduced, conditioned apnea response to the light/tone. In contrast, the unconditioned apnea (normal response to ammonia inhalation) was enhanced after irradiation, suggesting the performance capacity of the animal was intact. Another investigator (204) found reduced maze-learning behavior after up to 10 Gy of x-rays. Urmer and Brown (662) also reported a temporary reduction in the ability of rats to reorganize previously learned material after 4 Gy ^{60}Co gamma radiation.

These data support the notion of radiation's effects on some components of learning, and they are consistent with other results (90) suggesting that radiogenic disruptions in behavior may not merely reflect defects in nonassociative factors. Although the predominant work in this field concludes there are postirradiation learning deficits, improved or unaltered learning capacity after irradiation was observed under certain circumstances (for review see ref. 444).

Radiation exposure also may disrupt memory. For example, Wheeler and Hardy (697) reported a significant retrograde amnesia in rats after low doses of electron irradiation. Human memory may be impaired by radiation exposure as well. A few cases of acute retrograde amnesia were reported by people who survived the bombing of Hiroshima (320). Five years after the attack, deficits in memory and intellectual capacity were noted in individuals experiencing radiation sickness (138). Although there may be alternative explanations for these amnesias (e.g., psychological trauma), the data seem consistent with Soviet literature, which reported memory deficits in patients undergoing therapeutic irradiations (319).

Exposure to ionizing radiation is known to alter performance on behavioral tasks requiring nondemanding physical movements and the involvement of functional cognitive processes, such as timing, decision making, or concept formation. For example, Cynomolgus monkeys tested 2–3.5 months after a 20-Gy head-only exposure to X- or gamma rays showed a deficit on a series of discrimination problems (551). Cranial irradiation of rats with single doses of 20 or 25 Gy of x-rays produced delayed impairment of spatial learning and working memory (291). Chimpanzees exhibited a chronic inability to perform an oddity discrimination task after a whole-body ^{60}Co radiation of 4 Gy (551). Highly-trained complex behavior in laboratory rats can be disrupted with

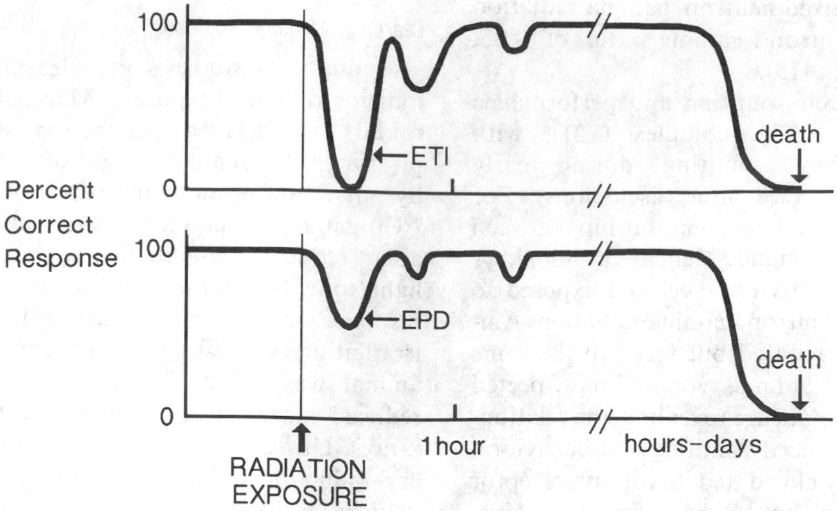

FIG. 15.6. Idealized performance time-courses for acute radiation-induced behavioral decrement. As shown, soon after a sufficiently large dose of radiation, several animal species exhibit an early transient incapacitation (ETI; *upper panel*) or an early performance decrement (EPD; *lower panel*). Subsequent smaller transient deficits may occur approximately 45 min and 4 h later. From References 210, 595, 723.

sublethal levels (4.5–6.75 Gy) of ^{60}Co gamma radiation (433–435,705,706). Typically, radiation-induced disruptions in rates and patterns of responding became evident within 1 day of exposure, with a duration of 24–96 h, before returning to pre-exposure levels (435).

Early, Transient Performance Deficits

Transient performance deficits were observed in animals and humans after a large, rapidly delivered dose of ionizing radiation. This response was termed early transient incapacitation (ETI) (590). An idealized, individual ETI profile is shown in the upper part of Figure 15.6. As shown, 5–10 min after radiation exposure, performance rapidly fell to near zero, followed by partial or total recovery 10–15 min later. Delayed ETIs also occurred about 45 min and 4 h after irradiation.

A less severe variant of ETI is early performance decrement (EPD), in which performance is significantly degraded rather than totally suppressed. ETI and EPD were presumed to occur only after supralethal radiation doses in which, following behavioral recovery, death occurred in hours or days. However, some data suggest lower doses may also produce these effects (70).

Early transient performance decrements are modulated by several factors. For instance, the radiation dose required to disrupt behavior is directly related to the requirements of the task being performed. Demanding/complex tasks and tasks that require rapid responding are most disrupted after radiation exposure (for review, see ref. 444). Radiation dose and dose rate can also influence behavioral deficits. When 10 Gy ^{60}Co gamma radiation was given at dose rates from 0.3–1.8/min, it produced 7–81% ETI, respectively (82).

The type of radiation can also differentially influence early transient behavioral deficits. The median effective doses required to disrupt rat performance on an accelerating rotating rod were 61 Gy for 18.6 MeV electrons, 81 Gy for 18.1 MVp Bremsstrahlung, 89 Gy for 1.25 MeV gamma photons, and 98 Gy for 1.67 MeV neutrons. Thus, in contrast to typical lethality data, electrons are significantly more effective than neutrons in producing motor deficits (69).

Several human accidents have involved very large doses of ionizing radiations sufficient to produce behavioral incapacitation. One of these exposures occurred in the early days of fissionable material production at Los Alamos Scientific Laboratory (United States) and resulted in the fatal radiation injury of a worker known as Mr. K. The accident victim received a rapid total body dose of 45 Gy and an estimated upper abdominal dose of 120 Gy of mixed neutrons and gamma radiations (606). During the event, Mr. K either fell or was knocked to the floor. For a short period, he was apparently dazed as he turned his plutonium-mixing apparatus off and then back on again. He was able to run to another room but soon became ataxic and disoriented. He could not stand unaided, was incapacitated, and drifted in and out of consciousness for more than a half hour before he was rushed to a local hospital. Later, Mr. K regained consciousness and coherence. From 2–30 h after the accident he showed significant behavioral recovery, at some points experiencing euphoria, although his clinical signs were grave. The few hours before his death (35 h postirradiation) were characterized by irritability, uncooperativeness, mania, and eventually coma. This case is consistent with the animal literature suggesting that a supralethal dose of radiation can produce early transient performance deficits. The physiological and behavioral symptoms associated with acute radiation effects in humans following exposure to doses of 0.5–30 Gy were summarized by Anno and his colleagues (17).

The Chernobyl (Ukraine) nuclear reactor accident in 1986 also produced behavioral deficits in personnel attempting to perform duties in high-radiation environments. A firefighter who fought the blaze of the burning reactor core suffered performance deficits and eventually had to withdraw because of radiation exposure (L. Telyatnikov, personal communication, 1987). Another individual exposed to an estimated 2.0–3.5 Gy radiation during the accident was reported to have permanent headaches and vision impairment (64). These human accidents add to the animal literature suggesting sublethal doses of radiation can also induce performance decrements.

Protection Against Radiogenic Behavioral Disruption

Few studies have attempted to normalize behavioral changes observed immediately (up to 24 h) after irradiation. However, as described earlier, antihistamines (i.e., chlorpheniramine) (183,442) and opiate antagonists (e.g., naloxone) may offer behavioral radioprotection under certain circumstances (446). Other data suggest that estrogens, already known for their ability to reduce the lethal effects of ionizing radiation (642), can reduce the intensity and duration of radiation-induced early transient behavioral deficits in castrated rats trained to perform an avoidance task (441). Currently, no definitive data identify agents capable of completely restoring normal behavior after irradiation-induced changes.

Separate experiments evaluated behavioral toxicity of radioprotectants used for their ability to reduce the lethal effects of irradiation (for reviews, see ref. 87,411,695). Most of these radioprotectants act as free-radical scavengers. Early studies administered *n*-decylaminoethanethiosulfuric acid, WR-1607 (10 mg/kg, IV) to monkeys and reported some protection against ETI (598,659). WR-1607 also extended the life of the subjects beyond that of controls. Today, the leading radioprotective drug is amifostine, formerly known as WR-2721 (635). Although amifostine is available for clinical use in conjunction with radiotherapy (72, 636,683), the drug's side effects (emesis, hypotension) limit its use (694). Unfortunately, in all species and tasks studied, WR-2721 alone at the best radioprotective doses was behaviorally toxic (that is, it disrupted trained behavior or it reduced locomotor activity), and it potentiated rather than attenuated radiation-induced performance decrements (372,373,376,423). In general, the behavioral toxicity of each of a variety of radioprotective compounds increases in parallel with the radioprotective properties (374,375).

Psychological Factors of Radiation Exposure

Compared to what we know about the physiological changes brought about by ionizing radiation exposure, we know little about the psychological changes that may also be exhibited. The information we do have is derived from the Japanese atomic bomb experience, human radiation accidents, clinical radiation exposures, and selected animal studies. The data from animal studies reflects behavioral changes resulting from direct effects of radiation on nervous system functioning. The human data reflect additional social, cognitive, and cultural factors that modulate human emotional and psychological phenomena (443).

The animal data have shown, for example, that we can expect motivational changes after sufficiently large doses of ionizing radiation. Rats that initially exerted similar amounts of work to receive rewarding brain stimulation of several different brain nuclei, following exposure to 100 Gy high-energy electrons, stopped working for stimulation of some nuclei (e.g., septum) but continued working for stimulation of the lateral hypothalamus (452). Although these irradiated subjects maintained the capacity to perform barpressing, there was selective modification of their motives such that they chose to exert work to obtain a selected subset of the incentives that were previously all rewarding.

In addition to the physiologically mediated changes in psychological variables that might be revealed by animal studies, human perceptions, interactions, and expectations can combine to produce distinct changes in emotional responses after radiation exposure (136). For example, the nuclear reactor accident in 1979 at Three Mile Island (United States) produced virtually no radiation exposure above background levels. Still, the perceived radiation hazard and the public's "nuclear phobia" evoked long-term emotional, behavioral, and physiological signs of stress (41,135). The particular fear associated with potential radiation exposure from nuclear power plants seems to be heightened by the fact that ionizing radiation presents an invisible, unfamiliar, man-made (and therefore "unnatural") hazard (572). Interestingly, fear and dread of radiation is lessened when the radiation source is natural and the individual may encounter it in a familiar setting (e.g., his/her own basement), as is the case with radon (693).

Psychological symptoms that have been reported following radiation accidents have been quite dramatic. Fear, anxiety, stress, depression, neurasthenia, and hypochondria were reported as part of the clinical course of persons exposed to radiation during the Chernobyl nuclear power plant accident (150,151,244,336,651,676). Deficits in memory, attention, and sensorimotor activities were also observed in these patients (116). Many individuals, and children in particular, reported symptoms of fatigue, pallor, inattention, abdominal pain, and headache as a result of the Chernobyl accident. Ukrainian doctors have labeled this syndrome "vegetative dystonia" (412,625).

In one of the most highly contaminated areas of Belarus, the results of a large health survey found that the Chernobyl accident caused long-standing loss of health-related quality of life, psychological well-being, and changes in illness behavior (276). Even immigrants from the former Soviet Union were found to have various stress-related disorders many years after leaving the Chernobyl-contaminated areas (151). As might be expected, one of the highest risk groups for these effects were the Chernobyl liquidators, the large number of people who were involved in cleaning up after the accident (676). The clinical significance of this well-documented psychological stress due to the Chernobyl accident, however, is still unknown (240,277,677).

The reaction of the public, and even the medical establishment, to radiation accident victims is often characterized as fearful (167). Following the radiation accident in Goiânia, Brazil, in 1987, the radiation exposure victims were subjected to chronic stress (137) and intense ostracism (167). Everyone fled from them, including doctors and nurses who were afraid they would become contaminated themselves (167). These fears are not totally unrealistic. Although the intrinsic radiation produced by a single patient may not be life threatening under these circumstances (139), care of many of these individuals may produce some risk to medical staff.

Summary

Radiation doses below the LD_{50} (whole body) do not produce permanent sensory changes; however, transient alterations were reported in several modalities at doses from 1–5 Gy. High radiation doses can cause more permanent sensory and perceptual impairments. Radiogenic damage to mature brain morphology may occur after an exposure of less than 15 Gy and is an accepted finding at higher doses.

The developing CNS is significantly more sensitive than the mature nervous system to radiation-induced changes in a variety of histological, morphological, and behavioral parameters. Likewise, indicators of brain functioning (e.g., electrophysiology, neurochemistry) are more radiosensitive than are neuroanatomical end points.

Under many circumstances, exposure to ionizing radiations can significantly impede performance. This conclusion is supported by extensive research on experimental animals and limited human experiences. At low to intermediate doses of radiation (up to 10 Gy), performance deficits may be slow in developing and relatively long-lasting. After high doses, the behavioral effects are often rapid (within minutes) and usually abate before the debilitation of chronic radiation sickness begins. These rapid effects can also occur at intermediate doses under certain circumstances.

Not all task performance is equally radiosensitive. Tasks with complex, demanding requirements are more easily disrupted than simple ones. The exception may be found in certain naturalistic behaviors (e.g., eating and drinking behavior) that are also quite radiosensitive. Postirradiation deficits in memory, cognitive ability, and motor performance have been reported. Radiation parameters such as dose, dose rate, and radiation quality can all influence the degree of performance decrement observed.

Many of the pharmacological compounds that protect animals from the lethal effects of ionizing radiation also have severe behavioral effects. In addition to the well-studied physiological and behavioral effects of ionizing radiations, psychological changes (e.g., motivational deficits, anxiety, depression) may also accompany radiation exposure.

CONCLUSION

To assess the average exposure of residents of the United States to ionizing radiation, the National Council on Radiation Protection and Measurements obtained the collective effective dose equivalent from each of six main radiation source categories (492). The collective effective dose equivalent is calculated by multiplying the average per capita effective dose equivalent by the estimated number of people exposed (34). The average effective dose equivalent was then calculated by dividing the collective effective dose equivalent by the total U.S. population. The dose equivalent accounts for differences in relative biological effectiveness by multiplying the absorbed dose by the quality factor while the effective dose equivalent relates the dose equivalent to risk.

As seen in Table 15.2, natural radiation sources contribute 82% of the total average annual effective dose equivalent of 3.6 mSv. By far the largest contribution (55%) is made by radon and its decay products. Radon in domestic water supplies is also the chief contributor to radiation exposure from consumer products (34).

Although much is written about radiation exposure from nuclear power production and nuclear weapons testing fallout, their contributions are negligible compared to the importance of environmental radon, the largest source of human exposure to ionizing radiation.

Unfortunately, the exception to the rule occurred on April 26, 1986, when the graphite-moderated reactor of Unit No. 4 of the Chernobyl nuclear power station of the former Soviet Union exploded, distributing a large amount of a variety of radionuclids throughout the northern hemisphere in what has been estimated to be the single most costly industrial accident in history (20,122,196,214,310,355,596,661). One result of the accident is that the contaminated areas of Belarus, Ukraine, and Russia have become a living laboratory of the consequences of radioactive contamination. The ecotoxicological effects of the Chernobyl accident have provided unprecedented observations of radionuclides in the environment and the human health effects are only now becoming evident with additional reports appearing each year. Many of these late reports have been included in this chapter because they are changing what is known about the toxicity of ionizing radiation.

QUESTIONS

1. What processes are involved in the amplification of a single exposure of ionizing radiation to a final end point of biological expression (injury, cancer, or death)?
2. The most important sensitizer of biological tissues to ionizing radiation is ________.
3. Describe how radiation is thought to affect the cell cycle. In which phase of the cell cycle are cells more sensitive to ionizing radiation? In which phase are they more sensitive?
4. Why is a 20 cGy dose of neutron radiation able to result in cataract formation, but not a 20 cGy dose X-radiation? What is the difference between a high LET radiation and a low LET radiation? How are RBE and LET related?
5. The "Law of Bergonie and Tribondeau" put forth in 1906 describes basically why some cells are more sensitive to ionizing radiation than other cells. Why are bone marrow cells and cancer cells sensitive to ionizing radiation?
6. What is the difference between *ionization* and *excitation*? What is a thiol, and how does it interact with a free radical?
7. What is the estimated lethal dose of ionizing radiation for humans? What are the lethality syndromes induced by ionizing radiation? Why can an organism tolerate a larger dose if it is protracted or fractionated, whereas a smaller, acute exposure dose can be lethal?
8. What is the role of apoptosis in response to radiation injury?
9. What have we learned about the effects of human populations living in the relatively highly contaminated areas around the Chernobyl reactor?
10. What is the reality of the actual incidence of birth defects from human exposure to environmental (not medical) radiation?
11. Discuss the behavioral alterations that can occur as a result of prenatal irradiation.
12. What is radiation-induced "early transient incapacitation"?
13. Explain the relatively high incidence of thyroid cancer in Belarus, Ukraine, and Russia in the 1990s.
14. How would a diet high in Brazil nuts contribute to a high body-burden of radionuclides and where in the body would they be concentrated?
15. Explain the difference in the risk of consuming clams, oysters, or scallops from an area contaminated with ^{60}Co and from one contaminated with ^{90}Sr.
16. Explain why denudation of the gastrointestinal mucosa may not be seen with death occurring from the neurovascular syndrome associated with the acute radiation syndrome.
17. Why does the conceptus exhibit the lowest irradiation LD_{50} of any stage of an organism's life?
18. How does irradiation depress both the specific and nonspecific immune responses?

REFERENCES

1. Abayomi, O. K. (1996): Pathogenesis of irradiation-induced cognitive dysfunction. *Acta. Oncol.*, 35:659–663.
2. Abbas, B., Boyle, F. C., Wilson, D. J., et al. (1990): Radiation induced changes in the blood capillaries of rat duodenal villi: A corrosion cast, light and transmission electron microscopical study. *J. Submicrosc. Cytol. Pathol.* (*BOLOGNA*), 22:63–70.
3. Abbas, B., Hume, S. P., McCullough, J. S., et al. (1990): Early morphological changes in blood capillaries of mouse duodenal villi induced by X-irradiation. *J. Submicrosc. Cytol. Pathol.* (*BOLOGNA*) 22:609–614.
4. Abdullin, G. Z. (1962): Study of comparative radiosensitivity of different parts of brain in terms of altered function. *Atomic Energy Commission TR-5141.* OTS/Department of Commerce, Washington, DC.
5. Akil, H., Madden, J., Patrick, R. L. III, and Barchas, J. D. (1976): Stress-induced increase in endogenous opioid peptides: Concurrent analgesia and its reversal by naloxone. In: *Opiates and Endogenous Opiate Peptides*, edited by H. W. Kosterlitz, p. 63. Elsevier North-Holland, Amsterdam.
6. Akiyama, M. (1995) Late effects of radiation on the human immune system: An overview of immune response among the atomic-bomb survivors. *Int. J. Radiat. Biol.*, 68:497–508.

7. Alaoui, F., Pratt, J., Trocherie, S., et al. (1995): Acute effects of irradiation on the rat brain: Protection by glutamate blockade. *Eur. J. Pharmacol.*, 276:55–60.
8. Alman, R. W., Rosenberg, M., and Fazekas, J. F. (1952): Effects of histamine on cerebral hemodynamics and metabolism. *A.M.A. Arch. Neurol. Psychiat.*, 67:354–356.
9. Al-sarraf, M., LeBlanc, M., Giri, P. G. S., et al. (1998): Chemoradiation therapy versus radiation therapy in patients with advanced nasopharyngeal cancer: Phase III randomized Intergroup study 0099. *J.C.O.*, 16:1310–1317.
10. Alter, W., Mickley, G. A., Catravas, G., et al. (1980): Role of histamine and beta-endorphin in radiation-induced hypotension and acute performance decrement in the rat. In: *Proceedings of the 51st Annual Meeting of the Aerospace Medical Association*, pp. 225–226. Anaheim, CA; 7–11 May 1980.
11. Alter, W. A., Catravas, G. N., Hawkins, R. N., and Lake, C. R. (1984): Effect of ionizing radiation of physiological function in the anesthetized rat. *Radiat. Res.*, 99:394–409.
12. Altman, K. I., Gerber, G. B., and Okada, S. (1970): *Radiation Biochemistry*. Academic Press, New York.
13. Anderson, V., Godber, T., Smibert, E., and Ekert, H. (1997): Neurobehavioural sequelae following cranial irradiation and chemotherapy in children: An analysis of risk factors. *Pediatr. Rehabil.*, 1:63–76.
14. Andrew, F. D., and Lytz, P. S. (1981): Biochemical disturbances associated with developmental toxicity. In: *Developmental Toxicology*, edited by C. Kimmel and J. Buelke-Sam, pp. 145–165. Raven Press, New York.
15. Andrushchak, L. I., Gol'Dshmid, B. Y., Nikitchenko, V. V., et al. (1993): Morphological and ultrastructural changes in small intestine of rats under long-term constant action of low doses of ionizing radiation (in Russian). *Tsitologiya I Genetika*, 27:13–19.
16. Andrykowski, M. A., Altmaier, E. M., Barnett, R. L., et al. (1990): Cognitive dysfunction in adult survivors of allogeneic marrow transplantation: Relationship to dose of total body irradiation. *Bone Marrow Transplant*, 6:269–276.
17. Anno, G. H., Baum, S. J., Withers, H. R., and Young, R. W. (1989): Symptomatology of acute radiation effects in humans after exposure to doses of 0.5-30 =Gy. *Health Phys.*, 5:821–838.
18. Anscher, M. S., Kong, F.-M., and Jirtle, R. L. (1998): The relevance of transforming growth factor *B*1 in pulmonary injury after radiation therapy. *Lung Cancer*, 19:109–120.
19. Antonellia, A., Silvano, G., Bianchi, F., et al. (1995): Risk of thyroid nodules in subjects occupationally exposed to radiation: A cross-sectional study. *Occup. Environ. Med.*, 52:500–504.
20. Aoyama, M., Hirose, K., Inoue, H., et al. (1989): 30 years records of the radioactive fallout in Japan. *J. Radiat. Res.* (*Tokyo*) 30:11.
21. Apanasenko, Z. I. (1967): Combined effect of double exposure to vibration and chronic irradiation on the functional state of vestibular apparatus. In: *NASA Technical Translation, F-413*, pp. 212–228. National Aeronautic and Space Administration, Washington, DC.
22. Archambeau, J. O. (1987): Relative radiation sensitivity of the integumentary system: Dose response of the epidermal, microvascular, and dermal populations. In: *Advances in Radiation Biology, Vol. 12, Relative Radiation Sensitivities of Human Organ Systems*, edited by J. T. Lett and K. I. Altman, pp. 147–203. Academic Press, San Diego.
23. Arena, V. (1971): *Ionizing Radiation and Life*. Mosby, St. Louis.
24. Arnold, A., Bailey, P., and Harvey, R. A. (1954): Intolerance of primate brain stem and hypothalamus to conventional high energy radiations. *Neurology*, 4:575–585.
25. Arnold, M., and Kummermehr, J. (1988): Radiation induced damage to the regenerative capacity of surgically traumatized rat femur after single doses of x-rays. In: Terrestrial Space Radiation and its Biological Effects, edited by P. D. McCormack, C. E. Swenberg, and H. Bücker, pp. 475–486. Plenum Press, New York.
26. Arsenian, M. A. (1991): Cardiovascular sequelae of therapeutic thoracic radiation. *Prog. Cardiovasc. Dis.*, 33:299–311.
27. Asfandiyarova, N. S., Romadin, A. E., Kolcheva, N. G., et al. (1998): Immunity system in residents of territories contaminated with radionuclides after the Chernobyl accident (in Russian). *Terapevticheskii Arkhiv.*, 70:55–59.
28. Astakhova, L. N., Anspaugh, L. R., Beebe, G. W., et al. (1998): Chernobyl-related thyroid cancer in children of Belarus: A case-control study. *Radiat. Res.*, 150:349–356.
29. Astor, M. B., Anderson, M. E., and Meister, A. (1988): Relationship between intracellular GSH levels and hypoxic cell radiosensitivity. *Pharmac. Ther.*, 39:115–121.
30. Auerbach, C. (1958): Radiomimetic substances. *Radiat. Res.*, 9:33–47.
31. Babadzhanova, Sh. A., and Busakov, B. S. (1997): Radiation as a risk factor for nerve system diseases. *Uzbekiston Tibbiet Zhurnali*, 5-7:41–43.
32. Bachofer, C. S. (1957): Enhancement of activity of nerves by x-rays. *Science*, 125:1140–1141.
33. Bachofer, C. S., and Gautereaux, M. E. (1959): X-ray effects on single nerve fibers. *J. Gen. Physiol.*, 42:723–735.
34. Bachofer, C. S., and Gautereaux, M. E. (1960): Bioelectric activity of mammalian nerves during X-irradiation. *Radiat. Res.*, 12:575–586.
35. Bachofer, C. S., and Gautereaux, M. E. (1960): Bioelectric response in situ of mammalian nerves exposed to x-rays. *Am. J. Physiol.*, 198:715–717.
36. Baetcke, K. P., Sparrow, A. H., Nauman, C. H., and Schwemmer, S. S. (1967): The relationship of DNA content to nuclear and chromosome volumes and to radiosensitivity (LD_{50}). *Proc. Natl. Acad. Sci. U.S.A.*, 58:533–540.
37. Baisakhatov, R., and Khanson, K. P. (1971): Comparison of the content of adenylic nucleotides and the activity of the process of oxidative phosphorylation in the rat thymus after total X-irradiation. *Radiobiologiya*, 11:155–159.
38. Baker, D. G., and Krochak, R. J. (1989): The response of the microvascular system to radiation: A review. *Cancer Invest.*, 7:287–294.
39. Barcellos-Hoff, M. H. (1993): Radiation-induced transforming growth factor *B* and subsequent extracellular matrix reorganization in the murine mammary gland. *Cancer Res.*, 53:3880–3886.
40. Bassant, M. H., and Court, L. (1978): Effects of whole-body irradiation on the activity of rabbit hippocampal neurons. *Radiat. Res.*, 75:593–606.
41. Baum, A., Gatchel, R. J., and Schaeffer, M. A. (1983): Emotional, behavioral, and physiological effects of chronic stress at Three Mile Island. *J. Consult. Clin. Psychol.*, 51:565–572.
42. Baum, S. J., Anno, G. H., Young, R. W., and Withers, H. R. (1984): Nuclear weapon effect research at PSR-1983: Vol.10, Symptomatology of acute radiation effects in humans after exposure to doses of 75 to 4500 Rads (cGy) free-in-air. *DNA TR-85-50*. Defense Nuclear Agency, Washington, DC.
43. Bayraktar, M., Gedik, O., Akalin, S., et al. (1990): The effect of radioactive iodine treatment on thyroid C cells. *Clin. Endocrinol., 33:625–630.*
44. Beard, C. M., Heath, H., 3d, O'Fallon, W. M., et al. (1989): Therapeutic radiation and hyperparathyroidism. A case-control study in Rochester, Minn. *Arch. Intern. Med.*, 149:1887–1890.
45. Becciolini, A. (1987): Relative radiosensitivities of the small and large intestine. In: *Advances in Radiation Biology. Vol. 12, Relative*

Radiation Sensitivities of Human Organ Systems, edited by J. T. Lett and K. I. Altman, pp. 83–128. Academic Press, San Diego.

46. Bedford, J. S., and Mitchell, J. B. (1973): Dose rate effects in synchronous mammalian cells in culture. *Radiat. Res.*, 54:316–327.
47. Beetz, A., Messer, G., Oppel, T., et al. (1997): Induction of interleukin 6 by ionizing radiation in a human epithelial cell line: Control by corticosteroids. *Int. J. Radiat. Biol.*, 72:33–43.
48. BEIR III. (1980): The effects on populations of exposure to low levels of ionizing radiation. Report of the Committee on the Biological Effects of Ionizing Radiations, National Research Council. National Academy Press, Washington, DC.
49. BEIR IV. (1988): Health risks of radon and other internally deposited alpha-emitters. Report of the Committee on the Biological Effects of Ionizing Radiations, National Research Council. National Academy Press, Washington, DC.
50. BEIR V. (1990): Health effects of exposure to low levels of ionizing radiation. Report of the Committee on the Biological Effects of Ionizing Radiations, National Research Council. National Academy Press, Washington, DC.
51. Belkacemi, Y., Ozsahin, M., Pene, F., et al. (1996): Total body irradiation prior to bone marrow transplantation: Efficacy and safety of granisetron in the prophylaxis and control of radiation-induced emesis. *Int. J. Radiat. Oncol. Biol. Phys.*, 36:77–82.
52. Bengtsson, G. (1991): Introduction: Present knowledge on the effects of radioactive contamination on pregnancy outcome. *Biomed. Pharmacother.*, 45:221–223.
53. Benline, T. A., and French, J. (1997): Anti-emetic drug effects on cognitive and psychomotor performance: granisetron vs. ondansetron. *Aviat. Space Environ. Med.*, 68:504–511.
54. Benline, T. A., French, J., and Poole, E. (1997): Anti-emetic drug effects on pilot performance: Granisetron vs. ondansetron. *Aviat. Space Environ. Med.*, 68:998–1005.
55. Berg, N. O., and Lindgren, M. (1958): Time dose relationship and morphology of delayed radiation lesions of the brain of the rabbit. *Acta Radiol.*, 167:1–118.
56. Berger, N. A., Sims, J. L., Catino, D. M., and Berger, S. J. (1983): Poly(ADP-ribose)polymerase mediates the suicide response to massive DNA damage: Studies in normal and DNA-repair defective cells. In: *ADP-Ribosylation, DNA Repair and Cancer*, edited by M. Miwa, O. Hayaisha, S. Shall, M. Smulson, and T. Sugimura, pp. 219–226. Japan Sci Soc Press, Tokyo.
57. Bergonie, J., and Triblondeau, L. (1906): De quelques resultats de la radiotherapie et essai de fixation d'une technique rationannelle. *Comptes rendus des seances de l'acadenie des sciences*, 143:983–985. English translation by Fletcher G. H. (1959): Interpretation of some results of radiotherapy and an attempt at determining a logical technique of treatment. *Radiat. Res.*, 11:587–588.
58. Bermudez, J., Boyle, E. A., Miner, W. D., and Sanger, G. J. (1988): The anti-emetic potential of the 5-hydroxytryptamine$_3$ receptor antagonist BRL 43694. *Br. J. Cancer*, 58:644–650.
59. Biaglow, J. E., Varnes, M. E., Clark, E. P., and Epp, E. R. (1987): Role of glutathione and other thiols in cellular response to radiation and drugs. In: *Radiation Research. Proceedings of the 8th International Congress of Radiation Research, Vol. 2, Edinburgh, July 1987*, edited by E. M. Fielden, J. F. Fowler, J. H. Hendry, and D. Scott, pp. 677–682. Taylor and Francis, New York.
60. Biard, D. S. F., Saintigny, Y., Maratrat, M., et al. (1997): Enhanced expression of the Kin17 protein immediately after low doses of ionizing radiation. *Radiat. Res.*, 147:442–450.
61. Bigbee, W. L., Jensen, R. H., Veideaum, T., et al. (1996): Glycophorin A biodosimetry in Chernobyl cleanup workers from the Baltic countries. *B.M.J.*, 312:1078–1079.
62. Bigbee, W. L., Jensen, R. H., Veidebaum, T., et al. (1997): Biodosimetry of Chernobyl cleanup workers from Estonia and Latvia using the glycophorin A in vivo somatic cell mutation assay. *Radiat. Res.*, 147:215–224.
63. Billen, D. (1987): Free radical scavenging and the expression of potentially lethal damage in X-irradiated repair deficient *Escherichia coli. Radiat. Res.*, 111:354–360.
64. Birioukov, A., Meurer, M., Peter, R. U., et al. (1993): Male reproductive system in patients exposed to ionizing irradiation in the Chernobyl accident. *Arch. Androl.*, 30:99–104.
65. Blank, K. R., Rudolz, M. S., Kao, G. D., et al. (1997): The molecular regulation of apoptosis and implications for radiation oncology. *Int. J. Radiat. Biol.*, 71:455–466.
66. Bleuer, J. P., Averkin, Y. I., and Abelin, T. (1997): Chernobyl-related thyroid cancer: What evidence for role of short-lived iodines? *Environ. Health Perspect.*, 105:1483–1486.
67. Bogo, V. (1988): Radiation: Behavioral implications in space. *Toxicology*, 49:299–307.
68. Bogo, V., Boward, C., Fiala, N., et al. (1989): Zacopride: A nonbehaviorally toxic radiation antiemetic. In: *Proceedings of the 60th Annual Meeting of the Aerospace Medical Association*, A31. Washington, DC; 12–15 May, 1989.
69. Bogo, V., Dennison, B. A., and Mulvihill, M. (1989): Motor performance, radiation and mortality in rats. In: *Proceedings of the 37th Annual Meeting of the Radiation Research Society*, 1:139. Seattle, WA; 18–23 March 1989.
70. Bogo, V., Franz, C. F., and Young, R. W. (1987): Effects of radiation on monkey visual discrimination performance. In: *Proceedings of the 8th International Congress of Radiation Research, Edinburgh, July 1987*, edited by E. M. Fielden, J. F. Fowler, J. H., Hendry, and D. Scott, p. 259. International Association for Radiation Research, Edinburgh.
71. Bogo, V., Zeman, G. H., and Dooley, M. (1989): Radiation quality and rat motor performance. *Radiat. Res.*, 118:341–352.
72. Bohuslavizki, K. H., Brenner, W., Klutmann, S., et al. (1998): Radioprotection of salivary glands by amifostine in high-dose radioiodine therapy. *J. Nucl. Med.*, 39:1237–1242.
73. Bornhausen, M. (1986): Analysis of behavioral changes induced by prenatal irradiation. In: *Radiation Risks to the Developing Nervous System*, edited by H. Kriegel, W. Schmahl, G. B. Gerber, and F.-E. Stieve, pp. 283–293. Gustav Fischer Verlag, Stuttgart.
74. Bossola, M., Merrick, H. W., Eltaki, A., et al. (1990): Rat liver tolerance for partial resection and intraoperative radiation therapy: Regeneration is radiation dose dependent. *J. Surg. Oncol.*, 45:196–200.
75. Breiter, N., Trott, K. R., and Sassy, T. (1989): Effect of X-irradiation on the stomach of the rat. *Int. J. Radiat., Oncol. Biol. Phys.*, 17:779–784.
76. Brent, R. L. (1984): The effects of ionizing radiation, microwaves, and ultrasound on the developing embryo: Clinical interpretations and applications of the data. *Curr. Prob. Pediatr.*, 14:1–87.
77. Brent, R. L., Beckman, D. A., and Jensh, R. P. (1987): Relative radiosensitivity of fetal tissues. In: *Advances in Radiation Biology, Vol. 12, Relative Radiation Sensitivities of Human Organ Systems*, edited by J. T. Lett, and K. I. Altman, pp. 239–256. Academic Press, San Diego.
78. Breuer, R., Tochner, Z., Conner, M. W., et al. (1992): Superoxide dismutase inhibits radiation-induced lung injury in hamsters. *Lung*, 170:19–29.
79. Brizzee, K. R., and Ordy, J. M. (1986): Effects of prenatal ionizing radiation on neural function and behavior. In: *Radiation Risks to the Developing Nervous System*, edited by H. Kriegel, W. Schmahl, G. B. Gerber, and F.-E. Stieve, pp. 255–282. Gustav Fischer Verlag, Stuttgart.

80. Brown, J. M., and Kovacs, M. S. (1993): Visualization of nonreciprocal chromosome exchanges in irradiated human fibroblasts by fluorescence in situ hybridization. *Radiat. Res.*, 136:71–96.
81. Brown, R. G., and Segal, D. S. (1980): Alterations in beta-endorphin-induced locomotor hyperactivity in morphine tolerant rats. *Neuropharmacology*, 19:619–621.
82. Bruner, A. (1977): Immediate dose-rate effects of ^{60}Co on performance and blood pressure in monkeys. *Radiat. Res.*, 70:378–390.
83. Bruni, J. E., Persaud, T. V., Froese, G., et al. (1994): Effects of in utero exposure to low dose ionizing radiation on development in the rat. *Histol. Histopathol.*, 9:27–33.
84. Bruni, J. E., Persaud, T. V., Huang, W., et al. (1993): Postnatal development of the rat CNS following in utero exposure to a low dose of ionizing radiation. *Exp. Toxicol. Pathol.*, 45:223–231.
85. Bucky, G., Blank, F., and Distelheim, I. H. (1950): Influence of genz rays on histamine-induced manifestations. *Arch. Derm. Syph.*, 62:319–322.
86. Buell, M. G., and Harding, R. K. (1989): Proinflammatory effects of local abdominal irradiation on rat gastrointestinal tract. *Dig. Dis. Sci.*, 34:390–399.
87. Bump, E., and Malaker, K. (1998): *Radiprotectors: Chemical, Biological, and Clinical Perspectives*. CRC Press, Washington, DC.
88. Burger, A., Loeffler, H., Bamburg, M., and Rodemann, H. P. (1998): Molecular and cellular basis of radiation fibrosis. *Int. J. Radiat. Biol.*, 73:401–408.
89. Burghardt, W. F., and Hunt, W. A. (1984): The interactive effects of morphine and ionizing radiation on the latency of tail withdrawal from warm water in the rat. In: *Proceedings of the 9th Symposium on Psychology in the Department of Defense*, edited by G. E. Lee, T. E. Ulrich, pp. 73–76. USAFA Technical Report No. 84-2. U.S. Air Force Academy, Colorado Springs, CO.
90. Burt, D. H., and Ingersoll, E. H. (1965): Behavioral and neuropathological changes in the rat following X-irradiation of the frontal brain. *J. Comp. Physiol. Psychol.*, 59:90–93.
91. Byelorussia and Chernobyl. (1991): The delegation of the Byelorussian SSR at the 45th session of the UN General Assembly: A review, pp. 6–52. Minsk Belarus Publishers, Minsk, Belarus.
92. Calvo, W. (1993): Experimental radiation damage of the central nervous system. *Recent Results Cancer Res.*, 130:175–188.
93. Carlson, R. G., Mayfield, W. R., Normann, S., and Alexander, J. A. (1991): Radiation-associated valvular disease. *Chest*, 99:538–545.
94. Carpenter, D. O. (1979): Early transient incapacitation: A review with considerations of underlying mechanisms. *AFRRI Scientific Report, SR 79-1*. Armed Forces Radiobiology Research Institute, Bethesda, MD.
95. Carter, S., Auer, K. L., Reardon, D. B., et al. (1998): Inhibition of mitogen activated protein (MAP) kinase cascade protentiates cell killing by low dose ionizing radiation in A431 human squamous carcinoma cells. *Oncogene*, 16:2787–2796.
96. Cassaret, G. W. (1980): *Radiation Histopathology*. CRC Press, Boca Raton, FL.
97. Castillo, L. A., Craft, A. W., Kernahan, J., et al. (1990): Gonadal function after 12-Gy testicular irradiation in childhood acute lymphoblastic leukaemia. *Med. Pediatr. Oncol.*, 18:185–189.
98. Catravas, G. N., and McHale, C. G. (1973): Activity changes of brain enzymes in rats exposed to different qualities of ionizing radiation. *AFRRI Scientific Report, SR 73-19*. Armed Forces Radiobiology Research Institute, Bethesda, MD.
99. Catterall, W. A. (1984): The molecular basis of neuronal excitability. *Science*, 223:653–661.
100. Caveness, W. F. (1977): Pathology of radiation damage to the normal brain of the monkey. *Natl. Cancer. Inst. Monogr.*, 46:57–76.
101. Caveness, W. F. (1980): Experimental observations: Delayed necrosis in normal monkey brain. In: *Radiation Damage to the Nervous System*, edited by H. A. Gilbert and A. R. Kagen, pp. 1–38. Raven Press, New York.
102. Cerveny, T. J., and Cockerham, L. G. (1986): Medical management of internal radionuclide contamination. *Med. Bull. U.S. Army Eur.*, 43:24–27.
103. Cerveny, T. J., MacVittie, T. J., and Young, R. W. (1989): Acute radiation syndrome in humans. In: *Medical Consequences of Nuclear Warfare*, edited by R. I. Walker and T. J. Cerveny, pp. 15–36. TMM Publications, Falls Church, VA.
104. Chaillan, F. A., Devigne, C., Diabira, D., et al. (1997): Neonatal gamma-ray irradiation impairs learning and memory of an olfactory associative task in adult rats. *Eur. J. Neurosci.*, 9:884–894.
105. Champlin, R. (1988): Treatment for victims of nuclear accidents: The role of bone marrow transplantation. *Radiat. Res.*, 113:205–210.
106. Chapman, P. H., and Young, R. J. (1968): Effect of cobalt-60 gamma irradiation on blood pressure and cerebral blood flow in the Macaca mulatta. *Radiat. Res.*, 35:78–85.
107. Chapman, P. H., and Young, R. J. (1968): Effect of head versus trunk fission-spectrum radiation on learned behavior in the monkey. *USAF SAM Technical Report, TR 68-80*. Brooks Air Force Base: School of Aerospace Medicine. San Antonio, TX.
108. Chapman, P. H., and Young, R. J. (1968): Effect of high energy X-irradiation of the head on cerebral blood flow and blood pressure in the Macaca mulatta. *Aerosp. Med.*, 3:1316–1321.
109. Chaput, R. L., and Wise, D. (1970): Miniature pig incapacitation and performance decrement after mixed gamma-neutron irradiation. *Aerosp. Med.*, 41:290–293.
110. Charlton, D. E., Nikjoo, H., and Humm, J. L. (1989): Calculation of initial yields of single- and double-strand breaks in cell nuclei from electrons, protons and alpha particles. *Int. J. Radiat. Biol.*, 56:1–19.
111. Chaterjee, J., De, K., Basu, S. K., and Das, A. K. (1994): Low-level x-ray exposures on rat skin: Hyperkeratinization and concomitant changes in biometal concentration. *Biol. Trace Element Res.*, 46:203–210.
112. Chen, A. Y., Okunieff, P., Pommier, Y., and Mitchell, J. B. (1997): Mammalian DNA topoisomerase I mediates the enhancement of radiation cytotoxicity by camptothecin derivatives. *Cancer Res.*, 57:1529–1536.
113. Cherkasova, L. S., and Mironova, T. M. (1976): Effects of ionizing radiation on enzymes of carbohydrate metabolism. *Radiobiologiya*, 16:657–664.
114. Chesser, R. K., Sugg, D. W., Lomakin, M. D., et al. ^{134,137}Cesium, ^{90}Strontium and partial dose rate estimates in small mammals at Chernobyl. *J. Environ. Toxicol. Chem.*, 2000; 19:305–312..
115. Chieng, P. U., Huang, T. S., Chang, C. C., et al. (1991): Reduced hypothalamic blood flow after radiation treatment of nasopharyngeal cancer: SPECT studies in 34 patients. *A.J.N.R. Am. J. Neuroradiol.*, 12:661–665.
116. Chinkina, O. V. (1991): Psychological characteristics of patients exposed to accidental irradiation at the Chernobyl atomic-power station. In: *The Medical Basis for Radiation-Accident Preparedness III: The Psychological Perspective*, edited by R. C. Ricks, M. E. Berger, and F. M. O'Hara, pp. 93–103. Elsevier, New York.
117. Chiu, S.-M., Xue, L.-Y., Friedman, L. R., and Olenik, N. L. (1992): Chromatin compaction and the efficiency of formation of DNA-protein cross-links in γ-irradiated mammalian cells. *Radiat. Res.*, 129:184–191.
118. Chmura, S. J., Nodzenski, E., Beckett, M. A., et al. (1997): Loss of ceramide production confers resistance to radiation-induced apoptosis. *Radiat. Res.*, 57:1270–1275.

119. Christensen, H. D., Flesher, A. M., and Haley, T. J. (1969): Changes in brain self-stimulation rates after exposure to X-irradiation. *J. Pharm. Sci.*, 58:128–129.
120. Cilliers, G. D., Harper, I. S., and Lochner, A. (1989): Radiation-induced changes in the ultrastructure and mechanical function of the rat heart. *Radiother. Oncol.*, 16:311–326.
121. Clarke, R. H. (1987): Dose distributions in western Europe following Chernobyl. In: *Radiation and Health. The Biological Effects of Low-Level Exposure to Ionizing Radiation*, edited by R. Jones, and R. Southwood, pp. 251–264. John Wiley & Sons, New York.
122. Clarke, R. H. (1989): Current radiation risk estimates and implications for the health consequences of Windscale, TMI and Chernobyl accidents. In: *Medical Response to Effects of Ionizing Radiation*, edited by W. A. Crosbie, and J. H., Gittus, pp. 103–118. Elsevier Science, New York.
123. Cockerham, L. G., Arroyo, C. M., and Hampton, J. D. (1988): Effects of 4-hydroxypyrazolo (3,4-d) pyrimidine (Allopurinol) on postradiation cerebral blood flow: Implications of free radical involvement. *Free Radic. Biol. Med.*, 4:279–284.
124. Cockerham, L. G., Cerveny, T. J., and Hampton, J. D. (1986): Postradiation regional cerebral blood flow in primates. *Aviat. Space Environ. Med.*, 57:578–582.
125. Cockerham, L. G., Doyle, T. F., Donlon, M. A., and Gossett-Hagerman, C. J. (1985): Antihistamines block radiation-induced increased intestinal blood flow in canines. *Fundam. Appl. Toxicol.*, 5:597–604.
126. Cockerham, L. G., Doyle, T. F., Donlon, M. A., and Helgeson, E. A. (1984): Canine postradiation histamine levels and subsequent response to Compound 48/80. *Aviat. Space Environ. Med.*, 55:1041–1045.
127. Cockerham, L. G., Doyle, T. F., Paulter, E. L., and Hampton, J. D. (1986): Disodium cromoglycate, a mast-cell stabilizer, alters postradiation regional cerebral blood flow in primates. *J. Toxicol. Environ. Health*, 18:91–101.
128. Cockerham, L. G., and Forcino, C. D. (1995): Effect of antihistamines, disodium cromoglycate (DSCG) or methysergide on post-irradiation cerebral blood flow and mean systemic arterial blood pressure in primates after 25 Gy, whole-body, gamma irradiation. *J. Radiat. Res.* (*Tokyo*), 36:77–90.
129. Cockerham, L. G., Forcino, T. C., Pellmar, T. C., and Smart, S. W. (1987): Effect of methysergide on postirradiation hypotension and cerebral ischemia. In: *Proceedings of the Cerebral Hypoxia and Stroke Symposium*. Budapest, Hungary, August 22–24.
130. Cockerham, L. G., Hampton, J. D., and Doyle, T. F. (1986): Dose dependent radiation-induced hypotension in the canine. *Life Sci.*, 39:1543–1547.
131. Cockerham, L. G., and Hawkins, R. N. (1987): Radiation injury and the splanchnic circulation. In: *Pathophysiology of the Splanchnic Circulation*, Vol. II, edited by P. R. Kvietys, J. A. Barrowman, and D. N. Granger, pp. 55–66. CRC Press, Boca Raton, FL.
132. Cockerham, L. G., Pautler, E. L., Carraway, R. E., et al. (1988): Effect of disodium cromoglycate (DSCG) and antihistamines on postirradiation cerebral blood flow and plasma levels of histamine and neurotensin. *Fundam. Appl. Toxicol.*, 10:233–242.
133. Cockerham, L. G., and Prell, G. D. (1989): Prenatal radiation risk to the brain. *Neurotoxicology*, 10:467–474.
134. Cockerham, L. G., Prell, G. D., and Cerveny, T. J., et al. (1991): Effects of aminoguanidine on pre- and postirradiation regional cerebral blood flow and systemic blood pressure in the primate. *Agents Actions*, 32:237–244.
135. Collins, D. L. (1991): Stress at Three Mile Island: Altered perceptions, behaviors, and neuroendocrine measures. In: *The Medical Basis for Radiation-Accident Preparedness III: The Psychological Perspective*, edited by R. C. Ricks, M. E. Berger, and F. M. O'Hara, pp. 71–79. Elsevier, New York.
136. Collins, D. L. (1992): Behavioral differences of irradiated persons associated with the Kyshtym, Chelyabinsk, and Chernobyl nuclear accidents. *Mil. Med.*, 157:548–552.
137. Collins, D. L., and de Carvalho, A. B. (1993): Chronic stress from the Goiania 137Cs radiation accident. *Behav. Med.*, 18:149–157.
138. Committee for the Compilation of Materials on Damage Caused by the Atomic Bombs in Hiroshima and Nagasaki. (1981): Psychological trends among A-bomb victims. In: *Hiroshima and Nagasaki: Physical, Mental and Social Effects of the Atomic Bombings*, translated by E. Ishikawa, and D. Swain, pp. 485–500. Basic Books, New York.
139. Conklin, J. J., and Walker, R. I. (1987): Diagnosis, triage, and treatment of casualties. In: *Medical Radiobiology*, J. J. Conklin, and R. I. Walker, pp. 231–240. Academic Press, Orlando, FL.
140. Cooper, J. S. (1997): Classic and acquired immunodeficiency syndrome (AIDS)-related Kaposi's sarcoma. In: *Principles and Practice of Radiation Oncology*, 3rd ed, edited C. A. Perez, and L. W. Brady, pp. 745–762. Lippincott-Raven Publishers, Philadelphia.
141. Cox, A. B., Lee, A. C., and Lett, J. T. (1988): Delayed effects of proton irradiation in the lens and integument: A primate model. In: *Terrestrial Space Radiation and its Biological Effects*, edited P. D. McCormack, C. E. Swenberg, and H. Bücker, pp. 415–422. Plenum Press, New York.
142. Cristaldi, M., D'Arcangelo, E. D., and Leradi, L. A., et al. (1990): ^{137}Cs determination and mutagenicity tests in wild Mus musculus domesticus before and after the Chernobyl accident. *Environ. Pollut.*, 64:1–9.
143. Cristaldi, M., Leradi, L. A., Mascanzoni, D., and Mattei, T. (1991): Environmental impact of the Chernobyl accident: Mutagenesis in bank voles from Sweden. *Int. J. Radiat. Biol.*, 59:31–40.
144. Croft, J. R. (1989): The Goiânia accident. In: *Medical Response to Effects of Ionizing Radiation*, edited by W. A. Crosbie and J. H. Gittus, pp. 83–101. Elsevier Science, New York.
145. Crompton, M. R., and Layton, D. D. (1961): Delayed radionecrosis of the brain following therapeutic X-irradiation of the pituitary. *Brain*, 84:85–101.
146. Cross, F. T., Palmer, R. F., Busch, R. H., et al. (1981): Development of lesions in Syrian Golden hamsters following exposure to radon daughters and uranium ore dust. *Health Phys.*, 41:135–153.
147. Cross, F. T., Palmer, R. F., Filipy, R. E., et al. (1982): Carcinogenic effects of radon daughters, uranium ore dust and cigarette smoke in beagle dogs. *Health Phys.*, 42:33–52.
148. Currey, J. D., Foreman, J., Laketic, I., et al. (1997): Effects of ionizing radiation on the mechanical properties of human bone. *J. Orthopaedic Res.*, 15:111–117.
149. Cust, M. P., Whitehead, M. I., Powles, R., Hunter, M., and Milliken, S. (1989): Consequences and treatment of ovarian failure after total body irradiation for leukaemia. *B.M.J.*, 299:1494–1497.
150. Cwikel, J. (1997): Comments on the psychosocial aspects of the International Conference on Radiation and Health. *Environ. Health Perspect.*, 105:1607–1608.
151. Cwikel, J., Abdelgani, A., Goldsmith, J. R., et al. (1997): Two-year follow up study of stress-related disorders among immigrants to Israel from the Chernobyl area. *Environ. Health Perspect.*, 105:1545–1550.
152. Dafny, N., and Pellis, N. R. (1986): Evidence that opiate addiction is in part an immune response: Immune system destruction by irradiation altered opiate withdrawal. *Neuropharmacology*, 25:815–818.

153. Dahlstrom, A., Haggendal, J., and Rosengren, B. (1973): The effect of Roentgen irradiation on monoamine containing neurons of the rat brain. *Acta Radiol. Ther. Phys. Biol.*, 12:191–200.
154. Dallas, C. E. (1993): Aftermath of the Chernobyl Nuclear Disaster: Pharmaceutical needs in the Republic of Belarus. *Am. J. Pharm. Ed.*, 57:182–185.
155. Dallas, C. E., Jagoe, C. H., Fisher, S. K., et al. (1995): Evaluation of genotoxicity in wild organisms due to the Chernobyl Nuclear Disaster. *Ecol. Ind. Regions*, 1:44–54.
156. Dallas, C. E., Lingenfelser, S. F., Lingenfelser, J. T., et al. (1998): Flow cytometric analysis of leukocyte and erthrocyte DNA in fish from Chernobyl-contaminated ponds in the Ukraine. *Ecotoxicology*, 7:211–219.
157. D'Amato, C. J., and Hicks, S. P. (1980): Development of the motor system: Effects of radiation on developing corticospinal neurons and locomotor function. *Exp. Neurol.*, 70:1–23.
158. Danquechin-Dorval, E., Mueller, G. P., Eng, R. R., et al. (1985): Effect of ionizing radiation on gastric secretion and gastric motility in monkeys. *Gastroenterology*, 89:374–380.
159. Danylash, M. M., Voshchepynets, H. A., Urban, V. I., and Fekiishgazi, S. B. (1996): Immune status parameters and renal function in subjects with prior ionizing radiation exposure (in Ukranian). *Likars'Ka Sprava*, 1-2:18–20.
160. Darby, S. C., and Weiss, H. A. (1995): Human studies in radiation leukaemogenesis. In: *Radiation Toxicology: Bone Marrow and Leukaemia*, edited by J. H. Hendry, and B. I. Lord, pp. 335–353. Taylor & Francis, Washington.
161. Dare, A., Hachisu, R., Yamaguchi, A., et al. (1997): Effects of ionizing radiation on proliferation and differentiation of osteoblast-like cells. *J. Dental Res.*, 76:658–664.
162. d'Avella, D., Cicciarello, R., Albiero, F., et al. (1992): Quantitative study of blood-brain barrier permeability changes after experimental whole-brain radiation. *Neurosurgery*, 30:30–34.
163. d'Avella, D., Cicciarello, R, Angileri, F. F., et al. (1998): Radiation-induced blood-brain barrier changes: Pathophysiological mechanisms and clinical implications. *Acta Neurochir. Suppl.* (*Wien*), 71:282–284.
164. Davidoff, L. M., Dyke, C. G., Elsberg, C. A., and Tarlov, I. M. (1938): The effect of radiation applied directly to brain and spinal cord. I. Experimental investigations on Macaca rhesus monkeys. *Radiology*, 31:451–463.
165. Davydov, B. I. (1961): Acetylcholine metabolism on the thalamic region of the brain of dogs after acute radiation sickness. *Radiobiologiia*, 1:550–554.
166. Day, R., Gorin, M. B., and Eller, A. W. (1995): Prevalence of lens changes in Ukrainian children residing around Chernobyl. *Health Phys.*, 68:632–642.
167. de Carvalho, A. B. (1991): The psychological effects of the Goiania radiological accident on the emergency responders. In: *The Medical Basis for Radiation-Accident Preparedness III: The Psychological Perspective*, edited by R. C. Ricks, M. E. Berger, and F. M. O'Hara, pp. 132–141. Elsevier, New York.
168. Deininger, M. W. N., Bose, S., Gora-Tybor, J., et al. (1998): Selective induction of leukemia-associated fusion genes by high-dose ionizing radiation. *Cancer Res.*, 58:421–425.
169. Deng, C., Zhang, P., Harper, J. W., et al. (1995): Mice lacking p21(CIP1/WAF1) undergo normal development, but are defective in G1 checkpoint control. *Cell*, 82:675–684.
170. Deroo, J., Gerber, G. B., and Maes, J. (1986): In: *Radiation Risks to the Developing Nervous System*, edited by H. Kriegel, W. Schmahl, G. B. Gerber, and F.-E. Stieve, pp. 211–219. Gustav Fischer Verlag, Stuttgart.
171. DeRyck, M., Schallert, T., and Teitelbaum, P. (1980): Morphine versus haloperidol catalepsy in the rat: A behavioral analysis of postural support mechanisms. *Brain Res.*, 201:143–172.
172. Deshmukh, B. D., and Suryawanshi, S. A. (1989): Effects of gamma irradiation on histomorphology of some endocrine glands of the rain quail, Coturnix coromandelica (Gmelin). *Ind. J. Exp. Biol.*, 27:780–784.
173. de Toledo, S. M., Azzam, E. I., Gasmann, Mk., and Mitchell, R. E. (1995): Use of semiquantitative transcription polymerase chain reaction to study gene expression in normal human skin fibroblasts following low dose-rate irradiation. *Int. J. Radiat. Biol.*, 67:135–143.
174. Dewey, W. C., Ling, C. C., and Meyn, R. E. (1995): Radiation-induced apoptosis: Revelance to radiotherapy. *Int. J. Radiat. Oncol. Biol. Phys.*, 33:781–796.
175. Di Cicco, D., Antal, S., and Ammassari-Teule, M. (1991): Prenatal exposure to gamma/neutron irradiation: Sensorimotor alterations and paradoxical effects on learning. *Teratology*, 43:61–70.
176. Donlon, M. A., and Walden, T. L., Jr. (1988): The release of biologic mediators in response to acute radiation injury. *Comments Toxicol.*, 2:205–216.
177. Dopico, A. M., and Zieher, L. M. (1993): Neurochemical characterization of the alterations in the noradrenertic afferents to the cerebellum of adult rats exposed to X-irradiation at birth. *J. Neurochem.*, 61:481–489.
178. Dorr, R. T. (1998): Radioprotectants: Pharmacology and clinical applications of amifostine. *Semin. Radiat. Oncol.*, 4(Suppl 1):10–13.
179. Dörr, W., and Schultz-Hector, S. (1992): Early changes in mouse urinary bladder function following fractionated X irradiation. *Radiat. Res.*, 131:35–42.
180. Douglas, W. W. (1985): Histamine and 5-hydroxytryptamine (serotonin) and their antagonists. In: *Goodman and Gilman's The Pharmacological Basis of Therapeutics*, edited by A. G. Gilman, L. S. Goodman, T. W. Rall, and F. Murad, pp. 605–615. Macmillan, New York.
181. Doull, J. (1967): Pharmacological responses in irradiated animals. *Radiat. Res.*, 30:334–341.
182. Doyle, T. F., Curran, C. R., and Turns, J. E. (1974): The prevention of radiation-induced early transient incapacitation of monkeys by an antihistamine. *Proc. Soc. Exp. Biol. Med.*, 145:1018–1024.
183. Doyle, T. F., and Strike, T. A. (1977): Radiation-released histamine in the rhesus monkey as modified by mast cell depletion and antihistamine. *Experientia*, 33:1047–1049.
184. Doyle, T. F., Turns, J. E., and Strike, T. A. (1971): Effect of antihistamine on early transient incapacitation of monkeys subjected to 4000 rads of mixed gamma-neutron radiation. *Aerosp. Med.*, 42:400–403.
185. Dubois, A. (1988): Effect of ionizing radiation on the gastrointestinal tract. *Comments Toxicol.*, 2:233–242.
186. Dubois, A., Fiala, N., Boward, C. A., and Bogo, V. (1988): Prevention and treatment of the gastric symptoms of radiation sickness. *Radiat. Res.*, 115:595–604.
187. Dubrova, Y. E., Nesterov, V. N., Krouchinsky, N. G., et al. (1996): Human minisatellite mutation rate after the Chernobyl accident. *Nature*, 380:683–686.
188. Dubrova, Y. E., Nesterov, V. N., Krouchinsky, N. G., et al. (1997): Further evidence for elevated human minisatelllite mutation rate in Belarus eight years after the Chernobyl accident. *Mutat. Res. Fundam. Mol. Mech. Mutagenesis*, 38:267–278.
189. Dulic, V., Kaufmann, W. K., Wilson, S. J., et al. (1994): p53-dependent inhibition of cyclin-dependent kinase activities in human fibroblast during radiation-induced G1 arrest. *Cell*, 76:1013–1023.
190. Dygalo, N. N., Sakharov, D. G., and Shishkina, G. T. (1997): Corticosterone and testosterone in the blood of adult rats: The effects of low doses and the times of the action of ionizing radiation

during intrauterine development (in Russian). *Radiat. Biol. Radioecol.*, 37:377–381.

191. Dynes, J. B., and Smedal, M. J. (1960): Radiation myelitis. *Am. J. Roentgenol. Radium Ther. Nuc. Med.*, 83:78–87.
192. Edwards, A. A. (1997): The use of choromosomal aberrations in human lymphocytes for biological dosimetry. *Radiat. Res.*, 148:S39–S44.
193. Edwards, J. C., Cramp, W. C., Chapman, D., and Yatvin, M. B. (1984): The effects of ionizing radiation on biomembrane structure and function. *Prog. Biophys. Mol. Biol.*, 43:71–93.
194. Egana, E. (1962): Some effects of ionizing radiations on the metabolism of the central nervous system. *Int. J. Neurol.*, 3:631–647.
195. Ehrhart, E. J., Segarini, P., Tsang, M. L.-S., et al. (1997): Latent transforming growth factor B1 activation in situ: Quantitative and functional evidence after low-dose gamma-irradiation. *F.A.S.E.B. J.*, 11:991–1002.
196. Eisenbud, M. (1987): *Environmental Radioactivity From Natural, Industrial, and Military sources*, 3rd Academic Press, New York.
197. Elliott, T. B., Brook, I., and Stiefel, S. M. (1990): Quantitative study of wound infection in irradiated mice. *Int. J. Radiat. Biol.*, 58:341–350.
198. Faure, E., Cavard, C., Zider, A., et al. (1995): X-irradiation-induced transcription from HIV type 1 long term repeat. *AIDS Res. Hum. Retroviruses*, 11:41–43.
199. Feldman, J. E. (1989): Ovarian failure and cancer treatment: Incidence and interventions for premenopausal women. *Oncol. Nurs. Forum*, 16:651–657.
200. Ferguson, J. L., Kandasamy, S. B., Harris, A. H., et al. (1996): Indomethacin attenuation of radiation-induced hyperthermia does not modify radiation-induced motor hypoactivity. *J. Radiat. Res. (Tokyo)*, 37:209–215.
201. Fetter, S. A., and Tsipis, K. (1981): Catastrophic releases of radioactivity. *Sci. Am.*, 244:41–47.
202. Feyerabend, T., Kapp, B., Richter, E., et al. (1990): Incidence of hypothyroidism after irradiation of the neck with special reference to lymphoma patients. A retrospective and prospective analysis. *Acta Oncol.*, 29:597–602.
203. Fici, G. J., Althaus, J. S., and von Voigtlander, P. F. (1997): Effects of lazaroids and a peroxynitrite scavenger in a cell model of peroxynitrite toxicity. *Free Radic. Biol. Med.*, 22:223–228.
204. Fields, P. E. (1957): The effect of whole-body X-irradiation upon activity drum, straight runway, and maze performances of white rats. *J. Comp. Physiol. Psychol.*, 50:386–391.
205. Fischbein, A., Zabludovsky, N., Eltes, F., et al. (1997): Ultramorphological sperm characteristics in the risk assessment of health effects after radiation exposure among salvage workers in Chernobyl. *Environ. Health Perspect.*, 105:1445–1450.
206. Flam, F. (1992): Quasars: Ablaze with gamma rays. *Science*, 256:311.
207. Fornace, A. J. (1992): Mammalian genes induced by radiation: Activation of genes associated with growth control. *Annu. Rev. Genet.*, 26:507–526.
208. Francois, A., Aigueperse, J., Gourmelon, P., et al. (1998): Exposure to ionizing radiation modifies neurally-evoked electrolyte transport and some inflammatory responses in rat colon in vitro. *Int. J. Radiat. Biol.*, 73:93–101.
209. Franke, T. F., and Lewis, C. C. (1997): A bad kinase makes good. *Nature*, 390:116–117.
210. Franz, C. G. (1985): Effects of mixed neutron-gamma total body irradiation on physical activity performance of rhesus monkeys. *Radiat. Res.*, 101:434–441.
211. Freud, A., Canfi, A., Sod-Moriah, U. A., and Chayoth, R. (1990): Neonatal low-dose gamma irradiation-induced impaired fertility in mature rats. *Isr. J. Med. Sci.*, 26:611–615.
212. Freud, A., and Sod-Moriah, U. A. (1990): Progesterone and estradiol plasma levels in neonatally irradiated cycling rats. *Endocr. Res.*, 16:221–229.
213. Fritzell, J. A., Narayanan, L., Baker, S. M., et al. (1997): Role of DNA mismatch repair in the cytotoxicity of ionizing radiation. *Cancer Res.*, 57:5143–5147.
214. Fry, F. A. (1987): Doses from environmental radioactivity. In: *Radiation and Health. The Biological Effects of Low-Level Exposure to Ionizing Radiation*, edited by R. Jones, and R. Southwood, pp. 9–17. John Wiley & Sons, New York.
215. Fujiwara, S., Sposto, R., Ezaki, H., et al. (1992): Hyperparathyroidism among atomic bomb survivors in Hiroshima. *Radiat. Res.*, 130:372–378.
216. Fukuda, T., Setoguchi, M., Inaba, K., et al. (1991): The antiemetic profile of Y-25130, a new selective 5-HT3 receptor antagonist. *Eur. J. Pharmacol.*, 196:299–305.
217. Furchtgott, E. (1963): Behavioral effects of ionizing radiations: 1955–61. *Psychol. Bull.*, 60:157–199.
218. Furchtgott, E. (1971): Behavioral effects of ionizing radiations. In: *Pharmacology and Biophysical Agents and Behavior*, edited by E. Furchgott, pp. 1–64. Academic Press, New York.
219. Furchtgott, E. (1975): Ionizing radiations and the nervous system. In: *Biology of Brain Dysfunction*, Vol. 3, edited by G. E. Galli, pp. 343–379. Plenum Press, New York.
220. Fushiki, S. (1997): Pathogenesis of the neuronal migration disorder, with special reference to the animal model of prenatal exposure to low-dose ionizing radiation (in Japanese). *No To Hattatsu*, 29:102–107.
221. Fushiki, S., Hyodo-Taguchi, Y., Kinoshita, C., et al. (1997): Short- and long-term effects of low-dose prenatal X-irradiation in mouse cerebral cortex, with special reference to neuronal migration. *Acta Neuropathol. (Berlin)*, 93:443–449.
222. Gaffey, C. T. (1962): Bioelectric effects of high energy irradiation on nerve. In: *Response of the Nervous System to Ionizing Radiation*, edited by T. J. Haley, and R. S. Snider, pp. 277–296. Academic Press, New York.
223. Gaichenko, V. A., Kryzhanovsky, V. I., and Stovbchaty, V. N. (1994): Post-accident state of the Chernobyl Nuclear Power Plant Alienated Zone faunal complexes. *Radiat. Biol. Ecol.*, Special Issue:27–32.
224. Gal, D., Strickland, D. M., Lifshitz, S., et al. (1984): Effect of radiation on prostaglandin production by human bowel in vitro. *Int. J. Radiat. Oncol. Biol. Phys.*, 10:653–657.
225. Gallegos, A., Berggren, M., Gasdaska, J. R., and Powis, G. (1997): Mechanisms of the regulation of thioredoxin reductase activity in cancer cells by the chemopreventive agent selenium. *Cancer Res.*, 57:4965–4970.
226. Gangloff, H. (1962): Acute effects of X-irradiation on brain electrical activity in cats and rabbits. In: *Effects of Ionizing Radiation on the Nervous System; Proceedings*, pp. 123–138. International Atomic Energy Agency, Vienna. Vienna, Austria; 5–9 June 1961.
227. Gangloff, H., and Haley, T. J. (1960): Effects of X-irradiation on spontaneous and evoked brain electrical activity in cats. *Radiat. Res.*, 12:694–704.
228. Ganong, W. F. (1989): *Review of Medical Physiology*, 14th ed. Appleton and Lange, San Mateo, CA.
229. Gasteiger, E. L., and Campbell, B. (1962): Alteration of mammalian nerve compound action potentials by beta irradiation. In: *Response of the Nervous System to Ionizing Radiation*, edited by T. J. Haley and R. S. Snider, pp. 597–605. Academic Press, New York.
230. Geist, B. J., Lauk, S., Bornhausen, M., and Trott, K. R. (1990): Physiologic consequences of local heart irradiation in rats. *Int. J. Radiat. Oncol. Biol. Phys.*, 18:1107–1113.

231. Geist, B. J., and Trott, K. R. (1992): Radiographic and function changes after partial lung irradiation in the rat. *Strahlenther. Onkol.*, 168:168–173.
232. Gembicki, M., Stozharov, A. N., Arinchin, A. N., et al. (1997): Iodine deficiency in Belarusian children as a possible factor stimulating the irradiation of the thyroid gland during the Chernobyl Catastrophe. *Environ. Health Perspect.*, 105:1487–1490.
233. George, A. M., and Cramp, W. A. (1987): The effects of ionizing radiation on structure and function of DNA. *Prog. Biophys. Mol. Biol.*, 50:121–169.
234. Geraci, J. P., Mariano, M. S., and Jackson, K. L. (1991): Hepatic radiation injury in the rat. *Radiat. Res.*, 125:65–72.
235. Geraci, J. P., Mariano, M. S., and Jackson, K. L. (1992): Radiation hepatology of the rat: Microvascular fibrosis and enhancement of liver dysfunction by diet and drugs. *Radiat. Res.*, 129:322–332.
236. Gershey, E. L., Klein, R. C., Party, E., and Wilkerson, A. (1990): *Low-Level Radioactive Waste. From Cradle to Grave*. Van Nostrand Reinhold, New York.
237. Gersterner, H. B. (1956): Effect of high-intensity X-irradiation on the A group fibers of the frog sciatic nerve. *Am. J. Physiol.*, 184:333–337.
238. Giambarresi, L., and Jacobs, A. J. (1987): Radioprotectants. In: *Military radiobiology*, edited by J. J. Conklin and R. I. Walker, pp. 265–301. Academic Press, San Diego, CA.
239. Gibson, D. P., DeGowin, R. L., and Knapp, S. A. (1982): Effect of X irradiation on release of prostaglandin E from marrow stromal cells in culture. *Radiat. Res.*, 89:537–545.
240. Giel, R. (1991): The psychosocial aftermath of two major disasters in the Soviet Union. *J. Traumatic. Stress*, 4:381–393.
241. Gillette, S. L., Gillette, E. L., Powers, B. E., et al. (1989): Ureteral injury following experimental intraoperative radiation. *Int. J. Radiat. Oncol. Biol. Phys.*, 17:791–798.
242. Gillette, S. M., Powers, B. E., Orton, E. C., and Gillette, E. L. (1991): Early radiation response of the canine heart and lung. *Radiat. Res.*, 125:34–40.
243. Gilmore, S. A., Sims, T. J., Davies, D. L., et al. (1997): Microglial development is altered in immature spinal cord by exposure to radiation. *Int. J. Dev. Neurosci.*, 15:1–14.
244. Ginzburg, H. M. (1993): The psychological consequences of the Chernobyl accident—findings from the International Atomic Energy Agency Study. *Public. Health Rep.*, 108:184–192.
245. Girinsky, T., Baume, D., Socie, G., et al. (1991): Blood cell kinetics after a 385 cGy total body irradiation given to a CML patient for bone marrow transplantation. *Bone Marrow Transplant.*, 7: 317–320.
246. Giwercman, A., von der Maase, H., Berthelsen, J. G., et al. (1991): Localized irradiation of testes with carcinoma in situ: Effects on Leydig cell function and eradication of malignant germ cells in 20 patients. *J. Clin. Endocrinol. Metab.*, 73:596–603.
247. Gluzman, D. F., Moutet, A., Simmonet, M.-L., et al. (1994): Oncohematological aspects of ionizing radiation exposure on human embryo and fetus (in Russian). *Eksperimental'Naya Onkologiya*, 16:279–287.
248. Gobbel, G. T., Seilhan, T. M., and Fike, J. R. (1992): Cerebrovascular response after interstitial irradiation. *Radiat. Res.*, 130:236–240.
249. Goldman, M. (1997): The Russian radiation legacy: Its integrated impact and lessons. *Environ. Health Perspect.*, 105:1385–1392.
250. Goncharova, R. I., and Ryabokon, N. I. (1995): Dynamics of cytogenetic injuries in natural populations of bank vole in the republic of Belarus. *Radiat. Protect. Dosim.*, 62:37–40.
251. Gonzales, S. (1982): Host rocks for radioactive-waste disposal. *Am. Sci.*, 70:191–200.
252. Goud, S. N. (1995): Effect of irradiation of lymphocyte proliferation and differentiation: Potential of IL-6 in augmenting antibody responses in cultures of murine spleen cells. *Int. J. Radiat. Biol.*, 67:461–468.
253. Graham, M. M., Evans, M. L., Dahlen, D. D., et al. (1990): Pharmacological alteration of the lung vascular response to radiation. *Int. J. Radiat. Oncol. Biol. Phys.*, 19:329–339.
254. Grevert, D., and Goldstein, A. (1977): Some effects of naloxone on behavior in the mouse. *Psychopharmacology (Berlin)*, 53:111–113.
255. Grosch, D. S., and Hopwood, L. E. (1979): *Biological Effects of Radiation*. Academic Press, New York.
256. Gueneau, G., Baille, V., Dubos, M., and Court, L. (1986): Protracted postnatal neurogenesis and radiosensitivity in the rabbit's dentate gyrus. In: *Radiation Risks to the Developing Nervous System*, edited by H. Kriegel, W. Schmahl, G. B. Gerber, and F.-E. Stieve, pp. 133–140. Gustav Fischer Verlag, Stuttgart.
257. Guinee, V. F., Guido, J. J., Pfalzgraf, K. A., et al. (1985): The incidence of herpes zoster in patients with Hodgkin's Disease. *Cancer*, 56:642–648.
258. Gunter-Smith, P. J. (1987): Effect of ionizing radiation on gastrointestinal physiology. In: *Military Radiobiology*, edited by J. J. Conklin and R. Walker, pp. 135–151. Academic Press, San Diego.
259. Gunter-Smith, P. J. (1989): Gamma radiation affects active electrolyte transport by rabbit ileum. II. Correlation of alanine and theophylline response with morphology. *Radiat. Res.*, 117:419–432.
260. Gupta, M. L., and Umadevi, P. (1990): Response of reptilian liver to external gamma irradiation. *Radiobiol. Radiother. (Berlin)*, 31:285–288.
261. Gupta, M. L., and Umadevi, P. (1990): Response of piscine liver to external gamma irradiation. *Radiobiol. Radiother. (Berlin)*, 31:289–292.
262. Guyton, A. C. (1986): *Textbook of Medical Physiology*, 7th ed. W. B. Saunders, Philadelphia.
263. Hagen, U. (1989): Biochemical aspects of radiation biology. *Experientia*, 45:7–12.
264. Haimovitz-Friedmann, A., Kolesnick, R. N., and Fuks, Z. (1996): Modulation of the apoptotic response: Potential for therapeutic applications in radiation oncology. *Semin. Radiat. Oncol.*, 6:273–283.
265. Hakem, R., Hakem, A., Duncan, G. S., et al. (1998): Differential requirement for caspace 9 in apoptotic pathway in vivo. *Cell*, 94:339–352.
266. Haley, T. J. (1962): Changes induced in brain activity by low doses of X-irradiation. In: *Effects of Ionizing Radiation on the Nervous System; Proceedings*, pp. 171–185. International Atomic Energy Agency, Vienna. Vienna, Austria; 5–9 June 1961.
267. Hall, E. C., and Cox, J. D. (1989): Physical and biologic basis of radiation therapy. In: *Radiation Oncology. Rationale, Technique, Results*, 6th ed., edited by M. T. Moss, and J. D. Cox, pp. 1–57. C. V. Mosby, St. Louis.
268. Hall, E. J. (1984): *Radiation and Life*, 2nd ed. Pergammon Press, New York.
269. Hall, E. J. (1994): *Radiobiology for the Radiologist*, 4th ed. J. B. Lippincott, New York.
270. Hallahan, D. E. (1996): Radiation-medicated gene expression in the pathogenesis of the clinical radiation response. *Semin. Radiat. Oncol.*, 6:250–267.
271. Halpern, J., Kishel, S. P., Park, J., et al. (1984): Radiation-induced brain edema in primates, studies with sequential brain CAT scanning and histopathology. *Res. Commun. Chem. Pathol. Pharmacol.*, 45:463–470.
272. Hamdorf, G., Shahar, A., Cervos-Navarro, J., et al. (1992): Irradiation neurotoxicity assessed in organotypic cultures of rat hippocampus. *Neurotoxicology*, 13:165–170.

273. Hancock, S. L., Cox, R. S., McDougall, I. R. (1991): Thyroid diseases after treatment of Hodgkin's disease. *N. Engl. J. Med.*, 325:599–605.

274. Hansen, P. V., Trykker, H., Svennekjaer, I. L., and Hvolby, J. (1990): Long-term recovery of spermatogenesis after radiotherapy in patients with testicular cancer. *Radiother. Oncol.*, 18:117–125.

275. Harley, N. H., Cross, F. T., and Stuart, B. O. (1984): Evaluation of occupational and environmental exposures to radon and radon daughters in the United States. *NCRP Report No. 78*. National Council on Radiation Protection and Measurement, Washington, DC.

276. Havenaar, J., Rumyantzeva, G., Kasyanenko, A., et al. (1997): Health effects of the Chernobyl disaster: Illness or illness behavior? A comparative general health survey in two former Soviet regions. *Environ. Health Perspect.*, 105:1533–1538.

277. Havenaar, J. M., van den Brink, W., Kasyanenko, A. P., et al. (1995): Mental health problems in the Gomel Region (Belarus). An analysis of risk factors in an area affected by the Chernobyl disaster. *Psychol. Med.*, 26:845–855.

278. Hawkins, R. N., Alter, W. A., Jr, Doyle, T. F., and Catravas, G. N. (1983): Radiation-induced cardiovascular dysfunction in the rhesus monkey. *Radiat. Res.*, 94:654.

279. Hawkins, R. N., and Cockerham, L. G. (1987): Postirradiation cardiovascular dysfunction. In: *Military Radiobiology*, edited by J. J. Conklin and R. Walker, pp. 153–163, Academic Press, San Diego.

280. Hawkins, R. N., and Forcino, C. D. (1988): Effects of radiation on cardiovascular function. *Comments Toxicol.*, 2:243–252.

281. Haymaker, W. (1962): Morphological changes in the nervous system following exposure to ionizing radiation. In: *Effects of Ionizing Radiation on the Nervous System; Proceedings*, pp. 309–358. International Atomic Energy Agency, Vienna. Vienna, Austria; 5–9 June 1961.

282. Henderson, E. E., Tudor, G., and Yang, J. Y. (1992): Inactivation of the human immunodeficiency virus type 1 (HIV-1) by ultraviolet and X irradiation. *Radiat. Res.*, 131:169–176.

283. Herman, B. H., and Panksepp, I. (1978): Effects of morphine and naloxone on separation distress and approach attachment: Evidence for opiate mediation of social effect. *Pharmacol. Biochem. Behav.*, 9:213–220.

284. Hewitt, M., Cornish, J., Pamphilon, D., and Oakhill, A. (1991): Effective emetic control during conditioning of children for bone marrow transplantation using ondansetron, a 5-HT3 antagonist. *Bone Marrow Transplant.*, 7:431–433.

285. Hienz, R. D. (1992): Effects of ionizing radiation on auditory and visual thresholds. *DNA-TR-91-47*. Defense Nuclear Agency, Alexandria, VA.

286. Highfield, D. A., Hu, D., and Amsel, A. (1998): Alleviation of x-irradiation-based deficit in memory-based learning by D-amphetamine: Suggestions for attention deficit-hyperactivity disorder. *Proc. Natl. Acad. Sci. U.S.A.*, 95:5785–5788.

287. Hill, J. M., Kornblith, A. B., Jones, D., et al. (1998): A comparative study of the long term psychosocial functioning of childhood acute lymphoblastic leukemia survivors treated by intrathecal methotrexate with or without cranial radiation. *Cancer*, 82:208–218.

288. Hirata, Y., Matsukado, Y., Mihara, Y., and Kochi, M. (1985): Occlusion of the internal carotid artery after radiation therapy for the chiasmal lesion. *Acta Neurochir.* (*Wien*), 74:141–147.

289. Hoar, R. M., and Monie, I. W. (1981): Comparative development of specific organ systems. In: *Developmental Toxicology*, edited by C. A. Kimmel and J. Buelke-Sam, pp. 13–33. Raven Press, New York.

290. Hobbs, C. H., and McClellan, R. O. (1986): Toxic effects of radiation and radioactive materials. In: *Casarett and Doull's Toxicology, 3rd ed.*, edited by C. D. Klaassen, M. O. Amdur, and J. Doull, pp. 669–750. Macmillan, New York.

291. Hodges, H., Katzung, N., Sowinski, P., et al. (1998): Late behavioural and neuropathological effects of local brain irradiation in the rat. *Behav. Brain Res.*, 91:99–114.

292. Hoekstra, H. J., Mehta, D. M., Oosterhuis, J. W., et al. (1990): The short- and long-term effect of single high-dose intra-operative electron beam irradiation of retroperitoneal structures—an experimental study in dogs. *Eur. J. Surg. Oncol.*, 16:240–247.

293. Hofer, M., Viklicka, S., Tkadlecek, L., and Karpfel, Z. (1989): Haemopoiesis in murine bone marrow and spleen after fractionated irradiation and repeated bone marrow transplantation. II. Granulopoiesis. *Folia Biol.* (*Praha*), 35:418–428.

294. Hohwieler, M. L., Lo, T. C., Silverman, M. L., and Freiberg, S. R. (1986): Brain necrosis after radiotherapy for primary intracerebral tumor. *Neurosurgery*, 18:67–74.

295. Hole, E. D., Nelson, W. H., Sagstuen, E., and Close, D. M. (1992): Free radical formation in single crystals of 2′-deoxyguanosine 5′-monophosphate tetrahydrate disodium salts: An EPR/ENDOR study. *Radiat. Res.*, 129:119–138.

296. Hollahan, E. V., Jr. (1987): Cellular radiation biology. In: *Military Radiobiology*, edited by J. J. Conklin, and R. I. Walker, pp. 87–110. Academic Press, Orlando.

297. Hollinden, G. E., and Pellmar, T. C. (1989): Attenuation of synaptic transmission in hippocampal slices following whole animal exposure to ionizing radiation. *Soc. Neurosci. Abstr.*, 15:134.

298. Holloman, K., Dallas, C. E., Jagoe, C. H., et al. (1998): Interspecies differences in oxidative stress response and radiocesium uptake in rodents inhabiting areas highly contaminated by the Chernobyl nuclear disaster. *J. Environ. Toxicol. Chem. 2000*; (In Press).

299. Hopewell, J. W. (1979): Late radiation damage to the central nervous system: A radiobiological interpretation. *Neuropathol. Appl. Neurobiol.*, 5:329–343.

300. Hopewell, J. W., and Wright, E. A. (1970): The nature of latent cerebral irradiation damage and its modification by hypertension. *Br. J. Radiol.*, 43:161–167.

301. Hopewell, J. W., and Wright, E. A. (1975): The effects of dose and field size on late radiation damage to the rat spinal cord. *Int. J. Radiat. Biol.*, 28:325–333.

302. Huang, T. S., Chen, S. T., Lui, L. T., et al. (1990): Early effects of cranial irradiation on hypothalamic pituitary function. *Taiwan I Hsueh Hui Tsa Chih*, 89:541–547.

303. Hunt, W. A., Dalton, T. K., and Darden, J. H. (1979): Transient alterations in neurotransmitter activity in the caudate nucleus of rat brain after a high dose of ionizing radiation. *Radiat. Res.*, 80:556–562.

304. Hunter, A. E., Prentice, H. G., Pothecary, K., et al. (1991): Granisetron, a selective 5-HT3 receptor antagonist, for the prevention of radiation induced emesis during total body irradiation. *Bone Marrow Transplant.*, 7:439–441.

305. Hwang, A., and Muschel, R. J. (1998): Radiation and the G_2 phase of the cell cycle. *Radiat. Res.*, 150(Suppl):S52–S59.

306. Hyer, M., and Nielsen, O. S. (1992): Influence of dose on regeneration of murine hematopoietic stem cells after total body irradiation and 5-fluorouracil. *Oncology*, 49:166–172.

307. Ibrahim, M. Z. M., Haymaker, W., Miquel, J., and Riopelle, A. J. (1967): Effects of radiation on the hypothalamus in monkeys. *Archiv für Psychiatrie und Zeitschrift f.d. ges. Neurologie*, 210:1–15.

308. Il'enko, A. I., and Krapivko, T. P. (1994): Radioresistance of populations of bank voles Clethrionomys glareolus in radionuclide-contaminated areas. *Doklady Biological Sciences*, 336:262–266.

309. Iliakis, G., Wang, Y., Pantelias, G. E., and Metzger, L. (1992): Mechanism of radiation sensitization by halogenated pyrimidines: Effect of BrdU on repair of DNA breaks, interphase chromatin breaks, and potentially lethal damage in plateau-phase CHO cells. *Radiat. Res.*, 129:202–211.

310. Imanaka, T., Seo, T., and Koide, H. (1988): Radioactivity release from the Chernobyl–4 accident and its cancer consequences. *J. Radiat. Res. (Tokyo)*, 29:80.

311. Inano, H., Suzuki, K., Ishii-Ohba, H., et al. (1989): Steroid hormone production in testis, ovary, and adrenal gland of immature rats irradiated in utero with ^{60}Co. *Radiat. Res.*, 117:293–303.

312. Innes, J. R., and Carsten, A. (1961): Demyelination or malacic myelopathy. *Arch. Neurol.*, 4:190–199.

313. Ito, M., Patronas, N. J., Di Chiro, G., et al. (1986): Effect of moderate level X-radiation to brain on cerebral glucose utilization. *J. Comput. Assist. Tomogr.*, 10:584–588.

314. Iverson, S. D., and Iverson, L. L. (1981): *Behavioral Pharmacology*, Oxford University Press, New York.

315. Izrael, Yu. A., Petrov, V. A., Avdjushin, S. I., et al. (1987): Radioactive pollution of the natural environment in the zone of the accident of the Chernobyl Atomic Power Plant (in Russian). *Meterologiya Hydrologiya*, 2:5–18.

316. Jacobs, A. J., Maniscalco, W. M., Parkhurst, A. B., and Finkelstein, J. N. (1986): In vivo and in vitro demonstration of reduced myelin synthesis following early postnatal exposure to ionizing radiation. *Radiat. Res.*, 105:97–104.

317. Jaenke, R. S., and Angleton, G. M. (1990): Perinatal radiation-induced renal damage in the beagle. *Radiat. Res.*, 122:58–65.

318. Jagoe, C. H., Chesser, R. K., Smith, M. H., et al. (1998): Radiocesium, mercury and lead in fish, and sediment radiocesium in waters near Chernobyl, Ukraine. *Ecotoxicology*, 7:202–210.

319. Jammet, H., Mathe, G., Pendic, B., et al. (1959): Study of six cases of accidental whole-body irradiation. *Rev. Fr. Etud. Clin. Biol.*, 4:210–225.

320. Janis, I. L. (1951): *Air War and Emotional Stress*. McGraw-Hill, New York.

321. Jensh, R. P., Eisenman, L. M., and Brent, R. L. (1995): Postnatal neurophysiologic effects of prenatal X-irradiation. *Int. J. Radiat. Biol.*, 67:217–227.

322. Jirtle, R. L., Anscher, M. S., and Alati, T. (1990): Radiation sensitivity of the liver. In: *Advances in Radiation Biology, Vol. 14, Relative Radiation Sensitivities of Human Organ Systems, Part II*. edited by K. I. Altman and J. T. Lett, pp. 269–311. Academic Press, San Diego.

323. Johnsson, J. E., Owman, C. H., and Sjoberg, N. O. (1970): Tissue content of noradrenaline and 5-hydroxytryptamine in the rat after ionizing radiation. *Int. J. Radiat. Biol.*, 18:311–316.

324. Jones, D. C., Kimeldorf, D. J., Rubadeau, D. O., et al. (1954): Effects of X-irradiation on performance of volitional activity by the adult male rat. *Am. J. Physiol.*, 177:243–250.

325. Jones, G. D. D., Ward, J. F., Limoli, C. L., et al. (1995): Mechanisms of radiosensitization in iododeoxyuridine-substituted cells. *Int. J. Radiat. Biol.*, 67:647–653.

326. Joseph, J. A., Erat, S., Rabin, B. M. (1998): CNS effects of heavy particle irradiation in space: Behavioral implications. *Adv. Space Res.*, 22:209–216.

327. Joseph, J. A., Hunt, W. A., Rabin, B. M., and Dalton, T. K. (1992): Possible "accelerated striatal aging" induced by ^{56}Fe heavy particle irradiation: Implications for manned space flight. *Radiat. Res.*, 130:88–93.

328. Joseph, J. A., Kandasamy, S. B., Hunt, W. A., et al. (1988): Radiation-induced increases in sensitivity of cataleptic behavior to haloperidol: Possible involvements of prostaglandins. *Pharmacol. Biochem. Behav.*, 29:335–341.

329. Jung, M., and Dritschilo, A. (1996): Signal transduction and cellular responses to ionizing radiation. *Semin. Radiat. Oncol.*, 6:268–272.

330. Kader, H. A., and Rostom, A. Y. (1991): Follicle stimulating hormone levels as a predictor of recovery of spermatogenesis following cancer therapy. *Clin. Oncol.*, (*R. Coll. Radiol.*), 3:37–40.

331. Kameyama, Y., and Hoshino, K. (1986): Sensitive phases of CNS development. In: *Radiation Risks to the Developing Nervous System*, edited by H. Kriegel, W. Schmahl, G. B. Gerber, and F.-E. Stieve, pp. 75–92. Gustav Fischer Verlag, Stuttgart.

332. Kandasamy, S. B., Hunt, W. A., and Mickley, A. G. (1988): Implications of prostaglandins and histamine H_1 and H_2 receptors in radiation-induced temperature responses of rats. *Radiat. Res.*, 114:42–53.

333. Kaplan, M. I., and Morgan, W. F. (1998): The nucleus is the target for radiation-induced chromosomal instability. *Radiat. Res.*, 150:382–390.

334. Karaoglou, A., Desmet, G., Kelly, G. N., and Menzel, H. G. (1995): The radiological consequences of the Chernobyl accident. In: *Proceedings of the First International Conference*, Minsk, Belarus. Office for Official Publications of the European Communities, Luxembourg. May 1995.

335. Katz, R. J., Carroll, B. J., and Baldright, G. (1978): Behavioral activation by enkephalins in mice. *Pharmacol. Biochem. Behav.*, 8:493–496.

336. Kaul, A., Landfermann, H., and Thieme, M. (1996): One decade after Chernobyl: Summing up the consequences. *Health Phys.*, 71:634–640.

337. Kekcheyev, K. (1941): Changes in the threshold of achromatic vision of man by the action of ultrashort, ultraviolet and x-ray waves. *Probl. Fisiol. Optics*, 1:77–79.

338. Kemper, T. L., O'Neill, R., and Caveness, W. F. (1977): Effects of single dose supervoltage whole brain radiation in Macaca mulatta. *J. Neuropathol. Exp. Neurol.*, 36:916–940.

339. Kent, C. R. H., Eady, J. J., Ross, G. M., and Steel, G. G. (1995): The comet moment as a measure of DNA damage in the comet assay. *Int. J. Radiat. Biol.*, 67:655–660.

340. Kerr, J. F. R., Wyllie, A. H., and Currie, A. R. (1972): Apoptosis: A basic biological phenomenon with wide-ranging implications in tissue kinetics. *Br. J. Cancer*, 26:239–256.

341. Keyse, S. M. (1998): Protein phosphatases and the regulation of MAP kinase activity. *Cell Dev. Biol.*, 9:143–152.

342. Khodarev, N. N., Sokolova, I. A., and Vaughan, A. T. M. (1998): Mechanisms of induction of apoptotic DNA fragmentation. *Int. J. Radiat. Biol.*, 73:455–467.

343. Kim, J. H., Mandell, L. R., and Leeper, R. (1990): Radiation effects on the thyroid gland. In: *Advances in Radiation Biology, Vol. 14, Relative Radiation Sensitivities of Human Organ Systems, Part II*, edited by K. I. Altman and J. T. Lett, pp. 119–156. Academic Press, San Diego.

344. Kimeldorf, D. J., and Hunt, E. L. (1965): *Ionizing Radiation: Neural Function and Behavior*, Academic Press, New York.

345. Kimeldorf, D. J., and Jones, D. C. (1951): The relationship of radiation dose to lethality among exercised animals exposed to Roentgen rays. *Am. J. Physiol.*, 167:626–632.

346. Kimeldorf, D. J., Jones, D. C., and Castanera, T. J. (1953): Effect of X-irradiation upon the performance of daily exhaustive exercise by the rat. *Am. J. Physiol.*, 174:331–335.

347. Kimler, B. F. (1998): Prenatal irradiation: A major concern for the developing brain. *Int. J. Radiat. Biol.*, 73:423–434.

348. Kimler, B. F., Vidal-Pergola, G. M., Peterson, S. L., et al. (1994): Effect of in utero radiation dose fractionation on rat postnatal

development, behavior and brain structure: 3-hour interval. *Neurotoxicology*, 15:183–189.

349. King, G. L. (1988): Characterization of radiation-induced emesis in the ferret. *Radiat. Res.*, 114:599–612.
350. King, G. L., and Landauer, M. R. (1990): Effects of Zacopride and BMY25801 (Batanopride) on radiation-induced emesis and locomotor behavior in the ferret. *J. Pharmacol. Exp. Ther.*, 253:1026–1033.
351. Kinsella, T. J. (1989): Effects of radiation therapy and chemotherapy on testicular function. *Prog. Clin. Biol. Res.*, 302:157–177.
352. Klatzo, I., Suzuki, R., Orzi, F., et al. (1989): Pathomechanisms of ischemic brain edema. In: *Recent Progress in the Study and Therapy of Brain Edema*, edited by K. G. Co and A. Raathmann, pp. 1–17. Plenum Press, New York.
353. Kligerman, M. M., Liu, T., Scheffler, B., et al. (1992): Interim analysis of a randomized trial of radiotherapy of rectal cancer with/without WR-2721. *Int. J. Radiat. Oncol. Biol. Phys.*, 22:799–802.
354. Klouwen, H. M., and Betel, I. (1963): Radiosensitivity of nuclear ATP synthesis. *Int. J. Radiat. Biol.*, 6:441–461.
355. Koga, T., Morishima, H., Niwa, T., and Kawai, H. (1991): Tritium precipitation in European cities and in Osaka, Japan owing to the Chernobyl nuclear accident. *J. Radiat. Res.* (*Tokyo*), 32:267–276.
356. Kondakova, N. V., Lisakovskii, S. V., Sakharova, V. V., et al. (1994): Effect of ionizing radiation on human muscle tissue (in Russian). *Voprosy Meditsinskoi Khimii*, 40:46–50.
357. Konings, A. W. T. (1987): Role of membrance lipid composition in radiation-induced death of mammalian cells. In: *Prostaglandin and Lipid Metabolism in Radiation Injury*, edited by T. L. Walden, Jr, and H. N. Hughes, pp. 29–43. Plenum Press, New York.
358. Konoplyannikov, A. G. (1997): Molecular and cellular mechanisms of late radiation damages. *Radiatsionnaya Biologiya Radioekologiya*, 37:621–628.
359. Koshurnikova, N., Buldakov, L., Bysogolov, G., et al. (1994): Mortality from malignancies of the hematopietic and lympathic tissue among personnel of the first nuclear plant in the USSR. *Sci. Total Environ.*, 142:19–23.
360. Koshurnikova, N. A., Bysogolov, G. D., Bolotnikova, M. G., et al. (1996): Mortality among personnel who worked at the MAYAK complex in the first years of its operation. *Health Phys.*, 71:90–93.
361. Kossenko, M. M. (1996): Cancer mortality among Techa river residents and their offspring. *Health Phys.*, 71:77–82.
362. Krabbe, A. A., and Olesen, J. (1982): Effect of histamine on regional cerebral blood flow in man. *Cephalalgia*, 2:15–18.
363. Krapivko, T. P., and Il'enko, A. I. (1988): First features of radioadaptation in a population of red-backed voles (Clethrionomys glareolus) in a radiation biogeocenosis. *Doklady Akademii Nauk SSR*, 302:1272–1274.
364. Krobel, W., and Kroem, G. (1959): Die Wirkung geringer strahlungsdosen auf die Signalerzeugungs und Fortleitungs eigenshaftens-eigenschaften in Froschnerven. *Atomkernergie*, 4:280– 286.
365. Kryshev, I. I. (1992): *Radioecological Consequences of the Chernobyl Accident.* Nuclear Society International, Moscow.
366. Kuettle, M. R., Thraves, P. J., Jung, M., et al. (1996): Radiation-induced neoplastic transformation in human prostate epithelial cells. *Cancer Res.*, 56:5–10.
367. Kulinski, V. I., and Semenov, L. F. (1965): Content of catecholamines in the tissues of macaques during the early periods after total gamma irradiation. *Radiobiologiia*, 5:494–500.
368. Kumar, K. S., Vaishnav, Y. N., and Weiss, J. F. (1989): Radioprotection by antioxidant enzymes and enzyme mimetics. *Pharma. Ther.*, 39:301–309.
369. Kundurovic, Z., Scepovic, M., Causevic, A., and Mornjakovic, Z. (1991): Histochemical aspects and fine structural characteristics of thyreocytes in pinealectomized and melatonin treated rats prior to irradiation. *Acta Med. Croatica*, 45:347–355.
370. Lam, K. S., Tse, V. K., Wang, C., et al. (1991): Effects of cranial irradiation on hypothalamic-pituitary function—a 5-year longitudinal study in patients with nasopharyngeal carcinoma. *Q. J. Med.*, 78:165–176.
371. Landauer, M. R., Davis, H. D., Dominitz, J. A., and Weiss, J. F. (1987): Effects of acute gamma radiation exposure on locomotor activity of Swiss-Webster mice. *Toxicologist*, 7:253.
372. Landauer, M. R., Davis, H. D., Dominitz, J. A., and Weiss, J. F. (1987): Dose and time relationships of the radioprotector WR-2721 on locomotor activity in mice. *Pharmacol. Biochem. Behav.*, 27:573–576.
373. Landauer, M. R., Davis, H. D., Dominitz, J. A., and Weiss, J. F., (1988): Long-term effects of radioprotector WR-2721 on locomotor activity and body weight of mice following exposure to ionizing radiation. *Toxicology*, 49:315–323.
374. Landauer, M. R., Davis, H. D., Kumar, K. S., and Weiss, J. F. (1992): Behavioral toxicity of selected radioprotectors. *Adv. Space Res.*, 12:273–283.
375. Landauer, M. R., McChesney, D. G., and Ledney, G. D. (1997): Synthetic trehalose dicorynomycolate (S-TDCM): Behavioral effects and radioprotection. *J. Radiat. Res.* (*Tokyo*), 38:45–54.
376. Landauer, M. R., Walden, T. L., and Davis, H. D., (1990): Behavioral effects of radioprotective agents in mice: Combination of WR-2721 and 16,16-dimethyl prostaglandin E2. In: *Frontiers in Radiation Biology*, edited by E. Riklis, pp. 199–207. VCH Publishers, New York.
377. Langlois, R. G., Ariyama, M., Kusunoki, Y., et al. (1993): Analysis of somatic cell mutations at the glycophorin A locus in atomic bomb survivors: A comparative study of assay methods. *Radiat. Res.*, 136:111–117.
378. Lauk, S., Bohm, M., Feiler, G., et al. (1989): Increased number of cardiac adrenergic receptors following local heart irradiation. *Radiat. Res.*, 119:157–165.
379. Law, M. P., and Ahier, R. G. (1989): Vascular and epithelial damage in the lung of the mouse after X rays or neutrons. *Radiat. Res.*, 117:128–144.
380. Le, X. C., Xing, J. Z., Lee, J., et al. (1998): Inducible repair of thymine glycol detected by an ultrasensitive assay for DNA damage. *Science*, 280:1066–1069.
381. Leadon, S. A. (1996): Repair of DNA damage produced by ionizing radiation: A minireview. *Semin. Radiat. Oncol.*, 6:295–305.
382. Lebedinsky, A. V., Grigoryev, U. G., and Demirchoglyan, G. G. (1958): On the biological effect of small doses of ionizing radiation. In: *Proceedings of Second United Nations International Conference on Peaceful Uses of Atomic Energy*, pp. 17–28. Geneva, Switzerland; 1982.
383. Lenoir, A. (1944): Adaptation and rontgenbestrahlung. *Radiol. Clin.*, (*Basel*), 13:264–276.
384. Liebster, J., and Kopoldova, J. K. (1964): The radiation chemistry of amino acids. *Adv. Radiat. Biol.*, 1:157–226.
385. Lindgren, M. (1958): On tolerance of brain tissue and sensitivity of brain tumors to irradiation. *Acta Radiol.*, 170:5–75.
386. Lingenfelser, S. K., Dallas, C. E., Jagoe, C. H., et al. (1997): Variation in blood cell DNA content in *Carassius carrassius* from ponds near Chernobyl, Ukraine. *Ecotoxicology*, 6:187–203.
387. Little, J. B., McGrandy, R. B., and Kennedy, A. R. (1978): Interactions between polonium-210, alpha-radiation, benzo(a)pyrene, and 0.9% NaCl solution instillations in the induction of experimental lung cancer. *Cancer Res.*, 38:1929–1935.
388. Littley, M. D., Shalet, S. M., and Beardwell, C. G. (1990): Radiation and hypothalamic-pituitary function. *Baillieres Clin. Endocrinol. Metab.*, 4:147–175.

389. Littley, M. D., Shalet, S. M., and Beardwell, C. G. (1991): Radiation and the hypothalamic-pituitary axis. In: *Radiation Injury to the Nervous System*, edited by P. H. Gutin, S. A. Leibel, and G. E. Sheline, pp. 303–324. Raven Press, New York.

390. Littley, M. D., Shalet, S. M., Morgenstern, G. R., and Deakin, D. P. (1991): Endocrine and reproductive dysfunction following fractionated total body irradiation in adults. *Q. J. Med.*, 78:265–274.

391. Livingston, G. K., Jensen, R. H., Silberstein, E. B., et al. (1997): Radiobiological evaluation of immigrants from the vicinity of Chernobyl. *Int. J. Radiat. Biol.*, 72:703–713.

392. Lo, E. H., Frankel, K. A., Steinberg, G. K., et al. (1992): High-dose single-fraction brain irradiation: MRI, cerebral blood flow, electrophysiological, and histological studies. *Int. J. Radiat. Oncol. Biol. Phys.*, 22:47–55.

393. Lomat, L., Galburt, G., Quastel, M. R., et al. (1997): Incidence of childhood disease in Belarus associated with the Chernobyl accident. *Environ. Health Perspect.*, 105:1529–1532.

394. Lott, J. R. (1962): Changes in ventral root potentials during X-irradiation of the spinal cord in the cat. In: *Effects of Ionizing Radiation on the Nervous System; Proceedings*, pp. 85–92. International Atomic Energy Agency, Vienna. Vienna, Austria; 5–9 June 1961.

395. Lucas, J. N. (1997): Dose reconstruction for individuals exposed to ionizing radiation using chromosome painting. *Radiat. Res.*, 148:S33–S38.

396. Lundbeck, F., Uls, N., and Overgaard, J. (1989): Cystometric evaluation of early and late irradiation damage to the mouse urinary bladder. *Radiother. Oncol.*, 15:383–392.

397. Lundin, J., Clemedson, C. J., and Nelson, A. (1957): Early effects of whole-body irradiation on cholinesterase activity in guinea pig's blood with special regard to radiation sickness. *Acta Radiol.*, 48:52–64.

398. Luxin, W., Yongru, Z., Zufan, T., et al. (1990): Epidemiological investigation of radiological effects in high background radiation areas of Yangjiang, China. *J. Radiat. Res. (Tokyo)*, 31:119–136.

399. Lyman, R. S, Kupalov, R. S., and Scholz, W. (1933): Effects of roentgen rays on the central nervous system. Results of large doses on the brains of adult dogs. *A.M.A. Arch. Neurol. Psychiat.*, 29:56–87.

400. Macklis, R. M., Bellerive, M. R., and Humm, J. L. (1990): The radiotoxicology of Radithor. Analysis of an early case of iatrogenic poisoning by a radioactive patent medicine. *J.A.M.A.*, 264:619–621.

401. MacNaughton, W. K., Aurora, A. R., Bhamra, J., et al. (1998): Expression, activity and cellular localization of inducible nitric oxide synthase in rat ileum and colon post-irradiation. *Int. J. Radiat. Biol.*, 74:255–264.

402. MacNaughton, W. K., and Prud'Homme-LaLonde, L. (1995): Exposure to ionizing radiation alters vasoreactivity in rat jejunum ex vivo. *Can. J. Physiol. Pharmacol.*, 73:699–705.

403. MacNaughton, W. K., Leach, K. E., Prud'Homme-LaLonde, L., and Harding, R. K. (1997): Exposure to ionizing radiation increases responsiveness to neural secretory stimuli in the ferret jejunum in vitro. *Int. J. Radiat. Biol.*, 72:219–226.

404. MacNaughton, W. K., Leach, K. E., Prud'Homme-LaLonde, L., et al. (1994): Ionizing radiation reduces neurally evoked electrolyte transport in rat ileum through a mast cell-dependent mechanism. *Gastroenterology*, 106:324–335.

405. MacVittie, T. J., Monroy, R. L., Patchen, M. L., and Souza, L. M. (1990): Therapeutic use of recombinant human G-CSF (rhG-CSF) in a canine model of sublethal and lethal whole-body irradiation. *Int. J. Radiat. Biol.*, 57:723–736.

406. MacVittie, T. J., Monroy, R. L., Vigneulle, R. M., et al. (1991): The relative biological effectiveness of mixed fission-neutron-γ radiation on the hematopoietic syndrome in the canine: Effect of therapy on survival. *Radiat. Res.*, 128:S29–S36.

407. Maier, D. M., and Landauer, M. R. (1989): Effects of acute sublethal gamma radiation exposure on aggressive behavior in male mice: A dose-response study. *Aviat. Space Environ. Med.*, 60:774–778.

408. Maier, D. M., and Landauer, M. R. (1990): Onset of behavioral effects in mice exposed to 10 Gy ^{60}Co radiation. *Aviat. Space Environ. Med.*, 61:893–898.

409. Maier, D. M., Landauer, M. R., Davis, H. D., and Walden, T. L. (1989): Effect of electron radiation on aggressive behavior, activity, and hemopoiesis in mice. *J. Radiat. Res. (Tokyo)*, 30:255–265.

410. Maisin, J. R. (1988): Acute radiation syndromes in man. In: *Terrestrial Space Radiation and Its Biological Effects*, edited by P. D. McCormack, C. E. Swenberg, and H. Bücker, pp. 445–463. Plenum Press, New York.

411. Maisin, J. R. (1998): Chemical radioprotection: Past, present, and future prospects. *Int. J. Radiat. Biol.*, 73:443–450.

412. Malysheva, O. A., and Shirinskii, V. S. (1998): Seasonal changes of secondary immunodeficiency in patients with vascular dystonia (in Russian). *Klin. Med. (Mosk.)*, 76:34–36.

413. Margules, D. L. (1979): Beta-endorphin and endoloxone: Hormones of the autonomic nervous system for the conservation of expenditure of bodily resources and energy in anticipation of famine or feast. *Neurosci. Biobehav. Rev.*, 3:155–162.

414. Marks, J. E., and Wong, J. (1985): The risk of cerebral radionecrosis in relation to dose, time and fractionation. *Prog. Exp. Tumor Res.*, 29:210–218.

415. Martin, C., Roman, V., Agay, D., and Fatome, M. (1998): Antiemetic effect of ondansetron and granisetron after exposure to mixed neutron and gamma irradiation. *Radiat. Res.*, 149:631–636.

416. Martin, S., Stratford, M. R. L., Watfa, R. R., et al. (1992): Collagen metabolism in the murine colon following X irradiation. *Radiat. Res.*, 130:38–47.

417. Martin, S., Vojnovic, B., Murray, J. C. (1991): Determination of x-ray-induced damage to the murine colon using tissue compliance measurements. *Int. J. Radiat. Biol.*, 59:503–515.

418. Maruyama, Y., and Feola, J. M. (1987): Relative radiosensitivities of the thymus, spleen, and lymphohemopoietic systems. In: *Advances in Radiation Biology, vol. 14, Relative Radiation Sensitivities of Human Organ Systems, Part II*, edited by K. I. Altman and J. T. Lett, pp. 1–82. Academic Press, San Diego.

419. Mastaglia, F. L., McDonald, W. I., Watson, J. V., and Yogendran, K. (1976): Effects of X-irradiation on the spinal cord: An experimental study of the morphological changes in central nerve fibers. *Brain*, 99:101–122.

420. Mattsson, A., Ruden, B.-I., Hall, P., et al. (1993): Radiation-induced breast cancer: Long-term follow-up of radiation therapy for benign breast disease. *J. Natl. Cancer Inst.*, 85:1679–1685.

421. Mattsson, A., Ruden, B.-I., Palmgren, J., et al. (1995): Dose- and time-response for breast cancer risk after radiation therapy for benign breast disease. *Br. J. Cancer*, 72:1054–1061.

422. Mattsson, J. L., and Yochmowitz, M. G. (1980): Radiation-induced emesis in monkeys. *Radiat. Res.*, 82:191–199.

423. McDonough, J. H., Mele, P. C., and Franz, C. G. (1992): Comparison of behavioral and radioprotective effects of WR-2721 and WR-36-89. *Pharmacol. Biochem. Behav.*, 42:233–243.

424. McFarland, W. L., and Levin, S. G. (1974): Electroencephalographic responses of 2500 rads of whole-body gamma-neutron radiation in the monkey Macaca mulatta. *Radiat. Res.*, 58:60–73.

425. McKay, M. J., Bull, C. A., Houghton, C. R., and Langlands, A. O. (1990): Persisting cyclical uterine bleeding in patients treated with

radical radiation therapy and hormonal replacement for carcinoma of the cervix. *Int. J. Radiat. Oncol. Biol. Phys.*, 18:921–925.

426. McMahon, T., and Vahora, S. (1986): Radiation damage to the brain. *Neuropsychiatr. Aspects*, 8:437–441.
427. Mechanick, J. I., Hochberg, F. H, and LaRocque, A. (1986): Hypothalamic dysfunction following whole brain irradiation. *J. Neurosurg.*, 65:490–494.
428. Medvedev, Z. A. (1979): *Nuclear Disaster in the Urals.* W. W. Norton, New York.
429. Medvedev, Z. A. (1990): *The Legacy of Chernobyl*, p. 187. W. W. Norton, New York.
430. Medvedev, Z. A. (1994): Chernobyl: Eight years after. *TREE*, 9:369–371.
431. Mefferd, J. M., Donaldson, S. S., and Link, M. P. (1989): Pediatric Hodgkin's disease: Pulmonary, cardiac, and thyroid function following combined modality therapy. *Int. J. Radiat. Oncol. Biol. Phys.*, 16:679–685.
432. Meistrich, M. L., and van Beek, M. E. A. B. (1990): Radiation sensitivity of the human testis. In: *Advances in Radiation Biology, Vol. 14, Relative Radiation Sensitivities of Human Organ Systems, Part II*, edited by K. I. Altman and J. T. Lett, pp. 227–268. Academic Press, San Diego.
433. Mele, P. C., Franz, C. G., and Harrison, J. R. (1988): Effects of sublethal doses of ionizing radiation on schedule-controlled performance in rats. *Pharmacol. Biochem. Behav.*, 30:1007–1014.
434. Mele, P. C., Franz, C. G., and Harrison, J. R. (1990): Effects of ionizing radiation on fixed-ratio escape performance in rats. *Neurotoxicol. Teratol.*, 12:367–373.
435. Mele, P. C., and McDonough, J. H. (1995): Gamma radiation-induced disruption in schedule-controlled performance in rats. *Neurotoxicology*, 16:497–510.
436. Melkonyan, H. S., Ushakova, T. E., and Umansky, S. R. (1995): Hsp 70 gene expression in mouse lung cells upon chronic gamma-irradiation. *Int. J. Radiat. Biol.*, 68:277–280.
437. Mettler, F. A., Jr., and Moseley, R. D., Jr. (1985): *Medical Effects of Ionizing Radiation.* Grune and Stratton, New York.
438. Meyerson, F. G. (1962): Effect of damaging doses of gamma-radiation on unconditioned and conditioned respiratory reflexes. In: *Works of the Institute of Higher Nervous Activity, Pathophysiological Series*, vol. 4, pp. 25–41. Izvestia Akademi USSR, Moscow, 1958; Israel Program Scientific Translation.
439. Michailov, M. C., Neu, E., Tempel, K., et al. (1991): Influence of X irradiation on the motor activity of rat urinary bladder in vitro and in vivo. *Strahlenther. Onkol.*, 167:311–318.
440. Michel, C. (1989): Radiation embryology. *Experientia*, 45:69–77.
441. Mickley, G. A. (1980): Behavioral and physiological changes produced by a supralethal dose of ionizing radiation: Evidence for hormone-influenced sex differences in the rat. *Radiat. Res.*, 81:48–75.
442. Mickley, G. A. (1981): Antihistamine provides sex-specific radiation protection. *Aviat. Space Environ. Med.*, 52:247–250.
443. Mickley, G. A. (1991): Can animals serve as useful models for research on the psychological effects of radiation exposure? In: *The Medical Basis for Radiation-Accident Preparedness III: The Psychological Perspective*, edited by R. C. Ricks, M. E. Berger, and F. M. O'Hara, pp. 25–38. Elsevier, New York.
444. Mickley, G. A., Bogo, V., and West, B. (1989): Behavioral and neurophysiological changes with exposure to ionizing radiation. In: *Textbook of Military Medicine*, edited by R. Zajtchuck, D. P. Jenkins, R. F. Bellamy, V. M. Ingram, R. I. Walker, and T. J. Cerveny, pp. 105–151. U.S. Army, Washington, DC.
445. Mickley, G. A., Ferguson, J. L., Mulvihill, M. A., and Nemeth, T. J. (1989): Progressive behavioral changes during the maturation of rats with early radiation-induced hypoplasia of fascia dentata granule cells. *Neurotoxicol. Teratol.*, 11:385–393.
446. Mickley, G. A., Ferguson, J. L., and Nemeth, T. J. (1992): Serial injections of MK 801 (Dizocilpine) in neonatal rats reduce behavioral deficits associated with x-ray-induced hippocampal granule cell hypoplasia. *Pharmacol. Biochem. Behav.*, 43:785–793.
447. Mickley, G. A., Sessions, G. R., Bogo, V., and Chantry, K. H. (1983): Evidence for endorphin-mediated cross-tolerance between chronic stress and the behavioral effects of ionizing radiation. *Life Sci.*, 33:749–754.
448. Mickley, G. A., Stevens, K. E., Burrows, J. M., et al. (1983): Morphine tolerance offers protection from radiogenic performance decrements. *Radiat. Res.*, 93:381–387.
449. Mickley, G. A., Stevens, K. E., Moore, G. H., et al. (1983): Ionizing radiation alters beta-endorphin-like immunoreactivity in brain but not blood. *Pharmacol. Biochem. Behav.*, 19:979–983.
450. Mickley, G. A., Stevens, K. E., White, G. A., and Gibbs, G. L. (1983): Changes in morphine self-administration after exposure to ionizing radiation: Evidence for the involvement of endorphins. *Life Sci.*, 33:711–718.
451. Mickley, G. A., Stevens, K. E., White, G. A., and Gibbs, G. L. (1983): Endogenous opiates mediate radiogenic behavioral change. *Science*, 220:1185–1187.
452. Mickley, G. A., and Teitelbaum, H. (1978): Persistence of lateral hypothalamic-mediated behaviors after a supralethal dose of ionizing radiation. *Aviat. Space Environ. Med.*, 49:863–873.
453. Mickley, G. A., Teitelbaum, H., Parker, G. A., et al. (1982): Radiogenic changes in the behavior and physiology of the spontaneously hypertensive rat: Evidence for a dissociation between acute hypotension and incapacitation. *Aviat. Space Environ. Med.*, 53:633–638.
454. Middleton, G. R., and Young, R. W. (1975): Emesis in monkeys following exposure to ionizing radiation. *Aviat. Space Environ. Med.*, 46:170–172.
455. Miki, T., Fukiu, Y., Hisano, S., et al. (1996): Histogenetic abnormalities of the hippocampus in prenatally gamma-irradiated rats. *Teratology*, 54:15A.
456. Miletich, D. J., and Strike, T. A. (1970): Alteration of postirradiation hypotension and incapacitation in the monkey by administration of vasopressor drugs. *AFRRI Scientific Report, SR70-1.* Armed Forces Radiobiology Research Institute, Bethesda, MD.
457. Miller, D. S. (1962): Effects of low level radiation on audiogenic convulsive seizures in mice. In: *Response of the Nervous System to Ionizing Radiation*, edited by T. J. Haley and R. S. Snider, pp. 513–531. Academic Press, New York.
458. Miller, R. W. (1990): Effects of prenatal exposure to ionizing radiation. *Health Phys.*, 59:57–61.
459. Minamisawa, T., Hirokaga, K., Sasaki, S., and Noda, Y. (1992): Effects of fetal exposure to gamma rays on aggressive behavior in adult male mice. *J. Radiat. Res.* (*Tokyo*), 33:243–249.
460. Minamisawa, T., and Hirokaga, K. (1995): Long term effects of prenatal exposure to low level gamma rays on spontaneous circadian motor activity of male mice. *J. Radiat. Res.* (*Tokyo*), 36:179–184.
461. Minamisawa, T., and Hirokaga, K. (1995): Long-term effects of prenatal exposure to low levels of gamma rays on open-field activity in male mice. *Radiat. Res.*, 144:237–240.
462. Mintz, M., Yovel, G., Gigi, A., and Myslobodsky, M. S. (1998): Dissociation between startle and prepulse inhibition in rats exposed to gamma radiation at day 15 of embryogeny. *Brain Res. Bull.*, 45:289–296.
463. Mitchell, J. B., and Russo, A. (1987): The role of glutathione in radiation and drug induced cytotoxicity. *Br. J. Cancer*, 55:96–104.
464. Mitchell, J. B, Wink, D. A., DeGraff, W., et al. (1993): Hypoxic mammalian cell radiosensitization by nitric oxide. *Cancer Res.*, 53:5845–5848.

465. Miyachi, Y. (1997): Analgesia induced by repeated exposure to low dose x-rays in mice, and involvement of the accessory olfactory system in modulation of the radiation effects. *Brain Res. Bull.*, 44:177–182.

466. Miyachi, Y., Kasai, H., Ohyama, H., and Yamada, T. (1994): Changes of aggressive behavior and brain serotonin turnover after very low-dose X-irradiation of mice. *Neurosci. Lett.*, 175:92–94.

467. Miyachi, Y., Koizumi, T., and Yamada, T. (1994): Immediate arousal response and adaptation to low-dose x-rays in mouse and its disappearance by olfactory bulbectomy and nitric oxide inhibitor. *Neurosci. Lett.*, 177:32–34.

468. Miyachi, Y., and Yamada, T. (1994): Low-dose x-ray-induced depression of sexual behavior in mice. *Behav. Brain Res.*, 65:113–115.

469. Miyachi, Y., and Yamada, T. (1996): Head-portion exposure to low-level x-rays reduces isolation-induced aggression of mouse, and involvement of the olfactory carnosine in modulation of the radiation effects. *Behav. Brain Res.*, 81:135–140.

470. Mole, R. H. (1986): Problems related to prenatal exposure of the nervous systems: History and perspective. In: *Radiation Risks to the Developing Nervous System*, edited by H. Kriegel, W. Schmahl, G. B. Gerber, and F.-E. Stieve, pp. 1–20. Gustav Fischer, Stuttgart, Germany.

471. Mole, R. H. (1990): Severe mental retardation after large prenatal exposures to bomb radiation. Reduction in oxygen transport to fetal brain: A possible abscopal mechanism. *Int. J. Radiat. Biol.*, 58:705–711.

472. Mole, R. H. (1992): Expectation of malformations after irradiation of the developing human in utero: The experimental basis for predictions. In: *Advances in Radiation Biology, Vol. 15, Relative Radiation Sensitivities of Human Organ Systems, part III*, edited by K. I. Altman and J. L. Lett, pp. 217–301. Academic Press, San Diego.

473. Molostovov, G. S., and Shavrova, E. N. (1997): Immunophenotyping of peripheral blood lymphocytes in children and adolescents with Hashimoto's thyroiditis (in Russian). *Vyestsi Akademii Navuk Byelarusi Syeryya Biyalahichnykh Navuk*, 1:93–100.

474. Monnier, M., and Krupp, P. (1962): Action of gamma radiation on electrical brain activity. In: *Response of the Nervous System to Ionizing Radiation*, edited by T. J. Haley, and R. S. Snider, pp. 607–617. Academic Press, New York.

475. Monroy, R. L. (1987): Radiation effects on the lymphohematopoietic system: A compromise in immune competency. In: *Military Radiobiology*, edited by J. J. Conklin and R. I. Walker, pp. 113–134. Academic Press, San Diego.

476. Monson, R. R., and MacMahon, B. (1984): Prenatal x-ray exposure and cancer in children. In: *Radiation Carcinogenesis: Epidemiology and Biological Significance*, edited by J. D. Boice, Jr, and J. F. Faumeni, Jr, pp. 97–105. Raven Press, New York.

477. Mooibroek, J., Trieling, W. B., and Konings, W. T. (1982): Comparison of the radiosensitivity of unsaturated fatty acids, structured as micelles or liposomes, under different experimental conditions. *Int. J. Radiat. Biol.*, 42:601–609.

478. Moore, I. M., Kramer, J. H., Wara, W., et al. (1991): Cognitive function in children with leukemia. Effect of radiation dose and time since irradiation. *Cancer*, 68:1913–1917.

479. Morse, D. E., and Mickley, G. A. (1988): Interaction of the endogenous opioid system and radiation in the suppression of appetite behavior. *Soc. Neurosci. Abstr.*, 14:1106.

480. Moulder, J. E., Fish, B. L., Holcenberg, J. S., and Sun, G. X. (1990): Hepatic function and drug pharmacokinetics after total body irradiation plus bone marrow transplant. *Int. J. Radiat. Oncol. Biol. Phys.*, 19:1389–1396.

481. Mtskhvetadze, A. V., and Kucherenko, T. M. (1968): Direct and indirect effect of irradiation on the transmission of the stimulus in the upper neck sympathetic ganglion of cats. *Radiobiologiia*, 8:624–627.

482. Mukherjee, S. K., Goel, H. C., Pant, K., and Jain, V. (1997): Prevention of radiation induced taste aversion in rats. *Ind. J. Exp. Biol.*, 35:232–235.

483. Mullenix, P. J., Kernan, W. J., Schunior, A., et al. (1994): Interactions of steroid, methotrexate, and radiation determine neurotoxicity in an animal model to study therapy for childhood leukemia. *Pediatr. Res.*, 35:171–178.

484. Mullenix, P. J. (1998): Radiation protection in the developing central nervous system: Investigation of a biological approach. In: *Radiprotectors: Chemical, Biological, and Clinical Perspectives*, edited by E. Bump, pp. 349–371. CRC Press LLC, Washington, DC.

485. Mullin, M. J., Hunt, W. A., and Harris, R. A. (1986): Ionizing radiation alters the properties of sodium channels in rat brain synaptosomes. *J. Neurochem.*, 47:489–495.

486. Munro, T. R. (1970): The relative radiosensitivity of the nucleus and cytoplasm of Chinese hamster fibroblasts. *Radiat. Res.*, 42:451–470.

487. Muscel, R. J., Zhang, H. B., and McKenna, W. G. (1993): Differential effect of ionizing radiation on the expression of cyclin A and cyclin B in Hela cells. *Cancer Res.*, 53:1128–1135.

488. Myers, J. H., Blackwell, L. H., and Overman, R. R. (1972): Early functional hemodynamic impairment in baboons after 1000 R or less of gamma radiation as revealed by hemorrhagic stress. *Radiat. Res.*, 52:564–578.

489. Nagata, S., and Golstein, P. (1995): The fas death factor. *Science*, 267:1449–1456.

490. Nam, S. Y., Kim, J. H., Cho, C. K., et al. (1997): Enhancement of radiation-induced hepatic microsomal epoxide hydrolase gene expression by oltipraz in rats. *Radiat. Res.*, 147:613–620.

491. Nandchahal, K. (1990): Mitotic figures and pyknotic nuclei and necrotic cells in the mouse jejunum during injury and repair after whole-body gamma irradiation. *Radiobiol. Radiother.* (*Berlin*), 31:333–336.

492. National Council on Radiation Protection and Measurements (NCRP). (1987): Ionizing radiation exposures of the population of the United States. *NCRP Report No. 93*. National Council on Radiation Protection and Measurements, Washington, DC.

493. National Council on Radiation Protection and Measurements (NCRP). (1990): The relative biological effectiveness of radiations of different quality. *NCRP Report 104*. National Council on Radiation Protection and Measurements, Bethesda, MD.

494. Neta, R., and Okunieff, P. (1996): Cytokine-induced radiation protection and sensitization. *Semin. Radiat. Oncol.*, 6:306–320

495. Nicklas, J. A., O'Neill, J. P., and Albertini, R. J. (1986): Use of T-cell receptor gene probes to quantify the in vivo hprt mutations in human T-lymphocytes. *Mutat. Res.*, 173:67–72.

496. Nikiforov, Y. E., Nikiforova, M., and Fagin, A. (1998): Radiation-induced post-Chernobyl pediatric thyroid carcinomas. *Oncogene*, 17:1983–1988.

497. Nokta, M., Belli, J., and Pollard, R. (1992): X-irradiation enhances in vitro human immunodeficiency virus replication. Correlation with cellular levels of cAMP. *Proc. Soc. Exp. Biol. Med.*, 200:402–408.

498. Norton, S., and Kimler, B. F. (1988): Comparison of functional and morphological deficits in the rat after gestational exposure to ionizing radiation. *Neurotoxicol. Teratol.*, 10:363–371.

499. Norton, S., Kimler, B. F., and Mullenix, P. J. (1991): Progressive behavioral changes in rats after exposure to low levels of ionizing radiation in utero. *Neurotoxicol. Teratol.*, 13:181–188.

500. Norton, S., Mullenix, P., and Culver, B. (1976): Comparison of the structure of hyperactive behavior in rats after brain damage from X-irradiation, carbon monoxide and pallidal lesions. *Brain Res.*, 116:49–67.

501. Nozue, M., and Ogata, T. (1989): Correlation among lung damage after radiation, amount of lipid peroxides, and antioxidant enzyme activities. *Exp. Mol. Pathol.*, 50:239–252.

502. Obe, G., Johannes, I., Johannes, C., et al. (1997): Chromosomal aberrations in blood lymphocytes of astronauts after long-term space flights. *Int. J. Radiat. Biol.*, 72:727–734.

503. O'Connel, J. F. A., and Brunschwig, A. (1937): Observations on the Roentgen treatment of intracranial gliomata with special reference to the effects of irradiation upon the surrounding brain. *Brain*, 60:230–258.

504. Odum, E. P. (1971): *Fundamentals of Ecology*, 3rd ed. W. B. Saunders, Philadelphia.

505. Ogilvy-Stuart, A. L., Shalet, S. M., and Gattamaneni, H. R. (1991): Thyroid function after treatment of brain tumors in children. *J. Pediatr.*, 119:733–737.

506. Okada, S., Okeda, R., Matsushita, S., and Kawano, A. (1998): Histopathological and morphometric study of the late effects of heavy-ion irradiation on the spinal cord of the rat. *Radiat. Res.*, 150:304–315.

507. Oleinick, N. L., and Rustad, M. (1976): Interrelationships between ionizing radiation, protein synthesis, and the physiological expressions of radiation damage. *Adv. Radiat. Biol.*, 6:107–160.

508. Olinski, R., Nackerdien, Z., and Dizdaroglu, M. (1992): DNA-protein cross-linking between thymine and tyrosine in chromatin of gamma-irradiated or H_2O_2-treated cultured human cells. *Arch. Biochem. Biophys.*, 297:139–143.

509. Olschowka, J. A., Kyrkanides, S., Harvey, B. K., et al. (1997): ICAM-1 induction in the mouse CNS following irradiation. *Brain Behav. Immunol.*, 11:273–285.

510. Onoda, J. M., Piechocki, M. P., and Honn, K. V. (1992): Radiation-induced increase in expression of the alpha IIb beta 3 integrin in melanoma cells: Effects on metastatic potential. *Radiat. Res.*, 130:281–288.

511. Ord, M. G., and Stocken, L. A. (1968): Variations in the phosphate content and thiol/disulfide ratio of histones during the cell cycle. *Biochem. J.* 107:403–410.

512. Ortin, T. T., Shostak, C. A., and Donaldson, S. S. (1990): Gonadal status and reproductive function following treatment for Hodgkin's disease in childhood: The Stanford experience. *Int. J. Radiat. Oncol. Biol. Phys.*, 19:873–880.

513. Otake, M., and Schull, W. J. (1984): In utero exposure to A-bomb radiation and mental retardation; a reassessment. *Br. J. Radiol.*, 57:409–414.

514. Otake, M., and Schull, W. J. (1998): Radiation-related brain damage and growth retardation among prenatally exposed atomic bomb survivors. *Int. J. Radiat. Biol.*, 74:159–171.

515. Overgaard, J., and Matsui, M. (1990): Effect of radiation on glucose absorption in the mouse jejunum in vivo. *Radiother. Oncol.*, 18:71–77.

516. Pallis, C. A., Louis, S., and Morgan, R. L. (1961): Brain myelopathy. *Brain*, 84:460–479.

517. Parshkov, E. M., Chebotareva, I. V., Sokolov, V. A., and Dallas, C. E. (1998): Additional thyroid dose factor from transportation sources in Russia following the Chernobyl disaster. *Environ. Health Perspect.*, 105:1491–1496.

518. Patchen, M. L., MacVittie, T. J., Solberg, B. D., and Souza, L. M. (1990): Therapeutic administration of recombinant human granulocyte colony-stimulating factor accelerates hemopoietic regeneration and enhances survival in a murine model of radiation-induced myelosuppression. *Int. J. Cell Cloning*, 8:107–122.

519. Patchen, M. L., MacVittie, T. J., Solberg, B. D., and Souza, L. M. (1990): Survival enhancement and hemopoietic regeneration following radiation exposure: Therapeutic approach using glucan and granulocyte colony-stimulating factor. *Exp. Hematol.*, 18:1042–1048.

520. Patchen, M. L., MacVittie, T. J., and Souza, L. M. (1992): Postirradiation treatment with granulocyte colony-stimulating factor and preirradiation WR-2721 administration synergize to enhance hemopoietic reconstitution and increase survival. *Int. J. Radiat. Oncol. Biol. Phys.*, 22:773–779.

521. Patchen, M. L., MacVittie, T. J., Williams, J. L., et al. (1991): Administration of interleukin-6 stimulates multilineage hematopoiesis and accelerates recovery from radiation-induced hematopoietic depression. *Blood*, 77:472–480.

522. Peimer, S. I., Dudkin, A. O., and Swerdlov, A. G. (1986): Response of hippocampal pacemaker-like neurons to low doses of ionizing radiation. *Int. J. Radiat. Biol.*, 49:597–600.

523. Pellmar, T. C., and Lepinski, D. L. (1993): Gamma radiation (5–10 Gy) impairs neuronal function in the guinea pig hippocampus. *Radiat. Res.*, 136:255–261.

524. Pellmar, T. C., Schauer, D. A., and Zeman, G. H. (1990): Time- and dose-dependent changes in neuronal activity produced by X radiation in brain slices. *Radiat. Res.*, 122:209–214.

525. Peter, R. U., Braun-Falco, O., Birioukov, A., et al. (1994): Chronic cutaneous damage after accidental exposure to ionizing radiation: The Chernobyl experience. *J. Am. Acad. Dermatol.*, 30(5 Part 1):719–723.

526. Peterson, L. M., Evens, M. L., Graham, M. M., et al. (1992): Vascular response to radiation injury in the rat lung. *Radiat. Res.*, 129:139–148.

527. Petridou, E., Trichopoulos, D., Dessypris, N., et al. (1996): Infant leukaemia after in utero exposure to radiation from Chernobyl. *Nature*, 382:352–353.

528. Philpott, D. E., Sapp, W., Miquel, J., et al. (1985): The effect of high energy (HZE) particle radiation (40 Ar) on aging parameters of mouse hippocampus and retina. In: *Scanning Electron Microspy*, III, edited by A. M. F. O'Hare, pp. 1177–1182. SEM, Inc, Chicago, IL.

529. Pineau, C., Velez de la Calle, J. F., Pinon-Lataillade, G., and Jegou, B. (1989): Assessment of testicular function after acute and chronic irradiation: Further evidence for an influence of late spermatids on Sertoli cell function in the adult rat. *Endocrinology*, 124:2720–2728.

530. Pinon-Lataillade, G., Viguier-Martinez, M. C., Touzalin, A. M., et al. (1991): Effect of an acute exposure of rat testes to gamma rays on germ cells and on Sertoli and Leydig cell functions. *Reprod. Nutr. Dev.* 31:617–629.

531. Pollack, A., and Zagars, G. K. (1998): Androgen ablation in addition to radiation therapy for prostate cancer. Is there a true benefit? *Semin. Radiat. Oncol.*, 8:95–106.

532. Pollack, M., and Timiras, P. S. (1964): X-ray dose and electroconvulsive responses in adult rats. *Radiat. Res.*, 21:111–119.

533. Pourquier, H., Baker, J. R., Giaux, G., and Benirschke, K. (1958): Localized roentgen-ray beam irradiation of the hypophysohypothalamic region of the guinea pig with a 2 million volt van de Graaf generator. *Am. J. Roentgenol. Radium Ther. Nucl. Med.*, 80:840–850.

534. Powers, D. A., Kress, T. S., and Jankowski, M. W. (1987): The Chernobyl source term. *Nuclear Safety*, 28:10.

535. Prasad, A. V., Mohan, N., Chandrasekar, B., and Meltz, M. (1995): Induction of transcription of "immediate early genes" by low-dose ionizing radiation. *Radiat. Res.*, 143:263–272.

536. Priestman, T., Challoner, T., Butcher, M., and Priestman, S. (1987): Control of radiation induced emesis with GR38032F (GR). *Proc. Am. Soc. Clin. Oncol.*, 7:281.

537. Quastel, M. R., Goldsmith, J. R., Cwikel, J., et al. (1997): Commentary: Lessons learned from the study of immigrants to Israel from areas of Russia, Belarus, and Ukraine contaminated by the Chernobyl accident. *Environ. Health Perspect.*, 105:1523–1528.

538. Quastel, M. R., Goldsmith, J. R., Mirkin, L., et al. (1997): Thyroid-stimulating hormone levels in children from Chernobyl. *Environ. Health Perspect.*, 105:1497–1498.

539. Rabin, B. M. (1996): Free radicals and taste aversion learning in the rat: Nitric oxide, radiation and dopamine. *Prog. Neuropsychopharmacol. Biol. Psychiatry*, 20:691–707.

540. Rabin, B. M., Hunt, W. A., Joseph, J. A., et al. (1991): Relationship between linear energy transfer and behavioral toxicity in rats following exposure to protons and heavy particles. *Radiat. Res.*, 128:216–221.

541. Rabin, B. M., Joseph, J. A., and Erat, S. (1998): Effects of exposure to different types of radiation on behaviors mediated by peripheral or central systems. *Adv. Space Res.*, 22:217–225.

542. Rakic, P. (1986): Normal and abnormal neuronal migration during brain development. In: *Radiation Risks to the Developing Nervous System*, edited by H. Kriegel, W. Schmahl, G. B. Gerber, and F.-E. Stieve, pp. 35–44. Gustav Fischer Verlag, Stuttgart.

543. Raleigh, J. A. (1987): Radiation peroxidation in model membranes. In: *Prostaglandin and Lipid Metabolism in Radiation Injury*, edited by T. L. Walden, Jr. and H. N. Hughes, pp. 1–27. Plenum Press, New York.

544. Randolph, M. L., and Brewen, J. G. (1980): Estimation of whole-body doses by means of chromosome aberrations observed in survivors of the Hiroshima A-bomb. *Radiat. Res.*, 82:393–407.

545. Reinhold, H. S., Fajardo, L. F., and Hopewell, J. W. (1990): The vascular system. In: *Advances in Radiation Biology, Vol. 14, Relative Radiation Sensitivities of Human Organ Systems, Part II*, edited by K. I. Altman and J. T. Lett, pp. 177–226. Academic Press, San Diego.

546. Reiter, R., Tang, L., Garcia, J. J., and Munoz-Hoyos, A. (1997): Pharmacological actions of melatonin in oxygen radical pathophysiology. *Life Sci.*, 60:2255–2271.

547. Reyners, H., Gianfelici de Reyners, E., and Maisin, J. R. (1982): The beta-astrocyte: A newly recognized radiosensitive glial cell type in the cerebral cortex. *J. Neurocytol.*, 11:967–983.

548. Reyners, H., Gianfelici de Reyners, E., and Maisin, J. R. (1986): Early cell regeneration processes after split-dose X-irradiation of the cerebral cortex of the rat. *Br. J. Cancer Suppl VII*, 53:218–220.

549. Reyners, H., Gianfelici de Reyners, E., and Maisin, J. R. (1986): The role of the glia in late damage after prenatal irradiation. In: *Radiation Risks to the Developing Nervous System*, edited by H. Kriegel, W. Schmahl, G. B. Gerber, and F.-E. Stieve, pp. 117–131. Gustav Fischer Verlag, Stuttgart.

550. Riches, A. C. (1995): Experimental radiation leukaemogenesis. In: *Radiation Toxicology: Bone Marrow and Leukaemia*, edited by J. H. Hendry and B. I. Lord, pp. 311–334. Taylor & Francis, Washington, DC.

551. Riopelle, A. J. (1962): Some behavioral effects of ionizing radiation on primates. In: *Response of the Nervous System to Ionizing Radiation*, edited by T. J. Haley, and R. S. Snider, pp. 719–728. Academic Press, New York.

552. Robbins, M. E., Bywaters, T., Rezvani, M., et al. (1991): Residual radiation-induced damage to the kidney of the pig as assayed by retreatment. *Int. J. Radiat. Biol.*, 60:917–928.

553. Robbins, M. E., Campling, D., Rezvani, M., et al. (1989): Nephropathy in the mature pig after the irradiation of a single kidney: A comparison with the immature pig. *Int. J. Radiat. Oncol. Biol. Phys.*, 16:1519–1528.

554. Robbins, M. E., Campling, D., Rezvani, M., et al. (1989): Radiation nephropathy in mature pigs following the irradiation of both kidneys. *Int. J. Radiat. Biol.*, 56:83–98.

555. Robertson, J. B. (1989): Toxicology of ionizing radiation. In: *A Guide to General Toxicology*, 2nd ed., edited by J. K. Marquis, pp. 141–156. S. Karger AG, New York.

556. Rodvall, Y., Pershagen, G., Hrubec, Z., et al. (1990): Prenatal x-ray exposure and childhood cancer in Swedish twins. *Int. J. Cancer*, 46:362–365.

557. Roizin, L., Akai, K., Carsten, A., et al. (1976): Post-x-ray myelinopathy (pathogenic mechanisms). In: *International Symposium on the Aetiology and Pathogenesis of Demyelinating Diseases*, edited by T. Yonawa, pp. 29–57. Japan Press Co, Heiho-Sha, Japan.

558. Romanova, L. K., and Zhorova, E. S. (1994): The effect of irradiation at small doses on human embryos and fetuses (in Russian). *Ontogenez*, 25:55–65.

559. Ron, E., Lubin, J. H., Shore, R. E., et al. (1995): Thyroid cancer after exposure to external radiation: A pooled analysis of seven studies. *Radiat. Res.*, 141:259–277.

560. Rosenthal, F., and Timiras, P. S. (1961): Changes in brain excitability after whole-body X-irradiation in the rat. *Radiat. Res.*, 18:648–657.

561. Rosenthal, F., and Timiras, P. S. (1961): Threshold and pattern of electroshock seizures after 250 R whole-body X-irradiation in rats. *Proc. Soc. Exp. Biol. Med.*, 208:267–270.

562. Ross, J. A. T., Levitt, S. R., Holst, E. A., and Clemente, C. D. (1954): Neurological and electroencephalographic effects of X irradiation of the head in monkeys. *A.M.A. Arch. Neurol. Psychiatry*, 71:238–249.

563. Rothenberg, M. A. (1950): Studies on permeability in relation to nerve function. II. Ionic movements across axonal membranes. *Biochim. Biophys. Acta*, 4:96–114.

564. Rowland, R. E., and Lucas, H. F., Jr. (1984): Radium-dial workers. In: *Radiation Carcinogenesis: Epidemiology and Biological Significance*, edited by J. D. Boice, Jr., and J. F. Faumenir, Jr., pp. 231–240. Raven Press, New York.

565. Rubin, P., Johnston, C. J., Williams, J. P., et al. (1995): A perpetual cascade of cytokines postirradiation leads to pulmonary fibrosis. *Int. J. Radiat. Biol. Phys.*, 33:99–110.

566. Rudoltz, M. S., Kao, G., Blank, K. R., et al. (1996): Molecular biology of the cell cycle: Potential for therapeutic applications in radiation oncology. *Semin. Radiat. Oncol.*, 6:284–294.

567. Russel, D. S., Wilson, C. W., and Tansley, K. (1949): Experimental radionecrosis in the brains of rabbits. *J. Neurol. Neurosurg. Psychiatry*, 12:187–195.

568. Russo, I. H., and Russo, J. (1996): Mammary gland neoplasia in long-term rodent studies. *Environ. Health Perspect.*, 105:938–967.

569. Rytomaa, T. (1996): Ten years after Chernobyl. *Ann. Med.*, 28:83–87.

570. Sabine, J. C. (1956): Inactivation of cholinesterases by gamma radiation. *Am. J. Physiol.*, 187:280–282.

571. Sadekova, S., Lehnert, S., and Chow, T. Y. (1997): Induction of PBP74/mortalin/Grp75, a member of the hsp 70 family, by low doses of ionizing radiation: A possible role in induced radioresistance. *Int. J. Radiat. Biol.*, 72:653–660.

572. Saenger, E. L., and Hinnefeld, J. (1991): Perception of radiation injury versus radiogenic effect. In: *The Medical Basis for Radiation-Accident Preparedness*, III: *The Psychological perspective*, edited by R. C. Ricks, M. E. Berger, and F. M. O'hara, pp. 39–50. Elsevier, New York.

573. Sakuma, S., Saya, H., Ijichi, A., and Tofilon, P. (1995): Radiation induction of the receptor tyrosine kinase gene Ptk-3 in normal rat astrocytes. *Radiat. Res.*, 143:1–7.

574. Samaan, N. A. (1990): Hypothalamic-pituitary failure after radiotherapy for tumors of the head and neck. In: *Advances in Radiation Biology, Vol. 14, Relative Radiation Sensitivities of Human Organ Systems, Part II*, edited by K. I. Altman and J. T. Lett, pp. 111–117. Academic Press, San Diego.

575. Sanders, C. L. (1986): *Toxicological Aspects of Energy Production*. Battelle Press, Columbus, OH, and Richland, WA.

576. Sarri, Y., Conill, C., Verger, E., et al. (1991): Effects of single dose irradiation on pancreatic beta-cell function. *Radiother. Oncol.*, 22:143–144.

577. Sato, M. (1978): Electrophysiological studies on radiation-induced changes in the adult nervous system. In: *Advances in Radiation Biology, Vol. 7, Relative Radiation Sensitivities of Human Organ Systems*, edited by J. T. Lett and H. Adler, pp. 181–221. Academic Press, New York.

578. Sato, M., and Austin, G. (1964): Acute radiation effects on mammalian synaptic activities. In: *Response of the Nervous System to Ionizing Radiation*, edited by T. J. Haley and R. S. Snider, pp. 279–289. Little, Brown and Co, Boston.

579. Sato, M., Austin, G. M., and Stahl, W. (1962): The effects of ionizing radiation on spinal cord neurons. In: *Response of the Nervous System to Ionizing Radiation*, edited by T. J. Haley and R. Snider, pp. 561–671. Academic Press, New York.

580. Sato, M., Austin, G. M., and Stahl, W. (1962): Delayed radiation effects on neuronal activity in the spinal cord of the cat. In: *Effects of Ionizing Radiation on the Nervous System; Proceedings of the Symposium on the Effects of Ionizing Radiation on the Nervous System*. pp. 93–110. International Atomic Energy Agency, Vienna. Vienna, Austria; 5–9 June 1961.

581. Sato, M., Stahl, W., and Austin, G. M. (1963): Acute radiation effects on synaptic activity in the mammalian spinal cord. *Radiat. Res.*, 18:307–320.

582. Scheid, W., Weber, J., Petrenko, S., and Traut, H. (1992): Chromosome aberrations in human lymphocytes apparently induced by Chernobyl fallout. *Health Phys.*, 64:531–534.

583. Schmidt-Ullrich, R. K., Mikkelsen, R. B., Dent, P., et al. (1997): Radiation-induced proliferation of the human A431 squamous carcinoma cells is dependent on EGRF tyrosine phosphorylation. *Oncogene*, 15:1191–1197.

584. Schmidt-Ullrich, R. K., Valerie, K. C., Chan, W., and McWilliams, D. (1994): Altered expression of epidermal growth factor receptor and estrogen receptor in MCF-7 cells after single and repeated radiation exposure. *Int. J. Radiat. Oncol. Biol. Phys.*, 29:813–819.

585. Schmitt, G., and Zamboglou, N. (1990): Radiation effects on bone and cartilage. In: *Advances in Radiation Biology, Vol. 14, Relative Radiation Sensitivities of Human Organ Systems, Part II*, edited by K. I. Altman and J. T. Lett, pp. 157–176. Academic Press, San Diego.

586. Scholz, W., Ducho, E. G., and Breit, A. (1959): Experimentelle Roentgenspatschaden am ruchenmark des erwachsenen kaninchens. Ein weiterer beitrag zur wirkungsweise ionisierender strahlen auf das zentralnervose gewebe. *Psychiat. Neurol. Japan*, 61:417–442.

587. Scholz, W., Schlote, W., and Hirschberger, W. (1962): Morphological effect of repeated low dosage and single high dosage of X-irradiation to the central nervous system. In: *Response of the Nervous System to Ionizing Radiation*, edited by T. J. Haley and R. S. Snider, pp. 211–232, Academic Press, New York.

588. Schrag, S. D., and Dixson, R. L. (1985): Occupational exposures associated with male reproductive dysfunction. *Ann. Rev. Pharmacol. Toxicol.*, 25:567–592.

589. Schull, W. J. (1995): *Effects of Atomic Radiation: A Half Century of Studies From Hiroshima and Nagasaki*. Wiley-Liss, New York.

590. Schull, W. J., and Otake, M. (1986): Neurological deficit among the survivors exposed in utero to the atomic bombing of Hiroshima and Nagasaki: A reassessment and new directions. In: *Radiation Risks to the Developing Nervous System*, edited by H. Kriegel, W. Schmahl, G. B. Gerber, and F.-E. Stieve, pp. 399–419. Gustav Fischer Verlag, Stuttgart.

591. Schultz-Hector, S., Böhm, M., Blöchel, A., et al. (1992): Radiation-induced heart disease: Morphology, changes in catecholamine synthesis and content, β-adrenoceptor density, and hemodynamic function in an experimental model. *Radiat. Res.*, 129:281–289.

592. Schwartz, G. N., Neta, R., Vigneulle, R. M., et al. (1988): Recovery of hematopoietic colony-forming cells in irradiated mice pretreated with interleukin 1 (IL-1). *Exp. Hematol.*, 16:752–757.

593. Scott, B. R., and Dillehay, L. E. (1990): A model for hematopoietic death in man from irradiation of bone marrow during radioimmunotherapy. *Br. J. Radiol.*, 63:862–870.

594. Segerstahl, B. (1991): The Costs. In: *Chernobyl: A Policy Response Study*, edited by B. Segerstahl, p. 59. Springer-Verlag, New York.

595. Seigneur, L. J., and Brennan, J. T. (1966): Incapacitation in the monkey (Macaca Mulatta) following exposure to a pulse of reactor radiation. *AFRRI Scientific Report SR 66-2*. Armed Forces Radiobiology Research Institute, Bethesda, MD.

596. Severa, J., and Bár, J. (1991): *Hand Book of Radioactive Contamination and Decontamination*. Elsevier Science, New York.

597. Shalet, S. M., Tsatsoulis, A., Whitehead, E., and Read, G. (1989): Vulnerability of the human Leydig cell to radiation damage is dependent upon age. *J. Endocrinol.*, 120:161–165.

598. Sharp, J. C., Kelly, D. D., and Brady, J. V. (1986): The radio-attenuating effects of n-decylaminoethanethiosulfuric acid in the rhesus monkey. In: *Use of Nonhuman Primates in Drug Evaluation*, edited by H. Vagtborg, pp. 338–346. Southwest Foundation for Research and Education, San Antonio, TX.

599. Sharplin, J., and Franko, A. J. (1989): A quantitative histological study of strain-dependent differences in the effects of irradiation on mouse lung during the intermediate and late phases. *Radiat. Res.*, 119:15–31.

600. Shaw, E. G., Gunderson, L. L., Martin, J. K., et al. (1990): Peripheral nerve and ureteral tolerance to intraoperative radiation therapy: Clinical and dose-response analysis. *Radiother. Oncol.*, 18:247–255.

601. Sheline, G. E., Wara, W. M., and Smith, V. (1980): Therapeutic irradiation and brain injury. *Int. J. Radiat. Oncol. Biol. Phys.*, 6:1215–1228.

602. Shenkin, H. A. (1951): Effects of various drugs upon cerebral circulation and metabolism in man. *J. Appl. Physiol.*, 3:465–471.

603. Shevchenko, V. A., Pomerantseva, M. D., Ramaiya, L. K., et al. (1992): Genetic disorders in mice exposed to radiation in the vicinity of the Chernobyl nuclear power station. *Sci. Tot. Environ.*, 112:45–56.

604. Shigematzu, I. (1991): *The International Chernobyl Project. An Overview. Assessment of Radiological Consequences and Evaluation of Protective Measures*. Report by an International Advisory Committee. International Atomic Energy Agency, Vienna.

605. Shimada, Y., Yasukawa-Barnes, J., Kim, R. Y., et al. (1994): Age and radiation sensitivity of rat mammary clonogenic cells. *Radiat. Res.*, 137:118–123.

606. Shipman, T. L., Lushbaugh, C. C., Peterson, D. F., et al. (1961): Acute radiation death resulting from an accidental nuclear critical excursion. *J. Occup. Med.*, 3:146–192.

607. Shubik, V. M., Zaitseva, M. B., and Kositskaya, L. S. (1996): Role of immune deviations in some diseases observed in areas contaminated with radionuclides after the accident in Chernobyl NPP (in Russian). *Radiatsionnaya Biologiya Radioekologiya*, 36:332–337.

608. Sich, A. R. (1994): Chernobyl accident management actions: Implications for source term estimates. *Nuclear Safety*, 35:1–24.

609. Sienkiewicz, Z. J., Haylock, R. G., and Saunders, R. D. (1994): Prenatal irradiation and spatial memory in mice: Investigation of dose-response relationship. *Int. J. Radiat. Biol.*, 65:611–618.

610. Sklar, C. A., Kim, Th., and Ramsay, N. K. C. (1982): Thyroid dysfunction among long-term survivors of bone marrow transplantation. *Am. J. Med.*, 73:668–694.

611. Sklar, C. A., Robison, L. L., Nesbit, M. E., et al. (1990): Effects of radiation on testicular function in long-term survivors of childhood acute lymphoblastic leukemia: A report from the Children Cancer Study Group. *J. Clin. Oncol.*, 8:1981–1987.

612. Sloan, S. R., Newconb, E. W., and Pellicer, A. (1990): Neutron radiation can activate K-ras via a point mutation in codon 146 and induce a different spectrum of ras mutations than does gamma irradiation. *Mol. Cell. Biol.*, 10:405–408.

613. Sokolov, V. E., Rjabov, I. N., Ryabtsev, I. A., et al. (1993): Ecological and genetic consequences of the Chernobyl atomic power plant accident. *Vegetatio*, 109:91–99.

614. Southwood, R. (1987): Opening remarks. In: *Radiation and Health. The Biological Effects of Low-Level Exposure to Ionizing Radiation*, edited R. Jones and R. Southwood, pp. 3–6. John Wiley & Sons, New York.

615. Spotheim-Maurizot, M., Gardier, F., Sabattier, R., and Charlier, M. (1992): Metal ions protect DNA against strand blockage induced by fast neutrons. *Int. J. Radiat. Biol.*, 62:659–666.

616. Stapleton, G. E., and Curtis, H. J. (1946): The effects of fast neutrons on the ability of mice to take forced exercise. *US Atomic Energy Report No. 9. MDDC-696*. Oak Ridge National Laboratory, Oak Ridge, TN.

617. Stather, J. W., Dionian, J., Brown, J., et al. (1987): Assessing risks of childhood leukaemia in Seascale. In: *Radiation and Health. The Biological Effects of Low-Level Exposure to Ionizing Radiation*, edited by R. Jones and R. Southwood, pp. 65–80. John Wiley & Sons, New York.

618. Stephan, G., and Oestreicher, U. (1989): An increased frequency of structural chromosome aberrations in persons present in the vicinity of Chernobyl during and after the reactor accident: Is this effect caused by radiation exposure? *Mut. Res.*, 223:7–12.

619. Stevenson, M. A., Pollock, S. S., Coleman, N. C., and Calderwood, S. K. (1994): X-irradiation, phorbolesters, and H_2O_2 stimulate mitogen activated protein kinase activity in NIH-3T3 cells through the formation of reactive oxygen intermediates. *Cancer Res.*, 54:12–15.

620. Stewart, F. A., Lundbeck, F., Oussoren, Y., and Luts, A. (1991): Acute and late radiation damage in mouse bladder: A comparison of urination frequency and cystometry. *Int. J. Radiat. Oncol. Biol. Phys.*, 21:1211–1219.

621. Stewart, F. A., Luts, A., and Lebesque, J. V. (1989): The lack of long-term recovery and reirradiation tolerance in the mouse kidney. *Int. J. Radiat. Biol.*, 56:449–462.

622. Stewart, F. A., Oussoren, Y., and Luts, A. (1990): Long-term recovery and reirradiation tolerance of mouse bladder. *Int. J. Radiat. Oncol. Biol. Phys.*, 18:1399–1406.

623. Stewart, F. A., Soranson, J. A., Alpen, E. L., et al. (1984): Radiation-induced renal damage: The effects of hyperfractionation. *Radiat. Res.*, 98:407–420.

624. Stieve, F.-E. (1986): Experiences with accidents and consequences for treatment. *Br. J. Radiol.*, 59(Suppl 19):18–22.

625. Stiehm, E. R. (1992): The psychologic fallout from Chernobyl. *Am. J. Dis. Child.*, 146:761–762.

626. Stryker, J. A., Robins, D. B., and Velkley, D. E. (1990): Relative radiosensitivity of the urinary bladder in cancer therapy. In: *Advances in Radiation Biology, Vol. 14, Relative Radiation Sensitivities of Human Organ Systems, Part II*, edited by K. I. Altman and J. T. Lett, pp. 1–21. Academic Press, San Diego.

627. Stuart, B. O., Palmer, R. F., Filipy, R. E., et al. (1977): Respiratory tract carcinogenesis in large and small experimental animals following daily inhalation of radon daughters and uranium ore dust. In: *Proceedings of the IVth Congress of the International Radiation Protection Association*. pp. 104–117. Foutenay, Aux Roses, France. IRPA.

628. Sugg, D. W., Bickham, J. W., Brooks, J. A., et al. (1996): DNA damage and radiocesium in channel catfish from Chernobyl. *Environ. Toxicol. Chem.*, 15:1057–1063.

629. Suzuki, K., Takahashi, M., Ishii-Ohba, H., et al. (1990): Steroidogenesis in the testes and the adrenals of adult male rats after gamma-irradiation in utero at late pregnancy. *J. Steroid. Biochem.*, 35:301–305.

630. Suzuki, R., Yamaguchi, T., Kirno, T., et al. (1983): The effects of 5-minute ischemia in mongolian gerbils. I. Blood-brain barrier, cerebral blood flow, and local cerebral glucose utilization changes. *Acta Neuropathol. (Berlin)*, 60:207–216.

631. Switzer, R. C., Bogo, V., and Mickley, G. A. (1991): High energy electron and proton irradiation of rat brain induces degeneration detectable with the cupric-silver stain. *Soc. Neurosci. Abstr.*, 17:1460.

632. Szekely, J. E., Ronai, A. Z., Duna-Kovacs, Z., et al. (1977): Cross tolerance between morphine and beta-endorphin in vivo. *Life Sci.*, 20:1259–1264.

633. Tamaki, Y., and Inouye, M. (1988): Go/No-go discriminated avoidance learning in prenatally X-irradiated rats. *Neurotoxicol. Teratol.*, 10:35–38.

634. Tanimura, H. (1957): Changes of the neurosecretory granules in hypothalamo-hypophysical system of rats by irradiating their heads with x-rays. *Acta Anat. Nippon*, 32:529–533.

635. Tannehill, S. P., and Mehta, M. P. (1996): Amifostine and radiation therapy: Past, present, and future. *Semin. Oncol.*, 23:69–77.

636. Tannehill, S. P., Mehta, M. P., Larson, M., et al. (1997): Effect of amifostine on toxicities associated with sequential chemotherapy and radiation therapy for unresectable non-small-cell lung cancer: Results of a phase II trial. *J. Clin. Oncol.*, 15:2850–2857.

637. Tateno, H., and Mikamo, K. (1989): Effects of neonatal ovarian X-irradiation in the Chinese hamster. I. Correlation between the age of irradiation and the fertility span. *J. Radiat. Res. (Tokyo)*, 30:185–190.

638. Taylor, G. M. (1995): Genetic effects of ionising radiation with respect to leukaemia. In: *Radiation Toxicology: Bone Marrow and Leukaemia*, edited by J. H. Hendry and B. Lord, pp. 275–310. Taylor & Francis, Washington, DC.

639. Taylor, J. A., Watson, M. A., Devereux, T. R., et al. (1994): p53 mutation hotspot in radon-associated lung cancer. *Lancet*, 343:86–87.

640. Teicher, B. A., Holden, S. A., Al-Achi, A., and Herman, T. S. (1990): Classification of antineoplastic treatments by their differential toxicity toward putative oxygenated and hypoxic tumor subpopulations in vivo in the FSaIIC murine fibrosarcoma. *Cancer Res.*, 50:3339–3344.

641. Teicher, B. A., Lazo, J. S., and Sartorelli, A. C. (1981): Classification of antineoplastic agents by their selective toxicities toward oxygenated and hypoxic tumor cells. *Cancer Res.*, 41:73–81.

642. Teskey, G. C., and Kavaliers, M. (1984): Ionizing radiation induces opioid-mediated analgesia in male mice. *Life Sci.*, 35:1547–1552.

643. Thacker, J., and Stretch, A. (1985): Responses of four x-ray-sensitive CHO cell mutants to different radiations and to irradiation conditions promoting cellular recovery. *Mut. Res.*, 146:99–108.

644. Thomas, D. B., Rosenblatt, K., Jimenez, L. M., et al. (1994): Ionizing radiation and breast cancer in men (United States). *Cancer Causes & Control*, 5:9–14.
645. Thorne, M. C., ed. (1986): Developmental effects of irradiation on the brain of the embryo and fetus. *ICRP Publication 49.*. Pergamon Press, Oxford.
646. Tillman, B. F., Loyd, J. E., Malcolm, A. W., et al. (1989): Unilateral radiation pneumonitis in sheep: Physiological changes and bronchoalveolar lavage. *J. Appl. Physiol.*, 66:1273–1279.
647. Timmermans, R., and Gerber, G. B. (1984): The effect of X-irradiation on cardiac β-adrenergic receptors following local heart irradiation. *Radiat. Res.*, 100:510–518.
648. Timmermans, R., Maes, J., Deroo, J., and Gerber, G. B. (1986): Serotonin receptors, vascular functions and lipids in rat brain after prenatal irradiation. In: *Radiation Risks to the Developing Nervous System*, edited by H. Kriegel, W. Schmahl, G. B. Gerber, and F.-E. Stieve, pp. 221–230. Gustav Fischer Verlag, Stuttgart.
649. Tolliver, J. M., and Pellmar, T. C. (1987): Ionizing radiation alters neuronal excitability in hippocampal slices of the guinea pig. *Radiat. Res.*, 112:555–563.
650. Torii, Y., Shikita, M., Saito, H., and Matsuki, N. (1993): X-irradiation-induced emesis in Suncus murinus. *J. Radiat. Res. (Tokyo)*, 34:164–170.
651. Torubarov, F. S. (1991): Psychological consequences of the Chernobyl accident from the radiation neurology point of view. In: *The Medical Basis for Radiation-Accident Preparedness. III: The Psychological Perspective*, edited by R. C. Ricks, M. E. Berger, and F. M. O'Hara, pp. 81–91. Elsevier, New York.
652. Trabalka, J. R., Eyman, L. D., and Auerbach, S. I. (1980): Analysis of the 1957–1958 Soviet Nuclear disaster. *Science*, 209:345–353.
653. Trakhtenbrot, L., Kelman, Z., Rotter, V., and Haaran-Ghera, N. (1990): Chromosomal mapping of the murine c-abl proto-oncogene by in situ hybridization. *Leukemia*, 4:136–137.
654. Travis, E. L. (1987): Relative radiosensitivity of the human lung. In: *Advances in Radiation Biology, Vol. 12, Relative Radiation Sensitivities of Human Organ Systems*, edited by J. T. Lett, pp. 205–238. Academic Press, San Diego.
655. Trnovec, T., Kallay, Z., and Bezek, S. (1990): Effects of ionizing radiation on the blood brain barrier permeability to pharmacologically active substances. *Int. J. Radiat. Oncol. Biol. Phys.*, 19:1581–1587.
656. Trnovec, T., Volenec, K., Bezek, S., et al. (1991): The effect of high energy electron irradiation on blood-brain barrier permeability to haloperidol and stobadin in rats. *Radiat. Environ. Biophys.*, 30:277–287.
657. Trotti, A. (1998): Toxicity antagonists in head and neck cancer. *Semin. Radiat. Oncol.*, 8:282–291.
658. Turbyfill, C. L., Roudon, R. M., and Kieffer, V. A. (1972): Behavior and physiology of the monkey (Macaca mulatta) following 2500 rads of pulse mixed gamma-neutron radiation. *Aerosp. Med.*, 7:41–45.
659. Turbyfill, C. L., Roudon, R. M., Young, R. W., and Kieffer, V. A. (1972): Alteration of radiation effects by 2-(n-decylamino) ethanethiolsulfuric acid (WR-1607) in the monkey. *AFRRI Scientific Report SR72-3*. Armed Forces Radiobiology Research Institute, Bethesda, MD.
660. Turns, J. E., Doyle, T. F., and Curran, C. R. (1971): Norepinephrine effects on early post-irradiation performance decrement in the monkey. *AFRRI Scientific Report SR71-16*. Armed Forces Radiobiology Research Institute, Bethesda, MD.
661. Uchiyama, M., Nakamura, Y., Kobayashi, S., et al. (1989): Radiocesium body burden of Japanese who returned from European countries following the Chernobyl accident. *J. Radiat. Res.*, 30:51.
662. Urmer, A. H., and Brown, W. L. (1960): The effect of gamma radiation on the reorganization of a complex maze habit. *J. Gen. Psychol.*, 97:67–76.
663. U.S. Environmental Protection Agency (USEPA). (1986): *Citizen's Guide to Radon*. U.S. Environmental Protection Agency, Washington, DC.
664. USSR State Committee on the Utilization of Atomic Energy. (1986): *The Accident at Chernoyl Nuclear Power Plant and its Consequences*. Information compiled for the IAEA Experts' Meeting, 24–9 August, 1986, Vienna. Working Document for the Post-Accident Review Meeting. Draft. Part I: General Material. Part II: Annexes 1–7, August 1986 (hereafter referred to as The Accident ... Soviet IAEA Report). Part I was subsequently published in Russian in *Atomnaya Energiya*, 61(5), Moscow.
665. Utley, J. F. (1987): Relative radiosensitivities of the oral cavity, larynx, pharynx, and esophagus. In: *Advances in Radiation Biology, Vol. 12, Relative Radiation Sensitivities of Human Organ Systems*, edited by J. T. Lett and K. I. Altman, pp. 129–146. Academic Press, San Diego.
666. Vahakangas, K. H., Samet, J. M., Metcalf, R. A., et al. (1992): Mutations of p53 and *ras* genes in radon-associated lung cancer from uranium miners. *Lancet*, 339:576–580.
667. Valk, P. E., and Dillon, W. P. (1991): Radiation injury of the brain. *Am. J. Neuroradiol.*, 12:45–62.
668. van Bekkum, D. W., Jongeiper, H. J., Nieuwerkerk, H. T. M., and Cohenm, J. A. (1954): The oxidative phosphorylation by mitochondria isolated from the spleen of rats after total body exposure to x-rays. *Br. J. Radiol.*, 27:127–130.
669. van der Kogel, A. J. (1986): Radiation-induced damage in the central nervous system: An interpretation of target cell responses. *Br. J. Cancer Suppl VII*, 53:207–217.
670. van der Meer, Y., Huiskamp, R., Davids, J. A. G., et al. (1992): The sensitivity of quiescent and proliferating mouse spermatogonial stem cells to X irradiation. *Radiat. Res.*, 130:289–295.
671. van der Meer, Y., Huiskamp, R., Davids, J. A. G., et al. (1992): The sensitivity to X rays of mouse spermatogonia that are committed to differentiate and of differentiating spermatogonia. *Radiat. Res.*, 130:296–302.
672. Van Dongen-Melman, J. E., De Groot, A., Van Dongen, J. J., et al. (1997): Cranial irradiation is the major cause of learning problems in children treated for leukemia and lymphoma: A comparative study. *Leukemia*, 11:1197–1200.
673. Varagic, V., Stepanovic, S., Svecenski, N., and Hajdukovic, S. (1967): The effect of X-irradiation on the amount of catecholamines in heart atria and hypothalamus of the rabbit and in brain and heart of the rat. *Int. J. Radiat. Biol.*, 12:113–119.
674. Verger, P. (1997): Down syndrome and ionizing radiation. *Health Phys.*, 73:882–893.
675. Vidal-Pergola, G. M., Kimler, B. F., and Norton, S. (1993): Effect of in utero irradiation on the postnatal development, behavior, and brain structure of rats: Dose fractionation with a 6-h interval. *Radiat. Res.*, 134:369–374.
676. Viel, J. F., Curbakova, E., Dzerve, B., et al. (1997): Risk factors for long-term mental and psychosomatic distress in Latvian Chernobyl liquidators. *Environ. Health Perspect.*, 105:1539–1544.
677. Viinamäki, H., Kumpusalo, E., Myllykangas, M., et al. (1995): The Chernobyl accident and mental well being—a population study. *Acta Psychiat. Scand.*, 91:396–401.
678. Vijayalaxmi, Reiter, R. J., Sewerynek, E., et al. (1995): Marked reduction of radiation-induced micronuclei in human blood lymphocytes pretreated with melatonin. *Radiat. Res.*, 143:102–106.

679. Voevodskaya, N. A., and Vanin, A. F. (1992): Gamma-irradiation potentiates L-arginine-dependent nitric oxide formation in mice. *Biochem. Biophys. Res. Commun.*, 186:1423–1428.

680. von Sonntag, C. (1987): *The Chemical Basis of Radiation Biology*. Taylor and Francis, New York.

681. von Sonntag, C. (1991): The chemistry of free-radical-mediated DNA damage. *Basic Life Sci.*, 58:287–317.

682. Vyatleva, O. A., Katargina, T. A., Puchinskaya, L. M., and Yurkin, M. M. (1997): Electrophysiological characterization of the functional state of the brain in mental disturbances in workers involved in the clean-up following the Chernobyl atomic energy station accident. *Neurosci. Behav. Physiol.*, 27:166–172.

683. Wagner, W., Prott, F., and Schonekas, K. (1998): Amifostine: A radioprotector in locally advanced head and neck tumors. *Oncol. Rep.*, 5:1255–1257.

684. Wakeford, R. (1995): The risk of childhood cancer from intrauterine and preconceptional exposure to ionizing radiation. *Environ. Health Perspect.*, 103:1018–1025.

685. Walden, T. L., Jr. (1989): Long-term and low level effects of ionizing radiation. In: *Medical Consequences of Nuclear Warfare*, edited by R. I. Walker and T. J. Cerveny, pp. 171–126. TMM Publications, Falls Church, VA.

686. Walden, T. L., Jr., and Farzaneh, N. K. (1990): *Biochemistry of Ionizing Radiation*, Raven Press, New York.

687. Walden, T. L., Jr., and Farzaneh, N. K. (1991): Biochemical response of normal tissues to ionizing radiation. In: *Radiation Injury to the Nervous System*, edited by P. H. Gutin, S. A. Leibel, and G. E. Sheline, pp. 17–36. Raven Press, New York.

688. Walden, T. L., Jr., Farzaneh, N. K., and Richards, L. (1989): Lipoxygenase products in radiation injury and protection. *New Trends Lipid Mediators*, 3:154–160.

689. Walker, D. I., and Eisen, V. (1979): Effect of ionizing radiation on 15-hydroxy prostaglandin dehydrogenase (PGDH) activity in tissue. *Int. J. Radiat. Biol.*, 36:399–407.

690. Wallace, W. H., Shalet, S. M., Crowne, E. C., et al. (1989): Ovarian failure following abdominal irradiation in childhood: Natural history and prognosis. *Clin. Oncol.* (*R. Coll. Radiol.*), 1:75–79.

691. Wallace, W. H., Shalet, S. M., Hendry, J. H., et al. (1989): Ovarian failure following abdominal irradiation in childhood: The radiosensitivity of the human oocyte. *Br. J. Radiol.*, 62:995–998.

692. Ward, J. F. (1990): The yield of DNA double-strand breaks produced intracellularly by ionizing radiation: A review. *Int. J. Radiat. Biol.*, 57:1141–1150.

693. Weinstein, N. D. (1991): Public response to home radon exposure. In: *The Medical Basis for Radiation-Accident Preparedness. III: The Psychological Perspective*, edited by R. C. Ricks, M. E. Berger, and F. M. O;'Hara, pp. 173–178. Elsevier, New York.

694. Weiss, J. F. (1997): Pharmacologic approaches to protection against radiation-induced lethality and other damage. *Environ. Health Perspect.*, 105(Suppl 6):1473–1478.

695. Weiss, J. F., Kumar, K. S., Walden, T. L., et al. (1990): Advances in radioprotection through the use of combined agent regimens. *Int. J. Radiat. Biol.*, 57:709–722.

696. Weshler, Z., Ligumsky, M., Brufman, G., et al. (1987): Functional and morphological alterations following isolated rat stomach irradiation. A model for estimation of radiation injury. *In Vivo*, 1:357–361.

697. Wheeler, T. G., and Hardy, K. A. (1985): Retrograde amnesia produced by electron beam exposure: Causal parameters and duration of memory loss. *Radiat. Res.*, 101:74–80.

698. Wheeler, T. G., and Tilton, B. M. (1983): Duration of memory loss due to electron beam exposure. *USAF SAM Technical Report TR 83-33*. USAF School of Aerospace Medicine, Brooks AFB, TX.

699. Whicker, F. W. (1989): Impact on plant and animal populations. In: *Health Impacts of Large Releases of Radionuclides. Ciba Foundation Symposium No. 203*, pp. 74–93. The Ciba Foundation, London.

700. Whicker, F. W., Pinder, J. E. III, Bowling, J. W., et al. (1990): Distribution of long-lived radionuclides in an abandoned reactor cooling reservoir. *Ecol. Monogr.*, 60:471–496.

701. Whicker, F. W., and Schultz, V. (1982): *Radioecology: Nuclear Energy and the Environment*, Vols. I and II. CRC Press, Boca Raton, FL.

702. Wientroub, S., Weiss, J. F., Catravas, G. N., and Reddi, A. H. (1990): Influence of whole body irradiation and local shielding on matrix-induced endochondral bone differentiation. *Calcif. Tissue Int.*, 46:38–45.

703. Williams, D. (1994): Chernobyl, eight years on. *Nature*, 371:556.

704. Winkler, H. (1957): Untersuchungen uber die Wirkung von Roentgensstrahlen auf die bluthirschranke mit hilfe von P32 Zbl allg. *Pathol. Anat.*, 97:301–307.

705. Winsauer, P. J., Bixler, M. A., and Mele, P. C. (1995): Differential effects of ionizing radiation on the acquisition and performance of response sequences in rats. *Neurotoxicology*, 16:257–269.

706. Winsauer, P. J., and Mele, P. C. (1993): Effects of sublethal doses of ionizing radiation on repeated acquisition in rats. *Pharmacol. Biochem. Behav.*, 44:809–814.

707. Wishkerman, Y. V., Quastal, M. R., Douvdevani, A., and Goldsmith, J. R. (1997): Somatic mutations at the glycophorin A (GPA) locus measured in red cells of Chernobyl liquidators who immigrated to Israel. *Environ. Health Perspect.*, 105(Suppl 6):1451–1454.

708. Withers, R. H. (1975): The four R's of radiotherapy. *Adv. Radiat. Biol.*, 5:241–271.

709. Wixon, H. N., and Hunt, W. A. (1983): Ionizing radiation decreases veratridine stimulated uptake of sodium in rat brain synaptosomes. *Science*, 220:1073–1074.

710. Wolfle, G., Bleyer, H., Muller, D., and Klinger, W. (1991): The influence of the radiation syndrome on cytochrome P450-dependent monooxygenation in rat liver. *Exp. Pathol.*, 43:89–95.

711. Wondergem, J., van der Laarse, A., van Ravels, F. J., et al. (1991): In vitro assessment of cardiac performance after irradiation using an isolated working rat heart preparation. *Int. J. Radiat. Biol.*, 59:1053–1068.

712. World Health Organization. (1995): *Health Consequences of the Chernobyl Accident. Results of the IPHECA Pilot Projects and Related National Programmes*. World Health Organization, Geneva.

713. Wright, E. G. (1995): The pathogenesis of leukaemia. In: *Radiation Toxicology: Bone Marrow and Leukaemia*, edited by J. H. Hendry and B. I. Lord, pp. 245–274. Taylor & Francis, Washington, DC.

714. Yaes, R. J. (1992): Radiation damage to the kidney. In: *Advances in Radiation Biology, Vol. 15, Relative Radiation Sensitivities of Human Organ Systems, Part III*, edited by K. I. Altman and J. T. Lett, pp. 1–35. Academic Press, San Diego.

715. Yamada, T., and Ohyama, H. (1988): Radiation-induced interphase cell death of rat thymocytes is internally programmed (apoptosis). *Int. J. Radiat. Biol.*, 53:65–75.

716. Yamamoto, M., Ueno, K., Igarashi, Y., et al. (1990): Determination of low-level Ra-226 in human bone by α-spectrometry. *J. Radiat. Res.*, 31:85.

717. Yamashita, H., and Miyasaka, T. (1952): Effects of beta rays upon a single nerve fiber. *Proc. Soc. Exp. Biol. Med.*, 80:375–377.

718. Yamashita, S., Namba, H., and Nagataki, S. (1993): Thyroid and radiation (in Japanese). *Folia Endocrinol. Jpn.*, 69:1035–1043.

719. Yeung, T. K., Lauk, S., Simmonds, R. H., et al. (1989): Morphological and functional changes in the rat heart after X irradiation: Strain differences. *Radiat. Res.*, 119:489–499.

720. Yoshii, Y., Maki, Y., Tsunemoto, H., et al. (1981): The effect of total-head irradiation C3H/He of X irradiation of the head in monkeys. *Radiat. Res.*, 86:152–170.

721. Young, R. W. (1986): Mechanisms and treatment of radiation-induced nausea and vomiting. In: *Nausea and Vomiting: Mechanisms and Treatment*, edited by C. J. Davis, G. V. Lake-Bakaar, and G. V. Grahame-Smith, pp. 94–109. Springer-Verlag, New York.

722. Young, R. W. (1987): Acute radiation syndrome. In: *Military Radiobiology*, edited by J. J. Conklin and R. I. Walker, pp. 165–190. Academic Press, New York.

723. Young, R. W., and Myers, P. H. (1986): The human response to nuclear radiation. *Med. Bull.*, 43:20–23.

724. Yuhas, J. M. (1970): Biological factors affecting the radioprotective efficiency of S-2-(3-aminopropylamino)ethylphosphorothioic acid (WR-2721): LD 50/30 doses. *Radiat. Res.*, 44:621–628.

725. Yuhas, J. M. (1980): Active versus passive absorption kinetics as the basis for selective normal tissue protection by S-2-(3-aminopropylamino) ethylphosphorothioic acid. *Cancer Res.*, 40:1519–1524.

726. Zaman, M. S., Lancaster, F. E., and Hupp, E. W. (1997): Physical and motor development in male and female rat offspring prenatally exposed to gamma radiation. *J. Environ. Sci. Health B*, 32:313–325.

727. Zamora, M. L., Tracy, B. L., Zielinski, D., et al. (1998): Chronic ingestion of uranium in drinking water: A study of kidney bioeffects in humans. *Toxicol. Sci.*, 43:68–77.

728. Zaridze, D. G. (1997): Epidemiology of leukemias in children (in Russian). *Arkhiv Patologii*, 59:65–70.

729. Zeman, W. (1963): Disturbances of nuclei acid metabolism preceding delayed radionecrosis of nervous tissue. *Proc. Natl. Acad. Sci. U.S.A.*, 50:626–630.

730. Zhavoronkova, L. A., Kholodova, N. B., Zubovskii, G. A., et al. (1995): Electroencephalographic correlates of neurological disturbances at remote periods of the effect of ionizing radiation (sequelae of the Chernobyl' NPP accident). *Neurosci. Behav. Physiol.*, 25:142–149.

731. Ziboh, V. A., Mallia, C., Mohart, E., and Taylor, L. (1982): Induced biosynthesis of cutaneous prostaglandins by ionizing radiation. *Proc. Soc. Exp. Biol. Med.*, 169:386–391.

732. Zmudzka, B. Z., and Beer, J. Z. (1990): Activation of human immunodeficiency virus by ultraviolet radiation. *Photochem. Photobiol.*, 52:1153–1162.

Principles and Methods of Toxicology, Fourth Edition, edited by A. Wallace Hayes.
Taylor & Francis, Philadelphia © 2001.

Chapter 16

The Use of Laboratory Animals in Toxicologic Research

William J. White

This chapter provides an overview of laboratory animal science and medicine as it pertains to the use of laboratory animals in toxicologic research. The purpose of this chapter is to familiarize the toxicologist with a number of important issues involving the use of laboratory animals. It is not possible to explore all subjects that pertain to this topic nor to comprehensively review the subjects in this chapter. The reader is urged to seek more detail in the references provided and to consult specialists in the field for more information.

Veterinarians with specialized training in laboratory animal medicine have played important supporting roles in institutions conducting toxicologic research. Much of the information used by them, as well as by other laboratory animal professionals and toxicologists, has been developed as a direct result of studies initiated in the basic sciences and in toxicology. By their very nature, toxicologic studies have required an understanding of the biological characteristics and needs of laboratory animals as well as an understanding of those variables that impact the performance of laboratory animals in research studies. Our understanding of laboratory animals is far from complete and is further complicated by the fact that there is a wide variety of species from which the toxicologist may choose. Species such as mice and rats are extensively used with vast amounts of background data available and whose biological characteristics have been well explored. Less commonly used species, such as guinea pigs, hamsters, and gerbils, have proportionally less known about them and much less published background data available. Recent efforts by a number of organizations to collect, analyze, and publish background data on a continuing basis in a variety of disciplines is helping to extend the knowledge of certain laboratory animal species (48,191).

Like any field, the quality of published information can vary widely. Moreover, a lot of dogma and unsubstantiated opinion still remain in the literature. A number of recommended practices still cannot be well substantiated in the peer-reviewed literature. In designing experimental protocols, the toxicologist should familiarize himself with the important variables associated with the animals that will be used in the study and put in place measures to control or to account for these variables.

In today's society the use of animals for research purposes has become a subject of much public discussion. Over the last century, economically developed countries in which most biomedical research takes place have moved further and further away from extensive public involvement with agricultural use of animals and replaced that exposure with zoos, family pets, and stylized animal characters in the media. This has caused society to reexamine their relationship with animals both in agriculture and in research. This has resulted in the development of laws, regulations, and guidelines that address responsible animal use. As with any controversial subject, there are those who find the measures taken to be insufficient and who advocate even further change through dialogue, protest, or terrorism. In many cases, radical views and actions are based on misinformation and a basic distrust of large organizations and governments. There are, however, a large number of individuals concerned with animal welfare who are open-minded and seek to strike an appropriate balance in their use in biomedical research. They, like the members of the research community, are focused on responsible animal usage, including, where appropriate, refinement, reduction, and replacement (the three Rs) of laboratory animals (278).

Responsible animal usage has stimulated interest in in vitro alternatives, computer-simulated models, and computer structure-activity analyses to screen for appropriate drug candidates. These efforts have had some limited success in the initial stages of the drug discovery process. They have not yet led to suitable in vitro replacements for most animal usage in toxicologic studies, especially product registration studies, nor do they appear likely to in the near future. This failure to develop complete substitutes for intact living organisms used in research is likely due to the complex interactions that exist on organ, cellular, and subcellular levels. A suitable replacement for animals will need to reliably predict biological phenomena, including being at least as good and consistent a model for risk assessment in humans as animals. Such systems will need to be extensively validated and accepted by regulatory bodies as suitable substitutes.

The use of animals in toxicologic research cannot be taken for granted. With their use comes responsibilities not only to adherence to institutional, governmental, and scientific principles, policies, laws, regulations, and guidelines, but also an ethical and moral responsibility for the lives of the animals used in research or product manufacture. Each researcher is also responsible for the quality of the care that they receive, the appropriateness of their use, and the minimization or relief of pain.

REGULATIONS, LAWS, POLICIES, AND GUIDELINES

The use of animals in research, as well as the assurance that provisions for appropriate animal welfare and care have been made, is controlled by a number of mechanisms. These can be subdivided into two general categories: (1) guidelines and recommendations and (2) laws and regulations. In addition, policies can be developed for either of these two categories. For example, guidelines or recommendations that are not regulated by law can be included in an overall policy that governs institutional activities or eligibility for receiving funding. Moreover, policies may also be created and used as accepted interpretations of regulations developed in response to laws.

Laws and regulations require mandatory compliance. Failure to meet the requirements imposed by laws or regulations usually is attended by legal actions that may culminate in fines, revocation of the ability to conduct animal-related activities, or imprisonment. In the case of laboratory animals in the United States, laws and regulations are administered by the U.S. Department of Agriculture (USDA). The regulatory body is charged with conducting regular inspections and registering all facilities using laboratory animals. Within the USDA, the Animal Plant and Health Inspection Service (APHIS) is charged with making such inspections. Within APHIS, the Regulatory Enforcement and Animal Care (REAC) unit is responsible for enforcing regulations developed in response to legislation governing the use of laboratory animals in research.

Guidelines and recommendations usually are developed by independent groups with expertise in one or more aspects of laboratory animal science and medicine. Compliance with guidelines or recommendations is voluntary; however, failure to do so may be accompanied by undesirable consequences, such as denial of funding by government institutions, inability to have data accepted for publication, or inability to use data in submissions filed in response to mandated regulatory processes (81,95). Compliance with such guidelines or recommendations may need to be assured through filing of legally binding statements, submission of regular reports to agencies tracking such activities, or by participation in a voluntary accreditation program, such as the one conducted by the Association for Assessment and Accreditation of Laboratory Animal Care-International (AAALAC), who uses a combination of regular reports and periodic site visits to evaluate programs, facilities, and animal care.

INTERNATIONAL ASSURANCE AND REGULATION OF LABORATORY ANIMAL CARE AND USE

The existence and complexity of laws, regulations, guidelines, and recommendations governing the care and use of laboratory animals varies significantly between countries. In general, nonindustrial countries commonly do not have laws governing the use of animals in research, teaching, or product production. Some international guidelines or recommendations may be followed, but only to the extent that they impact the suitability of work or products for registration in other countries.

Countries within the European Economic Union use certain minimal standards developed through the council of Europe and subsequently ratified by member states. These standards are used as the basis for individual country laws and regulations that meet or exceed these standards. Variation between countries can exist. Within an individual country, standards may be different for different aspects of animal production and use. These laws and standards may apply not only to research use of animals, but also to transportation of animals, as well as their exhibition and sale for other purposes. A comprehensive review of all of these items, including regulatory oversight and reporting requirements, are beyond the scope of this text. There are, however, a few important considerations that should be mentioned.

Protocol review at either a regional or national level is a common component of the regulations governing animal care and use in European countries. Protocols must fulfill certain guidelines and provide a detailed description of the proposed study as well as supporting rationale. There can be a significant time lag from the submission of a protocol until a decision is made by reviewers.

Licensing of researchers to perform specific procedures is often a component of the regulatory process. Guidelines for credentials and training are specified and licensing is often done on an individual procedure basis.

Evaluation of programs and unannounced inspection of facilities is often done through a government agency. Activities can be suspended based on findings of inspections, and licensure can be revoked. Other penalties can be imposed, depending on the country.

Unlike the United States, all species used in research conducted in Europe are covered by guidelines and regulations. Differences can exist between countries in terms of acceptable care and use practices, and there should be no assumption that all of these standards are similar to ones in the United States or elsewhere. The level of detail and the emphasis on various topics can differ substantially from United States standards.

The Federated European Laboratory Animal Science Associations (FELASA) is a European consortium of laboratory animal science associations. FELASA has developed a number of recommendations for health monitoring, accreditation of animal diagnostic laboratories, and other topics that can impact the quality of laboratory animals used in toxicologic research. Adherence to these recommendations is voluntary, and in some cases the recommendations may differ from accepted practices in other parts of the world.

In Canada, the Canadian Council on Laboratory Animal Care has produced guidelines for the care and use of laboratory animals. Inspection of research facilities is conducted on a voluntary basis by this organization (46,47). In Japan, efforts are underway to develop voluntary guidelines similar to those in the United States, Canada, and Europe. Laws governing the use of laboratory animals in research are not present.

UNITED STATES LAWS, REGULATIONS, GUIDELINES, RECOMMENDATIONS, AND POLICIES

The Animal Welfare Act

Regulation of laboratory animals used in research is governed by the Laboratory Animal Welfare Act of 1966, Public Law (P.L. 89-544) (308). The USDA administers the Animal Welfare Act. The act establishes legal requirements for research facilities to provide certain minimum standards for the care of animals in research. In 1970, the Laboratory Animal Welfare Act was amended (P.L. 91-579), at which time its name was changed to the Animal Welfare Act because the term *animal* was changed to include all warm-blooded animals except those used for food or fiber (308). The 1970 Act required registration of research facilities as well as annual reporting requirements. Animals used for other purposes, such as exhibition or as pets, were also extended coverage.

The Act was again amended in 1976 (P.L. 94-279) in order to include more rigorous standards for transportation of animals (308). The Act was last amended in 1985 (P.L. 99-198) to include requirements for exercising dogs, the psychological well being of nonhuman primates, the consideration of alternative procedures to ones causing pain or distress, training of personnel, and the establishment of an institutional animal care and use committee of specified composition (308).

In response to the Act and its amendments, a series of regulations and policies were developed. Significant additions to the regulations were added in, August of 1989, April of 1990, and February of 1991 that refined definitions and terms: set standards for humane handling, care, treatment, and transportation; set space requirements for primary enclosures for guinea pigs, rabbits, and hamsters; set standards for humane handling, care, treatment, and transportation of dogs, cats, and nonhuman primates (188,280). The regulations promulgated by the USDA in response to the Animal Welfare Act are published in the Code of Federal Regulations (CFR, Title 9, Chapter A, Parts I, II, and III) (71).

Currently, the Animal Welfare Act covers dogs, cats, nonhuman primates, hamsters, guinea pigs, rabbits, marine mammals, and any other domestic animal, as well as those animals normally found in the wild, used in research, testing, exhibition, experimentation, or kept as pets. The term *animal*, as defined in the Animal Welfare Act, has excluded rats, mice, and birds, as well as horses and other farm animals used or intended for use as food or fiber or for the use in improving animal nutrition, breeding, or production. Farm animals, including horses, are covered under the Animal Welfare Act if they are used for nonagricultural research or exhibition, which includes biomedical research (167).

Extension of the USDA's regulation of laboratory animals to include rats, mice, and birds is viewed by some as being inevitable. This exclusion was still in place as of 2000 and reflects a balancing of public and private resources with the perceived benefits to regulating these excluded species. The effects on toxicologic research in the United States of extension of regulation to these species is hard to predict, as these species represent the bulk of all animals used in such research, and hence the limited degree of experience with the present regulatory process may not be predictive of the consequences of extended coverage. Given the USDA's broad mandate for regulation, which includes transportation, the cost to the government and feasibility of providing the appropriate level of regulation of this activity may be difficult to accurately estimate.

The Guide for the Care and Use of Laboratory Animals

In the United States, the primary set of guidelines for the care and use of laboratory animals is *The Guide for the Care and Use of Laboratory Animals* (*The Guide*) which was developed by the National Academy of Sciences (243). *The Guide* is used as the primary reference for voluntary assurance and accrediting bodies, such as National Institutes of Health's Office for Laboratory Animal Welfare (OLAW) and AAALAC. This document was first prepared and published in 1963 and has been revised many times since. The last revision (1996) made substantial changes in the overall approach to laboratory animal care and use.

The Guide cannot be appropriately used without an institutional animal care and use committee (222,243). The institutional animal care and use committee (IACUC) is appointed by the chief executive officer of the institution and is advisory to him. The committee, in order to comply with both the requirements of *The Guide* and USDA regulations, should include a doctor of veterinary medicine who is certified or has training or experience in laboratory animal science and medicine or in the use of the species used in research at the institution. The committee should also have at least one practicing scientist experienced in research involving animals as well as one non-scientist who may or may not be employed by the institution. The committee should also include at least one public member to represent community interest with respect to care and use of laboratory animals. The public member should not be affiliated with the institution, should not be an immediate family member of anyone affiliated with the institution, and should not be involved in the use of laboratory animals.

The IACUC is responsible for the evaluation and oversight of the institution's animal care and use program and all related issues set forth in *The Guide*. The IACUC must inspect all animal facilities used by the institution's research program as well as carry out a programmatic review of the research program every 6 months. The committee subsequently analyzes the findings of their inspection and review and prepares a written report for the responsible institutional official that details their findings and any recommendations for action. The institutional official, in turn, must address any major deficiencies detailed in the report by providing a reasonable plan for corrective action and a timetable. The committee must maintain written records of their meetings and all decisions taken. Meetings should be held as frequently as necessary to accomplish their designated tasks, but it should meet at a minimum of twice a year. A mechanism for documenting minority views must also be provided.

An essential component of the IACUC's activity is the review and approval of animal use protocols prior to the initiation of research or other animal-related activities. Protocols submitted for committee review should be complete with respect to their description of the animal care and use components. To prepare a protocol that covers all of the areas and issues posed both by the USDA regulations and *The Guide* recommendations, the IACUC often requires the researcher to place the protocol in a standard format that may take the form of a questionnaire. Topics such as surgery, anesthesia, provision of analgesics during painful procedures, determination of acceptable alternatives to painful procedures, methods of euthanasia, criteria for ending an animal's participation in a study or procedure, and assurance of appropriate housing and care practices are some of the many issues that are considered in the review of any protocol.

The Guide charges the users of research animals with the responsibility of achieving specific outcomes with respect to the care and use of animals, but by using a performance-based approach, provides latitude as to how these outcomes are achieved (222). Performance standards define an outcome in detail and provide criteria for assessing that outcome. They do not restrict the method by which this outcome is achieved. This is in contrast to engineering standards that do not provide for interpretation and modification of prescribed methods or procedures in the event that acceptable alternative methods are available or usual circumstances occur. The IACUC is charged with developing additional performance standards to evaluate alternative methods to achieve specified outcomes and is given the latitude to modify recommendations set forth in *The Guide* based on performance data generated by researchers to establish the adequacy of alternative methods.

Public Health Service Policy

The administration and coordination of the Public Health Services' (PHS) policy on Humane Care and Use of Laboratory Animals (The Policy) is administered by the OLAW (264). This policy requires institutions to establish and maintain proper measures to assure the appropriate care and use of all animals involved in research, research training, and biological testing activities conducted or supported by the PHS. The policy also endorses a set of principles developed by the Interagency Research Animal Committee (IRAC) that covers the use and care of vertebrate animals used in testing, research, and training (140).

The Policy applies to all research supported by PHS and places a heavy emphasis on training of all personnel involved in the care and use of animals in a research setting. The Policy requires the biannual preparation and evaluation of reports by the IACUC on the institution's programs and facilities that involve animal activities. The Policy requires the filing of an assurance statement with OLAW binding the institution to The Policy as well as to the use of *The Guide* as a basis for developing and implementing institutional programs for activities involving animals. OLAW also requires the filing of annual reports by the institution. Achieving and maintaining such assurance is a prerequisite for consideration for funding of activities supported by the PHS, and, by extension, may be adopted by agencies as an essential criteria for consideration for funding.

THE ASSOCIATION FOR ASSESSMENT AND ACCREDITATION OF LABORATORY ANIMAL CARE–INTERNATIONAL

The Association for Assessment and Accreditation of Laboratory Animal Care-International is a voluntary organization that was founded in 1965. AAALAC is a United States–based nonprofit corporation with national and international representation from scientific and educational organizations and whose goal is to promote responsible and high-quality animal care and use by research institutions through the use of a peer-review process. The organization assists institutions in developing and improving programs and facilities for animal care and use.

The accreditation process is designed to assess the institution's conformance with appropriate locally applicable guidelines, recommendations, laws, regulations, and policies, as well as evaluate the program's ability to ensure that animals' health and well-being is safeguarded by institutional processes and operational procedures. In the United States, AAALAC uses *The Guide* as its primary standard, outside of the United States, applicable regulations, laws, and other standards are used that are relevant to that country and the institution's activities.

The accreditation process is confidential. It is initiated by the submission of a comprehensive application that is designed to provide a detailed description of the institution's animal programs and facilities. An initial site visit is made by two or more individuals representing AAALAC, one of whom may be an ad hoc consultant with special expertise in programmatic areas that are relevant to the institution applying for accreditation. Following the initial site visit, a written report is filed along with recommendations. This is then considered by AAALAC's Council on Accreditation to determine if the facility should be granted accreditation. Facilities that have obtained accreditation are revisited every 3 years to determine eligibility to maintain continued accreditation. Annual reports of activities that include programmatic changes and animal usage must be filed.

The achievement of AAALAC accreditation may reduce the level of some reporting requirements for organizations such as OLAW but does not substitute for assurances filed with OLAW or with other requirements set forth in laws, or regulations. AAALAC does not publish separate guidelines or recommendations nor set other standards that are at variance with existing guidelines, laws, or regulations. Lists of institutions that have obtained full accreditation status are regularly published by AAALAC; however, details of an institution's accreditation history are not made available.

DESIGN AND CONSTRUCTION OF ANIMAL HOUSING FACILITIES

The design of animal facilities for biomedical research has evolved over time, as have housing methods for research animals. Key design concepts that have survived the test of time relate to practical matters, such as waste handling, sanitation, investigator access, disease control, and the size of the animal species being used. There is no universally accepted design for animal facilities, nor is it likely that any one given design for animal holding rooms will be appropriate for all species of animals that could be used in toxicologic research. Some reviews on the subject of animal facilities design have been prepared, as have design process considerations for specialized support facilities for research animals (9,17,45,61, 64,79,113,128,130,139,174,189,222,223,258,281,297,345).

The process of animal facility design requires, first and foremost, a clear documentation of the intended type and extent of use of the facility based on past and present toxicologic research programs, as well as a reasonable expectation of the growth of these programs over a period of 5–10 years (345). In considering the intended facility use, the numbers and types of animals by species must be determined. While studies involving small rodent species often consume the bulk of toxicologic research that use animals, other larger species are frequently used and may have to be provided for within a facility. As an alternative, facilities may be designed to accommodate only a limited range of species, with housing and usage of other species being outsourced to other facilities that are more well suited to their maintenance.

Once the level of usage has been determined, specialized requirements—such as the use of biohazardous material requiring biocontainment facilities, a surgical program requiring facilities for aseptic procedures, specialized radiographic or imaging facilities, diet preparation facilities, specialized equipment or procedures facilities, diagnostic laboratory or necropsy facilities, or other specialized spaces requiring specific types of equipment or housing for animals used in toxicologic research—need to be identified, as well as the level of activity that will occur in such facilities. Because these types of facilities often represent a significant cost to construct and operate, as well as consume considerable amounts of floor space, it is important to carefully assess the realistic level of activity projected for such facilities.

The animal care program itself must also be carefully described, and details of the program should be well worked out before the design process is started. The reason for this is that the location of various components of the animal facility will depend greatly on the methodology and equipment to be used in the animal care program. For example, caging and racking within an animal facility must move to and from cage washing facilities. The amount of labor involved in performing these tasks is directly related to the distance of various components of the animal housing facility from the cage washing facilities, as is the opportunity for transmission of adventitious microorganisms potentially infecting one group of animals spreading to others through the cage sanitation process. The frequency of cage changing, as well as the location in which cages are changed and the equipment required for such cage changing, will also influence the amount of storage space and operational space within individual animals rooms and storage space within the cage washing facility.

The type of caging and the level of bioexclusion of microorganisms to be achieved for certain groups of animals maintained within the animal research facility will also dictate many aspects of the design (344). Facilities housing large numbers of rodents in microisolation cages or in flexible or semirigid isolators will require different designs and operational practices, as compared to facilities that use conventional opencage housing.

Animal holding rooms can be classified into two general types. The first *rodent housing*, is characterized by smaller rooms with few fixtures whose design is orientated toward removal of caging from the room for sanitation and perhaps sterilization (204,222,223,344). Such rooms usually have a small sink for hand washing and, if microisolation caging is used, will often be outfitted with a laminar flow hood designed for cage changing using aseptic technique. When microisolation caging is used, such rooms commonly have only a single access door to minimize traffic through the room. Such rooms generally do not contain floor drains or specialized equipment for spraying water under pressure during cleaning of the room or equipment.

The second type of animal holding room is designed to handle larger caging or runs/pens to house animals the size of rabbits or larger (222). Such rooms are equipped with floor drains or some form of trough-drain system to allow in-the-room cleaning of cage components or, in the case of rabbits, the frequent spillage of liquids onto the floor (222). While some caging may be removed from the room and taken to the cage washing area for more complete sanitation, certain components of daily cleaning are carried out within the room itself.

With the exception of some aspects of cage washing, most routine animal care activities are conducted manually, making the animal facility labor intensive. Moreover, the use of the animal facility by researchers also involves regular and often complex manual manipulations of the animals for study purposes. For this reason, distances between support facilities and the animal holding areas need to be minimized and provisions often need to be made within the design for strategic location of procedural rooms and, where appropriate, critical laboratory facilities necessary to conduct determinations that cannot be adequately conducted at great distances from the animal facility. The final design of an animal facility needs to be analyzed for efficient traffic flow of both personnel and equipment. It is important that both users of the animal facility, as well as the animal care staff, analyze the design with respect to day-to-day tasks that need to be accomplished and the distances that need to be traversed by both people and equipment to accomplish these tasks.

Over time, two common arrangements of rooms within animal facilities have been developed (129). These have evolved from considerations of material and personnel flow patterns and from the use of specialized equipment and practices to control the spread of adventitious organisms and contaminants within animal facilities (288). The most common facility is one with a single corridor design. Often, these are a result of renovation of existing space originally designed for laboratory use in which a single corridor that provides both entrance and exit from individual animal rooms was necessitated by the available space and location or, in some cases, by the need to isolate specialized animal facilities, such as microbiological barriers, in which shower and clothing change for people and decontamination of supplies are required. Such barriered animal facilities have become popular in support of some forms of toxicologic research, especially those programs using transgenic or immunologically deficient animals (344).

The other common animal facility arrangement is the dual-corridor system orientated toward cage-washing facilities. In such a system, one or more corridors (i.e., supply or clean) that exit the clean side of the cage wash connect with one of two entrance doors to each animal room. The second door in each room is used to remove caging and other material for return through a second corridor (i.e., return or dirty) to the cage wash by a separate entrance in which soiled caging is collected for subsequent sanitation. This design addresses logical flow of personnel and equipment through animal rooms so as not to have crossing of equipment within common corridors. It is unlikely that such a design provides any realistic measure of disease control by preventing cross contamination, given the many other opportunities for movement of microorganisms through a facility (344). Commonly, there is an air pressure gradient maintained across the two-corridor system such that the supply corridor (clean) is at the highest pressure, with the next highest air pressure being maintained in the animal room and the lowest pressure in the return (dirty) corridor (222,223).

Because toxicologic research programs are dynamic and requirements can change dramatically over time, most animal facility designs try to maintain some degree of flexibility (113). Animal rooms designed for large or small animals usually are designed with a minimum of fixed equipment or specialized mechanical systems. This allows easy conversion from use of one species to another within the categories of large or small animal holding areas. Because most caging and racking is more efficiently located along the perimeter of the room, rectangular designs for animal holding rooms are common, as they maximize wall space while minimizing the relatively unused center of the room space. It is the usual practice to keep the center of the room clear in order to allow the orderly movement of equipment, supplies, and personnel through the room and for the conduct of animal care and research functions. For this reason, common designs, whether on a one- or two-corridor system, usually have rooms with widths ranging from 12–14 feet and lengths of 18–20 feet.

Room sizes are also often dictated by building support structures which, in the case of multiple story buildings, result in support columns that must be maintained throughout the structure. The spacing of these columns is done at fixed intervals, and hence room dimensions must conform to these constraints in order to prevent columns being placed within the room itself rather than in the walls.

Animal rooms, as well as support areas, are often grouped by function in order to minimize the distance traveled between related functions and to minimize the runs of piping and other mechanical services between areas that have higher use of mechanical services (e.g., cage washing, operating rooms, and holding rooms containing dogs rooms, etc.).

In considering the design of animal research facilities, provisions must be made for future expansion (113). Certain items, such as cage washing facilities, specialized laboratories, and surgical facilities, are expensive components of new construction, and during the initial construction of animal facilities may be able to be designed with sufficient capacity to support larger animal populations through logical expansion of the existing building. In developing a design for an animal facility, planners often include provisions for future expansion that must be considered in the animal facility design so that architectural and mechanical barriers are not put in place.

An overriding concern in the construction of animal facilities is the need to frequently clean and disinfect surfaces within the facility. In some cases, specialized components of the animal facility, such as biocontainment facilities or bioexclusion facilities, must also have the capability of being totally disinfected or sterilized using aggressive agents that would be unsuitable for use in the rest of the animal facility. Many of the construction guidelines presented below are directed at making such tasks and routine cleaning/sanitization easier to accomplish on a regular basis, as well as preventing the deterioration of the physical facilities by conducting such practices. By their very nature, these guidelines are quite general and are based on common practices and equipment.

Floors

Opinion varies greatly on the best type of flooring to use for animal facilities. Each type of flooring has its advantages and disadvantages, and it is likely that no perfect flooring exists for animal facilities. Those materials showing the greatest chemical resistance often have difficulties withstanding impact with sharp or heavy objects, whereas those showing the greatest resistance to mechanical damage may have difficulty in resisting the action of chemicals and urine. To withstand repeated sanitation and spillage of urine and water, floors must be moisture resistant and nonabsorbent (222). They should be resistant to the action of hot water, cleaning, agents, disinfectants, urine, and other biological materials. They should be relatively smooth for ease of cleaning, although they may need to have textured surfaces, especially in high moisture areas, where injury to personnel could occur from slipping or to animals, such as hoof stock kept in pens that are regularly cleaned with water.

Floors need to be impact resistant and capable of supporting equipment, cage racks, and other stored items without becoming cracked, pitted, or gouged. To facilitate cleaning, there should be a minimum number of joints in which debris can become entrapped. Materials that have proved particularly satisfactory in many applications are epoxy aggregates, sealed concrete, and other hardened synthetic-based aggregates. Correct surface preparation of subflooring and experienced installation of the flooring itself is essential to its satisfactory performance.

Drains

Drains in animal facilities are a source of contention, but in some areas they are a necessity. Facilities housing large animals require drains. Floors in such areas should be gently sloped toward the drain, and in the case of pens and runs, a dedicated trough for draining should be considered. In such applications, drainage should be designed to allow rapid removal of water and the drying of surfaces to minimize elevation of humidity. Where waste is to be flushed down drains along with water, larger-diameter drains (4 inches or greater) should be considered (222). To facilitate this process, rim-flush drains that sweep waste collected from trough drainage systems down into drain pipes through coarse basket strainers fitted in the drains minimize maintenance considerations. It is critical in the sanitation program for animal facilities that drain traps be kept filled with liquid and that drains that are not in use for long periods of time be capped and sealed to prevent backflow of sewage, gases, and other contaminants into the animal holding areas.

Floor drains are not essential in all animals rooms. Rooms containing rodents can be sanitized better by using alternative cleaning methods, such as wet vacuuming or mopping with cleaning compounds and disinfectants.

Walls and Ceilings

Walls within animal facilities need to be frequently sanitized and therefore should be moisture resistant and nonabsorbent. They also should be free of cracks or holes, such as those created by unsealed utility penetrations. Junctions of the walls with the ceiling and floors, as well as to themselves, should be adequately caulked or otherwise sealed to prevent build-up of debris and harborage for insects. The construction of the walls can take a variety of forms, with masonry being the most durable; however, other wall construction materials may be more appropriate in certain situations. The surface coating of walls should be resistant to the chemical actions of disinfectants and cleaning agents and should have significant resistance to abrasion and impact. Common wall materials acceptable in other applications, such as painted gypsum board, may not prove satisfactory in some animal facility applications given their low impact resistance and significant damage when exposed to moisture. Some of the difficulties associated with certain wall construction materials can be overcome by protecting the wall surfaces through the use of strategically placed guard rails or bull-nosed curbing on the wall to floor junction in order to minimize the impact of equipment on the walls (222).

Like walls, ceilings should be smooth and moisture resistant. Their surfaces should be capable of withstanding detergents and disinfectants and be free of imperfect junctions that would allow the build-up of debris and harborage of insects. Generally, suspended ceilings are undesirable in animal facilities unless they are constructed in such a way as to be readily sanitizable and free of imperfect junctions or penetrations. Gypsum board that has been appropriately sealed and finished with a durable coating or concrete that has been smoothed and sealed or painted are the most appropriate and long-lasting choices for ceilings.

Doors to Animal Rooms

Doors to animal rooms should be constructed of and/or coated with materials that resist corrosion and are amenable to disinfection. They should be appropriately sealed/gasketted and fitted with door sweeps to ensure adequate sealing with the floor and the door frames. This is critical in preventing the incursion of pests and the uncontrolled movement of air and particulates beneath and around the door. Doors should be self-closing and should open into animal rooms to prevent injury to personnel or damage to equipment moving in hallways. For safety reasons, viewing windows often are appropriate, but the ability to cover the viewing windows in certain instances where close control of lighting is required must be considered.

Doors should be equipped with recessed or shielded handles (to prevent damage from equipment) and equipped with metal or plastic strike plates to prevent equipment damage to the surfaces. Generally, doors that are 42 in × 84 in accommodate most animal equipment; however, larger doors may be required in certain portions of the animal facilities. Consideration of room level security is important in order to limit access to animals on study or in areas in which bioexclusion or biocontainment is required. This is best accomplished with mechanical or electrical locks; however, it is important that doors be designed to be opened from the inside without a key for emergency egress purposes.

Corridors

Corridors within the animal facility are the principal means of access to animal rooms and support areas. For this reason, they should be wide enough to accommodate the movement of equipment and personnel and be amenable to cleaning and disinfection. Generally, a width of 6–8 feet is sufficient for most purposes (45,130,222). All of the considerations reviewed for floors, walls, and ceilings generally apply to corridors; however, suspended ceilings are more commonly used in corridors due to the need to access mechanical fixtures, such as electrical conduits and plumbing. It is good practice to ensure that access to water lines, drain pipes, and other utilities supporting animal rooms is available through panels or chases in the corridor outside of the animal rooms. Wall-mounted equipment in the corridors, such as, telephones, fire extinguishers, fire alarms, and record–keeping stations, should be recessed or installed high enough to prevent damage from movement of equipment and personnel through the corridors.

Support Areas

In addition to the basic animal rooms, animal facilities must incorporate certain facilities and equipment to support the basic day-to-day investigational and animal care needs, including locker rooms often coupled with shower facilities and restrooms, break areas, cage-washing facilities, feed and bedding storage, waste handling and storage areas, supply rooms, general storage areas, administrative offices, and procedural rooms for use by researchers. Although a comprehensive treatment of these areas will not be addressed in this chapter, information regarding their essential features and construction can be found elsewhere (222). A few essential points, however, bear emphasizing.

In designing animal facilities, it is a common error to undersize these facilities in comparison to the intended animal populations or types of research to be conducted. This is especially true of support areas that experience cyclic levels of activity during their normal function. For example, locker rooms where clothing change occurs are intensively used at the beginning and end of work days and, depending on the type of facility, may also experience significant activity at lunch time or during designated break periods. Commonly, the size of these areas are designed to only allow a few individuals to use them at a single time, requiring adaptation of schedules and difficulty in access to the facility during certain times throughout the day.

Such areas must be large enough to accommodate reasonable numbers of employees and to provide sufficient locker space for clothing and storage of uniforms and other supplies. If mandatory showering is required, as is the case in some barriered facilities, sufficient capacity for showers or other clothing change functions must be provided. From a programmatic standpoint, the necessity of certain types of clothing change or the use of certain items of disposable clothing, such as face masks or shoe covers, must be carefully considered. The more complex the clothing change, the more complex the support area for it needs to be. Similarly, if reusable garments are used, adequate storage space and provisions for laundering/disinfection must be made. If clothing changes are to be made at the level of the animal holding room, such changing must be provided for in the design of the facility and must be logical if it is to be routinely followed. Human use support areas, such as lockers rooms and break areas or administrative offices, should be separated from animal areas. They are often located at the periphery of the animal facility and are used as control points for entrance into the animal facility.

The location of support areas is dictated by the location of utilities and certain architectural features in the animal facility. For example, cage-washing facilities are usually located at the end of corridors servicing groups of animal rooms. These facilities usually are located near storage areas for bedding, feed, and building utility runs in order to minimize distances traveled and construction costs. Waste-handling facilities are commonly located near cage-washing facilities, and such facilities usually are located within a convenient distance of loading docks or other exterior entrances.

Cage-washing facilities are designed to allow the use of chemical detergents, and disinfectants, and large amounts of hot water. Regular cleaning of room surfaces is an essential part of their operation, and the facility must be designed to allow this to be easily done. Large amounts of equipment are moved in and out of these facilities and they must be big enough to accommodate such equipment both in process and for short periods of storage. Substantial quantities of heat and moist air are generated within the cage-washing facility, and Heating, Ventillation, and Air Conditioning (HVAC) systems must be designed to accommodate these loads.

Often the locations of support areas are selected to decrease the amount of unwanted noise and traffic passing by animal rooms (222). Noise-producing areas, such as, mechanical rooms, waste processing areas, and cage washers, are often grouped together and separated from animal holding areas by noise traps, such as air locks or sound-proofing surfaces. Commonly, species of animals such as dogs, nonhuman primates, and swine that produce loud vocalizations as part of their normal behavior are also separated from other holding areas that contain more noise-sensitive animals, such as rodents, by using similar building concepts. Housing for these noise-producing species is commonly located near support areas that produce noise, although the two functions usually are separated by air locks, doors, or other means.

Areas used for storage of feed are kept at lower environmental temperatures than other areas to inhibit decomposition of liable ingredients and the development of immature forms of insect pests that may contaminate the packaging or the feed.

Specialized Components of Animal Facilities

Within animal facilities there is often a need for specialized structures and equipment to support toxicologic research. Such facilities include, but are not limited to, barrier facilities for maintenance of animals in defined microbiological states, bio-containment facilities for housing and manipulation of animals exposed to biohazardous materials, surgical facilities, imaging facilities, necropsy facilities, and facilities for conducting diagnostic tests on animals.

Barrier Facilities/Barrier Rooms

Barrier facilities or individual barrier rooms may be used in toxicologic research for either bioexclusion or biocontainment purposes (344). Most commonly, they are used for bioexclusion. In this role, the room or series of rooms (facility) is separated from other components of the animal facility using a variety of construction methodologies in a manner to prevent undesirable microorganisms from entering the room whether carried on personnel, equipment, or materials. Barrier rooms are composed of durable materials that are impervious to liquids and free of unsealed penetrations. Personnel entry is usually through a lock system requiring progressive decontamination of personnel by shower and/or clothing change. Air to the room is independently supplied and HEPA (high efficiency particulate air) filtered. Water supplied to the area is independently decontaminated or sterilized, and provisions are available to provide sterilized feed, bedding, and other supplies for use in the room. Waste is removed using processes designed to prevent the incursion of unwanted microorganisms during the removal process.

Most commonly, multiple methods of introducing supplies and equipment are built into the barrier room. Generally, a through-the-wall autoclave is provided with sufficient capacity to handle reasonably large loads of materials. For maintenance purposes, the autoclave should be able to be serviced from the outside of the barrier. It is essential that the autoclave be calibrated and validated based on material types and load configurations. This calibration and validation should be done on a regular basis, usually yearly. The use of cumulative heat-sensitive or biological indicators placed at one or two points in a load to be autoclaved is not sufficient to confirm adequate disinfection or sterilization.

In addition to autoclaves for processing large volumes of materials that are unaffected or marginally affected by heat, alternative means of disinfection need to be provided for introduction of heat-sensitive materials into the barrier room. This is accomplished by using a double-door chamber into which materials that have been immersed in disinfectants can be placed and additional disinfectants sprayed into the port before it is closed and the materials held for an appropriate contact time. Once this chemical disinfectant process has taken place, materials can be removed from the chamber using the inside door for subsequent use in the barrier. As with autoclaving procedures, the use of chemical disinfectants must be calibrated so that adequate application procedures, concentrations and contact times are maintained. Materials processed by this method must be wrapped in coverings that can withstand the application of the disinfectants, and the materials inside of the packaging must be already disinfected by alternative means. For example, vacuum-packed containers of paper products that have been previously gamma irradiated could be introduced using this spray-port method.

Introduction of personnel into barrier rooms poses the greatest risk to the microbiological integrity of the barrier room. Because it is impossible to adequately disinfect the external surfaces of people, it is necessary to place a barrier between them and the animals maintained within the room. This is accomplished in an entry lock system by an orderly removal of clothing and a re-gowning in attire that covers the body surfaces using materials that are known to be free of organisms of concern (344).

The entry lock system usually is composed of four compartments. The first compartment, often referred to as an insect lock or air pressure lock, is used for static pressure control between other areas of the animal facility and the lock system. This first lock also serves to inhibit the passage of insects into the other more critical areas of the lock system. It is also used in some instances for storage of external clothing, such as jackets or for depositing of shoes worn elsewhere in the animal facility. The next component of the lock system is an undress lock, where all clothing is removed and placed in lockers or other suitable receptacles. Presumably, most, if not all, of the contamination that might be associated with personnel resides on such clothing.

At this point in the lock system there are two possible configurations. The first is termed the *wet entry system* and involves personnel taking a water shower. Depending on the rigors of the barrier facility, an electromechanical system may be placed in this portion of the lock system to assure that a wet shower is actually taken. This consists of interlocking doors with timers requiring a wait period within the shower area and an electrical interface with the water supply to the showers such that the release timers are only activated if water has run for a certain period of time. In the end, even such rigorous measures do not necessarily guarantee that the shower taken is adequate or consistent (344).

Although some decontamination of external surfaces of a person's body may occur to varying degrees with a shower, the principal rationale for the use of the water shower is to ensure that street clothing has been removed. There are a number of disadvantages associated with a shower in a lock entry system, including the time constraints associated with the entry procedure and the considerable requirements for expendable supplies used in the showering procedure. Following the shower, a separate room is provided for drying off and putting on a sterile/disinfected uniform, including components such as a cap, mask, gloves, and dedicated footwear. Once these procedures have been conducted, entrance into the barrier room can be made. Leaving the barrier room, the employee reverses the process; however, often the showering step is omitted.

Because the wet entry system is quite cumbersome and limits the number of employees that can enter the barrier facility at any given time, a new methodology, the *dry entry system*, has gained increasing favor in many research settings. This latter method involves the elimination of the wet shower and a direct change in a separate room from the de-gowning portion of the lock into clean, disinfected clothing as occurs in the last step of the wet entry system. Once clothed in appropriate attire, the employee enters an air shower that blows high-velocity HEPA-filtered air across all surfaces, removing particulates that may contain any contaminants imparted to the external surfaces of the gown during the changing process. Doors to the air shower are electrically interlocked, requiring that a full cycle be completed before the employee can enter the barrier room. Upon exiting the barrier room, all aspects of the process, including the air shower, are again used by the employee in reverse order.

In addition to time savings, the air shower also provides a very positive interlock between the barrier room and the lock system, preventing escape of any animals that have left their cages and any potential incursion of insects or other pests into the barrier room through the lock system. The air shower also greatly decreases the amount of particulates that are brought out of the barrier room serving as a safeguard for the general animal facility should a contamination occur within the barrier (344).

As a general rule, cage washing and other sanitation procedures are done within the barrier facilities rather than bringing caging materials out of the barrier. This is because each transport of materials across the barrier entails some degree of risk of introduction of unwanted microorganisms. Movement of caging from the barrier through common animal facility hallways and cage-washing facilities also poses a risk of contamination that may or may not be eliminated by the disinfection processes used to re-enter such materials into the barrier. Similarly, rigidly operated barrier rooms generally do not provide for personnel break areas or other administrative support facilities within the barrier. Such areas tend to encourage removal of protective clothing and inappropriate activities given the microbiological status of the barrier.

Barrier rooms are expensive to operate and are best used to house large numbers of animals or to house large animals under defined microbiological conditions. Due to their large size and the large amount of materials that must be passed across the barrier to maintain it, failure of the barrier, as measured by changes in the microbiological status of the animals maintained within the barrier, are common. Once an unwanted microorganism gains entrance, all animals within the barrier room are at risk of becoming contaminated unless some form of secondary containment/bioexclusion system (e.g., microisolation cages) is also used within the barrier (344). This practice is seldom done, given the high cost of such secondary bioexclusion practices.

Biohazard Containment Facilities

Toxicologic research often requires the use of biohazardous materials in conjunction with animals. Such materials, whether they be toxic, carcinogenic, radioactive, or infectious, must be contained within a very

Table 16.1
Comparison of conventional animal care strategies with strategies for containing biohazards

	Recommended Animal Care Practices Strategies[a]	Biocontainment Strategies[b]	Rationale
Air flow	High	Low	A
Cage cleaning	Frequent	Infrequent	A
Bedding change	Frequent	Infrequent	A
Equipment/supplies	Reusable	Disposable	B
Animal handling	Frequent	Infrequent	C

[a] Practices or approaches commonly used to provide a clean, healthful environment for animals.
[b] Practices or approaches designed to minimize the release of hazardous materials from animals or their environment.
A—The more potentially contaminated material generated, the more that has to be decontaminated and the greater chance for error; B—processing materials for reuse while assuming proper decontamination is costly, logistically difficult, and has the potential for error; C—the more handling, the greater risk for personnel injury and contamination.

defined space and handled appropriately so as not to contaminate other animals or personnel (287,288). It is a popular misconception that barrier facilities or certain other bioexclusion systems, such as microisolation cages, provide, in normal operation, the necessary level of biocontainment to meet most research needs. In general, good biocontainment practices are at odds with recommended animal husbandry and bioexclusion techniques (Table 16.1).

The type of biocontainment facilities required when using biohazardous materials in animals depends on the nature of the hazard and the level of risk posed by it. In the case of infectious materials, the Centers for Disease Control and Prevention (CDC) has published classification systems for microorganisms and have described biological containment facilities of four increasingly secure types designated BL I through BL IV (49,50). These safety practices and equipment used in conjunction with these increasing levels of hazards are designed to prevent inadvertent transmission or release of contaminants from the work area. These guidelines set standards for reducing aerosol generation, hazards associated with sharp objects, the use of protective clothing, and the operational standards for hoods and other devices used to manipulate infected materials, including animals.

Biocontainment facilities are resource intensive, and their complexity increases with the size of the animals that must be contained at the various biosafety levels. Laboratory animals the size of rabbits or larger require considerable housing space and generate large amounts of waste material that is potentially contaminated. Normal operations of cleaning and disinfection, as well as removal of biological materials, including animal carcasses, may require complex systems, making such facilities expensive to construct and to operate. For this reason, those institutions conducting limited work in larger species involving biohazardous materials may choose to subcontract these tasks to more specialized institutions in which the volume of such work is sufficient to justify the cost of constructing and maintaining these facilities.

Most institutions, however, use cage-level biocontainment practices for studies involving rodents and other small mammals. Studies up through biosafety level III can be conducted in small, dedicated facilities using these systems, along with appropriate safety practices.

Surgical Facilities

The use of surgically altered animals is common in toxicologic research. Traditionally, the complexity of surgical procedures performed and the nature of the surgical facilities required was directly proportional to the body size of the animals being used. Small laboratory animals, such as rats and mice, were often used in studies in which relatively simple procedures involving organ removal was required. The facilities to support these operative procedures were not complex in nature, and often a portion of a multipurpose area could be used on a temporary basis for conducting them. Larger, more complex procedures were usually reserved for animals the size of dogs or domestic farm animals in which the operative field was much larger, and techniques used in human surgery, as well as the necessary support equipment, such as specialized gas anesthesia machines, bypass equipment, and specialized imaging equipment used in human or traditional veterinary practice, could be employed. Such procedures require a much larger, dedicated surgical facility.

A few guidelines for the design and construction of surgical facilities for use in biomedical research have been published (222,345). In general, such facilities should have certain basic components, including the following:

an operating room in which the surgical procedure is conducted, a postoperative care area separated from the rest of the surgical facility in which animals can recover from the surgical procedure, an animal preparation area in which the animal can be anesthetized and other preoperative procedures conducted, an instrument and supply preparation area in which materials can be assembled, cleaned, and sterilized, and a surgeon preparation area in which personnel can decontaminate their hands and then become suitably attired for the surgical procedure. A number of support facilities may also be associated with the surgical facility, including a diagnostic laboratory, imaging facilities, and specialized procedure rooms to study instrumented animals.

Existing guidelines for surgical facilities endeavor to separate the various functions to be performed by physical barriers, distance, or by separating the functions in time (222). Surfaces and construction materials used in surgical suites are designed to be easily cleaned and disinfected (222). Air provided to surgical facilities should be highly filtered to remove microorganisms and should be appropriately conditioned in order to minimize temperature loss or gain during the surgical procedure. Such facilities are utility intensive and often require access to medical gases and emergency power.

Over the last decade there has been a trend toward miniaturization, and complex surgical procedures in support of toxicologic research can now be performed on small laboratory rodents. The increasing commercial availability of vascular catheterized rodents, coupled with numerous types of telemetry devices for continuous recording of a variety of parameters from nonrestrained animals, has provided new possibilities in drug discovery research. If sufficient numbers of such procedures are to be done, a dedicated surgical facility for rodents may be appropriate. In general, many of the same components used in traditional large-animal surgical facilities are present in such a dedicated rodent surgical facility but may not be separated by physical barriers, such as walls.

Due to the small size of the operative field in small laboratory animals, the use of sterile instrument tip procedures can be coupled with chemical disinfectants and table-top dry heat sterilizers to allow large numbers of rodents to be instrumented aseptically during a single surgical session (38,68,69). To facilitate these procedures, horizontal laminar-flow hoods may be used to minimize the chance of cross-contamination between animals during surgery and to reduce bacteriologic contamination of the operative site.

Unlike traditional operative procedures on larger animals, most rodent surgery is done in a sitting position and may require the use of magnification and focused, point-source illumination. For this reason, provision needs to be made for adequate counter space and electrical power. Because multiple groups of animals may be used in the surgical facility over a short period of time, preoperative and postoperative housing is often done in cage-level bioexclusion systems to prevent the chance of cross-contamination between projects when animals are used from either different sources of supply or from different locations employing different housing methods.

It is important to remember that the size of the animal or the species of the animal does not diminish the need to maintain appropriate aseptic procedures during the course of the surgical manipulation (20,32), however, due to the small size of rodents and the relatively small operative field, the risk of postoperative infection and the need for maintaining large areas of a facility in an aseptic fashion is greatly reduced (68,69).

CAGING AND HOUSING SYSTEMS

The environment of the laboratory animals used in toxicologic research is classified by levels of enclosure. A cage, pen, or stall is the immediate limit of an animal's environment in a research facility and is designated as its *primary* enclosure. The room or space in which the primary enclosure is located is termed the *secondary enclosure* (222).

The environmental conditions in the secondary enclosure influence, but do not control, the environment in the primary enclosure (26,354,355). The animal's primary enclosure needs to allow the animal to remain clean and dry, securely contain the animal so that it cannot escape and cannot injure itself while residing in the enclosure, and provide adequate ventilation in order to allow the animal a sufficient supply of fresh air that is appropriately conditioned to meet its needs. The primary enclosure should also provide for normal physiologic and behavioral requirements of the animals, including reproduction, movement, urination, and defecation. It should allow for investigator access and observation of the animal with minimal disturbance. In addition to these criteria, primary enclosures may also be used to maintain the animal and its environment in a specified microbiological status. This bioexclusion function requires a heavy reliance on aseptic techniques and personnel training, as well as significant support facilities, including autoclaves and laminar flow work stations (222,344).

Primary Enclosures

Microisolation Cages

A microisolation cage consists of a plastic cage bottom with stainless steel wire top that is covered by a fitted plastic lid containing a filter. The filter usually is comprised of a polyester material that can be fabricated to different thickness and average pore sizes. In principle, by the lid remaining on the cage, all ventilation occurs through the filter, which excludes particulates that may contain infectious organisms. As long as all manipulations are done in a laminar flow work station and all materials are adequately disinfected/sterilized, unwanted organisms should be excluded from the cage environment (72). For this to occur, all manipulations must be done using aseptic technique. Such systems can be effective in maintaining a particular microbiological status of animals, but manipulation of the animals may be cumbersome for researchers and requires that all research equipment and materials undergo rigorous and frequent decontamination/sterilization to ensure the microbiological status of the animals.

Microisolation caging does provide some disadvantages in terms of the environmental conditions surrounding the animals. Because static microisolation caging does not allow for significant air exchange through the filter, the concentration of water vapor, gases, and heat may build up to levels well above that in the secondary enclosure (161,298). Another difficulty may be related to the adequacy of the fit of the filtered top to the cage itself. Studies have shown that in some designs of microisolator caging, ventilation occurs under the lip of the cage, allowing unfiltered air to migrate across cage surfaces and other areas into the sterilized environment of the microisolation cage (202,203). This makes practices such as the exterior disinfection of the cage before manipulation in the change station an important consideration. In addition, when manipulating such caging in a laminar flow change station, it is important to minimize the amount of materials in the change station, as laminar flow air upon striking objects will eddy for a distance of at least three times the diameter of the object struck, causing unwanted movement of air between materials in the station, resulting in airborne cross-contamination (349).

Ventilated Microisolation Caging

To address some of the difficulties associated with poor ventilation of static microisolation caging, specialized racks designed to hold the microisolation caging have been developed. These racks contain a source of HEPA-filtered air that is discharged either through a nozzle directly into the cage or through small openings above the filter cage top such that the air moves directly into the cage. Ventilated racks usually have a mechanism for removing air from the cage, often through a port located directly above the filter top in another area of microisolation cage. This exhaust air is either HEPA filtered and discharged into the room or directly discharged into the room exhaust system. These racks usually are equipped with individual blowers to pass air through the HEPA filters and generate the necessary static pressure. Like static microisolation caging, ventilated microisolators must be handled and managed in the same manner as static microisolation caging using aseptic technique, sterilized materials, and laminar flow change stations (344).

By supplying relatively large volumes of conditioned fresh air to each cage, heat, moisture, and gas contaminant build-up is minimized. Bedding materials often stay drier than in unventilated cages, improving the animal's environment and allowing longer intervals between bedding changes (222). In the case of the ventilated microisolation cage, it is important to remember that the cage itself is maintained under positive pressure with respect to the secondary enclosure. As such, if hazardous or unwanted microorganisms are present within any given cage, the possibility exists of leakage of contaminants to surfaces outside of the cage through leakage in individual filter tops. For this reason, ventilated microisolation cages must be used with caution in research involving the use of hazardous materials (344).

Conventional Caging

By far the most commonly used type of caging in toxicologic research is conventional open caging. In the case of rodents, this is of two types. The first is solid bottom plastic or metal caging with contact bedding. The cage body is covered with a lid that often contains an integrated feeder for holding feed pellets and a space for a water bottle. As an alternative, water may be provided by automatic watering systems, in which case a small hole is found in one end of the cage, through which a small water valve is introduced.

The most common type of cage is constructed of plastic with a solid bottom. These can be opaque or transparent. Transparent materials have the advantage of allowing easy visualization of the animals, whereas opaque materials provide a more sheltered environment for the animals by decreasing the amount of light striking them. The type of plastic materials used in the construction of the caging is important, as procedures such as frequent autoclaving and washing with high-temperature water and chemical compounds that are designed to disinfect can rapidly deteriorate some forms of plastic (58,177). In addition, animal urine, which contains significant quantities of minerals and proteinaceous material, can cling tenaciously to plastic, requiring the use of mineral acids or other compounds to remove them (222). Over time, all plastic caging will deteriorate and need to be replaced. Cracks or other deficits in the plastic make sanitation difficult and may affect the structural integrity of the caging, requiring replacement.

A second type of caging is referred to under the general classification of *suspended caging*. Such caging usually is constructed of metal, most commonly stainless steel. The floors usually are of wire mesh, containing either two or four wires per inch. Some types of suspended caging have punched metal floors that have been electropolished or otherwise smoothed to prevent injury to feet. Punched metal flooring is commonly used for housing rabbits, as it provides greater support for their feet. As an alternative, some suspended caging is constructed of heavy duty plastics. Floors may also be constructed of the same plastic using the same principle as the punched metal flooring. Suspended cages for larger animals, such as dogs, cats, or swine, commonly use coated wire or coated, metal punched flooring to minimize the chance of damage to the animal's feet.

The mesh size of any suspended cage flooring is important. It must be sufficiently wide to allow the passage of feces while still providing sufficient support to the feet to prevent pressure injuries. In theory, suspended caging should allow feces and urine to pass onto catch pans containing sheet or loose bedding or, in some cases, onto catch pans that can be flushed into trough drain systems. Because most animals, including rodents, are coprophagic, if feces pass through the flooring, the animals will have limited access to it. Many species may consume feces as it is being defecated and before it can drop through the cage floor. Coprophagy is critical for normal health of some species, such as rabbits.

Larger suspended caging usually is cleaned in place, whereas caging for rodents and other small mammals usually is taken to a wash area for cleaning. Watering can be provided to suspended caging by means of automatic watering devices, water bottles, or, in the case of some large animals, water bowls. Feed usually is dispensed either in feeders that hang on the cages or within it or, for some larger animals, by use of feed bowls. Caging for some larger animals, such as nonhuman primates, cats, and dogs, often contain a resting board or perch that is suspended off of the floor. This allows the animals to express normal behaviors and provides them an elevated place on which to rest.

Neither solid-bottom nor suspended conventional caging is designed to prevent the airborne or fomite transmission of adventitious microorganisms. Control of such organisms when these cages are used is at the secondary enclosure level.

Pens and Runs

Domestic farm animals and dogs often are maintained in either runs or pens. A pen is a large indoor enclosure whose floor usually is the floor of the secondary enclosure. In the case of those animals that do not exhibit climbing behavior, indoor pens may be constructed such that the top of the pen is open. Most commonly, however, pens form a complete enclosure. Pens usually have an incorporated drainage system either by the use of a slanted floor underneath a raised pen floor that allows liquids to drain toward the back of the pen into a trough drain system or through the incorporation of a trough drain system in the floor of the pen itself. Pens are cleaned using water under pressure and detergent/disinfectants. Pens may also be bedded with loose bedding, which is removed and replaced on a regular basis. Whenever in-place cleaning of pens is done, it is important that the design of the pens be such that floor drains are large enough to accommodate fecal material and other items, such as bedding that may be flushed down the drainage system.

In theory, pens provide large animals the ability to move about normally and to acquire some exercise (131). Studies have shown, however, that such exercise is rarely spontaneous and usually is associated with the presence of humans (42,43,134). For this reason, components of some legislation, as well as certain guidelines, require regular periods of exercise for certain penned animals (308). Special provisions must be made to allow such exercise to occur.

The term *run* is often reserved for pens that have both an indoor and outdoor component. In such cases, the indoor component of the run often has a smaller floor area than the outdoor component. The indoor component usually is in a conditioned space or has other provisions for the thermal comfort of the animal, such as heated flooring. Access to the outdoor portion of the run may be limited through the use of animal-operated doors or doors that must be opened by animal facility personnel. Feeding and provision of water to animals housed in runs usually are done in the indoor portion of the run. Cleaning is done using water under pressure accompanied by detergents or disinfectants. Care must be taken during the process of cleaning such enclosures so as not to unduly stress or cause the animals to become wet during the process (222).

Housing of animals in pens or runs requires that consideration be given to handling and training of animals housed in such enclosures (256). Toxicologic research often requires repeated sampling or other manipulations. Removing animals from such enclosures, as well as protection of implanted sampling ports or catheters while animals are in the enclosures, must be given adequate attention. Many problems can be overcome by conditioning periods during which the animals are handled and trained to respond in certain ways.

SECONDARY ENCLOSURES

The construction of typical animal holding rooms has been previously discussed. A number of specialized secondary enclosures other than the conventional animal holding rooms have been developed for the purpose of minimizing transmission of adventitious microorganisms between groups of animals. In contrast to individual primary enclosure bioexclusion systems, these secondary enclosure systems provide some increased flexibility in animal handling and some decreased reliance on maintaining strict technical practices. They also pose an additional advantage of allowing the use of existing caging systems.

Cubicles

A cubicle is a small room partitioned off within another larger room and is used to decrease the chance of airborne cross-contamination between groups of animals housed in adjacent cubicles. The air supplied to the cubicle may come from a separate air supply within the cubicle or from the room in which the cubicle is located. In the latter instance, a negative pressure is created within the cubicle by an exhaust system, usually located in the ceiling of the cubicle, which pulls air into the cubicle through a space under the doors to the cubicle in a fashion similar to a fume hood. The cubicle is entered by opening the doors, at which point all directional control of air movement is lost (347). Unlike cage-level containment systems, cubicles only address airborne cross-contamination between cubicles, not fomite transmission, as might occur on dust particles or by manipulation by investigators or by animal care personnel. Due to the low face velocity associated with the air movement underneath the door to the cubicle, absolute prevention of airborne cross-contamination cannot be assured (344,347).

Cubicles have been shown to be useful in some applications where separation of species is required in limited space, and they apparently can limit the spread of certain microorganisms under the right conditions (171). They are probably best used in conjunction with cage-level bioexclusion systems if reliable prevention of microbiological contamination is required.

Ventilated Cabinets

Ventilated cabinets consist of a cabinet with one or more doors. The cabinet has a small fan and HEPA-filter that extracts air from the room and releases it into the cabinet. Air is exhausted either between the doors to the cabinet or through an exhaust duct into the room. The exhaust air may or may not be filtered (185). Like cubicles, when the cabinet door is opened, caging within the cabinets no longer receives the benefit of the HEPA-filtered air supply. Airborne cross-contamination between cages within the system is not controlled unless a cage-level bioexclusion system is also used. Fomite transmission is not prevented by ventilated cabinets. Their use in toxicologic studies is limited.

Mass Air Displacement and Laminar Air Flow Rooms

These secondary enclosure bioexclusion systems are designed to decrease the airborne transfer of microorganisms between groups of animals. Both systems use a HEPA filter and blower to supply air to either diffusers or a plenum located in the ceiling of an animal room. In the case of mass air displacement rooms, large volumes of appropriately filtered air is released through a series of diffusers located in the ceiling in an attempt to wash any airborne contaminants to the floor and out through exhaust ducts located at floor level at several locations in the room (186,194). By contrast, laminar air flow rooms pressurize a space above the ceiling (plenum) and discharge air out through the thousands of tiny holes in the ceiling, creating laminar movement of air (19). In theory, particles released from individual cages will be caught up in the laminar air stream and drop to the floor (65). In practice, once the laminar air flow strikes caging or other objects within the room, it eddies for distances of three or more times the diameter of any object that it strikes, causing mixing and producing an effect similar to mass air displacement (349).

Both of these room types do not effectively address airborne cross-contamination between adjacent cages and do not address fomite or other means of transmission of microorganisms. By themselves they are not a complete bioexclusion system (344). Depending on the design of the ventilation equipment, these rooms can be quite noisy and may be prone to excessive heat build up. Prior to the advent of cage-level bioexclusion systems, mass air displacement and laminar flow rooms were a common feature in toxicological research facilities using animals. They are less commonly used today.

ILLUMINATION

Light is an important environmental factor that can affect biological and behavioral processes in animals and the conduct of routine animal care duties. Numerous studies have documented effects of light on the morphology, physiology, and behavior of various animals (33,82,233,316,338). Not all of these effects have been adequately explored in all species or in sufficient detail to predict the magnitude and the extent of impact on various toxicologic studies.

There are three factors that characterize lighting: (1) lighting spectrum (wavelength), (2) light intensity as measured in foot candles (English) or lux (metric), and (3) photoperiodicity (light/dark cycle) (22,300). In addition, factors such as the light history of the animal, animal pigmentation, time of light exposure during the circadian cycle, species, sex, age, body temperature, hormonal status, and stock or strain of the animal can alter the influence of specific characteristics of the light on an animal (33,76,240,285,294,331).

The one characteristic of light that has the most profound effect on animals is photoperiodicity. It regulates circadian (one day in length) and ultradian (greater than one day) biological rhythms in animals. These, in turn, can alter a variety of basic processes. Photoperiodicity is a critical regulator of reproduction and behavior (118,196,268,339), including a behavioral influence on processes such as feed consumption and resulting body weight gain, nutrient intake, and hormone secretion (34,54,316). It appears that in most species, a period of 10–14 hours of light is required to maintain normal biological rhythms (200). Some species such as rats and mice are more tolerant of light cycle length than are species such as hamsters, which require at least 14 hours of daylight for normal reproductive function (54,99). Continuous daylight, which can occur with malfunctioning light timers or inadvertent overriding of light timing devices, can have serious consequences for some toxicologic studies (28). For this reason, it is important to regularly assess the function of light timing devices and to build in safeguards to any light timer overriding mechanism to ensure that a consistent photoperiodicity is maintained (222).

A consistent photoperiodicity with adequate dark cycles is also essential to allow for the regular daily renewal of rods and cones in the eye, especially in nocturnal and crepuscular species (60). Without adequate dark periods, retinal degeneration cannot occur and can magnify the effects of retinal degeneration associated with high light intensity (236). Every effort should be made to minimize disruption of the dark cycle of the photoperiod. When procedures need to be conducted during the dark cycle, infrared illumination, low-intensity red lighting, and the use of point source low-intensity lighting, such as hand-held flashlights, may allow the necessary procedures to be performed without significant disruption. Alternatively, light cycles can be adjusted to fit work required (reverse light cycles), or the necessary procedures may need to be rescheduled into the light cycle.

Consistency in the photoperiod is important, and for this reason the use of windows in animal rooms needs to be carefully considered. Exterior windows allow seasonal ambient lighting conditions to alter photoperiodicity. This may not be important in certain species, such as nonhuman primates, dogs, and some agricultural or other large mammals, and may be considered a form of enrichment. In small rodents in which reproduction may be a study parameter, this lack of control may be an important variable (222).

Other significant concerns posed by exterior windows may be difficulties in temperature regulation within the animal holding room because of heat loss or gain through the windows and difficulties in providing adequate security for exterior windows (222).

Light intensity is another important characteristic of light that can dramatically affect certain laboratory animals. Many commonly used laboratory animals, including rats and mice, are nocturnal. Moreover, many of these species have been developed on albino backgrounds, thereby lacking pigment in their eyes, skin, and other tissues that provide some protection from the effects of light intensity. The most damaging effect appears to be phototoxic retinal atrophy, which occurs in albino rats and mice (175,172,271).

Because light intensity is affected by the type, location, and number of lighting fixtures in a room, considerable variation can occur between toxicologic research facilities. The age of the light-producing fixture (i.e., bulbs/tubes) is also important, as the output intensity will vary with length of use. It is unclear whether the effects reported for light intensity are related to a single wavelength/group of wavelengths or occurs equally over the whole spectrum. Light intensity is also affected by caging type and location as well as the reflective ability of other room surfaces (234,339). Studies have shown that the position of mice in cages at various levels on the caging rack can influence the incidence of retinal atrophy, with an incidence of affected animals as high as 30.2% being recorded for animals housed in upper cages, as compared to 0.7% incidence for animals housed in lower cages (28,115). For this reason, randomization of caging, as well as rotation of cages, is an important consideration if such effects are to be equally distributed between test and control groups (116).

When specifying light intensity, it is important that a uniform point of measure be used. In recent studies, as well as recommendations by various organizations, a measuring point of 1 m off of a floor in the center of the animal holding room has been used and is considered to be the standard point of measure for intensity (22,59,222). This is used only to set an overall room intensity level for the purposes of comparing animal rooms and does not reflect the actual intensity experienced by the animals.

The light exposure history of individual animals can alter their sensitivity to phototoxicity. At least one study suggests that light intensities that are 130 to 270 lux above the intensity under which the animal was raised may be the point at which retinal damage may begin to occur (294). Young albino and pigmented mice appear to have the ability to reverse some of the retinal damage associated with elevated light intensities (331,341). Current recommendations suggest that a light level of 325 lux (30-foot candles) at 1.0 m (3.4 feet) above the floor is sufficient for routine sanitation while still avoiding significant retinal degeneration in albino animals (22). Other recommendations exist and are based on cage-level lighting intensities but are difficult to assess and administer (201).

The spectral distribution of light as it relates to adverse effects on laboratory animals has not been extensively studied. No artificial light has exactly the same spectrum as sunlight. Some fluorescent bulbs have a much wider spectrum with more output in the ultraviolet and infrared ranges than others. This can be partially compensated for by mixing standard fluorescent fixtures produced by different manufacturers in the same lighting fixture. Because different fluorescent compounds may be used by different manufacturers, this procedure can produce greater spectral diversity than bulbs from a single manufacturer. Overall, there is no definitive evidence to suggest that a wide spectral diversity in artificial lighting provides any direct enhancement of animal health or well being.

Some species of new-world primates are capable of synthesizing certain forms of vitamin D from dietary constituents and sunlight. Because it is common practice to provide enriched diets for these species that contain the appropriate forms of already converted vitamin D, access to full-spectrum artificial sunlight would not appear to be necessary.

A number of practical issues should be considered with respect to lighting in animal facilities. Many of these are covered in recommendations produced by the Illuminating Engineering Society of North American (IESNA) Handbook, which provides practical information on selection and installation of lighting (153,154). It is generally recommended that light bulbs or fixtures have protective covers to ensure the safety of both the animals and animal care staff. Cleaning operations and the use of water in animal husbandry procedures can pose hazards from breakage and electrical shock.

NOISE

There is little doubt that extreme levels of acoustic energy (80–120 decibels of sound pressure) can, under the right circumstances, produce auditory and extra-auditory changes in laboratory animals (18, 92,107,108,224,249,250,251,358). The assessment of sound-related interaction and injury in laboratory animals is complex, as the potential effects of noise on animals not only must take into consideration the intensity of the sound but also the frequency pattern of sound presentation, including rate of onset, duration, and vibration effects (12,59,241,252,255). The hearing range, noise-exposure history, and susceptibility to adverse effects of sound based on species, age, and strain further complicate any analyses (37,145,197,199,266, 284,328). Many diverse effects have been reported in the literature and could pose unwanted variation in any toxicologic study. There are no comparative damage risk criteria for each of the common laboratory animal species, making it difficult to know what sound presentation is harmful (22).

In general, noise-producing animals and animal care activities should be separated from species and activities that do not generate noise (103,222,252,283). This can be done by careful consideration of facility design and operational practices (11,245). Physical barriers such as doors, air locks, and sound-absorbing materials can be useful in minimizing the effect of sound (245). Excessive and unpredictable noise patterns can be minimized through personnel training and the use of alternative practices and equipment in routine animal care duties.

VENTILATION

The purpose of ventilating an animal holding room is to dilute gaseous and particulate contaminants, supply adequate oxygen, remove thermal loads caused by animal respiration, lights, and equipment, adjust the moisture content of room air, and, where appropriate, create static-pressure differentials between adjoining areas (58,222). It is, unfortunately, a common mistake to place heavy reliance on a ventilation system as the primary mechanism to prevent the movement of undesirable microbiological organisms from one location within a room or a facility to another. Other factors, including, movement of personnel between areas, movement of equipment, and transfer of animals within a facility, can quickly overcome any benefits associated with well-controlled ventilation. In theory, high ventilation rates should dilute out particulate and gaseous contaminants including undesirable microorganisms and allergens (104,301,307). Because, it is difficult to control the movement of air within secondary enclosures, viable particulates can easily escape any containment, provided strictly on the basis of ventilation.

As a general rule, air supplied to any secondary or primary enclosure should be free of contaminants and be properly conditioned. HEPA filtration is recommended to provide some assurance that supplied air is free of particulates that could potentially harbor infectious organisms (189). HEPA filters are given efficiency ratings that can exceed 99% for particulate exclusion within certain particle size ranges (5). Average pore diameters of HEPA filters are designed to exclude particulates the size of bacteria or larger but may not be small enough to exclude individual viral particles. Because viruses and other organisms tend to travel on particulates due to their high electrostatic charge, HEPA filters are effective in excluding them. Unfortunately, large volumes of air are processed by HEPA filters, and becasue their efficiency rating is not 100%, a certain amount of infectious particles will pass HEPA filters over time. Given the dilution in the air stream, this small amount of passage may not pose a significant threat in most situations. Moreover, because incoming air is seldom challenged with high concentrations of infectious particles, this deficiency usually is not a problem.

If HEPA filters become wet or excessively laden with particulates, bacteria associated with such particles may grow through the HEPA filters and be discharged on the clean side (77). Clogging of HEPA filters usually is monitored by measuring the static pressure across the HEPA filter. Increases in static pressure indicate that the HEPA filter is becoming laden with particulates and at some predetermined static pressure reading, should be changed.

Correct installation of HEPA filters is critical. If they are incorrectly mounted, untreated air can pass by the HEPA filters, producing the same effect as if they contained a large hole. For this reason, HEPA filters should be tested in place using particulate generation equipment (e.g., DOP testing) (77). It is important that such testing be done on a regular basis and should be thoroughly done when the HEPA filter is first mounted. It is critical that such testing be done by individuals experienced in the intricacies of the testing procedure, as inappropriate testing can fail to reveal difficulties in the mounting or construction of the HEPA filter. HEPA filters should be protected by pre-filters designed to catch the majority of particulates of large to intermediate size. This usually is accomplished by a series of pre-filters of different efficiencies. Such pre-filters should be changed regularly.

Air exhausted from animal holding rooms may or may not be filtered prior to discharge to the environment. In the case of toxicologic research involving hazardous agents, exhaust air usually is filtered using filters that are capable of excluding the material in question from the air stream. If the nature and level of hazard is low enough, dilution with large volumes of air by discharge into combined exhaust or into the environment directly may be sufficient.

Facility design guidelines emphasize the need for regulating air-pressure differentials either within animal holding facilities as a whole or within specialized support facilities, such as surgical, procedural, service, housing, or quarantine areas. In general, areas maintained under negative pressure with respect to adjacent areas are designed to prevent the escape in the air stream of unwanted materials from the area maintained under negative pressure (99,287,288). This would be most appropriate, for example, in an animal holding area being used for quarantining of animals. Conversely, maintenance of an animal holding area under positive pressure with respect to the surrounding areas would be undertaken under those circumstances where animals within the positive pressure area are free of certain microorganisms and whose exposure to particulates from other adjacent areas might increase their risk of contamination. Such positive pressure housing might be used in areas maintaining specific pathogen-free animals or used for surgery. While maintenance of static pressure differentials may pose some advantage with respect to contamination control, it should not be relied on for containment of chemical or infectious agents that could be transferred between areas. Most air handling systems have neither the capacity nor the necessary control mechanisms to maintain pressure differentials when doors, pass-throughs, or other structures are opened even for brief periods (222).

For years the ventilation rate for animal holding rooms and primary enclosures has been an important focus of many recommendations for research animal facilities. The ventilation rate or air exchange rate in the context of animal facilities refers to the number of times the total volume of air in the room is exhausted and resupplied with appropriately conditioned air per unit of time. This often is expressed in air exchanges per hour. Rules of thumb have been developed based on experience and limited data. These guidelines have suggested the air exchange rates of 10–15 changes per hour are generally satisfactory for animal facilities (45,222). Unfortunately, they do not take into account the range of possible heat loads, the type of bedding or frequency of cage cleaning; the species and number and size of animals housed; differences in room dimensions; or the efficiency of air distribution linking the secondary and primary enclosures (192,193, 198,222,355). Given these variables, either under- or overventilation can occur, with resulting problems in heat and odor accumulation (58).

Instead of using general guidelines, such as 10–15 air changes per hour, more recent recommendations suggest that the heat generated by animals be calculated using an average total heat gain formula as developed by the American Society of Heating, Refrigerating and Air Conditioning Engineering (6). Using this, the minimum ventilation required can be calculated from the total cooling load necessary to control heat generated by the animals and other heat sources. This, in turn, will allow determination of ventilation rates.

Additional ventilation capacity may be added as a margin of safety and to address any unusual odor generation (222).

The adequacy with which air is distributed within a room is an important consideration (193). If it is inadequately distributed, heat and water vapor build-up may occur unevenly. The coupling of secondary enclosure to the primary enclosure environments may also vary within the room (354). The use of computational fluid dynamic modeling has revealed that supply and exhaust diffuser placement, as well as type, can have a profound effect on air distribution (136, 137,269). This has important implications not only for the environment of the animals with the resulting effect on studies, but also for researchers and technicians working in the animal room.

The concept of drafts as they relate to human comfort has been explored (192,193). Unfortunately, little work has been done with animals to demonstrate whether or not there are biological consequences or if there is discomfort associated with the detection of movement of air. In the case of small laboratory rodents and rabbits, caging designs, and cage placements are unlikely to allow significant air movement within these enclosures to affect the animals contained therein. The one exception may be individually ventilated cages where high air exchange rates can be produced. Even so, there is no evidence to suggest that harmful effects occur. Similarly, larger species kept in pens, runs, or open cages have not been reported to have any ill effects associated with the detection of air movement.

Current guidelines allow the use of recycled air under certain conditions (222). In general, no less than 50% fresh air should be mixed with recycled air for reuse in animal holding areas. Recycled air must be appropriately conditioned and mixed with sufficient fresh air to control temperature, and humidity and other appropriate conditioning should be applied to remove particulates. Mixing recycled air from different animal holding areas is discouraged (222). Recycling of animal room air or the use of appropriately conditioned air from human use areas for animal rooms can provide energy cost savings and be an adjunct to other energy recovery efforts.

Ventilation should not be used as a substitute for good husbandry practices. Adjusting cage densities and bedding, or cage cleaning frequencies may prove a better solution to odor generation problems than trying to increase the capacity of air handling systems. The conditions within animal holding rooms should be regularly monitored to ensure that the ventilation system is working correctly. Plans should be made for action in the event of conditions that may affect the operation of the air handling system such as power failures, failure of mechanical parts, or failure of air filters.

TEMPERATURE AND HUMIDITY

The maintenance of body temperature within certain critical ranges is essential for animals if they are to maintain normal metabolic and physiologic processes (162,263,337). Thermal regulation has been extensively studied in some species (110,111). Clinically observable effects can occur in unadapted animals that have been exposed to temperatures above 85°F (29.4°C) or below 40°F (4.4°C) that are denied access to shelter or other protective mechanisms (110,162,265,343). Depending on the extent and length of time that the animals are exposed to temperatures outside of these ranges, the effects produced can vary from changes in reproductive ability to loss of life. In general, animals are quite adaptable to temperature changes and use behavioral, morphologic, and physiologic mechanisms to maintain body temperature (106,110,111,121,246,343). Unfortunately, such adaptation takes time and can affect the animal's performance in toxicologic studies.

For the most common laboratory animals, a dry bulb temperature range from 61°F (16°C) to 84°F (29°C) has been suggested as acceptable (222). Within this range, depending on species, clinical effects are unlikely to occur, and experience has shown that there is little likelihood of toxicologic interaction. Of the common laboratory animals, rabbits are generally kept in a somewhat cooler environment because of their dense hair coat. The recommended temperature range for rabbits is 61°F (16°C) to 72°F (22°C) (222). Close control of temperatures within this recommended range may reduce some variation in certain studies. Unfortunately, very close control of temperature is not always possible within animal facilities, and some fluctuation during the course of any 24-hour period is to be expected. It has also been demonstrated that temperature will stratify within an animal room, especially one containing many cages. Temperature fluctuations of 2°F to 6°F within any given animal room as measured from the floor to the ceiling are not uncommon (26,27). This is another reason that rotation of cages within any given animal room may be valuable. Variables such as cage construction, population density, the use of filter tops, and animal activity can also cause variations in temperature and humidity between the cage, the room, and between cages (4,27,234,295,298,354).

Some means of regularly assessing the temperature within individual animal holding rooms should be used. Most commonly, temperature sensors placed in the return air ducts or mounted at a height of approximately 5 feet off the floor near the door are used to monitor room temperature.

In addition to temperature, humidity may add additional stress to animals and can affect an animal's ability to efficiently lose heat. Many animals, such as rats, mice, dogs, and certain domestic farm animals, cannot sweat and as such cannot take advantage of evaporative cooling (26,337). These animals must use insensible heat loss through the respiratory track or alterations in blood supply to heat radiating structures, such as the tail, soles of the feet, and tips of the ears to dissipate excess heat or to protect against excessive heat loss (110,111). Some animals, such as dogs, can increase the frequency of their respiration (panting) to further lose heat. If the humidity in the environment is high, evaporative heat loss through insensible means is decreased and internal temperatures build. At very low humidities there is significant, insensible water loss that must be compensated for in order to maintain adequate fluid balance. Within recommended temperature ranges, however, the effects of relative humidity appear to be minimal. There is some human epidemiological evidence relating low relative humidity to increased susceptibility to certain respiratory diseases (16). Unfortunately, convincing evidence relating humidity to respiratory disease in animals is not available.

In rodents, low relative humidity has been suggested to cause ringtail (an annular notching of the tail that can lead to necrosis) in young rats and mice. Studies conducted on this condition indicate that it occurs at a high environmental temperature (81°F) with a low relative humidity (less than 30°) (93,235,314). While possible, these conditions are unlikely to occur under most laboratory animal housing conditions. Moreover, in those studies that have been reported, a variety of other factors, including diet and caging type, can effectively eliminate the condition (93,235). When the condition is seen, there generally are very few animals affected and often there is no correlation to relative humidity.

The concept of thermal neutrality as a desirable state in which to maintain animals on study has been explored (35,336). In theory, a temperature or temperature range exists for any given animal species in which oxygen consumption is minimal and no energy is expended to heat or cool the animal in order to maintain a constant body temperature. Ambient temperatures above the range result in increases in metabolism, physiologic alterations, and behavioral changes that favor heat loss. Conversely, temperatures below the range result in adjustments in the same systems designed to produce or conserve heat. Ambient temperatures outside of the thermal neutral zone can result in observable changes, such as alternations in feed consumption, activity, reproduction, and growth. When coupled with relative humidity, climatograms can be constructed in which it is presumed that animals are most comfortable (336). In practice, such optimal conditions are hard to determine for various species of animals, and there is evidence that climatograms may vary significantly with age, reproduction, and other factors (336).

BEDDING

Although many toxicologic studies are conducted on animals housed on suspended wire flooring with no contact bedding, there is increased use of contact bedding for many studies. This is due principally to the increase in bioexclusion housing that uses cage level containment. Even in the case of animals housed on suspended wire flooring, bedding often is placed below the flooring to absorb the moisture from urine and feces. Bedding can influence experimental data and animal well being (41,239,253,254,312).

Bedding is constructed of natural products, most commonly wood, paper, or corncobs. No bedding is ideal for all occasions and all species, but must be chosen based upon its characteristics. There have been a number of descriptions of the desirable characteristics of different types of bedding, as well as methods for evaluating various bedding types based upon these characteristics (27,149,169,261,309,335). Of all the characteristics of bedding, absorbency would seem to be the most important. It is the purpose of bedding to absorb moisture to keep the environment dry and thereby minimize the growth of microorganisms that would otherwise flourish on the organic material and moisture within the cage. Moreover, by diluting feces and urine with bedding, the animals within the cage have less contact with excreta and hence have less chance of being soiled by it.

Wood products, although probably the most common form of bedding, are not the most absorbent, with their absorbency being directly related to their total surface area. The finer the wood product bedding, the more surface area and hence the more moisture it can retain. Paper product bedding, unlike wood product, tends to absorb large amounts of water directly into the material, which cause it to swell. The absorbency of paper product bedding can be much greater than wood product bedding. Unfortunately, some forms of paper product bedding lose their structural integrity when wet, making them difficult to manipulate, which can be a problem if used under suspended catch pans. To address this, some types of paper product bedding have a thin plastic backing, which makes them easier to remove from catch pans.

Another important factor with respect to bedding is its potential for introducing contaminants. Wood product bedding is obtained as a waste product from the milling of lumber. Wood chip bedding is composed of the small wood chips produced by sawing lumber with coarse saws. Prior to processing, it may contain a range of chip sizes, including very coarse and very fine materials, such as saw dust. Wood from which bedding is produced may come from a variety of locations with different histories of exposure to compounds and microorganisms. Raw wood chips are processed by first screening out large debris and then heating them to a temperature of 140°F to 150°F in an air convection furnace for approximately 20 minutes. This dries the product, which reduces bacterial contamination and the potential for growth, and also drives off volatile oils. The wood chip bedding is then run through a series of screens to develop products of varying sizes. After being screened, it is placed in bags and made available for animal housing.

Wood shavings are the product of planing kiln-dried lumber. Lumber is dried in large ovens maintained at a temperature of 140°F for periods of up to 14 days. The lumber is then run through shaping planes that produce shavings. These shavings are then bagged and used for bedding.

Both hardwood and softwood bedding are available as processed products. Storage conditions for these products are critical to preventing contamination. Certain softwoods, such as cedar, are no longer used for bedding for laboratory animals, with their use being relegated primarily to bedding for pets. Studies using softwood bedding have shown that volatile oils in them have the ability to induce liver microsomal enzymes, which can alter drug metabolism (56,86,320,321,322,324,334) and increase the incidence of neoplasia (146,323). Softwood bedding that is kiln dried and hardwood bedding are both much less likely to produce hepatic microsomal effects, as essential oils associated with these inductive effects are driven off in the drying process. Hardwood beddings have not been shown to induce liver microsomal enzymes but may have other effects (309). If autoclaving or other heat treatments are applied to the bedding after receipt, the chance of essential oils producing any inductive effect are even further reduced (70,260). In general, any such induction takes 3 or more days to occur and is rapidly lost when animals are removed from bedding materials, such as unprocessed cedar.

Paper bedding can come in a variety of shapes and sizes. Flat cardboard-like sheets, as well as plastic-backed absorbent pads, are commonly used in bedding trays under suspended wire cages. Paper chips and shredded paper products that may be bleached or unbleached provide a highly absorbent, contaminant-free contact bedding. Recently, compressed pads of paper that are cut to the size of individual cages have been introduced. These materials can come presterilized and are inserted into the cage at changing. When placed in the cages bedded with this material, animals scratch up the paper product into a loose bedding that is highly absorbent. This activity by the animals is considered by some to be a form of psychological enrichment. Similarly, the ability to burrow in contact bedding is also considered to be beneficial to some rodents.

Corn cob bedding is produced from coarsely ground corn cobs that have been heat treated. Their absorbency is similar to wood product bedding. The bedding itself is of irregular shape, is not easily compressed, and retains its structure when wet. There has been little indication that this bedding can cause significant research interactions; however, it is not widely used (259).

Larger animals, such as swine, dogs, cats, and other species, may also benefit from the use of contact bedding. In general, the use of such bedding is designed primarily to aid in cleaning of the cages, however, in the case of swine, it may assist in providing for their natural routing behavior.

A number of problems have been associated with varying types of bedding. Nude mice and SKH-1 mice that do not have eyelashes have a tendency to collect debris under their eyelids. This effect is less noticeable with screened wood product bedding; however, paper product bedding appears to release many more fines that are capable of lodging under the eyelids and causing swelling, and in the presence of the right microorganism, produce abscesses. Corn cob bedding seems to be similar to wood product bedding in this regard.

The ingestion of bedding can be problematic for newborn animals. If the particles are too small or do not easily pass the GI tract, newborn animals can ingest the bedding and develop fatal gastrointestinal tract obstructions.

It is important to periodically assess bedding materials for the presence of toxic and carcinogenic materials. Whereas some of these materials may be driven off during the processing of the bedding, others may be more stable.

Bedding, especially contact bedding, needs to be changed frequently based on a variety of factors, including the wetness of the bedding, the amount of feces present, the number of animals in the cage, and a variety of other factors. In the case of large animals or group-housed animals, bedding change often is required several times a week. Smaller animals or individually-housed animals may require less frequent bedding change. Failure to change the bedding and replace it with new bedding can result not only in an unhealthful environment, but can also increase the concentration of materials excreted in the feces and urine within the animal's environment, making ingestion or inhalation much more likely. There is also evidence that a soiled environment may also affect liver metabolism, which could interfere with toxicologic research (322).

WATER

Access to a sufficient quantity of clean, potable water is essential for normal hydration of the animal and for the maintenance of normal physiologic and metabolic processes. Water consumption and drinking patterns of laboratory animals vary with the species (311). Water supplied to toxicologic laboratories may be either from municipal sources or from privately owned wells. In either case, the potential exists for contaminants to be introduced into animal holding facilities or for significant variation to occur in water quality over time.

To address this problem, animal facility drinking water, as well as water used for other husbandry tasks, is treated in order to adjust chemical and biologic characteristics. Water treatments may include one or more of the following: filtration, ion exchange, ultraviolet (UV) disinfection, halogenation (chlorination or iodination), reverse osmosis, or ozonization. At the local or room level, water may be acidified using mineral acids. Acidification usually is reserved for treatment of water used in water bottles although it is occasionally used in automatic drinking water systems.

Water filtration can be done using either depth or membrane filters. Depth filters are used for coarse filtration and involve passage of water through a coarse medium, such as sand. Finer filtration, down to 0.1 μm, can be obtained using a series of membrane filters often constructed out of paper or synthetic materials. These filters are only reliable for removing nonviable particulates, as many bacteria that collect on such filters can grow through them. If membrane filters are to be used for bacterial filtration, some regular means of disinfecting the filters must be employed. Some chemical components in water, such as suspended gases and certain organic compounds, can be removed by charcoal filters. These filters consist of canisters of activated charcoal that have varying degrees of retentivity for different compounds. These filters must be changed regularly and suffer from similar problems with respect to microbiological growth as membrane filters. Ion exchange resins can be used to remove inorganic compounds but offer no biological treatment.

Often, reverse osmosis is applied to animal water supplies. This treatment involves placing water under pressure on one side of a membrane that is designed to exclude all but a few types of molecules and collecting the water that passes through the membrane in an area of lower pressure on the opposite side of the membrane. To be effective in animal facilities, the capacity of the reverse osmosis equipment must be large enough to accommodate the necessary water usage. This entails either many such units or very large units. Water produced by reverse osmosis is devoid of all minerals and hence is chemically very aggressive to surfaces. Over time, water treated by reserve osmosis can recapture metal from stainless steel surfaces and other materials. Because the reverse osmosis process depends on an intact membrane, absolute bacteriologic or viral exclusion is only possible if there are no deficits in the membrane that might allow untreated water to pass through. Although water produced by reverse osmosis, in theory, should be free of microorganisms, in practice this is not always the case.

UV disinfection is a common and rapid means of killing a variety of microorganisms that might be found in water supplies. Because the process involves the exposure of water to UV light, the water must be reasonably free of minerals so that deposits do not form inside the exposure chambers. Moreover, light intensities of UV-producing fixtures decrease over time, and hence the effectiveness of the process. For this reason, regular measurements of the irradiance level of the light source, as well as regular replacement of the light source, must be done.

Halogenation, most commonly chlorination, is a relatively simple but effective means of disinfecting water supplies (133). Chlorine is effective against a wide range of microorganisms (21). Depending on the chlorine species being measured, ranges of effective concentrations have been established that will not adversely affect animals but still accomplished disinfection. It is important to realize that a certain minimum contact time is required for the chlorine or any chemical disinfectant to be effective. For this reason, chlorination usually is done centrally with the treated water being held in a contact tank for a period of several minutes to several hours in order to ensure adequate disinfection.

Depending on the form of chlorine being used, the chlorine reacts in variable fashion with organic materials present in the water, causing the generation of halogenated organic compounds (225). The importance and the likelihood of such occurrence is difficult to assess. It should be noted, however, that chlorine-based compounds are the most commonly used disinfectants for water and for husbandry practices in animal facilities, as well as for the treatment of drinking water for humans. The use of chlorine to disinfect drinking water has an important advantage over filtration and reverse osmosis methods in that it provides residual disinfection within watering systems. This prevents build up of bacteria in the watering systems as the result of back flow into water bottles or automatic watering devices of saliva and feed debris during drinking.

Ozonization is another means of assuring microbiological decontamination of water supplies and the destruction of dissolved organic compounds in the water. Such systems use an ozone generator to produce ozone gas and bubble it into a water contact tank. Contact periods of less than 90 seconds are required in order to adequately sterilize water. The resulting water is highly aggressive to pipes and surfaces, requiring that the ozone be broken down into less aggressive oxygen-containing compounds. This is done either by exposure to UV light or by the addition of chlorine-containing compounds (sometimes both). Water that has been ozonated is devoid of any residual disinfection capacity and hence must be treated with halogen-containing compounds (e.g., chlorine) in order to have residual disinfection capabilities.

Acidification of drinking water was first used to control the growth of pseudomonas in the drinking water in water bottles used for mice that had been irradiated (94,184, 187). Water of a low pH (acidic) is bacteriostatic to certain vegetative forms of some bacteria. To be most effective, acidification should be at pH 2.3 or lower (127). Usually this is done with mineral acids; however, such acids have little buffering capacity, and hence the addition of saliva or other alkaline containing compounds may rapidly increase the pH of the drinking water.

The use of acidification, as well as other forms of water treatment, are not without potential research effects (91,119). Any water treatment should be considered an experimental variable and should be well-understood by the toxicologist (58,127). Usually it is necessary to group together a number of different water treatments in order to provide a water system that is capable of not only adjusting the chemical composition of the water, but also to ensure that it is free from harmful microorganisms.

FEED

Feed is considered by some to be one of the principal uncontrolled variables in toxicology today. Many textbooks and articles, as well as guidelines, have been written on nutrition for laboratory animals (209,210, 211, 212,213,214,215,216,217,218,220,221,230,226). There are numerous examples of how diet composition or administration can affect the outcome of toxicological research either directly or indirectly (30,57,144,227, 232,237,292,340). There also are examples of individual nutrients either in excess or deficiency producing a wide range of metabolic, morphologic, or physiologic conditions that have influenced the outcome of studies (8,44,229,231,330). It is not the purpose of this review to cover all of these. The reader is encouraged to pursue such information from available texts, reports, and journal articles, as well as seek the advice of those skilled in laboratory animal nutrition for specific recommendations. Subcommittees of the National Research Council's Committee on Animal Nutrition have published reviews of the nutrient requirements of laboratory animals that can be used as a guide in assessing the adequacy of specific formulations (209,210,211, 212,213,214,215,216,217,218, 220,221).

Feed provided to laboratory animals should be palatable, nutritionally complete, and free of contaminants unless the lowering or removal of a nutrient or the addition of other compounds is required by the study design. The feed should be provided in sufficient quantity and be of the necessary quality to assure normal growth and provide for the overall health of the animal (46,222). Increased demands of reproduction and lactation may require slightly different feed formulations. Many commercially available diets are calorie dense, protein rich, and often are fed ad libitum. Such practices encourage feed wastage and may adversely affect some toxicology studies (159).

The physical and taste characteristics of laboratory animal feed can be important variables in study design. Some common laboratory animal species, such as nonhuman primates, guinea pigs, and rabbits, have well-developed taste and dietary consistency preferences. Guinea pigs, for example, do not easily accept changes in the texture of the diet or in its taste. These animals may need to be habituated to changes in diet by gradual introduction of the new diet during the course of feeding a previously accepted diet. This can prove challenging when artificial diets need to be substituted for natural ingredient diets.

Laboratory animal feeds can be classified as natural ingredient diets, semipurified (or purified) diets, or chemically defined diets (273). These classifications are based on the ingredients used to construct the feed. Natural ingredient diets are composed of unprocessed or crudely processed materials, such as cereal grains, milk products, and animal product meals, such as fishmeal or meatmeal. Semi-purified diets (also referred to as synthetic, semi-synthetic, and purified) are constructed of processed ingredients that are refined so as to be uniform in content. Examples of such ingredients include casein, dextran, soy protein, hemicellulose, and fats, such as corn oil. Chemically defined diets are composed of chemically pure compounds, including specific amino acids, fatty acids, inorganic salts, vitamins, and sugars, such as glucose and fructose (351).

Natural ingredient diets can be pelletized (extruded), expanded (baked), or processed as a meal (powdered). They can also be suspended in agar or other types of hydrocolloids, providing both feed and a source of water. Semi-purified and chemically defined diets are provided in either a powdered or liquid form. Experimental compounds can be incorporated in any of these physical forms, but as a rule are usually fed as a gel or in liquid or powdered form.

The exact formulation of specific feeds may or may not be available to the toxicologist. Open-formula diets are diets that are manufactured to published specifications based on quantities of specific ingredients (165,166). The quantitative and often qualitative ingredient compositions of open-formula diets are readily available from the manufacturer. Open-formula diets usually are made from natural ingredients, and as such may easily suffer from variability due to differences in source of ingredient supply, harvest times, and storage conditions (234). Detailed ingredient analysis prior to manufacture in both open- and closed-formula diets is seldom done, and when analysis is conducted, it usually is done for only a few key constituents. For this reason, open-formula diets can still exhibit significant variability between suppliers and within any given supplier.

Closed-formula diets are those manufactured by feed companies who hold the exact composition of the diet in terms of the quantities of specific ingredients as proprietary information. They will provide a list of the ingredients used and usually will provide a calculated analysis. Closed-formula diets are often less costly than open-formula diets, as the manufacturer can adjust the formula periodically, based on the availability and costs of various ingredients. It must be remembered that like open-formula diets, closed-formula diets may have variable nutrient levels. The calculated analysis on such products is not the same as a laboratory analysis of an individual batch of closed-formula diet.

Recently, the concept of constant nutrition or variable-ingredient diets has been introduced. This is a natural extension of closed-formula diets in that the manufacturer is allowed to select the type and quantity of various natural product ingredients to be used in a diet formulation based on availability and cost. The maximum percentage that any given ingredient can constitute in the diet is limited by published specifications; however, the final product must have analyzed nutrient levels that fall within prescribed ranges. Generally, constant nutrition diets are coupled with regular analysis by the manufacturer of the product for an extensive list of nutrients in order to assure that the product provides the specified levels of such nutrients as set forth in the diet specifications. Given the inherent variability with both open- and closed-formula diets, as well as the lack of regular laboratory analysis for specific nutrients in such diets, constant nutrition diets provide a means for standardizing diets between locations as well as suppliers.

Certain basic analyses are required for interstate shipment of dietary ingredients in the United States. Analyses for up to five constituents, including protein, are made, and certain minimal levels based on the guaranteed analysis stated on the feed container must be met (17). It is important to realize that the actual level of these nutrients is not guaranteed, only that the level is not less than that listed. Similarly, diets can be certified with respect to levels of certain toxic and carcinogenic compounds. This process involves holding in a secured location a batch of feed from which samples are taken for analysis of 15 or more toxic or carcinogenic compounds. The analysis for that particular lot of feed is used to certify the diet as containing specific levels of these compounds which may interfere with some toxicologic research (80,100,227,230,296,350). Certification of feed does not imply a laboratory analysis for specific nutrients, only that the material does not contain more than a stated level of certain compounds as determined by the analyses. Hence, a certified diet could be deficient in nutrients and yet still be certified (57,117,228,267,352,353).

For convenience in feeding and to minimize wastage, diets often are pelletized (97). During this process, the diets are briefly exposed to temperatures exceeding 60°C. The process of pelletizing diets is one of compression and extrusion. The amount of time that the pellet is exposed to elevated temperatures is very brief, and hence there is no assurance that vegetative or nonnegative forms of bacteria or other microorganisms are consistently killed.

Expanded diets undergo a process of prolonged mixing and heating with added liquid in a manner similar to mixing a cake batter. This material is mixed with air and expanded through a die into pellets that are dried with heated air. This process forms a much harder and durable product. The process also exposes the mixture to temperatures in excess of 100°C for periods of 15 minutes or more. This causes some reduction in microorganisms; however, the product itself is not sterile. Contamination can occur in both pelletized and expanded diets after processing. Expanded diets have a lower specific gravity, and hence a lower caloric density than pelletized or powered diets of equal volume. Hence, to obtain the same caloric intake, animals will consume greater volumes of an expanded diet.

A number of applications in toxicological research require the decontamination or sterilization of feed (204). If true reductions in bacteria and viruses are to be achieved in feed products, feed can be treated by application of steam under pressure (autoclaving), dry heat, or irradiation. Heat applied in these processes can destroy certain labile ingredients within the diets (62,96,242). Irradiation produces very little elevation in temperature and hence is less likely to require additional fortification if sterilization is contemplated (66,356).

Any process used to sterilize feed must be calibrated and carefully controlled. Minor items, such as variation in stacking patterns of bags of feed within an autoclave or the magnitude and number of vacuum pulses, can yield significant differences in the total reduction of microorganisms during the autoclaving process (222). Equipment used for such feed treatment must be regularly calibrated. The use of indictor tapes or other sterilization indicators in a single spot does not assure the adequacy of the process. Moreover, cycles designed for pelletized feed seldom are effective in processing powdered feed or other forms of diet.

When irradiation is used, it is important to specify dosages based on the minimum dosage received throughout the entire load or container. Once an item has been treated, it should be labeled as to the date of treatment so that judgments can be made as to the appropriate time in which the product should be used. Feed should be sealed in durable and preferably water-resistant packaging prior to irradiation.

With or without heat or radiation treatment, certain liable components within diets will degrade over time (102,242). Diet manufacturers place milling dates on containers of diet using either sequential dating codes or Julian dating. As a general rule, natural ingredient, dry laboratory–animal diets that have been stored properly can be used for 180 days after manufacture (222). Some diets that contain supplemental vitamin C or other very labile ingredients should be used in approximately 3 months from milling unless special stabilized forms of these especially labile nutrients are added to extend the shelf life (222). Supplemental vitamins and other labile ingredients can be provided separately through the use of drinking water supplements, sprayed on dietary additives, or in the case of nonhuman primates and certain other species, by the feeding of fruits and vegetables.

Feeding can also be used as part of a psychological enrichment program for certain species of animals. In the case of nonhuman primates, specialized feeders, the use of a variety of different types of food items, and the presentation of feed in a way that foraging is required can all be used to stimulate these animals and reinforce natural behaviors. For the purposes of toxicologic research, maintaining constancy in a diet is important. Varying the diet with a wide selection of unbalanced foods, as might occur through nonstructured supplementation of diets, can cause health-related problems (195). It is also important to minimize abrupt changes in diet because in many species these can lead to digestive and metabolic disturbances.

The storage of feed and other dietary ingredients should be done in areas that are regularly cleaned and enclosed to prevent entry of pests. In general, feed should be stored off of the floor and care should be taken to prevent exposure of these items to temperatures above 70°F for prolonged periods of time (102,228,272). Containers used to hold loose feed should be covered and constructed of materials that prevent the entrance of vermin and other pests.

The presentation of feed to animals is another important variable. With few exceptions, feed should be administered to animals in feeders that allow easy access to the feed while minimizing the possibility of contamination with feces or urine. Feeders should also minimize wastage, which is particularly important with powdered diets. The size and number of openings in feeders, as well as the location of the feeder, can affect the animals' consumption of feed. Some designs of feeders can actually restrict an animal's access to the feed, resulting in caloric restriction.

Dogs, cats, nonhuman primates, and certain other species are commonly "meal" fed such that feed is provided one to three times a day in limited quantities (178). Rodents are more commonly fed *ad libitum*. Feed consumption can be influenced by the light cycle, with some species preferring to consume more feed in the dark part of the light cycle than others. Rodents consume feed both in the light and dark portions of the light cycle, with more feed being consumed during the dark part of the cycle than the light. Poultry consume feed primarily during the light cycle, as do many other nonrodent species.

Hamsters characteristically horde feed, and for that reason will tend to remove feed from feeders in order to form feed piles on the floor. To minimize injury associated with this behavior, hamsters are commonly fed off of the floor when pelletized diets are used (122). The ready availability of a water source is also important in feeding behavior for many animals. Many species eat and drink at the same time.

Of all the variables associated with feed, perhaps that which has the greatest impact on toxicologic studies, other than outright nutritional deficiency, is overfeeding (159). Animals will consume feed until an internal caloric limit is reached. The imposition of mild to moderate caloric restriction in all species, including rodents, can increase longevity, postpone the development of spontaneously occurring neoplasms, decrease the incidence of background lesions in the kidneys, cardiovascular, and endocrine systems, and cause other changes that in aggregate can produce a more consistent model for toxicologic research (3,23,24,52,53,183,319). To adequately interpret data from long-term studies on animals using caloric restriction, other primary studies, including range-finding studies for dosages, need to be conducted in calorically restricted animals.

Caloric restriction or limited feeding is not a new concept (225,226,227,274,302,303,304,305,306,317). The effects produced by this procedure have been recognized for decades (63,150,182). A number of publications have reviewed various segments of this relatively large body of literature (123,124,156,157,158,357). The phenomena appears to be closely correlated with total calories and not with specific nutrient concentrations, such as protein levels (170). The technique appears to be most easily applied to those studies in which compounds are administered by gavage; however, there is little reason to believe that it could not be applied to studies in which the compound was administered by other routes. Errors associated with administering compounds incorporated into the diet and administered under a caloric restriction regimen may not pose any greater error than those associated with similar administration using *ad lib* feeding, which assumes a consistent intake on a daily basis and a consistent level of wastage.

The usefulness of caloric restriction in group-housed animals, however, still needs to be explored (55). It has been assumed that any dominance hierarchy established within a group would lead to significant differences in diet consumption between members of the group with, perhaps, the introduction of unwanted variation, however, any such dominance hierarchy that already exists within the group will still result in variation even when feed is available *ad libitum*. This problem could be further magnified if one or more members of the group died during the course of a study. The interaction of group size, sex, and caloric restriction still needs additional investigation.

The decision of the toxicologist to use caloric restriction as a means of decreasing the variability encountered in product registration studies using rodents must be based on a careful examination of the literature and a dialogue with regulatory authorities. Caloric restriction in rodents is used by a growing number of pharmaceutical companies and has gained acceptance by regulatory bodies, provided that adequate control data are provided.

HEALTH AND HEALTH MONITORING

Animals used in toxicologic research come from several different categories of sources. A limited number of animals are occasionally obtained from either wild populations or open colonies in which there is little attempt to control the introduction of adventitious organisms. Such conventional or random source animals have the potential for significant interindividual variability with respect to health status.

A second-source classification are closed colonies of animals in which the introduction of new animals is minimized or eliminated and certain control measures are put in place either by means of vaccination, antimicrobial therapy, or anthelminthic treatment to control and, in some cases, eliminate a limited number of microorganisms. Interindividual variability in health profiles may still exist; however, the maintenance of these control measures at the toxicology laboratory can provide some assurance that certain organisms have been eliminated.

The last source classification of animals are animals from colonies that have originated through procedures designed to totally eliminate unwanted microorganisms and parasites, usually caesarean section or embryo transfer. These animals are maintained within bioexclusion systems, such as barrier production facilities, that are designed to prevent contamination with species-specific pathogens and, in the case of some bioexclusion systems, even common opportunistic organisms that could pose unwanted research interference (315).

The availability of any species in any one of these source categories may be limited or even nonexistent. Larger domestic animals, such as dogs, cats, and farm animals, and nondomestic animals, such as nonhuman primates, generally are not available in a highly defined microbiological status. Health programs designed to control or improve the health status of these animals will not eliminate the possibility of species-specific or opportunistic disease that may interfere with toxicologic research using these animals.

Health monitoring programs for nonbarrier-maintained or random source animals depend heavily upon a comprehensive initial quarantine and screening process that is supplemented by individual and/or colony health data available from the supplier (84,85). Some organisms that are seldom found in barrier-reared animals are not uncommon in many research facilities (147). Routine vaccination and anthelmintic therapy, as well as the application of antimicrobial agents, may all be used to control or eliminate undesirable organisms. The toxicologist must be aware that during the course of a study, individual animals may develop clinical illness or may exhibit individual variation as a result of underlining infectious processes. The frequency of such occurrences cannot be predicted, and allowances must be made for this in the study design when using such animals.

To minimize the impact of health issues on toxicologic research, each institution must develop an institutional philosophy with respect to the impact of certain organisms in their research animals. Not all organisms have a significant impact on research, and those that do may not interfere with certain types of research. Simplistically, organisms can be divided in terms of their relative importance and the amount of peer-reviewed information available to support their impact on research (Figure 16.1).

A number of reviews of microorganisms affecting laboratory animals have been assembled (29,205, 206,120,247). Unfortunately there is no universally accepted list of organisms that should be excluded from all animals under all circumstances. Many adventitious organisms do not cause clinical disease. Instead they cause subclinical infections that do not produce histologic changes associated with their presence. In some cases they may have only limited or subtle research effects that are self-limiting and cease after protective antibodies are formed (344). In a few instances more significant effects occur only when the organism is first introduced into a naïve population (epizootic phase of infection). After the organism becomes established and protective antibodies are present either through maternal transfer or the development of a controlled infection, clinical signs or research effects may disappear. Often, agents that are commonly recommended to be screened for have been selected on a historical basis rather than through an analysis of their potential to cause effects or the prevalence of the organism.

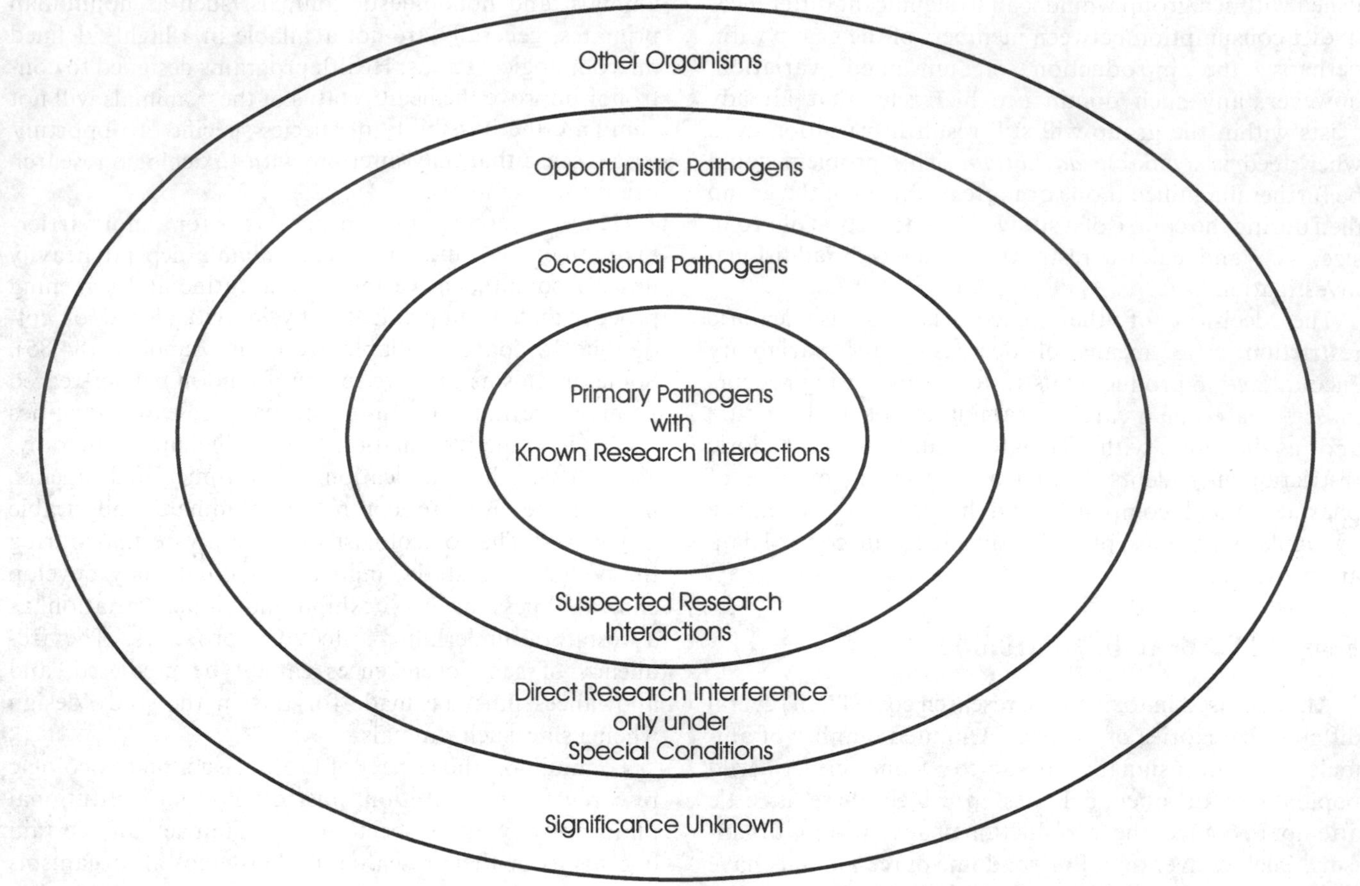

FIG. 16.1. Classification of organisms by their significance and impact on research.

Suppliers of barrier-produced animals have developed exclusionary lists of organisms that define the status of the animals that they produce. These exclusionary lists set forth microorganisms that are to be screened for on a regular basis and whose presence is deemed to be a cause for the supplier to eliminate that colony of animals from production. In some cases, an additional group of opportunistic microorganisms may be screened for by suppliers to document the presence of these organisms in the event that they might interfere with certain types of research. These opportunistic organisms may have little potential to cause research interaction and are not a cause to eliminate colonies. These organisms may be common human or environmental commensals that can only be excluded by very specialized bioexclusion housing techniques that may be impractical in the toxicologic research environment.

Animals free of one or more specified microorganisms are termed *specific pathogen free* (SPF) (206). There is no universal definition of SPF with respect to what organisms are to be excluded from each common laboratory species. Proprietary terms or abbreviations may be used to designate a particular supplier's or research institution's definition of SPF.

In developing an institutional health standard for laboratory animals to be used in toxicologic research, the advice of a competent veterinary professional with experience in laboratory animal medicine science should be sought. Decisions on which organisms to exclude and to test for will need to be based on the nature of the research being conducted, species being utilized, a realistic assessment of the facilities and equipment available for maintaining animals, and a thorough review of peer-reviewed literature with respect to the disease-causing potential, host range, and research interactions posed by specific microorganisms. Table 16.2 lists a number of organisms that may infect common laboratory animal species. This table includes species-specific organisms and some common environmental and human commensals whose exclusion might require extraordinary efforts although their presence may have little research impact; however, such opportunistic organisms may be considered for inclusion in the screening program if their presence would need to be documented in order to help

Table 16.2
Organisms capable of infecting laboratory rodents[a]

	Mice	Rats	Guinea Pigs	Hamsters
Sendai virus	X	X	X[b]	X
Pneumonia virus of mice	X	X	X	X
Mouse hepatitis virus	X			
Minute virus of mice	X			
GD-VII[c]	X			
Reo-3 virus	X	X	X	X
Epizootic diarrhea of infant mice	X			
Lymphocytic chroiomeningitis virus	X	X	X	X
Polyoma virus	X			
Mouse cytomegalovirus	X			
Ectromelia virus	X			
Mouse parvovirus	X			
K virus	X			
Mouse thymic virus	X			
Hanta viruses	X	X		
Sialodacryoadenitis virus		X		
Rat coronavirus		X		
Rat parvovirus		X		
Kilham rat virus		X		
H-1 virus		X		
Mouse adenovirus	X	X		
Guinea pig adenovirus			X	
Cilia associated respiratory bacillus	X	X		
Bordetella bronchiseptica	X	X	X	X
Citrobacter Freundii 4248	X			
Corynebacterium kutscheri	X	X	X	X
Salmonella spp.	X	X	X	X
Mycoplasma pulmonis	X	X	X	X
Mycoplasma spp.		X		
Streptobacillus moniliformis	X	X		
Helicobacter hepaticus	X	X		
Helicobacter bilis	X	X		
Helicobacter spp.	X	X	X	X
Klebsiella oxytoca	X	X	X	X
Klebsiella pneumoniae	X	X	X	X
Pasteurella pneumotropica	X	X	X	X
Pasteurella multocida	X	X	X	X
Pasteurella spp.	X	X	X	X
Pseudomonas aeruginosa	X	X	X	X
Pseudomonas spp.	X	X	X	X
Staphylococcus aureus	X	X	X	X
Streptococcus pneumoniae	X	X	X	X
β Hemolytic Streptococcus spp.	X	X	X	X
Streptococcus spp.	X	X	X	X
Streptococcus zooepidemicus			X	
Encephalitozooan cuniculi	X	X	X	X

[a] Infection does not imply disease or interference with research results.
[b] Also referred to as Theiler's Murine Encephalomyelitis Virus
[c] Probably is not really infected with this virus; can acquire other Parainfluenza viruses that cross-react serologically.

explain unexpected variation in certain specialized studies (84). It is unrealistic for most toxicologic research facilities, however, to set as a goal the exclusion of all the organisms on this list, as the likelihood of long-term success, unless extraordinary measures are used, is quite low (344).

No matter what institutional exclusionary list is decided upon, each organism on the list should have documentation in the peer-reviewed literature to support its inclusion. Moreover, in developing an exclusionary list, consideration should be given to the formulation of a plan to address the potential discovery of positive findings in research populations within the institution. Development of an exclusionary list presumes that some method is available to limit the spread of the organism if it gains entrance into the facility and that some course of action, such as elimination of infected animals or the imposition of some form of control measures, such as drug therapy, will be used to eliminate it (344). Because the toxicologist will be impacted by the health and health monitoring program at the institution, it is important that he/she participate in the formulation of that program.

There are a number of microorganisms that can be carried by animals that have health implications for man. Zoonotic organisms that can be transmitted from animals to man are often included in the screening and control processes that are part of the health program for laboratory animals. Many of these organisms, such as herpes B virus (nonhuman primates), *Salmonella*, *Shigella*, Hantaan virus, and Lymphocytic Choriomeningitis virus, may be included in screening programs not because of their possible research effects, but because of their ability to cause disease in people who work with the animals (101,138,289).

Health monitoring programs require consideration of sample size and frequency; the type, availability, sensitivity, and specificity of assays for various microorganisms; biological characteristics of the microorganisms; sampling procedures and preparation; and the interpretation of results. Discussions of these subjects are beyond the scope of this review but are available elsewhere (10,75,84,85,176,293,325,342). In light of all of these considerations, as well as the limitations of the health monitoring techniques currently available, it is imperative that no single set of results be used to make a determination of the health status of any group of animals used in toxicologic research. Any positive findings should be confirmed with alternative tests or additional samples. False-positive and false-negative results do, in fact, occur, and drastic actions taken without confirmatory data can cause irreparable damage to ongoing studies (342).

Special problems are imposed when immunocompromised animals are used in pharmacological research. The very property that makes these animals unique (i.e., defects in their immune system) makes them susceptible to many organisms that would not be of concern to animals with an intact immune system. Manipulation of these animals requires the use of aseptic technique and rigorous attention to detail to assure that they are not exposed to even common opportunistic organisms that could set up life-threatening infections or cause research interactions. Health monitoring programs for these animals often require the use of immunocompetent sentinel animals that are housed either on soiled bedding obtained from the immunocompromised animals or in direct contact with the animals themselves (73,310,342). Such animals must be obtained from suppliers in a microbiologically defined status that limits the microorganisms to which the animals are exposed to a small number of commensals that have no disease-causing capacity or research implications. Maintenance of these animals requires very special bioexclusion housing practices and modification of research techniques.

The collection of background data can be incorporated into the health monitoring program. In addition to documenting the presence or absence of various microorganisms, samples may also be collected for histopathology, clinical chemistry, and hematology using representative animals obtained from the same populations as the animals participating in the study.

In some instances it may be necessary to eliminate one or more microorganisms from a group of animals in order to make it acceptable for introduction into a toxicologic research facility if alternatives to the use of these animals are not available. This process is referred to as rederivation and can be accomplished either by caesarean section with cross-fostering of young onto lactating females of the correct microbiological status or by hand rearing the young using the appropriate milk substitute. As an alternative, embryos collected from donor females can be transferred, after washing, to recipient mothers of the appropriate health status. Both of these techniques require considerable technical skill and extensive health monitoring after the procedures to assure that the appropriate health status of the rederived animals has been obtained. Each technique has advantages and disadvantages. Both of these procedures are expensive and time consuming, especially if they are to be applied to outbred animals that require relatively large founding populations.

In the case of a few viral agents, cessation of breeding and the elimination of naive individuals for a period of 6 weeks or more, coupled with environmental disinfection, has been shown to eliminate certain viruses from infected populations (342). With some bacteria and parasites, medications can be used but usually are only practical when applied to small numbers of animals, as such therapies are seldom 100% effective.

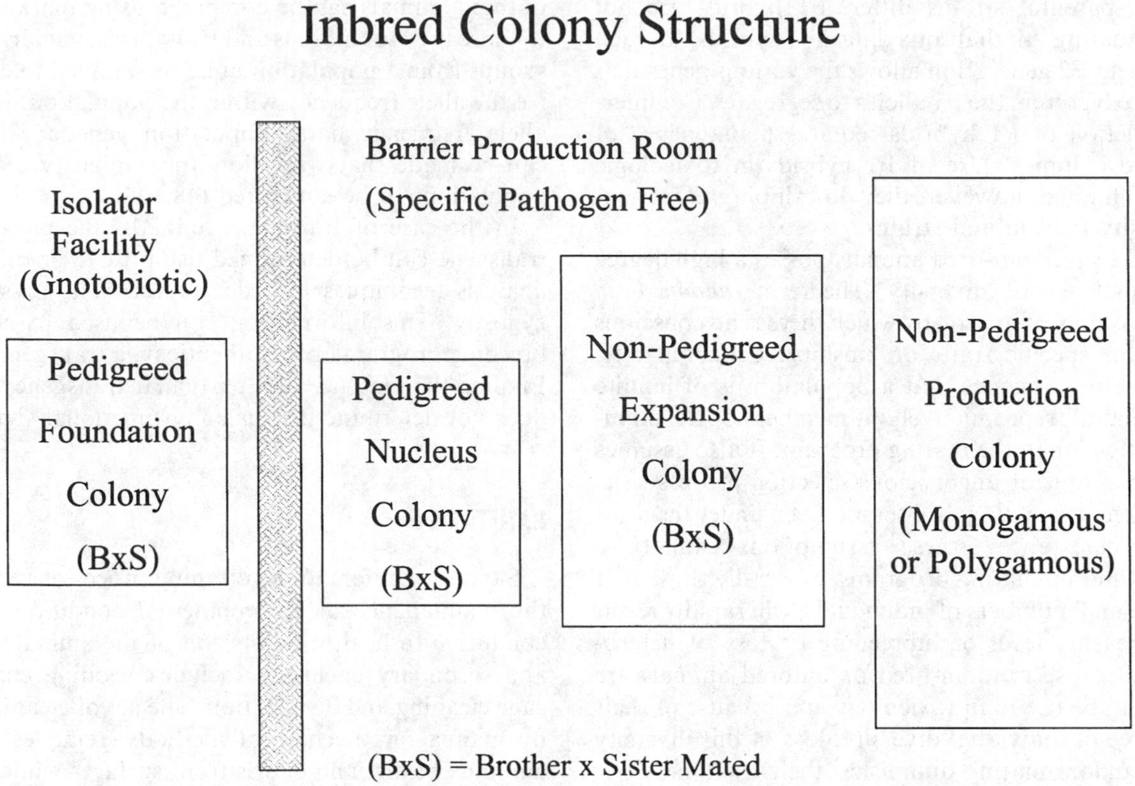

FIG. 16.2. Schematic representation of the segments of an inbred production colony.

GENETICS AND GENETIC MONITORING

Laboratory animals need to be appropriately identified in terms of nomenclature and genetics if studies are to be confirmed either at the same institution or at other institutions. Laboratory animals may be referred to by their common names as well as their scientific names for the purposes of description. In the case of laboratory rodents, specific rules of nomenclature exist for stock and strain designations that cover the genetic classification of the animal and identify its origins and its methods of derivation (87,90,142,143,207,208). Listing of various stocks and strains, as well as other genetic classifications of animals, are periodically published (88,89). The correct designation of the animals used should be included in any reports or publications as well as other information regarding the source of supply.

The majority of rodents used in toxicologic research fall into three general genetic classifications: outbred/random bred, inbred, and F1 hybrid. Transgenic animals can be produced on any of these backgrounds and represent a rapidly growing segment of rodents used in toxicologic research.

Inbred animals are produced as the result of 20 generations or more of brother–sister mating and possess more than 98% genetic homozygosity. They are produced by most breeders by means of a colony structure that allows breeding of large numbers of these animals that are, at most, separated from a brother–sister mating by no more than one generation (Figure 16.2). A gnotobiotic foundation colony is maintained in isolators or other bioexclusion systems and is periodically used to replace the pedigreed nucleus colony of animals within the production facility. The nucleus colony animals are brother–sister mated with pedigrees being maintained. The progeny from these matings form nonpedigreed brother–sister matings in an expansion colony that produces breeders for either a pair-mated or polygamous-mated production colony, the offspring of which are used in research.

Inbred animals are useful in toxicologic research in which genetic homogeneity is required. Inbred strains may differ significantly in their response to various compounds due to variations in their genotype and phenotype. They are particularly useful when studying pharmacological mechanisms. Conclusions drawn using a single inbred strain should be verified using other inbred strains or outbred stocks if the findings are to be applied to more genetically diverse populations, such as domestic animals or man.

F1 hybrids are produced from the mating of two inbred strains. Offspring are genetically identical at all alleles at which the parental strains differ. F1 hybrids are not self-perpetuating in that breeding F1 hybrids to each other to yield F2 generation allows the various genes that were heterozygous in the F1 alleles to segregate. Commercial production of F1 hybrids requires maintenance of two inbred colonies. Use of F1 hybrids in toxicologic research is limited; however, they do exhibit greater genetic diversity than inbred strains.

Outbred or random-bred animals posses a high degree of individual genetic diversity. The term *random bred* refers to a system of mating by which there is no conscious selection for specific traits or kinships. Unfortunately, random mating assumes that a population is of infinite size and that all reproductively fit members of the population participate in the mating program. It also assumes that no conscious or unconscious selection process issue is used when new matings are set up. Even under the most careful circumstances, these assumptions cannot be fulfilled. Random mating programs, especially those that start with small numbers of individuals, will rapidly result in an increasing level of inbreeding or loss of heterozygosity. Because random-bred or outbred animals are presumed to be useful in toxicology and because of their great degree of individual diversity, loss of this diversity through random mating diminishes their usefulness.

Outbred animals are produced using a purposeful system of mating that seeks to retain the heterozygosity within a group of animals. A number of rotational systems for outbreeding have been devised, as have systems based on the coefficient of inbreeding of pedigreed groups of breeders (114,163,257). The latter system provides the greatest assurance of continued genetic diversity, provided that the colony is started with a sufficiently large number of genetically unrelated individuals.

Because established colonies of outbred animals undergo independent genetic assortment of polymorphic alleles and will independently fix certain nondeleterious mutations, different colonies of outbred animals separated by time as well as by geographic location will undergo genetic divergence even if they were started from the same colony of animals. To minimize this genetic divergence, breed stock can be traded between colonies of the same stock within the same supplier's organization. Systems for linking colonies in this fashion have been described. These rely on well-established population genetic techniques (125).

The genetic authenticity of inbreds and F1 hybrids can be monitored by assaying a variety of polymorphic alleles located on multiple chromosomes (126,238). If mismatings occur, variations in this allelic profile will be found indicating a genetic contamination. Any polymorphic marker can be used, including biochemical, immunologic, and DNA assays.

The authenticity of outbred stocks or of individual outbred animals cannot be determined. Populations of outbred animals can be compared using markers similar to those used for inbreds and F1 hybrids, but large enough groups from a population must be sampled to characterize the allele frequency within the population. Using this allele frequency data, population genetic calculations can be made that will allow the similarity of different populations to be compared (48,125).

In the case of transgenic animals, the presence of a transgene can be determined using PCR or other DNA analysis techniques in order to verify its presence and zygosity. This information can be used to adjust the breeding program or to authenticate a transgenic animal. Finding the presence of a particular transgene, however, does not determine if it has any functional significance.

SANITATION

Sanitation refers to the cleaning processes required for the maintenance of environmental conditions that are conducive to health. Sanitation of the animal's primary and secondary enclosure includes bedding change and cage cleaning and disinfection. The act of cleaning, either by manual or mechanical methods, removes excessive amounts of dirt and debris from surfaces while disinfection reduces or eliminates unacceptable concentrations of microorganisms that can interfere with toxicologic studies (222). The frequency with which these processes of cleaning and disinfection are done, as well as the methods used, depends on a number of factors, including species, age, and size of the animals; the type, construction, and size of the enclosure; the nature and quantity of the feces, urine, or debris soiling the environment; the temperature and relative humidity; the rate at which the surfaces of the enclosure becomes soiled; and the normal behavioral and physiological characteristics of the animals housed in the enclosure (222,322).

To facilitate cleaning, the surfaces of both the secondary and primary enclosures should be impervious to liquids and smooth to allow easy application of cleaning materials and disinfectants. The surfaces should also be capable of withstanding scrubbing and should be free of cracks or other deficits that may inhibit the cleaning process (177). The use of agents designed to mask animal odors should not be used in animal facilities designed to support toxicologic research. Such agents expose the animals to chemical compounds that may interact with metabolic or physiologic processes involved in drug uptake and metabolism. Such agents simply obscure poor sanitation practices or inadequate ventilation. Conversely, characteristic animal odors released from the decomposition of urine or feces cannot be used as the sole criteria for the adequacy of sanitation practices or ventilation. Some studies suggest a relationship between certain decomposition products of urine and feces (principally ammonia) and the potentiation of the effects of certain disease-causing organisms (36,104,179).

The sanitation of cages and associated equipment, such as watering devices and feed containers, can be done either manually or with mechanical equipment. The frequency of cleaning is dictated by cage type and the husbandry program. The use of wire-bottom or perforated-bottom cages, the use of regularly changed contact or noncontact bedding, and regular flushing of catch pans suspended under certain types of caging, coupled with the number, size, and type of animals in the cage, will influence how often the cage will need to be washed and sanitized. Hamsters, guinea pigs, and rabbits produce urine that contains high concentrations of minerals and proteins that can adhere to caging equipment. Regular cleaning will minimize the build up of such materials on the caging; however, pretreatment with acid solutions prior to cleaning may be required in order to remove such deposits from cages housing these species of animals (223).

Disinfection of caging can be accomplished, with hot water or chemicals applied either singly or in combination. The conditions under which these disinfection regimens are used must be adjusted so that they adequately kill vegetative forms of common bacteria and other organisms to be controlled by the sanitation program. It must be remembered that cage-washing practices, including the use of disinfectants in the cage-washing regimen, will not necessarily produce sterilized equipment nor guard against contamination after the disinfectants have been rinsed off the surfaces. The process of disinfection with chemicals must be carefully controlled in terms of preparation of the agent, method of application, conditions of application, properties of the agent, and contact time (13,31,180).

The use of hot water to disinfect surfaces must also be done in a controlled fashion. It is the combination of the temperature of the water, coupled with the length of time that the surfaces are exposed to a given water temperature (cumulative heat factor), that must be controlled. The same total exposure in terms of time and temperature can be obtained by washing at lower water temperatures for longer periods of time (327). Water temperatures ranging from a 140°F to 180°F have been used effectively in mechanical cage washers for disinfection with hot water alone. If detergents and/or disinfectants are combined with the hot water washing process, it is important that these compounds be thoroughly rinsed from all surfaces, as residual materials may interfere with some types of studies. If manual washing of cages is undertaken, as might be necessary in some specialized housing facilities, special care must be given to standardize the washing process and to assure that personnel are provided with the necessary personal protection equipment to minimize their exposure to hot water or chemical agents (222).

Although conventional methods for washing cages may be satisfactory for most toxicologic studies, the use of specialized bioexclusion systems, such as microisolation caging, may require a greater level of assurance of disinfection. In such cases, wrapping caging after cleaning in steam-permeable materials and autoclaving may be required to achieve the necessary level of decontamination.

Runs and pens may be sanitized by using high-pressure water coupled with detergents and/or disinfectants. Some organisms, such as gastrointestinal parasites, may not be eliminated by such treatments and may require periodic application of chemical disinfectants for prolonged periods of time. In all cases, thorough rinsing of the enclosures is critical so that carry over of materials that might adversely affect the animals or research does not occur.

Secondary enclosures, such as animal holding rooms, hallways, and support areas, should also undergo regular cleaning and disinfection. These areas can easily become contaminated with infectious organisms that can reinfect clean and disinfected caging. Contamination of secondary enclosures can also allow the spread of organisms from one area of a facility to another. To break the cycle, it is necessary to regularly clean the floors, walls, and other surfaces in the room using agents similar to those used in the cage-washing process.

The choice of disinfectants to use in an animal facility is difficult, may not be limited to a single agent, and will rely on a variety of factors. Discussion of disinfection principles is beyond the scope of this text, but useful information that will aid in selecting agents can be found in a number of references (13,31,180). For general purpose disinfection, agents should be active both by direct contact and in the vapor phase. The agent should have a broad spectrum of activity, including the ability to kill spores and nonenveloped viruses. Halogen-based compounds, most commonly those containing chlorine, appear to have the widest range of activity and are commonly selected. Care must be taken when using such agents, as regular use of any aggressive disinfectant can also damage surfaces.

PEST CONTROL

Animal facilities by their very nature generate large amounts of waste and use significant amounts of feed and bedding. Their complex design and extensive mechanical systems provide excellent harborages for rodent and insect pests. Pests can serve as vectors for the introduction into research animal colonies of unwanted parasites and pathogenic microorganisms. Inappropriate application of materials designed to kill pests can pose a risk to toxicologic research either through direct toxic effects on the animals or by interaction on a molecular level with experimental protocols (98,155,329).

Pest control is best conducted by professionals who can design an integrated pest management system that puts in place control methods and monitoring systems to track the effectiveness of the program. The use of potentially toxic chemicals should be avoided whenever possible in favor of nonchemical control measures (73,105,109, 164,223). Application of pesticides should only be conducted with the knowledge of the animal care and research staff and done in compliance with federal, state, or local regulations (222).

WASTE DISPOSAL

Animal facilities generate large amounts of waste in either solid or liquid form. These wastes can either be nonhazardous or hazardous in nature. Depending on the country, wastes from animal facilities may be regulated and may have to be tracked and disposed of in a prescribed manner (244). In the United States, the Medical Waste Tracking Act (MWTA) of 1988 charged the EPA with tracking certain potentially hazardous wastes. Additional state and local regulations may also be imposed, causing the complexity of research waste management to vary from state to state (282). Although these regulations were designed to limit exposures to biohazardous wastes, all animal wastes may be subject to specific tracking and disposal procedures, depending on the interpretation of these regulations. For this reason, a local safety committee with expertise in these regulations should oversee the disposal process and ensure that all personnel handling waste are properly trained.

Some forms of waste may require special handling and may be incinerated on site. The operation of an on-site incinerator is heavily regulated in most countries and is not available at all research facilities. More commonly, contract waste handlers are used to dispose of research/medical waste using methods that comply with existing regulations. Waste water from cage washing, room cleaning, and flushing of pens and runs is flushed into drains to be subsequently treated either on site using local sewage treatment facilities or sent to municipal treatment systems.

Bedding constitutes the largest waste component in animal facilities. This is seldom treated on site and usually is removed either as bagged waste or in large containers for off-site disposal. Final disposal of noninfectious waste bedding is often by composting, land application, or landfills. Noninfectious animal carcasses and carcasses exposed to infectious or other hazardous materials are commonly refrigerated or frozen in plastic bags for subsequent incineration (222). Recently, cost-effective chemical digestion methods for carcasses and other solid biological wastes have become available, allowing on-site treatment of such items with minimal environmental impact. Wherever possible, waste that is known to contain infectious or heat-liable hazardous materials should be treated by autoclaving or other destructive methods prior to storage for final disposal. Care should be taken to ensure that biological materials with a high liquid content, such as carcasses, are placed in sturdy leak-proof containers that can be sealed to minimize the potential spread of contamination (222).

Areas in which wastes are stored should be adequately ventilated and appropriately labeled. Individual waste containers should also be labeled as to the contents and any hazardous materials that they might contain. In the case of biological materials that are being collected for disposal, refrigerated or freezer storage may be required; in such instances a properly labeled, dedicated refrigerator or freezer should be available.

ANESTHESIA, ANALGESIA, AND SURGERY

Some toxicologic research protocols involve the surgical modification of animals or may subject animals to procedures that are likely to cause pain. Such procedures have been an important focus of the animal use oversight processes in most countries that have legislation regulating the use of animals in research. The researcher bears ultimate responsibility for the use of the appropriate procedures and the administration of the necessary drugs in such circumstances to assure the welfare of animals. Many references are available to assist the toxicologist in developing an appropriate surgical, anesthetic, or analgesic regimen (39,68,69,152,168). Assistance in this process should be sought from veterinarians experienced in laboratory animal medicine. The conduct of surgery in a research setting usually is a team effort requiring advanced planning, training to acquire the necessary skills, the appropriate facilities and equipment, and regular evaluation of outcomes and objective oversight of the entire surgical process (39,40,69).

Because both infection or lack of appropriate materials to successfully complete the surgery can result in the failure of the surgical procedure with the subsequent loss of animals, it is important that all aspects of the surgical procedure, from the selection of the animal through its preparation, anesthesia, surgical manipulation, and postoperative recovery, be carefully planned in detail and all necessary supplies, equipment, and assistance be provided (14,15,222,291). It is well established that animals are no less susceptible to infection than humans (20,32,68,332,333). For this reason, any materials or equipment used in the operative procedure must be appropriately disinfected or sterilized and techniques be used to maintain the critical components of surgical supplies and equipment in aseptic condition throughout the surgical procedure (25,151,270,279,290).

The complexity of this task varies with the size and number of animals that must undergo a surgical procedure. Large animals often require a much larger surgical field from which hair is removed and the skin is scrubbed, disinfected, and covered by sterile drapes (132,348). Often the incision site is quite large and the procedures undertaken may be more complex and require more instrumentation than those conducted on small laboratory rodents (69). Personnel must be provided with appropriate operating attire that is decontaminated or sterile. The surgeon's hands and arms should be disinfected by scrubbing with an antibacterial soap and water, and the necessary clothing and gloves should be packaged in a manner that will allow them to be put on by the surgeon in a location and manner so they do not become contaminated. The extent of surgical clothing required will vary with species of animals being used and will be proportional to the size of the operative site and incision (51,248,348). In the case of surgery involving rodents, the use of sterile gloves, a face mask, and a clean garment that covers the upper torso including the arms may be all that is required, whereas surgery on larger animals, such as rabbits, dogs, or nonhuman primates, may require much more extensive coverage of the surgeon with disinfected/sterile attire (38,67,69).

It is critical to review in detail each component of the procedure to determine if assistance is needed either from a person who is in surgical attire and capable of manipulating instruments or tissues in the operative field or by personnel who are not in full surgical attire and can handle materials that have not been disinfected or sterilized, conduct anesthesia, or aseptically dispense surgical supplies.

To be qualified to conduct the surgical procedure, the toxicologist must undergo training. Most commonly, this is done using a combination of techniques, including assisting in similar surgical procedures, observing others performing the surgical procedure, practicing on cadavers, or in the case of basic surgical technique, using training aids to acquire the necessary skills to conduct the surgery (1). The surgeon should also be prepared to deal with possible complications, including anesthesia difficulties, hemorrhage, difficulties in wound closure, and other similar, unwanted occurrences that could be associated with the procedure.

The postoperative recovery of the animal should be carefully planned and the clinical parameters that would signal need for additional intervention, including supportive therapy, which might consist of supplemental heat, administration of fluids, use of parental drugs (antibiotics, analgesics), nutritional support, or resuscitative procedures, prepared for. The criteria for a successful surgical outcome should be determined, as should the criteria for terminating a process when the outcome is unsuccessful. The toxicologist should have planned for and be trained in appropriate methods of euthanasia if and when it is required (7,160,181).

When new procedures are being developed, veterinary assistance and oversight may be necessary to further refine techniques and minimize failures. If animals die unexpectedly or unfavorable outcomes occur, the process should be analyzed and steps taken to improve it. Often critical to this is a comprehensive diagnostic examination of the animals that have undergone the procedure, either at the end of the study or when unexpected deaths or failure of the procedure occurs. Postmortem examinations, including histopathology and, where appropriate, other diagnostic measures, are essential to this process.

Surgical procedures can be classified as either recovery or nonrecovery and further subdivided as major or minor (222). Each requires respect for the animals being used and provision of adequate anesthesia. There are many complex issues in selecting the appropriate anesthetic regimen for any surgical procedure. Anesthetic techniques, equipment, and drugs are constantly being refined. With few exceptions, most techniques that can be applied to man can be applied to animals. Most anesthetic regimens used in toxicologic research, however, tend to be relatively simple and effective. Commonly, only one or two drugs are administered, and agents are favored that are easy to administer and whose use is well characterized in the species selected.

Because most toxicologic research involves small rodent species, agents that can be given intraperitoneally or by inhalation are easiest to administer and are commonly used. Selecting a few anesthetic regimens and being skilled in their use in a particular species often proves to be the most successful approach for the toxicologist. Switching between new anesthetic regimens without adequate training can lead to undesirable outcomes. Conversely, if an anesthetic regimen does not work well in a particular species or for a specific procedure, the toxicologist should not be reticent to seek an alternative technique that is more successful.

If inhalational agents are used, care must be taken to minimize human exposure, especially to women of childbearing age. Simple systems have been devised to scavenge waste anesthetic gases, and devices exist to monitor personnel exposure. Many anesthetic agents and analgesics are categorized as controlled substances that require secure storage, record keeping, and licensure.

When administering anesthesia, it is necessary to be cognizant of the signs and reflexes used to gauge the depth of anesthesia and what dosages will be used to re-dose the animals should additional anesthesia be required.

Similarly, a number of important factors can influence the course of anesthesia, including the state of hydration of the animal, decreases in the animal's core temperature due to loss of heat into its surroundings, the route and site of administration of the agent, and variability in the depth of anesthesia associated with failure to fast the animal. Techniques have been described to address all of these issues as well as others (168,346).

Once an animal has recovered from anesthesia, there may be instances in the postoperative period where analgesics may be required. Similarly, in some studies, pain may result from nonsurgical procedures or conditions that may need to be relieved for the study to continue. The diagnosis of pain in animals is difficult and does not rely on any single clinical sign (135,299). Analgesics have not been well studied in laboratory animals. It is clear that animals can and do experience pain and that analgesics can provide relief from pain, as evidenced by alterations in parameters such as weight gain, feed consumption, and activity measurements (219). Determination of the presence or absence of pain in small laboratory animals is particularly difficult, as is the assessment of the effectiveness of various analgesics administered prior to or following the onset of pain. Because the information available for choosing analgesics is limited and in some cases relatively subjective, the toxicologist should seek to assess the effectiveness of any drug or regimen selected through measurement of clinical parameters that are affected by pain.

ACQUISITION, QUARANTINING, AND CONDITIONING ANIMALS

The choice of a particular species for use in toxicologic research may be based on past work using the species, evaluation of metabolic, physiologic, or morphologic characteristics of a given species, the incidence of the development of certain spontaneous lesions, conditions, or an assessment of other biologic parameters, including lifespan, reproductive cycles, and behavioral characteristics that would make them suitable for a particular type of toxicological study. Laws and guidelines in many countries require consultation of literature or other sources of information to verify the appropriateness of a particular species to assure unnecessary duplication of work and to determine if alternatives to painful procedures exists. Other factors, such as the availability of a particular species and its conservation status, may also impact the decision.

When ordering animals, the only truly verifiable specifications are weight and sex. With the exception of nonhuman primates, dogs, and cats, there are very few instances in which a complete clinical or historical record is kept on individual animals. In some cases, a vaccination history and records of preshipment conditioning programs, including dosing with anthelminthic and antimicrobial treatment, may also be available for cats, dogs, and nonhuman primates, as well as limited colony health history, as previously discussed.

Commercially bred rodents and rabbits maintained under defined microbiological conditions by large commercial breeders are easily obtainable, but care must be taken when ordering these animals. Most commercial breeders produce rodents and rabbits in large numbers, often using polygamous or harem mating systems. Stock animals are maintained after weaning either in weight groups or in age groups by week of birth. Animals are seldom held by day of birth unless specific arrangements are made to set aside groups of animals for this purpose.

When ordering, animals usually are specified by weight or age but seldom both. With outbred animals and, to a lesser extent, with inbred and F1 hybrid animals, the weight range at any given age can be relatively broad and significantly overlap weight ranges for other age groups. Hence, it is possible to have animals of two different ages have the same weight. These overlaps can span several weeks of growth. Suppliers construct growth charts that can be used to estimate age based on weight within specific weight ranges. These are useful when a specific weight range of animals is required for a particular study, but some assurance still needs to be given that this represents a certain age range. If both an exact age and a specific weight range are selected, only a small portion of an outbred population of animals (and to a lesser extent, inbred and F1 hybrid animals) will be represented, resulting in unconscious selection for certain traits associated with animals within the population that fall within this specific age/weight range. Such overselection can adversely skew study populations and can lead to circumstances where findings cannot be repeated. For these reasons, it is best to specify animals by either age or weight.

When selecting animals for a study, it is important that the toxicologist carefully determine the size of the study group to be used. If very small groups of outbred animals are used, it is possible to select, purely through sampling error, a nonrepresentative group of animals from a much larger population (125). Attempts to repeat the findings of the study with another small group or even with larger groups may yield different results purely due to inappropriate sampling. It is also a reason why care must be taken to adequately randomize the assignment of animals to both test and control groups.

Populations of animals are dynamic and constantly changing their profile of expressed phenotypes. This occurs to a much smaller degree with inbred animals and F1 hybrids but can occur, as previously described, through the process of fixation and assortment of natural mutations. The problem is magnified in outbred colonies due to random genetic drift (125). Hence, the toxicologist should expect that historical controls will vary over time in an unpredictable fashion and that such variation will occur regardless if the same colony is used for a source of animals for subsequent studies or if alternative colonies are selected. It is also important to appreciate that while different suppliers may produce strains or stocks of similar designations, perhaps derived from a common source, the longer the time interval from the point of stocking until the present, the more the groups of animals have likely drifted apart genetically and the more likely they are to have different phenotypic expressions, either through continual genetic reassortment and fixation or through the development of new allelic polymorphisms. Switching sources of supply of animals can cause changes in historical controls as well as in standardized assays. These changes usually are not dramatic but can be a source of concern for those assuming that there is some consistency between different populations of animals.

Animals are transported from suppliers to toxicology laboratories in shipping containers that are designed to meet national and certain international standards (141). Depending on the country, various regulations may be applicable to the control of animals in transport. Animals containing infectious agents or whose genetic material has been altered, and animals that have been exposed to hazardous materials of a noninfectious nature, must be shipped in conformance to regulations that can differ significantly between countries. Commercial animal suppliers are experienced in shipping animals in conformance with these requirements; however, if the toxicologist intends to ship animals between institutions, it is important to work with experienced brokers or other shipping agents who can assist in making the necessary arrangements and acquire the necessary shipping containers to legally conduct this process.

For the most part, animals are shipped in new, disposable containers that often are filtered to prevent the incursion of microorganisms. Containers are sometimes sterilized or disinfected, as may be the bedding, feed, and water used in shipping, depending on the supplier and the animals being transported. Most transportation either entirely or in part is done by truck. Most large laboratory animal suppliers maintain independent trucking routes and dedicated vehicles that are disinfected between shipments that transport animals. Some animal suppliers have only limited trucking capabilities and rely on air shipments. All suppliers ship some portion of their animals by air to supply customers not served by truck routes or to accommodate special conditions or orders that cannot be handled by truck. Unless very special shipping containers are used, shipment of animals by air allows the possibility of excessive stress and contamination during shipment (190,222,223). Moreover, the supplier does not have control of the shipment while it is being handled by the air carrier, and hence the control of environmental conditions may vary depending on the circumstances.

It is generally good practice to process animals immediately upon receipt at the research institution. Disinfection of the outside of the containers with solutions of general-purpose disinfectants is often a prudent step, especially if the animals have been shipped by air. Animals should be removed from their containers and examined upon arrival to confirm their clinical condition and to verify order specifications. They should be placed in appropriate caging that has been labeled to identify the animals, and they should be given access to feed and water as soon as possible after arrival. Most toxicologic research facilities provide a period of stabilization and/or quarantine for newly arrived animals. During quarantine periods, animals are observed for clinical signs of disease, samples are taken for health assessment, and in some cases, vaccinations, treatment with antimicrobials, or treatment with anthelminthics may also be undertaken (222). Other forms of diagnostic testing may also be conducted during the quarantine period. The length of quarantine can vary considerably, depending on the institutional exclusionary list of organisms for a particular species and health monitoring program.

A stabilization period differs from quarantine in that a stabilization period is designed to allow the animals time to recover from the stress of transportation, become rehydrated, and to gain back weight that may have been lost during transportation (2,74,78,148,326). This period of acclimation also allows the animal to become accustomed to using the water and feed sources and to adapt to any changes in diet (112,173,262,313). In the case of group-housed animals, it allows the establishment of both social hierarchies and other behavioral adaptations. Stabilization and quarantine should be done concurrently. Some institutions do not have a quarantine period in which health monitoring is conducted, but rather, health monitoring information from the animal supplier is used to determine the fitness of the animals for incorporation into the research program. A stabilization period, however, may be instituted for the group to allow the necessary acclimation to occur prior to use. Typical stabilization periods range from 3 to 7 days for most species and are based upon some limited work to suggest that periods of 48 or 72 hours are necessary to overcome the stress of transportation (173,286,318).

QUESTIONS

1. What housing systems can be used to minimize the risk of introduction and spread to animals of unwanted microorganisms that could alter toxicologic research?
2. What microorganisms that infect animals have the ability to alter toxicologic research results?
3. If outbred (non inbred) rodents are used in toxicologic research or product registration studies, what factors associated with their breeding methods and source colonies, as well as ordering specifications, can cause variation in research results?
4. What are the differences between closed formula, open formula, and constant nutrition natural ingredient diets used to feed research animals?
5. What laws, regulations, and guidelines affect the use of laboratory animals in toxicological and product registration research?
6. What constituents of the research animals' environment can cause variation in toxicologic research results?

REFERENCES

1. Academy of Surgical Research (ASR) (1989): Guidelines for training in surgical research in animals. *J. Invest. Surg.*, 2:263–268.
2. Aguila, H. N., Pakes, S. P., Lai, W. C., and Lu, Y. S. (1988): The effect of transportation stress on splenic natural killer cell activity in C57BL/6J mice. *Lab. Anim. Sci.*, 38:148–151.
3. Albanes, D. (1987): Total calories, body weight, and tumor incidence in mice. *Cancer Res.*, 47:1987–1992.
4. Allander, C., and Abel, E. (1973): Some aspects of the differences of air conditions inside a cage for small laboratory animals and its surroundings. *Z. Versuchstierkd, Bd.*, 15:20–34.
5. American Society of Heating, Refrigeration, and Air Conditioning Engineers, Inc. (ASHRAE) (1992): Air cleaners for particulate contaminants. In: *1992 ASHRAE Handbook: HVAC Systems and Equipment, I-P edition*. ASHRAE, Atlanta.
6. American Society of Heating, Refrigeration, and Air Conditioning Engineers, Inc. (ASHRAE) (1993): Environmental control of animals and plants. In: *1993 ASHRAE Handbook: Fundamentals, I-P edition*. ASHRAE, Atlanta.
7. American Veterinary Medical Association (AVMA) (1993): 1993 Report of the AVMA Panel on Euthanasia. *J. Am. Vet. Med. Assoc.*, 202:229–249.
8. Ames, B. N., Shigenaga, M. K., and Hagen, T. M. (1993): Review: Oxidants, antioxidants, and the degenerative disease of aging. *Proc. Natl. Acad. Sci. USA*, 90:7915–7922.
9. Animal Welfare Institute (1979): *Comfortable Quarters for Laboratory Animals*. Animal Welfare Institute, Washington, DC.
10. Anonymous (1976): Long-term holding of laboratory rodents. *ILAR News*, 19:L1–L25.
11. Anthony, A. (1962): Criteria for acoustics in animal housing. *Lab. Anim. Care*, 13:340–347.
12. Armario, A., Castellanos, J. M., and Balasch, J. (1985): Chronic noise stress and insulin secretion in male rats. *Physiol. Behav.*, 34:359–361.
13. Ascenzi, J. M. (1996): *Handbook of Disinfectants and Antiseptics*. Marcel Dekker, New York.
14. Association of Operating Room Nurses (AORN) (1982): Recommended practices for traffic patterns in the surgical suite. *Assoc. Oper. Room Nurs. J.*, 15:750–758.
15. Ayliffe, G. A. J. (1991): Role of the environment of the operating suit in surgical wound infection. *Rev. Infect. Dis.*, 13(suppl 10):S800–S804.
16. Baetjer, A. M. (1968): Role of environment temperature and humidity in susceptibility to disease. *Arch. Environ. Health.*, 16:565–570.
17. Barker, H. J., Lindsey, J. R., and Weisbroth, S. H. (1979): Housing to control research variables. In: *The Laboratory Rat, Volume 1: Biology and Diseases*, edited by H. J. Baker, J. R. Lindsey, and S. H. Weisbroth, pp. 169–192. Academic Press, Orlando.
18. Barrett, A. M., and Stockham, M. A. (1963): The effect of housing conditions and simple experimental procedures upon the corticosterone level in the plasma of rats. *J. Endocrinol.*, 26:97–105.
19. Beall, J. R., Torning, F. E., and Runkle, R. S. (1971): A laminar flow system for animal maintenance. *Lab. Anim. Sci.*, 21:206–212.
20. Beamer, T. C. (1972): Pathological changes associated with ovarian transplantation. In: *The 44th Annual Report of the Jackson Laboratory*, p. 104. Jackson Laboratory, Bar Harbor, Maine.
21. Beck, R. W. (1963): The control of *Pseudomonas aeruginosa* in mouse breeding colony by the use of chlorine in the drinking water. *Lab. Anim. Care*, 13:41–45.
22. Bellhorn, R. W. (1980): Lighting in the animal environment. *Lab. Anim. Sci.*, 30:440–450.
23. Berg, B. N., and Simms, H. S. (1960): Nutrition and longevity in the rat. II: Longevity and onset of disease with different levels of food intake. *J. Nutr.*, 71:255–263.
24. Berg, B. N., and Simms, H. S. (1961): Nutrition and longevity in the rat. III: Food restriction beyond 800 days. *J. Nutr.*, 74:23–32.
25. Berg, J. (1993): Sterilization. In: *Textbook of Small Animal Surgery, 2nd edition*, edited by D. Slatter, pp. 124–129. W. B. Saunders, Philadelphia.
26. Besch, E. L. (1975): Animal cage-room dry-bulk and dew-point temperatures differential. *ASHRAE Trans.*, 88:549–557.
27. Besch, E. L. (1980): Environmental quality within animal facilities. *Lab. Anim. Sci.*, 30:385–406.
28. Besch, E. L. (1990): Environmental variables and animal needs. In: *The Experimental Animal in Biomedical Research, Volume 1: A Survey of Scientific and Ethical Issues for Investigators*, edited by B. E. Rollin and M. L. Kesel, pp. 113–131. CRC Press, Boca Raton, FL.
29. Bhatt, P. N., Jacoby, R. O., Morse, H. C., III, and New, A. E. (1986): *Viral and Mycoplasmal Infections of Laboratory Rodents: Effects on Biomedical Research*. Academic Press, Orlando.
30. Birt, D. F., and Conrad, R. D. (1981): Weight gain, reproduction, and survival of Syrian hamsters fed five natural ingredients diets. *Lab. Anim. Sci.*, 31:149–155.
31. Block, S. S. (1991): *Disinfection, Sterilization and Preservation, 4th edition*, Lea & Febiger, Philadelphia.
32. Bradfield, J. F., Schachtman, T. R., McLaughlin, R. M., and Steffen, E. K. (1992): Behavioral and physiological effects of inapparent would infection in rats. *Lab. Anim. Sci.*, 42:572–578.
33. Brainard, G. C. (1989): Illumination of laboratory animal quarters: Participation of light irradiance and wavelength in the regulation of the neuroendocrine system. In: *Science and Animals: Addressing Contemporary Issues*, pp. 69–74. Scientists Center for Animal Welfare, Greenbelt, Maryland.
34. Brainard, G. C., Vaughan, M. K., and Reiter, R. J. (1986): Effect of light irradiance and wavelength on the Syrian hamster reproductive system. *Endocrinology*, 119:648–654.
35. Brewer, N. R. (1964): Estimating heat produced by laboratory animals: New data on animal heat and vapor transmission account

for activity and other factors to provide a more reliable basis for conditioning design calculations. *Heating Piping Air Cond.*, 36:139–141.

36. Broderson, J. R., Lindsey, J. R., and Crawford, J. E. (1976): The role of environmental ammonia in respiratory mycoplasmosis of rats. *Am. J. Pathol.*, 85:115–130.
37. Brown, A. M., and Pye, J. D. (1975): Auditory sensitivity at high frequencies in mammals. *Adv. Comp. Physiol. Biochem.*, 6:1–73.
38. Brown, M. J. (1994): Aseptic surgery for rodents. In: *Rodents and Rabbits: Current Research Issues*, edited by S. M. Niemi, J. S. Venable, and H. N. Guttman, pp. 67–72. Scientists Center for Animal Welfare, Bethesda, Maryland.
39. Brown, M. J., Pearson, P. T., and Tomson, F. N. (1993): Guidelines for animal surgery in research and teaching. *Am. J. Vet. Res.*, 54:1544–1559.
40. Brown, M. J., and Schofield, J. C. (1994): Perioperative care. In: *Essentials for Animal Research: A Primer for Research Personnel*, edited by B. T. Bennett, M. J. Brown, and J. C. Schofield, pp. 79–88. National Agricultural Library, Washington, DC.
41. Burkhart, C. A., and Robinson, J. L. (1978): High rat pup mortality attributed to the use of cedar-wood shavings as bedding. *Lab. Anim.*, 12:221–222.
42. Campbell, S. A. (1990): Effects of exercise programs on serum biochemical stress indicators in purpose-bred beagle dogs. In: *Canine Research Environment*, edited by J. A. Mench and L. Krulisch, pp. 77–82. Scientists Center for Animal Welfare, Bethesda, MD.
43. Campbell, S. A., Hughes, H. C., Griffin, H. E., Landi, M. S., and Mallon, F. M. (1988): Some effects of limited exercise on purpose-bred beagle dogs. *Am. J. Vet. Res.*, 49:1298–1301.
44. Campbell, T. C., and Hayes, J. R. (1974): Role of nutrition in the drug-metabolizing enzyme system. *Pharmacol. Rev.*, 26:171–197.
45. Canadian Council on Animal Care (1980): *Guide and Care and Use of Experimental Animals, Vol. 1.* Canadian Council on Animal Care, Ottawa, Canada.
46. Canadian Council on Animal Care (1984): *Guide and Care and Use of Experimental Animals, Vol. 2.* Canadian Council on Animal Care, Ottawa, Canada.
47. Canadian Federation of Humane Societies (1990): *Guidelines for Community Members of Animal Care Committees.* Experimental Animals Committee, Canadian Federation of Humane Societies, Nepean, Canada.
48. CD(SD)IGS Study Group (1998): Biological reference data on CD(SD)IGS rats—1998. Best Printing Co., Yokohama, Japan.
49. Centers for Disease Control and Prevention (CDC) and National Institutes of Health (NIH) (1993): *Biosafety in Microbiological and Biomedical Laboratories, 3rd edition.* HHS Publication No. (CDC) 93-8395, U.S. Government Printing Office, Washington, DC.
50. Centers for Disease Control and Prevention (CDC) and National Institutes of Health (NIH) (1995): *Primary Containment for Biohazards: Selection, installation and use of Biological Safety Cabinets.* U.S. Government Printing Office, Washington, DC.
51. Chamberlain, G. V., and Houang, E. (1984): Trial of the use of masks in gynecological operating theatre. *Ann. R. Coll. Surg.*, 66:432–433.
52. Cheney, K. E., Liu, R. K., Smith, G. S., Leung, R. E., Mickey, M. R., and Walford, R. L. (1980): Survival and Disease patterns in C57BL/6J mice subjected to undernutrition. *Exp. Gerontol.*, 15:237–258.
53. Cheney, K. E., Liu, R. K., Smith, G. S., Meredith, P. J., Mickey, M. R., and Walford, R. L. (1983): The effect of dietary restriction of varying duration on survival, tumor patterns, immune function, and body temperature in B10C3F$_1$ female mice. *J. Gerontrol.*, 38:420–430.
54. Cherry, J. A. (1987): The effect of photoperiod on development of sexual behavior and fertility in golden hamsters. *Physiol. Behav.*, 39:521–526.
55. Chvedoff, M., Clarke, M. R., Irisarri, E., Faccini, J. M., and Monro, A. M. (1980): Effects of housing conditions on food intake, body weight and spontaneous lesions in mice: A review of the literature and results of a 18-month study. *Food Cosmetics Toxicol.*, 18:517–522.
56. Cinti, D. K., Lemelin, M. E., and Christian, J. (1976): Induction of liver microsomal mixed-function oxidases by volatile hydrocarbons. *Biochem. Pharmacol.*, 25:100–103.
57. Clapp, M. J. L. (1980): The effect of diet on some parameters measured in toxicological studies in the rat. *Lab. Anim.*, 14:253–261.
58. Clough, G. (1976): The immediate environment of the laboratory animal. In: *Control of the Animal House Environment*, edited by T. McSheehy, pp. 77–94. Trevor Laboratory Animals, London.
59. Clough, G. (1982): Environmental effects on animals used in biomedical research. *Biol. Rev.*, 57:487–523.
60. Clough, G. (1987): The animal: Design, equipment and environmental control. In: *The UFAW Handbook on the Care and Management of Laboratory Animals, 6th edition*, edited by T. B. Poole, pp. 108–143. Longman Scientific & Technical, London.
61. Clough, G., and Gamble, M. R. (1976): *Laboratory Animal Houses: A Guide to the Design and Planning of Animal Facilities*, LAC Manual Series No. 4, Medical Research Council Laboratory Animals Council Laboratory Animals Centre, Abbey Press, Abingdon, Oxon.
62. Collins, T. F. X., Hinton, D. M., Welsh, J. J., and Black, T. N. (1992): Evaluation of heat sterilization of commercial rat diet for use in FDA toxicological studies. *Toxicol. Ind. Health.*, 8:9–20.
63. Conybeare, G. (1979): Effect of quality and quantity of diet on survival of tumour incidence in outbred Swiss mice. *Food Cosmetics Toxicol.*, 18:65–75.
64. Cooper, E. C. (1989): Design considerations for research animal facilities. *Lab. Anim.*, 18:23–26.
65. Coriell, L. L., and McGarrity, G. J. (1973): Biomedical applications of laminar airflow. In: *Germ-free Research Biological Effect of Gnotobiotic Environments*, edited by J. B. Henegham, p. 43. Academic Press, New York.
66. Cover, C. E., and Belcher, L. A. (1992): Effect of an irradiated rodent diet on growth and food consumption: A comparative study. *Contemp. Top. Lab. Anim. Sci.*, 31:13–17.
67. Cunliffe-Beamer, T. L. (1983): Biomethodology and surgical techniques. In: *The Mouse in Biomedical Research, Vol. III: Normative Biology, Immunology and Husbandry*, edited by H. L. Foster, J. D. Small, and J. G. Fox, pp. 419–420. Academic Press, New York.
68. Cunliffe-Beamer, T. L. (1990): Surgical techniques. In: *Guidelines for the Well-Being of Rodents in Research*, edited by H. N. Guttman, pp. 80–85. Scientists Center for Animal Welfare, Bethesda, Maryland.
69. Cunliffe-Beamer, T. L. (1993): Applying principles of aseptic surgery to rodents. *AWIC Newsl.*, 4:3–6.
70. Cunliffe-Beamer, T. L., Freeman, L. C., and Myers, D. D. (1981): Barbiturate sleeptime in mice exposed to autoclaved or unautoclaved wood beddings. *Lab. Anim. Sci.*, 31:672–675.
71. Department of Agriculture (1987): Animal and plant health inspection service: 9 CFR Parts 1 and 2; animal welfare; proposed rules. *Fed. Reg.*, 52:10292–10322.
72. Dillehay, D. L., Lehner, N. D. M., and Huerkamp, M. J. (1990): The effectiveness of a microisolator cage system and sentinel mice for controlling and detecting MHV and Sendai virus infections. *Lab. Anim. Sci.*, 40:367–370.

73. Donahue, W. A., VanGundy, D. N., Satterfield, W. C., and Coghlan, L. G. (1989): Solving a tough problem. *Pest Control*, August:46–50.
74. Drozdowicz, C. K., Bowman, T. A., Webb, M. L., and Lang, C. M. (1990): Effect of in-house transport on murine plasma corticosterone concentration and blood lymphocyte populations. *Am. J. Vet. Res.*, 51:1841–1846.
75. Dubin, S., and Zietz, S. (1991): Sample size for animal health surveillance. *Lab. Anim.*, 20:29–33.
76. Duncan, T. E., and O'Steen, W. K. (1985): The diurnal susceptibility of rat retinal photoreceptors to light-induced damage. *Exp. Eye Res.*, 41:497–507.
77. Dyment, J. (1976): Air filtration. In: *Control of the Animal Housing Environment*, edited by T. McSheehy, pp. 209–246. Laboratory Animals, London.
78. Dymsza, H. A., Miller, S. A., Maloney, J. F., and Foster, H. L. (1963): Equilibration of the laboratory rat following exposure to shipping stresses. *Lab. Anim. Care*, 13:60–65.
79. Eaton, P. (1987): Hygiene in the animal house. In: *The UFAW Handbook on the Care and Management of Laboratory Animals, 6th edition*, edited by T. B. Poole, pp. 144–148. Longman Scientific & Technical, London.
80. Edwards, G. S., Fox, J. G., Policastro, P., Goff, U., Wolf, M. H., and Fine, D. H. (1979): Volatile nitrosamine contamination of laboratory animal diets. *Cancer Res.*, 39:1857–1858.
81. Environmental Protection Agency (1978): Proposed guidelines for registering pesticides in the U.S. Hazard evaluation: Humans and domestic animals. *Fed. Reg.*, 43:37336–37403.
82. Erkert, H. G., and Grober, J. (1986): Direct modulation of activity and body temperature of owl monkeys (*Aotus lemurinus griseimembra*) by low light intensities. *Folia Primatol.*, 47:171–188.
83. Everett, R. (1984): Factors affecting spontaneous tumor incidence rates in mice: A literature review. *CRC Crit. Rev. Toxicol.*, 13:235–251.
84. Federation of European Laboratory Animal Science Associations (1994): Recommendations for the health monitoring of mouse, rat, hamster, guinea pig and rabbit breeding colonies. *Lab. Anim.*, 28:1–12.
85. Federation of European Laboratory Animal Science Associations, Supplement on Health Monitoring (1999): Health monitoring of non-human primate colonies. *Lab. Anim.*, 33(suppl. 1) S1:3–S1:18.
86. Ferguson, H. C. (1966): Effect of red cedar chip bedding on hexobarbital and pentobarbital sleep time. *J. Pharm. Sci.*, 55:1142–1143.
87. Festing, M., and Staats, J. (1973): Standardized nomenclature for inbred strains of rats: Fourth listing. *Transplantation*, 16:221–245.
88. Festing, M. F. W. (1993): *International Index of Laboratory Animals, 6th edition*. M. F. W. Festing, Leicester, United Kingdom (available from M. F. W. Festing, PO Box 301, Leicester LE1 7RE, UK).
89. Festing, M. F. W., and Greenhouse, D. D. (1992): Abbreviated list of inbred strains of rats. *Rat News Letter*, 26:10–22.
90. Festing, M. F. W., Kondo, K., Loosli, R., Poiley, S. M., and Spiegel, A. (1972): International standardized nomenclature for outbred stocks of laboratory animals. *ICLA Bull.*, 30:4–17.
91. Fidler, I. J. (1977): Depression of macrophages in mice drinking hyperchlorinated water. *Nature*, 270:735–736.
92. Fletcher, J. L., (1976): Influence of noise on animals. In: *Control of Animal House Environment—Laboratory Animal Handbooks, Vol. 7*, edited by T. McSheehy, pp. 51–62. Trevor Laboratory Animals, London.
93. Flynn, R. J. (1959): Studies of the etiology of ringtail of rats. *Proc. Anim. Care Panel*, 9:155–160.
94. Flynn, R. J. (1963): *Pseudomonas aeruginosa* infection and radiobiological research at Argonne National Laboratory: Effects, diagnosis, epizootiology, control. *Lab. Anim. Care*, 13:25–35.
95. Food and Drug Administration (1978): Nonclinical laboratory studies, good laboratory practice recommendations. *Fed. Reg.*, 43:59986–60025.
96. Ford, D. J. (1977): Effect of autoclaving and physical structure of diet on their utilization by mice. *Lab. Amin.*, 11:235–239.
97. Ford, D. J. (1977): Influence of diet pellet hardness and particle size on food utilization by mice, rats and hamsters. *Lab. Anim.*, 11:241–246.
98. Fouts, J. R. (1970): Some effects of insecticides on hepatic microsomal enzymes in various animal species. *Rev. Can. Biol.*, 29:377–389.
99. Fox, J. G. (1986): Interrelationships of disease and environmental variables in laboratory animals. In: *Safety Evaluation of Drugs and Chemicals*, edited by W. E. Lloyd, pp. 91–114. Hemisphere Publishing, Washington, DC.
100. Fox, J. G., Aldrich, F. D., and Boylen, G. W., Jr. (1976): Lead in animal foods. *J. Toxicol. Environ. Health*, 1:461–467.
101. Fox, J. G., Newcomer, C. E., and Rozmiarek, H. (1984): Selected zoonoses and other health hazards. In: *Laboratory Animal Medicine*, edited by J. G. Fox, B. J. Cohen, and F. M. Loew, pp. 614–648. Academic Press, New York.
102. Fullerton, F. R., Greenman, D. L., and Kendall, D. C. (1982): Effects of storage conditions on nutritional qualities of semipurified (AIN-76) and natural ingredient (NIH-07) diets. *J. Nutr.*, 112:567–473.
103. Gamble, M. R. (1979): Fire alarms and oestrus in rats. *Lab. Anim.*, 10:93–104.
104. Gamble, M. R., and Clough, G. (1976): Ammonia build-up in animal boxes and its effect on a rat tracheal epithelium. *Lab. Anim.*, 10:161–163.
105. Garg, R. C., and Donahue, W. A. (1989): Pharmacologic profile of methoprene, an insect growth regulator, in cattle, dogs and cats. *J. Am. Vet. Med. Assoc.*, 194:410–412.
106. Garrard, G., Harrison, G. A., and Weiner, J. S. (1974): Reproduction and survival of mice at 23°C. *J. Reprod. Fertil.*, 37:287–298.
107. Gerber, W. F., and Anderson, T. A. (1967): Cardiac hypertrophy due to chance audiogenic stress in the rat and rabbit. *Comp. Biochem. Physiol.*, 21:237.
108. Gerber, W. F., Anderson, T. A., and Van Dyne, B. (1966): Physiologic responses of the albino rat to chronic noise stress. *Arch. Environ. Health*, 12:751–754.
109. Gibson, S. V., Besch-Williford, C., Raisbeck, M. F., Wagner, J. E., and McLaughlin, R. M. (1987): Organophosphate toxicity in rats associated with contaminated bedding. *Lab. Anim.*, 37:789–791.
110. Gordon, C. J. (1990): Thermal biology of the laboratory rat. *Physiol. Behav.*, 47:963–991.
111. Gordon, C. J. (1993): *Temperature Regulation in Laboratory Animals*. Cambridge University Press, New York.
112. Grant, L., Hopkinson, P., Jennings, G., and Jenner, F. A. (1971): Period of adjustment of rats used for experimental studies. *Nature*, 232:135.
113. Graves, R. G., (1990): Animal facilities: Planning for flexibility. *Lab. Anim.*, 19:29–50.
114. Green, E. L. (1981): Breeding systems. In: *The Mouse in Biomedical Research, Vol. I: History, Genetics and Wild Mice*, edited by H. L. Foster, J. D. Small, and J. G. Fox, pp. 91–104. Academic Press, New York.
115. Greenman, D. L., Bryant, P., Kodell, R. L., and Sheldon, W. (1982): Influence of cage shelf level on retinal atrophy in mice. *Lab. Anim. Sci.*, 32:353–356.

116. Greenman, D. L., Kodell, R. L., and Sheldon, W. G. (1981): Association between cage shelf level and spontaneous and induced neoplasms in mice. *J. Natl. Cancer Inst.*, 73:107–113.

117. Greenman, D. L., Oller, W. L., Littlefield, N. A., and Nelson, C. J. (1980): Commercial laboratory animal diets: Toxicant and nutrient variability. *J. Toxicol. Environ. Health*, 6:235–246.

118. Halberg, F., Halberg, E., Barnum, C. P., and Bittner, J. J. (1959): Physiologic 24-hour periodicity in human beings and mice, the lighting regimen and daily routine. In: *Photoperiodism and Related Phenomena in Plants and Animals: Proceedings of a Conference on Photoperiodism*, edited by R. G. Withrow, pp. 803–879, Publ. No. 55. American Association for Advancement of Science, Washington, DC.

119. Hall, J. E., White, W. J., and Lang, C. M. (1980): Acidification of drinking water: Its effects on selected biologic phenomena in male mice. *Lab. Anim. Sci.*, 30:643–651.

120. Hamm, T. E. (1986): *Complications of Viral and Mycoplasmal Infections in Rodents to Toxicology Research and Testing*. Hemisphere Publishing, Washington, DC.

121. Hardy, J. D. (1961): Physiology of temperature regulation. *Physiol. Rev.*, 41:521–606.

122. Harkness, J. E., Wagner, J. E., Kusewitt, D. F., and Frisk, C. S. (1977): Weight loss and imparied reproduction in the hamster attributable to an unsuitable feeding apparatus. *Lab. Anim. Sci.*, 27:117–118.

123. Hart, R. W., Keenan, K., Turturro, A., Abdo, K. M., Leakey, J., and Lyn-Cook, B. (1995): Symposium overview: Caloric restriction and toxicity. *Fund. Apply. Toxicol.*, 25:184–195.

124. Hart, R. W., Leakey, J., Duffy, P. H., Feuers, R. J., and Turturro, A. (1996): The effects of dietary restriction on drug testing and toxicity. *Exp. Toxic. Pathol.*, 48:24–35.

125. Hartl, D. L. (1988): *A Primer of Population Genetics, 2nd edition*. Sinauer Associates, Sunderland, Massachusetts.

126. Hedrich, H. J., and Adams, M. (1990): *Genetic Monitoring of Inbred Strains of Rats: A Manual on Colony Management, Basic Monitoring Techniques, and Genetic Variants of the Laboratory Rat*. Gustav Fischer Verlag, Stuttgart.

127. Hermann, L. M., White, W. J., and Lang, C. M. (1982): Prolonged exposure to acid, chlorine, or tetracycline in the drinking water: Effects on delayed-type hypersensitivity, hemagglutination titers and reticuloendothelial clearance rates in mice. *Lab. Anim. Sci.*, 32:603–608.

128. Hessler, J. R., (1991): Facilities to support research. In: *Handbook of Facilities Planning: Volume 2—Laboratory Animal Facilities*, edited by T. Ruys, pp. 34–54. Van Nostrand Reinhold, New York.

129. Hessler, J. R. (1991): Single versus dual-corridor systems: Advantages, disadvantages, limitations, and alternatives for effective contamination control. In: *Handbook of Facilities Planning: Volume 2—Laboratory Animal Facilities*, edited by T. Ruys, pp. 59–66. Van Nostrand Reinhold, New York.

130. Hessler, J. R., and Moreland, A. F. (1984): Design and management of animal facilities. In: *Laboratory Animal Medicine*, edited by J. G. Fox, B. J. Cohen, and F. M. Loew, pp. 505–526. Academic Press, Orlando.

131. Hite, M., Hanson, H. M., Bohidar, N. R., Conti, P. A., and Mattis, P. A. (1977): Effect of cage size on patterns of activity and health of beagle dogs. *Lab. Anim. Sci.*, 27:60–64.

132. Hofmann, L. S. (1979): Preoperative and operative patient management. In: *Small Animal Surgery: An Atlas of Operative Technique*, edited by W. E. Wingfield and C. A. Rawlings, pp. 14–23. W. B. Saunders, Philadelphia.

133. Homberger, F. R., Pataki, Z., and Thomann, P. E. (1993): Control of *Pseudomonas aeruginosa* infection in mice by chlorine treatment of drinking water. *Lab. Anim. Sci.*, 43:635–637.

134. Hughes, H. C., Compbell, S., and Kenney, C. (1989): The effects of cage size and pair housing on exercise of beagle dogs. *Lab. Anim. Sci.*, 39:302–305.

135. Hughes, H. C., and Lang, C. M. (1983): Control of pain in dogs and cats. In: *Animal Pain: Perception and Alleviation*, edited by R. L. Kitchell and H. H. Erickson, pp. 207–216. American Physiological Society, Bethesda, Maryland.

136. Hughes, H. C., and Reynolds, S. (1995): The use of computational fluid dynamics for modeling air flow design in a kennel facility. *Contemp. Topics*, 34:49–53.

137. Hughes, H. C., Reynolds, S., and Rodriguez, R. (1996): Designing animal rooms to optimize air flow using computational fluid dynamics. *Pharm. Eng.*, Vol. 16(2):46–65.

138. Hugh-Jones, M. E., Hubbert, W. T., and Hagstad, H. V. (1995): *Zoonoses: Recognition, Control and Prevention*. Iowa State University Press, Ames, Iowa.

139. Institute of Laboratory Animal Resources (1978): *Laboratory Animal Housing*, proceedings of a symposium held at Hunt Valley, MD, September 22–23, 1976. National Academy of Sciences, Washington, DC.

140. Interagency Research Animal Committee (IRAC) (1985): U.S. Government Principles for Utilization and Care of Vertebrate Animals Used in Testing, Research, and Training. *Federal Register*, May 20, 1985, Office of Science and Technology Policy, Washington, DC.

141. International Air Transport Association (IATA) (1995): *IATA Live Animal Regulations*. International Air Transport Association (IATA), Montreal, Quebec. (Available from IATA, 2000 Peel Street, Montreal, Quebec H3A 2R4, Canada.)

142. International Committee on Standardized Genetic Nomenclature for Mice (1994): Rules for nomenclature of inbred strains. *Mouse Genome*, 92:xxviii-xxxii.

143. International Committee on Standardized Genetic Nomenclature for Mice (1994): Rules and guidelines for gene nomenclature. *Mouse Genome*, 92:viii–xxiii.

144. International Life Sciences Institute (1995): *Dietary Restriction: Implications for the Design and Interpretation of Toxicity and Carcinogenicity Studies*, edited by R. W. Hart, D. A. Neumann, and R. T. Robertson. ILSI Press, Washington, DC.

145. Iturrian, W. B. (1971): Effect of noise in the animal house on experimental seizures and growth of weanling mice. In: *Defining the Laboratory Animal*, Proceedings of the IVth International Symposium on Laboratory Animals, pp. 332–352. National Academy of Sciences, Washington, DC.

146. Jacobs, B. B., and Dieter, D. K. (1978): Spontaneous hepatomas in mice inbred from Ha : ICR swiss stock: Effects of sex, cedar shavings in bedding, and immunization with fetal liver or hepatoma cells. *J. Natl. Cancer Inst.*, 61:1531–1534.

147. Jacoby, R. O., and Lindsey, J. R. (1997): Health care for research animals is essential and affordable. *FASEB J.*, 11:609–614.

148. Jelinek, V. (1971): The influence of the condition of the laboratory animals employed on the experimental results. In: *Defining the Laboratory Animal*, pp. 110–120. National Academy of Sciences, Washington, DC.

149. Jones, D. M. (1977): The occurrence of dieldrin in sawdust used as bedding material. *Lab. Anim.*, 11:137.

150. Jose, D. G., and Good, R. A. (1973): Quantitative effects of nutritional protein and caloric deficiency on immune responses to tumors in mice. *Cancer Res.*, 33:807–812.

151. Kagan, K. G. (1992): Care and sterilization of surgical equipment. *Vet. Tech.*, 13:65–70.

152. Kagan, K. G., (1992): Aseptic technique. *Vet. Tech.*, 13:205–210.

153. Kaufman, J. E. (1984): *IES Lighting Handbook Reference Volume*. Illuminating Engineering Society, New York.

154. Kaufman, J. E. (1987): *IES Lighting Handbook Application Volume*. Illuminating Engineering Society, New York.
155. Keast, D., and Coales, M. F. (1967): Lymphocytopenia induced in a strain of laboratory mice by agents commonly used in treatment of ectoparasites. *Aust. J. Exp. Biol. Med. Sci.*, 45:645–650.
156. Keenan, K. P., Ballam, G. C., Dixit, R., Soper, K. A., Laroque, P., Mattson, B. A., Adams, S. P., and Coleman, J. B. (1997): The effects of diet, overfeeding and moderate dietary restriction on Sprague-Dawley rat survival, disease and toxicology. *J. Nutr.*, 127:851S–856S.
157. Keenan, K. P., Laroque, P., Ballam, G. C., Soper, K. A., Dixit, R., Mattson, B. A., Adams, S. P., and Coleman, J. B. (1996): The effects of diet, *ad libitum* overfeeding, and moderate dietary restriction on the rodent bioassay: The uncontrolled variable in safety assessment. *Toxicol. Pathol.*, 24:757–768.
158. Keenan, K. P., Laroque, P., and Dixit, R. (1998): Need for dietary control by caloric restriction in rodent toxicology and carcinogenicity studies. *J. Toxicol. Envior. Health* (Part B), 1:135–148.
159. Keenan, K. P., Smith, P. F., and Soper, K. A. (1994): Effect of dietary (caloric) restriction on aging, survival, pathobiology and toxicology. In: *Pathobiology of the Aging Rat, Vol. 2*, edited by W. Notter, D. L. Dungworth, and C. C. Capen, pp. 609–628. International Life Sciences Institute. Washington, DC.
160. Keller, G. L. (1982): Physical euthanasia methods. *Lab. Anim.*, 11(4): 20–26.
161. Keller, L. S. F., White, W. J., Snider, M. T., and Lang, C. M. (1989): An evaluation of intra-cage ventilation in three animal caging systems. *Lab. Anim. Sci.*, 39:237–242.
162. Keplinger, M. L., Lanier, G. E., and Deichmann, W. B. (1959): Effects of environmental temperature on the acute toxicity of a number of compounds in rats. *Toxicol. Appl. Pharmacol.*, 1:156–161.
163. Kimura, M., and Crow, J. F. (1963): On maximum avoidance of inbreeding. *Genet. Res.*, 4:399–415.
164. King, J. E., and Bennett, G. W. (1989): Comparative activity of fenoxycarb and hydroprene in sterilizing the German cockroach (Dictyoptera: Blattellidae). *J. Econ. Entomol.*, 82:833–838.
165. Knapka, J. J. (1983): Nurtition. In: *The Mouse in Biomedical Research, Vol. III*, edited by H. L. Foster, J. D. Small, and J. G. Fox, pp. 51–67. Academic Press, New York.
166. Knapka, J. J., Smith, K. P., and Judge, F. J. (1974): Effect of open and closed formula rations on the performance of three strains of laboratory mice. *Lab. Anim. Sci.*, 24:480–487.
167. Knauff, D. R. (1987): Revised laboratory animal policy, *Lab. Anim.*, 16:11.
168. Kohn, D. F., Wixson, S. K., White, W. J., and Benson, G. J. (1997): *Anesthesia and Analgesia In Laboratory Animals*. Academic Press, New York.
169. Kraft, L. M. (1980): The manufacture, shipping and receiving, and quality control of rodent bedding materials. *Lab. Anim. Sci.*, 30:366–376.
170. Krichevsky, D., Weber, M. M., and Klurfeld, D. M. (1984): Dietary fat versus caloric content in initiation and promotion of 7.12-dimethylbenz(a)anthracene induced mammary tumorigenesis in rats. *Cancer Res.*, 44:3174–3177.
171. Kuntz, M. J. (1989): Cubicles—Rational approach to specialized laboratory animal housing. *Anim. Technol.*, 40:203–209.
172. Kupp, R. P., Jr., Pinto, C. A., Rubin, L. F., and Griffin, H. E. (1989): Effects of ambient lighting on the eyes of rats. *Lab. Anim.*, 18:32–35,37.
173. Landi, M. S., Kreider, J. W., Lang, C. M., and Bullock, L. P. (1982): Effects of shipping on the immune function in mice. *Am. J. Vet. Res.*, 43:1654–1657.
174. Lang, C. M. (1983): Design and management of research facilities for mice. In: *The Mouse in Biomedical Research, Vol. III*, edited by H. L. Foster, J. D. Small, and J. G. Fox, pp. 37–50. Academic Press, New York.
175. Lanum, J. (1979): The damaging effects of light on the retina: Empirical findings, theoretical and practical implications. *Surv. Ophthalmol.*, 22:221–249.
176. LaRegina, M. C., and Lonigro, J. (1988): Serologic screening for murine pathogens: Basic concepts and guidelines. *Lab. Anim.*, 17:40–47.
177. LeBlanc, D. A., and Danforth, D. D. (1992): Substrate compatibility of animal cage wash products. *Contemp. Top. Lab. Anim. Sci.*, 31:13–16.
178. Leveille, G. A., and Hanson, R. W. (1966): Adaptive changes in enzyme activity and metabolic pathways in adipose tissue from meal-fed rats. *J. Lipid Res.*, 7(1):7–46.
179. Lindsey, J. R., and Conner, M. W. (1978): Influences of cage sanitation frequency on intracage ammonia (NH_3) concentration and progression of murine respiratory mycoplasmosis in the rat. *Zentralbl. Bakteriol. Parasitenkd. Infektionskr. Hyg.*, 241:215–216.
180. Linton, A. H., Hugo, W. B., and Russell, A. D. (1987): *Disinfection in Veterinary and Farm Animal Practice*. Blackwell Scientific Publications, Oxford.
181. Lumb, W. V., and Moreland, A. F. (1982): Chemical methods for euthanasia. *Lab. Anim.*, 11:29–35.
182. Maeda, H., Gleiser, C. A., Masoro, E. J., Murata, I., McMahan, C. A., and Yu, B. P. (1985): Nutritional influences on aging of Fischer 344 rats. II: Pathology. *J. Gerontol.*, 40:671–688.
183. Masoro, E. J., (1992): Aging and proliferative homeostasis: modulation by food restriction in rodents. *Lab. Anim. Sci.*, 42:132–137.
184. McDougall, P. T., Wolf, N. S., Stenback, W. A., and Trentin, J. J. (1967): Control of *Pseudomonas aeruginosa* in an experimental mouse colony. *Lab. Anim. Care*, 17:204–214.
185. McGarrity, G. J., and Coriell, L. L. (1973): Mass airflow cabinet for control of airborne infection of laboratory rodents. *Appl. Micro.*, 26:167–172.
186. McGarrity, G. J., and Coriell, L. L. (1976): Maintenance of axenic mice in open cages in mass air flow. *Lab. Anim. Sci.*, 26:746–750.
187. McPherson, C. W. (1963): Reaction of *Pseudomonas aeruginosa* and coliform bacteria in mouse drinking water following treatment with hydrochloric acid or chlorine. *Lab. Anim. Care*, 13:737–744.
188. McPherson, C. W. (1984): Laws, regulations, and policies affecting the use of laboratory animals. In: *Laboratory Animal Medicine*, edited by J. G. Fox, B. J. Cohen, and F. M. Loew, pp. 19–30. Academic Press, Orlando.
189. Megna, V. A. (1984): Engineering needs and trends of a toxicology laboratory. *Concepts Toxicol.*, 1:118–137.
190. Meskin, L. H., and Shapiro, B. L. (1971): Teratogenic effect of air shipment on A/Jax mice. *J. Dent. Res.*, 50:169.
191. Middle Atlantic Reproduction and Teratology Association (MARTA) and Midwest Teratology Association (MTA) (1996): *Historical Control Data (1992–1994) for Developmental and Reproductive Toxicity Studies Using the CRL : CD®(SD)BR Rat.* Charles River Laboratories, Wilmington, Massachusetts.
192. Miller, P. L., and Nash, R. T. (1971): A further analysis of room air distribution performance. *ASHRAE Trans.*, 77:205–215.
193. Miller, P. L., and Nash, R. T. (1979): Analysis, evaluation and comparison of room air distribution performance: A summary. *ASHRAE Trans.*, 78:235–242.
194. Miller, P. L., and Nevins, R. G. (1969): Room air distribution with an air distribution ceiling: Part II. *ASHRAE Trans.*, 75:118–131.
195. Moore, B. J. (1987): The California diet: An inappropriate tool for studies of thermogenesis. *J. Nutr.*, 117:227–231.

196. Mulder, J. B. (1971): Animal behavior and electromagnetic energy waves. *Lab. Anim. Sci.*, 21:389–393.

197. Mulligan, S. R., et al. (1993): Sound levels in rooms housing laboratory animals: An uncontrolled daily variable. *Physiology & Behav.*, 53:1067–1076.

198. Murakami, H. (1971): Differences between internal and external environments of the mouse cage. *Lab. Anim. Sci.*, 21:680–684.

199. Murata, M., and Takigawa, H. (1989): Teratogenic effects of noise in mice. *J. Sound Vibration*, 132:11–18.

200. Nair, V., and Casper, R. (1969): The influence of light on daily rhythm in hepatic drug metabolizing enzymes in rat. *Life Sci.*, 8(Part I):1291–1298.

201. National Aeronautics and Space Administration (NASA) (1988): Summary of conclusions reached in workshop and recommendations for lighting animal housing modules used in microgravity related projects. In: *Lighting Requirements in Microgravity: Rodents and Nonhuman Primates: NASA Technical Memorandum 101077*, edited by D. C. Holley, C. M. Winget, and H. A. Leon, pp. 5–8. Ames Research Center, Moffett Field, California.

202. National Institutes of Health Office of the Director, Division of Engineering Services, F. Memarzadeh Principal Investigator (1998): *Ventilation Design Handbook on Animal Research Facilities Using Static Microisolator, Vol. I.* National Institutes of Health, Bethesda, Maryland.

203. National Institutes of Health Office of the Director, Division of Engineering Services, F. Memarzadeh Principal Investigator (1998): *Ventilation Design Handbook on Animal Research Facilities Using Static Microisolator, Vol. II.* National Institutes of Health, Bethesda, Maryland.

204. National Research Council (1989): *Immunodeficient Rodents: A Guide to Their Immunobiology, Husbandry, and Use.* National Academy Press, Washington, DC.

205. National Research Council (1991): *Companion Guide to Infectious Diseases of Mice and Rats.* National Academy Press, Washington, DC.

206. National Research Council (1991): *Infectious Diseases of Mice and Rats.* National Academy Press, Washington, DC.

207. National Research Council (NRC), Institute of Laboratory Animal Resources, Committee on Rat Nomenclature (1992): Definition, nomenclature, and conservation of rats strains. *ILAR News*, 34:S1–S26.

208. National Research Council (NRC), Institute of Laboratory Animal Resources, Committee on Transgenic Nomenclature (1992): Standardized nomenclature for transgenic animals. *ILAR News*, 34:45–52.

209. National Research Council (NRC) (1977): *Nutrient Requirements of Rabbits: A Report of the Committee on Animal Nutrition.* National Academy Press, Washington, DC.

210. National Research Council (NRC) (1978): *Nutrient Requirements of Nonhuman Primates: A Report of the Committee on Animal Nutrition.* National Academy Press, Washington, DC.

211. National Research Council (NRC) (1981): *Nutrient Requirements of Cold Water Fishes: A Report of the Committee on Animal Nutrition.* National Academy Press, Washington, DC.

212. National Research Council (NRC) (1981): *Nutrient Requirements of Goats: A Report of the Committee on Animal Nutrition.* National Academy Press, Washington, DC.

213. National Research Council (NRC) (1982): *Nutrient Requirements of Mink and Foxes: A Report of the Committee on Animal Nutrition.* National Academy Press, Washington, DC.

214. National Research Council (NRC) (1983): *Nutrient Requirements of Warm Water Fishes and Shellfishes: A Report of the Committee on Animal Nutrition.* National Academy Press, Washington, DC.

215. National Research Council (NRC) (1985): *Nutrient Requirements of Dogs: A Report of the Committee on Animal Nutrition.* National Academy Press, Washington, DC.

216. National Research Council (NRC) (1985): *Nutrient Requirements of Sheep: A Report of the Committee on Animal Nutrition.* National Academy Press, Washington, DC.

217. National Research Council (NRC) (1986): *Nutrient Requirements of Cats: A Report of the Committee on Animal Nutrition.* National Academy Press, Washington, DC.

218. National Research Council (NRC) (1988): *Nutrient Requirements of Swine: A Report of the Committee on Animal Nutrition.* National Academy Press, Washington, DC.

219. National Research Council (NRC) (1992): *Recognition and Alleviation of Pain and Distress in Laboratory Animals: A Report of the Institute of Laboratory Animals Resources Committee on Pain and Distress in Laboratory Animals.* National Academy Press, Washington, DC.

220. National Research Council (NRC) (1994): *Nutrient Requirements of Poultry: A Report of the Committee on Animal Nutrition.* National Academy Press, Washington, DC.

221. National Research Council (NRC) (1995): *Nutrient Requirements of Laboratory Animals: A Report of the Committee on Animal Nutrition.* National Academy Press, Washington, DC.

222. National Research Council, Commission on Life Sciences, Institute of Laboratory Animal Resources (1996): *Guide for the Care and Use of Laboratory Animals.* National Academy Press, Washington, DC.

223. National Research Council, Commission of Life Sciences, Institute of Laboratory Animals Resources, Committee on Rodents (1996): *Laboratory Animal Management—Rodents.* National Academy Press, Washington, DC.

224. Nayfield, K. C., and Besch. E. L. (1981): Comparative responses of rabbits and rats to elevated noise. *Lab. Anim. Sci.*, 31:386–390.

225. Newall, G. W. (1980): The quality, treatment and monitoring of water for laboratory rodents. *Lab. Anim. Sci.*, 30:377–384.

226. Newberne, P. M. (1975): Diet: The neglected experimental variable. *Lab. Anim.*, 4:20–24.

227. Newberne, P. M. (1975): Influence on pharmacological experiments of chemicals and other factors in diets of laboratory animals. *Fed. Proc.*, 34:209–218.

228. Newberne, P. M., and Fox, J. G. (1980): Nutritional adequacy and quality control of rodent diets. *Lab. Anim. Sci.*, 30:352–365.

229. Newberne, P. M., and McConnell, R. G. (1979): Nutrition of the Syrian golden hamster. *Prog. Exp. Tumor Res.*, 24:127–138.

230. Newberne, P. M., and McConnell, R. G. (1980): Dietary nutrients and contaminants in laboratory animal experimentation. *J. Environ. Pathol. Toxicol.*, 4:105–122.

231. Newberne, P. M., and Rogers, A. E., (1973): Rat colon carcinomas associated with aflatoxin in marginal vitamin A. *J. Natl. Cancer Inst.*, 50:439–448.

232. Newberne, P. M., Rogers, A. E., and Wogan, G. N. (1968): Hepatorenal lesions in rats fed a low lipotrope diet and exposed to aflatoxin. *J. Nutr.*, 94:331–343.

233. Newbold, J. A., Chapin, L. T., Zinn, S. A., and Tucker, H. A. (1991): Effects of photoperiod on mammary development and concentration of hormones in serum of pregnant dairy heifers. *J. Dairy Sci.*, 74:100–108.

234. Newton, W. M. (1978): Environmental impact on laboratory animals. *Adv. Vet. Sci. Comp. Med.*, 22:1–28.

235. Njaa, L. R., Utne, F., and Braekkan, O. R. (1957): Effect of relative humidity on rat breeding and ringtail. *Nature*, 180:290–291.

236. Noell, W. K., and Albrecht, R. (1971): Irreversible effects of visible light on the retina: Role of vitamin A. *Science*, 172:76.

237. Nolen, G. A., and Alexander, J. C. (1966): Effects of diet and type of nesting material on the reproduction and lactation of the rat. *Lab. Anim. Care*, 16:327–336.

238. Nomura, T., Esaki, K., and Tomita, T. (1984): *ICLAS Manual for Genetic Monitoring of Inbred Mice*. University of Tokyo Press, Tokyo.

239. Noris, M. L., and Adams, C. E. (1976): Incidence of pup mortality in the rat with particular reference to nesting material, maternal age and parity. *Lab. Anim.*, 10:165–169.

240. O'Steen, W. K. (1980): Hormonal influences in retinal photodamage. In: *The Effects of Constant Light on Visual Processes*, edited by T. P. Williams and B. N. Baker, pp. 29–49. Plenum Press, New York.

241. Ogle, C. W., and Lockett, M. F. (1968): The urinary changes induced in rats by high pitched sound (20 kcyc/sec). *J. Endocrinol.*, 42:253–260.

242. Oller, W. L., Greenman, D. L., and Suber, R. (1985): Quality changes in animal feed resulting from extended storage. *Lab. Anim. Sci.*, 35:646–650.

243. Orlans, F. B., Simmonds, R. C., and Dodds, W. J. (1987): Consensus recommendations on effective institutional animal care and use committees. *Lab. Anim. Sci.*, 37(special issue):11–13.

244. Party, E., and Wilkerson, A. (1991): Implications of new medical waste regulations on laboratory animal research. *Lab. Anim.*, 20(8):28–36.

245. Pekrul, D. (1991): Noise control. In: *Handbook of Facilities Planning: Volume 2—Laboratory Animal Facilities*, edited by T. Ruys, pp. 166–173. Van Nostrand Reinhold, New York.

246. Pennycuik, P. R. (1967): A comparison of the effects of a range of high environmental temperatures and of two different periods of acclimatization on the reproductive performances on male and female mice. *Aust. J. Exp. Biol. Med. Sci.*, 45:527–532.

247. Percy, D. H., and Barthold, S. W. (1993): *Pathology of Laboratory Rodents and Rabbits*. Iowa State University Press, Ames Iowa.

248. Pereira, L. J., Lee, G. M., and Wade, K. J. (1990): The effect of surgical handwashing routines on the microbial counts of operating room nurses. *Am. J. Inf. Control*, 18:354–364.

249. Peterson, E. A. (1980): Noise and laboratory animals. *Lab. Anim. Sci.*, 30:422–436.

250. Peterson, E. A., Augenstein, J. S., Tanis, D. C., and Augenstein, D. G. (1981): Noise raises blood pressure without impairing auditory sensitivity. *Science*, 211:1450–1452.

251. Pfaff, J. (1974): Noise as an environmental problem in the animal house. *Lab. Anim.*, 8:347–354.

252. Pfaff, J., and Stecker, M. (1976): Loudness levels and frequency content of noise in the animal house. *Lab. Anim.*, 10:111–117.

253. Pick, J. R., and Little, J. M. (1965): Effect of type of bedding material on thresholds of pentylenetetrazol convulsions in mice. *Lab. Anim. Care*, 15:29–33.

254. Plank, S. J., and Irwin, R. (1966): Infertility of guinea pigs on sawdust bedding. *Lab. Anim. Care*, 16:9–11.

255. Poche, L. B., Jr., Stockwell, C. W., and Ades, H. W. (1969): Cochlear hair cell damage in guinea-pigs after exposure to impulse noise. *J. Acoust. Soc. Am.*, 46:947–951.

256. Podberscek, A. L., Blackshaw, J. K., and Beattie, A. W. (1991): The effects of repeated handling by familiar and unfamiliar people on rabbits in individual cages and group pens. *Appl. Anim. Behav. Sci.*, 28:365–373.

257. Poiley, S. M. (1960): A systematic method of breeder rotation for non-inbred laboratory animal colonies. *Proc. Anim. Care Panel*, 10:159–166.

258. Poiley, S. M. (1974): Housing requirements-general consideration. In: *Handbook of Laboratory Animal Science, Vol. 1*, edited by E. C. Melby, Jr., and H. H. Altman. CRC Press, Cleveland.

259. Port, C. D., and Kaltenbach, J. P. (1969): The effect of corncob bedding on reproductivity and leucine incorporation in mice. *Lab. Anim. Care*, 19:46–49.

260. Porter, G., and Lane-Petter, W. (1965): The provision of sterile bedding and nesting materials with their effects on breeding mice. *J. Anim. Technol. Assoc.*, 16:5–8.

261. Potgieter, F. J., and Wilke, P. I. (1991): Laboratory animal bedding: A review of specifications and requirements. *J.S. Afr. Vet. Assoc.*, 62:143–146.

262. Prasad, S., Gatmaitan, B. R., and O'Connell, R. C. (1978): Effect of a conditioning method on general safety test in guinea pigs. *Lab. Anim. Sci.*, 28:591–593.

263. Prychodko, H. (1958): Effect of aggregation of laboratory mice (*Mus Cusculus*) on food intake at different temperatures. *Ecology*, 39:500.

264. Public Health Service (PHS) (1996): Public Health Service Policy on Human Care and Use of Laboratory Animals. U.S. Department of Health and Human Services, (PL 99-158, Health Research Extension Act 1985), Washington, DC.

265. Pucak, G. J., Lee, C. S., and Zaino, A. S. (1977): Effects of prolonged high temperature on testicular development and fertility in the male rat. *Lab. Anim. Sci.*, 27:76–77.

266. Ralls, K. (1967): Auditory sensitivity in mice: *Peromyscus and Mus musculus. Anim. Behav.*, 15:123–128.

267. Rao, G. N., and Knapka, J. J. (1987): Contaminant and nutrient concentrations of natural ingredient rat and mouse diet used in chemical toxicology studies. *Fundam. Appl. Toxicol.*, 9:329–338.

268. Reiter, R. J. (1973): Comparative effects of continual fighting and pinealectomy on the eyes, the Harderian glands and reproduction in pigmented and albino rats. *Comp. Biochem. Physiol.*, 44:503–509.

269. Reynolds, S. D., and Hughes, H. C. (1994): Design and optimization of air flow patterns. *Lab. Anim.*, 23:46–49.

270. Ritter, M. A., and Marmion, P. (1987): The exogenous sources and controls of microorganisms in the operating room. *Orthopaedic Nursing*, 7:23–28.

271. Robison, W. G., Jr., and Kuwabara, T. (1976): Light-induced alterations of retinal pigment epithelium in black, albino, and beige mice. *Exp. Eye Res.*, 22:549–557.

272. Rogers, A. E. (1985): Factors influencing the results of animal experiments in toxicology. In: *Basic Toxicology: Fundamentals, Target Organs, and Risk Assessment*, edited by F. C. Lu, pp. 254–267. Hemisphere Publishing, Washington, DC.

273. Rose, R. J. (1990): Practical aspects of formulating research diets. *Lab. Anim.*, 19:47–49.

274. Ross, M. H., and Bras, G. (1971): Lasting influences of early caloric restriction on prevalence of neoplasma in the rat. *J. Natl. Cancer Inst.*, 47:1095–113.

275. Ross, M. H., and Bras, G. (1973): Influence of protein under- and over-nutrition on spontaneous tumor prevalence in the rat. *J. Nutr.*, 103:944–963.

276. Ross, N. H., Bras, G., and Ragbeer, N. S. (1970): Influence of protein and caloric intake upon spontaneous tumor incidence of the anterier pituitary gland and the rat. *J. Nutr.*, 100:177–189.

277. Ross, N. H., Lustbader, E. D., and Bras, G. (1983): Body weight, dietary practices, and tumor susceptibility in the rat. *J. Natl. Cancer Inst.*, 71:1041–1046.

278. Russell, W. M. S., and Burch, R. L. (1959): The principles of human experimental techniques. Methuen & Co., London (reprinted as a special edition in 1992 by the University Federation for Animal Welfare).

279. Rutala, W. A. (1990): APIC guideline for selection and use of disinfectants. *Am. J. Inf. Control*, 18:99–117.

280. Ruys, T. (1991): Codes, regulations and standards: Appendix E: Comments on the federal animal welfare regulations dealing with

dogs, cats and nonhuman primates (9 CFR Part 3. Subpart A. Feb. 15, 1991). In: *Handbook of Facilities Planning, Volume 2: Laboratory Animal Facilities*, edited by T. Ruys, pp. 398–405. Van Nostrand Reinhold, New York.

281. Ruys, T. (1991): The effect of animal species and types of the design of animal facilities. In: *Handbook of Facilities Planning, Volume 2: Laboratory Animal Facilities*, edited by T. Ruys, pp. 55–59. Van Nostrand Reinhold, New York.
282. Ruys, T. (1991): Waste. In: *Handbook of Facilities Planning, Volume 2: Laboratory Animal Facilities*, edited by T. Ruys, pp. 241–244. Van Nostrand Reinhold, New York.
283. Sales, G. D. (1991): The effect of 22 kHz calls and artificial 38 kHz signals on activity in rats. *Behav. Processes*, 24:83–93.
284. Sales, G. D., Wilson, K. J., and Spencer, K. E. V. (1988): Environmental ultrasound in laboratories and animal houses: A possible cause for concern in the welfare and use of laboratory animals. *Lab. Animals*, 22:369–375.
285. Saltarelli, D. G., and Coppola, C. P. (1979): Influenced of visible light on organ weights of mice. *Lab. Anim. Sci.*, 29:319–322.
286. Sanhouri, A. A., Jones, R. S., and Dobson, H. (1989): The effects of different types of transportation on plasma cortisol and testosterone concentrations in male goats. *Br. Vet. J.*, 145:446–450.
287. Sansone, E. G., and Losikoff, A. M. (1979): Potential contamination from feeding test chemicals in carcinogen bioassay research: Evaluation of single- and double-corridor animal housing facilities. *Toxicol. Appl. Pharmacol.*, 50:115–121.
288. Sansone, E. G., Losikoff, A. M., and Pendleton, R. A. (1977): Potential hazards from feeding test chemicals in carcinogen bioassay research. *Toxicol. Appl. Pharmacol.*, 39:435–450.
289. Schnurrenberger, P. R., and Hubbert, P. R. (1981): *An Outline of Zoonoses*. Iowa State University Press, Ames, Iowa.
290. Schofield, J. C. (1994): Principles of aseptic technique. In: *Essentials for Animal Research: A Primer for Research Personnel*, edited by B. T. Bennett, M. J. Brown, and J. C. Schofield, pp. 59–77. National Agricultural Library, Washington, DC.
291. Schonholtz, G. J. (1976): Maintenance of aseptic barriers in the conventional operating room. *J. Bone and Joint Surg.*, 58-A:439–445.
292. Schroeder, H. A., Balassa, J. J., and Vinton, W. H., Jr. (1965): Chromium, cadmium and lead in rats: Effects on life span, tumors and tissue levels. *J. Nutr.*, 86:51–66.
293. Selwyn, M. R., and Shek, W. R. (1994): Sample sizes and frequency of testing for health monitoring in barrier rooms and isolators. *Cont. Topics*, 33:56–60.
294. Semple-Rowland, S. L., and Dawson, W. W. (1987): Retinal cyclic light damage threshold for albino rats. *Lab. Anim. Sci.*, 37:289–298
295. Serrano, L. J. (1971): Carbon dioxide and ammonia in mouse cages: Effect of cage covers, population and activity. *Lab. Anim. Sci.*, 21:75–85.
296. Silverman, J., and Adams, J. D. (1983): *N*-nitrosamines in laboratory animal feed and bedding. *Lab. Anim. Sci.*, 33:161–164.
297. Simmonds, R. C. (1991): Characteristics of laboratory animal facilities. In: *Handbook of Facilities Planning, Volume 2: Laboratory Animal Facilities*, edited by T. Ruys, pp. 1–33. Van Nostrand Reinhold, New York.
298. Simmons, M. L., Robie, D. M., Jones, J. B., and Serrano, L. J. (1968): Effect of a filter cover on temperature and humidity in a mouse cage. *Lab. Anim.*, 2:113–120.
299. Soma, L. R. (1987): Assessment of animal pain in experimental animals. *Lab. Anim. Sci.*, 37:71–74.
300. Stoskopf, M. K. (1983): The physiological effects of psychological stress. *Zoo Biology*, 2:179–190.
301. Swanson, M. C., Campbell, A. R., O'Hollaren, M. T., and Reed, C. E. (1990): Rate of ventilation, air filtration, and allergen product rate in determining concentrations of rat allergies in the air of animal quarters. *Am. Rev. Respir. Dis.*, 141:1578–1581.
302. Tannebaum, A. (1942): The genesis and growth of tumors. II: Effect of caloric restriction per se. *Cancer Res.*, 2:460–467.
303. Tannenbaum, A., (1942): The genesis and growth of tumors. III: Effects of a high-fat diet. *Cancer Res.*, 2:468–475.
304. Tannenbaum, A. (1945): The dependence of tumor formation on the degree of caloric restriction. *Cancer Res.*, 5:609–615.
305. Tannenbaum, A. (1945): The dependence of tumor formation on the composition of the calorie-restricted diet as well as on the degree of restriction. *Cancer Res.*, 5:616–625.
306. Tannebaum, A. (1959): Nutrition and cancer. In: *The Physiopathology of Cancer 2nd edition*, edited by F. Homberger, pp. 517–562. Hoeber-Harper, New York.
307. Teelman, K., and Weihe, W. H. (1974): Microorganism counts and distribution patterns in air-conditioned animal laboratories. *Lab. Anim.*, 8:109.
308. The Animal Welfare Act of 1966. PL 89-544; as amended by Animal Welfare Act of 1970. PL 91-579; by the 1976 Amendments to the Animal Welfare Act. PL 94-297; and by the 1985 Food Security Act. PL 99–198.
309. Thigpen, J. E., Lebetkin, E. H., Dawes, M. L., Clark, J. L., Langely, C. L., Amyx, H. L., and Crawford, D. (1989): A standard procedure for measuring rodent bedding particle size and dust content. *Lab. Anim. Sci.*, 39:60–62.
310. Thigpen, J. E., Lebetkin, E. H., Dawes, M. L., et al. (1989): The use of dirty bedding for detection of murine pathogens in sentinel mice. *Lab. Anim. Sci.*, 39:324–327.
311. Thompson, R. (1971): The water consumption and drinking habits of a few species and strains of laboratory animals. *J. Inst. Anim. Technol.*, 22:29–36.
312. Torronen, R., Pelkonen, K., and Karenlampi, S. (1989): Enzyme-inducing and cytotoxic effects of wood-based materials used as bedding for laboratory animals: Comparison by a cell culture study. *Life Sci.*, 45:559–565.
313. Toth, L. A., and January, B. (1990): Physiological stabilization of rabbits after shipping. *Lab. Anim. Sci.*, 40:384–387.
314. Totton, M. (1958): Ringtail in new-born Norway rats: A study of the effect of environmental temperature and humidity on incidence. *J. Hyg.*, 56:190–196.
315. Trexler, P. C. (1987): Animals of defined microbiological status: Animal production and breeding methods. In: *The UFAW Handbook on the Care and Management of Laboratory Animals, 6th edition*, edited by T. B. Poole, pp. 85–98. Longman Scientific and Technical, London.
316. Tucker, H. A., Petitclere, D., and Zinn, S. A. (1984): The influence of photoperiod on body weight gain, body composition, nutrient intake and hormone secretion. *J. Anim. Sci.*, 59:1610–1620.
317. Tucker, M. J. (1979): The effect of long-term food restriction on tumours in rodents. *Int. J. Cancer*, 23:803–807.
318. Tuli, J. S., Smith, J. A., and Morton, D. B. (1995): Stress measurements in mice after transportation. *Lab. Anim.*, 29:132–138.
319. Turnbull, G. J., Lee, P. N., and Roe, F. J. C. (1985): Relationship of body-weight gain to longevity and to risk of development of nephropathy and neoplasia in Sprague-Dawley rats. *Food Chem. Toxicol.*, 23:355–361.
320. Vesell, E. S. (1967): Induction of drug-metabolizing enzymes in liver microsomes of mice and rats by softwood bedding. *Science*, 157:1057–1058.
321. Vesell, E. S., Lang, C. M., White, W. J., Passananti, G. T., Hill, R. N., Clemens, T. L., Liu, D. K., and Johnson, W. D. (1976): Environmental and genetic factors affecting the response of laboratory animals to drugs. *Fed. Proc.*, 35:1125–1132.

322. Vesell, E. S., Lang, C. M., White, W. J., Passananti, G. T., and Tripp, S. L. (1973): Hepatic drug metabolism in rats: Impairment in a dirty environment. *Science*, 179:896–897.
323. Vlahakis, G. (1977): Possible carcinogenic effects of cedar shavings in bedding of C3H-A^{vyf}B mice. *J. Natl. Cancer Inst.*, 58:149–150.
324. Wade, A. E., Holl, J. E., Hilliard, C. C., Molton, E., and Greene, F. E. (1968): Alteration of drug metabolism in rats and mice by an environment of cedarwood. *Pharmacology*, 1:317–328.
325. Waggie, K., Kagiyama, N., Allen, A. M., and Nomura, T. (1994): *Manual of Microbiologic Monitoring of Laboratory Animals, 2nd edition*. NIH Pub. No. 94-2498, U.S. Department of Health and Human Services, Washington, DC.
326. Wallace, M. E. (1976): Effect of stress due to deprivation and transport in different genotypes of house mouse. *Lab. Anim.*, 10:335–347.
327. Wardrip, C. L., Artwohl, J. E., and Bennett, B. T. (1994): A review of the role of temperature versus time in effective cage sanitation program. *Contemp. Topics*, 33:66–68.
328. Warfield, D. (1973): The study of hearing in animals. In: *Methods of Animal Experimentation, IV*, edited by W. Gay, pp. 43–143. Academic Press, London.
329. Wassermann, M., Wassermann, D., Gershon, Z., and Zellermayer, L. (1969): Effects of organochlorine insecticides on body defense systems. *Ann. N. Y. Acad. Sci.*, 160:393–401.
330. Wattenberg, L. W. (1975): Effects of dietary constituents on the metabolism of chemical carcinogens. *Cancer Res.*, 35:3326–3331.
331. Wax, T. M. (1977): Effects of age, strain, and illumination intensity on activity and self-selection of light-dark schedules in mice. *J. Comp. Physiol. Psychol.*, 91:51–62.
332. Waynforth, H. B. (1980): *Experimental and Surgical Technique in the Rat*. Academic Press, London.
333. Waynforth, H. B. (1987): Standards of surgery for experimental animals. In: *Laboratory Animals: An Introduction for New Experimenters*, edited by A. A. Tuffery, pp. 311–312. Wiley-Interscience, Chichester.
334. Weichbrod, R. H., Cisar, C. F., Miller, J. G., Simmonds, R. C., Alvares, A. P., and Ueng, T. H. (1988): Effects of cage beddings on microsomal oxidative enzymes in rat liver. *Lab. Anim. Sci.*, 38:296–298.
335. Weichbrod, R. H., Hall, J. E., Simmonds, R. C., and Cisar, C. F. (1986): Selecting bedding material. *Lab. Anim.*, 15(6):25–29.
336. Weihe, W. H. (1965): Temperature and humidity climatograms for rats and mice. *Lab. Anim. Care*, 15:18–28.
337. Weihe, W. H. (1973): The effect of temperature on the action of drugs. *Annu. Rev. Pharmacol.*, 13:409–425.
338. Weihe, W. H. (1976): The effect of light on animals. In: *Control of the Animal House Environment: Laboratory Animal Handbooks, Vol. 7*, edited by T. McSheehy, pp. 63–76. Trevor Laboratory Animals, London.
339. Weihe, W. H., Schidlow, J., and Strittmatter, J. (1969): The effect of light intensity on the breeding and development of rats and golden hamsters. *Int. J. Biometerol.*, 13:69–79.
340. Weindruch, R., and Walford, R. L. (1988): *The Retardation of Aging and Disease by Dietary Restriction*. Charles C. Thomas, Springfield, Illinois.
341. Weis, I., Stotzer, H., and Seitz, R. (1974): Age- and light-dependent changes in the rat eye. *Vichows Arch. A Pathol. Anat. Histopathol.*, 362:145–156.
342. Wesibroth, S. H., Peters, R., Riley, L. K., and Shek, W. (1998): Microbiological assessment of laboratory rats and mice. *ILAR Jour.*, 39:272–290.
343. White, W. J. (1990): The effect of cage space and environmental factors. In: *Guidelines for the Well-being of Rodents in Research*, edited by H. N. Guttman, pp. 29–45. Scientists Center for Animal Welfare, Bethesda, Maryland.
344. White, W. J., Anderson, L. C., Geistfeld, J., and Martin, D. C. (1998): Current strategies for controlling/eliminating opportunistic microorganisms. *ILAR Jour.*, 39:291–305.
345. White, W. J., and Blum, J. R. (1997): Design of surgical suites and postsurgical care units. In: *Anesthesia and Analgesia in Laboratory Animals*, edited by D. F. Kohn, S. K. Wixson, W. J. White, and G. J. Benson, pp. 149–163. Academic Press, New York.
346. White, W. J., and Field, K. J. (1987): Anesthesia and surgery of laboratory animals. *Vet. Clin. North Am.*, 17:989–1017.
347. White, W. J., Hughes, H. C., Singh, S. B., and Lang, C. M. (1983): Evaluation of a cubicle containment system in preventing gaseous and particulate airborne cross-contamination. *Lab. Anim. Sci.*, 33:571–576.
348. Whyte, W. (1988): The role of clothing and drapes in the operating room. *J. Hosp. Inf.*, 11(Suppl C): 2–17.
349. Whyte, W., and Shaw, B. H. (1974): The effect of obstructions and thermals in laminar-flow systems. *Journal of Hygiene*, 72:415–423.
350. Williams, G. M. (1984): The significance of environmental chemicals as modifying factors in toxicity studies. In: *Concepts in Toxicology, Volume 1: Toxicology Laboratory Design and Management for the 80's and Beyond*, edited by A. S. Tegeris, pp. 14–19. S. Kargar AG, Basel.
351. Wise, A. (1982): Interaction of diet and toxicity: The future role of purified diet in toxicological research. *Arch. Toxicol.*, 50:287–299.
352. Wise, A., and Gilburt, D. J. (1980): The variability of dietary fiber in laboratory animal diets and its relevance to the control of experimental conditions. *Cosmet. Toxicol.*, 18:643–648.
353. Wise A., and Gilbert, D. J. (1981): Variation of minerals and trace elements in laboratory animal diets. *Lab. Anim.*, 15:299–303.
354. Woods, J. E. (1975): Influence of room air distribution on animal cage environments. *ASHRAE Trans.*, 81:559–571.
355. Woods, J. E., Nevins, R. G., and Besch, E. L. (1975): Experimental envaluation of heat and moisture in metal dog cage environments. *Lab. Anim. Sci.*, 25:425–433.
356. Wostman, B. S. (1975): Nutrition and metabolism of the germfree mammal. *World Rev. Nutr. Diet*, 22:40–92.
357. Yu, B. P. (1990): Food restriction research: Past and present status. *Rev. Biol. Res. Aging*, 4:349–371.
358. Zondek, B., and Tamari, I. (1964): Effect of audiogenic stimulation on genital function and reproduction. III: Infertility induced by auditory stimuli prior to mating. *Acta Endocrinol.*, 45(Suppl. 90):227–234.

Principles and Methods of Toxicology,
Fourth Edition, edited by A. Wallace Hayes.
Taylor & Francis, Philadelphia © 2001.

Chapter 17

Genetic Toxicology

David Brusick

Genetic toxicology, as a subspecialty of toxicology, involves the identification and analysis of agents with toxicity directed toward the hereditary components of living organisms. A large proportion of human disease is either directly or indirectly associated with genetic dysfunction. Many agents are able to produce genetic damage at high exposure concentrations following the induction of acute, nonspecific cytotoxic effects across a wide range of cellular processes, however, the ultimate objectives of genetic toxicologists are to detect and access genetic hazard from agents that are highly specific for nucleic acids and are capable of producing genetic damage at subtoxic concentrations. Such agents are classified as *genotoxic*.

The term *genotoxic* is a general descriptor and is used to distinguish chemicals that have an intrinsic affinity for DNA from those that do not. Genotoxic substances have several common chemical or physical properties facilitating their interaction with nucleic acids (i.e., electrophilicity). A report of the International Commission for Protection Against Environmental Mutagens and Carcinogens (ICPEMC) provides a more detailed definition of genotoxic and emphasizes that categorization of a chemical as genotoxic is not a priori indication of a health hazard (46).

Mutagens comprise a subset of genotoxicants and are characterized by their ability to induce specific classes of stable changes in (a) the nucleotide sequence of genes, (b) chromosome structure, or (c) chromosome number. Changes in nucleotide sequence are described as point mutations, and chromosomal damage is referred to as clastogenicity. These two major classes of genetic damage are responsible for a large proportion of the array of human genetic diseases and contribute significantly to congenital malformations.

Because the original goal of genetic toxicology was to protect the human gene pool from increases in mutational load, the discipline of genetic toxicology initially focused on transmissable damage. Test methods employed during this early period were primarily in vivo and focused on measuring damage to mammalian germ cells. Later, reports from several independent groups of investigators were published showing a correlative relation between mammalian carcinogens and mutagens (3,14,18,60,93).

Table 17.1
Basic biochemical characteristics of all double-standard DNA

DNA consists of two purines (guanine, adenine) and two pyrimidines (thymine and cytosine).
A nucleotide pair consists of one purine and one pyrimidine (adenine/thymine (AT) or guanine/cytosine (GC)).
Nucleotide pairs are connected to a double helix molecule by sugar-phosphate backbone linkages and hydrogen bonding.
The AT base pair is held by two hydrogen bonds and the GC is held by three hydrogen bonds (see Figure 17.2).
The distance between each base pair in a molecule is 3.4 Å, producing 10 nucleotide pairs per turn of the DNA helix.
The number of adenine molecules must equal the number of thymine molecules in a DNA molecule. The same relation exists for guanine and cytosine molecules. The ratio at AT to GC base pairs, however, may vary in DNA from species to species.
The two strands of the double helix are complementary and antiparallel with respect to the polarity of the two sugar-phosphate backbones, one strand being 3′–5′ and the other 5′–3′ with respect to the terminal OH group on the ribose sugar.
DNA replicates by a semiconservative method in which the two strands separate, and each is used as a template for the synthesis of a new complementary strand.
The rate of DNA nucleotide polymerization during replication is approximately 600 nucleotides per second. The helix must unwind to form templates at a rate of 3600 rpm to accommodate this replication rate.
The DNA content of cells is variable (1.8×10^9 daltons for *Escherichia coli* to 1.9×10^{11} daltons for human cells).

Thus, genetic toxicology has evolved to play a dual role in safety evaluation programs. One role is the implementation of testing and risk assessment methods to determine the impact of genotoxic agents found in the environment on the integrity of the human gene pool. The second role is the application of genetic test methods to the detection and mechanistic understanding of carcinogenic processes.

BASIC GENETIC CONCEPTS

Gene Structure

The hereditary informational molecules of all living systems, with the exception of some viruses that use RNA, are composed of DNA, and those organisms which store their hereditary information in RNA go through a DNA intermediate during replication. Some common characteristic features of DNA molecules are listed in Table 17.1. The mechanisms of information storage and gene expression are similar for all organisms with DNA composition.

The simplest complete functional unit in a DNA molecule is termed a *gene*. Most of the early knowledge concerning structure and operation of genes was acquired from studies with bacteria or bacteriophages. During the past 10 years, development in molecular biology of mammalian cells has resulted in equivalent information in this cell type. The differences between the genes of prokaryotic (bacteria) and eukaryotic (plant and animal cells) organisms center primarily on the number, location of the respective chromosome, and mechanisms of gene regulation (Table 17.2). In prokaryotic cells there is a single *chromosome* with little or no differentiation along the DNA molecule so far as function is concerned. Eukaryotic cells, on the other hand, have DNA with nonfunctional, repeated sequences of some genes; these cells also have regions of noncoding DNA, called *introns*, inserted between coding sequences called *exons*. The exact function of repeated DNA sequences and intron regions is not known.

The nucleotide composition and the mechanisms by which information encoded in a gene is transformed into gene products is universal. Universality was confirmed by recombinant DNA genetic engineering studies in which genes continue to function properly after having been transplanted from human cells to bacterial cells or from bacterial cells to plant cells (15,53).

In eukaryotic cells, the process of gene expression follows the pattern shown in Figure 17.1. Enzymes located in the nucleus of the cell excise intron regions and splice the coding sequence back together. The resulting mRNA is then transported to ribosomes outside the nucleus for translation. Intron regions are not present in prokaryotic cells, and the gene is read in one sequence. DNA repair processes are also influenced by transcription activity. Important to a full appreciation of the functions of genes coding for structural proteins and enzymes is the identification of regulatory genes that control gene expression.

Somatic and Germ Cell Characteristics

From a genetic perspective, multicellular eukaryotic organisms are composed of two cell types: somatic cells and germ cells. Somatic cells constitute the major portion

Table 17.2
Characteristics of DNA in prokaryotic and eukaryotic cell types

Prokaryotic Cells	Eukaryotic Cells
Primarily haploid	Primarily diploid
DNA uncomplexed	DNA complexed with proteins forming chromosomes
DNA nonlocalized in the cell cytoplasm	DNA localized primarily within the nucleus of the cell
No morphologic stages in DNA replication	DNA replication described by mitotic cycle consisting of specific cytologic stages
DNA often found as a closed circle	DNA found in linear chromosomes
Replication not associated with cellular organelles	Replication and separation of chromosome associated with cellular organelles called centrioles
All genes encoded in the DNA are functional	Repetitive, nonfunctional gene sequences are common
Spacer sequences have not been identified	Noncoding spacer sequences identified as introns occur along the DNA molecule

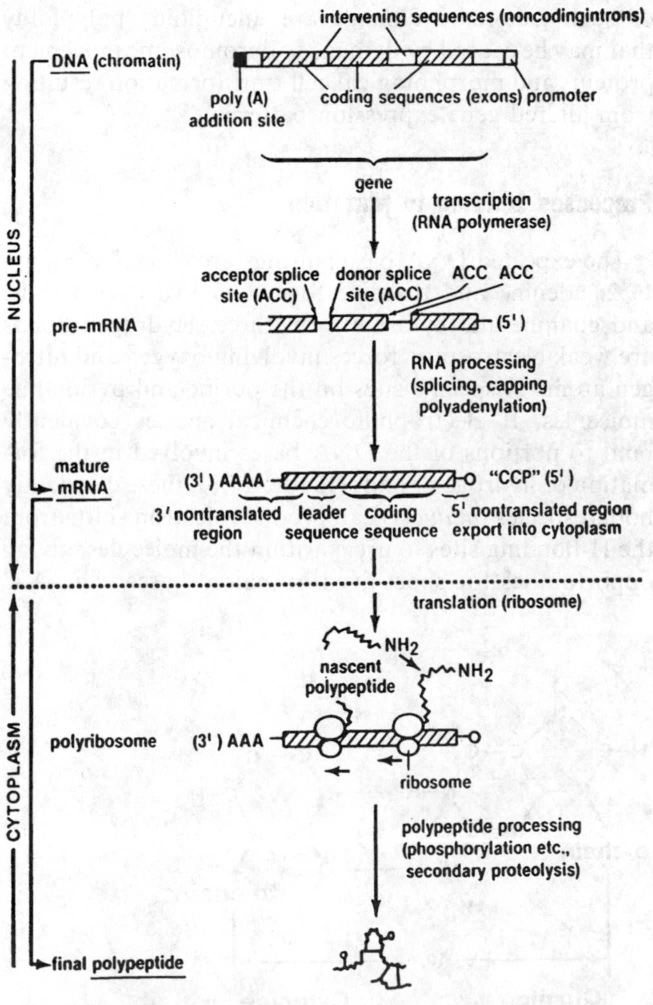

FIG. 17.1 Transcription and translocation of mammalian genes.

of the mammalian organism. The *genomes* of most somatic cells are *diploid* (two complete sets of chromosomes), and genetic alterations in somatic cells are not transmissible to subsequent generations. Virtually all in vitro mammalian cell assays used in genetic toxicology employ somatic cell types. Germ cells (sperm and eggs) are a special cell population in multicellular organisms. Their function is to form the next generation. Mutations carried in these cells produce a broad array of heritable genetic diseases, congenital malformations, and other disorders. Germ cells are derived from diploid stem cells in gonadal tissues following meiosis and carry a *haploid* set of chromosomes. *Mutations* carried in germ cells are classified as recessive or dominant, dependent on their expression in the diploid state. A large proportion of human genetic diseases are associated with recessive mutant genes that are expressed only when two mutant alleles (one contributed by each parent) are present in the homozygous condition. Recessive mutations are maintained at a constant level in the gene pool in the heterozygous state and are carried in that configuration by individuals who appear phenotypically normal. The inability to identify heterozygous from normal individuals is one of the primary reasons that the human genetic burden has not been reduced. Table 17.3 summarizes the spectra of mutations in humans for germ cell and somatic cell effects.

DNA ALTERATIONS RESULTING IN GENOTOXIC EFFECTS IN CELLS

DNA synthesis and replication are not flawless processes, and in rare instances, genetic alterations occur

Table 17.3
Mutational spectrum in humans[a]

Mutation Type	Examples of Inherited Effects	Examples of Somatic Effects
Single base changes	Sickle cell disease, Phenylketonuria	Epithelial cancers, activation of *ras* oncogenes
Small deletions and/or translocations	Haemophilias, Duchenne muscular dystrophy	Lymphomas, leukemias, enhanced activation of *myc, abl* oncogenes
Whole chromosome losses or gains	Down's syndrome, Turner's syndrome	Loss of tumor suppressor genes, retinoblastoma, Wilms' tumor, breast cancer

[a]From Reference 35.

spontaneously during normal cell division. In addition, endogenous oxidative metabolism produces reactive species capable of damaging DNA. The occurrence of intrinsic damage follows a predictable rate per gene and forms the basis of "background" or "spontaneous" mutation frequencies. In addition to errors in replication or repair, the origin of spontaneous mutations may arise from unavoidable environmental exposures (e.g., background radiation, diet).

Classification Scheme for Genotoxic Effects

DNA damage may be classified into several broad categories based on the nature (presumed mechanism) of the DNA change. The following is one type of such classification:

A. DNA disruption damage involves the breakage of and/or interchange of DNA segments between chromosomal structures. This type of damage may be visible through cytologic analysis of condensed chromosomes. Although genotoxicants such as alkylating agents induce DNA disruption damage, a characteristic of DNA disruption damage is that it may also be caused by secondary mechanisms (e.g., processes that result in cell stress such as high temperature) that do not target nucleic acids specifically (43,16).

B. DNA microlesions are nonvisible alterations occurring at the nucleotide level. Nucleotide damage generally produces point mutations through base-pair substitution or insertion/deletion or it may induce recombination between sister chromatids. Microlesions generally are induced by agents that specifically target nucleic acids (e.g., electrophilic agents).

In addition, some genotoxic effects may be induced by other mechanisms that do not fall readily into either of the two mechanisms defined previously. Examples of such genotoxic damage are aneuploidy/polyploidy that may be caused by damage to chromosome movement proteins and morphological cell transformation resulting from altered gene expression patterns.

Processes Leading to Mutation

The expected DNA base pairings are shown in Figure 17.2: adenine and thymine form two hydrogen bonds, and guanine and cytosine form three. Hydrogen bonds are weak electrostatic forces involving oxygen and nitrogen atoms at specific sites on the purine and pyrimidine molecules. If electrophilic chemical species covalently bind to portions of the DNA bases involved in the formation of hydrogen bonds (Figure 17.3), these covalently bound species (*adducts*) can produce electron shifts from the H-bonding sites to areas within the molecules, giving opportunities for short-lived mispaired bases (e.g., A:C

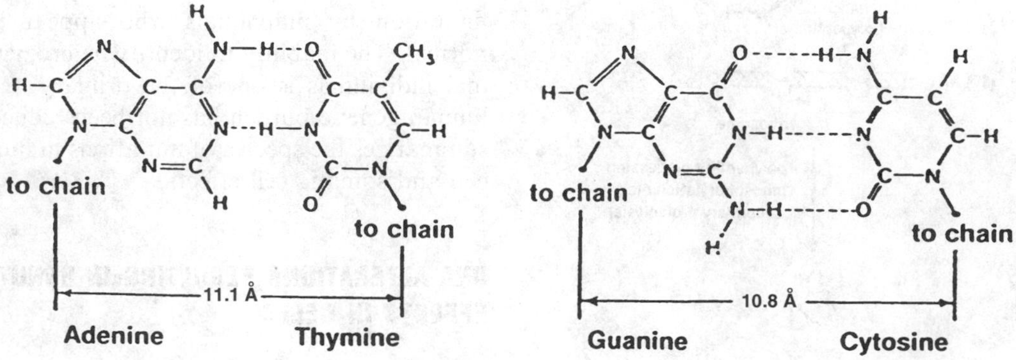

FIG. 17.2. Hydrogen bonding of nucleotides normally found in DNA.

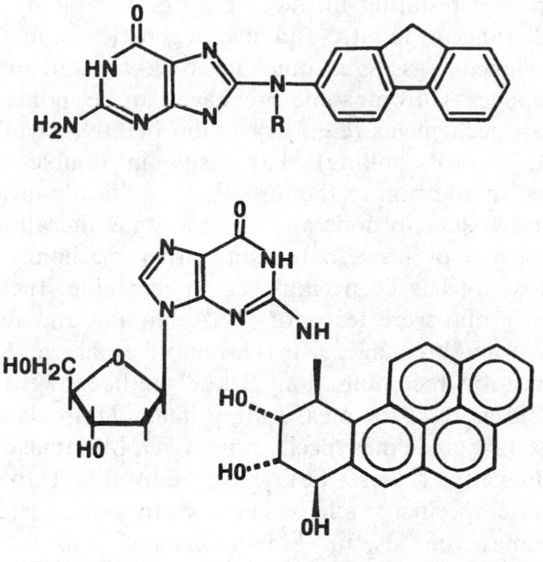

FIG. 17.3. Two examples of DNA chemical adducts. (Top) an aromatic amine adduct to guanine. (Bottom) a benzo[a]pyrene metabolite adduct to guanine.

or G:T). If this mispairing occurs before or during a DNA replication cycle, the result may be the substitution of an incorrect base pair for the original pair. The cycle of DNA replication to fix base-pair substitution mutations is called the "expression period" in in vitro mutation assays.

Base-pair addition-deletion mutations, also called *frameshift mutations*, result from the addition or deletion of one or a few nucleotide pairs from the nucleotide sequence in an exon or gene. Because the codon sequence reads in one direction and is nonpunctuated, the loss or gain of a single base pair changes the reading frame of the gene—hence frameshift mutation. This type of mutagenic mechanism is illustrated in Figure 17.4. Both frameshift and *basepair substitution* gene mutations result in alterations in translation of mRNA into the proper sequence of amino acids in the gene products (See Figure 17.1) and produce a mutant cell or organism. Mutations or DNA methylation in regulatory genes are capable of modulating the production of functional gene products (44).

DNA is visible microscopically as a chromosome. Figure 17.5 illustrates the generalized anatomy of a chromosome. The chromosome illustrated is typical of a metaphase structure and the anatomy shows distinctive bands as a result of giemsa staining. Mammalian chromosomes have a constriction known as the *centromere*. To either side of the centromere are the chromosome arms that terminate in structures called *telomeres*. The dark G+ bands represent highly condensed DNA and are areas of little or no gene expression (transcription). The light G– bands represent active genomic areas where gene expression (transcription) is occurring. The telomeric regions at the ends of the chromosome struc-

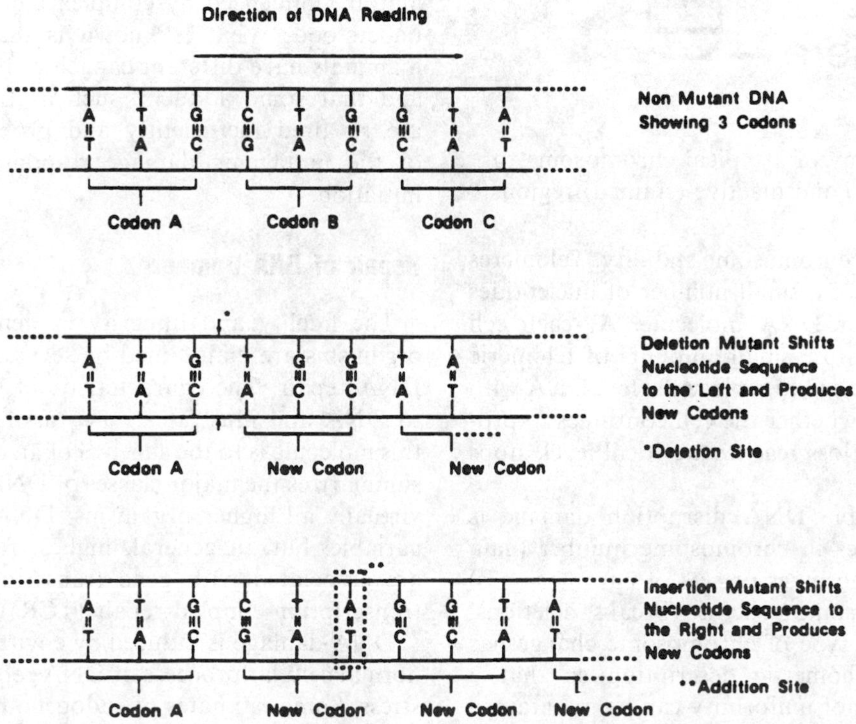

FIG. 17.4. The base pair changes involved with frameshift mutations. An insertion or deletion of a base pair results in the shift of the gene or exon reading frame.

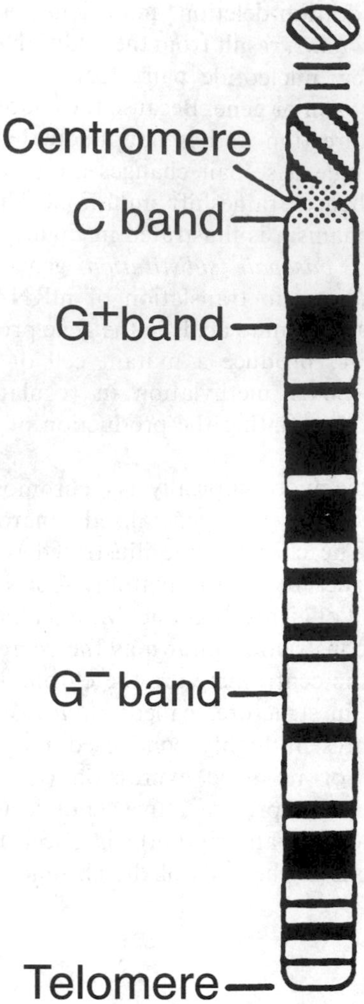

FIG. 17.5. The anatomy of a typical chromosome to show active (unstained) and inactive (stained) regions.

tures are important for chromosome stability. Telomeres consist of repeat units of a small number of nucleotides that stabilize the linear DNA molecule. At each cell division, chromosomes lose small amounts of telomeric DNA. The ability of the cell to replace the lost DNA with telomerase determines whether the cell continues to proliferate or, if the DNA loss reaches a critical level, stops dividing (28).

Microscopically visible DNA disruption damage is subdivided into changes in chromosome number (gain or loss of single chromosomes or sets of chromosomes) and changes in chromosome structure (breaks, deletions, rearrangements). Each type of chromosome change has a characteristic morphometric description so that a reasonably high degree of uniformity can be maintained when scoring them microscopically. Variations in chromosome number can result from incomplete dissociation of single or entire sets of chromosomes at metaphase, resulting in aneuploidy or polyploidy (34). A wide range of in vitro and in vivo genetic test methods are designed to assess chromosome breakage and numerical changes. Chromosome breakage can be induced by several mechanisms (e.g., disruption of DNA synthesis or DNA cross-linking) that result in double-strand breaks. In addition to the tests that specifically measure nucleotide substitutions and chromosome alterations, a third group of tests to measure other mechanisms of genotoxicity has been employed in screening. Included in this group were tests for DNA binding and repair, DNA strand breakage, sister chromatid exchange (SCE), and mitotic recombination. These methods were categorized as tests for measuring primary DNA damage. Few testing guidelines specify primary DNA damage tests any longer, as these tests have been found to lack adequate specificity and sensitivity. In some instances they may be useful biomarkers of exposure to genotoxicants.

A significant amount of research has focused on the induction and measurement of DNA adducts. The initial hope of this technology was to use adduct formation as a method to demonstrate exposure and calculate cancer risk. To date, that hope has not been fulfilled. Adduct formation remains a sensitive method to demonstrate exposure; however, we still do not know enough about adduct processing and repair to use this information to define genetic or cancer risk except for a small number of agents. Binding sites on DNA vary with the compound and are influenced by complex factors that are not yet understood. What is known is that organs/tissues in mammals have different capacities for repairing adducts and that some adducts, such as the O-alkyl adducts, are repaired inefficiently and probably produce most of the mutagenic damage responsible for tumor cell initiation.

Repair of DNA Damage

The fidelity and integrity of genetic information in organisms are maintained by several types of enzymatic DNA repair. The characteristic of self repair is unique to DNA and illustrates how important the integrity of this molecule is to the survival of an organism. Table 17.4 summarizes the major classes of DNA repair that exist in virtually all higher organisms. DNA repair kinetics are variable, but, in general, highest rates of DNA repair are associated with gene transcription processes (i.e., transcription-coupled-repair (TCR)).

DNA damage is induced by environmental agents and normal cellular proceses of DNA replication or oxidative stress. Some estimates of endogenous damage and repair capacities for human cells are given in Table 17.5. As indicated, endogenous cellular repair capacities are more than adequate to compensate for background DNA

Table 17.4
Classification and properties of DNA repair processes

Class	Properties
Base excision repair	Elimination of single nucleotide through cleavage of the glycosyl bond connecting the altered base to the deoxyribose sugar, resulting in an abasic site in the DNA followed by resynthesis using the opposite strand as template.
Nucleotide excision repair	Removal of bulky DNA adducts from DNA. Process involves 20 proteins that remove up to 100 nucleotides associated with damaged region. Repair synthesis using the opposite strand as template fills in repair patch.
Mismatch repair	A "second chance" repair system that corrects mismatch base pairs post-DNA replication. This process catches lesions missed by nucleotide excision repair and base excision repair (BER) processes.
Recombinational repair	This process acts on double-strand DNA breaks and/or DNA crosslinks, where both DNA strands are damaged.

damage; however, massive or frequent exposures to exogenous genotoxic agents may saturate the DNA repair capacity leading to human genetic disease, aging, and cancer (83).

The most important feature of most repair processes is the ability to enzymatically remove and replace damaged segments of DNA with higher fidelity. If a DNA lesion can be repaired prior to mutation fixation, the net effect of the DNA damage to an organism may be nil. This is especially true following intermittent, low-level exposures to genotoxicants, where repair enzymes are not fully saturated by excessive numbers of damaged DNA sites. DNA adducts are not all recognized or repaired equally by excision repair. The size and effect that an adduct has on the conformation of DNA determines how readily it is detected by the repair enzymes and is excised. As a consequence of this situation, it is not advisable to use the number of adducts per cell as a predictor of damage or genetic hazard unless definitive information is available about the elimination kinetics for the specific adducts (99).

Test systems measuring some parameter of the DNA repair process have been used as genotoxicity screens for detection of primary DNA damage (80,103). Normal organisms are capable of some type of DNA repair

Table 17.5
Estimates of human endogenous DNA damage and repair processes[a]

Type of Damage	Estimated Occurrences of Damage per Hour per Cell[b]	Maximal Repair Rate, Base Pairs per Hour per Cell
Depurination	1000	—[c]
Depyrimidination	55	—[c]
Cytosine Deamination	15	—[c]
Single-stranded breaks	5000	2×10^5
N^7-methylguanine	3500	Not reported
O^6-methylguanine	130	10^4
Oxidation products	120	10^5

[a] Modified from data in Reference 69.
[b] Might be higher or lower by a factor of 2.
[c] Not reported, but the rates are at least 10^4, based on concentration of repair activities in cell extracts.

activity following chemical insult; thus, stimulation or induction of repair activity following chemical treatment at sublethal concentrations is a good indicator that the target organism has experienced DNA-directed toxicity. These tests are generally identified as measures of unscheduled DNA synthesis (UDS).

Studies of DNA repair kinetics indicate that once permutational lesions have been induced in the DNA, both error-prone and error-free repair processes are activated. Error-prone repair processes generate nucleotide mismatches (i.e., A:C or G:T) that produce mutations de novo. Error-free repair replaces the damaged DNA site with a correct nucleotide sequence. The fidelity of repair depends on the degree to which the two different processes are involved. Factors that determine whether error-prone or error-free pathways predominate include (a) the target species, (b) cell type involved, (c) chemical mutagen, and (d) the specific DNA lesion induced. Some data suggest that the error-free repair pathways predominate at low exposure levels, and error-prone pathways come into play only following saturation of the error-free enzymes.

The basic processes of Nucleotide Excision Repair (NER) and Base Excision Repair (BER), the primary repair mechanisms for chemical damage, are shown in Figure 17.6. The enzyme complex responsible for NER of bulky adducts requires more than 20 proteins and consists of several steps (63). One step is an endonuclease activity that cleaves the DNA at the site of the damage; an exonuclease cuts out the damaged region, including nucleotides to either side. The correct bases are replaced by a DNA polymerase using an editing function to ensure that the correct bases are incorporated into the repair patch. DNA ligase seals the repair patch. Occasionally, even in error-free repair, incorrect bases are incorporated

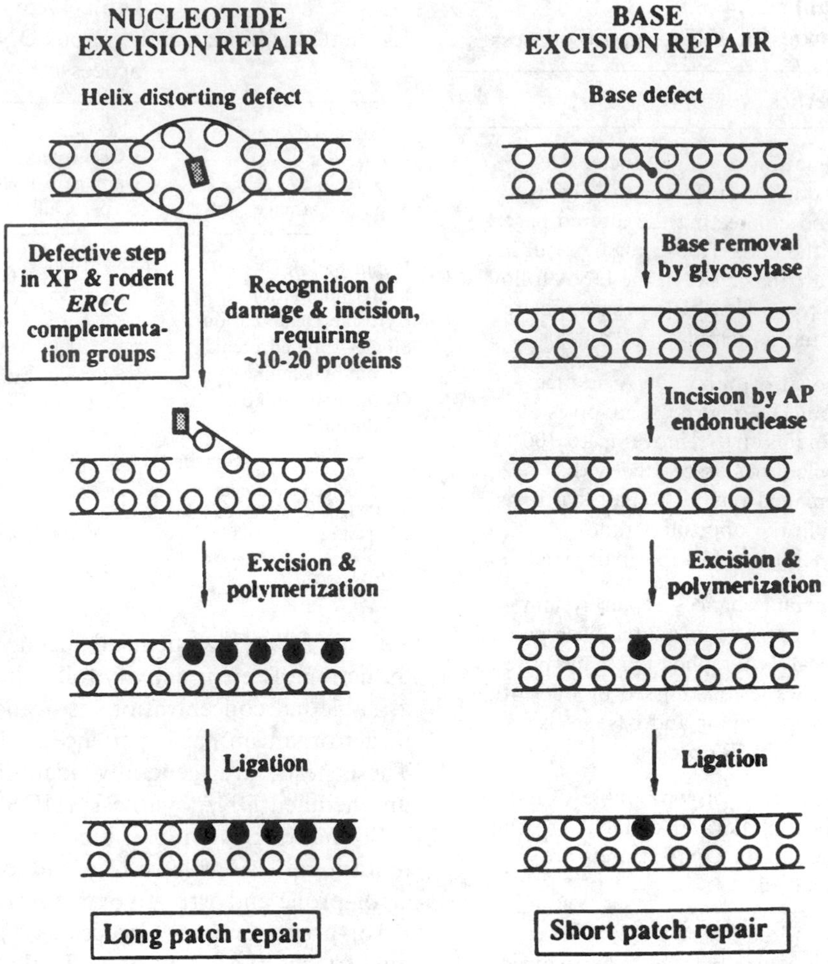

FIG. 17.6. Long and short patch excision repair processes.

by the polymerase, resulting in mismatched bases that do not properly hydrogen bond. In BER, a number of different glycosylases catalyze release of the inappropriate base, followed by replacement and ligation (38).

Mismatch repair (MR) enzymes recognize non-hydrogen bonding base pairs. A short segment of the DNA duplex is excised and filled by the repair polymerase. This is a second-chance repair process that occurs after BER and NER and improves the accuracy of those processes. Finally, recombinational repair acts on double-strand breaks and interstrand cross links, resulting in damage to both strands of the DNA. Collectively, these processes maintain integrity of DNA against endogenous and exogenous sources of damage.

Repair of mutational damage has been shown to be inducible by low-level exposures to DNA-damaging agents (79,105). Inducibility of repair processes above constitutional levels will increase the magnitude of exposure required to exceed the intrinsic capacity producing a "threshold" for mutation and produce a protective effort for subsequent exposures. Theoretical assumptions and data from studies of repair support the belief that at background or low-exposure levels, an error-free removal of alkyl groups from DNA can be virtually 100% effective. Thus, one observes survival shoulders and nonlinear kinetics for mutation induction in repair-proficient cells and the loss of apparent "no effect" regions in repair-deficient cells.

Because of the influence that species- and cell-specific genetic background have on repair capacity, an appreciation of the variability of DNA repair in somatic and germ cells of humans as well as the animal models is essential in assessing genetic risk (36,71). Several general characteristics of mammalian DNA repair are summarized in Table 17.6.

RELATIONSHIP OF GENOTOXIC DAMAGE TO TOXICITY

The proposed sequence of events from DNA interaction to the expression of human toxicity is represented

Table 17.6
DNA repair characteristics

DNA repair is tissue- and species-specific (e.g., human capacity approximately 10-fold greater than mouse)
DNA repair is increased in genes involved in transcription (e.g., chromosome loops)
DNA adducts are repaired with different efficiency (e.g., bulky > small)
Effects of DNA repair are tied closely to cell stringency and apoptosis (e.g., cell lines with low cycling stringency have higher error rates)

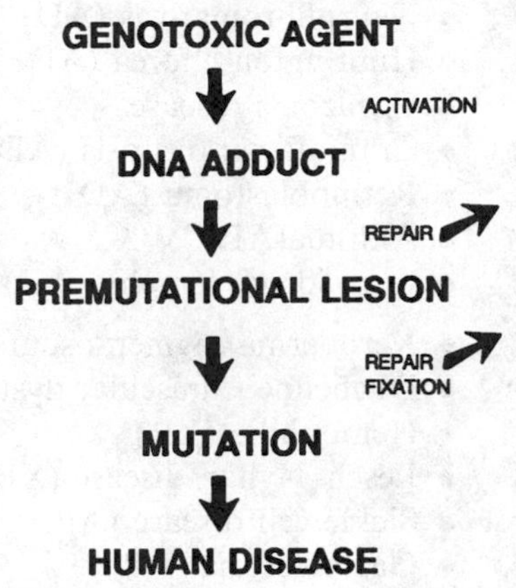

FIG. 17.7. The hypothetical process from exposure to genotoxin to the induction of genetic disease in humans. Repair processes can eliminate the formation of mutations that produce disease.

in Figure 17.7. The nature of the toxicity or disease is dependent on which cells or tissues and genes are altered by the mutation.

Because of the fundamental role genes play in all aspects of organisms, the mutational basis for many human disorders and anomalies is well documented (61). The genetic disease burden in humans is estimated to be approximately 5% (Table 17.7), and its effects contribute significantly to the health care costs of most developed countries. The origin of the mutations in the gene pool is unknown, but Table 17.8 provides several probable sources. Animal experiments offer convincing evidence that environmental agents are capable of inducing permanent, transmissible mutations in either somatic or germ cells and support the assumption that humans are susceptible to genetic risk factors in the environment (76,77). Other types of toxic phenomena appear to be determined or influenced by somatic cell genotoxicity. Among these endpoints are the following:

1. Oncogenesis-inherited and induced forms (12,54).
2. Teratogenesis (49).
3. Sterility or semisterility (23).
4. Atherosclerosis (47).
5. Aging (20).

Tests for DNA binding and repair, point mutation, and clastogenicity have been used to monitor human populations, putatively exposed to genotoxic agents, for evidence of somatic cell genotoxicity (27). In many studies there have been strong associations between somatic cell toxicity and the production of primary DNA damage (10,43). PAH exposure, DNA adducts, and tumor incidences are highly associated in human populations, but DNA adducts are not general predictors of carcinogenesis (57); however, the consistency between cancer and other types of DNA damage, such as chromosome aberrations, SCEs, or micronuclei in humans exposed to carcinogens, is not sufficient for routine human monitoring (11).

Carcinogens and Mutagens

During the early 1970s, the introduction of a *Salmonella* assay detecting reverse mutation, combined with an in vitro metabolic activation system, appeared to offer a rapid, inexpensive solution to the identification of chemical carcinogens (4,58). The Ames test was the forerunner for an array of submammalian and mammalian cell assays proposed as rapid screens for carcinogens (73,74). The rationale for the use of these methods consisted of several investigations demonstrating that properties associated with the transformed (malignant) cell phenotype were encoded in the DNA. During the late 1970s, studies were published showing that DNA isolated from transformed mouse cells could be purified of other contaminants, cut into discrete fragments by bacterial restriction enzymes, transfected into "normal" cells resulting in the conversion of "normal" cells into a transformed phenotype (101). Investigators conducting these experiments ultimately identified a series of genes in the restriction fragments (proto-oncogens) responsible for transforming the cells (12,75). Proto-oncogens are highly conserved genes found in most eukaryotic organisms, and some, such as the *ras*, *myc*, and *neu* genes, are known to be activated by base-pair substitution mutations or chromosome aberrations (34). Additional loci have been discovered that code for tumor suppressor molecules. The suppressor molecules, which prevent cell proliferation, become inactive following mutation in the genes coding for them (45). *Oncogenes* and *tumor suppressor* have been studied in humans and in rodents used for experimental carcinogenesis studies (7). It has been established that some strains of animals carry activated oncogenes in their germ line and are predisposed, therefore, to specific tumor types following exposures to promoting agents alone (55). Apoptosis is an important cellular process that functions

Table 17.7
Examples of genetic disorders in humans[a]

Category of Genetic Alteration	Estimated Frequency/10^3 Population	Typical Examples[b]
Chromosome abnormalities	6.86	• Down's syndrome (trisomy) • Klinefelter's syndrome (XXY) • Turner's syndrome (XO) • Cri du chat (deletion of chromosome) • Numerous other trisomies (XYY)
Dominant mutations	1.85–2.64	• Familial polyposis (AD) • Neurofibromatosis (AD) • Huntington chorea (AD) • Crouzon's disease • Craniofacial dystosis (AD) • Retinoblastoma (AD) • Anitidia(AD) • Chrondrodystrophy (AD)
Recessive mutations	2.23–2.54 0.78–1.99	• Xeroderma pigmentosum (AR) • Duchenne's muscular dystrophy (XR) • Hemophilia (XR) • Lesch–Nyhan disease (XR) • Sickle cell disease (AR) • Galactosemia (AR) • Phenylketonuria (AR) • Diabetes mellitus (AR) • Fanconi's syndrome (AR) • Albinism (AR) • Cystic fibrosis (AR)
Polygenic (complex inheritance)	26.00–32.00	• Cleft lip • Anencephaly • Spina bifida • Clubfoot • Idiopathic epilepsy • Congenital heart defects

[a] From Reference 109.
[b] AD—autosomal dominant; AR—autosomal recessive; XR—X-linked recessive.

in the immature and adult animals. In adult animals it is responsible for elimination of potentially preneoplastic cells by nuclear degredation (97). The p53 tumor suppressor gene is a major apoptosis-inducing protein. Elimination or reduction in the expression of p53 by mutation is believed to be a critical step in the process of neoplasia.

Support for genotoxicity as a means of carcinogen detection was derived from studies correlating the results of specific genotoxicity tests (or batteries of tests) on chemicals with tumor responses, for the same chemicals, in long-term tests using mice or rats. The animal cancer classifications were usually consensus responses derived from multiple tests employing several rodent species or strains. During the early 1970s, concordance between rodent carcinogenicity and results reported for chemicals in the Ames test ranged from 90% to 95% (89); however, by 1984 the concordance on a wider base of data had dropped to just over 60%. There are several reasons for this reduction in concordance (9); however, the factor that had the most influence was the selection of chemicals

Table 17.8
Origin of mutations in the human gene pool

- The majority are inherited
- A small number arise from spontaneous events that occur during normal DNA replication and repair
- Unavoidable environmental exposures (radiation, products of combustion, mycotoxin, pesticides, manufacturing emissions, etc.)
- Therapeutic treatments that are directly mutagenic (e.g. radiation)
- Successful treatment of individuals with lethal genetic diseases, thereby elevating the gene frequency in the reproducing population

used in the comparisons (17). Reports in the early to mid-1970s showing high concordance employed groups of chemicals highly biased toward electrophilc carcinogens (72). Reports with lower concordance employed groups of chemicals (a) not selected for electrophilicity and (b) with a greater proportion of noncarcinogens. A good comparison of the two approaches is summarized in Table 17.9, which compares the results of the EPA Gene-Tox analysis of concordance and the National Institute of Environmental Health Sciences (NIEHS) National Toxicology Program (NTP) analysis of concordance (52). The EPA Gene-Tox analysis, which demonstrated high positive correlations between mutagens and carcinogens, used published data heavily skewed toward positive responses in both the cancer and genotoxicity tests (Table 17.10). Consequently, it is impossible to exclude chance as an explanation for the high concordance found in the EPA Gene-Tox assessment.

Another outcome of the cancer concordance analyses has been the use of genotoxicity tests to help interpret the mechanism of rodent carcinogens. Carcinogens with positive effects in genetic tests are considered to act through direct genotoxic effects on DNA in contrast to carcinogens with predominantly negative results in genetic tests. Thus, a classification scheme of genotoxic and nongenotoxic carcinogens has been proposed by some individuals as a method to interpret the mechanisms of tumor initiation and aid in the selection of the most appropriate data extrapolation model for cancer risk assessment (84). A genotoxic mechanism implies a no-threshold mechanism, and risk data would be analyzed with more conservative methods than would data from nongenotoxic carcinogens. While conceptually this scheme appears reasonable, a better understanding of carcinogenic processes is necessary to support its general appreciation to risk assessment. With the correlation between carcinogens and mutagens averaging about 70%, the appropriate integration of genetic toxicology results into toxicological assessments is less than certain.

The use of genetic tests as part of an assessment for carcinogenic potential may be justified by mechanistic considerations alone and may not have to be supported by high correllations. New mutation models, such as the in vivo *transgenic* models developed for measuring

Table 17.9
A comparison of the sensitivities and specificities of several short-term tests used in carcinogen screening trials[a]

Assay	Sensitivity[b] (%) Gene Tox[c]	NTP[d]	Specificity[b] (%) Gene Tox[c]	NTP[d]
Ames/*Salmonella*	175/23 (78)	20/44 (45)	29/47 (62)	25/29 (86)
		66/119 (54)		51/73 (70)
Mouse lymphoma	45/54 (87)	31/44 (70)	0/5 (0)	13/29 (45)
CHO/HGPRT	40/41 (98)	—	1/1 (100)	—
V79/HGPRT	84/104 (81)	—	3/3 (100)	—
Drosophila SLRL	77/106 (73)	4/18 (22)	9/16 (60)	9/9 (100)
In vitro cytogenetics	40/54 (74)	24/44 (55)	2/6 (33)	20/29 (69)
In vivo cytogenetics	8/9 (89)	9/15 (60)	0/0 (—)	11/12 (92)
In vitro SCE	100/101 (99)	31/44 (70)	0/10 (0)	13/29 (45)
In vivo SCE	21/21 (100)	10/15 (67)	0/0 (—)	5/12 (42)
UDS in hepatocytes	19/22	6/30 (20)	0/0 (—)	13/14 (93)

[a] From Reference 53
[b] Sensitivity—proportion of positive results for carcinogens; specificity—proportion of negative results for noncarcinogens.
[c] Combined results for sufficient and limited evidence carcinogens and noncarcinogens.
[d] Assumes equivocal evidence compounds are noncarcinogens.

Table 17.10
Relative distribution of positive and negative agents among several types of bioassays reviewed under the EPA Gene-Tox program

	Chemicals with Either Sufficient Negative or Positive Responses	Positive Agents (%)	Negative Agents (%)
Rodent cancer tests	413	351 (85)	62 (15)
Ames test	1262	820 (65)	442 (35)
Mouse lymphoma test	138	114 (83)	24 (17)
In vitro cytogenetics	116	81 (70)	35 (30)
Micronucleus test	63	60 (95)	3 (5)
Drosophila (SLRL)	345	238 (69)	107 (31)

mutation, may offer a much more relevant assessment of carcinogenicity than in vitro assays (78). Two transgenic models for mutation detection employing transgenes from the bacteria *lac* operon have been developed and partially validated (64,85). Other transgenic mouse models with altered tumor suppressor genes (p53 heterozygote) or activated proto-oncogenes (TG:AC) are currently under validation in short-term bioassays for chemical carcinogens. The p53 model is used for genotoxic agents as the mode of action for enhanced tumorigenesis is inactivation of the normal p53 allele by chemical-induced mutation, deletion, or rearrangement (98).

EFFECTS OF MUTAGENS ON THE HUMAN GENE POOL

Induction of damage to the germ-line DNA of plant and animal species has the potential to create serious adverse consequences for the health and survival of those organisms. In humans, genetic damage is a cause of hereditary diseases, cancer, congenital anomalies, and even reduced life expectancy (94).

The genes needed to produce the current human population were all acquired from the previous generation's *gene pool*. The gene pool is the sum total of genes, at a given point in time in the reproductively active population of a species, available for transmission to the next generation. Deleterious genes are present in the gene pool at a set frequency, as evidenced by predictable rates of recurring genetic diseases in the human species. The origin of this genetic burden (genetic load) is not known, but it is imperative that the current caretakers of the gene pool use all precautions to transmit it to the next generation in no worse shape than it was received.

Genetic disease in humans appears to be produced by the same types of mutations identified in animal models:

Table 17.11
Examples of human diseases and conditions caused by mutations in germs cells[a]

Genetic Disease or Condition	Estimated No. of Cases in the United States
Dyslexia	15,000,000
Manic depression	2,000,000
Schizophrenia	1,500,000
Juvenile diabetes	1,000,000
Adult polycystic kidney disease	500,000
Familial Alzheimer's disease	250,000
Multiple sclerosis	250,000
AAT deficiency (emphysema)	120,000
Myotonic muscular dystrophy	100,000
Fragile X chromosome syndrome	100,000
Sickle cell anemia	65,000
Duchenne muscular dystrophy	32,000
Cystic fibrosis	30,000
Huntington's chorea	25,000
Hemophilia	20,000
Phenylketonuria	16,000
Retinoblastoma (childhood eye cancer)	10,000

[a]From Reference 96

(a) chromosome abnormalities resulting in stable changes in chromosome number or structure, (b) dominant gene mutations in which only a single mutant allele (of the normal gene pair) is required to produce the disease, (c) recessive gene mutations in which both alleles of the pair must be mutant for expression of the trait, or (d) polygenic mutations in which the mutant trait is determined by the interaction of several genes.

Table 17.11 provides examples of human genetic diseases as well as the frequency of these disorders in the United States population. The examples given in the table represent only a small portion of the total human diseases and defects known to be of genetic origin (61). It is estimated that the human genome consists of approximately 140,000 genes controlling all aspects of an organism's biology and behavior. Of the total number of genes, we currently know the function for about 1500 to 2000 genes (30). The current human genome project plans to complete sequencing the entire human genome by 2001; however, it will be many more years before all gene functions are mapped to a physical structure.

The degrees of impact to the gene pool from the separate categories of germ cell alterations (listed in Table 17.7) are not equivalent; for example, most of the chromosome abnormalities, other than balanced translocations, result in cell lethality, and if induced in either the ova or sperm, generally produce dominant lethal effects not transmitted to the next generation.

Dominant viable mutations will be expressed in the first generation after induction and may contribute only moderately to the genetic burden. The impact of these mutations on the gene pool may be limited because the affected individuals are aware that they are carrying the mutant form of the gene and that there will be a 50% probability of transmitting the trait to their children if married to an unaffected (normal) individual. Thus, depending on the severity of the effect, the parents can decide, prior to reproducing, if the risk associated with transmission is acceptable.

Recessive mutations are not expressed unless both alleles of the gene in a diploid organism are defective or if the mutation is on the X chromosome in male offspring. Therefore, two normal-appearing heterozygous carriers for an autosomal mutant allele could produce offspring (25% incidence) exhibiting a recessive disease. Consequently, increases in new recessive mutations pose the most serious threat to the gene pool because they would tend to accumulate, over time, in the gene pool as expressed heterozygotes. Due to this latent period, the ultimate expression of a new recessive mutation in the population will have no apparent association with the environmental exposure that induced it. This situation severely limits the opportunity to use human epidemiological studies for proof of human genetic risk.

Intrinsic Differences Affecting Susceptibility to Genotoxic Effects

Unlike the genetic uniformity intrinsic in the animals used as experimental models in toxicology testing, humans exhibit a broad range of variability in their capacity to process and repair DNA damage (30,41,63). Studies on DNA repair capacity in mice also indicate a substantial decrease in global DNA repair capacity compared with humans (40).

As described previously, DNA repair in organisms, including humans, is controlled by a complex genetic system of structural and regulatory genes involving almost 50 different proteins. Human *polymorphisms* exist for many of these genes. Individual DNA repair capacity may range as low as 65% of the normal average level (63), placing such individuals at a different risk to mutagens than most of the population.

Additional information about repair genes comes from studies of human genetic diseases, such as xeroderma pigmentosum (XP). Diseases such as XP are caused by mutations in NER genes. Individuals with XP lack one of the enzymes in the repair process, and affected individuals, with as little as 1%–2% of the normal repair capacity, usually experience high levels of intrinsic DNA damage (63). Cancer susceptibility among XP cases is believed to be a consequence of the genetic damage and can be as much as 1000 times greater than non-XP individuals. Other human syndromes associated with reduced repair capacity (e.g., ataxiatclangicctasia, Bloom Syndrome, and Fanconi anemia) are inherited traits that also exhibit increased cancer risk (64). Thus, it is unlikely that genetic damage induced in genetically homogenous animal models with uniform repair will be easily extrapolated to human populations because factors such as DNA repair exhibit such broad response ranges. It is also clear from this illustration that quantitative estimates of hazardous or safe exposures to genotoxic chemicals based on results from animal data are likely to have large margins of error.

Pharmacogenetics

In addition to DNA repair polymorphisms, other allele variations confer important differences that will influence the impact of genotoxic agents. Some of these differences affect metabolic conversion kinetics. Individuals genetically predisposed to be either a fast or slow metabolizer of specific chemicals may be at higher risk from the parent compound or metabolite. Determination of an individual's genotype can be made with only a small sample of their DNA (15).

Identification of single gene polymorphisms (one nucleotide change), which influence the susceptibility of an individual to the pharmacologic/toxic effects of therapeutic agents, has developed into a major field of medical genetics (107). Institutions have assembled alleles from hundreds of polymorphic genes, and large human populations can be screened for single gene polymorphisms with automated high through-put screening systems employing techniques such as DNA binding and transcription activation. Integration of such information into a genetic profile may eventually be used to direct an individual's lifestyle optimization. Studies in humans exposed to carcinogenic hydrocarbons documented a genotypic influence on the level of adducts. Polymorphism in GSTMI 2 (gluthathione transferase), CYP1A1, and CYP2D6 alleles all affected the formation of DNA adducts found in white blood cells of exposed individuals (21).

Life Style and Exposure to Genotoxicants

There are numerous examples of heritable cancer, where acquisition of specific genes confer a high risk of cancer (e.g., retinoblastoma, colon cancer, breast cancer). These alleles may contribute to as much as 5% of the total cancer incidence, the other 95% is a product of life style. It is well documented that occupation and life style can influence genetic hazard (48,86).

Table 17.12
Foods and mutagenic activity in the Ames assay

Coffee
Tea
Broiled beef and pork
Broiled fish
Pickled vegetables (Japanese)
Flavanoids in many edible plants
Mushrooms (Agaricus bisporus)
Salted fish (Chinese)
Caramelized sugars (glucose/fructose)
Pyrolysates of onion and garlic
Aflatoxin and other mycotoxins (food contamination)
Safrole

See References 2, 66, 67, and 68 for general discussion.

Tobacco smoke contains a broad range of mutagenic agents detectable in human lymphocytes and urine (51). Consumption of alcoholic beverages has been associated with genetic alterations in humans (69). Diet is also an important source of mutagens. The average human consumes about 10 tons (dry weight) of food by the age of 50 (92), and the list in Table 17.12 illustrates that many food items normally consumed by humans contain substances found to be mutagenic in microbial assays. Many of these agents are also mutagenic when tested in mammalian cell systems.

Other ubiquitous materials that have been reported to produce positive effects in mutagenicity tests include cosmetic ingredients, drugs, food additives, and pesticide residues (1,5,6,87). At present, it is not possible to assess, in quantitative terms, the relevance, if any, of these agents to the mutational or cancer risk in humans.

In addition to tobacco smoke, alcoholic beverages, and consumption of preformed mutagens in or on food products, other life style factors that may be important are less subject to individual control. Exposure to ultraviolet light and ionizing radiation are common. Ambient air contains carbonaceous particles coated with agents producing mutagenic responses in a range of assays (57). The level of particle loading is location dependent, and exposures encountered in urban areas or in certain occupations (e.g., coke oven workers) are considerably higher than exposures in more rural areas.

Ames (2) hypothesized that endogenously formed mutagens and intermediates found in various plants are significant contributors to genotoxic risk. He reported the formation of numerous mutagens resulting from lipid peroxidation of fatty acids. The agents include aldehydes, peroxides, and other free radicals.

Considerable efforts are currently under way to evaluate the relative contributions of dietary, environmental, and endogenously formed mutagens to the human disease burden, as well as the modulating influence of antimutagenic agents (e.g., antioxidants) on mutation expressions and cancer (48,91).

Methods for Assessing Genetic Hazard and Risk

Observations of "new" dominant mutations in human populations and experimental induction of mutations in the germlines of mice indirectly document the fact that mammalian species, including humans, are susceptible to induced mutation. The ability to demonstrate genetic toxicity to human populations through epidemiological methods has been limited by

1. the small number of instances in which sufficient induced sentinel mutations were induced that could be detected in an epidemiology study;
2. the small number of genetic diseases or marker genes identified with specific genetic diseases;
3. the difficulty in identifying reproductively active populations exposed to biologically significant levels of mutagenic agents.

In 1992, the United Nations Environment Program (UNEP) reviewed the status of and methods available for genetic risk assessment (95). The report outlined the situations in which genetic risk assessment might be appropriate and the criteria for selection of risk assessment strategies. Risk information can be developed using qualitative methods resulting in the assignment of a classification, such as "human mutagen" and "probable human mutagen," based on a set of test results criteria. This classification method has been proposed for environmental health uses due to the absence of sufficient in vivo germ cell data to perform quantitative assessments.

When information is limited or when only a general characterization of risk is required, a qualitative assessment can be made. The results are expressed as a ranking for classification based on the test results from a predetermined scheme in which exposure and intrinsic bioactivity are known (Figure 17.8). In most cases, this type of classification is adequate for making risk management decisions (90).

When essential, quantitative risk analysis for genetic damage can be performed using dose response results from animal models such as the mouse-specific locus test or the mouse heritable translocation assay. From these data, the population incidence of mutation can be calculated for anticipated exposure levels and expressed as the probability of new disease occurrence in the population. The same problems that confound the production of cancer risk estimates from animal studies affect the ability to generate accurate genetic risks (i.e.,

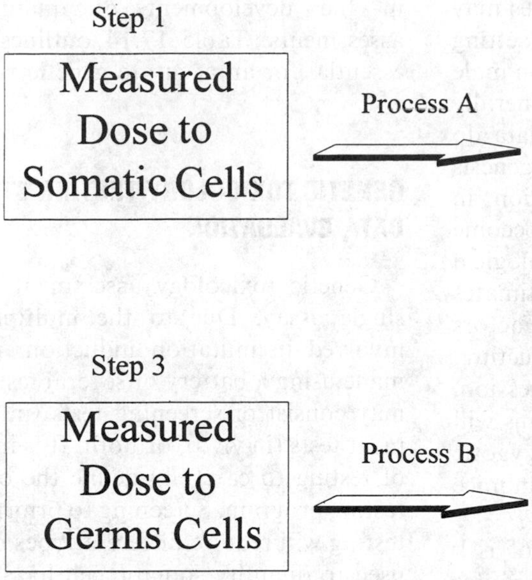

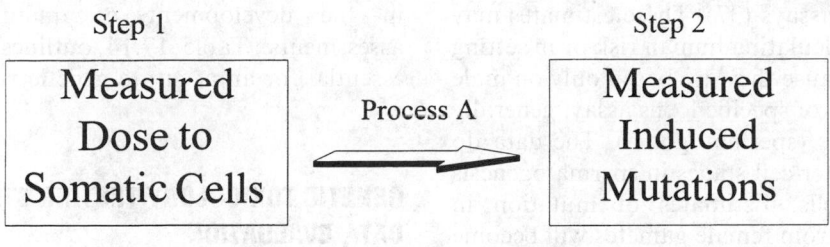

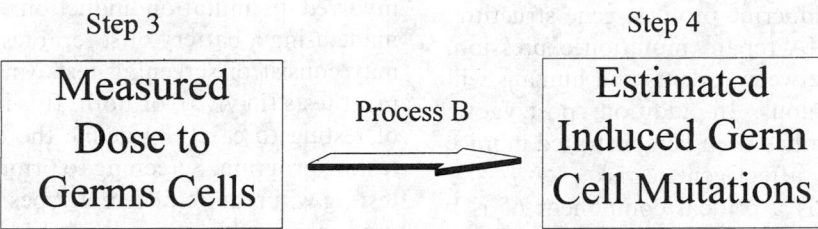

FIG. 17.8. Diagrammatical representation of the parallelogram method of estimating germ cell risk using somatic results and target site dosimetry. This method has been used with rodent and human data to develop probable mutation risks.

Table 17.13
Risk estimates for somatic and germ cell mutations for selected mammalian mutagens[a]

	Dose (mg/kg) required to double the spontaneous background			
	Germ Cell			
Compound	Stage	Gene	Chromosomal	Somatic Cell
Cyclophosphamide	pg	8	69	nt
	g	320	nt	
Methylmethane sulfate	pg	2	4	7
	g	17	nt	
Procarbazine	pg	43	33	11
	g	110	nt	
Mitomycin C	pg	nt	4	0.3

g = gonial stages; pg = postgonial stages; nt = not tested.
[a]From Reference 23

understanding the dose response kinetics, species differences in susceptibility, and factors that influence the phenotypic expression of new mutations). A few quantitative genetic risk assessments have been made (30) using data from mouse models for mutation and clastogenesis (Table 17.13). The major deficiencies in current risk assessment models are the lack of accurate methods to extrapolate animal mutation data to estimates of anticipated new disease incidences in exposed human populations. Mutagens are not as site specific (i.e., organ or tissue) as carcinogens.

INTERPRETING THE RESULTS OF GENETIC RISK ASSESSMENTS

Assessing human germ cell risk to mutagenic substances represents a formidable task, and no chemicals have been proven to induce new mutations in offspring of exposed individuals. Animal mutagens have been detected in rodent germ cells, and quantitative estimates of induced mutation rates per gene locus or the dose required to double a specific mutation rate have to be calculated from results of the in vivo–specific locus or heritable translocation assays (37). These estimates may be of limited value in calculating human risk or in setting safe exposure levels because they are based only on male gametes and, in the case of specific locus assay, generally on premeiotic stem cells (spermatogonia). The data do not reflect the risk to later cell stages in spermatogenesis or in female germ cells. Estimates of mutation in postmeiotic sperm and from female gametes will become available; but even so, other important biological variables would interfere with reliable risk estimates and extrapolation across species boundaries. Factors such as differences in endocrine profiles, gene structure, mutation specificity, DNA repair, mutation expression, and disease homology between rodents and humans will make extrapolation tenuous. In addition, postzygotic repair of damaged sperm has been demonstrated in mice and is a factor that may affect genetic risk.

Exposure assessment is a critical component of risk assessment. Exposure may occur by different routes and duration; however, most in vivo mutagenicity studies used in hazard assessment are dosed acutely by oral or intraperitoneal routes. Information derived from the physical/chemical properties of the agent, its concentration in environmental matrices, and exposure modeling are important factors that must be included in the development of quantitative genetic risk assessments. Table 17.14 outlines the variable factors essential for an accurate genetic risk assessment.

GENETIC TOXICOLOGY TESTING STRATEGIES AND DATA EVALUATION

Genetic toxicology assessments seldom consist of a single assay. Due to the multiplicity of mechanisms involved in mutation induction, most evaluations are made using a battery of several tests (102). Test batteries may consist of screening tests (in vitro), hazard assessment tests (in vivo), or both. It is important at the outset of testing to carefully define the objectives desired in a testing program. Screening to prioritize agents for further testing will require different types of tests than would be used to quantify somatic cell hazard to humans.

After conducting the tests, the more complex task is that of interpreting the results generated from the test battery. A genotoxic compound may be defined as

> "an agent that produces a positive response in a bioassay measuring any genetic endpoint (e.g., mutation, unscheduled DNA synthesis (UDS) or chromosome breakage)."

Table 17.14
A list of required information for genetic risk analysis[a]

Endogenous DNA Repair: Capacities and mechanisms for repairing damaged DNA differ among organisms.

Metabolic Specificity: Many agents are not mutagenic themselves but require conversion to a chemical form that can react with DNA and cause mutation. This conversion is called metabolic activation and is accomplished by enzymes which vary in specificity and amount among (a) species (b) individual organisms within a species, and (c) different tissues in an organism.

Background Mutation Rate: All organisms and genes have an inherent background rate of mutations. Genetic factors that alter normal error rates in repair will alter this among individuals.

Age: Somatic mutations may accumulate during the lifetime of an organism. An older organism may thus be more vulnerable to disease, due to a greater body burden of background and induced mutations, than a younger organism.

Diet: Deficiencies in the levels of some vitamins, such as folate, may increase susceptibility to chromosomal mutations. Many foods contain both mutagens and antimutagens. Consumption of large quantities of mutagenic foods may account for the occurrence of certain types of cancer.

Economic and Sound Factors: Poor diet, inadequate health care, prevalence of infectious diseases, and excess exposure to known environmental mutagens, such as cigarette smoke and sunlight, could interact to increase susceptibility to mutagens.

Duration of Exposure: Duration of exposure to a mutagenic substance may affect the resulting genetic risk, depending on the form of the dose-response curve and the specificity of the agent for particular stages of germ-cell development.

Germ Cell Specificity: Acute exposure to chemicals that induce mutation in late stages of germ-cell growth will result in a transitory genetic risk, confined to conceptions resulting from the gametes exposed during the sensitive stage. Acute exposure to chemicals that induce mutation in early stages of germ-cell growth will result in a permanent genetic risk.

[a]From Reference 96

Although this definition considers virtually all forms of damage to DNA to classify an agent as genotoxic, genotoxicity should not be interpreted, a priori, as an indication of hazard/risk. The label genotoxic is only a convenient method of classifying chemicals, according to their DNA reactivity, into genotoxic or nongenotoxic subgroups. Additional experimental information beyond this initial classification is necessary to resolve concerns of genetic hazard to somatic or germ cells.

Test results are interpreted on both an individual test basis (i.e., positive or negative in a specific assay) and on a test battery basis. Most decisions made for regulatory purposes are based on the response profile from a battery of tests specified by regulations or guidelines. The international scientific community has proposed a number of genetic test batteries for the evaluation of new chemicals, pesticides, food additives, and pharmaceutical products.

CONSIDERATIONS FOR ASSAY SELECTION

Regulatory Guidelines

Standard study designs for the routine genetic toxicology assays have been published by the EPA (32), Organization for Economic Co-operation and Development (OECD) (70), Canadian Health and Welfare (22), and European Economic Community (EEC) (29). Table 17.15 summarizes many of the recommended testing schemes for nonpharmaceuticals. Most test batteries include, at a minimum, (a) the Ames test, (b) a test for in vitro cytogenetic analysis, and usually (c) an in vivo test for cytogenetic damage. Other tests may be included to expand the profile on the agent if there were positive results or if human exposure was anticipated to be very high. It is also possible to add tests that may be particularly informative for special chemical classes. The EPA (33) has proposed guidelines for the interpretation of data, including in vivo tests. These guidelines provide a general framework for qualitative evaluation of results using a weight-of-evidence approach but do not define criteria to class agents as nonmutagenic.

A standard core battery of tests for pharmaceuticals has been developed under the ICH (officially, the International Conference on Harmonization of Technical Requirements for Registration of Pharmaceuticals for Human Use). The ICH process resulted in two guidelines: (1) guidance and recommendations for the conduct of genetic tests and (2) establishment of a standard genotoxicity test battery. This battery consists of the Ames test modified by the addition of an *Escherichia coli* tester strain, the mouse micronucleus test, and either the Mouse Lymphoma test (with colony sizing) or an in vitro test for chromosome aberrations (Table 17.16). Adoption of the battery has been completed by the European Union, Japanese *MHW* (Ministry of Health & Welfare), and the U.S. Food and Drug Administration.

Development of a standard core battery of the type recommended by ICH has raised a number of issues regarding which genotoxic endpoints are relevant to hazard assessment, and which tests should be conducted. The two tests agreeable to all participants in the harmonization process were the Ames test for gene

Table 17.15
Testing requirements and guidelines other than for pharmaceuticals

AGENCY	AMES	IN VITRO	IN VIVO	OTHER
U.S. EPA FIFRA	+		+	Mouse lymphoma[a]
U.S. FDA				
Devices/Implants[b]	+	+		Mouse lymphoma[a]/UDS
Drug or Food Additive	+	+		
EUROPEAN COMMUNITY				
Industrial Chemicals	+	+		
Food Additive	+	+	+	Mouse lymphoma
JAPAN				
Industrial Chemicals	+	+		

[a] The mouse lymphoma must be conducted with colony sizing. Alternatively, the mouse lymphoma or CHO/HGPRT assay plus in vitro cytogenetics may be used.
[b] Usually conducted on extracts.
In most instances, where the mouse lymphoma is designated, the CHO cell HGPRT assay may be substituted.
Protocol designs for the tests in Table 17.16 follow the most recent OECD guidelines except for the mouse lymphoma assay, which should follow the ICH design.

Table 17.16
ICH test battery

Study	OECD Guideline Design	Testing Expectations
Bacteria reverse mutation assay	471/472	*Salmonella* and *Escherichia* tester strains Maximum concentration of 5 mg/plate or 5 μl/plate Equivocal response requires further testing Negative response confirmed on a case-by-case basis
In vitro chromosome aberration test	473	Maximum concentration of 5 mg/ml or 10 mM Test into the insoluble range Toxicity should exceed LC_{50} One harvest time at 1.5 × normal cell cycle length If negative/–S9, do continuous treatment for 1.5 cycles Record polyploidy and endo replication when seen Equivocal responses require further testing Negative response/–S9 need to be confirmed on a case-by-case basis
Mouse lymphoma assay	476	Maximum concentration of 5 mg/ml or 10 mM Test into the insoluble range Toxicity should achieve 80%–90% Duplicate treatments or eight concentrations Sizing of mutant colonies required Equivocal responses require further testing Negative results must be confirmed on a case-by-case basis
Rodent micronucleus assay (mouse or rat)	474	Maximum dose of 2 g/kg Single sex is sufficient, if toxicity is similar in both May do acute or multiple dosing regimen Three dose levels For acute dosing, harvest high dose at 48 h; the rest at 24 h Must have 5 scorable animals/group Score 2000 PCE/animal Equivocal results should be clarified by further testing

mutation and the in vivo micronucleus for chromosome breakage. The use of in vitro tests for chromosome analysis and gene mutation were more controversial. The use of the mouse lymphoma assay was accepted, in part, because it could serve as both an in vitro measure of gene mutation and chromosome aberrations, and because induction of mutation at the target gene (thymidine kinase) can be induced by either base-pair substitution mutation at the mutant site on the normal chromosome or by deletions of the allele through chromosome breakage. The former mechanism results in large colony mutants and the latter mechanism produces small mutant colonies. Consequently, use of the mouse lymphoma assay for ICH purposes requires colony sizing. Chromosome analysis using cultured cell lines or human lymphocytes is an acceptable alternate to the mouse lymphoma assay.

NEW TECHNOLOGY AND ITS PLACE IN GENETIC TESTING

Limitations of Current Testing Strategies

By 1980, over 150 different tests for genotoxicity had contributed data to scientific journals. Many of the tests were redundant (i.e., measured same endpoint in a different organism or cell type) but each method had a champion who attempted to define the unique value of the particular technique or target organism. The following decade saw extensive efforts to validate and evaluate the best test or set of tests for the purposes of detecting relevant genotoxicant (carcinogens and/or germ cell mutagens). In the process, several valuable lessons were learned:

1. Many test methods are very sensitive and respond positively to rodent carcinogens; however, the tests do not discriminate agents based on DNA reactivity and they also respond to agents that are not carcinogenic or mutagenic. Examples of such tests are (a) in vitro SCE measures and (b) alkaline elution and other measures of single- and double-strand breakage. The use of these tests in genetic toxicology evaluations has dropped dramatically.
2. Several test methods worked extremely well in the laboratory of the inventor but did not reliably transfer to other testing laboratories. Some of the most difficult methods to transfer from lab to lab are the in vitro morphological cell transformation assays. Currently, only the Syrian hamster embryo (SHE) assays are used as a short-term test for carcinogenicity, and extensive standardization is required to acheive interlaboratory agreement on scoring colonies.
3. The array of mechanisms detected by the available tests may not include mechanisms that are relevant to genetic hazard in mammals. Examples of such deficiencies are tests that reliably measure aneuploidy, induction of tandom repeat errors, transposons, or effects from DNA methylation.
4. Commonly used tests, such as in vitro cytogenetic analysis and the Mouse Lymphoma assay, are susceptible to false-positive responses generated by (a) nonphysiological treatment conditions; (b) chemical-induced cytoxicity, and (c) reactive oxidation species generated by S9 mix chemistry (19).

Several actions were taken in an attempt to resolve the issues listed. The most dramatic was a reduction in test methods requested by regulatory agencies. Genetic toxicology testing schemes were simplified for the purposes of regulatory toxicology safety testing. Most agencies now expect to see the results from a limited test battery consisting of tests for gene mutation and chromosome aberrations before asking for further tests. The ICH core battery of tests is an example of this approach, and this battery is expected, over time, to become the international standard for most testing requirements. Other tests, such as in vitro cell transformation, DNA breakage and repair, mitotic recombination, and DNA adduct formation, are now used in research or as supplemental methods to support or explain findings from core battery assessments. Finally, treatment conditions and confirmatory testing were spelled out in more detail and have been structured to minimize false-positive responses.

Weight-of-evidence methods have been developed to evaluate complex response patterns from test batteries. Some of the methods, such as the Mutagenic Activity Profiles created by ICPEMC, have been validated with large data sets and encoded into computer software (62).

The technological deficiencies indicated in the prior list have not been resolved. The tests included in the ICH battery do not provide a full coverage of mechanisms known to operating in higher mammals and can potentially fail to detect agents that may be relevant to elements of the human genome. In addition, there are no routine methods capable of detecting gene mutation in vivo. This is a serious deficiency when attempting to confirm or extrapolate the results from the Ames test to organisms with eukaryotic DNA and chromosome structure.

Use of alternative methods for carcinogenicity testing, such as the p53 and TG:AC transgenic mice, may tend to reduce reliance on genotoxicity tests because these tests detect tumor endpoints and are both faster and more information rich than conventional rodent cancer bioassays, however, there will continue to be a need to assess the hazard to somatic and germ cell DNA from exposure to new products.

Proposed New Methods for Genetic Testing

Table 17.17 lists several technologies that have become widely available during the past 5 years and appear to be directly applicable to gaps identified in the existing methods used in genetic toxicology. Specific tests have been developed as a consequence of the technology. These new methods are currently being evaluated and validated as either replacements or additions to the current test batteries. Their primary advantage is that they allow more testing to be conducted in vivo using DNA from virtually any tissue.

Transgenic Models for in vivo Mutation Analysis

Transgenic animals for mutation detection were developed in 1990 using shuttle vector technology (40,86). The two models that are commercially available today are summarized in Table 17.18. A third model that is based on the *lac Z* gene integrated in plasmid DNA was developed by Boerringter and co-workers (13) and is in commercial development. In all commercial models, a gene from the lactose operon of *E. coli* was combined with DNA sequences from lambda phage to form a recoverable shuttle vector (Figure 17.9). The transgenic animals were generated following micro-injection of the vectors into fertilized mouse ova that were subsequently replaced back into the uteri of psuedo-pregnant dams. Founder animals with integrated shuttle vectors were recovered and used to develop stable homozygous strains of mice (and rats) from which the target *lac* genes can be recovered and analyzed for mutation following

Table 17.17
Technologies leading to the development of new genetic testing methods

Method	Properties	In Vivo Test Developed
Polymerase chain reaction (PCR)	Specific gene amplification which permits isolation, amplification, and analysis of specific endogenous mammalian genes	Gene mutation at the HGPRT gene in mice and rats
Shuttle vectors	Engineer-specific DNA sequences into a rescuable vector that can integrate into the host organism's genomic DNA	Transgenic mice and rat models for gene mutation
DNA gel electrophoresis	The use of various types of gels to separate DNA on the basis of size or base composition	COMET assay for DNA strand breakage; gene mutation using single strand conformated polymorphism
Flourescent immunochemical straining combined with in situ hybridization	The use of fluorescent stains attached to specific nucleotide sequences to identify gene locations	Highly specific chromosome mapping and tests to detect small delection and rearrangements

Table 17.18
Characteristics of commercially available transgenic model systems

MUTAMOUSE
80 copies of the *gt10lac* Z shuttle vector
40-merconcameters (head-to-tail) chromosome 3
lac Z target DNA is 3126 base pairs in length
Nontranscribed target gene
Positive selection system for mutant identification
BIG BLUE MOUSE
80 copies of *lac* I reported gene per diploid genome
lac I target DNA is 1080 base pairs in length
Nontranscribed target gene
Visual selection of mutants
Rat model also available

in vivo exposure. This technology offers an ideal model for in vivo mutation detection and molecular analysis (Figure 17.10).

The recoverable shuttle vector containing the *lac* gene can be isolated from virtually any cell type in the treated animal (Table 17.19). Validation studies with transgenic models have demonstrated that they generally are reliable. For example, studies of known rodent carcinogens have demonstrated tissue-specific mutation associated with the target organs associated with induced tumors (98). Both transgenic models show very close concordance with the Ames test for known genotoxic carcinogens (>90%), and may, therefore, serve as a confirmatory test for the Ames or other in vitro gene mutation screens.

All of the currently available models employ either *lac I* or *lac Z* target genes. The genes are not transcribed but appear to respond in a similar fashion to endogenous genes (96). The primary difference is associated with the ability of the transgenes to detect large deletions. Approximately 1%–1.5% of the spontaneous mutants from Big Blue or MutaMouse models are deletions of 50 base pairs or larger (98, personal communication); however, the *lac Z* plasmid model developed by Borringter and co-workers (13) is able to detect large deletions, and approximately 50% of the spontaneous mutations are due to deletions of 50 base pairs or larger. Recent development of positive selection methods for target genes has made the transgenic models faster and much less expensive to conduct.

Transgenic models for mutation have been used to show that many organ-specific carcinogens show a parallel organ specificity for mutation induction (35). These models are excellent models for the study of mutagenic specificity, as both *lac I* and *lac Z* genes can be sequenced. They may also prove to be good models to investigate the mechanisms of antimutagens and tumor promotors. Transgene sequences can be easily recovered from germinal tissue, making these models potentially ideal for genetic risk assessments. Validation studies for heritable risk analysis have not been conducted with transgenic models.

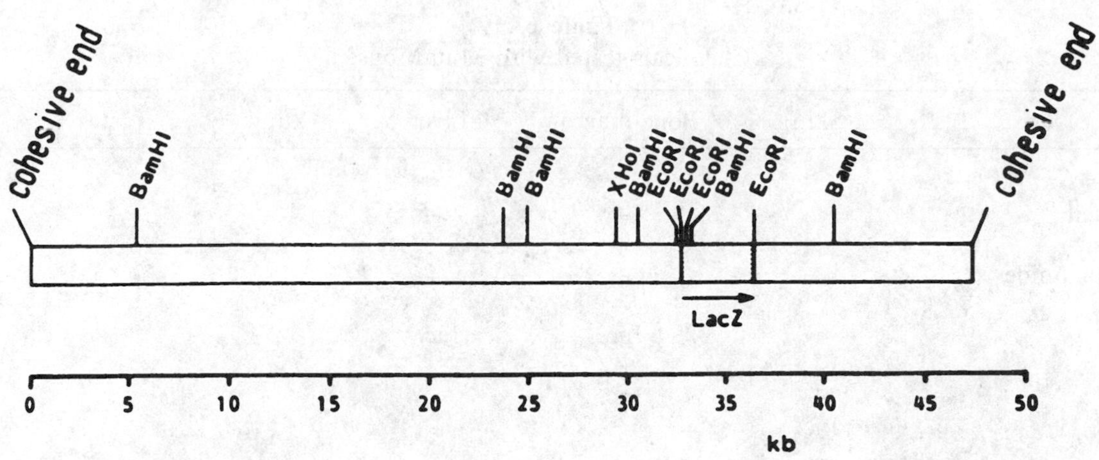

FIG. 17.9. The shuttle vector used to produce the MutaMouse transgenic model for mutation detection. The vector consists of the *lac* Z gene from *E. coli* with Lambda phage genes on either end. The vector is rescuable from mammalian DNA with lambda packaging extracts.

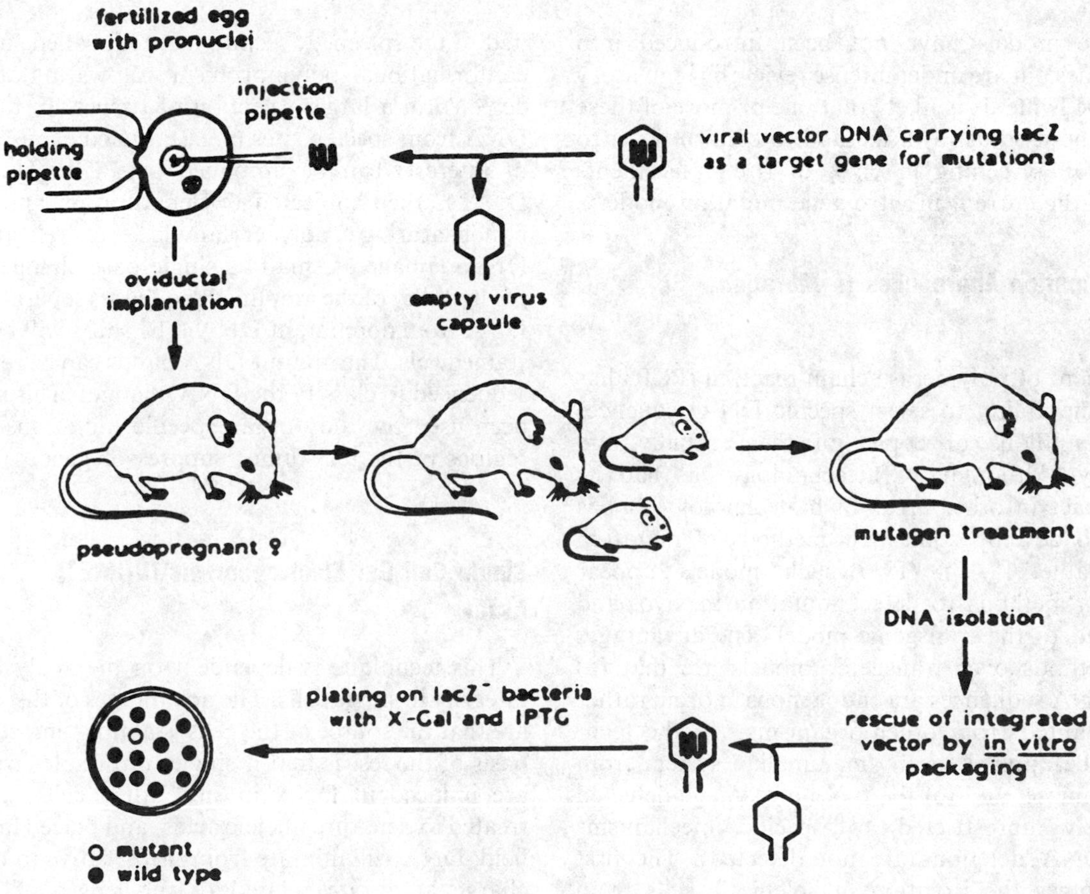

FIG. 17.10. The steps involved in the use of the MutaMouse transgenic mutation model. Exposure can be by any desired route. DNA can be recovered and analyzed from any tissue. The mutation detection part of the process is an in vitro technique.

Table 17.19
Chemicals tested with MutaMouse

Chemicals	Skin	Bone marrow	Liver	Lung	Testes	Other
ENU		+	+	+	+	Brain
Chlorambucil		+	+		+	
Procarbazine		+				
Cyclophosphamide		+				
Acrylamide		+				
Benzene		Inc.	Inc.			
MNNG	+					
DMBA	+	Inc.				
Acetic acid	Inc.					
TPA	−					
Diethyl nitrosamine		−	+			
Ethylmethane sulfonate		+				
Mitomycin C		+	Inc.			
1,3-Butadiene		−	−	+		

+—mutagenic effects reported; −—no mutagenic effect using conventional study design; Inc.—mutagenic effects reported but inconclusive based on small sample sizes.

Transgenic models have not been introduced into testing schemes but are under intense review by regulatory agencies worldwide. It is likely that one or more of these models will be used as (a) a method to confirm in vitro gene mutation screening in vivo, or (b) replacements for many of the current in vitro gene mutation models.

Gene Amplification Approaches to Mutation Detection

Development of polymerase chain reaction (PCR) has resulted in the ability to select specific DNA sequences and create millions of copies of them rapidly and inexpensively. Although PCR technology has had its greatest impact in other areas of biotechnology, it has been used to develop some new methods of mutation analysis (Table 17.17). Two such models appear promising as methods to detect mutation in vivo, and are compared to the transgenic model. The advantages of these methods over transgenic models are that (a) the target DNA sequences are endogenous in orgin rather than transplanted from other organisms, (b) the technology can be applied to any mammalian system from mouse to primate, and (c) the types of damage detected are relatively unrestricted to specific mechanisms (although DNA deletions are not detected). The first method involves the isolation of splenic T cells from treated rodents and subjecting these cells to 6-thioguanine resistant cells, amplification of the DNA by PCR, and classification of the mutations by sequence analysis. This technique works very well, but the mutation target is limited to the spleen. A second method, called single-strand conformational polymorphism, allows mutations to be detected in a larger selection of tissues. In this method, DNA from specific sites (e.g., targeted exons of the gene of interest) can be amplified by PCR. The amplified DNA is then subjected to denaturation and placed on nondenaturing polyacrylamide gel electrophoresis. DNA damage as small as single base changes will alter the mobility of the amplified sequences separating mutant DNA from nonmutant DNA. The shifts will be visible on stained gels. The mutant DNA bands can be removed and sequenced to classify the DNA changes. This method has been used to study organ-specific mutations in various regions of the p53 tumor suppressor gene.

Single Cell Gel Electrophoresis (COMET) Assay

This technique is dependent on the analysis of DNA integrity in single cells. The advantages of this technology are that the source of the cells is almost unrestricted. The basis of the test is that if single- or double-strand breaks are induced in DNA in situ, when cells are isolated, treated to denature nucleic acids, and placed in an electric field, DNA will migrate from the negative to the positive charge at a rate related to the length of the DNA. Fragmented DNA pieces migrate rapidly and, when stained, form a tail on the cells similar to that of a comet (Figure 17.11). The COMET assay is a very versatile technique that can be used in vitro or in vivo (88).

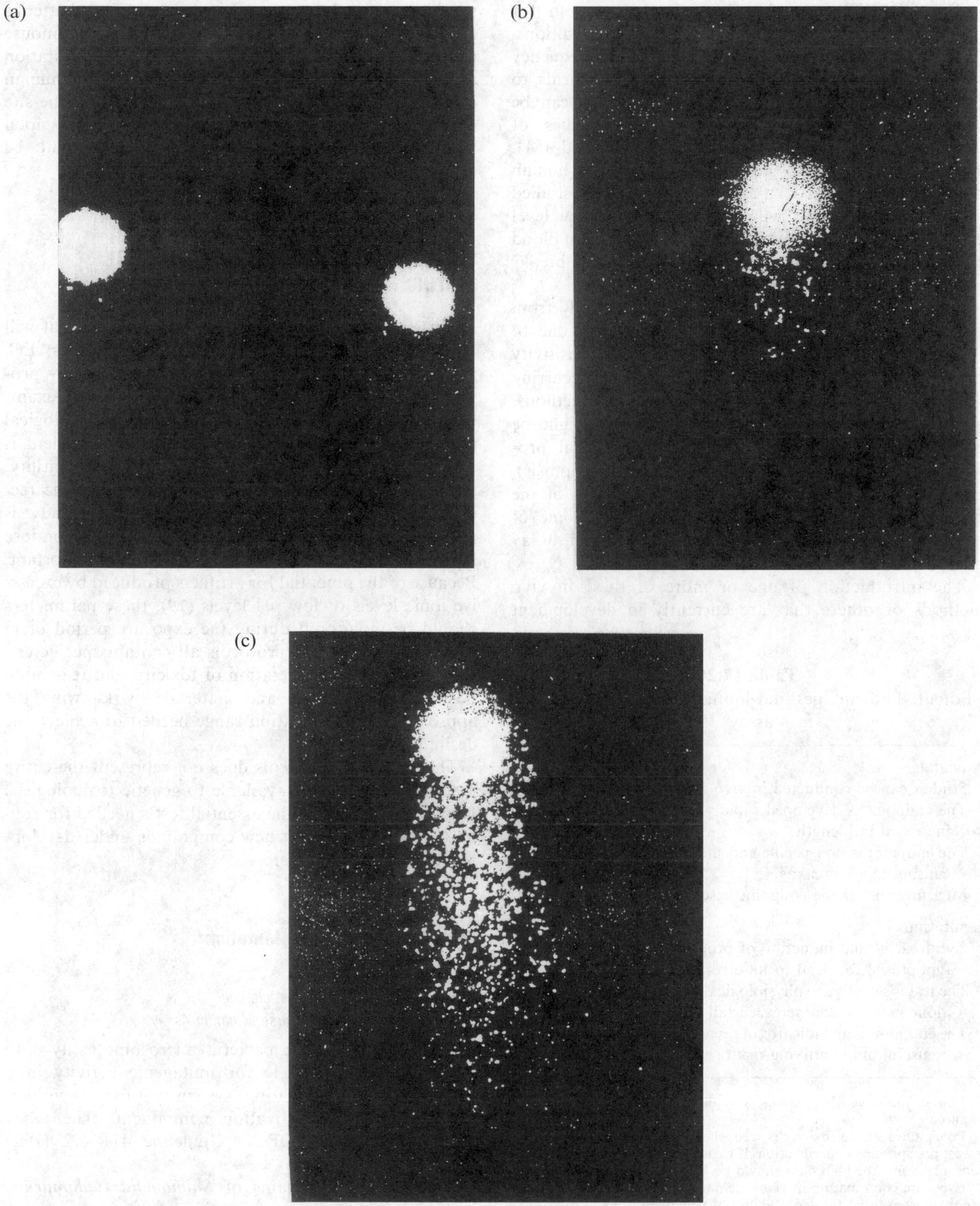

FIG. 17.11. Development of a "tail" in the COMET assay. A normal nucleus (a), followed by some leakage of broken DNA (b) forming ultimately a "tail" of DNA (c). The length of the tail is indicative of the amount of DNA damage.

The COMET assay has been used to screen for genotoxicity under the in vivo exposure conditions. The types of exposures have ranged from radio frequency radiation and agricultural and industrial chemicals to pharmaceutical products. Because the analysis can be conducted with small cell populations, studies of tissue-specific genotoxicity have been published (81). The method may also be applied directly to human populations. Wojewodzka and co-workers (104) studied a group of men and women with chronic low level exposure to radiation and reported that cells from blood cultures showed significant increases in DNA breaks compared to matched controls.

The use of this method increased dramatically from 1994 through 1996, but has slowed somewhat due to the technical problems associated with the sensitivity of the method to stress-induced positive effects occurring during the isolation and fixation steps of the methods. Interpretation of the results from this test might be compromised by cytotoxic effects from normal processes, such as programmed cell death (apoptosis). Extreme care must be taken during these steps of the procedure to eliminate false-positive effects. Some of the limitations and advantages of the COMET assay are listed in Table 17.20.

The introduction of one or more of these in vivo methods or others that are currently in development would significantly improve the relevance of test batteries such as the ICH core battery. In vivo data from the mouse micronucleus and, for example, a transgenic mutation assay conducted using the anticipated route of human exposure, coupled with toxicokinetic data from the site of cell harvest, could provide a realistic set of results upon which quantitative hazard/risk decisions might be developed.

Table 17.20
Potential advantages and limitations of the COMET assay[a]

Advantages
Studies can be conducted in vivo in almost any tissue
The endpoint is developed rapidly and seen visually as increased tail length
The endpoint is nonspecific and should respond to any agent causing DNA breakage
Measurement of the endpoint is sensitive and quantitative
Limitations
Cytotoxicity and induction of programmed cell death (apoptosis) can lead to false responses
The test is sensitive to physiological changes in vivo and stress alone may induce increased tail lengths
The endpoint is an indicator of reparable damage and may not be useful in quantifying risk or impact on germ cell DNA

[a] Either the mouse lymphoma assay or in vitro cytogenetics is required

Precipitates—if no toxicity is seen, the highest dose may use the lowest precipitating concentration. If toxicity is evident at precipitating concentrations, the high dose should be based on toxicity.

Exposure confirmation in vivo—demonstration of bone marrow exposure is essential for acceptability of negative results.

Mouse lymphoma repeat tests—if the results of the initial trial are negative, the treatment time in a repeat test (–S9) should be increased to 24 h.

SELECTED STUDY DESIGNS AND GENETIC TESTING

This section contains a set of study designs that will meet the ICH guideliness for the United States, EC, and Japan. Although not fully described in every protocol, it is recommended that each test article be examined for several chemical, physical, and biological parameters. Included in this preliminary assessment is an examination of the test article's solubility, volatility, and light sensitivity, as well as its stability in the recommended solvent. A preliminary toxicity study is performed to establish a maximum concentration or dose level. Careful selection of concentrations is important. Because of the potential for artifacts produced by excessive ionic levels or low pH levels (19), these parameters should be monitored during the exposure period of in vitro procedures. The protocols all contain specific criteria related to interpretation of toxicity, but it is often possible to save time and materials by knowing the approximate concentration range needed to achieve the desired toxicity.

This group of protocols does not represent the entire repertoire of methods available to genetic toxicologists. It provides, however, the essential test's needed for routine screening for most new compounds under development for use in commerce.

Tests Measuring Gene Mutation

Protocol 1: Salmonella-Eschericia coli/ mammalian-microsome Reverse Mutation Assay

The objective of the bacteria/microsome assay is to evaluate the test article for mutagenic activity in a bacterial reverse mutation system with and without a mammalian S9 activation component. The assay design is based on OECD Guideline 471–472 (1997 version).

Materials. The strains of *Salmonella typhimurium* and *E. coli* that are used routinely in the plate assay are described in the following table:

Table 17.21
Strains used in the plate assay

Tester Strains	*Target Group*	*Additional Mutations*		
Salmonella				
TA1535	*his* G46	*rfa*	*uvrB*	–
TA1537	*his* C3076	*rfa*	*uvrB*	–
TA98	*his* D3052	*rfa*	*uvrB*	+ R
TA100	*his* G46	*rfa*	*uvrB*	+ R
Escherichia				
WP_2	*trp*		*uvrA*	–

An S9 homogenate is used as the activation system. The 9000 × g supernatant fluid is prepared from Sprague–Dawley adult male rat liver induced by Aroclor 1254 (5). The components of the S9 mix are described in (4).

Test procedures. An appropriate number of tubes of molten overlay agar (at least three per control or concentration level) are prepared. An equivalent number of Vogel Bonner plates also are prepared and properly labeled.

The test article is weighed or measured and diluted in a solvent to set up the stock solutions. The test article and other components are prepared fresh and added to the overlay. The contents then are mixed and poured on the surfaces of the Vogel Bonner plates. For activation studies, 0.5 ml of the S9 mix is added to each overlay tube. For highly reactive chemicals that might have short half-lifes in aqueous environments, a liquid preincubation method has been developed (107). The entire test consists of nonactivation and activation (+ S9 mix) test conditions, each with appropriate negative and positive controls.

The plates (once the overlay has solidified) are incubated at 37°C for 36 to 72 h and scored for numbers of revertants per plate. Colonies are selected at random for verification of histidine independence by growth on minimal agar medium.

For the standard plate test, at least five dose levels of the test article, dissolved in a suitable solvent, are added to the test system. Triplicate plates per dose per strain are used in all standard assays. The test concentrations should be based on preliminary toxicity dose selection tests conducted both with and without S9 mix at 10 concentrations × 1 plate each. When no toxicity is observed, concentrations of up to 50 μl or 5000 to 10,000 μg per plate should be employed.

The chemicals that may be used as positive control agents are given in Table 17.22.

Assay acceptance criteria. Several methods for statistical analysis of the Ames test are suggested in the EPA Gene-Tox work group report for *S. typhimurium* mutation assay (50). Plate test data consist of direct revertant colony counts obtained from a set of selective agar plates seeded with populations of mutant cells suspended in a semisolid overlay. Because the test article and the cells are incubated in the overlay for 36 to 72 h, and because a few cell divisions occur during the incubation period, the test is semiquantitative in nature. Although these features of the assay reduce the quantitation of results, they provide certain advantages not contained in a quantitative suspension test:

1. The small number of cell divisions permits potential mutagens to act on replicating DNA, which is often more sensitive than nonreplicating DNA.
2. The combined incubation of the test article and the cells in the overlay permits constant exposure of the indicator cells for 36 to 72 h.

Surviving populations. Plate test procedures do not permit exact quantitation of the number of cells surviving chemical treatment. At low concentrations of the test article, the surviving populations on the treatment plates are essentially the same as that on the negative control plate. At high concentrations, the surviving population usually is reduced by some unknown fraction. This protocol normally employs several doses ranging over two or three log concentrations; the highest of these doses is selected to show toxicity as determined by subjective criteria, such as background clearing or a reduction in

Table 17.22
Positive control agents for the standard plate test

Assay	*Chemical*	*Solvent*	*Concentration per plate (μg)*	*Responding* Salmonella *strains*
Nonactivation	Sodium azide	Water	1	TA-1535, TA-100
	2-Nitrofluorene	DMSO	10	TA-1538, TA-98
	9-Aminoacridine	Ethanol	50	TA-1537
	4-Nitroquinoline	Oxide	1	*E. coli*
Activation	2-Anthramine	DMSO	2.5	All strains of *Salmonella*
	2-Anthramine	DMSO	25	*E. coli*

the number of spontaneous colonies on treated plates compared with the solvent control.

Dose-response phenomena. The demonstration of a dose-related increase in mutant counts is an important criterion for establishing mutagenicity. A factor that might modify dose-response results for a mutagen is the selection of doses that are too low (usually mutagenicity and toxicity are related). If the highest dose is far lower than a toxic concentration, no increase may be observed over the dose range selected. Conversely, if the lowest dose employed is highly cytotoxic, the test article may kill any mutants that are induced, and thus does not appear to be mutagenic. Occasionally, high levels of toxicity produce microcolonies (not mutants), which can be confused for revertants by inexperienced investigators.

Control tests. Positive and negative control assays are conducted with each experiment and consist of direct-acting mutagens for nonactivation assays and mutagens that require metabolic biotransformation in activation assays. Negative controls consist of the test article solvent in the overlay agar together with the other essential components. The negative control plates for each strain give a reference point to which the test data can be compared. The positive control assay is conducted to demonstrate that the test systems are functional with known mutagens.

Replication. OECD guidelines require independent repeat of all tests for confirmation of both negative and equivocal responses.

Assay Evaluation acceptance criteria. Because the procedures used to evaluate the mutagenicity of the test article are semiquantitative, the criteria used to determine positive effects are inherently subjective and based primarily on a historical database. Most data sets are evaluated using the following criteria:

1. Strains TA-1535 and TA-1537. If the solvent control value is within the typical range for the laboratory, a test article that produces a positive dose response over three concentrations, with the highest increase equal to three times the solvent control value, is considered mutagenic.
2. *Strains TA-98, TA-100, and WP2uvrA.* If the solvent control value is within the normal range for the laboratory, a test article that produces a positive dose response over three concentrations, with the highest increase equal to twice the solvent control value, is considered mutagenic. Occasionally, a doubling is not necessary for TA-100 if a clear dose-related pattern is observed over several concentrations.
3. *Pattern.* Because TA-1535 and TA-100 are derived from the parental strain (G-46), and because TA-1538 and TA-98 are derived from the same parental strain (D3052), to some extent there is a built-in redundancy in the microbial assay. In general, the two strains of a set respond to the same mutagen, and such a pattern is sought. Generally, if a strain responds to a mutagen in nonactivation tests, it does so in activation tests.

The preceding criteria are not absolute, and other extenuating factors may enter into a final evaluation decision, however, these criteria can be applied to most situations and are presented to aid individuals not familiar with this procedure. It must be emphasized that modifications of the procedure involving preincubation conditions or source of S9 mix are necessary for evaluation of specific chemicals or classes of chemicals. Attached to reports should be results of analytical chemical analyses for stability and dose-verification. Laboratory historical control ranges should also be included.

Protocol 2: Forward Mutation at the TK Locus in L5178Y Mouse Lymphoma Cells

This method is developed from OECD protocol 473 (1997 version). The objective of the mouse lymphoma assay is to evaluate a test article for its ability to induce forward mutation in the L5178Y TK +/– mouse lymphoma cell line, as assessed by colony growth in the presence of 5-trifluorothymidine (TFT).

Thymidine kinase (TK) is a cellular enzyme that allows cells to salvage thymidine from the surrounding medium for use in DNA synthesis. If a thymidine analog such as TFT is included in the growth medium, the analog is phosphorylated via the TK pathway and incorporated into DNA, eventually resulting in cellular death. Cells that are heterozygous at the TK locus (TK +/–) may undergo a single step forward mutation to the TK–/– genotype, in which little or no TK activity remains. Such mutants are as viable as the heterozygotes in normal medium because DNA synthesis proceeds by *de novo* synthetic pathways that do not involve thymidine as an intermediate. The basis for selection of the TK–/– mutants is the lack of any ability to use toxic analogs of thymidine, which enable only TK–/– mutants to grow in the presence of TFT. Cells that grow to form colonies in the presence of TFT are therefore assumed to have mutated to the TK–/– genotype either spontaneously or by the action of a test article.

Materials.

Indicator cells. The mouse lymphoma cell line used in this assay, L5178Y TK +/–, is derived from the Fischer L5178Y line. Stocks are maintained in liquid nitrogen and laboratory cultures are periodically checked for the absence of *Mycoplasma* contamination and karyotype stability. To reduce the negative control frequency (spontaneous frequency) of TK–/– mutants to as low a level as possible, cell cultures are exposed to conditions that select against the TK–/–phenotype and then returned to normal growth medium for 3 days or more before use.

Media. The cells are maintained in RPMI 1640 or Fischer's mouse leukemia medium supplemented with L-glutamine, sodium pyruvate, and horse serum (10% by volume). Cloning medium consists of the preceding growth medium with the addition of agar to achieve a semisolid state. Selection medium is cloning medium containing 3 μg/ml of TFT (25).

Control articles. A negative control consisting in assay procedures performed on cells exposed to solvent in the medium is assayed as the solvent-negative control article to determine any effects on survival or mutation caused by the solvent alone. For test articles assayed with activation, the solvent-negative control articles include the activation mixture.

Reference substances for use as positive control articles should be based on the historical data from the laboratory performing the assay. The positive control articles listed below are chosen because of the large database available and because both chemicals detect both small and large colonies (108).

Methyl methanesulfonate (MMS) can be used at concentrations of 10.0 to 15 nl/ml as a positive control for nonactivation studies. Ethylmethane sulfonate is highly mutagenic via alkylation of cellular DNA and may be used at 0.25 to 0.50 μl/ml as a positive control article for nonactivation studies. 3-Methylcholanthrene requires metabolic activation by microsomal enzymes to become mutagenic and may be used at 1.0 to 4.0 μg/ml as a positive control article for assays performed with activation.

Sample forms. All types of test articles can be evaluated in the mouse lymphoma assay. Solid articles can be dissolved in water, if possible, or in dimethylsulfoxide (DMSO), ethanol, or acetone unless another solvent is requested. Liquids can be tested by direct addition to the test system at predetermined concentrations or following dilution in a suitable solvent.

Experimental design.

Dose selection. The solubility of the test article in water or an organic solvent is determined first, and then a wide range of test article concentrations are tested for cytotoxicity, starting with a maximum applied dose of 1 to 5 mg/ml for a solid test article or 1 to 5 μl/ml for a liquid test article and using twofold dilution steps. After an exposure time of 4 h, the cells are washed and a viable cell count is obtained the next day. Relative cytotoxicities expressed as the reduction in growth compared to the growth of negative control cells are used to select 7 to 10 doses that cover the range from 0–50% to 80%–90% reduction in 24-h growth. These selected doses subsequently are applied to cell cultures prepared for mutagenicity testing, but only five or six of the doses may be carried through the mutant selection process. This procedure compensates for daily variations in cellular cytotoxicity and ensures the choice of five or six doses spaced from little or no survival to no apparent effect on cell growth.

Mutagenicity testing. The procedure used for the nonactivation assay is based on that which has been reported (1,24,25). Cultures exposed to the test article for 4 h at the preselected doses are washed and placed in growth medium for 2 to 3 days to allow recovery, growth, and expression of the induced TK–/– phenotype. Cell counts are determined daily and appropriate dilutions made to allow optimal growth rates.

At the end of the expression period 3×10^4 cells for each selected dose are seeded in soft agar plates with selection medium, and resistant (mutant) colonies are counted after 10 to 14 days incubation. To determine the number of cells capable of forming colonies, a portion of the cell suspension is also cloned in normal medium (nonselective). The ratio of resistant colonies to total viable cell number is the mutant frequency.

The activation assay can be run concurrently with the nonactivation assay. The only difference is the addition of the S9 fraction of rat liver homogenate and necessary co-factors (CORE) during the 4-h treatment period. CORE consists of NADP (sodium salt) and isocitric acid. The final concentrations of the activation system components in the cell suspension should be 2.4 mg NADP (sodium salt)/ml, 4.5 mg isocitric acid/ml, and S9/ml. The optimal concentration of S9 (usually 10 to 50 μl S9/ml) should be determined in a pretest with control and MCA-treated cells.

Preparation of 9000g supernatant fluid (S9). Sprague- Dawley or Fischer 344 male rats are normally used as the source of hepatic microsomes; the S9 can be obtained commercially. Briefly, induction with Aroclor 1254 or another agent is performed by injection 5 days prior to killing. After decapitation and bleeding, the liver is immediately dissected from the animal using aseptic technique and placed in ice-cold buffer at pH 7.4. When an adequate number of livers are obtained, the collection is washed twice with fresh buffer and completely homogenized. The homogenate is centrifuged for 10 min at 9000g in a refrigerated centrifuge, and the supernatant fluid (S9) from this centrifuged sample is retained and frozen at –80°C until used in the activation system.

Test materials identified as mutagenic should have representative control and mutagenic selection plates recounted to permit mutant colony sizing. Selection plates are recounted using the Artek colony counter at size settings between 0.0 to 4.0 in increments of 0.2.

If the initial trial is determined to be negative or equivocal, a report test of the nonactivation portion of the assay is conducted with a 24-h exposure period. It is suggested that the activation portion be repeated using a different dose range.

Assay acceptance criteria. An assay is considered acceptable for evaluation of test results only if all of the criteria in the following list are satisfied. The activation and nonactivation portions of the mutation assays usually are performed concurrently, but each portion is in fact an independent assay with its own positive and negative controls. The activation or nonactivation assays are repeated independently to satisfy general acceptance and evaluation criteria:

1. The average absolute cloning efficiency of the negative controls (average of the solvent and untreated controls) is 100%±30%. Assay variables can lead to artificially low cloning efficiencies in the range of 50%–70% and still yield internally consistent and valid results. Assays with cloning efficiencies in this range are conditionally acceptable and dependent on the scientific judgment of the investigator. All assays below 50% cloning efficiency are unacceptable.
2. The average negative control suspension growth factor is not less than about eight. The optimal value is 25, which corresponds to fivefold increases in cell number for each of the 2 days following treatment of the experimental cultures.
3. The background mutant frequency (average of the solvent and untreated negative controls) is calculated separately for concurrent activation and nonactivation assays, even though the same population of cells is used for each assay. For both conditions, the normal range of background frequencies for assays performed with different cell stocks is 20 to 120×10^{-6}. Assays with backgrounds outside this range are not necessarily invalid and should be considered in the context of the historical data in the laboratory performing the assay.
4. A positive control is included with each assay to provide confidence in the procedures used to detect mutagenic activity. The normal range of mutant frequencies induced by MMS (nonactivation assay) is 200×10^{-6} to 800×10^{-6}; for MCA 4.0 μg/ml (activation assay), the normal range is 200×10^{-6} to 1000×10^{-6}. An assay is considered acceptable in the absence of a positive control (loss due to contamination or technical error) only if the test article clearly shows mutagenic activity as described in the evaluation criteria.
5. For test articles with little or no mutagenic activity, an assay must include applied concentrations that reduce the relative growth to between 10% and 20% of the average solvent control or reach the maximum applied concentrations given in the evaluation criteria. This requirement is waived if a dose increment of about 1.5 or less causes excessive toxicity.
6. An experimental treatment that results in fewer than 3.0×10^{-6} cells by the end of the 2-day growth period is not cloned for mutant analysis.
7. An experimental mutant frequency is considered acceptable for evaluation only if the relative cloning efficiency is 10% or greater and the total number of viable clones exceeds 20.
8. Mutant frequencies are derived normally from sets of three dishes for both the mutant and the viable colony count. To allow for contamination losses, an acceptable mutant frequency can be calculated from a minimum of two dishes per set.
9. The mutant frequencies for six treated cultures are normally determined in each assay. A required number of various concentrations cannot be explicitly stated, although a minimum of four analyzed cultures is considered necessary under the most favorable test conditions to accept a single assay for evaluation of the test article.

Assay evaluation criteria. The minimum condition considered necessary to demonstrate mutagenesis for any given treatment is a mutant frequency that is at least two times the concurrent background frequency. *Background frequency* is defined as the average mutant frequency of the solvent controls. The minimum increase is based on extensive experience that indicates that the calculated minimum increase is often a repeatable result.

The observation of a mutant frequency that meets the minimum criterion for a single treated culture within a range of assayed concentrations is not sufficient evidence to evaluate a test article as a mutagen. The following test results must be obtained to reach this conclusion for either activation or nonactivation conditions:

1. A dose-related or toxicity-related increase in mutant frequency is observed. It is desirable to obtain this relation for at least three doses, but it depends on the concentration steps chosen for the assay and the toxicity at which mutagenic activity appears.
2. An increase in mutant frequency may be followed by only small or no further increases at higher concentrations or toxicities; however, a decrease in mutant frequency to values below the minimum criterion is not acceptable in a single assay to classify the test article as a mutagen. If the mutagenic activity at lower concentrations or toxicities is large, a repeat assay is performed to confirm the mutagenic activity.
3. If an increase of at least four times the background mutant frequency is observed for a single dose near

the highest testable toxicity, as defined in the Assay Acceptance Criteria section, the test article is considered mutagenic. Smaller increases at a single dose near the highest testable toxicity require confirmation by a repeat assay.

4. For some test articles the correlation between toxicity and applied concentration is poor. The proposition of the applied article that effectively interacts with the cells to cause genetic alterations is not always repeatable or under control. Conversely, measurable changes in the frequency of induced mutants may occur with concentration changes that cause only small changes in observable toxicity. Therefore, either parameter—applied concentration or toxicity (percent relative growth)—can be used to establish if the mutagenic activity is related to an increase in effective treatment. A negative correlation with dose is acceptable only if a positive correlation with toxicity exists. An apparent increase in mutagenic activity as a function of decreasing toxicity is not acceptable evidence for mutagenicity.

A test article is evaluated as nonmutagenic in a single assay only if the minimum increase in mutant frequency is not observed for a range of applied concentrations that extends to toxicity causing 10%–20% relative suspension growth. If the test article is relatively nontoxic, the maximum applied concentrations are normally 5 mg/ml (or 5 μl/ml) unless limited by solubility. If a repeat assay does not confirm an earlier, minimal response as discussed previously the test article is evaluated as nonmutagenic in this assay system.

Tests Detecting Chromosome-Breaking (Clastogenic) Agents

Protocol 4: Chromosome Aberrations in Chinese Hamster Ovary Cells

This design meets the OECD Guideline 473 (1997 version). The objective of the Chinese hamster in vitro assay is to evaluate the ability of a test article to induce chromosome aberrations in Chinese hamster ovary (CHO) cells.

Indicator cells. Cells to be used in this assay can be obtained from the American Type Culture Collection Repository No. CCL61 (Rockville, MD). The original cells were obtained from an ovarian biopsy of a Chinese hamster. It is a permanent cell line with an average cycle time of 10–12 h.

The CHO cells for this assay are grown in Ham's F12 medium supplemented with 10% fetal calf serum. The cells are split back to 3×10^5 per 75 cm^2 plastic flask and fed 24 h prior to treatment with 10 ml of fresh medium.

Control articles. The solvent for the test article is used as the solvent vehicle for the control article.

Ethylmethane sulfonate, a known mutagen and chromosome-breaking (clastogenic) agent, may be dissolved in the culture medium and used as a positive control article for the nonactivation studies at a final concentration of 0.5 μl/ml.

Experimental design. Toxicity and dose determination. The solubility, toxicity, and doses for the test article are determined prior to screening. The effect of each test article on the survival of the indicator cell is determined by exposing the cells to a wide range of article concentrations in complete growth medium. Toxicity is measured as the loss in growth potential of the cells induced by a 4-hour expression period in growth medium. Doses are selected from the range of concentrations by bracketing the highest dose that shows no loss in growth potential with at least one higher and three lower doses. Otherwise, a half-log series of doses are employed, with the highest dose being perhaps limited by solubility, but in any case not to exceed 5 mg/ml. The doses cover at least four orders of magnitude, and all doses that yield sufficient numbers of scorable metaphase cells are considered in the analysis. Alternatively, inhibition of cell cycling (BrdU staining, discussed later) can be used to set dose levels.

Cell treatment. For the nonactivation assay, approximately 10^6 cells are treated with the test article at predetermined doses for 3 h at 37°C in growth medium. The exposure period is terminated by washing the cells twice with saline. Four replicate cultures per dose are employed in this assay; all receive fresh medium after washing, and 5-bromo-2′-deoxyuridine (BrdU) is added to two of the four replicates (10 μM final concentration). Incubation is continued in the dark for 20 h. Colcemid is added for the last 3 h of incubation (2×10^{-7} M final concentration), and metaphase cells are collected by mitotic shake-off. These cells are swollen with 0.075 M KCl hypotonic solution, washed three times in fixative (methanol/acetic acid, 3:1), dropped onto slides, and air dried.

For the activation assay, the test article is tested in the presence of an S9 rat liver activation system. This assay differs from the nonactivation assay in that the S9 reaction mixture is added to the growth medium, together with the test article, for 3 h. The S9 mix is the same as that used in the mouse lymphoma assay. The exposure period is terminated by washing the cells twice with saline. From this point, they are treated as described for the nonactivation assay.

If the 3-h exposure studies are equivocal or negative, a repeat nonactivation study employing a 17.5-h exposure will be conducted to confim the negative results. It is suggested that the activiation test also be repeated using a different dose range.

Staining and scoring of slides. Slides are stained with 10% Giemsa at pH 6.8 for subsequent scoring of chromosome aberration frequencies. About 50 to 100 cells are scored from each of two replicate cultures per dose.

Standard forms are used to score and record gaps, breaks, fragments, and reunion figures, as well as numerical aberrations such as polypoid cells. The complete list of aberrations to be scored are as follows:

Chromatid gap
Chromosome break
Chromosome gap
Chromosome break
Chromatid deletion
Fragment
Acentric fragment
Translocation
Pulverized chromosomes
Pulverized chromosomes
Pulverized cells
Complex rearrangement
Ring chromosome
Dicentric chromosome
Minute chromosome
More than 10 aberrations
Triradial
Quadradial
Polypoid
Hyperdiploid

For control of bias, all slides are coded for scoring.

Assay evaluation criteria. A number of general guidelines have been established to aid in determining the meaning of CHO chromosome aberrations. Basically, an attempt is made to establish if a test article or its metabolites can interact with chromosomes to produce gross lesions or changes in chromosome numbers and if these changes are of a type that can survive more than one mitotic cycle of the cell. All aberration figures detected by this assay result from breaks in the chromatin that either fail to repair or repair in atypical combinations.

It is anticipated that many of the cells bearing breaks or reunion figures would be eliminated (i.e., fail to divide again) after their first mitotic division and, as a corollary, that those cells that survive the first division would primarily bear balanced lesions. The detection of these lesions, and hence a complete risk evaluation usually must rely on additional testing. In general, a cell bearing configurations such as small deletions or reciprocal translocations may be perpetuated and therefore constitutes a greater risk to an individual than one with large deletions or complex rearrangements.

Data are summarized in tabular form and evaluated. Gaps are not counted as significant aberrations unless they are present at a much higher than usual frequency. Open breaks are considered indicators of genetic damage, as are configurations resulting from the repair of breaks. The latter includes, for example, translocations, multiradials, rings, and multicenters. Reunion figures such as these are weighed higher than breaks and may lead to stable configurations.

The number of aberrations per cell are also considered significant. Cells with more than one aberration indicate more genetic damage than those containing evidence of single events. Frequently, one is unable to locate sufficient suitable metaphase spreads. Possible causes appear to be related to cytoxic effects, which alter the duration of the cell cycle, kill the cell, or cause clumping of the chromosomes. Additional information can be gained from the mitotic index, which appears to reflect cytotoxic effects, as well as from the frequencies of M1, M2, and M3 cells.

Comparison with a concurrent negative control that shows an unusually low frequency of aberrations can suggest undue statistical significance. Therefore, treatment data are considered against historical control data. In either event, the type of aberration, its frequency, and its correlation to dose trends within a given time period are all considered when evaluating a test article as being mutagenically positive or negative.

Statistical analysis employs a two-tailed t-test. This test can be performed on the number of breaks per chromosome in treated and control samples. Dose regression analysis also is useful.

Protocol 5: Rodent Bone Marrow Micronucleus Assay

This assay design is based on OECD Guideline 474 (1997 version). The objective of the mouse micronucleus assay is to evaluate a test article for clastogenic activity in polychromatic erythrocyte (PCE) stem cells in treated mice. The micronucleus test can serve as a rapid screen for clastogenic agents and test articles that interfere with normal mitotic cell division (42,82). Micronuclei are believed to be formed from chromosomes or chromosome fragments left behind during anaphase and scored during interphase because they persist. Thus, the time involved in searching for metaphase spreads in treated cell populations is eliminated. Test articles affecting spindle fiber function or formation, as well as clastogenic agents, can be detected through micronucleus induction.

Materials (This design will describe a study in mice). Adult male and/or female mice, strain CD-1, from a randomly bred closed colony may be used as well as other strains or species. A healthy, random-bred strain is selected to maximize genetic heterogeneity and at the same time ensure access to a common source. Animals usually are 8–10 weeks old at the time of dosing.

Trimethylene melamine (TEM) at 1.0 mg/kg may be used as the positive control article and is administered via a split-dose intraperitoneal injection. The negative control consists of the solvent or vehicle used for the test article and is administered by the same route as, and concurrently with, the test article in volumes equal to the maximum amount administered to the experimental animals.

Experimental design.

Animal husbandry. Animals are group-housed 7 mice per cage. A commercial diet and water are available *ad libitum* unless contraindicated by the particular experimental design.

Five animals per dose level are uniquely identified and assigned to study groups at random. Prior to study initiation, animals are weighed to calculate dose levels. The volume of test article administered per animal is established using a mean weight unless there is significant variation among individuals; in this case, individual calculations are made.

Sanitary cages and bedding are used. Personnel handling animals or working within the animal facilities are required to wear suitable protective garments. When appropriate, individuals with respiratory or other overt infections are excluded from the animal facilities.

Dose selection. If acute toxicity information (e.g., LD_{50}) is available, it can be used to determine dose levels. If it is not available, dose levels can be determined using five groups of six animals each in a toxicity study. For nontoxic agents, a limit dose of 2000 mg/kg is employed. For toxic agents, the high dose is selected based on some evidence of toxicity (e.g., clinical signs, death, depression in bone marrow cell maturation). Two lower doses at 1/2 and 1/4 of the high dose will be selected. An attempt is made in mutagenesis studies, as well as other toxicology work, to evaluate the extremes of dosage as well as values close to the use level.

Dosing schedule and route of administration. The test article administered may be in one of two groups: (1) animals may be treated once or (2) two or more daily doses are given 24 h apart. The single-dose administration is the most common. In the event that test article characteristics preclude oral gavage, intraperitoneal injection may be employed. These routes of administration are the ones most commonly used for this test procedure.

Extraction of bone marrow. For the single-dose regimen, sampling times will be at 24 and 48 hours after compound administration. Animals are killed with CO_2 and the adhering soft tissue and epiphyses of both femurs removed. The marrow is aspirated from the bone and transferred to centrifuge tubes containing 5 ml fetal calf serum (one tube for each animal).

Preparation of slides. After centrifugation to pellet the tissue, the supernatant fluid is drawn off and portions of the pellet spread on slides and air-dried. The slides are then stained in May–Gruenwald solution and Giemsa, followed by clearing in distilled water.

Screening the slides. One thousand PCEs per animal are scored. The frequency of micronucleated cells is expressed as percent micronucleated cells based on the total PCEs present in the scored optic field. The frequencies of other bone marrow cell types are recorded for analysis of cytotoxic effects (reduced production of specific blood cell types).

Evaluation criteria. In tests performed for this evaluation, only PCEs are scored for micronuclei. Mature erythrocytes and other cells in the field are recorded but not scored. Loss of nucleated cells is an indication of cytotoxicity. The dose levels are established to ensure that a nontoxic level of the test article is scored. Dose-response data are not necessary to define a test article as active. Responses considered active are assumed to reflect clastogenic and related activities of test articles. Agents that break chromosomes and induce nondisjunction, as well as other events that produce structural or numerical changes in chromosomes, can produce micronuclei.

The data generated in this study may be analyzed by a two-tailed t-test. Individual animal results are used as data points in the analysis. The set of micronuclei frequencies among the controls are compared to the set for each treatment level. Male and female animal data are combined unless there appears to be a sex difference, in which case the data are analyzed separately. Increases above the negative control frequency that are significant at $p < 0.01$ are considered indicative of an active agent.

For control of bias, all slides are coded prior to scoring and scored blind.

QUESTIONS

1. Would transcription-coupled DNA repair (TCR) be more active in an exon or an intron?
2. Which type of gene mutation would be corrected by mismatch repair: a basepair substitution or a frameshift mutation?
3. Which part of a chromosome is believed to influence cell mortality: the centromere, the telomere, or the centriole?
4. Which short-term test shows the best overall concordance with animal carcinogenicity: SCEs, the Ames test, or the mouse micronucleus test?

5. The p53 gene is a member of which class of genes: an oncogene, a dominant gene, or a tumor suppressor gene?
6. A disruption in the nucleotide sequence of which of the following is likely to result in a mutation: a codon, a gene, or a chromosome?
7. Which of the following technologies was critical to the development of the transgenic mouse models for mutation: shuttle vector, PCR, or gel electrophoresis?
8. Chemically-induced heritable mutations have not been documented in which of the following species: fruit fly, mouse, or human?

REFERENCES

1. Amacher, D. E., Paillet, S. C., Turner, G. N., Ray, V. A., and Salsburg, D. S.: Point mutations at the thymidine kinase locus in L5178Y mouse lymphoma cells II. Test validation and interpretation. *Mutation Research* 72:447–474.
2. Ames, B. N. (1984): Dietary carcinogens and anti–carcinogens. *Clin. Toxicol.*, A 22:291–301.
3. Ames, B. N. (1979): Indentifying environmental chemicals causing mutations and cancer. *Science*, 204:587–593.
4. Ames, B. N., Durston, W. E., Yamasaki, E., and Lee, F. D. (1973): Carcinogens are mutagens: A simple test system combining liver homogenates for activation and bacteria for detection. *Proc. Natl. Acad. Sci. USA*, 70:2281.
5. Ames, B. N., Kammen, H. L., and Yamasaki, E. (1975): Hair dyes are mutagenic: Identification of a variety of mutagenic ingredients. *Proc. Natl. Acad. Sci. USA*, 72:2423–2427.
6. Ames, B. N., McCann, J., and Yamasaki, E. (1975): Methods for detecting carcinogens and mutagens with the *Salmonella* mammalian microscome mutagenicity test. *Mutation Res.*, 31:347–364.
7. Anderson, M. W., Maronpot, R. R., and Reynolds, S. H. (1988): Role of oncogenes in chemical carcinogenesis: Extrapolation from rodents to humans. In: *Methods for Detecting DNA Damaging Agents in Humans*, edited by H. Bartsch, K. Hemminki, and I. K. O'Neill, pp. 477–485. IARC Scientific Publications No. 89, Lyon.
8. Ashby, J., de Serres, F. J., Draper, M., Ishidate, M., Margolin, B., Matter, B., and Shelby, M. D. (1985): *Short-Term Tests for Carcinogens: Results of the IPCS Study*. Elsevier, Amsterdam.
9. Ashby, J., and Purchase, I. F. H. (1988): Reflections on the declining ability of the *Salmonella* assay to detect rodent carcinogens as positive. *Mutation Res.*, 205:51–58.
10. Ashby, J., and Richardson, C. R. (1985): Tabulation and assessment of 113 human surveillance cytogenetics studies conducted between 1965 and 1984. *Mutation Res.*, 154:111–133.
11. Au, W. W., Cajas-Salazar, N., and Salama, S. (1998): Factors contributing to discrepancies in population monitoring studies. *Mutation Res.*, 400:467–478.
12. Barbacid, M. (1987): Mutagens, oncogenes and cancer. In: *Oncogenes and Growth Factors*, edited by R. A. Bradshaw and S. Prentis, pp. 90–99. Elsevier, Amsterdam.
13. Boerringter, M., Dolle, M., Martus, H., Gossen, J., and Vijg, J. (1995): Plasmid-based transgenic mouse model for studying in vivo mutations. *Nature*, 377:657–659.
14. Bridges, B. A. (1976): Short-term screening tests for carcinogens. *Nature*, 261:195–200.
15. Brousseau, R., Scarpulla, R., Sung, W., Hsing, H. M., Narang, S. A., and Ulu, R. (1982): Synthesis of a human insulin gene. V: Enzymatic assembly, cloning and characterization of the human proinsulin DNA. *Gene*, 17:279–289.
16. Brusick, D., Albertini, R., McRee, D., Peterson, D., Williams, G., Hanawalt, P., and Preston, J. (1998): Genotoxicity of Radiofrequency Radiation. Environmental and Molecular Mutagenesis. 32:1–16.
17. Brusick, D. (1983): Mutagenicity and carcinogenicity correlations between bacteria and rodents. In: *Cellular Systems for Toxicity Testing 407*, reprinted from Annals of the New York Academy of Sciences, pp. 164–176.
18. Brusick, D. J. (1978): The role of short-term testing in carcinogen detection. *Chemosphere*, 5:403–417.
19. Brusick, D. J. (1987): Implications of treatment-condition-induced genotoxicity for chemical screening and data interpretation. *Mutation Res.*, 189:1–6.
20. Burnet, F. M. (1974): *Intrinsic Mutagenesis: A Genetic Approach to Aging*. Medical & Technical Publishing, Lancaster, England.
21. Butkiewicz, D., Grzybowska, E., Hemminki, K., Ovrebo, S., Haugen, A., Motykiewicz, G., and Chorazy, M. (1998): Modulation of DNA adduct levels in human mononuclear white blood cells and granulocytes by CYP1A1, CYP2D6 and GSTM1 genetic polymorphisms. *Mutation Res.*, 415:97–108.
22. Canadian Health and Welfare (1986): Guidelines on the use of mutagenicity tests in the toxicological evaluation of chemicals. *Environ. Molec. Mutagen.*, 11:261–304.
23. Cacheiro, N. L. A., Russell, L. B., and Swartout, M. S. (1974): Translocations, the predominant cause of total sterility in sons of mice treated with mutagens. *Genetics*, 75:73–91.
24. Clive, D., Caspery, W., Kirby, P. E., Krehl, R., Moore, M., Mayo, J., and Oberly, T. J. (1987): Guide for performing the mouse lymphoma assay for mammalian cell mutagenicity. *Mutation Res.*, 189:143–156.
25. Clive, D., Johnson, K. O., Spector, J. F. S., Batson, A. G., and Brown, M. M. M. (1979): Validation and characterization of the L5178Y TK + / − mouse lymphoma mutagen assay system. *Mutation Res.*, 59:61–108.
26. Counter, C. (1996): The roles of telomeres and telomerase in cell life span. *Mutation Res.*, 366:45–63.
27. Perera., F., Dickey, C., Santella, R., O'Neill, J., Albertini, R., Ottman, R., Tsai, W., Mooney, L., Savela, K., and Hemminki, K. (1994): Carcinogen—DNA adducts and gene mutation in foundry workers with low-level exposure to polycyclic aromatic hydrocarbons. *Carcinogenesis*, 15:2905–2910.
28. deLange, T. (1994): Activation of telomerase in a human tumor. *Proc. Natl. Acad. Sci. USA*, 91:2882–2885.
29. EEC (European Economic Community) Official Journal of the European Communities, 6th Amendment to Directive 67/548/EEC, Annex VII, 15.10.79, and Annex V, EEC Directive 79-831, part B, Toxicological Methods of Annex VIII, Draft, July 1983.
30. Ehling, U. H. (1988): Quantification of the genetic risk environmental mutagens. *Risk Analysis*, 8:45–56.
31. Ehling, U. H., Averby, D., Cerutti, P. A., Friedman, J., Greim, H., Kolbye, A. C., Jr., and Mendelsohn, M. L. (1983): Review of the evidence for the presence or absence of thresholds in the induction of genetic effects by genotoxic chemicals. *Mutation Res.*, 123:281–341.
32. EPA (Environmental Protection Agency) Office of Pesticides and Toxic Substances (1982): *Health Effects Test Guidelines*. EPA Publication 560/682-001. National Technical Information Service, Springfield, Virginia.
33. EPA (1986): EPA guidelines for mutagenicity risk assessment. *Fed. Register*, 51:34006–34012.

34. Evans, H. J.: Cytogenetics: Overview. In: *Mutation and the Environment*, Part B, edited by M. L. Mendelsohn, and R. J. Albertini, pp. 301–323. Wiley-Liss, Inc., New York.
35. Fletcher, K., Tinwell, H., and Ashby, J. (1998): Mutagenicity of the human bladder carcinogen 4–aminobiphenyl to the bladder of MutaMouse transgenic mice. *Mutation Res.*, 400:245–250.
36. Generoso, W. M., Cain, K. I., and Banby, A. J. (1983): Some factors affecting the mutagenic response of mouse germ cells to chemicals. In: *Utilization of Mammalian Specific Locus Studies in Hazard Evaluation and Estimation of Genetic Risk*, edited by F. J. de Serres, and W. Sheridan, pp. 227–239. Plenum Press, New York.
37. Generoso, W. M., Cain, K. T., Huff, S. W., and Gosslee, D. G. (1978): Heritable translocation test in mice. In: *Chemical Mutagens: Principles and Methods for Their Detection, Vol. 5*, edited by A. Hollandaer and E. I. de Serres. Plenum Press, New York.
38. Glassner, B. J., Posnick, M., and Samson, L. D. (1998): The influence of DNA glycosylases on spontaneous mutation. *Mutation Res.*, 400:33–44.
39. Gossen, J., deleeuw, W., Tan, C., Zwarthoff, E., Berends, F., Lohman, P., Knock, D., and Viig, J. (1989): Efficient rescue of integrated shuttle vectors from transgenic mice: A model for studying mutations in vivo. *Proc. Nat. Acad. Sci. USA*, 86:7971–7975.
40. Hanawalt, P. (1998): Genomic instability: Environmental invasion and the enemies within. *Mutation Res.*, 400:117–125.
41. Harris, C. C. (1998): Interindividual variation among humans in carcinogen metabolism, DNA adduct formation and DNA repair. *Carcinogenesis*, 10:1563–1566.
42. Heddle, J. (1973): A rapid in vitro test for chromosomal damage. *Mutation Res.*, 18:187–190.
43. Hilliard, C., Armstrong, M., Bradt, C., Hill, R., Greenwood, S., and Galloway, S. (1998): Chromosome aberrations in vitro related to cytotoxicity of nonmutagenic chemicals and metabolic poisons. *Environmental and Molecular Mutagenesis*, 31:316–326.
44. Holliday, R., and Ho, T. (1988): Gene silencing in mammalian cells by uptake of 5-methyl deoxycytidine 5′ phospate. *Somatic Cell Mol. Genet.*, 17:537–542.
45. Horowitz, J., Yandell, D., and Park, S. (1989): Point mutational inactivation of the retinoblastoma antioncogene. *Science*, 243:937–940.
46. ICPEMC (1988): Testing for mutagens and carcinogens: The role of short-term genotoxicity assays. *Mutation Res.*, 205:3–12.
47. ICPEMC (1990): The possible involvement of somatic mutations in the development of atheriosclerotic plaques. *Mutation Res.*, 239:143–148.
48. Inger-Lise, H. (1990): Occupational and lifestyle factors and chromosomal aberrations of spontaneous abortions. In: *Mutation and the Environment*, Part B, pp. 467–475. Wiley-Liss, Inc., New York.
49. Kalter, H. (1977): Correlation between teratogenic and mutagenic effects of chemicals in mammals. In: *Chemical Mutagens: Principles and Methods for Their Detection, Vol. 6*, edited by A. Hollandaer. Plenum Press, New York.
50. Kier, L. D., Brusick, D. J., Auletta, A. E., Von Halle, E. S., Brown, M. M., Simmon, V. F., Dunkel, V., McCann, J., Mortelmans, K., Prival, M., Rao, T. K., and Ray, V. (1986): The *Salmonella typhimurium*/mammalian microsomal assay: A report of the U.S. EPA Gene-Tox Program. *Mutation Res.*, 168:69–240.
51. Kier, L. D., Yamasaki, E., and Ames, B. N. (1974): Detection of mutagenic activity in cigarette smoke condensates. *Proc. Natl. Acad. Sci. USA*, 71:4159–4163.
52. Kier, L. D. (1988): Comments and perspectives on the EPA workshop on the relationship between short-term test information and carcinogenicity. *Environ. Molec. Mutagen.*, 11:147–157.
53. Kleinhofs, A., and Behki, R. (1977): Prospects for plant genome modification by nonconventional methods. *Annu. Rev. Genet.*, 11:79–101.
54. Knudsen, A. G., Jr. (1973): Mutation and human cancer. *Adv. Cancer Res.*, 17:317–352.
55. Kopelovich, L., Bias, N. E., and Helson, L. (1979): Tumor promotor alone induces neoplastic transformation of fibroblasts from humans genetically predisposed to cancer. *Nature*, 282:619–621.
56. Kriek, E., Rojas, M., Alexandrov, K., and Bartsch, H. (1998): Polycyclic aromatic hydrocarbon-DNA adducts in humans: Relevance as biomarkers for exposure and cancer risk. *Mutation Res.*, 400:215–231.
57. Lewtas, J. (1986): A quantitative cancer risk assessment methodology using short-term genetic bioassays: The comparative potency method. In: *Risk and Reason: Risk Assessment in Relation to Environmental Mutagens and Carcinogens*, edited by P. Oftedal and A. Bragger, pp. 107–120. Alan R. Liss, New York.
58. Malling, H. V. (1971): Dimehthylnitrosamine: Formation of mutagenic compounds by interation with mouse liver microsomes. *Mutation Res.*, 13:425–429.
59. Maron, D. M., and Ames, B. N. (1983): Revised methods for the *Salmonella* mutagenicity test. *Mutation Res.*, 113:173–215.
60. McCann, J., Choi, E., Yamasaki, E., and Ames B. N. (1975): Detection of carcinogens as mutagens in the *Salmonella*/microsome test: Assay of 300 chemicals. *Proc. Natl. Acad. Sci. USA*, 72:5135–5139.
61. McKusick, V. A. (1978): *Mendelian Inheritance in Man: Catalogs of Autosomal Dominant, Autosomal Recessive and X-linked Phenotypes, 5th ed.* Johns Hopkins University Press, Baltimore.
62. Mendelsohn, M. L., Moore, D. H., II, and Lohman, P. H. M. (1992): A method for comparing and combining short-term genotoxicity test data: Results and interpretation. *Mutation Res.*, 266:43–60.
63. Mohrenweiser, H. W., and Jones, I. M. (1998): Variation in DNA repair is a factor in cancer susceptibility: A paradigm for the promises and perils of individual and population risk estimation. *Mutation Res.*, 400:15–24.
64. Myhr, B. (1991): Validation studies with MutaMouse: A transgenic mouse model for detection mutations in vivo. *Environ. Molec. Mutagen.*, 18:308–315.
65. Nagao, M., Sugimura, T., and Matsushima, T. (1978): Environmental mutagens and carcinogens. *Annu. Rev. Genet.*, 12:117–159.
66. Nagao, M., Takahashi, Y., Yamanaka, H., and Sugimura, T. (1979): Mutagens in coffee and tea. *Mutation Res.*, 68:101–106.
67. Nagao, M., Yahagi, T., Kawachi, T., Seino, Y., Honda, M., Matsukura, N., Sugimura, T., Wakabayashi, K., Tsuji, K., and Kosuge, T. (1977): Mutagens in foods, and especially pyrolysis products of protein. In: *Progress in Genetic Toxicology*, edited by D. Scott, B. A. Bridges, and F. H. Sobels, pp. 259–264. Elsevier/North-Holland, New York.
68. NAS (1989): Biological significance of DNA adducts and protein adducts. In: *Drinking Water and Health, Volume 9*, pp. 6–37. National Academy Press, Washington, D.C.
69. Obe, G., and Anderson, D. (1987): Genetic effects of ethanol. *Mutation Res.*, 186:177–200.
70. OECD (Organization for Economic Co-operation and Development) (1981, revised May 1983): *Guidelines for Testing of Chemicals*.
71. Pedersen, R. A., and Brandriff, B. (1980): Radiation- and drug-induced DNA repair in mammalian occytes and embryos. In: *DNA Repair and Mutagenesis in Eukaryocytes*, edited by W. M. Generoso, M. D. Shelby, and F. J. de Serres, pp. 389–410. Plenum Press, New York.

72. Pet-Edwards, J., Chankong, V., Rosenkranz, H. S., and Haimes, Y. Y. (1985): Applications of the carcinogenicity prediction and battery selection (CPBS) method to the Gene-Tox data base. *Mutation Res.*, 153:187–200.
73. Pienta, R. J., Kuschner, L. M., and Russell, L. S. (1984): The use of short-term tests and limited bioassays in carcinogenicity testing. *Regul. Toxicol. Pharmacol.*, 4:249–260.
74. Ray, V. A. (1979): Application of microbial and mammalian cells to the assessment of mutagenicity. *Pharmacol. Rev.*, 30:537–546.
75. Reedy, E. P., Reynolds, R. K., Santos, E., and Barbacid, M. (1982): A point mutation is responsible for the acquisition of transforming properties by the T24 human bladder carcinoma oncogene. *Nature*, 300:145–152.
76. Russell, L. B., Aaron, C. S., de Serres, F., Generoso, W. M., Kannan, K. L., Shelby, M., Springer, J., and Voytele, P. (1984): Evaluation of mutagenicity assays for purposes of genetic risk assessment. *Mutation Res.*, 134:143–157.
77. Russell, L. B., Selby, P. B., van Halle, E., Sheridan, W., and Valcovic, L. (1981): The mouse specific locus test with agents other than radiation: Interpretation of data and recommendations for future work. *Mutation Res.*, 86:329–354.
78. Saffer, J. D. (1992): Transgenic mice in biomedical research. *Lab. Animal*, 21:30–38.
79. Samson, L., and Schwartz, J. L. (1980): Evidence for an adaptive DNA repair pathway in CHO and human skin fibroblast cell lines. *Nature*, 287:861–863.
80. San, R. H. C., and Stich, H. F. (1975): DNA repair synthesis of cultured human cells as a rapid bioassay for chemical carcinogens. *Int. J. Cancer*, 16:284–291.
81. Sasaki, Y., Saga, A., Yoshida, K., Su, Y. Q., Ohta, T., Matsusaka, N., and Tsuda, S. (1998): Colon-specific genotoxicity of heterocyclic amines detected by the modified alkaline single cell gell electrophoresis assay of multiple mouse organs. *Mutation Res.*, 414: 9–14.
82. Schmid, W. (1975): The micronucleus test. *Mutation Res.*, 31:9–15.
83. Setlow, R. B. (1978): Repair deficient human disorders and cancer. *Nature*, 271:713–717.
84. Shelby, M. D. (1988): The genetic toxicity of human carcinogens and its implications. *Mutation Res.*, 204:3–15.
85. Short, J. M., Kohler, S. W., Provost, G. S., Ferik, A., and Kretz, P. L. (1990): The use of lambda phage shuttle vectors in transgenic mice for development of a short-term mutagenicity assay. In: *Mutation and the Environment*, Part A, edited by M. Mendelsohn, and R. Albertini, pp. 355–367. Wiley-Liss, Inc., New York.
86. Simic, M. C., and Bergtold, D. S. (1991): Dietary modulation of DNA damage in human. *Mutation Res.*, 250:17–24.
87. Simmon, V. F., Mitchell, A. D., and Jorgenson, T. A.: Evaluation of selected pesticides as chemical mutagens, in vivo and in vivo studies. EPA–600/1-77-028. National Technical Information Center, Springfield, Virginia.
88. Singh, N. P., McCoy, M. T., Tice, R. R., and Schneider, E. L. (1988): A simple technique for quantitation of low levels of DNA damage in individual cells. *Exp. Cell. Res.*, 175:184–191.
89. Slater, E. E., Anderson, M. D., and Rosenkranz, H. S. (1971): Rapid detection of mutagens and carcinogens. *Cancer Res.*, 31:970–973.
90. Sobels, F. H. (1982): Extrapolation from experimental test systems for evaluation of genetic risks in man. In: *Progress in Mutation Research, Vol. 3*, edited by K. C. Bora, et al., pp. 323–327. Elsevier, Amsterdam.
91. Stich, H. F. (1991): The beneficial and hazardous effects of simple phenolic compounds. *Mutation Res.*, 259:307–324.
92. Sugimura, T. (1978): Let's be scientific about the problem of mutagens in cooked food. *Mutation Res.*, 55:149–152.
93. Sugimura, T., Sato, S., Nagao, M., Yahagi, T., Matsushima, T., Seino, Y., Takeurchi, M., and Kawachi, T. (1976): Overlapping of carcinogens and mutagens. In: *Fundamentals in Cancer Prevention*, edited by P. N. Magee, T. Matsushima, T. Sugimura, and S. Takayama, pp. 191–215. University of Tokyo Press, Tokyo, and University Park Press, Baltimore.
94. Turturro, A., and Hart, R. W. (1984): DNA repair mechanisms in aging. In: *Comparative Pathology of Major Age-Related Diseases*, edited by D. G. Scarpelli and G. Migaki, p. 1946. Mark R. Liss, New York.
95. UNEP (1992): *Assessing the Risk of Genetic Damage*, edited by D. J. Brusick, W. B. Gopalon, E. Hesletine, J. W. Huismans, and P. H. M. Lohman. Lewis Press, Boca Raton.
96. van Delft, J., Bergmans, A., van Dam, F., Tates, A., Howard, L., Winton, D., and Baan, R. (1998): Gene-mutation assays in lacZ transgenic mice: Comparison of lacZ with endogenous genes in splenocytes and small intestinal epithelium. *Mutation Res.*, 415:85–96.
97. Venkatachalam, S., and Donehower, L. A. (1998): Murine tumor suppressor models. *Mutation Res.*, 400:391–407.
98. Vijg, J., and van Steeg, H. (1998): Transgenic assays for mutations and cancer: current status and future perspectives.
99. Vrieling, H., van Zeeland, A., and Mullenders, L. H. F. (1998): Transcription coupled repair and its impact on mutagenesis. *Mutation Res.*, 400:135–142.
100. Waters, M., and Auletta, A. (1981): The Gene-Tox program. *J. Chem. Inf. Comput. Sci.*, 21:35–38.
101. Weinberg, R. A. (1981): Use of transfection to analyze genetic information and malignant transformation. *Biochem. Biophys. Acta*, 651:25–35.
102. Weisburger, J. H., and Williams, G. M. (1981): The decision point approach for systematic carcinogen testing. *Food Cosmet. Toxicol.*, 19:561–566.
103. Williams, G. M. (1977): The detection of chemical carcinogens by unscheduled DNA synthesis in rat liver primary cell cultures. *Cancer Res.*, 37:1845–1851.
104. Wojewodzka, M., Kruszewsk, M., Iwanenko, T., Collins, A., Szumiel, I. (1998): Application of the comet assay for monitoring DNA damage in workers exposed to chronic low-dose irradiation I: Strand breakage. *Mutation Res.*, 416:21–35.
105. Wolff, S., Afzal, V., and Olivieri, G. (1990): Inducible repair of cytogenetic damage to human lymphocytes: Adaption to low-level exposures to DNA-damaging agents. In: *Mutation and the Environment*, Part B, pp. 397–405. Wiley-Liss, Inc., New York.
106. Woychik, R. P., Klebig, M. L., Justice, M. J., Magnuson, T. R., and Avrer, E. D. (1998): Functional genomics in the post-genome era. *Mutation Res.*, 400:3–14.
107. Yahagi, T., Nagao, M., Seino, Y., Matsushima, T., Sugimura, T., and Oleada, M. (1977): Mutagenicities of N-nitrosamines on *Salmonella*. *Mutation Res.*, 48:121–130.
108. Young, R., Oveisistork, F., Harrington-Brock, K., Schalkowsky, S., Moore, M., and Myhr, B. (1991): Quantitative size analysis of L5178Y TK +/– mutant colonies in soft agar: An interlaboratory comparison. *Environ. Molec. Mutagenesis*, 17(Suppl. 19):79.
109. Department of Health and Social Security (1979): *Committee on Mutagenicity, Committee on Mutagenicity of Chemicals in Food, Consumer Products, and the Environment. A consultative document on guidelines for the testing of chemicals for mutagenicity*. Department of Health and Social Security, Great Britain.

Principles and Methods of Toxicology, Fourth Edition, edited by A. Wallace Hayes.
Taylor & Francis, Philadelphia © 2001.

Chapter 18

Acute Toxicity and Eye Irritancy

Louis C. DiPasquale and A. Wallace Hayes

The methods and principles of evaluating two categories of hazards, acute systemic toxicity and eye irritation, both resulting from a single or very short-term exposure, are described in this chapter. In recent years, economics and concerns over animal welfare have raised many issues in animal testing. Alternate methods for acute toxicity and eye irritation are being developed and, in some cases, accepted by regulatory agencies for hazard assessment purposes. This chapter describes the classical methods for determining acute systemic toxicity and eye irritation, and the more modern methods requiring fewer animals are also discussed. In addition, criteria have been put in place for the validation and regulatory acceptance of alternative tests and these will be reviewed.

PRINCIPLES OF ACUTE TOXICOLOGY

Acute toxicity testing began nearly a century ago when physicians and pharmacologists were concerned with potent poisons and drugs. In 1927, Trevan (355) introduced the concept of a median lethal dose (LD_{50}) for the standardization of digitalis extracts, insulin, and diphtheria toxin. He recognized that the precision of the value was dependent on many factors such as seasonal variation and the number of animals used in a test. High-precision LD_{50} values can only be established with a large number of animals.

The list of extraneous factors that affect the precision of the LD_{50} has increased since Trevan's work and now includes, among other factors, sex, species, strain, age, diet, nutritional status, general health conditions, animal husbandry, experimental procedures, route of administration, stress, dosage formulation (vehicle), and intra- and inter-laboratory variations. In spite of the many variables affecting the LD_{50} determination, many government agencies still regard the LD_{50} as the sole measurement of the acute toxicity of all materials, though a change in this attitude has emerged.

It is important to obtain a sound measurement of the killing power of highly toxic substances because a small difference in exposure can distinguish a safe from a lethal situation. However, a precise LD_{50} is not necessary for less toxic materials such as pesticides and consumer household products. For these substances, an approximate measurement of the killing ability is sufficient and still desirable, since overexposure to these products is possible and lethal cases are not uncommon. There are errors inherent in the determination of LD_{50} values, some of which cannot be controlled by the experimenter, and it is therefore not scientifically sound to obtain a precise LD_{50} on low to moderate toxic substances. Many methods have been developed over the years to calculate LD_{50} values and to evaluate the acute toxicity of chemicals with a small number of animals. These methods are discussed later in this chapter.

Many scientists have advocated changes in the emphasis of acute toxicity testing. To date, there is a general consensus among toxicologists in academia, industry, and government that a change in the emphasis of acute toxicity testing is needed (24,122,132,208,227,262, 321,339). The value of a precise LD_{50}, except for highly toxic substances, is being de-emphasized and the focus is now on obtaining as much information as possible on the toxic manifestation and mechanism with the smallest number of animals. Undoubtedly, such information will be for physicians more useful than the LD_{50} in treating overexposure.

Even though the emphasis of acute toxicity testing is changing, the principles of dose-response and development of signs of toxicity remain the basis of the science of toxicology. This section refreshes the knowledge of the experienced and introduces the novice to these general concepts.

Definition of Acute Toxicity

Toxicity is defined as the harmful effect of a chemical or a drug on a living organism. Various expert groups have defined acute and subchronic toxicities. The Organization for Economic Cooperation and Development (OECD) defines acute toxicity as "the adverse effects occurring within a short time of (oral) administration of a single dose of a substance or multiple doses given within 24 hours" (275). In terms of human exposure, this definition of acute toxicity refers to life-threatening crises such as accidental catastrophes, overdoses, and suicide attempts.

Dose-Response Relationship

Toxicologists often obtain two types of data, quantal and graded. The quantal response is called the "all-or-none" response; it either happens or it does not happen. On the other hand, the graded response can be determined quantitatively and it is continuous. Mortality and incidences of pharmacotoxic signs are examples of quantal data, whereas enzyme activity, protein concentration, body weight, feed consumption, and electrolyte concentration are quantitative parameters. However, many apparently quantal responses are quantitative. If technical measurements permit, they may be graded. For example, the severity of a pharmacotoxic sign can be graded if detection methods are available.

At the molecular level, the graded dose-response relationship often can be explained by the receptor, a relatively old concept but still a valid one. Let S be a particular substance that produces a specific response by interacting with a target protein molecule, the receptor R, in the body to form a substance-receptor complex, SR. Assuming the reaction is reversible and there is only one binding site on every target receptor molecule, this process can be described by the following expression:

$$S + R \underset{K_2}{\overset{K_1}{\rightleftarrows}} SR$$

and the mass equation for this reversible process is

$$\frac{K_2}{K_1} = k_d = \frac{[S][R]}{[SR]} \qquad (1)$$

where [S] [R], and [SR] are the concentrations of the substance, the receptor, and the substance-receptor complex at any particular time, respectively, and K_d is the dissociation constant of the process. Let [R]O be the initial concentration of the receptor, which is usually very small and constant in number when compared with the concentration of the substance. Then

$$[R]\,0 = [R] = [SR]$$

thus

$$[R] = [R]\,0 - [SR]$$

Substituting the above into the mass equation [(Eq. (1)]

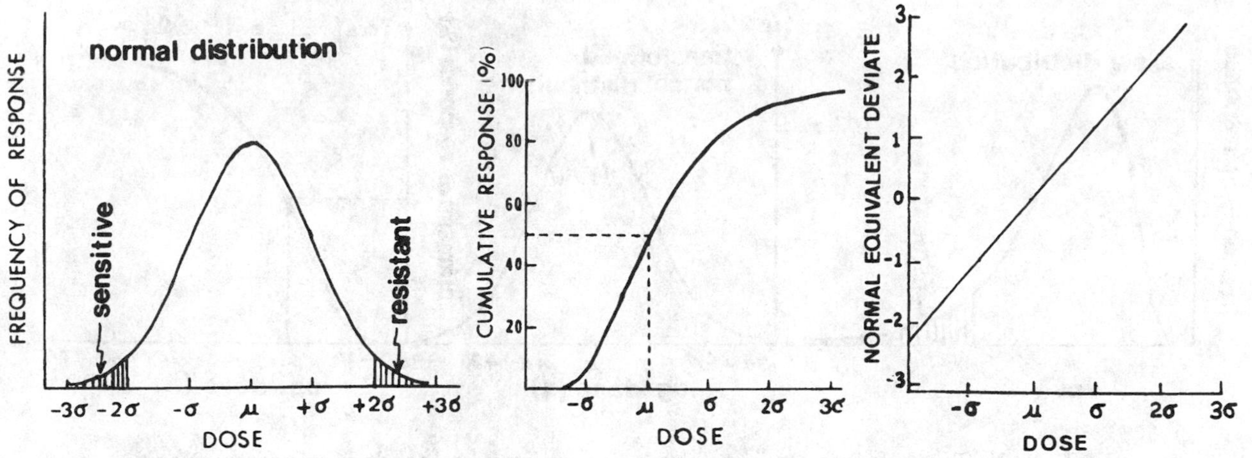

FIG. 18.1. Normal distribution of dose-response relationships: frequency of response, cumulative response, and cumulative response in terms of normal equivalent deviate.

and rearranging:

$$[SR]K_d = [S]([R]0 - [SR])$$

or

$$[SR](K_d + [S]) = [R]0[S]$$

which can be rearranged to

$$\frac{[SR]}{[R]0} = \frac{[S]}{k_d + [S]} \quad (2)$$

SR/[R]O is the fraction of receptor that has reacted with the substance to form the substance-receptor complex. If we assume that the response (E) resulting from the interaction of the substance with the receptor is dependent on the fraction of total receptor concentration that has reacted with the substance, then

$$E = \frac{[S]}{k_d + [S]} \quad (3)$$

Equation (3) is a hyperbolic function; therefore, the response (E) is related to the concentration of the substance in a hyperbolic function relationship. If the concentration of the substance at the receptor site is dependent on the dose, then the response is dependent on the dose administered. This phenomenon is perhaps the simplest version of the receptor kinetic concept relating the dose of the chemical to a biological response. The kinetics of the receptor–substrate interaction may be more complicated, and different dose-response relationships could be drawn based on these complicated kinetics. Readers who are interested in different receptor–substance kinetics are referred to Ferdinard (135).

The quantal dose-response relationship often is difficult to conceptualize based on the receptor theory. However, quantal response also can be viewed as a graded response if the whole population is considered as an individual. This relationship can best be explained in terms of a probability distribution. For a particular response, members of a population, for example, all the rats in the world, respond differently to a particular stimulus such as exposure to a chemical. Some rats will be highly sensitive and others will be very resistant. If these different responses are distributed normally within the population (i.e., with most members of the population being neither extremely sensitive nor resistant), the well-known bell-shaped population distribution curve results. If the probability of dose-response is expressed in terms of cumulative response, a sigmoidal curve can be obtained, as shown in Figure 18.1. However, most biological response distributions are not exactly normal and tend to be skewed to the higher dose, that is, extreme resistors have a larger *range of dose* to response than the extremely sensitive portion of the population. In general, a logarithmic dose transformation can normalize the distribution (i.e., convert the skewed distribution to a normal distribution) (Figure 18.2). After this logarithmic dose transformation, if the probability of the log dose-response is expressed cumulatively, the sigmoidal response curve is obtained (Figure 18.2). How is this lognormal transformation related to a regular dose-response curve? Is there justification or basis for a log dose transformation? To answer these questions, let us again look at Eq. (3). This equation can be arranged to

$$E = \frac{[S]}{k_2/k_1 + [S]}$$

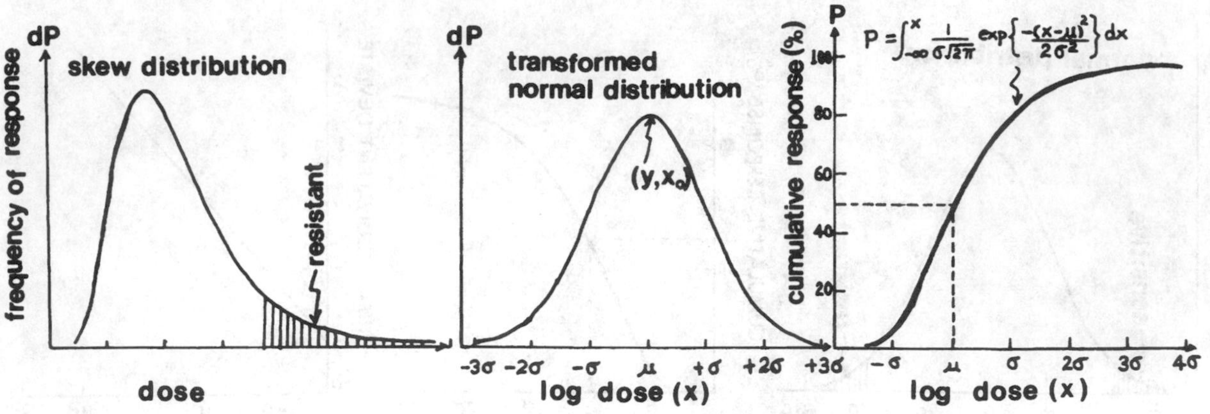

FIG. 18.2. Skew of dose-response can be normalized by log–dose transformation.

which can be rearranged to

$$E = \frac{k_1[S]}{k_2 + k_1[S]} \tag{4}$$

Over a certain concentration range, Eq. (4) will produce a curve very similar to the logarithmic function $E = K_1 \log (k_2\,[S] + 1)$ (77). Therefore, there may be justification for the log transformation besides simply a mathematical convenience.

Because a sigmoidal curve is more difficult to analyze than a straight line, many experts feel that further transformation of the log dose-response hyperbolic function is necessary to obtain a *straight-line* function curve. Perhaps the most widely used transformation is the normal equivalent deviate (NED) or the similar probit transformation (34,78,82,95,105,138,242). This technique involves the log dose transformation and the transformation of the cumulative response probability to the NED or probit. After both the probability and the dose are transformed, their transformed values are directly related to each other. A brief derivation of the straight-line direct function relationship between the log-dose and NED or probit is presented later in this chapter.

LD_{50} and Its Determination

Definition

The LD_{50} in its simplest form is the dose of a compound that causes 50% mortality in a population. A more precise definition has been provided by the OECD panel of experts as the "statistically derived single dose of a substance that can be expected to cause death in 50% of the animals" (275). In other words, an LD_{50} of a compound is not a constant, even though it has been treated that way by many; rather, it is a statistical term designed to describe the lethal response of a compound in a particular population under a discrete set of experimental conditions.

The significance of LD_{50} values has been examined by many scientists (24,122,132,208,227,262,321,339) who have arrived at similar conclusions: the LD_{50} is an imprecise value, it is not a biological constant and should be de-emphasized for most materials. They agree, furthermore, that approximate LD_{50} values often are sufficient for all practical purposes and that more emphasis should be placed on signs of toxicity, target organs, and other factors.

The numeric value of the LD_{50} has been used to classify and compare toxicity among chemicals. The extent of involvement of the LD_{50} in safety evaluation has almost reached a level of abuse. Although determining the LD_{50} under a set of experimental conditions can provide valuable information about the toxicity of a compound, the numeric LD_{50} per se is not equivalent to acute toxicity. One must always remember that lethality is only one of many reference points in defining acute toxicity. The slope (response/dose) of the dose-response curve, the time to death, pharmacotoxic signs, and pathological findings are all vital or even more critical than the LD_{50} in the evaluation of acute toxicity. Therefore, defining acute toxicity based only on the numeric value of an LD_{50} is inappropriate.

As pointed out previously, lethality is a quantal response, and the probability of a cumulative response is related to dose in a hyperbolic (sigmoidal) function. The cumulative probability of response is directly related to the standard deviates of a log dose population (Figure 18.1). Therefore, the slope of the log dose-response curve will indicate the relationship between the range of dose and the lethal response. This relationship is more important in risk assessment than the numeric value of the LD_{50} because more insight is available about the intrinsic toxic characteristics of a compound.

Sometimes the slope can give a clue to the mechanism of toxicity. For example, a steep slope may indicate rapid onset of action or faster absorption. A large margin of safety is predicted when a compound has a flat slope, that is, only a small increase in response with a large increase in dose. With the slope, it often is possible to extrapolate the response to a low dose (e.g., LD_0, LD_1) or even to a no-observed-effect level. It is especially important to know the slope when comparing a set of compounds. Two compounds may have identical LD_{50} values but different slopes and thus have quite different toxicological characteristics depending on the range of doses. Parallel dose-response curves may indicate a similar mechanism of toxicity, kinetic pattern, and probably similar prognosis. Neither the LD_{50} nor the slope can reveal absolutely a specific mechanism, but with pharmacokinetic and other biochemical studies elucidation of the mechanism of toxicity may be possible.

Determination of LD_{50}

Many methods are available for the determination of the LD_{50}. They can be grouped into two categories, the *normal population assumption* and *the normal population assumption-free* methods. The former usually can be analyzed by graphic procedures.

The normal population assumption-free methods are represented by Thompson's moving average interpolation (353,372) and the "up-and-down" method (51–54,77,98). The former method is widely accepted, and convenient tables (105,372) are available for estimation of the value of the LD_{50} with confidence limits when either 0 or 100% mortality incidences are observed. However, there are some restrictions on the use of this method, that is, four doses at equal log dose intervals and the number of animals per dose level must be equal. The up-and-down or the pyramid method is designed to estimate the LD_{50} with a small number of samples. It has a relative cost advantage because fewer animals are needed, but the test may be time-consuming and require excessive test material. Because of the advantage of using only a few animals, this method is popular when the test has to be conducted in large animals such as cows or sheep or expensive animals such as monkeys. A study comparing LD_{50} values obtained by the up-and-down method and other methods revealed an excellent agreement (52). There are apparently two shortcomings for this method—it is not adequate for estimating the incidence of delayed deaths, and a dose-response of mortality or signs of toxicity cannot easily be obtained. However, Weil (373) has adapted the up-and-down method to calculate the slope of acute toxicity response.

The normal population assumption method is represented by the probit analysis approach, which can be performed either by graphic means (138) or by mathematical calculation (139). Because the probit analysis is used widely in evaluating acute toxicity data, the priniciples are discussed briefly. This method involves the transformation of both the cumulative response probability and the dose.

When the dose is transformed into a log dose (x), the frequency of response versus log doses follows a normal distribution (Figure 18.2), which can be expressed mathematically as

$$dP = \frac{1}{\sigma\sqrt{2\pi}}\exp\left(\frac{-(x-u)^2}{2\sigma^2}\right) \tag{5}$$

where σ^2 and u are the variance and the mean of the population, respectively, and P is the probability corresponding to each value of x (Figure 18.2). The LD_{50} is defined as the log dose that can produce 50% mortality in a population (i.e., $P = 0.5$ or 50% cumulative response). Let x be the log LD_{50}; then $P = 0.5$ will correspond to the area under the log normal distribution curve from $-\infty$ to x_0; or $P = 0.5$ will correspond to the integration of Eq. (5) from $-\infty$ to x_0: That is,

$$P = 0.5 = \int_{-\infty}^{x_0} \frac{1}{\sigma\sqrt{2\pi}}\exp\left(\frac{-(x-u)^2}{2\sigma^2}\right)dx \tag{6}$$

The solution of Eq. (6) is $x = u$, the true mean or the median of the log normal distribution. One way to solve this equation is by a graphic method. The integration of Eq. (5) from $x = -\infty$ to $+\infty$ can be represented graphically by a sigmoidal curve as illustrated in Figure 18.2. Analysis of the sigmoidal curve is more difficult than a straight line. One way to transform the sigmoidal curve to a straight line is by NED analysis or, similarly, by probit analysis. For a detailed description of this analysis, the reader should consult Finney's text (138). A brief derivation of the straight-line function between log dose and the transformed probability of response is described below.

Probability (P) is normally expressed in terms of percentage or with values between 0 and 1; but Gaddum (152) has proposed to measure the probability of response on a transformed scale called the normal equivalent deviate (NED), or the standard deviation of a normal distribution, which can be described mathematically by Eq. (5). In a particular case, the normal distribution of response with mean equal to 0 and the standard deviation equal to 1, Eq. (5) can be written as

$$dP = \frac{1}{\sqrt{2\pi}}\exp\left(\frac{-x^2}{2}\right)dx$$

Similarly, if this distribution of response is plotted on the

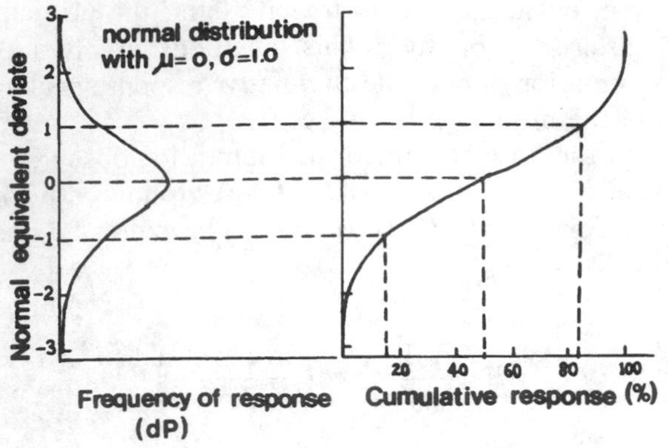

FIG. 18.3. Probability of response can be expressed in terms of percentage of the population or the NED of a normal distribution with mean = 0 and standard deviation = 1.

y axis (Figure 18.3), then

$$dP = \frac{1}{\sqrt{2\pi}} \exp\left(\frac{-y^2}{2}\right) dx \tag{7}$$

The probability in such a case is defined by a value on the y axis of Figure 18.3, that is, the integration of Eq. (7) from $-\infty$ to y:

$$P = \frac{1}{\sqrt{2\pi}} \int_{-\infty}^{y} \exp \frac{-y}{2} dy \tag{8}$$

In other words, for each value of y (from $-\infty$ to $+\infty$) expressed in terms of the standard deviation of a normal distribution with the mean equal to 0 and the standard deviation equal to 1, there is a corresponding value of probability (P) expressed in terms of percentage or having a value ranging from 0 to 1. Thus, equivalent values on the y axis can be used to define the value of P or vice versa; y and P define each other. This relationship is illustrated in Figure 18.3.

The particular probability of response to a particular log dose value x, as described in Eq. (6), will be

$$P = \int_{-y}^{-x} \frac{1}{\sigma\sqrt{2\pi}} \exp\left(\frac{-(x-u)^2}{2\sigma^2}\right) dx \tag{9}$$

where u and σ are the mean and standard deviation of the log dose, respectively.

If P is expressed by a value of y on the y axis (standard deviations), then

$$P = \frac{1}{\sqrt{2\pi}} \int_{-\infty}^{y} \exp\left(\frac{-y^2}{2}\right) dy$$
$$= \int_{-\infty}^{x} \frac{1}{\sigma\sqrt{2\pi}} \exp\left(\frac{-(x-u)^2}{2\sigma^2}\right) dx$$

The solution of this equation is $x = u + \sigma y$ or

$$y = \frac{(x-u)}{\sigma} - \frac{1}{\sigma} x - \frac{u}{\sigma} \tag{10}$$

Therefore, the probability when expressed in terms of y (the NED scale) is related linearly to x, the log dose. If x is plotted against the corresponding y, a straight line with slope $= 1/\sigma$ will be obtained. To further facilitate calculation, Bliss (33) suggested a slightly different NED unit called the probit, such that the new y value is equal to $[(x-u)/\sigma] + 5$. This procedure eliminates the negative values of NED when P has a value of less than 50%. Therefore, the probit is equal to the NED plus 5. The linear relationship between probits and log dose is similar to the relationship between NED and log dose. Thus, when $y = 5$, from Eq. (10),

$$5 = \frac{(x-u)}{\sigma} + 5$$

and $x = \mu$ (i.e., the median log dose which has a probability of response of 50%).

Logistic Transformation

Waud (371) suggested a logistic approach to calculate the LD_{50}. Thus

$$P = \frac{D^E}{(D^E + K^E)}$$

where P is the probability of response, D is the dose, E and K are scale and location parameters, respectively, and K corresponds to the LD_{50}. With the procedure of iteration, K and E can be estimated with a range of confidence. The derivation of this equation is beyond the scope of this chapter, and interested readers are referred to the original article by Waud (371).

Nonlethal Parameters

Although the LD_{50} and the slope of the dose-response curve can provide valuable information on the toxicity of a compound, the LD_{50} *is not equivalent to toxicity*. Chemicals can induce damage to the physiological, biochemical, immunological, neurological, or anatomical systems. Depending on the severity and the extent of the disturbance of the normal biological functions, the animal may survive the toxic response but some irreversible damage may occur. These nonlethal, adverse effects are as undesirable as lethality and certainly should be taken into consideration in the risk assessment of a chemical.

The major problem in the analysis of nonlethal responses is that the data often are not quantal. For example, dermal toxicity ranges from slight to severe.

These polychotomous data may be handled by RIDIT analysis, which was designed to analyze quantal responses with more than two outcomes (2,50,176).

Although toxic effects may contribute to lethality, any attempt to correlate a particular nonlethal response to mortality may be irrational (340) unless that response is the only one responsible for the eventual death of the animal. Identification of the response or responses related to mortality is not often a straightforward matter. Nonlethal responses that affect the general well-being of an animal should be considered in the risk assessment of a compound. If nonlethal responses can be viewed as true quantal data, the *median effective dose* (ED_{50}) and the corresponding dose-response curve may apply. The ED_{50}, which often is used in the standardization of a biologically active compound such as a drug, has a meaning similar to the LD_{50} except that it is designated to examine nonlethal parameters such as pharmacological responses and other nonlethal adverse effects. The ED_{50} is defined as a statistically derived single dose of a substance that can be expected to cause a particular effect to occur in 50% of the animal population. The therapeutic index (TI), defined by the ratio of LD_{50}/ED_{50} or LD_1/ED_{99}, has been applied to establish the safety margin of some biologically active drugs. The higher the index, the greater the margin of safety with the drug, that is, a large difference exists between the amount of compound predicted to kill 50% of the animals and the amount of compound predicted to elicit a particular response in 50% of the animals. The TI gives an even greater estimate of safety when the LD_1 is compared with the ED_{99}.

Reversibility of Nonlethal Parameters

In general, reversible responses are those that diminish with elimination of the chemical from the body. A true reversible response will cause no residual effects when the chemical is completely eliminated from the body. Such responses are commonly seen in drugs used at therapeutic dose levels. As the amount of drug in the body increases, the magnitude of the effect also increases. If it is truly reversible, the effect will wear off when the drug is completely eliminated.

The reversibility of a particular response is dependent on the organ or system involved, the intrinsic toxicity of the chemical, the length of exposure, the total amount of the chemical in the body at a specific time, and the age and general health of the animal. If the amount of chemical in the body is high enough, the intensity of the response may overwhelm a particular organ. Effects indicated through hormonal imbalance such as thyroid effects generally are reversible unless the threshold is surpassed. Damage in rapidly regenerating organs such as the liver is usually more likely to be reversible than damage in nonregenerating tissues such as nerves. A good example is the delayed onset of neuropathy caused by many organophosphate insecticides. The chemical may be completely eliminated from the body before the effect manifests itself. Animals with renal or liver diseases are often more susceptible to damage (reversible or irreversible) by a chemical insult because of their decreased ability to eliminate the chemical. Exposure to a chemical at an early age may induce irreversible damage more easily than at an older age because of the limited development of the kidneys and/or functional capacity of other organs such as the liver.

In risk assessment, it is important to know whether a toxic effect is reversible. Irreversible effects seen in animals obviously are weighted more heavily in reaching a conclusion on the toxicity and hazard a chemical may pose for humans.

ACUTE TOXICITY TESTING

The objectives of acute toxicity testing are to define the intrinsic toxicity of the chemical, predict hazard to nontarget species or toxicity to target species, determine the most susceptible species, identify target organs, provide information for risk assessment of acute exposure to the chemical, provide information for the design and selection of dose levels for prolonged studies, and, most important and practical of all, provide valuable information for clinicians to predict, diagnose, and prescribe treatment for acute overexposure (poisoning) to chemicals. Acute studies often are called the "first line of defense" in the absence of data from long-term studies. These data help industrial, government, and academic institutions formulate safety measures for their researchers and for limited segments of their worker population during the early stage of the development of a chemical. From a regulatory standpoint, acute toxicity data are essential in the classification, labeling, and transportation of a chemical. From an academic standpoint, a carefully designed acute toxicity study can often provide important clues on the mechanism of toxicity and the structure–activity relationship for a particular class of chemicals.

Many acute toxicity studies have been conducted solely for the purpose of determining the LD_{50} of a chemical. However, the reader is reminded that acute toxicity is not equivalent to the LD_{50}, and that the LD_{50} is not an absolute biological constant to be equated, as many investigators have, with such chemical constants such as pH, pK_a, melting point, and solubility. The LD_{50} is only one of many indices used in defining acute toxicity. A well-designed acute toxicity study should include consideration of the dose-response relationship of both lethal and nonlethal parameters, as discussed above. Sometimes biochemical measurements in an acute test can aid in elucidating the mechanism of toxic actions. Histopathology of organs may be helpful in determining the cause of death and identifying the target organs.

Types of Acute Testing

Because acute toxicity data may provide the first line of defense, a battery of tests under different conditions and exposure routes should be considered. In general, these tests should include oral, dermal, and inhalation toxicities, and skin and eye irritation studies. Other tests such as acute pre-neonatal and neonatal exposure, dermal contact sensitization, and phototoxicity should be considered. Depending on sound scientific factors, which may vary from one chemical to another, the number and kind of acute tests needed to establish the initial toxicity database may not be the same. For example, when inhalation exposure is not expected to occur because of the physical properties of the chemical, inhalation testing may not be needed. Such a case is not uncommon if respirable particles cannot be generated, even under the most favorable laboratory conditions. Nonetheless, for most purposes, oral, dermal, skin, and eye tests should be considered in the initial acute investigation. These four tests are often sufficient for regulatory purposes, labeling, and classification of a chemical, although increasing concerns also are placed on inhalation and skin sensitization studies. This chapter is concerned only with acute oral and dermal toxicity and eye irritation.

Acute Oral Toxicity

Principles

The test substance, undiluted or diluted with the appropriate solvent or suspending vehicle, is given to several groups of animals by gavage with a feeding needle or by gastric intubation. A vehicle control group is included if needed, but generally this group is not necessary if the toxicity of the vehicle is known. Clinical signs, morbidity, and mortality are observed at specific intervals. Animals that die or become extremely moribund during the study are subjected to necropsies. Animals that survive the test period are killed and necropsied at the end of the observation period. Tissues may be saved for histopathological examination to facilitate the understanding of the acute toxicity of the compound. To increase the reproducibility of the study, all experimental conditions and procedures should be standardized, and the study should be conducted according to generally recognized good laboratory practices (GLP) outlined by the U.S. Environmental Protection Agency (EPA) and the OECD (120,121,281).

Animal Species

The responses elicited by a compound often vary greatly among species. Ideally, toxicity tests should be conducted with an animal that will elicit compound-related toxic responses similar to those that occur in humans, that is, an animal that metabolizes the compound identically to humans and that has the same susceptible organ system(s). Under such conditions, the animal data may be extrapolated to humans. Unfortunately, finding such an ideal animal is a difficult if not impossible task.

A less ideal but more manageable approach is to conduct acute toxicity studies in a variety of animal species under the assumption that if the toxicity of a compound is consistent in all the species tested, then a greater chance exists that such a response may also occur in humans. Even though the response in different species is not consistent, it generally is considered better to err on the safe side with the risk assessment being based on the most sensitive species unless there is justification that such responses are less likely to occur in humans, for example, because of dissimilarity in metabolism between the less sensitive animal species and humans. Although these are logical assumptions and generally quite reliable, the danger of underestimating or overestimating the response in humans still exists. Therefore, there is no absolute criterion for selecting a particular animal species. However, priority should be given to species with metabolism or other physiological and biochemical parameters similar to humans. Animal species also should be selected on the basis of convenience, economic factors, and the existing database for the animal. Rats, mice, rabbits, and guinea pigs are most commonly chosen for acute toxicity studies.

Other Animal Variations

Acute toxicity, even within a particular species, can vary with health conditions; age; sex; genetic makeup; body weight; differences in absorption, distribution, metabolism, and excretion of the compound; and the influence of hormones (101). A conscientious investigator should be aware of the possible interaction of chemical treatment with these parameters. For example, immature animals may lack an effective drug-metabolizing enzyme system; this may contribute to higher toxicity of the compound in an immature animal if an enzyme is responsible for detoxification of the compound, or to decreased toxicity if an enzyme is responsible for activation of the compound. Obesity may affect the distribution and storage of a compound, especially when it is highly lipophilic. Sex hormones may be the target, or sex hormones may modify a particular toxic response which then may account for different toxic responses between sexes. Liver and renal diseases associated with old age may contribute to higher toxicity. Variations in genetic makeup among different strains may alter metabolism or other parameters, which may affect the toxicity of a particular compound. It is therefore important to document all data on animals: age, sex, body weight, strain, general health condition, and source. In general, healthy, young adults should be used. For example, if a rat is the test animal, then young adults weighing between 150 and 250 g should be used. The weight variation among animals should not exceed $\pm 20\%$ of the mean body weight.

Animal Numbers and Sex

The precision of the acute test is dependent to a large extent on the number of animals employed per dose level. Historically, 10 rats (5 male and 5 female) have been recommended in most regulatory guidelines (109,124, 125,275,337), although more recently modified protocols are acceptable using as few as three animals per dose level (278,279). The degree of precision needed and, in turn, the number of animals per dose group needed depend on the purpose of the study. In screening tests or tests designed to define the range of toxicity, fewer animals per dose level or fewer numbers of dose levels may be considered. In rare situations where a fairly precise LD_{50} is needed, the number of dose levels (at least three dose levels) and animals per dose group may need to be increased. The number of animals and dose levels should be based on sound scientific judgement.

In 1986, the OECD updating committee recommended that acute toxicity studies be conducted first in the male and at one dose level in females. If a marked sex difference appears when one dose level is used, then the test should be cross-checked. This approach reduces the number of animals used in acute toxicity testing. The more recent guideline (279), which is even more effective in reducing the number of animals used, specifies that in the absence of information suggesting that males are more sensitive, only females should be used. Literature surveys have shown that when there are sensitivity differences between the sexes, females, in general, are more sensitive (225).

Animal Housing and Environment

Studies should be conducted in a controlled environment. The temperature ($22 \pm 3°C$), relative humidity (30–70%), light and dark cycle (12 h dark, 12 h light), diet, and quality of drinking water should be standardized and maintained continuously. Animals may be caged in groups by sex or caged individually, depending on the species and size of the animals and on the needs of the particular study. Rodents can be caged in groups, usually not more than three per cage, but larger animals such as rabbits and dogs should be housed individually.

Dose levels. In general, the dose levels should be sufficient in number to allow a clear demonstration of a dose-response relationship and to permit an acceptable determination of the LD_{50}, if required. Three dose levels generally are sufficient. The selected dose levels should bracket the expected LD_{50} value with at least one dose level higher than the expected LD_{50} but not causing 100% mortality, and one dose level below the expected LD_{50} value but not causing 0% mortality, when the probit analysis method is applied to estimate the LD_{50}. However, with a method such as the moving average under some specific conditions (at least four dose levels with equal logarithmic intervals between each dose level, and with equal numbers of animals in each dose group), the LD_{50} can be estimated even with 0% mortality at the lower dose levels and 100% mortality at the two higher dose levels.

In any event, three or more dose levels with a wide range of toxicity responses are recommended if no other toxicity data are available. A pilot study may be needed for the selection of dose levels. Fewer animals per dose level and wider logarithmic intervals between dose levels usually are selected for the pilot study to ensure bracketing of the expected LD_{50} value. For example, if one desires an equal log interval of 0.6 between dose levels, and if the lowest dose is 1 mg/kg (log dose = 0), the next log doses would be $0+0.6$, $0.6+0.6$, $1.2+0.6$, and so on, corresponding to dose levels of antilogs 0.6, 1.2, 1.8 (i.e., the dose levels are: 1, 4, 16, 64, etc., in a geometric progression ratio of 4).

Dosages. If necessary, the test substance should be dissolved or suspended in a suitable vehicle, preferably in water, saline, or an aqueous suspension such as 0.5% methyl cellulose in water. If a test substance cannot be dissolved or suspended in an aqueous medium to form a homogeneous dosage preparation, corn oil or another solvent can be used. If the toxicity of the vehicle is not known, a vehicle control group should be included in the test. The animals in the vehicle control group should receive the same volume of vehicle given to animals in the highest dose group.

The test substance can be administered to animals at a constant concentration across all dose levels (i.e., varying the dose volume) or at a constant dose volume (i.e., varying the dose concentration). However, the investigator should be aware that the toxicity observed by administration in a constant concentration may be different from that observed when given in a constant dose volume. For instance, when a large volume of corn oil is given orally, the gastrointestinal motility is increased, causing diarrhea and decreasing the time for absorption of the test substance in the gastrointestinal tract. This situation arises when a highly lipid-soluble chemical is tested. A large fraction of such a material may quickly pass through the gastrointestinal tract and remain unabsorbed. Local irritation of a test substance generally decreases when the material is diluted. If the objective of the study is to establish systemic toxicity, the test substance should be administered in a constant volume (diluted concentration) to minimize gastrointestinal irritation that may in turn affect the absorption of the test substance. On the other hand, the test substance should be administered undiluted to assess the irritation potential of the test substance. The choice of constant concentration versus constant dose volume should be based on sound scientific judgment. The OECD guideline suggests a constant dose volume approach (275). The maximum dose volume in rodents should not exceed 10 ml/kg body weight for non-aqueous vehicles or 20 ml/kg body weight for aqueous solution or suspension. In any event, for scientific and humane reasons the dose volume should be as small as possible.

Observation. As has been discussed previously, the emphasis in acute toxicity studies is on the determination of the dose-response and the onset of toxic signs. The observation period should be flexible depending on the purpose of the study. This period should be based on the onset of signs, the nature of the toxicity, time to death, and the rate of recovery. For most highly toxic substances, the onset of toxic signs and the time to death may be very short, and prolonged observation may not be necessary. The slope of the dose-response curve for such test substances is usually very steep, and the treated animals either die or survive within a very short time. For other substances, the onset of signs and the time to death may be delayed for a few days to a few weeks or longer. Obviously, a longer observation period is needed to detect these delayed acute effects. The observation period also should be long enough for the determination of reversibility or the recovery of an adverse effect. Under specific circumstances the observation period might be longer, but it normally does not exceed 14 days.

Test limit. All chemicals can produce toxicity under some experimental conditions; for instance, if a sufficiently large dose is given. It is therefore scientifically misleading and inhumane to conduct acute toxicity studies at unreasonably high dose levels for the sake of demonstrating lethality and/or toxicity, which may be irrelevant to the compound itself. For example, an extremely high dose of a practically nontoxic compound can cause gastrointestinal blockage, which, in turn, can result in gastrointestinal tract dysfunction. Toxicity in this case is not related to the intrinsic characteristic of the test substance, because it is a direct result of the physical blockage caused by the biologically inert substance. There must be a point, however, at which an investigator can conclude that a test substance is practically nontoxic or nonlethal after an acute exposure. The traditional test limit for acute oral toxicity was considered to be 5.0 g/kg body weight. If no mortality was observed at this dose level, a higher dose level generally was not necessary. The more recently accepted protocols for acute toxicity (277–279) have a test limit of 2.0 g/kg-body weight.

Testing methods and procedures. The purpose of this section is to describe practical experimentation in detail, but it is not the authors' intention to list all technical procedures. A manual is available that describes technical procedures such as handling and dosing animals (286). Since the Good Laboratory Practices Act has been implemented in both the United States and most OECD countries, all experimental procedures should be documented and the studies conducted by trained personnel. For more details on GLP guidelines, the reader may consult several EPA, OECD, and Japanese publications (120, 121,281,337). The Japanese guidelines contain some unique requirements that are not duplicated by other countries.

Grouping, randomization, and preparation of animals. Animals not previously treated with test substances in other studies should be identified individually by coded marks, metal ear tags, or tattoos. The animals then should be quarantined for at least a week prior to dosing to acclimatize them to the conditions of the animal room. The animals should be fasted prior to administration of the test substance if the route of administration is oral. The purpose of fasting the animal is to eliminate feed in the gastrointestinal tract, which may complicate absorption of the test substance. Rats usually are fasted overnight. Because mice have a higher metabolic rate, withholding feed for 3–4 h may be adequate. Over-fasting small animals with a high metabolic rate may induce undesirable effects.

The animals should be randomly assigned to dose groups. Randomization, needed not only in acute toxicity studies but also in subchronic and chronic studies, ensures a homogeneous population and can minimize errors due to sampling bias. All animals with body weights and health conditions out of the normal range should be eliminated prior to the randomization procedure. With computer-generated random digit numbers or with tables of random digit numbers such as the one below, animals can be randomly assigned to groups by cage number or by individually assigned animal number.

Random numbers

	00–04	05–09	10–14	15–19	20–24
00	01826	72696	67261	13748	57834
01	70371	12890	90395	45245	71282
02	46616	84522	17249	78172	14197
	25–29	30–34	35–39	40–44	45–49
00	27748	47492	43428	85524	19311
01	15960	02749	86763	80564	02631
02	84272	53226	96719	83462	05628

For example, by using a random number table, 30 rats from a total of 60 rats are assigned to 3 dose groups of 10 rats each. Assume that 12 rats will be excluded from the study because of overweight, underweight, or other health problems; this leaves 48 rats, from which 30 would be chosen. One method of randomization is to arbitrarily number the 48 rats from 1 to 48. The random number table gives the following series of random numbers (row 00): 01826, 72696, 67261, 13748, 57834, 27748, 47492, and 43428. Because there are only 48 rats, the numbers should be two-digit numbers. The first group of rats would be rat numbers 01, ***82***, ***67***, 26, ***96***, ***67***, ***26***, 11, 37, 48, ***57***, ***83***, 42, ***77***, ***48***, 47, ***49***, 24, 34, and 28. The italicized numbers should be discarded because they are either repeated numbers or greater than 48. The second group of rats would be chosen similarly. The same procedure is repeated until 30 rats have been assigned to the 3 dose groups.

When the number of animals to be grouped is small, a large number of random numbers may be required to complete the grouping. Another way to use the random number table under such circumstances is by cycling. For example, 6 rabbits are assigned to 2 groups of 3 rabbits each from a total of 10 rabbits. From the second row of the same random digit number table, the first 3 two-digit numbers are 70, 73, and 11. Dividing these numbers by the total number of rabbits (i.e., 10), the remainders of these three numbers are 0, 3, and 1. If the remainder is zero, the denominator (in this case 10) will remain. Therefore, the 3 rabbits in the first group would be rabbit numbers 10, 3, and 1. Again, if the remainder numbers are repeated, they would be discarded. Also, if the number is smaller than the total number of animals, the number would be used and no division is needed. For the second group, the next series of numbers from the table are 28, 90, 90, 39, 54, 52, 45, 71, 28, 21, 59, 60, 02, 74, 98, and 67, and the corresponding numbers are 8, 0, 0, 9, 4, 2, 5, 1, 8, 1, 9, 10, 2, 4, 8, and 7. Therefore, the 3 rabbits in the second dose group would be rabbit numbers 8, 9, and 4. If a third group is needed, the 3 rabbits in this group would be rabbit numbers 2, 5, and 7. In general, the following rules apply when using the cycling method:

1. When the number from the random number table is less than the total number of animals to be chosen from, no division is needed.
2. When the number is greater than the total number of animals, the random number is divided by the total number of animals, and the remainder is used.
3. When the remainder is zero, the denominator is used.
4. No numbers or remainders should be allowed to repeat: any repeated numbers should be discarded.

The entry (the starting point) in the random number table should *not* be consistent. Thus, the entry should be made at a different point each time the random number table is used (one can start along the rows or the columns).

Calculation and Preparation of Doses

Doses in general are based on the body weight of the animal (expressed as weight of the test substance per kilogram of body weight of the animal), although for larger animals, the surface area may be more appropriate. The weight (or dose) of the test substance often is expressed in milligrams or grams of active ingredient if the test substance is not 100% pure. Ideally, only 100% pure sample should be tested; however, impurity-free samples are difficult to obtain. Although some toxicologists strongly advocate the use of pure samples in toxicity testing, others see the appropriateness of using technical samples, formulations, or crude products. It is acceptable to study the test substance in its pure form or in its technical or product form; however, the toxicity of impurities should be examined separately if the investigator feels that the impurities may contribute significantly to the toxicity of the test substance.

Selection of doses often is based on a pilot study, on existing toxicity data in other species, or on data obtained with a similar analog of the test substance. In an example based on the traditional LD_{50} determination, if 0 of 3 and 3 of 3 rats died at dose levels of 500 and 1000 mg/kg, respectively, in the pilot study, the expected LD_{50} numeric value would be between these two dose levels. If the investigator decides to select five doses that will bracket the expected LD_{50}, the logical approach would be to set the LD_{50} at 750 mg/kg for the definitive study with the following dose levels: 520, 625, 750, 900, and 1080 mg/kg. The dose levels progress by a value of the antilog 0.08 (i.e., multiplied or divided by 1.2 of the assumed LD_{50}). Although more modern methods may require fewer dose levels, the following procedure for calculation and preparation of doses is similar.

If the test substance contains only 75% active ingredient and the investigator chooses a constant dose volume of 10 ml/kg body weight across all dose levels, it will be more convenient to prepare a stock solution so that when 10 ml/kg of this stock solution is given to the animal, the dose will be 1080 mg/kg (active ingredient). The concentration of this stock solution would be

$$(1080\ \text{mg}/10\ \text{ml}) \div 0.75 = 144\ \text{mg of test substance/ml.}$$

Aliquots of the test substance for other dose levels can be prepared by dilution of the stock solution. For example, the solution concentration for the 900 mg/kg dose is

$$(900\ \text{mg}/10\ \text{ml}) \div 0.75 = 120\ \text{mg of test substance/ml.}$$

This solution can be prepared by diluting the stock solution 1.2 times, that is, for each ml of the 120 mg/ml solution to be prepared,

$$\frac{120\ \text{mg/ml} \times 1\ \text{ml}}{144\ \text{mg/ml}} = 0.833\ \text{ml of the stock solution should be diluted to a final volume of 1 ml with the vehicle.}$$

The vehicle should be one with limited or no toxicity. In preparing dosage solutions or suspensions, the vehicle of choice is water; other choices include an aqueous suspending vehicle such as 0.5% (w/v) methyl cellulose (Methocel) in water; corn oil; or other solvents such as aqueous ethanol, propylene glycol, or diluted DMSO in 5.0% $NaHCO_3$ solution. Magnetic stirring bars, micromills, or homogenizers can be used in preparing suspensions. Sometimes a small amount of a surfactant such as Tween 80, Span 20, or Span 60 is helpful in obtaining a homogeneous suspension. If surfactants are used, one must be aware of the potential effect of these surfactants on the absorption of the test substance.

On many occasions, it is desirable to prepare the dosage in an aqueous medium because of the undesirable effect of corn oil or other vehicles on the animals. In this case, one may try to prepare the dosage in a simple, water-suspensible, uniform formulation even though the test material is not soluble or cannot be suspended in aqueous medium. For example, a formulation can be prepared by dissolving a specific amount of the test material in an adequate amount of acetone, followed by mixing the acetone solution with a known amount of small particle size and biologically inert dispensing agent such as HiSil, and evaporating to dryness under a hood. In the resulting formulation, the test material is uniformly coated on the small particles. Then, a dosage in a uniform suspension can be prepared from the formulated test substance. This procedure has been used successfully in many studies.

Administration of the Dose

The test substance can be administered as a solution or suspension as long as it is homogeneous. The solution or suspension is gavaged to the animal with a suitable stomach tube or feeding needle attached to a syringe. For most acute oral toxicity studies with a test limit of 2.0 g/kg, the dose can be administered with one treatment. If unusual circumstances require a total dose that is too large to be administered at a single time, it should be divided into equal doses with 3 or 4 h between each administration. Feed should be withheld until the last dose, which should be within 24 h of the first dose.

Observations

Clinical examination, observation, and mortality checks should be made shortly after dosing, at frequent intervals over the next 4 h, and at least once daily thereafter. The intervals and frequency of observation should be flexible enough to determine the onset of signs, onset of recovery, and the time to death. The mortality checks should be frequent enough to minimize unnecessary loss of animals due to autolysis or cannibalism. The cage side observation should include any changes in the skin, fur, eyes, mucous membranes, circulatory system, autonomic and central nervous systems, somatomotor activities, behavior, and so on. Any pharmacotoxic signs such as tremor, convulsions, salivation, diarrhea, lethargy, sleepiness, morbidity, fasciculation, mydriasis, miosis, droppings, discharges, or hypotonia should be recorded. The most common pharmacotoxic signs are listed in Tables 18.1–18.3.

Individual body weights should be determined just prior to dosing, once weekly, and at death or at termination. The body weights of animals found dead generally are not as useful as the body weights of live animals. Necropsies should be performed on animals that are moribund, found dead, and killed at the conclusion of the study. All changes in the size, color, or texture of any organ should be recorded. Any gross change observed at necropsy should be described according to the size, color, and position of the lesion. Definitive pathological diagnostic terms should be avoided. Even though a complete microscopic examination of tissues and organs is ideal and would be helpful in defining acute toxicity, economic and time factors may preclude such a study. If the investigator feels that microscopic examination of a lesion is essential, tissues from the lesion should be preserved in an appropriate fixative such as 10% buffered formalin.

Table 18.1
Common signs and observations in acute toxicity tests

Clinical observation	Observed signs	Organs, tissues, or systems most likely to be involved
I. Respiratory blockage in the nostril, changes in rate and depth of breathing, changes in color of body surface	A. Dyspnea: difficult or labored breathing, essentially gasping for air, respiration rate usually slow	
	1. Abdominal breathing: breathing by diaphragm, greater deflection of abdomen upon inspiration	CNS respiratory center, paralysis of costal muscles, cholinergic
	2. Gasping: deep labored inspiration, accompanied by a wheezing sound	CNS respiratory center, pulmonary edema, secretion accumulation in airways, increased cholinergic
	B. Apnea: a transient cessation of breathing following a forced respiration	CNS respiratory center, pulmonary–cardiac insufficiency
	C. Cyanosis: bluish appearance of tail, mouth, foot pads	Pulmonary–cardiac insufficiency, pulmonary edema
	D. Tachypnea: quick and usually shallow respiration	Stimulation of respiratory center, pulmonary–cardiac insufficiency
	E. Nostril discharges: red or colorless	Pulmonary edema, hemorrhage
II. Motor activities: changes in frequency and nature of movements	A. Decrease or increase in spontaneous motor activities, curiosity, preening, or locomotions	Somatomotor, CNS
	B. Somnolence: animal appears drowsy, but can be aroused by prodding and resumes normal activities	CNS sleep center
	C. Loss of righting reflex, loss of reflex to maintain normal upright posture when placed on the back	CNS, sensory, neuromuscular
	D. Anesthesia: loss of righting reflex and pain response (animal will not respond to tail and toe pinch)	CNS, sensory
	E. Catalepsy: animal tends to remain in any position in which it is placed	CNS, sensory, neuromuscular, autonomic
	F. Ataxia: Inability to control and coordinate movement while animal is walking with no spasticity, epraxia, paresis, or rigidity	CNS, sensory, autonomic
	G. Unusual locomotion: Spastic, toe walking, pedaling, hopping, and low body posture	CNS, sensory, neuromuscular
	H. Prostration: immobile and rests on belly	CNS, sensory, neuromuscular
	I. Tremors: involving trembling and quivering of the limbs or entire body	Neuromuscular, CNS
	J. Fasciculation: involving movements of muscles, seen on the back, shoulders, hind limbs, and digits of the paws	Neuromuscular, CNS, autonomic
III. Convulsion (seizure): marked involuntary contraction or seizures of contraction of voluntary muscle	A. Clonic convulsion: convulsive alternating contraction and relaxation of muscles	CNS, respiratory failure, neuromuscular, autonomic
	B. Tonic convulsion: persistent contraction of muscles, attended by rigid extension of hind limbs	CNS, respiratory failure, neuromuscular, autonomic
	C. Tonic–clonic convulsion: both types may appear consecutively	CNS, respiratory failure, neuromuscular, autonomic
	D. Asphyxial convulsion: usually of clonic type but accompanied by gasping and cyanosis	CNS, respiratory failure, neuromuscular, autonomic
	E. Opisthotonos: tetanic spasm in which the back is arched and the head is pulled toward the dorsal position	CNS, respiratory failure, neuromuscular, autonomic

Table 18.1
Continued

Clinical observation	Observed signs	Organs, tissues, or systems most likely to be involved
IV. Reflexes	A. Corneal eyelid closure: touching of the cornea causes eyelids to close	Sensory, neuromuscular
	B. Primal: twitch of external ear elicited by light stroking of inside surface of ear	Sensory, neuromuscular
	C. Righting: ability of animal to recover when placed dorsal side down	CNS, sensory, neuromuscular
	D. Myotact: ability of animal to retract its hind limb when limb is pulled down over the edge of a surface	Sensory, neuromuscular
	E. Light (pupillary): constriction of pupil in presence of light	Sensory, neuromuscular, autonomic
	F. Startle reflex: response to external stimuli such as touch, noise	Sensory, neuromuscular
V. Ocular signs	A. Lacrimation: excessive tearing, clear or colored	Autonomic
	B. Miosis: constriction of pupil regardless of the presence or absence of light	Autonomic
	C. Mydriasis: dilation of pupils regardless of the presence or absence of light	Autonomic
	D. Exophthalmos: abnormal protrusion of eye in orbit	Autonomic
	E. Ptosis: dropping of upper eyelids, not reversed by prodding animal	Autonomic
	F. Chromodacryorrhea: red lacrimation	Autonomic, hemorrhage, infection
	G. Relaxation of nictitating membrane	Autonomic
	H. Corneal opacity, iritis, conjunctivitis	Irritation of the eye
VI. Cardiovascular signs	A. Bradycardia: decreased heart rate	Autonomic, pulmonary–cardiac insufficiency
	B. Tachycardia: increased heart rate	Autonomic, pulmonary–cardiac insufficiency
	C. Vasodilation: redness of skin, tail, tongue, ear, foot pad, conjunctivae, sac, and warm body	Autonomic, CNS, increased cardiac output, hot environment
	D. Vasoconstriction: blanching or whitening of skin, cold body	Autonomic, CNS, decreased cardiac output, cold environment
	E. Arrhythmia: abnormal cardiac rhythm	CNS, autonomic, pulmonary–cardiac insufficiency, myocardiac infraction
VII. Salivation	A. Excessive secretion of saliva: hair around mouth becomes wet	Autonomic
VIII. Piloerection	A. Contraction of erectile tissue of hair follicles resulting in rough hair	Autonomic
IX. Analgesia	A. Decrease in reaction to induce pain (e.g., hot plate)	Sensory, CNS
X. Muscle tone	A. Hypotonia: generalized decrease in muscle tone	Autonomic
	B. Hypertonia: generalized increase in muscle tension	Autonomic
XI. Gastrointestinal signs:		
Droppings (feces)	A. Solid, dried, and scant	Autonomic, constipation, GI motility
	B. Loss of fluid, watery stool	Autonomic, diarrhea, GI motility
Emesis	A. Vomiting and retching	Sensory, CNS, autonomic (in rat, emesis absent)
Diuresis	A. Red urine	Damage in kidney
	B. Involuntary urination	Autonomic sensory
XII. Skin	A. Edema: swelling of tissue filled with fluid	Irritation, renal failure, tissue damage, long-term immobility
	B. Erythema: redness of skin	Irritation, inflammation, sensitization

Table 18.2
Autonomic signs

Sympathomimetic	Piloerection Partial mydriasis
Sympathetic block	Ptosis Diagnostic if associated with sedation
Parasympathomimetic	Salivation (examined by holding blotting paper) Miosis Diarrhea Chromodacryorrhea in rats
Parasympathomimetic block	Mydriasis (maximal) Excessive dryness of mouth (detect with blotting paper)

Table 18.3
Toxic signs of acetylcholinesterase inhibition

Muscarinic effects[a]	Nicotinic effects[b]	CNS effects[c]
Bronchoconstriction	Muscular twitching	Giddiness
Increased bronchoconstriction	Fasciculation	Anxiety Insomnia
Nausea and vomiting (absent in rats)	Cramping Muscular weakness	Nightmares Headache
Diarrhea		Apathy
Bradycardia		Depression
Hypotension		Drowsiness
Miosis		Confusion
Urinary incontinence		Ataxia
		Coma
		Depressed reflex
		Seizure
		Respiratory depression

[a] Blocked by atropine.
[b] Not blocked by atropine.
[c] Atropine might block early signs.

Other Nonroutine Determinations

The cause of death in acute poisoning generally involves the nervous, cardiovascular, or respiratory systems. Effects on other organs such as the liver or kidney sometimes are masked by lethality or cannot be detected without special determinations. Clinical laboratory studies (hematology, clinical chemistry, or specific functional tests) may be needed to identify these adverse effects. Because these laboratory tests are costly, they are only justifiable when there is evidence indicating that a particular laboratory test would be helpful in identifying the target organ or mechanism of toxic action. For example, if the test substance has a chemical structure that belongs to a class of hepatotoxins, clinical chemistry measurements may be conducted to verify its hepatotoxicity.

Histopathology can be very valuable in identifying a target organ. Like clinical laboratory tests, histopathological examination of organs is expensive. However, the cost should not be the limiting factor in deciding whether histopathological examination is needed; rather the limiting factor should be whether there is evidence that a particular organ is involved.

Data Processing

All signs of toxicity, onset of signs, time to recovery, time to death, mortality, and necropsy findings can be summarized in tabular form. If a defined LD_{50} is required, it may be determined by an acceptable method (226,353,373). Although most laboratories are equipped with calculators or computer programs to facilitate the estimation of LD_{50} values, fiducial limits, and the slopes of the dose-response curve, the reader is advised to review the manual estimation procedure for two widely adopted methods, the probit analysis and the moving average method. The graphic procedure of the probit analysis is rapid and is sufficient for most purposes. But for a more precise estimate of the LD_{50}, mathematical calculation may be necessary, and the reader is referred to the maximum likelihood estimation described in Finney's text (138).

Graphic estimation of LD_{50} by probit analysis. The basic linear equation for the probit analysis as described in the previous section is

$$y = 5 + \frac{1}{\sigma}(x - u)$$

where y is the probit, (σ is the standard deviation of a log normal distribution with mean u, and x is the log dose. This equation is linear with respect to y and x often can be expressed as a linear equation, for example, $y = \alpha + \beta x$, where $\beta = 1/\sigma =$ slope, and $\alpha = 5 - (u/\sigma)$. When $y = 5$, $(x - u)/\sigma = 0$; thus $x = \mu$ (the median log dose). Further, y is related to P (the probability of response which has a value of 0 to 1 by the following equation:

$$P = \frac{1}{\sqrt{2\pi}} \int_{-x}^{y} \exp\left(\frac{-y}{2}\right) dy$$

The reader should bear in mind that both the u and x are in log dose scale.

The following steps should be taken for graphic estimation of LD_{50} by probit analysis.

1. Convert response probabilities to probit units by a probit transformation table (96, pp. 54–55).
2. Convert all doses into log dose units (e.g., $\log_{10}$ dose $= x$). (Steps 1 and 2 may be eliminated if probit-log graphic paper is available.)
3. Using the probit as the abscissa and $\log_{10}$ dose as the ordinate, plot the response probit units against the $\log_{10}$ dose.
4. Draw a straight line such that the vertical deviations of points (the probits) at each x value are as small as possible. Extreme probits, for example, those outside the range of probit 7 and 1, carry little weight in the fitting of the probit–log dose-response line and thus should be excluded.
5. From the regression of the probit–log dose line, extrapolate the log dose corresponding to probit units of 5, which also correspond to the $P = 0.5$. Thus, this extrapolated dose should be the median lethal *log dose*, and the LD_{50} value would be the *antilog* of this log dose value.
6. Calculate the slope of the probit–log dose line. This slope, $\beta = 1/\sigma$, is defined as the number of increases in probit units for a unit increase in log dose. The slope defined by Litchfield and Wilcoxon (226) is equal to

$$\frac{1}{2}\left(\frac{LD_{84}}{LD_{50}} + \frac{LD_{50}}{LD_{16}}\right) = \sigma$$

   This slope is different but related to the slope described here, thus, the larger the slope value, the steeper the probit–log dose response. The opposite is true in the Litchfield and Wilcoxon definition.
7. A x^2 test should be conducted to determine if the fitted line is adequate. A small value of x^2 statistic (within the limits of random variation) may indicate satisfactory agreement between the theoretically expected line and the fitted line. A significantly large x^2 statistic may indicate either that the animals do not respond independently or that the fitted line (probit–log dose) does not adequately describe the dose-response relationship of the test substance. If the latter is true, forms of the dose-response curve other than the probit–log dose linearity may exist, and further transformation may be needed (138). If the former is the case, then precision of the line is reduced.
8. Determination of precision is by weighting the coefficient. The standard deviation of a binomial distribution is, $\sqrt{PQ/n}$, where P and Q are the mean probabilities, P equals $(1 - Q)$, and n is the number of test subjects. Thus, the variance is PQ/n, the square of the standard deviation. It is obvious that the variance (i.e., the spread of a distribution) is inversely related to n. This relationship means that the larger the number of test subjects, the smaller the variance and the better the precision. The reciprocal of the variance is invariance, which measures the weight, nW. Here, W (weighting coefficient) $= Z^2/PQ$, where $Z = (1/\sqrt{2\pi})\exp(-y^2/2)$ and is related to the normal frequency function corresponding to the NED. A table of weighting coefficients (see 96, p. 53) corresponding to probits (y) is available (139). The standard error for the log LD_{50} is given by

$$\sigma/\sqrt{\Sigma nW}$$

if the estimated log LD_{50} does not greatly differ from the true mean log LD_{50}, because this estimation does not take into consideration the error in the estimation of σ for the probit–log dose-response line. A better equation for the estimation of the variance of the estimated log LD_{50} is given by

$$V(m) = \sigma^2\left(\frac{1}{\Sigma nW} + \frac{(m - \bar{x})^2}{\Sigma nW(x - \bar{x})^2}\right)$$

where $V(m)$ is the variance of LD_{50}, $\bar{x}$ is the weighted mean log dose, m is the median log dose, x is the log dose, and $1/\sigma = 1/1\Sigma nW\,(x - \bar{x})$. If the χ^2 is large, indicating that the test subjects do not respond independently to the dose, the estimation of variance of log LD_{50} may not apply, and adjustment due to the sampling variation of the slope $(1/\sigma)$ of the probit–log dose line may have to be made (138). For a quick estimation of the LD_{50} this adjustment may be dropped, and the standard error would be the square root of the variance, i.e., $\sqrt{V(m)}$. One must remember that the dose is expressed in log dose; therefore, the estimation of the standard error (SE) for the LD_{50} in the original dose unit (e.g., mg/kg) is impossible. However, an approximation is given:

$$SE(LD_{50}) = (10^m) \cdot ([\log_e(10) \cdot (S_m)]$$

where S_m (which equals $\sigma/\sqrt{\Sigma nW}$ or $\sqrt{V(m)}$) is the estimated standard error for the median log dose m (i.e., $m = \log LD_{50}$ or $10^m = LD_{50}$).

A more rapid approximation of the standard error of log LD_{50} was given by Litchfield and Wilcoxon (226) as

$$S_m = \frac{S}{N'/2}$$

where S is the difference between two log doses of expected effects (as indicated by the probiting dose line) that differ by one unit of probit and N' is the total number of animals between the log dose limits, corresponding to the expected probit 4.0–6.0 (i.e., the 16% and 80% responses).

9. *Fiducial limits*. The concept of fiducial limit is similar to the confidence limit. The value of the two may be the same, but they are not always identical. The fiducial probability F (e.g., 95%) can be defined as the situation when the true value of a parameter lies between the calculated upper and lower limits, which would not be contradicted by a significance test at the $1/2\,(1-F)$ probability level. These higher and lower limits are called the fiducial limits. For rapid analysis, the fiducial limits at the $F=95\%$ level can be estimated by $\log LD_{50} \pm 1.96\,(S_m)$. A more detailed estimation can be obtained by the maximum likelihood estimation (138).

   Another simple approximation of the fiducial limits is given by Litchfield and Wilcoxon (226) as LD_{50}/fLD_{50} or $LD_{50} \times fLD_{50}$ for the lower and upper limit, respectively, where LD_{50} is defined as the LD_{50} factor equal to $(s)\,(2.77/\sqrt{N'})$. Here s is the slope, which is defined as

$$\frac{1}{2}\left(\frac{LD_{54}}{LD_{50}}+\frac{LD_{50}}{LD_{16}}\right)=\frac{1}{2}(3.55+3.55)=3.55$$

   in this example, and N' is the total number of animals used between response probabilities 16% and 84% (i.e. probit 4 and 6, equal to 30 in this example). Then fLD_{50} equals 1.896. Therefore, the lower fiducial limit is equal to $8.91/1.896=4.70$, and the upper fiducial limit is equal to $8.96 \times 1.896=16.90$.

For all practical purposes, the graphic method should be sufficient to estimate the LD_{50}. Nonetheless, because computer programs are available to handle the mathematics, the more detailed maximum likelihood estimation (98,138) is used in many laboratories. Indeed the up-and-down procedure (52–54,279) (See Alternative Methods for Oral LD_{50} Test), which is one of the more modern methods of estimating the LD_{50}, is based on the maximum likelihood method. Calculations can be performed using either SAS (316) or BMDP (99) computer program packages which are available to many toxicology laboratories. Other examples of programming for the estimation of the LD_{50} with a small computer have been reported (223,311).

Acute Dermal Toxicity

Dermal exposure is an important route of exposure. The objective of conducting an acute dermal toxicity study is the same as an acute oral toxicity study. Such testing may provide information on the adverse effects resulting from a dermal application of a single dose of a test substance. The acute dermal test also provides the initial toxicity data for regulatory purposes, labeling, classification, transportation, and subsequent subchronic and chronic dermal toxicity studies. Comparison of acute toxicity by the oral and dermal routes may provide evidence of the relative penetration of a test material.

Although the general experimental design and principles of acute dermal toxicity testing are similar to those of acute oral testing, there are differences. These differences include selection of the animal species, number of animals per dose level, preparation of animals, dosage, and administration of the test substance. Only differences in the acute dermal test are described in this section.

Animals

The same concern about animal factors raised in connection with acute oral toxicity testing, such as species, age, health conditions, body weight, sex, and housing environment, can affect the outcome of an acute dermal test. The three most commonly used animal species are young, healthy adult rabbits (2–3 kg), rats (200–300 g), and guinea pigs (350–450 g). Other species can be used. The animals should be housed individually in a controlled environment. Quarantine, acclimatization, and randomization are as described for acute oral studies. The back of the animal or a band around the trunk should be clipped free of hair. When clipping the hair, care must be taken not to abrade the skin. If abraded skin is called for, a needle may be used, but care must be taken not to damage the dermis. Increasingly, investigators have come to question the value of conducting tests on abraded skin, and many consider such tests to be irrelevant. To date, almost all testing guidelines call for conducting the dermal test only on intact skin (109,124,125,275,337). Fasting the animals overnight is not necessary for the dermal test. Generally, five animals per dose level per sex is sufficient to allow for an acceptable estimation of the dermal LD_{50}. Smaller numbers of animals can be used.

Doses

Dose selection is similar to the acute oral test. Higher doses do not need to be tested when a test substance at 2000 mg/kg has not produced test substance-related mortality.

While a control group generally is not needed, a vehicle control group should be included in the study if the toxicity of the vehicle is not known. Its influence on dermal penetration of the test substance should be fully established prior to the study.

Preparation of Dosage and Dosing Procedure

The test substance should be applied uniformly to approximately 10% of the body surface of the animal (e.g., 4 cm × 5 cm for rats, 12 cm × 14 cm for rabbits, 7 cm × 10 cm for guinea pigs). This area may vary. For example, the area of application for highly toxic substances may be small because a smaller volume is applied. Liquid test substances generally are applied undiluted. If the test substance is a solid, it should be pulverized, weighed, placed on a plastic sheet or porous gauze dressing, moistened to a paste with normal saline (one part test substance for one part saline) or with the appropriate solvent, and spread evenly on the closely clipped skin to ensure uniform contact with the skin. Grinding of the solid test substances may not be needed under some conditions. For example, when a granular formulation is tested, it may be more relevant to test the substance in its formulation state than to destroy the formulation by grinding.

Because rabbits are the most widely used animal for acute dermal testing, the dosing procedure for the rabbit is detailed, especially for liquid substances. Dermal application of the test substance ranges from occlusive to semiocclusive to unocclusive.

The choice of the application method depends on what the most likely exposure pattern is in humans. Skin irritation is usually the worst after occlusive exposure, followed by semiocclusive and unocclusive exposure. Skin irritation may not only cause stress to the animal but also may increase dermal penetration. For unocclusive application, the application site remains uncovered but the volume of liquid test substance that can be applied to the skin may be limited depending on the volatility of the liquid. Immobilizing the animal or using a device such as a collar is needed to prevent ingestion through licking the application site. For occlusive or semiocclusive application, the application site is covered with an impervious material such as a plastic sheet, or with a porous gauze dressing as described in the following paragraph. The volume that can be applied with the occlusive or semiocclusive patch generally is larger than that of the unocclusive method.

Dosing procedures for liquid test substances. Rabbits are clipped free of hair with an electric animal hair clipper. The rabbit may have to be restrained by tightening the hind legs to a secured post and holding the nape of the neck during clipping. The area of skin to be clipped should be based on the need of the experiment and generally involves the entire band around the trunk between the flank and the shoulders if the dose exceeds 5.0 mg/kg. If abraded skin is to be tested (generally not required), abrasions to the stratum corneum may be made with a hypodermic needle (201/2 G) 2–3 cm apart longitudinally over the application site. A plastic cuff in a cylindrical shape (approximately 12–15 in. long and 10 in. in diameter) open at both ends can be used. The cuff is put on the trunk of the rabbits, covering the application site. With the help of another investigator, the plastic cuff is folded around the trunk and secured at the thorax and flank of the rabbit with surgical adhesive tape. Care should be exercised so that the cuff is sufficiently secured but not too tight to affect breathing. Using a long feeding needle, the correct amount of the liquid test substance is drawn into a syringe of appropriate size. The needle then is placed under the cuff and half of the dose is delivered evenly on each side of the vertebral column. After withdrawal of the needle, the test substance is evenly distributed over the application site by gently rubbing the top of the plastic cuff. A piece of cloth of appropriate size is then wrapped around the plastic cuff and taped in place to absorb any test substance that may spill off the cuff. After dosing, the investigator should observe the animal for a moment to see if breathing is affected, prior to putting the animal back into the cage. In the semiocclusive method, a porous gauze dressing replaces the plastic cuff. In unocclusive exposure, the test substance is applied uniformly over the skin: care must be taken to minimize run off from the skin, especially for aqueous dosing solutions. Applying the test substance in small amounts at a time may help.

Dosing procedure for solid test substances. If the test substance is a solid, it should be ground with a mortar and pestle unless there is justification not to pulverize it. The correct dose of the ground solid is weighed, placed in the center of a plastic sheet of appropriate size, and moistened with sufficient normal saline or another appropriate vehicle. If a vehicle other than saline or water is used, the effect of the vehicle on the skin penetration of the test substance should be considered, and its toxicity should be known. The type of vehicle selected should be based on the expected mode of exposure of the test substance and should be mixed into a paste. The paste then is spread evenly around the center of the plastic sheet. With one person holding the rabbit by grasping it at the back, another person moistens its belly and its back with paper towels soaked with saline. Then the rabbit is placed with its belly on the test substance paste on the plastic sheet, and another investigator wraps the sheet around the trunk of the rabbit. The plastic cuff is secured in place with surgical tape at the thorax and the flank. A piece of cloth of appropriate size then is wrapped around the plastic cuff and secured in place in the same manner. In the semiocclusive method, a porous gauze dressing replaces the plastic sheet.

Dosing procedures for rats and guinea pigs. Similar dosing procedures can be applied to rats and guinea pigs. Liquid samples should be placed on the back instead of the belly or on the lateral trunk. If unocclusive exposure is called for in rats, the test substance should be applied to the skin as near to the head as possible to prevent ingestion by preening of the application site. A plastic collar may be used to further limit access to the treatment site. Generally, the plastic collar produces more stress in the rat, as indicated by chromodacryorrhea (red stain around the eye), than in the rabbit. To minimize stress in rats, small collars can be handmade from light cardboard. The collar is lined with cut rubber tubing around the neck area and stapled in place. The cardboard collar is lighter and easier to place on small animals. It can readily be replaced if needed (the collar placed on the neck usually will last about three days), and it is more economical than the commercially available plastic collars.

Exposure Period and Removal of Cuff

Almost all testing guidelines (109,124,125,275,337) call for 24-h continous exposure. After the 24-h exposure, the cuff is removed and the application site is gently wiped with a paper towel soaked with saline, water, or any appropriate solvent to remove residual test substance remaining on the application site.

Observation Period

As in the acute oral toxicity test, the observation period and intervals should be flexible enough to establish onset of signs, time to death, and time to recovery, but should be frequent enough such that the loss of animals due to autolysis and cannibalizing is minimal. In addition, skin irritation should be assessed according to a scoring system such as the one described by Draize et al. (102).

Data Processing

Data should be analyzed and handled as in the acute oral toxicity test. Because the exposure period in a dermal toxicity study is longer than in a skin irritancy test, the skin irritation resulting from the 24-h exposure may not be relevant for assessing the skin irritancy potential of the test substance but may be considered as the worst case if the occlusive or semiocclusive method is used.

Test Limit

If no test substance-related mortality is observed at 2000 mg/kg, testing at higher doses may not be necessary because additional test substance may only be applied on top of the test substance layer already present. This layering may form a physical barrier to prevent further absorption of the test substance from the application site.

ALTERNATIVE METHODS FOR ORAL LD_{50} TEST

Animal testing has been widely debated. Many regard the issue as no more than animal protectionism and solely

Table 18.4
Summary of current recommendations on acute oral toxicity testing

Provisions	EEC and OECD	U.S. EPA	U.S. CPSC	U.S. FDA	U.S. DOT
Use of LD_{50}	Discourages	Same as OECD	Strongly discourages	Does not require	Same as OECD
Limit test (2 g/kg Dose)	Recommends	Same as OECD[a]	Same as OECD	Refers to	Recommends
Defined test (if limit>2 g/kg)	Test guideline 401 Test guideline 420 Test guideline 423 Test guideline 425	Same as OECD	NS	NS	NS
Endpoint evaluations	Onset, nature, reversibility of effects, gross necropsy, histopathology	Same as OECD	NS	NS	NS
Alternatives	NS	Structurally related activities (SAR)	Existing animal data Prior human experience Expert opinion	Accepts alternatives	Existing animal data Prior human experience

NS, not specified.

[a] Under current policy and regulations for pesticide products, precautionary statements may still be required unless there are data to indicate the LD_{50} is greater than 5 g/kg.

based on humanitarian reasons. Aside from valid scientific concerns on the usefulness of classic LD_{50} values (e.g., uncertainty in species extrapolation, seldom needed for potent drug standardization), there are broader issues on animal testing, some political in nature and others economically based. The cost of animal testing has been increasing at a skyrocketing rate over the last decades, and even without animal rights activism, the scientific community will need less costly alternatives to cope with the increasing demand for safety evaluation of a vast number of existing and new chemicals.

The approach to animal testing today is being altered by the so called Three Rs: reduction, refinement, and replacement. Reduction of the number of animals used in testing and refinement of existing testing methods to minimize pain and suffering of animals represent the short-term objective. Replacement of animal testing with non-animal-based methods, e.g., in vitro ("in glass," i.e., test tube) methods, is the ultimate goal. However, genuine, validated, and regulatory accepted nonanimal alternative methods to replace whole animal acute toxicity testing are still more of a goal than a reality, even though the concept has been widely accepted by scientists from industry, professional societies, and certain regulatory bodies (10,240,338,339).

As far as the oral LD_{50} test is concerned, a number of these classical, precise tests, using large number of animals, have been conducted for the purpose of labeling and classification of chemicals. Recently, there have been many positive developments in the reduction and refinement of acute oral toxicity tests. For example, the limit test (151), the British Society of Toxicology method (49), the up-and-down method (52–54), the fixed dose procedure (359), and the acute toxic class method (309), can achieve reduction in the number of animals. These methods, in general, have been endorsed by the scientific and regulatory communities and animal advocates alike (10,240,338,339), and some have been adopted as regulatory guidelines for the testing of chemicals (277–279). However, the classification and labeling schemes of many regulatory bodies around the world still use the LD_{50} value, and it may be some time before the classical, more precise test, using large numbers of animals, is eliminated. Perhaps it is time for regulatory bodies to redefine the scheme for classification and labeling of chemicals on the basis of reduced and refined acute toxicity testing results. An international study using the fixed dose procedure has shown that this is possible (359).

Modified LD_{50} Tests

The aim of these tests is to obtain adequate information on toxic signs, approximate LD_{50} values, and, in some, the slope of the dose-response. Many studies have shown that adequate acute toxicity and lethality information can be obtained by using fewer animals than in the classical LD_{50} studies. DePass (93) and Lipnick et al. (225) have reviewed several modified LD_{50} tests. Although the main endpoint remains lethality, these tests generally fulfill the goal of reducing the number and suffering of animals and in some cases provide adequate information for hazard classification and labeling. The key alternative tests are described below.

Table 18.5
Approximate lethal dose (ALD) versus conventional rat LD_{50} (g/kg)

	Conventional		Approximate	
Chemical	n	LD_{50}	n	ALD
Tetraethyllead	36	20	5	26
Methomyl	53	40	5	26
Hexachlorophene	46	165	11	90
Adiponitrite	65	301	7	300
Caffeine	40	483	8	450
N-Butylhexamethylene amine	35	536	7	1000
Hexamethylene diamine	92	1127	5	1500
Bromobenzene	35	3591	8	3400
Carbon tetrachloride	105	10,054	5	7500

Adapted from Reference 208.

Approximate Lethal Dose Method

This method involves sequential dosing until the lowest lethal dose is obtained. Initially, an arbitrary dose is given to an animal. If the animal survives, a second animal is given 1.5 times the initial dose, and, sequentially, several animals are given increasing doses in the same manner until a lethal dose is achieved. This dose is the approximate lethal dose (ALD). In general, only 6–10 animals are required to achieve the ALD. Comparison of classical LD_{50} values and the ALD indicates that the ALD can be used to closely predict the LD_{50} (Table 18.5).

The Up-and-Down Method

Animals are dosed one at a time, starting at an estimated LD_{50} dose. If the first animal survives, the next one receives a higher dose. If the first animal dies, the next one receives a lower dose. The spacing of doses generally is adjusted by a factor of 1.3 up or down depending on the outcome of the previous animal. Comparison of classical LD_{50} values to the up-and-down-derived LD_{50} shows close agreement (Table 18.6). This test has been adopted by the OECD as an alternative to the more traditional methods of LD_{50} determination (279). The

Table 18.6
Up-and-down method versus conventional rat Oral LD_{50} (g/kg)

Chemical no.	Conventional n	Conventional LD_{50}	Up-and-down n	Up-and-down LD_{50}
1	50	0.273	6	0.388
2	40	0.344	9	0.421
3	40	3.490	8	4.120
4	40	3.520	6	4.020
5	40	4.040	6	3.520
6	40	5.560	6	5.700
7	40	9.280	6	8.770
8	20	>10.00	3	>10.10
9	50	10.11	7	11.09
10	10	>20.00	8	22.40

Adapted from Reference 54.

OECD guideline also contains the provision for a limit test. The upper-limit dose is 2000 mg/kg (5000 mg/kg). If the first animal survives the upper-limit dose, then the second animal receives the same dose. If three animals survive the limit dose, then three animals of the other sex are tested at the limit dose. If all survive, the test is terminated.

The British Society of Toxicology (BST) Protocol

This protocol starts with three doses (5, 50, and 500 mg/kg) with five animals per sex per group, to minimize pain and suffering observed typically at the higher doses. The three initial doses generally will produce toxicity but no mortality. Depending on the response from the initial doses, subsequent doses can be increased or decreased by a factor of 10. Based on survival and toxic signs at a given dose, substances are placed into one of four categories. At least one study showed that classification of chemicals based on the BST protocol and the standard OECD protocol produced good agreement, but only use 74% of the animals and produce 87% less mortality than the OECD protocol (360).

The Fixed Dose Procedure

This modification of the BST protocol has been described by Van den Heuvel et al. (359). Basically, this procedure calls for testing at a dose selected from a series of pre-set doses (5, 50, 500, and 2000 mg/kg) for discriminating classification of the test substance into toxicity categories. The selected dose (discriminating dose) should be nonlethal, nonpainful, nonstressful, but toxicity-evident. It could be selected by using available information, or by conducting a "sighting study" using three or four animals. The focus of the test should not be limited to mortality (found dead or killed for humane reasons), but should include other toxicity endpoints such as time course of signs of toxicity and necropsy findings. These data and the "discriminating dose" should provide adequate data for hazard assessment, comparative reference, and labeling classification (Table 18.7).

A multinational validation study in 33 laboratories with 20 materials using the fixed dose approach produced consistent results on the time course of signs of toxicity which was adequate for acute toxicity risk assessment and acute toxicity classification based on the European Economic Community (EEC) criteria. Fewer animals were used and less stress occurred (359). This test has been adopted by the OECD as an alternative acute oral toxicity method (277).

The Acute Toxic Class Method

This method has been described by Roll et al. (309) and is based on the assumption that using a minimum number of animals in a stepwise procedure will provide enough information on the acute toxicity of a substance to allow classification according to the most commonly used classification schemes. Three animals of one sex are used for each step; either sex can be used. The initial dose is selected from one of three fixed levels, 25, 200, or 2000 mg/kg body weight, and should be chosen to produce some mortality. If existing information suggests that mortality is unlikely at the 2000 mg/kg dose, then a limit test at that level may be conducted with three animals of each sex. If deaths occur, further testing at the lower dose levels may be necessary. This method was evaluated in national and international validation studies (319,320), and has been adopted by the OECD as an alternative acute oral toxicity method (278).

Current Regulatory Status of Acute Oral Toxicity Testing

The current regulatory status of acute oral toxicity testing is in a state of flux. Although some form of acute toxicity information is required, most international regulatory agency guidelines are being revised to accept alternative methods based on the principles of reduction and refinement. A new regulatory philosophy is emerging which discourages the use of the classical LD_{50} test except when specifically justified for reasons of scientific necessity. Indeed, the OECD has agreed to phase out its Guideline 401—Acute Oral Toxicity, which requires an LD_{50} with 95% confidence interval, dose-mortality curve and slope, and to replace it with the more recently approved Acute Oral Toxicity Guidelines (277–279).

Various regulatory agency recommendations on acute oral toxicity testing are compared in Table 18.4. For specific information on regulatory agency requirements,

Table 18.7
Investigation of acute oral toxicity using the fixed-dose method of interpretation of results

Fixed dose	Results	Interpretation
5 mg/kg[a]	Less than 100% survival[b]	Compounds that may be very toxic if swallowed
	100% survival but evident toxicity	Compounds that may be toxic if swallowed
	100% survival; no evident toxicity	Retested at 50 mg/kg if not already tested at that level
50 mg/kg	Less than 100% survival[b]	Compounds that may be toxic or very toxic if swallowed; retested at 5 mg/kg if not already tested at that level
	100% survival but evident toxicity	Compounds that may be harmful if swallowed
	100% survival; no evident toxicity	Retested at 500 mg/kg if not already tested at that level
500 mg/kg	Less than 100% survival[b]	Compounds that may be toxic or harmful if swallowed; retested at 50 mg/kg if not already tested at that level
	100% survival but evident toxicity	Compounds that do not present a significant acute toxic risk if swallowed
	100% survival; no evident toxicity	Retested at 2000 mg/kg if not already tested at that level
2000 mg/kg[c]	Less than 100% survival[b]	Compounds that may be harmful if swallowed; retested at 500 mg/kg if not already tested at that level
	100% survival with or without evident toxicity	Compounds that do not present a significant acute toxic risk if swallowed

Adapted from Reference 359.
[a] Where a dose of 5 mg/kg produces significant mortality, or where a sighting study suggests that mortality will result at that dose level, the substance should be investigated at a lower dose level. The level chosen should be one that is likely to produce evident toxicity but no mortality.
[b] Includes compound-related mortality and humane kills but not accidental deaths.
[c] Testing mortality at this dose level is carried out primarily for risk assessment purposes. However, where no evident toxicity is seen at 500 mg/kg its results are relevant to classification if there is greater than 50% mortality (including humane kills).

the reader is encouraged to check the most recent regulatory guidelines that apply.

Refining the Acute Oral Toxicity Test

Humane Endpoints

Refinement of the acute oral toxicity test to minimize pain and suffering of animals, is an area that is also receiving considerable attention. Current OECD Test Guidelines require that animals which are moribund or in obvious pain and distress should be humanely killed. An ad hoc working group has been established to develop an OECD guidance document to provide a more humane perspective on when to euthanize animals used in toxicity studies. The final document will give specific criteria to determine when an animal is in moribund condition or experiencing significant pain and distress. Although the guidance document has not been finalized, the working group has agreed that a harmonized approach to defining humane endpoints in acute toxicity testing is essential. For additional information, the reader is referred to the accumulating literature on the subject of humane endpoints (217, 252–256,319,359).

Quantitative Structure–Activity Relationship (QSAR) Analysis

Analysis of the structure–activity relationships within a class of chemicals can yield valuable information and may reduce the number of bioassays conducted. QSAR analysis is particularly useful during the discovery stage for selection of chemicals for further development. QSAR also can be used for prioritization of chemicals for various actions related to health and safety and environmental assessment. The elements generally needed for QSAR include: a verified bioassays database for the endpoint to be predicted; a set of chemical–physical parameters which describe the chemical structures so that the endpoint can be modeled in terms of these parameters; statistical techniques, that is, principally multivariate regression and discriminant analysis for weighing these parameters in a near-optimum fashion for the explanation of the endpoint; and computer technology to make it all practical (119). Using QSAR, Enslein (119) has analyzed 2066 chemical structures and found that the oral rat LD_{50} of almost 50% of the compounds examined was predicted within a factor of 2, and 95% within a factor of 8.

Obviously there are limitations for the QSAR approach to predict a complex toxic response in whole animals. These include a limited database on which to base a QSAR model, the temptation to extrapolate beyond the confines of the model, and the noise inherent in the bioassays on which the models are based (119). The results from QSAR have to be used with caution, and at this stage, QSAR is useful during the discovery stage and for prioritizing chemicals.

Cytotoxicity Tests

Recent interest has focused on the use of in vitro cytotoxicity assays as predictors of human acute toxicity. The relationship between acute toxicity and cytotoxicity is not only intuitively appealing, but its relevance may be explained by the *basal cytotoxicity concept* (113). This concept derives from classifying all chemical toxicity to humans into three categories:

(1) organizational or extracellular toxicity;
(2) organ-specific cytotoxicity; or
(3) basal cell toxicity or chemical injury to structures and functions which are common to all human cells.

Because the mechanism of action of most toxic chemicals is related to basic biochemical processes found in all cells, it is postulated that there should be some correlation between toxic concentrations determined in vitro as well as in vivo.

An international program, the Multicenter Evaluation of In Vitro Cytotoxicity (MEIC), organized by the Scandinavian Society of Cell Toxicology, was designed to evaluate the relevance of in vitro toxicity assays for human acute toxicity (36,112,114,366). In this program, 29 laboratories tested 50 reference chemicals with known human toxicity (acute lethal blood concentrations as taken from clinical and forensic medicine handbooks) in 61 different in vitro assays (116). These assays comprised human and animal cell lines and primary cultures, fish cell cultures, other ecotoxicological systems, and cell free systems. In vitro IC_{50} values (geometric average 50% inhibitory concentrations) were compared to human mean lethal serum concentrations using multivariate partial least squares (PLS) analysis. To provide a benchmark for measuring the predictivity of in vitro assays to animal tests, rodent and human toxicity data were compared (115) and an evaluation of rodent LD_{50} values contrasted to human acute lethal dose was also conducted (116). Results indicated that rat and mouse LD_{50} values predicted human acute lethal doses with correlation coefficients (r^2) of 0.61 and 0.65, respectively. In contrast, the various in vitro assay predictions of human lethal blood concentrations ranged from $r^2 = 0.69$ (all human cell lines combined) to $r^2 = 0.34$ (all plant systems combined). These correlative findings show that for the 50 reference chemicals studied, in vitro tests using human cell lines are equivalent to rodent LD_{50} determinations in predicting human lethal blood concentrations.

Although this simplistic approach ignores most metabolic and toxicokinetic aspects operative in the intact organism, the results support the continued evaluation of the basal cytotoxicity concept and suggest that the use of human cell lines in in vitro cytotoxicity assays as predictors of human acute toxicity should be given serious further consideration as alternative methods to acute lethality studies in rodents.

Although substantial gains have been made, in vitro replacement methods for acute toxicity testing are difficult to define. Some investigators have proposed a battery of in vitro tests as a strategy to replace whole-animal acute toxicity tests (266).

ASSESSMENT OF EYE IRRITATION INDUCED BY CHEMICALS

The eye captures visible energy and converts the energy to neurosignals, which are transmitted to the intricate central nervous system in which they form neuroimages (vision). The importance of having this ability to perceive the external environment through vision is a giant step in the evolutionary process. In humans, vision along with hearing is vital for the development of speech, learning, and intelligence. Loss of vision can greatly curtail normal living.

There are three basic components of vision: optics, photoreceptors, and conducting nerves. All three components must function properly to form a clear and sharp neuroimage in the visual cortex. The optics of the eye (cornea, aqueous humor, iris, lens, and vitreous humor) must remain transparent and be able to refract and focus light on the right position on the photoreceptors. The photoreceptors (the cones and rods) of the retina must be able to undergo photolysis and convert light energy to neuropotential impulses. The optic nerves must be able to carry these neuroimpulses to the visual cortex.

Because the eye is constantly exposed to the external environment, the cornea must be protected from drying, dust, and microorganisms. The eyelids, the lacrimal system, and the somatosensory response of the cornea all work together to protect this outermost structure of the eye. Like other organs, the major portion of the eye is nourished by blood vessels. The retinal, circumcorneal, and uveal vessels also nourish and help maintain the eye. These vessels are so arranged and constructed that they normally do not alter the transparency of the ocular optics. Nutrients reach the transparent

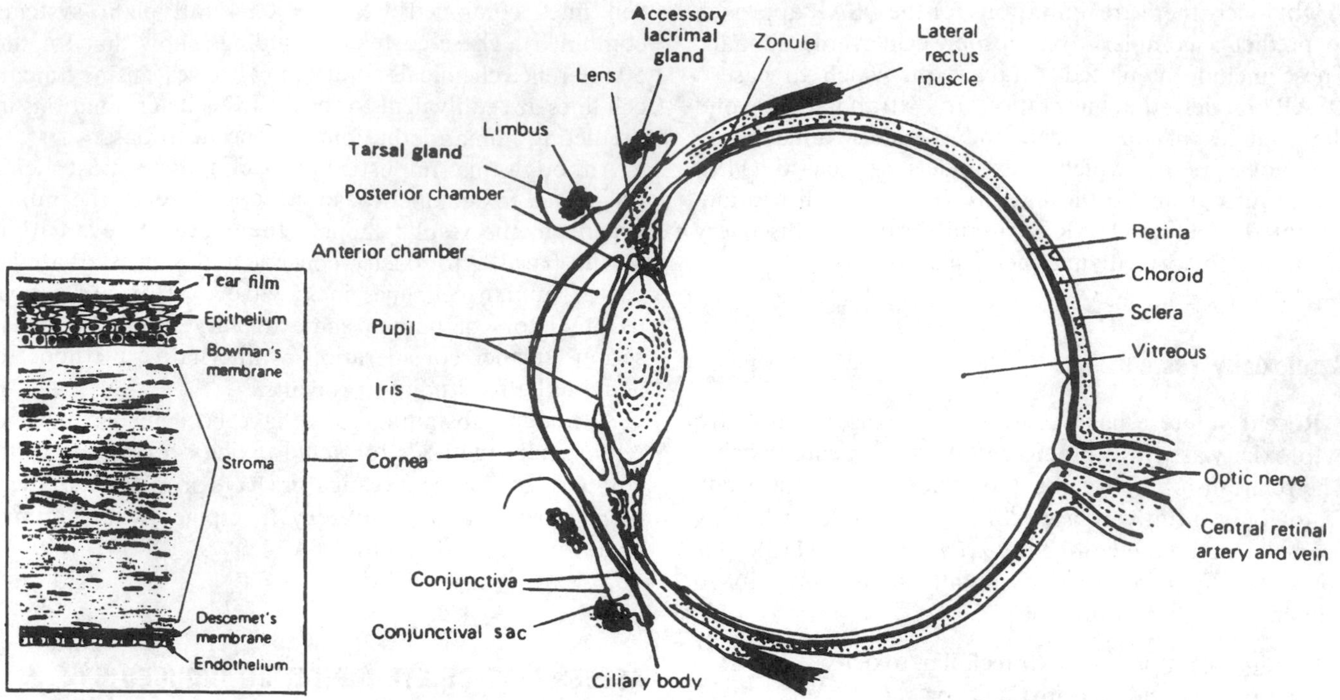

FIG. 18.4. Schematic illustration of the eye.

tissues of the eye via tears, the aqueous humor, and vitreous fluids.

Normal ocular functions are in delicate balance and are interdependent. Any traumatic insult, chemical or physical, can upset one or many of these ocular functions, thus creating a disturbance in vision. Depending on the extent of the traumatic injury (ranging from drying of the tear film to corneal ulceration or optic nerve damage), partial or complete loss of vision can result. Ocular injury not only can result from accidental physical trauma, but, also, from radiation and chemicals.

Chemicals can cause ocular damage locally by accidental exposure to the eye, or systemically by ingestion of chemicals such as food contaminants and drugs. Because many chemicals can produce ocular damage either locally or systemically (170,180,241,308), it is important to test products for ocular effects before exposing workers during manufacturing and, ultimately, before subjecting consumers to products on the market. Ocular effects resulting from systemic exposure are beyond the scope of this chapter. This section focuses on eye irritation resulting from direct ocular contact.

Conducting ocular tests in humans is not only impractical but also unethical. Consequently, many methods and techniques have been developed over the years for testing ocular effects in animals. This section describes the methods for detecting potential eye irritants and discusses their limitations. In recent years, in vitro methods intended to replace eye irritancy tests in animals have evolved. The pros and cons of alternative methods are discussed.

Testing for potential eye irritancy is required for labeling and classification of chemicals by most regulatory agencies worldwide. The test protocol, interpretation of results, and classification scheme vary among countries. The differences among major industrial countries also are discussed.

Definition of Chemically Induced Eye Irritation and Corrosion

Irritation can be defined as reversible inflammatory changes in the eye and its surrounding mucous membranes following direct exposure to a material on the surface of the anterior portion of the eye. Corrosion is irreversible ocular tissue damage following exposure to a material. From a practical point of view, the distinction between reversible and irreversible changes sometimes is limited by the length of the observation period. Therefore, the term "eye corrosion" should be reserved for gross tissue destruction of the eye, which generally occurs rapidly following exposure. When interpreting results from an eye irritation study, one must take into consideration the biological significance of the ocular changes. For example, redness of the conjunctiva is considered a mild ocular effect. Even if it does not disappear completely within a specific time period (e.g., 21 days), one can hardly justify classifying the material as corrosive.

Normal Physiology and Anatomy of the Eye

A brief description of the normal physiology and anatomy of the eye is essential for understanding the development of eye irritation. Details can be found in a variety of textbooks and reviews (137,238,298).

Functionally, the eye can be divided into three basic parts (Figure 18.4). From posterior to anterior, they are:

- *Photoreceptors* (*retina*): The part of the eye that connects to the central nervous system via the optic nerve
- *Optics*: Structure that focuses visible light (image) onto the retina; it includes (from anterior to posterior) the cornea, iris, aqueous humor in the anterior chamber, the lens, and its related organelles such as the zonules and ciliary body (muscles), and the vitreous in the posterior chamber
- *Protective, lubricating, and nutritional structures*: These include the anterior eyelids and conjunctiva and associated secretory glands, the sclera and its outside layer (the fibrous tunic) and inside layer (uvea-vascular), and the ciliary body (secretory).

For chemically induced eye irritation, the main concern is generally on the directly exposed organelles such as the cornea, conjunctiva, and the iris. Effects on these structures can easily be detected by gross observation. If the chemical can penetrate deeper into the eye, other organelles also can be affected. Detection of the effects on these deeper structures requires special aids.

Cornea

The cornea is composed of, from anterior to posterior, the epithelium, Bowman's membrane, stroma, Descemet's membrane, and endothelium. The epithelium is about five cells deep in the transitional zones at the periphery. The basal cells are columnar, the other cells are squamous, and the cells between the two layers are polygonal (wing cells). The Bowman's membrane (12 μm) is an acellular layer of collagen and ground substance which provides a functional interface between the stroma and epithelium. An intact Bowman's membrane and the epithelial basal cell layer are vital to the regeneration of damaged epithelium. Damage to Bowman's membrane may predispose the cornea to fibrosis. The stroma consists of lamellae of collagen fibrils and fibroblasts supported by ground substances. The stroma forms most (nine-tenths) of the cornea and is limited on its inner surface by Decemet's membrane.

In addition to the organization of sheets of fibrils, other unique features such as proper hydration also contribute to corneal transparency. The Descemet's membrane (5–10 μm), like the Bowman's membrane, is an acellular layer which is the basement membrane of the endothelium. The endothelium is a single layer of cells which completely covers the posterior surface of the cornea. The cells are hexagonal with large nuclei. This layer of the cornea is particularly rich in the active transport enzyme adenine triphosphatase (ATPase). The maintenance of proper hydration of the cornea has been attributed to the activity of this enzyme, which catalyzes an active sodium–potassium pump (38,203,228). The limbus is a transitional region between the cornea and the sclera. This region, rich in vascularization, is the source of fluid and infiltration cells during corneal injury.

The epithelium and the overlying tear film provide the intrinsic protection for the cornea. Other layers have almost no intrinsic resistance to injury. Penetration into deeper layers of the cornea and other structures of the eye is limited by chemicals' solubility and lipophilicity. Chemicals that are lipophilic and water-soluble penetrate more rapidly and probably deeper into the eye than other chemicals.

The cornea is always covered with a film of tears, which consists of several oily and aqueous layers. Proper tear formation and drainage as well as the stability of the precorneal tear film are important for a normal precorneal optical surface, proper lubrication, nutrition for the cornea, removal of bacteria and debris from the cornea, and activity on the cornea. Reduction of tear formation can lead to a dry eye, mechanical friction, irritation, or infection. A discussion of the assessment of tear film formation, stability, and drainage is available (73).

The cornea is a powerful refractive biological optic. Its refractive power is dependent on its being transparent and on proper hydration. Maintenance of proper transparency and hydration is dependent on many mechanisms, for example, proper tear flow, absence of deposits and blood vessels, proper arrangement of collagen fibrils, unimpaired nutritional supply for the metabolic active pump (Na^+-K^+), and proper intraocular pressure. Decreased transparency or hydration can be a result of corneal scars (decreased corneal thickness) or corneal edema (increased corneal thickness). Corneal edema can be caused by epithelial damage, endothelial damage, increased intraocular pressure, lack of oxygen, or inhibition of the electrolyte balance pump (Na^+-K^+-activated ATPase), which is located mainly in the endothelial membrane, but is also found in the epithelium. Methods for measuring corneal curvature, corneal thickness, intraocular pressure, blood/aqueous humor barrier, and corneal endothelium damages have been reviewed (73).

Conjunctiva

The conjunctiva is part of the eyelid. It is the delicate membrane that lines the eyelid (palpebral conjunctiva) and covers the exposed surface of the eyeball (bulbar conjunctiva). Histologically, the conjunctiva is an aqueous, nonkeratinized epithelium with numerous mucus-secreting cells. Accessory lacrimal glands are present in the conjunctiva, which contribute to the aqueous layer of a precorneal tear film. The Meibomian gland, a specialized sebaceous gland in the eyelid, secretes the outer oily layer of the tear film.

The main function of the eyelid is to protect the eye, especially the cornea, from external trauma through proper blinking reflexes and secretion of tears. Normal secretory and excretory functions of the tear are also important for normal optical function of the eye. The precorneal tear film can form an optically uniform layer over the microscopically irregular surface of the corneal epithelial cells. The tear flow continuously flushes cellular debris or foreign bodies from the eye, lubricates the corneal surface from mechanical friction caused by blinking, provides nutrients to the cornea, and induces antibacterial activities by proteolytic enzymes and immunoglobulin. All of these functions are important to maintain an optically intact corneal surface. Substances that affect the stability of the precorneal tear film by interfering with the secretory/excretory functions or with the blinking mechanism can cause serious damage to the cornea and may even cause corneal ulceration.

The nictitating membrane or the third eyelid is an important and prominent structure in many species of animals, including the rabbit, but is not as important in humans and nonhuman primates. It aids in protecting the conjunctiva and the cornea when the eyeball is retracted. The nictitating membrane, like the conjunctiva, also contains lacrimal glands and its secretion contributes to the aqueous layer of the precorneal tear film. In addition, the nictitating membrane helps to support the position of low eyelids and forms the lacrimal lake in the medial canthus. Vascularization in the conjunctiva generally consists of superficial and deep groups, mainly in the bulbar conjunctiva.

Three endpoints generally are associated with irritation in the conjunctiva: redness, chemosis, and discharge. In response to an irritant, the eyelids blink, the tear secretion increases, and the conjunctiva vessels dilate. Blinking and tearing (discharge) aid in removing the irritant from the eye, and tear flow also may reduce the acidity or basicity of the irritant. Vessel dilation may be triggered by histamine, prostaglandins, or other inflammatory mediators, resulting in an apparent increase in vascularity (redness) in the conjunctiva. If irritation is severe, the dilation of the vessel increases and vascular fluid and proteins leak into the conjunctiva resulting in edema (chemosis). If the edema is severe, bulging may hinder normal functioning of the eyelids.

Iris

The iris forms the pupil and functions in regulating the amount of light that may reach the retina. High-intensity light causes constriction of the diameter of the pupil and low-intensity light dilates it. It does so by two sets of muscles acting opposite each other to control the diameter of the pupil. These muscles, circulatory and radiating, are innervated by both the autonomic and sympathetic nervous systems. The set of muscles forms the distinct characteristic of iridic furrows of the iris.

The iris is anatomically located posterior to the cornea, and is a very vascular structure made of loose connective tissues, muscle, and pigmented cells. The amount of pigment in the iris varies. Heavily pigmented cells are found in most species, except albinos. Only a small amount of pigment is found in the albino rabbit eye. This is an advantage in ocular studies because it allows easier and better examination of the iridal vessels, lens, and retina.

The observation endpoints of local iridic injury are increased vascularity, edema (increased thickness of the stroma/swelling), reaction to light, aqueous flare, and gross destruction of tissue. These are the manifestations of an inflammatory process (iritis) responding to an irritant. Like the conjunctival vessels, the iridic vessels dilate and leak vascular fluid in response to irritants. Dilation of vessels and leakage cause edema and apparent changes in vascularity such as injection of iridic vessels (hyperemia). Aqueous flare is a result of protein leaking from the iridic vessels into the aqueous humor of the anterior chamber. Protein leakage into the anterior chamber alters the refractive index of the aqueous humors. Light beams entering the anterior chamber are scattered, giving the anterior chamber a cloudy appearance which contrasts with a clear appearance in normal eyes as a light beam passes through the pupil and the anterior chamber, for example, during examination with a slit lamp. This is called the aqueous flare or Tyndall phenomenon which is usually not noted during routine gross examination of the eye. In a more severe form of iritis, tissue destruction may result and nerve innervation may be disrupted, causing the pupil to be unresponsive to light. Failure to react to light, from a practical standpoint, is the most reliable observation of a severe iridic reaction since severe iritis is usually accompanied by severe opacity in the cornea, which may obscure the visible detection of changes on the iris.

THE DRAIZE TEST

The Draize test was developed in 1944 by Draize et al. to study eye irritation (102). The test was based on the original work of Freidenwald et al. (148). For years, the Draize test has been used as the animal test to identify human eye irritants. It is a simple and generalized test. It is easy to conduct and requires no special instruments. Even though simplicity is probably the main reason for its popularity, it is also the limitation of the test per se. Undeniably, the Draize test can adequately identify most of the moderate-to-severe human eye irritants, but the test may fail to detect mild or subtle ocular irritation even with proper modification.

In the original Draize test, a standard 0.1 ml or 0.1 g of test substance is applied to the conjunctival sac of an albino rabbit's eye. The eyelid is held together for a few seconds and then released. The degree or extent of opacity on the cornea, the redness on the iris, and the chemosis and discharge on the conjunctiva are scored subjectively according to an arbitrary scale at preselected intervals (1, 24, 48, and 96 h) after exposure. Scoring is based on the degree of effects caused by the testing substance. More emphasis is placed on the opacity of the cornea, which has a maximum score of 80, whereas emphasis is progressively less with other effects: conjunctival changes (maximum score of 20) and iritis (maximum score of 10) (62,165, 232).

The Draize test has been a subject of controversy among animal rights groups (178,313) and even in the scientific community (28,62,165,172,181,232,304,374). It has been criticized on the bases of dose volume, use of animals as models, methods of exposure, irrigation, number of animals, observation and scoring including laboratory procedure variability, and interpretation of results, all of which are discussed below.

Dose Volume

The 0.1 ml dose volume used in the original test was based on the volume used earlier by Friedenwald et al. (148) to study the mechanism of acid- and base-induced ocular damage. This dose volume was selected arbitrarily as a standard volume for intraocular injection. Draize et al. (102) adopted it solely for convenience which unfortunately has set a seemingly unchangeable doctrine for years even though the 0.1 ml dose volume lacks a scientific basis and, in conjunction with the conjunctival dosing method, often overpredicts the eye irritancy of a chemical.

Proponents of the 0.1 ml dose volume argue that this dose is a maximized test for the worst case and that it can better predict human eye irritants. The Draize test is basically a safety test. Its main purpose is to predict what would happen to human eyes *within* the expected range of exposure. The 0.1 ml dose is out of the range of human exposure. The maximal volume the cul-de-sac of a rabbit's eye can hold is only 30–50 μl (246); thus, even though one desires a maximal test, the dose volume should not be more than 50 μl. Any volume over this absolute maximum simply falls from the eye. Furthermore, the worst case is not necessarily the best case. Constantly overrating eye irritation will have a desensitizing effect on consumers' and workers' awareness of potential eye irritation. This will defeat the purpose of eye irritancy testing which is to protect them.

There are no data to substantiate the argument that the 0.1 ml dose can better predict human eye irritants. On the contrary, in at least one survey, there was little correlation between human accidental exposure experience and data generated by the traditional 0.1 ml maximal dose. The survey did not support the general presumption that rabbit eyes are more sensitive than human eyes (68). Simply reducing the dose volume has produced data closer to eye irritation experienced in humans. For example, comparison of human eye irritation resulting from accidental exposure to many consumer products has revealed that lower dose volume predicts the eye irritancy potential much better than the 0.1 ml dose volume (147,172). In one of the studies, the time needed for recovery from eye irritation in consumers or factory workers is compared with animal tests in monkeys and rabbits (147). This survey clearly demonstrated the modified Draize test (Federal Hazardous Substances Act (FHSA) protocol with a dose volume of 0.1 ml) was the poorest predicting test, whereas the low dose volume and the monkey tests were better predictors even though all three animal tests overpredicted the eye irritancy experienced in humans.

In 1977, a panel on eye irritancy test of the National Academy of Sciences (NAS), formed at the request of the Consumer Product Safety Commission (CPSC), recommended lowering the dose volume (267). Subsequently, even smaller dose volumes ranging from 0.003 to 0.03 ml were proposed by others because they predict human eye irritants more accurately, cause less pain to animals, and can discriminate slight-to-moderate eye irritants (172,174,380). Williams et al. (380) showed that direct corneal application in a dose volume of 0.01 ml increased the response on the cornea when compared with the standard 0.1 ml dose but did not change the response on the conjunctiva. These results in the absence of compounding effects of a high dose volume suggest that the lower dose volume is just as sensitive a method for eye irritancy testing as the higher dose volume.

Animal Models

As with other toxicological tests in animals, the primary issue of testing for ocular irritancy in animals is predictability for humans. Recognizing that there are anatomical, physiological, and biochemical differences between human and animal eyes, researchers are confronted with the difficult task of selecting the appropriate animal model and suitable test conditions to identify potential human eye irritants. The corneal thickness of dogs and rhesus monkeys is similar to that of humans (approximately 0.5 mm) (232,236,247); rabbit corneal thickness is somewhat thinner (0.37 mm) (232). There is a lack of a recognizable Bowman's membrane in rabbits, but they have a well-developed nictitating membrane (an additional target tissue), thick fur around the eyes, loose eyelids susceptible to mild irritants, an ineffective tear drainage system, and a poorly developed blinking mechanism (267). There are also species differences in biochemistry (e.g., variation in enzyme content (216)) and different penetration rates of various substances (231).

Even though there are shortcomings and exceptions in predictability, the rabbit has been used for most eye irritancy studies. There are some obvious advantages for choosing the rabbit: a wide database, economy, availability, ease of handling, and large, unpigmented eyes suitable for various ophthalmological examinations. With some exceptions (171,304), the rabbit eye is generally more sensitive to irritating materials than human or monkey eyes (25,63). Thus, there are built-in safety factors for making extrapolation and assessment of hazard to humans.

In addition to rabbits, dogs and primates sometimes are used for ocular testing. Eye irritancy in primates generally is more closely correlated with the exposure experience in humans, although dogs also are suitable under certain circumstances (29). Because they are more expensive and less available, dogs and primates are only used occasionally to assess eye irritancy.

Regardless of which animal is used, the investigator should always have a good understanding of the animal eye being observed. Background ocular findings, if not observed prior to exposure, can be recorded falsely as chemically induced damage.

Methods of Exposure

Basically, there are two ways of applying a test substance to the eye: (a) applying the test material into the cul-de-sac of the conjunctiva or (b) applying it directly onto the cornea. The conjunctival exposure method has been adopted historically because of the ease of application. It also has been perceived as being accurate in dosing. However, some have experienced (29,172) that conjunctival exposure is inappropriate under many circumstances, especially when the test material is a solid powder. The possibility exists that the test material will be trapped in the conjunctival sac, producing some undesirable mechanical effects and making the interpretation of the results more difficult. It is also evident that a considerable amount of the standard 0.1 ml or 0.1 g dose (especially as a solid powder) either falls or is blinked from the eye once the animal's eyelids are released. The claim that conjunctival dosing is more accurate may not be valid.

The corneal exposure method, on the other hand, mimics more closely the actual accidental exposure experience in humans. When assessing the hazard of most chemical accidents, this method should be considered except when the chemical is intended for pharmaceutical use (267). Applicators developed for the corneal exposure method have been used in some studies (25,63). A more uniform corneal lesion was observed, resulting in less observation variability (25). For a study as specific as corneal wound healing, a corneal applicator is recommended (258). However, for hazard assessment, it is desirable to apply the test substance directly onto the cornea while the lids of the test eye are gently held open. The eyelids are closed for a second and then released to allow blinking; this action more closely mimics actual human exposure (172).

Irrigation

Washing the eye is a typical emergency remedy after accidental exposure to chemical substances. In experimental studies, the treated eye usually is irrigated 20–30 sec after exposure to the test substance. Water is rapidly but gently squeezed from a plastic bottle to produce a constant gentle stream of water irrigating the entire treated eye. Irrigation should last for at least 1 min.

The effect of irrigation on the interpretation of test results has been the subject of many studies (25,27,28,37,89,140,171,173,285,322). While irrigation of the treated eye right after exposure can prevent or minimize eye irritation in rabbits, the effectiveness of irrigation is dependent on the chemical, the concentration, the time lag between exposure and initiation of the irrigation, and the volume of irrigation. Early washing (less than 1 min) generally is recommended to reduce irritation (89,140,173,322), but in some cases, increased irritation has been observed after irrigation with water (153,322). In other cases, ocular damage was almost instantaneous if irrigation did not begin after a few seconds (89).

Number of Animals

It is generally true in experimental studies that the larger the group size the more precise the test results. Sometimes, the desired precision may be offset by animal-to-animal variabilities. Economic considerations also are important in determining the number of animals used in a test group. A balance between economic considerations and reliability of test results should determine the number of animals tested in a study.

For eye irritation studies, a group size of 9 rabbits was recommended in the original Draize test, and group sizes of at least 6, 3, 3, and 4 rabbits have been recommended by the FHSA, Interagency Regulatory Liaison Group (IRLG), OECD, and NAS, respectively. The relationship of variability, classification, and group size is addressed in the literature (27,173,375). With larger group size, smaller variability has been noted (375), whereas with a decreased group size, lesser differentiation of irritancy has been suggested (27). Recognizing these facts, Guillot et al. (173) suggested a compromised approach. They suggested that with 3 rabbits in an initial study, there was a 96% chance that a positive or negative eye irritation result would be obtained. A similar conclusion was obtained in another study conducted with 67 petroleum products each with 6 rabbits (94). The eye irritation scores for the petroleum products based on all 6 rabbits were compared statistically with the scores from 2, 3, 4, or 5 animals. The comparison showed that a subsample size of 2, 3, 4, and 5 rabbits correctly classified (compared with the original 6 rabbits/test classification) the chemicals at 88, 93, 95, and 96% accuracy, respectively.

Observation and Scoring

Reversibility and severity are the two major criteria used to measure eye irritancy in the Draize test. Reversibility refers to the time needed for the ocular effects to disappear and for the eye to return to its normal state. To determine this reference time, treated eyes are examined periodically at 24-h intervals, on day seven after exposure, or at longer intervals if needed to establish reversibility (102). The observation period varies for different guidelines. For example, the FHSA uses 24-, 48-, and 72-h time spans (136); the OECD uses 1-, 24-, 48-, and 72-h, and, if needed, extended observations (276); and the NAS recommends 1, 3, 7, 14, and 21 days (267). The observation period should be flexible so that one can confidently assess the persistence of ocular effects and fully characterize the degree of involvement, because the onset and healing of ocular effects often are unpredictable (171).

The assessment of severity of different ocular effects is subjective. This subjective evaluation is the major source of error for intra- and inter-laboratory variation (374). Therefore, to minimize at least the intra-laboratory variability in scoring, uniformity in scoring techniques must exist among investigators regardless of which scoring system is followed. Pictorial references such as those prepared by the FDA (131) and the Consumer Product Safety Commission (CPSC) (85) can be extremely helpful in the standardization of scoring eye irritation.

The types of ocular effects observed in the Draize test involve the cornea, iris, nictitating membrane, and conjunctiva. A grading system (Table 18.8) was originally

Table 18.8

Scale of weighted scores for grading the severity of ocular lesions

Lesion	Score[a]
I. Cornea	
A. Opacity—degree of density (area which is most dense is taken for reading)	
Scattered or diffuse area—details of iris clearly visible	1
Easily discernible translucent areas, details of iris clearly visible	2
Opalescent areas, no details of iris visible, size of pupil barely discernible	3
Opaque, iris invisible	4
B. Area of cornea involved	
One-quarter (or less) but not zero	1
Greater than one-quarter—less than one-half	2
Greater than one-half—less than three-quarters	3
Greater than three-quarters—up to whole area	4
Score equals A × B × 5	
Total maximum = 80	
II. Iris	
A. Values	
Folds above normal, congestion, swelling, circumcorneal injection (any one or all of these or combination of any thereof), iris still reacting to light (sluggish reaction is positive)	1
No reaction to light; hemorrhage, gross destruction (any one or all of these)	2
Score equals A × 5	
Total maximum = 10	
III. Conjunctivae	
A. Redness (refers to palpebral conjunctivae only)	
Vessels definitely injected above normal	1
More diffuse, deeper crimson red, individual vessels not easily discernible	2
Diffuse beefy red	3
B. Chemosis	
Any swelling above normal (includes nictitating membrane)	1
Obvious swelling with partial eversion of the lids	2
Swelling with lids about half closed	3
Swelling with lids about half closed to completely closed	4
C. Discharge	
Any amount different from normal (does not include small amounts observed in inner canthus of normal animals)	1
Discharge with moistening of the lids and hairs just adjacent to the lids	2
Discharge with moistening of the lids and considerable area around the eye	3
Score equals (A + B + C) × 2	
Total maximum = 20	

From Reference 62.

[a] The maximum total score is the sum of all the scores obtained for the cornea, iris, and conjunctivae.

Table 18.9
Grades for ocular lesions

Lesion	Grades	Lesion	Grades
Cornea		Conjunctivae	
No ulceration or opacity	0	Redness (refers to palpebral and bulbar conjunctivae excluding cornea and iris)	
Scattered or diffuse areas of opacity (other than slight dulling of normal luster), details of iris clearly visible	1[a]	Vessels normal	0
		Some vessels definitely injected	1
Easily discernible translucent areas, details of iris slightly obscured	2	Diffuse, crimson red, individual vessels not easily discernible	2[a]
Nacreous areas, no details of iris visible, size of pupil barely discernible	3	Diffuse, beefy red	3
		Chemosis	
Complete corneal opacity, iris not discernible	4	No swelling	0
Iris		Any swelling above normal (includes nictitating membrane)	1
Normal	0	Obvious swelling with partial eversion of lids	2[a]
Markedly deepened folds, congestion, swelling, moderate circumcorneal Injection (any of these separately or combined); iris still reacting to light (sluggish reaction is positive)	1[a]	Swelling of lids about half closed	3
		Swelling of lids more than half closed	4
No reaction to light, hemorrhage, gross destruction (any or all of these)	2		

[a] Lowest grade considered positive.

proposed by Draize et al. (102), and subsequently a number of modifications were proposed (85,131,267). In the Draize system, the intensity and area of involvement on the cornea are graded separately on a scale of 0–4. The product of the two scores is multiplied by 5 to obtain a weighted corneal score. The congestion, swelling, circumcorneal injection, hemorrhage, and iridic failure of reactions to light are graded collectively on a scale of 0–2, and the score is multiplied by 5 to obtain a weighted iridic score. The redness, chemosis, and discharge of the conjunctivae are graded on scales of 0–3, 0–4, and 0–3, respectively. The sum of the conjunctival scores is multiplied by 5 to obtain a weighted conjunctival score. Other lesions also are recorded, such as pannus (corneal neovascularization), phylyctena, and rupture of the eyeball.

In the guidelines set forth by the EPA, CPSC, FHSA, OECD, EEC, and Japan's Ministry of Agriculture, Forestry and Food (MAFF) (85,109,124,136,337), only the degree (intensity of cornea damage, iritis, and redness and chemosis [swelling]) of the conjunctivitis is scored (Table 18.9). The area involved on the cornea as well as the discharge of the conjunctiva are not taken into consideration in scoring. Various aids are used at times to facilitate or increase the resolution power of these observations. These aids include fluorescein staining and ophthalmoscopic or slit lamp microscopic examinations. A scoring system has been developed for the slit lamp and fluorescein staining examination (267) (Table 18.10). Other scoring systems have been proposed for lacrimation, blepharitis, chemosis, injection of conjunctival blood vessels, iritis, kerectasis, and corneal neovascularization (9).

Interpretation of Results

There are essentially four categories of data, generated by the Draize test, to be considered when interpreting the results of ocular testing:

(a) kind of ocular effects,
(b) severity,
(c) reversibility, and
(d) rate of incidence.

Weighting the scores in the original Draize test has, to some extent, to take the first category into consideration, yet it biases toward the cornea, one of the most critical ocular tissues. Severity is measured according to a graded scoring system, and reversibility is expressed as the time needed for the affected ocular tissue to return to the normal state. Incidence is the number of animals that show some kind of ocular effect during the study. Interpretation of the data is a multiple and factorial undertaking. All four categories of data

Table 18.10
Scoring criteria for ocular effects observed in slit lamp microscopy

Location of observations	Grades	Location of observations	Grades
Corneal observations		*Iridal observations (cont'd)*	
Intensity		Aqueous flare (Tyndall effect)	
Only epithelial edema (with only slight stromal edema or without stromal edema)	1	Slight	1
		Moderate	2
		Marked	3
Corneal thickness 1.5 × normal	2	Iris hyperemia	
Corneal thickness 2 × normal	3	Slight	1
Cornea entirely opaque so that corneal thickness cannot be determined	4	Moderate	2
		Marked	3
Area involved		Pupillary reflex	
≤25% of total corneal surface	1	Sluggish	1
>25% but ≤50%	2	Absent	2
>50% but ≤75%	3	Maximal iridal score	11
>75%	4	*Conjunctival observations*	
Fluorescein staining		Hyperemia	
≤25% of total corneal surface	1	Slight	1
>25% but ≤50%	2	Moderate	2
>50% but ≤75%	3	Marked	3
>75%	4	Chemosis	
Neovascularization and pigment migration		Slight	1
≤25% of total corneal surface	1	Moderate	2
>25% but ≤50%	2	Marked	3
>50% but ≤75%	3	Fluorescein staining	
>75%	4	Slight	1
Perforation	4	Moderate	2
Maximal corneal score	20	Marked	3
Iridal observations		Ulceration	
Cells in aqueous chamber		Slight	1
A few	1	Moderate	2
A moderate number	2	Marked	3
Many	3	Maximal conjunctival score	12

are somewhat interrelated; the individual scores do not represent an absolute standard for the irritancy of a material (273).

In one study, interpretation of eye irritation was not considered to be the major factor contributing to interlaboratory variability (374). This finding is not surprising, if one assumes that everyone adheres to the same interpretation criteria. However, the question is what are the appropriate criteria for interpreting eye irritation results that would have an impact on placing eye irritants into different categories? The individual scores do not represent an absolute standard for the irritancy of a material (275).

Many classification systems for eye irritants have been proposed. Some have been published in the literature (171,173,202,267), and in various testing guidelines (109,136,337), and many others are used in individual laboratories. There is general agreement among investigators on how to classify test substances when no irritation is observed or when severe irritation or corrosion is seen, but there is little agreement on how to classify irritancy that falls between these two extremes. The manner in which data are evaluated directly affects the conclusions reached.

Because of the complexity of eye irritancy data and their interdependence, some investigators have chosen to simplify the interpretation to a pass-or-fail approach. For example, in the FHSA guideline (136), if four or more of the six test rabbits show ocular effects within 72 h after a conjunctival sac exposure (0.1 ml or 100 mg of the test material), the test material is considered to be a positive eye irritant. The ocular effects in consideration are "ulceration of the cornea (other than a fine stippling), corneal opacity (other than a slight deepening of the normal luster), inflammation of the iris (other than deepening of folds), an obvious swelling with partial eversion of the lids, or a diffuse crimson red with individual vessels but not easily discernible." If only one of the six tested animals shows ocular effects within 72 h, the test is considered negative. If two or three of the six tested animals show ocular effects, the test is repeated. The test substance is considered to be a positive irritant if three or more animals show ocular effects in the repeated test; otherwise, the test is repeated. Any positive ocular effect observed in the third test automatically classifies the test substance as an irritant. A similar approach has been adopted in the IRLG guideline (192), but an option is given that declares a test positive when two or three of six rabbits tested show a positive ocular effect and the test is not repeated. The pass-or-fail interpretation is too simplistic, however, and it does not separate eye irritants, especially those that fall between the two extreme irritancy categories (from nonirritating to severely irritating). Gradation of potential eye irritation is important to denote an anticipated hazard and to convey to consumers or workers that a specific degree of precaution should be exercised whenever a potential exposure to the substance exists.

Green et al. (171) used a different approach. Eye irritancy was classified into four easily recognizable categories based on the most severe responder in a group:

- *Nonirritation*: Exposure of the eye to the material under the specified conditions causes no significant ocular changes. No tissue staining with fluorescein was observed. Any changes that did occur cleared within 24 h and were no greater than those caused by normal saline under the same conditions.
- *Irritation*: Exposure of the eye to the material under the specified conditions causes minor, superficial, and transient changes of the cornea, iris, or conjunctiva as determined by external or slit lamp examination with fluorescein staining. The appearance at any grading interval of any of the following changes was sufficient to characterize a response as an irritation: opacity of the cornea (other than a slight dulling of the normal luster), hyperemia of the iris, or swelling of the conjunctiva. Any changes cleared within 7 days.
- *Harmfulness*: Exposure of the eye to the material under specified conditions causes significant injury to the eye, such as loss of the corneal epithelium, corneal opacity, iritis (other than a slight infection), conjunctivitis, pannus, or bullae. The effect healed or cleared within 21 days.
- *Corrosion*: Exposure of the eye to the material under specified conditions results in the types of injury described in the previous category and also results in significant tissue destruction (necrosis) or injuries that adversely affect the visual process. Injuries persisted for 21 days or more.

This classification system has taken into consideration the kinds of ocular effects, the reversibility, and, to a certain extent, the qualitative severity, but not the incidence. The committee that revised the NAS publication 1138 (267) put forward a system of classification similar to that of Green et al. (171). The categories are named differently: inconsequential or complete lack of irritation, moderate irritation, substantial irritation, and severe or corrosive irritation. The classification also is based on the most severe responder, and incidence is not considered. A provision for repeating the test is given as an option to increase the confidence level in making a judgment in some borderline cases. This eye irritancy classification system has been widely adopted. One shortcoming of the NAS system is that too wide a spectrum is created for moderate irritancy, which may lead to overutilization of the cautionary term, *moderate*. Many investigators have experienced problems in interpreting results from fluorescein staining of the cornea when the NAS gradation system is used. The confusion arises mainly from the occasional artifacts inherent in fluorescein staining. Experience and sound scientific judgment are needed to properly interpret the fluorescein staining results (see the discussion on ophthalmological techniques).

Griffith et al. (172) disagreed with using the most severe responder for classification of eye irritancy, claiming that there was no epidemiological evidence to suggest that the most severe rabbit responder would correlate with the worst possible case of human exposure. Instead, these investigators used the median time for recovery for classification according to the same temporal criteria as in the NAS system. The underlying logic is that the incidence of responders is being considered indirectly.

The classification systems of Green et al. (171), Griffith et al. (172), and NAS (267) apparently have not taken into account the severity of irritancy. Although there is a perception of a direct relationship between severity and reversibility, if one examines the data of Griffith et al. (172), indeed, it can be shown that a direct correlation of median time to recovery and the severity of irritancy does occur.

Kay and Calandra (202) proposed yet another rating system based on the Draize scores, taking into account the extent and persistence of irritation and the overall consistency of the data. Another system was proposed by Guillot et al. (173). Here, the greatest mean irritation score within an observation period is identified. On the basis of this score, the test substance is classified into six categories, ranging from nonirritating to maximum or extremely irritating. To maintain this initial rating, the data also must meet the arbitrary criteria for reversibility and frequency of occurrence, otherwise the rating is upgraded one category. The Kay and Calandra system has not been verified for correlation to human exposure experience, nor has it been compared with other classification systems. Guillot et al. (173) made an attempt to compare their rating with the OECD protocol. They claimed that one-third of the 56 materials tested could be classified into a lower category by the OECD protocol.

The most current modification of the OECD protocol (276) is an effort to minimize the number of animals used to produce data suitable for hazard classification. In this simplified scheme, a Draize eye test is conducted using one animal if severe effects are expected, or three animals if no severe eye irritation is anticipated. Scoring is based on ocular lesions that occur within 72 h of exposure and results are expressed in terms of the lesions and their reversibility (eye irritation) or irreversibility (eye corrosion). The EPA has recently revised its health effects test guidelines for acute eye irritation (126) to be more consistent with the OECD protocol. A revised EEC directive, based on the OECD approach, provides hazard classification corresponding to risk phrases (R 36—Irritating to eyes and R 41—Risk of serious damage to eyes). These risk phrases are assigned to the label of a chemical when two or more of the three animals exhibit scores within certain arbitrary numbers (110).

A summary of the current international classification systems and major features for eye irritancy testing is shown in Table 18.11. Despite such a range of classification schemes, there is little difference in the actual scoring system (basically adhering to the original Draize) (102).

SPECIAL OPHTHALMOLOGICAL TECHNIQUES

The Draize test is a generalized test concentrating on the effects of the material on the cornea, iris, and conjunctiva. Examination usually is performed under a hand light. Accurate observations are limited by the experience and training of the investigator. Subtle ocular changes may be missed. If these subtle changes are to be detected and ambiguous gross observations resolved, or if internal tissues (e.g., the lens and the retina) are to be examined, the investigator must rely on special techniques. Many such techniques have been developed over the years, most of which are more objective than the gross examination itself. A few comments on the fluorescein staining technique and several of the more objective methods are presented.

Fluorescein Staining for Corneal Damage

Fluorescein is a weak organic acid (Figure 18.5) and is only slightly soluble in water, but its sodium salt is moderately soluble in water. It is very efficient in absorbing ultraviolet light and emitting fluorescent light. The maximum absorption is 490 nm (excitation) in the violet region, and its maximum emission is 520 nm in the green region of the spectrum. Its un-ionized form is less fluorescent than its ionized form. At pH 7.4, fluorescein does not seem to bind to tissue and is nontoxic in animals, making it an ideal marker for an ocular fluid dynamics study. Because fluorescein is a deeply colored and highly fluorescent chemical, it can be detected at very low concentrations in biological tissues or fluid; however, its detection sensitivity often is limited by the background fluorescence of biological tissues.

Because sodium fluorescein is a polar molecule, it does not readily traverse lipophilic membranes but easily diffuses into aqueous medium. For example, if ulceration occurs on the cornea, the lipophilic membrane barrier is broken down and the fluorescein diffuses freely through the ulcerated area of the cornea and either is dissolved or suspended in the aqueous medium of the stroma. More detailed information on the chemical and biological properties of fluorescein is provided in two excellent reviews (235,249).

Since its first use in studying the origin of aqueous humor secretion a century ago (111), fluorescein has become an important aid in ophthalmology. It has been used as a marker in detecting obstructions in the nasolacrimal drainage systems, for studying changes in the flow dynamics of different ocular fluids, for demonstrating leakage of retinal vessels in angiography, for estimating permeability of the cornea and lens, and for identifying ulcerations on the cornea (235). Among these, its use in detecting subtle changes on the corneal epithelium (80,183) has been a routine procedure in animal eye irritation studies.

The corneal epithelium is a lipophilic barrier to sodium fluorescein, but such a barrier is broken when there is an ulceration or change in membrane structure. Some amount of fluorescein applied on the cornea will penetrate into the intercellular spaces of the stroma, which constitute a water-soluble layer of the stroma. When light is cast on the cornea, fluorescence is detected on the damaged area of the epithelium. Once the fluorescein enters the stroma, it eventually will pass through Descemet's membrane and the endothelium into the aqueous humor.

Fluorescein staining usually is accomplished by solution or impregnated paper strips. Fluorescein is commercially available in 2, 1, or 0.25% sodium salt solutions. Preservatives to minimize bacterial contamination are common in these commercially available sol-

Table 18.11
Major feature of eye irritation tests and international classification schemes

Methodology	FHSA (CPSC, FDA, OSHA)	OECD	EPA (Modified OECD)	Canada (Modified OECD)	EU (EEC)
Initial considerations					
Screen for pH (<2 or >11.5)	NS	Yes	Same as OECD	Same as OECD	Same as OECD
Results from skin irritation	NS	Yes	Same as OECD	Same as OECD	Same as OECD
Results from validated alternatives	NS	Yes	Same as OECD	Same as OECD	Same as OECD
Number of animals:					
Screen for severe effects	NS	1	Same as OECD	Same as OECD	Same as OECD
Main Test	≥ 6	≥ 3	Same as OECD	Same as OECD	3
Volume administered	0.1 ml or 100 mg	0.1 ml or ≤ 100 mg	Same as OECD	Same as OECD	Same as OECD
Scoring times	1,2,3 d	1 h, 1,2,3 d (may be extended to assess reversibility)	1 h, 1,2,3 d (may be extended to assess reversibility ≤ 21 d)	1 h, 1,2,3 d (may be extended to assess reversibility)	1 h; 1,2,3 d
Minimal positive response:					
Corneal opacity	1	NS[a]	1	2.0^b	≥ 2.0, $<3.0^c$
Iritis	1	NS[a]	1	1.0^b	≥ 1.0, $<1.5^c$
Conjuctival					
redness	2	NS[a]	2	2.5^b	2.5^c
chemosis	2	NS[a]	2	2.5^b	2.0^c
Positive test	≥ 4 positive of 6 animals	NS	NS[a]		≥ 2 positive of 3 animals
Number of classes/label categories:					
Irritant	1 (reversible inflammatory effect)	Same as FHSA	Same as FHSA	1 (positive response requires labeling as a poisonous and infectious material)	1(R 36: irritating to eyes) based on minimum positive response
Corrosive	1 (visible destruction or irreversible alterations)	Same as FHSA	Same as FHSA	NS	NS
Severe irritant	NS	NS	NS		1 (R 41: risk of serious damage to eyes) based on corneal opacity $\geq 3.0^c$ and/or iritis $\geq 1.5c$

NS, not specified.
[a] Individual scores do not represent an absolute standard for the irritant properties of a material.
[b] Mean of at least three animals.
[c] Mean of three scoring intervals and scores representing two or more animals.

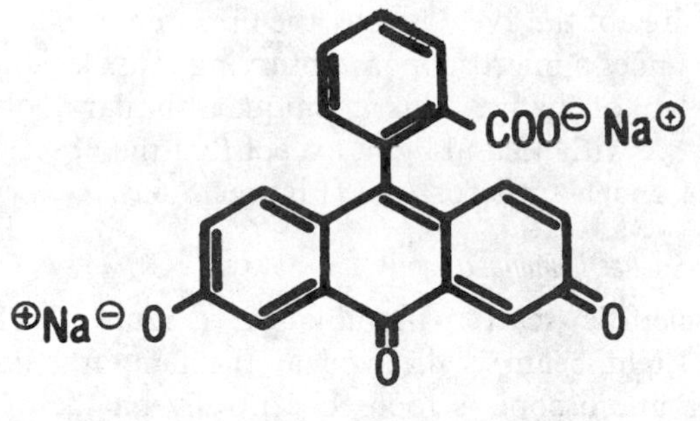

FIG. 18.5. Structure of fluorescein.

utions (71). A drop of the solution is instilled onto the eye and excessive fluorescein is flushed immediately with a sufficient amount of water. The eye then can be examined under a cobalt-filtered UV light for epithelial defects.

Fluorescein also is available in impregnated paper strips (210). These strips are free of contamination and easy to use. Moistened with collyria, a strip is touched lightly to the dorsal bulbar conjunctiva. The small amount of fluorescein should distribute uniformly on the cornea by either diffusion or blinking. Flushing is not usually necessary with the strips if applied properly. Nonetheless, if the strip touches the cornea, it becomes necessary for the cornea to be flushed with water before examination. Better results are obtained with the fluorescein-impregnated strip when examination is by slit lamp microscopy.

Fluorescein staining has two valuable applications in a routine eye irritation test. It can be used for screening eyes prior to the study to ensure that healthy eyes are being used. The other application is for the determination of total recovery from grossly observed damage on the cornea. Slight epithelial effects still can be detected by fluorescein even though they are not visible during gross observation. Even though most of these subtle effects on the cornea will disappear in a relatively short period of time, prolonged effects detected by fluorescein staining, but not by gross examination, should raise a concern over the healing process. However, when no gross lesions are detected at any time during a study (except for a few incidences of minor fluorescein staining on the cornea) one should not be overly concerned. If there are any effects on the cornea, they must be extremely minimal ones on the superficial epithelium for eye irritation to rate as nonirritating or inconsequential. If the staining is not an artifact, the minimal ocular effects detected under such circumstances should be readily reversible.

Although fluorescein staining can detect very subtle corneal epithelial changes, one can easily be misled by some very noticeable background staining. In addition, artifacts are quite common. For example, the apparent staining of the cornea can result from incomplete flushing of excessive fluorescein with water or even from reflected light. A strong jet of water during irrigation can cause mild damage to the cornea. Damage also can occur if the eye is not handled properly during gross examination. These changes are not related to the test compound but may be detected with fluorescein staining. Sometimes one may see haziness on the cornea after fluorescein staining even though a clear cornea is seen prior to fluorescein staining. Whether the hazy appearance of the cornea is a reflection of mild change or artifact depends on several factors. If the hazy appearance is also visible under a cobalt filter and is preceded by grossly visible lesions, it generally is considered to be a residual effect of mild severity that will disappear within a short time. However, if the hazy appearance is seen intermittently or is not preceded by ocular effects, it is likely an artifact. Proper training and experience are necessary to recognize artifacts and to obtain reliable, reproducible, and consistent results from fluorescein staining. In general, it is not necessary to stain lesions that are obvious and grossly evident. It is when lesions would otherwise go undetected by gross examination that fluorescein staining is of value.

Slit Lamp Microscopy

The slit lamp biomicroscope is an important instrument for studying ocular tissues, especially the cornea. As its name suggests, a slit lamp consists of a microscope that views optical sections of different layers of the cornea made by an intense light beam acting as a surgical knife or microtome, cutting through different layers of the eye. Many lesions that would remain undetected by gross examination can be observed with the slit lamp biomicroscope. Using recent models of slit lamp microscopes, one can observe not only the different layers of the cornea but, also, other transparent parts of the eye such as the aqueous humor, lens, and vitreous body.

The slit lamp biomicroscope consists of an illuminating light source and a microscope. Both components are movable and adjustable, allowing the eye to be illuminated and observed from different angles and with different width and height adjustments of the slit light beam. An area of the cornea can simultaneously be illuminated and magnified by aligning the incidence of the light beam and the focus of the microscope. The light beam also can be directed at the area from different angles, providing several views of the same area.

Two types of slit images are used for illumination: parallelepiped and optical section (239). For the parallelepiped slit image, a rectangular light beam (approximately 1–2 mm wide and 5–10 mm high) is projected onto the cornea. The shape of the illuminated area is similar to a parallelepiped prism where the outer

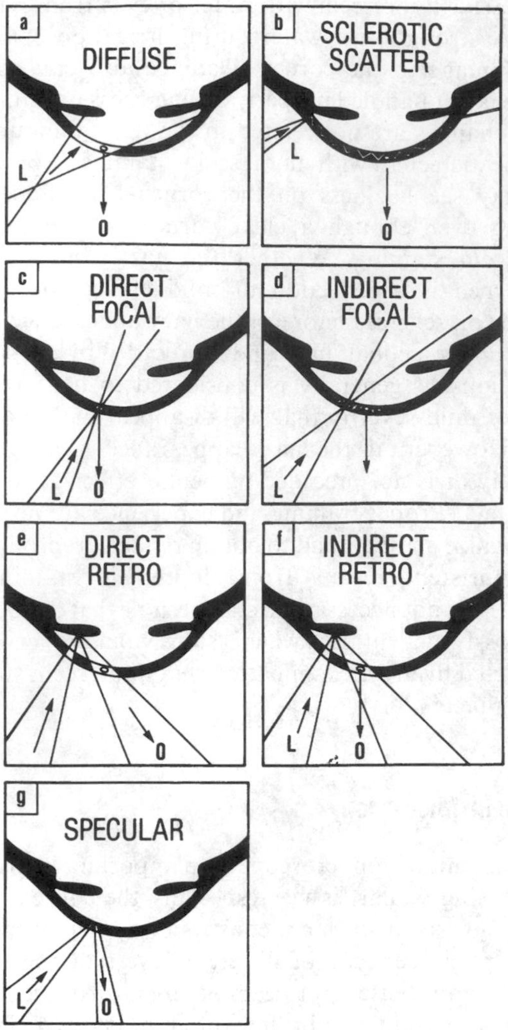

FIG. 18.6. Seven basic methods of illumination in slit lamp microscopy: (a) diffuse; (b) sclerotic scatter; (c) direct focal; (d) indirect focal; (e) direct retroillumination; (f) indirect retroillumination; (g) specular reflection. O = observer; L = illuminator light. Modified from Reference 239, with permission.

and inner surfaces are bent because of the shape of the cornea. For the optical section slit image, the width (20 μm) of the light beam is narrowed to its minimum and is projected onto the cornea, providing a sagittal view that is similar to a thin histological section.

There are several basic illumination techniques (Figure 18.6): diffuse illumination, sclerotic scatter illumination, direct and indirect focal illumination, direct and indirect retroillumination, and specular reflection (247,346).

Diffuse Illumination

In diffuse illumination, a slightly out-of-focus wide beam is used to scan and localize any gross lesions of a large area of the eye. Usually the first step in examining the eye under a microscope is observing gross lesions and their extent of change. This technique is similar to observing the eye with a hand light, except that the observation is made under a microscope (Figure 18.6a).

Sclerotic Scatter Illumination

In sclerotic scatter illumination (Figure 18.6b), a narrow light beam is directed at the temporal limbus, and the microscope is focused centrally on the area of the cornea to be examined. The light reflected from the sclera will transmit within the cornea by total reflection. Under normal conditions nothing will be seen, but if even minor changes are present the reflected light will be obstructed and the damaged area (e.g., mild corneal edema) will be illuminated. This technique is useful for detecting minimal changes in the cornea.

Direct Focal Illumination

In direct focal illumination, the light beam and the microscope are focused sharply at the same point of interest in the same plane (Figure 18.6c). If a rectangular slit image is used for illumination and focused on the cornea, three general areas are seen when the parallelepiped is formed on the cornea: the epithelium (the anterior bright line), the stroma (the central clear marble-like area), and the endothelium (the posterior thin, bright line). If an optical section slit image is used for illumination, the corneal layers seen from anterior to posterior are a thin, bridge layer, a thin dark layer, a granular layer, and another thin bright layer. These correspond to the tear film, the epithelium, the stroma, and the endothelium, respectively. Altering the angle of incidence of the light beam decreases or increases the reflection. This allows for the detection of depth of the lesion. Opacities on the different layers can be detected easily as obstructions of the incident light beam.

Indirect Focal Illumination

Indirect focal illumination (Figure 18.6d) is accomplished by a narrow beam of light directed at an opaque area of the cornea. For example, changes in blood vessels at the cornea adjacent to the opaque area are illuminated and can be detected by focusing the microscope at these areas.

Direct and Indirect Retroillumination

In direct (Figure 18.6e) and indirect (Figure 18.6f) retroillumination, the light beam is directed at tissues behind the cornea, e.g., the iris or the fundus. The reflected light illuminates the area of interest of the corneal tissue and can be focused under the microscope. The microscope can be located directly on the path of the reflected light (direct retroillumination), thus permitting subtle changes to be observed against a contrasting background. Any optical obstruction by lesions such as scars, pigment, or vessels located along the reflection light path will appear as darker areas on a brighter background. Lesions such as corneal edema and precipitates that can scatter the reflection light will show up as a brighter area against a darker background. When the microscope is located off the reflection light path (indirect retroillumination), the corneal structure is observed against a dark background such as the pupil or iris. Indirect retroillumination is better for observing opaque structures, whereas direct illumination often is used to detect corneal edema and precipitates.

Specular Reflection Illumination

Specular reflection (Fig. 18.6g) is most useful in studying the endothelium and precorneal tear film. This technique makes use of the difference in refractive properties between the corneal surface and the adjacent medium of the posterior and anterior surfaces of the cornea. The microscope is focused on the cornea adjacent to the path of the incident slit light beam. By alternating the angle of incidence, a point can be reached such that a total reflection is obtained on the junction between the aqueous medium and the most posterior corneal surface, thus illuminating endothelial cell patterns and the Descemet's membrane. Similar techniques can be performed on the anterior corneal surface to visualize precorneal tear film.

Scoring System for Slit Lamp Examinations

By using slit lamp microscopic techniques, many subtle changes can be observed that would not otherwise be evident from the Draize test. A different scoring system must be developed to reflect such subtle changes. Baldwin et al. (8) proposed a scoring system for the cornea, anterior chamber, iris, and lens. Subsequently, NAS (267) developed a scoring system for slit lamp examinations that is similar to the Draize system in placing emphasis on the cornea, iris, and conjunctiva. Basically, in the NAS system, the intensity and the area involved are the two main criteria for scoring. Using this scoring system, the investigator must have a good understanding of the physiology of the normal eye. Like the Draize score, the NAS system is based on corneal effects; total maximal corneal score is 20 as compared with 11 and 15 for iridic and conjunctival scores, respectively. A detailed scoring scale and criteria are listed in Table 18.10.

Corneal Pachymetry

Because corneal transparency is so important to vision (over 70% of the Draize score is derived from assessment of damage to the cornea) objective procedures to quantify corneal effects are an important element in eliminating intra- and inter-laboratory variability in assessing the effects of ocular exposure to exogenous agents. Corneal transparency, thickness, and hydration are related in a linear fashion (179). Therefore, changes in corneal thickness can be used as an indicator of irritant affects, which may impair normal corneal hydration and transparency. When corneal thickness is measured appropriately, it can be used to objectively quantify swelling of the corneal stroma, which is a typical early irritant response. The measurement of corneal thickness is called pachymetry, which comes from the Greek words *pachys* (thick) and *metry* (the process of measuring).

One method for measuring corneal thickness uses an optical pachometer attached to a slit lamp microscope. Optical pachometers provide essentially indirect measurements of apparent corneal thickness based on displacement of light beams bouncing off the endothelial and epithelial surfaces of the cornea. The principles of this method have been described previously (73).

Various investigators (66,81,207,251), using a variety of substances from different chemical classes, have reported that corneal thickness is significantly correlated with the Draize corneal score. Moreover, Kennah et al. (207) clearly demonstrated a substantial reduction in the coefficient of variation when comparing corneal swelling to Draize scores for various surfactants, alcohols, ketones, acetates, and aromatic chemicals.

Recent advances in human ophthalmological procedures to correct visual acuity (i.e., radial keratotomy, eximer-laser photorefractive keratectomy) have resulted in the development of improved devices to measure corneal thickness which guide the practitioner both before and after the procedure, and provide a means to measure the effectiveness of the treatment. The ultrasonic pachymeter is such a device (35,264,352,363) and it may have useful application to in vivo ocular irritation testing.

The ultrasonic pachymeter is an instrument with a hand-held probe that emits an ultrasonic signal of fixed velocity. The probe is placed directly on the anterior surface of the cornea and after signal emission, a sensor directly measures the time difference between echoes of signal pulses reflected from the front and back surfaces of the cornea. This time differential is directly proportional to the thickness of the cornea via a function that is computed as the product of the time delay between the two echoes (in seconds) and the velocity of sound in the corneal tissue (in meters/second). The optical pachometer indirectly equates displacement of incident light to corneal thickness, and the ultrasonic pachymeter provides a direct measurement.

Comparative evaluations of the sources of variability in human corneal thickness measurements using optical and ultrasonic (162,182,224,289,315) or between various ultrasonic devices (377) have been reported and discussed.

Salz et al. (315) found that sources of variation include intra- and inter-session variation, inter-observer variation, left/right eye variation, and variations due to alternate settings of ultrasonic sound frequency. They reported that the optical pachymeter had significant inter-session variation, significant inter-observer variation, and significant differences in left and right eye thickness measurements, while the ultrasonic pachymeter demonstrated high reproducibility, no inter-observer variation, and no left/right eye variation.

The ultrasonic pachymeter has many desirable features such as a relatively low cost, portability, ease of operation, and use requiring less operator skill and training than the optical pachometer. When used in humans, a topical anesthetic is employed, because the tip of the measuring probe must be in contact with the corneal surface before a measurement can be taken. However, it has been reported that because of a lower corneal sensitivity in rabbits (75,243) an anesthetic is not necessary before taking corneal thickness measurements.

Because the velocity of sound can vary in different tissue, accurate readings for absolute corneal thickness require that the ultrasonic sound frequency of the instrument be matched to the tissue of interest. The velocity of sound in human corneal tissue has been variously reported as 1502 m/s (265), 1586 m/s (307), and 1610 m/s (272). Salz et al. (315), in their human cornea comparison of optical to ultrasonic pachymetry, used an approximate velocity of 1590 m/s and found good agreement between the two measurement methods. The velocity of sound in cat (224), rabbit (74), and bovine (283) corneal tissue was found to be 1590 m/s, 1580 m/s, and 1550 m/s, respectively. Empirical methods to determine the velocity of sound in corneal tissue have been described (224,283).

The utility of ultrasonic pachymetry in measuring corneal thickness changes in rabbits (230,263) and rats (230), after treatment with ocular irritants, has been reported. The findings, albeit limited to a small number of chemicals, support the continued pursuit of this method as a relatively inexpensive, objective way to measure corneal irritant effects.

Confocal Microscopy

The confocal microscope is another instrument that can be used to measure corneal thickness, as well as provide high-resolution microscopic images to study the cellular structure within corneal tissue. The first confocal microscope was described by Minsky (244,245) in a 1957 patent application. This device had a pinhole and a lens (objective and condenser) located on either side of the specimen to be viewed. The intent of the design was to eliminate any scattered light that might pass through the specimen, thus concentrating all light at a point source that was the focal point. The term confocal originated because the objective lens and the condenser lens were focused on the same specimen point.

The image seen in a conventional light microscope includes the in-focus image in the x,y (horizontal) plane and the out-of-focus image above and below in the z (vertical) plane, the confocal microscope only focuses in the x,y plane. Indeed, de-focusing a confocal microscope makes the image totally disappear rather than appear blurred. Reducing the out of focus signal above and below the focal plane results in enhanced resolution. In contrast to the light microscope, which is focused by moving the objective, moving the specimen focuses the confocal microscope. This feature provides an optical sectioning capability that allows thick tissue sections such as the cornea to be viewed in vivo or in vitro in both the horizontal and vertical planes. Because of the point source light illumination, however, scanning the specimen is necessary to produce a full field of view with the confocal microscope. Scanned images can be viewed through a video monitor on a real-time basis, imported into a video cassette recorder, or stored as a digital image (291) for later viewing and analysis. For a complete review of the principles and applications of the scanning confocal microscope see Petroll et al. (292).

By successively scanning the cornea and capturing a series of optical sections it is possible to reconstruct a three-dimensional image of the tissue. Methods for three-dimensional imaging of rabbit cornea in vitro (196,233,293) and in vivo (129,196,250,290), have been described. These methods have been used to characterize the changes in area and depth of corneal injury of surfactant-induced eye irritation in the rabbit (234) and to examine the relationship between area and depth of injury to corneal cell death (195).

Mauer et al. (234) used in vivo scanning confocal microscopy to qualitatively and quantitatively characterize the initial changes occurring after treatment with surfactants known to produce slight, mild, moderate, and severe corneal irritation. Materials were applied directly to the corneas of 6 rabbits per group at a dose of 10 μl with macroscopic (Draize) and microscopic evaluations beginning at 3 h after treatment and continuing periodically through day 35. Microscopic three-dimensional images were obtained from the surface epithelium to the endothelium and measurements made for surface epithelial cell size, epithelial layer thickness, total corneal thickness, and depth of keratocyte necrosis. The average Draize scores at 3 h for the slight, mild, moderate, and severe irritants were 6.0, 39.3, 48.5, and 68.7, respectively. Confocal microscopic images at 3 h showed that corneal injury with the slight irritant was limited to the epithelium (cell size and thickness 59 and 82% of control). The mild irritant had removed the surface epithelium, increased the corneal thickness to 158% of control, and produced keratocyte necrosis to a depth of 4.3 μm. With the moderate irritant the epithelium was markedly attenuated, the corneal thickness was 156% of controls, and keratocyte necrosis extended to a depth of 19 μm. For the severe irritant, the epithelium was significantly thinned, the corneal thickness was 166% of controls and keratocyte necrosis extended to a depth of 391 μm.

The use of confocal microscopy in studies designed to provide semi-quantitative information on the nature and depth of injury to the cornea after chemical treatment has the potential to serve as an important link to the development of physiologically relevant and mechanistically based in vitro alternatives to the Draize eye test (234).

LOCAL ANESTHETICS

For humane and scientific reasons, guidelines such as those established by the IRLG and the OECD provide options for using local anesthetics in eye irritation studies. Tetracaine, lidocaine, butacaine, proparacaine, and cocaine have all been examined for their usefulness in eye irritation studies, with the results being mixed and inconclusive. Most of these anesthetics can alleviate pain, but they also can inhibit or reduce the somatosensory area of the eye and the blinking reflex. Tear flow is reduced, causing the test substance to be trapped and remain undiluted on the cornea instead of being blinked from the eye or diluted and flushed away by the tear flow. Especially among higher primates, the blinking and tearing reflexes are important defense mechanisms against accidental exposure to any substance (181). Some local anesthetics can cause delay in corneal epithelial regeneration and loss of surface cells from the cornea (174). Some such as procaine, lignocaine, piperocaine, amylocaine, amethocaine, and cinchocaine are cytotoxic to cultured human cells, including conjunctival cells (90). However, at least one study has shown that a 0.5% tetracaine solution apparently had no effect on corneal healing (294). Further research is needed to reveal the interaction of local anesthetics and chemically induced ocular effects. Local anesthesia is sometimes useful to induce akinesia of the eyelid during eye examination.

Local anesthetics are desirable to alleviate pain, but one must be aware of the potential physical, chemical, physiological, and toxicological incompatibilities before considering their use.

HISTOLOGICAL APPROACHES

Histological examination of the eyes has been included routinely in subchronic and chronic toxicity studies, but because it is time-consuming and costly, it is performed only occasionally in eye irritation studies. Results may be no more informative than those from observations and measurements by other techniques. However, histological examination of ocular tissue can reveal the type of damage, tissues involved, and certain subtle changes in ocular tissue.

Both electron and light microscopic examinations have been used to evaluate local ocular injury (171, 197,198,308,350,354,367, see Henkes and Canta [1973] (180) for review). Although such methods sometimes can reveal morphological changes of different parts of the cornea, conjunctiva, lens, and retina, as well as visual nerve degeneration, shortcomings are not uncommon. Among the problems are sectioning the precise lesion, problems in slide preparation, and subjective interpretation of observations. Another problem is that histological examination generally is made on dehydrated tissue (65), which makes some lesions, such as corneal edema, difficult to detect. However, histological examination of ocular tissues in local eye irritation studies has been considered an objective method because of its high sensitivity in detecting very mild ocular effects (181).

ALTERNATIVE METHODS FOR THE ASSESSMENT OF EYE IRRITATION

Humane and scientific concerns regarding the use of animals in toxicology have prompted development of many in vitro methods as potential alternatives for animal tests. One area that has seen considerable activity is the development of new methods for use as alternatives in the assessment of eye irritation. The use of first-generation screening tests (26,30,42,46,106–108,127, 184,205,206,248,258,261,300,317,331,344,364) has laid the foundation for continuing research with more sophisticated methods, many of which use human ocular cells as their basis (31,32,130,149,150,156,191,199,209, 219,222,268,295,310,312,336,348,356,357,368,381). Although the majority of procedures that use human cells are employed in studies of ocular disease, some are finding applications in eye irritation hazard assessment. For a review of this research, see Kruszewski (214).

Organizations such as the Johns Hopkins Center for Alternatives to Animal Testing, the European Center for the Validation of Alternative Methods (ECVAM), the Fund for Replacement of Animals in Medical Research in England (FRAME), and the U.S. Interagency Coordinating Committee on the Validation of Alternative Methods (ICCVAM) have been active in promoting development of such alternative methods for animal testing.

Research on alternatives for assessing ocular irritancy has focused on development and validation of a number of in vitro tests. These methods can be grouped into functional categories according to test endpoint (146), which includes morphology, cell toxicity, cell and tissue physiology, inflammation/immunity, recovery/repair, and others (e.g., protein denaturation, computer-based structure-activity relationships, *Tetrahymena thermophila* motility, etc.). Most of these endpoints are indicators of cellular membrane integrity and/or cytotoxicity. Detailed reviews of these methods are beyond the scope of this chapter but are available (60,306).

For the following discussion, the above classes of methods are grouped into four broad categories: ex vivo methods, cell-based assays, inflammation/immunity, and other methods.

Ex Vivo Methods

Several methods have been investigated which are based on morphological alterations to either whole eye tissue or isolated corneas. The enucleated perfused rabbit eye, enucleated chicken eye test, or isolated bovine or porcine cornea methods (17,67,117,186–190,237,259, 260,296,382), are based on visible alterations of tissues as the endpoints. The effect of a chemical on the tissue is measured by corneal opacity, corneal thickness, or corneal fluorescein retention. These methods are complex, lack good correlation with in vivo results, and still require killing animals; however, eye tissue can be obtained from slaughterhouses, from animals processed for food (299).

The bovine corneal opacity and permeability (BCOP) test, developed by Gautheron et al. (154), is a more recent modification of the original isolated bovine procedure (260). In the bovine corneal opacity method, freshly excised bovine eyes obtained from a slaughterhouse are used. The test material is placed on the cornea for 30 sec, after which corneal lesions are scored. In the BCOP test two endpoints are determined:

(1) opacity, which is measured by change in light transmission passing through the cornea; and
(2) permeability to fluorescein dye, a measure of barrier function. This method is an improvement over the earlier procedures and has been used with a variety of chemicals and consumer product formulations to produce results that compare favorably when extrapolated to corneal effects in the rabbit eye test (69,83,155,159,302,335,358,362). An expert working group has reported on the state of the art of the BCOP test (335).

Cell-Based Assays

Cytotoxicity Methods

These methods are based on cytotoxicity. Frazier et al. (146) grouped these methods under three categories according to the indicator of cytotoxicity. These are adhesion/cell proliferation (cellular growth), membrane integrity, and cell metabolism. Chemically induced cytotoxicity will interfere with cell growth and proliferation, which can be quantified by counting the number of viable cells, by assessing the adhesion or colony-forming ability of the cells, or by measuring the amount of macromolecules such as DNA, RNA, or protein. The endpoints investigated under the category of adhesion/cell proliferation include growth inhibition (BHK cells), colony-formation efficiency (BHK cells and SIRC cells), cell detachment (BHK cells), total protein (Balb/c 3T3 cells, BCL DI cells) (20,270, 305,330,342,370), or binding of certain dyes (the FRAME Kenacid Blue Test in 3T3-L1 cells) (79,211), and a plant cell-derived pollen tube test (201). The cell lines generally are well characterized; some are corneal cell lines. Several of these procedures are discussed below.

Adhesion and proliferation. The *colony-formation efficacy test* involves establishing good viability and growth of cells, exposing BHK or SIRC cells to a test substance for a predetermined period of time (e.g., 1 h), washing the exposed cells, and reincubating for the time needed for cellular proliferation. After reincubation, the effect of the test substance on the ability of the cells to adhere and/or form colonies is determined by fixing and staining the cells. The number of functionally viable cells (i.e., with the ability to adhere and proliferate) in the chemically exposed group is compared with an unexposed control group. Ranking of ocular irritancy often is based on the IC_{50}, the concentration of chemical at which functionally viable cells are only 50% of the unexposed control group. The correlation in ranking of irritancy of various surfactant and cosmetic formulations has been reported between this test and the in vivo rabbit eye irritancy test (39,40,158,161, 271,325).

The FRAME *Kenacid Blue* (*KB*) *Test* is based on the principle of a direct correlation between cell number, total protein, and the binding of certain dyes such as Kenacid Blue (Coomassie brilliant blue) (18,79,211,330). Proliferating 3T3-L1 cells are exposed to a low concentration of chemical for 72 h (at least two cell cycles). Then exposed and unexposed cells are removed from the growth medium and dried in the air for 72 h, and the amount of protein in the cells is measured by the KB dye-binding assay. The method involves treating cells with a fixative (glacial acetic acid/ethanol/distilled water 1 : 50 : 49), then staining with freshly prepared Kenacid Blue R solution, washing the cells, and releasing the dye into a desorbing solution (approximately 10% potassium acetate in water/ethanol solution). The absorbency of the dye is measured at 570 nm against a cell-free desorbing solution. Absorbency correlates linearly with the amount of protein and the number of cells. This method has been used in projects sponsored by Cosmetic Toiletries and Fragrance Association (CTFA) and the Commission of European Communities (CEC). Correlation between in vitro ranking and in vivo Draize test ranking of salts, chlorides, and certain cosmetic formulations has been reported (9,18,158,161).

The *pollen tube test* employs plant cells (201). It is essentially a cell proliferation assay. The endpoint is the amount of tube wall biomass (*Nicotiana sylvestris*) produced (through germination and growth) in vitro. After exposure to the test substance, the amount of biomass is determined by measuring optical density at 500 nm. Results are expressed as the concentration of test substance, which causes a 50% growth inhibition. Correlations between in vitro ranking and the in vivo Draize test ranking for certain cosmetic formulations and surfactant chemicals have been reported (158,159, 161,213).

Membrane integrity. Damaged membranes can cause a host of toxic responses including cell lysis and cell death, leakage of enzymes such as LDH, loss of certain cofactors such as Ca^{2+}, K^{+}, and NADPH, and alterations in substances being actively or passively transported across the membrane. Endpoints include dual-dye/fluorescent dye staining (LS cells, thymocytes), chromium isotope (^{51}Cr) release (RCE, SIRC, P815, YAC-1 cells), cell viability (L929 cells), hemolysis (bovine red blood cells), and transepithelial barrier integrity (MDCK or HCE-T cells) (100,199,206,261,317,324,325,368). Alteration in the ability of substances being actively or passively transported across the membrane barrier (release or uptake) indicates membrane toxicity.

The *chromium isotope* (^{51}Cr) *release assay* has been used in several studies (39,40,161,324,325). In the presence of excess Cr in the growth medium, normal cells take up Cr, which binds to intracellular macromolecules. After changing to isotope-free growth medium, Cr-labeled macromolecules are transported actively across the membrane of normal cells into the extracellular medium at a slow rate. In cells exposed to cytotoxic agents (and if membrane integrity is altered), Cr-labeled macromolecules will diffuse passively across the membrane into the extracellular medium at a much higher rate. The increased release rate (difference between release rate of normal and chemically treated cells) of Cr-labeled macromolecules indicates membrane toxicity. Correlations have been reported between in vitro ranking and in vivo Draize test ranking for several surfactant (39,40,146) and certain cosmetic formulations (161).

The *Neutral Red Release* (*NRR*) *Test* also measures the cellular membrane integrity (303). It is based on the principle that living cells accumulate the dye (2-amino-3-methyl-7-dimethyl aminophenazonium chloride) in lysosomes by an active metabolic process. If the membranes are damaged, the accumulated intracellular neutral red dye will be released into the extracellular medium. In this method, confluent 3T3-L1 cells are preloaded with neutral red dye, washed, replaced with fresh growth medium, and exposed to a high dose of the toxic substance for 1 min. The test substance is removed; the exposed and unexposed cells are washed and fixed with PBS, destained, and fixed with a glacial acetic acid/ethanol/distilled water (1 : 50 : 49) solution. The absorbance of the destained solution is measured at 540 nm against a cell-free destain reference solution. Results are expressed as NRR_{20}, NRR_{50}, or NRR_{80} (i.e., concentration of test substance, that causes 20%, 50%, or, 80% of the preloaded dye to be released). Correlations between in vitro ranking of certain classes of chemicals and certain cosmetic formulations and the in vivo Draize test ranking have been reported (158,159,161,303).

A neutral red release method to test solid materials has been reported (365). The *agarose diffusion assay* uses a confluent monolayer of culture cells preloaded with the neutral red dye. The cells are overlaid with agarose. Test material placed on the agarose can diffuse through the agarose to the cells. Any damage caused by the test material to the cellular membrane will release the dye into the agarose. Scoring is based on the presence of a dye zone. (The size of the zone may or may not correlate with the degree of cytotoxicity). Correlations between in vitro ranking of certain cosmetic formulations or ingredients and the in vivo Draize test ranking have been reported (158,159,161,365).

Membrane tight junctions between epithelial cells form a barrier for water movement across the corneal epithelium. When this barrier is damaged, water moves into the cornea, resulting in edema. The FRAME *fluorescein leakage* (*FL*) *test* is based on the principle that a damaged epithelial cell barrier will be more permeable to the nontoxic dye fluorescein than an undamaged barrier (327,351). Canine kidney cells (MDCK cells, an epithelial cell line) are grown to confluence in tissue culture inserts. The confluent cell layer is washed, exposed to 100 μl of test substance for 1 min, and then the test substance is removed by washing with distilled water. The washed cells are placed in clean wells containing PBS medium. Fluorescein (500 μl) in PBS (0.02%) is added to each cell insert. Cells are incubated for 1 h, and the leakage of fluorescein from the cells into the well is measured by absorbence at 492 nm. Results are expressed as FL_{20} and FL_{50} (concentration of test substance, which causes 20% and 50% of maximum leakage from inserts containing no cells) (327). A modification of this method expresses results as FL10 and FL20 (concentration of test substance which causes 10% and 20% of maximum leakage) and measures recovery at 4, 24, 48, and 72 h after treatment (84). Comparison of in vitro response to the in vivo irritancy classification of various chemicals has been reported (84,159,327).

The *transepithelial permeability* (*TEP*) *and the transepithelial resistance* (*TER*) *assays* are barrier function tests based in the human corneal epithelial cell line, 10.014 pRSV-T (HCE-T cells) (199,368,369). This cell line has been used to develop a three-dimensional in vitro model of the human corneal epithelium (HCE-T model). HCE-T cells form a stratified culture when grown in serum-free medium on a collagen membrane at the air–liquid interface. Because it is a multilayer model, barrier function is a well-developed property in the HCE-T model which can be quantitatively measured by its retention of fluorescein (TEP assay) and the maintenance of high electrical resistance (TER assay). For these procedures, HCE-T cells are grown in 24 well plates to confluence (3–4 days) in low-calcium (0.15 mM $CaCl_2$) keratinocyte growth medium (KGM), then airlifted in high-calcium (1.15 mM $CaCl_2$) KGM until Day 7, when they are treated. Treatment consists of 100 μl of test substance in KGM for 5 min and then the test substance is removed by washing three times with D-PBS. The washed cells are placed in clean 24-well plates containing high-calcium KGM.

For the *TEP assay*, fluorescein (200 μl) in high-calcium KGM (0.02%) is added to each well. Cells are incubated for 30 min, and the leakage of fluorescein into the well is measured by absorbance at 490 nm. Results are expressed as FR_{85} (concentration of test substance, which causes fluorescein retention to decrease to 85% of control) (215).

For the TER assay, resistance measurements are taken using an epithelial voltohmeter, EVOM (World Precision Instruments) after treatment of the cells as per the TEP assay. The instrument probe is inserted into the culture insert and a reading is recorded after a 20-sec instrument stabilization period. Resistance is calculated based on an area of 0.64 cm^2, which is the area of the culture insert. Results are expressed as R_{50} (concentration of test substance that causes the electrical resistance to decrease to 50% of control) (215). Correlations between these tests and the in vivo Draize test for various chemicals and certain cosmetic formulations have been reported (215).

Cellular metabolism. Even in viable cells, toxic substances can cause subtle metabolic changes in such cellular endpoints as plasminogen activator activity, ATP production, lysosomal activity, basic metabolic rate (measured as changes in acidic by-products), and amount of light produced by luminescent bacteria (43,44, 64,72,204,303,328,331). These changes can be quantified by techniques ranging from simple neutral red dye or 3-(4,5-dimethylthiazol-2-yl)-2,5-biphenyltetrazolium bromide (tetrazolium MTT) uptake into lysosomes (41,43,44,200), silicon microphysiometer sensor for detecting changes in pH caused by acidic metabolic by-products (177), or output of light by luminescent bacteria (64).

The *neutral red uptake* (*NRU*) test is based on the principle that living cells absorb the dye and accumulate it in the lysosomes. Cytotoxic agents can disrupt the metabolic energy required for dye accumulation and thus decrease dye uptake. Such a change can be quantified by a simple method. A culture cell line (BALB/c3T3 mouse fibroblasts) is grown and exposed to various concentrations of the test substance for 24 h. After exposure, the medium is removed, and cells are washed with fresh growth medium. The neutral red dye is added and the cells are incubated for 3 h at 37°C. The medium is removed and the cells are washed and fixed with a formaldehyde-based fixative. The dye is extracted into an acetic acid/ethanol solution and the concentration of dye is measured spectrophotometrically at 540 nm. Results are expressed as either NR_{50}, the concentration of test substance, that inhibits dye update by 50% compared to untreated cells, or HTD, the highest tolerated dose (41,43,44,200). Correlations between in vitro ranking of several surfactant and certain cosmetic formulations and the in vivo Draize test ranking have been reported (39,40,120,158,159,161).

The *MTT assay* measures the metabolic activity of mitochondria. It is based on the principle that only cells with respiring mitochondria can reduce significant amounts of MTT, a soluble, pale yellow dye, to the insoluble dark blue metabolite, MTT formazan (41). After incubating metabolically active cells (BALB/c3T3 mouse fibroblasts) with various concentrations of the test material for 24 h, cells are incubated with MTT for 3 h at 37°C in 96-well tissue culture plates. MTT formazan is solubilized in isopropanol and quantified by colorimetry. The concentration of MTT formazan as measured at 550 nm is related to the number of viable cells. Results are expressed as percentage difference from untreated cells. Correlations between in vitro ranking of certain cosmetic formulations and the in vivo Draize test ranking have been reported (158,159,161). MTT measurement in human epidermal keratinocytes after treatment with various chemicals, or personal care and cosmetic products has also been correlated to Draize test results (3,128,159, 301,302).

The *microphysiometer* measures changes in the cellular metabolic rate. The changes are detected as small changes in the physical properties of the growth medium as a result of accumulation of acidic metabolic by-products (57,177,287). The results are expressed as concentration of test material, which causes a 50% drop in metabolic rate. Preliminary results are encouraging but limited to acidic metabolic by-products. Correlation between this test and the in vivo Draize test for various surfactants, household cleaning products, and cosmetic formulations has been reported (4,57,58,70,159).

The *luminescent bacteria test* (*LBT*) is based on the principle that light emission occurs in certain strains of bacteria during metabolic activity. Thus, the amount of light produced by the bacteria reflects its metabolic rate. Cytotoxic agents which decrease the metabolic rate of the bacteria also will decrease light production. Light output from the luminescent bacteria *Phytobacterium phosphoreum* is measured after incubation of the bacteria with various concentrations of the test material. Results are expressed as the concentration of the test material that causes a 50% reduction in light output. Correlation between this test and the in vivo Draize test for a few chemicals and certain cosmetic and toiletry formulations has been reported (64,91,159,161).

Cellular morphology. The *Balb/c3T3 cell/morphological assay* (43–45,329) is a simple method that measures morphological changes in cultured cells. In this assay, chemicals are ranked on the basis of the highest tolerated dose (concentration) at which no morphological change associated with exposure to the chemical is observed by phase contrast microscopy.

Other cytotoxicity tests. Cell or tissue physiology also has been used as an endpoint for screening ocular irritants. Examples include electrical conductivity of epidermal tissue slices (284) and inhibition of contraction in rabbit ileum (258). In general, these tests have not been as extensively studied as the other methods because they all require killing animals. Some investigators have reported correlation with in vivo eye irritation tests for a few materials.

Inflammation/Immunity

Because ocular irritation is an inflammation process, inflammation/immunity has been evaluated as an endpoint for alternative irritancy tests (146). These tests include morphological observations of inflammatory/morphological changes in the chorioallantoic membrane (CAM) of developing chick embryos (212, 218,220,221,297), in vitro macrophage dynamics (chemotaxis method using Balb/c3T3 cells and leukocyte chernotactic factors using the bovine corneal cup model) (344), and quantitative measurement of release of inflammation mediators such as histamine (rat peritoneal mast cells and bovine eye cup), serotonin (rat peritoneal mast cells) (76,193), prostaglandins (rat vaginal tissue) (103,104), and leukotriene C4 (bovine eye cup) (118).

Chorioallantoic Membrane

In these methods, the endpoints are the subjective evaluation of vascular changes (hemorrhage or obstruction) and necrosis of the CAM, the vascularized, respiratory membrane just underneath the egg shell. This membrane was suggested to be equivalent to the conjunctiva of the eye (220). It enjoys the advantage of a viable membrane with the vasculature needed for an inflammatory response. However, recent studies have shown that responses to irritants in the CAM methods are morphological, rather than inflammatory, alternations. There are three variations of the CAM method: the CAM, the CAM vascular assay (CAMVA), and the hen's egg test–CAM (HET–CAM) method. Using a method similar to Leighton et al. (220) for acids, alkali, and surfactants, Parish (288) reported a correlation between CAM and Draize results. Correlation between this test and the in vivo Draize test for various chemicals, surfactants, household cleaning products, cosmetic formulations, and pesticides has been reported (3–7, 39,40,47,61,158,159,161,163). However, these methods require living embryos and results in ranking irritants have been mixed due to false positives probably attributable to embryo toxicity rather than local irritancy. The HET–CAM test has also been used in combination with the BCOP test (39,40,57,361,376). Irritancy is ranked according to the most severe response from the two tests. Correlation between this test and the in vivo Draize test for various surfactants, household cleaning products, and cosmetic formulations has been reported (39,40,57). A modification of the HET–CAM test (HET–CAM–TSA), which uses microscopic evaluation and a special test substance applicator, has also been reported (164).

Macrophage Chemotaxis

The underlying principle of this method is that leukocytes migrate to the site of inflammation. Cultured Balb/c3T3 cells are treated with potential irritants for different periods. The treated cells are washed and re-fed with fresh medium. The chemotactic factors in the re-fed medium are detected by placing the medium in the bottom wells of a microchemotaxis chamber, covering the wells with a polycarbonate membrane (5 μm pore size), and adding about 10^5 mouse peritoneal macrophages in the upper wells. The system is incubated for 4 h at 37°C. After staining, the number of macrophages that migrated through the membrane are counted. This method has not been routinely used and no information is available regarding extensive correlation to the in vivo Draize test.

Other Alternative Methods

Other approaches include the *Tetrahymena* motility assay (332), protein denaturation (168,169), ocular wound healing test (197,333), and quantitative structure–activity relationship analysis (119).

Tetrahymena Motility Assay

The motility assay evaluates the effect of the test material on the characteristic swimming pattern of the fresh water protozoa *Tetrahymena thermophila.* Motility is examined under a microscope following exposure to the test material for 2 min at 21°C. Results are expressed as the highest tolerated dose, the concentration or dilution of the test material, that is characterized by 90% normal cell motility (332). Correlations between this test and the in vivo Draize test for various chemicals, household cleaning products, and cosmetic formulations have been reported (3,39,40,158,159,161,332).

Protein Denaturation Test

Protein denaturation is the basis of the commercially available Irritection (Eytex) system. The test is based on the principle that opacity (precipitation of the specially organized protein in the cornea) is the major contribution to ocular irritancy in the Draize test. The degree of opacity and irritancy can be predicted by assessing the degree of aggregation of a synthetic (nonanimal) aqueous protein matrix that mimics the protein matrix of the cornea (168,169). The Irretection (Eytex) assay tests solutions and insoluble, immiscible, or opaque materials by using a special semi-permeable membrane bullet over the responding protein matrix. Correlation between Eytex results and the in vivo rabbit eye test for various chemicals and cosmetic formulations has been reported (92,97,158,159,161,229,314).

Ocular Wound Healing Test

Although reversibility is a key criterion in the Draize test, only a few in vitro studies have evaluated healing and repair of ocular lesions (197,333). In such studies cultured rabbit corneal cells are grown to multilayer confluency. A wound is created using a liquid nitrogen chilled probe and the test substance is added to the wounded cells. After 24 h of incubation, the cells are fixed and healing assessed by measuring the size (using computerized planimetry) of the remaining wound area not covered by cells as compared to the initial wound size (333). Although these tests may give information on cell migration and proliferation at the wound, a process needed for initial wound closure, the multilayer cell culture is not the same as an intact corneal epithelium with a basement membrane. This method has not been routinely used and no information is available regarding extensive correlation to the in vivo Draize test.

Quantitative Structure–Activity Relationship (QSAR)

Quantitative structure–activity relationship (QSAR) analysis, widely used to predict various physiological and biochemical activities of novel chemicals, also has been used to predict eye irritancy of structurally related chemicals. Using QSAR, Sugai et al. (345) examined the eye irritancy (opacity and conjunctivitis) of 131 chemically heterogeneous chemicals. The accuracy was 86.3% for classifying irritancy of the chemicals. In another study, overall accuracy of 91% was reported (119). More recent research involving QSAR analysis for eye irritancy has been reported (21,22,86,87). Although this approach may provide useful information on structurally related chemicals, its current utility for formulated products is questionable. The same limitations that impact the use of QSAR for acute toxicity applications are also applicable to acute ophthalmic irritation (See Alternative Methods for LD_{50} Test, Quantitative Structure–Activity Relationship [QSAR] Analysis).

Evaluation and Validation Programs

Since eye irritation is a process involving multiple mechanisms (347), it is not surprising that development of alternative in vitro tests for eye irritancy is an extremely complex issue. Although the current thrust in method development and validation is encouraging, many issues remain. The Johns Hopkins Center for Alternatives to Animal Testing (CAAT)/European Research Group for Alternatives in Toxicity Testing (ERGATT) Workshop on Validation of Toxicity Testing Procedures recognized the need for mechanistic similarity between an in vitro assay and the in vivo animal model (14). For screening purposes, mechanistic similarity may not be necessary if the empirical correlation/predictability criterion is met. However, mechanistic similarity is generally required if the alternative method is to be a replacement test.

Important issues must be addressed before alternative ocular irritancy test methods can replace current in vivo animal tests. For example, insolubility of certain chemicals remains an issue. Testing extracts may partially resolve this problem. Many in vitro assays are not suitable for testing materials that change the physiological pH of the test system. A major problem is the lack of correlation between in vitro and in vivo data. Correlation appears to be good only within certain classes of chemicals. Predictability is further confounded when testing complex mixtures and total product formulations. A battery of assays could possibly minimize these issues. Most in vitro techniques do not establish reversibility, which is extremely important in classification of eye irritants (123,202). These and other issues are apparent when reviewing the results of recent multi-laboratory evaluation/validation studies with alternative methods for ocular irritancy.

In the United States, a number of programs have been launched to evaluate alternative tests. Two such programs organized by the Soap and Detergent Association (SDA) and the Cosmetic Toiletry and Fragrance Association (CTFA) have reported on their findings (3,39,40,158,159,161). The CTFA program was designed to evaluate the performance (correlation with Draize test results) of a set of in vitro tests on materials used in the cosmetic and toiletry industry.

In Phase I of the CTFA program, 25 alternative tests (representing 12 different endpoints) were used to test 10 different hydroalcoholic cosmetic and toiletry products (161). Results indicated that 6 of the 25 assays demonstrated the least disagreement with the Draize test for these products. Predictability generally was better for materials with low, rather than high, irritancy potential.

In CTFA Phase II, 30 alternative tests (representing 14 different endpoints) were used to test 18 different oil/water emulsion cosmetic and toiletry products (158). Results indicated that 16 of the 30 assays demonstrated the least disagreement with the Draize test for these products. As in Phase 1, predictability generally was better for materials with low, rather than high, irritancy potential.

In CTFA Phase III, 23 alternative tests (representing 41 different endpoints) were used to test 25 different surfactant-containing cosmetic and toiletry products (159). Results indicated that no single in vitro endpoint exhibited relative superiority with regard to prediction of the Draize test results for these products. Overall, predictability of the in vitro assays was better in Phase I (hydroalcoholic products) than in Phase II (oil/water emulsion products) or in Phase III (surfactant-containing products).

In Phase I of the SDA program, 14 alternative tests (mostly cytotoxicity) were used to test 8 household cleaning product ingredients or formulations (39). Six assays were selected as having the best agreement with Draize test results.

In SDA Phase II, 9 in vitro assays were used to test 23 household cleaning product ingredients or formulations, 8 of which were tested in Phase I (40). Phases I and II results indicated that the combination of product alkalinity and in vitro data provide useful information on the ocular irritancy potential of alkaline and acidic household cleaning product ingredients or formulations.

In SDA Phase III, 9 in vitro assays were used to test 22 household cleaning product ingredients or formulations (3). When only nonalkaline materials were considered, the correlation coefficients of the 9 methods were not significantly different from one another, although none of the tests could accurately predict the relative irritation potential of the irritant materials. Various evaluation and validation programs also have been conducted in Europe and Japan, all with mixed results (17,48, 155,282,341).

A formal validation study on the HET–CAM and NRU cytotoxicity test was conducted in Germany to determine whether these tests were capable of identifying chemicals that are severe eye irritants (341). The study was carried out in 10 laboratories with 200 test materials under blind conditions. Results suggested that this combination of methods was adequate to identify severe irritants.

An evaluation of the BCOP test was sponsored by the European Directorate General (DGXI) (155). The study included 12 laboratories testing 52 chemicals with a wide range of structure, physical form, and irritancy potential. Results indicated that the BCOP correctly predicted whether a material would be an irritant or nonirritant for 44 of the 52 materials.

A European validation study was coordinated by the European Commission/British Home Office (EC/HO) (17). In this study, 9 Draize test alternatives were evaluated in 37 laboratories using 60 coded chemicals. The goal was to establish whether any of the alternative methods could replace the Draize test for all severely irritating materials, all severely irritating materials belonging to a specific chemical class, or materials with or without regard to chemical class. With the possible exception of predicting the irritancy potential of surfactants, none of the 9 tests met any of the pre-defined performance criteria.

In Phase I of a Japanese Cosmetic Industry Association validation trial, 12 Draize test alternatives in 20 laboratories were used to evaluate 9 cosmetic ingredients (282). Many of the assays handled the surfactant materials adequately.

The European Cosmetics Association (COLIPA) conducted a validation study evaluating 10 alternative methods in 34 laboratories using 55 test substances (23 ingredients, 32 formulations) selected as representative of those commonly used in the cosmetics industry (48). Using the criteria of reliability and relevance as defined in the study, preliminary results indicated that none of the methods could be considered a valid replacement for the Draize test across the full irritation scale, although several satisfied at least one criterion of reliability or relevance.

At present, none of the in vitro techniques appears able to replace eye irritation testing in animals. However, some methods are useful in screening for ocular irritancy potential and can aid in selection of a final product for further development. In fact, many of the tests described above have been adopted as routine screening tests for product development and are well documented in the scientific literature.

As efforts continue to develop appropriate alternatives, prudent science necessitates continued use of animals in safety testing. Nonetheless, protocol refinements and reduction in the number of animals should continue where appropriate while validated alternative methods are sought.

Protocol Refinement

Because it is generally agreed that in vitro techniques will not replace animal testing immediately, efforts should be made to reduce the number of animals used and to minimize their pain. The precision of an eye irritancy test is a function of the number of animals used. The question arises as to whether it is justified to use a large number of animals to increase precision. The answer is no, because there is seldom an advantage to testing eye irritancy with more than three to six animals. The largest variable in an eye irritancy test is among animals, and the test itself is designed to be a bioassay. Therefore, to use a large number of animals in hopes of achieving a higher level of precision is neither realistic nor scientifically sound. A statistical analysis of 155 Draize irritancy studies with six-rabbit scores has shown that reducing the number of animals to five-, four-, three-, or two-animal scores retains, respectively, a 98, 96, 94, or 91% agreement with an irritant classification of these chemicals based on the six-rabbit scores (349). The correlation coefficients for randomly selected subsets of five, four, three, or two scores were 0.998, 0.996, 0.992, and 0.984, respectively. The results of this study show that sufficient accuracy can be obtained by reducing the number of animals used in the Draize test. A combination of lower test substance dose volume (one-tenth the Draize test dose volume) and fewer animals (three) also has yielded good correlation with the standard Draize test (59).

Another proposal is to test only for skin irritation. If the material causes severe skin irritation, it is presumed to be severely irritating to the eye as well. Thus, the argument concludes, an eye irritation test is not needed. Extrapolation from skin to eye is not always valid. In at least one study of 60 severe skin irritants, only 39 also caused severe eye irritation; 15 caused mild or no ocular effects, and the other 6 caused moderate eye irritation (378,379). Nonetheless, this approach has been proposed as one element of a tier system to prevent conducting an eye irritancy test when other potentially relevant information is available (194).

Many company guidelines specify that materials with extremely high or low pH do not need to be tested for eye irritancy. This approach is fully justified, especially for highly basic compounds. Alkali compounds generally cause more severe eye irritation than acidic compounds.

Tier Testing Strategies

A variety of tier testing strategies have been proposed to reduce the number of animals in eye irritation testing (23,175,185,194). These strategies usually begin with a weight-of-evidence approach, in an effort to review existing information that would allow classification and labeling a material as a severe ocular irritant without animal testing, or to conduct testing with a reduced number of animals. An example of this approach is shown in Figure 18.7, a tier testing scheme proposed by the OECD to support the harmonization of eye irritation testing and classification (280). Stages 1–3 involve information on the physicochemical characterization of the test material and use decision points to preclude animal testing such as: if the test material has a high or low pH (<2 or >11.5); is a known corrosive or severe dermal irritant; or if relevant information from structure–activity relationships (SAR) is available. If the weight-of-evidence suggests that the test material is a severe irritant, it should be so labeled. If information suggests that the test material is not a severe eye irritant, conducting an alternative test is the next step. If the results of the alternative test are indicative of a severe response, the material is classified as a severe irritant. If not, then testing in one or two animals is necessary before a final evaluation can be made.

Current Regulatory Status of Eye Irritation Testing

As in acute oral toxicity testing, the current regulatory status of eye irritation testing is in a state of flux. Most international regulatory agencies are attempting both to reduce the number of animals necessary to assess the ocular hazard of a new substance and to harmonize classification and labeling schemes to accommodate some of the more modern testing approaches. For example, the use of the tier testing strategy (280) is a realistic approach that could minimize pain and suffering, reduce the number of animals without significantly compromising the safety of consumers and workers, and be harmonized to fit existing regulatory classification and labeling schemes.

The OECD has taken a lead role in coordinating the effort to harmonize regulatory strategies through its Program on Harmonization of Classification and Labeling Systems. Case studies are being conducted using existing rabbit eye irritation information submitted to various regulatory agencies under chemicals notification procedures. The data are then used to compare the sensitivity of various classification schemes. This ongoing project is attempting to define criteria for various degrees of eye irritation that are in the range of sensitivity of existing classification systems, and to explore ways to subdivide the effects for those systems that require such for labeling purposes (280).

For specific information on regulatory agency requirements for eye irritation testing, the reader is encouraged to check the most recent regulatory guidelines that apply.

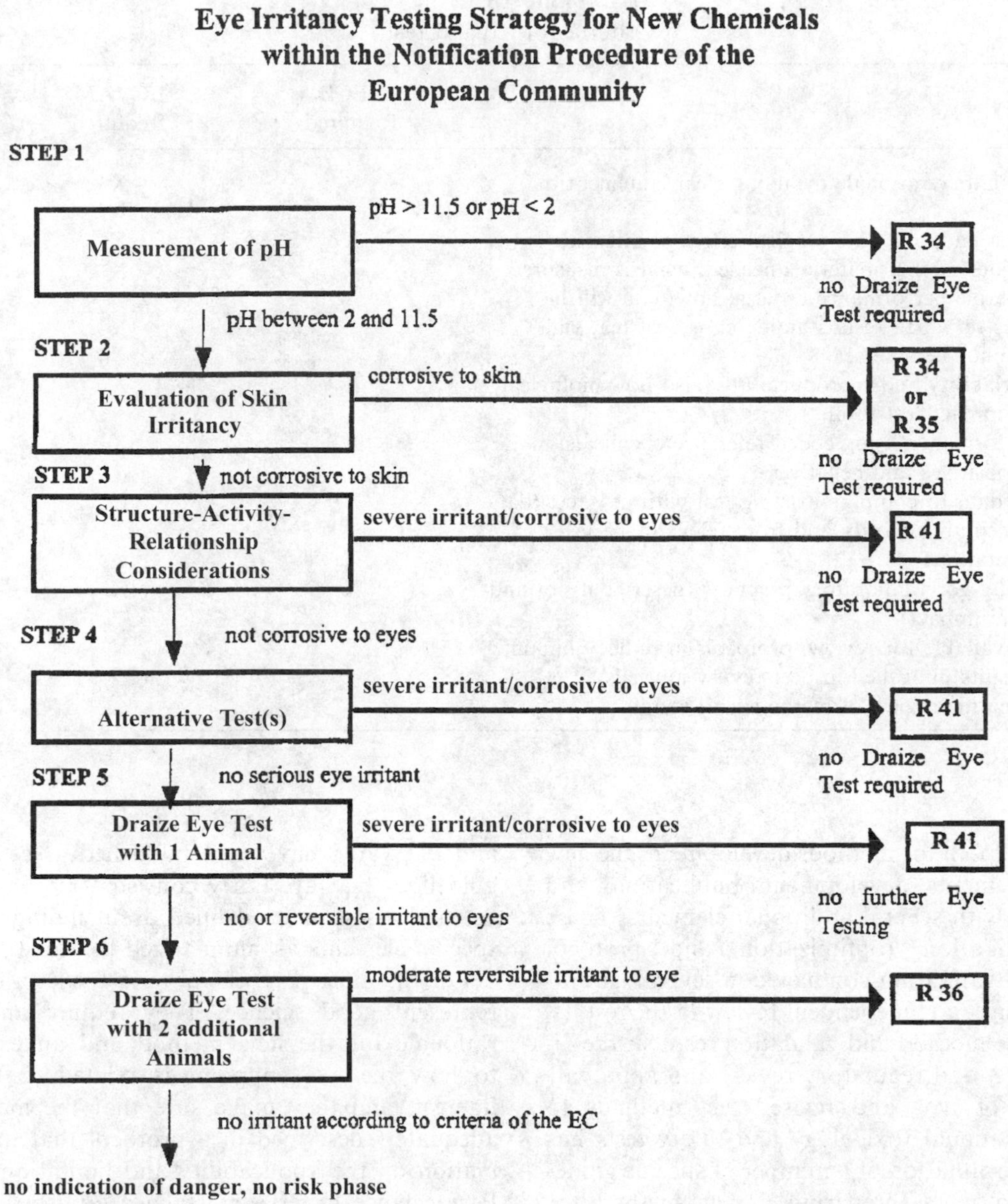

FIG. 18.7. Tier scheme for eye irritation testing. From Reference 280, with permission.

VALIDATION AND REGULATORY ACCEPTANCE OF ALTERNATIVE METHODS

The typical path for the emergence of new methods has historically comprised development and intra-laboratory assessment, peer review and publication, and, ultimately, peer acceptance of the method. Although this process has served us well, continued advancements in basic science, biotechnology, and engineering will undoubtedly result in a plethora of new methods intended as replacements for traditional animal tests such as acute toxicity and eye irritancy. The implementation of new and revised toxicological test methods should occur only if such methods have the capability to provide improved assessment of the potential toxic effects of chemicals and other agents on human and animal health and the environment. One way to assure that new methods represent an improvement over existing tests is through the process of formal validation followed by regulatory acceptance.

Validation has been described as *the process whereby the reliability and relevance of a procedure are established for a particular purpose* (15,141). In this context, validation encompasses a number of inherent criteria and features that are necessary preliminaries to regulatory acceptance of an alternative method. In contrast

Table 18.12
Criteria for a valid test

Necessary criteria	OECD Required	ECVAM Required	ICCVAM Required
Scientific and regulatory rationale including clear statement of proposed use	X	X	X
Relationship of test endpoint to biological effect of interest	X	X	X
Detailed protocol describing: materials needed; what is measured and how; acceptable performance criteria; how data will be analyzed; species to which results apply; classes of materials that can and cannot be assessed	X	X	X
Description of variability and reproducibility (also how biological variability may impact test results)	X	X	X
Demonstrated performance using coded reference chemicals; should include positives and negatives	X	X	X
Sufficient toxicity data to compare existing test with new test (data should be of acceptable quality and from relevant species)	X	X	X
Description of limitations	X		X
Data obtained using good laboratory practices (describe if not and indicate potential impact)	X	X	X
Supporting data available for review: protocols in public domain; methods and results published in peer-review journals; independent scientific review of methods and results	X	X	X

to the traditional path for methods development, the new paradigm supplements development, publication, and peer acceptance with several additional elements. These include pre-validation (optimization and protocol transfer), formal validation conducted in several laboratories (a blind trial), an independent review of the results, submission of the method and validation results to regulatory authorities, and regulatory review and approval.

Development of new and revised test methods to replace existing animal toxicology and safety tests has resulted in the formulation of a number of specific guidelines to be used when preparing a new method for validation and regulatory acceptance (11–13,15,56, 134,141,142–145,166,167). There has been recent movement by the OECD, ECVAM, and ICCVAM to formalize these guidelines and to put them into a harmonized, international regulatory context (16,269,274). A discussion of the guidelines follows.

Criteria for a Valid Test

Compliance with comprehensive criteria designed to assure that alternative test methods will meet the standards established for a proper validation study is the first and, unquestionably, the most important step in gaining regulatory acceptance for a new test. In recognizing the importance of such criteria, the OECD, ECVAM, and ICCVAM have each published a set of validation guidelines that are fairly consistent among the groups. A valid test can be defined as including a number of specific elements as summarized in Table 18.12.

For the most part, the criteria for a valid test simply represent good science. They require an appropriate rationale for the new method and an explanation as to how the test endpoint is related to the effect of interest, and they make sure that the methodology is adequately described in a protocol that includes information on the applicability and limitations of the test. Performance criteria must be established to allow an assessment of the inherent variability of the test and its performance in evaluating the chemical class of interest. Relevant in vivo data of sufficient quantity and quality must also be available to permit a comparison of the existing method to the new test. All data generation, collection, and reporting associated with the new test should be performed with adherence to GLP. Scientific credibility can be ensured through peer review of the test methodology, testing results, and subsequent published reports that place details of the new test and the attendant validation activities in the public domain.

If proper attention is given to these criteria and to their utilization in validation programs, appropriate recognition of new test methods by the scientific community will be facilitated. Having accomplished that, the poten-

VALIDATION PROCESS

I. Test Development

II. Prevalidation/Test Optimization
- A. Preliminary planning
  1. Define basis and purpose of test
  2. Develop protocol
  3. Develop control values
  4. Develop data/outcome prediction model
- B. Activities
  1. Qualify and train laboratories
  2. Measure intra- and inter-laboratory reproducibility
  3. Identify limitations of test

III. Determine Readiness for Validation
- A. Analyze test development and prevalidation data
- B. Standardize protocol

IV. Test Validation
- A. Form steering committee/management team
  1. Define purpose of validation study
  2. Design study
  3. Select participating laboratories
  4. Establish management evaluation and oversight procedures
- B. Pretest Procedures
  1. Implement data record keeping procedures
  2. Select reference chemicals
  3. Code and distribute reference chemicals
- C. Test Coded Chemicals
  1. Measure inter-laboratory performance
  2. Compile and evaluate data
- D. Evaluate Test
  1. Analyze and summarize test results
  2. Challenge data with prediction model
  3. Peer review of protocol and data
  4. Accept, revise, or reject model

V. Submission of Test for Regulatory Approval
- A. Prepare report
- B. Make supporting data available
- C. Prepare results for publication

FIG. 18.8. ICCVAM validation process. From Reference 269, with permission.

tial for assuring international regulatory acceptance as later described will be greatly enhanced.

Validation Process

The OECD and ICCVAM have also made recommendations on what fundamental elements should be contained within the validation process. Figure 18.8 summarizes the validation process as described by ICCVAM.

The validation process starts with the development of a new test method for a relevant biological endpoint and proceeds through a step called prevalidation. The role of prevalidation in the devclopment, validation, and acceptance of alternative methods has been described by Curren et al. (88). It is during the prevalidation phase that information is developed that defines the basis and purpose of the test, establishes its capabilities, limitations, and transferability between laboratories, and provides sufficient data to confirm whether the method correctly predicts the toxic endpoint of interest.

The tool used to predict the toxic endpoint of interest is called the prediction model. The requirements for an adequate prediction model have been described by Bruner et al. (55,56) as containing:

1. A definition of the specific purpose for which the alternative method is to be used.
2. A definition of all the possible results that may be obtained from the alternative method.
3. An algorithm that defines how to convert results from the alternative method into a prediction of the in vivo toxicity.
4. An indication of the accuracy and precision of the in vivo toxicity endpoint obtained from the model.

Essentially, a prediction model converts the results from an alternative method into a prediction of in vivo toxicity. For an alternative method to be considered reliable and relevant, it is important that the prediction model has high predictive power and is relatively insensitive to sources of variability. If these criteria are not met, the alternative method should not be pursued through the validation process because it will have little or no value to the toxicologist in making safety assessment decisions. Once the reliability and relevance of the new test method have been established, and the appropriate prediction model developed, a standardized protocol can be prepared and the test validation study initiated. For additional information on prediction models see Archer et al. (1).

The success of any validation study can be directly linked to the incorporation of several key elements into the study design. A number of these have been listed by Balls et al. (19) including:

1. A clear and unequivocal statement of what the validation study is designed to accomplish.
2. A well-defined plan for the study.
3. A sufficiently large set of test substances covering the relevant chemical classes, and the range of toxic endpoints to be evaluated.
4. Comparative in vivo data of high quality on all test substances to be used.
5. A clear description of how the alternative method can be used to predict an in vivo endpoint (the prediction model).

6. Agreed statistical procedures for testing whether the method can predict the in vivo endpoint of interest.
7. Agreed criteria to be met in order to show that an alternative method could successfully and safely replace the animal test.

Perhaps the most important of the listed elements are those which address sufficiency of test samples, quality of the in vivo data, and adequacy of the prediction model and subsequent statistical analysis of the resultant data. Without appropriate attention to these critical elements, a validation study can be doomed to failure.

Once a validation study has been completed, the results are put into the form of a report with supporting data and submitted for regulatory approval. Test method submissions must contain sufficient information for an independent peer-review panel to determine the validation status of the method, that is, its reproducibility, relevance, and limitations, and for agencies to assess the acceptability of the method for providing useful information for hazard or risk assessment.

Criteria for Regulatory Acceptance

Completion of a validation study does not automatically imply that a new test method is ready for regulatory acceptance. It is extremely important that the test fit into an existent regulatory structure and that it has a suitable regulatory rationale. The best way to ensure this is to involve regulatory agencies as early as possible in the design of any validation program. The importance of early liaison with regulators cannot be overemphasized.

The OECD and ICCVAM also provide guidance on the criteria and considerations for regulatory acceptance (Table 18.13). Once again, peer review is considered a significant element, along with adequately detailed information on the test method protocol and supporting documentation. Demonstrating linkage between the new test and the existing method is critical, and must be put into the context of specific regulatory programs and agency authorities. Technical transfer of the new test method should be relatively straightforward and at a reasonable cost, and the test should be amenable to regulatory harmonization and international acceptance. The new test also should provide some advantage in the reduction, refinement, or replacement of animal usage.

Because regulatory acceptance is an integral part of the successful implementation of new test method development, all reasonable efforts should be made to accommodate dialogue with the appropriate regulatory authorities and to take whatever measures are necessary to ensure that new methods can be harmonized into current regulatory testing strategies.

Table 18.13
Criteria for regulatory acceptance

Necessary criteria	OECD Required	ICCVAM Required
Independent scientific review (by experts with knowledge of method and no financial interest)		X
Detailed protocol with SOPs and criteria to judge performance and results		X
Data adequately measures desired endpoint; links new test to existing test or effects in target species	X	X
Data adequately represents products or chemicals of interest to agency or regulatory program	X	X
Method generates data useful for risk assessment purposes	X	X
Data is as useful (or better) than that from existing methods	X	
Method is robust and able to transfer between properly staffed and equipped labs	X	X
Method is time- and cost-effective	X	X
Method can be harmonized with requirements of other agencies or international groups		X
Method is suitable for international acceptance		X
Method provides consideration for reduction, refinement, and replacement of animal use	X	X

Regulatory Approaches to Alternatives Acceptance

International health regulatory agencies often have unique responsibilities in their mission to protect human and animal health and the environment. Because an agency usually carries out its responsibility through activities that are specific to the nature of its regulatory authority, the information requirements for data to make hazard or risk assessments are primarily driven by regulatory mandate, and many times directly linked to the regulated entity, that is, industrial chemicals, pesticides, biologics, human or veterinary drugs, cosmetics, consumer products, or chemicals in transport.

Most U.S. agencies have unique regulatory considerations that often result in different approaches to the way in which they request and use information to make hazard or risk assessments. These unique considerations will ultimately have an effect on the criteria used by an agency to approve new test methods. Moreover, other international organizations that require toxicological testing have their own special considerations regarding test method acceptance and use. Because of these differences, cooperation among all health regulatory agencies is a critical link to the development and acceptance of new alternative methods.

There is no agreed upon international process for health regulatory agencies to coordinate the review and acceptance of new alternative test methods. Further complicating the issue, in certain OECD member countries there is neither an understanding nor even a legal obligation that once an alternative test has been considered as sufficiently validated, it must be adopted for use.

ICCVAM recognizes that regulatory agency harmonization of approaches to test method acceptance is a critical aspect of the entire alternatives development process, and includes recommendations to enhance and facilitate the regulatory acceptance and use of new methods in its guidelines (269). Recommendations are provided in five areas: development and validation, regulatory review of new methods, intra- and interagency coordination and harmonization, communication, and international harmonization. The significant aspects of these recommendations are summarized below.

Development and Validation

As previously indicated, criteria for validation and regulatory acceptance must be taken into account in the planning and design stages of validation studies, and in so doing there should be continuing communication with the relevant regulatory agencies that will be asked to review and accept the methods. Likewise, regulatory agencies should be expected to evaluate new test methods using consistent, though flexible, validation criteria and should be involved in encouraging the development of new and innovative methods. Although both correlative and mechanistic tests can be validated and accepted, mechanistically based methods relevant to the biological effects of concern should be encouraged.

Regulatory Review of New Methods

An efficient and effective process that involves communicating with regulators at all stages prior to regulatory acceptance of alternative methods needs to be set up. As part of this process, agencies should establish internal central clearing systems for the evaluation of new or revised methods and for the periodic review of methods recommended by an agency to ensure their continued relevance. If agency personnel are not familiar with new methods, training should be instituted so that current efforts to incorporate validated alternatives into regulatory testing strategies can be continued and expanded. When questions arise about the acceptability of new or revised test methods, input from the relevant scientific community should be solicited. Many times, concurrent submission of data from new and existing methods will help facilitate regulatory acceptance and preclude these kinds of questions from being raised. If not, an agency-sponsored workshop is the best venue to exchange information.

Intra- and Interagency Coordination and Harmonization

Various regulatory agencies should be consistent in their processes and criteria for acceptance of new and revised toxicological test procedures. Interagency coordination is especially important for those test methods used by more than one agency. This coordination could be ensured by the formation of an interagency committee on test methods which would be a forum for information exchange and the vehicle for consistency in the review, evaluation, and acceptance of alternative test methods. When modifying existing test guidelines, each regulatory agency should solicit input from other agencies in an effort to harmonize testing guidelines to the extent possible. Such harmonization of testing guidelines may first require the harmonization of disparate hazard classification schemes.

Communication

Agency regulations and guidelines should be available to the public to facilitate a consistent and coordinated process of involvement and communication among researchers, method users, regulators, and the public. Exchange of information among these stakeholders will encourage the validation and acceptance of new alternative methods. Scientific journals, workshops, government publications (e.g., the *Federal Register*), and other means should be used to communicate the acceptance of new and revised test methods by regulatory agencies.

International Harmonization

Regulatory agencies in the United States should encourage international harmonization and make attempts to harmonize testing guidelines through international organizations. Where appropriate, this could be done by working with the OECD, the United Nations Committee of Experts on the Transport of Dangerous Goods organization, and other international groups.

From a regulatory perspective, the pieces are in place to foster the development of new and innovative methods that can be used to generate information to support the protection of human and animal health and the environment. Through the continued efforts of researchers working with informed regulators the future of alternative methods development is encouraging; there now exists a recognized pathway for moving appropriately validated new methods from their inception stage to regulatory acceptance.

ACKNOWLEDGEMENTS

The authors acknowledge the contributions of Ping Kwong (Peter) Chan to the development of this chapter.

QUESTIONS

1. What is the importance of acute toxicity testing and is a precise LD_{50} value necessary to adequately define acute toxicity?

   Answer: Acute toxicity testing is the way in which we define the intrinsic toxicity of a chemical, identify target organs, provide information for risk assessment of acute exposure, provide information for the design and selection of dose levels for more prolonged studies (i.e., subchronic, chronic), and, most importantly, provide information to clinicians for use in treatment of acute chemical poisoning. Information from acute toxicity testing is also used to provide insight into the mechanism of action of a chemical, to formulate safety measures during the early stages in the development of a new chemical, and for categorization and labeling purposes for handling and shipping chemicals. One should not confuse the concept of acute toxicity with the term, LD_{50}. The LD_{50} is a statistically defined measure of acute toxicity but is only one of many ways to define it. Indeed, a precise LD_{50} is seldom required in acute toxicity testing, and its use is being de-emphasized to reduce the total number of animals and pain and suffering involved in their use. The LD_{50} is being replaced by more modern methods. The Up-and-Down Procedure and the Acute Toxic Class Method are alternatives to the LD_{50} test that can be used to estimate the median lethal dose and to provide hazard classification for labeling, respectively.

2. The following mortality data were obtained from an acute oral toxicity study:

Dose (mg/kg)	1	2	4	8	16	32
Mortality	0/10	1/10	3/10	4/10	7/10	10/10

   Calculate the LD_{50}, the SE of the LD_{50}, the fiducial limits, and the slope of the dose-response curve.

Log dose (x)	n	Probits Observed	Probits Expected	Probabilities expected (P)	Responses Observed	Responses Expected	χ^2
0.30	10	3.72	3.82	11.9	1	1.19	0.0344
0.60	10	4.48	4.36	26.1	3	2.61	0.0344
0.90	10	4.75	4.75	46.4	4	4.64	0.0789
1.20	10	5.52	4.45	67.4	7	6.74	0.1646
1.50	10	—	—	—	10	—	0.0307

$\Sigma\chi^2 = 0.386$
$df = 2$

Answer: Procedure

1. Log dose 0 0.3 0.6 0.9 1.2 1.5
2. Probits — 3.72 4.48 4.75 5.52 —

3., 4. Plot log dose versus probits (Figure 18.9) and fit the best point(s) to a straight line.

5. From the log-dose probit line, extrapolate the log $LD_{50} = 0.95$; then $LD_{50} = $ antilog $0.95 = 8.91$ mg/kg body weight.
6. From the same line, calculate the slope as: (numbers of probit units)/unit log dose $= 2/11 = 1.818$.

$$\text{Thus, } \sigma = \frac{1}{\text{slope}} = 0.55 \text{ (Figure 18.9)}$$

7. χ^2 *test of goodness-of-fit*. Expected probability is converted from the expected probits. The test is conducted by converting each expected probit (y) back to the expected probability (P) and then to the number of expected responses (E) (i.e., multiply the expected probability P by n). The difference between expect-

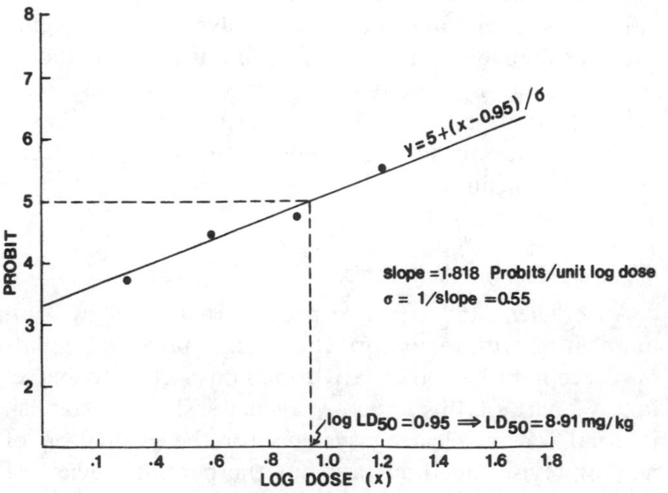

plot.

FIG. 18.9. Example of probit versus log–dose plot.

ed and observed number of responses will be used to calculate the χ^2 statistic, but instead of using $\Sigma[(E-0)^2/E]$, the weighted value will be used, i.e., $\Sigma[(E-0)^2/E(1-P)]$. The degrees of freedom (df) are $N-2$, where N is the number of dose levels used in the calculation of χ^2. The critical χ^2 for $(4-2)=2$ degrees of freedom is 6.0 at a $p=0.05$, and the calculated $\chi^2=0.386$, which is less than the critical value, indicating that the fitted line is adequate.

8. *Determination of precision of LD₅₀ by weighting*. The SE of log $LD_{50} = S_m = \sigma/\sqrt{\Sigma m W} = 0.55/\sqrt{18.5} = 0.129$. The approximation of SE $(LD_{50}) = (10^m)\cdot(S_m) = 8.91 \times 2.302 \times 0.129 = 2.646$. The precision of $LD_{50} = 8.91 \pm 2.646$ mg/kg.

Dose (mg/kg)	2	4	6	16
W	0.277	0.423	0.541	0.564
nW	2.77	4.23	5.41	5.64
nW			18.05	

9. *Fiducial limits*. Using the approximation formula, the fiducial limit calculated at the $F=95\%$ level is given by log $LD_{50} \pm 1.96\,(S_m)$. Thus the lower log LD_{50} limit $= 0.5 - 1.96 \times 0.129 = 0.697$, and the antilog $0.697 = 4.977$. The upper log LD_{50} limit $= 0.95 + 1.96 \times 0.129 = 1.20 = 15.849$. Antilogs of 0.697 and 1.2 give the fiducial LD_{50} limit 4.98 to 15.85 mg/kg.

3. Describe the basic elements needed to perform Quantitative Structure–Activity Relationship (QSAR) analysis and list the limitations of this method.

Answer: Basic elements needed to perform QSAR analysis include a reliable bioassay database for the predicted endpoint, a set of physical–chemical parameters that describe the chemical, structures of interest so the bioassay endpoint can be modeled in terms of these parameters, appropriate statistical methods to weigh these parameters in terms of the explanation of the endpoint, and associated computer technology to carry out the computations. Limitations of QSAR analysis in acute toxicity testing and eye irritancy include a limited database on which to base a QSAR model, uncertainties associated with extrapolating beyond the confines of the model, and biological variability (noise) in the bioassays on which the models are based.

4. Compare and contrast eye irritation and eye corrosion including in the discussion a description of the observation endpoints usually associated with irritancy in the three major tissues of the eye.

Answer: Eye irritation can be defined as reversible inflammatory changes in the eye and its surrounding mucous membranes following exposure to a material on the surface of the anterior portion of the eye. In contrast, corrosion represents irreversible tissue damage to the eye following exposure to a material. The amount of damage to each of the three major eye tissues, the cornea, the conjunctiva, and the iris, is what differentiates irritancy from corrosion. Gross tissue destruction that follows rapidly after exposure and persists for an extended period in any or all of these tissues is usually an indication of eye corrosion. Irritancy, however, can occur to various degrees. Assessment of injury is based on the presence and severity of: cloudiness (opacity) and swelling of the cornea; redness, edema (chemosis) and discharge in the conjunctiva; and increased vascularity, edema, absence of reaction to light, and cloudiness (aqueous flair) in the iris.

5. What are the Three Rs and how have they been implemented in acute toxicity and eye irritancy testing?

Answer: Three Rs refers to the reduction in the number of animals used, the refinement of testing methods to reduce the pain and suffering of animals, and the replacement of animals by other methods in testing procedures. Varying degrees of progress in the Three Rs have been made for acute toxicity and eye irritancy testing. Protocols requiring as few as six rats for acute toxicity or three rabbits for eye irritancy are being used in hazard assessment, although larger group sizes are usually required in regulatory requirements for labeling and classification of chemicals. At least one acute toxicity method, the fixed dose procedure, is based on classifying toxicity hazard using a pre-selected dose that is intended to be non-lethal, non-painful, and non-stressful, but toxicity-evident. Many company guidelines specify that materials with extremely high or low pH, e.g., <2 or >11.5, or which are severely irritating or corrosive to skin, do not need to be tested for eye irritancy, and the use of topical eye anesthetics before testing is also common practice. Quantitative Structure–Activity Relationship (QSAR) analysis and various in vitro tests are being researched as replacement methods, but at the present, none appears able to replace in vivo testing in animals for acute toxicity and eye irritancy.

6. What are the basic requirements for the development, validation, and regulatory acceptance of new alternative methods?

Answer: An understanding of the nature and use of the animal or other test intended for replacement is a prerequisite to the development of a new method. The new method is built around this knowledge, which must include supporting information that explains how the new test endpoint is related to the effect of interest. If the new method is intended for regulatory approval, there should be early dialog with the appropriate regulators to assure the method fits the existing regulatory scheme. Once a new test has been developed for a specific use it undergoes a prevalidation (optimization) phase. During prevalidation, the purpose and basis of the test are defined, a test protocol is standardized, a database is developed, inter- and intra-laboratory reproducibility is assessed, and a prediction model is generated from the database. The prediction model must explain the toxic endpoint of interest in terms of the new test output(s). Next, a validation study is designed to test the new method with a sufficiently large set of coded substances covering a relevant chemical class and a range of toxic endpoints. High-quality in vivo data should be available on these substances for comparative purposes. The validation study should be conducted among a sufficient number of laboratories to further assess inter- and intra-laboratory variability of the standardized protocol. Testing results should be analyzed using appropriate statistical methods that challenge the data with the prediction model. All methods, results, and supporting data should be peer reviewed, prepared for publication, and submitted for regulatory approval.

REFERENCES

1. Archer, G., Balls, M., Bruner, L. H., Curren, R. D., Fentem, J. H., Holzhutter, H., Liebsch, M., Lovell, D. P., and Southee, J. A. (1997): The validation of toxicological prediction models. *ATLA*, 25:505–516.
2. Ashford, J. R. (1959): An approach to the analysis of data for semiquantal responses in biological assay. *Biometrics*, 156:573–581.
3. Bagley, D., Booman, K. A., Bruner, L. H., Casterton, P. L., Demetrulias, J., Heinze, J. E., Innis, J. D., McCormick, W. C., Nuen, D. J., Rothenstein, A. S., and Sedlak, R. I. (1994): The SDA alternatives program phase III: Comparison of in vitro data with animal eye irritation data on solvents, surfactants, oxidizing agents and prototype cleaning products. *J. Toxicol. Cutan. Ocul. Toxicol.*, 13:127–155.
4. Bagley, D. M., Bruner, L. H., DeSilva, O., Cotton, M., O'Brien, K. A. F., Uttley, M., and Walker, A. P. (1992): An evaluation of five potential alternatives in vitro to the rabbit eye irritation test in vivo. *Toxicol. in Vitro*, 6:275–284.
5. Bagley, D. M., Rizvi, P. Y., Kong, B. M., and DeSalva, S. J. (1988): In: *Alternative Methods in Toxicology, Vol. 6, Progress in In Vitro Toxicology*, edited by A. M. Goldberg, pp. 131–138. Mary Ann Liebert, New York.
6. Bagley, D. M., Rizvi, P. Y., Kong, B. M., and DeSalva, S. J. (1991): Factors affecting use of the hens' egg chorioallantoic membrane as a model for predicting eye irritation potential. I. *J. Toxicol. Cutan. Ocul. Toxicol.*, 10:95–104.
7. Bagley, D. M., Rizvi, P. Y., Kong, B. M., and DeSalva, S. J. (1991): Evaluation of the vascular components of the chorioallantoic membrane assay as a model for eye irritation potential. II. *J. Toxicol. Cutan. Ocul. Toxicol.*, 10:105–114.
8. Baldwin, H. Q., McDonald, T. D., and Beasley, C. H. (1973): Slit-lamp examination of experimental animal eyes. 11. Grading scales and photographic evaluation of induced pathological conditions. *J. Soc. Cosmet. Chem.*, 24:181–195.
9. Ballantyne, B., and Swanston, D. W. (1974): The irritant effects of dilute solutions of dibenzoxyazepine(CR) on the eye and tongue. *Acta Pharmacol. Toxicol.*, 35:412–423.
10. Balls, M. (1991): Why modification of the LD_{50} test will not be enough. *Lab. Animals*, 25:198–206.
11. Balls, M. (1995): Scientific validation: A crucial and unavoidable prerequisite to the acceptance of new tests and testing strategies. *ATLA*, 23:474–479.
12. Balls, M. (1995): Defining the role of ECVAM in the development, validation and acceptance of alternative tests and testing strategies. *Toxicol. in Vitro*, 9:863–869.
13. Balls, M., and Blaauboer, B. J. (1994): The validation of replacement alternative methods. In: Proceedings of the ECVAM opening symposium, edited by M. Balls and B. J. Blaauboer. *Toxicol. in Vitro*, 9:789–869.
14. Balls, M., Blaauboer, B. B., Brusick, D., Frazier, J., Lamb, D., Pemberton, M., Reinhardt, C., Roberfroid, M., Rosenkranz, H., Schmid, B., Speilemann, H., Stammati, A. L., and Walum, E. (1990). Report and recommendations of the CAAT/ERGATT workshop on the validation of toxicity test procedures. *ATLA*, 18:313–328.
15. Balls, M., Blaauboer, B., Brusick, D., Frazier, J., Lamb, D., Pemberton, M., Reinhardt, C., Roberfroid, M., Rosenkranz, H., Schmid, B., et al. (1990): Report and recommendations of the CAAT/ERGATT workshop on the validation of toxicity test procedures. *ATLA*, 18:313–337.
16. Balls, M., Blaauboer, B., Fentem, J. H., Bruner, L., Combes, R. D., Ekwall, B., Fielder, R. J., Guillouzo, A., Lewis, R. W., Lovell, D. P., et al. (1995): Practical aspects of the validation of toxicity test procedures. The report and recommendations of ECVAM Workshop 5. *ATLA*, 23:129–147.
17. Balls, M., Botham, P. A., Bruner, L. H., and Spielman, H. (1995): The EC/HO international validation study on alternatives to the Draize eye irritation test. *Toxicol. in Vitro*, 9:871–929.
18. Balls, M., and Clothier, R. H. (1992): *Cytotoxicity Assays for Intrinsic Toxicology*, edited by G. Jolles and A. Cordier, pp. 31–52. Academic Press, New York.
19. Balls, M., De Klerck, W., Baker, F., van Beek, M., Bouillon, C., Bruner, L., Carstensen, J., Chamberlain, M., Cottin, M., Curren, R., et al. (1995): Development and validation of non-animal tests and testing strategies: The identification of a coordinated response to the challenge and the opportunity presented by the 6th Amendment to the Cosmetic Directive (76/768/EEC). The report and recommendations of ECVAM Workshop 7. *ATLA*, 23:398–409.
20. Balls, M., and Homer, S. A. (1985): The FRAME Inter-Laboratory Programme on In Vitro Cytotoxicology. *Food Chem. Toxicol.*, 23:209–213.
21. Barratt, M. D. (1995): A quantitative structure–activity relationship for the eye irritation potential of neutral organic chemicals. *Toxicol. Lett.*, 80:69–74.
22. Barratt, M. D. (1997): QSARS for the eye irritation potential of neutral organic chemicals. *Toxicol. in Vitro*, 11:1–8.

23. Barratt, M. D., Castell, J. V., Chamberlain, M., Combes, R. D., Dearden, J. C., Fentem, J. H., Gerner, I., Giuliani, A., Gray, T. J. B., Livingston, D. J., et al. (1995): The integrated use of alternative approaches for predicting toxic hazard. *ATLA*, 23:410–429.
24. Bass, R., Gunzel, P., Henschler, D., et. al. (1982): LD_{50} versus acute toxicity. *Arch. Toxicol.*, 51:183–186.
25. Battista, S. P., and McSweeney, E. S. (1965): Approaches to a quantitative method for testing eye irritation. *J. Soc. Cosmet. Chem.*, 16:199–301.
26. Baum, J. L., Niedra, R., Davis C., and Yoe, D. (1979): Mass culture of human corneal endothelial cells. *Arch. Ophthalmol.*, 97:1136–1140.
27. Bayard, S., and Hehir, R. M. (1976): Evaluation of proposed changes in the modified Draize rabbit irritation test. *Toxicol. Appl. Pharmacol.*, 37:186.
28. Beckley, J. H. (1965): Comparative eye testing: Man versus animal. *Toxicol. Appl. Pharmacol.*, 7:93–101.
29. Beckley, J. H. (1965): Critique of the Draize eye test, now and then: Eighteen, nine or six rabbits. *Am. Perf. Cosmet.*, 80:51–54.
30. Bell, M., Holmes, P. M., Nisbet, T. M., Uttley, M., and Van Abbe, N. J. (1979): Evaluating the potential eye irritancy of shampoos. *Int. J. Cosmet. Sci.*, 1:123.
31. Benson, M. T., Shepherd, L., Rees, R. C., and Rennie, I. G. (1992): Production of interleukin-6 by human retinal pigment epithelium in vitro and its regulation by other cytokines. *Curr. Eye Res.*, 1:173–179.
32. Bernstein, P. S., Lloyd, M. B., O'Day, W. T., and Bok, D. (1992): Effect of phytanic acid on cultured retinal pigment epithelium: An in vitro model for Refsum's disease. *Exp. Eye Res.*, 55:869–878.
33. Bliss, C. I. (1934): The method of probits-A correction. *Science*, 79:409–410.
34. Bliss, C. I. (1964): Insecticide assays. In: *Statistics and Mathematics in Biology*, edited by O. Kempthorne, T. A. Bancroft, J. W. Gowen, and J. L. Lush, pp. 345–360. Hofner, New York.
35. Bohnke, M., Chavanne, P., Gianotti, R., and Salathe, R. P. (1996): High-precision, high-speed measurement of eximer laser keratectomies with a new optical pachymeter. *Ger. J. Ophthalmol.*, 5:338–342.
36. Bondesson, I., Ekwall, B., Hellberg, S., Romert, L., Stenberg, K., and Walum, E. (1989): MEIC. A new international multicenter project to evaluate the relevance to human toxicity of in vitro cytotoxicity tests. *Cell Biol. and Toxicol.*, 5:331–347.
37. Bonifield, C. T., and Scala, R. A. (1965): The paradox in testing for eye irritation. A report on thirteen shampoos. *Proc. Sci. Sect. Toilet Goods Assoc.*, 43:34–43.
38. Bonting, S. L., Simon, K. A., and Hawkins, N. M. (1961): Studies on sodium-potassium-activated adenosine triphosphatase. 1. Quantitative distribution in several tissues of the rat. *Arch. Biochem.*, 95:416–423.
39. Booman, K. A., Cascieri, T. M., Demetrulias, J., Driedger, A., Griffith, J. F., Grochoski, G. T., Kong, B., McCormick, W. C. 3rd, North-Root, H., Rozen, M. G., and Sedlak, R. I. (1988): In vitro methods for evaluating eye irritancy of cleaning products. Phase 1: preliminary assessment. *J. Toxicol. Cutan. Ocul. Toxicol.*, 7:173–185.
40. Booman, K. A., De Prospo, J., Demetrulias, J., Driedger, A., Griffith, J. F., Grochoski, G. T., Kong, N., McCormick, W. C. 3rd, North-Root, H., Rozen, M. G., and Sedlak, R. I. (1989): The SDA alternatives program: Comparison of in vitro data with Draize test data. *J. Toxicol. Cutan. Ocul. Toxicol.*, 8:35–49.
41. Borenfreund, E., Babich, H., and Martin-Alguacil, N. (1988): Comparison of two in vitro cytotoxicity assays—The neutral red (NR) and tetrazolium MTT tests. *Toxicol. in Vitro*, 2:1–6.
42. Borenfreund, E., and Borrero, O. (1984): In vitro cytotoxicity assays: Potential alternatives to the Draize ocular irritancy test. *Cell Biol. Toxicol.*, 1:33–39.
43. Borenfreund, E., and Puerner, J. A. (1984): A simple quantitative procedure using monolayer culture for cytotoxicity assays (HTD/NR90). *J. Tissue Culture Meth.*, 9:7–9.
44. Borenfreund, E., and Puerner, J. A. (1985): Toxicity determined in vitro by morphological alterations and neutral red absorption. *Toxicol. Lett.*, 24:119–124.
45. Borenfreund, E., and Shopsis, C. (1984): Toxicity monitored with a correlated set of cell culture assays. *Xenobiotica*, 15:705–712.
46. Borenfreund, E., Shopsis, C., Barrero, O., and Sathe, S. (1983): In vitro alternative irritancy assays: Comparison of cytotoxic and membrane transport effects of alcohols. *Ann. NY Acad. Sci.*, 407:416–419.
47. Boue-Grabot, M., Bernardin, G., Chaumond, S., and Pinon, J. F. (1995): Alternative methods: Hen's egg chorioallantoic membrane and in vitro cytotoxicity—Complementary approach. *Int. J. Cosmet. Sci.*, 17:207–215.
48. Brantom, P. G., Bruner, L. H., Chamberlain, M., De Silva, O., Dupuis, J., Earl, L. K., Lovell, D. P., Pape, W. J. W., Uttley, et al. (1997): A summary report of the COLIPA international validation study on alternatives to the Draize rabbit eye irritation test. *Toxicol. in Vitro*, 11:141–179.
49. British Toxicology Society (1984): A new approval to classification of substances and preparations on the basis of their acute toxicology. *Human Toxicol.*, 3:85–92.
50. Bross, I. D. J. (1958): How to use RIDIT analysis. *Biometrics*, 14:18–38.
51. Brownlee, K. A., Hodges, J. L., and Rosenblatt, M. (1953): The up-and-down method with small samples. *J. Am. Stat. Assoc.*, 48:262–277.
52. Bruce, R. D. (1984): An up-and-down procdure for acute toxicity testing. In: *Acute Toxicity Testing: Alternative Approaches*, edited by A. M. Goldberg, p. 184. Mary Ann Leibert, New York.
53. Bruce, R. D. (1985): An up-and-down procedure for acute toxicity testing. *Fund. Appl. Toxicol.*, 5:151–157.
54. Bruce, R. D. (1987): A confirmatory study of the up-and-down method for acute toxicity testing. *Fund. Appl. Toxicol.*, 8:97–100.
55. Bruner, L. H., Carr, G. J., Chamberlain, M., and Curren, R. D. (1996): Validation of alternative methods for toxicity testing. *Toxicol. in Vitro*, 10:479–501.
56. Bruner, L. H., Carr, G. J., Chamberlain, M., and Curren, R. D. (1996): No prediction model, no validation study. *ATLA*, 24:139–142.
57. Bruner, L. H., Kain, D. J., Roberts, D. A., and Parker, R. D. (1991): Evaluation of seven in vitro alternatives for ocular safety testing. *Fund. Appl. Toxicol.*, 17:136–149.
58. Bruner, L. H., Miller K. R., Owicki, J. C., Paree, J. J. W., and Muir, V. C. (1991): Testing ocular irritancy in vitro with silicon microphysiometer. *Toxicol. in Vitro*, 5:277–284.
59. Bruner, L. H., Parker, R. D., and Bruce, R. D. (1992): Reducing the number of rabbits in the low-volume eye test. *Fund. Appl. Toxicol.*, 19:330–335.
60. Bruner, L. H., Shadduck, J., and Essex-Sorlie, D. (1991): Alternative methods for assessing the effects of chemicals in the eye. In: *Dermal and Ocular Toxicology: Fundamentals and Methods*, edited by D. W. Hobson. pp. 585–606. CRC Press. Boca Raton, FL.
61. Budai, P., Somlyay, I. M., Varnagy, L. E., and Varga, T. (1995): Comparison of in vitro (HET–CAM) and in vivo (Draize) irritation tests using different pesticides. *Meded Fac. Landbouwkd. Toegepaste Biol. Wetenschap Univ. Gent.*, 60:593–597.

62. Buehler, E. V. (1974): Testing to predict potential ocular hazards of household chemicals. In: *Toxicology Annual*, edited by C. L. Winek, pp. 53–69. Marcel Dekker, New York.
63. Buehler, E. V., and Newman, E. A. (1964): A comparison of eye irritation in monkeys and rabbits. *Toxicol. Appl. Pharmacol.*, 6:701–710.
64. Bulich, A. A., Tung, K. K., and Scheibner, G. (1990): The luminescent bacteria toxicity test: Its potential as an in vitro alternative. *J. Biolumin. Chemilumin.*, 5:71–77.
65. Burnstein, N. L. (1980): Corneal cytotoxicity of topically applied drugs, vehicles, and preservatives. *Surv. Ophthalmol.*, 25:15–30.
66. Burton, A. B. G. (1972): A method for the objective assessment of eye irritation. *Food Cosmet. Toxicol.*, 10:209–217.
67. Burton, A. B. G., York, M., and Lawrence, R. S. (1981): The in vitro assessment of severe eye irritant. *Food Cosmet. Toxicol.*, 19:471–480.
68. Calabrese, E. J. (1983): Ocular toxicity. In: *Principles of Animal Extrapolation*, p. 400. John Wiley, New York.
69. Casterton, P. L., Potts, L. F., and Klein, B. D. (1996): A novel approach to assessing eye irritation using the bovine corneal opacity and permeability assay. *J. Toxicol. Cutan. Ocul. Toxicol.*, 15:147–163.
70. Catroux, P., Rougier, A., Dossou, K. G., and Cottin, M. (1993): The silicon microphysiometer for testing ocular toxicity in vitro. *Toxicol. in Vitro*, 7:465–469.
71. Cello, R. M., and Lasmanis, J. (1958): *Pseudomonas* infection of the eye of the dog resulting from the use of contaminated fluorescein solution. *J. Am. Vet. Med. Assoc.*, 132:297.
72. Chan, K. Y. (1986): Chemical injury to an in vitro ocular system differential release of plasminogen activator. *Curr. Eye Res.*, 5:357–562.
73. Chan, P. K., and Hayes, A. W. (1985): Assessment of chemically induced ocular toxicity: A survey of methods. In: *Toxicology of the Eye, Ear and Other Special Senses*, edited by A. W. Hayes. Raven Press, New York.
74. Chan, T., Payor, S., and Holden, B. A. (1983): Corneal thickness profiles in rabbits using an ultrasonic pachymeter. *Invest. Ophthalmol. Vis. Sci.*, 24:1408–1410.
75. Chan-Ling, T., Tervo, K., Tervo, T., Vannas, A., Holden, B. A., and Eranko, L. (1987): Long-term neural degeneration in the rabbit following 180° limbal incision. *Invest. Ophthalmol. Vis. Sci.*, 28:2083–2088.
76. Chasin, M., Scott, C., Shaw, C., and Persico, F. (1979): A new assay for the measurement of mediator release from rat peritoneal mast cells. *Int. Srch. Allergy Appl. Immunol.*, 58:1–10.
77. Choi, S. C. (1971): An investigation of Wetherill's method of estimation for the up-and-down experiment. *Biometrics*, 27:961–970.
78. Clark, A. J. (1933): *Mode of Action of Drugs on Cells*. Williams and Wilkins, Baltimore.
79. Clothier, R. H., Hulme, L., Ahmed, A. B., Reeves, A. L., Smith, M., and Balls, M. (1988): In vitro cytotoxicity of 150 chemicals to 3T3-L1 cells, assessed by the FRAME Kenacid Blue method. *ATLA*, 16:84.
80. Cohen, I. J. (1983): Use of fluorescein in eye injuries. *J. Occup. Med.*, 5:540.
81. Conquet, P. H., Durand, G., Laillier, J., and Plazonnet, B. (1977): Evaluation of ocular irritation in the rabbit: Objective versus subjective assessment. *Toxicol. Appl. Pharmacol.*, 39:129–131.
82. Cornfield, J. (1964): Measurement and composition of toxicities: The quantal response. In: *Statistics and Mathematics in Biology*, edited by O. Kempthorne, T. A. Bancroft, J. W. Gowen and J. L. Lush, pp. 327–344. Hofner, New York.
83. Cottin, M., Dossou, K. G., DeSilva, O., Tolle, M., Roguet, R., Cohen, C., Catroux, P., Delabarre, I., Sicard, C., and Rougier, A. (1994): Relevance and reliability of in vitro methods in ocular safety assessment. *In Vitro Toxicol.*, 7:277–282.
84. Cottin, M., and Zanvit, A. (1997): Fluorescein leakage test: A useful tool in ocular safety assessment. *Toxicol. in Vitro*, 11:399–405.
85. Consumer Product Safety Commission (CPSC) (1976): Illustrated guide for grading eye irritation by hazardous substances. Directorate for Engineering and Science, Washington, D.C.
86. Cronin, M. T. (1996): The use of cluster significance analysis to identify asymmetric QSAR data sets in toxicology. An example with eye irritation data. *SAR QSAR Environ. Res.*, 5:167–175.
87. Cronin, M. T., Basketter, D. A., and York, M. A. (1994): Quantitative structure–activity relationship (QSAR) investigation of a Draize eye irritation database. *Toxicol. in Vitro*, 8:21–28.
88. Curren. R. D., Southee, J. A., Spielmann, H., Liebsch, M., Fentam, J. H., and Balls, M. (1995): The role of prevalidation in the development, validation and acceptance of alternative methods. *ATLA*, 23:211–217.
89. Davies, R. G., Kynoch, S. R., and Liggett, M. P. (1976): Eye irritation tests—An assessment of the maximum delay time for remedial irrigation. *J. Soc. Cosmet. Chem.*, 27:301–306.
90. Dawson, M., and Mustafa, A. F. (1985): Use of cultured human conjunctival and other cells to assess the relative toxicity of six local anesthetics. *Food Chem. Toxicol.*, 23:305–308.
91. Decker, D., Harper, R., and Rehfeldt, T. (1994): Evaluation of the Microtox system as a predictor of ocular irritancy of toiletry products. *In Vitro Toxicol.*, 7:83–88.
92. Decker, D., Stemp, M., and Harper, R. (1993): Evaluation of the Eytex system for use as a predictor of ocular irritancy: II Conditioners and styling aids. *J. Toxicol. Cutan. Ocul. Toxicol.*, 12:371–380.
93. DePass, L. R. (1989): Alternative approaches in median lethality (LD_{50}) and acute toxicity testing. *Toxicol. Lett.*, 49:159–170.
94. DeSousa, D. J., Rosue, A. A., and Smolon, W. J. (1984): Statistical consequences of reducing the number of rabbits utilized in eye irritation testing. Data on 67 petrochemicals. *Toxicol. Appl. Pharmacol.*, 76:234–242.
95. Dews, P. B., and Berkson, J. (1964): On the error of bioassay with quantal response. In: *Statistics and Mathematics in Biology*, edited by O. Kempthorne, T. A. Bancroft, J. W. Gowen, and J. L. Lush, pp. 361–370. Hofner, London.
96. Diem, K. (1968): *Documenta Geigy Scientic Tables*, 6th ed. Geigy Pharmaceutical Division, Geigy Chemical Corp., Ardsley, New York.
97. Dierickx, P. J. and Gordan, V. C. (1990): The EYTEX- system and the neutral red uptake inhibition assay in cultured Hep G2 cells as alternative methods for in vivo eye irritation following the EEC protocol. *ATLA*, 17:325–333.
98. Dixon, W. J. (1965): The up-and-down method for small samples. *J. Am. Stat. Assoc.*, 60:967–978.
99. Dixon, W. J., ed., (1981). BMDP Statistics Software. University of California Press, Berkeley.
100. Douglas, H. J., and Spillman, S. D. (1983): Product safety testing. In: *Alternative Methods in Toxicology. Vol. 1* pp. 205–230, edited by A. M. Goldberg. Mary Ann Liebert, New York.
101. Doull, J. (1980): Factors influencing toxicology. In: *Cassarett and Doull's Toxicology: The Basic Science of Poisons*, edited by J. Doull, C. D. Klaassen, and M. O. Amdur, pp. 70–83. Macmillan, New York.
102. Draize, J. H., Woodward, G., and Calvery, H. O. (1944): Methods for the study of irritation and toxicity of substances applied topically to the skin and mucous membranes. *J. Pharmacol. Exp. Ther.*, 82:377–390.
103. Dubin, N. H., Diblasi, M. C., Thomas, C. L., and Wolff, M. C. (1984): Development of an in vitro test for cytotoxicity in vaginal

tissue effect of ethanol on prostanoid release. In: *Alternative Methods in Toxicology, Vol. 2. Acute Toxicity Testing Alternative Approaches*, edited by A. M. Goldberg, pp. 127–137. Mary Ann Liebert, New York.

104. Dubin, N. H., Wolff, M. C., Thomas, C. L., and DiBlasi, M. C. (1985): Prostaglandin production by rat vaginal tissues in vitro in response to ethanol, a mild mucosal irritant. *Toxicol. Appl. Pharmacol.*, 78:458–463.
105. Dunnett, C. W. (1968): Biostatistics in pharmacological testing. In: *Selected Pharmacological Testing Methods*, edited by A. Burger, pp. 7–18. Edward Arnold, London.
106. Edelhauser, H. F., Gonnerings, R., and Van Horn, D. L. (1978): Intraocular irrigation solutions: A comparative study of BBS plus and lactated Ringer's solution. *Arch. Ophthalmol.*, 93:516.
107. Edelhauser, H. F., Van Horn, D. L., Hundink, R. A., and Schultz, R. O. (1975): Intraocular irrigating solutions: Their effect on the corneal endothelium. *Arch. Ophthalmol.*, 93:648.
108. Edelhauser, H. F., Van Horn, D. L., Schultz, R. O., and Hundink, R. A. (1976): Comparative toxicity of intraocular irrigating solution on the corneal endothelium. *Am. J. Ophthalmol.*, 81:473–481.
109. EEC (1983): Methods for the determination of toxicity. EEC Directive 79/831 Annex V, Part B. Brussels.
110. EEC (1992): Acute toxicity (eye irritation). EEC guideline for testing of chemicals No. B.5. Brussels.
111. Ehrlich, P. (1882): Uber provocirte flurescenzer-Scheinungen am Auge. *Dtsch. Med. Wochenschr.*, 2:21.
112. Ekwall, B. (1992): Features and prospects of the MEIC cytotoxicity evaluation project. *AATEX*, 1:231–237.
113. Ekwall, B. (1994): The basal cytotoxicity concept. In: *Alternative Methods in Toxicology and the Life Sciences, Vol. 11, The World Congress on Alternatives and Animal Use in the Life Sciences, Education, Research, Testing*, edited by A. M. Goldberg and A. F. M. van Zupthen. Mary Ann Liebert, New York.
114. Ekwall, B., Bondesson, I., Castell, J. V., Gomez-Lechon, M. J., Hellberg, S., Hogberg, J., Jover, R., Ponsoda, X., Romert, L., Stenberg, K., and Walum, E. (1989): Cytotoxicity evaluation of the first ten MEIC chemicals: acute lethal toxicity in man predicted by cytotoxicity in five cellular assays and by oral LD_{50} tests in rodents. *ATLA*, 17:83–100.
115. Ekwall, B., Clemedsen, C., Crafoord, B., Ekwall, B., Hallander, S., Walum, E., and Bondesson, I. (1998): MEIC evaluation of acute systemic toxicity. Part V: Rodent and human toxicity data for the 50 reference chemicals. *ATLA*, 26(Suppl. 2):571–616.
116. Ekwall, B., Walum, E., Clemedsen, C., Barile, F. A., Castano, A., Clothier, R. A., Dierickx, P., Ekwall, B., Ferro, M., Fiskesjo, G., Garza-Ocanas, L., Gomez-Lechon, M. J., Gulden, M., Hall, T., Isomaa, B., Kahru, A., Kerszman, G., Kristen, U., Kunimoto, M., Karenlampi, S., Lewan, L., Loukianov, A., Ohno, T., Persoone, G., Romert, L., Sawyer, T. W., Shrivastava, R., Segner, H., Stammati, A., Tanaka, N., Valentino, M., Walum, E., and Zucco, F. (1998): MEIC evaluation of acute systemic toxicity. Part IV: Prediction of human toxicity by rodent LD_{50} values and results from 61 in vitro tests. *ATLA*, 26(Suppl. 2):617–658.
117. Elgebaly, S. A., Gilles, C., Forouhar, F., Hashem, M., Baddour, M., O'Roucke, J., and Kreuter, D. L. (1988): An in vitro model of leukocyte mediated injury to the corneal epithelium. *Curr. Eye. Res.*, 7:403–410.
118. Elgebaly, S. A., Nabawi, K., Kerbert, N., O'Tourke, J., and Kruetzer, D. L. (1985): *Invest. Ophthalmol. Vis. Sci.*, 26:320.
119. Enslein, K. (1988): An overview of structure–activity relationships as an alternative to testing in animals for carcinogenicity, mutagenicity, dermal and eye irritation and acute oral toxicity. *Toxicol. Ind. Health*, 4:479–498.
120. EPA (1983): Pesticide programs: Good laboratory practice standards: Final rule. *Fed. Register*, 48(230):53945–53969, November 29.
121. EPA (1983): Toxic substance control: Good laboratory practice standards: Final rule. *Fed. Register*, 48(230):53921–53944, November 29.
122. EPA (1984): EPA fact sheet: Background on acute toxicity testing for chemical safety, August 1984.
123. EPA (1984): Data requirements for pesticide registration: Final rule. 40 CFR Part 158. *Fed. Register*, Oct. 24:42855–42905.
124. EPA/FIFRA (1982): Pesticide Assessment Guidelines. Subdivision F, Hazard evaluation: Human and domestic animals. PB83-153916. Office of Pesticide Programs. U.S. EPA. Reproduced by the National Technical information Service, U.S. Department of Commerce, Springfield, VA.
125. EPA/TSCA (1984): Health effects test guidelines. PB84 Office of Pesticides and Toxic Substances, U.S. EPA. Reproduced by NTIS, U.S. Department of Commerce, Springfield, VA.
126. EPA/OPPTS (1998): Health effects test guidelines. Acute eye irritation. 870.2400. Office of Prevention, Pesticides and Toxic Substances. U.S. EPA, Washington, D.C.
127. Ernst, R., and Ardetti, J. (1980): Biological effects of surfactants IV. Effects of non-ionic and amphoterics on Hela cells. *Toxicology*, 15:233.
128. Esperson, R. J., Olsen, P., Nicolaisen, G. M., Jensen, B. L., and Rasmussen, E. S. (1997): Assessment of recovery from ocular irritancy using a human tissue equivalent model. *Toxicol. in Vitro*, 11:81–88.
129. Essepian, J. P., Rajpal, R. K., Azar, D. T., New, K., Antonacci, R., Shields, W., and Stark, W. (1994): The use of confocal microscopy in evaluating corneal wound healing after eximer laser surgery. *Scanning*, 16:300–304.
130. Eurell, T. E., and Meacham, S. H. (1994): In vitro evaluation of ocular irritants using tissue isoelectric focusing protein profiles from human, rabbit, and bovine corneal specimens. *Toxicol. Methods*, 4:66–75.
131. FDA (1976): Illustrated guide for grading eye irritation by hazardous substances. FDA, Washington, D.C.
132. FDA (1983): Final report on acute studies workshop. Sponsored by the U.S. Food and Drug Administration on November 9, 1983.
133. *Federal Register* (1980): 45:33063, May 19.
134. Fentem, J. H., Prinsen, M. K., Spielmann, H., Walum, E., and Botham, P. A. (1995): Validation-lessons learned from practical experience. *Toxicol. in Vitro*, 9:857–862.
135. Ferdinard, W. (1976): *The Enzyme Molecule*. John Wiley, New York.
136. FHSA (1979): Regulations under the Federal Hazardous Substance Act. Chapter 11. Title 16. Code of Federal Regulations.
137. Fine, B. S., and Yanoff, M. (1972): *Ocular Histology: A Text and Atlas*. Harper and Row, New York.
138. Finney, D. J. (1971): *Probit Analysis*, 3rd ed. Chapters 3 and 4, Cambridge University Press, Cambridge, United Kingdom.
139. Fisher, R. A., and Yates, F. (1963): *Statistical Tables for Biological, Agricultural and Medical Research*, 6th ed., edited by Oliver and Boyd Ltd., Edinburgh, Scotland.
140. Floyd, E. P., and Stockinger, H. G. (1958): Toxicity studies of certain organic peroxides and hydroperoxides. *Am. Ind. Hyg. Assoc. J.*, 19:205–212.
141. Frazier, J. M. (1990): OECD environment monograph no. 36: Scientific criteria for validation of in vitro toxicology tests. OECD, Paris.
142. Fraizer, J. M. (1990): Validation of in vitro models. *J. Am. Coll. Toxicol.*, 9:355–359.

143. Fraizer, J. M. (1992): Validation of in vitro toxicity tests. In: *In Vitro Toxicity Testing: Applications to Safety Evaluations*, edited by J. M. Frazier. Marcel Dekker, New York.
144. Frazier, J. M. (1994): The role of mechanistic toxicology in test methods validation. *Toxicol. in Vitro*, 8:787–791.
145. Frazier, J. M. (1995): Interdisciplinary approach to toxicity test development and validation. *Toxicol. in Vitro*, 9:8925–8949.
146. Frazier, J. M., Gad, S. C., Goldberg, A. M., and MaCulley, J. P. (1987): A critical evaluation of alternatives to acute irritation testing. In: *Alternative Methods in Toxicology, Vol. 4*, edited by J. M. Frazier, S. C. Gad, A. M. Goldberg, and J. P. MaCulley. Mary Ann Liebert, New York.
147. Freeberg, F. E., Griffith, J. F., Bruce, R. D., and Bay, P. H. S. (1984): Correlation of animal test methods with human experience for household products. *J. Toxicol. Cutan. Ocul. Toxicol.*, 1(3):53.
148. Friedenwald, J. S., Hughes, W. F., and Hermann, H. (1944): Acid-base tolerance of the cornea. *Arch. Ophthalmol.*, 31:279–283.
149. Fulcher, S., Foulks, G. N., Wilkerson, M., Cobo, L. M., Houston, L. L., and Hatchell, D. (1993): Suppression of human corneal epithelial proliferation with breast carcinoma immunotoxin. *Cornea*, 12:391–396.
150. Gabourel, J. D., Bradley, J. M. B., and Acott, T. S. (1990): Antagonism of retinol-induced RNA synthesis: Assessment of retinoid toxicity in cultured retinal pigment epithelium. *J. Toxicol. Cutan. Ocul. Toxicol.*, 9:251–263.
151. Gad, S. C., Smith, A. C., Cramp, A. L., Gavigan, F. A., and Derelanko, M. J. (1984): Innovative designs and practices for acute systemic toxicity studies. *Drug Chem. Toxicol.*, 7:423–434.
152. Gaddum, J. H. (1983): Reports on biological standards III. Methods of biological assay depending on a quantal response. *Spec. Rep. Ser. Med. Res.*, No. 813, London.
153. Gaunt, I. F., and Harper, K. H. (1964): The potential irritancy to rabbit eye mucosa of certain commercially available shampoos. *J. Soc. Cosmet. Chem.*, 15:209–230.
154. Gautheron, P., Dukic, M., Alix, D., and Sina, J. (1992): Bovine corneal opacity and permeability test: An in vitro assay of ocular irritancy. *Fund. Appl. Toxicol.*, 18:442–449.
155. Gautheron, P., Giroux, J., Cottin, M., Audegond, L., Morilla, A., Mayordomo-Blanco, L., Tortajada, A., Haynes, G., Vericat, J. A., Pirovano, R., Gillio Tos, E., Hagemann, C., Vanparys, P., Deknudt, G., Jacobs, G., Prinsen, M., Kalweit, S., and Spielmann, H. (1994): Interlaboratory assessment of the bovine corneal opacity and permeability (BCOP) assay. *Toxicol. in Vitro*, 8:381–392.
156. Geppetti, P., Del Bianco, E., Cecconi, R., Tramontana, M., Romani, A., and Theodorsson, E. (1992): Capsaicin releases calcitonin gene-regulated peptide from the human iris and ciliary body in vitro. *Regul. Pept.*, 41:83–92.
157. Gettings, S. D. (1991): The current status of in vitro test validation (evaluation) in the United States. *ATLA*, 19:432–436.
158. Gettings, S. D., DiPasquale, L. C., Bagley, D. M., Casterton, P. L., Chudkowski, M., Curren, R. D., Demetrulias, J. L., Feder, P. I., Galli, C. L., Gay, R., Glaza, S. M., Hintze, K. L., Janus, J., Kurtz, P. J., Lordo, R. A., Marenus, K. D., Moral, J., Muscatiello, M., Pape, W. J. W., Renskers, K. J., Roddy, M. T., and Rozen, M. G. (1994): The CTFA evaluation of alternatives program: An evaluation of in vitro alternatives to the Draize primary eye irritation test. (Phase II) oil/water emulsions. *Food Chem. Toxicol.*, 32:943–976.
159. Gettings, S. D., Lordo, R. A., Hintze, K. L,. Bagley, D. M., Casterton, P. L., Chudkowski, M., Curren, R. D., Demetrulias, J. L., DiPasquale, L. C., Earl, L. K., Feder, P. I., Galli, C. L., Glaza, S. M., Gordon, V. C., Janus, J., Kurtz, P. J., Marenus, K. D., Moral, J., Pape, W. J. W., Renskers, K. J., Rheins, L. A., Roddy, M. T., Rozen, M. G., Tedeschi, J. P., and Zyracki, J. (1996): The CTFA Evaluation of Alternatives Program: An evaluation of potential in vitro alternatives to the Draize primary eye irritation test. (Phase III) Surfactant-based formulations. *Food Chem. Toxicol.*, 34:79–117.
160. Gettings, S. D., and McEwen, Jr., G. N. (1990): Development of potential alternatives to the Draize eye test: The CTFA evaluation of alternatives program. *ATLA*, 17:317–324
161. Gettings, S. D., Teal, J. J., Bagley, D. M., Demetrulias, J. L., Dipasquale, L. C., Hintze, K. L., Rozen, M. G., Weise, S. L., Chudkowski, M., Marenus K. D., Pape, J. W., Roddy, M. T., Schnetzinger, R., Silber, P. M., Glaza, S. M., and Kurtz, P. J. (1991): The CTFA Evaluation of Alternatives Program: An evaluation of in vitro alternatives to the Draize primary eye irritation test (Phase 1) hydroalcoholic, formulations: (Part 2) Data analysis and biological significance. *In Vitro Toxicol.*, 4:247–288.
162. Giasson, C., and Forthomme, D. (1992): Comparison of central corneal thickness measurements between optical and ultrasound pachymeters. *Optom. Vis. Sci.*, 69:236–241.
163. Gilleron, L., Coecke, S., Sysmans, M., Hansen, E., Van Oproy, S., Marzin, D., Van Cauteren, H., and Vanparys, P. (1996): Evaluation of a modified HET–CAM assay as a screening test for eye irritancy. *Toxicol. in Vitro*, 10:431–446.
164. Gilleron, L., Coecke, S., Sysmans, M., Hansen, E., Van Oproy, S., Marzin, D., Van Cauteren, H., and Vanparys, P. (1997): Evaluation of the HET–CAM–TSA method as an alternative to the Draize eye irritation test. *Toxicol. in Vitro*, 11:641–644.
165. Giovacchini, R. P. (1972): Old and new issues in the safety evaluation of cosmetics and toiletries. *CRC Crit. Rev. Toxicol.*, 1:361–378.
166. Goldberg, A. M., Frazier, J. M., Brusick, D., Dickens, M. S., Flint, O., Gettings, S. D., Hill R. N., Lipnick, R. L., Renskers, K. J., Bradlaw, J. A., et al. (1993): Framework for validation and implementation of in vitro toxicity tests. *In Vitro Cell. Dev. Biol.*, 29A:688–692.
167. Goldberg, A. M., Epstein, L. D., and Zurlo, J. (1995): A modular approach to validation: A work in progress. *In Vitro Toxicol.*, 8:431–435.
168. Gordon, V. C., and Bergman, H. C. (1987): EYTEX: An in vitro method for evaluation of ocular irritancy. In: *Alternative Methods in Toxicology, Vol. 5, Approaches to Validation*, edited by A. M. Goldberg, pp. 293–302. Mary Ann Liebert, New York,
169. Gordon, V. C., and Kelly, C. P. (1989): An in vitro method for determining ocular irritation. *Cosmet. Toilet.*, 104:69–73.
170. Grant, W. M. (1974): *Toxicology of the Eye*, 2nd ed. Charles C. Thomas, Springfield, Illinois.
171. Green, W. R., Sullivan, J. B., Hehir, R. M., et al. (1978): A systematic comparison of chemically-induced injury in the albino rabbit and rhesus monkey. Soap and Detergent Association, New York.
172. Griffith, J. F., Nixon, G. A., Bruce, R. D., et al. (1980): Dose-response studies with chemical irritants in the albino rabbit eye as a basis for selecting optimum testing conditions for predicting hazard to human eye. *Toxicol. Appl. Pharmacol.*, 55:501–513.
173. Guillot, J., Gonnet, J. F., and Clement, C. (1982): Evaluation of the ocular irritation potential of 56 compounds. *Food Chem. Toxicol.*, 20:573–582.
174. Gunderson T., and Liebman, S. D. (1944): Effect of local anesthetics on regeneration of corneal epithelium. *Arch. Ophthalmol.*, 31:29–33.
175. Gupta, K. C., Chambers, W. A., Green, S., Hill, R. N., Hurley, P. M., Lambert, L. A., Liu, P. T., Lowther, D. K., Seabaugh, V. M., Springer, J. A., and Wilcox, N. L. (1993): An eye irritation test protocol and an evaluation and classification system. *Food Chem. Toxicol.*, 31:117–121.

176. Gurland, J., Lee, L., and Dahm, P. A. (1960): Polychotomous quantal response in biological assay. *Biometrics*, 16:382–398.
177. Hafeman, D. G., Parce, W. J., and McConnell, H. M. (1988): Light addressable potentiometric sensor for biochemical system. *Science*, 240:1182–1185.
178. Harriton, L. (1981): Conversation with Henry Spira: Draize test activist. *Lab. Anim.*, 10:16–22.
179. Hedbys, R. O., and Mishima, S. (1966): The thickness–hydration relationship of the cornea. *Exp. Eye Res.*, 5:221–228.
180. Henkes, H., and Canta, L. R. (1973): Drug-induced disorders of the eye. In: *Proceedings of the European Society for the Study of Drug Toxicity*, edited by W. A. M. Duncan, pp. 146–153. Elsevier, North-Holland, New York.
181. Heywood, R., and James, R. W. (1978): Towards objectivity in the assessment of eye irritation. *J. Soc. Cosmet. Chem.*, 29:25–29.
182. Hitzenberger, C. K., Drexler, W., and Fercher, A. F. (1992): Measurement of corneal thickness by laser doppler interferometry. *Invest. Ophthalmol. Vis. Sci.*, 33:98–103.
183. Holland, M. C. (1964): Fluorescein staining of the cornea. *JAMA*, 188:81.
184. Hull, D. S. (1979): Effects of epinephrine, benzalkonium chloride, and intraocular miotics on corneal endothelium. *S. Afr. Med. J.*, 2:1390–1381.
185. Hurley, P. M., Chambers, W. A., Green, S., Gupta, K. C., Hill, R. N., Lambert, L. A., Lee, C. C., Lee, J. K., Liu, P. T., Lowther, D. K., Roberts, C. D., Seabaugh, V. M., Springer, J. A., and Wilcox, N. L. (1993): Screening procedures for eye irritation. *Food Chem. Toxicol.*, 31:87–94.
186. Igarashi, H. (1987): The opacification of bovine isolated cornea by surfactants and other chemicals: A process of protein denaturation. *ATLA*, 15:8–19.
187. Igarashi, H., Katsuta, Y., Matsuno, H., Nakazato, Y., and Kawasaki, T. (1989): Carbachol-induced opacity of porcine isolated corneas. *ATLA*, 16:322–330.
188. Igarashi, H., Katsuta, Y., Matsuno, H., Nakazato, Y., and Kawasaki, T. (1989): Opacification test by using pig isolated cornea and its application to a test of corneal opacity induced by befunolol hydrochloride. *J. Toxicol. Sci.*, 14:91–103.
189. Igarashi, H., Katsuta, Y., Nakazato, Y., and Kawasaki, T. (1991): The opacifying effects of carteolol HCI and benzalkonium chloride on porcine isolated corneas. *ATLA*, 19:344–351.
190. Igarashi, H., and Northover, A. M. (1987): Increase in opacity and thickness induced by surfactants and other chemicals in the bovine isolated cornea. *Toxicol. Lett.*, 39(2–3):249–254.
191. Immonen, I., Siren, V., Stephens, R. W., Lietso, K., and Vaheri, A. (1993): Retinoids increase urokinase-type plasminogen activator production by human retinal pigment epithelial cells in culture. *Invest. Ophthalmol. Vis. Sci.*, 34:2062–2067.
192. IRLG (Interagency Regulatory Liaison Group) (1981): Recommended guidelines for acute eye irritation test.
193. Jacaruso, R. B., Bartlett, M. A., Carson, S., and Trombetta, L. D. D. (1985): Release of histamine from rat peritoneal cells as an in vitro index of irritation potential. *J. Toxicol. Cutan. Ocul. Toxicol.*, 4:39–48.
194. Jackson, J., and Rutty, D. A. (1985): Ocular tolerance assessment-integrated tier policy. *Food Chem. Toxicol.*, 23: 309–310.
195. Jester, J. V., Li, H., Petroll, W. M., Parker, R. D., Cavanagh, H. D., Carr, G. J., Smith, B., and Maurer, J. K. (1998): Area and depth of surfactant-induced corneal injury correlates with cell death. *Invest. Ophthalmol. Vis. Sci.*, 39:922–936.
196. Jester, J. V., Petroll, W. M., Garana, R. M. R., Lemp, M. A., and Cavanagh, H. D. (1992): Comparison of in vivo and ex vivo cellular structure in rabbit eyes detected by scanning confocal microscopy. *J. Microsc.*, 165:169–181.
197. Jumblatt, M. M., Fogle, J. A., and Neufeld, A. H. (1980): Cholera toxin stimulates adenosine 3′5′-monophosphate synthesis and epithelial wound closure in the rabbit cornea. *Invest. Ophthalmol. Vis. Sci.*, 19:1321–1329.
198. Jumblatt, M. M., and Neufeld, A. H. (1981): Characterization of cyclic AMP-mediated wound closure of the rabbit corneal epithelium. *Curr. Eye Res.*, 1:189–195.
199. Kahn, C. R., Young, E., Lee, I. H., and Rhim, J. S. (1993): Human corneal epithelial primary cultures and cell lines with extended life span. *Invest. Ophthalmol. Vis. Sci.*, 34:3429–3441.
200. Kalweit, S., Gerner, I., and Spielmann, H. (1987): Validation project of alternatives for the Draize eye test. *Mol. Toxicol.*, 1:579–603.
201. Kappler, R. and Kristen, U. (1987): Photometric quantitation of in vitro pollen tube growth: A new method suited to determine the cytotoxicity of various environmental substances. *Environ. Exp. Bot.*, 27:305–309.
202. Kay, J. H. and Calandra, J. C. (1962): Interpretation of eye irritation tests. *J. Soc. Cosmet. Chem.*, 13:281–289.
203. Kaye, G. I., and Tice, L. W. (1966): Studies on the cornea. V Electron microscopic localization of adenosine triphosphatase activity in the rabbit cornea in relation to transport. *Invest. Ophthalmol.*, 5:22–32.
204. Kemp, R. B., Cross D. M., and Meredith R. W. J. (1986): Adenosine triphosphate as an indicator of cellular toxicity. *Food Chem. Toxicol.*, 24:465–466.
205. Kemp, R. B., Meredith , R. W., and Gamble, S. H. (1985): Toxicity of commercial products on cells in suspension culture: A possible screen for the Draize eye irritation test. *Food Chem. Toxicol.*, 23:267–270.
206. Kemp, R. B., Meredith, R. W., Gamble, S., and Frost, M. (1983): A rapid cell culture technique for assessing the toxicity of detergent-based products in vitro as a possible screen for eye irritancy in vivo. *Cytobios*, 36:153.
207. Kennah, H. E., Hignet, S., Laux, P. E., Dorko, J. D., and Barrow, C. S. (1989): An objective procedure for quantitating eye irritation based on changes in corneal thickness. *Fundam. Appl. Toxicol.*, 12:258–268.
208. Kennedy, G. L., Jr., Ferenz, R., and Burgess, B. A. (1986): Estimation of acute oral toxicity in rats by determination of the approximate lethal dose rather than the LD_{50}. *J. Appl. Toxicol.*, 6:145–148.
209. Khaw, P. T., Sherwood, M. B., MacKay, S. L. D., Rossi, M. J., and Shultz, G. (1992): Five-minute treatments with fluorouracil, floxuridine, and mitomycin have long-term effects on human tendon's capsule fibroblasts. *Arch. Ophthalmol.*, 110:1150–1154.
210. Kimura, S. J. (1951): Fluorescein paper: Simple means of insuring use of sterile fluorescein. *Am. J. Ophthalmol.*, 34:466.
211. Knox, P., Uphill, P. F., Fry, J. R., Benford, J., and Balls, M. (1986): The FRAME multicentre project on cytotoxicology. *Food Chem. Toxicol.*, 24:457–463.
212. Kong, B. M., Viau, C. J., Rizvi, P. Y., and DeSalva, S. J. (1987): The development and evaluation of the chlorioallantoic membrane (CAM) assay. In: *Alternative Methods in Toxicology, Vol. 5, Approach to Validation*, edited by A. M. Goldberg, pp. 59–73. Mary Ann Liebert, New York.
213. Kristen, U., Hoppe, U., and Pape, W. (1993): The pollen tube growth test: A new alternative to the Draize eye irritation test. *J. Soc. Cosmet. Chem.*, 44:153–162.
214. Kruszewski, F. H. (1998): Human cells as in vitro alternatives for ocular toxicity studies. *Comm. Toxicol.*, 6:221–233.
215. Kruszewski, F. H., Walker, T. L., and DiPasquale, L. C. (1997): Evaluation of a human corneal epithelial cell line as an in vitro model for assessing ocular irritation. *Fundam. Appl. Toxicol.*, 36:130–140.

216. Kuhlman, R. E. (1959): Species variation in the enzyme content of corneal epithelium. *J. Cell. Comp. Physiol.*, 53:313–326.
217. Kuijpers, M. H. M., and Walvoort, H. C. (1991): Discomfort and distress in rodents during chronic studies. In: *Animals in Biomedical Research*, edited by C. F. M. Hendriksen and H. W. B. M. Koeter, pp. 281–285. Elsevier, Amsterdam.
218. Lawrence, R. S., Groom, M. H., Ackroyd, D. M., and Parish, W. E. (1986). The chorioallantoic membrane in irritation testing. *Food Chem. Toxicol.*, 24:497–502.
219. Lee, D. A., Shapourifar-Tehrani, S., Stephenson, T. R., and Kitada, S. (1991): The effects of fluorinated pyrimidines FUR, FudR, FUMP, and FdUMP on human tendon's fibroblasts. *Invest. Ophthalmol. Vis. Sci.*, 32:2599–2609.
220. Leighton. J., Nassaurer, J., and Tehoa, R. (1985): The chick embryo in toxicology, An alternative to the rabbit eye. *Food Chem. Toxicol.*, 23:293–298.
221. Leupke, N. P. (1985): Hen's egg chorioallantoic membrane test for irritation potential. *Food Chem. Toxicol.*, 23:287–291.
222. Li, L., and Hoffman, R. M. (1991): Eye tissues grown in 3-dimensional histoculture for toxicological studies. *J. Cell. Pharmacol.*, 2:311–316.
223. Lieberman, H. R. (1983): Estimating LD_{50} using the probit technique: A basic computer program. *Drug Chem. Toxicol.*, 6:111–116.
224. Ling, T., Ho, A., and Holden, B. A. (1986): Method of evaluating ultrasonic pachymeters. *Am. J. Optom. Physiol Optics*, 63:462–466.
225. Lipnick, R. L., Cotruvo, J. A., Hill, R. N., Bruce, R. D., Stitzel, K. A., Walker, A. P., Chu, I., Goddard, M., Segal, L., Springer, J. A., and Myers, R. C. (1995): Comparison of the up-and-down, conventional LD_{50}, and fixed dose acute toxicity procedures. *Food Chem. Toxicol.*, 33:223–231.
226. Litchfield, J. T., and Wilcoxon, F. (1949): A simplified method of evaluating dose–effect experiments. *J. Pharmacol. Exp. Ther.*, 96:99–115.
227. Lorke, D. (1983): A new approach to practical toxicity testing. *Arch. Toxicol.*, 54:275–287.
228. Maeda, K., and Sakagudin, K. (1965): Studies on sodium–potassium-activated adenosine triphosphatase in the cornea. Electron-microscopic observations on the rat cornea. *Jpn. J. Ophthalmol.*, 9:195–199.
229. Martin, S. A., Roy, T. A., Saladdin, K. A., Fleming, B. A., and Mackerer, C. R. (1994): Safety evaluation of petroleum products using an in vitro eye irritation test battery. *Toxicol. in Vitro*, 8:715–717.
230. Martins, T., Pauluhn, J., and Machemer, L. (1992): Analysis of alternative methods for determining ocular irritation. *Food Chem. Toxic.*, 30:1061–1067.
231. Marzulli, F. N. (1965): New data on eye and skin tests. *Toxicol. Appl. Pharmacol.*, 7:79–85.
232. Marzulli, F. N., and Simmon, M. E. (1971): Eye irritation from topically applied drugs and cosmetics: Preclinical studies. *Am. J. Optom.*, 48:61–79.
233. Masters, B., and Paddock, S. (1990): In vitro confocal imaging of the rabbit cornea. *J. Micros.*, 158:267–274.
234. Mauer, J. K., Li, H., Petroll, W. M., Parker, R. D., Cavanagh, H. D., and Jester, J. V. (1997): Confocal microscopic characterization of initial corneal changes of surfactant-induced eye irritation in the rabbit. *Toxicol. Appl. Pharmacol.*, 143:291–300.
235. Maurice, D. M. (1967): The use of fluorescein in ophthalmological research. *Invest. Ophthalmol.*, 6:465–477.
236. Maurice, D. M., and Giardini, A. A. (1951): A simple optical apparatus for measuring the corneal thickness, and the average thickness of the human cornea. *Br. J. Ophthalmol.*, 35:169–177.
237. Maurice, D. M., and Singh, T. (1986): A permeability test for acute corneal toxicity. *Toxicol. Lett.*, 31:125–130.
238. McCaa, C. S. (1985): Anatomy, physiology and toxicology of the eye. In: *Toxicology of the Eye, Ear, and Other Special Senses*, edited by A. Wallace Hayes, pp. 1–15. Raven Press, New York.
239. McDonald, T. O., Baldwin, H. A., and Beasley, C. H. (1973): Slit-lamp examination of experimental animal eyes. I. Techniques of illumination and the normal eye. *J. Soc. Cosmet. Chem.*, 24:163–180.
240. Mehlman, M. A., Pfitzer, E. A., and Scala, R. A. (1989): A report on methods to reduce, refine, and replace animal testing in industrial toxicology laboratories. *Cell Biol. Toxicol.*, 5:349–357.
241. Meier-Ruge, W. (1973): Eye toxicity. In: *Proceedings of the European Society for the Study of Drug Toxicity, Vol. 14*, edited by W. A. M. Duncan, pp. 133–145. Elsevier, North Holland, New York.
242. Miller, L. C. (1964): The quantal response in toxicity tests. In: *Statistics and Mathematics in Biology*, edited by O. Kempthorne, T. A. Bancroft, J. W. Gowen, and J. L. Lush, pp. 315–326. Hofner, New York.
243. Millodot, M., Lim, C. H., and Ruskell, G. L. (1978): A comparison of corneal sensitivity and nerve density in albino and pigmented rabbits. *Ophthal. Res.*, 307.
244. Minsky, M. (1988): Memoir on inventing the confocal scanning microscope. *Scanning*, 10:128–138.
245. Minsky, M. (1961): U.S. patent no. 30313467. Microscopy Apparatus. December 19, 1961.
246. Mishima, S. (1981): Clinical pharmacokinetics of the eye. *Invest. Ophthalmol. Vis. Sci.*, 21:504.
247. Mishima, S., and Hedbys, B. O. (1968): Measurement of corneal thickness with the Haag–Streit pachometer. *Arch. Ophthalmol.*, 80:710–713.
248. Mishima, S., and Kudo, T. (1967): In vitro incubation of rabbit cornea. *Invest. Ophthalmol. Vis. Sci.*, 6:329–339.
249. Mishima, S., and Maurice, D. M. (1971): In vivo determination of the endothelial permeability to fluorescein. *Acta Soc. Ophthalmol. (Japan)*, 765:236–243.
250. Moller-Pedersen, T., Li, H. F., Petroll, W. M., Cavanagh, H. D., and Jester, J. V. (1998): Confocal microscopic characterization of wound repair after photorefractive keratectomy. *Invest. Ophthalmol. Vis. Sci.*, 39:487–501.
251. Morgan, R. L., Sorenson, S. S., and Castles, T. R. (1987): Prediction of ocular irritation by corneal pachymetry. *Food Chem. Toxicol.*, 25:609–613.
252. Morton, D. B. (1995): The post-operative care of small experimental animals and the assessment of pain by score sheets. In: *Proceedings of Animals in Science Conference Perspective on their Use, Care and Welfare*, edited by N. E. Johnston, pp. 82–87. Monash University, Victoria, Australia.
253. Morton, D. B. (1997): A scheme for the recognition and assessment of adverse effects. In: *Animal Alternatives, Welfare and Ethics*, edited by L. F. M. van Zutphen and M. Balls, pp. 235–241. Elsevier, Amsterdam.
254. Morton, D. B., Burghardt, G., and Smith, J. A. (1990): Critical anthropomorphism, animal suffering and the ecological context. *Science and Ethics*, 20:13–19.
255. Morton D. B., and Griffiths, P. H. M. (1985): Guidelines on the recognition of pain, distress and discomfort in experimental animals and an hypothesis for assessment. *Veterinary Record*, 116:431–436.
256. Morton, D. B., and Townsend, P. (1995): Dealing with adverse effects and suffering during animal research. In: *Laboratory Animals an Introduction for Experimenters*, edited by A. A. Tuffery, pp. 215–231. John Wiley & Sons, Ltd., Chichester, United Kingdom.

257. Moses, R. A., Parkinson, G., and Schuchardt, R. (1979): A standard large wound of the corneal epithelium in rabbits. *Invest. Ophthalmol. Vis. Sci.*, 18:103–106.

258. Muir, C. K. (1983): The toxic effect of some industrial chemicals on rabbit ileum in vitro compared with eye irritancy in vivo. *Toxicol. Lett.*, 19:309.

259. Muir, C. K. (1984): A simple method to assess surfactant-induced bovine corneal opacity in vitro: Preliminary findings. *Toxicol. Lett.*, 22:199–203.

260. Muir, C. K. (1985): Opacity of bovine cornea in vitro induced by surfactants and industrial chemicals compared with ocular irritancy in vivo. *Toxicol. Lett.*, 24:157–162.

261. Muir, C. K., Flower, C., and Van Abbe, N. J. (1983): A novel approach to the search for in vitro alternatives to in vivo eye irritancy testing. *Toxicol. Lett.*, 18:1–5.

262. Muller, H., and Kley, H. P. (1982): Retrospective study on the reliability of an "approximate LD_{50}" determined with a small number of animals. *Arch. Toxicol.*, 51:189–196.

263. Myers, R. C., Ballentyne, B., Christopher, S. M., and Chun, J. S. (1998): Comparative evaluation of several methods and conditions for the in vivo measurement of corneal thickness in rabbits and rats. *Toxicol. Meth.*, 8:219–231.

264. Nagy, Z. Z., Suveges, I., and Nemeth, J. (1995–1996): Interoperative pachymetry during eximer photorefractive keratectomy. *Acta Chir. Hung.*, 35:217–223.

265. Nakajima, A., Kimura, T., and Yamazaki, M. (1967): Applications of ultrasound in biometry of the eye. In: *Ultrasonics in Ophthalmology Diagnostic and Therapeutic Applications*, edited by R. E. Goldberg and L. K. Sarin, pp. 124–144. W. B. Saunders, Philadelphia.

266. Nardone, R. M. (1989): The LD_{50} test and in vitro toxicology strategies. *Acta Pharmacol. Toxicol.* (*Copenhagen*), 52(Suppl 2):65–79.

267. NAS Committee for Revision of NAS Publication 1138 (1977): Dermal and eye toxicity tests. In: *Principles and Procedures for Evaluating the Toxicity of Household Substances*, pp. 41–54. National Academy of Sciences, Washington, D.C.

268. Nguyen, K. D., and Lee, D. A. (1993): In vitro evaluation of antiproliferative potential of topical cyclo-oxygenase inhibitors in human tendon's fibroblasts. *Exp Eye Res.*, 57:97–105.

269. NIEHS. (1997): Validation and regulatory acceptance of toxicological test methods: A report of the ad hoc Interagency Coordinating Committee on the Validation of Alternative Methods. NIH Publ. No. 97-3981. Research Triangle Park, North Carolina.

270. North-Root, H., Yackovich, F., Demetrulias, J., Gacula, M., Jr., and Heinze, J. E. (1982): Evaluation of an in vitro cell toxicity test using rabbit corneal cells to predict the eye irritation potential of surfactants. *Toxicol. Lett.*, 14:207–212.

271. North-Root, H., Yackovich, F., Demetrulias, J., Gacula, M., Jr., and Heinze, J. E. (1985): Prediction of the eye irritation potential of shampoo using the in vitro SIRC cell toxicity test. *Food Chem. Toxicol.*, 23:271–273.

272. Nover, A., and Glanschneider, D. (1965): Untersuchungen uber die fortpflanzungsgeschwindigkeit und absorptiondes ultraschalls im Gewebe. Experimentelle beitrage zur ultraschalldiagnostik intraocular tumoren. *Albtecht von Graefes Arch. Klin. Exp. Ophthamol.*, 168:304–321.

273. OECD (1984): Data interpretation guides for initial hazard assessment of chemicals. OECD, Paris.

274. OECD (1996): Final report of the OECD workshop on harmonization of validation and acceptance criteria for alternative toxicological test methods. ENV/MC/CHEM/TG(96)9. OECD, Paris.

275. OECD (1981): OECD guidelines for testing of chemicals. OECD, Paris.

276. OECD (1987): OECD guideline for testing of chemicals. Guideline 405: Acute eye irritation/corrosion. OECD, Paris.

277. OECD (1992): OECD guideline for testing of chemicals. Guideline 420: Acute oral toxicity—Fixed dose method. OECD, Paris.

278. OECD (1996): OECD guideline for testing of chemicals. Guideline 423: Acute oral toxicity—Acute toxic class method. OECD, Paris.

279. OECD (1998): OECD guideline for testing of chemicals. Guideline 425: Acute oral toxicity—Up and down procedure. OECD, Paris.

280. OECD (1999): OECD series on testing and assessment. Detailed review on classification systems for eye irritation/corrosion in OECD member countries. ENV/JM/MONO(99)4. OECD, Paris.

281. OECD Test Guidelines (1981): Decision of the council concerning mutual acceptance of data in the assessment of chemicals. Annex 2. OECD Principles of Good Laboratory Practices. OECD, Paris.

282. Ohno, Y., Kaneko, T., Kobayaashi, T., Inoue, T., Kuroiwa, Y., Yoshida, T., Momma, J., Hayashi, M., Akiyama, J., Atsumi, T., Chiba, K., Endo, T., Fujii, A., Kakishima, H., Kojima, H., Masamoto, K., Masuda, M., Matsukawa, S., Ohkoshi, K., Okada, J., Sakamoto, K., Takano, K., and Tanaka, A. (1994): First-phase validation of the in vitro eye irritation tests for cosmetic ingredients. *In Vitro Toxicol.*, 7:89–94.

283. Oksala, A., and Lehtinen, A. (1958): Measurement of the velocity of sound in some parts of the eye. *Acta Ophthalmologica*, 36:633–639.

284. Oliver, G. J. A., and Pemberton, M. A. (1985): An in vitro epidermal slice technique for identifying chemicals with potential for severe cutaneous effects. *Food Chem. Toxicol.*, 23:229–232.

285. Olson, K. J., Dupree, R. W., Plomer, E. T., and Rerve, V. (1962): Toxicological properties of several commercially available surfactants. *J. Cos. Cosmet. Chem.*, 13:469–476.

286. Paget, G. E., and Thomson, R. (1979): *Standard Operation Procedures in Toxicology*. MTP Press, Lancaster, United Kingdom.

287. Parce, J. W., Owicki, J. C., Keresco, K. M., Sigal, G. B., Wada, H. G., Muir, V. C., Bouse, L. J., Ross, K. I., Sikie, B. I., and McConnell, H. M. (1989): Detection of cell healing agents with a silicon biosensor. *Science*, 246:243–247.

288. Parish, W. E. (1985): Ability of in vitro (corneal injury-eye organ-and chorioallantoic membrane) tests to represent histopathological features of acute eye inflammation. *Food Chem. Toxicol.*, 23:215–227.

289. Patel, S., and Stevenson, R. W. W. (1994): Clinical evaluation of a portable ultrasonic and a standard optical pachometer. *Optom Vis. Sci.*, 71:43–46.

290. Petroll, W. M., Cavanagh, H. D., and Jester, J. V. (1993): Three-dimensional imaging of corneal cells using in vivo confocal microscopy. *J. Micros.*, 170:213–219.

291. Petroll, W. M., Cavanagh, H. D., Lemp, M. A., Andrews, P. M., and Jester, J. V. (1992): Digital image acquisition in in vivo confocal microscopy. *J. Micros.*, 165:61–69.

292. Petroll, W. M., Jester, J. V., and Cavanagh, H. D. (1994): In vivo confocal imaging: General principles and applications. *Scanning*, 16:131–149.

293. Petroll, W. M., Jester, J. V., and Cavanagh, H. D. (1996): Quantitative three-dimensional confocal imaging of the cornea in situ and in vivo: System design and calibration. *Scanning*, 18:45–49.

294. Pfister, R. R., and Burstein, N. (1976): The effects of ophthalmic drugs, vehicles, and preservatives on corneal epithelium: A scanning electron microscope study. *Invest. Ophthalmol.*, 15:246–258.

295. Polansky, J. R., Fauss, D. J., Hydorn, T., and Bloom, E. (1990): Cellular injury from sustained versus acute hydrogen peroxide exposure in cultured human corneal endothelium and human lens epithelium. *CLAO J.*, 16:S23–S28.

296. Price. J. B., and Andrews, I. J. (1985): The in vitro assessment of eye irritancy using isolated eyes. *Food Chem. Toxicol.*, 23:313–315.

297. Price, J. B., Barry, M. P., and Andrews, I. J. (1986): The use of the chick chorioallantoic membrane to predict eye irritants. *Food Chem. Toxicol.*, 24:503–505.

298. Prince, J. H., Diesem, C. D., Eglitis, I., and Ruskell, G. L. (1960): *Anatomy and Histology of the Eye and Orbit in Domestic Animals*. Charles C Thomas, Springfield, Illinois.

299. Prinsen, M. K., and Koeter, H. B. W. M. (1993): Justification of the enucleated eye test with eyes of slaughterhouse animals as an alternative to the Draize eye irritation test with rabbits. *Food Chem. Toxicol.*, 31:69–76.

300. Protty, C., and Ferguson, T. F. M. (1976): The effects of surfactants upon rat peritoneal mast cells in vitro. *Food Cosmet. Toxicol.*, 14:425.

301. Rachui, S. R., Robertson, W. D., Duke, M. A., and Heinze, J. (1994): Predicting the ocular irritation potential of surfactants using the in vitro Skin^2 model ZK 1200. *J. Toxicol. Cutan. Ocul. Toxicol.*, 13:215–220.

302. Rachui, S. R., Robertson, W. D., Duke, M. A., Paller, B. S., and Ziets, G. A. (1994): Predicting the ocular irritation potential of cosmetics and personal care products using two in vitro models. *In Vitro Toxicol.*, 7:45–52.

303. Reader, S. J., Blackwell, V., O'Hara, R., Clothier, R. H., Griffin, G., and Balls, M. (1989): A vital dye release method for assessing the short-term cytotoxic effects of chemicals and formulations. *ATLA*, 17:28–33.

304. Reiger, M. M., and Battista, G. W. (1964): Some experiences in the safety testing of cosmetics. *J. Soc. Cosmet. Chem.*, 15:161–172.

305. Reinhardt, C. A., Pelli, D. A., and Zbinden, G. (1985): Interpretation of cell toxicity data for the estimation of potential irritation. *Food Chem. Toxicol.*, 23:247–252.

306. Rhode, B. H. (1992): In vitro methods in ophthalmic toxicology. In: *Ophthalmic Toxicology*, edited by G. C. Y. Chiou, pp. 106–165. Raven Press, New York.

307. Rivera, A., and Sanna, G. (1962): Determiniazione della velocita degli ultrasuoni nei tessuti oculari di uomo et di maiale. *Annali di Ottalmologia e Clinica Oculistics*, 88:675–682.

308. Roeig, D. L., Hasegawa, A. I., Harris, G. J., Lynch, K. L., and Wang, R. I. H. (1980): Occurrence of corneal opacities in rats after acute administration of 1-alpha-acetylmethadol. *Toxicol. Appl. Pharmacol.*, 56:155–163.

309. Roll, R., Hoffer-Bosse, T., and Kayser, D. (1986): New perspectives in acute toxicity testing of chemicals. *Toxicol. Lett.*, (Suppl. 31):86.

310. Romani, A., Puccioni, M., Tramontana, M., Del Bianco, E., and Geppetti, P. (1992): Release of proinflammatory neuropeptide (calcitonin gene-regulated) from capsaicin-sensitive, nerve fibers of the iris and ciliary body in humans. *Chibret Int. J. Ophthalmol.*, 9:3–9.

311. Rosiello, A. P., Essigmann, J. M., and Wogan, G. N. (1977): Rapid and accurate determination of the median lethal dose (LD_{50}) and its error with a small computer. *J. Toxicol. Environ. Health*, 3:797–809.

312. Rothman, B., Despins, A., Webb, D., Taylor, D., Sundarraj, N., O'Rourke, J., and Kreutzer, D. (1991): Cytokine regulation of C3 and C5 production by human corneal fibroblasts. *Exp. Eye Res.*, 53:353–361.

313. Rowan, A. (1981): The Draize test: Political and scientific issues. *Cosmet. Tech.*, 3(7):32–48.

314. Roy, T. A., Saladdin, K. A., and Mackerer, C. R. (1994): Evaluation of the EYTEX system as a screen for eye irritatancy of petroleum products. *Toxicol. in Vitro*, 8:197–198.

315. Salz, J. J., Azen, S. P., Berstein, J., Caroline, P., Villasenor, R. A., and Schanzlin, D. J. (1983): Evaluation and sources of variability in the measurement of corneal thickness with ultrasonic and optical pachymeters. *Ophthal. Surg.*, 14:750–754.

316. SAS User's Guide: Statistics. SAS Institute Inc. Cary, North Carolina.

317. Scaife, M. C. (1982): An investigation of detergent action on cells in vitro and possible correlations with in vivo data. *Int. J. Cosmet. Sci.*, 4:179.

318. Scaife, M. C. (1985): An in vitro cytotoxicity test to predict the ocular irritation potential of detergents and detergent products. *Food Chem. Toxicol.*, 23:253–258.

319. Schlede, E., Mischke, U., Diener, W., and Kayser, D. (1994): The international validation study of the acute toxic class method (oral). *Arch. Toxicol.*, 69:659–670.

320. Schlede, E., Mischke, U., Roll, R., and Kayser, D. (1992): A national validation study of the acute toxic class method—An alternative to the LD_{50} test. *Arch. Toxicol.*, 66:455–470.

321. Schutz, E., and Fuchs, H. (1982): A new approach to minimizing the number of animals used in acute toxicity testing and optimizing the information of test results. *Arch. Toxicol.*, 51:197–220.

322. Seabaugh, V. M., Osterberg, R. E., Hoheisel, C. A., Murphy, J. C., and Bierboer, G. W. (1976): A comparative study of rabbit ocular reactions of various exposure times to chemicals. *Society of Toxicology, Fifteenth Annual Meeting*, Atlanta.

323. Selling, J., and Ekwall, B. (1985): Screening for eye irritancy using cultured Hela cells. *Xenobiotica*, 15:8–9.

324. Shadduck, J. A., Everitt, J., and Bay, P. H. S. (1985): Use of in vitro cytotoxicity to rank ocular irritation of six surfactants. In: *Alternative Methods in Toxicology, Vol. 3, In Vitro Toxicology*, edited by A. M. Goldberg, pp. 641–649. Mary Ann Liebert, New York.

325. Shadduck, J. A., Render, I., Everitt, J., Meccoli, R. A., and Essex-Sorlie, D. (1987): An approach to validation: Comparison of six materials in three tests. In: *Alternative Methods in Toxicology, Vol. 5, In Vitro Toxicology*, edited by A. M. Goldberg, pp. 75–78. Mary Ann Liebert, New York.

326. Shapiro, H. (1956): Setting and dissolution of the rabbit cornea in alkali. *Am. J. Ophthalmol.*, 42:292–298.

327. Shaw, J. A., Clothier, R. H., and Balls, M. (1990). Loss of trans-epithelial impermeability of a confluent monolayer of Madin–Darby canine kidney (MDCK) cells as a determinant of ocular irritancy potential. *ATLA*, 18:145–151.

328. Shopsis, C. (1984): Inhibition of uridine uptake in cultured cells: A rapid, sublethal cytotoxicity test. *J. Tissue Culture Meth.*, 9:19.

329. Shopsis, C., Borenfreund, E., Walberg, J., and Stark, D. M. (1985): A battery of potential alternatives to the Draize test: Uridine uptake inhibition, morphological cytotoxicity, macrophage chemotaxis, and exfoliative cytology. *Food Chem. Toxicol.*, 23:259–266.

330. Shopsis, C., and Eng, B. (1985): Rapid cytotoxicity testing using a semi-automated protein determination on cultured cells. *Toxicol. Lett.*, 26:1–8.

331. Shopsis, C., and Sathe, S. (1984): Uridine uptake inhibition as a cytotoxicity test: Correlation with the Draize test. *Toxicology*, 29:195–206.

332. Silverman, J. T., and Pennisi, S. (1987): Evaluation of *Tetrahymena thermophila* as an in vitro alternative to ocular irritation studies in rabbits. *J. Toxicol. Cutan. Ocul. Toxicol.*, 6:33–42.

333. Simmons, S. J., Jumblatt, M. M., and Neufeld, A. H. (1987): Corneal epithelial wound closure in tissue culture. An in vitro model of ocular irritancy. *Toxicol. Appl. Pharmacol.*, 88:13–23.

334. Sina, J. (1994): Validation of the bovine corneal opacity–permeability assay as a predictor of ocular irritation potential. *In Vitro Toxicol.*, 7:283–289.

335. Sina, J., Gautheron, P., Casterton, P., Evans, M. G., Harbell, J. W., Curren, R. D., Earl, L., and Bruner, L. (1998): Report from

the bovine corneal opacity and permeability technical workshop, November 3–4, 1997, Gaithersburg, Maryland. *In Vitro and Molec. Toxicol.*, 11:315–353.
336. Smyth, R. J., Nguyen, K., Ahn, S. S., Panck, W. C., and Lee, D. A. (1993): The effects of Photofrin on human tendon's capsule fibroblasts in vitro. *J. Ocular Pharmacol.*, 9:171–178.
337. Society of Agricultural Chemical Industry (1985): Agricultural Chemicals Laws and Regulations. Japan(II) (English translation).
338. Society of Toxicology Animal in Research Committee (1989): SOT position paper comments on LD_{50} and acute eye and skin irritation tests. *Fund. Appl. Toxicol.*, 13:621–623.
339. Society of Toxicology of Canada (1985): Position paper on the LD_{50}. Adopted at the STC annual meeting on December 3, 1985.
340. Sperling, F. (1976): Nonlethal parameters as indices of acute toxicity: Inadequacy of the acute LD_{50}. In: *New Concepts in Safety Evaluation*, edited by M. A. Mehlman, R. E. Shapiro, and H. Blumenthal, pp. 177–191. Hemisphere, Washington, D.C.
341. Spielmann, H., Kalweit, S., Liebsch, M., Wirnsberger, T., Gerner, I., Bertram-Neis, E., Krauser, K., Kreiling, R., Miltenburger, H. G., Pape, W., and Steiling, W. (1993): Validation study of alternatives to the Draize eye irritation test in Germany: Cytotoxicity testing and HET–CAM test with 136 industrial chemicals. *Toxicol. in Vitro*, 7:505–510.
342. Stark, D. M., Borenfreund, E., Walberg, J., and Shopsis, C. (1985): Comparison of several alternative assays for measuring potential toxicants. In vitro toxicology: A progress report from the Johns Hopkins Center for Alternatives to Animal Testing. In: *Alternative Methods in Toxicology, Vol. 3*, edited by A. M. Goldberg, pp. 371–390. Mary Ann Liebert, New York.
343. Stark, D. M., Shopsis, C., Borenfreund, E., and Babich, H. (1986): Progress and problems in evaluating and validating alternative assays in toxicology. *Food Chem. Toxicol.*, 24:449–455.
344. Stark, D. M., Shopsis C., Borenfreund, E., and Walberg, J. (1983): *Alternative Approaches to the Draize Assay: Chemotoxicity, Cytology, Differentiation and Membrane Transport Studies in Product Safety Evaluation*, edited by A. M. Goldberg, p. 179. Mary Ann Liebert, New York.
345. Sugai, S., Murata, K., Kitagaki, T., and Tomita, I. (1990): Studies on eye irritation caused by chemicals in rabbits. I. A quantitative structure–activity relationship approach to primary eye irritation of chemicals in rabbits. *J. Toxicol. Sci.*, 15:245–262.
346. Sugar, J. (1980): Corneal examination. In: *Principles and Practice of Ophthalmology, Vol. 1*, edited by G. A. Peyman, D. R. Sanders, and M. F. Goldberg, pp. 393–395. W. B. Saunders, Philadelphia.
347. Swanton, D. W. (1983): Eye irritancy testing. In: *Animals and Alternatives in Toxicity Testing*, edited by M. Balls, R. J. Ridell, and A. N. Worden, p. 337. Academic Press, London.
348. Takahashi, N., and Ikoma, N. (1990): The cytotoxic effect of 5-fluorouracil on cultured human conjunctival cells. In: *Ocular Toxicology*, edited by S. Lerman and R. C. Tripathi, pp. 157–166. Marcel Dekker, New York.
349. Talsma. D. M., Leach, C. L., Hatoum, N. S., Gibbons, R. D., Roger, J. C., and Garvin, P. J. (1988). Reducing the number of rabbits in the Draize eye irritancy test: A statistical analysis of 155 studies conducted over 6 years. *Fund. Appl. Toxicol.*, 10:146–153.
350. Tanaka, N., Ohkawa, T. , Hiyama, T., and Nakajima, A. (1982): Evaluation of ocular toxicity of two beta blocking drugs, cereteolol and practolol, in beagle dogs. *J. Pharmacol. Exp. Ther.*, 224:424–430.
351. Tchao, R. (1988): Trans-epithelial permeability of fluorescein in vitro as an assay to determine eye irritants. In: *Alternative Methods in Toxicology, Vol. 6. Progress in In Vitro Toxicology*, edited by A. M. Goldberg, pp. 271–283. Mary Ann Liebert, New York.
352. Terry, M. A., and Ousley, P. J. (1996): Variability in corneal thickness before, during, and after radial keratotomy. *J. Refract. Surg.*, 12:700–704.
353. Thompson, W. R. (1947): Use of moving averages and interpolation to estimate median effective dose. *Bacterial. Rev.*, 11:115–145.
354. Tonjum, A. M. (1975): Effects of benzalkonium chloride upon the corneal epithelium: Studies with scanning electron microscopy. *Acta Ophthalmol.*, 53:358–366.
355. Trevan, J. W. (1927): The error of determination of toxicity. *Proc. R. Soc. Lond.*, 101B:483–514.
356. Tripathi, B. J., Tripathi, R. C., and Kolli, S. P. (1992): Cytotoxicity of ophthalmic preservatives on human corneal epithelium. *Lens Eye Toxicol. Res.*, 9:361–375.
357. Tripathi, B. J., Tripathi, R. C., and Millard, C. B. (1990): Epinephrine-induced toxicity of human trabecular cells in vitro. In: *Ocular Toxicology*, edited by S. Lerman and R. C. Tripathi, pp. 141–156. Marcel Dekker, New York.
358. Ubels, J. L., Erickson, A. M., Zylstra, U., Kreulen, C. D., and Casterton, P. L. (1998): Effect of hydration on opacity in the bovine corneal opacity and permeability (BCOP) assay. *J. Toxicol. Cutan. Ocul. Toxicol.*, 17:197–220.
359. Van den Heuvel, M. J., Clark, D. G., Fielder, R. J., Koundakjian, P. P., Oliver, G. J. A., Pelling, D., Thomlison, N. J., and Walker, A. P. (1990). The international validation of a fixed dose procedure as an alternative to the classical LD_{50} test. *Food Chem. Toxicol.*, 28:469–482.
360. Van den Heuvel, M. J., Dayan, A. D., and Shillaker, R. O. (1987): Evaluation of the BTS approach to the testing of substances and preparations for their acute toxicity. *Human Toxicol.*, 6:279–291.
361. Van Erp, Y. H. M., and Weterings, P. J. (1990): Eye irritancy screening for classification of chemicals. *Toxicol. in Vitro*, 4:267.
362. Vanparys, P., Deknudt, G., Sysmans, M., Teuns, G., Coussement, W., and VanCauteren, H. (1993): Evaluation of the bovine opacity–permeability assay as an in vitro alternative to the Draize eye irritation test. *Toxicol. in Vitro*, 7:471–476.
363. Villasenor, R. A., Santos, V. R., Cox, K. C., Harris, D. F., Lynn, M., and Waring, G. O. (1986): Comparison of ultrasonic corneal thickness measurements before and during surgery in the prospective evaluation of Radial Keratotomy (PERK) Study. *Ophthalmol.*, 93:327–330.
364. Walberg, J. (1983): Exfoliative cytology as a refinement of the Draize eye irritancy test. *Toxicol. Lett.*, 18:49.
365. Wallin, R. F., Hume R. D., and Jackson, E. M. (1987): The agarose diffusion method for ocular irritancy screening: Cosmetic products. Part 1. *J. Toxicol. Cutan. Ocul. Toxicol.*, 6:239–250.
366. Walum, E., Clemedsen, C., and Ekwall, B. (1994): Principles for the validation of in vitro toxicology test methods. *Toxicol. in Vitro*, 8:807–812.
367. Waltman, S. R., and Kaufman, H. E. (1970): In vivo studies of human corneal and endothelial permeability. *Am. J. Ophthalmol.*, 70:45–47.
368. Ward, S. L., Kahn, C. R., Walker, T. L., and Dimitrijivch, S. D. (1994): Response and recovery of a human corneal epithelial cell line to chemical insult. *Invest. Ophthalmol. Vis. Sci.*, 35:1942.
369. Ward, S. L., Walker, T. L., and Dimitrijivch, S. D. (1997): Evaluation of chemically induced toxicity using an in vitro model of human corneal epithelium. *Toxicol. In Vitro*, 11:121–139.
370. Watanabe, M., Watanabe K., Zuzuki, K., Nikaide, O., Ishii, I., Konishi, H., Tanaka, N., and Sugahara, T. (1989): Use of primary rabbit cornea cells to replace the Draize rabbit eye irritancy test. *Toxicol. in Vitro*, 3:329–334.
371. Waud, D. R. (1972): On biological assays involving quantal responses. *J. Pharm. Exp. Ther.*, 183:577–607.

372. Weil, C. S. (1952): Tables for convenient calculation of median effective dose (LD_{50} or ED_{50}) and instruction in their use. *Biometrics*, 8:249–263.

373. Weil, C. S. (1983): Economical LD_{50} and slope determinations. *Drug Chem. Toxicol.*, 6:595–603.

374. Weil, C. S., and Scala, R. A. (1971): Study of intra- and interlaboratory variability in the results of rabbit eye and skin irritation tests. *Toxicol. Appl. Pharmacol.*, 19:276–360.

375. Weltman, A. S., Sharber, S. B., and Jurtshuk, T. (1968): Comparative evaluation and influence of various factors on eye irritation tests. *Toxicol. Appl. Pharmacol.*, 7:308–319.

376. Weterings, P. J., and Van Erp, Y. H. M. (1987): In vitro toxicology approaches to validation. In: *Alternative Methods in Toxicology, Vol. 5*, edited by A. M. Goldberg. Mary Ann Liebert, New York.

377. Wheeler, N. C., Morantes, C. M., Kristensen, R. M., Petit, T. H., and Lee, D. A. (1992): Reliability coefficients of three corneal pachymeters. *Am. J. Ophthalmol.*, 113:645–651.

378. Williams. S. J. (1984): Prediction of ocular irritancy potential from dermal irritation test results. *Food Chem. Toxicol.*, 22: 157–161.

379. Williams, S. J. (1985): Changing concepts of ocular irritation evaluation: Pitfalls and progress. *Food Chem. Toxicol.*, 23:189–193.

380. Williams, S. J., Grapel, G. J., and Kennedy, G. I. (1982): Evaluation of ocular irritancy: Potential intralaboratory variability and effect of dosage volume. *Toxicol. Lett.*, 12:235–241.

381. Williams, D. E., Nguyen, K. D., Shapourifar-Tehrani, S., Kitada, S., and Lee, D. A. (1992): Effects of Timolol, Betaxolol, and Levobunolol on human tendon's fibroblasts in tissue culture. *Invest. Ophthalmol. Vis. Sci.*, 33:2233–2241.

382. York, M., Lawrence, R. S., and Gibson, G. B. (1982): An in vitro test for the assessment of eye irritancy in consumer products—preliminary findings. *Int. J. Cosmet. Sci.*, 44:223.

Principles and Methods of Toxicology, Fourth Edition, edited by A. Wallace Hayes.
Taylor & Francis, Philadelphia © 2001.

Chapter 19

SHORT-TERM, SUBCHRONIC, AND CHRONIC TOXICOLOGY STUDIES

Nelson H. Wilson, Jerry F. Hardisty, and Johnnie R. Hayes

REPEATED DOSE STUDIES AND HAZARD (SAFETY) ASSESSMENT

Repeated dose toxicity studies are conducted to screen for potential adverse effects of a chemical, using laboratory animals as surrogates for a target species, most often the human. Repeated dose studies may be of varying duration, generally 1 to 4 weeks for short-term studies, 3 months for subchronic studies, and 6–12 months for chronic studies. Many variables associated with the health of the test species are monitored in short-term, subchronic, and chronic toxicity studies, resulting in the ability to detect a variety of adverse effects. Sometime during their career, most toxicologists are involved in the design, performance, or review of data from these toxicology studies. This results from the central role played by these studies in the safety assessment of pharmaceuticals, pesticides, food additives, and other chemicals. It has been suggested that subchronic data alone may be sufficient to predict the hazard of long-term, low-dose exposure to a compound (50). Even though this may be true for compounds where adequate structure-activity relationships exist, it generally is not true when compounds have completely unknown toxicity or when structure-activity relationships predict a potential adverse effect. For certain chemicals or mixtures, results from a short-term or a subchronic toxicity study may represent the most sophisticated toxicology data available. With many chemicals, a subchronic study is critical to the design of longer-term hazard assessment studies.

It is essential that toxicologists become familiar with the scientific principles upon which repeated dose toxicology studies are based and understand the methodology used to perform these studies. This chapter provides an introduction to these studies and some of the principles upon which they are based.

A typical hazard assessment program is illustrated in Figure 19.1. However, in the practice of toxicology, there is no such thing as a "typical" hazard assessment

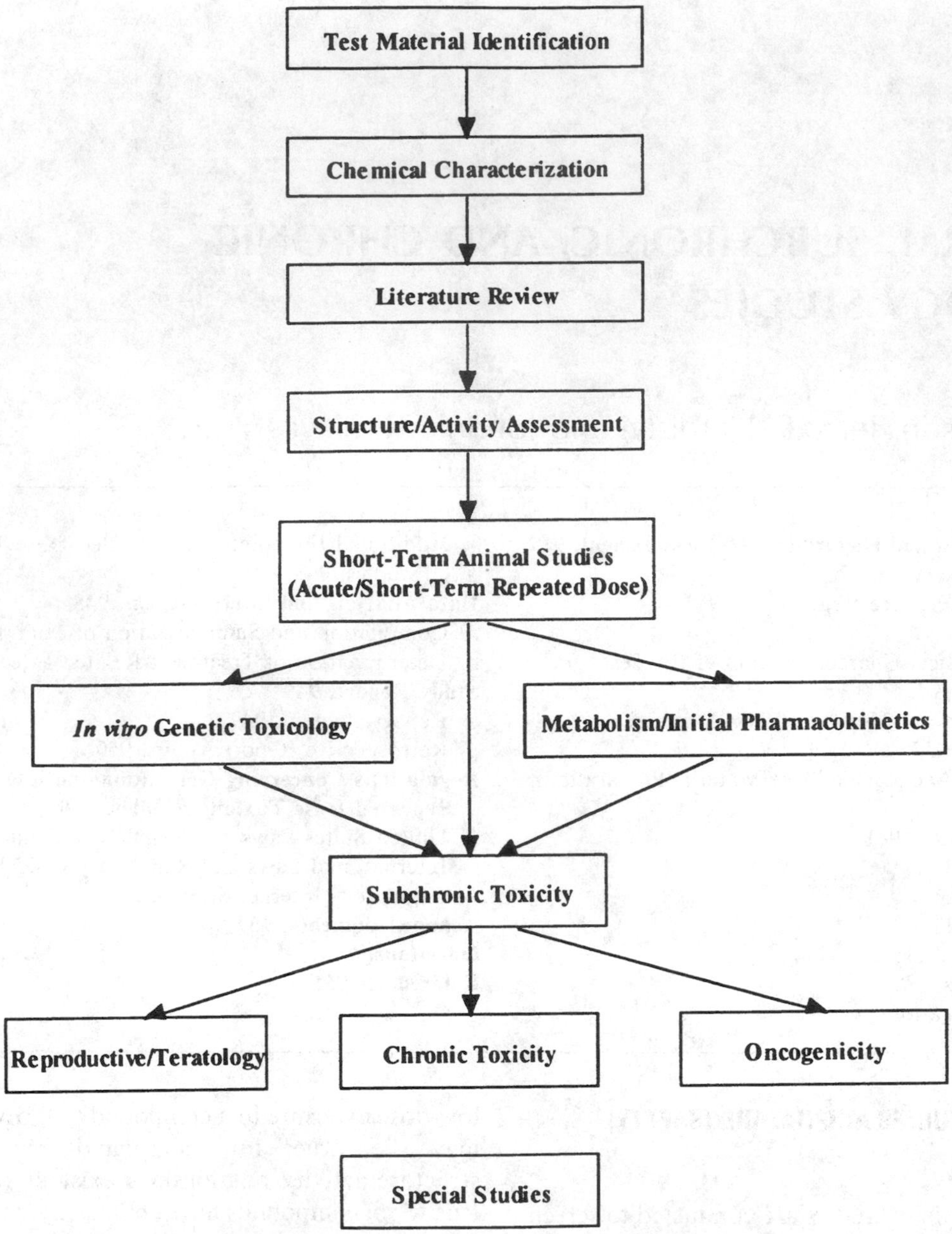

FIG. 19.1. Schematic representation of a typical hazard assessment program illustrating a step-by-step, tiered approach and the interactions between the various elements. The approach presented here is not the only approach that could be used.

program. Each program is unique, based upon the individual material being tested and its intended use.

The first step in any hazard assessment is determination of the material to be studied and the purpose of the assessment. Both these factors will influence the final design of the program. At the time of selection of the material to be tested, its intended use in the marketplace will have been defined, dictating, in most cases, factors such as exposure route and the types of studies required.

The next step is the chemical and physical characterization of the material or mixture to be investigated. Knowledge of the major component(s) and any associated contaminants is required for almost every phase of the hazard assessment program. The more detailed the chemical and physical characterization, the greater the assurance that there will not be unexpected interferences from impurities.

Once the toxicologist has information concerning the chemical nature of the *test material*, the scientific literature is searched to determine what, if anything, is known about its biological activity. If no information is available, then the potential biological activity of

Table 19.1
Objectives of short-term repeated dose studies

- Determine adverse effects of the test compound at doses low enough to allow survival of most animals, as opposed to acutely toxic doses
- Determine adverse effects over a longer exposure (dosing) period than used in acute studies
- Determine dose response for adverse effects following repeated dosing and identify no observable adverse effect level (NOAEL)
- Identify target organs
- Provide data concerning species differences, if any, in sensitivity to potential adverse effects
- Provide initial data for comparative risk assessment
- Determine need for specialized endpoints to be assessed in longer-term studies

chemicals with similar chemical structure should be ascertained. Based upon the chemical characterization data and any toxicology information available in the scientific literature, the toxicologist can then perform a structure-activity assessment. This will aid in developing the hazard assessment program and the specific designs for each of the toxicology studies.

In most cases, the first series of studies will be short-term toxicity studies. The initial short-term toxicity study is generally a single dose, *acute* toxicity study. Results from acute toxicity studies are used to estimate dosages to be used in short-term repeated dose studies and obtain initial data useful in assessing relative toxicity. A number of regulatory agencies have made recommendations concerning designs for acute studies as discussed in the acute toxicity chapter of this text. Additional variables may be added to these recommended designs based upon the structure-activity assessment and literature review, if warranted.

Data obtained from short-term repeated dose studies are generally required for the successful design of subchronic toxicity studies. Similarly, data from subchronic studies are essential for design of chronic studies. Table 19.1 lists objectives for short-term repeated dose toxicity studies. Table 19.2 lists examples of data obtained from these studies that are useful in the design of subsequent toxicity studies. As is discussed later, one of the difficult decisions for a toxicologist designing a toxicology study is selection of the dose range to be used. Dose response relationships for toxicological endpoints evaluated in short-term toxicology studies are critical to the successful design of subsequent toxicity studies.

Although not always available, data from genetic toxicology and metabolism studies are useful adjuncts to data from short-term repeated dose studies. For

Table 19.2
Data obtained from short-term repeated dose studies that are useful in the design of subsequent studies

- Palatability of test material/diet mixture, if dosing is by feed
- Body weight response patterns
- Physical observations
- Observed behavior changes
- Clinical pathology
- Gross necropsy
- Histopathology
- Identification of target organs
- Dose responses

instance, if the in vitro phase of the genetic toxicology program has indicated that the test material has genotoxic potential, it may be dropped from consideration for further development and further testing may be unnecessary. On the other hand, in vivo genetic toxicology studies can be added to the design of subchronic or chronic toxicology studies. This can, in many cases, reduce the number of animals used in the overall safety assessment and conserve other resources. If information concerning the metabolism and pharmacokinetics of the test material is known, it should be used in the design of repeated dose toxicity studies. For example, if pharmacokinetic studies indicate a potential for accumulation of the test material from multiple dosing, this is an important consideration in deciding the most appropriate dose range. Also, because different species may metabolize the test material differently, this information is important in selection of appropriate animal species and strains for subsequent testing. The major objectives of subchronic toxicity studies are presented in Table 19.3.

In some cases, subchronic toxicity testing may complete the data required for a hazard assessment. In other cases, as illustrated in Figure 19.1, data from subchronic studies are used in the design of additional studies, including chronic toxicity studies. Data from subchronic toxicity studies are useful in the design of oncogenicity and reproduction studies as well as any "special" studies that may be either warranted by the results of other studies or requested by a regulatory agency.

As noted above, data from a short-term repeated dose study should be available before initiation of subchronic toxicity testing and, generally, data should be available from a subchronic study before proceeding with chronic testing. The major utility in progression from shorter-term to longer-term studies is to insure, to the extent possible, that proper dose ranges are selected. Requirements for a scientifically valid short-term repeated dose study are similar to those of subchronic

Table 19.3
Objectives of subchronic toxicology studies

- Identify adverse effects not detected in shorter-term acute or repeated dose studies
- Provide additional information on adverse effects identified in short-term studies
- Identify observable effect level and the NOAEL
- Provide data for dose selection and other study design features for chronic toxicity and other longer-term studies
- Confirm and/or identify target organs or sites of action
- Provide data to determine if specialized endpoints are required
- Provide a basis for species selection for additional studies, if required, and for data extrapolation to humans
- Provide information for regulatory agencies in support of the safety of the test material
- Provide risk assessment data

toxicity studies. Therefore, the general aspects of short-term studies will not be discussed separately. However, three aspects of short-term repeated dose studies need to be mentioned.

First, as implied by the description "short-term repeated dose study," these studies are of shorter duration than subchronic toxicity studies. Generally, the duration of these studies is either 14 or 28 days with compound administered daily. A 28-day study can produce more valuable information than a 14-day study because the longer-term exposure increases the probability of detecting more slowly developing adverse effects, assuming the dose-range tested is similar.

Second, dose selection is somewhat dependent upon the purpose of the study. If the short-term dosing is designed to produce information to be used in the design of a subchronic study, then dosing should be high enough to ensure any potential adverse effect is observed. Higher doses are generally used in short-term studies to determine target organs and it may not be as critical to ascertain a no observable adverse effect level (NOAEL). However, it is always useful to have a NOAEL in a toxicology study. If no further studies are anticipated with the compound, a dose range that includes a NOAEL becomes more important. Because little information other than acute toxicity data is generally available, it may be necessary to run a more comprehensive range of dose levels in short-term repeated dose studies. Four, five, or more dose groups are generally used in short-term studies. This increases the chances of defining the dose response and should increase the confidence of dose range selection for subsequent studies.

A third aspect of short-term studies that is different from subchronic studies is the number of animals per group. Although fewer animals may be used, 10 animals of each gender in each dose group is the recommendation for short-term rodent studies. Additional animals may be required for non-routine endpoints, such as a group added to ascertain the reversibility of an adverse effect upon cessation of dosing. Additional animals also may be added to the high-dose group if potential compound-related mortality is expected.

Many other factors influence the design of all repeated dose toxicity studies. Before initiation of a study, it must be decided if the specific chemical or chemical mixture—that is, the test material—to be used in the study is appropriate based on its purity and other chemical characteristics. Appropriate animal models must be chosen, the correct route of exposure must be selected, and the study duration must be decided. Control and treatment groups and their doses have to be selected. Variables to be evaluated must be selected to maximize the probability of detecting potential adverse effects.

Regulatory Requirements

National and international regulatory bodies have issued guidelines for the design and conduct of repeated dose toxicity studies. Even though study designs proscribed by these various guidelines have similar characteristics, some differences between the requirements have existed within and between regulatory agencies. This has resulted, in some cases, in the duplication of studies to ensure guidelines of different agencies are satisfied. The agencies themselves and the regulated community have considered this duplication of the use of animals and other resources undesirable. As a result, regulatory authorities worldwide are attempting to harmonize their guidelines to ensure toxicity studies conducted under a single set of regulations will be universally acceptable. In the United States, the Environmental Protection Agency (EPA) issued a single set of harmonized toxicity testing guidelines in 1997 (17) to blend the requirements of the separate guidelines previously promulgated through the Federal Insecticide, Fungicide and Rodenticide Act (FIFRA), the Toxic Substances Control Act (TSCA), and the Organization for Economic Cooperation and Development (OECD).

OECD, an international organization of 29 countries including the United States, has issued its own toxicity testing guidelines (54). Each member country has agreed to accept studies conducted according to these guidelines. In 1991, regulatory authorities and trade organizations from the United States, Japan, and the European Union initiated a cooperative effort through the International Conference on Harmonization (ICH) to produce guidance documents concerning requirements for safety studies with pharmaceutical products. ICH guidance documents generally address specific issues related to toxicity testing, for example, the duration of chronic toxicity testing (43), and are not detailed guidelines for protocol design.

Each regulatory harmonization effort discussed above has been useful. However, a well-planned, scientifically valid, adequately conducted, repeated dose study should satisfy the requirements of any regulatory agency. The scientific foundation for toxicological hazard assessment is continually expanding and to compromise this foundation by pursuing standard checklist protocols is irrational, wasteful, and unscientific. Today, regulations generally recognize the importance of scientific judgment and encourage discussions between the regulated community and the regulator about alternative study designs. Investigator and regulator each share in the obligation to do a scientifically sound study.

This chapter focuses on hazard assessment for chemicals that are small molecules. Today, biotechnology is a rapidly developing field. Hazard assessments for biologicals—for example, recombinant proteins—are a special case that will not be discussed in detail in this chapter. Suffice it to say that guidelines for testing such materials are under development. The hazard assessment for a biological is tailored specifically to the compound and may be more or less comprehensive than a classical assessment with a small-molecule compound. However, many of the principles and methods of individual studies with small molecules are applicable to testing with biotechnology products. The toxicologist responsible for investigating the safety of these materials should become familiar with the current guidelines and suggestions for their testing.

The balance of this chapter relates to the typical design and conduct of subchronic and chronic repeated dose toxicity studies. The information provided should suffice to satisfy most regulatory guidelines. Variables determined in subchronic and chronic toxicity studies are essentially identical, the major difference being the schedule for data collection. Table 19.4 compares the minimum requirements for subchronic and chronic toxicity studies using rodents as described in the EPA (17), U.S. Food and Drug Administration (FDA) (23), and OECD (54) testing guidelines. For repeated dose study designs intended to satisfy guidelines of a particular regulatory authority, it is recommended that the reader:

(1) use the testing guidelines of that authority as a starting point during the design of a study,
(2) refine the design based upon the compound of interest,
(3) document the design in a detailed, written protocol, and
(4) discuss the protocol with a representative of the regulatory authority prior to initiating a study.

Good Laboratory Practice Regulations

In addition to regulations and guidelines concerning the design of repeated dose studies, U.S. and international regulatory authorities have issued good laboratory practice (GLP) regulations or principles concerning the manner in which all nonclinical hazard assessment studies (e.g., animals studies) are to be conducted, documented, and reported (11,19,36,46–48,56,60). These GLPs are designed to ensure the quality of the study data and report. Requirements from each of the regulatory agencies are similar. GLPs set standards for the *test system*, laboratory organization, personnel, facilities, equipment, operations, and record keeping. They require that studies be conducted according to written protocols (see Table 19.5) and validated, written standard operating procedures (SOPs). Chemical analyses are required to characterize the *test article* and control article administered during the studies, and study procedures and data must be clearly and completely documented and reported. Regulatory agencies inspect testing laboratories to assure GLP compliance. Safety studies not conducted according to GLPs will not be accepted by regulatory agencies, and some versions of GLPs, including those of the U.S. regulatory agencies, provide for disqualification of laboratories that are in major noncompliance with GLP requirements. For these reasons, laboratories conducting studies for regulatory submission generally take great care to comply with GLPs.

STUDY DESIGN

Chemical and Physical Characterization of the Test Material

It may seem that selection of the test material for repeated dose toxicity testing should require little involvement by the toxicologist because it is usually provided by a chemist or product manager. However, several important factors must be considered by the toxicologist to insure that a study will adequately assess the potential toxicity of the chemical and be accepted by regulatory agencies. Obviously, one of these factors is that the batch or lot of test material should be representative of the chemical intended to be tested. Adequate chemical and physical characterization is essential for this determination. Several regulatory agencies and organizations have issued guidelines to describe the information needed and some of the methodology to be used to characterize a chemical (16,24,42,55).

Table 19.4
Subchronic and chronic rodent oral toxicity studies based on various regulatory guidelines

	EPA OPPTS Guidelines		FDA Redbook		OECD Guidelines	
	Subchronic (14)	Chronic (15)	Subchronic (22)	Chronic (23)	Subchronic (57)	Chronic (53)
Study Duration	≥90 days	≥12 mo.	≥90 days	≥12 mo.	≥90 days	≥12 mo.
No. of Treated Groups						
standard study	≥3	≥3	≥3	≥3	≥3	≥3
limit test[a]	1	1	NA	NA	1	NA
No. of Negative Control Groups[b]						
untreated control	1	1	1	1	1	1
vehicle control	1	1	1	1	1	1
No. of Animals/Gender/Group[c]	≥10	≥20	≥20	≥20	≥10	≥20
Age of Animals (at start of study)	≤8–9 weeks	≤8 weeks	≤6 weeks	~6 weeks	<9 weeks	asap[f]
Body Weight Measurement						
frequency through 13 weeks	weekly	weekly	weekly	weekly	weekly	weekly
frequency after 13 weeks	NA	every 4th wk	NA	monthly	NA	every 4th wk
Feed Consumption Measurement						
frequency through 13 weeks	weekly	weekly	weekly	weekly	weekly	weekly
frequency after 13 weeks	NA	monthly	NA	monthly	NA	every 3rd mo
Observations						
for mortality and morbidity (times/day)	2	2	2	2	2	2
for general condition (times/day)	1	1	n	n	1	1
for detailed clinical findings (frequency)	weekly	weekly	daily	daily	weekly	daily
Neurotoxicity Evaluation (at term)[d]	y	y	n	n	y	n
Ophthalmology						
no. animals pretest	AA	AA	AA	AA	AA	n
no. animals/gender/high dose and control every 3 months[e]	NA	n	NA	AS	NA	n
no. animals/gender/high dose and control at term[e]	AS	10	AS	AS	AS	n
Hematology and Clinical Chemistry (no./gender/group)	AS	10	10	10	AS	10
intermediate time(s)	n	6 mo	n	every 3rd mo	n	3 & 6 mo[g]
term	y	y	y	y	y	y
Urinalysis (no./gender/group)	AS	10	NA	NA	AS	10
intermediate time(s)	n	n	n	n	n	3 & 6 mo
term	o	y	n	n	o	y

Table 19.4
Continued

	EPA OPPTS Guidelines		FDA Redbook		OECD Guidelines	
	Subchronic (14)	Chronic (15)	Subchronic (22)	Chronic (23)	Subchronic (57)	Chronic (53)
Gross Necropsy and Tissue Collection	AA	AA	AA	AA	AA	AA
Organ Weights (no/gender/group at term)	AS	AS	AS	AS	AS	10
adrenals, kidneys, liver	y	y	y	y	y	y
brain	y	y	n	n	y	y
testes/ovaries	y/y	y/y	y/n	y/n	y/y	y/y
epididymides, heart, uterus	y	y	n	n	y	n
spleen	y	y	n	n	y	n
thymus	y	n	n	n	y	n
Histopathology						
all tissues (all high-dose and control animals)	y	y	y	y	y	y
all tissues (all animals killed or died on study)	y	y	y	y	n	y
target tissues and gross lesions (All animals)	y	y	y	y	y	y
selected tissues (all intermediate–dose animals)	n	n	n	y	n	n

NA = not applicable; y = yes/required; n = no/not required; o = optional; AA = all animals; AS = all survivors

[a] If a test at one dose level of at least 1000 mg/kg body weight/day produces no observed adverse effects and if toxicity would not be expected based upon data from structurally related compounds, then a full study using three dose levels may not be considered necessary.

[b] Contingent upon the route of exposure in the test article treated groups.

[c] Extra animals must be added for interim sacrifices.

[d] Not required if similar data are available from other studies or if other clinical signs are noted to an extent that would interfere with evaluation.

[e] Animals in intermediate groups are to be evaluated if treatment related findings are noted in the high-dose group.

[f] As soon as possible after weaning and acclimation, e.g. $\leq$6–8 weeks of age.

[g] No clinical chemistry at three months.

Table 19.5
Protocol contents required by FDA good laboratory practices regulations

- Title and study objective
- Identification of test and control articles
- Identification of sponsor and testing facility
- Justification of test system (animal model)
- Test system information (number, body weight, gender, source, species/strain, age, method of identification, etc.)
- Description of study design and methods for control of bias, such as random assignment of animals to treatment groups, processing of clinical pathology samples in replicates, etc.
- Animal husbandry information
- Dosing information, including dose form preparation and route of administration
- Methods by which degree of absorption of the test and control articles by the test system will be determined, if necessary
- Types and frequencies of assays, analyses, and measurements to be made
- Description of statistical methods
- Records to be maintained

A safety assessment should include a partnership between the toxicologist and a chemist who understands the chemical characteristics of the test material. An adequate chemical characterization of the test material should be provided to the toxicologist, including methods of synthesis, precursors used in the synthesis and any solvents and manufacturing aids used in the manufacturing process. In addition, the methods of purification should be provided, to allow the toxicologist to determine the potential for occurrence of residues and impurities that could produce adverse effects. This provides the toxicologist with information needed to determine if any specific residues or impurities should be specifically targeted for additional analytical determinations.

The specific information required by the toxicologist may vary with each test material, and the required data may be different from that used to establish manufacturing and quality control specifications. It is essential, however, that the manufacturing and quality control specifications and procedures meet the specific regulatory requirements for toxicity testing. For instance, good manufacturing practices (GMP), which are somewhat similar to GLPs, are required for some chemicals (21,30,32,33,40). The chemist should insure that adequate GMP records exist, if they are required.

Prior to initiation of a repeated dose study, the toxicologist should carefully review the chemical and physical characterization data. Chemical characterization should include a quantitative assessment of the major components, with associated accuracy and precision information, and at least a qualitative analysis of minor components. Ideally, the toxicologist should be provided with a mass balance for the test material.

Before initiation of a repeated dose toxicity study, chemical analyses should be conducted to ensure that the test material, in bulk form and after mixing with any carrier, is stable over the range of anticipated concentrations and for the maximum period of use during the study. According to GLPs, this evaluation can be conducted concurrently with the study, but detection of instability during the study could invalidate the results. If the material is stable only under certain conditions—for example, frozen storage—special arrangements for its storage should be made to eliminate instability problems with the test material, resulting in lower than expected doses and exposure of the animals to degradation products. The products of degradation may either have their own unique toxicity or alter the toxicity of the test material. This may make it impossible to correctly interpret data from the study.

The toxicologist will have assessed the chemical characterization of the test material at the initial stages of the hazard assessment. More complete information may become available before initiation of repeated dose toxicity studies. Sometimes the chemical synthesis or other production methods may change between the initial assessment and the start of subchronic or chronic studies, and, it may be necessary to reassess the chemical characterization before initiation of these studies. Unanticipated changes in the chemistry of the test material or mixture may necessitate changes in the toxicity study design.

The test material should be as similar as possible to the chemical to which humans will be exposed, with every attempt made to ensure the test material is either identical to the final commercial product or representative of the anticipated final product. This may not always be possible with commercial products because large-scale production facilities are usually not available during this phase of a safety assessment. When such facilities become available, it may be possible to bridge between the final commercial product and the test material by chemical analysis. "Bridge chemistry" should identify any differences between the chemical that was tested and the commercial product, allowing a determination of the toxicological bioequivalence of the test material and final commercial product.

If a "new" impurity of unknown toxicity is detected in a drug product after chronic animal studies have been conducted, the second International Conference on Harmonization (42) has proposed the following:

1. If intended human use is short term:
   - Single-dose toxicology comparison of old and new test substance
   - Repeated dose, four-week comparison of old and new test substance
   - Mutagenicity tests
2. If intended use is long term, with a high dose of the active compound:
   - Single-dose toxicology comparison of old and new test substance
   - Repeated dose, three-month subchronic comparison of old and new test substance
   - Mutagenicity tests (if results of the mutagenicity test are positive, carcinogenicity testing of the impurity may be considered)
3. If the product is to be given to women of childbearing age:
   - Consider the need for a comparative embryotoxicity and teratogenicity (segment II) study in one suitable species

The test material should have not only the same chemical characteristics as the material of commerce, but should also have the same physical characteristics. If the test material is a solid intended to be used as a powder, it should be administered to the test animals in powder form. Particle size of the powder should be similar for the test material and the material to which humans will be exposed. If humans will be exposed to the material in solution, a solution of the material should be used in the repeated dose study. Analyses should be conducted to ensure that the composition of the test material falls within the limits of anticipated or known product specifications. Physical specifications will allow the toxicologist, often in consultation with the chemist, to determine the most appropriate method of adding the test material to the dosing matrix, such as the diet or drinking water (see Route of Exposure discussion).

It is important for the toxicologist to ensure an adequate supply of test material is available before initiating a toxicity study. A single lot of the test material should be used throughout the subchronic or chronic study, whenever possible. If the repeated dose study is part of a series of studies in a safety assessment program, it is desirable to use a single lot of test material for the entire program. This reduces the probability of encountering inconsistent results in different studies with the same test material, resulting from inter-lot differences in chemical/physical characteristics. If a single lot of test material is not available in sufficient quantity to complete a study or studies, multiple lots may be used, with chemical characterization of each new lot required to insure it meets all specifications and reasonably duplicates previous lots.

The FDA has issued guidelines addressing the chemistry data requirements for direct food additives and generally recognized as safe (GRAS) petitions (24). ICH has issued guidelines for chemistry requirements for drug candidates during preclinical hazard assessment (42). Although the toxicologist may not have as complete a data package as described above before the initiation of a repeated dose study, sufficient data must be available to meet GLP regulations.

FDA GLPs state that, "The identity, strength, purity, and composition or other characteristics which will appropriately define the test or control article shall be determined for each batch and shall be documented. Methods of synthesis, fabrication, or derivation of the test and control articles shall be documented. . . ." (35).

EPA GLP statements concerning the requirements for chemical characterization of the test material are essentially identical to those of FDA (12). The OECD GLP guidelines for chemical characterization state, "For each study, the identity, including batch number, purity, composition, concentrations, or other characterizations to appropriately define each batch of the test or reference items should be known" (56).

Further information on the chemical characterization of the test material is provided by the FDA in its proposed revision to the guidelines for toxicity studies, "The composition of the test substance should be known: Information should include the name and quantities of all major components, known contaminants and impurities, and the percentage of unidentifiable materials. The test substance in toxicology studies should be the same substance that the petitioner intends to market" (25).

Route of Exposure and Method of Test Material Administration

The anticipated human route of exposure to the test material dictates the route of exposure for most subchronic and chronic toxicity studies. Unintended routes of human exposure also should be considered during selection of exposure route. The most common routes of exposure in these studies are dietary, oral (gavage or capsule), dermal, and inhalation. Less frequently, test materials are administered in the drinking water or parenterally by intravenous, subcutaneous, intraperitoneal or other types of injection. Other types of administration include direct implant and *parenteral* infusion using implanted or external pumps.

Frequently, there are several potential routes of human exposure to a single chemical. For example, consumer exposure to a pesticide may occur by dietary consumption of food crops containing residues of the chemical. Farm worker exposure to the same pesticide may occur by either inhalation or dermal routes during application and harvesting. In such cases, subchronic testing may be required to assess the effects of exposure by all three routes. Emphasis is generally placed upon the route by which the most widespread human exposure would occur, with chronic testing usually conducted using only that route of exposure. Several of the more common routes of exposure are discussed in detail below.

Capsule Administration

If expected human exposure is by the oral route, a solid test material (e.g., a dry powder) can be administered by capsule. Unformulated bulk test material can be given to some large animals, such as dogs and cats, in gelatin capsules inserted into the esophagus manually or with the aid of a mechanical device designed to prevent the animal from biting the individual administering the capsule. Capsules are available in a wide range of sizes and can hold, depending on the density of the test material, as much as 1.5 g. The amount of test material that can be administered is limited by the capacity of each capsule and the practical number of capsules that can be administered at one time. For smaller species, such as rodents, this method is impractical and the test material must be administered orally as a solution or suspension in an appropriate vehicle.

Oral Gavage

Another common route of oral administration is oral *gavage* by *intubation*. This technique may be used for rodent and nonrodent species. For oral gavage, a solution or suspension of the test material is deposited into the stomach via the esophagus using an intubation tube attached to a graduated syringe or other device. A test material is added to an appropriate vehicle, usually aqueous. If the material is not readily soluble, a suspension may be prepared. For suspensions, a thickener such as methylcellulose, carboxymethylcellulose, or gum tragacanth is added to water to increase the viscosity, and the test material is homogeneously suspended in the vehicle. A wetting agent such as Tween 80 can be used to increase the suspendability of the material. Although aqueous vehicles are preferred, it is possible to use an oil vehicle for lipid-soluble materials. Food oils, such as corn oil, may be used but mineral oils must be avoided. It should be remembered that food oils add to normal dietary caloric intake and, at high volumes, oils may interfere with absorption of fat-soluble nutrients, such as fat-soluble vitamins. Also, absorption of the test material may be quite different with an oil vehicle compared to an aqueous vehicle and this may be highly volume-dependent.

The volume of test solution or suspension administered can influence gastric emptying time. Because gastric emptying time may affect gastrointestinal uptake and bioavailability, it generally is preferred that the dose levels of the test substance be administered on a constant-volume (ml/kg), variable-concentration (mg/ml) basis. For dosing using a constant volume, 10 ml/kg body weight is most commonly used as the upper limit. At 10 ml/kg, a 260 g rat would receive a dose volume of 2.6 ml, a 35 g mouse would receive 0.35 ml, and a 10 kg dog would receive 100 ml. Dosing usually is conducted once daily but may be performed more frequently to mimic the intended human dosing regimen or if concentration and/or pharmacokinetics considerations limit the achievable single-dose exposure to less than the amount desired.

Daily exposure by oral gavage results in a *bolus dose*. Administration via the diet or drinking water results in a more constant exposure throughout the duration of the study that is more dependent on feeding patterns than dosing schedule. Because rodents are nocturnal, the peak periods for activity and feeding behavior are the end of the light and dark periods (i.e., just before lights-on or just after lights-off). If high volumes of dosing solution (i.e., 20–50 ml/kg) are to be administered to rodents and/or if the presence of feed may interfere with the absorption of the test substance, consideration should be given to dosing animals during late morning or in the afternoon. For nonrodents, timing of dosing relative to feeding (i.e., before or at a certain time after daily feeding) accomplishes the same purpose. In any case, the timing of gavage dose(s) in relation to feeding should be stated clearly in the study protocol.

Administration of a test chemical as an undiluted liquid, as a diluted liquid, as a dissolved solid, or as a solid in suspension generally results in accurate delivery of the intended dose to each of the animals in a repeated dose study when exposure is by oral gavage. To deliver an accurate dose of test chemical in solution or suspension, the chemical must be mixed with solvent or suspending agent at the proper concentration which can be calculated using the intended dose level and the dose volume of the solution/suspension to be administered to the animals. This calculation is illustrated in Figure 19.2. Obviously, this same calculation applies to solutions or suspensions for other exposure routes, for example, administration by capsule, dermally, or parenterally.

Use of a vehicle to carry the test material into the animal has been mentioned several times in the preceding discussion. Choice of vehicle is a critical decision for toxicology studies. Obviously, the vehicle should be nontoxic at the dose (volume) administered, and should not act in an additive or synergistic manner to enhance the toxicity of the test material, nor should it interfere with the expression of any potential toxicity. Because such interactions are not always predictable, it is

- **Formula**

CONCENTRATION (mg test material/ml solution or suspension) =

$$\frac{\text{INTENDED DOSE LEVEL (mg test material/kg body weight/interval)}}{\text{DOSE VOLUME (ml solution or suspension/kg body weight/interval)}}$$

- **Example**

The concentration of a solution intended to deliver a daily 1500 mg/kg dose level of test material A to rats at a dose volume of 5 ml/kg body weight (BW) is calculated as follows:

$$\text{Concentration (mg A/ml)} = \frac{\text{1500 mg A/kg BW/day}}{\text{5 ml solution/kg BW/day}}$$

$$= \text{300 mg A/ml solution}$$

As indicated in the following, a 300 gram rat would receive 1.5 ml of this solution each day and, therefore, would receive the intended daily dose level. First, calculating the volume of solution administered to the rat:

0.3 kg body weight x 5 ml solution/kg BW/day = 1.5 ml/day

Then, calculating the amount of test material A in that volume:

1.5 ml of solution/day x 300 mg A/ml solution = 450 mg A/day

Finally, calculating the dose level resulting from administration of that amount of test material:

450 mg A/day ÷ 0.3 kg BW = 1500 mg A/kg BW/day

FIG. 19.2. Calculation of test material concentration in a solution or suspension.

imperative that vehicle controls be used in all oral gavage toxicology studies (and in virtually every other type of administration). However, even use of a vehicle control may not always compensate for the administration of vehicle in the groups receiving the test material. Interactions between vehicle and test materials can be encountered and must be considered during the design of studies because vehicles may produce physiological/nutritional alterations that may affect the toxicity of the test material, especially in longer-term studies. For instance, an oil vehicle may result in poor absorption of fat-soluble nutrients; food oil vehicles add to the caloric intake of the animal and may produce effects in longer-term studies; absorption of fat-soluble materials from oil vehicles can be slower than when the same material is administered in an aqueous matrix. The resulting change in the toxicokinetics of the test material can produce profound differences in toxicity. Because toxicity testing generally uses exaggerated doses compared to human exposure, it is sometimes difficult to obtain solutions. In such cases, suspensions are sometimes used, which, again, can affect toxicokinetics and influence toxicity. For these reasons, among others, great care must be utilized in selecting an appropriate vehicle for administration of test materials to animals.

Dermal Application

For a drug, cosmetic, industrial chemical, or pesticide with dermal exposure potential for humans, dermal application is the most appropriate exposure route for repeated dose studies. The test material is applied to a defined area of skin from which the hair has been removed. Removal of hair by both shaving and depilatories can alter skin permeability to applied materials. Because the test animal can ingest some of a dermal dose during grooming, it is common practice to cover the test material application site by wrapping the trunk of the animal with a semi-occlusive material (e.g., gauze strips) during the exposure period. Occasionally, if exaggerated dermal absorption is desired, the application site is covered with an occlusive material (e.g., rubber dam). Either method of wrapping, occlusion or semi-occlusion, maintains the test material in contact with the skin. Wrapping also increases the accuracy of the administered dose because on unoccluded animals, dry test materials may fall off the application site and liquid materials may run off or evaporate from the site. Restraint and/or "Elizabethan" collars are also sometimes used to prevent tampering with the wrap or to prevent oral ingestion if the application site is unoccluded. However, use of restraint or collars stresses the animals and, therefore, may alter the outcome of a study. To avoid unnecessary stress, the animals should be trained to accept such procedures before actual dosing is initiated.

Parenteral Administration

A pharmaceutical intended for administration to humans by injection should be administered to the test animals by the same parenteral route. A common type of parenteral exposure is subcutaneous injection. To avoid irritation and other potential effects, such as fibrotic reactions, the specific site of injection should be changed daily. It is recommended that the dosing vehicle be aqueous since oil vehicles may track back along the needle path and be deposited in the lipophilic skin and hair. As with oral gavage exposure, absorption from an oil vehicle may differ compared with an aqueous vehicle. For subcutaneous administration, care must be taken to ensure the material is deposited subcutaneously rather than intradermally or intramuscularly. This can be accomplished by lifting the skin of the animal to form a pocket and injecting the dosage into the subcutaneous pocket.

Other common routes of parenteral exposure include intravenous (iv), intramuscular (im), and intraperitoneal (ip) injection. Special considerations are required for each of these routes. For iv administration, the test material must be soluble in an aqueous vehicle since physiological saline is the usual vehicle. Air bubbles must be cleared from the delivery system—the needle, catheter and/or syringe, before injecting the material intravenously. The dosing solution for iv administration must be at a physiological pH and must not be extremely irritating or corrosive. Repeated use of the same injection site must be avoided. To prevent inadvertent delivery of the test material into the muscle or other surrounding tissue, care must be taken to insure that the needle tip is in the lumen of the vein before injecting the test material. Proper placement of the needle can be assessed by drawing a small amount of blood back into the delivery device. If no blood is observed, the needle is not located in the lumen of the vein. For im and ip routes of exposure, proper placement of the needle tip also must be assessed before administering the dose material. In contrast to iv exposure, drawing back on the delivery device without obtaining blood is required prior to administering material by the im route. Similarly, drawing back on the device without obtaining blood or intestinal contents prior to injecting test material is necessary for correct ip adminstration. Most other considerations for im and ip exposure are similar to those for iv administration for example, the material must not be corrosive or irritating, repeated injections at the same site should be avoided, and so on.

Continuous infusion may be used to simulate a constant human exposure or, for intravenous infusion of poorly soluble test substances, to deliver a sufficiently large daily dose for safety assessment. Infusions may be administered using either implanted or external pumps. Implanted pumps may be battery-operated mechanical pumps (nonrodents) or osmotic pumps (rodents and nonrodents); both of which permit unrestricted movement of the animal. Practical considerations of volume and weight of implanted pumps restrict their use to very soluble and/or potent test substances that can be administered slowly over a long period. External pumps may be connected to rodents and nonrodents using tethers and swivels or affixed to nonrodents as "back packs." External pumps allow for infusion of larger volumes of test substance but also require more waste substance because of the larger "dead space" of the tether catheter. Their use may be problematic for subchronic or chronic studies because of their relatively long duration. The patency of the catheter for implanted and external pumps must be confirmed. The dose received by each animal can be determined by measuring the weight of the pump and solution prior to initiation and following completion of exposure, or by direct measurement of the infused volume by syringe markings or by using calibrated pumps displaying the infusion rate. Study designs often incorporate measurement of blood concentrations of the test material and its metabolytes.

Implantation

Subcutaneous or intramuscular implantation is often used for evaluating biopolymers for medical devices or prostheses. In addition, test materials have been embedded in special matrices that allow continuous, sustained release for weeks or months after subcutaneous implantation. Demonstration of the stability of the test substance in the matrix, both during preparation of the pellet and after implantation, is required when using this technology. Determination of plasma concentrations of the test material and/or its metabolites can be used to confirm proper dosing. Because of size limitations, these pellets are useful only for delivery of very potent substances, such as hormones and biological proteins.

Dietary Administration

Dietary administration would be appropriate for a food additive or a pesticide that has potential to become a residue in or on food crops. This type of administration, although frequently used in subchronic and chronic toxicity studies, is less accurate than most other routes of dose delivery primarily because of differences between body weight and feed consumption of individual animals, which result in variable compound consumption. A further complication in rodent studies is that these animals tend to add body fat and not lean body mass as they age. Therefore, lipophilic compounds have a larger mass of fat into which they can partition. This may actually decrease the effective dose. In addition, fat does not have significant detoxication enzymes. Therefore, as dose is increased to account for increased body weight in older rodents, detoxication capacity may be stressed resulting in unanticipated toxicity. This complication is not unique to dietary exposure studies and will affect the effective dose of a test material in rodents exposed by most other routes. Although potential variability in effective dose is important to interpretation of the results of a study, no attempt is generally made to compensate for this variability during preparation of the test diet or calculation of the administered dose in repeated dose toxicity studies. Spillage or soiling of feed, which occurs fairly frequently with some test animals, is a factor that contributes variability to the calculation of dietary dose. Significant spillage or soiling must be considered when measuring feed consumption to be used in calculation of dietary concentration or compound consumption. Dietary administration can be conducted by either of two methods:

(1) adjusting the dietary concentration of the test material to account for changing body weight and feed consumption, or
(2) feeding a constant concentration in the diet.

Routinely adjusting the dietary concentration of a test material based upon the changing body weight and feed consumption of the animal provides reasonably good control over the delivered dose during a repeated dose study. Dietary concentration is usually adjusted weekly during a subchronic study. In a chronic study, diet concentration is usually adjusted weekly during the first 13–14 weeks (especially for rodents because of the rapid growth of the animals during this period) and biweekly or sometimes monthly thereafter. Using this method, the mean feed consumption and body weight of a dose group during a given study interval are used to calculate the dietary concentration to be fed to that group during the following interval. There are several ways to calculate the concentration. One formula for this calculation and an example of its use are presented in Figure 19.3. A caution in using this approach in quickly growing, young rats is that the concentration may increase dramatically during the study. Sometimes the target concentrations become too high to formulate the mix homogeneously or they reach a level that becomes unpalatable to the animals.

Feeding a constant concentration of the test material in the diet throughout the study is the second form of dietary administration. This method provides less control over the administered dose level because it is a function of the amount of feed (and, therefore, test material) consumed and body weight gained by each animal. The consumed dose, or compound consumption, of each individual animal can be calculated using its feed consumption and body weight. The mean of the individual animal compound consumptions represents the compound consumption for each dose group. A commonly used formula for the calculation of individual compound consumption is illustrated in Figure 19.4.

When feeding a constant concentration in a rodent study, the toxicologist must be aware that the compound consumption may vary significantly for an individual animal or group of animals during the course of the study. For example, compound consumption during the first week of a 13-week rat study in which the test compound is fed at a constant dietary concentration is frequently more than twice the compound consumption during the last week of the study. This variation results from the rapid decrease in feed consumption relative to body weight (g feed/kg body weight/day) by young rats during the first several months of life. This variability in compound consumption is illustrated in the example given in Figure 19.4.

Drinking Water

Water-soluble test substances can be offered as a mixture in the drinking water, providing adequate dosage can be achieved. This route may be preferred when it mimics human exposure conditions of constant exposure, compared with event-oriented exposure such as pill taking. Spillage can be a significant problem when administering material in drinking water and recovery of spilled water is usually not feasible. Another complication with drinking water administration is that evaporation of water and/or volatilization of the test material can occur from the tip of the drinking (sipper) tube, resulting in alteration of the concentration of the material in the water. Use of a sipper tube containing a ball bearing tip minimizes this problem.

Assessment of the Adequacy of Test Material Preparations

Whatever the route of exposure, it is critical to determine if the test material is delivered to the animals at the intended doses. For dietary studies, test diets should be prepared before initiation of a repeated dose study, using the intended diet preparation method. It must be shown that this preparation method yields diets containing the appropriate amounts of homogeneously mixed test material. Chemical analysis of samples taken from several locations in each test diet preparation should be conducted to determine if the proper concentrations of test material have been achieved and to assess the

- **Formula**

CONCENTRATION (mg test material/kg diet) =

$$\frac{\text{INTENDED DOSE LEVEL (mg test material/kg body weight/day)}}{\text{PROJECTED FEED CONSUMPTION (kg feed /kg body weight/day)}}$$

where projected feed consumption (PFC) for a study week is based on body weight (BW) and absolute feed consumption (AFC) data from the previous week and is calculated as follows:

PFC (kg/kg/day) for week$_n$ =

$$\frac{\text{AFC week}_{n-1}\text{ (kg)}}{7\text{ days}} \div \left[\text{BW end of week}_{n-1}\text{ (kg)} + \frac{\text{BW gain during week}_{n-1}\text{ (kg)}}{2}\right]$$

- **Example**

In a subchronic rat study, the mean body weight of the males in the 15 mg/kg/day dose group at the beginning of week 11 is 520 g. At the end of week 11, the mean weight for these males is 540 g. Mean feed consumption of these animals is 154 g during the 7 days of week 11. The dietary concentration intended to deliver a 15 mg/kg/day dose level of compound A to this group of rats during week 12 of the study is calculated as follows:

$$\text{PFC (week 12)} = \frac{0.154\text{ kg feed}}{7\text{ days}} \div \left[0.540\text{ kg BW} + \frac{0.020\text{ kg BW gain}}{2}\right]$$

$$= 0.04\text{ kg feed/kg BW/day}$$

and, therefore

$$\text{Concentration (week 12)} = \frac{15\text{ mg A/kg BW/day}}{0.04\text{ kg feed/kg BW/day}}$$

$$= 375\text{ mg A/kg feed}$$

Note that, because their body weight and feed consumption differ, the diet concentrations for males and females in the same dose group will generally differ throughout the study.

FIG. 19.3. Calculation of adjusted diet concentration to yield constant dose level.

homogeneity of the dietary admixtures. If the results of these analyses indicate the anticipated concentrations were not achieved or the distribution of test material in the diet was not homogenous, the diet preparation method should be revised and retested. Diet preparation must be validated before the study can be initiated.

During the pre-study homogeneity determinations, additional diet samples should be collected and analyzed to show that, within the range of concentrations to be used in the study, the test material is stable in the diet. These samples should be stored under animal room conditions and under frozen conditions for the maximum period of time during which the diet will be used or stored. For a study in which dietary admixtures will be prepared and fed once per week, stability of the test material in the diet would commonly be assessed for samples stored under animal room conditions for at least seven and fourteen days. This allows estimation of the degradation rate at room temperature. Analysis of frozen diet samples stored for several intervals is also advisable. Demonstration of stability under frozen storage conditions makes chemical analysis of diet samples immediately after collection during the toxicity study unnecessary and also validates the possibility of confirming analytical results by reanalysis of stored frozen samples, if needed. Adequate stability of the test material in the diet should be demonstrated prior to initiation of the study.

Even though the adequacy of the diet preparation method and stability of the test material in the diet have been demonstrated, it is important to monitor diet preparation during the study. For each diet preparation

Formula

COMPOUND CONSUMPTION (mg test material/kg body weight/day) =

$$\frac{\text{CONCENTRATION}}{\text{(mg test material/kg feed)}} \times \frac{\text{RELATIVE FEED CONSUMPTION}}{\text{(kg feed/kg body weight/day)}}$$

where relative feed consumption (RFC) for a study week is based on body weight (BW) and absolute feed consumption (AFC) during that week and is calculated as follows:

RFC (kg/kg/day) =

$$\frac{\text{AFC (kg)}}{\text{7 days}} \div \left[\text{BW start of week (kg)} + \frac{\text{BW gain during week (kg)}}{2}\right]$$

Example

In a subchronic rat study, a group of males is fed test material A at a constant dietary concentration of 2% (w/w). The body weight of one animal in this group is 175 g at the start of week 1 and 225 g at the end of week 1. Its feed consumption during the 7 days of week 1 is 168 g. Subsequently, this rat weighs 490 g at the start and 510 g at the end of week 13; and its feed consumption during that week is 196 g. The compound consumption of this rat for each week is calculated as follows:

$$\text{RFC (week 1)} = \frac{\text{0.168 kg feed}}{\text{7 days}} \div \left[\text{0.175 kg BW} + \frac{\text{0.050 kg BW gain}}{2}\right] = \text{0.120 kg feed/kg BW/day}$$

$$\text{RFC (week 13)} = \frac{\text{0.196 kg feed}}{\text{7 days}} \div \left[\text{0.490 kg BW} + \frac{\text{0.020 kg BW gain}}{2}\right] = \text{0.056 kg feed/kg BW/day}$$

and, therefore:

Compound Consumption (week 1) = 2% test material A x RFC (week 1)
= 2 g A/100 g feed x 0.120 kg feed/kg BW/day
= 20,000 mg A/kg feed x 0.120 kg feed/kg BW/day
= 2400 mg A/kg BW/day

Compound Consumption (week 13) = 2% test material A x RFC (week 13)
= 20,000 mg A/kg feed x 0.056 kg feed/kg BW/day
= 1120 mg A/kg BW/day

FIG. 19.4. Calculation of compound consumption resulting from constant diet concentration.

during the first several weeks of the study, concentrations of the test material in the diets should be assessed. Subsequent analysis of diet preparations every two to four weeks will add assurance that diets were prepared properly. More frequent analysis, for example, weekly throughout the study, is even more desirable.

For routes of exposure other than dietary, the principles cited above also apply. Concentration, homogeneity and stability of the test material in solvents or suspending agents must be determined for studies using oral, dermal, inhalation, or other routes of exposure when the test material is to be administered in solution, suspension, or as an aerosol. Suspensions represent a special case because care must be taken to ensure that the suspensions do not settle and become nonhomogenous during administration to the test species. For inhalation studies, the concentration of gas, aerosol, or particulates to which the animals are exposed should also be assessed using appropriate analytical methods.

Duration of Exposure

As stated previously, the duration of subchronic toxicity studies involves exposure of the test species to a chemical during a significant portion of its lifetime. Classically, these studies are conducted for 90 consecutive days or approximately 13 weeks. Chronic toxicity studies in rodents most commonly involve exposure for a major portion of their life span, generally 12 months, although studies of shorter duration (i.e., 6–9 months) are considered acceptable by some groups (43). Rodent chronic toxicity studies are sometimes combined with lifetime oncogenicity studies to achieve efficiencies during some of the study procedures, for example, diet preparation. During these combination studies, the animals in the chronic toxicity segment are generally studied during the first 6–12 months, and then are terminated. Those in the oncogenicity segment continue on study generally for at least 24 months. In nonrodents—for example, dogs and non-human primates, which are longer lived than rodents—6–12 months represent a significantly smaller portion of their life span but is currently considered an adequate duration of exposure to detect chronic effects.

Daily test material administration during a repeated dose toxicity study can be continuous, intermittent, or repeated. In most dietary and drinking water studies, the animals have free access to diets or water containing the test material throughout the study and exposure is essentially continuous, although influenced by diurnal variation. In dermal or inhalation studies, exposure to the test material is intermittent, generally four to six hours per day. When the route of administration is intravenous infusion, exposure may be either continuous or intermittent. With bolus dose parenteral administration or oral gavage, test material administration is generally once or, at most, a few times each day. Labor-intensive methods of administration, such as oral gavage, are sometimes done only during the standard work week, that is, five days per week. This is not recommended because two days of non-exposure each week during the study may be sufficient to allow modification or reversal of toxic responses.

Dose Groups

The minimum number of groups receiving test material in a repeated dose toxicity study is generally three (low, mid-, and high dose). The high-dose level should produce evidence of toxicity, but should not result in more than 10 percent mortality. The mid-dose level should produce no more than slight toxicity and the low-dose level should produce no toxicity yielding a NOAEL. As previously stated, a short-term (two to four weeks) repeated dose study should be conducted to aid in the selection of doses for subchronic testing. For test materials where a dose response has not been well defined during a short-term repeated dose study, additional dose groups may be required in the subchronic study to insure the range of desired responses—that is, no toxicity to significant toxicity—is achieved. However, it is sometimes difficult to completely satisfy these criteria. Before selecting doses for a chronic toxicity study, a subchronic study that defines no-effect and effect levels should be completed.

Limit Studies

For test materials that possess very low potential for toxicity, the inclusion of only one test material dose group in a repeated dose study is sometimes acceptable. A study with this design is termed a *limit study*. Limit testing is inappropriate for materials with anticipated high human exposure. The dose level for the test material group in dietary and dermal limit studies is normally at least 1000 mg/kg/day. Another type of limit study involves utilization of the maximal exposure level under the conditions of the study. For example, suppose the majority of toxicology data concerning a lipophilic drinking water contaminant has been collected using oral administration in a corn oil vehicle and additional data are desired using a water vehicle. The limited water solubility of the test material may result in the maximal dose being significantly lower than the dose used in the corn oil gavage studies. However, the test material can be tested as a saturated water solution and such a study may reveal the test material to be either more or less toxic in water than in the oil vehicle. The data are relevant to the assessment of hazard associated with exposure in the drinking water because the maximal possible exposure by this route of administration was tested. Thus, while a limit study may not define the "complete" toxicology of a test material, it can define the "practical" toxicology of the material.

Control Groups

Adequate controls are essential to successful toxicity studies of all types, including repeated dose studies. Studies should contain at least one control group for comparison with the groups receiving the test material. The control group should be treated identically to the treated groups except the control group should receive no test material. Control groups can be either negative or positive controls.

Negative control groups are intended to demonstrate the normal state of the animal for comparison to data from the groups treated with the test material. They also provide an opportunity to compare baseline data for the current study to baseline data from previous studies. There are several types of negative controls. If the test material is dissolved or suspended in a vehicle for administration, a vehicle control group should receive, by the same route of exposure, the maximum amount of solvent or suspending agent administered to any of the test material groups. If the test material is administered in the diet, an untreated control group should receive the same diet without test material. For test materials administered undiluted, a sham control group should receive the same physical treatment as the treated groups, for example, insertion of an intubation tube with or without delivery of an innocuous substance like water, administration of empty capsules, or injection of physiological saline.

Positive control groups are intended either to demonstrate susceptibility of the animal to a specific toxicity or to compare the response of test material-treated animals to that of animals treated with a chemical that produces a known toxicity similar to the test material. If a positive control group is included in a study design, at least one negative control group should also be included. Positive control groups are infrequently used in repeated dose toxicity testing. However, if the chemical structure of a test material suggests that it may possess a specific toxicity—for example, neurotoxicity—it may be important to demonstrate that the species and strain selected for testing is susceptible to that toxicity.

A positive control that is sometimes useful in repeated dose studies is the reference control. This control consists of a material that is chemically or physically similar to the test material but has either a comprehensive toxicology database associated with it or a history of use without adverse effects. Inclusion of a reference control group allows a comparison between reference and test material within the same study. This can assist in identifying any effects related to the general characteristics of the reference material. For instance, oral administration of a poorly absorbed oil can decrease the absorption of fat-soluble vitamins. If the test material is known or suspected to produce this effect, use of a reference material, such as mineral oil, can be useful. This would distinguish effects related to vitamin depletion from effects produced directly by the test material. Additionally, if the test material were to add substantially to the caloric intake, a reference control diet isocaloric to the test diet would be useful, especially in longer-term studies. A reference control group also may be useful to compare the degree of anticipated toxicity of the test material to a reference material of known toxicity. For example, it could be important to demonstrate that the hepatotoxicity of a test material intended for use as an anesthetic is significantly less severe than that produced by an anesthetic already in use.

Animal Models

To increase the probability of testing in a species that may respond to the test material in a manner similar to humans, two species are generally used. Routinely, one rodent species and one nonrodent species are utilized. Rats and dogs are the generally preferred species for most routes of exposure. The rabbit is preferred for dermal exposure. Mice, hamsters, miniature swine, guinea pigs, non-human primates, and a few other species are used on occasion in these studies. Many factors should be carefully considered during the selection of the most appropriate species and strain for testing with a specific chemical. Some of these factors are summarized in Table 19.6.

Table 19.6
Selection criteria for species and strain in repeated dose studies

- Requirements by regulatory agencies
- Metabolism of test material in a manner similar to humans
- Availability of historical control data
- Most sensitive species and strain
- Responsiveness of particular organs and tissues to specific toxicities
- Availability of the species and strain
- Availability of appropriate animal housing and husbandry
- Experience of the laboratory in the use of the species and strain

Toxicokinetics

Ideally, selection of an animal model for repeated dose toxicity studies should be based upon the similarity between toxicokinetics of the test chemical in that species and strain to its toxicokinetics in humans. This selection criterion assumes that these factors are known in potential test animals and in humans, though often, these data are unavailable during the initial phase of a hazard assessment. Although the metabolism of a chemical may be understood in one strain of one species of laboratory animal before initiation of repeated dose testing, it is seldom known in several species and strains. With the exception of pharmaceuticals, the metabolism of a chemical in humans is almost never known before initiation of a subchronic or chronic study. Consequently, similarity in metabolism between humans and animal models is seldom the initial basis for selection of test species and strain. This may change, however. Currently, human microsomes and systems that express specific human detoxification enzymes are commercially available. This opens the possibility of having in vitro data concerning human metabolism before initiating a hazard assessment.

Sensitivity to Test Material

Another commonly used criterion for selection of the animal species and strain for repeated dose testing is sensitivity to the test material. As a conservative approach to the extrapolation of toxic effects seen in animals to humans, the animal model selected should be the most sensitive to the effects of the chemical. Data required for this decision are often not available until a significant portion of the total hazard assessment program for the chemical has been completed. Acute and short-term repeated dose studies may reveal information concerning species sensitivity. However, relative sensitivity of different species and strains frequently only can be determined following completion of longer-term studies with their more comprehensive endpoints. Nevertheless, sensitivity to the chemical should be considered during selection of the test animal. For example, differences in the sensitivity of particular organs and tissues to toxic compounds among different species should be considered, and strains that have aberrant metabolic pathways, especially those associated with detoxification, should not be used except in special cases. For instance, the Gunn rat does not produce certain glucuronides (63) and would not be an appropriate animal model for a hazard assessment. Cats are deficient in their ability to produce glucuronides but can produce sulfate conjugates.

Although the concurrent control is the most important source of data for comparison, availability of historical control data for the variables evaluated during repeated dose toxicity testing is an important consideration in selecting the test species and strain. These data are frequently useful in determining the significance of a finding when comparison of data from treated and concurrent control groups suggests a potential treatment-related effect. Historical data concerning growth, feed consumption, clinical pathology, and other variables are often useful in interpreting findings from a subchronic or chronic study. Historical histopathology data are of particular importance due to their subjective nature. Although published data can be useful, historical data from the laboratory at which the study is being conducted are more applicable. Most laboratories have historical databases for commonly used species and strains. If less common species are being considered, the availability of historical data should be assessed before final selection.

Other Animal Model Considerations Involved in Study Design

After consideration of the above criteria, pragmatic considerations are necessary during selection of a species and strain. The animals should be obtained from a reputable, reliable supplier who will guarantee their health and will arrange expeditious and controlled shipment of the animals to the laboratory. The supplier should maintain careful records concerning the animal colony and maintain a healthy colony, providing disease-free animals because it is often not possible to treat for disease once a study has begun. The quantity of available test material may influence the selection of the animal model. For example, it may be necessary to select a rodent species if the amount of test material available is insufficient for long-term administration to a larger species such as the dog or non-human primate. Capabilities of the testing laboratory should be considered during test animal selection. The laboratory must have appropriate caging and other equipment and must be able to maintain the proper environmental conditions in the animal room. In addition, the laboratory conducting the study should have experience with use of the chosen species in toxicology studies. This can avoid problems associated with species specific physiology and anatomy.

Age of Animals

Age of animals used in subchronic and chronic toxicity studies is relatively standard. For rodents, initiation of test material administration at six weeks of age will satisfy virtually all guidelines for testing. Dogs should be approximately four to six months of age at initiation of exposure to the chemical. Precise age of non-human primates is frequently not known; however, age can be approximated by experienced suppliers. For non-human primates and other less commonly used species, young animals generally should be used.

Pre-study Health Assessment

To the extent possible, it should be ensured that each animal included in a repeated dose study is in good health. The animals must not have been previously used for any other type of experimental procedures. An exception is sometimes made for non-human primates, which may occasionally be used for more than one study, with a reasonable period between studies to ensure any residual test material is absent. These animals should undergo extensive health screening, including clinical pathology, between studies.

For rodent studies, enough animals of each gender should be obtained to allow culling of those with conditions that could either interfere with completing the study or be interpreted as treatment related at completion of the study. It is good practice to obtain at least 10% more animals than will be required to fill the study groups. Minimally, pre-test physical examination and body weight measurement should be conducted to assess the health of each animal before study initiation. Pre-test ophthalmological examination and clinical pathology evaluations are advisable. Animals in poor health or exhibiting ocular or other defects should be eliminated from consideration for the study.

To insure the toxicologist is aware of any infection that the animals may be exposed to during the study, a sentinel group is often maintained in the room with the study animals. For rodents, this group normally contains five to ten animals of each gender. Serum antibody titers are assessed at the initiation of the study and at the termination of the in-life phase of the study. If necessary, antibody titers and/or other evidence of infection can also be obtained from these animals during the study without

Table 19.7
Serum antibody analyses in rodents

Rat	Mouse
Sendai virus	Sendai virus
Pneumonia virus of mice	Pneumonia virus of mice
Reovirus type III	Reovirus type III
Mycoplasma pulmonis	*Mycoplasma pulmonis*
Lymphocytic choriomeningitis virus	Lymphocytic choriomeningitis virus
Mouse adenovirus FL/K87	Mouse adenovirus FL/K87
Mouse polio virus	Mouse polio virus
Hantaan virus	Hantaan virus
Encephalitozoon cuniculi	*Encephalitozoon cuniculi*
Cilia associated respiratory bacillus	Cilia associated respiratory bacillus
Rat parvovirus-IFA	Mouse parvovirus-IFA
Rat coronavirus/ sialodacryoadenitis virus	Murine hepatitis virus
Kilham rat virus	Minute virus of mice
Toolan H-1 virus	Ectomelia virus
	Mouse pneumonitis virus
	Polyomavirus
	Mouse thymic virus
	Epizootic diarrhea of infant mice virus
	Mouse cytomegalovirus

disturbing the animals on test. A relatively complete list of antibody analyses used in rodent species is presented in Table 19.7.

Health assessment of nonrodent species by the supplier is generally more comprehensive than rodents. This reduces the need to obtain many extra nonrodents. However, it is good practice to conduct procedures after receipt of nonrodents to make sure their health has not changed before use in a subchronic or chronic toxicity study.

Number of Animals

To satisfy most regulatory guidelines, a minimum of 10–20 rodents of each gender should be included in each control and test material dosed group in a repeated dose study. For nonrodents, the minimum number of animals of each gender in each group is four. However, the minimum number of animals is frequently exceeded in an attempt to allow for unexpected mortality or to increase the sensitivity of the study. Twenty rodents or four-to-six nonrodents of each gender per group are often used as the base number of animals for the study. Some study designs include an interim necropsy at one or more intervals for detection and evaluation of the progression of potential effects during the study. Other designs may contain treated animals that will be maintained without exposure after the termination of the main study groups to determine the reversibility of any adverse effects. Still other designs include satellite groups for special purposes, for example, toxicokinetic determinations or untreated sentinel animals used to monitor the health of the study animals. The base number of animals placed on study at its initiation should be increased by the number of animals to be used for these enhanced study designs.

Individual Animal Identification

Before assignment to the repeated dose toxicity study, each animal must be provided a unique identification number. This number will be associated with the animal throughout the study and will be used to identify specimens, tissues, and data from the animal after the in-life portion of the study is completed. Therefore, this number must stay with the animal continuously during the study so that there is no chance of misidentification. It is not adequate to simply attach the animal identification to each cage because animals may escape from their cages or may be placed in the wrong one during cage-changing operations. Unique identification numbers can be placed on the animals by a number of methods. Whatever the identification method, it should remain permanent and readable for the duration of the study. Older methods used for rodents included toe clipping, where a small portion of the toe was removed in a specified coded manner, and ear punching, where holes were punched through the ears in a specified coded manner. These methods are less acceptable today because more precise and humane methods have become widely available. Currently, the use of a numbered tag attached to an ear or tattoos placed on the tail or ear are commonly used methods for large and small animal identification. A newer method that has gained considerable acceptance in recent years involves subcutaneous implantation of a miniature electronic device that can be read by a hand held scanner.

Randomization of Animals

After culling all animals that do not meet the study criteria, such as those that do not pass physical examination or are not within specified body weight boundaries, and assigning unique identification numbers to the remaining animals, the next step is to randomize them into the various study groups. This is a critical step in the study to ensure the greatest ability to detect statistical differences between the groups in the study without bias. Although a number of randomization methods have been devised, some more appropriate than others, one of the most popular is the utilization of random number tables. After randomization into the various study groups, some method should be employed to determine if the animals are truly randomized based upon a variable critical to the study. The most commonly used variable is body weight. Statistical analysis of mean body weight data is conducted to show that there are no statistically significant intergroup differences in mean body weight, and, hopefully, other variables, at the initiation of the study. It is not uncommon to find that the mean body weight of the animals in one of the study groups is significantly different from one or more of the other groups. In cases where there may be a significant difference between the mean body weights of any of the study groups, the animals are again randomized into study groups and the process repeated. Randomization must be conducted independently for each gender because of body weight differences between males and females.

Animal Husbandry

Proper care and maintenance of animals in a repeated dose toxicity study is essential not only for ethical reasons but also to minimize mistakenly attributing adverse findings to the test material. The Animal Welfare Act (AWA), enforced by the Animal, Plant and Health Inspection Service (APHIS) of the U.S. Department of Agriculture, mandates standards for acceptable handling, care, treatment, and transportation of many species, including most laboratory species except mice, rats, and birds (61). In its *Guide for the Care and Use of Laboratory Animals*, the Institute of Laboratory Animal Resources (ILAR) of the National Research Council has published guidelines that are widely accepted as standards for laboratory animal husbandry (44). From their arrival at the laboratory, animals must be maintained in an appropriately controlled environment and provided an adequate quantity and quality of feed and water and housed in clean cages of appropriate design. They should be acclimated to the study room conditions for at least one week before study initiation (see Chapter 16).

Environmental Factors

Temperature and humidity should be controlled within limits specified in the documents referenced above. Table 19.8 is taken from the ILAR document and contains the recommended temperature ranges for various laboratory animal species (44). Low humidity can result in drying of the mucous membranes and eyes of laboratory animals, and high humidity can result in growth of bacterial and fungal populations that result in respiratory distress and dermal involvement, such as ringworm. In addition, urine and excreta may not dry as readily, thereby increasing room odor. Relative humidity of 30–70% is considered acceptable by ILAR for most laboratory species (44).

Adequate ventilation is a key factor in maintaining good animal health during a toxicology study. Establishing a positive room air pressure reduces possible exposure of animals to test materials being used in other animal rooms. When more air is forced into a room than can be completely cleared by exhaust systems, it flows through the cracks, around the door, and the partial pressure of air in the room becomes positive with respect to the hallway or area outside the room. Ventilation should be homogeneous throughout the room; this generally is controlled by adjustable diffusers and the ventilation of all rooms in a facility must be "balanced" periodically to provide the same relative airflow and positive pressure with regard to hallways. In general, 10–15 fresh air changes per h is considered acceptable but this range is highly dependent on a number of factors, for example, the number of animals in the room.

Common lighting schedules used are 12 h of continuous light and 12 h of darkness for rats, mice, dogs, and monkeys, and 14 h of light and 10 h of dark for hamsters. This schedule allows the animals to become acclimated to a light cycle. This stimulates a constant pattern of secretion of thyroid hormones, ACTH, and growth hormone. Regulated lighting cycles are necessary in reproduction studies because rodents enter continuous estrus under conditions of constant light without darkness. Because high-intensity fluorescent light can cause blindness in albino rodents, current practice is to limit their exposure to high-intensity light to times when observations are collected by providing dual-intensity (high–low) lighting systems.

Animal Caging

In the United States, rodents are commonly housed one per cage during subchronic and chronic toxicity studies. In other countries, rodents are frequently multiply housed during these studies because it is believed that multiple housing increases survival and decreases background pathology. Multiple caging of animals can produce problems associated with unique identification and trauma to the animals from fighting, and multiply housed rodents are more susceptible to transmitted disease and other health concerns. Furthermore, a multiply caged rodent that dies on study may sustain tissue destruction from cannibalism. It also is not possible to determine individual feed consumption when multiple animals are housed in a single cage, resulting in the loss of important data

Table 19.8
ILAR recommended dry-bulb temperatures for common laboratory species

	Dry-Bulb Temperature	
	°C	°F
• Mouse, rat, hamster, gerbil, guinea pig	18–26	64–79
• Rabbit	16–22	61–72
• Cat, dog, non-human primate	18–29	64–84
• Farm animals and poultry	16–27	61–81

because it is not possible to correlate body weight with individual feed intake. In addition, if the test material is fed as part of the diet, it is not possible to calculate actual exposure doses for individual rodents in the absence of individual feed consumption data. Although some of the same problems exist for nonrodents, multiple housing of some species (e.g., non-human primates and dogs) on a regular or continuous basis during the study is accepted practice to permit the social interaction and exercise considered necessary for these species.

Rodents generally are housed in metal (stainless or galvanized steel) or plastic (polyethylene, polypropylene, or polycarbonate) cages. Metal caging or floor pens are used for dogs. Minimum cage sizes for all species are stipulated in the ILAR publication (44) and, for nonrodents, in the AWA (61). Compliance is monitored by federal and state health agencies. Because minimum sizes for cages are stipulated, only caging type remains to be decided between solid floor cages or pens and suspended-floor cages.

Solid floor caging requires bedding to be added to the cage to absorb and contain waste materials; this may introduce dust. Sawdust and chips of some conifers induce hepatic cytochrome P450 monooxygenase activity, which may affect the outcome of the study. In addition, this type of caging allows animals to have access to their waste. Shoebox-style cages used for rodents may clear the atmosphere at a slower rate than suspended wire cages.

Cages with suspended wire floors also have disadvantages. Traumatic foot and leg injuries can occur, particularly with smaller animals. Plantar foot pad lesions are common in long-term studies of rats housed in wire bottom cages, especially in heavy males. This type of cage also exposes the animal to room drafts.

Most gradients in light, temperature, or airborne products in an animal room will occur vertically. Animals within groups should be distributed in cage racks so that members of each study group are present equally at all vertical caging levels. This practice, and the practice of periodically changing the relative position of each cage rack within the room, avoids confounding treatment group with cage position. Documentation of environmental conditions and of cage/rack rotation is essential.

Cleaning cages at frequent intervals is essential. Poor husbandry may result in skin lesions, alopecia, or the appearance of signs and behavior that may be interpreted as a possible effect of the test article.

Diets

The influence of diet and nutrition on the toxicity of xenobiotics is another important aspect of the design of toxicology studies. Because the diet fed the animals during toxicology studies can influence the results, the decision made by the toxicologist concerning what diet to feed the animals may have a profound impact upon the outcome of the studies. The diet fed during a study should have been designed for the study species. Although diets can be custom-made, they are generally obtained from commercial suppliers who should be reputable and capable of supplying information concerning basic diet composition and nutritional information. Although not feasible for a long-term study (e.g., 12 months), the same lot of diet should be used for the entire study whenever possible, and used before its expiration date. It should be stored under appropriate conditions to maintain nutritional value, minimize insect and rodent infestations, and ensure it is not contaminated by environmental chemicals.

Commercial diets are available in either ground "powder" or pelleted form. When the test material is to be incorporated into the feed, a powdered diet is generally used. Use of powdered diet also facilitates the determination of feed consumption. Pelleted diets are most frequently used when test material administration is by routes other than dietary. A powdered diet can be pelleted after a test material has been added, which reduces the dust from the diets. Pelleted diets also decrease the potential exposure of animal room personnel to the test material. However, the heat and pressure involved during the pelleting process may cause degradation of test materials sensitive to these conditions.

Diets used in toxicology studies are of two basic compositions. Currently, diets made from natural ingredients are most commonly used, but semi-purified diets made from refined macronutrients, such as protein and carbohydrate, and micronutrients, such as vitamin and mineral mixes, are sometimes used. Each has particular advantages and disadvantages that must be carefully considered by the toxicologist.

Natural diets are formulated from unrefined plant and animal products to meet the nutritional requirements of a particular species. In closed formula diets, the manufacturer does not provide the exact proportions of the constituents. The diets are formulated based upon nutritional specifications without emphasis on consistency of specific ingredients between lots. Plant materials contain a number of "non-nutritive" components that can effect various physiological and biochemical functions, including detoxification and metabolic activation, in the test animal. Because these components may vary with plant species, strain, growing conditions, and site, individual lots of closed-formula diets may differ in these constituents. Open-formula diets are formulated with constant quantities of specified ingredients, resulting in a more consistent composition than closed-formula diets. An example is the NIH-07 rodent diet, which has been relatively well characterized (59). Open-formula diets have advantages for long-term studies because of their consistent formulation. An additional consideration concerning both open- and closed-formula natural diets is their potential to contain contaminants, such as pesticides, heavy metals, and mycotoxins. To overcome this problem, some manufacturers provide diets that have been assayed for certain potential contaminants to insure they are below stated specifications. It is highly recommended that these "certified" diets be used in toxicology studies. A disadvantage of natural commercial diets is that their nutritional composition cannot be readily altered. It is possible to supplement these diets but not to remove constituents. An important advantage of natural diets is their long history of use and the resulting large quantities of historical control data.

Semi-purified diets are made from refined macroconstituents such as protein, carbohydrate and fiber, and micronutrient mixes containing individual minerals and vitamins and a defined fat source such as corn oil. Their constituents can be varied to design diets for specific nutritional purposes and allow for the inclusion of test materials that may provide nutrient activity or result in nutritional deficits. Nutrient composition can be reproduced exactly from lot to lot of semi-purified diet. As opposed to natural ingredient diets, semi-purified diets do not contain pesticides, mycotoxins, and other constituents that may alter the animal's response to the test material. However, a major problem with semi-purified diets is a lack of historical data from their use in long-term studies. A large number of different dietary compositions are currently in use and data obtained from one semi-purified diet may not extrapolate to another. Even with the most commonly used semi-purified diet, the AIN-76A (1), there are insufficient data to determine its impact on long-term toxicology studies, especially carcinogenicity studies (26). Although these diets can be utilized in subchronic toxicity studies, the data obtained may not be as useful as that from studies with natural diets, especially when these data are used to design longer-term studies with natural diets. While it may be necessary to use semi-purified diets with specific test materials, care must be taken if they are to be used in a safety assessment.

Dietary restriction has been shown to prolong the life of rats and mice. There is some interest in employing restricted food intake (~20%) in chronic toxicity and carcinogenicity studies to prolong the lifespan, and therefore the exposure period, of the animals. If feed restriction is planned, it may be appropriate to employ this regimen in the shorter-term studies also. Utilization of feed restriction in toxicity studies should be discussed with the appropriate regulatory agency before it is included in a safety assessement program.

Drinking Water

Drinking water free of contaminants that could interfere with the objectives of the study should be available to the animals during repeated dose toxicity studies. Water is frequently provided to the rodent and nonrodent animals through automatic watering systems in which a common water supply is piped to the animal cages and each cage contains a valve that allows the animal ad libitum access to the water. Water bottles are another, more labor-intensive method of providing water to the rodents and some nonrodents. For this method, each bottle is fitted with a stopper containing a sipper tube through which the animal can drink and, which, is suspended on the cage. A third method, generally only used with nonrodents, is to provide the animals with water in a drinking bowl. Any of these is acceptable as long as procedures are in place to insure that the animals are provided an adequate supply of potable water.

In-Life Evaluations

Physical Examination

Several variables are routinely evaluated during the treatment phase of subchronic toxicity studies. Each animal should be observed twice daily at least four hours apart (A.M. and P.M.) for overt signs of toxicity, moribundity, and mortality. During these A.M. and P.M. observations, the cage of each animal should be opened to permit unobstructed observation. In addition, each animal should be removed from its cage for a complete physical examination at least once a week. These examinations should include detailed observations for approximate time of onset of any changes, degree and duration of changes involving the skin, fur, eyes, mucous membranes, respiratory function, circulatory system, autonomic and central nervous systems, somatomotor function, and general behavior. A study-specific or SOP-specific glossary of clinical terms and descriptive criteria for each finding is recommended, with simple and descriptive terms, and using a minimum of medical or diagnostic terminology.

Body Weight Measurement

It is recommended that body weight be measured at least once a week, even though biweekly or monthly measurement after the first three months of a chronic toxicity study is acceptable to most regulatory agencies. Weekly measurement is recommended because body weight is one of the most sensitive indicators of the condition of an animal if it is monitored frequently and carefully during a study. Rapid and/or marked body weight loss is usually a harbinger of ill health or death. Rapid body weight loss can be due to either decreased feed or water consumption, disease, or specific toxic effects.

Feed Consumption

In rodents, feed consumption generally is measured once a week during subchronic studies and the first three months of chronic studies. After the third month of a rodent chronic study, feed consumption may be measured less frequently, that is, biweekly or monthly. For nonrodents, in which the quantity of feed required usually does not allow weekly feeding, feed consumption is evaluated for shorter intervals, often once or twice per day. Accurate measurement of feed consumption is essential for studies in which the test material is administered in the diet. As discussed earlier in this chapter, feed consumption and the dietary concentration of the test material are used to calculate the dose of test material consumed by the animals in such studies. Some species, especially the mouse and the non-human primate, frequently soil or waste feed; which makes accurate measurement of consumption difficult. In these species, feed consumption measurement can be attempted using either a feed container designed to minimize wastage or by attempting to estimate feed wastage. Limitations of such data should be considered in evaluating test material consumption and the significance of any apparent differences between feed consumption in test material-treated and control animals. Feed consumption measurement is another means of monitoring animal well-being. Animals that are ill or suffering adverse effects from exposure to the test material frequently will exhibit significantly decreased feed intake.

Ophthalmological Examination

Ophthalmological examination of all test animals should be conducted before initiation and at the completion of the test material administration period. This evaluation should be conducted by a veterinary ophthalmologist experienced in the observation of the species used for the study.

Clinical Pathology

Clinical pathology variables such as hematology, clinical chemistry, and urinalysis are important indicators of general health and toxicity and are assessed at termination of a subchronic or chronic study. In addition, pretest and interim (typically at 4 weeks in subchronic studies and at 13 weeks in chronic studies) clinical pathology may be conducted to allow evaluation of progression of any treatment-related effects noted at termination of the study. In rodents, clinical pathology determinations are usually conducted for 10 animals of each gender in each group. For nonrodents, clinical pathology should be done for all animals.

Sample collection. Proper sample collection and handling are critical to completion of a meaningful clinical pathology evaluation. Whenever possible, the method of sample collection should be the same throughout the study and should be one that distributes variance—such as run-to-run variation in an enzyme assay—equally across groups. Samples generally are collected according to either a totally random design or a stratified random design. A stratified random design ensures that approximately the same number of animals of each gender and from each group are sampled within any block of time or during any set of assays.

Repeated blood sampling of rodents can be accomplished by serial collection from the same animals by non-terminal procedures (such as puncture of the orbital sinus or jugular vein), or by collection from the abdominal aorta or vena cava at termination of subgroups of animals. Because of practical restraints on the frequency and volume of blood collection in rodents, pretest studies often are not performed. Repeated collection of adequate volumes of blood usually is not a problem for nonrodents and pretest clinical pathology is often included in studies using these animals.

The effect of repeated blood sampling on the animals and on the sample volume that can be reliably obtained at each sampling interval should be considered. Sample volumes should be sufficient both to conduct the assays indicated in the protocol and, if possible, to provide a reserve sample for any necessary repeat test. However, significant reduction of blood volume (more than 10%) by blood collection should be avoided.

Plasma or serum to be used for clinical evaluation should be clear and straw-colored. Red or pink plasma suggests that some hemolysis has occurred either as a result of pathology or as an artifact of the sample collection/preparation procedures. Severe artifactual hemolysis may alter the results for some of the clinical variables to be evaluated. Slight hemolysis, commonly observed in serum and plasma collected from rodents by orbital sinus or jugular venipuncture, generally is acceptable for clinical pathology studies as long as historical laboratory ranges have been established for blood collected by these methods. If unusual or unexpected results are obtained, aliquots of serum or plasma can be "spiked" with ascending amounts of test material to determine if it interferes with the assay.

Clinical chemistry, hematology, and urinalysis. Clinical pathology should include determination of a number of serum or plasma chemistry and hematology variables which should assess electrolyte balance, protein and carbohydrate metabolism, and organ function. An acceptable list of clinical chemistry variables is shown in Table 19.9. Additional variables should be assessed, as appropriate, to address other anticipated effects of the test material, for example, serum cholinesterase levels in the case of carbamate or organophosphate insecticides. Assays designed for assessment of clinical chemistry in humans must be validated for use with the species used in the toxicology studies. Typical hematological variables assessed during repeated dose testing are shown in Table 19.10. The reader is referred to the chapter concerning clinical pathology in

Table 19.9
Clinical chemistry variables normally obtained in repeated dose studies[a,b]

• glucose*	• potassium*
• urea nitrogen*	• chloride*
• creatinine*	• bilirubin (total)
• total protein*	• cholesterol
• albumin	• triglycerides
• globulin	• alkaline phosphatase*
• albumin/globulin ratio	• aspartate aminotransferase
• inorganic phosphorus	• alanine aminotransferase*
• calcium	• gamma glutamyl transferase*
• sodium*	• ornithine carbamyl transferase*

[a] Based, in part, upon the recommendations of Referene 23.
[b] This list does not include all clinical chemistry variables that could be obtained. Additional variables could be added dependent upon the test material. When the blood volume obtained for analysis is small, the FDA recommends priority be given those assays marked with an asterisk (*).

Table 19.10
Hematology and urinalysis variables generally determined in a repeated dose study

Hematology	Urinalysis
• hematocrit	• appearance
• hemoglobin	• urine volume
• erythrocyte count	• specific gravity
• mean corpuscular volume	• pH
• mean corpuscular hemoglobin	• glucose
• mean corpuscular hemoglobin concentration	• protein
• total leukocyte count	• microscopic evaluation of urinary sediment
• differential leukocyte count	
• reticulocyte count	
• platelet count	
• prothrombin time	

this text for a more detailed discussion of these clinical chemistry and hematology determinations, and two excellent veterinary texts available for further reference (45,49).

Urinalysis is often included in the clinical pathology evaluation and may be important, especially for test materials that are nephrotoxins. Urinalysis variables typically evaluated are listed in Table 19.10. Urinalysis however, is frequently of limited value because collection of satisfactory urine samples is fraught with technical difficulties. Urine generally is collected in containers or tubes from troughs or trays placed below the cages in which the animals are housed and, therefore, steps must be taken to minimize fecal contamination. Because urine is frequently collected during an extended period, for example, overnight, bacterial growth in the sample is a concern. Collection of the sample on ice can reduce bacterial growth but presents its own technical challenges. Care should be taken that water be either freely available to the animals throughout the urine collection period or withdrawn at the appropriate time before collection, and the sample must not be inadvertently contaminated by feed or drinking water spilled by the animal. Because of these difficulties, the utility of urinalysis should be discussed with an experienced veterinary clinical pathologist prior to its inclusion in the design of a repeated dose toxicity study. If urinalysis is conducted, its limitations must be kept in mind when the data are reviewed.

Post-Mortem Evaluations

One of the more definitive assessments of toxicological effects conducted during a repeated dose study is the macroscopic and microscopic examination of tissues and organs from treated and control animals. In typical subchronic and chronic studies, samples of approximately 50 tissues and organs are collected during the necropsy of each animal. Table 19.11 presents a list of tissues that are commonly collected for potential histopathological examination.

Necropsy

Necropsy of an animal is conducted when it dies during the study, when it is killed during the study for humane reasons (e.g., in cases of moribundity), or when it is killed at a scheduled interval (interim sacrifice or termination of the study). Necropsy should be completed as quickly as possible after the death of an animal to avoid *autolysis* that can interfere with the subsequent microscopic examination of its tissues. Autolysis is defined as the enzymatic self-digestion of cells or tissues that occurs after death. It is an especially important consideration for animals that die during the study because their death may not be discovered for a significant period of time. Animals found to be moribund (i.e., about to die) during the study should be terminated for humane reasons and to avoid tissue autolysis.

During necropsy, tissues and organs are systematically removed and macroscopically visible abnormalities are noted, including changes in color, shape, size, or consistency of a tissue. The documentation of an abnormality in the necropsy records should include its location and a clear description of the change, using nondiagnostic terminology. Completeness of the examination during necropsy and the quality of the description of abnormalities are critical to the determination of pathological effects. An abnormality in a tissue can only be prepared for microscopic examination if it was collected and accurately described during necropsy. Because of the central role that the necropsy plays in detecting effects in a repeated dose toxicity study, it is extremely important that necropsy technicians are highly trained and experienced in the necessary techniques.

After collection, tissue samples are usually preserved by immersion in an appropriate fixative, commonly 10% neutral buffered formalin. In some cases, particularly for organs such as testes or eyes, special fixatives may be used (62). To ensure adequate fixation, the volume of fixative should be at least 10 times the volume of tissues. Certain organs, for example, the lung and urinary bladder, are frequently filled with fixative prior to immersion to improve fixation. During collection of large numbers of tissues from many animals, it is possible to inadvertently miss a tissue. Therefore, it is highly advisable to inventory and document the samples as they are placed into the fixative containers. This inventory will be invaluable during subsequent preparation of the tissues for microscopic examination and in reconstructing the study during post-study auditing of the data. In addition, it must be ensured that the identity of each tissue is clearly maintained while in fixative. This is not a problem for tissues that are large or have distinctive morphology. To ensure subsequent identification of extremely small tissues and those with indistinct morphology, they are frequently placed in labeled plastic cassettes or cloth bags prior to being placed in the fixative container.

Organ Weights

Collection of terminal body weight and organ weights for all animals during necropsy is normal practice in repeated dose toxicity studies. Minimally, weights should be recorded for the brain, liver, kidneys, testes, and adrenal glands. Frequently, other organs such as the thyroid/parathyroid, ovaries, spleen, thymus, uterus, epididymis, heart, or lungs are also weighed. Consideration should be given to the residual blood that may remain in organs such as the spleen, heart, and lungs, which may be variable between animals due to the method of sacrifice and blood collection. Organs should be weighed as soon as possible after removal from the animal and trimmed free of fat and connective tissue prior to weighing and placed into fixative immediately thereafter.

It is common practice to normalize organ weights by expressing them relative to body weight and brain weight. Relative organ weights are used to eliminate the influence of normal variation in animal growth on the interpretation of organ weight data. However, normalized organ weight data should be reviewed with the knowledge that they have some limitations. Expressing organ weights relative to body weight can yield apparent, but artificial, treatment-related effects on organ weights in studies where the test material affects body weight gain, although organ weights normalized to brain weights help overcome this problem because test materials that alter body weight generally do not alter brain weight. The best practice is to consider all three types of data, that is, actual organ weight and organ weight relative to body and brain weight. Histopathological data are often used to help assess the significance of apparent differences between organ weights of test material-treated and control animals.

Microscopic Pathology

Microscopic examination of the tissues and organs of treated and control animals is one of the most time-consuming laboratory functions in toxicity studies. In nonrodent studies, sections of all tissues and organs from all animals should be prepared for microscopic examination. Generally, in rodent studies, only tissues and organs from the controls and high-dose group animals and animals that were killed or died during the study are examined microscopically. For the other treatment groups, only a few major organs (e.g., liver and kidney, and any other organs in which macroscopic abnormalities were noted at necropsy or in which test material-related effects are detected in high-dose animals) are examined. Although initial histopathological examination of control and high-dose tissues followed by examination of other doses is typical in rodent studies, simultaneous histopathological examination of all tissues from all animals is not uncommon. This practice yields the most expeditious completion of the histopathological evaluation phase of a study because sequential examinations are not required. Simultaneous examination also reduces the inter-group variability in diagnoses that might occur when tissues from intermediate groups are examined considerably after completion of the evaluation of the control and high-dose groups. Such variability can lead to incorrect conclusions concerning treatment relationship of lesions noted in the intermediate dose groups. In a draft of its guidelines for safety studies, the FDA has proposed that tissues from all dose groups, not just the high-dose and controls, be subjected to histopathological examination (27).

Routinely, tissues are prepared for light microscopic examination by embedding in paraffin, sectioning at 5–7 microns, and staining with hematoxylin and eosin (H&E) stain (Figure 19.5). Special stains, such as stains for the presence of fat (Oil Red O) or connective tissue (trichrome stain) may be used for some tissues. Use of a protein-specific stain (Mallory–Heidenhain) is illustrated in Figure 19.6. If desired, representative samples of selected tissues may be frozen at necropsy and stored for biochemical or immunohistochemical analyses or specially prepared for electron microscopy. In the histology laboratory, it is important that tissues be prepared according to standardized procedures especially with respect to type of section (i.e., cross, longitudinal), location, and orientation on the microscope slide. The histology technician must review the observations recorded during necropsy of the animals to ensure that all grossly observed lesions are properly sectioned and mounted on the slide for subsequent microscopic examination. Whenever possible, samples of lesions prepared for examination should include the lesion and portions of surrounding "normal" tissue.

Histopathological examination of the tissues requires specialized training and is performed by a pathologist trained and experienced in the evaluation of toxicologic pathology. The pathologist must be familiar with the normal features and naturally occurring lesions that can be observed microscopically in tissues from laboratory animals. The pathologist's responsibility, however, is more than evaluation of the tissues and accounting for all the lesions reported at necropsy. The pathologist should be an integral part of the protocol design team to provide input into many factors, for example, selection of the species/strain to be used, clinical pathology variables to be evaluated, and others. The pathologist should also provide guidance concerning the list of tissues to be collected to ensure that they are processed, stained, and evaluated in a manner that satisfies the study objective.

It is critical that the pathologist review the data generated during the in-life and necropsy phases of the study before proceeding with the histopathological evaluation. Results of clinical observations, clinical chemistry and hematology determinations, organ weight measurements, and necropsy examinations can lead the pathologist to focus on particular organs as potential targets for toxicity during the microscopic examination. For example, increased liver weight should lead to a more careful examination for hepatocellular hyperplasia or hypertrophy, and elevated serum creatinine along with a necropsy description of the surface of the kidneys as "rough" should result in a more thorough examination for nephropathy.

Some have suggested that knowledge of in-life and necropsy findings will bias the pathologist, causing a more stringent examination of the potentially affected tissue. Similarly, some are concerned that knowledge of the dose level administered to the animal during the study will bias the pathologist, resulting in a more thorough examination of the tissues from animals that received the test material. The second situation, in particular, could result in a higher incidence and/or severity of microscopic findings in treated animals compared with controls, a higher incidence that is simply an artifact of the thoroughness of the microscopic examination. One way to prevent potential bias is to keep the pathologist ignorant of other study findings and of the identity of the animal until histopathological examination of the tissues has been completed. Because this so-called "blinded reading" does prevent bias but may also prevent the pathologist from identifying certain subtle, dose-related changes, blinded reading is not recommended for routine histopathological evaluations and should only be conducted in special situations.

Pathological changes in cellular or subcellular structure can occur either spontaneously, such as with aging, or as a result of exposure to a chemical. Deciding which changes are significant and what severity should be assigned to a change during histopathological examination is quite subjective.

Because of this, it is possible that different pathologists looking at the same tissues will produce different diagnoses. It is even possible that, during histopathological evaluation of a large number of tissues that extends over a number of months, the criteria for diagnosis of the same finding by a single pathologist will change somewhat. The variability that results from the subjective nature of histopathological evaluation is unavoidable. To minimize its effect on the results of toxicity studies, several procedures can be useful. First, during each "reading period," the pathologist should examine tissues from a small subset of the study animals. Each subset should contain approximately equal numbers from each control and treated group to be examined. Second, if a potential target organ is identified over an extended period of time, the pathologist should re-examine that organ from all animals during a compressed reading period of a few days or less to assess to what extent, if any, "diagnostic drift" occurred over time. Third, informal peer consultation concerning unusual or subtle tissue changes observed during examination of the tissues can be conducted to arrive at a consensus diagnosis. In addition, a formal peer review process involving

(1) re-examination of target organs,
(2) reexamination of a representative percentage of other tissues from the study, and
(3) review of interpretation of the pathology findings can be conducted by a second pathologist to ensure consistency in diagnosis and grading of tissue changes and accuracy of the pathology conclusions (37).

The objective of the histopathological evaluation is the same as the objective of all other determinations during a repeated dose toxicity study—to detect adverse effects that could be relevant to humans or any other target species exposed to the test compound. Because of certain idiosyncrasies, some animals and strains are not useful for this purpose. In some cases, the animal exhibits a high spontaneous rate of pathology in a particular organ that prevents detection of any compound-induced increase in that rate. For example, severe testicular pathology occurs spontaneously in a very high percentage of old

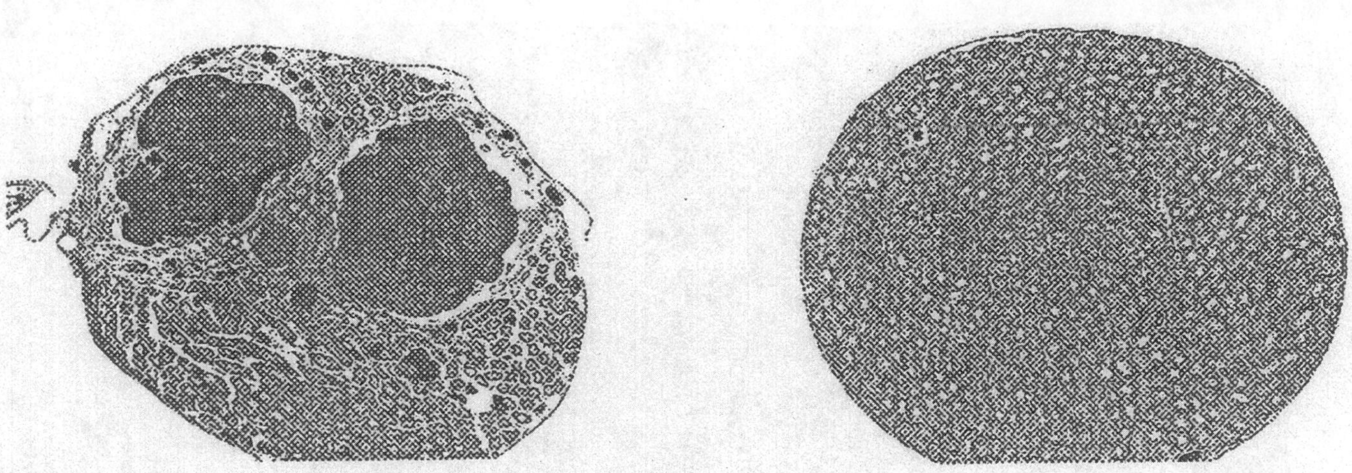

FIG. 19.5. Photomicrographs of Hematoxylin & Eosin stained testes from Fischer 344 rats (2.5 × magnification). The testis on the left exhibits an interstitial cell tumor. The testis on the right is without pathological changes.

male Fischer 344 rats (see Figure 19.5). Therefore, this strain of rat is generally not useful for the detection of testicular effects. In other cases, a pathological change occurs in the laboratory animal only in response to test-compound exposure, but that pathology would not be expected to occur in the target species. An example of this is light hydrocarbon nephropathy that occurs only in male rats. Many hydrocarbons produce this nephropathy, for example, d-Limonene and unleaded gasoline. It is caused by accumulation of a male rat-specific protein, alpha-2-microglobulin, in the renal tubule following exposure to these chemicals. This nephropathy is characterized by hyaline droplets in the cytoplasm (Figure 19.6), granular casts in the lumen (Figure 19.7) and cellular regeneration in the tubules. Because humans do not produce alpha-2-microglobulin, this gender- and species-specific pathological finding has no relevance to human hazard assessment and the male rat is not a suitable model for human renal effects related to light hydrocarbon exposure. For both examples cited, however, the test animal is perfectly acceptable for use as a human surrogate in toxicity testing as long as the limitations imposed by its idiosyncrasies are taken into account.

Even though the idiosyncratic situations discussed above do occur occasionally, the pathology that occurs in most laboratory animals and most tissues is considered relevant to the assessment of hazard in humans. The histopathological examination of tissues in a subchronic or chronic toxicity study can yield a vast array of diagnoses. A detailed discussion of possible chemical-related pathological findings is beyond the scope of this chapter. For detailed descriptions of methods for and diagnosis of veterinary toxicological pathology, the reader is referred to a review by Hardisty (37) and two comprehensive texts on the subject (2,38).

Additional Endpoints for Repeated Dose Toxicology Studies

Evaluation of special endpoints can be added to repeated dose toxicology studies to maximize the utilization of animal resources, minimize the time and cost of a hazard assessment, and obtain additional data. Care should be used in selecting these endpoints to ensure valid methodology is used and that the data will be accepted by regulatory agencies. Draft guidelines for safety assessment of direct food additives and color additives suggest data concerning the immunotoxic and neurotoxic potential of the test material should be generated during subchronic toxicity studies (27). To insure the methodology and data presentation is acceptable to the regulatory agencies, meetings should be held with the appropriate agency during design of the study.

It is possible, through the addition of special determinations, to make a subchronic or chronic toxicity study so complicated that the main objectives are jeopardized. All the ramifications of the addition of special endpoints to a study design, including practical considerations such as daily workload, should be considered to ensure that basic study endpoints are not compromised. Rather than overwhelming the capabilities of the testing laboratory, conduct of a separate study designed to evaluate the special endpoints may be preferable. This is not to say that special evaluations should never be added to subchronic or chronic studies; with appropriate consideration of the possible complications, they can be and often are.

If a question still remains whether additional endpoints should be added to short-term repeated dose study or to longer-term studies, the following should be considered. If these endpoints were added to short-term studies, then the data would be available to aid in design of longer-term

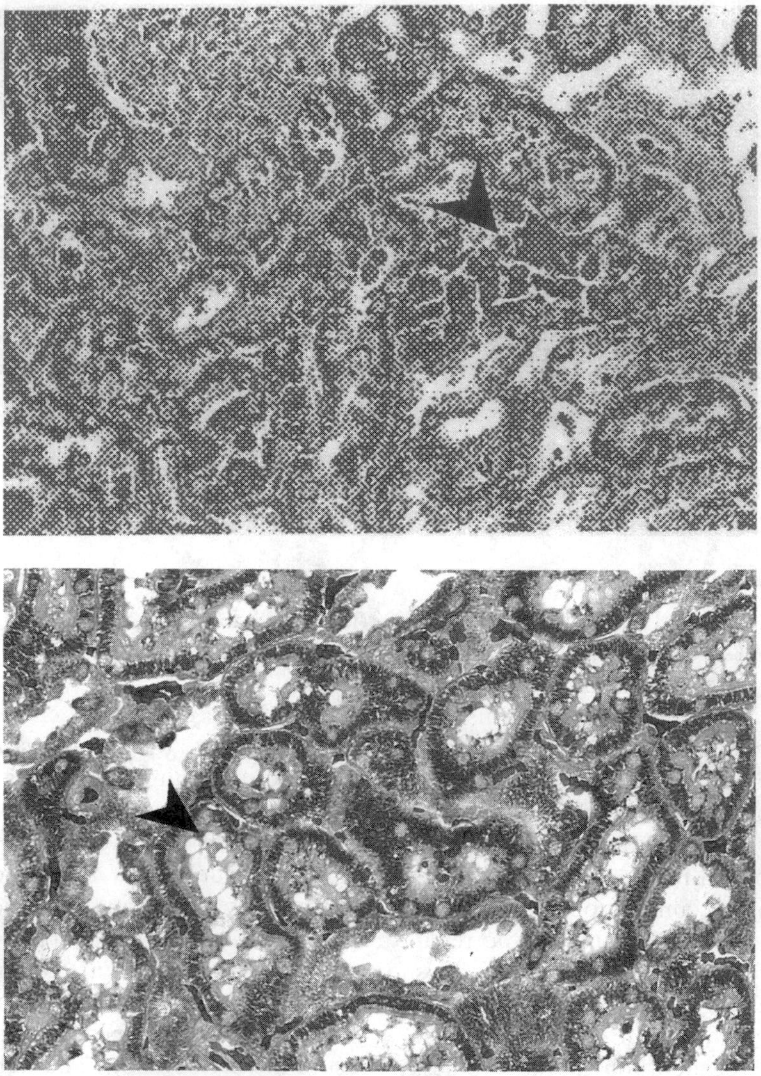

FIG. 19.6. Photomicrographs of kidneys from Fischer 344 male rats stained for protein using Mallory–Heidenhain stain (100 × magnification). The kidney tubules on the top are stained heavily and contain many hyaline droplets (arrow). The kidney tubules on the bottom exhibit normal levels of protein staining (arrow).

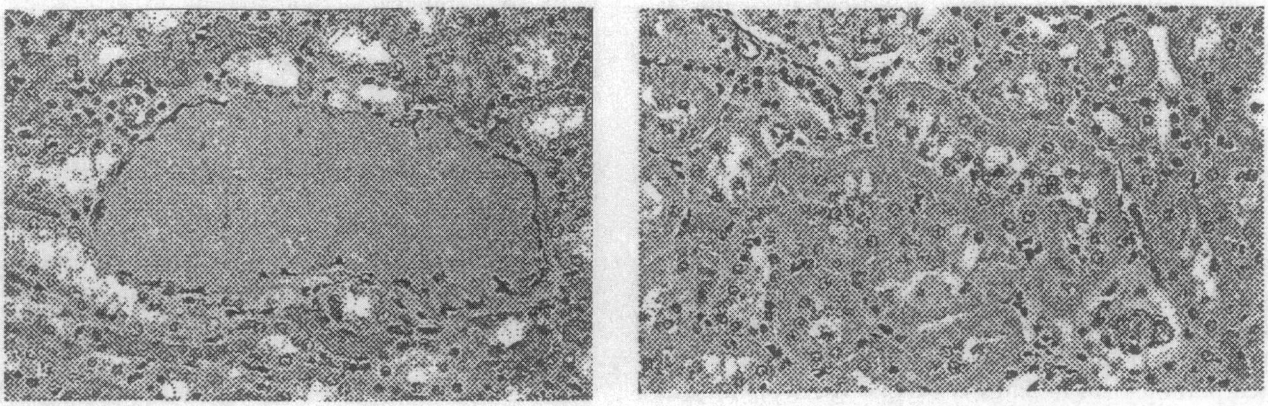

FIG. 19.7. Photomicrographs of Hematoxylin & Eosin stained kidneys from Fischer 344 male rats (100 × magnification). The lumen of one tubule in the kidney on the left is obstructed by a large accumulation of granular casts. The kidney on the right is without pathological changes.

studies. However, if the particular variable to be evaluated appears only after longer exposure periods, any change might not occur in short-term studies. The most conservative approach is to add the endpoints to each study type. The following paragraphs provide examples of how data concerning non-standard toxicological endpoints may be obtained from classical repeated dose toxicity study designs.

Genetic Toxicology

Certain in vivo and in vivo/in vitro genetic toxicology data may be obtained during or at the termination of a repeated dose toxicity study. Addition of these endpoints to a study could decrease the number of animals used in a hazard assessment and shorten its duration. In vivo genetic toxicology studies increase the value of a hazard assessment. Because they use the route of administration by which humans are exposed to the test material and all processes of absorption, distribution, metabolism, excretion, and DNA repair are intact, these in vivo studies provide important information that cannot be obtained from in vitro studies using cellular systems.

A number of in vivo genetic toxicology assays are in use, some of which are suitable for incorporation into repeated dose toxicity assays. For example, the authors have incorporated the bone marrow micronucleus assay into a classic subchronic study design. During most repeated dose toxicity studies, bone marrow smears are made (see Table 19.11), in essentially the same manner as those used for the in vivo micronucleus assay (39). These slides can be stained with acridine orange and the polychromatic erythrocytes analyzed for micronuclei. Use of bone marrow slides from the repeated dose study has several advantages:

(1) it incurs no additional time and cost for collecting the samples,
(2) it allows the assay to be conducted on animals exposed to the test material for long periods of time,
(3) it eliminates the need for resources to conduct an independent study, and
(4) it does not interfere with the histopathological assessment of the tissues.

It may be possible to use bone marrow slides from repeated dose toxicity studies for the bone marrow chromosomal aberration assay (4). This is another in vivo genetic toxicology assay that could provide additional data without an independent study being conducted. Another such genetic toxicology assay is the in vivo/in vitro unscheduled DNA synthesis assay (51), in which freshly isolated hepatocytes are used to determine unscheduled DNA synthesis. Although this assay is not compatible with histopathological use of the liver, as few as two to three extra animals per group are all that are required. One problem associated with incorporation of additional endpoints, such as genetic toxicology, into a repeated dose study design is that the laboratory conducting the study must have valid assay methodology. This is not always the case.

Table 19.11
Tissues collected for histopathology in repeated dose studies

Adrenals	Mammary gland (females)
Aorta	Muscle (thigh)
Bone marrow smear	Nose
Brain	Ovaries
Cecum	Pancreas
Colon	Pharynx
Duodenum	Pituitary
Epididymides	Prostate
Esophagus	Rectum
Eyes	Salivary gland (submandibular)
Femur and bone marrow	Sciatic nerve
Gallbladder (when present)	Seminal vesicles
Heart	Skin
Ileum	Spinal cord (cervical, thoracic, lumbar)
Jejunum	Spleen
Kidneys	Sternum and bone marrow
Lacrimal gland	Stomach
Larynx	Testes
Lesions	Thymus
Liver	Thyroid with parathyroid
Lungs	Trachea
Lymph nodes (mandibular and mesenteric)	Urinary bladder
	Uterus

Not all in vivo genetic toxicology assays are completely suitable for incorporation into repeated dose studies. For instance, the in vivo sister chromatid exchange assay requires the administration of deoxybromouridine to the animals. This compound can compromise the classical endpoints used in toxicity studies, including histopathology. It is possible, however, to incorporate extra animals to assess specific endpoints while not compromising the main study animals.

Neurotoxicity

It is possible to incorporate neurotoxicity screening into repeated dose toxicity study designs. In fact, in its draft version of its food additive toxicology testing recommendations, the FDA has suggested that neurotoxicity screening be incorporated into these study designs (27). EPA has similar recommendations (14,15).

Neurotoxicity screening is designed to determine if the test material has the potential to produce adverse effects on the nervous system. Screening is conducted to determine if additional, more sophisticated, neurotoxicity testing is required. The first indication of a requirement for neurotoxicity testing may come from the structure-activity assessments. However, the database for neurotoxicity structure activity assessments is not as extensive as for certain other types of toxicity and may not provide useful insight into the need for neurotoxicity testing. Drugs and pesticides that target the nervous system are a well-known exception. For instance, there is no question that a new organophosphate insecticide will require neurotoxicity testing. For most compounds, it will be necessary to develop data through empirical testing.

Most classical repeated dose study designs contain elements that may provide some information on neurotoxicity potential. These include cage-side observations of the animals, physical examinations, and measurement of variables, such as food consumption, that may relate to behavior modifications during the in-life phase of the study. Additional information is obtained during histopathological examination of the structures of the nervous system collected at necropsy, such as the brain and spinal cord. The FDA believes, however, that these procedures, as well as others, should be specifically included into the design of repeated dose toxicity protocols (27). Table 19.12 lists the design elements recommended by the FDA for a neurotoxicity screen. Specific behavioral and neurotoxicity tests exist to provide most of the requested data, and the particular test designs should be chosen based upon their validity, history of use, lack of undue stress to the animal, and the experience of the laboratory with the specific test. Care should be taken to perform these procedures on all the treatment groups and controls in the study. A concern is that some of these tests may stress the animals and produce changes in the traditional variables measured during a toxicity study. If this were to happen, it is assumed that the control group would also demonstrate these changes, which may or may not be true. Therefore, a conservative approach would be the addition of extra animals to the study that would be subjected to the manipulative procedures for neurotoxicity screening and not be used in the traditional phases of the study. For a more complete discussion of the FDA recommendations, the reader is referred to the draft guidelines for safety of direct food additives (27).

Table 19.12
FDA draft criteria for a neurotoxicity screen as a component of short-term and subchronic studies

- Histopathological examination of tissues representative of the nervous system, including the brain, spinal cord, and peripheral nervous system
- Quantitative observations and manipulative test to detect neurological, behavioral, and physiological dysfunctions. These may include:
  - general appearance
  - body posture
  - incidence and severity of seizure
  - incidence and severity of tremor, paralysis, or other dysfunction
  - level of motor activity and arousal
  - level of reactivity to stimuli
  - motor coordination
  - strength
  - gait
  - sensorimotor response to primary sensory stimuli
  - excessive lacrimation or salivation
  - piloerection
  - diarrhea
  - polyuria
  - ptosis
  - other signs of neurotoxicity deemed appropriate

Immunotoxicity

Rapid advances have been made during the last 20 years in respect to detection of immunotoxicity. The two major forms of immunotoxicity are immunosuppression and hyperactivity of the immune system. Immunosuppression results in a reduction in the animal's resistance to infection and potential increase in susceptibility to tumorigenesis by a suppression of critical immunological responses. Hyperactivity of the immune system can result in autoimmune diseases and increased sensitivity to allergic disorders. Determination of the mechanisms associated with these disorders can be extremely complex because of the large number of biochemical, cellular, and physiological factors that can be effected as well as the cellular interactions required to mount an immunological defense. The detection of potential immunological changes is less complex and a number of tests exist that can provide warning of a potentially immunotoxic compound.

The FDA has published draft recommendations for the inclusion of immunotoxicity evaluations in repeated dose toxicity studies (27). It suggests that such evaluations be conducted in rodents. Immunotoxicology testing procedures were divided into two broad categories—Type I tests are those assays that do not require the study animals to be treated with an agent that presents an immunological challenge. Type II Tests are assays that require the study animals to be challenged with an agent that elicits an immune response, such as antigens, vaccines, infectious agents, or tumor cells. Because Type I tests do not require manipulation of animals, they can be included in the routine assays done during a repeated dose toxicity study. Because Type II tests do require treatment of the animals with an immunological challenge, these animals are not suitable for evaluations conducted during toxicity studies. Therefore, additional animals must be included in the study design.

Table 19.13 lists the immunotoxicology evaluations that the FDA suggests should be included in Type I tests.

Table 19.13
FDA draft recommendation for type I immunotoxicity test that can be included in repeated dose toxicity studies

Type I Test

Hematology
- white blood cell counts
- differential white blood cell counts
- lymphocytosis
- lymphopenia
- eosinophilia

Clinical Chemistry
- total serum protein
- albumin
- albumin-to-globulin ratio
- serum transaminases

Histopathology
- lymphoid tissues
- spleen
  - lymph nodes
  - thymus
  - Peyer's patches in gut
  - bone marrow
- cytology (if needed)[a]
  - prevalence of activated macrophages
  - tissue prevalence and location of lymphocytes
  - evidence of B-cell germinal centers
  - evidence of T-cell germinal centers
- necrotic or proliferative changes in lymphoid tissues

[a] More comprehensive cytological evaluation of the tissues would not be done unless there is evidence of potential immunotoxicity from the preceding evaluations.

Table 19.14
FDA draft recommendation for expanded type I immunotoxicity test that can be included in repeated dose toxicity studies

Hematology
- Flow cytometric analysis
  - B-lymphocytes
  - T-lymphocytes
  - T-lymphocyte subsets
    - TH & TS
  - Immunostaining of blood or spleen fraction
    - B-lymphocytes
    - T-lymphocytes

Serum Chemistry
- Serum protein electrophoresis
  - albumin
  - α-globulin
  - β-globulin
  - γ-globulin
    - Quantification of γ-globulin
  - IgG, IgM, IgA, IgE
- Complement
  - Cytokines
  - ·IL-2, IL-1, γ-interferon
  - Auto-antibodies
  - Anti-parietal cell antibodies

Histopathology
- Immunostaining of B-lymphocytes in spleen and lymph nodes with polyclonal antibodies to IgG
- Immunostaining of T-lymphocytes and subsets with monoclonal or polyclonal antibodies
- Micrometric measurements of germinal centers and periarteriolar lymphocyte sheath of the spleen and follicles and germinal centers of lymph nodes

In vitro analysis of functional capacity of specific immune cells
- Activity of natural killer cells
- Mitogenic stimulation of B- and T-lymphocytes
- Macrophage phagocytic index
- Stem cell assays

Generally, these evaluations are those currently recommended for repeated dose toxicity studies with the exception of a more comprehensive histopathology of lymphoid tissues. Inclusion of these evaluations into current study designs should have no impact on the validity of the study. Inclusion of the expanded Type I tests listed in Table 19.14 would require more planning during the study design phase and assurance that the laboratory performing the study would be capable of performing the assays. The expanded Type I test generally would only be conducted after consultation with the FDA. Type II immunotoxicity tests recommended by FDA could be done as a component of a repeated dose toxicity study, but they appear to be more appropriately conducted as independent studies and are beyond the scope of this discussion.

Miscellaneous Other Endpoints

There are a wide variety of additional endpoints that could be evaluated in repeated dose studies. In part, any additional endpoints would depend upon the questions to be addressed and the creativity of the toxicologist designing the studies. For instance, the increased availability of electron microscopy makes this endpoint a more viable option today than in previous decades. Development of an increased number of histochemical assays, especially those employing specific antibodies, makes the preserved wet tissues, embedded tissues, and the histopathology slides obtained from these studies valuable for future use. In many cases, the need for additional endpoints is unknown until the initial results of the study are known, at which point the preserved materials then become a valuable resource. For instance, if it is found that the liver from a study contains vacuoles and the toxicologist suspects these to be fat vacuoles, it is possible to use special lipid stains to determine if the vacuoles are lipid. Other special stains exist for a variety of purposes. An example of a protein-specific stain, Mallory–Heidenhain, is illustrated in Figure 19.6.

If the toxicologist believes the histopathological data indicate a particular compound is producing cellular proliferation, there are a number of approaches to investigate this hypothesis. A standard method to determine cellular proliferation is by injecting the animal with ^{3}H-thymidine and measuring the incorporation of the radiolabel into cellular DNA by methods such as radioautography. However, if the study has been terminated, this is not possible. Also, the toxicologist may not want to administer radiolabel to the animals for a number of reasons, even if the in-life portion of the study has not been terminated. If the evidence of increased cellular proliferation occurs in tissues with a relatively high rate of normal proliferation, such as the gut mucosa, it is possible to determine the mitotic index by counting mitotic figures in cells from slides previously prepared for histopathological analysis. Alternatively, it is now possible to immunostain for specific proteins associated with cellular proliferation in preserved tissues. Again, the particular additional endpoints added to the toxicology study should address a specific issue.

DATA ANALYSIS AND INTERPRETATION

Compilation and Summarization of Study Data

Once the data have been collected from a repeated dose toxicity study, the next steps involve data analysis, interpretation, and reporting. These data are derived either from the measurement of a variable associated with the test animal—for example, body weight, feed consumption, serum enzyme activity—or from observation of the animal, for example physical examination findings, macroscopic and microscopic pathology, and so on. The frequency, number, and variety of these measurements and observations in repeated dose toxicity studies yield an extremely large volume of data that must be organized and summarized prior to analysis. Historically, individual animal data were recorded manually and then were compiled either manually or following entry into a computer. Some specialized data are still handled manually today; however, most routine data are collected, compiled, and statistically analyzed electronically using custom or commercially available computer programs.

For quantitative data such as body weights and feed consumption, individual animal data are used to calculate the mean values with a measure of statistical variation for each treated or control group. For other types of quantitative data such as the number of animals exhibiting a behavioral effect or the number of animals in which a particular finding is determined histopathologically, the incidence of the observation in each treated and control group—that is, the number of animals affected as a fraction of the total number of animals observed—is presented. Some data, like leukocyte differential counts and results of microscopic examination of urinary sediment, cannot be effectively summarized using a group mean or incidence value. Summarization of these types of data involves listing the individual animal data in their appropriate groups.

Determination of Treatment-Related Effects

Data from the treatment groups are compared with data from the control group to determine if any treatment related effects have occurred. In virtually all cases, the data from one group of animals will differ somewhat from the data for any other group. Therefore, differences between the sets of data that are potentially related to treatment must be differentiated from spurious occurrences and from normal biological variation. This is accomplished by two methods. The first is simple examination of the data and detection of differences worthy of further consideration based upon the experience of the toxicologist and comparison with historical data. The second method uses statistical tests to detect differences for which the probability that the difference occurred by chance is low. These methods should always be used in combination. Although it is an extremely powerful and useful tool, statistical analysis alone should not be used to detect treatment-related effects because, as stated by the FDA, "... statistical outliers are not always biological outliers and a "significant" statistical test ($p \leq 0.05$) does not always indicate biological significance" (27).

Differences between the data from the control and treated animals that are detected using the methods cited above may indicate either an adverse effect associated with the test material, physiological adaptation to the test material, or normal biological variation unrelated to the test material. Determination of the significance of differences between treated and control groups is based on a number of factors that are frequently considered in combination with each other. These are listed in Table 19.15 and discussed in the following paragraphs.

Dose-related Trend

One of the best indicators of an effect related to treatment is the presence of a dose-related trend in the data, that is, the magnitude of the effect varies directly with the dose level. Such an effect is reflective of the basic principle of toxicology stated by Paracelsus in the 16th century and often paraphrased as, "The dose makes the poison" If a difference from controls is noted in two or more dose groups and the severity or incidence of the difference increases as the dose level of the test material increases, it is probably a treatment-related effect. When a difference from controls is noted only

Table 19.15
Factors considered to determine the significance of differences between treated and control groups

- Dose-related trends
- Reproducibility
- Related findings
- Magnitude and type of difference
- Occurrence in both genders

in animals receiving the highest dose level of the test material, it may or may not be treatment-related and other factors must be considered in determining its significance. Differences from control data in test material-treated animals are probably not associated with treatment if a dose-related trend is not observed. Because of this, as stated previously, selection of an appropriate range of dose levels is extremely important and facilitates data interpretation.

Reproducibility of Effect

Another reliable indicator of a treatment-related effect is its reproducibility. If a difference from controls is noted in the treated animals at multiple intervals during a study, the difference is likely related to treatment. Further weight is given to the determination of the treatment relationship if the same difference is noted in other independent studies in which the test material was administered to the same species and, even more weight is given if the difference is observed in a second species. The absence of reproducibility, especially in the same species, is an indication that the difference may have occurred by chance.

Correlated Findings

Another consideration in the assessment of significance of an intergroup difference is the presence of related findings. For example, an elevation in the activity of serum alanine aminotransferase in treated animals when compared with the control group is probably related to treatment if there is an elevation in serum aspartate aminotransferase with concomitant hepatic necrosis. If no correlation with other findings is observed, the elevation may be of no significance or, at least, its significance must be determined considering other factors.

Magnitude and Type of Inter-group Difference

The magnitude and type of difference observed between treated and control data may also give an indication of its potential association with test material administration. For example, a doubling of an organ weight in treated animals compared with controls should be considered more likely to be treatment-related than a 10% increase, even if the smaller increase is statistically significant. Furthermore, a fairly large decrease in the activity of serum alanine aminotransferase in treated animals is generally assigned limited clinical significance whereas an increase of the same magnitude in the activity of this enzyme may be considered indicative of a toxic effect. It is obvious that the assessment of the significance of a change on the basis of its magnitude or type requires knowledge of normal trends and ranges for the data.

Gender Differences

Determination of the significance of an apparently treatment-related effect is also influenced by whether or not the difference occurs in animals of both genders. Since treatment-related effects often occur in both genders, a difference from controls that is noted only in treated animals of one gender may not be associated with the test material. It must be remembered, however, that there are cases where one gender or the other is more sensitive to the toxicity of a chemical and, therefore, only the sensitive gender will exhibit the effect at a given dose. For this reason, a difference should not be considered insignificant solely on the basis of its absence in one gender. Male rats are well known for their greater capacity to detoxify certain compounds because of their higher activity of P450-dependent monooxygenases. Therefore, they may demonstrate less toxicity to these compounds than females. However, if the metabolic product is more toxic than the parent compound, they may demonstrate higher sensitivity than females (see Chapter 3). This gender difference is not seen in a number of other species, including humans (52).

STUDY REPORT

After the data from a study have been analyzed, a report is prepared. Depending upon the intended use of the report, it may contain various levels of detail. For example, reports prepared for submission to a regulatory agency in support of the safety of a chemical will generally contain much more detail (including all individual animal data) than research reports intended for publication or that will be used by an organization or individual only to give guidance for future testing. Whatever the purpose of the report, it should be written in sufficient detail to permit peer review of the conduct and conclusions of the study and to allow the study to be reproduced.

Report Content

All reports, regardless of their purpose, should contain certain common elements that are essential to adequately describe the conduct and results of a study. The report should clearly state the objective(s) of the study. It should precisely define the test material, indicate the test species used, and describe the methods and equipment employed to collect and analyze the data. Protocol deviations and an assessment of their impact upon the study should be presented. The report should present the data pertinent to the study objective(s) in a form that facilitates its review and should discuss these data in the depth required to support the conclusion(s) of the study. The discussion should describe any treatment-related effects observed and should explain how the various factors described above were used to determine the significance of any differences between treated and control animals in the study. Finally, the conclusion(s) drawn from the results of the study should be clearly and concisely stated.

Retrospective Report Audits

After the study has been completed and reported, retrospective audits of the study are frequently conducted. The manufacturer of the test material may audit the study prior to submitting it to a regulatory agency in support of registration or approval of the test material for its intended use. The regulatory agency to which the study report was submitted may also conduct an audit. Regulators also audit study reports to assess compliance of the testing laboratory with GLP regulations. Whatever the reason for retrospective auditing of the study, the process is essentially the same. The raw data are inventoried to ensure that they have been properly maintained. They are reviewed and compared with the study report to ensure the report accurately and completely presents the methods used and the data collected. Any deviations from laboratory standard operating procedures, the study protocol, or GLP regulations that occurred during conduct and documentation of the study should have been clearly explained in the report. Individual animal data should support summary tables and discussion of the results should be consistent with the individual and summary data.

Retrospective auditing is of great value to all parties involved. The manufacturer of the test material can feel comfortable that it will receive no surprises during a subsequent audit by the regulatory agency. The regulator will be more confident about the quality of the study if the data have been audited. If the regulator is confident about the data, his or her review will proceed more smoothly and, therefore, regulatory decisions will be expedited.

REGULATIONS CONCERNING GENERATION AND USE OF DATA FROM REPEATED DOSE TOXICITY STUDIES

Almost every industrialized country in the world has regulations governing the introduction, transportation, and use of new pesticides, food additives, human and animal drugs, and other chemicals. Many of these countries also have regulations governing medical devices, workplace exposure to chemicals, the introduction of industrial chemicals into commerce, and the disposition of chemical waste.

There is general uniformity in the objectives of these laws, that is, not to impede the beneficial use of chemicals, but at the same time to ensure their safety in use. Even though the regulatory agencies can agree, in broad terms, on one framework of toxicity testing guidelines, the toxicologist must become familiar with the details of particular guidelines to fulfill his or her role as a bridge between scientific and regulatory concerns. Several regulations governing repeated dose toxicity and other types of toxicity testing are briefly described below.

United States Laws and Regulatory Guidelines

Federal Food, Drug and Cosmetic Act (FFDCA)

FFDCA (29) as amended by the Food and Drug Administration Modernization Act of 1997 (38), controls the introduction of human and animal drugs, direct food additives, indirect food additives (such as packaging materials), and components of cosmetics. In the case of new human or animal drugs, safety and efficacy must be established for a particular therapeutic application before the FDA grants approval for marketing. The approval process is comprehensive and involves two sequential phases. For the investigational new drug (IND) phase, industry is required to file preclinical toxicity data with the FDA before investigation of the safety and potential therapeutic value of a drug in limited numbers of humans. When the efficacy and safety of the drug in the treatment of a particular disease is established through extensive clinical trials, these data together with additional animal toxicity data are provided to the agency as part of a new drug application (NDA) or new animal drug application. The NDA is reviewed by the FDA with respect to safety and claims of efficacy of the drug, and is either approved or disapproved, or deficiencies in the data cited.

The summary of a NDA must address benefit/risk relationships, clinical data, nonclinical pharmacology and toxicology, human pharmacokinetics, bioavailability, and microbiology. It must also contain information on pharmacological class, scientific rationale and clinical benefits, and chemistry and manufacturing (34).

For food additives, industry must show that a material either intended for direct addition to food, such as a preservative or flavoring agent, or having indirect contact with food, such as a packaging or can-coating material, is safe for its intended use. Results from a hazard assessment are submitted to the FDA for review as part of a food additive petition. If the data demonstrate the safety of the chemical, a regulation is published allowing the chemical to be used for a particular purpose in food or in contact with food. In 1982, the FDA published *Toxicological Principles for the Safety Assessment of*

Direct Food Additives and Color Additives Used in Food (23). A revised version of this document has recently been released by the FDA (Toxicological Principles for the Safety of Food Ingredients, Redbook 2000) (27). This so-called "Redbook" delineates the nature of evaluations necessary to determine food additive safety and provides a basic scheme for scientifically sound decisions for the development of the safety assessment. These guidelines include a priority-setting system that increases the efficiency of the food additive safety assessment.

FFDCA also provides an alternative method by which materials can be approved for use in or on food, the generally recognized as safe (GRAS) process (31). For a material to be considered GRAS, its safety evaluation must satisfy three basic requirements. First, a group of experts qualified by scientific training and experience must conclude that the material, when used as intended, is safe for human consumption. The sponsor of the potential additive convenes this expert group and the group operates without regulatory oversight. Second, the information considered by the expert group during the GRAS review must be common knowledge, that is, available in the scientific literature. Third, within the scientific community there must be general agreement with the conclusion of the expert group. Final GRAS approval does not require regulatory review; however, many producers of such materials petition FDA to affirm their GRAS status prior to marketing them.

There are no requirements for the FDA to review cosmetic formulations for safety prior to marketing. Even though the FFDCA only requires that the cosmetics be free of any "poisonous and deleterious" substances, responsible suppliers of ingredients for use in cosmetics and manufacturers of final products conduct toxicity studies relevant to the specific cosmetic.

FFDCA also addresses the concentrations of pesticides permitted in foods in the United States. Under FFDCA Section 408, the EPA establishes maximum allowable concentrations for pesticide residues in raw agricultural commodities—food crops, eggs, raw milk, and meat. Under FFDCA Section 409, EPA also establishes a maximum allowable concentration for a pesticide in processed food, if processing concentrates the residue of the pesticide in the raw agricultural commodity. These maximum concentrations are referred to as *tolerance levels* or tolerances. Human exposure resulting from consumption of foods containing tolerance levels of a pesticide must not exceed the maximum permissible intake of the pesticide established by EPA under the Federal Insecticide, Fungicide and Rodenticide Act (FIFRA). Tolerances for most foods are enforced by FDA, and those for meat, poultry, and some egg products are enforced by the Food Safety and Inspection Service (FSIS) within the U.S. Department of Agriculture (USDA).

Federal Insecticide, Fungicide and Rodenticide Act

FIFRA was administered initially by USDA and is now administered by the EPA (10). Under FIFRA, EPA is responsible for registration of pesticides for use in the United States. This act requires extensive toxicity testing to be conducted in mammalian, avian, and aquatic species to support the safety of a pesticide. Detailed guidelines for toxicity study design and reporting have been issued by EPA (17). Toxicity data submitted in an application for registration of a pesticide are reviewed by toxicologists in the Office of Pesticide Programs at EPA. Other data specifically required by FIFRA as a condition of pesticide registration include product chemistry, residue chemistry, environmental fate, reentry protection, spray drift, plant protection, non-target insects, and product performance.

Food Quality Protection Act

The Food Quality Protection Act (FQPA) was signed into law in 1996 and amends sections of both FFDCA and FIFRA (13). It is intended to establish more consistent regulation of pesticides and to protect human health using an approach that places increased emphasis on the scientific evaluation of pesticide safety data. Among other provisions affecting pesticide registration and tolerance setting, it

(1) mandates special considerations for protection of infants and children,
(2) requires determination of aggregate pesticide exposure from all sources (e.g., food, home use, drinking water, etc.),
(3) requires summation of exposures from multiple chemicals that exhibit a common mechanism of toxicity,
(4) expedites approval of pesticides considered to be most safe, and
(5) requires periodic reevaluation of tolerances for registered pesticides to be certain that the data supporting registration remain acceptable and complete by current standards.

The methods to be used for implementation of several of the provisions of the FQPA are still being developed, and some (such as the means for special protection of children) are the subject of considerable controversy within the scientific community. EPA is considering input concerning resolution of these controversial issues from pesticide manufacturers, agricultural trade organizations, academia, consumer protection groups, and the public prior to finalizing their approach. Significant progress must be made soon, however, because FQPA mandates that EPA complete review of the tolerances for 33% of all currently registered pesticides by August 1999, of an additional 33% by August 2002, and of the balance by August 2006.

Toxic Substances Control Act

The Toxic Substances Control Act (TSCA) is administered by the Office of Pollution Prevention and Toxics within EPA and is a complex and far-reaching law that affects industrial chemicals existing in commerce as well as new chemicals in the United States (20). One of the first requirements of TSCA was the compilation of an inventory of chemicals that were active in commerce in the years 1977–1979 and determination of the need for toxicity testing of these chemicals.

Manufacturers or importers of industrial chemicals that are considered new under the TSCA definition are required to notify the EPA at least 90 days before the manufacture or import of a new chemical. The act requires that certain information regarding the new chemical be submitted to the EPA for review in a premanufacture notification (PMN). Although the act does not require toxicity testing to be conducted on a new chemical prior to manufacture, it does require submission of all existing health and safety data for the new chemical so that its risk to health or the environment can be assessed. If the EPA determines in its review that the new chemical does present an unreasonable risk, one of several actions it may take is to require that the chemical be tested for specific toxic effects. The EPA may also issue a testing rule requiring that a specified chemical or chemical mixture be tested for certain toxic effects. The EPA has issued test standards for the conduct of toxicity studies on chemicals or chemical mixtures for which testing will be required under TSCA. These standards are the same guidelines used for pesticide testing under FIFRA (17).

Transportation Act

Regulations promulgated by the U.S. Department of Transportation (DOT) require that materials shipped in interstate commerce be labeled and contained in a manner consistent with the degree of hazard they present (5). DOT requires that acute toxicity data for chemicals be used to place them into "packing groups," with labeling requirements for chemicals based upon this packing group.

The Coast Guard

Prior to importing a chemical into the United States, the Coast Guard requires a set of acute mammalian toxicity data for the chemical (6). This acute toxicity profile should minimally include the following: acute oral toxicity, acute dermal toxicity, and skin and eye irritation studies.

Consumer Product Safety Act

Prior to passage of the Consumer Product Safety Act (CPSA), the classification and testing for acute toxicity of household products was conducted under regulations promulgated by the FDA, which administered the Federal Hazardous Substances Act (FHSA). The function of administering FHSA now resides with the Consumer Product Safety Commission (CPSC). If results obtained in acute oral or dermal toxicity tests conducted using methods outlined in the *Code of Federal Regulations* (CFR) for hazardous substances meet prescribed criteria of toxicity, labeling and packaging as prescribed in the regulation must be used (3).

Occupational Safety and Health Act

This law, administered by the Occupational Safety and Health Administration (OSHA) of the U.S. Department of Labor, is designed to assure safety in the workplace (58). No requirements exist in this law for manufacturers to test substances for toxicity prior to their use in the workplace. The impact of the TSCA has an overlapping effect, in that occupational exposure to new chemicals is considered in premanufacture notices. As indicated previously, specific test requirements under TSCA affect new or existing chemicals that are manufactured or processed in the United States.

Resource Conservation and Recovery Act

The Resource Conservation and Recovery Act (RCRA) authorizes the EPA to institute a national program to control hazardous waste defined as "solid, liquid, semi-solid or gaseous waste that may cause increased mortality or serious illness, or may cause substantial hazard to the health or the environment when improperly managed" (18). The main purpose of these regulations is to control the generation, storage, treatment, transportation, disposal, record-keeping, and reporting of hazardous waste. RCRA places the primary responsibility of identifying and managing hazardous waste on the waste generators. Other persons or institutions involved in waste disposal and management also have an obligation to know if the waste is hazardous. The degree of toxicity, concentration, migration to the environment, persistence or degradation in the environment, bioaccumulation in the ecosystem, types of improper management, quantities of waste, past human and environmental damage records, and other factors are all taken into consideration.

International Laws and Regulatory Guidelines

The United States has not been alone in developing laws to protect humans and their environment from possibly dangerous effects of new industrial chemicals in the marketplace. In the European Union, the Council of Ministers of the European Economic Community (EEC) has issued a directive concerning laws, regulations, and administrative procedures which relate to the classification, packaging, and labeling of dangerous substances (7). An amendment to this directive was adopted later to protect humans and their environment from potential risks that might arise through the marketing of new chemicals (8). It requires that a new chemical be subjected to a base set of tests to define its physical and chemical properties, mammalian toxicity, and ecotoxicological effects. The base set of mammalian studies consists of the following: acute oral LD_{50}, acute dermal LD_{50}, acute inhalation LC_{50} (if applicable), skin and eye irritation, and dermal sensitization. A manufacturer or importer is required to furnish the appropriate authorities in his or her EEC member state with a notification containing, in part, the results of these tests with the new chemical. Such notification must be filed 45 days before marketing in the member state in which it is to occur.

The amendment to the EEC directive is the counterpart of the U.S. TSCA. There are, however, some differences, not the least of which is in the approach to toxicity testing. The EEC requires only notification of a new chemical prior to marketing whereas TSCA demands that the notification, in the case of a domestic manufacturer, be given to the EPA at least 90 days before manufacture.

The EEC has also provided guidance on the evaluation of safety and efficacy of drugs. It has now adopted guidance notes for efficacy, testing of pharmacokinetics in humans, and bioavailability of drugs for long-term use, as well as a number of more specific activity groups including cardiac glycosides, oral contraceptives, topical corticosteroids, nonsteroidal anti-inflammatories, antimicrobials, anticonvulsants, antianginals, and chronic peripheral arterial disease agents. Safety guidance notes also were adopted for single-dose and repeated dose toxicity, pharmacokinetic metabolism, mutagenic potential, carcinogenic potential, and reproduction studies (9).

As discussed earlier in this chapter, with many countries establishing their own regulations for safety assessment, it became more likely that manufacturers would have to perform several different versions of the same tests to satisfy the requirements of different countries. In an attempt to avoid unnecessary and wasteful duplication of work, the Organization for Economic Cooperation and Development (OECD) produced a set of toxicity testing guidelines that allow tests to be carried out in a similar manner in different countries (54). The OECD package, which has been revised 10 times to implement improvements to individual study designs, includes guidelines on acute oral, dermal, and inhalation studies; eye and skin irritation and skin sensitization studies; subchronic oral, dermal, and inhalation studies; and teratogenicity, carcinogenicity, and chronic and combined chronic/carcinogenicity studies. Results from studies conducted according to OECD guidelines are generally fully acceptable to the various regulatory bodies throughout the world.

To facilitate more universal acceptance of data generated to support approval and use of pharmaceutical products, the International Conference on Harmonization (ICH) has developed guidance documents concerning the efficacy, quality, and safety of these drugs. The ICH is made up of regulatory authorities and trade organizations from the United States, Japan, and the European Union. Instead of providing detailed instructions for study design or conduct, the ICH guidances address specific issues related to testing, for example, the duration of chronic toxicity testing, definition of an acceptable battery of genotoxicity studies, required elements of chemical stability testing of new drug products, and so on (41). Because of ICH efforts, many hindrances to the approval and use of valuable pharmaceuticals around the world have been removed.

Regulatory Internet Sites

Many of the regulatory agencies and organizations worldwide that have responsibility for protection of humans from the hazardous effects of chemicals maintain Internet websites. These websites usually include information concerning the history, structure, and specific responsibilities of these organizations. The sites also generally contain or reference the statutes and guidelines under which the organizations operate. Internet addresses for a number of informative regulatory sites are listed in Table 19.16.

ACKNOWLEDGMENTS

The third edition of this text contained one chapter concerning short-term and subchronic toxicity studies and a second concerning chronic toxicity studies. Because many elements of short-term, subchronic, and chronic toxicity testing are similar, the decision was made to combine these subjects into a single chapter in the fourth edition. Some information in this chapter is derived entirely or only with slight modification from the chronic toxicity chapter in the third edition. This note is written to acknowledge the efforts of the authors of that chapter, Drs. Kent R. Stevens and Louis Mylecraine.

QUESTIONS

1. *BetterBelly* is a new drug entity intended to mitigate the irritating properties of aspirin in the human gut. Because of its intended use, human exposure to this

Table 19.16
Internet Addresses for regulatory websites

Regulatory Subject	Site Address (http://)
International:	
European Union	www.eurunion.org/legislat/index.htm
EU Testing Guidelines for Medicinal Products	dg3.eudra.org/eudralex/index.htm
Organization for Economic Cooperation and Development	www.oecd.org
OECD Testing Guidelines	www.oecd.org/ehs/test/testlist.htm
International Conference on Harmonization	www.ich.org
ICH Guidance Documents	www.ich.org/ich5.html
United States:	
Food and Drug Administration	www.fda.gov
FDA Center for Food Safety and Applied Nutrition	vm.cfsan.fda.gov/list.html
FDA Center for Drug Evaluation and Research	www.fda.gov/cder
Environmental Protection Agency	www.epa.gov
EPA Office of Pollution Prevention and Toxic Substances	www.epa.gov/internet/oppts
EPA Office of Pesticide Programs	www.epa.gov/pesticides
Toxic Substances Control Act	www4.law.cornell.edu/uscode/15/ch53.html
Federal Insecticide, Fungicide and Rodenticide Act	www.law.cornell.edu/uscode/7/ch6.html
Federal Food, Drug and Cosmetic Act	www.fda. gov/opacom//laws/fdcact/fdctoc.htm
Food Quality Protection Act	www.epa.gov/oppfead1/fqpa
Food and Drug Administration Modernization Act of 1997	www.fda.gov/opacom/backgrounders/modact.htm
EPA Testing Guidelines	www.epa.gov/opptsfrs/home/guidelin.htm
FDA Guidance Documents	www.fda.gov/cder/guidance/index.htm

compound will range from a few days to a few months. The intended treatment population includes males and females from 4 to 90 + years of age. You are designated to be the toxicologist responsible for generating the toxicity data necessary to get *BetterBelly* to the marketplace. What steps/studies would you include in the hazard assessment program for this compound? When you propose your plan to FDA, what questions would you ask them concerning approval of this compound?

2. It has been determined that the hazard assessment program for *BetterBelly* should include subchronic toxicity testing. In a short-term, repeated dose study with this compound in rats at 500 mg/kg/day, oral gavage administration resulted in mortality in 40% of the animals. These rats also exhibited marked body weight loss, convulsions followed by prostration, urinary incontinence, and enlarged and discolored kidneys. At 100 mg/kg/day, no mortality occurred in the study and the only adverse signs observed were mild and reversible body weight loss, lethargy, urinary incontinence, and twitching of the extremities. At 20 mg/kg/day, neither mortality nor adverse signs were noted. Efficacy testing revealed that *BetterBelly* is effective for its intended use at 2 mg/kg/day. Pharmacokinetic determinations indicate that *BetterBelly* is excreted almost entirely in the urine and its serum half-life is 120 minutes. What dose levels would you select for the subchronic toxicity study? Why? What concentrations of dosing solutions would be required to accurately deliver these dose levels to the rats? In addition to the standard variables, what special endpoints would you include for investigation during the subchronic study?

Table 19.17
Selected results from the subchronic toxicity study of *BetterBelly* in rats

	Treatment Group—Males				Treatment Group—Females			
Variable/Finding/Interval	Control	Low	Mid	High	Control	Low	Mid	High
Body weight (g)								
Week 4	200 ± 7	205 ± 11	192 ± 10	173 ± 9[a]	112 ± 8	105 ± 8	110 ± 5	98 ± 6[a]
Week 13	403 ± 13	410 ± 15	371 ± 11[a]	350 ± 17[a]	201 ± 12	202 ± 10	198 ± 13	175 ± 10[a]
Hepatocellular hypertrophy (rats with finding/total rats)								
Week 4	0/10	2/10	0/10	6/10[a]	1/10	0/10	1/10	4/10
Week 13	3/20	8/20[a]	2/20	15/20[a]	2/20	3/20	1/20	12/20[a]
Renal tubule hyperplasia (rats with finding/total rats)								
Week 4	1/10	2/10	4/10	7/10[a]	0/10	0/10	2/10	2/10
Week 13	4/20	5/20	12/20[a]	17/20[a]	3/20	2/20	3/20	12/20[a]

[a] Statistically significantly different from controls ($p < 0.05$).

3. The results in Table 19.17 were obtained during the subchronic study with *BetterBelly*. In what dose groups is there a treatment-related effect on body weight? Are liver and kidney target organs for *BetterBelly* toxicity? If so, in which dose groups is there a treatment-related effect? Based on the data in the table, what is the NOAEL for this study?

REFERENCES

1. American Institute of Nutrition (1977): Report of the American Institute of Nutrition Ad Hoc Committee on Standards for Nutritional Studies. *J. Nutr.*, 107:1340–1348.
2. Boorman, G. A., Eustis, S. L., Elwell, M. R., Montgomery, C. A., Jr., and MacKenzie, W. F. (1990): *Pathology of the Fischer Rat—Reference and atlas.* Academic Press, San Diego.
3. Consumer Products Safety Commission (CPSC): 16 CFR Parts 1015–1402, *Consumer Product Safety Act.* Office of the Federal Register, National Archives and Records Administration, U.S. Government Printing Office, Washington DC.
4. Datta, P. K., Friger, H., and Schleiermacher, E. (1970): The effect of chemical mutagens on the mitotic chromosomes of the mouse in vivo. In: *Chemical Mutagenesis in Mammals and Man*, edited by F. Vogel and G. Rohrborn, pp. 194–213, Springer-Verlag, New York.
5. U.S. Department of Transportation (DOT): 49 CFR Part 173, *Shippers-General Requirements for Shipments and Packaging.* Office of the Federal Register, National Archives and Records Administration, U.S. Government Printing Office, Washington DC.
6. DOT: 49 CFR Part 176, *Carriage by Vessel.* Office of the Federal Register, National Archives and Records Administration, U.S. Government Printing Office, Washington, DC.
7. European Economic Community (EEC) (1967): Council Directive 67/548/EEC, Official Journal of the European Community, Brussels.
8. EEC (1979): Sixth Amendment to Council Directive 79/831/EEC, Official Journal of the European Community, Brussels.
9. EEC (1987): Council Recommendation 87/176/EEC, Official Journal of the European Community. Brussels.
10. U.S. Environmental Protection Agency (EPA)/FIFRA: 40 CFR 152–186, *Federal Insecticide, Fungicide and Rodenticide Act*, Office of the Federal Register. National Archives and Records Administration, U.S. Government Printing Office, Washington DC.
11. EPA/FIFRA: 40 CFR Part 160, *Good Laboratory Practice Standards.* Office of the Federal Register, National Archives and Records Administration, U.S. Government Printing Office, Washington, DC.
12. EPA/FIFRA: 40 CFR Part, *Good Laboratory Practice Standards*, p. 150, Office of the Federal Register, National Archives and Records Administration, U.S. Government Printing Office, Washington, DC.
13. EPA/FQPA: Public Law 104–170, *Food Quality Protection Act.* Office of the Federal Register, National Archives and Records Administration, U.S. Government Printing Office, Washington, DC.
14. EPA/OPPTS (1998): *90-Day Toxicity in Rodents*, OPPTS Test Guideline 870–3100. U.S. Government Printing Office, Washington, DC.
15. EPA/OPPTS (1998): *Chronic Toxicity*, OPPTS Test Guideline 870–4100. U.S. Government Printing Office, Washington, DC.
16. EPA/OPPTS (1998): *OPPTS Test Guidelines*, Series 830, Physical Chemical Properties. U.S. Government Printing Office, Washington, DC.
17. EPA/OPPTS (1998): *OPPTS Test Guidelines*, Series 870, Health Effects U.S. Government Printing Office, Washington, DC.
18. EPA/RCRA: 40 CFR Parts 240–271, *Resource Conservation and Recovery Act.* Office of the Federal Register, National Archives and Records Administration, U.S. Government Printing Office, Washington, DC.
19. EPA/TSCA: 40 CFR Part 792, *Good Laboratory Practice Standards.* Office of the Federal Register, National Archives and

Records Administration, U.S. Government Printing Office, Washington, DC.

20. EPA/TSCA: 40 CFR Parts 700–799, *Toxic Substances Control Act*. Office of the Federal Register, National Archives and Records Administration, U.S. Government Printing Office, Washington, DC.
21. European Union (EU) (1991): *Good Manufacturing Practices—Medicinal and Veterinary Products*. Directives 91/356/EEC and 91/412/EEC. Commission of the European Communities, Brussels.
22. U.S. Food and Drug Administration (FDA) (1982): *Toxicological Principles for the Safety Assessment of Direct Food Additives and Color Additives Used in Food*, Appendix II, pp. 19–21. Bureau of Foods, FDA. National Technical Information Service, Springfield, Virginia.
23. FDA (1982): *Toxicological Principles for the Safety Assessment of Direct Food Additives and Color Additives Used in Food*. Center for Food Safety and Applied Nutrition, FDA, Washington, DC.
24. FDA (1983): *FDA Guidelines for Chemistry and Technological Data Requirements for Direct Food Additives and GRAS Food Ingredients*. Bureau of Foods, FDA, Washington, DC.
25. FDA (1993): *Toxicological Principles for the Safety Assessment of Direct Food Additives and Color Additives Used in Food "Redbook II,"* p. 61. Center for Food Safety and Applied Nutrition, FDA, Washington, DC.
26. FDA (1993): *Toxicological Principles for the Safety Assessment of Direct Food Additives and Color Additives Used in Food*, "Redbook II," p. 86. Center for Food Safety and Applied Nutrition, FDA, Washington, DC.
27. FDA (2000): *Toxicological Principles for the Safety of Food Ingredients, Redbook 2000*, Center for Food Safety and Applied Nutrition, FDA, Washington, DC.
28. FDA (1997): Public Law 105–115, *Food and Drug Administration Modernization Act of 1997*. U.S. Department of Health and Human Services, Public Health Service, FDA, Rockville, Maryland.
29. FDA: 21 USC 301 et seq., *Federal Food Drug and Cosmetic Act, as Amended, and Related Laws*. U.S. Department of Health and Human Services, Public Health Service, FDA, Rockville, Maryland.
30. FDA: 21 CFR 110, *Current Good Manufacturing Practice in Manufacturing, Packaging or Holding Human Food*. Office of the Federal Register, National Archives and Records Administration, U.S. Government Printing Office, Washington, DC.
31. FDA: 21 CFR 170, *Food Additives*. Office of the Federal Register, National Archives and Records Administration, U.S. Government Printing Office, Washington, DC.
32. FDA: 21 CFR 210, *Current Good Manufacturing Practice in Manufacturing, Processing, Packaging or Holding of Drugs; General*. Office of the Federal Register, National Archives and Records Administration, U.S. Government Printing Office, Washington, DC.
33. FDA: 21 CFR 211, *Current Good Manufacturing Practice for Finished Pharmaceuticals*. Office of the Federal Register, National Archives and Records Administration, U.S. Government Printing Office, Washington, DC.
34. FDA: 21 CFR 314, *Applications for FDA Approval to Market a New Drug or an Antibiotic Drug*. Office of the Federal Register, National Archives and Records Administration, U.S. Government Printing Office, Washington, DC.
35. FDA: 21 CFR Part 58, *Good Laboratory Practice for Nonclinical Laboratory Studies*, p. 253. Office of the Federal Register, National Archives and Records Administration, U.S. Government Printing Office, Washington, DC.
36. FDA: 21 CFR Part 58, *Good Laboratory Practice for Nonclinical Laboratory Studies*. Office of the Federal Register, National Archives and Records Administration, U.S. Government Printing Office, Washington, DC.
37. Hardisty, J. F., and Eustis, S. L. (1990): Toxicological pathology: A critical stage in study interpretation. In: *Progress in Predictive Toxicology*, edited by D. B. Clayson, I. C. Nunro, P. Shubik, and J. A. Swenberg, Elsevier Science Publishers, New York.
38. Haschek, W. M., and Rousseaux, C. G. (1991): *Handbook of Toxicologic Pathology*. Academic Press, San Diego, California.
39. Heddle, J. A., Hite, M., Kirkhart, B., Larson, K., MacGregor, J. T., Newell, G. W., and Salamone, M. F. (1983): The induction of micronuclei as a measure of genotoxicity. *Mutat. Res.*, 123:61–118.
40. HPB (1998): *Good Manufacturing Practices (GMP) Guidelines—1998 Edition*. Health Protection Branch, Ottawa, Canada.
41. ICH (1994–1998): *Harmonized Tripartite Guidelines*. ICH Secretariat, Geneva.
42. ICH (1996–1997): *Harmonized Tripartite Guideline—Quality*. ICH Secretariat, Geneva.
43. ICH (1998): *Harmonized Tripartite Guideline—Duration of Chronic Toxicity Testing in Animals (Rodent and Non-Rodent Toxicity Testing)*. ICH Secretariat, Geneva.
44. ILAR (1996): *Guide for the Care and Use of Laboratory Animals*. National Academy Press, Washington, DC.
45. Jain, N. C. (1986): *Schalm's Veterinary Hematology*, 4 ed., edited by N. C. Jain. Lea & Febiger, Philadelphia.
46. Japan/MAFF (1984): *Good Laboratory Practice Standards for Toxicological Studies in Agricultural Chemicals*. Agricultural Production Bureau, Ministry of Agriculture, Forestry and Fisheries, Japan.
47. Japan/MITI (1984): *Good Laboratory Practice Standards Applied to Industrial Chemicals*. Basic Industries Bureau, Ministry of International Trade and Industry, Japan.
48. Japan/MOHW (1982): *Good Laboratory Practice Standards for Safety Studies on Drugs*. Pharmaceutical Affairs Bureau, Ministry of Health and Welfare, Japan.
49. Loeb, W. F., and Quimby, F. W. (1989): *The Clinical Chemistry of Laboratory Animals*. Pergamon Press, New York.
50. McNamara, B. P. (1976): Concepts in health evaluation of commercial and industrial chemicals. In: *New Concepts in Safety Evaluation*, edited by M. A. Mehlman, R. E. Shapiro, and H. Blumenthal, pp. 61–140. Hemisphere, Washington, DC.
51. Mirsalis, J. C., and Butterworth, B. E. (1980): Detection of unscheduled DNA synthesis in hepatocytes isolated from rats treated with genotoxic agents: An In Vivo-In Vitro assay for potential carcinogens and mutagens. *Carcinogenesis*, 1:621–625.
52. Mugford, C. A., and Kedderis, G. L. (1998): Sex-dependent metabolism of xenobiotics. *Drug Metab. Rev.*, 30:441–498.
53. OECD (1981): *Chronic Toxicity Studies—OECD Guidelines for Testing of Chemicals*. Test Guideline 452. OECD, Paris.
54. OECD (1981–1998): *OECD Guidelines for Testing of Chemicals*, Section 4. Health Effects. OECD, Paris.
55. OECD (1981–1998): *OECD Guidelines for Testing of Chemicals*, Section 1, Physical Chemical Properties. OECD, Paris.
56. OECD (1997): *OECD Principles of Good Laboratory Practice*. OECD, Paris.
57. OECD (1998): *Repeated Dose 90-Day Oral Toxicity Study in Rodent—OECD Guidelines for Testing of Chemicals*, Test Guideline 408, OECD. Paris.
58. Occupational Safety and Health Administration (OSHA): 29 CFR Parts 1910, 1915, 1918 and 1926, *Occupational Safety and Health Act*. Office of the Federal Register, National Archives and Records Administration, U.S. Government Printing Office, Washington, DC.

59. Rao, G. N., and Knapka, J. J. (1987): Contaminant and nutrient concentrations of natural ingredient rat and mouse diet used in chemical toxicology studies. *Fund. and Appl. Tox.*, 9:324–238.

60. UK/DHSS (1986): *Good Laboratory Practice—The United Kingdom Compliance Programme*. Department of Health and Social Security, London.

61. U.S. Department of Agriculture (USDA): 9 CFR 1–3, *Animal Welfare Act*. Office of the Federal Register, National Archives and Records Administration, U.S. Government Printing Office, Washington, DC.

62. World Health Organization (WHO) (1978): *Principles and Methods for Evaluating the Toxicity of Chemicals*, part 1, pp. 178–198, WHO, Geneva.

63. Zakim D., Hochman, Y., and Vessey, D. A. (1985): Methods for characterizing the function of UDP-Glucuronyltransferases. In: *Biochemical Pharmacology and Toxicology, Vol. 1*, edited by D. Zakim and D. A. Vessey, p. 189. John Wiley & Sons, New York.

Principles and Methods of Toxicology,
Fourth Edition, edited by A. Wallace Hayes.
Taylor & Francis, Philadelphia © 2001.

Chapter 20

Principles of Testing for Carcinogenic Activity

Gary M. Williams and Michael J. Iatropoulos

CHEMICALS WITH CARCINOGENIC ACTIVITY

Cancer is one of the leading causes of death, and it can result from exposure to exogenous chemicals (275). Thus, in the toxicological assessment of chemicals, testing for carcinogenicity constitutes one of the most important evaluations (Table 20.1).

A large database on the carcinogenic activities of chemicals in rodents has accrued (87,177) as a consequence of over 80 years of basic research and the output from national testing programs in several countries, particularly the United States and Japan. Under the aegis first of the U.S. National Cancer Institute (NCI), and subsequently of the U.S. National Toxicology Program

Table 20.1
Regulations or agreements under which carcinogenicity testing may be required

Legislation/guidance	Agency	Agents of concern
Commission Directive 414 EEC (1991)	EU	Plant protection products
Commission Directive 67 EEC (1993)	EU	Risk assessment for new notified substances
Commission Regulation 1488 EEC (1994)	EU	Risk assessment for existing substances
Dangerous Substances Directive (1967; amended 1992)	EU	Industrial chemicals
Food, Drug and Cosmetics Act (1906, 1938, amended 1992)/FDA Red Book II	US FDA	Food, medicines, cosmetics, food additives, color additives, animal and feed additives, medical devices
Federal Hazardous Substances Act (1960; amended 1988)	US CPSC	Toxic household products
Federal Insecticide, Fungicide and Rodenticide Act (FIFRA) (1948, amended 1978)	US EPA	Pesticides
Guidance on Toxicology Study Data for Application of Agriculture Chemical Registration (1985)	MAFF, Japan	Agricultural chemicals
Guideline for Toxicity Testing of Chemicals (1990)	MHW, Japan	Chemicals
Pharmaceutical Affairs Law (1980)/Guidelines for Toxicity Studies of Drugs Manual (1990)	MHW, Japan	Medicines
Guidelines for Toxicity Studies of New Animal Drugs (1988)	MHW, Japan	Animal medicines
Pesticide Registration Directive (1991)	EU	Pesticides
Technical Requirements for the Registration of Pharmaceuticals for Human Use (1995)	ICH	Medicines
Toxic Substances Control Act (TCSA) (1976, amended 1992)	US EPA	Hazardous chemicals not covered by other laws, includes premarket review

Note. EEC, European Economic Communities; EU, European Union; MAFF, Ministry of Agriculture, Forestry and Fisheries; MHW, Ministry of Health and Welfare; ICH, International Conference on Harmonizations; US CPSC, U.S. Consumer Product Safety Commission; US EPA, U.S. Environmental Protection Agency; US FDA, U.S. Food and Drug Administration.

(NTP), routine rodent cancer bioassays (RCBs), mainly in mice and rats, have been conducted on about 300 chemicals (106).

The definitive test for animal carcinogenic activity is the RCB, which in its various forms is detailed here and elsewhere (115,168,207,260,261,274). The present method for the RCB is exemplified by that currently in use by the NTP (16). This method was refined from basic procedures developed in the 1960s largely by the pharmaceutical industry under guidance from the U.S. Food and Drug Administration (U.S. FDA) and by the NCI Bioassay Program (33,34,48,273). The extensive use of the RCB has led to the recognition that its results cannot be unquestioningly extrapolated to humans (172,274), for which, of course, carcinogenic activity is established by epidemiological studies. Available mechanistic procedures to be discussed assist in assessment of potential human hazard.

Carcinogenic Activity

A committee of the International Federation of Societies of Toxicologic Pathologists has adopted the definition of a chemical carcinogen as a "substance that causes a cell or group of normal cells, which would not otherwise have shown this property, to change its biological behavior and demonstrate progressive growth of a malignant character" (66). Thus, the carcinogenic or oncogenic activity of chemicals is best defined by the finding of unequivocal evidence in a strain of animal of either gender that a test substance (TS) causes types of malignant neoplasms not seen in controls, clearly indicating ab initio induction of neoplasia. A marginal increase of a very rare malignancy of a certain type and site under some circumstances may incriminate a chemical substance. Another generally used criterion is an increase in the incidence of the types of malignant

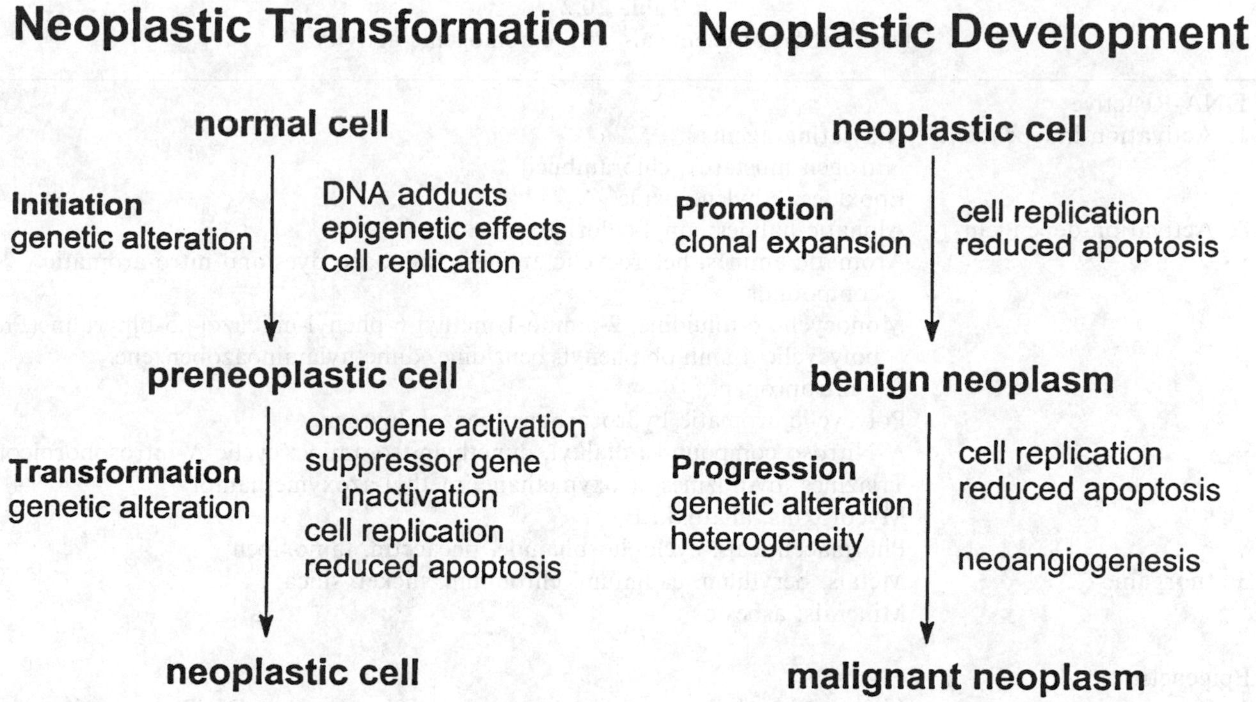

FIG. 20.1. Sequences of oncogenesis.

neoplasms that occur in controls. The malignant neoplasms can be of any histological type, epithelial or mesenchymal, and while a clear increase in malignant neoplasms is most persuasive, a combination of malignant and benign neoplasms of the same cell type of origin is generally accepted as reflecting carcinogenic activity (114,164). The evidence of malignancy is best established by the presence of invasion or metastasis, but for most rodent neoplasms, the diagnosis of malignancy is made histologically on evidence of cellular atypia; thus some diagnoses are controversial, as discussed in the sections on anatomic pathology and on cancer hazard evaluation. The finding of an increase in only benign neoplasms, especially if the type of neoplasm is not established to be premalignant, does not constitute sufficient evidence for carcinogenicity, but does provide limited evidence. In addition to these criteria, an increase in the multiplicity of neoplasms above that in controls or a reduction in the latency period for development of neoplasms has also been considered. While these may indicate an influence of the chemical on tumor development, they are less definitive evidence of carcinogenic activity. Rarely, an increase in the overall incidence of neoplasms without increase in any specific type of neoplasm has been proposed as evidence of carcinogenic activity, but this is highly questionable (115). These criteria apply to findings in any species/strain/gender. A strong effect in one gender of one species may be sufficient to implicate a chemical as a carcinogen, but obviously findings in more than one gender or species strengthen the evidence.

Of course, each expert body applies criteria as it sees fit, often influenced by a concern for hazard identification in the interests of public health protection. Ultimately, in assessing human risk, the reason for which animal tests are done, scientific judgment must be used in evaluating all the information available, including importantly mechanism (or mode) of action.

Types of Carcinogens

Widely varied chemical structures have exhibited carcinogenic activity in rodents (87,116,121,122). This reflects the fact that the multistep process of oncogenesis (Figure 20.1) can be influenced by chemicals in various ways, mainly involving either chemical reactivity in producing neoplastic transformation or epigenetic modulation of cell growth facilitating neoplastic development. Thus, chemicals can give rise to increases in neoplasms through a variety of mechanisms, which have been broadly characterized as DNA reactive or epigenetic (283,288). The types of chemicals that can be assigned to these categories are given in Tables 20.2 and 20.3 and have been discussed in detail elsewhere (288). Carcinogens are, of course, both naturally occurring and man-made.

Table 20.2
Classification of chemicals with carcinogenic activity

A. DNA-Reactive	
1. Activation-independent	Alkylating agents
	Nitrogen mustards, chlorambucil
	Epoxides: ethylene oxide
2. Activation-dependent	Alphatic halides: vinyl chloride
	Aromatic amines, heterocyclic amines, aminoazo dyes and nitro-aromatic compounds:
	Monocyclic *o*-toluidine, 2-amino-1-methyl-6-phenyl-imidazo[4,5-b]pyridine(PhIP), polycyclic 4-aminobiphenyl, benzidine, dimethylaminoazobenzene, 1-nitropropane
	Polycyclic aromatic hydrocarbons: benzo[a]pyrene
	N-Nitroso compounds: dialkyl, dimethylnitrosamine; cyclic-*N*-nitrosonornicotine
	Triazines, hydrazines, azoxymethane, methyl-azoxymethamol
	Mycotoxins: aflatoxin B_1
	Pharmaceuticals: cyclophosphanide, pheacetin, tamoxipen
3. Inorganic[a]	Metals: beryllium, cadmium, chromium, nickel, silica
	Minerals: asbestos
B. Epigenetic	
1. Promoter	Liver enzyme-inducer type hepatocarcinogens; chlordane, DDT, pentachlorophenol, phenobarbital, polybrominated biphenyls, polychlorinated biphenyls
	Saccharin
2. Endocrine modifier	Hormones: estrogens, diethylstilbestrol, atrazine, cholor-S-triazines
	Estrogens
	Atrazine
	Diethylstilbestrol
	Antiandrogens: finasteride, vinclozolin
	Antithyroid thyroid tumor enhancers
	Thyroperoxidase inhibitors: amitrole, sulfamethazine
	Thyroid hormone conjugation enhancers: phenobarbital, spironolactone
	Gastrin-elevating inducers of gastric neuroendocrine tumors: omeprazole, lansoprazole, pantoprazole
3. Immunosuppressor	Purine analogs
	Cyclosporin
4. Cytotoxin	Mouse forestomach toxicants: butylated hydroxyanisole, propionic acid, diallyl phthalate, ethyl acrylate
	Rat Nasal toxicants: chloracetanilide herbicides
	Rat renal toxicants: potassium bromate, nitrilotriacetic acid
	$\alpha_{2\mu}$-Globulin nephropathy inducers: *d*-limonene, *p*-dichlorobenzene
5. Peroxisome proliferator	Hypolipidemic fibrates: ciprofibrate, clofibrate, gemfibrozil
	Phthalates: di(2-ethylhexyl)phthalate(DEHP), di(isononyl)phthalate(DINP)
	Lactofen
C. Unclassified	Acrylamide, acrylonitrile, dioxane, furfural, methapyrilene, sugar alcohols

[a] Some are categorized as genotoxic because of evidence for damage of DNA; others may operate through epigenetic mechanisms such as alterations in fidelity of DNA polymerase.

Table 20.3
Classification of chemicals and mixtures judged to be carcinogenic to humans by the International Agency for Research on Cancer

DNA-Reactive	
Aflatoxins	Cyclophosphamide
4-Aminobiphenyl	Ethylene oxide[a]
2-Aminonaphthalene	Melphalan
5-Azacytidine	MOPP (nitrogen mustard, vincristine, procarbazine, and prednisone)
Benzidine	
Betel quid with tobacco	
N,*N*-Bis(2-chloroethyl)-2-naphthylamine (chlornaphazine)	Nickel and nickel compounds
	Phenacetin-containing analgesic mixtures
Bis(chloromethyl) ether	
1,4-Butanediol dimethanesulfonate (myleran)	Soot
	Sulfur mustard
Chlorambucil	Tamoxifen
1-(2-Chloroethyl)-3-(4-methylcyclo hexyl)-1-nitrosourea (methyl-CCNU)	Thiotepa
	Tobacco smoke and products
Chromium compounds, hexavalent	Triethylenethiophos-phoramide (treosulphan)
Coal tars	
	Vinyl chloride
Epigenetic	
Azathioprine	Oral contraceptives, combined
Cyclosporin A	2,3,7,8-Tetrachloro-dibenzo-*p*-dioxin (TCDD)
Postmenopausal therapy	
Unclassified	
Alcoholic beverages	Diethylstilbestrol
Arsenic and arsenic compounds	Mineral oils
Benzene	Nickel and nickel compounds
	Shale oils

[a] Based on evidence for a relevant mechanism in humans.

Of the many chemicals with carcinogenic activity in RCBs, few are associated with cancer in humans (Table 20.3). Most of these are of the DNA-reactive type, indicating the importance of this mechanism in human hazard. In support of this, several DNA-reactive carcinogens have been active in primates (237), including transplacentally (203). Apart from cigarette smoke and mycotoxins, virtually all DNA-reactive carcinogens occur as occupational or therapeutic exposures, which are substantial compared to general environmental exposures. The few human epigenetic carcinogens are mainly pharmaceuticals, and these are associated with cancer increase only at therapeutic exposures that produce the cellular effect that underlies their carcinogenicity in rodents, mainly immunosuppression or hormonal effects. Thus, a primary objective of cancer hazard assessment is to identify chemicals with DNA reactivity (289).

Because of the significance of DNA reactivity and the reliability with which it is identified, few agents of this type are proposed for uses in which there is any appreciable human exposure, apart from chemotherapeutic alkylating agents. In contrast, agents that elicit rodent tumor increases by epigenetic mechanisms are widely used; for example, more than 80 medicines in current use are tumorigenic in the RCB (46). Importantly, no epigenetic carcinogen has been active in primates (224,237). Accordingly, an important aspect of carcinogen testing is to elucidate any mode of action that might lead to a tumor increase in an RCB in order to guide mechanistic research for informed hazard evaluation (289).

Potency

The magnitude of the carcinogenic activity in rodents of chemicals with respect to dose varies more than 10-million-fold (87). The most extensive system for expressing numerical indices of carcinogenic potency is the Carcinogenic Potency Data Base (87), which uses TD50 values, defined as the daily dose rate required to halve the probability of an experimental animal of remaining tumor free at the end of its standard life span (196). A simplified method proposed for use in the regulatory setting is the T25, defined as the chronic dose rate in milligrams per kilogram body weight per day that will give 25% of the animals tumors at a specific site, after correction for the spontaneous incidence, within the standard lifetime of that species (55). Also, for DNA-reactive carcinogens, there is a general relationship between carcinogenicity and DNA binding, which can be expressed as the chemical binding index (CBI) (157).

REQUIREMENTS FOR TESTING

Testing of chemicals in experimental animals for carcinogenic activity is done to assess potential human cancer hazard under conditions to which humans might be exposed. The U.S. federal government has enacted numerous laws covering requirements for carcinogenicity testing of substances for which there is human or environmental exposure (Table 20.1). Other countries have similar provisions (Table 20.1).

For pharmaceuticals and food additives, both direct and indirect, circumstances requiring carcinogenicity studies have been agreed upon by the International Conference on Harmonization (available on FDA/Center for Drug Evaluation and Research web site, http://www.fda.gov/cder), which applies in the United States, European Union, and Japan. Cosmetics, as with foods, usually do not require carcinogenicity testing.

The requirements for testing of biopharmaceuticals present specific issues (223), for which FDA/Center for Biologics Evaluation and Research has provided guidance (http://www.fda.gov/cber). Growth factors and immunosuppressive antibodies are noted as raising concern for carcinogenic potential. Normal hormones or growth factors that are intended to correct deficiency states, such as insulin, may not need to be tested, unless they are administered by a route that results in substantial exposure of tissues that would not be exposed to the endogenous protein. Modified proteins with new biologic properties may require testing, since, for example, it is known that a modified insulin with affinity for the insulin-like growth factor-1 receptor produced mammary tumors in rats (51). Also, a fragment of parathyroid hormone with bone-trophic activity is widely rumored to have produced bone neoplasms in rats. Certain modifications of proteins to improve bioavailability, such as with conjugation to polyethylene glycol, have not raised carcinogenicity issues. As yet, carcinogenicity testing of transgenes used in gene therapy is not required.

An emerging aspect of regulatory concern is photochemicalcarcinogenicity (129). Indications for the possible need for photochemicalcarcinogenicity testing are (a) long-term exposure of the skin to chemicals that can undergo photoactivation, (b) alteration of the structure of the epidermis, (c) sensitization of the skin to ultraviolet radiation (UVR), and (d) exacerbation of suspected UVR-induced carcinogenesis (75).

Thus, for the use of many types of chemicals, proscribed RCBs are required. Nevertheless, expedited approaches to assessment of potential carcinogenic activity are valuable to obtain data quickly and cheaply with minimal use of experimental animals in order to appreciate potential hazard before extensive development or exposures of humans.

SYSTEMATIC APPROACH TO TESTING

The goal of a systematic approach to testing is to obtain reliable data for hazard assessment and evaluation of the TS at the earliest possible stage. An approach that incorporates the mechanistic concepts described above is the decision-point approach (DPA) (274), which is presented here as a general framework for the concept (Table 20.4). An expedited approach to testing is needed not only for the large reservoir of existing untested chemicals, but also for the host of new molecular (or chemical) entities (NMEs), both small and large (e.g., protein) molecules, that are being synthesized, particularly in the pharmaceutical industry, using combinatorial chemical synthesis.

Table 20.4
Decision point approach in carcinogen testing

Stage A. *Structure of chemical*
1. Possible electrophiles
2. Relation to known carcinogens

Stage B. *Short-term genotoxicity assays*
1. Bacterial mutagenesis hepatocyte, DNA repair
2. Other

Decision point 1: Evaluation of findings in stages A and B.

Stage C. *Assays for epigenetic effects*
1. Cultured cells
   Mitogenesis
   Induction of cytochrome P450
   Peroxisome proliferation
   Gap junction protein downregulation
   Inhibition of cell–cell communication
   Altered gene expression
2. In vivo
   Increased cell proliferation
   Induction of cytochrome P450
   Peroxisome proliferation
   Hormone perturbation
   Gap junction protein downregulation
   Enhancement of preneoplastic lesions
   Immunosuppression

Decision point 2: Evaluation of results from stages A through C.

Stage D. *In vivo assays*
1. Genotoxicity
   DNA binding
2. Limited bioassays: Preneoplastic lesions—rat liver, mouse skin, mouse lung, rat breast; transgenic mice

Decision point 3: Evaluation of results from stages A–C and selected tests in stage D.

Stage E. *Carcinogenicity bioassays*
1. Accelerated bioassays
2. Long-term bioassays

Decision point 4: Final evaluation of all results and cancer hazard assessment.

Implications of Chemical Structure

From the classes of DNA-reactive carcinogens given in Table 20.2, the types of electrophiles that are involved in chemical reactivity and hence DNA binding are well known (Figure 20.2). Such molecular features also have

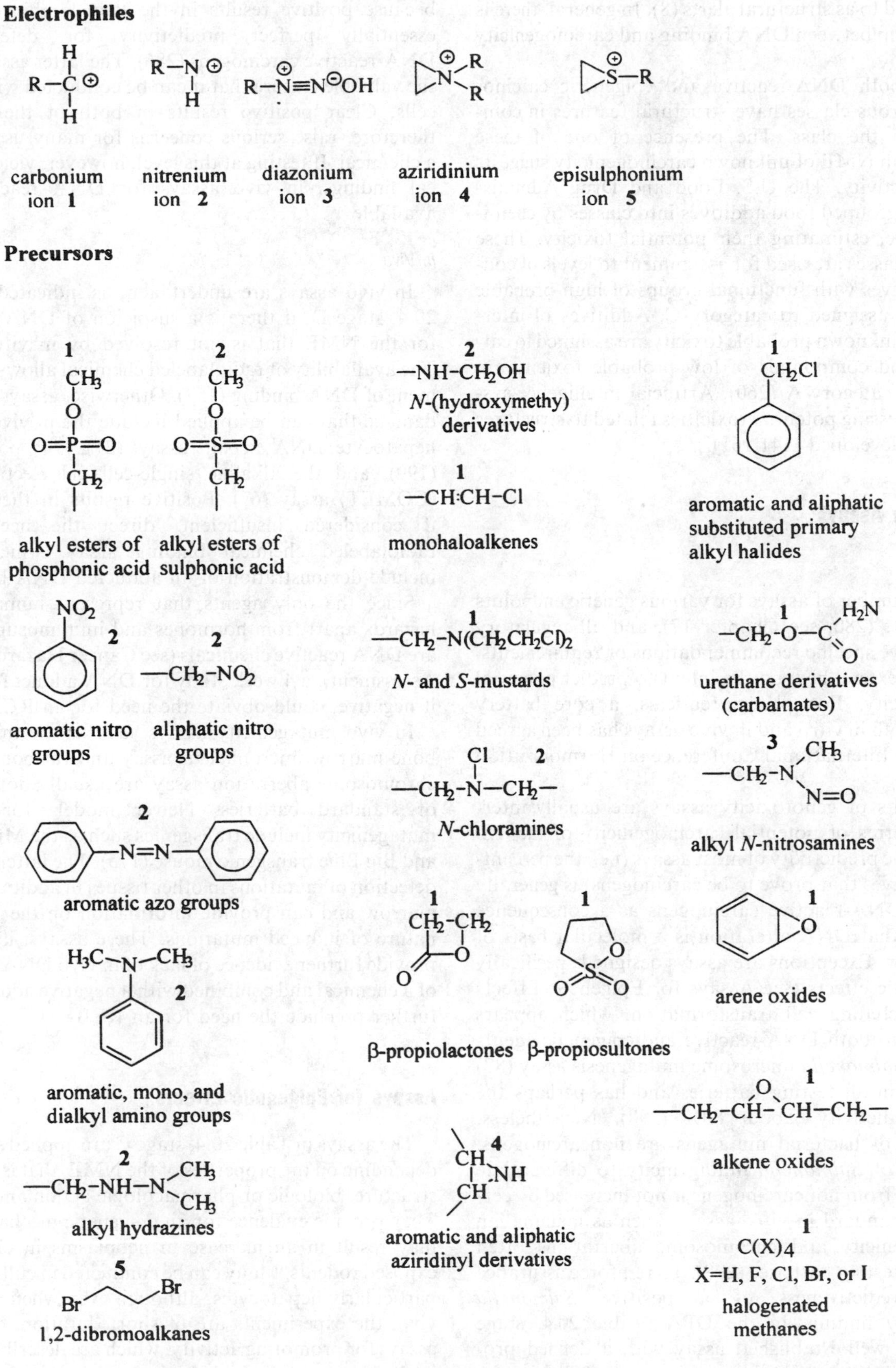

FIG. 20.2. Structure of reactive electrophiles and precursors.

been referred to as structural alerts (8). In general, there is a relationship between DNA binding and carcinogenicity (157).

Among both DNA-reactive and epigenetic carcinogens, numerous classes have structural features in common within the class. The presence of one of these features in an NME of unknown carcinogenicity suggests potential activity. The U.S. Food and Drug Administration has grouped food additives into classes by chemical structure, estimating their potential toxicity. These structural classes are used for assignment to levels of concern. Additives with functional groups of high probable toxicity are assigned to category C. Additives of intermediate or unknown probable toxicity are assigned to category B, and compounds of low probable toxicity are assigned to category A (260). Artificial intelligence systems for assessing potential toxicities related to structures have been developed (141,161).

Genotoxicity Assays

In Vitro

A large number of assays for various genetic endpoints are available (280, see Chapter 17), and all regulatory agencies have specific recommendations or requirements, which may extend beyond the intent to predict potential carcinogenicity. For pharmaceuticals, a core battery including both in vitro and in vivo assays has been agreed upon by the International Conference on Harmonization (ICH) (44).

The results of genotoxicity assays are usually interpreted in terms of potential carcinogenicity of the TS. However, the predictivity of most assays (i.e., the percentage of positives that prove to be carcinogens) is generally limited to DNA-reactive carcinogens as a consequence of the fact that DNA alteration is a molecular basis of mutagenicity. Exceptions are assays designed specifically for epigenetic effects (see Assays for Epigenetic Effects section), including cell transformation, which appears to respond to both DNA-reactive and epigenetic agents (150). The *Salmonella* microsome mutagenesis assay (87) is required in all testing batteries and has perhaps the highest predictivity, about 80% (298). Nevertheless, about 20% of bacterial mutagens are noncarcinogens. The ability of *Salmonella* mutagenicity to differentiate carcinogens from noncarcinogens is not increased by certain other standard in vitro assays, such as mammalian cell mutagenicity and chromosome aberrations often included in testing batteries (298). To reinforce assurance of the predictiveness of a positive *Salmonella* mutagenicity finding, in the DPA (Table 20.4, stage B), another well-established assay with a defined protocol, the hepatocyte/DNA repair assay (287), is recommended in addition to *Salmonella* mutagenesis because positive results in the two combined provide essentially perfect predictivity for detection of DNA-reactive carcinogens (286). The latter assay affords the valuable feature that it can be conducted with human cells. Clear positive results in both of these assays, therefore, raise serious concerns for many uses of such a chemical. If testing at this level, however, yields equivocal findings, in vivo assays for DNA reactivity are available.

In Vivo

In vivo assays are undertaken, as indicated in Table 20.4, stage D, if there is a suspicion of DNA reactivity for the NME that is not resolved by in vitro assays. The availability of radiolabeled chemical allows measurement of DNA binding (157). Otherwise, assays for DNA damage that can be applied include the in vivo/in vitro hepatocyte/DNA repair assay (21), ^{32}P postlabeling (199), and the alkaline single-cell gel electrophoresis (COMET) assay (67). Positive results in these assays, if considered insufficient, direct the need for a radiolabeled chemical binding assay, which should include demonstration of an adducted DNA base.

Since the only agents that represent human cancer hazards apart from hormones and immunosuppressants are DNA reactive chemicals (see Cancer Hazard and Risk Assessment), a 4 week study for DNA adduct formation, if negative, could obviate the need for an RCB.

In vivo mutagenicity assays such as the mouse (rat) bone marrow micronucleus assay and rat bone marrow chromosome aberration assay are usually done as part of standard batteries. Newer models for in vivo mutagenicity include transgenics such as the Muta mouse and Big Blue transgenic mouse (175). The latter allow for detection of mutations in other tissues in addition to bone marrow and can provide information on the molecular nature of induced mutations. These assays, if negative, provide further evidence of lack of in vivo DNA reactivity of a chemical and combined with a negative adduct study, further preclude the need for an RCB.

Assays for Epigenetic Effects

The assays in Table 20.4, stage C are applied selectively depending on the properties of the NME, that is, chemical structure, biologic or pharmacologic action and toxicity. They provide evidence for an epigenetic mechanism that may result in an increase in neoplasms in chronically exposed rodents. Many can be conducted in cultured cells, particularly hepatocytes, although even when applied in vivo, the experiments are of short duration, except for assays for promoting activity, which are described further in the section on limited carcinogenicity bioassays. Positive results for the TS indicate a potential tumorigenic

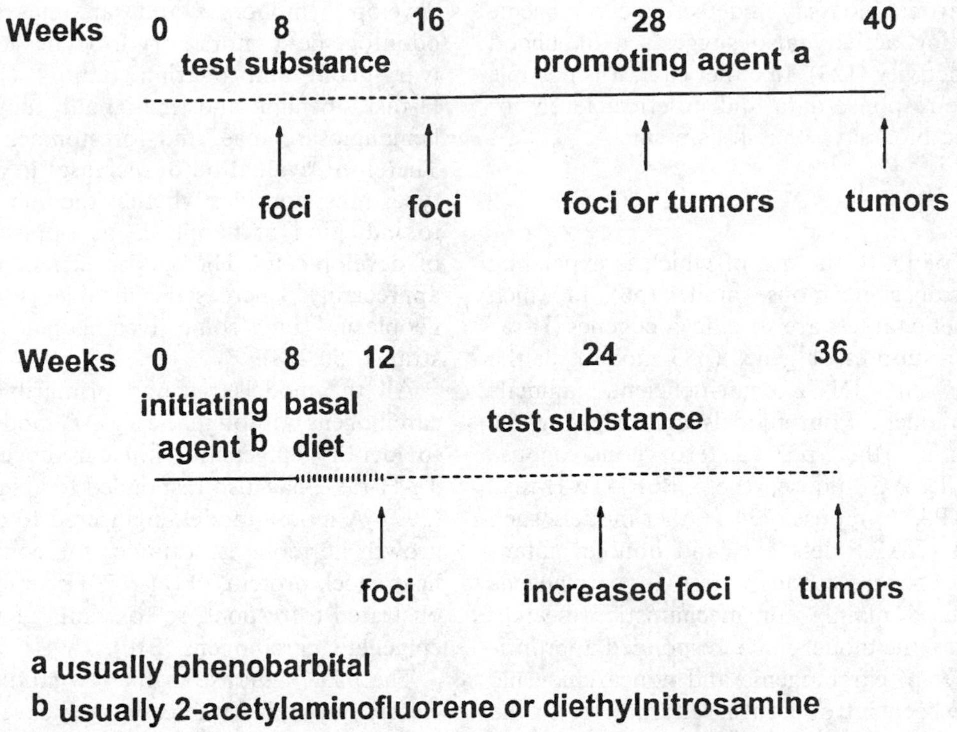

FIG. 20.3. Limited bioassays for initiation and promotion in rodent liver.

effect, in which case the carcinogenic potency of established tumorigens with a similar mechanism and organotropism provides a guide to whether a favorable risk assessment can be made for the NME.

Genomic technologies are becoming available for screening for effects on gene expression and function, including microarray hybridization methods ("DNA Chips") and proteomics. If expression of specific genes, such as acyl coenzyme A (CoA) oxidase (peroxisome proliferators) or cytochrome P450s (liver promoters), can be linked to epigenetic carcinogenesis, then these methods will have utility for screening.

Limited Carcinogenicity Bioassays

Limited carcinogenicity bioassays (LCB) are based on either neoplasms or established pre-neoplastic lesions as their endpoint (60,61,284). These can be applied as initiation assays, in which the TS is tested for its ability to induce the endpoint lesion, or as promotion assays, in which the TS is administered after an agent known to induce the endpoint lesion to determine the ability of the TS to enhance development of the lesion (240).

Initiation/Promotion

In early experimental studies of initiation of skin carcinogenesis, initiation was achieved with a single exposure (11). Although this is possible with potent DNA-reactive agents, repeated exposure is required for an adequate assay for initiation. Since promotion requires an even longer time for expression, more extensive exposure, up to 6 months, is required for an adequate bioassay. Essentially, an assay for initiating activity is directed largely toward assessing potential in vivo genetic activity of the TS, whereas the assay for promoting activity assesses an epigenetic mechanism. Accordingly, assays for promoting activity are also appropriate in the DPA at stage C in vivo assays for epigenetic effects (Table 20.4).

The most extensively validated and used model for an LCB is rat liver (53,60,61,226). This is a consequence of the extensive capability of chemical biotransformation in the liver and the availability of sensitive and reliable markers for preneoplastic lesions. A typical study design for initiation and promotion is shown in Figure 20.3.

Other commonly used LCBs are the mouse skin papilloma, the mouse lung adenoma, and the rat mammary-gland tumor assays (274). These have advantages for specific types of agents; for example, mouse skin is very responsive to polycyclic aromatic hydrocarbons.

Positive findings for initiation are highly indicative of potential carcinogenic activity (123). In fact, Williams et al. (294) calculated that initiation/promotion can be as sensitive as chronic bioassay in detecting carcinogenic activity. Promoting activity also suggests a likelihood of carcinogenic activity (123). In either case, it is possible to establish dose-response data and no-effect levels for design of chronic bioassays or risk assessment.

Transgenic Mice

Another type of LCB, the use of which is expanding rapidly, is the transgenic mouse model (56), in which the principal genetic targets are specific oncogenes (H-ras model) or tumor suppressor genes (p53 model), or the entire genome in DNA-repair-deficient animals (XPA-deficient model). Four models are receiving the greatest attention: the p53 heterozygous mouse ($p53^{+/-}$), the Tg-AC mouse, the CB6F1-Tg-H-ras2 mouse and the $XPA^{-/-}$ mouse (234). Other models, such as Min, Eμ-pim-1, ARF-deficient, and double mutant p53/XPC, have shown responsiveness to carcinogens but are being used mainly for mechanistic research. The studied transgenic models have responded appropriately to a number of carcinogenic and noncarcinogenic agents and have been introduced as alternatives to the RCB in mice and accepted as providing evidence of carcinogenicity (35,234).

Three of the commonly used models are based upon alterations in genes that are relevant to many human and rodent neoplasms—the p53 tumor suppressor gene and the H-ras oncogene—while the $XPA^{-/-}$ model provides an enhanced response to DNA damage as a consequence of the absence of nucleotide excision repair. Each model has specific features. Mice heterozygous for p53 differ in response depending upon the strains used as parents. For example, the C57BL, which is most widely used (52), is resistant to hepatocarcinogenesis, whereas the C3H is highly susceptible. The Tg-AC model carries a v-Ha-ras oncogene fused to the promoter of ζ-globin gene in the FVB/N mouse strain (151), a strain not commonly used in toxicology and that is susceptible to audiogenic seizure. The Tg-H-ras2 mouse carries five to six copies of human c-Ha-ras gene integrated in tandem array in the genome of F_1 mice of transgenic male C57BL/6J mice and normal female BALB/*c*ByJ mice (212), which again are strains not very susceptible to hepatocarcinogenesis. Currently, the $p53^{+/-}$ and Tg-AC mice are widely available, whereas the Tg-H-ras2 is available only in Japan where it was developed. Although any route of exposure can be used with these models, most data have been obtained by the oral route for the $p53^{+/-}$ and Tg-H-ras2 , whereas skin painting is the preferred route for the Tg-AC. In these models, tumors can be elicited within 6 months with few or no tumors in controls. Beyond 6 months, these animals begin to develop genetically determined tumors in high incidence as follows: the $p53^{+/-}$ with a C57BL parent develops lymphomas and sarcomas (159); the Tg-AC, odontogenic tumors, erythrocytic leukemia, and salivary-gland and ovarian tumors (158,159); and the H-ras2, benign and malignant lung tumors, splenic hemangiosarcomas, and forestomach papillomas (212). Therefore, evaluation of increases in any of these tumor types must consider whether the increase is attributable to induction of neoplasia as opposed to acceleration of development. The XPA-deficient mice do not show appreciably increased incidences of spontaneous neoplasms (only some liver neoplasms in C3H-derived strain) (50,268).

All the models respond primarily to DNA-reactive carcinogens, although the Tg-AC model has the potential to identify epigenetic skin carcinogens (230), and the Tg-H-ras-2 has also responded to epigenetic carcinogens (297). A mouse model engineered to contain the human growth hormone gene under the control of the human heat-shock protein 70 (Hsp 70) promoter has been demonstrated to respond to toxicants of which some act as epigenetic carcinogens (210).

The $p53^{+/-}$ mouse in the few studies available so far clearly responds with accelerated development of thymic lymphomas (e.g., phenolphthalein), but compared to the wild-type background has not exhibited an accelerated response to DNA-reactive carcinogens targeting liver (e.g., diethylnitrosamine) (139), mammary gland (e.g., 7,12-dimethylbenz[a]anthracene) (131a), or colon (e.g., 1,2-dimethylhydrazine). This may reflect the fact that p53 mutation is not an early event in murine carcinogenesis for some tissues. If established, this situation strongly diminishes the usefulness of the p53 model for chemical screening.

For all these models, evaluation may be enhanced by measurement of cell proliferation in critical target organs.

Other Models

The newborn mouse is also used as an LCB (70). In this model, newborn mice of any strain are administered intraperitoneal injections or oral intubations of TS at days 8 and 15 after birth and then held for observation for up to 1 year of age. The model exhibits high sensitivity to DNA-reactive carcinogens, but is unlikely to respond to epigenetic agents because of the limited exposure that is provided.

An interesting new approach is the use of avian eggs for an in ovo carcinogenicity assay (IOCA) (61). TS is injected into the egg white of fertilized turkey or quail eggs prior to incubation. The embryonic liver is removed 3–4 days before hatching for the evaluation of preneoplastic lesions. This assay has the advantage of being defined as an in vitro method for carcinogenicity testing.

Table 20.5
Accelerated carcinogenicity bioassay

Initiation segment (IS)		Promotion segment (PS)		
Control, 16 weeks		Control, 24 weeks		
TS, 16 weeks		Promoter, 24 weeks		
			Liver	PB
			Kidney	NTA
			Bladder	NTA
			Stomach	BHA
			Lung	BHT
			Breast	DES
Initiator, 10 weeks		TS, 24 weeks		
Liver	DEN			
Kidney	EHEN			
Bladder	BHBN			
Stomach	MNU			
Lung	DMN			
Breast	DMBA			
TS, 16 weeks		TS, 24 weeks		

Note. TS, test substance; DEN, diethylnitrosamine; EHEN, *N*-ethyl-hydroxy-ethylnitrosamine; BHBN, *N*-butyl-*N*-(4-hydroxybutyl)nitrosamine; MNU, methylnitrosourea; DMN, dimethylnitrosamine; DMBA, 7,12-dimethylbenz[a]anthracene; PB, phenobarbital; NTA, nitrilotriacetic acid; BHA, butylated hydroxyanisole; BHT, butylated hydroxytoluene; DES, diethylstilbestrol.

Accelerated Cancer Bioassay

The accelerated cancer bioassay (ACB) model can be used to develop data on carcinogenicity when (a) there is not a requirement for a RCB, (b) there is an urgent need to obtain data, or (c) as an alternative RCB for one species.

The ACB is essentially a composite of six or more LCBs for rodent organs in which carcinogenicity has been found for known human carcinogens: the liver, lung, kidney, urinary bladder, stomach, and mammary gland. The protocol involves two segments, a first in which the TS is administered for 16 weeks in an initiating segment followed by promoters for the target organs and a second part in which the TS is administered in a promotion segment for 24 weeks after exposure to initiating agents for the target organs (Table 20.5). The TS is also given alone for 40 weeks, to assess carcinogenicity.

The ACB has a number of advantages as follows: (a) It takes less time than the RCB, as the name implies; (b) it provides mechanistic data on initiation/promotion; and (c) the animals exhibit much less age-related pathology at termination because they are less than 1 year of age. Of course, the chief limitation is that the ACB is not as comprehensive as the RCB, although it has been calculated that because of the promoting stimulus, initiation is as sensitive as a chronic bioassay (294).

RODENT CANCER BIOASSAY

Historically, the RCB has been conducted in rats and mice, although other species may be used, as discussed in the section on animals and their environment. For pharmaceuticals, experts in Europe question the value of a mouse RCB (267). Alternatives to the mouse RCB that are now being evaluated are the transgenic or neonatal mouse bioassays and the ACB in mice, as discussed in the section on limited bioassays.

The RCB was developed for testing of small molecules, but also is being used for testing of large biological molecules. Such biomolecules were introduced into medicine beginning with the hormone insulin and now include oligodeoxynucleotides, genes, recombinant human proteins, humanized monoclonal antibodies, blood products, vaccines, and cellular therapies. Each of these presents specific issues in application of the RCB. The International Conference on Harmonization has produced a framework for preclinical safety evaluation of biotechnology-derived pharmaceuticals (223,265). In the systematic approach discussed here, genetic toxicology studies unfortunately are not particularly informative for biopharmaceuticals because the large molecules may not enter the cells used in assays, particularly bacteria. Moreover, it is exceedingly unlikely that such macromolecules would be genotoxic.

Customized approaches are usually required for chronic preclinical safety assessment of biotechnology-derived pharmaceuticals and genetically engineered food products (265). Some of these products are intended for intravenous administration, which is a difficult route of administration for an RCB. Immunogenicity presents an additional complication with proteins, since with the development of neutralizing antibodies the biological activity of the protein can be abrogated, and the chronic antigenic stimulation can compromise carcinogenicity testing. Guidances concerning the design of chronic/carcinogenicity studies are generally based on the clinical indication or in-use exposure. Exceptional with these products is the possibility of using relevant but nontraditional species or the use of animal models of disease (223). Any testing should, of course, be done in a species in which the molecule has biological activity. For an immunogenic protein, one solution to this problem is to test a homologous rodent molecule in the corresponding species.

Design

Most RCBs are done to meet regulatory requirements, as listed in Table 20.1; otherwise, there are more efficient approaches to carcinogen identification, as discussed in the section on systematic approach to testing. An RCB performed for regulatory requirements must follow guidelines (63,66,261,265), and, in particular, the regulations for Good Laboratory Practices (described below), although those conducted by the NTP do not strictly meet this criterion. Detailed descriptions of standard procedures for an RCB with chemicals have been published (168,207,274). Aspects of the design, conduct, analysis, evaluation, reporting, and interpretation are given next.

Feeding Procedures

During the past 20 years, increased variability in body weights, survival and incidences of spontaneous tumors in Sprague-Dawley and Fischer 344 strain rats and CD-1 and $B6C3F_1$ mice have been noted (3,29,137). Specifically, increased body weights, decreased survival, and increased spontaneous tumor incidence can confound and even jeopardize the interpretation of an RCB (19,135,137,183,200,222,238).

Thus far, most RCBs have been conducted using ad libitum (AL) feeding. To overcome the problem of overeating with AL feeding, two solutions have been proposed (29,137,183,238); one is referred to as caloric optimization diet (COD) and consists of limiting caloric intakes to 50–80% of AL consumption (29,94,95), while the other is called the diet-restricted (DR) model, in which animals are given diets limited in offered quantity of feed sufficient to produce a 15% reduction in body weight compared to the AL controls (1,183). In addition to these procedures, the use of weight-matched groups that are fed in such a way that their mean body weight is matched with that of the high exposure AL group has been evaluated (1,183) but is not currently being used. The COD and DR procedures clearly improve the health and survival of animals, reducing the occurrence of age-related pathology, such as chronic progressive nephropathy and myocardiopathy in rats (113) and incidence of certain spontaneous neoplasms (113). Another approach to overcoming the overeating problem is simply to use a strain that does not present this difficulty (see the section on species and strain).

In the past, dietary control was routinely used in testing of oral contraceptives (132). Recently, an emphasis has been placed on the use of dietary control for all medicinal and chemical products (3). Differences in the incidence of neoplasia between AL-fed and DR rodents are shown in Table 20.6 for the two commonly used rat strains, Sprague-Dawley and Fischer 344, and the $B6C3F_1$ hybrid mouse. In both rats and mice, and especially the latter, hepatocellular neoplasia in both genders is reduced in DR groups. Similarly, pancreatic (both acinar and islet) neoplasia (especially in male rats), pituitary (especially in female rats) neoplasia, and adrenomedullary (especially in male Sprague-Dawley rats) neoplasia reduction with DR was present in both species. In general, these decreases in DR groups are due to changes in metabolism and hormonal homeostasis induced by DR. In addition, certain decreases in the DR groups are only present in one species (thyroid C-cell, mammary gland, pulmonary, ovarian, uterine, and hematopoietic), one strain (thyroid C-cell neoplasia in male F344 rats), or one gender (pulmonary adenoma in male mice). The mechanism of these decreases cannot be explained currently. Available information, however, on the impact of either COD or DR on response to well-studied carcinogens generally reveals a reduced response. Accordingly, detection of carcinogenic effects may be masked at sites sensitive to tumor reduction by body weight gain inhibition. Analyzing tumor incidence within body weight strata can reduce bias introduced by weight differences (see the section on statistical analyses).

Groups

Animals must be assigned to groups using randomization procedures. Randomization eliminates bias, but if there is another source of variation, such as gender, cage position, and order of euthanasia at termination, then a stratified randomization is more appropriate. This involves separate randomization within each level of stratifying variable, such as body weight or cage position (152). For further information, see the section on statistics.

The use of two independent control groups helps to control for biological variability in incidences of commonly occurring cryptogenic neoplasms that may occur in only one group. The usual group size is 50–60, which permits detection of neoplasms with incidences in the range of 5–10%. Groups of 75 can be used to allow for an interim kill, as described later in the statistical analyses section. An interim kill of control and exposed animals is useful in that it provides information on time to tumor. This information is not otherwise available when the neoplasia is not life-threatening and there are no resultant unscheduled deaths with neoplasms (80,152). Finally, since the diagnosis of proliferative lesions can be controversial, a short recovery segment (1–3 months) is desirable, because induced neoplastic lesions should progress while nonneoplastic proliferative lesions may regress. To monitor for intercurrent diseases (see the section on animals and their environment), a satellite group of six or nine is used.

The groups typically consist of a high-dose group (see the section on dose selection) and one or two lower doses. Many laboratories, including the NTP, favor a second group at half the high dose to provide sufficiently exposed animals in the event that the high dose impairs adequate long-term survival. Other laboratories space doses by

Table 20.6
Comparative percent incidence of neoplasia under conditions of ad libitum (AL) feeding and diet restriction (DR) regimens in 104-week-old rodents

	F344 rats				S-D rats				$B6C3F_1$ Mice			
	AL[a]		DR[a]		AL[b]		DR[c]		AL[d]		DR[e]	
Types of neoplasia	Males	Females	Males	Females	Males	Females	Males	Females	Males	Females	Males	Females
Hepatocellular adenoma	4	<1	2	0	5	<1	0	2	29	30	16	14
Hepatocellular carcinoma	2	0	0	0	2	0	2	0	26	16	12	4
Pancreatic acinar adenoma	6	0	0	0	1	0	0	0	2	0	0	0
Pancreatic islet adenoma	12	2	4	0	8	9	4	4	2	0	0	0
Pheochromocytoma	21	4	5	0	23	5	2	0	0	2	0	0
Pituitary adenoma	49	42	12	15	62	85	45	77	2	8	0	2
Thyroid C-cell adenoma	17	8	8	2	7	6	4	8	0	0	0	0
Thyroid follicular adenoma	0	0	0	0	4	2	0	0	2	6	4	2
Mammary-gland fibroadenoma	4	57	6	0	2	54	0	15	0	0	0	0
Mammary-gland carcinoma	0	4	0	0	<1	26	0	30	0	0	0	0
Skin papilloma	6	0	2	0	2	0	0	0	0	0	0	0
Skin fibroma	10	2	2	2	2	1	0	1	1	2	1	0
Pulmonary adenoma	4	4	2	0	<1	1	0	0	22	6	12	4
Leydig-cell adenoma	89	NA	61	NA	7	NA	6	NA	0	NA	0	NA
Ovarian cystadenoma	NA	2	NA	0	NA	0	NA	0	NA	6	NA	0
Ovarian granulosa neoplasia	NA	4	NA	0	NA	1	NA	0	NA	0	NA	0
Uterine polyps	NA	14	NA	8	NA	6	NA	0	NA	1	NA	0
Mononuclear-cell leukemia	62	42	26	0	0	0	0	0	0	0	0	0
Lymphoma	0	0	0	0	2	1	0	0	14	24	4	10

Note. F344, Fischer 344 rats; S-D, Sprague-Dawley rats; $B6C3F_1$ mice $(C57BL/6N+C3H/Hen)F_1$; NA, nonapplicable; the average number used by species/strain/gender was in excess of 750 animals; AL, ad libitum; DR, diet restriction (see text).

[a] Modified from References 183 and 29.
[b] Modified from References 167 and 29.
[c] Modified from Reference 29.
[d] Modified from References 232 and 183.
[e] Modified from Reference 183.

one-third or one-fourth. Since generally only TSs that are not DNA reactive should advance to an RCB, a valuable third group is one at the no-effect level (NEL) for any epigenetic effect identified at higher doses that may lead to tumorigenesis. This NEL should yield a cancer NEL, which is valuable for risk assessment. If quantitative risk assessment is envisioned, even more dose levels may be needed.

Duration

With the commonly used strains of rats the anticipated life span is 24–30 months, and 18–24 months for mice. The usual duration for both a rat and mouse RCB is 24 months, although for a mouse RCB, 18 months is acceptable, especially if survival is compromised (33). Exposure should be daily (7 days/week) and should start shortly after weaning. Exposure groups are not allowed to live longer than control groups. If a high-dose group experiences high mortality (greater than 50%) due to exposure, it should be terminated; the other exposure groups and controls should continue until 24 months are completed. In general, survival should not be less than 50% for mice at 15 months and rats at 18 months, or 25% for mice at 18 months and rats at 24 months (33).

GOOD LABORATORY PRACTICE

As regards the RCB, the main intent of Good Laboratory Practice (GLP) is the maintenance of integrity of a complex system of data management. This presupposes that the study is designed, conducted, evaluated, and reported according to standard operating procedures and that records are maintained in a manner that ensures a comprehensive and independent review (251,259). GLP must be conducted in such a way that all data can be validated.

GLP is a global process, which is internationally harmonized, with de facto reciprocal recognition of national GLP programs. This occurs through planned publications of the International Conference on Harmonization (ICH) since 1990 (43,231). The purpose of ICH is to make continuous recommendations on ways to achieve harmonization of technical guidelines and requirements for medicinal product approval. In addition, the U.S. Food and Drug Administration (FDA) and the U.S. Environmental Protection Agency (EPA) have relied in the past on bilateral memoranda of understanding (MOU). Currently, both agencies are negotiating a mutual recognition agreement (MRA) with the European Union. It is conceivable that all MOUs will be replaced by MRAs. At the time of this writing, MRAs exist between Germany, Netherlands, and the United Kingdom. In a GLP study, the study director plays the critical roles of moderator, catalyst, and gatekeeper, responsible for the integrity of study data. As with any process, the management of the GLP process has three components; these are planning (organizing, goal setting, prioritizing, and scheduling), operating (implementing, conducting), and controlling (monitoring, evaluating, and taking of remedial action). Here the importance of the test facility manager is crucial. The test facility manager has the ultimate responsibility for ensuring that all work from all studies is carried out in accordance with GLP principles. The specific responsibilities of the test facility manager include appointment and, if needed, replacement of the study director, the commitment of adequate and trained human resources to each study, the appropriateness of housing for the experimental animals, and scientists and equipment dedicated to the conduct of a study and the assurance of the integrity of the TS.

At the core of the GLP process are information transfer and data acquisition systems and programs. Documented and validated performances (using a standard data set) of these systems and programs are requirements in GLP. Manual systems are subject to standard operating procedures (SOP) review and approval. Computer-based systems (both hardware and software) are subject to validation. The validation methods must address common features relating to system definition, documentation and management. These methods must be clear, specific, operational, and must be periodically reviewed. Validation is the responsibility of the end user. The validation control system includes (a) system definition, (b) test protocol, (c) validation testing, (d) performance evaluation, (e) operational procedures, and (f) validation report. The basic objectives of the test protocol should include determination of accuracy, reliability, performance, and reporting of activities and errors. There are systems such as statistical analysis system (SAS), vendor-supplied graphics, word processor, spreadsheet applications, and calculator programs, which ordinarily have a validation control system provided by the vendor. For these, documentation is needed of the source of codes and formulas. For other programs requiring a control system, validation of hardware, the manufacturer's name, model, serial number, configuration options, peripheral devices, memory boards sensors, interface boards, controlling devices, communication links, and references to system documentation are needed. For other software, development resources (e.g., compilers), function libraries, source-code management tools, and debugging utilities are needed.

All raw data must be properly identified and stored, eventually in study notebooks that ensure the integrity of the data. All data must be entered in a permanent and legible manner. Any changes to data must be dated and identified as changes, with reasons noted for any change, as well as the identification of the scientist making the change. Further, the professionals responsible for data entry, verification, and review should also be identified. Finally, the documentation of the data so described must be maintained at all times, and secure audit trails must be created for authorized changes in the database and also in the study notebook (251). In histopathology, raw data are by definition the tissues on glass slides and their respective blocks, requiring a specific trail leading from sampling records during necropsy and trimming records after necropsy (15,259). To achieve proper material, tissues are prepared according to standardized procedures with respect to location, type of section (e.g., cross), and orientation on the slide. In addition, slides of lesions should include both lesion and surrounding "normal tissue." Any failure to adhere to this regimen is a form of censorship and results in noncompliance. It is the duty of the study pathologist to integrate clinical (cage-side observation), structural (gross and microscopic), and functional (cellular and biochemical) data. Failure to integrate the three types of data will result in compromise of data and loss of data integrity. The pathologist must keep the study director apprised of events as they occur. The responsibilities of the study pathologist include keeping account of all the lesions reported at necropsy and performing microscopic evaluation of the normal and abnormal tissue changes. Thus, the pathologist ensures that appropriate tissues are collected, processed, and evaluated in a manner that satisfies the objective of the study. The pathologist also functions in a quality control capacity for the morphologic aspects of a carcinogenicity study (e.g., if a compound discolors adipose tissue, the pathologist ascertains whether all adipose tissues of exposed animals are discolored or whether the intensity is more pronounced in the high-dose group, etc.). Finally, the pathologist ensures consistency in diagnosis, integration of data, and grading of pertinent lesions, avoiding diagnostic drifts and censorship, as discussed in the section on pathology.

For a facility to be GLP compliant, specified environmental conditions (see the section on animals and their environment) must be maintained and monitored through a program applied at appropriate intervals.

The final regulatory end-product for every study is the compliance statement of the final report, which is signed by the study director. In this section of the report, all modifications, deviations, and amendments to the protocol should be listed. A second page with a quality assurance (QA) statement is signed by the QA auditor. During the last 20 years of GLP implementation, several common findings of importance (listing deficiencies in form FD-483) have been compiled by various agencies. The deficiencies noted were in all subparts of the FDA regulations (subparts A–J, 21 Code of Federal Regulation (CFR) 58.10–58.190). Those pertaining to pathology are detailed in the section on anatomic pathology.

Clearly, implementation of GLPs has benefited the conduct of chronic toxicity and carcinogenicity studies in many ways. These include (a) improved documentation, (b) refinement in bioavailability/bioequivalance information, (c) crystallization of the thinking process in safety assessment, and (d) strong, science-based regulated professionalism.

HEALTH AND SAFETY PROCEDURES

A comprehensive, rigorously followed health and safety plan is necessary for the proper conduct of an RCB. The fact that the substance is being tested for such activity makes it, in effect, a suspect carcinogen, although information in the Material Safety Data Sheet (MSDS) (e.g., genotoxicity, reproductive toxicity) influences the stringency of the handling procedures instituted, from receipt of the chemical through disposal of animal waste and processing of tissues for histopathological examination. All measures are subject to quality control.

The safety plan (178,190) must address the responsibility within management for development and adherence of the plan; medical surveillance for employees; employee training; safe handling practices for the chemical; animal handling; general laboratory safety; safe personnel practices; safe work-area practices (e.g., spill control and decontamination); handling of air, liquid, and solid wastes; monitoring of workers and physical equipment; emergency control; record keeping; the design of facilities; and the pollution potential. Applicable regulations of the Occupational Safety and Health Administration (OSHA) provide only a minimum structure from which to work, and lessening of the hazard within the particular facility must be addressed individually and with ingenuity. Laboratory directors must appreciate that chemicals may penetrate protective clothing and travel a considerable distance from their point of use (189,214,215,216,254,257).

No safety measure is unique to an RCB; it is the degree of adherence to such procedures that distinguishes the conduct of these studies from all others. It is beyond the scope of this section to address each individually. A few examples of aspects that are often inadequately addressed include the following: (a) use of a properly ventilated cage dumping area or an enclosed animal bedding disposal cabinet to prevent inhalation of contaminated dust and aerosols by employees; (b) an air-handling system that provides decreasing gradations of air pressure from clean corridor to the animal rooms to the dirty corridor and that is periodically tested under such stress as several doors being opened at one time or with all possible chemical hoods in operation; (c) maintenance personnel as well as scientific supervisors that follow the same rules as technicians for personal protection; (d) storage facilities that protect the integrity of the chemicals over an extended period of time during which unused material may be held and the immediate containers checked for deterioration; (e) a "breathable air" line available for use with an air-supplied respirator in the TS preparation areas; and (f) workers, including weekend staff, who are familiar with emergency safety instructions within the laboratory and know whom to notify in the event of various types of potential emergency situations.

ANIMALS AND THEIR ENVIRONMENT

The use of animals in research is subject to national regulations. In the United States, the use of rats, mice, and birds is not regulated. Guidelines for other animal use have been provided by the U.S. Department of Health and Welfare for Care and Use of Laboratory Animals (178,179,249), the latest amendment of the U.S. Congress Animal Welfare Act (245), the U.S. Public Health Service Policy of Humane Care and Use of Laboratory Animals (179), the U.S. Department of Agriculture Animal Welfare Rules (248), the Animal Welfare Act of the National Research Council (182), and the U.S. EPA Health Effects Test Guidelines (258). Institutional responsibilities include making available all protocols for review by a committee and providing veterinary care. More extensive coverage is provided in Chapter 16.

Species and Strain (Genotype)

For the rat RCB, several strains have been widely used. The NTP generally uses the inbred Fischer F344, while the pharmaceutical and chemical industries have favored the outbred Sprague-Dawley or Wistar. For the mouse RCB, industry generally favors the CD-1 strain, whereas the NTP uses the $B6C3F_1$ hybrid, which is the first-generation cross between male C_3H and female C57BL/6 strains.

Both rat and mouse strains differ substantially in their background of tumors and their susceptibility to induction of tumors (30). For example, the F344 has very high incidence of several neoplasms (Table 20.7). Among mouse strains, those derived from the C3H, that is, $B6C3F_1$, have a high incidence of liver tumors. Thus, male C3H/HeJ mice are highly susceptible to induction of liver cancer whereas those of the C57BL strain (6J or 10J sublines) are resistant; the $B6C3F_1$ hybrid is intermediate. Furthermore, when A/J mice (high lung tumor susceptibility) were crossed with C3HeB/FeJ (C3H) mice (high liver tumor susceptibility), the relative frequency of lung tumors was A/J>Hybrid>C3H and of liver tumors was C3H>Hybrid>A/J. For both tumor types, the incidences were higher in males than in females. The comparative percent incidence of the principal spontaneous neoplasms from five different strains of rats and mice is given in Table 20.7.

Several factors that influence response to carcinogens differ among genotypes. Notably, biotransformation activities differ considerably for certain chemicals. In addition, gender-dependent differences in xenobiotic metabolism are most pronounced in rats. The differences involve mainly cytochrome P450s (CYP), sulfotransferases, glutathione transferases, and glucuronyltransferases (176,184).

A troublesome feature of the F344 rat and $B6C3F_1$ mouse is that their average survival has progressively decreased and increases have occurred in the incidences of liver tumors in female and male mice, pituitary tumors in female mice and thyroid tumors, adrenal pheochromocytomas and leukemias in male rats, and mammary tumors in female rats (201,243). Some of these tumor increases are positively correlated with excessive body weight (243), due to overeating. A detailed discussion of this issue is presented earlier in this chapter, in the feeding procedures section. Likewise, in Charles River Sprague-Dawley rats decreases in survival have been reported (136,137). These problems may be due to breeding practices. Currently, the Wistar strain does not appear to present this problem (197).

Feed and Water

Four major types of diets are available, as follows: (a) natural-product, unrefined, largely cereal-based formulations unusually referred to as "chow-type" diets, such as NIH-07 (Purina 5018 or Purina 5001); (b) semipurified diets, formulated from refined nutrient ingredients, such as AIN76A (with sucrose) or modified AIN 76A (with dextrose); (c) open-formula diets, such as NIH-31 (Purina 7017), which are formulated to contain researcher-specified quantities of nonproprietary ingredients; and (d) chemical-defined diets, which are individually specialized (142,182). Industry generally favors the open formula diet. The NTP has introduced a new diet, NTP-2000, designed to reduce certain spontaneous pathologies in the F344 rat.

Details about various regimens of feed availability are given earlier, in the discussion of Feeding Procedures.

Caging and Stratification

Following randomization (see section on groups), animals can be caged individually or with more than one animal in each cage, each having advantages and disadvantages. Individually caged animals tend to

Table 20.7
Comparative percent incidence of pertinent neoplasia in different strains of rats and mice (104 weeks old)

	F344 rats[a]		S-D rats[b]		Wistar rats[c]		$B6C3F_1$ mice[d]		CD-1 mice[e]	
Types of neoplasia	Males	Females	Males	Females	Males	Females	Males	Females	Males	Females
Hepatocellular adenoma	4	<1	5	<1	1	2	29	30	26	5
Hepatocellular carcinoma	2	0	2	0	<1	<1	26	16	10	1
Pancreas islet adenoma	12	2	8	9	4	2	2	0	<1	<1
Pancreas islet carcinoma	3	0	<1	5	<1	<1	0	0	0	0
Pancreas acinar adenoma	6	0	1	0	13	<1	2	0	<1	0
Pheochromocytoma	21	4	23	5	10	2	0	2	<1	<1
Adrenocortical adenoma	0	2	3	0	8	9	<1	0	1	<1
Pituitary adenoma	49	42	62	85	34	55	2	8	0	5
Thyroid C-cell adenoma	17	8	7	6	6	8	0	0	0	0
Thyroid follicular adenoma	0	0	4	2	2	1	2	6	1	<1
Mammary-gland fibroadenoma	4	57	2	54	3	36	0	0	<1	1
Mammary-gland carcinoma	0	4	<1	26	1	13	0	0	0	6
Skin fibroma	10	2	2	<1	5	1	1	2	<1	<1
Skin papilloma	6	0	2	0	2	<1	0	0	<1	0
Pulmonary adenoma	4	4	<1	<1	<1	0	22	6	15	15
Preputial-gland neoplasia	10	NA	>1	NA	<1	NA	<1	NA	<1	NA
Leydig-cell neoplasia	89	NA	7	NA	11	NA	0	NA	1	NA
Clitoral-gland neoplasia	NA	14	NA	<1	NA	<1	NA	<1	NA	0
Uterine polyps	NA	14	NA	6	NA	16	NA	1	NA	<1
Ovarian neoplasia	NA	6	NA	1	NA	8	NA	6	NA	1
Mononuclear-cell leukemia	62	42	0	0	<1	<1	0	0	2	2
Lymphoma	0	0	2	1	3	5	14	24	8	22
Forestomach papilloma	0	2	<1	<1	0	<1	4	2	<1	<1
Scrotal mesothelioma	5	NA	1	NA	2	NA	0	NA	0	NA

Note. F344, Fischer 344 rats; S-D, Sprague-Dawley rats; $B6C3F_1$, mice $(C57BL/6N{+}C3H/HeN)F_1$; CD-1, 1CRCr: CD-1 mice; NA, nonapplicable; the average number used by species/strain/gender was in excess of 750 animals.

[a] Modified from References 183 and 29.
[b] Modified from References 167 and 29.
[c] From References 271, 14, and 197.
[d] Modified from References 232 and 183.
[e] Modified from Reference 160.

overeat. Multiple-animal caging leads to a conflict for hierarchy in the cage and consequent cage differences. Group-caged female mice develop pseudopregnancy, which results in uterine decidual reactions. Also, group caging of mice produces almost a doubling of the lymphoma incidence in both males and females (236). In general, group-caged rodents demonstrate higher survival rates and lower background pathology (206). For inhalation and dermal administration studies, single housing is required.

All cages used should be either metallic (stainless or galvanized steel) or plastic (polycarbonate, polyethylene, or polypropylene), with a minimum stipulated cage size (249). The floor of the cages can either be solid or suspended. Solid-floor cages require bedding, that should not possess enzyme induction properties, such as hardwood bedding (269).

Rotation of cages and racks periodically should be used to balance known confounding sources of variability such as proximity to dual-intensity fluorescent light (148,202). Consequently, rodents within groups should be distributed in cage racks in such a way as to be present equally at all vertical levels of caging. A thorough documentation of such cage and rack rotation is mandated.

Ventilation, Temperature, Humidity, and Emergency Power

Environmental stress to test animals must be minimized, particularly with mice, which are easily stressed even when maintained under conventional housing conditions and handled in the usual manner. The incidence of tumors in mice infected with viruses can be increased by chronic stress (205,221).

Standards for care are detailed in the *Guide for the Care and Use of Laboratory Animals* (182). These include (a) 10–15 fresh air changes per hour in each animal room; (b) air pressure adjusted so that the animal rooms are slightly positive to the "dirty" corridor and negative to the "clean" one, with minimal crossovers between the corridors; (c) all air adequately filtered before it enters the animal facility, and diluted or filtered after it leaves to prevent possibly toxic concentrations of the test chemical from entering the outside air (a process that is particularly important with inhalation studies because of the large amounts of chemical used); (d) temperature and humidity maintained within those ranges reported to be optimal, that is, 23.3±1.1°C (74±2°F) and a relative humidity of 40±5% in rat and mouse rooms; and (e) automatic control systems that record both temperature and humidity at least three or four times per day. Control of lighting is essential. Usually, a 12-h continuous light interval per day is used for both rats and mice (14-h light day for hamsters). Moreover, high (only during cage-side observation time of approximately 4 h)–low (20 h) intensity of fluorescent light is recommended in order to avoid blindness caused by high-intensity light. In addition, because the light and temperature gradients occur vertically, a cage-rack rotation is mandated (182). An emergency power source is essential to maintain operation of storage freezers and refrigerators, lighting, tissue processors, and some degree of air-conditioning, as well as air handling, during power failure or when personnel are unable to reach the facility. The emergency power and alarm systems should be tested on a regular schedule. In a GLP-compliant facility, all these conditions must be monitored.

Also important is control of pests by adequate facility design and sanitary procedures. Pesticides must not be allowed to contaminate the animal rooms, feed rooms, or cage washing areas and accordingly should be dispensed only in closed traps in limited areas. Detergents and cleaning agents for use on floors, cage washers, and other equipment must be nonvolatile and must not leave a residue.

DOSE SELECTION STUDIES FOR BIOASSAY

Dose Selection: The Maximum Tolerated Dose

Dose setting can be based upon a number of end-points, including toxicity, toxicokinetics, saturation of absorption, and maximum feasible dose (73). Generally, it has been expected that the high dose level in an RCB should be a toxicity-based dose, the maximum tolerated dose (MTD) (229), which is also referred to as the minimum toxic dose (or the minimally toxic dose used by NTP) (100). The various methods for selection of the high-dose level have been reviewed by a working group on dose selection convened by the International Life Sciences Institute (73). Testing at the MTD has the virtue that a negative outcome is compelling, but creates problems in the interpretation of positive findings, because of specific high-dose effects, as discussed with rodent cancer bioassay evaluation.

The first widely used definition of the MTD was formulated by the National Cancer Institute (229) as follows: "The MTD is defined as the highest dose of the test agent during the chronic study that can be predicted not to alter the animals' normal longevity from effects other than carcinogenicity." This definition does not stipulate that any toxicity be produced, and hence a slight, but significant, reformulation was introduced by the U.S. Interagency Staff Group on Carcinogens (181,262) as follows: The MTD is "the highest dose which when given for the duration of the chronic study is just high enough to elicit signs of minimal toxicity without significantly altering animals' normal lifespan due to effects other than carcinogenicity." The MTD so defined is a dose used in the chronic study (7), which, of necessity, is selected from subchronic studies (normally 90-day). The ICH defines the MTD as the dose predicted from a range finding study to produce minimum toxicity over the course of the carcinogenicity study (262). Such toxicity may be predicted from alterations in physiological function that would be expected to alter survival, toxicity to target organs, significant alterations in clinical pathological parameters or suppression of weight gain of no more than 10% relative to controls calculated as the difference between the starting weights and those at the end of the study (181,262). A fortuitously selected target MTD should in the RCB study suppress weight gain by 10% or slightly greater and produce only minimal other toxicities. This, however, infrequently happens, and issues arise when the high dose is either below or above what is considered by a regulatory agency to be an MTD.

Toxicokinetic endpoints have gained acceptance for dose setting for pharmaceuticals (42,76). A dose that produces saturation of absorption is considered an MTD, and a dose that produces a plasma concentration that is 25 times greater than human exposure is considered pragmatic (124). The endpoints are easier to establish.

Toxicodynamic endpoints can be used to establish a high dose that will produce a cellular effect beyond which the validity of the study would be compromised. An example is induced toxicity, which would be expected to become more severe with aging in rats as they develop chronic progressive nephropathy.

To identify the target MTD or high dose, subchronic studies are performed, as described next. If the target MTD (or the high dose) cannot be established on the criteria discussed, it is usually recommended that the high dose level or limit dose not exceed 5% in the feed (115,169,191), which translates into approximately 3–4 g/kg/day for rats and 7–8 g/kg/day for mice. This limit appears to be based upon concern for the nutritional impact of high proportions of TS. Certainly, some TSs at high exposure interfere with nutritional elements, such as impairment of vitamin K function by butylated hydroxytoluene (37,127), but such problems can be overcome by nutritional supplements. Nevertheless, reduced feed intake, and hence caloric intake, will affect the outcome of the RCB, usually reducing tumor incidence (1,29,183).

In the United States, for pharmaceuticals, the dose selection should be submitted to the FDA Center for Drug Evaluation and Research Carcinogenicity Assessment Committee, which strongly favors a toxicity-based endpoint. Such consultation is not yet practiced in Europe.

The selection of other dose levels is discussed in the section on rodent cancer bioassay groups.

Subchronic Study

The MTD is usually identified from results of a 90-day study, using the route of administration to be used in the RCB. It is unusual that a tested dose would qualify as the predicted MTD, and therefore interpolation is usually made. When genders show different MTDs, then based on kinetic study results, different sets of doses are administered.

Kinetic Studies

Before starting an RCB, it is helpful, and in the case of medicinal products, it is a requirement (76,124), to determine the time course of exposure and the relationship between the concentration of exposure and effect. For this purpose, multiple-dose toxicokinetic studies are conducted (23,42,124). Plasma protein binding of the TS in rodents and humans should be determined before initiation of the carcinogenicity studies. Should binding exceed 80%, it is advisable to express exposure (plasma TS concentration) in terms of the free fraction (26,276). In addition, tissue distribution and accumulation data can be valuable (25,198,225), but this is more difficult and requires other techniques. Furthermore, accurate and useful extrapolation from rodents to humans presupposes understanding of histokinetic and xenodynamic considerations. For example, smaller species (e.g., rodents) have a higher xenobiotic metabolic rate per kilogram of body weight, faster rate of tissue distribution, and shorter tissue half-life (111). Tissue volume directly affects the volume of distribution of xenobiotics, bioavailability, half-life, and systemic clearance (13,130, 140). In general, with increasing age, as will occur over the course of a carcinogenicity study, body weight increases, as does the proportion of adipose tissue, which has a lower metabolic rate than skeletal muscle mass (82). Both influence the outcome of kinetic studies. In dose-proportional linear kinetics, half-life and clearance are independent of xenobiotic concentration. In contrast, in nonlinear kinetics, these parameters are dependent, because the various processes (e.g., absorption, distribution, metabolism, and excretion) can become saturated (153).

The toxicokinetic component of a carcinogenicity study often entails satellite groups run in parallel and consists of at least three rodents per group per gender per time interval, with interim kills at least every 6 months. The time-course factor is very important in explaining how the various concentrations accumulate and relate to different exposures (76). The animals are maintained and exposed under identical conditions with the main study. Approximately 4 blood samples are taken from each animal over the duration of the RCB, with the blood removed not exceeding 15% of the total blood volume.

The parameters examined may include (a) the maximum achieved concentration (C_{max}), the minimum concentration (C_{min}), the time to C_{max} (T_{max}), and the area under the flood concentration versus time curve (AUC) for TS and all metabolites (109). Only the AUC is required to establish exposure (124). In an RCB, together with measuring the systemic concentration of exposure (AUC), determination of the total (cumulative) amount of exposure over time is also essential so that exposure can be related to induced effects (124,198). In addition, if indicated from chronic toxicity data, target site (tissue) compound levels (or major metabolites) can be measured, but, as noted, this requires separate assay validation and a more extensive study design to acquire appropriate tissues. Target site compound levels potentially connect the target site of both chronic toxicity and carcinogenicity. For accurate extrapolation of exposure over time, human time equivalent (HTE) values are employed. These values amount at 12 months of exposure to a HTE of 38 years for the mouse and 34 years for the rat, and at 24 months to a HTE of 76 and 64 years for the mouse and rat, respectively (109,111).

Pharmacokinetic data are critical, not only for delineating blood levels, but also for understanding the effects of exposure—that is, if the parent or a metabolite is the main active moiety, or even if the plasma concentration reflects the cellular site of action, and which is the interspecies concentration (blood)–response (site) relationship (109,171,193). Furthermore, metabolism can also distort concentration-response homeostasis. Here, at high exposures, together with absorption and elimination being saturable (i.e., capacity limited), intermediary metabolism can also significantly target tissue bioavailability through transformation, which is especially important in interspecies extrapolation (27,86,225,296). Moreover, metabolic saturation and activation of secondary routes of metabolism should also be taken into consideration (25,47,85,93). Knowledge of metabolic behavior (e.g., species differences in biotransformation enzymes) of the xenobiotic under test is the best foundation for interpreting the mechanism(s) of neoplasia and for extrapolating to humans.

QUALITY CONTROL OF THE TEST SUBSTANCE

The test substance should be of a high quality and stability, and should be manufactured in the same way and contain the same concentration of impurities as the final product. Impurities in excess of 0.1% should be individually identified. For pharmaceuticals, the preclinical and clinical final product tested should be preferably the same. The product should have a well-defined and described scale-up process (125).

Most medicines will be formulated with excipients and, accordingly, the noncarcinogenicity of these must be established. In other situations, as with agricultural chemicals and cosmetics, the technical-grade product or a representative technical grade of active ingredients is tested. In some instances, complex mixtures are tested, as with polychlorinated biphenyls. This aspect is discussed further with complex mixtures.

Test Substance

Chemicals or Small Molecules

In some situations, it is desirable or necessary to test pure chemicals, as with candidate medicines or food additives. With isomeric compounds, if the two enantiomers exhibit inversion in vivo or have the same biological activity, they are considered one entity and carcinogenicity of the racemate is appropriate. If the biological activity is not the same, then carcinogenicity testing of the active enantiomer is indicated.

Biopharmaceuticals

Biopharmaceuticals include recombinant human proteins, humanized monoclonal antibodies, oligodeoxynucleotides, and genes. Recombinant human proteins are being produced by a variety of techniques, often in bacteria where glycosylation does not occur. Quality control of biopharmaceuticals, as with small molecules, is necessary to establish that they are actually what they are expected to be at all times during the study. For this purpose, all relevant information, such as synonyms, trade names, and structural and molecular formulas and weights, as well as methods of analysis and chemical and physical properties of the pure substance, should be provided.

Impurities or Contaminants

It is highly recommended that all TS should be pure chemicals of analytical grade, since even traces of impurities of <1% can have confounding effects resulting in neoplasms. An example of this would be *o*-toluenesulfonamide (OTS), an impurity of saccharin, present in the early carcinogenicity studies (173). Impurities can occur in the starting materials to be used in the formulation, or in materials used in the manufacturing process of the TS (69,131,266). Impurities in excess of 0.1% should be thoroughly identified. If the TS with the identified impurity is intended for long-term use, such as with a high dose of active compound, then multiple-dose toxicity (up to 3 months) and mutagenicity studies should be performed. If the results of the mutagenicity assays are positive, carcinogenicity testing of the impurity may be considered (125).

Preparation of Dose

The most essential aspects in preparing a TS for dosing are identity of all ingredients, homogeneity of the product, particle size, stability of all active ingredients, and vehicle (carrier) to be used (69,131). All batches of dosage preparations must be analyzed for concentration to confirm accurate preparation prior to use.

Homogeneity of the TS–diet mixture and stability of the TS in diet under the intended in-study conditions should be established prior to the start of RCB. During the conduct of the RCB, samples of the TS–diet mixture are taken approximately every 6 months for analysis and correction if necessary. It is recommended that the same batch be used for the entire RCB. This presupposes that there is a complete method of analysis for the active ingredients at hand. Quality control data as described earlier should be provided, and monitoring should continue throughout the duration of the study.

TEST SUBSTANCE OF ADMINISTRATION

The route of administration should be appropriate to potential human exposure and reflect knowledge about comparative bioavailability. Thus, comparative absorptive, dispositional, metabolic, and excretion data are essential and should be used in designing the 2-year RCB.

The most common route is the oral, followed by parenteral exposure and inhalation. The selection of a delivery system is crucial for all routes, as it has the potential to significantly affect bioavailability. Second, producing uniform and homogenous TS exposure throughout the bioassay is equally important. This requires the availability of a validated analytical methodology (124,225).

For some TS there is a rationale for prenatal exposure, but generally exposure is begun postweaning at 4–6 weeks of age.

Oral

The oral route of administration is most frequently used, especially for medicines and food additives for which ingestion is the usual route of exposure of humans. For oral administration, the TS can be admixed in the feed or given by intragastric (ig) instillation (gavage). Comparable systemic exposures can be achieved with either, but with the ig route, the bolus dose results in a higher blood $C_{\max}$ (143).

The concentration of TS in diet is adjusted to compensate for changes in body weight. During the rapid growth phase the concentrations are adjusted biweekly at first, then weekly, and later monthly after the growth plateau has been reached. Here TS stability and homogeneity data are essential. Periodically during the study, samples of TS–diet mixtures should be analyzed to confirm desirable concentrations and enable corrective action to be implemented. In general, this is the most cost-efficient mode of exposure with most TS.

Intragastric (ig) administration affords the most precise oral delivery of TS. For this route of administration, a vehicle is required, such as corn or olive oil. For a TS that cannot be dissolved in water or oils, a suspension in Tween 80 or carboxymethylcellulose can be used. For a TS that is unstable or volatile in diet, microencapsulation can be used. Oils as vehicle will prolong residence time in the stomach compared to water (23). Corn oil given ig is reported to increase the body weights of male rats, but to have an opposite effect on females (99). Also, the incidence of some background tumors, such as mononuclear-cell leukemia and pancreatic acinar-cell tumors, can be affected. For this reason, a second control group (without gavage) is strongly recommended. For more details, see the section on feeding procedures. In general, the TS volume in rats is 3–5 ml/kg body weight. In mice a volume of up to 10 ml/kg has been shown to be desirable, as this enables more accurate measurement of the dose. In addition, dilution enhances absorption and decreases local irritation, especially with weak bases or acids, which comprise the majority of TS (17). Unscheduled deaths should be closely monitored at necropsy by inspection of the lungs and trachea for TS. If deaths are due to gavage accidents, then a monitoring program should be implemented. In general, the baseline rate for accidents per technician should not exceed 1 per 10,000 gavages.

Dermal

Under certain circumstances of dermal human exposure, TS are delivered via this route either by topical application or injection. The sensitivity of this route of exposure depends on the fact that the skin is also capable of biotransformation, albeit not to the same degree as that of the liver or intestinal tract (23).

Dermal application is usually to the superior dorsal area of the back (interscapular), where the skin is clipped at least weekly, 24 h prior to application (149). In dermal studies, animals are routinely housed singly to minimized ingestion by other cage mates. TS (0.25–1 ml) is applied topically over the clipped area at intervals (e.g., 2 times or 3 times weekly) to allow for recovery (especially when the TS is irritating). Skin penetration varies with species, chemistry of TS, and vehicle (219). Thus, one should consider, in dermal dosing by weight or surface area, to the fact that rats are large enough to vary significantly in size, whereas mice are not. Moreover, effects at the site of dermal injection should be monitored carefully.

Inhalation (Intratracheal)

With some TS, chronic inhalation is indicated. Routinely, under these conditions, animals are exposed 6 h/day during the day (104). After exposure, the animals can either remain in the chamber or be taken to another room. Either way, constant airflow through the chamber during and after exposure prevents build up of ammonia. Single cage occupancy is recommended to avoid grooming and licking-based ingestion. The cages should be rotated within the chamber periodically. Inhalation exposure is an expensive, labor-intensive route of administration, requiring frequent monitoring of achieved air concentrations. Sampling should be done from several fixed locations in the chamber after documenting homogeneity of the test atmosphere (162).

Nose-only or head-only exposure units are available for rodents (228). Their major advantages include minimization of external contamination and effective monitoring of respiratory parameters. The major disadvantages include restraining the animals, leading to alteration of many physiological parameters and entailing excessive manpower requirements.

Intratracheal exposure can be conducted under anesthesia to permit chronic delivery (up to 2 years) directly into the bronchial passages. Here, a second control group (with the anesthetic) should be added and exposure should be limited to once or twice weekly (227).

Parenteral

In special cases, or when the TS is destroyed in the gastrointestinal tract, intraperitoneal, intramuscular, or subcutaneous routes of administration are employed. Here, new factors such as molecular size and pH have the potential to affect absorption and cause irritation (9). Again, if a carrier is used, then a second control group without carrier is needed. The exposure regimen here is limited to two or three times per week. In using these routes, the potential exists for local tumor formation due to physical factors (207).

Multigenerational/Transplacental/Perinatal

Experimental transplacental carcinogenesis has been extensively studied, mainly in rats and mice (239), but also in primates (203,237). The design of experiments ranges from multigenerational, involving exposure of germ cells of one or both parents and subsequently the progeny, to exposure of embryonal or fetal cells (4,239). It has frequently been discussed whether such exposures should be included in an RCB, but so far, it is accepted that a conventional RCB beginning at 4 to 6 weeks of age can identify carcinogens that might have activity in developmental stages.

CLINICAL AND PATHOLOGICAL EXAMINATION

The RCB is not an extended chronic toxicity study; standard chronic toxicity assays (i.e., 6 and 9 or 12 months, depending upon requirements) involve more clinical observations than are necessary or appropriate for the RCB. In the RCB, animals should be observed at the beginning and at the end of each work day so that unwell animals can be euthanized before they become moribund or are lost to autolysis (or cannibalization, if multiple caging is used). Real-time automated programs for carcinogenicity studies have been developed (188), allowing for monitoring, at least biweekly, the appearance, location, and growth of palpable cutaneous or subcutaneous masses.

Standard parameters measured in the RCB include body weight, health status, and mortality.

Body Weight and Survival

In RCBs using an MTD, controls frequently show greater weight gain and often poorer survival than the high-dose group, in which body weight is reduced both by toxicity as well as secondary effects resulting in reduced feed consumption or energy utilization (156).

Intercurrent Diseases

Laboratory strains of rats and mice are susceptible to a variety of diseases, both genetic and acquired. The genetically determined conditions include predisposition to development of neoplasms, as discussed with species and strain. Also, pathologies such as amyloidosis in mice and chronic progressive nephropathy in rats are common. These conditions increase with age and complicate long-term studies. Acquired diseases, such as sialoadenitis and murine hepatitis, can be minimized by proper animal husbandry. Many strains of mice harbor *Helicobacter hepaticus* in the gastrointestinal tract. Infection with this organism can lead to an increased incidence of liver neoplasms, particularly in male mice (91). Satellite sentinel animals are included in all chronic studies to effectively monitor intercurrent acquired diseases.

Clinical Pathology

Several regulatory agencies have suggested the monitoring of continuous variables, including hematology, clinical chemistry, urinalysis, and organ weights (128,260). It must be realized that, in spite of initial randomization, aged rodents are no longer homogeneous because of nonrandom attrition and development of diseases in the latter portion of the in-life phase. Although such measures may be helpful at times, they need not be implemented without a specific reason; for example, hematology smears assist in the diagnosis of leukemia.

Anatomic Pathology

Pathology is not only an integral part of the protocol design, but plays a pivotal role throughout the conduct, evaluation, and interpretation of carcinogenicity studies (16), as discussed in Good Laboratory Practice. In general, emphasis is placed on routine methods, but special pathology methods may be required depending on the target organs. Whatever can be anticipated from previous subchronic and chronic studies should be utilized in the protocol for pathology. Furthermore, the pathologist must correlate clinical observations, body weight gain and survival patterns, clinical pathology data, and other data with gross and microscopic changes. The general and specific GLP and statistical considerations are given in separate sections elsewhere in this chapter.

All animals euthanized for humane reasons and those found dead should be submitted to a complete necropsy. At scheduled necropsies, the pathology team should be prepared for potential outcomes by participating in a prenecropsy briefing, where all known clinicopathological correlations are discussed. At necropsy, body weights are obtained. Examination of all recorded palpable masses constitutes an initial procedure with examination of all body orifices and skin. A ventral midline incision, with reflection of the skin so that subcutaneous tissues are exposed, initiates the opening of the abdominal cavity, followed by the thoracic and finally the cranial cavities. All gross lesions are described as to their location, size, shape, consistency, and color. In general, organs should be examined in situ as well as after removal from the animal. Any artifactual tissue damage (e.g. crushing or tearing of tissues) must be avoided, but if this is not possible, damage should be minimized and noted. Tissues should be cleaned by rinsing in physiologic saline solution (tap water is not acceptable because the low osmolarity damages cells). Alimentary-tract hollow organs (because of their rapid rate of autolysis) are opened to avoid tissue autolysis and examined (their anatomic integrity if possible should be maintained). Lungs are instilled (with 10% neutral buffered formalin, ~4 ml in rats and ~2 ml in mice) with care not to overinflate, and if indicated, also the urinary bladder (with formalin ~0.2–0.5 ml), after which the trachea and urethra, respectively, are ligated to maintain the inflated state. Lesions/neoplasms are dissected to include regional lymph nodes, if possible, and a small portion of surrounding (normal) tissue. At least 55 standard tissues and lesions are sampled, trimmed, and processed for histopathological examination, including brown adipose tissue, blood and bone marrow smears (28,79,163,207). Any significant deviation from any of these procedures amounts to censoring, which potentially compromises the integrity of the study (see GLP and statistical analyses sections). Organ weights are usually not taken in carcinogenicity studies because of variability of weights caused by disease, neoplasms, or body-weight fluctuations. In some cases selected organs are weighed (260,261), usually the adrenals, brain, heart, kidneys, liver, lungs, spleen, testes (with epididymides), and uterus (including horns). Where organ weights are taken, organ-to-body-weight percentage values are recommended (79).

The preparation of routine microscopic slides should be in accordance with a standard operating procedure (SOP). Each slide should be matched with blocks and routinely taken tissues or grossly observed findings. Special methods (e.g., quantification of proliferating cell nuclear antigen [PCNA]), compatible with formalin fixation, should be either described in detail in the protocol or be part of an SOP. Recently, these methods have shown utility, since they are capable of identifying proliferation (PCNA) and preneoplasia and early neoplasia (112,294). During microscopic examination, an "open" slide evaluation is recommended (107,108,186). It consists of evaluation of the concurrent control group(s) first and, subsequently, the high-exposure groups. After this the rest of the exposure groups are evaluated and the presence or absence of an exposure response pattern is established. Lastly, the findings can be compared to in-house historical or published control data to minimize subjectivity and diagnostic drift. "Open" evaluation is preferably conducted by one pathologist. If the study entails more than 1000 animals, then one pathologist may read the males and a second the females, to reduce the length of time to complete the histopathologic evaluation. "Open" evaluation is also performed when quantitation is performed (e.g., PCNA). Under certain circumstances, a re-evaluation of certain tissue-specific lesions is needed. Then a "blinded" microscopic examination of selected target tissues may be performed, in which all slides are reevaluated by the pathologist in a blinded manner in a random sequence. Also, the valuable practice of peer review can be utilized. This consists of an independent examination by a second pathologist of all tissues from a representative sampling of randomly selected animals of both genders from the control and high-dose groups and a representative sampling of proliferative lesions to substantiate the data from the initial evaluation for neoplasms and other proliferative lesions. Here it is also recommended that the evaluation be "open," and that all changes (not only microscopic) are taken into consideration.

It is vital that all pathology data are recorded in a consistent manner and are depicted as individual data in appendices. A summary of all exposure-related data should be in tables. An appendix depicting all missing tissues is highly desirable. Neoplastic diagnoses should adhere to an accepted nomenclature of histopathologic terms, according to recommendations made by the Society of Toxicologic Pathologists (Guides for Toxicologic Pathology, STP/ARP/AFIP, Washington, DC), with particular care to distinguish between proliferative non-neoplastic lesions, benign neoplasms, and malignant neoplasms (65,66,88,90,164). The pathologist must integrate all clinical, structural (gross and microscopic), and functional (cellular and biochemical) data. Moreover, the pathologist ensures proper accounting of gross and microscopic lesions and changes, as detailed in the sections covering Good Laboratory Pratice and statistical analyses. In pathology, the most common deficiencies in Good Laboratory Practice are as follows: (a) Gross observations are not fully available and the exposure related ones are not compared side-by-side with microscopic findings; (b) gross microscopic pathology data do not match and no explanation is provided; (c) organ weights in notebook and report do not match; (d) termination dates before completion of the study are not in the final report and no explanation is given; (e) differences between forms of data recording by the pathologist and the SOPs are not explained; (f) individual animal data in the notebook and data in tabular form in the report on the corresponding animal are not the same and no explanation is provided; (g) there is a lack of uniformity in pathology nomenclature and no explanation is provided; (h) there is lack of lesion accountability and important tissues are missing without any explanation being given; (i) the method of slide evaluation is not stated (e.g., open, peer-reviewed, etc.); and (j) lack of initialing and dating in various records such as gross data, tissue trimming, microscope evaluation, tissue recuts, and so on. Each of these is important and, if no explanation is provided, can compromise the RCB.

RODENT CANCER BIOASSAY EVALUATION

Tumor Increases or Decreases

If the RCB has been conducted properly, it should provide adequate evidence to assess whether exposure has lead to increases or decreases in the incidence of specific well-defined neoplasms. A conclusion of lack of carcinogenic activity requires survival of adequate numbers of animals given sufficient relevant exposures, usually the MTD, with no evidence of tumor increases according to the criteria discussed in the section on chemicals with carcinogenic activity.

A conclusion for a positive outcome is generally less rigorous. That is, in the interest of conservative hazard identification, a clear increase in tumors is often accepted as valid in spite of artifacts in the study such as excessively reduced weight gain or poor survival. Nevertheless, the possibility must be considered that the tumor increases are a consequence of the toxicity of the treatment conditions (89), and not a chemical action of the TS.

A critical aspect in the evaluation is the interpretation of pathological diagnoses. Findings of increases in malignant neoplasms are universally accepted as evidence of carcinogenic activity. Combining malignant and benign neoplasms of the same cell type of origin is also widely accepted, and guidelines have been published for the NTP procedures (164). In evaluating tumor increases, attention must be paid to pathology in the tissue that is the site of tumors because cell injury and compensatory cell proliferation can facilitate tumor development (see the section on cancer hazard and risk assessment).

The most appropriate comparison of an experimental group is with its matched control or controls, where two groups are used (83). Nevertheless, in arriving at a conclusion of tumor increase, it is important to consider historical control data (98), especially if control groups differ. Differences between controls and exposed groups can be analyzed by a variety of statistical methods, as discussed next. Whether any true increases in neoplasms have relevance for human cancer hazard is discussed in the section on cancer hazard and risk assessment.

A controversial issue is the interpretation of tumor decreases in the RCB (45), which are quite frequent (101). One consideration is that the reduction should not be attributable to nonspecific weight gain suppression, as discussed in the feeding procedures section. A variety of mechanisms for specific anticarcinogenesis have been delineated, as discussed in the section on anticarcinogenesis.

Statistical Analyses

An expert biostatistician should be involved in the RCB. The methods ultimately employed can be diverse and only some general guidance is provided here. More extensive coverage is provided in Chapter 7.

Statistics are employed in all aspects of the study, that is, design, conduct, evaluation, analysis, and interpretation. The object of statistics is to aid an investigator in the interpretation of RBC results by providing a quantitative measure (p value) of the likelihood that an increased tumor incidence is due to random variability. Other than exposure, two other factors can underlie an increase in neoplasia: One is bias, which is a systematic difference other than what is caused by exposure, and the other is chance, a random difference. It is indeed highly desirable to avoid bias and to minimize (and control) chance, although it cannot be completely excluded (i.e., identically exposed animals do not respond identically—the biological reality). The probability of chance can be statistically measured: the smaller the probability, the higher the confidence (152). A further complicating factor is that the multiplicity of tumor sites examined in a typical RCB increases the likelihood that an increased tumor incidence at any single given site is due to chance.

A one-sided (one-tailed) p value, is the probability of getting by chance an exposure effect in a specified direction as great as or greater than that observed (68). A two-sided (two-tailed) p value is the probability of getting by chance an exposure difference (effect) in either direction that is as great as or greater than that observed. The calculation of a p value of <0.05 implies that the effect could have occurred by chance less than 1 time in 20. Theoretically at least, randomization eliminates nonsystematic bias. But if there is another major source of variation (e.g., gender of the same strain, or batch of the same strain), then a stratified randomization is more appropriate. To achieve that, separate randomization within each level of the stratifying variable (e.g., cage position, order of weighting, or order of killing at termination) must be performed (152). The power of any statistical measurement refers to the probability that the subject test will correctly detect a difference, when such a difference truly exists (80).

There are three aspects that determine the nature of collected data: the biological system, the study design instrumentation, and methodologies applied. Censoring any of these must be minimized. In general, exposure variables are independent, while effect variables are dependent. (80,152). Representative samples should be appropriately collected and be of sufficient size. In addition, samples should be accurate (of high quality) and precise (reproducible). The pattern of distribution of data in the sample is very important, because it shows their central tendency and dispersion. There is the Gaussian distribution (the most common), in which two-thirds of all values are within one standard deviation. Others include binomial and chi-square patterns of distribution. In order to successfully combine data for analysis, stratification is applied (e.g., early, late, or total deaths).

In order to enhance detection exposure effects, the exposure-related trend is employed (233). Furthermore, if there are differences in survival, there is a need for age adjustment to avoid bias. Certain statistical procedures used in the analysis of tumor data require specification of the context of observation is taken into account—that is, whether the condition (neoplasm) is assumed to have caused death, or death was an incidental finding (195). If the study pathologist concludes that it is not possible to determine the context of observation, then alternative methodology must be used (78). Because of the multiplicity of tumor sites examined it may also be necessary in certain cases to employ a statistical adjustment for multiple comparisons.

When animal weights differ across dose groups, as is usually the case with high-dose testing, such differences can contribute to differences in tumor incidence (see feeding procedures). Analyzing tumor incidence within body weight strata can reduce the bias resulting from weight differences (84).

In the past, the single most important statistical consideration in the analysis of bioassays was a simple quantal response: that is, either neoplasia did occur or it did not occur. Presently, the mechanisms underlying neoplasia induced by chemicals are more fully understood and must be given individual consideration. These mechanisms include effects on survival rate, body weight gain, age at first tumor, time-to-tumor, patterns (trends) of tumor incidence, tumor multiplicity, rates of proliferation at target sites, presence of markers of preneoplasia or early neoplasia, and exposure response. As recommended in the study design section, at least one interim kill should be included, and possibly also a short (1–3 months) recovery segment before final termination.

In an RCB, the time course of adverse effects (or risks) is of importance. Consequently, life-table methods are employed to compare survival curves and/or survival time until neoplasms develop (40,41,195). For continuous, normally distributed outcome measures, group means are typically compared against the control mean using a one-way analysis of variance (ANOVA) followed by Dunnett's method for multiple comparisons, which is a powerful post hoc test (54). Moreover, a square-root transformation may be necessary in some cases to stabilize the variance. To make all possible pairwise comparisons, Tukey's multiple-comparison procedure may be used (72). To assess the course of exposure response (its linearity), ordinary least-squares regression analysis can be used, fitting the outcome level versus exposure and squared exposure terms. For incidence of specific site neoplasia comparing all test groups, the Pearson chi-square test followed by pairwise comparisons of each exposure group with control, adjusted for multiple comparisons, can be applied (77). For incidence trend analysis, the Cochran–Armitage test, partitioning the chi-square statistic into the overall trend and departure from linearity (p nonlinear), can be tested (71). Furthermore, survival data can be used by applying log-rank test for both homogeneity and exposure-related trend (96,97). Neoplastic data can be analyzed using a survival-adjusted trend test discriminating fatal, incidental, and palpable neoplasms (195). For rare neoplasms, a p value of <0.025 and for common neoplasms

Table 20.8
Classification of carcinogens

IARC	HWC	EPA	IFSTP
Group 1	Group I	Group A	Group 1
Group 2A	Group II	Group B_1	Group 2a
Group 2B	Group III	Group B_2	Group 2b
—	—	Group C	—
Group 3	Group IV	Group D	Group 3a
—	—	—	Group 3b
—	—	—	Group 3c
Group 4	Group V	Group E	—

Note: IARC=International Agency for Research on Cancer, (116). HWC=Health and Welfare Canada, (103). EPA=U.S. Environmental Protection Agency (250). IFSTP=International Federation of Societies of Toxicologic Pathologists, Faccini et al. (66). —, not applicable. Group 1=Group I=Group A=Group 1=The agent is carcinogenic to humans; there is sufficient evidence in man showing a positive relationship between cancer and human exposure; chance, bias, and confounding variables can be reasonably ruled out. Group 2A=Group II=Group B_1=Group 2a=The agent is probably carcinogenic to humans; there is limited evidence in man showing a positive relationship between cancer and human exposure; but chance, bias, and confounding variables cannot be ruled out; there is sufficient evidence of carcinogenicity in animals, i.e., the genotoxic agent is sufficiently in strong evidence of carcinogenicity in animals, i.e., the agent has caused benign and malignant neoplasms in two independent studies or there is a positive relation between cancer and animal exposure. Group 2B=Group III=Group B_2=Group 2b=The agent is possibly carcinogenic to humans; there is either limited evidence or absence of data in man; there is either sufficient or limited and weak evidence of carcinogenicity in animals, i.e. presence of other relevant data, genotoxic agents that cause only benign tumors or increases in certain spontaneous neoplasms; Group C=The agent is possibly carcinogenic to humans, there is either absence of data in man, or limited evidence of carcinogenicity in animals, i.e., agents that cause only benign tumors, or neoplasm incidence increases are marginal and not consistent; Group 3=Group IV=Group D=Group 3a=The agent is not classifiable as to its carcinogenicity in man; in Group V the data are inadequate for evaluation, or these agents cannot be classified in other groups; in IFSTP Group 3a, the experimental data of epigenetic carcinogens show threshold level within the range of human exposure. Group 3b=The experimental data of epigenetic carcinogens show threshold level beyond the range of human exposure. Group 3c=The experimental data of epigenetic carcinogens show that their mechanism of action is not applicable in humans. Group 4=Group IV=Group E=The agent is probably not carcinogenic to humans; there is evidence suggesting lack of carcinogenicity in man (even if it is inadequate) and animals (negative animals studies); in IFSTP Group 4, the suspected carcinogens have not been sufficiently tested.

a p value of <0.05 are appropriate levels of significance (Table 20.7) (96).

The interpretation of analyzed data is the final critical step of the whole process. Of importance here is the existence of extensive historical control data, both published and unpublished, for the specific species and strains used (97,99,147,189). The operational concepts here involve the biological and statistical data differences between control and exposed groups. Important here is the nature of these differences and the main reason for the differences. The final interpretation should be based on both biological and statistical consideration (66,265). If a statistical test falsely detects a significant neoplastic effect when none truly exists, a false positive outcome is the result. This constitutes a type 1 error. Conversely, if a statistical test fails to identify a true biological effect (e.g. a small increase in the incidence of a rare tumor), then a type 2 error has occurred. In both cases, by providing an explanation for the differences (causality) and demonstrating the proof for the underlying mechanism, both types of error are minimized. Statistical considerations are very important, but they should not be a substitute for sound biological judgement.

Finally, any statistical evaluation of RCB data should take into account the following eight factors: (a) exposure-effect relationship; (b) incidence of proliferation and preneoplastic and early neoplastic markers at the target site of neoplasia; (c) presence of gender and species similarities or differences at the target sites; (d) convergence in target sites of nonproliferative chronic toxicity and neoplasia; (e) combined neoplasia increases in tissues affected by chronic toxicity; (f) neoplasms of similar histogenetic target sites in other genders or species; (g) concurrent and historical control data, and (h) relative survival of control and exposed groups.

BIOASSAY REPORTING

The final critical step of the RCB is the study final report. The final report consists first of an introductory section containing the compliance statement signed by the study director, followed by the quality assurance and study identification statements. The study identification statement contains the study title and number, the test substance, the testing facility, the sponsor, the study director, and the principal investigator of all study aspects, the exact specific study timetable, and approved signatures from all final report authors. This should include the study director and the investigators of all aspects of the study (e.g., analytical, toxicokinetic, during-life, pathologist, etc.). The first part of the final report itself consists of the summary. This is an abstract of the entire study. It contains, in this order, an introduction, a listing of the materials and methods, the results, and the conclusions. The summary is followed by a summary table that depicts all pertinent findings in tabular form.

After the summary section, there is an extensive introduction into the origin and purpose of the RCB, followed by listings of test animals, test materials, methods, results, discussion, conclusions, and references. All sections should fully describe all methods used and all data obtained. All individual data should be in appropriate appendices (e.g., analytical, body weight, necropsy, and microscopic data). All relevant summary data should be in tables (e.g., analytical, body weight, etc.). Numerical incidences should precede percent incidences. Tables and graphs presenting special issues and arguments are recommended in the text (text tables or text graphs). Appropriate statistical analysis of correlation of survival patterns, clinical observations, body weight gain pattern, and toxicokinetic data with gross and microscopic findings should be conducted. All of these considerations have been discussed in other sections in detail.

An effective way of summarizing the findings is a format used in Europe known as the tabulated study report (TSR). All relevant data are presented in standardized tabular form without narrative. This corresponds to the tables of the final report described here.

CLASSIFICATION OF EVIDENCE OF CARCINOGENICITY

Completed RCBs must be reported to the regulatory agency under whose purview they were performed (33,48,63,255). The results are then subject to evaluation and classification.

In the United States, the results of RCBs on pharmaceuticals tested under Investigational New Drug applications (INDs) approved by FDA Center for Drug Evaluation and Research (CDER) are submitted to the Reviewing Division, which then evaluates them often through the CDER Carcinogenicity Assessment Committee (CAC). The final interpretation of the results will appear in the labeling of the medicine, if approved. The FDA normally describes the RCB data without comment on human relevance, except to note multiples of exposure in the rodents compared to humans. The CAC consists of a chair, an executive secretary, and members from several divisions: The Office of Epidemiology and Biostatistics, the Office of Testing and Research, and the Office of Pharmaceutical Sciences. The Reviewing Division (of the FDA) notifies the sponsor when a CAC meeting is scheduled after all RCB studies are submitted.

The U.S. Environmental Protection Agency (EPA) has been using an alphabetical/numerical classification ranging from group A, human carcinogen (based on animal data), to group E, noncarcinogen (192,255,258), but has proposed to convert to a narrative classification (257,258), which allows incorporation of mechanistic data, similar to the International Federation of Societies of Toxicologic Pathologists (IFSTP) classification, described later. At the U.S. EPA, an ad hoc CAC of the EPA Science Advisory Committee evaluates the submitted dossier.

RCBs conducted by the NTP are reviewed by a peer review panel and published as technical reports, which are submitted to the National Institute of Environmental Health Sciences (NIEHS) and subsequently to the U.S. EPA, FDA, and OSHA for regulatory action (255,256). The NTP uses a classification system of no, limited (some), or clear evidence of carcinogenicity (183). The NTP also publishes a biennial report on carcinogenesis, the most recent of which appeared in 2000 (249a).

In Europe and Japan, similar classification schemes are used by various health boards and the Commission for Proprietary Medicinal Product of the European Medicine Evaluation Agency (48,55,62,64).

The International Agency for Research on Cancer (IARC) convenes working groups several times each year to evaluate groups of chemicals with published carcinogenicity data. The findings are published as monographs with evaluations of the experimental and human data. The grouping ranges from group 1, carcinogenic to humans, to group 4, evidence suggesting lack of carcinogenicity.

The IFSTP (66) has proposed a classification as follows: 1, carcinogens for man based on epidemiological data; 2, genotoxic carcinogens for animals based on experimental data; 3, epigenetic carcinogens for animals based on experimental data; and 4, suspected carcinogens insufficiently tested. This is the only classification that explicitly incorporates mechanistic distinction.

Some of the classification schemes are depicted in Table 20.8. The IARC reviews are the most comprehensive, since they include all chemicals with published reports, and review all chemical and biologic data relevant to risk assessment.

CANCER HAZARD AND RISK ASSESSMENT

In cancer risk assessment, the first step is hazard identification, which involves the RCB to identify exposure-related tumors (see the section on rodent cancer bioassay evaluation). Using dose-response data from the bioassay and potential human exposure, a cancer risk is assessed (180), often involving allomorphic scaling (253). To identify a potential human cancer hazard, as for example following the IFSTP recommendations, the RCB results must be interpreted together with other mechanistic data. If the agent is clearly genotoxic, that implies a potential hazard (279), as discussed later in the section on types of cancer hazards. On the other hand, as discussed earlier, it is now recognized that epigenetic carcinogens may elicit their effects only in particular rodent species, as for $\alpha_{2\mu}$-globulin nephropathy inducers, or only at high toxic doses, as for nitrilotriacetic acid. Such effects are considered irrelevant to human hazard (252) or can be subjected to a margin-of-exposure (MOE) risk assessment (256,258).

The mechanism of carcinogenesis for epigenetic (nongenotoxic) agents is complex, involving a variety of secondary organ and tissue target sites, with indirect interference with the organ/tissue homeostasis. Disruption of endocrine, paracrine, nervous, and immune systems is often involved in the pathogenesis of neoplasia induced by such agents. Accordingly, the carcinogenetic effects of these agents are species, gender, and tissue specific.

Table 20.9
Examples of neoplastic effects in rodents with limited significance for human safety

Neoplastic effect	Pathogenesis (agents)
Renal tubular neoplasia in male rats	$\alpha_{2\mu}$-Globulin nephropathy/hydrocarbons (*d*-limonene, *p*-dichlorobenzene)
Hepatocellular neoplasia in rats and mice	Peroxisome proliferation (clofibrate, phthalate esters, phenoxy agents) Phenobarbitol-like promotion
Urinary-bladder neoplasia in rats	Crystalluria, carbonic anhydrase inhibition, urine pH extremes, melamine, saccharin, carbonic anhydrase inhibitors, dietary phosphates
Hepatocellular neoplasia in mice	Enzymatic–metabolic activation (in part unknown)/phenobarbital-like promotion
Thyroid follicular-cell neoplasia in rats	Hepatic enzyme induction, thyroid enzyme inhibition/oxazepam, amobarbital, sulphonamides, thioureas
Gastric neuroendocrine-cell neoplasia mainly in rats	Gastric secretory suppression, gastric atrophy induction (cimetidine, omeprazole, butachlor)
Adenohypophysis neoplasia in rats	Feedback interference/neuroleptics (dopamine inhibitors)
Mammary-gland neoplasia in female rats	Feedback interference/neuroleptics, antiemetics, antihypertensives (calcium channel blockers), serotonin agonists, anticholinergics, exogenous estrogens
Pancreatic islet-cell neoplasia in rats	Feedback interference/neuroleptics
Harderian-gland neoplasia in mice	Feedback interference/misoprostol (PGE_1), nalidixic acid, aniline dyes
Adrenal medullary neoplasia in rats	Feedback interference (lactose, sugar alcohols)
Forestomach neoplasia in rats and mice	Stimulation of proliferation/butylated hydroxyanisole, phthalate esters, proprionic acid
Lymphomas in mice	Immunosuppression/cyclosporin
Mononuclear-cell leukemia in rats (mainly F344)	Immunosuppression (in part unknown)/furan, iodinated glycerol
Splenic sarcomas in rats	Methemoglobinemia (in part unknown)/dapsone
Osteomas in mice	Feedback interference (calcineurin, in part unknown)/cyclosporin, misoprostol, proestrogens
Leydig-cell testicular neoplasia in rats	Feedback interference/lactose, sugar alcohols, H2 antagonists, carbamazepine, vidarabine, isradipine, dopaminergics, finasteride
Leydig-cell testicular neoplasia in mice	Feedback interference (proestrogens, finasteride, methoxychlor, cadmium)
Endometrial neoplasia in rats	Feedback interference (proestrogens, dopamine agonists)
Uterine leiomyoma in mice	Feedback interference (β_1-antagonists)
Mesovarial leiomyoma in rats (occasionally in mice)	Feedback interference (β_2-agonists)
Ovarian tubulostromal neoplasia in mice	Feedback interference (cytotoxic agents, nitrofurantoin)

Most of these secondary mechanisms involve interference with proliferation, disruption of hormonal feedback pathways, inhibition of the trophic activity in tissues including long-standing tissue ischemia, immune surveillance dysfunction, sustained exaggerated pharmacological effect, inhibition of enzymatic reaction/activation in cells, modulation of apoptosis, and sustained accumulation of normally low occurring level of endogenous products. All these effects result in sustained cellular toxicity, leading to compensatory proliferation, which is a common pathway through which agents with diverse cellular effects ultimately induce neoplasia (31,38,112). The effects that lead to compensatory cellular proliferation usually require high levels of exposure and exhibit thresholds. It is perhaps for this reason that of the NCI/NTP rodent carcinogens tested, 6% had increased tumor rates that were limited to the top dose for all sites of carcinogenicity (100). Examples of neoplastic effects with limited significance for human hazard are given in Table 20.9, and some mechanisms and tumor findings are described in more detail next.

Mechanisms Not Indicative of Cancer Hazard to Humans

For several neoplastic responses in rodents, sufficient mechanistic information has accrued to support the general conclusion that the underlying mechanisms for agents that are not DNA reactive in the target tissue are species specific and do not operate in humans.

Rat Kidney $\alpha_{2\mu}$-Globulin Nephropathy-Mediated Increases in Kidney Neoplasms

Various xenobiotics induce kidney tumors in male rats, mainly F344, which excrete $\alpha_{2\mu}$-globulin in the urine. This protein is associated with hyaline droplet formation, atypical hyperplasia of the epithelium of the P_2 segment of the proximal tubules and neoplasia. Male rats (especially F344) are very proteinuric compared to humans, and no human renal protein is similar to $\alpha_{2\mu}$-globulin (252). Accordingly, the U.S. EPA (252) concluded that renal tubule tumors produced as a result of the $\alpha_{2\mu}$-globulin accumulation mechanism are not an appropriate endpoint for human hazard identification. Likewise, an IARC working group concluded that an agent that acts solely through $\alpha_{2\mu}$-globulin nephropathy in the production of renal cell tumors alone in male rats is not a cancer hazard to humans (204).

Rat Stomach Acid Secretion Suppression-Mediated Neuroendocrine Neoplasm (Carcinoid)

Hyperplasia and neoplasia of gastric neuroendocrine cells (enterochromaffin-like cells) are stimulated by gastrin in rats and to a lesser degree in mice. Elevations of gastrin are elicited by reduced hydrochloric acid production, which can be caused either by gastric antisecretory medicines such as proton pump inhibitors (lansoprazole, omeprazole, pantoprazole) or H_2 antagonists (loxtidine or cimetidine) (18,170). Agents that cause gastric atrophy—for example, alachlor and butachlor—have also elicited this neoplasm (235). Rats have a high density of gastric neuroendocrine cells (NE), achieve high levels of gastrin (over 1000 pg/ml), and are very responsive to elevation of gastrin (241). With most of the agents, female rats are more susceptible than males.

NE cell tumors have been observed in patients with multiple endocrine neoplasia syndrome (MEN-1), associated with elevated gastrin, but not with antiulcer therapy (170). Significant NE cell proliferation in humans is seen only with gastrin levels above 400 pg/ml, and this can be controlled.

Rat Urinary Bladder Luminal-Milieu-Modification-Based Increases in Transitional Cell-Neoplasms

Many studies have used rat models for urothelial neoplasia. Rats have been shown to be more sensitive than mice to urothelial damages, apparently because the rat bladder lacks tight junctions, rendering the superficial urothelial layer ineffective as an intraluminal barrier, leaving the underlying layers vulnerable to chronic stimulation (110,144). Moreover, rats have more intraluminal proteins, silicate precipitation, crystal formation, and urolithiasis than humans. In particular, rats, unlike humans, develop calcium phosphate urinary precipitates (204). Thus rats are more prone to chronic cell damage to the bladder urothelium, which results in cell proliferation and neoplasia (31). This effect does not occur in humans (31,57,291). An IARC working group has concluded that production of bladder cancer in rats under conditions of formation of calcium phosphate-containing urinary precipitates is not predictive of cancer hazard to humans (204).

Rodent Liver Peroxisome Proliferator-Mediated Increases in Liver Neoplasms

Widely varied xenobiotics elicit increases in rodent liver tumors associated with increased numbers of peroxisomes (120). Rodents are more susceptible to induction of hepatic peroxisome proliferation than primates or humans (120,290), apparently because of high expression of the peroxisome proliferator activated receptor of the class ($PPAR_{\alpha}$) in rodent liver (242). Perhaps related to this, it has been reported that in rat hepatocytes, peroxisome proliferators enhance DNA synthesis and suppress apoptosis, whereas in human hepatocytes, DNA synthesis was suppressed and apoptosis enhanced (194). While the mechanisms of carcinogenicity of these agents is not fully understood, none is associated with cancer in humans, and an IARC group has recommended that a tumor response in mice or rats secondary only to peroxisome proliferation could modify the evaluation of carcinogenicity (120).

Rodent Thyroid–Pituitary Disruption-Mediated Thyroid Tumor

Few DNA-reactive carcinogens elicit thyroid tumors, probably because bioactivation is minimal in this gland. On the other hand, thyroid–pituitary disruption is a common mechanism of thyroid carcinogenesis in rodents, particularly rats (236). Reduced thyroid hormone levels, through either inhibition of synthesis by antithyroid agents (e.g., amitrole) or increased clearance as a result of enhanced conjugation (e.g., phenobarbital), can lead to feedback increase of thyroid stimulating hormone levels, which produce thyroid follicular-cell hypertrophy, hyperplasia, and eventually neoplasia. Species differ in their susceptibility to this disruption, with the rat being particularly sensitive (59). Several inducers of liver thyroid hormone conjugation (which often is associated with increased liver tumors) in rats do not affect mice (270). No nonradioactive chemical exposure is known to cause thyroid follicular neoplasms in humans (204). Accordingly, it has been concluded that chemical-specific data on thyroid effects in rodents can be applied to risk assessment (105), and that agents that cause thyroid neoplasia through an adaptive hormonal mechanism belong to a different category from those acting through genotoxic effects or involving pathological response to tissue injury (204).

Mechanisms Probably Not Indicative of Cancer Hazard to Humans

Several mechanisms of epigenetic tumorigenesis in rodents appear not to be relevant to human cancer hazard (6).

Rat Testes Hormone Disruption-Mediated Leydig-Cell Neoplasms

Leydig- or interstitial-cell neoplasms occur spontaneously in high incidence (>80%) in aged F344 rats

(102). These tumors are invariably benign. The human counterpart is extremely rare, and no agent that produces increases in rat testicular tumors (i.e., cimetidine, hydralazine, gemfibrozil, carbamazepine, vidarabine, isradipine, exogenous gonadotropins, luteinizing-hormone releasing hormone [LHRH] analogs, flutamide, ergolines, and finasteride) has been associated with induction of this or any other neoplasm in humans. Therefore, the data suggest that nongenotoxic compounds that induce Leydig-cell neoplasms in rats do not indicate a human cancer hazard (36).

Rodent Hormone Disruption-Mediated Mammary and Adenohypophysis Neoplasia

The occurrence of mammary neoplasms and prolactinomas in female rats (mainly) and mice after exposure to neuroleptics, antiemetics, antihypertensives, calcium channel blockers, serotonin agonists, exogenous estrogens, or anticholinergics is species specific (185,217,277,289). The triggering mechanism for this consists of sustained prolactin (PRL) elevation. PRL is controlled by dopamine. In contrast to its action in humans, PRL is luteotrophic in rats and mice, leading to progesterone elevation and sustained stimulation of proliferation of mammary epithelium (209). These neoplasms are accompanied by an increase in serum PRL, contrary to mammary neoplasia in humans (208,220).

Tumors of Questionable Significance to Human Cancer Hazard

Tumors of questionable significance for hazard assessment (6) are those whose pathogenesis may be unique to rodents, in some cases due to their cell type of origin, and for which no association with human cancer hazard has been established. If one of these is the only tumor increased in the RCB, such a finding should not be taken as evidence of human cancer hazard.

Mouse Bladder "Mesenchymal Lesion"

This lesion occurs in the trigone area of the bladder and has been known under various names for sometime (133). Recently the lesion was called "mesenchymal tumor" (20,92). The lesion has been found in mice given agents that bind to progesterone receptors (165). Persuasive evidence has been provided (133,134) that the lesion represents a decidual reaction of mesenchymal cells carrying or developing progesterone receptors. No known counterpart of this lesion has ever been described in humans, and therefore its significance is questionable.

Mouse Histiocytic Sarcoma

This neoplasm of histiocytes affects mainly the liver and uterus in mice. A comparable lesion has not been reported in humans and no agent established to produce an increase in only this neoplasm is associated with cancer development in humans (244).

Mouse Ovary Tubular Adenoma

This is a benign neoplasm with tubular, stromal, or mixed components, and occurs mainly in mice (5,24). Tubulostromal adenomas have been observed with cytotoxic agents but are not seen in other laboratory animals or humans and are considered irrelevant for human safety assessment (5,24).

Rat Granular-Cell Tumor

A proliferative lesion of "granular" cells with granular eosinophilic cytoplasms occurs in the vaginal–cervical regions of female Sprague-Dawley, Donryu, and Wistar rats (39,218). This lesion is probably under hormonal influence, mainly estrogen. Granular cell aggregates occur rarely in the vulva of women, but there is no evidence to suggest that the pathogenesis is similar to that of rat granular-cell tumors. Thus, this lesion is considered probably not relevant for humans.

Rat Mammary-Gland Fibroadenoma

This is a benign neoplasm with a minor glandular epithelial component and a predominant pericanalicular type of proliferation of connective tissue. It bears no resemblance to the common intracanalicular type of fibroadenoma seen in women (208,209), which is hormonally responsive (10). Fibroadenoma is the most common breast neoplasm in all the major rat strains and does not progress to malignancy. Thus, combining fibroadenomas and carcinomas is inappropriate and the tumor by itself is of questionable significance.

Rat Mesovarial Leiomyoma

Smooth-muscle tumors of the ovarian suspensory ligament have developed in female rats after long exposures to beta$_2$-adrenoceptor stimulant medicines (138). This neoplasm is rare in humans, and the agents that have induced it in rats (i.e., soterenol, mesuprine, zinterol, terbutaline, reproterol, salbutamol) are not associated with cancer in humans.

Rat Mononuclear-Cell Leukemia

This neoplasm occurs in high incidence (about 60% in males and 40% in females) in F344 rats (102). Mononuclear-cell leukemia (MCL), also referred to as large granular lymphocyte leukemia (LGL), is a spontaneously occurring lethal neoplasm that first develops in the spleen and then in the liver, lungs, lymph nodes, and bone marrow. It occurs at over 18 months of age. No agent has been demonstrated to reproducibly induce this neoplasm and hence nothing is known about its pathogenesis. MCL is induced by DNA-reactive agents such as elthylene oxide. In addition, a number of chemicals that are not implicated in human cancer (furan, C.I. direct blue 15, iodinated glycerol, diisononyl phthalate, and dimethylmorpholinophosphoramidate) are known to be associated with increased incidences (58,155).

Rodent Forestomach Squamous-Cell Carcinoma

A number of DNA-reactive agents have induced neoplasms of the forestomach in rodents (146), usually through a direct effect. The rodent forestomach is a portion of the stomach between the esophagus and glandular stomach, lined by squamous epithelium, and does not exist in humans. Nongenotoxic agents such as butylated hydroxyanisole, propionic acid, and HMG CoA-reductase inhibitors have produced increases in this neoplasm. The epigenetic mechanism appears to involve chronic irritation leading to a promoting action, which requires high exposure, as shown for butylated hydroxyanisole (291,293). None of these epigenetic agents has been associated with cancer in humans.

Rat Scrotal Tunica Vaginalis Mesothelioma

This mesenchymal lesion, which includes hyperplasia and neoplasia (166), arises from the serous membranes of the scrotal tunica vaginalis testes. It is common (about 3%) in F344 rats, (102). Since the scrotal lesion often arises in association with testicular tumors, especially Leydig-cell tumors, which assume large size, there may be an element of physical initiation involved in the pathogenesis. Chemicals that produce increases in this tumor (e.g., acrylamide, potassium bromate, pentachlorophenol) are chemically diverse and no mode of action has been established. None of these is associated with mesothelioma in humans or with any other cancer.

Types of Cancer Hazards

Formerly, all rodent carcinogens were considered to be potential human cancer hazards. This concept was embodied in the Delaney clause to the 1958 Federal Food, Drug, and Cosmetic Act, section 409(3)(A), which provided that no chemical determined to be carcinogenic in either humans or animals could be allowed as a food or color additive, regardless of concentration. Likewise, the U.S. EPA cancer principles of 1970 stated that no level of exposure to a chemical carcinogen should be considered toxicologically insignificant for humans. Subsequently, expanded understanding of mechanisms of carcinogenesis has led to refinements of hazard assessment. Notably, in Europe, governmental agencies have not been required by legislatures to impose standards of no exposure for carcinogenic agents and have used more flexible approaches than those imposed in the United States (278). Beginning in 1992, the IARC accepted data on mechanisms as being relevant to evaluation of the carcinogenic risk of an agent to humans (118), and this is being elaborated upon (204). Recently, the distinction between DNA-reactive and epigenetic carcinogens has been explored in detail by an international group of experts, drawing on comprehensive reviews of mechanisms of 10 prototype carcinogens (126).

Currently, in assessing potential human cancer hazard, regulatory agencies often refer to findings implicating an agent as a "genotoxic carcinogen" usually with only an operational definition (32) that the chemical produced positive results in genotoxicity tests. All chemicals that are reliably positive in a variety of tests are in fact DNA reactive and thus belong to that category of carcinogen, as discussed in the section on types of carcinogens. Most chemicals, however, are positive in some tests, like phenobarbital and DES (116,123), sometimes because of intrinsic spurious positive results (19), and thus the issue becomes the question of which tests are to be accepted as evidence of genotoxicity. A scientifically sound approach is to define genotoxicity as a mechanism of carcinogenesis; that is, a genotoxic carcinogen is one that forms molecular lesions (such as DNA adducts) that lead to mutations or one that produces mutations in the cells that are the precursors of tumors induced by the agent. Under this definition, genotoxic carcinogens would likely be confined to DNA-reactive agents fulfilling the criterion for carcinogenic activity of an agent that induces malignant tumors not seen in controls. Such chemicals are generally multispecies carcinogens, which induce tumors in high yield with short latent periods and often in several organs. For agents of this type, assumption of human hazard is well founded (279), although evidence is accruing that even DNA-reactive carcinogens have thresholds (294). Moreover, some of the underlying mechanisms of these agents are species specific and do not operate in humans because of functional or toxicokinetic differences. Epigenetic carcinogens, in contrast, are generally not relevant to human hazard, as evidenced by the few associated with human cancer (Table 20.3), in spite of the large number to which humans are regularly exposed (87,122). The lack of relevance stems from the fact that their effects are either rodent specific or require high and long-duration exposure in rodents in order to elicit the cellular effect leading to carcinogenicity. Epigenetic mechanisms that are either not indicative of a cancer hazard to humans or probably not indicative have been discussed already. These should be taken into account in formulating any risk assessment.

Cancer Risk Assessment

It is becoming increasingly accepted that for epigenetic agents, even if some cancer hazard is presumed, a safety margin can be established. For plasma concentration versus time pharmaceuticals, this has been referred to as the safety factor, which is the ratio of the area under the concentration vs. time curve (AUC) in rodents for the highest noncarcinogenic dose (nontumorigenic effect level, i.e., NTEL) to the human AUC at the therapeutic dose (12,32). In 1996, the Federal Food, Drug, and Cosmetic Act was amended by removing the zero-risk provision of the Delaney clause and replacing it with a new standard of "a reasonable certainty of no harm" (33). The new standard applies to pesticide residues in both raw and processed foods, allowing the presence of some residues that have been shown to cause cancer in animals (246,247). In the new U.S. EPA draft cancer assessment guidelines, the safety margin is referred to as margin of exposure (MOE) (192). The FDA Center for Food Safety and Nutrition has published a "threshold of regulation" procedure for indirect food additives (263,264). In an analysis of human risk for carcinogenic veterinary drugs present as tissue residues, Galer and Monro (81) argue that human intake of up to 100 μg/person/day presents no cancer risk, similar to the assessments of Williams (282) and Munro et al. (174). In a further refinement, Williams (285) proposed a carcinogen safe exposure level (SEL) as the no-effect level for the molecular/cellular effect that is the basis for carcinogenicity divided by a safety margin, similar to uncertainty factors. This is actually more conservative than using the NTEL, since the NEL for molecular effects is lower.

For genotoxic or DNA-reactive agents, authorities regulate such agents either by prohibiting human exposure or using a linear no-threshold model for quantitative risk assessment (250,255,295). In the European Union, it is proposed to incorporate potency considerations, including T25 values, and to classify all carcinogens in three potency groups (55). However, evidence is accruing that even DNA-reactive carcinogens have thresholds (294), and accordingly, the SEL concept just described can also be applied to DNA-reactive carcinogens using a NEL for DNA binding (285).

INTERACTIVE CARCINOGENESIS

Interactive carcinogenesis comprises the enhancement or inhibition of carcinogenesis by combined, concurrent, or sequential exposures to more than one carcinogen or a carcinogen and noncarcinogen (281). Various types of interaction between chemicals have been described, including syncarcinogenesis, tumor promotion, cocarcinogenesis, and anticarcinogenesis. In the testing of complex mixtures, these types of interactions can influence the outcome (Figure 20.4).

Syncarcinogenesis

Syncarcinogenesis is the enhancement of carcinogenesis produced by concurrent or sequential administration of two carcinogens, usually of the DNA-reactive type. This interaction in the case of DNA-reactive carcinogens represents a summation of the genetic effects of the agents. Usually the enhancement occurs in a target organ where both carcinogens produce a tumor effect.

Promotion

Tumor promotion is the enhancement of tumor development by a second agent given after an initiating carcinogen (11), when a sufficient interval has been allowed for acute molecular effects, such as DNA adducts, to be processed. If the second agent is administered when molecular lesions are still present, the enhancement may be due to cocarcinogenesis (discussed next). Promoting agents essentially facilitate clonal expansion of initiated cells and their evolution into neoplasms. The selective growth of preneoplastic populations can be achieved either by an enhanced rate of cell proliferation in the tissue or a decreased rate of apoptosis in incipient neoplasms.

Promoting agents are usually assumed to be noncarcinogens, but in fact, most are weak carcinogens under some circumstance, probably because they facilitate tumor development from cryptogenically initiated cells that are the source of spontaneous tumors. Thus, most, if not all, promoters are epigenetic carcinogens (Table 20.2). An essential characteristic of a promoting agent is that it is not DNA reactive and is not an initiating agent; otherwise, the enhancement is likely to be due to syncarcinogenesis.

Cocarcinogenesis

Cocarcinogenesis is the enhancement by a noncarcinogen of the carcinogenicity of a carcinogen when administered prior to or concurrently with the carcinogen or when given shortly after a carcinogen at a time when molecular damage is still present. Cocarcinogens may enhance the uptake of the carcinogen, enhance its tissue localization, increase the proportion that is bioactivated, or enhance the induced neoplastic transformation, usually by transiently increasing cell proliferation. Cocarcinogens do not act as pro-

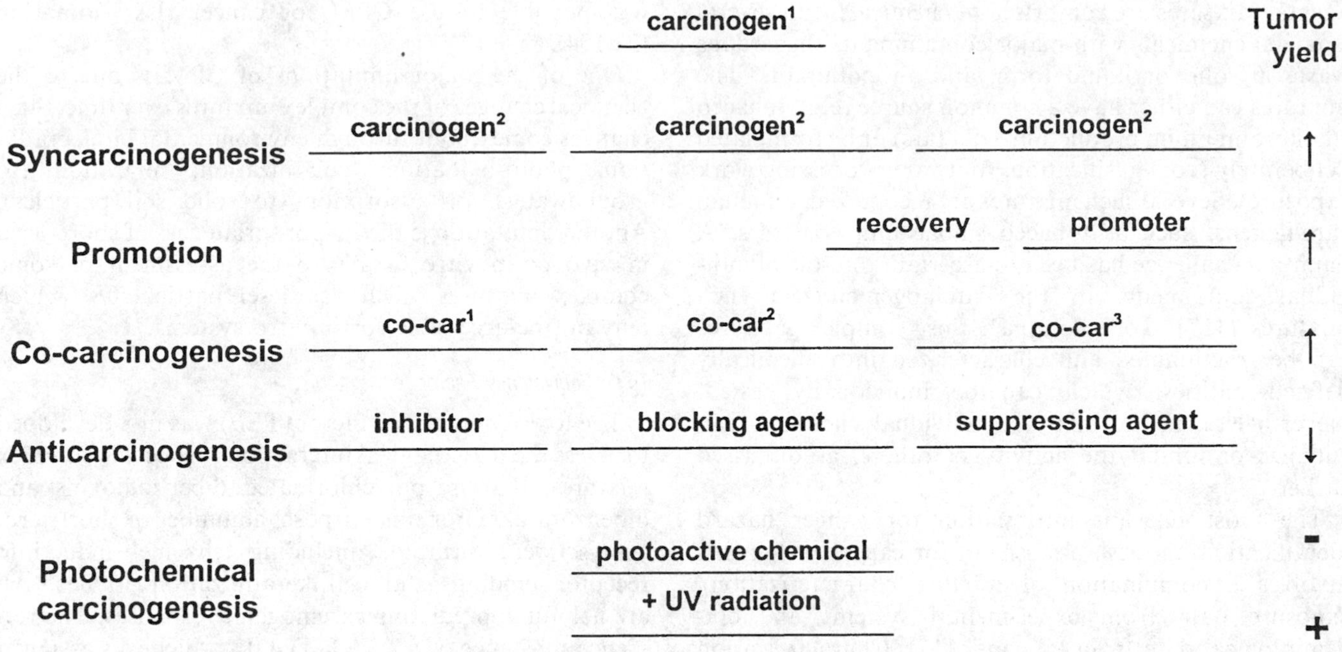

FIG. 20.4. Types of interactive carcinogenesis.

moters, although most promoters have cocarcinogenic activity, often due to enhancement of cell proliferation.

Anticarcinogenesis

Anticarcinogenesis is the reduction of the carcinogenicity of an agent by a previously, concurrently, or subsequently administered agent, usually a noncarcinogen, although certain epigenetic carcinogens, such as phenobarbital, are effective anticarcinogens. Three operational pathways are recognized as follows: inhibitors that prevent formation of carcinogens, blocking agents that counteract effects of carcinogens, and suppressing agents that suppress tumor development (272).

Photochemical Carcinogenesis

A specific type of interactive carcinogenesis is photochemical carcinogenesis, which is the combined skin carcinogenicity of a chemical and ultraviolet light (75,129). Photochemical carcinogenicity can result from several types of interaction between the chemical, ultravioltet radiation (UVR), and the skin. Some chemicals, such as psoralens, can be photoactivated to DNA-reactive chemical species. Others, such as fluoroquinolones, can undergo photoactivation to generate secondary reactive molecular species such as reactive oxygen (230a). Also, some chemicals can affect the structure of skin, for example, thinning of the epidermis in the case of retinoids, to sensitize the skin to effects of UVR radiation. Finally, immunosuppression can enhance skin carcinogenesis (145).

Photochemical carcinogenicity studies are often required for topically applied medicines and even for some oral medicines, as well as for topically applied cosmetics and consumer products. The test species is usually the SKH1 albino hairless mouse, which has the advantage that it does not require hair clipping and allows easy detection of UVR-induced squamous-cell papillomas and carcinomas. In a typical protocol (49,74,213), the test substance is applied before UVR (at 290–400 nm by a UV solar simulator) on Monday, Wednesday, and Friday and after UVR on Tuesday and Thursday for 40 weeks, followed by a 12-week observation period without exposure. This pattern of exposure allows detection of photoactivated chemicals, as well as those that may modulate photocarcinogenesis. Typically, separate groups are administered low and high UVR in addition to the TS. The endpoints of evaluation include tumor incidence (prevalence), multiplicity (yield), and latency (time to tumor).

Complex Mixtures

Most chemical exposures involve mixtures rather than single agents. Yet the scientific data for these mixtures are generated almost entirely from studies of individual agents. Mixtures are comprised of chemicals with several isomers, chemicals with major contaminants, hazardous waste in solid or liquid form, and air pollutants. The mixtures can either have a common source (e.g., tobacco smoke, aluminum production, coal tars) or be formulated deliberately (coal gasification, footware processing work exposure). Several such mixtures are recognized as human carcinogens, such as tobacco smoke and coal tars. A daunting challenge has been to ascertain the role of individual components in the carcinogenicity of such mixtures (117). To accomplish this, complex mixtures can be fractionated and characterized into chemically defined entities, which can be individually tested. Nevertheless, in the mixture, individual chemicals can enhance or inhibit the activity of others, as discussed earlier.

The most relevant information for cancer hazard identification and risk assessment for cancer of humans involves a combination of mixture characterization/exposure data from experimental systems and epidemiological data from humans (117). Characterization and definition of exposure, identification of the source, and distribution and occurrence of the mixture, as well as its composition and physicochemical properties, are essential. Here the most common method of fractionation is the one that partitions complex mixtures into organic and inorganic constituents. This is followed until active agents are separated from inactive ones. Chemical characterization of all biologically active ingredients is pursued. Important in experimental systems is the identification of in vitro/in vivo effects and rodent carcinogenicity data. In addition, definitions of dosimetry, toxicokinetics, bioavailability, disposition, and molecular and biochemical effects are also needed. The comparative potency method (CPM) is one that is based on data correlation from all in vitro and in vivo experimental assays, with human potency estimates (2,22). What is being compared is a known human risk complex mixture with a CPM from a similar complex with incomplete data (154). CPM for cancer risk estimation is not validated yet, and consequently its utility is still limited.

Comparative Potency Method

The comparative potency method (CPM) has been applied to estimate human lung cancer risk from coke oven emissions, roofing tar, and cigarette smoke condensate, all combustion products of complex mixtures. Each of these complex mixtures was compared using standard protocols, which included an in vivo mouse skin initiation/promotion study, and two in vitro studies, such as mouse lymphoma and *Salmonella typhimurium* (Ames) mutagenicity assays. The result of the three mixtures showed agreement among assays (Ames activity was highest with cigarette smoke condensate), and thus it was possible to use CPM for cancer risk estimation (22,154).

One of the major limitations of CPM is due to the chemical changes of the complex mixtures over time. Such changes come about through environmental biodegradation, photo-oxidation, volatilization, migration (to groundwater), or adsorption (to solid soil particles). Another limitation is the inappropriateness of short-term in vivo or in vitro assays to the assessment of some complex mixtures, such as diesel particulates, which may not be accessible for in vitro systems.

Toxic Equivalency Factor

The toxic equivalency factor (TEF) was first developed to assess the toxicological interactions of specific complex mixtures, that is, polychlorinated dibenzodioxins and dibenzofurans. For this purpose, a number of short-term assays were utilized, including enzyme induction, receptor binding, and cell keratinization studies. All are helpful in predicting carcinogenic responses. The reference substance was 2,3,7,8-TCDD, which was assigned the value of 1 (22).

Based on this, the TEF was determined by multiplying the substance concentration with the relative toxicity from the short-term assays for each mixture ingredient—that is, the product is the TEF. The TEF is very helpful with chemically related compounds in a mixture. The process has been applied to polycyclic aromatic hydrocarbons and polychlorinated biphenyls. However, results of several studies have also shown that for specific responses, the TEFs for some halogenated aromatic hydrocarbon mixtures are nonadditive (211).

ACKNOWLEDGMENTS

We thank Barbara Iatropoulos and Katey Bateman for preparation of the text. Also, we gratefully acknowledge the thoughtful comments by many colleagues in the chemical and pharmaceutical industries. The preparation of this chapter was made possible by support provided to the Medicine, Food, and Chemical Safety Program at New York Medical College.

QUESTIONS

1. What are the pertinent mechanisms of carcinogenesis operational in rodents and man?
2. What are the mechanisms of carcinogenesis operational only for rodents? Explain why.
3. Which neoplasms are of questionable significance to human cancer hazard? Explain why.
4. What are the types of cancer hazard?
5. What constitutes adequate exposure in a rodent cancer bioassay?

REFERENCES

1. Abdo, K. M., and Kari, F. W. (1996): The sensitivity of the NTP bioassay for carcinogen hazard evaluation can be modulated by dietary restriction. *Exp. Toxicol. Pathol.*, 48:129–137.
2. Albert, R. E. (1985): The comparative potency method: An approach to quantitative cancer risk asessment. In: *Methods for Estimating Risk of Chemical Injury: Humans and Non-Human Biota and Ecosystems*, edited by V. B. Vonk, G. C. Butler, D. G. Hoel, and D. B. Peakall, pp. 281–287. John Wiley and Sons, New York.
3. Allaben, W. T., Turturro, A., Leakey, J. E. A., Seng, J. E., and Hart, R. W. (1996): FDA Points-to-consider documents: The need for dietary control for the reduction of experimental variability within animal assays and the use of dietary restriction to achieve dietary control. *Toxicol. Pathol.*, 24:776–781.
4. Alexandrov, V. A., Popovich, I. G., Anisimov, V. N., and Napalkov, N. P. (1989): Influence of hormonal disturbances on transplacental and multigeneration carcinogenesis in rats. In: *Perinatal and Multigeneration Carcinogenesis*, edited by N. P. Napalkov, J. M. Rice, L. Tomatis and H. Yamasaki, pp. 35–49. IARC Science Publ. No. 96, Lyon, France.
5. Alison, R. H., and Morgan, K. T. (1987): Ovarian neoplasms in F344 rats and B6C3F$_1$ mice. *Environ. Health Perspect.*, 73:91–106.
6. Alison, R. H., Capen, C. C., and Prentice, D. E. (1994): Neoplastic lesions of questionable significance to humans. *Toxicol. Pathol.*, 22:179–186.
7. Apostolou, A. (1990). Relevance of maximum tolerated dose to human carcinogenic risk. *Regul. Toxicol. Pharmacol.*, 11:68–80.
8. Ashby, J., and Tennant, R. W. (1991): Definitive relationships among chemical structure, carcinogenicity and mutagenicity for 301 chemicals tested by the U.S. NTP. *Mutat. Res.*, 257:229–306.
9. Ballard, B. E. (1968): Biopharmaceutical consideration in subcutaneous and intramuscular drug administration. *J. Pharm. Sci.*, 57:357–378.
10. Bartow, S. A. (1994): The breast. In: *Pathology*, edited by E. Rubin and J. L. Farber, pp. 73–992, J.B. Lippincott, Philadelphia.
11. Berenblum, I. (1974): *Frontiers of Biology: Carcinogenesis as a Biological Problem*, edited by A. Neuberger and E. L. Tatum. North Holland, Amsterdam.
12. Bergman, K., Olofsson, I.-M., and Sjoeberg, P. (1998): Dose selection for carcinogenicity studies of pharmaceuticals: Systemic exposure to phenacetin at carcinogenic dosage in the rat. *Regul. Toxicol. Pharmacol.*, 28:226–229.
13. Bischoff, K. B. (1975): Some fundamental considerations of the applications of pharmacokinetics to cancer chemotherapy. *Cancer Chemother. Rep.*, 59:777–793.
14. Bomhard, E., and Rinke, M. (1994). Frequency of spontaneous tumours in Wistar rats in 2-year studies. *Exp. Toxicol. Pathol.*, 46:17–29.
15. Boorman, G. A., Montgomery, C. A., Jr., Eustes, S. L., Wolfe, M. J. McConnell, E. E., and Hardesty, J. F. (1985): Quality Assurance in pathology for rodent carcinogenicity studies. In: *Handbook of Carcinogen Testing*, edited by H. Milman and E. Weisburger, pp. 345–357. Noyes, Park Ridge, NJ.
16. Boorman, G. A., Maronpot, R. R., and Eustis, S. L. (1994): Rodent carcinogenicity bioassay: Past, present and future. *Toxicol. Pathol.*, 22:105–111.
17. Borowitz, J. L., Moore, P. F., Yim, G. K. W., and Miya, T. S. (1971): Mechanism of enhanced drug effects produced by dilution of the oral dose. *Toxicol. Appl. Pharmacol.*, 19:164–168.
18. Brunner, G. H. G., Lamberts, R., and Creutzfeldt, W. (1990): Efficacy and safety of omeprazole in the long-term treatment of peptic ulcer and reflux oesophagitis resistant to ranitidine. *Digestion*, 47:64–68.
19. Brusick, D., Albertini, R., McRee, D., Peterson, D., Williams, G., Hanawalt, P., and Preston, J. (1998): Genotoxicity of radio frequency radiation. *Environ. Mol. Mutagen.*, 32:1–16.
20. Butler, W. H., Cohen, S. H., and Squire, R. A. (1997): Mesenchymal tumors of the mouse urinary bladder with vascular and smooth muscle differentiation. *Toxicol. Pathol.*, 25:268–274.
21. Butterworth, B. E., Ashby, J., Bermudez, E., Casciano, D., Mirsalis, J., Probst, G., and Williams, G. (1987): A protocol and guide for the in vivo rat hepatocyte DNA repair assay. *Mutat. Res.*, 189:123–133.
22. Calabrese, E. J. (1991): *Multiple Chemical Interactions*. Lewis, Chelsea, MI.
23. Caldwell, J., Gardner, I., and Swales, N. (1995): An introduction to drug disposition: The basic principles of absorption, distribution, metabolism and excretion. *Toxicol. Pathol.*, 23:148–157.
24. Capen, C. C., Beamer, W. G., Tennent, B. J., and Stitzel, K. A. (1995): Mechanisms of hormone-mediated carcinogenesis of the ovary in mice. *Mutat. Res.*, 333:143–151.
25. Cayen, M. N. (1995): Considerations in the design of toxicokinetic programs. *Toxicol. Pathol.*, 23:148–157.
26. Cayen, M. N., and Black, H. E. (1993): Role of toxikokinetics in dose selection for carcinogenicity studies. In: *Drug Toxicokinetics*, edited by P. G. Welling and F. A. de la Iglesia, pp. 69–83. Marcel Dekker, New York.
27. Chappell, W. R., and Mordenti, J. (1991): Extrapolation of toxicological and pharmacological data from animals to humans. *Adv. Drug Res.*, 20:2–116.
28. Chengelis, C. P., Gad, S. C., and Holston, J. (1995): *Regul. Toxicol.* Raven Press, New York.
29. Christian, M. S., Hoberman, A. M., Johnson, M. D., Brown, W. R., and Bucci, T. J. (1998): Effect of dietary optimization on growth, survival, tumor incidences and clinical pathology parameters in CD Sprague-Dawley and Fischer-344 rats: A 104-week study. *Drug Chem. Toxicol.*, 21:97–117.
30. Clayson, D. B., and Kitchin, K. T. (1999): Interspecies differences in response to chemical carcinogens. In: *Carcinogenicity*, edited by K. T. Kitchin, pp. 837–880. Marcel Dekker, New York.
31. Cohen, S. M., and Ellwein, L. B. (1991): Genetic errors, cell proliferation, and carcinogenesis. *Cancer Res.*, 51:6493–6505.
32. Contrera, J. F., Jacobs, A. C., Prasanna, H. R., Mehta, M., Schmidt, W. J., and DeGeorge, J. J. (1995): A systemic exposure-based alternative to the maximum tolerated dose for carcinogenicity studies of human therapeutics. *J. Am. Coll. Toxicol.*, 14:1–10.
33. Contrera, J. F., Jacobs, A. C., DeGeorge, J. J., Chen, C., Choudary, J., DeFelice, A., Fairweather, W., Farrelly, J. Fitzgerald, G., Goheer, A., Jordan, A., Lin, D., Lin, K., Kelly, R., Meyers, L., Osterberg, R., Prasanna, H. R., Resnick, C., Sheevers, H., and Sun, J. (1996): Carcinogenicity testing and the evaluation of regulatory requirements for pharmaceuticals. *Fed. Reg.*, U.S. Department of Health and Human Services, Public Health Service, Docket No. 96D-0235.
34. Contrera, J. F., Jacobs, A. C., and DeGeorge, J. J. (1997): Carcinogenicity testing and the evaluation of regulatory requirements for pharmaceuticals. *Regul. Toxicol. Pharmacol.*, 25:130–145.
35. Contrera, J. F., and DeGeorge, J. J. (1998): In vivo transgenic bioassays and assessment of the carcinogenic potential of pharmaceuticals. *Environ. Health Perspect.*, 106(suppl. 1):71–80.
36. Cook, J. C., Klinefelter, G. R., Hardisty, J. F., Sharpe, R. M., and Foster, P. M. D. (1999): Rodent Leydig cell tumorigenesis: A review of the physiology, pathology, mechanisms, and relevance to humans. *Crit. Rev. Toxicol.*, 29:169–261.
37. Cottrell, S., Andrews, C. M., Clayton, D., and Powell, C. J. (1994): The dose-dependent effect of BHT (butylated hydroxytoluene) on

vitamin K-dependent blood coagulation in rats. *Food Chem. Toxicol.*, 32(7):589–594.

38. Counts, J. L., and Goodman, J. I. (1995): Principles underlying dose selection for, and extrapolation from, the carcinogen bioassay: Dose influences mechanism. *Regul. Toxicol. Pharmacol.*, 21:418–421.
39. Courtney, C. L., Hawkins, K. L., Meierhenry, E. F., and Graziano, M. J. (1992): Immunohistochemical and ultrastructural characterization of granular cell tumors of the female reproductive tract in two aged Wistar rats. *Vet. Pathol.*, 29:86–89.
40. Cox, D. R. (1972): Regression models and life tables. *J. R. Stat. Soc.*, 13:187–220.
41. Cutler, S. J., and Ederer, F. (1958): Maximum utilization of life table method in analyzing survival. *J. Chron. Dis.*, 8:699–712.
42. Dahlem, A. M., Allerheiligen, S. R., and Vodicnik, N. J. (1995): Concomitant toxicokinetics: Techniques for interpretation of exposure data obtained during the conduct of toxicology studies. *Toxicol. Pathol.*, 23:170–178.
43. D'Arcy, P. F., and Harron, D. W. G. (1992): *Proceedings of the First International Conference of Harmonization*. Brussels, Belgium, 1991.
44. D'Arcy, P. F., and Harron, D. W. G. (1996): *Proceedings, Third International Conference on Harmonization*. Yokohama, Japan, 1995, Greystone Books, Antrim, North Ireland.
45. Davies, T. S., and Monro, A. (1994): The rodent carcinogenicity bioassay produces a similar frequency of tumor increases and decreases: Implications for risk assessment. *Regul. Toxicol. Pharmacol.*, 20:281–301.
46. Davies, T. S., and Monro, A. (1995): Marketed human pharmaceuticals reported to be tumorigenic in rodents. *J. Am. Coll. Toxicol.*, 14:90–107.
47. Dedrick, R. L. (1986): Interspecies scaling of regional drug delivery. *J. Pharmaceut. Sci.*, 175:1047–1052.
48. DeGeorge, J. J., and Contrera, J. F. (1996): A regulatory perspective of the guidance on the utility of two rodent species. In: *Proceedings, Third Internatinal Conference on Harmonization*. Yokohama, Japan, 1995, edited by P. F. D'Arcy and D. W. G. Harron, pp. 274–277, Greystone Books, Antrim, North Ireland.
49. De Gruijl, F. R., and Forbes, P. D. (1995): UV-induced skin cancer in a hairless mouse model. *BioEssays*, 17:651–660.
50. De Vries, A., von Oostrom, C. T. M., Dortant, P. M., Beems, R. B., van Kriejl, C. F., Capel, P. J. A., and van Steeg, H. (1997): Spontaneous liver tumours and benzo[a]pyrene-induced lymphomas in XPA-deficient mice. *Mol. Carcinogen.*, 19:46–53.
51. Dideriksen, L. H., Joregensen, L. N., and Drejer, K. (1992): Carcinogenic effect on female rats after 12 months administration of the insulin analogue B (10)Asp. *Diabetes*, 41(suppl. 1):143A (abstr.).
52. Donehower, I., Harvey, M., Slagle, B. L., McArthur, M. J., Montgomery, C. A., Jr., Butel, J. S., and Bradley, A. (1992): Mice deficient for p53 are developmentally normal but susceptible to spontaneous tumors. *Nature*, 356:215–221.
53. Dragan, Y. P., Rizvi, T, Xu, Y.-H., Hully, J. R., Bawa, N., Campbell, H. A., Maronpot, R. R., and Pitot, H. C. (1991): An initiation-promotion assay in rat liver as a potential complement to the 2-year carcinogenesis bioassay. *Fundam. Appl. Toxicol.*, 16:525–547.
54. Dunnett, C. W. (1955): A multiple comparison procedure for comparing several treatments with a control. *J. Am. Stat. Assoc.*, 50:1096–1122.
55. Dybing, E., Sanner, T., Roelfzema, H., Kroese, D., and Tennant, R. W. (1997) T25: A simplified carcinogenic potency index: Description of the system and study of correlations between carcinogenic potency and species/site specificity and mutagenicity. *Pharmacol. Toxicol.*, 30:272–279.
56. Eastin, W. C., Haseman, J. K., Mahler, J. F., and Bucher, J. R. (1998): The National Toxicology Program evaluation of genetically altered mice predictive models for identifying carcinogens. *Toxicol. Pathol.*, 26:461–584.
57. Ellwein, L. G., and Cohen, S. (1990): The health risk of saccharin revisted. *Crit. Rev. Toxicol.*, 20:311–326.
58. Elwell, M. R., Dunnick, J. K., Hailey, J. R., and Haseman, J. K. (1996): Chemicals associated with decreases in the incidence of mononuclear cell leukemia in the Fischer rat. *Toxicol. Pathol.*, 24:238–245.
59. Emerson, C. H., Cohen, J. H. III., Young, R. A., Alex, S., and Fan, S.-L. (1990): Gender-related differences of serum thyroxine-binding proteins in the rat. *Acta Endocrinol.*, 123:72–78.
60. Enzmann, H., Bomhard, E., Iatropoulos, M. J., Ahr, H. J., Schlueter, G., and Williams, G. M. (1998): Short- and intermediate-term carcinogenicity testing—A review: Part 1—The prototypes mouse skin tumour assay and rat liver focus. *Food Chem. Toxicol.*, 36:979–995.
61. Enzmann, H., Iatropoulos, M. J., Brunnemann, K. D., Bomhard, E., Ahr, H. J., Schlueter, G., and Williams, G. M. (1998): Short- and intermediate-term carcinogenicity testing—A review: Part 2—Available experimental models. *Food Chem. Toxicol.*, 36:997–1013.
62. European Economic Communities. (1967): Directive 67/548/EEC with amendments and adaptions: Annex VI. *Criteria for Classification of Carcinogenic Substances*, Brussels, Belgium.
63. European Economic Communities. (1983): *Note for Guidance Concerning the Application of Chapter I (E) of Part 2 of the Annex to Directive 75/398/EEC, With a View to the Granting of a Marketing Authorization of a New Drug*. Brussels, Belgium.
64. European Economic Communities. (1988): *Directive 88/379/EEC With Amendments: Annex I Criteria for Classification of Carcinogenic Substances*. Brussels, Belgium.
65. Faccini, J. M., Abbott, D. P., and Paulus, G. J. J. (1990): *Mouse Histopathology, A Glossary for Use in Toxicity and Carcinogenicity Studies*. Elsevier, Amsterdam.
66. Faccini, J. M., Butler, W. R., Friedmann, J.-C., Hess, R., Reznik, G. K., Ito, N., Hayashi, Y., and Williams, G. M. (1992): IFSTP guidelines for the design and interpretation of the chronic rodent carcinogenicity bioassay. *Exp. Toxicol. Pathol.*, 44:443–456.
67. Fairbairn, D. W., Olive, P. L., and O'Neill, K. L. (1995): The comet assay: A comprehensive review. *Mutat. Res.*, 339:37–59.
68. Feinstein, A. R. (1975): Clinical biostatistics. *Clin. Pharmacol. Ther.*, 17:499–513.
69. Fitzgerald, J. M., Boy, V. F., and Manus, A. G. (1984). Formulation of insoluble and inmiscible test agents in liquid vehicles for toxicity testing. In: *Chemistry for Toxicity Testing*, edited by C. W. Jameson and D. B. Walters, pp. 83–90. Butterworth, Stoneham, MA.
70. Flammang, T. J., von Tungeln, L. S., Kadlubar, F. F., and Fu, P. P. (1997): Neonatal mouse assay for tumorigenicity: Alternative to the chronic rodent bioassay. *Regul. Toxicol. Pharmacol.*, 26:230–240.
71. Fleiss, J. L. (1981): *Statistical Methods for Rates and Proportions*, 2nd ed., pp. 145–146. John Wiley and Sons, New York.
72. Fleiss, J. L. (1986): *The Design and Analysis of Clinical Experiments*, pp. 58–59. John Wiley and Sons, New York.
73. Foran, J. A. (Ed.). (1997): *Principles for the Selection of Doses in Chronic Rodent Bioassays*. ILSI Press, Washington, DC.
74. Forbes, P. D., Sambuco, C. P., and Davies, R. E. (1993): Photocarcinogenesis safety testing. *J. Am. Coll. Toxicol.*, 12:417–424.
75. Forbes, P. D., and Sambuco, C. P. (1998): Assays for photocarcinogenesis: Relevance of animal models. *Int. J. Toxicol.*, 17:577–588.

76. Frantz, S. W., Beatty, P. W., English, J. C., Hundley, S. G., and Wilson, A. G. E. (1994): The use of pharmacokinetics as an interpretive and predictive tool in chemical toxicology testing and risk assessment: A position paper on the appropriate use of pharmacokinetics in chemical toxicology. *Regul. Toxicol. Pharmacol.*, 19:317–337.

77. Gabriel, K. (1966). Simultaneous test procedures for multiple comparisons on categorical data. *J. Am. Stat. Assoc.*, 61:1081–1096.

78. Gabriel, K. R. (1978): A simple method of multiple comparison of means. *J. Am. Stat. Assoc.*, 73:724–729.

79. Gad, S. C. (1996): Histologic and clinical pathology in the safety assessment and development of new therapeutic agents. *Scand. J. Lab. Anim. Sci.*, 13:325–334.

80. Gad, S. C., and Weil, C. S. (1986): *Statistics and Experimental Design for Toxicologists*, pp. 1–17. Telford Press, Caldwell, NJ.

81. Galer, D. M., and Monro, A. M. (1998): Veterinary drugs no longer need testing for carcinogenicity in rodent bioassays. *Regul. Toxicol. Pharmacol.*, 28:115–123.

82. Garby, L., Garrow, J. S., Jorgensen, B., Lammert, O., Madsen, K., Sorensen, P., and Webster, J. (1988): Relationship between energy expenditure and body composition in man: Specific energy expenditure in vivo of fat and fat-free tissue. *Eur. J. Clin. Nutrition*, 42:301–305.

83. Gart, J. J., Chu, K. C., and Tarone, R. E. (1979): Statistical issues in the interpretation of chronic bioassay tests for carcinogenicity. *JNCI*, 62:957–974.

84. Gaylor, D. W., and Kodell, R. I. (1999): Dose-response trend tests for tumorigenesis, adjusted for body weight. *Toxicol. Sci.*, 49:318–323.

85. Gehring, P. J., Watanabe, P. G., and Park, C. N. (1978): Resolution of dose response toxicity data for chemicals requiring metabolic activation. Example—Vinyl chloride. *Toxicol. Appl. Pharmacol.*, 44:581–591.

86. Gillette, J., Weisburger, E. K., Kraybill, H., and Kelsey, M. (1985): Strategies for determining the mechanisms of toxicity. *Clin. Toxicol.*, 23(1):1–78.

87. Gold, L. S., and Zeiger, E. (1996): *Handbook of Carcinogenic Potency and Genotoxicity Data Bases*. CRC Press, Boca Raton, FL.

88. Gopinath, C., Prentice, D. E., and Lewis, D. J. (1987): *Atlas of Experimental Toxicological Pathology*. MTP, Lancaster, UK.

89. Grasso, P., Sharratt, M., and Cohen, A. J. (1991): Role of persistent, non-genotoxic tissue damage in rodent cancer and relevance to humans. *Annu. Rev. Pharmacol. Toxicol.*, 31:253–287.

90. Greaves, P. C. (1990): *Histopathology of Preclinical Toxicity Studies*. Elsevier, Amsterdam.

91. Hailey, J. R., Haseman, J. K., Bucher, J. R., Raadovsky, A. E., Malarkey, D. E., Miller, R. T., Nyska, A., and Maronpot, R. R. (1998): Impact of *Helicobacter hepaticus* infection in B6C3F$_1$ mice from twelve National Toxicology Program two-year carcinogenesis studies. *Toxicol. Pathol.*, 26:602–611.

92. Halliwell, W. H. (1998): Submucosal mesenchymal tumors of the mouse urinary bladder. *Toxicol. Pathol.*, 26:128–136.

93. Halpert, J. R., Guengerich, F. P., Bend, J. R., and Correia, M. A. (1994): Selective inhibitors of cytochrome P450. *Toxicol. Appl. Pharmacol.*, 124:163–175.

94. Hart, R. W., Keenan, K. P., Turturro, A., Abdo, K. M., Leakey, J., and Lyn-Cook, L. (1995): Caloric restriction and toxicology. *Fundam. Appl. Toxicol.*, 25:184–195.

95. Hart, R. W., Neumann, D. A., and Robertson, R. T. (Eds.). (1995): *Dietary Restriction: Implications for the Design and Interpretation of Toxicity and Carcinogenicity Studies*. ILSI Press, Washington, DC.

96. Haseman, J. K. (1984): Statistical issues in the design analysis and interpretation of animal carcinogenicity studies. *Environ. Health Perspect.*, 58:385–392.

97. Haseman, J. K. (1990): Use of statistical decision rules for evaluating laboratory animal carcinogenicity studies. *Fundam. Appl. Toxicol.*, 14:637–648.

98. Haseman, J. K., Huff, J., and Boorman, G. A. (1984): Use of historical control data in carcinogenicity studies in rodents. *Toxicol. Pathol.*, 2:126–135.

99. Haseman, J. K., and Rao, G. N. (1992): Effects of corn oil, time-related changes, and inter-laboratory variability on tumor occurrence in control Fischer 344 (F344/N) rats. *Toxicol. Pathol.*, 20:52-60.

100. Haseman, J. K., and Lockhart, A. (1994): The relationship between use of the maximum tolerated dose and study sensitivity for detecting rodent carcinogenicity. *Fundam. Appl. Toxicol.*, 22:382–391.

101. Haseman, J. K., and Johnson, L. (1996): Analysis of National Toxicology Program rodent bioassay data for anticarcinogenic effects. *Mutat. Res.*, 350:131–141.

102. Haseman, J. K., Hailey, J. R., and Morris, R. W. (1998): Spontaneous neoplasm incidences in Fischer 344 rats and B6C3F$_1$ mice in two-year carcinogenicity studies: A National Toxicology Program update. *Toxicol. Pathol.*, 26:428–441.

103. Health and Welfare Canada. (1989): *Guidelines for Canadian Drinking Water Quality: Supporting Documentation*, Part 1, pp. 1–5. Health and Welfare, Ottawa, Canada.

104. Hesseltine, G. R., Wolff, R. K., Hanson, R. L., Mauderly, J. L., and McClellan, R. O. (1984): *Effect of day versus night inhalation exposure on lung burdens of gallium oxide in rats*. Inhalation Toxicology Research Institute Annual Report, Albuquerque, NM.

105. Hill, R. N., Crisp, T. M., Hurley, P. M., Rosenthal, S. L., and Singh, D. V. (1998): Risk assessment of thyroid follicular cell tumors. *Environ. Health Perspect.*, 106:447–457.

106. Huff, J. (1999): Value, validity, and historical development of carcinogenesis studies for predicting and confirming carcinogenic risks to humans. In: *Carcinogenicity*, edited by K. T. Kitchin, pp. 21–123. Marcel Dekker, New York.

107. Iatropoulos, M. J. (1984): Appropriateness of methods for slide evaluation in the practice of toxicologic pathology. *Toxicol. Pathol.*, 12:4–5.

108. Iatropoulos, M. J. (1988): Society of Toxicologic Pathologists position paper: "Blinded" microscopic examination of tissues from toxicologic or oncogenic studies. In: *Carcinogenicity*, edited by H. C. Grice and J. L. Ciminera, pp. 133–135, Springer Verlag, New York.

109. Iatropoulos, M. J. (1993): Comparative histokinetic and xenodynamic considerations in toxicity. In: *Drug Toxicokinetics*, edited by D. G. P. Welling and F. A. de la Iglesia, pp. 245–266. Marcel Dekker, New York.

110. Iatropoulos, M. J., Newman, A. J., Dayan, A. D., Brughera, M., Scampini, G., and Mazue, G. (1994): Urinary bladder hyperplasia in the rat: Non-specific pathogenetic considerations using a beta-lactam antibiotic. *Exp. Toxicol. Pathol.*, 46:265–274.

111. Iatropoulos, M. J., Williams, G. M., Wang, C.-X., and Karlsson, S. H. (1996): New histopathologic and histokinetic methods in preclinical safety studies. *Scand. J. Lab. Anim. Sci.*, 13:339–343.

112. Iatropoulos, M. J., and Williams, G. M. (1996): Proliferation markers. *Exp. Toxicol. Pathol.*, 48:175–181.

113. Imai, K., Yoshimura, S., Yamaguchi, K., Matsui, E., Isaka, H., and Hashimoto, K. (1990): Effects of dietary restriction on age-associated pathological changes in F-344 rats. *J. Toxicol. Pathol.*, 3:209–221.

114. Interdisciplinary Panel on Carcinogenicity (IPC/AIHC). (1984): Criteria for evidence of chemical carcinogenicity. *Science*, 225:682–687.
115. International Agency for Research on Cancer. (1980): *Long-Term and Short-Term Screening Assays for Carcinogens: A Critical Appraisal*, IARC Monographs, Supplement 2, Lyon, France.
116. International Agency for Research on Cancer. (1987): *IARC Monographs on the Evaluation of Carcinogenic Risks to Humans: Preamble*. IARC Tech. Rep. No. 87/001, Lyon, France.
117. International Agency for Research on Cancer. (1990): *Complex Mixtures and Cancer Risk*. IARC Science Publ. No. 104, Lyon, France.
118. International Agency for Research on Cancer. (1992): *Mechanisms of Carcinogenesis in Risk Identification*. IARC Science Publ. No. 116, Lyon, France.
119. International Agency for Research on Cancer. (1992): *Solar and Ultraviolet Radiation*. IARC Tech. Rep. No. 55, Lyon, France.
120. International Agency for Research on Cancer. (1995): *Peroxisome Proliferation and Its Role in Carcinogenesis, Views and Expert Opinions of an IARC Working Group*. IARC Tech. Rep. No. 24, Lyon, France.
121. International Agency for Research on Cancer. (1996): *Directory of Agents Being Tested for Carcinogenicity*. IARC Science Publ. No. 134, Lyon, France.
122. International Agency for Research on Cancer. (1997): *IARC Monographs on the Evaluation of Carcinogenic risks to Humans*, vols. 1–69. IARC, Lyon, France.
123. International Agency for Research on Cancer. (1999): *The Use of Short- and Medium-Term Test for Carcinogens and Data on Genetic Effects in Carcinogenic Hazard Evaluations*. IARC Tech. Rep. No. 146, Lyon, France.
124. International Conference on Harmonization. (1994): *Guideline III/5081 on Toxicokinetics*. Commission of the European Communities, Directorate-General III, Industry: Industrial Affairs III: Consumer Goods Industries-Pharmaceuticals, Brussels, Belgium.
125. International Conference on Harmonization. (1996): *Impurities in New Drug Products: ICH Harmonized Tripartite Guideline*. Washington, DC.
126. International Expert Panel on Carcinogen Risk Assessment (IEPCRA). (1996): The use of mechanistic data in the risk assessments of ten chemicals: An introduction to the chemical-specific reviews. *Pharmacol. Ther.*, 71:1–5.
127. International Programme on Chemical Safety (IPCS). (1996): Butylated hydroxytoluene. *Toxicological Evaluation of Certain Food Additives and Contaminants*, pp. 3–86. Prepared by the Expert Committee on Food Additives (JECFA) at the 4th joint meeting of FAO/WHO. WHO, Geneva.
128. International Workshop. (1992): Clinical pathology testing in preclinical safety assessment. *Toxicol. Pathol.*, 20:469–543.
129. Jacobs, A., Avalos, J., Brown, P., and Wilkin, J. (1999): Does photosensitivity predict photococarcinogenicity? *Int. J. Toxicol.*, 18:191–198.
130. Jain, R. K., Gerlowski, L. E., Weissbrod, J. M., Wang, J., and Pierson, R. N., Jr. (1981): Kinetics of intake, distribution and excretion of zinc in rats. *Ann. Biomed. Eng.*, 9:345–361.
131. Jameson, C. W. (1984): Analytical chemistry requirements for toxicity testing of environmental chemicals. In: *Chemistry for Toxicity Testing*, edited by C. W. Jameson and D. B. Walters, pp. 3–14. Butterworth, Stoneham, MA.
131a. Jerry, D. J., Butel, J. S., Donehower, L. A., Paulson, E. J., Cochran, C., Wiseman, R. W., and Medina, D. (1994): Infrequent p53 mutations in 7,12-dimethylbenz(a)anthracene induced mammary tumors in BALB/c and p53 hemizygous mice. *Mol. Carcinog.*, 9:175–183.
132. Jordan, A. (1992): FDA requirements for nonclinical testing of contraceptive steroids. *Contraception*, 46:499–509.
133. Karbe, E. (1999): "Mesenchymal tumor" or "decidual-like reaction"? *Toxicol. Pathol.*, 27:354–362.
134. Karbe, E., Hartmann, E., George, C., Wadsworth, P., Harleman, J., and Geiss, V. (1998): Similarities between the uterine decidual reaction and the "mesenchymal lesion" of the urinary bladder in aging mice. *Exp. Toxicol. Pathol.*, 50:4–6.
135. Keenan, K. P. (1996): The uncontrolled variable in risk assessment: Ad libitum overfed rodents—Fat, facts and fiction. *Toxicol. Pathol.*, 24:376–383.
136. Keenan, K., Smith, P., Hertzog, P., Soper, K., Ballam, G., and Clark, R. (1994): The effects of overfeeding and dietary restriction on Sprague-Dawley rat survival and early pathology biomarkers of aging. *Toxicol. Pathol.*, 22:300–331.
137. Keenan, K. P., Laroque, P., Ballam, G. C., Soper, K. A., Dixit, R., Mattson, B. A., Adams, S. P., and Coleman, J. B. (1996): The effects of diet, ad libitum overfeeding, and moderate dietary restriction on the rodent bioassay: The uncontrolled variable in safety assessment. *Toxicol. Pathol.*, 24:757–768.
138. Kelly, W. A., Marler, R. J., and Weikel, J. H. (1993): Drug-induced mesovarial leiomyomas in the rat—A review and additional data. *J. Am. Coll. Toxicol.*, 12:13–22.
139. Kemp, C. J. (1995): Hepatocarcinogenesis in p53-deficient mice. *Mol. Carcinogenesis*, 12:132–136.
140. King, F. G., Dedrick, R. L., and Farris, F. F. (1986): Physiological pharmacokinetic modeling of cisdichlorodiamine platinum(II) (DDP) in several species. *J. Pharmacokin. Biopharmaceut.*, 14:131–155.
141. Klopman, G., and Rosenkranz, H. S. (1994): Approaches to SAR in carcinogenesis and mutagenesis. Prediction of carcinogenicity/mutagenicity using MULTICASE. *Mutat. Res.*, 305:33–46.
142. Knapka, J. J. (1979): Laboratory animal feed. *Science*, 204:1367–1368.
143. Komulainen, H. (1996): Pharmacokinetic experiments in animals—Needs and application of data. *Scand. J. Lab. Anim. Sci.*, 23:315–316.
144. Kunze, E., and Chowaniec, J. (1990): Tumors of the urinary bladder. In *Pathology of Tumours in Laboratory Animals*, vol. I, *Tumors of the Rat*, pp. 345–373. IARC Science Publ. No. 99, Lyon, France.
145. Kripke, M. L. (1994): Ultraviolet radiation and immunology: Something new under the sun—Presidential address. *Cancer Res.*, 54:6102–6105.
146. Kroes, R., and Wester, P. W. (1986): Forestomach carcinogens: Possible mechanisms of action. *Food Chem. Toxicol.*, 24:1083–1089.
147. Krewski, D., Smythe, R. T., Dewanji, A., and Colin, D. (1988): Statistical tests with historical controls. In: *Carcinogenicity*, edited by H. C. Grice and J. L. Ciminera, pp. 23–38. Springer Verlag, New York.
148. Lai, Y. L., Jacoby, R., and Jonas, A. (1978): Age related and light associated retinal changes in Fischer rats. *Invest. Ophthalmol. Visual Sci.*, 17:634–638.
149. Lavbelin, G., Roba, J., Roncucci, R., and Parmentier, R. (1975): Carcinogenicity of 6-aminochrysene in mice. *Eur. J. Cancer*, 11:327–334.
150. Le Boeuf, R. A., Kerckaert, G. Aardema, M., Gibson, D., Brauninger, R., and Isfort, R. (1996): The pH 6.7 Syrian hamster embryo cell transformation assay for assessing the carcinogenic potential of chemicals. *Mutat. Res.*, 356:85–127.
151. Leder, A., Kuo, A., Cardiff, R. D., Sinn, E., and Leder, P. (1990) v-Ha-ras transgene abrogates the initiation step in mouse skin

tumorigenesis: Effects of phorbol esters and retinoic acid. *Proc. Natl. Acad. Sci. USA*, 87:9178–9182.

152. Lee, P. (1988): Assumptions in analyses of the bioassay; A statistician's view. In: *Carcinogenicity*, edited by H. C. Grice and J. L. Ciminera, pp. 1–10. Springer Verlag, New York.
153. Leung, H. W., and Paustenbach, D. J. (1988): Application of pharmacokinetic to derive biological exposure indexes from threshold limit values. *Am. Ind. Hyg. Assoc.*, 49:445–450.
154. Lewtas, J. (1988): Genotoxicity of complex mixtures: Strategies for the identification and comparative assessment of airborne mutagens and carcinogens from combustion sources. *Fundam. Appl. Toxicol.*, 10:571–589.
155. Lington, A. W., Bird, M. G., Plutnick, R. T., Stubblefield, W. A., and Scala, R. A. (1997): Chronic toxicity and carcinogenic evaluation of diisonoyl phthalate in rats. *Fundam. Appl. Toxicol.*, 36:79–89.
156. Long, G. G., Symanowski, J. T., and Roback, K. (1998): Precision in data acquisition and reporting of organ weights in rats and mice. *Toxicol. Pathol.*, 26:316–318.
157. Lutz, W. K. (1986): Quantitative evaluation of DNA binding data for risk estimation and for classification of direct and indirect carcinogens. *J. Cancer Res. Clin. Oncol.*, 112:85–91.
158. Mahler, J. F., Stokes, W., Mann, P. C., Takaoka, M., and Maronpot, R. R. (1996): Spontaneous lesions in aging FVB/N mice. *Toxicol. Pathol.*, 24:710–716.
159. Mahler, J. P., Flagler, N. D., Malarkey, D. E., Mann, P. C., Haseman, J. K., and Eastin, W. (1998): Spontaneous and chemically-induced proliferative lesions in Tg.AC transgenic and p53-heterozygous mice. *Toxicol. Pathol.*, 26:501–511.
160. Maita, K., Hirano, M., Harada, T., Mitsumori, K., Yoshida, A., Takahashi, K., Nakashima, N., Kitazawa, T., Enomoto, A., Inui, K., and Shirasu, Y. (1988): Mortality, major cause of moribundity, and spontaneous tumors in CD-1 mice. *Toxicol. Pathol.*, 16:340–349.
161. Matthews, E. J., and Contrera, J. F. (1998): A new highly specific method for predicting the carcinogenic potential of pharmaceuticals in rodents using enhanced MCASE QSAR-ES software. *Regul. Toxicol. Pharmacol.*, 28:242–264.
162. McClellan, R. O., and Hobbs, C. H. (1986): Generation, characterization and exposure systems for test atmospheres. In: *Safety Evaluation of Chemicals*, edited by W. E. Lloyd, pp. 41–48. Hemisphere, Washington, DC.
163. McConnell, E. E. (1983): Pathology requirements for rodent two year studies. I. A review of current procedures. *Toxicol. Pathol.*, 11:60–64.
164. McConnell, E. E., Solleveld, H. A., Swenberg, J. A., and Boorman, G. A. (1986): Guidelines of combining neoplasms for evaluation of rodent carcinogenesis studies. *JNCI*, 76:283–289.
165. McConnell, R. F. (1989): General observations on the effects of sex steroids in rodents with emphasis on long-term oral contraceptive studies. In: *Safety Requirements for Contraceptive Steroids*, edited by F. Michael, pp. 211–229. Cambridge University Press, New York.
166. McConnell, R. F., Westen, H. H., Ulland, B. M., Bosland, M. C., and Ward, J. M. (1992): Proliferative lesions of the testes in rats with selected examples from mice. In: *Guides for Toxicologic Pathology*, pp. 1–25. STP/ARP/AFIP, Washington, DC.
167. McMartin, D. N., Sahota, P. S., Gunson, D. E., Hsu, H. H., and Spaet, R. H. (1992): Neoplasms and related proliferative lesions in control Sprague-Dawley rats from carcinogenicity studies. Historical data and diagnostic considerations. *Toxicol. Pathol.*, 20:212–225.
168. Milman, H. A., and Weisburger, E. K. (1985): *Handbook of Carcinogen Testing*. Noyes, Park Ridge, NJ.
169. Ministry of Health and Welfare. (1989): *Guidelines for toxicity studies required for applications for approved to manufacture (import) drugs: Carcinogenicity study*. Tokyo, Japan.
170. Modlin, I. M., and Sachs, G. (1998): *Age Related Diseases: Biology and Treatment*, pp. 242–245. Schnetztor-Verlag, Konstanz, Germany.
171. Monro, A. (1992): What is an appropriate measure of exposure when testing drugs for carcinogenicity in rodents? *Toxicol. Appl. Pharmacol.*, 112:171–181.
172. Monro, A. (1993): How useful are chronic (life-span) toxicology studies in rodents in identifying pharmaceuticals that pose a carcinogenic risk to humans? *Adv. Drug React. Toxicol. Rev.*, 12:5–34.
173. Munro, I. C. (1977): Considerations in chronic testing: The chemical, the dose, the design. *J. Environ. Pathol. Toxicol.*, 1:183–197.
174. Munro, I. C., Ford, R. A., Kennepohl, E., and Sprenger, J. G. (1996): Thresholds of toxicological concern based on structure–activity relationships. *Drug Metab. Rev.*, 28:209–217.
175. Morrison, V., and Ashby, J. (1994): A preliminary evaluation of the performance of the Muta mouse (bac Z) and Big Blue (bac I) transgenic mouse mutation assays. *Mutagenesis*, 9:367–376.
176. Mulder, G. J. (1986): Sex differences in drug conjugation and their consequences for drug toxicity. Sulfation, glucuronidation and glutathione conjugation. *Chem. Biol. Interact.*, 57:1–15.
177. National Cancer Institute. (1994): *Survey of Compounds Which Have Been Tested for Carcinogenic Activity*. NIH Publ. No. 94-3765, Washington, DC.
178. National Institutes of Health. (1981): *NIH Guidelines for the Laboratory Use of Chemical Carcinogens*. NIH Publ. No. 81-2385, Washington, DC.
179. National Institutes of Health. (1986): *Humane Care and Use of Laboratory Animals*. NIH Publ. No. 86-23, Washington, DC.
180. National Research Council. (1983): *Risk Assessment in the Federal Government: Managing the Process*. National Academy Press, Washington, DC.
181. National Research Council. (1993): *Use of Maximum Tolerated Dose in Animal Bioassays for Carcinogenicity*. National Academy Press, Washington, DC.
182. National Research Council. (1996): *Guide for the Care and Use of Laboratory Animals*. National Academy Press, Washington, DC.
183. National Toxicology Program. (1997): *Effect of dietary restriction on toxicology and carcinogenesis studies in F344/N rats and B6C3F$_1$ mice*. NTP Tech. Rep. 460. NIH Publ. No. 97-3376. Research Triangle Park, NC.
184. Nelson, D. R., Koymans, L., Kamatski, T., Stegeman, J. J., Feyereisen, R., Waxman, D. J., Waterman, M. R., Gotoh, O., Coon, M. J., Estabrook, R. W., Gunsalus, I. C., and Nebert, D. W. (1996). P450 superfamily: Update on new sequences, gene mapping ascession numbers and nomenclature. *Pharmacogenetics*, 6:1–42.
185. Neumann, F. (1991): Early indicators for carcinogenesis in hormone sensitive organs. *Mutat. Res.*, 248:341–356.
186. Newberne, P. M., and dela Iglesia, F. A. (1985): Philosophy of blind slide reading in toxicologic pathology. *Toxicol. Pathol.*, 13:225.
187. Newberne, P. M., and Sotnikov, A. V. (1996): Diet: the neglected variable in chemical safety evaluations. *Toxicol. Pathol.*, 24:746–756.
188. Noble, J. F. (1984): Automated data acquisition systems in the 80s and beyond. II. Operation. In: *Toxicology Laboratory Design and Management for the 80s and Beyond*, edited by A. Tegeris, pp. 143–158. Karger, New York.

189. Office of Science and Technology Policy. (1985): Chemical carcinogens: A review of the science and its associated principles. *Fed. Reg.*, March 14:10371–10442.
190. Office of Technology Assessment. (1987): *Identifying and Regulating Carcinogens, A Background Paper*. U.S. Congress, Washington, DC.
191. Organization for Economic Cooperation and Development. (1981): *Adopted Guidelines for Testing of Chemicals*, Section 4—Health effects, Number 451—Carcinogenicity Studies. Paris.
192. Page, N. P., Singh, D. V., Farland, W., Goodman, J. I., Conolly, R. B., Anderson, M. E., Clewell, H. J., Frederick, C. B., Yamasaki, H., and Lucier, G. (1997): Implementation of EPA revised cancer assessment guidelines: Incorporation of mechanistic and pharmacokinetic data. *Fundam. Appl. Toxicol.*, 37:16–36.
193. Peck, C. C., Barr, W. H., and Benet, L. Z. (1992): Opportunities for integration of pharmacokinetics, pharmacodynamics and toxicokinetics in rational drug design. *J. Pharm. Sci.*, 81:605–610.
194. Perrone, C. E., Shao, L., and Williams, G. M. (1998): Effect of rodent hepatocarcinogenic peroxisome proliferatiors on fatty acyl-CoA oxidase, DNA synthesis, and apoptosis in cultured human and rat hepatocytes. *Toxicol. Appl. Pharmacol.*, 150:277–286.
195. Peto, R., Pike, M. C., Day, N. E., Gray, R. G., Lee, P. N., Parish, S., Peto, J., and Wahrendorf, J. (1980): Guidelines for simple, sensitive significance tests for carcinogenic effects in long-term animal experiments. In: *Long-Term and Short-Term Screening Assays for Carcinogens: A Critical Appraisal*, edited by R. Montesano, H. Bartsch, and L. Tomatis, pp. 311–426. IARC Monographs on the Evaluation of the Carcinogenic Risk of Chemicals to Humans, Suppl. 2. Lyon, France.
196. Peto, R., Pike, M. C., Bernstein, L., Gold, L. S., and Ames, B. N. (1984): A proposed general convention for the numerical description of carcinogenic potency of chemicals in chronic-exposures animal experiments. *Environ. Health Perspect.*, 58:1–8.
197. Poteracki, J., and Walsh, K. M. (1998): Spontaneous neoplasms in control Wistar rats: A comparison of reviews. *Toxicol. Sci.*, 45:1–8.
198. Powles, P. (1996): Interpretation of data from toxicokinetic studies. *Scand. J. Lab. Anim. Sci.*, 23:317–323.
199. Randerath, K., Reddy, M. V., and Gupta, R. C. (1981): ^{32}P-postlabeling test for DNA damage. *Proc. Natl. Acad. Sci. USA*, 78:626–6129.
200. Rao, G. N., Piegorsch, W. W., and Haseman, J. K. (1987): Influence of body weight on the incidence of spontaneous tumors in rats and mice of long-term studies. *Am. J. Clin. Nutr.*, 45:252–260.
201. Rao, G., Haseman, J., Grumbein, S., Crawford, S., and Eustis, S. (1990): Growth, body weight, survival and tumor trends in (C57B1/6 × C3H/NeN) F1 (B6C3F1) mice during a nine year period. *Toxicol. Pathol.*, 18:71–77.
202. Reuter, J., and Hobbelen, H. (1977): The effect of continuous light exposure on the retina in albino and pigmented rats. *Physiol. Behav.*, 18:939–944.
203. Rice, J. M., Williams, G. M., Palmer, A. E., London, W. T., and Sly, D. L. (1981): Pathology of gestational choriocarcinoma induced in patas monkeys by ethylnitrosourea given during pregnancy. *Placenta Suppl.*, 3:223–230.
204. Rice, J. M., Baan, R. A., Blettner, M., Genevois-Charneau, C., Grosse, Y., McGregor, D. B., Partensky, C., and Wilbourn, J. D. (1999): Rodent tumors of urinary bladder, renal cortex, and thyroid gland in IARC monographs evaluation of carcinogenic risk to humans. *Toxicol. Sci.*, 49:166–171.
205. Riley, V. (1975): Mouse mammary tumors: Alteration of incidence as apparent function of stress. *Science*, 189:465–467.
206. Riley, V. (1981): Psychoneuroendocrine influences on immune-competence and neoplasia. *Science*, 212:1100–1109.
207. Robens, J. F., Calabrese, E. J., Piegorsch, W. W., Schueler, R. L., and Hayes, A. W. (1994): Principles of testing for carcinogenicity. In: *Principles and Methods of Toxicology*, 3rd ed., edited by A. W. Hayes, pp. 697–728. Raven Press, New York.
208. Rosai, J. (1981): Breast. In: *Ackerman's Surgical Pathology*, pp. 1098–1149, C.V. Mosby, St. Louis, MO.
209. Russo, J., Russo, I. H., Rogers, A. E., Van Zwieten, M. J., and Gusterson, B. (1990): Tumours of the mammary gland. In: *Pathology of Tumours in Laboratory Animals*, vol. I, *Tumors of the Rat*, edited by V. S. Turusov and U. Mohr, pp. 47–78. IARC Science Publ. No. 99, Lyon, France.
210. Sacco, M. G., Zecca, L., Bagnasco, L., Chiesa, G., Parotini, C., Bromley, P., Cato, E. M., Roncucci, R., Clerici, L. A., and Veggoni, P. (1997): A transgenic mouse model for the detection of cellular stress inducted by toxic inorganic compounds. *Nature Biotechnol.*, 15:1392–1397.
211. Safe, S. (1997/1998): Limitations of the toxic equivalency factor approach for risk assessment of TCDD and related compounds. *Teratogen. Carcinogen. Mutagen.*, 17:285–304.
212. Saitoh, A., Kimura, M., Takahashi, R., Yokoyama, M., Nomura, T., Izawa, M., Sekiya, T., Nishimura, S., and Katsuki, M. (1990): Most tumors in transgenic mice with human c-Ha-ras gene contained somatically activated transgenes. *Oncogene*, 5:1195–1200.
213. Sambuco, C. P., Davies, R. E., Forbes, P. D., and Hoberman, A. M. (1991): Photocarcinogenesis and consumer product testing: Technical aspects. *Toxicol. Methods*, 1:75–83.
214. Sansone, E. B., and Losikoff, A. M. (1978): Contamination from feeding volatile test chemicals. *Toxicol. Appl. Pharmacol.*, 46:703–708.
215. Sansone, E. B., and Tewari, Y. B. (1978): Penetration of protective clothing materials by 1,2-dibromo-3-chloropropane, ethylene dibromide, and acrylonitrile. *J. Am. Ind. Hyg. Assoc.*, 39:921–922.
216. Sansone, E. B., and Tewari, Y. B. (1978): The permeability of laboratory gloves to selected solvents. *J. Am. Ind. Hyg. Assoc.*, 39:169–174.
217. Sarkar, D. K., Gottschall, P. E., and Meites, J. (1982): Damage to hypothalamic dopaminergic neurons associated with development of prolactin-secreting pituitary tumors. *Science*, 218:684–686.
218. Sasahara, K., Ando-Lu, J., Nishiyama, K., Takahashi, M., Yoshida, M., and Maekawa, A. (1998): Granular cell foci of the uterus in Donryu rats. *J. Comp. Pathol.*, 119:195–199.
219. Scheuplein, R. J., and Blank, I. H. (1971): Permeability of the skin. *Physiol. Rev.*, 51:702–743.
220. Schyve, P. M., Smithline, F., and Metzger, H. Y. (1978): Neuroleptic-induced prolactin level elevation and breast cancer. *Arch. Gen. Psychiatry*, 35:1291–1301.
221. Seifter, E., Rettura, G., Zisblatt, M., Levenson, S. M., Levine, N., Davidson, A., and Seigter, J. (1973): Enhancement of tumor development of physically-stressed mice inculated with an oncogenic virus. *Experientia*, 29:1379–1882.
222. Seilkop, S. K. (1995): The effect of body weight on tumor incidence and carcinogenicity testing in B6C3F$_1$ mice and F344 rats. *Fundam. Appl. Toxicol.*, 24:247–259.
223. Serabian, M. A., and Pilaro, A. M. (1999): Safety assessment of biotechnology-derived pharmaceuticals: ICH and beyond. *Toxicol. Pathol.*, 27:27–31.
224. Sieber, S. M., and Adamson, R. H. (1978): Long-term studies on the potential carcinogenicity of artificial sweeteners in non-human primates. In: *Health and Sugar Substitutes*, edited by B. Guggenheim, pp. 266–271. Karger, Basel, Switzerland.
225. Shah, V. P., Midha, K. K., Dighe, S., McGilveray, I. J., Skelly, J. P., Yacobi, A., Layloff, T., Viswanathan, C. T., Cook, C. E., McDowall, R. D., Pittman, K. A., and Spector, S. (1992): Analytical methods validation—Bioavailability, bioequivalence and pharmacokinetic studies. *J. Pharmaceut. Res.*, 81:309–312.

226. Shirai, T., Hirose, M., and Ito, N. (1999): Medium-term bioassays in rats for rapid detection of the carcinogenic potential of chemicals. In: *The Use of Short- and Medium-Term Tests for Carcinogenic Hazard Evaluation*, edited by D. B. McGregor, J. M. Ricc, and S. Venitt, pp. 251–271. IARC Publ. No. 146, Lyon, France.
227. Smith, D. M., Rogers, A. E., and Newberne, P. M. (1975): Vitamin A and benzo(a)pyrene carcinogenesis in the respiratory tract of hamsters fed a synthetic diet. *Cancer Res.*, 35:1485–1488.
228. Smith, D. M., Ortiz, L. W., Archuleta, R. F., Spalding, J. F., Tillery, M. I., Ettinger, H. J., and Thomas, R. G. (1981): A method of chronic nose-only exposures of laboratory animals to inhaled fibrous aerosols. In: *Inhalation Toxicology and Technology*, edited by H. P. Leong, pp. 89–105. Ann Arbor Science, Ann Arbor, MI.
229. Sontag, J. R., Page, N. P., and Safiotti, U. (1976): *Guidelines for Carcinogen Bioassay in Small Rodents*. DHHS Publication (NIH) 76-801, National Cancer Institute, Bethesda, MD.
230. Spalding, J. W., French, J. E., Tice, R. R., Furedi-Machek, M., Haseman, J. K., and Tennant, R. W. (1999): Development of a transgenic mouse model for carcinogenesis bioassays: Evaluation of chemically induced skin tumors in Tg.AC mice. *Toxicol. Sci.*, 49:241–254.
230a. Spratt, T. E., Schultz, S. S., Levy, D. E., Chen, D., Schlüter, G., and Williams, G. M. (1999): Different mechanisms for the photo-induced production of oxidative damage by fluoroquinolones differing in photostability. *Chem. Res. Toxicol.*, 12:805–815.
231. Stringer, C. (1992): Safety workshop-ICH 1. *Regul. Affairs J.*, 3:350–356.
232. Tamano, S., Hagiwara, A., Shibata, M., Kurata, Y., Fukushima, S., and Ito, N. (1988): Spontaneous tumors in aging B6C3F$_1$ mice. *Toxicol. Pathol.*, 16:321–326.
233. Tarone, R. E. (1975): Tests for trend in life table analysis. *Biometrika*, 62:679–682.
234. Tennant, R. W., Stasiewicz, S., Mennear, J., French, J. E., and Spalding, J. W. (1999). Genetically altered mouse models for identifying carcinogens: In: *The Use of Short- and Medium-Term Tests for Carcinogens and Data on Genetic Effects in Carcinogenic Hazard Evaluation*, edited by D. B. McGregor, J. M. Rice, and S. Venitt, pp. 23–148. IARC Science Publ. No. 146, Lyon, France.
235. Thake, D. C., Iatropoulos, M. J., Hard, G. C., Hotz, K. J., Wang, C.-X., Williams, G. M., and Wilson, A. G. E. (1995): A study of the mechanism of butachlor-associated gastric neoplasms in Sprague-Dawley rats. *Exp. Toxicol. Pathol.*, 47:107–116.
236. Thomas, G. A., and Williams, E. D. (1991): Evidence for and possible mechanisms of non-genotoxic carcinogenesis in the rodent thyroid. *Mutat. Res.*, 248:357–370.
237. Thorgiersson, U., Dalgard, D., Reeves, J., and Adamson, R. (1994): Tumor incidence in a chemical carcinogenesis study of nonhuman primates. *Regul. Toxicol. Pharmacol.*, 19:130–151.
238. Thurman, J. D., Bucci, T. J., Hart, R. W., and Torturro, A. (1994): Survival, body weight, and spontaneous neoplasms in ad libitum—fed and food-restricted Fischer-344 rats. *Toxicol. Pathol.*, 22:1–9.
239. Tomatis, L. (1989): Overview of perinatal and multigeneration carcinogenesis. In: *Perinatal and Multigeneration Carcinogenesis*, edited by N. P. Napalkov, J. M. Rice, L. Tomatis, and H. Yamasaki, pp. 1–15. IARC Science Publ. No. 96, Lyon, France.
240. Tsuda, H., Park, C. B., and Moore, M. A. (1999): Short- and medium-term carcinogenicity tests. In: *The Use of Short- and Medium-Term Tests for Carcinogenic Hazard Evaluation*, edited by D. B. McGregor, J. M. Rice, and S. Venitt, pp. 203–249. IARC Publ. No. 146, Lyon, France.
241. Tuch, K., Ockert, D., Hauschke, D., and Christ, B. (1992): Comparison of the ECL-cell frequency in the stomachs of 3 different rat strains. *Pathol. Res. Pract.*, 188:672–675.
242. Tugwood, J. D., and Elcombe, C. R. (1999): Predicting carcinogenicity: Peroxisome proliferators. In: *Carcinogenicity*, edited by K. T. Kitchin, pp. 337–360. Marcel Dekker, New York.
243. Turturro, A., Duffy, P., Hart, R., and Allaben, W. T. (1996): Rationale for the use of dietary control in toxicity studies—B6C3F1 mouse. *Toxicol. Pathol.*, 24:769–775.
244. Turusov, V. S. (1994): Histiocytic sarcoma. In: *Pathology of Tumours in Laboratory Animals*, vol. II, *Tumors of the Mouse*, edited by V.S. Turusov and U. Mohr, pp. 671–680. IARC Science Publ. No. 111, Lyon, France.
245. U.S. Congress. (1985): *Animal Welfare Act*. CFR 9, Parts 1, 2, 3, Washington, DC.
246. U.S. Congress. (1996): *Food Quality Protection Act*. Public Law 104-170 of August 3, 1996. Washington, DC.
247. U.S. Congress. (1998): *Food Quality Protection Act Amendment*. Public Law 105-324 of October 30, 1998. Washington, DC.
248. U.S. Department of Agriculture. (1989): *Animal Welfare Rules*. CFR 9, Parts 1, 2. Washington, DC.
249. U.S. Department of Health and Welfare. (1977): *Guide for Care and Use of Laboratory Animals*. Publ. No. NIH 77-23. Washington, DC.
249a. U.S. Department of Health and Human Services (2000): *Ninth Report on Carcinogens*. PHS, NTP, Research Triangle Park, NC.
250. U.S. Environmental Protection Agency. (1986): Guidelines for carcinogen risk assessment. *Fed. Reg.*, 51:33992–34005.
251. U.S. Environmental Protection Agency. (1990): *Good Automated Practices*, Draft 12-28-90. Scientific Systems Staff, Office of Information Resources Management. U.S. EPA, Washington, DC.
252. U.S. Environmental Protection Agency. (1991): *Alpha 2μ-globulin: Association with chemically induced renal toxicity and neoplasia in the male rat. Risk Assessment Forum*. EPA/625/3-91/019F. U.S. EPA, Washington, DC.
253. U.S. Environmental Protection Agency. (1992): A cross-species scaling factor for carcinogen risk assessment based on equivalence of mg/kg$^{3/4}$/day: Notice. *Fed. Reg.*, 57:24152–24173.
254. U.S. Environmental Protection Agency. (1992): Guidelines for exposure assessment. *Fed. Reg.*, 57:22888–22938.
255. U.S. Environmental Protection Agency. (1996): Proposed guidelines for carcinogen risk assessment. *Fed. Reg.*, 61:17960–18011.
256. U.S. Environmental Protection Agency. (1996): Proposed guidelines for ecological risk assessment; Notice. *Fed. Reg.*, 61:47052–47631.
257. U.S. Environmental Protection Agency. (1997): *Exposure Factors Handbook*. Office of Research and Development, EPA/600/P-95-002A, Washington, DC.
258. U.S. Environmental Protection Agency. (1998): *Health Effects Test Guidelines*. OPPTS 870.4200 and OPPTS.4300, EPA 712-C-98-211 and 212. Washington, DC.
259. U.S. Food and Drug Administration. (1978): Good Laboratory Practices for Nonclinical Laboratory Studies, Code of Federal Regulations, Title 21, Part 58. *Fed. Reg.*, 43:59986–60025.
260. U.S. Food and Drug Administration. (1993): *Toxicological Principles for the Safety Assessment of Direct Food Additives and Color Additives Used in Food*. Redbook II. Washington, DC.
261. U.S. Food and Drug Administration. (1993): Advisory committee for protocols for safety evaluation, panel on carcinogenesis: Report on cancer testing in the safety of food additives and pesticides. *Toxicol. Appl. Pharmacol.*, 20:419–438.
262. U.S. Food and Drug Administration. (1994): International Conference on Harmonization; Draft guideline on dose selection for carcinogenicity studies of pharmaceuticals. *Fed. Reg.*, 59:9752–9760. Available at http://www.ifpma.org/ich5s.html
263. U.S. Food and Drug Administration. (1994): *General Principles for Evaluating the Safety of Compounds Used in Food-Producing Animals*. Center for Veterinary Medicines, Washington, DC.

264. U.S. Food and Drug Administration. (1995): Food additives: Threshold of regulation for substances used in food contact articles. *Fed. Reg.*, 60:36582–36596.
265. U.S. Food and Drug Administration. (1997): International Conference on Harmonization: Guidance on preclinical safety evaluation of biotechnology-derived pharmaceuticals. *Fed. Reg.*, 62:61515–61519. available at http://www.iben.gov
266. U.S. Food and Drug Administration. (1997): International Conference on Harmonization: Guidelines on impurities in new drug products. *Fed. Reg.*, 62:27454–27461.
267. van Oosterhout, J. P. J., van der Laan, J. W., de Waal, E. J., Olejniczak, K., Hilgenfeld, M., Schmidt, V., and Bass, R. (1997): The utility of two rodent species in carcinogenic risk assessment of pharmaceuticals in Europe. *Regul. Toxicol. Pharmacol.*, 25:6–17.
268. van Steeg, H., Klein, H., Beems, R. B., and van Kreijl, C. F. (1998): Use of DNA repair-deficient XPA transgenic mice in short-term carcinogenicity testing. *Toxicol. Pathol.*, 26:742–749.
269. Vessel, E. S. (1967): Induction of drug metabolizing enzymes in liver microsomes of mice and rats by softwood bedding. *Science*, 157:1057–1058.
270. Viollon-Abadie, C., Lassere, D., Debruyne, E., Nicod, L., Carmichael, N., and Richert, L. (1999): Phenobarbital, β-napthoflavone, clofibrate, and pregnenolone-16α-carbonitrile do not affect hepatic thyroid hormone UDP-glucuronosyl transferase activity, and thyroid gland function in mice. *Toxicol. Appl. Pharmacol.*, 155:1–12.
271. Walsh, K. M., and Poteracki, J. (1994): Spontaneous neoplasms in control Wistar rats. *Fundam. Appl. Toxicol.*, 23:65–72.
272. Wattenberg, L. W. (1985): Chemoprevention of cancer. *Cancer Res.*, 45:1–8.
273. Weisburger, E. K. (1983): History of the bioassay program of the National Cancer Institute. *Prog. Exp. Tumor Res.*, 26:187–201.
274. Weisburger, J. H., and Williams, G. M. (1984): Bioassay of carcinogens: In vitro and in vivo tests. In: *Chemical Carcinogenesis*, ACS Monograph 182, 2nd ed., vol. 2, pp. 1323–1373. American Chemical Society, Washington, DC.
275. Weisburger, J. H., and Williams, G. M. (1995): Causes of cancer. In: *American Cancer Society Textbook of Clinical Oncology*, edited by G. P. Murphy, W. Lawrence, Jr., and R. E. Lenhard, Jr., pp. 10–39. ACS, Atlanta, GA.
276. Welling, P. G. (1993): Pharmacokinetic principles. In: *Drug Toxicokinetics*, edited by P. G. Welling and F. A. de la Iglesia, pp. 69–83. Marcel Dekker, New York.
277. Welsch, C. W., and Nasagawa, H. (1977). Prolactin and murine mammary tumorigenesis: A review. *Cancer. Res.*, 37:951–963.
278. Whysner, J., and Williams, G. M. (1992): International cancer risk assessment: The impact of biologic mechanisms. *Regul. Toxicol. Pharmacol.*, 15:41–50.
279. Williams, G. M. (1987): Definition of a human cancer hazard. In: *Nongenotoxic Mechanisms in Carcinogenesis*, Banbury Report 25, pp. 367–380. Cold Spring Harbor Laboratory, Cold Spring Harbor, NY.
280. Williams, G. M. (1989): Methods for evaluating chemical genotoxicity. *Annu. Rev. Pharmacol. Toxicol.*, 29:189–211.
281. Williams, G. M. (1989): Interactive carcinogenesis in the liver. In: *Liver Cell Carcinoma*, Falk Symposium 51, edited by P. Bannasch, D. Keppler, and G. Weber, pp. 197–216. Kluwer, Boston. MA.
282. Williams, G. M. (1990): Screening procedures for evaluating the potential carcinogenicity of food-packaging chemicals. *Regul. Toxicol. Pharmacol.*, 12:30–40.
283. Williams, G. M. (1992): DNA reactive and epigenetic carcinogens. *Exp. Toxicol. Pathol.*, 44:457–464.
284. Williams, G. M. (1999): Chemical-induced preneoplastic lesions in rodents as indicators of carcinogenic activity. In: *The Use of Short- and Medium-Term Tests for Carcinogens and Data on Genetic Effects in Carcinogenic Hazard Evaluations*, edited by D. B. McGregor, J. M. Rice, amd S. Venitt, pp. 185–202. IARC Publ. No. 146, Lyon, France.
285. Williams, G. M. (1999): Mechanistic considerations in cancer risk assessment. *Inhal. Toxicol.*, 11:549–554.
286. Williams, G. M., Laspia, M. F., and Dunkel, V. C. (1982): Reliability of the hepatocyte primary culture/DNA repair test in testing of coded carcinogens and non carcinogens. *Mutat. Res.*, 97:359–370.
287. Williams, G. M., Mori, H., and McQueen, C. A. (1989): Structure–activity relationships in the rat hepatocyte DNA-repair test for 300 chemicals. *Mutat. Res.*, 221:263–286.
288. Williams, G. M., and Weisburger, J. H. (1991): Chemical carcinogenesis. In: *Toxicology, The Basic Science of Poisons*, edited by M. O. Amdur, J. Doull, and C. D. Klaassen, pp. 127–200. Pergamon, New York.
289. Williams, G. M., Iatropoulos, M. J., and Weisburger, J. H. (1996): Chemical carcinogen mechanisms of action and implications for testing methodology. *Exp. Toxicol. Pathol.*, 48:101–111.
290. Williams, G. M., and Perone, C. (1996): Mechanism-based risk assessment of peroxisome proliferating rodent hepatocarcinogens. In: *Peroxisomes: Biology and Role in Toxicology and Disease*, edited by J. K. Reddy, T. Suga, G. P. Mannaerts, P. B. Lazarow, and S. Subramani, pp. 554–572. New York Academy of Sciences, vol. 804, New York.
291. Williams, G. M., Karbe, E., Fenner-Crisp, P., Iatropoulos, M. J., and Weisburger, J. H. (1996): Risk assessment of carcinogens in food with special consideration of non-genotoxic carcinogens. *Exp. Toxicol. Pathol.*, 48:209–215.
292. Williams, G. M., Iatropoulos, M. J., Jeffrey, A. M., Luo, F. Q., Wang, C.-X., and Pittman, B. (1999): Diethylnitrosamine exposure-response for DNA ethylation, hepatocellular proliferation and initiation of carcinogenesis in rat liver display non-linearities and thresholds. *Arch. Toxicol.*, 73:394–402.
293. Williams. G. M., Iatropoulos, M. J., and Whysner, J. (1999): Safety assessment of butylated hydroxyanisole and butylated hydroxytoluene as antioxidant in food additives. *Food Chem. Toxicol.*, 37:1027–1038.
294. Williams, G. M., Iatropoulos, M. J., and Jeffrey, A. M. (2000): Mechanistic basis for nonlinearity and thresholds in rat liver carcinogenesis by the DNA-reactive carcinogens 2-acetyl aminofluorene and diethylnitrosamine. *Toxicol. Pathol.*, 28:388–395.
295. Wiltse, J., and Dellarco, V. L. (1996): U.S. Environmental Protection Agency guidelines for carcinogen risk assessment: Past and future. *Mutat. Res.*, 365:3–15.
296. Wolfe, F. J. (1980): Effect of overloading pathways on toxicity. *J. Environ. Pathol. Toxicol.*, 3:113–134.
297. Yamamoto, S., Urano, K., Koizumi, H., Wakana, S., Hioki, K., Mitsumori, K., Kurokawa, Y., Hayashi, Y., and Nomura, T. (1998): Validation of transgenic mice in carrying the human prototype c-Ha-ras gene as a bioassay model for rapid carcinogenicity testing. *Environ. Health Perspect.*, 106:57–69.
298. Zeiger, R. (1998): Identification of rodent carcinogens and non-carcinogens using genetic toxicity tests: Premises, promises, and performance. *Regul. Toxicol. Pharmacol.*, 28:85–95.

Principles and Methods of Toxicology, Fourth Edition, edited by A. Wallace Hayes.
Taylor & Francis, Philadelphia © 2001.

Chapter **21**

Principles of Clinical Pathology for Toxicology Studies

Robert L. Hall

Clinical pathology is an integral component of preclinical safety assessment and toxicity studies designed to identify target organs and establish dose-response relationships. In the context of these studies, clinical pathology usually consists of relatively routine hematology, clinical chemistry, and urinalysis tests. The majority of the parameters evaluated are identical to those used in human and veterinary medicine because the fundamental physiology and pathophysiology of blood and major organ systems are similar in most mammalian species. There are, of course, species differences for reference ranges, some methodologies, the value or appropriateness of individual tests, and interpretation of findings. Selection of tests for a toxicology study is dependent upon several factors, including study objectives, test species, regulatory requirements, and characteristics of the test material.

Clinical pathology tests are best characterized as screening tools to identify general metabolic or pathologic processes and target tissues. Although specific diagnoses and precise mechanisms for a toxic effect are infrequently identified, test results narrow the possibilities and help direct further studies. Clinical pathology tests also provide one measure for determining the biological importance of effects associated with administration of a test material. Alterations in clinical pathology test results are typically not the only evidence of adverse or pathologically significant toxicologic effects. In-life clinical observations and/or anatomical pathology findings usually corroborate pathologically meaningful laboratory findings.

Interpretation of clinical pathology data from a toxicology study is considerably different from the assessment of data from an individual patient suffering from an unknown illness. The most obvious difference is that data from groups of treated subjects, receiving increasing dose levels of a test material, are compared with data from a group of age-, weight-, and sex-matched control subjects that are concurrently exposed to the same environmental and experimental conditions. For larger laboratory animals (e.g., rabbits, dogs, monkeys), pretreatment clinical pathology data for each individual are also available for comparison with posttreatment results. Finally, clinical pathology results from a toxicology study can be correlated with carefully recorded in-life observations, necropsy observations, organ weight data, and histopathologic findings for an extensive list of tissues. Given the uniformity of the animals studied and the analytical precision of modern clinical pathology instrumentation, identification of very subtle effects on clinical pathology results, which would not be apparent for an individual patient, is the norm. One of the most challenging aspects of data interpretation for a toxicology study is differentiating potentially harmful toxic effects from minor changes representing subtle homeostatic or metabolic responses to benign effects of the test material or to study-related procedures. Proper interpretation of clinical pathology results from a toxicology study requires not only an understanding of the tests themselves, but knowledge of species differences, study design, unique study-related procedures, clinical observations, anatomical pathology findings, and the test material. Interpretation of one test result is frequently dependent upon the results of another test, and pattern recognition is essential.

This chapter addresses (a) experimental design considerations including test selection, timing and frequency of testing, sources of variability in clinical pathology test results with emphasis on preanalytical factors, and quality control, (b) basic principles of clinical pathology data interpretation including the use and misuse of reference ranges, and (c) the characteristics and interpretation of routine hematology, clinical chemistry, and urinalysis tests used in toxicology studies. For in-depth descriptions of clinical pathology tests, including methods, the reader is referred to references 8, 14, 63, 68, 72, 73, and 84.

EXPERIMENTAL DESIGN CONSIDERATIONS

The value of clinical pathology in toxicology studies is heavily influenced by the experimental design. Selection and timing of appropriate tests, consideration of unique study procedures, reduction of sources of variation, proper sample collection and handling, and controlled analytical technique are all factors that ultimately determine the worth of clinical pathology test results.

Test Selection

The selection of appropriate clinical pathology tests for a toxicology study is first dependent upon the objective or purpose of that study. If the objective is simply to screen a number of similar chemical entities for potential hepatocellular toxicity, it may be sufficient to limit the laboratory evaluation to a single test such as alanine aminotransferase activity. On the other hand, if the study is part of the package of studies required to support governmental approval of a new drug or other chemical entity with potential human exposure (e.g., food additives, pesticides, chemicals used in manufacturing), there are several tests required or recommended in study guidelines published by the presiding governmental regulatory agencies (e.g., U.S. Food and Drug Administration, FDA; U.S. Environmental Protection Agency, EPA; Japanese Ministry of Health and Welfare) or professional standards organization (e.g., the European Organization for Economic Co-operation and Development, OECD) (60). Although there are many similarities between the various published guidelines with respect to recommended clinical pathology tests, there are also several differences and instances of ambiguous or inappropriate testing requirements.

In an effort to encourage global harmonization of regulatory guidelines, a Joint Scientific Committee for International Harmonization of Clinical Pathology Testing was formed in 1992 to provide recommendations for clinical pathology testing of laboratory animals used in regulated safety assessment and toxicity studies. The committee was comprised of representatives from ten different professional organizations, located throughout the world, with scientific expertise in animal clinical pathology and was independent of the International Conference on Harmonization of Technical Requirements for Registration of Pharmaceuticals for Human Use. The committee prepared a document (135) listing minimum recommendations for clinical pathology testing in regulated safety assessment and toxicity studies. These recommendations are described in the following paragraphs.

With respect to hematology, the core recommended tests are total white blood cell (WBC) count, absolute differential WBC count, red blood cell (RBC) count, hemoglobin concentration, hematocrit (or packed cell volume), mean corpuscular volume (MCV), mean corpuscular hemoglobin (MCH), mean corpuscular hemoglobin concentration (MCHC), evaluation of RBC morphology, and platelet count. The importance of calculating absolute WBC differential counts from the total WBC count and the relative (%) WBC differential counts was stressed. The method for evaluation of RBC morphology was not defined, but most laboratories prepare blood smears and examine the RBCs microscopically for morphologic characteristics such as variations in size (anisocytosis, microcytosis, or macrocytosis), color (polychromasia), shape (poikilocytosis), and hemoglobin content (hypochromasia). Other laboratories may choose to evaluate RBC morphology with the use of automated measurements such as MCV, MCH, MCHC, red cell distribution width (RDW), and hemoglobin distribution width (HDW). For those laboratories using automated measurements, it is prudent to routinely prepare blood smears in the event the data indicate a need to examine the cells microscopically.

Although not routinely recommended, absolute reticulocyte counts and bone marrow cytologic examinations may be indicated by other hematology findings. For example, test material-induced anemia is an indication for performing absolute reticulocyte counts to assess whether the anemia is regenerative or nonregenerative. Unexplained nonregenerative anemia, leukopenia, thrombocytopenia, and pancytopenia are indications for performing bone marrow cytologic examinations. It was therefore recommended that blood smears be prepared for possible reticulocyte counts and bone marrow smears be made at termination for possible cytologic examination. If a laboratory has the ability to perform automated reticulocyte counts, it may wish to do these routinely as an alternative to preparing reticulocyte count smears.

Prothrombin time (PT) and activated partial thromboplastin time (APTT) [or appropriate alternatives such as the Thrombotest (55)] and platelet count are the core recommended tests for assessment of hemostasis. If blood volume limitations are a concern (e.g., multiple blood collections for a rat study), it may be necessary to perform PT and APTT only at study termination.

Current regulatory guidelines recommend performing limited hematology tests on some or all animals at set intervals during a carcinogenicity/oncogenicity study (e.g., weeks 26, 52, 78, and 104). This approach to identifying leukemogenic test materials is very insensitive compared with the microscopic examination of multiple tissues from animals that died during the study, were terminated because of poor health, or survived to the terminal kill. For carcinogenicity/oncogenicity studies, the only procedure recommended by the Joint Scientific Committee is to make blood smears for all animals at unscheduled kills (e.g., moribund animals) and at the terminal kill. If necessary, the smears can be used as an adjunct to histopathology for the identification of hematopoietic neoplasia. For example, if the histopathologist is unsure whether leukocytic infiltrates in multiple tissues from an animal represent leukemia or a leukemoid response (i.e., marked leukocytosis secondary to an inflammatory stimulus), the blood smear can be examined to help differentiate between the two conditions. It may also be possible to diagnose a specific type of leukemia from the blood smear (e.g., lymphocytic leukemia versus granulocytic leukemia).

With respect to clinical chemistry, the core recommended tests are glucose, urea nitrogen, creatinine, total protein, albumin, globulin (calculated from total protein and albumin), cholesterol, calcium, sodium, potassium, and selected tests of hepatocellular and hepatobiliary health and function. Measurement of at least two scientifically appropriate tests for hepatocellular evaluation (e.g., alanine aminotransferase, aspartate aminotransferase, sorbitol dehydrogenase, glutamate dehydrogenase, or total bile acids) and at least two scientifically appropriate tests for hepatobiliary evaluation (e.g., alkaline phosphatase, gamma glutamyltransferase, 5′-nucleotidase, total bilirubin, or total bile acids) was recommended. Because there are several acceptable tests used to evaluate hepatic health and function, the Joint Scientific Committee decided it was appropriate to give each laboratory the freedom to choose those tests that best met their individual needs and with which they had the most experience. For example, glutamate dehydrogenase is commonly evaluated in Europe, but no commercial kit for this enzyme assay is available in the United States.

The core recommended urinalysis tests, performed on an overnight sample (i.e., approximately 16-h collection), are an assessment of urine appearance (color and turbidity), volume, specific gravity or osmolality, pH, and either the quantitative or semiquantitative determination of total protein and glucose.

The Joint Scientific Committee listed several tests that are specifically not recommended for routine use in animal toxicity and safety studies. These tests include ornithine decarboxylase, ornithine carbamoyltransferase, lactate dehydrogenase, creatine kinase, serum or plasma protein electrophoresis, microscopic examination of urine sediment, and urinary mineral and electrolyte excretion (e.g., urine sodium, potassium, chloride, calcium, or inorganic phosphorus excretion). Although ornithine decarboxylase appears in the test lists of several regulatory guidelines, it has no value as a diagnostic clinical chemistry test (19). This enzyme may have been included in the original FDA guidelines by mistake, and the error was repeated by other organizations. The FDA may have intended to include ornithine carbamoyltransferase, a liver-specific enzyme involved in the urea cycle that enjoyed limited popularity as a diagnostic test in the late 1970s. This enzyme never demonstrated a clear diagnostic advantage over other more common liver enzymes (e.g., alanine aminotransferase) and is rarely measured in today's laboratories. Lactate dehydrogenase is very similar to aspartate aminotransferase, and the use of another nonspecific enzyme is not considered beneficial. Creatine kinase may be helpful for evaluating test materials that cause muscle injury but is not considered necessary for the great majority of test materials, especially if aspartate aminotransferase is already part of the clinical chemistry test list. Blood collection techniques that potentially damage muscle and contaminate the blood sample (e.g., cardiac puncture and retro-orbital plexus collection) can diminish the value of measuring muscle enzyme activities by increasing variability. As a diagnostic test for patients, serum or plasma protein electrophoresis is used to evaluate large, unexplained increases or decreases in globulin concentration. With respect to increased globulin concentration, the goal of protein electrophoresis is to rule out a monoclonal gammopathy caused by some cancers of lymphoid origin (e.g., plasma cell myeloma). Monoclonal gammopathies and large, unexplained decreases in globulin concentration are rare in toxicity and safety studies, and the routine use of protein electrophoresis is inappropriate. Microscopic examination of urine sediment may be helpful for screening test materials that are known to cause severe renal or bladder toxicity, but histopathology is a more sensitive tool for detecting lesions of the kidney and bladder. In part, this is because the collection of high-quality urine specimens from many animals at one time is very difficult. On rare occasions, examination of urine sediment may be valuable for detecting the presence of crystals specific for a test material. Measurement of urinary mineral or electrolyte excretion may be appropriate for test materials that are known to affect renal function (e.g., diuretics) or bone metabolism (e.g., parathyroid hormone), but as routine screening tests, these are inappropriate. If serum/plasma mineral and electrolyte concentrations are greatly affected by a test material and other causes for these findings are ruled out (e.g., vomiting, diarrhea, renal failure), an assessment of the renal handling of the mineral or electrolyte in question may then be valuable.

The recommendations of the Joint Scientific Committee and the requirements listed in the various regulatory guidelines should be viewed as a minimum database for screening the potential toxicity of a test material that will undergo extensive evaluation in studies of varying duration with multiple species before regulatory approval. There are many additional tests that may be appropriate to perform, depending upon the study objectives and known characteristics of the test material. Platelet function tests (e.g., platelet aggregation and bleeding times) may be appropriate for evaluating drugs that target platelets. Analysis of methemoglobin concentration or the enumeration of erythrocyte Heinz bodies can be valuable for assessing oxidative injury caused by a compound. Activity of plasma or red blood cell cholinesterase is a measure of exposure to organophosphates or carbamates. Activity of brain cholinesterase is a measure of the toxic effect of these compounds. Determination of urinary enzyme activities and characterization of urinary protein excretion can be used for screening related compounds known or suspected to cause renal toxicity (29,77,117). Various hormones may be measured when endocrine dysfunction is suspected, and lipoprotein analysis may help define effects on lipid metabolism. Serum inorganic phosphorus and chloride concentrations are commonly measured as part of standard chemistry profiles in the United States and can be helpful when assessing changes in calcium and sodium concentrations, respectively. Determination of alkaline phosphatase and creatine kinase isoenzyme activities may help differentiate the origin of increases in total activity of these enzymes. The list of potentially valuable clinical pathology tests is long and growing. The key is to use the tests judiciously. That is, a nonstandard test should be used for a specific purpose and only after the test has been proven useful for the species in question.

Frequency and Timing of Testing

Frequency and timing of clinical pathology testing are dependent upon study objectives, study duration, the biological activity of the test material, and the species tested. The Joint Scientific Committee made minimum recommendations (135) that may be modified because of these factors.

With respect to regulated, acute, or single-dose toxicity studies, it is interesting to note that the regulatory guidelines have no clinical pathology requirements. Traditionally in these studies, the animals are dosed once and killed and necropsied following a 2-week observation period. Although the purpose of many of these studies is to determine appropriate dose levels for future repeated-dose studies, a great deal can be learned about potential toxicities of the test material because the dose levels are frequently higher than those administered in the repeated-dose studies. If clinical pathology tests are utilized, it is a mistake to wait until the end of the observation period to obtain samples. Two weeks following the administration of near-lethal doses of carbon tetrachloride or mercuric chloride to rats, standard clinical pathology tests will fail to recognize the effects of these compounds on the liver and kidney, respectively, because of the regenerative capacity and large functional reserve of these tissues. Although there is no single optimal time for all test materials, a general guideline for clinical pathology testing following an acute dose is to obtain samples between 24 and 72 h postdose. Occasionally, specific clinical pathology tests may be most appropriate within hours postdose because the test material has a very short half-life or a limited duration of action (e.g., some cytokines, peptides, and organophosphates). Following administration of acute renal toxins, urinary enzyme activities tend to be greatest in the first 24 to 48 h postdose. Alternatively, the effects of some test materials (e.g., cytotoxic chemotherapeutic agents) may take longer to reach their peak. For these test materials, it may be best to wait several days before performing clinical pathology tests or to take samples at multiple times in order to distinguish the time of greatest effect (e.g., days 4, 7, 10, and 14).

Limited blood volume in mice dictates that blood sample collection is usually practical only when the animals are killed. Because the blood volume of a 30-g mouse is less than 2 ml, it is difficult to acquire a full milliliter of blood from a single mouse, regardless of the blood collection technique. If several tests are required or desired (e.g., full hematology and clinical chemistry profiles), it may be necessary to specify certain animals for hematology tests and others for clinical chemistry tests. A preferred alternative is to limit the number of clinical chemistry tests to those that are the most relevant as screening tools for major organ toxicity (e.g., urea nitrogen or creatinine, alanine aminotransferase or another liver-specific enzyme, total protein, and albumin). Pooling of blood samples is inappropriate for clinical pathology testing.

Prestudy clinical pathology testing is not recommended for rats because of the relatively large number of animals per group, the homogeneity of the population, and the risk of adversely affecting the health of young animals due to blood loss or the blood collection procedure. For repeated-dose studies in rats, testing should at least be done at study termination. Interim testing may not be necessary for long-duration studies (e.g., a 13-week study) if testing were done in short-duration studies (e.g., a 4-week study) that used dose levels not substantially lower than those of the long-duration studies. On the other hand, interim testing (e.g., a week 6 testing point during a 13-week study) can be beneficial for interpretation of subtle effects. Clinical pathology testing is not recommended for rodents after 52 weeks because naturally occurring geriatric disease conditions (e.g., ulceration and infection of mammary gland tumors, chronic progressive nephropathy, pituitary tumors disrupting normal endocrine function) obscure meaningful interpretation of laboratory data.

For repeated-dose studies in dogs and monkeys, testing should be done before initiation (i.e., prestudy or baseline), at least once during the study, and at study termination. Animals shipped from a supplier should have several days to acclimate to the new environment before baseline testing is performed. The baseline data are important for screening out animals with potential health problems or results that are notably different from those of their peers. Findings that may signal possible subclinical health problems and that are commonly cited for eliminating animals from study consideration include low values for erythrocyte parameters (e.g., red blood cell count, hemoglobin concentration, hematocrit, and mean corpuscular volume), high white blood cell and neutrophil counts, low total protein and albumin concentrations, high globulin concentration, and high liver enzyme activities. There may be a specific need to eliminate otherwise healthy animals because they have findings that might complicate interpretation of test material-related effects. For example, beagles that are heterozygotes for factor VII deficiency have slightly prolonged prothrombin times. Even though these animals are clinically normal, it may be inappropriate to include one in a study evaluating a product that targets coagulation. One might choose to exclude an animal with a normally low neutrophil count from a study of a chemotherapeutic drug because it may be more difficult to determine if, or how much, the drug is impacting neutrophil production. By the same token, if an animal has an unusually high neutrophil count at a baseline interval simply because of excitement or fear during blood collection (i.e., physiological leukocytosis), then a subsequent postdose decrease in the neutrophil count, when the animal is less fearful of various procedures, could be overinterpreted as caused by the test material.

The advantage of using test animals such as dogs and monkeys with greater blood volume enabling more frequent clinical pathology evaluations is offset by the low number of animals in each treatment group (often four or less per sex per group) and the increased variability between animals for many tests. The lower the number of animals studied, the more desirable it is to have more than one baseline interval. Because monkeys tend to exhibit greater variability than dogs, it can be helpful for data interpretation to have more than one baseline interval for studies using monkeys, regardless of the number of animals per sex per group. An additional benefit to multiple baseline intervals is that the animals become more accustomed to the blood collection procedures, and variability caused by excitement or fear is generally reduced. In some range-finding studies, it is not unusual to have only one animal per sex per group. In essence, each animal serves as its own control. Using at least two baseline intervals affords an appreciation for normal day-to-day, intra-animal variability. Finally, two baseline intervals are generally desirable for animals that have been surgically manipulated (e.g., placement of indwelling intravenous catheters) to avoid using animals with iatrogenic complications.

The timing and number of clinical pathology intervals for repeated-dose studies in dogs and monkeys are often dictated by the test material. For studies of 6 weeks duration or less, an interim testing interval is sometimes recommended within 7 days of initiation of dosing. The primary purpose for this early interval is to detect transient increases in serum enzyme activities that may be absent at later intervals (34). This information can be very important for the clinical trials. For studies with cytotoxic chemotherapeutic agents, the number and frequency of hematology intervals are often considerable because one common objective is to identify the nadir for circulating leukocyte counts and the timing of hematopoietic recovery. For example, a single-dose study of a chemotherapeutic agent in dogs might require hematology tests twice before initiation of treatment and at days 4, 7, 10, 14, 21, and 28 and clinical chemistry tests twice before initiation of treatment and at days 7 and 28.

Urinalysis testing should be conducted at least once during a repeated-dose study. It is best to conduct the urinalysis testing at the same time as other clinical pathology tests. Although not stated in the Joint Scientific Committee's document, urinalysis testing for mice is impractical and not recommended as a routine test.

Sources and Control of Preanalytical Variation

Although most toxicology studies are relatively well controlled, there are many study design and procedural factors that affect variability of the data and impact clinical pathology evaluation and interpretation. In order to identify subtle (and in some cases, not so subtle) effects on clinical pathology test results, preanalytical sources of variation should be reduced whenever possible within the limitations of the study. Sources of variation can be loosely categorized as physiological, procedural, and artifactual. Physiological sources of variation include differences associated with age, strain, sex, diet, fasted condition, excitement or fear, stress, and time of blood collection. Procedural sources of variation include order of sample collection (i.e., group order versus randomization), blood collection site and technique, and anesthesia. Causes of artifactual or spurious results include poor-quality specimens (e.g., partially clotted hematology samples; hemolyzed serum/plasma samples), inappropriate use of an anticoagulant, improper sample storage, and iatrogenic blood loss.

Initiation of treatment for most regulated toxicology studies occurs when the animals are relatively young and still in a growth phase (e.g., rats 6–8 weeks old and beagles 4–6 months old). As the animals mature, several clinical pathology parameters are affected. Typical changes in most species include increasing red blood cell count, hemoglobin concentration, hematocrit, absolute neutrophil count, total protein and globulin concentration and decreasing reticulocyte count, mean corpuscular volume, absolute lymphocyte count, alkaline phosphatase activity, and inorganic phosphorus concentration. Although these and other age-related changes may be subtle, they are sufficient to evoke false conclusions if interpretation of posttreatment data were based solely on comparisons with pretreatment or baseline data collected more than a week or two earlier. Age-related changes are just one of many factors that make concurrent control groups an absolute necessity for most toxicology studies. As previously mentioned, the variability of a number of parameters becomes much greater for aging rodents, especially those over 1 year of age. This variability significantly reduces the likelihood of drawing meaningful conclusions from clinical pathology data collected in the latter half of chronic rodent studies.

Strain differences, especially for rodents, are important to consider when evaluating clinical pathology data. Differences for hematology parameters tend to be the most obvious. For example, Fischer 344 rats tend to have lower leukocyte counts than those of Sprague-Dawley rats but are also more predisposed to developing large, granular lymphocytic leukemia (86,119). An important difference has recently been identified for red blood cells of cynomolgus monkeys (*Macaca fasicularis*) based on geographical origin. Cynomolgus monkeys from China and contiguous areas such as Vietnam have much larger, but fewer, red blood cells than cynomolgus monkeys from Indonesia, the Philippines, or Mauritius (16). The differences are so great that reference ranges for red blood cell count and mean corpuscular volume for these animals may not overlap. Interpretation of hematologic effects could easily be compromised if monkeys from these different geographical origins were used in the same toxicology study or perhaps different studies of the same test material. Although not yet reported, it is likely that there are other differences for clinical pathology test results between these populations of cynomolgus monkeys.

Diet clearly affects many clinical pathology parameters, and standard diets are necessary to avoid small differences that might be misinterpreted. Comparison of data from animals fed purified or unusual diets with data from animals fed standard diets (e.g., historical reference ranges) should be done with caution. Some species, such as the rabbit, are prone to the effects of atherogenic diets and exhibit very high cholesterol concentrations when fed these diets. The amount of protein in the diet is known to affect urea nitrogen concentration but likely has subtle effects on other parameters over time. Because some diets, especially for dogs, are more prone than others to cause false positive results for fecal occult blood, diet can be an important factor when assessing the potential of a test material to cause gastrointestinal ulceration or hemorrhage.

Much has been published on the effects of fasting animals prior to blood collection for clinical pathology (1,76,85,87,124), and differences of opinion exist concerning this practice, especially with respect to rodents. While most laboratories routinely fast dogs and monkeys overnight prior to blood collection, procedures for rodents differ among laboratories. Historically, fasting has been encouraged in clinical practice as a means of reducing the variability of certain parameters, most conspicuously glucose concentration, so that the physician can more readily compare the results from a single patient with reference ranges in order to formulate a differential diagnosis. In toxicology studies, because the concurrent control group is much more relevant for comparison purposes than are historical reference ranges, the key principle is to treat all of the groups the same with respect to conditions prior to blood collection.

Fasting of mice for longer than a few hours is not encouraged because mice reduce their water consumption when fasted and rapidly become dehydrated. Not only does dehydration affect many clinical pathology parameters (e.g., erythrocyte count, serum protein concentrations, urea nitrogen concentration), it makes blood collection more difficult and reduces the volume of blood collected. Because some laboratories prefer to fast animals before killing (in part to reduce hepatocyte glycogen stores and improve histopathologic detection of hepatocellular injury or change) and because blood collection from mice is often a terminal procedure prior to sacrifice, mice are sometimes fasted for a limited time before blood collection and kill (e.g., four h). If this is done, care must be taken to keep the period of fasting similar for all animals even though the killing of many animals may take several hours because of necropsy procedures.

Most laboratories in the United States prefer to fast rats overnight. Although one frequently cited reason for this is to reduce variability for certain parameters such as glucose, perhaps the most important reason is to "standardize" the conditions for all animals. If animals in the high-dose group are eating poorly, providing all animals with access to feed before blood collection can have the effect of comparing fed animals (i.e., the control animals) to fasted animals (i.e., the high-dose animals). Since there are several differences for clinical pathology parameters between fed and fasted animals, it is more difficult to determine if differences between the control and high-dose groups are due to an effect of the test material or simply to differences in overnight feed consumption. When compared with rats having access to feed, fasted rats tend to have lower white blood cell counts; lower urea nitrogen, cholesterol, triglyceride, calcium, and bilirubin concentrations; and lower alanine aminotransferase and alkaline phosphatase activities (76,87).

Excitement/fear and stress can have pronounced effects on clinical pathology test results. Excitement and fear are associated with acute endogenous catecholamine release ("fight or flight" phenomenon), and stress is associated with endogenous corticosteroid release. Effects of catecholamines are immediate but short-lasting (e.g., less than 30 min). Effects of corticosteroids tend to be more gradual and long-lasting. The most obvious changes observed in very excited or frightened animals are increased leukocyte counts and glucose concentrations. These changes are observed occasionally with the overexcited beagle and with unanesthetized monkeys that are not used to handling for blood collection. Monkeys may also react to the presence of several people in the animal room performing additional study-related procedures at the same time as blood collections. Endogenous corticosteroids affect leukocyte counts, but somewhat differently than catecholamines. Whenever possible, clinical pathology testing should be delayed for at least a week following shipping or surgical procedures to avoid stress-related changes.

Blood samples should be collected in a manner that minimizes the possibility of temporal biases. Examples of time-related biases include differences between morning and afternoon results (circadian effects), differences caused by delayed separation of serum from clotted blood, and day-to-day differences (may be preanalytical or analytical). These biases can be eliminated or at least minimized by randomization of the animals for blood collection and the use of procedures that enable blood collection and sample processing over the shortest reasonable amount of time. An alternative to true randomization is a structured pattern of bleeding such that one animal from each group is bled in succession. Once samples have been collected, they should be analyzed in the same order as the blood collection. Rearranging the samples back to group order has the potential of causing false positive findings that are actually due to analytical drift. For example, a small drift in the analysis of chloride by ion-selective electrode (e.g., an increase of 2 mmol/L over 60 samples) may be sufficient to produce a statistically higher mean chloride concentration for the high-dose animals if the groups are sufficiently large (e.g., 15 animals/sex/group), the control animals are analyzed first, and the high-dose animals are analyzed last. If animals must be bled over 2 days because of laboratory or necropsy capacity issues, the problem of day-to-day variability can be reduced by collecting and analyzing samples from the males on one day and the females on the other.

Randomization of animals for blood collection is occasionally impractical (e.g., if timed collections must follow intravenous administration of the test material). When animals must be sampled by group, it is better to sample the high-dose group immediately before or after the control group than to sample the animals in consecutive group order (i.e., control, low-dose, mid-dose, high-dose). If it is necessary to sample the animals in consecutive group order, then procedures must be in place to analyze or process the samples in a similar time frame. When control animals are bled 1 h or more before the high-dose animals, analysis of the hematology samples and separation of the chemistry samples should not be delayed until all of the groups are bled. Such a delay can result in differences between the control and high-dose groups that are due solely to time-related, in vitro changes. This is most likely to occur for rodents when blood collection is one of the terminal procedures and several hours are necessary to bleed, sacrifice, and necropsy all of the animals. If hematology analysis of whole blood from the control animals is delayed, it is possible that the last group bled will appear to have increased platelet counts relative to those of the control group because platelet counts decrease over time as a result of spontaneous platelet aggregation. If clotted blood from the control group is allowed to stand 1 or 2 h longer than that from the high-dose group before separation of serum, the high-dose group will often have statistically significant differences for several chemistry parameters, including higher glucose concentration, lower potassium and inorganic phosphorus concentrations, and lower aspartate aminotransferase and lactate dehydrogenase activities. These differences result from changes in the control animal samples—that is, the consumption of glucose by erythrocytes, and the release of cell constituents by erythrocytes, leukocytes, and platelets. Circadian effects are another potential source of variation when blood collection is protracted. For example, rodents bled early in the morning can have slightly higher leukocyte counts than those bled in the afternoon during their normal period of inactivity.

Collection site, collection technique, and use of anesthesia are perhaps the most commonly cited procedural influences on clinical pathology test results. Many investigators have analyzed differences in data resulting from these variables (6,33,75,76,86,88,92,94,104,112,118, 121,126), especially for the rat. But while differences in the results do exist (e.g., total leukocyte counts in samples from the retro-orbital venous plexus are higher than those from larger vessels such as the abdominal aorta or posterior vena cava; glucose concentrations in samples from the abdominal aorta are higher than those from other sources), the principal message from these works is that laboratories should use the technique with which they have had good success obtaining high-quality samples and with which they are most comfortable. Use of an unfamiliar or unpracticed blood collection technique introduces unnecessary variability and spurious results. With appropriate instruction and practice, any of the commonly used techniques can generate adequate results. To optimize the value of the data, however, a single method of collection should be used throughout a study or series of comparable studies. For example, anesthesia tends to decrease interanimal variability for clinical pathology results from monkeys, especially their cell counts and electrolyte concentrations. If pretreatment or baseline blood collection is performed on animals anesthetized for physical examinations or other baseline procedures, the relatively heterogeneous data obtained from unanesthetized animals during treatment may cause confusion or be misinterpreted. Similar problems can occur when interim blood samples from rodents are collected from the tail or retro-orbital venous plexus, and terminal blood samples are collected from the heart or posterior vena cava. Small differences observed between control and treated animals at one interval may be masked at another interval because of increased preanalytical variability. The cause of the variability is often related to differences in bleeding technique proficiency and not the method itself (88).

Blood collection from dogs, monkeys, and rabbits is facilitated by relatively easy access to large vessels (e.g., jugular, cephalic, and saphenous veins for dogs; femoral, cubital, and saphenous veins for monkeys; ear and jugular veins for rabbits). Blood collection from mice is complicated by size and volume limitations, and terminal procedures are often used (e.g., cardiac puncture or sampling of the posterior vena cava or abdominal aorta at necropsy). There are many acceptable methods for blood collection from rats, and the choice of technique depends on a number of factors, not the least of which is frequency of opportunities to collect blood from rats. If a laboratory performs enough studies on rats to require blood collection every day or two, then it is probably worthwhile for some of the technical staff to become proficient at collecting blood from the jugular vein (105). Although every bleeding technique has procedural advantages and disadvantages, this technique offers the greatest number of advantages if mastered. Several high-quality blood samples can be collected from one animal, directly from a large vessel with needle and syringe, without anesthesia or expensive equipment, and without damaging important structures such as the eye or heart. Because there are no time-consuming ancillary procedures (e.g., warming the tail to dilate the tail vein or anesthesia), samples can be collected quickly, and it is possible to accurately collect timed samples (e.g., at 1, 5, 10, and 15 min postdose) from a single animal. As with most techniques, blood collection from the jugular vein requires regular practice to remain proficient.

Inappropriately collected or prepared samples increase variability of the data by introducing spurious or artifactual results. Fibrin or clot formation in a hematology sample always results in a spuriously low platelet count but may also cause low erythrocyte and leukocyte counts. Small clots may form because of an insufficient amount of anticoagulant (potassium ethylenediamine tetraacetic acid [K EDTA] is the anticoagulant of choice for hematology samples), inadequate mixing of the blood with anticoagulant, or poor blood collection technique with exposure of the blood to substances from traumatized tissue. Excessive anticoagulant can cause dilutional errors for cell counts and prolonged coagulation times. In addition to the dilutional error, manual packed cell volumes are further lowered because of shrinkage of the erythrocytes. The use of an inappropriate anticoagulant can cause spurious results and must be avoided. Intentional or accidental exposure of clinical chemistry samples to K EDTA results in very high potassium concentrations, very low calcium and magnesium concentrations due to chelation, and very low activities of enzymes such as alkaline phosphatase and creatine kinase that use magnesium as a cofactor (41). Trisodium citrate, the anticoagulant of choice for the coagulation assays, also chelates divalent cations and would additionally increase sodium concentration if incorrectly used for the clinical chemistry sample.

Hemolysis can be caused by poor technique for sample collection, sample transport, or serum/plasma separation, and hemolysis can result in spuriously increased or decreased test results by two principle mechanisms: release of erythrocyte constituents, and interference with test methodology (41,50,53,80,81).

Techniques and procedures should be chosen that eliminate in vitro hemolysis to the greatest extent possible.

As previously indicated, prolonged contact between serum and clotted blood causes spurious changes that can be controlled by prompt separation of the serum (143). Although most analytes are relatively stable for a reasonable amount of time (73,97,125), unnecessary delay or storage of samples before analysis should be avoided. Ideally, hematology samples should be analyzed within a few hours of collection and no later than 24 h after collection. If samples for coagulation tests cannot be run on the day of collection, the plasma should be frozen at $-20°C$ and thawed only once before analysis (38). If samples for clinical chemistry tests cannot be run on the day of collection, the serum or plasma (lithium heparin is the recommended anticoagulant when plasma is used for clinical chemistry) should be refrigerated or frozen overnight. If there will be a long delay before analysis or if a desired analyte is relatively labile, then the samples should be frozen at $-70°C$.

There are several other sources of variation for clinical pathology data, but the impact of each on data interpretation in toxicology studies is generally minimized by the inclusion of age and sex-matched control groups exposed to the same environmental conditions and undergoing the same experimental procedures. Occasionally overlooked are the effects of procedures that may differ between the control and treated groups. Because toxicology studies in larger animals frequently include blood collections for analyses other than clinical pathology (e.g., toxicokinetic measurements or detection of antibody directed at a peptide test material), it is imperative that control animals be bled in a similar manner to the treated animals. The number and volume of blood samples for these tests can have a significant effect on hematology and clinical chemistry results (108), and data interpretation is seriously compromised if control animals do not undergo the same procedures. Even when control animals are bled in a like manner, iatrogenic blood loss can complicate data interpretation (67).

Analytical Variation and Quality Control

In addition to sources of variation that occur before sample analysis, the analytical procedure itself is a source of variation. Analytical variation is minimized by an active quality control system within the clinical pathology laboratory. Detailed discussions of quality control systems are available in many textbooks (14,100,138). At a minimum, the quality control system should include initial verification that a new method satisfies the goals of the laboratory for accuracy and precision for the analyte being measured; standard operating procedures for all laboratory functions necessary for analysis and reporting of test results; documentation of routine instrument calibration procedures; documentation of routine and nonroutine instrument maintenance; documentation of appropriate personnel training; proper labeling of all reagents, controls, standards, calibrators, and other chemicals in the laboratory; routine analysis of quality control specimens and review of quality control data for detection of systematic errors; routine review of "patient" data for detection of random errors; standard procedures for responding to and documenting "out-of-control" situations; and participation in some form of external quality control or proficiency testing with "unknown" samples for analysis.

Analytical variation is affected by the accuracy and precision of a test procedure. Accuracy is a measure of the extent to which the mean estimate of a quantity approaches its true value, and precision is a measure of the agreement among replicate measurements (i.e., the reproducibility of a test result). Accuracy is generally determined in a formal way when a new method is introduced into the laboratory, and it is continually reassessed, albeit somewhat crudely, by means of proficiency testing. Most analytical procedures exhibit a small amount of systemic bias or inaccuracy that is either constant or proportional. In other words, the mean estimate of the quantity of analyte is always in error in the same direction, either higher or lower, than the true quantity. Precision of a test can be assessed within a single run (e.g., 20 consecutive analyses of the same sample for within-run precision) or from day to day (e.g., the same sample analyzed several days in a row for between-run precision) and is reflected by a test's coefficient of variation (CV). The CV expresses the error or variability of replicate test results as a percentage of the mean value (i.e., [standard deviation/mean] $\times$ 100); the lower the CV, the greater is the test's precision or repeatability.

Although accuracy and precision are both desirable, test procedures can be accurate but imprecise or inaccurate but precise. In the context of most toxicology studies, where results from groups of treated animals are compared with results from concurrent control groups and their own pretreatment results, good precision is more valuable than good accuracy. This is in contrast to the clinical setting, where the physician or veterinarian evaluates individual patients under less controlled conditions and uses, by necessity, broad historical reference ranges for making decisions. An imprecise test, regardless of accuracy, is less able to detect small differences between the control and treated groups. If the true mean glucose concentrations for 4 control dogs and 4 treated dogs are 100 and 115 mg/dl, respectively, but the standard deviations for the groups are large because of imprecision, then it is unlikely that the observed difference between the means (i.e., 15 mg/dl) will be considered a real difference. A precise test, regardless of a systemic bias or inaccuracy, is better able to identify small test material-related differences between the groups. In the same example, if the glucose test had a positive bias but was more precise, the means of the two groups might be 110 and 125 mg/dl with lower standard deviations. The improved precision permits a more accurate interpretation of the same 15-mg/dl difference between group means.

Clinical pathology laboratories that test animal samples frequently use tests, especially standard clinical chemistry tests found in routine chemistry panels, that are optimized for accuracy using human samples. It is likely that many of these tests have small systemic biases when used for animal specimens. In most cases, however, the excellent precision afforded by using standardized commercial reagent kits, standards, and calibrators is preferable to time-consuming, costly efforts to optimize the accuracy of a test for different animal species by using "home-brew" materials that undermine precision. Occasionally there are standard chemistry tests that do not work well for certain species, such as albumin for rabbits, and these tests require specialized methods. Immunoassays utilizing monoclonal or polyclonal antibodies raised against human substances (such as hormones) are frequently inappropriate for use on animal specimens, and hematology analyzers that enumerate and differentiate blood cells must be modified for animal blood because of differences in cell morphology.

For human hospital laboratories, federal regulations allow each laboratory to set its own policies for assaying control materials as long as at least 2 control samples of different concentrations (i.e., normal and abnormal levels) are assayed every 24 h. The data from each quality-control analysis are used to make decisions about the validity of the patients' data. In the setting of preclinical toxicology studies, it is advisable to assay at least two control samples with each study run. In other words, if a laboratory is scheduled to run samples from two or more regulated toxicology studies (e.g., studies needed to make submissions to regulatory agencies and using Good Laboratory Practices), then quality control samples should be assayed with each of the studies, and the results should be maintained with the study data. If results from a control sample are found to exceed the allowable limits for one or more analytes, then steps must be taken to resolve the problem. Actions that may be taken include, but are not limited to, the following: check for obvious problems such as reagent levels, clots, or mechanical fault; repeat the assays on control samples using fresh aliquots; repeat the assays using newly reconstituted control samples; recalibrate the instrument for the analyte(s) in question, then reassay the control samples; change the reagents, recalibrate, and reassay the control samples; and perform maintenance, recalibrate, and reassay the control samples.

PRINCIPLES OF DATA INTERPRETATION

Interpretation of data from toxicology studies begins with the identification of differences between control and treated groups and ends with an assessment of toxicological or biological relevance. Or in other words, are there real differences between the groups, and if so, are those differences bad? Interpretation of clinical pathology data requires an understanding of each test's characteristics, species differences, and principles of internal medicine. Factors that influence the interpretation of a potential effect include study design and conditions, clinical observations, other clinical pathology results, anatomical pathology findings, and the test material itself. Interpretations of many clinical pathology findings are interdependent, and pattern recognition is critical. After range-finding studies have been conducted, appropriate dose selection usually precludes large, dramatic effects on clinical pathology test results. The most common effects are relatively mild and often appear to be secondary to small alterations in metabolic or homeostatic mechanisms. However, test materials causing significant damage to liver, kidney, or hematopoietic tissue can produce marked changes in clinical pathology results. Effects on clinical pathology results are rarely the only evidence of biologically important or adverse toxic effects. Clinical observations or anatomical pathology findings usually corroborate biologically important laboratory findings.

Statistical Comparisons

Statistical analysis of clinical pathology data is commonly performed in toxicology studies, and it often results in identification of several statistically significant differences between control and treated groups. However, all effects caused by a test material need not be statistically significant, and all statistically significant differences do not necessarily represent true or toxicologically significant effects. If used, statistical tests should be viewed simply as a tool to help identify differences between groups and not as the principal justification for decisions concerning potential test material effects (20,26). It is important to remember that the power of a statistical test is affected by the number of animals per group. Fewer test subjects increases the likelihood that statistical tests will fail to identify a true effect. Since the number of animals/per group is usually quite small for studies with dogs or monkeys (e.g., 4/sex/group, or less), it is imperative that the data for each animal at the different test intervals be examined to look for patterns of change over time among the treated animals that are absent among the control animals. As the number of animals per group increases, the frequency of identifying statistically significant differences of very small magnitude increases. In rat studies with 15 or more animals per sex per group, it is common to observe statistically significant differences that have little or no effect on the health of the animals and are not toxicologically relevant.

Is an Apparent Difference Real?

When faced with an apparent difference between control and treated groups, the first answer the investigator must determine is whether or not that difference represents a true effect of the test material or is an incidental finding. Many factors can influence the answer, not the least of which is the size of the difference. A large difference is obviously more likely to be real than a small one. Additional factors that favor a difference being test material-related include dose dependency, consistency over time, consistency between sexes, correlation with clinical observations (e.g., low chloride concentration and emesis), correlation with other clinical pathology findings (e.g., low hematocrit and high reticulocyte count), correlation with anatomical pathology findings (e.g., high globulin concentration and lymph-node hyperplasia), presence in a large number of animals (e.g., 15/sex/group versus 3/sex/group), and consistency with previously identified effects of the test material or related compounds. With large animals, it is necessary to make certain that an apparent difference was not present before treatment was initiated. The chronology of an apparent difference is also important for interpretation. For example, following a single administration of most test materials, it is more likely that a real difference will occur within a few days rather than only after 2 weeks. Following repeated administration of most test materials, it is more likely that a real difference will occur after a few months of treatment rather than only after several months. In other words, it is somewhat unusual that a real difference at 6 months will be completely absent at 3 months.

With regard to specific tests and test species, the amount of expected analytical, interanimal, and intra-animal variability can influence the interpretation of apparent differences. For example, because alanine aminotransferase activity has much greater interanimal and intra-animal variability for monkeys than for dogs, a relatively modest difference for this enzyme between control and treated groups is less likely to be a true effect for monkeys. Interanimal variability increases dramatically for older rodents (e.g., >52 weeks of age) because of naturally occurring disease conditions, and small differences between groups are less likely to represent true effects. Procedural factors such as the route of test material administration, blood collection technique, and randomization for blood collection also affect variability and must be considered. For example, continuous intravenous infusion increases interanimal variability for several tests (e.g., white blood cell count, hematocrit, serum proteins), and interpretation of small differences in results of these tests is difficult. Blood collection by cardiac puncture affects variability of muscle enzymes such as creatine kinase and aspartate aminotransferase. The potential for spurious findings associated with lack of randomization for blood collection was discussed previously.

Is a Real Difference Bad?

If a difference between control and treated groups is clearly real, the next answer the investigator must determine is whether or not that difference represents a bad or adverse effect. Does the finding itself (e.g., low hemoglobin concentration) or the condition that caused the finding (e.g., blood loss from gastrointestinal erosions/ulcerations) represent a toxic effect that compromises the animal's health? The answer is often ambiguous and quite subjective. Many of the factors previously considered are important, and the size of the difference is clearly a focal point. Although a large difference for a given parameter is more likely to be adverse than a small difference, it is clearly not that simple, and it is not possible to define set limits for each test that represent an adverse effect. The same magnitude of change for a given test can have completely different connotations depending upon the mechanism for that change, correlative findings, the test species, the study design and procedures, and the test material itself (e.g., a clinical pathology parameter may be the target for the pharmacological activity of a drug). Urea nitrogen may be markedly increased because of dehydration (e.g., mice that have been fasted too long before blood collection or animals that refuse to drink water containing test material), but only mildly increased in the early stages of renal toxicity. Increased alanine aminotransferase activity associated with histopathological evidence of hepatocellular degeneration and necrosis is likely to be more toxicologically important than the same level of increase for which there are no correlative findings. Because of species differences for interanimal variability, a threefold increase for alanine aminotransferase activity for dogs (i.e., treated vs. control group means) is more likely to represent an adverse condition than the same increase for monkeys. A 10% decrease in hemoglobin concentration is less likely to represent an adverse condition in animals that were bled repeatedly during a study or that received the test material by continuous intravenous infusion than in animals that were not bled repeatedly or were treated by oral gavage. Very high neutrophil counts would normally reflect an adverse condition, but if the test material was a granulocyte colony-stimulating factor, the high counts would be a desirable effect.

Some tests measure analytes that are critical to good health (e.g., neutrophil count, hemoglobin concentration, glucose concentration, calcium concentration, potassium concentration), and correlative in-life observations (e.g., bacterial infections, lethargy, weakness, weight loss) may help determine whether an observed effect on such a test has impacted the animals' health. Other tests measure analytes that are markers for effects best evaluated by histopathological examination (e.g., alkaline phosphatase, urea nitrogen). All routine tests can be altered by more than one process or mechanism, and some mechanisms have worse implications than others. For example, increased urea nitrogen in mice associated with poor feed and water consumption is likely of less concern than increased urea nitrogen because of proximal tubular necrosis. When determining the biological or toxicological significance of an effect on a clinical pathology test result, consideration must be given to the analyte's normal function for maintaining health, correlative findings that may better define the overall impact of the test material on health, and the mechanism that brought about the change.

Reference Intervals

Like statistical comparisons, historical reference intervals can be used as a tool when assessing apparent differences between control and treated groups. Unfortunately, the value of reference intervals for data interpretation is sometimes overestimated, and the potential for their improper use is great (61,131,134). It is tempting to invoke historical reference intervals when trying to decide whether apparent differences for clinical pathology results are true effects or whether they are adverse effects. While historical reference intervals can be helpful for establishing some perspective concerning what is typical or expected, the conditions of every toxicology study are unique, and it is inappropriate to use a reference interval as the primary reason for dismissing an apparent difference between control and treated animals as being incidental or biologically insignificant. It can be equally inappropriate to use a reference interval as the primary reason for determining that an apparent difference is real or adverse. As detailed in the previous sections, there are many other factors to consider when evaluating the nature of an apparent test material effect.

Reference intervals (often incorrectly referred to as reference ranges or normal ranges) are constructed with values obtained from reference individuals. In most clinical pathology laboratories used for toxicology studies, the reference individuals are control animals from previous studies and clinically healthy animals that have not received treatment (e.g., monkeys or dogs that have clinical pathology tests performed before initiation of dosing). In human medicine, the National Committee for Clinical Laboratory Standards recommends that reference intervals be estimated by the nonparametric method and that a minimum of 120 values from reference individuals be used (93). Test results from the reference individuals are subjected to statistical treatment such that rare values at both ends of the distribution are eliminated. For example, if the lowest and highest 2.5% of the values are eliminated, the resulting reference interval represents the central 95% of the distribution of values. If the distribution is gaussian, the interval corresponds to the mean$\pm$1.96 SD. By definition, when the central 95% is used as the reference interval, 5% of the results from "normal" individuals (1 of 20) are outside of the reference interval for any given test. Clearly, a value outside of the reference interval does not necessarily indicate an abnormality (36).

The suitability of a historical reference interval for data interpretation for a given study is a function of the parameters or *partitioning factors* that define the reference population used to construct the interval. There are many potential partitioning factors with respect to toxicology studies, and their importance is sometimes overlooked. The most commonly used partitioning factors are species, strain, sex, and age. In other words, a typical reference population might be defined as male Fischer 344 rats from 8 to 10 weeks of age. However, many other partitioning factors can influence the reference interval and make it broader, narrower, higher, or lower. These factors include animal supplier, site of blood collection, use of anesthetic, type of anesthetic, diet, fasting status, time of sample collection, and sample matrix (e.g., serum or plasma). If control animals are used for the reference population, additional partitioning factors include route of administration (e.g., dietary, oral gavage, or intravenous infusion), vehicle or control material administered (e.g., sterile water or corn oil in a gavage study; sterile saline or 5% dextrose in an intravenous infusion study), and whether or not the animals were bled repeatedly for toxicokinetic analyses or multiple clinical pathology intervals. Finally, there are laboratory considerations including instrumentation or technique used to analyze the specimen and sample storage conditions (e.g., storage temperature and time interval between collection and analysis). Ideally, whenever a new instrument or reagent system is introduced, a new reference interval is constructed. In practice, laboratories often rely on evidence that demonstrates relative consistency between the old and new analytical methods to avoid complete replacement of old intervals.

The number of partitioning factors used obviously has a direct impact on the number of reference individuals available for each reference interval. With the exceptions of reference intervals for dogs and monkeys tested before treatment is initiated (e.g., male beagles, 4 to 6 months old, XYZ supplier, jugular vein, no anesthetic, fasted), it can be very difficult obtaining enough data for meaningful reference intervals. Because of this problem, laboratories often ignore many of the partitioning factors and "lump" together the data from control animals of dissimilar types of studies or from samples that have been handled differently. The result is broader reference intervals with less relevance to data interpretation.

Even when reference intervals are appropriate for a given study (i.e., the partitioning factors match the study animals, conditions, and procedures), it is wrong to assume that a difference between control and treated groups represents a true effect or an adverse effect simply because the mean of the treated group falls outside of the reference interval. Concurrent control animal data for a given study are never a perfect reflection of the historical reference data; that is, they do not exhibit the same means and distribution. The mean for the control group may fall anywhere within the reference interval, and the distribution of results for the control group is almost always narrower than that of the reference interval. Depending on the location of the control group data within the reference interval, a very small, incidental difference for the treated group may fall outside of the reference interval and a relatively large, adverse test material-induced difference may fall within the reference interval. There are many situations when a small difference, within the reference interval, represents a very significant adverse effect. For example, anemia and hypoproteinemia can be masked by dehydration, and the loss of an entire subpopulation of lymphocytes is not necessarily enough to cause absolute lymphocyte count to fall below the reference interval. When reference intervals are broad, as occurs when few partitioning factors are used or normal interanimal variability is great (e.g., alkaline phosphatase activity for monkeys), significant toxicity can occur without test results exceeding the limits of the intervals. Investigators must understand the limitations of reference intervals with respect to data interpretation. By themselves, reference intervals do not determine whether or not an apparent difference is real or adverse. They are simply an adjunct to sound scientific judgment.

Regardless of the many pitfalls affecting their use for data interpretation, historical reference intervals do have other important functions. They serve as a nonspecific measure of quality control that can detect changes over time in assays, study conditions, or animal characteristics. For example, it may be noticed that liver enzyme activity in mice has increased over time. The cause of this finding might be traced to changes in handling practices or animal supplier. Reference intervals also serve as a nonspecific measure of analyte variability. The cause of seemingly excessive variability might be inadequate assay precision, nonstandardized preanalytical procedures, or true interanimal variability. Finally, reference intervals can be valuable when very few animals are used for small investigational studies with no concurrent control group. Although pretreatment baseline data are more relevant to interpretation of potential effects, it may be discovered that the few animals acquired for the study have preexisting problems or are atypical with respect to historical data.

HEMATOLOGY TESTS AND INTERPRETATION

The hematology tests recommended and most often performed for toxicology studies evaluate erythrocytes, leukocytes, platelets, and coagulation. Technological advances by manufacturers of hematology and coagulation analyzers, along with a growing interest in supporting customers who must evaluate samples from a variety of animal species, have increased the availability of highly sophisticated instruments to perform these tests with precision and accuracy suitable for preclinical safety assessment studies. The automated methods are a necessity. Manual methods are unacceptably imprecise, labor-intensive, and slow. Many currently marketed hematology instruments are capable of measuring or calculating all of the routinely recommended tests and more from less than 150 μl of anticoagulated whole blood. The instruments typically utilize a combination of two or more principles including electrical aperture impedance, laser light scatter, and differential staining characteristics to determine cell number (RBC, WBC, and platelet counts), cell size and size distribution (MCV, RDW, mean platelet volume [MPV], and platelet distribution width [PDW]), and cell type (WBC differential count). They measure hemoglobin concentration directly and calculate MCH and MCHC; some also calculate HDW. Because the blood cells of laboratory animal species differ morphologically from human blood cells, instruments and the instrument software used for human samples are generally inappropriate for use without modifications. Fortunately, instrument manufacturers are producing instruments with the necessary modifications to permit accurate and precise analysis of blood from a variety of laboratory animals species. Modifications have also been made for coagulation analyzers that measure the time required for fibrin clot formation in a plasma sample, to which reagent has been added, by detecting changes in conductivity, physical resistance, light scatter, or optical density. Most instruments can now be programmed to permit detection of clot formation at times much faster (e.g., prothrombin time for dogs) or slower (e.g., prothrombin time for guinea pigs) than are typically observed for human samples.

Erythrocytes

Effects on erythrocyte parameters typically reflect a change in the balance between red blood cell production and red blood cell loss or destruction. In addition, changes in plasma volume (e.g., dehydration or volume expansion) can indirectly affect erythrocyte parameters. Although mechanisms for effects on erythrocyte parameters may be obvious, such as hemorrhage from gastric ulceration, they are often relatively obscure. But even when the exact mechanism is unclear, the effects can usually be described in terms of broad mechanistic categories and impact on health.

Anemia

Anemia is defined clinically as the condition characterized by a hemoglobin concentration below the lower reference limit. RBC count and hematocrit may or may not be proportionately lower, depending on the cause of the anemia and whether or not cell size and hemoglobin content are affected. Low hemoglobin concentration reduces the oxygen-carrying capacity of blood, which in turn may result in clinical signs such as pallor, weakness, exercise intolerance, tachycardia, or tachypnea. In many toxicology studies, a treated group has lower means for RBC count, hemoglobin concentration, and hematocrit than those for the control group, but the differences are less than those necessary to cause clinical signs and are not indicative of anemia. For example, reductions from control values for these parameters up to approximately 10% are relatively mild and probably do not have an adverse effect on the health of the animal. Reductions from approximately 10% to 25% may be considered a moderate effect and may or may not be clinically adverse. Reductions of more than 25% are marked and clearly represent a clinically adverse anemic condition. Keep in mind that while a 5% reduction in hemoglobin concentration may be insufficient to adversely affect health, the cause of the reduction (e.g., liver toxicity) may be very adverse. Unless the differences for RBC count, hemoglobin concentration, and hematocrit are quite large, it is preferable to simply discuss the magnitude of the differences between the control and treated groups and avoid using the term *anemia*. In this chapter, however, *anemia* is used for the purposes of discussing mechanisms.

Anemias are broadly categorized as regenerative or nonregenerative. Regenerative anemias are characterized by an appropriate erythropoietic response to reduced circulating erythrocyte mass or hemoglobin concentration, and nonregenerative anemias are characterized by the absence of an appropriate erythropoietic response.

Regenerative anemias result from two general causes: abnormal blood loss (hemorrhage), and accelerated erythrocyte destruction (hemolysis). Following acute blood loss or hemolysis, it takes approximately 3 to 4 days for new erythrocytes, called reticulocytes, to increase in number in peripheral blood. Reticulocytes are larger and slightly more basophilic than mature erythrocytes when stained with the Romanowsky-type stains (e.g., Wright or Giemsa stain) typically used for assessing red blood cell morphology and doing manual WBC differential counts. During a strong regenerative response, erythrocyte morphology is described by the terms *anisocytosis* (variable size) and *polychromasia* (variable color) because of the increased numbers of reticulocytes. Greater numbers of nucleated red blood cells, also called metarubricytes, and Howell–Jolly bodies (small pieces of nuclear material not cleared from the erythrocyte) may be observed during a regenerative response, but these may also increase with some nonregenerative conditions. Reticulocytes can be counted with an automated reticulocyte counter or counted manually by staining blood with a vital stain such as new methylene blue before making a blood film. For proper interpretation, the absolute reticulocyte count (i.e., reticulocytes/μl) should always be determined by multiplying the relative reticulocyte count (i.e., percent of erythrocytes) by the RBC count. Relative reticulocyte counts can be increased in severely anemic animals even though the absolute reticulocyte counts are no different than for normal animals. In this case, the erythropoietic response is not appropriate for the degree of anemia and indicates inadequate RBC production is at least partially responsible for the anemic condition. During a strong regenerative response, the increased number of "young" erythrocytes will usually result in higher MCV and lower MCHC because these relatively large cells have lower hemoglobin concentration. In practice, higher MCV is more commonly observed than lower MCHC. During a strong regenerative response, erythrocyte production can increase six- to eightfold over normal levels. As long as the accelerated erythropoiesis is able to match the erythrocyte loss or destruction, the anemia will not become worse. If erythropoiesis exceeds the loss or destruction, or if their cause is eliminated, the anemia will be reversed.

In toxicology studies, mild nonregenerative anemias are more common than regenerative anemias. If normal erythrocyte production is reduced for any reason, or if erythropoiesis does not increase in response to decreased erythrocyte survival, circulating erythrocyte mass will decrease over time. In nonregenerative anemia, erythrocyte morphology is characterized by the absence of anisocytosis and polychromasia. Most often, the erythrocytes appear normocytic (normal size) and normochromic (normal color). Absolute reticulocyte count is unchanged or decreased, depending on whether the problem is simply an inability to adequately respond to increased needs or, more significantly, failure of erythropoiesis. Mean corpuscular volume is typically unchanged or mildly decreased.

The most common hematology findings in preclinical toxicology studies are mildly decreased RBC count, hemoglobin concentration, and hematocrit without a corresponding increase in absolute reticulocyte count and without an obvious mechanism for the effect. The decreases are usually no more than about 10% from the values for the respective control group (e.g., mean control group hematocrit = 44%; mean high-dose group hematocrit = 40%) and less than what would be classified as anemia. Slightly lower MCV (e.g., control mean = 56 fl; high-dose mean = 54 fl) may also be observed, especially in rodents. In conjunction with these minor effects, the animals may exhibit mild reductions in body weight or body weight gain and less frequently, feed consumption. They may have other clinical signs of poor health, including dull haircoat, poor grooming habits, and decreased activity. Potential concurrent effects on other clinical pathology test results include mildly decreased total protein and albumin. Although specific mechanisms for these changes are typically not identified, they suggest a generalized reduction of anabolic processes. Anything that affects the normally brisk pace of RBC production (in humans, approximately 100 billion new cells/day), will ultimately be reflected in the test results. It is possible that decreased physical activity and correspondingly decreased tissue oxygen demand may contribute to reduced erythropoiesis. These relatively mild, nonspecific findings for circulating erythrocyte mass are identified most frequently in rat studies where the number of animals per sex per group is usually high (e.g., 10 animals per sex per group), the dose levels used are typically higher than those for dog or monkey studies, and the normal interanimal variability of hematology data is relatively low. In addition, because the circulating life spans of mouse and rat erythrocytes (approximately 25 to 40 and 45 to 65 days, respectively) (68) are shorter than those for dogs (approximately 100 to 120 days) and nonhuman primates (varies with species; for rhesus monkeys, approximately 85 to 100 days) (68), similar reductions in RBC production will first become apparent for mice and rats.

Nonregenerative Anemias

There are several other causes of reduced RBC production, and they are distinguished from one another by their severity, the presence of morphologically distinct erythrocytes, and other findings that identify the etiology. Test materials may affect RBC production directly or indirectly. Direct inhibition of erythropoiesis, if sustained, will result in a gradually developing, severe anemia because senescent erythrocytes are not replaced. Indirect effects on erythropoiesis are more common in toxicology studies and result from toxic effects on other tissues or organ systems. Indirect effects on the erythron tend to be relatively mild and are not as toxicologically important as the effects on the primary target tissue.

Direct injury to pluripotent hematopoietic stem cells or their stromal microenvironment causes failure of blood cell production, resulting in the condition called *aplastic anemia* (109,137). Aplastic anemia is characterized by varying degrees of pancytopenia (i.e., decreased erythrocytes, leukocytes [primarily neutrophils], and platelets) and hypocellular bone marrow. If the animal survives long enough, the anemia becomes severe. Typically, however, decreased resistance to bacterial infections causes severe illness or death before the anemia is life-threatening. Irradiation is a classic model of stem cell injury and is used therapeutically as part of the process for bone marrow transplantation. In addition to irradiation, several chemicals and drugs are known to cause aplastic anemia in humans. These include benzene, toluene, lindane, pentachlorophenol, chloramphenicol, phenylbutazone, penicillamine, gold salts, and acetazolamide. Chemotherapeutic drugs such as alkylating agents (e.g., busulfan and cyclophosphamide), antimetabolites (e.g., fluorouracil and methotrexate), and cytotoxic antibiotics (e.g., doxorubicin and daunorubicin) have the potential to cause aplastic anemia because of their pharmacological activity. Normally, however, their effects are reversible following completion of each treatment cycle. In toxicology studies with test materials such as these, decreased WBC and platelet counts are typically recognized earlier in the study (generally 7–10 days after initiation of treatment) than decreased RBC counts because the circulating life spans for neutrophils (12–24 h) and platelets (7–10 days) are much shorter than that for erythrocytes. On the other hand, reticulocyte counts can be a sensitive indicator of hematopoietic injury and may be better than WBC or platelet counts for identifying the onset of toxic effect and subsequent recovery. The value of assessing reticulocyte counts when testing antineoplastic drugs is most apparent in rodent studies because the normally high reticulocyte counts for young rodents facilitate identification of decreases while their normally low neutrophil counts make neutropenia more difficult to recognize. Furthermore, reticulocyte counts are not compromised by poor blood collection technique that may cause increased interanimal variability for platelet count. The timing of sample collection following administration of a test material that temporarily interrupts hematopoiesis will dictate the findings in peripheral blood and can impact interpretation. During the peak effect, reticulocytes, neutrophils, monocytes, eosinophils, platelets, and often lymphocytes are decreased in number, and histopathologic examination of the bone marrow reveals hypocellularity. Once the effect ends, hematopoietic tissue usually mounts a strong recovery, sometimes called a rebound effect, that is characterized peripherally by reticulocytosis, thrombocytosis, and sometimes neutrophilia. Increased extramedullary hematopoiesis in the spleen, especially for rodents, is often apparent before the bone marrow repopulates. Because the time to peak effect and the duration of effect vary for different test materials, it is necessary to perform hematology tests at multiple intervals for proper interpretation.

Pure red cell aplasia is rarely observed in toxicology studies, even though several drugs are known to cause the disorder in humans (46). Because drug-induced pure red cell aplasia is usually an idiosyncratic condition and may be immune mediated, recognition of this toxic effect is low in animal studies using a limited number of test subjects. Furthermore, it would be very difficult to prove that uncomplicated, nonregenerative anemia in a single animal was a direct effect of the test material.

Chronic inflammatory diseases (44,48,49) and significant kidney (23), liver (99), and endocrine dysfunction (e.g., hypothyroidism and hypoadrenocorticism) (45) negatively affect erythropoiesis and erythrocyte survival, and all of these conditions can be associated with a mild to moderate, normochromic, normocytic anemia. With chronic inflammatory conditions, the principle cause of reduced erythropoiesis is thought to be decreased availability or transfer of iron to developing erythrocytes. True iron deficiency, most commonly associated with chronic blood loss or inadequate dietary iron, is relatively rare in toxicology studies, and, in contrast to the anemia of chronic disease, is characterized by microcytic (low MCV), hypochromic (low MCHC) erythrocytes. With renal disease, reduced erythropoiesis is attributed to decreased renal production of erythropoietin and the effects of "uremic toxins." Liver failure is sometimes associated with acanthocytosis, a morphological abnormality of erythrocytes characterized by several blunt cytoplasmic projections resembling pseudopodia. The acanthocytes are thought to result from accumulation of free, nonesterified cholesterol in the RBC membrane. Acanthocytes are relatively inflexible and are eventually removed from circulation by cells of the mononuclear phagocyte system. Small reductions in circulating erythrocyte mass are observed with hypothyroidism and may result from reduced basal metabolic rate and cellular requirements for oxygen. Changes in thyroid metabolism may play a role in the mild erythrocyte effects observed in some animals with reduced food consumption because caloric malnutrition can result in decreased T_3 and decreased responsiveness to T_3, which may in turn lead to reduced production of erythropoietin.

Megaloblastic anemia is a nonregenerative anemia characterized by macrocytic erythrocytes, asynchronous maturation of cytoplasm and nucleus in hematopoietic precursors, and hypersegmented or "giant" neutrophils (2). In humans, it is associated with a variety of disorders that cause folate or vitamin B_{12} deficiency (e.g., sprue, alcoholic cirrhosis, and pernicious anemia) and drugs (e.g., methotrexate) that impair DNA synthesis. Macrocytosis results because developing erythrocytes undergo fewer divisions before maturation. Megaloblastic anemia is rarely identified in laboratory animals, perhaps due to differences in uptake and metabolism of folate and vitamin B_{12}. On the other hand, nonhuman primates have been used frequently as animal models for folate and vitamin B_{12} deficiency (142).

Finally, nonregenerative anemia is usually a feature of leukemia because the proliferating neoplastic hematopoietic cells compete with normal hematopoietic cells for nutrients and space in the bone marrow and spleen. It is not unusual in carcinogenicity studies to observe severe anemia secondary to naturally occurring leukemia in a few animals.

Regenerative Anemias

Blood loss can occur secondary to a variety of conditions or study-related procedures and should always be considered when a decrease in circulating erythrocyte mass is accompanied by a similar decrease in serum protein concentration. The source of the blood loss may be identified by clinical observations (e.g., dermal ulceration, melena, epistaxis), necropsy findings (e.g., gastrointestinal ulceration, cystitis), or other laboratory tests (e.g., fecal and urine occult blood tests). Blood loss associated with serial blood collection for pharmacokinetic investigations, clinical pathology tests, or other study-specific requirements must always be accounted for when interpreting changes in erythrocyte parameters. Blood loss typically results in increased polychromasia, MCV, and reticulocyte count unless the condition is very acute (i.e., less than the 3–4 days necessary for the regenerative response to build up) or there are complicating factors affecting erythropoiesis.

There are a number of potential mechanisms for test material-induced hemolysis, but the three most common mechanisms observed in toxicology studies are direct damage to the red blood cell membrane, oxidation of hemoglobin resulting in Heinz body formation, and immune-mediated red blood cell destruction (90). Each has specific characteristics, and they are relatively easy to differentiate.

Test materials administered intravenously are those most likely to be associated with direct damage to the red blood cell membrane. The lipid bilayer of the cell membrane is sensitive to test materials with detergent-like properties, and intravascular hemolysis can occur rapidly during treatment when the red blood cells are exposed to high concentrations of the test material at the site of injection or infusion. If the amount of released hemoglobin exceeds the carrying capacity of circulating haptoglobin, unbound hemoglobin passes through the glomerulus and is excreted in the urine. Visible hemoglobinuria (red-tinged urine) may be observed within a few hours of treatment, and a regenerative response is detectable in the blood within 3 or 4 days of treatment. Intravenously administered test materials that cause extensive intravascular hemolysis are usually associated with local damage to endothelium. The effect of the vascular damage may be observed grossly (e.g., tail lesions in rodents treated via the tail vein) or histologically. Additional histological evidence of intravascular hemolysis is the presence of hemoglobin pigment within renal tubular epithelial cells and hemoglobinuric nephrosis. Administration of a very hypotonic solution, as might occur if sterile water is inappropriately chosen as the vehicle for a low concentration solution, is another potential cause of acute intravascular hemolysis. Water passively enters red blood cells because of the ionic concentration gradient, and the cells swell and rupture. Hypertonic solutions typically do not cause hemolysis.

Heinz bodies are particles of irreversibly denatured hemoglobin attached to the interior of the red blood cell membrane. They result when test materials with oxidative properties cause disulfide bonds to form from the sulfhydryl groups of hemoglobin. Red blood cells containing Heinz bodies may be removed from circulation by cells of the mononuclear phagocyte system (extravascular hemolysis), or they may become morphologically distinct (e.g., ghost cells and blister cells) following selective removal of the Heinz bodies. Although Heinz bodies can be difficult to detect with the Romanowsky-type stains, they stain prominently with vital stains such as methylene blue, crystal violet, or brilliant cresyl blue used for manual reticulocyte counts, and the number of affected cells can be determined in the same manner as that for manual reticulocyte counts. The size and number of Heinz bodies are dependent on the causative agent, the dose, and the time after exposure. Acute exposure to a potent oxidative agent typically causes an acute anemia characterized by the observation of many affected red blood cells containing a single, large Heinz body, or, less frequently, multiple, small Heinz bodies. Ghost cells, blister cells, and other morphologic abnormalities may be present. Reticulocytosis develops after 3 to 4 days. As is true for most causes of significant, acute extravascular hemolysis, splenomegaly and extramedullary hematopoiesis are common findings. Bilirubinemia and bilirubinuria are possible but less common correlative findings. Chronic, low-level exposure to an oxidizing agent usually does not cause anemia. Although absolute reticulocyte count and MCV may be slightly increased, hematocrit and hemoglobin concentration are relatively unchanged or only slightly reduced. The number of red blood cells containing Heinz bodies is low, and they may go unrecognized if not looked for specifically. Identification of test materials that cause Heinz body formation is particularly important clinically because the most common human erythrocyte enzyme deficiency, glucose-6-phosphate dehydrogenase deficiency, makes affected individuals particularly susceptible to oxidant-induced hemolysis (7).

Test materials that cause Heinz body formation have the potential to cause methemoglobinemia and vice versa (91). Methemoglobin is hemoglobin in which the iron has been reversibly oxidized from the ferrous state (Fe^{2+}) to the ferric state (Fe^{3+}); it is incapable of carrying oxygen. The clinical signs of methemoglobinemia, therefore, are those of hypoxia. Mucous membranes become cyanotic at methemoglobin concentrations above 10%. Lethargy and weakness occur at concentrations of approximately 30% or more. At greater than 80%, methemoglobinemia may be fatal. Blood containing a high concentration of methemoglobin appears brown. Accurate and efficient measurement of methemoglobin concentration can be accomplished with dedicated instruments called hemoximeters. These multiwavelength, microprocessor-controlled photometers are designed to measure hemoglobin pigments such as carboxyhemoglobin and methemoglobin as well as the percentage of hemoglobin oxygenation. Samples collected for methemoglobin determination should be analyzed quickly (e.g., within 30 to 60 min) because methemoglobin is normally reduced by the erythrocyte enzyme methemoglobin reductase. The combination of a sensitive, precise instrument and a well-executed toxicology study allows detection of test material-induced methemoglobin formation at concentrations well below those necessary to cause clinical signs (35). Among laboratory animals, the mouse is a poor model for studying the potential of test materials to cause methemoglobinemia because it has very high activity of methemoglobin reductase (115). Test material-induced methemoglobin in mice is quickly reduced to hemoglobin and therefore more difficult to detect.

Immune-mediated red blood cell destruction has been associated with many drugs (98) but is largely an idiosyncratic phenomenon and is therefore detected infrequently in preclinical toxicology studies. When it is observed, there are typically only one or two animals affected, and they may or may not be in the high-dose group. In contrast to hemolytic conditions that occur immediately upon exposure to the test material, immune-mediated hemolysis is typically not observed until the test material has been administered for at least a week. There are three general mechanisms for immune-mediated hemolysis: The test material acts as a hapten bound to the red blood cell membrane; the test material elicits an antibody response and the resulting antigen–antibody complex binds to the red blood cell; and the test material causes the immune system to mistakenly recognize normal red blood cell membrane antigens as foreign, and true autoantibodies are produced. On rare occasion, immune-mediated hemolysis is complement mediated and intravascular. More commonly, cells of the mononuclear phagocyte system, especially in the spleen, recognize antibody-coated red blood cells and either phagocytize the entire cell (extravascular hemolysis) or remove a portion of its membrane, creating morphologically distinct cells called spherocytes. In a blood film, spherocytes appear smaller and denser than other red blood cells; they are perfectly round and lack central pallor. While small numbers of spherocytes can be observed with other conditions, they are the predominant morphologic feature of immune- mediated hemolytic anemia. Autoagglutination of red blood cells will sometimes occur, especially if the antibody response is primarily immunoglobulin M (IgM), and may be observed in the blood film. Alternatively, autoagglutination may be detected in a wet mount of fresh blood diluted with saline. Direct antiglobulin tests may be used to confirm the presence of antibody or complement on red blood cells, but species-specific anti- immunoglobulin or anticomplement must be used. Animals with test material-induced immune-mediated hemolytic anemia become severely anemic with repeated administration of the test material. However, they usually exhibit a strong regenerative response and will nearly always recover if administration of the test material is stopped. Confirmation that the anemia was induced by the test material can be accomplished by rechallenging the animal following recovery. Upon rechallenge, hemolysis should be evident within a day or two. Immune-mediated hemolytic anemia, unrelated to test material administration, is a common sequela of the large granular lymphocyte leukemia observed in a high percentage of Fischer 344 rats older than 1 year of age (119).

Whenever regenerative anemia is identified in a nonhuman primate study, consideration must be given to the possibility of hemolysis associated with the hemotropic parasite *Plasmodium*. Many imported monkeys, even though they are captive bred, harbor subclinical infections with the organism that causes malaria (39). The readily identifiable intracellular organism is frequently observed in blood films from healthy animals that have no signs of anemia. Parasitemia, however, is inconsistent or cyclical, and multiple blood samples may be examined from an animal before the organism is identified. On rare occasion, administration of a test material or the stress of shipment and study-related procedures precipitates a hemolytic crisis. When this occurs, the parasitemia is usually quite obvious.

An infrequent cause of hemolysis in toxicology studies is mechanical fragmentation or microangiopathic hemolysis. This form of hemolysis typically occurs when red blood cells are forced to pass through small, fibrin-obstructed vessels in highly vascular tissue. The resulting fragmented red blood cells are called schizocytes (helmet cells) and are easily identified microscopically. Disseminated intravascular coagulation (DIC) is the best example of a condition causing microangiopathic hemolysis, but widespread vascular injury in tissues such as lung, liver, or intestine also causes some degree of fragmentation. These conditions, especially DIC, are generally so severe that an animal may fail to mount a significant regenerative response before it dies or is humanely killed.

Leukocytes

The differential WBC count enumerates neutrophils, lymphocytes, monocytes, eosinophils, and basophils in peripheral blood. Increased numbers of these cells in circulation are termed neutrophilia, lymphocytosis, monocytosis, eosinophilia, and basophilia, respectively. Neutropenia, lymphopenia, monocytopenia, and eosinopenia refer to decreases; normal basophil numbers are so low that decreases are not recognized. Leukocytosis and leukopenia are less specific terms that indicate increased and decreased total WBC count, respectively. When interpreting and reporting differential WBC count results, it is essential to evaluate the absolute cell counts (i.e., cells/μl). Relative or percent counts are simply a means for determining the absolute counts and have little or no inherent value for assessing an animal's condition. A 50% neutrophil count in a dog could be normal or represent neutrophilia or neutropenia, depending on the total WBC count.

Neutrophils and lymphocytes are the most numerous cell types in peripheral blood, and toxicological effects on leukocytes usually involve them. While direct effects on these two cell lines can and do occur (136), indirect effects, in response to study-related procedures or test material effects on other tissues, are much more common.

Physiological Leukocytosis

Excited or frightened animals may exhibit a physiological leukocytosis secondary to endogenous catecholamine release. Increased heart rate, blood pressure, and muscular activity shift cells from the marginal leukocyte pool (i.e., cells that adhere to the endothelium of small vessels or are sequestered in vascular beds of tissues like the spleen) to the circulating leukocyte pool. The total WBC count may double in number. The specific cell type responsible for the majority of the increase varies with species because of species-dependent differences in normal distribution of leukocyte types. Neutrophilia is the most obvious change for dogs, while lymphocytosis is most conspicuous for rats. The physiological leukocytosis observed for primates is fairly evenly distributed between neutrophils and lymphocytes. Because physiological leukocytosis is most frequently observed in animals that are not accustomed to handling or blood collection, it is not unusual for a few animals to have notably high WBC counts only at the first blood collection interval for a study. Recognition of this phenomenon is critical in studies using few animals (usually dogs or monkeys) and only one pretreatment interval. Overinterpretation of the data might lead to the false conclusion that a test material has a myelosuppressive effect because posttreatment WBC counts, determined when the animal is less excited, may be much lower than pretreatment counts. By the same token, if the test material is an antineoplastic drug, and myelosuppression is a critical endpoint, strong consideration should be given to acquiring at least two pretreatment hematology samples to facilitate proper data interpretation.

Steroid- or Stress-Induced Leukocyte Response

This leukocyte pattern occurs following exogenous corticosteroid administration or when stressful conditions result in increased production of endogenous corticosteroids. It is characterized primarily by mature neutrophilia (immature neutrophils, such as bands, are absent), lymphopenia, and eosinopenia. Monocytosis may or may not be present. It is relatively unusual to observe this pattern for an entire group of animals on study, even though study-related procedures or administration of the test material appear to create conditions typically considered stressful. However, individual animals, especially those in moribund condition resulting from toxicity, often exhibit this pattern.

Neutrophilia and Neutropenia

Although their primary function is to protect the host from bacterial infections, neutrophils are a common component of many nonseptic inflammatory lesions as well. It is therefore not unusual to observe increased neutrophil counts secondary to a variety of inflammatory conditions resulting from test material toxicity or study-related procedures (e.g., chronic catheterization or repeated injections), with or without the involvement of an infectious agent. If severe enough, degeneration and necrosis of most tissues result in inflammation and a systemic neutrophil response. Hemolysis, for example, can be a potent stimulus for neutrophilia. In addition, various cytokines with therapeutic potential have been identified and produced that affect neutrophil kinetics directly and may result in mild to marked neutrophilic leukocytosis. The term *left shift* refers to an increased number of immature neutrophils (e.g., band ncutrophils) in circulation, usually in response to an inflammatory lesion with a significant demand for neutrophils. Lesions that cause left shifts or marked neutrophilia are almost always easily identified, either by physical examination or at necropsy, and often involve invasion of damaged tissues by bacteria. The term *degenerative left shift* describes the combination of a normal or decreased absolute neutrophil count with more immature than mature neutrophils. It generally reflects a very severe infection as might occur with aspiration pneumonia, gastrointestinal perforation, or septicemia associated with bacterial contamination of an indwelling intravenous catheter. In conditions such as these, "toxic neutrophils" may be observed. These neutrophils have distinct morphological characteristics including cytoplasmic basophilia, vacuolation, and granulation and the presence of Döhle bodies (small, bluish-gray cytoplasmic inclusions made of aggregated rough endoplasmic reticulum).

Unless the test material is a potent cytotoxic agent (e.g., a conventional chemotherapeutic), the observation of severe neutropenia, with or without a left shift or toxic neutrophils, is generally limited to one or two individuals that have severe complications secondary to test material toxicity or study-related procedures. Leukocyte effects of cytotoxic agents, on the other hand, are typically observed in most or all of the animals in groups receiving toxic dose levels. Because mice and young rats normally have very low neutrophil counts (e.g., less than $1000/\mu l$), recognition of neutropenia is more difficult for these species than for others. In addition, while a neutrophil count below $500/\mu l$ is generally considered an indicator of great risk for bacterial infection in humans, monkeys, and dogs, the same is not true for rodents.

Single or short-term administration of a potent cytotoxic agent is usually characterized by neutropenia within a few days to a week of treatment, followed by a recovery that may include the presence of immature neutrophils for a short time and may result in a rebound neutrophilia. Detection of these changes is dependent on the timing and frequency of hematology testing. Similarly, the appearance of the bone marrow, whether hypocellular or hypercellular, is also dependent on timing of sample collection. Hematology findings for test materials that directly injure pluripotent stem cells or rapidly dividing committed precursor cells are usually characterized by decreased numbers of reticulocytes, platelets, neutrophils, monocytes, eosinophils, and possibly lymphocytes. Selective damage of granulocyte precursors without affecting erythropoiesis or thrombopoiesis is unusual.

Lymphocytosis and Lymphopenia

Lymphocytes are responsible for a wide variety of immune system functions. There are several subpopulations of lymphocytes, but they are indistinguishable by light microscopy. Lymphocytes are relatively long-lived compared with other leukocytes and have the ability to leave the vascular system through venules in lymph nodes and eventually reenter the blood via the thoracic duct. Lymphocytosis is an uncommon test material-related effect, although it may be observed in conjunction with chronic inflammatory lesions, especially in rodents, or with administration of test materials that are antigenic and elicit an immune response by the test animals. Physiological leukocytosis should be considered whenever lymphocytosis is present in only a few animals.

Lymphopenia is most frequently observed as part of the stress- or steroid-induced leukocyte response. Moribund animals are commonly lymphopenic. Cytotoxic test materials often cause decreased absolute lymphocyte count, but the magnitude of the decrease is usually less prominent than that for neutrophils. In rodents, however, it may be easier to detect the effect on lymphocytes because of the normally high number of lymphocytes compared with neutrophils. During recovery from effects of cytotoxic test materials, lymphocyte counts may remain decreased longer than neutrophils and typically do not exhibit a prominent rebound response. Because of the many subpopulations of lymphocytes, it is difficult to gauge the biological importance of small decreases in absolute lymphocyte count. Selective reduction or elimination of a subpopulation may occur (e.g., the human immunodeficiency virus effect on CD4+ lymphocytes) without greatly affecting the total lymphocyte count. Evaluation of the overall health of the animals and findings that might suggest immunosuppression are essential correlates that help to place the importance of small changes into context.

Monocytes, Eosinophils, and Basophils

Absolute counts for these cell types are generally quite low (e.g., $<1000/\mu l$), and effects on these cells are infrequently observed in toxicology studies. As with neutrophils and lymphocytes, increases in circulating numbers of these cells are generally secondary phenomena unless the test material is a hematopoietic growth factor or other cytokine (e.g., interleukin-5 increases eosinophil count) that directly stimulates cell production. Eosinophils are part of the body's defense against helminthic parasite infections, and eosinophilia is occasionally observed in nonhuman primates with a heavy parasite load. Eosinophilia is also observed secondarily to some hypersensitivity reactions. A primary function of monocytes is phagocytosis and digestion of large particulate matter, such as senescent cells and necrotic cell debris. Monocytosis may occur secondarily to any condition with substantial tissue destruction, such as widespread inflammation, tumor-associated necrosis, or hemolytic anemia. Because of their normally low circulating numbers, decreases in these cell types are often difficult to detect. However, eosinopenia and monocytopenia are sometimes identified following administration of chemotherapeutic agents, and eosinopenia is occasionally observed as part of the stress-induced leukocyte pattern. Effects on basophil counts are extremely rare.

Leukemia

In most, if not all, 2-year carcinogenicity studies using rodents, a small percentage of the animals will develop leukemia, a neoplastic proliferation of a hematopoietic cell line. Although leukemias are often characterized by markedly elevated white blood cell counts and the presence of neoplastic cells (e.g., blasts) in circulation, some animals with leukemia exhibit neither of these prominently, and the diagnosis is best made by histopathological examination of tissues infiltrated with the neoplastic cells. The odds of correctly identifying animals with leukemia are much greater by doing routine histopathology than by doing periodic examinations of the blood at regularly scheduled intervals. Even when neoplastic cells are present in peripheral blood, it is often difficult to determine from which cell line they were derived (e.g., granulocytic, lymphocytic, myelomonocytic, etc.) because immature, anaplastic, or blast-stage cells from different cell lines can be indistinguishable by light microscopy using standard staining techniques.

The most commonly observed leukemia in laboratory animals is large granular lymphocyte leukemia of Fischer 344 rats (119). As many as 30–40% of Fischer 344 rats may develop this leukemia, also known as mononuclear cell leukemia, in the second year of a carcinogenicity study. The neoplasm appears to arise in the spleen and commonly infiltrates other tissues, particularly the liver. Affected rats consistently develop an immune-mediated hemolytic anemia and often exhibit hyperbilirubinemia and elevated liver enzyme activities in the serum. Neoplastic cells in peripheral blood appear as large, immature lymphocytes and may contain prominent azurophilic granules. Erythrophagocytosis by the neoplastic cells is occasionally observed.

Platelets

When blood vessels are damaged, platelets quickly adhere to the subendothelium, undergo a shape change, and begin to aggregate, forming a primary platelet plug that is sufficient to control bleeding from minor injuries to small vessels. These activated platelets secrete a variety of substances that stimulate vasoconstriction and promote fibrin formation. Fibrin serves to cement the aggregated platelets into a stable hemostatic plug. Healthy endothelial cells in close proximity to the damaged vessel release inhibitors of platelet aggregation and fibrin formation in order to limit the size of the clot.

Thrombocytosis is typically asymptomatic, although extremely high platelet counts may increase the risk of thrombosis. Signs of thrombocytopenia include petechial and ecchymotic hemorrhages, most commonly observed in mucous membranes or at mucocutaneous sites, epistaxis, melena, menorrhagia, and prolonged bleeding from small wounds such as venipuncture sites. These signs typically do not occur spontaneously unless the platelet count is very low (e.g., less than 20,000/μl) or there is some type of hemostatic challenge (e.g., surgery) (9). Test materials that affect platelet function have the potential to cause the same clinical signs as marked thrombocytopenia, but the tendency to do so is much less because of the complexity of platelet function and the presence of alternative or redundant pathways in vivo for the various platelet functions. Platelet function tests such as bleeding time and platelet aggregation may be beneficial when evaluating safety of therapeutic agents related to coagulation and platelet function, but it is important to recognize the considerable analytical and interanimal variability for these tests. Group results may be less meaningful than assessment of results from individual animals before and after test material administration.

Thrombocytosis

Unless the test material is a hematopoietic growth factor (e.g., thrombopoietin), increased platelet count is almost never a primary effect. The terms *reactive* or *secondary thrombocytosis* have been used to describe the increased platelet count observed in conjunction with generalized bone marrow stimulation as observed with hemolytic anemia, blood loss, and many types of acute and chronic inflammation. Release of cytokines such as interleukin-6 and interleukin-11 may be at least partially responsible for the increased platelet production (141) in some of these conditions. Acute, transient thrombocytosis may occur in association with physiological leukocytosis because catecholamine-induced splenic contraction releases platelets into circulation that were sequestered within the sinusoids of the spleen. A rebound thrombocytosis typically follows significant thrombocytopenia caused by test materials such as chemotherapeutic agents that reversibly inhibit platelet production or injure megakaryocytes. The increased platelet counts observed in toxicology studies are generally small and not likely to have any biological significance.

Thrombocytopenia

Decreased platelet count is a relatively common spurious finding associated with difficult venipuncture or inadequate anticoagulation of the blood sample and subsequent in vitro platelet aggregation. When this occurs, platelet clumps can usually be observed at the feathered edge of the blood film. Although most typically a problem detected for individual mice and rats, spuriously low platelet counts can sometimes appear group related because animals receiving the test material may be more difficult to bleed as a result of poor health, dehydration, or small size relative to the control animals.

When not a spurious finding, decreased platelet count results from decreased production or increased consumption of platelets. Test materials that reduce erythroid and myeloid cell production, such as chemotherapeutic agents, frequently inhibit platelet production as well. Moderately to markedly reduced platelet counts tend to occur a few days after obvious reductions in neutrophil and reticulocyte counts because the circulating life span of platelets is about 7 to 10 days. Thrombocytopenia due to increased consumption of platelets can occur secondarily to acute lesions of highly vascular tissues such as the gastrointestinal tract or result from extensive hemorrhage, especially from multiple sites. If lesions affecting blood vessels are severe and widespread, disseminated intravascular coagulation may develop, and platelet counts will be markedly decreased. Immune-mediated thrombocytopenia, like immune-mediated hemolytic anemia, has been associated with many drugs (54) but is largely an idiosyncratic phenomenon and is therefore detected infrequently in preclinical toxicology studies. When observed, there are typically only one or two animals affected, and these animals may or may not be in the high-dose group. Immune-mediated thrombocytopenia and immune-mediated hemolytic anemia may occur together. Antiplatelet antibody is very difficult to detect, and the best evidence that thrombocytopenia is immune mediated may come from a rechallenge exposure with the test material following cessation of treatment and recovery. Upon rechallenge, platelet count should drop acutely if the mechanism is immune-mediated destruction.

Bone-Marrow Smear Evaluation

The most important aspect of bone marrow smear evaluation is understanding when it is indicated. Although preparation of smears is advisable for most regulated, repeated-dose toxicology studies, evaluation of those smears is usually unnecessary. The standard hematology tests provide considerable information concerning bone marrow function, and if results from these tests are unaffected, it is very unlikely that bone marrow evaluation will provide any additional knowledge concerning potential significant test material effects on the hematopoietic system. Even when results of hematology tests are affected by administration of a test material, bone marrow evaluation has no benefit if mechanisms for the hematology findings are already evident. For example, regenerative anemias indicate a normal erythropoietic response to hemorrhage or hemolysis, and bone marrow evaluation would simply confirm the presence of erythroid hyperplasia. Neutrophilic leukocytosis in response to an inflammatory condition is normal, and bone marrow evaluation would only confirm granulocytic hyperplasia. The main indications for bone marrow smear evaluation in toxicology studies are moderate to marked nonregenerative anemia, leukopenia, or thrombocytopenia (or any combination of the three) with no apparent etiology. If the effects observed in peripheral blood are relatively small, it is less likely that bone marrow smear evaluation will be beneficial. The primary objective of the bone marrow smear evaluation is to assess the relative numbers of precursor cells, their morphologic appearance, and whether they are developing or maturing normally. Miscellaneous findings such as increased iron stores, plasma cell hyperplasia, or excessive cytophagia may also be recognized.

There are multiple approaches to bone marrow smear evaluation. Regardless of the approach taken, the findings must be interpreted in conjunction with peripheral blood test results. The most simplistic and least informative bone marrow evaluation is to determine the myeloid:erythroid (M:E) ratio by counting at least 500 cells and differentiating the granulocytic cells from the erythroid cells. An increased M:E ratio may indicate granulocytic hyperplasia, erythroid hypoplasia, or both. If the animal has a high neutrophil count and its hematocrit is normal, then an increased M:E ratio likely indicates granulocytic hyperplasia. If the animal has a normal neutrophil count and a nonregenerative anemia, then an increased M:E ratio likely indicates erythroid hypoplasia. In both cases, the outcome of the M:E ratio could have been predicted from the peripheral blood results. If the animal is neutropenic and has a nonregenerative anemia, an increased M:E ratio only indicates that there are relatively more granulocytic cells than erythroid cells. It does not help to understand the underlying problem.

The most time-consuming and labor-intensive bone marrow evaluation is to perform a bone marrow cell differential count by differentiating the cell type of at least 500 cells. When completed, the M:E ratio can be calculated from the results. This evaluation yields more information but at a very high cost. Differential counts provide numerical information concerning the relative numbers of different precursor cells and whether a cell line is maturing normally. Unusual or abnormal morphological characteristics of the cells must be described separately.

The most cost-effective and informative approach to bone marrow evaluation is the subjective cytological examination. In this approach, the bone marrow smear is examined in much the same manner as a morphologic pathologist examines a histologic section of liver, and a diagnosis or interpretation is recorded. The person performing the examination, usually a veterinary pathologist or clinical pathologist, assesses the quality and cellularity of the smear, the presence and relative number of precursors for each of the three major cell lines (erythrocytes, granulocytes, and platelets), and the maturation of each of the cell lines. Abnormal morphology is noted, as well as unusual numbers or characteristics of other cell types such as lymphocytes, plasma cells, monocytes, macrophages, and mast cells. A diagnosis or interpretation is rendered based on the examination of the smear and the results of the peripheral blood tests. Because bone marrow smears are relatively poor indicators of the actual cellularity of the bone marrow, it is also prudent to consider the histopathological findings for sections of sternum, rib, or possibly femur. While these sections are inadequate for evaluating individual cell types and abnormal cell morphology, they can provide a good assessment of overall cellularity.

Ultimately, the goal of the bone marrow smear evaluation is to determine if administration of the test material has negatively impacted the number and/or maturation of hematopoietic cell precursors (103). For example, the absence of megakaryocytes indicates thrombocytopenia is due to failure of platelet production rather than increased platelet consumption peripherally. Increased numbers of normal-appearing megakaryocytes indicate thrombocytopenia is due to a consumptive process.

Coagulation

The clotting mechanism or "cascade" has traditionally been divided into two pathways. In vivo, the intrinsic pathway begins with the activation of zymogen factor XII following exposure to negatively charged subendothelial components such as collagen. Factors XI, IX, and VIII are also part of the intrinsic pathway. The extrinsic pathway begins with the activation of zymogen factor VII following exposure to tissue factor (also called tissue thromboplastin) expressed by cells deep in the vessel wall. Both pathways share the same terminal sequence of events including activation of factor X, conversion of prothrombin to thrombin, and conversion of fibrinogen to fibrin. It is thought that the extrinsic pathway is the primary initiator of coagulation in vivo (70). The intrinsic and extrinsic pathways are routinely evaluated by the activated partial thromboplastin time (APTT) and one-stage prothrombin time (OSPT or PT), respectively. The activated coagulation time (ACT) test is a simple, rapid measure of the intrinsic pathway that does not require a coagulation analyzer (17,107,140). These coagulation assays are relatively insensitive and nonspecific. Activity of a single clotting factor must be reduced to approximately 30% of normal before noticeably prolonged times are detected for an individual animal. When the results from groups of animals are compared, statistically significant differences are occasionally observed that are smaller than what would generally be considered an important change for an individual animal (e.g., less than 2 s of difference between the means for the control and high-dose groups). The toxicological significance of differences such as these is sometimes difficult to determine. While they clearly do not represent an effect likely to be associated with a bleeding diathesis for individual animals, they may be an indication of an important change in coagulation homeostasis. It may be valuable to design a longer study or increase the dose level to see if the effect is repeatable, dose-related, and associated with clinical signs.

Under the conditions of most toxicology studies, where animals are exposed to high concentrations of a test material for a prolonged period of time, any major effect on the production of a clotting factor will likely result in a clinically obvious bleeding diathesis. The administration of vitamin K antagonists such as dicumarol or the ingestion of synthetic or poorly absorbed fat substitutes is associated with bleeding and prolonged APTT and PT because the fat-soluble vitamin K is required by the liver for production of functional forms of factors II, VII, IX, and X. In theory, PT will be affected before APTT because factor VII has the shortest half-life of the clotting factors. Although nearly all the clotting factors are synthesized by the liver, APTT and PT are insensitive measures of liver function. Because of the liver's large functional reserve, liver injury must be relatively severe before coagulation times are noticeably affected. In addition to the previously mentioned thrombocytopenia, disseminated intravascular coagulation is characterized by depletion of all clotting factors, including fibrinogen, and moderately to markedly prolonged coagulation times. In many cases of disseminated intravascular coagulation, the plasma samples fail to clot during the coagulation assays.

Similarly to platelet count, coagulation times can be spuriously prolonged by difficult blood collection or poor collection technique. The combination of low platelet count and prolonged coagulation times, in an otherwise healthy animal, is an indication of poor sample quality. Inherited factor VII deficiency affects a small number of laboratory beagles (38). These animals can usually be distinguished during pretreatment screening by a PT that is 2 or 3 s longer than those of the other animals acquired for the study. Although the deficiency rarely causes a clinical problem, it would be inappropriate to use these animals if the test material is known or suspected to affect coagulation. PT and APTT can both be artifactually prolonged because of excessive sodium citrate anticoagulant in the plasma sample (79,96). This could occur if insufficient blood volume is added to standardized collection tubes or if the animal's hematocrit is elevated because of hemoconcentration (e.g., dehydration) or drug-induced polycythemia. Normal coagulation times vary from one laboratory animal species to another. Among the notable differences are the relatively fast PTs for dogs (e.g., 6 to 8 s) and slow PTs for guinea pigs (e.g., 30 to 40 s).

CLINICAL CHEMISTRY TESTS AND INTERPRETATION

Routinely performed clinical chemistry tests provide information concerning hepatocellular and biliary integrity and function, renal function, carbohydrate, lipid, and protein metabolism, and mineral and electrolyte balance. Modern clinical chemistry analyzers require very small sample volumes, and complete biochemical profiles can be obtained from rats at multiple intervals within a study without compromising the health of the animals because of excessive blood collection. Less than 250 μl of serum is needed to perform as many as 20 tests. Few of the common test methods require modification for testing animal samples.

Hepatocellular and Hepatobiliary Integrity and Function

Many routine clinical chemistry tests can be affected by liver toxicity because of the liver's critical metabolic, synthetic, and excretory functions and the abundant enzymatic machinery needed to perform these functions (110,120). Conversely, a significant loss of liver tissue with little or no detectable change in routine tests is possible because of the liver's large functional reserve. No single test is superior for detecting all of the various types of liver toxicity, but the pattern of abnormal findings in a battery of tests may help characterize the location and severity of liver lesions (21).

Liver Enzymes

Many enzymes normally present within hepatocytes exhibit increased serum activity following hepatocellular injury with degeneration and necrosis. The utility of a particular enzyme depends on factors such as relative specificity to liver, intrahepatic location, intracellular location, the concentration gradient between cell and serum, serum half-life, in vitro stability, and economy of measurement (12,13,74). The most frequently used enzymes to assess hepatocellular injury are alanine aminotransferase (ALT), aspartate aminotransferase (AST), sorbitol dehydrogenase (SDH), glutamate dehydrogenase (GDH), and lactate dehydrogenase (LDH). Each has advantages and disadvantages. The aminotransferases, ALT and AST, were formerly referred to as serum glutamic pyruvic transaminase (SGPT) and serum glutamic oxaloacetic transaminase (SGOT), respectively, and are the most commonly measured of all serum enzymes. Although sometimes included under the heading of liver function tests, serum activities of hepatic enzymes do not evaluate liver function.

In general, ALT is the most useful enzyme for detection of hepatocellular injury in the majority of laboratory animal species. Although the enzyme is present in many tissues, its greatest concentration in most species is within hepatocytes, and for practical purposes, significant elevations of serum ALT activity result only from release of ALT by hepatocytes. Species for which ALT is less useful because of relatively low hepatocyte concentrations include the guinea pig (28) and large domestic animals such as pigs, goats, sheep, cows, and horses (13,30,78). Because the enzyme is primarily cytosolic, and its concentration within the cell is up to 10,000 times greater than that in the serum, ALT may enter the serum in any condition that sufficiently alters cell membrane permeability. In addition to simple leakage from degenerating or necrotic cells, there may be other mechanisms for movement of the enzyme across the cell membrane because high serum activities of ALT are occasionally observed with no apparent cell death. The magnitude of serum activity elevation is proportional to the number of affected hepatocytes and is not necessarily indicative of the reversibility of the lesion. However, the greatest elevations result from severe lesions affecting a large portion of the liver. As a general guideline, activities for ALT in excess of 200 IU/L are usually accompanied by histopathologic evidence of hepatocellular injury, while activities below this level may or may not have correlative findings.

Following an acute but reversible hepatotoxic event, serum ALT activity rises relatively rapidly, peaks within 1 or 2 days, and then declines over the next few days. Significant hepatotoxicity can go undetected if clinical pathology tests are delayed for 1 or 2 weeks following a single administration of test material. Prolonged elevations following a single insult may reflect increased production of ALT in regenerative liver tissue or continued loss of ALT from cells in close proximity to the primary lesion that undergo degenerative changes as a result of the altered microenvironment.

Increased serum ALT activity does not always indicate primary hepatocellular injury. Biliary disease or toxicity and bile duct obstruction may cause increased serum ALT activity at least in part due to the effect of retained bile salts on the cell membranes of neighboring hepatocytes. Muscle damage, if severe and extensive, can increase serum ALT activity in the absence of hepatic injury (123,133). Increased intracellular activity of ALT as a result of induction will cause serum ALT activity to increase proportionately. Drugs such as corticosteroids and anticonvulsants appear to induce ALT production. Because these drugs may also have pathologic effects on hepatocytes, it may be difficult to determine whether an elevation is due to enzyme induction or drug-induced disease.

Interpretation of potential effects on serum ALT activity in monkeys may be complicated by the presence of subclinical, enzootic hepatitis A infection (111). Transiently increased serum ALT activity correlates with seroconversion to the virus and periportal inflammation. Because animals entering a facility may not have been exposed to the virus previously, it is possible to observe sporadic, high ALT activities (e.g., up to approximately 300 IU/L) for a few individual monkeys during the course of a toxicology study. Some facilities choose to bank serum collected from monkeys before a study is initiated for possible serologic testing to help clarify ambiguous study findings for ALT activity. Interpretation of serum ALT activities for mice is complicated by considerable interanimal variability, much of which is probably due to the effects of handling (122). In toxicology studies using mice, it is not unusual for a few animals, including the control animals, to have much higher serum ALT activities than those of the majority (e.g., 200 IU/L vs. 40 IU/L). The cause of these high activities is thought to be physical damage to the liver, especially when mice are handled by grasping the body. Unfortunately, if the only animals affected happen to belong to the high-dose group, it may be difficult to rule out an effect of the test material.

Serum AST and LDH activities tend to parallel serum ALT activity with respect to liver damage, but these enzymes are much less liver specific because of high concentrations in other tissues, especially muscle. Rodents tend to exhibit increased interanimal variability for these enzymes, some of which may be due to contamination with muscle tissue during blood collection procedures such as cardiac puncture and rupture of the retroorbital plexus. There is little advantage to determining both of these enzyme activities, and AST is generally preferred. Elevations in serum AST activity caused by hepatotoxicity are usually less pronounced than concurrent elevations in serum ALT activity. Since a portion of intracellular AST is located in mitochondria, a more severe injury may be necessary for release of like quantities of AST. As with ALT, drugs such as corticosteroids and anticonvulsants may induce production of AST.

Decreased serum activities of ALT and AST are occasionally observed in toxicology studies. Among the potential causes for these findings are decreased hepatocellular production or release of the enzymes, inhibition or reduction of the enzymes' activity, and interference with the enzyme assay. The most widely recognized of these causes involves an effect on pyridoxal 5′-phosphate (vitamin B_6), a coenzyme cofactor required for full catalytic activity of the aminotransferases. If a test material negatively affects this cofactor, directly or indirectly, serum aminotransferase activities decrease (31,37,132). Because the aminotransferase assays can be run with or without additional pyridoxal 5′-phosphate, a test material-related effect on pyridoxal 5′-phosphate can be identified by correction of an apparent decrease in aminotransferase activity when the assay is repeated with additional cofactor. Regardless of the mechanism involved, decreased serum activities of the aminotransferases have not been shown to correlate with toxicologically significant effects on the liver.

Serum SDH and GDH activities have been recommended as good indicators of hepatic toxicity in laboratory animal species (21,40,135) because increased serum activities are liver specific and relatively sensitive. SDH is a cytosolic enzyme, and GDH is mitochondrial. Elevations in serum SDH activity generally return to baseline levels faster than for other liver enzymes because of a short serum half-life. The addition of either of these tests to a standard clinical chemistry profile is a good choice if potential liver toxicity is of particular interest. The major drawback for both, however, is the assay. Although GDH is commonly used in Europe and both enzymes have been used in veterinary medicine for assessing liver injury in large domestic animals, simple test kits and standard automated procedures are unavailable because these enzymes lack popularity in human medicine in the United States.

Several enzymes that originate from hepatocytes and biliary epithelial cells are increased in serum as a result of increased production following intrahepatic or extrahepatic cholestasis or in conjunction with biliary hyperplasia. These include serum alkaline phosphatase (ALP), gamma-glutamyltransferase (GGT), leucine aminopeptidase (LAP), and 5′-nucleotidase (5′-N). Of these, the most commonly measured are ALP and GGT.

Serum ALP activity results from a mixture of membrane-localized isoenzymes, the product of different genes, and isoforms, the product of posttranslational modifications. In humans, at least four genes have been identified that code for different ALP isoenzymes: tissue nonspecific (found in liver, bone, and kidney), intestinal, placental, and germ cell. In most laboratory animals, only two genes have been identified: tissue nonspecific and intestinal. Although the ALP activities originating in liver, bone, and kidney are the product of the same gene and therefore are isoforms, they can be distinguished because of differences in degree of posttranslational glycosylation and tissue of origin and have classically been referred to as isoenzymes (64,65). Dogs have a unique isoform, known as the corticosteroid-induced ALP isoenzyme, that is a hyperglycosylated form of the intestinal ALP isoenzyme. The contribution of each isoenzyme to the total serum ALP activity is dictated by tissue production and serum half-life.

In normal dogs, serum ALP activity is a combination of the liver, bone, and corticosteroid-induced isoenzyme activities. The relative amount of corticosteroid-induced ALP activity is small compared with the others, and it is completely absent for most dogs. In young puppies, the bone isoenzyme may be responsible for up to 95% of total serum ALP activity, while in adult dogs, the liver isoenzyme is the predominant form. Intestinal and kidney ALP isoenzymes are virtually absent in dog serum because of extremely short serum half-lives, and diseases affecting these tissues do not increase serum ALP activity. In normal rats, serum ALP activity is a combination of the liver, bone, and intestinal isoenzyme activities. The intestinal isoenzyme activity increases after feeding and is reduced with fasting (130). Because toxicology studies are routinely initiated with young, growing animals, it is common for total serum alkaline phosphatase to decrease during the course of the study as a result of reduced osteoblast activity (the origin of bone ALP) in the maturing animals.

In spite of the number of ALP isoenzymes, serum ALP activity is most frequently considered a measure of cholestasis. It is a sensitive indicator of cholestasis in the dog and usually increases well before other markers such as GGT and total bilirubin. Because of cell swelling and pressure obstruction of small bile ductules, primary hepatocellular toxicities often cause enough intrahepatic cholestasis to elevate serum ALP activity. Periportal lesions result in higher activities than do centrilobular lesions. Extrahepatic cholestasis, as might occur with pancreatitis, biliary calculi, or complications of bile duct cannulation, stimulates higher serum ALP activity than intrahepatic cholestasis. The degree of elevation, however, is rarely sufficient for differentiating primary hepatocellular toxicity from primary biliary toxicity. In contrast to the dog, the value of serum ALP activity for distinguishing cholestatic lesions in monkeys is reduced because of marked interanimal variability.

Although the lack of specificity is sometimes considered a fault of ALP, the potential for detecting increases in serum ALP activity due to effects on bone is actually a benefit of this test. Elevations of serum ALP activity can be the first indication of a toxic effect on bone formation. Elevations of serum ALP activity due to increased osteoblast activity tend to be less pronounced than those due to cholestasis (e.g., no greater than two- to threefold higher than control animals). If the test material is administered for sufficient duration, the effect on ALP activity is usually accompanied by clinical or histopathological evidence of effects on bone.

Drugs such as anticonvulsants and corticosteroids can induce production of the liver ALP isoenzyme, with or without evidence of hepatobiliary disease. Following corticosteroid administration to dogs, liver ALP activity increases within a few days, while the corticosteroid-induced ALP activity does not increase noticeably for about 10 days (113). Although an increase in corticosteroid-induced ALP activity has been observed in dogs with a variety of chronic disease conditions (65) and may be related to increased endogenous corticosteroid release, this isoenzyme has not been closely evaluated in toxicology studies using dogs.

The measurement of serum GGT activity has gained popularity because it is more specific than ALP and was shown to be effective in certain models of biliary toxicity in the rat (82). Although the highest tissue concentrations of this membrane-localized enzyme are in the kidney and pancreas, serum elevations have been reported only with hepatobiliary toxicity and following induction by drugs that stimulate microsomal enzyme production (56,110). Unlike ALP, GGT is not affected by bone growth or disease. Furthermore, its serum activity is less likely to increase secondary to primary hepatocellular toxicity or intrahepatic cholestasis due to hepatocellular swelling. In rodents, serum GGT activity is often undetectable, and even small increases may be significant.

Serum LAP and 5′-N activities have been investigated as alternatives to ALP and GGT but have not found general acceptance. In some models of liver toxicity, 5′-N appears to be more sensitive than ALP or GGT (21,22).

The sensitivity or predictive value of any liver enzyme is largely dependent on the models of hepatotoxicity used to make those determinations. Acknowledgment of this fact is at least partially responsible for the practice of including multiple liver enzymes in the clinical chemistry test panels for toxicology studies. The absence of change in liver enzyme activities does not necessarily rule out the possibility of hepatotoxicity or hepatic dysfunction. Elevations may be missed because of poor timing for clinical pathology testing, and excessive variability within the control group (especially for mice and monkeys) may obscure an effect on treated groups. Furthermore, serum liver enzyme activities are not hepatic function tests. The liver can be dysfunctional in the absence of significant cholestasis or ongoing hepatocellular degeneration and necrosis. Animals with end-stage liver cirrhosis, for example, can exhibit normal serum enzyme activities. In contrast to the liver enzymes, serum total bilirubin concentration is primarily a liver function test. In the absence of hemolysis, hyperbilirubinemia indicates liver dysfunction.

Bilirubin

Bilirubin results from the breakdown of heme by cells of the mononuclear phagocyte system. Hemoglobin from senescent erythrocytes accounts for approximately 85% of all serum bilirubin. When macrophages release bilirubin into circulation, it is known as free, unconjugated, prehepatic, or indirect bilirubin. It is water insoluble and circulates bound to albumin. Hepatocytes efficiently remove unconjugated bilirubin from plasma and prepare it for removal from the body by a four-step process that includes uptake, conjugation, secretion, and excretion. Secretion of conjugated bilirubin across the canalicular membrane is the rate-limiting step in the process, and small amounts of conjugated or direct bilirubin escape into plasma. Conjugated bilirubin is not bound to albumin and is freely filtered through the glomerulus. In most species, conjugated bilirubin is completely reabsorbed by renal tubular epithelial cells unless the amount of filtered bilirubin is excessive. In the dog, the renal threshold is low and traces of bilirubin are normal in concentrated urine.

Even though the liver is a frequent target organ, increased total bilirubin concentration, whether due to conjugated bilirubin, unconjugated bilirubin, or both, is a relatively uncommon finding in toxicology studies because of the large functional reserve of the liver. In the dog, a 70% hepatectomy will not increase total bilirubin concentration.

Conjugated hyperbilirubinemia occurs as a result of impaired secretion of bilirubin, cholestasis, or both. Because bilirubin secretion is the rate-limiting step, any disease that damages enough hepatocytes can potentially increase serum conjugated bilirubin concentration. Periportal lesions cause higher serum bilirubin concentrations than do centrilobular lesions, and extrahepatic cholestasis causes higher serum bilirubin concentration than does intrahepatic cholestasis. When increased bilirubin concentration results from a cholestatic process, particularly in the dog, serum ALP activity is elevated.

Unconjugated hyperbilirubinemia occurs almost exclusively as a result of relatively severe, acute hemolysis. If hepatocytes cannot process the large amount of unconjugated bilirubin produced by macrophages during a hemolytic episode, serum bilirubin concentration increases. A hemolytic event sufficient to overload a normal liver always produces other findings indicative of hemolysis. It is possible, however, for relatively modest hemolysis to cause unconjugated hyperbilirubinemia if hepatic function is already compromised. Although a number of nonhemolytic, unconjugated hyperbilirubinemia syndromes are known, these syndromes are usually due to hereditary defects in the uptake and conjugation of free bilirubin.

Unconjugated (or indirect) bilirubin can be differentiated from conjugated (or direct) bilirubin by the Van den Bergh test. The test is used clinically to help distinguish prehepatic causes of hyperbilirubinemia, such as hemolysis, from hepatic or posthepatic causes such as hepatitis or biliary obstruction. In well-designed toxicology studies, the combination of clinical observations, other laboratory data (e.g., hematocrit or liver enzyme activities), and anatomical pathology findings (e.g., hemosiderin accumulations in splenic macrophages or periportal hepatocellular necrosis) are usually more than sufficient to determine the primary mechanism for any observed hyperbilirubinemia. Laboratory determination of direct and indirect bilirubin is rarely necessary and should not be included as part of the routine panel of tests performed in toxicology studies.

Decreased serum bilirubin concentration is occasionally associated with administration of test materials that induce microsomal enzyme production (56). Human patients receiving phenobarbital therapy have lower serum bilirubin levels than the general population as a whole (69). Enzyme induction apparently enhances the metabolism and excretion of bilirubin and could potentially mask an otherwise elevated bilirubin level.

Bile acids are synthesized from cholesterol by hepatocytes, conjugated to an amino acid, secreted into the biliary system, and excreted into the intestine where they facilitate fat absorption. There is an efficient enterohepatic circulation of bile acids with most of the reabsorption occurring at the level of the ileum. Portal blood conveys the bile acids to the liver for uptake, reconjugation, and resecretion. Any toxicity of the liver has the potential to alter one of the steps in bile acid metabolism and cause increased serum bile acid concentration. Like bilirubin concentration, bile acid concentration is a measure of a hepatic function. Although not commonly used in toxicology studies, serum bile acid concentration is considered a sensitive and specific test for hepatobiliary disease (24). Alone, however, increased serum bile acid concentration does not discriminate between different types of hepatic lesions.

Miscellaneous Parameters

The liver is wholly or partially responsible for the synthesis of many substances including glucose, cholesterol, urea nitrogen, and a variety of proteins. Severe hepatocellular dysfunction can cause decreased serum urea nitrogen concentration, hypoglycemia, hypocholesterolemia, hypoproteinemia (especially hypoalbuminemia), and prolonged coagulation times. On the other hand, liver disease can also result in hypercholesterolemia and hyperglobulinemia. The patterns of change caused by different types of liver toxicity, whether primary or secondary (e.g., hypoxia-induced centrilobular necrosis), are varied, but often overlapping. Examination of the entire biochemical profile, along with other clinical pathology and anatomical pathology findings, is necessary to properly evaluate potential liver toxicity.

Renal Function

Serum urea nitrogen and creatinine concentrations, in conjunction with urine specific gravity or urine osmolality, are the most common tests used to evaluate renal function (10,52,83,101,116). Although easy and inexpensive to perform, these tests are relatively insensitive to small effects on the kidney, and there are a number of nonrenal causes for changes in their results.

Urea is synthesized by the liver from ammonia that is absorbed from the intestine or produced by endogenous protein catabolism. Urea is freely filtered through the glomerulus and excreted in urine. Some urea is reabsorbed passively with water at the level of the proximal tubule; the amount reabsorbed is inversely related to rate of urine flow through the tubule. Serum urea nitrogen concentration is therefore affected by the rate of urea production, the glomerular filtration rate (GFR), and flow rate of urine through the renal tubule. Increased serum urea nitrogen concentration, termed azotemia, is categorized as prerenal, renal, or postrenal.

Prerenal azotemia occurs as a result of increased urea synthesis or decreased renal blood flow. Increased urea synthesis results from consumption of high-protein diets or conditions that increase protein catabolism such as starvation, fever, infection, tissue necrosis, and high gastrointestinal hemorrhage. Decreased renal blood flow, which decreases GFR, results from conditions such as dehydration (the most common cause of increased urea nitrogen in toxicology studies), cardiovascular disease, or shock. Changes in serum urea nitrogen concentration caused by increased urea synthesis are typically small. Changes caused by decreased renal perfusion may also be small, but if GFR is severely affected, the increase in urea nitrogen is indistinguishable from that which would occur due to primary renal failure. The causes of prerenal azotemia typically do not affect the ability of the kidney to concentrate urine. If dehydration is the cause of increased serum urea nitrogen concentration, urine specific gravity and urine osmolality will usually be increased, and urine volume will be decreased, because the kidneys attempt to conserve water. It is not unusual to observe very small, but statistically significant, differences for urea nitrogen concentration (e.g., 2 or 3 mg/dl) between control and treated animals, particularly in rat studies with several animals per sex per group. These differences nearly always have a prerenal cause, and over-interpretation of renal toxicity should be avoided.

Renal azotemia is caused by diseases or toxicity of the renal parenchyma. Like the liver, kidneys have a large functional reserve capacity. Serum urea nitrogen concentration does not increase notably until approximately 75% of the kidneys' nephrons are nonfunctional. If the cause of azotemia is primary renal disease, renal concentrating ability is usually impaired, and urine specific gravity is isosthenuric (i.e., the same as the glomerular filtrate; approximately 1.008 to 1.012). Renal azotemia is accompanied by histopathological evidence of renal toxicity (e.g., proximal tubular nephrosis), and the animals nearly always exhibit signs of poor health such as inappetence, weight loss, or inactivity.

Postrenal azotemia results from obstruction of the urinary outflow tract. Although it is a rare occurrence in toxicology studies, test materials that promote urinary calculi formation might cause this condition.

Creatinine is a nonprotein nitrogenous waste product that is formed at a relatively constant rate by the nonenzymatic breakdown of creatine, a molecule that stores energy in muscle as phosphocreatine. Serum creatinine concentration is therefore influenced by muscle mass and conditioning, but it is relatively independent of dietary influences and protein catabolism. Creatinine is freely filtered by the glomerulus, but unlike urea, it is not reabsorbed by the tubules. Following alterations in renal blood flow, renal function, or urine outflow, the changes in serum creatinine concentration tend to parallel those for serum urea nitrogen concentration. The timing and magnitude of the changes for serum creatinine may lag behind those for serum urea nitrogen as a result of the tubular reabsorption of urea, especially when urine flow is slow, or there is increased formation of urea. Because it is influenced by fewer secondary factors, serum creatinine is usually a better reflection of glomerular filtration. Unfortunately, the most commonly used method for determining serum creatinine concentration, the Jaffé reaction, is not specific, and interfering compounds called noncreatinine chromagens affect its accuracy. Noncreatinine chromagens are typically of insufficient quantity to complicate data interpretation. However, if serum creatinine concentrations are increased in the absence of correlative effects on serum urea nitrogen or renal histopathology, enzymatic creatinine methods are available to investigate the possibility of analytical interferences.

Other clinical chemistry findings often observed when renal function is significantly impaired include increased serum inorganic phosphorus concentration and decreased serum sodium and chloride concentrations. Endogenous creatinine clearance is sometimes used as a noninvasive measure of GFR because blood levels of creatinine are relatively stable over short intervals, creatinine is freely filtered, and creatinine is not significantly secreted or reabsorbed (10,11).

Proteins, Carbohydrates, and Lipids

Serum Proteins

Serum total protein concentration is a measure of all plasma proteins with the exception of those consumed in clot formation such as fibrinogen and the other clotting factors. Serum total protein concentration is therefore about 0.3 to 0.5 g/dl lower than plasma total protein concentration. Albumin is the most abundant protein and is largely responsible for maintaining intravascular osmotic pressure. Albumin serves as a storage reservoir of amino acids and as a transport protein for plasma constituents that do not have a specific transport protein. Globulins are a heterogeneous population of proteins that include specific transport proteins (e.g., transferrin for iron, lipoproteins for lipids, haptoglobin for hemoglobin, and thyroxine-binding globulin for thyroxine), mediators of inflammation (e.g., complement and C-reactive protein), clotting factors, enzymes, and immunoglobulins. Globulins are loosely categorized by their electrophoretic migration pattern as α, β, and γ globulins; there are several different proteins in each category or region of the electrophoretic pattern (71). The regions can be further subdivided (e.g., most species have two α regions), but serum protein electrophoresis cannot distinguish specific globulins. Immunoglobulins are generally thought of as γ globulins, but some, particularly IgM, extend into the β regions of the electrophoretogram. The liver synthesizes albumin and most of the globulins; the major exception is the immunoglobulins. Serum total protein and albumin concentrations are measured directly; serum globulin concentration is calculated by subtraction. Hydration status is always an important consideration for proper interpretation of changes in serum protein concentrations. Hypoproteinemia, like anemia, can be masked by dehydration.

In toxicology studies, the most frequent reason for increased serum total protein concentration is reduced hydration of the treated animals relative to the control animals. If the cause of the difference in hydration status is relatively uncomplicated, serum albumin and serum globulin concentrations increase proportionately. The effect on hydration status of the treated animals may or may not be detectable as clinical dehydration. Possible correlative clinical observations include gastrointestinal fluid losses (e.g., vomiting, diarrhea, excessive salivation), polyuria, and reduced water consumption. Since water consumption in rodents is closely associated with food consumption, any cause of decreased food consumption in rodents has the potential to cause relative dehydration. In short-term dietary studies, for example, palatability problems may result in higher serum protein and urea nitrogen concentrations because of differences in hydration. On the other hand, if decreased feed consumption is protracted and body weights or body weight gains are affected, serum protein concentrations will typically decrease over time.

The only other relatively common causes for increased serum total protein concentration in toxicology studies are inflammatory conditions that stimulate the production of acute-phase proteins (e.g., fibrinogen, haptoglobin, α_2-macroglobulin, and C-reactive protein) and immunoglobulins (15,114). Often with inflammatory conditions, however, there is a concurrent decrease in serum albumin concentration that serves to negate the globulin effect on serum total protein concentration. This pattern is commonly observed in animals affected by complications of long-term indwelling intravenous catheterization. Albumin is sometimes referred to as a negative acute-phase protein.

Decreased serum protein concentrations result from either decreased protein synthesis or increased protein loss. Protein synthesis can be negatively affected by decreased feed consumption, maldigestion or malabsorption, and hepatic dysfunction. Although the functional reserve capacity of the liver is quite substantial and hepatic injury must be relatively severe before protein synthesis is notably diminished for individual patients, small differences between control and treated groups in large studies may be apparent with relatively modest hepatotoxicity. Loss of protein, both albumin and globulin, occurs with hemorrhage and exudative lesions such as burns or severe dermal toxicity. Because of its relatively small size, albumin is the principal protein lost as a result of protein-losing enteropathies and glomerulopathies. Globulin concentrations may actually increase secondarily to enteropathies because of inflammation and increased systemic exposure to gastrointestinal toxins and bacterial flora. Decreased globulin concentration, without a concurrent or proportional decrease in albumin concentration, may be indicative of decreased synthesis of immunoglobulins. Concurrent histopathological evidence of an effect on lymphoid tissue strengthens this interpretation. Reduced serum globulin concentrations have been observed following prolonged administration of antibiotics (e.g., $\geq$4 weeks) to young animals, perhaps as a result of inhibition of normal bacterial flora and subsequently reduced antigenic stimulation.

Effects on serum albumin concentration are more commonly observed for rodents than for the larger species. Although this may be due simply to the increased numbers of animals per group, it may also be a function of differences among species for the circulating half-life of albumin. Smaller species tend to have faster turnover than larger species (71). For example, the half-life of albumin is approximately 2 days for mice, 8 days for dogs, and 16 days for baboons. A small decrease in serum albumin concentration is one of the most frequent findings in toxicology studies for animals given poorly tolerated dose levels of a test material. Like the small decreases for other parameters (e.g., hematocrit, glucose concentration, cholesterol concentration, body weight, and body weight gain) that may or may not occur concurrently, the effect on albumin is usually considered an indication of the overall poor condition of the animals rather than evidence of a specific toxic mechanism.

Serum Glucose

Serum glucose concentration is a reflection of intestinal glucose absorption, hepatic glucose production, and tissue uptake of glucose. The balance between hepatic production and tissue uptake is influenced by many hormones, including insulin, glucagon, corticosteroids, adrenocorticotropic hormone, growth hormone, and catecholamines. In oversimplified terms, insulin promotes uptake of glucose by tissues, glucocorticoids and glucagon stimulate hepatic gluconeogenesis, and catecholamines and glucagon stimulate glycogenolysis.

The most frequently encountered causes of increased serum glucose concentration in toxicology studies are failure to fast an animal and catecholamine release secondary to excitement or fear. Moribund animals occasionally exhibit marked hyperglycemia, probably as a result of both corticosteroid and catecholamine release. If blood collection is performed in group order rather than random order, and the samples are not processed promptly, the last group bled (usually the high-dose group) will appear to have higher serum glucose concentrations than those of the first group (usually the control group) because of greater glucose consumption by erythrocytes in the samples of the first group. When serum is not separated from the blood clot, glucose concentration decreases at a rate of approximately 7 to 10 mg/dl/h. Infrequent causes of increased serum glucose concentration in toxicology studies include some relatively common clinical conditions such as diabetes mellitus, pancreatitis, hyperadrenocorticism, and steroid therapy.

In toxicology studies, test material-related decreases in serum glucose concentration are most commonly observed in animals that fail to thrive and gain body weight, with or without a concurrent decrease in food consumption. When this occurs, the difference for serum glucose concentration between the control and treated animals is usually no more than 10 or 15 mg/dl and likely does not adversely affect the animals. Although a precise mechanism for the effect is typically not determined, the difference appears to reflect the overall process that has caused the animals to do poorly and is frequently accompanied by small decreases in circulating erythrocyte mass and serum protein concentrations. Clinical conditions that cause hypoglycemia include intestinal disease with malabsorption, severe hepatic disease, endotoxemia, and some tumors, in particular insulinomas and hepatomas.

Serum Lipids

Cholesterol is required for the synthesis of bile acids, corticosteroids, and sex steroids, and triglycerides are an important source of energy. Serum cholesterol and triglycerides are derived from dietary intake and endogenous synthesis, primarily by the liver. In circulation, cholesterol and triglycerides are components of chylomicrons and the lipoproteins: very-low-density lipoprotein (VLDL), low-density lipoprotein (LDL), and high-density lipoprotein (HDL) (3). Chylomicrons are produced by intestinal cells after a fatty meal and are rich in triglycerides. Hepatocytes synthesize VLDLs, which have less triglyceride, but more cholesterol, than chylomicrons. The triglycerides in chylomicrons and VLDLs are broken down to free fatty acids and monoglycerides by lipoprotein lipase attached to the surface of endothelial cells, especially in the capillaries of adipose tissue and muscle. Adipocytes tend to reesterify the fatty acids for storage as triglycerides. Muscle tends to oxidize the fatty acids for energy. The loss of triglyceride transforms VLDL to LDL. In humans, about two-thirds of serum cholesterol is transported by LDL. In contrast, HDL is responsible for the great majority of cholesterol transport in most laboratory animal species. Species differences in lipid metabolism make it difficult to correlate effects in animal models with those in humans (4).

Effects on serum cholesterol and triglyceride concentrations, both increases and decreases, are relatively frequent findings in toxicology studies. The changes are usually small and are generally believed to represent minor alterations in lipid metabolism that do not adversely affect the health of the animals. Unfortunately, exact mechanisms for the changes are rarely identified. Factors to consider include food consumption and assimilation, body weight and composition, liver function, and hormone balance. Serum triglyceride concentration is elevated postprandially, while serum cholesterol concentration is relatively stable. When fat is mobilized to meet energy requirements because of significant anorexia, starvation, malabsorption, or maldigestion, serum triglycerides are usually increased, sometimes markedly; cholesterol levels, however, are variable. Clinical conditions that increase both serum cholesterol and serum triglycerides include hypothyroidism and diabetes mellitus. Hypercholesterolemia is more prominent in hypothyroidism, and hypertriglyceridemia is more prominent in diabetes mellitus. In both diseases, lipoprotein lipase activity is reduced. Cholestasis and other forms of liver disease can increase serum cholesterol concentration because the liver is the major excretory pathway for cholesterol. On the other hand, liver disease may also be associated with hypocholesterolemia. Nephrotic syndrome is characterized by increased urinary protein excretion because of glomerular disease, hypoalbuminemia, and hypercholesterolemia. Although serum cholesterol and triglyceride concentrations are extremely variable for older rats because of a number of naturally occurring diseases such as pituitary tumors that affect hormone balance, younger rats (e.g., 7 to 20 weeks of age) usually exhibit less interanimal variability than dogs and monkeys. It is therefore more common to detect subtle effects on serum lipid concentrations in short-term rat studies, versus dog or monkey studies, especially since the number of animals per group is typically much higher for rat studies.

Minerals and Electrolytes

Serum Calcium and Inorganic Phosphorus

Serum calcium concentration is controlled primarily by parathyroid hormone, calcitonin, and vitamin D and represents a balance between intestinal absorption, bone formation and reabsorption, and urinary excretion (18). Serum inorganic phosphorus concentration is affected by the same hormones but is more sensitive to changes in dietary intake and urinary excretion. Approximately 50% of serum calcium is in its biologically active, ionized form. Ionized calcium is critical for neuromuscular activity, bone formation, coagulation, and other biochemical mechanisms. Approximately 40% of serum calcium is bound to albumin, and the remainder is complexed to anions such as phosphate and citrate.

Although there are many disease conditions associated with hypercalcemia (18), increased serum calcium concentration is relatively uncommon in toxicology studies unless the test material is specifically designed to target calcium metabolism or has properties of either parathyroid hormone or vitamin D. Because approximately one-half of serum calcium is bound to albumin, mildly increased serum calcium concentration is occasionally observed when serum albumin concentration is increased due to dehydration. Rare causes of hypercalcemia in toxicology studies include primary hyperparathyroidism, pseudohyperparathyroidism (a paraneoplastic syndrome), hypervitaminosis D, and renal disease.

Mildly decreased serum calcium concentration, as a result of decreased serum albumin concentration, is a frequent finding in toxicology studies. Signs of hypocalcemia, such as neurological and neuromuscular abnormalities, are absent because ionized calcium is relatively unaffected. Rare causes of hypocalcemia in toxicology studies include hypoparathyroidism, nutritional hyperparathyroidism, acute pancreatitis, and renal disease.

Young, rapidly growing animals have high serum inorganic phosphorus concentrations (e.g., greater than or equal to serum calcium concentration) that decrease as the animals mature. Serum inorganic phosphorus concentration is very sensitive to GFR, and increased concentrations are most commonly associated with azotemia, whether prerenal, renal, or postrenal. Rare causes of hyperphosphatemia in toxicology studies include hypoparathyroidism, nutritional hyperparathyroidism due to excess dietary phosphorus, and hypervitaminosis D. Perhaps the most common cause of decreased serum inorganic phosphorus concentration observed in toxicology studies is significantly reduced food consumption.

Serum Sodium, Potassium, and Chloride

Sodium, the major cation in serum, is the principal determinant of extracellular fluid volume (i.e., hydration status). Chloride, the major anion in serum, supports fluid homeostasis and balances cation secretion. Potassium is the major intracellular cation and has a critical role in neuromuscular and cardiac excitability. Reference ranges for electrolyte concentrations tend to be much wider than the range of values obtained from animals in a well-controlled study. It is not unusual to observe very small, but statistically significant, differences between control and treated groups with no apparent mechanism or effect on animal health. Many of these differences are likely incidental, while others probably represent subtle homeostatic effects. Changes in serum sodium and chloride concentrations tend to parallel each other when they are associated with relative water content, but serum chloride concentrations are disproportionately affected when alterations are associated with disorders affecting acid–base balance.

Significant hypernatremia is rare in toxicology studies, but hyperchloremia is occasionally observed secondarily to metabolic acidosis resulting from diarrhea. In this condition, renal tubular reabsorption of chloride is increased because of decreased availability of bicarbonate. Relatively proportional decreases in serum sodium and chloride concentrations can occur with gastrointestinal losses (e.g., vomiting or diarrhea), polyuric renal losses (e.g., renal failure), diuretic effects, and hypoadrenocorticism (rare in toxicology studies). Vomiting may cause decreased serum chloride concentration in the absence of an effect on sodium because stomach secretions are rich in chloride.

Increased serum potassium concentration is an uncommon finding in toxicology studies, but it may be observed with a variety of conditions causing acidosis because extracellular hydrogen ions are exchanged for intracellular potassium ions. Severe tissue necrosis and anuric or oligouric renal failure are infrequent causes of hyperkalemia. Serum potassium concentration may be falsely elevated because of hemolysis in species that have high intraerythrocytic potassium (e.g., nonhuman primates). Marked thrombocytosis and thrombocytopenia can be associated with increased and decreased serum potassium concentrations, respectively, because potassium is released from platelets during clot formation. Serum potassium concentration is very sensitive to potassium intake, and decreased concentrations are often associated with anorexia. Similar to the effects on sodium and chloride, decreased serum potassium concentrations are sometimes associated with gastrointestinal losses and polyuric renal losses. Disorders resulting in alkalosis (e.g., persistent vomiting) may cause hypokalemia because intracellular hydrogen ions are exchanged for extracellular potassium ions.

Miscellaneous Serum Chemistry Tests

Creatine kinase (CK) activity is measured primarily as a marker for skeletal muscle toxicity. In cases of true skeletal muscle toxicity, which are relatively rare, increased CK activity can be detected if complicating factors or study-related procedures do not obscure results. For example, intramuscular injections, surgical procedures, and poor venipuncture technique can all give rise to marked elevations in CK that preclude identification of meaningful differences between control and treated animals.

Several tests have been used with varying degrees of success in human medicine as markers of acute myocardial injury (27), and a few of these tests, such as CK-MB (one of the isoenzymes of creatine kinase), troponin I, and troponin T, appear to have limited application in acute, exploratory toxicology studies (5,32,47,66,95). It is unknown whether any of these tests are sensitive or specific enough to detect subclinical myocardial toxicity in standard repeated-dose toxicity studies.

Amylase and lipase activities are measured clinically to diagnose diseases causing acute pancreatic necrosis. These enzymes have limited value in toxicology studies, especially repeated-dose studies, because toxin-induced pancreatitis will cause severe illness in the animals and have prominent, unmistakable morphologic consequences. Amylase and lipase are not sufficiently sensitive to be markers for test materials with specific action against pancreatic islet cells.

URINALYSIS AND URINE CHEMISTRY TESTS AND INTERPRETATION

Urinalysis

Urinalysis has traditionally been considered part of the minimum laboratory data base for evaluating patients. Although it provides specific information about the urogenital tract and general information regarding some systemic conditions, urinalysis is not particularly well suited for most toxicology studies. The cost:benefit ratio is poor because sample collection and analysis are labor-intensive and relatively few toxicities produce detectable effects on urinalysis parameters. In addition, there are technical difficulties associated with collecting a large number of urine specimens from small laboratory animals or "uncooperative" large animals that impact the accuracy of the test results. If a test material is known or suspected to affect the urinary system, then measures can be taken to provide appropriate specimens for urinalysis (e.g., by catheterization, cystocentesis, or carefully collected voided samples). Usually, however, when a large number of animals are being tested with a test material of unknown toxic potential, the most efficient method of urine collection (i.e., in a collection vessel at the bottom of a metabolic cage) produces many artifacts that affect the test results and complicate interpretation. Because voided urine traverses the urethra, vagina or prepuce, and perineal or preputial hairs, it acquires both cells and bacteria that are not indicative of toxicity. Given time to "incubate" overnight with contaminants at the bottom of the cage (e.g., feces, bacteria, food, hair, and cleaning chemicals), it is understandable that urinalysis data from timed collections in a metabolic cage can produce questionable results. Preservatives and methods for keeping the urine chilled may help limit artifactual changes, but these procedures are not without cost.

The standard urinalysis has two components: measurement of physicochemical properties, and microscopic evaluation of urine sediment. The physicochemical properties include volume (for timed collections), color, clarity, specific gravity or osmolality, and the reagent strip tests (pH, protein, glucose, ketones, bilirubin, urobilinogen, and occult blood). Some reagent strips have additional tests for nitrite (indicates presence of nitrite-producing bacteria) and leukocyte esterase, but these are not particularly valuable for animal specimens, especially those collected overnight (127). Urinary sediment evaluation is a semiquantitative microscopic measure of the presence of cells, casts, bacteria, and crystals. This is the most expensive component of the urinalysis and, in most instances, the least informative or necessary (51). In general, disorders that increase the number of cells or casts in urine sediment will be better characterized by histopathological examination of the kidneys and bladder. Occasionally, test material-specific crystals that might otherwise go undetected are identified by urine sediment examination.

Urine Volume and Concentration

Timed urine volume and urine specific gravity or osmolality are measures of renal function because they demonstrate the concentrating ability of the kidneys. Loss of urine-concentrating ability usually precedes the development of azotemia as a consequence of chronic renal disease. If water contamination is avoided, timed urine volume (e.g., 16 or 24 h) and urine specific gravity are probably the most beneficial of the routine urinalysis tests.

Urine specific gravity, as determined by refractometry, is an approximation of solute concentration, and usually varies inversely with urine volume. Animals with decreased ability to concentrate urine have decreased urine specific gravity and increased urine volume. Isosthenuria (i.e., urine specific gravity from approximately 1.008 to 1.012; also referred to as "fixed" specific gravity) occurs with advanced renal disease. Isosthenuria and hyposthenuria (urine specific gravity below 1.008) are particularly meaningful when serum urea nitrogen concentration is elevated. If the urine sample is free of water contamination, this combination indicates primary renal dysfunction. Test materials with diuretic activity also produce dilute urine and increased urine volume, but serum urea nitrogen is usually unaffected. Artifactual hyposthenuria is observed frequently in toxicology studies as a result of water leakage from faulty sipper tubes and animals that habitually "play" with their water source. Dehydrated animals with functional kidneys should have concentrated urine (e.g., urine specific gravity >1.020) as the animals attempt to conserve water. In toxicology studies, urine specific gravity is sometimes high in treated animals that are anorectic and consequently not drinking normally. This is particularly true of rodents.

Reagent Strip Tests

Urine pH is affected by diet. Animals consuming high-protein meat diets tend to produce urine of lower pH than do animals consuming cereal or vegetable diets. If administered in large enough quantities, an acid or alkaline test material can affect urine pH. Urine pH is not, however, a good indicator of acid–base balance. Urine pH is often artifactually elevated in samples collected overnight for two reasons: urease-producing bacteria cause ammonia formation, and carbon dioxide is lost from open containers.

A small amount of protein is a normal finding in the urine of most animals, especially if the urine is concentrated. A large amount of protein is abnormal, especially in dilute urine. Increased urine protein, proteinuria, may result from glomerular injury, defective tubular reabsorption, hemorrhage, inflammation, or proteinaceous secretions from the lower urogenital tract in voided specimens. The sediment findings may help to identify the cause of proteinuria. Older rats, particularly males, develop marked proteinuria as a consequence of chronic progressive nephropathy, a common, naturally occurring disease of rats. Highly alkaline urine and quaternary ammonium compounds commonly used as disinfectants can cause false-positive findings for urine protein measured by reagent strips.

Glucosuria is an abnormal finding. Under normal conditions, the renal tubules reabsorb all glucose that is filtered through the glomerulus. If the glucose load is excessive as a result of marked hyperglycemia (e.g., >180 mg/dl for the dog), glucosuria results. While diabetes mellitus is the most frequent disease associated with glucosuria, it is rarely observed in toxicology studies. Glucosuria may be observed with renal toxins that target proximal tubular epithelial cells because of failure to adequately reabsorb filtered glucose. If urine glucose is considered an important endpoint for a study, precautions should be taken to avoid false-negative findings resulting from proliferation of bacteria that consume glucose.

Ketonuria is occasionally observed in anorectic animals and animals that have been fasted for a prolonged period of time. Ketonuria indicates that energy metabolism has shifted to incomplete oxidation of fatty acids. Diabetic animals often have ketonuria. False-negative findings for urine ketones occur as a result of bacterial degradation and the loss of volatile ketones from open containers.

Bilirubinuria is a normal finding in the dog, especially in concentrated urine, but an abnormal finding in other species. Increased urine bilirubin occurs as a result of the same conditions that cause increased serum bilirubin, and it may precede the change in blood. False-negative findings for urine bilirubin occur from prolonged exposure to light, which oxidizes the bilirubin to biliverdin.

Theoretically, urine urobilinogen tests for patency of the bile duct. Intestinal bacteria convert conjugated bilirubin to urobilinogen, a portion of which is reabsorbed by the intestine. Because a small amount of the reabsorbed urobilinogen is normally excreted in the urine, a negative urine urobilinogen is supposed to indicate an obstructed bile duct, an extremely rare occurrence in toxicology studies. The test has little value and is generally determined simply because it exists on the same reagent strip as the other tests.

Positive findings for urine occult blood occur frequently in normal animals. Although the origin of the blood is usually not known, estrus is a common source in female animals. Reagent strips do not discriminate well between erythrocytes, hemoglobin, and myoglobin, and examination of the sediment may help to differentiate hematuria from hemoglobinuria. Hematuria may result from bleeding disorders or inflammation, trauma, or neoplasia of the urogenital tract.

Urine Sediment Evaluation

Small numbers of erythrocytes, leukocytes, and epithelial cells are normal findings in urine sediment obtained from voided urine specimens. Large numbers of these cells may or may not be abnormal, and histopathological correlates are necessary to determine their origin. Increased numbers of large epithelial cells (i.e., squamous and transitional cells) generally do not indicate a significant abnormality, but increased numbers of small epithelial cells (i.e., renal tubular cells), especially in conjunction with granular or cellular casts, are indicative of kidney disease.

A cast is the cylindrical mold of a segment of renal tubule formed by protein alone or protein and cells. Hyaline casts are made of protein alone, and increased numbers are sometimes observed with glomerular disorders that cause excessive proteinuria. An occasional hyaline cast is normal. Cellular casts (erythrocyte, leukocyte, or epithelial) usually indicate severe renal lesions but are rarely observed in animal urine. If not moved rapidly into the urine, cellular casts become granular casts as the cells degenerate and take on a granular appearance. Waxy casts represent the final stage of degeneration of the cellular cast and indicate prolonged, intrarenal urine stasis. Granular and waxy casts, therefore, may also be an indication of renal disease. Broad casts are identified by their width and represent casts formed in collecting ducts or pathologically dilated portions of the nephron. Broad casts also indicate intrarenal urine stasis. While cells can originate from lesions all along the urogenital tract, cylindruria (increased number of casts) implicates a renal disorder.

Given the methods normally used to collect urine during toxicology studies, bacteria are a consistent finding. If the test material is an antibiotic, there may be a test material-related decrease in the number of bacteria observed.

Crystals are common in the urine of laboratory animals and are pH dependent. Crystals observed frequently in alkaline urine include triple phosphate, amorphous phosphate, calcium carbonate, and ammonium urate crystals. Urate and oxalate crystals are associated with acid urine. Test material-specific crystals will occasionally form when a test material is highly concentrated in the urine. These crystals may be pathologically significant if they obstruct renal tubules or lead to the development of calculi. Ammonium biurate crystals, a rare finding, are associated with liver failure.

Cells, casts, and crystals are poorly preserved in urine during overnight or 24-h collections. For example, it is common to find no erythrocytes in the urine sediment even though the reagent strip occult blood test is positive and hemolysis has been ruled out. This is a significant problem with prolonged, timed urine collections. If sediment detail is deemed an important endpoint for a study, other means of urine collection (e.g., cystocentesis) should be considered.

Urine Chemistry Tests

Because serum tests such as urea nitrogen and creatinine and standard urinalysis tests are relatively insensitive markers of renal injury, several urine chemistry tests have been proposed as better methods for identifying and quantifying early renal injury or dysfunction. For the most part, these tests are impractical as part of the general screen in routine, regulated toxicology studies. However, they may be valuable as tools for assessing early renal toxicity at dose levels below those which cause histopathological lesions and for determining the intrarenal location of the earliest toxic insult. Some of these tests are also well suited for acute studies to determine the relative nephrotoxicity of different analogues of a parent compound with known nephrotoxic action in order to select the least toxic analogue for further development.

Urinary Enzyme Activity

Many urinary enzymes have been evaluated for use as early markers of nephrotoxicity (29,102), and several have been proven effective in specific models of nephrotoxicity (42,43,57,59,89,117). Perhaps the two most frequently measured urinary enzymes are GGT and *N*-acetyl-β-glucosaminidase (NAG) because they are relatively stable at room temperature and have somewhat different cellular locations; GGT is located in the brush border of proximal tubular epithelial cells, and NAG is a lysosomal enzyme with apparently greater distribution along the nephron. Other urinary enzymes that have been evaluated include ALP, another brush border enzyme, and LDH, ALT, and AST, primarily cytosolic enzymes. Urinary enzyme activities should be corrected for variations in urine concentration by calculating the total activity excreted per unit time or the ratio of urinary enzyme activity to urinary creatinine concentration. Urinary enzyme activities are most effective for assessing acute renal injury. They appear to have much less utility for assessing chronic conditions (e.g., repeated-dose studies of several weeks duration), and they do not provide information concerning renal function.

Urinary Proteins

Quantitative measurement of urinary protein excretion has historically been used to evaluate protein-losing nephropathies that occur primarily from disorders affecting the glomerulus but are also seen with a variety of chronic renal diseases (25,58,62,139). Nephrotoxins that produce readily identifiable proteinuria typically exhibit correlative histopathologic findings for glomeruli, tubules, or both. As with urinary enzyme activities, urine protein excretion should be corrected for urine concentration by calculating the total amount excreted per unit time (e.g., mg/16 h) or the ratio of urinary protein concentration to urinary creatinine concentration. Although glomerular disorders (increased protein filtration) tend to exhibit greater proteinuria than tubular disorders (decreased protein reabsorption), the exact source of the protein loss cannot be determined by simply quantifying total protein loss.

An immunoassay for urinary β_2-microglobulin, a low-molecular-weight serum protein that is freely filtered through glomeruli and almost completely reabsorbed (>99%) by proximal tubular epithelial cells, has been used to differentiate glomerular from tubular protein loss and to assess tubular function (106,128,129). Unfortunately, antibodies specific for animal β_2-microglobulin are not commercially available, and the structure of the protein appears to be highly species specific (83). The use of sodium dodecyl sulfate–polyacrylamide gel electrophoresis has been proposed as a means of classifying renal injury by the molecular weight pattern of excreted urinary proteins (77). An increase in high-molecular-mass proteins (e.g., >69,000 D) is associated with glomerular injury, and an increase in low-molecular-mass proteins (e.g., 12,000 to 60,000 D) is associated with tubular injury.

Urinary Electrolytes

Urinary electrolyte concentrations (e.g., sodium, potassium, and chloride) from timed urine collections are the most commonly performed urine chemistry tests for regulated toxicology studies because they have been listed in the study guidelines for preclinical evaluation of new pharmaceutical products by Japan's Ministry of Health and Welfare (60). Unfortunately, these tests have a very poor cost–benefit ratio as screening tools for nephrotoxicity. If only the concentrations are assessed, they offer little advantage or information beyond that obtained from urine specific gravity or osmolality. Additional information can be obtained by calculating the total amount of each electrolyte excreted per unit time (e.g., mmol/16 h) or the fractional clearance of each electrolyte. However, in contrast to effects on urinary enzyme activities or protein concentrations, effects on urinary electrolyte excretion are most often a reflection of the normal homeostatic mechanisms required to maintain electrolyte and fluid balance in the face of changes in intake (e.g., anorexia) and output (e.g., gastrointestinal losses from diarrhea) and are not specific measures of renal injury or dysfunction. Increased excretion of urinary electrolytes can of course occur secondarily to administration of many nephrotoxins and test materials with diuretic activity, but more standard tests are typically more sensitive and cost-effective. One reason for the relative insensitivity of urinary electrolyte measurements is that they tend to exhibit considerable interanimal variability. With respect to the effect of diuretic agents on urinary electrolyte excretion, the period of time for which the urine is collected has a major impact upon the results obtained. For example, if a diuretic is administered in the morning, fluid and electrolyte excretion may be quite high during the first several hours postdose. But if the urine sample collection is performed overnight, after the effect of the diuretic has subsided, electrolyte excretion may appear decreased because of compensatory electrolyte reabsorption to counteract the loss of fluid during the day.

QUESTIONS

1. Time-related biases are sources of preanalytical variation. Give at least three examples of time-related bias, and describe how these biases might affect interpretation of several different clinical pathology test results.
2. Describe how reference intervals are constructed, and compare their uses with those of concurrent control groups and correlative findings for a given toxicology study.
3. Differentiate regenerative anemia from nonregenerative anemia, and give examples of each type.
4. Describe how the common tests of hepatocellular and hepatobiliary integrity and function are used to characterize hepatic toxicity.

REFERENCES

1. Apostolou, A., Saidt, L., and Brown, W. R. (1976): Effect of overnight fasting of young rats on water consumption, body weight, blood sampling, and blood composition. *Lab. Anim. Sci.*, 26:959–960.
2. Babior, B. M. (1995): The megaloblastic anemias. In: *Williams Hematology*, 5th ed., edited by E. Beutler, M. A. Lichtman, B. S. Coller, and T. J. Kipps, pp. 471–489. McGraw-Hill, New York.
3. Bartley, J. C. (1989): Lipid metabolism and its diseases. In: *Clinical Biochemistry of Domestic Animals*, 4th ed., edited by J. J. Kaneko, pp. 106–141. Academic Press, San Diego.
4. Bauer, J. E. (1996): Comparative lipid and lipoprotein metabolism. *Vet. Clin. Pathol.*, 25(2):49–56.
5. Beck, M. L., Dameron, G. W., Kang, Y. J., Erickson, B. K., Di Battista, T. H., Miller, K. E., Jackson, K. N., Mittelstadt, S., and O'Brien, P. J. (1997): Cardiac troponin T is a sensitive and specific biomarker of cardiac injury in laboratory animals. *Clin. Chem.*, 43(6):S192.
6. Bennett, J. S., Gossett, K. A., McCarthy, M. P., and Simpson, E. D. (1992): Effects of ketamine hydrochloride on serum biochemical and hematological variables in rhesus monkeys (*Macaca mulatta*). *Vet. Clin. Pathol.*, 21(1):15–18.
7. Beutler, E. (1995): Glucose-6-phosphate dehydrogenase deficiency and other enzyme abnormalities. In: *Williams Hematology*, 5th ed., edited by E. Beutler, M. A. Lichtman, B. S. Coller, and T. J. Kipps, pp. 564–581. McGraw-Hill, New York.
8. Beutler, E., Lichtman, M. A., Coller, B. S., and Kipps, T. J. (1995): *Williams Hematology*, 5th ed. McGraw-Hill, New York.
9. Boon, G. D. (1993): An overview of hemostasis. *Toxicol. Pathol.*, 21(2):170–179.
10. Bovee, K. C. (1986): Renal function and laboratory evaluation. *Toxicol. Pathol.*, 14(1):26–36.
11. Bovee, K. C., and Joyce, T. (1979): Clinical evaluation of glomerular function: 24-Hour creatinine clearance in dogs. *J. Am. Vet. Med. Assoc.*, 174(5):488–491.
12. Boyd, J. W. (1983): The mechanisms relating to increases in plasma enzymes and isoenzymes in diseases of animals. *Vet. Clin. Pathol.*, 12(2):9–24.
13. Boyd, J. W. (1988): Serum enzymes in the diagnosis of diseases in man and animals. *J. Comp. Pathol.*, 98:381–404.
14. Burtis, C. A., and Ashwood, E. R. (1998): *Tietz Textbook of Clinical Chemistry*, 3rd ed. W. B. Saunders, Philadelphia.
15. Burton, S. A., Honor, D. J., Mackenzie, A. L., Eckersall, P. D., Markham, R. J., and Horney, B. S. (1994): C-reactive protein concentration in dogs with inflammatory leukograms. *Am. J. Vet. Res.*, 55(5):613–618.
16. Butterfield, L. (1997): Are there just "races" (subspecies) of cynomolgus monkeys or should the name of *Macaca irus* be revived? *Lab. Primate Newslett.*, 36(1):19.
17. Byars, T. D., Ling, G. V., Ferris, N. A., and Keeton, K. S. (1976): Activated coagulation time (ACT) of whole blood in normal dogs. *Am. J. Vet. Res.*, 37(11):1359–1361.
18. Capen, C. C., and Rosol, T. J. (1989): Calcium-regulating hormones and diseases of abnormal mineral (calcium, phosphorus, magnesium) metabolism. In: *Clinical Biochemistry of Domestic Animals*, 4th ed., edited by J. J. Kaneko, pp. 678–752. Academic Press, San Diego.
19. Carakostas, M. C. (1988): What is serum ornithine decarboxylase? *Clin. Chem.*, 34(12):2606–2607.
20. Carakostas, M. C., and Banerjee, A. K. (1990): Interpreting rodent clinical laboratory data in safety assessment studies: Biological and analytical components of variation. *Fundam. Appl. Toxicol.*, 15:744–753.
21. Carakostas, M. C., Gossett, K. A., Church, G. E., and Cleghorn, B. L. (1986): Evaluating toxin-induced hepatic injury in rats by laboratory results and discriminant analysis. *Vet. Pathol.*, 23:264–269.
22. Carakostas, M. C., Power, R. J., and Banerjee, A. K. (1990): Serum 5′-nucleotidase activity in rats: A method for automated analysis and criteria for interpretation. *Vet. Clin. Pathol.*, 19(4):109–113.
23. Caro, J., and Erslev, A. J. (1995): Anemia of chronic renal failure. In: *Williams Hematology*, 5th ed., edited by E. Beutler, M. A. Lichtman, B. S. Coller, and T. J. Kipps, pp. 456–462. McGraw-Hill, New York.
24. Center, S. A., Baldwin, B. H., Erb, H. N., and Tennant, B. C. (1985): Bile acid concentrations in the diagnosis of hepatobiliary disease in the dog. *J. Am. Vet. Med. Assoc.*, 187(9):935–940.
25. Center, S. A., Wilkinson, E., Smith, C. A., Erb, H., and Lewis, R. M. (1985): 24-Hour urine protein/creatinine ratio in dogs with protein-losing nephropathies. *J. Am. Vet. Med. Assoc.*, 187(8):820–824.
26. Chanter, D. O., Tuck, M. G., and Coombs, D. W. (1987): The chances of false negative results in conventional toxicology studies with rats. *Toxicologist*, 43:65–74.
27. Christenson, R. H., and Azzazy, H. M. E. (1998): Biochemical markers of the acute coronary syndromes. *Clin. Chem.*, 44(8B):1855–1864.

28. Clampitt, R. B., and Hart, R. J. (1978): The tissue activities of some diagnostic enzymes in ten mammalian species. *J. Comp. Pathol.*, 88:607–621.
29. Clemo, F. A. S. (1998): Urinary enzyme evaluation of nephrotoxicity in the dog. *Toxicol. Pathol.*, 26(1):29–32.
30. Cornelius, C. E. (1989): Liver function. In: *Clinical Biochemistry of Domestic Animals*, 4th ed., edited by J. J. Kaneko, pp. 338–363. Academic Press, San Diego.
31. Cornish, H. H. (1969): The role of vitamin B_6 in the toxicity of hydrazines. *Ann. NY Acad. Sci.*, 166:136–145.
32. Dameron, G. W., Beck, M. L., Brandt, M. A., and O'Brien, P. J. (1997): Tissue and species specificity of two generations of cardiac troponin-T immunoassays. *Clin. Chem.*, 43(6):S192.
33. Dameron, G. W., Weingand, K. W., Duderstadt, J. M., Odioso, L. W., Dierckman, T. A., Schwecke, W., and Baran, K. (1992): Effect of bleeding site on clinical laboratory testing of rats: Orbital venous plexus versus posterior vena cava. *Lab. Anim. Sci.*, 42(3):299–301.
34. Davies, D. T. (1992): Enzymology in preclinical safety evaluation. *Toxicol. Pathol.*, 20(3):501–505.
35. Davis, J. A., Greenfield, R. E., and Brewer, T. G. (1993): Benzocaine-induced methemoglobinemia attributed to topical application of the anesthetic in several laboratory animal species. *Am. J. Vet. Res.*, 54(8):1322–1326.
36. Desbiens, N. A., Turney, S. L., and Gani, K. S. (1990): Multichannel 18-test panels: Are 60% of the panels abnormal by chance? *J. Lab. Clin. Med.*, 115(3):292–297.
37. Dhami, M. S. I., Drangova, R., Farkas, R., Balazs, T., and Feuer, G. (1979): Decreases in aminotransferase activity of serum and various tissues in the rat after cefazolin treatment. *Clin. Chem.*, 25:1263–1266.
38. Dodds, W. J. (1989): Hemostasis. In. *Clinical Biochemistry of Domestic Animals*, 4th ed., edited by J. J. Kaneko, pp. 274–315. Academic Press, San Diego.
39. Donovan, J. C., Stokes, W. S., Montrey, R. D., and Rozmiarek, H. (1983): Hematologic characterization of naturally occurring malaria (*Plasmodium inui*) in cynomolgus monkeys (*Macaca fascicularis*). *Lab. Anim. Sci.*, 33(1):86–89.
40. Dooley, J. F. (1984): Sorbitol dehydrogenase and its use in toxicology testing in lab animals. *Lab. Anim.*, May/June:20–21.
41. Dufour, D. R. (1996): Sources and control of analytical variation. In: *Clinical Chemistry: Theory, Analysis, Correlation*, 3rd ed., edited by L. A. Kaplan and A. J. Pesce, pp. 65–82. Mosby, St. Louis, MO.
42. Ellis, B. G., Price, R. G., and Topham, J. C. (1973): The effect of papillary damage by ethyleneimine on kidney function and some urinary enzymes in the dog. *Chem. Biol. Interact.*, 7:132–142.
43. Ellis, B. G., Price, R. G., and Topham, J. C. (1973): The effect of tubular damage by mercuric chloride on kidney function and some urinary enzymes in the dog. *Chem. Biol. Interact.*, 7:101–113.
44. Erslev, A. J. (1995): Anemia of chronic disease. In: *Williams Hematology*, 5th ed., edited by E. Beutler, M. A. Lichtman, B. S. Coller, and T. J. Kipps, pp. 518–524. McGraw-Hill, New York.
45. Erslev, A. J. (1995): Anemia of endocrine disorders. In: *Williams Hematology*, 5th ed., edited by E. Beutler, M. A. Lichtman, B. S. Coller, and T. J. Kipps, pp. 462–466. McGraw-Hill, New York.
46. Erslev, A. J. (1995): Pure red cell aplasia. In: *Williams Hematology*, 5th ed., edited by E. Beutler, M. A. Lichtman, B. S. Coller, and T. J. Kipps, pp. 448–456. McGraw-Hill, New York.
47. Evans, G. O. (1990): Biochemical assessment of cardiac function and damage in animal species. *J. Appl. Toxicol.*, 11(1):15–21.
48. Feldman, B. F., Kaneko, J. J., and Farver, T. B. (1981): Anemia of inflammatory disease in the dog: Clinical characterization. *Am. J. Vet. Res.*, 42:1109–1113.
49. Feldman, B. F., Kaneko, J. J., and Farver, T. B. (1981): Anemia of inflammatory disease in the dog: Ferrokinetics of adjuvant-induced anemia. *Am. J. Vet. Res.*, 42:583–588.
50. Feldman, B. F., and O'Neil, S. (1988): Hemolysis as a factor in clinical chemistry and hematology of the dog. *Vet. Clin. Pathol.*, 17:20.
51. Fettman, M. J. (1987): Evaluation of the usefulness of routine microscopy in canine urinalysis. *J. Am. Vet. Med. Assoc.*, 190(7):892–896.
52. Finco, D. R., and Duncan, J. R. (1976): Evaluation of blood urea nitrogen and serum creatinine concentrations as indicators of renal dysfunction: A study of 111 cases and a review of related literature. *J. Am. Vet. Med. Assoc.*, 168(7):593–601.
53. Frank, J. J., Bermes, E. W., Bickel, M. J., and Watkins, B. F. (1978): Effect of in vitro hemolysis on chemical values for serum. *Clin. Chem.*, 24:1966–1970.
54. George, J. N., El-Harake, M., and Aster, R. H. (1995): Thrombocytopenia due to enhanced platelet destruction by immunologic mechanisms. In: *Williams Hematology*, 5th ed., edited by E. Beutler, M. A. Lichtman, B. S. Coller, and T. J. Kipps, pp. 1315–1355. McGraw-Hill, New York.
55. Godsafe, P. A., and Singleton, B. K. (1992): The use of the whole blood thrombotest (1/51) as a routine monitor of vitamin K-dependent blood coagulation factor levels in the rat. *Comp. Haematol. Int.*, 2:51–55.
56. Goldberg, D. M. (1980): The expanding role of microsomal enzyme induction, and its implications for clinical chemistry. *Clin. Chem.*, 26(6):691–699.
57. Grauer, G. F., Greco, D. S., Behrend, E. N., Mani, I., Fettman, M. J., and Allen, T. A. (1985): Estimation of quantitative enzymuria in dogs with gentamicin-induced nephrotoxicosis using urine enzyme/creatinine ratios from spot urine samples. *J. Vet. Intern. Med.*, 9:324–327.
58. Grauer, G. F., Thomas, C. B., and Eicker, S. W. (1985): Estimation of quantitative proteinuria in the dog, using the protein-to-creatinine ratio from a random, voided sample. *Am. J. Vet. Res.*, 46(10):2116–2119.
59. Greco, D. S., Turnwald, G. H., Adams, R., Gossett, K. A., Kearney, M., and Casey, H. (1985): Urinary γ-glutamyl transpeptidase activity in dogs with gentamicin-induced nephrotoxicity. *Am. J. Vet. Res.*, 46(11):2332–2335.
60. Hall, R. L. (1992): Clinical pathology for preclinical safety assessment: Current global guidelines. *Toxicol. Pathol.*, 20(3):472–476.
61. Hall, R. L. (1997): Lies, damn lies, and reference intervals (or hysterical control values) for clinical pathology data. *Toxicol. Pathol.*, 25(6):647–649.
62. Hall, R. L., Wilke, W. L., and Fettman, M. J. (1986): The progression of adriamycin-induced nephrotic syndrome in rats and the effect of captopril. *Toxicol. Appl. Pharmacol.*, 82:164–174.
63. Hasegawa, A., and Furuhama, K. (1998): *Atlas of the Hematology of the Laboratory Rat*. Elsevier, Amsterdam.
64. Hoffman, W. E., Everds, N., Pignatello, M., and Solter, P. F. (1994): Automated and semiautomated analysis of rat alkaline phosphatase isoenzymes. *Toxicol. Pathol.*, 22(6):633–638.
65. Hoffman, W. E., and Solter, P. F. (1994): Alkaline phosphatase isoenzymes: Biochemistry and clinical evaluation in domestic and laboratory animals. *Curr. Top. Vet. Res.*, 1:171–178.
66. Hossein-Nia, M., Suter, K. E., Heining, P., Zwanenburg, S. B., and Holt, D. W. (1996): Creatine kinase MB isoforms and troponins T and I: Sensitive markers of myocardial damage in pre-clinical studies. *Clin. Chem.*, 42(6):S241.
67. Hulse, M., Feldman, S., and Bruckner, J. V. (1981): Effect of blood sampling schedules on protein drug binding in the rat. *J. Pharmacol. Exp. Ther.*, 218:416–420.

68. Jain, N. C. (1986): *Schalm's Veterinary Hematology*, 4th ed. Lea & Febiger, Philadelphia.
69. Jaynes, P. K. (1984): Antiepileptic drug therapy: The laboratory effects on enzyme induction. *Lab. Manage.*, March:40–46.
70. Jesty, J., and Nemerson, Y. (1995): The pathways of blood coagulation. In: *Williams Hematology*, 5th ed., edited by E. Beutler, M. A. Lichtman, B. S. Coller, and T. J. Kipps, pp. 1227–1238. McGraw-Hill, New York.
71. Kaneko, J. J. (1989): Serum proteins and the dysproteinemias. In: *Clinical Biochemistry of Domestic Animals*, 4th ed., edited by J. J. Kaneko, pp. 142–165. Academic Press, San Diego.
72. Kaneko, J. J., Harvey, J. W., and Bruss, M. L. (1997): *Clinical Biochemistry of Domestic Animals*, 5th ed. Academic Press, San Diego.
73. Kaplan, L. A., and Pesce, A. J. (1996): *Clinical Chemistry: Theory, Analysis, Correlation*, 3rd ed. Mosby, St. Louis, MO.
74. Keller, P. (1981): Enzyme activities in the dog: Tissue analyses, plasma values, and intracellular distribution. *Am. J. Vet. Res.*, 42(4):575–582.
75. Khan, K. N. M., Komocsar, W. J., Das, I, Lazzaro, N. C., Senese, P. B., Hamilton, P., Roth, A., and Smith, P. F. (1996): Effect of bleeding site on clinical pathologic parameters in Sprague-Dawley rats: Retro-orbital venous plexus versus abdominal aorta. *Contemp. Top.*, 35(5):63–66.
76. Kimball, J. P., Eitzen, B. H., Lewandowski, A. D., Kirk, J. F. E., Sansone, J., and Johnson, A. N. (1995): Short-term carbon dioxide/oxygen anesthesia for laboratory rats and mice. *Clin. Chem.*, 41(6):S163.
77. Kolaja, G. J., VanderMeer, D. A., Packwood, W. H., and Satoh, P. S. (1992): The use of sodium dodecyl sulfate-polyacrylamide gel electrophoresis to detect renal damage in Sprague-Dawley rats treated with gentamicin sulfate. *Toxicol. Pathol.*, 20(4):603–607.
78. Kramer, J. W. (1989): Clinical enzymology. In: *Clinical Biochemistry of Domestic Animals*, 4th ed., edited by J. J. Kaneko, pp. 338–363. Academic Press, San Diego.
79. Kurata, M., Noguchi, N., Kasuga, Y., Sugimoto, T., Tanaka, K., and Hasegawa, T. (1998): Prolongation of PT and APTT under excessive anticoagulant in plasma from rats and dogs. *J. Toxicol. Sci.*, 23(2):149–153.
80. Laessig, R. H., Hassemer, D. J., Paskey, T. A., and Schwartz, T. H. (1976): The effect of 0.1 and 1.0% erythrocytes and hemolysis on serum chemistry values. *Am. J. Clin. Pathol.*, 66:639–644.
81. Leard, B. L., Alsaker, R. D., Porter, W. P., and Sobel, L. P. (1990). The effect of haemolysis on certain canine serum chemistry parameters. *Lab. Anim.*, 24:32–35.
82. Leonard, T. B., Neptun, D. A., and Popp, J. A. (1984): Serum gamma glutamyl transferase as a specific indicator of bile duct lesions in the rat liver. *Am. J. Pathol.*, 116:262–269.
83. Loeb, W. F. (1998): The measurement of renal injury. *Toxicol. Pathol.*, 26(1):26–28.
84. Loeb, W. F., and Quimby, F. W. (1989): *The Clinical Chemistry of Laboratory Animals*. Pergamon Press, Oxford.
85. Maejima, K., and Nagase, S. (1991): Effect of starvation and refeeding on the circadian rhythms of hematological and clinico-biochemical values and water intake of rats. *Exp. Anim. Jpn.*, 40:389–393.
86. Matsuzawa, T., Nomura, M., and Unno, T. (1993): Clinical pathology reference ranges of laboratory animals. *J. Vet. Med. Sci.*, 55(3):351–362.
87. Matsuzawa, T., and Sakazume, M. (1994): Effects of fasting on haematology and clinical chemistry values in the rat and dog. *Comp. Haematol. Int.*, 4:152–156.
88. Matsuzawa, T., Tabata, H., Sakazume, M., Yoshida, S., and Nakamura, S. (1994): A comparison of the effect of bleeding site on haematological and plasma chemistry values of F344 rats: The inferior vena cava, abdominal aorta, and orbital venous plexus. *Comp. Haematol. Int.*, 4:207–211.
89. McAuley, F. T., Simpson, J. G., Thomson, A. W., and Whiting, P. H. (1986): The predictive value of enzymuria in cyclosporin A-induced renal toxicity in the rat. *Toxicol. Let.*, 32:163–169.
90. McGrath, J. P. (1993): Assessment of hemolytic and hemorrhagic anemias in preclinical safety assessment studies. *Toxicol. Pathol.*, 21(2):158–163.
91. McGrath, J. P., Meador, V. P., Swain, R. R., and Jensen, C. B. (1993): Oxidative erythrocytic injury in preclinical toxicity testing. *Vet. Pathol.*, 30(5):429.
92. Millis, D. L., Hawkins, E., Jager, M., and Boyle, C. R. (1995): Comparison of coagulation test results for blood samples obtained by means of direct venipuncture and through a jugular vein catheter in clinically normal dogs. *J. Am. Vet. Med. Assoc.*, 207(10):1311–1314.
93. National Committee for Clinical Laboratory Standards. (1995): *How to define and determine reference intervals in the clinical laboratory: Approved guideline*. NCCLS document C28-A, Villanova, PA.
94. Neptun, D. A., Smith, C. N., and Irons, R. D. (1985): Effect of sampling site and collection methods on variations in baseline clinical pathology parameters in Fischer-344 rats. I. Clinical chemistry. *Fundam. Appl. Toxicol.*, 5:1180–1185.
95. O'Brien, P. J., Landt, Y., and Ladenson, J. H. (1997): Differential reactivity of cardiac and skeletal muscle from various species in a cardiac troponin I immunoassay. *Clin. Chem.*, 43(12):2333–2338.
96. O'Brien, S. R., Sellers, T. S., and Meyer, D. J. (1995): Artifactual prolongation of the activated partial thromboplastin time associated with hemoconcentration in dogs. *J. Vet. Int. Med.*, 3:163–170.
97. Ono, T., Kitaguchi, K., Takehara, M., Shiba, M., and Hayami, K. (1981): Serum-constituents analysis: Effect of duration and temperature of storage of clotted blood. *Clin. Chem.*, 27(1):35–38.
98. Packman, C. H., and Leddy, J. P. (1995): Drug-related immune hemolytic anemia. In: *Williams Hematology*, 5th ed., edited by E. Beutler, M. A. Lichtman, B. S. Coller, and T. J. Kipps, pp. 691–697. McGraw-Hill, New York.
99. Palek, J. (1995): Acanthocytosis, stomatocytosis, and related disorders. In: *Williams Hematology*, 5th ed., edited by E. Beutler, M. A. Lichtman, B. S. Coller, and T. J. Kipps, pp. 557–563. McGraw-Hill, New York.
100. Passey, R. B. (1996): Quality control for the clinical chemistry laboratory. In: *Clinical Chemistry: Theory, Analysis, Correlation*, 3rd ed., edited by L. A. Kaplan and A. J. Pesce, pp. 382–401. Mosby, St. Louis, MO.
101. Perrone, R. D., Madias, N. E., and Levey, A. S. (1992): Serum creatinine as an index of renal function: New insights into old concepts. *Clin. Chem.*, 38(10):1933–1953.
102. Price, R. G. (1982): Urinary enzymes, nephrotoxicity, and renal disease. *Toxicologist*, 23:99–134.
103. Rebar, A. H. (1993): General responses of the bone marrow to injury. *Toxicol. Pathol.*, 21(2):118–129.
104. Roncaglioni, M. C., de Gaetano, G., and Donati, M. B. (1982): Some aspects of hematological toxicity in animals. In: *Animals in Toxicological Research*, edited by I. Bartosek, pp. 77–89. Raven Press, New York.
105. Sawyer, M. L., Douglas, S. E., and Mielke, P. M. (1997): Blood collection via the jugular vein in rats. *Contemp. Topics*, 36(4):64.
106. Schardijn, G. H. C., and van Eps, L. W. S. (1987): β_2-Microglobulin: Its significance in the evaluation of renal function. *Kidney Int.*, 32:635–641.
107. Schiffer, S. P., Gillett, C. S., and Ringler, D. H. (1984): Activated coagulation time for rhesus monkeys (*Macaca mulatta*). *Lab. Anim. Sci.*, 34(2):191–193.

108. Scipioni, R. L., Diters, R. W., Meyers, W. R., and Hart, S. M. (1997): Clinical and clinicopathological assessment of serial phlebotomy in the Sprague Dawley rat. *Lab. Anim. Sci.*, 47(3):293–299.

109. Shadduck, R. K. (1995): Aplastic anemia. In: *Williams Hematology*, 5th ed., edited by E. Beutler, M. A. Lichtman, B. S. Coller, and T. J. Kipps, pp. 238–251. McGraw-Hill, New York.

110. Sherwin, J. E., and Sobenes, J. R. (1996): Liver function. In: *Clinical Chemistry: Theory, Analysis, Correlation*, 3rd ed., edited by L. A. Kaplan and A. J. Pesce, pp. 505–527. Mosby, St. Louis, MO.

111. Slighter, R. G., Kimball, J. P., Barbolt, T. A., Sherer, A. D., and Drobeck, H. P. (1988): Enzootic hepatitis A infection in cynomolgus monkeys (*Macaca fascicularis*). *Am. J. Primatol.*, 14:73–81.

112. Smith, C. N., Neptun, D. A., and Irons, R. D. (1986): Effect of sampling site and collection methods on variations in baseline clinical pathology parameters in Fischer-344 rats. II. Clinical hematology. *Fundam. Appl. Toxicol.*, 7:658–663.

113. Solter, P. F., Hoffman, W. E., Chambers, M. D., Schaeffer, D. J., and Kuhlenschmidt, M. S. (1994): Hepatic total 3α-hydroxy bile acids concentration and enzyme activities in prednisone-treated dogs. *Am. J. Vet. Res.*, 55(8):1086–1092.

114. Solter, P. F., Hoffman, W. E., Hungerford, L. L., Siegel, J. P., St. Denis, S. H., and Dorner, J. L. (1991): Haptoglobin and ceruloplasmin as determinants of inflammation in dogs. *Am. J. Vet. Res.*, 52(10):1738–1742.

115. Stolk, J. M., and Smith, R. P. (1966): Species differences in methemoglobin reductase activity. *Biochem. Pharmacol.*, 15:343–351.

116. Stonard, M. D. (1990): Assessment of renal function and damage in animal species. *J. Appl. Toxicol.*, 10(4):267–274.

117. Stonard, M. D., Gore, C. W., Oliver, G. J. A., and Smith, I. K. (1987): Urinary enzymes and protein patterns as indicators of injury to different regions of the kidney. *Fundam. Appl. Toxicol.*, 9:339–351.

118. Stringer, S. K., and Seligmann, B. E. (1996): Effects of two injectable anesthetic agents on coagulation assays in the rat. *Lab. Anim. Sci.*, 46(4):430–433.

119. Stromberg, P. C. (1985): Large granular lymphocyte leukemia in F344 rats. *Am. J. Pathol.*, 119(3):517–519.

120. Sturgill, M. G., and Lambert, G. H. (1997): Xenobiotic-induced hepatotoxicity: Mechanisms of liver injury and methods of monitoring liver function. *Clin. Chem.*, 43(8):1512–1526.

121. Suber, R. L., and Kodell, R. L. (1985): The effect of three phlebotomy techniques on hematological and clinical chemical evaluation in Sprague-Dawley rats. *Vet. Clin. Pathol.*, 14(1):23–30.

122. Swaim, L. D., Taylor, H. W., and Jersey, G. C. (1985): The effect of handling techniques on serum ALT activity in mice. *J. Appl. Toxicol.*, 5(3):160–162.

123. Swenson, C. L., and Graves, T. K. (1997): Absence of liver specificity for canine alanine aminotransferase. *Vet. Clin. Pathol.*, 26(1):26–28.

124. Thompson, M. B. (1986): Avoiding pitfalls in clinical chemistry—Quality control is not quality assurance. In: *Managing Conduct and Data Quality of Toxicology Studies. Sharing Perspectives Expanding Horizons*, Conference Proceedings, pp. 199–206. Princeton Scientific, Princeton, NJ.

125. Thoreson, S. I., Harve, G. N., Morberg, H., and Mowinckel, P. (1992): Effects of storage time on chemistry. Results from canine whole blood, heparinized whole blood, serum, and heparinized plasma. *Vet. Clin. Pathol.*, 21(3):88–94.

126. Upton, P. K., and Morgan, D. J. (1975): The effect of sampling technique on some blood parameters in the rat. *Lab. Anim.*, 9:85–91.

127. Vail, D. M., Allen, T. A., and Weiser, G. (1986): Applicability of leukocyte esterase test strip in detection of canine pyuria. *J. Am. Vet. Med. Assoc.*, 189(11):1451–1453.

128. Viau, C., Bernard, A., and Lauwerys, R. (1986): Determination of rat β_2-microglobulin in urine and in serum. I. Development of an immunoassay based on latex particles agglutination. *J. Appl. Toxicol.*, 6:185–189.

129. Viau, C., Bernard, A., Ouled, A., and Lauwerys, R. (1986): Determination of rat β_2-microglobulin in urine and in serum. II. Application of its urinary measurement to selected nephrotoxicity models. *J. Appl. Toxicol.*, 6:191–195.

130. Waner, T., and Nyska, A. (1994): The influence of fasting on blood glucose, triglycerides, cholesterol, and alkaline phosphatase in rats. *Vet. Clin. Pathol.*, 23(3):78–81.

131. Waner, T., Nyska, A., and Chen, R. (1991): Population distribution profiles of the activities of blood alanine and aspartate aminotransferase in the normal F344 inbred rat by age and sex. *Lab. Anim. Sci.*, 25:263–271.

132. Waner, T., Nyska, A., Nyska, M., Sela, M., Pirak, M., and Galiano, A. (1988): Gingival hyperplasia in dogs induced by oxodipine, a calcium channel blocker. *Toxicol. Pathol.*, 16:327–332.

133. Watkins, J. R., Gough, A. W., and McGuire, E. J. (1989): Drug-induced myopathy in beagle dogs. *Toxicol. Pathol.*, 17(3):545–548.

134. Weil, C. S., and Carpenter, C. P. (1969): Abnormal values in control groups during repeated–dose toxicologic studies. *Toxicol. Appl. Pharmacol.* 14:335–339.

135. Weingand, K., Brown, G., Hall, R., Davies, D., Gossett, K., Neptun, D., Waner, T., Matsuzawa, T., Salemink, P., Froelke, W., Provost, J., Dal Negro, G., Batchelor, J., Nomura, M., Groetsch, H., Boink, A., Kimball, J., Woodman, D., York, M., Fabianson-Johnson, E., Lupart, M., and Melloni, E. (1996): Harmonization of animal clinical pathology testing in toxicity and safety studies. *Fundam. Appl. Toxicol.*, 29:198–201.

136. Weiss, D. J. (1993): Leukocyte response to toxic injury. *Toxicol. Pathol.*, 21(2):135–140.

137. Weiss, D. J., and Klausner, J. S. (1990): Drug-associated aplastic anemia in dogs: Eight cases (1984–1988). *J. Am. Vet. Med. Assoc.*, 196(3):472–475.

138. Westgard, J. O., and Klee, G. G. (1987): Quality assurance. In: *Fundamentals of Clinical Chemistry*, 3rd ed., edited by N. W. Tietz, pp. 238–253. W. B. Saunders, Philadelphia.

139. White, J. V., Olivier, N. B., Reimann, K., and Johnson, C. (1984): Use of protein-to-creatinine ratio in a single urine specimen for quantitative estimation of canine proteinuria. *J. Am. Vet. Med. Assoc.*, 185(8):882–885.

140. Wilkerson, R. D., Conran, P. B., and Greene, S. L. (1984): Activated coagulation time test: A convenient monitor of heparinization for dogs used in cardiovascular research. *Lab. An. Sci.*, 34(1):62–65.

141. Williams, W. J. (1995): Secondary thrombocytosis. In: *Williams Hematology*, 5th ed., edited by E. Beutler, M. A. Lichtman, B. S. Coller, and T. J. Kipps, pp. 1361–1363. McGraw-Hill, New York.

142. Wixson, S. K., and Griffith, J. W. (1986): Nutritional deficiency anemias in nonhuman primates. *Lab. Anim. Sci.*, 36(3):231–236.

143. Zhang, D. J., Elswick, R. K., Miller, W. G., and Bailey, J. L. (1998): Effect of serum-clot contact time on clinical chemistry laboratory results. *Clin. Chem.*, 44(6):1325–1333.

Principles and Methods of Toxicology, Fourth Edition, edited by A. Wallace Hayes.
Taylor & Francis, Philadelphia © 2001.

Chapter 22

Dermatotoxicology

Howard Maibach and Esther Patrick

Adult human skin constitutes approximately 10% of normal body weight. Its functions include regulation of body temperature and water loss, temporary storage of nutrients, vitamin synthesis, and its major function, protection (256,257,307,347). Resiliency and tensile strength protect against physical injury, pigmentation protects against ultraviolet light, barrier properties protect against environmental chemicals' entry into the body, and the growth pattern and surface characteristics protect against microbial colonization and invasion. The regenerative capacity following wounding, and the number of processes by which skin can deal with environmental insults, provides strong evidence of the importance of healthy skin to the organism. The psychological value of healthy skin has led in part to the development of multibillion dollar cosmetic and personal care industries.

The policies of agencies such as OHSA (Occupational Health and Safety Administration), DOT (Department of Transportation), CPSC (Consumer Product Safety Commission), and FDA (Food and Drug Administration) in the United States, and OECD (Organization for Economic Co-operation and Development) and EEC (European Economic Community) internationally, indicate that the identification of chemicals hazardous to the skin and the protection of society from exposure to those chemicals should be given high priority. These agencies mandate specific assays to evaluate the effects of skin exposure prior to registration, transport, and marketing of chemicals of formulated products. The adverse skin responses associated with repetitive, low-dose exposure to industrial chemicals and consumer products all too often are not accurately predicted by the required assays. The need to market products with low risk of producing dermal and systemic injury in order to increase consumer satisfaction has led to the development of numerous assays to rank chemicals for their ability to injure the skin. Although these assays are not mandated by regulatory agencies, the frequency with which they are conducted and their utility warrants attention.

The field of dermatotoxicology includes measurement of absorption of materials and assays that evaluate the development of neoplasms, trigger an immune response, directly destroy the skin (corrosion), irritate the skin, produce urticaria (hives), and produce noninflammatory painful sensations. The inflammatory responses of skin are the most common chemically-induced diseases in man.

SKIN STRUCTURE AND FUNCTION

To understand the variety of adverse responses to skin and the basis for the predictive assays for skin injury, some understanding of skin anatomy and physiology is necessary. Approximately 20,000 to 23,000 cm^2 of skin

Table 22.1
Regional variation of skin thickness[a] in man

Region	Thickness (μm)	Reference
Stratum corneum of abdomen	8.2	Holbrook and Odland, (156)
Abdomen	46.6	Whitton and Ewell, (379)
Stratum corneum of back	9.4	Holbrook and Odland, (156)
Back	43.2	Bergstressor et al., (23)
Stratum corneum of thigh	10.9	Holbrook and Odland, (156)
Thigh	54.3	Bergstressor et al., (23)
Stratum corneum of forearm	15.0	Holbrook and Odland, (156)
Forearm	60.9	Bergstressor et al., (23)
Cheek	38.8	Whitton and Ewell, (379)
Forehead	50.3	Whitton and Ewell, (379)
Back of hand	84.5	Whitton and Ewell, (379)
Fingertip	369.0	Whitton and Ewell, (379)

[a] Values are for full thickness skin unless stratum corneum is specified.

cover the body of an adult human. Skin is heterogeneous; the number of appendages (i.e., sweat glands, hair follicles, sebaceous glands, the thickness of skin) vary by body region (156,379). For example, thickness of skin of the eyelid is approximately 0.51 mm whereas that of the palm and sole are approximately 4.1 mm (Table 22.1).

A film composed of triglycerides, phospholipids, esterified cholesterol, and other materials released by holocrine sebaceous glands, and salts and water released by eccrine sweat glands, normally covers the outer surface (264). This surface film has been referred to as an acid mantle, pH of the skin normally varying between 4.2 and 5.6. Micrococciae, and *Corynebacterium* species normally colonize the skin surface (217,256). Changes in surface film composition, for example, changes caused by inflammatory conditions of occlusion, may result in a 1000-fold increase in absolute number of microorganisms colonizing the area and in a shift in flora present (33,34). The surface film penetrates the outermost cellular layers of the skin.

Based on structure and embryonic origin, the cellular layers of the skin are divided into two distinct regions (Figure 22.1): the epidermis and the dermis. The outer region, the epidermis, develops from embryonic ectoderm and covers the connective tissue; the dermis is derived from the mesoderm (155,157,248). The epidermis comprises approximately 5% of full-thickness skin (216,257). For descriptive purposes, the epidermis is subdivided into five to six layers based on cellular characteristics (Figure 22.2). Note that these layers of keratinocytes are formed by ordered differentiation of cells from one layer of mitotic basal cells. The number of distinguishable layers varies by anatomical site.

Basal layer keratinocytes are metabolically active cells with the capacity to divide. Some daughter cells of the basal layer move upward and differentiate. Cells adjacent

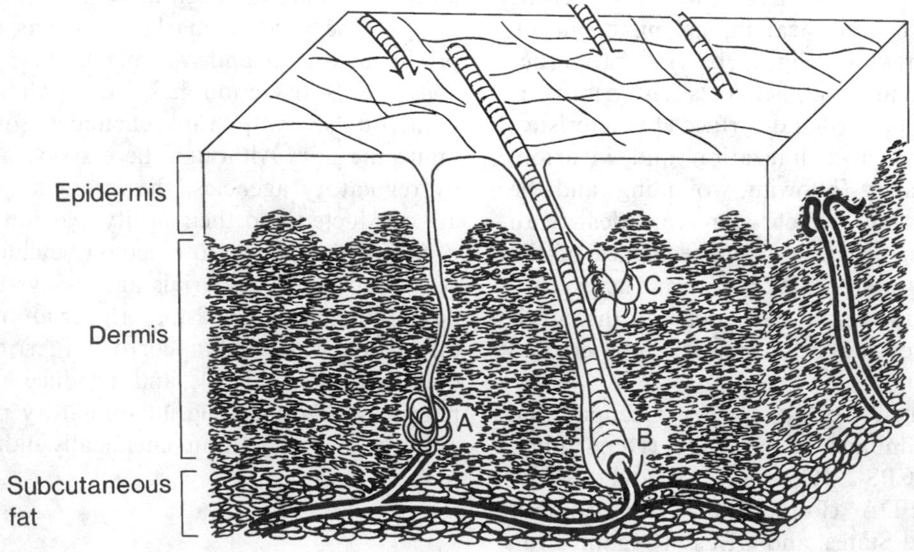

FIG 22.1. A Schematic of Human Skin. Eccrine sweat glands (A) are located in the dermis; a duct transports sweat through the epidermis to the surface. Hair follicles (B) are located deep in the dermis. Each hair extends through the skin via an epithelized channel. Contents of sebaceous glands (C) are released into the follicular channel as the sebocytes die. Each skin appendage has its own blood supply. Plexuses formed in the upper dermis (shown in the drawing to the far right) supply nutrients to the upper epidermis and upper dermis.

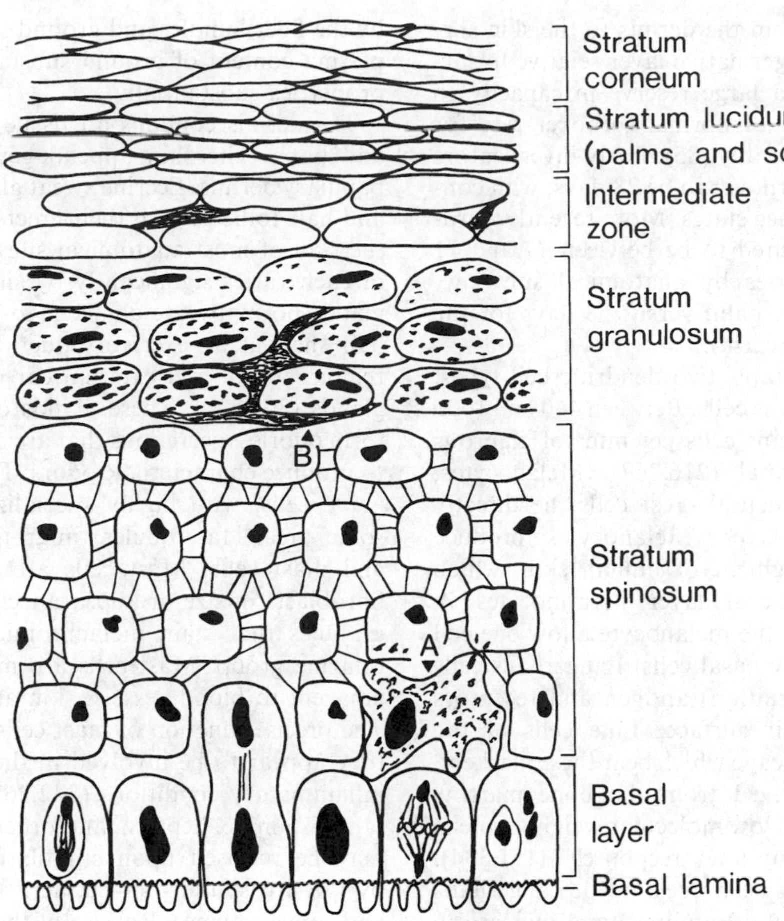

FIG 22.2. The Epidermis. All possible cell layers and the locations of the two dendritic cell types, melanocytes (A) and Langerhans cells (B), are shown.

to the basal layer contain large mitochondria; the golgi apparatus and rough endoplasmic reticulum (RER) are well developed. These cells produce lamellar granules, intracellular organelles, which later fuse to the cell membrane to release neutral lipids believed to form a barrier to penetration through the epidermis (95,96,338,374). Microscopically, the desmosomes and bridges connecting adjacent cells resemble spines, and the three- to four-cell thick layer of cells above the basal layer is referred to as the stratum spinosum. The spines connecting adjacent cells are temporary structures; keratinocytes dissociate from neighboring cells and form new associations as they move upward, individually, in the epidermis (257). Cells of the third subdivision of the epidermis, the stratum granulosum, are characterized by the presence of keratohyalin granules, polyribosomes, large golgi apparatus, and RER. Cells of the granular layer are the uppermost viable cells of the epidermis. Here the lamellar granules are released at the cell surface. An intermediate zone of cells separates the cornified layers of the outer epidermis from the viable granulosum. In the palms and soles, the stratum lucidum, or clear cell layer, lies above the stratum granulosum. This layer is indistinguishable in skin sections from other areas. Cells of the intermediate zone may contain enzymes capable of metabolizing exogenous chemicals but have lost the ability to synthesize proteins. The outermost cornified layer, the stratum corneum, consists of cells that have lost their nucleus and all capacity for metabolic activity. The dominant constituent of these cells is keratin, a scleroprotein with chains linked by both disulfide and hydrogen bonds that were synthesized and stored in the deep epidermal layers. The intracellular attachments between these cells gradually break and the outermost cells are sloughed.

In addition to the visible intercellular and metabolic changes observed during keratinocyte differentiation, their size and shape have also changed. Cells derived from basal cuboidal cells approximately 5 μm in diameter have elongated and flattened to approximately 30 μm (216). Four differentiated cornified cells of the stratum corneum (2 × 2) cover the same area as 100 basal keratinocytes (10 × 10). Each basal cell has the capacity to cover itself many times with modest mitotic rates. The pattern of papillae (ridges and grooves) of the basal layer formed by accessory structures from the dermis to the skin surface increases the area of germative layer relative to surface area. This provides a large reserve in capacity to cover the area. Estimates of normal turnover rate for keratinocytes vary considerably (85). Early investigators (292) estimated normal turnover to be 28 days, with considerable increases in disease states. More recently, turnover rate has been calculated to be between 17 and 71 days (103). Turnover varies by anatomical site (e.g., 32–36 days for the human palm versus 58 days for the anterior surface of the forearm).

The epidermis also contains two dendritic cell types: melanocytes and Langerhans cells. Between 460 and 1000 melanocytes and Langerhans cells per mm^2 of glabrous nonspecified skin is normal (216,267). Melanocytes, derived from embryonic neural crest cells, lie directly adjacent to the basal layer. Melanocytes produce melanin, the principal pigment of human skin, which is then transferred to basal layer keratinocytes in granules. The dendrites of the melanocyte allow one cell to supply melanin to many basal cells. Langerhans cells express Ia (immune recognition) antigen and receptors for IgG and C3 on their surface. Like cells of the monocyte/macrophage lineage which bear these markers, Langerhans cells are derived from the bone marrow mesenchyme. They process low molecular weight haptens during induction of immune responses (151,334). Although this function has been questioned, Langerhans cells take up small molecules (nonlipid) and increase in number in areas that have developed allergic reactions (333). Note that Langerhans cells lie in epidermal layers containing enzymes that can metabolize exogenous chemicals. In some cases, metabolites of the agent applied to the skin cause allergic contact dermatitis.

The dermis and epidermis are separated by a basal lamina. The dermis is attached to this membrane by fine fibers of connective tissue. Cells of the basal layer are anchored to the lamina by radicles. This area of attachment, called the marginal layer, is identified histologically by periodic acid Schiff reaction. There are occasional breaks in the attachments. Large breaks are observed in exfoliative skin conditions (43,216). The dermal connective tissue enclosed by the epidermal papilla is referred to as papillary dermis; the area below the papilla is the stratum subpapillare, or reticular dermis. The fibers of the papillary dermis are finer than fibers of the reticular dermis. The reticular dermis contains thick collagen bundles, especially in areas adjacent to blood vessels and skin appendages. Connective tissue fibers are separated by the ground substance, an amorphous material consisting of proteins and glycosaminoglycans, such as chrondroitin A sulfate and hyaluronic acid. The constituents of ground substance are derived from both fibrocytes and blood plasma. The physical behavior of the dermis, including elasticity, is determined by the fiber bundles and ground substance. Variations in plasma content of ground substance may alter physical properties substantially.

The dermis contains all tissue types, except cartilage and bone. The skin appendages originate in the subpapillary dermis. Eccrine sweat glands, sebaceous glands, and hair follicles with their erector muscles are found in the skin of most anatomical sites; however, the number of each varies significantly by site (309,336). Sebaceous glands normally are adjacent to hair follicles, using the hair shaft as an excretory duct. The axillae, anogenital region, eyelid, and external ear contain apocrine sweat glands (301,328). These glands develop at puberty and form odorless secretions that are decomposed by bacteria to produce characteristic odors. The dermis also contains nerve cells, with highly specialized sensory endings in some areas, fat lobules, migratory white blood cells, and mast cells. Mast cells are indistinguishable from fibroblasts in size or appearance; however, they contain granules that stain metachromically with agents of a thiazine group. Mast cells are most numerous in areas adjacent to blood vessels, skin appendages, and nerves. The precise function of mast cells is unknown; however, they appear to be involved in the pathogenesis of some inflammatory conditions (342,368). Their granules contain histamine, heparin, and other vasoactive agents that may be released upon stimulation of the cell surface by IgE crosslinking 48–80, activated serum compounds, and some enzymes. Release of these mediators is accompanied by formation of other agents, such as the metabolites of arachidonic acid (342), which are inflammatory mediators in some conditions.

The dermis and fascia of muscles are separated by the subcutis, a layer of fatty tissue. The extent and development of subcutis depends on sex, age, diet, and body region. Blood vessels supplying the skin arise from the subcutis. Vascular plexuses are formed in the transition zone of the subcutis and dermis adjacent to coils of the eccrine sweat gland. Arteries extend upward to mid-dermis, forming anastomoses there. Similar, but independent, plexuses form at the base of the hair shaft and sebaceous glands. A third vascular network is formed from arteries branching off from vessels at the level of eccrine sweat glands that branch into finer vessels that form plexuses in the papillary dermis. Plexuses of the papillary dermis supply the upper dermis, including the upper hair shaft, and the epidermis with nutrients. The adjacent but separate vascular units in the dermis sometimes react differently in pathological processes (i.e., follicular rash).

A simple visual comparison allows one to conclude that the skin of man and animals vary considerably. The most obvious difference is hair coat covering the skin. In lower mammals, each hair shaft may contain several follicles, a large follicle arising from the subpapillary dermis, and several accessory follicles arising from the papillary dermis. In man, sebaceous gland density varies from 100 to 900 glands per cm^2; in other mammals, sebaceous glands are more evenly distributed (328). Human sweat is produced by eccrine sweat glands. Apocrine sweat glands are the dominant sweat gland of animals. Eccrine sweat glands open directly to the skin surface, whereas apocrine glands empty into the hair shaft. Apocrine sweat is less acidic than eccrine sweat, and the pH of the skin surface of animals usually is somewhat higher than that of man (203). The thickness of skin also varies extensively by species and body site. Differences in content of granules of mast cells from different species have been reported (368), as have differences in sensitivity to various inflammatory mediators applied to skin. These differences undoubtedly contribute to the lack of correlation between the results of some animal and human predictive assays (285). The lack of correlation justifies predictive skin testing in man after preliminary screening in animals if the risks to subjects are minimal.

PHARMACOKINETICS FOLLOWING APPLICATION OF CHEMICALS TO THE SKIN

Until the beginning of the 20th century, skin was considered a relatively inert barrier to chemicals that might enter the body (312). We now know that this view is incorrect. Although the skin's barrier properties are impressive, many chemicals penetrate the skin, and the skin can metabolize exogenous compounds. Because of its large surface area, skin may be a major route of entry into the body for some exposure situations. Delivery of drugs through the skin to treat systemic conditions has become almost commonplace. Interest in cutaneous pharmacokinetics has increased as the skin has been reconsidered to be a route for systemic administration of drugs and chemicals, as well as a route of entry for toxins. A variety of assays, both in vivo and in vitro, for measuring absorption through the skin have been developed (11,12,376,377), and many factors that govern absorption through the skin have been determined (Table 22.2).

The stratum corneum is a major diffusion barrier of the skin (146,308). Removal of the stratum corneum by tape stripping increases the rate of absorption of some chemicals (34). Absorption of chemicals through shunts, openings of skin appendages, and gaps in the stratum corneum associated with these structures have been considered (137,311,346,380). Because of the relative surface area of these shunts (0.1%–1.0% of the total area) they do not play a decisive role in absorption (311); however, they may be important initially after application of the penetrant (313), and sebaceous glands may act as a drug reservoir for some materials (146,159,308). The stratum

Table 22.2
Factors determining percutaneous absorption

Release from Vehicle
Varies with solubility in vehicle
Varies with concentration
Varies with pH
Kinetics of Skin Penetration
Influenced by anatomical site
Influenced by degree of occlusion
Influenced by intrinsic skin condition
Influenced by animal age
Influenced by concentration of dosing solution
Influenced by surface area dosed
Influenced by frequency of dosing
Tissue distribution
Excretion kinetics
Substantivity to the skin
Volatility
Wash and rub resistance
Binding to skin components
Cutaneous metabolism
Anatomic pathways

Adapted from Reference 377.

corneum is nonviable and has no capacity for active transport processes. Therefore, absorption can be described as passive diffusion across this membrane by the equation $J = Km \times Cv \times Dm \times y$ (89), Rate of absorption = Partition coefficient between vehicle and stratum corneum times concentration times diffusion constant of penetrant in stratum corneum times thickness of stratum corneum. It is obvious that skin from different animals or sites of different thickness from the same animal will vary in barrier properties to absorption.

The concentration term is concentration at the skin surface. Application of suspensions of penetrant with slow dissolution rates, or of emulsions, or of penetrants in vehicles in which diffusion rate is slow will alter surface concentration and may control the fate of penetration (48,56,65,154). This principle has been used in designing slow-release transdermal delivery devices. Other factors that affect thermodynamic activity of the solution at the skin surface, such as pH and temperature, may vary the absorption rate (312,313). Vehicle influence cannot be overstated for a specific concentration of drug; thermodynamic activity may vary by 1000-fold from one vehicle to another. Some vehicles may promote penetration by altering the characteristics of the stratum corneum (196). Other factors that affect percutaneous absorption include condition of the skin (110), age (149,230,304), surface area to which the material is applied (377), penetrant volatility, temperature and humidity (119), substantivity, and wash and rub resistance to removal from the skin, and binding to the skin (277). Skin may become saturated by a penetrant and thus resist penetration from subsequent applications.

In an intuitive sense, it has been assumed that multiple applications would provide significantly greater mass transfer; however, dermatopharmacokinetics (DPK) studies demonstrate that in any one given day, multiple applications may add little transfer. This may explain why many dermatologic drugs can be successfully dosed on a once-daily basis. Over many days the above phenomea does not appear to occur (80,375).

Once a chemical has gained access to the viable epidermal layers, it may initiate a local effect, it may be absorbed into the circulation and produce an effect, or it may produce no local or systemic effects. The viable epidermis contains many enzymes capable of metabolizing exogenous chemicals (24–27,239,266), including cytochrome P450 isoenzymes, mixed function oxidases and glucuronyl transferases. Enzymes have been identified in three compartments (10,71). Skin enzymes are inducible by systemic phenobarbital, rifampicin, and 3-methyl cholanthrene (360) and topical 2,3,7,8-tetrachlorodibenzo (p) dioxin (TCDD) (293), 3 methyl cholanthrene and Aroclor 1254 (79).

Early studies indicated that enzymatic activity in skin was only a fraction of the activity of the liver. Those studies were conducted in vitro using whole skin; the enzymatic activity is in the epidermis, which makes up less than 5% of whole skin (266). When enzymatic activities of the epidermis were calculated, activities ranged from 80% to 240% of those in liver. In some cases, different metabolites are formed in liver and skin from the same parent compound.

While the list of enzymes isolated from skin continues to grow, the skin does not have the capacity to metabolize all chemicals. For example, topically applied hexachlorophene does not appear to be metabolized. At present, it is not possible to predict metabolic pathways or rates following topical application; these must be determined experimentally. Comprehensive reviews of the metabolic capability of skin have been published recently (10,177).

In Vivo Percutaneous Absorption Assays

Percutaneous absorption can be determined by applying a known amount of chemical to a specified surface area and then measuring the level of the chemical in the urine and/or feces. To correct for excretion of the material through the lungs, sweat (of retention in the body) levels measured following topical administration usually are expressed as a percentage of levels following parenteral administration of the chemical (46,376). Because the analytical techniques to measure the chemical are not always available, and because some chemicals may be metabolized, radioactive-labeled chemicals, usually carbon 14 or tritium, are customarily used in these assays. Although studies with radiolabeled compounds accurately reflect absorption, they may not provide accurate estimates of bioavailability. For example, comparison of bioavailability from nitroglycerin (unmetabolized drug) level and level of radioactive tracer indicates that use of the tracer overestimates available drug by as much as 20%. This corresponds to the metabolism of the drug to an inactive form.

In vivo studies have been conducted in man and in a number of species (11,12). Comparison of absorption fates of a number of compounds showed that absorption rates in the rat and rabbit tend to be higher than in human and that the skin permeability of monkeys and swine more closely resembles humans (Table 22.3). Although these differences are not predicted by any single factor,

Table 22.3
Species differences in in vivo absorption (% dose absorbed)

Compound	Rat	Rabbit	Pig	Squirrel Monkey	Man	Reference
Haloprogin	95.8	113.0	19.7	—	11.0	Bartek et al., (11)
Acetylcysteine	3.5	2.0	6.0	—	2.4	Bartek et al., (11)
Cortisone	24.7	30.3	4.1	—	3.4	Bartek et al., (11)
Caffeine	53.1	69.2	32.4	—	47.6	Bartek et al., (11)
Butter yellow	48.2	100.0	41.9	—	21.6	Bartek et al., (11)
Testosterone	47.4	69.6	29.4	—	13.2	Bartek et al., (11)
DDT	46.3	—	43.4	1.5	10.4	Bartek and LaBudde, (12)
Lindane	51.2	—	37.6	16.0	9.3	Bartek and LaBudde, (12)
Parathion	97.5	—	14.5	30.3	9.7	Bartek and LaBudde, (12)
Malathion	64.6	—	15.5	19.3	8.2	Bartek and LaBudde, (12)

such as epidermal thickness, they are not unexpected in light of differences in skin characteristics. There are interspecies differences in routes of excretion of some chemicals as well. This may be due in part to metabolism of the chemical, and the metabolic capabilities of the species should be considered when selecting an animal model and designing the experiment. Ingestion of the test material by the animal must be prevented, and this may require restraint of the animal or design of specialized protective apparatus for the site of application. Because urine and feces are collected for analysis, specialized cages are also required.

The difficulties in conducting these types of pharmacokinetic assays—collecting excrement for relatively long period of time (24 h), requirements for specialized cages and specialized protective apparatus, and the increased space requirements for housing animals individually—has led to the use of other in vivo assays and to the development of in vitro models. Loss of radioactive material from the skin surface has been used to estimate in vivo percutaneous absorption (234). The difference in applied dose and residue on the skin is assumed to be absorbed. The characteristics of the radioisotope, penetrant, and vehicle may limit the usefulness of this procedure. Volatile materials leave the surface without penetrating, and it is difficult to recover all material from the skin surface. In addition, skin may retain a reservoir of the penetrant that has not entered the circulation.

There is a clear relationship between the mass of a chemical residing in the strateum corneum that has been washed 30 min after application and the eventual penetration that can be measured in urine and/or blood. This principle has led to a facile method for estimating percutaneous absorption in animals and man. One samples and measures stratum corneum content with cellophane tape sampling. This method is used also for bioequivalence determination (46).

In vivo biological responses, such as vasoconstriction assays estimating absorption of corticosteroids (245) and changes in blood flow to study penetration through various types of skin and under diverse conditions (144,145), have been used to estimate rate of penetration. These endpoints are complicated biological processes and may vary with the tissue's ability to produce the response. For example, application of histamine produces increased blood flow, however, the degree of change would depend not only on the rate of penetration, but on the reactivity of receptors at that time. Most exogenous chemicals produce their vascular effects by triggering formation and release of endogenous mediators. Thus, the usefulness of penetration studies using biological endpoints is limited to comparisons between closely related chemical structures that can be assumed to trigger the same process.

In Vitro Percutaneous Absorption Assays

The excised skin of humans or animals can be used to measure penetration of chemicals. In vitro assays using excised skin use specially designed diffusion cells (12,47,117). The skin is stretched over the opening of a collecting receptacle, epidermal side up. The chemical to be studied is applied to the epidermis, and fluid from the receptacle is assayed to measure the penetration of the chemical. Chemicals usually are radioactively labeled. Some investigators have used diffusion cells in which the epidermis was covered with fluid containing the chemical; however, the preferred method for toxicological relevance is a one-chambered cell in which the stratum corneum is exposed to the air and the underside of the skin is bathed in saline or other receptacle fluid. Because diffusion through a membrane depends on relative concentrations on each side, some chambers have been designed to allow periodic replacement of the receptacle fluid. Fluid in the receptacle base usually is constantly stirred and maintained at a physiological temperature. Either full-thickness skin or epidermis alone may be used in in vitro assays. With relatively hairless skin, epidermis can be separated from the dermis by heat treatment.

This type of in vitro assay offers advantages over in vivo assays. Highly toxic compounds can be studied in human skin. Large numbers of cells can be run simultaneously. Diffusion through the membrane, eliminating other pharmacokinetic factors, can be studied. In addition, these assays may be cheaper and easier to conduct; however, these assays do not mimic human exposure in some important areas. Because excised skin must often be stored prior to use, it cannot be assumed that the skin will retain full enzymatic activity. This may alter the metabolic profile of compounds entering the receptacle. In intact skin, chemical penetrating the epidermis would enter the circulation through vessels and lymphatics located just below the epidermis. In excised full-thickness skin, the dermis is also involved in the absorptive process. The influence of the dermis can be minimized by using heat-separated epidermis, or by removal of the skin with a dermatome at the level of the upper dermis. In the intact animal, the chemical enters the peripheral circulation in plasma; the collecting fluid of diffusion chambers is usually saline or water. The relative solubility of hydrophobic and hydrophilic chemicals in these collecting fluids may alter the fate at which they leave the skin. Surface conditions of excised skin may vary from normal skin; changes in the surface emulsion occurring during storage have not been studied. Storage conditions and procedures for preparing the tissue may affect skin absorption and metabolism. It has been proposed that the suitability of each specimen of excised skin be verified by measurement of penetration of a standard, tritiated water through the tissue prior to its use to study penetration of other chemicals. Comparisons of penetration rates obtained from in vitro and in vivo assays have been made (12,47). Often a good correlation between the two methods was obtained; however, with some compounds, correlation of the methods was poor. Differences between in vivo and in vitro results for some compounds can be explained because of solubility in the receptacle fluid and blood. Differences observed for other compounds cannot be explained.

In vitro penetration rates through skin of various species have also been compared (Table 22.3). Skin of the weanling pig and miniature swine appear to be good in vitro models for most compounds (11). The skin of monkeys appears to be a good model as well (376). For most compounds, mouse and hairless mouse skin appears more permeable than skin of other species. Rat skin appears to be a good model for some compounds; however, when differences have been noted, they have been large.

A few investigators have estimated percutaneous absorption using 'model' membranes, including excised stratum corneum, and physiochemical data have been used to predict absorption. Lipid/water partition coefficients have been correlated with skin permeability. Smaller molecules (molecular weight $\sim$400) are more readily absorbed than large molecules. Molecules with polar groups, in general, do not penetrate as well as nonpolar molecules (307). The addition of hydroxyl groups also lowers the permeability. Substitutions that increase lipid solubility may increase penetration, depending upon the vehicle in which the chemicals are applied (312). Electrolytes do not penetrate the skin well (313); shunt diffusion through skin appendages for these molecules may be important.

The presumed simplicity of in vitro penetration assays has led to their universal acceptance for preclinical and other screening purposes. This acceptance and wide-scale use resulted in many variations in how studies were conducted. It is not surprising that confusion about interpretation of the data generated by the variations of the method occurs. Bronaugh (47) collated the experimental variables leading to discrepancies. His text provides a catalogue of variables that, properly considered, can lead to experimental designs that may have in vivo relevance, especially for hydrophilic materials.

NEOPLASTIC RESPONSE OF SKIN

The skin is the most common site of cancer in humans. Both benign and malignant tumors may be derived from viable keratinocytes and melanocytes of the epidermis, and rarely from skin appendages, blood vessels, peripheral nerves, and lymphoid tissue of the dermis (216,390). Historically, basal cell and squamous cell carcinomas, which develop from keratinocytes, account for 60% and 30%, respectively, of all skin cancer. The remainder includes malignant melanoma and the rare tumors developing from other cell types; however, the incidence of malignant melanomas appears to be increasing. Melanomas often metastasize, and prognosis for patients with this disease is poor. Only 4%–5% of squamous cell carcinomas are metastatic, and basal cell tumors rarely metastasize. The relatively noninvasive nature of the common forms of skin cancer accounts for a cure rate of over 95%. Skin cancer accounts for less than 0.3% of all cancer deaths.

The association between exposure to environmental carcinogens and the development of basal cell and squamous cell carcinomas is strong (326). Epidemiological studies have demonstrated a strong correlation between exposure to ultraviolet radiation and development of skin cancer (99). Clinical experience leaves little doubt that radiographs can also produce cancer of the skin. Both forms of radiation have induced tumors in experimental animals (44). The association between environmental chemicals and skin cancer was first demonstrated by Sir Percival Potts in 1775. Following Potts' association between skin cancer of the scrotum and soot exposure, experimental studies in animals have shown that polycyclic aromatic hydrocarbons such as benzo(a)pyrene are the carcinogens in soot, coal tar, pitch, and various cutting oils (107). The same types of experiments demonstrated that skin cancer development is a multistage process (43,44).

Despite abundant experimental evidence that chemicals can produce skin cancer, few chemicals have been associated with increased incidences of skin cancer in man. Epidemiological studies have demonstrated associations between polycyclic aromatic hydrocarbons and arsenic and increased incidence of benign, precancerous lesions and basal cell and squamous cell carcinomas (166). The ability to establish relationships between chemical exposure and the development of skin cancer by epidemology is minimized by many confounding factors, including exposure to ultraviolet light, high background incidence rates, long latency periods for development of cancer (107), and incomplete reporting due to the nonlethal nature of the disease. Even without strong epidemological evidence, the experimental evidence that exposure of the skin can lead to tumor development and the degree of dermal exposure to chemicals in the workplace justifies the practice of evaluating carcinogenic potential by dermal exposure. Furthermore, it is likely that certain internal tumors (bladder cancer from occupational aniline exposure) result from chemicals absorbed through the skin.

In vivo skin carcinogenesis studies are generally conducted using Sprague–Dawley rats; mice have also been used frequently. Differences in species sensitivity to various agents have been demonstrated (44,280), and a review of the data suggested that when differences in species sensitivity were noted, rats tended to be more sensitive. The design of carcinogenesis assays has been reviewed in other texts (164,220,276,115,116) and is described in Chapter 20. The method, in brief, is daily application of the test material to the clipped skin of up to 6 groups of animals (untreated, vehicle control, and up to 4 dose groups) for 104 weeks. The dose is generally administered as a constant volume of 1.0 ml/kg body weight to 5%–10% of the animal's body surface. Typically, 70 male and 70 female animals are included in each group, with additional groups dosed on the same schedule used for periodic blood analysis and for evaluating the toxicokinetics of the test material. Two variations of standardized skin carcinogenicity studies have also been reported. In the first, the skin is treated with the chemical of interest. Then, a promoting agent, such as tetradecanoyl phorbol acetate (TPA), may be applied to reduce the latency period. In the second, the skin is treated with a noncarcinogenic dose of a carcinogen, such as dimethyl benzanthracene (DMBA), followed by repeated doses of the agent under study. These approaches may be helpful in elucidating the mechanism of the chemicals' action.

Numerous factors may influence the outcome of dermal carcinogenic assays, and the choice of what to test is crucial in such assays. Although it is tempting to evaluate pure chemicals, it should be remembered that other agents in mixtures could act as promoting agents. For example, coal tar and pitch may contain catechol and pyrogallol, which are promoters of the carcinogen benzo(a)pyrene found in these mixtures. Wounding increases the number of tumors that spontaneously develop, and severe inflammatory responses may cause tissue destruction. Care should be taken in selecting an appropriate nonirritant dose.

Epidemiology and experimental studies have shown that sunlight (ultraviolet light) is a skin carcinogen (101,102). Various investigators (352) have shown that exposure to some chemicals in combination with a dose of ultraviolet light increases the number of tumors or decreases the latency period for tumor development following exposure to the chemical or ultralviolet (UV) light alone. No standard protocol has yet been put forth by any regulatory agency, and typically, regulatory agencies request to review specific protocols prior to study conduct (164,115,116). In general, the studies have involved repeated intercurrent exposures to simulated sunlight and the test article. The endpoint is time required for UV radiation (UVR) to produce skin cancer. Two doses of UVR are used as control: a high dose that will result in a short latency period for tumor development, and a weaker dose that would result in a lower tumor yield and longer latency period. The interaction of the test article and the weaker dose of UVR is compared to each control and to a vehicle control group irradiated with the lower dose of UVR. Complete details of a typical protocol have been published by Forbes et al. (115,116)

The FDA has recently expressed concern that some topical drugs and cosmetic ingredients may potentiate (promote?) neoplastic changes in skin induced by other agents, such as sunlight. Although to date there is no epidemiological evidence for such an occurence, the exploration of this possiblity will necessitate new approaches to conventional assays for carcinogenicity.

A number of in vitro assays for studying chemical carcinogenesis have been developed (165). Of particular interest for dermal carcinogenesis is the ability to cultivate epidermal keratinocytes of rats and mice and, more recently, humans (204). Cultured human keratinocytes can metabolize polycyclic aromatic hydrocarbons, and chemical transformation using human fibroblasts has been achieved (204). The establishment of human epidermal lines for in vitro carcinogenesis testing will provide an important new predictive tool. Chapter 17 reviews the relationship of mutagenicity and carcinogenicity.

SKIN ALLERGY (DELAYED-TYPE HYPERSENSITIVITY)

Since the turn of the century, certain forms of eczema have been recognized as allergic in nature. Joseph Jadassohn demonstrated that in some patients, dermatitis was due to increased sensitivity following repeated contact with a substance, not the toxic (irritant) properties of the material (166,167). By 1930, a procedure for producing this hypersensitivity to chemicals in guinea pigs had been developed (35). The pioneering work of Landsteiner and his colleagues demonstrated that low molecular weight chemicals conjugate with proteins to form an antigen that stimulates the immune system to form a hyperreactive state (214). They demonstrated that immunogenicity is related to chemical structure (213) and that two types of immunologic response exist, one transferable by serum and another transferred by suspensions of white blood cells (212).

It is now known that most cases of allergic contact dermatitis are of the cell-mediated type, transferable by lymphocytes. This type of skin response is often referred to as delayed contact hypersensitivity because of the relatively long period (approximately 24 h) required for the development of the inflammation following exposure.

Some understanding of the processes by which this hypersensitivity develops is helpful in selecting and interpreting results of predictive sensitization tests. During ontogenesis, stem cells from the yolk sac, fetal liver, and bone marrow migrate to the central lymphoid organs, the thymus, and bone marrow in mammals. After birth, stem cells derive from bone marrow. In the central lymphoid organs, stem cells differentiate into immunocompetent lymphocytes. This results in two classes of lymphocytes: thymus-processed T lymphocytes and B lymphocytes processed in bone marrow. B lymphocytes are precursors of antibody-producing cells responsible for immune responses transferable by serum. T lymphocytes are responsible for producing delayed-type hypersensitivity (DTH) and for regulation of the immune system. This regulation is accomplished by subsets of T cells (i.e., T helper and T suppressor cells). Lymphocytes leaving the lymphoid organs are "programmed" to recognize a specific chemical structure via receptor molecules. If during circulation through body tissues a cell encounters the structure it is programmed to recognize, an immune response may be induced. The ability to develop and express a hypersensitivity response is determined by the relative activities of the T helper and T suppressor cell types (294).

To stimulate an immune response, a chemical must be presented to lymphocytes in an appropriate form (213,214). Chemicals usually are haptens that must conjugate with proteins in the skin or other tissues in order to be recognized by the immune system. Haptens conjugate with multiple proteins to form a number of different antigens that may stimulate an allergic response by stimulating T lymphocytes with different recognition capabilities (295).

Hapten-protein conjugates are processed by macrophages, Langerhans cells, or other cells expressing immune response Ia proteins on their surface. Although the exact nature of this process is not completely understood, it is known that physical contact between macrophage and T cells is required (70,350), suggesting that receptor interactions are necessary. Physical interaction is accompanied by the release of interleukins, a family of soluble, regulatory proteins, which stimulate cell division, act as growth factors, and increase expression of immune proteins on the surface of some cells (109, 161,253,258).

Following antigen stimulation in the skin, lymphocytes enter the lymphatic system and migrate to the draining lymph nodes. Disruption of lymphatic drainage prevents sensitization of an animal (118). Stimulated cells settle in the paracortical regions of the lymph nodes, and T lymphocytes differentiate into immunoblasts. This differentiation involves interaction with other cell types. Immunoblasts eventually give rise to T-effector cells, which enter the systemic circulation and, upon encountering the antigen which they are programmed to recognize, release lymphokines that initiate a local inflammatory response. Immunoblasts also give rise to memory cells that enter the systemic circulation. These memory cells are capable of similar activities as the T-processed lymphocytes; they recognize antigen and can be stimulated to divide. Memory cell production is essentially an expansion of the number of cells capable of recognizing a given antigen. The lymphokines, which are released by primed effector cells that encounter their stimulating antigen directly, and indirectly, by stimulation of other white blood cells, produce a local inflammatory response. Actions of lymphokines include direct tissue damage, chemotactic factors, stimulation of mitosis, increased phagocytic activity of macrophages, and factors that inhibit migration of some cell types from the area (77). Only a small percentage of lymphocytes in an area of skin exhibiting a delayed hypersensitivity response are specifically stimulated by antigen (261). Most cells in the lesion are "recruited" by lymphokines. Histologically, the response has been described as a hyperproliferative epidermis with intracellular edema, spongiosis, intraepidermal vesiculation, and mononuclear cell infiltrate by 24 h. The dermis shows perivenous accumulation of lymphocytes, monocytes, and edema. No reaction occurs if the local vascular supply is interrupted, and the appearance of epidermal changes follows the invasion of monocytes. Vascular changes (i.e., increased blood flow) occur early (2–6 h) in the response.

The histology of the response varies somewhat by species. For example, a higher proportion of polymorphonuclear cells in the cellular infiltrate has been observed in DTH reaction sites of mice than in guinea pigs or man (169). These differences may be due, in part, to mixed immune responses. Mice develop both antibody and DTH responses to haptens applied to the skin (6). Exposure via the skin is believed to preferentially lead to DTH in guinea pigs and man.

The biological processes necessary for producing hypersensitivity in predictive tests are often grouped into two phases: induction of the capability to respond and elicitation of a response. Induction has been referred to as the afferent phase, the initial exposures through clonal expansion, and the release of memory cells that enter the system circulation. Elicitation as the efferent phase, consists of local recognization of the antigen by the memory cells, their release of lymphokines, and the activity of inflammatory mediators that are generated locally which produce the dermatitis. All standardized predictive tests in guinea pigs and some early tests in mice (6,128,233) use the efferent phase response as an indication of immune reactivity to the chemical. The local lymph node assay (LLNA) in mice uses stimulation of lymphocytes (185–187) in local draining lymph nodes during the afferent phase as the endpoint.

Modulation of development of DTH in experimental animals and in humans is complex. The intrinsic biological variables controlling sensitization can be influenced by selection of animals likely to be capable of mounting an immune response to the hapten. The extrinsic variables of dose, vehicle, route of exposure, adjuvant, etc., can be manipulated to develop sensitive predictive assays. The method of skin exposure is important. Keratinocytes produce interleukins (77), important regulatory proteins for induction of DTH. Langerhans cells express Ia antigen and may act as antigen-presenting cells (70,303,350). Intradermal injection in animals bypasses these processes but assures entry of the chemical into the skin.

Vehicle plays an important role in percutaneous penetration, and hence presumably in sensitization. The theory, at least in regard to flux, should be simple: maximum solubility leads to maximum thermodynamic activity and enhanced flux. The experimental literature only partially documents this presumed truth. Analysis of the relevant literature provides a partial interpretative key to this fundamental area (229). Increasing the dose per unit area increases the sensitization rate. Recently, Upadhye and Maibach (351) reviewed in detail the influence of area of application on the development of human sensitization. Early publications viewed as dogma, when examined with statistical methods, failed to be significant, yet, dose/unit area and occlusion (224,225) appear to be highly important variables.

Application of haptens to damaged skin (i.e., irritated, tapestripped) increases the sensitization fate. Although effects of vehicle, dose level, and damaged tissue have been studied more extensively in guinea pigs and man than in mice, until conclusive studies are reported, it is prudent to consider their influence in the design of all studies. Repeated applications to the same site is more effective for inducing sensitization than application to new sites each time (104,224). The incidence of sensitization increases with increased numbers of exposures (224). An interval between exposures of 2 to 6 days increases the sensitization rate (6,187,224). This may be due to the "booster-effect" of memory cells. Materials such as Freund's complete adjuvant nonspecifically enhance development of immune responses but may selectively trigger humoral immunity in some species (54). Treatment of animals with adjuvant, either simultaneously or shortly after hapten exposure, increases sensitization rates (225–227). The development of DTH is under genetic control; within the human and guinea pig populations all individuals do not have the capability to respond to a given hapten (224). The status of the immune system will determine if an immune response can be induced. For example, animals may become tolerant to a hapten, and pregnancy may suppress expression of the allergy (200).

Appropriate planning and execution of predictive sensitization assays is critical. All too often, techniques are discredited when, in fact, the performance of the tests was inferior or study design (i.e., choice of vehicle or dose) was inappropriate. The first priority is to choose an appropriate experimental design. Often the assay to be used is chosen on a pro forma basis without realizing the inherent weaknesses and strengths of the method. A common error in choosing an animal assay is using Freund's complete adjuvant when one wishes to set dose response relationships. The adjuvant provides such sensitivity that dose effect relationships are muted.

Choice of dose and vehicle appropriate to the assay and the study question is the second priority. Although dose must be sufficient to assure penetration, it must be below the irritation threshold at challenge to avoid misinterpretation of irritant inflammation as allergic. For instance, quaternary ammonium compounds, such as benzalkonium chloride, rarely sensitize, but they have been identified as allergens in some guinea pig assays. Knowing the irritation potential of compounds allows the investigator to appropriately design and execute these studies. Vehicle choice determines, in part, the absorption of the test material and can influence sensitization rate, ability to elicit response at challenge, and the irritation threshold. Inappropriate selection of vehicle and dose effectively invalidates studies.

Sensitization assays often are assigned to the novitiate when they should be performed and read by persons experienced with the method being used. Experienced investigators will recognize marginal reactions that should be further investigated, positives that may be irritant in nature, and will be able to assist in the estimation of risk associated with the proposed use of the material. Working with laboratories and personnel with extensive experience greatly decreases errors and increases the reliability and relevance of all standard assays described below (158,180,181,191,300).

Data from various sensitization assays have been broadly used to determine the likelihood of induction of clinical allergic contact dermatitis in populations to be exposed. Interpretation of these assays requires experience, judgement, and sophistication because each assay has its own strengths, weaknesses, and limitations. Central to the issue of interpretation is definition of allergic contact dermatitis in man and animals. For instance, in the mouse the endpoint is only documented reliably by measuring ear swelling. In man the patch test, albeit a highly valuable bioassay, has often been misinterpreted. Guidance for proper interpretation is found in the original references for many of the assays discussed below, and for human repeat insult patch tests, guidance is found in a review article by Stotts (235). Several authors and groups are refining criteria for allergic contact dermatitis that are operational rather than mechanistic. Fundamentally, each of the systems acknowledges the complexity of the biological process: each parameter is qualitative or quantitative and is multifactoral. For instance, in humans one needs a pertinent history, carefully performed patch test results with appropriate virgin controls, and sufficient follow-up to define that removal of the allergen improved clinical status (175,365).

Guinea Pig Sensitization Tests

Predictive animal tests to determine the potential of substances to induce delayed hypersensitivity in man are conducted most often in guinea pigs. Several tests have been described. Each offers its own advantages and disadvantages; most have many features in common. All use young (1–3 months old or 250–550 g), randomly bred albino guinea pigs. To reduce the possibility of seasonal variability in reactivity, animals are maintained in facilities with temperature of approximately 20±1°C, 40%–50% relative humidity, 12-h automatic light cycle, a standard vitamin C–supplemented chow, and water available at all times. Test sites are clipped free of hair with electric clippers; some assays specify chemical depilation as well. Almost all evaluate the response as production of visible dermatitis, using descriptive scales for erythema and edema. Because of genetic influences, sensitivity to a common chemical, such as dinitrochlorobenzene, is usually confirmed periodically for animals from each vendor. There is disagreement as to which sex, if either, is more susceptible to sensitization. Males are more aggressive and may damage the skin of cagemates. Some assays specify use of one sex or one half of each sex. The tests differ significantly in route of exposure, use of adjuvants, induction interval, and number of exposures. The principal features of the most commonly used assays and assays acceptable to regulatory agencies (67,100,105,170,262,300) to predict sensitization are summarized in Table 22.4.

The Draize Test

The Draize sensitization test (DT) (87,171,188) was the first predictive sensitization test accepted by regulatory agencies, and is still widely used. One flank of 20 guinea pigs is shaved and 0.05 ml of a 0.1% solution of test material in saline, paraffin oil, or polyethylene glycol is injected into the anterior flank on day 0. The next day, and every other day through day 20, 0.1 ml of the test solution is injected into a new site on the same flank. Challenge follows a 2-week rest period. The opposite untreated flank is shaved and 0.05 ml of test solution is injected into each animal. Twenty previously untreated controls are injected at the same time. The test site is visually evaluated 24 and 46 h after injection. The intensity of the responses of test animals is compared with that of controls. A larger or more erythematous response than that of controls is considered a positive response. Results are expressed as the percentage of animals positive or as the ratio of positive animals to the number tested.

Open Epicutaneous Test

The open epicutaneous test (OET) (180,188,189) simulates the conditions of human use by using topical application of the test material. The procedure determines the dose required to induce sensitization and to elicit a response in sensitized animals. The irritancy profile is evaluated by testing various concentrations (typically, undiluted, 30%, 10%, 3%, and 1%) in ethanol, acetone, water, polyethylene glycol, or petrolatum. In six to eight guinea pigs, 0.025 ml of the dosing solutions are applied to 2 cm^2 areas of the shaved flanks. Vehicle solubility and use conditions (e.g., direct application to skin or dilution during normal use) is considered in selecting the concentrations to be tested. Test sites are visually evaluated 24 h after application of test solutions for the presence or absence of erythema. The dose not causing a reaction in any animal (maximal nonirritant concentration) and the dose causing a reaction in 25% of the animals (minimal irritant concentration) are determined. During induction, 0.10 ml of test solution is applied to an 8 cm^2 area of flank skin of 6 to 8 guinea pigs for 3 weeks, or 5 times a week for 4 weeks. As many as six groups of animals are treated with different doses; a control group is treated with vehicle only. The highest dose tested usually is the minimal irritant concentration; lower doses are based on usage concentration or a stepwise reduction (e.g., 30-10-3-1). Solutions are applied to the same site each day unless a moderate inflammatory response develops. A new site on the same flank is treated when inflammation develops. Twenty-four to 72 h after the last induction treatment, each animal is challenged on the previously untreated flank. The minimal irritant concentration, the maximum nonirritant concentration (from irritancy screen), and five solutions of lower concentrations are applied, 0.025 ml to a 2 cm^2 area. Skin reactions are read on an all or none basis at 24, 48, and 72 h after application of the solutions. The maximum nonirritating concentration in the vehicle-treated group is calculated. Animals in test groups that develop inflammatory responses to lower concentrations are considered sensitized. The dose required to sensitize is determined by comparing the number of positive animals in the test groups. The minimal concentration necessary to elicit a positive response in a sensitized animal is apparent from the challenge responses.

Buehler Test

The Buehler test (52–54,121,188) also employs topical application of the test material. An absorbent patch, 20 × 20 mm Webril, backed by Blenderm tape and saturated with 0.4 ml of the test material, is placed on the shaved flanks of 10 to 20 guinea pigs. Test concentration

Table 22.4
Principle features of guinea pig sensitization assays

Feature of Test	Draize	Open Epicutaneous Test (OET)	Buehler Assay	Freund's Complete Adjuvant Test (FCA)	Optimization Test	Split Adjuvant	Guinea Pig Maximization (GPMT)
Number in test group	20	6–8	10–20	8–10	20	10–20	20–25
Number in control group	20	6–8	10–20	8–10	20	10–20	20–25
INDUCTION							
Exposure route	id	Open epicutaneous	Patch	id	id	Patch	id and patch
Number of exposures	10	20–21	3	3	9	4	1 id; 1 topical
Duration of each patch	No patch	Continuous (no patch)	6 hours	—	—	48 h each	48 h patch
Concentration	0.2	Non-irritating	Slightly irritating	5–50%	0.1%	0.1–0.2 ml	Maximum tolerated
Test group(s)	TS	TS	TS	TS in FCA	TS in FCA	TS, FCA	TS, TS + FCA, FCA
Control group	None	Vehicle only	Vehicle only	FCA only	—		FCA, FCA + V, V
Site for dosing	Left flank	Right flank	Left flank	Shoulder	Back (flank 1st injection)	Mid-back	Shoulder
Frequency of exposure	Every 2nd day	Daily	Every 5–7 days	Every 4 days	Every other day	Day 0, 2, 4, 7	0 (id); day 7 patch
Duration (days)	1–18	0–20	0–14	0–9	0–21	0–9	0–9
Misc.			9 exposure version			Day 0 dry ice treatment FCA (id) day 4	Irritant dose or SLS pretreatment
Rest Period (days)	19–34	21–34	15–27	9–21; 22–34	22–34	10–21	9–20
CHALLENGE							
Exposure Route	id	Open	Patch	id; patch	id	Patch	Patch
Number of exposures	1	2	1	2	2	1	1
Duration of exposure	—	—	24 h			24 h	24 h
Exposure day(s)	35	21 and 35	28	22; 35	14–28	22	21

FCA—Freund's complete adjuvant; SLS—sodium lauryl sulfate; TS—test substance; V—vehicle; id—interdermal.

varies from undiluted to usage levels. An optimum concentration that produces slight erythema is selected based on an irritancy screen conducted in other animals. The patch is held in place by wrapping the animal with an occlusive wrapping, then placing the animal in a special restrainer fitted with a rubber dam to maintain even pressure over the patch for a 6-h exposure period. This procedure is repeated 7 and 14 days after the initial exposure. A control group of 10 to 20 animals is patched with vehicle only. Two weeks after the last induction patch, animals are challenged with patches saturated with a nonirritating concentration of test material applied to both flanks and with the vehicle (if other than water or acetone). Wrapping and restraint are as during induction. After 6 hours, the patch is removed and the area depilated. Test sites are visually evaluated 24 and 48 h after patch removal. Animals developing erythematous responses are considered sensitized (if irritant control animals do not respond). The incidence of positive reactions and the average intensity of the response are calculated.

Freund's Complete Adjuvant Test

Freund's complete adjuvant test (FCAT) is an intradermal technique incorporating test material in a 50/50 mixture of FCA and distilled water. The test has been significantly modified since originally described (188). The latest published description (189) is summarized here. A 6 × 2 cm area across the shoulders of two groups of 10 to 20 guinea pigs is shaved and used as the injection site. Animals of one group are injected with a 5% solution of the test material in FCA/water; injection volume is 0.1 ml. Control animals are injected with FCA/water. Injections are repeated every 4 days until three injections are given. The minimal irritating and maximum nonirritating concentration following topical application of 0.025 ml solutions to a 2 cm^2 area of skin is determined on a minimum of four naive guinea pigs (see OET procedure). Twenty-one days after the first induction injection, 0.025 ml of the minimal irritant concentration, the maximum nonirritant concentration, and two lower concentrations are applied to 2 cm^2 areas of the shaved flank. Test sites are not covered and are evaluated for the presence of erythema at 24, 46, and 72 h after application. The minimum nonirritating concentration in FCA/water-treated controls is determined. Animals injected with the test material during induction that respond to lower doses are considered sensitized. The incidence of sensitization and the threshold concentration for elicitation of the response in these animals are calculated.

Optimization Test

The optimization test resembles the DT but incorporates the use of adjuvant for some induction injections and both intradermal and topical challenges (188,189,244). Injections during induction are 0.1 ml of 0.1% concentration of test material in 0.9% saline or in 50/50 FCA/saline. In total, 10 injections are given. On day 1 of the first week, 1 injection into the shaved flank and 1 into a shaved area of dorsal skin are given. Two and 4 days later, 1 injection into a new dorsal site is given. The test material is administered in saline during the first week. During the second and third weeks, test material is administered in FCA/saline every other day to a shaved area over the shoulders. Twenty test animals are treated; 20 controls are injected with saline during week 1 and FCA/saline during weeks 2 and 3. The intensity of the 24-h responses during week 1 is calculated as reaction volume. Thickness of a skin fold over the injection site is measured with a caliper (mm), and the two largest diameters of the erythematous reaction are recorded (mm). The reaction volume is calculated by multiplying fold thickness times both diameters and is expressed as microliters. The mean reaction volume of each animal to the intradermal injections using saline as a vehicle (week 1) is calculated. Thirty-five days after the first injection, animals are challenged with 0.1 ml of 0.1% test material in saline. The challenge reaction volume for each animal is calculated and compared to the mean reaction volume for that animal. Any animal developing a reaction volume at challenge greater than the mean plus one standard deviation during induction is considered sensitized. Vehicle control animals are injected with saline at challenge. A second challenge is conducted 45 days after the first injection. A nonirritating concentration of the test material in a suitable vehicle is applied to the flank skin, away from injection sites; 0.05 ml is applied to an area of approximately 1 cm^2.

The area is covered with a 2 × 2 cm piece of filter paper backed by an occlusive dressing, which remains in place for 24 h. Reactions are visually evaluated using the four-point erythema scale of the Draize primary irritancy scale (see Table 22.9). The control animals are patched with vehicle alone. The number of positive animals in the test group is statistically compared with the number of "pseudo-positive" animals in the control groups using the exact Fisher test. Separate comparisons of intradermal and epicutaneous challenges are made. A p value of ≤ 0.01 is considered significant. To classify materials as strong/moderate/weak/nonsensitizer, a classification scheme has been devised using results of exact Fisher test and number of positives detected (Table 22.5).

The Split Adjuvant Test

The split adjuvant test (188,226,227) uses skin damage and FCA as adjuvants; application of the test material is topical. An area of back skin just behind the scapulas of 10–20 guinea pigs is clipped, shaved to glistening, then treated with dry ice for 5–10 sec. A dressing of a layer

Table 22.5
Classification scheme for the optimization test

% interdermal positive animals	% epidermal positive animals	Classification
N.S., 0–30	N.S., 0	No sensitizer
S., 30–50	N.S., 0–30	Weak sensitizer
S., 50–75	S., 30–50	Moderate sensitizer
S., >75	S., >50	Strong sensitizer

S—statistically significant; N.S.—not statistically significant by exact Fisher test.

of loose mesh gauze and stretch adhesive with a 2 × 2 cm opening over the shaved area is placed around the animal and secured with adhesive tape. This dressing remains in place throughout induction. Approximately 0.2 ml of creams or solid test material, 0.1 ml if liquid, is spread over the test site and covered with two layers of #2 filter paper backed by occlusive tape and attached to the dressing by adhesive tape. The concentration tested varies by irritancy potential, use conditions, etc. Two days later, the filter paper is lifted from the test site, the test material is reapplied, and the filter paper covering is replaced. On day 4, the filter paper cover is removed; two injections of 0.075 cc FCA are given into the edges of the test site, the test material is reapplied, and the site is resealed. On day 7, the test material is reapplied, and on day 9 the dressing is removed. Twenty-two days after the initial treatment, animals are challenged by topical application of 0.5 ml of test material to a 2 × 2 cm area of the shaved mid-back. The test site is covered by filter paper backed with adhesive tape, held in place by wrapping the animal with an elastic adhesive bandage secured with adhesive tape. A group of naive controls, 10–20 animals, is treated by the same procedure at challenge. Twenty-four h after application, the dressing is removed and the test site is evaluated at 24, 48, and 72 h, visually using a seven-point descriptive visual scale. Sensitization of individual animals is indicated by significantly stronger reactions than reactions of controls.

Guinea Pig Maximization Test

The Guinea Pig Maximization Test (GPMT) (188,224,225,364) combines FCA, irritancy, intradermal injection, and occlusive topical application during the induction period. The shoulder region of two groups of 20–25 guinea pigs is shaved. Two identical sets of intradermal injections of 0.1 ml 50/50 FCA/water, test material in water, paraffin oil, or propylene glycol, and the same dose of test material in FCA/vehicle, are placed in a 2 × 4 cm area. Seven days later the test article is placed on filter paper over the injection site. The filter paper is covered with approximately 4 × 8 cm occlusive surgical tape and secured in place with an elastic bandage wrapped around the animal. If the test material is nonirritating, the test site is pretreated with 10% sodium lauryl sulfate in petrolatum on day 6 to provoke an irritant reaction. If a vehicle other than petrolatum is used for topical application of the test material, the filter is saturated with the solution. Control animals are patched with the vehicle alone. The dressing is removed from the animals 48 h after application. Test and control animals are challenged on the shaved flank with the highest nonirritating concentration, with approximately one half of the highest nonirritating concentration, and with the vehicle. Solutions are applied to 1 × 1 cm pieces of filter paper secured in place as during induction; patches are removed 24 h later. The challenge area is shaved, if needed, 21 h after patch removal. Reactions are evaluated visually 24 and 48 h after patch removal. The intensity of responses to test material and vehicle in the test group is compared to the responses in controls. Reactions are considered positive when they are more intense than the response to vehicle and the responses to the test material in controls. Based on the incidence of positives in the test group, test materials are rated as a weak to extreme sensitizer (Table 22.6).

Sensitization Tests In Mice

Although guinea pigs have been the animal of choice for predictive sensitization assays for 40 years, interest and activity in developing and validating standardized predictive assays in mice has been intensive during the last 10 years. Classical guinea pig sensitization assays are relatively costly and time consuming. All use subjective endpoints, and data interpretation is prone to difficulties. Manipulations of the animals are sufficiently stressful in some assays to alter normal physiological parameters. With development of new techniques for studying DTH (41) and evaluating cellular response (130), it has become possible to study the response in other laboratory animals (6,74,75) in shorter time frames. Numerous less subjective techniques for

Table 22.6
Classification of materials by maximization test

Sensitization rate (% responding at challenge)	Grade	Classification
0–8	I	Weak
9–28	II	Mild
29–64	III	Moderate
65–80	IV	Strong
81–100	V	Extreme

evaluating the allergic response have been proposed, including change in water content of challenged ears (41), measurement of the ear thickness with an engineer's micrometer (8,354), and responses of lymphocytes (8,251,252,288). Although numerous approaches to developing a predictive sensitization assay in mice have been proposed, only two methods have been sufficiently developed to warrant consideration as standardized assays. The test site for each is the mouse ear, yet they employ distinctively different approaches. The mouse ear swelling test (MEST) uses both topical and injection exposures for induction and a topical challenge of the pinnea in which visual evaluation is replaced by measuring ear thickness with an engineer's micrometer. The Local Lymph Node Assay (LLNA) consists of a topical induction followed by measurement of the mitotic activity of the draining lymph node. LLNA is unique of all predictive assays in evaluating the response of the efferent phase of the response. In a third mouse sensitization assay, the vitamin A enhancement test (VAET) has been used for the evaluation of ingredients of consumer products but has not been used by a sufficient number of laboratories to be considered standard. In the VAET, the reactivity of the immune system is heightened by maintaining animals on a diet with high doses of vitamin A for a preconditioning period and throughout induction and challenge. Challenge is topical and is assessed by measuring ear thickness. The three assays are contrasted in Table 22.7.

Local Lymph Node Assay

Kimber and his colleagues (182,185,186,269) investigated measuring lymphocyte proliferation as an alternative approach to visual evaluations or measurement of edema of the mouse ear. They found that exposure of the dorsum of the ear pinnea to sensitizers produced hyperplasia of T cells in auricular lymph nodes. A doses divided into three exposures over three consecutive days produced a more intense response than the same dose delivered in a single exposure (187). In a limited trial, Balb-C mice were shown to be more sensitive than other strains (186). Initial studies used 24-hour cultures of excised lymph node cells labelled with ^{3}H thymidine, with or without exogenous IL-2 (185–186); however, to simplify the assay, the method was modified to expose proliferating cells to ^{3}H thymidine in situ via intravenous injection. The method described is the final method used in intralaboratory validation studies that have been reported (15,314). A complete list of references is available in an independent review evaluation of the method sponsored by the Interagency Coordinating Committee on the Validation of Alternative Methods (IACCVAM) (263).

LLNA employees multiple topical in vivo doses of the material of interest to the mouse ear. This is followed by in vitro evaluation of mitotic activity of cells from the draining lymph nodes. At least three dose levels are evaluated in separate groups of four CBA/ca mice. Experimental animals between 8–12 weeks of age are used. Either males or females may be used, but each assay should use only a single sex.

Vehicle selection and test concentration is based primarily on solubility and viscosity of the solution/suspension. Investigators should be sure the doses selected are nontoxic to the animals. Vehicles shown to be acceptable include 4 : 1 acetone/olive, methyl ethyl ketone, dimethylformamide, propylene glycol, dimethyl sulphoxide, and 2.5% hydroxypropyl cellulose in methanol. Investigators have proposed that three consecutive concentrations from the series 100%, 50%, 25%, 10%, 5%, 2.5%, 1.0%, 0.5%, 0.25%, 1.0%, 0.05%, and 0.001% are tested.

Twenty-five μl of the appropriate test solution or the vehicle alone is applied to the dorsal surface of the pinnea each day for three consecutive days. Five days after the first exposure, 250 ml phosphate buffered saline (PBS) containing 20 μci methyl thymidine is injected via the tail vein of each animal. Five hours after injection, animals are euthanized by carbon dioxide asphyxiation. Draining auricular lymph nodes are excised and pooled with nodes from other animals in the same group. A single-cell suspension is prepared by gently passing the nodes though stainless steel, 200-mesh gauze with the plunger of a syringe. The cell suspension is centrifuged at $190 \times g$ for 10 min, and then the pellet is washed twice with 10 ml PBS. Cells are resuspended in 3 ml of 5% trichloroacetic acid (TCA) and incubated overnight at 4°C. The precipitated macromolecules are recovered by centrifugation, the supernate is removed, and then the precipitate is resuspended in 1 ml 5% TCA. The suspension is transferred to 10 ml scintillation fluid, and disintegrations/min are counted using a β scintillation counter. Disintegrations per lymph node is calculated for each experimental group and the control group. The ratio of ^{3}H TdR incorporation into the test group and the control is calculated for each dose. Some investigators prefer to pool the lymph nodes from all animals in the dosage group. If the ratio is 2–3 for any dose, the material is considered a sensitizer.

Several groups of workers have reported comparisons of the LLNA with various guinea pig assays and have suggested variations of the method (13,14,181,182, 162,314). It is clear that LLNA is not as stringent as some guinea pig assays; however, it is expected to retain utility as a rapid screening assay for materials with strong sensitization potential—it offers advantages in the low number of animals used, lower cost, and less time required for conducting the assay. A validation meeting to review the strengths and weaknesses of the assay has been reported (263). Certain materials, such as

Table 22.7
Principal features of human sensitization assays

Feature	Complete Schwartz–Peck	Shelanski/Shelanski	Repeat Insult Patch Tests Draize	Griffith–Voss–Stotts	Modified Draize	Human Maximization
Number of subjects	200	200	200	200	100–200	25
Induction						
Exposure site	Upper arm	Upper arm, same site	Upper arm or back; naïve site for each exposure	Upper arm, same site	Upper arm or back, same site	Upper arm or lower back, same site
Number of exposures	1	15	10	9	10	5
Duration of exposure	24–72 h	24 h	24 h	24 h	48–72 h	48 h
Frequency of exposure	—	3 per week	3 per week	3 per week	3 per week	24 h between patches
Evaluation schedule	At removal, 24, 48 h	At removal	At removal	48–72 h	30 minutes are removal	Before each application
Miscellaneous	4-week usage period	Fatiguing index		Pilot group	Continuous exposure	SLS/irritation as adjuvant
Rest period duration		14–21 days	10–14 days	14 days	14 days	14 days
Challenge						
Exposure site	Upper arm	Upper arm	Upper arm or back	Upper arm	Upper arm or back	Lower back, upper arm
Duration of exposure	24–72 h	48 h	48 h	24 h	72 h	SLS 1 h; 48 h
Evaluation schedule	At removal, 24, 48 h	At removal	At removal	48 and 96 h	At removal, 24 h	At removal, 24, 48 h
Miscellaneous			Naïve test site	Original and naïve sites	Naïve test site; may use two 48-h exposures	Sensitization index

SLS—sodium lauryl sulfate 5% for induction adjuvancy and 10% at challenge.

metals, have not been reliably identified as allergens. The validation attempt matched LLNA results with guinea pig Buehler and maximization assays. Both have false-positives and false-negatives. No attempt was made to determine the clinical relevance of the LLNA data nor the benchmarks used. Furthur experience will be needed to place this assay in toxicologic relevance.

Mouse Ear Swelling Test (MEST)

Gad and his co-workers (128,129) used ear thickness measured with a caliper-type engineer's micrometer to evaluate the response of mice after challenge with potential sensitizers. They optimized a protocol in which tape-stripped skin sites that had been injected with Freund's complete adjuvant were topically exposed to the test material each day for 4 days.

Seven days after the last topical exposure, animals were challenged by topical application of the test material to one ear. Early work also showed that Balb/c, CF-1, or SW mice could be used in the assay. Females were selected because their less aggressive behavior allows group housing with minimally damaged ears. Responses of animals less than 5 weeks old or more than 13 weeks old were weaker than animals 6–10 weeks of age. Administration of induction doses to the stomach region yielded a higher rate of sensitization than application to the back of the animals. The efficacy of the induction method was increased somewhat by both tape stripping and preinjection of the test site with Freund's complete adjuvant. Preliminary work showed that exposure via occlusive patches during induction did not increase the sensitivity of the assay, and in some cases, the response was diminished when the patching system was employed. Their final protocol incorporated these findings.

For the MEST, 6- to 8-week old female CF-1, Balb/c, or SW female mice are gang housed in direct bedding cages. Following a 5–7 day quarantine period, the fur of the abdomen is shaved by electric clippers from 10–15 test animals and 5 controls. Animals with damaged pinea are excluded from testing at this time. After shaving, the area is tape stripped with Dermaclear, a surgical adhesive tape, until the skin appears glossy. Then a divided dose of 0.05 ml Freund's complete adjuvant is injected intradermally with a tuberculin syringe fitted with a 30-gauge needle. The Freund's complete adjuvant is injected into two sites within the shaved area but along the borders. Following the injection of adjuvant, 100 μl of vehicle containing the test material or vehicle alone (controls) is applied to the center of the shaved area. The abdomen is allowed to dry, and then the mouse is returned to its cage. The tape stripping and application of appropriate material to the abdomen is repeated each day for the next 3 days.

Vehicle is chosen based on solubility and chemical compatibility with the test substance. Acetone, methyl ethyl ketone or 70%, 80%, and 95% ethanol in water have been shown to be acceptable vehicles. Mixed ethanol/olive oil systems were not satisfactory. The dose selection is based on dermal irritation toxicity range finding studies prior to testing each compound. Four groups of two mice each were subjected to the induction procedure, including shaving, tape stripping, and application of the test material, and then the ears exposed as during challenge. At least four concentrations are evaluated in the range study. Minimally irritating or nonirritating concentrations are selected for the induction application. The highest nonirritating concentration is used at challenge.

Seven days after the last topical induction application, challenge is performed by applying 20 μl of the test material in vehicle to one ear of each animal (test and control) and 10 μl of the vehicle to the opposite ear. Ear thickness is measured before application of the challenge dose and 24 and 48 h after challenge application. Animals are lightly anesthetized with ether, and the thickness of both pineas is measured with an Oditest engineers micrometer. Positive respondents are defined as animals in which the ear dosed with the test material shows at least a 2–3 fold greater increase in thickness than the vehicle-treated control ear. The control group should not show greater than a 10% increase in ear thickness for the test to be considered valid.

If the control groups show more than a 10% increase, the study should be repeated using lower doses. The percentage of respondents is calculated. In addition, the degree of ear swelling is calculated by dividing the thickness of the ear to which the test material was applied by the thickness of the vehicle treated control ear. Measurements from all animals in the test group are included. No additional explanations or examples of the use of the degree of ear swelling in interpreting results has been provided. A later paper proposed that data generated by MEST (and classical guinea pig assays) could be used to calculate a potency index of sensitization (127).

Gad and co-workers' original paper (128) included validation studies of 72 compounds. They reported a false-negative rate of only 2% and no false-positives when MEST was compared to GPMT data on the same materials. The incidence of sensitization in MEST was consistently lower than that produced by GPMT. Similar findings were reported for comparisons between the Buehler assay and MEST in the same paper; however, published guinea pig data used for comparisons included data from other topical guinea pig techniques that did not employ the restraint procedure specified by Buehler. Intralaboratory validation of the method includes a comparison of test results for eight materials tested in five laboratories (129). That report indicates that MEST did not identify weak sensitizers in two of three laboratories. More recent publications have confirmed that the incidence of positive response in MEST is consistently lower than that in GMPT, and weak and moderate sensitizers are not identified correctly (73,91). The MEST has been accepted by the Environmental Protection Agency for registration of chemicals under the Toxic Substances Control Act (TSCA) (68).

Although not reported in papers describing this method, the type of micrometer used may affect interpretation of the test results. Van Loveren (354) compared the use of spring-loaded caliper-type instruments with screw and friction thimble micrometers. Spring-loaded instruments were best. Electronic instruments have been used in other types of immunological investigations. In our experience, the use of anesthetic can be eliminated by operator training and prior handling of animals.

The Vitamin A Enhancement Test (VAET)

Miller and her colleagues decreased the dose of strong sensitizers required to induce sensitization by maintaining the animals on diet supplemented with high levels of vitamin A acetate (233–236,250). The mechanism of the increase in response was studied using radioisotopes, but because of ease in performing the assay, ear thickness measurement was selected for use in the predictive assay. Principal features of the test included a preconditioning period of the diet of 28 days, 6 exposures to the shaved abdomen and thorax during the 12-day induction period, and challenge 4 days later. Results from the test group were compared statistically to that of controls, with a 50% increase over the response to controls, indicating sensitization. The minimally irritating concentration was used for induction, and the highest nonirritating dose was used at challenge (determined by dose response in separate groups of mice). The vehicle was selected based on nonirritancy and solubility of the test substance. An obvious difficulty with the method was the long conditioning period required prior to the study. General comments concerning choice of micrometer for MEST also apply to VAET. The test was never widely adopted or submitted to formal validation procedures.

Human Sensitization Assays

Chemicals can be tested for their ability to induce contact hypersensitivity in panels of human volunteers from whom informed consent is obtained. Human studies should be undertaken only after the results of predictive tests in animals are available if the test material is a new compound, or if it contains significantly increased levels of common ingredients. Testing higher doses in animals provides some margin of safety for potential human subjects. Generally, materials identified as sensitizers in animals are not tested on humans; however, if the potential benefit of the material warrants, a small group of human subjects may be tested with materials inducing sensitization in animals. Such situations should be reviewed by an Institutional Review Board. Test subjects should be informed of the increased risks, and the number of subjects used should be limited (additional subjects can be exposed if members of a small group do not respond).

Subjects should be randomly selected; however, some precautions are indicated. Some investigators believe intact draining lymph nodes adjacent to the application site is necessary to induce sensitization, and patches should not be placed on areas adjacent to mastectomies. Persons with a unilateral mastectomy who wish to participate may be tested by applying patches to the opposite side of the body. Tests should not be performed on scar tissue. Recurrence of skin conditions in remission (i.e., psoriasis, eczema) has been associated with patch testing and other minor physical traumas. Subjects at risk should be informed of this possibility and encouraged to consult their dermatologist prior to testing. Subjects should not be tested with materials to which they are known to be allergic (demonstrated by diagnostic patch test or in previous predictive assays). It is prudent to routinely question potential subjects concerning their history of dermatologic disease and allergies. Allergic contact dermatitis to materials already in commerce is sometimes detected by early induction patches. This indicates that under patch conditions, the material may elicit a response in presensitized individuals. Although the incidence of preexisting sensitization to the material should be considered in risk assessment decisions regarding marketing, detection of preexisting sensitization is not helpful in evaluating a material's ability to induce sensitization. Records of previous responses of individuals participating in multiple predictive assays should be reviewed prior to testing to eliminate subjects presensitized to components of the products.

Although numerous variations have been reported, there are four basic predictive human sensitization tests in current use: (1) single induction/single challenge patch tests; (2) repeated insult patch tests (RIPT); (3) RIPT with continuous exposure (modified Draize); and (4) the maximization test. Principal features of human sensitization assays are summarized in Table 22.7. As originally described, all methods used customized patches. Patch selection was governed by available adhesive systems. Description of customized patches would be of historical interest only; as currently conducted, all human assays use similar patches. Occlusive patches, consisting of a nonwoven pad, usually Webril, of four-ply gauze sponges, backed by a good occlusive surgical tape, such as Blenderm, are available commercially or may be custom made in strips of four or five pads. Acceptable alternatives include the Hilltop Chamber (176), which contains a Webril pad inside an occlusive plastic disc backed by a porous tape, the Duhring Chamber (124), a stainless steel disc which contains a

Table 22.8
Draize scoring system[a] in albino rabbits

Description	Score[b] assigned
Erythema and Eschar Formation	
No erythema	0
Very slight erythema (barely perceptible)	1
Well-defined erythema	2
Moderate to severe erythema	3
Severe erythema (beet redness) to slight eschar formation (injuries in depth)	4
Edema formation	
No edema	0
Very slight edema (barely perceptible)	1
Slight edema (edges of area well defined by definite raising)	2
Moderate edema (raised approximately 1 mm)	3
Severe edema (raised more than 1 mm and extending beyond the area of exposure)	4

[a] The scale as defined by Draize and adopted by various regulatory agencies.
[b] The PII (primary irritation index) is calculated by averaging the erythema values and averaging the edema values from all animals and then combining the averages (maximum PII = 8).

Webril pad, and the large Finn Chamber. Duhring and Finn chambers usually are secured in place by porous surgical tape. Occasionally, semiocclusive patches made of Webril backed by porous tape may be used. Semiocclusive patches are decidedly inferior to occlusive patches in induction of sensitization.

For assays other than maximization, usually 150–200 subjects are tested. Henderson and Riley (145) showed statistically that if no positive reactions are observed in 200 randomly selected subjects, as many as 15/1000 of the general population may react (95% confidence). As sample size is reduced, the likelihood that the test will not correctly predict adverse reactions in the general population increases.

Results of RIPT, modified Draize test, and human maximization tests have been accepted as valid by regulatory agencies; however, some sponsors routinely use one of the methods described and defend its use as the "standard of the industry"; this is a simplistic view of the methods and their strengths and weaknesses. As for all toxicity endpoints, *the method used should provide a reasonable exaggerated exposure over the anticipated exposure from use of the product*. The device group of the FDA held several meetings to review details of sensitization procedures. These deliberations led to a guidance document (63) for evaluating skin sensitization to chemicals in natural rubber products. The modified Draize procedure is recommended. Tests for the transdermal products are currently being evaluated by the FDA.

Schwartz–Peck Test (and Modifications)

A single application induction patch followed by a single application patch test was described by Schwartz (316–318) and Schwartz and Peck (318) with a usage test of 1 month after challenge to verify patch results. The test has been modified by some to eliminate the usage test (50), to eliminate patching altogether, and to place a usage period between induction and challenge patches (345). The term complete Schwartz–Peck refers to a single induction patch, usage period, and single challenge patch test. This may also be referred to as the Traub–Tusing–Spoon method. Incomplete Schwartz–Peck tests do not incorporate a usage period. A patch saturated with the test material, diluted if necessary, is applied to the outer upper arm of 200 test subjects and remains in place for 24–72 h. The dose tested and duration of patch contact varies with intended use. Cosmetics may be tested without a covering (open application), or with semi-occlusive patches. The test site is visually evaluated at patch removal and at 24 and 48 h after removal for erythema and edema. A 4-week normal usage period follows the induction patch in the complete Schwartz–Peck test, with a challenge patch applied to the same site on the upper arm at the conclusion of the usage period. For the incomplete Schwartz–Peck test, a second patch procedure is performed 10–14 days after the induction patch. Duration of contact and evaluation of site is performed as during induction. The development of dermatitis at challenge that is much stronger than during induction signifies sensitization.

Schwartz originally described the incomplete Schwartz–Peck test. A usage test was to be conducted after the challenge patch using 1000 different subjects. Although Schwartz and Peck referred to their assay as a "prophetic patch" test, experience has shown that only potent haptens will induce sensitization in this assay (191). In fairness, it should be noted that the test was originally designed to evaluate the effect of nylon garments on the skin. It was intended to detect adverse effects, irritation, and "secondary irritation" (sensitization). The mechanism of skin allergy was not understood when the test was designed. Although the test was useful for its original purpose, unfortunately its use was expanded without considering new information generated by immunologists. Clearly, the assay is inferior to all other predictive human sensitization assays; however, a few groups continue to use the method.

Repeat Insult Patch Test (RIPT)

Three major variations on the RIPT are in common use: (1) the Draize human sensitization test (86,87); (2) the Shelanski/Shelanski test (320–322); and (3) the Voss/Griffith test (52,138,139,362). Although the

Shelanskis first published a description of a RIPT, they based its development on a verbal description of a method Draize was devising (322). Voss modified the Shelanski/Shelanski test (362), and his assay was later modified by Griffith (138). As one would expect, the three assays have much in common. There are some significant differences in the assays as originally described, however.

In the Draize human sensitization test, an occlusive patch containing the test material is applied to the upper arm or upper back of 200 volunteers. The patch remains in place for 24 h and is then removed. The test site is evaluated at patch removal for erythema and edema. A second patch test is applied to a new site 24 h after the first patch is removed. This process is repeated until 10 patches are applied. For convenience, the test may be run on a Monday–Friday schedule, with subjects removing their own patches Saturday (72 h between Friday and Monday applications). Ten to 14 days after application of the last induction patches, subjects are challenged via a patch applied to a new site. Duration of contact is 24 h; sites are visually evaluated at removal of the patch. The response at challenge is compared to the response to patches applied early in induction. The incidence of sensitization is reported.

Like the Draize RIPT, the Shelanski/Shelanski test employs occlusive patches that remain in contact with the skin of the upper arm for 24 h. The patching cycle is the same; however, patches are placed on the same test site each time, and a total of 15 sets of patches is applied during induction. The test site is evaluated before application of a new patch to the site. If inflammation has developed, the patch is placed on an adjacent uninflamed site. Two to 3 weeks after the induction period, subjects are challenged by application of a patch, which remains in place for 48 h. Test sites are evaluated at patch removal for erythema and edema. The incidence of positive response is reported. Patch responses during induction were considered by Shelanski and Shelanski to be evidence of "skin fatigue" (cumulative irritation); the time to development (i.e., number of patches) was reported as a fatiguing index. Voss (362) reduced the number of 24-h patch exposures to 9 over a 3-week period. At challenge 2 weeks after the last induction patch, duplicate patches applied to the original test site are worn for 24 h. Patch sites are evaluated 48 and 96 h after patch application. A pilot group of 10 to 12 subjects was tested prior to exposing the full panel of 60 to 70 subjects. Griffith later published more details of the method (138,139). A maximum of four dissimilar materials was tested simultaneously and duplicate challenges were applied to the sites of induction and to the opposite arm, thus testing on areas drained by different regional lymphatics. The concept of a rechallenge of subjects with reactions difficult to interpret was also introduced. The number of subjects was increased to 200 by conducting tests on multiple panels. Stotts (335) presented detailed examples of proper interpretation of human repeat insult patch tests. Sensitization is characterized by challenge reactions stronger than reactions early in the induction phase, by persistence of responses through delayed readings, by delayed appearance of a response, or by weak responses in a few subjects when the material has not produced irritation in the panel. Examples of patterns of responses indicating presensitization and weak responses that warrant rechallenge were also presented.

As currently conducted, the differences in Draize and Voss/Griffith RIPT are minimal. Many investigators apply patches to the same site during induction and refer to the procedure as a Draize RIPT. The value of multiple grades at challenge is widely recognized and used. Multiple test materials are tested simultaneously in all RIPT for reasons of efficiency and economy. Although the distinctions between Draize and Voss/Griffith procedures have blurred with common usage, the Shelanski/Shelanski test, with five to six more induction applications, remains distinct.

Human Maximization Test

Kligman (191) reviewed the common human predictive sensitization test methods in use in 1966 and found them to be unsatisfactory in inducing sensitization to nine clinical allergens. In panels of 200 subjects, the Shelanski/Shelanski method induced sensitization to four materials; the original Draize test and the complete Schwartz/Peck test induced sensitization to two allergens each; and the incomplete Schwartz/Peck test failed to induce sensitization to any allergen. He concluded

> Emphasis must shift from prophecy to the more practical objective of identifying potential allergens. Once the allergenic potential is known with reasonable certainty, a judgement of risk might be ventured after examining all the pertinent variables. (193)

This represented a profound change in the intent of predictive sensitization assays. Based on his studies of factors affecting rates of sensitization in predictive assays (190,197), Kligman designed the Human Maximization Test (197). He later modified the procedure somewhat to reduce difficulties in performing the test and in interpreting the test (197). The maximization test uses irritancy as an adjuvant. During induction, irritating compounds are tested at a concentration that produces a moderate erythema within 48 h. If materials are nonirritating, the test site is pretested with a 24-h patch of 5% sodium lauryl sulfate (SLS). Additional pretreatment SLS patches may be applied before each patch application until a brisk erythema is produced. Induction concentrations are at least five times higher than use levels; petrolatum is the preferred vehicle. Often, custom-made Webril/Blenderm patches or Duhring Chambers are used. Patches are applied to either the outer aspect of the arm or lower back, and up to four dissimilar materials may be tested at one time. Wrapping with extra tape is often necessary to ensure occlusion. Bandage sprays may be used to assure sealing of the test site. Five sets of patches are worn on the same site for 48 h each, with a 24-h rest period between removal and reapplication. Following a 2-week rest period, an SLS provocative patch is applied to prepare the skin for challenge. A patch saturated with a 2.5–5.0 solution of SLS is applied to previously untreated sites on the lower back. SLS concentration is based on the season and on individual subject response. The SLS patch is removed after 1 hour, and a patch containing the test material is applied. A control site is patched with SLS (1 h) and petrolatum (48 h) to aid in interpretation of the results. Forty-eight h after application, the patch is removed and test sites are evaluated. Test sites are reexamined 24 and 48 h after patch removal. The number of subjects developing a positive response is reported and a sensitization index based on percentage of subjects responding is assigned to the test material. In common practice, the human maximization procedure is performed on either the outer upper arm or the back. Although it is clear that the maximization test is a sensitive tool for detection of allergenicity, the skin damage produced is dramatic and unacceptable to many subjects.

Modified Draize Human Sensitization Test

The RIPT procedure was modified to provide for continuous patch exposure. Materials are applied to the outer upper arm each Monday, Wednesday, and Friday until 10 patches have been applied during a 3-week period (240,241). Patches remain in place until approximately 30 min before application of a fresh patch. This brief rest period allows some clearing of responses to tape and facilitates grading. Fresh patches are applied to the same site unless moderate inflammation has developed; the patches are placed on adjacent noninflamed skin, should inflammation become pronounced. This produces a continuous exposure of 504 to 552 h (some investigators apply only nine patches), compared to a total exposure period of 216 to 240 h for RIPT of comparable induction applications. In addition, induction concentration was increased to levels above usage exposure. Two weeks after induction, subjects are challenged by exposure of a new site to a patch of 72 h,' duration at a nonirritating concentration. Test sites are evaluated at patch removal and 24 h after removal. Jordan and King (173) proposed modifying the challenge procedure to two consecutive 48-h patch periods. The modified Draize test has recently been selected as the test of choice for chemicals in natural rubber products (63).

In Vitro Assays For Allergic Contact Dermatitis

As our understanding of the cell biology of delayed contact hypersensitivity has increased, in vitro assays to replace diagnostic patch testing and as early-screening predictive assays have been proposed. Much of the work toward diagnostic procedures has centered on measuring the effect of cytokines released by sensitized lymphocytes on target cells as a marker for allergy. Proposals for in vitro predictive assays have focused on the afferent phase of antigen binding and stimulation of target cells. To date, neither approach has proved satisfactory, but some limited experimental successes have been reported.

Migration inhibition of peritoneal exudate cells from capillary tubes has been reported to be inhibited by the antigen to which donor guinea pigs were sensitized (131). Inhibition of macrophage migration is mediated by soluble factors produced by sensitized lymphocytes in the presence of sensitizing antigen (88). This factor, identified as migration inhibition factor (MIF), has been shown to aggregate macrophages, increase macrophage adherence to glass, and decrease macrophage mobility (81). Rocklin (303) reported that MIF was produced by highly purified populations of proliferating T cells. Morehead (258) later demonstrated that MIF production is dependent on Ia–T-cell subsets. Mitogenic factors, such as phytohemagglutinin, initiate mitotic activity and transformation of lymphocytes in their blast forms. Pearmain (289) demonstrated that tuberculin produced the same effect in peripheral blood leukocyte cultures from sensitive patients but not from unsensitized patients. Similar work experiments were conducted in nickel-sensitive subjects (7). Lymphocytes from unsensitized controls also underwent blast transformation when exposed to nickel. Nonspecificity of nickel and mercury transformation was confirmed by numerous other investigators (281,288,294). Using ^{14}C thymidine uptake to measure blast transformation, MacLeod (218) demonstrated transformation in over half of nickel-sensitive subjects and no unsensitized controls.

Experimental studies of blast transformation in which animal or human subjects were intentionally sensitized have been somewhat more successful. At least two investigators (130,251) demonstrated that lymphocytes from guinea pigs sensitized with dinitrochlorobenzene (DNCB) and incubated with dinitroflurobenzene (DNFB) (a dinitrophenyl group would attach to protein using either material) were transformed to a greater degree than cells from unsensitized controls. Tritiated thymidine was used to measure blast formation when exposed to DNFB conjugated to epidermal protein. Similar responses were demonstrated using human volunteers and epidermal extracts for conjugation (252). Miller and Levy (249) produced the same effect using leukocyte and erythrocyte membranes for conjugation.

Cytotoxicity consistent with that produced by lymphotoxin has been demonstrated in experimentally induced allergic contact dermatitis (84). Peripheral lymphocytes from DNFB-sensitized guinea pigs were incubated with DNFB-coated radiolabeled chick erythrocytes. Increased radioisotope leakage was produced by lymphocytes from sensitized animals than produced by controls. Similar effects were demonstrated using epidermal cells (341).

The use of exclusively in vitro assays for predicting sensitization potential of schemes has been proposed. In one hypothetical system (41), binding to Langerhans cells would be measured. If no binding occurred, the activation state of the Langerhans cell would be evaluated. If no activation was detected, the material would not be considered to induce sensitization. If Langerhans cells were activated, an autologous lymphocyte blastogenesis assay would be performed. Although this approach has not been supported experimentally, current commercial activity in producing skin recombinants may make this type of approach feasible. Blomberg et al. (36) recently reviewed the use of in vitro assays to study mechanisms of contact dermatitis.

SKIN IRRITATION AND CORROSION

Historically, skin irritation has been described by exclusion as localized inflammation not medicated by sensitized lymphocytes or antibodies (e.g., that which develops by a process not involving the immune system). Application of some chemicals destroys tissues directly, producing skin damage, including necrosis at the site of application. Chemicals producing necrosis that result in the formation of scar tissue are described as corrosives. Chemicals producing inflammation after a single exposure are termed acute irritants. Some chemicals do not produce acute irritation from a single exposure but may produce inflammation following repeated application to the same area of skin. The cumulative irritation from repeated exposures was originally called skin fatigue (320). Because of the possibility of skin contact during transport and the use of many chemicals, regulatory agencies have mandated that chemicals be screened for their ability to produce skin corrosion and acute irritation. These studies have been conducted in animals using standardized protocols; however, recent efforts to replace animal studies with in vitro or human assays have had some success. It is not appropriate to conduct screening studies for corrosion in humans. Acute irritation can be evaluated in humans after animal studies have shown that the risk of systemic toxicity is low and if the material is known to be noncorrosive. Tests for cumulative irritation in both animals and humans have been reported. In general, cumulative irritation is evaluated in man unless the toxicity of the material necessitates testing in animals (pesticides, industrial chemicals).

The processes that result in any form of skin irritation are not well understood. In addition to destroying tissue directly, chemicals can disrupt cell functions and/or trigger the release, formation, or activation of autocoids. Autocoids that are generated following exposure of tissue to some chemicals produce local increases in blood flow, increase vascular permeability, attract white blood cells in the area, and damage cells indirectly. The additive effects of the autocoid mediators would result in local skin inflammation. No agent has yet met all the criteria to establish it as a mediator of skin irritation (297); however, histamine, 5-hydrotryptamine, prostaglandins, leukotrienes, kinins, complement, reactive oxygen species, and products of white blood cells (278) have been strongly implicated as mediators of some irritant reactions.

We have studied the process by which chemicals produce acute skin irritation following open topical applications to the ear of the mouse (283,285,258). The time course of the development of inflammatory responses varied from compound to compound and was independent of vehicle and applied dose. Because the differences in time course could not be attributed to differing rates of penetration, this suggested that the materials tested triggered different inflammatory processes. Differences in the irritation process triggered by three chemicals were confirmed by histology, albumin leakage, and changes in rate of blood flow. Using a series of pharmacological antagonists of putative mediators of irritation, enzyme inhibitors to prevent formation of suspected mediators, and agents that deplete the body of serum mediators, we confirmed that different pathways of mediator involvement existed for skin irritation. The implications for this finding are clear: a battery of in vitro assays would be needed to screen materials for skin irritation; no single assay would be effective.

Many factors may modulate the development of skin irritation (see Table 22.12). As with delayed contact hypersensitivity (DCH), these factors have been classified as extrinsic or intrinsic (210,232,243,381). Some extrinsic factors have been experimentally shown to be important considerations in designing predictive tests for skin irritation. A few investigators have also considered intrinsic variables when designing studies.

Like other toxic responses, skin irritation is related to dose. If the duration of contact and the dosing procedure are held constant, intensity of response increases as concentration of the solution increases. Under patch test conditions, the rate of increase in intensity decreases as the concentration increases (383). The type of appliance, chamber, and tape used to secure patches in place have been shown to influence the intensity of irritant responses (67,191,202). More intense inflammatory responses are produced as the degree of occlusion is increased. The search for good techniques of occlusion ultimately led to the development of the Prilia (Finn), Duhring, and Hilltop Chambers now routinely used in patch testing.

Increases in occlusion usually are accompanied by local increases in surface temperature, and increased temperature is believed to predispose subjects to irritation. The temperature of solutions used in immersion assays is usually around 105°F (140,174,273). Although systematic studies demonstrating that those temperatures were necessary were not presented, increased temperature has been shown to be necessary to reproduce irritant dermatitis in some instances (305).

The influence of vehicle in diagnostic patch testing for allergy is well recognized. Similar effects are seen when irritation is studied. These effects are demonstrated convincingly in open systems (e.g., a dose of croton oil that produces no measurable edema in the mouse ear when applied in olive oil produces the maximum response when applied in acetone) (285). Patch occlusivity and interactions between vehicles and adhesives used in patch systems also influence the intensity of response and make it more difficult to demonstrate vehicle effects under patch conditions. In most predictive irritation tests, the choice of solvent is related to use conditions, and water is the solvent often used.

Dosing schedules have been developed that maximize the development of the responses of interest. In general, the longer the duration of contact to the same dose of a given chemical, the greater the intensity of the response. Multiple exposures at frequent intervals are the basis for most cumulative irritation assays, although there is some disagreement on the optimal time between exposures. In developing the soap chamber test (discussed later), Frosch and Kligman (125) varied both the frequency and duration of exposure in order to produce a more sensitive test.

The seasonal variability in human response to normal exposure to irritants is well documented (148). Conducting usage studies in late fall and winter increases the test's discriminating ability (62). Some investigators have demonstrated similar effects using patch test procedures (190,383) and small-scale exaggerated exposure tests (174). Although the basis for this variability is not well understood, it is believed to be due in part to changes in the barrier properties of the skin. Many investigators have experimentally altered the barrier properties of skin in order to develop assays that are more sensitive. Alteration varies from the abrasion of Draize-type tests (88) and the chamber scarification test (121) to tape stripping to remove the outer surface of the epidermis (194). Pretreating the test sites with damaging agents has been shown to increase the skin's reactivity to other chemicals (111,112,284). Although these extrinsic factors modify barrier function, intrinsic factors governing barrier properties are also important (238). Barrier function would be expected to contribute to responses observed in screening tests used to identify sensitive subjects (122,126). The demonstration that persons with some skin diseases develop more intense response to irritants (30,325) and had diminished barrier function (356) was not unexpected. Susceptibility to development of irritant responses is believed to be under genetic control. The prevalence of irritant responses in atopic individuals supports this theory. The response to identical patches applied to different sites is convincing evidence that there is regional variation in susceptibility to irritants. The reactivity of the various sites appears to correlate to the ability of chemicals to penetrate the skin in that area. Regional differences in skin response is not limited to man (358).

Susceptibility to irritation is believed to vary by age, sex, and race. Children have been shown to develop inflammatory responses to lower levels of a variety of chemicals than adults (302). The inflammatory response to some materials is decreased in the elderly (195,340). Some investigators have suggested that the skin of women is more sensitive to irritants than men (363); however, sex differences in reactivity were not confirmed by other investigators (31). Investigators have reported that higher doses of irritants are required to produce inflammation of the skin of blacks (370,371). This difference in reactivity disappeared when black skin was tape stripped, leading some investigators to hypothesize that black skin forms a more efficient barrier. Berardesca (21) recently questioned whether these differences are more real than apparent.

The principles of general toxicology should be remembered when one designs and interprets any animal (and human) assay for skin irritation. One should consider dose-response relationships. Draize scores require careful interpretation; they are best interpreted by comparison to related compounds or formulations with a history of human exposure. Knowledge of intended human use (and foreseeable misuse) permits a more rational interpretation. With occlusive application techniques, one should remember that occlusion increases the permeability of some but not all moieties. Although there is a consistent, reasonably good correlation between responses in rabbits and humans, occasional inconsistencies have ocurred (133). Investigators (179,285) have found that different species exhibit widely varying reactivity under identical test conditions, especially in substances with only minor irritant potential. Thus, the accuracy of the Draize test and other animal testing as it relates to humans has been called into question (152). In addition, results from the animal methods currently used differ due to the subjective visual test scoring. These differences occur most frequently in the assessment of the toxicity of mild irritants and colored material (272). Wise investigators conduct carefully planned and executed tests in humans when rabbit tests indicate that materials are possible irritants. This is particularly true when one wishes to compare the irritancy potential of mild irritants. One should follow the guidelines of the National Academy of Science (NAS) committee (262) when this course of action is taken.

There is sufficient interest in irritant dermatitis to support an international symposium approximately every 3 years. Recent textbooks summarize current advances (98,355).

Irritation Tests In Animals

Draize-Type Tests

Primary irritation and corrosion are most often evaluated by modifications of the method described by John Draize and his colleagues in 1944 (88). The Federal Hazardous Substance Act (FHSA) adopted one modification as a standard procedure (66). The backs of six albino rabbits are clipped free of hair. Each material is tested on two 1-in square sites on the same animal; one site is intact and one is abraded in such a way that the stratum corneum is opened but no bleeding produced. Abrasion can be performed using the tip of a hypodermic needle drawn across the skin repeatedly or commercial instruments such as the Berkeley Scarifier (147). Materials are tested undiluted, and 0.5 ml liquid, or 0.5 g solid or semisolid material is applied. In some cases the skin may be moistened to help solids adhere to the site, or an equal volume of solvent may be used to moisten the material. Each test site is covered with two layers of 1-in square surgical gauze secured in place with tape. The entire trunk of the animal is then wrapped with rubberized cloth or other occlusive impervious material to retard evaporation of the substances and hold the patches in one position. Twenty-four hours after application, the wrappings are removed and the test sites are evaluated for erythema and edema using a prescribed scale (Table 22.8). Evaluations of abraded and intact sites are recorded separately. Test sites are evaluated again 48 h later (72 h after application) using the same scale.

The reproducibility of the FHSA procedure (358,372) and the relevance of test results to human experience (82,158,243,296,331) have been questioned. Numerous modifications to the Draize procedure have been proposed to improve its prediction of human experience. Modifications that have been proposed include changing the species tested (260), reduction of exposure period, use of fewer animals, and testing on intact skin only (93,142,265). A few investigators have supplemented visual evaluation with other techniques (247,248), but these additions have not been considered for the standard method. Several governmental bodies have used their own modification of the Drake procedure for regulatory decisions. The Consumer Product Safety Commission (CPSC), Department of Transportation (DOT), Environmental Protection Agencies (EPA), and Organization for Economic Co-operation and Development (OECD) guidelines are contrasted to the original Draize methods in Table 22.9. Cruzan et al. (76) proposed a composite test that meets requirements of major agencies.

Summaries and evaluations of the scores vary somewhat. Draize reported values for individual animals at each time point, combined the erythema and edema values at each time point, and then averaged the 24- and 72-h evaluations for intact and abraded sites separately. He also calculated a primary irritation index (PII) that was the average of the intact and abraded sites. Agents producing PII of 2 were considered only mildly irritating, 2–5 moderately irritating, and more than 5 severely irritating. The primary irritation calculated for the FHSA is essentially the PII of Draize. A minimum PII of 5 defines an irritant by CPSC standards. The method of the National Institute of Occupational Safety and Health (NIOSH) does not combine responses of abraded sites and includes probable effects on normal and damaged skin in their evaluation.

Although vesiculation, ulceration, and severe eschar formations are not included in the Draize Scoring Scales, all Draize-type tests are used to evaluate corrosion as well as irritation. When severe reactions, which may not be reversible, are noted, test sites are observed for a longer period. Delayed evaluations usually are made on days 7 and 14; however, evaluations have been made as late as 35 days after application. EPA bases interpretations on 7-day observations. The basic exposure procedures for skin irritation/corrosion of OECD guidelines have been further modified to test for corrosion during shorter periods (275). Under a directive of the European Economic Community, a shorter, 3-min exposure was added (with no wrapping procedure). The United Nations' recommendations for the Transport of Dangerous Goods is based on exposure times of 4 h, 1 h, and 3 min, with the recommendation that the 1-h exposure be conducted first. Evaluations are made 1, 24, 48, and 72 h, and 7 days after dosing.

It should be noted that the Draize method has generally erred on the side of safety in that it overpredicts the severity of skin damage produced by chemicals, thus providing a safety factor for those exposed. One criticism, which is often repeated, is that the test is not sensitive enough to separate mild from moderate irritants. The purpose when designing the Draize test was to identify chemicals that posed a severe hazard to the public, not to compare products. Criticisms of the Draize test have been embraced by groups supporting abolition of animal

Table 22.9

Comparison of skin irritation tests based on the Draize method

Feature	Draize	FHSA	DOT	FIFRA	OECD[a]
Number of animals	3[b]	6	6	6	3
Abrasion	Abraded and intact	Abraded and intact	Intact	2 abraded and 2 intact	Intact
Dose liquids	0.5 ml undiluted	0.5 ml undiluted	0.5 ml	0.5 ml undiluted	0.5 ml
Dose solids	0.5 g	0.5 g in solvent	0.5 g	0.5 g moistened	0.5 g moistened
Wrapping materials	Gauze and rubberized cloth	Impervious material			Semiocclusive
Length of exposure	24 h	24 h	4 h	4 h	4 h
Evaluated at[c]	24, 72 h	24, 72 h	4, 48 h	0.5, 1, 24, 48, 72 h.	0.5, 1, 24, 48, 72 h
Treatment at removal	Not specified	Not specified	Skin washed	Skin wiped, not washed	Skin washed
Excluded from testing				Materials pH ≤2 or ≥11.5	Materials pH ≤2 or ≥11.5

[a] Although other species are acceptable, the albino rabbit is the preferred species.
[b] Draize tested four materials on six rabbits. Three abraded and three intact sites were tested with each material.
[c] Times listed are after removal for FIFRA and OECD. Times listed for Draize, FHSA, and DOT are after application of the test material.
DOT—Department of Transportation; FHSA—Federal Hazardous Substance Act; FIFRA—Federal Insecticide, Fungicide, and Rodenticide Act; OECD—Organization for Economic Cooperation and Development.

testing as demonstrating that use of the method is unwarranted. These criticisms overlook the tremendous value the test has provided in warning consumers, workers, and manufacturers of potential dangers associated with specific chemicals so that appropriate precautions could be taken. Although Draize-type tests will be replaced by in vitro assays at some time in the future, we have no validated in vitro substitute at present (297).

Non-Draize Animal Studies

Animal assays to evaluate the ability of chemicals to produce cumulative irritation have been developed (291); however, they are not required by any regulatory agency. The impetus for their use is largely development of products that are better tolerated by consumers and industrial workers. Although many such tests have been described, only a few are used extensively enough to summarize. Even those used more often are not as well standardized as Draize-type tests, and many variables have been introduced by multiple investigators.

Repeat application patch tests in which diluted materials are applied to the same site each day for 15–21 days have been reported, using several species (291); the guinea pig or rabbit is most commonly used. Patches used vary considerably, with gauze-type dressings and metal chambers being the extremes. Some authors recommend testing the materials with no covering, presumably with a restraining collar to prevent grooming of the area and ingestion of the material. A material of similar use or that produces a known effect in man is included in almost all repeat application patch procedures as a control. The degrees of inflammation produced by the materials in a single assay are compared. Test sites are evaluated for erythema and edema using the scales of the Draize-type tests or more descriptive scales developed by the investigator. Although interpretation ratings such as "slight", "moderate", or "severe" irritant are not usually made, the data from cumulative irritancy assays in rabbits have been used to predict reactions in man. Other investigators have used multiple application with shorter periods of time to evaluate materials (174).

A 5-day dermal irritation test in rabbits was used to compare consumer products of various types (219). After shaving the animals' backs 0.5 ml of test materials was spread over a 5 × 4.5 cm area of skin. The test sites were protected from grooming by placing the animal in a leather harness or Elizabethan collar. After 4 hours, sites were cleaned and graded using the Draize scoring system. This procedure was repeated each day for 5 days. The authors showed good agreement between this assay and 21-day human patch tests of liquid detergents, after bath colognes and hair preparations; the technique was less satisfactory for other types of materials.

The guinea pig immersion assay has been used to evaluate the irritancy of aqueous detergent solutions (58,273,274). Ten guinea pigs are placed in restraining devices that are immersed in a 40°C test solution for 4 h. The apparatus is designed to maintain the guinea pig's head above the solution. Immersion is repeated daily for three treatments. Twenty-four hours after the final immersion, the flank is shaved and the skin is evaluated for erythema, edema, and fissures. A photographic grading scale for this assay was presented in MacMillan et al. (219). Only materials of limited toxic potential are suitable for this assay because systemic absorption of a lethal dose is possible. Concentration of test materials varies somewhat but is usually below 10% to limit systemic toxicity of the agents. A second group of animals is usually tested with a reference material as a control for the material of interest.

An open application procedure in guinea pigs uses microscopic examination of skin biopsies of sites treated with weak irritants to rank materials (5). Biopsies are taken after three daily applications of 10% of solvent or 5% aqueous test solutions to 1 cm^2 areas of the shaved flank. Sites are evaluated visually for erythema and edema, and microscopically, 3 μm histological sections a stained with May–Grunward–Giemsa under oil immersion for epidermal thickness and dermal infiltration. A composite score reflecting the macroscopic evaluation, number of applications before development of visible response, the epidermal thickness, and the cellular response is used to rank chemicals. Although this method provides information on pathogenesis of the response to each chemical, the extensive processing may limit its application to special studies.

Uttley and Van Abbey (353) developed a mouse ear test in which undiluted shampoos were applied to one ear daily for 4 days. The degree of inflammation was quantified visually as vessel dilation, erythema, and edema. The degree of inflammation produced by materials of interest was compared to that produced by a reference material tested on another group of mice. One confounding factor with this assay may be the use of anesthetics that may alter development of inflammation to facilitate performance of the procedure.

To distinguish between mild and moderate irritants in an acute exposure test, Finkelstein and colleagues (111,112) used pretreatment of test sites with an irritant and enhanced visualization of the response by injection of trypan blue to increase test sensitivity. The technique was performed in anesthetized rabbits, rats, or guinea pigs. A circular area of the shaved abdomen was painted with a 20% solution of formaldehyde and then was allowed to dry for 5 min. This was repeated three times and then 1-in cotton flannel pads saturated with test material were applied to each site. A control substance of known irritancy was tested in each study. Pads were secured in place and then the entire trunk was wrapped in polyethylene. A solution of trypan blue was injected into subcutaneous tissue away from the dosage sites. The dye was absorbed and served as a marker for plasma leakage because it spontaneously binds to albumin. After 16 h, patches were removed and the degree of bluing at each site was evaluated on a 0 to 100% scale. In light of more recent work comparing the reactivity of dorsal and abdominal animal skin (358), one wonders if the enhanced sensitivity was due in part to choice of test site. Another recent study reported quantitating the amount of the dye Evans blue recovered from rat skin after exposing the skin to inflammatory agents (160).

A few tests in which material is not applied topically have been developed, claiming to evaluate the intrinsic irritancy of test materials. The persistence of edema in the skin of depilated juvenile white mice following intracutaneous injection of solutions has been used to assess local irritation (51,367). The number of wrinkles observed on reefing the skin with thin pincers is counted before and at selected timepoints through 6 h after injection of 0.01 ml test solution. Although the number of test animals has varied between 8 and 25, the developers considered 20–25 optimal. An obvious limitation of this method is that materials must be administered as iso-osmotic solutions, which requires substantial pretest formulation. Although the developers claim this procedure has good predictive power for eye, skin, and mucosal irritation, it has not been adopted extensively, and no validation studies comparing this method to the standard assays have been published.

Justice et al. (174) described a Repeat Animal Patch (RAP) test for comparing irritation potential of surfactants. Solutions were applied to the clipped back of immobilized albino mice with a saturated cotton-tipped applicator. The test site was covered with a rubber dam to prevent evaporation. This process was repeated seven times at intervals of 10 min. The skins were evaluated microscopically for epidermal erosion.

Brown (49) used both open and closed exposures to rank surfactants for skin irritation potential. Tests ranged from 6-h patch exposures each day for 3 consecutive days in rabbits to daily open application to the skin of rabbits, guinea pigs, or hairless mice for up to 4.5 weeks. Good agreement among the test methods was not obtained, and none of the methods gained wide acceptance, although they are similar to techniques developed by others later.

We have used an assay in which dilute solutions of surfactants and other chemicals are applied to one ear of 5 or 6 mice each day for 4 days (284). Ear thickness was measured at various timepoints after each treatment was used to quantify the degree of inflammation. Multiple groups (at least four) were tested with different doses of the material. The dose producing a 50% maximum response following a single treatment and the slope of the dose response lines for the chemicals were compared. Pretreating the ear with croton oil or TPA 72 h before application of the material of interest increased the sensitivity of the assay. Although the procedure was useful for most surfactant-based products, it was not suitable for oily and highly perfumed materials because animals attempt to remove the materials by grooming. Maloney and Teal (255) also used ear thickness to quantify inflammatory changes produced by n-alkanes applied to ears of mice. They dosed animals twice per day for 4 days in order to produce inflammation. More recently, dithranol-induced skin irritation and the modulating effects of different pharmacological agents, like the corticosteroids and the lipoxygenase and cyclooxygenase inhibitors studies, were studies using the mouse ear model (357).

Human Irritation Tests

Because only a small area of skin need be tested, it is possible to conduct predictive irritation assays in man, provided that systemic toxicity (from absorption) is low and informed consent is obtained. Although regulatory agencies do not routinely require testing in man, human tests are preferred to animal tests in some cases because of the uncertainties of interspecies extrapolation. New materials, those of unknown or unfamiliar composition, should be tested on animal skin first to determine if application to man is warranted (263). Patch test responses generally heal rapidly, within a week or so. More severe reactions should be evaluated periodically over a longer period to determine how the inflammatory response is resolved. Some subjects may develop changes in pigmentation level at the test site following severe responses. It is prudent to prearrange for medical consultation whenever human clinical tests are undertaken.

Single-Application Irritation Patch Tests

Many forms of single-application patch tests have been published. Duration of patch exposure has varied between 1 and 72 h. Custom-made apparatus to hold the test material have been designed (221,321,323). A variety of adhesives that are no longer commercially available have been used (223). Although the individual assays provided important information to the investigators of the period, they were never standardized or gained wide acceptance.

The single-application patch procedure outlined by the NAS (262) incorporates important aspects of assays used by many investigators. The procedure is similar to FHSA tests in rabbits. Commercial patches, chambers, gauze squares, or cotton bandage material, such as Webril,

Table 22.10
Human patch test grading scales

A.	*SIMPLE PATCH TEST GRADING SCALE*
0	Negative, normal skin
±	Questionable erythema not covering entire area
1	Definite erythema
2	Erythema and induration
3	Vesiculation
4	Bullous reaction
B.	*DETAILED HUMAN PATCH TEST GRADING SCALE*
0	No apparent cutaneous involvement
$\frac{1}{2}$	Faint, barely perceptible erythema or slight dryness (glazed appearance)
1	Faint but definite erythema, no eruptions or broken skin ***OR*** No erythema but definite dryness; may have epidermal fissuring
$1\frac{1}{2}$	Well-defined erythema or faint erythema with definite dryness; may have epidermal fissuring
2	Moderate erythema, may have a *few* papules or deep fissures, moderate-to-severe erythema in the cracks
$2\frac{1}{2}$	Moderate erythema with barely perceptible edema ***OR*** Severe erythema not involving a significant portion of the patch (halo effect around the edges), may have a few papules ***OR*** Moderate to severe erythema
3	Severe erythema (beet redness), may have generalized papules ***OR*** Moderate to severe erythema with slight edema (edges well defined by raising)
$3\frac{1}{2}$	Moderate to severe erythema with moderate edema (confined to patch area) ***OR*** Moderate to severe erythema with isolated eschar formations or vesicles
4	Generalized vesicles ***OR*** Eschar formations ***OR*** Moderate to severe erythema and/or edema extending beyond the patched area

applied to either the intrascapular region of the back or to the dorsal surface of the upper arms are expected to produce equivalent reactions (196). Patches are secured in place with surgical tape without wrapping the trunk of the arm. For new volatile materials, a relatively nonocclusive tape, such as Micropore, Dermical, or Scanpore, should be used. Increasing the degree of occlusion with occlusive tapes such as Blenderm or chamber devices such as the Duhring or Hilltop Chamber generally increases the severity of responses. A 4-hour exposure period was suggested by the NAS panel; however, it is desirable to test new materials and volatiles for shorter periods—30 min to 1 hour—and many investigators apply materials intended for skin contact for 24 to 48 hour periods. Subjects should routinely be instructed to remove patches immediately if any unusual discomfort develops. After the period of exposure, the patches should be removed, the area cleaned with water to remove any residue, and the test site marked by study personnel.

Responses are evaluated 30 min to 1 h after patch removal (to allow hydration and pressure effects to subside), and again 24 h after the patch is removed. Persistent reactions may be evaluated for 3 to 4 days. The Draize scales for erythema and edema (Table 22.8) have been used for grading human skin responses; however, they have no provision for scoring papular, vesicular, or bullous responses. Integrated scales ranging from 4 to 16 points have been published (Table 22.10) and are generally preferred to the Draize scales. Up to 10 materials can be tested simultaneously on each subject. Skin reactivity differs by body region, and some patch sites may receive more pressure from chairs, clothing, etc. Therefore, the position that the materials are placed on the skin (i.e., upper right back, lower left back, etc.) should be systematically varied within each study. Each study should include at least one reference material. Scores from all subjects are averaged for each material, and comparisons between standards and other test materials are made. Some investigators have accepted an average difference of one unit on the grading scale as meaningful. Other investigators analyze the data by standard nonparametric statistical tests. It is also possible to test multiple doses and calculate ID_{50} (199).

Wooding and Updyke (383) investigated the effects of modifying some test parameters on intensity of the response, and the intensity of inflammation has been shown to increase after removal of patches in some cases (77,299). Kooyman and Snyder (202) used 6-h exposures to 8% solutions of bar soaps and evaluated test sites 24 h after patch application. Griffith et al. (140) reported using single-application patch tests with exposures of less than 24 h to evaluate laundry detergents containing enzymes. Justice et al. (174) varied exposure time between 18 and 24 h to test bar soaps, liquid detergents, and laundry detergents. Others have suggested that 48-h patch exposures are more suitable for some products (305).

A standardized procedure for evaluating the irritation potential of new chemicals in man as a replacement for the Draize rabbit test has been proposed (16,17,92,141,385,386). The method has been tested in several different laboratories and results seem to be reasonably reproducible. The classification of irritancy is based on comparison of the length of exposure to the chemical being tested versus the length of exposure producing irritation following application of a 20% solution of sodium laurel sulfate (SLS). Chemicals producing irritation after shorter exposures than used for SLS are considered irritants and would be labeled as such. Each test subject is exposed to the undiluted test material in occlusive chambers (Hill Top Chambers) and to a 20% solution of sodium laurel sulfate. Length of exposure begins with a 15-min exposure with evaluation at removal and at 24 and 48 h. If no response is observed, then another set of patches are applied and worn for 30 min. This process of patching, evaluation, and patching for a longer exposure interval is repeated until the subject responds to the SLS exposure or until a 4-h exposure has been completed. The test was developed for chemicals but may have use for evaluating consumer products as well. For most household chemicals and cosmetics, this cycle can probably be shortened considerably. Nixon et al. (265) have used a 4-hour FHSA-type procedure (including abrasion) to evaluate a range of household products.

Repeat Application Irritation Patch Tests

The term skin fatigue was used to explain the development of inflammation late in the induction phase of sensitization tests without positive responses at challenge (320). The phenomenon was also referred to as secondary irritation and later as cumulative irritation. The HRIPT for skin allergy was modified to evaluate skin irritation. As with single-application patch tests, many investigators developed their own version of the repeat application patch test. Most were patterned after human sensitization studies with 24-h exposures with or without a rest period between patches. Kligman and Wooding (199) applied the Litchfield and Wilcoxon probit analysis to cumulative irritation testing with calculation of IT_{50} and ID_{50} values, and statistical comparison of those values for different

Table 22.11
Grading scale for the chamber scarification tests

0	Scratch marks barely perceptible
1	Erythema confined to scratches
2	Broader bands of erythema with or without rows of vesicles, pustules, or erosions
3	Severe erythema with partial confluence with or without other lesions
4	Confluent, severe erythema sometimes with edema, necrosis, or bulla

materials. Their early work forms the basis for the 21-day cumulative irritation assay, which is currently widely used.

The cumulative irritation assay, as described by Lanman and his co-workers (215), was developed to compare antiperspirants, deodorants, and bath oils to provide guidance for product development. A 1-in square of Webril was saturated with liquid, or up to 0.5 g of viscous substances, and applied to the surface of the pad to be applied to the skin. The patch was applied to the upper back and sealed in place with occlusive tape. After 24 h the patch was removed, the area evaluated, and a fresh patch applied. The procedure was repeated daily for up to 21 days. The sensitivity of the assay was increased by increasing the number of test subjects from 10 to 24. The IT_{50}, as described by Kligman and Wooding (199), was used to evaluate and compare test materials.

Modifications of the cumulative irritation assay have been reported. Intensity of response has been evaluated using other evaluation schemes, the interval between application of fresh patches has been varied, and other methods of data evaluation have been proposed (22,61,298). The newer chamber devices have replaced Webril with occlusive tape in some laboratories. Some investigators currently use cumulative scores to compare test materials and do not calculate an IT_{50}. The necessity of 21 applications has recently been questioned (22). Although the procedure came to be known as the 21-day cumulative irritation assay, the number of applications used was varied by Lanman, depending on the types of materials to be tested. Twenty-one days was the maximum period of testing. Kligman and Wooding performed their studies on surfactants in 10 days. Lanman needed 21 applications to discriminate between baby lotions. The number of applications used to rank materials should be chosen based on the class of material being studied.

Numerous other human repeated application schedules have been used successfully for comparing commercial products. Finkelstein et al. (111,112) described tests using either a 5–6 or a 17–18 h exposure each day for 4 days.

Test sites were evaluated 1 hour after patch removal. Modifications of this procedure have also been used to evaluate shaving creams and toilet soaps (327).

Repeated-application patch tests on intact skin fail to predict some adverse reactions due to repeated application of materials to damaged skin (i.e., acne, shaved underarms, or sensitive areas such as the face) (18). The chamber scarification test (121,123,125) was developed to evaluate materials that would normally be applied to damaged skin. Light-skinned whites who developed severe erythema with edema and vesicles following a 24-h exposure to 5% sodium lauryl sulfate in Duhring Chambers applied to the inner forearm are preselected as subjects. Six to eight 10 mm^2 areas on the mid-volar forearm are scarified with eight crisscross scratches made with a 30-gauge needle. Four scratches are parallel, with another four at right angles. In scarifying the tissue, the bevel of the needle is to the side and is drawn across the tissue at a 45-degree angle with enough pressure to scratch the epidermis without drawing blood. Duhring Chambers containing the test material, 0.1 g for ointments, creams, powders or Webril saturated with 0.1 ml for liquids, are placed over the scarified areas and are secured in place with nonocclusive tape wrapped around the forearm. Fresh chambers containing the same materials are applied daily for 3 days. Thirty minutes after removal of the last set of chambers, the test sites are evaluated on a 0 to 4 scale (Table 22.12). The responses are averaged and materials are classified as low (0 to 0.41), slight (0.5 to 1.4), moderate, (1.5 to 2.4), or severe irritants. A scarification index (S.I.) may be calculated by dividing the score on intact skin by the score from the scarified site. The S.I. is used to estimate the relative risk for damaged and normal tissue. It is not used to rank test materials.

Although bar soaps produce erythema when tested by conventional patch test techniques, the typical clinical response is dryness and flaking with occasional erythema and fissuring. Frosch and Kligman (125) developed the soap chamber test to compare the "chapping" potential of bar soaps. Sensitive subjects were preselected as described for the chamber scarification test or by ammonium hydroxide blistering time (102). Duhring Chambers fitted with Webril pads are used to apply 0.1 ml of an 8% solution of soap to the forearm. Chambers are secured in place by encircling the arm with porous tape. Patch contact time is 24 h on day 1 (Monday) and 6 h each day for the next 4 days (Tuesday through Friday). Test sites are monitored each day before application of fresh solutions. If severe erythema is noted, dosing is discontinued. Unless treatment was discontinued before the fifth exposure, skin reactions are evaluated on day eight (Monday). This test showed good agreement with skin washing procedures but overpredicted irritant responses to some materials (120).

Exaggerated Exposure Irritation Tests

Although patch tests have been useful in detecting differences in the irritation potential of some materials, in some cases predicted differences were not apparent when the materials were used by consumers. Exaggerated exposure tests have been developed to bridge the gap between responses occurring during product use and patch tests. Perhaps the oldest nonpatch irritancy test still in use is the arm immersion technique (202) in which the relative irritancy of two soap or detergent products is compared. As originally described, soap solutions of up to 8% were prepared in troughs. Temperature was maintained at 105°F while subjects immersed one hand and arm to just above the elbow in one test solution and the other arm in a solution containing a second product. The period of exposure varied between 10 and 15 min 3 times each day for 5 days or until observable irritation was produced on both arms.

In most volunteers, the first sign of irritation was erythema of the anticubital surface of the arm (174,202). Later the hands developed dryness and cracking. These observations led to the development of separate assays on the anticubital area and the hands. Numerous versions of the anticubital washing test (also know as flex washing test and elbow crease washing test) have been used. Published methods compare two products; however, dosing regimes differ somewhat. Investigators have used two (120) or three (140,337) washing procedures per day, and some specify that lather is allowed to remain on the skin for a brief period. Erythema and edema are evaluated as endpoints in all studies. Frosch (120) used a similar procedure on the cheeks to evaluate toilet soaps. Simple 1–4 (i.e., slight, moderate, severe, very severe) grading scales are used to evaluate the severity of the response. Products can be compared in terms of the average grades or the number of washes producing an effect. Some investigators have tested up to 4 samples per forearm by washing in glass cylinders then rinsing the area (162).

At least two types of hand immersion procedures have been used. In small studies (i.e., 10 subjects), relatively concentrated solutions (up to 2%) of two materials are tested. Up to four hand dishwashing products have been compared at near use concentration in studies on 64 subjects using a Latin square dosing pattern (9). Exposure conditions have varied from two or three 10–15 min immersions each day (140) to a single 30-min exposure each day (9). Grading scales for this type of assay focus on scaling and cracking as well as erythema.

Evaluation of skin condition before and after use in the home has also been used to compare the irritation potential of various products. These tests represent skin tolerance studies, as either irritation or allergy could be detected. The clinical method published by Johnson

Table 22.12
Factors influencing sensitivity of skin to development of irritation

Extrinsic Variables	References
Degree of occlusion	Magnusson and Hersle (221, 222)
Choice of vehicle	Patrick et al., (287)
Frequency of dosing	Kligman and Wooding, (199)
	Frosch and Kligman, (124)
Duration of exposure	Wooding and Opdyke, (383)
Dose (concentration)	Patrick et al., (287)
	Kligman and Wooding, (199)
Temperature	Rothenberg et al., (306)
Environmental conditions	Hannuksela et al., (148)
	Carter and Griffith, (62)
Altered barrier function (including abrasion)	Draize-type tests
	Frosch and Kligman, (121)
Chemical damage	Finkelstein et al., 1963, (111, 112)
	Patrick and Maibach, (284)
Tape stripping	Kligman, (194)
Intrinsic Variables	
Anatomical site	Magnusson and Hersle, (221, 222)
Concomitant disease	Skog, (325); Bjomberg, (30)
Species differences	Davies et al., (82)
Age	Rockl et al., (302)
Gender (effect disputed)	Wagner and Purschel, (363)
	Bjornberg, (31)
	Frosch and Kligman, (122)
Race	Weigand et al., (371)
	Weigand and Gaylor, (370)

et al. (172) has been varied to include tests of bar soaps, laundry soaps and detergents, and dishwashing detergents. Essentially the method is a double-blind crossover study with usage periods of 2 weeks (62). Skin condition is evaluated by a dermatologist before the study and after use of each product. Magnification of the area is used to facilitate grading using a 0 to 10 scale. Tests are conducted using large panels, more than 300 housewives per product, and up to eight materials can be evaluated simultaneously using a Latin square design. The principles used in conducting this type of large-scale usage study have been applied to laundry powders for diapers and bar soaps used in infants (97,140) and to fabric softeners in adult populations (369). Special emphasis should be placed on statistical design of clinical trials of this type to assure validity of the study (1).

Use of Bioengineering Devices in Irritancy Evaluations

Measurements of biophysical parameters of skin function have been proposed as adjuncts to visual evaluations of the inflammatory response (237,239,343,344,382). In many instances, investigators constructed their own instruments to perform these measurements. As availability of commercial instruments increases, assessment of the biophysical changes in skin has become widely used to supplement visual evaluations. The benefits of the methods vary and include more objective measurement of erythema (as change in blood flow), more precise determination of the color change, and measurement of parameters of damage that cannot be evaluated visually. When combined with various techniques of exposure, it is possible to vastly decrease the number of subjects and probable clinical relevance of the studies.

Laser Doppler velocimetry has been used to quantify the increased blood flow to inflamed tissue. This device is an optical technique for estimation of microcirculation, based on the Doppler principle. When the laser beam, a 632-nm He–Ne (helium–neon) laser source, is directed toward the tissue, reflection, transmission, absorption, and scattering occur. Laser light back-scattered from moving particles, such as red cells, is shifted in frequency according to the Doppler principle, whereas radiation that is back-scattered from nonmoving structures remains at the same frequency. Detailed guidelines for using this device are reported by the Standardization Group of the European Society of Contact Dermatitis (28).

Skin reflectance spectrophotometery has been used to measure the color change in skin associated with inflammation. Polychromatic light is directed into the skin. The reflected light is collected in an integrating sphere and guided to a monochromator, where the light is split into 5 bands in the spectral range of 355–700 nm. Melanin content and oxygenized and deoxygenized hemoglobin are analyzed at different spectra, and the relative changes are expressed as a percentage of chromophore content in control skin (3,29).

Changes in transepidermal water loss (TEWL) and electrical resistance have been detected before inflammatory changes are apparent. Early investigations have clearly established that chemicals that provoked inflammation increased TEWL. TEWL reflects the integrity of the water-barrier function of stratum corneum and an evaporimeter (open chamber method), using a skin capsule that is open to the atmosphere. TEWL is calculated from the slope provided by two hygrosensors precisely oriented in the chamber. Air movement and humidity are the drawbacks of this method. A report reviewing interindividual, environmental, and instrument-related variables with respect to Evaporimeter EPI (ServoMed), its use, and good practice guidelines can be obtained from Pinnagoda et al. (292). Malten and Thiele (238) showed that increase in TEWL occurred before visible inflammation when ionic, polar, water-soluble substances (e.g., sodium hydroxide, soaps, detergents) were used as irritants. Unionized, polar irritants, like dimethyl sulfoxide, and unionized, nonpolar, water-soluble irritants, like hexanediol diacrylate and butanediol diacrylate, did not induce increased water loss until visible inflammation occurred. This method thus seems to be valuable for detecting irritancy with no perceivable irritancy possibly for ionizable, polar, water-soluble substances. These techniques have been used to compare the irritancy potential of soaps tested at near use level (150).

Water content of the skin can be estimated by electrical measurements of skin resistance and capacitance. Subtle degrees of skin damage can be measured using skin resistance before skin inflammation occurs (343). The corneometer is used to register the electrical capacitance of the skin surface. The principle of this instrument is to decipher distinctly different dielectric constants of water and other constitutional materials (less than 7), with a probe applied to the skin at constant pressure. Another instrument working on similar principle is the skin hygrometer, which measures conductance of the skin using high-frequency electric current of 3.5 MHz with the help of a sensitive probe (341). Several other devices using different frequencies and technologies have been developed to measure water content, including instruments that measure impedance, resistance, phase angle, microwave transmission, and photoacoustic methods. Noninvasive bioengineering techniques, like colorimetry, remittance spectroscopy, measurement of surface pH, and skin surface topography, have been reviewed by Berardesca and Maibach (20,21). One unique new way of evaluating irritancy uses in vivo measurements of the water-binding capacity of the stratum corneum after occlusion (20). Bioinstrumentation techniques have now been used in in vitro studies too. These techniques permit more clinically realistic bioassays that more closely mimic use experience.

In Vitro Assays of Skin Irritation and Corrosion

Since 1980, much effort has been expended in attempting to develop in vitro alternatives to Draize-type tests for both eye and skin irritation. Approaches to development of an in vitro model include cell toxicity (37,39), measurement of inflammatory mediators, effect on cell recovery and survival (94,201,259), effect on cellular physiology (282), cell morphology (37–39), biochemical endpoints (254), and effect on membranes (32) and artificial membranes (134–136) constructed to release dye indicator. Some investigators have included metabolic activators in their system (40). Nonmammalian cells (55) have also been used.

In vitro assays for skin irritation are being explored as tools in toxicologic research and as aids in formulating mild products, as well as for replacement of the Draize-type tests. This mirrors the overall use of in vitro assays during the last 15 years (17). Numerous proposals for validation of the methods have been put forth; however, currently tests in intact animals or man are the only means of assessing the potential irritation hazard from skin exposure (329). In vitro assays for skin corrosion are near acceptance and validation.

Although it is possible to conduct assays using most endpoints using laboratory cultures, two commercial systems, Skin2 and EpiDerm, have been used extensively for skin irritation testing. Skin2 (114,348,349) is a three-dimensional co-culture of human fibroblasts and keratinocytes. In Skin2, human neonatal fibroblasts are seeded on a nylon mesh to which they attach and lay down collagen. When the proper degree of confluence is reached, human keratinocytes are seeded onto the fibroblast culture. The epidermis is exposed to air and a partially differentiated stratum corneum develops. Several cytotoxicity assays and assays for release of inflammatory mediators are available for use with these systems. EpiDerm (59) consists of a multilayered cornified epithelium with no dermal element. It appears to have a well-differentiated stratum corneum. Perkins et al. (290) used these systems to evaluate skin corrosion in vitro using dimethyltriazoldiphenyl tetrazolium-formazan (MTT) (60) cell viability assay with some success.

Skintex and Corrositex (116–119) are described as membrane barrier/protein matrices. They are two component systems consisting of a barrier matrix that contains an indicator dye. Dye release is expected to correlate with protein disruption and denaturation. The second compartment is a reagent system that increases in turbidity when exposed to irritants. Corrositex has been accepted by the DOT as an alternative to the Draize test for skin corrosion (163) and has been validated for limited purposes by IACCVAM (391).

Several European investigators have reported success in using excised rat or human skin to access skin corrosivity (16,270,271,366,378) using change in transcutaneous electrical resistance (TER). A rubber "O" ring is used to secure full thickness (including dermis) skin, epidermal surface uppermost, onto the top of small tubes. These tubes are then suspended in a larger tube containing an electrolyte solution in distilled water. Applied to the surfaces of at least three discs is 150 μg of the test material. After 24 h the skin is rinsed and the surface is treated with ethanol, and electrolyte solution is added to the skin surface. The TER is then measured using a commercial instrument. Values above 11–12.5 kohms/disc are indicative of corrosivity (varies by investigator and source of skin). With the judicial use of reference materials to set the threshold values for classifying materials as corrosive, this method appears to be reproducible. Full validation of the method has not yet been completed.

CONTACT URTICARIA AND URTICARIA-LIKE SYNDROMES

Circumscribed, erythematous, evanescent areas of edema involving the epidermis and superficial portions of the dermis are referred to as urticaria (361). Classically the reaction has been described as the wheal-and-flare response, which develops within 30 to 60 min after exposure of the skin to certain agents. Symptoms of immediate contact reactions can be classified according to their morphology and severity, itching, tingling, and burning with erythema is the weakest type of immediate contact reaction. Local superficial wheal-and-flare with tingling and itching represents the prototype reaction of contact urticaria. Generalized urticaria after local contact is rare but can occur from strong urticants. Signs in other organs appear with the skin symptoms in cases of immunologic contact urticaria syndrome. Urticaria and angioedema, lesions with edematous processes in the deep dermis, subcutaneous, of submucosal layers that may persist for up to 72 h (72). The strength of the reactions may vary greatly, and often the whole range of local signs—from slight erythema to strong edema and erythema—can be seen from the same substance if different concentrations are used in skin tests (205). Not only the concentration, but also the site of the skin contact affects the reaction. A certain concentration of contact urticant may produce strong edema and erythema reactions on the skin of the upper back and face, but only erythema on the volar surfaces of the lower arms or legs. In some cases, contact urticaria can be demonstrated only on slightly or previously eczematous skin, and it can be part of the mechanism responsible for maintenance of chronic eczemas (2,228,268). Some agents, such as formaldehyde, produce urticaria on healthy skin following repeated but not single applications to the skin. Diagnosis of immediate-contact urticaria is based on a thorough history and skin testing with suspected substances (72). Skin tests for human diagnostic testing have been summarized (361). Because of the risk of systemic reactions, such as anaphylaxis, human diagnostic tests should be performed only by experienced personnel with facilities for resuscitation on hand.

Contact urticaria has been divided into two main types: immunologic and nonimmunologic contact urticaria (207). Recent reviews list agents suspected to cause each type of urticarial response (208,209,361). A few common urticants are listed in Table 22.13. Nonimmunologic contact urticaria occurs without previous exposure in most individuals, and is the most common type. The reaction remains localized and does not cause systemic symptoms or spread to become generalized urticaria. Typically, the strength of this type of contact urticaria reaction varies from erythema to a generalized urticarial response, depending on the concentration, skin site, and substance. The mechanism of nonimmunologic contact urticaria has not been delineated, but a direct influence upon dermal vessel walls and nonimmunologic release of mast cell mediators are possible mechanisms (319). Recent reports suggest that nonimmunologic urticaria produced by different agents may involve different combinations of mediators (207).

The most potent and best studied substances producing nonimmunologic contact urticaria are benzoic acid, cinnamic acid, cinnamic aldehyde, and nicotinic esters. Under optimal conditions, more than half of a random sample of individuals shows local edema and erythema reactions within 45 min of application of these substances if the concentration is high enough. Benzoic acid and sodium benzoate are used as preservatives for cosmetics and other topical preparations at concentrations from 0.1% to 0.2% and are capable of producing immediate contact reactions at the same concentrations. Cinnamic aldehyde at a concentration of 0.01% may elicit an

Table 22.13
A few agents reported to cause urticaria in man

Immunologic Mechanism	
	Grains
	Nuts
	Bacitracin
	Parabens
	Seafood (protein extracts)
	Penicillin
	Butylated hydroxy toluene
Non-immunologic Mechanism	
	Asprin
	Balsam of Peru
	Benzoic Acid
	Cayenne pepper
	Cinnamic aldehyde
	Codine
	Dimethyl sulfoxide
Unknown Mechanisms	
	Lettuce/endive
	Cassia oil
	Formaldehyde
	Ammonium persulfate
	Neomycin

More comprehensive lists and the original references can be found in Reference 2.

erythematous response associated with a burning or stinging feeling in the skin (242). Mouthwashes and chewing gums contain cinnamic aldehyde at concentrations high enough to produce a pleasant tingling or "lively" sensation in the mouth that enhances the sale of the product. Higher concentrations produce lip swelling of typical contact urticaria in normal skin. Eugenol in the mixture inhibits contact sensitization to cinnamic aldehyde and inhibits nonimmunologic contact urticaria from this same substance. The mechanism of the quenching effect is not certain, but a competitive inhibition at the receptor level may be the explanation (124).

Immunologic contact urticaria is an immediate type 1 allergic reaction in people previously sensitized to the causative agent (361). The molecules of a contact urticant react with specific IgE molecules attached to mast cell membranes. The cutaneous signs are elicited by vasoactive substances, including histamine, released from mast cells. The role of histamine is conspicuous, but other mediators of inflammation (i.e., prostaglandins, leukotrienes, kinins) may influence the degree of response. Immunologic contact urticaria reactions can extend beyond the contact site, and generalized urticaria may be accompanied by other symptoms, such as rhinitis, conjunctivitis, asthma, and even anaphylactic shock. The term contact urticaria syndrome was therefore suggested by Maibach and Johnson (231). The name has been accepted for a symptom complex where local urticaria occurs at the contact site with symptoms in other parts of the skin or in target organs, such as the nose and throat, lung, and gastrointestinal and cardiovascular systems. Fortunately, the appearance of systemic signs is rare, but it may be seen in cases of strong hypersensitivity or in a widespread exposure and abundant percutaneous absorption of an allergen.

Foodstuffs are the most common causes of immunologic contact urticaria. The otolaryngeal area is a site where immediate contact reactions frequently are provoked by food allergens, most often in atopic individuals. The actual antigens are proteins or protein complexes. As a proof of immediate hypersensitivity, specific IgE antibodies against the causative agent typically can be found in the patient's serum using the RAST technique and skin test for immediate allergy. The passive transfer test (Prausnitz–Kustner test) also often gives a positive result.

Predictive assays for evaluating the ability of materials to produce nonimmunologic contact urticaria have been developed. No predictive assays for immunologic contact urticaria have been published. Lahti and Maibach (206) developed an assay in guinea pigs using materials known to produce urticaria in man. One tenth of a milliliter of the material is applied to one ear of the animal; it is applied to the opposite ear as a control. Ear thickness is measured prior to application and then every 15 min for 1 or 2 h after application. The swelling response is dependent on the concentration of the eliciting substance. The maximum response is about a 100% increase in ear thickness, and it appears within 50 min after application of a contact urticant. In histologic sections, marked dermal edema and intra- and perivascular infiltrate of heterophilic granulocytes appear 40 min after application of test substances. This assay is the predictive test of choice for nonimmunologic contact urticaria if animals are to be tested. Guinea pig body skin reacts with quick-appearing erythema to cinnamic aldehyde, methyl nicotinate, and dimethyl sulfoxide, but not benzoic acid, sorbic acid, or cinnamic acid. Analogous reactions can be elicited in the earlobes of other animal species. Cinnamic aldehyde and dimethyl sulfoxide produce a swelling reaction in the guinea pig, rat, and mouse. Benzoic acid, sorbic acid, cinnamic acid, diethyl fumafate, and methyl nicotinate produce no response in the rat or mouse, but the guinea pig ear reacts to all of them (207). This suggests that either there are several mechanisms of nonimmunologic contact urticaria or that differences are due to relative sensitivity of the species to the mediators.

Materials can also be screened for nonimmunologic contact urticaria in man. A small amount of the test material is applied to a marked site on the forehead, and the vehicle is applied to a parallel site. The areas are evaluated at approximately 20–30 min after application for erythema and/or edema (361). Differentiating between nonspecific irritant reactions and contact urticaria may be difficult. Strong irritants, such as hydrochloric acid, lactic acid, cobalt chloride, formaldehyde, and phenol, can cause clear-cut immediate whealing if the concentration is high enough, but the reactions usually do not fade away within a few hours. Instead, they are followed by signs of irritation; erythema and scaling or crusting are seen 24 h later. Some substances have only urticant properties (e.g., benzoic acid, nicotinic acid esters), some are pure irritants (e.g, sodium lauryl sulfate), and some have both of these features (formaldehyde, dimethyl sulfoxide). Contact urticaria reactions are much less frequently encountered than either skin irritation or skin allergy (209); however, increasing awareness of contact urticaria has expanded the list of etiologic agents and hopefully will lead to the development of adequate predictive assays for detecting causative agents of other forms of urticaria.

SUBJECTIVE IRRITATION AND PARAESTHESIA

Cutaneous application of some chemicals elicits sensory discomfort, tingling, and burning without visible inflammation. This noninflammatory painful response has been termed *subjective irritation* (122,126). Materials reported to produce subjective irritation include dimethyl sulfoxide, some benzoyl peroxide preparations, and the chemicals salicylic acid, propylene glycol, amyl-dimethyl-paramino benzoic acid, and 2-ethoxyethyl-p-methoxy cinnamate, which are ingredients of cosmetics and over the counter (OTC) drugs. Pyrethroids, a group of broad-spectrum insecticides, produce a similar condition that may lead to temporary numbness that has been called paraesthesia (57,11,200). As in subjective irritation, the nasolabial folds, cheeks, and periorbital areas are frequently involved. The ear is also sensitive to the pyrethroids.

Only a portion of the human population seems to develop nonpyrethroid subjective irritation. Frosh and Kligman (122) found they needed to prescreen subjects to identify "stingers" for conducting predictive assays. Only 20% of subjects exposed to 5% aqueous lactic acid in a hot humid environment developed stinging response (122). All stingers in their series reported a history of adverse reactions to facial cosmetics, soaps, etc. A similar screening procedure by Lammintausta et al. (211) identified 18% of their subjects as stingers. Prior skin damage, such as sunburn, pretreatment with surfactants, and tape stripping, increases the intensity of responses in stingers. Persons not normally experiencing a response report pain upon exposure to lactic acid or other agents that produce subjective irritation (122). Attempts to identify reactive subjects by association with other skin descriptions (i.e., atopy, skin type, degree of skin dryness) have not yet been fruitful; however, recent data show that stingers develop stronger reactions to materials, causing nonimmunologic contact urticaria and some increase in transepidermal water loss and blood flow following application of irritants via patches than those of "nonstingers" (211).

The mechanisms by which materials produce subjective irritation have not been investigated extensively. Pyrethroids act directly on the axon by interfering with the channel-gating mechanism and impulse firing (359). It has been suggested that agents causing subjective irritation act via a similar mechanism because no visible inflammation is present. An animal model was developed to rate paraesthesia to pyrethroids and may be useful for other agents (57,113). The test site is the flank of 300–450 g guinea pigs. Both flanks are shaved, and animals are housed individually in observation cages. A volume of 100 μl of the test material is spread over approximately 30 mm^2 on one flank. The same amount of the vehicle is applied to the other flank. The animal's behavior is monitored by an unmanned video camera for 5 min and at 0.5, 1, 2, 4, and 6 h after application of the materials. Subsequently, the film is analyzed for the number of full turns of the head made to the control and pyrethroid-treated flank. Head turns were usually accompanied by attempted licking and biting of the application sites. It was possible to rank pyrethroids for their ability to produce paraesthesia using this technique. The ranking corresponded to the ranking available from human exposure.

As originally published, the human subjective irritation assay required the use of a 110°F environmental chamber with 80% relative humidity (122). Volunteers were seated in the chamber until a profuse facial sweating was observed. Sweat was removed from the nasolabial fold and cheek. A 5% aqueous solution of lactic acid was then rubbed briskly over the area. Those who reported stinging for 3 to 5 min within the first 15 min were designated as stingers and used for subsequent tests. Subjects were asked to evaluate the degree of stinging as 0 = no stinging, 1 = slight stinging, 2 = moderate stinging, 3 = severe stinging. Stinging was evaluated 10 sec and 2.5, 5, and 8 min after application of the test material. Other investigators (211) used a 15-min treatment with a commercial facial sauna to produce facial sweating. The subjects turn away from the sauna for application of the test materials, then turn back to face the sauna for the observation period. The facial sauna technique is less stressful to both subjects and investigators and produces similar results.

Advances in understanding the somatosensory processes in humans is leading to the development of more objective methods for evaluating skin sensory effects (384,387). Although these approaches are not yet sensitive enough to warrant use in predictive assays, they have been used to study pain and itch responses to histamine (389) and to some solvents (388). In time these techniques will undoubtedly be applied to predictive testing.

QUESTIONS

1. A chemically exposed occupational worker developed generalized urticaria and shortness of breath at the work site. Differential diagnosis includes
   A. Photoirritation
   B. Allergic contact dermatitis
   C. Contact urticaria syndrome (answer)
2. On introduction of a revised topical formulation, telephone complaint of acute burn, sting and itch increase beyond the expected level. Likely diagnostic possibilities include
   A. Photoallergic contact dermatitis
   B. Sensory irritation (answer)
   C. Photoirritation
3. Topical formulations may be contraindicated during pregnancy because of concern regarding
   A. Irritant dermatitis
   B. Allergic contact dermatitis
   C. Percutaneous penetration (answer)

REFERENCES

1. Allen, A. M. (1978): Clinical trial design in dermatology: Experimental design part I. *Int. J. Dermatol.*, 17:42–51.
2. Amin, S., Lahti, A., and Maibach, H. I. (1998): Contact urticaria syndrome. In: *Dermatotoxicology Methods: The Laboratory Worker's Vade Mecum*, edited by F. N. Marzulli and H. I. Maibach, pp. 161–176. Taylor & Francis, Washington D.C.
3. Anderson, P. Y., and Bjerring, P. (1990): Non invasive computerized analysis of skin chromophores in vivo by reflectance spectroscopy. *Photodermatol. Photoimmunol. Photomed.*, 7:249–257.
4. Andersen, K. E., and Maibach, H. I. (1983): Multiple-application delayed-onset contact urticaria: Possible relation to certain unusual formalin and textile reactions. *Contact Dermatitis*, 10:227–234.
5. Anderson, C., Sundberg, K., and Groth, O. (1986): Animal model for assessment of skin irritancy. *Contact Dermatitis* 15:143–151.
6. Asherson, G. L., and Ptak, W. (1968): Contact and delayed hypersensitivity in the mouse 1: Active sensitization and passive transfer. *Immunology* 15:405–416.
7. Aspergren, N., and Rorsman, H. (1962): Short-term culture of leucocytes in nickel hypersensitivity. *Acta. Derm. Venereol. (Stocklholm.)*, 42:412–417.
8. Back, O., and Larsen, A. (1982): Contact sensitivity in mice evaluated by means of ear swelling and a radiometric test. *J. Invest. Dermatol.*, 78:309–312.
9. Bannan, E. A. (1975): Personal communication.
10. Baron, J., Voigt, J. M., Whitter, T. B., Kawabata, T., Knipp, S. A., Gruengerich, F. P., and Jacoby, W. B. (1986): Identification of intratissue sites for xenobiotic activation and detoxication. *Adv. Exp. Biol. Med.*, 197:119–144.
11. Bartek, M., LaBudde, J. A., and Maibach, H. I. (1972): Skin permeability in vivo comparison in rat, rabbit, pig and man. *J. Invest. Dermatol.*, 58:114–123.
12. Bartek, M. J., and LaBudde, J. A. (1975): Percutaneous absorption in vitro. In: *Animal Models in Dermatology*, edited by H. I. Maibach, pp. 103–120. Churchill Livingston, New York.
13. Basketter, D. A., Robertts, D. W., Cronin, M., and Scholes, E. W. (1992): The value of the local lymph node assay in quantitative structure-activity investigation. *Contact Dermatitis*, 26:137–142.
14. Basketter, D. A., and Scholes, E. W. (1992): Comparison of the local lymph node assay with the guinea pig maximization test for the detection of a range of contact allergens. *Food Chem. Toxic.*, 30:65–69.
15. Basketter, D. A., Scholes, E. W., and Kimber. I., et al. (1991): Interlaboratory evaluation of the local lymph node assay with 25 chemicals and comparison with guinea pig test data. *Toxicol. Methods*, 1:30–43.
16. Basketter D. A., Whittle, E., and Chamberlain, M. (1994): Identification of irritation and corrosion hazard in skin: An alternative strategy to animal testing. *Food and Chemical Toxicology*, 32:539–542.
17. Basketter D. A., Whittle, E., Griffiths, H. A., and York, M. (1994): The identification and classification of skin irritation hazard by a human patch test. *Food and Chemical Toxicology*, 32:769–775.
18. Battista, C. W., and Rieger, M. M. (1971): Some problems of predictive testing. *J. Soc. Cosmet. Chem.*, 22:349–359.
19. Benvenuto, A. J., and Cohen, A. (1990): A realistic role for non-animal tests. *Pharmaceutical Executive*, June.
20. Berardesca, E., and Maibach, H. I. (1989): Physical anthropology of skin. In: *Models in Dermatology, Volume 4*, edited by H. I. Maibach and N. Lowe, pp. 202–206. Karger, New York.
21. Berardesca, E., and Maibach, H. I. (1989): Effect of nonvisible damage on the water-holding capacity of the stratum corneum, utilizing the plastic occlusion stress test (POST). In: *Current Topics in Contact Dermatitis*, edited by P. Frosch, et al., pp. 554–559. Springer-Verlag, New York.
22. Berger, R. S., and Bowman, J. P. (1962): A reappraisal of the 21-day cumulative irritation test in man. *J. Toxicol: Cutaneous and Ocular. Toxicol.*, 1:109–115.
23. Bergstressor, P. R., Paniser, R. J., and Taylor, J. R. (1978): Counting and sizing of epidermal cells in human skin. *J. Invest. Derm.*, 70:280–284.
24. Bickers, D. R. (1991): Xenobiotic metabolism in skin. In: *Physiology, Biochemistry, and Molecular Biology of the Skin, 2nd edition*, edited by L. A. Goldsmith, pp. 205–236. Oxford University Press, New York.
25. Bickers, D. R., Dutta-Choudhury, T., and Mukhtar, H. (1982): Epidermis: A site of drug metabolism in neonatal rat skin: Studies on cytochrome P450 content and mixed-function oxidase and epoxide hydrolase activity. *Mol. Pharmacol.*, 21:241–249.
26. Bickers, D. R., Eiseman, J., Kappas, A., and Alvares, A. P. (1975): Microscope immersion oils: Effects of skin application on cutaneous and hepatic drug-metabolizing enzymes. *Biochem. Pharmacol.*, 24:779–783.
27. Bickers, D. R., Kappas, A., and Alvares, A. P. (1974): Differences in inducibility of cutaneous and hepatic drug metabolizing enzymes and cytochrome P450 by polychlorinated biphenyls and 1,1,1-trichloro-2, 2-bis(p-chlorophenyl) ethane (DDT). *J. Pharmacol. Exp. Ther.*, 188:300–309.
28. Bircher, A., De Boer, E. M., Agner, T., Wahlberg, J. E., and Serup, J. (1994): Guidelines for measurement of cutaneous blood flow by

laser doppler flowmetery: A report from the standardization group of the European Society of Contact Dermatitis. *Contact Dermatitis*, 30:65–72.

29. Bjerring, P., and Anderson, P. H. (1990): Skin reflectance spectrophotometry. *Photodermatol. Photoimmunol. Photomed.*, 4:167–171.
30. Bjornberg, A. (1974): Skin reactions to primary irritants and predisposition to eczema. *Br. J. Dermatol.*, 91:425.
31. Bjornberg, A. (1975): Skin reactions to primary irritants in men and women. *Acta. Derm. Venereol. (Stockh.)*, 55:191.
32. Blake-Haskins, J. C., Scala, D., Rhein, L. D., et al. (1986): Predicting surfactant irritation from the swelling response of a collagen film. *J. Soc. Cosmet. Chem.*, 317:199–210.
33. Blank, H. I. (1952): Water content of stratum corneum. *J. Invest. Dermatol.*, 18:433–440.
34. Blank, H. I. (1953): Further observations on factors which influence the water content of the stratum corneum. *J. Invest. Dermatol.*, 21:259–269.
35. Bloch, B., and Steiner-Wourlisch, A. (1930): Die Sensibilisierung des Meerschweinchens gegen prirneln. *Arch. Dermatol. Syph.*, 162:349–378.
36. Blomberg, B. M. E., Bruynzeel, D. P., and Scheper, R. J. (1991): Advances in mechanisms of allergic contact dermatitis in vitro and in vivo research. In: *Dermatotoxicity, 4th Edition*, edited by F. N. Marzulli and H. I. Maibach, pp. 255–362. Hemisphere Publishing Co., New York.
37. Borenfreund, E., Babich, H., and Martin-Alguacil, N. (1988): Comparison of two in vitro cytotoxicity assays: The neutral red (NR) and tetrazolium MTT tests. *Toxicology In Vitro*, 2:1–6.
38. Borenfreund, E., and Puerner, J. A. (1984): A simple quantitative procedure using monolayer cultures for cytotoxicity assays. *J. Tissue Culture Meth.*, 9:7–9.
39. Borenfreund, E., and Puerner, J. A. (1985): Toxicity determined in vitro by morphological alterations and neutral red absorption. *Toxicology Letters*, 24:119–124.
40. Borenfreund, E., and Puerner, J. A. (1987): Short-term quantitative in vitro cytotoxicity assay involving an S-9 activatin system. *Cancer Lett.*, 34:243–248.
41. Bos, J. D. (1984): A new approach to contact allergenicity screening. *Med. Hypotheses*, 15:103–108.
42. Botham, P. A., Hall, T. J., Dennett, R., McCall, J. C., Basketter, D. A., Whittle, E., Cheeseman, M., Esdaile, D. J., and Gardner, J. (1992): The in vitro skin corrosivity tests: Results of a interlaboratory trial. *Toxicology In Vitro*, 6:191–194.
43. Boutwell, R. K. (1981): Chemical carcinogenesis. a: Biochemical role. In: *Biology of Skin Cancer (Excluding Melanomas)*, edited by D. D. Laerum and O. H. Iverson, pp. 134–150. International Union Against Cancer, Geneva.
44. Boutwell, R. K., Urbach, F., and Carpenter, G. (1981): Chemical carcinogenesis. b: Experimental models. In: *Biology of Skin Cancer (Excluding Melanomas)*, edited by D. D. Laerum and O. H. Iverson, pp. 109–123. International Union Against Cancer, Geneva.
45. Briggaman, R. A., Toshliki, R., Cronce, D. J. (1991): The epidermal-dermal junction and genetic disorder of this area. In: *Physiology, Biochemistry, and Molecular Biology of the Skin, 2nd edition*, edited by L. A. Goldsmith, pp. 1243–1265. Oxford University Press, New York.
46. Bronaugh, R., and Maibach, H. I. (1999): *Percutaneous Absorption. 3rd Edition*. Marcel Dekker, New York.
47. Bronaugh, R., and Maibach, H. I. (1991): *In Vitro Percutanesous Absorption*. CRC Press, Boca Raton, FL.
48. Bronaugh, R. L., Congolon, E. R., and Scheuplein, R. J. (1981): The effect of cosmetic vehicles on the penetration of N-nitrodiethanolarnine through excised skin. *J. Invest. Dermatol.*, 76:94–96.
49. Brown, V. K. H. (1971): A comparison of predictive irritation tests with surfactants on human and animal skin. *J. Soc. Cosmet. Chem.*, 22:411–420.
50. Brunner, M. J., and Smiljanic, A. (1952): Procedure for evaluation of skin sensitizing power of new materials. *Arch. Derm. (Chicago)*, 66:703–705.
51. Bucher, K., Bucher, K. B., and Walz, D. (1981): The topically irritant substance: Essentials-bio-tests-predictions. *Agents and Actions*, 11:515–519.
52. Buehler, E. V. (1964): A new method for detecting potential sensitizers using the guinea pig. *Toxicol. Appl. Pharmacol.*, 6:341.
53. Buehler, E. V. (1965): Experimental skin sensitization in the guinea pig and man. *Arch. Dermatol.*, 91:171.
54. Buehler, E. V. (1985): A rationale for the selection of occlusion to induce and elicit delayed contact hypersensitivity in the guinea pig: A prospective test. In: *Contact Allergy Predictive Tests in Guinea Pigs*, edited by K. E. Andersen and H. I. Maibach, pp. 38–58. Karger, Basel.
55. Bulich, A. A., Greene, M. W., and Isenberg, D. L. (1981): Reliability of bacterial luminescence assay for determination of the toxicity of pure compounds and complex effluents. In: *Aquatic Toxicology and Hazard Assessment, 4th Conference*, edited by D. R. Branson and K. L. Dickson, pp. 338–347. American Society for Testing and Materials, Washington, D.C.
56. Busse, M. J., Hunt, P., Lees, K. A., Maggs, P. N. D., and McCarthy, T. M. (1969): Release of betamethasone derivatives from ointments: In vivo and in vitro studies. *Br. J. Dermatology*, 81:103.
57. Cagen, S. Z., Malloy, L. A., Parker, C. M., Gardiner, T. H., Van Celder, C. A., and Jud, V. A. (1964): Pyrethroid mediated skin sensory stimulation characterized by a new behavorial paradigm. *Toxicol. Appl. Pharmacol.*, 6:270–279.
58. Calandra, J. (1971): Comments on the guinea pig immersion test. *CTFA Cosmet. Journal*, 3:47.
59. Cannon, C. L., Neal, P. J., Kubilus, J., Klausner, M., Swartzendruber, D. C., Squier, C. A., and Wertz, P. W. (1994): Lipid ultrastructure and barrier function characterization of a new in vitro epidermal model. *J. Invest. Dermatol.*, 102:600.
60. Carmichael, J., Degraff, W. G., Gazdar, A. F., Minna, J. D., and Mitchell, J. B. (1987): Evaluation of a tetrazolium-based semiautomated colorimetric assay: Assessment of chemosensitivity testing. *Cancer Res.*, 47:936–942.
61. Carabello, F. B. (1985): The design and interpretation of human skin irritation studies. *J. Toxicol: Cutaneous and Ocular. Toxicol.*, 4:61–71.
62. Carter, R. O., and Griffith, J. F. (1965): Experimental basis for the realistic assessment of safety of topical agents. *Toxicol. Appl. Pharmacol.*, 7:60–73.
63. Center for Devices and Radiological Health (1999): Guidance for Industry and FDA Reviewers/Staff: Premarket notification [510(K)] Submissions for Testing for Skin Sensitization to Chemicals in Natural Rubber Products. U.S. Department of Health and Human Services, FDA.
64. Choman, B. R. (1963): Determination of the response of skin to chemical agents by an in vitro procedure. *J. Invest. Dermatol.*, 44:177–182.
65. Christie, O. A., and Moore-Robinson, M. (1970). Vehicle assessment: Methodology and results. *Br. J. Dermatol.*, 82:93.
66. Code of Federal Regulations (1997): Office of the Federal Registrar, National Archives of Records Service. General Services Administration Title 16, part 1500.40, part 1500.41, part 1500.42.

67. Code of Federal Regulations (1998): Office of the Federal Registrar, National Archives of Records Service. General Services Administration Title 40, part 162.10, part 163.31, part 771.
68. Code Federal Regulations (1998): Office of the Federal Registrar, National Archives of Records Service. General Services Administration Title 49 Part 173, Appendix A.
69. Code of Federal Regulations (1998): Office of the Federal Registrar, National Archives of Records Service. General Services Administration Title 49, part 173.240.
70. Cohen, P. J., and Katz, S. I. (1992): Cultured human Langerhans cells process and present intact protein antigens. *J. Invest. Dermatol.*, 99:331–336.
71. Coomes, M. W., Norling, A. M., Pohl, R. J., Muller, D., and Fouts, J. R. (1983): Foreign compound metabolism by isolated skin cells from the hairless mouse. *J. Pharmacol. Exp. Ther.*, 225:770–777.
72. Cooper, K. D. (1991): Urticaria and angioedema: Diagnosis and evaluation. *J. Am. Acad. Dermatol.*, 25:166–175.
73. Cornacoff, J. B., House, R. V., and Dean, J. H. (1988): Comparision of a radioisotopic incorporation method and the mouse ear swelling test (MEST) for contact sensitivity to weak sensitizers. *Fund. Appl. Toxicol.*, 10:40–44.
74. Crowle, A. J. (1975): Delayed hypersensitivity in the mouse. *Advances Immunol.*, 20:197–264.
75. Crowle, A. J., and Crowle, C. M. (1961): Contact hypersensitivity in mice. *J. Immunol.*, 32:302–320.
76. Cruzan, G., Dalbey, W. E., D'Aleo, C. J., and Singer, E. J. (1986): A composite model for multiple assays of skin irritation. *Toxicology and Indust. Health*, 2:309–320.
77. Cunningham-Rundles, S. (1981): Cell-mediated immunity. In: *Immunodermatology*, edited by B. Safai and R. A. Good, pp. 1–33. Plenum Medical Book Co., New York.
78. Dahl, M. V., and Trancik, R. J. (1977): Sodium lauryl sulfate irritant patch test: Degree of inflammation at various times. *Contact Dermatitis*, 3:263–266.
79. Das, M., Bickers, D. R., and Mukhtar, H. (1986): Epidermis: The major site of cutaneous benzo(a)pyrene 7,8-diol metabolism in neobatal Balb/c mice. *Drug Metab. Disp.*, 14:637–642.
80. Dash and Maibach, Single versus multiple treatments with corticosteriods. *British Journal of Dermatology*, 1997 or 1998
81. David, J. R., and Remold, H. G. (1976): Macrophage activation by lymphocyte mediators and studies on the interaction of macrophage inhibitory factor (MIF) and its target cell. In: *Immunology of the Macrophage*, edited by D. S. Nelson, pp. 401–427. Academic Press, New York.
82. Davies, R. E., Harper, K. H., and Kymoch, S. R. (1972): Interspecies variation in dermal reactivity. *J. Soc. Cosmet. Chem.*, 23:371–381.
83. DeLeo, V., Harber, L. C., Kong, B. M., and DeSalva, S. J. (1987): Surfactant induced alteration of arachadonic acid metabolism of mammalian cells in culture. *Proc. Soc. Exp. Biol. Med.*, 184:477–482.
84. Delescluse, J., and Turk, J. L. (1970): Lymphocyte cytotoxicity: A possible in vitro test for contact dermatitis. *Lancet*, 2:75–77.
85. Dover, R., and Wright, N. A. (1991): The cell proliferation kinetics of the epidermis. In: *Physiology, Biochemistry, and Molecular Biology of the Skin, 2nd editon*, edited by L. A. Goldsmith, pp. 1480–1501. Oxford University Press, New York.
86. Draize, J. H. (1955): Procedures for the appraisal of the toxicity of chemicals in foods, drugs, and cosmetics. VIII: Dermal Toxicity. *Food Drug Cosmet. Law J.*, 10:722–731.
87. Draize, J. H. (1959): Dermal toxicity. In: *Assoc. Food and Drug Officials. U.S. Appraisal of the Safety of Chemicals in Food. Drugs and Cosmetics*, pp. 46–59. Texas State Department of Health, Austin, Texas.
88. Draize, J. H., Woodard, G., and Calvery, H. O. (1944): Methods for the study of irritation and toxicity of substances applied topically to the skin and mucous membrane. *J. Pharmacol. Exp. Ther.*, 82:377–390.
89. Dugard, P. J. (1983): Skin permeability theory in relation to measurements of percutaneous absorption. In: *Dermatotoxicology, 2nd edition*, edited by F. N. Marzulli and H. I. Maibach, pp. 91–115. Hemisphere Publishing Corporation, Washington D.C.
90. Dumonde, D. C., Wolstencroft, R. A., Panayi, G. S., et al. (1969): Lymphokines: Non-antibody mediators of cellular immunity generated by lymphocyte activation. *Nature* (London), 224:38–43.
91. Dunn, B. J., Rusch, G. M., Siglin, J. C., and Blaszcak, D. L. (1990): Variability of a mouse ear swelling test (MEST) in prediction of weak and moderate contact sensitizers. *Fundam. Appl. Toxicol.*, 15:242–248.
92. Dykes, P. J., Black, D. R., York, M., Dickens, A. D., and Marks, R. (1995): A stepwise procedure for evaluating irritant materials in normal volunteer subjects. *Human and Experimental Toxicology*, 14:204–211.
93. Edwards, C. C. (1972): Hazardous substances: Proposed revision of test for primary skin irritants. *Fed. Reg.*, 37:27635–27636.
94. Ekwal, B. (1963): Screening of toxic compounds in mammalian cell cultures. *Ann N.Y. Acad. Sci.*, 407:64–77.
95. Elias, P. M. (1987): Lipids and the epidermal permeability barriers. *Arch. Derm. Research*, 270:95–117.
96. Elias, P. M., Cooper, E. R., Korc, A., and Brown, B. E. (1981): Percutaneous transport in relation to stratum corneum structure and lipid composition. *J. Invest. Dermatol.*, 76:297–301.
97. Ellickson, B. E., and Jungermann, E. (1987): Comparative soap mildness test on infants. *Current Therap. Res.*, 9:441–446.
98. Elsner, P., and Maibach, H. I. (1995): Irritant dermatitis: New clinical and experimental aspects. In: *Current Problems in Dermatology*, Basel, Karger.
99. Emmett, E. A. (1975): Occupational skin cancer: A review. *J. Occupational Med.*, 17:44–49.
100. Environmental Protection Association (1982): Pesticides registrations: Proposed data reguirements. Sec. 158.135, Toxicology data requirements. *Fed. Reg.*, 47:53192.
101. Epstein, J. H. (1965). Comparison of the carcinogenic and cocarcinogenic effects of ultraviolet light on hairless mice. *J. Nat. Cancer Inst.*, 34:741–745.
102. Epstein, J. H. (1985). Animal models for studying photocarcinogenesis. In: *Models in Dermatology. Vol. 2*, edited by H. I. Maibach and N. Lowe, pp. 303–312. Karger, Basel.
103. Epstein, W., and Maibach, H. I. (1965): Cell renewal in human epidermis. *Arch. Dermatol.*, 92:462–468.
104. Epstein, W. L., Kligman, A. M., and Senecal, L. P. (1963): Role of regional lymph nodes in contact sensitization. *Arch. Dermatol.*, 88:789.
105. European Economic Community (1963): Sixth amendment to the council directive on the classification and labelling of dangerous substances, Annex VI. *Official Journal of the European Communities*, L257:13–33.
106. Everall, J. D. (1981): Chemical carcinogenesis. A: Environmental Carcinogens. In: *Biology of Skin Cancer (Excluding Melanomas)*, edited by D. D. Laenum and O. H. Iverson, pp. 105–108. International Union Against Cancer, Geneva.
107. Everall, J. D., and Dowd, P. M. (1978): Influence of environmental factors excluding ultraviolet radiation on the incidence of skin cancer. *Bull. Cancer*, 65:241–248.
108. Fare, G. (1966): Rat skin carcinogenesis by topical applications of some azo dyes. *Cancer Res.*, 26:2466–2408.
109. Farrar, J. J., Benjamin, W. R., Hilficker, M. L., Howard, M., Farrar, W. V., and Fuller-Farrar, J. F. (1982): The biochemistry,

biology, and role of interleukin in the induction of cytotoxic T-cell and antibody-forming B-cell responses. *Immunological Rev.*, 63:129–166.

110. Feldman, R. J., and Maibach, H. I. (1967): Regional variation in percutaneous penetration of C^{14}cortisone in man. *J. Invest. Dermatol.*, 48:151–183.

111. Finkelstein, P., Laden, K., and Meichowski, W. (1963): New methods for evaluating cosmetic irritancy. *J. Invest. Dermatol.*, 40:11–14.

112. Finkelstein, P., Laden, K., and Miechowski, W. (1965): Laboratory methods for evaluating skin irritancy. *Toxicol. Appl. Pharmacol.*, 7:74–78.

113. Flannigan, S. A., and Tucker, S. B. (1986): Variation in cutaneous sensation between synthetic pyrethroic insecticides. *Contact Dermatitis*, 13:140–147.

114. Fleischmajer, R., Contard, P., Schwartz, E., et al. (1991): Elastin-associated microfibrils in a three-dimensional fibroblast culture. *J. Invest. Dermatol.*, 97:638–643.

115. Forbes, P. D. (1997): Carcinogenesis and photocarcinogenesis test methods. In: *Dermatotoxicology, 5th edition*, edited by F. N. Marzulli and H. I. Maibach, pp. 535–544. Taylor & Francis, Washington D.C.

116. Forbes, P. D., Sambuco, C. P., Dearlove, G. E., Parker, R. M., Kiorpes, A. L., and Wedig, J. H. (1997): Sample protocols for carcinogenesis and photocarcinogenesis. In: *Dermatotoxicology Methods: The Laboratory Worker's Vad Mecum*, edited by F. N. Marzulli and H. I. Maibach, pp. 281–302. Taylor & Francis, Washington D.C.

117. Franz, T. J. (1975): Percutaneous absorption: On the relevance of in vitro data. *J. Invest. Dermatol.*, 64:190–195.

118. Frey, J. R., and Wenk, P. (1957): Experimental studies on the pathogenesis of contact eczema in the guinea pig. *Int. Arch. Allergy*, 11:81–100.

119. Fritsch, W. C., and Stoughton, R. B. (1963): The effect of temperature and humidity on the penetration of [^{14}C] acetylsalicylic acid in excised human skin. *J. Invest. Dermatol.*, 41:307.

120. Frosch, P. J. (1982): Irritancy of soap and detergent bars. In: *Principles of Cosmetics for the Dermatologist*, edited by P. Frost and S. N. Howitz, pp. 5–12. C.V. Mosby, St. Louis.

121. Frosch, P. J., and Kligman, A. M. (1976): The chamber scarification test for irritancy. *Contact Dermatitis*, 2:314–324.

122. Frosch, P. J., and Kligman, A. M. (1977): A method for appraising the stinging capacity of topically applied substances. *J. Soc. Cosmet. Chem.*, 25:197–207.

123. Frosch, P. J., and Kligman, A. M. (1977): The chamber scarification test for assessing irritancy of topically applied substances. In: *Cutaneous Toxicity*, edited by V. A. Drill and P. Lazar, pp. 127–144. Academic Press, New York.

124. Frosch, P. J., and Kligman, A. M. (1979): The Duhring chamber: An improved technique for epicutaneous testing of irritant and allergic reactions. *Contact Dermatitis*, 5:73.

125. Frosch, P. J., and Kligman, A. M. (1979): The soap chamber test: A new method for assessing the irritancy of soaps. *J. American Acad. Dermatol.*, 1:35–41.

126. Frosch, P. J., and Kligman, A. M. (1982): Recognition of chemically vulnerable and delicate skin. In: *Principles of Cosmetics for the Dermatologist*, edited by P. Frost and S. N. Howitz, pp. 287–296. C.V. Mosby, St. Louis, Toronto, London.

127. Gad, S. C. (1988): A scheme for the prediction and ranking of relative potencies of dermal sensitizers based on data from several systems. *J. Appl. Toxicol.*, 8:361–368.

128. Gad, S. C., Dunn, B. J., Dobbs, D. N., et al. (1986): Development and validation of an alternative dermal sensitization test: The mouse ear swelling test (MEST). *Toxicol. Appl. Pharmacol.*, 84:93–114.

129. Gad, S. C., Dunn, B. J., Gavigan, F. A., Reilly, C., and Walsh, R. D. (1987): Development, validation, and transfer of a new test system technology in toxicology. In: *New Test System in Toxicology*, edited by A. M. Goldberg, pp. 275–292. Mary Ann Liebert, New York.

130. Geczy, A. F., and Baumgarten, A. (1970): Lymphocyte transformation in contact sensitivity. *Immunology*, 19:189–203.

131. George, M., and Vaughan, J. H. (1962): In-vitro cell migration as a model for delayed hypersensitivity. *Proc. Soc. Exp. Biol. Med.*, 111:514–521.

132. Gibson, W. T., and Teall, M. R. (1983): Interactions of C 12 surfactants with the skin: Changes in enzymes and visible and histological features of rat skin treated with sodium laurel sulfate. *Food Chem. Toxicol.*, 21:587–593.

133. Gilman, M. E., Evans, R. A., and DeSalva, S. J. (1978): The influence of concentration, exposure duration, and patch occlusivity upon rabbit primary dermal irritation indices. *Drug Chem. Toxicol.*, 1:391–400.

134. Gordon, V. C. (1990): An in vitro dermal safety test. *Drug Cosmet. Ind.*, pp. 32.

135. Gordon, V. C., Kelly, C. D., and Bergman, H. C. (1989): SkinTEX^{TM}: An in vitro method for determining dermal irritation. Presented at the V International Congress of Toxicology.

136. Gordon, V. C., Kelly, C. D., and Bergman, H. C. (1990): Evaluation of Skintex^{TM}: An in vitro method for determining dermal irritation. *The Toxicologist*, 10:75.

137. Grasso, P. (1971): Some aspects of the role of skin appendages in percutaneous absorption. *J. Soc. Cosmet. Chem.*, 22:523–534.

138. Griffith, J. F. (1969): Predictive and diagnostic test for contact sensitization. *Toxicol. Appl. Pharmacol.*, S3:90–102.

139. Griffith, J. F., and Buehler, E. (1976): Prediction of skin irritancy and sensitization potential by testing with animals and man. In: *Cutaneous Toxicity*, edited by V. Drill and P. Lazer, pp. 155–173. Academic Press, New York.

140. Griffith, J. F., Weaver, J. E., Whitehouse, H. S., Poole, R. L., Newman, E. A., and Nixon, C. A. (1969): Safety evaluation of enzyme detergents: Oral and cutaneous toxicity, irritancy and skin sensitization studies. *Food Cosmet. Toxicol.*, 7:501–573.

141. Griffiths, H. A., Wilhelm, K. P., Robinson, M. K., Wang, S. M., McFadden, J., York, M., and Basketter, D. A. (1997): Interlaboratory evaluation of a human patch test for the identification of skin irritation potential/hazard. *Food Chem. Toxicol.*, 35:255–260.

142. Guillot, J. P., Gonnet, J. F., Clement, C., Caillard, L., and Truhaut, R. (1982): Evaluation of the cutaneous-irritation potential of 56 compounds. *Food Chem. Toxicol.*, 20:563–572.

143. Guin, J. D., Meyer, B. N., Drake, R. D., and Haffley, P. (1984): The effect of quenching agents on contact urticaria caused by cinnamic aldehyde. *J. Am. Acad. Dermatol.*, 10:45–51.

144. Guy, R. H., Tur, E., Bugatto, B., Gaebel, C., Sheiner, L., and Maibach, H. I. (1984): Pharmaco-dynamic measurements of methyl nicotinate percutaneous absorption. *Pharm. Res.*, 1:76–51.

145. Guy, R. H., Wester, R. C., Tur, E., and Maibach, H. I. (1983): Noninvasive assessments of the percutaneous absorption of methyl nicotinate in humans. *J. Pharm. Sci.*, 72:1077–1079.

146. Hadgraft, J. (1979): The epidermal reservoir: A theoretical approach. *Int. J. Pharm.*, 2:265–274.

147. Haley, T., and Hunziger, J. (1974): Instrument for producing standardized skin abrasions. *J. Pharm. Sci.*, 63:106.

148. Hannuksela, M., Prilia, V., and Salo, O. P. (1975): Skin reactions to propylene glycol. *Contact Dermatitis*, 1:112.

149. Harpin, V. A., and Rutter, N. (1983): Barrier properties of the newborn infant's skin. *J. Pediatr.*, 102:419–425.

150. Hassing, J. H., Nater, J. P., and Bleumink, E. (1982): Irritancy of low concentrations of soap and synthetic detergents as measured by skin water loss. *Dermatologica*, 164:312–314.

151. Hauser, C., Elbe, A., and Stingl, G. (1991): The Langerhans cell. In: *Physiology, Biochemistry, and Molecular Biology of the Skin, 2nd edition*, edited by L. A. Goldsmith, pp. 1144–1164. Oxford University Press, New York.

152. Helman, R. G., Hall, J. W., and Kao, J. Y. (1986): Acute dermal toxicity: In vivo and in vitro comparisons in mice. *Fundam. Appl. Toxicol.*, 7:94–100.

153. Henderson, C. R., and Riley, B. C. (1945): Certain statistical considerations in patch testing. *J. Invest. Dermatol.*, 6:227–230.

154. Higuchi, T. (1960): Physical chemical analysis of percutaneous absorption process from creams and ointments. *J. Soc. Cosmet. Chem.*, 11:85–97.

155. Holbrook, K. A. (1991): Structure and function of the developing human skin. In: *Physiology, Biochemistry, and Molecular Biology of the Skin, 2nd edition*, edited by L. A. Goldsmith, pp. 64–111, Oxford University Press, New York.

156. Holbrook, K. A., and Odland, G. F. (1974): Regional differences in the thickness (cell layers) of the human stratum corneum: An ultrastructural analysis. *J. Invest. Dermatol.*, 62:415–422.

157. Holbrook, K. A., and Smith, L. T. (1981): Ultrastructural aspects of human skin during the embryonic, fetal, premature, neonatal, and adult periods of life. In: *Morphogenesis and Malforming of the Skin*, edited by R. J. Blandau, pp. 9–38. Alan R Liss, New York.

158. Hood, D. B., Neher, R. J., Reinke, R. E., and Zapp, J. A. (1965): Experience with the guinea pig in screening primary irritants and sensitizers. *Toxicol. Appl. Pharmacol.*, 7:455–456.

159. Hueber, F., Wepierre, J., and Schaefer, H. (1992): Role of transepidermal and transfollicular routes in percutaneous absorption of hydrocortisone and testosterone: In vivo study in the hairless rat. *Skin Pharmacol.*, 5:99–107.

160. Humphrey, D. M. (1993). Measurement of cutaneous microvascular exudates using Evans blue. *Biotechnic Histochem.*, 68:342–349.

161. Ihle, J. N., Rebar, K., Keller, J., Lee, J. C., and Hapel, A. J. (1982): Interleukin 3: Possible roles in the regulation of lymphocyte differentiation and visual assessment. *Br. J. Dermatol.*, 92:131–142.

162. Imokowa, G., Sumura, K., and Katsumi, M. (1975): Study on skin roughness caused by surfactants. I: A new method in vivo for evaluation of skin roughness. *J. Am. Oil Chem. Soc.*, 52:479–483.

163. In vitro International (1993): Application for Exemption (49 CFR 173.136 and 173.137) for the Corrositex™ Test to the U.S. Department of Transportion. Exemption E-11082m, April 28.

164. IRAC (1992): *Solar and Ultraviolet Radiation: Monographs on the Evaluation of Carcinogenic Risks to Humans, Vol. 55.* IRAC, Lyon France.

165. Iverson, O. H. (1981): Chemical carcinogenesis. e: Short term tests for carcinogens. In: *Biology of Skin Cancer (Excluding Melanomas)*, edited by D. D. Laerum and O. H. Iverson, pp. 151–163. International Union Against Cancer, Geneva.

166. Jackson, R., and Grainge, J. W. (1975): Arsenic and cancer. *Can. Med. Assoc.*, 113:396–401.

167. Jadassohn, J. (1896): Zur Kenntniss der medicamentosen Dermatosen. *Verhdlg. Deutsch. Derm. Gesellsch. 5. Congress*, pp. 103–129.

168. Jadassohn, J. (1896): A contribution to the study of dermatoses produced by drugs. In: *Selected Essays and Monographs* (transl. L. Elking, 1900), pp. 207–229. New Sydenham Society, London.

169. Jaffee, B. D., and Maguire, H. C., Jr. (1981): Delayed-type hypersensitivity and immunological tolerance to contact allergens in the rat. *Fed. Proc.*, (abstract 4312), 40:991.

170. Japan/MAFF (1985): Testing Guidelines for Evaluation of Safety of Agriculture Chemicals. The Ministry of Agriculture, Forestry and Fisheries, Japan.

171. Johnson, A. W., and Goodwin, B. F. J. (1985): The Draize test and modifications. In: *Contact Allergy Predictive Tests in Guinea Pigs*, edited by K. E. Andersen and H. I. Maibach, pp. 31–38. Karger, Basel.

172. Johnson, S. A. M., Kile, R. L., Kooyman, D. J., Whitehouse, H. S., and Brod, J. S. (1953): Comparison of effects of soaps and detergents on the hands of housewives. *Arch. Dermatol. Syph.*, 68:643–650.

173. Jordan, W. P., and King, S. E. (1977): Delayed hypersensitivity in females during the comparison of two predictive patch tests. *Contact Dermatitis*, 3:19–26.

174. Justice, J. D., Travers, J. J., and Vinson, L. J. (1961): The correlation between animal tests and human tests in assessing product mildness. *Proceedings of the Scientific Section of the Toilet Goods Association*, 35:12–17.

175. Kanerva L. (2000): Handbook of occupational dermatology, Springer Verlag, Berlin.

176. Kaminsky, M., Szivos, M. M., and Brown, K. R. (1986): Application of the Hill Top patch Test Chamber to Dermal Irritancy Testing in the Albino Rabbit. *J. Toxicol. Cut. Ocular Toxicol.*, 5:81–87.

177. Kao, J., and Carver, M. P. (1991): Skin metabolism. In: *Dermatotoxicity, 4th edition*, edited by F. N. Marzulli and H. I. Maibach, pp. 143–200. Hemisphere Publishing Co., New York.

178. Kao, J., Hall, T., and Holland, T. M. (1983): Quantitation of cutaneous toxicity: An in vitro approach using skin organ culture. *Toxicol. Appl. Pharmacol.*, 65:206–217.

179. Kastner, D. (1977): Irritancy potential of cosmetic ingredients. *J. Soc. Cosmet. Chem.*, 28:741–754.

180. Kero, M., and Hannuksela, M. (1980): Guinea pig maximization test, open epicutaneous test and chamber test in induction of delayed contact hypersensitivity. *Contact Dermatitis*, 6:341–344.

181. Kimber, I., and Basketter, D. A. (1992): The murine local lymph node assay: A commentary on collaborative studies and new directions. *Food Chem. Toxicol.*, 30:165–169.

182. Kimber, I., Hilton, J., and Botham, P. A. (1990): Identification of contact allergens using the murine local lymph node assay: Comparisons with the Buehler occluded patch test in guinea pigs. *J. Appl. Toxicol.*, 10:173–180.

183. Kimber, I., Hilton, J., Botham, P. A., et al. (1991): The murine local lymph node assay. Results of an inter-laboratory trial. *Toxicol. Lett.*, 55:203–213.

184. Kimber, I., Hilton, J., and Weisenberger, C. (1989): The murine local lymph node assay for identification of contact allergens: A preliminary evaluation in in situ measurement of lymphocyte proliferation. *Contact Dermatitis*, 21:215–220.

185. Kimber, I., Mitchell, J. A., and Griffin, A. C. (1986): Development of a murine local lymph node assay for the determination of sensitizing potential. *Food Chem. Toxicol.*, 24:481–494.

186. Kimber, I., and Weisenberger, C. (1989): A murine local lymph node assay for the identification of contact allergens: Assay development and results of an initial validation study. *Arch. Toxicol.*, 63:274–282.

187. Kimber, I., and Weisenberger, C. (1991): Anamnestic responses to contact allergens: Application in the murine local lymph node assay. *J. Appl. Toxicol.*, 11:129–133.

188. Klecak, G. (1983): Identification of contact allergens: Predictive tests in animals. In: *Dermatotoxicology*, edited by F. N. Marzulli and H. I. Maibach, pp. 193–236. Hemisphere, New York.

189. Klecak, G. (1985): The Freund's complete adjuvant test and the open epicutaneous test. In: *Contact Allergy Predictive Tests in*

Guinea Pigs, edited by K. E. Andersen and H. I. Maibach, pp. 152–171. Karger, Basel.

190. Kligman, A. M. (1964): Quantitative testing of chemical irritants. In: *Evaluation of Therapeutic Agents and Cosmetics*, edited by M. Steinberg, et al., pp. 186–192. McGraw-Hill, New York.
191. Kligman, A. M. (1966): The identification of contact allergens. *J. Invest. Dermatol.*, 47:369–374.
192. Kligman, A. M. (1966): The identification of contact allergens by human assay. II: Factors influencing the induction and measurement of allergic contact dermatitis. *J. Invest. Dermatol.*, 47:375–392.
193. Kligman, A. M. (1966): The identification of contact allergens by human assay. III: The maximization test: A procedure for screening and rating contact sensitizers. *J. Invest. Dermatol.*, 47:393–409.
194. Kligman, A. M. (1969): Evaluation of cosmetics for irritancy. *Tox. Appl. Pharmacol.*, 53:30–44.
195. Kligman, A. M. (1976): Perspectives and problems in cutaneous gerontology. *J. Invest. Dermatol.*, 73:39–46.
196. Kligman, A. M. (1983): A biological brief on percutaneous absorption. *Drug Dev. Ind. Pharmacol.*, 521–560.
197. Kligman, A. M., and Epstein, W. (1959): Some factors affecting contact sensitization in man. In: *Mechanism of Hypersensitivity*, edited by H. Shaffer, et al., pp. 713–722. Little Brown, Boston.
198. Kligman, A. M. and Epstein, W. (1975): Updating the maximization test for identifying contact allergens. *Contact Dermatitis*, 1:231–239.
199. Kligman, A. M., and Wooding, W. M. (1967): A method for the measurement and evaluation of irritants on human skin. *J. Invest. Dermatol.*, 49:75–94.
200. Knox, J. M., Tucker, S. B., and Flannigan, S. A. (1984): Paraesthesia from cutaneous exposure to synthetic pyrethroid insecticide. *Arch. Dermatol.*, 120:744–746.
201. Knox, P., Uphill, P. F., Fry, J. R., Benford J., et al. (1986): The FRAME multicentre project on in vitro cytotoxicology. *Food Chem. Toxicol.*, 24:457–463.
202. Kooyman, D. J., and Snyder, F. M. (1942): Tests for the mildness of soaps. *Arch. Dermatol. Syph.*, 46:846–855.
203. Kral, F., and Schwartzman, R. M. (1964): *Veterinary and Comparative Dermatology*. J.B. Lippincott, Philadelphia.
204. Kuroki, T., Nemoto, N., and Kitano, Y. (1980): Use of human epidermal keratinocytes in studies on chemical carcinogenesis. In: *Carcinogenesis: Fundamental Mechanisms and Environmental Effects*, edited by B. Pullman, P. O. P. Tso, and H. Gelboin, pp. 417–426. Reidel Publishing, Boston.
205. Lahti, A. (1980): Non-immunologic contact urticaria. *Acta. Derm. Venereol. Stockholm*, 605:1–49.
206. Lahti, A., and Maibach, H. I. (1984): An animal model for non-immunologic contact urticaria. *Toxicol. Appl. Pharmacol.*, 76:219–224.
207. Lahti, A., and Maibach, H. I. (1985): Species specificity of non-immunologic contact urticaria: Guinea pig, rat and mouse. *J. Am. Acad. Dermatol.*, 13:66–69.
208. Lahti, A., and Maibach, H. I. (1991): Immediate contact reactions: Contact urticaria and the contact urticaria syndrome. In: *Dermatotoxicity, 4th edition*, edited by F. N. Marzulli and H. I. Maibach, pp. 473–495. Hemisphere Publishing, New York.
209. Lahti, A., von Krogh, G., and Maibach, H. I. (1985): Contact urticaria syndrome: An expanding phenomenon. In: *Dermatologic Immunology and Allergy*, edited by J. Stone, pp. 379–390. C.V. Mosby, St. Louis.
210. Lammintausta, K., and Maibach, H. I. (1988): Exogenous and endogenous factors in skin irritaton. *Int. J. Dermatol.*, 27:213–222.
211. Lammintausta, K., Maibach, H. I., and Wilson, D. (1988): Mechanisms of subjective (sensory) irritation: Propensity of non-immunologic contact urticaria and objective irritation in stingers. *Dermatosen in Beruf und Umwelt*, 36:45–49.
212. Landsteiner, K., and Chase, M. W. (1937): Studies on the sensitization of animals with simple chemical compounds. IV: Anaphylaxis induced by picryl chloride and 2 : 4 dinitrochloro-benzene. *J. Exp. Med.*, 66:337–351.
213. Landsteiner, K., and Jacobs, J. (1935): Studies on the sensitization of animals with simple chemical compounds. *J. Exp. Med.*, 61:643–648.
214. Landsteiner, K., and Jacobs, J. (1936). Studies on the sensitization of animals with simple chemical compounds. II: *J. Exp. Med.*, 64:625–629.
215. Lanman, B. M., Elvers, W. B., and Howard, C. S. (1968): The role of human patch testing in a product development program. In: *Proceedings of the Joint Conference on Cosmetic Sciences*, pp. 135–145. The Toilet Goods Association, Washington, D.C.
216. Lever, W. F., and Schaumburg-Hevor, C. (1983). *Histopathology of the Skin, 6th edition*. Lippincott, Philadelphia.
217. Leyden, J. J., Nordstrom, K. M., and McGinley, K. J. (1991): Cutaneous microbiology. In: *Physiology, Biochemistry, and Molecular Biology of the Skin, 2nd edition*, edited by L. A. Goldsmith, pp. 1403–1423. Oxford University Press, New York.
218. MacLeod, T. M., Hutchinson, F., and Raffle, E. F. (1970): The uptake of labelled thymidine by leucocytes of nickel sensitive patients. *Br. J. Dermatol.*, 82:487–492.
219. MacMillan, F. S. K., Rafft, R. R., and Elvers, W. B. (1975): A comparison of the skin irritation produced by cosmetic ingredients and formulations in the rabbit, guinea pig, beagle dog to that observed in the human. In: *Animal Models in Dermatology*, edited by H. I. Maibach, pp. 12–22. Churchill-Livingstone, Edinburgh.
220. Magee, P. N. (1970): Tests for carcinogenic potential. In: *Methods in Toxicology*, edited by G. E. Paget, pp. 158–196. Davis Publishers, Philadelphia.
221. Magnusson, B., and Hersle, K. (1965): Patch Test Methods I: A comparative study of six different types of patch tests. *Acta Dermatol.*, 45:123–128.
222. Magnusson, B., and Hersle, K. (1965): Patch test methods II: Regional variations of patch test responses. *Acta Dermatol.*, 45:257–261.
223. Magnusson, B., and Hersle, K. (1966): Patch test methods. III: Influence of adhesive tape on test response. *Acta Dermatol.*, 46:275–278.
224. Magnusson, B., and Kligman, A. M. (1969): The identification of contact allergens *by* animals assay: The guinea pig maximization test. *J. Invest. Dermatol.*, 52:268–276.
225. Magnusson, B., and Kligman, A. M. (1970): *Allergic Contact Dermatitis in the Guinea Pig*. Charles C. Thomas, Springfield.
226. Maguire, H. C. (1973): Mechanism of intensification by Freunds complete adjuvant of the acquisition of delayed hypersensitivity in the guinea pig. *Immunol. Commun.*, 1:239–246.
227. Maguire, H. C. (1974): Alteration in the acquisition of delayed hypersensitivity with adjuvant in the guinea pig. *Monogr. Allergy*, 8:13–26.
228. Maibach, H. I. (1976): Immediate hypersensitivity in hand dermatitis: Role of food contact dermatitis. *Arch. Dermatol.*, 112:1289–1291.
229. Maibach, H. (1994): Role of vehicle in allergic contact dermatitis, *Contact Dermatis*, .
230. Maibach, H., and Boisits, E. (1982): *Neonatal Skin*. Marcel Dekker, New York.
231. Maibach, H. I., and Johnson, H. L. (1975): Contact urticaria syndrome: Contact urticaria to diethyltoluamide (immediate-type hypersensitivity). *Arch. Dermatol.*, 111:726–720.

232. Maibach, H. I., Lamminatusta, K., Berardesca, E., and Freeman S. (1989): Tendency to irritation: Sensitive skin. *J. Am. Acad. Dermatol.*, 21:833–835.

233. Maisey, J., and Miller, K. (1986): Assessment of the ability of mice fed on vitamin A supplemented diet to respond to a variety of potential contact sensitizers. *Contact Dermatitis*, 15:17–23.

234. Malkinson, F. D. (1958): Studies on the percutaneous absorption of C^{14} labeled steroids by use of the gas-flow cell. *J. Invest. Dermatol.*, 31:19.

235. Malkovsky, M., Dore, C., Hunt, R., Palmer, L., Chandler, P., and Medawar, P. B. (1983): Enhancement of specific antitumor immunity in mice fed a diet enriched in vitamin A acetate. *Proc. Nat. Acad. Sci. USA*, 80:6322–6326.

236. Malkovsky, M., Edwards, A. J., Hunt, R., Palmer, L., and Medawar, P. B. (1983): T-cell-mediated enhancement of host-versus-graft reactivity in mice fed a diet enriched in vitamin A acetate. *Nature*, 302:338–340.

237. Malten, K. E., and Thiele, F. A. J. (1973): Evaluation of skin damage. II: Water loss and carbon dioxide release measurements related to skin resistance measurements. *Br. J. Dermatol.*, 89:565–569.

238. Malten, K. E., and Thiele, F. A. J. (1973): Some theoretical aspects of orthoergic (=irritant) dermatitis. *Arch. Belges Dermatol.*, 28:9–22.

239. Martin, R., Denyer, S., and Hadgraft, J. (1987): Skin metabolism of topically applied compounds. *Int. J. Pharm.*, 39:23–32.

240. Marzulli, F. N., and Maibach, H. I. (1973): Antimicrobials: Experimental contact sensitization in man. *J. Soc. Cosmet. Chem.*, 24:399–421.

241. Marzulli, F. N., and Maibach, H. I. (1974): The use of graded concentration in studying skin sensitizers: Experimental contact sensitization in man. *Food Cosmet. Toxicol.*, 12:219–227.

242. Mathias, C. G. T., Chappler, R. R., and Maibach, H. I. (1980): Contact urticaria from cinnamic aldehyde. *Arch. Dermatol.*, 116:74–76.

243. Mathias, C. G. T., and Maibach, H. I. (1978): Dermatoxicology monographs. I: Cutaneous irritation: Factors influencing the response to irritants. *Clin. Toxicol.*, 13:333–346.

244. Maurer, T., Thomann, P., Weirich, E. G., and Hess, R. (1975): The optimization test in the guinea pig: A method for the predictive evaluation of the contact allergenicity of chemicals. *Agents Actions*, 5:174–179.

245. McKenzie, A. W., and Stoughton, R. M. (1962): Method for comparing the percutaneous absorption of steroids. *Arch. Dermatol.*, 86:608–610.

246. McKillop, C. M., Brock, J. A. C., Oliver, C. J. A., and Rhodes, C. (1987): A quantitative assessment of pyrethroid-induced paresthesia in the guinea pig flank model. *Toxicol. Lett.*, 36:1–7.

247. Mezei, M. (1970): Dermatitic effect of nonionic surfactants. V: The effect of nonionic surfactants on rabbit skin as evaluated by radioactive tracer techniques in vivo. *J. Invest. Dermatol.*, 54:510–516.

248. Mezei, M., Sager, R. W., Stewart, W. D., and DeRuyter, A. L. (1966): Dermatitic effect on nonionic surfactants I: Gross, microscopic, and metabolic changes in rabbit skin treated with nonionic surface-active agents. *J. Pharm. Sci.*, 55:584–590.

249. Miller, A. E., and Levis, W. R. (1973): Studies on the contact sensitization of man with simple chemicals. I: Specific lymphocyte transformation in response to dinitrochlorobenzene sensitiztion. *J. Invest. Dermatol.*, 61:261–269.

250. Miller, K., Maisey, J., and Malkovsky, M. (1984): Enhancement of contact sensitization in mice fed a diet enriched in vitamin A acetate. *Int. Arch. Allergy Appl. Immunol.*, 75:120–125.

251. Milner, J. E. (1970): In vitro lymphocyte response in contact hypersensitivity. *J. Invest. Dermatol.*, 55:34–38.

252. Milner, J. E. (1971): In vitro lymphocyte response in contact hypersensitivity II. *J. Invest. Dermatol.*, 56:349–352.

253. Mizel, S. B. (1982): Interleukin 1 and T cell activation. *Immuno Rev.*, 63:51–72.

254. Mol, M. A. E., Van de Ruit, A. B. C., and Kluivers, A. W. (1989): NAD^+ levels and glucose uptake of cultured human epidermal cells exposed to sulfur mustard. *Toxicol. Appl. Pharmacol.*, 98:159–165.

255. Moloney, S. J., and Teal, J. J. (1988): Alkane-induced edema formation and cutaneous barrier dysfunction. *Arch. Dermatol. Res.*, 280:375–379.

256. Montagna, W. (1962): *The Structure and Function of Skin*. Academic Press, New York.

257. Montagna, W., and Lobitz, W. C. (1964): *The Epidermis*. Academic Press, New York.

258. Moorehead, J. W., Murphy, J. W., Harvey, R. P., et al. (1962): Soluble factors in tolerance and contact sensitivity to 2,4-dinitrofulurobenzene in mice IV. *Eur. J. Immunol.*, 12:431–436.

259. Mosman, T. (1983): Rapid colorimetric assay for cellular growth and survival: Application to proliferation and cytotoxic assays. *J. Immunol. Methods*, 65:55–63.

260. Motoyoshi, K., Toyoshima, Y., Sato, M., and Yoshimura, M. (1979): Comparative studies on the irritancy of oils and synthetic perfumes to the skin of rabbit, guinea pig, rat, miniature swine and man. *Cosmet. Toiletries*, 94:41–42.

261. Najarian, J. S., and Feldman, J. D. (1963): Specificity of passive transfer or delayed hypersensitivity. *J. Exp. Med.*, 118:341–352.

262. National Academy of Sciences, Committee for the Revision of NAS Publication 1138 (1977): *Principles and Procedures for Evaluating the Toxicity of Household Substances*, pp. 23–59. National Academy of Sciences, Washington D.C.

263. National Toxicology Program (1999): *The murine local lymph node assay: A test method for assessing the allergic contact dermatitis potential of chemicals/compounds*. National Institutes of Health Publication 99-4494, Research Triangle Park, NC.

264. Nicolaides, N. (1963): Human skin surface lipids: Origins, composition and possible function. In: *Advances in Biology of Skin, Vol. IV, The Sebaceous Glands*, edited by W. Montagna, R. A. Ellis, and A. F. Silver, pp. 167–187. Pergamon Press, Oxford.

265. Nixon, G. A., Tyson, C. A., and Wertz, W. C. (1975): Interspecies comparisons of skin irritancy. *Toxicol. Appl. Pharmacol.*, 31:481–490.

266. Noonan, P. K., and Wester, R. C. (1983): Cutaneous biotransformations and some pharmacological and toxicological implications. In: *Dermatotoxicology, 2nd edition*, edited by F. N. Marzulli and H. I. Maibach, pp. 71–90. Hemisphere, New York.

267. Odland, G. F. (1991): Structure of the skin. In: *Physiology, Biochemistry and Molecular Biology of the Skin, 2nd edition*, edited by L. A. Goldsmith, pp. 3–62. Oxford University Press, New York.

268. Odom, R. B., and Maibach, H. I. (1976): Contact urticaria: A different contact dermatitis. *Cutis*, 18:672–676.

269. Oliver, G. J. A., Botham, P. A., and Kimber, I. (1986): Models for contact sensitization: Novel approaches and future developments. *Br. J. Dermatol.*, 115:53–62.

270. Oliver, G. J. A., Pemberton, M. A., and Rhodes, C. (1986): An in vitro skin corrosivity test-modification and validation. *Food Chem. Toxicol.*, 24:507–512.

271. Oliver, G. J. A., Pemberton, M. A., and Rhodes, C. (1986): The identification of corrosive agents for human skin in vitro. *Food Chem. Toxicol.*, 24:513–515.

272. Oliver, G. J. A., Pemberton, M. A., and Rhodes, C. (1988): An in vitro model for identifying skin-corrosive chemicals. I: Initial validation. *Toxicol. In Vitro*, 2:7–17.

273. Opdyke, D. (1971): The guinea pig immersion test: A 20 year appraisal. *CTFA Cosmetic J.*, 3:46–47.
274. Opdyke, D. L., and Burnett, C. M. (1965): Practical problems in the evaluation of the safety of cosmetics. *Proceedings of the Scientific Section, Toilet Goods Association*, 44:3–4.
275. OECD (1993). Acute dermal irritation/corrosion. In: *OECD Guidelines for Testing of Chemicals*. Section 4, #404. Organization for Economic Cooperation and Development, Paris, France.
276. OECD (1981): *Guidelines for testing of chemicals: Carcinogenicity studies* (#451) *and Combined chronic toxicity/carcinogenicity studies* (#453). Organization for Economic Cooperation and Development, Paris, France.
277. Ostrenga, J., Steinmetz, C., Poulsen, B., and Yett, S. (1971): Significance of vehicle composition II: Prediction of optimal vehicle composition. *J. Pharm. Sci.*, 60:1180–1183.
278. Page, A. R., and Good, R. A. (1958): A clinical and experimental study of the function of neutrophils in the inflammatory response. *Am. J. Pathol.*, 34:645–656.
279. Page, N. P. (1977): Concepts of a bioassay program in environmental carcinogenesis. In: *Environmental Cancer, Vol. 3: Advances in Modern Toxicology*, edited by H. F. Kraybill and M. A. Mehlman, pp. 87–171. Hemisphere Publishing, Washington, D.C.
280. Palotay, J. L., Adachi, K., Dobson, R. L., and Pinto, J. S. (1986): Carcinogen-induced cutaneous neoplasms in non-human primates. *J. Nat. Cancer. Inst.*, 97:1269–1272.
281. Pappas, A., Orfanos, C. E., and Bertram, R. (1970): Non-specific lymphocyte transformation in vitro by nickel acetate. *J. Invest. Dermatol.*, 55:198–200.
282. Parce, J. W., Owicki, J. C., Kercso, K. M., Sigal, G. B., et al. (1989): Detection of cell-affecting agents with a silicon biosensor. *Science*, 246:243–247.
283. Patrick, E., Burkhalter, A., and Maibach, H. I. (1987): Recent investigations of mechanisms of chemically induced skin irritation in laboratory mice. *J. Invest. Dermatol.*, 88:24s–31s.
284. Patrick, E., and Maibach, H. I. (1987): A novel predictive irritation assay in mice. *The Toxicologist*, vol 84.
285. Patrick, E., and Maibach, H. I. (1989): Comparision of the time course, dose response, and mediators of chemically induced skin irritation in three species. In: *Current Topics in Contact Dermatitis*, edited by P. Frosch, A. Dooms-Goossens, R. Lachapelle, R. Rycroft, and R. Scheper, pp. 399–404. Springer-Verlag, Berlin.
286. Patrick, E., and Maibach, H. I. (1991): Predictive skin irritation tests in animal and humans. In: *Dermatotoxicity, 4th edition*, edited by F. N. Marzulli and H. I. Maibach, pp. 201–222. Hemisphere, New York.
287. Patrick, E., Maibach, H. I., and Burkhalter, A. (1985): Mechanisms of chemically induced skin irritation I: Studies of time course, dose response, and components of inflammation in the laboratory mouse. *Toxicol. Appl. Pharmacol.*, 81:476–490.
288. Pauly, J. L., Caron, G. A., and Suskind, R. R. (1969): Blast transformation of lymphocytes from guinea pigs, rats, and rabbits induced by mercuric chloride in vitro. *J. Cell Biol.*, 40:847–850.
289. Pearmain, G. E., Ltcette, R. R., and Fitzgerald, P. H. (1963): Tuberculin induced mitoses in peripheral blood lymphocytes. *Lancet*, 1:637–638.
290. Perkins, M. A., Osborne, R., and Johnson, G. R. (1996): Development of an in vitro method for skin corrosion testing. *Fund. Appl. Toxicol.*, 31:9–18.
291. Phillips, L., Steinberg, M., Maibach, H. I., and Akers, W. A. (1972): A comparison of rabbit and human skin response to certain irritants. *Toxicol. Appl. Pharmacol.*, 21:369–382.
292. Pinnagoda, J., Tupker, R. A., Agner, T., and Serup, J. (1990): Guidelines for transepidermal water loss (TEWL) measurements: A report from the standardization group of the European society of contact dermatitis. *Contact Dermatitis*, 22:164–178.
293. Pohl, R. J., Philpot, R. M., and Fouts, J. R. (1976): Cytochrome P450 content and mixed function oxidase activity in microsomes isolated from mouse skin. *Drug Metab. Dis.*, 4:442–450.
294. Polak, L. (1977): Immunological aspects of contact sensitivity. In: *Dermatotoxicology and Pharmacology*, edited by F. N. Marzulli and H. I. Maibach, pp. 225–288. Hemisphere, Washington, D.C.
295. Polak, L., Polak, A., and Frey, J. R. (1974): The development of contact sensitivity to DNFB in guinea pigs genetically differing in their response to DNP-skin protein conjugate. *Int. Arch. Allergy*, 46:417–426.
296. Potokar, M. (1985): Studies on the design of animal tests for the corrosiveness of industrial chemicals. *Food Chem. Toxicol.*, 23:615–617.
297. Prottey, C. (1978): The molecular basis of skin irritation. In: *Cosmetics, Vol. 1*, edited by M. M. Breuer, pp. 275–349. Academic Press, London.
298. Rapaport, M., Anderson, D., and Pierce, U. (1978): Performance of the 21-day patch test in civilian populations. *J. Toxicol Cut. Ocular Toxicol.*, 1:109–115.
299. Rietschell, R. L. (1982): Advances and pitfalls in irritant and allergen testing. *J. Soc. Cosmet. Chem.*, 33:309–313.
300. Ritz, H. L., and Buehler, E. V. (1980): Planning conduct and interpretation of guinea pig sensitization patch tests. In: *Current Concepts in Cutaneous Toxicity*, edited by V. A. Drill and P. Lazar, p. 25. Academic Press, New York.
301. Robertsaw, D. (1991): Apocrine sweat glands. In: *Physiology, Biochemistry, and Molecular Biology of the Skin, 2nd edition*, edited by L. A. Goldsmith, pp. 763–775. Oxford University Press, New York.
302. Rockl, H., Muller, E., and Haltermann, W. (1966): Zum aussagewert positiver epicutantest bei sauglingen and kindern. *Arch. Klin. Exp. Dermatol.*, 226:407.
303. Rocklin, R. E., MacDermott, R. P., Chess, L., et al. (1974): Studies on mediator production by highly purified human T and B lymphocytes. *J. Exp. Med.*, 140:1303–1316.
304. Roskos, K., and Maibach, H. (1992): Percutaneous absorption and age: Implications for therapy. *Drugs and Aging*, 2:432–449.
305. Rostenberg, A. (1961): Methods for the appraisal of the safety of cosmetics. *Drug Cosmet. Ind.*, 88:592.
306. Rothenborg, H. W., Menne, T., and Sjolin, K. E. (1977): Temperature dependent primary irritant dermatitis from lemon perfume. *Contact Dermatitis*, 3:37.
307. Rothman, S. (1954): *Physiology and Biochemistry of the Skin*. The University of Chicago Press, Chicago.
308. Rouigier, A., Dupuis, D., Lotte, C., Roguet, R., and Schafer, H. (1983): In vivo correlation between stratum corneum reservoir function and percutaneous absorption. *J. Invest. Dermatol.*, 81:275–278.
309. Sato, K., Kang, W. H., and Sato, F. (1991): Eccrine sweat glands. In: *Physiology, Biochemistry, and Molecular Biology of the Skin, 2nd edition*, edited by L. A. Goldsmith, pp. 741–762. Oxford University Press, New York.
310. Sauder, D. N. (1991): Interleukens. In: *Physiology, Biochemistry, and Molecular Biology of the Skin, 2nd edition*, edited by L. A. Goldsmith, pp. 1188–1198. Oxford University Press, New York.
311. Scheuplein, R. J. (1967): Mechanism of percutaneous absorption II: Transient diffusion and the relative importance of various routes of skin penetration. *J. Invest. Dermatol.*, 48:79–88.
312. Scheuplein, R. J. (1978): Permeability of skin: A review of major concepts. *Curr. Probl. Dermatol.*, 7:58–68.
313. Scheuplein, R., and Bronough, R. L. (1983): Percutaneous absorption. In: *Biochemistry and Physiology of the Skin*, edited

by L. A. Goldsmith, pp. 1255–1295. Oxford University Press, New York.

314. Scholes, E. W., Basketter, D. A., Saril, A. E., et al. (1992): The local lymph node assay: Results of a final inter-laboratory validation under field conditions. *J. Appl. Toxicol.*, 12:217–222.

315. Schopf, E., Schulz, K. H., and Isensee, I. (1969): Untersuchungen uber den lymphocyten trans formationstest be: Quecksilberallerge. *Arch. Klin. Exp. Dermatol.*, 234:420.

316. Schwartz, L. (1951): The skin testing of new cosmetics. *J. Soc. Cosmet. Chem.*, 2:321–324.

317. Schwartz, L. (1969): Twenty-two years experience in the performance of 200,000 prophetic patch tests. *South. Med. J.*, 53:478–484.

318. Schwartz, L., and Peck, S. M. (1944): The patch test in contact dermatitis. *Public Health Rep.*, 59:546–557.

319. Schwartz, L. B. (1991): Mast cells and their role in urticaria. *J. Am. Acad. Dermatol.*, 25:190–204.

320. Shelanski, H. A. (1951): Experience with and considerations of the human patch test method. *J. Soc. Cosmet. Chem.*, 2:324–331.

321. Shelanski, H. A., and Shelanski, M. V. (1953): A new technique of human patch tests. *The Proceedings of the Scientific Section of the Toilet Goods Association*, 19:46–49.

322. Shelanski, H. A., and Shelanski, M. V. (1953): New technique of patch tests. *Drug Cosmet. Ind.*, 73:186.

323. Shellow, W. V. R., and Rapaport, M. J. (1981): Comparison testing of soap irritancy using aluminum chamber and standard patch methods. *Contact Dermatitis*, 7:77–79.

324. Simpson, W. L., and Cramer, W. (1943): Fluorescence studies of carcinogens in skin. *Cancer Res.*, 3:362–369.

325. Skog, E. (1960): Primary irritant and allergic eczematous reactions in patients with different dermatoses. *Acta Derm. Venerol.*, 40:307–312.

326. Slaga, T. J., Klein-Szanto, A. J. P., Boutwell, R. K., Stevenson, D. E., Spitzer, H. L., and D'Motto, B. (1989): *Skin Carcinogenesis: Mechanisms and Human Relevance*. Alan R. Liss, New York.

327. Smiles, K. A., and Pollack, M. E. (1977): A quantative human patch testing procedure for low level skin irritants. *J. Soc. Cosmet. Chem.*, 26:755–764.

328. Sokolov, U. E. (1962): *Mammal Skin*. University of California Press, Berkeley.

329. SOT Position Paper (1989): Comments on the LD5O and acute eye and skin irritation tests. *Fund. Appl. Toxicol.*, 13:621–623.

330. Soter, N. A. (1991): Acute and chronic urticaria and angioedema. *J. Am. Acad. Dermatol.*, 25:146–154.

331. Steinberg, M., Akers, W. A., Weeks, M., McCreesh, A. H., and Maibach, H. I. (1975): A comparison of test techniques based on rabbit and human skin responses to irritants with recommendations regarding the evaluation of mildly or moderately irritating compounds. In: *Animal Models in Dermatology*, edited by H. I. Maibach, pp. 1–11. Churchill-Livingston, Edinburgh.

332. Stephens, T. J., Silber, P. M., Recce, B., et al. (1990): Testskin™: An in vitro model for detecting cytotoxicity and inflammation. *The Toxicologist*, 10:78.

333. Stingl, G., and Abever, W. (1983): The Langerhans cell. In: *Biochemistry and Physiology of the Skin*, edited by L. A. Goldsmith, pp. 907–921. Oxford University Press, New York.

334. Stingl, G., Katz, S. I., Clement, L., Green, I., and Shevach, E. (1978): Immunologic functions of Ia-bearing epidermal Langerhans cells. *J. Immunol.*, 121:2005–2013.

335. Stotts, J. (1980): Planning, conduct, and interpretation: Human predictive sensitization patch tests. In: *Current Concepts in Cutaneous Toxicity*, edited by V. A. Drill and P. Lazar, pp. 41–53. Academic Press, New York.

336. Strauss, J. S., Downing, D. T., Ebling, F. J., and Stewart, M. E. (1991): Sebaceous glands. In: *Physiology, Biochemistry, and Molecular Biology of the Skin, 2nd edition*, edited by L. A. Goldsmith, pp. 712–740. Oxford University Press, New York.

337. Strube, D. D., Koontz, S. W., Murahata, R. I., and Theiler, R. F. (1989): The flex wash test: A method for evaluating the mildness of personal washing products. *J. Soc. Cosmet. Chem.*, 40:297–306.

338. Sweeney, T. M., and Downing, D. T. (1970): The role of lipids in the epidermal barrier to water diffusion. *J. Invest. Dermatol.*, 55:135–140.

339. Swisher, D. A., Johnson, J., and Ledger, P. W. (1987): A method for screeing in vitro cytotoxicity of agents toward human keratinocytes. *J. Invest. Dermatol.*, 88:520.

340. Tagami, H. (1971): Functional characteristics of aged skin. *Acta Dermatol. Venereol. (Stockholm)*, 66:19–21.

341. Tagami, H., Masatoshi, O., and Iwatsuki, K. (1986): Evaluation of the skin surface hydration in vivo by electrical measurements. *J. Invest. Dermatol.*, 75:500–597.

342. Tharp, M. D. (1991): The mast cell and its mediators. In: *Physiology, Biochemistry, and Molecular Biology of the Skin, 2nd edition*, edited by L. A. Goldsmith, pp. 1019–1083. Oxford University Press, New York.

343. Thiele, F. A. J., and Malten, K. E. (1973): Evaluation of skin damage I: Skin resistance measurements with alternating current (impedance measurements). *Br. J. Dermatol.*, 89:373–382.

344. Thiele, F. A. J., and Malten, K. E. (1973): Some measuring methods for the evaluation of orthoergic contact dermatitis. *Arch. Belges Dermatol.*, 28:23–46.

345. Traub, E. F., Tusing, T. W., and Spoor, H. J. (1954): Evaluation of dermal sensitivity: Animal and human tests compared. *Arch Derm (Chicago)*, 69:399–409.

346. Tregear, R. T. (1964): Relative penetrability of hair follicles and epidermis. *J. Physiol. (London)*, 156:303–313.

347. Tregear, R. T. (1966): *Physical Function of Skin*. Academic Press, New York.

348. Triglia, D., Braa, S. S., Donnelly, T., Kidd, I., and Naughton, G. K. (1991): A three dimensional human dermal model substrate for in vitro toxicological studies. In: *In Vitro Toxicology: Mechanisms and New Technology*, edited by A. M. Goldberg, pp. 351–362. Mary Ann Lieber, New York.

349. Triglia, D., Braa, S. S., Yonan, C., and Naughton, G. K. (1991): In vitro toxicity of various classes of test agents using the neutral red assay on a human three-dimensional physiologic skin mode. *In Vitro Cell Dev. Biol.*, 27A:239–244.

350. Unanue, E. R. (1984): Antigen-presenting function of the macrophage. *Annu. Rev. Immunol.*, 2:395–428.

351. Upadhye, M., and Maibach, H. (1992): Influence of area of application of allergens in contact dermatitis. *Contact Dermatitis*, 27:186.

352. Urbach, F., Davies, R. E., and Forbes, P. D. (1988): Chemical modifiers of photocarcinogenesis. *Arch. Toxicol.*, 12(Supp.): 47–51.

353. Uttley, M., and Van Abbe, N. J. (1973): Primary irritation of the skin: Mouse ear test and human patch test procedures. *J. Soc. Cosmet. Chem.*, 24:217–227.

354. Van Loveren, H., Kato, K., Ratzlaff, R. E., Meade, R., Ptak, W., Askenase, P. W. (1984): Use of micrometers and calipers to measure various components of delayed-type hypersensitivity ear swelling reactions in mice. *J. Immunol. Methods*, 67:311–319.

355. Van der Valk, P. G. M., and Maibach, H. I. (1996): *The Irritant Contact Dermatitis Syndrome*. CRC Press, Boca Raton, FL.

356. Van der Valk, P. O. M., Nater, J. P. K., and Bleumink, E. (1985): Vulnerability of the skin to surfactants in different groups of eczema patients and controls as measured by water vapor loss. *Clin. Exp. Dermatol.*, 101:98.

357. Viluksela, M. (1991): Characteristics and modulation of dithranol (anthralin)-induced skin irritation in the mouse ear model. *Arch. Dermatol. Res.*, 283:262–268.
358. Vinegar, M. B. (1979): Regional variation in primary skin irritation and corrosivity potentials in rabbits. *Toxicol Appl. Pharmacol.*, 49:63–69.
359. Vivjeberg, H. P., and VandenBercken, J. (1979): Frequency dependent effects of the pyrethroid insecticide decamethrin in frog myelinated nerve fibers. *Eur. J. Pharmacol.*, 58:501–504.
360. Vizethum, W., Ruzicka, R., and Goetz, G. (1980): Inducibility of drug-metabolizing enzymes in the rat skin. *Chem. Biol. Interact.*, 31:215–219.
361. Von Krogh, G., and Maibach, H. I. (1982): The contact urticaria syndrome. *Sem. Dermatol.*, 1:59–66.
362. Voss, J. G. (1958): Skin sensitization by mercaptans of low molecular weight. *J. Invest. Dermatol.*, 31:273–279.
363. Wagner, G., and Purschel, W. (1962): Klinisch-analytische studie die zum neuroderm-itisproblem. *Dermatologica*, 125:1.
364. Wahlberg, J. E., and Boman, A. (1985): Guinea pig maximization test. In: *Contact Allergy Predictive Tests in Guinea Pigs*, edited by K. E. Andersen and H. I. Maibach, pp. 9–106. Karger, Basel.
365. Wahlberg, J., and Menne, T. in scanavian government equalent to WHO.
366. Walker, A. P., Basketter, D. A., Baveral, M., Diembeck, W., Matthies, W., Mougin, D., Paye, M., Rothlisberg, R., and Dupuis, J. (1996): Test guidelines for assessment of skin compatability of cosmetic finished products in man. *Food Chem. Toxicol.*, 34:651–660.
367. Walz, D. (1985): Quantitative assessment of irritation in the mouse skin test. *Food Chem. Toxicol.*, 23:199–203.
368. Wasserman, S. J. (1983): The mast cell and its mediators. In: *Biochemistry and Physiology of the Skin*, edited by L. A. Goldsmith, pp. 878–898. Oxford University Press, New York.
369. Weaver, J. E. (1976): Dermatologic testing of household laundry products: A novel fabric softener. *Int. J. Dermatol.*, 15:297–300.
370. Weigand, D. A., and Gaylor, J. R. (1976): Irritant reaction in negro and caucasian skin. *South. Med. J.*, 67:548–551.
371. Weigand, D. A., Haygood, C., and Gaylor, J. R. (1974): Cell layer and density of negro and caucasian stratum corneum. *J. Invest. Dermatol.*, 62:563–568.
372. Weil, C. S., and Scala, R. A. (1971): Study of intra- and inter laboratory variability in the results of rabbit eye and skin irritation tests. *Toxicol. Appl. Pharmacol.*, 19:276–360.
373. Werner, Y., Lindberg, M., and Forslind, B. (1982): The water binding capacity of stratum corneum in dry non-eczematous skin of atopic eczema. *Acta Derm. Venereol.* (*Stockholm*), 62:334–336.
374. Wertz, P. W., and Downing, D. T. (1991): Epidermal lipids. In: *Physiology, Biochemistry, and Molecular Biology of the Skin, 2nd edition*, edited by L. A. Goldsmith, pp. 205–236. Oxford University Press, New York.
375. Wester, R. C., and Maibach, H. I. (1999): In vivo percutaneous absorption effect of repeated application versus single dose. (new percutaneous penetration book)
376. Wester, R. C., and Maibach, H. I. (1975): Rhesus monkey as a animal model for percutaneous absorption. In: *Animal Models In Dermatology*, edited by H. I. Maibach, pp. 133–137. Churchill Livingstone, New York.
377. Wester, R. C., and Maibach, H. I. (1983): Cutaneous pharmacokinetics: 10 steps to percutaneous absorption. *Drug Metab. Rev.*, 14:169–205.
378. Whittle, E., and Basketter, D. A. (1993): The in vitro skin corrosivity test: Development of a method using human skin. *Toxicol. In Vitro*, 7:265–268.
379. Whitton, J. T., and Ewell, J. D. (1973): The thickness of epidermis. *Br. J. Dermatol.*, 89:467–478.
380. Wiechers, J. (1989): The barrier function of the skin in relation to percutaneous absorption of drugs. *Pharm. Week.* (*Sci.*), 11:185–198.
381. Wilhelm, K. P., and Maibach, H. I. (1990): Factors predisposing to cutaneous irritation. *Contact Dermatitis*, 8:17–22.
382. Wilhelm, K. P., Surber, C., and Maibach, H. I. (1989): Quantification of sodium lauryl sulfate irritant dermatitis in man: Comparision of four techniques: Skin color reflectance, transepidermal water loss, laser doppler flow measurement and visual scores. *Arch. Dermatol. Research*, 281:293–295.
383. Wooding, W. H., and Opdyke, D. L. (1967): A statistical approach to the evaluation of cutaneous responses to irritants. *J. Soc. Cosmet. Chem.*, 16:809–829.
384. Yarnitsky, D., and Fowler, C. J. (1994): Quantitative sensory testing. In: *Manual of Clinical Neurophysiology*, edited by J. W. Osselton, pp. 253–320. Butterworths, London.
385. York, M., Basketter, D. A., Cuthbert, J. A., and Neilson, L. (1995): Skin irritation testing in man for hazard assesssment-evaluation of four patch systems. *Human and Exper. Toxicol.*, 14:729–734.
386. York, M., Griffiths, H. A., Whittle, E., and Basketter, D. A. (1996): Evaluation of a human patch test for the identification and classification of skin irritation potential. *Contact Dermatitis*.
387. Yosipovitch, G., and Yarnitsky, D. (1997): Quantitative sensory testing. In: *Dermatotoxicology Methods: The Laboratory Worker's Vad Mecum*, pp. 313–318. Taylor & Francis, Washington, D.C.
388. Yosipovitch, G., Szolar, C., Hui, X. Y., and Maibach, H. I. (1996): Effect of topically applied menthol on thermal pain and itch sensations and biophysical properties of the skin. *Arch. Dermatol. Res.*, 288:245–248.
389. Yosipovitch, G., Szolar, C., Hui, X. Y., and Maibach, H. I. (1996): High potency corticosteroid rapidly decreases histamine induced itch but not thermal sensation and pain in man. *J. Am. Acad. Dermatol.*, 55:118–120.
390. Yuspa, S. H., Blugosz, A. A. (1991): Cutaneous carcinogenesis. In: *Physiology, Biochemistry, and Molecular Biology of the Skin, 2nd edition*, edited by L. A. Goldsmith, pp. 1365–1401. Oxford University Press, New York.
391. National Toxicology Program (1999): Corrositex®: An in vitro test method for assessing dermal corrosivity potential of chemicals. National Institutes of Health. Publication 99-4495. Research Triangle Park, N.C.

Principles and Methods of Toxicology,
Fourth Edition, edited by A. Wallace Hayes.
Taylor & Francis, Philadelphia © 2001.

Chapter 23

Inhalation Toxicology

Rudolph Valentine and Gerald L. Kennedy, Jr.

The interactions between humans and the materials that make up our environment occur continually, often unavoidably, with each having an influence on the other. There are three main routes of contact: a material can land on one's body surface (dermal exposure), it can be swallowed after contact with the mouth and oral cavity (oral exposure), and it can be breathed through the nose or mouth into the lungs (inhalation exposure). With each route of exposure, some of the substance or its metabolites may be available for interaction with body cells, tissues, organs, and organ systems. Each exposure route can contribute to the total amount and form of chemical substance that gets into our system. Thus, the ultimate response of the organism will depend on the integrated amount and form of the chemical or foreign substance in the body from all three routes of exposure.

Because the respiratory tract forms a critical link between the blood supply of the body and the external environment, an understanding of the factors that can modify the integrity or function of nose, upper airways, or lungs is of great importance to the inhalation toxicologist. By virtue of the rich vasculature of the lungs, inhaled substances entering this organ gain ready access to the internal milieu of the body. External influences that interfere with the operation of the respiratory system may have profound effects on the organism, which in turn can be reflected by a broad spectrum of untoward responses ranging from upper respiratory tract irritation to pulmonary edema and death. Today, more and more chemical substances are undergoing inhalation testing to better define the interactions of these materials throughout the respiratory system.

The chapter is intended to give the reader an overview of the principles and methods used by the inhalation toxicologist and some of the recent scientific developments in this area. We will focus on the methods used in measuring the effects of chemical substances on the respiratory system following their inhalation. The emphasis is not on describing the many types of physical or toxicological changes that can be produced by agents, but on providing selected examples of these interactions that demonstrate applications of the experimental methodologies. A selected bibliography is provided at the end of the chapter for the reader who is interested in a more in-depth treatment of the topics presented here.

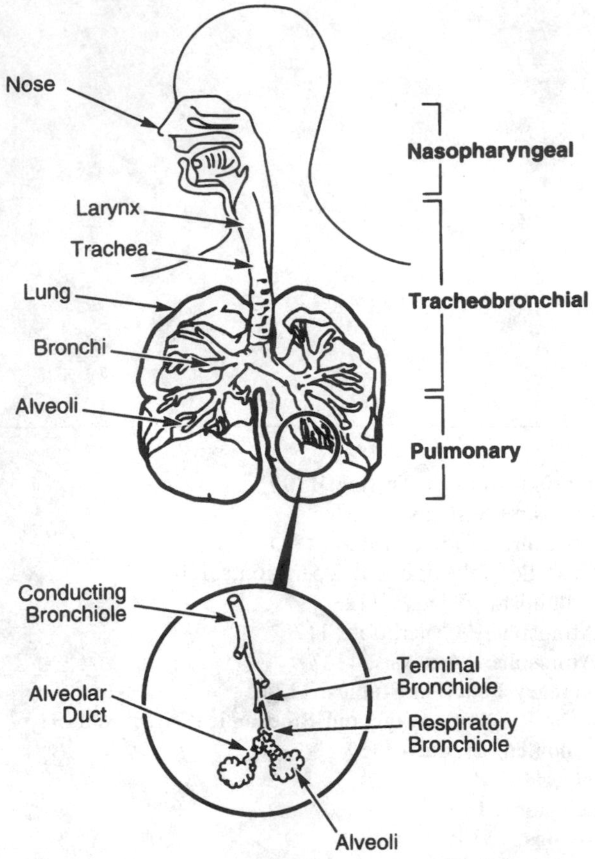

FIG. 23.1. Compartmental model of the human respiratory tract.

ANATOMY AND FUNCTION OF THE RESPIRATORY TRACT

An overview of the anatomy, function, and physiology of the mammalian respiratory system is presented to clarify some of the issues that face the inhalation toxicologist. The respiratory system can be simplified into three major components: (a) nasopharyngeal, (b) tracheobronchial, and (c) pulmonary. Although this is not the only description that can be used to compartmentalize the respiratory organs (e.g., the physician might think in terms of large airways, small airways, the acinus, and the blood vessels), it does serve to anatomically distinguish the various components of the respiratory tract that are of importance to the inhalation toxicologist (Figure 23.1).

Nasopharyngeal Region

The nasopharyngeal region includes the nasal turbinates, epiglottis, glottis, pharynx, and larynx. As the entry port for inspired air, the nares and nasal cavity serve to remove the larger inhaled particles (through impaction in the turbinates and filtration by nasal hairs) and to condition (by moderating the temperature and raising the humidity) the incoming air. The importance of this area has been previously overlooked, but because the nose is exposed to the highest chemical concentrations within the respiratory tract, the nasopharyngeal region is now the subject of considerable investigation.

The nasopharyngeal region also plays an important role in the physiological response to inhaled irritants. There are three basic types of irritants (13): (a) sensory irritants that act on the trigeminal nerve; (b) pulmonary irritants that act on irritant or stretch receptors of the airways; and (c) mixed sensory and pulmonary irritants.

The initial response to an inhaled irritant may involve an immediate burning or stinging sensation in the eyes, nose, or throat. Such stimuli may range from unpleasant to extreme pain and are mediated by interaction of irritants with chemoreceptive nerve endings from the trigeminal nerve in the cornea, nose, tongue, oral cavity, and upper respiratory tract. Once stimulated, these nerve endings can cause systemic responses, resulting not only in a burning sensation of the nose and eyes, but also a reflex reduction in respiratory rate. This response occurs once a threshold concentration at the irritant receptor is exceeded and develops immediately or within a few minutes of exposure. These sensory irritants may also evoke other physiological responses, including laryngeal and bronchial spasm, decreases in pulmonary ventilation and pulse, and increases in blood pressure. All of these responses are generally protective in nature, limiting further exposure of the offending chemical especially to the lower respiratory tract. Although the effects of sensory irritants per se are not usually life threatening, some irritants have the capacity to cause respiratory tract epithelial injury, possibly producing fatal lung edema hours to days after exposure.

In our environment, there are many different types of respiratory tract irritants. Chlorine, for example, has been used as a war gas and methyl isocyanate was associated with massive accidental human exposures in India. Chemical irritants act on specific targets. For example, formaldehyde acts primarily on respiratory epithelial cells, chlorine acts on the nasal cilia and bronchial functions, dimethylamine acts on olfactory sensory cells, and cigarette smoke affects the laryngeal epithelium. Furthermore, a number of disease states, including acute asphyxiation, chronic bronchitis, emphysema, pulmonary fibrosis, and pneumoconioses, can be induced or exacerbated by exposure to irritants. Some of the toxicological effects of inhaled materials on the nose are shown in Table 23.1.

Table 23.1
Effects of inhaled materials on the nose

Effect	Agent/example
Restrict airflow	Temperature changes—cold air; irritants—acids, bases
Mucociliary flow	Slowing by sulfur dioxide, formaldehyde, methyl amines
Cellular	
Olfactory degeneration	Chloroform, aliphatic esters, methyl bromide
Respiratory/olfactory irritation	Chlorine, sulfur dioxide, formaldehyde
Nasal tumors	Hexamethyl phosphoramide, acetaldehyde, formaldehyde, dimethyl sulfate

Nose

The nasal airway is divided into two passages by the nasal septum. Each passage extends from the nostrils to the nasopharynx. The nasopharynx is the airway posterior to the termination of the nasal septum and proximal to the determination of the soft palate. Air moves through the nostril openings (nares) into the vestibule which is just before the main chamber of the nose. The main chamber is defined by a lateral wall, a septal wall, a roof, and a floor. Turbinates (bony structures lined by well-vascularized respiratory or olfactory mucosal tissue) project into the airway lumen from the lateral walls into the main chamber of the nose (Figure 23.2).

As the initial site of entry, the nasal passages are an important target site for a wide range of inhaled agents. For the epithelial mucosa in the nose, squamous tissue is the target of glutaraldehyde toxicity (1), transitional epithelial tissue is attacked by ozone (2), respiratory mucosal tissue by formaldehyde (3), and the olfactory region by β,β-iminodipropionitrile (4). The effects produced at these locations may be attributable to the local dose of the agents reaching the site, site-specific tissue susceptibility, or a combination of these factors.

Importantly, the location and proper characterization of nasal lesions play a role in assessing the mode of action and for interspecies comparisons. Techniques have been developed and optimized to describe the location and nature of effects seen in this anatomically complex tissue. The very complexity of the structure makes it a challenge to properly interpret chemically induced changes. Young (5) proposed a set of four standard transverse sections from the rat nasal cavity be prepared for histopathological examination. These included sections taken at the following landmarks: (i) immediately posterior to the upper incisor teeth; (ii) at the incisive papilla; (iii) at the second palatal ridge; and (iv) at the level of the first upper molar teeth. Young's method is applicable to both short-term and chronic toxicity studies and allows

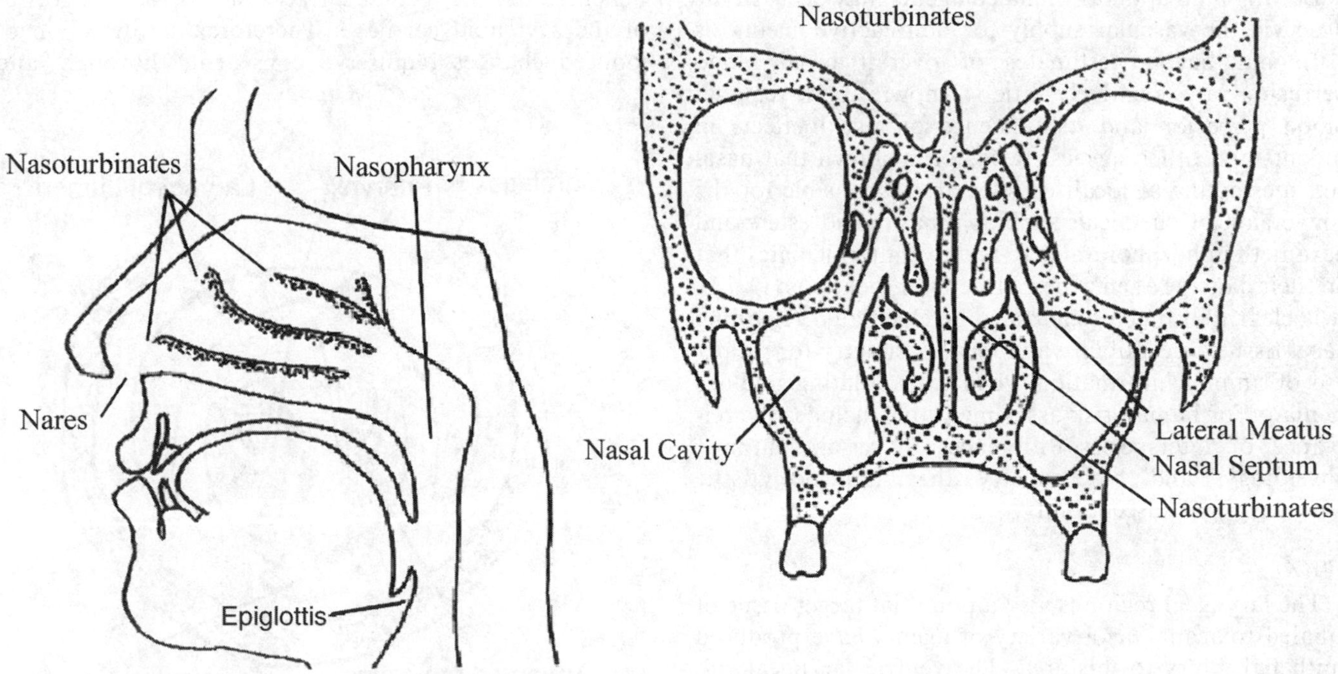

FIG. 23.2. Schematic diagram of the human nasal cavity.

for a thorough examination of the nasal cavity without destructive invasion at the time of necropsy. Other sampling strategies includes that of the National Toxicology Program (6,7), which uses three sites for sectioning while others (2,8) propose more numerous sections. Regardless, section level selection is a critical issue and availability of anatomically similar sections is essential for comparing the extent, severity, and relevance of the lesions characterized.

A series of diagrams designed for mapping nasal lesions of both the Fischer-344 rat and the B6C3F1 mouse has been published by Mery et al. (9). The diagrams present each of the major cross-sectional airway profiles and provide space for recording nasal mucosal lesions. Sagittal diagrams are also provided to permit transfer of data from transverse sections onto the long axis of the nose. The use and application of these diagrams help unify and make the collection and presentation of data more consistent.

It should be emphasized that recording the lesion distribution is only the first step in the process of identifying patterns of nasal toxicity. Because the lesion distribution results from the interplay of local dose and tissue susceptibility, the researcher needs to keep in mind their relative influence and the relevance of such responses to humans. For example, the airflow-driven local dose of highly reactive water-soluble chemicals such as formaldehyde accounts for the lesion distribution but airflow is not likely to be a major factor in the lesions produced by less water soluble substances like ozone, chloroform, and methyl bromide.

Locally high uptake of inhaled agents may occur in the nose via the vascular supply for nonreactive chemicals (10), but beyond estimates of overall nasal blood perfusion rates relatively little is known about regional blood perfusion and its influence on nasal effects in rodents and other species. It has been shown that nasal enzymes acting at localized sites are responsible for the conversion of chemicals such as dibasic acid esters and hexamethylphosphoramide to reactive intermediates that do their damage at enzyme-rich cellular locations (11,12). It is clear that much remains to be elucidated regarding nasal tissue susceptibility and local dosimetry for proper use of animal information when extrapolating findings to man. For human risk assessment this includes the relevance of interspecies differences in nasal anatomy, physiology, and biochemistry that influence tissue dosimetry and susceptibility.

Larynx

The laryngeal region is also a potential target tissue of inhaled toxicants, as a variety of agents have produced epithelial injury to this area. The ventral laryngeal epithelium of rats and mice is highly responsive to inhaled materials such as cobalt sulfate (14), tobacco smoke (15), and a wide variety of industrial chemicals, pharmaceuticals, and aerosol propellants (16). The rat larynx contains five types of epithelium and two forms of pseudostratified cuboidal epithelium. Each epithelial type has a specific location within the relatively complex anatomic configuration of the larynx. There also are interspecies differences among laboratory rodents in the microscopic anatomy of these sensitive areas of the laryngeal mucosa. In Sprague–Dawley rats, the mucosa covering the epiglottis differs from that of the Syrian golden hamsters in that in rats it is thinner and composed of a mixture of cell types. In contrast, the cartilage of the hamster is much more prominent and forms a distinct protrusion into the lumen at the base of the epiglottis. These anatomic differences can play a role in the use of this information in extrapolating these findings to man (17) (Figure 23.3).

Laryngeal lesions commonly involve degeneration of the epithelium with subsequent regeneration, hyperplasia, and squamous metaplasia. In more severe reactions, the larynx may have epithelial ulceration with exudation. To some extent, the changes commonly observed are dependent upon the duration of the study and the exposure concentration rather than the individual compound. Recovery or regression from induced changes is variable and dependent upon the time scale involved and severity or type of initial lesion (18). Specific areas of the rodent laryngeal mucosa appear to be more sensitive to inhaled materials and more likely to contain cellular changes in response to injury. These sites include the epithelium covering the base of the epiglottis, ventral pouches, and the medial surfaces of the vocal processes of the arytenoid cartilage. Therefore, the detection of induced changes requires a consistent, thorough, and

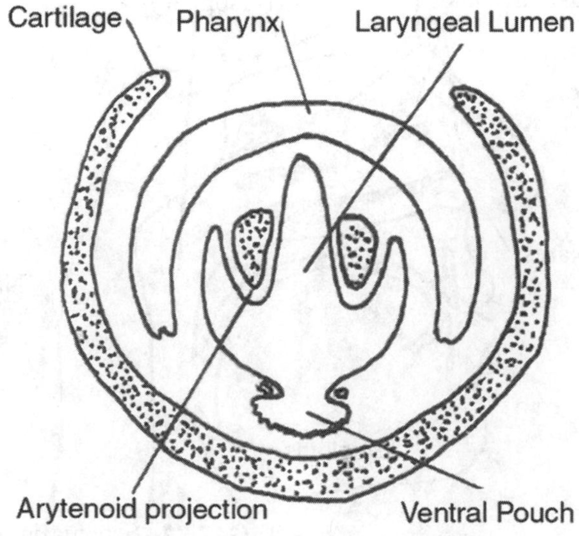

FIG. 23.3. Schematic diagram of the rat larynx.

detailed histological examination in order to identify the often subtle changes in the distribution of epithelial injury. Renne et al. (17) has proposed embedding and sectioning techniques to optimize histopathological evaluation of this region.

Tracheobronchial Airways

The tracheobronchial region is responsible for delivering the inspired air to the deeper portions of the lung; it includes a series of branching ducts that begin at the trachea and end at the terminal bronchioles. Surfaces of the tracheobronchial region are covered with a layer of mucus-secreting goblet cells and ciliated columnar cells that form a protective and functional mucociliary blanket. The mucus that covers the luminal surfaces is continuously propelled toward the oral region (it is often referred to as the mucociliary "escalator") and serves to carry particulate material that deposits in the mucus covering the bronchi and trachea to the back of the mouth whereupon this material can be swallowed or expectorated. The series of branching ducts of the tracheobronchial region further condition the inspired air by warming it to body temperature and saturating it with water vapor.

Pulmonary Region

The pulmonary region is composed of respiratory bronchioles, alveolar ducts, and alveoli. The alveolus is the functional gas exchange unit of the lung. Oxygen diffuses from the inspired air to the lung through the extremely thin alveolar epithelial and capillary endothelial membranes into the blood stream. After dissolution in plasma, oxygen then diffuses into the red blood cells, where, after binding to hemoglobin, it can be transported and released to tissues. Concurrently, diffusion of carbon dioxide from the blood also occurs for presentation to and removal from the body in the expired air.

A number of special cells and tissues of the respiratory tract have evolved to protect the delicate tissues of the distal respiratory tract and are critical to homeostasis. The anterior portions of the nose, larynx, trachea, bronchi, and bronchioles are lined by ciliated mucosa. Interspersed between these cells are columnar goblet cells that manufacture and secrete mucus. The cilia and mucus work together in a coordinated fashion to propel particulate material entrained in the mucus away from the lungs. The alveolus itself has walls formed by epithelial cells. Two such cell types have been described, the type I and type II cells. The type I cell is very thin, has a smooth surface, and covers the greatest part of the respiratory epithelium. The type II cell contains numerous microvilli and manufactures and secretes surfactant(s), which, by reducing surface tension at the air–liquid interface of the alveolus, reduces the tendency for alveoli to collapse.

Another major cell type found in the lung is the alveolar macrophage. This is a large, mononucleated cell that functions in part to engulf foreign particulate materials depositing in this region. These cells are very efficient scavengers of inhaled particulate material by the process of phagocytosis and their location on the alveolar surfaces preserves the sterility of the deep lung by keeping inhaled bacteria and particles from accumulating. The function of macrophages can be affected by cytotoxic airborne substances, such as quartz and heavy metals, thereby compromising their ability to protect the lung. This response is not limited to cytotoxic particles; for example, the instillation of 4 mg of carbon particles (considered by some a "nuisance" dust by its relative lack of cytotoxicity) into the lung of a mouse induces a massive macrophage response within a few hours and by 24 h, the number of macrophages increases 10-fold (19). A spectrum of responses, resulting in alterations in macrophage numbers, viability, morphology, and changes in phagocytic capacity, can be produced by chemical insult (20). The effects of inhaled gases and particles on macrophage responses are of major concern because the integrity and function of these pivotal cells are important to the homeostasis of the lung and ultimately, survival. Indeed, some of the pioneering studies of macrophage function describe the injurious effects of gases on macrophage bacteriocidal activity. In these early infectivity models, animals first preexposed to ozone had higher mortality if subsequently exposed to pathogenic bacteria, ostensibly by impairing macrophage phagocytosis and lysosomal enzyme activity (20–22).

Wide variations in respiratory tract anatomy are known to exist among the various mammalian species commonly used as human surrogates for testing or modeling purposes. The nasal cavity of the dog, for example, can be many times longer than that of a human and contains up to 25 turbinates (23); in addition, the nasal cavities of rodents or other laboratory animals are highly convoluted and more complex than those of humans (24,25). Species differences also exist in the structure of the tracheobronchial region. Typically, the branching patterns of the tracheobronchial tree are either monopodal or regular dichotomous. The monopodal pattern is characterized by long tapering airways with asymmetric, smaller lateral branches that leave the main tube at a shallow ($<60^\circ$) angle as seen in cats, dogs, hamsters, horses, mice, monkeys, pigs, rabbits, and rats. In contrast, regular dichotomous branching, typical of humans, involves division of a tube into nearly identical, equal-diameter smaller tubes with approximately equal branching angles. These variations in symmetry of branching, airway diameters and lengths, and number of airway generations become important when considering species differences in the deposition of particles in the respiratory tract.

McLaughlin et al. (26) classified mammalian lungs on the basis of pleural characteristics, such as the presence or absence of respiratory bronchioles and the nature of the blood supply. Lung type I, characterized by a thick pleura, well-developed secondary lobulation, and marked interlobular septa, is found in the cow, pig, and sheep. Lung type II has a very thin pleura, no secondary lobulation, and poorly defined interlobular sepia and is found in the cat, dog, and rhesus monkey. Lung type III, which is found in horses and humans, is intermediate. After considering all the anatomical features and classifications, and recognizing that there are definable differences, the similarities in terms of tissues and functions between humans and other mammals are remarkable.

The functional performance of the respiratory system can be estimated by measurement of lung volume and capacities. Measurement of breathing pattern, lung flows and volumes, lung capacities, forced expirograms, and blood gas and pH are important in determining not only the functional ability of the lung but also the actual dose of chemical received under experimental conditions. Obtaining reliable values for these parameters in many laboratory animals is difficult because of size restrictions and the need for cooperation in maximal effort respiratory maneuvers. The use of masks, mouthpieces, or anesthesia to obtain this information may alter normal breathing patterns. Species such as the dog, horse, and sheep as well as some rodents, have been trained to wear masks, or alternatively, appropriate correction factors have been applied, to describe pulmonary function under normal conditions. A comparison of typical breathing characteristics of a number of commonly studied species is shown in Table 23.2.

Table 23.2
General breathing characteristics of commonly studied species

Species	Mass (g)	Frequency (breaths/min)	Tidal volume (ml)	Minute ventilation (ml)
Human	70,000			
Rest		12	750	9000
Light exercise		17	1700	28,900
Dog	10,000	20	200	3600
Monkey	3000	40	21	840
Guinea pig	500	90	2.0	180
Rat	350	160	1.4	240
Mouse	30	180	0.25	45

Allometric scaling factors ($Y = kM^x$; M in kg)[a]

	Frequency *k*	Frequency *x*	Tidal volume *k*	Tidal volume *x*	Minute ventilation *k*	Minute ventilation *x*
	53.5	−.26	7.69	1.04	411	.78

[a] From Reference 296.

The size and structural complexity of the respiratory tract and the diversity of its response to inhaled toxicants impose strict requirements to properly complete a thorough examination. The anatomic variations in the tract make necessary wide and careful sampling. The nonhomogeneity of response within any given anatomic compartment means that there must be careful sampling of specific sites. This is particularly important for ultrastructural and morphometric evaluations. Further considerations in this area are found in reviews by Dungworth, et al. (27), Pinkerton and Crapo (28), and Schwartz (29).

DEPOSITION AND CLEARANCE OF INHALED TOXICANTS

Gases and Vapors

Inhaled gases and vapors can be absorbed throughout the respiratory tract. Depending largely on their physiochemical characteristics (e.g., concentration, water solubility, partition coefficient) and individual respiratory tract physiological characteristics (e.g., airflow, tissue perfusion, local metabolism), inhaled gases or vapors produce either local injury or systemic toxicity.

The net driving force for absorption of inhaled gases or vapors is diffusion, that is, the net movement of molecules from a region of high concentration to one of lower concentration. Vapor absorption continues until the vapor concentrations in the airspace and tissue are the same. At this point, the system is at equilibrium and no further transport of vapor occurs. However, additional absorption may occur if the absorbed vapor is removed by transport into the bloodstream, metabolism to a different chemical, or chemical reaction with tissue macromolecules. These processes effectively lower the vapor concentration of the chemical in the tissue so that further diffusion into the tissue may again proceed. Conversely, once the vapor concentration is higher in tissue than the inspired air, the net diffusive force is external, that is, from tissue to air. Passive diffusion is the mode by which carbon dioxide, a by-product of aerobic metabolism, is conducted from the tissue to the bloodstream, then to the alveolar airspace, and ultimately removed in the expired breath.

Inhaled gases or vapors may be absorbed directly within the nasal cavity, thereby sparing the lung from direct exposure, although exposing the nose to potentially injurious concentrations of inhaled substances. Vapors may be either physically absorbed within nasal tissues, a reversible process driven in part by the relative solubilities of the vapor in air or tissue, or irreversibly bound to tissue components. Vapors that are highly soluble in aqueous solutions, such as the mucus covering the epithelial surfaces of the upper respiratory tract, generally tend to be absorbed within these regions. Highly water-soluble agents, such as hydrogen fluoride and propylene glycol monomethylether, exhibit nearly complete deposition (39,40), within the nose. In contrast, gases or vapors with low water solubility, such as nitrogen dioxide or methylene chloride, are not well absorbed in the upper respiratory tract but are absorbed deeper in the respiratory tract (41,42). Although applicable for some gases, these generalizations oversimplify respiratory tract vapor absorption, as reliable models of absorption have not yet been developed that are based on simple physical/chemical properties such as water solubility and blood/water-to-air partition coefficients. An additional determinant of vapor absorption is the upper respiratory tract vascular blood flow and tissue metabolism or binding (40,42). Indeed, irreversible binding to nasal tissues may occur if the inhaled vapor is reactive or is metabolized within nasal epithelium, with subsequent formation of covalent bonds with tissue macromolecules.

Although vapors may be absorbed continuously along the respiratory tract, in general, vapors with low chemical reactivity and water solubility bypass the nasal cavity and are transported into the conductive airways. Although vapors may be absorbed in the conducting airways, because gas exchange does not occur in these airways, this region represents a respiratory "dead space," amounting to approximately 30% of the resting tidal volume (i.e., about 150 ml in humans). Once past this dead space, the inhaled vapor may enter the alveolar (gas exchange) region and diffuse across a very thin epithelial or endothelial membrane (typically 0.1 μm thick) into the tissue or blood.

Aerosols

The physical/chemical and aerodynamic properties of the aerosol, the anatomic characteristics of the respiratory tract, and the breathing pattern are the major determinants of aerosol deposition. As will be noted later, aerosols have intrinsic physical properties (e.g., size, density, shape) that govern their aerodynamic behavior. The interaction between the individual's respiration pattern and respiratory tract anatomy and the aerodynamic properties of the aerosol dictate the amounts and sites of aerosol deposition. Breathing pattern characteristics affect deposition through changes in breathing rate (with its attendant effect on air velocity through the airways), tidal volume, inspiratory capacity, distribution within conducting airways, and breath-holding. The anatomy of the nasal, oral, and pharyngeal areas; nasal hairs; dimensions and geometry of the conducting airways from the nasal turbinates to the lower respiratory tract; the size and shape of openings throughout the tract; and mucus distribution further define the respiratory tract characteristics that govern particle deposition.

Some description of the physical characteristics of aerosols is necessary to understand particle deposition. Particle size is the single most important determinant of aerosol deposition. Because "size" may be expressed as either some physical attribute (e.g., measured physical diameter) or its aerodynamic size, it must be clearly specified to avoid confusion. Particle size may be reported based on several physical attributes such as diameter, length, light scattering properties, surface area, volume, number, or electrical charge. Although particle number or surface area may be better correlated in some cases with toxicity, it is aerosol mass that is most often associated with particle toxicity and thus represents the most important physical attribute of the particle size population.

As particles are rarely of uniform size (or mass), a description of the particle population's average size and uniformity is needed. By convention, particles are defined by their median size (e.g., mass median diameter) and a measure of the variability of particle sizes (e.g., geometric standard deviation, GSD). The lognormal distribution most commonly describes particle size data from most inhalation studies, although Gaussian and bimodal or multimodal distributions may better describe the size characteristics of some aerosols, especially mixtures. Lognormal particle distributions are described completely by their median diameter and geometric standard deviation.

Lognormal particle populations are visualized readily if the frequency or mass of particles with a given size (measured either with size selective atmospheric samplers, such as the impactor cut point, or physical diameters; both in μm) is plotted against the measured particle size using linear axes. Using representative data from a six-stage cascade impactor (Table 23.3), cut points for each impactor stage are plotted against the aerosol mass collected on each stage (Figure 23.4A); the resulting distribution curve is typically skewed. If the data are replotted using a logarithmic scale for particle size (impactor cut point), a symmetric normal distribution curve is produced (Figure 23.4B). By replotting the same data, but expressing the frequency as the cumulative percentage of particles less than a given size (such as the impactor cut point), again using a log-

Table 23.3
Cascade impactor data

Impactor stage	Impactor cut point (Dpc) (μm)	Aerosol mass per stage (mg)	% Mass per stage	Cumulative mass < Dpc
1	9	0.08	0.6	99.4
2	5.1	0.90	7.3	92.1
3	3	2.96	24.0	68.1
4	1.6	4.50	36.5	31.6
5	0.9	3.18	25.8	5.8
6	0.4	0.70	5.7	0.2
Final	0	0.02	0.2	0.0

arithmic scale for particle size, a relatively linear central region with curvilinear tails is obtained (Figure 23.4C). A straight line results if the cumulative mass data on the abscissa are transformed and graphed using a probability scale for the cumulative frequency (Figure 23.4D). The mass median diameter (MMD) may be read directly from this plot and it represents the size where 50% of the particles are larger (or smaller) than the median size. The GSD (σ_g) is simply derived from the lognormal data as follows:

$$\sigma_g = \frac{\text{size at 84.1\% mass}}{\text{size at 50\% mass}} \text{ or } \frac{\text{size at 50\% mass}}{\text{size at 15.9\% mass}}$$

A particle population with uniform size (i.e., all the particles comprising the aerosol are relatively uniform in size) is referred to as monodisperse and has σ_g values less than approximately 1.2. In contrast, a polydisperse particle population encompasses a broad range of particle sizes and has σ_g values greater than approximately 1.8.

The simplest aerosols have spherical shapes and may also be characterized by their physical diameter; generally this attribute is measured by either optical or scanning electron microscopy techniques. Using the same graphic method of presentation as described above, using the number of particles as a function of a given size, the count median diameter and GSD of a particle population may be determined. For a given lognormal distribution, the mean mass-, surface area-, or volume-equivalent diameters of these spheres may be calculated according to the equations developed by Hatch and Choate (43). The interrelationships between mass median diameter, surface area mean diameter, volume mean diameter, and count median diameter may be calculated knowing one of these values and the distribution's geometric standard deviation.

Most aerosols however, are not simple spheres and exist in various and often complex shapes. Indeed, aerosols may be fibrous (defined as particles with length-to-width ratios greater than 3), globular, flake, crystal-like, or irregular agglomerates. The "size" of these aerosols, although again dependent on diameter, is more difficult to characterize based solely on physical diameter. However, the nonspherical shape of these aerosols may be accounted for if the "size" of these aerosols is expressed as the aerodynamic equivalent diameter (AED), defined as the diameter of a spherical particle of unit density (1 g/ml), which has the same terminal settling velocity as the particle in question. The AED accounts for differences in the shape, size, mass, density, and aerodynamic drag of particles with different shapes and is used as a means for comparing the dynamic behavior of different aerosols. This aerodynamic property is advantageously utilized in some of the particle sizing equipment frequently used in inhalation toxicology experimentation (refer to Table 23.13).

Fibers

A special type of aerosol, and one of increasing significance to human health, is fibers. Because of the association of naturally occurring (e.g., asbestos and erionite) and man-made synthetic fibers with the development of pulmonary carcinogenesis and fibrosis in humans (44), interest in the pulmonary hazards of inhaled fibers has heightened. Toxicologists today have identified major differences in the nature and persistence of lung injury based on fiber composition, fiber durability (a factor determining biological persistence in the lung), fiber size (another factor governing fiber penetration and reactivity into the lung), and fiber exposure concentration.

For the purposes of describing the physical dimensions of fibers of toxicological concern, general size characteristics of fibers have emerged from both animal and occupational exposure studies. In the animal studies, a variety of particle types and dimensions were instilled or injected into the pleura or abdominal cavities (45–48). Although these methods of fiber introduction into the body are artificial and by no means reflective of normal exposure pathways (in terms of both the rate and location of fiber deposition and quantitative aspects of the cellular response), this early research provided fundamental insights into the physical bases for the biological reactivity of fibers. Based on this work, a general relationship between the fiber dimension and tumor response emerged. Notably, Stanton and Wrench (48) found that intrapleural sarcomas were likely to develop upon fiber exposure and occurred with the highest potency if the implanted fibers were >8 μm in length and had diameters

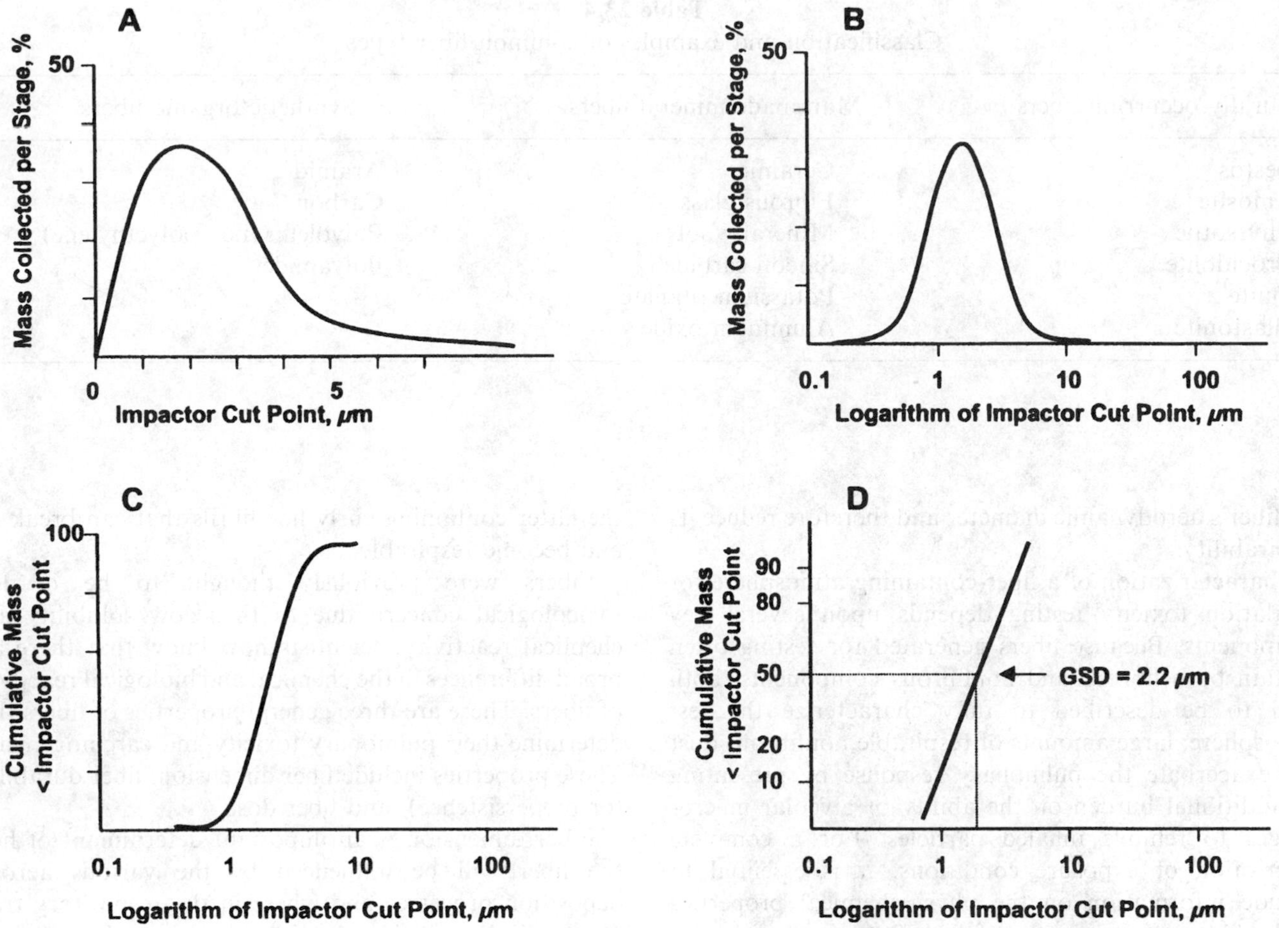

FIG. 23.4. A: Cascade impactor data from Table 23.3 plotted on arithmetic axes. B, Size distribution data from A, replotted using logarithmic scale for impactor cut point. C, Size distribution data from B, replotted using cumulative mass less than cut point diameter. D, Size distribution data from C, replotted using probability scale for cumulative mass. Geometric standard deviation is 2.2 μm.

of <1.5 μm. In contrast, nonfibrous preparations of these same materials had a much less severe pulmonary response (49). Walton (50) has suggested that asbestos fibers >5–10 μm in length and <1.5–2 μm in diameter, with an aspect ratio (length-to-width ratio) of >5, are most hazardous. A considerable body of evidence has accumulated supporting the hypothesis that fibers that are especially long and thin present the greatest health hazard. Recognizing that there are not necessarily clear distinctions between fiber dimension and pathogenicity, the U.S. Environmental Protection Agency has defined a fiber as a particle with a length of >5 μm and an aspect ratio of at least 3 (51).

In terms of respirability, the diameter, length, and shape of fibers are key determinants of deposition. Fiber diameter is recognized as the most important factor in determining fiber respirability; the thinner the fiber, the more respirable and penetrating it becomes for the lung. The probability of fiber impaction and sedimentation is governed by the aerodynamic diameters of the fibers, which is approximately three times their physical diameter (52–54). In humans, aerosols with limited deposition in the lung are considered around 10 μm aerodynamic diameter so that fibers with actual diameters exceeding about 3.5 μm are nonrespirable; conversely, fibers with diameters under 3.5 μm but which are very long (50–100 μm) are highly respirable. Timbrell and Skidmore (54) showed that finite limits exist for fiber respirability so that fibers with lengths exceeding about 200 μm and diameters greater than about 3.5 μm would not penetrate the airways and deposit in distal alveoli to a significant amount. This generalization does not readily apply to nonstraight fibers as any curvature, bends, or twists in the fiber would necessarily increase

Table 23.4
Classification and examples of common fiber types

Naturally occurring fibers	Man-made mineral fibers	Synthetic organic fibers
Asbestos	Ceramic	Aramid
Amosite	Fibrous glass	Carbon
Chyrsotile	Mineral wool	Polyolefin (i.e., polyethylene)
Crocidolite	Silicon carbide	Polyamide
Erionite	Potassium titanate	
Wollastonite	Aluminum oxide	

the fiber's aerodynamic diameter and therefore reduce its respirability.

Characterization of a fiber-containing atmosphere for inhalation toxicity testing depends upon several key components. Because fibers generated for testing often contain both fibrous and nonfibrous components, both need to be described to fully characterize the test atmosphere; large amounts of respirable nonfibrous dust can exacerbate the pulmonary response by presenting an additional burden on the ability of alveolar macrophages to remove inhaled particles. For a complete description of exposure conditions, it is essential to include information on the physiochemical properties of the fiber, measurements of aerodynamic particle size and mass, and expression of fiber concentrations as count, length, and width distributions per unit volume of air.

There are three general fiber categories, based on their origin. These include naturally occurring fibers, man-made synthetic mineral fibers, and synthetic organic fibers (Table 23.4). The most well known and studied naturally occurring fiber is asbestos, which has been grouped into serpentine asbestos (e.g., chrysotile, a hydrated magnesium silicate) and amphibole asbestos (e.g., amosite and crocidolite, both hydrated metal silicates). The surface morphology of the two are very distinct; whereas chrysotile is a curly fiber comprised of fibrillar subunits, amosite fibers have a straight, rodlike structure. Of the man-made mineral fibers, fibrous glass is perhaps the most studied. Unlike the naturally occurring fibers, fibrous glass doesn't possess a crystalline structure. They are produced by drawing molten glass through an orifice, and yield very fine diameter fibers typically 3–10 μm in diameter, with some as fine as 1 μm. The synthetic organic fibers are becoming commercially more prevalent, with some having high tensile strength and chemical and flame resistance. Aramid fibers, for example, have been used as asbestos replacements. These exist as either a continuous filament or as pulped material, the latter containing curly fine fibrils that can break off and become respirable.

Fibers were previously thought to be of low toxicological concern due to their low solubility and chemical reactivity, scientists now know that there are broad differences in the chemical and biological reactivity of fibers. There are three general properties of fibers that determine their pulmonary toxicity and carcinogenicity. These properties include fiber dimension, fiber durability (or biopersistence), and fiber dose.

Fiber dimension is an important determinant of how the fiber will be influenced by the various aerosol deposition processes and where in the respiratory tract fibers will deposit (just as with other aerosols, the deposition site will impact bioavailability of the fiber due to site-dependent processes responsible for facilitating fiber clearance). Fiber diameter has already been noted to be the most important factor for fiber respirability with fiber length having a comparatively minor influence. In general, fibers with lengths longer than 200 μm and diameters wider than ~ 3 μm are considered to be the upper boundaries for fiber penetration to the deep lung in humans. An early clue to the importance of fiber length in the pathogenicity of inhaled fibers was the observation of Stanton and Wrench (48) that fibers, regardless of composition, longer than about 8 μm were associated with the development of mesothelial tumors. Coincidentally, the lymphatic stromata of this region have the same approximate dimension, offering a possible anatomic explanation for why fibers might be retained in the mesothelium. In addition, when fibers are larger than alveolar macrophages (about 10–20 μm), they can no longer be readily engulfed and subsequently cleared, thereby enhancing fiber retention and increasing the potential for adverse pulmonary response. Besides fiber dimension, other factors can influence deposition; notably, those factors that change aerodynamic size, including fiber density, shape, and orientation of the fiber within the airstream, will also affect deposition sites and amounts.

Fiber durability is another critical determinant of fiber toxicity and it is believed that fibers that biopersist in the lung or other organs of the body represent the greatest health concern. Thus, those properties of a fiber that impart a chemical or mechanical resistance to fiber disintegration or fragmentation in the lung will tend to prolong its persistence and therefore increase the potential for causing potentially adverse biochemical/pathological responses in the target tissue. This property of fibers to disintegrate in tissues was first noted when natural and man-made fibers of different compositions were found to have different toxicological properties and lung retention characteristics (55–57). Investigators found lower residual concentrations of some fibers in chronically exposed lungs than expected based on the exposure concentration of fibers and in general, this correlated with a less severe spectrum of pulmonary pathological effects (58). Indeed, a sizeable body of data has accumulated relating the biological effects of inhaled fibers not so much to their composition but rather to their durability and resistance to disintegration in the lung (59).

There are two general pathways by which fiber degradation may proceed. In the first, the fiber dissolves and is completely solubilized within the lung milieu. In the second, the physical dimensions of the fiber (either diameter or length) may be altered by the action of lung fluids on the fiber surface. If solubilization alters the mechanical integrity of the fiber such that the fiber breaks along its longitudinal axis, both the dimensions and number of subsequent fibers change. Notably, by breaking, an additional fiber or particle is produced and the overall length of the fiber is reduced; this can result in facilitated clearance, especially if the fiber fragments are now of a size that may be readily engulfed and removed from the lung by macrophages. Conversely, some fiber types are especially prone to mechanical disruption, releasing more fibers. Chrysotile asbestos deposited in the lung, for example, may split longitudinally, releasing numerous fine fibrils and increasing the lung fiber burden as demonstrated by Bellmann et al. (60). Dissolution processes that only affect particle diameter are less effective in reducing the likelihood of adverse lung effects, because the particle is essentially unchanged in overall size and its ability to be cleared from the lung. The various factors influencing fiber durability has been reviewed by Searl (61) and experimental methods for the evaluation of fiber solubility in vitro and in vivo has been reviewed by Hesterberg et al. (58,62).

Experimental demonstration of fiber degradation in the lung has been reported by measuring fiber dimensions recovered from the lungs of animals. Techniques vary, but predominant lung digestion methods utilize either thermal or microwave ashing techniques, chemical digestion with strong alkali, and oxidizing agents (63,64). It is imperative to determine the effects of the lung digestion method on the fibers alone to ensure that artefactual reductions in fiber size or number do not occur. This consideration may be bypassed with in situ observations of fiber dimensions by using histological techniques and scanning/transmission electron microscopy (65).

Fine and Ultrafine Particles

Most of the above descriptions of the physical properties of fibrous or particulate aerosols center around relatively coarse particles, approximately 1–10 μm (AED). These particles are of general toxicological relevance because they are of a size range produced by many commonly encountered mechanical processes (e.g., grinding, spraying, etc.), but more importantly are able to penetrate and deposit throughout the respiratory tract (Figure 23.5). However, a growing interest in the health hazards of fine ($\sim$0.1–1 μm) and ultrafine ($<$0.1 μm) particles (UFP) is emerging based on scientific data showing increased pulmonary toxicity in rodents and epidemiological data linking the fine particle modes with acute morbidity and mortality in humans. More information on the toxicological hazards of these particles is discussed in the section on Ultrafine Particle Effects.

UFP are formed by high temperature processes that create an atmosphere saturated with the vapor of the test material or its degradation products (refer to Figure 23.5). A common example of UFP is the metal oxide combustion fumes produced during welding. Once below the substance's vapor saturation point for ambient conditions, the vapors can condense on molecular clusters, forming nucleation sites (condensation nuclei). Upon condensing, high number concentrations of these ultrafine primary particles may be created. UFP are characterized by an extremely small particle size, typically 1–100 nm (1–100 $\times$ 10^{-9} m) in diameter. Given their small size, UFP have vanishingly low masses but have relatively high surface areas with respect to their mass. Although combustion processes may produce particle number concentrations of 10^8–10^9 particles per cubic centimeter of air (p/cm^3) or more, the physical process of coagulation (agglomeration of primary particles) renders such aerosols unstable. Because the distance between these particles is very small, individual particles readily collide with and adhere to other particles, rapidly forming a particle cluster of much larger size (often up to several micrometers diameter) known as a chain agglomerate; soot is a visible example of such chain agglomerates. Because agglomeration is proportional to the square of the particle concentration, UFP at a low number concentration remain stable indefinitely, whereas a high number

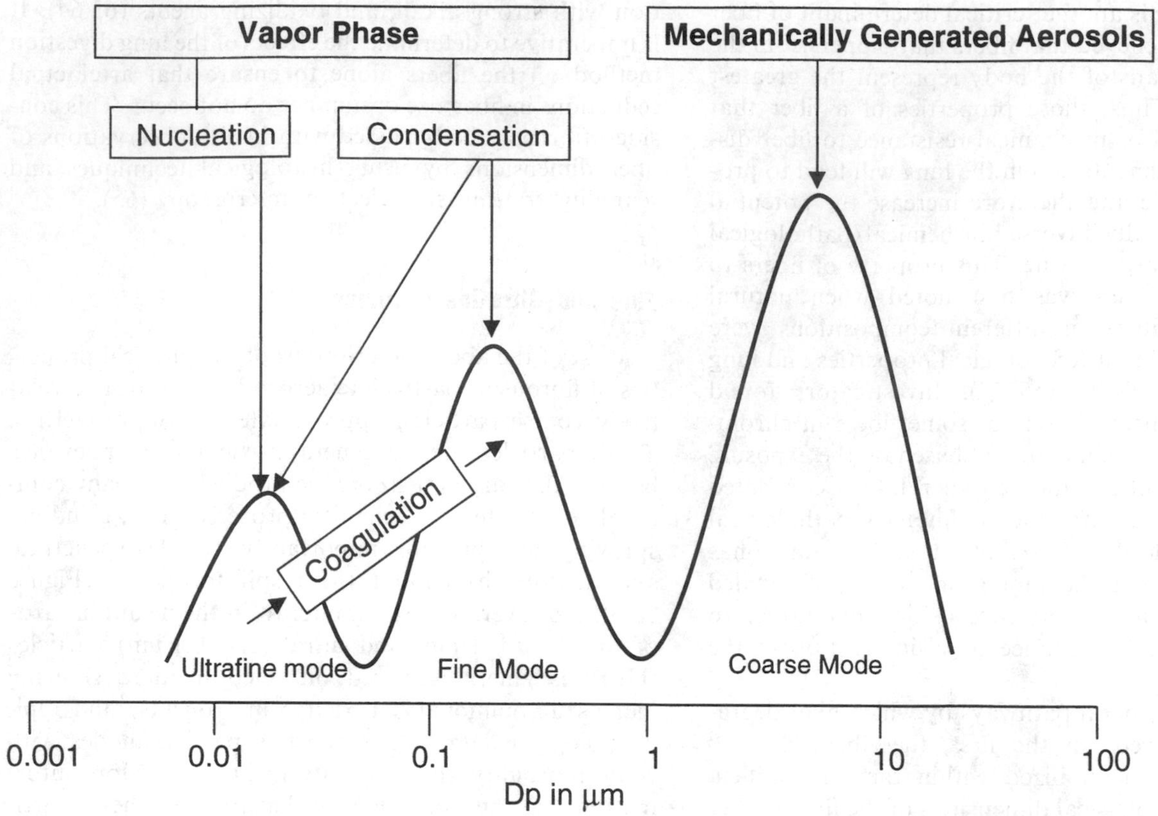

FIG. 23.5. Particle size regimes and formation mechanisms for aerosols. Adapted from References 66 and 67.

concentration of UFP will rapidly agglomerate in a time scale measured in milliseconds to minutes. For example, the time required to reduce the initial particle concentration by half due to particle coagulation is estimated to be around 0.2 s for 10^{10} p/cm^3, 20 s for 10^8 p/cm^3, and 33 min for 10^6 p/ cm^3. This topic is more thoroughly covered in general reference books on aerosol technology (68,69).

Deposition Processes

Enroute to the lungs, inhaled air follows a tortuous pathway. Inspired air has a relatively high velocity in the nose and follows the convoluted pathways of the upper respiratory tract. Once in the conducting airways, air velocity has moderated, but the airstream must change direction frequently as it flows into and out of a series of bifurcating airways. Finally, in the pulmonary region, air velocity has slowed greatly because the total cross-sectional airway area increases with each additional airway bifurcation. Different deposition mechanisms exist within each of these regions and are influenced by the aerodynamic diameter of the aerosol, breathing characteristics, and respiratory tract anatomy. These deposition mechanisms are shown schematically in Figure 23.6 and include sedimentation, impaction, interception, and diffusion.

1. *Impaction.* When airflow changes direction, the inertia of any suspended particle will cause it to continue in its original direction for some finite time before changing direction. Thus impaction occurs when the inertial characteristics of the particles are such that they cannot follow the airstream. The particles depart from the airstream and impact the airway surface downstream from the directional change. Impaction is dependent on the velocity and angular change in the airstream direction, particle density, and the aerosol diameter squared. Impaction is the predominant deposition mechanism for particles larger than 1 μm and in regions of the respiratory tract where air velocities are high and airstream directional changes are abrupt.
2. *Sedimentation.* Particles suspended in a gas will slowly settle under the influence of gravity. The speed at which particles settle is proportional to the density of the particle and its diameter squared. Sedimentation is also an important deposition mechanism for particles larger than 1 μm and in

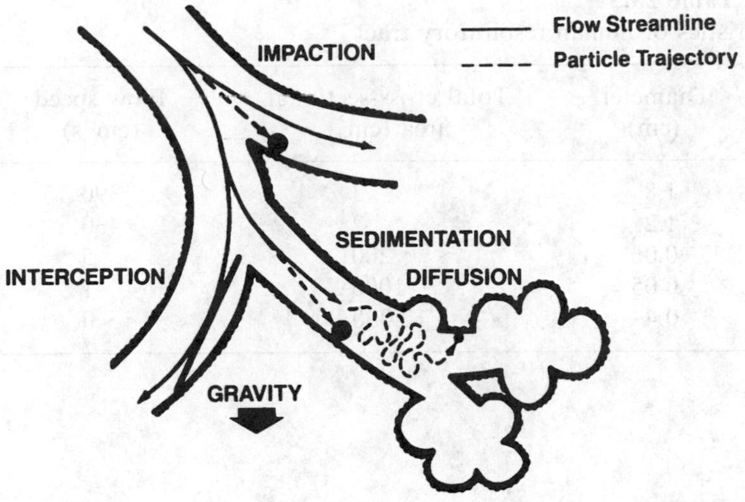

FIG. 23.6. Mechanisms of particle deposition.

regions of the respiratory tract where air velocity is low, particle residence times are high, and airway diameters are small.

3. *Interception.* Interception occurs when the trajectory of the particles brings them sufficiently close to airway walls such that the particle contacts the airway wall. Interception is an important deposition mechanism for fibers, especially for fibers with higher aspect ratios (i.e., length to width). These longer fibers will have a greater chance of airway contact compared to those with lower aspect ratios. Fibers normally align themselves with the airflow; however, when airflow direction suddenly changes such as where airways branch, fiber deposition can occur at the transition, that is, the ridge where the airways diverge. Interception increases as airway turbulence increases and as airway diameter decreases.
4. *Brownian diffusion.* The gas molecules that surround aerosols continuously bombard these airborne particles, inducing random particle movement. This process is inversely proportional to particle diameter but is independent of their density. Diffusion is not an important deposition mechanism for particles larger than about 0.5 μm but represents the major mode of particle deposition in the alveoli where airflow is low. Diffusion may occur throughout the respiratory tract.

Physiological and anatomic factors also influence aerosol deposition. Air may be inhaled through the nose, mouth, or both. Air entering the nose must flow through a series of convoluted passages. Compared to humans, the nasal passages in rodents are more complex and tortuous (70), resulting in comparatively higher particle deposition in the nose of rodents than humans. In contrast, mouth breathing effectively bypasses the nasal particle deposition processes and results in a higher proportion of particles that may reach the lower respiratory tract.

The branching pattern of the tracheobronchial tree influences airflow dynamics and the amount and location of particle deposition in three fundamental ways. First, the diameter of the conducting airways becomes progressively smaller with each successive division. In humans, the major bronchi have diameters of about 1 cm whereas bronchioles and alveolar ducts are about 1 mm in diameter. Thus the chances of particle deposition in a given period of time due to diffusion or sedimentation are much higher in smaller airways because aerosols have a greater chance of contacting airway walls in this area. The probability of particle deposition by these two mechanisms increases the farther the particle travels into the respiratory tract. Second, the total number of airways increases with each airway branch. Although the airway branches become progressively smaller, the number of such airways is so great that the total cross-sectional area increases. A given volume of air thus moves more and more slowly as it enters the deep lung (Table 23.5). Third, variations in airway branching patterns can have considerable effect on the amount of particle deposition. In humans, for example, the branching pattern is dichotomous (symmetrical) whereas in rodents the branching pattern is monopodal (asymmetric). The flow in dichotomous airways is highest toward the airway centerline and results in localized areas of particle deposition, primarily at bifurcations due to the higher velocity around the centerline, favoring deposition by impaction and local turbulence. In contrast, little change in either airstream direction or velocity occurs in animals with monopodal branching patterns because the branching angle of the daughter airways is much

Table 23.5
Generalized characteristics of human respiratory tract

Respiratory region	Number	Diameter (cm)	Total cross-sectional area (cm^2)	Flow speed (cm/s)
Trachea	1	1.8	3	390
Main bronchus	2	1.2	2	430
Terminal bronchioles	60,000	0.06	200	5
Respiratory bronchioles	500,000	0.05	1000	1
Alveoli	8,000,000	0.4	12,000	~0

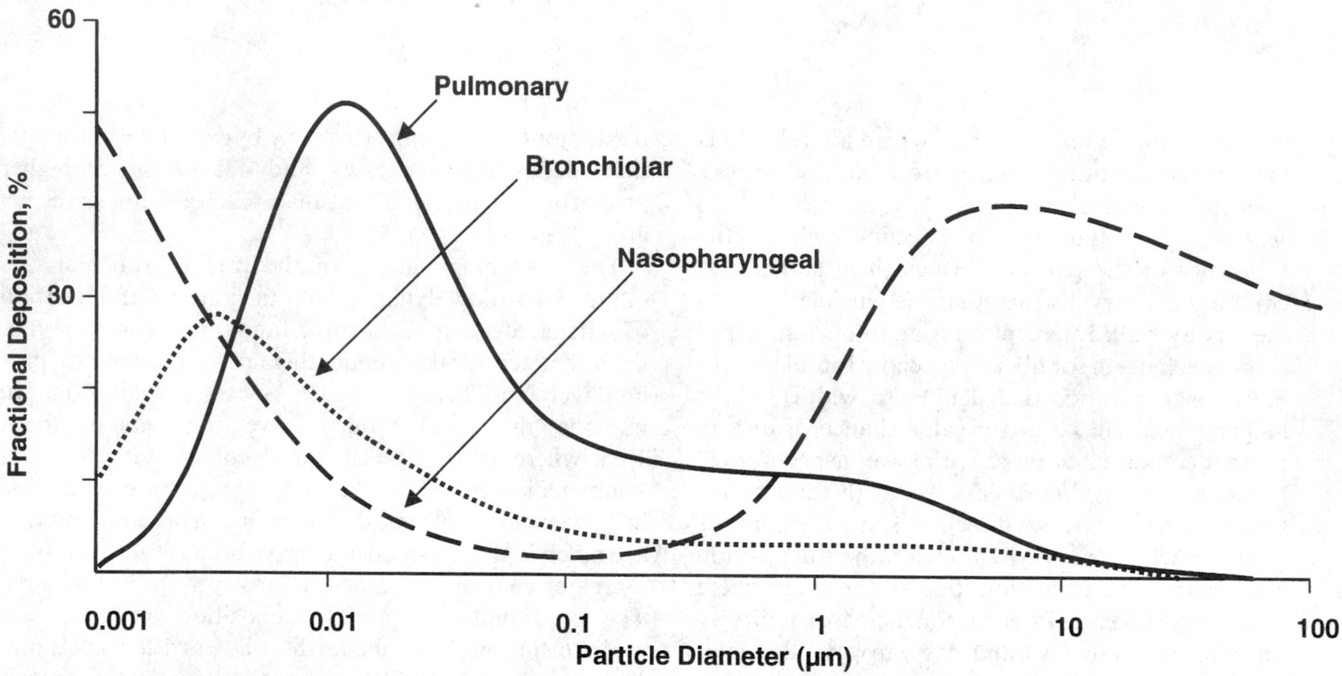

FIG. 23.7. ICRP model of aerosol regional deposition with indicated aerodynamic diameter.

shallower compared to dichotomous branching. As a consequence, relatively lower particle deposition occurs in animals with monopodal compared to dichotomous branching.

Quantitative particle deposition studies have been conducted in both humans and animals by numerous investigators. Due to the variability in the experimental techniques, airway anatomy, and physiological characteristics of individuals, however, aerosol deposition models for humans have not been defined precisely. Nevertheless, a widely cited model was developed by the International Commission on Radiologic Protection (ICRP) (71) for regional aerosol deposition in humans (Figure 23.7). This model has been found to be in general agreement with experimental deposition data for humans (72). Although the latest ICRP aerosol deposition model includes several improvements over previous ICRP models, such as accounting for oral and nasal cavity deposition and deposition of UFP, the model still represents "average" deposition behavior and cannot fully describe the range of regional particle deposition due to intersubject variability.

The collective deposition data for humans show that deposition in the respiratory tract is at a minimum with approximately 0.3–0.5 μm (AED) aerosols. Particles in this size range are minimally affected by Brownian diffusion, sedimentation, and impaction processes and consequently are mostly expired. However, total deposition increases markedly with aerosols either larger or smaller than those at the deposition minimum. With smaller particle sizes, diffusion dominates the deposition process so that particles in the ultrafine size range behave aerodynamically similarly to gas molecules. In addition, diffusion is not affected by particle density so that aerodynamic diameters do not apply to UFP. Although actual deposition data for UFP in the various compartments of the respiratory tract are scarce, modeling studies indicate that UFP have very high deposition efficiencies in the alveolar region of the lung; recent predictions suggest lung deposition as much as 50% for 10 = nm particles in humans (73). Interestingly, studies by Cheng et al. (74,75) and Swift et al. (76) show that ultrafine aerosols (<0.2 μm) do not preferentially target the lower respiratory tract, but can have relatively high nasal deposition efficiency. In this work, upper airway and nasal deposition was found to increase markedly when particles <0.2 μm were tested. For very small UFP (below 2 nm), deposition in the nose was found to predominate, with deposition approaching 80%, presumably via a turbulent diffusional mechanism. As described earlier, UFP can have relatively short atmospheric lifetimes because UFP may agglomerate, growing in size to a fine particle size regime (~1 μm diameter). In addition to their comparatively lower biological activity, these agglomerates would not present as high an exposure burden in the respiratory tract as primarily UFP because the deposition processes of diffusion and sedimentation are not very efficient in the 0.1–1 μm size range. In comparison with model data for humans, ultrafine aerosol deposition was predicted to be approximately 20%–30% higher in rats (75). Aerosols larger than about 0.5 μm deposit predominantly in the nasopharyngeal region by impaction and/or interception processes. In general, however, particles larger than approximately 30–80 μm are not inhalable through the nose (77). Yet when mouth breathing, a somewhat different deposition pattern emerges. It has been shown that the inhalable particle diameter when mouth breathing may increase and total deposition decreases with particles greater than 0.2 μm compared to nose breathing due to the higher collection efficiency of particles within the nose. For the same size aerosol, the net effect of nose breathing is to lower the total amount of aerosol available for delivery to the lung relative to mouth breathing.

Aerosol deposition has also been investigated in experimental animals (78,79). Due to differences in respiratory tract anatomy and physiological factors, the doses of inhaled particulate matter to the various regions of the respiratory tract will differ among species. In the upper respiratory tract, total aerosol deposition is minimal in most species between approximately 0.5 and 1 μm. The nasal deposition profile with increasing particle size is similar among dogs and humans, although the amount deposited in the nose is lower in dogs compared to humans. The data also suggest that the human nose has a higher deposition efficiency than rodents for particles greater than 1 μm. Given the anatomic complexity of the rat nose, this unexpected observation may result from the experimental conditions used (i.e., decreased inertial impaction in rodents from an anesthesia-related reduction in breathing rate and airflow velocity). In the tracheobronchial region, deposition among test animals is minimal but relatively constant with 0.1–5-μm particles; by comparison, deposition efficiency in humans is generally higher than dogs or rodents. In the pulmonary region, aerosol deposition is similar for rats and hamsters, but is considerably lower than for humans and dogs; alveolar deposition efficiencies for dogs and nasal-breathing humans are comparable. Although peak deposition efficiencies in animals occur with about 1–2-μm aerosols, most alveolar deposition in humans occurs with approximately 2–4-μm particles.

Overall, the relative deposition efficiencies within various portions of the human and nonhuman respiratory tract are quite similar, with somewhat lower deposition efficiencies for rodents compared to humans. However, when differences in lung size, body size, and ventilation rates are considered, smaller animals inhaling an aerosol with a given size and the same atmospheric concentration will receive a greater dose (for a given exposure time) per unit of lung or body weight than humans. For particles of approximately 1 μm in diameter, the rat can be expected to get a dose roughly 5–10 times, and the dog about 3 times, that of humans on a per unit lung mass basis (80).

The practical implications of aerosol size in inhalation toxicology centers on the need to generate an aerosol respirable for the species under investigation. The aerosol generation system, connecting ductwork, and exposure chamber conditions must be evaluated and optimized, if necessary, so that particles of respirable size are produced and delivered to the animals; there is no point in conducting inhalation toxicity studies where the particles are nonrespirable. For rodents, two general schools of thought have emerged. For acute studies, the goal is to expose animals to an aerosol that can deposit throughout the respiratory tract and without selective deposition in any one area. The objective in this case is to ensure that every anatomic compartment of the respiratory tract has some exposure to the test substance. In this way, potentially sensitive elements of the upper and lower respiratory tract receive a portion of the inhaled test substance. This topic was investigated by an ad hoc group with the recommendation that for acute studies, aerosols with a 1–4 μm mass median aerodynamic diameter which deposit in both upper and lower portions of the rat respiratory tract be used (81). This recommendation was based on the fact that because aerosols may be toxic to specific anatomic regions (i.e., the nose), testing should not be conducted with aerosols having a size range that might preclude deposition at other, perhaps more sensitive, tissue sites. Therefore to maximize the likelihood of detecting an adverse response when testing a material of unknown toxicity, it was recommended that aerosols be tested in a range that would deposit throughout the respiratory tract for acute toxicity studies. On the other hand, for subchronic or chronic inhalation studies, the emphasis is on detecting functional or pathological changes in the respiratory tract such as alterations in lung clearance, pulmonary function, or chronic disease (fibrosis or cancer). Thus, with consideration to detecting adverse lung effects in repeated-exposure inhalation studies, a comparatively smaller size aerosol (i.e., 1–3 μm) is recommended for testing (82).

Ultrafine Particle Effects

There is increasing toxicological interest in the mechanisms and potential health impacts of fine particle inhalation. This interest is based on two general, but widely researched, observations linking first the very fine particle fraction with an exacerbation of pulmonary injury compared to larger particles and second, epidemiological studies reporting associations between low ambient particle concentrations and sickness and deaths in elderly populations.

Experimentally, very fine particles have been observed to produce a more severe pulmonary response compared to larger particles of the same material. Oberdoerster et al. (83) described differences in the inflammatory response between fine (0.25 μm) and ultrafine (0.02 μm) TiO_2 particles following instillation in rat lungs. Only the instillation of the ultrafine TiO_2 produced inflammatory changes described as an increase in total number of cells recovered, primarily polymorphonuclear leukocytes, and increased protein in the bronchial lavage fluid. Similar studies showed that release of pro-inflammatory mediators might be exaggerated following exposure to UFP. Driscoll and Maurer (84), for example, showed that ultrafine (0.02 μm) TiO_2 produced a greater number of alveolar macrophages and polymorphonuclear leukocytes, as well as an increase in inflammatory cytokines in lavage fluid, and increased interstitial inflammation and collagen compared to fine (0.3 μm) TiO_2. These authors have also reported that the pulmonary burden of ultrafine TiO_2 was greater than the equivalent mass of fine TiO_2. Taken together, these authors have offered that UFP, even those of inherently low cytotoxicity and solubility like TiO_2, have greater pulmonary inflammatory activity and toxicity than larger particles through one or more processes. The plausibility that UFP are comparatively more reactive and toxic to the lung has received some support from the work with UFP from the combustion of the perfluoropolymer, polytetrafluoroethylene. Studies begun by Waritz and Kwon (85) and later pursued by Seidel et al. (86), Warheit et al. (87), and Oberdoerster et al. (88) indicated that exposure to freshly generated polytetrafluoroethylene UFP (approximately 30 nm diameter) was lethal to rats at aerosol concentrations of approximately 100 $\mu g/m^3$ (approximately 1×10^6 particles/cm^3 in 30 min); conversely, allowing the aerosol to age for 5 min significantly reduced toxicity, ostensibly by allowing the particles to agglomerate to a larger size (86). Although there is no exposure to perfluoropolymer UFP in ambient air, studies with such particles provide a tool to explore mechanistic bases to the possible activity of UFP in the lung. Overall, the various hypotheses proposed suggest that: UFP are comparatively more reactive, perhaps by their comparatively greater surface area and larger particle concentration per unit of aerosol mass; and may be more toxic by either translocating more rapidly through the epithelium and into the interstitium (89); by causing greater impairment of alveolar macrophage clearance processes (90); or by enhancing activation of alveolar macrophages to release inflammatory mediators (91).

In the early 1990s, a series of epidemiological studies were conducted that described associations between the levels of ambient particulate matter and the incidence and severity of health effects in humans (92–98). Although UFP were not specifically monitored, the association of adverse health outcomes with aerosol size was generally stronger with fine particle modes (< 2.5 μm) than coarser (10 μm) particles (94,98). Specifically, these epidemiology studies indicated that inhalation of particles less than 10 μm in diameter (PM-10) at levels below the federally established ambient air quality standard of 150 $\mu g/m^3$ (24 h average), was associated with increased daily mortality. Other workers have also found an association between PM-10 inhalation and increased hospital admissions and emergency room visits for respiratory distress (99), increased incidence of asthma attacks (100), increased use of asthma medications (101), and reduced pulmonary function (101). Where deaths were reported, they were primarily in those individuals whose health status was compromised, that is, people typically over 60 years old and with preexisting cardiovascular and/or chronic pulmonary diseases. Interestingly, the data did not suggest that ambient particle concentrations were a cause of death among healthy individuals. The severity of the health effects also differed among the cities evaluated, suggesting that the physiochemical properties of the aerosol at a given location impacts the shape of the exposure response curve (102). Although these epidemiological findings suggest an association of adverse health effects with the inhalation of ambient fine particle matter based on statistical relationships, epidemiological studies alone do not prove causality; although the inferential data may be compelling, they cannot discount other possible mechanisms or copollutants not evaluated in these reports (103).

What also makes these epidemiological observations so intriguing is that acute health effects are reported to occur below current regulatory standards, sparking debate over whether and to what extent the standard should be reduced. More importantly, scientists question what mechanism(s) would be invoked to explain health effects at such low levels. Several hypotheses have been forwarded although none have been sufficiently evaluated to fully describe all reported health effects. These include (a) reduced integrity of the pulmonary epithelial and/or endothelial barriers; (b) impaired pulmonary host defense mechanisms; (c) release of inflammatory mediators to produce either local or systemic effects; (d) impaired particle clearance with airway hypersecretion of mucus; (e) aggravation of preexisting airway occlusion; and (f) direct or indirect effects on cardiovascular function.

Biological Mechanisms of Particle Injury

There are several mechanisms whereby inhaled particles can impair the integrity of the pulmonary epithelial barrier and injure the respiratory tract (30). In one, deposited particles are directly cytotoxic, causing the transudation of serum proteins from alveolar capillaries. The mechanism whereby this occurs may involve peroxidation of membrane lipids by free radical, resulting in defects in membrane integrity and, function, and subsequently, cell death. If injury is sufficiently severe, the airways and alveoli fill with fluid, causing pulmonary edema and ultimately death. The source of these radicals may be membrane-based oxidases (31).

Some metal containing particles, especially those that either contain or can complex the ferric form (Fe^{+3}) of iron, are particularly active in inducing membrane peroxidation through a reduction–oxidation pathway, producing hydroxyl radical ($OH^{\cdot}$)(32); inclusion of chelators markedly reduces the oxidant-generating capacity of the particles (33). In a second, related mechanism, particles can activate pulmonary alveolar macrophages, stimulating the release of such reactive oxidant species (ROS) as hydrogen peroxide (H_2O_2), superoxide anion (O_2^-), or hydroxyl radical. These radicals may cause either direct tissue injury or genetic damage. A variety of metal-containing dusts have been shown to stimulate production of ROS from macrophages (34), with iron being among the most active metals, whereas other metal dusts such as titanium dioxide are either inactive or minimally active (35–37). Interestingly, oxidant production may also degrade cellular inhibitor proteins, activating nuclear transcription factor nuclear factor kappa B (NF-κB). NF-κB activation has been associated with the secretion of various inflammatory cytokines, a class of chemical messengers that regulate cellular homeostasis. In turn, initiating cytokines, such as tumor necrosis factor-α (TNF-α) and interleukin-1 (IL-1), can induce production of other cytokines that are responsible for the recruitment of inflammatory cells such as neutrophils to sites of particle deposition (38), with subsequent activation of those recruited cells to produce ROS, providing further toxic insult to airway epithelium integrity.

Particle Clearance

Depending on the anatomic site of aerosol deposition within the respiratory tract, different particle clearance mechanisms exist, that affect both the rate and route of particle removal. In the anterior nose, for example, the coarse nasal hairs filter out larger particles, so that any particles that deposit on the mucus layer overlying the nonciliated respiratory epithelium are generally removed by sneezing or nose wiping; some may also be carried anteriorly by mucus traction to the ciliated regions. Particles that deposit in the more distal regions of the nasal cavity are cleared on a mucus film overlying a ciliated epithelium. The coordinated movement of cilia facilitates mucus flow in this region, which propels the mucus toward the nasopharynx; subsequent removal of insoluble particles is through swallowing or expectoration. In contrast, soluble particles may be absorbed into the bloodstream by diffusion into the mucus and through the nasal epithelium.

The tracheobronchial region, like much of the nasopharyngeal region, is lined with a mucus-covered, ciliated epithelium. Insoluble particles that deposit in this area are cleared via mucociliary transport, a process where mucus-entrained particles are swept toward the oral cavity for removal by swallowing or expectoration. Clearance in this region is generally faster in the larger rather than the smaller airways (104). Agents such as sulfur dioxide (SO_2) may produce an increase in mucus secretion, which acts to slow net ciliary movement and subsequently delay clearance (105). Also, particles may directly enter the peribronchiolar regions by crossing bronchial epithelium or be absorbed into the circulation after dissolution in the mucus layer.

Depending on the amount of particles deposited and the physiochemical properties of the particles, several processes exist to clear particles entering the alveolar (gas exchange) region. These clearance processes include dissolution, macrophage phagocytosis, direct passage, uptake by the vascular system, or movement into the lymphatic system. Dissolution of particles is a process whose rate is generally inversely related to particle size and may occur within the fluid lining the alveoli, the interstitium, the alveolar macrophages, or the lymphatic system; the solute may subsequently be absorbed through the epithelium into tissue or blood.

Macrophages serve important roles in particle clearance from the alveoli because secretory mucous cells and a ciliated epithelium are absent in alveoli. As mobile phagocytic cells of alveolar surfaces, macrophages are thought to deliver engulfed particles or fibers to the terminal bronchioles, where mucociliary transport may proceed or pass directly through alveolar epithelium to the interstitium for bronchiolar or lymphatic system removal. Of these two processes, particle clearance from the alveoli is believed to proceed primarily along the former pathway (106). Free or macrophage-associated particles that enter the lymphatic system may be translocated to tracheobronchial lymph nodes, where they may accumulate (if the particles are insoluble) or, alternatively, enter the blood stream. Particles that are not removed by the lymphatic or bronchiolar clearance routes may eventually migrate within the interstitium toward the pleura. Finally, particles may directly cross capillary endothelium and enter the blood (107). Failure to remove particles from the alveoli by one of these processes may result in particle accumulation or sequestration, a condition known as pneumoconiosis.

The clearance rates or kinetics of inhaled, insoluble particles from the respiratory tract vary depending on the anatomic location. Particle clearance kinetics may be described in five phases, each with a different clearance rate (Table 23.6). As considerable interindividual variations in the rapidity of clearance can exist within species, these phases describe idealized depictions of generally accepted clearance mechanisms within the respiratory tract. The first phase reflects the removal of particles deposited in the nasopharyngeal region. Here, the clearance rate is dependent on regional variations in mucus transport velocity, a process that can vary widely among individuals (108). Typically, particle clearance from the nasopharynx occurs with a removal time of approximately 10 min (109). A second phase of particle clearance involves removal of particles from the tracheobronchial tree. Again, clearance proceeding via the tracheobronchial mucociliary transport system will occur at rates dependent on mucus transport velocities. Regional differences in transport velocity are well known, although clearance rates are highest in the trachea and diminish toward the terminal bronchioles; this regional dependency is due to the reduced thickness and velocity of the mucus blanket toward the peripheral airways (110). Although particle transport from the tracheobronchial region is relatively rapid, with clearance of most particles occurring within approximately 24 h, particle clearance is not always complete even when evaluated weeks later. Indeed, prolonged retention of insoluble particles has been shown with particles instilled in the upper respiratory tract (111), an observation that may represent particle translocation into tissues. Particle clearance from the alveolar region represents the third, fourth, and fifth phases. The third phase is believed to represent particle transport by the alveolar macrophages to the ciliated epithelium or the lymphatic system; this phase proceeds at variable rates but has a clearance half-time of approximately 2–6 weeks. The fourth phase represents particle removal by interstitial pathways. This has been found to be especially true for UFP, which migrate readily into interstitial tissues, largely escaping phagocytosis and elimination by alveolar macrophage. The fifth phase represents removal by particle dissolution. Clearance half-times for these last two processes is generally measured in months and years, respectively. The efficiency of alveolar macrophage-mediated particle clearance may be greatly reduced if the particles are cytotoxic so that macrophages do not have an opportunity to participate in particle transport. Although clearance is dependent on several factors, including particle solubility, the physical removal of particles from the lung to the gastrointestinal tract and/or the regional lymph nodes appears independent of particle size for mono- or poly-disperse 0.7-2.8 μm aerosols (112).

Table 23.6
Particle clearance phases

Anatomic region	Clearance mechanism	Approximate clearance half-time
Nasopharynx	Mucociliary transport	Minutes
Tracheobronchial	Mucociliary transport	Minutes to hours
Alveolar	Macrophages	Days to weeks
Pulmonary	Interstitial migration	Months
Pulmonary	Dissolution	Months to years

Alveolar Macrophages

Due to the absence of a mucociliary transport apparatus in alveoli, alveolar macrophages play an important role in particle clearance from this region. Ordinarily, large numbers of macrophages may be attracted to particles that deposit in the lung. The mechanisms whereby macrophages are attracted to sites of particle deposition are not fully understood. However, Warheit et al. (113,114) demonstrated that several different types of particles might activate complement and that complement-derived factors are liberated from particle deposition sites. These factors are chemotactic for alveolar macrophages, which respond by migrating, within hours, to the deposition sites. Recruited macrophages may then engulf particles and either migrate toward the terminal bronchioles or enter the interstitium.

Phagocytosis constitutes another important function for alveolar macrophages. Once within the phagosome, the particle is subjected to a diverse array of hydrolysases and other lysosomal enzymes, as well as activated oxygen species including superoxide anions and hydroxyl radicals. These bioactive substances are involved in killing inhaled microorganisms but may also play a role in several particle-induced diseases, possibly through altering the biochemical microenvironment near the macrophage. Pulmonary emphysema, for example, is thought to be related to a protease and protease inhibitor imbalance; the secretion of excessive amounts of protease by macrophages or neutrophils and an insufficient amount of protease inhibitor are factors leading to the hydrolysis of lung connective tissues. Alternatively, the phagocytosis of asbestos fibers may either be incomplete so that the phagolysosome does not encapsulate the fiber, or result in injury to the macrophage membranes so that the macrophage releases lysosomal enzymes directly into the alveoli, causing local tissue injury. Macrophages may also become activated upon particle phagocytosis, releasing: inflammatory mediators such as ROS, macrophage and neutrophil chemotactic factors, prostaglandins, and platelet-activating factors that play roles in smooth muscle contraction and vascular permeability; growth factors for fibroblasts and collagen production; and various cytokines, such as TNF-α and IL-1, which modulate the inflammatory process. Particles that are readily cleared or rapidly dissolved may only transiently activate macrophages; however, continued macrophage activation by certain cytotoxic dusts such as silica or asbestos is thought to be responsible for chronic lung diseases ostensibly by initiating a prolonged inflammatory response within the lung (115).

As cytokines are critical messengers for maintaining homeostasis, they play an important role in the response of the lung to inhaled toxicants by modulating the recruitment and activation of inflammatory cells and the integrity of the pulmonary connective tissue matrix. Cytokines are low-molecular-weight proteins that govern intercellular communication by interaction with membrane receptors on target cells. Low levels are normally expressed in the body and are necessary for cell replication, differentiation, and tissue maintenance; however, as cytokines modulate these functions, agents that reduce or amplify cytokine levels can have major effects on the outcome of the body's response to the inhaled material.

For the purposes of classifying effects of cytokines on lung homeostasis, Driscoll et al. (116) describes three main categories of cytokines. One category is the initiating cytokines, generally acknowledged to be pivotal in moderating the initial host response to inhaled materials. Prototypic cytokines are TNF-α and IL 1 and are involved in triggering a secondary cascade of responses through additional cytokine networks. Although peripheral blood monocytes and alveolar macrophages are primary sources of TNF-α and IL-1, alveolar macrophages appear to contribute more TNF-α than blood monocytes and relatively more TNF-α than IL-1 (117). The presence of pathogenic dusts, such as crystalline silica, serves as a chronic stimulus for TNF-α and IL-1 expression because the cytotoxic silica cannot be readily cleared from the lung (118). A second category is the recruitment cytokines, which govern the recruitment of certain inflammatory cell populations to sites of TNF-α and IL-1 release. This class of cytokines also contains chemokines because they regulate influx of neutrophils and other immune system cells. The source of these chemokines is not clear but recent work suggests that pulmonary epithelial cells, alveolar type II cells, fibroblasts, and alveolar macrophages can all release the chemokine macrophage inflammatory protein-2 (MIP-2) in response to cytotoxic dusts (119). There appears to be marked specificity in the types of leukocytes responding to a given recruitment cytokine. Thus, whereas MIP-1α is chemotactic for monocytes, neutrophils, and lymphocytes, MIP-2 is chemotactic for neutrophils. Finally, there is a third class of cytokines known as resolution cytokines. These cytokines can both moderate fibroblast proliferation and production of collagen and also downregulate expression of the initiating cytokines. In so doing, these resolution cytokines ultimately terminate or resolve the inflammatory response to inhaled substances by affecting repair of damaged tissues. Examples of resolution cytokines include transforming growth factor (TGF)-α, TGF-β, IL-4, IL-6, and IL-10. Overall, a considerable body of evidence has accumulated implicating the central role cytokines have in the pathophysiology of fibrotic lung disease by regulating inflammatory cell recruitment, fibroblast and epithelial cell replication, and ultimately tissue repair.

A consequence of the inability of alveolar macrophages to effectively remove inhaled particles may result in a phenomenon known as "dust overloading." This condition arises when the normal clearance processes become less effective with high particle exposures, leading to accumulation of particles within the lungs (120). Overloading has been observed pathologically as an increased uptake of particles in the interstitium, increased numbers of macrophages that are swollen with ingested particles, chronic inflammation, and increased alveolar cell hyperplasia with the subsequent development of alveolitis, granulomas, fibrosis, and pulmonary tumors

(121). More importantly, the particle over-loaded lung has exhibited pathological changes with particles that previously have been considered benign; that is; the same particles would have not caused pathological changes if lung clearance processes had not been overwhelmed. The functional decrements in clearance due to dust overloading are apparent if the clearance kinetics is measured; overloaded lungs exhibit a marked increase in particle retention compared to the nonoverloaded lung. The mechanism for the overload phenomenon is believed to be due to a saturation of the capability of alveolar macrophages to ingest particles. The available data suggest that alveolar macrophages become overloaded not by the total mass of ingested particles but by the cumulative volume of particles within macrophages. Morrow (121) estimated that overloading may occur when the average volumetric load of particles exceeds 60 μm^3/macrophage and that macrophage-mediated clearance ceases when the volumetric load exceeds 600 μm^3/macrophage. Once the phagocytic activity of macrophages is reduced by large numbers of particles within alveoli, the mobility of macrophages also diminishes even if the particles are not inherently cytotoxic. The immobilization of alveolar macrophages within the lung results in two detrimental effects: first, subsequent clearance is greatly slowed, and second, the macrophages may continue to elaborate bioactive substances (e.g., proteases, cytokines, growth factors, oxidants, and immunomodulating agents) within the lungs. The overall effect is to increase the likelihood for a prolonged inflammatory response and subsequent pulmonary tissue injury.

To summarize, particle deposition and clearance are dependent on a complex series of interactions between particle behavior and the physiological attributes of the respiratory tract. Our understanding of these processes is important in the toxicological assessment of inhaled particulate materials.

EXPERIMENTAL INHALATION TOXICOLOGY

The potential toxic effects that need to be appreciated following inhalation exposure include irritation of the respiratory tract, behavioral changes, pathological changes to vital organs or tissues distal to the respiratory tract, immune system responses, pulmonary function alterations, metabolic disturbances, carcinogenicity, and even death. Studies to measure the effects of chemical and physical agents on the biological system after entering the respiratory tract must follow carefully designed protocols and be well described so that the intricacies of aerosol generation and measurement can be replicated by others. Indeed, the process of establishing constant and reproducible exposure conditions is considerably more complex than that required for other portals of entry such as oral or dermal. This is a direct result of the type of equipment needed to generate, maintain, and measure experimentally-produced atmospheres in a form that can be inhaled by the test species. Furthermore, there are inherent difficulties in measuring the dose; that is, relating the quantity of inhalable materials to that absorbed or retained in the test system. The total dose received depends on the physical and chemical properties of the material, the physiological characteristics of the test animal, and the numerous factors involved in deposition and clearance. One must also remember that inhalation exposures often result in simultaneous chemical exposures via the skin and the gastrointestinal tract from aerosol deposition and subsequent animal grooming.

Animal Models

The choice of an animal species for an inhalation study is an important one. It is apparent that there is no one ideal human surrogate and that each species presents its own advantages and disadvantages. Most commonly, rodents including the rat, mouse, guinea pig, and hamster (probably in that order) are used. As a consequence of the extensive use of rodents in inhalation toxicology, investigators have generated a large body of background and historical information on responses. Rodents have been used in toxicological tests as models for vapor and particle deposition and clearance, mechanisms of toxicant-induced lung and airway injury, and as models for infectivity and immunological function. Due to their relatively short life span, the use of rodents affords a practical and reasonably cost-effective animal model for studying chronic toxicity and carcinogenesis. When extrapolating from experimental animal data to humans, factors that need to be considered include the comparative anatomy of the respiratory tract, presence or absence of concurrent diseases or infections, and similarities of the physical, biochemical, and physiological responses to the intended species.

In practice, however, selection of the test species is more often based on criteria such as the size and availability of the test animals, the number of such animals needed to differentiate chemically induced changes from background or incidental changes, and the expense involved in obtaining and maintaining large numbers of animals needed to ensure statistical validity for various periods up to and including their lifetime.

The guinea pig has been used in studies of immune function and respiratory sensitization and has been particularly useful in determining the relative potencies of isocyanates (122,123). The guinea pig's unusually abundant bronchial smooth muscle makes this species a useful model to study airway hyperresponsiveness or bronchoconstriction in asthma models.

The hamster, having a relatively low spontaneous lung tumor rate and resistance to pulmonary infections, has been used in respiratory tract cancer studies. Some investigators feel that the hamster is the best animal model for the study of experimental lung cancer (124).

There are several disadvantages in using rodents to predict effects in humans. Because the nasal/pharyngeal anatomy of rodents is unlike that of humans, the amounts and sites of particle deposition are quite different. Rodents are also obligate nose breathers, with superior nasal filtering efficiency compared to humans especially for submicron particles. Assessment of pulmonary function in nonanesthetized rodents is difficult, although recent miniaturization of probes and detectors has allowed success here (125). The most serious problems with rodents, especially rats, are those involving spontaneous respiratory infections and their sequelae. Rats appear to be uniquely susceptible to chronic inflammation, pulmonary fibrosis, and cancer from insoluble, noncytotoxic particles through a process believed to involve overwhelming of lung clearance mechanisms ("particle overload"). Because rats appear to be the most susceptible to particle overloading, their selection for some types of particle inhalation studies often complicates extrapolation of the results to humans (126). In oncogenicity studies, rats appear to be less susceptible to fiber-induced mesothelioma, a malignant tumor of the pleural lung surface. Conversely, hamsters appear to be more susceptible to the development of fiber-induced mesothelioma but less sensitive to induction of lung tumors than rats. Despite these considerations, rats remain the most favored animal model for both short- and long-term inhalation studies.

There also exists a great deal of background data from inhalation toxicity studies on the dog, especially the beagle. The dog is a convenient size for a number of laboratory measurements, including evaluation of pulmonary function. Several natural disease states exist in the dog, making it a good model for evaluating the impact of the agent on conditions such as asthma. The cost and facilities needed to properly care for dogs represent a minor disadvantage. The dog also may be relatively insensitive to certain inhaled gases such as ozone (127).

Because the nasal anatomy of monkeys is similar to humans, monkeys are sometimes used in inhalation experiments. Lung function can readily be determined. However, considerable cost is involved in obtaining and maintaining monkey colonies and their lack of general availability is becoming a major problem limiting their use. A potentially more serious limitation to the use of monkeys is the extreme care that must be taken to prevent the transmission of disease from monkeys to humans. Note that within the species identified as "monkey," serious intraspecies differences do exist. Also, the subgross pulmonary anatomy differs between types of monkeys and humans (128).

Other species such as the ferret, horse, donkey, sheep, cat, rabbit, and pig have been suggested for use in inhalation studies. Each of these species has been used for special applications, which may take advantage of a particular anatomic feature, chemical sensitivity, or research curiosity.

Although the choice of animal model is seldom obvious, a compromise for general screening purposes is to use multiple species (129). This approach has been used in testing radionuclides, (130,131), ozone (127), sulfur oxides (132), polychlorinated biphenyls (133), chlorinated hydrocarbons (134), and ethylene oxide/propylene oxide copolymers (135). In the selection of an appropriate animal species, one must consider the available background information; the unique functional or structural characteristics, if any, of the species that make it a good (or bad) animal model; what the anticipated response might be that would enable the investigator to most accurately determine the number of animals needed for the duration of the study; and, finally, appropriate controls. The use of small rodents predominates because their small size allows testing of larger groups; their relatively short lifetime allows testing over the entire life span (a large body of data already exists on these species); and, finally, the cost of their acquisition and upkeep is relatively low.

Study Types

Evaluating the inhalation toxicity of chemical substances includes determining chemically-induced changes, following both short- and long-term exposures. Acute studies generally define both the amount of chemical needed to produce a given response (most often death) and the clinical signs potentially suggestive of target organ toxicity associated with high levels of exposure. Longer-term studies (up to and including life-span studies) are conducted to determine the target organ(s) for repeated exposures and carcinogenic potential (Table 23.7).

Acute studies generally involve a single, 4- or 6-h exposure of small groups of rodents to the test chemical at a series of concentrations ranging from those producing little or no signs of response (e.g., clinical signs, body weight changes) to those producing death. Studies may also be conducted at shorter durations (i.e., 1 h) to help assess responses arising from very short-term exposure (e.g., accidental releases requiring population evacuation). The practice of using many groups and relatively many animals per group to define the LC_{50} (i.e.,

Table 23.7
Study types for evaluating inhalation toxicity

To determine	Duration (number of exposures)	Examples
Acute response	Generally 1	LC_{50} (4–6 h, sometimes shorter) Approximate lethal concentration (ALC) Sensory irritation (RD_{50})
Target organ	>1 but ≤90 days	2-, 4-, 13-week studies
Effects of chronic exposure (carcinogenic potential)	>90 days to lifetime	2-year studies (rodents)
Biochemical response	Any of above	Bronchoalveolar lavage studies
Morphological changes	Any of above	Quantitative morphometry, special staining, cell proliferation
Functional capability	Any of above	Pulmonary function parameters

the concentration calculated to kill half of the exposed animals under the particular set of experimental conditions) has been replaced to some extent by the determination of the approximate lethal concentration (the lowest concentration at which the first death is observed). This protocol dramatically reduces the number of animals needed per study (from an average of 56 to 7) (136) and may find value in toxicity screening; however, regulatory agencies still require formal LC_{50} determinations with multiple groups of animals. To minimize animal use and improve the utility of inhalation screening assays, more detailed examinations of respiratory tract histopathology and analysis of bronchoalveolar lavage fluid for evaluation of cellular injury may be useful in mechanistic evaluations. Another major purpose of the acute study is to help define the exposure concentrations that should be used for further repeated-exposure studies.

A special variation of the acute toxicity study is based on the fact that a large number of chemicals are sensory irritants (i.e., depression of respiratory rate through stimulation of irritant receptors in the upper respiratory tract) and that animal models can be used to predict both the degree of irritancy and their relative potency. The majority of chemicals for which occupational exposure limits (i.e., American Conference of Governmental Industrial Hygienists Threshold Limit Values [TLV] have been established are based on sensory irritation. In these cases, no clear target organ toxicity other than irritation to the eyes, nose, or upper respiratory tract has been identified from either animal studies or reports of human experiences in the workplace. Efforts to refine exposure limits based solely on the use of sensory irritation data from animal testing have been proposed by several investigators (137,138). Although equating exposure limits to sensory irritation levels simplifies exposure limit setting in one regard, caution must be exercised in the use of sensory irritation data alone (139). Some workers have found that pathological changes may occur in the respiratory tract below acutely irritating levels in rodents, limiting the usefulness of sensory irritating assays by themselves for exposure limit setting (140,141).

In sensory irritation studies, changes in respiratory rate and depth are recorded in response to known concentrations of test substances (142,143). Animals (usually rats or mice) are placed in small cylindrical tubes with the head protruding through a rubber dam. The neck fitting forms a relatively airtight seal, which, with appropriate attachments, allows the unit to be used as a body plethysmograph. The animal in the tube is then placed with the head protruding into the exposure chamber. Following an acclimatization period, the animal is exposed to pre-equilibrated concentrations of either vapors or aerosols (Figure 23.8) and the changes in respiratory rate and pattern are determined. Each animal is exposed to a given concentration for approximately 10–30 min. This technique allows determination of the upper respiratory tract irritation potential in a simple and reproducible manner. The data are expressed as the RD_{50}, the calculated concentration expected to reduce the normal respiratory rate by 50%.

Despite their utility, there is some debate regarding the role that sensory irritation assays play in occupational exposure limit setting. Some have stated that the RD_{50} (a) is, by itself, insufficient to prevent systemic or portal-of-entry toxicity; and (b) should be used over no-observed-adverse-effect levels (NOAELs) from histopathological evaluation of the respiratory tract only if actual animal RD_{50} data exist and sensory irritation is the critical endpoint (139,144).

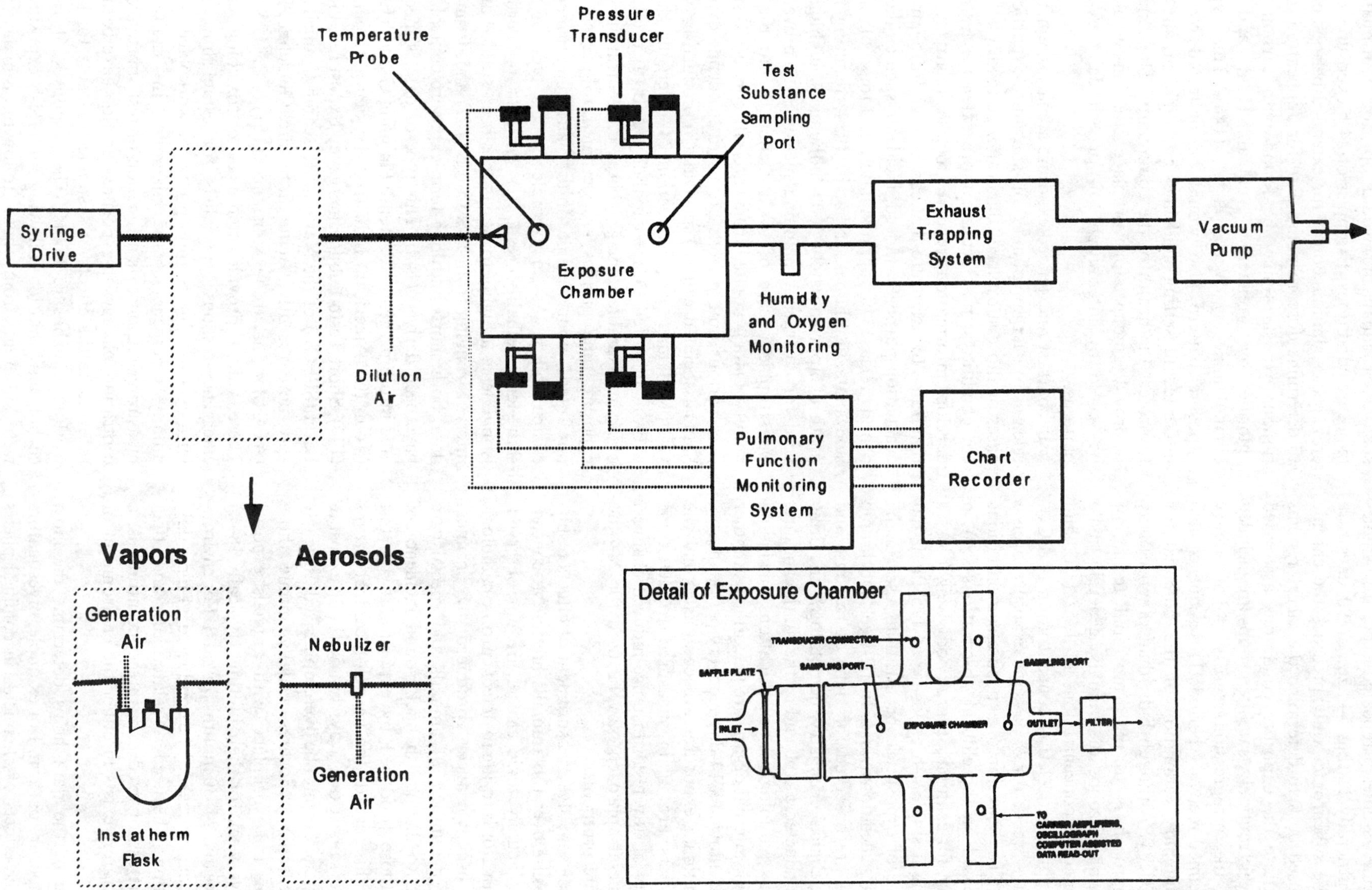

FIG. 23.8. Apparatus for determination of sensory irritation properties of vapors or aerosols. *Insert*: Details of exposure chamber.

Beyond acute studies, repeated-exposure studies (subchronic—generally lasting 14, 28, or 90 days) are conducted. The subchronic study precedes the chronic study and is used both to determine the target systems and to quantitate the exposure conditions associated with the changes; routinely, satellite groups are included to monitor the progression/regression of injury following a defined recovery period. This sequence also allows a preliminary estimation of the potential for cumulative toxicity. Although individual practices may vary, our approach is to perform initial testing of 2-weeks duration. Groups of animals, generally male rats, are exposed to concentrations of 1/5, 1/15, and 1/50 of the approximate lethal concentration or LC_{50}, 6 h/day, 5 days/week, for 9 days of exposure over a 2-week period. The selection of exposure concentrations can also be based on the clinical observations seen in the acute study; for example, if large body weight losses occur following a single 4-h exposure at 1/5 the lethal dose, the range of exposure concentrations used in the study would be scaled downward. In a 2-week subchronic study, animals are observed for signs of response and weighed daily; clinical chemistry, hematology, and urine analysis are conducted at the end of the ninth exposure; and complete pathological examinations including weights of major internal organs are performed. Another group of rats is allowed a 14-day recovery period, during which no additional exposures are conducted and the above parameters are again measured to determine the reversibility of any test substance-induced changes. This same general approach may be used for 28- and 90-day exposure protocols.

Chronic studies involve measurement of effects resulting from exposure over the animal's lifetime at concentrations where acutely toxic effects are not observed. Here the investigator is trying to detect chronic pathological changes, usually cancer, produced by chemical exposure. Large numbers of animals and special care must be taken to distinguish background incidence of effects from those produced by exposure to the test substance. In this regard, the need for control groups handled in the same exact way, but without exposure to the test substance, cannot be overemphasized. In nearly all studies, chronic exposures usually mimic those encountered in the workplace with animals exposed 6 h/day, 5 days/week for their lifetime (typically 18–24 months for mice and 24–30 months for rats). For environmental agents, exposures may be conducted 24 h per day. In both situations, the need to relate cause and effect necessitates the use of fixed exposure concentrations, a situation that rarely exists in either the environment or the workplace.

The end-use of the data helps determine the most appropriate exposure pattern. For example, investigators interested in the effects of chemicals in confined places such as a submarine would opt for continual 24-h exposure conditions. Examples of 24-h exposures of several species simultaneously for extended periods of time to determine dose–response data for application to continuous exposures may be found with carbon tetrachloride by Prendergast et al. (134) and with ethanolamine by Weeks et al. (146). This type of exposure pattern also would be preferred by those interested in setting guidelines for ambient, air levels to protect the health of the community. Those needing to provide guidance for workplace situations would best be served by intermittent, 6- or 8-h daily exposure patterns.

In contrast to extended exposure scenarios, emergency releases of large volumes of substances, particularly gases or those substances that vaporize readily at ambient conditions, may require more extensive testing to develop information relative to the relatively short timeframe for exposure that can be used for community evacuation purposes. Indeed, incidents such as the accidental release of approximately 50 tons of methyl isocyanate in Bhopal, India, in 1984, resulting in the death of approximately 3000 individuals, highlight the need for emergency planning measures to prevent the catastrophic release of toxic chemicals into the community. Data generated from carefully conducted studies over various time periods are useful to define exposure limits associated with (a) survival, (b) production of irreversible damage, (c) production of reversible damage without impaired escape capability, and (d) production of no measurable damage. These concentration versus exposure time profiles are designed to prevent both unwanted, nonreversible injury and impairment of escape ability. As an example of this type of work, short-term lethality responses of rats to perfluoroisobutylene, a highly toxic gas, has been studied at time intervals ranging from 15 s to 6 h (147) and, from these data, both short- and long-term exposure control limits have been derived (148). This type of data is incorporated into Emergency Response Planning Guides (ERPG) (from the American Industrial Hygiene Association) (149), Short Term Public Emergency Exposure Guideline Level (SPEGL) of the National Research Council (150), and more recently, Acute Exposure Guideline Levels (AEGL) for hazardous substances (151) of the U.S. EPA. These values provide guidance to toxicologists and emergency-response specialists for establishing short-term exposure limits appropriate for workplace or community emergency-escape planning. In addition to measuring response as a function of test substance concentration, changes in exposure duration have been used to evaluate the effects of systemic toxicants for setting workplace exposure limits. The responses of rats to carbon tetrachloride following an 11.5-h exposure/day were different from those following 8 h/day (152).

Altering exposure schedules of rats from 8 h/day for 5 days to 12 h/day for 4 days produced both concentration- and time-dependent responses to aniline (153). Burgess et al. (154) found that concentration was the primary determinant of toxicity in a study where three aniline concentrations were tested in rats using three times periods, either 3, 6, or 12 h/day.

INHALATION TOXICITY TESTING

Domestic and international regulatory agencies have implemented testing guidelines regarding the conduct of inhalation toxicity studies. These guidelines attempt to formalize and more recently, standardize testing procedures so that toxicity data may be obtained and compared using similar protocols. Test data generated in this fashion may be used in a variety of ways: (i) to investigate the relationship between exposure concentration and adverse effects; (ii) to provide information on the mechanism of toxicity and permit a reasoned extrapolation of the experimental animal data to potential human health risks; (iii) to form the basis for dose-level selection for repeated-exposure studies; or (iv) to categorize the inhalation toxicity of a test material relative to other chemicals. Such data are the foundation for establishing defensible exposure limits for the protection of workers and the general population from possible adverse effects of airborne chemicals.

Regulatory agencies have adopted standardized protocols for both short-term and long-term inhalation testing and recently have begun to harmonize protocols internationally. In Tables 23.8–23.10, general study design, exposure conditions, and measurement frequencies required for data submission to the U.S. EPA (Federal Insecticide, Fungicide, and Rodenticide Act [FIFRA] and Toxic Substances Control Act [TSCA]), the Organization for European Economic Co-operation and Development (OECD), and the Japanese Ministry of Agriculture, Forestry, and Fisheries (MAFF) are shown for acute, subchronic, and chronic (carcinogenicity) inhalation toxicity testing.

Acute inhalation studies frequently are required by regulatory agencies for the classification of test material toxicity for labeling purposes. The subchronic inhalation study is useful for determining target organ toxicity and establishing a no-observable-effect level associated with repeated exposure (i.e., periods up to approximately 90 days). Depending on the toxicity of the test substance, additional groups may be added to assess the reversibility or persistence of injury using a battery of clinical chemical and anatomic pathology endpoints. Subchronic testing is also necessary to select appropriate exposure levels for chronic studies. Chronic inhalation testing provides information on the cumulative toxicity of test materials over the lifetime of the animal; modified protocols exist for evaluating both the chronic toxicity and oncogenic potential of test materials. Further information on the protocols and methods used in inhalation testing may be found in Gardner and Kennedy (155) and Morrow and Mermelstein (156).

Concurrent with exposure to aerosols, some measure of particle clearance (such as the lung particle burden or the clearance rate of a radiolabeled tracer particle) is highly recommended. Indeed, an important but often overlooked principle in designing inhalation toxicology experiments to evaluate potential biological sequelae of chemical exposure is that tolerated doses (i.e., exposure concentrations) be defined and employed. This is particularly important with particles that are relatively insoluble and have a low order of systemic and respiratory tract toxicity. If particle clearance from the lung is impaired, particle burdens in the lung will exceed those predicted based on data developed at lower exposure rates (157). Once the normal clearance mechanism(s) are saturated, biological effects may ensue from the unusually high lung burdens. Some recent experiments using titanium dioxide (158), antimony trioxide (159), talc (161), toner (162), carbon black (163,164), and diesel soot (165,166) point out the importance of not saturating the lung clearance mechanisms, which otherwise may lead to dust overloading (82,167,168).

Indeed, a considerable body of evidence implicates the development of lung fibrosis and tumors not from the inhalation of inherently cytotoxic or genotoxic particles but from the prolonged inflammatory response induced by high particle concentrations (either from high exposure levels or inability to remove inhaled particles) in the lung (169). This overload phenomenon can produce similar pathological lesions in the lung as more cytotoxic dusts such as quartz (170). The impetus for the overload theory lies, in part, from rodent chronic inhalation bioassays with diesel soot, carbon black, titanium dioxide, and talc. As a class, these particles have low solubility, low cytotoxicity, and with the exception of diesel soot are nongenotoxic although genotoxicity per se is not a rigid requirement for tumor development with these particles (171). Consistent with all, however, is the observation that high levels of chronic exposure is associated with an increasing lung burden of particles; at some level above the threshold capacity of alveolar macrophages to remove particles, lung overload occurs (172). In rats, characteristic sequelae of the overloaded lung may include accumulation of particle-filled alveolar macrophages in airspaces or interstitium, particle translocation to regional lymph nodes, chronic inflammation, fibrosis, cellular metaplasia, and tumor development. Although impaired macrophage clearance and chronic inflammation may arise in the overloaded lung, tumor

Table 23.8
Testing guidelines for acute inhalation toxicity studies

Criteria	US EPA OPPTS 870.130[a]	Europe OECD 401[b]	Japan MAFF[c]
Study design			
Species[d]	Rat	Rat	Rat
Sex and number per group	≥5 of each sex[e]	5 male, 5 female	5 male, 5 female
Age	Young adult, 8–12 weeks	Young adult	Young adult
Weight range	<±20% of mean weight per sex	<±20% of mean weight per sex	Not specified
Exposure time	4 h after equilibration of chamber concentration	4 h after equilibration of chamber concentration	4 h
Observation period	14 days	14 days	14 days
Limit test[f]	2 mg/L	5 mg/L	5 mg/L
Exposure conditions			
Chamber temperature	22±2°C	22±2°C	22±2°C
Relative humidity	30–70%	30–70%	40–60%
Airflow	≥10 air changes/h	12–15 air changes/h	Not specified
Chamber oxygen concentration	At least 19%	At least 19%	At least 19%
Particle size distribution	1–4 μm MMAD	Not specified	Not specified
Chamber loading	Total animal volume ≤5% chamber volume	Total animal volume ≤5% chamber volume	Not specified
Frequency of measures			
Airflow	Monitor continuously, record ≥3 times/exposure	Prefer continuously	Not specified
Particle size	2–4 times/exposure	As needed to determine consistency	As needed to determine consistency
Exposure concentration	2–4 times/exposure	Not specified	Not specified
Temperature and humidity	Monitor continuously, record ≥3 times/exposurc	Prefer continuously	Not specified
Nominal concentration[g]	Required but frequency not specified	Once/exposure	Not specified
Endpoints			
Morbidity and mortality	Yes; daily	Yes; daily	Yes
Clinical observations	Yes; daily	Yes; daily	Yes
Body weights	Yes; weekly	Yes; daily	Yes
Gross pathology	Yes; at termination	Recommended	Recommended
Histopathology	Optional; in animals with gross changes at necropsy	Discretionary	Discretionary

[a] This harmonized guideline was developed by the Office of Prevention, Pesticides and Toxic Substances to blend the testing requirements for the Federal Insecticide, Fungicide, and Rodenticide Act (FIFRA) and the Toxic Substances Control Act (TSCA) with the Organization for Economic Cooperation and Development (OECD).
[b] OEDC Guideline for Testing for Chemicals, Acute Inhalation Toxicity, Section 403, 1–4, 1981. At the time of publication a revised, harmonized OECD guideline had not been issued.
[c] Requirements for Safety Evaluation of Agricultural Chemicals. Testing guidelines for Toxicology Studies, Ministry of Agriculture, Forestry and Fisheries (Japan), Acute Inhalation Toxicity Study, 1985.
[d] Mammals are specified in the test guidelines but rats are generally preferred.
[e] At least five experimentally naive animals are used of each concentration and they should be of one sex. After completion of the study in one sex, at least one group of five animals of the other sex is exposed to establish that animals of this sex are not markedly more sensitive to the test substance.
[f] If exposure at the limit concentration (LC) (or where this is not possible due to the physical characteristics of the test substance) produces no observable toxic effects, a full study may not be necessary.
[g] Amount of test material delivered to the generation system divided by the air volume used during the exposure.

development may not always arise. Conversely, lung tumors have not been reported where particle clearance and pulmonary inflammation did not result, suggesting a threshold-related phenomenon.

There are several other notable features of the overload phenomenon that impacts risk assessment. First, species differences are known in the levels at which overloading and the pathological sequelae occur, complicating the extrapolation of results from test animals to humans. For example, rats have developed lung tumors whereby mice or hamsters, exposed to similar particle concentrations and producing impaired alveolar macrophage clearance, did not (171,173). Second, expression of concentration is important because the dose metric (i.e., par-

Table 23.9
Testing guidelines for subchronic inhalation toxicity studies

Criteria	US EPA OPPTS 870.3465[a]	Europe OECD 413[b]	Japan MAFF[c]
Study design			
Species[d]	Rat	Rat	Rat
Sex and number	10 male and 10 female	10 male and 10 female	10 male and 10 female
Age	Young adult, 8–9 weeks old	Young adult	Young adult
Weight range	<±20% of mean weight/sex	<±20% of mean weight/sex	Not specified
Exposure time	6 h/day, 5 or 7 days/weeks for 90 days	6 /day (after equilibrium), 5 days/week for 90 days	6 h/day, 5 days/week for 90 days
Exposure groups	3 tests and 1 control	3 tests and 1 control	3 tests and 1 control
Satellite groups	Optional; control and high level for 90 days with ≥28 days' recovery	Optional; high level for 90 days with ≥ 28 days' recovery	Optional; high level for 90 days with ≥ 28 days' recovery
Limit test[e]	1 mg/L	Not specified	Not specified
Exposure conditions			
Chamber temperature	22±2°C	22±2°C	Not specified
Relative humidity	40–60%	30–70%	Not specified
Airflow	Dynamic, ≥10 air changes/h	12–15 air changes/h	Not specified
Chamber oxygen concentration	≥19%0	≥19%	Not specified
Particle size distribution	1–3 μm MMAD	Not specified	Not specified
Chamber loading	Total animal volume ≤5% of chamber volume	Total animal volume ≤5% of chamber volume	Not specified
Frequency of measures			
Airflow	Monitor continuously; record ≥3 times/exposure	Prefer continuously	Not specified
Particle size	2–4 times/exposure, depending upon consistency	As needed to determine consistency	Not specified
Exposure concentration	2–4 times/exposure, depending upon consistency	Not specified	Not specified
Temperature and humidity	Monitor continuously; record ≥3 times/exposure	Prefer continuously	Not specified
Nominal concentration	Required but frequency not specified	Required but frequency not specified	Required but frequency not specified
Endpoints			
Morbidity and mortality	Yes; twice daily	Yes, daily	Yes
Clinical observations	Yes; once weekly	Yes; once weekly	Yes
Functional observational battery[g]	Yes, once	No	Yes
Body weights	Yes; weekly	Yes; weekly	Yes
Feed consumption	Yes; weekly	Yes; weekly	Yes
Ophthalmology	Yes; prior to study and at termination	Yes; prior to study and at termination	Yes
Hematology and clinical chemistry	Yes; at termination	Yes; at termination	Yes
Gross necropsy	Yes; at termination	Yes; at termination	Yes
Histopathology[h]	Yes; at termination	Yes; at termination	Yes
Urinalysis	Discretionary	Discretionary	Discretionary

[a] This harmonized guideline was developed by the Office of Prevention, Pesticides and Toxic Substances to blend the testing requirements for the Federal Insecticide, Fungicide, and Rodenticide Act (FIFRA) and the Toxic Substances Control Act (TSCA) with the Organization for Economic Cooperation and Development (OECD).
[b] OEDC Guideline for Testing of Chemicals, Section 4, Health Effects Test, Subchronic Inhalation Toxicity: 90-day, Section 413, 1981. At the time of publication a revised, harmonized OECD guideline had not been issued.
[c] Requirements for Safety Evaluation of Agricultural Chemicals. Testing Guidelines for Toxicology Studies, Ministry of Agriculture, Forestry and Fisheries (Japan), Subchronic Inhalation Toxicity Study, 1985.
[d] Mammals are specified in the test guidelines but rats are generally preferred.
e If exposure at the limit concentration (LC) (or where the LC is not possible due to the physical characteristics of the test substance) produces no observable toxic effects, a full study may not be necessary.
[f] Amount of test material delivered to the generation system divided by the air volume used during the exposure.
[g] A functional observational battery should consist of assessment of motor activity, grip strength, and sensory reactivity to different stimuli.
[h] Histopathology of the respiratory tract is needed for all high-dose and control groups and for lungs, target organs, and gross lesions of all animals.

Table 23.10
Testing guidelines for inhalation toxicity studies to evaluate carcinogenicity

Criteria	US EPA OPPTS 870.4200[a]	Europe OECD 451[b]
Study design		
Species[c]	Rat and mouse	Rat and mouse
Sex and number per group	50 male, 50 female	50 male, 50 female
Age	6–8 weeks	6–8 weeks
Weight range	< ± 20% of mean weight/sex	< ± 20% of mean weight/sex
Exposure time	6 h/day, 5 days/week for 18 months (mice) or 24 months (rats)	6 h/day, 5 days/week for 18 months (mice) or 24 months (rats)
Observation Period	24–30 months (rats) 18–24 months (mice)	24–30 months (rats) 18–24 months (mice)
Survival	Not less than 25% at 18 months (mice) or 25% at 24 months (rats)	Not less than 50% at 18 months (mice) or 50% at 24 months (rats)
Exposure groups	At least 3 tests and 1 control	At least 3 tests and 1 control
Exposure conditions		
Chamber temperature	22 ± 2°C	22 ± 2°C
Relative humidity	40–60%	30–70%
Airflow	At least 10 air changes/h	12–15 air changes/h
Chamber oxygen concentration	At least 19%	At least 19%
Particle size distribution	1–3μm MMAD	Not specified
Frequency of measures		
Airflow	Monitor continuously; record ≥3 times/exposure	Monitor continuously
Particle size	2–4 times/exposure, depending on consistency	As needed to determine consistency
Exposure concentration	2–4 times/exposure, depending on consistency	Not specified
Temperature and humidity	Monitor continuously, record every 30 min	Prefer continuously
Nominal concentration[d]	Once/exposure	Not specified
Endpoints		
Morbidity and mortality	Yes	Yes
Clinical observations	Yes	Yes
Body weights	Yes	Yes
Feed consumption	Yes	Yes
Hematology (smear)	Yes	Yes
Gross pathology	Yes	Yes
Histopathology	Yes	Yes

[a] This harmonized guideline was developed by the Office of Prevention, Pesticides and Toxic Substances to blend the testing requirements for the Federal Insecticide, Fungicide, and Rodenticide Act (FIFRA) and the Toxic Substances Control Act (TSCA) with the Organization for Economic Co-operation and Development (OECD).

[b] OEDC Guideline for Testing of Chemicals, Section 4, Health Effects, Oncogenicity Studies, Section 451, 1981. At the time of publication a revised, harmonized OECD guideline had not been issued.

[c] At least two mammalian species should be tested; rats and mice are generally preferred due to their comparatively short life span, low cost, ready availability, and ease of handling.

[d] Amount of test material delivered to the generation system divided by the air volume used during exposure.

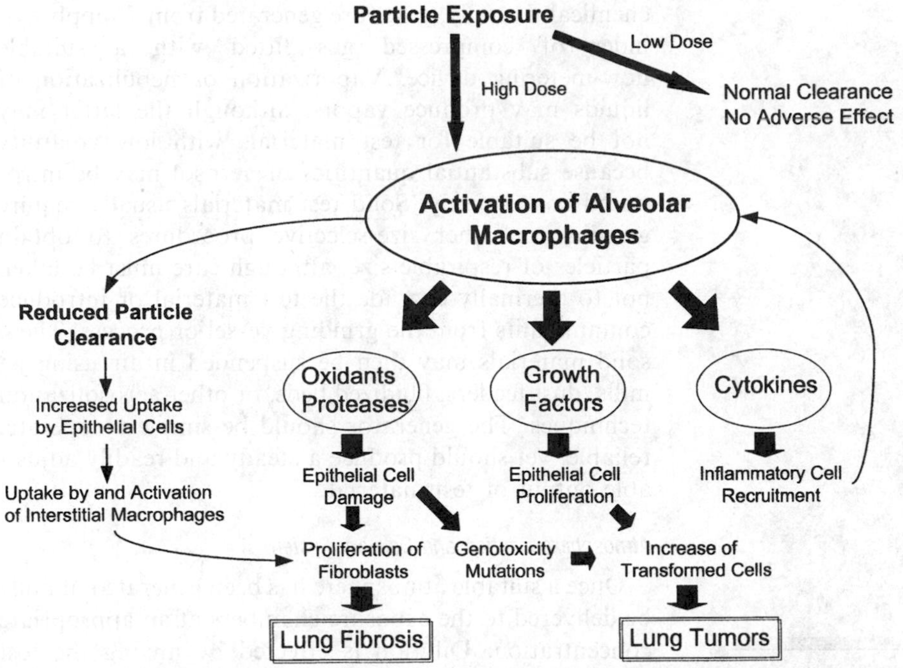

FIG. 23.9. Relationships between particle exposure, macrophage activation, and development of lung fibrosis and cancer. Adapted from Reference 126.

ticle concentration expressed on either a mass, count, volume, or surface area basis) may differ, depending upon the species, for overload to occur. The available data suggest that particle surface area is the particle characteristic most closely associated with pulmonary inflammation, fibrosis, and lung tumor development (90,174). By whatever metric, the most important outcome of overload is the persistent inflammatory response produced by the particles. The consequences of this have an important bearing on the mechanism of tumor development. Notably, at 7.1 mg/m^3 or greater, corresponding to exposure levels producing marked impairment of particle clearance in rats, Driscoll (175) reported that carbon black produced lung injury, chronic inflammation, epithelial hyperplasia and fibrosis; these changes were not seen in a 13-week study at 1.1 mg/m^3. Most importantly, Driscoll reported a significant, dose-dependent increase of *hprt* mutations in alveolar epithelial cells at these inflammatory concentrations. He postulated that inflammatory cell products, including ROS and cytokines, provide the conditions, including induction of cellular mutations and cell proliferation, that are necessary for tumor development. Driscoll's observation that particle-elicited rat inflammatory lung cells can be directly mutagenic suggests that there will be an exposure level that does not induce persistent inflammatory changes and therefore mutations should not occur for nongenotoxic particles (175). On the other hand, at inflammatory concentrations, both the inherent genotoxicity of the particle and the resultant genotoxicity of the particle-elicited inflammatory cells may influence tumor development. The proposed theory relating these observations is shown in Figure 23.9. Overall, these data provide an important mechanistic link for the development of lung tumors from low cytotoxicity, low solubility nongenotoxic dusts.

Exposure Systems

Inhalation exposure systems involve the harmonious integration of several subsystems whose design and construction are critical to an efficient, functional system. The various subsystems are shown schematically in Figure 23.10 and include a conditioned air supply system, a suitable vapor or aerosol generator for the test chemical, an atmosphere dilution and delivery system, one or more exposure chambers, an atmosphere sampling and analytical system, and an exhaust/scrubbing system. Whereas there may be differences in the mode of exposure to test substances (i.e., nose-only or whole-body), the design, operational parameters, testing objectives, and technical requirements for these subsystems are similar. Components typically used for test substance generation and analysis and animal exposure are shown in more detail in Figure 23.11.

Conditioned Air Supply

Some means must be provided for supplying a sufficient amount of clean, conditioned air for chamber operation. The availability of high quality, particle-free, and organic vapor-free air for chamber supply is essential, especially for long-term inhalation studies. Ordinarily, ambient air is dried, filtered, and purged of organic vapors prior

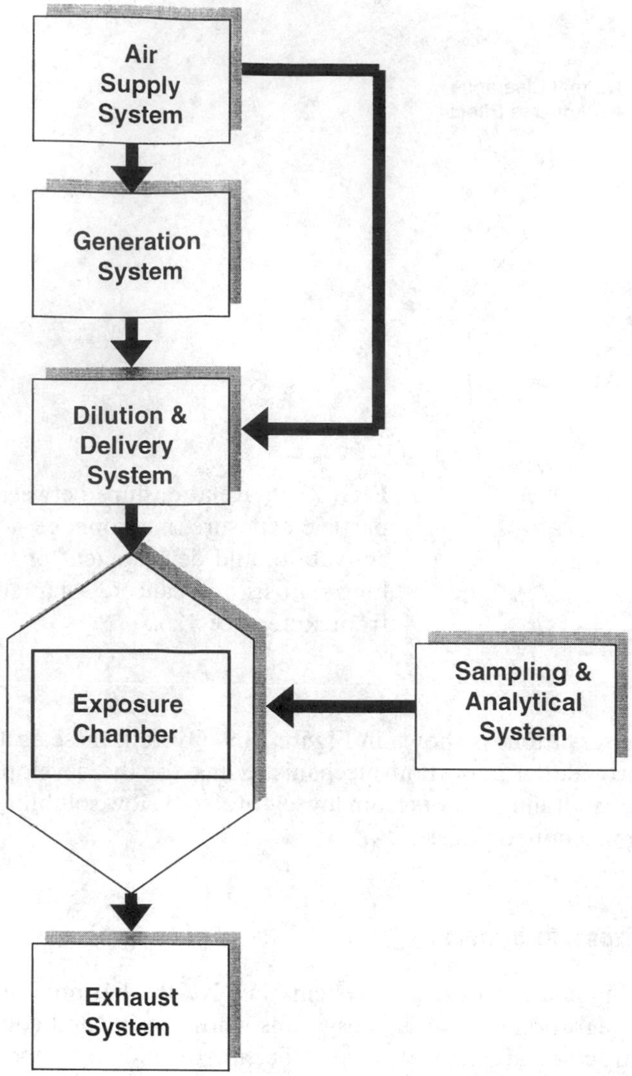

FIG. 23.10. Components of an inhalation exposure system.

to adjusting its temperature and humidity to the desired levels. Where this is not available for very small, low airflow chambers with limited numbers of animals, a commercial source of compressed purified air may be utilized. The size of the air-conditioning equipment should be scaled to allow some excess flow capacity for the required number of chambers operating at the desired flow rates.

The design should permit adjustments of the airflow rate, temperature, and humidity to maintain these parameters within the specified ranges. Automated airflow, temperature, and humidity measurement systems are commercially available and greatly reduce the need for manual measurements.

Generation of Test Atmospheres

The type of atmosphere generator depends on the nature, physical properties, and availability of the test chemical. Usually, gases are generated from a supply cylinder of compressed gas fitted with a suitable flow-metering device. Vaporization or nebulization of liquids may produce vapors, although the latter may not be suitable for test materials with low volatility because substantial quantities of aerosol may be introduced concurrently. Solid test materials usually require grinding or other size-selective procedures to obtain particles of respirable size, although care must be taken not to thermally degrade the test material or introduce contaminants from the grinding vessel or process. These solid materials may then be suspended in air using jet mills, dust feeders, fluidized beds, or other aerosolization techniques. The generator should be simple to operate, reliable, yet should produce a steady and readily adjustable output of test material

Atmosphere Dilution and Delivery System

Once a suitable atmosphere has been generated, it must be delivered to the exposure chambers at an appropriate concentration. Dilution is effected by mixing the test atmosphere with conditioned, filtered air before its introduction into the exposure chamber. It is important that the delivery system be fabricated with materials that minimize wall losses, either through absorptive or reactive processes, and designed to minimize physical losses through aerosol deposition within ductwork. The former situation may be avoided by using nonreactive materials and the latter by minimizing the number of bends and maintaining laminar flow in the ductwork. In general, the delivery system should be nonreactive with tubing as wide, short, and straight as practical to minimize test material losses and pressure drop. It is especially important to use conductive materials in the choice of tubing materials. Substantial aerosol deposition can occur in areas of high electrostatic charge, leading to excessive and variable aerosol losses along transfer lines. A broad selection of mechanical and electrical valves and flow measurement devices are available to measure and control the flow of test material and dilution air.

Exposure Chambers

The selection of a suitable exposure chamber depends on the exposure mode (e.g., nose-only or whole-body), reactivity of the test material, available resources (supply of conditioned air and test material), number of animals to be exposed, and efficiency in delivering test material to the animals. Apart from the obvious difference in size, the design objectives for nose-only or whole-body exposure chambers are similar. Chambers should be constructed of nonreactive materials such as stainless steel, glass, or plastic. Although stainless steel is durable and nonreactive toward many materials, it is comparatively expensive. In contrast, glass or plastic chambers are less expensive and permit ready observation of ani-

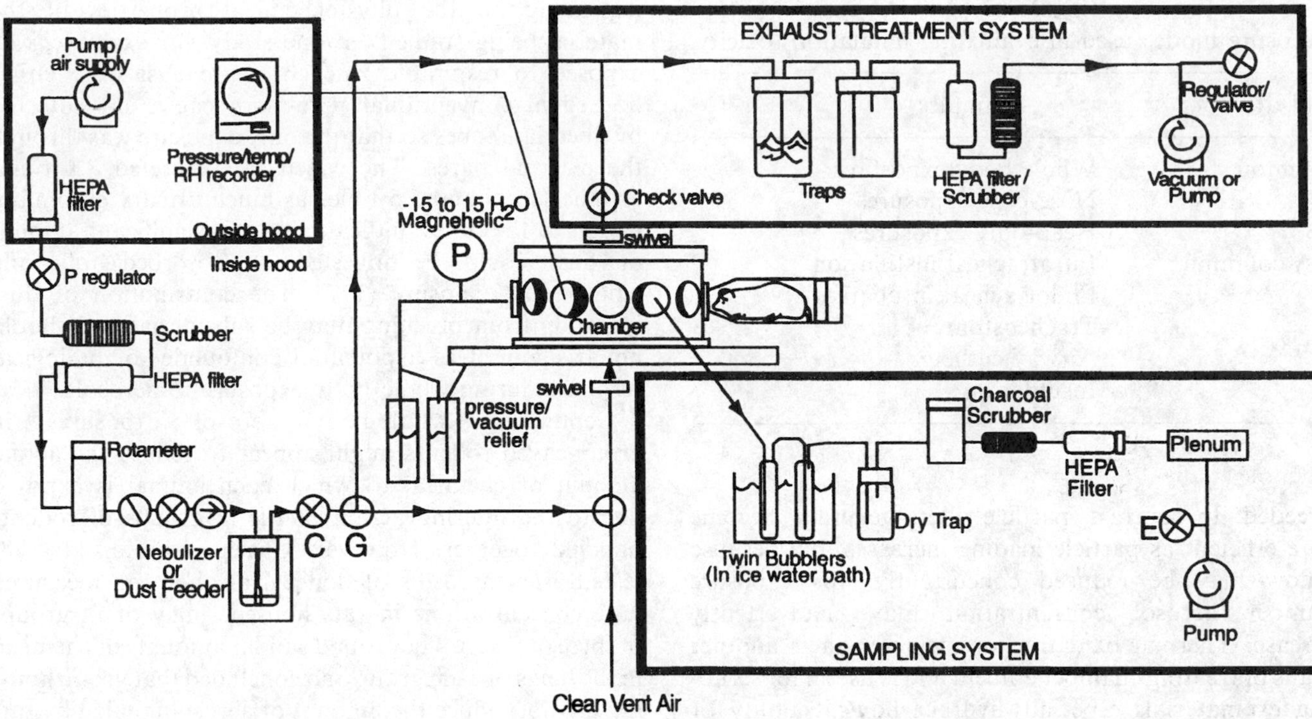

FIG. 23.11. Details of components used for air supply and test atmosphere generation, dilution and sampling, and exhaust in a nose-only inhalation exposure system.

mals but are electrically nonconductive. This may allow charge differences to accumulate within the chamber, causing variable test aerosol losses through electrostatic attraction, and can contribute to unacceptable spatial and temporal variations in chamber aerosol concentrations.

Normally, chambers are operated under dynamic exposure conditions (i.e., a continuous supply of air is flowing through the chamber) with a slight negative pressure within the chamber to prevent leakage of test material into the exposure room. The size of the chamber should be optimized to minimize heat build-up due to animal loading; typically, animal loading should be approximately 5% or less (176).

Atmosphere Sampling and Analytical System

Once the test atmosphere has been generated and delivered to the chambers, a means for collecting and analyzing the chamber air for test substance concentration must be developed. This information is essential to adjust exposure conditions as necessary so that the desired exposure concentrations are maintained. Additionally, sampling must be conducted to ensure that chamber temperature, airflow, and relative humidity are within the desired ranges, thereby minimizing the potential for biological effects from extremes in the environmental conditions. As with the selection of construction materials for the chamber, and generation and dilution systems, the test atmosphere sampling lines should not alter the concentration or composition of the species being analyzed. Ideally, sampling should be conducted from the breathing zone of the animals and with sufficient frequency during the exposure to determine the variability in test parameters (i.e., exposure concentrations and environmental conditions).

Exhaust/Scrubbing System

Exhaust systems are included in chamber design not only to assist in the flow of air through the exposure chambers but also to minimize discharge of test material into the environment. Federal, state, and local regulations on air emissions are becoming more stringent such that adequate abatement systems must be incorporated as a condition for study conduct. Depending on the physical properties of the test material, liquid or solid absorbents (e.g., water for water-soluble solvents and activated charcoal for low levels of organics) may be employed to remove gases or vapors, whereas porous filtering material may be appropriate for aerosols. However, liquid or solid absorbents can become saturated with test material and must be monitored with sufficient frequency to ensure that the adsorbent capacity has not been

Table 23.11
Exposure modes used in evaluating inhalation toxicity

Utilization	Examples
Common	Whole-body exposures
	Nose-only exposures
	Head-only exposures
Less common	Intratracheal instillation
	Endotracheal intubation
	Tracheostomy
	Airway catheter
	Insufflation

exceeded. In contrast, particle filters generally become more efficient as particle loading increases, but because airflow may be reduced concurrently, the exposure chamber aerosol concentration may inadvertently increase. Thermal oxidation or incineration is another means of treating chamber effluent and is useful for scrubbing test materials, especially hydrocarbons; its utility for halogen-containing substances has been limited by the additional difficulty and expense needed to dispose/treat the acids formed during oxidation.

Exposure Modes

A variety of exposure modes have been used to evaluate the effect of substances following inhalation (Table 23.11). The whole-body exposure mode is encountered most frequently in the human situation; that is, the exposed individual may freely move about in an atmosphere containing the chemical such that systemic absorption occurs through the lung following inhalation, through the skin following contact with aerosols or vapors, and through the gastrointestinal tract after swallowing readily cleared materials that initially deposited in the upper respiratory tract.

Whole-body inhalation exposures will result in a substantial portion of the chemical being ingested regardless of physical form. Gases or vapors can dissolve in the mucus fluid lining the respiratory tract and, via the mucociliary escalator, reach the pharynx, where they are swallowed. Droplets or solid particles also reach the gastrointestinal tract via this mechanism. Further contributions to total absorbed dose can occur by dermal absorption of the test agent. The normal grooming and preening activities of rodents both during and after inhalation exposures can deliver the chemical to the gastrointestinal tract. The quantitative contributions of dermal and oral absorption have not been studied adequately but would be expected to vary greatly depending on the physiochemical properties of the material being studied. In one study, for example, rats exposed to respirable zinc chromate dust were either housed in conventional wire-mesh cages or protected by fiberglass tubes so that the only exposure was through the external nares. The caged rats excreted 8.4 times as much fecal and 5.5 times as much urinary chromium as rats in the tubes, indicating that a significant amount of dust could be ingested or absorbed following whole-body exposure (177). The contribution of dust ingestion from preening may be substantial and should not be ignored as a potential confounder of biological response during whole body exposure to aerosols.

Conducting whole-body aerosol exposures in group-caged rodents might appear to reduce the actual amount of chemical to which each animal is exposed due to the filtering action of fur in groups of rodents huddled together. However, Ulrich and Marold (178) tested 3-μm aerosols of dodecyl alcohol and measured lung concentrations in rats housed singly or in groups of three or seven. They found similar amounts of chemical in the lungs of each group and concluded that group housing did not reduce the amount of aerosol inhaled by rats during a 6-h whole-body exposure.

Head-only exposures are useful for repeated brief exposures, where the amount of test agent is somewhat limited, and for restricting the route of entry of the material into the animal to the respiratory tract. Because nose-only systems limit exposure of the test substances to the respiratory tract and not the entire body, the amount of test material needed is considerably reduced. This feature facilitates testing highly toxic and/or limited-availability test substances. In addition, nose-only units simplify test substance containment and subsequent clean-up and allow the chamber concentrations to be more easily and readily altered. Disadvantages of this system include loss of material to the fur of the head, difficulty in obtaining a proper seal at the neck without impairing circulation, the possibility of restraint-induced stress to the animals, time and difficulty in handling the animals, and the relatively limited number of animals that can be tested simultaneously.

All of the above disadvantages can be dealt with in a manner that makes this type of testing useful in safety evaluation programs. To ensure uniformity of exposure conditions on an animal-to-animal basis, a relatively large airflow is needed. This prevents animals from inhaling chemical-depleted atmospheres. For larger animals such as the dog and monkey, helmet exposures can be conducted that also requires high airflow to prevent condensation. Pressure fluctuations in these systems may be great and records of breathing patterns during exposure may be needed to accurately measure the exposure doses. In addition, the fitting at the neck must be comfortable and easy to manipulate. Designs including both inflatable collars and thin rubber membranes have been used successfully.

Kirk et al. (179) describe a system for exposing guinea pigs to radioactive gases. The animals were placed in plethysmographs to record breathing patterns, and a rubberseal isolated the head inside the exposure area; the animals also could be exposed body-only while breathing fresh air if desired. Thomas and Lie (180) describe a similar system for aerosol testing in rats and mice. Dogs (181) and monkeys (182) have been tested using head-only techniques.

A typical nose-only exposure unit employs an animal exposure cylinder, generally constructed from rigid plastic. This tube is connected to an enclosure or exposure chamber that allows introduction and evacuation of test atmospheres and contains sampling probes to determine test concentrations, particle-size distributions, temperature, and humidity. Rodent holders are usually fabricated of polymethylmethacrylate, polycarbonate, or stainless steel cylinders to conform to the general shape of the animals, and are fitted with conical headpieces projecting into the plenum of the exposure chamber. Some nose-only systems minimize rebreathing of test atmospheres by attempting to have a constant flow of fresh test atmosphere into the face of the animal while having a local exhaust near the nose as shown in Figure 23.12. The animal holder needs to be of varying sizes to accommodate rodents of differing sizes to minimize stress, supported carefully to minimize discomfort to the animal, and adequately ventilated to minimize heat retention within the tubes.

Both physical restraint and inadequate temperature control within the chamber can subject the test animals to additional stresses not well understood. This seems to be especially true for inhalation developmental and/or reproductive studies. Pathological effects on the male reproductive system, independent of the inhaled test substance, have been reported in restrained male rats where inadequate temperature control occurred, leading to excessive body temperature (183). Inhalation developmental toxicity studies conducted with restrained pregnant rodents have produced slight increases in maternal toxicity and either slight (184) or no (185) increases in fetal anomalies when dams were restrained during the period of organogenesis. To minimize confinement induced stress in inhalation developmental toxicity studies in mice, Dorman et al. (186) utilized a rat restrainer tube to expose an unrestrained pregnant mouse, making essentially a whole-body exposure chamber for individual mice. Poorly understood effects on metabolism may also exist as restraint has a reportedly greater effect on slowing metabolism and energy balance in rats when restraint occurs in the morning (187). Overall, the selection of the nose-only exposure mode can affect the outcome of some inhalation toxicity studies and represents a decision that investigators should properly control for in experimental design. Nonetheless, high-capacity nose-only exposure systems, such as those described by Cannon et al. (188), are widely used for various acute and subchronic inhalation studies. A thorough description of the components used in a nose-only inhalation system, with details on automated collection

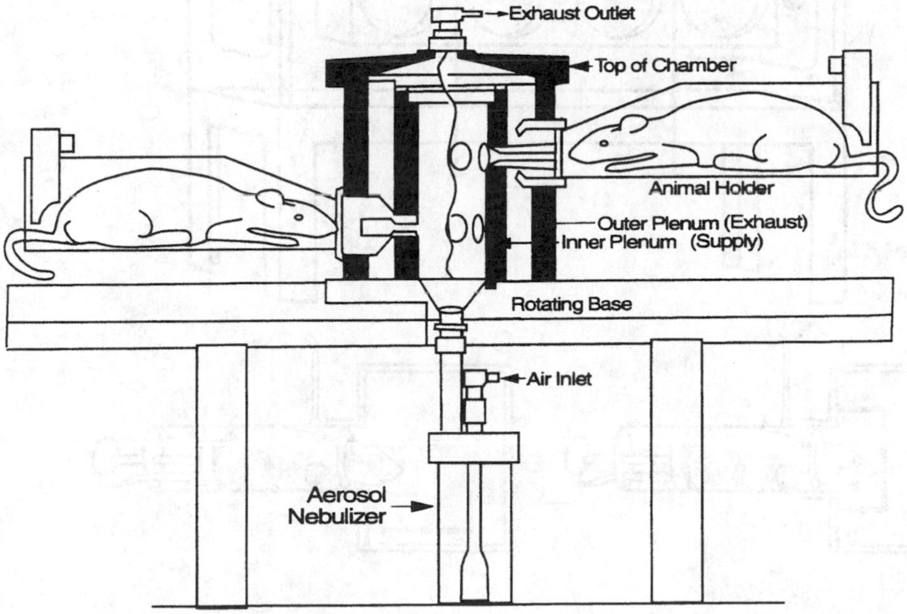

FIG. 23.12. Exposure chamber and rodent holder designed for nose-only exposures to aerosols or vapors.

methods for airflow regulation and test atmosphere analysis, was presented by Pauluhn (189).

Design considerations of head-only units are identical to those of nose-only units. Mask designs represent a unique kind of nose-only exposure and usually are limited to relatively large animals. Masks for dogs (190), monkeys (191), ponies (192), donkeys (193), chickens (194) and also rats (195) have been used successfully.

It may be necessary to conduct brief or instantaneous exposure to airborne materials. This might be required when developing data to deal with setting emergency exposure limits or when only small quantities of materials are available. Approaches include airlock and very low internal volume nose-only exposure chambers. To evaluate the lethal doses of highly toxic perfluoroisobutylene in rats with exposure times from 0.25–10 min, a low volume chamber was designed. A 1.5-L cylindrical Plexiglas chamber (75 cm × 5 cm diameter) with 10 staggered animal ports was developed using three equidistant sampling ports to monitor gas uniformity. With a 10 L/min airflow rate, chamber equilibrium was rapidly achieved in less than 1 min.

Sliding or dropping airlock mechanisms have also been used to achieve essentially instantaneous exposures. One simple design is the drop-away headspace compartment shown in Figure 23.13. Here animals are restrained and placed in slots, which allow their heads to protrude into the exposure chamber. Prior to exposure, a headspace compartment is held in place over the head, allowing circulation of fresh air to the animals. Atmospheres are premixed to the desired concentration and the flap is dropped away for instantaneous exposure. This design is inexpensive, easy to construct, and has been used to compare the irritating and lethal concentrations of stannic chloride. Stannic chloride reacts with moisture in the air to form an irritant smoke, which has been proposed to test for respirator fit in workers. In rats given a 1-min exposure (similar to the duration of an actual fit test), marked respiratory irritation but no mortalities were observed. With a 10-min exposure interval, respiratory irritation and mortality occurred—more importantly, in overlapping concentration ranges. On this basis, it was decided that an insufficient safety margin existed for general use of stannic chloride irritant smoke to test respirator fit in workers (196).

Large-scale testing using head-only exposures has been conducted (197) in 0.5-m^3 pyramidal, vertical flow chambers that accommodated up to 60 rats per chamber. Rats were exposed to fibrous aerosols for 6 h/day, 5 days/week for up to 24 months with relatively little test condition-related stress as measured by growth, body temperature, and plasma corticosteroid levels. The

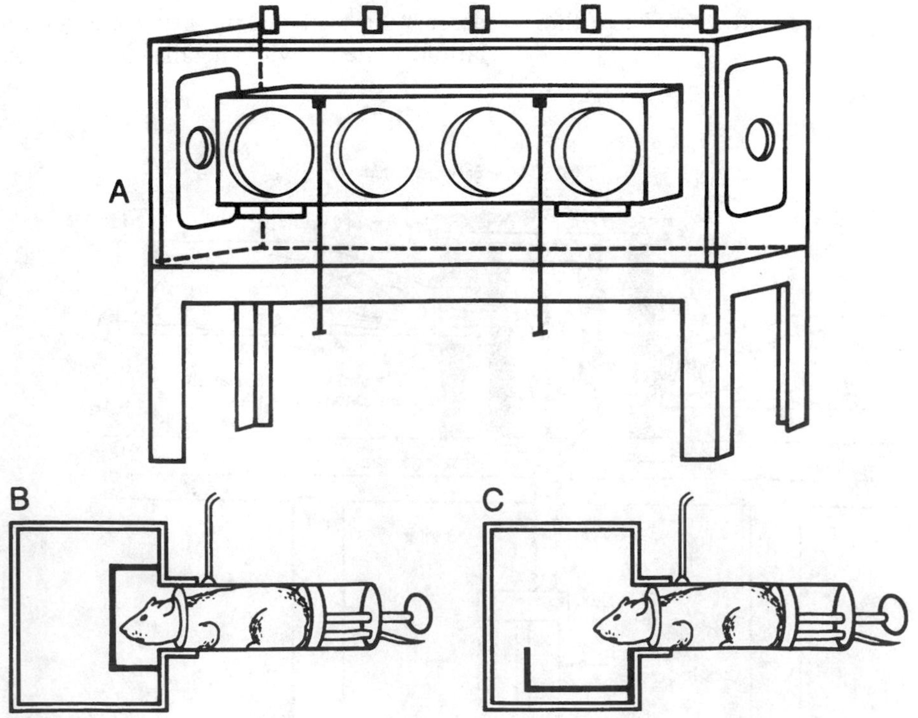

FIG. 23.13. Airlock exposure chamber for instantaneous exposures. A, Front view. B, End view, atmosphere preequilibrated while rats breathe fresh air. C, Airlock dropped for instantaneous exposure.

number of personnel needed to accomplish these exposures, following appropriate training so that the tasks became routine, was not considered excessive.

Alternative Exposure Techniques

Endotracheal intubation, tracheostomies, and airway catheters can be used to bypass the upper airway and expose only the lung to aerosols and gases. Endotracheal tubes are made of a flexible polymer and are passed through the mouth to the trachea and are sealed by inflation of a balloon placed at the tip of the tube. A high degree of control of total dose delivered can be obtained, which is helpful when studying extremely toxic or expensive materials. Several disadvantages, including bypassing natural upper respiratory tract defense mechanisms, mechanical complications, and interference with normal airflow characteristics, lead to a relatively nonphysiological animal preparation that makes extrapolation of these data tenuous.

Tracheostomy generally has the same applications, advantages, and disadvantages. Airway catheters allow deep penetration into the lung and can be used to deliver very exact doses to specific localized sites. Examples of experiments involving endotracheal tubes include studies with exposure to radioactive metal fume aerosols (198), to fresh cigarette smoke (199), and to radioactive tantalum dust (200).

The use of intratracheal instillation as an alternative to exposure of animals by inhalation deserves some comment. Conditions exist in which the pulmonary effects of a chemical cannot be easily evaluated by inhalation. Although not entirely valid reasons, space, time, and/or economic reasons can sway the decision not to use inhalation as the route of test material exposure, but rather to use intratracheal instillation techniques to get the material directly into the respiratory tract. The reason for choosing intratracheal instillation over inhalation can also rest on nonavailability of sufficient quantities of test material or on safety issues (extreme toxicity, flammability, explosivity). Using this method, the actual dose delivered to the lung of the experimental animal can be directly and precisely measured. This technique is inexpensive in that very small amounts of chemical are needed while expensive chambers, generating apparatus, and support personnel are avoided. Also, because the technique is contained and uses relatively little material, exposure hazards to laboratory workers are greatly reduced compared to that of an inhalation study. Finally, materials that are not readily respirable in rodents can be introduced to the lungs with this technique; notably, long fibers that can be inhaled by man but not by rodents can be tested via this route. The problem that limits the usefulness of intratracheal instillation as an exposure technique relative to inhalation is that the dose to the respiratory tissues can be variable, highly artificial, and does not accurately reflect the lung distribution of chemical following inhalation exposure. Additionally, intratracheal instillation techniques focus on the lower respiratory tract and, as such, cannot evaluate responses that would occur in the nasopharyngeal region by inhalation exposure.

Intratracheal instillation involves a suspension of particles in a carrier liquid that is injected directly into the lumen of the trachea or nebulized as very fine droplets into the airway. Gravity causes the fluid and particles to flow into the dependant areas of the lung. The carrier liquid is then rapidly absorbed into the pulmonary circulation, leaving the particles on the internal surfaces of the lung. This technique permits the introduction of a wide range of doses and substances to the lung in a short period of time. In larger animals, localized exposures to specific areas or lobes of the lung are possible, often allowing the contralateral lung to serve as a control (for nonsystemically acting agents). The technique was first applied by Kimura (201), using rabbits and guinea pigs and looking at the response to various coal tars. Early works have described in detail the methodologies found to be useful in the mouse (202,203), in the rat (204), and in the hamster (205). The procedures used in these studies are quite similar, with the main difference in the maximal amount of total liquid that can be used to deliver the test agent to the lung without killing the animal.

In small rodents, intratracheal instillation is accomplished by inserting a catheter or needle transorally through the mouth and epiglottis into the tracheal lumen. In larger species (including human), a fiberoptic bronchoscope can be used to more precisely visualize the instillation site. Because the animal must not move during the procedure, the choice of anesthetic is important, with short-acting materials that suppress reflexes for a minimal period of time being preferred. Saline is the vehicle most frequently used to suspend or solubilize the test substance, although even this may evoke a mild transient inflammatory response. Surfactants can be used to improve the suspension properties, but the effect on the lung tissue needs to be considered. In addition, dosage volumes need to be adjusted for the body weight of the animal; some evidence suggests that larger volumes might distribute the agent more evenly in the lung; however, excessive volumes will suffocate the animal. The rate of instillation must be controlled.

Although intratracheal instillation enables administration of large amounts and nonrespirable sizes of particulate matter that would otherwise not be able to gain access to the lung, highly localized deposition of particle usually results. Indeed, the major obstacle for routine use of intratracheal instillation as a replacement for inhalation bioassays lies in the fact that the patterns of particle distribution in the lung following instillation are uneven and are unlike those resulting from inhalation. Particle deposition by inhalation is focal, that is, inhaled particles deposit at selected sites in the lung depending upon their size. Brain and co-workers (207) showed that intratracheal instillation of particles produced nonuniform deposition patterns, largely dependent on gravitational settling. These investigators studied the distribution of particles labeled with ^{99}Tc in both rats and hamsters following either intratracheal injection or aerosol inhalation. Particle distribution patterns in the lung following inhalation were distributed evenly within a given lobe; among lung lobes, most of the dust deposited in the apical lobes (208). Pritchard et al. (209) found that variability in the deposition of cerium oxide particles in rats within a specific lobe was considerably greater following instillation than inhalation with little penetration of instilled particles to the peripheral lung. Similarly, greater peripheral lung loading was seen following inhalation of ferric oxide particles than following instillation (210). Using electron microscopic techniques, Brody and Roe (208) have shown that inhaled particles and fibers, which are small enough to pass through the conducting airways, deposit at selective sites (i.e., alveolar duct bifurcations) in the distal lung. This preferential deposition pattern has been confirmed by Warheit et al. (211) in several rodent species and substantiates the idea that the initial distribution pattern of inhaled particles appears to be focal. In contrast, the distribution of both short and long glass fibers in rats was reportedly similar using either inhalation or instillation (212). Drew (213) and Muller (214) and their colleagues found that both routes produced the same relative lobular distribution of uranium oxide particles. Despite these issues, other studies showed comparable levels of pulmonary injury for instilled or inhaled quartz dust, although animals that inhaled quartz developed granulomas whereas the instilled animals did not (215).

As a consequence of these differences in cellular and biochemical reactions, intratracheal instillation is a relatively nonphysiological approach with respect to the deposition patterns and can create an artefactual series of cellular (macrophage) reactions that do not accurately reflect the events that occur following inhalation exposure to dusts. The utility and limitations of intratracheal instillation methods for evaluating respiratory tract toxicity were recently reviewed and several recommendations for its use were provided (reference). As a screening tool, intratracheal instillation should prove to be useful to test potency differences between substances and to evaluate injury to the lower respiratory tract. The method would be particularly valuable as a screening tool if the substances to be tested were similar to a substance which already had extensive inhalation data. Intratracheal instillation was also considered useful to expose animals to particles of a size range that, if administered by inhalation, would have limited respirability or deposition in the rodent lung. In this case, instillation would provide an alternative dosing method for the distal lung to study pulmonary responses or particle retention characteristics. Acknowledged limitations of intratracheal instillation include: the potential for a localized inflammatory response arising from high local doses of instilled particles; the difficulty in extrapolating the instilled lung dose of substance to that derived by inhalation; the inability to duplicate particle deposition patterns from inhalation given the nonphysiologic nature of particle delivery; the possible interaction with vehicle/suspending agents; and potential interference of normal mucociliary transport rates.

Nonetheless, intratracheal instillation methods are being refined and used for some applications. Recently, exposure studies were completed to validate intratracheal instillation methodology and its applicability to more traditional inhalation studies (216). Rather than using an injected liquid bolus, liquid suspensions were injected with a bolus of air to form aerosol droplets within the airway. In this way, aerosol droplets were more uniformly distributed throughout the respiratory tract. These studies also indicated that particle size of the test suspension was not critical to the distribution of test particles into the lower respiratory tract and that this intratracheal nebulization method would be suitable for pulmonary absorption and disposition studies where knowing the precise dose administered is the primary concern (216). Ultimately, such methodology may find applications in acute toxicity screening studies or mechanistic studies where inhalation exposure doesn't necessarily provide any advantages.

Chamber Selection and Operation

Early inhalation experimentation utilized chambers that consisted of glass walls in a wooden frame (217), plywood and metal coated with a chemically resistant plastic (133), or made entirely of sheet metal (218). Acrylic chambers were developed from commercially available stock items and used by Gage (219), Montgomery et al. (220), and Laskin and Drew (221). The Laskin and Drew chamber was portable, permitted feed and water consumption determinations, and could accommodate up to 25 rats in a chamber with total volume of about 90 L.

Larger units were described by Fraser et al. (176) who introduced solid aerosols through the bottom of the chamber and exhausted them at the top. A plastic hexagonal chamber with a volume of 2.7 m^3 was used for dust studies and included a turntable allowing animals to be brought to the access windows for observation during the exposures. Wedge-shaped cages contained in plastic hemispheres were used to minimize loss of airborne agent by physical adsorption on the walls.

Conventional chambers are constructed of stainless steel and have transparent observation ports of plastic or glass. Both stainless steel and glass are well suited as chamber construction materials due to their excellent chemical resistance and their low adsorption characteristics. The Rochester chamber design described by Leach et al. (222) consists of a hexagonal chamber fitted at the bases with hexagonal pyramids. This design was shown to have a good airflow pattern (i.e., no stagnant areas) and uniform distribution of test substance within the chamber. As originally designed, the chamber also allows for good visibility of the test animals and could simultaneously house eight dogs, four monkeys, or 40 rats. Hinners et al. (223) found the hexagonal construction to be unnecessary and obtained satisfactory performance using chambers with a square cross-section, thereby simplifying design and reducing manufacturing costs. This design provides a large access door for efficient animal loading, large windows for animal observations, appropriate sampling ports, control of air and contaminant flows, signal devices for equipment failure, and temperature and humidity control, and has interior surfaces of stainless steel to prevent corrosion and to facilitate cleaning. A more modern exposure chamber design is described by Moss et al. (224). This vertical flow chamber of approximately 2 m^3 has an offset pyramidal inlet with three levels of caging and solid sheet catch pans below the cages. By incorporating offset catch pans, this design creates multiple areas of turbulence and promotes more uniform aerosol distribution within the chamber.

Horizontal flow chambers seem to be comparable to vertical feed chambers in concentration gradient characteristics but require higher flow rates to maintain uniform aerosol concentrations. A system described by Hemenway and MacAskill (225) utilized a unique inlet and outlet diffuser/plenum configuration, which, along with premixing of the test agent, allowed achievement of uniform exposure concentrations. These chambers also allow a higher animal packing density due to the lack of large inlet and outlet cones, and can fit into most conventional animal rooms without major modification. Ferin and Leach (227) describe a horizontal flow unit comprised of separate modules for air supply, contaminant addition, animal exposure, and exhaust. High airflow rates may cause laminar flow entering the module to become turbulent as it passes through the animal cages.

Most inhalation experiments utilize dynamic exposure conditions. That is, the test atmosphere, comprising test substance diluted with fresh air, is continually replenished; the test atmosphere flows through the exposure chamber and is then exhausted. Once the generation apparatus is turned on, the concentration in the chamber rises to a theoretical equilibrium value, which is the ratio of the flow of the agent to the total flow in the chamber. The equation describing the concentration–time curve is

$$C_t = f/F[1 - e^{-(F/V)t}]$$

where C_t is concentration after t min, f is the flow of agent, F is total flow through the chamber, and V is the chamber volume. Usually, this equation is converted to an expression that defines the time required to attain a given percentage of the equilibrium concentration ultimately attained:

$$t_x = K \times V/F$$

where t_x is the time required to attain x% of the equilibrium concentration and K is a constant whose value depends on x. Most frequently, the concentration–time relationship is described by t_{90} or t_{99}, the time needed to attain 90 or 99% of the theoretical equilibrium concentration. For determination of t_{90}, $K = 2.303$, whereas to calculate t_{99}, $K = 4.605$. At this time point, the concentration in the chamber may be considered constant, assuming no changes in air or test substance supply rates. The concentration–time characteristics of a given chamber are described by the values of V and F, which are preferred and more descriptive than the outdated practice of giving air changes per hour (228,229).

The duration of exposure is defined as the interval from the start of flow of test agent to the point where delivery is discontinued. The exposure is terminated by stopping the flow of agent to the atmosphere generator, which leads to the decline in the chamber concentration on an exponential curve that is the inverse of the rising curve (Figure 23.14). Animals are not removed from the chamber, nor are the chamber doors opened to observe the animals, until at least t_{99} min to allow sufficient time for the chamber contents to be fully eliminated. For longer-term exposures, the rising and falling sections of the curves can be neglected and the exposure profile becomes a square-wave form. For short exposures, where t is less than $13 \times t_{99}$, the system should include an airlock mechanism or some other instant exposure/nonexposure mechanism (230).

Chambers should be operated at a slight negative pressure (e.g., -2 cm H_2O) with respect to room pressure to protect personnel against leaks in the system. Chamber pressure should be monitored continually, especially in older units. The distribution of test substance within the exposure chamber is determined by taking repeated samples from different areas of the chamber in relation to a reference sampling location, using statistically valid sampling strategies to avoid the possibility of concentration variations. After homogeneous distribution of test substance within the chamber has been established, the

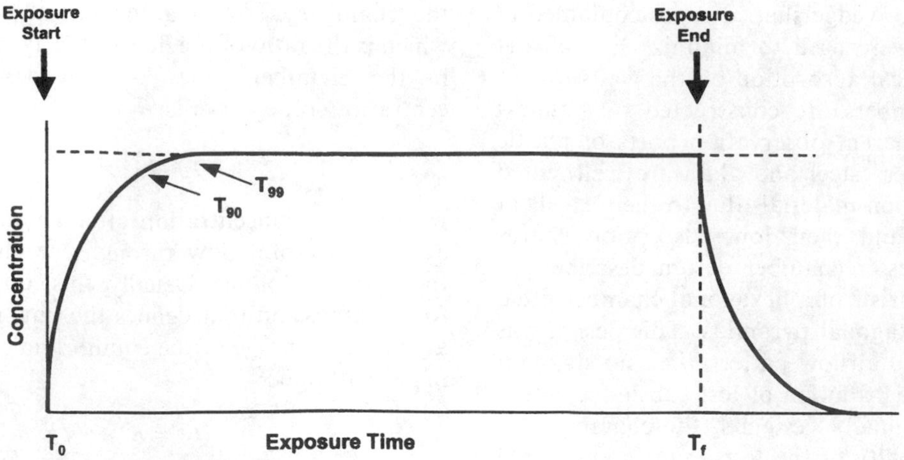

FIG. 23.14. Concentration and time relationship in a dynamic exposure chamber.

actual concentration should be measured several times during the exposure. For exposures of 4- to 6-h duration, a common practice is to sample every 0.5 h (or at least hourly), although for regulatory purposes much less frequent sampling (i.e., 2–4 times per exposure) may be acceptable; the frequency of sampling should be dictated by the temporal stability of the test atmosphere generation and airflow supply systems. Continuous readout monitoring and control instruments are especially useful in long-term studies, because they are capable of preventing concentration excursions when appropriate alarms are integrated into the system. This type of instrumentation can prevent many weeks or months of effort from being destroyed by sudden elevations in test substance concentration.

Inhalation chambers operated in a dynamic mode should have a reasonably uniform distribution of test chemical to avoid differential animal exposures. Due to their comparatively higher diffusion rates, it is generally acknowledged that gas and vapor concentrations show less intrachamber variations than aerosols. Aerosols are also subject to size-dependent impaction and sedimentation losses, compounding the difficulty in maintaining uniform chamber concentrations. However, MacFarland (231) calculated the percentage differences in concentrations between aerosols and gases/vapors. He considered the deviations encountered under normal test conditions to be similar and within ±15% suggesting that there is little difference in the chamber uniformity for aerosoles or gases/vapors. Examples from the literature concerning the degree of variability encountered are presented in Table 23.12. Because variations exist in all chamber types and airflow control operating systems, the investigator is well advised to carefully characterize the exposure chamber distribution of test substance under actual generation conditions to prevent concentration-gradient errors from complicating the study.

The actual concentrations measured in the chamber may vary within any single exposure or between exposure days. The control of vapor concentration is somewhat more readily achieved than that of aerosols and, after a few trials with most vapor generator systems, the standard deviation for a series of measurements through the day and from day to day should not vary by more than 10%. Variations of as much as 20–30% are commonly encountered with aerosols, particularly solid aerosols; in general, variability increases with particle size. Although this variation may be considered acceptable, greater control is generally possible (232).

Table 23.12
Intrachamber concentration variations reported in inhalation studies

Test chemical	Physical form	Difference (%) from average concentration
Ammonium fluorescein	Aerosol	3.0–7.6
Asbestos	Fiber	3.3–7.4
Carbon monoxide	Gas	0.7
Chlorine	Gas	2.1
Cobalt metal	Aerosol	11.7
Diesel exhaust	Aerosol	14.3–16.7
Formaldehyde	Gas	5.1
Methane	Gas	4.3
Nitrogen dioxide	Gas	4.3
Ozone	Gas	7.4
Sulfuric acid	Aerosol	3.4–18.0
Sulfur colloid of technetium	Aerosol	9
Sulfur dioxide	Gas	14.9

As described earlier, the actual dose delivered to the target tissue depends on factors other than concentration. Variations in breathing rates, respiratory volumes, and anatomic variations, for example, can be greater than the variation of agent concentration in terms of the delivered dose. In long-term studies, if a chamber reached only 60–70% of the target value for one particular exposure day, this does not suggest that the study is invalid in terms of the quantitative dose. The total accumulated exposure (concentration × time) should approach that specified in the experimental design, but an occasional value of 40% or even 50% above or below the target value is not sufficient reason to terminate or invalidate a study (233).

Airflow to a chamber can vary from approximately 10–60 changes per hour. This is understood as the addition and withdrawal of a volume of air equal to the volume of the chamber. Because added air mixes with that already present, a complete change of air has not occurred. The term "air change" is misleading and the dynamics of mixing in inhalation chambers has been described by the statistical considerations first put forward by Silver (229). As already discussed, a more descriptive term for chamber airflow is the t_{90} or t_{99}.

Although used infrequently, static exposures can generate some useful comparative toxicity information. In this method, animals are exposed in a sealed chamber without supplemental airflow and, therefore, offer a potentially useful method of experimentation for the investigator when the availability of the test chemical is limited. Indeed, because the air can be readily and repeatedly sampled for test substance and volatile metabolite concentrations, static exposure systems are finding increasing use in pharmacokinetic studies to measure the rates of test substance uptake and metabolism in experimental animals (234). Only materials that are gases or vapors at room temperature may be studied in this fashion, as aerosol deposition will likely reduce chamber aerosol concentrations with time. In static exposures, the substance is either injected through a sealable port or released from within the chamber (235), with the concentration increasing rapidly to a peak. Of necessity, the exposures can be at most 30–60 min in duration because oxygen depletion will occur and carbon dioxide and internal temperatures can rise rapidly, depending on both the size of the chamber and the number of animals contained therein. If the test substance is physically or chemically adsorbed to the internal surfaces of the test system, gradual losses of test substance will occur, gradually decreasing its concentration. Despite these limitations, static exposure systems have undergone improvements over the years through the use of soda lime traps to remove carbon dioxide, periodic injection of oxygen to replenish depleted oxygen, and better temperature control through use of cooling systems; these changes have greatly improved the versatility of this exposure mode (236). Further improvements in this methodology have included recirculation of the exposure atmosphere after passage through carbon dioxide and water traps and oxygen supplementation as necessary (237).

Control of the relative humidity but more importantly, the internal temperature, of inhalation chambers is crucial to the integrity and interpretation of animal inhalation studies. As already noted, elevated temperatures can alter animal physiology, affect metabolic rates, and increase the rate and type of chemical interactions. Ideally, the total volume of animals in a chamber should not exceed 5% of the chamber volume to avoid heat-induced artefacts among test animals (176). Coincidentally, chamber loading also affects the test substance equilibrium concentration in the exposure chamber. Silver (229) reported, for example, that when the animal loading (total animal weight to chamber volume) exceeded 5%, excessive losses of test substance occurred, presumably by absorption to body surfaces. Temperature should be monitored regularly during the exposure. In some instances, such as when chamber loadings exceed this recommendation, chambers may require that inlet air be cooled to maintain normal interior temperatures. Heat-balance studies with rats in stainless steel or glass chambers of equal size and using a room air intake of 100 L/min showed that the chamber walls were effective at removing approximately 90% of the animal body heat as compared with the heat loss through the airstream. If conducting studies in chambers with low airflow rates, heat transfer to the surrounding environment can be increased by painting the chambers, by attaching cooling coils to the chamber walls, or by directing air-conditioning ducts directly onto the chamber (238). In addition, control of relative humidity is essential for proper heat balance in rodents. Although it is generally acknowledged that relative humidity should be controlled within relatively narrow limits (e.g., 40–60%) to minimize adverse effects on feed consumption and behavior on study outcome (239), recent work by Pauluhn and Mohr show that rats tolerated humidity levels of either 3, 40, or 80% without effects on body weights, feed or water consumption, or respiratory tract histopathology (240).

Administered Dose

The fundamental concept of dose (i.e., the amount of substance introduced into the test system) is not excluded from the domain of inhalation toxicology. Yet due to the difficulty in measuring individual respiratory parameters and the test substance's physical/chemical properties (two direct primary characteristics that affect the respiratory tract deposition of inhaled materials), determination of the internalized dose is much more complex by inhalation compared to other exposure routes. Of the total amount of test material inhaled, a variable fraction may actually be deposited, absorbed, and reach target tissues. This absorbed fraction is, in turn, dependent on the local absorptive, metabolic, and clearance processes that may modify the chemical properties and/or its concentration of the inhaled substance within the lung, the target tissue, or the body. Although these processes are not easily determined and have restricted the ability of inhalation toxicologists to provide quantitative measures of inhaled dose, progress in the area of dose determination has evolved in the related areas of biomarkers and mathematical modeling. Increasingly sophisticated models are being used to estimate toxicant concentrations in the blood and organs by treating the uptake, distribution, metabolism, and excretion of toxicants as a series of independent processes occurring at experimentally determined rates (241).

The administered dose in inhalation studies is most often characterized in terms of the exposure conditions, that is, the exposure concentration and duration according to certain conventions. For example, "rats were exposed to *x* ppm (or *y* mg/m^3) of chemical *z* for 6 h/day, 5 days/week for 13 weeks." For gases and vapors, concentration may be expressed on a volume basis (i.e., mole *x*/total moles, parts per million [ppm], or parts per billion [ppb]) or on a weight basis (milligrams per liter [mg/L] or milligrams per cubic meter [mg/m^3]). For solid or liquid aerosols, concentrations are generally expressed on a weight basis (milligrams per liter [mg/L]), or for fibrous materials, on a number basis (number of fibers per cubic centimeter [fibers/cm^3]). Furthermore, for fibrous aerosols, consideration should be given to expressing concentration on both a respirable mass (mg/m^3) and a particle count (fibers/cm^3) basis; with some low density fibers, the number count may be extremely high but the mass concentration may be very low. It must be understood that these conventions do not convey any information about the actual amount internalized but are conventions that merely reflect the conditions under which the study was conducted.

A fundamental interrelationship exists for many inhaled substances between exposure concentration and time. Haber (242), for example, determined that the response of an animal to a gas could be related to the product of the concentration and the exposure time. This relationship, known as Haber's law, states that the product of the concentration (C) and exposure time (T) required to produce a specific physiological or toxicological effect is equal to a constant, $C \times T = K$. The specific effect can be something other than death, but death is a commonly applied endpoint. Haber's law has been used to predict response for exposure conditions that have not been described experimentally, for example, predicting the expected 1-h LC_{50} value for a chemical agent where only 4-h data exist. There are short but finite time periods during which the specific endpoint may never be attained (i.e., death may not occur at practically attainable concentrations in short [e.g., 0.1-, 1-, or 10-min] time periods). At the other extreme, some exposure levels exist where substances do not produce measurably adverse effects despite continuous, prolonged exposures. For these reasons, Haber's law does not apply to all chemicals but generally is applicable when extrapolated to $C \times T$ values that differ by a factor of about 3 to 4 for a given $C \times T$ product. Rinehart and Hatch (243) and Kelly et al. (244) have shown, for example, that Haber's law applies for phosgene gas and titanium tetrachloride aerosol when evaluated for respiratory rate and lethality endpoints, respectively. Gelzleichter et al. (245) also showed that Haber's law applied for nitrogen dioxide or ozone in rats exposed for 3 days over a fourfold range of exposure concentrations. However, if rats were exposed to mixtures of ozone and nitrogen dioxide, lung damage was found to be related to the peak concentration rather than the cumulative dose of the gases; this observation was related to the synergistic, adverse effects of the mixture of these two gases (245). A quantitative assessment of the temporal and concentration relationships for lethality with several irritant and systemically acting substances was evaluated by ten Berge et al. (294). These authors reported that for the substances evaluated, the $C \times T$ relationship does not always represent the dose response data over the exposure periods reported. They reported that $C^n \times T$, where the exponent n may vary from 0.8 to 3.5, is often a better predictor of mortality. However, recent work by Pauluhn et al. (246) to explore $C \times T$ relationships from acute inhalation testing for product classification purposes suggests that 4-h exposure data provide essentially the same projected acute lethality value as would 1-h testing; where only 4-h data were available, a default value of 4 should be used for conversion of 4-h LC_{50} values to 1-h LC_{50} values, independent of the physical state of the test substance.

The internalized dose is related to the atmospheric concentration of the test substance, the duration of exposure, the individual's respiratory volume and frequency, and the deposition efficiency within the individual. These parameters are related according to the following general equation:

$$D = E_d V_m C T$$

where

D = deposited dose (mg)
E_d = deposition efficiency for the substance within the respiratory tract

V_m = minute volume (L/min)
C = concentration of the test substance (mg/L)
T = time of exposure (min)

Use of this equation presupposes that the above parameters are well characterized for the species and chemical substance under investigation and a given set of experimental conditions. In practice, such data are not generally available, especially for gases or vapors and other methods of dose estimation have been used. For a series of vapors, the internalized dose has been estimated by measuring the net decrease in test substance concentration in the exhaled air compared to the concentration in the inhaled air (40); similar methodology has been used to measure deposition of ultrafine aerosols in the human respiratory tract (247). Alternative methods to estimate the deposited dose have included chemical assays for the total amount of test substance or its metabolite in excreta, a useful technique for radioactively labeled materials. Measurement of metabolite levels and DNA or protein adducts in biological fluids or tissues represents another means of assessing chemical exposure and internalized dose (248–250). In related studies, the amount and formation rate of DNA and protein cross-links in nasal mucosa following exposure to formaldehyde (251), the formation of DNA adducts from polycyclic aromatic hydrocarbon exposure (252), butadiene monoepoxide levels in tissues (253), complex mixtures such as tobacco smoke (254), and the dose-dependent differences in benzene (255) metabolic formation (256) have been measured. An advantage of measuring DNA adducts in evaluating dose–response relationships is the comparatively higher sensitivity associated with the measurement of such biomarkers. In contrast to the comparatively high exposure concentrations employed in cancer bioassay studies, changes in the amount of metabolite–DNA adducts may be measured at much lower exposure concentrations compared to those associated with changes in tumor incidences: This method thus provides a better estimation of the shape of the dose–response curve at low concentrations.

For refinements of dosimetry in the human population, current work is focusing on development of a quantitative description of representative lung forms and breathing patterns, especially for potentially more sensitive subpopulations. Also, aerosol dosimetry within the respiratory tracts of susceptible subpopulations as a function of particle size, water-solubility, and breathing rates requires more research. Finally, the mathematical relationships for predicting regional and local deposition in the respiratory tracts in the aged and diseased need to be modeled and verified.

The importance of quantifying the internalized dose, particularly as it relates to human risk assessment, has encouraged research in the area of physiologically based pharmacokinetic (PBPK) modeling (257). Use of PBPK modeling is finding wide acceptance among risk assessors and regulatory agencies for estimating thc dosc of toxicant to a given tissue under various exposure conditions. This approach describes the kinetic relationships between physiological factors (such as organ and body weights, respiratory rate, and blood flow), biochemical factors (such as substrate affinity for an enzyme and reaction velocity), and physiochemical factors (such as the extent of chemical partitioning into air, blood, or tissue) on the disposition of that chemical within the body. Pharmacokinetic modeling is based on a thorough understanding of these processes in an experimental animal, and then extrapolating these parameters, with appropriate validation in experimental animals, to predict target tissue doses and toxic effects in humans. Validated PBPK models, using accepted physiological values, may then be useful in predicting expected tissue levels of a chemical (and thus organ toxicity) under various exposure regimens (Figure 23.15). Indeed, PBPK models have been developed to describe the expected tissue doses of chemicals in rodents or humans for vapors such as butadiene (258), benzene (259), halogenated hydrocarbons (260), butoxyethanol (261), as well as particulate matter such as powdered fire suppressants (262) or diesel soot, titanium dioxide (263), and quartz dust (264). The utility of PBPK modeling is not limited to inhalation exposures; McDougal et al. (265) described a model to predict dermal absorption of vapors, which is based on permeability constants. When PBPK modeling is employed, due caution must be exercised with respect to the applicability of the animal model and experimental techniques used and their relationship to human values for the data to be useful in human health risk assessment.

A practical example of the utility of PBPK modeling was presented in a recent study evaluating the hazard of formaldehyde to humans (266). These workers developed a PBPK model to predict the concentration of formaldehyde–DNA cross-links based on minute volume and amount of nasal mucosal DNA in rats. After predicting the expected cross-link formation rates, the PBPK model was verified experimentally in monkeys. The PBPK model, verified in both rats and monkeys, was then offered as a more realistic predictor of the delivered doses of formaldehyde to human nasal tissue. Use of such PBPK models may reduce the uncertainty for human cancer risk assessment by decreasing the uncertainty in interspecies extrapolations.

Atmosphere Generation

Gases are the simplest atmospheres to generate. They can be metered by flowmeters, syringe drives, diffusion

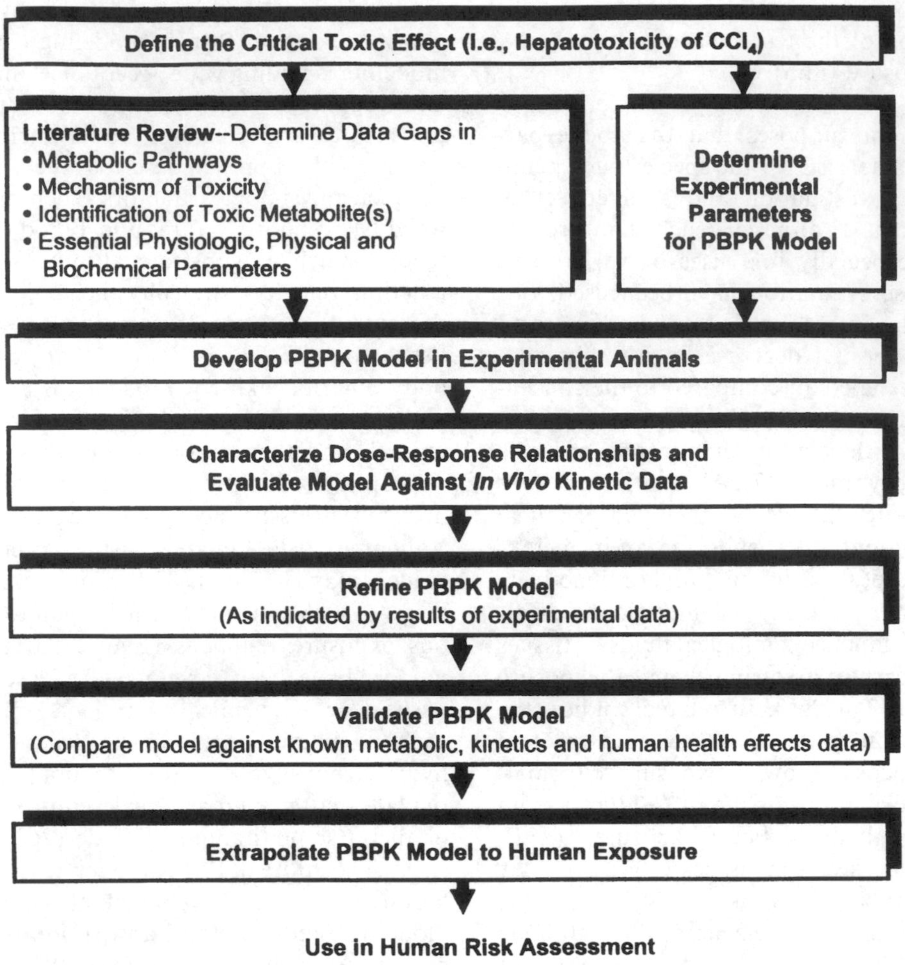

FIG. 23.15. Steps in developing a physiologically based pharmacokinetic (PBPK) model for use in predicting human health risks from exposure to chemicals in test animals (see Chapter 5).

tubes, or some other suitable technique into a dilution airstream, allowed to mix, then introduced into the exposure chamber. A number of flow dilution devices are available.

Vapors of either liquid or solid compounds can be formed by heating within a temperature-controlled heating device (care must be taken to prevent chemical decomposition or reaction with air or water at elevated temperatures used to generate vapor). Another technique, depending on physical properties such as viscosity and chemical purity, is to use an infusion pump to meter the liquid test substance onto a heated surface. A variation of this technique is the "J-tube" developed by Miller et al. (267). This device uses a heated J-shaped tube filled with glass beads to increase the available surface area for compound vaporization. This unit works well with substances that decompose at temperatures near their boiling point. Other liquid materials may be vaporized in fritted-glass bubblers. Frequently, nitrogen is used to vaporize the test substance to minimize chemical reaction or oxidation at elevated temperatures. The saturated airstream can then be diluted with filtered air to raise the oxygen concentration to 19–21% and to adjust the test substance level to the desired concentration. Special care must be taken when generating vapors from mixtures of test substances with low boiling points. If test atmospheres are generated from the liquid mixture followed by flash evaporation, the composition of the resulting vapor will be representative of the composition of the liquid mixture. In contrast, if the headspace of the liquid mixture is tapped, the resulting vapor composition will reflect the partial pressures of the components with a disproportionate amount of the component with the highest vapor pressure relative to the other components. This is a problem in longer-term inhalation studies, because the concentration will vary from day to day as the higher vapor pressure components of the mixture are depleted.

The generation of particulate materials in a uniform manner is considerably more difficult than that for vapors. Particulate materials may be generated from dry powders or from liquids and the resultant particles may vary greatly in size. Dispersions of liquids in air are called aerosols and occur in sizes ranging between colloidal (nm) and macroscopic (μm). Examples that occur in industrial processes include dusts, fumes, smokes, mists, clouds, and fogs. Their physical properties, particle size range, and source distinguish these various aerosol forms.

The generation of aerosols using dry dispersion techniques presents problems that are unique to each dust being studied. In toxicological testing, particle concentration and size distribution need to remain constant over long periods of time. The powder being tested must be dispersed into unitary particles of respirable size rather than agglomerates. This requires a means of continuously metering a powder into the aerosol generator at a constant rate, a means of disrupting particle clumps or aggregates, and a way of suspending the resulting discreet particles in an airstream. Most materials contain particles of irregular size and shape, which means that monodisperse aerosols are rarely produced and that, in the generating system, the particle size distribution will differ from that occurring in the original powder.

Simple dust metering systems use gravity feed of loose powder into an airstream, usually assisted by screw driven conveyors, agitators, or vibrators. Systems such as volume feeders deliver specific amounts from a reservoir or hopper to an aerosol generator. The Wright dust feed uses a scraping mechanism to remove a finely ground powder from the surface of a packed cylinder of test substance. Other metering systems use metal screws or brushes to move small amounts of powder to the generator. These systems are described in more detail by Hinds (68) and Cohen (268).

Aerosol generation involves the dispersion of a powder by supplying sufficient energy, such as a high velocity airstream, to a relatively small volume of the bulk powder in order to separate the particles by overcoming their own attraction forces. Hydrophobic materials such as talc are more easily dispersed than hydrophilic materials such as limestone or quartz because particle agglomeration or clumping is minimal. Thus, dry powders are considerably easier to disperse than humidified ones. The metered powder may be dispersed and agglomerates broken up directly by a turbulent air jet, or the dust-laden airstream can be passed through an impactor or fluidized bed. Elutriators, used to selectively remove large agglomerates, are also useful in dispersion. Clean, dry air can be used to generate aerosols but it should be noted that extremely dry air (relative humidity less than 50%) can cause strong electrostatic forces among particles, reducing their dispersibility.

Willeke et al. (269) describe fluidized-bed aerosol generators that are capable of very stable output of particles from 0.5–3 μm. This generator uses a fluidized bed of glass or metallic beads (100–200 μm) into which the powdered test substance is added. The mechanism of dispersion involves the agitation of particles by the beads and their subsequent entrainment into the airstream from both the particle impaction, as the beads collide with one another, and aerodynamic turbulence. The entire system also acts as an elutriator, preventing large particles and agglomerates from leaving the system. This means of generation can only be used for dry, nonadhering powders and produces electrically charged aerosols, which need to be neutralized upon leaving the fluidized bed.

Lee et al. (270) used a high pressure air-impingement device (microjet) to separate the finer fibrils from a Kevlar fiber matrix. Once separated from the bulk fiber matrix, the smaller fibers pass through a cyclone into the exposure chamber (Figure 23.16). This system was used to generate fiber mass concentrations as high as 18 mg/m^3 or fiber count concentrations as low as 2.5 fibers/cm^3 for periods ranging from 2 weeks to 2 years. The microjet is a versatile aerosol generator, finding practical applications for both fibrous and nonfibrous materials. By increasing airflow to the secondary high pressure air jets, the microjet can be adjusted to either disrupt particle aggregates or to effect some reduction in particle size through trituration in the oval inner chamber (Figure 23.17). Other examples of the use of this technology for particle dispersal are described by Cheng et al. (271) and Bernstein et al. (272). Bernstein et al. (272) described a brush feed micronizing jet mill that produces a relatively wide concentration range of respirable particles. Test concentrations from 0.22–7.48 mg/L were attained and maintained with particles less than 3 μm. Only at higher aerosol concentrations were these small particle sizes not attainable.

Atmosphere Analysis

The sampling system used in determining chamber concentrations should be designed to transmit a representative air sample (from the breathing zone of the animal) to the sensor or collection medium without significant losses. The sampling train should be designed to contain as few impaction locations (bends, reducers, and turns) as possible. It is not necessary that the collection efficiency be 100%, but the efficiency should be known and consistent to be useful. Rarely are aerosols monodisperse and because most particle entrapment mechanisms are size dependent, the collection characteristics of a given sampler will change with particle size. Also, the collection efficiency will change in response

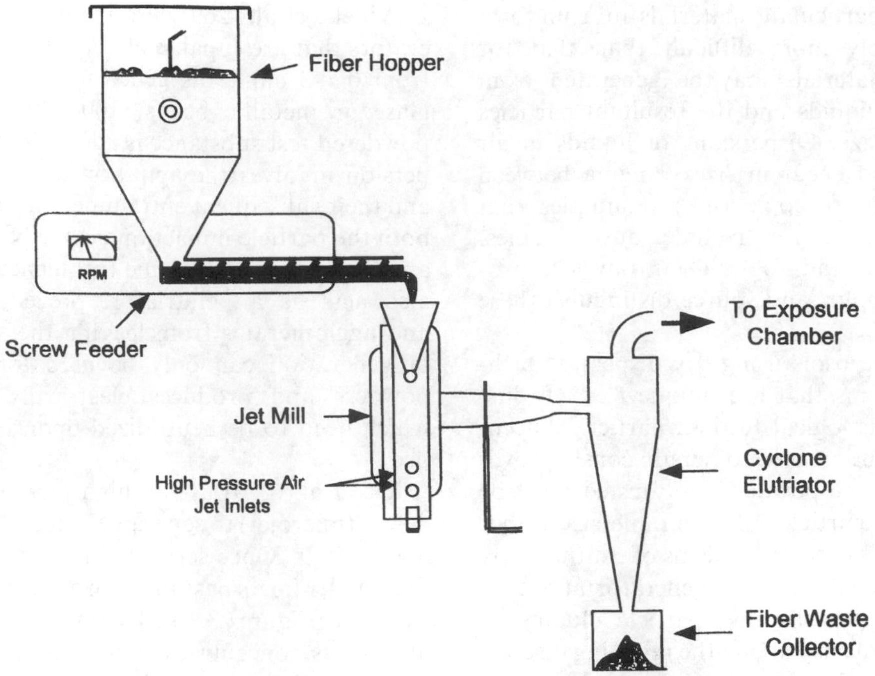

FIG. 23.16. Generation system used to produce air-borne Kevlar fibrils using a commercially available jet mill.

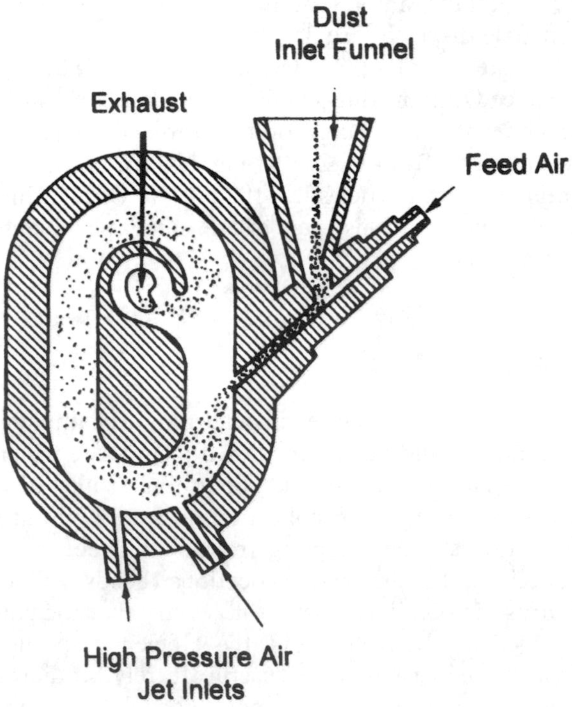

FIG. 23.17. Cross-section of jet mill used for fiber and particle generation.

to particle loading. A filter will be more efficient as dust collects on the surface. In contrast, the efficiency of an electrostatic precipitator will drop as a resistive layer of particles accumulates on the collection electrode.

Sampling errors generally reflect the contribution of many small errors in the system rather than any single large source of error. The items that need to be carefully considered and examined in any such system include sampling train leakage and losses, variations in flow rate and sample volumes, collection efficiency, sample stability, extraction efficiency from the sampling substrate, and analytical background or interferences introduced by the sampling substrate.

Gases and vapors offer the least difficulty in sampling as they follow the normal laws of diffusion, mix freely with the general atmosphere, and equilibrate rapidly. Direct reading instruments that have response times of seconds or less can be used to conduct sampling. Sensors in these instruments utilize infrared and ultraviolet radiation, flame and photoionization, and chemiluminescence.

Direct samples may be instantaneous or continuous in nature. If grab sampling is conducted, samples should be taken with sufficient frequency to identify fluctuations in chamber concentration. Such samples may be collected in evacuated glass or metal containers, inflatable flexible polymer bags, or by gas-tight syringe. Alternatively samples may be taken remotely by directing the sample through sample lines using a vacuum pump and by injecting aliquots of the stream directly into the analytical instrument. Continuous samples can be taken by pumping (or drawing) a constant stream of gas directly through a detector.

Extractive sampling involves removal of the chemical from air by scrubbing through a solvent or reagent, adsorption to a collection surface, or condensation on a cold surface. This type of collection involves use of a sample collector that may include sampling lines, a scrubbing device, an airflow or volume meter, and a vacuum pump.

Instantaneous or integrated sampling may be used to collect particulate matter. Instantaneous sampling involves removing a small volume of the atmosphere and impacting it against a solid substrate on which the deposited particles are later characterized (counted and sized). For continuous sampling, physical forces such as gravity, impaction, electrophoresis, thermophoresis, and diffusion techniques may be employed. Instrumentation for determining the mass and size of particulate matter in inhalation chambers are listed in Table 23.13.

Filters represent the most commonly used method for determining aerosol mass concentration in the chamber. The filtering material should be chemically unreactive with the test aerosol, have good collection efficiency, have low pressure loss, and should allow quick and quantitative desorption of test substances for possible chemical

Table 23.13
Features of some aerosol monitoring instrumentation

Instrument	Aerosol size (μm)	Response time	Measured parameter	Factors affecting response	Advantages	Disadvantages
Photometer	0.3–15	Continuous	Total light scattering	Density, size distribution, refractive index	Continuous readout	Response changes with dust type
β-Attenuation monitor	1–15	1–30 min	Absorption of β-radiation	Atomic number	Direct mass measurement	Low sensitivity
Optical particle counter	0.3–15	0.1–10 min	Light scattering, size, and count	Density, refractive index	Indication of size, high sensitivity	Low resolution and accuracy
Piezobalance	0.02–10	0.5–2 min	Mass	Particle size	Direct mass measurement	Sensor cleaning
Piezobalance cascade impactor	0.05–25	1–60 min	Mass	Particle size	Direct mass measurement, size distribution	Sensor cleaning, internal losses
Condensation nucleus counter	0.01–1	0.5–30 s	Particle count	Particle count	Small particle sensitivity	Alcohol emission
Diffusional mobility particle sizer	0.003–1	<1–5 min	Size based on electrical mobility	Electrical charge	Real time display of ultrafine particle size	Measures only fine particles
Fibrous aerosol monitor	Optically visible fibers	1–1000 min	Light scattering "size" of fibers	Fiber length, size	Specific for fibers	Nonfibrous interferences
Aerodynamic particle sizer	0.8–15	2–10 min	Aerodynamic size	Density	Direct measure of aerodynamic diameter	Coincidence and density effects
Tapered element oscillating microbalance	0.002–15	0.01–30 min	Mass	Absorbed water	Direct mass measurement	Frequent Filter replacement

Adapted from Reference 295.

analysis. Filters made from superfine glass fibers with diameters below 1 μm are available, for collecting virtually all suspended particles. These have low airflow resistance and interfere negligibly with most subsequent chemical analyses. Low volatility liquid particles such as sulfuric acid mist may be collected on glass filters with good results. Membrane filters with different flow and particle collection efficiencies are also available, and have been used widely in characterizing atmospheres of mineral dusts by both optical and electron microscopy. Some of the different filter media available include polytetrafluoroethylene, cellulose acetate, or polycarbonate.

Complementary to aerosol mass monitoring by filtration, real-time aerosol monitors can be used to provide continuous analytical data for concentration adjustments. Cheng and colleagues (273) describe the application of one such system. The detector is a photometer that collects scattered light from the aerosol cloud within a 55–95° envelope prior to detection with a silicon photodetector. The system has worked well at lower (<50 mg/m^3) aerosol concentrations.

Impingers and impactors rely on the inertial properties of particles for sample collection. An impinger consists of a glass nozzle submerged in water or alternative liquid media. For particle sizing, cascade impactors are used. These contain a number of impingement stages in series with graduated nozzle velocities and impaction distances to effect a progressive separation of smaller and smaller particles as aerosol progresses through the unit. Particles deposited on each stage can be weighed and/or examined microscopically. The aerodynamic median size of an aerosol may be determined with the cascade impactor by calculating the percentage by weight on each stage using weight, radioactivity, or chemical analysis to determine the amount of material deposited on each stage. This process is shown in Table 23.3 and in Figure 23.4.

Electrostatic precipitators involve the use of an open tube with collection of airborne particles directly on the inside of the tube, on an inserted foil of transparent or opaque material, or on glass microscope slides placed between the collecting tube and a central ionizing wire. Thermal precipitators are limited in use because the dust-free zone around the hot body can be maintained only at very slow airflow sampling rates. Settling chambers, centrifugal devices, and scrubbers are used infrequently but do have certain specialized applications for aerosol size classification.

PULMONARY FUNCTION STUDIES

Although less frequently used in animal toxicology, tests of pulmonary function are useful tools for evaluating the hazards of inhaled materials. Reviews of this topic which are very useful in gaining additional insight have been presented by Costa (274) and O'Neil and Raub (275). Reviews allowing fuller appreciation of the total body responses are well covered in respiratory physiology reviews by Green (276) and West (277) and in cardiovascular physiology reviews by Gross (278) and Gibson (279). Another valuable chapter that covers the majority of types of pulmonary function tests commonly applied to laboratory animals was prepared by Anthonisen (280).

Pulmonary function tests are a nondestructive means of assessing the functional impact of alterations in lung structure. The tests supply information on the presence, nature, and extent of functional loss. The application of these tests to inhalation toxicology can provide indicators of response, characterize the pathogenesis of lung disease, and be used in the extrapolation of information from animal tests to human.

It must be understood that functional changes themselves do not describe structural changes but they do imply that something is happening. Because these tests evaluate the integrated function of the entire organ, focal lesions can exist without measurably affecting organ function. These pulmonary function tests are clearly not substitutes for histopathological evaluation. Although changes in pulmonary function are not pathognomonic for specific lesions, with experience much information about lung structure can be implied from functional changes.

Ventilation involves the movement of air into and out of the lung in a reciprocal manner via the conducting airways in response to the chest wall and diaphragm. Physiological parameters that are important here include the rate at which the air is being moved, the portion reaching the gas-exchange membrane, the work required to move the air, and the uniformity of distribution at the gas exchange membrane. Breathing patterns (respiratory frequency, tidal volume, and minute volume as measured parameters), lung volumes (total lung capacity, vital capacity, residual volume), static and quasistatic lung compliance (measurements of the elastic property of the lung), dynamic lung mechanics (airflow resistance), and forced exhalation tests (forced vital capacity, forced expiratory volume) are parameters commonly applied to evaluation of lung function.

Gas distribution within the lung is affected by the mechanical properties of the airways and lung parenchyma. Hence, the uniformity of the intrapulmonary gas distribution is often measured as an index of lung mechanical properties. These tests include single- and multiple-breath gas washouts as well as those involving radiolabeled gas.

The efficient exchange of carbon dioxide and oxygen across the alveolar–capillary membrane is the ultimate result of normal pulmonary function. Derangements of this process can be used as a marker of disease. Oxygen and carbon dioxide exchange is usually measured by collecting expired air over a short period of time. Some useful indices of distribution of inspired gases among ventilated compartments such as anatomic dead space, perfused alveoli, and alveolar dead space can be calculated if inspired, expired, and alveolar gas concentrations, carbon dioxide output, and arterial oxygen are measured. Blood gas determinations are key to these endpoint functional determinations.

BRONCHOALVEOLAR LAVAGE AND BIOCHEMICAL STUDIES

Bronchoalveolar lavage (BAL) is playing an increasingly valuable role for the inhalation toxicologist in the investigation of pulmonary injury. Cytological analysis of BAL fluid has been used in animals and humans for the diagnosis of lung disease for many years. Relatively recently, not only the compositional and functional characteristics of the cellular fraction but also the biochemical components of BAL fluids have been used to detect, define, and quantify the type and severity of airway injury (281–285). In its simplest form, BAL is a procedure in which the airway surfaces of the bronchial and alveolar regions of the lung are washed or lavaged with an isotonic salt solution. It is a method of sampling the fluid and free cells covering bronchoalveolar epithelium. In analyzing selected cytological, functional, and biochemical parameters of BAL fluids, the investigator has a powerful tool to detect the presence of an inflammatory response in the bronchoalveolar region of the lung, to follow sequentially the progress of a disease, and to elucidate pathological mechanisms.

BAL can be performed in vivo or in the excised lung. In small laboratory animals, multiple lavages are performed on the entire lung and the recovered BAL fluids are pooled. If used for biochemical evaluations, the lavage fluid from the first lavage is utilized to avoid dilution of protein and enzyme activity. Repeated lavages are essential for maximizing cell yield. In larger animals, lavages are typically performed on a single segmental lung lobe using a bronchoscope. Lavage fluids are slowly instilled and withdrawn via a catheter with the airway sealed off to prevent leakage of fluid. The lavage fluids must be isotonic to avoid cellular and tissue lysis, with physiological saline being most commonly used. An important consideration is whether to have Ca^{2+} and Mg^{2+} in the fluid; these cations are necessary for the adherence of macrophages to surfaces, thus the use of calcium- and magnesium-containing BAL fluids will result in fewer cells being collected.

The major cellular component of BAL fluid is the macrophage; these cells typically represent 95–100% of the cell types found in lavage fluids from animals with normal lungs. These cells can be isolated by centrifugation and subjected to various morphological evaluations or functional assays for migration, phagocytosis, or cell killing activities. Lymphocytes are a minor component from larger animals including humans and are rarely seen in BAL from laboratory rodents. Polymorphonuclear neutrophils (PMN) are associated with inflammatory processes and are rarely observed in the normal lung. Small amounts of protein (primarily albumin) and low levels of enzyme activities (such as β-glucuronidase, acid phosphatase, or lactate dehydrogenase) are present in control animals. The source of protein is typically from injury to epithelial and/or endothelial membranes, resulting in leakage of serum from the blood into the airspace. Macrophages can release the lysosomal enzymes, acid phosphatase and β-glucuronidase, when damaged. If the inhaled material is an insoluble particle, the resident macrophages will be activated as a consequence of particle phagocytosis by the cell membrane. This results in the release of reactive forms of oxygen, cytokines, growth factors, arachidonate metabolites, and hydrolysases.

A typical use of BAL is to detect and quantify inflammatory responses in the lungs of animals exposed to potential toxicants (286). Good examples of this application comes from work ranking the pulmonary toxicity of a series of nickel compounds (287), rare earth metals such as gallium (288), environmental contaminants such as diesel soot and fly ash, and minerals such as quartz. Quantitative as well as qualitative estimates of the inflammatory potential and potency of dusts can be made depending on the test substance, the experimental design, and the endpoints affected (Table 23.14).

In addition, examination of BAL fluids has been extremely useful in predicting the long-term consequences of particle inhalation. Attempts have been made to correlate early findings in BAL parameters with histopathological changes such as fibrosis for a series of fibrogenic materials, such as quartz and other mineral particles. For example, quartz produced a rapid increase in lactate dehydrogenase (LDH) and in the acid hydrolase β-*N*-acetylglucosminidase, which was distinguishable from the nonfibrogenic particles of aluminum and ferric oxide. Sequential BAL samplings can be used to follow the progression of chemically initiated lung disease. In rodents, the sequential response to soot form diesel exhaust was described following time-spaced BAL evaluations (289).

In considering BAL as a tool in inhalation toxicity studies, it is important to look carefully at relative advantages and disadvantages. One of the greatest advantages is that BAL can detect early cellular and biochemical

Table 23.14
Cellular and biochemical indicators of lung damage

Agent	Injury	Cellular or Biochemical marker
Beryllium	Granuloma	Eosinophilia
Cadmium	Diffuse alveolitis	LDH, protein, PMN
Cyclophosphamide	Upper respiratory	Aniline hydroxylase
Diesel exhaust soot	Focal chronic alveolitis	LDH, protein, PMN, lysosomal enzymes, glutathione reductase
Sulfuric acid	Upper respiratory tract	Not useful
Mineral dusts	Focal alveolitis	LDH, protein, PMN, lysosomal enzymes
Nitrogen dioxide	Terminal bronchioles	Protein, PMN
Oxygen	Endothelial tissue	Protein, PMN
Silica	Alveolar proteinosis	Phospholipids, PMN

Note: LDH = lactate dehydrogenase; PMN = polymorphonuclear leukocytes.

changes in response to inhaled toxicants. Compared to traditional nonmorphometric techniques, BAL can provide a quantitative measure of lung condition. Also, because BAL samples primarily lung surfaces, it is less subject to focal airway injury and reflects the total integrated changes of inflammatory responses located throughout the luminal areas of the bronchoalveolar region. Finally, it provides insights into the mechanisms of disease development. On the other hand, BAL is an invasive procedure that cannot be done routinely in humans. In addition, although it is a validated procedure, the increase or decrease in measurable parameters is not easily interpreted in terms of toxicological significance. For example, it is difficult to distinguish between a normal physiological response directed toward lung defense and repair, and the more significant changes reflective of frank injury.

PATHOLOGICAL STUDIES

Detailed structural analysis of the respiratory tract tissues at the most elemental level can be helpful in assessing the amount and degree of lung damage produced (or not produced) by chemical agents. Morphometric techniques are available to obtain quantitative data regarding changes in lung structure. These techniques allow the investigator to focus on specific regions of interest and to determine quantitatively the changes in lung tissue or in lung cellular population patterns (291). Clearly, further structural evaluation of the respiratory system in toto needs to be conducted. Table 23.15 presents the recommendations regarding the structural evaluation of the respiratory system.

SAFETY

The safety of persons working in an experimental area dealing with the generation and maintenance of airborne chemicals must be protected. The basic measures employed that prevent contact with chemicals or their spread within the laboratory must be reinforced continually. Specifically, to prevent the inhalation of test agents by those working on an experiment, a number of additional considerations apply. Dust masks provide only minimal protection, and only from larger dust particles including animal dander and hair. For somewhat greater chemical protection, half-face cartridge respirators may be used against certain organic vapors and dusts during times of potential exposure (e.g., transfer of test agents, removing animals from exposure chambers, observing animals following whole-body inhalation exposures). Positive pressure air-supplied respirators afford a much higher level of protection and should be used when handling open containers of highly toxic materials; additionally, such transfers should be made within a functional laboratory hood. All respirators should be fit-tested regularly and personnel should be trained to use them properly. Air-supplied respirators should also be used when handling animals exposed to these agents.

Provisions to isolate animals following exposure to test agents should be made (e.g., walk-in storage areas for animal racks, portable hoods). The type of monitoring needed in any experimental situation must be geared

Table 23.15
Pulmonary function studies that can be used in evaluating inhalation toxicity[a]

Parameter	Tests available
Blood gases	Several to determine O_2, CO_2, CO, pH, etc.
Diffusion	Several using blood-gas electrodes, tracer gases
Distribution of ventilation	Closing volume
	Single or multibreath nitrogen (or ^{133}Xe) washout, regional pulmonary function
Pulmonary circulation	Cardiovascular pressure
	Cardiovascular volumes, flow resistance and work distribution of perfusion
	Edema determine (wet/dry weights, gas transfer, radioisotopes)
	Histamine, fibrinopeptide B, bradykinin analysis
	Matching of ventilation and perfusion
	Right-to-left pulmonary vascular shunt during O_2 breathing
Regional ventilation/perfusion matching	Several using arterial blood and alveolar gas measurements
Respiratory mechanics	Airway flow resistance
	Dynamic lung compliance
	Flow-volume; maximum inspiratory
	Flow-volume; maximum expiratory
	Lung and thoracic cage flow resistance
	Small airway flow resistance
	Spirometry—forced expired volume versus time
	Static lung and thoracic cage compliance
	Static volume pressure curves of saline-filled exercise lungs
	Work of breathing
Lung volumes	Expiratory reserve volume
	Functional residual capacity
	Inspiratory capacity
	Residual volume
	Total lung capacity
	Vital capacity
Ventilatory exchange	Minute ventilation
	Respiratory rate
	Tidal volume

[a]From Reference 292.

to that particular chemical. Area-monitoring should be conducted before, during, and after daily exposures to establish operating conditions that will avoid human exposure and to ensure that acceptable workplace exposure levels are not exceeded.

The best practice to follow when conducting experimental inhalation tests is to remember that the subjects of the test must be isolated. The working area itself should be isolated so that only those directly involved with the experiment have access to the facility. Any potential for human contact should be minimized prior to initiation of the experiment. This often is best accomplished by enclosing the entire generation and exposure system (including the exhaust) within a laboratory hood. The specific measures taken will follow from the type of test, the amount of chemical being handled during the test, and the toxicity of the chemical.

CONCLUSIONS

It is important to recognize that the evaluation of the inhalation toxicity of a material is generally more complex, technically challenging, and resource intensive compared to testing by other routes of exposure. The effects of a given agent when inhaled must be understood so that appropriate control measures can be applied in the workplace and in the community to prevent the occurrence of adverse health effects. Both the qualitative and the quantitative aspects of these potential responses need to be considered. The tools for such evaluation exist, even though the area of inhalation toxicology is continually making technical advances. The basic methodologies available to the investigator for studying the effects of chemicals as they enter the respiratory tract have been reviewed in this chapter, and these approaches remain constant in the face of technological advances. It is important that information from several differing endpoints be integrated to ensure that the proper conclusions are reached. Inhalation toxicologists must continue to be receptive to new procedures and ideas so that the work of protecting the community at large from the adverse effects of inhaled agents can be conducted with appropriate, up-to-date tools. The proper design and conduct of inhalation studies are essential, as this route of exposure is a major way that humans and chemical agents have the possibility to interact.

QUESTIONS

1. In the design of inhalation experiments for hazard identification purposes, what are a few of the main factors that need to be considered so that the information can best be applied to man?
2. If a test material, by virtue of its physical properties, is difficult to get into the atmosphere, is there any reason to develop inhalation-specific information? Explain why.
3. What are the key pieces of information obtained from both acute- and repeated-exposure inhalation studies? Describe how they need to be applied in the context of human risk assessment.
4. Describe special considerations that may need to be dealt with in the generation of test atmosphere, that are (A) gases, (B) low boiling liquids, and (C) fibers.
5. What are some of the biochemical and molecular changes that can be measured in experimental animals and used to indicate the presence (or absence) of pulmonary toxicity?

REFERENCES

1. Gross, E. A., Mellick, P. W., Kari, F. W., Miller, F. J., and Morgan, K. T. (1994): Histopathology and cell replication responses in the respiratory tract of rats and mice exposed by inhalation to glutaraldehyde for up to thirteen weeks. *Fundam. Appl. Toxicol.*, 23:348–362.
2. Morgan, K. T. (1991): Approaches to the identification and recording of nasal lesions in toxicology studies. *Toxicol. Pathol.*, 19:337–351.
3. Morgan, K. T., Kimbell, J. S., Monticello, T. M., Patra, A. L., and Fleishman, A. (1991): Studies of inspiratory airflow patterns in the nasal passages of the F344 rat and rhesus monkey using nasal molds: Revelance to formaldehyde toxicity. *Toxicol. Appl. Pharmacol.*, 110:223–240.
4. Genter, M. B., Llorens, J., O'Callaghan, J. P., Peele, D. B., Morgan, K. T., and Crofton, K. M. (1992): Olfactory toxicity of β,β-iminodiproprionitrile (IDPN) in the rat. *J. Pharma. Exp. Ther.*, 263:1432–1439.
5. Young, J. T. (1981): Histopathologic examination of the rat nasal cavity. *Fundam. Appl. Toxicol.*, 1:309–312.
6. Uriah, L. C., and Maronpot, R. R. (1990): Normal histology of the nasal cavity and application of special techniques. *Environ. Health Perspect.*, 85:187–208.
7. Uriah, L. C., Morgan, K. T., and Maronpot, R. R. (1990): Symposium in toxicologic pathology of the upper respiratory system. *Environ. Health Perspect.*, 85:161–352.
8. Reuzel, P. G. J., Wilmer, J. W. G. M., Woutersen, R. A., Zwart, A., Rombout, P. J. A., and Feron, V. J. (1990): Interactive effects of ozone and formaldehyde on the nasal respiratory lining epithelium in rats. *J. Toxicol. Environ. Health*, 29:279–292.
9. Mery, S., Larson, J. L., Butterworth, B. E., Wolf, D. C., Harden, R., and Morgan, K. T. (1994): Nasal toxicity of chloroform in male F344 rats and female B6C3F1 mice following one week inhalation exposure. *Toxicol. Appl. Pharmacol.*, 125:214–227.
10. Morris, J. B., Hassett, D. N., and Blanchard, K. T. (1993): A physiologically based pharmacokinetic model for nasal uptake and metabolism of nonreactive vapors. *Toxicol. Appl. Pharmacol.*, 123:120–129.
11. Bogdanffy, M. S. (1990): Biotransformation enzymes in the rodent nasal mucosa: The alue of a histochemical approach. *Environ. Health Perspect.*, 85:177–186.
12. Dahl, A. R., and Hadley, W. H. (1991): Nasal cavity enzymes involved in xenobiotic metabolism: Effects on the toxicity of inhalants. *CRC Crit. Rev. Toxicol.*, 21:345–372.
13. Alarie, Y. (1973): Sensory irritation by airborne chemicals. *CRC Crit. Rev. Toxicol.*, 2:299–363.
14. Bucher, J. R., Elwell, M. R., Thompson, M. B., Chou, B. J., Renne, R., and Ragan, H. A. (1990): Inhalation toxicity studies of cobalt sulfate in F344/N rats and $B6C3F_1$ mice. *Fundam. Appl. Toxicol.*, 15:357–372.
15. Sagartz, J. W., Madarasz, A. J., Forsell, M. A., Burger, G. T., Ayres, P. H., and Coggins, C. E. (1992): Histological sectioning of the rodent larynx for toxicity testing. *Toxicol. Pathol.*, 20:118–121.
16. Gopinath, C., Prentice, D. E., and Lewis, D. J. (1987): The respiratory system. In: *Atlas of Experimental Toxicologic Pathology Current Histopathology*, Vol. 13, edited by G. A. Gresham, pp. 22–42. MTP Press, Norwell, MA.
17. Renne, R. A., Wehner, A. P., Greenspan, B. J., DeFord, H. S., Ragan, H. A., Westerburg, R. B., Buschhom, R. L., Burger, G. T., Hayes, A. W., Suber, R. L., and Mosberg, A. T. (1993): 2-Week and 13-week inhalation studies of aerosolized glycerol in rats. *Inhal. Toxicol.*, 4:95–111.
18. Lewis, D. J. (1991): Morphological assessment of pathological changes within the rat larynx. *Toxicol. Pathol.*, 19:352–357.
19. Bowden, D. H., and Adamson, I. Y. R. (1978): Adaptive responses of the pulmonary macrophagic system to carbon. I. Kinetic studies. *Lab. Invest.*, 42:422–429.
20. Gardner, D. E. (1984): Alterations in macrophage functions by environmental chemicals. *Environ. Health Perspect.*, 55:343–358.

21. Coffin, D. L., Gardner, D. E., Holzman, R. S., and Walock, F. S. (1968): Influence of ozone on pulmonary cells. *Arch. Environ. Health*, 16:633–636.
22. Goldstein, E., Bartlema, H. C., Van der Ploeg, M., van Duijn, P., Van der Stap, J. G., M. M., and Lippert, W. (1978): Effect of ozone on lysosomal enzymes of alveolar macrophages engaged in phagocytosis and killing of inhaled *Staphylococcus aureus*. *J. Infect. Dis.*, 138:299–311.
23. Miller, M. E. (1964): *Anatomy of the Dog*, Chap. 14. W. B. Saunders, Philadelphia.
24. Schlesinger, R. B., and McFadden, L. (1981): Comparative morphometry of the upper bronchial tree in six mammalian species. *Anat. Rec.*, 199:99–108.
25. Schreider, J. P. (1986): Comparative anatomy and function of the nasal passages. In: *Toxicology of the Nasal Passages*, edited by C. S. Barrow, pp. 1–25. Hemisphere, Washington, DC.
26. McLaughlin, R. F., Jr., Tyler, W. S., and Canada, R. O. (1961): A Study of the subgross pulmonary anatomy in various mammals. *Am. J. Anat.*, 108:149–166.
27. Dungworth, D. L., Tyler, W. S., and Plopper, C. G. (1985): Morphological methods for gross and microscopoic pathology. In: *Toxicology of Inhaled Materials*, edited by H. P. Witschi and J. D. Brain, pp. 229–258. Springer–Verlag, New York.
28. Pinkerston, K. E., and Crapo, J. D. (1985): Morphometry of the alveolar region of the lung. In: *Toxicology of Inhaled Materials*, edited by H. P. Witschi and J. D. Brain, pp. 259–258. Springer–Verlag, New York.
29. Schwartz, L. W. (1987): Pulmonary responses to inhaled irritants and the morphological evaluation of those responses. In: *Inhalation Toxicology Research Methods, Applications, and Evaluation*, edited by H. Salem, pp. 293–348. Marcel Dekker, New York.
30. Castranova, V. (1998): Particulates and the airways: Basic biological mechanisms of pulmonary pathogenicity. *Appl. Occup. Environ. Hyg.*, 13:613–616.
31. Vallyathan, V., Mega, J. F., Shi, X., and Dalal, N. S. (1992): Enhanced generation of free radicals from phagocytes induced by mineral dusts. *Am. J. Respir. Cell. Mol. Biol.*, 6:404–413.
32. Ghio, A. J., Kennedy, T. P., Whorton, A. R., Crumbliss, A. L., Hatch, G. E., and Hoidal, J. R. (1992): Role of surface complexed iron in oxidant generation and lung inflammation induced by silicates. *Am. J. Physiol.*, 263:L511–L518.
33. Ghio, A. J., Zhang, J., and Piantadosi, C. A. (1992): Generation of hydroxyl radical by crocidolite asbestos is proportional to surface [Fe^{3+}]. *Arch. Biochem. Biophys.*, 298:646–650.
34. Berg, I., Schluter, T., and Gercken, G. (1993): Increase of bovine alveolar macrophage superoxide anion and hydrogen peroxide release by dusts of different origin. *J. Toxicol. Environ. Health*, 39:341–354.
35. Nyberg, P., and Klockars, M. (1990): Measurement of reactive oxygen metabolites produced by human monocyte-derived macrophages exposed to mineral dusts. *Int. J. Exp. Pathol.*, 71:537–544.
36. Goodglick, L. A., and Kane, A. B. (1986): Role of reactive oxygen metabolites in crocidolite asbestos toxicity to mouse macrophages. *Cancer Res.*, 46:5558–5566.
37. Blackford, J. A., Antonini, J. M., Castronova, V., and Dey, R. D. (1994): Intratracheal instillation of silica upregulates inducible nitric oxide synthase gene expression and increases nitric oxide production in alveolar macrophages and neutrophils. *Am. J. Respir. Cell. Mol. Biol.*, 11:426–431.
38. Driscoll, K. E. (1996): The Role of interleukin-1 and tumor necrosis factor α in the lung's response to silica. In: *Silica and Silica-Induced Lung Disease*, edited by V. Castranova, V. Vallyathan, and W. E. Wallace, pp. 163–184. CRC Press, Boca Raton, FL.
39. Morris, J. B., and Smith, F. A. (1982): Regional deposition and absorption of inhaled hydrogen fluoride in the rat. *Toxicol. Appl. Pharmacol.*, 62:81–89.
40. Stott, W. T., and McKenna, M. J. (1984): The Comparative absorption and excretion of chemical vapors by the upper, lower, and intact respiratory tract of rats. *Fundam. Appl. Toxicol.*, 4:594–604.
41. Chang, L., Graham, J. A., Miller, F. J., Ospital, J. J., and Crapo, J. D. (1986): Effects of subchronic inhalation of low concentrations of nitrogen dioxide. I. The proximal alveolar region of juvenile and adult rats. *Toxicol. Appl. Pharmacol.*, 83:46–61.
42. Morris, J. B. (1990): First-pass metabolism of inspired ethyl acetate in the upper respiratory tracts of the F344 rat and Syrian hamster. *Toxicol. Appl. Pharmacol.*, 102:331–345.
43. Hatch, T., and Choate, S. P. (1929): Statistical description of the size properties non-uniform particulate substances. *J. Franklin Inst.*, 29:66–78.
44. IPCS. (1986): *IPCS Environmental Health Criteria, EHC 53: Asbestos and Other Natural Mineral Fibers*. International Programme on Chemical Safety, World Health Organization, Geneva.
45. Pott, F. (1978): Some aspects o nthe dosimetry on the carcinogenic potency of asbestos and other fibrous dusts. *Staub-Reinhalt Luft*, 38:486–490.
46. Wagner, J. C., Berry, G., and Timbrell, V. (1973): Mesothelioma in rats after innoculation with asbestos and other materials. *Br. J. Cancer*, 28:175–185.
47. Davis, J. M. G. (1974): Pathological aspects of the injections of glass fibers into the pleural and peritoneal cavities of rats and mice. In: *Occupational Exposure to Fibrous Glass*, U.S. Dept. of Health, Education and Welfare, NIOSH Publication No. 76-151, pp. 141–149. College Park, MD, June 1974.
48. Stanton, M. F., and Wrench, C. (1972): Mechanisms of mesothelioma induction with asbestos and fibrous glass. *J. Natl. Cancer Inst.*, 48:797–821.
49. Wright, G. W., and Kuschner, M. (1977): The Influence of varying lengths of glass and asbestos fibers on tissue response in guinea pigs. In: *Inhaled Particles*, IV, edited by W. H. Walton, pp. 455–474. Pergamon, New York.
50. Walton, W. H. (1982): The Nature, hazards, and assessment of occupational exposure to airborne asbestos dust: A review. *Ann. Occup. Hyg.*, 25:115–247.
51. U.S. EPA. (1986): *Airborne Asbestos Health Assessment Update*. EPA/600/8-84/003F. US EPA, Washington, DC.
52. Stober, W., Flachsbart, H., and Hochrainer, D. (1970): Der Aerodynamische durchmesser von Latexaggregaten und Asbestifasern. *Staub-Reinhalt Luft*, 30:277–285.
53. Timbrell, V. (1965): The inhalation of fibrous dusts. *Ann. N.Y. Acad. Sci.*, 132:255–273.
54. Timbrell, V., and Skidmore, J. W. (1970): The effect of shape on particle penetration and retention in animal lungs. In: *Inhaled Particles*, III, edited by W. H. Walton, pp. 49–57. Unwin Bros Ltd., Surrey, England.
55. Morgan, A., Holmes, A., and Davison, W. (1982): Clearance of sized glass fibers from the rat lung and their solubility in vivo. *Ann. Occup. Hyg.*, 25:317–331.
56. Morgan, A., and Holmes, A. (1984): The deposition of MMMF in the respiratory tract of the rat, their subsequent clearance,

solubility in vivo and protein coating. In: *Biological Effects of Man-Made Mineral Fibers*, Vol. 2, pp. 1–17. WHO/IARC Conference, Copenhagen, Denmark. April 1982.

57. Johnson, N. F., Griffiths, D. M., and Hill, R. J. (1984): Size distributions following long-term inhalation of MMMF. In: *Biological Effects of Man-Made Mineral Fibers*, Vol. 2, pp. 102–125. WHO/IARC Conference, Copenhagen, Denmark. April 1982.
58. Hesterberg, T. W., Chase, G., Axten, C., Miller, W. C., Musselman, R. P., Kamstrup, O., Hadley, J., Morscheidt, C., Bernstein, D. M., and Thevenaz, P. (1998): Biopersistence of synthetic vitreous fibers and amosite asbsestos in the rat lung following inhalation. *Toxicol. Appl. Pharmacol.*, 151:262–275.
59. Lippmann, M. (1990): Man-made mineral fibers MMMF: Human exposures and health risk assessment. *Toxicol. Ind. Health*, 6:225–246.
60. Bellmann, B., Konig, H., Muhle, H., and Pott, F. (1986): Chemical durability of asbestos and of man-made mineral fibres in vivo. *J. Aerosol Sci.*, 17:341–345.
61. Searl, A. (1994): A Review of the durability of inhaled fibres and options for the design of safer fibers. *Ann. Occup. Hyg.*, 38:839–855.
62. Hesterberg, T. W., Miller, W. C., Musselman, R. P., Kamstrup, O., Hamilton, R. D., and Thevenaz, P. (1996): Biopersistence of man-made vitreous fibers and crocidolite asbestos in the rat lung following inhalation. *Fundam. Appl. Toxicol.*, 29:267–279.
63. Kelly, D. P., Williams, S. J., Kennedy, G. L., and Lee, K. P. (1985): Recovery and characterization of of lung-deposited Kevlar aramid fibers in rats. *Toxicologist*, 5:129.
64. Warheit, D. B., Hwang, H. C., and Achinko, L. (1991): Assessments of lung digestion methods for recovery of fibers. *Environ. Res.*, 54:183–193.
65. Brody, A. R., Hill, L. H., Adkins, B., and O'Connor, R. W. (1981): Chrysotile asbestos inhalation in rats: Deposition patterns and reaction of alveolar epithelium and pulmonary macrophages. *Am. Rev. Respir. Dis.*, 123:670–679.
66. Whitby, K. T. (1978): The physical characteristics of sulfer aerosol. *Atmos. Environ.* 12:135–159.
67. Whitby, K. T., Killelson, D. B., Cantrell, B. K., Barsic, N. J., Dolon, D. F., Tarvestad, L. D., Nieken, D. J., Wolf, J. L., and Wood, J. R. (1976): Aerosol size distributions and concentrations measured during the General Motors Proving Grounds sulfate study, In: *The General Motors/Environmental Protection Agency Sulfate Dispersion Experiment*, edited by R. K. Stevens, P. J. Lamothe, W. E. Wilson, J. L. Durham, and T. G. Dzubay, pp. 29–80. EPA-600/3-76-035. EPA, Research Triangle Park, NC.
68. Hinds, W. C. (1982): *Aerosol Technology. Properties, Behavior, and Measurement of Airborne Particles*. John Wiley and Sons, New York.
69. Hidy, G. M. (1984): *Aerosols: An Industrial and Environmental Science*. Academic Press, Orlando, FL.
70. Schreider, J. P. (1986): Comparative anatomy and function of the nasal passages. In: *Toxicology of the Nasal Passages*, edited by C. S. Barrow, pp. 1–25. Hemisphere, Washington DC.
71. Task Group of the International Commission on Radiological Protection (ICRP). (1994): *Human Respiratory Tract Model for Radiological Protection*. Pergamon, Tarrytown, NY.
72. Mercer, T. T. (1975): The deposition model of the Task Group on Lung Dynamics: A comparison with recent experimental data. *Health Phys.*, 29:673–680.
73. International Commission of Radiological Protection. (1994): *Human Respiratory Tract Model for Radiological Protection*. A Report of Committee 2 of the ICRP. Pergamon Press, Oxford, UK.
74. Cheng, Y. S., Yamada, Y., Yeh, H. C., and Swift, D. L. (1988): Diffusional deposition of ultrafine aerosol in a human nasal cast. *J. Aerosol Sci.*, 19:741–751.
75. Cheng, Y. S., Hansen, G. K., Su, Y. F., Yeh, H. C., and Morgan, K. T. (1990): Deposition of ultrafine aerosols in rat nasal molds. *Toxicol. Appl. Pharmacol.*, 106:222–233.
76. Swift, D. L., Montassier, N., Hopke, P. K., Karpen-Haves, K., Cheng, Y. S., Su, Y. F., Yeh, H. C., and Strong, J. C. (1992): Inspiratory depositon of ultrafine particles in human nasal replicate cast. *J. Aerosol Sci.*, 23:65–72.
77. Vincent, J. H., and Armbruster, L. (1981): On the quantitative definition of the inhalability of airborne dust. *Ann. Occup. Hyg.*, 24:245–248.
78. Schlesinger, R. B. (1985): Comparative deposition of inhaled aerosols in experimental animals and humans: A review. *J. Toxicol. Environ. Health*, 15:197–214.
79. Schlesinger, R. B. (1995): Deposition and clearance of inhaled particles. In: *Concepts in Inhalation Toxicology*, 2nd ed., edited by R. O. McClellan and R. F. Henderson, pp. 191–224. Taylor and Francis, Washington, DC.
80. Phalen, R., Kenoyer, J., and Davis, J. (1977): Deposition and clearance of inhaled particles: comparison of mammalian species. In: *Proceedings of the Annual Conference on Environmental Toxicology*, Vol. 7, AMRL-TR-76-125, pp. 159–170. National Technical Information Service, Springfield, VA. Conference in Dayton, OH, October 1976.
81. Kennedy, G. L., Jr., Morris, J. B., Roloff, M. V., Salem, H., Ulrich, C. E., Valentine, R., and Wolff, R. K. (1992): Recommendations for the conduct of acute inhalation limit tests. *Fundam. Appl. Toxicol.*, 18:321–327.
82. Lewis, T. R., Morrow, P. E., McClellan, R. O., Raabe, O. G., Kennedy, G.L., Jr., Schwetz, B. A., Goehl, T. J., Roycroft, J. H., and Chhabra, R. S. (1989): Establishing aerosol exposure concentration for inhalation toxicity studies. *Toxicol. Appl. Pharmacol.*, 99:377–383.
83. Oberdoerster, G., Ferin, J., Gelein, R., Soderholm, S. C., and Finkelstein, J. (1992): Role of the alveolar macrophage in lung injury: Studies with ultrafine particles. *Environ. Health Perspect.*, 97:193–199.
84. Driscoll, K. E., and Maurer, J. K. (1991): Cytokine and growth factor release by alveolar macrophages: Potential biomarkers of pulmonary toxicity. *Toxicol. Pathol.*, 19:398–405.
85. Waritz, R. S., and Kwon, B. K. (1968): The inhalation toxicity of pyrolysis products of polytetrafluoroethylene heated below 500 degrees centigrade. *Am. Ind. Hyg. Assoc. J.*, 68:19–26.
86. Seidel, W. C., Scherer, K. V., Cline, D. T., Olson, A. H., Bonesteel, J. K., Church, D. F., Nuggehalli, S., and Pyror, W. A. (1991): Chemical, physical, and toxicological characterization of fumes produced by heating polytetrafluoroethylene homopolymer and its copolymers with hexafluoropropylene and perfluoro(propyl vinyl ether). *Chem. Res. Toxicol.*, 4:229–236.
87. Warheit, D. B., Seidel, W. C., Carakostas, M. C., and Hartsky, M. A. (1990): Attenuation of perfluoropolymer fume pulmonary toxicity: Effects of filters, combustion method and aerosol age. *Exp. Mol. Pathol.*, 52:309–329.
88. Oberdoerster, G., Gelein, R. M., Ferin, J., and Weiss, B. (1995): Association of particulate air pollution and acute mortality: Involvement of ultrafine particles? *Inhal. Toxicol.*, 7:111–124.

89. Ferin, J., Oberdoerster, G., and Penny, D. P. (1992): Pulmonary retention of ultrafine and fine particles in rats. *Am. J. Respir. Cell. Mol. Biol.*, 6:535–542.

90. Oberdoerster, G., Ferin, J., and Lehnert, B. E. (1994): Correlation between particle size, in vivo particle persistence and lung injury. *Environ. Health Perspect.*, 102(suppl.):173–179.

91. Driscoll, K. E., Strzelecki, J., Hassenbein, D., Janssen, Y. M. W., Marsh, J., Oberdoerster, G., and Mossman, B. T. (1994): Tumor necrosis factor (TNF): Evidence for the role of TNF in increased expression of manganese superoxide dismutase after inhalation of mineral dusts. In: *Proceedings of the 7th International Symposium on Inhaled Particles*, pp. 375–382.

92. Fairly, D. (1990): The relationship of daily mortality to suspended particulates in Santa Clara County, 1980–1986. *Environ. Health Perspect.*, 89:159–168.

93. Schwartz, J. (1991): Particulate air pollution and daily mortality in Detroit. *Environ. Res.*, 56:204–213.

94. Dockery, D. W., Schwartz, J., and Spengler, J. D. (1992): Air pollution and daily mortality: Associations with particulates and acid aerosols. *Environ. Res.*, 59:362–273.

95. Pope, C. A., Schwartz, J., and Ransom, M. R. (1992): Daily mortality and PM-10 pollution in Utah Valley. *Arch. Environ. Health*, 47:211–217.

96. Schwartz, J., and Dockery, D. W. (1992): Increased mortaliy in Philadelphia associated with daily air pollution concentrations. *Am. Rev. Respir. Dis.*, 145:600–604.

97. Schwartz, J., and Dockery, D. W. (1992): Particulate air pollution and daily mortality in Steubenville, Ohio. *Am. J. Epidemiol.*, 135:12–19.

98. Dockery, D. W., Pope, C. A., Xiping, X., Spengler, J. D., Ware, J. H., Fay, M. E., Ferris, B. G., and Speizer, F. E. (1993): An association between air pollution and mortality in six US Cities. *N. Engl. J. Med.*, 329:1753–1759.

99. Samet, J. M., Bishop, Y., Speizer, F. E., Spengler, J. D., and Ferris, B. G. (1981): The relationship between air pollution and emergency room visits in an industrial community. *J. Air Pollut. Control Assoc.*, 31:236–240.

100. Whittemore, A., and Korn, E. (1980): Asthma and air pollution in the Los Angeles area. *Am. J. Public Health*, 70:687–696.

101. Pope, C. A., Dockery, D. W., Spengler, J. D., and Raizenne, M. E. (1991): Respiratory health and PM-10 pollution. A daily time series analysis. *Am. Rev. Respir. Dis.*, 144:668–674.

102. Spurney, K. R. (1993): Atmospheric, anthropogenic aerosol and its toxic and carcinogenic components. *Wiss. Unwelt.*, 2:139–151.

103. Valberg, P. A., and Watson, A. Y. (1998): Alternative hypotheses linking outdoor particulate matter with daily morbidity and mortality. *Inhal. Toxicol.*, 10:641–662.

104. Morrow, P. E. (1970): Models for the study of particle retention and elimination in the lung. In: *Inhalation Carcinogenesis*, (CONF-691001), edited by M. G. Hanna, Jr., P. Nettesheim, and J. R. Gilbert, pp. 103–115. U.S. Atomic Energy Commission, Division of Technical Information, Oak Ridge, TN.

105. Schlesinger, R. B., Chen, L. C., and Driscoll, K. E. (1984): Exposure-response relationship of bronchial mucociliary clearance in rabbits following acute inhalations of sulfuric acid mist. *Toxicol. Lett.*, 22:249–254.

106. Bowden, D. H., and Adamson, I. Y. R. (1984): Pathways of cellular efflux and particulate clearance after carbon instillation to the lung. *J. Pathol.*, 143:117–125.

107. Holt, P. F. (1981): Transport of inhaled dust to extrapulmonary sites. *J. Pathol.*, 133:123–129.

108. Proctor, D. F. (1980): The upper respiratory tract. In: *Pulmonary Diseases and Disorders*, edited by A. P. Fishman, pp. 209–223. McGraw-Hill, New York.

109. Rutland, J., and Cole, P. J. (1981): Nasal mucociliary clearance and ciliary beat frequency in cystic fibrosis compared with sinusitis and bronchiectasis. *Thorax*, 36:654–658.

110. Morrow, P. E., Gibb, F. R., and Gazioglu, K. M. (1967): A study of particulate clearance from the human lungs. *Am. Rev. Respir. Dis.*, 96:1209–1221.

111. Patrick, G., and Stirling, C. (1977): The retention of particles in large airways of the respiratory tract. *Proc. R. Soc. Lond. Serv. V.*, 198:455–462.

112. Snipes, M. B., Boecher, B. B., and McClellan, R. O. (1983): Retention of monodisperse or polydisperse aluminosilicate particles inhaled by dogs, rats, and mice. *Toxicol. Appl. Pharmacol.*, 69:345–362.

113. Warheit, D. B., Hill, L. H., George, G., and Brody, A. R. (1986): Time course of chemotactic factor generation and the corresponding macrophage response to asbestos inhalation. *Am. Rev. Respir. Dis.*, 134:128–133.

114. Warheit, D. B., Overby, L. H., George, G., and Brody, A. R. (1986): Pulmonary macrophages are attracted to inhaled particles through complement activation. *Exp. Lung Res.*, 14:51–66.

115. Driscoll, K. E. (1995): Role of cytokines in pulmonary inflammation and fibrosis. In: *Concepts in Inhalation Toxicology*, edited by R. O. McClellan and R. F. Henderson, pp. 471–503. Taylor and Francis, Washington, DC.

116. Driscoll, K. E., Higgins, J. M., Leytart, M. J., and Crosby, L. L. (1990): Differential effects of mineral dusts on the in vitro activation of alveolar macrophages eicosanoid and cytokine release. *Toxicol. In Vitro*, 4:284–288.

117. Driscoll, K. E., Lindenschmidt, R. C., Maurer, J. K., Higgins, J. M., and Ridder, G. (1990): Pulmonary responses to silica or titanium tioxide: Inflammatory cells, alveolar macrophage-derived cytokines and histopathology. *Am. J. Resp. Cell. Mol. Biol.*, 2:381–390.

118. Driscoll, K. E., Howard, B. W., Carter, J. M., Asquith, T., Johnston, C., Detilleux, P., Kunkel, S. L., and Isfort, R. J. (1996): Alpha-quartz-induced chemokine expression by rat lung epithelial cells: Effects of in vivo and in vitro particle exposure. *Am. J. Pathol.*, 149:1627–1637.

119. Driscoll, K. E. (1994): Macrophage inflammatory proteins: Biology and role in pulmonary inflammation. *Exp. Lung Res.*, 20:473–490.

120. Morrow, P. E. (1992): Dust overloading of the lungs: Update and appraisal. *Toxicol. Appl. Pharmacol.*, 113:1–12.

121. Morrow, P. E. (1988): Possible mechanisms to explain dust overloading of the lungs. *Fundam. Appl. Toxicol.*, 10:369–384.

122. Weyel, D. A., and Schaeffer, R. B. (1985): Pulmonary and sensory irritation of diphenylmethane–4,4′- and dicyclohexylmethane-4,4′-diisocyanate. *Toxicol. Appl. Pharmacol.*, 77:427–433.

123. Wong, K. L., and Alarie, Y. (1982): A Method for repeated evaluation of pulmonary performance in unanesthetized, unrestrained guinea pigs and its application to detect effects of sulfuric acid mist inhalation. *Toxicol. Appl. Pharmacol.*, 63:72–90.

124. Saffiotti, U. (1970): *Morphology of Experimental Respiratory Carcinogenesis, A.E.C. Symposium Series 21*, pp. 2, 45–250. U.S.A.E.C. Division of Technical Information, Washington, DC.

125. Costa, D. L., Schafrank, S. N., Wehner, R. W., and Jellett. E. (1985): Alveolar permeability to protein in rats differentially susceptible to ozone. *J. Appl. Toxicol.*, 5:18–186.

126. Oberdoerster, G. (1995): Lung particle overload: Implications for occupational exposure to particles. *Reg. Toxicol. Pharmacol.*, 27:123–135.
127. Stockinger, H. E. (1957): Evaluation of the hazards of ozone and oxides of nitrogen-factors modifying toxicity. *Arch. Ind. Health*, 15:181–190.
128. McLaughlin, R. F., Jr., Tyler, W. S., and Canada, R. O. (1961): A study of the subgross pulmonary anatomy in various mammals. *Am. J. Anat.*, 108:149–166.
129. Hammond, P. B. (1979): *The Use of Animals in Toxicological Research*. National Library of Medicine, Bethesda, MD.
130. Leach, L. J., Spiegl, C. J., and Wilson, R.H., et al. (1959): A multiple chamber exposure unit designed for chronic inhalation studies. *Am. Ind. Hyg. Assoc. J.*, 20:13–22.
131. Stockinger, H. E. (1949): Toxicity following inhalation. In: *Pharmacology and Toxicology of Uranium Compounds*, edited by C. Voegtlin and H. C. Hodge, p. 423. McGraw-Hill, New York.
132. Stockinger, H. E. (1957): Evaluation of the hazards of ozone and oxides of nitrogen-factors modifying toxicity. *Arch. Ind. Health*, 15:181–190.
133. Treon, J. F., Cleveland, F. P., Cappel, W. J., and Atchley, R. W. (1956): The toxicity of the vapors of Aroclor 1242 and Aroclor 1254. *Am. Ind. Hyg. Assoc. Q.*, 17:204–213.
134. Prendergast, J. A., Jones, R. A., Jenkins, L. J., and Siegel, J. (1967): Effects on experimental animals of long-term inhalation of trichloroethylene, carbon tetrachloride, 1,1,1-trichloroethane, dichlorodifluoromethane, and 1,1-dichloroethylene. *Toxicol. Appl. Pharmacol.*, 10:270–289.
135. Hoffman, G. M., Newton, P. E., Thomas, W. C., Birnbaum, H. A., and Kennedy, G. L., Jr. (1991): Acute inhalation toxicity studies in several animal species of an ethylene oxide/propylene oxide copolymer (Ucon 50-HB-5100). *Drug Chem. Toxicol.*, 14:243–256.
136. Kennedy, G. L., Jr., Ferenz, R. L., and Burgess, B. A. (1986): Estimation of acute oral toxicity in rats by determination of the approximate lethal dose rather than the LD_{50}. *J. Appl. Toxicol.*, 6:145–148.
137. Alarie, Y. (1981): Bioassay for evaluating the potency of airborne sensory irritants and predicting acceptable levels of exposure in man. *Food Cosmetic Toxicol.*, 19:623–626.
138. Schaper, M. (1993): Development of a database for sensory irritants and its use in establishing occupational exposure limits. *Am. Ind. Hyg. Assoc. J.*, 54:488–544.
139. Bos, P. M. J., Zwart, A., Ruezel, P. G. J., and Bragt, P. C. (1992): Evaluation of the sensory irritation test for the assessment of occupational health risk. *CRC Crit. Rev. Toxicol.*, 21:423–450.
140. Buckley, L. A., Jiang, X. Z., James, R. A., Morgan, K. T., and Barrow, C. S. (1984): Respiratory tract lesions induced by sensory irritants at the RD50 concentration. *Toxicol. Appl. Pharmacol.*, 74:417–429.
141. Zissu, D. (1995): Histopathological changes in the respiratory tract of mice exposed to ten families of airborne chemicals. *J. Appl. Toxicol.*, 15:207–213.
142. Alarie, Y. (1973): Sensory irritation by airborne chemicals. *CRC Crit. Rev. Toxicol.*, 2:299–363.
143. Amdur, M. O. (1957): The influence of aerosols upon the respiratory response of guinea pigs to sulfur dioxide. *Am. Ind. Hyg. Assoc. Q.*, 18:149–155.
144. Calabrese, E. J., and Kenyon, E. M. (1991): An approach for the rapid development of scientifically defensible AALs. In: *Air Toxics and Risk Assessment*, p. 71. Lewis Publishers, Chelsea, MI.
145. Calandra, J. C., and Fancher, O. E. (1979): Target organ studies. In: *New concepts In Safety Evaluation*, part 2, edited by M. A. Mehlman, R. E. Shapiro, and H. Blumenthal, pp. 170–186. Wiley, New York.
146. Weeks, W. M., Downing, T. O., Musselman, N. P., Carson, B. S., and Groff, W. A. (1960): The effects of continuous exposure of animals to ethanolamine vapor. *Am. Ind. Hyg. Assoc. J.*, 21:374–381.
147. Smith, L. W., Gardner, R. J., and Kennedy, G. L., Jr. (1982): Inhalation toxicity of perfluoroisobutylene. *Drug Chem. Toxicol.*, 5:295–303.
148. Kennedy, G. L., Jr., and Geisen. R. J. (1985): Setting occupational exposure limits for perfluoroisobutylene, a highly toxic chemical following acute exposure. Joint Conference Occupational Health, Orlando, FL, October 1985. *J. Occup. Med.*, 27:675.
149. AIHA. (1998): *The AIHA 1998 Handbook: Emergency Response Planning Guidelines and Workplace Environmental Exposure Level Guides*. American Industrial Hygiene Association, Fairfax, VA.
150. National Research Council, Committee on Toxicology. (1986): *Criteria and Methods for Preparing Emergency Exposure Guidance Level (EEGL), Short Term Public Emergency Guidance Level (SPEGL) and Continuous Exposure Guidance Level (CEGL) Documents*. National Academy Press, Washington, DC.
151. US EPA. (1997): National Advisory Committee for Acute Exposure guideline levels for hazardous substances. *Fed. Reg.*, 62:58840–58851.
152. Paustenbach, D. J., Christina, J. E., Carlson, G. P., and Born, G. S. (1986): The effect of an 11.5 hr/day exposure schedule on the distribution and toxicity of inhaled carbon tetrachloride in the rat. *Fundam. Appl. Toxicol.*, 6:472–483.
153. Kim, Y. C., and Carlson, G. P. (1986): The effect of an unusual workshift on chemical toxicity—II. Studies on the exposure of rats to aniline. *Fundam. Appl. Toxicol.*, 7:144–152.
154. Burgess, B. A., Pastoor, T. P., and Kennedy, G. L., Jr. (1984): Aniline-induced methemoglobinemia and hemolysis as a function of exposure concentration and duration. *Toxicologist*, 4:64.
155. Gardner, D. E., and Kennedy, G. L., Jr. (1993): *Toxicology of The Lung*, 2nd ed. Raven Press, New York.
156. Morrow, P. E., and Mermelstein, R. (1988): Chronic inhalation toxicity studies: Protocols and pitfalls. In: *Inhalation Toxicology: The Design and Interpretation of the Inhalation Studies and Their Use in Risk Assessment*, U. Mohr, Ed. pp. 103–117. Springer–Verlag, New York.
157. Drew, R. T. (1987): Inhalation toxicology—a status report. *Appl. Ind. Hyg.*, 2:213–217.
158. Lee, K. P., Trochimowicz, H. J., and Reinhardt, C. F. (1985): Pulmonary response of rats exposed to titanium dioxide (TiO_2) by inhalation for two years. *Toxicol. Appl. Pharmacol.*, 79:179–192.
159. Drew, R. T., Terrill, J. B., Daly, I. W., and Sheldon. A. (1986): Dose-dependent clearance of antimony from rat lungs. *Toxicologist*, 6:141.
160. Wilze, R. R., Henderson, R. F., Edison, A. F., and Hahn, F. F. (1987): Inhaled gallium oxide particles may be of comparable toxicity to quartz. In: American Industrial Hygiene Conference Abstract, Montreal, Canada.
161. National Toxicology Program. (1993): Toxicology and carcinogenesis studies of talc in F344/N rats and B6C3F mice. Technical Report Series No. 421, NIH Publication No. 93-315. National Toxicology Program, Research Triangle Park, NC.
162. Muhle, H., Bellmann, B., Creutzenberg, O., Dasenbrock, C., Ernst, H., Klipper, R., MacKenzie, J. C., Morrow, P., Mohn, U., Takenaka, S., and Mermelstein, R. (1991): Pulmonary response to toner upon chronic inhalation exposure in rats. *Fundam. Appl. Toxicol.*, 17:280–299.

163. Nikula, K. J., Snipes, M. B., Barr, E. B., Griffith, W. C., Henderson, R. F., and Mauderly, J. L. (1995): Comparative pulmonary toxicities and carcinogenicities of chronically inhaled diesel exhaust and carbon black in F344 rats. *Fundam. Appl. Toxicol.*, 25:80–94.

164. Heinrich, U., Dungworth, D. L., Pott, F., Peters, L., Dasenbrock, C., Levsen, K., Kock, W., Creutzenberg, O., and Schulte, A. (1994): The carcinogenic effects of carbon black particles in rats and tar-pitch condensation aerosol after inhalation exposure in rats. *Occup. Hyg.*, 38:351–356.

165. Mauderly, J. L., Jones, R. K., Griffith, W. C., Henderson, R. F., and McClellan, R. O. (1987): Diesel exhaust is a pulmonary carcinogen in rats exposed chronically by inhalation. *Fundam. Appl. Toxicol.*, 9:208–221.

166. McClellan, R. O. (1985): Health effects of diesel exhaust—a case study in risk assessment. *Am. Gov. Ind. Hyg.*, 12:3–12.

167. Lewis, T. R., Morrow, P. E., McClellan, R. O., Raabe, O. G., Kennedy, G. L., Jr., Schwetz, B. A., Goehl, T. J., Roycroft, J. H., and Chhabra, R. S. (1989): Establishing aerosol exposure concentration for inhalation toxicity studies. *Toxicol. Appl. Pharmacol.*, 99:377–383.

168. Mauderly, J. L., and McCunney, R. J., eds. (1996): *Particle Overload in the Rat Lung and Lung Cancer; Implications for Human Risk Assessment*. Proceedings of a conference at the Massachussetts Institute of Technology in March, 1995. Taylor and Francis, Washington, DC.

169. Morrow, P. E., Haseman, J. K., Hobbs, C. H., Driscoll, K. E., Vu, V., and Oberdoerster, G. (1996): The maximun tolerated dose for inhalation bioassays: Toxicity vs. overload. *Fundam. Appl. Toxicol.*, 29:155–167.

170. Oberdoerster, G. (1988): Lung clearance of inhaled insoluble and soluble particles. *J. Aerosol Med.*, 1:289–330.

171. Heinrich, U., Fuhst, R., Rittinghausen, S., Creutzenberg, O., Bellmann, B., Koch, W., and Levsen, K. (1995): Chronic inhalation exposure of Wistar rats and two different strains of mice to diesel engine exhaust, carbon black, and titanium dioxide. *Inhal. Toxicol.*, 7:533–556.

172. Warheit, D. B., Hansen, J. F., Yuen, I. S., Kelly, D. P., Snajdr, S., and Hartsky, M. A. (1997): Inhalation of high concentrations of low toxicity dusts in rats results in impaired pulmonary clearance mechanisms and persistent inflammation. *Toxicol. Appl. Pharmacol.*, 145:10–22.

173. Brightwell, J., Fouillet, X., Cassano-Zoppi, A. L., Bernstein, D., Crawley, F., Duchosal, F., Gatz, R. S., and Pfeifer, H. (1989): Tumours of the respiratory tract in rats and hamsters following chronic inhalation of engine exhaust emissions. *J. Appl. Toxicol.*, 9:25–31.

174. Oberdoerster, G., Ferin, J., and Lehnert, B. E. (1994): Correlation between particle size, in vivo particle persistence and lung injury. *Environ. Health Perspect.*, 102(suppl 5):173–179.

175. Driscoll, K. E. (1996): The role of inflammation in the development of rat lung tumors in response to chronic particle exposure. *Inhal. Toxicol.*, 8:139–153.

176. Fraser, D. A., Bales, R. E., Lippmann, M., and Stockinger, H. E. (1959): *Exposure Chambers for Research in Animal Inhalation, Public Health Monograph 357*. U.S. Government Printing Office, Washington, DC.

177. Langard, S., and Nordhagen, A. L. (1980): Small animal inhalation chambers and the significance of dust ingestion from the contaminated coat when exposing rats to zinc chromate. *Acta Pharmacol. Toxicol.*, 46:43–46.

178. Ulrich, C. E., and Marold, B. W. (1979): Pulmonary deposition of aerosols in individual and group-caged rats. *Am. Ind. Hyg. Assoc. J.*, 40:633–636.

179. Kirk, W. P., Rennberg, B. F., and Morken, D. A. (1975): Acute lethality in guinea pigs following respiratory exposure to ^{85}Kr. *Health Phys.*, 28:275–284.

180. Thomas, R. G., and Lie, R. (1963): *Procedures and Equipment Used in Inhalation Studies on Small Animals*. U.S. Atomic Energy Commission Research and Development Report, Lovelace Foundation Report No. LF-11. Albuquerque, NM.

181. Stuart, B. O., Willard, D. H., and Howard, E. B. (1971): Studies of inhaled radon daughters, uranium ore dust, diesel exhaust and cigarette smoke in dogs and hamsters. In: *Inhaled Particles III*, edited by W. H. Walton, pp. 543–553. Unwin. Surrey, England.

182. Scheimberg, J., McShane, O. P., and Carson, S. (1973): Inhalation of a powdered aerosol medication by non-human primates in individual space-type exposure helmets. *Toxicol. Appl. Pharmacol.*, 25:478.

183. Brock, W. J., Trochimowicz, H. J., Farr, C. H., Millischer, R. J., and Rusch, G. M. (1996): Acute, subchronic, and developmental toxicity and genotoxicity of 1,1,1-trifluoroethane (HFC-143a). *Fundam. Appl. Toxicol.*, 31:200–209.

184. Miller, D. B., and Chernoff, N. (1995): Restraint-induced stress in pregnant mice—degree of immobilization affects maternal indices of stress and developmental outcome in offspring. *Toxicology*, 98:177–186.

185. Tyl, R. W., Ballantyne, B., Fisher, L. C., Fait, D. L., Savine, T. A., Pritts, I. M., and Dodd, D. E. (1994): Evaluation of exposure to water aerosol or air by nose-only or whole-body inhalation procedures for CD-1 mice in developmental toxicity studies. *Fundam. Appl. Toxicol.*, 23:251–260.

186. Dorman, D. C., Wong, B. A., Struve, M. F., James, R. A., LaPerle, K. M. D., Marshall, M., and Bolon, B. (1996): Development of a mouse whole body exposure systems from a directed flow, rat nose only system. *Inhal. Toxicol.*, 8:107–120.

187. Rybkin, I. I., Zhou, Y., Volaufova, J., Smagin, G. N., Ryan, D. H., and Harris, R. B. (1997): Effect of restraint stress on food intake and body weight is determined by time of day. *Am. J. Physiol.*, 273:1612–1622.

188. Cannon, W. C., Blanton, E. F., and McDonald, K. E. (1983): The flow-past chamber: An improved nose-only exposure system for rodents. *Am. Ind. Hyg. Assoc. J.*, 44:923–928.

189. Pauluhn, J. (1994): Validation of an improved nose-only exposure system for rodents. *J. Appl. Toxicol.*, 14:55–62.

190. Bair, W. J., Porter, N. S., Brown, D. P., and Wehner, A. P. (1969): Apparatus for direct inhalation of cigarette smoke by dogs. *J. Appl. Physiol.*, 26:847–850.

191. Greenberg, H. L., Avol, E. L., Bailey, R. M., and Bell, K. A. (1977): Effects of sulfate aerosols upon cardiopulmonary function in squirrel monkeys, PB, 279–393. National Technical Information Service, Springfield, VA.

192. Mauderly, J. L. (1974): Evaluation of the female pony as a pulmonary function model. *Am. J. Vet. Res.*, 35:1025–1029.

193. Albert, R. E., Berger, J., Sanburn, K., and Lippmann, M. (1974): Effects of cigarette smoke components on bronchial clearance in the donkey. *Arch. Environ. Health*, 29:96–101.

194. Batista, S. P., Guerin, M. R., Gori, B. G., and Kensler, C. J. (1973): A new system for quantitatively exposing laboratory animals by direct inhalation. *Arch. Environ. Health*, 27:376–382.

195. Stavert, D. M., Archuleta, D. C., Behr, M. J., and Lehnert, B. E. (1991): Relative acute toxicities of hydrogen fluoride, hydrogen

chloride and hydrogen bromide in nose- and pseudo-mouth-breathing rats. *Fundam. Appl. Toxicol.*, 16:636–655.

196. Burgess, B. A., and Brittelli, M. R. (1981): Acute inhalation toxicity of stannic chloride lethality and sensory irritation in rats. *Toxicologist*, 1:77.

197. Smith, D. M., Ortiz, L. W., Archuleta, R., et al. (1981): A method for chronic nose-only exposures of laboratory animals to inhaled fibrosis aerosols. In: *Inhalation Toxicology and Technology*, edited by B. K. J. Leong, pp. 89–105. Ann Arbor Science Publishers, Ann Arbor, MI.

198. Phalen, R. F., and Morrow, P. E. (1973): Experimental inhalation of metallic silver. *Health Phys.*, 24:509–518.

199. Auerbach, D., Hammond, E. C., Kirman, D., and Garfinkel, L. (1970): Effects of cigarette smoking in dogs. *Arch. Environ. Health*, 21:754–768.

200. Bianco, A., Gibb, F. R., Kilpper, R. W., et al. (1974): Studies of tantalum dust in the lungs. *Radiology*, 112:549–556.

201. Kimura, T. (1923). Artificial production of a cancer in the lungs following intrabronchial insufflation of coal-tar. *Gann*, 7:15–21.

202. Kouri, R. E., Rude, T., Thomas, P. E., and Whitmire, C. J. (1976). Studies on pulmonary aryl hydrocarbon hydroxylase activity in inbred strains of mice. *Chem. Biol. Interact.*, 13:317–331.

203. Nettesheim, P., and Hammonds, A. S. (1971). Induction of squamous cell carcinoma in the respiratory tract of mice. *J. Natl. Cancer Inst.*, 47:697–701.

204. Blair, W. H. (1974). Chemical induction of lung carcinomas in rats. In: *Experimental Lung Cancer*, edited by E. Karbe and J. F. Park, pp. 199–206. Springer–Verlag, New York.

205. Saffiotti, U., Cefis, F., and Kolb, L. A. (1968): A method of the experimental induction of bronchogenic carcinoma. *Cancer Res.*, 28:104–124.

206. Warheit, D. B., George, G., Hill, L. H., et al. (1985): Inhaled asbestos activates a complement-dependent chemoattractant for macrophages. *Lab. Invest.*, 52:505–514.

207. Brain, J. D., Knudson, D. E., Sorokin, S. P., and Davis, M. A. (1976): Pulmonary distribution of particles given by intratracheal instillation or by aerosol inhalation. *Environ. Res.*, 11:13–33.

208. Brody, A. R., and Roe, M. W. (1983): Deposition pattern of inorganic particles at the alveolar level in the lungs of rats and mice. *Am. Rev. Respir. Dis.*, 128:724–729.

209. Pritchard, J. N., Holmes, A., Evans, J. C., Evans, N., Evans, R. J., and Morgan, A. (1985): The distribution of dust in the rat lung following administration by inhalation and by single intratracheal instillation. *Environ. Res.*, 36:268–297.

210. Dorries, A. M., and Valberg, P. A. (1992): Heterogeneity of phagocytosis for inhaled versus instilled material, *Am. Rev. Respir. Dis.*, 146:831–837.

211. Warheit, D. B., Hartsky, M. A., and Stefaniak, M. (1988): Comparative physiology of rodent pulmonary macrophages: in vitro functional responses. *J. Appl. Physiol.*, 64:1953–1959.

212. Henderson, R. F., Driscoll, K. E., Harkema, J. R., Lindenschmidt, R. C., Chang, I. Y., Maples, K. R., and Barr, E. B. (1995): A comparison of the inflammatory response of the lung to inhaled versus instilled particles in F344 rats. *Fundam. Appl. Toxicol.*, 24:183–197.

213. Drew, R. T., Kuschner, M., and Bernstein, D. M. (1987): The chronic effects of exposure of rats to sized glass fibres. *Ann. Occup. Hyg.*, 31:711–729.

214. Muller, H. L., Drosselmeyer, E., Hotz, G., Seidel, A., Thiele, H., and Pickering, S. (1989): Behaviour of spherical and irregular $(U_1,Pu)O_2$ diatomic oxygen particles after inhalation or intratracheal instillation in rat lung during in vitro culture with bovine alveolar macrophages. *Int. J. Radiat. Biol.*, 55:829–842.

215. Leong, B. K., Coombs, J. K., Sabaitis, C. P., Rop, D. A., and Aaron, C. S. (1998): Quantitative morphometric analysis of pulmonary deposition of aerosol particles inhaled via intratracheal nebulization, intratracheal instillation or nose-only inhalation in rats. *J. Appl. Toxicol.*, 18:149–160.

216. Sabaitis, C. P., Leong, B. K., Rop, D. A., and Aaron, C. S. (1999): Validation of intratracheal instillation as an alternative for aerosol inhalation toxicity testing. *J. Appl. Toxicol.*, 19:133–140.

217. Irish, D. D., and Adams, E. M. (1940): Apparatus and methods for testing the toxicity of vapors. *Am. Ind. Hyg. Assoc. Q.*, 1:1–5.

218. Treon, J. F., Dutra, F. R., Cappel, J. W., Sigmon, H., and Younker, W. (1950): Toxicity of sulfuric acid mist. *Arch. Ind. Hyg. Occup. Med.*, 2:716–734.

219. Gage, J. C. (1959): The toxicity of epichlorhydrin vapour. *Br. J. Ind. Med.*, 16:11–14.

220. Montgomery, M. R., Anderson, R. E., and Mortenson, G. A. (1976): A compact versatile inhalation exposure chamber for small animal studies. *Lab. Anim. Sci.*, 26:461–464.

221. Laskin, S., and Drew, R. T. (1970): An inexpensive portable inhalation chamber. *Lab. Anim. Sci.*, 26:645–646.

222. Leach, L. J., Maynard, E. A., Hodge, H. C., et al. (1970): A five-year inhalation study with natural uranium dioxide (UO_2) dust. I. Retention and biological effect in the monkey, dog, and rat. *Health Phys.*, 18:599–612.

223. Hinners, R. G., Burkart, J. K., and Punte, C. L. (1968): Animal inhalation exposure chambers. *Arch. Environ. Health*, 16:194–204.

224. Moss, O. R., Decker, J. R., and Cannon, W. C. (1982): Aerosol mixing in an animal exposure chamber having three levels of caging with excreta pans. *Am. Ind. Hyg. Assoc. J.*, 43:244–249.

225. Hemenway, D. R., and MacAskill, S. (1982): Design, development and test results of a horizontal inhalation toxicology facility. *Am. Ind. Hyg. Assoc. J.*, 43:874–879.

226. Moss, O. R., Decker, J. R., and Cannon, W. C. (1982): Aerosol mixing in an animal exposure chamber having three levels of caging and excreta pans. *Am. Ind. Hyg. Assoc. J.*, 43:244–249.

227. Ferin, J., and Leach, L. J. (1980): Horizontal air flow inhalation exposure chambers. In: *Generation of Aerosols and Facilities for Exposure Experiments*, edited by K. Willeke, pp. 517–523. Ann Arbor Science Publishers, Ann Arbor, MI.

228. MacFarland, H. N. (1981): A Problem and a non-problem in chamber inhalation studies. In: *Inhalation Toxicology and Technology*, edited by B. K. J. Leong, pp. 11–18. Ann Arbor Science Publishers, Ann Arbor, MI.

229. Silver, S. D. (1946): Constant flow gassing chambers: principles influencing design and operation. *J. Lab. Clin. Med.*, 31:1153–1161.

230. MacFarland, H. N. (1976): Respiratory toxicology, In: *Essays in Toxicology*, Vol 7, edited by W. J. Hayes, pp. 121–154. Academic Press, New York.

231. MacFarland, H. N. (1983): Designs and operational characteristics of inhalation exposure equipment—a review. *Fundam. Appl. Toxicol.*, 3:603–613.

232. Cheng, Y. S., Barr, E. B., Carpenter, R. I., Benson, J. M., and Hobbs, C. H. (1989): Improvement of aerosol distribution in whole-body inhalation exposure chambers. *Inhal. Toxicol.*, 1:153–166.

233. Drew, R. T. (1985): Design of inhalation exposure systems. Society of Toxicology Refresher Course, 24th Annual Meeting of the Society of Toxicology, San Diego. March, 1985.

234. Anderson, M. E., Gargas, M. L., Jones, R. A., and Jenkins, L. J. (1980): Determination of the kinetic constants for metabolism of inhaled toxicants in vivo using gas uptake measurements. *Toxicol. Appl. Pharmacol.*, 54:100–116.

235. MacFarland, H. N. (1968): The Pyrolysis products of plastics—problems in defining their toxicity. *Am. Ind. Hyg. Assoc. J.*, 29:7–9.

236. Bolt, H. M., Kappus, H., Buchter, A., and Bolt, W. (1976): Disposition of [^{12}C]vinyl chloride in rats. *Arch. Toxicol.*, 35:153–162.

237. Jaeger, R. J., Shoner, L. G., and Coffman, L. (1977): 1,1-Dichloroethylene hepatotoxicity: Proposed mechanism of action and distribution and binding of ^{14}C radioactivity following inhalation exposure in rats. *Environ. Health Perspect.*, 21:113–119.

238. Bernstein, D. M., and Drew, R. T. (1980): The major parameters affecting temperature inside inhalation chambers. *Am. Ind. Hyg. Assoc. J.*, 41:420–426.

239. Rao, G. N. (1986): Significance of environmental factors on the test system. In: *Managing Conduct and Data Quality of Toxicology Studies*, B. K. Hoover, Ed. pp. 173–185. Princeton Scientific, Princeton, NJ.

240. Pauluhn, J., and Mohr, U. (1999): Repeated 4-week inhalation exposure of rats: Effect of low-, intermediate- and high-humidity chamber atmospheres. *Exp. Toxicol. Pathol.*, 51:178–187.

241. Crapo, J. D., Smolko, E. D., Miller, F. J., Graham, J. A., and Hayes, A. W. (1989): *Extrapolation of Dosimetric Relationships for Inhaled Particles and Gases*. Academic Press, San Diego.

242. Haber, F. (1924): *Funf Vortrage aus den Jahren 1920–1923*. Springer–Verlag, Berlin.

243. Rinehart, W. E., and Hatch, T. (1964): Concentration product (Ct) as an expression of dose in sublethal exposures to phosgene. *Am. Ind. Hyg. Assoc. J.*, 25:545–553.

244. Kelly, D. P., Lee, K. P., and Burgess, B. A. (1981): Inhalation stoxicity of titanium tetrachloride atmospheric hydrolysis products. *Toxicologist*, 1:76–77.

245. Gelzleichter, T. R., Witschi, H., and Last, J. A. (1992): Concentration-response relationships of rat lungs to exposure to oxidant air pollutants: A critical test of Haber's law for ozone and nitrogen dioxide. *Toxicol. Appl. Pharmacol.*, 112:73–80.

246. Pauluhn, J., Bury, D., Fost, U., Gamer, A., Hoernicke, E., Hofmann, T., Kunde, M., Neustadt, T., Schlede, E., Schnierle, H., Wettig, K., and Westphal, D. (1996): Acute inhalation toxicity testing: Considerations of technical and regulatory aspects. *Arch. Toxicol.*, 71:1–10.

247. Schiller, C. F., Gebhart, J., Heyder, J., Rudolf, G., and Stahlhofen, W. (1986): Factors influencing total deposition of ultrafine aerosol particles in the human respiratory tract. *J. Aerosol. Sci.*, 17:328–332.

248. Bond, J. A., Wallace, L. A., Osterman-Golkar, S., Lucier, G. W., Buckpitt, A., and Henderson, R. F. (1992): Assessment of exposure to pulmonary toxicants: Use of biologic markers. *Fundam. Appl. Toxicol.*, 18:161–174.

249. Dahl, A. R., Schlesinger, R. B., Heck, H. D., Medinski, M. A., and Lucier, G. W. (1991): Comparative dosimetry of inhaled materials: Differences among animal species and extrapolation to man. *Fundam. Appl. Toxicol.*, 16:1–13.

250. Lucier, G. W., Belinsky, S., and Thompson, C. (1989): Molecular dosimetry of chemical carcinogens: Implications for epidemiology and risk assessment. In: *Assessment of Inhalation Hazards*, edited by D. V. Bates, D. L. Dungworth, P. N. Lee, R. O. McClellan, and F. J. C. Roe, pp. 85–101. Springer–Verlag, New York.

251. Casanova, M., Deyo, D. F., and Heck, H. D'A. (1989): Covalent binding of inhaled formaldehyde to DNA in the nasal mucosa of Fischer 344 rats: Analysis of formaldehyde and DNA by high-performance liquid chromatography and provisional pharmacokinetic interpretation. *Fundam. Appl. Toxicol.*, 12:397–417.

252. Bond, J. A., Harkema, J. R., Henderson, R. F., Mauderly, J. L., McClellan, R. O., and Wolff, R. K. (1989): Molecular dosimetry of inhaled diesel exhaust. In: *Assessment of Inhalation Hazards*, edited by D. V. Bates, D. L. Dungworth, P. N. Lee, R. O. McClellan, and F. J. C. Roe, pp. 315–324. Springer–Verlag, New York.

253. Thorton-Manning, J. R., Dahl, A. R., Allen, M. L., Bechtold, W. E., Griffith, W. C., and Henderson, R. F. (1998): Disposition of butadiene epoxides in Sprague Dawley rats following exposures to 8000 ppm 1,3-butadiene: Comparisons with tissue epoxide concentrations following low level exposures. *Toxicol. Sci.*, 41:167–173.

254. Scherer, G., and Richter, E. (1997): Biomonitoring exposure to environmental tobacco smoke: A critical reappraisal. *Hum. Exp. Toxicol.*, 16:449–459.

255. Medeiros, A. M., Bird, M. G., and Witz, G. (1997): Potential biomarkers of benzene exposure. *J. Toxicol. Environ. Health*, 51:519–539.

256. Henderson, R. F., Sabourin, P. J., Bechtold, W. E., Griffith, W. C., Medinsky, M. A., Birnbaum, L. S., and Lucier, G. W. (1989): The effect of dose, dose rate, route of administration and species on tissue and blood levels of benzene metabolites. *Environ. Health Perspect.*, 82:9–18.

257. Anderson, M. E. (1987): Tissue dosimetry in risk assessment or what's the problem here anyway? In: *Pharmacokinetics and Risk Assessment, Drinking Water and Health*, Vol. 8, pp. 8–26. National Academy Press. Washington, DC.

258. Himmelstein, M. W., Acquavella, J. F., Recio, L., Medisnky, M. A., and Bond, J. A. (1997): Toxicology and epidemiology of 1,3-butadiene. *CRC Crit. Rev. Toxicol.*, 27:1–108.

259. Roy, A., and Georgopoulos, P. G. (1998): Reconstructing week-long exosures to volatile organic compounds using physiologically based pharmacokinetic models. *J. Exp. Anal. Environ. Epidemiol.*, 8:407–422.

260. Vinegar, A., Jepson, G. W., and Overton, J. H. (1998): PBPK modeling of short term (0–5 min) human inhalation exposures to halogenated hydrocarbons. *Inhal. Toxicol.*, 10:411–429.

261. Lee, K., Dill, J. A., Chou, B. J., and Roycroft, J. H. (1998): Physiologically based pharmacokinetic model for chronic inhalation of 2-butoxyethanol. *Toxicol. Appl. Pharmacol.*, 153:211–226.

262. Kimmel, E. C., Carpenter, R. L., Smith, E. A., Reboulet, J. E., and Black, B. H. (1998): Physiologic models for comparison of inhalation dose between laboratory and field-generated atmospheres of a dry powder fire suppressant. *Inhal. Toxicol.*, 10:905–922.

263. Stöber, W., Morrow, P. E., and Morawietz, G. (1990): Alveolar retention and clearance of insoluble particles in rats simulated by a new physiology-oriented compartmental kinetics model. *Fundam. Appl. Toxicol.*, 15:329–349.

264. Stöber, W. (1999): Pock model simulation of pulmonary quartz dust retetnion data in extended inhalation exposures of rats. *Inhal. Toxicol.*, 11:269–292.

265. McDougal, J. N., Jepson, G. W., Clewell, H. J., MacNaughton, M. G., and Anderson, M. E. (1986): A physiological pharmacokinetic model for dermal absorption of vapors in the rat. *Toxicol. Appl. Pharmacol.*, 85:286–294.

266. Casanova, M., Morgan, K. T., Steinhagen, W. H., Everitt, J. I., Popp, J. A., and Heck, H. D'A. (1991): Covalent binding of inhaled

formaldehyde to DNA in the respiratory tract of rhesus monkeys: Pharmacokinetics, rat-to-monkey interspecies scaling, and extrapolation to man. *Fundam. Appl. Toxicol.*, 17:409–428.

267. Miller, R. R., Leto, R. L., Potts, W. J., and McKenna, M. T. (1980): Improved methodology for generating controlled test atmospheres. *Am. Ind. Hyg. Assoc. J.*, 41:844–846.

268 Cohen, B. S. (1995): Air sampling instruments for evaluation of atmospheric contaminants. In: *American Conference of Governmental Industrial Hygiensists*, 8th ed. Cincinnati.

269. Willeke, K., Lo, C. S. K., and Whitby, K. J. (1974): Dispersion characteristics of a fluidized bed. *J. Aerosol Sci.*, 5:449–455.

270. Lee, K. P., Kelly, D. P., and Kennedy, G. L., Jr. (1983): Pulmonary response to inhaled Kevlar aramid synthetics fibers in rats. *Toxicol. Appl. Pharmacol.*, 71:242–253.

271. Cheng, Y. S., Marshall, T. C., Henderson, R. F., and Newton, G. J. (1985): Use of a jet mill dispersing dry powder for inhalation studies. *Am. Ind. Hyg. Assoc. J.*, 46:449–454.

272. Bernstein, D. M., Moss, O. R., Fleissner, H., and Bretz, R. (1984): A brush feed micronising jet mill powder aerosol generator for producing a wide range of concentrations of respirable particles. In: *Aerosols: Science, Technology, and Industrial Application of Airborne Particles*, edited by B. Y. H. Liu, D. Y. H. Pui, and H. Fissan, pp. 721–724. Elsevier, New York.

273. Cheng, Y. S., Barr, E. B., Benson, J. M., et al. (1988): Evaluation of a real-time aerosol monitor (RAM-5) for inhalation studies. *Fundam. Appl. Toxicol.*, 10:321–328.

274. Costa, D. L. (1985): Interpretation of new techniques used in the determination of pulmonary function in rodents. *Fundam. Appl. Toxicol.*, 5:423-434.

275. O'Neil, J. J., and Raub, J. A. (1984): Pulmonary function testing in small laboratory animals. *Environ. Health Perspect.*, 56:1–22.

276. Green, J. F. (1997): *Mechanical Concepts in Cardiovascular and Pulmonary Physiology*. Lea and Feibiger, Philadelphia.

277. West, J. B. (1994): *Respiratory Physiology—The Essentials*, 5th ed. Williams and Wilkins, Baltimore, MD.

278. Gross, D. R. (1995): *Animal Models in Cardiovascular Research*. Martinus Nijhoff, Dordecht, the Netherlands.

279. Gibson, G. J. (1989): *Clinical Tests of Respiratory Function*. Raven Press, New York.

280. Anthonisen, N. R. (1986): Tests of mechanical function. In: *Mechanics of Breathing, Handbook of Physiology, Section 3: The Respiratory System*, edited by P. T. Macklem and J. Mead. American Physiology Society, Bethesda, MD.

281. Beck, B. D., Brain, J. D., and Bohannon, D. E. (1982): An in vivo hamster bioassay to assess the toxicity of particles for the lungs. *Toxicol. Appl. Pharmacol.*, 66:9–29.

282. Henderson, R. F., Benson, J. M., Hahn, F. F., et al. (1985): New approaches for the evaluation of pulmonary toxicity: bronchioalveolar lavage fluid analysis. *Fundam. Appl. Toxicol.*, 5:451–458.

283. Moores, S. R., Black, A., Evans, J. C., et al. (1981): The short-term cellular and biochemical response of the lung to toxic dusts: An in vivo cytotoxicity test. In: *The In Vitro Effect of Mineral Dusts*, edited by R. C. Brown, I. P. Gormley, M. Chamberlain, and R. Davis, pp. 297–303. Academic Press, New York.

284. Henderson, R. F. (1991): Commentary on "Cellular and biochemical indices of bronchoalveolar lavage for detection of lung injury following insult by airborne toxicants." *Toxicol. Lett.*, 58:235–238.

285. Khan, M. F., and Gupta, G. S. D. (1991): Cellular and biochemical indices of bronchoalveolar lavage for detection of lung injury following insult by airborne toxicants. *Toxicol. Lett.*, 58:239–255.

286. Henderson, R. F. (1984): The use of bronchoalveolar lavage to detect lung damage. *Environ. Health Perspect.*, 56:115–129.

287. Benson, J. M., Henderson, R. F., McClellan, R. O., Hanson, R. L., and Rebar, A. H. (1986): Comparative acute toxicity of four nickel compounds to F344 rat lung. *Fundam. Appl. Toxicol.*, 7:340–347.

288. Wolff, R. K., Henderson, R. F., Eidson, A. F., Pickrell, J. A., Rothenberg, S. J., and Hahn, F. F. (1998): Toxicity of gallium oxide particles following a 4-week inhalation exposure. *J. Appl. Toxicol.*, 8:191–200.

289. McClellan, R. O. (1986): Health effects of diesel exhaust: A case study in risk assessmesnt. *Am. Ind. Assoc. J.*, 471:1.

290. Fabbri, L. M., Aizawa, H., O'Byrne, P. M., Bethel, R. A., Walters, E. H., Holtzman, M. J., and Nadel, J. A. (1985): An anti-inflammatory drug (BW755C) inhibits airway hyperresponsiveness induced by ozone in dogs. *J. Allergy Clin. Immunol.*, 76:162.

291. Barry, B. E., and Crapo, J. D. (1985): Application of morphometric methods to study diffuse and focal injury in the lung caused by toxic agents. *CRC Crit. Rev. Toxicol.*, 14:1–32.

292. Tyler, E. S., Dungworth, D. L., Plopper, C. G, et al. (1985): Structural evaluation of the respiratory system. *Fundam. Appl. Toxicol.*, 5:405–422.

293. Driscoll, K. E., Costa, D. L., Hatch, G., Henderson, R., Oberdorster, G., Salem, H., and Schlesinger, R. B. (2000). Intratracheal instillation as an exposure technique for the evaluation of respiratory tract toxicity: Uses and limitations. *Toxicological Sciences*, 55:24–35.

294. ten Berge, W. F., Zwart, A., and Appelman, L. M. (1986). Concentration-time mortality response relationship and systemically acting vapors and gases. *J Hazardous Mater.*, 13:301–309.

295. Baron, P. A. (1988): Modern real-time aerosol samplers. *Appl. Ind. Hyg.*, 3:97–103.

296. Boggs, D. F. (1992): In *Treatise on Pulmonary Toxicology, Vol 1, Comparative Biology of the Normal Lung* (Richard Parent, Editor). CRC Press, Boca Raton, FL.

ADDITIONAL READINGS

Barrow, C. S. (1986): *Toxicology of the Nasal Passages*. Hemisphere, New York.

Baum, G. L., and Wozinsky, E. (1983): *Textbook of Pulmonary Diseases*, 3rd ed. Little, Brown and Co., Boston.

Brain, J. D., Proctor, D. F., and Reid, L. M. (1977): *Respiratory Defense Mechanisms*, Vols. I and II. Elsevier, New York.

Brown, S. S., and Davies, D. S. (1981): *Organ-Directed Toxicity: Chemical Indices and Mechanisms*. Pergamon Press, New York.

Dail, D. H., and Hammar, S. P. (1994): *Pulmonary Pathology*, 2nd ed. Springer–Verlag, New York.

Derelenko, M. J., and Hollinger, M. A., eds. (1995): *CRC Handbook of Toxicology*. CRC Press, Boca Raton, FL.

Fiserova-Bergerova, V. (1983): *Modeling of Inhalation Exposure to Vapors: Uptake, Distribution and Elimination*. CRC Press, Boca Raton, FL.

Gardner, D. E., and Kennedy, G. L., Jr. (1993): Methodologies and technology for animal inhalation toxicology studies. In: *Toxicology of the Lung*, 2nd ed., edited by D. E. Gardner, J. D. Crapo, and R. O. McClellan, pp. 1–30. Raven Press, New York.

Hook, G. (1984): Monograph on pulmonary toxicology. *Environ. Health Perspect.*, 55:1–416.

Jenkins, P. G., Kayser, D., Muhle, H., Rosner, G., and Smith, E. M. (1994): *Respiratory Toxicology and Risk Assessment*. Wissenschaftliche Verlagsgesellschaft, Stuttgart.

Kennedy, G. L., Jr. (1988): Techniques for evaluating hazards of inhaled products. In: *Product Safety Evaluation Handbook*, edited by S. C. Gad, pp. 259–290. Marcel Dekker, New York.

Lenfant, C. (1996): *Inhalation Aerosols: Physical and Biological Basis for Therapy in Lung Biology in Health and Disease*, Vol. 94. Marcel Dekker, New York.

Leong, B. K. J. (1981): *Inhalation Toxicology and Technology*. Ann Arbor Science Publishers, Ann Arbor, MI.

McClellan, R. O., and Henderson, R. E. (1995): *Concepts in Inhalation Toxicology*, 2nd ed. Taylor & Francis, Washington, DC.

Menzel, D. B., and Amdur, M. O. (1960): Toxic responses of the respiratory system. In: *Casarett and Doull's Toxicology*, edited by C. D. Klaassen, M. O. Amdur, and J. Doull, pp. 330–358. Macmillan, New York.

Mohr, U. (Editor-in-Chief). (1989): Assessment of Inhalation Hazards: Integration and Extrapolation Using Diverse Data. ILSI Press, Washington, DC.

National Research Council. (1989): *Biologic Markers in Pulmonary Toxicology*. National Academy Press, Washington, DC.

Parkes, W. R. (1994): *Occupational Lung Disorders*, 3rd ed. Butterworth-Heinemann, Boston.

Phalen, R. F. (1997): *Methods in Inhalation Toxicology*. CRC Press, Boca Raton, FL.

Salem, H. (1986): *Inhalation Toxicology: Research Methods, Applications, and Evaluation*. Marcel Dekker, New York.

Warheit, D. B. (1993): *Fiber Toxicology*. Academic Press, San Diego.

Walton, W. H. (1982): Inhaled particles. In: *Proceedings of Symposium on Inhaled Principles and Vapours*, Cardiff, England, September 1980. Pergamon Press, New York.

Weibel, E. R. (1963): *Morphometry of the Human Lung*. Springer–Verlag, Berlin.

Willeke, K. (1980): *Generation of Aerosols and Facilities for Exposure Experiments*. Ann Arbor Science, Ann Arbor, MI.

Witschi, H. P., and Brain, J. D. (1985): *Toxicology of Inhaled Materials*. Springer–Verlag, New York.

World Health Organization (WHO). (1983): *Biological Effects of Man-Made Mineral Fibres*. WHO, Geneva.

Principles and Methods of Toxicology, Fourth Edition, edited by A. Wallace Hayes. Taylor & Francis, Philadelphia © 2001.

Chapter 24

Detection and Evaluation of Chemically Induced Liver Injury

Gabriel L. Plaa and Michel Charbonneau

Liver injury induced by chemicals has been recognized as a toxicological problem for more than 100 years. During the late 1800s, scientists were concerned about the mechanisms involved in the hepatic deposition of lipids following exposure to yellow phosphorus. Hepatic lesions produced by arsphenamine, carbon tetrachloride, and chloroform were also studied in laboratory animals during the first 40 years of the 20th century. During the same period the correlation between hepatic cirrhosis and excessive ethanol consumption was recognized.

"Liver injury" is not a single entity; the lesion observed depends not only on the chemical agent involved but also on the period of exposure. After acute exposure, one usually finds lipid accumulation in the hepatocytes, cellular necrosis, or hepatobiliary dysfunction, whereas cirrhotic or neoplastic changes are usually considered the result of chronic exposures. Different biochemical alterations may lead to the same endpoint; no single mechanism governs the appearance of hepatocellular degenerative changes or alterations in function. Some forms of liver injury are reversible, whereas others result in a permanently deranged organ. The mortality associated with various forms of liver injury is variable. The incidence of injury can differ among species, and the presence of a dose-dependent relation may not always be apparent.

The marked vulnerability of the liver to chemically induced damage is a function of:

(a) its anatomical proximity to the blood supply from the digestive tract,
(b) its ability to concentrate and biotransform foreign chemicals, and
(c) its role in the excretion of xenobiotics or their metabolites into the bile.

The diverse nature of the functional activity of the liver and its varied response to injury makes the selection of appropriate testing procedures a difficult task.

This chapter discusses the major tests that are useful in the detection and evaluation of liver injury in laboratory animals.

CLASSIFICATION OF CHEMICALLY INDUCED LIVER INJURY

The morphological changes observed following hepatic injury produced by chemical and biological agents can be classified according to two parameters: location and type of lesion produced.

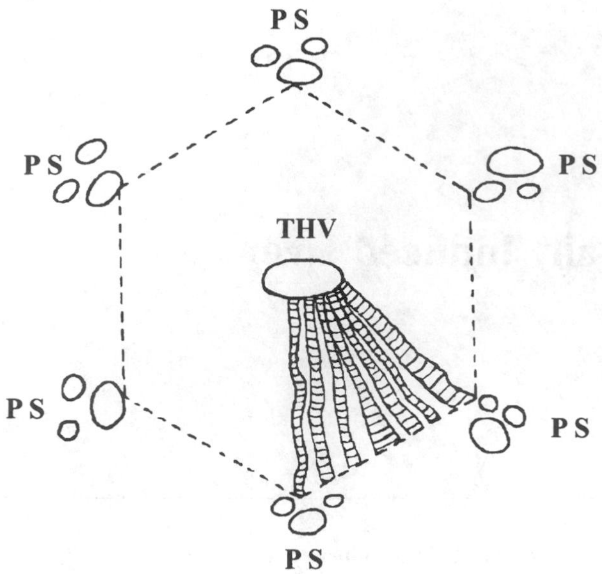

FIG. 24.1. Schematic representation of the traditional hexagonal lobule. (*PS*) portal space, consisting of a branch of the portal vein, hepatic arteriole, and a bile duct; (*THV*) terminal hepatic venule (central vein) (From Plaa [249] with permission).

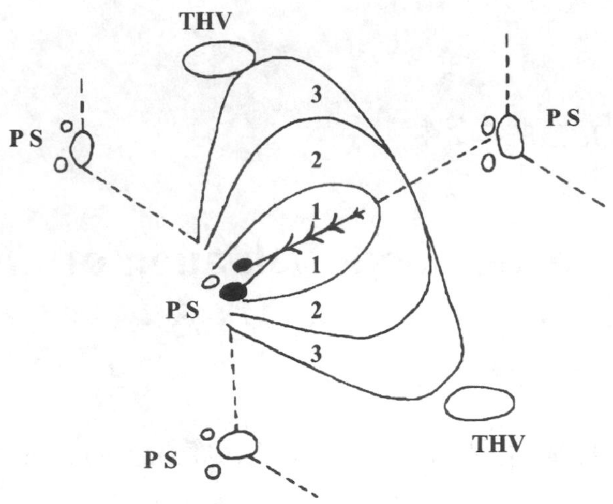

FIG. 24.2. Schematic representation of a simple hepatic acinus, according to A. M. Rappaport. (*PS*) portal space, consisting of a branch of the portal vein, hepatic arteriole, and a bile duct; (*THV*) terminal hepatic venule (central vein); (1, 2, 3) zones draining off the terminal afferent vessel (in black) (From Plaa [249] with permission).

Location Within the Hepatic Parenchyma

An early system of describing pathological lesions of the liver originated from the concept of the hexagonal lobule introduced by Kiernan in 1833 (162) (Figure 24.1). This configuration, the classical manner of presenting the relations among the hepatic cell, its vascular supply, and the biliary system, was considered to represent the functional unit of the liver. The terminal hepatic venule (central vein) is found in the center of the lobule; and the portal space, containing a branch of the portal vein, a hepatic arteriole, and a bile duct, is located at the periphery of the lobule. Based on this configuration, lesions of the hepatic parenchyma have been classified as centrilobular, midzonal, or periportal.

The hexagonal lobule configuration does not correspond to the functional unit of the liver. The hexagonal lobule is not conspicuous under microscopic examination. Injection of colored gelatin mixtures in the portal vein or hepatic artery shows that terminal afferent vessels supply blood only to sectors of adjacent hepatic lobules. These sectors are situated around terminal portal branches and extend from the terminal hepatic venule of one hexagon to the terminal hepatic venule of an adjacent hexagon. Rappaport defined the parenchymal mass in terms of functional units called the liver acini (262,263); the concept has undergone some re-evaluation (115,190). A simple liver acinus consists of a small parenchymal mass that is irregular in size and shape and is arranged around an axis consisting of a terminal portal venule, a hepatic arteriole, a bile ductule, lymph vessels, and nerves (Figure 24.2). This acinus lies between two or more terminal hepatic venules with which its vascular and biliary axis interdigitates. There is no physical separation between two liver acini. The hepatic cells of the simple acini are in cellular and sinusoidal contact with the cells of adjacent or overlapping acini. Even with this extensive communication, the hepatic cells of one particular acinus are preferentially supplied by their parent vessels. Three relatively discrete circulatory zones appear within each acinus (Figure 24.2). Hepatocytes in close juxtaposition to the terminal afferent vessel constitute zone 1. These cells are the first to be supplied with fresh blood, rich in oxygen and nutrients. The higher order of zones 2 and 3 is indicative of the greater distance between the cells comprising these zones and the supply of fresh blood.

One of the interesting correlates of the concept of zonal acinar circulation is the growing realization that not all hepatic parenchymal cells within the liver lobule have the same kind of functional specificity. Rappaport's acinar concept has been modulated by others (115,190) to account for differences in enzyme distribution and redox state. Areas of differing metabolic activity exist within the liver (157). Respiratory enzyme activity is particularly high in the zone closest to the terminal afferent vessel (zone 1) (Figure 24.2), whereas the most distant zone (zone 3) is particularly rich in cytochrome P450–dependent enzyme systems. The perivenous (zone 3) cells are relatively rich in some NADPH-dependent enzymes, and periportal cells (zone 1) are relatively poor (115). The concept of "metabolic zonation" is based on differences observed between enzyme activities in periportal and perivenous regions (157). Thurman and Kauffmann (310) reported on the lobular distribution of maximal enzyme activities measured by immunohistochemical or microchemical techniques; these parameters do not always correlate with metabolic flux rates as measured by microfluorometry and miniature O_2 electrodes. Periportal–perivenous gradients are described for cytochrome P450s, sulfatation, glucuronidation, and glutathione *S*-transferases (115). Functional gradients are also reported for hepatobiliary activity (131). The implications of such findings are not well understood. Zonal and cellular enzymatic specificity and metabolic heterogeneity may, however, permit the rationalization of differing mechanisms of action in the development of hepatic lesions associated with hepatotoxic agents.

The classical hexagonal descriptions of focal, midzonal, periportal, and centrilobular lesions, although functionally incorrect, are compatible with Rappaport's zonal acinar configuration. Centrilobular necrosis, for example, occurs in cells located in the distal acinar zone (zone 3) (Figure 24.2). When several such zones are affected, a concentric lesion can be visualized. Regeneration is said to occur from cells located in the midzonal region of the hexagonal representation, which corresponds to the acinar zone closest to the terminal afferent vessel (zone 1), a zone shown to be particularly high in cytogenic activity. Therefore, it appears that the acinal circulatory concept of the hepatic lobule does not come into serious conflict with the earlier descriptions of pathological lesions.

Morphological Classification

Morphologically, liver injury can manifest itself in different ways (249). The acute effects can consist of an accumulation of lipids (steatosis) and the appearance of degenerative processes, leading to cell death (necrosis). The necrotic process can affect small groups of isolated parenchymal cells (focal necrosis), groups of cells located in zones (centrilobular, midzonal, or periportal necrosis), or virtually all of the cells within a hepatic lobule (massive necrosis). The accumulation of lipids can also be zonal or more diffuse in nature. Although acute injury may consist in both necrosis and fat accumulation, it is not necessary that both features be present. The cholestatic type of lesion, resulting in diminution or cessation of bile flow with retention of bile salts and bilirubin, is also an important form of liver injury (235,245,254); this lesion leads to the appearance of jaundice. A type of massive necrosis that resembles a viral infection (335) is produced by certain chemicals. A number of drugs are also associated with a mixed type of lesion, that is, one that possesses both cholestatic and viral-like hepatic components (335). Chemically induced liver injury resulting from chronic exposure can produce marked alteration of the entire liver structure, with degenerative and proliferative changes observed in the various forms of cirrhosis. Neoplastic changes may be another endpoint of chemical liver injury.

Through the years a number of classification systems have evolved to describe the chemicals involved. The schemes are beyond the scope of this chapter. In brief, however, some are based on morphological changes (249), and others deal with the postulated mechanisms of action or the circumstances of exposure (335).

In the morphological classifications, one finds those chemicals (e.g., carbon tetrachloride [CCl_4], chloroform [$CHCl_3$], phosphorus, tannic acid, ethionine, ethanol) that produce zonal hepatocellular alterations (necrosis, steatosis). Intrahepatic cholestasis is a lesion produced by a number of drugs (e.g., phenothiazine derivatives, antimicrobial agents, anabolic steroids, oral hypoglycemics) and is characterized by biliary dysfunction. In addition, massive hepatocellular necrosis is produced by other drugs (e.g., iproniazid, monoamine oxidase inhibitors, halothane).

In the classification schemes based on mechanism of action, one finds differences of opinion regarding which categories to include and how the various chemicals fit in these categories. It is clear, however, that in a number of instances the hepatic injury is an expression of individual susceptibility rather than the intrinsic toxicity of an offending agent; hypersensitivity (allergic reactions) and reactions involving an aberration in the metabolic handling of the chemical are important components in the elucidation of such lesions.

From these classifications, one sees that there are a variety of pathological processes involved in what is called, in general terms, "liver injury." Furthermore, many different substances can cause injury. Although classification schemes assist in conceptualizing what is occurring, with additional knowledge of the events actually involved in the elaboration of the biochemical lesion, changes in the classifications certainly occur. Regardless of this fact, the pathological types of injury produced by hepatotoxicants largely determine the biochemical and functional manifestation of injury and thus the battery of toxicological tests needed to detect and evaluate "liver injury."

EVALUATION OF HEPATIC INJURY IN VIVO

The major tests that have proved useful for evaluation of experimental hepatic injury in laboratory animals can be placed in four primary categories:

(a) serum enzyme tests,
(b) hepatic excretory tests,
(c) alterations in the chemical constituents of the liver, and
(d) histological analysis of liver injury.

Two important processes, that is, repair and recovery of liver parenchyma and apoptosis of hepatocytes, also are the bases for tests to study the effects of chemicals on the liver. This chapter covers methods used to detect hepatic dysfunction or injury, but does not address biochemical approaches employed to define the different mechanisms involved. The reader is referred to Kodavanti and Mehendale (177) for additional biochemical techniques not covered in the present chapter.

Serum Enzyme Techniques

Determination of the activity of hepatic enzymes released into the blood by the damaged liver is one of the most useful tools in the study of hepatotoxicity. The application of serum enzyme methodology to the detection of liver injury was introduced during the 1930s and 1940s with the demonstration of abnormal serum activities of alkaline phosphatase (281) and cholinesterase (39). However, the discovery during the 1950s that the activity of several serum aminotransferases was increased by tissue destruction represents the true advent of the serum enzyme methods. Subsequently, a number of other enzymes were identified in blood, several of which demonstrate abnormal activity in the presence of liver injury.

Zimmerman (335) identified four major categories of serum enzymes based on their specificity for and sensitivity to different types of liver injury. The first group contains enzymes such as alkaline phosphatase (AP), 5′-nucleotidase (5′-NT), and γ-glutamyltranspeptidase (γ-GT). Elevated serum activities of these enzymes appear to reflect cholestatic injury more effectively than necrogenic injury. In contrast, the second group of enzymes includes those that are more sensitive to cytotoxic hepatic injury. This group has been further subdivided into:

(a) enzymes that are somewhat nonspecific and can reflect injury to extrahepatic tissue, for example aspartate aminotransferase (AST) and lactic dehydrogenase (LDH);
(b) enzymes found mainly in the liver, for example, alanine aminotransferase (ALT); and
(c) enzymes that are almost exclusively located in the liver, for example, ornithine carbamyl transferase (OCT) and sorbitol dehydrogenase (SDH).

Assay of the latter, more hepatospecific subgroup of enzymes may be particularly useful when studying agents with unknown hepatotoxic potential. Although elevated serum activity of the aminotransferases may reflect injury to extrahepatic organs such as the heart, skeletal muscle, or kidney, elevated activities of OCT and SDH are reliable reflections of hepatic injury. The third and fourth serum enzyme categories contain, respectively, enzymes that are relatively insensitive to hepatic injury but are elevated with extrahepatic diseases, for example, creatine phosphokinase (CPK), and enzymes that demonstrate a depressed serum activity in liver disease, for example, cholinesterase (ChE).

Aminotransferases, Ornithine Carbamyl Transferase, and Sorbitol Dehydrogenase

The selection of a battery of enzymes for evaluating the hepatotoxic potential of an unknown chemical in laboratory animals is complicated by the varying sensitivity of the enzymes to different types of lesion. In an early series of experiments, Molander et al. (225) found that the measurement of serum AST provided a more sensitive index of hepatocellular injury in rats treated with CCl_4 than did the measurement of either ChE or AP. A number of experimentally induced necrotic states are also detectable by an elevation in the serum activity of ALT, a liver cytoplasmic enzyme. Balazs et al. (18) assessed serum ALT as a liver test in rats after treatment with ethionine, CCl_4, thioacetamide, dimethylnitrosamine, or allyl alcohol. Serum ALT elevation occurred following the acute administration of all of these agents, but with ethionine the elevation was not pronounced. This finding is understandable because ethionine does not produce extensive centrilobular necrosis but usually results in fatty infiltration.

Other investigators also found that ALT is an insensitive measure of hepatic steatosis (7,116). On the other hand, those agents that are associated with severe necrotic lesions produce pronounced elevation of serum ALT. Balazs et al. (17,18) found that when the gross pathological changes or the severity of the histopathology were compared to the elevation in ALT, there was a good correlation between the elevation in serum activity and the severity of the lesion. Others showed (197,252) that there was an excellent correlation between the severity of quantified histological damage produced by $CHCl_3$ or acetaminophen and the elevation in serum ALT activity in rats. Therefore, it seems with ALT that not only is it possible to detect the presence of liver injury, but under some circumstances the severity of the lesion can be estimated by the elevation in serum enzyme activity.

Aminotransferase activity in different tissues varies and distinct species differences occur (331). In most instances, AST activity is greater than ALT. High AST activity occurs in skeletal muscle, diaphragm, heart muscle, and liver tissue. ALT is not as widely distributed; in humans, the greatest activity is found in the liver. Cornelius (71) studied the hepatic distribution of ALT in various animals and found that a relation exists between body size and the amount of hepatic ALT. The smaller the animal is within the weight range studied, the greater the hepatic ALT activity. More than 90% of the ALT was found to be located within the liver of all mammals of small body size; this group includes the common laboratory animals used in toxicity studies. Cornelius et al. (73) showed that, whereas AST was present in almost all tissues of pigs, cattle, dogs, and horses, low ALT activity was found in horses, cattle, and pigs. When these species were subjected to CCl_4 intoxication, significant elevation of serum ALT occurred only in the dog. On the other hand, when serum AST activity was used for measuring hepatotoxicity, all species exhibited an increase in serum enzyme activity after CCl_4. In the rat, both serum AST and ALT activities are markedly elevated after experimental injury; either enzyme could probably be used for detecting injury in this species. Hemolysis, however, has a marked effect on serum AST in the rat, whereas its effect is practically negligible in the case of serum ALT (246). This fact should be kept in mind when one is using rats for assessing liver function. In addition, because the hepatic specificity of ALT is greater than AST, measurement of serum ALT activity, rather than AST, might be preferable for determining the status of the liver.

Ornithine carbamyl transferase is found predominantly in the mitochondrial fraction of liver cells (78,272,273) and normally occurs only in minute amounts in serum. The mucosa of the small intestine contains a small amount, 1 to 2% that of the liver, and tissue such as brain and kidney contains only trace amounts (273–275). OCT serum activity is markedly elevated in both acute and chronic liver disease in humans (229,275). With experimentally induced hepatotoxicity, Reichard (272) found that serum activity of OCT increased considerably more than those of the aminotransferases but followed a similar temporal phase. OCT was also as sensitive an index of liver injury as GDH and AST in cattle and sheep poisoned with CCl_4, dimidium bromide, or sporidesmin (103). Tegeris et al. (309) found that OCT activity was markedly elevated in dogs and swine poisoned with CCl_4, whereas the serum activity remained within normal limits in animals treated with uranyl nitrate, a nephrotoxicant. In addition, the peak serum activities of OCT (expressed as multiples of control values) in CCl_4-challenged animals were markedly greater that those of ALT, AST, LDH, or isocitric dehydrogenase (ICDH); the temporal pattern of OCT response was similar to that of the aminotransaminases. Serum OCT activity is a useful monitor of liver injury in rats treated with various hepatotoxicants (78,89, 90,181). Indeed, Drotman (89) described a dose-dependent relation between the amount of CCl_4 administered to rats and serum OCT activity. In addition, a sixfold increase in OCT activity was found at a CCl_4 dose that did not produce distinctive liver damage upon light microscopic examination of the tissue, suggesting that OCT may be as sensitive an index of liver injury as histopathological examination (90). The correlation between elevation in serum OCT activity and quantified histological changes following $CHCl_3$ administration is good (252).

Sorbitol dehydrogenase, a cytoplasmic enzyme, is also relatively specific for liver (8,78), and an increase in the serum activity of this enzyme is a relatively sensitive index of hepatocellular damage. In an elegant series of experiments, Korsrud et al. (180) determined the serum activity of nine hepatic enzymes in CCl_4-poisoned rats in an attempt to identify those enzymes that would respond quantitatively to varying CCl_4 doses and would indicate minimal liver damage. They placed the enzymes in three groups based on the lowest dose of CCl_4 required to elevate serum activity and concluded that SDH was the most sensitive enzymic index of liver injury. A group of four enzymes (ICDH, fructose-1,6-aldolase [F-1,6-ALD], ALT, and AST) were less sensitive to CCl_4 than SDH but were more responsive to liver injury than were alcohol dehydrogenase (ADH), 6-phosphodigluconase (6-PDG), LDH, and malic dehydrogenase (MDH). However, histological alterations were observed at CCl_4 doses that did not elevate serum enzyme activity. Subsequently, Korsrud et al. (181) studied thioacetamide and dimethylnitrosamine. As before, serum SDH was the most sensitive enzymic index of liver necrosis.

Sorbitol dehydrogenase, however, was not a preferentially sensitive index of liver injury in diethanolamine-treated rats. Six enzymes (SDH, ICDH, F-1,6-ALD, ALT, AST, and MDH) were equally responsive to diethanolamine hepatotoxicity, whereas a higher dose of this compound was required to elevate the serum activity of OCT, GDH, and LDH. Based on these observations Korsrud et al. (181) suggested that SDH was the best enzymic index of liver injury when minimal damage or minimal changes are being assessed. However, histological changes characteristic of each hepatotoxicant were noted at doses that did not result in an elevation of serum activity. Thus, the serum enzyme assays were less sensitive than histopathological examination for detecting liver damage.

Later work by Travlos et al. (314) compared the relative sensitivities of SDH, ALT, and histopathology as indices of liver injury in rats. When increases in both enzymes occurred simultaneously, terminal histopathological changes were very highly predictable (75–100%). They concluded that clinical chemistry evaluations could be useful for detecting potential treatment effects throughout a study, although histopathological evaluation can only be performed on termination.

Serum ALT activity is probably the most frequently used enzymic parameter to assess hepatic injury in laboratory animals. Because of the high sensitivity of OCT and SDH, however, it appears reasonable that one of these two enzymes could be used in conjunction with ALT when examining the hepatotoxic potential of an unknown chemical. In this manner, the battery of tests might better reflect the range of sensitivity encompassed by light microscopy.

Lactate Dehydrogenase Isoenzymes

In addition to serum enzyme activities, serum isoenzyme patterns have been utilized for the detection of organ damage in humans and laboratory animals (74,75,129,327). Isoenzymes are enzymatically active proteins that catalyze the same reactions and occur in the same species but differ in their physicochemical properties. The isoenzymes of LDH are used as diagnostic agents in clinical medicine (75) and in some instances have been evaluated for use in experimentally induced organ damage in laboratory animals. Cornish et al. (75) utilized LDH isoenzymes to detect specific organ damage in rats; they found that the serum isoenzyme patterns resulting from liver or kidney damage differed markedly and concluded that these differences could be utilized to distinguish the damaged organ. Liver damage resulted primarily in an increase in serum LDH-5 isoenzyme activity, whereas the activity of the LDH-1 and LDH-2 isoenzymes was elevated in rats with kidney injury. Grice et al. (129) treated rats with CCl_4, mercuric chloride, thioacetamide, or diethanolamine at doses that would produce either minimal or pronounced tissue damage. Although AST activity was a more sensitive indicator of organ damage than LDH, it did not provide isoenzyme patterns that could identify the specific target organ. In contrast, LDH isoenzyme patterns were capable of identifying the specific target organ; the LDH-5 bands indicative of liver injury were increased in rats poisoned with CCl_4, diethanolamine, and thioacetamide, whereas mercuric chloride, a potent nephrotoxicant, increased the activity of LDH-1 and LDH-2. Morphological damage generally occurred at dosage levels considerably below those producing detectable serum enzyme alterations. Thus, these authors concluded that serum enzyme activities and isoenzyme patterns are an important supplement to, but not a substitute for, histopathological examination of tissues.

A number of other enzymes of clinical interest occur in multiple forms, among them AST and alkaline and acid phosphatase. Although these enzymes may have well-established roles in experimental toxicology, the use of their isoenzyme patterns does not yet have a definitive role.

Enzymes Useful for Detecting Obstructive Disorders

Most of the preceding discussion concerns the use of serum enzymes to detect necrotic or degenerative processes following the administration of toxicants. In general, these enzymes are not as useful for detecting those types of hepatic alteration that are associated with diminution or cessation of bile flow. The degree of change in serum enzyme activities that one can obtain by the induction of experimental hepatotoxicity in mice is demonstrated in Table 24.1. Three hepatotoxic procedures were employed in this study (246). One group of animals received α-naphthylisothiocyanate (ANIT), another received CCl_4, and members of the third group had their bile ducts ligated. Serum enzyme activities (ALT and AP) were determined 24 h later. For comparative purposes, sulfobromophthalein (BSP) retention and serum bilirubin concentrations were also measured in these animals. It is evident (Table 24.1) that a necrotizing agent such as CCl_4 produces sufficient parenchymal

Table 24.1

Effect of various hepatotoxic procedures on four liver function tests in mice[a]

Hepatotoxic Procedure[b]	BSP Retention (mg/dl)	Alkaline Phosphatase (units)	Bilirubin Concentration (mg/dl)	ALT Activity (units/ml)
Control (no treatment)	0.3 ± 0.3	3.0 ± 0.5	0.2 ± 0.1	25 ± 5
ANIT (150 mg/kg po)	45.0 ± 23	5.6 ± 2.6	1.1 ± 0.4	282 ± 126
CCl_4 (1 mg/kg po)	13.0 ± 7	5.3 ± 1.3	0.4 ± 0.2	8510 ± 1930
Bile duct ligation	26.0 ± 3	19.0 ± 10	3.8 ± 0.8	655 ± 132

Data obtained from Reference 246.

[a] Values are expressed as means ± SE; each group contained 10 mice.
[b] Hepatotoxic procedure was performed 24 h before assessing function.

injury to cause a large increase in serum ALT activity, whereas those experimental procedures that markedly impair biliary excretion (ANIT treatment, bile duct ligation) cause only a mild increase in ALT activity. The reciprocal relation is obtained when serum AP activity is assessed; obstruction of biliary flow (bile duct ligation) markedly increases serum AP activity, whereas the necrotizing challenge (CCl_4) produces only a mild elevation.

Alkaline phosphatase is the prototype of those enzymes (Zimmerman's group 1) that reflect pathological reductions in biliary flow. In the rat, this enzyme is found in the liver and the intestine. After bile duct ligation, the activity in the liver increases due to de novo synthesis of the membranous form of the enzyme (158,291). The use of this enzyme in chemically induced liver dysfunction has been fairly extensively investigated. In the dog, the enzyme is useful for detecting biliary dysfunction. In the cat, however, ligation of the common bile duct results in only a slight increase in serum AP activity. The normal level of serum AP in the rat is exceptionally high, independent of growth, and unusually susceptible to variations in diet (137). Increases in serum AP activity were not remarkable in a comparative study of clinical chemistry and liver histopathology performed in a subchronic study in rats, although increases in serum total bile acid concentration were (314). Thus, serum AP activity may not be useful for detecting cholestatic changes in the rat.

In addition to AP, other enzymes, for example, 5′N, γ-GT, and leucine aminopeptidase (LAP), may be of use in assessing obstructive liver injury. The serum activity of these enzymes, which are localized in the membranes of hepatocytes and bile duct cells, is increased during extrahepatic cholestasis in humans (20,326). Kryszewski et al. (184) found a significant elevation in serum activity of AP, 5′N, and γ-GT 12 h after bile duct ligation in the rat; AP and 5′N peaked at 24 h and then gradually decreased, and γ-GT peaked at 48 h and remained elevated even 192 h after bile duct ligation. Fujii (111) found serum AP and γ-GT useful indicators of cholestasis in dogs. Thus, changes in the serum activities of these enzymes are useful for detecting toxicant-induced cholestatic changes in laboratory animals. A simplified electrophoretic method was developed to separate and quantify multiple forms of human serum 5′N (240); three isoforms were identified in normal subjects and hepatobiliary dysfunction resulted in the increased activity of only one form of serum 5′-nucleotidase. Comparable studies have not been performed in animals.

The increase in serum γ-GT activity during ANIT-induced cholestasis in rats appears to be of biliary cell origin and not from hepatocytes (44). In this respect, elevated serum γ-GT differs from serum AP increases in activity also observed during cholestasis; AP appears to originate from the canalicular pole of the hepatocyte (44).

Of interest is the observation of Moritz and Snodgrass (227) that acute obstruction of the bile duct in the rat produced a rapid rise in the serum activity of SDH and OCT. From 1 to 24 h following bile duct ligation, the activities of these two enzymes increased in serum to levels approximating those found after a single dose of CCl_4, even though the histological degree of hepatic necrosis was substantially less with obstruction than with CCl_4 poisoning. This finding confirmed and extended the observation of Hallberg et al. (140) that bile duct obstruction in dogs resulted in increased serum OCT activity. These observations, if confirmed in other models of experimentally induced obstructive disorders, suggest that OCT and SDH could serve to identify hepatic alterations associated with a diminution or cessation of bile flow.

Analytical Determination of Aminotransferase and Ornithine Carbamyl Transferase Activity

There are essentially two major techniques employed for the measurement of serum aminotransferase activity. For AST, one measures the conversion of aspartic acid and α-ketoglutaric acid to glutamic acid and oxaloacetic acid; for ALT, one measures the conversion of alanine and α-ketoglutaric acid to glutamic acid and pyruvic acid. With the ultraviolet method of analysis, the enzyme processes are coupled with ones in which nicotinamide adenine dinucleotide (NAD) is converted from its reduced form (NADH) to the oxidized form (NAD). The course of the reaction is followed by the decrease in absorbance at 340 nm produced by the oxidation of NADH.

The colorimetric procedure involves the reaction of the product (oxaloacetic or pyruvic acid) with dinitrophenylhydrazine to form a colored hydrazone. This product can be determined by its absorbance in the visible range. The principal advantages of the colorimetric method are that an ultraviolet spectrophotometer is not required and temperature control of the enzymic reaction is more easily attained.

There is a certain amount of controversy in the literature over the relative accuracies of both these procedures. Most of the argument, however, concerns the use of AST for the detection of coronary occlusion (3). For experimentally induced hepatic injury, these objections do not seem to be as pertinent as they might be for the diagnosis of coronary occlusion. If one is interested primarily in following the kinetics of the enzyme reaction, the ultraviolet method is probably preferred. With this procedure, the product of the enzyme reaction does not accumulate because it is converted to another product through the use of either MDH or LDH. It is also true that when AST is measured by the colorimetric procedure, one of the substrates (α-ketoglutaric acid) does interfere with the final colorimetric analysis. However, the use of serum aminotransferase activity in laboratory animals, generally, is to detect the presence or absence of liver injury. In this situation one is not interested primarily in the absolute value of activity but, rather, the degree of change. Therefore, the colorimetric procedure of Reitman and Frankel (277) is of sufficient accuracy. The relative ease of this procedure over the spectrophotometric method seems to make it more advantageous for use with laboratory animals, where large numbers of samples are to be analyzed. Wells and To (322) developed a microanalytical technique that allows repetitive plasma ALT measurements on tail vein blood from individual mice using the Reitman and Frankel procedure.

Alanine Aminotransferase Method

The colorimetric procedure of Reitman and Frankel (277) is described. For use in mice and rats, plasma or serum is prepared as desired.

Reagents.

1. Phosphate buffer (0.1 *M*, pH 7.4): Mix 420 ml of 0.1 *M* disodium phosphate (26.81 g of $Na_2HPO_4 \cdot 7 H_2O$/L) and 80 ml of 0.1 *M* potassium dihydrogen phosphate (13.61 g of KH_2PO_4/L). The pH should be 7.4.
2. α-Ketoglutarate-alanine substrate: Dissolve 29.2 mg of α-ketoglutaric acid and 1.78 g of alanine in a small amount (1–2 ml) of 1 *M* NaOH. Adjust pH to 7.4 and bring to a final volume of 100 ml in a volumetric flask using the 0.1 *M* phosphate buffer.
3. Color reagent: Dissolve 19.8 mg of 2,4-dinitrophenylhydrazine in 100 ml of 1 *N* hydrochloric acid.
4. Sodium hydroxide (0.4 N): Dissolve 16 g of NaOH in distilled water to make 1 L.
5. Pyruvate standard (2 m*M*): Dissolve 22 mg of sodium pyruvate in 100 ml of phosphate buffer.

Procedure.

1. Pipette 0.5 ml of the substrate in a test tube. Incubate at 37°C for 5 min in a Temp-Blok module heater (Lab-Line Instruments). Prepare an extra tube for a blank.
2. Pipette an aliquot (0.1 ml) of plasma into the tube, mix by swirling, and incubate for exactly 30 min at 37°C.
3. At the end of the incubation, remove the tube from the heater, add 0.5 ml of the color reagent, and mix.
4. After 30 min, add 5.0 ml of 0.4 *N* NaOH and mix.
5. The absorbance of this solution is determined at 505 nm 30 min after the addition of NaOH. The units of enzyme are read from a standard curve after subtraction of the blank. If activities are too high to read on the standard curve, repeat the entire assay with an appropriate dilution of plasma.

Standard Curve.

1. Set up a series of four tubes containing the amounts of the pyruvate standard, substrate, and water as indicated below:

Tube. No.	Pyruvate standard (ml)	Substrate (ml)	H_2O (ml)	Calculated ALT units/ml
1	0.0	1.0	0.2	0
2	0.1	0.9	0.2	28
3	0.2	0.8	0.2	57
4	0.3	0.7	0.2	97

2. Add 1.0 ml of the color reagent to each tube, mix, and allow to stand at room temperature for 30 min.
3. At 30 min after the NaOH is added, add 10 ml of 0.4 *N* NaOH, mix, and determine the absorbance of the solution at 505 nm.
4. Plot the curve on linear graph paper using the calculated ALT units given above and their respective absorbance values.

Note that comparative studies have been made using commercially prepared reagents, and the results were found to be comparable to those obtained with the individually prepared reagents.

Ornithine Carbamyl Transferase Methods

Mammalian OCT catalyzes the transfer of the carbamyl group from carbamyl phosphate to ornithine and results in the formation of citrulline. OCT activity may be measured directly by following the appearance of citrulline or indirectly by arsenolysis, in which the enzyme catalyzes the reverse reaction of citrulline to ammonia, carbon dioxide, and ornithine. In the forward reaction, citrulline is determined colorimetrically with diacetyl monoxime after destruction of serum urea with urease (51,52,317). In the reverse reaction, OCT activity is determined by production of $^{14}CO_2$ from (^{14}C-ureido)-L-citrulline (89,181,276) or by production of ammonia. The formation of ammonia can be analyzed by conversion to indophenol (179) or by a microdiffusion procedure in a Conway cell (271).

The isotopic method of Reichard (276) as modified by Korsrud et al. (181) and the colorimetric (indophenol) method of Konttinen (179,180) are described here. As in the assay of ALT activity, plasma or serum is prepared as desired.

Isotopic Method

Reagents.

1. (^{14}C)Citrulline-0.5 *M* arsenate reagent: Dissolve 0.44 g of L-citrulline and 3.9 g of dibasic sodium arsenate ($Na_2HAsO_4 \cdot 7\ H_2O$) in 20 ml of distilled water, adjust pH to 7.1 with 1 *N* hydrochloric acid (approx. 2–3 ml), then complete to 25 ml with distilled water. Add 15 μCi of (^{14}C-ureido)-L-citrulline (15 μl of 100 μCi/ml commercial solution).
2. Sulfuric acid (9 *N*): Add 25 ml of concentrated H_2SO_4 to 75 ml of distilled water.
3. Hyamine hydroxide (1 *M*): Obtain commercially.
4. Scintillation fluid: Dissolve 4 g of Omnifluor (New England Nuclear) containing 98% 2,5-diphenyloxazole and 2% *p*-bis-(O-methylstyryl)-benzene in 1000 ml of toluene.

Procedure.

1. Add 0.5 ml of the (^{14}C)citrulline–arsenate reagent and plasma (up to 0.5 ml) to a 25 ml Erlenmeyer flask.
2. Immediately cap the flask with a one-hole rubber septum stopper containing a polypropylene center well.
3. Remove 15 ml of air from the flask (using a syringe and needle).
4. Incubate the flask, with gentle agitation, for 18 h at 37°C.
5. At the end of the incubation period, stop the reaction by adding 0.5 ml of 9 *N* sulfuric acid (1.0 ml syringe fitted with a 20 gauge [1.5 inch] needle).
6. Add 0.25 ml of hyamine hydroxide to the center well (syringe and needle).
7. Incubate the flask for an additional 60 min to trap the evolved $^{14}CO_2$.
8. At the end of the trapping period, remove the center well and stopper from the flask, wipe the well free of condensation, and place it in a counting vial containing 15 ml of scintillation fluid.
9. Determine the activity of $^{14}CO_2$ by liquid scintillation spectrophotometry, correct for quench, and subtract the activity of the blank (flask containing all components minus plasma).
10. Divide net dpm (sample-background) by 13.17 dpm/nmol and divide by 0.25 ml of plasma to express results as nanomoles citrulline converted per minute per milliliter of plasma.

The formation of $^{14}CO_2$ from (^{14}C-ureido)-L-citrulline is linear over a period of 24 h. Drotman (89) used a modification of this method with success.

Colorimetric Method

With the colorimetric method, citrulline is decomposed by arsenolysis catalyzed by OCT. The liberated ammonia is determined as indophenol after reaction with phenol–nitroprusside and alkaline hypochlorite (179).

Reagents.

1. Citrulline–arsenate reagent: Dissolve 3.5 g of DL-citrulline and 15.6 g dibasic sodium arsenate ($Na_2HAsO_4 \cdot 7\ H_2O$) in distilled water. Adjust the pH to 7.1 and dilute to 100 ml. This reagent can be obtained commercially.
2. Phenol-nitroprusside reagents: Dissolve 10 g of phenol and 50 mg of sodium nitroprusside in distilled water and bring to a final volume of 400 ml. Store solution in an amber bottle at 4°C.
3. Alkaline hypochlorite: Dissolve 5 g of sodium hydroxide pellets in approximately 200 ml of distilled water. When cool, add 6 ml of sodium hypochlorite (10–14% Cl). Bring to a final volume of 400 ml with distilled water. Store in an amber bottle at 4°C.
4. Standard ammonia solution: Dissolve 464 mg of ammonium sulfate ($(NH_4)_2SO_4$) in approximately 600 ml of distilled water. Add 2 ml of concentrated sulfuric acid and dilute to a final volume of 1000 ml with distilled water. Dilute 10 ml of this stock solution to a final volume of 50 ml with distilled water. This solution contains 1.4 μmol ammonia/ml.

Procedure.

1. Prepare two tubes for each plasma sample. The first tube (S) is used to measure OCT activity, and the second tube (A) is used to determine endogenous plasma ammonia concentrations.
2. Add plasma (0.2–0.5 ml) to tubes S and A.
3. Add an equivalent volume of the citrulline–arsenate reagent to tube S, mix, and cap both tubes S and A.
4. Incubate the tubes for 24 h at 37°C.
5. At the end of the incubation period, add the requisite volume of the citrulline–arsenate reagent to tube A and mix.
6. Transfer 0.05 ml of the reaction mixtures from tubes S and A to separate tubes; add 2.0 ml of the phenol–nitroprusside solution and mix.
7. Add 2.0 ml of the alkaline hypochlorite solution to each tube, mix, and incubate at 37°C for 15 min.
8. Prepare a blank and a standard by adding 0.05 ml of distilled water and the standard ammonia solution, respectively, to separate tubes. The color reaction is performed as in steps 6 and 7.
9. The absorbance of the colored solutions is determined at 630 nm.

10. The results are expressed as international units (IU) per liter of plasma according to the equation:

$$(Abs_S - Abs_A)/(Abs_{std} - Abs_B) \times 1.94 = IU/L \text{ of plasma}$$

where Abs_S is the absorbance of tube S (NH_3 production from OCT activity), Abs_A is the absorbance of tube A (endogenous NH_3 in plasma), Abs_{std} is the absorbance of the standard, and Abs_B is the absorbance of the blank. One international unit (IU) is the activity of OCT that catalyzes the transformation of 1 μmol of citrulline to ornithine per minute.

This colorimetric determination of OCT activity has the advantage of not requiring a liquid scintillation spectrophotometer, and it eliminates the use of radiolabeled chemicals and scintillation mixtures.

Hepatic Excretory Function

Chemicals entering the systemic circulation may be excreted by the liver unchanged or after modification within the hepatocyte. Compounds that undergo biliary excretion have been divided arbitrarily into three classes (A–C) based on the bile/plasma concentration ratios obtained during their excretion (36,176). Examples of class A substances include sodium, potassium, and chloride ions as well as glucose; these compounds have a bile/plasma ratio of about 1.0. Class B substances, for example, bile salts, bilirubin, BSP, and many xenobiotics, achieve a bile/plasma ratio of more than 1.0, usually between 10 and 1000. Among class C substances, which have a bile/plasma ratio of less than 1.0, are macromolecules such as inulin, phospholipids, mucoproteins, and albumin.

In terms of detecting and quantifying hepatic damage, the compounds of class B are of particular interest. Their biliary excretion is mediated by several multicomponent transport systems (34). For example, most organic acids, such as bilirubin and BSP, are believed to be excreted by a common transport system in the liver; however, a distinct system may exist for bile acids. In addition to the organic acid system, two other carrier systems—one for organic bases, for example, procaineamide ethobromide (PAEB), and one for neutral organic molecules, for example, ouabain—exist in the liver. Finally, (a) transport system(s) may exist for the biliary excretion of metals such as lead (169,176).

The molecular mechanisms of bile formation are now being identified (228,313). Transport systems in the sinusoidal and canalicular membranes of hepatocytes have been characterized: sodium-taurocholate cotransporter (NTCP), organic anion-transporting polypeptide (OATP), organic cation transporter (OCT1), multidrug-resistance 1 P-glycoprotein (MDR1), multidrug-resistance 3 P-glycoprotein (MDR3), multidrug-resistance-associated protein (MRP2), canalicular bile salt-export pump (BSEP), and glutathione transporter. NTCP is associated with the uptake of conjugated bile salts from portal blood, and OATP is a multispecific carrier for sodium-independent uptake of bile salts, organic anions, and other amphipathic organic solutes. MRP2 is linked to ATP-dependent excretion of multispecific organic anions (including bilirubin diglucuronide, glutathione-*S* conjugates, and sulfate conjugates), while MDR3 is associated with phospholipid transport; MDR1 is involved with the canalicular excretion of bulky lipophilic cations. BSEP (sister of P-glycoprotein, SPGP) is associated with ATP-dependent canalicular transport of bile salts.

Sulfobromophthalein Retention

The most common class B chemical used in the detection of liver injury is BSP. This anionic phthalein dye was introduced into clinical medicine by Rosenthal and White in 1925 after preliminary tests with other phthalein dyes proved less satisfactory (285,286). Since its introduction, this substance has been used extensively for the assessment of liver function in humans and laboratory animals. After intravenous injection, BSP is present in the cardiovascular compartment. Its disappearance from the circulatory system depends on its uptake by the liver. The use of BSP to assess liver function is based on the observation that dye removal from blood is delayed by hepatic dysfunction. Commonly, BSP concentration in plasma is determined at a specific time after a standard dose of dye (per unit of body weight) is administered intravenously. Selection of the optimal dose of BSP is essential for correct interpretation of functional impairment.

The removal of BSP from the plasma is dependent on the simultaneous operation of a number of hepatic processes, for example, active transport across the plasma membrane into a storage compartment, metabolic transformation, and ATP-dependent transport across the canalicular membrane (334). The most critical step in this process is thought to be the transfer of BSP from liver to bile. Most important in terms of selecting an optimal BSP dose is that its biliary excretion can be saturated and a transport maximum (Tm) exists; the clearance of BSP by laboratory animals is dose-dependent (171). Usually one observes that small doses are rapidly removed from the circulation; this rate of removal continues as one increases the dose, until a dosage level of BSP is reached where the rate of disappearance becomes longer. For example, with the isolated perfused rat liver (253), 5, 10, and 20 mg of BSP are cleared at the same exponential rate; the capacity of the liver to extract

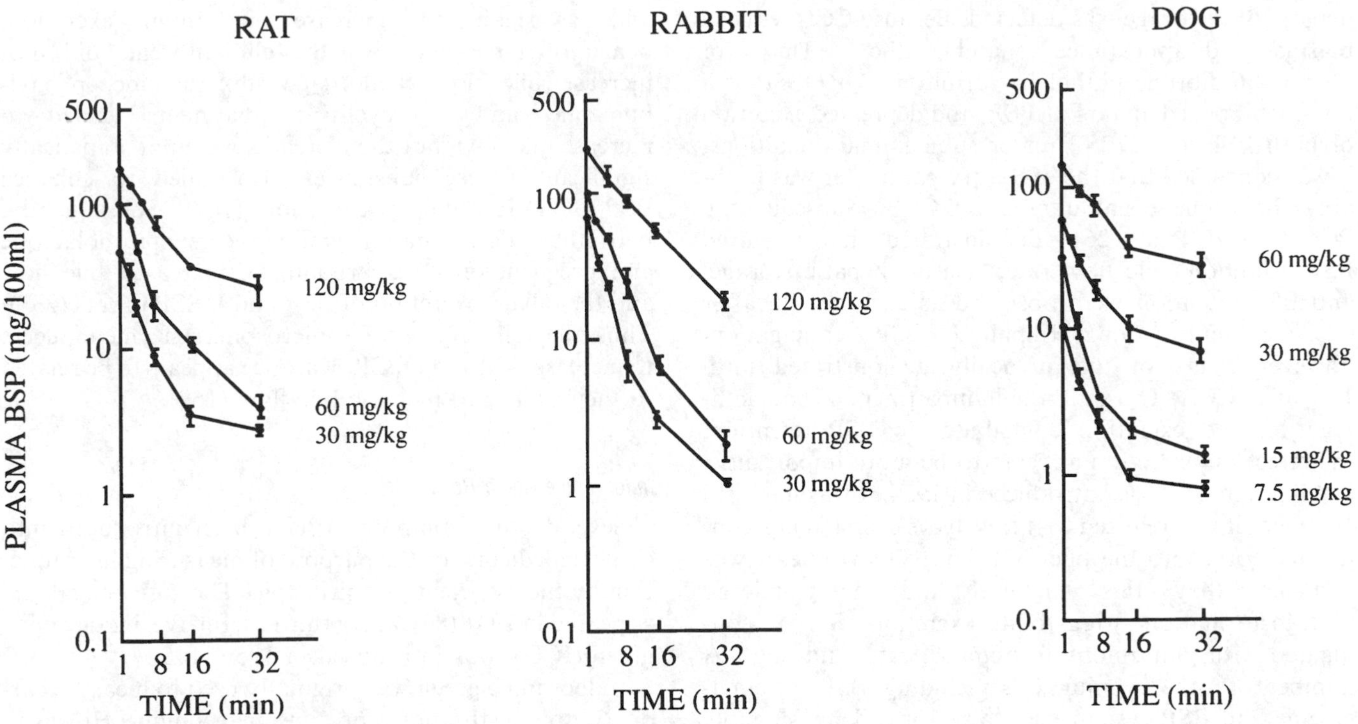

FIG. 24.3. Plasma disappearance curves for BSP administered in varying doses in the rat, rabbit, and dog (From Klaassen and Plaa [171] with permission).

BSP from the perfusate, however, becomes saturated when 30 or 40 mg is injected. With the latter dose, the rate of disappearance becomes zero order, which indicates that the maximal capacity of the transport system is reached. This same type of phenomenon occurs in mice in vivo (92).

A marked species difference exists in the ability of the rat, rabbit, and dog to remove BSP from the plasma; this difference can be readily discerned by administering varying BSP doses to these laboratory animals (Figure 24.3). Both the rat and the rabbit have a remarkable ability to clear BSP from the plasma; the dog has a relatively poor capacity (171). If the overall BSP Tm for biliary excretion is measured, large differences are observed (171). The rat and rabbit excrete BSP at a rate of about 1 mg/min/kg; the dog excretes it at a rate of about 0.2 mg/min/kg.

The significance of these findings is that the optimal dose of BSP for measuring liver function depends on the species employed. The dose should be one that is relatively close to the one that indicates BSP clearance capacity is being exceeded. For the rabbit, dog, and rat, these dosages are about 75, 15, and 50 mg/kg, respectively (171). In mice, the optimal dosage depends on the strain employed but it is somewhere between 75 and 100 mg/kg (246). The dose selected should result in about 2 to 3% retention at 30 min in normal animals.

Determination of the BSP Tm has been used as an index of hepatic function in humans. Wheeler et al. (325) devised a procedure that can be employed in unanesthetized dogs. With this technique, one infuses BSP at three different rates and measures the serum concentration at varying times. From the data, one can calculate the Tm and the relative storage capacity (S) for BSP. In addition, methods have been devised for making similar measurements in the rabbit and rat (170). Use of these techniques has not been widespread in laboratory animals. However, they are useful for assessing excretory capacity and are employed in mechanistic studies to determine specific functional lesions involved in the reduction of BSP clearance. For example, defects in

(a) transfer of BSP from plasma to liver,
(b) storage of BSP within the hepatocyte,
(c) conjugation of BSP with glutathione, or
(d) transfer of BSP from the liver cell into the bile could participate in the CCl_4-induced depression of BSP clearance.

When these possibilities were evaluated, it appeared that the major effect of CCl_4 was to decrease the transfer of BSP from the hepatocyte to the bile (172,261). Klaassen and Plaa (172) found that 24 h after a single intraperitoneal dose of CCl_4 both the BSP Tm and hepatic BSP conjugating activity were depressed; no change in hepatic BSP storage was detected. Because CCl_4 reduced plasma disappearance and the Tm of phenol-3,6-dibromophthalein disulfonate (DBSP), a non-metabolized analog of BSP, and depressed excretion of both BSP and DBSP under submaximal conditions, it was concluded that the excretory parameter was probably the prime event altered by CCl_4. Subsequently, Priestly and Plaa (261) demonstrated that impaired BSP excretion, bile flow rate, relative hepatic storage, and BSP retention were observed as early as 3 h after CCl_4 administration. Impaired BSP conjugation, however, was not unequivocally demonstrated until 12 h after CCl_4. Thus, although impairment of both conjugation and excretion contributes to BSP retention, the effect on excretion appears to be more important.

Although BSP was introduced in 1924, it was not until 1950 that it was realized that this dye is excreted in a conjugated form into the bile (37). Up to that time, it was assumed that this material did not undergo biotransformation prior to its excretion. BSP is conjugated with glutathione in humans, rats, and dogs. A number of other conjugates, including BSP-cysteinyl-glycine and BSP-cysteine, are also formed, presumably by cleavage of glutamic acid and glycine from the glutathione moiety. BSP conjugation, catalyzed by a glytathione *S*–transferase, is a cytoplasmic process. Under certain conditions, impairment of BSP conjugation with hepatic glutathione can lead to depression of BSP excretion in the bile without impairment of general excretory function (35,67,259,260).

Although BSP is a useful and sensitive test of liver function, a variety of events can cause BSP retention. Diffuse and severe hepatocellular damage is associated with an increase in dye retention (141). Liver injury of the cholestatic type, however, usually decreases biliary excretion to a greater extent than does parenchymal cell injury (169,332). For example, using ANIT, Becker and Plaa (21) showed that the amount of BSP retained following such treatment is much greater than that observed after the necrotic effects of CCl_4. In this instance, ANIT affects BSP retention by decreasing the biliary excretion of BSP (250). In rabbits, treatment with anabolic steroids can result in BSP retention owing to a decrease in excretory capacity (196). In contrast, bunamiodyl [sodium 3-(3-butyramide-2,4,6-triiodophenyl)-2-ethylacrylate] seems to diminish uptake of BSP by the hepatocyte (29). Decreased hepatic blood flow can also cause BSP retention (92).

Phenobarbital markedly enhances the excretion of BSP (173,247). This effect is apparently not related to an increase in BSP conjugation, as phenobarbital pretreatment also enhances the biliary excretion of DBSP (247). Klaassen showed (163–167) that when seven microsomal enzyme inducers were examined only phenobarbital produced a significant increase in bile flow and a significant increase in anion excretion; benzo(*a*)pyrene and 3-methyl-cholanthrene did not increase bile flow. Chlordane, nikethamide, phenylbutazone, and chlorcyclizine treatments tended to increase bile flow, but the increases were not statistically significant. These substances also failed to enhance BSP or DBSP biliary excretion (167). Subsequently, two other microsomal enzyme inducers, spironolactone and pregnenolone-16α-carbonitrile, increased bile flow and the biliary excretion of BSP and DBSP in rats (337). Thus, the ability of various microsomal enzyme inducers to increase BSP and DBSP clearance appears to be related to their ability to increase bile flow (169).

Indocyanine Green Retention

Several other compounds have been introduced into clinical medicine for the purpose of measuring liver function by the dye-clearance principle. The rose bengal test appeared in 1931 (83), and a third useful dye, indocyanine green (ICG), was introduced in 1959 (195).

Indocyanine green was originally used to measure cardiac output by the indicator-dilution technique. However, it was subsequently found (324) in the dog that 97% of the administered dose was eventually recovered from the bile in an unaltered form. No dye was found in the urine. ICG has about the same spectrum of sensitivity and specificity as BSP, but it has a number of properties that make it more desirable to employ under certain circumstances. Cherrick et al. (59) found the following:

(a) ICG is rapidly and completely bound to plasma protein, of which albumin is the principal carrier;
(b) the dye is excreted in bile in an unconjugated form;
(c) there seems to be no extrahepatic mechanism for removing the material;
(d) ICG is nonirritating when inadvertently introduced subcutaneously, and it produces no untoward reactions upon single or repeated intravenous injections; and
(e) the plasma disappearance of ICG is similar to that of BSP.

In laboratory animals, ICG is usually employed to supplement BSP tests. In the dog, Hunton et al. (151) found that:

(a) the plasma disappearance rate of ICG is exponential for at least 15 min and usually for 30 to 60 min;
(b) the amount removed per minute seems to be inversely related to the dose administered;
(c) the maximal rate of excretion of ICG into the bile is about 0.4 mg/min/kg; and
(d) substances such as bilirubin, rose bengal, and BSP interfere with ICG excretion.

Table 24.2
ICG plasma disappearance rates in rats, rabbits, and dogs

ICG Dose (mg/kg)	T1/2 (min)	K (% removed/min)
Rat		
4	2.5	28
8	4.0	17
16	6.5	11
32	8.5	8
64	18.0	4
Rabbit		
8	1.5	46
16	3.5	20
32	7.0	10
Dog		
1	7.0	10
2	17.0	4
4	30.0	2

Klaassen and Plaa (175) found that over a 32-min period the rate of disappearance of ICG was exponential in the rat, rabbit, and dog (Table 24.2). The rabbit exhibited a greater capacity to remove ICG from plasma than did the rat, and the dog had the lowest capacity. It appears that the optimal dosage for ICG clearance in the dog is about 1.5 to 2.0 mg/kg; in the rat, approximately 16 mg/kg; and in the rabbit, 25 to 30 mg/kg.

Biliary excretory maximum and hepatic storage values for ICG could not be determined (175), as infusion rates sufficient to produce a biliary excretory Tm produced a marked decrease in bile flow. Decreased bile flow was observed in all three species but was most pronounced in the rat and least in the dog. Rapid administration of ICG, as used in plasma clearance experiments, does not produce marked alterations in bile flow. Other investigators (142) reported maximal biliary excretion rates for rats given ICG that were comparable to the peak excretion rates obtained by Klaassen and Plaa (175).

The major advantage of ICG in the detection and evaluation of hepatic function is that the material is not biotransformed prior to excretion. In addition, ICG is directly determined in plasma, without chemical treatment. In practice, it simply involves diluting an aliquot of plasma (0.1–1.0 ml) with water and determining the absorbance at 805 nm, the wavelength for peak ICG absorption. ICG, however, is unstable in aqueous solutions; this instability can be prevented by mixing ICG directly with serum or with an albumin solution. The dye is unstable when mixed with heparin solutions containing bisulfite (65), indicating that preservatives of the same type may also have an effect on ICG.

Other Anionic Chemicals

Although rose bengal was introduced before ICG, it has not been extensively employed in laboratory animals; in humans the dye is used to diagnose hepatic disorder, especially in children. Rose bengal, like ICG, has the advantage that it is apparently not biotransformed before excretion into the bile (168,185). It is available commercially in a radioactive form, so its concentration can be quantified in small blood samples. Its uptake in isolated hepatocytes is similar to that of BSP (334). Klaassen (168) examined the pharmacokinetics of rose bengal in four species (rat, rabbit, dog, and guinea pig) and found that, with the exception of biotransformation, the dye appears to be handled by the liver in a manner similar to BSP; it is a class B anion that is actively excreted into the bile. A marked species variation in the rate of biliary excretion of rose bengal exists (168). The rat and rabbit excrete rose bengal into the bile at comparable rates, and the guinea pig is much more efficient and the dog much less efficient.

Like BSP, the removal of rose bengal from the blood is altered by changes in hepatic excretory function (168,219,308), and Klaassen indicated that the dye could be used as a measure of hepatic excretory function in laboratory animals. Because it is not biotransformed, alterations in its clearance would reflect changes in its uptake into the liver or its excretion into the bile. However, if used as a hepatic function test by measuring the concentration of rose bengal in the blood at only one time after its administration, the selection of this time interval is critical; a blood sample at 15 to 20 min after administration appears optimal (168). Additional studies are needed to determine if rose bengal is as sensitive an index of hepatic dysfunction in laboratory animals as BSP.

Other agents exist for monitoring hepatic excretory function. Mehendale and co-workers (215,216,218) used phenolphthalein glucuronide (PG), imipramine (IMP), and the polar metabolites of imipramine (PMIMP) as model compounds to characterize the hepatobiliary dysfunction produced by mirex. This pesticide did not suppress hepatic uptake and metabolism of IMP but inhibited the movement of PMIMP from the hepatocyte to bile; it also inhibited the biliary excretion of PG, a model anionic substrate that does not undergo biotransformation. These model substrates allowed the investigators to localize the site of mirex-induced dysfunction. In another report (77), they suggested that PG may be a more sensitive model compound than BSP for detection of hepatobiliary dysfunction. CCl_4 at 100/μl/kg depressed biliary excretion of PG in rats; hepatobiliary dysfunction was undetectable with BSP at this dosage of CCl_4 (38,172). The plasma disappearance and biliary excretion kinetics of PG in the rat have been described (217).

Endogenous Cholephiles

At least one endogenous substance, bilirubin, has been used to evaluate chemically induced hepatic injury. Normally, bilirubin is excreted into the bile. Elevation of serum bilirubin concentration accompanies sufficiently severe parenchymal injury, but it is a relatively insensitive measure of chemically induced hepatic injury. The degree of change in serum bilirubin that one obtains with experimental hepatotoxicity in mice is summarized in Table 24.1. CCl_4, although producing sufficient parenchymal injury to cause a large increase in serum ALT activity, does not affect bilirubin concentrations greatly. On the other hand, bile duct occlusion does elevate serum bilirubin considerably. ANIT also elevates serum bilirubin but not to the extent of bile duct occlusion. The BSP retention values indicate that those experimental procedures that markedly impair biliary excretion also affect BSP retention, whereas CCl_4 causes a lesser degree of retention. However, if one assumes that BSP retention and bilirubin concentrations measure relatively the same type of liver function, it is evident that the changes occurring with BSP are considerably greater that those occurring with bilirubin. A likely explanation is that the measurement of endogenous concentrations of bilirubin may not assess the total capacity of the liver to clear bilirubin, as does a load of BSP selected to be a near-capacity dose for the particular species of animal employed. Indeed, if one does administer exogenous amounts of bilirubin and follows its plasma disappearance, as with BSP, the sensitivity of the bilirubin clearance procedure can be increased. Nevertheless, BSP clearance is simpler and more sensitive than bilirubin and is therefore preferred for measurement of hepatocellular injury.

Bile acids, a second group of endogenous chemicals that are normally excreted into bile, have been used to assess some hepatotoxicants (72). Unlike serum bilirubin retention, elevation of serum bile acid concentrations, presumably because of decreased biliary secretion, appears to be a highly responsive index of hepatobiliary dysfunction (15,105). At least following $CHCl_3$ and CCl_4 treatments in rats, elevation of serum bile acids occurred at dosages that exerted no effect on serum enzyme activity or bilirubin concentration (15). Furthermore, elevations of individual serum bile acids occurred at dosages of CCl_4 that produced no consistent histological change. Neghab and Stacey (231) recently demonstrated that toluene, a nonhalogenated aromatic hydrocarbon, also results in increases of serum bile acids in rats in a dose-dependent manner; the elevations occur in the absence of other abnormal liver enzyme findings. Xylene also results in toluene-like interference of hepatocellular uptake of bile acids in isolated hepatocytes (230). Even though these findings are consistent with toluene and xylene actions on hepatocellular bile acid transport, they are not necessarily indicative of liver injury. The specificity of serum bile acid elevations and the role of such events in the evaluation of hepatotoxicity are yet to be determined.

Biliary Secretory Function

Techniques designed to assess bile secretory function are also available; however, these methods lend themselves more to specific research problems than to overall toxicological assessment. The methods applicable in vivo were reviewed by Fujimoto (112). The so-called bile acid-dependent and bile acid-independent fractions of total bile flow (94,176,235) have been studied extensively in several species; secretin-sensitive bile flow is thought to be small in the rat but more important in the rabbit and dog.

Fujimoto (112) developed a number of new techniques where marker substances are injected retrogradely into the biliary tree to assess the permeability characteristics of the biliary system. ANIT, which produces intrahepatic cholestasis in rats, and bile duct ligation increase the distended capacity of the biliary tree, whereas another cholestatic agent, taurolithocholate, decreases the distended capacity; CCl_4 seems to exert no effect (110,239,244).

The retrograde technique has been modified to become the "segmented retrograde intrabiliary injection" (SRII) procedure (238). With the use of radioactive marker substances of varying molecular weights (D-glucose, mannitol, sucrose, inulin, or dextran), one can assess the "membrane" characteristics of the biliary tree (canalicular and tight-junction complexes). This procedure was used to study the hepatobiliary dysfunction produced by *Amanita phalloides* (110), taurolithocholate (112), colchicine (16), S,S,S-tributylphosphorotrithioate (16), manganese and manganese-bilirubin combinations (11), and sequential treatments with ketones and chloroform (144). These studies have been useful for discerning the site and possible mechanisms of action involved in their hepatobiliary effects.

Determination of Biliary Function

Sulfobromophthalein clearance procedure: Reagents.

1. BSP injection solution: prepare a solution (50 mg/ml) of BSP in 0.9% NaCl.
2. Acidified NaCl: 100 ml of 0.9% NaCl plus 5 ml of 10% HCI.
3. Alkalinized NaCl: 100 ml of 0.9% NaCl plus 5 ml of 10% NaOH.

Sulfobromophthealein clearance procedure: Procedure.

1. Inject mice with BSP (75 mg/kg) via the tail vein.
2. Lightly anesthetize each mouse with ether and obtain a blood sample (0.6 ml) 30 min after BSP injection. A syringe rinsed with 1.6% sodium oxalate is used.
3. Add blood to a small test tube containing 1 mg of sodium oxalate, and centrifuge to separate plasma.
4. After centrifugation, place aliquots (0.1 ml) of the plasma into two tubes. Add 1.0 ml of acidified NaCl to one tube and 1.0 ml of alkalinized NaCl to the second tube. Mix each tube.
5. Determine the absorbance of the two solutions at 580 nm.
6. The concentration of BSP in plasma is determined by the difference between the absorbance of the alkalinized tube and that of the acidified tube followed by comparison with a BSP standard curve.

The test dose of BSP employed should be one that normal animals can readily clear in a 30 min period. Thus, the amount of BSP retained by the mouse at 30 min is about 1% of the dose administered. As noted above, this procedure can be successfully used in several other species simply by altering the dose of BSP administered.

Biliary sulfobromophthalein transport maximum procedure:

1. Anesthetize rats with sodium pentobarbital (50 mg/kg, ip).
2. Restrain the rat in the supine position on a surgical board and cannulate the bile duct (PE-10 tubing) and a femoral vein (PE-50 tubing). The rectal temperature of the anesthetized rat is maintained at 37°C with a heat lamp to prevent hypothermic alterations in Tm (280).
3. A BSP solution in 0.9% NaCl is prepared to give an infusion of 2.5 mg BSP/kg/min at an infusion rate of 0.03 ml/min.
4. The infusion is continued for a period of 60 min, and bile is collected at 15-min intervals.
5. Measure the bile volume and determine the total biliary BSP concentration by alkalinizing an aliquot (50 μl) of bile with 0.01 *M* NaOH. The absorbance is determined at 580 nm.
6. The amount of BSP excreted (min^{-1} kg^{-1}) is calculated; the maximum value attained is the Tm. In the Sprague–Dawley rat, the BSP Tm is about 1.0 mg/kg/min.

SRII method: Reagents.

1. (^{3}H(G))Inulin (133.0 mCi/g), diluted with 0.9% NaCl to give a 15 nmol/ml, 10 μCi/ml solution.
2. D-(I-^{3}H)Mannitol (27.4 Ci/mmol), diluted with 0.9% NaCl to give a 0.4 nmol/ml, 10 μCi/ml solution.

SRII method: Procedure.

1. Anesthetize rats with sodium pentobarbital (60 mg/kg, ip).
2. Restrain the rat in the supine position on a surgical board and cannulate the bile duct with a 10-cm length of PE-20 tubing just distal to the bifurcation of the biliary tree. Attach this tubing (via a stainless steel 26-gauge needle) to a longer piece of PE-20 tubing capable of containing exactly 40 μl of solution. The rectal temperature of the anesthetized rat should be maintained at 37°C with a heat lamp to prevent hypothermic alterations in bile flow (280).
3. Inject a "segment" (40 μl) of solution containing the radioactive marker compound (~0.4 μCi/ animal; 0.60 nmol (^{3}H)inulin or 0.02 nmol (^{3}H) mannitol) into the bile duct, followed by 70 μl of 0.9% NaCl. A 200 μl-Hamilton syringe attached to a Harvard infusion pump is used for the injection; the infusion rate is 2.3 μl/sec. The total volume injected is 110 μl.
4. Immediately after completion of the SRII, reestablish bile flow by disconnecting the 10-cm bile duct cannula from the infusion pump.
5. Collect 20 separate drops of bile serially (7.6 μl/drop, 152 μl of bile total) in vials containing 5 ml of Aquasol (New England Nuclear Corp.) scintillation medium.
6. Calculate the bile flow rate by determining the time required to form each drop, assuming a volume of 7.6 μl/drop.
7. Determine radioactive content of each drop by liquid scintillation spectrometry.
8. Express the radioactive content of each drop as a percentage of the total radioactivity administered by SRII. Plot the percentage of marker recovered in each drop versus the cumulative volume of bile collected. Calculate the percentage of total marker recovered in the 152 μl of bile collected.
9. The volume of the distended biliary tree can also be evaluated by the SRII method (112,244).

Alterations in Chemical Constituents of the Liver

In addition to producing elevations in serum enzyme activities and altering hepatocyte transport processes, chemical hepatotoxicants can produce changes in structural and functional hepatic constituents that have been found useful for detecting and quantifying the degree

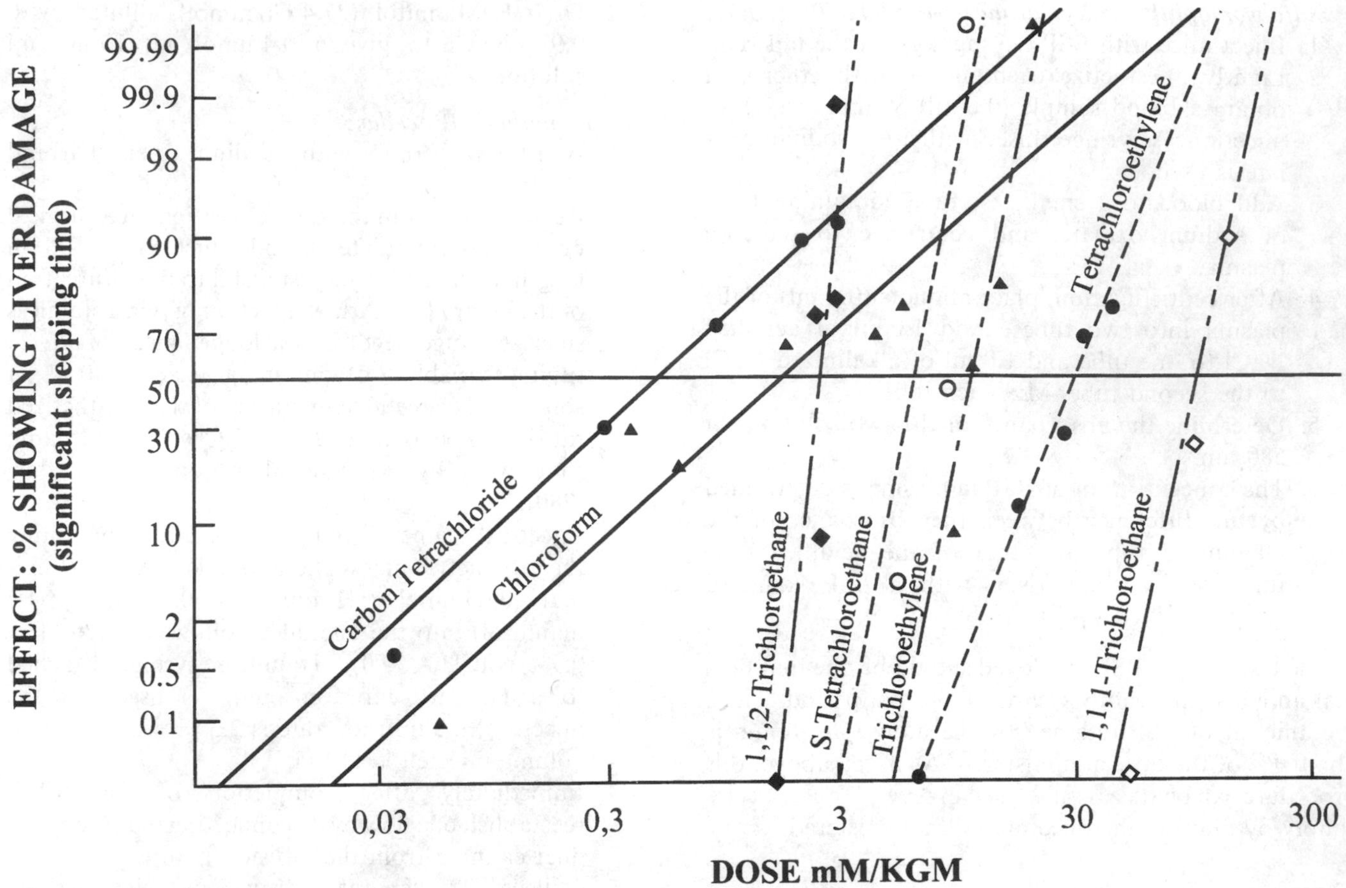

FIG. 24.4. Dose-response curves for the effect of seven halogenated hydrocarbons on the prolongation of pentobarbital sleeping time in mice (From Reference 251 with permission).

of liver injury produced, as well as elucidating the mechanism(s) involved in producing the lesions.

Alterations in the pharmacological effects of drugs can be used to detect and in some instances quantify liver dysfunction. Plaa et al. (251) demonstrated that prolongation of pentobarbital sleeping time could be used to quantify the relative hepatotoxicity of seven haloalkanes (Figure 24.4). Pentobarbital sleeping time is directly dependent on the ability of the liver to biotransform the barbiturate. Hepatocellular injury can lead to decreased activity of hepatic drug metabolizing enzymes, and, therefore, a prolongation of pentobarbital hypnosis. In these experiments, the upper limit of normalcy (mean sleeping time +2 SD) for pentobarbital sleeping time was established in a large number of control mice. Subsequently, mice were administered various doses of one of the seven haloalkanes, and the pentobarbital sleeping time was determined 24 h later. The frequency of abnormal sleeping times was then plotted against the haloalkane dose as one normally plots lethality data. These data permit comparison of dose-response curves, tests for parallelism, and statistical analyses of potency differences. Thus, the relative hepatotoxic potential of these agents could be assessed. Kutob and Plaa (187) also used pentobarbital sleeping time in conjunction with BSP retention and liver succinic dehydrogenase activity to study the ability of ethanol to potentiate $CHCl_3$-induced liver damage in mice. Dingell and Heimburg (87), Lal et al. (189), Jaeger et al. (155), and Anderson et al. (4) have made use of barbiturate sleeping time to assess chemically induced hepatotoxicity.

Hepatic Lipid Content

A number of agents that produce liver injury also cause the accumulation of abnormal amounts of fat, predominantly triglycerides, in the parenchymal cells. In general, triglyceride accumulation can be thought of as resulting from an imbalance between the rate of synthesis and the rate of release of triglyceride by the parenchymal cells into the system circulation. Nonesterified fatty acids (NEFAs) removed from the circulation or synthesized endogenously are processed through two major pathways in the liver:

(a) mitochondrial β-oxidation for production of metabolic energy; and
(b) incorporation into complex lipids, especially triglycerides, phospholipids, cholesteryl esters, and glycolipids (84).

Once synthesized, the complex lipids may be used for production of cellular membranes (structural lipids) or be continuously secreted from the liver into the blood. The latter pathway appears to be of greatest interest in the triglyceride accumulation observed in steatosis.

Blockage of the secretion of hepatic triglyceride into the plasma is the basic mechanism underlying the fatty liver induced in the rat by CCl_4, ethionine, phosphorus, puromycin, or tetracycline, by feeding a choline-deficient diet, or by feeding orotic acid (84,149,205). When released into the plasma, hepatic triglyceride is not released as such but, instead, as a lipoprotein. The very low-density fraction of the lipoproteins (VLDL) is the major transport vehicle for endogenously synthesized triglyceride; there is some evidence indicating that CCl_4 and ethionine cause a fall in the level of circulating lipoprotein, principally VLDL. The composition of VLDL by weight is 8 to 10% protein and 90 to 92% lipid. Of the lipids, triglyceride is the most abundant component (56%); the average content of phospholipid is 19 to 21% and cholesterol, 17% (154).

Elevated triglyceride could result because of an increase in the rate of synthesis of this substance. There is evidence that the rate of synthesis is directly proportional to the concentration of the substrates present (NEFAs and glycerophosphate) and so it is theoretically possible that increased hepatic triglyceride synthesis could occur because of increased NEFAs or increased glycerophosphate. Increased NEFAs could result from decreased oxidation, increased synthesis, or increased mobilization from peripheral stores. In the case of ethanol-induced fatty liver, impaired mitochondrial oxidation of NEFAs appears to be the primary abnormality seen in humans (149) due to a shift in redox potential (increased NADH/NAD ratio). It may be accompanied, however, by other abnormalities (153). There is little evidence to support the idea that fatty acid synthesis is involved in the development of fatty liver.

In humans, two types of steatosis, macrovacuolar and microvacuolar, have been characterized as hepatic lesions. With macrovacuolar steatosis, the hepatocyte contains a single, large, vacuole of fat and the nucleus is displaced to the periphery of the cell. In microvacuolar steatosis, the lipid exists in the hepatocyte as numerous small lipid vesicles and the nucleus remains in the center of the cell. Impaired mitochondrial β-oxidation of NEFAs has received more attention as a possible explanation for the presence of microvacuolar steatosis (109). Among the drugs reported to be associated with such a lesion, one finds salicylates, hypoglycin, valproic acid, amineptine, 2-arylpropionic acids, tetracyclines, zidovudine, and fialuridine.

Determination of hepatic fat content remains a reliable technique for demonstrating alterations by agents that produce steatosis with little or no necrosis (ethionine, phosphorus, tetracycline) and that are poorly reflected by serum enzyme measurement (335). Alterations in hepatic triglyceride content have also been used as one of a battery of tests to determine the relative hepatotoxic potential of various halogenated hydrocarbons in rats (174) and to determine the ability of various alcohols to potentiate the hepatotoxic actions of CCl_4 (312) (Table 24.3).

Lipid Peroxidation and Oxidative Stress

It is generally accepted that the toxicity of CCl_4 depends on the cleavage of a carbon-chlorine bond to generate a trichlormethyl free radical ($\cdot CCl_3$); this free radical reacts rapidly with oxygen to form a trichlormethyl peroxy radical ($\cdot CCl_3O_2$), which may contribute to the

Table 24.3
Effect of alcohol pretreatment on CCl_4-induced hepatotoxicity in rats[a]

Treatment	ALT Activity (units/ml)	Triglycerides (mg/g liver)	G-6-Pase Activity (mg Pi/g liver/20 min)
Ethanol (5.0 ml/kg)	50	8	6.7
Isopropanol (2.5 ml/kg)	50	6	6.2
CCl_4 (0.1 ml/kg)	100	9	6.0
CCl_4 (1.0 ml/kg)	500	17	3.8
Isopropanol + CCl_4 (0.1 ml/kg)	2250[b]	22[b]	2.8[b]
Ethanol + CCl_4 (0.1 ml/kg)	500[b]	13[b]	4.8[b]

Data were obtained from Reference 312.
[a] Alcohol given po 18 h before ip CCl_4; tests run 24 h after CCl_4 in 10 rats.
[b] Significantly different from group given alcohol alone ($p<0.05$).

toxicity (58). The work of a number of investigators (58,224,266,267) demonstrates that:

(a) the cleavage occurs in the endoplasmic reticulum and is mediated by the cytochrome P450 mixed function oxidase system;
(b) the product of the cleavage can bind irreversibly to hepatic proteins and lipids; and
(c) the CCl_4-derived free radical(s) can initiate a process of autocatalytic lipid peroxidation by attacking the methylene bridges of unsaturated fatty acid side chains of microsomal lipids.

The peroxidative process initiated by the $\cdot CCl_3$ radical, for example, is thought to result in early morphological alteration of the endoplasmic reticulum, loss of activity of the cytochrome P450 xenobiotic metabolizing system, loss of glucose-6-phosphatase activity, loss of protein synthesis, loss of the capacity of the liver to form and excrete VLDL, and eventually, through as yet unidentified pathways, to cell death (58,68,266,267). Alterations in these parameters have been used to monitor the course and extent of CCl_4-induced hepatic damage, and furthermore, have been applied to the evaluation of other hepatotoxicants.

Normal cellular metabolism can result in the production of reactive oxygen species (superoxide, hydrogen peroxide, singlet oxygen, and hydroxyl radical) and all cells contain defense systems to prevent or limit damage; glutathione is the major component of this system, but α-tocopherol and ascorbic acid play important roles (200). The imbalance between prooxidants and antioxidants is known as oxidative stress (270).

Three groups of agents have been described to characterize the toxicants associated with the induction of lipid peroxidation or oxidative stress in liver cells (69,270). One group consists of agents biotransformed to reactive free radicals that promote membrane lipid peroxidation directly; CCl_4 and $CBrCl_3$ are examples of this group. A second group consists of chemicals that are biotransformed to electrophilic intermediates, that then conjugate with glutathione and result in glutathione depletion; bromobenzene and acetaminophen are examples. The third group consists of substances that are converted to nonalkylating intermediates that generate reactive oxygen species by redox cycling; diquat and menadione serve as examples.

It is now established that nonparenchymal cells can be involved in oxidative stress responses leading to hepatotoxicity (192). Reactive oxygen intermediates are generated by macrophages, as well as endothelial cells and stellate cells (Ito cells), but under physiological conditions, cellular antioxidants normally present prevent the intermediates from producing cytotoxicity. Enhanced formation of oxygen intermediates was demonstrated with CCl_4, galactosamine, and 1,2-dichlorobenzene. With the latter agent, recent evidence indicates that Kupffer-cell-derived oxygen species are largely responsible for the lipid peroxidation (147), while with ANIT, neutrophils appear to be involved (178).

Several procedures have been developed for the detection and quantification of lipid peroxidation in tissue samples or whole animals (255,268). The reaction of malonaldehyde, a degradation product of peroxidized lipids, with thiobarbituric acid (TBA) to produce a TBA-malonaldehyde chromophore has been taken as an index of lipid peroxidation and is the most widely used method for detecting lipid peroxidation in vitro. Because malonaldehyde is rapidly metabolized in whole animals (255) and in whole liver homogenates (265), the failure to detect TBA-reacting material is not an indication of the absence of lipid peroxidation.

The determination of conjugated dienes in lipid extracts of hepatic subcellular fractions is a second approach for detecting lipid peroxidation (268). The ultraviolet difference spectra of peroxidized lipids show an absorption maximum at 233 nm with a secondary absorption maximum between 260 and 280 nm due to the presence of ketone dienes. The appearance of conjugated dienes after treatment in vivo with toxicants is an unmistakable indication that lipid peroxidation has taken place.

Several other methods for the measurement of lipid peroxidation have been described. For example, the iodometric procedure of Bunyan et al. (45) has been employed. A comparatively new approach is to measure the presence of fluorescent products. A variety of molecules that occur commonly in tissue may react with malonaldehyde and yield characteristic fluorescent chromophores (62). Malonaldehyde undergoes decomposition, and the decomposition products may also lead to fluorescent products when they react with proteins (295). Measurement of these fluorescent products seems to offer a workable way for detecting lipid peroxidation in biological systems and tissues (268).

A second interesting approach is the measurement of hydrocarbon gases. These gases appear early in the course of autoxidation of edible fats (106,148). Two gases, ethane and pentane, are useful for measuring the peroxidative process in vitro and in vivo. Ethane is the predominant gas produced during autoxidation of linolenic acid (199), and pentane is the major gaseous hydrocarbon arising during thermal decomposition (95,96) and iron-catalyzed decomposition of linoleic and arachidonic acid hydroperoxides (91). Riely et al. (279) initiated the use of ethane analysis in biological systems. They observed that ethane production was a characteristic of spontaneously peroxidizing mouse tissue (liver and brain) and was found in mice injected with CCl_4. In addition, they found that CCl_4-induced ethane evolution in vivo was potentiated by prior administration of phenobarbital and diminished by α-tocopherol, an antioxidant.

Several other groups of investigators used ethane production to monitor the course of lipid peroxidation in vivo (46,139,182,201). Dillard et al. (86) suggested that pentane expiration was a more sensitive index of lipid peroxidation than ethane in rats fed a vitamin E–deficient diet containing a high content of linoleic acid. Pentane production has also achieved considerable use as an index of the lipoperoxidative process (202,287,288). A method has been devised for monitoring lipid peroxidation in humans by quantifying the excretion of ethane and pentane in exhaled breath during a 2-h period (319). Although the measurement of hydrocarbon gas production is an alternate procedure for the determination of lipid peroxidation, this technique cannot identify the tissue or subcellular organelle from which these substances arise. In addition, precautions must be taken to prevent or estimate the evolution of hydrocarbon gases by microorganisms in the gastrointestinal tract when in vivo studies are undertaken.

Prostglandin F2-like compounds (F2-isoprostanes) are produced by peroxidation of arachidonic acid in phospholipids and released into the circulation (69,294). The presence of lipid peroxidation in rats exposed to halothane has been demonstrated by the quantification of F2-isoprostane in plasma and liver (9). The measurement of F2-isoprostanes in vivo is said to represent a promising method for detection of lipid peroxidation because of its reliability and sensitivity (10,69), but its utility in various forms of chemical-induced lipid peroxidation remains to be investigated.

Hepatic Glucose-6-Phosphatase Activity

Regardless of the mechanism by which a chemical exerts its hepatotoxic effect, the biochemical sequelae may be useful in detecting and quantifying the damage produced. Glucose-6-phosphatase (G-6-Pase) is associated with the endoplasmic reticulum, and depression of its activity appears to specifically reflect injury to this organelle (266). The functional integrity of the enzyme is dependent on the presence of phospholipid, and peroxidative decomposition of microsomal lipids, as occurs with CCl_4, results in a significant loss of G-6-Pase activity (266,267,269).

Feuer et al. (99) administered a series of 19 compounds, including 10 known hepatotoxicants, to rats and monitored their effects on 8 hepatic enzymes. The enzymes selected represented the mitochondrial, microsomal (G-6-Pase), lysosomal, and cytoplasmic fractions. These investigators found that each of the 10 known hepatotoxicants decreased hepatic G-6-Pase activity. Most of the other compounds, not known to affect the liver, did not alter G-6-Pase. Two compounds not considered to be hepatotoxicants, however, also reduced the activity of this enzyme. Based on these and other data, Grice (128) suggested that alterations in G-6-Pase activity might serve as an indicator of incipient liver damage and might occur in advancc of histologically detectable organ damage. However, other data suggest that reduction of G-6-Pase is not the most sensitive test for detecting minimal hepatic damage. Klaassen and Plaa (174) found a significant depression of G-6-Pase in rat liver only at CCl_4 dosages of 0.3 mg/kg or greater, whereas hepatic triglyceride accumulation occurred at dosages of CCl_4 below 0.3 ml/kg; BSP retention occurs in rats after a CCl_4 dosage of 0.1 ml/kg (172); with light microscopy, morphological changes are observed in rats treated with 0.13 ml CCl_4/kg (191).

Regardless of the relative sensitivity of this enzyme, it can be used as a diagnostic tool to quantify the effects of experimental maneuvers designed to increase or reduce the toxicity of known hepatotoxicants. An example is found in Table 24.3. This study (312) was designed to determine the ability of ethanol and isopropanol to potentiate CCl_4-induced hepatotoxicity. It is evident that the two alcohols themselves had no significant effect on ALT activity, triglyceride accumulation, or G-6-Pase activity. However, when pretreatment with either of these alcohols occurred 18 h before the administration of the challenge dosage of CCl_4 (0.1 ml/kg), the response was greatly increased; it was evident using all three parameters of hepatotoxicity. The challenge dose of CCl_4 merely caused a slight hepatotoxic response when it was given alone. Increasing the challenge dose of CCl_4 tenfold (1.0 ml/kg) resulted in a response that was less than that produced with isopropanol plus CCl_4 (0.1 ml/kg). Ethanol plus CCl_4 resulted in a response that was about equal to the response exerted by the tenfold dose of CCl_4 given alone.

G-6-Pase has also been used to study mechanisms of CCl_4 and $CHCl_3$ liver injury. $CHCl_3$, which causes pathological changes similar to those produced by CCl_4, does not alter hepatic G-6-Pase activity or the formation of conjugated dienes in hepatic microsomal lipids (174). These observations, along with others (255), suggest that $CHCl_3$ does not exert its hepatotoxic action by initiation of lipid peroxidation. Subsequently, $CHCl_3$ was found to produce conjugated dienes (41) and depress G-6-Pase activity (193) in phenobarbital-pretreated rats. Because $CHCl_3$-induced liver injury is more severe in phenobarbital-pretreated rats, the possibility exists that peroxidation is not the primary pathway by which $CHCl_3$ produces injury; rather, the putative initial lesion induced by $CHCl_3$ in these animals is only aggravated by the appearance of lipid peroxidation. Similarly, Jaeger et al. (155), using differences in the temporal sequences of serum (ALT) and hepatic (G-6-Pase) enzyme changes, found that CCl_4 and 1,1-dichloroethylene (1,1-DCE) have different modes of action. In conjunction with an analysis of the ability of 1,1-DCE to initiate lipid peroxidation, the enzyme data suggest that:

(a) the initial site of injury differs for CCl_4 and 1,1-DCE; and
(b) 1,1-DCE does not act through a lipoperoxidative mechanism.

Thus, as part of an integrative approach, G-6-Pase activity aided in distinguishing separate mechanisms of action for these hepatotoxicants.

Depression of G-6-Pase activity has been used to document microsomal damage produced by addition of agents to in vitro incubation systems. Glende et al. (122) and Benedetti et al. (24) used this enzyme (among other parameters) to demonstrate that the key event in CCl_4-induced alteration of microsomal enzyme activity is lipid peroxidation and not covalent binding of CCl_4-derived free radicals to microsomal lipids. Similarly, reduction of activity of this enzyme in vitro was used to document the destructive properties of degradation products of the lipoperoxidative process (31,150).

Formation and Binding of Reactive Metabolites

Although the concept of lipid peroxidation is one of the truly important concepts of current experimental pathology and toxicology, it does not appear to serve as a universal mechanism of liver injury. A number of drugs and chemicals, for example, acetaminophen (118,223), furosemide (118,223), 1,1-dichloroethylene (155,211, 212), trichloroethylene (1), bromobenzene (118,278), and dimethylnitrosamine (118), produce hepatic damage but do not appear to promote lipid peroxidation. Rather, these agents are thought to be converted to highly reactive, electrophilic metabolites by the hepatic mixed function oxidase (MFO) system. Following formation, the metabolites, which are considered to be the ultimate toxicants, can interact with hepatic constituents (e.g., protein, lipid, RNA, DNA) to form alkylated or arylated derivatives. Various investigators postulate that the binding of reactive metabolites to hepatic macromolecules can initiate cellular damage through processes as yet unidentified. This can result in intrinsic or idiosyncratic liver injury (159,305,336).

A detailed discussion of the formation and detoxification of reactive metabolites and their interaction with hepatic constituents is beyond the scope of this chapter, and the reader is referred to several excellent reviews (58,118,119,210,220–224,297). However, the experimental work carried out to unravel the mechanisms by which several toxicants produce liver injury has led to some important observations that need to be discussed. One is that hepatotoxicity need not be correlated with the pharmacokinetics of the parent substance or even its major metabolites, but may be correlated with the formation of quantitatively minor, highly reactive intermediates. Assuming that a relation exists between the severity of the lesion and the amount of covalently bound metabolite, the covalent binding of the metabolite can be used as an index of its formation. Indeed, this parameter might well be the most reliable estimate of the availability of the metabolite for production of damage at the target site, as most of the metabolite may undergo decomposition or further metabolism before it can be isolated in body fluids or urine (220). Thus, one widely used maneuver to assess the contribution of formation and binding of metabolites in chemically induced hepatotoxicity is to determine if radiolabeled chemicals administered to animals over a wide dosage range are covalently bound to macromolecular constituents in tissues that subsequently become necrotic (220).

A second concept is that a threshold tissue concentration of the metabolite must be attained before liver injury is elicited; if it is not attained, injury does not occur. Endogenous substances such as glutathione play an essential role in protecting hepatocytes from injury by chemically reactive metabolites. The mechanism that establishes a dose threshold, however, may vary from compound to compound. Finally, other enzymic pathways, for example, glutathione *S*-transferase and epoxide hydrolase, also play a role in protecting the hepatocyte by catalyzing the further degradation of the toxic reactive intermediates.

The studies mentioned above have provided relatively straightforward biochemical strategies for uncovering the possible existence of potentially toxic chemically reactive metabolites in new compounds (220). In general, a dose-response study employing the radiolabeled compound over a wide dosage range is perhaps the single most important facet of the overall study because it can provide information relating to a dose threshold for toxicity, possible mechanisms for the threshold response (e.g., glutathione depletion), and the degree of covalent binding of metabolites to target organs or constituents with the target organ. This latter information, in conjunction with dose-response studies documenting the dosages required to produce necrosis (or other endpoint), provides strong presumptive evidence favoring toxicity mediated by a reactive metabolite.

Subsequent efforts should include the use of inducers (e.g., phenobarbital, 3-methylcholanthrene) and inhibitors (e.g., SKF-525A, $CoCl_2$, piperonyl butoxide) of the MFO system. Enhancement of in vivo or in vitro covalent binding of the radiolabeled compound, as well as toxicity by an inducing agent, can provide support for the contention that a reactive metabolite mediates toxicity. A similar conclusion can be drawn if an inhibitor of the MFO system depresses covalent binding and toxicity. However, the observation that inhibitors increase the response or that inducers decrease the response does not preclude the possibility that the toxicant exerts its effect through the formation of chemically reactive metabolite (220). For example, an inducing agent may stimulate the activity of a detoxifying pathway to a greater extent than a toxifying pathway. In addition, manipulation of the concentration of hepatoprotective substances such as glutathione (e.g., depression of hepatic GSH concentration by diethyl maleate administration) can alter covalent binding or toxicity of a compound and support the likelihood that the toxic effects are mediated by a metabolite. Correlation of the data from several of these studies with a pharmacokinetic analysis can delineate the participation of a chemically reactive metabolite in the production of toxicity. For a more detailed discussion of these concepts, the reader is referred to the reviews cited above.

Liver Fibrosis

Fibrosis—the accumulation of collagen—represents a key phenomenon in chronic liver disease (256,283). Septal fibrosis is the principal feature of experimentally induced liver cirrhosis. CCl_4 and ethanol have been the toxicants most frequently used to induce liver fibrosis and cirrhosis. In the rat, twice weekly administrations of CCl_4 for 7 to 12 weeks have been shown to produce cirrhosis (50,56,143). Ito cells (also called lipocytes, fat-storing cells, or stellate cells) acquire characteristics of myofibroblasts (282) and play an important role in the formation of collagen in liver fibrosis (307). Ito cells isolated from fibrotic livers have significant increases in mRNA levels of type I, III, and IV procollagen compared to normal cells (320). Serum concentration of the aminoterminal propeptide of procollagen type III (PIIIP) can be used as a fibrogenic marker for the period progressing to cirrhosis, but its use in cirrhosis seems to be limited by factors other than liver fibrogenesis (143).

High concentrations of the amino acid 4-hydroxy-L-proline are found only in collagen. Determination of hepatic hydroxyproline content represents a valuable marker to evaluate total collagen content and thus fibrosis in liver tissue (283). The hepatic levels of hydroxyproline are well corrolated with the degree of liver fibrosis measured histologically (56,143,160,236). Figure 24.5 illustrates the effect of repeated CCl_4 gavage on hepatic hydroxyproline concentrations in corn oil- and acetone-pretreated rats; after 10 weeks of treatment, acetone $+ CCl_4$-treated animals showed a fully developed cirrhosis, whereas a much less severe lesion was observed in corn oil $+ CCl_4$-treated rats (37±2% and 16±3% of the liver occupied by fibrous connective tissue, respectively). Finally, the serum activity of immunoreactive prolyl hydroxylase, the enzyme responsible for proline hydroxylation, is elevated in rats with fibrotic livers, but Okuno et al. (236) suggested that these elevations should be carefully evaluated when being used

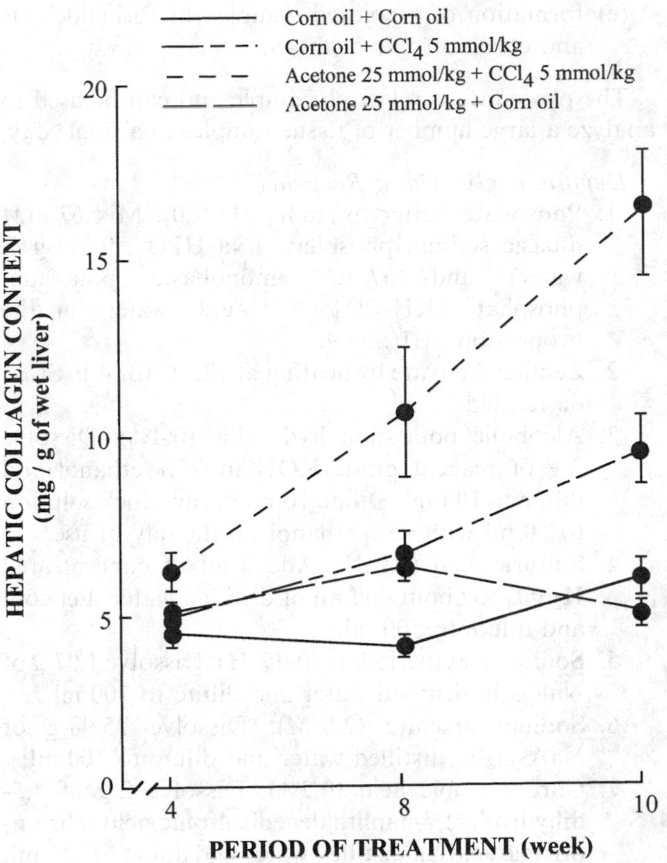

FIG. 24.5. Temporal progression of hepatic collagen content in rats treated with corn oil or acetone twice weekly (Tuesday and Thursday) and challenged with corn oil or CCl_4 18 h later. Values represent the mean±SE determined in eight rats. Data obtained from Reference 56.

as a parameter to estimate the activity of fibrogenesis in the liver.

Analytical Determination of Hepatic Triglyceride, Hepatic Malonaldehyde, and Hepatic Collagen Contents

Hepatic triglycerides. The hepatic triglyceride assay described by Butler et al. (48) is an adaptation of the method of Van Handel and Zilversmit (316), originally developed for the direct determination of serum triglycerides. The procedure consists of five steps:

(a) homogenization of tissue;
(b) adsorption of phospholipids onto zeolite, followed by extraction of triglycerides into chloroform;
(c) hydrolysis of triglycerides to fatty acids and glycerol;
(d) oxidation of glycerol with $NaIO_4$ to formic acid and formaldehyde; and

(e) formation of a colored complex of formaldehyde and chromotropic acid (48).

The procedure is relatively simple and can be used to analyze a large number of tissue samples in a single day.

Hepatic triglycerides: Reagents.

1. Phosphate buffer (67 m*M*, pH 7.0): Mix 67 m*M* dibasic sodium phosphate (Na_2HPO_4, 9.513 g/L water) and 67 m*M* monobasic potassium phosphate (KH_2PO_4, 9.118 g/L water) in the proportion 61.1 : 38.9.
2. Zeolite: Activate by heating at 125°C for 4 h. Store desiccated.
3. Alcoholic potassium hydroxide (0.4%): Dissolve 2 g of reagent grade KOH in 95% ethanol and dilute to 100 ml. Dilute 10 ml of this stock solution to 50 ml with 95% ethanol on the day of use.
4. Sulfuric acid (0.2 *N*): Add 3 ml of concentrated H_2SO_4 to about 400 ml of distilled water. Let cool and dilute to 500 ml.
5. Sodium metaperiodate (0.05 *M*): Dissolve 1.07 g of $NaIO_4$ in distilled water and dilute to 100 ml.
6. Sodium arsenite (2.0 *M*): Dissolve 25.98 g of $NaAsO_2$ in distilled water and dilute to 100 ml.
7. Chromotropic acid (0.2%): Dissolve 2 g of 4,5-dihydroxy-2,7-naphthalenedisulfonic acid (chromotropic acid) in distilled water and dilute to 200 ml. Separately, add 600 ml of concentrated H_2SO_4 to 300 ml of distilled water chilled in an icebath. When cool, add the diluted H_2SO_4 to the chromotropic acid solution. Store in an amber bottle and prepare fresh every 2 to 3 weeks.
8. Triglyceride standard solution (0.05 mg/ml): Dissolve 0.5 g of commercial corn oil in chloroform and dilute to 100 ml with chloroform. Dilute this stock solution 1 : 100 with chloroform to prepare the working standard.

Hepatic triglycerides: Procedure.

1. Remove the liver from an anesthetized rat, rinse in cold phosphate buffer, blot, and weigh.
2. Prepare a 10% (w/v) homogenate of liver in phosphate buffer using a minimum of 200 mg of liver.
3. Immediately after homogenization, add 1 ml of the homogenate to a 25-ml glass-stoppered tube containing 4 g activated zeolite moistened with 2 ml of chloroform.
4. Add 18 ml of chloroform and shake intermittently for at least 10 min.
5. Filter through Whatman No. 2 paper.
6. Transfer 0.5 ml (0.125–1.000 ml may be used) aliquots of the filtrate to each of three glass-stoppered tubes. Similarly, add aliquots (10 ml) of the corn oil standard to each of three glass-stoppered tubes.
7. Evaporate the chloroform from all tubes by heating at 80°C for about 30 min in a dry block heater.
8. Add 0.5 ml of alcoholic KOH to two of each three standards and unknowns (saponified sample). The third standard and unknown tube receives 0.5 ml of 95% ethanol (unsaponified sample). For each set of three standards, two samples will be saponified and one will be unsaponified. For each set of three unknowns, two samples will be saponified and one will be unsaponified.
9. Incubate all tubes at 65°C for 20 min.
10. Add 0.5 ml of 0.2 *N* H_2SO_4, mix, and heat tubes at 95°C for approximately 15 min to remove the ethanol.
11. After cooling, add 0.1 ml of the sodium metaperiodate to each tube and mix. Wait 10 min.
12. Add 0.1 ml of the sodium arsenite solution, mix, and wait 10 min.
13. Add 5.0 ml of the chromotropic acid reagent to each tube, mix, and incubate in the dark for 30 min at 95°C.
14. Determine the absorbance at 570 nm after the tubes have cooled.

Calculations are carried out as follows:

Triglyceride content (mg/g tissue)

$$= (A_{su} - A_{nsu})/(A_{ss} - A_{nss}) \times 0.05 \times (200/F)$$

where A_{su} is the average absorbance of saponified unknowns, A_{nsu} is the average absorbance of unsaponified unknowns, A_{ss} is the average absorbance of saponified standards, A_{nss} is the average absorbance of unsaponified standards, and F is the volume (ml) of chloroform extract used.

Hepatic malonaldehyde. The procedure is based on the reaction of malonaldehyde with thiobarbituric acid (TBA) to produce a fluorescent complex. The assay is adapted from the method of Buege and Aust (43) using fluorescent measurements as described by Yagi (333) with the exception that excitation wavelength was 532 nm. A calibration curve was prepared using 1,1,3,3-tetraethoxypropane (TEP), a chemical releasing MDA in acidic conditions, as performed by Sinnhuber and Yu (296).

Hepatic malonaldehycle: Reagents.

1. TBA-solution: Dissolve 0.375 g of TBA in approximately 60 ml of distilled water. Add 2.1 ml of 12 N hydrochloric acid, 15 g of trichloroacetic acid, then agitate and heat (45°C) the solution until dissolution of solids. Complete to 100 ml with distilled water.

2. Phosphate buffer: Add 19 ml of 200 mM NaH_2PO_4 to 81 ml of 200 mM Na_2HPO_4 to obtain a buffer solution at pH 7.4. Dissolve 13.0375 g of potassium chloride in buffer and complete to 1 liter with distilled water.

Hepatic malonaldehycle: Procedure.

1. Prepare 5 to 6 solutions of TEP ranging from 0.15 to 2.5 μM (in buffer) to construct a calibration curve.
2. Place 2 ml of TBA solution in 10-ml glass test tubes (2 tubes per sample). Add 1 ml of standard or biological sample (e.g. mitochondrial fraction, cytosol, or homogenate prepared to be at a protein concentration of 4–6 mg/ml in phosphate buffer). Cover samples with a cap without screwing it tight and mix vigorously by swirling them for 10 sec.
3. Incubate samples at 100°C for 10 min using a water bath. Cool samples by leaving them at room temperature for approximately 7 min.
4. Add 4 ml of n-butanol and mix vigorously by swirling samples for 10 sec.
5. Centrifuge samples at 1000 g for 10 min.
6. Collect the organic phase layering on top of the aqueous phase for fluorescence measurement. Use 532 nm and 553 nm for excitation and emission wavelengths, respectively (excitation and emission slits can be adjusted to 10 and 14, respectively).
7. The concentration of MDA in sample is calculated from fluorescence values using the calibration curve and then divided by the protein concentration to express results as pmol of MDA per mg of protein.

Hepatic collagen. Liver content of hydroxyproline is measured by the colorimetric method of Edwards and O'Brien (93), and total collagen content is calculated assuming 12.5% of collagen is constituted of hydroxyproline residues. Hydroxyproline is liberated from collagen by acid hydrolysis, oxidized to pyrrole with chloramine-T, then transformed into a red chromogen using a p-dimethyl-aminobenzaldehyde solution, commonly called Ehrlich reagent.

Hepatic collagen: Reagents.

1. Hydroxyproline standards: Dissolve 500 mg of trans-4 L-proline in 1 L of distilled water, then dilute this 500 μg/ml solution to prepare standards at 1, 2, and 4 μg/ml.
2. Citrate buffer: Place 133 g of monohydrate citric acid, 320 g of sodium acid trihydrated, 91 g of NaOH in 32 ml of glacial acetic acid, and 800 ml of 1-propanol, then complete to 3 L with distilled water. Adjust pH to a value ranging from 6.0 to 6.5 and complete volume to 4 L with distilled water. Add 1 or 2 ml of toluene as preserving agent.
3. Chloramine-T solution: Dissolve 1.76 g of chloramine-T hydrate into 125 ml of distilled water.
4. Ehrlich reagent: Dissolve 18.75 g of p-dimethyl-aminobenzaldehyde into 75 ml of 1-propanol and 32.5 ml of 70% perchloric acid, then complete to 125 ml with distilled water.

Hepatic collagen: Procedure.

1. Prepare a 1% liver homogenate in HCl: Excised liver from an anesthetized animal, take 1 g of the left lobe, and homogenize it into 9 ml of 6 N HCl. Put 1 ml of this 10% homogenate into 9 ml of 6 N HCl and rehomogenize.
2. For each sample, put 2.5 ml of the 1% homogenate in four conical pyrex (12 ml) tubes and cover them with a glass ball to prevent evaporation. Place tubes in an autoclave kept at 120°C under 210 KPa (2.07 atm) for 3 h.
3. Put the uncovered tubes in a dessicator maintained at 50 to 60°C (internal temperature) under a moderate vacuum and containing a layer of calcium sulfate. Dried hydrolysates are obtained in approximately 18 to 24 hs.
4. Resuspend hydrolysates with citrate buffer to obtain a solution with a concentration ranging from 0.1 to 4.0 μg hydroxyproline/ml (needs to be adjusted according to animal species and treatment). For each sample, transfer 2 ml of this solution in a clean test tube.
5. Add 1 ml of citrate buffer to tube 1, and 1 ml of the 1, 2, and 4 μg/ml standards to tubes 2, 3, and 4, respectively. A reference tube for the spectrophotometric analysis is prepared by putting 3 ml of citrate buffer in a tube.
6. Add 1.5 ml of the chloramine-T solution to each tube and incubate at room temperature for 22 min. Prepare the Ehrlich reagent during this incubation period.
7. Add 1.5 ml of Ehrlich reagent to each sample and incubate tubes in a water bath maintained at 60°C for 15 min.
8. Cool samples and measure absorbance at 500 nm using the reference tube to calibrate the instrument.
9. Calculations: Compute a standard curve of the absorbance (y) in relation to the added hydroxyproline concentration (x). The abscissa at the origin is the concentration of hydroxyproline in the 2-ml aliquot of resuspended hydrolysate. Multiply this value by the total volume of resuspended hydrolysate to obtain the total amount of hydroxyproline in the hydrolysate; divide the total amount by 0.025 g to obtain the concentration

of hydroxyproline in wet liver. Assuming 12.5 g of hydroxyproline per 100 g of collagen, the concentration of hydroxyproline in wet liver is divided by 0.125 to obtain the concentration of collagen in liver.

Repair and Recovery

Although various forms of chemical-induced liver injury have been studied extensively in terms of biochemical events for over 50 years, interest generally has focused on the early initiating effects leading to the appearance of hepatocellular dysfunction, rather than on the later recovery phase of the lesion. In the rat, organ recovery after acute hepatotoxic insult is largely dose-dependent; recovery time is longer when the lesion is more extensive. As the lesion progresses, hepatocellular regeneration appears; it appears within six hours after administration of a low dose of CCl_4 in the rat, even though the centrilobular necrosis is just becoming evident (203,204). When the hepatic lesion is enhanced by the introduction of another agent, however, recovery time can be an important consideration for assessing possible mechanisms of action involved in the potentiations (248). With the combination of CCl_4 and several potentiating agents (*n*-hexane, 2-hexanone, 2,5-hexanedione, isopropanol, and acetone), this relationship was assessed using both biochemical indices (serum ALT and OCT activities) and morphological patterns (quantitative histology) of liver injury; appropriate dose-response curves were established from the percentage of animals affected (55). Time of recovery was shown to be due to the maximal severity of the lesion, regardless of the potentiation. Although pretreatment with the potentiator resulted in an enhanced hepatotoxic response from a low dose of CCl_4, the dose-response curve for the enhanced response was no different than that produced by a higher, but equitoxic dose of CCl_4 administered alone. These data were interpreted as an indication that the five potentiators did not alter the temporal progression of CCl_4-induced liver injury.

Mehendale and his collaborators (49,301) have performed an extensive series of experiments to assess the role of tissue repair in potentiated liver injury. The studies originated from the observation that chlordecone-potentiated CCl_4 hepatotoxicity in rats was quantitatively quite remarkable and resulted in enhanced lethality. Two tissue repair responses were observed after exposure to a low dose of CCl_4 (49); the early phase regeneration (EPR) response (arrested G_2 hepatocytes activated to proceed through mitosis) occurs quickly (peaks about 6 h) and is followed (about 24 h) by the secondary phase regeneration (SPR) response (hepatocytes mobilized from G_0/G_1 to proceed through mitosis). During chlordecone potentiation of CCl_4 hepatotoxicity, the EPR phase is thought to be eliminated and the SPR phase decreased; thus, the progression of the severe injury is facilitated and leads to lethality. There is evidence that induction of EPR may accelerate SPR. Interestingly enough, large doses of CCl_4 given alone also result in regeneration responses similar to those obtained with chlordecone and a small dose of CCl_4. Experiments performed with colchicine, partial hepatectomy, CCl_4 autoprotection, nutritional factors, and different animal species have provided data consistent with the purported roles attributed to EPR, SPR, and liver injury (49,301).

The role of tissue repair has been assessed with other hepatotoxicants (301). Dose-response studies indicate that thioacetamide when given alone affects hepatic tissue regeneration (measured with ^{3}H-thymidine incorporation into DNA; proliferating nuclear cell antigen) in a manner not unlike that observed with CCl_4. Comparable observations were obtained with o-dichlorobenzene and trichloroethylene, although the dose-dependent relationships were not as evident with these agents. Increased lethality was not observed with isopropanol-potentiated CCl_4 liver injury. Mehendale and his collaborators (301) have proposed a two-stage model for chemical-induced hepatotoxicity. Stage one would involve initiation and infliction of injury; stage two would lead to recovery or progression to massive injury depending on the effects of the toxicant on cellular regeneration (enhancement would lead to recovery; inhibition would lead to massive injury). Although various aspects of the repair-recovery process are still hypothetical or speculative, the concept as such is thought-provoking and certainly an important contribution to the understanding of chemical-induced liver injury. It will be interesting to see how it evolves.

Apoptosis

Previous sections highlighted the fact that necrosis of hepatocytes is a common type of cell death occuring after chemical exposure. There exists, however, another type of cell death, called apoptosis (from the Greek "apo" meaning away from and "ptosis" meaning falling—cells "falling away from" a tissue) (70) that has been recognized as an important process in chemically induced effects in the liver. In a landmark article, Kerr et al. (161) defined a form of cell death morphologically distinct from necrosis, which they called apoptosis. Apoptotic cells exhibited nuclear and cytoplasmic condensation followed by dissociation of the cell into membrane-bound fragments in a process similar to the events observed in a phenomenon previously described by embryologists as programmed cell death; for this reason apoptosis has been inappropriately used as a synonym for programmed cell death. Apoptosis is defined as an active mode of cell death because it requires RNA and protein synthesis, is controlled by pro- and antiapoptotic genes, and is induced by physiological stimuli in addition to the typical pathological stimuli associated with necrosis (66). On the other hand, necrosis is considered to be a form of "passive" cell death.

Apoptosis is morphologically defined by a progressive condensation of the chromatin to the inner face of the nuclear membrane (DNA hyperchromicity and cresenteric caps), convoluted cell shape ("blebbing/budding"), dilatation of the endoplasmic reticulum, cell shrinkage with consequent loss of membrane contact with neighboring cells, and fragmentation of the cell with formation of membrane-bound acidophilic globules (apoptotic bodies), often containing nuclear material. The latter are frequently found within the cytoplasm of intact cells, indicating that they are phagocytized by adjacent cells (66,80). In addition, apoptosis is not commonly associated with the inflammatory response that accompanies necrosis (161). Other morphological criteria specific for necrotic cells are cell and nuclear swelling, patchy chromatin condensation, swelling of mitochondria, vacuolization in cytoplasm, plasma membrane rupture ("ghost-like" cells), and dissolution of DNA (karyolysis). Histological criteria of cell death, such as pyknosis and karyorrhexis, can be applied to both apoptosis and necrosis at certain stages and thus cannot distinguish between these two modes of cell death (243). Finally, from the above, it is apparent that apoptosis involves only scattered single cells, whereas necrosis affects large areas of liver lobules. In the normal liver, apoptosis is predominant in acinar zone 3 and is thought to subserve the elimination of senescent cells (23).

Apoptosis and mitosis play complementary contrasting roles in tissue homeostasis—the former leads to cell removal and tissue hypoplasia, the latter causes tissue hyperplasia. Because apoptosis plays a critical role in deleting cells from tissues, it is not surprising that failure of apoptosis leads to imbalanced cell proliferation and is now recognized as a phenomenon associated carcinogenesis. Tumor promoters and nongenotoxic carcinogens inhibit active cell death, thereby increasing the accumulation of (pre)neoplastic cells and accelerating the development of cancer (289). Acute and chronic treatment with 2,3,7,8-tetrachlorodibenzodioxin (TCDD) decreased apoptosis in GST-P-positive liver foci to about 60% and 10% of control level, respectively (303); in normal liver tissue, apoptosis was only slightly reduced by TCDD treatment suggesting that the promoting activity of TCDD is mediated by selective inhibition of apoptosis in the enzyme-altered cell population.

The peroxisome proliferator nafenopin can suppress rat hepatocyte apoptosis both in vivo and in vitro; experiments indicate it suppresses apoptosis in mouse, hamster, guinea pig, and rat hepatocytes and induces S-phase in mouse and rat hepatocytes (156). Species differences in response to the nongenotoxic hepatocarcinogens assessed in this study correlated with the induction of DNA synthesis rather than with suppression of apoptosis.

Examples of Chemically Induced Liver Apoptosis

In addition to being present in various viral, immunological, malignant, or drug-induced human liver diseases, hepatocyte apoptosis in animals can be triggered either in vivo or in vitro by many toxic agents (98). Histopathological features of apoptosis are frequently observed in chronic cholestatic disorders as a result of accumulation of toxic bile salts within hepatocytes (243). Hydrophobic bile salts, such as glycodeoxycholate, glycochenodeoxycholate, or taurochenodeoxycholate cause apoptosis in isolated hepatocytes (61,243). The hydrophilic bile acid, tauroursodeoxycholic acid, significantly reduced glycochenodeoxycholate-induced hepatocyte apoptosis (25). Bile salt-induced apoptosis occurs in a concentration-dependent manner at concentrations that are far smaller than those critical for micelle formation and that do not cause cell necrosis (242).

Increases in the number as well as changes in the distribution of apoptotic bodies within the liver were observed in ethanol-fed rats and mice (22,124). When compared with normal livers, the increased apoptosis was more pronounced as the duration of ethanol exposure increased and was reversed by ethanol withdrawal. All the putative mechanisms for alcohol-induced hepatocellular damage, such as oxidative stress, toxic acetaldehyde adduct formation, hypoxia, or immunologically mediated destruction, can induce apoptosis, suggesting it may represent a final common mechanism mediating heptocellular damage by ethanol (243).

Mice injected with 5–60 μmol/kg ip of cadmium showed both a time- and dose-dependent increase in liver apoptotis, which peaked at 9–14 h after cadmium administration, then decreased (138). The time course of apoptotic DNA fragmentation index, monitored by quantification of oligonucleosomal DNA fragments, correlated with the results obtained by histopathological analysis and a commercial in situ apoptotic DNA detection kit. An interesting conclusion of this work is that apoptosis is a major mode of elimination of critically damaged cells in acute cadmium hepatotoxicity in the mouse and that it precedes necrosis. An organic metal, tributyltin, which is a highly toxic water contaminant, also induces apoptosis in rainbow trout hepatocytes through a step involving Ca^{2+} efflux from the endoplasmic reticulum or other intracellular pools and by a mechanism involving cysteine proteases, such as calpains, as well as the phosphorylation of apoptotic proteins, such as Bcl-2 homologues (264).

Assessment of Apoptosis

Measurement of apoptosis is limited by the rapidity of the process. Using a model of apoptosis-driven regression of rat liver hyperplasia induced by cyproterone acetate, the mean duration of the histological stages of apoptosis was found to be approximately 3 h (47). Because apoptosis occurs in isolated single cells and does not stimulate persistent tissue changes, such as inflammation and scarring that characterize necrosis, procedures based on biochemical endpoints, such as DNA cleavage patterns, have been developed as complementary tools for the analysis of cell morphology. Internucleosomal DNA cleavage caused by a Ca^{2+}/Mg^{2+}-dependent endonucleases is a prominent feature of apoptosis (6). During apoptosis, DNA is cleaved in a nonrandom manner into 50–300 kilobases, then into 180 base pair fragments. Several techniques are based on the analysis of DNA fragments. Separation of nuclear DNA from apoptotic cells on agarose gel yields a typical "ladder" appearance of fragments, whereas DNA from necrotic cells produces a smear on electrophoresis. It is not recommended to use DNA electrophoresis as the sole criterion for apoptosis, because DNA ladders can be observed in cells with necrotic-type of morphology, and cells with ultrastructural characteristics of apoptotis can fail to produce DNA ladders.

Individual cell electrophoresis can be performed using the so-called "comets" assay (80); the apoptotic cells appear as "comets" having characteristic "heads," which represent the cells' remains containing high molecular weight DNA, and "tails," which represent a fraction of the degraded DNA. Commonly used techniques involve in situ labeling of DNA strand breaks such as the TUNEL (TdT-mediated dUTP-digoxigenin Nick End Labeling) assay; deoxynucleotides can be either fluorochrome- or enzyme (phophatase or peroxidase)-tagged. For a description of this procedure used in the context of liver toxicity assessment see Habeebu et al. (138). Wheeldon et al. (323) suggested that further validation is required before in situ end labeling can be used confidently alone, because they observed variation in apoptotic body indices after cyproterone acetate withdrawal between in situ end labeling and hematoxylin and eosin staining techniques. Similarly, Grasl-Kraupp et al. (127) concluded that DNA fragmentation is common to different kinds of rat liver cell death and that its detection in situ should not be considered a specific marker of apoptosis.

Several techniques rely on flow or laser scanning cytometry (for a review see pp. 49–61 in Darzynkiewicz and Traganos [80]. Dive et al. (88) proposed a rapid multiparameter flow cytometric assay, which discriminates and quantifies viable, apoptotic, and necrotic cells via measurement of forward- and side-light scatter (proportional to cell diameter and internal granularity, respectively) and the DNA-binding fluorophores Hoechst 33342 and propidium. For a comparison of approaches for quantifying hepatocyte apoptosis see Goldsworthy et al. (125), and for a discussion on the selection of methods and the inappropriate uses of methodology see pp. 61–69 in Darzynkiewicz and Traganos (80).

Apoptosis and necrosis both involve the activation of calcium-dependent endonucleases (which might differ from one process to the other) and early degradation of cellular DNA, so that elevation of intracellular calcium concentrations is a salient biochemical feature of cell death by both processes (159). The major qualitative difference in biochemical pathways between cell death by apoptosis and necrosis appears to be in their molecular control points and extracellular signals (159).

In contrast to other cells, the mechanisms leading to liver cell apoptosis, however, remain poorly understood. Two proteins could play an important role; the fa/apo-1 protein present at the surface of hepatocytes and the bcl-2 protein localized in biliary cells (98). Bcl-2 protein appears to be a marker of cholangiocarcinoma but not of hepatocellular carcinoma and could help distinguish between these two primary liver tumors (57). Bcl-2 is a protein acting as an inhibitor of cell death. Apoptosis was increased in hepatocytes from bcl-2-null mice, which indicated that the bcl-2 family contributes to hepatocyte apoptosis regulation (64). Bcl-2, as well as the functionally related bcl-x and bax proteins, are modulated at the transcript and protein level during liver regeneration, suggesting a role for the proteins in normal liver growth (183). Caspases are a family of at least cysteine proteases. Activation of caspases during apoptosis results in the cleavage of critical cellular substrates.

Apoptosis clearly represents an important physiological process which can be perturbed by chemicals. It is best confirmed with morphological evidence by light, fluorescence or electron microscopy, or by flow cytometry. Apoptosis is increasingly being recognized as an important mechanism in hepatobiliary diseases (243,290).

Measurement of Apoptosis

The following procedure describes a simple cytological method routinely used in different laboratories for evaluating apoptosis. The assay can be applied to tissue slices, primary cells, cell lines, or freshly isolated cells, and can be performed with cells of virtually any origin. The method has been extensively used for evaluating the apoptotic rate of human neutrophils (120,121,188), because these cells are known to spontaneously undergo apoptosis without any stimulation and are recognized as an excellent model for studying this biological process. Furthermore, observations made using this technique correlate well with the results obtained by conventional Hoechst 3342 and propidium iodide cytofluorimetric analyses (120). This is a simple and low-cost histologically based procedure.

Procedure. The assay is performed at room temperature. Other techniques to measure apoptosis can be used in parallel. For new applications using isolated or cultured cells, it is strongly recommended that cell viability be verified by trypan blue exclusion before performing the assay. Apoptotic, but not necrotic, cells exclude trypan blue. The level of nonviable cell loss can also be monitored by such an approach.

1. For isolated cells, an aliquot of 250–300 μl (from a suspension of 10×10^6 cells/ml) is loaded into a cytospin chamber and gently spun at ~600 rpm for 1 min to adhere the cells onto a microscope slide using a cytocentrifuge (such as the Cyto-Tec centrifuge from Miles Scientific). For adhering cells, the cells can be directly grown on glass coverslips; for tissues, 5-μm thick slices are used.
2. A rapid coloration procedure is performed using the Diff-Quick staining kit (Baxter, Miami, FL) according to the manufacturer's instruction. This kit consists of three different solutions: Solutions I (fixative: 1.8 mg/L triarylmethane in methyl alcohol), II (1.0 g/L xanthene dye in sodium azide 0.01%), and III (1.25 g/L thiazine dye mixture: 0.625 g/L azure A and 0.625 g/L methylene blue). About 3–5 ml of the solutions are successively poured onto each slide placed over a recovery container (10 sec for each solution is recommended).
3. The slides are rinsed with distilled water, then air dried, and a coverslip is gently placed on each slide and the slide sealed with warm parafilm or nail varnish. (The sealed slides can be kept for several days).
4. Cells are observed under a light microscope at a magnification of 400 × or 1000 ×; nuclei appear as dark purple structures. Apoptotic cells can be easily distinguished from normal cells by examining morphological changes: cell shrinkage, nuclear collapse (crescent shape or small dot profiles), dense white inner cell vacuoles, and apoptotic bodies (plasma membrane blebs/buds or granules). It is recommended that a minimum of 100 cells from different fields be counted in two replicate slides. Results are expressed as the percentage of cells in apoptosis (100 × the number of apoptotic cells/the total number of cells).

EVALUATION OF HEPATIC INJURY IN VITRO

In vitro systems offer the possibility of assessing liver injury in the absence of extrahepatic factors, such as the absorption, distribution, and extrahepatic metabolism of the chemical, humoral factors, and toxic effects caused at other sites. For this reason, they are especially valuable for studying specific mechanisms involved in chemically induced liver injury. In the present chapter, however, we focus on the use of these systems to detect and evaluate hepatotoxic properties of chemical agents.

The in vitro approaches available to assess hepatotoxic properties of chemical agents encompasses different levels of organization ranging from isolated hepatocytes and cell cultures to precision-cut liver slices and isolated livers. Liver cell organization is not disrupted in these four in vitro systems, so the injury caused by a chemical results from the overall effects of phase I and II biotransformation reactions, defense and repair systems, and cellular processes. Zonal architecture of the liver, normal polarity of hepatocytes (biliary and plasmatic poles), and presence of all liver cell types are present only with the liver slice system and the isolated perfused liver. Isolated hepatocytes, however, offer the following advantages: they are relatively easy to prepare without sophisticated equipment; a large number of experiments with the liver of one animal, serving as its own control, can be performed; and sampling throughout the experiment is feasible. Selection of a particular in vitro approach depends on specific research needs; xenobiotic biotransformation is generally comparable from one system to another as exemplified by similar metabolic profiles for caffeine biotransformation in liver slices, hepatocyte cultures, and microsomes, with a rate of metabolite formation close to that calculated from in vivo caffeine elimination (30).

Technical aspects and applications of the isolated perfused liver system are well covered in chapter 33 by Mehendale on isolated organs and will not be discussed here. For additional reading on the use of the isolated perfused liver as a model for studying drug- and chemical-induced hepatotoxicity, the reader can consult a monograph edited by Ballet and Thurman (19) and a review by Sweeny and Diasio (306).

Isolated Hepatocytes

The liver is constituted of six different cell populations—the hepatocytes, biliary epithelial cells, endothelial cells, Kupffer cells, Ito cells (lipocytes, fat-storing cells), and pit cells. The cells other than the hepatocytes are designated the nonparenchymal cells. The hepatocytes (or parenchymal cells) constitute 60% of the liver cell population and occupy 80% of the total liver volume. Much of the effort in isolation of liver cells has focused on viable hepatocytes because they are the main metabolic unit of the liver. Procedures, however, are also available for isolating nonparenchymal cells (108).

The literature on preparation, properties, and application of isolated hepatocytes is abundant, and excellent monographs and reviews have been published (26,135,213,214,306). The in situ two-step procedure is the most commonly used technique to isolate hepatocytes. It is derived from the pioneering work of Berry and Friend (27), who introduced in situ liver perfusion with digestive enzymes, and from the subsequent work of Seglen (292,293) who enhanced the recovery of isolated viable cells by initially perfusing the liver with a calcium-free buffer and then placing the digestive enzymes in a calcium-supplemented buffer. In current techniques, buffers containing a chelating agent and collagenase as the digestive enzyme are used for the first and second steps; suspensions exhibiting greater than 90% viability are usually obtained. Nonviable hepatocytes can be separated from viable ones using a dibutyl phthalate separation technique (97).

Hepatocytes are most commonly isolated from rat liver; the two-step procedure, however, has been successfully adapted to other species such as the mouse, rabbit, and guinea pig (213,214). Specialized techniques are also available for preparing suspensions enriched with periportal or perivenous hepatocytes (28). Increasing interests in toxicological risk assessment have prompted the development of procedures, such as the biopsy perfusion methods (2), to isolate hepatocytes from human liver samples. Successful approaches have also been achieved to optimize cryopreservation procedures for human hepatocytes (60,194,207).

Isolated hepatocytes have been extensively employed for studies on chemical (including drugs) biotransformation and toxicity. Over the years, the bulk of the reports published on chemical metabolism in isolated hepatocytes has defined the capabilities and limits of this system. There is no doubt that isolated cells have proved valuable for investigating biotransformation (26,28,135). The activity of Phase I or Phase II metabolizing enzymes in viable cells is maintained for a few hours (133). However, in standard metabolic/toxicological studies the incubation period of the cells with the chemical is relatively short (less than 3 h), so the losses in activity do not generally invalidate these experiments. The substrate metabolic rates are often similar or slightly slower in isolated hepatocytes than in corresponding 9000*g* supernatant or microsomes (133).

Cytotoxicity of chemicals in freshly isolated hepatocyte suspensions is a valuable tool when screening xenobiotics for hepatotoxic properties. As with the in vivo tests, the major cytotoxicity parameters studied are based on the structural integrity of the cell membrane. The uptake of normally nonpermeable dyes, such as trypan blue and neutral red, is one of the most common tests; the percentage of nonviable colored cells requires a cell counting analysis under a light microscope. Leakage into the medium (separated from the cells) of the cytosolic enzyme LDH is a biochemical test that is as frequently common as the dye exclusion assay. The former, however, is more convenient to perform than the dye assay, and it also offers the advantage of summing up the release of all damaged cells, including disintegrated hepatocytes. For some chemicals, decreases in intracellular concentrations of LDH have been reported at dosages where LDH leakage into the medium could not be detected (208).

Measurement of intracellular potassium, sodium, or calcium content is a more sensitive marker of cell membrane integrity. Fariss et al. (97) observed a decrease in potassium level 3 h prior to LDH leakage in cells treated with adriamycin in combination with 1,3-bis(2-chloroethyl)-1-nitrosourea or ethyl methanesulfonate. Indices of cellular metabolic competence are also sensitive markers; modulation of glycogen deposits and protein synthesis have been shown to detect early changes in isolated cells treated with chlorpromazine, promethazine, bromobenzene, acetaminophen, and isoniazid (123).

Frazier (107) reported that cellular potassium concentration was the most sensitive toxicity index, with inhibition of protein synthesis second, and trypan blue staining last, to evaluate cadmium, copper, and zinc toxicity. In addition, morphological changes in isolated cells can be assessed by electron microscopy.

The isolation procedure inevitably introduces changes and renders cells more susceptible to the effect of chemicals compared to the intact liver. When studying the hepatotoxic properties of organic solvents, care should be given to the selection of concentrations used, because these agents are thought to exert direct solvent effects (26). In addition, it is preferable to use equilibration techniques in stoppered flasks to study volatile chemicals with low water solubility.

Studies have shown that known in vivo hepatotoxicants tested in isolated cell suspensions are cytotoxic in vitro; individual chemicals such as acetaminophen, ethanol, methotrexate, fentanyl, bromobenzene, and chlorinated aliphatic compounds (133,315,318), as well as mixtures like $CCl_4/CHCl_3$ (233) and combinations of trichloroethylene, tetrachloroethylene, and 1,1,1-trichloroethane (302) are hepatotoxicants in vivo and in vitro. There are also examples of species and strain differences observed in vivo that also occur in vitro (226,328).

Differences between in vivo and in vitro hepatotoxic potency, however, were observed on several occasions. Dimethylnitrosamide and thioacetamide are not as potent in the isolated cell system as expected from their in vivo hepatotoxicity (304). Rankings of relative toxicity for different haloalkanes or bile salts in isolated hepatocytes differ from those observed in vivo (79,126,302). The ability of isolated cell suspensions to accurately detect the hepatotoxic properties for chemicals with unknown in vivo effects remains to be fully demonstrated, in particular for chemicals found to be weak or moderate hepatotoxicants.

Cholestatic responses per se cannot be seen in isolated hepatocytes. However, it is possible to evaluate chemical interference with processes involved in the transport of endogenous substances into and out of hepatocytes. Such approaches have been successful for thioacetamides and cyclosporin A (42,186). Hepatocyte couplets (two adjacent hepatocytes surrounding a lumen or vacuole) represent the primary bile secretory unit and are thought to be the equivalent of the bile canaliculus (33). Secretory polarity is retained in hepatocyte couplets and methods that permit the isolation of these couplets, as well as their utility for assessing canalicular function, have been perfected. The functional aspects include: the excretion of fluid, organic anions and cations, lipids, and proteins; the regulation of cellular and canalicular pH; transcytosis and protein transport; cytoskeletal function and canalicular contractility; signal transduction, calcium signaling, and paracellular permeability; and electrophysiological events (33). The effects of cholestatic agents on tight junctional permeability in isolated rat hepatocyte couplets have been assessed by monitoring the retention of a fluorescent bile acid analogue (cholyl-lysyl-fluoresein) or the penetration of horseradish peroxidase (284). Incubation of couplets in the presence of taurolithocholic acid, cyclosporin A, estradiol 17β-glucuronide, menadione, or t-butyl hydroperoxide (substances known to affect hepatobiliary function in vivo) resulted in a quantifiable dose-dependent decrease in canalicular retention.

Hepatocyte Cultures

Hepatocyte cell cultures represent an extension of the isolated hepatocyte assay that permits longer test periods by attaching cells to a matrix placed in a periodically refreshed medium to keep them viable. The comprehensive review prepared by Grisham (130) in 1979 is one indicator of the long-standing popularity of hepatic cell cultures to detect and evaluate the mechanisms of actions of toxic chemicals. More recently, Berry et al. (26) reviewed (pp. 265–354) the subject in their excellent monograph on the use of isolated hepatocytes for in vitro studies. Technical aspects of culturing hepatocytes are presented in a recent monograph: methods for preparing primary monolayer cultures of postnatal rat liver cells to assess xenobiotic hepatotoxicity (81); the preparation of human hepatocyte cultures (132); and the culturing hepatocytes from different laboratory species (213). Factors such as matrix used for cell attachment, culture medium, addition of hormones, oxygen tension, cell density, and presence of other cell types determine enzyme and gene expression and affect cell viability in monolayer cultures of hepatocytes (213).

Biochemical parameters used to measure liver injury in isolated cells also apply to hepatocyte cultures. CCl_4-induced biochemical changes in cultured hepatocytes followed nearly the same continuum as observed in vivo, although the progression was much more rapid in vitro (206); leakage of ALT was increased and G-6-Pase activity was decreased in intact liver and cultured cells, and 5′-nucleotidase activity was unaffected in either preparation. In hepatocyte cultures incubated with tetracycline or norethindrone, Anuforo et al. (5) found that the leakage into the medium of arginossuccinate lyase, ALT, or LDH was more pronounced than that for AP and AST. Chao et al. (54) reported that intracellular LDH content is a better indicator of the number of viable hepatocytes than LDH released into the medium.

Cultures of viable hepatocytes can be maintained for several days. Xenobiotic biotransformation enzyme activities decrease, however, after one or two days in culture (133,214,298). For this reason, assessment of cytotoxicity in hepatocyte cultures is routinely performed during the first two days of culturing. Hepatocytes cultured in hormone-supplemented, serum-free medium maintain, however, high biotransformation enzyme activities for several days (85,136,214). Long-term cultures of functional hepatocytes can be achieved by co-culturing hepatocytes with another rat liver cell type and represent a promising tool to investigate chronic liver toxicity (136). Human hepatocytes, particularly when mixed with rat liver epithelial cells, may provide a valuable tool for predicting hepatotoxicity of new drugs in humans (134). In addition, there is evidence for the reconstruction of functionally intact biliary polarity in hepatocytes in culture, indicating the possible utility of this system for studies on intrahepatic cholestasis (114).

Toxicity studies involving cultured hepatocytes usually assess three types of effects: cytotoxicity, genotoxicity, and enzyme induction (198). For cytotoxicity, one can follow morphology and dye permeation (trypan blue), as well as release of cytoplasmic enzymes (ALT, AST, LDH). Promutagen activation and induction of unscheduled DNA synthesis can be used to assess genotoxicity. Finally, enzyme induction effects can be discerned by following peroxisomal induction or cytochrome P450 induction. Cultured hepatocytes are considered useful for the study of peroxisome proliferation, because the cells can be used for screening new chemicals, for evaluating the sequence of events involved in their mechanism of action, and for assessing the potential for producing such effects in humans (104).

Liver Slices

Liver slices maintained for short periods of time have been used with success in biochemical and pharmacological research for over 50 years. For hepatotoxicity, Weldon et al. (321) reported in 1965 a clear dose-dependent reduction in the metabolism of L-leucine by liver slices incubated with CCl_4. Smuckler (300) subsequently observed a marked reduction in amino acid incorporation into proteins by liver slices from animals that had received CCl_4, as well as in control slices incubated with CCl_4. Marsh and Bizzi (209) concluded that the rat liver slice was a valid and useful system for the study of the action of drugs on lipid and lipoprotein metabolism.

In a discussion of techniques for studying drug metabolism in vitro, Gillette (117) presented the liver slice system in the following terms:

> Since the circulation of nutrients and oxygen through the capillaries is lost, the transfer of these substances from the medium to the innermost cells must depend on passive diffusion. It is therefore imperative that the slices be thin because the rate of diffusion is inversely related to the square of the distance the substances must traverse. Even with slices as thin as 0.5 mm, the concentrations of the nutrients and other substrates which are rapidly utilized by cells in the slice may not be identical throughout the slice.

In recent years, technological improvements in the preparation of precision-cut rat liver slices have allowed this system to assess liver injury in a reproducible fashion. Precision-cut liver slice technology was pioneered at the University of Arizona, and a review of the tissue slice technology was published by Brendel et al. (40). Their dynamic organ culture system allows both the upper and lower surfaces of the cultured slice to be exposed to the gas phase during the course of incubation to overcome disintegration of the slice-medium interface in long-term incubation of tissue slices. One advantage the liver slice system offers over isolated or cultured hepatocytes is the fact that tissue architecture is preserved. The liver slice procedure also appears to be more efficient for the collection of serial data than the perfused liver preparation.

As with isolated hepatocytes, the parameters measured to evaluate liver injury include LDH leakage, decreased protein synthesis, decreased intracellular potassium content, and histological alterations. Pig and human liver slices have also been cryopreserved with success and used for future toxicological and metabolic studies (102). Fisher et al. (100) observed that three dichlorobenzene isomers were more toxic to human liver slices when the incubation medium was Krebs–Henseleit buffer compared to Waymouth's medium.

More recent reviews (113,241) have described various isolation and maintenance conditions for performing such studies. Two different tissue slicers (Krumidieck/Alabama Research and Development Tissue Slicer, Brendel/Vitron Slicer) have been described (241). Both slicers appear to readily produce liver slices that are adequate for biotransformation or toxicity studies (257). Thickness of the liver slice is very critical for slice viability, the optimum being 200–250 μm. The slicing buffer medium should be similar in inorganic composition to the culture medium used in liver cultures; HEPES is recommended.

The slices are pooled and transferred to culture vessels (stainless steel screens located in cylindrical Teflon cradles, loaded horizontally in glass scintillation vials containing culture medium to wet the screen from the underside). Waymouth's medium is recommended as the culture medium, and a viability of 120 h is claimed for liver slices. A roller culture system is claimed to be most effective for the extended viability of precision-cut tissue slices.

The parameters for assessing viability of liver slices originally described by the Arizona group include: enzyme (LDH) leakage, intracellular potassium content, non-protein sulfhydril content, lipid peroxidation, protein synthesis, gluconeogenesis, phase I and II biotransformation, and histological evaluation. Olinga et al. (237) compared different methods (magnetically stirred 24-well, full immersed system; shaker-stirred, 6-well, fully immersed system; rocker platform, 6-well culture plate system; roller incubation-vial, partially immersed system) for incubation of liver slices for periods of 1.5–24.5 h; in terms of cell viability, the stirred systems, generally, fared the worst, whereas the rocker and roller methods appeared to be superior. In another study (311), where precision-cut liver slices were incubated in either a shaking platform or a roller incubation system for 72 h, the roller system was reported as the better one for preserving histological and functional integrity of the slices.

Assessing the relative toxicities of ortho-substituted bromobenzenes, *o*-bromobenzonitrile, *o*-bromobenzene, *o*-bromoanisole, *o*-bromotoluene, and *o*-bromo-benzomethyltrifluoride, Fisher et al. (101) concluded that results obtained with precision-cut liver slices appear to be more representative of those observed in vivo than do results obtained from isolated hepatocytes. Wormser et al. (329,330) observed species and age differences in toxicity and reported that the relative toxicities of various chemicals in the liver slice system were similar to those reported in vivo. The hepatotoxicities of CCl_4 and $CHCl_3$ in precision-cut liver slices have suggested this system is a useful tool for the investigation of site-specific toxicants

(12–14); future studies with other chemicals are necessary before this property of the system is fully demonstrated.

In rats, bromobenzene produces centrilobular necrosis in vivo, whereas allyl alcohol produces periportal lesions. In liver slices, centrilobular lesions following bromobenzene exposure were observed, but the expected periportal lesion with allyl alcohol was not (113). The lack of the expected site-specific response with allyl alcohol is attributed to the absence of circulatory influences in the tissue slice system. Indications of oxidative stress (GSH : GSSG ratio), as a mechanism of action to explain the hepatotoxic properties of atractyloside, was reported in studies using precision-cut liver slices obtained from rats and domestic pigs (234). The hepatotoxic properties of coumarin, menadione, and allyl alcohol on protein synthesis, potassium content, and mitochondrial dimethylthiazoldiphenyl tetrazolium-formazan production (MTT assay) were assessed in liver slices prepared from different species (rats, guinea pigs, cynomolgus monkeys, and humans) and incubated for 24-h periods (258). Menadione toxicity was evident in all four species, while allyl alcohol toxicity was less evident in rats; coumarin concentration-dependent toxicity was evident in guinea pigs and rats, but less effective in monkeys or humans. These interesting species-dependent observations demonstrate the utility of the liver slice technique for evaluating species differences in chemical-induced hepatotoxicity.

The application of the precision-cut slice technique to the biotransformation of xenobiotics in liver, including the coupling of phase I and II metabolic pathways, has been extensive (113,241). Liver slices from several species (rats, dogs, guinea pigs, and humans) have been employed with success. Liver slices also were shown to respond to several known different metabolic situations: peroxisome proliferation, hormone-regulated glucose metabolism, unscheduled DNA synthesis, and formation of neoantigens after halothane exposure. Recently, other applications of the technique have been demonstrated. The live-time evaluation of cell toxicity by following production of specific fluorescent dyes in liver slices by confocal microscopy was studied after exposing precision-cut slices to 1,1-dichloroethylene and then examining them microscopically; very few dead cells were observed at 2 h, progressively more were seen after 3–7 h (76). Apoptosis (detected by DNA fragmentation, amplification of the Bax gene, and histology) in liver slices was assessed after incubating slices in the presence of staurosporine, a protein kinase C inhibitor (63); features of apoptosis were successfully detected even in the presence of necrosis.

Since its original introduction in 1985 by Smith et al. (299), the diverse utility of precision-cut liver slice technique for evaluating liver function and injury is now well established. Furthermore, it is readily adaptable to the evaluation of human tissue. One advantage the system offers over isolated or cultured hepatocytes is the fact that tissue architecture is preserved and multiple analyses coupled with morphological examination are possible. Thus, detailed mechanistic toxicological investigations seem achievable in vitro with the technique.

HISTOLOGICAL ANALYSIS OF LIVER INJURY

Analysis of the hepatotoxic potential of a chemical agent is incomplete without a histological description of the lesion produced. The characteristic hepatic lesions defined by light microscopy are mentioned above. The reader is referred to Zimmerman (335) and Newberne (232) for a more detailed discussion of the various expressions of hepatotoxicity as observed by light microscopy.

Quantification of the degree of injury observed by light microscopy can be achieved using the method of Chalkley (53), essentially as described by Mitchell et al. (222). One ocular of a microscope is fitted with a micrometer eyepiece containing a grid on which 16 points of reference are chosen. A section of suitably stained liver tissue is selected from each animal and examined at $400\times$ magnification. In a study of acetaminophen hepatotoxicity in mice, Mitchell et al. (222) found that a single section of liver could be considered representative of the entire organ. Each section is evaluated by scanning a series of 25 microscopic fields chosen at random. In each field, the tissue element immediately underneath each of the 16 points of reference is termed a "hit"; thus, 16 hits are examined per field. A total of 400 hits are examined in each section. The hits are categorized as:

(a) normal parenchymal hepatocyte;
(b) degenerated parenchymal hepatocyte;
(c) necrotic parenchymal hepatocyte; and
(d) other cellular structure (146).

Hits on each of the first three categories are recorded and expressed as a percentage of the total number of hepatocytes examined in that section. Accumulation of the data from three to five animals in each treatment group provides a database of sufficient size for statistical analysis.

This type of quantitative histological analysis was useful for determining the relative ability of various solvents to potentiate $CHCl_3$-induced hepatotoxicity (Table 24.4). In this study (146) rats were pretreated with an equimolar dose of *n*-hexane (H), acetone (A), 2,5-hexanedione (2,5-HD), or methyl *n*-butyl ketone (MBK); 18 h later the rats received a small challenging dose of $CHCl_3$, calculated to produce minimal signs of liver injury. Hepatic damage was assessed 24 h after $CHCl_3$ administration.

Table 24.4
Histological evaluation of the effects of pretreatment with various agents on $CHCl_3$-induced hepatotoxicity in male rats[a]

Treatment	Normal Hepatocytes (%)	Degenerated Hepatocytes (%)	Necrotic Hepatocytes (%)	ALT Activity (units/ml)	Total Bilirubin (mg/dl)
$CHCl_3$	99.7±0.1	0.3±0.1	0	37±3	0.18±0.01
n-Hexane + $CHCl_3$	97.9±2.3	5.8±0.9	6.3±2.2	347±3.1	0.24±0.01
Acetone + $CHCl_3$	76.2±4.7	9.2±2.1	14.6±3.0	1177±534	0.26±0.02
2,5-Hexanedione + $CHCl_3$	51.9±5.0	13.5±2.6	34.7±3.1	2228±477	0.82±0.32
Methyl n-butyl ketone + $CHCl_3$	45.2±2.0	17.5±2.0	27.2±1.8	4910±631	1.35±0.17

Data were obtained from References 146.
[a] $CHCl_3$ (0.5 ml/kg ip) given 18 h after agent (15 mmol/kg po); rats killed 24 h later. Values are mean±SE of 4–15 rats.

Although each of the solvents was capable of potentiating the hepatotoxic effects of $CHCl_3$, it is clear (Table 24.4) that a marked difference exists in the severity of the potentiation produced. Normal hepatocytes accounted for approximately 88, 75, 52, and 45% of the total of $CHCl_3$-challenged rats pretreated with H, A, 2,5-HD, or MBK, respectively. Degenerated hepatocytes accounted for approximately 6% of the total in rats receiving the combination of H + $CHCl_3$, and rose to approximately 18% in rats treated with MBK + $CHCl_3$. The percentage of necrotic hepatocytes was greatest in rats treated with MBK + $CHCl_3$ (37%) and decreased in the following order: 2,5-HD + $CHCl_3$ (35%), A + $CHCl_3$ (15%), and H + $CHCl_3$ (6%).

These results indicate that this method for quantifying histological alterations provides an index of toxicity sensitive enough to discern the varying potentiating capacities of the four solvents tested. It is also noteworthy that the use of histological criteria to rank these solvents in order of increasing potentiating ability (H<A< 2,5-HD ≈ MBK) provided results similar to those obtained via determination of serum ALT (Table 24.4) and serum OCT (146) activity. Furthermore, the quantitative histological analysis provided a greater degree of discrimination between the solvents tested than did determination of total plasma bilirubin content (Table 24.4). In general, this procedure for quantifying histological abnormalities correlates well with other indices of liver injury (252).

An example of correlations between histopathological alterations and changes in functional indices of liver injury is given in Table 24.5. The severity of the hepatic lesion, expressed as the percentage of degenerated hepatocytes, the percentage of necrotic hepatocytes, or the percentage of abnormal hepatocytes (necrotic plus degenerated) is compared to alterations in ALT and OCT or to the plasma content of bilirubin. Regardless of the parameters assessed, a linear correlation was observed between the extent of the lesion as quantified by light microscopy and the severity of the biochemical alteration. Marked differences, however, were observed in the strength of correlation between the different combinations of parameters examined. In general, elevations in the serum activity of ALT were most strongly correlated with the histopathological alterations. The correlations between the severity of the lesion and alterations in relative liver weight, however, were not strong.

Minor modifications of this method have been used. Mitchell et al. (222) used an eyepiece containing 8 points of reference and examined 50 random microscopic fields to collect 400 hits. It appears that the arrangement and number of reference points examined per field are of little consequence as long as a sufficient number of hits are collected for analysis. In one study (145), 30 points of reference per field and 50 fields were examined for a total of 1500 hits/section. However, Miyajima (unpublished observations) found no statistical difference between the results obtained by examining 1500 versus 400 hits per section. Thus, for routine usage, it appears that collection of 400 hits per section is satisfactory.

The quantitative method described above does not allow one to visualize the lobular distribution relative to the zonal configuration of the hepatic lobule. Iijima et al. (152) devised a semiquantitative morphological method that permits such visualization. To evaluate the morphological patterns, 10 hexagonal lobules are chosen randomly for each liver section. The distance of the injured area from the hepatocytes adjacent the terminal hepatic venule (THV; central vein) to the portal area is measured in one fixed direction per lobule using a micrometer ocular disc (5 mm divided into 100 parts). This distance is measured at a magnification of 100 ×.

Table 24.5.
Linear regression analysis of the relation between histological evaluation of severity of liver injury and alterations in various parameters of hepatic damage

Correlation Coefficient (r)	x-Axis (% hepatocytes)	y-Axis (parameter)	Regression Line [y = m(x) + (b)]	Points/Line
0.959	Abnormal	Log (ALT activity)	y = 0.0397(x) + (1.5538)	49
0.950	Necrotic	Log (ALT activity)	y = 0.0566(x) + (1.5881)	49
0.926	Degenerated	Log (ALT activity)	y = 0.1186(x) + (1.5386)	49
0.922	Necrotic	ALT activity	y = 99(x) + (− 74)	49
0.903	Abnormal	ALT activity	y = 67(x) + (− 106)	49
0.885	Abnormal	Log (OCT activity + 1)	y = 0.0550(x) + (0.5728)	47
0.879	Degenerated	Log (OCT activity + 1)	y = 0.1691(x) + (0.5281)	47
0.865	Necrotic	Log (OCT activity + 1)	y = 0.0773(x) + (0.6331)	47
0.830	Necrotic	Bilirubin concentration	y = 0.0025(x) + (0.15)	49
0.820	Abnormal	Bilirubin concentration	y = 0.017(x) + (0.14)	49
0.816	Degenerated	OCT activity	y = 116(x) + (− 64)	47
0.813	Degenerated	ALT activity	y = 188(x) + (− 69)	49
0.799	Abnormal	OCT activity	y = 37(x) + (19)	47
0.770	Necrotic	OCT activity	y = 51(x) + (27)	47
0.755	Degenerated	Bilirubin concentration	y = 0.049(x) + (0.14)	49
0.650	Abnormal	Relative liver weight[a]	y = 0.016(x) + (4.22)	49
0.645	Necrotic	Relative liver weight	y = 0.023(x) + (4.23)	49
0.628	Degenerated	Relative liver weight	y = 0.049(x) + (4.21)	49

Data obtained from Reference 252.
[a] Relative liver weight = liver wt/body wt × 100.

The sections are then examined at a magnification of 400 × to classify the cellular changes observed. The damage is classified using six categories:

(a) necrosis;
(b) ballooning of hepatocytes;
(c) swelling of hepatocytes;
(d) inflammatory cell infiltration;
(e) presence of lipid droplets; and
(f) normal hepatocytes.

The results are expressed in absolute mean distances (micrometers) from the THV. The mean distance for each category observed in a treatment group is calculated for four to six animals (total of 40–60 hexagonal lobules). The graphic representation of such an analysis is depicted in Figure 24.6, where the lesions produced by two dosages of CCl_4 (0.1 and 1.0 ml/kg, ip) were monitored over a 120-h period (55). It is evident that the severity of the lesion and recovery were dose-dependent. The major advantage of this semiquantitative morphological procedure is that it permits the investigator to prepare a graphic representation of what is visualized after examination of many microscopic sections. It can be particularly useful for the preparation of toxicological reports.

Electron microscopy is also of value in toxicological studies, because it permits a correlation between the ultrastructural and functional changes induced by foreign chemicals. Grice (128) delineated several of the advantages and disadvantages encountered in the application of electron microscopic techniques to the study of chemically induced liver injury. In general, electron microscopy provides a much earlier demonstration of hepatocyte injury and is of value for detecting minimal and often reversible pathological changes that may be evident before they are detectable by light microscopy. The ability to detect subtle ultrastructural defects early in the course of poisoning often permits identification of the initial site of the lesion and thus can provide clues to possible biochemical mechanisms involved in the pathogenesis of liver injury. In addition, the power of these techniques can be enhanced through a quantitative, morphometric analysis of chemical effects (32,82). However, serious restrictions involving proper fixation techniques, sampling procedures, and the complexity of sample preparation argue against the routine use of electron microscopy in the initial evaluation of the hepatotoxic potential of a new chemical. Rather, this technique is probably of greatest use for confirming a

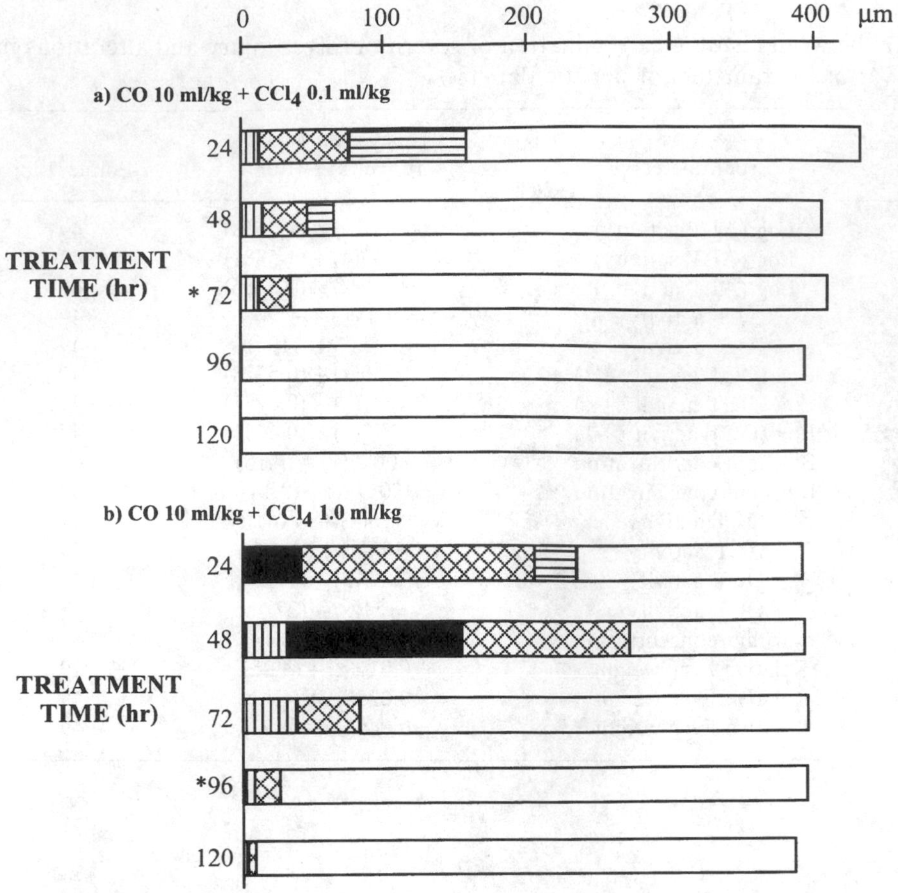

FIG. 24.6. Lobular morphological patterns of CCl_4-induced liver injury for a 120-h posttreatment period, according to the technique of Iijima et al. (152). The left side (0 μm) of the figure corresponds to the centrilolubar region, whereas the right side (400 μm) corresponds to the periportal space of the hepatic lobule. ■, necrosis; ▥, inflammatory cell infiltration; ▤, swollen hepatocytes; ▩, accumulation of lipid droplets; and □, normal hepatocytes. (From Charbonneau et al. [55] with permission).

suspected alteration or defining a pathological event (128).

CONCLUSION

Although techniques for determination of chemically induced liver injury in laboratory animals are readily available, no single one is satisfactory for the detection and quantification of all forms of injury. Instead, a battery of procedures consisting of one or more of the biochemical/functional techniques coupled with a histological analysis of the liver is essential for the correct evaluation of the hepatotoxic potential of a chemical agent.

QUESTIONS

1. If interested in a general screen to assess the possible hepatotoxic properties of a new medicinal agent currently in development, what battery of tests would you perform? Defend your choices.
2. What specific tests would you use to assess if a new therapeutic agent possesses cholestatic properties? Defend your choices.
3. A new industrial chemical is suspected of potentially interacting with other solvents in the workplace and resulting in hepatotoxic responses in exposed workers. Design an exploratory experimental study in laboratory animals to assess this possibility.
4. How best can liver histological studies be integrated with biochemical evaluation of hepatic dysfunction?
5. A chemical agent is suspected of resulting in hepatic oxidative stress in rats. Design an experimental study in rats to assess this possibility.

REFERENCES

1. Allemand, H., Pessayre, D., Descatoire, V., Degott, C., Feldman, G., and Benhamou, J.-P. (1978): Metabolic activation of trichloroethylene into a chemically reactive metabolite toxic to the liver. *J. Pharmacol. Exp. Ther.*, 204:714–723.
2. Allen, K. L., and Green, C. E. (1993): Isolation of human hepatocytes by biopsy perfusion methods. In: *In Vitro Biological Systems*, edited by C. A. Tyson and G. N. Frasier, pp. 262–270. Academic Press, New York.

3. Amador, E., Frany, R. J., and Massod, M. F. (1966): Serum glutamic-oxaloacetic transaminase activity: Diagnostic accuracy of the revised spectrophotometric and the dinitrophenylhydrazine methods. *Clin. Chem.*, 12:475–481.
4. Anderson, M. E., French, J. E., Gargas, M. L., Jones, R. A., and Jenkins, L. J. J. (1979): Saturable metabolism and the acute toxicity of 1,1-dichloroethylene. *Toxicol. Appl. Pharmacol.*, 47:385–393.
5. Anuforo, D. C., Acosta, D., and Smith, R. V. (1978): Hepatotoxicity studies with primary cultures of rat liver cells. *In Vitro*, 14:981–988.
6. Arends, M. J., Morris, R. G., and Wyllie, A. H. (1990): Apoptosis: The role of the endonuclease. *Am. J. Pathol.*, 136:593–608.
7. Asada, M. (1958): Transaminase activity in liver damage. 1. Study on experimental liver damage. *Med. J. Osaka Univ.*, 9:45–51.
8. Asada, M., and Galambos, R. J. (1963): Sorbitol dehydrogenase and hepatocelluar injury: An experimental and clinical study. *Gastroenterology*, 44:578–587.
9. Awad, J. A., Horn, J. L., Roberts, L. J., and Franks, J. J. (1996): Demonstration of halothane-induced hepatic lipid peroxidation in rats by quantification of F2-isoprotanes. *Anesthesiology*, 84:910–916.
10. Awad, J. A., Roberts, L. J., Burk, R. F., and Morrow, J. D. (1998): Isoprotanes—Prostaglandin-like compounds formed in vivo independently or cyclooxygenase: Use as clinical indicators of oxidant damage. *Gastroenterol. Clin. NA*, 25:409–427.
11. Ayotte, P., and Plaa, G. L. (1986): Modification of biliary tree permeability in rats treated with a manganese-bilirubin combination. *Toxicol. Appl. Pharmacol.*, 84:205–303.
12. Azri, S., Gandolfi, A. J., and Brendel, K. (1990): Carbon tetrachloride toxicity in precision-cut rat liver slices. *In Vitro Toxicol.*, 3:127–138.
13. Azri, S., Mata, H. P., Reid, L. L., Gandolfi, A. J., and Brendel, K. (1992): Further examination of the selective toxicity of CCl_4 in rat liver slices. *Toxicol. Appl. Pharmacol.*, 112:81–86.
14. Azri-Meehan, S., Mata, H. P., Gandolfi, A. J., and Brendel, K. (1992): The hepatotoxicity of chloroform in precision-cut rat liver slices. *Toxicology*, 73:239–250.
15. Bai, C. L., Canfield, P. J., and Stacey, N. H. (1992): Individual serum bile acids as early indicators of carbon tetrachloride- and chloroform-induced liver injury. *Toxicology*, 75:221–224.
16. Bajwa, R. S., and Fujimoto, J. M. (1983): Effect of colchicine and S,S,S,-tributyl phosphorotrithioate (DEF) on the biliary excretion of sucrose, mannitol and horseradish peroxidase in the rat. *Biochem. Pharmacol.*, 32:85–90.
17. Balazs, T., Airth, J. M., and Grice, H. C. (1962): The use of serum glutamic pyruvic transaminase test for the evaluation of hepatic necrotropic compounds in rats. *Can. J. Bichem. Physiol.*, 40:1–6.
18. Balazs, T., Murray, R. K., McLaughlan, J. M., and Grice, H. C. (1961): Hepatic tests in toxicity studies on rats. *Toxicol. Appl. Pharmacol.*, 3:71–79.
19. Ballet, F., and Thurman, R. G. (1991): *Research in Perfused Liver*. INSERM/John Libbey, Paris.
20. Batsakis, J. G., Kremers, B. J., Thiessen, M. M., and Shilling, J. M. (1968): Biliary tract enzymology—a clinical comparison of serum alkaline phosphatase, leucine aminopeptidase, and 5′-nucleotidase. *Am. J. Clin. Pathol.*, 50:485–490.
21. Becker, B. A., and Plaa, G. L. (1965): Quantitative and temporal delineation of various parameters of liver dysfunction due to α-naphthylisothiocyanate. *Toxicol. Appl. Pharmacol.*, 7:708–718.
22. Benedetti, A., Brunelli, E., Risicate, R., Cilluffo, T., Jezequel, A.-M., and Orlandi, F. (1988): Subcellular changes and apoptosis induced by ethanol in rat liver. *J. Hepatol.*, 6:137–143.
23. Benedetti, A. A., Jezaquel, M., and Orlandi, F. (1988): Preferential distribution of apoptotic bodies in acinar zone 3 or normal human and rat liver. *J. Hepatol.*, 7:319–324.
24. Benedetti, A., Casini, A. F., Feralli, M., and Comporti, M. (1977): Studies on the relationships between carbon tetrachloride-induced alterations of liver microsomal lipids and impairment of glucose-6-phosphatase activity. *Exp. Mol. Pathol.*, 27:309–323.
25. Benz, C., Angermüller, S., Töx, U., Klöters-Plachky, P., Riedel, H. D., Sauer, P., Stremmel, W., and Stiehl, A. (1998): Effect of tauroursodeoxycholic acid on bile-acid-induced apoptosis and cytolysis in rat hepatocytes. *J. Hepatol.*, 28:99–106.
26. Berry, M. N., Edwards, A. M., and Barritt, G. J. (1991): *Isolated Hepatocytes. Preparation, Properties and Applications*. Elsevier, New York.
27. Berry, M. N., and Friend, D. S. (1969): High-yield preparation of isolated liver parenchymal cells. A biochemical and fine structural study. *J. Cell Biol.*, 43:506–520.
28. Berry, M. N., Halls, H. J., and Grivell, M. B. (1992): Techniques for pharmacological and toxicological studies with isolated hepatocyte suspensions. *Life Sci.*, 51:1–16.
29. Berthelot, P., and Billing, B. H. (1966): Effect of bunamiodyl on hepatic uptake of sulfobromophthalein in the rat. *Am. J. Physiol.*, 211:395–399.
30. Berthou, F., Ratanasavanh, D., Riche, C., Picart, D., Voirin, T., and Guillouzo, A. (1989): Comparison of caffeine metabolism by slices, microsomes and hepatocyte cultures from adult human liver. *Xenobiotica*, 19:401–417.
31. Bertone, G., and Dianzani, M. U. (1977): Inhibition by aldehydes as a possible further mechanism for glucose-6-phosphatase inactivation during CCl_4-poisoning. *Chem. Biol. Interact.*, 19:91–100.
32. Bolender, R. P. (1978): Morphometric analysis in the assessment of the response of the liver to drugs. *Pharmocol. Rev.*, 30:429–443.
33. Boyer, J. L. (1997): Isolated hepatocyte couplets and bile duct units—Novel preparations for the in vitro study of bile secretory function. *Cell Biol. Toxicol.*, 13:289–300.
34. Boyer, J. L., Graf, J., and Meier, P. J. (1992): Hepatic transport systems regulating pH_i, cell volume, and bile secretion. *Ann. Rev. Physiol.*, 54:415–438.
35. Boyland, E., and Grover, P. L. (1967): The relationship between hepatic glutathione conjugation and BSP excretion and the effect of therapeutic agents. *Clin. Chim. Acta*, 16:205–213.
36. Brauer, R. W. (1959): Mechanisms of bile secretion. *JAMA*, 169:1462–1466.
37. Brauer, R. W., Krebs, J. S., and Pessotti, R. L. (1950): Bromosulfophthalein as a tool for study of liver physiology. *Fed. Proc.*, 9:259.
38. Brauer, R. W., Pessotti, R. L., and Krebs, J. S. (1955): The distribution and excretion of S^{35} labeled sulfobromophthalein sodium administered to dogs by continuous infusion. *J. Clin. Invest.*, 34:35–43.
39. Brauer, R. W., and Root, M. A. (1946): The effect of carbon tetrachloride induced liver injury upon the acetylcholine hydrolyzing activity of blood plasma of the rat. *J. Pharmacol. Exp. Ther.*, 88:109–118.
40. Brendel, K., Fisher, R. L., Krumdieck, C. L., and Gandolfi, A. J. (1993): Precision-cut rat liver slices in dynamic organ culture for structure–toxicity studies. In: *In Vitro Biological Systems*, edited by C. A. Tyson and G. N. Frasier, pp. 222–230. Academic Press, New York.
41. Brown, B. R., Sipes, I. G., and Sagalyn, A. M. (1974): Mechanisms of acute hepatic toxicity: Chloroform, halothane and glutathione. *Anesthesiology*, 41:554–561.

42. Brown, D. J., and Hunter, A. (1984): The effect of thioacetamide on sulfobromophtalein and ouabain transport in isolated rat hepatocytes. *Toxicology*, 32:165–176.
43. Buege, J. A., and Aust, S. D. (1978): Microsomal lipid peroxidation. *Methods Enzymol.*, 53:302–310.
44. Bulle, F., Mavier, P., Zafrani, E. S., Preaux, A.-M., Lescs, M.-C., Siegrist, S., Dhumeaux, D., and Guellaen, G. (1990): Mechanism of gamma-glutamyl transpeptidase release in serum during intrahepatic and extrahepatic cholestasis in the rat: A histochemical, biochemical and molecular approach. *Hepatology*, 11:545–550.
45. Bunyan, J., Murrell, E. A., Green, J., and Diplock, A. T. (1969): On the existence and significance of lipid peroxides in vitamin E-deficient animals. *Br. J. Nutr.*, 21:475–495.
46. Burk, R. F., and Lane, J. M. (1979): Ethane production and liver necrosis in rats after administration of drugs and other chemicals. *Toxicol. Appl. Pharmacol.*, 50:467–478.
47. Bursch, W., Paffe, S., Putz, B., Barthel, G., and Schulte-Hermann, R. (1990): Determination of the length of the histological stages of apoptosis in normal liver and in altered hepatic foci of rats. *Carcinogenesis*, 11:847–853.
48. Butler, W. N., Maling, H. M., Horning, M. G., and Brodie, B. B. (1961): The direct determination of liver triglycerides. *J. Lipid Res.*, 2:95–96.
49. Calabrese, E. J., and Mehendale, H. M. (1996): A review of the role of tissue repair as an adaptive strategy: Why low doses are often non-toxic and why high doses can be fatal. *Fd. Chem. Toxicol.*, 34:301–311.
50. Cameron, G. R., and Karunaratne, W. A. E. (1936): Carbon tetrachloride cirrhosis in relation to liver regeneration. *J. Pathol. Bacteriol.*, 92:1–21.
51. Ceriotti, G., and Gazzaniga, À. (1966): A sensitive method for serum ornithine carbamyltransferase determination. *Clin. Chim. Acta*, 14:57–62.
52. Ceriotti, G., and Gazzaniga, A. (1967): Accelerated micro and ultramicro procedure for ornithine carbamyltransferase (OCT) determination. *Clin. Chim. Acta*, 16:436–439.
53. Chalkley, H. W. (1943): Method for the quantitative morphologic analysis of tissues. *J. Natl. Cancer Inst.*, 4:47–53.
54. Chao, E. S., Dunbar, D., and Kaminsky, L. S. (1988): Intracellular lactate dehydrogenase concentration as an index of cytotoxicity in rat hepatocyte primary culture. *Cell Biol. Toxicol.*, 4:1–11.
55. Charbonneau, M., Iijima, M., Côté, M. G., and Plaa, G. L. (1985): Temporal analysis of rat liver injury following potentiation of carbon tetrachloride hepatotoxicity with ketonic or ketogenic compounds. *Toxicology*, 35:95–112.
56. Charbonneau, M., Tuchweber, B., and Plaa, G. L. (1986): Acetone potentiation of chronic liver injury induced by repetitive administration of carbon tetrachloride. *Hepatology*, 6:694–700.
57. Charlotte, F., L'Herminé, A., Martin, N., Geleyn, Y., Nollet, M., Gaulard, P., and Zafrani, E. S. (1994): Immunohistochemical detection of bcl-2 protein in normal and pathological human liver. *Am. J. Pathol.*, 144:460–465.
58. Cheeseman, K. H., Albano, E. F., Tomasi, A., and Slater, T. F. (1985): Biochemical studies on the metabolic activation of halogenated alkanes. *Environ. Health Perspect.*, 64:85–101.
59. Cherrick, G. R., Stein, S. W., Leevy, C. M., and Davidson, C. S. (1960): Indocyanine green: Observations on its physical properties, plasma decay and hepatic extraction. *J. Clin. Invest.*, 39:592–600.
60. Chesne, C., Guyomard, C., Grislain, L., Cleerc, C., Fautrel, A., and Guillouzo, A. (1991): Use of cryopreserved animal and human hepatocytes for cytotoxicity studies. *Toxicol. in Vitro*, 5:479–482.
61. Chieco, P., Romagnoli, E., Aicardi, G., Suozzi, A., Forti, G. C., and Roda, A. (1997): Apoptosis induced in rat hepatocytes by in vivo exposure to taurochenodeoxycholate. *Histochem. J.*, 29:875–883.
62. Chio, K. S., and Tappel, A. L. (1969): Synthesis and characterization of the fluorescent products derived from malonaldehyde and amino acids. *Biochemistry*, 8:2821–2827.
63. Chitkara, M. K., Petrick, J. S., Parrish, A. R., and Gandolfi, A. J. (1999): Generation and detection of apoptosis in rat liver slices. *Toxicologist*, 48(1S):90.
64. Christensen, J. G., Gonzales, A. J., Cattley, R. C., and Goldworthy, T. L. (1998): Regulation of apoptosis in mouse hepatocytes and alteration of apoptosis by nongenotoxic carcinogens. *Cell Growth Differ.*, 9:815–825.
65. Cobb, L. A. (1965): Effects of reducing agents on indocyanine green dye. *Am. Heart J.*, 70:145–146.
66. Columbano, A. (1995): Cell death: Current difficulties in discriminating apoptosis from necrosis in the context of pathological processes in vivo. *J. Cell. Biochem.*, 58:181–190.
67. Combes, B. (1965): The importance of conjugation with glutathione for sulfobromophthalein sodium (BSP) transfer from blood to bile. *J. Clin. Invest.*, 44:1214–1224.
68. Comporti, M. (1985): Lipid peroxidation and cellular damage in toxic liver injury. *Lab. Invest.*, 53:599–623.
69. Comporti, M. (1998): Lipid peroxidation as a mediator of chemical-induced hepatocyte death. In: *Toxicology of the Liver, 2nd ed.*, edited by G. L. Plaa and W. R. Hewitt, pp. 221–257. Taylor & Francis, Washington, D.C.
70. Corcoran, G. B., Fix, L., Jones, D. P., Treinen Moslen, M., Nicotera, P., Oberhammer, F. A., and Buttyan, R. (1994): Apoptosis: Molecular control point in toxicity. *Toxicol. Appl. Pharmacol.*, 128:169–181.
71. Cornelius, C. E. (1963): Relation of body weight to hepatic glutamic pyruvic transaminase activity. *Nature*, 200:580–581.
72. Cornelius, C. E. (1991): Liver function tests. In: *Hepatotoxicology*, edited by R. G. Meeks, S. D. Harrison, and R. J. Bull, pp. 181–213. CRC Press, Boca Raton, FL.
73. Cornelius, C. E., Bishop, J., Switzer, J., and Rhode, E. A. (1959): Serum and tissue transaminase activities in domestic animals. *Cornell Vet.*, 49:116–126.
74. Cornish, H. H. (1971): Problems posed by observations of serum enzyme changes in toxicology. *CRC Crit. Rev. Toxicol.*, 1:1–32.
75. Cornish, H. H., Barth, M. L., and Dodson, V. N. (1970): Isoenzyme profiles and protein patterns in specific organ damage. *Toxicol. Appl. Pharmacol.*, 16:411–423.
76. Cromey, D., Lantz, C., Parrish, A. R., and Gandolfi, A. J. (1999): Live-time evaluation of cell toxicity in precision-cut tissue slices using confocal microscopy. *Toxicologist*, 48(1S):71.
77. Curtis, L. R., Williams, W. L., and Mehendale, H. M. (1979): Potentiation of the hepatotoxicity of carbon tetrachloride following preexposure to chlordecone (Kepone) in the male rat. *Toxicol. Appl. Pharmacol.*, 51:283–293.
78. Curtis, S. J., Moritz, M., and Snodgrass, P. J. (1972): Serum enzymes derived from liver cell fractions. I. The response to carbon tetrachloride intoxication in rats. *Gastroenterology*, 62:84–92.
79. Dahlström-King, L., Couture, J., Lamoureux, C., Vaillancourt, T., and Plaa, G. L. (1990): Dose-dependent cytotoxicity of chlorinated hydrocarbons in isolated rat hepatocytes. *Fund. Appl. Pharmacol.*, 14:833–841.
80. Darzynkiewicz, Z., and Traganos, F. (1998): Measurement of apoptosis. In: *Apoptosis*, edited by M. Al-Rubeai, pp. 33–73. Springer-Verlag, New York.
81. Davilla, J. C., and Acosta, D. (1993): Preparation of primary monolayer cultures of postnatal rat liver cells for hepatotoxic assessment of xenobiotics. In: *In Vitro Biological Systems*, edited by C. A. Tyson and G. N. Frasier, pp. 244–254. Academic Press, New York.

82. De la Iglesia, F. A., Sturgess, J. M., and Feuer, G. (1982): New approaches for the assessment of hepatotoxicity by means of quantitative functional–morphological interrelationships. In: *Toxicology of the Liver*, edited by G. L. Plaa and W. R. Hewitt, pp. 47–102. Raven Press, New York.
83. Delprat, G. D., and Stowe, W. P. (1931): The rose bengal test for liver function. *J. Lab. Clin. Med.*, 16:923–925.
84. Dianzani, M. U. (1978): Biochemical aspects of fatty liver. In: *Biochemical Mechanisms of Liver Injury*, edited by T. F. Slater, pp. 45–96. Academic Press, New York.
85. Dich, J., Vind, C., and Grunnet, N. (1988): Long-term culture of hepatocytes: Effect of hormones on enzyme activities and metabolic capacity. *Hepatology*, 8:39–45.
86. Dillard, C. J., Dumelin, E. E., and Tappel, A. L. (1977): Effect of dietary vitamin E on expiration of pentane and ethane by the rat. *Lipids*, 12:109–114.
87. Dingell, J. F., and Heimburg, M. (1968): The effects of aliphatic halogenated hydrocarbons on hepatic drug metabolism. *Biochem. Pharmacol.*, 17:1269–1278.
88. Dive, C., Gregory, C. D., Phipps, D. J., Evans, D. L., Milner, A. E., and Wyllie, A. H. (1992): Analysis and discrimination of necrosis and apoptosis (programmed cell death) by multiparameter flow cytometry. *Biochim. Biosphys. Acta*, 1133: 275–285.
89. Drotman, R. B. (1975): A study of kinetic parameters for the use of serum ornithine carbamoyltransferase as an index of liver damage. *Food Cosmet. Toxicol.*, 13:649–651.
90. Drotman, R. B., and Lawhorn, G. T. (1978): Serum enzymes as indicators of chemically induced liver damage. *Drug Chem. Toxicol.*, 1:163–171.
91. Dumelin, E. E., and Tappel, A. L. (1977): Hydrocarbon gases produced during in vitro peroxidation of polyunsaturated fatty acids and decomposition of preformed hydroperoxides. *Lipids*, 12:894–900.
92. Eckhardt, E. T., and Plaa, G. L. (1963): Role of biotransformation, biliary excretion and circulatory changes in chlorpromazine-induced sulfobromophthalein retention. *J. Pharmacol. Exp. Ther.*, 139:383–389.
93. Edwards, C. A., and O'Brien, W. D. J. (1980): Modified assay for the determination of hydroxyproline in tissue hydrolyzate. *Clin. Chim. Acta*, 104:161–167.
94. Erlinger, S. (1982): Bile flow. In: *The Liver: Biology and Pathobiology*, edited by I. Arias, H. Popper, D. Schacter, and D. A. Shafritz, pp. 407–427. Raven Press, New York.
95. Evans, C. D., List, G. R., Doles, A., McConnell, D. G., and Hoffman, R. L. (1967): Pentane from thermal decomposition of lipoxidase-derived products. *Lipids*, 2:432–434.
96. Evans, C. D., List, G. R., Hoffman, R. L., and Moser, H. H. (1969): Edible oil quality as measured by thermal release of pentane. *J. Am. Oil Chem. Soc.*, 46:501–504.
97. Fariss, M. W., Brown, M. K., Schmitz, J. A., and Reed, D. J. (1985): Mechanism of chemical-induced toxicity. I. Use of a rapid centrifugation technique for the separation of viable and nonviable hepatocytes. *Toxicol. Appl. Pharmacol.*, 79:283–295.
98. Feldmann, G. (1997): Liver apoptosis. *J. Hepatol.*, 26:1–11.
99. Feuer, G., Golberg, L., and LePelley, J. R. (1965): Liver response tests. I. Exploratory studies on glucose-6-phosphatase and other liver enzymes. *Food Cosmet. Toxicol.*, 3:235–249.
100. Fisher, R., Barr, J., Zukoski, C. F., Putnam, C. W., Sipes, I. G., Gandolfi, A. J., and Brendel, K. (1991): In-vitro hepatotoxicity of three dichlorobenzene isomers in human liver slices. *Hum. Exp. Toxicol.*, 10:357–363.
101. Fisher, R., Hanzlik, R. P., Gandolfi, A. J., and Brendel, K. (1991): Toxicity of ortho-substituted bromobenzenes in rat liver slices: A comparison to isolated hepatocytes and the whole animal. *In Vitro Toxicology*, 4:173–186.
102. Fisher, R., Putman, C. W., Koep, L. J., Sipes, I. G., Gandolfi, A. J., and Brendel, K. (1991): Cryopreservation of pig and human liver slices. *Cryobiology*, 28:131–142.
103. Ford, E. J. H. (1965): Changes in the activity of ornithine carbamyltransferase (OCT) in the serum of cattle and sheep with hepatic lesions. *J. Comp. Pathol.*, 75:299–308.
104. Foxworthy, P. S., and Eacho, P. I. (1994): Cultured hepatocytes for studies of peroxisome proliferation: methods and applications. *J. Pharmacol. Toxicol. Methods*, 31:21–30.
105. Franco, G. (1991): New perspectives in biomonitoring liver function by means of serum bile acids: Experimental and hypothetical biochemical basis. *Br. J. Indust. Med.*, 48:557–561.
106. Frankel, E. N., Nowakowska, J., and Evans, C. D. (1961): Formation of methyl azelaaldehydate on autoxidation of lipids. *J. Am. Oil Chem. Soc.*, 318:161–162.
107. Frazier, J. M. (1990): Multiple endpoints measurements to evaluate the intrinsic cellular toxicity of chemicals. *In Vitro Toxicol.*, 3:349–357.
108. Friedman, S. L. (1993): Isolation and culture of hepatic non parenchymal cells. In: *In Vitro Biological Systems*, edited by C. A. Tyson and G. N. Frasier, pp. 292–310. Academic Press, New York.
109. Fromenty, B., and Pessayre, D. (1995): Inhibition of mitochondrial beta-oxidation as a mechanism of hepatotoxicity. *Pharmacol. Ther.*, 67:101–154.
110. Fuhrman-Lane, C. L., Erwin, C. P., Fujimoto, J. M., and Dibben, M. J. (1981): Altered hepatobiliary permeability induced by *Amanita phalloides* in the rat and the protective role of bile duct ligation. *Toxicol. Appl. Pharmacol.*, 58:370–378.
111. Fujii, T. (1997): Toxicological correlation between changes in blood biochemical parameters and liver histopathological findings. *J. Toxicol. Sci.*, 22:161–183.
112. Fujimoto, J. M. (1982): Some in vivo methods for studying sites of toxicant action in relation to bile formation. In: *Toxicology of the Liver*, edited by G. L. Plaa and W. R. Hewitt, pp. 121–145. Raven Press, New York.
113. Gandolfi, A. J., Wijeweera, J., and Brendel, K. (1996): Use of precision-cut liver slices as an in vitro tool for evaluating liver function. *Toxicol. Pathol.*, 24:58–61.
114. Gebhardt, R. (1983): Primary cultures of rat hepatocytes as a model system of canalicular development, biliary secretion, and intrahepatic cholestasis. *Gastroenterology*, 84:1462–1470.
115. Gebhardt, R. (1992): Metabolic zonation of the liver: regulation and implications for liver function. *Pharmacol. Ther.*, 53:275–354.
116. Ghoshal, A. K., Porta, E. A., and Hartroft, W. S. (1969): The role of lipoperoxidation in the pathogenesis of fatty livers induced by phosphorous poisoning in rats. *Am. J. Pathol.*, 54:275–291.
117. Gillette, J. R. (1971): Techniques for studying drug metabolism in vitro. In: *Fundamentals of drug metabolism and drug disposition*, edited by B. N. La Du, H. G. Mandel, and E. L. Way, pp. 400–418. Williams & Wilkins, Baltimore.
118. Gillette, J. R. (1975): Mechanisms of hepatic necrosis induced by halogenated aromatic hydrocarbons. In: *The Pathogenesis and Mechanisms of Liver Cell Necrosis*, edited by D. Keppler, pp. 239–254. MTP Press, Lancaster, United Kingdom.
119. Gillette, J. R. (1977): Kinetics of reactive metabolites and covalent binding in vivo and in vitro. In: *Biological Reactive Intermediates*, edited by D. J. Jollow, J. J. Kocsis, R. Snyder, and H. Vanio, pp. 25–41. Raven Press, New York.
120. Girard, D., Paquet, M. E., Paquin, R., and Beaulieu, A. D. (1996): Differential effects of interleukin-15 (IL-15) and IL-2 on human neutrophils: Modulation of phagocytosis, cytoskeletal rearrangement, gene expression, and apoptosis by IL-15. *Blood*, 88:3176–3184.

121. Girard, D., Paquin, R., and Beaulieu, A. D. (1997): Responsiveness of human neutrophils to interleukin-4: Induction of cytoskeletal rearrangements, de novo protein synthesis, and delay of apoptosis. *Biochem. J.*, 325:147–153.

122. Glende, E. A., Jr., Hruszkewycz, A. M., and Recknagel, R. O. (1976): Critical role of lipid peroxidation in carbon tetrachloride-induded loss of aminopyrine demethylase, cytochrome P450 and glucose-6-phosphatase. *Biochem. Pharmacol.*, 25:2163–2170.

123. Goethals, F., Krack, G., Deboyser, D., Vossen, P., and Roberfroid, M. (1984): Critical biochemical functions of isolated hepatocytes as sensitive indicators of chemical toxicity. *Fund. Appl. Toxicol.*, 4:441–450.

124. Goldin, R. D., Hunt, N. C., Clark, J., and Wickramasinghe, S. N. (1993): Apoptotic bodies in a murine model of alcoholic liver disease: Reversibility of ethanol-induced changes. *J. Pathol.*, 171:73–76.

125. Goldsworthy, T. L., Fransson-Steen, R., and Maronpot, R. R. (1996): Importance of and approaches to quantitation of hepatocyte apoptosis. *Toxicol. Pathol.*, 24:24–35.

126. Gottschall, D. W., Wiley, R. A., and Hanzlik, R. P. (1983): Toxicity of ortho-substituted bromobenzenes to isolated hepatocytes: Comparison to in vivo results. *Toxicol. Appl. Pharmacol.*, 69:55–65.

127. Grasl-Kraupp, B., Ruttkay-Nedecky, B., Koudelka, H., Bukowska, K., Bursch, W., and Schulte-Hermann, R. (1995): In situ detection of fragmentated DNA (TUNEL assay) fails to discriminate among apoptosis, necrosis, and autolytic cell death: A cautionary role. *Hepatology*, 21:1465–1468.

128. Grice, H. C. (1972): The changing role of pathology in modern safety evaluation. *CRC Crit. Rev. Toxicol.*, 1:119–152.

129. Grice, H. C., Barth, M. L., Cornish, H. H., Foster, G. V., and Gray, R. H. (1971): Correlation between serum enzymes, isoenzyme patterns and histologically detectable organ damage. *Food. Cosmet. Toxicol.*, 9:847–855.

130. Grisham, J. W. (1979): Use of hepatic cell cultures to detect and evaluate the mechanisms of action of toxic chemicals. *Internat. Rev. Exp. Pathol.*, 20:123–210.

131. Groothuis, G. M. M., and Meijer, D. K. F. (1992): Hepatocyte heterogeneity in bile formation and hepatobiliary transport of drugs. *Enzyme*, 46:94–138.

132. Guguen-Guillouzo, C., and Guillozo, A. (1993): Human hepatocyte cultures. In: *In Vitro Biological Systems*, edited by C. A. Tyson and G. N. Frasier, pp. 271–278. Academic Press, New York.

133. Guguen-Guillouzo, A. (1986): Use of isolated and cultured hepatocytes for xenobiotic metabolism and cytotoxicity studies. In: *Research in Isolated and Cultured Hepatocytes*, edited by A. Guillouzo and C. Guguen-Guillouzo, pp. 314–331. John Libbey Eurotext Ltd./INSERM, Paris.

134. Guillouzo, A., Begue, J.-M., Campion, J. P., Gascoin, M.-N., and Guguen-Guillouzo, C. (1985): Human hepatocyte culture: A model of pharmaco-toxicological studies. *Xenobiotica*, 15:635–641.

135. Guillouzo, A., and Guguen-Guillouzo, C. (1986): *Research in Isolated and Cultured Hepatocytes*. John Libbey Ltd./INSERM, Paris.

136. Guillouzo, A., Morel, F., Ratanasavanh, D., Chesne, C., and Guguen-Guillouzo, C. (1990): Long-term culture of functional hepatocytes. *Toxicol. In Vitro*, 4:415–427.

137. Gutman, A. D. (1959): Serum alkaline phosphatase activity in diseases of the skeletal and hepatobiliary systems: A consideration of the current status. *Am. J. Med.*, 27:875–901.

138. Habeebu, S. S. M., Liu, J., and Klaassen, C. D. (1998): Cadmium-induced apoptosis in mouse liver. *Toxicol. Appl. Pharmacol.*, 149:203–209.

139. Hafeman, D. G., and Koekstra, W. G. (1977): Protection against carbon tetrachloride-induced lipid peroxidation in the rat by dietary vitamin E, selenium and methionine as measured by ethane evolution. *J. Nutr.*, 107:656–665.

140. Hallberg, D., Jonson, G., and Reichard, H. (1960): Serum alkaline phosphatases, transaminases and ornithine carbamoyl transferase in biliary obstruction. *Acta Chir. Scand.*, 120:251–257.

141. Hallesy, D., and Benitz, K. F. (1963): Sulfobromophthalein sodium retention and morphological liver damage in dogs. *Toxicol. Appl. Pharmacol.*, 5:650–660.

142. Hargreaves, T. (1966): Bilirubin, bromosulfophthalein and indocyanine green excretion in bile. *Q. J. Exp. Physiol.*, 51:184–195.

143. Hayasaka, A., Koch, J., Schuppan, D., Maddrey, W. C., and Hahn, E. G. (1991): The serum concentrations of the aminoterminal propeptide of procollagen type III and the hepatic content of mRNA for the alpha chain of procollagen type III in carbon tetrachloride-induced rat liver fibrogenesis. *J. Hepatol.*, 13:328–338.

144. Hewitt, L. A., Ayotte, P., and Plaa, G. L. (1986): Modifications in rat hepatobiliary function following treatment with acetone, 2-butanone, 2-hexanone, mirex, or chlordecone and subsequently exposed to chloroform. *Toxicol. Appl. Pharmacol.*, 83:465–473.

145. Hewitt, W. R., Miyajima, H., Côté, M. G., and Plaa, G. L. (1979): Acute alteration of chloroform-induced hepato- and nephrotoxicity by mirex and kepone. *Toxicol. Appl. Pharmacol.*, 48:509–527.

146. Hewitt, W. R., Miyajima, H., Côté, M. G., and Plaa, G. L. (1980): Acute alteration of chloroform-induced hepato- and nephrotoxicity by acetone, n-hexane, methyl n-butyl ketone and 2,5-hexanedione. *Toxicol. Appl. Pharmacol.*, 53:230–248.

147. Hoglen, N. C., Younis, H. S., Hartley, D. P., Gunawardhana, L., Lantz, R. C., and Sipes, I. G. (1998): 1,2-Dichlorobenzene-induced lipid peroxidation in male Fischer 344 rats is Kupffer cell dependent. *Toxicol. Sci.*, 45:376–385.

148. Horvat, R. J., Lane, W. G., Ng, H., and Shepherd, A. D. (1964): Saturated hydrocarbons from autooxidizing metyl linoleate. *Nature*, 203:523–524.

149. Hoyumpa, A. M., Greene, H. L., Dunn, D. D., and Schenker, S. (1975): Fatty liver: Biochemical and clinical considerations. *Dig. Dis.*, 20:1142–1170.

150. Hruszkewycz, A. M., Glende, E. A., Jr., and Recknagel, R. O. (1978): Destruction of microsomal cytochrome P450 and glucose-6-phosphatase by lipids extracted from peroxidized microsomes. *Toxicol. Appl. Pharmacol.*, 46:695–702.

151. Hunton, D. B., Bollman, J. L., and Hoffman, H. N., II (1961): The plasma removal of indocyanine green and sulfobromophthalein: Effect of dosage and blocking agents. *J. Clin. Invest.*, 40:1648–1655.

152. Iijima, M., Côté, M. G., and Plaa, G. L. (1983): A semiquantitative morphologic assessment of chlordecone-potentiated chloroform hepatotoxicity. *Toxicol. Lett.*, 17:307–314.

153. Isselbacher, K. J. (1977): Metabolic and hepatic effects of alcohol. *N. Engl. J. Med.*, 296:612–626.

154. Jackson, R. L., Morissett, J. D., and Gotto, A. M., Jr. (1976): Lipoprotein structure and metabolism. *Physiol. Rev.*, 56:259–316.

155. Jaeger, R. J., Trabulus, M. J., and Murphy, S. D. (1973): Biochemical effects of 1,1-dichloroethylene in rats: dissociation of its hepatotoxicity from a lipoperoxidative mechanism. *Toxicol. Appl. Pharmacol.*, 24:457–467.

156. James, N. H., and Roberts, R. A. (1996): Species differences in response to peroxisome proliferators correlate in vitro with

induction of DNA synthesis rather than suppression of apoptosis. *Carcinogenesis*, 17:1623–1632.

157. Jungermann, K., and Katz, N. (1989): Functional specialization of different hepatocyte populations. *Physiol. Rev.*, 69:708–764.
158. Kaplan, M. M. (1986): Serum alkaline phosphatase—Another piece is added to the puzzle. *Hepatology*, 6:526–528.
159. Kedderis, G. L. (1996): Biochemical basis of hepatocellular injury. *Toxicol. Pathol.*, 24:77–83.
160. Kent, G., Fels, G., Dubin, A., and Popper, H. (1959): Collagen content b-524.
161. Kerr, J. F. R., Wyllie, A. H., and Currie, A. R. (1972): Apoptosis: A basic biological phenomenon with wide ranging implications in tissue kinetics. *Br. J. Cancer*, 26:239–257.
162. Kiernan, F. (1833): The anatomy and physiology of the liver. *Philos. Trans. R. Soc. London*, 123:711.
163. Klaassen, C. D. (1969): Biliary flow after microsomal enzyme induction. *J. Pharmacol. Exp. Ther.*, 168:218–223.
164. Klaassen, C. D. (1970): Effects of phenobarbital on the plasma disappearance and biliary excretion of drugs in rats. *J. Pharmacol. Exp. Ther.*, 175:289–300.
165. Klaassen, C. D. (1970): Plasma disappearance and biliary excretion of sulfobromophthalein and phenol-3,6-dibromophthalein disulfonate after microsomal enzyme induction. *Biochem. Pharmacol.*, 19:1241–1249.
166. Klaassen, C. D. (1971): Does bile acid secretion determine canalicular bile production in rats? *Am. J. Physiol.*, 220:667–673.
167. Klaassen, C. D. (1971): Studies on the increased biliary flow produced by phenobarbital in rats. *J. Pharmacol. Exp. Ther.*, 176:743–751.
168. Klaassen, C. D. (1976): Pharmacokinetics of rose bengal in the rat, rabbit, dog, and guinea pig. *Toxicol. Appl. Pharmacol.*, 38:85–100.
169. Klaassen, C. D. (1977): Biliary excretion. In: *Handbook of Physiology, Sect. 9: Reactions to Environmental Agents*, edited by D. H. K. Lee, H. L. Falk, S. D. Murphy, and S. R. Geiger, pp. 537–553. Williams & Wilkins, Baltimore.
170. Klaassen, C. D., and Plaa, G. L. (1967): Determination of sulfobromophthalein storage and excretory rate in small animals. *J. Appl. Physiol.*, 22:1151–1155.
171. Klaassen, C. D., and Plaa, G. L. (1967): Species variation in metabolism, storage, and excretion of sulfobromophthalein. *Am. J. Physiol.*, 213:1322–1326.
172. Klaassen, C. D., and Plaa, G. L. (1968): Effect of carbon tetrachloride on the metabolism, storage and excretion of sulfobromophthalein. *Toxicol. Appl. Pharmacol.*, 12:132–139.
173. Klaassen, C. D., and Plaa, G. L. (1968): Studies on the mechanism of phenobarbital-enhanced sulfobromophthalein disappearance. *J. Pharmacol. Exp. Ther.*, 161:361–366.
174. Klaassen, C. D., and Plaa, G. L. (1969): Comparison of the biochemical alterations elicited in livers from rats treated with carbon tetrachloride, chloroform, 1,1,2-trichloroethane and 1,1,1-trichloroethane. *Biochem. Pharmacol.*, 18:2019–2027.
175. Klaassen, C. D., and Plaa, G. L. (1969): Plasma disappearance and biliary excretion of indocyanine green in rats, rabbits and dogs. *Toxicol. Appl. Pharmacol.*, 15:374–384.
176. Klaassen, C. D., and Watkins, J. B. (1984): Mechanisms of bile formation, hepatic uptake, and biliary excretion. *Pharmacol. Rev.*, 36:1–67.
177. Kodavanti, P. R. S., and Mehendale, H. M. (1991): Biochemical methods of studying hepatotoxicity. In: *Hepatotoxicology*, edited by R. G. Meeks, S. D. Harrison, and R. J. Bull, pp. 241–325. CRC Press, Boca Raton, FL.
178. Kongo, M., Ohta, Y., Nishida, K., Sasaki, E., Harada, N., and Ishiguro, I. (1999): An association between lipid peroxidation and alpha-naphthylisothiocyanate-induced liver injury in rats. *Toxicol. Lett.*, 105:103–110.
179. Konttinen, A. (1968): A further simplified method of ornithine carbamoyltransferase measurement. *Clin. Chim. Acta*, 21:29–32.
180. Korsrud, G. O., Grice, H. C., and McLaughlan, J. M. (1972): Sensitivity of several serum enzymes in detecting carbon tetrachloride-induced liver damage in rats. *Toxicol. Appl. Pharmacol.*, 22:474–483.
181. Korsrud, G. O., Grice, H. G., Goodman, R. K., Knipfel, J. E., and McLaughlan, J. M. (1973): Sensitivity of several serum enzymes for the detection of thioacetamide-, dimethylnitrosamine- and diethanolamine-induced liver damage in rats. *Toxicol. Appl. Pharmacol.*, 26:299–313.
182. Köster, U., Albrecht, D., and Kappus, H. (1977): Evidence for carbon tetrachloride- and ethanol-induced lipid peroxidation demonstrated by ethane production in mice and rats. *Toxicol. Appl. Pharmacol.*, 42:639–648.
183. Kren, B. T., Trembley, J. H., Krajewski, S., Behrens, T. W., Reed, J. C., and Steer, C. J. (1996): Modulation of apoptosis-associated genes bcl-2, bcl-x, and bax during liver regeneration. *Cell Growth Differ.*, 7:1633–1642.
184. Kryszewski, A. J., Neale, G., Whitfield, J. F., and Moss, D. W. (1973): Enzyme changes in experimental biliary obstruction. *Clin. Chim. Acta*, 47:175–182.
185. Kubin, R. H., Grodsky, G. M., and Carbone, J. V. (1960): Investigation of rose bengal conjugation. *Proc. Soc. Exp. Biol. Med.*, 104:650–653.
186. Kukongviriyapan, V., and Stacey, N. H. (1991): Chemical-induced interference with hepatocellular transport. Role in cholestasis. *Chem. Biol. Interact.*, 77:245–261.
187. Kutob, S. D., and Plaa, G. L. (1962): The effect of acute ethanol intoxication on chloroform-induced liver damage. *J. Pharmacol. Exp. Ther.*, 135:245–251.
188. Labbé, P., Pelletier, M., Omara, F. O., and Girard, D. (1998): Functional responses of human neutrophils to sodium sulfite (Na_2SO_3) in vitro. *Hum. Exp. Toxicol.*, 17:600–605.
189. Lal, H., Puri, S. K., and Fuller, G. C. (1970): Impairment of hepatic drug metabolism by carbon tetrachloride inhalation. *Toxicol. Appl. Pharmacol.*, 16:35–39.
190. Lamers, W. H., Hilberts, A., Furt, E., Smith, J., Jonges, G. N., van Noorden, C. J. F., Janzen, J. W. G., Charles, R., and Moorman, A. F. N. (1989): Hepatic enzymic zonation: A reevaluation of the concept of the liver acinus. *Hepatotoxicology*, 10:72–76.
191. Larson, R. E., Plaa, G. L., and Crew, L. M. (1964): The effect of spinal cord transection on carbon tetrachloride hepatotoxicity. *Toxicol. Appl. Pharmacol.*, 6:154–162.
192. Laskin, D. L., and Gardner, C. R. (1998): The role of nonparenchymal cells and inflammatory macrophages in hepatotoxicity. In: *Toxicology of the Liver, 2nd ed.*, edited by G. L. Plaa and W. R. Hewitt, pp. 297–320. Taylor & Francis, Washington, D.C.
193. Lavigne, J. G., and Marchand, C. (1974): The role of metabolism in chloroform hepatotoxicity. *Toxicol. Appl. Pharmacol.*, 29:312–326.
194. Lawrence, J. N., and Benford, D. J. (1991): Development of an optimal method for the cryopreservation of hepatocytes and their subsequent monolayer culture. *Toxicol. In Vitro*, 5:39–50.
195. Leevy, C. M., Stein, S. W., Cherrick, G. R., and Davidson, C. S. (1959): Indocyanine green clearance: A test of liver excretory function. *Clin. Res.*, 7:290.
196. Lennon, H. D. (1966): Relative effects of 17α-alkylated anabolic steroids on sulfobromophthalein (BSP) retention in rabbits. *J. Pharmacol. Exp. Ther.*, 151:143–150.
197. Leonard, T. B., Hewitt, W. R., Dent, J. G., and Morgan, D. G. (1986): Serum alanine aminotransferase (ALT) as a quantitative indicator of hepatocyte necrosis. *Toxicologist*, 6:184.

198. Li, A. P. (1994): Primary hepatocyte culture as an in vitro toxicological system of the liver. In: *In Vitro Toxicology*, edited by S. C. Gad, pp. 195–220. Raven Press, New York.

199. Lieberman, M., and Mapson, L. W. (1964): Genesis and biogenesis of ethylene. *Nature*, 204:343–345.

200. Liebler, D. C., and Reed, D. J. (1997): Free-radical defense and repair mechanisms. In: *Free Radical Toxicology*, edited by K. B. Wallace, pp. 141–171. Taylor & Francis, Washington, D.C.

201. Lindstrom, R. D., and Anders, M. W. (1978): Effect of agents known to alter carbon tetrachloride hepatotoxicity and cytochrome P450 levels on carbon tetrachloride-stimulated lipid peroxidation and ethane production in the intact rat. *Biochem. Pharmacol.*, 27:563–567.

202. Litov, R. E., Irving, D. H., Downey, J. E., and Tappel, A. L. (1978): Lipid peroxidation: A mechanism involved in acute ethanol toxicity as demonstrated by in vivo pentane production in the rat. *Lipids*, 13:305–307.

203. Lockard, V. G., Mehendale, H. M., and O'Neal, R. M. (1983): Chlordecone-induced potentiation of carbon tetrachloride hepatotoxicity: A light and electron microscopic study. *Exp. Molec. Pathol.*, 39:230–245.

204. Lockard, V. G., Mehendale, H. M., and O'Neal, R. M. (1983): Chlordecone-induced potentiation of carbon tetrachloride hepatotoxicity: A morphometric and biochemical study. *Exp. Molec. Pathol.*, 39:246–256.

205. Lombardi, B. (1966): Considerations on the pathogenesis of fatty liver. *Lab. Invest.*, 15:1–20.

206. Long, R. M., and Moore, L. (1988): Biochemical evaluation of rat hepatocyte primary cultures as a model for carbon tetrachloride hepatotoxicity: Comparative studies in vivo and in vitro. *Toxicol. Appl. Pharmacol.*, 92:295–306.

207. Loretz, L. J., Li, A. P., Flye, M. W., and Wilson, A. G. E. (1989): Optimization of cryopreservation procedures for rat and human hepatocytes. *Xenobiotica*, 15:489–498.

208. Malledant, Y., Siproudhis, L., Tanguy, M., Clerc, C., Chesne, C., and Saint-Marc, C. (1990): Effects of halothane on human and rat hepatocyte cultures. *Anesthesiology*, 72:526–534.

209. Marsh, J. B., and Bizzi, A. (1972): Effects of amphetamine and fenfluramine on the net release of triglycerides of very low density lipoproteins by slices of rat liver. *Biochem. Pharmacol.*, 21:1143–1150.

210. Mazel, P., and Pessayre, D. (1976): Significance of metabolite-mediated toxicities in the safety evaluation of drugs and chemicals. In: *Advances in Modern Toxicology*, edited by M. A. Mehlman, R. E. Shapiro, and H. Blumenthal, pp. 307–343. Hemisphere, New York.

211. McKenna, M. J., Zempel, J. A., Madrid, E. O., Braun, W. H., and Gehring, P. J. (1978): Metabolism and pharmacokinetic profile of vinylidene chloride in rats following oral administration. *Toxicol. Appl. Pharmacol.*, 45:821–835.

212. McKenna, M. J., Zempel, J. A., Madrid, E. O., and Gehring, P. J. (1978): The pharmacokinetics of [^{14}C]vinylidene chloride in rats following inhalation exposure. *Toxicol. Appl. Pharmacol.*, 45:599–610.

213. McQueen, C. A. (1993): Isolation and culture of hepatocytes from different laboratory species. In: *In Vitro Biological Systems*, edited by C. A. Tyson and G. N. Frasier, pp. 255–270. Academic Press, New York.

214. McQueen, C. A., and Williams, G. M. (1987): Toxicology studies in cultured hepatocytes from various species. In: *The Isolated Hepatocyte. Use in Toxicology and Xenobiotic Biotransformations*, edited by E. J. Rauckman and G. M. Padilla, pp. 51–67. Academic Press, New York.

215. Mehendale, H. M. (1977): Mirex-induced impairment of hepatobiliary function: Suppressed biliary excretion of imipramine and sulfobromophthalein. *Drug Metab. Disp.*, 5:56–62.

216. Mehendale, H. M. (1979): Modification of hepatobiliary function by toxic chemicals. *Fed. Proc.*, 38:2240–2245.

217. Mehendale, H. M. (1990): Assessment of hepatobiliary function with phenolphthalein and phenolphthalein glucuronide. *Clin. Chem. Enzyme Comm.*, 2:195–204.

218. Mehendale, H. M., Ho, I. K., and Desaiah, D. (1979): Possible molecular mechanisms of mirex-induced hepatobiliary dysfunction. *Drug Metab. Disp.*, 7:28–33.

219. Meurman, L. (1960): On the distribution and kinetics of injected ^{131}I-rose bengal. *Acta Med. Scand.* [*Suppl. 354*], 167:7–85.

220. Mitchell, J. R., and Boyd, M. R. (1978): Dose thresholds, host susceptibility, and pharmacokinetic considerations in the evaluation of toxicity from chemically reactive metabolites. In: *Proceedings of the First International Congress on Toxicology*, edited by G. L. Plaa and W. A. Duncan, pp. 169–175. Academic Press, New York.

221. Mitchell, J. R., and Jollow, D. J. (1975): Metabolic activation of drugs to toxic substances. *Gastroenterology*, 68:392–410.

222. Mitchell, J. R., Jollow, D. J., Potter, W. Z., Davis, D. C., Gillette, J. R., and Brodie, B. B. (1973): Acetaminophen-induced hepatic necrosis. I. Role of drug metabolism. *J. Pharmacol. Exp. Ther.*, 187:185–194.

223. Mitchell, J. R., Nelson, S. D., Thorgeirsson, S. S., McMurty, R. J., and Dybing, E. (1976): Metabolic activation: Biochemical basis for many drug-induced liver injuries. *Prog. Liver Dis.*, 5:259–279.

224. Mitchell, J. R., Smith, C. V., Lauterburg, B. H., Hughes, H., Corcoran, G. B., and Horning, E. C. (1984): Reactive metabolites and the pathophysiology of acute lethal cell injury. In: *Drug Metabolism and Drug Toxicity*, edited by J. R. Mitchell and M. G. Horning, pp. 301–319. Raven Press, New York.

225. Molander, D. W., Wroblewski, F., and LaDue, J. S. (1955): Serum glutamic oxalacetic transaminase as an index of hepatocellular injury. *J. Lab. Clin. Med.*, 46:831–839.

226. Moldeus, P. (1978): Paracetamol metabolism and toxicity in isolated hepatocytes from rat and mouse. *Biochem. Pharmacol.*, 27:2859–2863.

227. Moritz, M., and Snodgrass, P. J. (1972): Serum enzymes derived from liver cell fractions. II. Responses to bile duct ligation in rats. *Gastroenterology*, 62:93–100.

228. Muller, M., and Jansen, P. L. M. (1998): The secretory function of the liver: New aspects of hepatobiliary transport. *J. Hepatology*, 28:144–154.

229. Musser, A. W., Ortigoza, C., Vazquez, M., and Riddick, J. (1966): Correlation of serum enzymes and morphologic alterations of the liver; with special reference to serum guanase and ornithine carbamyl transferase. *Am. J. Clin. Pathol.*, 46:82–88.

230. Neghab, M., and Stacey, N. H. (1997): In vitro interference with hepatocellular uptake of bile acids by xylene. *Toxicology*, 120:1–10.

231. Neghab, M., and Stacey, N. H. (1997): Toluene-induced elevation of serum bile acids: Relationship to bile acid transport. *J. Toxicol. Environ. Health*, 52:249–268.

232. Newberne, P. (1982): Assessment of the hepatocarcinogenic potential of chemicals: Response of the liver. In: *Toxicology of the Liver*, edited by G. L. Plaa and W. R. Hewitt, pp. 243–290. Raven Press, New York.

233. O'Hara, T. M., Sheppard, M. A., Clarke, E. C., Borzelleca, J. F., Gennings, C., and Condie, L. W. J. (1991): A $CCl_4/CHCl_3$ interaction study in isolated hepatocytes: Non-induced and phenobarbital-pretreated cells. *J. Appl. Toxicol.*, 11:147–154.

234. Obatomi, D. K., Brant, S., Anthonypillai, V., and Bach, P. H. (1998): Toxicity of atractyloside in precision-cut rat and porcine

renal and hepatic tissue slices. *Toxicol. Appl. Pharmacol.*, 148:35–45.

235. Oelberg, D. G., and Lester, R. (1986): Cellular mechanisms of cholestasis. *Annu. Rev. Med.*, 37:297–317.

236. Okuno, M., Muto, Y., Kato, M., Moriwaki, H., Noma, A., Tagaya, O., and Tanabe, Y. (1991): Changes in serum and hepatic levels of immunoreactive prolyl hydroxylase in two models of hepatic fibrosis in rats. *J. Gastroenterol. Hepatol.*, 6:271–277.

237. Olinga, P., Groen, K., Hof, I. H., De Kanter, R., Koster, H. J., Leeman, W. R., Rutten, A. A. J. J. L., Van Twillert, K., and Groothuis, G. M. M. (1997): Comparison of five incubation systems for rat liver slices using functional and viability parameters. *J. Pharmacol. Toxicol. Methods*, 38:59–69.

238. Olson, J. R., and Fujimoto, J. M. (1980): Evaluation of hepatobiliary function in the rat by the segmented retrograde intrabiliary injection technique. *Biochem. Pharmacol.*, 29:205–211.

239. Olson, J. R., Fujimoto, J. M., and Peterson, R. E. (1977): Three methods for measuring the increase in the capacity of the distended biliary tree in the rat produced by α-naphthylisothiocyanate treatment. *Toxicol. Appl. Pharmacol.*, 42:33–43.

240. Panteghini, M. (1994): Electrophoretic fractionation of 5′-nucleotidase. *Clin. Chem.*, 40:190–196.

241. Parrish, A. R., Gandolfi, A. J., and Brendel, K. (1995): Precision-cut tissue slices: Applications in pharmacology and toxicology. *Life Sci.*, 57:1887–1901.

242. Patel, T., Bronk, S., and Gores, G. (1994): Increases of intracellular magnesium promote glycodeoxycholate-induced apoptosis in rat hepatocytes. *J. Clin. Invest.*, 94:2183–2192.

243. Patel, T., and Gores, G. J. (1995): Apoptosis and hepatobiliary disease. *Hepatology*, 21:1725–1741.

244. Peterson, R. E., Olson, J. R., and Fujimoto, J. M. (1976): Measurement and alteration of the capacity of the distended biliary tree in the rat. *Toxicol. Appl. Pharmacol.*, 36:353–368.

245. Phillips, M. J., Poucell, S., and Oda, M. (1986): Mechanisms of cholestasis. *Lab. Invest.*, 54:593–608.

246. Plaa, G. L. (1968): Evaluation of liver function methodology. In: *Selected Pharmacological Testing Methods, Medical Research Series*, edited by A. Burger, pp. 255–288. Marcel Dekker, New York.

247. Plaa, G. L. (1977): Factors influencing biliary excretion and apparent T_m for bilirubin and related anions. In: *Chemistry and Physiology of Bile Pigments*, edited by P. D. Berk and N. I. Berlin, pp. 396–403. National Institutes of Health, Bethesda, Maryland.

248. Plaa, G. L. (1988): Experimental evaluation of haloalkanes and liver injury. *Fundam. Appl. Toxicol.*, 10:563–570.

249. Plaa, G. L. (1991): Toxic responses of the liver. In: *Casarett and Doull's Toxicology: The Basic Science of Poisons, 4th ed.*, edited by M. O. Amdur, C. D. Klaassen, and J. Doull, pp. 334–353. Pergamon Press, New York.

250. Plaa, G. L., and Becker, B. A. (1965): Demonstration of bile stasis in the mouse by a direct and an indirect method. *J. Appl. Physiol.*, 20:534–537.

251. Plaa, G. L., Evans, E. A., and Hine, C. H. (1958): Relative hepatotoxicity of seven halogenated hydrocarbons. *J. Pharmacol. Exp. Ther.*, 123:224–229.

252. Plaa, G. L., and Hewitt, W. R. (1982): Quantitative evaluation of indices of hepatotoxicity. In: *Toxicology of the Liver*, edited by G. L. Plaa and W. R. Hewitt, pp. 103–120. Raven Press, New York.

253. Plaa, G. L., and Hine, C. H. (1960): The effect of carbon tetrachloride on isolated perfused rat liver function. *Arch. Industr. Health*, 21:114–123.

254. Plaa, G. L., and Priestly, B. G. (1976): Intrahepatic cholestasis induced by drugs and chemicals. *Pharmacol. Rev.*, 28:207–273.

255. Plaa, G. L., and Witschi, H. (1976): Chemicals, drugs and lipid peroxidation. *Annu. Rev. Pharmacol. Toxicol.*, 16:125–141.

256. Popper, H., and Udenfriend, S. (1970): Hepatic fibrosis—Correlation of biochemical and morphological investigations. *Am. J. Med.*, 49:707–721.

257. Price, R. J., Ball, S. E., Renwick, A. B., Barton, P. T., Beamand, J. A., and Lake, B. G. (1998): Use of precision-cut rat liver slices for studies of xenobiotic metabolism and toxicity—Comparison of the Krumdieck and Brendel tissue slicers. *Xenobiotica*, 28:361–371.

258. Price, R. J., Mistry, H., Wield, P. T., Renwick, A. B., Beamand, J. A., and Lake, B. G. (1996): Comparison of the toxicity of allyl alcohol, coumarin and menadione in precision-cut rat, guinea-pig, Cynomolgus monkey and human liver slices. *Arch. Toxicol.*, 71:107–111.

259. Priestly, B. G., and Plaa, G. L. (1969): Effects of benziodarone on the metabolism and biliary excretion of sulfobromophthalein and related dyes. *Proc. Soc. Exp. Biol. Med.*, 132:881–885.

260. Priestly, B. G., and Plaa, G. L. (1970): Sulfobromophthalein metabolism and excretion in rats with iodomethane-induced depletion of hepatic glutathione. *J. Pharmacol. Exp. Ther.*, 174:221–231.

261. Priestly, B. G., and Plaa, G. L. (1970): Temporal aspects of carbon tetrachloride-induced alteration of sulfobromophthalein excretion and metabolism. *Toxicol. Appl. Pharmacol.*, 17:786–794.

262. Rappaport, A. M. (1969): Anatomic considerations. In: *Diseases of the Liver*, edited by L. Schiff, pp. 1–49. J. B. Lippincott, Philadelphia.

263. Rappaport, A. M. (1979): Physioanatomical basis of toxic liver injury. In: *Toxic Injury of the Liver*, edited by E. Farber and M. M. Fisher, pp. 1–57. Marcel Dekker, New York.

264. Reader, S., Moutardier, V., and Denizeau, F. (1999): Tributyltin triggers apoptosis in trout hepatocytes: The role of Ca^{2+}, protein kinase C and proteases. *Biochim. Biophys. Acta*, 1448:473–485.

265. Recknagel, R. O., and Ghoshal, A. K. (1966): New data on the question of lipoperoxidation in carbon tetrachloride poisoning. *Exp. Mol. Pathol.*, 5:108–117.

266. Recknagel, R. O., and Glende, E. A., Jr. (1973): Carbon tetrachloride hepatotoxicity: An example of lethal cleavage. *CRC Crit. Rev. Toxicol.*, 2:263–297.

267. Recknagel, R. O., and Glende, E. A., Jr. (1977): Lipid peroxidation: A specific form of cellular injury. In: *Handbook of Physiology, Sect. 9: Reactions to Environmental Agents*, edited by D. H. K. Lee, H. L. Falk, S. D. Murphy, and S. R. Geiger, pp. 591–601. Williams & Wilkins, Baltimore.

268. Recknagel, R. O., Glende, E. A., Jr., Waller, R. L., and Lowrey, K. (1982): Lipid peroxidation: Biochemistry, measurement, and significance in liver cell injury. In: *Toxicology of the Liver*, edited by G. L. Plaa and W. R. Hewitt, pp. 213–241. Raven Press, New York.

269. Recknagel, R. O., and Lombardi, B. (1961): Studies of biochemical changes in subcellular particles of rat liver and their relationship to a new hypothesis regarding the pathogenesis of carbon tetrachloride fat accumulation. *J. Biol. Chem.*, 236:564–569.

270. Reed, D. J. (1998): Evaluation of chemical-induced oxidative stress as a mechanism of hepatocyte death. In: *Toxicology of the Liver, 2nd ed.*, edited by G. L. Plaa and W. R. Hewitt, pp. 187–220. Taylor & Francis, Washington, D.C.

271. Reichard, H. (1957): Determination of ornithine carbamyl transferase with microdiffusion technique. *Scand. J. Clin. Invest.*, 9:311–312.

272. Reichard, H. (1959): Ornithine carbamoyl transferase in dog serum on intravenous injection of enzyme, choledochus ligation and carbon tetrachloride poisoning. *J. Lab. Clin. Med.*, 53:417–425.

273. Reichard, H. (1960): Ornithine cabamoyl-transferase activity in human tissue homogenates. *J. Lab. Clin. Med.*, 56:218–221.

274. Reichard, H. (1961): Ornithine carbamyl transferase activity in human serum in diseases of the liver and biliary system. *J. Lab. Clin. Med.*, 57:78–87.

275. Reichard, H. (1962): Studies on ornithine carbamoyl transferase activity in blood and serum. *Acta Med. Scand.* [*Suppl. 390*], 172:1–8.

276. Reichard, H. (1964): Determination of ornithine carbamoyl transferase in serum: a rapid method. *J. Lab. Clin. Med.*, 63:1061–1064.

277. Reitman, S., and Frankel, S. (1957): A colorimetric method for the determination of serum oxaloacetic and glutamic pyruvic transaminases. *Am. J. Clin. Pathol.*, 28:56–63.

278. Reynolds, E. S. (1972): Comparison of early injury to liver endoplasmic reticulum by halomethanes, hexachloroethane, benzene, toluene, bromobenzene, ethionine, thioacetamide and dimethylnitrosamine. *Biochem. Pharmacol.*, 21:2555–2561.

279. Riely, C. A., Cohen, G., and Lieberman, M. (1974): Ethane evolution: A new index of lipid peroxidation. *Science*, 183:208–210.

280. Roberts, R. J., Klaassen, C. D., and Plaa, G. L. (1967): Maximum biliary excretion of bilirubin and sulfobromophthalein during anesthesia-induced alteration of rectal temperature. *Proc. Soc. Exp. Biol. Med.*, 125:313–316.

281. Roberts, W. M. (1933): Blood phosphatase and the Van Den Bergh reaction in the differentiation of the several types of jaundice. *Br. Med. J.*, 1:734–738.

282. Rockey, D. C., Boyles, J. K., Gabbiani, G., and Friedman, S. L. (1992): Rat hepatic lipocytes express smooth muscle action upon activation in vivo and in culture. *J. Submicrosc. Cytol. Pathol.*, 24:193–203.

283. Rojkind, M., and Dunn, M. A. (1979): Hepatic fibrosis. *Gastroenterology*, 76:849–863.

284. Roma, M. G., Orsler, D. J., and Coleman, R. (1997): Canalicular retention as an in vitro assay of tight junctional permeability in isolated hepatocyte couplets: Effects of protein kinase modulation and cholestatic agents. *Fund. Appl. Toxicol.*, 37:71–81.

285. Rosenthal, S. M. (1922): An improved method for using phenotetrachlorphthalein as a liver function test. *J. Pharmacol. Exp. Ther.*, 19:385–391.

286. Rosenthal, S. M., and White, E. C. (1925): Clinical application of the bromosulphalein test for hepatic function. *JAMA*, 84:1112–1114.

287. Sagai, M., and Tappel, A. L. (1978): Effect of vitamin E on carbon tetrachloride-induced lipid peroxidation as demonstrated by in vivo pentane production. *Toxicol. Lett.*, 2:149–155.

288. Sagai, M., and Tappel, A. L. (1979): Lipid peroxidation induced by some halomethanes as measured by in vivo pentane production in the rat. *Toxicol. Appl. Pharmacol.*, 49:283–291.

289. Schulte-Hermann, R., Bursch, W., Grasl-Kraupp, B., Török, L., Ellinger, A., and Müllauer, L. (1995): Role of active cell death (apoptosis) in multi-stage carcinogenesis. *Toxicol. Lett.*, 82–83:143–148.

290. Searle, J., Harmon, B. V., Bishop, C. J., and Kerr, J. F. R. (1987): The significance of cell death by apoptosis in hepatobiliary disease. *J. Gastroenterol. Hepatol.*, 2:77–96.

291. Seetharam, S., Sussman, N. L., Komoda, T., and Alpers, D. H. (1986): The mechanism of elevated alkaline phosphatase activity after bile duct ligation in the rat. *Hepatology*, 6:374–380.

292. Seglen, P. O. (1972): I. Effect of calcium on enzymatic dispersion of isolated, perfused liver. *Exp. Cell Res.*, 74:450–454.

293. Seglen, P. O. (1976): Preparation of isolated rat liver cells. In: *Methods in Cell Biology*, edited by D. M. Prescott, pp. 29–83. Academic Press, New York.

294. Sevanian, A., and McLeon, L. (1997): Formation and biological reactivity of lipid peroxidation products. In: *Free Radical Toxicology*, edited by K. B. Wallace, pp. 47–70. Taylor & Francis, Washington, D.C.

295. Shin, B. C., Huggins, J. W., and Caraway, K. L. (1972): Effects of pH, concentration and aging on the malonaldehyde reaction with proteins. *Lipids*, 7:229–233.

296. Sinnhuber, R. O., and Yu, T. C. (1958): 2-Thiobarbituric acid method for the measurement of rancidity in fishery products. *Food Technology*, 12:9–12.

297. Sipes, I. G., and Gandolfi, A. J. (1982): Bioactivation of aliphatic organohalogens: Formation, detection, and relevance. In: *Toxicology of the Liver*, edited by G. L. Plaa and W. R. Hewitt, pp. 181–212. Raven Press, New York.

298. Sirica, A. E., and Pitot, H. C. (1980): Drug metabolism and effects of carcinogens in cultured hepatic cells. *Pharmacol. Rev.*, 31:205–228.

299. Smith, P. F., Gandolfi, A. J., Krumdieck, C. L., Putnam, C. W., Zukoski, C. F. I., Davis, W. M., and Brendel, K. (1985): Dynamic organ culture of precision liver slices for in vitro toxicology. *Life Sci.*, 36:1367–1375.

300. Smuckler, E. A. (1966): Studies on carbon tetrachloride intoxication IV. Effect of carbon tetrachloride on liver slices and isolated organelles in vitro. *Lab. Inves.*, 15:157–166.

301. Soni, M. G., and Mehendale, H. M. (1998): Role of tissue repair in toxicologic interactions among hepatotoxic organics. *Environ. Health Persp.*, 106(suppl 6):1307–1317.

302. Stacey, N. H. (1989): Toxicity of mixtures of trichloroethylene, tetrachloroethylene and 1,1,1-trichloroethane: Similarity of in vitro and in vivo responses. *Toxicol. Indus. Health*, 5:441–450.

303. Stinchcombe, S., Buchmann, A., Bock, K. W., and Schwarz, M. (1995): Inhibition of apoptosis during 2,3,7,8-tetrachlorodibenzo-p-dioxin-mediated tumour promotion in rat liver. *Carcinogenesis*, 16:1271–1275.

304. Story, D. L., Gee, S. J., Tyson, C. A., and Gould, D. H. (1983): Response of isolated hepatocytes to organic and inorganic cytotoxins. *J. Toxicol. Environ. Health*, 11:483–501.

305. Sturgill, M. G., and Lambert, G. H. (1997): Xenobiotic-induced hepatotoxicity: Mechanisms of liver injury and methods of monitoring hepatic function. *Clin. Chem.*, 43:1512–1526.

306. Sweeny, D. J., and Diasio, R. B. (1991): The isolated hepatocyte and isolated perfused liver as models for studying drug- and chemical-induced hepatotoxicity. In: *Hepatotoxicology*, edited by R. G. Meeks, S. D. Harrison, and R. J. Bull, pp. 215–239. CRC Press, Boca Raton, FL.

307. Szende, B., Lapis, K., Kovalszky, I., and Timar, F. (1992): Role of the modified (glycosaminoglycan producing) perisinusoidal fribroblasts in the CCl_4-induced fibrosis of the rat liver. *In vivo*, 6:355–361.

308. Taplin, G. V., Meredith, O. M., and Kade, H. (1955): The radioactive (I^{13L}-tagged) rose bengal uptake-excretion test for liver function using external gamma ray scintillation counting techniques. *J. Lab. Clin. Med.*, 45:655–678.

309. Tegeris, A. S., Smalley, H. E., Jr., Earl, F. L., and Curtis, J. L. (1969): Ornithine carbamoyl transferase as a liver function test: Comparative studies in dog, swine and man. *Toxicol. Appl. Pharmacol.*, 14:54–66.

310. Thurman, R. G., and Kauffmann, F. C. (1985): Sublobular compartmentation of pharmacologic events (SCOPE): Metabolic fluxes in periportal and pericentral regions of the liver lobule. *Hepatology*, 5:144–151.

311. Toutain, H. J., Moronvalle-Halley, V., Sarsat, J. P., Chelin, C., Hoet, D., and Leroy, D. (1998): Morphological and functional integrity of precision-cut rat liver slices in rotating organ culture

and multiwell plate culture—Effects of oxygen tension. *Cell Biol. Toxicol.*, 14:175–190.

312. Traiger, G. J., and Plaa, G. L. (1971): Differences in the potentiation of carbon tetrachloride in rats by ethanol and isopropanol pretreatment. *Toxicol. Appl. Pharmacol.*, 20:105–112.
313. Trauner, M., Meier, P. J., and Boyer, J. L. (1998): Molecular pathogenesis of cholestasis. *New Engl. J. Med.*, 339:1217–1227.
314. Travlos, G. S., Morris, R. W., Elwell, M. R., Duke, R., Rosenblum, S., and Thompson, M. B. (1996): Frequency and relationships of clinical chemistry and liver and kidney histopathology findings in 13-week toxicity studies in rats. *Toxicology*, 107:17–29.
315. Tyson, C. A., Gee, S. J., Hawk-Prather, K., Story, D. L., and Milman, H. A. (1989): Correlation between in vivo and in vitro toxicity of some chlorinated aliphatics. *Toxicol. in Vitro*, 3:145–150.
316. Van Handel, E., and Zilversmit, D. B. (1957): Micromethod for the direct determination of serum triglycerides. *J. Lab. Clin. Med.*, 50:152–157.
317. Vassef, A. A. (1978): Direct micromethod for colorimetry of serum ornithine carbamoyltransferase activity, with use of a linear standard curve. *Clin. Chem.*, 24:101–107.
318. Vonen, B., and Mørland, J. (1984): Isolated rat hepatocytes in suspension: Potential hepatotoxic effects of six different drugs. *Arch. Toxicol.*, 56:33–37.
319. Wade, C. R., and van Rij, A. M. (1985): In vivo lipid peroxidation in man as measured by the respiratory excretion of ethane, pentane, and other low-molecular-weight hydrocarbons. *Anal. Biochem.*, 150:1–7.
320. Weiner, F. R., Shah, A., Biempica, L., Zern, M. A., and Czaja, M. J. (1992): The effects of hepatic fibrosis on Ito cell gene expression. *Matrix*, 12:36–43.
321. Weldon, P. R., Rubenstein, B., and Rubenstein, D. (1965): The direct action of CCl_4 on the metabolism of liver slices. *Can. J. Biochem.*, 43:647–659.
322. Wells, P. G., and To, E. C. A. (1986): Murine acetaminophen hepatotoxicity: Temporal interanimal variability in plasma glutamic-pyruvic transaminase profiles and relation to in vivo chemical covalent binding. *Fund. Appl. Toxicol.*, 7:17–25.
323. Wheeldon, E. B., Williams, S. M., Soames, A. R., James, N. H., and Roberts, R. A. (1995): Quantitation of apoptotic bodies in rat liver by in situ end labeling (ISEL): Correlation with morphology. *Toxicol. Pathol.*, 23:410–415.
324. Wheeler, H. O., Cranston, W. I., and Meltzer, J. I. (1958): Hepatic uptake and biliary excretion of indocyanine green in the dog. *Proc. Soc. Exp. Biol. Med.*, 99:11–14.
325. Wheeler, H. O., Meltzer, J. I., and Bradley, S. E. (1960): Biliary transport and hepatic storage of sulfobromophthalein sodium in the unanesthetized dog, in normal man, and in patient with hepatic disease. *J. Clin. Invest.*, 39:1131–1144.
326. Whitfield, J. B., Pounder, R. E., Neale, G., and Moss, D. W. (1972): Serum γ-glutamyl transpeptidase activity in liver disease. *Gut*, 13:702–708.
327. Wilkinson, J. H. (1970): Clinical application of isoenzymes. *Clin. Chem.*, 16:733–739.
328. Willson, R. A., Hart, J., and Hall, T. (1991): The concentration and temporal relationships of acetaminophen-induced changes in intracellular and extracellular total glutathione in freshly isolated hepatocytes from untreated and 3-methylcholanthrene pretreated Sprague–Dawley and Fischer rats. *Pharmacol. Toxicol.*, 69:205–212.
329. Wormser, U., Ben Zakine, S., Stivelband, E., and Eizen, O. (1990): The liver slice system: A rapid in vitro acute toxicity test for primary screening of hepatotoxic agents. *Toxicol. in Vitro*, 4:783–789.
330. Wormser, U., and Ben-Zakine, S. (1990): The liver slice system: An in vitro acute toxicity test for assessment of hepatotoxins and their antidotes. *Toxicol. in Vitro*, 4:449–451.
331. Wroblewski, F. (1959): The clinical significance of transaminase activities of serum. *Am. J. Med.*, 27:911–923.
332. Yaari, A., Sikuler, E., Keyman, A., and Ben-Zvi, Z. (1992): Bromosulfophthalein disposition in chronically bile duct obstructed rats. *Hepatology*, 15:67–72.
333. Yagi, K. (1984): Assay for blood plasma or serum. *Methods Enzymol.*, 105:328–331.
334. Yamazaki, M., Suzuki, H., Sugiyama, Y., Iga, T., and Hanano, M. (1992): Uptake of organic anions by isolated rat hepatocytes. A classification in terms of ATP-dependency. *J. Hepatology*, 14:41–47.
335. Zimmerman, H. J. (1978): *Hepatotoxicity*. Appleton-Century-Crofts, New York.
336. Zimmerman, H. J. (1998): Drug-induced hepatic disease. In: *Toxicology of the Liver, 2nd ed.*, edited by G. L. Plaa and W. R. Hewitt, pp. 3–60. Taylor & Francis, Washington, D.C.
337. Zsigmond, G., and Solymoss, B. (1972): Effect of spironolactone, pregnenolone-16α-carbonitrile and cortisol on the metabolism and biliary excretion of sulfobromophthalein and phenol-3,6-dibromophthalein disulfonate in rats. *J. Pharmacol. Exp. Ther.*, 183:499–507.

Principles and Methods of Toxicology,
Fourth Edition, edited by A. Wallace Hayes.
Taylor & Francis, Philadelphia © 2001.

Chapter 25

Renal Methods for Toxicology

Mary E. Davis and William O. Berndt

This chapter presents methods of interest to the renal toxicologist. It exposes the reader to the state of the art with respect to renal function techniques as they apply to toxicology, including observations on data interpretation and pitfalls of the procedures. Specific detailed procedures are not given when they involve standard methods of renal physiology; these techniques can be found in well-known renal physiology texts (e.g., Smith [34]).

Background material on renal physiology and anatomy is given only briefly, because many excellent, detailed text and reference books are available (4,32,41). A thorough background in renal physiology is essential for understanding the techniques and their application to renal toxicology.

It is not the intent of this chapter to be a "cookbook" of laboratory procedures. The focus is on evaluation of the techniques as they apply to toxicology and the interpretation of data generated from the various relevant procedures.

RENAL PHYSIOLOGY AND ANATOMY

The kidneys function to maintain water and electrolyte balance by removing large quantities of solutes and solvent from the plasma by filtration, and then selectively returning to the plasma the needed chemicals, including water (reabsorption), and further adding some chemicals to the tubular fluid (secretion). Despite processing a large volume of fluid, overall balance is maintained. The vascular tissue and tubular epithelia constitute the major tissue types of the kidneys. The anatomical relationships between the blood vessels and the nephron are depicted in Figure 25.1.

The blood supply to the kidney comes from the renal artery, which supplies the arcuate and interlobular arteries within the renal mass. The glomeruli arise from the interlobular arteries via the afferent arterioles. The glomeruli are unusual in that their capillaries are specialized for filtration and are the first of two capillary beds in series within the kidney. Blood leaves the glomerulus via the efferent arterioles and then branches into capillary networks around the nephrons. The capillary networks are in the same general region as their parent glomeruli (the glomeruli from whence they arose); that is, efferent arterioles of glomeruli in the superficial cortex form the peritubular capillary network around the nephron tubules in the cortex, and efferent arterioles from glomeruli in the midcortical area give rise to the peritubular capillaries in the midcortical area. Most of the glomeruli at the junction of the cortex and medulla (the juxtamedullary nephrons) have efferent arterioles that descend into the medulla, branching at various depths within the medulla to form capillary beds around the loop of Henle, the vasa rectae.

The glomerulus is a capillary bed specialized for filtering large amounts of water, electrolytes, and small molecules yet retaining proteins and formed elements within the vasculature (Figure 25.2A). The physical bar-

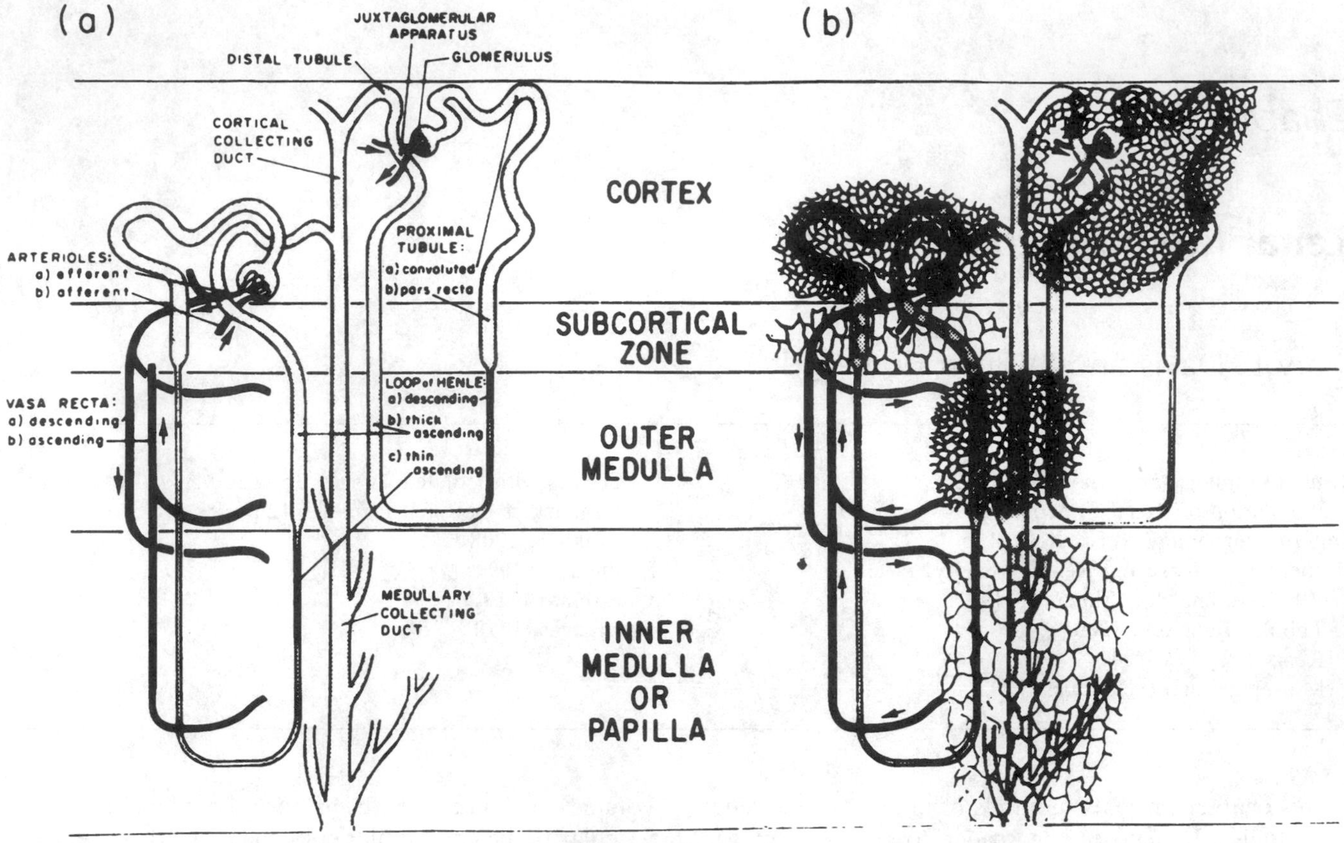

FIG. 25.1. (a) Two major nephron types: superficial cortical and juxtamedullary nephrons. The early distal tubule segment near the glomerulus is the juxtaglomerular apparatus. (b) The capillary networks surround all segments of the nephrons, including the collecting ducts. From Reference 39.

rier separating plasma from urine is composed of three parts. The first is the fenestrae within the capillary endothelial cells. Fenestrae occupy approximately 20% of the endothelial wall; they are large (50–100 nm in diameter), and unlike other capillary fenestrae, they do not have a diaphragm. The fenestrae have a negative charge; so although they are large in diameter, they can obstruct molecules, for example, albumin, that have a negative charge. Dextran molecules of the same size as albumin cross the glomerulus, whereas anionic dextran sulfate molecules of the same size are trapped at the capillary fenestrae and do not reach the tubular urine (19,36). The second barrier to filtration is the basement membrane, a hydrated gel that excludes molecules based on size. The last barrier is the filtration slit formed by the interdigitation of finger-like processes of the epithelial cells that form the nephron capsule. The space between the two processes retards cationic molecules, and the slit constitutes the major hydraulic barrier.

Filtration occurs because the forces moving the fluid out of the capillary (hydrostatic pressure) exceed the forces preventing movement out of the capillary (oncotic pressure, due to the plasma proteins) and into the Bowman's space (hydraulic pressure within Bowman's capsule). The hydrostatic pressure derives from arterial blood pressure and decreases slightly over the length of the capillary, which permits the flow of blood through the glomerular capillary. As water is filtered out of the capillary, the proteins remaining behind are concentrated, and the plasma oncotic pressure increases. In most mammals the oncotic pressure exceeds the hydraulic pressure, and filtration stops before the blood reaches the end of the capillary; the remaining length of capillary can be thought of as a functional reserve.

The rate of filtration (glomerular filtration rate, or GFR) is affected by changes of blood pressure, plasma protein concentration, and the ultrafiltration coefficient (K_f). GFR varies directly with blood pressure and inversely with protein concentration in the afferent arteriole. Increasing the rate of blood flow within the capillary increases the amount of water to be filtered, and the point of pressure equilibrium moves closer to the end of the capillary. In this way more filtration occurs. Conversely, decreasing the rate of glomerular blood flow allows more water to be filtered early along the length

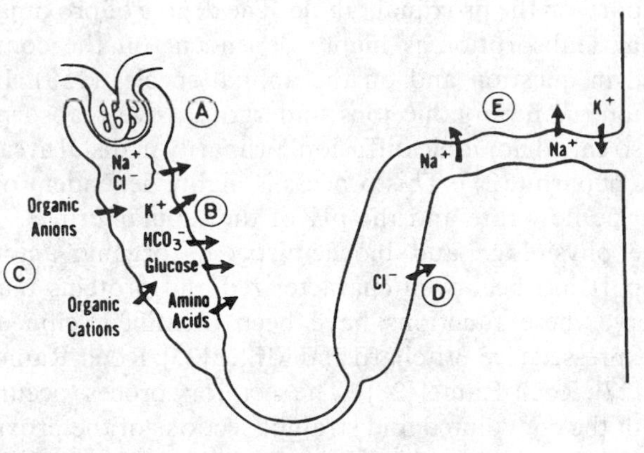

FIG. 25.2. Various transport functions of the nephron.

of the capillary, and less total fluid is filtered. Whereas GFR is highly blood flow-dependent, renal blood flow is normally independent of systemic blood pressure. Blood flow to the kidney is autoregulated, that is, maintained approximately constant, as long as blood pressure is above about 80 mm Hg. Thus, flow dependence occurs only when blood pressure falls, autoregulation fails, or intrinsic feedback mechanisms constrict the afferent arterioles (glomerular–tubular balance; see below).

The ultrafiltration coefficient K_f expresses the intrinsic permeability of the glomerulus and the surface area available for filtration. The coefficient is not constant but changes in response to such agents as angiotensin II, vasopressin, and norepinephrine. There are contractile elements within the connective tissue of the glomerulus (the glomerular mesangium), and contraction of these elements reduces the K_f (99). Decreases of K_f have been reported in acute renal failure caused by uranyl nitrate or gentamicin (50,139). The reduction of K_f is thought to be a major factor in the decrease of GFR but is not suggested as a mechanism of tubular toxicity (59). Alterations of K_f may be important in glomerular damage.

In addition to playing an important role in the regulation of GFR, plasma proteins also influence the rate of excretion of toxic chemicals and the effects of these chemicals on the kidneys. Only those substances of relatively small molecular weight and in free solution pass the glomerular filter. If a chemical is partially bound to plasma proteins, only that portion not bound is filtered at the glomerulus. Therefore, binding to plasma proteins can decrease excretion of the chemical and extend the duration of action (on the kidneys or other organs). The extent of binding is important when determining the concentration to which tubular cells are actually exposed as well because materials bound to plasma proteins are neither filterable nor active while they are bound.

The distribution of glomeruli decreases from the outer cortical to the inner cortical area. The rate of blood flow per glomerulus and the filtration rate per glomerulus are approximately equal throughout the cortex. Therefore, the rate of blood flow parallels the distribution of glomeruli, being greater in the outer cortex and decreasing to the inner cortex. Still lesser amounts of blood are distributed to the medulla, renal papilla, perirenal fat, and connective tissue. Data from krypton or xenon washout studies suggest that as much as 85% of the total renal blood flow is associated with the cortical regions of the kidney. Total renal blood flow and distribution of blood within the kidney can be altered by chemical substances. The renal vasculature is a possible site of action for nephrotoxic chemicals or for chemicals that influence (either increase or decrease) nephrotoxicity.

The nephron tubule is a chain of segments that have different functions supported by different ultrastructure and enzymology (29). The proximal segments of the tubule can be differentiated by their gross appearance as either convoluted or straight. Ultrastructural studies have demonstrated three areas. The first segment (S1) is contained entirely within the proximal convoluted tubule and the last segment (S3) entirely within the straight segment. The second segment (S2) includes the end of the convoluted section and the beginning of the straight section. Both classification schemes are used because junctions between segments can be discerned only by ultrastructural techniques. The proximal convoluted tubule is a leaky epithelium that allows movement of solute between the cells, the paracellular path, as well as through cells, the transcellular route (Figure 25.2B). Approximately 60–70% of the filtrate is reabsorbed by the proximal convoluted tubule. Solutes are reabsorbed by transport processes, and water follows, passively, down the osmotic gradient; the tubular urine remains isosmotic to plasma (i.e., this process is an isosmotic reabsorptive one). The energy for this work is derived primarily from oxidation of fatty acids; both the convoluted and straight sections of the proximal tubule have relatively high concentrations of the enzymes of gluconeogenesis and low concentrations of those of glycolysis. Na^+,K^+-ATPase activity drives reabsorption and is found in all parts of the proximal tubules. The proximal tubule has glutathione and glutathione *S*-transferase activity.

The cells of the S1 segment are tall and have a prominent brush border, extensive infoldings of the basal membrane, and interdigitations of lateral borders of adjacent cells. The interdigitating cell processes are filled with mitochondria, characteristic of Na^+-transporting epithelia. Sodium diffuses into the tubular cells and is actively extruded by Na^+,K^+-ATPase localized in the basolateral membrane. Within the S1 segment other osmolytes are cotransported with Na^+, including glucose, amino acids, and phosphate. Failure to reabsorb these osmolytes prevents reabsorption of an isosmotic amount of water, which is the cause of polyuria in patients with diabetes mellitus. In hyperglycemia the amount of glucose filtered overwhelms the capacity of the kidneys to reabsorb glucose, and glucose remains in the final urine. Each gram of glucose retains 21 ml of water in the urine. Glucosuria occurs in nephrotoxicity; in this situation the plasma glucose concentration is normal, but the damaged cells are not able to reabsorb the amount of glucose filtered. Amino acid reabsorption is handled by several transport systems that are selective for charge (acidic, basic, or neutral amino acids) or other structural features (imino acids, amino acids). Some amino acids are substrates for more than one system. Normally, most (99%) of the filtered amino acids are reabsorbed; this percent is less in nephrotoxicity and certain congenital disorders, that is, cystinurias (32).

The cells of the S2 segment are less complex than those of S1; the S2 cells have a shorter, less dense brush border and less basolateral interdigitation. Phosphate-dependent glutaminase (PDG), one of the enzymes catalyzing ammonia formation, is present in S2, and its activity is increased in the presence of acidosis (71). Glucose transport capability is about half that of S1; there are fewer glucose transporters available, but their affinity for glucose is greater, which is important because the concentration of glucose decreases along the length of the proximal tubule. The presence of high-affinity transporters allows the remaining glucose to be reabsorbed more readily. A similar situation exists for glycine transport.

The rate of volume reabsorption is thought to decrease from S1 to S2, although in vitro studies using perfused tubules have demonstrated that S2 cells have approximately the same capacity as S1 cells. The rate decreases in vivo because the concentrations of the electrolytes driving volume reabsorption (Na^+, glucose, etc.) have been greatly decreased by reabsorption in the S1 segment. In contrast, transport of organic anions is much greater in S2.

The transport of organic anions and cations represents two types of secretory process (Figure 25.2C). Although both are found within the proximal tubule and both are active secretory processes, they are functionally distinct; that is, each transport system has its own transporters, substrates, competitors, and inhibitors. Transport of organic anions is not affected by organic cations; similarly, organic cation transport is not decreased in the presence of either substrates or inhibitors of the organic anion transport system. The organic anion and cation transport systems are similar in that both require expenditure of energy, either directly or indirectly, and, therefore, both are subject to inhibition by metabolic inhibitors such as cyanide or iodoacetate. Tissue concentrations in excess of tenfold can be achieved by the organic ion transport system.

Many of the organic ions also undergo reabsorption in the proximal segment; that is, they undergo "bidirectional transport" in the proximal tubule. The degree of proximal tubular reabsorption is highly dependent on the compound in question and on the animal species (150). In addition, many organic ions undergo passive reabsorption, so called nonionic diffusion, primarily in distal areas of the nephron (27). This process is highly dependent on the urine flow rate and the pH of the tubular urine.

The physiology and biochemistry of organic anion transport has been well characterized and proteins that subserve these functions have been identified, cloned, and expressed (see Pritchard and Miller [25]; Roch-Ramel et al. [27]; Roch-Ramel [28]). The secretory process occurs in both the convoluted and straight sections of the proximal tubule; the specific segment having the highest activity depends on the species. The classical model substrate for the organic anion transport system is *p*-aminohippurate (PAH); model inhibitors are probenecid and penicillin. On the basal surface of the cell, PAH enters the cell by countertransport with an endogenous carboxylic acid (such as lactate or α-ketoglutarate). The carboxylic acid enters the cell on both the basal and luminal sides, by cotransport with Na^+. PAH exits on the luminal side. Energy is required to pump Na^+ out of the cell, maintaining the gradient for carboxylic acid transport. A protein that matches the basolateral organic anion transporter (OAT 1; ROAT-1) has been cloned, expressed, and characterized (140,146). It has properties identical to those of the basolateral PAH transporter, including countertransport of α-ketoglutarate, inhibition by probenecid, and organic anion transport substrates. It has 551 amino acid residues in 12 transmembrane domains and is a member of the major facilitator superfamily. It is found exclusively in the basolateral region and is limited to the S2 segment of the proximal tubule.

Three organic anion transporters have been localized to the brush border. Mrp2 transports reduced and oxidized glutathione and glutathione conjugates (and derivatives), including leuokotrienes C4 and D4, glucuronide conjugates of bilirubin, and estradiol. It is an ATP binding cassette transporter and is found in the proximal tubule, particularly the S3 segment, where it functions as an export pump (136). The organic anion transport peptide (oatp) is found in the proximal tubule brush border as well as in the basolateral region of liver cells (77). It transports taurocholate and bromosulfophthalein, but not PAH. Also in the brush border is OAT-K1. This protein is 669 amino acids and is 72 percent identical to liver OATP (134). It transports methotrexate; transport is inhibited by nonsteroidal antiinflammatory drugs, folate, and BSP. It does not transport taurocholate. Finally, sodium-dependent dicarboxylate cotransporter has been found in the brush border as well (121).

In many species, PAH is so effectively transported that its clearance is equal to, and used for measurement of, total renal blood flow. PAH excretion can be used to measure renal blood flow because filtration at the glomerulus and secretion by the tubule remove virtually all the PAH from the renal arterial blood. Actual measurements of PAH extraction (as the arteriovenous difference) in humans and dogs have shown PAH extraction to be 80–90 percent complete. Renal clearance of PAH is dependent on normal blood flow to the kidneys as well as a functioning transport system and intact tubule (maintaining normal imperviousness to passive reabsorption of PAH in the tubular urine). A nephrotoxic agent may affect PAH clearance by altering any of these three, that is, decreasing renal blood flow, interfering with the organic anion transport system, or rendering the tubule leaky to PAH so that secreted PAH does not remain in the urine. Integrity of the transport system is readily assessed using in vitro techniques described later. With severe damage, the tubular epithelium is permeable to inulin (a polysaccharide with MW of 5000 D), and leakiness can sometimes be assessed as the increased concentration of inulin in tissue.

Organic cations, such as tetraethylammonium (TEA) or *N*-methylnicotinamide (NMN), also are secreted actively (see Koepsell et al. [14]; Pritchard and Miller [25]). This process occurs in the proximal tubule, as demonstrated with a variety of techniques (42,115,116). Cations are transported across the basolateral surface by organic cation transporters 1 and 2 (OCT1 and OCT2) (65,86). Transport is electrogenic and dependent on the potential difference across the membrane; transport is independent of Na^+ and H^+. The substrate specificities are species-dependent; both transport TEA and the endogenous monoamines norepinephrine, epinephrine, dopamine and serotonin, and other cationic drugs. OCT1 and 2 are members of the same major facilitator superfamily as OAT1 and 2. Transport across the brush border occurs in both influx and efflux directions. ATP-dependent P-glycoprotein drug efflux pumps, members of the mdr1 subfamily, have been localized in the brush border. Another member of the major facilitator superfamily, OCTN1, exhibits pH-dependent, potential independent, bi-direction flux that is similar to the efflux step of organic cation secretion (157). OCTN1 is found in the proximal convoluted tubule; however, its location within the cell has not yet been determined.

In general, metabolic inhibitors do not show selectivity for one transport system over the other, for example, cyanide or iodoacetate blocks transport of both anions and cations. However, some selective effects of nephrotoxic substances have been reported (54,89).

There is little transition between the S2 and S3 segments, and the ultrastructure of S3 is different in rats and rabbits. In rabbits, S3 cells are shorter and show less complexity than S2 cells; there are minimal lateral interdigitations and basal infoldings, and microvilli of the brush border are short and sparse. The S3 cells of rats have a well-developed brush border that is longer than the other proximal segments. Glucose reabsorptive capacity is about one-tenth that of S1. Organic anion and cation transport is high in S3. Xenobiotic biotransformation activity is localized to the S3 segment. Induction of renal cytochrome P450 activity by TCDD is accompanied by proliferation of the smooth endoplasmic reticulum (SER) in the S3 segment (81). Fluorescence from NADPH-cytochrome P450 reductase is more intense in S3 (63). Catabolism and synthesis of glutathione (GSH) occurs to a much greater extent in S3; γ-glutamyl transpeptidase is present in greater amounts in S3 than S1 or S2, and γ-glutamylcysteinylsynthetase is localized to the S3 segment. γ-Glutamyl transpeptidase is attached to the brush border membrane, which juts into the lumen and catalyzes the first step in the breakdown of GSH or GSH conjugates that are present in the tubular urine. This action prevents excessive excretion of GSH precursors (GSH itself does not cross membranes). γ-Glutamyl transpeptidase is identical to phosphate-independent glutaminase (72); glutaminase activity predominates at low pH (~ 6). Overall, the S3 segment has greater activity of enzymes associated with biotransformation of chemicals and high capacity to concentrate chemicals intracellularly. Moreover, the S3 segment exists in the medullary region in which low blood flow, low hematocrit, and countercurrent exchange of O_2 combine to create a relatively hypoxic environment. These factors may contribute to apparent sensitivity of this region to nephrotoxic chemicals.

Juxtamedullary nephrons have long, hairpin-like loops of Henle that extend into the medulla and papilla. In contrast, the loop of Henle segments of superficial nephrons do not descend into the medulla. The tubular epithelia of the descending and ascending portions have different permeabilities to water, urea, sodium, and chloride. These selective permeabilities allow the urine to become concentrated relative to plasma (4,32,41). In the kidneys of an animal producing concentrated urine, a gradient of tissue osmolality develops from the cortex (isosmotic with plasma) to the medulla (up to four times plasma osmolality). This gradient is initiated by reabsorption of chloride in the thick segment of the ascending limb (Figure 25.2D) and is magnified by counterflow exchange between the loop of Henle and the vasa recta, the vasa recta removing excess water during times of urine concentration. As the tubular fluid travels to the distal tubule, osmolytes are extruded and remain trapped in the interstitium. High tissue osmolality is achieved and maintained within the inner reaches of the medulla and papilla, and the urine is again concentrated as it passes through the collecting duct to the ureter. The chloride reabsorptive process results in movement of chloride ion against an electrochemical gradient (128).

In vitro studies have shown that the rate of chloride transport is increased in the presence of sodium or potassium. The thick ascending limb has the highest Na^+, K^+-ATPase activity and highest density of mitochondria of all the nephron segments. Energy for this work is derived from glycolysis (8). Chloride reabsorption is inhibited by the "high-ceiling" diuretics (61,62); and the result, excretion of large volumes of relatively dilute urine, is a common finding in chemical-induced acute failure. Inhibition of Cl transport by nephrotoxic agents has not been identified as a mechanism of nephrotoxicity; however, the osmotic gradient crucial to elaboration of concentrated urine may be "washed out" by high urine flow rates, possibly contributing to failure to concentrate urine. Furthermore, evidence suggests that most nephrotoxicants act on proximal tubule segments.

The distal tubule is a heterogeneous segment anatomically and functionally (Figure 25.2E). It appears to include as many as four distinct regions between the macula densa and the first confluence of the "distal" segment with another tubule segment (36). This complex distal segment has been referred to as the cortical diluting segment, partly because active sodium transport occurs essentially independently of fluid movement, leading to formation of a dilute tubular fluid.

Late in the distal tubule (or perhaps in the collecting duct) potassium ion enters the tubular fluid. Although net secretion of potassium can occur, the overwhelming body of evidence suggests that potassium entry into the nephron is largely a passive event. However, details of the mechanisms are not absolutely certain. Classically, potassium secretion was associated with a sodium reabsorptive process and referred to as a sodium–potassium exchange. Although the concept of a one-for-one exchange has been useful, there is little doubt that the active sodium reabsorptive component is not linked directly to the passive potassium secretory process. Apparently, the major role of the sodium reabsorption is to generate a favorable electrochemical gradient for potassium entry from the distal tubular cell, which has a high intracellular potassium concentration. Blockade of the sodium reabsorption, with an appropriate diuretic or by the presence of a nonreabsorbable anion, reduces or eliminates potassium secretion (155).

It is also in the distal segment of the nephron that urinary acidification occurs. This consideration is important because alterations in tubular fluid pH may greatly affect passive reabsorption (nonionic diffusion) of organic compounds in this nephron segment. Hence, a nephrotoxic substance with an appropriate pK might be recycled in the distal segment of the nephron through passive reabsorption of the un-ionized chemical moiety, which might then allow enhanced exposure of the distal tubular cells to an undesirable chemical, as well as permit a prolonged stay of the substance in the blood. Despite the potential exposure of distal tubular cells to nephrotoxic compounds, it is noteworthy that the proximal tubular segments are those most often affected.

Regulation of Renal Function

In addition to the extrinsic mechanisms that determine the rate of glomerular filtration, the kidneys have intrinsic feedback mechanisms that control GFR. The distal tubule of each nephron loops back and makes contact with the afferent and efferent arterioles of its own glomerulus. This area is called the juxtaglomerular apparatus (JGA) and is composed of specialized cells of the distal tubular epithelium called the macula densa cells, Goormaghtigh cells (which contain contractile fibrils), and granular cells, near the arterioles. The Goormaghtigh cells are between the macula densa and granular cells and are in contact with both. The macula densa cells sense a change in the composition of the distal tubular fluid associated with a change in the rate of fluid flow.

The exact nature of the signal and the mechanism of decreased glomerular filtration are the subjects of some controversy. Feedback control is blunted by inhibition of angiotensin II (AII) synthesis or blocking of its receptors. An increased release of AII causes contraction of the afferent arteriole, decreasing blood flow and therefore the rate of filtration in that nephron. The overall result is that the rate of filtration is decreased when the quantity of tubular fluid is increased; thus, tubuloglomerular feedback can be thought of as a means for preventing massive fluid loss when the tubule cannot reabsorb the quantity of fluid delivered to it by filtration. Normally, approximately 99.6 percent of the glomerular filtrate is reabsorbed by the tubule. If filtration were to continue at normal rates when reabsorptive capacity is impaired, fluid losses and derangements of selectivity and balance would occur. Nephrotoxic chemicals generally impair tubular function without affecting the glomeruli; yet decreased GFR is often observed (either directly or indirectly). When it occurs, GFR is decreased by feedback mechanisms. With severe damage, feedback regulation either is not complete or is impaired, and the urine output is increased even though the GFR is decreased. In this situation the reabsorption of water may fall to 80 percent of the filtered load (as happens with the tubular toxicant hexachloro-1,3-butadiene). If feedback regulation is perfect, the amount of filtrate formed, relative to the amount of plasma delivered (the filtration fraction, GFR/RPF [renal plasma flow]), is constant. Inhibition of glomerulotubular feedback allows excessive fluid losses and occurs with nephrotoxic agents (potassium dichromate) and diuretics. (It is probably

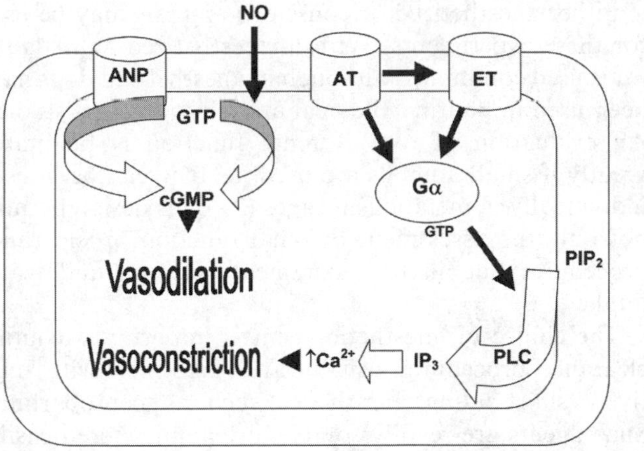

FIG. 25.3. Signal transduction mechanisms for control of renal blood flow by factors. Atrial natriuretic peptide (ANP), angiotensin (AT) and endothelin (ET) receptors are shown. The ANP receptor includes guanyl cyclase activity nitric oxide (NO) activates, soluble guanyl cyclase. AT and ET receptors activate a G protein that then activates membrane-bound phospholipase C, eventually resulting in increased intracellular Ca^{2+}.

important for the large diuresis seen with furosemide and other "high-ceding" diuretics.) Because of this feedback, it is possible to see either an increase or a decrease of urine volume after damage to the tubule.

The kidneys are influenced by an array of hormones, peptides, and factors that either constrict or relax the renal vasculature (Figure 25.3). The effects of angiotensin II, bradykinin, epinephrine, norepinephrine, dopamine, and various arachidonic acid metabolites have been well studied and do not appear to initiate acute renal failure. Dopamine agonists have the potential to decrease renal vascular resistance and so increase renal blood flow and glomerular filtration. Clinical experience has been disappointing; however, the more specific agonists for dopamine-1 receptor hold promise (33).

More recently, interest has focused on atrial natriuretic peptide (ANP) (9,66,111) and endothelial-derived vasoactive factors that mediate either dilation (endothelial-erived relaxing factor, EDRF) (15,133) or constriction (9,21,133). ANP is a 24-amino-acid peptide that was first found in extracts of atrial muscle. Administration of ANP causes a dramatic increase of GFR and sodium excretion. The effect on renal blood flow is variable; however, there is dilation of the afferent arterioles which, with the increase of K_f, accounts for the natriuresis. Analogs of ANP are beneficial in experimental ischemic and nephrotoxic acute renal failure. EDRF is nitric oxide (NO), synthesized from arginine by nitric oxide synthase (NOS). Kidneys are under tonic influence of NO and blocking its synthesis decreases renal perfusion and glomerular filtration (49). The kidneys are able to synthesize arginine from aspartate and citrulline, and kidneys are an important source because arginine synthesized in the liver is mostly further metabolized (107,108).

Lack of arginine production may be an important component of kidney damage. NO and ANP both produce vasodilation by stimulating guanylate cyclase, resulting in formation of cGMP. Endothelin is a 21-amino-acid peptide that occurs as three isoforms; the most prevalent is ET-1. It causes renal vasoconstriction and decreases GFR and likely works in a paracrine manner. Endothelin is short-lived but its effects on the vasculature are prolonged. Endothelin vasoconstriction is mediated by G-protein-linked receptors that have seven transmembrane domains. Activation of the receptor activates the phospholipase C–inositol trisphosphate cascade to increase intracellular Ca^{2+}, and causing constriction of vascular smooth muscle (6,9). Angiotensin II causes vasoconstriction by the same signal transduction pathway and ET receptor antagonists block angiotensin II-induced vasoconstriction, indicating that angiotensin II effects are mediated, in part, by endothelin (47,126).

Normal renal function requires a delicate balance amongst these factors and the sequelae of altering one depend on appropriate compensatory adjustments in the others (18). Endothelin stimulates release of ANP, which counteracts endothelin effects. Activation of ET_B receptors stimulates a brief release of NO and resultant transient decrease of blood pressure. NO also diminishes the magnitude of the Ca^{2+} transient and causes endothelin to be released from its receptor (83). Experimental studies suggest roles for these factors in various forms of acute and chronic renal failure (15,21).

The control of renal function is an integral part of kidney activity, and the control mechanisms are possible targets for the action of toxic agents. The ability of the kidney to modulate renal hemodynamics complicates assessment of the actions of nephrotoxicants. Because the kidneys compensate for their own deficiencies, one must use relatively sophisticated, and usually invasive, techniques to monitor the early phases of renal failure. Only detection of relatively massive impairment is possible with routine screening procedures. Furthermore, the effect of nephrotoxicant action on renal control mechanisms has been relatively infrequently evaluated.

ROLE OF MORPHOLOGICAL STUDIES

It is accepted that all functional studies in toxicology should be coupled with appropriate histological studies. Although this approach is commonplace, it is important to know if information that is not available from the physiological or biochemical experiments, can be gained from morphological studies.

Appropriate morphological studies are useful, especially for anatomical localization of the action of a nephrotoxin. Studies by Oliver and others (98) have demonstrated localization of the chromium ion in the proximal convoluted tubule of the kidney, whereas mercury produces its greatest morphological damage in the pars recta. These morphological observations were not helpful in understanding the mechanisms underlying the acute renal failure syndrome produced by these metals. In general, routine morphological studies with light microscopy are most useful for corroborating the data from appropriately planned physiological or biochemical studies. For example, if the action of a nephrotoxicant was thought to depend on renal metabolism of the chemical to a reactive form, evidence of damage to S3 cells would support that supposition and would be seen as damage to the corticomedullary junction (36).

Electron microscopic studies may prove more useful than routine light microscopy studies. With adequate sophistication, for example, it might be possible to identify a toxin effect on the plasma membrane before changes in other subcellular organelles were observed. Although not directly indicative of a mechanism of action, such studies might help localize toxin effects on specific cell types. In addition, subcellular sites of action might be observed with electron microscopy.

METHODS FOR MEASURING RENAL TOXICITY

To properly assess renal dysfunction as related to the toxic effects produced by xenobiotics, it is necessary to utilize a battery of techniques. The complexity and diversity of function at various sites along the nephron (sometimes referred to as intranephron heterogeneity) precludes the use of a single technique for examination of renal function, whether the assessment is for normal physiological function or renal toxicology. Under most circumstances more than one of the procedures discussed below is necessary to determine adequately the presence of renal toxicity.

Whole-Animal Experiments

In general, studies involving whole animals utilize one or another form of "clearance experiment." The exact procedures vary from traditional clearance measurements to the use of micropuncture techniques. Some of the routine procedures discussed here also are useful with other experimental approaches and are not repeated subsequently.

Either anesthetized or conscious animals may be used for these experiments. With unanesthetized animals the rat is used commonly, although unanesthetized dogs have been used in pharmacological and physiological studies. An evaluation of overall renal function is facilitated greatly if small animals are used, as they can be housed individually in metabolism cages (2). This design permits not only the assessment of renal function by clearance procedures but also measurements of feed and water intake.

The choice of anesthetic agent is important. Routine clearance procedures usually are performed with relatively short-acting anesthetics such as pentobarbital. Such agents are readily soluble, are administered easily, and are relatively inexpensive. Once injected (usually 30–60 mg/kg ip, depending on species), the level of anesthesia remains relatively constant without frequent supplementation. If "minute-to-minute" control over the anesthesia is desired, volatile or gaseous agents can be administered with anesthesia machines. Such devices are available for small animals (69). However, less information concerning effects on renal function is available for the volatile agents.

Although it is generally suggested that anesthetics do not alter blood flow to vital organs, caution should be taken with respect to the kidney. Walker et al. (149) studied the effects of anesthesia in trained, conscious, chronically catheterized rats. Pentobarbital and inactin each produced an approximately 25% reduction in renal blood flow and GFR. Furthermore, in experiments where ether anesthesia was used, these same parameters failed to recover for several days after recovery from the anesthesia. These observations should be considered when anesthetized rats are used for renal function studies.

Because anesthetic agents may significantly affect renal function such an experimental design may complicate a study of the effect of xenobiotics on renal function; that is, interaction of anesthetics with compounds that adversely affect renal function is possible. Little or no information is available concerning such interactions, but they may be important in renal toxicology studies.

The use of anesthetized animals permits greater precision in the conduct of clearance experiments, better control with respect to problems of fluid balance, achievement and maintenance of desired blood levels of a given test substance, assessment of early and direct toxic events, and so forth. Although precision with respect to the above parameters is greatly enhanced by the use of anesthetized animals, to some extent flexibility in experimental design is lost.

Clearance Experiments

A procedure fundamental to whole-animal studies is the clearance technique. Details of clearance calculations as applied to renal physiology are discussed in any number of references (e.g., Brenner [4], Pitts [24]). These procedures involve the accurate assessment of the blood (P_x) and urine (U_x) concentrations of the substance under study, as well as urine flow rates (V). Either glomerular or tubular function can be quantified with the clearance techniques depending on which test substance is used. The renal clearance calculation is the same regardless of whether glomerular or tubular function is being determined. The classical clearance equation is:

$$C_x = \frac{U_x V}{P_x}$$

and defines the clearance (C) of compound x. The clearance represents the quantity of blood or plasma cleared of the substance per unit time and has units of volume (usually milliliters) $\times t^{-1}$.

The renal physiologist routinely uses the clearance procedure to calculate GFR by monitoring the renal handling of inulin or creatinine (Figure 25.4). The effective renal plasma flow also can be measured if a marker is used that is excreted not only by filtration but by active tubular secretion as well. PAH is a good example of a substance whose clearance can be equated to the effective renal plasma flow if the organic anion transport system is intact.

The basic methodology of clearance experiments requires that the test substances be administered so that a relatively constant concentration of the substance is maintained in the plasma. Urine samples are collected over a set period of time, and blood samples are taken contemporaneously (either at the midpoint of the urine collection or before and after the urine collection period). If anesthetized animals are used, a vein and an artery are cannulated for infusion of test substance and collection of blood, respectively. Urine is obtained from either a large-diameter catheter placed in the bladder or by cannulating the ureters. (For a detailed discussion of clearance methods for the rat, see Simmons [142]). For conscious animals, inulin can be administered as a subcutaneous bolus in gelatin (32% w/v) (76). The solution is viscous and serves as a depot for inulin. The clearance period is begun 60 min after the injection; the rats are stimulated to urinate prior to placing them in metabolism cages to collect urine. Usually a 60-min collection period is sufficient to obtain an adequate sample. At the end of the period, a blood sample is taken from either the tail vein or the abdominal aorta (if the rat is to be killed).

The same clearance procedures can be applied to an analysis of the renal handling of any substance. If the clearance of substance x is greater than that calculated for a glomerular marker such as inulin, that is, greater than the GFR, it may be concluded that substance x is added to the tubular fluid by mechanisms other than just filtration. Clearance values as large as those for PAH are suggestive of active tubular secretion, as well as glomerular filtration, with little or no reabsorption. Clearance values that are less than those for glomerular filtration suggest that tubular reabsorption may have occurred. The reabsorptive process may be either active or passive. Passive reabsorptive processes (nonionic diffusion) are highly pH- and flow-dependent. For example, salicylate excretion can be greatly reduced by acidification of the urine or greatly increased by alkalinization. Excretion of a substance such as PAH is not affected by changes in urine pH.

Before the significance of clearance data can be determined, it is important to know about the plasma protein binding of the test substance. As indicated earlier, small molecular weight substances bound to plasma proteins are not filtered at the glomerulus. The magnitude of the protein binding is important for interpretation of clearance data, and several routine procedures are available for such measurements. Ultrafiltration procedures utilizing filter cones (Amicon Corporation, Lexington, MA) yield good results. These cones do not prevent the passage of all plasma proteins. However, the leakage is small and does not complicate the overall analysis. Furthermore, these cones have a loose matrix and relatively larger surface area, which permit rapid filtration. Analysis of the ultrafiltrate and the original plasma for the compound under study gives information about binding. Equilibrium dialysis also is used for analysis of plasma protein binding. The method of McMenanry (117) is more rapid than older procedures and gives results comparable to those for ultrafiltration or older equilibrium dialysis procedures. Unquestionably, ultrafiltration is technically simpler and more rapid; and although somewhat expensive to initiate, it is preferred for routine use.

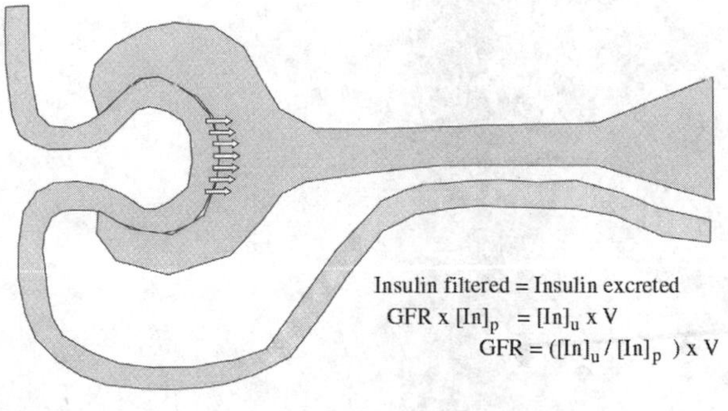

FIG. 25.4. Glomerular filtration process and calculation the glomerular filtration rate in the physiology of the kidney.

Computation of the GFR based on the clearance of a substance such as inulin is an important technique for assessing glomerular integrity. Substances such as inulin—which are not reabsorbed by the renal tubules, are not bound to plasma proteins, are small enough to pass the glomerular filter, and have no pharmacological effects—are ideal for the measurement of GFR. If inulin clearance values are below the expected normal, glomerular function may be compromised. Several chemical analyses for inulin are available and are discussed below and described in detail elsewhere (34). Inulin clearance also can be assessed with radiochemical procedures. Both [^{3}H]-inulin and [^{14}C]-inulin are available for use in experimental animals. Radioactivity in urine and plasma samples can be determined easily by standard liquid scintillation techniques.

Other ways to assess glomerular function involve the measurement of some normally occurring constituents of the blood. Blood urea nitrogen (BUN) may be the most commonly used procedure for assessing glomerular function. As filtration slows or ceases, BUN rises. The relation between BUN and glomerular function has been studied by many, and an example of this relation is seen in Figure 25.5. The plasma creatinine level parallels that of BUN and frequently is used as a marker for glomerular filtration. The relation depicted in Figure 25.5 allows accurate assessment of remaining renal function for a given value of BUN. Figure 25.5 also shows that substantial loss of renal function can occur before BUN or plasma creatinine concentrations rise above normal; that is, BUN or plasma creatinine determinations do not detect a modest impairment of renal function. Control values for BUN are well established for every commonly used laboratory animal, and often a single value considerably in excess of known controls is predictive of renal dysfunction. These analyses are effective for both the chronic renal failure patient and the subject or animal that has ingested a nephrotoxic xenobiotic and is experiencing acute renal failure.

In general, elevations of BUN or plasma creatinine can be used as an index of decreased glomerular filtration. Ordinarily, the BUN/creatinine ratio is about 10 : 1. Hence, a BUN measurement of 50 mg/dl or a creatinine measurement of about 5 mg/dl suggests that the GFR was approximately 25% of normal, as indicated in Figure 25.5. Under some circumstances the BUN/creatinine ratio can be altered. For example, any situation that would increase the amount of protein that is metabolized to urea (e.g., high protein intake, increased catabolism) may cause a selectivc risc in BUN. Dehydration may also do it but not because of an effect on urea synthesis. Dehydration results in a decreased tubular fluid flow rate, and under these conditions the percentage of the filtered urea reabsorbed is increased (31), a situation that does not occur with creatinine. Care should be taken in toxicological studies to ensure that these extraneous events are not disrupting the BUN or the BUN/creatinine ratio, either of which might be misleading with respect to glomerular function.

Plasma creatinine concentrations can be determined routinely and simply by a variety of methods, as can PAH and inulin. The details of these chemical analyses are presented elsewhere (34). PAH is determined by the method of Bratton and Marshall (61), as modified by Smith (34), which involves a diazotization of PAH with *N*-(2-naphthyl)ethylenediainine dihydrochloride after nitrite reduction in acid. The color formed is stable for relatively long periods of time, and the color intensity,

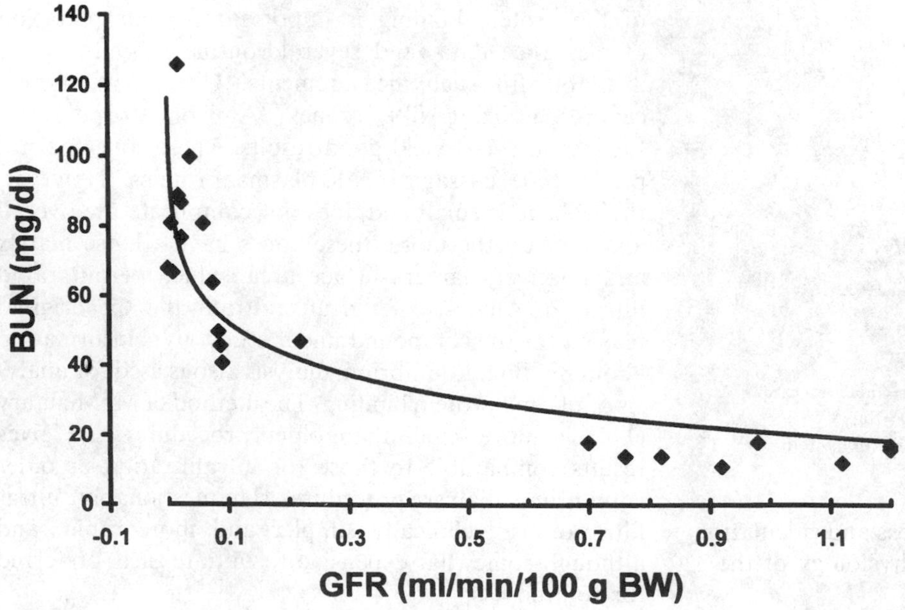

FIG. 25.5. Relation between BUN and glomerular filtration rate in the Spraguc–Dawley rat.

which can be determined spectrophotometrically, is directly related to PAH concentration.

The inulin analyses, in general, involve hydrolysis of the polysaccharide followed by determination of the fructose by colorimetric analysis. Several methods are available (see Smith [34] for details) and are of approximately equal utility. Specific techniques for measurement of BUN are somewhat more complicated (51) but are used routinely. Indeed, some of these analyses have been developed into commercial kits intended for routine use. Although these kits are cookbook-like, there has been no loss of precision or sensitivity.

Although not strictly speaking a clearance procedure, measurement of the urinary excretion of proteins is important for the assessment of glomerular integrity (1,16). The selective permeability of the glomerular membranes is an important aspect of normal renal function (62). In general, the selectivity of the barrier is decreased by renal disease and by the actions of various nephrotoxic xenobiotics. Hence, a common occurrence in renal failure is the excretion of excessive amounts of plasma proteins into the urine.

However, not all proteinurias should be interpreted as evidence of glomerular dysfunction. The so-called tubular proteinurias (1,16,67,112) probably are indicative of normal filtration of relatively small molecular weight proteins coupled with the failure of the tubular uptake mechanisms for these proteins. Protein also enters urine as a consequence of proximal tubule necrosis and loss of the brush border. The microvilli are sloughed into the lumen (and may coalesce, forming casts); this debris contains cellular protein and is excreted in the urine. Frequently, to resolve this problem it is necessary to use electrophoretic analyses of the urinary proteins, so that the specific proteins can be identified. However, any time an experimental animal excretes large amounts of protein in the urine after the administration of a suspected nephrotoxicant, one should be concerned about the possibility of glomerular dysfunction.

The renal clearance of PAH or similar organic ions is a quantitative expression of renal tubular secretory activity (Figure 25.6) and is a measure of the effective renal plasma flow (if transport capacity has not been impaired by a tubular toxicant). However, renal extraction of PAH can be calculated from measurements of arterial and renal venous PAH concentrations and is used to correct the effective renal plasma flow. Correction of the plasma flow for hematocrit yields renal blood flow. Details of these procedures are given by Smith (34).

$$\textit{renal plasma flow} = \frac{C_{PAH}}{E_{PAH}}$$

$$\textit{renal blood flow} = \frac{\textit{renal plasma flow}}{1 - \textit{hematocrit}}$$

where C_{PAH} is PAH clearance and E_{PAH} is PAH extraction by the kidney.

The intrarenal distribution of blood also may be altered by nephrotoxins. Whether such an action represents the primary disruption of renal function that leads to acute renal failure is unclear. Nonetheless, such effects might be important and suggest a vascular action of nephrotoxic compounds. Yarger et al. (159) examined procedures for measurement of both nutrient and glomerular blood flow, and their article should be reviewed for specific details. Rubidium-86 (^{86}Rb) distribution in the renal cortex and medulla gives an approximation of total renal blood distribution within the kidney. If a nephrotoxicant shunted blood flow from cortex to medulla, it might be expected that intrarenal ^{86}Rb distribution would become greater in medullary regions and lesser in cortical regions. The techniques involved are demanding. Injection of ^{86}Rb intravenously is followed immediately by the continuous collection of arterial blood samples to determine the arterial blood concentration curve. After 15–30 sec from the time of injection, the kidneys are removed and dissected into cortical and medullary regions. Blood and tissue samples are counted for radioactivity, and regional blood distribution is calculated as described by Yarger et al. (159).

The use of radioactive microspheres allows assessment of glomerular blood flow. The microspheres are tagged with a variety of short- and long-half-life γ-emitting isotopes and are of such a size as to lodge in the glomerular capillaries. Hence, by dissecting the renal cortex it is possible to learn whether glomerular flow has shifted, for example, to the inner cortical regions in response to a nephrotoxicant. Both renal blood flow (from microsphere clearance) and regional (cortical) blood flow can be calculated as indicated by Yarger et al. (159).

Although nutrient and glomerular blood flow measurements may be helpful in toxicological studies,

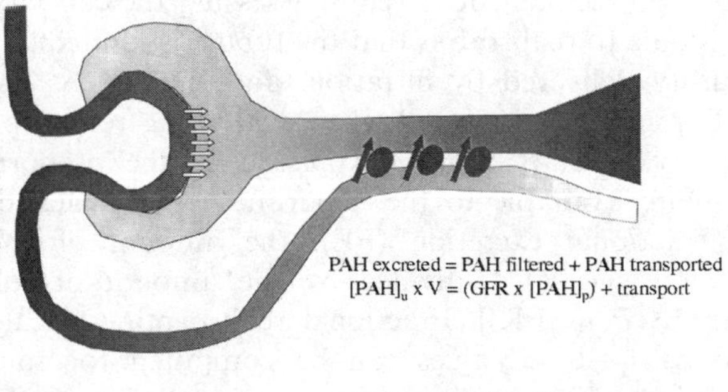

PAH excreted = PAH filtered + PAH transported
$[PAH]_u \times V = (GFR \times [PAH]_p)$ + transport

FIG. 25.6. Renal handling of PAH as an example of tubular secretion.

these techniques have been used relatively little. Rather than being connected with toxicology, these procedures usually are associated with studies in renal physiology. Although studies of renal blood or plasma flow have been useful for examining toxin effects on renal vascular effects (e.g., a suspected primary mechanism of action), emphasis should be placed on more standard clearance procedures.

Alterations in the ability of the kidney to concentrate the urine are important. Frequently, potential nephrotoxins reduce the ability of an animal to concentrate the urine (54,57). Even in those situations where urinary volume is reduced significantly by the nephrotoxin, the ability to concentrate urine still fails. Changes in urine osmolality occur early after administration of a nephrotoxin and frequently warn of more serious consequences to ensue. Measurements of urine osmolality are technically simple. Most commercially available osmometers measure osmolality by freezing point depression and provide "direct reading" (milliosmoles per liter) capability. Measurement of specific gravity yields similar information but not with as much accuracy or precision.

An important point with respect to effects on urine osmolality is that these actions are not nephrotoxicant-specific. Regardless of the xenobiotic (e.g., metals, solvents, drugs), decreased urinary osmolality occurs, usually as a prelude to other events. Thus, nephrotoxin-induced alteration of urine-concentrating ability has not proved useful for analyses of mechanisms of action.

Tubular Function

The variety of functions subserved by the tubular segments of the nephron are readily accessible to examination by the investigator. These tests can evaluate tubular secretory as well as tubular reabsorptive activities and, at least in part, may give insights into mechanisms of action.

One problem encountered in assessing the capacity of the tubule to reabsorb is that the tubule is limited by the quantity delivered by filtration, and thus decreases of GFR must be considered when evaluating reabsorptive capacity. Results can be expressed as the proportion of solute available to the nephron; it is calculated as the fractional excretion (FE): the amount of solute excreted, $[(U_x)(V)]$, divided by the amount of solute filtered $[(P_x)(\mathrm{GFR})]$. Fractional reabsorption is calculated as $1-\mathrm{FE}$. Values can be computed for solutes or volume. The reabsorptive capacity of a nephron for glucose is well established (see above) (Figure 25.7). Frequently, a nephrotoxicant causes increased excretion in the urine of moderate to large amounts of glucose in the absence of an elevated blood glucose. Fractional excretion of glucose is normally zero and can be increased to 100% of the filtered load after a nephrotoxic agent. Of course, it is important to establish that the blood glucose has remained normal and that the glucosuria observed is not the result of the production of a diabetes mellitus-like syndrome. Glucose determinations are accomplished most readily by the specific glucose oxidase procedure. This technique has been adapted to commercially available kits for routine use. The specificity of the technique is such that other reducing sugars do not interfere.

Excretion of proteins in urine can be monitored as an index of renal function (1,16). Excretion of high molecular weight proteins (MW>40000 daltons) is considered to reflect increased permeability of the filtration barrier and is referred to as glomerular proteinuria. Small molecular weight proteins that are filtered at the glomerulus are normally reabsorbed by the proximal tubules and this function is compromised by damage to the tubules, resulting in tubular proteinuria. Normally, some albumin is filtered and reabsorbed as well. These proteins will be detected with urine dipsticks, as will proteins that have been shed into the urine following damage to tubules or other structures of the urinary tract. To determine the source of the protein, the MW of the proteins is estimated by electrophoretic separation and detection by staining (122).

Secretory activity of the nephron can be monitored by examining the excretion of PAH as noted above. The clearance of this compound can be used to measure total renal blood flow because it is actively secreted by the proximal tubular cells into the tubular lumen. Thus, the reduced excretion of PAH after the administration of a nephrotoxicant may be the result of interference with the active tubular secretory process or the direct disrup-

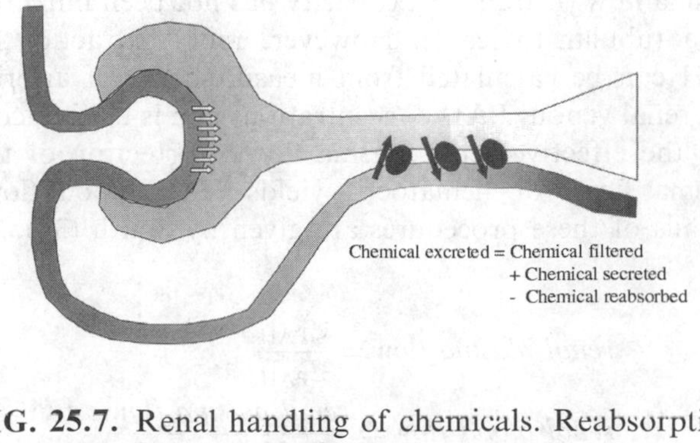

FIG. 25.7. Renal handling of chemicals. Reabsorption by passive diffusion also occurs.

tion of blood flow to prevent the delivery of blood to the proximal tubular cells. Experimental protocols other than clearance experiments are needed to distinguish between these possible actions. For example, measurement of PAH transport by renal cortical slices, determination of the renal extraction of PAH with in vivo experiments, or measurement of total renal blood flow with electromagnetic or Doppler flow probes help distinguish between these events. Animals (human, dog, rat) with normal renal function extract 80–90 percent of the PAH present in the arterial blood in a single passage through the kidney. Although PAH is filtered at the glomerulus, the major component in this extraction process is active tubular secretion (27). Measurement of renal extraction of PAH is facilitated by the use of large animals. Experiments can be done in rats, but care is required with the renal vein catheterization.

Another organic anion, phenolsulfophthalein (PSP), has been used by Plaa and Larsen (123) to assess tubular activity in mice. This anion is excreted in a manner similar to that for PAH; and although not used to assess renal blood flow as such, it has been useful in defining the functional integrity of the kidney. PSP is injected into control animals, and the rapidity of its urinary excretion by conscious, intact animals is compared to that of animals treated with the suspected nephrotoxicant. Although significant animal to animal variation occurs, this technique has proved useful for studies on certain nephrotoxic compounds. Although the procedure was first developed for studies in the mouse, it can be adapted to the rat. Its major utility is to allow the assessment of renal function in conscious, small animals. Details of the analytical procedures, described by Plaa and Larsen (123), essentially involve only urine collection on filter paper, extraction of the filter paper, and colorimetric determination of the PSP.

The effects of nephrotoxic compounds, particularly heavy metals, on renal tubular absorption of sodium and potassium also are in the assessment of renal function. Frequently, metals interfere with sodium reabsorption and may produce dramatic effects on potassium excretion as well (20). However, assessment of tubular dysfunction by urinary sodium and/or potassium analysis offers no advantages to testing for PAH excretion or glucose reabsorption. The sodium and potassium analyses (primarily by flame emission photometry), although not complex, offer no simplifications over routine colorimetric studies for glucose or PAH. Furthermore, no enhanced sensitivity with respect to the detection of renal dysfunction has been reported with measurements of urine concentration. Fractional excretion of sodium is an important index of renal reabsorptive capacity and can be used to demonstrate impaired reabsorptive capacity even in the presence of decreased urine output.

Renal Enzymes

Some investigators (16,118) have suggested that analysis of some "renal enzymes" might be useful in the early detection of nephrotoxicity induced by exogenous compounds or in identifying which specific tubular regions have been damaged. Specifically, maltase, *N*-acetyl-*β*-D-glucosaminidase, alanine aminopeptidase, lactate dehydrogenase, and alkaline phosphatase have been suggested as candidates (16,22).

Although investigations of urinary enzymes as markers for nephrotoxicity have not been pursued vigorously, several workers (118,145) have demonstrated the possible utility of such an approach. Stroo and Hook (145) found that mercury caused increased urinary enzyme activities at doses lower than those that elevated BUN. Although neither chromium nor uranium showed selectivity for the brush border enzymes, the early onset of an effect caused by chromium can be interpreted as evidence of the sensitivity of the technique. Nonmetallic substances known to produce nephrotoxicity (e.g., carbon tetrachloride) did not release brush border enzymes at doses lower than those that elevated BUN. Nomiyama et al. (118) reported that changes in urinary enzymes (alkaline phosphatase, glutamic oxaloacetic transaminase) occur early after administration of uranyl nitrate. Unfortunately, measurements earlier than 24 h after injection were not undertaken, so it is difficult to evaluate which urinary parameter (enzymes, inulin clearance, etc.) was first to respond. Enzymuria was found in rats treated with erythritol in a two-year feeding study. Enzymuria occurred in the absence of other signs of nephrotoxicity (histopathological, elevated BUN, or creatinine) and was attributed to diuresis (109).

Care must be taken to ensure that the enzymes being measured are not inactivated in the urine during urine collection, which may extend over several hours. To avoid this problem, technical arrangements may be needed, for example, that permit collection of the urine in an ice bath. Obviously, the collection of urine from rats in metabolism cages may be complicated if the collections are for more than a few hours. The presence of enzyme inhibitors in the urine may also prove troublesome. Frequently, however, this problem can be avoided by dialyzing the urine sample for 12 h or 24 h before making the enzyme measurement. Because the urinary concentration of some of the enzymes is relatively low, it may be necessary to concentrate the urine before the assays can be undertaken. Although all of the above technical difficulties are surmountable, they have contributed to a generalized lack of interest in this procedure for the routine assessment of urinary dysfunction.

In general, all the analytical procedures required for the renal function tests discussed above (except enzyme analyses) are relatively straightforward. The chemical analyses for glomerular filtration or tubular function markers (e.g., inulin, PAH) have been described in great detail elsewhere (34,61), and these specific chemical analyses have not been repeated here. All the procedures involve standard colorimetric or spectrophotometric analyses of relatively stable, colored products. In some instances, efforts have been made to utilize radiochemical analyses instead of colorimetric tests. Once again, these tests are routine.

Many of the above clearance-type procedures have considerable utility as screening methods for nephrotoxicity. Under these circumstances, individual animals are housed in metabolism cages, and urine samples are collected for 12–24 h. For screening purposes it may be sufficient to measure urinary excretion of protein, glucose, and other materials, by standard dipstick procedures that give a qualitative assessment of these substances in the urine. These procedures, coupled with assessment of urinary volume and urinary osmolality, reveal quickly the possibility of xenobiotic-induced nephrotoxicity. Although the dipstick methods yield primarily qualitative results, there is no loss of specificity. The colorimetric procedures used are in every case just as specific as the quantitative analytical analyses; indeed, in many cases (e.g., glucose), the same procedures have been adapted to the dipstick approach. These methods have been used for studies with metals (54) and various organic substances (55,56).

Micropuncture Techniques

Micropuncture methodology is used to determine tubular sites of action and to quantitate transport processes in the single nephron. These techniques allow direct assessment of tubular fluid concentration, tubular fluid flow rates, and other renal functions in an intact, anesthetized animal. Because of the sophistication of this technology, micropuncture is especially susceptible to the introduction of technical errors and misinterpretation of results. These techniques are not to be adopted by the casual investigator or to be planned for routine screening procedures. Renal micropuncture methodology is not used routinely by toxicologists to assess renal function; rather, some micropuncture experts have adapted their techniques to the study of toxic substances (e.g., Smith [34]; Baylis et al. [49]; Kramp et al. [98]; Rodeheaver [129]).

No attempt is made here to detail procedures or methods. Those interested in developing micropuncture techniques in their own laboratories would be required to train with a known micropuncturist. Only through such on-the-job training could one acquire the necessary skills and knowledge to develop the techniques in a new laboratory. Detailed descriptions of the methodology have been published (26,40,141). A few general comments, however, are in order.

Fundamental to many micropuncture procedures is the ability of the micropunctinist to collect measured samples of tubular fluid without influencing the formation of tubular fluid. Most workers try to obviate this problem by limiting their collections to very small volumes or collecting only a small fraction of the tubular fluid flow past a given point in the nephron. If these two restrictions are maintained, collections can be undertaken without the presence of an oil droplet. However, when these techniques are applied to the calculation of the single-nephron filtration rate, a difficulty may be that the volume of fluid collected is so small that accurate fluid concentrations of the glomerular marker cannot be determined.

The stationary, microperfusion, or split oil droplet technique has been popular. This procedure allows assessment of tubular function in a restricted area of the nephron; and, theoretically, it might be advantageous to the toxicologist looking at the effects of toxicants on tubular function. Gertz et al. (81) perfected this technique as follows: A droplet of castor oil is split by injection of the perfusion solution into the oil, and the change in the volume of the aqueous droplet is assessed photomicrographically as the two oil droplets approach each other. Because the osmolality of the proximal tubular fluid and proximal tubular reabsorbate are essential isosmotic, observations on the rate of disappearance of the droplet from between the oil plugs allow estimation of proximal tubular sodium chloride transport.

Tubular micropuncture and perfusion have been combined with capillary microperfusion to elucidate structural requirements for organic ion transport across the luminal or peritubular surface of the proximal tubule in situ (148). This technique has been applied to assess the relative sensitivities of the brush border and basolateral sides of the proximal tubule cell to cisplatin toxicity (43).

The tubular microinjection technique is one that has great utility for the assessment of tubular permeability characteristics and that should be of considerable value to those with an interest in toxicology (26,40). With this procedure, a small volume of fluid containing radioactive inulin or other isotopes is injected into some part of the nephron during a free-flow situation. Serial urine samples are collected from the injected and contralateral kidneys and assayed for the compound injected. This technique is a relatively simple one for micropuncture studies and avoids such problems as the effects of oil on tubular function. The effects of nephrotoxicants on tubular permeability could be assessed readily with such a technique. For example, if inulin recovery was greatly reduced after injection of a suspected nephrotoxin, it would probably mean that the inulin was leaking out of the injected nephron somewhere along its course. Although it would not prove that the nephrotoxicant was acting directly on the nephron as opposed to the vasculature, it would clearly indicate that the tubular permeability to inulin had been changed.

The value of all micropuncture technology depends to a large extent on the stability of the animal preparation. It is necessary to use an anesthetic that has minimal effects on renal blood flow, systemic blood flow, and so on. In addition, one should take all necessary precautions to ensure that the surgical procedures involved, which are extensive, are as atraumatic as possible so as to preserve the stability of the animal. Once again, these techniques are best learned at the hands of the masters in the field and are essential for successful experiments. Detailed reviews on this methodology, its pitfalls, and its utilities are available (26,40).

Studies with Isolated Tissues: In Vitro versus In Vivo

In general, studies with isolated tissues or subcellular fractions are directed at the mechanisms of action of nephrotoxic compounds rather than simply a description of a nephrotoxic event. Isolated tissue techniques offer several advantages over studies in intact animals. Specific transport studies can be undertaken without unwanted influences or alterations in GFR or renal blood flow, either of which may affect the availability of metabolites, substrates, and other material, to the functional cells of the nephron. Although some nephrotoxicants act at the level of the renal vasculature to produce their effects, frequently gross alterations in systemic circulation produce changes in renal blood flow that have only indirect effects on renal function. Noxious agents also may be tested in vitro without unwanted effects on other physiological systems. In addition, for the most part, precise control over the temperature, the gas atmosphere, and other factors can be maintained. Finally, and not insignificantly, a large number of experimental variables may be tested with the renal tissue from a single animal.

Specific transport studies can be accomplished for a variety of compounds using in vitro techniques. Organic substances (e.g., organic anions, organic cations, amino acids, sugars) can be examined with any number of the techniques discussed below. Furthermore, the transport of inorganic electrolytes can be monitored in certain experiments and their importance in supporting the transport of other substances tested. Finally, with most of the in vitro procedures to be described, the effects of toxicants added directly to fresh tissue preparations can be studied. Animals also can be pretreated with toxic substances and the effects of these pretreatment regimens on discrete transport processes examined subsequently.

With transport studies there seems to be little doubt concerning the correlation between in vivo and in vitro studies. Other in vitro procedures need the same correlative approach but, in general, can be accepted as valid expressions of the in vivo function. Certainly, the isolated perfused tubule, which in practice is a segment of the intact functional unit of the nephron, can be utilized to obtain fundamental in vivo information. Isolated membrane vesicles are somewhat more removed than even the renal slices, but they are designed to examine parameters other than strictly renal function parameters. This technique was developed to learn fundamental aspects of membrane function, and the evidence suggests that the behavior of the vesicles reflects what intact membranes do in the intact animal.

Recently, there has been a movement to use isolated cells (primary cultures or standard cell lines) for toxicological studies. Compared to other in vitro methods such as slices or tubules, cells eliminate the problem of closed lumens, a potential problem for slices or tubules if one attempts to address a toxic response on the brush border. Many cell preparations retain various biochemical and physiological properties observed with intact animals, for example, certain transport processes, GSH metabolism, and energy demands (101,102). These techniques have been useful in studying selected biochemical toxicological events (103) wherein they appear to mimic precisely what is observed in vivo and with other in vitro procedures. Although concerns remain about isolated cells as ideal for studying all toxicological events observed in vivo, it is clear that some activities can be examined quite reliably.

Renal Cortex Slices, Tissue Fragments, and Tubules

For screening of tubular toxicity, renal cortical slices or tissue fragments may be prepared conveniently and rapidly free hand with the aid of a Stadie–Rigg microtome or a McIlwain tissue slicer. Such slices can be prepared from dog, rabbit, rat, or mouse kidneys. The slices or fragments prepared by these procedures (0.2–0.5 mm in thickness) are incubated in a balanced salt solution at a known temperature and with appropriate oxygenation. Frequently, the Cross–Taggart medium (70) is used, although other solutions (e.g., modified Cross–Taggart medium [13] and bicarbonate-buffered medium [38]) are just as appropriate. Specific formulations are given by Umbriet et al. (38). As a rule, albumin or other proteins are not used. Approximately 100 mg of tissue per incubation flask (25-ml Erlenmeyer) or beaker (30 ml) each containing 3 or 4 ml of buffer is usually sufficient for most studies. Incubations usually are undertaken in temperature-controlled, shaking waterbath. Unless the flasks are stoppered, a continual flow of the gas needed to establish the gas atmosphere is essential. For bicarbonate buffers 95% $O_2 + 5\%$

CO_2 is used, whereas 100% O_2 is satisfactory for phosphate buffers. An adult 250-g rat supplies enough renal tissue for 10–12 such flasks or beakers. The tissue from a single rabbit is sufficient for as many as 25–30 such flasks or beakers.

After an appropriate period of incubation under prescribed conditions, the tissue slices are removed from the beaker with forceps, blotted on moist filter paper, and weighed. The tissue slices are then processed, along with an aliquot of bathing solution, to determine the extent of uptake of whatever test substance is under study. For example, if radioactive substances are used, and it can be established that these compounds are not metabolized by the renal tissue, uptake of radioactivity by the slice can be monitored as a measure of accumulation. The tissue is homogenized in distilled water and an aliquot of the whole homogenate counted with standard liquid scintillation procedures. Similarly, an aliquot of the bathing solution is counted. The data obtained from such an experiment can be expressed in terms of the slice/medium ratio (S/M ratio), that is, the amount of radioactivity per gram of tissue divided by the amount of radioactivity per milliliter of bathing solution. In general, it is agreed that S/M ratios of more than 1 are indicative of an active transport process. For example, with a substance such as PAH, the addition of a metabolic inhibitor can induce the S/M ratio to less than 1.

This technique is a sensitive one for both the addition of toxic substances in vitro and the assessment of effects on transport after pretreatment. Specificity of the transport process can be assessed using various competitive transport inhibitors: probenecid for the renal organic anion system, tetraethylammonium (TEA) and *N*′1-methylnicotinamide (NMN) for the organic base transport substrates, and the basic dye cyanine No. 863 is a specific inhibitor of this system (25).

Although high S/M ratios usually reflect active accumulation, care must be taken with renal slices to ensure that the high ratios do not reflect nonspecific binding by renal tissue. With some substances (e.g., 2,4-dinitrophenol), nonspecific binding and specific tubular transport have been demonstrated (56). Even in the absence of renal tubular transport, 2,4-dinitrophenol accumulated to S/M ratios as high as 5, which apparently reflected nonspecific binding to cellular proteins and other macromolecules. Direct measurements of binding by cortical homogenates supported this contention, as did the failure of metabolic inhibitors to reduce the dinitrophenol S/M ratios to 1 or below.

The general state of function of the renal tubular cells can be monitored by assessment of sodium and potassium concentrations of renal tissue, total tissue water, and intracellular–extracellular water distribution. Disruptions in cellular sodium and potassium content do not reflect changes in renal sodium or potassium reabsorption, or secretion by the nephron. Rather, alterations in the renal slice sodium or potassium content reflect changes in the general homeostatic function of the renal tubular epithelial cells. However, this analysis has utility because it may give insights into the mechanisms of action of toxins. The techniques involved are relatively simple. The slices are incubated with inulin until a steady-state distribution is achieved (60–90 min). The tissues are then weighed wet, dried to a constant weight, and reweighed. The differences in weight reflect total tissue water. After the tissue has been dried, it is extracted with dilute nitric acid for several days. The nitric acid extract is used for inulin analyses (liquid scintillation counting or colorimetry analysis) and flame emission photometric analysis for sodium and potassium. The inulin is used for measurement of extracellular space and intra- and extracellular water, and intracellular electrolyte concentrations can be calculated by standard procedures (13).

Finally, renal cortical slice viability can be studied by monitoring oxygen consumption. Once again, this procedure does not give specific data on renal transport or renal function. The use of an oxygen electrode (e.g., Clark electrode) offers the greatest flexibility for such studies. The tissue is added to a small volume of balanced salt solution in the electrode chamber. The oxygen electrode is placed in the chamber (excluding the gas phase completely) to monitor the decrease in oxygen in the bathing solution. The reduction in oxygen tension in the bathing solution can be used to calculate oxygen consumption by the tissue. A complete measurement can be accomplished in 5–10 min utilizing as little as 15–30 mg of tissue.

Slices with specific orientation can be prepared from rabbit kidneys. A cylinder of tissue is cored along the axis from the cortex to the papilla and then perpendicular slices ($\sim 300\ \mu m$) are prepared using a Krumdiek Tissue Slicer. The slices can be incubated for up to three days using dynamic culture techniques and for shorter times using suspension culture techniques (133). These positional slices feature tubule cross sections from different segments of the tubule and thus are particularly useful for assessing tubule segment selectivity or specificity of a nephrotoxicant; potassium dichromate and mercuric chloride showed the same selectivity as occurs in vivo (convoluted and straight segments, respectively) (132). Toxicity is assessed by loss of enzymes from tissue (γ-glutamyltranspeptidase for the straight section and alkaline phosphatase for the convoluted section), loss of tissue potassium, decreased O_2 consumption, depletion of ATP, and histological examination (154).

Fragments of tubules can be prepared by either enzymatic or mechanical disruption of tissue. Either preparation is longer and more involved than that for slices.

Tubules isolated by collagenase perfusion of the kidney are separated and purified by Percol gradient centrifugation. Mechanical separation involves use of iron oxide infusion, mechanical disruption, separation of tubules by sieving through mesh, and removal of iron-laden glomeruli with a magnet. The tubule suspension can be used similar to slices for characterizing the effects of toxicant exposure, either in vivo or in vitro, on transport processes and metabolic functions.

Collagenase disruption of tissue damages the basement membrane and this may alter cell function. Compared to slices, the resulting tubule preparation is a more homogenous preparation, the tubules maintain their tubular shape, and cells are well exposed to incubation medium. Tubules produced by mechanical disruption maintain their tubular morphology for up to a week and seem to have patent lumens (129). For transport studies, uptake is measured at increasing concentrations of radiolabeled substrate, in the presence and absence of excess nonlabeled substrate (to correct for tissue binding, etc.). The difference is analyzed kinetically to determine transport parameters (85).

It is important to have such assessments of tissue viability (electrolytes, oxygen consumption) so the investigator can distinguish between effects of toxins on specific renal transport processes and effects on the general metabolism within the tissue. Obviously, cessation of tissue metabolism would be expected to interfere with transport, but such an effect is not specific for one or another transport system. On the other hand, an action of a toxin on metabolism might represent an important mechanism of action.

Isolated Perfused Tubule

The isolated perfused tubule technique represents an attempt to develop an in vitro procedure that retains renal tubular function comparable to that in the intact animal. Furthermore, this technique can be used to analyze mechanisms of transport. Unlike the renal slice procedure, this approach allows assessment of transepithelial transport. Each of the tubule segments studied has been shown to retain nearly its normal physiological function. For example, the proximal tubule shows no measurable osmotic gradient across it, the cortical collecting tubule responds to vasopressin, and electrolyte transport across the proximal tubule is similar to that seen with other techniques.

As with the micropuncture procedure, this technique is sophisticated and requires some significant dedication to the technique itself. It is not one that can be learned casually, but it is powerful enough to provide an understanding of renal function. Details of the procedure are not given here because they have been defined thoroughly by Burg and Orloff (5) and various other workers (Lulrich and Greger [37], Schafer and Williams [137], Williams and Schafer [152], Wright et al. [156]). Some comments about advantages and disadvantages are appropriate, however. A preparation of the tubule segment for perfusion is perhaps the most complicated and difficult part of the whole procedure. At present, such tubule segments are prepared for perfusion by manual dissection with the aid of a microscope. Earlier procedures utilizing enzymes, for example, collagenase, have proved inappropriate because of damage to the basement membrane of the tubule segments. The rabbit kidney has proved the most useful for dissection of tubule segments, although kidneys from the dog, rat, mouse, hamster, frog, and human also have been studied.

The segment of nephron is suspended in a fluid bath of several milliliters between two such pipettes, one of which is the perfusion pipette and the other the collection pipette. Fluid transport out of the tubule segment is monitored by changes in the concentration of a nonpermeable marker in the perfusion solution. For example, $[^{131}I]$ albumin or $[^{14}C]$inulin may be included in the perfusion solution. The collection pipette is used to obtain small volumes of perfusate, and both samples can be taken directly.

The major advantages of this technique over other in vitro procedures is that the relation between the in vitro and in vivo procedures is clear. The technique has demonstrated significant utility for studying the effects of pharmacological agents and should be as useful for toxicological studies. Of course, a dissected tubule is not in a normal environment and may differ from the in vivo situation because of that. Nonetheless, studies to date suggest that this model is a good one to study in vivo renal function. Unfortunately, little use has been made of this technique for studies of toxicological agents. In many ways it would be ideal to determine the action of toxicological agents on tubular cells versus glomerular events and localization of critical tubule segments. It would permit isolation of a nephron segment and study of that segment separate from the vasculature, glomerular problems, or the influences of other nephron segments. Presumably both pretreatment studies and direct in vitro addition studies would be possible.

A word of caution is indicated. As noted above, to date many studies have been done with rabbit nephron segments. Micropuncture and other studies (summarized by Weiner [150]) indicate that large species differences exist with respect to organic anion transport (both secretory and reabsorptive) on a segment-by-segment analysis of nephron function. Consequently, broad generalizations based on the isolated perfused nephron segments of rabbit kidney should be avoided.

Renal Cells in Culture

The use of cultured renal cells for the study of nephrotoxicity has obvious advantages. Under ideal circumstances large populations of specific cell types could be studied in circumstances where control of the environment would be maximized. Potentially, short- and long-term studies could be undertaken. A major complication in nephrotoxicity studies relates to the cellular heterogeneity of the kidney. Ideally, this obstacle can be overcome with tissue culture studies. An important advantage of renal cell culture is the ability to assess toxicity in human tissue. Racusen and colleagues (125) have established a human proximal tubule line. There is an excellent review of these techniques (7), and cell injury has been covered by Wilson (153). More detailed procedures have been reviewed for primary culture of tubule cells (90) and established cell lines (142).

A major approach to the use of cultured cells has involved established cell lines. These established lines (e.g., MDCK, LLC-PK_1, OK) are available from tissue culture banks and are easily maintained in culture. The cells are not ideal, however, for studies of specific renal cell types. Often those cells were derived from cells of unknown origin, and all have been through many passages in culture. No doubt the cells have been modified from their original state as they adapted to tissue culture, and they continue to change, yielding subtypes with different characteristics. Even those cell lines that have been studied extensively and are well characterized do not perform ideally. The MDCK line (dog kidney) is thought of as a model for collecting duct or distal tubule epithelium and yet has some properties not normally associated with these cells. Furthermore, these cells may be tumorigenic in the nude mouse. The pig kidney cell line LLC-PK_1 does not behave under all circumstances as a proximal tubule cell line, which it is thought to represent, although it does retain some characteristics. For example, the OCT1 cation transporter was isolated from LLC-PK_1 cells. Sodium-dependent glucose transport occurs, but certain amino acid transport functions appear to be absent (124). In addition, the LLC-PK_1 cell line shows a considerable biochemical response to vasopressin, a substance normally thought to exert its physiological effect on distal or collecting duct cells (143). The OK line (American opossum) is also a model for proximal tubule cells and, like LLC-PK_1 cells, expresses glucose, amino acid, and organic cation transport capability; unlike the LLC-PK_1 cells it does not respond to vasopressin and does transport phosphate. Transfection of cell lines with organic ion transporters has been achieved (80,113,147).

Primary cultures also have been used, and they often overcome some of the difficulties associated with the long-term cell lines. Often the exact cells of origin are not known in these studies as well, but at least the region of the nephron involved can be established easily, that is, proximal tubule. In some studies, precise dissection of specific nephron segments has been undertaken and the cells explanted for further studies. Obviously these experiments are technically more complex than simple tissue culture studies with standard cell lines.

The establishment of primary cell cultures is not simple and straightforward. Nonetheless, many of the long-standing problems are being overcome. For example, enriched preparations of either proximal or distal tubular cells can be obtained by Percol gradient centrifugation and have been useful for establishing cell cultures that retain segment-specific biochemical parameters (104,105). Dedifferentiation of renal cells is one of the limitations to use of primary cells cultures. Manipulation of incubation media and culture conditions can serve to extend the differentiated state. Proximal tubule cells maintain their in vivo metabolic characteristics if grown in the presence of physiological concentrations of glucose and insulin, and the cultures are well oxygenated (120). A different approach is to leave the cells in tubule. Cultures of proximal tubules maintain their differentiated state and appearance, particularly those produced using mechanical, rather than enzymatic, disruption (129).

Several studies have been undertaken to study chemical effects on renal tissue culture cells and have been summarized by Wilson (153) and Pfaller and Gstraunthaler (23). Various drugs, metabolic inhibitors, and metals have been examined in an attempt to better understand specific mechanisms of cell injury. A wide variety of metabolic and membrane perturbations have been reported, although how the effects related directly to the production of nephrotoxicity is unclear. It is equally unclear if the effects observed on tissue culture cells explain target organ selectivity of some nephrotoxic compounds. For example, mercuric chloride is known to damage a variety of cells, and the selectivity of this metal for the kidney in vivo is not seen in tissue culture studies.

The use of renal cells in culture holds promise for the future. Because of the technical problems associated with tissue culture, specialized laboratories are essential. Furthermore, the dominant issue of target organ selectivity must be addressed if the events of nephrotoxicity are to be understood. Finally, procedures must be developed to permit specific cell types to retain the well-recognized functions characteristic of a renal cell. Mechanistic studies with cells in culture cannot be achieved if the cells do not behave like renal tubule cells.

Isolated Membrane Vesicles

Preparations of membranes isolated from either the brush border or basolateral sides of the tubule have been crucial to understanding the steps of transepithelial transport of molecules. Such preparations may be valuable for mechanistic studies aimed at signal transduction-mediated responses to nephrotoxicants and for assessing relative sensitivity of the brush border and basolateral sides of the cell to various nephrotoxicants.

First attempts to isolate brush border membranes separate from basolateral membranes involved density gradient centrifugation techniques and free flow electrophoresis (78,94,151). Kinsella et al. (95) modified previously known cation precipitation techniques for a more efficient separation of basolateral and luminal membranes. This procedure, coupled with density gradient separation, has successfully isolated both types of membrane. However, this procedure has the limitation of requiring many hours to complete the separation. Boumendil-Podevin and Podevin (60) reported a technique of density gradient separation of both membrane types on a Percoll gradient. This procedure can be accomplished in a matter of 4–5 h. Even with the best separation techniques, contamination of basolateral with luminal, and luminal with basolateral, membranes is unavoidable. Concern must be expressed as well about the orientation of the membranes. In every preparation some vesicles are "right side out" and some "inside out." Care must be taken to establish the extent of "right-sidedness" of the vesicles with each procedure.

To date, most of the efforts with isolated membrane preparations have dealt with the electrolyte-driven transport of organic substances, for example amino acids and glucose. Some studies with PAH, NMN, and other substances have been undertaken (90,96). Clearly, preparations of this sort have great utility for determining whether a toxicologically important substance has actions directly on membrane function as opposed to cellular metabolism, for example. Metabolism as a factor is eliminated with these preparations, and any effects that might be noted must be related to the specific membrane transport process.

Several examples can be given that demonstrate the utility of isolated membrane vesicles for toxicological studies. These examples represent not only purely in vitro studies, but experiments where vesicles were isolated from pretreated rats as well. Hori et al. (91), Yanase et al. (158), and Lee et al. (106) pretreated animals with various nephrotoxicants and isolated both brush border and basolateral vesicles at various times after treatment. Deficits in membrane transport were observed at the various times after treatment, but with these studies it was not possible to determine if membrane damage was an initiating or even very early event in the overall nephrotoxic response. Ansari et al. (44–46) used both in vitro and pretreatment studies to examine direct effects of nephrotoxicants on membrane function and to study early effects after treatment. Specific effects were observed on either basolateral or brush border membrane vesicles when added to the vesicles or when vesicles were isolated from treated rats. Furthermore, some toxicants exert their effects on membranes as early as 3 h after treatment, which suggests a very early role for membrane damage in the nephrotoxic process.

Biomarkers of Renal Damage

Because humans often are exposed to hazardous chemicals, a search for indicators of such exposure has been undertaken. These biomarkers would be useful in a number of ways including confirming exposures, perhaps quantifying the extent of exposure, and identifying those individuals most likely to be affected by such exposure. Ideally, biomarkers (i.e., measurements on biological specimens) will clarify the relationship between exposure to environmental chemicals and human diseases. If effective biomarkers can be identified, they can be used to develop dose-response relationships and to estimate risk associated with exposure. The use of biomarkers in renal toxicology is reviewed by the National Research Council (22).

Biomarkers of exposure, effect, and susceptibility are recognized and are useful to characterize the response of any organ system. A marker of exposure can be represented by measurement of a chemical in a biological sample. This may be a chemical, a metabolite of a chemical, or the product of an interaction between a chemical and a biological receptor or target. Usually markers of exposure are assayed in urine, blood, or some body tissue. Such measurements may be straightforward, but problems have been noted. For example, some xenobiotics have similar metabolites, which can complicate interpretation of the data. The extent of exposure can affect retention of the parent compound and its metabolites that may cause similar complications. Wherever possible, pharmacokinetic parameters should be considered in interpreting data generated from markers of exposure.

If alterations in cellular or organ function are observed, these serve as markers of effect. These may be determined by standard clinical laboratory measurements as used in the differential diagnosis of disease. Depending on the magnitude of alteration of a physiological or biochemical marker, there may be evidence for potential health impairment or disease. These markers may be signals of tissue dysfunction, for example, appearance of selected enzymes in blood or urine, elevation of waste products (e.g., urea) in blood, or alterations in physiological parameters (e.g., blood pressure). The presence of modulators associated with repair and regeneration, such as epidermal growth factor and insulin-like growth factor I, may indicate that damage has occurred. These have the potential to provide the sensitivity needed for a screening test, because they would be elevated when repair is occurring even if the extent of damage is not sufficient to have overwhelmed functional reserve capacity. The presence of DNA adducts also may reflect the potential for adverse health effects. A number of renal markers of effect are of interest, including those which reflect tubular damage, such as *N*-acetyl-*p*-glucosaminidase (NAG), α2-microglobulin, brush border antigen, low molecular weight proteinuria, and inability to concentrate the urine. The usefulness of these for predicting renal dysfunction after exposure to hazardous chemicals but before gross renal damage, needs to be examined (22).

If cellular, organ, and other measurements can identify individuals who are susceptible to certain toxic chemicals, these are markers of susceptibility. Such markers may indicate an inherited or acquired limitation of an individual's ability to produce a protective response after exposure to a particular chemical. A preexisting disease may contribute to an unusual response to a given chemical. In addition, normal events such as aging may influence evidence of susceptibility.

Although biological markers are relatively easy to define and describe, it is less clear how valid these are for the intended purposes. In particular, are the markers valid in epidemiological studies? Sensitivity and specificity are key issues for the use of biological markers. Furthermore, these attributes are different when applied to population rather than laboratory studies. Sensitivity reflects the ability to identify a "true positive." In population studies, sensitivity indicates the proportion of events that actually did occur. Specificity allows the identification of a "true negative," that is, an analytical test that will detect the chemical. For very rare events, even very good measures (i.e., markers) give poor positive predictability.

Ideal biological markers would be absent in all unexposed individuals but easily detected in all exposed individuals. However, no marker is known that fulfills these criteria. Variability among humans causes a significant overlap between and among human populations with regard to markers. In addition, extrinsic factors complicate this issue. For example, there may be circumstances or conditions that cause in some individuals the appearance of a marker that also is caused by exposure to specific chemicals. Analytical errors also can contribute to variability in population and individual sensitivity and specificity; that is, selection of a threshold value can greatly influence both selectivity and specificity.

The availability of highly sensitive and specific markers also raises ethical and practical issues. Issues of cost must be considered. What to do with marker data also must be considered. If a marker is found that demonstrates an unusual sensitivity of an individual or population to a particular chemical, will that individual or population no longer be allowed to work where that chemical exists? Are other positions available in the same industry? Are other opportunities available and who is responsible for finding those opportunities? How should subjects be notified of the potential consequences of such marker tests? Are the markers universally recognized as appropriate? These issues are important and bear directly on the utility of markers in the industrial setting.

THE FUTURE

A major commitment of modern renal toxicology is to understand the mechanisms by which chemical substances disrupt renal function, producing ultimately acute or chronic renal failure. Many insights have been gained from revealing the important role of xenobiotic metabolism as a prelude to nephrotoxicity, for example, formation of reactive intermediates. However, relatively few precise descriptions of toxic mechanisms exist. In some instances, attempts to understand mechanisms have been conducted for decades (e.g., with mercuric chloride) and although recent approaches are showing great promise, a precise definition of a cellular or subcellular process that results in renal damage is still lacking. Perhaps most striking is the issue of target organ selectivity exhibited by many xenobiotics and the absence of convincing explanations for this phenomenon for many compounds.

One solution to these unanswered questions may rest with a new look at the physiological response to injury. Nephrotoxic insults initiate sequences of responses that result in cell death, loss of cells, viable and nonviable, and regeneration or proliferation (see Safirstein [30]). The signal transduction paths for these responses are similar but differ in the specific enzymes or factors involved and understanding why a particular path is invoked for a particular insult may provide important information. Growth factors activate a proliferative pathway mediated by extracellular-regulated kinases whereas ischemia, oxidative stress, and toxic agents stimulate stress-activated protein kinases that are antiproliferative. Growth factors, for example, may play a crucial role in modifying the renal response (reviewed in Harris [10]; Hirschberg and Adler [11]). Several growth factors, for example, epidermal growth factor (EGF), the insulin-like growth factors (IGF-1), transforming growth factors, hepatocyte growth factor—have been found in renal tissue, among others, or have been shown to act on renal cells in culture. Some growth factors have been suggested to increase the regeneration of renal cells after injury in rats. For example, EGF and IGF-1 have been shown to hasten recovery from either ischemia or mercuric chloride-induced proximal tubular necrosis, however EGF is decreased and IGF-1 is expressed transiently. The beneficial effect of exogenous IGF-1 is due, in part, to improved renal blood flow from increased NO production. The expression of agents that code for small glycoproteins with cytokine-like properties is increased after renal ischemia (134). There also is increasing interest in heat shock proteins and their potential role in both ischemic and chemical-induced renal injury (77,84).

Transgenic approaches, especially selective disruption of a gene, the so-called knock-out models, have yielded important information on the role of specific proteins in kidney development and normal function. This approach offers the ability to determine the role of specific proteins in toxicity. For example, metallothionein knock-out mice still develop nephropathy after cadmium chloride exposure, suggesting that metallothionein is not necessary for cadmium toxicity (110). Mice lacking IL-1 receptors recover from ischemia more rapidly than their wildtype counterparts (88). The technique combines the ability to focus on a particular protein, and specific isoform of that protein, without uncertainties and non-specificities of drug or chemical inhibition of the protein, within the intact animal.

These and other observations point to a potentially important role for host-modifying factors in the nephrotoxic response and should be a focus for future studies, especially those directed toward an understanding of nephrotoxic mechanisms. Furthermore, this approach may contain a clue about target organ toxicity in that other organs may be useful as "controls" for the renal response. If these regulatory processes are selective for the renal response to known nephrotoxic chemicals, other organs would not be expected to yield the same qualitative response. The role of these and possibly other factors that modify the nephrotoxic response will no doubt give important insights into mechanisms of chemically induced renal tissue damage.

SUMMARY

The functional unit of the kidney, the nephron, is in reality a series of functional units. This complexity of renal anatomy is amplified by physiological and biochemical studies. The importance of these observations to renal toxicological evaluations is that there is no single technique or procedure that allows an investigator to assess renal toxicity. Furthermore, this issue will be more complicated as greater interest in biomarkers develops and new information becomes available regarding mechanisms of renal toxicity. Presently, a battery of renal tests is necessary to provide evidence of the existence of nephrotoxicity, although a standard screening procedure can be established to develop preliminary evidence. Such whole-animal screening procedures are best undertaken with small animals and with a balance study format.

Detailed clearance procedures on whole animals (conscious or anesthetized) can yield specific data about the time course of nephrotoxicity, glomerular versus tubular involvement, reversibility of the insult, and other processes. Experiments with anesthetized animals offer greater control and precision than those on conscious animals. On the other hand, studies conducted with metabolism cages offer greater flexibility. In either situation, however, the possibility of glomerular and/or tubular involvement can be assessed. All of the techniques utilized in these studies are standard and readily learned by the novice.

Micropuncture procedures are powerful (potentially) tests for the analysis of nephrotoxicity. However, the cost and sophistication of these procedures precludes routine use as a screening technique. Micropuncture cannot be used by the novice.

Studies with isolated tissues, tubules, cells, and so forth are most useful for evaluating mechanisms and sites of action. Such studies eliminate problems with renal blood flow, systemic effects of toxins, and so on. Although some investigators argue that in vitro procedures bear no relation to what occurs in vivo, this view is not shared by all. Renal slice studies are simple and easily learned. Isolated perfused tubule techniques are complicated and much more difficult to master but clearly resemble the in vivo situation more closely. Renal cells in culture hold promise for the future. The techniques are complex and many technical problems exist, but this approach may become ideal for an understanding of mechanisms of action. Isolated cell membranes are useful for studies on membrane mechanisms free of cellular influences, for example, energy production.

Overall, it is best first to apply a whole-animal screening procedure (Figure 25.8). This method allows a description of the time course of nephrotoxicity and its general characteristics. Subsequent studies with anesthetized animals allow more precise description of quantitative effects on renal function. Finally, studies with slices, tubules, cells, isolated perfused kidney, or isolated membranes possibly permit an assessment of mechanisms and specific sites of action. This generalized approach, depicted in Figure 25.8, offers an opportunity to acquire both in vivo and in vitro data from the same experiment.

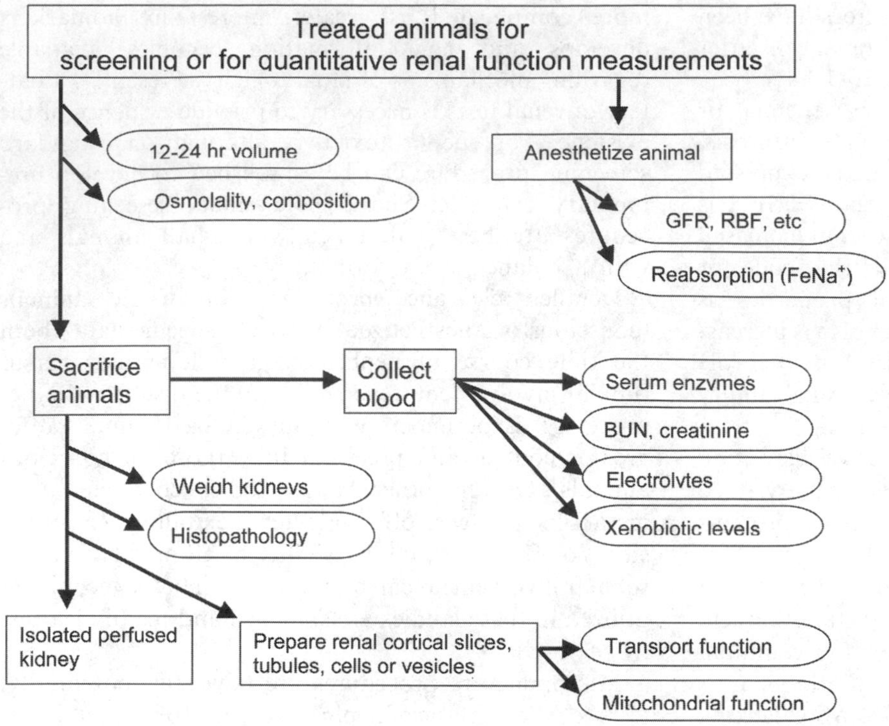

FIG. 25.8. Flow chart for in vivo and in vitro protocols for assessing effects of potential nephrotoxins on renal function.

QUESTIONS

1. What would be the consequences, in acute tubular necrosis, if glomerular filtration rate were not matched to tubular reabsorptive function?
2. What renal functions or parameters would be good candidates for sensitive biomarkers of renal toxicity?
3. What would be the characteristics for an in vitro screening technique to fully replace in vivo toxicity testing?

REFERENCES

Monographs, Reviews, and Texts

1. Bernard, A., and Lauwerys, R. R. (1991): Proteinuria: Changes and mechanisms in toxic nephropathies. *CRC Crit. Rev. Toxicol.*, 21:373–405.
2. Berndt, W. O. (1976): Renal function tests: what do they mean? A review of renal anatomy, biochemistry, and physiology. *Environ. Health Persp.*, 15:55–71.
3. Berndt, W. O. (1976): Use of the tissue slice technique for evaluation of renal transport processes. *Environ. Health Persp.*, 15:73–88.
4. Brenner, B. M. (1996): *Brenner and Rector's The Kidney*, 5th ed. W. B. Saunders, Philadelphia.
5. Burg, M. B., and Orloff, J. (1973): Perfusion of isolated renal tubules. In: *Handbook of Physiology, Sect. 8., Renal Physiology*, Chap. 7, edited by J. Orloff and R. W. Berliner. American Physiological Society, Washington, D.C.
6. Douglas, S. A., and Ohlstein, E. H. (1997): Signal transduction mechanisms mediating the vascular actions of endothelin. *J. Vasc. Res.*, 34:152–164.
7. Fine, L. G. (1986): Renal cells in culture. *Miner. Electrolyte Metab.*, 12:1–84.
8. Gullans, S. R., and Herbert, S. C. (1996): Metabolic basis of ion transport. In: *Brenner and Rector's The Kidney*, 5th ed., Chap. 5, edited by B. M. Brenner. W. B. Saunders, Philadelphia.
9. Gunning, M. E., Inglefinger, J. R., King, A. J., and Brenner, B. M. (1996): Vasoactive peptides and the kidney. In: *Brenner and Rector's The Kidney*, 5th ed., Chap. 16, edited by B. M. Brenner. W. B. Saunders, Philadelphia.
10. Harris, R. C. (1997): Growth factors and cytokines in acute renal failure. *Adv. Ren. Replace. Ther.*, 4:43–53.
11. Hirschberg, R., and Adler, S. (1998): Insulin-like growth factor system and the kidney: Physiology, pathophysiology, and therapeutic implications. *Am. J. Kidney Dis.*, 31:901–919.
12. Hirschberg, R., and Ding, H. (1998): Growth factors and acute renal failure. *Semin. Nephrol.*, 18:191–207.
13. Kleinzeller, A., Kostyuk, P. G,. Kotyk, A., and Lev, A. A. (1969): Determination of intracellular ionic concentrations and activities. In: *Laboratory Techniques in Membrane Biophysics*, edited by H. Passow and R. Stampfli, pp. 69–84. Springer-Verlag, New York.
14. Koepsell, H., Gorboulev, V., and Arndt, P. (1999): Molecular pharmacology of organic cation transporters in kidney. *J. Membr. Biol.*, 167:103–117.
15. Kone, B. C. (1997): Nitric oxide in renal health and disease. *Am. J. Kidney Dis.*, 30:311–333.
16. Lauwerys, R., Bernard, A., and Cardenas, A. (1992): Monitoring of early nephrotoxic effects of industrial chemicals. *Toxicol. Lett.*, 64–65:33–42.
17. Lazarus, J. M., and Brenner, B. M. (1993): *Acute Renal Failure*. Churchill-Livingstone, New York.

18. Lieberthal, W. (1997): Biology of acute renal failure: Therapeutic implications. *Kidney Int.*, 52:1102–1115.
19. Maddox, D. A., Deen, W. M., and Brenner, B. M. (1992): Glomerular filtration. In: *Handbook of Physiology, Sect. 8: Renal Physiology*, Chap. 13, edited by E. E. Windhager. Oxford University Press, New York.
20. Magos, L., and Clarkson, T. W. (1977): Renal injury and urinary excretion. In: *Handbook of Physiology, Sect. 9: Reactions to Environmental Chemicals*, Chap. 17, edited by D. H. K. Lee. American Physiological Society, Bethesda, Maryland.
21. Marsen, T. A., Schramek, H., and Dunn, M. J. (1994): Renal actions of endothelin: Linking cellular signaling pathways to kidney disease. *Kidney Int.*, 45:336–344.
22. National Research Council (1995): *Biologic Markers in Urinary Toxicology*, National Academy Press, Washington, D.C.
23. Pfaller, W., and Gstraunthaler, G. (1998): Nephrotoxicity testing in vitro—What we know and what we need to know. *Environ. Health Persp.*, 106 supplement 2:559–569.
24. Pitts, R. R. (1974): *Physiology of the Kidney and Body Fluids*, Chap. 13. Year Book, Chicago.
25. Pritchard, J. B., and Miller, D. S. (1992): Renal tubular transport of organic anions and cations. In: *The Kidney: Physiology and Pathophysiology*, 2nd ed. Chap. 84, edited by D. W. Seldin and G. Giebisch. Raven Press, New York.
26. Roch-Ramel, F., and Peters, G. (1979): Micropuncture techniques as a tool in renal pharmacology. *Annu. Rev. Pharmacol. Toxicol.*, 19:323–345.
27. Roch-Ramel, F., Besseghir, K., and Murer, H. (1992): Renal excretion and tubular transport of organic anions and cations. In: *Handbook of Physiology, Sect. 8: Renal Physiology*, Chap. 6, edited by E. E. Windhager. Oxford University Press, New York.
28. Roch-Ramel, F. (1998): Renal transport of organic anions. *Curr. Opin. Nephrol. Hypertens.*, 7:517–524.
29. Ross, B. D., and Guder, W. G. (1982): Heterogeneity and compartmentation in the kidney. In: *Metabolic Compartmentation*, edited by H. Sies, pp. 363–409. Academic Press, New York.
30. Safirstein, R. (1997): Renal stress response and acute renal failure. *Adv. Ren. Replace. Ther.*, 4:38–42.
31. Schreir, R. W., and Gottschalk, C. W. (1996): *Diseases of the Kidney*. 6th ed., Little, Brown and Co., New York.
32. Seldin, D. W., and Giebisch, G. (1985): The *Kidney, Physiology and Pathophysiology*. Raven Press, New York.
33. Singer, I., and Epstein, M. (1998): Potential of dopamine A-1 agonists in the management of acute renal failure. *Am. J. Kidney Dis.*, 31:743–755.
34. Smith, H. (1956): *Principles of Renal Physiology*. Oxford University Press, New York.
35. Sullivan, L. P. (1974): *Physiology of the Kidney*. Lea & Febiger, Philadelphia.
36. Tisher, C. C., and Madsen, K. M. (1996): Anatomy of the kidney. In: *Brenner and Rector's The Kidney*, 5th ed., Chap. 1, edited by B. M. Brenner. W. B. Saunders, Philadelphia.
37. Ullrich, K. J., and Greger, R. (1985): Approaches to the study of tubule transport functions. In: *The Kidney, Physiology and Pathophysiology, Vol. 1*, Chap. 20, edited by D. G. Seldin and G. Geibisch. Raven Press, New York.
38. Umbriet, W. W., Burris, R. H., and Stauffer, J. F. (1972): *Manometric and Biochemical Techniques*, 5th ed., pp. 146–147. Burgess, Minneapolis.
39. Valtin, H., and Schafer, J. A. (1995): *Renal Function*. 3rd ed. Little, Brown and Co., Boston.
40. Velazquez, H., and Wright, F. S. (1992): Renal micropuncture techniques. In: *Handbook of Physiology, Sect. 8: Renal Physiology*, Chap. 6, edited by E. E. Windhager. Oxford University Press, New York.
41. Windhager, E. E. (1992): *Handbook of Physiology, Sect. 8: Renal Physiology*. Oxford University Press, New York.

Research Articles

42. Acara, M., Roch-Ramel, F., and Rennick, B. (1979): Bidirectional renal tubular transport of free choline: A micropuncture study. *Am. J. Physiol.*, 236:F112–F118.
43. Ammer, U., Natochin, Y., David, C., Rumrich, G., and Ullrich, K. J. (1993): Cisplatin nephrotoxicity: Site of functional disturbance and correlation to loss of body weight. *Renal Physiol. Biochem.*, 16:131–145.
44. Ansari, R. A., Thakran, R. S., and Berndt, W. O. (1990): The effects of mercuric chloride on transport by brush border and basolateral membrane vesicles isolated from rat kidney. *Toxicol. Appl. Pharmacol.*, 106:145–153.
45. Ansari, R. A., Thakran, R. S., and Berndt, W. O. (1991): Effects of mercuric chloride on renal plasma membrane function after depletion or elevation of renal glutathione. *Toxicol. Appl. Pharmacol.*, 111:364–372.
46. Ansari, R. A., Thakran, R. S., and Berndt, W. O. (1991): The effects of potassium chromate and citrinin on rat renal membrane transport. *Fund. Appl. Toxicol.*, 16:701–709.
47. Balakrishnan, S. M., Wang, H. D., Gopalakrishnan, V., Wilson, T. W., and McNeill, J. R. (1996): Effect of an endothelin antagonist on hemodynamic responses to angiotensin II. *Hypertension*, 28:806–809.
48. Bank, N., Matz, E. F., and Aynedjian, H. S. (1967): The role of "leakage" of tubular fluid in anuria due to mercury poisoning. *J. Clin. Invest.*, 46:695–704.
49. Baylis, C., Mitruka, B., and Deng, A. (1992): Chronic blockade of nitric oxide synthesis in the rat produces systemic hypertension and glomerular damage. *J. Clin. Invest.*, 90:278–291.
50. Baylis, R., Rennke, H. R., and Brenner, B. M. (1977): Mechanisms of the defect in glomerular ultrafiltration associated with gentamicin administration. *Kidney Int.*, 12:344–353.
51. Beale, R. N., and Croft, D. N. (1961): A sensitive method for the colorimetric determination of urea. *J. Clin. Pathol.*, 14:418–424.
52. Bell, G. I, Fong, N. M., Stempien, M. M., Wormsted, M. A., Caput, D., et al. (1988): Human epidermal growth factor precursor: cDNA sequence, expression in vivo and gene organization. *Nucleic Acid Res.*, 14:8427–8446.
53. Bell, G. I, Gerhard, D. S., Fong, N. M., Sanchez-Pescador, R., and Rall, L. D. (1985): Isolation of the human insulin-like growth factor genes: Insulin-like growth factor II and insulin genes are contiguous. *Proc. Natl. Acad. Sci. USA*, 82:6450–6454.
54. Berndt, W. O. (1975): The effect of potassium dichromate on renal tubular transport processes. *Toxicol. Appl. Pharmacol.*, 32:40–52.
55. Berndt, W. O. (1977): A further characterization of cytembena-induced nephrotoxicity. *Toxicol. Appl. Pharmacol.*, 39:207–217.
56. Berndt, W. O., and Grote, D. (1968): The accumulation of C^{14}-dinitrophenol by slices of rabbit kidney cortex. *J. Pharmacol. Exp. Ther.*, 164:223–231.
57. Berndt, W. O., and Hayes, A. W. (1977): Effects of citrinin on renal tubular transport functions in the rat. *J. Environ. Pathol. Toxicol.*, 1:93–103.
58. Biber, T. U. L., Mylle, M., Baines, A. D., and Gottschalk, C. W. (1968): A study by micropuncture and microdissection of acute renal failure in rats. *Am. J. Med.*, 44:664–705.
59. Blantz, R. C., and Pelayo, J. C. (1983): In vivo actions of angiotensin II on glomerular function. *Fed. Proc.*, 42:3071–3074.
60. Boumendil-Podevin, E. F., and Podevin, R. A. (1983): Isolation of basolateral and brush-border membranes from the rabbit kidney cortex. *Biochim. Biophys. Acta*, 735:86–94.

61. Bratton, A. C., and Marshall, E. K. (1939): A new coupling component for sulfanilamide determination. *J. Biol. Chem.*, 128:537–550.

62. Brenner, B. M., Hostetler, T. H., and Humes, H. D. (1978): Glomerular permselectivity: Barrier function based on discrimination of molecular size and change. *Am. J. Physiol.*, 234:F455–F460.

63. Burg, M., and Green, N. (1973): Function of the thick ascending limb of Henle's loop. *Am. J. Physiol.*, 224:659–668.

64. Burg, M., Stoner, L., Cardinal, J., and Green, N. (1973): Furosemide effect on isolated perfused tubules. *Am. J. Physiol.*, 225:119–145.

65. Busch, A. E., Quester, S., Ulzheimer, J. C., Waldegger, S., Gorboulev, V., Arndt, P., Lang, F., and Koepsell, H. (1996): Electrogenic properties and substrate specificity of the polyspecific rat cation transporter rOCT1. *J. Biol. Chem.*, 271:32599–32604.

66. Carmines, P. K., and Fleming, J. T. (1990): Control of the renal microvasculature by vasoactive peptides. *FASEB J.*, 4:3300–3309.

67. Carone, F. A., Peterson, D. R., Oparil, S., and Pullman, T. N. (1979): Renal tubular transport and catabolism of proteins and peptides. *Kidney Int.*, 16:279–289.

68. Coimbra, T. M., Cresfinski, D. A., and Humes, H. D. (1990): Epidermal growth factor accelerates repair in mercuric chloride nephrotoxicity. *Am. J. Physiol.*, 259:F438–F443.

69. Cooke, W. J. (1976): Small inexpensive anesthetic apparatus for rats. *J. Appl. Physiol.*, 41:429–430.

70. Cross, R. J., and Taggart, J. V. (1950): Renal tubular transport: Accumulation of p-aminohippurate by rabbit kidney slices. *Am. J. Physiol.*, 161:181–190.

71. Curthoys, N. P., and Lowry, O. H. (1973): The distribution of glutaminase isoenzymes in the various structures of the nephron in normal, acidotic and alkalotic rat kidney. *J. Biol. Chem.*, 248:162–168.

72. Curthoys, N. P., and Kuhlenschmidt, T. (1975): Phosphate-independent glutaminase from rat kidney: Partial purification and identity with γ-glutamyl-transpeptidase. *J. Biol. Chem.*, 250:2099–2105.

73. Dees, J. H., Coe, L. D., Yasukochi, Y., and Masters, B. S. (1980): Immunofluorescence of NADPH-cytochrome C(-P450) reductase in rat and minipig tissues injected with phenobarbital. *Science*, 208:1473–1475.

74. Deryuck, R., Jarrett, J. A., Chen, E. Y., et al. (1995): Human transforming growth factor-β complementary DNA sequence and expression in normal and transformed cells. *Nature*, 316:701–705.

75. Deryuck, R., Rhee, L., Chen, E. Y., and Van Tilburg, A. (1987): Intron-exon structure of the human transforming growth factor-β precursor gene. *Nucleic Acid Res.*, 15:3188–3189.

76. Dicker, S. E., and Heller, H. (1945): The mechanisms of water diuresis in normal rats and rabbits analyzed by inulin and diodone clearances. *J. Physiol.* (*London*), 103:449–460.

77. Dubuisson, C., Cresteil, D., Desrochers, M., Decimo, D., Hadchouel, M., and Jacquemin, E. (1996): Ontogenic expression of the Na(+)-independent organic anion transporting polypeptide (oatp) in rat liver and kidney. *J. Hepatol.*, 25:932–940.

78. Ebel, H., Aulbert, E., and Merker, H. J. (1976): Isolation of the basal and lateral plasma membranes of rat kidney tubule cells. *Biochim. Biophys. Acta*, 443:531–546.

79. Emani, A., Schawartz, J. H., and Brokan, S. C. (1991): Transient ischemia or heat stress induces a cytoprotectant protein in rat kidney. *Am. J. Physiol.*, 260:F479–F485.

80. Evers, R., Kool, M., van Deemter, L., Janssen, H., Calafat, J., Oomen, L. C., Paulusma, C. C., Oude, E. R., Baas, F., Schinkel, A. H., and Borst, P. (1998): Drug export activity of the human canalicular multispecific organic anion transporter in polarized kidney MDCK cells expressing cMOAT (MRP2) cDNA. *J. Clin. Invest.*, 101:1310–1319.

81. Fowler, B. A., Hook, G. E. R., and Lucier, G. W. (1977): Tetrachlorodibenzo-p-dioxin induction of renal microsomal enzyme systems: Ultrastructural effects on pars recta (S3) proximal tubule cells of the rat kidney. *J. Pharmacol. Exp. Ther.*, 203:712–721.

82. Gertz, K. H., Brum-Schubert, G., and Brandis, M. (1969): Methode der Messung der filtrations rate einzelner nohe der nierenoberflache gelegener glomeruli. *Arch. Ges. Physiol.*, 310:109–115.

83. Goligorsky, M. S., Tsukahara, H., Magazine, H., Andersen, T. T., Malik, A. B., and Bahou, W. F. (1994): Termination of endothelin signaling: Role of nitric oxide. *J. Cell. Physiol.*, 158:485–494.

84. Goering, P. L., Fisher, B. R., Chaudhary, P. P., and Dick, C. A. (1992): Relationship between stress protein induction in rat kidney by mercuric chloride and nephrotoxicity. *Toxicol. Appl. Pharmacol.*, 113:184–191.

85. Groves, C. E., Morales, M., and Wright, S. H. (1998): Peritubular transport of ochratoxin A in rabbit renal proximal tubules. *J. Pharmacol. Exp. Ther.*, 284:943–948.

86. Grundemann, D., Babin-Ebell, J., Martel, F., Ording, N., Schmidt, A., and Schomig, E. (1997): Primary structure and functional expression of the apical organic cation transporter from kidney epithelial LLC-PK1 cells. *J. Biol. Chem.*, 272:10408–10413.

87. Hanks, S. K., Armour, R., Baldwin, J. H., Maldonado, F., Spliss, J., and Holley, R. W. (1988): Amino acid sequence of the BSC-I cell growth inhibitor (polyergin) deduced from the nuclemide sequence of the DNA. *Proc. Natl. Acad. Sci. USA*, 85:79–82.

88. Haq, M., Norman, J., Saba, S. R., Ramirez, G., and Rabb, H. (1998): Role of IL-1 in renal ischemic reperfusion injury. *J. Am. Soc. Nephrol.*, 9:614–619.

89. Hirsch, G. H. (1973): Differential effects of nephrotoxic agents on renal organic ion transport and metabolism. *J. Pharmacol. Exp. Ther.*, 186:593–599.

90. Holoban, P. D., Pessah, N. L, Pessah, I. N., and Ross, C. R. (1979): Reconstitution of *N*′-methylnicotinamide and p-aminohippuric acid transport in phospholipid vesicles with a protein fraction isolated from dog kidney membranes. *Mol. Pharmacol.*, 16:343–356.

91. Hori, R., Takano, M., Okano, T., and Inui, K.-L. (1985): Transport of *p*-aminohippurate, tetratethylammonium and D-glucose in renal brush border membranes from rats with acute renal failure. *J. Pharmcol. Exp. Ther.*, 233:776–781.

92. Horster, M., and Sone, M. (1990): Primary culture of isolated tubule cells of defined segmental origin. In: *Methods in Enzymology, Vol. 191*, edited by S. Fleischer and B. Fleischer, pp. 409–426. Academic Press, San Diego.

93. Jansen, M., Van Schaib, F. M. A., Ricker, A. T., Bullock, B., Woods, D. E., et al. (1983): Sequence of encoding human insulin-like growth factor I precursor. *Nature*, 306:1609–1611.

94. Kinne, R., Murer, H., Kinne-Saffran, E., Thees, M., and Sacks, G. (1975): Sugar transport by renal plasma membrane vesicles: Characterization of the system in the brush border microvilli and basal-lateral plasma membranes. *J. Membr. Biol.*, 21:375–395.

95. Kinsella, J. L., Holohan, P. D., Pessah, N. I., and Ross, C. R. (1969): Isolation of luminal and antiluminal membranes from dog kidney cortex. *Biochim. Biophys. Acta*, 552:468–477.

96. Kinsella, J. L., Holahan, P. D., Pessah, N. I., and Ross, C. R. (1979): Transport of organic ions in renal cortical luminal and antiluminal membrane vesicles. *J. Pharmacol. Exp. Ther.*, 209:443–450.

97. Kon, V., and Badr, K. F. (1991): Biological actions and pathophysiologic significance of endothelin in the kidney. *Kidney Int.*, 40:1–12.

98. Kramp, R. A., MacDowell, M., Gottschalk, C. W., and Oliver, J. R. (1974): A study in microdissection and micropuncture of the structure and the function of kidneys and the nephrons of rats with chronic renal disease. *Kidney Int.*, 5:147–176.

99. Kreisberg, J. I. (1983): Contractile properties of the glomerular mesangium. *Fed. Proc.*, 42:3053–3057.

100. Lash, L. H. (1990): Susceptibility to toxic injury in different nephron populations. *Toxicol. Lett.*, 53:97–104.

101. Lash, L. H. (1993): Purification of renal cortical cell populations by Percoll density-gradient centrifugation. In: *In Vitro Biological Systems: Preparation and Maintenance. Methods in Toxicology, Vol. 1*, edited by C. A. Tyson and J. M. Frazier. Academic Press, San Diego.

102. Lash, L. H. (1998): In vitro methods of assessing renal damage. *Toxicol. Pathol.*, 26:33–42.

103. Lash, L. H., and Anders, M. W. (1986): Cytotoxicity of S-(1,2-dichlorvinyl)glutathione and S-(1,2-dicholorovinyl)-L-cysteine in isolated rat kidney cells. *J. Biol. Chem.*, 261:13076–13081.

104. Lash, L. H., and Tokarz, J. J. (1989): Isolation of two distinct populations of cells from rat kidney cortex and their use in the study of chemical-induced toxicity. *Anal. Biochem.*, 182:271–279.

105. Lash, L. H., Tokarz, J. J., and Pegouske, D. M. (1995): Susceptibility of primary cultures of proximal tubular and distal tubular cells from rat kidney to chemically induced toxicity. *Toxicology*, 103:85–103.

106. Lee, H. Y., Kim, K. R., Won, J. S., Kim, Y. K., and Park, Y. S. (1990): Transport of organic compounds in renal plasma membrane vesicles of cadmium intoxicated rats. *Kidney Int.*, 37:727–735.

107. Levillain, O., Hus-Citharel, A., Morel, F., and Bankir, L. (1990): Localization of arginine synthesis along rat nephron. *Am. J. Physiol.*, 259:F916–923.

108. Levillain, O., Hus-Citharel, A., Morel, F., and Bankir, L. (1993): Arginine synthesis in mouse and rabbit nephron: Localization and functional significance. *Am. J. Physiol.*, 264:F1038–F1045

109. Lina, B. A. R., Bos-Kuijpers, M. H. M., Til, H. P., and Bär, A. (1996): Chronic toxicity and carcinogenicity study of erythritol in rats. *Regulat. Toxicol. Pharamcol.*, 24:S264–S279.

110. Liu, J., Liu, Y., Habeebu, S. S., and Klaassen, C. D. (1998): Susceptibility of MT-null mice to chronic $CdCl_2$-induced nephrotoxicity indicates that renal injury is not mediated by the CdMT complex. *Toxicol. Sci.*, 46:197–203.

111. Maack, T., Camargo, M. J. F., Kleinert, H. D., Laragh, J. H., and Atlas, S. A. (1985): Atrial natriuretic factor: Structure and functional properties. *Kidney Int.*, 27:607–615.

112. Maack, T., Johnson, V., Kau, S. T., Figueiredo, J., and Sigulem, D. (1979): Renal filtration, transport, and metabolism of low-molecular-weight proteins: A review. *Kidney Int.*, 16:271–278.

113. Masuda, S., Saito, H., and Inui, K. I. (1997): Interactions of nonsteroidal anti-inflammatory drugs with rat renal organic anion transporter, OAT-K1. *J. Pharmacol. Exp. Ther.*, 283:1039–1042.

114. Matejka, G. L., and Jennische, E. (1992): IGF-I binding and IGF-I mRNA expression in the postischemic regenerating rat kidney. *Kidney Int.*, 42:1113–1123.

115. McKinney, T. D., and Speeg, K. V., Jr. (1982): Cimetidine and procainamide secretion by proximal tubules in vitro. *Am. J. Physiol.*, 242:F672–F680.

116. McKinney, T. D., Myers, P., and Speeg, K. V., Jr. (1981): Cimetidine secretion by rabbit renal tubules in vitro. *Am. J. Physiol.*, 241:F69–F76.

117. McMenanry, R. H. (1968): Binding studies by dialysis equilibrium: A description of an accurate and rapid technique. *Anal. Biochem.*, 23:122–128.

118. Nomiyama, K., Yamamoto, A., and Sato, C. (1974): Assay of urinary enzymes in toxic nephropathy. *Toxicol. Appl. Pharmacol.*, 27:484–490.

119. Norman, J., Tsau, Y.-K., Bacay, A., and Fine, L. G. (1990): Epidermal growth factor accelerates functional recovery from ischemic acute tubular necrosis in the rat: Role of the epidermal growth factor receptor. *Clin. Sci.*, 78:445–450.

120. Nowak, G., and Schnellmann, R. G. (1995): Improved culture conditions stimulate gluconeogenesis in primary cultures of renal proximal tubule cells. *Am. J. Physiol.*, 268:C1053–C1061.

121. Pajor, A. M. (1995): Sequence and functional characterization of a renal sodium/dicarboxylate cotransporter. *J. Biol. Chem.*, 270:5779–5785.

122. Pesce, A. J., Boreisha, I., and Pollak, V. E. (1972): Rapid differentiation of glomerular and tubular proteinuria by sodium dodecyl sulfate polyacrylamide gel electrophoresis. *Clinica Chimica Acta*, 40:27–34.

123. Plaa, G., and Larsen, R. E. (1965): Relative nephrotoxic properties of chlorinated methane, ethane, and ethylene derivatives in mice. *Toxicol. Appl. Pharmacol.*, 7:37–44.

124. Rabito, C. A. (1986): Sodium cotransport processes in renal epithelial cell lines. *Miner. Electrolyte Metab.*, 12:32–42.

125. Racusen, L. C., Monteil, C., Sgrignoli, A., Lucksay, M., Marouillat, S., Rhim, J. G. S., and Morin, J.-P. (1997): Cell lines with extended in vitro growth potential from human renal proximal tubule: Characterization, response to inducers, and comparison with established cell lines. *J. Lab. Clin. Med.*, 129: 318–329.

126. Rajagopalan, S., Laursen, J. B., Borthayre, A., Kurz, S., Keiser, J., Haleen, S., Giaid, A., and Harrison, D. G. (1997): Role for endothelin-1 in angiotensin II-mediated hypertension. *Hypertension*, 30:29–34.

127. Richards, A. N. (1929): Direct observations of change in function of the renal tubule casued by certain poisons. *Trans. Assoc. Am. Physicians*, 44:64–73.

128. Rocha, A. S., and Kokko, J. P. (1973): Sodium and water transport in the medullary thick ascending limb of Henle: Evidence for active chloride transport. *J. Clin. Invest.*, 52:612–623.

129. Rodeheaver, D. P., Aleo, M. D., and Schnellmann, R. G. (1990): Differences in enzymatic and mechanical isolated rabbit renal proximal tubules: Comparison in long-term incubation. *In Vitro Cell. Dev. Biol.*, 26:898–904.

130. Ross, C. R., Pessah, N. I., and Farah, A. (1968): Inhibitory effects of β-haloalkylamines on the renal transport of NMN. *J. Pharmacol. Exp. Ther.*, 160:375–384.

131. Rubanyi, G. M. (1991): Endothelium-derived relaxing and contracting factors. *J. Cell. Biochem.*, 46:27–36.

132. Ruegg, C. E., Gandolfi, A. J., Nagle, R. B., and Brendel, K. (1987): Differential patterns of injury to the proximal tubule of renal cortical slices following in vitro exposure to mercuric chloride, potassium dichromate, or hypoxic conditions. *Toxicol. Appl. Pharmacol.*, 90:261–273.

133. Ruegg, C. E. (1994): Preparation of precision-cut renal slices and renal proximal tubular fragments for evaluating segment-specific nephrotoxicity. *J. Pharmacol. Toxicol. Methods*, 31:125–133.

134. Safirstein, R., Megyesi, J., Saggi, S. J., et al. (1991): Expression of cytokine-like genes JE and KC is increased during renal ischemia. *Am. J. Physiol.*, 261:F1095–F1101.

135. Safirstein, R., Price, P. M., Saggi, S. J., and Harris, R. C. (1990): Changes in gene expression after temporary renal ischemia. *Kidney Int.*, 37:1515–1521.

136. Saito, H., Masuda, S., and Inui, K. (1996): Cloning and functional characterization of a novel rat organic anion transporter mediating basolateral uptake of methotrexate in the kidney. *J. Biol. Chem.*, 271:20719–20725.

137. Schafer, J. A., and Williams, J. C. (1990): Flux measurements in isolated perfused tubules. In: *Methods in Enzymology, Vol. 191*, edited by S. Fleischer and B. Fleischer, pp. 354–370. Academic Press, San Diego.

138. Schaub, T. P., Kartenbeck, J., Konig, J., Vogel, O., Witzgall, R., Kriz, W., and Keppler, D. (1997): Expression of the conjugate export pump encoded by the mrp2 gene in the apical membrane of kidney proximal tubules. *J. Am. Soc. Nephrol.*, 8:1213–1221.

139. Schor, N., Ichikawa, I., Rennke, H. R., Troy, J. L., and Brenner, B. M. (1981): Pathophysiology of altered glomerular functions in aminoglycoside-treated rats. *Kidney Int.*, 19:288–296.

140. Sekine, T., Watanabe, N., Hosoyamada, M., Kanai, Y., and Endou, H. (1997): Expression cloning and characterization of a novel multispecific organic anion transporter. *J. Biol. Chem.*, 272:18526–18529.

141. Shafik, I. M., and Quamme, G. A. (1990): Micropuncture techniques in renal research. In: *Methods in Enzymology, Vol. 191*, edited by S. Fleischer and B. Fleischer, pp. 72–97. Academic Press, San Diego.

142. Simmons, N. L. (1990): Tissue culture of established renal cell lines. In: *Methods in Enzymology, Vol. 191*, edited by S. Fleischer and B. Fleischer, pp. 426–436. Academic Press, San Diego.

143. Skorecki, K. L., Verkman, A. S., and Ausiello, D. A. (1986): Vasopressin receptor-adenylate cyclase interactions: Studies in intact cultured renal epithelial cell line (LLC-PK_1). *Miner. Electrolyte Metab.*, 12:64–71.

144. Stitzer, S. A., and Martinez-Meldonado, M. (1978): Clearance methods in the rat. In: *Methods in Pharmacology, Vol. 4B*, edited by M. Martinez-Maldonado, pp. 23–40. Plenum Press, New York.

145. Stroo, W. E., and Hook, J. B. (1977): Enzymes of renal origin in urine as indicators of nephrotoxicity. *Toxicol. Appl. Pharmacol.*, 39:423–434.

146. Sweet, D. H., Wolff, N. A., and Pritchard, J. B. (1997): Expression cloning and characterization of ROAT1. The basolateral organic anion transporter in rat kidney. *J. Biol. Chem.*, 272:30088–30095.

147. Urakami, Y., Okuda, M., Masuda, S., Saito, H., and Inui, K. I. (1998): Functional characteristics and membrane localization of rat multispecific organic cation transporters, OCT1 and OCT2, mediating tubular secretion of cationic drugs. *J. Pharmacol. Exp. Ther.*, 287:800–805.

148. Ullrich, K. J., and Rumrich, G. (1991): Kidney: microperfusion-double-perfused tubule in situ. In: *Methods in Enzymology, Vol. 191*, edited by S. Fleischer and B. Fleischer, pp. 98–107. Academic Press, San Diego.

149. Walker, L. A., Buscemi-Bergin, M., and Gellai, M. (1983): Renal hemodynamics in conscious rats: Effects of anesthesia, surgery and recovery. *Am. J. Physiol.*, 245:F67–F74.

150. Weiner, I. M. (1979): Urate transport in the nephron. *Am. J. Physiol.*, 237:F85–F92.

151. Wilfong, R. F., and Neville, D. M. (1970): The isolation of the brash border membrane fraction from rat kidney. *J. Biol. Chem.*, 245:6106–6112.

152. Williams, J. C., and Schafer, J. A. (1990): Measurement of transmural water flow in isolated perfused tubule segments. In: *Methods in Enzymology, Vol. 191*, edited by S. Fleischer and B. Fleischer, pp. 232–252. Academic Press, San Diego.

153. Wilson, P. D. (1986): Use of cultured renal tubular cells in the study of cell injury. *Miner. Electrolyte Metab.*, 12:71–84.

154. Wolfgang, G. H. I., Gandolfi, A. J., Nagle, R. B., Brendl, K., and Stevens, J. L. (1990): Assessment of *S*-(1,2-dichlorovinyl)–cysteine induced toxic events in rabbit renal cortical slices. Biochemical and histological evaluation of uptake, covalent binding, and toxicity. *Chem.-Biol. Interactions*, 75:153–170.

155. Wright, F. S., and Giebisch, G. (1976): Renal potassium transport: Contributions of individual nephron segments and populations. *Am. J. Physiol.*, 235:F515–F527.

156. Wright, P. A., Burg, M. B., and Knepper, M. A. (1990): Microdissection of kidney tubule segments. In: *Methods in Enzymology, Vol. 191*, edited by S. Fleischer and B. Fleischer, pp. 226–231. Academic Press, San Diego.

157. Yabuuchi, H., Tamai, I., Nezu, J., Sakamoto, K., Oku, A., Shimane, M., Sai, Y., and Tsuji, A. (1999): Novel membrane transporter OCTN1 mediates multispecific, bidirectional, and pH-dependent transport of organic cations. *J. Pharmacol. Exp. Ther.*, 289:768–773.

158. Yanase, M., Orita, Y., Okada, N., et al. (1983): Decreased Na^+ gradient dependent D-glucose transport in brush border membrane vesicles from rabbits with experimental Fanconi syndrome. *Biochim. Biophys. Acta*, 733:95–101.

159. Yarger, W. E., Boyd, M. E., and Schrader, N. W. (1978): Evaluation of methods of measuring glomerular and nutrient blood flow in rat kidneys. *Am. J. Physiol.*, 235:H592–H600.

Principles and Methods of Toxicology, Fourth Edition, edited by A. Wallace Hayes. Taylor & Francis, Philadelphia © 2001.

Chapter 26

Methods in Gastrointestinal Toxicology

Carol T. Walsh

STRUCTURE AND FUNCTION OF THE GASTROINTESTINAL TRACT

The gastrointestinal tract is an organ of considerable complexity, which is comprised of numerous tissue types and serves multiple functions (77,182). There are consequently many possible loci for toxic effects by chemical substances (9,105,116). In addition, being the normal portal of entry of dietary substances, this organ has considerable potential for exposure to toxic agents. Sources of gastrointestinal toxicants include ingested contaminants of the diet and drinking water, pharmacologic agents taken orally or delivered to the gut in the blood or bile, and inhaled substances that are swallowed in secretions of the oral cavity or lungs.

Ingested substances may exert toxicity locally within the gastrointestinal tract or at other sites following absorption. The disposition of a toxicant in the gastrointestinal tract is a key determinant of the magnitude of its local or systemic toxicity and is dependent on its physiochemical characteristics in relation to the anatomical, physiological, and biochemical characteristics of the organ (183). Among key variables that influence the magnitude of toxicity are dissolution rates of ingested particulates; extent of dilution in luminal fluid from gastrointestinal secretions; residence times of the luminal contents in various sites of the organ; chemical characteristics that influence the extent and rate of absorption such as lipophilicity, pK_a, and molecular weight; and finally, clearance by biotransformation within the organ (21,70,86) or by fecal excretion (128).

The gastrointestinal tract can be equated to a continuous tube connecting the buccal cavity and the anus. Each portion of this tube is highly specialized in regards to both structure and function. Throughout the gastrointestinal tract a cross-section of the tissue consists of a series of layers. Epithelium lines the lumen. Directly beneath the epithelial layer lies an innervated and vascularly rich layer of connective tissue, the lamina propria. The muscularis mucosae is a thin layer of smooth muscle that separates the lamina propria from the underlying tissue. These first three layers comprise the mucosa. Below the mucosa is the submucosa, where larger blood vessels, lymphatics, and nerve plexi are located and branch to connect with the overlying mucosal or underlying musculature, the *muscularis externa*. The external muscle layer includes circular muscle that constricts the lumen and a longitudinal layer that shortens the tube. Coordinated contractions and relaxations of these muscles are required for the mixing, digestion, and propulsion of ingested substances through the gastrointestinal tract.

The five major subdivisions of the gastrointestinal tract, from the proximal to the distal end, include: the esophagus, which functions as a conduit; the stomach, a reservoir for mixing and digestion; the small intestine, a digestive and absorptive organ consisting of the duodenum, jejunum, and ileum; and the large intestine, which absorbs electrolytes and water from the luminal contents and processes them for elimination as feces.

Esophagus

Ingested feed and water move from the pharynx to the digestive reservoir of the stomach via the esophagus. The luminal cell layers in the esophagus are stratified squamous epithelia, continually renewed by mitosis of small, rounded cells in the deepest layer (69). As squamous cells migrate toward the luminal surface, they become flatter, acquire keratohyalin granules, lose nuclei and specialized cell junctions, and are sloughed off (167). The epithelial layer is protected by a coat of keratin, a protein that resists degradation by weak acids, alkalis, and proteolytic enzymes. The thickness of this keratinized epithelium is species dependent; for example, it is thicker in rodents than dogs. The surface area is increased by folds in the mucosal layer. During the passage of feed, these folds are able to stretch flat due to elasticity of tissue in the submucosal region. Mucous glands in the submucosal layer secrete mucins that lubricate the surface of the esophagus. The density of these glands are species dependent and are absent in rodents. The circular muscle adjacent to the submucosal layer is smooth muscle, whereas the outer longitudinal muscle begins as striated in proximal regions and then changes to smooth muscle. The muscle types and their neural regulation is species dependent. At the junction of the esophagus and stomach is the lower esophageal sphincter, a ring of circular muscle that helps prevent reflux of gastric contents into the esophageal lumen.

Stomach

There are important species differences in the anatomy of the stomach (41). In most species there are not marked separations between regions of the stomach, but rather, approximate subdivisions based on characteristics of the gastric glands. The cardiac region surrounds the esophageal junction, the fundus is the next most proximal, then the corpus, and a much smaller distal portion is the antral/pyloric region. At the junction of the stomach and the small intestine is the pyloric sphincter. Emptying of luminal solids is delayed by constriction of the sphincter which prevents back flux of duodenal contents into the stomach.

Unlike humans, rabbits, and dogs, the proximal portion of the stomach of rats and mice consists of nonglandular tissue referred to as the forestomach (14). A protruding layer called the limiting ridge separates the forestomach from the glandular tissue. Like the esophagus, the forestomach is lined with a stratified squamous epithelium (50–100 μm in rat), and the most luminal layer of cells are kerantinized. The forestomach lacks a protective mucus layer, the surface population of bacteria and yeast is more abundant (146), and the pH of the contents and mucosal surface is generally more basic than in the glandular acid-secreting portion of the stomach (17). In part because ingested materials tend to remain longer in the forestomach, this tissue is susceptible to the actions of both genotoxic and nongenotoxic carcinogens not seen in esophageal tissue under normal conditions (40,84). Furthermore, mice and rats lack the vomiting reflex, which in other species serves as a protective mechanism for eliminating compounds irritating to the stomach lining.

The prominent histological feature of the surface epithelium, columnar cells with short microvilli, is the high number of apical vacuoles that contain mucins. The secretory activity of these cells produces a gel-like layer of mucin, a high-molecular-weight polymer consisting of a protein backbone with carbohydrate side chains held together with disulfide bonds (38). A protective coating is provided by this mucous layer. For example, the pH between the mucus and surface cell is higher than the gastric lumen, suggesting that the mucus retards diffusion of hydrogen ions. There is also evidence that the sugar moieties can function as scavengers of cytotoxic, activated oxygen radicals (53). The passage of large molecules such as ferritin and gastric enzymes is inhibited by the mucus layer.

Interspersed in the surface of the glandular regions are pits (*foveolae*) lined with a single layer of mucus-secreting columnar cells with glands at the base (75). Cell types in the glands of the corpus include (i) parietal cells, responsible for the acid secretory properties of the stomach wall; and (ii) chief cells that secrete pepsinogen, the precursor of pepsin, the major proteolytic enzyme of the stomach. Enteroendocrine cells containing autacoids such as histamine, serotonin, substance P, and neurotensin play a role in regulation of acid secretion and gastric motility. Macrophages and plasma cells in the lamina propria may contain receptors for major regulators of acid secretion (107). In the antrum, a primary cell type in the gastric gland is the G cell which secretes gastrin, a parietal cell stimulant.

A major biochemical feature of the stomach is its acid secretory properties. Digestion of protein is facilitated by secreted acid through activation of pepsin. Emptying of the stomach and growth of microorganisms are inhibited by gastric acidity. The pH of the stomach affects the extent of ionization of toxicants which are weak electrolytes and is therefore an important determinant of their absorption kinetics. Gastric toxicity such as erosions and ulcerations induced by surface membrane-damaging agents may be enhanced by high levels of acid secretion because backflux of hydrogen ions into surface cells may be cytotoxic. The level of acid secretion therefore can be an important factor in the gastrointestinal disposition of toxic substances and in gastric toxicity. Acid secretion by parietal cells is controlled by the central nervous system (vagus nerve) and by gastrointestinal reflexes mediated through neural, autacoid, and hormonal input (151).

Small Intestine

The longest portion of the gastrointestinal tract is the small intestine. The small intestine mixes and propels chyme and passes unabsorbed solids and fluids to the large intestine. The primary function of the small intestine is absorption of ingested nutrient substances and water by specialized absorptive processes. The contractile patterns and propulsive action of the smooth muscles that envelope the small intestine facilitate contact between the luminal contents and the absorptive epithelial surface.

The surface area per unit length and total surface area are markedly greater in the small intestine than in the stomach or large intestine, which enhances the absorptive capacity of this organ. The surface consists of leaflike or fingerlike villi (about 0.8 mm high in humans) (100). The geometry of these surface projections varies somewhat with species. In humans there are submucosal foldings (folds of Kerckring, about 1×5 cm) that are covered with villi, which are most numerous in the duodenum and jejunum and are absent in the distal ileum (121). In humans, the surface area (approximately 200 m^2) is therefore greater in the more proximal region of the small intestine. The rat is unlike humans in this regard; villi project from the submucosa without additional foldings. The surface area is further enhanced, more than 40-fold, by microvilli which densely protrude from the apical luminal surface of the epithelium (35). Microvilli (0.5–1.5 μm in length) contain longitudinally oriented, actinlike microfilaments, which connect to the terminal web at the cell apex and may play a role in microvillar motility (100). The villar surface of the small intestine is composed of a single layer of columnar absorptive epithelium and mucus-secreting goblet cells. These cells originate from monoclonal stem cells in crypts at the base of the villi where mitoses occur (50). Cells migrate upward, differentiate, and are extruded from the villar tip. The rate of this process is species dependent.

The duodenum is the most proximal portion of the small intestine. It is characterized by the presence of Brunner's glands in the submucosa (110). A key physiological feature is the luminal influx of biliary and pancreatic secretions including bile salts, bicarbonate, and pancreatic digestive enzymes. A notable species difference is the absence of a gall bladder in the rat; bile flows into the duodenum at a relatively constant rate, unlike other species where flow depends more on meal-related reflex gall bladder contractions, such as those elicited by cholecystokinen.

The major pathways for absorption are through the columnar epithelium, 22–26 μm in height in man, into the capillaries in the lamina propria. Adjacent cells are joined by tight junctions at their apex which prevent intercellular transport of large molecules but may be a shunt pathway for water and electrolytes. The plasma membrane, a primary diffusion barrier, is wider than most eukaryotic membranes (10–11 nm) and has a relatively high protein-to-lipid ratio and unique lipid composition (100). Adherent to the membrane surface is an aqueous phase referred to as the "unstirred water layer" that is not in equilibrium with the bulk of the luminal fluid. For substances with limited aqueous solubility, diffusion through this layer may be a rate-limiting step in the overall absorption process (172). This layer has a more acidic pH than the bulk luminal contents and contains mucus secreted from goblet cells along the villus.

Transport of substances through the mucosal cell of the small intestine can occur by a variety of mechanisms. Passive diffusion, in which the concentration gradient from the lumen to the vasculature acts as a driving force, is one type of process and is the major mechanism for lipophilic substances. The small intestine is designed biochemically to enhance transport of nutrients at rates that kinetically exceed that attributable to passive transport. There are regional differences in maximal absorption rates of nutrients within the small intestine. These differences may result from the density of apical membrane transport carriers, membrane channels or receptors, digestive enzymes, cytoplasmic binding sites, or gradients generated by enzymes in the basolateral membrane.

Both the small and large intestine, under normal physiological conditions, are net water-absorbing organs. The primary driving force for water reabsorption is the osmotic gradients generated by the flux of electrolytes. The transport of the major electrolytes—sodium, potassium, chloride, and bicarbonate—results from biochemical mechanisms which differ in the apical and basolateral membranes of the mucosal cell (64). The basolateral membrane of the mucosal cells is enriched with sodium–potassium ATPase that pumps three sodium ions out of the mucosa into the serosal, or nonluminal border of the cell, in exchange for two potassium ions pumped into the cell. This enzyme generates a potential difference across the basolateral membrane and a concentration gradient for sodium that favors the influx of sodium from the lumen into the cell.

Sodium transport through the apical membrane occurs by a variety of mechanisms which differ in magnitude depending on intestinal region and species. One mechanism is via a carrier coupled to solutes such as monosaccharides, amino acids, and di- or tripeptides. This mechanism of sodium uptake is quantitatively most important in the jejunum, the primary absorptive site for products of carbohydrate and protein digestion. A second mechanism of sodium absorption, generally more important in the ileum, is an electrochemically neutral process, because it is associated with apical absorption of chloride, the major anion. These two uptake mechanisms are not linked biochemically; each is a separate mechanism with sodium uptake occurring in exchange for hydrogen secretion and chloride uptake with bicarbonate excretion. This transport process is modulated by neurotransmitters and autacoids that interact with receptors on the basolateral membranes. For example, agonists such as acetylcholine interact with muscarinic receptors and increase intracellular calcium binding to calmodulin, in abundance in the core of the microvilli. The calcium–calmodulin complex acts on the brush border surface to inhibit sodium chloride absorption (28).

Another determinant of net water and electrolyte flux in the small intestine as well as in the large intestine is the activity of the secretory mucosal cells that line the crypts at the base of the villi (188). These cells have a high capacity for chloride secretion, which can osmotically drive large-volume loss of water into the lumen. The basolateral membrane of these cells has a sodium–potassium–chloride cotransporter. The gradient generated by sodium–potassium ATPase favors influx of chloride with sodium via this cotransporter. The permeability of the apical membrane to chloride is rate limiting to the total flux of the ion and subject to modification by physiological and pathogenic factors. The major intracellular enhancer of increased chloride secretion is cyclic AMP, which can be increased by endogenous neuropeptides and inflammatory mediators such as vasoactive intestinal peptide, prostaglandins, and leukotrienes and by bacterial toxins such as those of *Vibrio cholerae* and heat labile *Esherichia coli*. Cyclic AMP activates kinases that phosphorylate proteins associated with the chloride channel in the apical membrane (28).

Another key biochemical feature of the apical membrane of the mucosa in the small intestine is the enzymes anchored into it and protruding into the lumen. These enzymes comprise the so-called glycocalyx or "fuzzy" coat of the microvilli, observed in high-power photomicrographs of the tissue (100). These enzymes, most abundant in the jejunum, include three major types of carbohydrases and a variety of peptidases which catalyze digestion of carbohydrates to the monosaccharides glucose and galactose and of peptides to di- and tripeptides and amino acids. Apical membrane carrier proteins for these monosaccharide and amino acid products facilitate their absorption. Carriers have been identified with specificity for each of the major monosaccharides and for several categories of amino acids.

Following transport through the mucosal cell, molecules pass through the basal lamina, a continuous sheet just below the mucosal cell layer; gaps, seen with scanning eletron microscopy, allow passage of chylomicrons and lymphocytes. Capillaries lie just below the basal lamina (within 2 μm) (51). Endothelial cells of capillaries are thinner on the mucosal cell side and contain diaphragmed fenestrations (500–600 nm) thought to be more permeable sites than the plasma membrane. The blood vessels of the lamina propria feed into the superior mesenteric vein. The major venous drainage from the gastrointestinal tissue courses into the portal vein, which flows through the liver. The appearance of substances in the systemic circulation, after absorption through the mucosa, is therefore dependent on the magnitude of clearance by the liver. Substances, highly susceptible to hepatic biotransformation, may have hepatic clearance values approaching hepatic blood flow and low bioavailability, despite substantial or even complete absorption through the intestinal mucosa, because of this extensive first-pass effect.

The absorption mechanism of dietary lipids possesses additional complexities (171) and may contribute to uptake of highly hydrophobic, lipophilic toxicants. The absorption of triglycerides is illustrative. Following partial digestion by pancreatic lipases, the resulting monoglycerides and free fatty acids are solubilized in the aqueous luminal contents by bile acids through micelle formation. Micelles facilitate the presentation of the lipids to the membrane surface where they diffuse out of the micelle and diffuse through the membrane. Within the cell, triglycerides are resynthesized and packaged within the Golgi apparatus into chylomicrons, also containing cholesterol esters, phospholipids, and apoproteins. Chylomicrons are contained within secretory vesicles that merge with the basolateral membrane and release their contents by exocytosis. These particles (750–6000 nm in diameter) pass between adjacent endotheolial cells in the central lacteal of the villus. Their size precludes uptake into capillaries. The lymph from the small intestine drains into the superior mesenteric lymphatic duct that flows into the thoracic duct. Lymph flow in the small intestine is considerably less than blood flow and therefore generally is not an important transport route for substances that can diffuse into capillaries (51).

Another transport mechanism in the small intestine is pinocytosis (179). The surface membrane invaginates, pinches off to form a vesicle, and may or may not coalesce with lysosomes containing degradative enzymes. The remaining contents may be released from the mucosal cell by exocytosis into the intercellular space. This transport mechanism is responsible for the duodenal absorption of maternal IgG in neonatal rats. This route is not quantitatively significant in most adult mucosal cells. Pinocytotic properties do persist, however, in the M cell, a specialized mucosal cell in the ileum. M cells overlay clusters of lymphatic cells in the submucosa referred to as Peyer's patches. They are distinguished morphologically by relatively short microvilli and by deep invaginations in the basolateral membrane in close proximity to lymphocytes. These cells are believed to deliver macromolecules and microorganisms to lymphocytes for immunological processing.

Large Intestine

The ileal contents are delivered to the large intestine, which includes the cecum, colon, and rectum. This region exhibits marked species differences in gross anatomical structure (22). The dog, for example, has a relatively simple tubelike large intestine. In humans and herbivores, such as the rabbit, the longitudinal muscle layer is arranged in three thick bands and the tissue has pouchlike outpocketings called haustra. Herbivores such as rats and rabbits have a large cecum between the small and large intestine; bacterial fermentation processes in this organ are of caloric importance in these species. These species-dependent variables may be of significance to the absorption and biotransformation of xenobiotics that are emptied into the large intestine.

The large intestine generally has no folds or villi and therefore appears smooth on the luminal surface. It is covered by a single layer of columnar epithelial cells interspersed by deep invaginations, the crypts of Lieberkuhn. The crypts are lined with epithelial cells in part, but primarily by mucus-secreting goblet cells. The surface cells are responsible for the high water-absorbing capacity of this organ. Sodium is actively transported by these cells as in the small intestine. In the rat, sodium transport is primarily an electroneutral process entailing exhange with hydrogen, linked to chloride–bicarbonate exchange. A major mechanism in the rabbit is via electrogenic transport, uncoupled to chloride or solutes. The transport of sodium is regulated by hormones as in the kidney; aldosterone, for example, increases the density of sodium channels in the apical membrane and the pump molecules in the basolateral membrane. Absorption rates of xenobiotics are generally lower from the large intestine than from the small intestine, in part because of the smaller surface area.

ASSESSMENT OF THE STRUCTURAL INTEGRITY OF THE GASTROINTESTINAL TRACT

Histology

Examination of gastrointestinal tissue by histological techniques is a useful approach for detection of toxic effects of some substances. Despite the importance of histological assessment, altered function of the organ may be induced without changes in the microanatomy of the tissue. In addition, microscopic lesions may be highly localized so that they are missed by selective sampling techniques.

Samples must be placed in fixative within 1–2 min after biopsy or death of an experimental animal because of the rapid autolysis of this tissue. In sectioning the stomach and small intestine, cuts should be made perpendicular to the longitudinal axis so that morphology of gastric pits and glands and intestinal villi can be inspected. Histological evaluation should include inspection of the vasculature, because ischemia and increased vascular permeability are associated with ulcerative lesions produced by some agents, such as ethanol (45). Examination of the lamina propria should include assessment of changes in numbers of eosinophils, plasma cells, neutrophils, macrophages, and lymphocytes. Increases in any of these cell populations, indicative of an inflammatory response, may play a role in mucosal cell injury. For example, recent evidence including in vivo assessment of leukocyte adherence to endothelium of mesenteric venules and extravasation into interstitium suggests a role for neutrophils in ethanol-induced gastritis (85).

The light microscopy of biopsies from the stomach, duodenum, jejunum, ileum, and colon in humans has been reviewed by Whitehead (189). The normal microanatomy of human small intestinal mucosal cells, including evaluation by electron microscopy, is described by Madara and Trier (100). Examples of depiction of the luminal surface of the gastrointestinal tract by scanning electron microscopy and cellular ultrastructure by transmission electron microscopy can be found in Pfeiffer et al. (117). This text covers the various regions of the gastrointestinal tract and includes discussion on tissue from several species of research animals including rat, mouse, and cat.

An important advance in clinical and experimental gastroenterology is the use of fiber optic instruments for visualizing the luminal surface of the gastrointestinal tract. In conjunction with endoscopy, biopsies of the gastrointestinal wall for histological evaluation can be obtained with instrument attachments such as forceps or suction capsules. Animals should be anesthetized before insertion of endoscopes or biopsy tools. The Olympus Bronchofibrescope Type BF-3C4 is suitable for use in rats (130).

Gross Evaluation: Extravasation of Nonerythrocytic Vascular Markers

Injury to the gastrointestinal wall may also be detected by killing the animal and inspecting the mucosa for lesions or the serosa for perforations or adhesions (15,16,143). These methods are based on observations of hemorrhagic sites resulting from damage to mucosal cells and underlying vasculature. An example of semiquantitative methodology for assessing chemically induced ulcerogenesis is provided in the work of Szabo (157). A *duodenal ulcer index* is generated as follows: The rat is killed and the duodenum is examined. The intensity of ulcerogenic effect, for example, by cysteamine, is rated 0 to 3, where 0 = no ulcer, 1 = superficial mucosal erosion, 2 = deep ulcer or transmural necrosis, 3 = perforated or penetrated (into the pancreas or liver) ulcer. The mean of this value in a group of animals is added to the incidence (positive/total) of ulcer formation × 2. In evaluation of gastric lesions (160), the animal is killed, and 4 ml of 10% aqueous-buffered formaldehyde is instilled into the stomach via a rubber stomach tube. After 5 min, the stomach is removed, opened along the greater curvature, and pinned out with additional formaldehyde. The fixative was found to prevent loss of hemorrhagic fluid from the mucosal surface and thereby improves detection of sites of gastric lesions. The number of lesions are counted. The intensity of effect is assessed as 0 = normal mucosa; 1 = one to four small petechiae; 2 = five or more petechiae or hemorrhagic streaks up to 4 mm; 3 = erosions larger the 5 mm or confluent hemorrhages. Szabo et al. (160) also developed a more quantitative approach for measuring gastric lesions by using planimetry to determine the total area of lesions. The glandular portion of the stomach is magnified with a stereomicroscope and projected onto the surface of the planimeter. The area of each lesion and total area involved are determined relative to the area of glandular tissue.

Visual inspection techniques can be made more sensitive by pretreating test animals with a nonerythrocytic vascular marker, followed by its visualization on the mucosal surface or its quantitation in the gut lumen. One such marker, found useful in the analysis of gastrointestinal effects of nonsteroidal anti-inflammatory agents, is the dye pontamine sky blue 6. This procedure, as applied by Brodie et al. (16), consists of injecting 1 ml of a 5% solution of the dye in 0.9% saline into the tail vein of 125–150-g rats. After 10 min, the animal is killed by intracardiac injection of pentobarbital. The gastrointestinal tract is then removed and opened, and the mucosal surface is inspected for foci of dark blue coloration. Under these conditions control animals are reported to have no sites of dye accumulation, whereas animals treated orally with aspirin 4 h previously exhibited dose-dependent incidences of these lesions. The sensitivity of animals to aspirin-induced lesions was markedly affected by 24-h feed deprivation. Fasting was found to increase the incidence of gastric lesions and to decrease the incidence of intestinal lesions.

A similar approach has been used with Evans blue dye administered intravenously in rats to characterize the pathological effects on the stomach and duodenum of ulcerogenic compounds, such as nonsteroidal anti-inflammatory agents (133) and ethanol (153). Just before killing the animals, 1 ml of a 1% Evans blue solution is injected via the tail vein or the jugular vein of lightly anesthetized animals. The stomach and small intestine are dissected and opened, along the greater curvature and antimesenteric side respectively, and pinned out. The length or area of lesions is determined using a dissecting microscope with a 1-mm square-grid eyepiece (10 ×) (133). Similarly, a 3% suspension of monastral blue B administered intravenously in doses of 0.1 ml/100 g body weight has been used as a marker to visualize and quantify vascular damage in the stomach induced by nonsteroidal anti-inflammatory agents, endothelin, hydrochloric acid, and ethanol (112,159,180).

An additional approach is to measure extravasation of a vascular dye into gastrointestinal tissue and the gastric lumen. Evans blue dye has been injected intravenously, animals killed after 15 min, and tissue and luminal content of the dye determined by spectrophotometry (159).

The blood-to-lumen clearance of ^{51}Cr-EDTA has also proven useful in assessing mucosal permeability (193). Transport of this radiolabeled chelate is normally inhibited by intercellular epithelial tight junctions. Agents that damage the epithelial layer, such as acetic acid instilled into the colon, significantly increase the flux of ^{51}Cr-EDTA into the lumen. The experimental technique entails injection of the radioisotope (e.g., 100 μCi in a 300–350-g rat) into the femoral vein of an anesthetized animal with ligated renal pedicles. The colon, cannulated at the splenic flexure and rectum, is perfused with Tyrode's solution. After a 1-h equilibration, aliquots of the distal perfusate and of blood are measured for radioactivity in order to compute the clearance of EDTA into the colon. Studies have also been carried out to assess leakage into the perfused jejunum of endogenous markers, such as albumin and hyaluronic acid, after exposure to agents such as ethanol (90).

It should be noted that in testing for ulcerogenic effects of chemicals, the magnitude and site of lesions are dependent on a variety of factors including species, diet and feeding procedures, and dose, route, and time following chemical administration. For example, lesions produced in humans by indomethacin are best mimicked in a rat model by fasting the animal for 48 h, feeding rat chow pellets, administering the drug subcutaneously 1 h later, and killing 6 h later (133). Ulcerative lesions occur in the antrum and are inhibited by the prostaglandins PGE_2 and $PGF_{2\alpha}$. Results differ from the fasted or fed rat in which indomethacin (as well as stress, other nonsteroidal anti-inflammatory drugs, and acid secretagogues) primarily produced erosions in the corpus, not ulcers in the antrum.

Fecal Blood Loss

Another approach for monitoring the integrity of the mucosal lining of the gastrointestinal tract, which has the advantage of being noninvasive, is based on the estimation of gastrointestinal bleeding by examination of the feces. This procedure entails the determination of occult blood in the feces by colorimetric or radioisotopic methods. The detection of fecal occult blood, a clinical diagnostic tool (145, 191), has application to the screening of substances for potential toxic effects on the gut and to the testing of agents with suspected or probable ulcerogenic properties, for example, non-steriodal anti-inflammatory agents.

There are a number of procedures available for assaying blood in the feces. Colorimetric techniques are based on the use of phenolic compounds, such as *o*-tolidine, benzidine, and guaiac, whose oxidation to color-emitting substances by hydrogen peroxide is catalyzed by hemoglobin (73). Commercially available formulations for clinical application primarily use guaiac as the reagent; for example, Hemoccult in which a slide is impregnated with guaiac (4).

There are numerous factors that affect a colorimetric assay (2). A primary variable is the fecal peroxidase activity originating from the diet rather than from gastrointestinal bleeding. Boiling the fecal sample eliminates some of this activity but not that from hemoglobin. Consequently, hemoglobin from dietary sources, such as red meat, remains active in the assay. In contrast, certain dietary substances, for example, ascorbic acid, decrease the reactivity of the colorimetric assay. In addition to interference from dietary factors, the results of this type of assay are dependent on the extent to which hemoglobin loses peroxidase activity by its metabolism in the gut lumen during transit from the site of bleeding (194). In addition, because bleeding may be intermittent, the results will depend on the extent of fecal hydration that affects the concentration of the hemoglobin in the sample (2).

The reagents used in colorimetric assays differ in several respects. For one, their sensitivities differ, with guaiac being relatively less sensitive and *o*-tolidine being among the most sensitive. A second factor affecting their use is their carcinogenic potential, a property that has been demonstrated for benzidine and *o*-tolidine, necessitating caution in their handling. Usually this technique is only semiquantitatively applied, with results reported as negative, weakly positive, or strongly positive for occult blood. This approach is the most reasonable because of the various problems, described above, in relating the colorimetric response in a fecal sample to the amount of hemoglobin present because of gastrointestinal bleeding. In setting up such an assay for a given experimental animal population, the reagent concentration may be adjusted such that feces from control animals give negative color reactions within the standard time. For example, Nakamura et al. (114) used the following procedure in assessing fecal blood loss in mice. Three fecal pellets were homogenized in 1 ml of 30% acetic acid and extracted with 2 ml ethyl ether. One volume of this extract was then added 1 min after combining 2 volumes of *o*-tolidine reagent and 1 volume of 3% $H2O_2$. This mixture was inspected 1 min later for color. Of 30 daily tests on each of seven control animals, all but two tests were reported as negative using this procedure.

An improved approach for measuring fecal blood is the HemoQuant assay (2,136). The advantages of this technique are its increased sensitivity (compared to Hemoccult) and its capacity to detect degraded hemoglobin. The assay measures the fluorescence of porphyrin after removal of iron from the molecule. Direct measurement of stool samples detects porphyrins already released from hemoglobin by the action of intestinal and bacterial enzymes. Distinction can be made, therefore, between total and degraded hemoglobin, which may prove useful in determining the site of bleeding. A greater fraction of hemoglobin that is lost from the proximal sites would be expected to be degraded than that lost distally. The procedure for this assay is to heat the stool sample, for example, 8 mg for 90 min at 43°C in reducing acid (2.0 ml of 2.5 M oxalic acid and 0.09 M ferrous sulfate), extract iron-free porphyrins with a series of solvent washes, measure fluorescence with excitation setting at 402 nm and emission at 653 nm, and compare to a standard curve to determine milligrams of hemoglobin.

A second approach for assessing gastrointestinal bleeding is based on quantitating radioactivity in the feces following radioisotopic labeling of erythrocytes with ^{59}Fe or ^{51}Cr. This procedure, which requires greater experimental intrusion than colorimetric methods, entails intravenous administration of ^{59}Fe sulfate for in vivo labeling of erythrocytes (118) or of erythrocytes prelabeled with ^{51}Cr in vitro (87). These techniques, being based on radioisotopes, require the experimenter to exercise considerably greater attention to the proper housing of animals, handling of excreta, disposal of carcasses, and other problems related to contamination and exposure. However, such approaches are more sensitive than older colorimetric methods and are not subject to invalid results caused by interference from dietary sources. In addition, metabolism of hemoglobin during its transit through the gut lumen has less of an effect on a radioisotopic assay than on the peroxidase-based colorimetric ones. Reabsorption of the ^{59}Fe liberated from erythrocytes metabolized in the gut lumen is believed, however, to explain the lower estimates of gastrointestinal bleeding obtained with this isotope as compared to those from ^{51}Cr studies (93).

An example of the application of ^{59}Fe in quantitating gastrointestinal bleeding in experimental animals has been detailed by Phillips (118). The procedure entails intravenous administration of 50 μCi of ^{59}Fe-labeled ferrous sulfate in 1.0 ml isotonic saline to 10-kg dogs. Complete 24-h fecal collections are made, diluted to a fixed volume (750 ml) in water, and homogenized. The entire sample is then assayed for radioactivity, using a gamma counter with a large-volume well. An estimate of the volume of 24-h fecal blood loss is then computed by dividing the radioactivity in the stool by that found per milliliter of whole blood. An initial equilibration period, for example 7 days, is necessary for the disposition of injected ^{59}Fe not associated with erythrocytes. Studies can then be carried out for as long as 68 days after ^{59}Fe administration.

Cell Shedding

Another approach for quantitating structural damage to the gastrointestinal surface is to monitor the rate of cell loss into the gastrointestinal lumen. Exfoliation of mucosal cells from the gastric surface and intestinal villar apex is a normal component of the epithelial proliferative process in these organs (see below). Chemicals that induce mucosal injury may directly increase cell loss from these structures into the lumen.

One technique for quantitating the rate of cell loss is measurement of the DNA content of the luminal fluid. This approach was met with limited success when colorimetric methods were used for assay of DNA; sensitivity was insufficient and was affected by other luminal contents, for example, mucous glycoproteins. The use of radioimmunoassay for DNA is reported to improve the feasibility of this procedure greatly (67). The assay is sufficiently sensitive that small samples of luminal fluid can be withdrawn at frequent intervals from an experimental animal or human subject. The procedure has been described for gastric and duodenal studies in anesthetized cats, dogs with exteriorized Pavlovian pouches, and patients intubated with multilumen gastroduodenal tubes. For example, with the anesthetized cat (previously fasted to reduce luminal DNA content from feed sources), cannulas are inserted through the duodenal wall to form a 16-mm closed duodenal segment. Initially, luminal contents are rinsed out through the cannula. Test solutions in a 20-ml volume are perfused over 30 min, and 1-ml samples are removed for DNA measurement. Aliquots (50 ml) are assayed for DNA content. The assay procedure quantitates the extent to which the experimental samples displace ^{125}Iododeoxyuridine DNA from DNA antibodies. In these studies, each animal must serve as its own control. For purposes of summarizing the data, an estimate of the area of the mucosal surface is obtained for each animal at the end of the experiments by planimetry of the dissected, opened organ. This procedure has demonstrated quantitative and qualitative differences in responses of the stomach and duodenum from different species to acid and ulcerative agents.

ANALYSIS OF PROLIFERATION OF MUCOSAL CELLS

A potential effect of toxic substances on the gastrointestinal tract is alteration of the proliferative process, which occurs in the deeper regions of the gastric pits and in the intestinal crypts (31). This effect may be a primary event, as occurs with antineoplastic agents that impair cell division. The effect may, however, be a secondary one that occurs in response to changes in one of the many factors regulating gastrointestinal renewal, for example, hormones, microorganisms, feed intake, and tissue injury (97). For a review of the proliferative characteristics of the many cell types in gastrointestinal tissue in normal and pathological states the reader is referred to Lipkin (96,97).

Alterations in intestinal crypt cell division and migration up the villar surface may in some cases be inferred from histological evaluation of cell morphology and villar height. More definitive assessment is based on techniques of cell kinetic analysis (19,20). These procedures are based on pulse exposure of cells to tritiated thymidine, which is incorporated into DNA of crypt cells undergoing DNA replication. Tissue is collected at various times after thymidine exposure, and thin sections are processed using autoradiography. Specifically, in animal studies, ^{3}H-thymidine, 1 μCi/g body weight, is injected via the tail vein after an overnight fast (31).

Bouin's solution is injected into the gastrointestinal lumen, and the tissue of interest is removed, cut open, flattened, and fixed in additional solution. After conventional alcohol dehydration and paraffin embedding, 5-mm sections are mounted on glass slides, dipped in Kodak NTB-2 or NTB-3 photographic emulsion (diluted 1 : 1 with distilled water), and enclosed in lightproof containers at 4°C for 2–4 weeks. Slides are then developed with Kodak D19, fixed, and stained (e.g., hematoxylin and eosin). From these samples, it is possible to determine the time for complete migration of newly formed cells from the crypt to the site of extrusion on the villar tip. In addition, by evaluation of the fraction of mitoses in the crypt that are labeled with ^{3}H-thymidine as a function of time, one can estimate the characteristics of the cell cycle, including the duration of the various phases as well as the complete cell cycle time. Other markers for assessing cell proliferation kinetics include antibodies to cell cycle-related antigens, such as proliferation cell nuclear antigen (PCNA), and to exogenously administered bromodeoxyuridine (195). These immunohistochemical approaches have the advantage of much more rapid processing time, hours rather than several weeks with autoradiography.

Methodology has been developed to analyze intestinal epithelial cell kinetics by flow cytometry. These procedures depend on separation and high recovery of crypt and villar cells from the intestinal wall (62). Cheng et al. (19,20) demonstrated the feasibility of incubation of intestinal tissue in calcium- and magnesium-free Hanks balanced salt solution containing 30 mM EDTA, followed by vibration, which removes the epithelial layer. Flow cytometry, which separates cells according to their DNA content, provides a much more rapid and precise approach to quantitation of cell kinetics than is possible with autoradiography.

As new columnar epithelial cells are formed in the intestinal crypts and subsequently migrate up the villus, they differentiate from proliferative, secretory cells to absorptive ones. There are numerous structural and functional indicators of this differentiation process (147). Several enzymes whose activities markedly differ in the crypt cells and fully differentiated villar cells have been used as markers to assess the differentiation process. These tools also have application in verification procedures for methods of separating crypt and villar cells. Examples include thymidine kinase, whose activity is highest in proliferating crypt cells (71); oligosaccharidases (25); fatty acid esterases (141); and cytochrome P-450s (78), whose activities are highest in differentiated villar cells. The activity of these enzymes is dependent not only on their rate of formation but also on their rate of degradation (52). This factor must be taken into account in interpretation of studies in which activity of mucosal enzymes is altered by xenobiotics.

DETERMINATION OF GASTRIC SECRETORY ACTIVITY

A primary function of the stomach is secretion of hydrogen ions by the parietal cells that line the gastric glands. Gastric acidity is required for optimum activation of pepsinogen, elaborated and secreted by the chief cells of the stomach. This enzyme is responsible for initial digestion of proteins present in the diet. The acid secretory activity of the stomach provides one index of the functional status of this organ. Numerous physiological factors affect basal and stimulated acid output, most notably neural and hormonal input to the parietal cell. The following are of importance to the toxicologist:

1. Agents with irritative effects on the gastric mucosa may, on chronic administration, produce gastritis characterized by inflammation, glandular atrophy, and reduction of secretory activity.
2. Agents that stimulate gastric acid secretion may cause acid-induced erosions and ulcers in the stomach and duodenum.

In Vivo Methods

One approach to measurement of gastric acid secretion is invasive. Animals are fasted for 24 h, and drinking water is withheld for 1 h. The animal is then briefly anesthetized, the abdomen opened, and a tie placed around the pylorus to prevent gastric emptying. The gastric content is removed through a syringe and a 22-gauge needle inserted through the gastric wall (158). The abdominal incision is sutured, and the animals are unrestrained. After a fixed interval, for example, 30 min, the animal is reanesthetized, the esophagus clamped, and the gastric contents aspirated again. After centrifugation to remove solid components, the fluid volume is determined. The sample is then assayed for the material under investigation. For determination of total titratable acidity, samples are titrated to pH 7.0 with 0.01 N NaOH, and results are usually expressed as millimoles per hour. (Use of pH 7.0 as an endpoint detects hydrogen ions associated with endogenous acidic compounds, e.g., mucoproteins.) Titration to pH 3.5 may provide a better estimate of hydrochloric acid (166). An interval longer than 30 min is not advisable because pyloric ligation induces acid secretion; after longer times a secretory effect of a chemical can be masked by the procedure itself (158).

An advance upon this procedure in anesthetized animals entails intravital microscopy of the gastric mucosal surface with a microfluorometric technique for measurement of intracellular pH. A small stainless steel disc with a 5 mm central aperture is affixed to an exposed gastric mucosal site for application of 5,6-carboxyfluorescein diacetate. The image intensity following loading with this dye is monitored at wavelengths that differ in their pH sensitivity. This methodology, which permits assessment of the intracellular surface cell pH, can be combined with determination of the local acid secretion rate, mucosal blood flow based on output from a laser Doppler instrument, and mucosal gel thickness based on microscopic analysis (163).

A noninvasive approach entails quantitation of the liberation of azure A from an azure A–resin complex in the stomach, a reaction that is pH dependent (138). Azure A is absorbed from the intestine only after release from the resin and is substantially cleared into the urine. With this technique, the dye (azuresin, Diagnex Blue) is administered by gavage in a dose of 20 mg/100 g in 2 ml of 4% gelatin. Animals are individually housed in metabolism cages, and urine is collected for 24 h. (Feed and water are withheld and the animals are subcutaneously injected with a total of 3 ml of 5% sucrose.) The 24-h urine volume is measured and concentration of azure A determined by spectrophotometry. In an experiment of this type, it is essential to verify that the experimental treatment does not affect the intestinal absorption or renal excretion of the unconjugated azure A. Azure A should therefore be administered to control and experimental animals to verify that once liberated from resin, its disposition is similar in the two groups.

A model that permits repeated study in an unanesthetized animal such as the dog is the use of the Heidenhain fundic pouch, which is surgically created with access to the body surface. The denervated preparation has the disadvantage of low basal acid secretory rate. The preparation, however, permits controlled exposure of the gastric surface to toxic substances and repeated measurement of volume changes, electrolyte concentrations, hemorrhage, and mucosal blood flow. This technique has been used to demonstrate the damaging effect of aspirin in acid solution on the mucosa (186). Characteristically, the drug induces a decrease in hydrogen concentration in the luminal solution (increased inward flux) and an increase in sodium, potassium, blood, and plasma protein efflux into the lumen.

In Vitro Methods

Significant advances in elucidating physiological mechanisms of gastric secretion have resulted from use of in vitro preparations (151). One approach is study of the epithelial tissue in a Ussing chamber. A segment of the stomach wall is removed from the animal, and the muscle layer is stripped off. The remaining tissue is mounted so as to separate two solutions. Acid secretion and electrolyte flux can be monitored.

For improved definition of the physiology of individual cell types in the stomach, techniques have been developed to isolate and culture gastric mucous cells (61) and the gastric gland and its individual cell types. The gastric gland preparation is obtained by treatment of the intact mucosa with pronase or collagenase. This material is primarily composed of parietal and peptic cells in greater concentration than in the intact tissue. Advantages of this approach include the relatively good viability of the glands and the relatively normal intercellular connections, including tight junctions.

Techniques have also been developed for isolation of parietal cells (151) and chief cells (177) from gastric glands. A calcium chelator, such as EDTA, increases dispersion of single cells from gastric glands (151). A Percoll step-gradient purification or centrifugal elutriation (131) can be effectively used to separate parietal cells from other cell types in the tissue, based on the difference in their mass. With these single-cell preparations, unlike the intact tissue, no anatomical barrier exists between mucosal and serosal surfaces. Alternative approaches must therefore be used for measuring hydrogen ion secretion. Two techniques include quantitating oxygen consumption of the cells and measuring their accumulation of aminopyrine. Several types of studies have shown a close correlation between oxygen consumption and the energy-dependent process of acid secretion. Measurement of oxygen consumption with a Clark-type polarographic electrode or Gilson respirometer is one index of secretory activity. Another approach is based on monitoring the uptake of a weak base, aminopyrine, into the intracellular vesicular space of the parietal cell (150). Aminopyrine, which has a pK_a of 5.0, readily traverses plasma membranes in its unionized form as it exists at neutral pH. In the parietal cell under conditions in which acid secretion is occurring, the compound becomes ionized in acid secretory vesicles and remains trapped in this acidic fluid. The cellular content of the compound relative to that in the medium can be used as an index of acid formation by the parietal cell. The conventional approach is to use the ^{14}C isotope of aminopyrine and measure radioactivity in cells separated from the media by filtration.

For review of procedures to assess gastric secretion of other substances that play a role in chemically induced ulcerogenesis, for example, mucins, prostaglandins, and bicarbonates, the reader is referred to texts by Harmon (56) and Allen et al. (3).

ASSESSMENT OF ABSORPTIVE FUNCTION OF THE GASTROINTESTINAL TRACT

The toxicologist is concerned with analysis of absorptive function of the gut for two primary reasons. One issue entails determination of the gastrointestinal absorption, metabolism, and excretion of toxic substances, and factors that affect this process (74,117,122,183). The second problem is understanding the effect of toxic substances on the absorption of normal dietary constituents or orally administered therapeutic agents. Similar methodology may be applied to analysis of both problems.

There are numerous approaches for studying gastrointestinal absorption, both in vivo and in vitro (1,78). The technique chosen for a particular study will depend on the aspect of the absorption process that is of primary interest. Broadly speaking, the methodology can be categorized according to the procedure for administering the test substance to the absorptive surface of the gut, and the technique for determining the extent and/or rate of absorption.

In Vivo Determination of Overall Extent of Gastrointestinal Absorption

One approach, permitting the most overall assessment of gastrointestinal absorption, is based on oral administration of a test substance, followed by determination of its concentration in systemic fluids as a function of time. This technique is the least precise approach to quantitating gastrointestinal absorption kinetics in that numerous variables may influence the results. However, this methodology provides the best measure of the bioavailability of a xenobiotic and the impact of its absorption kinetics on systemic exposure. This approach is also useful as a screening procedure for determining whether a test substance induces malabsorption of nutrients.

Dosing

Several techniques for administering a test substance in an absorption study may be relevant. In certain cases, such as in the determination of the gastrointestinal absorption of a toxic substance that may be a contaminant of the diet, the most meaningful analysis may entail appropriate incorporation of the substance into the diet of the experimental animal. Not only may the rate of absorption differ from that following oral intubation, but the extent of absorption may differ as well (175). Care must be exercised to ensure that the procedures required for dietary incorporation, especially into solid components of the diet, do not result in chemical modification of the test substance. Determination of the total ingested dose of the test substance must be made by careful measurement of the feedstuffs before and after presentation to the experimental animal. Such studies require use of metabolic cages that restrict the areas of the cage in which the animal has access to feed. As a consequence, unconsumed feed may be collected without contamination with urine, feces, or drinking water. Consideration must be made of the eating habits of the experimental animals. If consumption of the test substance over an extended period, for example, hours, is undesirable, animals may be fasted and then presented with the diet for a shorter interval. A fasting procedure, however, may alter both the rate and extent of absorption.

A second technique for oral administration of a test substance is its intubation into the stomach of experimental animals. This procedure permits more precise control of the administered dose and allows the investigator to give the same dose (in absolute terms or on a per kilogram basis) to each experimental animal. With this technique the test substance is administered in a fluid vehicle, either in solution or as a suspension. Intubations are readily carried out in small animals, for example, rats or mice, without use of sedative agents. The intubation needle must be passed into the stomach because delivery into the esophagus will often result in loss of dose by regurgitation or aspiration into the lungs. Intubation needles for animals of a variety of sizes are commercially available. Care must be taken to ensure that the volume of the dose administered does not exceed the capacity of the stomach. The eating habits of the animal should be taken into consideration because the maximum dosing volume must be smaller when feed is present in the stomach.

For many substances administered by the oral route, the rate of emptying from the stomach into the small intestine may be the determining factor in the overall rate and extent of systemic absorption (120). This phenomenon results from the generally lower rate of absorption of substances, whether acids, bases, or nonelectrolytes, from the stomach than from the small intestine, because of the smaller surface area of the gastric region and the larger intraluminal distances. Consequently, in studies in which the question of interest is the relative rate and extent of absorption of an agent through the intestinal mucosal barrier, dosing in feed or by intubation may be inappropriate. For such a study, the test substance should be directly administered into the intestinal lumen. This procedure has been extensively used in the study of intestinal transport in humans through use of small-bore intubating tubes localized through radiographic techniques (37). In studies with small animals, dosing into the intestine is readily achieved by lightly anesthetizing the animal, making a midline incision through the gut wall, and inserting a needle into the intestinal lumen through the gut wall opposite the attachment of the mesenteries. A tie should be made around the intestine to include the needle to prevent efflux of the injected substance at the site of insertion.

When administering a potentially toxic agent by the oral route to assess its absorption, the investigator must choose doses and their concentration with care. Preferably, a concentration range is achieved in the gastrointestinal lumen of the experimental animals, which includes levels likely to be reached during exposures in man. It is important to consider the possibility that an agent may produce direct effects on mucosal cells that alter its own absorption kinetics. Such a phenomenon would be expected to be highly dependent on the concentration of the agent in the gastrointestinal lumen. A similar consideration applies in choosing doses of nutrients when testing the effects of chemicals on absorption of dietary substances. Many nutrients are absorbed by concentration-dependent mechanisms, for example, facilitated diffusion and active transport. Effects of chemicals on absorption of a nutrient may therefore depend on the dose of both substances.

To quantitate the total amount of absorption from the oral route by sampling systemic fluids, the agent under study is also administered systemically (43). Ideally, the substance is given by the intravenous route, which provides a standard of complete systemic absorption for comparision to the situation after oral dosing. Where possible, the intravenous dose should be chosen to produce plasma concentrations in the range of those expected after oral administration. This adjustment is especially important in the case of substances likely to produce acute toxic effects, especially effects that might alter the distribution, metabolism, or elimination of the agent itself.

Quantitation of Absorption

Sampling Techniques and Experimental Design. In an investigation of the overall absorption of an agent following its acute oral administration, quantitation of the rate and extent of this process entails appropriate sampling and analysis of the concentration of the agent in a systemic fluid as a function of time. Relevant information may be derived from sampling not only systemic fluids such as plasma, but also saliva, urine, or breath. In addition, a more direct approach for analyzing absorption characteristics than the sampling of systemic or excreted body fluids entails the sampling of portal blood (115) or the collection of the mesenteric blood draining the sites of absorption of the test substances (7). These procedures require considerably more complicated surgical techniques and may necessitate transfusions of blood into the animal. An important advantage of this procedure is the capacity to determine the in vivo kinetics of biotransformation of a test substance by intestinal tissues. An analogous approach for studying perturbations in mucosal uptake and metabolism of triglycerides and cholesterol is to cannulate the mesenteric lymphatic vessel for sampling lymph that carries these lipids from their absorption site (57). To assess the contribution of enterohepatic circulation of a substance to its systemic concentrations, studies can be carried out in animals with biliary cannulas that are exteriorized for complete biliary diversion or that are forked to enter the gut lumen as well as provide an exterior sampling site (98).

Generally, collection of plasma samples is preferred as a relatively noninvasive procedure, which provides the most direct indication of systemic concentration of the agent under study. A number of considerations dictate aspects of experimental design and procedure. First of all, samples must be collected over a sufficiently long time to determine the area under the plasma concentration versus time curve. Second, the volume of each sample must be large enough to permit detection of the agent by the method of quantitation. Third, the amount of blood withdrawn from the animal must not be so large as to affect blood volume and the subsequent kinetics of the agent under study.

Data Analysis. Under most circumstances, the extent of gastrointestinal absorption of a substance after acute administration is proportional to the area under the curve (AUC) of its concentration in plasma as a function of time. Consequently, assessment of extent of absorption, or bioavailability, can be determined by comparing the area achieved after oral administration to that after intravenous administration in which absorption is complete. Similarly, to determine whether a chemical induces malabsorption of a nutrient, the AUC of the nutrient is computed under control and test conditions. It is critical to recognize that the AUC is also a function of the elimination kinetics of the substance, specifically its total plasma clearance. Changes in this parameter may therefore be a source of error in the assessment of oral absorption by this method.

The area under the plasma concentration–time curve can be calculated by several techniques. A simple approach entails performing this integration by the trapezoidal rule (43). Another more precise approach is the use of Simpson's rule (162). These techniques have the advantage of not requiring a mathematical model to describe the kinetics observed. The ratio of the area observed after oral administration to that after intravenous route is a measure of the systemic absorption of an agent, its bioavailability. The extent of absorption, as determined by this procedure, is dependent not only on the nature of the transport of a substance through the mucosal cell barrier but also on the magnitude of biotransformation that occurs during the absorption process (the first-pass effect) (42,55).

Malabsorption Tests for Dietary Substances

Monosaccharides: the D-Xylose Test. The functional integrity of the proximal small intestine can be assessed by quantitation of D-Xylose absorption. D-Xylose is a pentose monosaccharide that is absorbed by passive diffusion as well as by the Na^+-coupled carrier mechanism for dietary sugars, for example, glucose and galactose. D-Xylose has the advantage over glucose for testing purposes in that (a) its blood levels are insensitive to insulin, (b) its elimination pathway is primarily (although not exclusively) through renal excretion and not systemic metabolism, and (c) it is not normally present in blood or urine. Extensive injury to the luminal surface of the small intestine is reflected in reduction of the concentration of D-Xylose in the blood and urine after its oral administration. Xylose is absorbed intact and is not dependent on mammalian luminal or brush border enzyme activity. The xylose test would generally not be abnormal in cases in which malabsorption, for example, of fats or polysaccharides, results from defects in luminal or brush border enzyme activity. The test is carried out as follows: Animals are fasted, for example, for 12 h, to minimize variability in results associated with stomach emptying and interactions with dietary contents. D-Xylose is then administered by gavage (0.5 g/kg body weight) in an aqueous solution. Blood samples are obtained every 30 min for 180 min. The concentration of D-Xylose in plasma is determined by a spectrophotometric assay (166). A review of studies in dogs indicates that normal animals exhibit peak plasma levels of D-Xylose greater than 45 mg/dl between 60–90 min (140). Malabsorption is characterized by reduced peak levels and AUC. Possible errors of interpretation occur if: (i) gastric emptying is unusually slow, in which case the rate of absorption and therefore the peak plasma concentration will be low; (ii) marked bacterial overgrowth exists in the proximal small intestine, in which case bacterial metabolism of D-Xylose reduces its availability for absorption (168); (iii) renal clearance of D-Xylose is depressed, which elevates the plasma levels and may mask an absorption defect. These sources of error can be evaluated from urinary excretion data. The bladder must be empty at time of xylose administration and complete urine collections must subsequently be carried out.

Disaccharides. Disaccharides in the diet or released on starch digestion are absorbed only after cleavage into monosaccharides by the disaccharidases of the intestinal brush border (192). Malabsorption, including diarrhea and abdominal distension, may result from low activity of these enzymes, as occurs, for example, in lactase deficiency which is a genetically based phenomenon. In addition, the activity of disaccharidases may be selectively impaired by synthetic structural analogues of the endogenous substrates. Inhibition or deficiency of these enzymes can be assessed by oral administration of the disaccharide substrate and measurement of the subsequent rise in blood glucose. This rise is depressed under conditions of impaired disaccharidase activity. To prove the specificity of the abnormality, it is necessary to demonstrate that the absorption of glucose administered orally is normal. Numerous experimental variables can influence plasma glucose levels. In rats, for example, factors such as method and duration of restraint, method of blood collection, animal handling, and fasting can alter baseline values (10), which average 98–152 mg/dl in plasma and serum (123). Experiments should be designed to minimize variability from these sources. Verification of altered brush border enzyme activity can be carried out by in vitro assays using intestinal homogenates or brush border membrane preparations.

Fats. Under normal conditions, fat in the diet is nearly completely digested and absorbed. Lipids that are excreted in the feces are primarily associated with intestinal bacterial cells and mucosal cells sloughed from the intestinal surface. Structurally, these lipids include mono-, di-, and triglycerides, fatty acids, phospholipids, glycolipids, sterols, and cholesterol esters. Numerous factors affect the process of digestion and absorption of dietary lipids (172). Fat malabsorption can therefore result from a variety of different toxic mechanisms. A primary goal in determining the cause of fat malabsorption is to distinguish between defects in the intraluminal digestion of fats to fatty acids from impairment in fatty acid absorption. Impaired digestion of lipids suggests a reduction in pancreatic lipase activity, which may result from a lack of the cholecystokinin signal for release, exocrine pancreatic insufficiency, or presence of a lipase inhibitor. Absorption defects may result from impaired micelle formation because of bile salt deficiency, reduced mucosal cell uptake because of cell damage or villous atrophy, impaired reesterification and chylomicron formation caused by reduced enzyme activities in the mucosa, and reduced chylomicron transport into the lymphatics because of cellular infiltration of the lamina propria or systemic lymphatic disease.

Crude screening for fat malabsorption can be effectively carried out by examination of the feces. Steatorrhea, an increase in fecal fat, can be qualitatively detected by use of the Sudan III preparation stain. A fresh sample of feces is smeared on a microscope slide. Two drops of glacial acetic acid and two drops of Sudan III are then added and a cover slip is placed on top. The slide is heated until the sample boils. The specimen is then examined for the presence of refractile orange droplets, which are fat globules. With high-power magnification, the presence in a single field of many orange droplets the size of, or larger than, red blood cells is an indication of steatorrhea. Quantitative assessment of fecal lipid excretion can be accomplished gravimetrically or by titration of total fatty acids (32).

Once steatorrhea has been documented, additional tests are needed to determine the cause. The initial objective should be to distinguish maldigestion from malabsorption to isolate the mechanisms described above. One approach is oral dosing with a radiolabeled triglyceride, for example, triolein, and on a separate occasion, the fatty acid (oleic acid). In clinical studies the validity of this approach has been demonstrated by use of the ^{13}C- and ^{14}C-labeled compounds, with assay of the isotope in breath CO_2 at hourly intervals 3–6 h after ingestion of the lipid (135). Reduction in the absorption of triglyceride but not fatty acid is indicative of a defect in intraluminal metabolism. Impairment of fatty acid absorption, as well, suggests bile salt deficiency or mucosal injury.

In Vivo Intestinal Closed-Segment Technique

With the in vivo closed-segment technique, a solution of the agent under study is directly administered into the intestinal lumen (181). The region of the intestine of interest is identified, using landmarks such as the ligament of Trietz (just distal of the pylorus) and the ileocaecal junction. A segment is closed distally with a ligature. The needle for injection is then inserted at a more proximal site, and the gut lumen is closed around the needle with another tie. Care must be taken to ensure that the needle tip remains only within the lumen of the closed segment and does not puncture the gut wall. After the solution is injected, this tie is tightened and knotted as the needle is slowly withdrawn. To minimize variability in the results in a single experiment, segments should be located in the same part of the intestine in all the animals, the length of the segment should be approximately the same, and the volume of fluid administered into the lumen should be identical. After dosing, the incision in the abdomen should be sutured, and the animal permitted to regain consciousness to minimize any possible influence of the anesthetic agent.

Quantitation of Absorption

At a predetermined time after injection of the agent under study, the animal is anesthetized for removal of the entire closed intestinal segment. The amount of the injected substance remaining in this segment is then quantitated after homogenization of the sample. The extent of absorption is determined as the difference between the total amount injected and the amount remaining in the segment at the end of the absorption period. This approach has the advantage of directly determining the entire systemic absorption from both the intestinal lumen and the mucosal cell. This method differs in this respect from perfusion techniques in which the absorption of substances is quantitated from their loss out of the luminal fluid. Especially for substances that are highly bound in the intestinal mucosal cell, absorption out of the intestinal lumen cannot be equated with absorption into the systemic circulation.

The quantitation of absorption by determining the disappearance of a substance from a closed segment is only valid if loss does not occur because of metabolism of the substance in the intestinal lumen or tissue. If metabolism of the substance does occur, assay of the intestinal closed segment for the parent compound and metabolites alone is inadequate for description of its absorption kinetics, unless metabolites are poorly absorbed and are all completely recovered in the gut samples. Consequently, analysis should be carried out to determine whether metabolite formation and absorption would be likely to occur before choosing this technique to assess the absorption rate of a compound.

Intestinal Perfusion Techniques

Another in vivo procedure for quantitating intestinal transport is based on infusion of a solution at a constant rate into the intestinal lumen (95). The amount of the test substance in the effluent from a distal site is compared to the amount infused into the gut to determine its net absorption as a function of time. This technique, unlike the other in vivo procedures described above, is especially useful in studying the transport of water and its perturbations by toxicological compounds. Quantitation of the net flux of water into the gut caused by absorptive and secretory processes can be carried out by monitoring the change in intraluminal concentration of a nonabsorbable marker. ^{14}C-Polyethylene glycol 4000 (PEG) is a frequently used marker substance suitable for these purposes (149).

Before a perfusion study, animals should be fasted overnight to reduce luminal contents of the intestine. Animals are then anesthetized, and the proximal and distal ends of the region of the intestine of interest are cannulated. With rats, for example, PE-50 polyethylene tubing is inserted into the intestinal lumen of the anesthetized animals. The marker is then infused into the proximal tubing using a peristalic pump. The solution containing PEG, under most circumstances, should be made isotonic with the plasma of the species under study and should be heated to body temperature. An initial equilibrium period of PEG infusion must be carried out to obtain constant output rates from the distal end of the small intestine.

After equilibration, fluid from the distal cannula is collected for fixed intervals, for example, 10 min. Aliquots are removed for determination of the concentration of PEG in the effluent. The volume of the effluent can then be determined by computing the ratio of the amount of PEG infused during the collection period to its concentration in the collected fluid:

$$\text{Effluent volume} = \frac{\text{pump rate} \times \text{collection period} \times [\text{PEG in infused fluid}]}{[\text{PEG in collected fluid}]}$$

Comparison of the volume infused to that of the effluent then provides a measure of the net absorption or secretion of water by the intestinal segment.

A modification of this approach has been developed for studies in dogs (101). An exteriorized segment of the small intestine is opened and fixed in a plexiglass chamber with the vascular and neural supply still intact. The mucosal surface faces up into the chamber, which is perfused with test solutions. An advantage of this method is the ability to use videomicroscopic techniques to monitor villous motility.

In Vitro Methods

Numerous advances in the understanding of cellular mechanisms of electrolyte flux and nutrient absorption in the intestine have been made using in vitro, as opposed to in vivo, techniques. The review by Kimmich (83) documents the impact of in vitro techniques on elucidation of intestinal transport mechanisms of sugar. With in vitro procedures, physiological variables, for example, intestinal motility and mesenteric blood flow, can be eliminated or controlled. In addition, the experimenter has the option of control over factors such as the composition of the solution bathing both the mucosal and the serosal side of the intestine and the electrochemical potential difference between the mucosal and serosal surfaces. Another advantage of certain in vitro techniques is the ability to carefully control the stirring rate in the mucosal solution. The stirring rate influences the thickness of the unstirred water layer, which can impose significant resistance to the mucosal uptake of substrates such as long-chain fatty acids, bile acids, cholesterol, and monosaccharides (172). The layer of mucus that adheres to the mucosal cell surface can also impede the diffusion of nutrients, for example, disaccharides, small peptides (148), and cholesterol (104). The pronounced quantitative differences in the uptake rates of nutrients into various in vitro preparations of the small intestine (165) probably result, at least in part, from differences in the resistances conferred by the unstirred water layer and mucous coat. In vitro techniques include those analogous to in vivo methods already discussed. Investigators, for example, have studied the absorption of substances from isolated gut segments with perfusions of the lumen (81) and with perfusions of the vasculature (68).

One in vitro method with no in vivo analogue is the everted sac technique (190). This method has been useful in the characterization of energy-dependent carrier-mediated transport processes. In this procedure small lengths of the intestine are everted, filled with fluid, and tied at both ends. Absorption is quantitated by monitoring the appearance of a test substance inside the sac in the fluid bathing the serosal surface of the intestine. Unlike the in vivo condition, therefore, absorption of a test substance in this model is considered equivalent to its passage not only through the mucosa but also through the submucosa, the external muscle layers, and serosal tissue of the gut wall. Problems with the everted segment technique include inadequate oxygen diffusion into the tissue and distension and hydration of the gut segment. Consequently, the preparation of the tissue and the experimental incubations must be short in duration. Everted sacs of the duodenum from rats exhibit structural abnormalities after 5-min incubation at 37°C (94).

A further refinement has been the development of methods for isolating gut mucosal cells (6). Methods for recovering mucosal cells, for example, scraping the inner surface of the gut with a glass slide or vibrating a gut segment everted on a glass spiral, have been improved to reduce contamination from cells of the lamina propria (169), as well as to isolate crypt cells (58). In addition, of importance to analysis of nutrient digestion and absorption and alteration by xenobiotics (11) has been the isolation of brush border membranes, recovered as vesicles after differential centrifugation of tissue from intestinal segments (63,154) or biopsies (142). The preparation permits analysis of membrane transport kinetics uncontaminated by cytosolic metabolism of the permeant. Also, production of membrane vesicles is reported to remove adherent mucus (148) so that this preparation, unlike in vivo and other in vitro models, is devoid of this diffusion barrier. Basal–lateral membranes of mucosal cells have also been isolated by the use of differential and discontinuous sucrose-gradient centrifugation (29). Isolation of these membrane fractions has facilitated the biochemical, structural, and genetic characterization of membrane transport proteins, such as the Na–glucose transporter in the brush border membrane (8,33,80,153), and their regulation by signal transduction mechanisms. Methods based on use of lipid-soluble fluorophores and fluorescent spectroscopy have permitted assessment of alterations in the fluidity of brush border membranes induced by membrane-perturbing toxicants (30).

An additional in vitro preparation has been a major significance to the elucidation of mechanisms controlling electrolyte absorption and secretion (12). This procedure, the use of a Ussing chamber (173), entails in vitro short-term exposure of a segment of intestine to defined mucosal and serosal solutions. The electrical potential difference across the intestine is measured with a voltmeter, and short-circuit current with an external microamp source. Flux of electrolytes is determined by addition of an isotope to the solution bathing one surface of the intestinal segment and monitoring its accumulation in the tissue or solution bathing the other surface.

Similarly, the unidirectional flux chamber designed by Schultz et al. (134) exposes a defined area of luminal surface of the intestinal wall to solution containing the test permeant. Brief exposure times are used to permit measurement of influx through the mucosa. This methodology permits assessment of the integrity of brush border transport mechanisms. Studies of intact tissue, as compared to mucosa stripped of external muscle and enteric ganglia, permit assessment of neuroregulation and its modification by exogenous substances (124,139).

An in vitro preparation with the advantage of more prolonged viability is the organ culture of mucosal biopsies (65,111). This technique permits the in vitro maintenance of mucosal explants for 24–48 h, depending on the species and region of the intestine biopsied. Modification of culture conditions may permit even greater longevity of samples (36). Autrup (5), for example, reported maintenance of human colonic mucosa for 28 days. A major advantage of this approach is that the normal anatomical arrangement of the villus and its mucosal cell proliferation and differentiation can be studied. This preparation has been useful in the study of colonic carcinogenesis and chemotherapy. Toxicant accumulation and efflux can be characterized as well, and related to biological effects. This approach has been used to provide evidence of the role of P-glycoprotein encoded by the *mdr1* (multidrug resistance) gene in colonic transport of the alkaloid vincristine (72).

Development of mucosal cell lines in culture (CaCO-2, T_{84} and HT_{29}) has further enhanced in vitro techniques for studying electrolyte transport, its regulation, and perturbation by toxicants. Dharmsathaphorn et al. (27) described the structural and functional characteristics of the human colonic carcinoma cell line, T_{84}, which forms a confluent monolayer in culture. These cells, when grown in serum-supplemented medium, exhibit properties characteristic of the normal epithelum, including the presence of tight junctions, apical microvilli, and vectorial electrolyte transport. Transport by the monolayer, for example, of sodium, mannitol, and inulin, can be monitored in a modified low-turbulence Ussing chamber (59). A collagen-coated filter substrate is preferable to plastic (99). A subclone of the HT_{29} colon adenocarcinoma cell line (HT-29-18N2) has been developed with a phenotype like the intestinal goblet cell and provides a methodologic approach for study of alteration in mucus secretion by xenobiotics (92,119).

ROLE OF MICROFLORA IN GASTROINTESTINAL TOXICITY

A comprehensive review of model systems for in vivo and in vitro study of the gastrointestinal flora has been published by Rumney and Rowland (129). The entire length of the gastrointestinal tract is populated by a diversity of microorganisms (144,174). It is not uncommon to find 400 different species of bacteria in the feces of a single subject (46). The species composition and quantity of the microflora differ markedly in the various regions of the gastrointestinal tract. The stomach is relatively sparsely populated ($<10^3$ colony forming units [CFU]/ml) due to the gastric juices that destroy a vast majority of microorganisms (46). The population of microflora in the stomach consist primarily of gram-positive, aerobic microorganisms, for example, *Streptococci*, *Staphylococci*, and *Lactobacilli*. The concentration of microorganisms in the small intestine increases from 10^3–10^4 CFU/ml in the duodenum to 10^6–10^7 CFU/ml in the distal ileum (46). Along the small intestine the concentration of gram-positive microbes decreases as the concentration of gram-negative aerobes increases. The large intestine is densely inhabited by gram-negative anaerobes such that luminal contents may contain 10^{12} CFU/ml. Among the more prominent species are *Bacteroides*, *Bifidobacterium*, *Fusobacterium*, *Clostridium*, and *Eubacterium* (46). Studies with animals that are delivered and reared under germ-free conditions have clearly demonstrated that the indigenous microflora influence the structure and function of the gastrointestinal tract (23,34,39).

The gut microflora may mediate toxic effects on this organ by a variety of mechanisms. *Helicobacter pylori* is now recognized as a leading cause of gastritis and peptic ulcers (178). Pathogenic strains such as *Shigella* elicit damage in part by their capacity to invade the mucosal epithelium and produce necrosis and hemorrhagic effects (132). Microorganisms are also capable of elaborating toxins that cause diarrhea by perturbing mucosal cell electrolyte and water flux. The toxin of *Vibrio cholerae*, for example, has become an important tool for elucidation of biochemical mechanisms regulating cyclic AMP-dependent chloride efflux. Overgrowth of the indigenous bacterial population in the small intestine may also produce malabsorption, most notably of fats and vitamin B_{12} (103).

Another mechanism of toxicity mediated by intestinal microorganisms is an indirect one. The bacterial population is capable of catalyzing numerous chemical reactions that can alter the biologic activity of dietary substances and xenobiotics, especially in more distal portions of the gut (47,48,126,127). Many examples exist of bacterial activation of chemicals to a form that exerts toxicity in the gut. A classic case is that of cycasin, the β-glucoside of methylazoxymethanol (MAM), which is contained in nuts of cycad plants (108). The β-glucosidase activity of indigenous bacteria hydrolyzes cycasin and releases MAM, a mutagenic carcinogen that causes tumor formation in the colon, liver, and kidney (88).

Methods for Toxin Studies

A conventional technique for assessing the potential of a microorganism to perturb electrolyte and water flux in the gut is use of the rabbit ileal segment. Toxins of bacteria, for example, *V. cholerae*, *Clostridium difficile*, and *E. coli*, that produce diarrhea in humans and experimental animals, cause fluid accumulation when injected into a closed segment of the small intestine. This technique provides a simple experimental approach for identifying the potential of a toxin for inducing intestinal antiabsorptive and/or secretory activity and estimating its potency (76,79,170,171). Young (12–24-week-old) rabbits are fasted overnight. The ileum, which is more sensitive and gives more consistent results than jejunum, is tied into three or four closed segments each 3 inches long. Segments are separated by 6 inches. Cultures or supernatant are injected into the segments with a 22-gauge needle. The animal is allowed to recover from anesthesia and then reanesthetized to examine the ileal contents after 4–6 h. The experimenter can distinguish between toxicity induced by an exotoxin from that resulting from bacterial invasion of the mucosa. Experimental approaches that have permitted elucidation of the intestinal mucosal surface receptors for enterotoxins and their mechanism of activating chloride secretion by elevating mucosal adenylate cyclase in crypt cells or inhibiting sodium absorption in villous cells are illustrated in studies by Lencer et al. (91) and Keusch et al. (82), respectively.

Methods for Bacterial Metabolism Studies

An experimental approach for assessing the role of intestinal bacteria in mediating gastrointestinal or systemic toxicity is the use of germ-free animals. Rats, for example, that have been aseptically delivered by cesarean section and reared under germ-free conditions are available from animal suppliers. Procedures required for establishing and maintaining a germ-free animal colony are described by Foster (39). To test whether bacteria are responsible for metabolic alteration of a compound, comparison can be made of its urinary and fecal elimination in germ-free and conventional animals of the same strain. A difference in the composition of the metabolites of the compound in the urine or the feces may suggest participation of bacterially mediated reactions in the biotransformation process. Absence of a particular metabolite of an administered compound in the urine or feces from the germ-free animal is presumptive evidence that the reaction is only catalyzed by bacterial and not mammalian enzymes.

Support for such a hypothesis can be obtained by examining the in vitro metabolic capability of defined bacterial cultures or of homogenates of the luminal gut contents. In experiments of this type, the culture conditions can markedly affect the experimental outcome. With studies of large intestinal contents or bacterial isolates from this source, it is especially important to carry out experiments using anaerobic conditions because the majority of organisms from this site are obligate anaerobes that are highly sensitive to even brief exposure to aerobic conditions. Demonstration of a particular enzymatic activity in a bacterial strain in vitro provides additional evidence of a possible bacterial role. However, it has frequently been difficult to predict in vivo routes of intestinal metabolism from in vitro studies. One possible reason for discrepancies of this type is offered by the work of Tasich and Piper (164). Their studies demonstrate a synergistic interaction between an extract from *Bacteroides fragilis*, which populates the distal intestine, and the microsomal enzyme activity of the colonic mucosa. Each component alone had minimal capacity to transform 2-aminoanthracene into a mutagen (with respect to a *Salmonella* tester strain). However, in combination, a substantial increase in mutagen formation occurred. The mechanism of this activating effect of a heat-labile component of the bacteria on the colonic microsomes is not known. This observation illustrates the complex interaction between bacteria, intestinal tissue, and xenobiotics, and the potential limitations of in vitro studies.

ASSESSMENT OF THE PROPULSIVE FUNCTION OF THE GASTROINTESTINAL TRACT

A potential toxic effect of substances on the gastrointestinal tract is derangement of the propulsive function of this organ. Normal propulsion of the intraluminal contents of the gut is essential for the appropriate digestion of dietary constituents, delivery to their sites of absorption, and elimination of unabsorbed materials. In addition, a key variable in the gastrointestinal disposition of a toxicant is the motility of the organ, which affects transit of the luminal contents. Numerous studies with pharmacologic agents, for example, have demonstrated that changes in gastric emptying can alter the overall absorption half-life of the compound (120). Generally, increased delivery rate to the small intestine is associated with more rapid absorption because of the greater surface area and higher blood flow of this tissue compared to the stomach.

There are numerous factors that influence the propulsive function of the gut and consequently many mechanisms by which substances can interfere with this aspect of gut physiology. For coverage of this subject, the reader should consult the reviews of Hunt (66), Weisbrodt (187), Christensen (22), and Burks (18). The motility patterns of the gastrointestinal tract, that is, the frequency and time-course of contractions, differ throughout the organ. The major determinants are similar, however. One key component is the smooth muscle cells of the circular, longitudinal, and, in the stomach, oblique layers. These cells act as a syncytium and display a baseline electrophysiological pattern with associated baseline contractile activity that differs in various regions. A complex system of neurons in the gut wall, including the myenteric plexus between the longitudinal and circular muscles, plays a role in coordinated changes in motility. A key feature of propulsion in the stomach and small intestine are contractions that originate in the lower esophagus and pass distally to the ileum (187). This contractile pattern, important in propelling transit of luminal contents, is dependent on enteric neurons (not extrinsic). Among the neurotransmitters of the complex neuronal architecture of the gut wall are vasoactive intestinal peptide, enkephalin, substance P, gastrin-releasing peptide, neuropeptide Y, and somatotropin (24).

Extrinsic neurons affect motility as well (125). Cholinergic input from the vagus and distally from the pelvic nerve terminate in the myenteric plexus; post-ganglionic fibers innervating the muscle release acetylcholine which stimulates contraction. Sympathetic neural input from the celiac, superior mesenteric, and inferior mesenteric ganglia terminates in the myenteric plexus and norepinephrine release inhibits function of cholinergic neurons.

Gut motility is also subject to alteration by hormones synthesized in the stomach and duodenum such as gastrin, secretin, and cholecystokinin. Components of the diet are one regulator of their release. For example, an increase in fatty acids in the duodenum following a high fat meal stimulates release of cholecystokinen, which may then mediate in part an inhibition of gastric emptying.

Methods used in the analysis of gastrointestinal propulsive function are of several types. One approach entails study of the transit of unabsorbed marker substances, the most direct approach for assessment of changes in propulsion. Other techniques involve analysis of the pressure in the gut lumen with a variety of devices used in the monitoring of pressure changes. More direct analysis of the properties of the smooth muscle of the gut is achieved by quantitation of its contractile activity (187) or its electrical activity (44,161), which may be determined in vivo or in vitro.

Measurement of the Transit of Luminal Contents

The propulsive activity of the gastrointestinal tract can be assessed by monitoring the transit of a nonabsorbable intraluminal marker. Flow of the gut contents is influenced by a variety of factors, a critical one being contractile activity of the gastrointestinal circular and longitudinal smooth muscle. Substances affecting the resting tone or frequency of contraction of the smooth muscle would therefore be expected to affect the transit characteristics. A second important factor that affects transit is the volume and viscosity of the intraluminal content. Flow can also be altered by substances that act on mucosal cells of the gut and alter their absorptive and secretory activities. This technique can therefore serve as an effective screening device for substances that affect the gastrointestinal tract by numerous mechanisms.

The application of this method requires the choice of a valid marker. Among the characteristics of the ideal marker are lack of absorption from the gut, minimal adsorption onto the mucosal surface, lack of effect on gut function, and ease of precise quantitation. An additional consideration is the physical form of the marker. This factor is especially relevant to the study of gastric emptying, in which it has been shown that the contractile activity of the stomach has differing effects on solid as compared to liquid components of the stomach (89,106). Suitable markers for tracing flow of substances in solution include sodium chromate, labeled with ^{51}Cr, and polyvinyl pyrollidine, labeled with ^{125}I or ^{131}I (54). Markers used for solid components of the diet include ^{99m}technitium, incorporated into chicken liver meal (89). The use of gamma-emitting radioisotopes has the advantage of allowing assay of the gastrointestinal segment and contents directly without any processing of the sample. The composition and volume of the solution or test meal containing a marker must be strictly controlled to minimize potential variability from this source. An example of a liquid test solution is 0.1 M Krebs phosphate buffer (pH 7.4) containing 100 mg glucose, 2.0 mg polyethylene glycol, 0.5 mg phenol red, and 100 μCi of ^{51}Cr as Na_2CrO_4 per 100 ml of solution (156). For studies with 200–300 g rats, 1 ml of this solution is administered intragastrically or 0.5 ml intraduodenally.

A second critical factor in carrying out a transit study is the method of administering the marker. If the marker is administered by gastric intubation, the transit of the marker will be markedly affected by stomach emptying. If the experimenter is more interested in propulsion through the small intestine, the marker should be directly administered into the duodenum via an indwelling cannula (156). This technique avoids use of anesthesia or acute duodenal intubations, both of which would be expected to affect gastrointestinal contractility. The method entails anesthetizing the animal and making a midline incision. A no. 15 spinal needle is then inserted through the back of the neck and fed subcutaneously to a ventral site where it is passed through the abdominal muscles and forestomach into the duodenum. PE 50 polyethylene tubing is then threaded through the needle and held in the duodenum as the needle is removed. The stomach is sutured to the abdominal wall at the site where the tubing has passed. A blunt 22-gauge needle is placed in the tubing opening at the back of the neck and sutured to the skin. Animals are used in transit studies 5 days later. The marker is injected at the neck and then flushed with air in a volume equivalent to the dead space of the tubing. A similar procedure has been described in which the cannula is inserted directly through the duodenal wall (155).

A third variable in this methodology is the procedure for quantitation of the location of the marker in the gastrointestinal tract. The animal should be rapidly euthanized for removal of the gut. A report by Scott and Summers (137) indicated that no major differences are observed in transit patterns after use of various procedures for rapid sacrifice of the animal. A technique should then be used to prevent movement of the marker in the gut before its assay. One approach, for example, is to put ligatures at 3–5 cm lengths of the small intestine. The technique, introduced by Derblom et al. (26), permits detection of radioactivity along the continuous length of the gastrointestinal tract. The organ is placed on a device that is moved at a constant rate under a scintillation detector, and radioactive counts are continuously recorded. Integration of the radioactive counts in a particular region, either instrumentally or by planimeter, then permits reporting of marker content as a percentage of the total amount detected. One commonly used approach is to describe the small intestinal radioactivity for 10 equal segments. Without equipment for continuous recording, the gut can be cut into segments that are individually counted in a conventional well-type gamma counter (185).

Several procedures have been used for summarizing data on marker distribution in order to facilitate comparisons among treatments. In studies of gastric emptying, the percent of the marker remaining in the stomach is calculated, and the mean for control animals is compared to those in the experimental group by appropriate statistical methods. In studies of intestinal transit, one approach is to identify the most distal site that 50% of the marker has reached. This site can then be expressed as a percent of the total distance of the small intestine, a value that is then used in statistical analyses. Another approach is to compute the geometric center of marker distribution (109). For each segment assayed, the marker content is determined as a percent of the total recovered, and is multiplied by the segment number, 1 being the most proximal and n being the nth and most distal. These values are summed and divided by n to generate the geometric center.

Two additional points should be noted about the experimental design of a transit study. First of all, the time at which the animal is killed should be chosen so that in control animals, half the marker has been emptied from the stomach or has traversed to the midpoint of the small intestine after gastric or intraduodenal administration, respectively. This approach improves the likelihood of demonstrating inhibition or acceleration of transit by test substances. Second, in an investigation of the effect of a substance on gastrointestinal transit, studies should be carried out at a series of time points after various doses of the test substance. Because each animal provides only one measure of marker distribution, each experimental condition requires use of replicate animals.

Measurement of Contractility of Gastrointestinal Smooth Muscle In Vitro

Introduction

The contractile and electrophysiological properties of smooth muscle can be assessed with relative simplicity using in vitro preparations of this organ. Such in vitro techniques are of value in screening potentially toxic substances for effects on gastrointestinal smooth muscle and for elucidation of mechanisms of effects on propulsion observed with in vivo methodology. Use of in vitro techniques to study gastrointestinal motility has certain advantages over in vivo procedures. Generally, they are technically simpler to execute. They isolate the tissue from extrinsic neural and hormonal influences. The tissue can also be directly exposed to the test substance. These advantages are at the expense of loss of prediction of in vivo effects of a test substance.

The choice of a particular in vitro technique depends on the specific aim of the experimentation. Those techniques that are most commonly used differ in two ways. First, the species from which the gut segment is taken markedly affects the basal contractile activity. The rabbit jejunum, for example, maintains rhythmic contractions in vitro and is therefore especially useful for analysis of substances with inhibitory effects on gastrointestinal smooth muscle (152). The guinea pig ileum, in contrast, exhibits little spontaneous activity in vitro. This preparation is useful in the bioassay of agents causing contraction of smooth muscle. To test for depressant effects, the investigator must induce contraction of the tissue with electrical stimulation, potassium depolarization, or pharmacologic agonists. Second, there are differences in the responses of gastrointestinal smooth muscle depending on the site of the gut under investigation. This limits the ability of the investigator to generalize from an experiment carried out with a muscle preparation from a single region of the gut and reinforces the importance of strictly controlling the tissue region studied in a series of experiments.

In vitro study of gastrointestinal smooth muscle can be evaluated with isolation of myocytes and measurement of contractile and electrophysiological events of single cells (13,102,113). This approach permits assessment of the direct effects of chemicals on these cells in isolation from their intrinsic innervation via the myenteric and submucosal plexi that exist in situ. The isolated myocyte preparation has facilitated elucidation of membrane receptors, ionic channels, and excitation–contraction coupling mechanisms (113). This approach provides an additional tool in toxicological studies for precisely defining the mechanism of xenobiotic-induced altered gastrointestinal propulsion.

The Guinea Pig Ileum Preparation

The guinea pig ileum preparation has been extensively used in the study of the effects of chemicals on smooth muscle contractility. The guinea pig is euthanized without the use of drugs, because of their potential to alter responsivity of smooth muscles. Segments should be cut from the distal ileum, with care taken to avoid damaging the muscle layers with forceps. The location and length of these segments should be standardized in an experimental series; commonly, 1-cm segments are used, avoiding use of the most distal 10 cm of the ileum. The mesentery should be cut away from the gut segment, which is then placed in Tyrode's solution at 37°C. Once relaxed, the tissue should be gently flushed with solution at 37°C to remove the intraluminal contents. The segment will maintain its viability for several hours if held in Tyrode's solution at just below 20°C. For studies in a single muscle type, the longitudinal muscle layer is readily dissected from the ileal segment (184). When obtained from the guinea pig, this tissue retains the mesenteric plexus and is therefore useful for study of agents that affect neuronal conduction or neurotransmitter release, as well as smooth muscle contractility.

Threads are secured to the proximal and distal end of the segment without occluding the lumen. The tissue is mounted with the proximal end up, in an organ bath containing Tyrode's solution, maintained at 37°C and gassed with 95% O_2/5% CO_2. The thread tied to the proximal end of the tissue is attached to a device for quantitating the contractile response of the tissue. Commonly, this apparatus consists of a Statham force-displacement transducer connected to an amplifier and chart recorder permitting continuous monitoring of response under isometric conditions. Initially, tension, for example, 1.0 g, should be applied to the tissue followed by an equilibration period, for example, 30 min, before addition of test substances to the bath. The tension applied to the muscle should be chosen to stretch the tissue to a length that results in the greatest generated force on activation. This length, referred to as the optimum length, is determined by measuring the difference between passive and active tension for different lengths of the muscle with a maximally effective stimulus such as high potassium (110 mM)-induced depolarization (60). To reduce the contribution of spontaneous contractile activity and tone to "passive" tension, which may be confounding with intestinal muscle from some species, force–length relationships can be examined at low temperature (22°C), which minimizes this factor (49).

Modifications of this technique include electrical stimulation of the tissue and application of intraluminal pressure for eliciting peristaltic reflexes (176). The parameters chosen for electrical stimulation of tissue determine the mechanism and characteristics of the contractile response. For electric field stimulation, muscle is hung between platinum electrodes connected to a stimulator. Stimuli of 1-Hz frequency for 1 ms at 100 V are likely to induce contractions mediated by neural stimulation. These contractions are sensitive to inhibition of neural conduction by sodium channel inactivators, for example, tetrodotoxin (10^{-7} g/ml). Stimuli of higher frequency, for example, 60 Hz, are likely to depolarize the muscle membrane directly, to be unaltered by tetrodotoxin, and to reflect the mechanical properties of the muscle itself.

Substances tested with this preparation should be added in a broad concentration range with washing of the tissue after each application. When a concentration of the test substance is found to cause contraction, additional concentrations should be tested to permit construction of a concentration–response curve that will facilitate analyses by use of such parameters as the EC_{50}, the affinity, and the intrinsic activity. An additional consideration that may require evaluation is the development of tachyphylaxis to the test substance. This phenomenon may necessitate use of multiple tissue preparations, each exposed to only one concentration of the test substance, in order to describe the concentration–response relationship adequately.

QUESTIONS

1. Preclinical in vivo studies of a potential new therapeutic agent indicate that diarrhea is a side effect. What mechanisms might explain this observation, and what methods should be used to test the hypothesis?
2. In vitro studies of a potential new therapeutic agent indicate a marked dose-dependent increase in hydrogen ion secretion from parietal cells. What gastrointestinal toxicity might be expected in vivo, and how should that be tested?

REFERENCES

1. Acra, S. A., and Ghishan, F. K. (1991): Methods of investigating intestinal transport. *Jpn. J. Parenter. Enteral. Nutr.*, 15:93S–98S.
2. Ahlquist, D. A., McGill, D. B., Schwartz, S., Taylor, W. F., and Owen, R. A. (1985): Fecal blood levels in health and disease. A study using hemoQuant. *N. Engl. J. Med.*, 312:1422–1428.
3. Allen, A., Flemstrom, G., Garner, A., Silen, W., and Turnberg, L. A., eds. (1984): *Mechanisms of Mucosal Protection in the Upper Gastrointestinal Tract*. Raven Press, New York.
4. Anonymous. (1986): Tests for occult blood. *Med. Lett.*, 28:5–6.
5. Autrup, H. (1980): Explant culture of human colon. In: *Methods in Cell Biology*, edited by C. C. Harris, B. F. Trump, and G. D. Stoner, pp. 385–401. Academic Press, London.
6. Aw, T. Y., Bai, C., and Jones, D. P. (1993): Small intestinal enterocytes. In: *Methods in Toxicology. In Vitro Biological Systems*, edited by C. A. Tyson and J. M. Frazier, pp. 193–201. Academic Press, Boston.
7. Barr, W. H., and Reigelman, S. (1970): Intestinal drug absorption and metabolism. I. Comparison of methods and models to study physiologic factors of in vitro and in vivo intestinal absorption. *J. Pharm. Sci.*, 59:154–163.
8. Bell, G. I., Kayano, T., Buse, J. B., Burant, C. F., Takeda, J., Lin, D., Fukumoto, H., and Seino, S. (1990): Molecular biology of mammalian glucose transporters. *Diabetes Care*, 13:198–208.
9. Bertram, T. (1991): Gastrointestinal tract. In: *Handbook of Toxicologic Pathology*, edited by W. M. Haschek and C. G. Rousseaux, pp. 195–251. Academic Press, Boston.
10. Besch, E. L., and Chou, B. J. (1971): Physiological responses to blood collection methods in rats. *Proc. Soc. Exp. Biol. Med.*, 138:1019–1021.
11. Bevan, C., and Foulkes, E. C. (1989): Interaction of cadmium with brush border membrane vesicles from the rat small intestine. *Toxicology*, 54:297–309.
12. Binder, H. J., and Sandle, G. I. (1994): Electrolyte transport in the mammalian colon. In: *Physiology of the Gastrointestinal Tract*, Vol. 2, edited by L. R. Johnson, pp. 2133–2172. Raven Press, New York.
13. Bitar, K. N., and Makhlouf, G. M. (1982): Receptors on smooth muscle cells: Characterization by concentration and specific antagonists. *Am. J. Physiol.*, 242:G400–G407.
14. Bivin, W. S., Crawford, M. P., and Brewer, N. R. (1979): Morphophysiology. In: *The Laboratory Rat, Vol. I: Biology and Disease*, edited by H. J. Baker, J. R. Lindsey, and S. H. Weisbroth, pp. 74–103. Academic Press, New York.
15. Brodie, D. A., Cook, P. G., Bauer, B. J., and Dagle, G. E. (1970): Indomethacin-induced intestinal lesions in the rat. *Toxicol. Appl. Pharmacol.*, 17:615–624.
16. Brodie, D. A., Tate, C. L., and Hooke, K. F. (1970): Aspirin: Intestinal damage in rats. *Science*, 170:183–185.
17. Browning, J., Gannon, B. J., and O'Brien, P. (1983): The microvasculature and gastric luminal pH of the forestomach of the rat: A comparison with the glandular stomach. *Int. J. Microcirc. Clin. Exp.*, 2:109–118.
18. Burks, T. F. (1990): Central nervous system regulation of gastrointestinal motility. *Ann. N.Y. Acad. Sci.*, 597:36–42.
19. Cheng, H., and Bjerknes, M. (1982): Whole population cell kinetics of mouse duodenal, jejunal, ileal and colonic epithelia as determined by radioautography and flow cytometry. *Anat. Rec.*, 203:251–264.
20. Cheng, H., Bjerknes, M., and Amar, J. (1984): Methods for the determination of epithelial cell kinetic parameters of human colonic epithelium isolated from surgical and biopsy specimens. *Gastroenterology*, 86:78–85.
21. Chhabra, R. S., and Eastin, W. C., Jr. (1984): Intestinal absorption and metabolism of xenobiotics in laboratory animals. In: *Intestinal Toxicology*, edited by C. M. Schiller, pp. 145–160. Raven Press, New York.
22. Christensen, J. (1994): Motility of the colon. In: *Physiology of the Gastrointestinal Tract*, edited by L. Johnson, pp. 991–1024. Raven Press, New York.
23. Coates, M. E., and Gustafsson, B. E., eds. (1984): *The Germ-Free Animal in Biomedical Research*. Laboratory Animals Limited, London.
24. Costa, M., Furness, J. B., and Llewellyn-Smith, I. J. (1987): Histochemistry of the enteric nervous system. In: *Physiology of the Gastrointestinal Tract*, edited by L. R. Johnson, pp. 1–40. Raven Press, New York.
25. Dahlqvist, A., and Nordstrom, C. (1966): The distribution of disaccharidase activities in the villi and crypts of the small-intestinal mucosa. *Biochim. Biophys. Acta*, 113:624–626.
26. Derblom, H., Johansson, H., and Nylander, G. (1966): A simple method of recording quantitatively certain gastrointestinal motility functions in the rat. *Acta Clin. Scand.*, 132:154–165.
27. Dharmsathaphorn, K., McRoberts, J. A., Mandel, K. G., Tisdale, L. D., and Masui, H. (1984): A human colonic tumor cell line that maintains vectorial electrolyte transport. *Am. J. Physiol.*, 246:G204–G208.
28. Donowitz, M., and Welsh, M. J. (1986): Ca^{2+} and cyclic AMP in regulation of intestinal Na, K, and Cl transport. *Ann. Rev. Physiol.*, 48:135–150.
29. Douglas, A. P., Kerley, R., and Isselbacher, K. J. (1972): Preparation and characterization of the lateral and basal plasma membranes of the rat intestinal epithelial cell. *Biochem. J.*, 128:1329–1338.
30. Dudeja, P. K., Wali, R. K., Harig, J. M., and Brasitus, T. A. (1991): Characterization and modulation of rat small intestinal brush-border membrane transbilayer fluidity. *Am. J. Physiol.*, 260:G586–G594.
31. Eastwood, G. L. (1981): Epithelial renewal in gastrointestinal mucosal injury. In: *Basic Mechanisms of Gastrointestinal Mucosal Cell Injury and Protection*, edited by J. W. Harmon, pp. 49–66. Williams and Wilkins, Baltimore.
32. Ellefson, R. D., and Caraway, W. T. (1976): Lipids and lipoproteins. In: *Fundamentals of Clinical Chemistry*, edited by N. Tietz, pp. 474–541. W. B. Saunders, Philadelphia.
33. Elsas, L. J., and Longo, N. (1992): Glucose transporters. *Annu. Rev. Med.*, 43:377–393.
34. Falk, P. G., Hooper, L. V., Midtvedt, T., and Gordon, J. I. (1998): Creating and maintaining the gastrointestinal ecosystem: What we know and need to know from gnotobiology. *Microbiol. Mol. Biol. Rev.*, 62:1157–1170.
35. Ferraris, R. P., Lee, P. P., and Diamond, J. M. (1989): Origin of regional and species differences in intestinal glucose uptake. *Am. J. Physiol.*, 257:G689–G697.
36. Finney, K. (1993): Maintenance and characterization of an organ culture system for rat colonic mucosa. In: *Methods in Toxicology. In Vitro Biological Systems*, edited by C. A. Tyson and J. M. Frazier, pp. 202–221. Academic Press, Boston.
37. Fordtran, J. S., Rector, F. C. J., Ewton, M. F., Soter, N., and Kinney, J. (1965): Permeability characteristics of the human small intestine. *J. Clin. Invest.*, 44:1935–1944.
38. Forstner, J. F., and Forstner, G. G. (1994): Gastrointestinal mucus. In: *Physiology of the Gastrointestinal Tract*, Vol. 2, edited by L. R. Johnson, pp. 1255–1284. Raven Press, New York.
39. Foster, H. L. (1980): Gnotobiology. In: *The Laboratory Rat. Vol. II: Research Applications*, edited by H. J. Baker, J. R. Lindsey, and S. H. Weisbroth, pp. 43–57. Academic Press, New York.

40. Frederick, C. B., Hazelton, G. A., and Frantz, J. D. (1990): The histopathological and biochemical response of the stomach of male F344/N rats following two weeks of oral dosing with ethyl acrylate. *Toxicol. Pathol.*, 18:247–256.
41. Ghoshal, N. G., and Bal, H. S. (1989): Comparative morphology of the stomach of some laboratory mammals. *Lab. Animal*, 23:21–29.
42. Gibaldi, M., Boyes, R. N., and Feldman, S. (1971): Influence of first-pass effect on availability of drugs on oral administration. *J. Pharm. Sci.*, 60:1338–1340.
43. Gibaldi, M., and Perrier, D. (1982): *Pharmacokinetics*. Marcel Dekker, New York.
44. Gilbert, R. J., Sarna, S. K., and Harder, D. R. (1987): Effect of morphine on electrophysiological properties of circular and longitudinal muscles. *Am. J. Physiol.*, 252:G333–G338.
45. Glavin, G. B., and Szabo, S. (1992): Experimental gastric mucosal injury: Laboratory models reveal mechanisms of pathogenesis and new therapeutic strategies. *FASEB J.*, 6:825–831.
46. Goldin, B. R. (1986): In situ bacterial metabolism and colon mutagens. *Ann. Rev. Microbiol.*, 40:367–393.
47. Goldin, B. R. (1990): Intestinal microflora: Metabolism of drugs and carcinogens. *Ann. Med.*, 22:43–48.
48. Goldman, P. (1978): Biochemical pharmacology of the intestinal flora. *Ann. Rev. Pharmacol. Toxicol.*, 18:523–539.
49. Gordon, A. R., and Siegman, M. J. (1971): Mechanical properties of smooth muscle I. Length-tension and force-velocity relations. *Am. J. Physiol.*, 221:1243–1249.
50. Gordon, J. (1989): Intestinal epithelial differentiation: New insights from chimeric and transgenic mice. *J. Cell Biol.*, 108:1187–1194.
51. Granger, D. N., Kvietys, P. R., Perry, M. A., and Barrowman, J. A. (1987): The microcirculation and intestinal transport. In: *Physiology of the Gastrointestinal Tract*, edited by L. R. Johnson, pp. 1671–1697. Raven Press, New York.
52. Gray, G. (1981): Carbohydrate absorption and malabsorption. In: *Physiology of the Gastrointestinal Tract*, edited by L. R. Johnson, pp. 1063–1072. Raven Press, New York.
53. Grisham, M. R., VonRitter, C., Smith, B. F., Lamont, J. T., and Granger, D. N. (1987): Interaction between oxygen radicals and gastric mucin. *Am. J. Physiol.*, 253:G93–G96.
54. Gustavsson, S., Jung, B., and Nelsson, F. (1977): Simultaneous measurements of the propulsion and mixing of small bowel contents in the rat. *Acta Clin. Scand.*, 143:359–364.
55. Hall, S. D., Thummel, K. E., Watkins, P. B., Lown, K. S., Benet, L. Z., Paine, M. F., Mayo, R. R., Turgeon, D. K., Bailey, D. G., Fontana, R. J., and Wrighton, S. A. (1999): Molecular and physical mechanisms of first-pass extraction. *Drug Metab. Disposit.*, 27:161–166.
56. Harmon, J. W., ed. (1981): *Basic Mechanisms of Gastrointestinal Mucosal Cell Injury and Protection*. Williams and Wilkins, Baltimore.
57. Harnett, K. M., Walsh, C. T., and Zhang, L. (1989): Effects of Bay o 2752, a hypocholesterolemic agent, on intestinal taurocholate absorption and cholesterol esterification. *J. Pharmacol. Exp. Ther.*, 251:502–509.
58. Harrison, D. D., and Webster, H. L. (1969): The preparation of isolated intestinal crypt cells. *Exp. Cell Res.*, 55:257–260.
59. Hecht, G., Koutsouris, A., Pothoulakis, C., LaMont, J. T., and Madara, J. L. (1992): *Clostridium difficile* toxin B disrupts the barrier function of T_{84} monolayers. *Gastroenterology*, 102:416–413.
60. Herlihy, J. T., and Murphy, R. A. (1973): Length-tension relationship of smooth muscle of the hog carotid artery. *Circ. Res.*, 33:275–283.
61. Hiraishi, H., Terano, A., and Ivey, K. J. (1993): Gastric mucosal cell culture for toxicological study. In: *Methods in Toxicology. In Vitro Biological Systems*, edited by C. A. Tyson and J. M. Frazier, pp. 182–192. Academic Press, Boston.
62. Holt, P. R., and Koss, L. G. (1984): Flow cytometry-biologic and clinical application of a powerful methodology. *Gastroenterology*, 86:196–198.
63. Hopfer, U. (1977): Isolated membrane vesicles as tools for analysis of epithelial transport. *Am. J. Physiol.*, 233:E445–E449.
64. Hopfer, U., and Liedtke, C. M. (1987): Proton and bicarbonate transport mechanisms in the intestine. *Ann. Rev. Physiol.*, 49:51–67.
65. Howdle, P. D. (1984): Organ culture of gastrointestinal mucosa. *Postgrad. Med.*, 60:645–652.
66. Hunt, J. N. (1983): Mechanisms and disorders of gastric emptying. *Ann. Rev. Med.*, 34:219–229.
67. Hurst, B. C., Rees, W. D. W., and Garner, A. (1984): Cell shedding by the stomach and duodenum. In: *Mechanisms of Mucosal Protection in the Upper Gastrointestinal Tract*, edited by A. Allen, G. Flemstrom, A. Garner, W. Silen, and L. A. Turnberg, pp. 21–26. Raven Press, New York.
68. Hutchison, J. D., Undrill, V. J., and Porteous, J. W. (1991): The vascularly and luminally perfused small intestine in vitro: Dissection technique and model system. *Lab. Anim.*, 25:168–83.
69. Iatropoulos, M. J. (1986): Morphology of the gastrointestinal tract. In: *Gastrointestinal Toxicology*, edited by K. Rozman and O. Hänninen, pp. 246–266. Elsevier, New York.
70. Ilett, K. F., Tee, L. B. G., Reeves, P. T. et al. (1990): Metabolism of drugs and other xenobiotics in the gut wall. *Pharmacol. Ther.*, 46:67–93.
71. Imondi, A. R., Balis, M. E., and Lipkin, M. (1969): Changes in enzyme levels accompanying differentiation of intestinal epithelial cells. *Exp. Cell Res.*, 58:323–330.
72. Ince, P., Elliott, K., Appleton, D. R., Moorghen, M., Finney, K. J., Sunter, J. P., Harris, A. L., and Watson, A. J. (1991): Modulation by verapamil of vincristine pharmacokinetics and sensitivity to metaphase arrest of the normal rat colon in organ culture. *Biochem. Pharmacol.*, 41:1217–1225.
73. Irons, G. J., and Kirsner, J. (1965): Routine chemical tests of the stool for occult blood; an evaluation. *Am. J. Med. Sci.*, 249: 247–260.
74. Israili, Z. H., and Dayton, P. G. (1984): Enhancement of xenobiotic elimination: Role of intestinal excretion. *Drug Metab. Rev.*, 15:1123–1159.
75. Ito, S. (1987): Functional gastric morphology. In: *Physiology of the Gastrointestinal Tract*, edited by L. R. Johnson, pp. 817–851. Raven Press, New York.
76. Jenkin, C. R., and Rowley, D. (1959): Possible factors in the pathogenesis of cholera. *Br. J. Exp. Pathol.*, 40:474–481.
77. Johnson, L. R., ed. (1994): *Physiology of the Gastrointestinal Tract*, Vol. 1 & 2. Raven Press: New York.
78. Kaminsky, L. S., and Fasco, M. J. (1991): Small intestinal cytochromes P450. *Crit. Rev. Toxicol.*, 21:407–22.
79. Kandel, G., Donohue-Rolfe, A., Donowitz, M., and Keusch, G. T. (1989): Pathogenesis of *Shigella* diarrhea. VXI. Selective targeting of Shiga toxin to villus cells of rabbit jejunum explains the effect of the toxin on intestinal electrolyte transport. *J. Clin. Invest.*, 84:1509–1517.
80. Kayano, T., Burant, C. F., Fukumoto, H., Gould, G. W., Fan, Y. S., Eddy, R. L., Byers, M. G., Shows, T. B., Seino, S., and Bell, G. I. (1990): Human facilitative glucose transporters. Isolation, functional characterization, and gene localization of cDNAs encoding an isoform (GLUT5) expressed in small intestine, kidney, muscle, and adipose tissue and an unusual glucose transporter pseudogene-like sequence (GLUT6). *J. Biol. Chem.*, 265:13276–13282.

81. Kellett, G. L., and Barker, E. D. (1989): The effect of vanadate on glucose transport and metabolism in rat small intestine. *Biochim. Biophys. Acta*, 979:311–315.
82. Keusch, G. T., Jacewicz, M., Mobassaleh, M., and Donohue, R. A. (1991): Shiga toxin: Intestinal cell receptors and pathophysiology of enterotoxic effects. *Rev. Infect. Dis.*, 13:S304–S310.
83. Kimmich, G. A. (1981): Intestinol absorption of sugar. In *Physiology of the Gastrointestinal Tract*, edited by L. R. Johnson, pp. 1035–1062. Raven Press, New York.
84. Kroes, R., and Wester, P. W. (1986): Forestomach carcinogens: Possible mechanisms of action. *Food Chem. Toxicol.*, 24:1083–1089.
85. Kvietys, P. R., Perry, M. A., Gaginella, T. S., and Granger, D. N. (1990): Ethanol enhances leukocyte-endothelial cell interactions in mesenteric venules. *Am. J. Physiol.*, 259:G578–G583.
86. Laitinen, M., and Watkins, J. B. (1986): Mucosal biotransformation. In: *Gastrointestinal Toxicology*, edited by K. Rozman and O. Hänninen, pp. 169–192. Elsevier, New York.
87. Lanza, F. L., and Arnold, J. D. (1989): Etodolac, a new nonsteroidal anti-inflammatory drug: Gastrointestinal microbleeding and endoscopic studies. *Clin. Rheumatol.*, 8(Suppl 1): 5–15.
88. Laqueur, G. L., McDaniel, E. G., and Matsumoto, H. (1967): Tumor induction in germfree rats with methylazoxymethanol (MAM) and synthetic MAM acetate. *J. Natl. Cancer Inst.*, 39:355–371.
89. Lavigne, M. E., Wiley, Z. D., Meyer, J. H., Martin, P., and MacGregor, I. L. (1978): Gastric emptying rates of solid food in relation to body size. *Gastroenterology*, 74:1258–1260.
90. Lavo, B., Colombel, J. F., Knutsson, L., and Hallgren, R. (1992): Acute exposure of small intestine to ethanol induces mucosal leakage and prostaglandin E2 synthesis. *Gastroenterology*, 102: 468–473.
91. Lencer, W. I., Delp, C., Neutra, M. R., and Madara, J. L. (1992): Mechanism of cholera toxin action on a polarized human intestinal epithelial cell line: role of vesicular traffic. *J. Cell. Biol.*, 117:1197–1209.
92. Lencer, W. I., Reinhart, F. D., and Neutra, M. R. (1990): Interaction of cholera toxin with cloned human goblet cells in monolayer culture. *Am. J. Physiol.*, 258:G96–G102.
93. Leonards, J. (1963): Aspirin and gastrointestinal blood loss. *Gastroenterology*, 44:617–619.
94. Levine, R. R., McNary, W. F., Kornguth, P. J., and LeBlanc, R. (1970): Histological reevaluation of everted gut technique for studying intestinal absorption. *Eur. J. Pharmacol.*, 9:211–219.
95. Lewis, L. D., and Fordtran, J. S. (1975): Effect of perfusion rate on absorption, surface area, unstirred water layer thickness, permeability, and intraluminal pressure in the rat ileum in vivo. *Gastroenterology*, 68:1509–1516.
96. Lipkin, M. (1985): Growth and development of gastrointestinal cells. *Ann. Rev. Physiol.*, 47:175–197.
97. Lipkin, M. (1987): Proliferation and differentiation of normal and diseased gastrointestinal cells. In: *Physiology of the Gastrointestinal Tract*, edited by L. R. Johnson, pp. 145–168. Raven Press, New York.
98. Lipsky, M. H., and Berkley, S. (1977): Prolonged biliary fistulization in the rat without interruption of the enterohepatic cycle. *J. Surg. Res.*, 22:65–68.
99. Madara, J. L., Stafford, J., Dharmsathaphorn, K., and Carlson, S. (1987): Structural analysis of a human intestinal epithelial cell line. *Gastroenterology*, 92:1133–1145.
100. Madara, L., and Trier, J. S. (1994): Functional morphology of the mucosa of the small intestine. In: *Physiology of the Gastrointestinal Tract*, Vol. 2, edited by L. R. Johnson, pp. 1577–1622. Raven Press, New York.
101. Mailman, D., Womack, W. A., Kvietys, P. R., and Granger, D. N. (1990): Villous motility and unstirred water layers in canine intestine. *Am. J. Physiol.*, 258:G238–G246.
102. Makhlouf, G. M. (1987): Isolated smooth muscle cells of the gut. In: *Physiology of the Gastrointestinal Tract*, edited by L. R. Johnson, pp. 555–569. Raven Press, New York.
103. Mathias, J. R., and Clench, M. H. (1985): Review: Pathophysiology of diarrhea caused by bacterial overgrowth of the small intestine. *Am. J. Med. Sci.*, 289:243–248.
104. Mayer, R. M., Treadwell, C. R., Gallo, L. L., and Vahouny, G. V. (1985): Intestinal mucins and cholesterol uptake in vitro. *Biochem. Biophys. Acta*, 833:34–43.
105. McCuskey, R. S., and Earnest, D. L., eds. (1997): *Comprehensive Toxicology, Vol. 9, Hepatic and Gastrointestinal Toxicology. Comprehensive Toxicology*, Elsevier Science, New York.
106. Meyer, J. H. (1987): Motility of the stomach and gastroduodenal junction. In: *Physiology of the Gastrointestinal Tract*, edited by L. R. Johnson, pp. 613–629. Raven Press, New York.
107. Mezey, E., and Palkovits, M. (1992): Localization of targets for anti-ulcer drugs in cells of the immune system. *Science*, 258:1662–1665.
108. Mickelsen, O. (1972): Introductory remarks, symposium on cycads. *Fed. Proc.*, 31:1465–1546.
109. Miller, M. S., Galligan, J. J., and Burks, T. F. (1981): Accurate measurement of intestinal transit in the rat. *J. Pharmacol. Methods*, 6:211–217.
110. Misiewicz, J. J., Bartram, C. I., Cotton, P. B., Mee, A. S., Price, A. B., and Thompson, R. P. H. (1987): *Atlas of Clinical Gastroenterology*. Lea and Febiger, Philadelphia.
111. Moorghen, M., Chapman, M., and Appleton D. R. (1996): An organ-culture method for human colorectal mucosa using serum-free medium. *J. Pathol.*, 180:102–105.
112. Morales, R. E., Johnson, B. R., and Szabo, S. (1992): Endothelin induces vascular and mucosal lesions, enhances the injury by HCl/ethanol, and the antibody exerts gastroprotection. *FASEB J.*, 6:2354–2360.
113. Murthy, K., Grider, J., and Maklouf, G. (1992): Receptor-coupled G proteins mediate contraction and Ca^{++} mobilization in isolated intestinal muscle cells. *J. Pharmacol. Exp. Ther.*, 260:90–97.
114. Nakamura, W., Kankura, T., and Eto, H. (1971): Occult blood appearance in feces and tissue hemorrhages in mice after whole body x-irradiation. *Radiat. Res.*, 48:169–178.
115. Pelzmann, K. S., and Havemeyer, R. N. (1971): Portal, vein blood sampling in intestinal drug absorption studies. *J. Pharm. Sci.*, 60:331.
116. Pfeiffer, C. J. (1977): Gastroenterologic response to environmental agents-absorption and interactions. In: *Handbook of Physiology, Section 9: Reactions to Environmental Agents*, edited by D. H. K. Lee, H. L. Falk, S. D. Murphy, and S. R. Geiger, pp. 349–374. American Physiological Society, Bethesda, MD.
117. Pfeiffer, C. J., Rowden, G., and Weibel, J. (1974): *Gastrointestinal Ultrastructure: An Atlas of Scanning and Transmission Electron Microscopy*. Academic Press, New York.
118. Phillips, B. M. (1973): Aspirin-induced gastrointestinal microbleeding in dogs. *Toxicol. Appl. Pharmacol.*, 24:182–189.
119. Phillips, T. E., Huet, C., Biblo, P. R., Podolsky, D. K., Louvard, D., and Neutra, M. R. (1988): Human intestinal goblet cells in monolayer culture: Characterization of a mucus-secreting subclone cleaved from the HT-29 colon adenocarcinoma cell line. *Gastroenterology*, 94(6):1390–1403.
120. Prescott, L. F., and Nimmo, W. S., eds. (1981): *Drug Absorption*. Adis Press, New York.
121. Previte, J. J. (1983): *Human Physiology*. McGraw-Hill, New York.
122. Reinhardt, M. C. (1989): Macromolecular absorption of food antigens in health and disease. *Ann. Allergy*, 53:597–601.

123. Ringler, D. H., and Dabich, L. (1979): Hematology and clinical biochemistry. In: *The Laboratory Rat, Vol I: Biology and Disease*, edited by H. J. Baker, J. R. Lindsey, and S. H. Weisbroth, pp. 105–121. Academic Press, New York.
124. Rivière, P. J. M., Sheldon, R. J., Malarchik, M. E., Burks, T. F., and Porreca, F. (1990): Effects of bombesin on mucosal ion transport in the mouse isolated jejunum. *J. Pharm. Exp. Ther.*, 253:778–783.
125. Roman, C., and Gonella, J. (1987): Extinsic control of digestive tract motility. In: *Physiology of the Gastrointestinal Tract*, edited by L. R. Johnson, pp. 507–553, Raven Press, New York.
126. Rowland, I. R. (1988): Interactions of the gut microflora and the host in toxicology. *Toxicol. Pathol.*, 16:147–153.
127. Rowland, I. R., ed. (1988): *Role of the Gut Flora in Toxicity and Cancer*. Academic Press, London.
128. Rozman, K. (1988): Disposition of xenobiotics: Species differences. *Toxicol. Pathol.*, 16:123–129.
129. Rumney, C. J., and Rowland, I. R. (1992): In vivo and in vitro models of the human colonic flora. *Crit. Rev. Food Sci. Nutr.*, 31:299–331.
130. Salmon, G. K., and Leslie, G. B. (1985): The use of endoscopy in the induction and monitoring of gastric mucosal lesions in the rat. *Toxicologist*, 5:9.
131. Sanders, M. J., and Soll, A. H. (1989): Cell separation by elutriation: Major and minor cell types from complex tissues. *Methods Enzymol.*, 171:482–497.
132. Sansonetti, P. J. (1998): Molecular and cellular mechanisms of invasion of the intestinal barrier by enteric pathogens. *Folia Microbiol.*, 43:239–246.
133. Satoh, H., Inada, I., Hirata, T., and Maki, Y. (1981): Indomethacin produces gastric antral ulcers in the refed rat. *Gastroenterology*, 81:719–725.
134. Schultz, S. G., Curran, P. F., Chez, R. A., and Fuisz, R. E. (1967): Alanine and sodium fluxes across mucosal border of rabbit ileum. *J. Gen. Physiol.*, 50:1241–1260.
135. Schwabe, A. D., and Hepner, G. W. (1979): Breath tests for the detection of fat malabsorption. *Gastroenterology*, 76:216–218.
136. Schwartz, S., Dahl, J., Ellefson, M., and Ahlquist, D. A. (1983): The "HemoQuant" test: A specific and quantitative assay of heme (hemoglobin) in feces and other materials. *Clin. Chem.*, 29:2061–2067.
137. Scott, L. D., and Summers, R. W. (1976): Correlation of contractions and transit in rat small intestine. *Am. J. Physiol.*, 230:132–137.
138. Segal, H. L., Miller, L. L., and Plumb, E. J. (1955): Tubeless gastric analysis with an azure A ion-exchange compound. *Gastroenterology*, 28:402–408.
139. Sheldon, R. J., Malarchik, M. E., Fox, D. A., Burks, T. F., and Porreca, F. (1989): Pharmacological characterization of neural mechanisms regulating mucosal ion transport in mouse jejunum. *J. Pharm. Exp. Ther.*, 249:572–582.
140. Sherding, R. G. (1983): Diseases of the small bowel. In: *Textbook of Veterinary Internal Medicine. Diseases of the Dog and Cat*, edited by S. J. Ettinger, pp. 1278–1346. W. B. Saunders, Philadelphia.
141. Shiau, Y.-F., Boyle, J. T., Umstetter, C., and Koldovsky, O. (1980): Apical distribution of fatty acid esterification capacity along the villus-crypt unit of rat jejunum. *Gastroenterology*, 79:47–53.
142. Shirazi-Beechey, S. P., Davies, A. G., Tebbutt, K., Dyer, J., Ellis, A., Taylor, C. J., Fairclough, P., and Beechey, R. B. (1990): Preparation and properties of brush-border membrane vesicles from human small intestine. *Gastroenterology*, 98:676–685.
143. Shriver, D. A., Dove, P. A., White, C. B., Sandor, A., and Rosenthale, M. E. (1975): A profile of the gastrointestinal toxicity of aspirin, indomethacin, oxaprozin, phenylbutazone, and fentiazac in arthritic and Lewis normal rats. *Toxicol. Appl. Pharmacol.*, 42:75–83.
144. Simon, G. L., and Gorbach, S. L. (1984): Intestinal flora in health and disease. *Gastroenterology*, 86:174–193.
145. Simon, J. B. (1998): Fecal occult blood testing: Clinical value and limitations. *Gastroenterologist*, 6:66–78.
146. Smith, H. W. (1965): Observations on the flora of the alimentary tract of animals and factors affecting its composition. *J. Pathol. Bacteriol.*, 89:95–122.
147. Smith, M. W. (1985): Expression of digestive and absorptive function in differentiating enterocytes. *Ann. Rev. Physiol.*, 47:247–260.
148. Smithson, K. W., Millar, D. B., Jacobs, L. R., and Gray, G. M. (1981): Intestinal diffusion barrier: Unstirred water layer or membrane surface mucous coat. *Science*, 214:1241–1244.
149. Soergel, K. H. (1968): Inert markers. *Gastroenterology*, 54:449–452.
150. Soll, A. H. (1980): Secretagogue stimulation of ^{14}C-aminopyrine accumulation by isolated canine parietal cells. *Am. J. Physiol.*, 238:G366–G375.
151. Soll, A. H., and Berglindh, T. (1987): Physiology of isolated gastric glands and parietal cells: receptors and effectors regulating function. In: *Physiology of the Gastrointestinal Tract*, edited by L. R. Johnson, pp. 883–909. Raven Press, New York.
152. Staff of the Department of Pharmacology, University of Edinburgh. (1970): *Pharmacological Experiments on Isolated Preparations*. E & S Livingstone, Edinburgh.
153. Stevens, B. R., Fernandez, A., Hirayama, B., Wright, E. M., and Kempner, E. S. (1990): Intestinal brush border membrane Na^+/glucose cotransporter functions in situ as a homotetramer. *Proc. Natl. Acad. Sci. U.S.A.*, 87:1456–1460.
154. Stevens, B. R., Kavnitz, J. D., and Wright, E. M. (1984): Intestinal transport of amino acids and sugars: Advances using membrane vesicles. *Ann. Rev. Physiol.*, 46:417–433.
155. Stewart, J. J., Weisbrodt, N. W., and Burks, T. F. (1978): Central and peripheral actions of morphine on intestinal transit. *J. Pharmacol. Exp. Ther.*, 195:347–354.
156. Summers, R. W., Kent, T. H., and Osborne, J. W. (1970): Effects of drugs, ileal obstruction, and irradiation on rat gastrointestinal propulsion. *Gastroenterology*, 59:731–739.
157. Szabo, S. (1978): Duodenal ulcer disease. Animal model: Cysteamine-induced acute and chronic duodenal ulcer in the rat. *Am. J. Pathol.*, 93:273–276.
158. Szabo, S., Reynolds, E. S., Lichtenberger, L. M., Haith, L. R., and Dzau, V. J. (1977): Pathogenesis of duodenal ulcer. Gastric hyperacidity caused by propionitrile and cysteamine in rats. *Res. Commun. Chem. Pathol. Pharmacol.*, 16:311–323.
159. Szabo, S., Trier, J. S., Brown, A., and Schnoor, J. (1985): Early vascular injury and increased vascular permeability in gastric mucosal injury caused by ethanol in the rat. *Gastroenterology*, 88:228–236.
160. Szabo, S., Trier, J. S., Brown, A., Schnoor, J., Homan, H. D., and Bradford, J. C. (1985): A quantitative method for assessing the extent of experimental gastric erosions and ulcers. *J. Pharmacol. Methods*, 13:59–66.
161. Szurszewski, J. H. (1987): Electrophysiological basis of gastrointestinal motility. In: *Physiology of the Gastrointestinal Tract*, edited by L. R. Johnson, pp. 383–422. Raven Press, New York.
162. Tallarida, R. J., and Murray, R. B. (1987): *Manual of Pharmacologic Calculations With Computer Programs*, 2nd ed. Springer–Verlag, New York.
163. Tanaka, S., Akiba, Y., and Kaunitz, J. D. (1998): Pentagastrin gastroprotection against acid is related to H2 receptor activation but not acid secretion. *Gut*, 43:334–341.

164. Tasich, M., and Piper, D. W. (1983): Effect of human colonic microsomes and cell-free extracts of *Bacteroides fragilis* on the mutagenicity of 2-aminoanthracene. *Gastroenterology*, 85:30–34.

165. Thomson, A. B. R., and O'Brien, B. D. (1980): Uptake of homologous series of saturated fatty acids into rabbit intestine using three in vitro techniques. *Dig. Dis. Sci.*, 25:209–215.

166. Tietz, N. W. (1976): Gastric, pancreatic and intestinal function. In: *Fundamentals of Clinical Chemistry*, edited by N. W. Tietz, pp. 1063–1099. W. B. Saunders, Philadelphia.

167. Toner, P. G., Carr, K. E., and Wyburn, G. M. (1971): *The Digestive System—An Ultrastructural Atlas Review*. Appleton–Century–Crofts, New York.

168. Toskes, P. P., King, C. E., Spivey, J. C., and Lorenz, E. (1978): Xylose catabolism in the experimental rat blind loop syndrome. Studies including use of a newly developed *d*-[^{14}C]xylose breath test. *Gastroenterology*, 74:691–697.

169. Towler, C. M., Pugh-Humphreys, G. P., and Porteous, J. W. (1978): Characterization of columnar absorptive epithelial cells isolated from rat jejunum. *J. Cell. Sci.*, 29:53–75.

170. Triadafilopoulos, G., Pothoulakis, C., O'Brien, M. J., and LaMont, J. T. (1987): Differential effects of *Clostridium difficile* toxins A and B on rabbit ileum. *Gastroenterology*, 93:273–279.

171. Triadafilopoulos, G., Pothoulakis, C., Weiss, R., Giampaolo, C., and LaMont, J. T. (1989): Comparative study of *Clostridium difficile* toxin A and cholera toxin in rabbit ileum. *Gastroenterology*, 97:1186–1192.

172. Tso, P. (1994): Intestinal lipid absorption. In: *Physiology of the Gastrointestinal Tract*, Vol. 2, edited by L. R. Johnson, pp. 1867–1908. Raven Press, New York.

173. Ussing, H. H., and Zerahn, K. (1951): Active transport of sodium as the source of electric current in the short-circuited isolated frog skin. *Acta Physiol. Scand.*, 23:110–127.

174. Van der Waaij, D. (1991): The microflora of the gut: Recent findings and implications. *Dig. Dis. Sci.*, 9:36–48.

175. VanHarken, D. R., and Hottendorf, G. H. (1978): Comparative absorption following the administration of a drug to rats by oral gavage and incorporation in the diet. *Toxicol. Appl. Pharmacol.*, 43:407–410.

176. Van Neuten, J. M., Geivers, H., Fontaine, J., and Janssen, P. A. J. (1973): An improved method for studying peristalsis in the isolated guinea-pig ileum. *Arch. Int. Pharmacodyn.*, 203:411–414.

177. Vigna, S. R., Mantyh, C. R., Soll, A. H., Maggio, J. E., and Mantyh, P. W. (1989): Substance P receptors on canine chief cells: Localization, characterization, and function. *J. Neurosci.*, 9:2878–2886.

178. Walker, M. M., and Crabtree, J. E. (1998): Helicobacter pylori infection and the pathogenesis of duodenal ulceration. *Ann. N.Y. Acad. Sci.*, 859:96–111.

179. Walker, W. A. (1981): Intestinal transport of macromolecules. In: *Physiology of the Gastrointestinal Tract*, edited by L. R. Johnson, pp. 1271–1289. Raven Press, New York.

180. Wallace, J. L., Keenan, C. M., and Granger, D. N. (1990): Gastric ulceration induced by nonsteriodal anti-inflammatory drugs is a neutrophil-dependent process. *Am. J. Physiol.*, 259:G462–G467.

181. Walsh, C. T. (1982): The influence of age on the gastrointestinal absorption of mercuric chloride and methyl mercury chloride in the rat. *Environ. Res.*, 27:412–420.

182. Walsh, C. T. (1990): Anatomical, physiological, and biochemical characteristics of the gastrointestinal tract. In: *Principles of Route-To-Route Extrapolation for Risk Assessment*, edited by T. R. Gerrity and C. J. Henry, pp. 33–50. Elsevier Science, New York.

183. Walsh, C. T. (1997): Toxicokinetics: Oral exposure and absorption of toxicants. In: *Comprehensive Toxicology, Vol. 1, General Principles*, edited by J. Bond, pp. 51–62. Elsevier Science, New York.

184. Walsh, C. T., and Harnett, K. M. (1986): Inhibitory effect of lead acetate on contractility of longitudinal smooth muscle from rat ileum. *Toxicol. Appl. Pharmacol.*, 83:62–68.

185. Walsh, C. T., and Ryden, E. B. (1984): The effect of chronic ingestion of lead on gastrointestinal transit in rats. *Toxicol. Appl. Pharmacol.*, 75:485–495.

186. Warrick, M. W., and Lin, T.-N. (1977): Action of glucagon and aspirin on ionic flux, mucosal blood flow and bleeding in the fundic pouch of dogs. *Res. Commun. Chem. Pathol. Pharmacol.*, 16:325–335.

187. Weisbrodt, N. W. (1987): Motility of the small intestine. In: *Physiology of the Gastrointestinal Tract*, edited by L. R. Johnson, pp. 631–664. Raven Press, New York.

188. Welsh, M. J., Smith, P. L., Fromm, M., and Frizzell, R. A. (1982): Crypts are the site of intestinal fluid and electrolyte secretion. *Science*, 218:1219–1221.

189. Whitehead, R. (1979): *Mucosal Biopsy of the Gastrointestinal Tract*. W. B. Saunders, Philadelphia.

190. Wilson, T. H., and Wiseman, G. (1954): The use of sacs of everted small intestine for the study of the transference of substances from the mucosal to the serosal surface. *J. Physiol.*, 123:116–125.

191. Winawer, S. (1976): Fecal occult blood testing. *Am. J. Dig. Dis.*, 21:885–888.

192. Wright, E. M, Hirayama, B. A, Loo, D. D. F., Turk, E., and Hager, K. (1994): Intestinal sugar transport. In: *Physiology of the Gastrointestinal Tract*, Vol. 2, edited by L. R. Johnson, pp. 1751–1772. Raven Press, New York.

193. Yamada, T., Specian, R. D., Granger, D. N., Gaginella, T. S., and Grisham, M. B. (1991): Misoprostol attenuates acetic acid-induced increases in mucosal permeability and inflammation: role of blood flow. *Am. J. Physiol.*, 261:G332–G339.

194. Young, G. P., St. John, D. J., Rose, I. S., and Blake, D. (1990): Haem in the gut. Part II. Faecal excretion of haem and haem-derived porphyrins and their detection. *J. Gastroenterol. Hepatol.*, 5:194–203.

195. Yu, C. C., Woods, A. L., and Levison, D. A. (1992): The assessment of cellular proliferation by immunohistochemistry: A review of currently available methods and their applications. *Histochem. J.*, 24:121–131.

Principles and Methods of Toxicology,
Fourth Edition, edited by A. Wallace Hayes.
Taylor & Francis, Philadelphia © 2001.

Chapter 27

Cardiovascular Physiology and Methods for Toxicology

Thomas L. Smith, Louis Andrew Koman, Arnold T. Mosberg, and
A. Wallace Hayes

OVERVIEW OF CARDIOVASCULAR PHYSIOLOGY AND ANATOMY

The cardiovascular system may be viewed as having four major components: the *arterial* system, comprising the heart and the high-pressure distribution conduit arteries; the *venous* system, comprising the collection venules and capacitance veins; the *microcirculation*, the site of nutrient and metabolite exchange; and the *blood*, a complex tissue composed of plasma and cellular elements with many different functions. These four systems differ greatly in their anatomy and physiology.

Blood flow within the arterial system is initiated by contraction of the heart. This muscular organ is capable of uninterrupted fluid pumping for a century or longer. The heart's primary perfusion and nutrition is provided by coronary arteries that branch from the aorta immediately past the mitral valve. The arterial distribution system through which blood is pumped begins with the ascending aorta. The ascending aorta receives all of the output of the heart (the cardiac output) with the exception of the coronary blood flow. The aorta and the major arteries are thick-walled structures with vascular smooth muscle, elastic and connective tissue. As blood is pumped into the arterial system the aorta expands with the extra inflow. During diastole, the aorta constricts down to its previous size, propelling blood downstream. This is known as the "Wind-kessel" effect and serves to maintain a more constant arterial blood flow from a very periodic pump.

Blood is distributed to different regions and organ systems of the body via the major arteries that branch from the aorta. These arteries give rise to successively smaller branches. Repetitive branching leads to smaller and smaller arteries with the smallest vessels on the arterial side of the circulation being arterioles. The arterioles distribute oxygenated blood to the nutritive capillaries of the body.

The capillaries are the primary site for the exchange of nutrients and metabolites from the tissues. Capillaries are also the primary site for the exchange of oxygen and carbon dioxide. The walls of the capillaries are only one cell layer thick. This means that fluids with dissolved gases and solutes can pass easily from the vascular compartment to the interstitial compartment and vice versa. Exchange of solutes and dissolved gases also can occur across the vessel walls of small arterioles.

The capillaries drain into venules. The venules are the first stage of the venous circulation, which serves in the collection of blood from the body's tissues. The

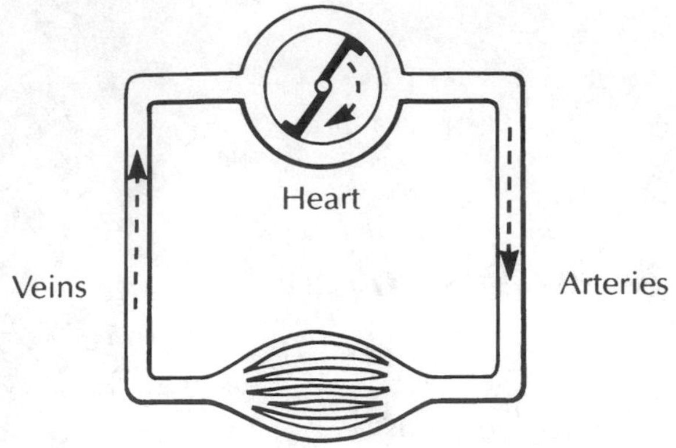

FIG. 27.1. Schematic representation of the cardiovascular system. Major components are listed and direction of blood flow follows the arrows.

venules are thin-walled and have a relatively large surface area for reabsorption of filtered plasma from the tissue. The venules and veins ultimately drain into the vena cava, which returns blood to the heart (Figure 27.1).

In addition to serving as a collection system for the return of blood to the heart, the venous system also serves an important capacitance function. This function allows the cardiovascular system to make rapid adjustments for maintaining perfusion to the tissues in the event of hemorrhage. The larger veins are invested with vascular smooth muscle which, when constricted, reduces the venous capacitance and moves more blood back to the heart. Since the heart can only pump the blood that is returned to it, a reduction in venous capacitance ultimately increases or maintains cardiac output (Figure 27.2).

The lymphatic system is a low-pressure system of vessels and channels for returning plasma that has not been reabsorbed by the venous system back to the circulation. Lymph is an acellular ultrafiltrate of plasma derived from the capillaries. The tiniest lymphatic vessels are blind tubes with poorly defined walls. The lymphatic walls are very permeable and once fluid is reabsorbed it is quickly moved through the lymphatics for return to the heart. All of the lymphatics ultimately drain into

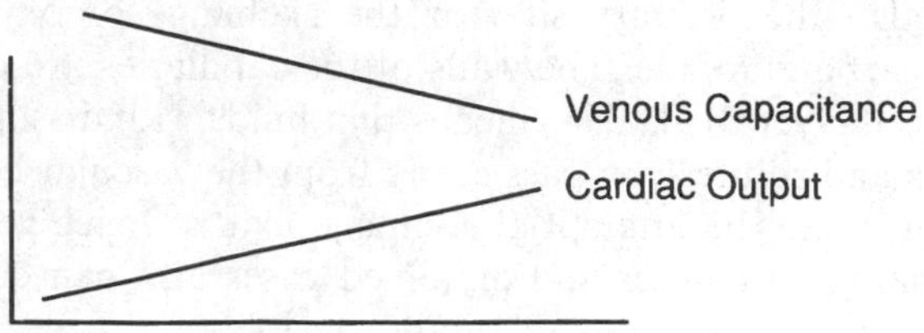

FIG. 27.2. Relationship of venous capacitance to cardiac output.

the vena cava. The function of lymphatics is to maintain a negative interstitial pressure by removing any excess fluid which could elevate interstitial pressures and lead to edema.

A final major component of the cardiovascular system is blood. This complex tissue serves a variety of functions. Blood is the carrier of oxygen and carbon dioxide, nutrients, metabolites, and hormones. It is composed of formed elements (erythrocytes, platelets, and lymphocytes) as well as plasma. The pattern of circulation of blood can either conserve heat or dissipate heat (thermoregulation). The blood also has crucial clotting properties to permit plugging of small and large leaks in the vascular system. The key participants in these clotting properties are the platelets. The platelets are small cellular fragments that respond chemically to disruptions in the endothelial lining of the blood vessels. This response consists of increased stickiness, adherence, and, in conjunction with fibrin, the formation of clots. Malfunction of the clotting system leads to hemorrhage and death such as that seen with warfarin rat poison. Coumarin is used clinically for therapeutic intervention of the clotting process following coronary bypass surgery. It minimizes clot formation in newly revascularized coronary supply arteries where factors that initiate clot formation such as prostaglandins and physical disruption of coronary artery blood flow are prominent. Aspirin is prescribed prophylactically to reduce platelet activation and lower thrombotic activity in situations where small focal cerebral infarcts are suspected. This is low-dose therapy with proven efficacy at minimal risk.

Chemicals can effect the blood in a variety of ways including anemia, hemolysis, and related disorders. Damage to bone marrow can lead to a decrease in the number of red and white cells and platelets (pancytopenia). Severe damage or outright destruction of stem cells prevent these cells from producing new cells (aplastic anemia). Chemicals including drugs such as chloramphenicol, insecticides (lindane), and commercial solvents such as benzene can cause pancytopenia or aplastic anemia. Chemicals that damage dividing cells (anticancer drugs) have the potential to produce frank bone marrow toxicity. Benzene under chronic exposure (100 ppm or higher) can produce a reversible pancytopenia or aplastic anemia. Benzene also has been linked to development of acute myelogenous leukemia.

In other cases, a chemical may effect one or more blood cell types specifically. Therapeutic agents have been designed to produce decreases in platelet number while others inhibit production of various classes of white blood cells. Blood cells can either be effected through the direct action of the chemical on the bone marrow or on circulating cells. Hemolytic anemia, the condition involving a decrease in the number of red blood cells circulating, is induced by oxidants such as phenylhydrazine or analine. Other toxicants, such as lead and mercury, cause red blood cell hemolysis. Lead, for example, increases hemolysis probably through damage to cell membranes. Lead also effects hemoglobin synthesis by inhibiting the enzyme ALA-D.

Carbon monoxide disrupts oxygen transport by interfering with the binding of oxygen molecules to hemoglobin. Carbon monoxide binds at the same site on the hemoglobin molecule but with an affinity 240 times greater than oxygen. Low concentrations of carbon monoxide can produce sufficient binding to hemoglobin with displacement of oxygen. Exposure to as low as 0.1% carbon monoxide can lead to symptoms such as headache, nausea, tachycardia, and even death from oxygen deprivation in a matter of hours. Nitrites, nitrates, aromatic amines, and other nitrogen-containing compounds also oxidize the heme molecule, converting the iron atom from ferrous to ferric which can no longer combine with oxygen rendering the hemoglobin molecule abnormal. Red blood cells, however, have an enzyme, methemoglobin reductase, which is capable of reducing methemoglobin.

The overall functions of the cardiovascular system may be addressed by examining the macrocirculation versus the microcirculation. Although some of the functions of these two major components have been alluded to, a more detailed examination of the cardiovascular system based on this classification would improve the understanding of both the physiology and pathophysiology associated with toxicology.

MACROCIRCULATION

The macrocirculation comprises the heart, the great vessels (both arterial and venous), and the larger arteries and veins. Control of the macrocirculation occurs predominantly through the autonomic portion of the central nervous system. The cardiovascular control centers in the brainstem integrate information from osmolarity receptors, chemoreceptors, thermoreceptors, and pressure receptors. This information is gathered from the different sensor areas of the cardiovascular and nervous systems and control of the circulation is adjusted to alter heart rate, perfusion patterns and overall blood flow, change ventilation rate, and adjust arterial pressure.

Control of arterial pressure is one aspect of cardiovascular physiology that is of interest to most people since arterial hypertension is such a widespread problem. Arterial pressure is controlled through several mechanisms of differing temporal domains. Moment-to-moment adjustments to arterial pressure are effected through baroreceptor reflex controls. The baroreceptors are stretch receptors whose nerves exhibit a tonic level of firing activity. When arterial pressure increases, nerve activity also increases, signaling the cardiovascular centers to decrease heart rate and reduce sympathetic nervous system outflow resulting in vasodilation. Pressure (P) is determined by arterial blood flow (Q) and vascular resistance (R) to flow ($P = QR$). Vasodilation reduces arterial pressure by reducing resistance (inversely related to blood vessel radius). The Poiseuille equation expresses this relationship as follows:

$$R = \frac{8\eta l}{\pi r^4}$$

where η = viscosity
l = length
π = pi
r = radius

This equation demonstrates the importance of adjustments in blood vessel radius in determining the overall resistance to blood flow. As one can see, the resistance to flow changes as a function of radius to the fourth power. Therefore, only small adjustments in radius are required to return arterial pressure to its previous value.

It is also important to realize that baroreceptor function is bidirectional. With decreases in arterial pressure, sympathetic activity increases, resulting in decreased arteriolar radius and increased heart rate. Baroreceptor activity is a powerful mechanism for controlling arterial pressure, but it is probably most effective in short-term control. Longer term control of arterial pressure is effected via hormonal control mechanisms.

Hormonal control of arterial pressure is predominantly through the renin-angiotensin-aldosterone system. This is another powerful regulatory system that controls arterial pressure not only through adjustments to vascular radius but through alterations in overall vascular volume. This system controls arterial pressure in concert with renal adjustments to overall fluid content in the vascular tree. By regulating both the plasma volume and the vascular tone, this control system is much more powerful than the baroreceptor system in maintaining a constant arterial pressure and is effective in long-term pressure control.

Although arterial pressure control is important, the *fundamental* function of the cardiovascular system is the delivery of oxygen and nutrients to the tissues of the body. The metabolic demands of the body therefore determine the cardiac output. The cardiac output is determined in its simplest terms by the stroke volume of the heart (milliters of blood pumped by the left ventricle with each heart beat) multiplied by the heart rate (beats per minute).

$$\text{Cardiac output} = \text{stroke volume} \times \text{heart rate}$$

Heart rate is determined both by intrinsic pacemakers in the heart and by autonomic influences on the heart. Sympathetic nervous system stimulation results in an increased heart rate while parasympathetic stimulation decreases heart rate. Heart rate under resting conditions is usually the result of a balance between sympathetic and parasympathetic influences. Cardiovascular changes that result in stimulation of baroreceptors or the cardiovascular control centers in the brainstem result in alterations in heart rate through the autonomic nerves to the heart.

Heart rate is an important consideration in myocardial perfusion. First, the heart provides the pumping power for its own perfusion. In addition, perfusion of the heart muscle occurs primarily during the relaxation phase of the heartbeat known as diastole. This becomes important when one considers conditions resulting in increases in heart rate known as tachycardia. With higher heart rates less time is spent in the period of diastole; therefore less time is available for myocardial perfusion. Second, increases in heart rate greatly increase the metabolic demands of the heart.

Stroke volume is determined by the intrinsic contractility of the heart and the filling of the heart. In general, the greater the filling of the heart and stretch of the myocardial walls, the greater the force of contraction and ejection of blood. The force of contraction also may be increased by sympathetic nervous system stimulation. Sympathetic stimulation not only enhances contractility but also results in the simultaneous release of epinephrine and norepinephrine from the adrenal gland. These powerful hormones then travel in the bloodstream to the heart and increase the force of contraction.

MICROCIRCULATION

If the macrocirculation is the delivery system for the body, then the microcirculation is the business end of the circulation where the delivery of oxygen and nutrients and the removal of carbon dioxide and metabolites takes place. The architecture of the microvasculature, particularly with regard to the endothelial wall structure, varies from tissue to tissue, depending on the function of the organ in question and the morphology of the tissue. Usually there is some capillary reserve available, meaning that a particular area of tissue can be perfused by more than one capillary. Under these conditions, not all of the capillaries are perfused at any given time. As metabolic demands of the tissue increase, more capillaries can open up to meet the increased demands. Similarly, if a thrombus should occur and occlude a capillary, sufficient capillaries are in close proximity so that tissue in the vulnerable area is not compromised. In some tissue, such as the brain, this capillary reserve does not appear to be present and only one arteriole and capillary supply a given area of tissue. Therefore, any occlusion of small arterioles or capillaries in the brain can be devastating due to the lack of any functional reserve.

The microcirculation is under four different types of control: (a) Neuronal control is provided by central nervous system influences (54); (b) humoral control is provided by endocrine influences; (c) metabolites produced by tissue metabolism provide local control of the microcirculation; and (d) the stretch of the muscles within the vessel walls of the microcirculation provides myogenic control. Taken together, all of these controls make the microcirculation exceptionally well regulated, with the tissue receiving neither more nor less flow than they require metabolically. The obvious exceptions to this control are the skin, where microvascular flow is used to maintain body temperature, and the kidney, where microvascular filtration is used to cleanse the blood of unwanted metabolites and solutes.

Microvascular flow also can be regulated by a process called autoregulation. Autoregulation is thought to be primarily under the control of local concentrations of metabolites that can produce vasodilation. If the tissue is underperfused, dilatory metabolite concentrations increase and allow more blood to enter the tissue. Conversely, if tissue perfusion is excessive, dilatory metabolites are washed away and the blood vessels constrict, thereby reducing perfusion until metabolite levels increase again. Some tissues such as the brain are powerful autoregulators and are neither overperfused nor underperfused.

The primary function of the nutritive capillaries is transcapillary exchange. This is the process by which oxygen dissociates from hemoglobin within the red blood cell and moves out of the capillary into the interstitium. Similarly, carbon dioxide moves from the interstitium into the capillary to be carried to the venous system. The capillaries are also the site for fluid and ion exchange. Fluid moves out of the capillary on the arteriolar side due to higher hydrostatic forces. This extravasated fluid moves into the interstitium and is reabsorbed into the capillary on its venular end. Reabsoprtion occurs due to a higher oncotic pressure within the venular end of the capillary. This elevation in oncotic pressure is generated by the movement of fluids out of the arteriolar end of the capillary leaving the plasma proteins behind. The capillary wall is permeable to water and dissolved ions but is impermeable to plasma proteins. The hydrostatic pressure in the venular end of the capillary is also lower than the arteriolar end. The total amount of water filtered from the capillary is usually slightly greater than the amount reabsorbed. This situation would eventually lead to edema, a buildup of water within the interstitial spaces if left unchecked. The lymphatic vessels serve an essential function in removing this excess fluid and maintaining a negative pressure within the interstitium. This negative pressure ensures that the interstitium will remain "dry."

IMPACT OF SYSTEM DYSFUNCTIONS

The impact of component failure in the above systems can be dramatic. Most of us are aware of component failure such as heart attacks and strokes but not everyone is aware of system participation in other pathological states.

Cardiac Dysfunction

The pumping function of the heart can be compromised both by tissue damage and by dysrhythmias of the contractile process. Tissue damage in the heart is usually the result of ischemic damage secondary to vascular occlusions. These occlusions generally follow atherosclerotic changes in the endothelium of the coronary arteries. These changes are characterized by the deposition of atherosclerotic material in the vascular wall that progressively impinges on the lumen of the blood vessel. When the lumen of the coronary artery has been compromised approximately 90%, the vessel can no longer carry enough blood to adequately perfuse the distal tissues when metabolic demand increases. When occlusion progresses beyond 90–95%, tissue ischemia and tissue death may occur. This death of tissue is accompanied by a loss of pumping function, particularly with respect to cardiovacular reserve. The person may be able to tolerate nonstressful activities but normal daily functions are severely compromised. Obviously if tissue damage is extensive, the heart will no longer function as a pump.

The heart muscle is a complex combination of obliquely arranged fibers whose contraction must be carefully controlled for maximum efficiency. Control of the heartbeat by electrical impulses is very complex and pumping function of the heart can be severely compromised by dysrhythmias in the electrical activity of the heart. The heart muscle is also a functional syncytium, meaning that electrical activity spreads through the tissue in a wavelike fashion once contraction is initiated. If the normal pathway for the spread of electrical activity in the heart is disrupted, then the muscle fibers of the heart will not contract in the complimentary fashion to propel blood from the cardiac chambers. The electrocardiogram (EKG) reflects the electrical activity of the heart as it is measured on the surface of the body. The EKG is a powerful diagnostic tool that is sensitive to disruption in the electrical activity of the heart itself. Many different substances can effect the heart and their effects are reflected in disruptions in the EKG. Typical EKG patterns that would lead to morbidity or mortality are (a) atrioventricular blockade in which the activity of the atria is dissociated from the activity of the ventricles; (b) ventricular tachycardia in which the heart beats normally and rapidly; (c) and ventricular fibrillation, a fatal dysrhythmia in which the normal conduction pattern of the heart is disrupted and the heart does not contract in a synchronous manner. A number of toxins disrupt normal electrical activity in the heart. Examples are digitalis glycosides such as belladonna or digitalis purpurea, oleander, cocaine, and potassium.

Heart failure is usually a complex series of changes specific to the heart and occurs when pumping performance of the heart is reduced such that (a) the total volume of venous blood returning to the heart is not pumped into the arterial side of the circulation, and (b) the pressure generated on the arterial side is reduced to the point that perfusion is compromised.

Treatment of heart failure is usually twofold. First, diuretics are administered to reduce blood flow volume and edema. Second, agents are administered to improve contractility of the heart. The cardiac glycosides are the benchmark pharmacological agents for treatment of heart failure. Interestingly, these compounds are represented by extracts of digitalis purpurea, or purple foxglove, a well-recognized toxic plant. This class of drugs is very effective for treatment of heart failure but also is characterized by a small margin of safety with therapeutic dosage being only slightly lower than toxic dosages. Anything that interferes with metabolism of these compounds can alter the pharmacokinetics of these drugs resulting in toxic plasma levels. Iatrogenic toxic reactions are a real possibility with these compounds and close supervision is required. Heart failure is a significant cause of morbidity and mortality and is another common reason for pump failure. Contractility is compromised in heart failure due to chronic diseases such as valvular heart disease, chronic overloading of the heart muscle due to hypertension, or ischemia following vasoocclusive disease such as atherosclerosis. Many clinical manifestations result from the failure of the heart to pump all of the blood that returns to it. Failure leads to an increase in venous pressures (either systemic or pulmonary) which in turn results in edema, ascites, or dyspnea, to name a few of the more commonly observed sequelae to heart failure.

Vasoocclusive Pathology

Although the impact of vasoocclusion is quickly apparent, we often do not think of this type of dysfunction from an organ systems point of view. Atherosclerosis is one of the most widely known diseases that result in vascular occlusion (49). This disease has traditionally been considered to be a large-vessel disease affecting the aorta, branches of the aorta, and coronary arteries. The resistance to blood flow produced by the encroachment of the atherosclerotic lesion on the lumen of the blood vessel results in a decreased perfusion of the vascular bed distal to the lesion. This type of lesion is often associated with an even higher resistance when blood flow increases. As blood moves more rapidly through the stenosis produced by the lesion, blood flow becomes turbulent. Turbulence per se greatly increases resistance so that the decrease in perfusion is proportionally greater under these circumstances when compared to the simple reduction in cross-sectional area imposed by the atherosclerosis.

The impact of occlusive diseases is to create a condition of chronic ischemia distal to the site of the occlusion. Ischemia is often associated with pain or a loss of organ function. An example of loss of organ function can be demonstrated in the cerebral circulation, where chronic ischemia can result in a loss of cognitive function. A toxicological example of peripheral vasoocclusive conditions is seen with ergot alkaloid toxicity. The fungus *Claviceps purpurea* produces these alkaloids and is found in grains such as rye. Many years ago, when a population was exposed to the alkaloids, a type of "dry" gangrene was observed in some individuals' fingers and toes. These alkaloids produce intense peripheral vasoconstriction and can damage the vascular endothelium resulting in ischemia and tissue death. A more common example of vasoocclusive disease seen today is atherosclerosis. The gradual incursion of plaque into vessel lumen eventually results in occlusion with ischemia peripheral to the lesion.

Microvascular Pathology

The microcirculation is a primary site of pathology in a number of illnesses and is ultimately involved in a wide variety of morbid conditions. Structural alterations in the integrity of the microcirculation can lead to pathologies. Diabetes mellitus is a common disease in which degeneration of the basement membrane of the capillaries results in destruction of the blood vessel, ischemia, and tissue death (40, 65). This process is responsible for diabetic retinopathies, skin necrosis, and gangrene of the toes.

Cold intolerance and Raynaud's phenomenon are other conditions in which microvascular disorders can result in tissue death. Under these conditions, an individual exhibits an abnormally intense response to cold or cool temperatures expressed as an exaggerated vasoconstrictor response to cold exposure. The pathology in this case appears to be an increased sensitivity to sympathetic nervous system stimulation. The condition usually responds to sympatholytic interventions such as pharmacological blockade or surgical transection of sympathetic innervation. Left untreated, the patient can develop ulcerations on the tips of the fingers with gangrenous lesions requiring amputation of the fingertip.

A final microvascular topic that must be addressed, particularly with regard to those agents that are carcinogenic, is microvascular angiogenesis (10). Angiogenesis is the process of increasing the number of microvessels through growth of additional vessels. This is a normal physiological response to growth, increased metabolic demand of a tissue, or hypoxic hypoxia (e.g., high altitude). Angiogenesis also is involved in most forms of inflammation and helps speed the healing of tissues (14). This type of angiogenesis is reversible and disappears after the tissue has healed. The process of angiogenesis also explains oxygen toxicity in newborns raised in an incubator with high levels of oxygen. When the infant is removed from the high-oxygen environment, the microvessels in the eye sense the relative hypoxia of going from an enhanced oxygen environment to one with a normal oxygen content and respond with an explosive growth of microvessels that obliterate the retina (retrolental hyperplasia). Angiogenesis is an essential factor for tumor growth. Any type of neoplastic tumor requires angiogenic activity to support increased tissue growth of the tumor. Normally this is accomplished by the tumor expression of growth factors (tumor growth factors) that stimulate and direct the growth of new blood vessels. If angiogenesis to a tumor is arrested, the tumor cannot grow.

Blood Pathologies

The blood itself also can demonstrate pathologies that affect normal function. Aside from leukemias and platelet disorders, one can have toxicological disorders that affect function. Carbon monoxide poisoning is one form of poisoning that has immediate effects on the body via changes in the blood. Carbon monoxide has a greater affinity than oxygen for the hemoglobin molecule and complexes tightly with the hemoglobin molecule. Oxygen is displaced from the oxyhemoglobin complex. The red blood cells cannot carry oxygen and the tissues then die from asphyxia even though the blood is bright red.

Another pathology of the blood is sickle cell anemia. In this condition the erythrocyte cell wall becomes rigid and distorted into a sickle shape. This reduces the ability of the distorted cells to move through the capillaries and creates thrombi. Conversely, an area of current research focuses on drugs that improve blood viscosity. The rationale behind this research is that by reducing viscosity one can improve microvascular perfusion since flow is inversely proportional to viscosity.

METHODS TO STUDY THE CARDIOVASCULAR SYSTEM

Temporal Considerations

The functional cardiovascular system is by definition very dynamic. When attempting to study this system one has to consider the proposed question in relationship to temporal considerations. Many examples can be considered. One may wish to know the effect of a particular compound on arterial pressure. One immediately needs to clarify whether the acute or the long-term effects of the compound are of interest. If only the acute effects are to be studied, one could easily measure arterial pressure immediately before, during, and after the administration of the compound in question. If, however, the longer term effects are of interest, then a more complicated approach has to be followed.

Arterial pressure on the long term varies diurnally with pressures being higher during the active cycle vs. the resting cycle (18). People are obviously diurnal (active during the day) and demonstrate higher blood pressures during the day than during the night. Conversely, rats are nocturnal and demonstrate higher pressures in the dark cycle than in the light cycle (Figure 27.3).

In either case, in order to study the effects of a compound over this entire period, many measurements would have to be performed. Furthermore, it has been demonstrated that a given compound may have apparent differing levels of potency depending on when within the nyctohemeral (day/night) cycle it is given (39). It is therefore important to be very consistent in the administration of a compound and very specific in interpretation of results. Longer term observations also can be helpful in validating measurement parameters. For example, Giorgiev (21) has shown that body core temperature, a reflection of metabolic rate, changes diurnally and that in laboratory animals it is often lower during the weekends than during the week. They also demonstrated that transient increases occur with external environmental changes such as thunderstorms.

Similarly, Popper et al. (50) demonstrated that the physical handling of animals can produce dramatic increases in plasma catecholamines and that these changes are reflected in the arterial pressure and heart rate. Therefore, if one performs a study of the cardiovascular system in conscious animals, one must work to minimize any psychogenic influences that could alter the arterial pressure or heart rate (18,35).

On the other end of the temporal spectrum one can use observation techniques that only demonstrate a very small portion of the actual sequence of events that is occurring. An example of this would be the use of 35mm photography to document microvascular changes over time. This technique could demonstrate the growth of new blood vessels over a period of days or weeks but would not necessarily reflect the diameter status of the arterioles being studied. The reason for this is that

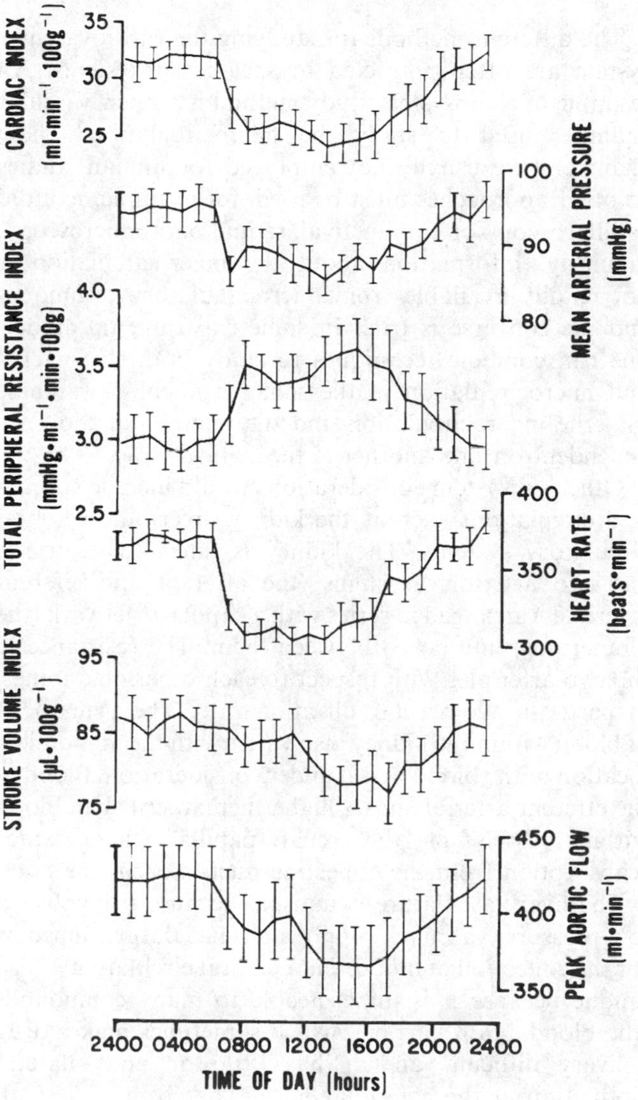

FIG. 27.3. Pattern of hemodynamic variability over a 24-h cycle in Sprague–Dawley rats. Lights-on at 0700 h, lights-off at 1900 h with 2400 h being midnight. Heart rate, total peripheral resistance, mean arterial pressure, and cardiac index were significantly lower during the light period (0700–1900) than the dark period. From Reference 55.

arterioles normally show a rhythmic increase and decrease in diameter that occurs 3–12 times/min. The maximal change in diameter that occurs can be quite large. The use of 35mm photography, however, limits one's observation period to the shutter speed of the camera. The information contained in the 1/250 of a second may or may not be indicative of the overall microvascular diameter. This type of study might better be performed using videomicroscopic techniques capable of recording dynamic events such as vasomotion.

Subsystem Considerations

The different methods for studying the cardiovascular system are often restricted to specific subsystems. An example of a subsystem study method is a microvascular chamber used to study the microcirculation. These chambers are usually not employed for human studies so other approaches must be used, for example, nailfold capillaroscopy or conjunctival/retinal photomicroscopy. Similarly, information about the macrocirculation is not readily available from microcirculatory techniques and the converse is true. In some experimental models one can combine techniques to study both the macro- and microcirculation in the same protocol. Awareness that the macrocirculation and the microcirculation are dependent on one another is the critical issue.

Other subsystem considerations would include specialized circulations such as the kidney, liver, and cerebral circulatory systems. The kidney is unusual because it has two arteriolar systems (the afferent and efferent arterioles) arranged in series with a capillary network (the glomerulus) interposed between them. The resistance in the two arterioles with respect to each other determines, in part, the glomerular filtration rate. The hematocrit of blood within the kidney also varies with the anatomical location of the blood vessel under consideration. Blood in the efferent arteriole has a higher hematocrit than blood within vessels of the renal papilla where water reabsorption from the collecting duct is occurring.

The liver vasculature is unusual because it involves a low-pressure vascular supply and has large sinusoids for the collection of blood. The cerebral circulation is also unique because it is impermeable to many compounds (the blood–brain barrier), which sometimes makes drug delivery difficult, and it has little or no collateral circulation at the arteriolar level. Therefore, if a small thrombus occurs at the arteriolar level, all tissues downstream become ischemic.

Limitations of Study Techniques

Obviously limitations exist in any techniques used for research. The cardiovascular system is particularly sensitive to alteration by external stimuli and observational errors are not uncommon in cardiovascular studies (45,52). For example, anesthetics themselves can have profound effects on the cardiovascular system (51). These effects can be dramatic and can vary with the anesthetic agent and the strain of animal studied (30,34,41). An example of these effects would be the difference between spontaneously hypertensive and Wistar-Kyoto rats in their response to ether anesthesia and to pentobarbital sodium anesthesia. (Figure 27.4A)

Similarly, one can note that the arterial pressure response of an animal to hemorrhage during pentobarbital sodium anesthesia differs from the response observed in the same animal that is conscious (Figure 27.4B, C). Some of the cardiovascular parameters affected by anesthetics include arterial pressure, cardiac output, regional perfusion patterns, ventricular performance, microvascular velocities, and cerebral perfusion (1,8,19,22,38,46,62,68) (Figure 27.5).

When one also considers that anesthesia can affect arterial pO_2 and pCO_2 and thereby alter cardiovascular parameters, it becomes apparent that anesthetics can make interpretation of experimental results very difficult.

Another source of error in cardiovascular studies can be the selection of specific sites for investigations. For example, one cannot readily extrapolate the results from a microvascular study of the mesentery to the microcirculation of the brain. The vascular beds of different organs have differing functions, architecture, anatomy, and control.

Finally, the experimental design should be sensitive to the limitations of acute vs. chronic experiments. Both types of experimental models have advantages and disadvantages. Obviously an acute experiment cannot evaluate the long-term cardiovascular effect(s) of an intervention. Conversely, a chronic experiment cannot incorporate drastic procedures that would inadvertently bias future observations. A common sense approach indicates that interpretation of cardiovascular studies must be confined to the context of the experimental conditions under which the data were collected.

SPECIFIC TECHNIQUES TO STUDY THE CARDIOVASCULAR SYSTEM

Flow Measurement Techniques

Flow measurement techniques are available for cardiovascular studies that allow one to investigate blood flow in vessels as large as the aorta and as small as the capillary. Knowledge of the flow information permits the investigator to determine not only the level of perfusion of tissue, but also calculate the derived hemodynamic variable of resistance. Interventions or

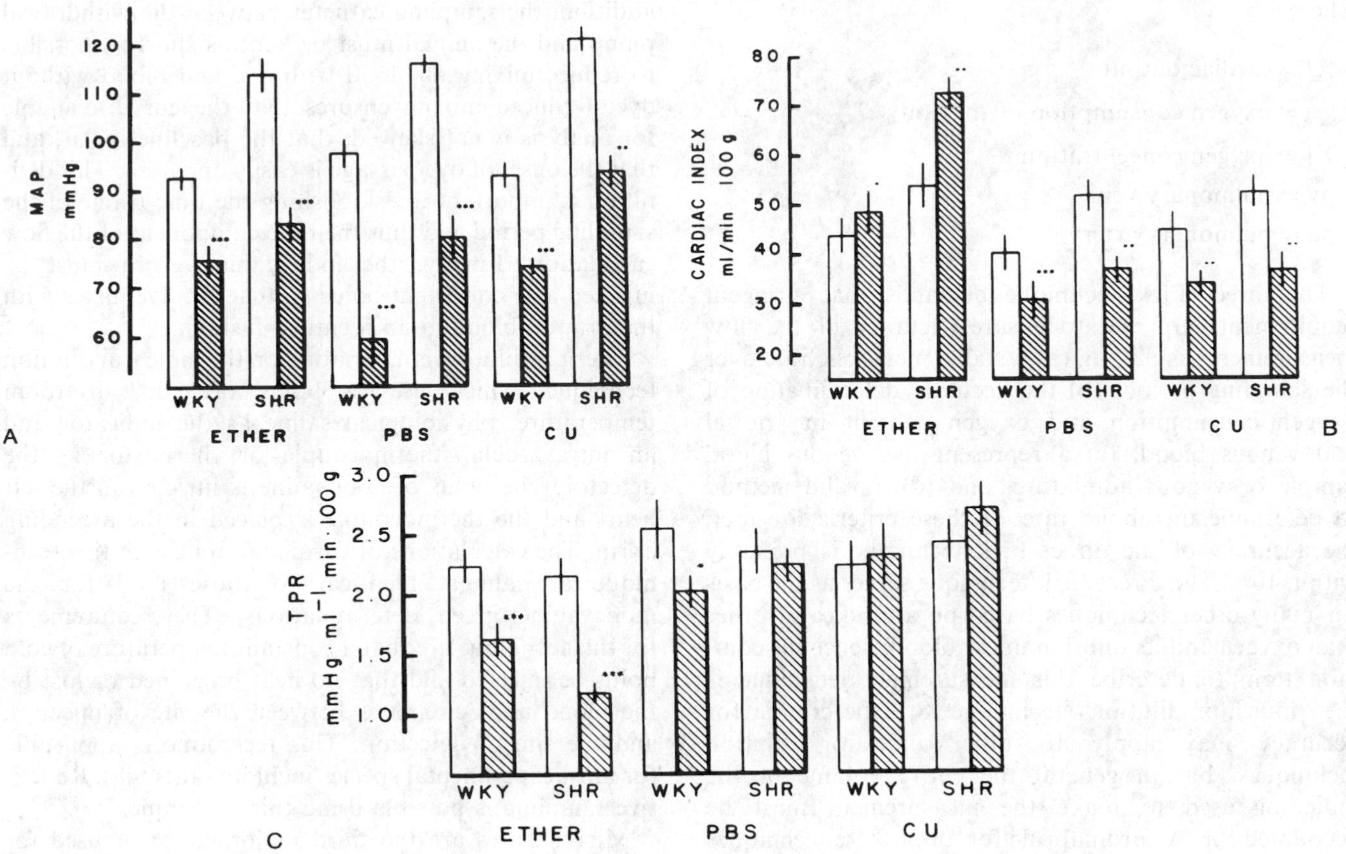

FIG. 27.4. A: Mean arterial pressure (MAP) in normotensive (Wistar-Kyoto, WKY) or hypertensive (spontaneously hypertensive rats, SHR) rats before (conscious, *clear bars*) or after (anesthetized, *hatched bars*) three different anesthetics. Anesthetics studied were diethyl ether (ether), pentobarbital sodium (PBS), or a mixture of α-chloralose and urethane. PBS and CU were administered intraperitoneally. ***$p < .001$, **$p < .01$, *$p = .05$. **B:** Cardiac index in rats before (*clear*) and after (*hatched*) anesthetics. Key is identical to that in Fig. 27.4A. **C:** total peripheral resistance (TPR) in rats before and after anesthetics. TPR calculated as MAP/cardiac index. Key is identical to that in 27.4A. From Reference 56.

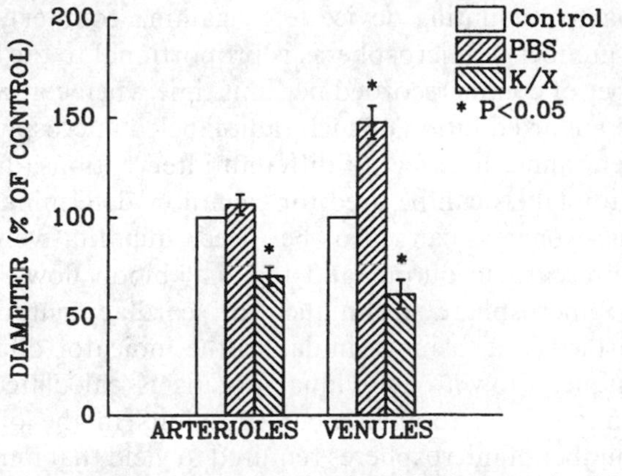

FIG. 27.5. Effects of anesthetics (PBS, pentobarbital sodium, K/X, ketamine/xylazine) on arteriolar and venular diameters when compared to control (conscious) values. Measurements were performed in male Sprague–Dawley rats ($n = 7$) chronically instrumented with microvascular chambers.

compounds that alter resistance then can be evaluated. The methodologies for measurement of flow are ingenious and varied. Selected representative techniques are discussed here but this discussion is not meant to be the definitive summary of all the techniques available to investigators.

The *direct Fick* technique was one of the earliest techniques used for the determination of cardiac output. This technique is based on a careful measurement of oxygen consumption of an individual and the determination of the amount of oxygen in the arterial and venous blood. By estimating the metabolic rate of the subject, one can determine the volume of blood that would be required to carry the volume of oxygen consumed in a finite period. This relationship yields some *volume flow* or measurement of flow in milliliters per min. The equation for calculating flow is given below:

$$Q = q^2/[O^2]pv - [O^2]pa$$

where

Q = cardiac output

q^2 = oxygen consumption of the body

$[O^2]$ = oxygen concentration

pv = pulmonary vein

pa = pulmonary artery

The direct Fick technique demands that stringent requirements are met to ensure accuracy of the flow measurements including (a) a stable metabolic rate over the sampling period, (b) the accurate determination of oxygen consumption and oxygen content in arterial and venous blood, (c) a representative venous blood sample or venous admixture, and (d) a valid method to determine metabolic rate. If these criteria are met, the accuracy of the direct Fick technique is probably within 10%. The direct Fick technique serves as the basis for many other techniques based on an indicator other than oxygen and its dilution in the blood; hence the common term to describe this measurement technique is the "indicator dilution" technique. Specific criteria for accuracy may apply to other indicator dilution techniques, but in general the entire volume of the indicator used to make the measurement must be accounted for. A cardinal rule for all of these techniques is that indicator is neither gained nor lost during the measurement period.

Indocyanine green has been used for many years for the determination of cardiac output using the Fick technique (64). A small amount of indocyanine green at a specific concentration is administered into the left heart (33). Arterial blood then is sampled, preferably from the aorta, by constant withdrawal through an optical cuvette sensitive to the specific absorption spectrum of indocyanine green. The concentration of indocyanine green in the blood is automatically determined as the sample is withdrawn through the cuvette, plotted graphically, and described by a curve. The investigator must truncate the tail end of the curve because the dye can recirculate and be sampled twice. By integrating the area under the curve and comparing this area to a sample standard of known concentration, the average concentration of dye is calculated over the length of the sampling period. Since the withdrawal rate is known, the volume of blood required to attain that dilution can be calculated and the amount of blood that must have been pumped over the sampling period to attain that concentration can be determined. The volume of blood pumped per unit time then equals the cardiac output. A stringent requirement for this technique is that the withdrawal rate of blood through the cuvette be constant and that the rate be fast enough to obtain a representative sample of blood before a recirculation of dye begins. In addition, the sampling catheter between the withdrawal pump and the animal must be kept as short as possible to reduce mixing of blood with dye and blood without dye. Reduced mixing ensures that the curve available for analysis is not skewed, that the baseline is flat, and that the onset of dye passage is easily apparent. This definition is important in establishing the time frame of the sampling period and thus the time component of the flow calculation. Finally, the indocyanine green must be injected as a consistent bolus so that the dye mixes with the arterial blood in an identical fashion.

Thermal dilution is a variation on the indicator dilution technique, which uses a bolus of cold, or room temperature, physiological saline as the indicator and an intravascular thermocouple or thermistor as the detector. The bolus of cool saline is injected in the left heart and the thermocouple is placed in the ascending aorta. The calculations of cardiac output with this technique are almost identical to those used for the indocyanine green determinations. The requirements for this technique are that a constant temperature of cold bolus be injected and that no heat be gained or lost by the blood as it circulates between the site of injection and the site of detection. This technique is applicable for most experimental species including rats (48). Repetitive sampling is possible using this technique.

Microspheres are the third major indicator used for the determination of blood flow. Microspheres are small, carbonized spheres, usually 15 μm in diameter, that flow evenly distributed within the bloodstream and are trapped in the circulation at the arteriolar level. The microspheres can be used to determine qualitative flow by examining the organ for the presence of microspheres. Since microspheres can be labeled with different radioactive tracers, tissue samples can be taken from the site in question to determine the radioactive level using a radioactive counting device (e.g., gamma counter). The total number of microspheres is proportional to the total number of counts recorded per unit time when compared to a standard dilution of such radiolabeled microspheres. To determine the effect of different interventions, different radiolabels can be used for each flow determination.

Microspheres can also be used quantitatively to measure cardiac output and regional blood flows. The basic microsphere technique for cardiac output is performed in a fashion similar to the indicator dilution technique. Flow to individual organs is calculated by determining the total number of counts in the organ, the number of microspheres required to yield that number of counts, and the percentage of cardiac output represented by that number (as a simple proportion) (58). The final data for organ blood flows are appropriately expressed in milliliters × minute^{-10} × gram of tissue. These techniques are detailed for use in rats in Stanek et al. (58).

Colored microspheres may also be used in the same manner as radiolabeled microspheres with the determination of actual counts of numbers of microspheres instead of radioactivity level determinations. For multiple observations, different colors of microspheres can be utilized. Automated counting techniques for colored microspheres are available using image-processing technology. Individual organ perfusions may be determined with this technique although it requires the retrieval of microspheres for counting. This process involves chemical digestion of the target tissue in order to count all the microspheres.

Regardless of the indicator dilution technique chosen, temporal constraints are imposed on the observation by the sampling technique. The determined flow value represents the average blood flow for the time period over which the arterial blood sample or oxygen consumption was measured. Therefore, it is important for the blood flow/ metabolism to be relatively stable during the measurement time period. Similarly, transient changes in blood flow may not be observable with the indicator dilution technique.

Electromagnetic flowmetry is a quantitative technique to measure the flow in a blood vessel that is placed within the lumen of the electromagnetic flow probe. This technique is based on the electronic principle of magnetic induction, that is, the generation of an electrical potential by the movement of a conducting material across the lines of force of a magnetic field. The probes used for this type of investigation consist of a cuff-like electromagnetic cast in a polymer. Electrodes for detecting the potential generated by the movement of plasma through the magnetic field are then cast within the lumen of the probe. The assumption is made that the probe will stay in position so that the axis of flow is perpendicular to the axis of the magnetic field. Calibration of the electromagnetic probe is performed by passing blood through the lumen at known flow rates and adjusting the voltage output of the flowmeter to a standard value. The concentration of erythrocytes can often affect the sensitivity of the measurement; therefore the hematocrit of the blood during calibration usually is changed to determine the impact of hematocrit on accuracy of flow measurement. Similarly, it is necessary to know the hematocrit of the subject in which flow is being measured so that the correct electronic gain may be used in blood flow measurements. Finally, good electrical contact must exist between the flow probe electrodes and the blood vessel. Flow probe manufacturers generally recommend a snug fit between the flow probe and the vessel reproducing approximately 10% constriction for acute experiments. For chronic experiments, a snug fit could eventually result in aortic rupture. Therefore a probe that does not constrict the vessel must be used. In this chronic application, several days must pass between implantation surgery and recording to allow for tissue growth to occur between the probe and vessel and to establish an electrical contact for correct electrical function of the flow probe.

The stability of the flow signal, and particularly the baseline measurements, was a source of problems in early flowmeter designs. These problems were overcome by the use of square wave alternating current excitation rather than sine wave or by careful selection of magnetic material. To verify that zero flow is accurate, a downstream occluder and static flow should be used to verify that electrical drift has not occurred. Chronic implantation of the electromagnetic probe can lead to the development of short circuit currents around the blood vessel, which can change the electronic value for zero flow. Chronic implantation of a downstream occluder can facilitate verification of zero flow or, if ascending aortic blood flow is being measured, the diastolic section of the flow waveform can be used to identify the zero flow portion of cardiac output at the aortic root. Baseline adjustments for zero flow values then can be made.

The frequency response of electromagnetic flow probes is excellent with minimal loss of fidelity at 100 Hz. The probes come in a wide assortment of diameters ranging from 1mm to several centimeters. Flowmeters are commercially available from several vendors, are easily operated, may be interfaced with microcomputers for automated data collection, and are dependable.

Pulsed Doppler flowmetry is a technique for velocity measurement of blood flow based on the principle of Doppler shift of ultrasound produced by the movement of blood exposed to the ultrasound (24). In this technique an ultrasonic crystal is placed against the blood vessel at approximately a 45 degree angle with acoustic gel filling the void between the crystal and the blood vessel. A burst of ultrasound is introduced from the crystal to the vessel for a brief period (25). The crystal then acts as a receiver for reflection of the ultrasound from the moving bloodstream. The frequency of the reflected ultrasound is shifted from the frequency introduced due to the Doppler effect. The magnitude of the frequency shift is proportional to the velocity of the moving bloodstream. Normally the operator adjusts the output of the probe so that the centerline of the bloodstream is being sampled for Doppler shift of reflected ultrasound. This sampling technique is thought to sample the highest velocity portion of the bloodstream. For these assumptions, the velocity profile of the bloodstream is assumed to be laminar and parabolic as shown in Figure 27.6. Construction techniques for miniature probe fabrication may be found in Haywood et al. (25).

If the vessel is assumed to be cylindrical, then changes in velocity are proportional to changes in flow (3). In fact, if the instantaneous diameter of the blood vessel could be measure simultaneously with velocity, volumetric flow could be determined. As presently configured, however,

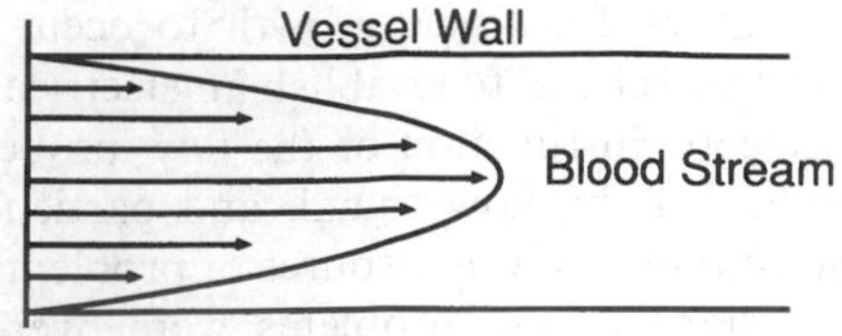

FIG. 27.6. Parabolic velocity profile of blood moving within the arterial vasculature. This profile would be representative of nonturbulent flow in a straight segment of blood vessel.

the output of the flowmeter is expressed as a kilohertz shift and is not a volumetric (milliliters per minute) flow measure. Validation studies in which volumetric and pulsed Doppler measurements were performed simultaneously found that the magnitude and directions of changes in kilohertz shift closely paralleled those in volumetric flow (3,25). Furthermore, the pulsed Doppler measurements were precise. Although these data do not validate the use of pulsed Doppler for the measurement of volumetric flow, they indicate that pulsed Doppler studies are valuable in assessing changes in perfusion within the same experiment. The results can be expressed as percent change from control values.

The pulsed Doppler device has several advantages over electromagnetic flowmetry. These advantages include the relatively low cost of flow probes, small probe size, and nonconstricting fit of the flow probe for increased longevity of animals instrumented with probes. The cost of the flow probes is very low. In fact, the probes can be easily made by the investigator. The small size of the flow probes allows them to be used chronically in small-vessel application (1 mm or less). The frequency response of the pulsed Doppler is excellent and is capable of following changes in perfusion at very high heart rates.

The primary limitation of pulsed Doppler flowmetry is its inability to accurately measure volumeric flow; the researcher does not know whether initial flow values are within normal range. Also, the velocity values and flow assumptions are based on measuring laminar, parabolic velocity profile within the vessel. If the velocity profile is nonparabolic, then the assumptions could be invalid. Furthermore, the velocity data are unobtainable under conditions of turbulent flow. Turbulence can be encountered immediately beyond a stenosis of bifurcation and is only apparent at higher velocities.

Transit time flowmetry also uses ultrasound generated by electrically excited crystals but the measurement principle is different. The transit time flowmeter uses a wide burst of ultrasound to cover the entire width of the vessel, thereby simultaneously encompassing all of the differing velocities within the blood vessels. The device measures the amount of time it takes for ultrasound to pass from a transmitting crystal to a downstream receiving crystal.

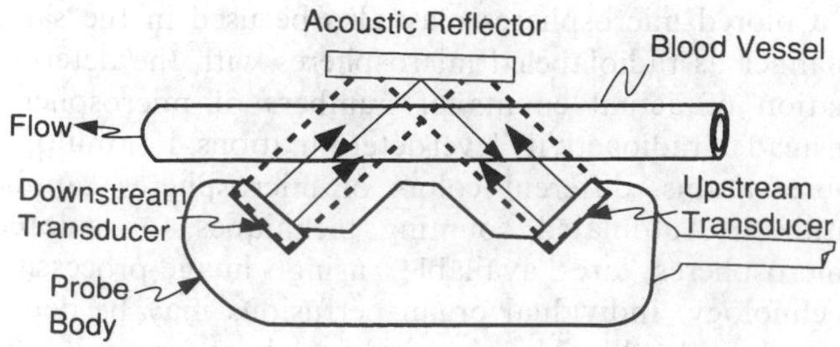

FIG. 27.7. Schematic of transit time flow probe orientation to a blood vessel. Pathway of ultrasound is indicated by straight arrows.

The transmitting and receiving crystals then change functions, with the transmitter becoming the receiver and vice versa, so that the amount of time required for ultrasound to be transmitted upstream is determined (Figure 27.7).

A highly accurate comparator circuit then analyzed the difference between the upstream and downstream transit times. This difference in transit times is directly proportional to the average bulk flow of blood through the vessel (12). Individual probes can be calibrated to determine the amount of amplification of signal required to successfully use these devices to measure volumetric flow. The frequency response to transit time flow probes is at least 100 Hz. Zero flow is electronically stable with little or no electronic drift over time.

Transit time flow probes are moderately priced, with their cost less than electromagnetic but more than pulsed Doppler devices. The probes may be used in acute applications as long as acoustical coupling between the probe and the blood vessel is accomplished. This can be done by injecting surgical lubricant or saline around the blood vessel and probe, making certain that no air bubbles are included in the lumen of the probe. Transit time devices can be implanted chronically in most animal models.

Transit time flowmetry has several advantages over other techniques when utilized in chronic applications. The stability of zero flow values makes long-term monitoring of blood flow possible. In addition, since the probes do not have to restrict the blood vessel to function properly, the longevity of the chronically implanted preparation is improved. The high-frequency response of the system means that transient alterations inflow can be measured. Finally, transit time flowmetry may be applied to small (1-mm-diameter) as well as large (48-mm-diameter) vessels.

Laser Doppler fluxmetry is a relatively new technique for evaluating microvascular perfusion. The laser Doppler fluxmetry technique is based on the Doppler principle of frequency shift by moving objects (53). The laser Doppler transmits monochromatic laser light into the tissue via fiberoptics. This light is reflected back into the laser Doppler probe head where a receiving optical fiber transmits the light back to the instrument. Some of the laser light is shifted in wavelength by the movement of erythrocytes within the tissue being examined. The amount of shifted light is proportional to both the total number of erythrocytes within the microvasculature in the illuminated area and the average velocity of the erythrocytes (23). Therefore, the technique is influenced by the hematocrit and by the total volume of blood within the tissue being illuminated. There is some debate concerning the quantitative nature of laser Doppler fluxmetry. Some investigators believe that the laser Doppler is capable of yielding values for quantitative blood flow in the tissue in milliliters per minute per cubic milliliter of tissue. Others believe that the technique is more qualitative in nature (11,59). This more conservative approach suggests that laser Doppler can be used in conjunction with visualization of microvessels to characterize and diagnose specific microvascular changes (66).

A source of disparate results in laser Doppler studies can be the specific type of laser light used. Some laser sources are helium neon tubes that produce laser light in the 620-nm wavelength. This wavelength of laser light does not penetrate the tissue as deeply as longer wavelengths of laser light. Other laser Dopplers employ laser diodes as the source of laser light. This approach is advantageous from a dependability point of view since the laser diode lasts for thousands of hours. The disadvantage is that this laser light is of a longer wavelength (730 nm) and penetrates more deeply into the tissue. This difference can become critical, for example, in studies of human skin. If a helium neon laser instrument is used to study human skin, it will detect the predominantly capillary (nutritive) flow. Conversely, a laser diode instrument also will detect deeper, thermoregulatory microvascular networks. Under certain circumstances the deeper microvascular structures can be adequately perfused while the skin nutritive vessels are ischemic. Under these conditions, the choice of laser Doppler instrument will affect the results of the microvascular perfusion study.

The laser Doppler has many advantages in studying microvascular perfusion. The technique is essentially noninvasive and nondestructive. Repeated measurements can be made over time but reproducibility of numbers can be difficult since it is hard to position the laser probe over exactly the same spot each time. In some applications one can leave the device in position for several days to monitor the progression of healing of skin flaps in reconstructive surgery. Other studies have been performed in which human subjects have been examined at regular intervals to assess the efficacy of treatment to improve cutaneous circulation (32, 66).

A modification of the laser Doppler technique is the laser scanner (63). This machine combines the laser Doppler effect with computerized scanning of a large field (12 × 12 cm). The large area that is examined allows one to evaluate cutaneous perfusion in an entire structure such as the hand or foot and permits detection and evaluation of focal aberrations. This technology holds promise for future studies. The applicability of this technique would allow one to evaluate the effects of toxicants on cutaneous circulation and the efficacy of countermeasures to treat that toxicity.

Microvascular methods for the flow measurement require videomicroscopic capabilities. These techniques require the separate measurement of microvascular diameter and velocity of the red cell column (2,27). These two parameters then are used to calculate flow within the microvessel, assuming that the capillary is cylindrical (12). The advent of newer technologies has greatly simplified these techniques and improved their accuracy. The two major techniques for determining microvascular velocity are the flying spot technique and the dual-slit technique. The dual-slit technique is the more accurate of the two methods. The dual slit is actually two photodensitometric windows created by the positioning of two photodiodes separated by a fixed distance over the same blood vessel. As a moving column of blood and plasma passes the first photodiode an optical "signature" based on a characteristic densitometric pattern is created. This signature can be recognized by the second photodiode a short time later as the moving column of blood passes down the vessel. The time between the recognition of the signatures between the two photodiodes serves as a basis for the calculation of velocity since the windows are separated by a known distance.

Diameter measurements can be performed by video image shearing. The latter technique is relatively simple. The operator can split the top and bottom of a video image along a raster line. The top image then can be displaced with respect to the bottom image by delaying the sweep of the video screen. The two walls of the microvessel can then be aligned so that the total displacement of the two images equals the diameter of the blood vessel (26) (Figure 27.8).

The unit can be calibrated in micrometers for any given magnification by video analysis of a stage micrometer image. The displacement information in milliseconds can be converted to linear units (micrometers). The restrictions on this technique are that a clear video image must be available for analysis and that the operator make the decision as to where the edges are aligned. This necessarily introduces a degree of subjectivity into the analysis. A similar technique can be used that recognizes the microvessel edge on a video image and determines how long it takes for the beam sweep to cross the dark area

FIG. 27.8. Diagrammatic representation of video image shearing for microvascular dimension analysis. The bottom image is displaced in time from the top image. The amount of temporal displacement is proportional to the distance across the red cell column and can be referenced to a stage micrometer for calibration purposes.

of the blood vessel. This technique requires a clear video image, good contrast, and a uniform background.

The techniques for microvascular analysis have broad applications, particularly in acute experiments. Chronic experiments also can utilize these techniques but the availability of microvascular beds for measurements is limited. A clear advantage of these techniques is that they are noninvasive. They also have the capability of yielding dynamic information about microvascular diameter and flow.

Pressures

The measurement of pressures within the cardiovascular system is one of the most commonly performed procedures available to the investigator. Pressure within the vascular system is determined both by blood flow to the tissue and by resistance to the flow within the tissue. This relationship is expressed by the equation:

$$\text{Pressure} = \text{flow} \times \text{resistance}$$

Arterial pressure decreases dramatically as measurements are taken from the heart down the vascular tree to the capillaries. A further decrease in pressure occurs between the capillaries and the right heart. Although the systemic arterial pressure is pulsatile, the microvascular pressure is relatively stable. The peak pulsatile arterial pressure is termed *systolic* whereas the minimal pulsatile arterial pressure is called *diastolic*.

Measurements of intravascular pressures may be performed either indirectly or directly. Indirect techniques utilize an external compression technique to completely occlude blood flow. External compression is applied to an appendage and then slowly released so that pressure within the occluder decreases. This technique may be applied to primate and human extremities (limbs and digits), and to dog and rat tails. Movement of blood past the occluder is detected using audio techniques or by detecting the change in temperature in the blood vessel distal to the occluder as arterial blood moves past the occluder. Audible detection of the movement of blood is possible because the turbulence accompanying the movement of blood through the partially compressed artery results in the generation of sound waves. Whichever detection technique is utilized, the systolic pressure is equivalent to the intravascular pressure that just exceeds the occlusion pressure. The accuracy of these techniques depends on the ratio of occluding cuff width to limb diameter. Inaccurate measurements will be obtained if an occluding cuff of too great or too little width is used (4,5). Diastolic pressure is somewhat more difficult to determine utilizing indirect techniques. In experimental animals, only systolic pressures can be measured with relative confidence under most conditions. All of the indirect techniques are capable of measuring only an average pressure (systolic or diastolic) over the entire sampling period. Little or no information about transient changes in pressure can be obtained using these techniques.

An additional significant source of error is inherent in the use of a thermoregulatory end organ, such as the rat tail, for performing indirect arterial pressure measurements. In order to perform measurements in this species, it is often necessary to warm the animal to obtain perfusion of the tail. Without warming, the tail arteries are constricted and measurements are impossible. With warming, however, rats often exhibit a psychogenically mediated increase in arterial pressure. This artificial elevation in pressure can mislead the investigator.

Direct measurement of intravascular pressures avoids many of the problems associated with indirect techniques but also imposes a new set of limitations. First among these is that direct measurement techniques are invasive. These techniques require surgical access to the vascular tree but also pose the risk of infection. Access to a major blood vessel requires some degree of trauma, and therefore this technique can result in increased arterial pressure. Measurements of arterial pressure obtained soon after catheter implantation surgery do not represent values that reflect the normal functional state of the animal. Four to five days are required for recovery from catheter implantation before pressure measurements can be obtained with confidence.

Another consideration in pressure measurements using direct techniques is the frequency response or fidelity of the pressure measurement system. The fidelity of the manometric system reflects the accuracy of the assembled components to measure the absolute magnitude of the arterial pressure as well as the temporal relationships. Therefore, not only can the absolute magnitude of the pressure being measured vary, but the relationship of the time-dependent components also may vary with the waveforms representing components of pressure being delayed in time when compared to the actual event (17). The ability of the manometric system to accurately follow these pressure changes is determined by the diameter of the catheter, the length of the catheter, the catheter material, the volume displacement utilized by the pressure transducer, and the electrical characteristics of fidelity utilized by the transducer/amplifier/recording system. Generally speaking, the manometer system should be capable of accurately recording up to 10 harmonics of the fundamental pressure frequency being studied. For example, to measure systolic and diastolic pressure in a rat with a heart rate of 360 (fundamental frequency 6 Hz), the manometer system should have a frequency response of at least 60 Hz. To obtain the greatest frequency response possible from the system being used, the following generalizations may be made. The manometric system should have low compliance in both catheter material and the pressure transducer. In addition, catheters should be kept as short as possible and have the largest diameter possible. Therefore, the pressure transducer and amplifier should be mounted as close as possible to the experimental subject. Finally, all air and gas bubbles must be purged from the system of the transducer, stopcock, and catheters. These small bubbles can dramatically reduce the performance of the manometer system.

One solution to many of the sources of error inherent in catheter-based pressure measurements is the use of solid state pressure transducers for intravascular use. These devices utilize a pressure-sensing element located on the tip of a catheter so that the pressure waveform is sampled within the blood vessel. These systems are characterized by high-frequency responses because the sensing element is relatively stiff and the long, narrow-bore cannulas are not involved in the measurement. Connection between the animal and the recording device is electrical only and is accomplished by hardwiring (electrical tether) or by telemetry. Some systems are available that are a hybrid between conventional catheter systems and completely solid state devices. These units have a short fluid-filled catheter that is placed intravascularly and that is connected to a transducer system also within the animal. The pressure signal that is monitored then is transmitted outside the animal via an FM transmitter. Advances in electronic miniaturization permit the transducer/amplifier/transmitter to be quite small (4.5 ml volume) and lightweight (9 g), permitting application of this technology in animals as small as rats (39). Studies that have used these devices find that the measured arterial pressures and heart rates are somewhat lower than those reported using catheter systems with or without chronic tethers. The rationale to explain these results is that the monitoring procedures utilizing tethers elicit sympathetic responses that elevate these cardiovascular parameters.

Microvascular pressures can be monitored by direct cannulation using micropipettes. The pressure transduction device that is applicable to such small displacement systems is the servo-null device (20). The servo-null system utilizes an electrolyte within the micropipette and circuitry to monitor electrical resistance within the pipette. As the electrical resistance within the pipette changes, a voltage is applied to an electrical bellows that pushes electrolyte into the pipette until the original resistance is restored. This system is extremely accurate and has quite a high-frequency response. Using this technique, pressure within microvessels down to the capillary level may be sampled.

Dimensions/Volume

Measurement of the internal diameter of vascular structures is often of interest. Such measurements can be used to calculate volumes if sufficient data are available. Usually one can make such estimates if two axes of the structure, such as the ventricular chambers, are accurately measured. Intravascular dimensions currently are measured using ultrasonic crystals transmitting at 15 kHz. The amount of time required for the pulse of ultrasound to traverse the chamber and be received at the opposite side by a receiving crystal is directly proportional to the distance traveled. The resolution of these devices is approximately 0.1 mm. The application of these devices is usually by suturing a pair of crystals to the myocardial wall in an opposed position. A second pair then is implanted at right angles to the first. For irregularly shaped structures it may be necessary to suture a third pair of crystals to the myocardial walls to obtain a Z axis in addition to X and Y.

External ultrasound also may be used to examine internal vascular dimensions, particularly of the carotid arteries of persons. These measurement techniques are well suited to clinical applications and can be used to assess long-term disease processes such as arteriosclerosis. The technique is similar to echocardiography or abdominal sonography in that it uses reflected ultrasound to measure the dimensions of internal structures. The overall resolution of this technique can be quite good and the technique can provide useful information about the underlying structures.

Microscopic techniques are available for the measurement of diameters or volume. These techniques can be very rudimentary, for example, the observer can measure the diameter of a microvessel using an eyepiece retical calibrated in micrometers for the specific objective being used. A map of the microvascular field is drawn and the dimensions of each branch are recorded. The technique has some degree of subjectivity associated with the observations, but the variance can be minimized for a given study by having a single, trained observer making the measurements. A modification of this technique would entail photomicrography of the microscopic field and subsequent enlargement of the photographic negative. The diameter and length of individual vessels then can be accurately established using a digitizing tablet interfaced with a microcomputer.

Another microscopic technique utilizes videoanalysis of the microvessels. Image shearing, as described previously, may be done continuously over time by the operator to record any transient changes in the diameter of the blood vessel. Such changes in diameter are termed vasomotion and are usually associated with rhythmic dilation and constriction occurring 5–12 times/min. The significance of vasomotion is not completely established but it appears to be a blood flow regulatory phenomenon found in most tissues. Vasomotion may be altered or eliminated by anesthesia. Video image analysis also may be performed using computer software to recognize the edge of the blood vessel as a change in the contrast of the video image. The opposite edge then is also identified and the diameter of the blood vessel determined either by countering the number of pixels between the two walls or by establishing the time required to go from one point in the video image to the next.

Electrocardiogram

The electrocardiogram or EKG is a bioelectric potential originating in the myocardium and recorded on the surface of the body. The EKG represents the sum of the electrical depolarizations of the myocardial syncytium as the wave of depolarization sweeps across the heart. The EKG is sensitive to disturbances and may be used as a good, noninvasive measurement to reveal underlying myocardial problems. The EKG can be monitored with relatively simple equipment and, in larger subjects, can be recorded for long periods on magnetic tape for later analysis. Alternatively, the data may be collected and transmitted to receivers close to the subject and stored on a device chosen by the investigator.

Telemetry vs. Hardwired

Measurement of cardiovascular parameters usually requires tethering of a physiological transducer, for example, a blood pressure transducer or an EKG electrode, to a meter and/or amplifier and recording device. This necessitates several sets of wires for studies entailing different simultaneous measurements. This collection of wires may be inconsequential for acute studies or for short-term measurements in chronically instrumented preparations. Long-term measurements may require tethering of the animal to the recording device. Tethering can be cumbersome, however, and may interfere with the design parameters of the experiment. Exercise studies, for example, can be complicated by tethering. In addition, tethering may impose a psychological stress on the experimental animal. The cardiovascular system is sensitive to psychological stress and therefore tethering may alter the cardiovascular parameters under investigation.

An alternative to tethering is radiotelemetry, more commonly termed telemetry. This technique incorporates the physiological sensor and amplifier on or within the animal. The signal then is transmitted on a carrier radiowave. This carrier wave is detected by an FM receiver, normally close to the subject. Usually only one signal can be carried on each transmitted frequency, but several different transmitters may be employed to relay different information. Alternatively, a multiplexer may be used to sequentially transmit different channels of information on a single carrier wave.

Telemetry offers many advantages over tethering but also has some disadvantages. The functional lifespan of the implanted device is normally limited by the longevity of the battery. Battery life can be extended a great deal by adding an on/off switch, either electromagnetic or radiofrequency-operated. However, when the battery is drained the implanted power source must be replaced. Alternatively, one can power the device using an implanted induction coil and a matching external coil. This requires manipulation of the experimental subject, however, which may produce the same psychological stress as tethering. An additional disadvantage to telemetry is the initial acquisition cost. The individual units are expensive and refurbishment costs between animals are also high. It can be argued, however, that the superior quality of the data obtained ultimately results in fewer animals required for study because of reduced variability in cardiovascular parameters with this type of instrumentation (39).

MICROCIRCULATION—ACUTE VS. CHRONIC

Microvascular studies allow evaluation of the "business end" of the circulation where tissue level delivery of nutrients and oxygen takes place and tissue metabolites and carbon dioxide are removed. At the microvascular level one can measure dimensions (lengths, static and dynamic diameters), velocities, vessel distribution patterns, and cellular components. Blood cellular components such as erythrocyte density (hematocrit), shape, and deformability can be studied. In addition, platelet adhesion, microemboli, and polymorphonuclear leukocyte activity can be evaluated directly. In acute experiments microelectrode measurements of tissue oxygen tension, carbon dioxide, pH, nitric oxide, and intravascular pressures (using micropipettes) can be made. One can readily appreciate the importance of those measurements from a toxicologist's point of view.

The microcirculation can be studied in many different experimental models and tissues. The earliest studies utilized models in which the skin was thin and transparent and the overall tissue was not thick. These models were the webs between frog toes and the thin skin between digits of the bat wing. As technical improvements were made in microscopy techniques, a much wider variety of tissues was studied. Table 27.1 identifies a few of those microvascular beds available for study.

The variety of tissues available for study challenge the investigator to develop microscopy and quantification techniques. Both acute and chronic microcirculatory techniques have been developed to pursue those studies. Acute, invasive techniques are often required for the study of some microvascular beds. Although acute studies in general require anesthesia, they may be advantageous in that more experimental variables can be controlled.

Table 27.1
Microvascular beds available for study

Tissue	Location	Species
Skeletal muscle	Spinotrapezius	Cat, rat
	Gracilis	Rat
	Cremaster	Rat
	Cutaneous maximus	Rat
	Cheek pouch	Hamster
Skin	Wing	Bat
	Back	Rat
	Ear	Rabbit, rat, mouse
	Tail	Rat
	Toe	Rat
	Finger	Human
Brain	Pial/cortex	Rat, cat
Gut	Bowel	Rat
Kidney	Glomeruli	Rat
Eye	Conjunctiva	Human
	Retina	Human, rat

An additional challenge for the investigator is to ensure that the experimental conditions for the research do not artificially alter the parameters they are studying. Interpretation of these studies must be conservative. Extrapolation of acute experimental results to other conditions may be made only when one is confident that criteria for acceptance are met.

Microcirculatory chambers that permit long-term microvascular observations to be made have been available for many years (45). There are two broad subtypes of chambers: one in which new blood vessels infiltrate the chamber and one in which preexisting blood vessels may be studied. Microvascular chambers for chronic study have been utilized for the rabbit ear (connective tissue and cartilage) (13), skeletal muscle (hamster and rat back flap), pial/cortex (rat, rabbit) (6,7,37,47), and bone (67) (Figure 27.9). Chambers that require in growth of new blood vessels must be implanted several weeks prior to the onset of studies. Chambers that examine preexisting vessels may be utilized 5–7 days after implantation. This recovery period allows the animal to recuperate from the implantation procedure (Figure 27.10).

One disadvantage of chamber techniques is that it is difficult to administer pharmacological agents directly into the chamber to affect only those vessels under observation. Opening of the chamber for direct application of pharmacological agents is not advised since this introduces a high probability of infection. The investigator usually has to administer compounds systemically. However, systemic administration of drugs may affect the microvascular bed indirectly via reflex systemic pressure changes.

Advantages of microvascular chambers include the ability to perform repeated observations of a microvascular bed for relatively long periods of time. This allows one to examine microvascular changes that accompany a disease process, such as renovascular hypertension, as well as those changes that follow an acute intervention such as a contusion. Changes that can be documented would include diameters of both arteries and veins, flow velocities, microemboli, and increases or decreases in vessel density (number per unit area). Changes in vessel density can be observed within 3 days of the initiation of a stimulus that could alter this parameter. Chronic microvascular chambers offer the toxicologist the opportunity to study the microvascular effects of compounds of interest longitudinally.

One can reduce systemic reflex changes in a few limited instances by administering a compound into the environment of the microcirculation. For example, one can study the effects of vasoactive compounds on the pial microcirculation by administering the drugs through an intracerebroventricular cannula (Figure 27.11).

Similarly, one can study the effects of hyperglycemia on the microcirculation of the gut by performing a sterile

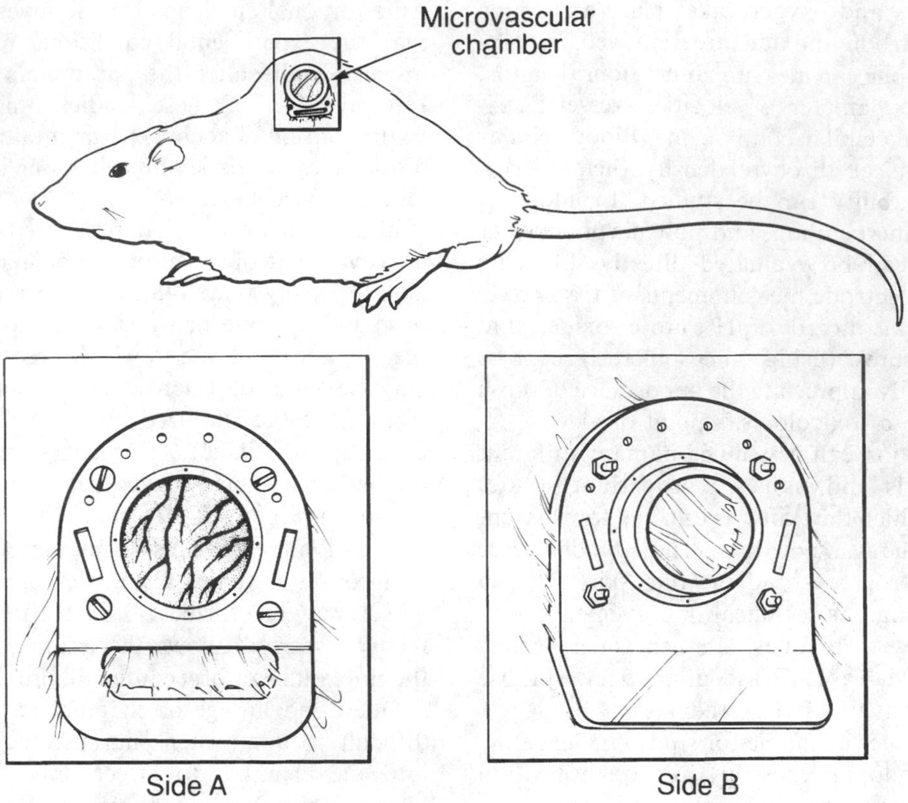

FIG. 27.9. Schematic drawing of a skeletal muscle microvascular chamber suitable for implantation in a rat. The chamber is made of polycarbonate and is very lightweight (approximately 2.3 g). Implantation described in Smith et al. (57).

laparotomy, examining the mesenteric circulation, and then administering hypertonic glucose by repeated intraperitoneal injection for several days. The animal then is studied again in an acute protocol in which the same microvascular bed is examined (60,61). The vascular density and morphology can then be documented.

Although not widely used to evaluate cardiovascular injury, there are a number of excellent in vitro approaches available for examining specific types of cardiovascular injury. The detection of cardiovascular dysfunction at the cellular level is beset by many difficulties, not the least of which is no in vitro method has been validated and/or accepted by regulatory authorities. Nonetheless, such systems have been advocated as a means of studying the direct effects of chemicals on isolated cells without the complex interaction of the physiological systems present in the intact animal. Functional, uniform cells of almost any specific type are available. The use of cultured cells allows for species-and-organ-specific comparisons of toxicity. Cell culture systems also provide useful approaches that can, in many cases, offer insight into a chemical mechanism underlying the toxicity observed in vivo. Such approaches include modification of subcellular macromolecules and enzymatic reaction, or the use of organelles as sensitive and specific indicators of toxicity. However, no single system or approach shows the whole picture.

Specific protocols for such in vitro systems are scattered throughout the biomedical literature (69, 70, 71). One of the earliest myocardial cell culture models used hearts obtained from two-to-four-day old rats (72). In the case of heart cell cultures, the heart can be segregated into single cells, which are grown in a chemically defined medium. These cells are capable of forming a confluent monolayer. When intact, cells in culture beat in unison and are sensitive to chemicals in a manner similar to the whole heart. There are, however, disadvantages to heart cell cultures. Myocytes in culture show variable contraction rates and electrical mechanical uncoupling caused by cell isolation procedures. These cells exhibit an action potential but do not visibly contract. The myofibrils also may not be in a highly differentiated state even though the cells may be highly differentiated electrically. Often cultured cells revert to the embryotic status; this limitation can be minimized if the cells are utilized shortly after monolayer formation. Metabolism may shift from aerobic to a more anaerobic state. Fibroblasts may be present in myocyte cultures.

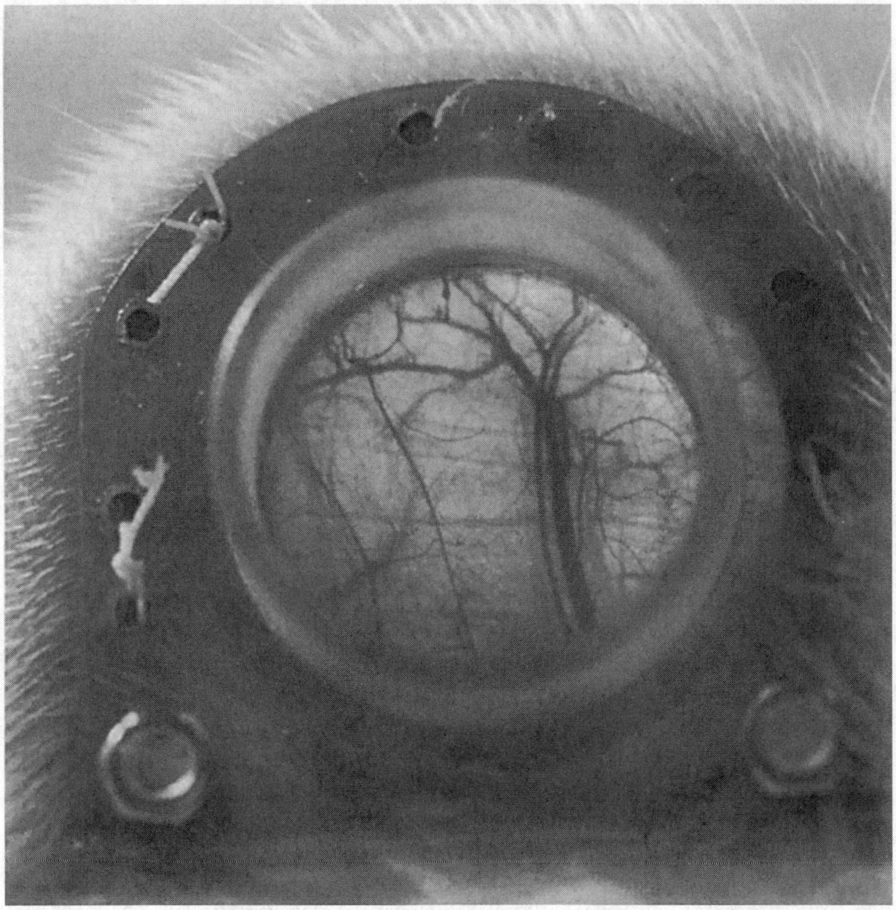

FIG. 27.10. Photograph of skeletal muscle microvessels within a chronically implanted chamber on the dorsum of a rat. Skeletal muscle fibers are oriented from left to right. Dorsum of rat is at top of picture. From Reference 57.

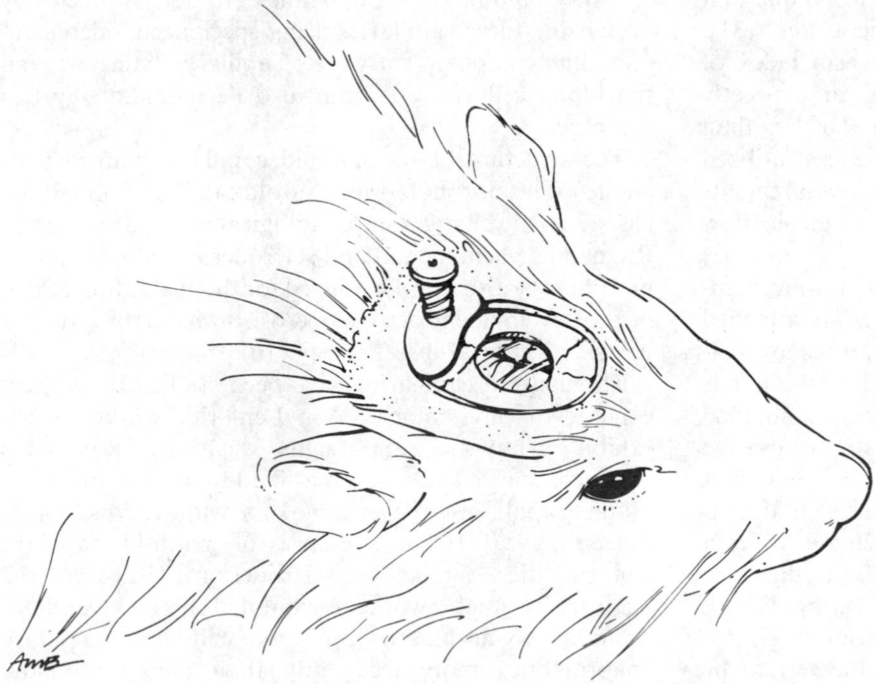

FIG. 27.11. Implanted pial/cortical window and IV intracerebro-ventricular cannula in a chronically instrumented rat. Cannula may be unplugged to administer agents into the cerebrospinal fluid bathing the pial vessels under observation. This technique allows one to administer agents that do not readily cross the blood–brain barrier.

Nonetheless, if reasonable precautions are taken, cultured heart cells can provide information not easily obtained from intact cardiac muscle preparations.

Clinical Microcirculation

Clinical microcirculation is the application of microvascular techniques to patients. The number of tissues available for study is fewer than that in animal models, but important information can be obtained. Nailfold and conjunctival capillaroscopy can be performed using intravital compound microscopy. This technique allows direct visualization of the microcirculation on the surface of the body. Laser Doppler fluxmetry may be used on the skin's surface to evaluate overall perfusion of the skin (both nutritive and thermoregulatory) as well as control of that circulation (through cold stress or invocation of sympathetic nervous system reflexes).

In order to obtain an adequate evaluation of extremity vascular perfusion it is necessary to apply a stress procedure. Controlled exposure to cold has been developed as a method to deliver a stress in order to assess the thermoregulatory capacity of a digit. Several different methods have been developed to produce a cold stress on the digits. These methods include ice water immersion of the hands (43), application of cold to the nape of the neck (28, 29), total-body cooling (43), and isolated cold stress testing (31). Of these methods, isolated cold stress testing (ICST) offers several advantages such as providing a non-immersion technique that employs relatively physiological temperatures (31). ICST utilizes skin surface temperature as an index of blood flow. Digital skin temperatures are directly proportional to blood flow at temperatures of less than 30°C (16). Temperature measurements are best utilized to measure trends over time since these measurements are not sensitive to rapid fluctuations in cutaneous flow (15).

In order to perform isolated cold stress testing, temperature probes interfaced with a computer are attached to the pulp of each digit. Digital temperatures are collected during a 5-min baseline period. Then the hands or feet are inserted through special portholes in a modified refrigeration unit to undergo a thermal stress (average 8°C) for 20 min. After the cold stress, the hands/feet are removed from the refrigeration unit and digital temperatures are monitored for an additional 20 min at room temperature to assess the vasculature of the digits to rewarming. Data are collected and stored during the test using specialized computer software that allow graphs of digital temperatures obtained during the test to be generated.

Laser Doppler fluxmetry (LDF) can be combined with ICST to evaluate digital microvascular perfusion and to assess rapid fluctuations in flow. LDF uses laser light and the Doppler principle to measure the relative movement of structures within the microvascular bed. Since most of the moving structures in the digital skin microcirculation are red blood cells, the laser Doppler produces an output signal that is proportional to the flux of red blood cells within the area illuminated by the laser light (44). LDF offers several advantages, including (a) sensitivity to rapid changes in flow, (b) simplicity in performance, and (c) noninvasiveness. In order to obtain laser Doppler measurements of microvascular flux, a laser Doppler probe is attached with double-side adhesive disks to the palmar or plantar surface of one or more digits. The combined ICST and LDF evaluation provides three measures of blood flow over time. First, the baseline measurements provide an index of resting blood flow. Resting blood flow is extremely variable in normal individuals. Second, ICST/LDF provides an assessment of the digital response to the 20-min cold stress and provides an index of vascular responsiveness to local cooling. Third, ICST/LDF provides a measure of microcirculatory recovery to a cold stress.

The nutritional capillaries of the skin are located in the skin papilla. These capillaries can be studied utilizing specialized microscopy techniques. Although the majority of capillaries are oriented in the skin papilla so that only the top of the loop is visible, the capillaries in the digital nailfold appear as long, hairpin-shaped loops (16). The vital capillaroscopy technique allows capillary blood flow dynamics to be studied by visualizing these capillaries using specialized video cameras and computer software. Capillary diameters and red blood cell velocities can also be measured by this technique.

The structure of the nailfold capillaries can also be studied. The morphology of nailfold capillaries undergoes characteristic changes in pathological conditions such as Raynaud's phenomenon and scleroderma (36). Capillary morphology also may be utilized for the evaluation of risk of the development of skin necrosis in patients with diabetes and arterial insufficiency (16).

The nailfold capillaries have been studied in workers exposed to vinyl chloride. Vinyl chloride workers often exhibit symptoms and signs such as Raynaud's phenomenon and scleroderma-like lesions. Examination of the capillaries of some wokers with vinyl chloride disease revealed the presence of nailfold capillary abnormalities similar to scleroderma. However, the majority of these workers exhibited limited capillary changes. Symptomatic workers exhibited capillary abnormalities more frequently than nonsymptomatic workers.

QUESTIONS

1. The cardiovascular system is composed of four major components. Name and describe each of these components.
2. What is the *fundamental* function of the cardiovascular system?
3. What are platelets? What is their function?
4. What controls/regulates macrocirculation? How is arterial pressure mediated?
5. Name and define five control systems involved in regulating microcirculation.
6. What is unusual about the vasculature of the kidney? The liver? The brain?
7. Name and define four techniques that can be used to determine blood flow.

REFERENCES

1. Altura, B. M., Altura, B. T., Carella, A., Turlapaty, P. D. M. V., and Weinberg, J. (1980): Vascular smooth muscle and general anesthetics. *Fed. Proc.*, 39:1584–1591.
2. Baker, M., and Wayland, H. (1974): On-line volume flow rate and velocity profile measurements for blood in microvessels. *Microvasc. Res.*, 7:131–143.
3. Benessiano, J. Levy, B. I., and Michel, J. B. (1985): Instaneous aortic blood flow measurement with range grated Doppler flowmeter in anesthetized rat. *J. Pharmacol. Meth.*, 14:99–110.
4. Bunag, R. D. (1973): Validation in awake rats of a tail-cuff method for measuring systolic pressure. *J. Appl. Physiol.*, 34(2):279–282.
5. Bunag, R. D., McCubbin, J. W., and Page, I. H. (1971): Lack of correlation between direct and indirect measurements of arterial pressure in unanesthetized rats. *Cardiovasc. Res.*, 5:24–31.
6. Byrom, F. B., and Cameron, D. A. (1955): Cranial windows in the rat. *Aust. J. Exp. Biol.*, 33:225–236.
7. Byrom, F. B., and Lond, M. D. (1954): The pathogenesis of hypertensive encephalopathy and its relation to the malignant phase of hypertension. *Lancet*, E201–211.
8. Chraemmer-Jorgensen, B., Hoilund-Carlsen, P. F., Marving, J., and Pedersen, J. F. (1985): Left ventricular performance monitored by radionuclide cardiography during induction of anesthesia. *Anesthesiology*, 62:278–286.
9. Conrad, M. C., and Green, H. D. (1963): "Blood-to-skin" heat transfer in peripheral vascular disease (abstract). *Circulation*, 28:705.
10. Dawson, J. M., and Hudlicka, O. (1989): The effects of long term administration of prazosin on the microcirculation in skeletal muscles. *Cardiovasc. Res.*, 23:913–920.
11. Dirnagl, Y., Kaplan, B., Jacewicz, M., and Pulsinelli, W. (1989): Continuous measurement of cerebral cortical blood flow by laser-Doppler flowmetry in a rat stroke model. *J. Cereb. Blood Flow Metab.*, 9:589–596.
12. Drost, C. J. (1978): Vessel diameter independent volume flow measurements using ultrasound. *Proc. San Diego Biomed. Symp.*, 17:299–302.
13. Dudar, T. E., and Jain, R. K. (1983): Microcirulatory flow changes during tissue growth. *Microvasc. Res.*, 25:1–21.
14. Dusseau, J. W., Hutchins, P. M., and Malbasa, D. S. (1986): Stimulation of angiogenesis by adenosine on the chick chorioallantoic membrane. *Circ. Res.*, 59:163–170.
15. Fagrell, B. (1986): Skin preparations: Advantages and disadvantages. In: *Microcirculatory Technology*, edited by C. A. Baker and W. L. Nostuk, pp. 19–42. Academic Press, Orlando, FL.
16. Fagrell, B. (1973): Vital capillary microscopy. A clinical method for studying changes of the nutritional skin capillaries in legs with arteriosclerosis obliterans. *Scand. J. Clin. Lab. Invest.*, 133(Suppl 31):10.
17. Falsetti, H. L., Mates, R. E., Carpoll, R. J., Gupta, R. L., and Bell, A. C. (1974): Analysis and correction of pressure wave distortion in fluid-filled catheter systems. *Circulation*, 49:165–172.
18. Forsyth, R. P., and Baireuther, R. (1967): Systemic arterial blood pressure and pulse rate in chronically restrained rhesus monkeys. *Am. J. Physiol.*, 212:1461–1463.
19. Forsyth, R. P., and Hoffbrand, B. I. (1970): Redistribution of cardiac output after sodium pentobarbital anesthesia in the monkey. *Am. J. Physiol.*, 218:214–217.
20. Fox, J. R., and Wiederhelm, C. A. (1973): Characteristics of the servo-controlled micro-pet pressure system. *Microvasc. Res.*, 5:324–335.
21. Georgiev, J. (1978): Influence of environmental conditions and handling on the temperature rhythm of the rat. *Biotel. Pat. Mon.*, 5:229–234.
22. Goldman, H., and Sapirstein, L. A. (1973): Brain blood flow in the conscious and anesthetized rat. *Am. J. Physiol.*, 224:122–126.
23. Haberl, R. L., Heizer, M. L., Marmarou, A., and Ellis, E. F. (1989): Laser-Doppler assessment of brain microcirculation; effect of systemic alterations. *Am. J. Physiol.*, 256:H1247–H1254.
24. Hartley, C. J., and Cole, J. S. (1974): An ultrasonic pulsed Doppler system for measuring blood flow in small vessels. *J. Appl. Physiol.*, 37:626–629.
25. Haywood, J. R., Shaffer, R. A., Fastenow, C., Fink, G. D., and Brody, M. J. (1981): Regional blood flow measurement with pulsed Doppler flowmeter in conscious rat. *Am. J. Physiol.*, 241:H273–H278.
26. Intaglietia, M., and Tompkins, W. R. (1973): Microvascular measurements by video image shearing and splitting. *Microvasc. Res.*, 5:309–312.
27. Intaglietia, M., Tompkins, W. R., and Richardson, D. R. (1970): Velocity measurements in the microvasculature of the cat omentium by on-line method. *Microvasc. Res.*, 2:462–473.
28. Jamieson, G. G., Ludbrook, J., and Wilson, A. (1971): Cold hypersensitivity in Raynaud's phenomenon. *Circulation*, 44:254.
29. Jamieson, G. G., Ludbrook, J., and Wilson, A. (1971): The response of hand blood flow to distant ice application. *Aust. J. Exp. Biol. Med. Sci.*, 49:145.
30. Jones, R. E., Linde, H. W., Deutsch, S., Dripps, R. D., and Price, H. L. (1962): Hemodynamic actions of diethyl ether in normal man. *Anesthesiology*, 23:299–305.
31. Koman, L. A., Nunley, J. A., Goldner, J. L., Seaber, A. V., and Urbaniak, J. R. (1984): Isolated cold stress testing in the assessment of symptoms in the upper extremity: Preliminary communication. *J. Hand Surg.*, 9A: 305.
32. Koman, L. A., Smith, B. P., and Smith, T. L. (1993) Stress testing in the evaluation of upper extremity perfusion. *Hand. Clin.*, 9(1):59–83.
33. Krovetz, L. J., and Goldbloom, S. (1972): Normal standards for cardiovascular data. Examination of the validity of cardiac index. *Hopkins Med. J.*, 130:174–186.
34. Kubota, Y., Schweizer, H. J., and Vandam, L. D. (1962): Hemodynamic effects of diethyl ether in man. *Anesthesiology*, 23:306–314.
35. Kvetnansky, R., Sun, C. L., Lake, C. R., Thoa, N., Torda, T., and Kopin, I. J. (1978): Effect of handling and forced immobilitation on rat plasma levels of ephedrine, norepinephrine, and dopamine-β-hydroxylase. *Endocrinology*, 103:1868–1874.

36. Lawrence, H. W. (1937): Collateral circulation in the hand after cutting radial and ulnar arteries at wrist. *Ind. Med.*, 6:410.
37. Leaf, N., and Zarem, H. A. (1970): Construction and use of a miniaturized rabbit ear chamber. *J. Vasc. Res.*, 2:77–85.
38. Longnecker, D. E., Ross, D. C., and Silver, I. A. (1982): Anesthetic influence on arteriolar diameters and tissue oxygen tension in hemorrhaged rats. *Anesthesiology*, 57:177–182.
39. Mattes, A., and Lemmer, B. (1991): Effects of amlodipine on circadian rhythms in blood pressure, heart rate, and motility: A telemetric study in rats. *Chronobiol. Int.*, 8(6): 526–538,
40. McMillan, D. E. (1975): Deterioration of the microcirculation in diabetes. *Diabetes*, 24:944–957.
41. Miller, R. A., and Morris, M. E. (1961): Sympatho-adrenal responses during general anesthesia in the dog and man. *Can. Anaeth. Soc. J.*, 8:356–386.
42. Navari, R. M., Wei, E. P., Kontos, H. A., and Patterson, J. L., Jr. (1978): Comparison of the open skull and cranial window preparations in the study of the cerebral microcirculation. *Microvasc. Res.*, 16:304–315.
43. Nielsen, P. E. (1976): Digital blood pressure in normal subjects and patients with peripheral arterial disease. Effect of change in temperature. *Scand. J. Clin. Lab. Invest.*, 36:725.
44. Nillson, G. E., Tenland, T., and Oberg, P. A. (1980): Evaluation of a laser Doppler flowmeter for measurement of tissue blood flow. *IEEE Trans., Biomed. Eng. BME*, 27:597.
45. Nims, J. C., and Irwin, J. W. (1973): Chamber techniques to study the microvasculature. *Microvasc. Res.*, 5:105–118.
46. Novelli, G. P. (1979): Effects of enflurane and halothane on the microcirculation. *Acta. Anaeth. Scand.*, S71:64–68.
47. Nugent, L. J., and Jain, R. K. (1982): Monitoring transport in the rabbit ear chamber. *Microvasc. Res.*, 5:105–118.
48. Osborn, J. W., Jr., Barber, B. J., Quillen, E. W., Jr., Abram, R. J., and Cowley, A. W., Jr. (1986): Chronic measurement of cardiac output in unanesthetized rats using miniature thermocouples. *Am. J. Physiol.*, 251 (*Heart Circ. Physiol.*, 20):H1365–H1765.
49. Owens, G. K. (1989): Control of hypertrophic versus hyperplastic growth vascular smooth muscle cells. *Am. J. Physiol.*, 257:H1755–H1765.
50. Popper, C. W., Chiueh, C., and Kopin, I. J. (1977): Plasma catecholamine concentrations in unanesthetized rats during sleep, wakefulness, immobilization and after decapitation. *J. Pharmacol. Exp. Ther.*, 202:144–148.
51. Salgado, M. C. O., and Kriger, E. M. (1976): Cardiac output in unrestrained conscious rats. *Clin. Exp. Pharm. Phys.*, S3:165–167.
52. Scharf, S. M., Brown, R., Saunders, N., and Green, L. H. (1980): Hemodynamic effects of positive-pressure inflation. *J. Appl. Physiol.: Resp. Environ. Exer. Physiol.*, 49: 124–131.
53. Shepherd, A. P. (1990): History of laser Doppler blood flowmetry. In: *Laser-Doppler Flowmetry*, edited by A. P. Shepherd and P. A. Oberg, pp. 3–12. Kluwer Academic, Dordrecht.
54. Shoukas, A. A., and Bohlen, G. (1990): Rat venular pressure-diameter relationships are regulated by sympathetic activity. *Am. J. Physiol.*, 259:H674–H680.
55. Smith, T. L., Coleman, T. G., Stanek, K. A., and Murphy, W. R. (1987): Hemodynamic monitoring for 24 h in unanesthetized rats. *Am. J. Physiol.*, 253 (*Heart Circ. Physiol.*,22): H1335–H1341.
56. Smith, T. L., and Hutchins, P. M. (1980): Anesthetic effects on hemodynamics of spontaneously hypertensive and Wistar-Kyoto rats. *Am. J. Physiol.*, 238 (*Heart Circ. Physiol.*, 7): H539–H544.
57. Smith, T. L., Osbourne, S. W., and Hutchins, P. M. (1985): Long-term micro- and macrocirculatory measurements in conscious rats. *Microvasc. Res.*, 29:360–370.
58. Stanek, K. A., Smith, T. L., Murphy, W. R., and Coleman, T. G. (1983): Hemodynamic disturbances in the rat as a function of the number of microspheres injected. *Am. J. Physiol.*, 245 (*Heart Circ. Physiol.*, 14): H920–H923.
59. Tamura, T., Togawa, T., and Yokoyama, K. (1992): Comparison of laser Doppler fluxmetry and the thermal diffusion method of measuring skin blood flow with hydrogen clearance. *Int. J. Microcirc.: Clin. Exp.*, 11:95–107.
60. Unthank, J. L., and Bohlen, H. G. (1988): Intestinal microvascular growth during maturation in diabetic juvenile rats. *Circ. Res.* 63:429–436.
61. Unthank, J. L., and Bohlen, H. G. (1987): Quantification of intestinal microvascular growth during maturation: Techniques and observations. *Circ. Res.*, 61: 616–624.
62. Vidt, D. G., Bredemeyer, A., Sapirstein, E., and Sapirstein, L. A. (1959): Effect of ether anesthesia on the cardiac output, blood pressure, and distribution of blood flow in the albino rat. *Circ. Res.*, 7:759–764.
63. Wardell, K. (1992): Laser Doppler Perfusion Imaging. Linkoping studies in science and technology. Thesis no. 308, Linkoping.
64. Weaver, P. C., Bailey, J. S., and Redding, V. J. (1970): A comparative study of cardiac outputs in dogs using indicator: Dilution curves and an electromagnetic flowmeter. *Cardiovasc. Res.*, 248–252.
65. Well, R. (1973): The microcirculation in diabetes mellitus. In: *The Microcirculation in Clinical Medicine*, pp. 47–59. Academic Press, New York.
66. Williams, S. A., and Tooke, J. E. (1992): Noninvasive estimation of increased structurally-based resistance to blood flow in the skin of subjects with essential hypertension. *Int. J. Microcirc: Clin. Exp.*, 11:109–116.
67. Winet, H. (1993): Local microcirculatory changes in healing bone: A preliminary study in the rabbit tibial bone champer. *Trans. Orthop. Res. Soc.*, 18(1):253.
68. Woodside, J. R., Jr., Beckman, J. J., Althaus, J. S., Peach, M. J., Longnecker, D. E., and Miller, E. D., Jr. (1984): Renovascular hypertension: Effect of halothan and enflurane. *Anesthesiology*, 60:440–447.
69. Acosta, D. Jr., (Editor) (1992): *Cardivascular Toxicology*, (2nd ed.) Raven Press.
70. Van Stee, E. W., (Ed.) (1982): *Cardiovascular Toxicity*, Raven Press.
71. Tyson, C. A., and Frazier, J. M., (Eds.) (1993): In Vitro Biological Systems, Methods in Toxicology, Academic Press.
72. Wenzel, D. G., Wheatley, J. W., and G. D. Byrd (1970): *Toxicol. Appl. Pharmacol.* 17:774.

Principles and Methods of Toxicology, Fourth Edition, edited by A. Wallace Hayes.
Taylor & Francis, Philadelphia © 2001.

Chapter 28

Assessment of Male Reproductive Toxicity

Eric D. Clegg, Sally D. Perreault, and Gary R. Klinefelter

Among the potential health risks associated with exposure to chemical or physical agents, a prominent concern is that agents may interfere with the functions of the reproductive system. Of particular concern for males are the potentials for reduced fertility and transmissible effects on sperm that can affect offspring normality. Estimated incidences of infertility include 8.4% in the United States (168) and 14.1% in France (236). Higher incidences have been measured in other studies. Among the infertile French couples, both the male and female presented with reproductive disorders in 39% of the cases, while the male alone was responsible for the infertility in 20% of the cases. Therefore, the males were at least partially responsible for the infertility in 59% of the couples. In addition, male-mediated effects on offspring have been demonstrated clearly (52,69,181,210). Thus, the potential for the male to contribute to reproductive failure and adverse pregnancy outcomes is significant.

While numerous environmental, occupational, and therapeutic agents have been identified as male reproductive toxicants in test species, relatively few have been shown to cause similar effects in human males. This discrepancy is likely due to the reduced resolving power that is inherent in many human studies, rather than lower susceptibility for humans. Agents that have been shown to cause male reproductive effects in humans include heavy metals, chemotherapeutic agents, radiation, dibromochloropropane, ethylene dibromide, carbon disulfide, chloroprene, and 2-ethoxyethanol (211,219). Many reviews are available that summarize information about various agents that cause male reproductive system effects in test species (25,123,143,146,147,189,193,200, 214,237,258,262,263). The outcomes of such exposures have included not only reduced fertility, but also embryo/fetal loss, birth defects, cancer, and other postnatal structural or functional deficits. The results have suggested that, for certain agents, the male reproductive system could be the first affected or the most sensitive target organ.

Compared to species used routinely in toxicity testing, fertility of the human male is particularly susceptible to agents that reduce the number or quality of sperm produced. Sperm production may have to be decreased by 70 to more than 90% in some strains of mice and rats to affect fertility with routine mating procedures (158,201). However, the distribution of number of normal sperm for human males appears to be much closer to the threshold for reduced fertility than that for the test species used routinely for fertility testing. With that being the case, smaller decreases in sperm production in men could have serious consequences on their reproductive potential. If the number of normal sperm per ejaculate is sufficiently low, fertilization is unlikely and an infertile condition exists. The incidence of infertility in men has been considered to increase at sperm concentrations below 20×10^6 sperm/ml ejaculate (267). However, some men with low sperm concentrations are able to achieve conception, and many subfertile men have concentrations greater than 20×10^6, illustrating the importance of

The views expressed in this chapter are those of the authors and do not necessarily reflect the views or policies of the U.S. Department of Defense or the U.S. Environmental Protection Agency. The U.S. government has the right to retain a nonexclusive royalty-free license in and to any copyright covering this chapter.

sperm quality. Results from a recent prospective study indicate that human conception rate may begin to decline below sperm concentrations of 60×10^6 sperm/ml (56); the average sperm concentration of ejaculates in that study was 65×10^6 with 36- to 48-h abstinence intervals. It is reasonable to assume that reductions in sperm production by a toxic agent may decrease further the human male reproductive potential.

Concerns about human male reproductive health have been elevated by reports of downward secular trends in sperm counts, as well as increases in incidences of male reproductive-tract malformations (e.g., hypospadias and testicular maldescent) observed during the latter half of the 20th century (47,172,238,254). It has been suggested that exposures during reproductive-system development to environmental agents that mimic or antagonize endogenous hormones may be causally related to such effects, sparking renewed interest in research strategies to address this hypothesis (120). Up-to-date information on the Endocrine Disruptors Research Initiative (EDRI) can be found on the Internet at www.epa.gov/endocrine, including links to a continually updated compilation of ongoing research on this topic (the Global Endocrine Disruptor Research Inventory), much of it relevant to male reproductive toxicology. Concern about this issue is having a significant impact on the testing approaches being used to identify reproductive hazards.

To ascertain the relationships between environmental exposures and male reproductive risks requires a systematic approach to obtaining appropriate data and evaluating the available data. The approach utilized by the U.S. Environmental Protection Agency (EPA) for male reproductive toxicity risk assessment (252) is presented in this chapter, with particular emphasis on a critical analysis of the strategies and endpoints that are available for male reproductive risk assessment. The chapter concludes with discussion of some of the current issues and recent advances in male reproductive toxicology. Male reproductive failure resulting from germ-cell mutation (i.e., genotoxicity), the role of the endocrine system in the support of reproductive function, and female reproductive and developmental toxicity are discussed elsewhere in this volume.

Although the focus of this chapter is on the assessment of male reproductive risk, the concept of exposure being limited to a single parent is most appropriate when applied to occupational or clinical settings. As one shifts to the general environment, the likelihood increases that both parents experience common exposures, although dose, duration, and periodicity may vary. Examples where this is the case include ambient outdoor and indoor air pollutants, drinking-water contaminants, residential and recreational pesticide contact, and potential exposure from neighborhood waste disposal sites. In these instances, discriminating between a male or female contribution to a reproductive problem or adverse developmental outcome may be difficult and inappropriate. Since a pregnancy that produces a healthy, normal child is the result of the reproductive competence of both parents, reproductive toxicity risk assessments must consider the couple as the unit for evaluation. Studies that focus solely on the contribution of one parent (paternal or maternal) to reproductive failure resulting from environmental exposures may either miss or substantially underestimate the true reproductive risk.

For background information, numerous reviews are available on the physiology, cell biology, and toxicology of the male reproductive system (35,116,126,139,140, 143,157,208,216,262,263).

RISK ASSESSMENT IN MALE REPRODUCTIVE TOXICOLOGY

Overview of the Risk Assessment Process

A paradigm for the risk assessment process has been described in detail in two publications prepared by the National Academy of Sciences (173,174). Although devised primarily for cancer risk assessment, many of the components also apply to the assessment of noncancer health effects such as reproductive toxicity. The major components of that paradigm are: (a) hazard identification, (b) dose-response assessment, (c) exposure assessment, and (d) risk characterization. U.S. EPA Guidelines for Reproductive Toxicity Risk Assessment (252) have modified the first two components to hazard characterization followed by quantitative dose-response analysis for risk assessments involving nonlinear low dose extrapolation with reproductive effects.

In the following sections, information relevant to the hazard characterization/quantitative dose-response assessment components is presented, including testing protocols and endpoints employed in assessing male reproductive toxicity. This material is then followed by a discussion of the current approaches used to derive estimates of male reproductive risk.

Hazard Characterization and Quantitative Dose-Response Assessment

Laboratory Protocols

Testing protocols describe the procedures to be used to provide data for risk assessments. The quality and usefulness of those data are dependent on the design and conduct of the tests, including endpoint selection and resolving power. A single protocol is unlikely to provide all of the information that would be optimal for conducting a comprehensive risk assessment. For example, the test design to study reversibility of adverse effects or mechanism of toxic action may be different from that needed to determine time of onset of an effect or for calculation of a safe level for repeated exposure over a long term. Ideally, results from several different types of tests should be available when performing a risk assessment. Typically, only limited data are available. Under those conditions, the limited data should be used to the extent possible to assess risk.

Integral parts of the hazard characterization and quantitative dose-response processes are the evaluation of the protocols from which data are available and the quality of the resulting data. In this section, design factors that are of particular importance in reproductive toxicity testing are discussed, followed by descriptions of standardized protocols that may provide useful data for reproductive risk assessments.

Selection of Species

If sufficient data are available, information from human studies should be used to estimate exposure levels below which there is no appreciable risk. When sufficient human data are not available, pharmacokinetic and response data from test species should be used to select the test species that appears most similar to humans for the agent under consideration. In the absence of such information, confidence in the results of testing for male reproductive toxicity is increased when multiple species have been examined. Under many circumstances, the rat or mouse is an appropriate test species. Advantages of the rat model are its widespread use and the resulting extensive database on reproductive characteristics, convenient size of both the intact animal and its reproductive organs, uniformity within strains, and consistently high reproductive performance. In addition, the basic mechanisms underlying male reproductive function in the rat are well researched and reasonably representative of those in human males.

For a second mammalian test species, the rabbit has specific advantages that make it a good choice. First, ejaculated semen can be collected from bucks using an artificial vagina, allowing longitudinal assessment of semen quality. Second, by collecting semen (as opposed to epididymal sperm), alterations in the accessory sex gland secretions can be assessed, and levels of xenobiotics present in seminal fluid can be measured. Finally, ejaculated semen samples can also be used for artificial insemination. Use of artificial insemination with a limited number of sperm can be a highly effective strategy for detecting adverse effects on sperm fertilizing ability in rabbits or rats.

Under some circumstances, data from other mammalian or nonmammalian species may be appropriate for incorporation into human health risk assessments. Use of other species is likely to become increasingly important as the ability to use mechanistic and molecular genetic information increases.

Dose Selection and Duration of Dosing

To ensure adequate detection of toxicity, it is important to use relatively high dose levels and a sufficient array of endpoints to be confident that a potential effect would not be missed. For such toxicity testing, the highest dose should produce systemic toxicity, but not mortality. Dose-response assessment requires the generation of dose-response curves that adequately describe the increments in degree of effect as well as any changes in pattern of endpoints affected with changing dose level. Dose-response data should also include sufficiently low dose levels that a low level of response or no effect is produced. Spacing between doses is especially critical in dose-response assessment. If the gaps between dose levels are too large, the estimate of the lowest-observed-adverse-effect level (LOAEL) could be too high, while the no-observed-adverse effect level (NOAEL) could be too conservative.

Adverse effects of an agent on the spermatogenic process may not be observed in semen evaluations or in fertility for a substantial time after initiation of treatment. Damage that is limited to spermatogonial stem cells would not appear in cauda epididymal sperm or in ejaculates for 8 to 14 weeks, depending on the species examined. To allow effects on spermatogonial stem cells to be expressed in all evaluations of cauda epididymal or ejaculated sperm in subchronic studies, treatment of adult males should be continued for a minimum of six cycles of the seminiferous epithelium (71) prior to mating or sample collection. For the more commonly used species, one cycle of the seminiferous epithelium requires the following number of days: rat, 12.9; mouse, 8.6; rabbit, 10.7; rhesus monkey, 9.5; human, 16.0 (71). Therefore, treatment for six cycles of the seminiferous epithelium for the test species requires from 52 to 78 days to ensure that all possible adverse effects are expressed in each endpoint observed. This recommendation assumes that levels and cumulative effects of the agent at the site(s) of attack reach steady state within one cycle of the seminiferous epithelium after initiation of treatment. If that assumption is not valid for an agent, the treatment period may need to be extended accordingly. In studies using shorter dosing periods, a prolonged follow-up may be necessary to detect effects on the earlier stages of spermatogenesis or to determine the persistence of an effect.

In these situations, knowledge of the relevant pharmacokinetic and pharmacodynamic data can facilitate selection of dose levels and treatment duration. Equally important is proper timing of examination of treated animals relative to initiation and termination of exposure to the agent.

Length of Mating Period

In fertility testing, pairs of animals may be allowed to cohabit for periods of varying length. If prolonged cohabitation (i.e., 8–10 days or longer) is allowed, each nonpregnant female rat may be in estrus two or more times during that period. Under those conditions, a large impact on sperm production is often necessary before an adverse effect on fertility can be detected, and reduced fertility in a male may be masked due to the multiple mating opportunities during each estrus and the multiple estrus periods.

During cohabitation, females should be examined daily for presence of seminal plugs and/or by vaginal lavage for evidence of mating. Females are usually separated from the male on the day following mating. This practice limits mating to one estrus, but still allows numerous copulations during that estrus. As a result, an adequate number of sperm may be ejaculated to insure fertility even with males that have been severely compromised. The hypothesis that restricting the number of copulations would increase the sensitivity of fertility testing has been tested (40). Male rats were exposed to a well-documented spermatotoxicant, ethoxyethanol (EE) (0 or 450 mg/kg/day), by gavage for 7 weeks. That dose level produced severe depressions in sperm counts and testis weight (Table 28.1). Each control and EE-treated male was mated initially, in a counterbalanced design, to a female in proestrus, with either a single mating or a minimum of three matings allowed. Three days later, each male was mated under the alternate condition. Despite the extreme reduction in sperm counts in EE males, no differences in fertility were observed relative to controls with multiple matings. However, a marked decrease in fertility was seen in the EE group when only a single copulation was allowed (Table 28.1). These results suggest that the sensitivity of breeding protocols may be enhanced by limiting the number of copulations that are allowed.

The observation and control of number of copulations is facilitated by maintaining the animals on a reverse light–dark schedule so that estrus and matings occur during normal working hours. If sexually experienced rats are used, copulatory behavior can be rapidly and accurately monitored, with several males observed simultaneously. Details of this mating procedure have been published previously (276,278).

Number of Animals

The number of animals per dose group that should be used in a toxicology study is determined by the number of animals expected to survive and yield data, the expected variation between animals in the endpoints to be examined, the magnitude of effect to be detected, and the level of probability selected for statistical significance. The number of animals needed per treatment should be calculated by standard statistical methods as part of the study design process (13). Estimates of the coefficients of variation for some parameters used for tests of the male reproductive system have been reported by several authors (12,16,82,83,166,167,215,266,277). Further discussion may be found in the subsection Endpoints for Evaluating Male Reproductive Toxicity. In general, when multiple endpoints will be used in a study of male reproductive toxicity, 20 males per treatment should be sufficient to detect effects. However, in tests designed to evaluate fertility, it is often necessary to start with more males per treatment group to obtain 20 pregnancies per treatment. Reducing the number of animals per treatment because a species (e.g., rabbit, dog) is more expensive to purchase or maintain is not justified scientifically.

Some protocols specify mating of two females per male. In such cases it is important to note that this practice does not double sample size for the statistical analysis. The male must be the unit of measure in the analysis. The

Table 28.1
Reproductive toxicity data from restricted mating study

Dose (mg/kg/day)	Testis weight (g)	Spermatid count (10^6)	Cauda sperm count (10^6)	Fertility[a]	
				$1 \times$ (%)	$\geq 3 \times$ (%)
0	1.78	149.7	143.3	60	80
450	1.23	32.4	28.4	22	72

Note. Rats were treated with ethylene glycol monoethyl ether for 7 weeks, given mating experience, then allowed either one copulation followed by separation or at least three copulations by overnight cohabitation with a female in estrus.
[a] Fertility index (number pregnant/number mated).

use of the number of pregnant females as the unit of analysis would inflate sample size artificially.

Protocols

There are many protocols that have been used to test for toxicity to the reproductive system. The standard protocols recommended in U.S. EPA and Food and Drug Administration (FDA) test guidelines for evaluating male reproductive toxicity include the single-generation reproduction test, the multigeneration reproduction test, and the dominant lethal test. In addition, acute and subchronic toxicity test protocols can provide information on potential male reproductive effects. The U.S. EPA has published revised guidelines for several of these tests recently (253). Several screening tests for reproductive toxicity have also been designed. In this subsection, these protocols, as well as other options, are described along with discussions of their strengths and limitations.

Single- and Multigeneration Reproduction Tests

Comprehensive reproductive toxicity studies in laboratory animals generally involve continuous exposure to a test substance and evaluation of reproductive capability for one or more generations. The objective is to detect effects on the integrated reproductive process as well as to study effects on the individual reproductive organs.

The single-generation reproduction test evaluates effects of subchronic exposure of peripubertal and adult animals. In the multigeneration reproduction protocol, F_1 and F_2 offspring are exposed continuously in utero from conception until birth and during the preweaning period. F_1 offspring exposures are continued beyond puberty. This allows detection of effects that occur from exposures throughout development, including the peripubertal and young adult phases. Because the parental and subsequent filial generations have different exposure histories, reproductive effects seen in any particular generation are not necessarily comparable with those of another generation. Also, successive litters from the same parents cannot be considered as replicates because of factors such as continuing exposure of the parents, increased parental age, sexual experience, and parity of the females.

In a single- or multigeneration reproduction test, rats are used most often. In a typical reproduction test with rats, dosing for 8 to 10 weeks is initiated at 5 to 8 weeks of age and continued through mating to allow effects on gametogenesis to be expressed and increase the likelihood of detecting histologic lesions. Three dose levels plus one or more control groups are usually included. Enough males and females are mated to ensure 20 pregnancies per dose group for each generation. Animals producing the first generation of offspring should be considered the parental (P) generation, and the subsequent offspring generations should be designated filial generations (e.g., F_1, F_2). Only the P generation is mated in a single-generation test, while both the P and F_1 generations are mated in a two-generation reproduction test.

In the P generation, both females and males are treated prior to and during mating, with treatment usually beginning around puberty. Cohabitation should be terminated when evidence of mating is detected. Females continue to be exposed during gestation and lactation. In the two-generation reproduction test, randomly selected F_1 male and female offspring continue to be exposed after weaning (day 21) and through the mating period. Treatment of mated F_1 females is continued throughout gestation and lactation. More than one litter may be produced from either P or F_1 animals. Depending on the route of exposure of lactating females, it is important to consider that offspring may be exposed to a chemical by ingestion of maternal feed or water (diet or drinking water studies), by licking of exposed fur (inhalation study), by contact with treated skin (dermal study), or by coprophagia, as well as via the milk.

In single- and multigeneration reproduction tests, reproductive endpoints evaluated in P and F generations should include visual examination of the reproductive organs. Weights and histopathology of the pituitary, testes, epididymides, male accessory sex glands, uterus, and ovaries should be evaluated, as well as histopathology of the vagina. Number and quality of sperm produced, estrous cycle normality, number of ovarian primordial follicles, and landmarks associated with normal development of the reproductive system should also be determined. Male and female mating and fertility results are evaluated. Litters (and often individual pups) are weighed at birth and examined for number of live and dead offspring, gender, gross abnormalities, and growth and survival to weaning.

Earlier standardized multigeneration test protocols did not require reproductive organ weights or evaluations of sperm number or quality, oocyte toxicity, estrous cycle normality or landmarks of reproductive system development. Data gathered using alternative test protocols have resulted in the U.S. EPA "harmonized" multigeneration reproduction test protocol in which dosing begins when animals are 5 to 9 weeks old (Figure 28.1). In this protocol, pubertal landmarks such as vaginal opening and preputial separation are monitored, and if developmental reproductive effects are indicated, anogenital distance is evaluated in the F_2 pups. This protocol also mandates enumeration of both testicular and epididymal sperm numbers and epididymal sperm quality measures, in addition to reproductive organ histology and weights.

If effects on fertility or pregnancy outcome are the only adverse effects observed in a study using one of these

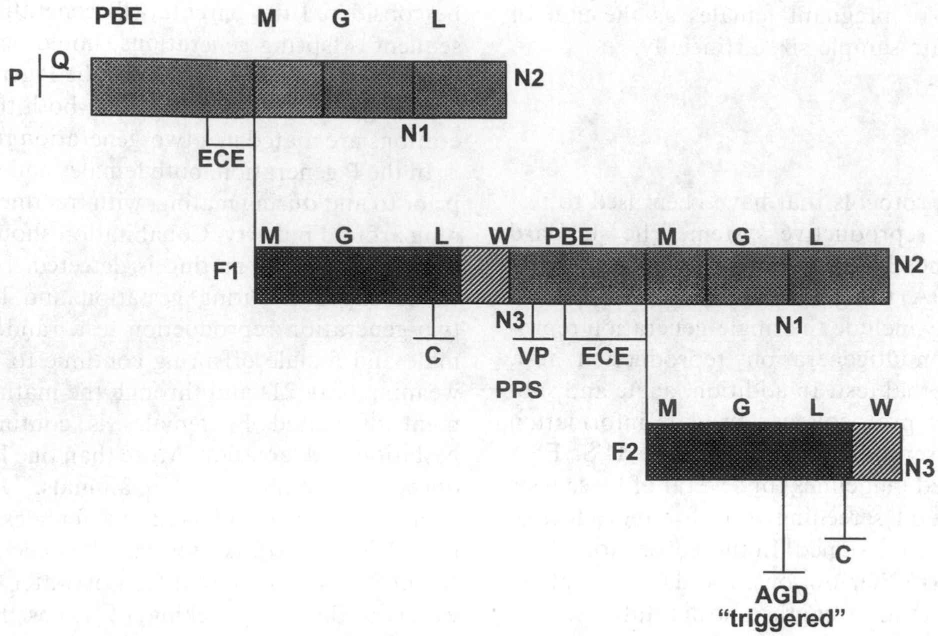

FIG. 28.1. Schematic depicting U.S. EPA harmonized multigeneration reproduction test. Q, quarantine; PBE, prebreeding exposure; M, a 2-week mating; G, gestation; L, lactation; VP, vaginal patency monitored in F1 females from postnatal day 22; PPS, preputial separation monitored in F1 males from postnatal day 35; W, weaning on postnatal day 21; N1, necropsy of the parental males (assessments include organ weights, histology, and sperm measures); N2, necropsy of the parental females (assessments include organ weights and histology); N3, necropsy of three weanlings per sex per litter (assessment is a macroscopic evaluation, and if indicated organs are weighed and preserved for histology); ECE, a 3-week evaluation of estrous cyclicity; C, litters are culled to 10 pups with equal numbers of males and females on postnatal day 4; AGD, ano-genital distance measured in the F2 pups at birth if pubertal landmarks are affected in the F1.

protocols, the contributions of male- and female-specific effects often cannot be distinguished. If testicular histopathology or sperm evaluations have been included, it may be possible to characterize a male-specific effect. Similarly, ovarian and reproductive-tract histology or changes in estrous cycle normality may be indicative of female-specific effects. However, identification of effects in one sex does not exclude the possibility that both sexes may have been affected adversely. Data from matings of treated males with untreated females and vice versa (crossover matings) are necessary to separate sex-specific effects.

A U.S. EPA workshop has considered the relative merits of one- versus two-generation reproductive effects studies (67). The participants concluded that a one-generation study is insufficient to identify all potential reproductive toxicants, because it would exclude detection of effects caused by prenatal and postnatal exposures (including the prepubertal period), as well as effects on germ cells that could be transmitted to and expressed in the next generation. A one-generation test might also miss adverse effects with delayed or latent onset because of the shorter duration of exposure for the P generation. These limitations are shared with the shorter term "screening" protocols described later. Because of these limitations, a comprehensive reproductive risk assessment should include results from a two-generation test or its equivalent.

In studies where parental and offspring generations are evaluated, there are additional risk assessment issues regarding the relationships of reproductive outcomes across generations. Increasing vulnerability of subsequent generations is often, but not always, observed. Qualitative predictions of increased risk of the filial generations could be strengthened by knowledge of the reproductive effects in the adult, the likelihood of bioaccumulation of the agent, and the potential for increased sensitivity resulting from exposure during critical periods of development (77). In addition to the sensitivity of the developing reproductive system to endocrine-active agents (47), many of the detoxifying enzyme systems and renal excretory mechanisms develop neonatally in the rodent, contributing to the increased vulnerability of generations exposed during this critical period (186). Qualitative predictions of the increased risk of the filial generations could be strengthened by knowledge of the nature of the reproductive effects in the adult, the metabolic pathways and the likelihood of bioaccumulation of the agent, and the potential for increased sensitivity resulting from exposure during critical periods of development (78).

Increasing vulnerability of subsequent generations may not always be observed; effects may be static or possibly even of decreasing severity. The latter situation may be the result of the animals in the F_1 and/or F_2 generations representing "survivors" who are (or become) more resistant to the agent than the P generation. Also, the males and females are more experienced breeders for the second litter within a generation. Therefore, results between generations or between sequential litters within a generation should not necessarily be compared directly. Significant adverse effects in any generation should be considered cause for concern unless inconsistencies in the data indicate otherwise.

A review of 20 "positive" multigeneration reproduction studies has provided some preliminary observations on the relationship of male toxicity to effects on offspring within a given generation and the relationships of reproductive outcomes across generations (37):

1. The presence of toxicity in the adult male, reproductive or otherwise, was not a prerequisite for the occurrence of effects on offspring.
2. Approximately one-half of the studies were classified as "positive-increasing." In these cases, the second generation (F_1) animals exhibited effects that were more severe than those in the first generation and/or occurred at equivalent or lower doses.
3. The increasing toxicity across generations is consistent for chemicals that bioaccumulate. However, exposure of sequential generations that involve different developmental stages (P versus F_1 adults) might also contribute to differential effects across generations.

As done usually, the multigeneration reproduction test does not address the issue of reversibility. However, inclusion of additional mated pairs in a study can provide additional animals for a reversibility test or developmental toxicity evaluation.

Alternative Multigeneration Protocols

A continuous breeding protocol, fertility (or reproductive) assessment by continuous breeding (FACB or RACB), has been developed by the National Toxicology Program (NTP) (88,142,165). As originally described, this protocol (FACB) was a one-generation test. However, the current protocol (RACB) extends dosing into the F_1 generation and features a 14-week continuous cohabitation of male–female pairs (in the P generation). Since up to five litters can be produced with the pups removed soon after birth, this protocol provides information on changes in the spacing, number, and size of litters over the 14-week dosing interval. Treatment (three dose levels plus controls) is initiated in postpubcrtal malcs and fcmales (11 weeks of age) 7 days before cohabitation and continues throughout the test. Offspring that are removed from the dam soon after birth are counted and examined for viability, litter and/or pup weight, sex, and external abnormalities and are then discarded. The last litter may remain with the dam until weaning to study the combined effects of in utero as well as perinatal and postnatal exposures. If effects on fertility are observed in the P or F generations, additional reproductive evaluations may be conducted, including crossover matings, to define the affected gender and site of toxicity.

The sequential production of litters from the same adults allows observation of the timing of onset of an adverse effect on fertility. In addition, it improves the ability to detect subfertility due to the potential to produce larger numbers of pregnancies and litters than in a standard single- or multigeneration reproduction study. With continuous treatment, a cumulative effect could increase the incidence or extent of expression with subsequent litters. In the more recent version of the RACB protocol (88), sperm measures (including sperm number, morphology, and motility) and vaginal smear cytology to detect changes in estrous cyclicity have been added at the end of the test period and their utility has been examined (34).

A protocol referred to as the alternative reproductive test (ART) combines the use of multiple endpoints in both sexes of rats with initiation of treatment at weaning (84). Morphologic and physiologic changes associated with puberty are included as endpoints. Both P sexes are treated (at least three dose levels plus controls) continuously through breeding, pregnancy, and lactation. Vaginal smears are recorded daily throughout the test period to evaluate estrous cycle normality and confirm breeding and pregnancy (or pseudopregnancy). Pregnancy outcome is monitored in both the P and F_1 generations at all doses, and terminal studies on both generations include comprehensive assessment of sperm measures (number, morphology, motility) as well as organ weights, histopathology, and the serum and tissue levels of appropriate reproductive hormones. Identification of pubertal effects makes this protocol particularly useful for detecting compounds eliciting endocrine-disruptive action (i.e., environmental estrogens or antiandrogens).

Subchronic Protocols May Provide Reproductive Data

Subchronic toxicity tests may have been conducted before a detailed reproduction study is initiated. In the subchronic toxicity test with rats, exposure usually begins at 6–8 weeks of age and is continued for 90 days (253).

Initiation of exposure at 8 weeks of age (compared with 6) and exposure for approximately 90 days allow the animals to reach a more mature stage of sexual development and assure an adequate length of dosing for observation of effects on the reproductive organs with most agents. Dosing is often done orally (i.e., gavage, in diet, or in drinking water), but may be by inhalation or dermal application. Animals are monitored for clinical signs throughout the test and are necropsied at the end of dosing.

The endpoints that are usually evaluated for the male reproductive system include visual examination of the reproductive organs, plus weights and histopathology for the testes, epididymides, and accessory sex glands. For the females, endpoints may include visual examination of the reproductive organs, uterine and ovarian weights, and histopathology of the vagina, uterus, cervix, ovaries, and mammary glands.

Scientists in the National Toxicology Program have examined the feasibility and value of incorporating some basic measures of reproductive toxicity into the protocols of their standard 13-week, prechronic toxicity studies to serve as a "reproductive screening" battery. The sperm morphology and vaginal cytology examination (SMVCE) includes evaluations of epididymal sperm motility, sperm concentration, sperm head morphology, and reproductive organ weights in the males, and average estrous cycle length and relative frequency of different estrous cycle stages in the females. Data were collected at the end of fifty 13-week studies, of which 25 were conducted in mice and the remainder in rats (167), and 25 RACB studies in mice (166). The authors observed significant interlaboratory variation as well as only moderate agreement (58%) in comparing data on rats and mice from the 13-week studies. Reproductive organ weights and sperm motility appeared to be the most statistically powerful endpoints. Seven days appeared to be an inadequate time frame for evaluating stages of the estrous cycle. Based on the results of these studies, the authors recommended that multiple endpoints of spermatotoxicity be evaluated in screening tests. This test may be useful to identify an agent as a potential reproductive hazard, but usually does not provide information about the integrated function of the reproductive systems (sexual behavior, fertility, and pregnancy outcomes), nor does it include effects of the agent on immature animals.

Specific Tests for Endocrine-Disruptive Chemicals

A battery of short term in vivo tests has been proposed to fulfill congressional mandates to screen for endocrine-disrupting chemicals (120). These are a logical extension of the alternative reproductive tests described earlier and capitalize upon the increased sensitivity of the developing reproductive system to chemicals that alter hormone production or function. One test, the Hershberger assay, is designed to detect environmental antiandrogens (or androgens) and is based on exposing young castrated male rats to the compounds in question and weighing the prostate gland (an androgen-dependent organ) 5–7 days later. A male pubertal assay would detect a wider array of endocrine disruptors by exposing male rats from weaning through puberty and then evaluating reproductive and thyroid organ weights and hormones, as well as assessing pubertal indices. A slightly longer protocol would initiate dosing during pregnancy and would continue through puberty. This assay would also detect reproductive-tract malformations such as cleft phallus, ectopic testes, retained nipples, and altered anal–genital distance. Finally, efforts are underway to ascertain whether addition of a few endpoints to the harmonized reproductive toxicity test described earlier would insure that it, too, would detect all endocrine disruptors. These assays are undergoing international validation in conjunction with the Organization for Economic Co-operation and Development (OECD). Information on the progress of this effort can be found at the following website: www.epa.gov/scipoly/oscpendo/index.htm.

Short-Term Reproductive Protocols

Although short-term tests (i.e., less than one full spermatogenic cycle for the species being evaluated) have been proposed to "screen" chemicals for testicular toxicity, the risk of false negatives due to insufficient duration of exposure is high. A serious limitation, especially when using them for chemicals with unknown toxicity, is that effects of exposures during development would not be evaluated. However, these tests may be appropriate when prior information exists about the target organ or if a chemical is suspected to be a testicular toxicant by structure–activity relationships. Short-term tests are also of value, if not essential, in the identification of target sites, affected cell types, and mechanisms of toxicity, delineation of which is often impossible after subchronic treatment. Because a wide variety of short-term tests has been used to assess reproductive toxicity, only a few examples are presented.

Protocol for toxicity in the epididymis. This protocol was developed to identify toxicants that alter the structure and/or function of the epididymis within 5 days of toxicant exposure (133). Based on the known transit rate of rat sperm through the epididymis, sperm that are within the proximal region of the epididymis at the onset of exposure (day 1) can be recovered from the proximal cauda epididymis, the first site in which fertile sperm can be found, 4 days later (day 5). By limiting the exposure period in this manner, sperm that would be within the testis at the onset of exposure are precluded from assessment. With toxicants that compromise testosterone production, it is possible to implant testosterone-filled Silastic capsules to clamp serum testosterone at control levels. Also, the efferent ducts can be ligated to prevent toxicant-induced perturbations in testicular fluid from altering the epididymis. This protcol has been used to identify epididymal toxicity resulting from exposure to chloroethylmethanesulfonate (130), as well as from epichlorohydrin and hydroxyflutamide (135). However, to detect antiandrogenic effects from a chemical such as hydroxyflutamide, it is necessary to castrate the animals to lower endogenous androgen levels to the extent that competition of test chemical for the androgen receptor is effective. To prevent loss of androgen-dependent function within the epididymis following castration, a testosterone-filled Silastic capsule can be implanted to maintain androgen status at a level that maintains epididymal sperm maturation over 4 days (131). A similar short exposure design has been used to identify sperm defects associated with cyclophosphamide-induced postimplantation loss (196), as well as the infertility of epididymal sperm that results from the metabolic inhibitors ornidazole (257) and alpha-chlorohydrin (222).

Importantly, one manifestation that seems to be common to the epididymal toxicants ethane dimethane sulfonate (EDS), chloroethylmethanesulfonate, hydroxyflutamide, and epichlorohydrin, as well as developmental exposure to tetrachlorodibenzo-*p*-dioxin (TCDD) and methoxychlor, was reduced epididymal sperm number without any concommitant reduction in testicular sperm number. This suggests that epididymal sperm transit is accelerated by certain chemical exposures. Indeed, when the short-term epididymal toxicity protocol was modified to test this hypothesis, accelerated transit was demonstrated (135). The acceleration appeared to be independent of androgen status, but was significantly correlated to several constitutive epididymal proteins. Accelerated sperm transit in humans, which have a much shorter period of epididymal transit, could have adverse effects on the process of sperm maturation.

Spermatoxicity test protocol. Linder et al. (152) originally proposed a short-duration test to screen chemicals for "spermatotoxicity" in structure–activity studies or to set priorities for chemicals requiring further evaluation. Depending on the duration of dosing and the day on which necropsies are performed, the protocol may cover a period of up to 2.5 weeks (e.g., dose for 5 days, necropsy 14 days later). The 14-day period allows for spermatids that are compromised at the onset of exposure to appear in the epididymis. In a validation study, groups of male rats were dosed for 1–5 days with 14 chemicals shown to produce minimal testicular effects in subchronic studies and necropsies were performed 2–3 days and 13–14 days after dosing was terminated. Reproductive organ weights (testis, epididymis, seminal vesicle, and prostate), sperm counts (testicular and epididymal), and sperm motion parameters (computer-assisted sperm analysis, CASA) were measured. Both the testes and epididymides were subjected to rigorous histopathologic evaluation. Spermatotoxicity was detected for the 10 most potent testicular toxicants. Results for the other four chemicals, which were judged to be minimally toxic in a subchronic test, were equivocal to negative. Thus, chemicals that produce moderate to severe damage to germ cells in latter stages of spermatogenesis are detectable with this short-duration test. More recently, this protocol has been abbreviated to encompass a 14-day exposure with a necropsy following administration of the last dose. With this, it has been established that the disubstituted haloacetic acid by-products of drinking-water disinfection [i.e., dibromoacetic acid (149), dichloroacetic acid (150), and bromochloroacetic acid (231)] produce lesions in the later stages of spermatogenesis. The histopathologic profile of these insults includes the formation of atypical residual bodies, fusion of sperm, and delayed spermiation.

35-Day reproductive assessment. Harris et al. (97) initiated a 21-day reproductive and developmental toxicity screen, which has subsequently been revised to a 35-day screen. This screen has been utilized increasingly to identify potential reproductive toxicants among the growing list of putative endocrine disruptors and by-products of drinking water disinfection. In the "male" portion of this protocol, animals (mice or rats) are dosed from study day (SD) 5 to 35 with one of three dosages of test chemical; the highest dose is selected as a dose that begins to inhibit drinking or feed consumption. These males are mated from SD 12 to 17 to females that are dosed with chemical from SD 1 to 35. At necropsy, testis and epididymal weights are obtained and cauda epididymal sperm concentration and motility are determined. In addition, the testis is subjected to a thorough histopathologic evaluation. This reproductive screen is likely to detect potent testicular toxicants, but subtle effects on early stages of spermatogenesis and effects on other organ systems (epididymis, central nervous system, sex accessory glands, and pituitary) may go undetected unless manifested rapidly.

OECD Reprotox protocol. The Organization for Economic Co-operation and Development (OECD) has developed a guideline protocol, ReproTox, to rapidly screen high priority chemicals for safety assessment (182). The protocol is designed to generate information on systemic toxic effects with repeated dosing along with data on reproductive and developmental toxicity in both sexes.

Tanaka et al. (233) have examined the ability of this protocol to confirm the effects of cyclophosphamide reported in the published literature. In their study, male rats were dosed for 42 to 43 days, including 14 days prior to mating. After 14 days of treatment, each male rat was paired with a treated female for 14 days, or until sperm were detected in the vaginal smear. Males were necropsied on days 43 or 44, and thymus, liver, kidneys, spleen, testes, and epididymal weights were measured. In addition, the brain, heart, liver, kidneys, adrenal glands, spleen, bone marrow, testes, and epididymides were subjected to histopathologic examination. The authors found that the ReproTox protocol identified most of the known toxicological properties of this chemical, except for the adverse effects on spermatogenesis and fertility.

Dominant lethal test protocol. The dominant lethal test is intended to detect mutagenic effects in the spermatogenic process that are lethal to the embryo or fetus. A review of this test has been published as part of the U.S. EPA Gene-Tox program (86). Dominant lethal protocols may utilize acute dosing (1–5 days) followed by serial matings with one or two females per male per week for the duration of the spermatogenic process. An alternative protocol may utilize subchronic dosing for the duration of the spermatogenic process followed by mating(s). Females are monitored for evidence of mating, killed at approximately midgestation, and examined for incidence of pre- and postimplantation loss.

The acute exposure protocol of the standard dominant lethal test, combined with serial mating, may allow identification of the spermatogenic cell types that are affected. However, acute dosing may not produce adverse effects at levels as low as with subchronic dosing because of factors such as bioaccumulation. Information from such studies can be useful for identifying site and potential mechanism of action and, thus, can facilitate design of subsequent studies.

Endpoints for Evaluating Male Reproductive Toxicity

This subsection describes various endpoints that can reflect male reproductive toxicity and their use in risk assessment (126,252). A comprehensive assessment of male reproductive toxicity requires information on multiple endpoints that are capable of detecting the range of potential adverse effects. These should include measures of the primary functions of fertility and reproductive behavior. Because the usual measures of fertility in rodents have limited sensitivity, endpoints should also be included that are capable of detecting effects on components of the male reproductive system that support those functions (e.g., production of normal spermatozoa and normal differentiation of the reproductive tract and external genitalia).

Alterations in these reproductive endpoints may be the result of direct or indirect toxicity to the male reproductive system. In either case, the exposure to the agent has caused a reproductive effect and there may be cause for concern. Careful evaluation of the dose-response curves for the various target organs and effects may provide insight into whether the reproductive effects are independent of these other toxicities. Seldom, however, is such a judgment possible. Estimating the dose levels at which these various target-organ effects occur has significance in predicting the effects of anticipated human exposure. Also, the likelihood that reproductive toxicity will be present in the absence of other systemic effects can be better characterized.

Statistical analyses are important in determining the effects of a particular agent, but the biological significance of data is most important. When many endpoints are investigated, statistically significant differences may occur by chance. On the other hand, apparent trends with dose may be relevant biologically even though pairwise comparisons do not indicate a statistically significant effect. In the following discussion, endpoints are identified in which significant changes may be considered adverse, but concordance of results and known biology should be considered in interpreting all results. All effects that may be considered as adverse are appropriate for use in establishing a NOAEL, LOAEL, or benchmark dose.

Although the measures discussed in this section may detect impairment to the various components of the reproductive process, they do not discriminate effectively between nonmutagenic and mutagenic mechanisms. If the effects seen in evaluation of male reproductive endpoints are the result of mutagenic events (e.g., interaction with DNA), then there is the potential for transmissible genetic damage. Approaches for evaluating potential germ cell mutagens are discussed in Chapter 17.

To facilitate discussion, the endpoints of reproductive toxicity can be separated into three categories: couple-mediated, female-specific, and male-specific. Couple-mediated endpoints are those in which both sexes can have a contributing role if both partners are exposed. In this chapter, couple-mediated endpoints are included along with male-specific endpoints because male exposures may result in effects on those endpoints.

The discussions of endpoints and the factors influencing results that are presented in this section are directed to evaluation and interpretation of results with test species. Many of those endpoints require invasive techniques that preclude routine use with humans. However, in some instances, related endpoints that can be used with humans are identified.

Table 28.2
Couple-mediated endpoints of reproductive toxicity

Multigeneration studies	Other reproductive endpoints
Mating rate, time to mating (time to pregnancy[a])	Ovulation rate
Pregnancy rate[a]	Fertilization rate
Delivery rate[a]	Preimplantation loss
Gestation length[a]	Implantation number
Litter size (total and live)	Postimplantation loss[a]
Number of live and dead offspring (fetal death rate[a])	Internal malformations and variations[a]
Offspring gender[a] (sex ratio)	Postnatal structural and functional development[a]
Birth weight[a]	
Postnatal weight[a]	
Offspring survival[a]	
External malformations and variations[a]	
Offspring reproduction[a]	

[a] Endpoints that can be obtained with humans.

Couple-Mediated Endpoints

Fertility and pregnancy outcomes. Breeding studies with test species are a major source of data on reproductive toxicants. Evaluations of fertility and pregnancy outcomes provide measures of the functional consequences of reproductive injury. Measures of fertility and pregnancy outcome that are often obtained are presented in Table 28.2. Many of the endpoints reflect developmental toxicity that may be male-mediated. Some of the endpoints identified earlier are used to calculate ratios or indices (42,55,142,215,235,249,250). While the presentation of such indices is not discouraged, the measurements used to calculate those indices should also be available for evaluation. Definitions of some of these indices in published literature vary substantially. Also, the calculation of an index may be influenced by the test design. Therefore, it is important that the methods used to calculate indices be specified. Some commonly reported indices are given in Table 28.3.

Reproductive testing often entails the cohabitation of treated males with treated females. Therefore, the influences of the male and female parents on changes in fertility or other reproductive outcome (e.g., reduced survival) may not readily be discriminated. Assignment to the male of at least some of the responsibility for a toxic effect on fertility may be possible from evaluation of data on other reproductive measures (organ weights, histopathology, sperm measures, cleft phallus). Data on mating behavior could also clarify effects on fertility by indicating whether or not the males were behaviorally competent.

If evaluation of mating success is included, useful data would include confirmation of the day of insemination (i.e., sperm plugs or sperm-positive vaginal lavages), plus analysis of the length of time required for each animal to achieve successful mating (time to mating). The data presented routinely from the majority of breeding tests affirm the occurrence of matings, but do not report the length of time required or any difficulties in achieving normal insemination. However, most laboratories conducting fertility studies obtain information on the number of days required for mating as part of their fertility record system. Although evidence of mating is not synonymous with successful impregnation and does not preclude undetected matings, such data could provide a more complete evaluation of reproductive competence.

Evaluations of time to mating might also help detect the presence of subfertility. Exposure to a reproductive toxicant may not produce a total absence of fertility (i.e., sterility), but rather a condition of subfertility seen as an increased time to conception. (Subfertility may also be reflected as a reduction in litter size in polytocous species.) The assessment of time to mating in reproductive studies might indicate the potential for increased time to conception in humans.

Data are available on the variability associated with some of these functional reproductive measures which allow evaluation of the power and group size requirements (215). Coefficients of variation range from approximately 10% for neonatal survival (to day 21) to 20% for fertility ratios. The background variability associated with rates of mating success may be mark-

Table 28.3
Selected indices that may be calculated from endpoints of reproductive toxicity in test species

MATING INDEX =

$$\frac{\text{Number of males or females mating}}{\text{Number of males or females cohabited}} \times 100$$

Note: Mating is used to indicate that evidence of copulation (observation or other evidence of ejaculation such as vaginal plug or sperm in vaginal smear) was obtained.

FERTILITY INDEX =

$$\frac{\text{Number of cohabited females becoming pregnant}}{\text{Number of nonpregnant couples cohabited}} \times 100$$

Note: Because both sexes are often exposed to an agent, distinction between sexes often is not possible. If responsibility for an effect can be clearly assigned to one sex (as when treated animals are mated with controls), then a female or male fertility index could be useful.

GESTATION (PREGNANCY) INDEX =

$$\frac{\text{Number of females delivering live young}}{\text{Number of females with evidence of pregnancy}} \times 100$$

LIFE BIRTH INDEX =

$$\frac{\text{Number of live offspring}}{\text{Number of offspring delivered}} \times 100$$

SEX RATIO =

$$\frac{\text{Number of male offspring}}{\text{Number of female offspring}} \times 100$$

4-DAY SURVIVAL INDEX (VIABILITY INDEX) =

$$\frac{\text{Number of live offspring at lactation day 4}}{\text{Number of live offspring delivered}} \times 100$$

Note: This definition assumes that no standardization of litter size is done until after the day 4 determination is completed.

LACTATION INDEX (WEANING INDEX) =

$$\frac{\text{Number of live offspring at day 21}}{\text{Number of live offspring born}} \times 100$$

Note: If litters were standardized to equalize numbers of offspring per litter, number of offspring after standardization should be used instead of number born alive. When no standardization is done, measure is called weaning index. When standardization is done, measure is called lactation index.

PREWEANING INDEX =

$$\text{Number of offspring born} - \frac{\text{Number of offspring weaned}}{\text{Number of live offspring born}} \times 100$$

Note: If litters were standardized to equalize numbers of offspring per litter, then number of offspring remaining after standardization should be used instead of number born.

edly reduced if experienced males are mated to females that have been determined to be in proestrus by vaginal cytology.

As noted earlier, dominant lethal assays, in which the female is killed in mid to late pregnancy, may also produce reproductive data. Endpoints examined from dominant lethal tests often include mating and fertility ratios and estimates of preimplantation loss [(number of corpora lutea – number of implantation sites)/number of corpora lutea] and postimplantation loss [(number of implantation sites – number of fetuses)/number of implantation sites]. The occurrence of pre- and/or postimplantation loss is often considered to provide sufficient evidence that the agent has gained access to the reproductive organs and has induced mutagenic damage to the sperm.

A genotoxic basis for postimplantation loss is accepted widely. However, current methods of assessing preimplantation loss provide little distinction between contributions of mutagenic events that cause embryo/fetal death and nonmutagenic factors that result in failure of fertilization (e.g., inadequate numbers of normal and motile sperm, failure in sperm transport or ovum penetration). The interpretation of an increase in preimplantation loss may require additional data on the agent's mutagenic and/or spermatotoxic potential (232). Approaches have been pursued that may prove useful in distinguishing these events. For example, oocytes can be recovered the day after mating and examined to evaluate fertilization (151,232), and they subsequently can be cultured in vitro to the blastocyst stage to evaluate preimplantation developmental potential (75). This approach makes it possible to discriminate between fertilization failure and early embryo mortality. That distinction is important since fertilization failure is predictive of reduced fertility, but does not increase the risk of transmissible genetic damage that is associated with mutagenic events.

Animal data on reproductive success (or the lack thereof) are difficult to verify in human populations. First, humans are characterized by low rates of conception. Thus, an insufficient number of pregnancies may occur in an exposed population to provide sufficient power to detect an effect. Moreover, both partners may be exposed to the toxicant(s), making it more difficult to ascribe reproductive failure solely to the male. Studies of gender-specific occupational work groups may provide some clarification as to the male's contribution. Such studies also provide the opportunity to study individuals with higher exposures than those encountered in the general population.

Data on fertility potential and other measures of reproductive outcomes provide the most comprehensive and direct insight into reproductive capability. In studies with male-only exposure, substantial weight can be placed on results that demonstrate that an agent acted on the male to impair those outcomes. However, fertility assessments are limited by their insensitivity as measures of reproductive injury. As noted earlier, normal males of most test species produce sperm in numbers that greatly exceed the minimum requirements for fertility as evaluated in current protocols that allow multiple matings. However, human males appear to function nearer to the threshold for the number of normal sperm needed to insure reproductive competence. This difference between test species and humans means that data that fail to demonstrate an effect on fertility in a study using a test species should not be the basis for concluding that the test agent poses no reproductive hazard to fertility in humans. In such instances, data from additional reproductive endpoints may provide clarification and should be examined.

A number of investigators have used the strategy, proposed by Amann (7), of employing artificial insemination (AI) with a limited number of sperm with control and treated males. Artificial insemination by in utero insemination does indeed increase the sensitivity of detection for toxicant-induced decreases in sperm number or function (49,129,131,136,149). Moreover, Robl and Dzuik (203) have successfully used in utero insemination in three strains of mice. Dose-response curves for fertility as a function of number of sperm inseminated intracervically have been developed for both mice (203) and rats (131). Robl and Dziuk (203) found that the ED_{50} sperm concentrations for fertility varied among the strains: 1.5×10^6 (DBA/2N), 3×10^6 (CF1), and 6.3×10^6 (C57BL/6N) sperm. Klinefelter et al. (131) reported that the ED_{50} for rat sperm was 2.5×10^6 inseminated per uterine horn. However, an insemination dose of 5.0×10^6 sperm per uterine horn was selected to evaluate toxicant-induced alterations in fertility as this concentration lies within the linear (i.e., sensitive) portion of the sperm dose-response curve; 2.5×10^6 sperm results in suboptimal control fertility and 10×10^6 sperm results in 100% fertility with no enhancement of sensitivity. Rather than oviductal flushing of eggs to enumerate the percentage of eggs containing a sperm tail and two pronuclei, it has now been established that the use of vasectomized males to cervically stimulate synchronized females provides sufficient uterine priming for implantation of the fertilized eggs. Thus, the number of postimplantation implants can be enumerated on gestation day 9 (129,136) or gestation day 20 (129) without any decrease in control fertility levels. These studies have been used to demonstrate the potential for by-products of drinking water disinfection to produce low experimental dose alterations in fertility, as well as identify a novel sperm protein biomarker of fertility (SP22).

Table 28.4
Male-specific endpoints of reproductive toxicity

Organ weights	Testes, epididymides, seminal vesicles, prostate, pituitary
Visual examination and histopathology	Testes, epididymides, seminal vesicles, prostate, pituitary
Sperm evaluation[a]	Sperm number (count) and quality (morphology, motility)
Sexual behavior[a]	Mounts, intromissions, ejaculations
Hormone levels[a]	Luteinizing hormone, follicle-stimulating hormone, testosterone, estrogen, prolactin
Developmental effects	Testis descent,[a] preputial separation, sperm production,[a] ano-genital distance, structure of external genitalia[a]

[a] Reproductive endpoints that can be obtained or estimated relatively noninvasively with humans.

Male-Specific Endpoints

This subsection describes various male-specific endpoints of reproductive toxicity that can be obtained (Table 28.4). Guidance is presented for interpretation of results involving these endpoints and their use in risk assessment. Effects are identified that should be considered as adverse reproductive effects if significantly different from controls.

Body weight and reproductive organ weights. Monitoring body weight during treatment provides an index of the general health status of the animals, and such information may be important for the interpretation of reproductive effects. Depression in body weight or reduction in weight gain may reflect a variety of responses, including rejection of chemical-containing feed or water because of reduced palatability, treatment-induced anorexia, or systemic toxicity. Less than severe reductions in adult body weight induced by restricted nutrition have shown little effect on the male reproductive organs or on male reproductive function (30,31). When a meaningful, biologic relationship between a body weight decline and a significant effect on the male reproductive system is not apparent, it is not appropriate to dismiss significant alteration of the male reproductive system as secondary to the occurrence of nonreproductive toxicity. Unless additional data provide the needed clarification, alteration in a reproductive measure that would otherwise be considered adverse should still be considered as an adverse male reproductive effect in the presence of mild to moderate body weight changes. In the presence of severe body weight depression or other severe systemic debilitation, it should be noted that an adverse effect on a reproductive endpoint occurred, but the effect may have resulted from a more generalized toxic effect.

The male reproductive organs for which weights may be useful for reproductive risk assessment include the testes, epididymides, pituitary gland, seminal vesicles (with coagulating glands), and prostate. Organ weight data may be presented both as absolute weights and as relative weights (i.e., organ weight to body weight ratios). Organ weight data may also be reported relative to brain weight since, subsequent to development, the weight of the brain usually remains quite stable (229). Evaluation of data on absolute organ weights is important, because a decrease in a reproductive organ weight may occur that was not necessarily related to a reduction in body weight gain. The organ weight to body weight ratio may show no significant difference if both body weight and organ weight change in the same direction, masking a potential organ weight effect.

Normal testis weight varies only modestly within a given test species (16,215). This relatively low interanimal variability suggests that absolute testis weight should be a precise indicator of gonadal injury. However, damage to the testes may be detected as a weight change only at doses higher than those required to produce significant effects in other measures of gonadal status (11,66,141). This contradiction may arise from several factors, including a delay before cell deaths are reflected in a weight decrease (due to preceding edema and inflammation, cellular infiltration) or Leydig-cell hyperplasia. Blockage of the efferent ducts by cells sloughed from the germinal epithelium or the efferent ducts themselves can lead to an increase in testis weight due to fluid accumulation (105,171), an effect that could offset the effect of depletion of the germinal epithelium on testis weight. Thus, while testis weight measurements may not reflect certain adverse testicular effects and do not indicate the nature of an effect, a significant increase or decrease is indicative of an adverse effect.

Pituitary-gland weight can provide valuable insight into the reproductive status of the animal. However, the pituitary contains cell types that are responsible for the regulation of a variety of physiologic functions, including some that are separate from reproduction. Thus, changes in pituitary weight may not necessarily reflect reproductive impairment. If weight changes are observed, gonadotroph-specific histopathologic evaluations may be useful in identifying the affected cell types. This information may be used then to judge whether the observed effect on the pituitary is related to reproductive system function and is therefore an adverse reproductive effect.

Prostate and seminal vesicle weights are androgen dependent and may reflect changes in the animal's endocrine status or testicular function. Separation of the seminal vesicles and coagulating gland (dorsal prostate) is difficult in rodents. However, the seminal vesicle and prostate can be separated and results may be reported for these glands separately or together, with or without their secretory fluids. Differential loss of secretory fluids prior to weighing could produce artifactual weights. Because the seminal vesicles and prostate may respond differently to an agent (endocrine dependency and developmental susceptibility differ), more information may be gained if the weights were examined separately.

Adverse effects. Significant changes in absolute or relative male reproductive organ weights may constitute an adverse reproductive effect. Such changes also may provide a basis for obtaining additional information on the reproductive toxicity of that agent. However, significant changes in other important endpoints that are related to reproductive function may not be reflected in organ weight data. Therefore, lack of an organ weight effect should not be used to negate significant changes in other endpoints that may be more sensitive.

Histopathologic evaluations. Histopathologic evaluations of test animal tissues have a prominent role in male reproductive risk assessment. Organs that are often evaluated include the testes, epididymides, prostate, seminal vesicles (often including coagulating glands), and pituitary. Tissues from lower dose exposures are often not examined histologically if the high dose produced no difference from controls. Histologic evaluations can be especially useful by (a) providing a relatively sensitive indicator of damage; (b) providing information on toxicity from a variety of protocols; (c) with short-term dosing, providing information on site (including target cells) and extent of toxicity; and (d) indicating the potential for recovery.

The quality of the information presented from histologic analyses of spermatogenesis is improved by proper fixation and embedding of testicular tissue. With adequately prepared tissue (24,104,208), a description of the nature and background level of lesions in control tissue, whether preparation induced or otherwise, can facilitate interpreting the nature and extent of the lesions observed in tissues obtained from exposed animals.

Many histopathologic evaluations of the testis only detect lesions if the germinal epithelium is severely depleted or degenerating, if multinucleated giant cells are obvious, or if sloughed cells are present in the tubule lumen. More subtle lesions, such as retained spermatids or missing germ cell types, that can significantly affect the number of sperm being released normally into the tubule lumen may not be detected when less adequate methods of tissue preparation are used. Also, familiarity with the detailed morphology of the testis and the kinetics of spermatogenesis of each test species can assist in the identification of less obvious lesions that may accompany lower dose exposures or lesions that result from short-term exposure (208). Several approaches for qualitative or quantitative assessment of testicular tissue are available that can assist in the identification of less obvious lesions that may accompany lower-dose exposures, including use of the technique of "staging." A book is available (208) that provides extensive information on tissue preparation, examination, and interpretation of observations for normal and high-resolution histology of the germinal epithelium of rats, mice, and dogs. Included is guidance for identification and quantification of the various cell types and associations for each stage of the spermatogenic cycle. Also, a decision-tree scheme for staging with the rat has been published (102).

Cell staging is based on the examination of cross sections of the seminiferous tubules. The proliferation and differentiation of germ cells is a highly ordered, time-locked process. Thus, the temporal and spatial relationships of the different spermatogenic cell types can be defined for the different stages of the spermatogenic cycle (Figure 28.2). Based on differences in light absorption of tubules containing different stages, transillumination has also proven useful for isolating specific cell stages for subsequent biochemical analyses (188). Knowledge of the cytoarchitecture of the testis can allow identification of specific lesions that have resulted from toxicity to the germ cell at a given stage of development.

Quantification of cell staging may include analysis of frequency distributions of the cell stages present or the proportion of tubules that have identifiable stages with all expected cell types (27,102,208). The cell-staging approach is being applied more frequently in the evaluation of environmental agents (27,36,44–46,103,228, 247,255,256).

Morphometry is a term applied to a variety of techniques to obtain quantitative data on cellular or organelle characteristics (11,164,208). The methods may be applied to measure diameters, areas, or volumes of testicular compartments (e.g., tubular versus interstitial), specific cell types, or subcellular structures (208). Cell counts may also be obtained, as well as ratios of one cell type to another (e.g., pachytene spermatocytes; Sertoli cell).

Analysis of cell stages might be applied in standard histopathological evaluations to establish the presence of testicular damage. Morphometric analyses, which can be done with the same slides, could be delayed until tentative mechanisms of action have been identified. In the absence of information on site or mechanism of action, it is difficult to state which of the many

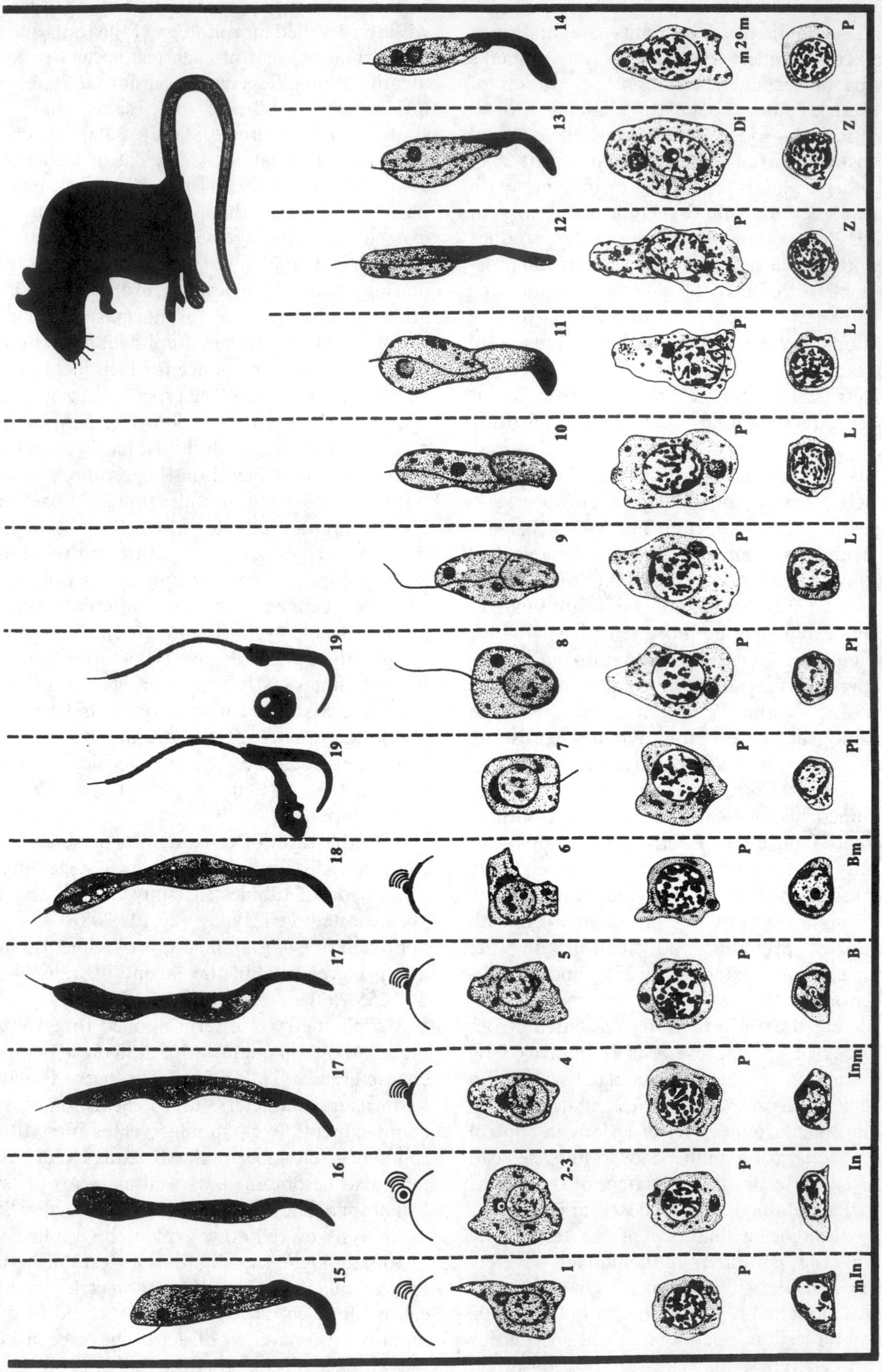

I
II-III
IV
V
VI
VII
VIII
IX
X
XI
XII
XIII
XIV
mIn
In
Inm
B
Bm
Pl
L
Z
P
Di
m2Om
1
2-3
4
5
6
7
8
9
10
11
12
13
14
15
16
17
18
19

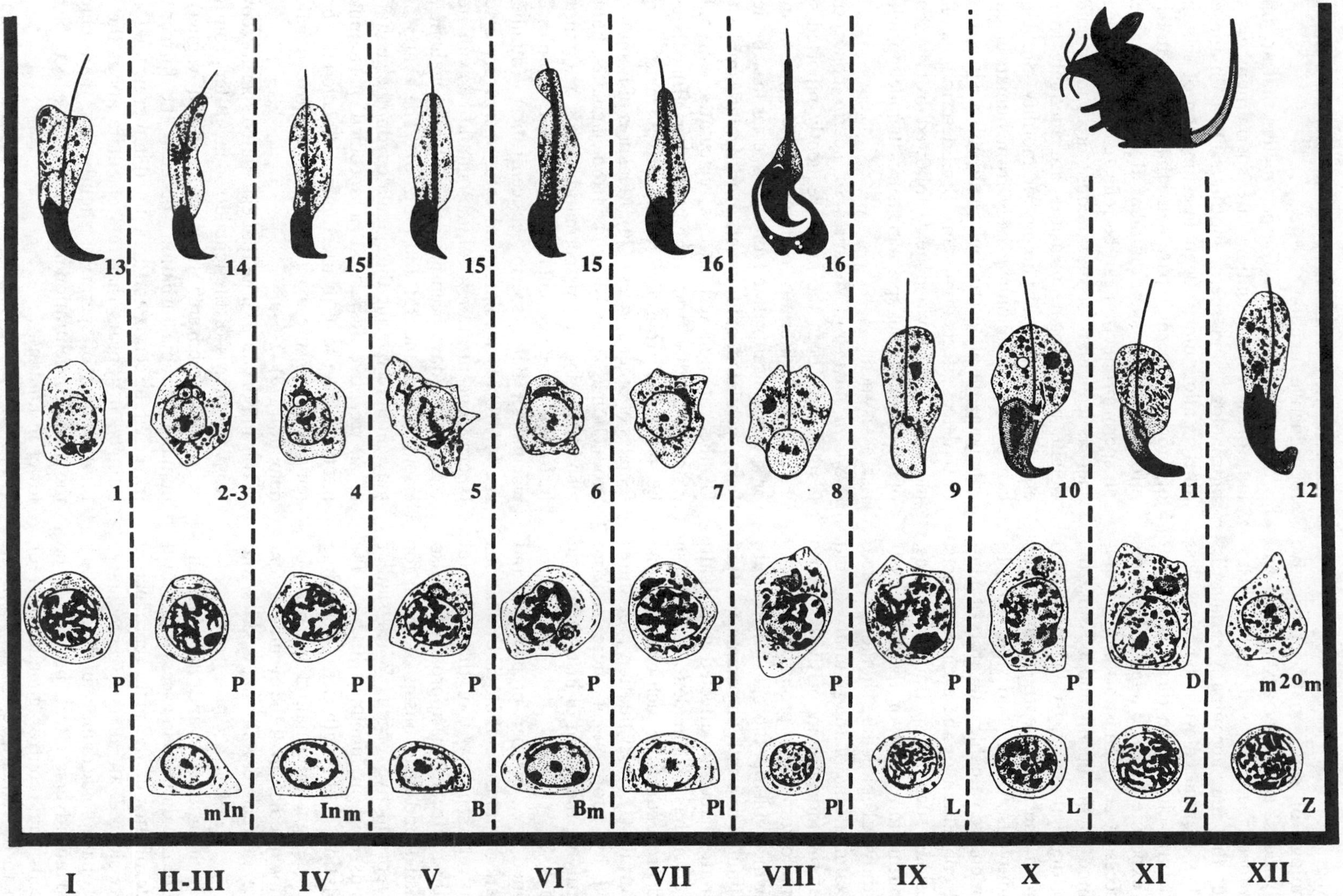

FIG. 28.2. Cycle maps of spermatogenesis for (A) the rat and (B) the mouse (208). The vertical columns, designated by Roman numerals, depict cell associations (stages). In the scheme provided, stages II and III are combined into a single stage called II–III. The developmental progression of a cell is followed horizontally until the right-hand border of the cycle map is reached. The cell progression continues at the left of the cycle map, one row up. The cycle map ends with the completion of spermiation. The symbols used designate specific phases of cell development.

morphometric analyses should be pursued. The strength of morphometry is in providing highly quantitative measurements that may add support for hypotheses generated in earlier studies.

The basic morphology of other male reproductive organs (e.g., epididymides, accessory sex glands, and pituitary) has been described, as well as the histopathologic alterations that may accompany certain disease states (62,98,117). Compared with the testes, less is known about structural changes in these tissues that are associated with exposure to toxic agents. With the epididymides and accessory sex glands, histologic evaluation is usually limited to the height and possibly the integrity of the secretory epithelium. Evaluation should include information on the caput, corpus, and cauda segments of the epididymis. Debris and sloughed cells in the epididymal lumen are valuable indicators of damage to the germinal epithelium or the excurrent ducts. The presence of lesions such as sperm granulomas, leukocyte infiltration (inflammation), or absence of clear cells in the cauda epididymal epithelium should be noted. Information from examinations of the pituitary should include evaluation of the morphology of the cell types that produce the gonadotropins and prolactin.

The degree to which histopathologic effects are quantified is usually limited to classifying animals, within dose groups, as either affected or not affected using qualitative criteria. Little effort has been made to quantify the extent of injury, and procedures for such classifications are not applied uniformly (151). Evaluation procedures would be facilitated by adoption of more uniform approaches for quantifying the extent of histopathologic damage per individual.

If properly obtained (i.e., proper preparation and analysis of tissue), data from histopathologic evaluations may provide a relatively sensitive tool that is useful for detection of low-dose effects. This approach may also provide insight into sites and mechanisms of action for the agent on that reproductive organ. When similar targets or mechanisms exist in humans, the basis for interspecies extrapolation is strengthened. Depending on the experimental design, information can also be obtained that may allow prediction of the eventual extent of injury and degree of recovery in that species and humans (207).

Adverse effects. Significant and biologically meaningful histopathologic damage in excess of the level seen in control tissue of any of the male reproductive organs should be considered an adverse reproductive effect. Significant histopathologic damage in the pituitary should be considered an adverse effect, but should be shown to involve cells that control gonadotropin or prolactin production to be called a reproductive effect. Although thorough histopathologic evaluations that fail to reveal any treatment-related effects may be quite convincing, consideration should be given to the possible presence of other testicular or epididymal effects that are not detected histologically (e.g., genetic damage to the germ cell, decreased sperm motility), but may affect reproductive function.

Sperm evaluations. The parameters that are important for sperm evaluations are sperm number, sperm morphology, and sperm motility. Data on those parameters allow more adequate estimation of the number of "normal" sperm, a parameter that is likely to be more informative than sperm number alone. Although effects on sperm production can be reflected in other measures such as testicular spermatid count or cauda epididymal weight, no surrogate measures are adequate to reflect effects on sperm morphology or motility. Similar data can be obtained noninvasively from human ejaculates, enhancing the ability to confirm effects seen in test species or to detect effects in humans. Brief descriptions of these measures are provided next, followed by a discussion of the use of various sperm measures in male reproductive risk assessment.

Sperm number. Measures of sperm concentration (count) have been the most frequently reported semen variable in the literature on humans (270). Sperm number or sperm concentration from test species may be derived from ejaculated, epididymal, or testicular samples (217). Of the common test species, ejaculates can only be obtained readily from rabbits or dogs. Ejaculates can be recovered from the reproductive tracts of mated females of other species (276). Measures of human sperm production are usually derived from ejaculates, but could also be obtained from spermatid counts or quantitative histology using testicular biopsy tissue samples. With ejaculates, both sperm concentration (number of sperm/mL of ejaculate) and total sperm per ejaculate (sperm concentration × volume) should be evaluated.

Strategies have been developed also to evaluate serial ejaculates in the rat (80,198,276). These approaches may entail recovering the ejaculate from the genital tract of a receptive female at a specified postcopulation interval. The use of ovariectomized, hormonally primed females can insure availability of receptive females on demand (278).

It is important to note that ejaculated sperm recovered from the uterus of the female rodent differ from those of rabbits (recovered from an artificial vagina) and humans (via masturbation) because the former have traversed the cervix and are diluted in uterine fluid. Interestingly, it appears that rats ejaculate about the same total number of sperm, or slightly less, than men, but the sperm concentration in the uterus appears to be much lower in humans.

Typically in the rat, 97% of the sperm are found in the uterus within 15 min of coitus (21). Treatments that reduce this number by approximately 90–95% are associated with infertility. For example, studies by Gray et al. (81) indicate that a single injection of cadmium chloride during pubertal development reduced ejaculated sperm counts and fertility without affecting mating behavior. In those studies, males with 1×10^7 sperm were fertile, while those with less than 1×10^6 were not. Hurtt and Zenick (110) demonstrated a dramatic shift in the dose-response curve following ethoxyethanol treatment by mating male rats more frequently to reduce epididymal sperm reserves both prior to and during the dosing period. All of the sperm endpoints were affected at lower doses in the mated group of animals. Although fertility was not assessed in this study, it seems likely that detection of toxicant-induced alteration in fertility would be enhanced by this design. More recently, enumeration of ejaculated sperm numbers has provided data implicating toxicant action at the level of mating behavior rather than decreased epididymal sperm numbers (123). In this study, chemical denervation by guanethidine produced infertility that was linked to insufficient deposition of sperm upon mating, rather than to alterations in sperm quality coincident with aging in the epididymis.

Assessment of samples collected through electroejaculation is not recommended. It is uncertain that such a sample is representative of an ejaculate that would be delivered through normal copulation. Variation in factors such as electrode placement and intensity and duration of stimulation can cause substantial differences in the nature and relative amounts of accessory sex gland secretions and effluent from the vas deferens. The possibility of contamination of the sample with urine also is increased. Therefore, semen volume, sperm concentration, and sperm quality can be compromised in electroejaculated samples.

Ejaculated sperm number from any species is influenced by several variables, including the length of abstinence and the ability to obtain the entire ejaculate. Intra- and interindividual variation are often high, but are reduced somewhat if ejaculates were collected at regular intervals from the same male (260). Such a longitudinal study design has improved detection sensitivity and thus requires a smaller number of subjects (272). In addition, if a preexposure baseline is obtained for each male (test animal or human studies when allowed by protocol), then changes during exposure or recovery can be better defined.

Epididymal sperm evaluations with test species usually use sperm from only the cauda portion of the epididymis, but the samples for sperm motility and morphology may be derived also from the vas deferens. Automation of counting has improved the efficiency with which this endpoint can be obtained (230). It has been customary to express the sperm count in relation to the weight of the cauda epididymis. However, because sperm contribute to epididymal weight, expression of the data as a ratio may actually mask declines in sperm number. The inclusion of data on absolute sperm counts can improve resolution. As is true for ejaculated sperm counts, epididymal sperm counts are influenced directly by level of sexual activity (6,110).

Sperm production data may be derived from counts of the distinctive elongated spermatid nuclei that remain after homogenization of testes in a detergent-containing medium (6,17,22,158). The elongated spermatid counts are a measure of sperm production from the stem cells and their ensuing survival through spermatocytogenesis and spermiogenesis (158,161). If evaluation was conducted when the effect of a lesion would be reflected adequately in the spermatid count, then spermatid count may serve as a substitute for quantitative histologic analysis of sperm production (208). However, spermatid counts may be misleading when duration of exposure is shorter than the time required for a lesion to be fully expressed in the spermatid count. Also, spermatid counts reported from some laboratories have large coefficients of variation that may reduce the statistical power and thus the usefulness of that measure.

The ability to detect a decrease in testicular sperm production may be enhanced if spermatid counts are obtained. However, spermatid enumerations only reflect the integrity of spermatogenic processes within the testes. Posttesticular effects or toxicity expressed as alterations in motility, morphology, viability, fragility, and other properties of sperm can be determined only from epididymal, vas deferens, or ejaculated samples.

Sperm morphology. Sperm morphology refers to structural aspects of sperm and can be evaluated in cauda epididymal, vas deferens, or ejaculated samples. A thorough morphologic evaluation identifies abnormalities in the sperm head and flagellum. Because of the suggested relationship between an agent's mutagenicity and its ability to induce abnormal sperm, sperm head morphology has been a frequently reported sperm variable in toxicologic studies on test species (271). The tendency has been to conclude that increased incidence of sperm head malformations reflects germ-cell mutagenicity. However, not every mutagen induces sperm head abnormalities, and other nonmutagenic chemicals may alter sperm head morphology. For example, microtubule poisons may cause increases in abnormal sperm head incidence, presumably by interfering with spermiogenesis, a microtubule-dependent process (209). Sperm morphology also may be altered due to degeneration subsequent to cell death. Thus, the link between sperm morphology and mutagenicity is not necessarily sensitive or specific.

An increase in abnormal sperm morphology has been considered evidence that the agent has gained access to the germ cells (251). Exposure of males to toxic agents may lead to sperm abnormalities in their progeny

(109,166,167,269). However, transmissible germ-cell mutations might exist in the absence of any warning morphologic indicator such as abnormal sperm. The relationships between these morphologic alterations and other karyotypic changes remains uncertain (53).

The traditional approach to characterizing morphology in toxicologic testing has relied on subjective categorization of sperm head, midpiece, and tail defects in either stained preparations by bright-field microscopy (64) or fixed, unstained preparations by phase-contrast microscopy (152,217). Such approaches may be adequate for mice and rats with their distinctly angular sperm head shapes. However, the observable heterogeneity of structure in human sperm and in nonrodent species makes it difficult for the morphologist to define clearly the limits of normality. More systematic, quantitative, and automated approaches have been offered that can be used with humans and test species (119,272). Data that categorize the types of abnormalities observed and quantify the frequencies of their occurrences are preferred to estimation of overall proportion of abnormal sperm. Objective, quantitative approaches that are done properly should result in a higher level of confidence than more subjective measures.

Sperm morphology profiles are relatively stable and characteristic in a normal individual (and a strain within a species) over time. Sperm morphology is one of the least variable sperm measures in normal individuals, which may enhance its use in the detection of spermatotoxic events. The majority of studies in test species and humans have suggested that abnormally shaped sperm may not reach the oviduct or participate in fertilization (176,199). The implication is that the greater the number of abnormal sperm or the smaller the number of normal sperm in the ejaculate, the greater is the probability of reduced fertility. A prospective human male fertility study (280) has reported that the number of normal sperm (by strict criteria; 162) in ejaculates was highly related to the probability of couples achieving pregnancy within 1 year.

Sperm motility. The biochemical environments in the testes and epididymides are highly regulated to assure the proper development and maturation of the sperm and the acquisition of critical functional characteristics (e.g., progressive motility and the potential to fertilize). With chemical exposures, perturbation of this balance may occur, producing alterations in sperm properties such as motility. Chemicals (e.g., epichlorohydrin) have been identified that selectively affect sperm motility and also reduce fertility. Studies have examined rat sperm motility as a reproductive endpoint (166,167,241,243), and sperm motility assessments are an integral part of some reproductive toxicity tests (84,165,253). While motility measurements are typically obtained on epididymal rat spermatozoa, sperm recovered from the vas deferens can be similarly analyzed (57). Rabbit sperm motility has been shown to be perturbed by ethylene dibromide (261) in the same fashion described for human sperm (213), although sperm morphology was affected in humans but not in rabbits.

Motility estimates may be obtained on ejaculated, vas deferens, or cauda epididymal samples. Standardized methods are needed because motility is influenced by a number of experimental variables, including abstinence interval, method of sample collection and handling, elapsed time between sampling and observation, the temperature at which the sample is stored and analyzed, the extent of sperm dilution, the nature of the dilution medium, and the microscopic chamber employed for the observations (29,212,217,225,239,259).

Sperm motility can be evaluated in fresh samples under phase-contrast microscopy, or sperm images can be recorded and stored in video or digital format and analyzed later, either manually or by computer-aided semen analysis (19,148,224,240,273). For manual assessments, the percentage of motile and progressively motile sperm can be estimated and a simple scale used to describe the vigor of the sperm motion.

The recent application of video and/or digital technology to sperm analysis allows a more detailed evaluation of sperm motion, including information about the individual sperm tracks. It also provides a permanent record of the sperm tracks that can be reanalyzed as necessary (manually or computer assisted). With computer-assisted technology, information about sperm velocity (straight-line and curvilinear) as well as the amplitude and frequency of the track are obtained rapidly and efficiently on large numbers of sperm. Using this technology, chemically induced alterations in sperm motion have been detected (130,226,240,242), and such changes have been related to the fertility of the exposed animals (178,223,241). These preliminary studies indicate that significant reductions in sperm velocity are associated with infertility, even when the percentage of motile sperm is not affected. The ability to distinguish between the proportion of sperm showing any type of motion and those with progressive motility is important (217).

Relationships between semen quality measures and fertility. Changes in endpoints that measure effects on spermatogenesis and sperm maturation have been related to fertility in several test species, but the ability to predict infertility from these data (in the absence of fertility data) for test species is not reliable. This is in part due to the observation, in both test species and humans, that fertility is dependent not only on having adequate numbers of sperm, but also on the degree to which those sperm are normal. If sperm quality is high, then sperm number must be reduced substantially before fertility is affected. For example, in a rat model that employs artificial insemination of differing numbers of good-quality sperm, sperm numbers can be reduced substantially before fertility is affected (131). Similarly, if sperm numbers are normal in rodents, a relatively large effect on sperm motility is required before fertility is affected. Rodent sperm velocity must be reduced substantially, in the presence of adequate numbers of sperm, before fertility is affected (223,241). Fertility may be impaired by smaller decrements in both number and motility (or other qualitative characteristics). These models show that relatively modest changes in sperm numbers or quality may not cause infertility in those species with relatively robust reproductive characteristics, but can nevertheless be predictive of infertility at higher exposure levels or in other species that do not have the same level of excess sperm production.

In humans, the distributions of sperm counts for fertile and infertile men overlap, with the mean for fertile men being higher (159). Recent prospective studies (18,280) have examined the influence of varying semen quality on human male fertility. Those studies have shown that number of sperm, percent motile sperm, and percent normal sperm were all significantly associated with fertility, with number of morphologically normal sperm using strict criteria being particularly strongly associated with fertility. These results with humans suggest that more detailed examination of the sperm of test species could provide more useful information than the approaches used currently.

For semen quality measures to be of value in predicting effects on male fertility, it is necessary that the variances associated with their application be sufficiently low to have adequate resolving power. The relative variability associated with a number of indices of spermatotoxicity in the rat is indicated in Table 28.5 (277). These data, for the most part, are in close agreement with values reported elsewhere in the literature (e.g., 16,266) and reflect the percent difference that can be detected statistically for a change in a given measure as a function of sample size. Similar data on endpoint sensitivity, including a variety of motility measures, are presented in Table 28.6. The motility measures were derived from computerized analyses of videomicrographic images (266) and are in agreement with previously published values (16).

Given that fertility tests with rodents may be relatively insensitive, reproductive risk assessment can benefit from the inclusion of data on additional variables such as sperm measures. Support for including such measures is provided by examining data on methyl chloride (264,265) and on ethylene glycol monomethyl ether (26,28). Both investigations incorporated high-quality histopathology (including cell staging), sperm measures, and fertility assessments. The results of those studies are summarized in Tables 28.7 and 28.8. For both agents, histopathological lesions and sperm alterations were seen either at lower doses and/or earlier in time than were effects on fertility or fetal outcomes. Similar relationships can be observed in reviewing the effects of dibromochloro-propane (DBCP) in rabbits (39,65,66). Thus, the process of reproductive risk assessment is facilitated by having information on a variety of sperm measures and reproductive organ histopathology in addition to fertility. Specific information about reproductive organ and gamete function can then be used to evaluate the occurrence and extent of injury, and the probable site of toxicity in the reproductive system. The more information that is available from supplemental endpoints, the more the risk assessment can be based on science rather than uncertainty.

Table 28.5
Relative sensitivity of testicular and epididymal sperm parameters for the rat

Parameter	Coefficient of variation	Percent difference detected ($n=10$)	($n=15$)	($n=50$)
Testis weight	4.65	6.08	4.96	4.31
Epididymal weight	9.40	12.30	10.03	8.70
Sperm production rate[a]	16.56	21.67	17.68	15.33
Sperm count/g epididymis	29.32	38.36	31.30	27.14
Percent motile	16.00	20.93	17.09	14.82
Swimming speed	7.24	9.47	7.73	6.70
Percent normal morphology[b]	2.70	3.53	2.88	2.49

Note. Data from Reference 16.
[a] Sperm rate production = spermatid enumeration/rat.
[b] Derived from literature on Long-Evans and Sprague-Dawley rats.

Table 28.6
Variability in testicular and sperm motility parameters in Fisher 344 rats

Indicator	n^a	Range	Mean±SD	CV[b] (%)
Testes weight (g)	30	2.3–2.9	2.6±.01	5.61
Sperm production rate ($\times 10^6$)				
Per testis/day	30	14.7–25.6	22.3±2.7	12.09
Per g testis/day	30	14.6–21.1	17.8±1.5	8.54
Cauda epididymal sperm number ($\times 10^6$)				
Per cauda epididymis[c]	50	55.2–153.2	86.1±20.8	24.16
Per g cauda epididymis	30	307.1–972.9	696.5±151.9	21.81
Cauda epididymal sperm motility				
Motile cells (%)	50	39–82	61±9	14.72
Curvilinear velocity (μm/s)	50	98.3–156.5	128.3±11.4	8.88
Straight-line velocity (μm/s)	50	41.8–93.5	69.2±10.2	14.68
Linearity	50	4.2–6.3	5.4±0.5	9.45

Note. From Reference 266, with permission.
[a] Number of animals examined for each indicator.
[b] Coefficient of variation = [(SD/mean) × 100].
[c] Regions 5, 6A, and 6B of the cauda epididymis.

Table 28.7
Effects of methyl chloride exposure on various endpoints of male reproductive toxicity

Endpoint	Dose (ppm)[a] 1000	3000
Fertility	—	D (wk 2,3)
Fetal loss		
Preimplant	I (wk 3)	I (wk 2–4, 6, 8)
Postimplant	—	I (wk 1)
Histopathology		
Epididymis	—	+ (wk 2)
Testis	—	+ (wk 1–8)
Spermatid counts	—	D (wk 2–8)
Vas deferens sperm measures		
Sperm count	—	D (wk 3–8)
Percent motile	—	D (wk 1–8)
Percent abnormal forms	—	I (wk 1–3)
Number of intact sperm	D (wk 3)	D (wk 2–8)

Note. Adapted from References 264 and 265.
[a] Five-day inhalation exposure: +, effect observed; —, no effects; D, decrease; I, increase.

Adverse effects. Due to the inherent inefficiency of spermatogenesis in humans and the increased incidences of abnormal sperm in a "normal" human ejaculate, human male fertility is generally lower than that of test species and may be more susceptible to damage from toxic agents. Therefore, the conservative approach should be taken that, within the limits indicated in the sections on those parameters, statistically significant changes in measures of sperm count, morphology, or motility, as well as number of normal sperm, should be considered adverse effects.

Additional markers of sperm function and integrity. The functional capacity of sperm can also be evaluated in vivo by recovering eggs at the appropriate time after copulation (species dependent) and determining whether fertilization and normal initial development (timing of cleavage divisions) occurred (e.g., 151,243). Alternatively, sperm can be collected and cultured in vitro under capacitating conditions and then cocultured with eggs. In vitro fertilization (IVF) assays have been used for years to study basic mechanisms of sperm maturation and function, but only recently have such methods been proposed for use in toxicology studies (51,190), where they may be applied after either in vitro or in vivo exposures. The latter approach has been used to evaluate sperm function in rats exposed acutely to the testicular toxicant 1,3-dinitrobenzene (106). Although labor-intensive, such methods may prove valuable in identifying the site of action of impaired gamete function.

In vitro fertilization tests, as well as the sperm cervical mucus penetration test, have proven useful clinically in assessing the functional competence of sperm (204). The diagnostic information obtained may identify subfertile men whose semen appears to be normal by other routine criteria. However, it is not feasible to implement these tests routinely for screening purposes in human

Table 28.8
Effects of ethylene glycol monomethyl ether on various endpoints of male reproductive toxicity

	Dose (mg/kg)[a]		
Endpoint	50	100	200
Fertility	—	D (wk 5)	D (wk 4–16) fetus loss
Preimplant	—	I (wk 5)	I (wk 3–16)
Live fetuses	—	D (wk 5)	D (wk 4–16)
Resorptions	—	—	I (wk 5–6)
Histopathology—testis[b]	+ (wk 4–7)	+ (wk 1–8)	+ (wk 1–8)
Accessory sex organ weight	—	—	—
Epididymal sperm measures			
Sperm count	D (wk 5)	D (wk 2–16)	D (wk 2–16)
Percent motile	—	D (wk 4–7)	D (wk 3–16)
Percent abnormal forms	D (wk 5)	D (wk 5–16)	D (wk 3–16)
Percent headless forms	—	I (wk 5–?)	I (wk 5–?)

Note. Adapted from References 26 and 28.
[a] Five-day oral exposure (po): +, effect observed; —, no effect; D, decrease; I, increase.
[b] Assessed for only 8 weeks.

populations or with test species. The techniques, which have not been standardized, are highly specialized and not readily established in every laboratory. Also, an adequate normative data base does not exist for these tests (183,184).

The extrapolation of in vitro fertilization data to predict the in vivo condition requires further exploration. The ease with which in vitro fertilization can be achieved varies across species, being readily accomplished in the mouse and hamster, but rather difficult in the rat. Such test systems do not reflect the dynamic role played by the female reproductive tract in sperm transport, survival, and capacitation prior to fertilization. The conditions required to achieve successful fertilization in vitro may, in some instances, bear little resemblance to the state that exists in vivo (73,220). For example, IVF typically employs far higher sperm concentrations than those found at the site of fertilization, in vivo.

Measures are also available to detect toxicant-induced alterations in the nuclear integrity, membrane integrity, and mitochondrial activity of sperm. These measures ultimately may be better predictors of fertilizing ability and normal development than the more traditional measures. Over the past few years much work has evolved in these areas. The stability of nuclear chromatin has been assayed extensively using acid-denatured, acridine orange-reacted sperm. This technique is referred to as the sperm chromatin structure assay (SCSA) (59). Briefly, the acridine orange dye intercalates differently into native and denatured DNA, resulting in green and red fluorescence, respectively. The relative abundance of red fluorescence is an indication of abnormal chromatin structure and DNA damage. The method has been applied successfully to detect toxicant-induced chromatin damage in test species and is predictive of infertility in humans (60). Other tests for detecting DNA damage in human and rodent sperm include the COMET assay, the TUNEL assay, and measurement of oxidative DNA adducts. These are undergoing intense investigation as tools for evaluating the effects of toxicants on the genetic integrity of sperm (reviewed in ref. 58). New assays for detecting aneuploidy and chromosome breakage in sperm are also beginning to be used in toxicology studies. These are based on the use of chromosome-specific fluorescent probes detected by fluorescence in situ hybridization (FISH) methods (10). For example, exposure to air pollution was recently reported to be associated with increased incidence of an extra Y chromosome (202), and a similar effect was found to be associated with smoking (205). Since these methods are also being developed for use with rat sperm (154), it should be possible in the near future to design studies to compare responses in humans and rats for this endpoint.

The plasma membrane of sperm can be examined for changes in oxidative status (218), sperm lipid composition (96), and sperm protein composition (133). Diminutions in specific sperm proteins have been linked to toxicant-induced effects, particularly chemicals thought to alter epididymal function such as EDS, chloroethanemethanesulfonate, epichlorohydrin, α-chlorohydrin, 6-chloro-6-deoxyglucose, ornidazole, and hydroxyflutamide (128). More recently, it has been demonstrated that toxicants such as brominated haloacids (136) and diethylhexylphthalate (Klinefelter, unpublished observation), which act on the testis, also produce alterations in the epididymal or ejaculated sperm protein profiles. It is noteworthy that a novel sperm protein (SP22) has now been implicated with fertility (137). This protein was initially identified as highly correlated with the fertility of sperm recovered from animals exposed to epididymal toxicants (129). Of 120 resolved proteins in a detergent extract of cauda epididymal sperm, this 28-kD protein was the only protein that was compromised by each of the epididymal toxicants and was significantly correlated with fertility. Moreover, the toxicant-induced diminutions in the levels of this protein proved to be more sensitive than other more typical measures of sperm quality, that is, sperm motion and sperm morphology. Upon discovery that this protein actually originates in the testis, its feasibility as a biomarker of effect following exposure to testicular toxicants was also tested, and once again, the observed diminutions were highly correlated with fertility (137). Antibodies to recombinant SP22 localize to the equatorial segment of the sperm head in rat, bull, and human. Studies are now underway to correlate SP22 immunostaining with fertility in hopes of using a diagnostic immunoassay of SP22 to screen human and laboratory animals alike for chemical-induced alterations in fertility.

The ability of mammalian sperm to undergo the acrosome reaction has been studied using a variety of techniques over the years (48), but perhaps the most exciting work has evolved recently. A plant lectin, *Pisum sativum* agglutinin, used alone or in conjunction with phospholipid, identifies acrosome-intact and acrosome-reacted sperm, respectively (76). When fluorescently-labeled lectin is added to sperm that have been incubated with dilauroylphosphatidylcholine, acrosomal staining results without the loss of rhodamine-123 staining of the mitochondria or the uptake of propidium iodide. Together, these results demonstrate that the sperm were acrosome reacted without compromising plasma membrane or mitochondrial integrity. This multi-compartment, flow-cytometric evaluation could be most useful in mechanistic studies when the fertilizing ability of sperm is altered.

In Vitro Systems

The following discussion highlights in vitro methods in use in male reproductive toxicology. In vitro methods can add a great deal of information about the action of a particular toxicant. However, the application of in vitro methodology is most practical when definitive effects linked to a specific tissue or cell type have been demonstrated following an in vivo toxicant exposure. Even if appropriate preliminary in vivo data are obtained, one may fail to demonstrate an effect in vitro. This may reflect the need for a toxicant to interact in vivo with another tissue or cell type, perhaps to form an active metabolite. Thus, it is advisable to ascertain both the metabolic fate and dosimetry of a toxicant and metabolite(s) within the putative target tissue.

Provided the target tissue or cell type has been identified correctly and the test compound is active in vitro, in vitro cultures can provide increased sensitivity by measuring cell functions not readily assessed in vivo. Data can also be obtained on the cellular site of action, characteristics of the toxic response (death versus injury and/or dedifferentiation), direct cross-species comparisons, and reversibility and mechanism(s) of action. Finally, these in vitro methods can be used to demonstrate that common mechanisms of action exist for specific toxicants. Knowing the mechanism of action of various groups of toxicants will enable more sensitive biomarkers of dysfunction to be generated. These biomarkers, if applied to humans, would greatly benefit human health risk assessment.

Hypothalamus and Pituitary

If a toxicant is suspected to disrupt either the pulsatile release of gonadotropin-releasing hormone (GnRH) from the hypothalamus or the release of luteinizing hormone (LH) and/or follicle-stimulating hormone (FSH) from the pituitary, a method is available to investigate the responsivity of these tissues in vitro following in vivo or in vitro exposure. For example, when chlordimeform was administered in vivo, and hypothalamic and pituitary fragments were incubated in vitro under maximal stimulation with norepinephrine and GnRH, respectively, GnRH secretion was significantly decreased while gonadotropin secretion was unaffected (74). These results suggested that chlordimeform interferes with the normal hypothalamic–adrenergic relationship.

Leydig Cell

Today, a variety of well-accepted methods are available to identify and characterize Leydig cell toxicity in vitro. The choice of method depends largely on the available in vivo data, the tissue availability, and the sensitivity desired. A perfused testis model, originally developed by Ewing et al. (61), is labor-intensive, but retains the natural cytoarchitecture of the testis, permits quantification of all steroidogenic substrates/products secreted into the effluent medium during LH stimulation, and perhaps most importantly reflects testosterone biosynthetic ability when paracrine-mediated modulations are still functioning. This method was used to confirm that, in vivo, TCDD compromises Leydig-cell steroidogenesis by inhibiting pregnenolone production (125). The perfused testis model was also used to demonstrate the differential sensitivity of adult and immature Leydig cells to EDS in vitro (121). This study provided convincing evidence that adult, but not immature, Leydig cells are sensitive to the cytotoxic effects of EDS.

An enzymatically dispersed, testicular interstitial cell preparation (144) can provide concentration-response data and information regarding the intracellular site of a steroidogenic lesion. Klinefelter et al. (132) used a highly purified Leydig cell preparation (127) to establish the dose-response, intracellular site of action, and morphological integrity following in vitro EDS exposure. Results from this study demonstrated clearly that the steroidogenic lesion induced by either in vivo or in vitro EDS exposure exists between the second-messenger cyclic AMP and cytochrome P450 side-chain cleavage enzyme. In another study, highly purified Leydig cells were incubated with increasing concentrations of EDS and with either a maximally stimulating concentration of LH or with [^{35}S]methionine, to discriminate between functional and cytotoxic effects (121). Similarly purified Leydig cells were used recently to study the interaction between Sertoli cells and Leydig cells during in vitro exposure to tri-*o*-cresyl phosphate (TOCP). This approach demonstrated that Leydig cells must first metabolize the toxicant for subsequent Sertoli cell toxicity to occur (33).

To evaluate the ability of the active metabolite of methoxychlor to produce differentiation-dependent alterations in the ability of the Leydig cell to produce testosterone during postnatal development, purified Leydig cells were isolated from rats on postnatal days 21, 35, and 90 when progenitor, immature, and adult Leydig-cell populations are present within the testis (4). Results indicated that the prepubertal Leydig cell was more sensitive than the adult Leydig cell to disrupted cholesterol side-chain cleavage activity and cholesterol mobilization. While most, if not all, of the discussion to date regarding Leydig cell hyperplasia and its assocation with Leydig cell adenoma formation has centered around mechanisms of toxicant-induced hyperplasia in the adult testis (38,43), it is possible that the fetal and/or prepubertal Leydig cell is uniquely capable of becoming hyperplastic, and that the mechanisms of initiation may differ. Transgenic mice that are deficient in anti-Mullerian hormone exhibit Leydig cell hyperplasia (197). In this regard, gestational exposure to dibutyl hexyl phthalate and dibutyl phthalate have been associated recently with an increased postnatal incidence of Leydig cell hyperplasia (187) and adenoma formation (170), respectively.

Another relatively simple approach involves the use of decapsulated testicular parenchyma incubated with or without LH stimulation to identify alterations in testosterone biosynthetic ability under stimulated or basal conditions, respectively. These incubations can be performed using parenchyma derived from testes exposed in vivo or in vitro. An advantage is that data can be easily obtained on a per animal basis, an important consideration when using species like the rabbit and hamster, which contain relatively few steroidogenically active Leydig cells following enzymatic dispersion. This technique has been used to identify chemical effects on both LH-stimulated and basal testosterone production. The effects of EDS on LH-stimulated testosterone production were compared in the rat and hamster (79). Testosterone production was linear over time in the testis incubations of both species, and the results demonstrated that the hamster Leydig cell is far less sensitive than the rat Leydig cell to the cytotoxic effects of EDS. Chloroethylmethanesulfonate is an example of a toxicant that resulted in significantly reduced basal testosterone production (130).

Seminiferous Tubule

Toxicology studies that have demonstrated a disruption in the process of spermatogenesis have implicated virtually every cell type in the seminiferous tubule. A toxicant may perturb either one of the early germ cell types in the basal compartment of the seminiferous epithelium or one of the more mature germ cell types in the adluminal compartment. To affect the more advanced germ cells, a toxicant might either exert its effects directly by passing through the blood–testis barrier or indirectly by perturbing Sertoli cell function.

The cell–cell interactions that occur normally within the seminiferous tubule, particularly the interactions between Sertoli cells and germ cells (111,179), justify the use of in vitro models in which the whole seminiferous tubule is studied. Seminiferous tubule cultures from rats have been used to study the in vitro effects of dinitrobenzene and methoxyacetic acid (MAA). These agents are toxic to Sertoli cells and pachytene spermatocytes, respectively (5). The amount of inhibin secreted by the seminiferous tubules in vitro was significantly increased by both compounds. More importantly, the stimulation in inhibin secretion was seen in rats exposed in vivo to doses resulting in intratesticular toxicant concentrations that approximated the effective in vitro concentrations. The seminiferous tubule culture reported by Allenby et al. (5) formed the basis of a series of elegant studies designed to determine the role germ cells play in the expression of androgen-dependent protein secretion (156,221). In the former study, seminiferous tubules were isolated 4, 18, and 30 days following exposure to MAA when pachytene spermatocytes, round spermatids, and elongating spermatids would be depleted selectively. Specific proteins were secreted selectively by these different germ cells. The effects of androgen depletion were assessed in the latter study 4 days following exposure to EDS, with or without exogenous androgen supplementation. Together these studies present evidence that specific androgen-dependent proteins are synthesized by seminiferous tubules when different germ cell types are present. This may explain why it has been impossible to demonstrate androgen-dependent proteins in isolated Sertoli-cell cultures. It is clear from this work that isolated seminiferous tubules can be used to identify in vitro effects on the seminiferous epithelium if a toxicant disrupts spermatogenesis in vivo. Short (overnight) culture of seminiferous tubules is also being used to evaluate the response of the spermiation process to testicular toxicants (32). Both the stimulation and release of spermatids can be evaluated with this system, and it is a promising tool for studying both the hormonal control of spermiation and the mechanisms by which toxicants may induce or inhibit this process.

It is clear that the disubstituted haloacid by-products of drinking-water disinfection produce alterations during the latter stages of spermatogenesis in adult rats (abnormal spermatid head morphology, delayed spermiation, spermatid fusion), implicating a defect during spermiogenesis that could be mediated through the Sertoli cell or directly through the late germ cells. Stage-isolated seminiferous tubules from adult rats have been used following a combination of ex vivo and in vitro exposures to explore the possibility that requisite Sertoli cell–germ cell interactions might be altered via changes in protein synthesis and secretion (108). At least three specific proteins are diminished by either in vivo or in vitro exposure to dibromoacetic acid.

In a study by Allenby et al. (5), a comparison was made between the response of optimized cultures of isolated seminiferous tubules and cultures of isolated Sertoli cells. The results clearly showed that inhibin production by isolated Sertoli cells was smaller and more variable in response to both toxicants. This may be attributed to the fact that the isolated Sertoli cells were derived from immature Sertoli cells. It would be useful to know whether the response of Sertoli cells from adult rats would better approximate the response of the isolated seminiferous tubules. Immature cells have been used in virtually all Sertoli cell culture/toxicological studies to date, although the effects of various phthalate esters have been compared in cultures of Sertoli cells obtained from both immature and young adult rats (99). Since differentiated function (transferrin and androgen binding protein secretion) of the Sertoli cell changes with sexual maturity (23,268), an in vitro study should use Sertoli cells that are at the same ontogenic stage as those affected in the in vivo studies. This is important if in vitro data are to be useful in risk assessment.

A detailed method for successful culture of mature rat Sertoli cells has been described (118). The adult Sertoli cells were cultured on an extracellular matrix to promote differentiated structure and function (90). When immature Sertoli cells are cultured at high density (91), tight junctions form between adjacent Sertoli cells. If Sertoli cells are cultured at high density on a semipermeable filter (113), the culture chamber becomes divided into basal and apical compartments and vectorial secretion by the cultured Sertoli cells occurs. To date, adult Sertoli cells have not been cultured under these conditions, but such an approach might be useful in toxicology.

Immature Sertoli cells cultured in the form of a monolayer on a semipermeable support have been used to study the toxicologic effects of cadmium chloride (112). This study assessed multiple endpoints over a wide range of toxicant concentrations administered at various culture time points. Measures included transepithelial electrical resistance (TER), a measure of junctional complex integrity; the MTT viability assay, a measure of mitochondrial activity; and inhibin secretion, a measure of Sertoli-cell function. The data showed that lower cumulative exposures to cadmium chloride in vitro compromised selectively the maintenance of tight junctions between Sertoli cells, while higher cumulative exposures decreased inhibin secretion and viability as well as tight junctional integrity.

To study the interaction between Sertoli cells and Leydig cells during in vitro exposure to tri-*o*-cresyl phosphate (TOCP), a similar Sertoli cell culture system was used. However, in this study, purified Leydig cells were placed in coculture beneath the semipermeable filter supporting the Sertoli cells (33).

As indicated earlier, the important cell–cell interactions that occur normally within the testis lend support for mixed cell cultures. Cocultures of immature Sertoli cells and germ cells have been used to study effects of testicular toxicants such as the phthalate esters and glycol ethers, which cause testicular atrophy via exfoliation of spermatocytes and spermatids in vivo (85). In vitro, these compounds resulted in a dose-dependent exfoliation of cocultured germ cells. Moreover, the significantly increased levels of inhibin produced in Sertoli cell–germ cell cocultures, compared to Sertoli cell cultures (5), permits increased sensitivity when Sertoli cell toxicity is assessed with this endpoint. To date, these Sertoli cell–germ cell cocultures have used cell aggregates comprised of Sertoli cells with adherent germ cells. To address specific mechanistic questions regarding a particular testicular toxicant, it might become necessary to isolate different germ cell types (180) and coculture one or more of these germ cells with the isolated Sertoli cells.

Epididymis

Since this is the organ that confers fertilizing ability to sperm, it is important that methods are developed which identify epididymal toxicity following in vivo exposure, and confirm any direct toxicant action on the epididymis following in vitro exposure. To establish direct toxicant action, a culture system must be used that is capable of maintaining facets of normal epididymal sperm maturation. This means that the culture system must: (a) preserve the morphological integrity of both epididymal epithelial cells and cocultured sperm; (b) support protein synthesis by the epididymal epithelial cells and the association of the secreted protein with cocultured sperm; and (c) promote the acquisition of progressive motility by the cocultured sperm. An in vitro model has been developed that meets these criteria. Using that model, the exposure of epididymal epithelial cells and sperm to EDS in vitro resulted in a significant decline in protein secretion by the epididymal epithelial cells during coculture and a decreased association of specific secretory proteins with the cocultured sperm. Moreover, EDS resulted in a dose-dependent decline in the progressive motility of cocultured sperm (134). It was concluded that EDS acts directly on epididymal epithelial cells to disrupt protein secretion, and this, in turn, disrupts facets of sperm maturation. Since the biomarker of fertility (SP22) was discovered using a protocol to identify toxicity within the epididymis, and is now known to originate in the testis around the time of round spermatid formation (137), it is likely that a protein(s) secreted by the epididymal epithelium serves to stabilize SP22 on the sperm surface. To explore this possibility, epididymal epithelial cell–sperm cocultures will be used. Recently, a human epididymal epithelial cell–sperm coculture has been successfully adapted (163). Finally, since it is known that gestational exposures to a variety of environmental chemicals perturb reproductive development, including the differentiation of the Wolffian ducts, it may be worthwhile to investigate the critical events (i.e., gene/protein expression) that imprint the development of the epididymis. For this, a system for the isolation and culture of the Wolffian ducts will be required.

In Vitro Tests of Reproductive Function

Numerous in vitro tests are available or under development to measure or detect chemically induced changes in various aspects of both male and female reproductive systems (124). These include in vitro fertilization using isolated gametes, whole organ (e.g., testis, ovary) perfusion, culture of isolated cells from the reproductive organs (e.g., Leydig cells, Sertoli cells, or epididymal epithelium), and coculture of several populations of isolated cells, quarter testes, and seminiferous tubule segments.

Tests of sperm properties and function that have been applied to reproductive toxicology include penetration of sperm through viscous medium (273), in vitro capacitation (including acrosome reaction), and fertilization assays (106,107,191,223). In addition, evaluation of human sperm function may include sperm penetration of cervical mucus, ability of sperm to undergo an acrosome reaction, and ability to penetrate zona pellucida-free hamster oocytes or bind to human hemi-zona pellucidae (68,153).

The diagnostic information obtained from such tests may help to identify potential effects on the reproductive system. However, each test bypasses essential components of the intact animal system and therefore, by itself, is not capable of predicting exposure levels that would result in toxicity in intact animals. While it is desirable to replace whole-animal testing to the extent possible with in vitro tests, the use of such tests currently is to screen for toxicity potential and to study mechanisms of action and metabolism (51,106,107,190).

Paternally Mediated Effects on Offspring

The concept is well accepted that exposure of a female to toxic chemicals during gestation or lactation may produce death, structural abnormalities, growth alteration, or postnatal functional deficits in her offspring. Sufficient data now exist with a variety of agents to conclude that male-only exposure also can produce deleterious effects in offspring (41,52,195,210). Agents for which such adverse effects in test species have been reported include lead (20), diethylstibesterol (248), urethane (177), cyclophosphamide (1,2,9,93,95,114,122,244–246), marijuana (50), and opiates (70). A number of human studies have reported associations between a variety of paternal occupations and the occurrence of birth defects or childhood cancer (e.g., 8,63,101,115,138,192,194). However, others have failed to observe such relationships (e.g., 100,185,274). Paternally mediated effects include pre- and postimplantation loss, growth and behavioral deficits, and malformations. A large proportion of the chemicals reported to cause paternally mediated effects have genotoxic activity, and are considered to exert this effect via transmissible genetic alterations (reviewed in ref. 94). Low doses of cyclophosphamide have resulted in induction of single strand DNA breaks during rat spermatogenesis which, due in part to absence of subsequent DNA repair capability, remain at fertilization (195). The results of such damage have been observed in F_2 generation offspring (92).

Other mechanisms of induction of paternally mediated effects also are possible. Xenobiotics present in seminal plasma or bound to the fertilizing sperm could be introduced into the female genital tract or into the oocyte directly, and might also interfere with fertilization or early development. With humans, the possibility exists that a parent could transport the toxic agent from the work environment to the home (e.g., on work clothes), exposing other adults or children. Further work is needed to clarify the extent to which paternal exposures may be associated with adverse effects on offspring. Regardless, if an agent is identified in test species or in humans as causing a paternally mediated adverse effect on offspring, the effect should be considered an adverse reproductive effect.

Sexual Behavior

Sexual behavior is a very complicated process involving neural and endocrine components of the central and peripheral nervous systems and the reproductive system. For humans, complex interactions of personality, social, and experiential factors also influence the initiation and performance of these behaviors. Similar factors may exist in other species, but they are more controlled by standardized laboratory conditions. However, the perturbation of sexual behavior in animals suggests the potential for similar effects on humans. Consistent with this position are data on central nervous system (CNS)-active drugs that have been shown to disrupt sexual behavior in both animals and humans (206,258).

Although the functional components of sexual performance can be quantified in rats (54), no direct evaluation of this behavior is done in most breeding studies. Rather, the presence of copulatory plugs or sperm-positive vaginal lavages has been taken as indirect evidence of successful mating. These markers do not demonstrate that male performance necessarily resulted in adequate sexual stimulation of the female. In rats, the degree of sexual preparedness of the female partner can strongly influence the site of semen deposition and subsequent sperm transport in her genital tract (3). Failure of the female to achieve sufficient stimulation may adversely influence these processes, thereby reducing the probability of successful impregnation. Such a "mating failure" would be reflected in the fertility index as reduced fertility and could erroneously be attributed to a spermatotoxic effect. There are other aspects of current breeding protocols that may serve to mask a decline in the fertility potential of a given male.

The need to directly evaluate sexual behavior routinely for all suspected reproductive toxicants is questionable. Likely candidates may be agents reported to exert neurotoxic effects, since several neurotoxicants have also been shown to produce disruptions in copulatory behavior [trichloroethylene (175); carbon disulfide (275); acrylamide (279)]. Chemicals possessing or suspected to possess androgenic or estrogenic properties (or antagonistic properties) also are potential candidates for the evaluation of copulatory behavior, separate from effects on reproductive organs (e.g., chlorinated hydrocarbon pesticides).

Structure–Activity Relationships

Structure–activity relationships have not been well studied in reproductive toxicology. Data are available that suggest structure–activity relationships for certain classes of chemicals (e.g., glycol ethers, phthalate esters, heavy metals). Yet, for other agents, nothing in their structure would have identified them as male reproductive toxicants (e.g., chlordecone). Bernstein (14) has reviewed the literature and has offered a set of classifications relating structure to reported male reproductive activity. Although limited in scope and in need of rigorous validation, such schemes do provide hypotheses that can be tested.

Comparison of the chemical or physical properties of an agent with those of known male reproductive toxicants may provide some indication of a potential for reproductive toxicity. Such information may be helpful in setting priorities for testing of agents or for the evaluation of potential toxicity when only minimal data are available.

Pharmacokinetic Considerations

Pharmacokinetic data are most useful for risk assessment when administration of the test agent has been done by the route(s) expected for human exposure. Differences in metabolic fates at the site of entry, absorption rate into the blood, initial absorption into the portal versus the systemic blood, and lipophilic properties can markedly affect the amount, form, and time course in which a toxic agent is delivered to a target site. Several major factors influence the pharmacokinetics of a given agent as related to gonadal toxicity, including: (a) the existence of a blood–testis barrier that may restrict access of a compound to the adluminal compartment of the seminiferous tubules, and (b) the metabolic capability (including DNA repair) of the different compartments of the testis and other reproductive system organs that determine the eventual disposition of the agent.

The reproductive organs appear to have a wide range of metabolic capabilities directed at both steroid and xenobiotic metabolism. These properties have been best characterized for the testis. The distributions of these enzymes and cytochrome P450 levels (multiple forms) in the testis differ between interstitial and germ cell compartments. Aryl hydrocarbon hydroxylase activity and cytochrome P450 levels in interstitial tissue are approximately twice as high as those in the seminiferous tubules. On the other hand, activities of some of the detoxifying enzymes in the germ cells such as epoxide hydrase and glutathione transferase are nearly double those in the interstitial compartment (169). High levels of glutathione transferase are seen in the neonatal rodent testis and rapidly approach adult levels (87), suggesting an early capacity to detoxify electrophilic agents.

The protective role of glutathione should not be underestimated since it may serve to prevent interactions between reactive electrophiles and critical cellular proteins and nucleic acids. For germ-cell mutagens such as ethylene oxide, ethyl methanesulfonate, and acrylamide, the level of mutagenic response may be directly related to the rate of glutathione depletion (155,227,234). Moreover, the concurrent exposure of an individual to a germ-cell mutagen and a nonmutagenic, glutathione depletor could significantly lower the dose-response threshold of the former. This has been demonstrated for the induction of dominant lethal mutations by ethyl methanesulfonate administered in combination with the glutathione depletor buthionine sulfoximine (15). The sensitivity of different species to germ-cell mutagens may also, in part, be a function of the concentration of glutathione (72,155).

The majority of pharmacokinetic studies have incompletely characterized the distribution of toxic agents and their subsequent metabolic fate within the testis. Generalizations based on hepatic metabolism are inadequate since the metabolic profile for a given agent may differ between the liver and the testes (145). As an example, the isoenzyme patterns for glutathione transferase are markedly different for these two systems (89). Detailed interspecies comparisons of the metabolic capabilities of the testis have not been conducted.

Attention should be directed toward delineating the relationship between the pharmacokinetic fate of an agent in the testes and the occurrence of spermatotoxicity. Of primary importance is determining the relationships between different exposure conditions (acute, intermittent, subchronic, chronic), pharmacokinetic status (e.g., bioaccumulation, steady state), and the nature of the response (i.e., transient, static, or progressive) as a function of site or mechanism of action (e.g., stem cell, mature sperm). Understanding these interactions is critical to more accurately assess the risks for different human exposure situations as well as to predict the degree of injury associated with prolonged exposures in humans. Such predictions currently must be based on test animal data from different exposure protocols.

FACTORING REVERSIBILITY INTO MALE REPRODUCTIVE RISK ASSESSMENT

When an agent has been identified as a male reproductive toxicant, it may be of interest to determine whether or not the effects are reversible. In the spermatogenic process, extensive damage to the spermatogonial stem cells is known to produce an irreversible effect. Even though an agent may affect only spermatocytes or spermatids at low dose levels, stem cells are often affected at higher doses. Damage to certain other cell types in the male reproductive system may also result in irreversible effects that are of concern (e.g., Sertoli cells).

While recovery from stem-cell damage is possible, the duration of the recovery period is determined by the time for regeneration (for stem cells) and repopulation of the affected spermatogenic cell type(s). To that must be added the time required for appearance of those cells as sperm in an ejaculate. The time required for these events varies with species, pharmacokinetic properties of the agent, the extent to which the stem cell population has been destroyed, and the degree of sublethal toxicity inflicted on the stem cells and/or Sertoli cells. When the stem cell population has been partially destroyed, humans require longer to attain the same degree of recovery than mice (160).

The design of a protocol to study reversibility of effects on spermatogenesis requires assessment of degree of damage at intervals after cessation of treatment. In the absence of ability to monitor ejaculates in a longitudinal design, necropsy of satellite groups at intervals during the recovery phase is needed to specify the time required for recovery. Even with the ability to obtain ejaculates, data on testis parameters (e.g., histopathology and/or spermatid count) at the end of dosing and at intervals during recovery are useful in determining the potential for and progress of recovery.

Under some conditions, the level of concern associated with a reversible male reproductive effect might be less than with an irreversible effect. However, that stance is not necessarily justified, for several reasons. First, reversibility assumes a discontinuation in exposure or a decrease in exposure below a critical (threshold) level. Thus, the assessment of reversibility must consider the exposure conditions. Second, an agent that produces a reversible effect with a low exposure level may produce an irreversible effect at a higher exposure level. Third, the potential for reversibility may vary greatly between individuals. Individuals who border on subfertility may have a reduced capability to compensate for spermatotoxicity. Therefore, the extent of an effect on fertility may be greater in those individuals and the probability of full recovery less likely. Fourth, exposures that occur prior to puberty may produce effects that are not reversible, even if they would be reversible in adults. Finally, even if the effect is fully reversible, a period of infertility may be disruptive to family and career planning, as well as psychological health. Unless those factors described here have been considered carefully and judged to be of lesser significance compared to other considerations for that agent, the same level of concern should be given to an apparent reversible effect as to an irreversible male reproductive effect.

QUESTIONS

1. Why is it necessary to evaluate so many different endpoints to assess adult male reproductive toxicity?

2. Why is it insufficient to only have data from a one-generation reproductive toxicity test and/or a subchronic toxicity test?
3. Under what testing conditions is it particularly important to use the technique of "staging" for testis histopathologic examination? Why?
4. To what extent do the endpoints in standardized multigeneration reproduction tests address the question of whether transmissible mutagenic alterations have occurred as a result of exposure to a test agent?
5. How should the appropriate number of animals per treatment group be determined for toxicity testing?

REFERENCES

1. Adams, P. M., Fabricant, J. D., and Legator, M. S. (1981): Cyclophosphamide-induced spermatogenic effects detected in the F1 generation by behavioral testing. *Science*, 211:80–82.
2. Adams, P. M., Fanini, D., and Legator, M. S. (1987): Neurobehavioral effects of paternal drug exposure on the development of offspring. In: *Functional Teratogenesis*, edited by T. Fujii and P. M. Adams, pp. 147–156. Teikyo University Press. Tokyo.
3. Adler, N. T., and Toner, J. P. (1986): The effect of copulatory behavior on sperm transport and fertility in rats. In: *Reproduction: Behavioral and Neuroendocrine Perspective*, edited by B. R. Komisaruk, H. I. Siegel, M. F. Chang, and H. H. Feder, pp. 21–32. New York Academy of Science, New York.
4. Akingbemi, B. T., Ge, R. S., Klinefelter, G. R., Gunsalas, G. L., and Hardy, M. P. (2000): A metabolite of methoxyclor, 2,2-bis(*p*-hydroxyphenyl)-1,1,1-trichlorethane, reduces testosterone biosynthesis in rat Leydig cells through the suppression of steady-state mRNA levels of the cholesterol side-chain cleavage enzyme. *Biol. Reprod.*, 62:571–578.
5. Allenby, G., Foster, P. M. D., and Sharpe, R. M. (1991): Evaluation of changes in the secretion of immunoactive inhibin by adult rat seminiferous tubules in vitro as an indicator of early toxicant action on spermatogenesis. *Fundam. Appl. Toxicol.*, 16:710–724.
6. Amann, R. P. (1981): A critical review of methods for evaluation of spermatogenesis from seminal characteristics. *J. Androl.*, 2:37–58.
7. Amann, R. P. (1986): Detection of alterations in testicular and epididymal function in laboratory animals. *Environ. Health*, 70:149–158.
8. Aschengrau, A., and Monson, R. R. (1990): Paternal military service in Vietnam and the risk of late adverse pregnancy outcomes. *Am. J. Public Health*, 80:1218–1224.
9. Auroux, M. R., Dulioust, E. M., Nawar, N. Y., and Yacoub, S. G. (1986): Antimitotic drugs (cyclophosphamide and vinblastine) in the male rat; Deaths and behavioral abnormalities in the offspring. *J. Androl.*, 7:378–386.
10. Baumgartner, A., VanHummelen, P., Lowe, X. R., Adler, I. D., and Wyrobek, A. J. (1999): Numerical and structural chromosomal abnormalities detected in human sperm with a combination of multicolor FISH assays. *Environ. Mol. Mutagen.*, 33:49–58.
11. Berndtson, W. E. (1977): Methods for quantifying mammalian spermatogenesis: A review. *J. Anim. Sci.*, 44:818–833.
12. Berndtson, W. E., and Clegg, E. D. (1992): Developing improved strategies to determine male reproductive risk from environmental toxins. *Theriogenology*, 38:223–237.
13. Berndtson, W. E., and Thompson, T. L. (1990): Age as a factor influencing the power and sensitivity of experiments for assessing body weight, testis size, and spermatogenesis in rats. *J. Androl.*, 11:325–335.
14. Bernstein, M. E. (1984): Agents affecting the male reproductive system: Effects of structure on activity. *Drug Metab. Rev.*, 15:941–996.
15. Bishop, J. B., and Teaf, C. M. (1985): A dominant lethal mutation study in male F-344 rat: Effects of ethyl methane sulfonate alone and in combination with agents perturbing the glutathione system in reproductive tissue. NCTR Final Report. Experiment 6298 and 6314.
16. Blazak, W. F., Ernst, T. L., and Stewart, B. E. (1985): Potential indicators of reproductive toxicity, testicular sperm production and epididymal sperm number, transit time and motility in Fischer 344 rats. *Fundam. Appl. Toxicol.*, 5:1097–1103.
17. Blazak, W. F., Treinen, K. A., and Juniewicz, P. E. (1993): Application of testicular sperm head counts in the assessment of male reproductive toxicity. In: *Methods in Toxicology: Male Reproductive Toxicology*, edited by R. E. Chapin and J. J. Heindel, pp. 86–94. Academic Press, San Diego.
18. Bonde, J. P. E., Ernst, E., Jensen, T. K., Hjollund, N. H. I., Kolstad, H., Henriksen, T. B., Scheike, T., Giwercman, A., Olsen, J., and Skakkebaek, N. E. (1998): Relation between semen quality and fertility: A population-based study of 430 first-pregnancy planners. *Lancet*, 352:1172–1177.
19. Boyers, S. P., Davis, R. O., and Katz, D. F. (1989): Automated semen analysis. *Curr. Prob. Obstet. Gynecol. Fertil.*, 12:173–200.
20. Brady, M., Herrera, Y., and Zenick, H. (1975): Influence of parental lead exposure on subsequent learning ability in offspring. *Pharmacol. Biochem. Behav.*, 3:561–565.
21. Carballada, R., and Esponda, P. (1992): Role of fluid from seminal vesicles and coagulating glands in sperm transport into the uterus and fertility in rats. *J. Reprod. Fertil.*, 95:639–648.
22. Cassidy, S. L., Dix, K. M., and Jenkins, T. (1983): Evaluation of a testicular sperm head counting technique using rats exposed to dimethoxyethyl phthalate (DMEP), glycerol alpha-monochlorohydrin (GMCH), epichlorohydrin (ECH), formaldehyde (FA), or methyl methanesulphonate (MMS). *Arch. Toxicol.*, 53:71–78.
23. Castellon, E., Janecki, A., and Steinberger, A. (1989): Influence of germ cells on Sertoli cell secretory activity in direct and indirect co-culture with Sertoli cells from rats of different ages. *Mol. Cell. Endocrinol.*, 64:169–178.
24. Chapin, R. E. (1988): Morphologic evaluation of seminiferous epithelium of the testis. In: *Physiology and Toxicology of Male Reproduction*, edited by J. C. Lamb and P. M. D. Foster, pp. 155–177. Academic Press, New York.
25. Chapin, R. E. (1997): Germ cells as targets for toxicants. In: *Comprehensive Toxicology*, edited by K. Boekelheide, R. E. Chapin, P. B. Hoyer, and C. Harris, pp. 139–150. Elsevier Science, New York.
26. Chapin, R. E., Dutton, S. L., Ross, M. D., and Lamb, J. C. (1985): Effects of ethylene glycol monomethyl ether (EGME) on mating performance and epididymal sperm parameters in F344 rats. *Fundam. Appl. Toxicol.*, 5:182–189.
27. Chapin, R. E., Dutton, S. L., Ross, M. D., Sumrell, B. M., and Lamb, J. C., IV. (1984): The effects of ethylene glycol monomethyl ether on testicular histology in F344 rats. *J. Androl.*, 5:369–380.
28. Chapin, R. E., Dutton, S. L., Ross, M. D., Swaisgood, R. R., and Lamb, J. C. (1985): The recovery of the testis over 8 weeks after short-term dosing with ethylene glycol monomethyl ether: Histology, cell-specific enzymes, and rete testis fluid protein. *Fundam. Appl. Toxicol.*, 5:515–525.
29. Chapin, R. E., Filler, R. S., Gulati, D., Heindel, J. J., Katz, D. F., Mebus, C. A., Obasaju, F., Perreault, S. D., Russell, S. R., Schrader, S., Slott, V., Sokol, R. Z., and Toth, G. (1992): Methods for assessing rat sperm motility. *Reprod. Toxicol.*, 6:267–273.

30. Chapin, R. E., Gulati, D. K., Barnes, L. H., and Teague, J. L. (1993): The effects of feed restriction on reproductive function in Sprague-Dawley rats. *Fundam. Appl. Toxicol.*, 20:23–29.
31. Chapin, R. E., Gulati, D. K., Fail, P. A., Hope, E., Russell, S. R., Heindel, J. J., George, J. D., Grizzle, T. B., and Teague, J. L. (1993): The effects of feed restriction on reproductive function in Swiss CD-1 mice. *Fundam. Appl. Toxicol.*, 20:15–22.
32. Chapin, R. E., Harris, M. W., Haseman, J. K., and Wine, R. N. (2000): The control of spermiogenesis in the rat. *J. Androl.*, 21(suppl.): 50.
33. Chapin, R. E., Phelps, J. L., Somkuti, S. G., Heindel, J. J., and Burka, L. T. (1990): The interaction of Sertoli and Leydig cells in the testicular toxicity of tri-*o*-cresyl phosphate. *Toxicol. Appl. Pharmacol.*, 104:483–495.
34. Chapin, R. E., Sloane, R. A., and Haseman, J. K. (1997): The relationships among reproductive endpoints in Swiss mice,using the reproductive assessment by continuous breeding database. *Fundam. Appl. Toxicol.*, 38:129–142.
35. Chapin, R. E., Stevens, J. T., Hughes, C. L., Kelce, W. R., Hess, R. A., and Daston, G. P. (1996): Endocrine modulation of reproduction. *Fundam. Appl. Toxicol.*, 29:1–17.
36. Chapin, R. E., White, R. D., Morgan, K. T., and Bus, J. S. (1984): Studies of lesions induced in the testis and epididymis of F-344 rats by inhaled methyl chloride. *Toxicol. Appl. Pharmacol.*, 76:328–343.
37. Christian, M. S. (1986): A critical review of multigeneration studies. *J. Am. Coll. Toxicol.*, 5:161–180.
38. Clegg, E. D., Cook, J. C., Chapin, R. E., Foster, P. M. D., and Foster, G. P. (1997): Leydig cell hyperplasia and adenoma formation: Mechanisms and relevance to humans. *Reprod. Toxicol.*, 11:107–121.
39. Clegg, E. D., Sakai, C. S., and Voytek, P. E. (1986): Assessment of reproductive risks. *Biol. Reprod.*, 34:5–16.
40. Clegg, E. D., and Zenick, H. (1988): Restricting mating trials enhanced the detection of ethoxyethanol-induced fertility impairment in rats. *Toxicologist*, 8:19.
41. Colie, C. F. (1993): Male mediated teratogenesis. *Reprod. Toxicol.*, 7:3–9.
42. Collins, T. F. X. (1978): Multigeneration reproduction studies. In: *Handbook of Teratology*, edited by J. G. Wilson and F. C. Fraser, pp. 191–214. Plenum Press, New York.
43. Cook, J. C., Klinefelter, G. R., Hardisty, J. F., Sharpe, R. M., and Foster, P. M. D. (1999): Rodent Leydig cell tumorigenesis: A review of the physiology, pathology, mechanisms, and relevance to humans. *Crit. Rev. Toxicol.*, 29:169–261.
44. Creasy, D. M., Ford, G. R., and Gray, T. J. B. (1990): The morphogenesis of cyclohexylamine-induced testicular atrophy in the rat: In vivo and in vitro studies. *Exp. Mol. Pathol.*, 52:155–169.
45. Creasy, D. M., Foster, J. R., and Foster, P. M. D. (1983): The morphological development of di-*n*-pentyl phthalate induced testicular atrophy in the rat. *J. Pathol.*, 139:309–321.
46. Creasy, D. M., Jones, H. B., Beech, L. M., and Gray, T. J. B. (1986): The effects of two testicular toxins on the ultrastructural morphology of mixed cultures of Sertoli and germ cells: A comparison with in vivo effects. *Fund. Chem. Toxicol.*, 24:655–656.
47. Crisp, T. M., Clegg, E. D., Cooper, R. L., Wood, W. P., Anderson, D. G., Baetcke, K. P., Hoffmann, J. L., Morrow, M. S., Rodier, D. J., Schaeffer, J. E., Touart, L. W., Zeeman, M. G., and Patel, Y. M. (1998): Environmental endocrine disruption: An effects assessment and analysis. *Environ. Health Perspect.*, 106(suppl. 1):11–56.
48. Cross, N. L., and Meizel, S. (1989): Methods for evaluating the acrosomal status of mammalian sperm. *Biol. Reprod.*, 41:635–641.
49. Cukierski, M. A., Sina, J. L., Prahalada, S., and Robertson, R. T. (1991): Effects of seminal vesicle and coagulating gland ablation on fertility in rats. *Reprod. Toxicol.*, 5:347–352.
50. Dalterio, S. L., Steger, R. W., and Bartke, A. (1984): Maternal or paternal exposure to cannabinoids affects central neurotransmitter levels and reproductive function in male offspring. In: *The Cannabinoids: Chemical, Pharmacologic and Therapeutic Aspects*, edited by S. Agurell, W. L. Dewey, and R. E. Willette, pp. 411–425. Academic Press, New York.
51. Darney, S. P. (1991): In vitro assessment of gamete integrity. In: *In Vitro Toxicology: Mechanisms and New Technology*, edited by A. M. Goldberg, pp. 63–75. Mary Ann Liebert, New York.
52. Davis, D. L., Friedler, G., Mattison, D., and Morris, R. (1992): Male-mediated teratogenesis and other reproductive effects: Biologic and epidemiologic findings and a plea for clinical research. *Reprod. Toxicol.*, 6:289–292.
53. de Boer, P., van der Hoeven, F. A., and Chardon, J. A. P. (1976): The production, morphology, karyotypes and transport of spermatozoa from tertiary trisomic mice and the consequences for egg fertilization. *J. Reprod. Fertil.*, 48:249–256.
54. Dewsbury, D. A. (1967): A quantitative description of the behavior of rats during copulation. *Behavior*, 29:154–178.
55. Dixon, R. L., and Hall, J. L. (1984): Reproductive toxicology. In: *Principles and Methods of Toxicology*, edited by A. W. Hayes, pp. 107–140. Raven Press, New York.
56. Dornan, W. A., Peterson, M., Matuszewich, L., and Malen, P. (1991): Ibotenic acid-induced lesions of the medial zona incerta decrease lordosis behavior in the female rat. *Behav. Neurosci.*, 105:210–214.
57. Dostal, L. A., Faber, C. K., and Zandee, J. (1996): Sperm motion parameters in vas deferens and cauda epididymal rat sperm. *Reprod. Toxicol.*, 10:231–235.
58. Evenson, D. P. (1999): Alterations and damage of sperm chromatin structure and early embryonic failure. In: *Towards Reproductive Certainty: Fertility and Genetics Beyond 1999*, edited by R. Jannsen and D. Mortimer, pp. 313–329. Parthenon, New York.
59. Evenson, D., and Jost, L. (1994): Sperm chromatin structure assay: DNA denaturability. In: *Methods in Cell Biology*, edited by L. Darzynkiewicz and J. P. Robinson, pp. 159–176. Academic Press, New York.
60. Evenson, D. P., Jost, L. K., Marshall, D., Zinaman, M. J., Clegg, E., Purvis, K., deAngelis, P., and Claussen, O. P. (1999): Utility of the sperm chromatin structure assay as a diagnostic and prognostic tool in the human fertility clinic. *Hum. Reprod.*, 14:1039–1049.
61. Ewing, L. L., Zirkin, B. R., and Chubb, C. (1981): Assessment of testicular testosterone production and Leydig cell structure. *Environ. Health Perspect.*, 38:19–27.
62. Fawcett, D. W. (1986): *Bloom and Fawcett: A Textbook of Histology*. W. B. Saunders, Philadelphia, PA.
63. Fedrick, J. (1976): Anencephalus in the Oxford record linkage study area. *Dev. Med. Child Neurol.*, 18:643–656.
64. Filler, R. (1993): Methods for evaluation of rat epididymal sperm morphology. In: *Methods in Toxicology: Male Reproductive Toxicology*, edited by R. E. Chapin and J. J. Heindel, pp. 334–343. Academic Press, San Diego.
65. Foote, R. H., Berndtson, W. E., and Rounsaville, T. R. (1986): Use of quantitative testicular histology to assess the effect of dibromocholoropropane (DBCP) on reproduction in rabbits. *Fundam. Appl. Toxicol.*, 6:638–647.
66. Foote, R. H., Schermerhorn, E. C., and Simkin, M. E. (1986): Measurement of semen quality, fertility, and reproductive hormones to assess dibromochloropropane (DBCP) effects in live rabbits. *Fundam. Appl. Toxicol.*, 6:628–637.
67. Francis, E. Z., and Kimmel, G. L. (1988): Proceedings of the workshop on one- versus two-generation reproductive effects studies. *J. Am. Coll. Toxicol.*, 7:911–925.

68. Franken, D. R., Burkman, L. J., Coddington, C. C., Oehninger, S., and Hodgen, G. D. (1990): Human hemizona attachment assay. In: *Human Spermatozoa in Assisted Reproduction*, edited by A. A. Acosta, R. J. Swanson, S. B. Ackerman, T. F. Kruger, J. A. VanZyl, and R. Menkveld, pp. 355–371. Williams & Wilkins, Baltimore, MD.
69. Friedler, G. (1996): Paternal exposures: Impact on reproductive and developmental outcome, an overview. *Pharmacol. Biochem. Behav.*, 55:691–700.
70. Friedler, G., and Wheeling, H. S. (1979): Behavioral effects in offspring of males injected with opioids prior to mating. *Pharmacol. Biochem. Behav.*, 11(suppl.):23–28.
71. Galbraith, W. M., Voytek, P., and Ryon, M. S. (1983): Assessment of risks to human reproduction and development of the human conceptus from exposure to environmental substances. In: *Advances in Modern Environmental Toxicology*, edited by M. S. Christian, W. M. Galbraith, P. Voytek, and M. A. Mehlman, pp. 41–153. Princeton Scientific, Princeton, NJ.
72. Gandy, J., Bates, H. K., Conder, L. A., and Harbison, R. D. (1992): Effects of reproductive tract glutathione enhancement and depletion on ethyl methanesulfonate-induced dominant lethal mutations in Sprague-Dawley Rats. *Teratogen. Carcinogen. Mutagen.*, 12:61–70.
73. Goeden, H., and Zenick, H. (1985): Influence of the uterine environment on rat sperm motility and swimming speed. *J. Exp. Zool.*, 233:247–251.
74. Goldman, J. M., Cooper, R. L., Laws, S. C., Rehnberg, G. L., Edwards, T. L., McElroy, W. K., and Hein, J. F. (1990): Chlordimeform-induced alterations in endocrine regulation within the male rat reproductive system. *Toxicol. Appl. Pharmacol.*, 104:25–35.
75. Goldstein, L. S. (1984): Use of an in vitro technique to detect mutations induced by antineoplastic drugs in mouse germ cells. *Cancer Treat. Rep.*, 68:855–858.
76. Graham, J. K., Kunze, E., and Hammerstedt, R. H. (1990): Analysis of sperm cell viability, acrosomal integrity, and mitochondrial function using flow cytometry. *Biol. Reprod.*, 43:55–64.
77. Gray, L. E. (1991): Delayed effects on reproduction following exposure to toxic chemicals during critical periods of development. In: *Aging and Environmental Toxicology: Biological and Behavioral Perspectives*, edited by R. L. Cooper, J. M. Goldman, and T. J. Harbin, pp. 183–210. Johns Hopkins University Press, Baltimore, MD.
78. Gray, L. E. (1992): Chemical-induced alterations of sexual differentiation: A review of effects in humans and rodents. In: *Advances in Modern Environmental Toxicology*, edited by T. Colburn and C. Clement, pp. 203–230. Princeton Scientific, Princeton, NJ.
79. Gray, L. E., Klinefelter, G., Kelce, W., Laskey, J., Ostby, J., Marshall, R., and Ewing, L. (1995): Hamster Leydig cells are less sensitive to ethane dimethane sulphonate when compared to rat Leydig cells both in vivo and in vitro. *Toxicol. Appl. Pharmacol.*, 130:248–256.
80. Gray, L. E., Klinefelter, G., Laskey, J., Ostby, J., Sigmon, R., and Ferrell, J. (1991): Effects of the Leydig cell toxicant ethane dimethane sulphonate (EDS) on ejaculated sperm counts, mating behavior and testosterone in rats. *Toxicology*, 41:246A.
81. Gray, L. E., Marshall, R., Ostby, J., and Setzer, R. W. (1992): Correlation of ejaculated sperm numbers with fertility in the rat. *Toxicology*, 42:433A.
82. Gray, L. E., Ostby, J., Ferrell, J., Sigmon, R., Cooper, R., Linder, R., Rehnberg, G., Goldman, J., and Laskey, J. (1989): Correlation of sperm and endocrine measures with reproductive success in rodents. In: *Sperm Measures and Reproductive Success*, Institute for Health Policy Analysis, Forum on Science, Health, and Environmental Risk, pp. 193–209. Alan R. Liss, New York.
83. Gray, L. E., Ostby, J., Linder, R., Goldman, J., Rehnberg, G., and Cooper, R. (1990): Carbendazim-induced alterations of reproductive development and function in the rat and hamster. *Fundam. Appl. Toxicol.*, 15:281–297.
84. Gray, L. E., Ostby, J., Sigmon, R., Ferrell, J., Linder, R., Cooper, R., Goldman, J., and Laskey, J. (1988): The development of a protocol to assess reproductive effects of toxicants in the rat. *Reprod. Toxicol.*, 2:281–287.
85. Gray, T. J. B. (1986): Testicular toxicity in vitro: Sertoli-germ cell co-cultures as a model system. *Fundam. Chem. Toxicol.*, 24:601–605.
86. Green, S., Auletta, A., Fabricant, R., Kapp, M., Sheu, C., Springer, J., and Whitfield, B. (1985): Current status of bioassays in genetic toxicology: The dominant lethal test. *Mutat. Res.*, 154:49–67.
87. Grosshans, K., and Calvin, H. I. (1985): Estimation of glutathione in purified populations of mouse testis germ cells. *Biol. Reprod.*, 33:1197–1205.
88. Gulati, D. K., Hope, E., Teague, J., and Chapin, R. E. (1991): Reproductive toxicity assessment by continuous breeding in Sprague-Dawley rats: A comparison of two study designs. *Fundam. Appl. Toxicol.*, 17:270–279.
89. Guthenberg, B., Alin, P., and Mannervik, B. (1983): Glutathione transferases in rat testis. *Acta Chem. Scand.*, 37:261–262.
90. Hadley, M. A., Byers, S. W., Suarez-Quian, C. A., Kleinman, H. K., and Dym, M. (1985): Extracellular matrix regulates Sertoli cell differentiation, testicular cord formation, and germ cell development in vitro. *J. Cell Biol.*, 101:1511–1522.
91. Hadley, M. A., Byers, S. W., Suarez-Quian, C. S., Djakiew, D., and Dym, M. (1988): In vitro models of differentiated Sertoli cell structure and function. *In Vitro Cell. Dev. Biol.*, 24:550–557.
92. Hales, B., Crosman, K., and Robaire, B. (1992): Increased post-implantation loss and malformations among the F2 progeny of male rats chronically treated with cyclophosphamide. *Teratology*, 45:671–678.
93. Hales, B. F., and Robaire, B. (1990): Reversibility of the effects of chronic paternal exposure to cyclophosphamide on pregnancy outcome in rats. *Mutat. Res.*, 229:129–134.
94. Hales, B. F., and Robaire, B. (1996): Paternally mediated effects on development. In: *Handbook of Developmental Toxicology*, edited by R. D. Hood, pp. 91–107. CRC Press, Boca Raton, FL.
95. Hales, B. F., Smith, S., and Robaire, B. (1986): Cyclophosphamide in the seminal fluid of treated males: Transmission to females by mating and effect on pregnancy outcome. *Toxicol. Appl. Pharmacol.*, 84:423–430.
96. Hall, J. C., Hadley, J., and Doman, T. (1991): Correlation between changes in rat sperm membrane lipids, protein, and the membrane physical state during epididymal maturation. *J. Androl.*, 12:76–87.
97. Harris, M. W., Chapin, R. E., Lockhart, A. C., Jokinen, M. P., Allen, J. D., and Haskins, E. A. (1992): Assessment of a short-term reproductive and developmental toxicity screen. *Fundam. Appl. Toxicol.*, 19:186–196.
98. Haschek, W. M., and Rousseaux, C. G. (1991): *Handbook of Toxicologic Pathology*. Academic Press, New York.
99. Heindel, J. J., and Powell, C. J. (1992): Phthalate ester effects on rat Sertoli cell function in vitro: Effects of phthalate side chain and age of animal. *Toxicol. Appl. Pharmacol.*, 115:116–123.
100. Hemminki, K., Mutanen, P., Luoma, K., and Saloniemi, I. (1980): Congenital malformations by the parental occupation in Finland. *Int. Arch. Occup. Environ. Health*, 46:93–98.
101. Hemminki, K., Saloniemi, I., and Salonen, T. (1981): Childhood cancer and paternal occupation in Finland. *J. Epidemiol. Commun. Health*, 35:11–15.

102. Hess, R. A. (1990): Quantitative and qualitative characteristics of the stages and transitions in the cycle of the rat seminiferous epithelium: Light microscopic observations of perfusion-fixed and plastic-embedded testes. *Biol. Reprod.*, 43:525–542.
103. Hess, R. A., Linder, R. E., Strader, L. F., and Perreault, S. D. (1988): Acute and long term sequelae of 1,3-dinitrobenzene on male reproduction in the rat. II. Quantitative and qualitative histopathology of the testis. *J. Androl.*, 9:327–342.
104. Hess, R. A., and Moore, B. J. (1993): Histological methods for evaluation of the testis. In: *Methods in Toxicology: Male Reproductive Toxicology*, edited by R. E. Chapin and J. J. Heindel, pp. 52–85. Academic Press, San Diego.
105. Hess, R. A., Moore, B. J., Forrer, J., Linder, R. E., and Abuel-Atta, A. A. (1991): The fungicide Benomyl (methyl 1-(butylcarbamoyl)-2-benzimidazolecarbamate) causes testicular dysfunction by inducing the sloughing of germ cells and occlusion of efferent ductules. *Fundam. Appl. Toxicol.*, 17:733–745.
106. Holloway, A. J., Moore, H. D. M., and Foster, P. M. D. (1990): The use of in vitro fertilization to detect reductions in the fertility of male rats exposed to 1,3-dinitrobenzene. *Fundam. Appl. Toxicol.*, 14:113–122.
107. Holloway, A. J., Moore, H. D. M., and Foster, P. M. D. (1990): The use of rat in vitro fertilization to detect reductions in the fertility of spermatozoa from males exposed to ethylene glycol monomethyl ether. *Reprod. Toxicol.*, 4:21–27.
108. Holmes, M., Suarez, J., and Klinefelter, G. (1999): Dibromoacetic acid perturbs protein synthesis in adult rat seminiferous tubules. *Biol. Reprod.*, 60(suppl. 1):146A.
109. Hugenholtz, A. P., and Bruce, W. R. (1983): Radiation induction of mutations affecting sperm morphology in mice. *Mutat. Res.*, 107:177–185.
110. Hurtt, M. E., and Zenick, H. (1986): Decreasing epididymal sperm reserves enhances the detection of ethoxyethanol-induced spermatotoxicity. *Fundam. Appl. Toxicol.*, 7:348–353.
111. Janecki, A., Jakubowiak, A., and Steinberger, A. (1988): Effect of germ cells on vectorial secretion of androgen binding protein and transferrin by immature rat Sertoli cells in vitro. *J. Androl.*, 9:126–132.
112. Janecki, A., Jakubowiak, A., and Steinberger, A. (1992): Effect of cadmium chloride on transepithelial electrical resistance of Sertoli cell monolayers in two-compartment cultures—A new model for toxicological investigations of the "blood-testis" barrier in vitro. *Toxicol. Appl. Pharmacol.*, 112:51–57.
113. Janecki, A., and Steinberger, A. (1986): Polarized Sertoli cell functions in a new two-compartment culture system. *J. Androl.*, 7:69–71.
114. Jenkinson, P. C., and Anderson, D. (1990): Malformed foetuses and karyotype abnormalities in the offspring of cyclophosphamide and allyl alcohol-treated male rats. *Mutat. Res.*, 229:173–184.
115. Johnson, C. C., Annegers, J. F., Frankowski, R. F., Spitz, M. R., and Buffler, P. A. (1987): Childhood nervous system tumors—An evaluation of the association with paternal occupational exposure to hydrocarbons. *Am. J. Epidemiol.*, 126:605–613.
116. Johnson, L., Welsh, T. H., and Wilker, C. E. (1998): Anatomy and physiology of the male reproductive system and potential targets for toxicants. In: *Reproductive and Endocrine Toxicology*, edited by K. Boekelheide, R. E. Chapin, P. B. Hoyer, and C. Harris, pp. 5–62. Elsevier Science, New York.
117. Jones, T. C., Mohr, U., and Hunt, R. D. (1987): *Genital System.* Springer-Verlag, New York.
118. Karzai, A. W., and Wright, W. W. (1992): Regulation of the synthesis and secretion of transferrin and cyclic protein-2/cathepsin L by mature rat Sertoli cells in culture. *Biol. Reprod.*, 47:823–831.
119. Katz, D. F., Diel, L., and Overstreet, J. W. (1982): Differences in the movement of morphologically normal and abnormal human seminal spermatozoa. *Biol. Reprod.*, 26:566–570.
120. Kavlock, R. J. (1999): Overview of endocrine disruptor research activity in the United States. *Chemosphere*, 39:1227–1236.
121. Kelce, W. R., Zirkin, B. R., and Ewing, L. L. (1991): Immature rat Leydig cells are intrinsically less sensitive than adult Leydig cells to ethane dimethanesulfonate. *Toxicol. Appl. Pharmacol.*, 111:189–200.
122. Kelly, S. M., Robaire, B., and Hales, B. F. (1992): Paternal cyclophosphamide treatment causes postimplantation loss via inner cell mass-specific cell death. *Teratology*, 45:313–318.
123. Kempinas, W. D., Suarez, J. D., Roberts, N. L., Strader, L. F., Ferrell, J. M., Goldman, J. M., Narotsky, M. G., Perreault, S. D., and Klinefelter, G. R. (1998): Fertility of rat epididymal sperm after chemically and surgically-induced sympathectomy. *Biol. Reprod.*, 59:897–904.
124. Kimmel, G. L., Clegg, E. D., and Crisp, T. M. (1995): Reproductive toxicity testing: A risk assessment perspective. In: *Reproductive Toxicology*, edited by R. J. Witorsch, pp. 75–98. Raven Press, New York.
125. Kleeman, J. M., Moore, R. W., and Peterson, R. E. (1990): Inhibition of testicular steroidogenesis in 2,3,7,8-tetrachlorodibenzo-*p*-dioxin-treated rats: Evidence that the key steroidogenic lesion occurs prior to or during pregnenolone formation. *Toxicol. Appl. Pharmacol.*, 106:112–125.
126. Klinefelter, G., and Gray, L. E. (1993): The clinical relevance of animal models: Animal studies that assess the potential for drugs and environmental agents to cause reproductive disorders in humans. In: *Reproductive Toxicology and Infertility*, edited by A. R. Scialli and M. J. Zinaman, pp. 219–282. McGraw-Hill, New York.
127. Klinefelter, G. R., Hall, P. F., and Ewing, L. L. (1987): Effect of luteinizing hormone deprivation in situ on steroidogenesis of rat Leydig cells purified by a multistep procedure. *Biol. Reprod.*, 36:769–783.
128. Klinefelter, G. R., and Hess, R. A. (1998): Toxicology of the male excurrent ducts and accessory glands. In: *Reproductive and Developmental Toxicology*, edited by K. S. Korach, pp. 553–591. Marcel Dekker, New York.
129. Klinefelter, G. R., Laskey, J. W., Ferrell, J., Suarez, J. D., and Roberts, N. L. (1997): Discriminant analysis indicates a single sperm protein (SP22) is predictive of fertility following toxicant exposure. *J. Androl.*, 18:139–150.
130. Klinefelter, G. R., Laskey, J. W., Kelce, W. R., Ferrell, J., Roberts, N. L., Suarez, J. D., and Slott, V. (1994): Chloroethylmethanesulfonate-induced effects on the epididymis seem unrelated to altered Leydig cell function. *Biol. Reprod.*, 51:82–91.
131. Klinefelter, G. R., Laskey, J. W., Perreault, S. D., Ferrell, J., Jeffay, S., Suarez, J., and Roberts, N. (1994): The ethane dimethanesulfonate-induced decrease in the fertilizing ability of cauda epididymal sperm is independent of the testis. *J. Androl.*, 15:318–327.
132. Klinefelter, G. R., Laskey, J. W., and Roberts, N. L. (1991): In vitro/in vivo effects of ethane dimethanesulfonate on Leydig cells of adult rats. *Toxicol. Appl. Pharmacol.*, 107:460–471.
133. Klinefelter, G. R., Laskey, J. W., Roberts, N. R., Slott, V., and Suarez, J. D. (1990): Multiple effects of ethane dimethanesulfonate on the epididymis of adult rats. *Toxicol. Appl. Pharmacol.*, 105:271–287.
134. Klinefelter, G. R., Roberts, N. L., and Suarez, J. D. (1992): Direct effects of ethane dimethanesulphonate on epididymal function in adult rats: an in vitro demonstration. *J. Androl.*, 13:409–421.

135. Klinefelter, G. R., and Suarez, J. D. (1997): Toxicant-induced acceleration of epididymal sperm transit: Androgen-dependent proteins may be involved. *Reprod. Toxicol.*, 11:511–519.

136. Klinefelter, G. R., Suarez, J., Roberts, N., and Strader, L. (1999): The sperm biomarker SP22 is highly correlated with infertility resulting from the testicular toxicant bromochloroacetic acid. *Biol. Reprod.*, 60(suppl. 1):187A.

137. Klinefelter, G. R., and Welch, J. E. (1999): The saga of a male fertility protein (SP22). *Annu. Rev. Biomed. Sci.*, 1:145–184.

138. Kluwe, W. M., Weber, H., Greenwell, A., and Harrington, F. (1985): Initial and residual toxicity following acute exposure of developing male rats to dibromochloropropane. *Toxicol. Appl. Pharmacol.*, 79:54–68.

139. Knobil, E., and Neill, J. D. (1998): *Encyclopedia of Reproduction*. Academic Press, New York.

140. Knobil, E., Neill, J. D., Greenwald, G. S., Markert, C. L., and Pfaff, D. W. (1994): *The Physiology of Reproduction*. Raven Press, New York.

141. Ku, W. W., Chapin, R. E., Wine, R. N., and Gladen, B. C. (1993): Testicular toxicity of boric acid (BA): Relationship of dose to lesion development and recovery in the F344 rat. *Reprod. Toxicol.*, 7:305–319.

142. Lamb, J. C., and Chapin, R. E. (1985): Experimental models of male reproductive toxicology. In: *Endocrine Toxicology*, edited by J. A. Thomas, K. S. Korach, and J. A. McLachlan, pp. 85–115. Raven Press, New York.

143. Lamb, J. C., and Foster, P. M. D. (1988): *Physiology and Toxicology of Male Reproduction*. Academic Press, New York.

144. Laskey, J. W., and Phelps, P. V. (1991): Effect of cadmium and other metal cations on in vitro Leydig cell testosterone production. *Toxicol. Appl. Pharmacol.*, 108:296–306.

145. Lee, I. P., and Nagayama, J. (1980): Metabolism of benzo(a)pyrene by the isolated perfused rat testis. *Cancer Res.*, 40:3297–3303.

146. Lewis, J. R. (1991): *Reproductively Active Chemicals: A Reference Guide*. Van Nostrand Reinhold, New York.

147. Li, L.-H., and Heindel, J. J. (1998): Sertoli cell toxicants. In: *Reproductive and Developmental Toxicology*, edited by K. S. Korach, pp. 655–691. Marcel Dekker, New York.

148. Linder, R. E., Hess, R. A., and Strader, L. F. (1986): Testicular toxicity and infertility in male rats treated with 1,3-dinitrobenzene. *J. Toxicol. Environ. Health*, 19:477–489.

149. Linder, R. E., Klinefelter, G. R., Strader, L. F., Narotsky, M. G., Suarez, J. D., Roberts, N. L., and Perreault, S. D. (1995): Dibromoacetic acid affects reproductive competence and sperm quality in the male rat. *Fundam. Appl. Toxicol.*, 28:9–17.

150. Linder, R. E., Klinefelter, G. R., Strader, L. F., Suarez, J. D., and Roberts, N. L. (1997): Spermatotoxicity of dichloroacetic acid. *Reprod. Toxicol.*, 11:681–688.

151. Linder, R. E., Strader, L. F., Barbee, R. R., Rehnberg, G. L., and Perreault, S. D. (1990): Reproductive toxicity of a single dose of 1,3-dinitrobenzene in two ages of young adult male rats. *Fundam. Appl. Toxicol.*, 14:284–298.

152. Linder, R. E., Strader, L. F., Slott, V. L., and Suarez, J. D. (1992): Endpoints of spermatotoxicity in the rat after short duration exposures to fourteen reproductive toxicants. *Reprod. Toxicol.*, 6:491–505.

153. Liu, D. Y., and Baker, H. W. G. (1992): Tests of human sperm function and fertilization in vitro. *Fertil. Steril.*, 58:465–483.

154. Lowe, X. R., de Stoppelaar, J. M., Bishop, J., Cassel, M., Hoebee, B., Moore, D., and Wyrobek, A. J. (1998): Epididymal sperm aneuploidies in three strains of rats detected by multicolor fluorescence in situ hybridization. *Environ. Mol. Mutagen.*, 31:125–132.

155. McKelvey, J. A., and Zemaitis, M. A. (1986): The effects of ethylene oxide (EO) exposure on tissue glutathione levels in rats and mice. *Drug Chem. Toxicol.*, 9:51–66.

156. McKinnell, C., and Sharpe, R. M. (1992): The role of specific germ cell types in modulation of the secretion of androgen-regulated proteins (ARPs) by stage VI–VIII seminiferous tubules from the adult rat. *Mol. Cell. Endocrinol.*, 83:219–231.

157. McPhaul, M. J. (1998): The biology of the male reproductive tract. In: *Reproductive and Developmental Toxicology*, edited by K. S. Korach, pp. 475–508. Marcel Dekker, New York.

158. Meistrich, M. L. (1982): Quantitative correlation between testicular stem cell survival, sperm production, and fertility in the mouse after treatment with different cytotoxic agents. *J. Androl.*, 3:58–68.

159. Meistrich, M. L., and Brown, C. C. (1983): Estimation of the increased risk of human infertility from alterations in semen characteristics. *Fertil. Steril.*, 40:220–230.

160. Meistrich, M. L., and Samuels, R. C. (1985): Reduction in sperm levels after testicular irradiation of the mouse: A comparison with man. *Radiat. Res.*, 102:138–147.

161. Meistrich, M. L., and van Beek, M. E. A. B. (1993): Spermatogonial stem cells: Assessing their survival and ability to produce differentiated cells. In: *Methods in Toxicology: Male Reproductive Toxicology*, edited by R. E. Chapin and J. J. Heindel, pp. 106–123. Academic Press, San Diego.

162. Menkveld, R., Stander, F. S. H., Kotze, T. JvW., Kruger, T. F., and van Zyl, J. A. (1990): The evaluation of morphological characteristics of human spermatozoa according to stricter criteria. *Hum. Reprod.*, 5:586–592.

163. Moore, H. D., Curry, M. R., Penfold, L. M., and Pryor, J. P. (1992): The culture of human epididymal epithelium and in vitro maturation of epididymal spermatozoa. *Fertil. Steril.*, 58:776–783.

164. Mori, H., and Christensen, A. K. (1980): Morphometric analysis of Leydig cells in the normal rat testis. *J. Cell Biol.*, 84:340–354.

165. Morrissey, R. E., Lamb, J. C., Morris, R. W., Chapin, R. E., Gulati, D. K., and Heindel, J. J. (1989): Results and evaluations of 48 continuous breeding reproduction studies conducted in mice. *Fundam. Appl. Toxicol.*, 13:747–777.

166. Morrissey, R. E., Lamb, J. C., Schwetz, B. A., Teague, J. L., and Morris, R. W. (1988): Association of sperm, vaginal cytology, and reproductive organ weight data with results of continuous breeding reproduction studies in Swiss (CD-1) mice. *Fundam. Appl. Toxicol.*, 11:359–371.

167. Morrissey, R. E., Schwetz, B. A., Lamb, J. C., Ross, M. D., Teague, J. L., and Morris, R. W. (1988): Evaluation of rodent sperm, vaginal cytology, and reproductive organ weight data from National Toxicology Program 13-week studies. *Fundam. Appl. Toxicol.*, 11:343–358.

168. Mosher, W. D., and Pratt, W. F. (1991): Fecundity and infertility in the United States: Incidence and trends. *Fertil. Steril.*, 56:192–193.

169. Mukhtar, H., Philpot, R. M., Lee, I. P., and Bend, J. R. (1978): Developmental aspects of epoxide-metabolizing enzyme activities in adrenals, ovaries, and testes of the rat. In: *Developmental Toxicology of Energy Related Pollutants*, edited by D. D. Mahlum, M. R. Sikov, P. L. Hackett, and F. D. Andrew, pp. 89–104. Technical Information Center, U.S. Department of Energy, Springfield, VA.

170. Mylchreest, E., Sar, M., Cattley, R. C., and Foster, P. M. D. (1999): Disruption of androgen-regulated male reproductive development by di(*n*-butyl) phthalate during late gestation in rats is different from flutamide. *Toxicol. Appl. Pharmacol.*, 156:81–95.

171. Nakai, M., Moore, B. J., and Hess, R. A. (1993): Epithelial reorganization and irregular growth following carbendazim-induced injury of the efferent ductules of the rat testis. *Anat. Rec.*, 235:51–60.

172. National Academy of Science. (1999): *Hormonally Active Agents in the Environment*. National Academy Press, Washington, DC.

173. National Research Council. (1983): *Risk Assessment in the Federal Government: Managing the Process*. National Academy Press, Washington, DC.

174. National Research Council. (1994): *Science and Judgment in Risk Assessment*. National Academy Press, Washington, DC.

175. Nelson, J. L., and Zenick, H. (1986): The effect of trichloroethylene on male sexual behavior. Possible opiate role. *Neurobehav. Toxicol. Teratol.*, 8:441–445.

176. Nestor, A., and Handel, M. A. (1984): The transport of morphologically abnormal sperm in the female reproductive tract of mice. *Gamete Res.*, 10:119–125.

177. Nomura, T. (1982): Parental exposure to x-rays and chemicals induces heritable tumors and anomalies in mice. *Nature*, 296:575–577.

178. Oberlander, G., Yeung, C. H., and Cooper, T. G. (1994): Induction of reversible infertility in male rats by oral ornidazole and its effects on sperm motility and epididymal secretions. *J. Reprod. Fertil.*, 100:551–559.

179. O'Brien, D. A., Froysa, A., and Rockett, D. (1986): Sertoli cell-conditioned medium increases viability and ATP levels of pachytene spermatocytes and round spermatids in vitro. *J. Cell Biol.*, 103:485a.

180. O'Brien, D. A., Gabel, C. A., Rockett, D. L., and Eddy, E. M. (1989): Receptor-mediated endocytosis and differential synthesis of mannose-6-phosphate receptors in isolated spermatogenic and Sertoli cells. *Endocrinology*, 125:2973–2984.

181. Olshan, A. F., and Faustman, E. M. (1993): Male-mediated developmental toxicity. *Reprod. Toxicol.*, 7:191–202.

182. Organization for Economic Cooperation and Development. (1990): Guideline for Testing of Chemicals: Extended Steering Group Document 3. OECD.

183. Overstreet, J. W. (1984): Laboratory tests for human male reproductive risk assessment. In: *Environmental Influences on Fertility Pregnancy and Development. Strategies for Measurement and Evaluation*, edited by M. S. Legator, M. Rosenberg, and H. Zenick, pp. 67–82. Alan R. Liss, New York.

184. Overstreet, J. W. (1986): Sperm penetration of cervical mucus. *Fertil. Steril.*, 45:324–326.

185. Papier, C. M. (1985): Parental occupation and congenital malformations in a series of 35,000 births in Israel. *Prog. Clin. Biol. Res.*, 163:291–294.

186. Park, D. V. (1984): Development of detoxication mechanisms in the neonate. In: *Toxicology and the Newborn*, edited by S. Kacew and M. J. Reason, pp. 1–32. Elsevier, New York.

187. Parks, L. G., Ostby, J. S., Lambright, C. R., Abbott, B. D., Klinefelter, G. R., and Gray, L. E. (1999): Perinatal butyl benzyl phthalate (BBP) and bis(2-ethylhexyl) phthalate (DEHP) exposures induce antiandrogenic effects in Sprague-Dawley rats. *Biol. Reprod.*, 60(suppl. 1):191A.

188. Parvinen, M., and Vanha-Perttula, T. (1972): Identification and enzymatic quantification of the stages of the seminiferous epithelial wave in the rat. *Anat. Rec.*, 174:435–449.

189. Perreault, S. D. (1997): The mature spermatozoon as a target for reproductive toxicants. In: *Comprehensive Toxicology*, edited by K. Boekelheide, R. E. Chapin, P. B. Hoyer, and C. Harris, pp. 165–179. Elsevier Science, New York.

190. Perreault, S. D. (1998): Gamete toxicology: The impact of new technologies. In: *Reproductive and Developmental Toxicology*, edited by K. S. Korach, pp. 635–654. Marcel Dekker, New York.

191. Perreault, S. D., and Jeffay, S. C. (1993): Strategies and methods for the functional evaluation of oocytes and zygotes. In: *Methods in Toxicology: Female Reproductive Toxicology*, edited by J. J. Heindel and R. E. Chapin, pp. 92–109. Academic Press, San Diego.

192. Peters, J. M., Preston-Martin, S., and Yu, M. C. (1981): Brain tumors in children and occupational exposure of the parents. *Science*, 213:235–237.

193. Peterson, R. E., Cooke, P. S., Kelce, W. R., and Gray, L. E. (1997): Environmental endocrine disruptors. In: *Comprehensive Toxicology*, edited by K. Boekelheide, R. E. Chapin, P. B. Hoyer, and C. Harris, pp. 181–192. Elsevier Science, New York.

194. Polednak, A. P., and Janerich, D. T. (1983): Use of available record systems in epidemiologic studies of reproductive toxicology. *Am. J. Ind. Med.*, 4:329–348.

195. Qiu, J., Hales, B. F., and Robaire, B. (1995): Damage to rat spermatozoal DNA after chronic cyclophosphamide exposure. *Biol. Reprod.*, 53:1465–1473.

196. Qui, J., Hales, B. F., and Robaire, B. (1992): Adverse effects of cyclophosphamide on progeny outcome can be mediated through post-testicular mechanisms in the rat. *Biol. Reprod.*, 46:926–931.

197. Racine, C., Rey, R., Forest, M. G., Louis, F., Ferre, A., Huhtaniemi, I., Josso, N., and diClemente, N. (1998): Receptors for anti-Mullerian hormone on Leydig cells are responsible for its effects on steroidogenesis and cell differentiation. *Proc. Natl. Acad. Sci. USA*, 95:594–599.

198. Ratnasooriya, W. D. (1979): A simplified method for measuring ejaculated sperm content of male rats. *J. Pharmacol. Methods*, 2:379–381.

199. Redi, C. A., Garagna, S., Pellicciari, C., Manfredi-Romanini, M. G., Capanna, E., Winking, H., and Gropp, A. (1984): Spermatozoa of chromosomally heterozygous mice and their fate in male and female genital tracts. *Gamete Res.*, 9:273–286.

200. Richburg, J. H., Boekelheide, K., and Blanchard, K. T. (1997): The Sertoli cell as a target for toxicants. In: *Comprehensive Toxicology*, edited by K. Boekelheide, R. E. Chapin, P. B. Hoyer, and C. Harris, pp. 127–150. Elsevier Science, New York.

201. Robaire, B., Smith, S., and Hales, B. F. (1984): Suppression of spermatogenesis by testosterone in adult male rats: effect on fertility, pregnancy outcome and progeny. *Biol. Reprod.*, 31:221–230.

202. Robbins, W. A., Rubes, J., Selevan, S. G., and Perreault, S. D. (1999): Air pollution and sperm aneuploidy in health young men. *Environ. Epidemiol. Toxicol.*, 1:125–131.

203. Robl, J. M., and Dziuk, P. J. (1984): Influence of the concentration of sperm on the percentage of eggs fertilized for three strains of mice. *Gamete Res.*, 10:415–422.

204. Rogers, B. J. (1985): The sperm penetration assay: Its usefulness reevaluated. *Fertil. Steril.*, 43:821–840.

205. Rubes, J., Lowe, X., Moore, D., Perreault, S., Slott, V., Evenson, D., Selevan, S. G., and Wyrobek, A. J. (1998): Smoking cigarettes is associated with increased sperm disomy in teenage men. *Fertil. Steril.*, 70:715–723.

206. Rubin, H. B., and Henson, D. E. (1979): Effects of drugs on male sexual function. In: *Advances in Behavioral Pharmacology*, pp. 65–86. Academic Press, New York.

207. Russell, L. D. (1983): Normal testicular structure and methods of evaluation under experimental and disruptive conditions. In: *Reproductive and Developmental Toxicity of Metals*, edited by T. W. Clarkson, G. F. Nordberg, and P. R. Sager, pp. 227–252. Plenum, New York.

208. Russell, L. D., Ettlin, R., Sinha Hikim, A. P., and Clegg, E. D. (1990): *Histological and Histopathological Evaluation of the Testis*. Cache River Press, Clearwater, FL.

209. Russell, L. D., Malone, J. P., and McCurdy, D. S. (1981): Effect of microtubule disrupting agents, colchicine and vinblastine, on seminiferous tubule structure in the rat. *Tiss. Cell*, 13:349–367.

210. Savitz, D. A., Sonnenfeld, N. L., and Olshan, A. F. (1994): Review of epidemiologic studies of paternal occupational exposure and spontaneous abortion. *Am. J. Ind. Med.*, 25:361–383.

211. Schrader, S. M. (1997): Male reproductive toxicants. In: *CRC Handbook of Human Toxicology*, edited by E. J. Massaro, pp. 961–980. CRC Press, New York.

212. Schrader, S. M., Chapin, R. E., Clegg, E. D., Davis, R. O., Fourcroy, J. L., Katz, D. F., Rothmann, S. A., Toth, G., Turner, T. W., and Zinaman, M. (1992): Laboratory methods for assessing human semen in epidemiologic studies: A consensus report. *Reprod. Toxicol.*, 6:275–279.

213. Schrader, S. M., Turner, T. W., and Ratcliffe, J. M. (1988): The effects of ethylene dibromide on semen quality: A comparison of short-term and chronic exposure. *Reprod. Toxicol.*, 2:191–198.

214. Schrag, S. D., and Dixon, R. L. (1985): Reproductive effects of chemical agents. In: *Reproductive Toxicology*, edited by R. L. Dixon, pp. 301–319. Raven Press, New York.

215. Schwetz, B. A., Rao, K. S., and Park, C. N. (1980): Insensitivity of tests for reproductive problems. *J. Environ. Pathol. Toxicol.*, 3:81–98.

216. Scialli, A. R., and Clegg, E. D. (1992): *Reversibility in Testicular Toxicity Assessment*. CRC Press, Boca Raton, FL.

217. Seed, J., Chapin, R. E., Clegg, E. D., Dostal, L., Foote, R. H., Hurtt, M. E., Klinefelter, G. R., Makris, S. L., Perreault, S. D., Schrader, S., Seyler, D., Sprando, R., Treinen, K. A., Veeramachaneni, D. N. R., and Wise, L. D. (1996): Methods for assessing sperm motility, morphology, and counts in the rat, rabbit and dog: A consensus report. *Reprod. Toxicol.*, 10: 237–244.

218. Seligman, J., Kosower, N. S., and Shalgi, R. (1992): Effects of caput ligation on rat sperm and epididymis: Protein thiols and fertilizing ability. *Biol. Reprod.*, 46:301–308.

219. Sever, L. E., Arbuckle, T. E., and Sweeney, A. (1997): Reproductive and developmental effects of occupational pesticide exposure: The epidemiological evidence. *Occup. Med.*, 12: 305–325.

220. Shalgi, R. (1984): Developmental capacity of rat embryos produced by in vivo or in vitro fertilization. *Gamete Res.*, 10:77–82.

221. Sharpe, R. M., Maddocks, S., Millar, M., Kerr, J. B., Saunders, P. T. K., and McKinnell, C. (1992): Testosterone and spermatogenesis: identification of stage-specific, androgen-regulated proteins secreted by adult rat seminiferous tubules. *J. Androl.*, 13:172–184.

222. Slott, V. L., Jeffay, S. C., Dyer, C. J., Barbee, R. R., and Perreault, S. D. (1997): Sperm motion predicts fertility in male hamsters treated with alpha-chlorohydrin. *J. Androl.*, 18:708–716.

223. Slott, V. L., Jeffay, S. C., Suarez, J. D., Barbee, R. R., and Perreault, S. D. (1995): Synchronous assessment of sperm motility and fertilizing ability in the hamster following treatment with alpha-chlorohydrin. *J. Androl.*, 16:523–535.

224. Slott, V. L., and Perreault, S. D. (1993): Computer-assisted sperm analysis of rodent epididymal sperm motility using the Hamilton–Thorne motility analyzer. In: *Methods in Toxicology: Male Reproductive Toxicology*, edited by R. E. Chapin and J. J. Heindel, pp. 319–333. Academic Press, San Diego.

225. Slott, V. L., Suarez, J. D., and Perreault, S.D. (1991): Rat sperm motility analysis: Methodologic considerations. *Reprod. Toxicol.*, 5:449–458.

226. Slott, V. L., Suarez, J. D., Simmons, J. E., and Perreault, S. D. (1990): Acute inhalation exposure to epichlorohydrin transiently decreases rat sperm velocity. *Fundam. Appl. Toxicol.*, 15: 597–606.

227. Smith, M. K., Zenick, H., Preston, R. J., George, E. L., and Long, R. E. (1986): Dominant lethal effects of subchronic acrylamide administration in the male Long-Evans rat. *Mutat. Res.*, 173:273–277.

228. Somkuti, S. G., Lapadula, D. M., Chapin, R. E., and Abou-Donia, M. B. (1991): Light and electron microscopic evidence of tri-*o*-cresyl phosphate (TOCP)-mediated testicular toxicity in Fischer 344 rats. *Toxicol. Appl. Pharmacol.*, 107:35–46.

229. Stevens, K. R., and Gallo, M. A. (1989): Practical considerations in the conduct of chronic toxicity studies. In: *Principles and Methods of Toxicology*, edited by A. W. Hayes, pp. 237–250. Raven Press, New York.

230. Strader, L. F., Linder, R. E., and Perreault, S. D. (1996): Comparison of rat epididymal sperm counts by IVOS HTM-IDENT and hemacytometer. *Reprod. Toxicol.*, 10:529–533.

231. Strader, L. F., Suarez, J. D., Roberts, N. L., and Klinefelter, G. R. (1998): Spermatotoxicity of bromochloroacetic acid (BCA) in the rat after 14 daily doses. *Toxicologist*, 47:511A.

232. Sublet, V., Zenick, H., and Smith, M. K. (1989): Factors associated with reduced fertility and implantation rates in females mated to acrylamide-treated rats. *Toxicology*, 55:53–67.

233. Tanaka, S., Kawashima, K., Naito, K., Usami, M., Nakadate, M., Imaida, K., Takahashi, M., Hayashi, Y., Kurokawa, Y., and Tobe, M. (1992): Combined repeat dose and reproductive/ developmental toxicity screening test (OECD): Familiarization using cyclophosphamide. *Fundam. Appl. Toxicol.*, 18:89–95.

234. Teaf, C. M., Harbison, R. D., and Bishop, J. B. (1985): Germ cell mutagenesis and GSH depression in reproductive tissue of the F-344 rat induced by ethyl methanesulfonate. *Mutat. Res.*, 144:93–98.

235. Thomas, J. A. (1991): Toxic responses of the reproductive system. In: *Casarett and Doull's Toxicology*, edited by M. O. Amdur, J. Doull, and C. D. Klaassen, pp. 484–520. Pergamon Press, New York.

236. Thonneau, P., Marchand, S., Tallec, A., Ferial, M. L., Ducot, B., Lansac, J., Lopes, P., Tabaste, J. M., and Spira, A. (1991): Incidence and main causes of infertility in a resident population (1,850,000) of three French regions (1988–1989). *Hum. Reprod.*, 6:811–816.

237. Toppari, J., Larsen, J. C., Christiansen, P., Giwercman, A., Grandjean, P., Guillette, L. J., Jegou, B., Jensen, T. K., Jouannet, P., Keiding, N., Leffers, H., McLachlan, J. A., Meyer, O., Muller, J., Rajpert-De Meyts, E., Scheike, T., Sharpe, R., Sumpter, J., and Skakkebaek, N. (1995): Male Reproductive Health and Environmental Chemicals with Estrogenic Effects. Miljoprojekt nr. 290. Danish Environmental Protection Agency. Copenhagen.

238. Toppari, J., Larsen, J. C., Christiansen, P., Giwercman, A., Grandjean, P., Guillette, L. J., Jegou, B., Jensen, T. K., Jouannet, P., Keiding, N., Leffers, H., McLachlan, J. A., Meyer, O., Muller, J., Rajpert-De Meyts, E., Scheike, T., Sharpe, R., Sumpter, J., and Skakkebaek, N. E. (1996): Male reproductive health and environmental xenoestrogens. *Envir. Health Perspect.*, 104(suppl. 4):741–803.

239. Toth, G. P., Stober, J. A., George, E. L., Read, E. J., and Smith, M. K. (1991): Sources of variation in the computer-assisted motion analysis of rat epididymal sperm. *Reprod. Toxicol.*, 5:487–495.

240. Toth, G. P., Stober, J. A., Read, E. J., Zenick, H., and Smith, M. K. (1989): The automated analysis of rat sperm motility following subchronic epichlorohydrin administration: Methodologic and statistical considerations. *J. Androl.*, 10:401–415.

241. Toth, G. P., Stober, J. A., Zenick, H., Read, E. J., Christ, S. A., and Smith, M. K. (1991): Correlation of sperm motion parameters with fertility in rats treated subchronically with epichlorohydrin. *J. Androl.*, 12:54–61.

242. Toth, G. P., Wang, S. R., McCarthy, H., Tocco, D. R., and Smith, M. K. (1992): Effects of three male reproductive toxicants on rat cauda epididymal sperm motion. *Reprod. Toxicol.*, 6:507–515.
243. Toth, G. P., Zenick, H., and Smith, M. K. (1989): Effects of epichlorohydrin on male and female reproduction in Long-Evans rats. *Fundam. Appl. Toxicol.*, 13:16–25.
244. Trasler, J. M., Hales, B. F., and Robaire, B. (1985): Paternal cyclophosphamide treatment of rats causes fetal loss and malformations without affecting male fertility. *Nature*, 316:144–146.
245. Trasler, J. M., Hales, B. F., and Robaire, B. (1986): Chronic low dose cyclophosphamide treatment of adult male rats: effect on fertility, pregnancy outcome and progeny. *Biol. Reprod.*, 34:275–283.
246. Trasler, J. M., Hales, B. F., and Robaire, B. (1987): A time course study of paternal cyclophosphamide treatment in rats: Effects on pregnancy outcome and the male reproductive and hematologic systems. *Biol. Reprod.*, 37:317–326.
247. Treinen, K. A., and Chapin, R. E. (1991): Development of testicular lesions in F344 rats after treatment with boric acid. *Toxicol. Appl. Pharmacol.*, 107:325–335.
248. Turusov, V. S., Trukhanova, L. S., Parfenov, Y. D., and Tomatis, L. (1992): Occurrence of tumours in the descendants of CBA male mice prenatally treated with diethylstilbestrol. *Int. J. Cancer*, 50:131–135.
249. U.S. Environmental Protection Agency. (1982): Reproductive and Fertility Effects. Pesticide Assessment Guidelines, Subdivision F. Hazard Evaluation: Human and Domestic Animals. Office of Pesticides and Toxic Substances, Washington, DC. EPA-540/9-82-025.
250. U.S. Environmental Protection Agency. (1985): Toxic Substances Control Act test guidelines: Final rules. *Fed. Reg.*, 50(188): 39426–39436.
251. U.S. Environmental Protection Agency. (1986): Guidelines for mutagenicity risk assessment. *Fed. Reg.*, 51(185):34006–34012.
252. U.S. Environmental Protection Agency. (1996): Guidelines for reproductive toxicity risk assessment. *Fed. Reg.*, 61(212):56274–56322.
253. U.S. Environmental Protection Agency. (1998): OPPTS Harmonized Test Guidelines. 870.3800. Reproduction and Fertility Effects. U.S. EPA, Washington, DC.
254. U.S. Environmental Protection Agency. (1999): Endocrine Disruptor Screening and Testing Advisory Committee (EDSTAC) Final Report. Available online: http//www.epa.gov/opptendo/finalrpt.htm.
255. van der Meer, Y., Huiskamp, R., Davids, J. A. G., van der Tweel, I., and Derooij, D. G. (1992): The sensitivity of quiescent and proliferating mouse spermatogonial stem cells to x-irradiation. *Radiat. Res.*, 130:289–295.
256. van der Meer, Y., Huiskamp, R., Davids, J. A. G., van der Tweel, I., and Derooij, D. G. (1992): The sensitivity to x-rays of mouse spermatogonia that are committed to differentiate and of differentiating spermatogonia. *Radiat. Res.*, 130:296–302.
257. Wagenfeld, A., Ching-Hei, Y., Strupat, K., and Cooper, T. G. (1998): Shedding of a rat epididymal sperm protein associated with infertility induced by ornidazole and α-chlorohydrin. *Biol. Reprod.*, 58:1257–1265.
258. Waller, D. P., Killinger, J. M., and Zaneveld, L. J. D. (1985): Physiology and toxicology of the male reproductive tract. In: *Endocrine Toxicology*, edited by J. A. Thomas, K. S. Korach, and J. A. McLachlan, pp. 269–333. Raven Press, New York.
259. Weir, P. J., and Rumberger, D. (1995): Isolation of rat sperm from the vas deferens for sperm motion analysis. *Reprod. Toxicol.*, 9:327–330.
260. Williams, J., Gladen, B. C., Schrader, S. M., Turner, T. W., Phelps, J. L., and Chapin, R. E. (1990): Semen analysis and fertility assessment in rabbits: Statistical power and design considerations for toxicology studies. *Fundam. Appl. Toxicol.*, 15:651–665.
261. Williams, J., Gladen, B. C., Turner, T. W., Schrader, S. M., and Chapin, R. E. (1991): The Effects of ethylene dibromide on semen quality and fertility in the rabbit: Evaluation of a model for human seminal characteristics. *Fundam. Appl. Toxicol.*, 16:687–700.
262. Witorsch, R. J. (1995): *Reproductive Toxicology*. Raven Press, New York.
263. Working, P. K. (1989): *Toxicology of the Male and Female Reproductive Systems*. Hemisphere, New York.
264. Working, P. K., Bus, J. S., and Hamm, J., T. E. (1985): Reproductive effects of inhaled methyl chloride in the male Fischer 344 rat II. Spermatogonial toxicity and sperm quality. *Toxicol. Appl. Pharmacol.*, 77:144–157.
265. Working, P. K., Bus, J. S., and Hamm, T. E. (1985): Reproductive effects of inhaled methyl chloride in the male Fischer 344 rat. *Toxicol. Appl. Pharmacol.*, 77:133–143.
266. Working, P. K., and Hurtt, M. (1987): Computerized videomicrographic analysis of rat sperm motility. *J. Androl.*, 8:330–337.
267. World Health Organization. (1992): *WHO Laboratory Manual for the Examination of Human Semen and Sperm-Cervical Mucus Interaction*. Cambridge University Press, Cambridge.
268. Wright, W. W., Zabludoff, S. D., Erickson-Lawrence, M., and Karzai, A. W. (1989): Germ cell–Sertoli cell interactions. *Ann. NY Acad. Sci.*, 564:173–185.
269. Wyrobek, A. J., and Bruce, W. R. (1978): The induction of sperm-shape abnormalities in mice and humans. In: *Chemical Mutagens: Principles and Methods for Their Detection*, edited by A. Hollander and F. J. de Serres. Plenum Press, New York.
270. Wyrobek, A. J., Gordon, L. A., Burkhart, J. G., Francis, M. W., Kapp, R. W., Letz, G., Malling, H. V., Topham, J. C., and Whorton, D. M. (1983): An evaluation of the mouse sperm morphology test and other sperm tests in nonhuman mammals. *Mutat. Res.*, 115:1–72.
271. Wyrobek, A. J., Gordon, L. A., Burkhart, J. G., Francis, M. W., Kapp, R. W., Jr., Letz, G., Malling, H., V, Topham, J. C., and Whorton, D. M. (1983): An evaluation of human sperm as indicators of chemically induced alterations of spermatogenic function. *Mutat. Res.*, 115:73–148.
272. Wyrobek, A. J., Watchmaker, G., and Gordon, L. (1984): An evaluation of sperm tests as indicators of germ-cell damage in men exposed to chemical or physical agents. In: *Reproduction: The New Frontier in Occupational and Environmental Health Research*, edited by J. E. Lockey, G. K. Lemasters, and W. R. Keye, pp. 385–407. Alan R. Liss, New York.
273. Yeung, C. H., Oberlander, G., and Cooper, T. G. (1992): Characterization of the motility of maturing rat spermatozoa by computer-aided objective measurement. *J. Reprod. Fertil.*, 96:427–441.
274. Zack, M., Cannon, S., Lloyd, D., Heath, C. W., Falleta, J. M., Jones, B., Housworth, J., and Crowley, S. (1980): Cancer in children of parents exposed to hydrocarbon-related industries and occupations. *Am. J. Epidemiol.*, 3:329–336.
275. Zenick, H., Blackburn, K., Hope, E., and Baldwin, D. J. (1984): An assessment of the copulatory, endocrinologic, and spermatotoxic effects of carbon disulfide exposure in rats. *Toxicol. Appl. Pharmacol.*, 73:275–283.
276. Zenick, H., Blackburn, K., Hope, E., and Baldwin, D. J. (1984): Evaluating male reproductive toxicity in rodents: A new animal model. *Terat. Carcin. Mutagen.*, 4:109–128.
277. Zenick, H., and Clegg, E. D. (1986): Issues in risk assessment in male reproductive toxicology. *J. Amer. Coll. Toxicol.*, 5:249–259.

278. Zenick, H., and Goeden, H. (1987): Evaluation of copulatory behavior and sperm in rats: role in reproductive risk assessment. In: *Physiology and Toxicology of Male Reproduction*, edited by J. C. Lamb and P. M. D. Foster, pp. 174–197. Academic Press, New York.

279. Zenick, H., Hope, E., and Smith, K. (1986): Reproductive toxicity associated with acrylamide treatment in male and female rats. *J. Toxicol. Environ. Health*, 17:457–472.

280. Zinaman, M. J., Brown, C. C., Selevan, S. G., and Clegg, E. D. (2000): Semen quality and human fertility: A prospective study with normal couples. *J. Androl.*, 21:145–153.

Principles and Methods of Toxicology,
Fourth Edition, edited by A. Wallace Hayes.
Taylor & Francis, Philadelphia © 2001.

Chapter 29

Test Methods for Assessing Female Reproductive and Developmental Toxicology

Mildred S. Christian

PURPOSE

The principal subject of this chapter will be presentation of practical methods used in performing reproductive (female) and developmental toxicity studies. In general, the methods reported are those used in studies conducted for regulatory use (i.e., in the process of identifying the safe use of pharmaceuticals, chemicals, pesticides, fungicides, direct and indirect food additives, and devices). Although many additional in vitro and elegant in vivo methods exist for screening agents and to identify mechanisms, in general, the methods described in this chapter will be limited to in vivo tests conducted for regulatory use in standard laboratory species. Tests used to evaluate reproductive toxicity in male animals are addressed elsewhere in this book, as are in vitro methods used to evaluate development and in vivo behavioral/functional tests. Mechanistic studies employing biotechnology techniques and methods for identifying the pharmacodynamics and kinetics of specific exposures will be alluded to but are also described in detail in other chapters.

INTRODUCTION

Although diseases and some agents, such as alcohol, historically had been considered to possibly affect reproductive performance or a given pregnancy before 1961, human birth defects were usually considered spontaneous or hereditary events (233). Jackson's definitive 1925 review (95) of the effects of malnutrition identified potential reduction in fertility, reduced birth weight, abortion, or death of the conceptus, but not congenital malformation, as a possible outcome. The relationship of maternal measles and congenital cataracts in humans was the first disease clearly identified to affect the outcome of a human pregnancy, (73) but this causal relationship was considered unique. Only after World War II, when the effects of malnutrition in Leningrad and Holland were reported, (3,194), was it identified that maternal malnutrition could result in congenital malformations in humans as well as other unfavorable outcomes, including reproductive failure, abnormal or absent menstrual cycles, increased abortion, small birth weight, and reduced postnatal survival.

Animal research in the first half of the 20th century generally focused on enhancing the reproductive performance of animals used for food and the adverse effects of malnutrition on these animals. Although a 1921 anecdotal report identified a congenital malformation associated with maternal malnutrition (238)—rudimentary limbs in four piglets born to a sow fed a deficient diet in a study of "fat-soluble factor"—it was not until Hale's studies of vitamin A deficiency in pigs (76,77) that it was definitively demonstrated that the observed anophthalmia was associated with a maternal dietary deficiency (vitamin A). The first publications of congenital malformations in a conventional laboratory species, the rat, were issued in 1940 and 1941 by Warkany and Nelson (231,232) who were also studying agents that might affect nutrition and subsequently affect reproduction. Once it was clearly proven that mammalian maternal organisms did not prevent teratogenic effects, considerable research into teratogenic agents and susceptibility to these agents followed (233).

Regulatory research and revision and development of testing guidelines were directly related to three human tragedies that resulted from in utero exposure to a drug: (1) 1961—congenital malformations (122,123); (2) early 1970s—cancer; (85) and (3) 1976—behavioral/functional alterations (115). The first event, the thalidomide tragedy, completely changed the perception of concern regarding consumption of a medicine and the potential adverse outcomes of a pregnancy. The second event, cancer resulting from in utero exposure to diethystilbesterol (DES), raised additional concerns regarding adverse effects that were not evident until after puberty. The third, Minimata disease, resulted in addition of tests for postnatal behavioral changes to the regulations.

As the result of increased concern, including regulatory requirements, a large body of research developed investigating the morphological changes resulting from teratogenic insult during the first trimester of gestation (237); however, many investigators continued to assume that susceptibility to teratogenesis (i.e., gross anatomical malformation) was limited to the period of organogenesis (104,236). It is now clearly evident the "all or nothing" law of recovery or death does not always apply to preimplantation embryos (i.e., surviving embryos may demonstrate growth retardation, malformation, and/or functional impairment), and that the fetal and perinatal stages of development are also susceptible to toxic insult (i.e., toxic exposure may result in death, retarded growth, and/or functional impairment).

Despite theoretical and practical efforts to separate exposures and effects in the maternal animal from those of the developing conceptus, it remains axiomatic that there are three dynamic populations at risk: the male, the female, and the conceptus (30). The very existence of any given pregnancy, as well as the outcome of that pregnancy, is dependent upon dynamic complex interactive systems. As shown in Figure 29.1, each pregnancy is dependent upon the entire reproductive process, including the development, genetic makeup, and nutritional status of the parental generation, as well as the genetic makeup, nutritional status during growth and development, and exposure of the offspring to perturbations in the macro- and microenvironments. Perturbations include, but are not limited to, primary and secondary toxic effects resulting from exposures to xenobiotics. Both sensitivity and response are sex, age, dose, and tissue dependent.

NORMAL REPRODUCTION AND DEVELOPMENT

Reproduction and production of offspring can occur multiple times in an individual's life within the interval beginning at puberty and ending at reproductive senility. During this process, two haploid chromosomes, one from each sex, are joined to produce a diploid state in a new individual. One phase of the reproductive cycle is the development of a new individual, which principally occurs within the uterus of the female in most mammalian species. Development of the conceptus from the fertilized ovum to birth is a complex process during which extremely rapid cell proliferation occurs, apoptosis is normal and required, and regulatory genes produce necessary products that are associated with cancers if produced in adult life. As noted by Klinefelter and Gray (110), the multiplicity of xenobiotic exposures, lesion sites, and potential reproductive disorders precludes simple

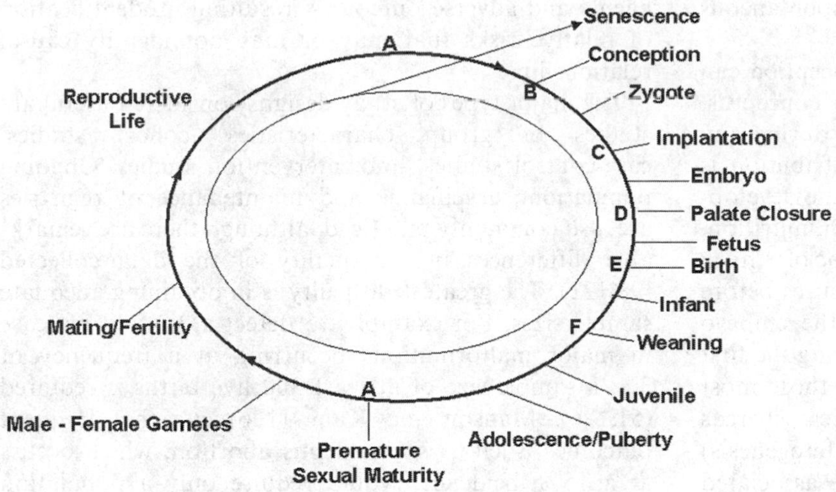

FIG. 29.1. Reproductive and developmental events.

screening of suspected reproductive toxicants in humans because the effects and the agents causing reproductive dysfunctions or altered development are often impossible to predict. The entire reproductive process is interactive, with the affected sex, organ, tissue, or cell having continually changing sensitivities in terms of the dose, duration, and timing (age) at insult (prenatal, in utero, and postnatal), and involves interactions of male and female animals and maternal animals and developing individuals.

Normal Reproductive Performance

As described later, under normal conditions, a high proportion of the population of all species, including humans, has remarkable reproductive and developmental risks; many couples are infertile, and spontaneous abortions are frequent in humans. Infertility occurs in approximately 11 million married couples in the United States, with noncontraceptive sterility occurring in at least one of the partners in 3 million of these couples (145); ovulatory problems have been reported to be the cause of infertility in approximately 40% of all infertile couples (198). Hertig (86) estimated that as many as 50% of all fertilized ova are lost within the first three weeks of human development. In 1970, the World Health Organization (238) estimated that 15% of all clinically recognizable pregnancies end in a spontaneous abortion and that 50–60% of the spontaneously aborted fetuses have chromosomal abnormalities (12,191). Prematurity occurs in approximately 7% of births (i.e., birth before the 37th week of gestation), and the most common developmental abnormality in humans is low birth weight (2.5 kg or less) (90,155), a finding often associated with functional/neurological defects and malformations. Of approximately 3 million liveborn infants annually, 13.1 per 1000 die before 1 year of age (151), and 2–3% of these liveborn infants are identified to have a congenital malformation within the first year postnatal (51,83). Although technical improvements for identifying defects will increase this number, based on the current relatively crude criteria, approximately 16% of live births have major or minor malformations that become apparent after the first year (35).

The cause of approximately 65%–75% of human congenital malformations is unknown (23,64,15,17,83). During the early 1900s, genetic causes were believed to be the predominant cause, with the remaining birth defects unsolved clinical problems. In 1976, Fraser (62) published the multifactorial/threshold hypothesis, which involved modulation of a continuum of genetic characteristics by intrinsic and extrinsic (environmental) factors. Modulating factors include, but are not limited to, placental blood flow, placental transport, site of implantation, maternal disease states, infections, drugs, chemicals, and spontaneous errors of development. Presently, genetic causes may continue to predominate, if Fraser's multifactorial/threshold hypothesis is modified to altered genetic expression and interaction of environmental factors, although the three traditional categories for the etiology of congenital malformations (i.e., unknown, genetic, and environmental factors) continue to be used. A large proportion of these congenital malformations is likely to be due to two or more genetic loci (23,124), or are polygenetic. Those with an increased recurrent risk (e.g., cleft lip and palate, anencephaly, spina bifida, certain congenital heart diseases, pyloric stenosis, hypospadias, inguinal hernia, talipes equinovarus, congenital dislocation of the hip) can be categorized as multifactorial disease, as well as polygenic inherited disease (23,62). Some malformations are probably spontaneous errors of development, without apparent abnormalities of the genome or environmental influence, similar to the concept of spontaneous mutations (62,14).

A mutation in either germ cell before conception can result in chromosome abnormalities in the conceptus. Mutations in the conceptus can also occur during any given pregnancy. The maternal genetic contribution is known to provide a greater contribution to the development of the embryo, although maternal health, nutrition, and toxic exposures can also affect the outcome of a given pregnancy. With few exceptions, toxic exposures before implantation generally result in death of the embryo or no observable effect. Toxic exposures during the first trimester of pregnancy (embryogenesis) are those most likely to produce gross morphological changes, whereas those during later stages of pregnancy (fetogenesis) and postpartum are those more likely to be associated with retarded growth, functional alterations, and reduced capacity of the various systems, including the cardiovascular, endocrine, reproductive, pulmonary, central nervous system (CNS), urinary tract, gastrointestinal, and immune systems (99,100,28,31,105,184, 64,154). Thus, the development of an organism is a life-long cycle characterized by changes in size, biochemistry, physiology, form, and functionality (108,102, 178).

Human Epidemiology Studies

Epidemiology has the potential to play central and imperative roles regarding identifying how developmental and reproductive toxicology affects human populations. This is particularly apparent when one considers that regardless of the results of studies in animals, for the purpose of human reproductive and developmental risks, the human is the ultimate species of interest (16). As noted by Erickson (54), several inherent problems exist in performing human epidemiology studies. First, they are time consuming and expensive, especially when dealing with rare disease states, as are most conditions that could conceivably result from reproductive or developmental toxicity. Second, reported findings are often based on anecdotal information, and logically, it is essentially impossible to prove the absence of an association. Third, studies may be either experimental (interventional) or observational, and the more scientifically useful type, interventional, are essentially precluded by ethical concerns that disallow direct testing of women of child-bearing potential. Thus, epidemiology studies in the area of reproduction and development usually are observational, (i.e., evaluation of events in two groups without intervention or random assignment of subjects to treatments). As a result, epidemiology studies usually involve statistical analyses of medical data to identify associations between toxic agents and adverse outcomes, resulting in identification of relative risks that may or may not identify causal relationships.

The major types of study designs considered useful are studies of group characteristics, cohort studies, case-control studies, and intervention studies. Ongoing population surveillance and maintenance of registries are also commonly practiced, although there are remarkable differences in the quality of the data collected (98,121). The greatest difficulty is in obtaining adequate sample sizes. For example, to detect a 3.2-fold increase in major malformations occurring at a frequency of 3%, a sample size of at least 300 live births is required (51,126). Manson and Kang (126) cite that frequent outcomes, such as spontaneous abortion, which occurs at a 15% incidence, would require only a population of 50 pregnancies to detect a three-fold increase. The importance of perceived risk versus actual risk is evident for the most well-studied risk of human exposure, environmental radiation. Despite well-characterized risks of exposure to environmental radiation (18), the perceived risk of any exposure remains high, perpetuating the nonscientific approach often taken regarding potential adverse effects of exposure to any agent during pregnancy. Thus, because of the difficulties and complexities associated with human clinical and epidemiological studies and the desire to prevent potential human exposures to agents at levels producing adverse effects, animal studies are those most frequently used to detect potential reproductive or developmental toxicants. Such studies are, for the most part, the subject of this chapter.

FEMALE REPRODUCTIVE TOXICOLOGY

Maturation of the Female Reproductive System

Gametogenesis and Ovulation

Each sex (male and female) of most multicellular animals produces specialized cells (gametes), which are joined (fertilization) to form a new individual (zygote/conceptus). The mammalian ovulatory cycle includes multiple interrelated events involving folliculogenesis, ovulation, and preparation of the reproductive tract for fertilization and implantation leading to pregnancy. Ovulation is the central event in the ovulatory cycle (13).

Ovulation results from interaction of multiple feedback systems, including the diencephalon and especially the hypothalamic regions, the anterior pituitary, and the ovary. The hypothalamus releases gonadotropin hormone-releasing hormone (GnRH), and through this process regulates anterior pituitary production and

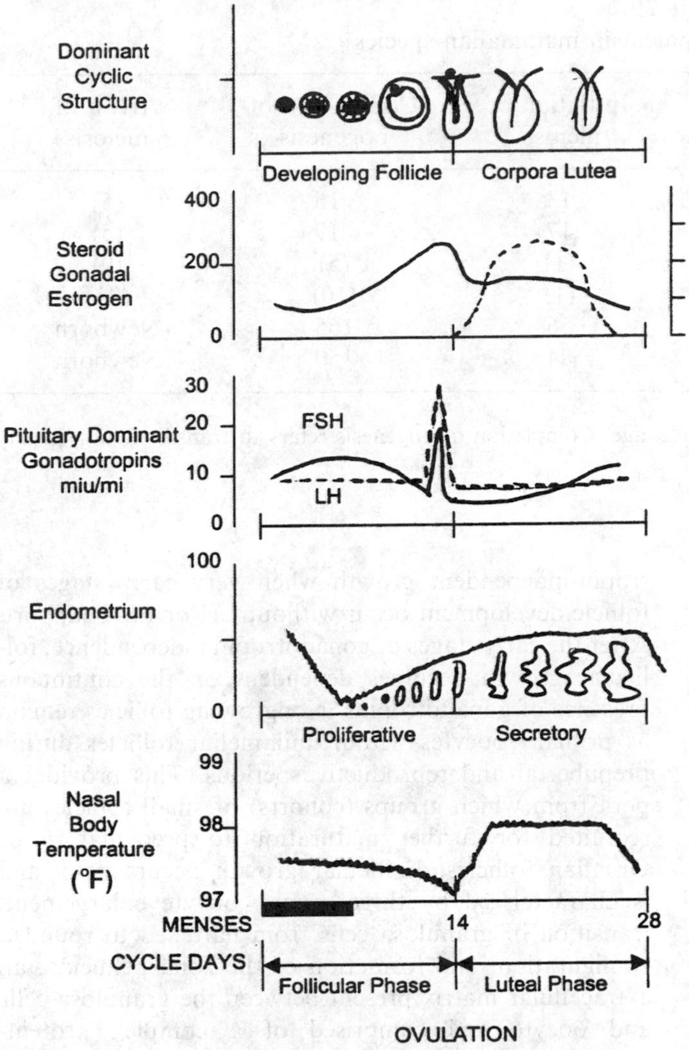

FIG. 29.2. Progression of ovulatory cycle in humans. Development of the dominant follicle of pituitary gonadotropins, endometrial proliferation, and basal body temperature are depicted. Adapted from References 79 and 129.

secretion of gonadotropin hormones, including luteinizing hormone (LH) and follicle-stimulating hormone (FSH). LH and FSH released from the anterior pituitary and transported to the ovary initiate and maintain ovarian follicle growth. Figure 29.2 demonstrates the progression of the ovulatory cycle in humans.

The initial phase of positive feedback is that in which the hypothalamic-anterior pituitary axis component signals the ovary to initiate growth of the follicles. Phase two of the cascade is initiated by the mature ovarian follicle, which signals readiness to ovulate through production and secretion of estradiol and progesterone. Estradiol and progesterone secreted by the ovary initiate a surge of GnRH, which is followed by a surge of the ovulating-inducing hormones, LH and FSH, which provide the stimulus initiating the cascade of events in the ovary ultimately resulting in ovulation (13).

Ovulation of a fertilizable ovum (oocyte, egg, or female gamete) requires formation of a *corpus luteum* and growth, maturation, and differentiation of three cell types. Each of these three cell types, the germ cell (oocyte), granulosa cells, and thecal endocrine cells, are susceptible to toxic effects, as also are the three major processes that occur during development of the mature oocyte: (1) mitosis of oogonia and granulosa cells during follicular growth; (2) meiosis of oogonia to form oocytes; and (3) differentiation of granulosa cells and theca cells, allowing response to a surge of luteinizing hormone (LH) and subsequent ovulation.

The inseparability of the reproductive process and development of the conceptus is most apparent when one considers that the female germ cells and follicles are formed during prenatal life. Primordial germ cells are first detectable in the yolk sac at 3 weeks of human development. These cells undergo mitosis, migrate to the urogenital ridge, populate the indifferent gonad, and then differentiate into oogonia or prespermatogonia. Approximately 1700 germ cells migrate to the gonads in a human embryo. These increase to approximately 600,0000 germ cells by 2 months of gestation and peak

Table 29.1
Ovarian germ cell development in mammalian species

Species	Days of gestation	Gonadal sex differentiation	Initiation of meiosis	Completion of oogenesis	Arrest of meiosis
Mice	19	12	13	16	(5)
Rats	21	13–14	17	19	(5)
Hamsters	16	11–12	(1)	(5)	(9)
Rabbits	31	15–16	(1)	(10)	(21)
Monkeys (rhesus)	165	38	56	165	Newborn
Humans	270	40–42	84	150	Newborn

Numbers in parentheses indicate days of gestation or postnatal age. Completion of oogenesis refers to transformation of all oogonia to primary oocytes.
Adapted from References 71 and 126.

at approximately 7,000,000 germ cells by 5 months of gestation. Oogonia begin to enter meiosis at month 3, with all oogonia in early prophase I by the end of month 5, at which time the oogonia are termed primary oocytes (71). From this point onward, atresia results in decline of oocyte numbers to less than 1,000,000 by birth, with continued reductions in numbers throughout the remainder of the reproductive life of the woman through atresia and ovulation (13).

There are four stages of meiotic divisions: prophase, metaphase, anaphase, and telophase. The first meiotic division (prophase) occurs during the fetal or neonatal period. Within 8 weeks after birth, human oocytes enter a resting phase (diakinesis) in which they stay until puberty begins (10). Sex differentiation and ovarian germ cell development occurs at different developmental ages in various mammalian species, as shown in Table 29.1.

Atresia

As noted previously, the majority of germ cells are lost to normal, physiological degeneration (atresia), which occurs during the oogonial and primary oocyte stages. Approximately 60% of the germ cells in a human fetus are lost between 5 months of gestation and birth, with three distinct waves of oogonial degeneration occurring. One wave affects oogonia in mitosis (final interphase), and the other two affect oocytes in the pachytene and diplotene stages of prophase I. This normal apoptosis is synchronous in oogonia connected by cytoplasmic bridges. After the meiotic prophase, simultaneous atresia no longer occurs, although individual oocytes spontaneously degenerate at all stages of development.

Folliculogenesis

Surviving oocytes in prophase are surrounded by granulosa cells and begin to form follicles (folliculogenesis). Initially there is a period of gonadotropin-independent growth when very early stages of follicle development occur without LH or FSH support. After the early stages of gonadotropin independence, follicular growth becomes dependent on the continuous presence of gonadotropins. Nongrowing follicles remain as primary oocytes within unilamellar follicles during prepubertal and reproductive periods. This provides a pool from which groups (cohorts) of small follicles are recruited for further maturation to preovulatory or Graafian follicles. Follicular growth occurs daily and is characterized by three events: oocyte enlargement, transition of granulosa cells from flattened to rounded configuration, and formation of the zona pellucida, an extracellular matrix present between the granulosa cells and oocyte and comprised of a complex protein-carbohydrate extracellular matrix. The first stage is characteristic of small type 2 follicles (167) that enter the pool of committed growing follicles. What triggers follicular growth remains unidentified, although it is known that follicle-stimulating hormone (FSH) and luteinizing hormone (LH) are not involved (174). Follicle growth requires five events: continued oocyte enlargement; rapid proliferation and increase in layers of granulosa cells; formation of basal lamina (extracellular matrix external to outer layer of granulosa cells); organization of endocrine thecal cells around a basal lamina; and formation of the antrum (fluid-filled cavity within the follicle). The majority of type 2 follicles grow into the preantral stage (Type 5–6). A large surge of gonadotropins in the cycle preceding ovulation results in selection of a few type 7–8 follicles (antral stage) from a pool of large preantral follicles.

The preovulatory surge in gonadotrophin includes the increase in LH, which stimulates conversion of progesterone to androstenedione in theca cells (175), which is then converted to estradiol in granulosa cells. The estradiol secreted by the growing follicles, in conjunction with FSH, effects differentiation of granulosa cells. Differentiation of the granulosa cells includes increased cellular content of FSH and LH receptors, increased aromatase activity, cholesterol side chain cleavage, and prostaglandin synthetase activity (174,175), which regulates the synthesis of the prostaglandins required for ovulation. Only follicles that can produce estradiol progress to preovulatory follicles. It should be noted that this scheme is well established in the rat ovary, but there is some question as to the importance of estrogen in proliferation of granulosa cells in the primate ovary (13). Atresia can be induced by any agent that inhibits either theca cell function (ability to synthesize androstenedione) or granulosa cell function (synthesis and action of estradiol). Atresia may also be caused by agents that alter gonadotropin receptor content or the functional coupling of the receptor to adenylate cyclase because FSH and LH act via cycle adenosine monophosphate (AMP).

After the rise in FSH and LH, primary oocytes in preovulatory follicles continue to form secondary oocytes through the first meiotic division and remain in metaphase of the second division. The first polar body, containing half of the chromosomes that were present in the primary oocyte, is extruded. In addition, as ovulation nears, the follicle vascularizes and swells on the ovary's surface, becoming a macroscopically visible blister-like protuberance. The secondary oocyte is ovulated at metaphase II and stays in this stage until fertilization. At fertilization, the second meiotic division is completed, the second polar body extruded, and the female pronucleus formed. Male and female pronuclei combine at fertilization to regain the diploid state (55).

Fertilization

Fertilization (union of a spermatozoon or "sperm" and an oocyte, or "egg") occurs in the female reproductive tract in birds and mammals. Restoring the diploid number of chromosomes, determines the genetic sex of the zygote and initiates cleavage (rapid mitotic division). It should be noted that maternal and paternal genomes are not functionally equivalent in their contributions to the zygotic genome due to imprinting. The process of imprinting occurs during gametogenesis, conferring differential expressivity to certain allelic genes, depending on whether they originate from the male or the female (78). Although imprinting is not well understood and there are no documented examples of toxicant effects on this process, such could conceivably play a role in paternally mediated developmental toxicity.

Implantation/Luteinization

Following ovulation, vascularization of the granulosa cell layer occurs and granulosa cells are transformed into luteal cells, which produce the progesterone required for preparation of the endometrial lining of the uterus for implantation of the conceptus (79). In the absence of fertilization, luteinization occurs. This process includes degeneration of the ovulated oocyte, continued LH stimulation, and luteinizing of the empty follicle into a corpus luteum, which secretes progesterone. The process continues to occur throughout reproductive life until all primordial follicles are depleted or menopause occurs.

Corpus Luteum

The function of the *corpus luteum* is dependent on LH, and withdrawal of LH leads to luteal failure, decreased estrogen and progesterone secretion, and failure to maintain the pregnancy. In a normal cycle without fertilization, corpus luteal failure occurs after approximately 10 days of functioning. This failure is believed to be associated with an increase in activity of prostaglandin $F_{2\alpha}$ ($PGF_{2\alpha}$) (63). $PGF_{2\alpha}$ is produced by the uterus in some animals, but the importance of endogenous prostaglandin from the uterus in the primate uterus has not been established, although exogenously administered $PGF_{2\alpha}$ is luteolytic in primates. When the oocyte is fertilized, the *corpus luteum* is maintained by secretion of human chorionic gonadotropin (HCG), which is an LH-like molecule synthesized by the trophoblastic tissue of the embryo. Under HCG stimulation, progesterone synthesis continues in the *corpus luteum* until this steroid is principally produced by the placenta. The *corpus luteum* also provides an important source of relaxin, oxytocin, GnRH-related molecules, and growth factors that function in pregnancy and parturition (13).

Ovulatory Cycles

Ovulatory cycles differ between laboratory animals, farm animals, nonhuman primates and humans (13), and even among humans (84,207). Two major categories exist: animals with spontaneous ovulation and animals with ovulation induced by mating. Spontaneous ovulators include laboratory rats, hamsters, mice, guinea pigs, sheep, pigs, rhesus monkeys, humans, and baboons, with cycle lengths ranging from 3–33 days. Rats, hamsters, and mice develop a functional *corpus luteum* only if mated, with vaginal stimulation resulting in pseudopregnancy or pregnancy. The remaining species always form an active *corpus luteum* that secretes progestoerone and is functional for 10–15 days. Reflex or induced ovulators include rabbits, cats, ferrets, short-tailed shrews, and voles. Mechanical or coital stimulation in these species results in a gonadotropin surge (primarily LH) within 1–2 h that results in ovulation of follicles that have reached maturity in the ovary. The FSH secreted in the surge may result in development of new ovarian follicles for estradiol production, which is essential for *corpus luteum* function.

At least two other neuroendocrine signals are important in regulating spontaneous ovulatory cycles, circadian rhythms in the gonadotropin surge, and seasonal variation. Humans and guinea pigs appear to be the species least affected by circadian rhythms and seasonal variations, although some circadian variations in LH levels have been reported in women during the follicular phase of the cycle (13). In rats, the suprachiasmatic nucleus (SCN) in the hypothalamus is identified as the site of signal transduction by light-dark cycles, and lesioning of this site or exposure to constant light terminates the estrous cycle. Seasonal reproduction is also known to be associated with the duration of the photoperiod, and for most laboratory species, a minimum of 10 h of light is required for reproduction to occur. In addition, diet, in particular, phytoestrogen content, is known to affect ovulatory cycles and fertility (phytoestrogens are naturally occurring diphenols found in many plants and have structural and functional similarities to 17β-estradiol) (84,111,112).

Ovarian Toxicology

During each menstrual cycle in humans, oocyte maturation, folliculogenesis, ovulation, and *corpus luteum* formation occurs. These processes are under the influence of gonadotropins that act on the ovarian cells to initiate morphologic changes, steroidogenesis, and induction of various receptors. Many of these events also occur in rodents, although factors other than gonadotropins appear to be involved in the initial stimulation of growth of the resting follicle; however, once the follicle is committed to growth, selection of antral, preovulatory follicles depends on the LH surge preceding the cycle (126).

Evaluation of follicular alterations is difficult because a sexually mature ovary contains a diverse population of resting, maturing, and mature follicles, and the female has only one cluster of follicles that is selected for maturation in each cycle. In addition, the oogonia enter meiosis during fetal life, after a specified number of mitotic divisions, and there is no mechanism to replace oocytes. Thus, the presence of reduced numbers of oocytes, which may occur in the fetus or result from subsequent destruction, has the potential to reduce reproductive life in the female. If the oocytes are subject to irreversible DNA damage, mutagenic manifestations may occur if the damaged oocyte is fertilized. During adulthood, each of the three components of the follicle may be uniquely susceptible to specific toxicants (129,131). For example, a xenobiotic agent might increase the progesterone/estradiol or testosterone/estradiol ratios in the granulosa cell stimulated by FSH or alter steroidogenesis and androgen production by the thecal cells, thus delaying follicle maturation and ovulation. DNA in the oocyte can be damaged during maturation and fertilization of the oocyte, depending upon the agent (68), and such damage is the probable mechanism by which antineoplastic agents deplete the oocyte pool and result in premature menopause in women (129).

Reproductive Endocrinology and Toxicologic Interactions

Interaction of Reproductive Hormones and Target Tissues

Estrogens increase oviduct secretions and muscular contractions, actions antagonized by progesterone. Thus, cyclic patterns of estrogen and progesterone levels that occur during the menstrual cycle in primates and humans play important roles in regulating sperm transport through the cervix, into the uterine lumen, and to the oviduct (120). Of 150–300 million sperm in an ejaculation, less than 500 reach the site of fertilization, with the greatest obstacle to sperm transport being the cervix and uterotubal junction, where most sperm loss occurs. Mammalian sperm undergo changes in the female reproductive tract to allow penetration of the ovum. This change, or capacitation, is normally induced by secretions in the female genital tract and requires one to several hours for completion. Capacitated sperm penetrate the layers of the granulosa cells and bind to a major glycoprotein (ZP3) in the zona pellucida, which is the main barrier to fertilization in mammals. Sperm binding to ZP3 induces the acrosomal reaction, releasing proteases and hyaluronidase, which are essential enzymes for sperm penetration of the zona. After penetration, contact of the sperm and oocyte membrane triggers the cortical reaction in the egg, releasing enzymes that act on the zona and oocyte membrane to prevent further binding and entry of sperm (120).

After fertilization, the ovum divides and slowly moves down the oviduct. Decreased motility in the oviduct is associated with rising progesterone levels secreted by the *corpus luteum* and prevents the ovum from prematurely reaching the uterus. Estrogen treatment during ovum migration accelerates movement of the embryo, resulting in the ovum reaching the uterus prematurely. This occurs with use of the "morning-after" pill, in which a synthetic estrogen, diethylstilbestrol (DES), is administered for five days. Similar effects have been observed with agents, such as methoxychlor, which mimic estrogens (34,45). Before implantation, which begins on day 7 and is completed on day 12 in humans, (timing differs slightly among species and strains [66]), the embryo floats free in the uterus, nourished by endometrial gland secretions, controlled by progesterone. Combined estrogen and progesterone action result in the uterine endometrium preparing for implantation of the blastocyst and the embryo invading the uterine endometrium. Implantation triggers a decidualization reaction in several rodent species ("placental sign") when the uterine stromal cells are actively converted to decidual cells. In humans, decidualization of the uterine lining normally occurs during the luteal phase of the menstrual cycle, whether or not implantation occurs. Decidualization of the uterine lining contributes the maternal portion of the placenta (120).

Estrogen and progesterone synthesis and secretion during normal human pregnancy are a cooperative effect of the mother, fetus, and placenta. Extremely large amounts of estrogens (estradiol, estrone, estriol) are produced during pregnancy, with the placenta being the primary source. Estriol excretion is a biomarker used to monitor fetal well-being because one of the precursors for estriol synthesis by the placenta is dehydroepiandrosterone, which is produced by the fetal adrenal gland (49). In addition, the placenta can synthesize estrogens de novo, although the exact role of the high levels of estrogen present during pregnancy is unclear (190).

Hormonal Interaction with the Placenta

The placenta also secretes human placental lactogen (HPL), which is similar to human growth hormone and human prolactin, does not appear to promote body growth, may be involved in fetal nutrition, and is probably involved in preparation of the mammary gland for lactation. This protein usually appears in the blood approximately 2 months after fertilization, increases until parturition, and provides a biomarker to monitor placental size and growth during pregnancy (204,120).

Mammary Development during Pregnancy

Mammary development in women is controlled by prolactin, which is secreted by the anterior pituitary gland. Prolactin levels increase during pregnancy from about 2 months after fertilization until parturition (120). Although the role of prolactin during pregnancy is unclear, it probably contributes to the profound mammary development that occurs during pregnancy.

Parturition

The exact mechanisms that initiate parturition in humans are unknown; however, most current evidence suggests that estrogen, progesterone, oxytocin, and prostaglandins may all be involved (25,195). Estrogen and oxytocin stimulate uterine contractility, which increases and becomes more coordinated as labor approaches. Progesterone antagonizes the effects of progesterone and oxytocin, and declining levels of progesterone may trigger initiation of uterine contractions, although peripheral progesterone concentrations do not fall before the onset of labor. It is hypothesized that a fall in tissue levels of progesterone could occur before detection of peripheral changes, and that local prostaglandin production may also be involved in initiating labor by direct or indirect means (25).

The role of oxytocin in labor is also unclear, although it is important once labor begins. Stretching of the uterine cervix and vagina stimulates reflex release of oxytocin from the posterior pituitary, resulting cyclically in increased uterine contractions and stretching, facilitating the delivery process. The increase in oxytocin receptors near term may be the cause of the increased sensitivity of the myometrial response to oxytocin (197). Physical factors also regulate myometrial activity in the human, of which the increase in uterine volume associated with fetal and placental growth resulting in stimulation of myometrial contractions, and the inhibition of myometrial contractions by progesterone, are the most important. Estrogens, oxytocin, and $PGF_{2\alpha}$ are stimulatory hormones additionally contributing to uterine contractility. They are inhibited by progesterone, which blocks estrogen action, oxytocin receptor production, and prostaglandin release. Autonomic innervation also contributes to increased or inhibited myometrial activity. Drugs, such as alcohol, can directly act on uterine smooth muscle or indirectly inhibit oxytocin release (120).

In summary, parturition in humans usually is effected by three major factors: myometrial stretch, maturation of the fetal adrenal gland, and sensitivity to oxytocin. Maturation of the fetal adrenal gland late in pregnancy causes increased secretion of cortisol, promoting myometrial contractility. Myometrial contractile activity is also stimulated by stretching of the uterine smooth muscle fibers as the result of growth of the fetus and placenta and by increased sensitivity to oxytocin as the result of increased numbers of oxytocin receptors.

Lactation

Various hormones also modulate the development and secretory capacity of the mammary gland. Prolactin is the primary hormone responsible for mammary growth. Estrogen works indirectly on the mammary gland via promoting prolactin synthesis and secretion by the anterior pituitary. Gonadotrophin hormones are also involved in that they stimulate ovarian estrogen secretion. Estrogens also directly stimulate mammary gland growth, but only in the presence of prolactin. Development of the breast is a major event at the onset of puberty; milk secretion usually is not initiated until after parturition and is inhibited by estrogen and progesterone secreted by the placenta, antagonizing prolactin's ability to stimulate milk secretion (97). Estrogens are the primary ovarian hormones responsible for mammary gland development and growth, although progesterone is important for alveolar development in some animals; however, there is no evidence that progesterone is required for alveolar development in humans (208). The milk secretion stimulatory effect of prolactin is different from prolactin's growth-promoting effects. Initiation of lactation normally involves withdrawal of an estrogen and progesterone block to the stimulatory effect of prolactin on milk secretion (120).

Milk secretion is initiated by suckling of the nipple; continued secretion requires continued suckling stimulus and the associated rapid release of prolactin from the pituitary gland. The prolactin release as the result of suckling does not cause the milk release at the time of suckling, but it is responsible for release of milk (milk letdown) during the subsequent nonsuckling interval. The young obtain this milk at the next suckling. Normal milk secretion also requires other hormones, including ACTH, provided the adrenals are intact. Insulin, growth hormone, parathyroid hormone, and thyroid hormones are also interactive stimulators of milk secretion (208). Milk letdown at suckling is a phenomenon affected by the suckling-induced release of oxytocin and contraction of the myoepithelial cells (97). In humans, this is a conditioned reflex that can be effected as a response to the presence or crying of a baby. Release of oxytocin apparently can be inhibited by higher levels of the CNS because emotional disturbances or pain during nursing reduces milk release.

Both LH and FSH secretion are reduced during lactation, apparently as the result of suckling (125), and lactating women may have a diminished response to GnRH, which suggests that the inhibition occurs at the level of the pituitary. The ovaries also seem refractory to gonadotropic stimulation during lactation, although the mechanisms resulting in lactational amenorrhea are not currently understood.

Several conditions are known to result in abnormal lactation associated with increased prolactin levels. For example, pituitary tumors can cause this effect as the result of increased prolactin levels. Hypothalamic lesions, abnormal afferent neural input into the hypothalamus, and tranquilizers can also raise prolactin secretion sufficiently to result in galactorrhea (97).

Test Systems and Endpoints for Detection of Toxic Effects on Female Reproductive Capacity

Ovarian Cyclicity

Despite the commonality of many features of ovarian cyclicity in humans and rodents, distinct differences exist that should be considered in designing toxicologic studies (110). For example, in most mammals, follicular growth continues through the luteal phase. Luteolysis is believed to be mediated by uterine prostaglandins in rats and nonhuman primates. In human females, follicular growth does not continue through the luteal phase, and estrogen, rather than prostaglandins, appears to be the luteolytic agent (110). Elger et al. (53) notes other important differences among species, including maintenance of progesterone production by the *corpora lutea* throughout pregnancy in the rat, whereas in humans and guinea pigs, placental progesterone contributes significantly to maintenance of pregnancy during mid and late gestation. In rats, progesterone levels must be remarkably reduced to induce parturition, whereas humans and guinea pigs have high progesterone levels until parturition. In rats, deciduoma formation is highly dependent on a correct progesterone/estrogen ratio, and abortion occurs when the serum estrogen level is increased, whereas humans and guinea pigs are estrogen-resistant. In contrast, prostaglandins have abortifacient properties in humans and guinea pigs. Thus, the hormonal similarities between guinea pigs and humans, in addition to the greater similarities in timing of fetal in utero development, suggests that the guinea pig may be a better model for human risk assessment than the rat, although this model has not been as extensively studied as the rat for evaluations of toxic effects in mid and late pregnancy.

Normal ovarian function is predicted based on appropriate interaction of various compartments of the ovary and the changes that occur in these individual compartments during the cycle. In vivo adverse effects may result from active intermediates or metabolites or through modulation of the hypothalamic-pituitary axis; such effects would not be identified by in vitro assays. In addition, in vitro screening techniques are appealing for use in assessment of effects on the ovary; effects identified in in vitro systems must be confirmed using in vivo methods.

Reproductive Behavior

Female reproductive behavior in vertebrates is dependent on the ovarian hormones, estrogen and progestins (8,237). A plethora of normal, neural and molecular mechanisms for female reproductive behaviors in the rat have been widely investigated, and on this basis, the rat is frequently considered the best model system to study CNS function and behavioral development. Unfortunately, little is known about the role of these processes in human and nonhuman primate reproductive behaviors.

Although not the model most used for basic research, female monkeys show clear changes in behavior during the menstrual cycle and following injection of steroid hormones. Copulation in nonhuman primates is restricted to the periovulation period. Similar findings have not been made in women, although the absence of clear findings may reflect methodological problems inherent in the conduct of such studies (169). It can be assumed that steroid hormone behavioral mechanisms are present in humans; however, other social and environmental factors appear to be more important. Humans clearly have sexual behaviors that begin and are dependent on steroid hormone secretion during puberty, and perceptual and sensory behaviors vary within the menstrual cycle (65), as well as the susceptibility to irritability, anxiety, and depression during the premenstrual period (180). Although it has been reported that women exposed to DES prenatally had reduced female sexual behavior (136), and that some masculization of girls can be induced by androgens prenatally (52), these studies remain equivocal.

Maternal behaviors are also hormonally dependent in the rat but have not been well investigated in nonhuman primates, although steroid hormones may facilitate maternal responsiveness to alien newborns in monkeys (156). The early postpartum period in humans is known to be an interval with emotional alterations in many women and severe disturbances in some women (181). Human and rodent studies suggest that serum prolactin may affect postpartum hostility (156).

Alteration of Hypothalmic-Pituitary Axis/Ovarian Feedback

As is evident in Table 29.2, effects on female reproduction generally are studied by evaluation of many endpoints also examined in developmental toxicity. Toxic effects may be produced by targeting the hypothalamic pituitary axis, the ovary, or any point in the complex feedback system. Examples of some agents known to adversely affect female reproductive performance are cited in Table 29.3.

Altered hypothalamic and pituitary secretions have been demonstrated to adversely affect fertility and estrous cyclicity in female rats (110). The mechanism by which such effects can occur can sometimes be identified through the use of in vitro perfusion systems. These can be used to evaluate specific functions of an organ system independently from other endocrine organs and sometimes provide less variable data. For example, Middleton et al. (138) demonstrated inhibition of ovarian estradiol synthesis by R151775, a triazole fungicide, with resultant delay in the LH surge and ovulation. Further study of this fungicide by Milne et al. (140) found that pituitaries from rats treated at midday on diestrus 2 had LH production after GnRH stimulation. This chemical was later identified as an aromatase inhibitor, preventing ovarian synthesis of estradiol (110).

Ovarian Morphometry

Ovarian compartments likely to be affected by xenobiotic exposure and of interest include oocyte number and follicular development, ovulation, estrous cycling, fertility, and maintenance of pregnancy. Models used to evaluate dose- and stage-dependent, as well as age-dependent, effects of xenobiotic exposures of the ovary generally use morphometry, which can be performed either as part of general toxicity evaluations or within the framework of the reproductive toxicity studies. Although the original methods were extremely time consuming and required that serial sections of the ovary are made and numbers of follicles (170) or oocyte size (192) be evaluated, current screening methods generally are restricted to every 10th or 20th section.

Corpora Lutea Count and Preimplantation Loss

Evidence of toxic activity at the ovarian level in in vivo studies is most frequently based on identification of reduced numbers of *corpora lutea*, often in combination with preimplantation loss, although these methods are not appropriate or equivalent for all species. An example of the complex nature of the ovarian endpoints is provided below regarding calculation of preimplantation loss in developmental toxicity studies in rabbits and in Table 29.4.

Preimplantation loss reflects the number of eggs ovulated, fertilized, and implanted, as well as the receptivity of the uterus. Rabbits are reflex (induced) ovulators, requiring stimulation of the cervix, which is essentially absent when artificial insemination procedures are used for breeding, and an intravenous injection of human chorionic gonadotropin (HCG) is generally administered to compensate for reduced natural cervical stimulation during mating (HCG injection is less frequently used in natural mating practices). Artificial insemination procedures result in greater variability in ovulation, numbers of *corpora lutea*, and preimplantation loss values than natural mating because of several factors.

First, release of ova depends on the number of mature follicles present when ovulation is induced by the stimulation of mating (natural mating) or injected HCG. One major consequence of HCG priming of the female is the possibility of "superovulation" (i.e., a large number of eggs ovulated), including ones not completely mature, and subsequent inability of these eggs to be fertilized

Table 29.2
Scheme for identifying effects on female reproductive process

Step	Treatment	Activity	Potential adverse effects examples
1	Pretreatment—14 days	Identify estrous cycling	Abnormal cycling—if incidence abnormally high, consider adverse environmental factors
2	Treatment—14 days precohabitation	Identify estrous cycling	Altered from pretreatment; assume hormonal changes
3	Treatment through cohabitation and gestation	Cohabit females with untreated males (1 : 1). Observe mating behavior (receptivity) and fertility (persistent diestrus, sperm in smear or plug; sperm/plug = day 0 of gestation—GD 0)	Reduced or absent copulatory behavior Irregular estrous cycling
4	Treatment through day before killed	Kill $\frac{1}{2}$ of pregnant animals/group at GD 21 (preselect, to preclude biasing results based on mating performance). Observe for gross lesions, corpora lutea, pregnancy, implantation numbers, early and late resorptions and live and dead fetuses, fetal body weights, and sexes.	Reduced corpora lutea, implantation sites, and/or live fetuses (timing indicates when effect occurred); reduced fetal body weight; altered sex ratios
5	Treatment through delivery and lactation	Allow remaining $\frac{1}{2}$ of animals in group to deliver. Observe durations of gestation and parturition, maternal behavior peripartum, pup number, viability, body weight, sex, and morphology at birth; pup viability, growth, clinical signs and interaction with dam to weaning, maternal implantation sites, and gross lesions.	Reduced implantation sites; altered duration of gestation; altered duration of parturition; reduced maternal care/lactation; reduced total litter size, live litter size, and/or pup viability; reduced or increased pup weight; altered pup sex ratio; altered pup morphology; reduced pup growth and viability; altered function

Adapted from Reference 26.

Table 29.3
Examples of agents producing female reproductive toxicity

General mechanism	Potential activity	Examples
Altered puberty, estrous/menstrual cycling	Altered ovarian activity and hypothalamic/pituitary feedback	Alcohol, o,ρ′DDT, isoflavones
Impaired ovulation	Altered endocrine signal	o,ρ′DDT, kepone
Altered mating behavior	Endocrine modulation	β-endorphin, naloxone
Altered gamete/embryo transport	Altered motility in oviduct	Progesterone, diethylstilbesterol, estrogens, methoxychlor
Suboptimal endometrial environment	Increased uterine contractions	Prostaglandins ($PGF_{2\alpha}$), PGE_1, PGE_2), RU 486
Ovarian toxicity/oocyte destruction/atresia	Mimic structure of naturally occurring hormones	Estrogens, DDt, methoxychlor, kepone, EGME
	General chemical reactivity	Alkylating agents, chemotherapeutic agents (e.g., prednisone, vincristine, vinblastine, 6-mercaptopurine, radiation, methotrexate, adriamycin), alcohol, polycyclic aromatic hydrocarbons, 4-vincyclohexene, cyclophosphamide
Altered steroid synthesis	Inhibition of sterioidogenic enzymes	Aminoglutethimide, 3-methoxybenzidine, cyanoketone, estrogens, azastene, danazol, spironolactone epostane triazole fungicide (L151775)
Antagonized steroid action	Inhibited steroid activity	Clomiphene citrate Cimetidine Spironolactone Opioid peptides
Inhibition of gonadotropins	Alterations at hypothalamic level	Marihuana (Δ-9-tetrahydrocannabinol)
Altered maternal behavior/lactation	Alterations of hypothalamic level	Tranquilizers
Impaired lactation	Altered prolactin levels	Tranquilizers

Developed from References 24, 45, 53, 79, 81, and 169.

Table 29.4
Comparative reproductive and placental parameters

Parameter	Mice	Rats	Rabbits	Hamsters	Guinea pigs	Rhesus monkeys	Humans
Estrous cycle (days)	3–9	4–6	None	4	16	28 (menstrual cycle)	28 (menstrual cycle)
Ovulation stimulus	Spontaneous	Spontaneous	Coitus	Spontaneous	Spontaneous	Spontaneous	Spontaneous
Uterus	Bicornuate	Bicornuate	Duplex	Bicornuate	Bicornuate	Simplex	Simplex
Implantation (days)	4.5–5	5.5–6	7–7.5	4.5–6	6–6.5	9	5–7.5
Implantation type	Eccentric—early Interstitial—late	Eccentric—early Interstitial—late	Superficial	Interstitial	Interstitial	Superficial	Interstitial
Fetal membranes in placental type	Early—inverted yolk sac Definitive Chorioallantoic	Early—Inverted yolk sac Definitive Chorioallantoic	Early—Inverted yolk sac Definitive Chorioallantoic	Early—Inverted yolk sac Definitive Chorioallantoic	Early—Inverted yolk sac Definitive Chorioallantoic	Chorioallantoic	Chorioallantoic
Placental shape	Discoid	Discoid	Discoid	Discoid	Discoid	Bidiscoid	Discoid
Internal placental shape	Labyrinthine	Labyrinthine	Labyrinthine	Labyrinthine	Labyrinthine	Villous	Villous
Placental relation to maternal tissues	Hemotrichorial	Hemotrichorial	Hemodichorial	Hemotrichorial	Hemomonochorial	Hemomonochorial	Hemomonochorial
Duration of gestation (days)	19	22	30–32	15.5	67–68	166	266
Expected no. of offspring	4–12	6–14	6–12	5–12	3–4	1	1

Adapted from Reference 47.

or implanted, resulting in a large percentage of preimplantation loss (209).

Second, fertilization depends on multiple factors, including the quality and quantity of both the eggs and sperm, as well as the timing of priming, ovulation, and insemination. Artificial insemination generally is performed using one introduction of diluted sperm into the primed female's vagina, with four to 20 does inseminated with sperm from the same buck. The angle of insertion of the insemination tube, handling of the female, and degree of priming of the female all affect the number of eggs fertilized and implanted. In contrast, in natural mating, generally only one buck inseminates any female on one day (bucks may inseminate multiple females used in the same study, but rabbit breeders generally allow matings of only the same pair on any single breeding day). Natural breeding may involve one or more intromissions and inseminations, generally increasing the number of sperm inseminated, cervical stimulation of the female, associated hormonal changes and ovulation of appropriately aged eggs, and the number of eggs fertilized and implanted.

Third, there are natural patterns associated with the number of *corpora lutea* ovulated and the success of a specific pregnancy. Feussner et al., (60) published data for 1463 control group rabbits artificially inseminated at Argus (98 studies, 1980–1989). Preimplantation loss was increased in does with high (15 or more *corpora lutea*, 90 does) or low (7 or fewer *corpora lutea*, 117 does) numbers of *corpora lutea* (numbers presumably associated with the development of the eggs in the ovary and degree of ovulation induced by hormonal stimulation). Preimplantation loss averaged 36.8% for the does with high numbers of *corpora lutea*, presumably reflecting superovulation of these animals resulting in ovulation of immature follicles. Preimplantation loss in the 177 does with low numbers of *corpora lutea* averaged 33.9%, numbers that probably resulted from either insufficient maturity of ovarian follicles or inadequate stimulation of the ovary by intravenously injected HCG. Preimplantation loss for the entire population averaged 27.8%, a value very similar to that reported for a smaller population by Tyl and Marr (209).

DEVELOPMENTAL TOXICOLOGY

As early as 1973, Wilson (236) expressed the concept of developmental toxicology in his statement, "The unborn is not only the embryo and the fetus in utero but also the as yet unconceived individuals whose potential for future development is represented in the germ cells residing in the parental gonads. Also of interest ... are those who have already been born but who are incompletely developed." This giant of the field of teratology also expanded the definition of teratology (study of congenital malformations) to "the study of the adverse effects of environment on developing systems, that is, on germ cells, embryos, fetuses, and immature postnatal individuals," and stated, "a more comprehensive definition is that teratology is the science dealing with the causes, mechanisms, and manifestations of developmental deviations of either structural or functional nature." (236) Based on these definitions, developmental toxicology can be considered to be the study of the entire reproductive process, with special emphasis on the developing conceptus, but including the development and function of that conceptus throughout its entire lifespan.

Wilson's basic principles remain valid, and all investigators in the field should be familiar with their details (discussed later; to comply with current usage, "teratogenesis" has been made synonymous with "developmental toxicity"):

I. Susceptibility to developmental toxicity depends on the genotype of the conceptus and the manner in which this interacts with adverse environmental factors.
II. Susceptibility to developmental toxicity varies with the developmental stage at the time of exposure to an adverse influence.
III. Developmental toxicants act in specific ways (mechanisms) on developing cells and tissues to initiate sequences of abnormal developmental events (pathogenesis).
IV. The access of adverse influences to developing tissues depends on the nature of the influence (agent).
V. The four manifestations of deviant development are death, malformation, growth retardation, and functional deficit.
VI. Manifestations of deviant development increase in frequency and degree as dosage increases from the no-effect to the totally lethal level.

Schmidt and Johnson (185) provided an elegant refinement of Wilson's principles, including that while "teratogenesis per se, has its primary focus on embryogenesis, developmental biology, and molecular genetics, the field of developmental toxicology also involves basic principles of toxicokinetics, dose-response relationships, target organ toxicity, and exposure assessment." Thus, for many investigators, the fields of embryology and teratology have been essentially replaced by molecular cell biology. We now use transgenic animal models (113), consider gene therapy a practical possibility (11,44), and are approaching deciphering the human genome. Despite these advances and the common use of molecular cell biology techniques by academic and pharmaceutical laboratories for mechanistic studies, such techniques are not commonly used in the first-line screening to identify doses causing general and specific toxicity in "normal" animals and their offspring, the principal subject of this chapter.

NORMAL DEVELOPMENT

The following information is provided as an overview of the complex process of normal development and also as an introduction to differences in developmental events in laboratory animal species and humans. For additional information on specific facets discussed, the reader is recommended to reviews by DeSesso, Klinefelter and Gray, Rogers and Kavlock, and Shield and Mirkes (47,110, 178,188), as well as to basic texts on embryology. Much of the information below is excerpted from these sources. For the interrelationship of the reproductive process in the maternal animal, vis a vis the developing conceptus, the reader is referred to the prior sections in this chapter.

As noted by Rogers and Kavlock (178), development is characterized by changes in size, biochemistry and physiology, and form and functionality. The overall process is orchestrated by a cascade of gene transcription regulating factors, the first of which are present in the egg before fertilization. These factors activate regulatory genes in the embryonic genome, with sequential gene activation continuing throughout development.

Development of the Conceptus

Preimplantation

From sperm penetration to first cleavage requires approximately 12 h in most laboratory species. As the fertilized oocyte (zygote) travels down the fallopian tube to the uterus, cleavage continues with growth to the morula stage. During this time, the zygote is surrounded by an acellular mucopolysaccharide layer, the zona pellucida, which previously prevented sperm penetration and now prevents premature implanting. In most mammals, the zona pellucida disappears at the blastocyst stage, and the morula cavitates between 5 and 8 days of gestation. The preimplantation embryo has remarkable regulative (restorative) growth potential (196), and it has been shown that one cell from an eight-celled rabbit embryo can produce a normal offspring (143). The preimplantation period is generally identified as a period during which toxic insult generally results in embryo death or absence of effect because of the regenerative powers of the embryo (237), although it has been shown that preimplantation exposure to some agents affect the ultimate growth and development of the embryo (e.g., actinomycin D and methotrexate, among others) (146,199).

Implantation and Placentation

Cavitation is followed by attachment of the blastocyst to the uterine wall (nidation), and subsequent invasion of the uterine wall (implantation) by the syncytiotrophoblast, which erodes the endometrium. Placental circulation is subsequently established (206).

Each blastocyst includes two different cell populations: the outer layer (trophoblast), which becomes the placenta and fetal membranes, and the inner cell mass (cluster of cells within the blastocyst), which becomes the embryo. Although sometimes not considered in the overall development of the embryo, the trophoblast serves an important function: the extraembryonic membranes protect the conceptus, whereas the placenta provides a means to supply nutrients and remove metabolic waste. There are multiple diverse mechanisms for placental transport of molecules, including both simple diffusion and carrier-mediated mechanisms (active transport, facilitated diffusion, receptor-mediated endocytosis). The placenta is clearly not a barrier, but rather a means by which a substance in the maternal system will, at some rate and by some mechanism, be transported into the embryo. Remarkable differences exist across species with respect to the layers of embryonic and maternal tissues interposed between the respective circulations and differences in the duration and functions of the yolk sac among species that can affect the rate and access of a test material to a conceptus. Comparative reproductive and placental parameters are provided in Table 29.5.

Embryogenesis

The rapid growth of the conceptus continues through embryonic, fetal and neonatal stages. The duration of these stages differs in various species, as shown in Table 29.6 (19). The period of embryogenesis (organogenesis) is generally identified as the interval between implantation (and formation of the neural plate in the ectoderm) and closure of the hard palate. Most organ systems are formed during this period, requiring cell proliferation, cell migration, cell-cell interactions, and morphogenetic tissue remodeling. Each forming structure has a period of maximum susceptibility, with peak susceptibility to insult coinciding with the time key developmental events occur in these structures. Wilson's classic diagram (Figure 29.3) (235) demonstrates the pattern for the rat embryo.

Shenefelt (186) demonstrated the varying susceptibilities in the hamster, (177,186), and provided similar observations in the mouse, and in the guinea pig (87). In toto, these investigations demonstrate that peak sensitivity may not only differ for a given tissue/organ, but also with the administered dose, reverting to Wilson's concepts (235,236,237). In addition, the same insult may affect the growth of concurrently developing systems.

Table 29.5
Historical values for mean % preimplantation loss in Hra:(NZW)SPF rabbits

Facility and mating procedure	Number of studies, time period, number of does	Mean, standard deviation, and range per study
Artificially Inseminated—HCG-Primed Rabbits		
RTI—Tyl and Marr (109)	88 does; years and number of studies not reported	30.90% ± 2.9 (range not reported)
Argus Research Laboratories Feussner (60)	98 studies—1980–1989, 1463 does	27.8% (standard deviation not reported) Range = 8.2% to 38.4%)
Naturally Mated Rabbits		
RTI—Tyl and Marr (209)	117 does; years and number of studies not reported	11.34±1.49%
Argus Research Laboratories (historical control data)	20 Studies—1998–1999, 378 Does	13.0% ± 7.8 (3.7%–39.0%)

Table 29.6
Timing of early development in some mammalian species

Mammal	Times of early development (days from ovulation)			
	Blastocyst formation	Implantation	Organogenesis period	Length of gestation
Mice	3–4	4–5	6–15	19
Rats	3–4	5–6	6–15	22
Rabbits	3–4	7–8	6–18	33
Sheep	6–7	17–18	14–36	150
Monkeys (rhesus)	5–7	9–11	20–45	184
Humans	5–8	8–13	21–56	267

Adapted from Reference 19.

Thus, insult during the period of organogenesis is that which is most likely to result in gross structural malformations (235,236), although all endpoints of developmental toxicology have been shown affected and the dose-response pattern for agents often differ (Figure 29.4), and the interrelationships of the responses often confound apparent dose-dependency. In general, the type of agent that is of most concern is that which causes malformation at doses that are lower than those associated with growth retardation or lethality. As discussed later, regardless of the dose response, current practice in risk assessment is to base the developmental toxicity effect level on the lowest of the four potential endpoints adversely affected, whether the effect occurs alone or in combination.

Fetogenesis

The fetal period is characterized by tissue differentiation, growth, and physiological maturation. Almost all organs are present and grossly recognizable, and further development of these organs proceeds with the fetus attaining required functions before birth, including fine structure morphogenesis (e.g., synaptogenesis, neural outgrowth, branching morphogenesis of the bronchial

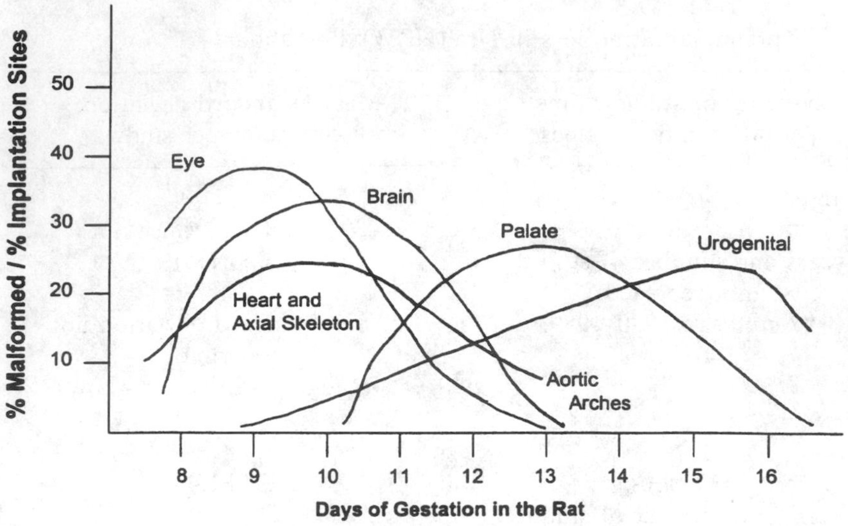

FIG. 29.3. Hypothetical pattern of susceptibility of embryonic organs to teratogenic insult. Adapted from Reference 235.

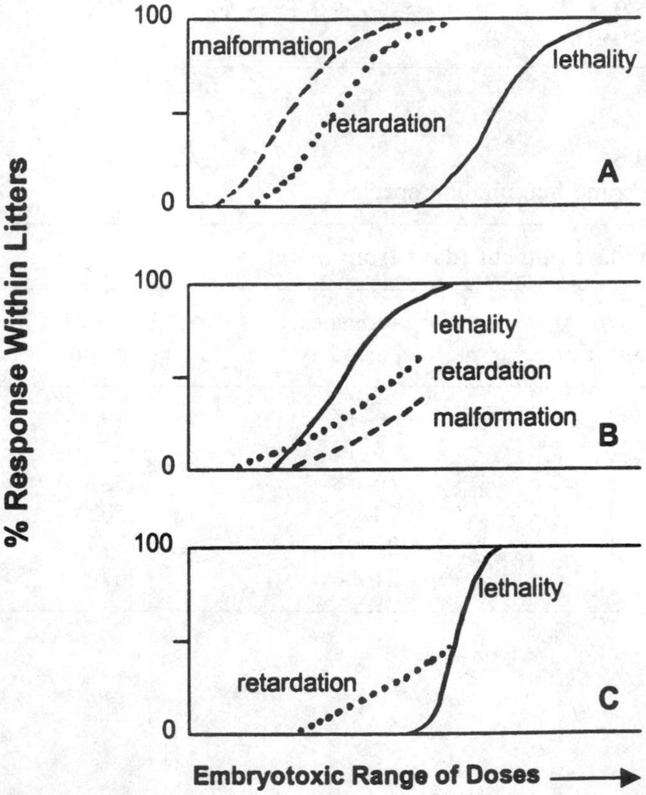

FIG. 29.4. Dose-response patterns (A–C) for different types of developmental toxicant. Adapted from Reference 153.

tree, renal cortical tubules) and biochemical maturation (e.g., induction of tissue-specific enzymes and structural proteins). Insult during the period of fetogenesis is most likely to affect growth and functional maturation of the central nervous system, reproductive organs (including behavioral and motor deficits and reductions in fertility), the pulmonary system, and the immune system. Although gross structural changes can occur during the fetal period, such observations are generally secondary to deformations (changes in previously normal structures, such as clubbed or bent limbs) rather than malformations (abnormal growth).

Endpoints of Developmental Toxicology

One or more endpoints of developmental toxicity, alone or in combination, have been identified as affected for scores of agents despite the fact that "teratogenicity" remains the endpoint of greatest interest. Compendiums of "animal teratogens" are regularly updated (183,187) and provide overviews of effects of test agents, generally in animal studies conducted at high multiples of human exposures. Despite the concept that most, and possibly all, agents are toxic to development when administered to the appropriate species, at the required dose, and during the appropriate period of sensitivity (103), researchers continue to perceive teratogenicity as a unique property of an agent and incorrectly categorize agents as "teratogenic" or "non-teratogenic" (101) or induced by "maternal toxicity" when only an association of toxicity at a given dose can be identified on the basis of the study design (106,107,46,89). It is hoped that current readers will understand that agents resulting in toxic effects in the maternal and paternal animals may be expected to result in adverse effects on the developing conceptuses from which the parents, but not necessarily the conceptuses, may recover, and that cross-species extrapolation of the affected developmental endpoint does not necessarily occur because of multiple timing, exposure, and species-specific differences.

Table 29.7
Examples of mechanisms for agents producing developmental toxicity

General mechanism	Potential activity	Examples
Mitotic interference	Inhibit DNA synthesis	Hydroxyurea, Cytosine arabinoside, 5-flurouracil—Faustman (58)
	Chromosome instability, single-strand breaks, double-strain breaks, DNA-protein cross-links, mitotic delay	Radiation—Brent (18)
	Perturbations in mitotic spindle resulting in cell cycle arrest, aneuploidy, altered cell division rate, and/or cell death	Antitubulin agents, e.g., benzimidazole carbamates, colchicine—Faustman (58)
	Inhibited cell cycling	Methylmercury—Faustman (58)
Altered membrane function/signal transduction	Instructive induction or permissive induction	Low level lead, methylmercury—Faustman (58)
Altered energy sources	Altered mitochondrial function	Riboflavin deficiency, iron deficiency, diphenylhydantoin, chloramphenicol, sodium phenobarbital, cocaine—Faustman (58)
Enzyme inhibition	Inhibition of enzymes critical for cell growth and proliferation	Methotrexate, 5-flurouracil, mevinolin—Faustman (58)
Nucleic acid interaction	Interference with normal synthesis and functioning of DNA and RNA	Hydroxyurea, cytosine arabinoside—Faustman (58)
Mutations	Alteration of DNA nucleotide sequence	Ionizing radiation, alkylating agents, aromatic amines—Faustman, et al., (58)
Altered gene expression	Induction or repression of transcription	Retinoic acid, Dioxin, Cocaine—Koebbe, et al., (114), Phenytoin—Gelineau-Van Waes (67)
Programmed cell death (apoptosis)	Alterations of normal apoptosis	Retinoic acid, Dioxin, DNA damaging agents—Faustman (58)

Mechanisms of Developmental Toxicity

As early as 1977, Wilson (237) identified six general categories for mechanisms resulting in developmental toxicity, including mitotic interference, altered membrane function/signal transduction, altered energy sources, enzyme inhibition, altered nucleic acid synthesis, and mutations. The current increased knowledge regarding molecular mechanisms of normal development results in addition of perturbations in gene expression and programmed cell death to Wilson's general categories (58). Examples of developmental toxins known to act by one or more of these mechanisms are identified in Table 29.7.

Apoptosis

Because of the relatively recent interest in apoptosis as a mechanism in carcinogenicity, the following information is provided to illustrate the occurrence of the phenomenon from conception to death. Although not previously emphasized, for almost 50 years, controlled cell death (apoptosis) has been recognized to be as important to development of the conceptus as are cell proliferation and differentiation (70,182,75,188). Apoptosis occurs in the developing embryo and in normal healthy adult tissues, as well as in many pathological settings. It is genetically directed and usually requires ongoing protein synthesis (2), continues through life, and provides the central mechanism for removal of surplus, unwanted, damaged, or aged cells. It is characterized by ultrastructural and biochemical features, including cytoplasmic and nuclear condensation, formation of membrane-bound apoptotic bodies, and oligonucleosomal DNA degradation into micronuclei and cytolysis into condensed apoptotic bodies. Apoptosis is not generally associated with an inflammatory cell infiltrate, a hallmark of necrosis (59). In contrast, changes associated with necrosis include cellular swelling, organelle dysfunction, mitochondrial collapse, and ultimately cellular disintegration, release of the cellular contents in the extracellular milieu, and a marked host inflammatory reaction (11).

Apoptosis occurs in normal tissue turnover, organ involution after withdrawal of trophic hormones, in distinct cells after deprivation of growth factors or specific stimuli, and in cells that have undergone sublethal damage (2,75,230). Interference with the interrelated cell functions that result in normal growth during embryogenesis can result in abnormalities during embryogenesis as well as cancers in adult life. For example, exaggerated or defective apoptosis can result in developmental abnormalities, such as cleft palate, neural tube defects, phocomelia and hypospadias, or a likelihood of tumorous growth, as occurred in daughters of mothers administered diethylstilbestrol during pregnancy (230). Among the multiple genetic events associated with tumor development are activation of antiapoptotic oncogenes, such as the BCL2 family, and inactivation of apoptosis inducing tumor suppressor genes including the retinoblastoma (Rb), p53 and BAX and BCL2 genes (59,166,188,232).

Apoptosis occurs in almost every tissue during development (36,139), including palate formation (228,189), body sculpting (e.g., digit formation (91)), gastrointestinal development (230), sexual organ development and gamete formation and number (2,5,22,75,96, 134,139,230), and in the homeostasis of normal tissues, especially the gastrointestinal tract, immune system, and skin (2,230).

Establishment of normal craniofacial pattern requires apoptosis of the neural crest (72), with apoptosis perhaps most well studied in development of the nervous system. It is critical in development of both neuronal and non-neuronal cells in the peripheral and central nervous systems (21,147) and occurs both pre- and postnatally. As noted by Mazarakisk et al. (134), apoptosis is seen in the developing nervous system as early as neural tube formation and persists throughout terminal differentiation of the neural network, with more than 50% of the neurons lost during development. These cell deaths occur in structures as diverse as sensory and autonomic ganglia, cranial motor nuclei, and spinal motor neuron pools, the retina, various brainstem nuclei, and the cerebral cortex during development of most regions of the central and peripheral nervous systems. Apoptosis is evident during transformation of the neural plate into the neural tube, in the suboptic death center at the junction between the diencephalon and telencephalon, and in the ventral midline of the embryonic retina and optic stalk. It is also a common phenomenon in the CNS during normal postnatal development (150).

Several mechanisms appear responsible for survival of developing neurons, including retrograde transport of trophic factors, of which nerve growth factor (NGF) is the best characterized (147). Unchecked apoptosis and failure of the apoptotic pathway contribute to nervous system pathology in both the developing embryo (150) and the adult (147), and can be caused by viruses, metabolic stress, damage to cell structures, and drug, chemical, and physical insults (75). Dysregulation of apoptosis has been shown to result in neurodegeneration and tumorigenesis (166). Failure to undergo apoptosis is also associated with low-grade follicular lymphoma (2).

Studies have identified association of apoptosis and tumor suppressor genes (230,234). For example, the retinoblastoma gene (Rb) and p53 genes are mutated in a wide range of sporadic human tumor types, and germ-line mutations in Rb and p53 result in a greatly increased cancer risk. The Rb gene encodes a nuclear phosphoprotein believed to act through protein-protein interactions as a regulator of the G_1 to S phase of cell cycle transition. The p53 gene encodes a transcriptional regulator, has been linked to cell cycle arrest and the induction of apoptosis (234), and has been termed the "guardian of the genome" because it plays an essential role in surveillance of DNA damage, regulation of the cell cycle, and a regulatory role in apoptosis.

The interrelationship of oncogenes, tumor suppressor genes, apoptosis, and normal growth and development is being actively studied but has not yet been defined (166). For example, apoptosis in the neural crest rhombomeres 3 and 5 and also in the interdigital mesenchyme appears to involve homeobox gene MSX-2 and the signaling molecule BMP 4 (72). Although the 5′-located HOXd genes are reported to be involved in patterning of the digital rays, Hurle et al. (91) found that experimental inhibition of interdigital cell death and formation of extra digits was not accompanied by a modified expression of these genes nor precocious modification of

MSX-1 and MSX-2 gene expression, even though these two genes exhibit a domain of expression relatively coincident with the interdigital cell death zones, indicating involvement of other unidentified genes. Studies of the BCL_2 gene identified a contradictory phenomenon. Although the BCL_2 gene is not expressed in areas of cell death in the developing limb but is expressed in the digital rays, transgenic mice with disruption of the BCL_2 gene have normal limbs. Transgenic embryo models have also been used to demonstrate that proper regulation of the p53 tumor suppressor gene is necessary for normal morphogenesis, that too little p53 makes the embryo susceptible to neural defects associated with instability of the genome or chromosomal damage, and that excessive p53 may result in cell death abnormalities, particularly in the eye (113).

Structure Activity and Agent Interaction Considerations

Although the cause of many investigations for developmental toxicity has been a relationship in structure to human teratogens [(e.g., to thalidomide, as occurred for the phthalic acids, to valproic acid, as occurred for di-(2-ethylhexyl) phthalate (DEHP)], structure-activity relationships remain weak for elucidating mechanisms of developmental toxicity (61). Considerable interest also lies in the potential for interaction of agents by the same or different mechanisms.

It is known that the potential for interaction of multiple chemicals exists for developmental and other toxicities, and that such interactions may enhance or reduce general toxicity of the agents and their potential developmental toxicity, although not necessarily equally or by the same mechanism. For example, early on it was identified that caffeine potentiates the activity of multiple agents (176), and although initial emphasis was on the pharmacologic activity of the putative agent, in this case, the vasoconstrictive effect of caffeine (48), studies now tend to investigate the interaction of the agent with gene expression. The US EPA has an active program for evaluating multiple chemical combinations that are potential water contaminants, often using modified reproductive or developmental toxicity protocols (69,74,82,148).

METHODS USED IN REPRODUCTIVE (FEMALE) AND DEVELOPMENTAL TOXICOLOGY

Testing Procedures and Guidelines for Regulatory Use

The purpose of this section is to provide an overview of the methods used in collection and interpretation of data obtained from reproductive and developmental toxicity studies when conducted for regulatory use. The methods described are those used in our laboratory and were developed from the literature and practical experience. Because it was not always practical to provide in-depth details, useful publications have been referenced, when possible. Multiple laboratory species are used in these types of studies; however, for practical reasons, most studies are performed using rats, rabbits, mice, or hamsters. In general, the described techniques can be applied to ferrets, guinea pigs, mini-pigs, dogs, and nonhuman primates using species-specific considerations. As previously noted, there are often special reasons to use alternative species (e.g., prolonged in utero development and comparable in utero CNS development in the guinea pig theoretically make this species ideal for evaluation of neural development). Important caveats are that studies conducted for regulatory use should provide evidence that the agent is pharmacologically/toxicologically active in the species, absorbed, if administered orally or topically, and, if possible, similarly handled metabolically by the test species and humans.

The Guidelines for Toxicity to Reproduction of Medicinal Products, an effort of the International Conference for Harmonization (ICH) (93), are accepted by the US Food and Drug Administration (FDA) (227,228), European Union (EU), and Japan. These guidelines address all elements of reproductive/developmental toxicity testing and provide an overview of the various study designs and the endpoints evaluated in the regulatory testing of pharmaceuticals, biotechnology products (224), indirect food additives and devices (226), chemicals (29,220,221,222), and pesticides, fungicides, and rodenticides (29,214,215,216). As harmonization progresses, it is likely that the guidelines will become more rather than less similar. For instance, the ICH guidelines (227,228) replace the former guidelines issued by the U.S. FDA Bureau of Drugs (224), EU countries (40,56) and Japan (141,142,205), and the Office of Prevention, Pesticides and Toxic Substances (OPPTS) replace the former EPA Toxic Substances Control Act (TSCA) guidelines (29,220,221,222) and Federal Insecticide, Fungicide and Rodenticide (FIFRA) guidelines (29,214, 215,216); harmonization efforts are currently ongoing between EPA and the Organization for Economic and Co-operation and Development (OECD).

Comprehensive comparisons of the ICH Guidelines with other guidelines have been published by Christian and Hoberman (33) and Collins (39). For complete details, it is recommended that the documents be obtained. They are available on the internet, in the Federal Register and from the various regulatory publishing houses. Practical updates on regulatory issues, shared experience, and access to historical databases can be obtained through access to the web sites cited in Table

Table 29.8
List of useful web sites

Organization	Web site
American College of Toxicology	http://actox.org/
Congenital Anomalies (Journal of the Japanese Teratology Society)	http://www.med.hiroshima-u.ac.jp/med/med/kiso/kaibo1/CongAnome/Welcome.html
EPA	http://www.epa.gov/epahome/Standards.html (this is a front page; i.e., one needs to select OPPTS.)
European Teratology Society	http://www.etsoc.com/
FDA—CDER	http://www.fda.gov/cder/guidance/index.htm (a front page for guidance documents; one can click on ICH from the column on the left.)
FDA—CFSAN	http://vm.cfsan.fda.gov/~redbook/red-toct.html
International Federation of Teratology Societies (IFTS) Atlas of Developmental Abnormalities	http://www.ifts-atlas.org/
Mid-Atlantic Reproduction and Teratology Society (MARTA)	Soon to be up; will be linked to Teratology Society
Midwest Teratology Association	http://www.midwest-teratology.org/
National Institute of Environmental Health Sciences (NIEHS)	http://ehpnet1.niehs.nih.gov/docs/1999/107p397-405fisher/abstract.html (effects of neonatal exposure to DES on excurrent ducts of the rat testis)
Neurobehavioral Teratology Society	http://nbts.bsbe.umn.edu/
Reproductive Toxicology (Journal—$850/year subscription; online)	http://www.elsevier.nl/inca/publications/store/5/2/5/4/8/9/
Society of Toxicology (SOT)	http://www.toxicology.org/
Teratology Society	http://www.teratology.org/
TERIS (Teratogen Information System; $1000/yr subscription price)	http://weber.u.washington.edu/~terisweb/teris/index.html

29.8. A listing of the majority of the regulatory guidelines currently in use is provided in Table 29.9.

For the purposes of this chapter, the ICH guidelines (93) were used as the reference for identifying the various stages and interrelationships of female reproductive functions and development of the offspring. These guidelines (227,228) segment the reproductive cycle into six "ICH STAGES" (ICH STAGES A through F) that may be tested separately or in combination, generally using a one-day overlap of treatment. As many publications describe tests using now outdated terms (Segment I, II, and III tests), as multigeneration evaluations, or as alternative tests, Table 29.10 is provided for use in identification of comparable intervals in the various guidelines and in academic research.

The ICH guidelines (227,228) cite recommendations that were often unidentified in other guidelines, including use of (1) scientific justification of flexible study designs; (2) kinetics; (3) expanded male reproductive toxicity evaluations; (4) a requirement for mechanistic studies; and (5) essentially equal emphasis on all endpoints of developmental toxicity (death, malformation, reduced weight, functional/behavioral alterations), rather than emphasizing malformation as the most important outcome. Flexible testing strategies are to be based on (1) anticipated drug use, especially in relation to reproduction; (2) the form of the substance and routes of administration intended for humans; and (3) consideration of existing data on toxicity, pharmacodynamics, kinetics, and similarity to other compounds in structure/activity. In toto, the purpose of these studies is to identify any effect of an active substance on mammalian reproduction, to compare this effect with all other pharmacologic and toxicologic data for the agent, and ultimately, to determine whether the human risk for reproductive and developmental effects is the same, increased, or reduced, in comparison with the risks of other toxic effects of the agent. As should occur for all toxicologic observations, additional pertinent information should be considered before the results of the ani-

Table 29.9
Current regulatory guidelines—ICH, FDA, OECD, EPA

Medical Agents	
ICH (93)	Detection of Toxicity to Reproduction for Medicinal Products. (Proposed Rule Endorsed by the ICH Steering Committee at Step 4 of the ICH Process, 24 June 1993.)
ICH (94)	Detection of Toxicity to Reproduction for Medicinal Products. (Proposed Rule Endorsed by the ICH Steering Committee at Step 4 of the ICH Process, 1995)
FDA (27)	International Conference on Harmonisation: Guideline on detection of toxicity to reproduction for medicinal products. Federal Register, September 22, 1994, Vol. 59, No. 183.
FDA (228)	International Conference on Harmonisation: Guideline on detection of toxicity to reproduction for medicinal products; Addendum on Toxicity to male fertility. Federal Register, April 5, 1996, Vol. 61, No. 67.
Indirect Food Additives	
FDA, Bureau of Foods (225)	Toxicological Principles and Procedures for Priority Based Assessment of Food Additives (Red Book), Guidelines for Reproduction Testing with a Teratology Phase
FDA, Center for Food Safety and Applied Nutrition (226)	Toxicological Principles for the Safety Assessment of Direct Food Additives and Color Additives Used in Food. (Red Book II), Guidelines for Reproduction and Developmental Toxicity Studies.
FDA, Center for Food Safety and Applied Nutrition (241)	Toxicological Principles for the Safety of Food Ingredients (Red Book 2000).
Chemicals	
EPA, OPPTS (217)	Health Effects Test Guidelines; Prenatal Developmental Toxicity Study. (OPPTS) 870.3700, August, 1998.
EPA, OPPTS (218).	Health Effects Test Guidelines; Reproduction and Fertility Effects.(OPPTS) 870.3800, August, 1998.
EPA, OPPTS (219).	Health Effects Test Guidelines; Developmental Neurotoxicity Study. (OPPTS) 870.6300, August, 1998.
EPA, Risk Assessment Forum (212)	Guidelines for Developmental Toxicity Risk Assessment, Dec. 5, 1991. Federal Register 56(234):63798–63826.
EPA (213).	Guidelines for Reproductive Toxicity Risk Assessment, September, 1996, NTIS PB No. PB97-100098
OECD (159)	Guidelines for Testing of Chemicals. Section 4, No. 414: Teratogenicity, adopted 12 May 1981.
OECD (160)	OECD Guidelines for Testing of Chemicals. Section 4, No. 415: One-Generation Reproduction Toxicity, adopted 26 May 1983.
OECD (161)	OECD Guidelines for Testing of Chemicals. Section 4, No. 416: Two-Generation Reproduction Toxicity Study, adopted 26 May 1983.
OECD (163)	OECD Guidelines for Testing of Chemicals. Section 4, No. 422: Combined Repeated Dose Toxicity Study with the Reproduction/Developmental Toxicity Screening Test, adopted 22 March 1996.

Table 29.10

Comparison of ICH stages and study types with similar observations made (bolded information indicates treatment interval)

ICH Stage	FDA Guidelines (224)	Great Britain (40) and EEC (56) Guidelines	Japanese Guidelines, (141,142) Tanimura (205)	EPA OPPTS, (217,218,219) OECD (159–163) and FDA Redbook Guidelines (225,226,227)	Alternate/Additional Evaluations Chernoff and Kavlock (27) Hardin (80) Lamb (116) Morrissey (144) Narotsky (148)
A—**Premating to Conception**: reproductive functions in adult animals, including development and maturation of gametes, mating behavior, and fertilization.	**Segment I**	**Segment I**	**Segment I**	**Multigeneration** **One-Generation**	**Continuous Breeding** **Modified Chernoff-Kavlock**
B—**Conception to Implantation:** reproductive functions in the adult female, preimplantation and implantation stages of the conceptus.	**Segment I**	**Segment I**	**Segment I**	**Multigeneration** **One-Generation** **Developmental Toxicity**	**Continuous Breeding** **Modified Chernoff-Kavlock**
C—**Implantation to Closure of the Hard Palate**: adult female reproductive functions and development of the embryo through major organ formation.	**Segment I** **Segment II**	**Segment I** **Segment II**	**Segment II**	**Multigeneration** **One-Generation** **Developmental Toxicity** **Developmental Neurotoxicity**	**Continuous Breeding** **Modified Chernoff-Kavlock**
D—**Closure of the Hard Palate to the End of Pregnancy:** adult female reproductive function, fetal development, and growth and organ development and growth.	**Segment I** **Segment II** **Segment III**	**Segment I** Segment II	**Segment II**	**Multigeneration** **One-Generation** **Developmental Toxicity** **Developmental Neurotoxicity**	**Continuous Breeding** **Modified Chernoff-Kavlock**
E—**Birth to Weaning**: adult female reproduction function, adaptation of the neonate to extrauterine life, including preweaning development and growth (postnatal age optimally based on postcoital age).	**Segment I** **Segment III** **Pediatric**	**Segment I** Segment II **Segment III**	Segment II **Segment III**	**Multigeneration** **One-Generation** **Developmental Toxicity** **Developmental Neurotoxicity**	**Modified Chernoff-Kavlock**
F—**Weaning to Sexual Maturity**: (pediatric evaluation when treated) postweaning development and growth, adaptation to independent life and attainment of full sexual development.	**Pediatric**	Segment I	Segment II Segment III	**Multigeneration** **Developmental Neurotoxicity** **Developmental Immunotoxicity**	

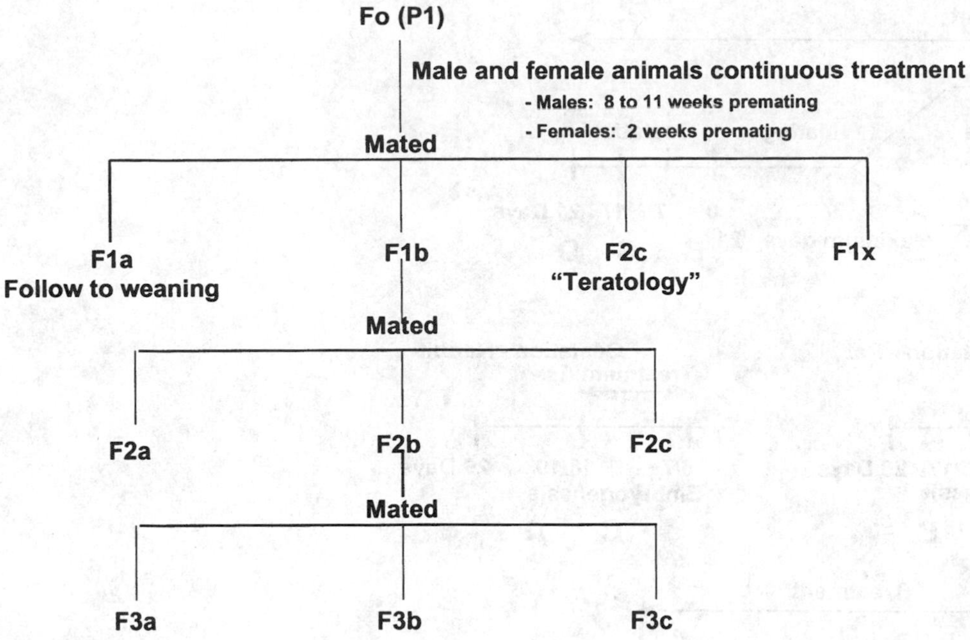

FIG. 29.5. Three generation multigeneration study in rats.

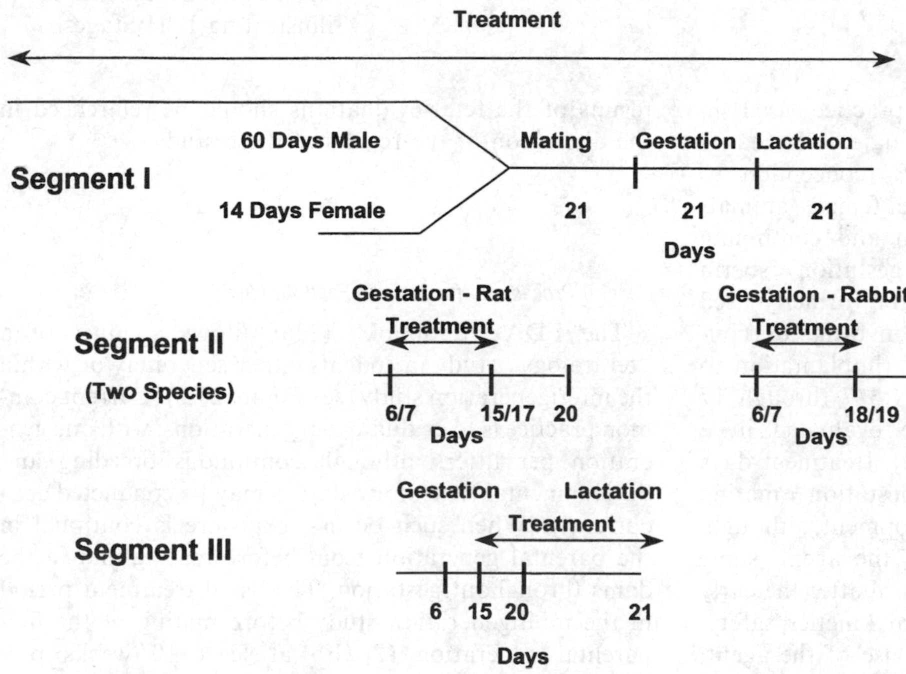

FIG. 29.6. Three segments – FDA.

mals studies are extrapolated to humans. This information includes human exposure considerations, comparative kinetics, and the mechanism of the toxic effect.

Because this chapter emphasizes toxic effects on the female animal and its offspring (through completion of the lactation period), sections of the ICH guideline (227,228) relevant to male reproductive performance and postnatal development of the offspring are discussed only when relevant to the primary subject area. Assessments of male reproductive effects, functional/behavioral effects in the offspring, and pediatric effects are more fully described in Chapter 28.

General Procedures for Pharmaceuticals

The ICH stages are identified in Figure 29.1. Conduct of a study including two full reproductive cycles is equivalent to a two-generation study. As previously noted, rodents and rabbits are the most commonly used laboratory animals. Common protocol designs used for evaluation of these species are provided in Figures 29.5

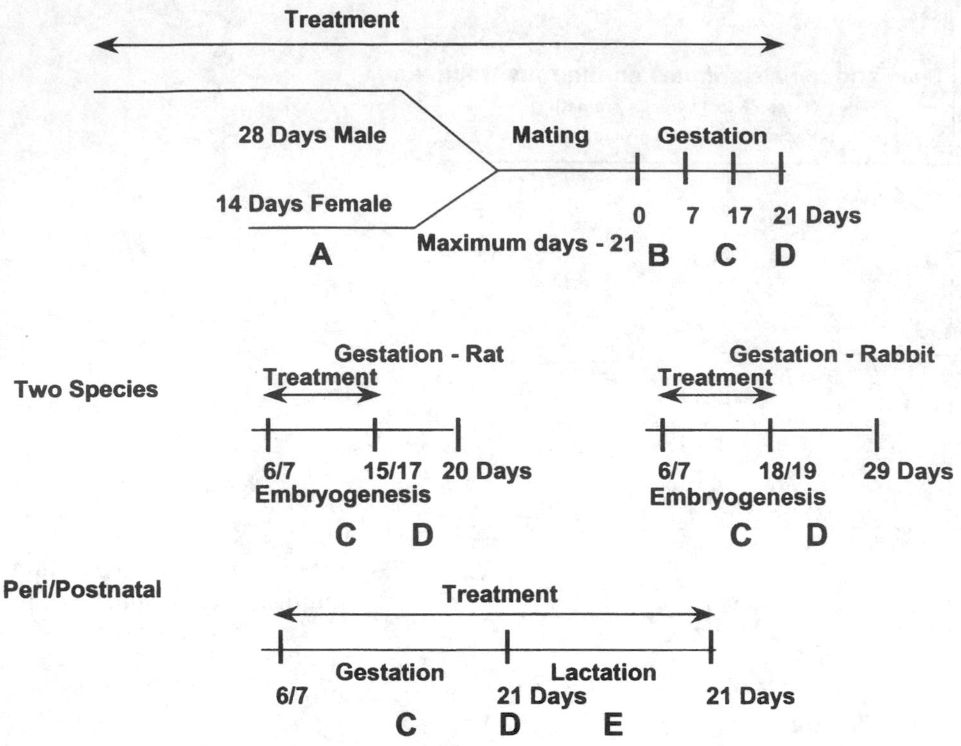

FIG. 29.7. Study designs illustrating ICH Stages.

through 29.8. The most common practice used in developing pharmaceuticals is to evaluate ICH Stages A (premating to conception) and B (conception to implantation), with treatment of the female animals initiated 2 weeks before cohabitation and continuing through day 7 of gestation (day 0 of gestation = sperm in smear), a protocol comparable to the formerly used Japanese Segment I design (141). Many investigators continue treatment through ICH stage C (implantation to closure of the hard palate; rats—days 6/7 through 17 of gestation). ICH stage C is also evaluated in a nonrodent species (generally the rabbit; treatment days 6/7 through 19 of gestation; day 0 of gestation = mating or insemination) early in product development, although, depending upon the proposed use of the agent, some investigators chose to delay this test until after the early clinical trials are completed (metabolism, kinetics, safety, and efficacy). Based on the proposed use of the agent, studies are also conducted that evaluate ICH stages C (implantation to closure of the hard palate), D (closure of the hard palate to parturition; rats—day 17 through 22 of gestation), E (birth to weaning; rats—day 0/1 through 21 postnatal), and F (without drug exposure—weaning to sexual maturity; rats day 22 through 60 postnatal), a design comparable to a combination of the former Japanese Segment II and Segment III designs. When these studies provide a second evaluation of stage C (embryogenesis), the female animals usually are permitted to naturally deliver all offspring, and the fetal evaluations not repeated, although the results of the fetal evaluations should be referenced in the discussion of the results of these studies.

General Procedures for Indirect Food Additives

The FDA "Redbook" (226) allows conduct of a "teratology" study in rodents either seperately or within the multigeneration study (see Figure 29.5). Current common practice is to evaluate two generations, with one generation per litter, although continuous breeding and developmental toxicology studies may be conducted concurrently. When such occurs, exposure is continual in the parental generation from before mating and in the dams throughout gestation. The usual treatment period in the multigeneration study before mating of the first parental generation (Po/Fo at least 10 weeks precohabitation in male and female rats). It continues through mating, gestation, and lactation and then in the selected weanlings identified as the second (P1/F1) gestation. These guidelines (226), have been issued, and include evaluations of estrous cycling as well as postnatal behavioral and functional assessments (including immune function).

It is acceptable to conduct the developmental toxicity studies in rats and rabbits separately. The current requirements identify the treatment period days 6 through 20 in rats and 6 through 29 in rabbits (from implantation to one day prior to the expected day of parturition).

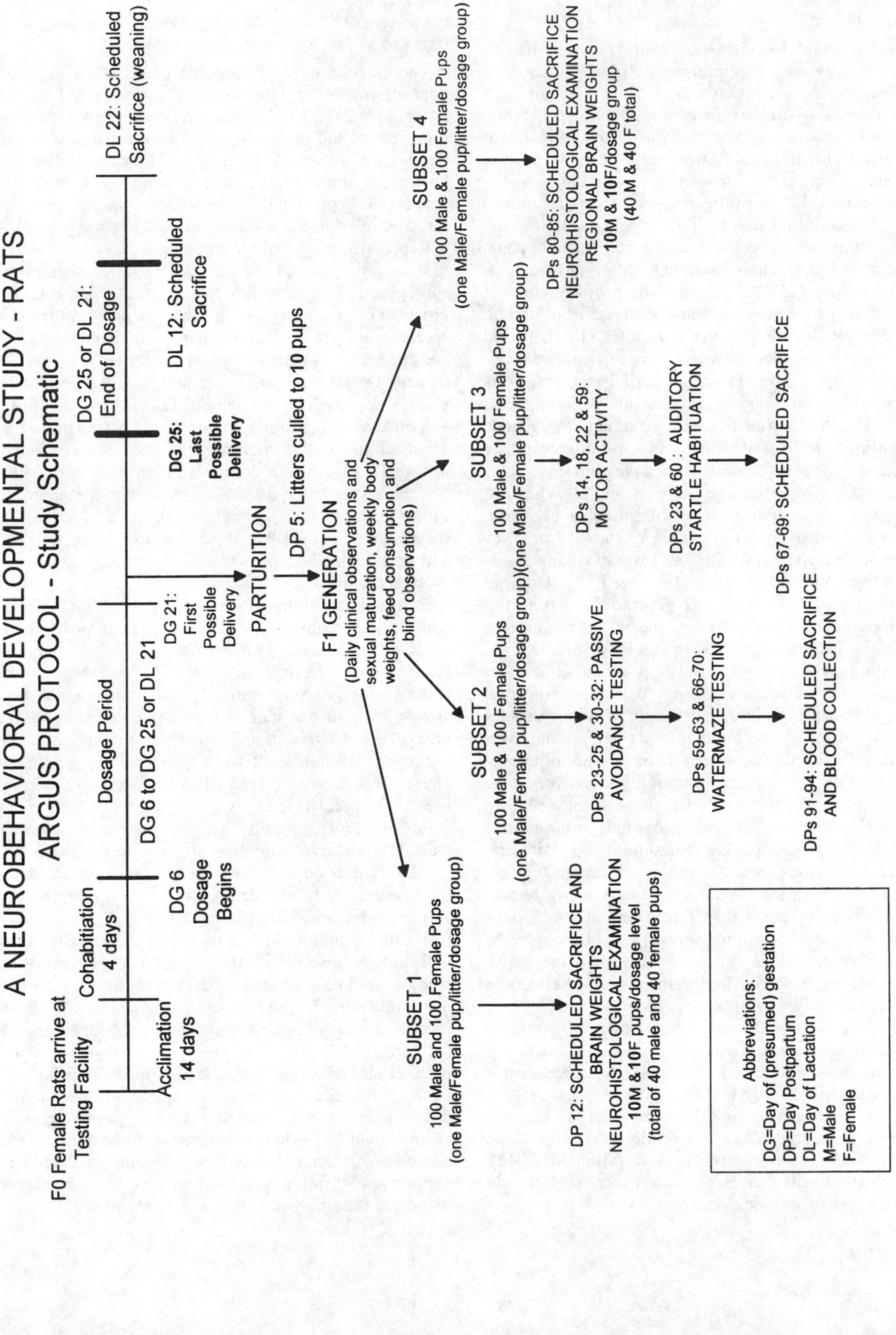

FIG. 29.8. Neurobehavioral developmental toxicity study – rats.

General Procedures Specific to EPA OPPTS Protocols (217,218,219)

Developmental toxicity studies are required in two species. Treatment is administered from implantation to delivery (gestation days 6 through 20 in rats; 6 through 29 in rabbits), with 20 pregnant animals per group assigned to study. It is acceptable to provide treatment throughout the entire gestation period (gestation days 0 through 20 in rats; 0 through 29 in rabbits).

The revised EPA multigeneration (two-generation) protocol has multiple new endpoints. As a result, it incorporates many endpoints traditionally performed in pharmaceutical development, although differing from the ICH guidelines (227,228) in that the protocols are set rather than open to scientific judgement regarding design. Treatment of the parental generation (Po/Fo male and female rats) is initiated 10 weeks before mating and continues through a 3-week mating period (the male rats can be terminated after the cohabitation period). Treatment of the Po/Fo and F1 generation male and female rats continues until termination. Endpoints not previously assessed include estrous cyclicity data (vaginal smears) for 3 weeks prior to mating, during mating, and at termination; sperm parameters (total number of sperm, percent progressively motile sperm, and sperm morphology); developmental milestones (age of vaginal opening and preputial separation for the F1 generation, anogenital distance for the F2 generation, if triggered by a treatment-related effect on the sexual maturation of the F1 generation); gross pathology and selected histopathology of weanlings and adult organ weight data (uterus, ovaries, testes, one epididymis, including the total weight and cauda epididymal weight, seminal vesicles with coagulating glands and fluids, prostate, brain, liver, kidneys, adrenal glands, spleen, thymus, and all known target organs). Histologic evaluation of the ovary is to include a minimum of 10 sections, randomly selected from one completely sectioned ovary per female in the control and high dosage groups. Examination of the intact epididymis is to include the caput, corpus, and cauda regions. For the F1 generation, organ weight data are to be collected for one pup per sex per litter from all dose groups for the ovaries, testes, brain, liver, kidney, adrenal glands, spleen, thymus, and known target organs, with histopathology triggered by treatment-related effects in the F1 high dosage group histopathology.

The EPA developmental neurotoxicology protocol (219) may be incorporated within the multigeneration study design or conducted separately. A schematic for this very complex study is presented as Figure 29.8. In this study, treatment occurs from implantation through postnatal development of the majority of the CNS (rats—gestation day 6 through lactation day 12), although treatment can be continued through lactation to day 21, when weaning occurs.

General Considerations Regarding Reproductive/Developmental Toxicology Studies Conducted for Submission to Regulatory Agencies

These studies should be conducted in conformance with appropriate Good Laboratory Practices (GLP) regulations (57,211,210,223,164). Whenever possible, the same species and strain of animal should be used as tested in other toxicology studies and in the kinetics studies. The kinetics, pharmacological, and toxicological data should support the position that the selected species provides a model relevant for use in human safety assessment.

Reproductive toxicology studies generally are conducted in one species (usually the rat), with some subsegments (e.g., ovarian toxicity, testicular toxicity) obtained from companion subchronic studies in the same species and strain. Developmental toxicology studies are generally conducted in two species, one rodent (usually the rat) and one nonrodent (usually the rabbit). Each study usually includes a vehicle control group and three or more groups administered dosages of the test agent at arithmetic multiples of the highest clinical dosage. Ideally, the low dosage is a multiple of the highest clinical dosage based on blood serum levels. Each group should include 16–20 animals or litters. It is axiomatic that animals should be at comparable ages, weights, and parity when assigned to a study.

Reproductive toxicology studies may be conducted by treating animals of only one sex and mating these animals with untreated animals of the opposite sex or by treatment of both male and female animals. A common refinement of the test is to use double-sized control and high dosage groups during the premating period, with cross-mating of one half of the animals in each dosage group, in order to determine whether administration of the agent to animals of only one sex causes different effects from those observed when both sexes are administered the agent (172).

Positive control groups are not considered necessary when reproductive toxicology studies are conducted for regulatory use because consistent sensitivity to xenobiotics has already been demonstrated in most laboratory species by historical experience; however, historical control data of abnormalities in fertility, fecundity, fetal morphology, resorption, and consistency from study to study should be available for comparative use with any new study data. Historical data for common laboratory species are available from many published sources (117,118,119,137,149), but the most relevant data are those generated at the testing facility in the same animal strains, using the same nomenclature and technical conditions (32,9). A rule of thumb is that a positive control agent should be evaluated before conducting a new test paradigm or examining a new endpoint to document appropriate training and expertise. GLP compliance mandates training and expertise of personnel.

In general, regulatory studies require that the high dosage be maternally and/or developmentally toxic and that the low dosage should be a no-observed-adverse-effect level (NOAEL). In the past, depending upon the regulatory body, no more than 10% mortality and/or 10% reduction in maternal body weight gain were usually considered sufficient to identify a maternally toxic dosage. Conformance with these criteria and the associated testing of excessively high dosages resulted in both maternal toxicity and developmental toxicity (135). In contrast, the ICH guidelines (227) indicate that the high dosage should produce minimal maternal (adult) toxicity and be selected on the basis of data from all available studies, including pharmacologic, acute, and subchronic toxicity and kinetic studies. These guidelines allow evidence of maternal toxicity to include reduced or increased weight gain, specific target organ toxicity, changes in hematology or clinical chemistry parameters, and exaggerated pharmacological response, which may or may not be reflected as marked clinical reactions (e.g., sedation, convulsions). Additional justification for high dosage selection include (1) physicochemical properties of the test substance or dosage formulation which, in combination with the route of administration, can limit the administered amount (generally 1–1.5 g/kg/day provides an adequate limit dosage); (2) kinetics, which can be very useful in determining exposure; and (3) a marked increase in embryo-fetal lethality in preliminary studies. Although often contested and infrequently pursued, the author's experience is that good science can also be used successfully to justify dosage selection and as a negotiating point with regulatory bodies.

METHODS FOR TESTING REPRODUCTIVE/DEVELOPMENTAL TOXICITY

This section describes the methods used to evaluate each ICH stage (see Figure 29.1). In the absence of information regarding effects on specific segments of the reproductive process, the most robust screen for evaluating female reproductive toxicity is an abbreviated multigeneration study, which ends at weaning of the second generation. This design is similar to the former UK Segment I design (40) and an extension of the FDA Segment I design (224) (see Figure 29.6) to include treatment beginning before cohabitation of the first generation and continuing through the delivery of offspring by the second generation. It screens for potential adverse effects on gonadal function and mating behavior in female animals, conception rates, early and late stages of gestation, parturition, lactation, and development of the offspring; however, when effects on specific female reproductive process are suspected or anticipated, a segmented approach may prove more appropriate. For example, evidence of LH inhibition in a pharmacology study, ovarian atresia in a chronic study, or abnormal estrous cycling in a subchronic toxicity study or preliminary reproductive toxicology screen may be predictive of potential reductions in mating and fertility in the parental generation and preclude production of adequate numbers of litters for further evaluation. Common protocols for use in evaluation of the various ICH segments are identified in Figure 29.7.

ICH STAGE A: Premating to Conception (Reproductive Functions in Adult Animals, including Development and Maturation of Gametes, Mating Behavior, and Fertilization)

Evaluation of the Ovary

Weight. Ovarian weights are recorded using the same techniques as those generally used for recording organ weights. The tissue should be trimmed and weighed close to the time removed from the animal to avoid dehydration. An alternate method is to weigh the ovaries after trimming and fixation.

Follicle number and size. Follicle number and size can be identified by histological evaluation of cross-sections of the ovary (170,193). This procedure is extremely time consuming and expensive (30–60 sections per ovary for mice and rats, resulting in 300 and 600 sections per group of 10 animals, respectively). A shorter screening method is described by Plowchalk (171) for potential use when indicated by observations in companion studies (e.g., pharmacologic action or reduced ovarian weight or atresia). After fixation of the ovaries in Bouin's solution, to prevent undue shrinkage, standard histologic techniques are used to prepare 6.0 μm serial sections. Five random sections are evaluated for primordial, growing, and antral follicles. Although this method reduces the statistical power of the assay, it allows assessment of loss of specific follicle types and changes in component volumes.

Corpora lutea number. Details regarding gross evaluation of *corpora lutea* at Caesarean sectioning of the female animal are provided later in this section. As previously discussed, the number of *corpora lutea* can be affected by many factors, including enhanced ovarian atresia, injection of hormones, a procedure common in mating rabbits, handling, especially in reflex ovulators, and litter size and hormonal feedback mechanisms, some of which are species specific (88,209). As a result, identification of preimplantation loss on the basis of comparison of the number of implants at caesarean-sectioning of the female animals is often quite imprecise, especially in mice and rabbits. Generally, in these types of studies, comparison of litter sizes is a more representative indicator of preimplantation loss. As regression of the *corpora lutea* occurs during lactation, inclusion of this parameter in postlactational evaluations is unnecessary.

Hormone integrity and function. Direct measurements of hormone levels usually are second-level evaluations. These can most effectively be performed by using commercially available antibody kits or by sending samples to contract laboratories for evaluation. Unfortunately, little historical experience with these assays exists with laboratory animal species. The expected background levels relevant to the specific strain and source should be developed before using these evaluations in a regulatory setting.

Collecting evaluation of the Uterus

Weight. Collecting uterine weight measurements is an historic method of measuring potential estrogenicity of a test material. Both juvenile and ovariectimized models are used, with the intact model demonstrating both primary and secondary effects and the ovariectimized model identifying uterine-specific effects. Despite the use and value of this assay for pharmacologic testing since 1939 (4), no standardized method is currently available (157,158,173), although the results of the Endrocrine Disruptor Screening and Testing Advisory Committee (EDSTAC) are expected to produce one for use in screening environmental contaminants. Regardless of the duration of the treatment period, responses can vary with the strain, source, and specific population and age tested, requiring characterization of historical data at the testing laboratory. The common use of only 10 animals per group often results in statistical significance between groups when outlier values (increased and reduced uterine weights) are included, with inappropriate identification of false-positives and false-negatives (24). Because of the sensitivity of the assay, the screen is a good predictor of absence of effect. When a positive effect is observed, it should be further characterized. When uterine weights are evaluated in animals in subchronic or chronic tests, it is helpful to identify the estrous cycle stage shortly before sacrifice, as cyclicity greatly affects uterine weight. The estrous stage identified from a vaginal lavage and the uterine estrous stage identified by histopathology will differ by approximately 1/2 day.

Evaluation of Estrous Cycling

Initial reprotoxicity screening studies usually are performed in rodent species, with the female animals treated for the first 14 days before cohabitation and then until mating occurs. Ideally, sexually mature female rodents are evaluated for estrous cycling (41) for 14 days before treatment to establish a baseline for regularity of cycling. Animals that irregularly cycle should be excluded from evaluation before the treatment phase. They can then be evaluated daily for one or more comparable intervals during the study to identify potential effects and possible reversal of effects. Animals housed in the same room tend to have synchronous estrous cycles, with resultant cyclic matings. Repeated use of this evaluation can be used to identify the onset of reproductive senility in chronic toxicity studies.

Estrous cycling in rodent species is evaluated by obtaining a sample of cells from the vagina by lavage and then examining the cytology. The regularity of the light cycle should be monitored, and vaginal smears should be collected from the animals at approximately the same time each day. Care should be taken in handling the animals to prevent effecting pseudopregnancy. It is also important to avoid contamination of the saline and pipette and to prevent potential infection of the animal and inappropriate sample collection.

Vaginal lavage samples are prepared from one or two drops of saline and delivered into and removed from the vagina with a dropping pipette. A new (clean) pipette should be used for each animal, and the tip of the pipette should always point downward when it contains a sample in order to avoid contaminating the bulb. After the pipette is removed from the vagina, the contents are delivered onto either a clean glass slide (identified with the animal number) or a ring slide containing designated areas for the placement of each sample. The smear of the vaginal contents is then examined (wet and unstained) by using a microscope at 100–200 × magnification. Ring slides should not be used for vaginal smears taken during cohabitation because it is difficult to wash sperm off this type of slide. After all daily smears are collected, the saline used in preparing the smears should be evaluated for potential contamination because carryover of sperm from an inseminated female could result in incorrect identification of mating.

The cellular characteristics of vaginal smears reflect structural changes of vaginal epithelium and follow a predictable course during the estrous cycle. The stage of the estrous cycle is determined by recognition of the predominant cell type present in the smear at each daily evaluation. An estrous cycle in rats and mice is typically 4–5 days and may be influenced by multiple factors, including light, temperature, humidity, noise, nutrition, and social relationship. In general, cycles are more easily influenced in mice than in rats.

Cycling changes usually are divided into four stages: estrus, metestrus, diestrus, and proestrus (Figure 29.9). Estrus lasts approximately 10–15 h in rats and approximately 21 h in mice; it is the only stage in the cycle when the female will copulate with the male. As shown in Figure 29.9a, cornified squamous epithelial cells are the dominant cell type in the vaginal smear and are few in number or absent. The squamous epithelial cells vary from flat (occur singly during early estrus) to curled (occur in large sheets in late estrus). Metestrus lasts from

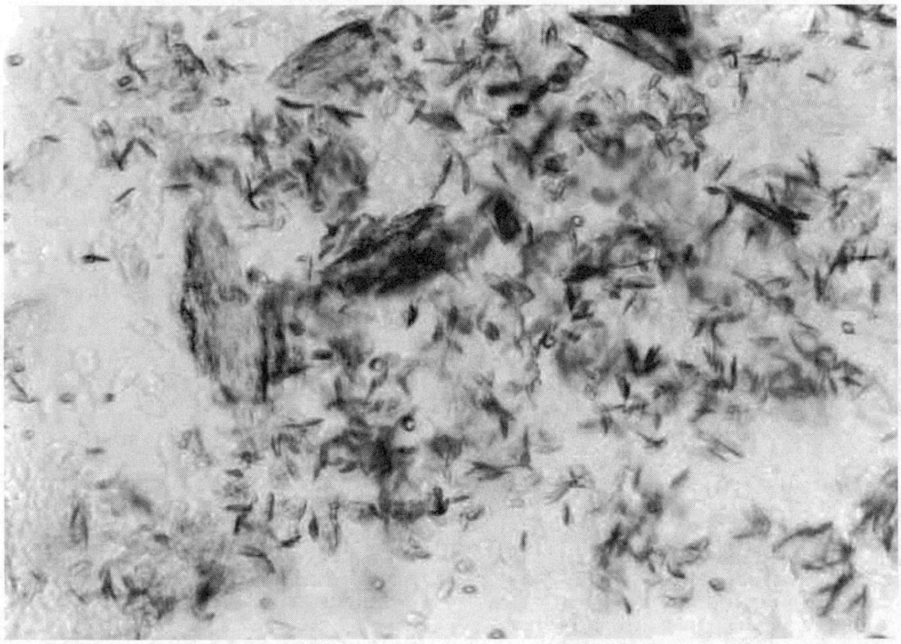

FIG. 29.9a. Estrous cycle stage 1: estrus.

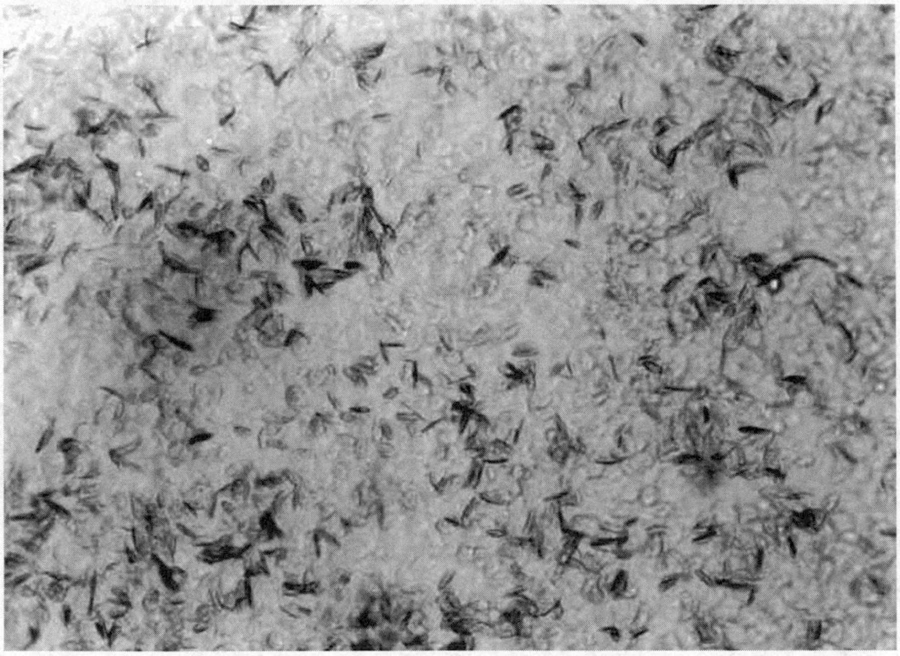

FIG. 29.9b. Estrous cycle stage 2: metestrus.

6–14 h in rats and approximately 22 h in mice. It is characterized by the presence of numerous cornified epithelial cells together with irregularly shaped nucleated epithelial cells. Leukocytes are present in considerable numbers (Figure 29.9b). Diestrus lasts 60–70 h (approximately half of entire cycle) in rats and 22–33 h in mice. It is dominated by leukocytes, although some nucleated epithelial cells may be present. In late diestrus, the nucleated epithelial cells become more spherical, and occasional cornified cells and erythrocytes are present (Figure 29.9c). Proestrus has a duration of 12–18 h in rats and approximately 21 h in mice and denotes the beginning of the next cycle. The vaginal smear is dominated by numerous nucleated epithelial cells, usually arranged in "grape-like" clusters (Figure 29.9d).

The duration of an estrus cycle is calculated for each animal based on the number of days between estrous stages per interval observed; these values are then averaged. When high variability is present in the averages or there are animals with persistent diestrus or estrus (more than 6 days), the abnormally cycling animals should be excluded from analyses and separately cited.

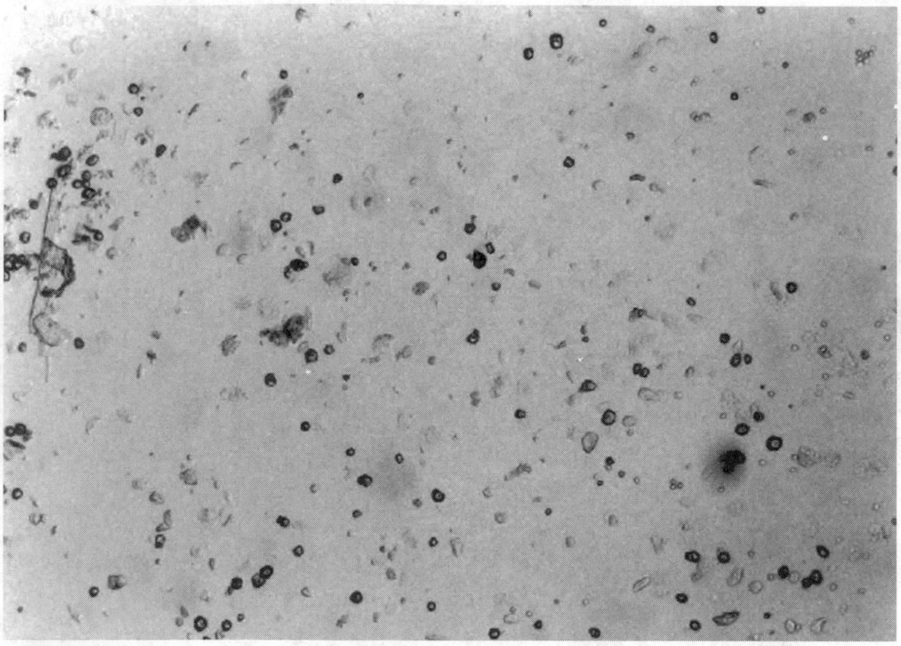

FIG. 29.9c. Estrous cycle stage 3: dietrus.

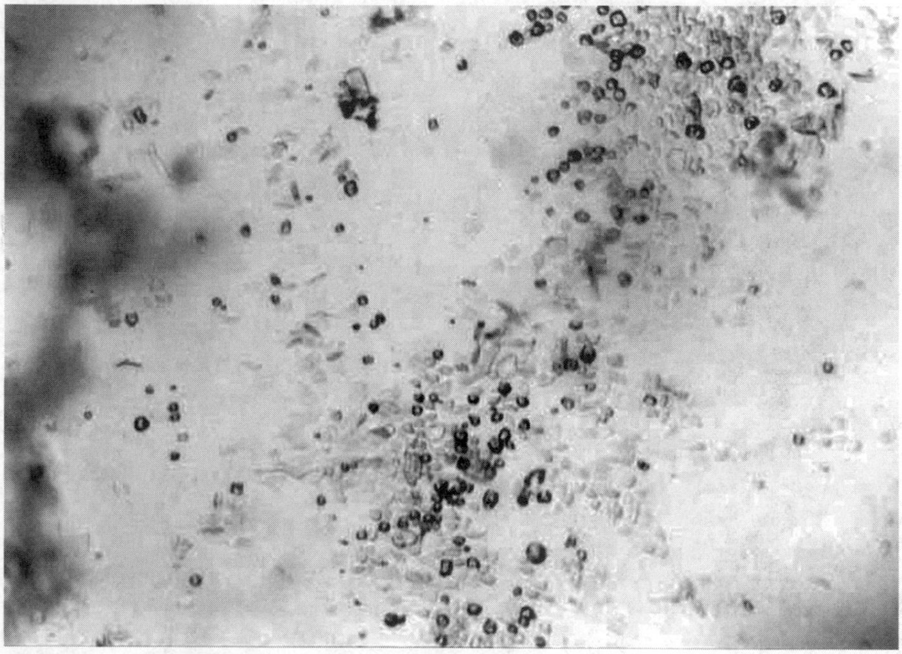

FIG. 29.9d. Estrous cycle stage 4: proestrus.

Such findings may reflect environmental or handling problems but may also be associated with effects of the test agent and should be evaluated for dose dependency.

Evaluation of Mating Behavior and Fertilization

Techniques for evaluating mating performance and fertility are used both for impregnating animals for use in developmental toxicity studies and when mating performance is evaluated in a reproductive toxicology evaluation. In the later case, treatment usually is begun in the female animal at least 2 weeks before cohabitation and continued until necropsy. The timing of necropsy is dependent on the endpoint to be evaluated, occurring at some interval within the gestation period. If the purpose of the screen is to observe mating behavior and any associated impairment of fertility or implantation, necropsy usually is performed at 13–15 days of presumed gestation. For alternate uses, treatment continues to the day before termination, either approximately 1 day before expected parturition, with Caesarean-sectioning and evaluation of uterine contents, or at completion of a 21–28 day lactation period, with evaluation of uterine contents and litter sizes and viability.

In general, mating ratios of one male per female are ideal for use in rodents because it allows easy identification of the sire and dam, history of reproductive performance, and excludes potential reductions in performance associated with excess use of the same male. The most effective way to produce pregnancies is to pair the animals when the female is in proestrus (usually late in the afternoon, dependent upon the light cycle used), as it will soon enter estrus and be receptive; however, assuming a large population of animals is available (approximately 125 breeder males and 125 virgin females), sufficient numbers (approximately 100 mated females) can be obtained within 4–5 days by simply cohabiting the entire population simultaneously.

Although estrous cycling usually is not evaluated when animals are bred for use in developmental toxicity studies, this parameter is very helpful in identifying potential effects in female animals in reproductive toxicity evaluations, when perturbations in estrous cycling may predict reduced female receptivity and fertility. Male mating performance should be considered in evaluation of any observed effects, as altered estrous cycling during cohabitation and reduced female fertility may reflect male-mediated effects (e.g., naivete, general health, altered/reduced mating performance, testicular lesions, abnormal sperm).

Rats and mice generally have multiple intromissions in one copulatory interval. If there is an indication that aberrant copulatory behavior may be present, the animals can be observed (videotaped), and graded for number of copulations, number of intromissions, duration of intromission, and expected female receptivity (lordosis). Mating (copulation) is confirmed by the presence of spermatozoa in the contents of the vaginal smear and/or the observation of a copulatory plug in situ; these findings designate day 0 of presumed gestation. It is prudent to note when less than 10 sperm are present in a smear because this information can assist in interpreting mating and fertility data. For mice, the presence of an expelled copulatory plug in the pan is often considered adequate proof of mating, although only approximately 85% of the mice identified in this fashion actually become pregnant.

Female mating performance can be measured by several endpoints, including identifying the number of days in cohabitation before mating, the number of mated (inseminated) female animals per group, and pregnancy incidences based on the total population per group (percentage pregnant/number cohabited) and on the inseminated population per group (percentage pregnant/number inseminated). The number of females assigned to an alternate male and the duration of cohabitation with the second male always should be identified. Care must be taken to ensure that all parameters based on group values are calculated on the basis of observations for the initial cohort pair. Data regarding any subsequent matings should be identified as such.

Artificial Insemination Procedures

Artificial insemination is an alternate method of mating rabbits. It has the advantages of better control over fewer male breeders and reductions in possible cross-infection and technical time requirements. The downside is a slightly reduced pregnancy rate and limited genetic background of the sires, although this can prove a benefit should a malformation be traceable to the sire.

The methodology, although not the subject of this chapter, can be easily adapted for use in male reproductive toxicity evaluations. Semen is collected in an artificial vagina that is lined with a condom from which the tip has been cut off. A collection cone is attached to the artificial vagina, which is then filled with warm water (approximately 50°C). The condom is then lubricated with a small amount of petroleum jelly (do not use a condom lubricated with a spermicide). The "teaser" female is introduced into the male's cage. The semen is collected when the buck attempts copulation with the doe.

Average spermatozoa concentration during a collection is $1.5–3.0 \times 10^8$/mL from a mature male breeder rabbit. Sperm concentration is determined by evaluation in a Neubauer RBC counting chamber to ensure appropriate quality. The mucus is removed and the volume recorded. A specimen sample is drawn to the 0.5 mark in an RBC counting pipette and then diluted with warm saline to the highest mark on the pipette, resulting in a dilution of 1 : 200. The pipette is shaken for thorough mixing, several drops are discarded from the tip of the pipette, and an appropriate amount of the sample is placed onto the Neubauer counting chamber. The number of sperm and the estimated percentage of motile sperm are then counted in the four corner squares and one of the middle squares of the lined area.

After determining that the sample has live, apparently normal spermatozoa, a count is calculated as follows:

$$\text{\# Live Spermatozoa} \times 1.0 \times 10^7 \times \text{Semen Volume} = \text{Spermatozoa Count.}$$

The standard sperm concentration used for insemination is 6.0×10^6 (0.6×10^7) spermatozoa per 0.25 mL. This concentration is obtained by using the following formula:

Spermatozoa Count / 2.4 (dilution constant) – mL semen
= mL saline to add.

The measured volume of saline is then used to dilute the semen sample by adding a portion of the saline to the collection cone. A glass bottle that has been warmed with normal saline is emptied and the diluted semen in the collection cone poured into the warmed bottle; this procedure is repeated several times, using the remaining saline from the graduated cylinder.

Before insemination, each doe is given an intravenous injection (ear vein) of 20 U.S.P. units/kg Human Chorionic Gonadotropin (HCG) to induce ovulation (larger dosages tend to result in superovulation and do not increase fertility or litter sizes). HCG is supplied as powder with 10,000 U.S.P. units per vial. These 10,000 U.S.P. units are diluted with normal saline to a volume of 50 mL (200 U.S.P. Units/mL). The same volume of diluted HCG is separated into labeled sterilized vials, one for each day of insemination (usually four or five consecutive days), and maintained refrigerated after preparation. At this concentration, each injection volume is 0.10 mL/kg of body weight (e.g., a rabbit weighing 5.0 kg is administered 0.50 mL for a dosage of 20 U.S.P. units/kg, which is a total dose of 100 U.S.P. units/animal).

Approximately 3 to 6 h after HCG-induced ovulation of the female rabbits, each is inseminated with approximately 0.25 mL of diluted semen. To do so, the technician holds the doe between his or her knees to gently restrain the rabbit, with the rabbit's head downward and facing away from the technician. A glass insemination tube with an inside diameter of 4 mm and length of 7.5 in is used. The tube is bent at a 45° angle 1.5 in from one end; a rubber bulb covers the opposite end. The tube is filled to the bend (which is the point at which it will contain 0.25 mL) with the diluted semen (this volume is a close approximation). The tail of the rabbit is pulled toward the technician, exposing the rabbit's vulva, which should be pink and glistening (evidence of receptivity). The glass tube containing 0.25 mL of diluted semen is held with the short end of the glass tube parallel to the rabbit's spine and guided into the vagina to the depth of the bend (at the pelvic brim). The tube is inserted until resistance is no longer felt because the tube has passed into the cervix. The tube bulb is squeezed, depositing the semen, and the tube is then gently rotated 90 degrees (stimulating the cervix) and subsequently removed (continued squeezing of the bulb occurs during removal).

Each day, after the insemination procedure is completed, a sample of the diluted semen is examined for apparent viability and continued motility. If the postinsemination count is estimated to have less than 60% motility, it is generally considered appropriate to inseminate the does again.

ICH Stage B: Conception to Implantation (Reproductive Functions in the Adult Female, Preimplantation and Implantation Stages of the Conceptus)

Evaluation of Preimplantation Loss and Impaired Implantation

This process is based on comparison of the number of *corpora lutea* with the number of uterine implantation sites identified at Caesarean sectioning of the female animals. As previously described, this parameter is highly variable and tends to be of minimal value in mice, rabbits, and guinea pigs, and is highly associated with fetal survival and hormonal feedback in rats.

ICH Stages B, C, and D

B: Conception to implantation—reproductive functions in the adult female, preimplantation and implantation stages of the conceptus;

C: Implantation to closure of the hard palate—adult female reproductive functions and development of the embryo through major organ formation;

D: Closure of the hard palate to the end of pregnancy—adult female reproductive function, fetal development and growth, and organ development and growth.

Caesarean-Sectioning Procedures

When the purpose of the reproductive or developmental toxicity study is to screen for preimplantation loss and early implantation, the animals are killed near the beginning of the fetal period, as this allows easy identification of viability based on a beating heart. In a full developmental toxicity screen, the animals are killed on the day before or the day parturition is expected, to preclude effects associated with delivery complications (e.g., prolonged gestation and associated pup mortality and maternal cannibalization of stillborn or malformed pups). Use of time-mated animals tends to increase the variability in gestational ages and viability of the conceptuses and should be considered as a potential confounding factor in data evaluation. Regardless of the day of gestation, balanced termination of animals across groups should occur to preclude differences associated with gestational ages. Termination of large populations of animals on the day parturition is expected tends to result in some female animals delivering litters. This is particularly common in mice and hamsters and occurs occasionally in rabbits. Such events produce complications in data capture because the animals can be included in some analyses (e.g., pregnancy incidence, implantation numbers) but should be excluded from others (e.g., fetal body weights, fetal ossification site observations). One benefit of termination of the female on the day parturition is expected is that there is less variability in the degree of skeletal ossification. General practice is to terminate mice, rats, rabbits, and hamsters on days 18, 20 or 21, 29, and 15 of gestation, respectively.

Gross Necropsy of Maternal Animals

Euthanasia of the dams is easily accomplished by asphyxiation with carbon dioxide gas, and animals are terminated at intervals ensuring that the time between death and necropsy is no more than 20 min. After external examination, the animal is placed on its dorsal surface and an incision made through the skin and/or musculature, extending from the inguinal area to the anterior portion of the neck. The abdominal viscera are exposed by making an incision through the abdominal muscles and peritoneum up to the sternum. The thoracic viscera are exposed by making an incision along one or both sides of the sternum up to the level of the clavicles.

Gross examination of the thoracic, abdominal, and pelvic viscera of the dam and retention of gross lesions in neutral buffered 10% formalin is a standard procedure that often provides evidence of maternal effects. When required, the brain may also be examined. In some cases, target organs (e.g., liver, kidneys, and brain) are weighed and retained for further evaluation. It is also common to collect maternal blood, placentas, amniotic fluid, and embryos or fetuses for use in pharmacokinetic evaluations at caesarean sectioning. Obviously, data from nonpregnant animals should be excluded in the pharmacokinetic studies relevant to pregnancy.

According to present ICH guidelines, pharmacokinetic studies should be conducted in pregnant animals to determine if pharmacokinetic differences occur in the pregnant state versus the nonpregnant state and whether the fetus is exposed to appreciable amounts of the test material. These studies, usually conducted twice (first and last dosage) during pregnancy in rats and rabbits, are most frequently performed as separate studies, in order to preclude the occurrence of developmental abnormalities that may be associated with the stress of multiple blood collections and/or unusually high dosages of test material in the dams assigned to full reproduction or developmental toxicity studies. Although it is occasionally appropriate to perform detailed kinetics studies, such usually is not done. Common practice in the kinetics animals is to identify only pregnancy (presence of live conceptuses) to avoid potential legal or liability actions based on the identification of possible fetal malformations associated with nondrug-related manipulations of the female animal.

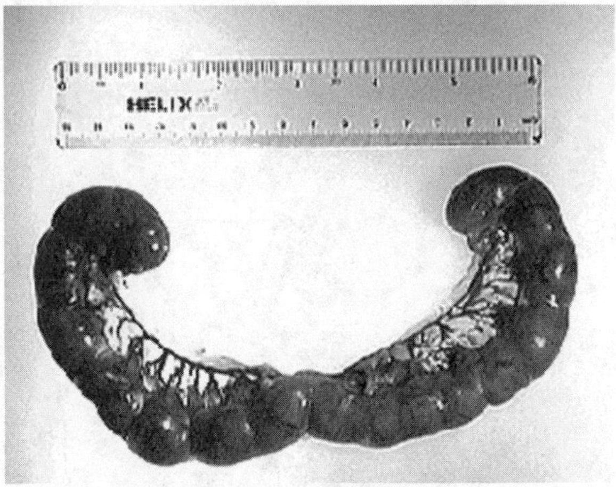

FIG. 29.10. Rat – Day 20 of gestation uterus.

Evaluation of Ovaries and Uterus

Evaluation of the uterus and its contents can be performed at any time during the gestation period, depending upon the purpose of the evaluation (Figure 29.10). The uterus with attached ovaries is removed from the abdominal cavity and placed on a dissection blotting paper. The number of *corpora lutea* in each ovary is counted (with ovaries attached to oviduct) and the number compared with the number of implantation sites, which can be identified through the uterine wall. Figures 29.11a and 29.11b show rat and rabbit ovaries with *corpora lutea*, respectively. The uterus of female rodents that do not appear pregnant can be examined effectively either by pressing the uterus between glass plates and examining it for the presence of implantation sites or staining it with ammonium sulfide (179).

Evaluation of Uterine Weight

When a uterine weight is desired, the right ovary is removed, and the left ovary remains on the oviduct of the uterine horn (for identification of right and left uterine horns). An alternate method is to remove both ovaries and attach a hemostat (weight tared before weighing) to the right uterine horn for identification. Care is taken throughout the process to not cut the uterus or express any fluid. The same procedure can be used to evaluate nonpregnant uterine weights of rats or mice used in assays for estrogenicity, as described previously.

Evaluation of Uterine Contents

After weighing, the uterine horns are opened along the greater curvature, and the number and distribution of implantation sites are recorded (Figures 29.12a and 29.12b). Each implantation site is consecutively numbered in both uterine horns, beginning with the ovarian end of the right horn and counting toward the

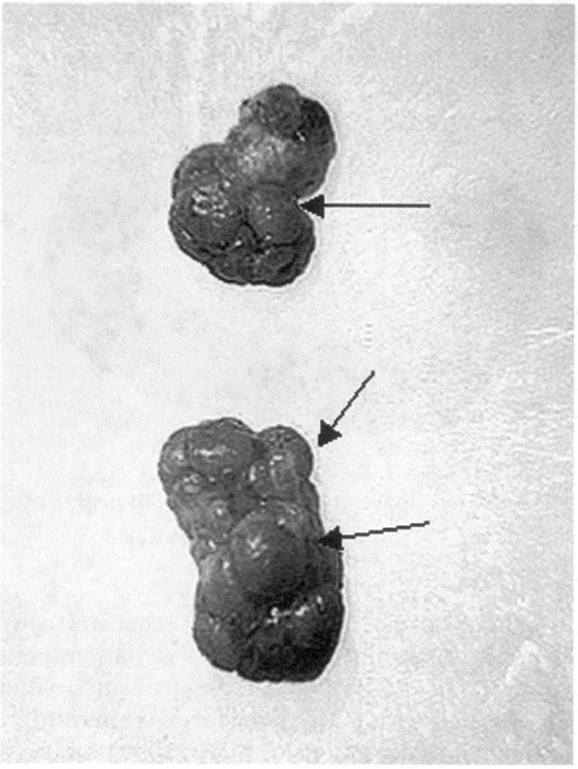

FIG. 29.11a. Rat Ovaries – Corpora lutea.

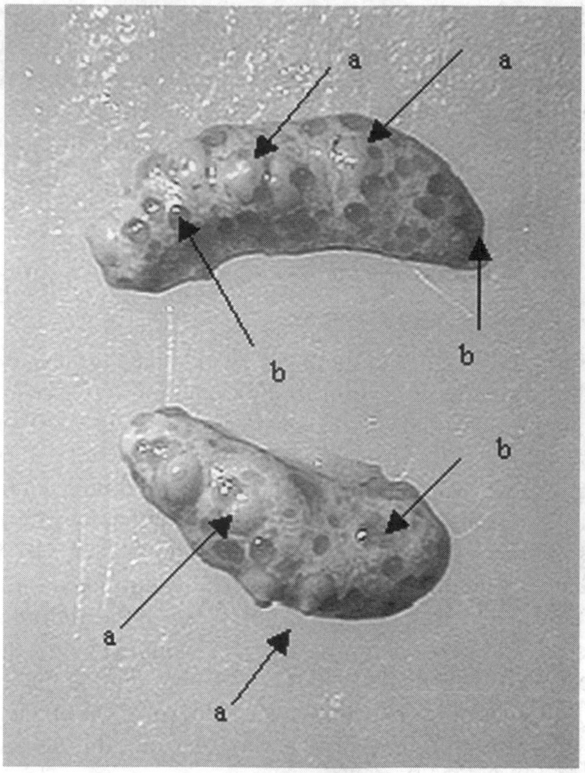

FIG. 29.11b. Rabbit ovaries (a) corpora lutea, (b) empty follicles.

cervix, and continuing with the ovarian end of the left uterine horn and again counting toward the cervix. Each implantation site is described as:

An early or late resorption. An early resorption is defined as a conceptus in which it is not grossly evident that organogenesis has occurred; a late resorption is defined as a fetus (day 16 of developmental age or later in the rat) in which it is grossly evident that organogenesis has occurred.

A live or dead fetus. A live fetus is defined as one that responds to stimuli; a dead fetus is defined as a term fetus not demonstrating marked to extreme autolysis. Fetuses with marked to extreme autolysis are considered to be late resorptions.

Viable or nonviable embryos (*day 10, 13, or 15 of gestation for rats*). A viable embryo is oval or crescent shaped, pink, firm, and enclosed in an amniotic sac filled with clear fluid. A nonviable embryo is amorphous, small, pale pink to tan or deep red to black, soft, and enclosed in an amniotic sac filled with clear or cloudy fluid; it is unnecessary to open the uterine horns to determine viability of day 10 or day 13 rat embryos.

Excess blood and amniotic fluid are removed from the fetus by rinsing and/or blotting on absorbent paper. Individual fetuses are deposited in multicompartmented boxes, each compartment of which contains a tag that will ultimately be tied to the fetus and will remain with the fetus throughout processing, evaluation, and archiving. The tag cites the study number, dam number, uterine placement of the fetus, and appropriate fixative to be used for further processing, if required. When evaluations are to be made without the investigator's knowledge of the dosage group of the fetus (i.e., "blind"), the box containing the fetuses is given a white label bearing only the study number and animal number and with a Caesarean-sectioning processing tag. Although some investigators believe that blind evaluations enhance the quality of the data, this procedure is not always valid. In many cases, knowledge regarding the specimen evaluated enhances the ability of an experienced investigator to identify alterations associated with treatment. In addition, conducting evaluations under blinded conditions increases the probability of error in data processing and storage of the specimens. It also increases the difficulties of data collection should an automated data collection system not be available.

Gross Examination and Weight of Placenta

The placenta and attached amniotic sac containing the fetus are removed from the uterine horn. The placenta

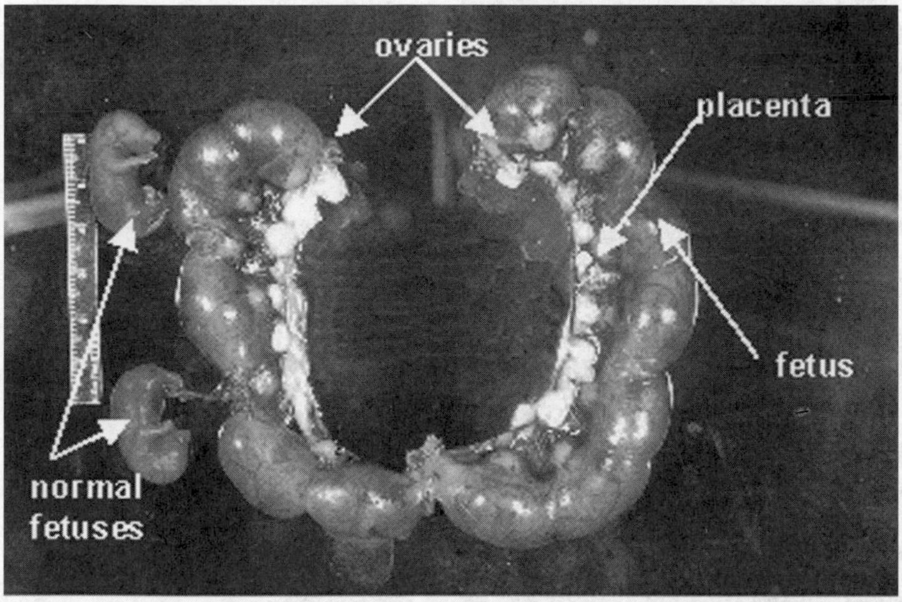

FIG. 29.12a. Rat uterus – Day 20 of gestation.

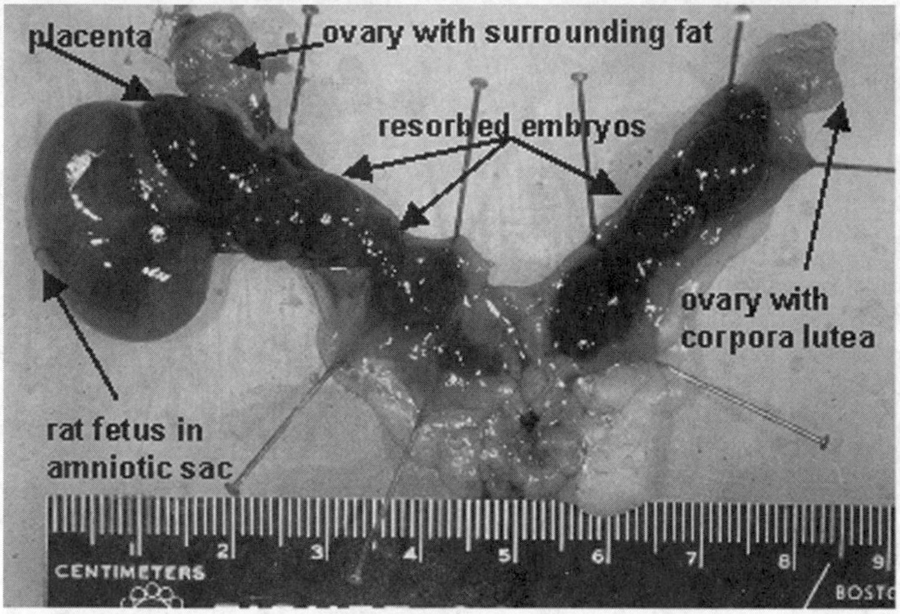

FIG. 29.12b. Rat uterine contents – Day 20 of gestation.

is separated from the amniotic sac, and the placenta and fetus are placed in the compartmentalized box for the litter. Each placenta is observed for gross changes (e.g., white spots, areas of necrosis, abnormal size). Individual weights are sometimes taken should an estrogenic effect be suspected, although the relatively high variability in placental weights is associated with fetal size and blood status at maternal death.

Fetal Evaluations

Experience and expertise are pivotal requirements for accurate evaluations of fetal specimens. Technical training should include evaluation of a positive control group (e.g., aspirin or vitamin A), as well as evaluation of several untreated control group litters (co-evaluation of two or three studies, with an experienced investigator), particularly for soft tissue and skeletal evaluations, to ensure comparable levels of expertise when multiple technicians perform these evaluations in the same laboratory. It is also recommended that identified alterations be confirmed by a senior level investigator to ensure comparable evaluation within a study as well as across studies. To the extent possible, observations made during gross external examination of the fetus should be confirmed in soft tissue

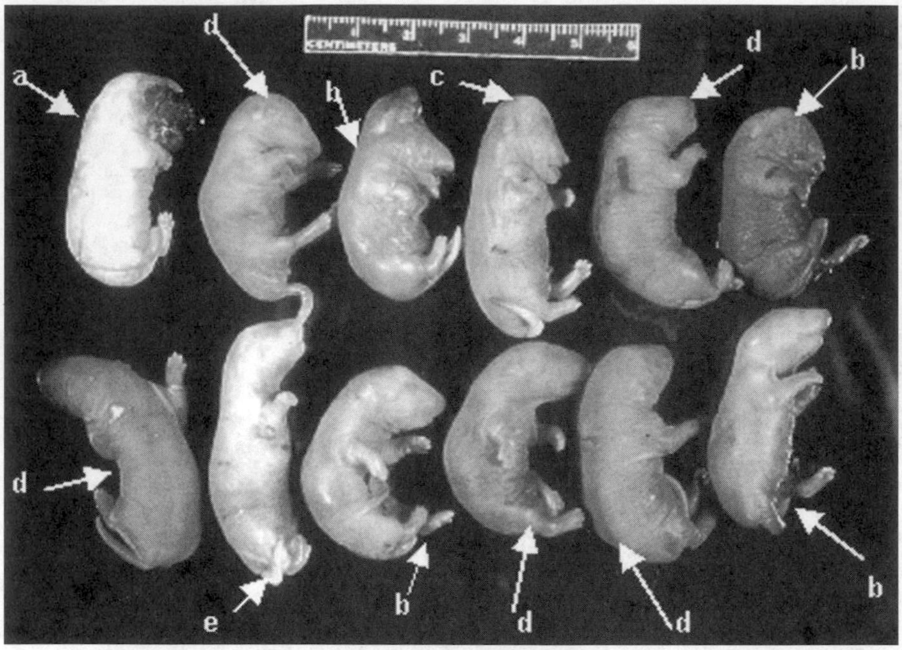

FIG. 29.13a. Rat fetuses – Day 20 of gestation – Example of differential effects on litter: a = dead, macerated; b = malformed; c = dead, compressed; d = live, externally normal; e = dead.

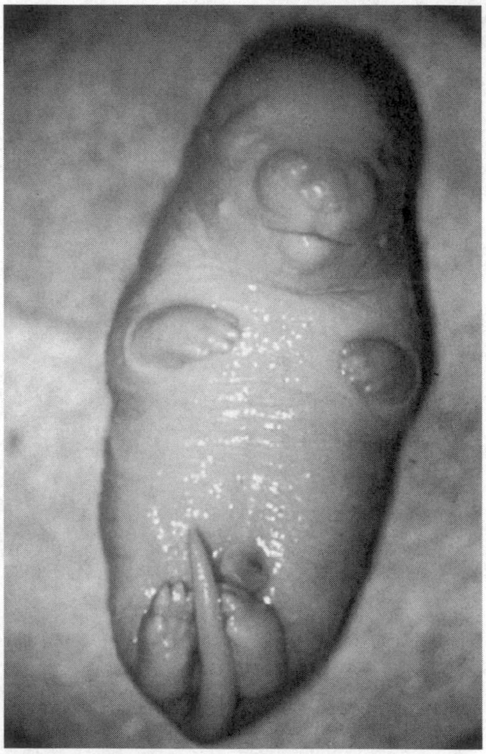

FIG. 29.13b. Rat fetus – Day 20 of gestation: anasarca (edema of entire body); note apparent clubbing of limbs.

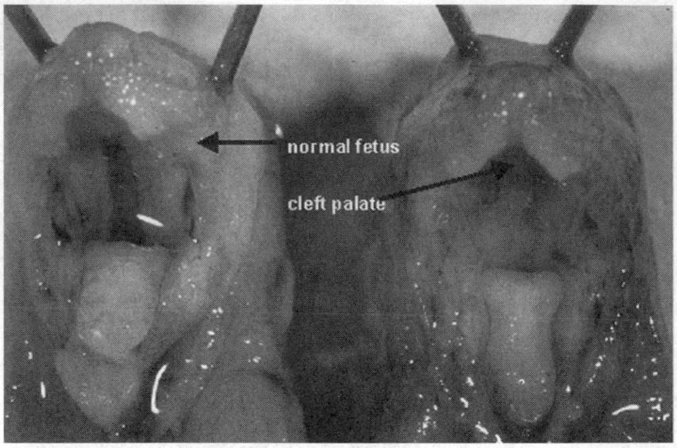

FIG. 29.13c. Rat fetuses – Day 20 of gestation – Cleft palate.

and skeletal examinations and the related changes described. Because the degree of ossification increases very rapidly shortly before birth, any errors regarding day 0 of gestation for the dam should result in exclusion of the litter from summarizations of delays in ossification.

Gross External Fetal Examination. Examples of typical externally identifiable abnormalities in rat fetuses are provided in Figures 29.13a through 29.13f. All fetuses are examined for gross external alterations, externally sexed (rabbit fetuses by internal inspection), weighed, and tagged. It should be noted that no truly adequate method for fetal euthanasia exists. Because of ethical animal care and use concerns, multiple new methods have been developed (e.g., chilling, carbon dioxide, oral administration of barbiturates). Each has associated problems, the most frequent of which is prolonged time between administration and fetal death, inadvertent production of artifacts (intrathoracic and intraperitoneal injections of barbiturates with associated deformations and occasional internal bleeding or apparent hemorrhage

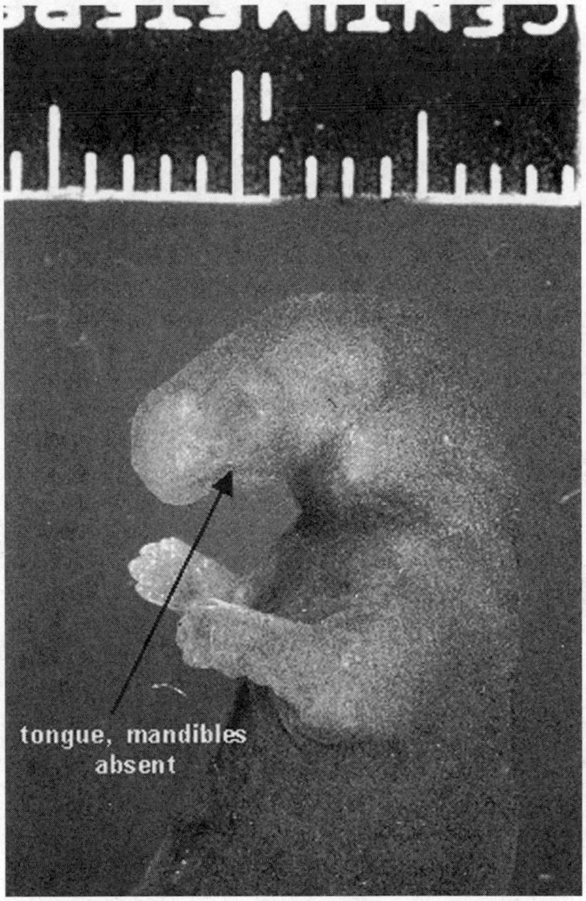

FIG. 29.13d. Mouse fetus – Day 18 of gestation – Agmathia (absence of tongue and mandibles).

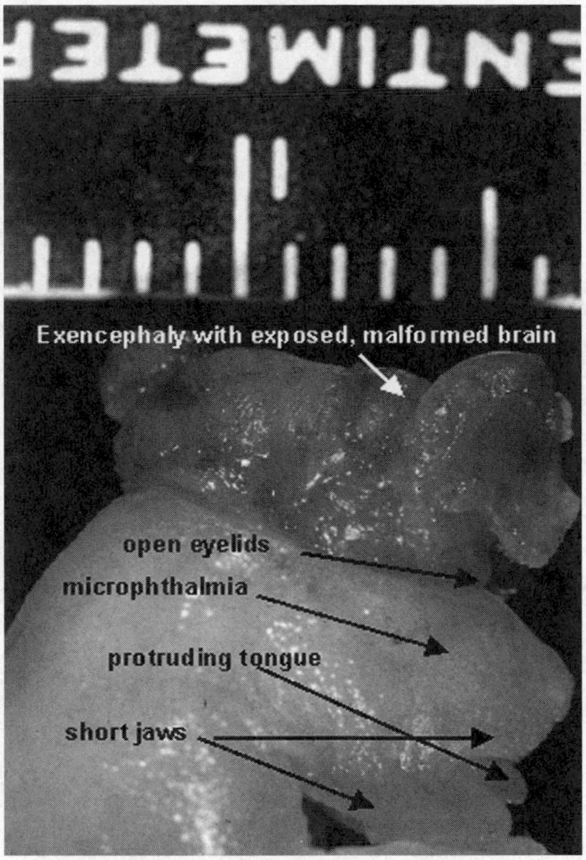

FIG. 29.13e. Rat fetus – Day 20 of gestation: exencephaly, short jaws, protruding tongue, microphthalmia.

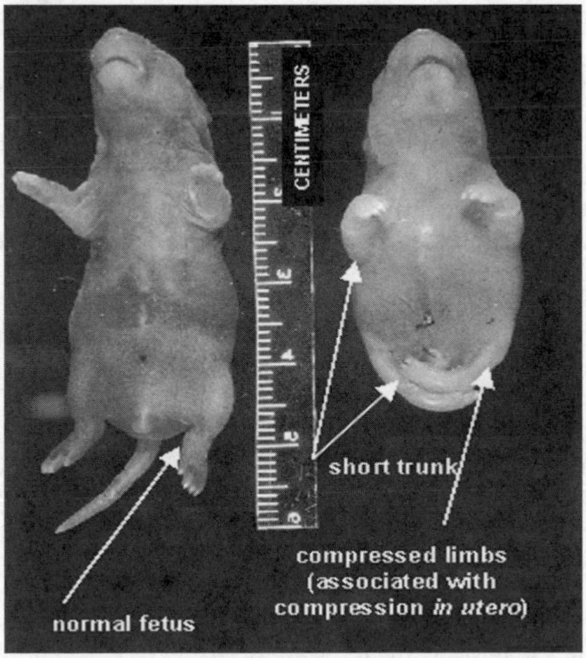

FIG. 29.13f. Rat fetuses – Day 20 of gestation – Normal fetus and fetus with short trunk and compressed limbs.

tracts) and potential employee health concerns associated with increased access to barbiturates in the laboratory. The investigator should be aware of the potential for artifact production, as many artifacts have been incorrectly diagnosed as findings by inexperienced technicians. The methods described in the following paragraphs are those generally used in our laboratory, although alternate methods are sometimes used.

Each fetus is euthanized by intraperitoneal injection of pentobarbital or euthanasia solution (preferred method of euthanasia for fetuses assigned to skeletal evaluation). Decapitation may be used and is preferred for fetuses assigned to evaluation using Wilson's free-hand sectioning technique (235) for the head and visceral dissection of the body (201). Hypothermia may be used alone or may be combined with one of the above methods to facilitate death.

After completion of the gross external fetal examinations, fetuses are placed in an appropriate fixative for subsequent processing when soft tissue evaluation is to be performed using Wilson's free-hand sectioning technique. Should all fetuses be evaluated for both soft

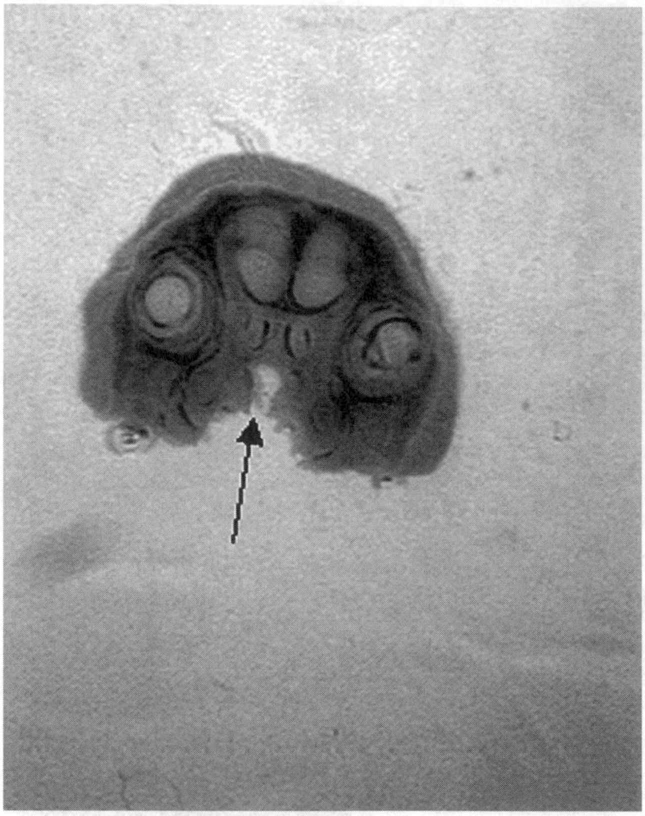

Fig. 29.14a. Rat fetus – Day 20 of gestation – Bouin's fixation – Cleft palate.

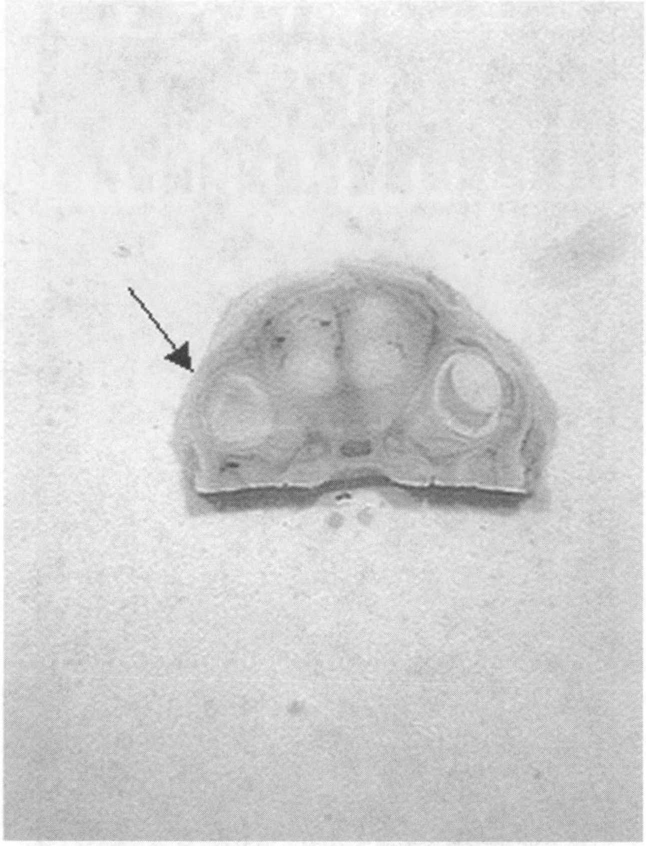

FIG. 29.14b. Rat fetus – Day 20 of gestation – Unilateral microphthalmia.

tissue and skeletal examinations, dissection procedures, such as those described by Staples (201) and Stuckhardt and Poppe (203), are performed before fixation of tissues and processing for skeletal examination.

The general practice for rabbits and other large mammals with relatively small litter sizes is to evaluate all fetuses for gross external, soft tissue, and skeletal alterations; for small rodents (rats, mice, hamsters; relatively large litter sizes), the usual practice is to evaluate half of the fetuses in each litter for soft tissue alterations and the remaining fetuses for skeletal alterations. Although some investigators recommend random assignment of fetuses to either evaluation, this procedure complicates an already technically difficult process. The most common practice is to assign fetuses to skeletal or soft-tissue evaluation on an every-other-fetus basis, beginning with the first fetus at the ovarian position of the right uterine horn and ending with the last fetus at the vaginal position of the left uterine horn. The first fetus is assigned to skeletal evaluation, although use of the reverse procedure would not affect the overall outcome of the evaluation. Occasionally it may be desirable to assign a fetus with a specific gross external alteration to the alternate fixative in order to achieve a more meaningful evaluation.

Soft Tissue Evaluation. All nonrodent fetuses are evaluated for soft tissue alterations by using gross dissection techniques. Soft tissue evaluation in rodents can be performed by using either Wilson's free-hand cross-sectioning (235) or gross dissection (201). Examples of normal sections and a few abnormalities in rat fetuses are provided as Figures 29.14a through 29.14j. Although debate has occurred as to which method is optimal, both are currently considered to be equivalent. The method selected should be based on the laboratory's personnel resources, training, historical experience, and scheduling requirements. Several of the senior and technical personnel in our laboratory had the honor of being trained by Dr. Wilson and/or Dr. Staples in their respective techniques. This author is particularly indebted to them both for access to their figures and descriptions of the procedures, some of which are presented in this volume.

As noted previously, approximately half of the rodent fetuses in each litter are generally assigned to soft tissue evaluation after gross external evaluation. Fixation of these specimens in Bouin's solution and subsequent evaluation by Wilson's method (235), rather than dissection of the fetuses directly after Caesarean-delivery, allows use

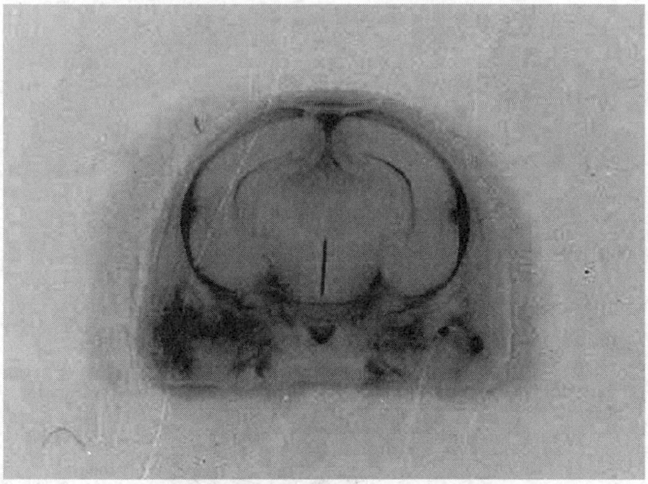

FIG. 29.14c. Rat fetus – Day 20 of gestation – Bouin's fixation – Normal brain.

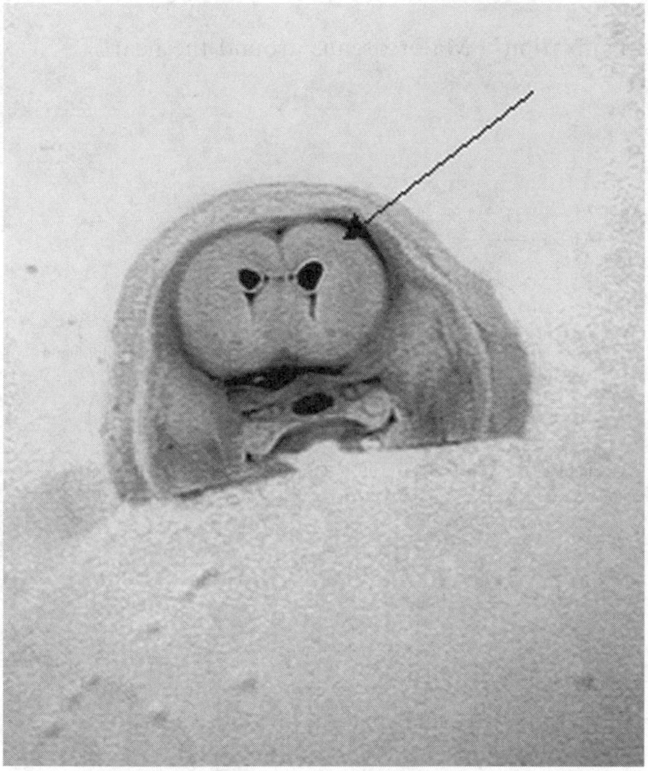

FIG. 29.14d. Rat fetus – Day 20 of gestion – Slight dilation lateral ventricles in brain.

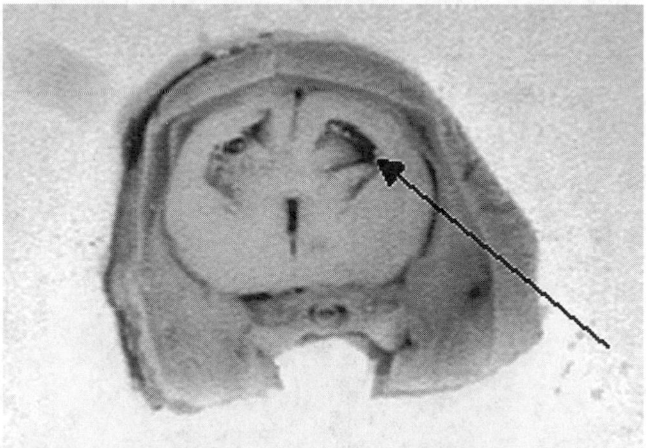

FIG. 29.14e. Rat fetus – Day 20 of gestion – Marked dilation of lateral ventricles in brain.

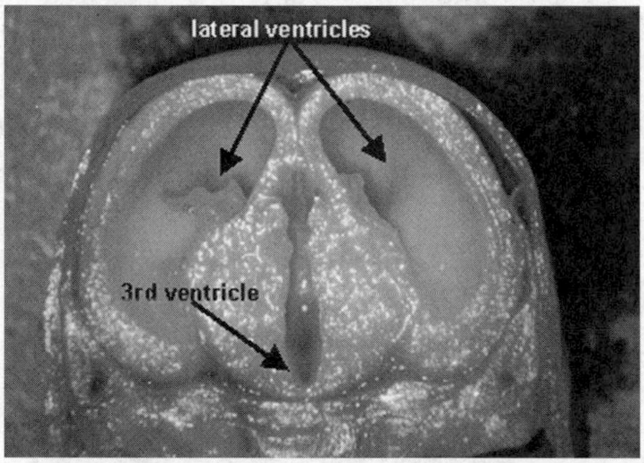

FIG. 29.14f. Rat fetus – Day 20 of gestation – Bouin's fixation – extreme dilation of lateral ventricles and moderate dilation of 3rd ventricle in brain.

of fewer personnel and reduces the time required to perform all observations associated with Caesarean-sectioning. Evaluation of the Bouin's-fixed fetuses can occur at any time after hardening and decalcification of the specimens (a process usually requiring approximately 1 week). In the absence of high incidences of multiple abnormalities in the fetuses, an experienced individual can generally evaluate all specimens (approximately 1000) from a study over 5 working days. The cross-sections are easily preserved and are ready for processing for histopathological evaluation, if required. The disadvantages of this method are that it tends to require more intensive training and experience than fresh dissection. This is because the evaluator must have an extensive knowledge of normal appearance of each cross-section, be aware of potential artifacts associated with fixation (e.g., potential shrinkage, tracks from slicing), biased slicing, and small differences in the thickness of the slices and the tissue present, events associated with individual fetal size.

In contrast, gross dissection (202) allows identification of both gross external and soft tissue alterations on the same day Caesarean-delivery occurs, shortening study time by approximately 1 week. It requires less training

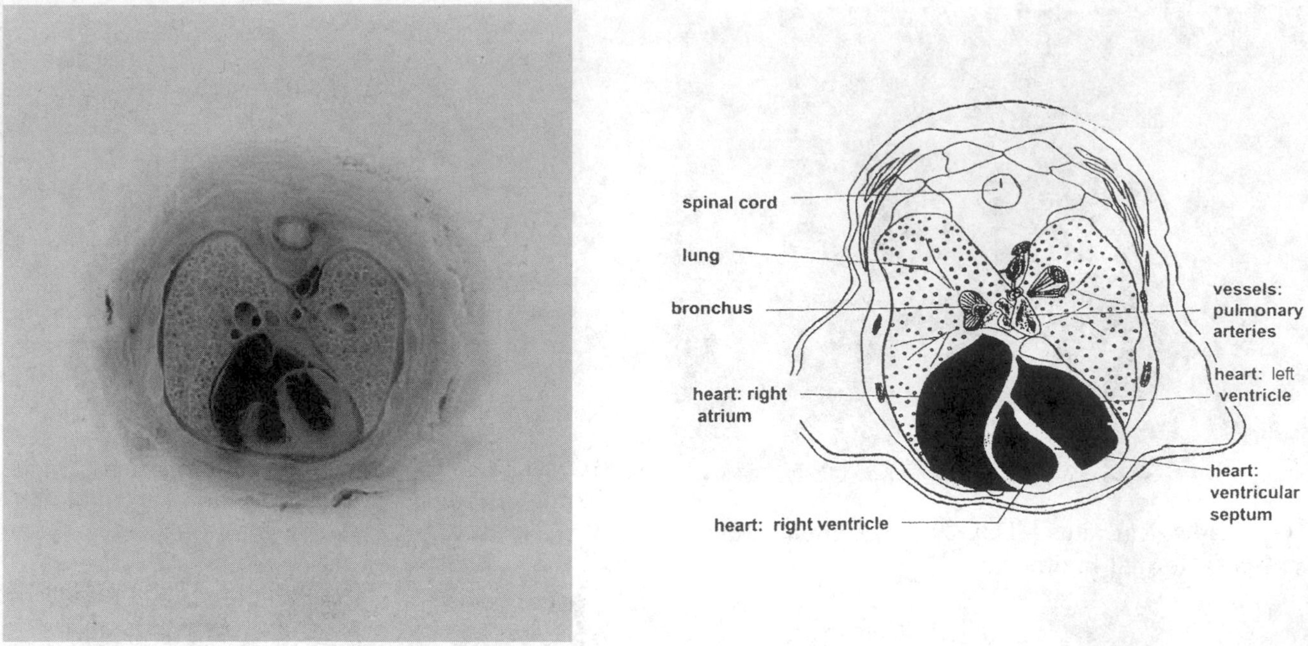

FIG. 29.14g. Rat fetus – Day 20 of gestation – Bouin's fixation – Major organs around the heart.

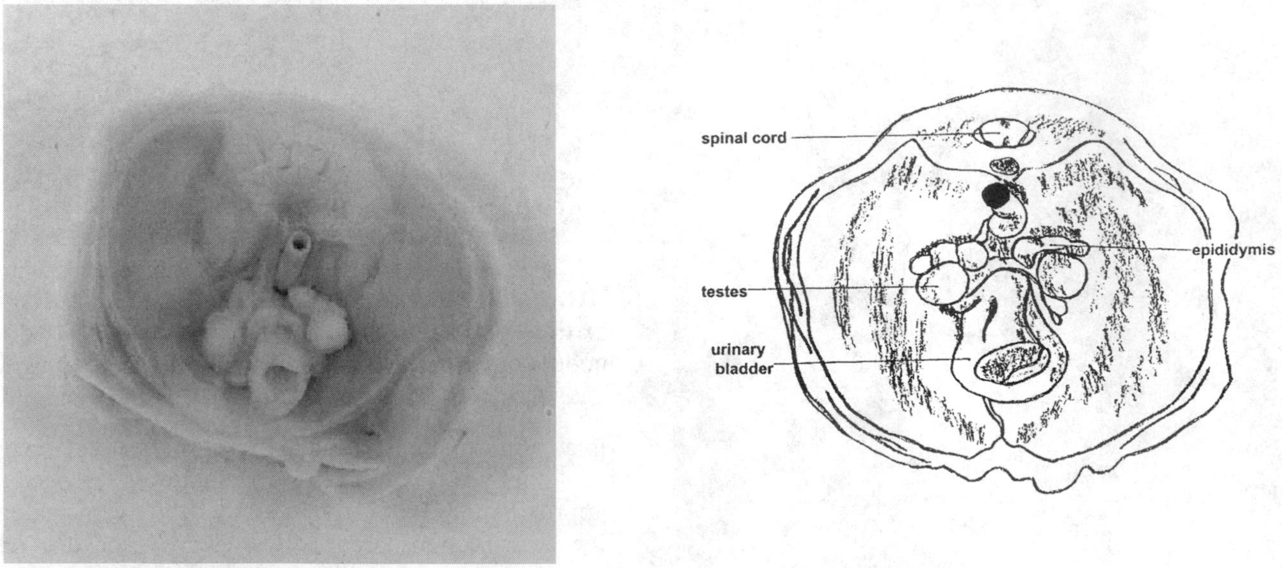

FIG. 29.14h. Rat fetus – Day 20 of gestation – Bouin's fixation – Normal male reproductive organs.

because the viscera are evaluated in situ, an aspect that is relatively easy to conceptualize. As originally described (beating heart preparation), gross dissection provides an overall view of the major organs, blood vessels, and the functioning heart, as well as a relatively easy identification of most common cardiac and great vessel alterations (for humane reasons, the fetuses are now killed before evaluation). It also eliminates artifacts associated with fixation and allows processing of all fetuses for skeletal examination. The disadvantage of this method is increased personnel requirements (generally four technicians are required to simultaneously evaluate the fetuses in order to complete all Caesarean-sectioning deliveries and evaluations within approximately 5 h, which greatly reduces interlitter variability) and, when initially introduced, absence of historical incidences.

Wilson's cross-sectioning technique (235). After the fetuses have been fixed in Bouin's solution long enough to harden soft tissues and decalcify the bones (but before sectioning), the fetus is re-examined for external

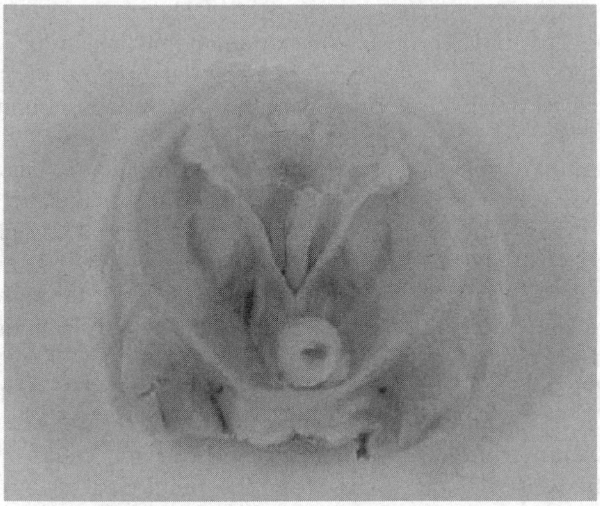

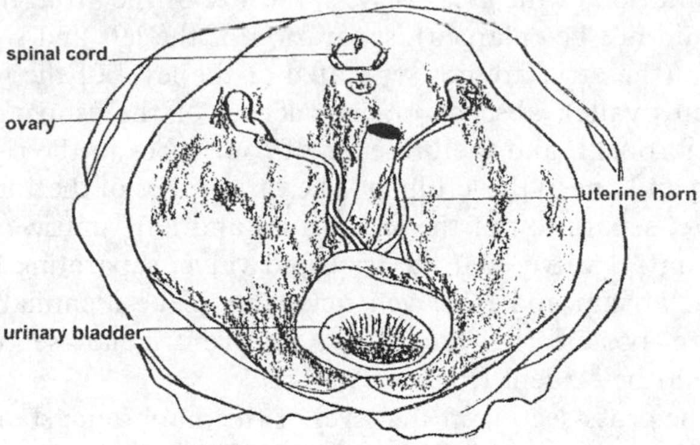

FIG. 29.14i. Rat fetus – Day 20 of gestation – Bouin's fixation – Normal female reproductive organs.

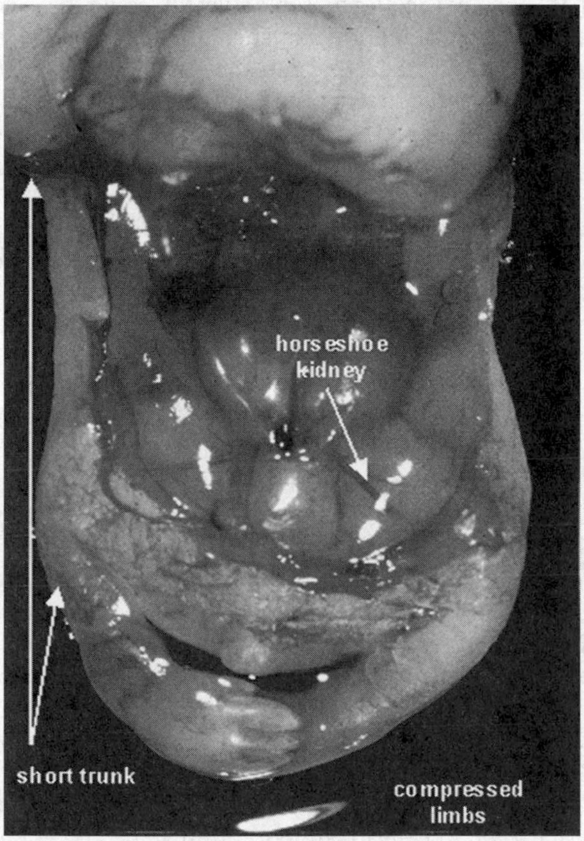

FIG. 29.14j. Rat fetus – Day 20 of gestation – Dissected – Short trunk, compressed limbs and horseshoe kidney.

abnormalities. Any previously noted abnormality is confirmed and any additional findings are noted. The fetal identification tag and the limbs and tail of the fetus are then removed, and the fetus is cross-sectioned. The actual number of cross-sections made is dependent on the size of the fetus. Keeping the sections moist with Bouin's solution, each section is examined with the aid of a stereo microscope at 7 × to 40 × magnification. Because so many diagrams and photographs of Wilson's procedure are available (235), for brevity, only a few representative sections (Figures 29.14a through 29.14i) are provided here, along with a description of expected observations.

The initial sections are made through the nasal passages, which should be open and unblocked throughout. The roof of the mouth should be continuous (Figure 29.14a) and separate the oral cavity from the nasal passages. The nasal septum should completely divide the nasal passage in anterior sections but lose its connection ventrally in more posterior sections. The cross section through the eyes should demonstrate the presence of two eyes of equal size (Figure 29.14b). The retina should be in one piece, without separation of the layers.

Cross-sections through the cerebral hemispheres should demonstrate presence of cranial nerves and minimal dilation of the lateral and third ventricles in the brian (Figures 29.14c through 29.14f). Both lobes of the pituitary should be identifiable, with minimal space between the lobes. The section through the inner ears should allow identification of the presence of the lumina of the cochlea, sacculus, and utriculus, and absence of obstruction of the lumina of the semicircular canals.

Cross-section through the upper neck should demonstrate that the esophagus is dorsal to the trachea and that both are unobstructed. The thyroid should be present on each side of the trachea, with lobes of equivalent and appropriate sizes. The cross-section through the lower neck should reveal the presence and size of the thymus, absence of obstruction of the esophagus and trachea, and presence of the trachea to the right of the esophagus.

Subsequent cross-sections through the upper thorax and great vessels should allow identification of the size and orientation of the great vessels, the size of the atria (they should not be enlarged), separation of the left and right atria (the atria are not separated at the level of the foramen ovalle), absence of obstruction of the esophagus and bronchi, and the presence of four lobes in the right lung and one in the left lung. The three cusps of the aortic valve, separation of the left atrium and left ventricle by the mitral valve, and the tricuspid valve, separating the right atrium and right ventricle, should be identifiable. More posteriorly, the intact interventricular septum should be evident (Figure 29.14g).

The cross-section at the level of the diaphragm should allow inspection of the surface of the diaphragm for any ruptures or herniations of abdominal viscera into the thoracic cavity. More posteriorly, the lobation of the liver should be evident, as well as the entry of the esophagus into the stomach. The mid-abdominal cross-section should be evaluated for any unusual patches or raised areas in the mucosa of the stomach. More posteriorly, it should be noted that the right kidney is slightly anterior to the left kidney; the size and shape of the kidneys and each pelvis should be checked for enlargement and papillary development and the spleen evaluated for size, shape, and texture. Should the adrenal glands not be transected, they should be examined separately and sectioned; normal adrenal glands appear as a solid mass of tissue.

The pelvic area should be examined for the ureters, located in the connective tissue of the lower back, and any deviations in the course or diameter noted. The sex of each fetus should be confirmed internally (Figures 29.14h and 29.14i), and any discrepancy from the externally identified sex noted. Bilateral testes and ovaries should be present, with the testes descended.

Staples' dissection technique (202). Unless also assigned to skeletal examination, the head of the rodent fetus is removed and stored in Bouin's solution for subsequent examination after cross-sectioning, as described by Wilson (325) or Barrow and Taylor (7). The fetus is placed on a board, and the limbs are restrained with elastic bands or dissection pins. Visceral examinations may be made using a binocular microscope or a magnifying lens and light when necessary (for the larger nonrodent fetuses, a microscope is not generally required). A longitudinal cut is made extending from below the umbilicus through the midline of the trunk. The diaphragm is examined for intactness, after which the cut is continued along one side of the sternum exposing the thoracic viscera. The trachea is detached from the surrounding tissues, and the supporting ligaments are separated from the viscera, after which the trachea, esophagus, and thymus are examined. The thymus is removed, and the heart and great vessels are examined for shape and position. The main arterial branches above the heart are examined, but sub-branches of these major vessels are not explored because of the extensive variability present in normal fetuses (Figure 29.15a). At the anterior portion of the heart, the semilunar values are present at the base of the pulmonary truncus. Also present are the ascending arch of the aorta, the innominate artery, the right carotid artery, the right subclavian artery, the left carotid artery, and the left subclavian artery. The heart is then pulled over to the right, revealing the pulmonary arteries leading to the lungs and the ductus arteriosis.

The heart is cut and examined for internal alterations (Figures 29.15b and 29.15c) as follows. The first cut is made anteriorly from the apex of the heart, enters the right ventricle, and exits from the pulmonary truncus without cutting the dorsal musculature of the heart. This cut reveals the papillary muscles, the tricuspid valve, and the three semilunar valves. In a beating heart preparation, a functional septal defect could be easily detected because blood would spurt through the septum. A second cut is made through the left ventricle, which will cross over the first incision and enter the ascending aorta. This cut will reveal the bicuspid valve, the papillary muscles, and the three semilunar values.

The lungs, liver, stomach, pancreas, spleen, and gallbladder (when appropriate) are examined for color, size, shape, position, and appropriate lobation. The color, size, and position of adrenals, kidneys, ureters, intestines, bladder, and genitalia are then evaluated (the rectum should contain meconium) (see Figure 29.14j). Particular attention is given to evaluation of the reproductive organs for gross integrity, size, shape, and position. During this procedure, gender (sex) is confirmed for rodent species and identified for rabbits (ferrets can be sexed either as fresh or fixed specimens). The ureters are observed for hydroureter, tortuousness, and obstruction, and it is noted whether urine is present in the urinary bladder. The kidneys are sectioned for a detailed examination of infrastructures (size of each renal pelvis, size and appearance of the renal papilla). The patency of the anus can be checked by use of a hair.

When the head is examined for skeletal alterations, the skull and brain may be sectioned at the level of the frontal-parietal suture and the brain examined in situ. Alternatively, the head and/or brain may be retained in Bouin's solution for later sectioning, as previously described. The eyes are removed and examined for color, size, and shape (nonrodent species).

Evisceration of fetuses. Fetuses are eviscerated to aid in clearing and staining of the skeleton. It is helpful to also remove the skin from nonrodent fetuses. Small scissors are used to make a longitudinal cut in rodent fetuses. This cut extends from below the umbilicus through the midline of the trunk and along one side of the sternum, severing

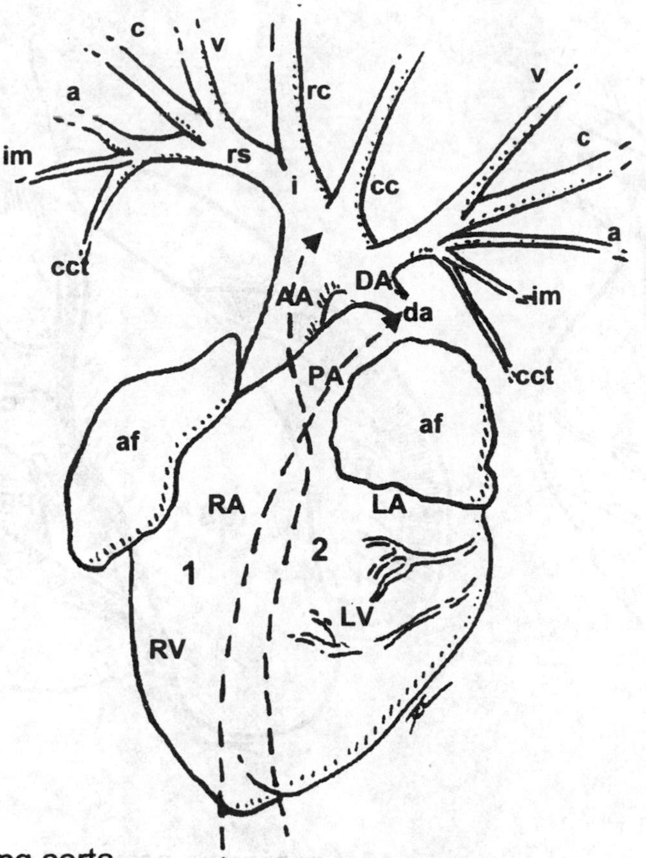

FIG. 29.15a. Major arteries above the heart.

costal cartilage, but not ribs, and avoiding the clavicle. Before further processing, the externally identified fetal sex is confirmed internally (evidence of testicles or uterine horns and ovaries). Similar procedures are then used to evaluate both rodent and nonrodent specimens, although small forceps are used for the rodent fetuses, and blunt forceps may be used for the larger nonrodent fetuses. Evisceration is performed by inserting the forceps into the thoracic cavity and pulling downward on the trachea and esophagus, removing these organs and the lungs and heart (thoracic viscera) as a unit. The diaphragm is gripped and pulled downward and abdominal viscera (liver, kidneys, intestines) are removed. Any remaining viscera in the abdomen or pelvis are then removed. Throughout this process, care must be taken to prevent damaging the skeleton.

For nonrodent fetuses, blunt forceps are used to remove as much of the skin and subcutaneous fat as possible, although skin can remain on the paws, tail, and snout to prevent damage to the underlying bones. Any damage occurring during processing should be noted to prevent the artifact from being potentially incorrectly identified as a skeletal anomaly. After checking that the fetal identification tag remains secure, that the eyes have been removed, and that the head was sectioned, the eviscerated, skinned fetus is returned to the holding tray containing 95–99% isopropyl alcohol or 70–95% ethanol.

Staining of fetal skeletons. Recently there has been an emphasis on the use of double-staining to identify changes in cartilage in term fetuses. In practice, this procedure has not been found to greatly assist in evaluation of late fetal development because most of the observed changes are of a transient nature. Retaining the cartilage by not overprocessing during clearing allows detection of whether apparent absence of an ossification site normally present is a developmental delay or a valid absence of the site.

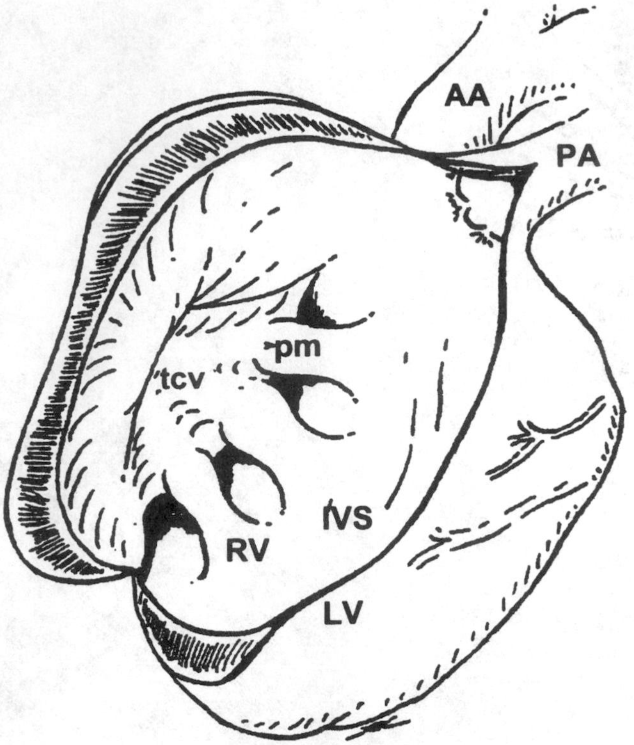

AA ascending aorta
IVS interventricular septum
LV left ventricle
PA pulmonary artery
pm papillary muscle
RV right ventricle
tcv tricuspid valve

FIG. 29.15b. First heart cut.

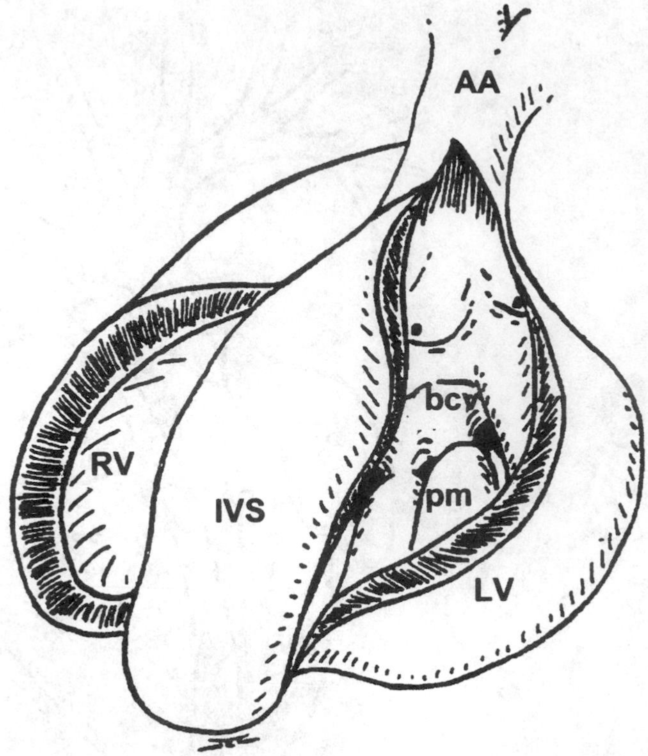

AA ascending aorta
bcv bicuspid valve
IVS interventricular septum
LV left ventricle
RV right ventricle

FIG. 29.15c. Second heart cut.

Double-staining may be of use if one is studying development of the skeleton earlier than the day before expected parturition or if a specific site (e.g., development of the cervical vertebrae) is being investigated. Although not described here, several references are available for double-staining (92,168,127). A description of age-related fetal observations in the rat skeleton can be found in Marr et al. (128).

A 1% KOH solution is recommended for clearing rodent fetuses; a 2% KOH solution is recommended for nonrodent fetuses. Although higher concentrations may be used, the speed of maceration is associated with fetal size, temperature and lighting conditions, and agitation, and small specimens can be easily and inadvertently dissolved. For optimal skeletal processing, minor changes should be made in any maceration/staining process, depending upon individual specimens. Inspection should be ongoing and the speed of the process modified depending upon the observed degree of completion of the maceration and staining of the individual specimen. It goes without saying that it is necessary to have full dissolution of the KOH pellets into a true solution. KOH is generally prepared or obtained in 1-gallon units, and alizarin red S is added (50.0 mg/1 gallon of 1% KOH solution) to stain the skeletons.

Several concentrations of glycerine are needed to clear and preserve the stained skeletal preparations during storage. As supplied by the manufacturers, glycerine is 99.5% pure. This should be diluted to 20%, 40%, 60%, and 80% concentrations and used sequentially so that the macerated, stained fetuses can be gradually brought up to the 80% or 99.5% glycerine concentration used for storage. Too rapid an increase of the glycerine concentration will result in compression of the fetal skull.

Processing can be performed using compartmentalized polystyrene utility boxes or alternate containers that do not react with the KOH or alizarin. Several commercial units are now available, although they are not recommended for use in staining very small fetuses, which should be observed during the processing to prevent inadvertent damage.

The procedure described is a modification of the method of Staples and Schnell (200) in which eviscerated, skinned (if appropriate) fetuses are fixed in plastic bottles filled with 99% isopropanol or 95% ethanol. Fixation of rodent fetuses generally requires at least 7 days, whereas nonrodent fetuses may require at least 14 days for fixation. After the alcohol fixation period, the fetuses are placed into individual compartmentalized plastic boxes and any remaining alcohol drained away. Each compartment is then filled with 1% (rodent) or 2% (nonrodent) KOH solution, and the fetuses allowed to mascerate for approximately 24 h. The KOH solution is then drained and replaced with 1% KOH solution containing the alizarin red S stain and the fetuses allowed to remain in the stain for approximately 24 h, after which this solution is drained and replaced with a fresh 1% KOH solution in which the specimens remain for another 24 h. The KOH solution is again drained, and the rodent fetuses are cleared with progressively higher concentrations of glycerine (20%, 40%, 60%, and 80% for rodents; 20%, 40%, and 80% for nonrodents). After completion of this process, the fetuses are stored, ultimately for archiving, in plastic jars to which 80% to 99.5% glycerine and a few crystals of thymol, a preservative, have been added.

Examination of Fetal Skeletons. We have found that calculation of ossification site averages for each litter is the most appropriate unit of evaluation for the hyoid (body), vertebrae (cervical, thoracic, lumbar, sacral, and caudal), ribs (pairs), sternum (manubrium, xiphoid, and sternal centra between these sites), forepaws (carpals, metacarpals, phalanges), and hindpaws (tarsals, metatarsals, and phalanges); it provides an easy method for identifying delays in ossification. Separate averages for the manubrium, 4 or 5 sternebrae, and xiphoid better identifies reduced ossification than citing retarded sternal ossification by site, to the exclusion of the interrelationship of the biological pattern of sternal development. Delays in ossification identified by using this method should be correlated with other evidence of retarded ossification that may be observed (e.g., a reduction in the litter average number of ossified sternebrae per fetus should be compared with nonsequential sternal ossification). This method also allows association of increases in rib numbers (supernumerary thoracic ribs) with increases in thoracic vertebrae and reductions in lumbar vertebrae, thus eliminating identification of supernumerary thoracic ribs as rudimentary, full, unilateral, or bilateral, which often obscures an increase in supernumerary ribs because the counts are recorded as separate findings rather than an overall response.

As stated previously, fetal processing (evisceration, skinning, clearing, and staining) and examination require considerable manipulation of the fetuses, and any artifacts (breakage or removal of a bone) should be recorded during the processing procedures because such can be misidentified as malformations by inexperienced investigators. During many years of consulting, it has been the author's experience that many "major malformations" were processing artifacts. For example, one agent was incorrectly labeled as a "teratogen" because multiple fetuses were missing portions of the digits. Reexamination of the digits identified that the small fetuses had the ends of the digits removed as the result of being caught in the screening of the cover of the tray used in the staining process, and were associated with poor technique. Unfortunately, to convince regulatory reviewers that this reported malformation was an artifact, it was necessary to repeat the study, as well as provide photographs that clearly demonstrated tissue loss.

Terminology remains a serious problem in the field of developmental toxicology, especially in the area of skeletal assessment. Because definitions differ among laboratories, comparative historical data or a glossary should be provided so that consistent terminology is, at the least, used in the same laboratory (32). It is highly recommended that technical personnel describe the observations using clear statements and that any summarization of associated alterations and classification as malformation or variation, should this archaic practice be used, occur only during higher level evaluations to prevent inappropriate summarization and statistical analyses. For example, the technical observations of fusion of the 8th and 9th right ribs, right arches and right aspects of the centra in the 8th and 9th thoracic vertebrae, and asymmetric and bifid centra in the 7th thoracic vertebra should be classified at the supervisory and data summarization levels as an interrelated vertebral-rib malformation, not as separate findings. The bifid thoracic vertebral centra in this malformation are part of the overall malformation, not a variation; however, bifid centra in the absence of other vertebral changes would generally be classified as a variation. Our practical definition of "absent" is that both bone and cartilage are not present in an expected site (e.g., when inadvertently removed in processing or associated with inappropriate development (e.g., anencephaly is associated with absence of the bones of the calvaria)).

Terms more relevant to human syndromology should be avoided when examining laboratory specimens, as they are often alarming to reviewers inexperienced in animal observations (e.g., frequently physicians) and often inappropriate. Interrelated alterations (external, soft tissue, and skeletal) in the same fetus should be described as one entity (e.g., external doming of the skull, dilation of the lateral and third ventricles in the brain and small

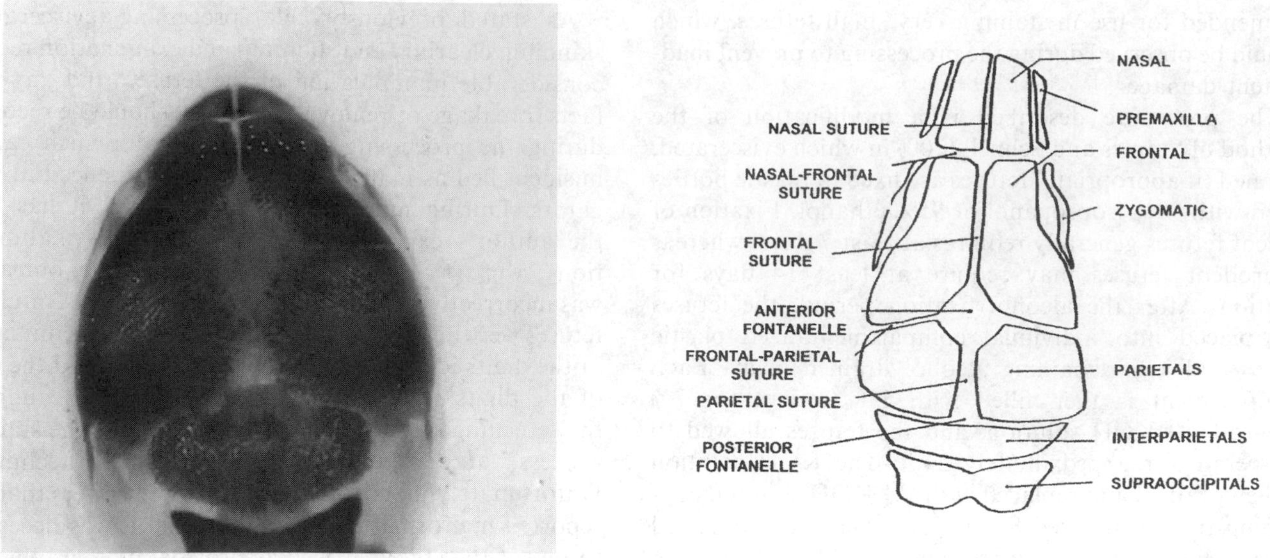

FIG. 29.16a. Rat fetus – Day 20 of gestation – Normal skull, dorsal view.

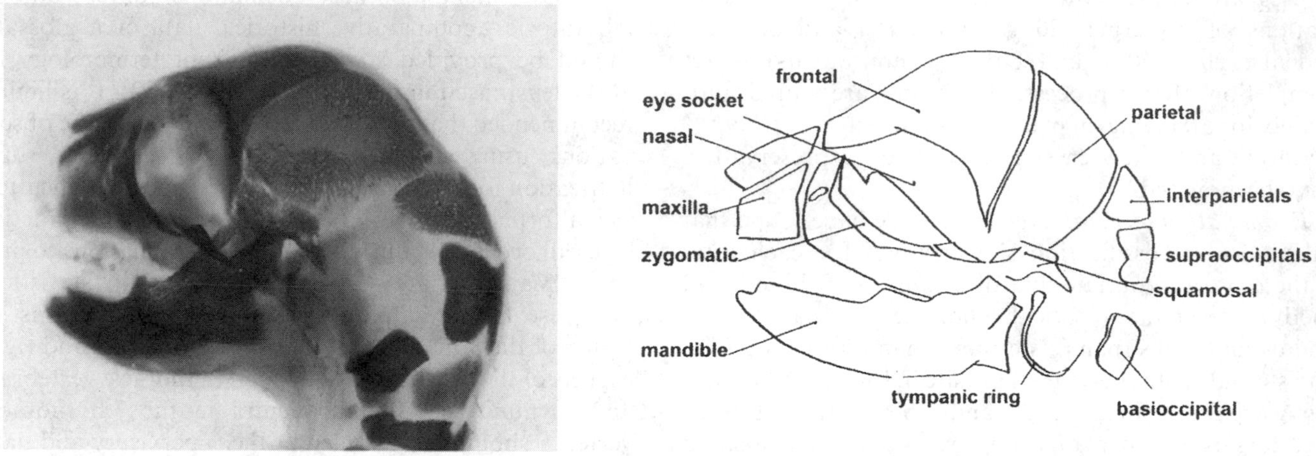

FIG. 29.16b. Rat fetus – Day 20 of gestation – Normal skull, lateral view.

holes in the skull bones, and enlargement of the fontanelles represent one malformation, not multiple malformations). Unfortunately, current use of computer data entry, proscribed terms, and inability of naive investigators to identify related changes in multiple organ systems often results in inappropriate conclusions, statistical findings that are not biologically relevant, and inappropriate assignment of site-specific findings to bimodal categorization, such as malformation and variation. Biologically based data interpretation and summarization is highly recommended.

Procedures. To perform a skeletal examination, each fetus is removed from the container holding the processed litter, checked for identification, and then placed in a petri dish and examined using a light source and magnification (5 × –10 ×). When fetuses are to be evaluated without the investigator's knowledge of the dosage group (i.e., blind), a white label bearing only the study number, maternal animal number, and fixative is affixed to the container holding the fetuses (see also section on Evaluation of Uterine Contents). Rat, mouse, hamster, and ferret fetuses are examined using a binocular microscope. All nonrodent fetuses (except ferrets) are examined using a magnifying light.

Each skeletal examination proceeds systematically from head to tail (diagrams and comparable photographs by Ms. Donna W. Lewis of our laboratory are provided in Figures 29.16a through 29.16s). Representa-

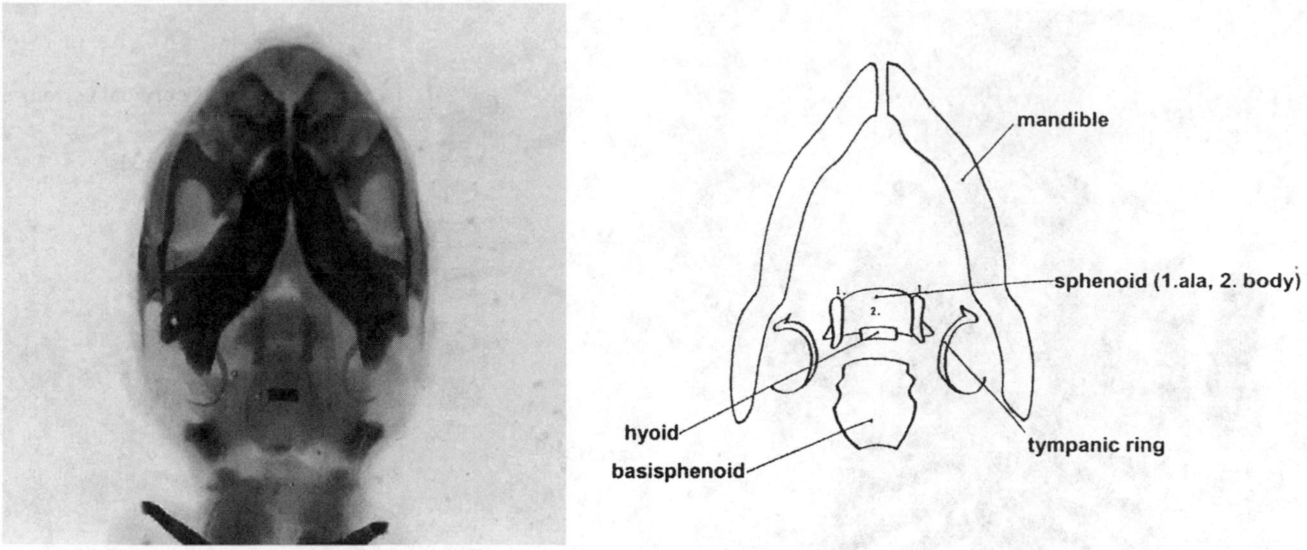

FIG. 29.16c. Rat fetus – Day 20 gestation – Normal skull, ventral view.

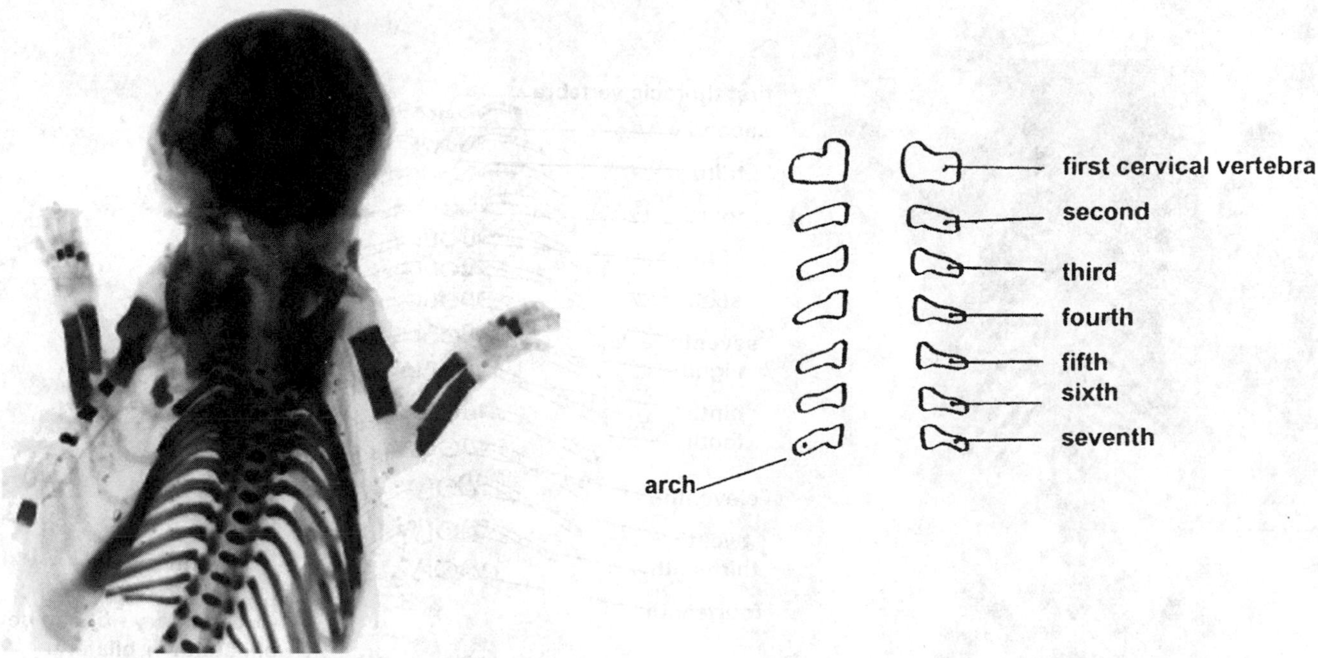

FIG. 29.16d. Rat fetus – Day 20 of gestation – Normal cervical vertebrae, ventral view.

tive abnormalities observed in day 20 of gestation rat fetuses are provided as Figures 29.17a through 29.17q. Representative abnormalities observed in day 29 of gestation rabbit fetuses are provided as Figures 29.18a through 29.18o.

The skull (Figures 29.16a through 29.16c) is examined for size, shape, and extent of ossification; each skull bone is examined for ossification appropriate to the specimen's gestational age. A listing of the skull bones as follows:

Singular	*Plural*
Nasal	Nasals
Frontal	Frontals
Parietal	Parietals
Interparietal	Interparietals
Supraoccipital	Supraoccipitals
Exoccipital	Exoccipitals
Premaxilla	Premaxillae
Maxilla	Maxillae

(Continued)

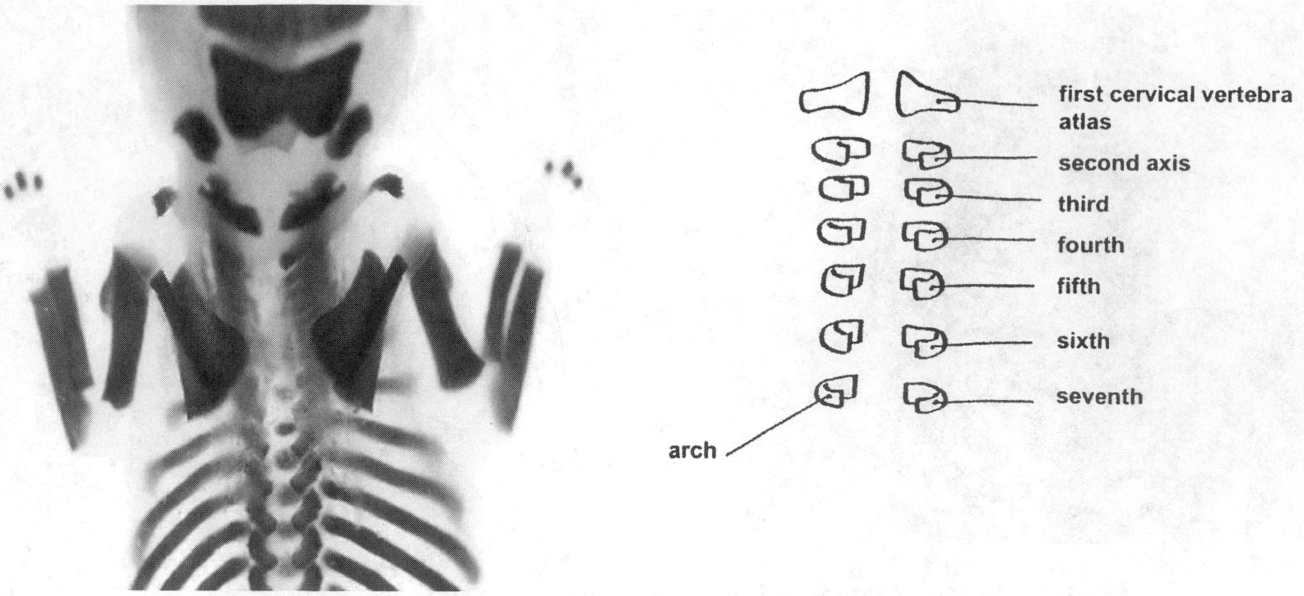

FIG. 29.16e. Rat fetus – Day 20 of gestation – Normal cervical vertebrae, dorsal view.

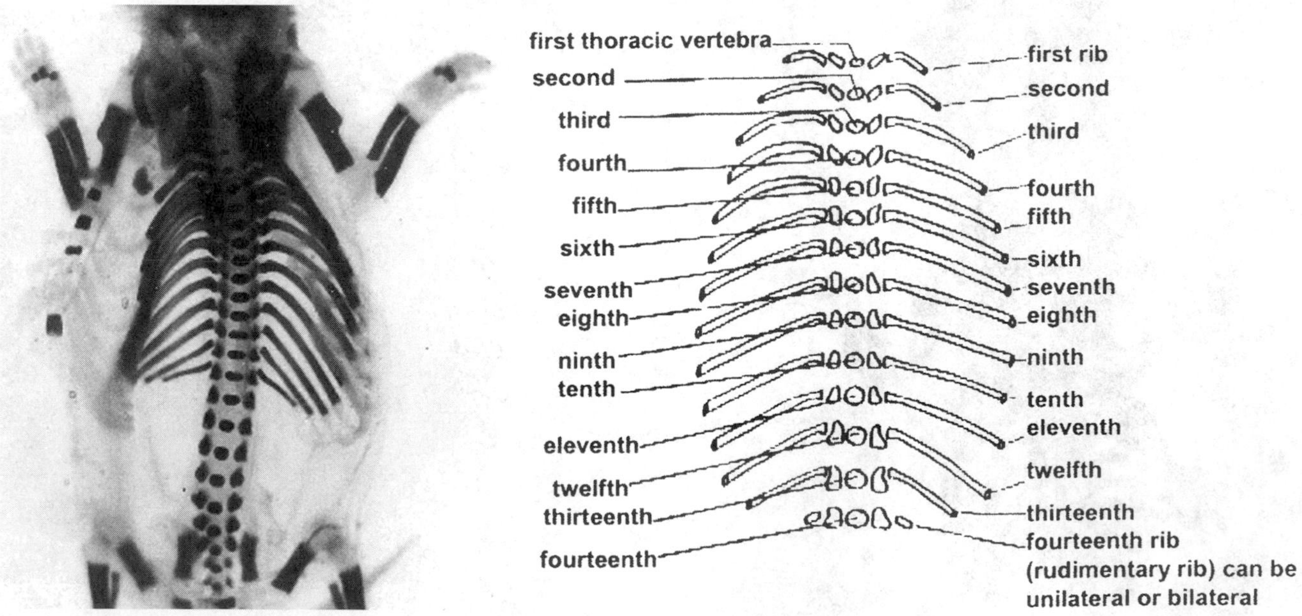

FIG. 29.16f. Rat fetus – Day 20 of gestation – Normal thoracic vertebrae and ribs, ventral view.

Singular	*Plural*
Zygomatic	Zygomatics
Squamosal	Squamosals
Eye socket	Eyesockets
Mandibula (Mandible)	Mandibulae (mandibles)
Hyoid (ala)	Hyoids (alae)
Basisphenoid	Basisphenoids
Basioccipital	Basioccipitals
Tympanic ring	Tympanic rings

Should the fetus have a domed skull associated with marked or extreme dilation of the lateral ventricles in the brain or be small and have retarded ossification, the anterior and posterior fontanelles are often enlarged and the parietals frequently contain holes. In such cases, the affected fontanelle and degree of dilation should be noted (1 = slight, 2 = moderate, 3 = marked, and 4 = extreme enlargement of the fontanelle). When holes are present (Figure 29.18a), the number, location, and

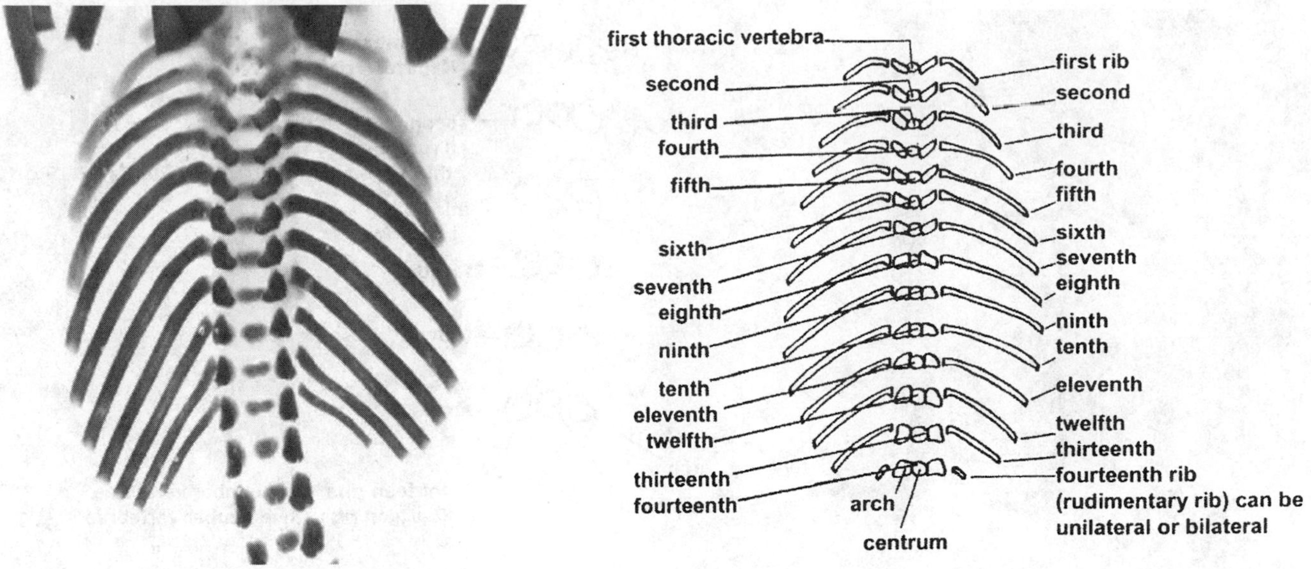

FIG. 29.16g. Rat fetus – Day 20 of gestation – Normal thoracic vertebrae and ribs, dorsal view.

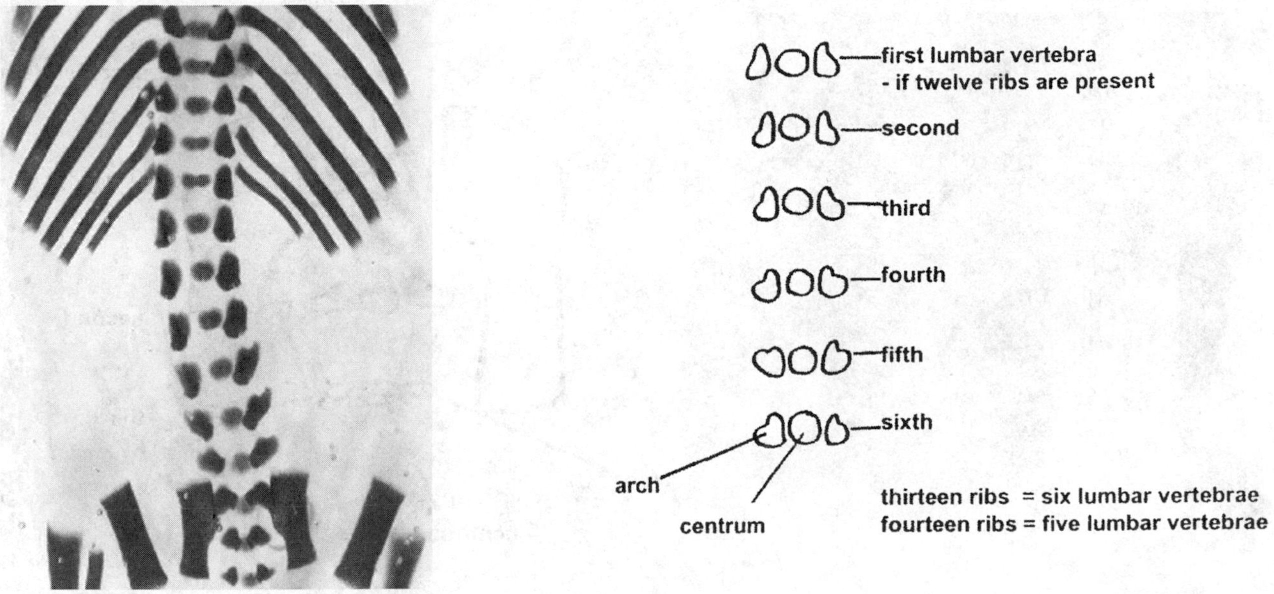

FIG. 29.16h. Rat fetus – Day 20 of gestation – Normal lumbar vertebrae, ventral view.

approximate size of each hole should be noted, as also should be intra- and interossification sites (Figure 29.18b).

The hyoid bone (Figure 29.16c) is observed to be present (1) or not ossified (0). Rabbit fetuses frequently have angulation of the hyoid alae (Figure 29.18d); the hyoid is not ossified (cartilage is present) in rat fetuses at 20 or 21 days of gestation (Figure 29.16c). Appropriate alignment and closure of the upper and lower jaws (mandibles and maxillae) should be present (teeth should be present in rabbit fetuses). The size and shape of each eye socket should be checked and correlated with reported findings of microphthalmia or apparent anophthalmia.

The vertebral column is next examined (see Figures 29.16d through 29.16k); each vertebra consists of three parts (the centrum and two arches) and is evaluated to determine whether areas other than those expected to have minor developmental alterations demonstrate

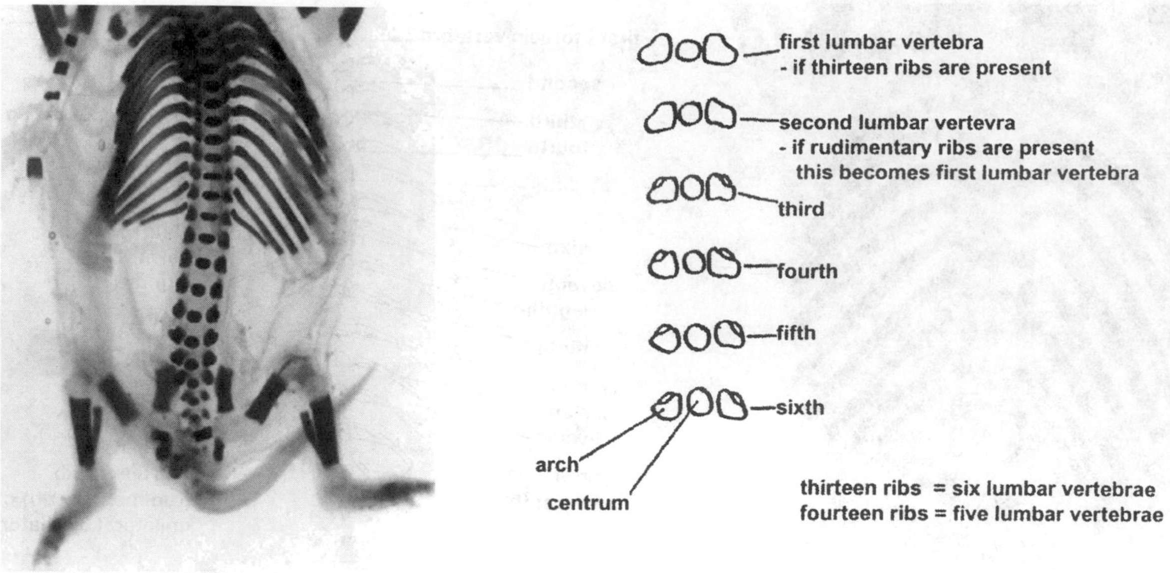

FIG. 29.16i. Rat fetus – Day 20 of gestation – Normal lumbar vertebrae, dorsal view.

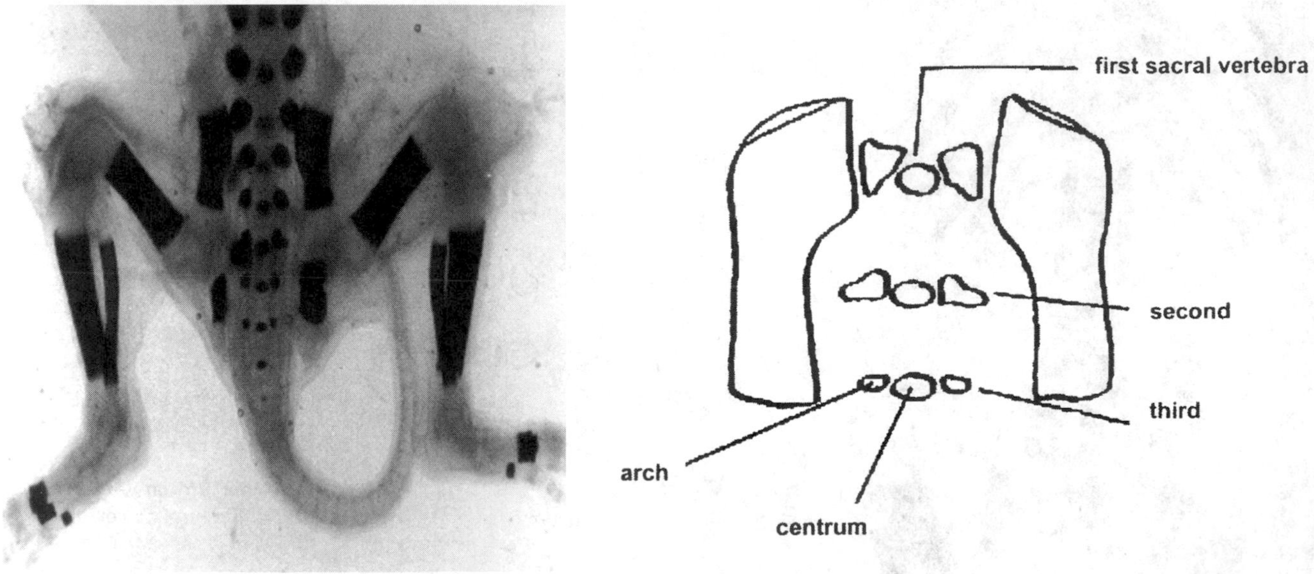

FIG. 29.16j. Rat fetus – Day 20 of gestation – Normal sacral vertebrae, ventral view.

changes. The total number of vertebrae present and the relationship of the subsections to the ribs and pelvis are considered in order to identify when there is an anterior-posterior shift in the number of thoracic and/or lumbar vertebrae. Although some laboratories identify only the number of presacral vertebrae, we have found that this method does not allow for correlation of increases in supernumerary thoracic ribs and the related increase in thoracic vertebrae and decrease in lumbar vertebrae. Occasionally there is a dose-dependent increase in both thoracic and lumbar vertebrae, which usually is a more severe expression of an increase in only thoracic ribs. Use of the following working definitions for numbers of vertebrae increases comparability across studies in the same species.

7 (C1–C7) Cervical vertebrae—(Figures 29.16d and 29.16e); thoracic vertebrae (Figures 29.16f and 29.16g) [rat—13 or 14 (T1–T13 or T14); rabbit—12 or 13 (T1–T12 or T13)]; lumbar vertebrae (Figures 29.16h and 29.16i) [rat—5 or 6 (L1–L5 or L6); rabbit—6 or 7 (L1–L6 or L7)];

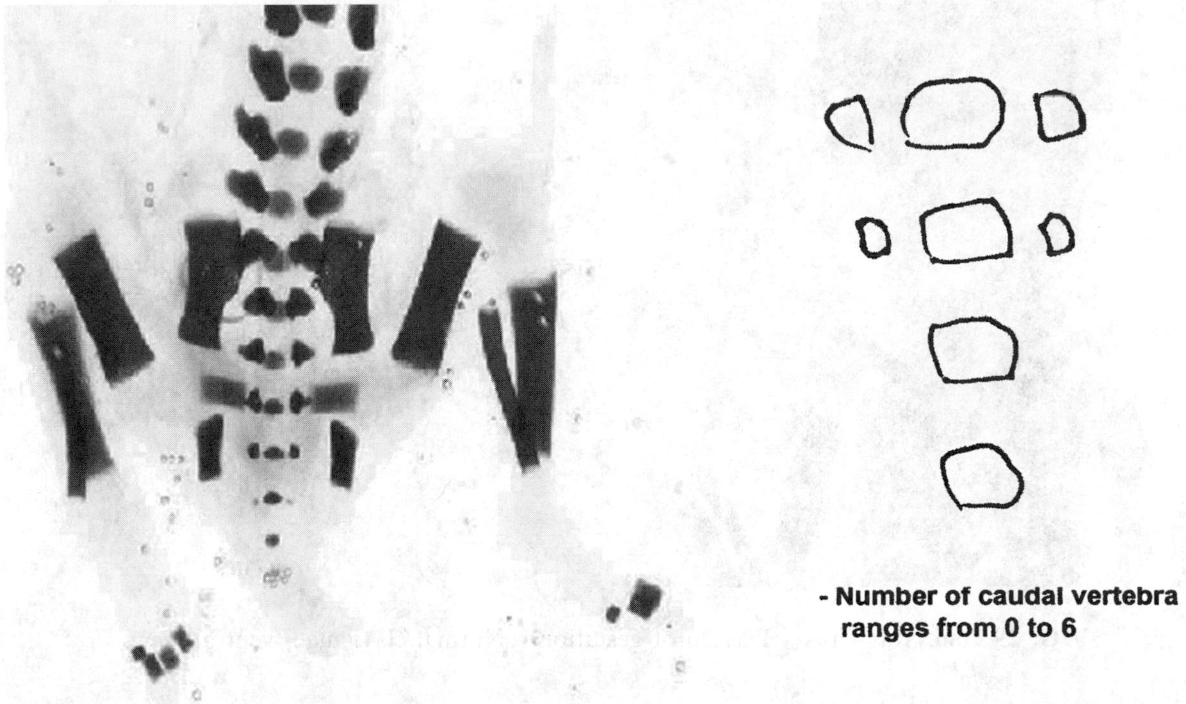

FIG. 29.16k. Rat fetus – Day 20 of gestation – Normal caudal vertebrae, dorsal view.

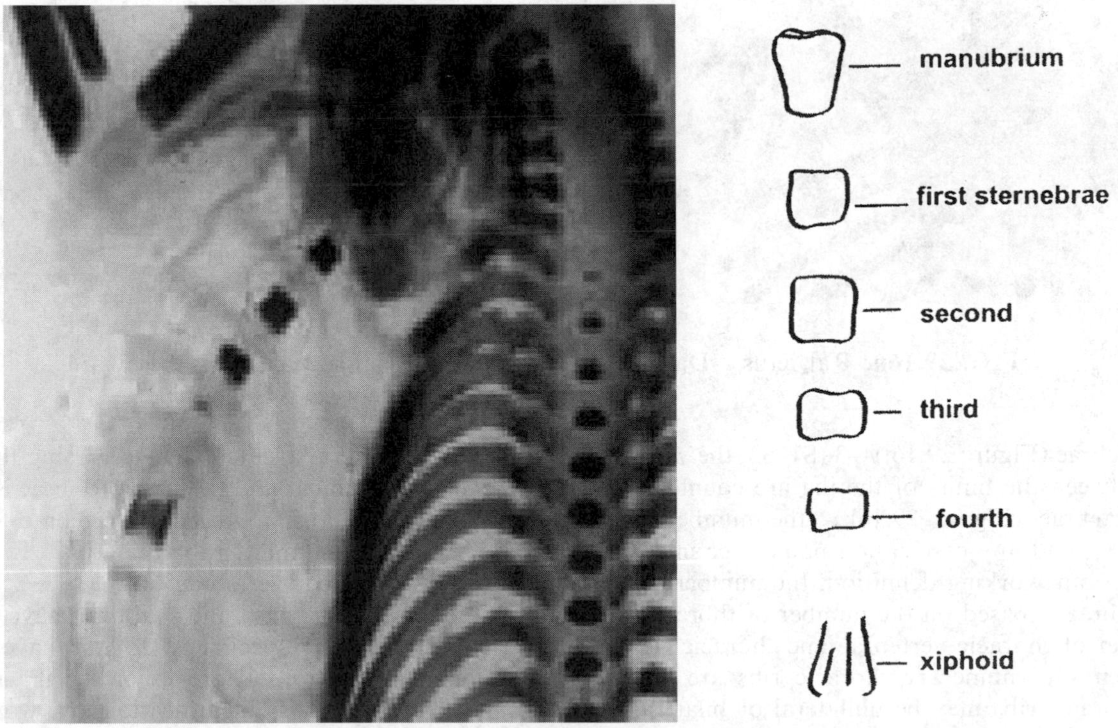

FIG. 29.16l. Rat fetus – Day 20 of gestation – Normal sternebrae, ventral view.

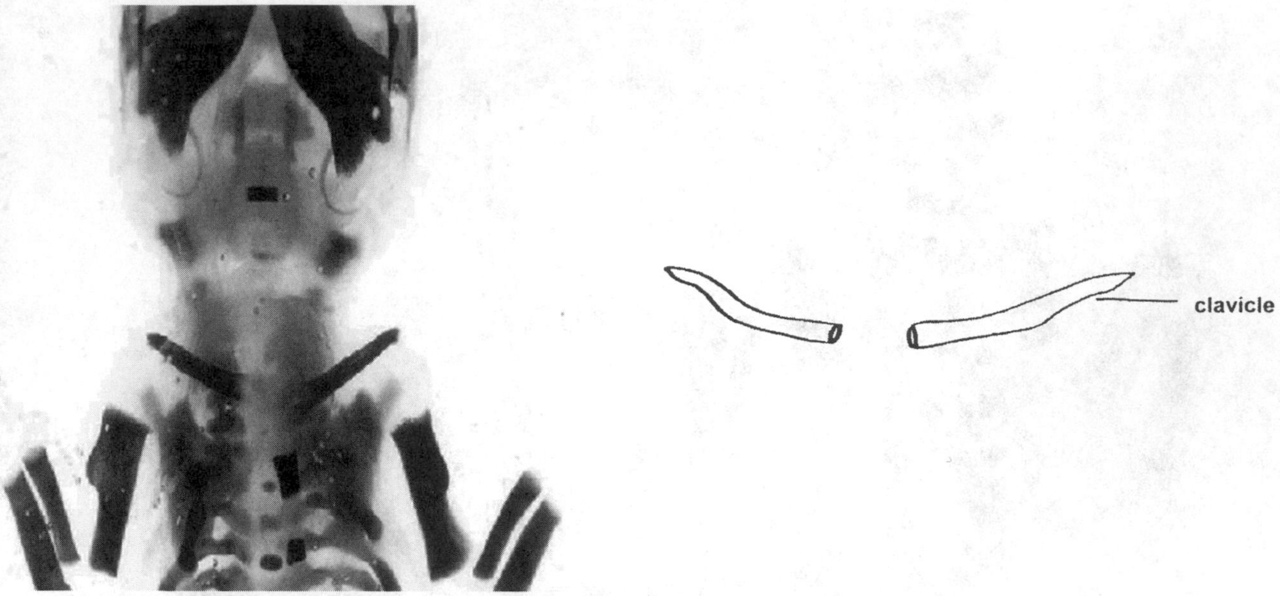

FIG. 29.16m. Rat fetus – Day 20 of gestation – Normal claviculae, ventral view.

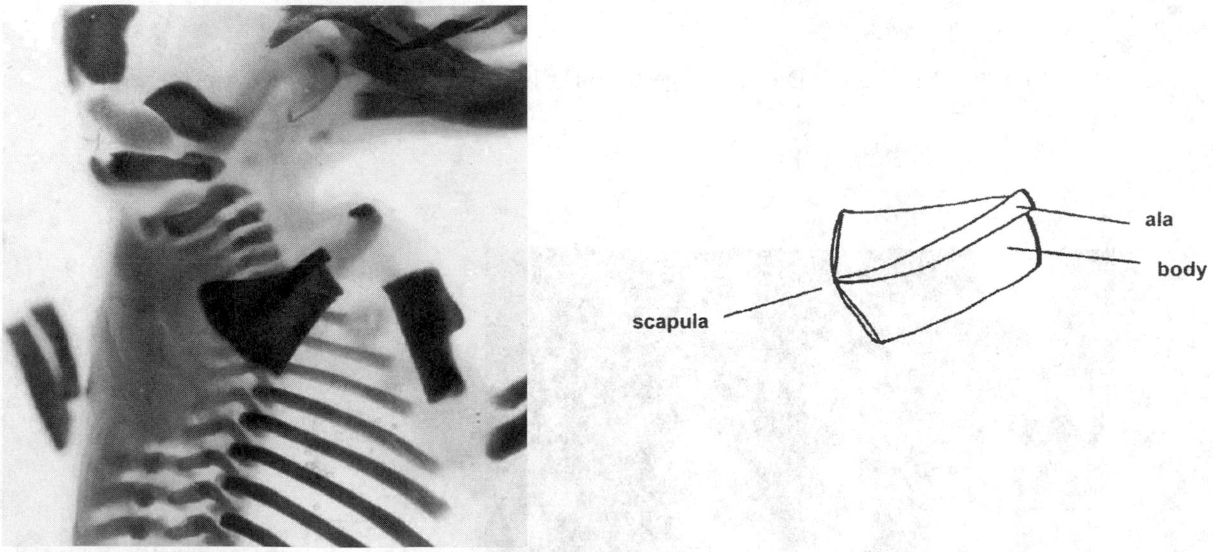

FIG. 29.16n. Rat fetus – Day 20 of gestation – Normal scapula, dorsal view.

sacral vertebrae (Figure 29.16j)—3 (S1–S3; the vertebrae present between the limits of the ilia are counted); and caudal vertebrae (Figure 29.16k)—the number varies (CA1–CAX), and any ossification point is counted.

Using on our working definition, the number of thoracic vertebrae is based on the number of thoracic ribs. The number of thoracic vertebrae and thoracic ribs are equal; when supernumerary thoracic ribs are present, the last thoracic ribs may be unilateral or bilateral. As previously noted, this counting procedure simplifies and more clearly identifies presence of supernumerary thoracic ribs and associated changes. Using this system, the sum of the lumbar and thoracic vertebrae is normally 19 (normal rat fetus: 13 thoracic vertebrae + 6 lumbar vertebrae = 19; normal rabbit fetus: 12 thoracic vertebrae + 7 lumbar vertebrae = 19).

Although adult rats and rabbits have 4 sacral vertebrae, the fetal specimens do not have complete development of vertebral arches or the ilia for use as landmarks. To simplify identification, our working definition for fetal specimens is that sacral vertebrae are those present between the cephalic and caudal limits

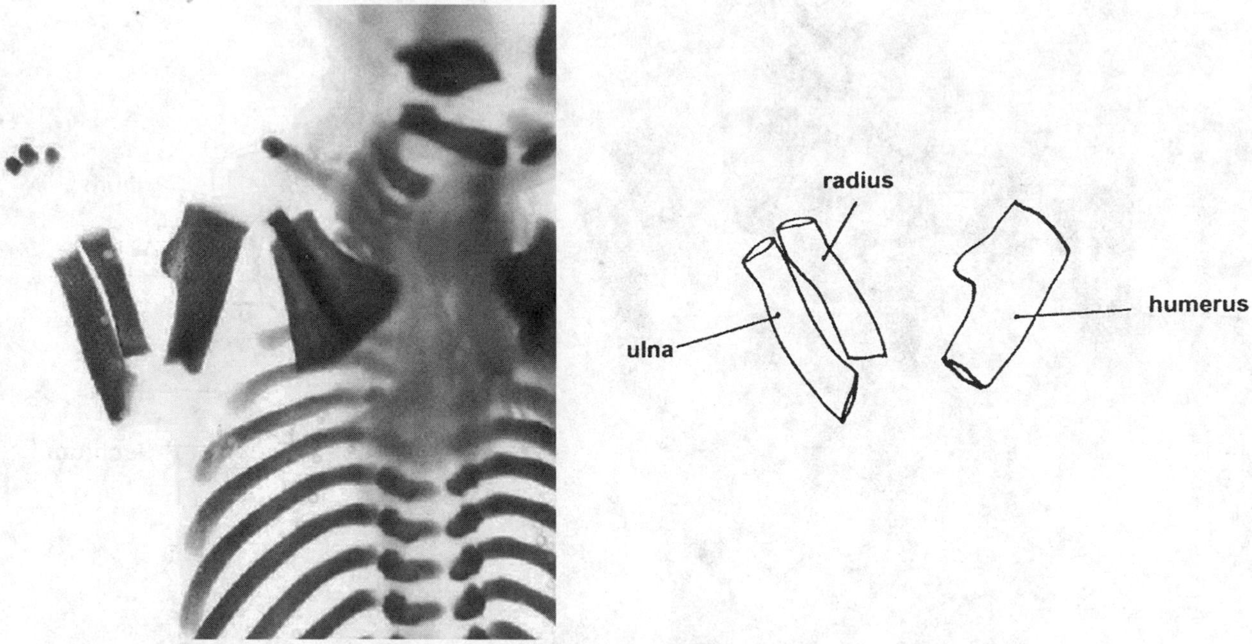

FIG. 29.16o. Rat fetus – Day 20 of gestation – forelimb, dorsal view.

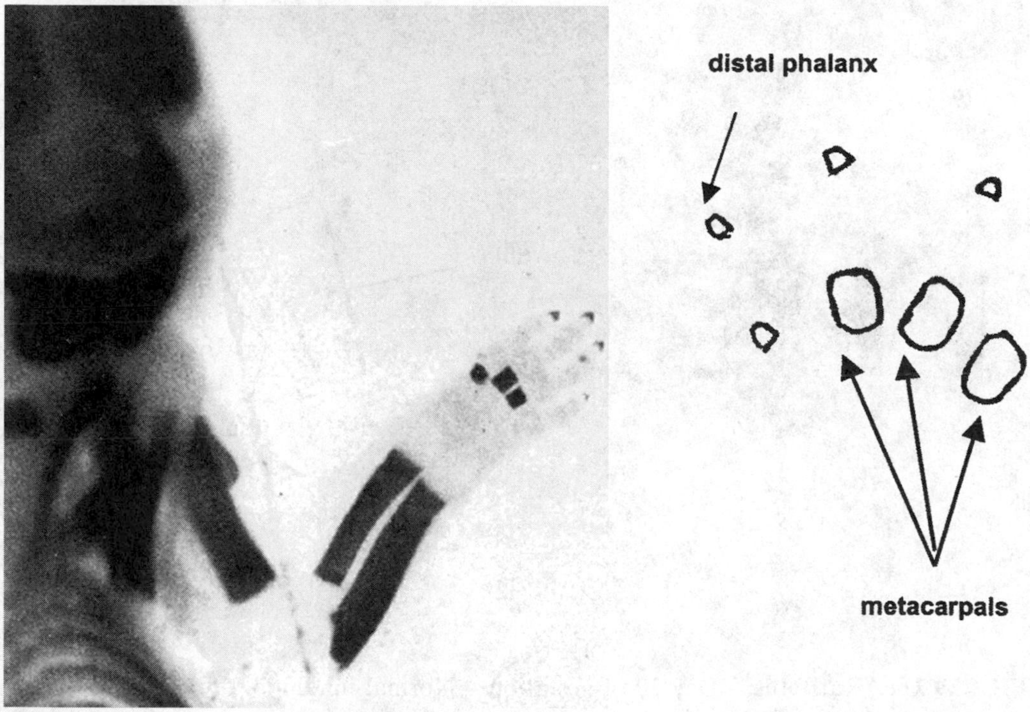

FIG. 29.16p. Rat fetus – Day 20 of gestation – Normal forewaw, dorsal view.

of the ilia, generally resulting in identification of 3 ossified sacral vertebrae. It is presumed that one of the vertebrae identified as caudal in the fetal specimen will be identified as sacral in the mature animal. This procedure eliminates the need to identify uneven ossification of the iliac crest and also more clearly identifies when an increase in thoracic-lumbar vertebrae has occurred.

An alternate method used in many laboratories is counting of the total number of presacral vertebrae

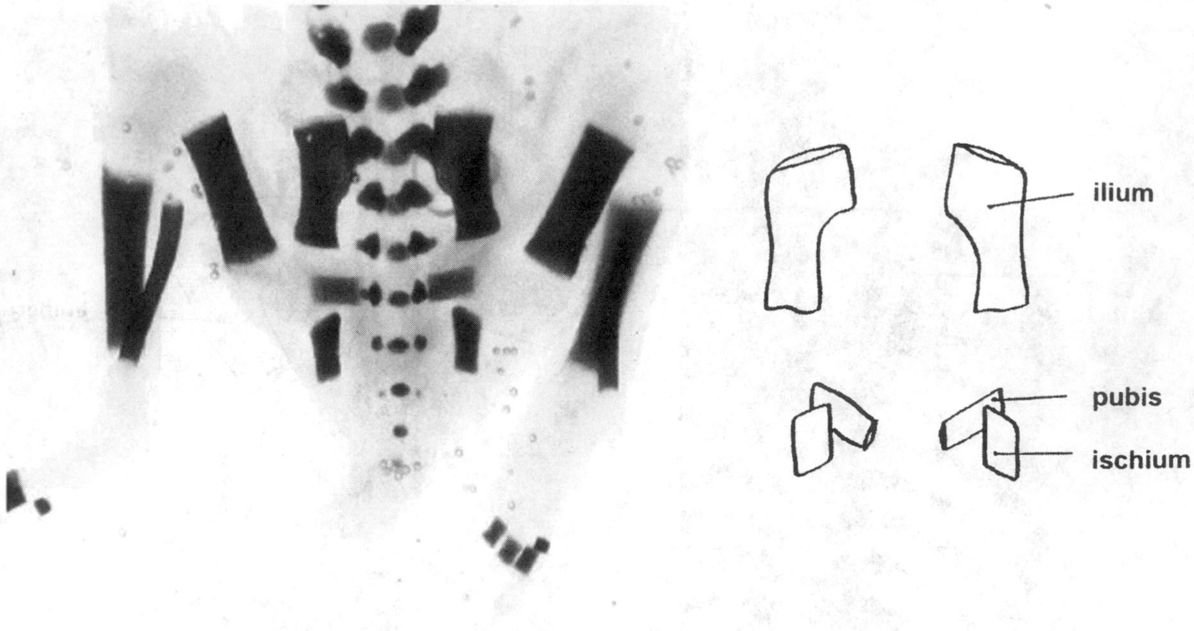

FIG. 29.16q. Rat fetus – Day 20 of gestation – Normal pelvis, dorsal view.

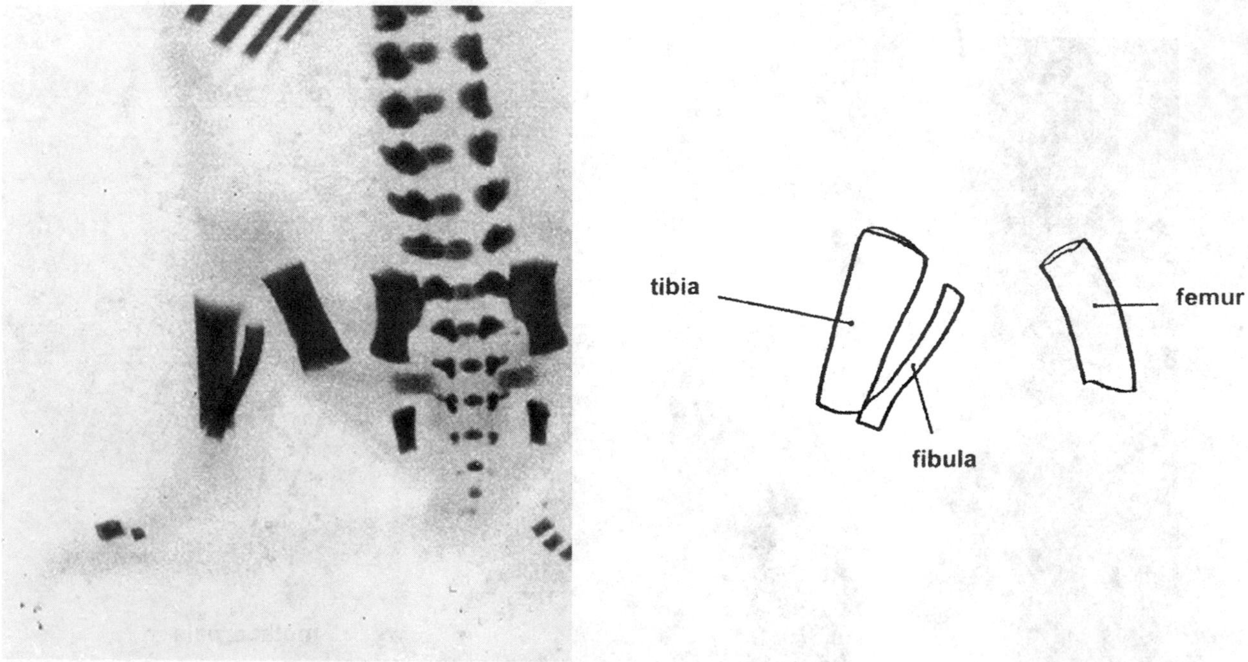

FIG. 29.16r. Rat fetus – Day 20 of gestation – Normal hindlimb, dorsal view.

(normally 26; rat fetus: 7 + 13 + 6 = 26; rabbit fetus: 7 + 12 + 7 = 26) and then identifying the number of fetuses with additional presacral vertebrae. This method is considered inferior because it fails to correlate the relationship of increased thoracic ribs with the number of vertebrae, and frequently, when remarkable increases occur, such as the presence of 28 presacral vertebrae, it misidentifies the number of fetuses with 27 presacral vertebra because those with 28 are incorrectly excluded from this category in subsequent statistical analyses. This method can serve well when it is biologically based and overall changes are integrated; however, experience has shown that presently this seldom occurs.

Any alterations in vertebral ossification are identified. This includes a bifid (split) centrum (Figures 29.17d and 29.18i); absent, asymmetric, or small centrum (Figure

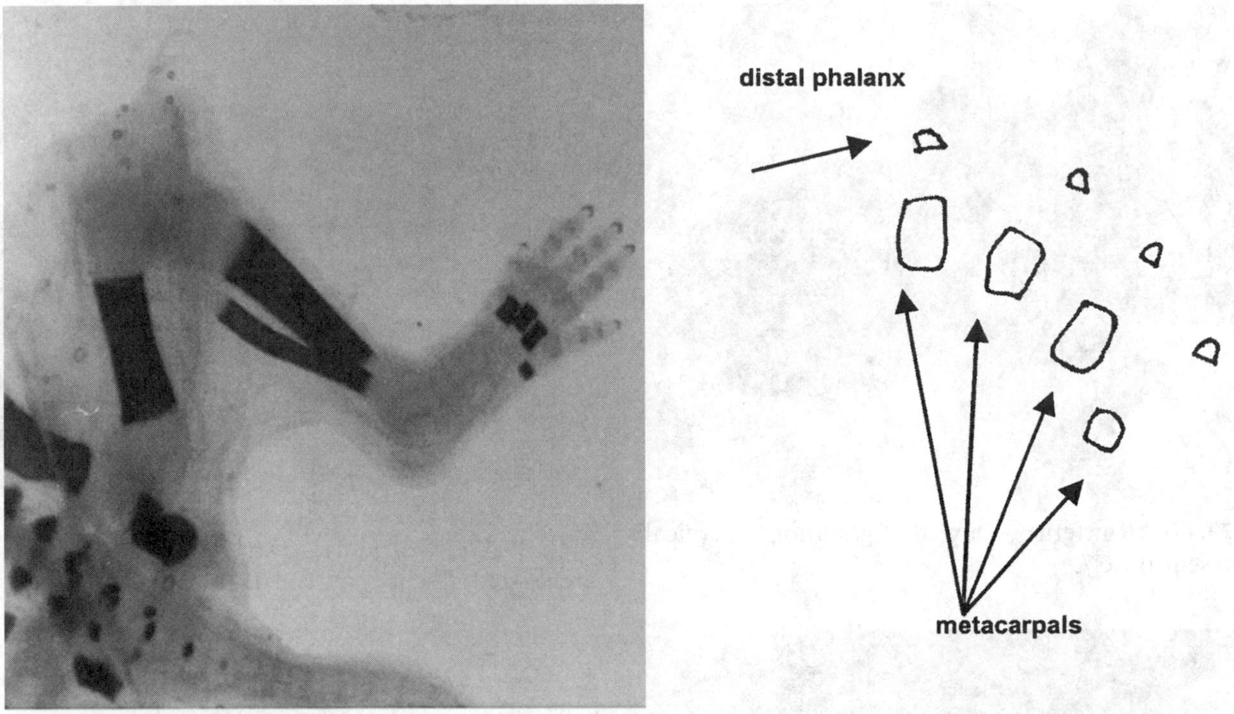

FIG. 29.16s. Rat fetus – Day 20 of gestation – Normal hindpaw, dorsal view.

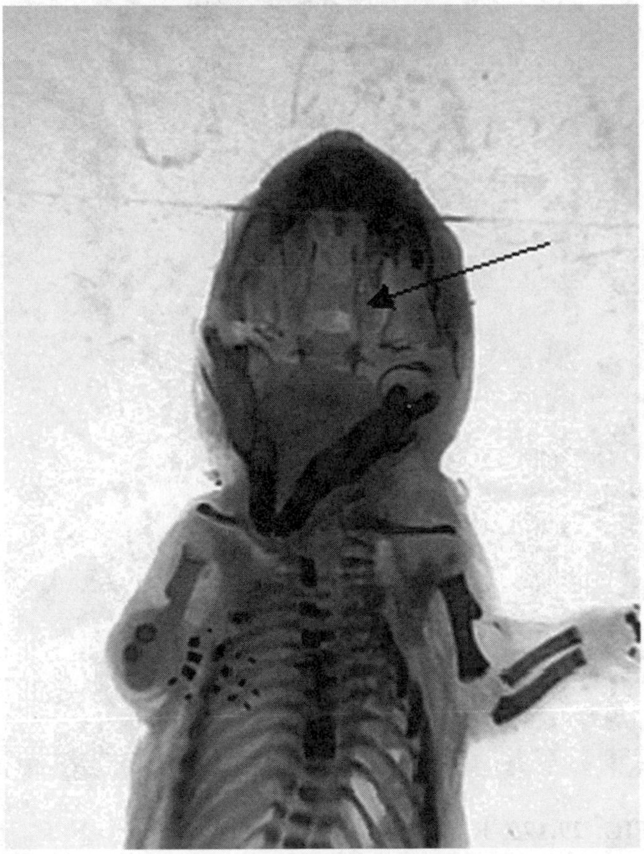

FIG. 29.17a. Rat fetus – Day 20 of gestation – Incomplete ossification of palantine shelves.

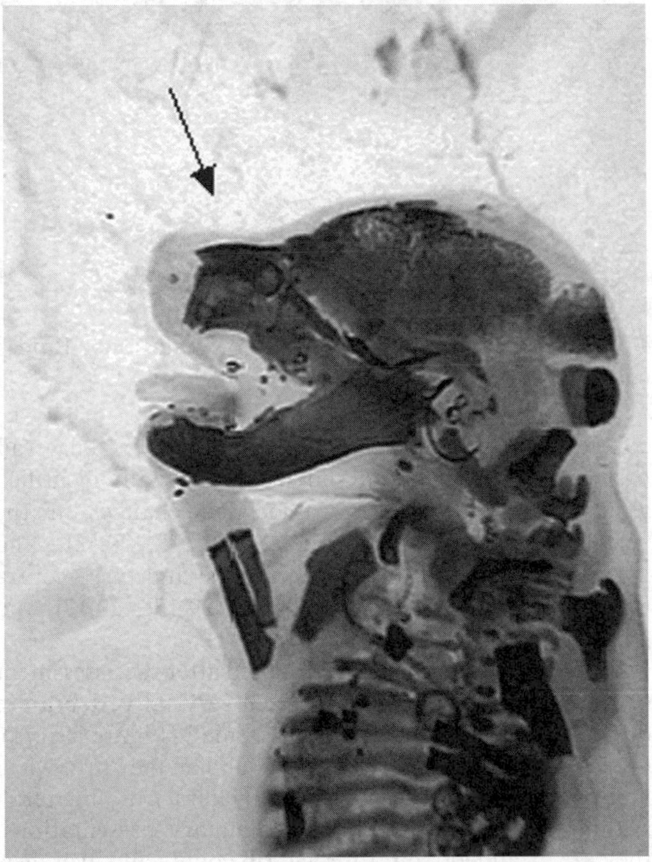

FIG. 29.17b. Rat fetus – Day 20 of gestation – Short nasal bones.

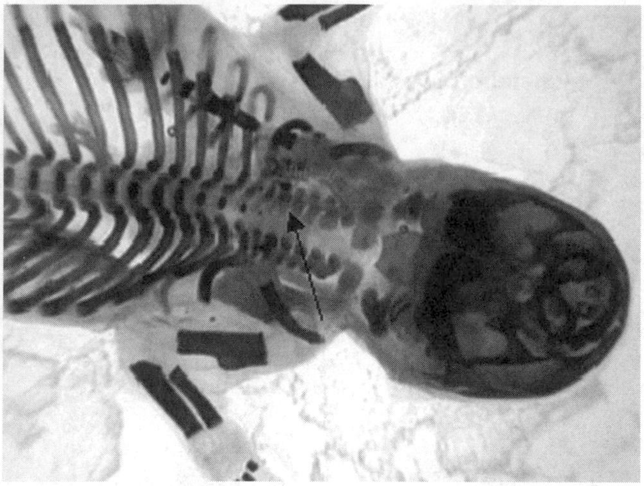

FIG. 29.17c. Rat fetus – Day 20 of gestation – Cervical ribs present on C7.

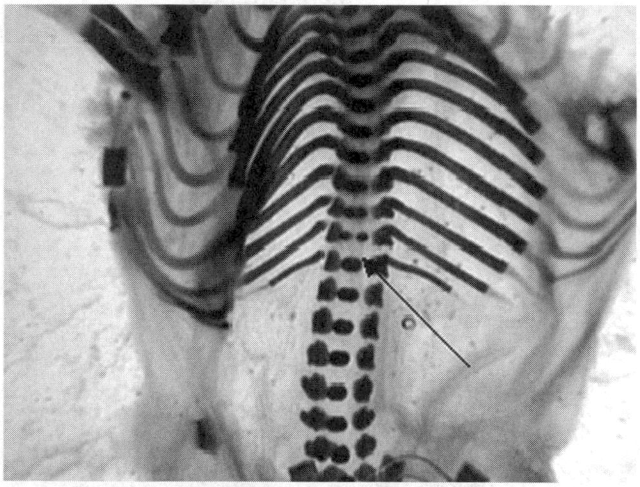

FIG. 29.17d. Rat fetus – Day 20 of gestation – Bifid centrum, T12.

29.17e, 29.17j); unilateral (left, right, or bilateral) ossification of a centrum and/or arch (usually identified as a hemivertebrae with associated changes in the vertebrae and ribs; see Figures 29.17f, 29.18f, and 29.18g); a small arch(es); open arches; and fused centra and/or arches of vertebrae (Figures 29.17e, 29.17j, and 29.18g).

The ribs are examined and counted after the assessment of the vertebral column. Ribs on a cervical vertebra are difficult to see and often are quite small (Figure 29.17c). Cervical ribs are most frequently found on the 7th cervical vertebra (C7) and may be unilateral or bilateral. Although tabulated as ribs in summary presentations, they are excluded from thoracic rib counts and averages. The total number of thoracic ribs (regardless of size) on each side is identified, with the highest number of tho-

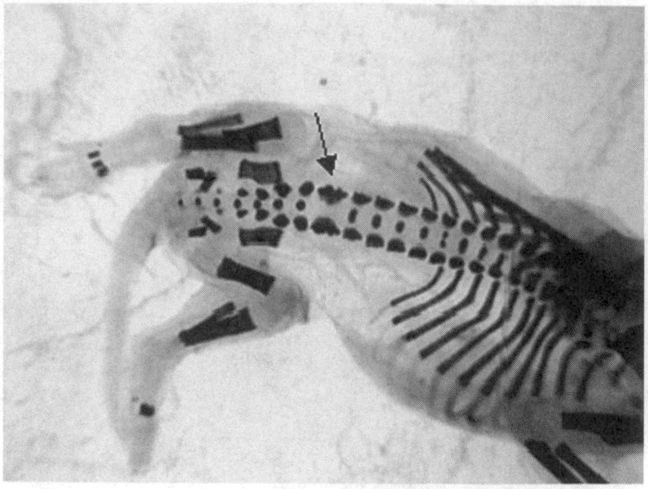

FIG. 29.17e. Rat fetus – Day 20 of gestation. Fused arches and absent centra of L4 and L5.

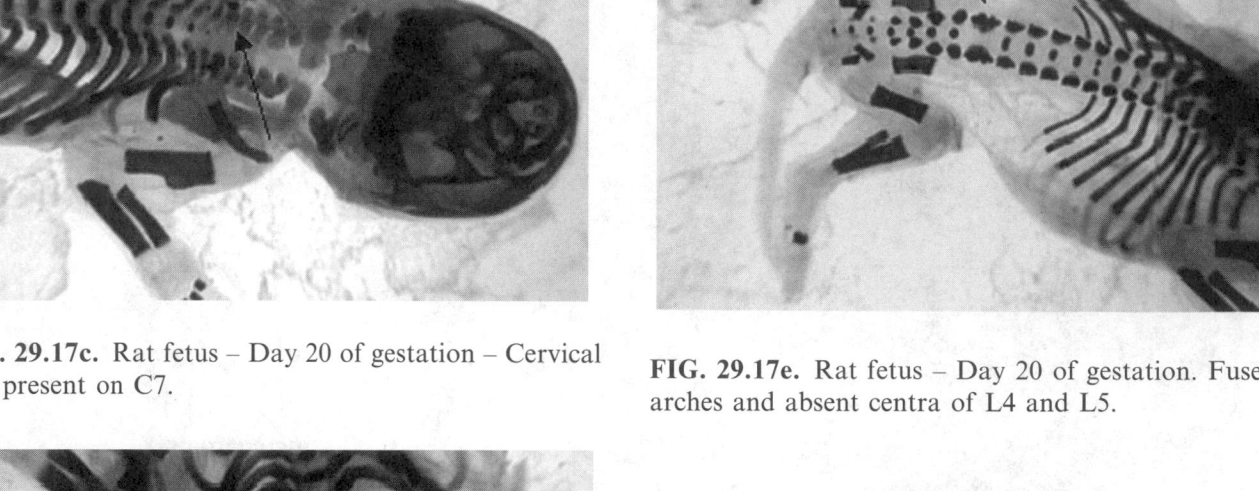

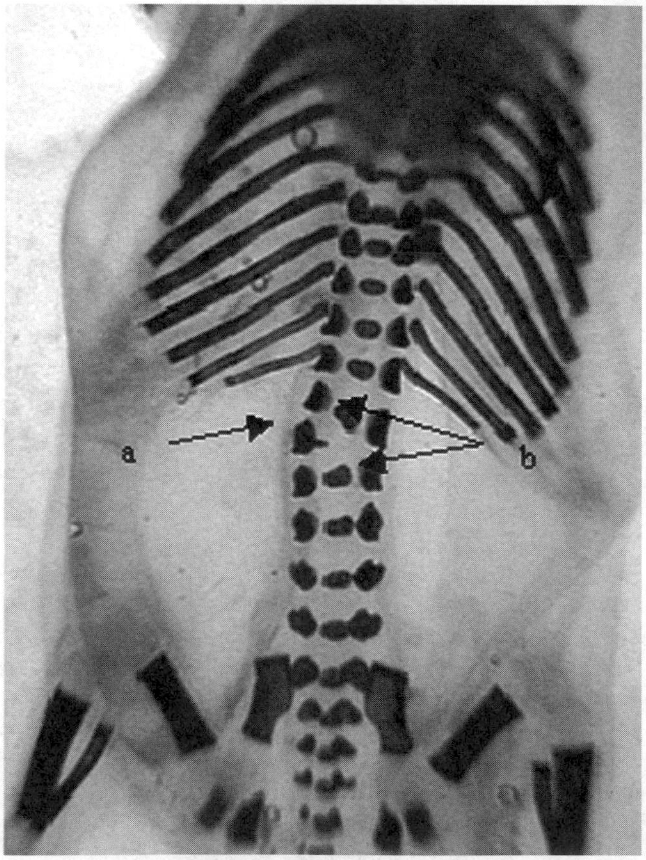

FIG. 29.17f. Rat fetus – Day 20 of gestation – Interrelated malformations of lumbar vertebrae [(a) L2 present as a left hemivertebra with (b) assymetry of centra of L1 and L3].

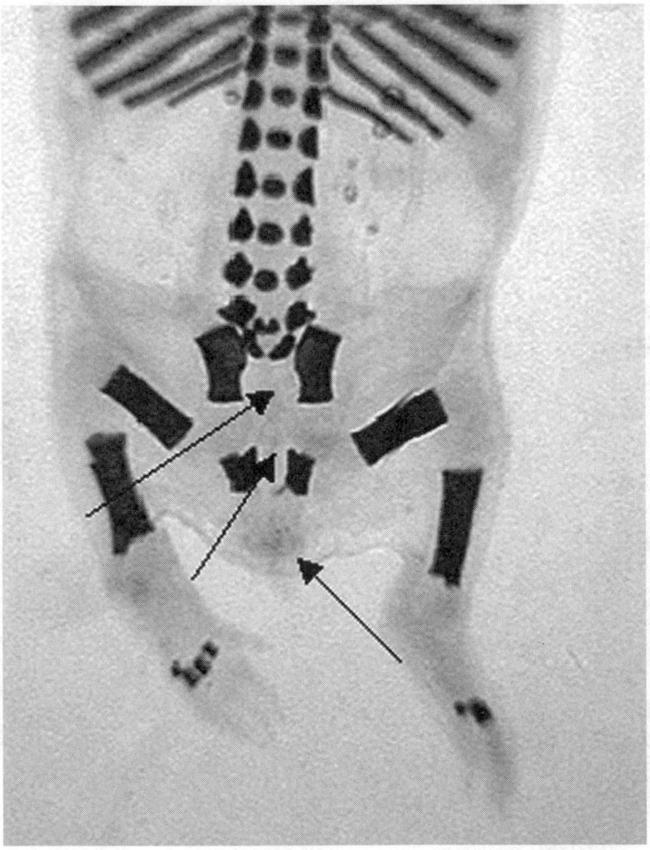

FIG. 29.17g. Rat fetus – Day 20 of gestation – Skeletal malformations associated with absence of tail (absence of lumbar, sacral and caudal vertebrae).

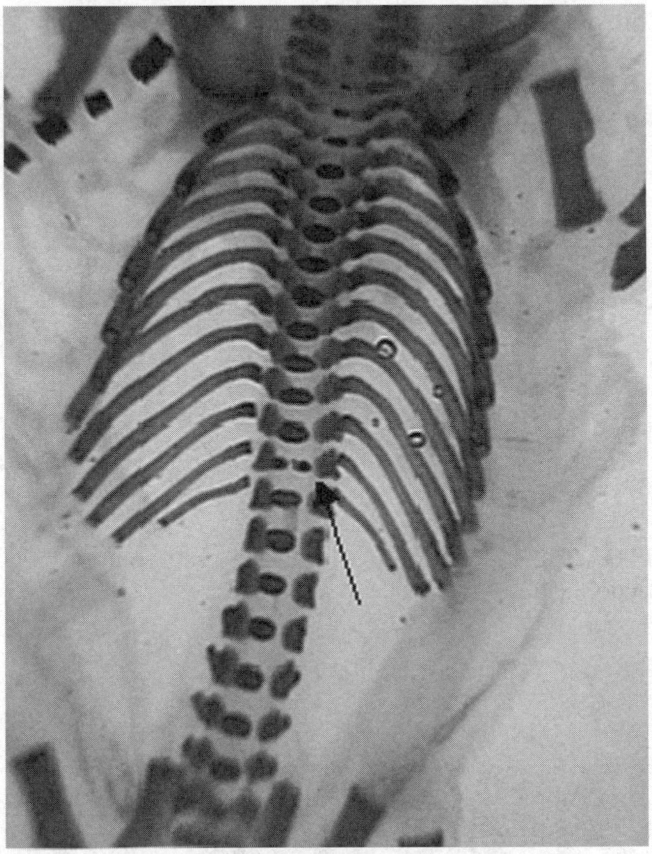

FIG. 29.17h. Rat fetus – Day 20 of gestation – Bifid vertebral centrum.

racic ribs on either side defining the number of thoracic vertebrae. For example, 13 ribs bilaterally (13 rib pairs) = 13 thoracic vertebrae; 14 ribs bilaterally (14 rib pairs) = 14 thoracic vertebrae; 13 ribs, right, 14 ribs, left (13.5 rib pairs) = 14 thoracic vertebrae. Any alterations in rib ossification are noted, such as a thickened area of ossification (Figure 29.18e), waviness (Figure 29.17i), splitting (branching), fusion, or misalignment (Figures 29.17k, 29.17m, and 29.18h). To the extent possible, interrelated vertebral-rib malformations are identified and this malformation counted as one finding (Figures 29.18f and 29.18g). Abnormal rib numbers (unilaterally increased or decreased) associated with increased or absent ribs and the presence of a hemivertebra are excluded from the litter average. Altered ribs are noted by number (T1–T13), affected area of ossification (proximal—beside the vertebral column; medial—middle of the ossified area; distal—near costochondral junction), and whether the alteration is unilateral (left or right) or bilateral.

Evaluation of the sternum then occurs (Figures 29.16l, 29.17n, 29.18m, 29.18n, and 29.18o). The adult sternum usually consists of 6 or 7 ossification sites (manubrium, 4 or 5 sternal centers and xiphoid). For the fetal examination, the manubrium and xiphoid are counted (0 = no ossification is present; 1 = any degree of ossification), followed by the intermediate sternal ossification sites, which may have degrees of delayed ossification (incompletely ossified or not ossified). For these sites, incompletely ossified centra are included in the count and unossified sites are excluded. Any alterations in sternal ossification are noted. For example, sternal ossification between the manubrium and xiphoid is nonsequential, and centra 2 and 3 normally ossify before centrum 1. Thus, delayed ossification (i.e., centrum 1 unossified and centra 2, 3, and 4 ossified) should be identified and incompletely ossified and not ossified sites noted individually. Incomplete ossification of the last (3rd, 4th, or 5th) centrum between the manubrium and xiphoid is not recorded because it is considered normal and identified as a delay based on the number of ossified sites present (i.e., 2, 3, or 4).

The pectoral girdle consists of two claviculae and two scapulae (Figure 29.16m and 29.16n). Any alterations in ossification, such as an irregular shape, waviness, bending, or small size are noted.

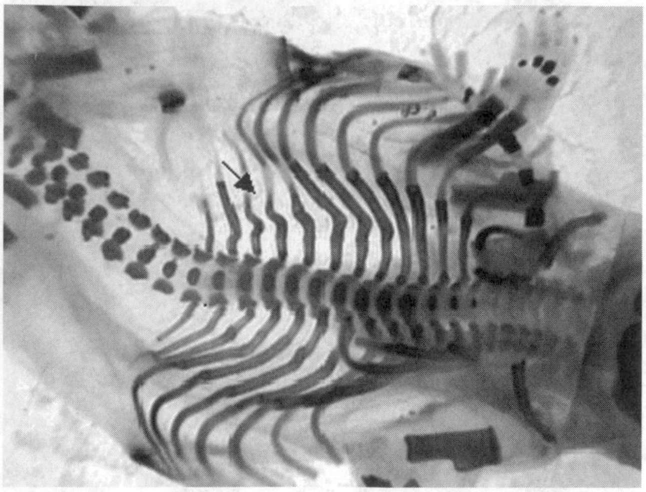

FIG. 29.17i. Rat fetus – Day 20 of gestation – Wavy, hypoplastic thoracic ribs.

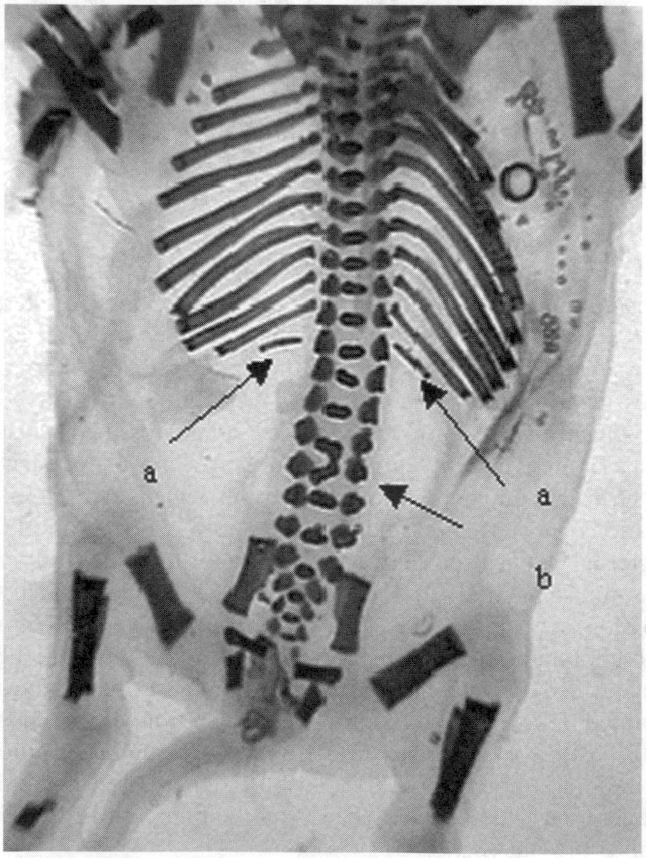

FIG. 29.17j. Rat fetus – Day 20 of gestation – a. Supernumary thoracic ribs; b. unilateral fusion of centra of L3 and L4.

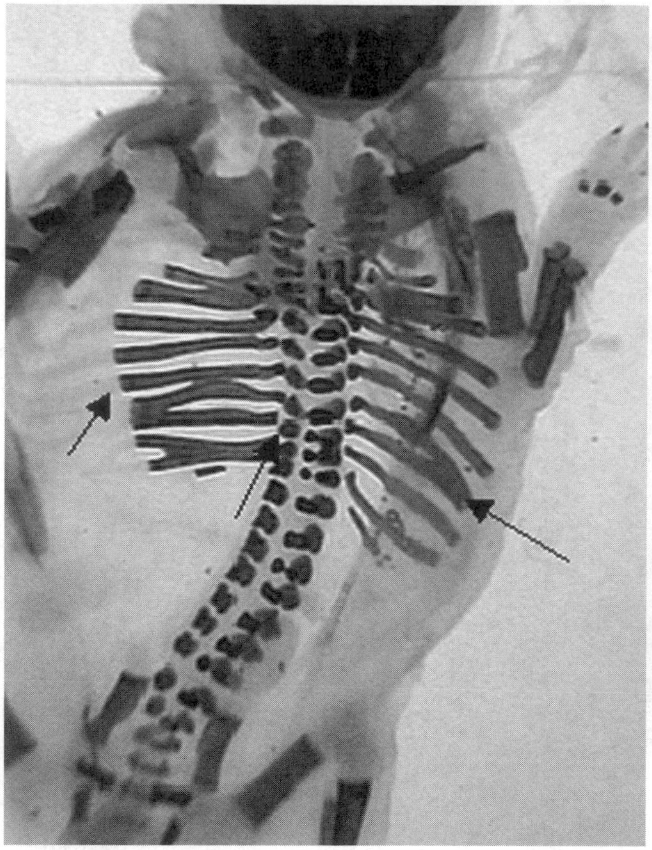

FIG. 29.17k. Rat fetus – Day 20 of gestation – Multiple interrelated vertebral/rib fusions.

Each forelimb (Figures 29.16o and 29.16p) consists of long bones (humerus, radius, and ulna) and the bones of the forepaws (metacarpals and phalanges). The number of carpals, metacarpals, and phalanges in each digit are counted on the basis of any point of ossification and incomplete ossification is not cited. Averaging these values identifies retarded ossification on a litter basis. Each paw is evaluated separately and between-paw differences noted. The carpals usually are not ossified; there are normally 4 or 5 metacarpals present in each forepaw. Because the preaxial metacarpal often is not ossified in fetuses, the presence of only 4 metacarpals indicates delayed ossification of the preaxial metacarpal unless the finding is associated with absence of the pollex (first preaxial digit), a relatively common finding in some rabbit strains. Each forepaw has 5 digits in most rodent and nonrodent species. The digit count begins at the preaxial digit, after which the phalanges in each digit are counted, including the distal phalanx (claw). Day 20 rat fetuses normally have 1, 1, 1, 1, and 1 ossified phalanges, and day 29 rabbit fetuses normally have 2, 3, 3, 3, and 3 ossified phalanges in the five respective digits. Counts excluded from the ossification site averages

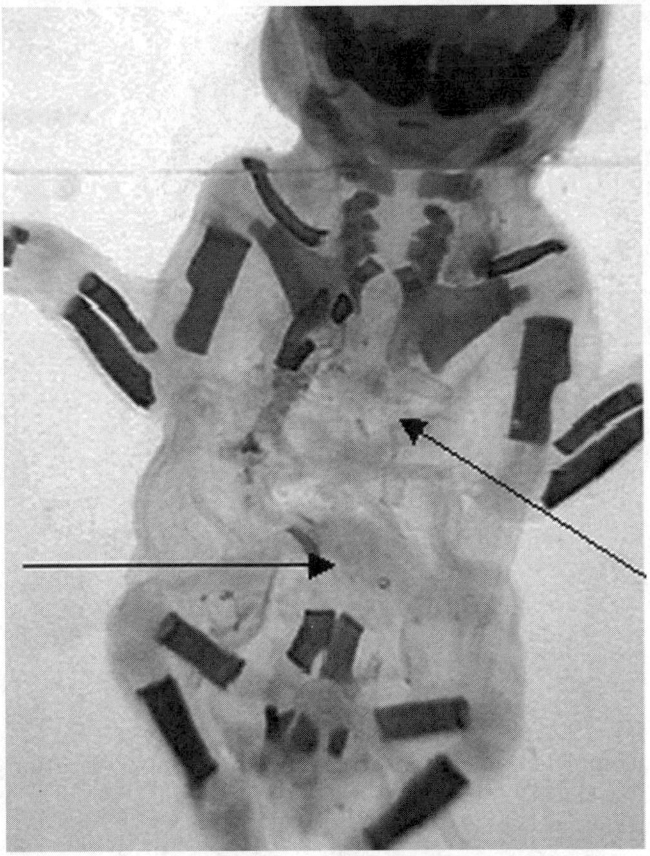

FIG. 29.17l. Rat fetus – Day 20 of gestation – Absence of vertebrae and ribs.

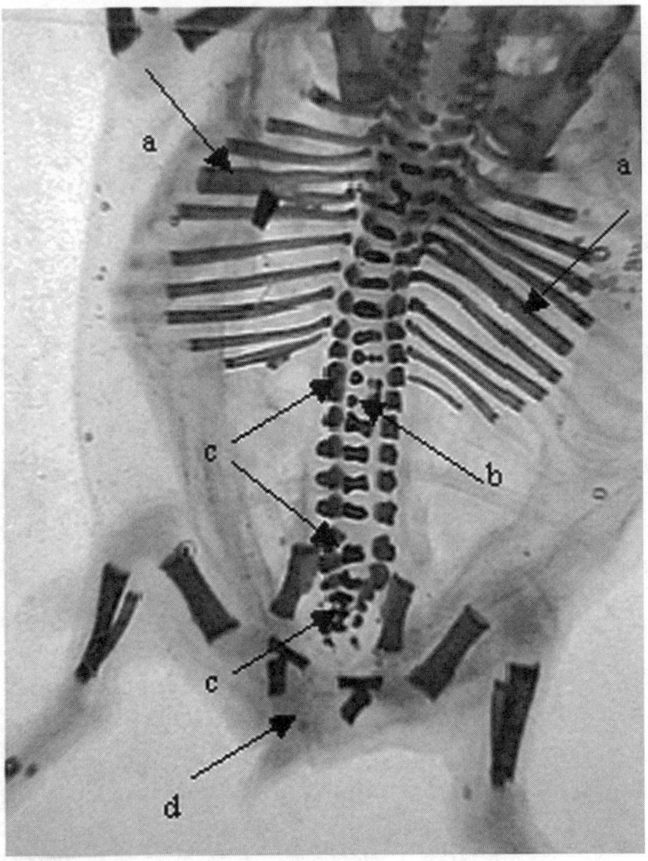

FIG. 29.17m. Rat fetus – Day 20 of gestation – Skeletal alterations associated with short trunk and short tail. a. fused ribs; b. bifid unilateral/incomplete ossification of vertebral centra; c. fused vertebral arches and centra; and d. absent caudal vertebrae.

are noted; (e.g., fused or absent digits and short, twisted, thick, bent, absent, or incompletely ossified long bones).

The pelvic girdle (pelvis) consists of two ilia, two ischia, and two pubes (Figure 29.16q). Any alterations in ossification are recorded, including incomplete, absent, or abnormal ossification (Figure 29.17o).

Each hindlimb (Figure 29.16r and 29.16s) consists of long bones (tibia and fibula) and the bones of the hindpaws (tarsals, metatarsals, and phalanges). Using the methods described to count the bones in the forepaws, the numbers of tarsals, metatarsals, and phalanges in each digit are counted. Normally 4 metatarsals are observable. Rat fetuses have 5 hindpaw digits, and when 4 metatarsals are present, the finding indicates delayed ossification of the preaxial metacarpal. Rabbit fetuses have only 4 hindpaw digits and 4 metacarpal bones. Beginning with the preaxial digit, the hindpaw phalanges are counted across. Normal day-20 of gestation rat fetuses have 1, 1, 1, 1, and 1 phalanges, and normal day-29 of gestation rabbit fetuses have 3, 3, 3, and 3 phalanges, including the distal phalanx, or claw (Figure 29.18p). Examples of reasons for exclusion of count values from averages include fused or absent digits, and short, thick, bent or absent long bones (Figure 29.17q).

Our practice is to have a senior level scientist confirm alterations identified at the technical level, with random evaluations of additional sites and/or specimens made to test for laboratory consistency across studies. These confirmations generally exclude sites included in ossification site averages and common variations in skull ossification (rabbits).

ICH STAGE E: Birth to Weaning

E: Adult female reproduction function, adaptation of the neonate to extrauterine life, including preweaning development and growth (postnatal age optimally based on postcoital age).

Observation and Timing of Parturition

Parturition, lactation, maternal-pup interaction, and pup growth and development until weaning are moni-

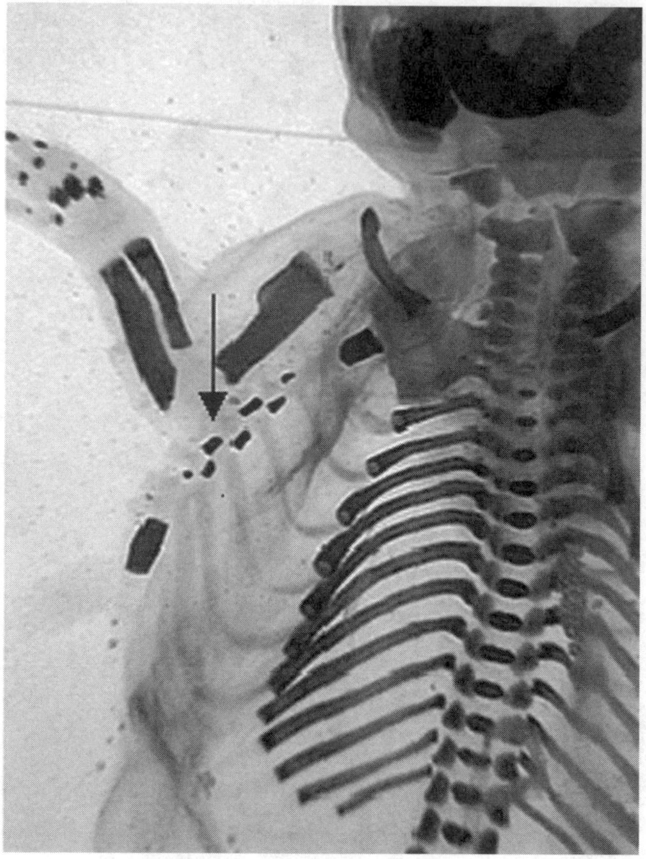

FIG. 29.17n. Rat fetus – Day 20 of gestation – Asymmetric, incompletely ossified sternebrae.

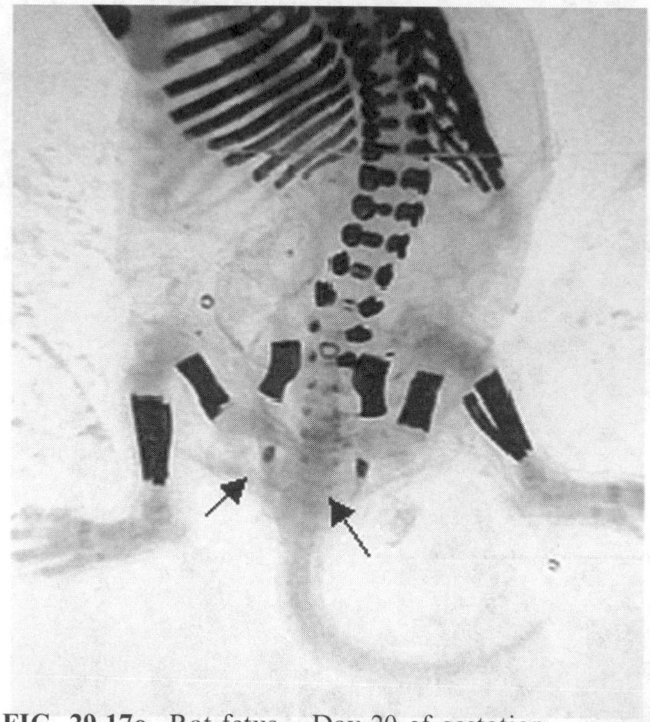

FIG. 29.17o. Rat fetus – Day 20 of gestation – Incomplete ossification of pubes and absent ossification of ischia.

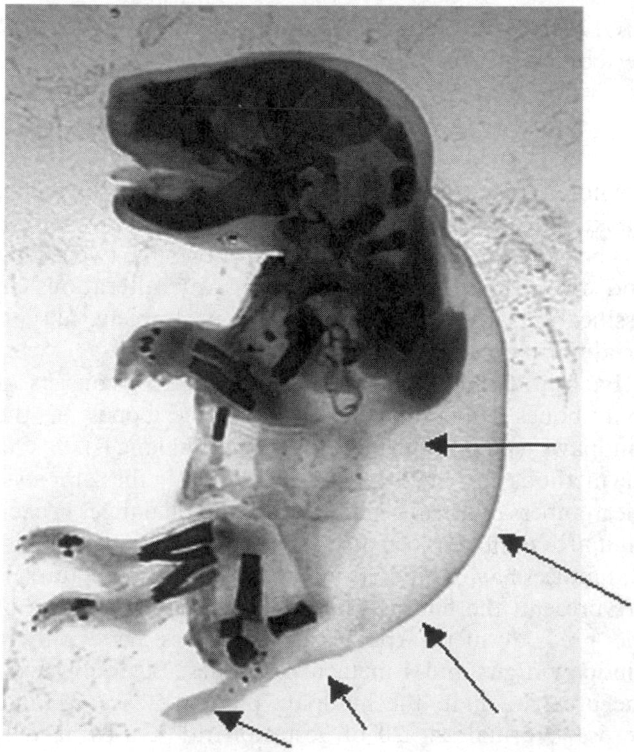

FIG. 29.17p. Rat fetus – Day 20 of gestation – Absence of thoracic vertebrae, ribs, lumbar, sacral and most caudal vertebrae.

tored during ICH Stage E. For some classes of compounds (e.g., nonsteroidal anti-inflammatory drugs, and sedatives), gestation will be prolonged and insufficient numbers of deliveries will occur during the normal 10- or 12-h light interval. The identified pharmacologic activity of the agent, in combination with a screening study, generally will identify whether the duration of gestation or parturition is affected and overnight observations will be needed. When continual observations are made (i.e., 24 h/day), the modification of the light cycle will lengthen the duration of gestation after approximately 3 days. Although this can be prevented by conducting the evaluations under "red light," this is sometimes considered to be detrimental to employee health and safety.

Presumed pregnant animals should be housed in a nesting box with bedding, beginning approximately 2 days before the expected day of delivery (hanging cages can be used before this time). They should be observed periodically for signs indicating onset of parturition, such as stretching, visible uterine contractions, vaginal

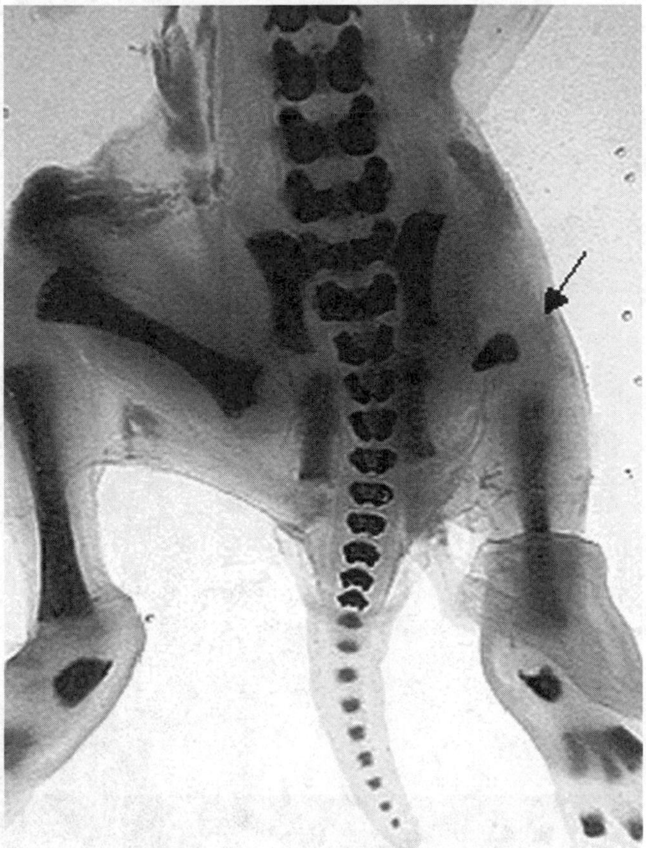

FIG. 29.17q. Rat fetus – Day 20 of gestation – Short femur.

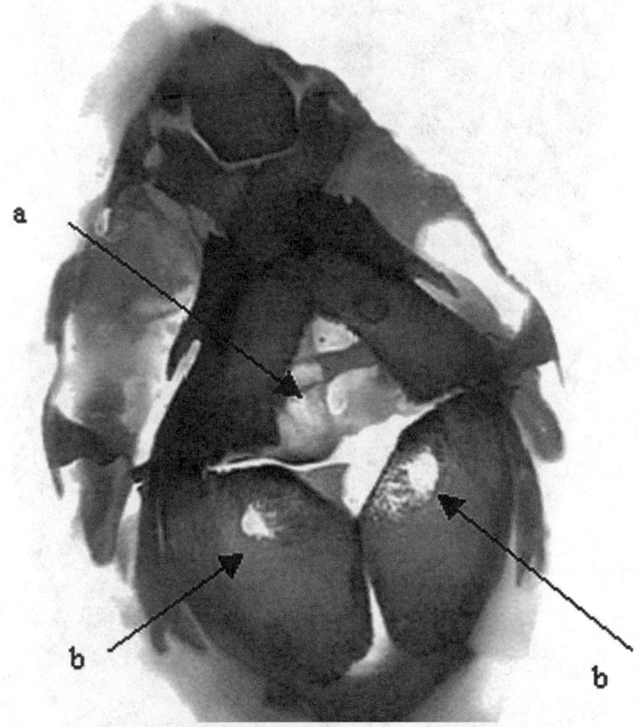

FIG. 29.18a. Rabbit fetus – Alternations associated with hydrocephaly and domed skull [(a) large anterior fontanelle; (b) holes in parietals].

bleeding, and the presence of pups or placentas in the nesting box.

After parturition begins, observations are made every few min for delivery of a pup (the dam may be gently lifted to verify the presence of pups) and the delivery time for each pup is recorded. Delivery complications (dystocia) and abnormal maternal behavior (e.g., failure to remove the placenta, groom and nest the litter, mutilization or cannibalization of pups) are noted. Pups that appear stillborn or die shortly after birth are removed from the nesting box to preclude cannibalization by the dam. Dams in the process of delivery are generally not treated until parturition is completed in order to prevent overdosing of the animal (rats generally lose 100 or more grams from the beginning to end of parturition, which would remarkably affect a dosage adjusted for body weight changes).

The day on which delivery is completed is functionally defined as day 0 or 1 postpartum, depending on the laboratory's historical use (our laboratory uses day 1). Appropriate maternal behavior is determined on the basis of examinations for maternal and pup nesting behavior. Criteria evaluated include pup appearance (clean and

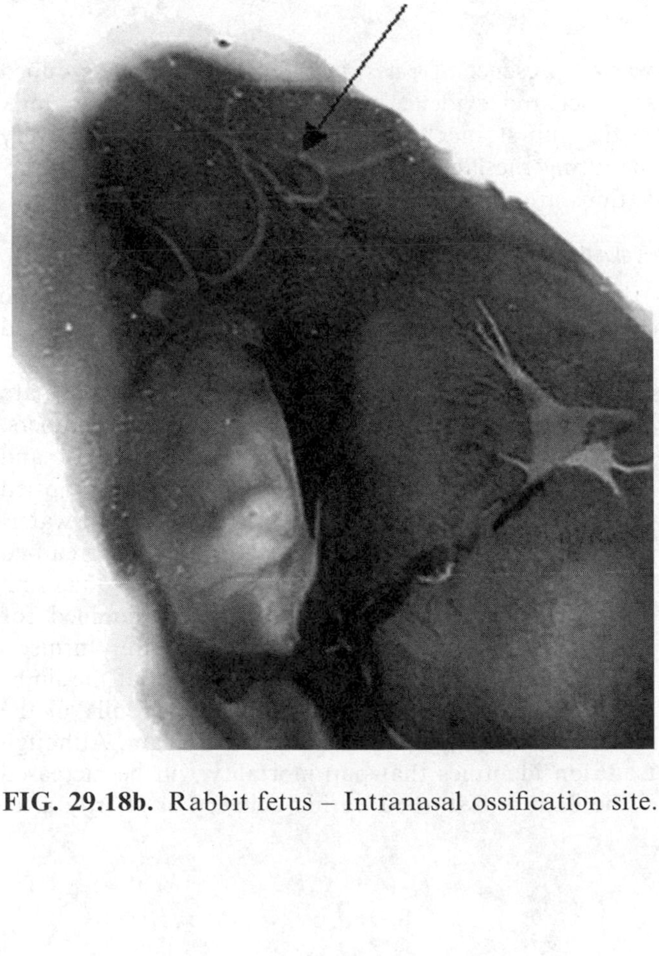

FIG. 29.18b. Rabbit fetus – Intranasal ossification site.

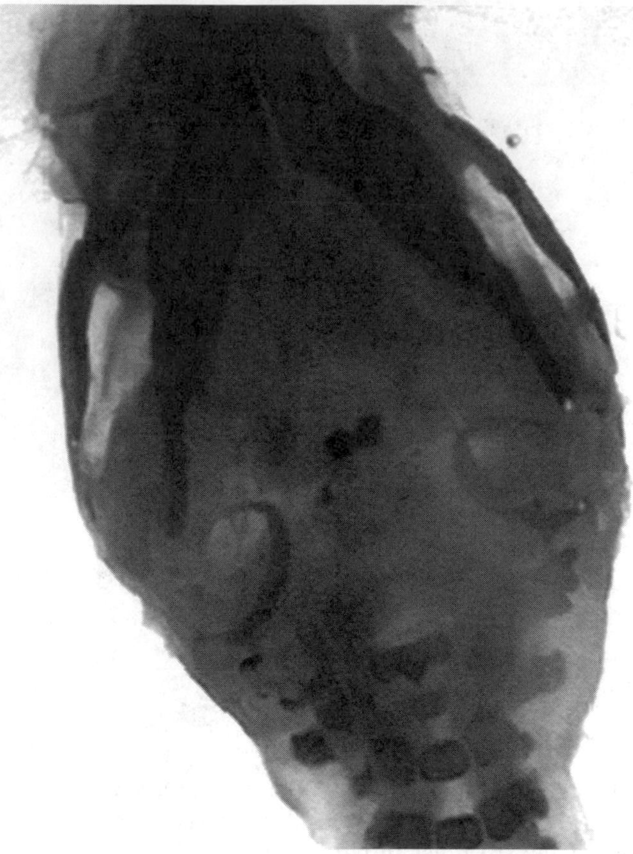

FIG. 29.18c. Rabbit fetus – Absent hyoid alae.

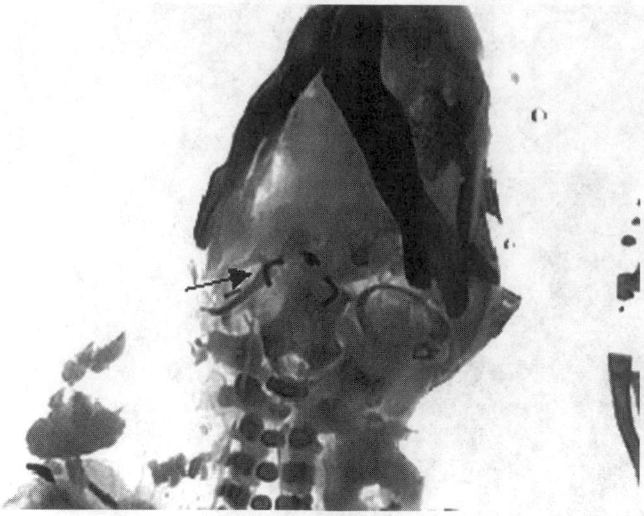

FIG. 29.18d. Rabbit fetus – bent hyoid alae.

warm), presence of a nest in which the pups are grouped together and evidence of nursing activity and/or milk in the pup stomach. Should a dam die during delivery or during the lactation period, no further in life observations are made on the litter.

Evaluation of Pups at Birth

The pups are further evaluated after removal from the nesting box. Gender is identified on the basis of observed anogential distance (longer in male than in female pups). For studies in which endocrine perturbations are expected, these observations are made using calipers. Any gross physical alterations and the viability and weight of each pup is identified. Dead pups are necropsied and a section of the lung placed in a container of water. Pups with lungs that float are assumed to have breathed and are considered liveborn. Pups with lungs that sink are identified as stillborn. Each pup is examined for the general shape of the head and features, bruises, lesions, number of digits, length and shape of the limbs and tail, presence of an anus, presence of milk in the stomach, and any injury inflicted by the dam. Although tradition identifies that pup mortality will be increased if the dam is disturbed during delivery or shortly after

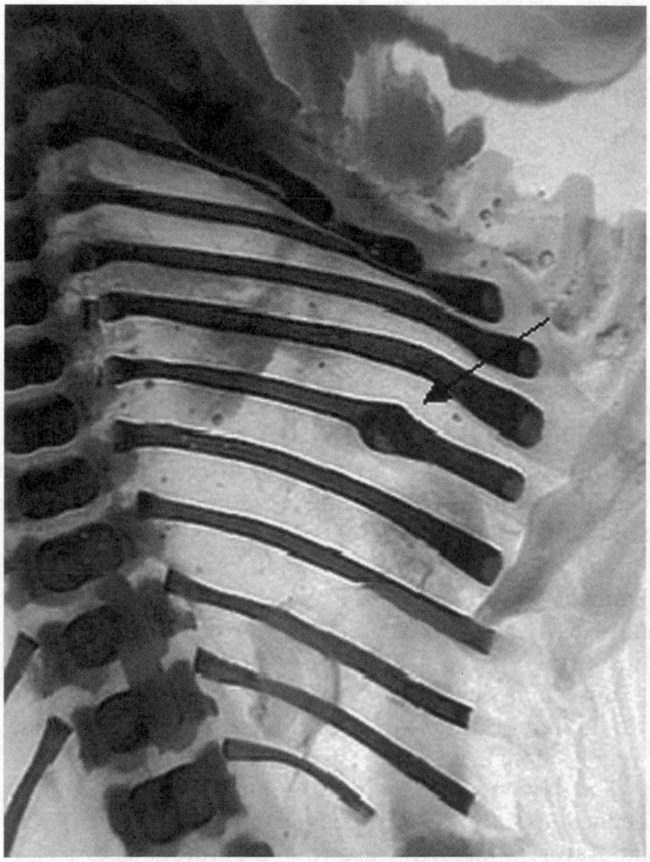

FIG. 29.18e. Rabbit fetus – thickened area of ossification in rib.

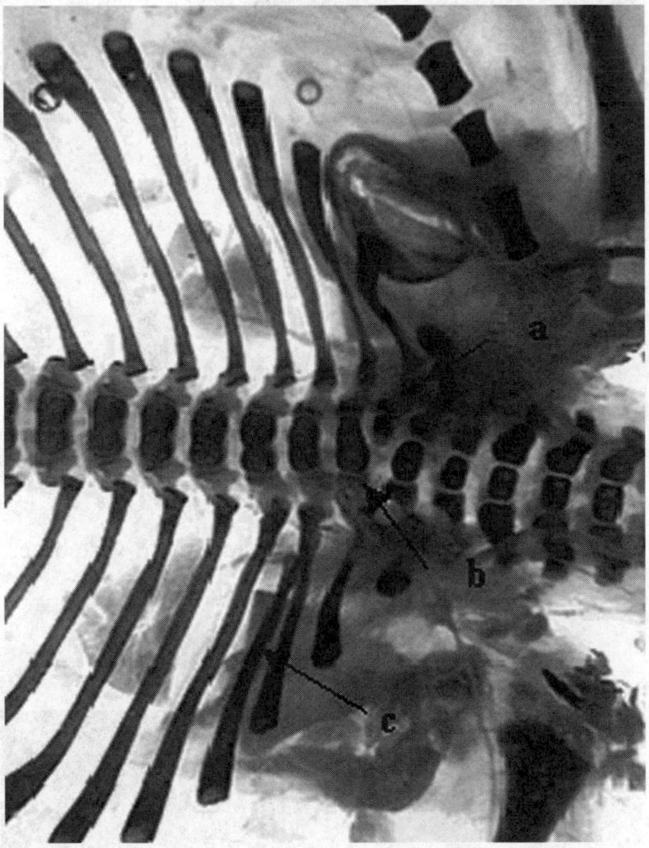

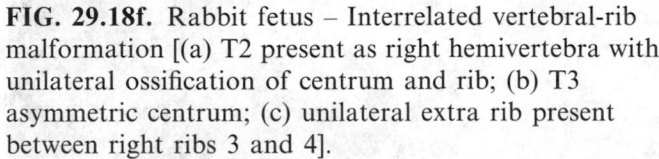

FIG. 29.18f. Rabbit fetus – Interrelated vertebral-rib malformation [(a) T2 present as right hemivertebra with unilateral ossification of centrum and rib; (b) T3 asymmetric centrum; (c) unilateral extra rib present between right ribs 3 and 4].

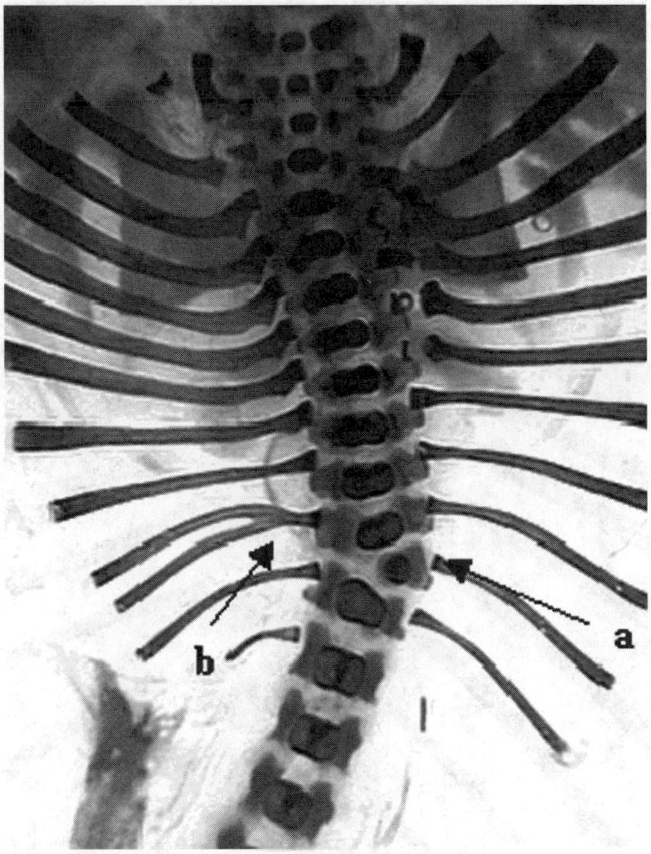

FIG. 29.18g. Rabbit fetus – Interrelated vertebral-rib malformations [(a) T12 present as left hemivertebra with unilateral centrum and rib; (b) forked right 10th rib, compensating for absence of 11th right rib].

parturition is completed, appropriately trained individuals can perform all of these activities without adverse effects.

Culling

Whether to cull is an area of debate (1,165). Its appropriateness is dependent upon the purpose of the study and the degree of control required for evaluation of the endpoint in question. Although culling is a common practice and required in some guidelines, this practice does increase the variability in litter values for viability and weight gain and has the potential to obscure late occurring effects because pups are removed from evaluation. It goes without saying that these comments also apply to selection of animals for continued evaluation in multigeneration studies.

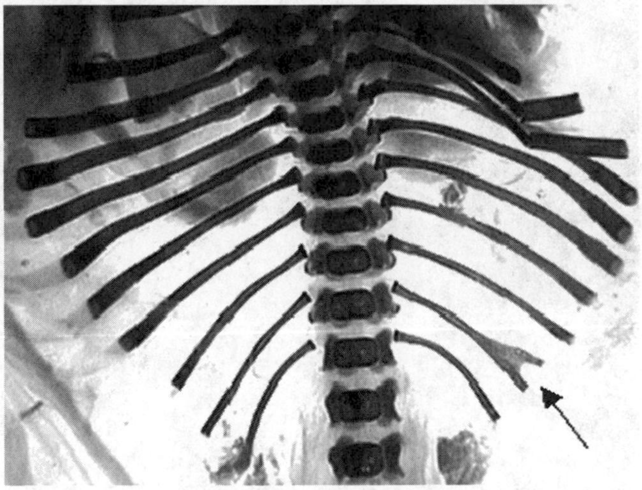

FIG. 29.18h. Rabbit fetus – Forked rib.

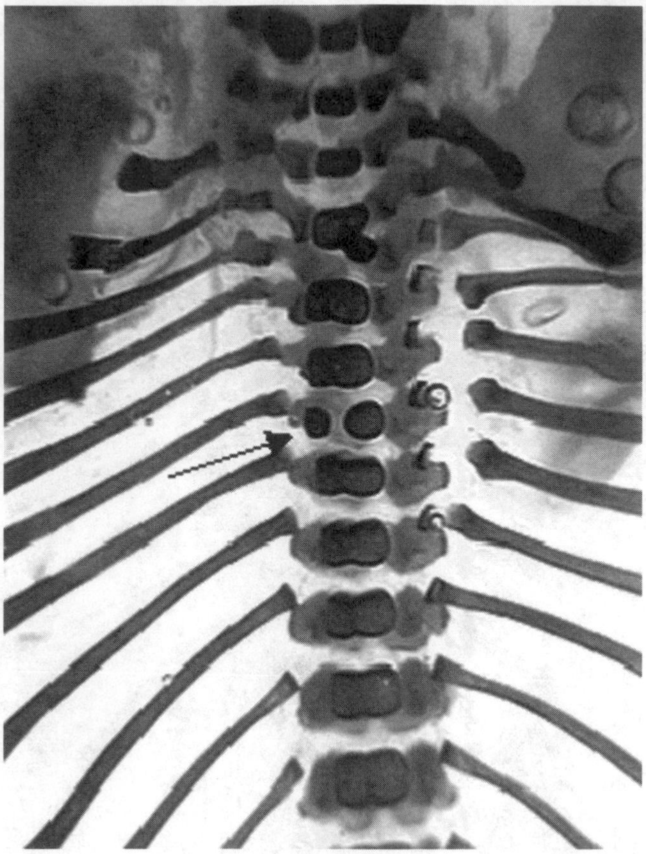

FIG. 29.18i. Rabbit fetus = Bifid centrum in T6.

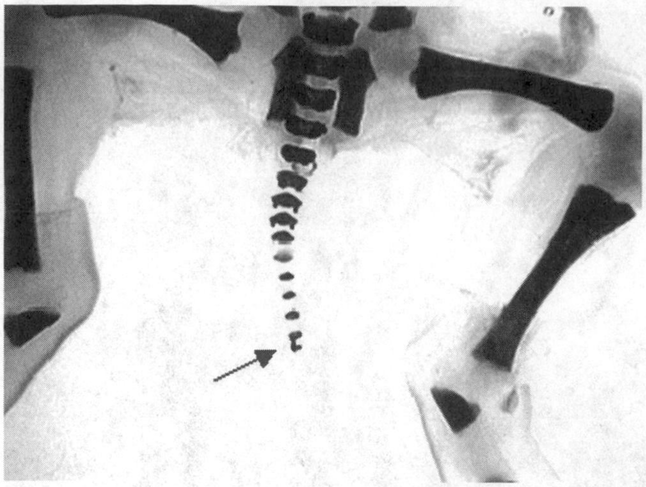

FIG. 19.18k. Rabbit fetus – fused caudal vertebrae.

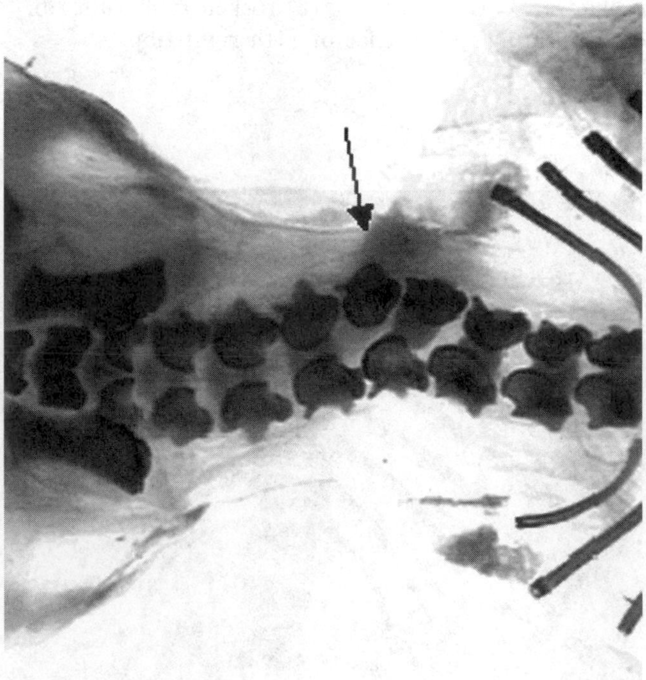

FIG. 29.18j. Rabbit fetus – Lumbar hemivertebra with associated scoliosis.

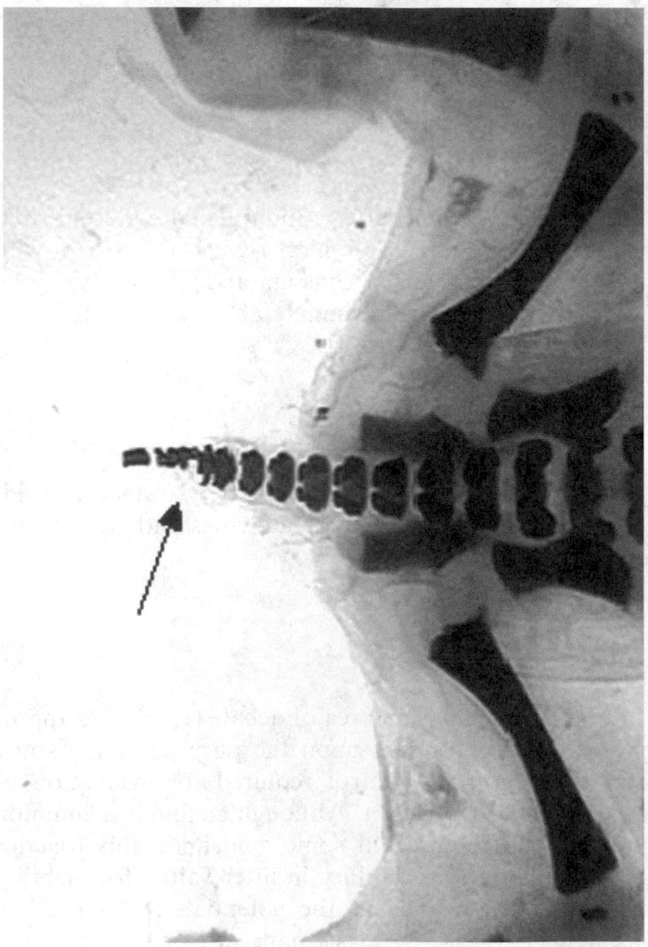

FIG. 29.18l. Rabbit fetus – Short tail with associated fusion of caudal vertebrae.

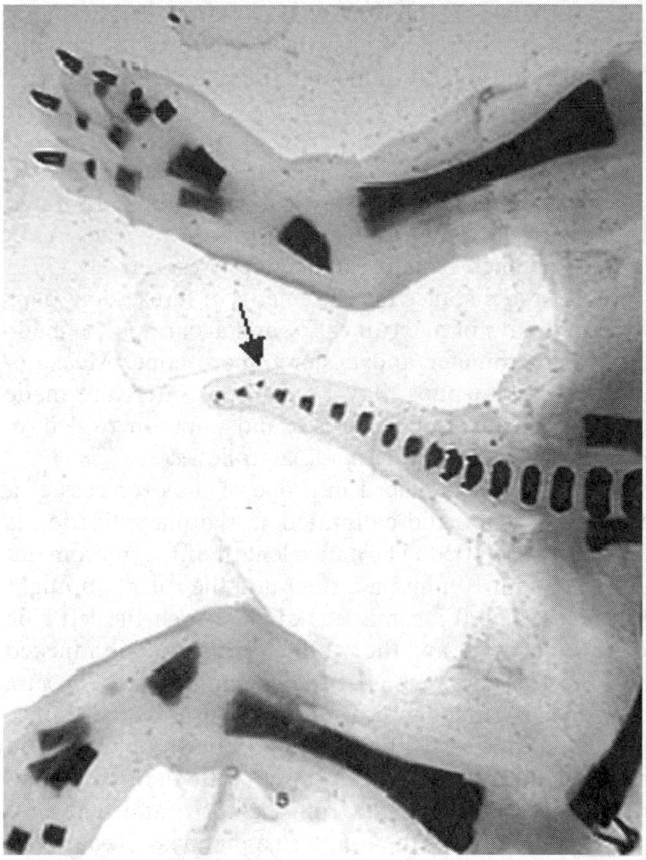

FIG. 29.18m. Rabbit fetus – Caudal vertebra misaligned.

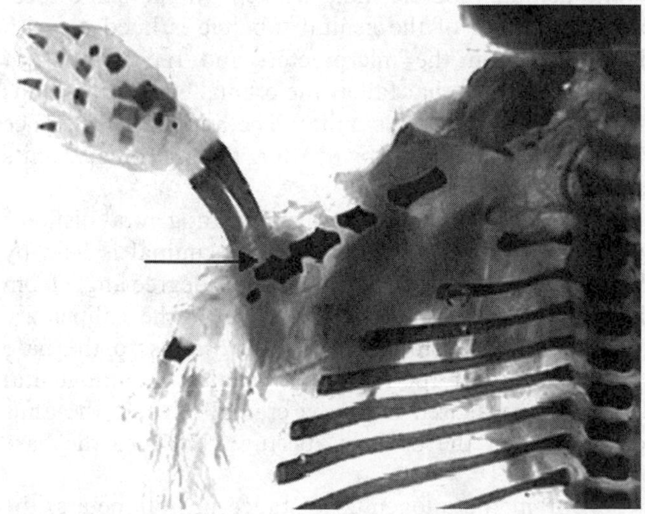

FIG. 29.18n. Rabbit fetus – Asymmetric fused sternebrae.

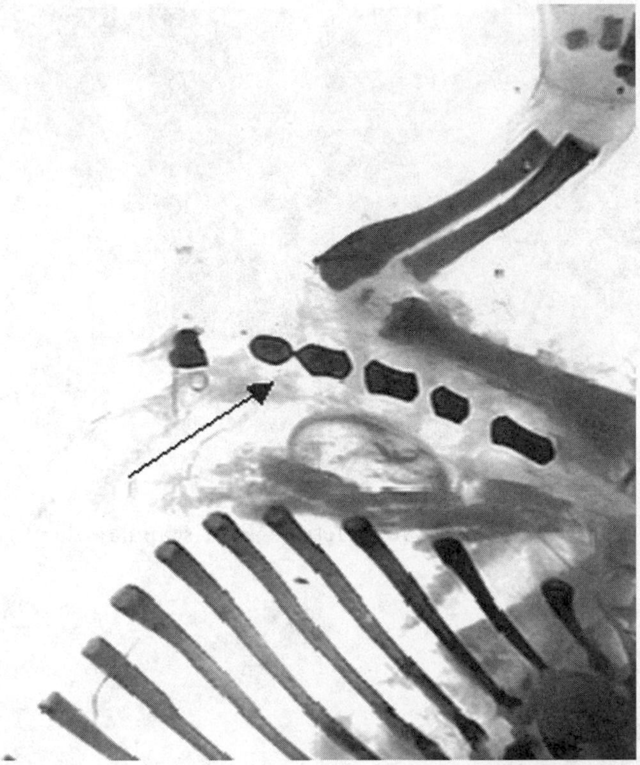

FIG. 29.18o. Rabbit fetus – Fused sternebrae 3 asnd 4.

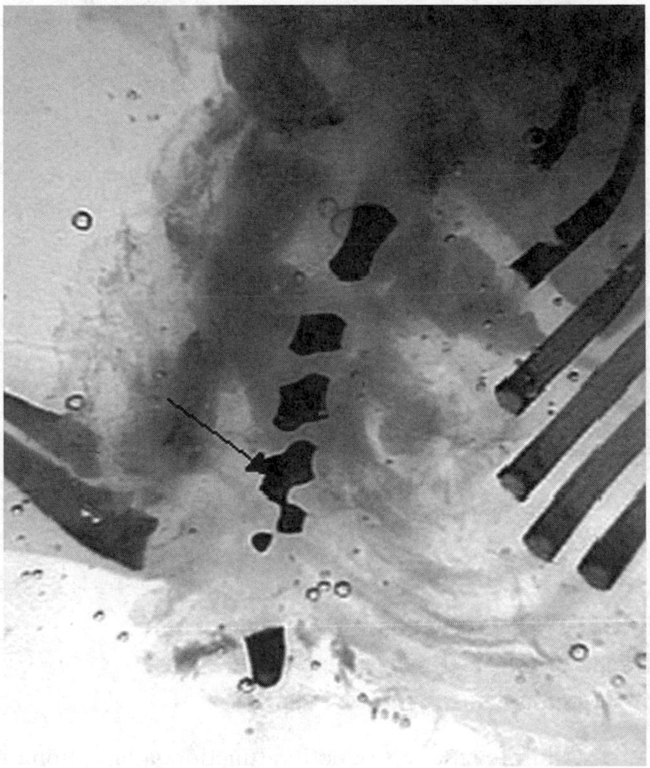

FIG. 29.18p. Rabbit fetus – Fused, asymmetric sternal centra.

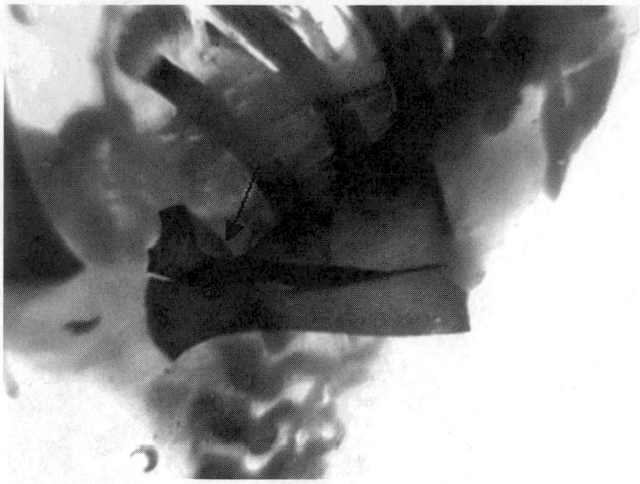

FIG. 29.18q. Rabbit fetus – Bent scapular ala.

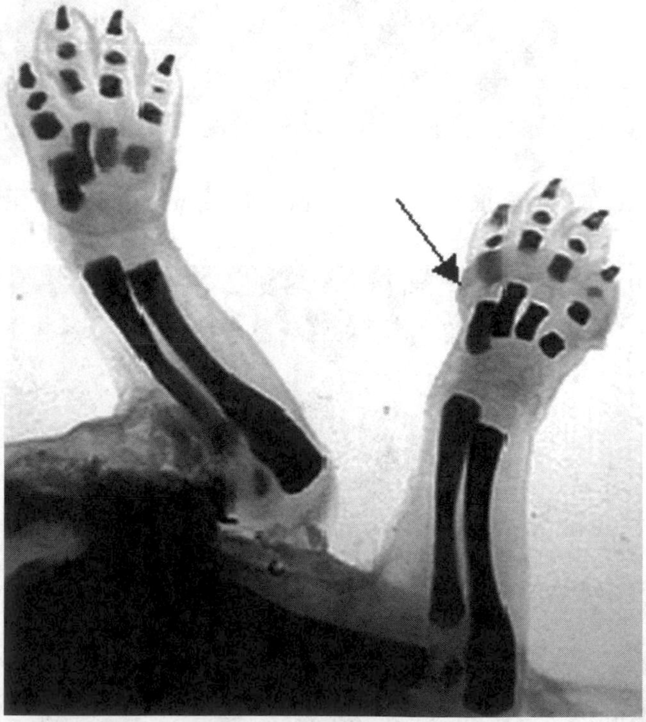

FIG. 29.18r. Rabbit fetus – Absent pollex.

ICH STAGES E (Postnatal Development to Weaning) and F (Postweaning Development of Reproductive Organs to Puberty)

E: Adult female reproduction function, adaptation of the neonate to extrauterine life, including preweaning development and growth (postnatal age optimally based on postcoital age).

F: Pediatric evaluation when treated; postweaning development and growth, adaptation to independent life and attainment of full sexual development.

Anogenital Distance

With the event of enhanced concern regarding estrogenic agents, many investigators have incorporated determination of anogenital distance at Caesarean-delivery or birth of fetuses and pups, respectively (37).

Anogenital distance measurements of fetuses and pups through 4 days of age can easily and accurately be made using a micrometer and a stereomicroscope. Measurements taken on pups, day 5 of age or later, are made by using a caliper. For fetuses and pups up to 4 days of age, the evaluation is made as follows.

A micrometer is placed into one of the eyepieces of a stereomicroscope and calibrated so the magnification is approximately 10 × . The entire length of the micrometer is aligned with 10 mm on a ruler and the ruler is brought into focus. The 0 μm mark is aligned with the left side of the 0 mm mark and the zoom magnification is adjusted until the 100 μm mark is at the beginning of the 10 mm mark. The zoom magnification may not be changed once the microscope is calibrated. The fetus or pup is held in one hand and the tail is raised with the other hand to a 80- or 90-degree angle from the horizontal. The anus is opened by raising the tail in this manner. Care should be taken to not pull the tail because this elongates the anogenital distance. The anogenital area is brought into focus and measured from the cranial edge of the anus (which comes to a point) to the base of the genital tubercle. Because the base of the tubercle is not clearly differentiated as it slopes into the anogenital area, it is necessary to visually estimate a base line between the distinct edges of the genital tubercle. The anus and the base of the genital tubercle must be kept in the same focal plane. The base of the genital tubercle is lined up with the 0 mark on the micrometer, and the number of micrometer units that fall at the cranial edge of the anus is recorded (micrometer units). The anogenital distance value in mm is obtained by dividing the micrometer units by the number 10.

When using a caliper to determine anogenital distance for pups 5 or more days of age, the animal is held by the tail, keeping the tail at an 80- to 90-degree angle from the horizontal. For males, the arms of the caliper are aligned from the cranial edge of the anus to the base of the anogenital aperture. For females, the anogenital distance is measured from the cranial edge of the anus to the base of the urinary aperture (NOT to the base of the vulva).

To obtain the anogenital distance in millimeters, the number of complete millimeters on the vernier scale is added to the number of millimeters indicated by the first coinciding line between the vernier and metric scales.

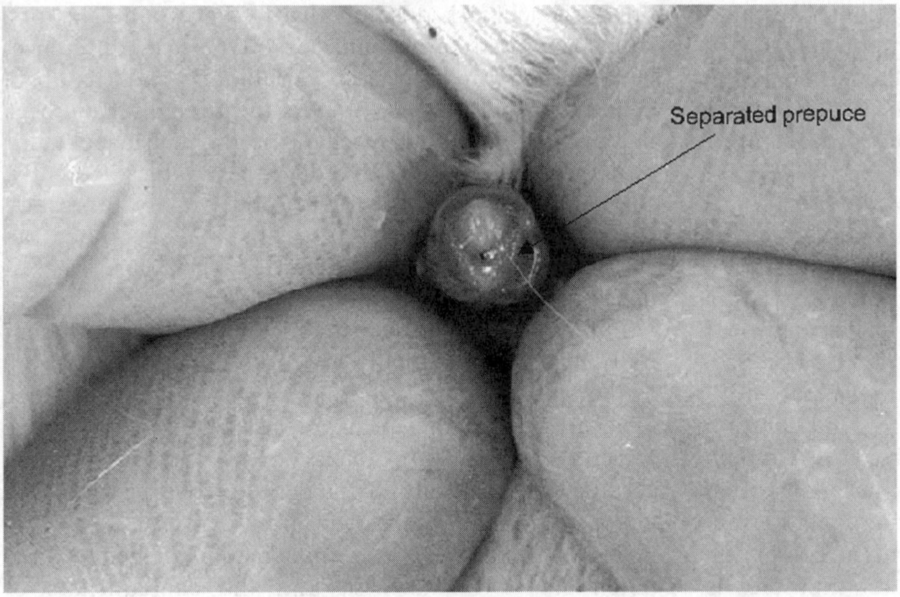

FIG. 29.19. Rat pup – preputial separation.

Nipple Evaluation

One physical landmark used to evaluate both estrogenicity of xenobiotics and physical development of female animals is to evaluate pups for nipple development. Beginning on day 12 postpartum, all pups in the litter are examined individually. Each pup is observed for any presence of nipples by brushing the hair coat against the nap. The criterion is met when a nipple is found. The number of pups of each sex that meet the criterion is recorded over the total number of pups of each sex tested. Testing continues until all animals identified as female have at least one nipple identified.

Balano–Preputial (Male Rodents) and Vaginal (Female Rodents) Opening (Sexual Maturation)

Evaluation of male rodents for balano–preputial separation is begun on day 22 (mouse), day 27 (hamster), or day 39 (rat) postpartum. Evaluation of female rodents for vaginal patency is begun on day 21 (mouse) or day 28 (rat) postpartum. The most appropriate way to perform this evaluation is to observe all animals daily until all animals (by sex) in the litter meet the appropriate criterion; however, as these evaluations may be begun after weaning of the litter and random selection of only one or two pups per sex for continued evaluation, this process has the potential to skew data distribution. Therefore, when differences occur on the basis of individual animal evaluations, litter analyses should be made. Evaluations are performed while the male or female rodent is held in a supine position. For male rodents, gentle digital pressure is applied to the sides of the rodent's prepuce. The criterion for balano– preputial opening is met when the prepuce completely retracts from the head of the penis (see Figure 29.19). The prepuce remains attached along the shaft of the penis but is not attached to the opening of the urethra.

RISK ASSESSMENT

Assessing the human risk of reproductive and developmental toxicities associated with exposure to pharmaceutical and chemical agents is a complex process involving the conduct of animal, and if possible, human studies evaluating all relevant data and then extrapolating the risk to humans. Although the endpoints that are used to identify reproductive and developmental toxicity are the same for both environmental and pharmaceutical agents, the methods used to identify the risk of exposure to these agents differ, based on the regulatory agency involved. A summary of current methodologies used by the FDA (food, drugs), EPA (chemicals), and California (Proposition 65) will serve to illustrate the differences in assessing reproductive or developmental risk for humans.

EPA

Guidelines for reproductive toxicity risk assessment were issued by the U.S. EPA in 1996 (213); those for developmental toxicity were issued in 1991 (212). These procedures provide guidance for interpreting, analyzing, and using the data from reprotoxicity and developmental toxicity studies conducted in conformance with the then issued guidelines, as well as information to be used in interpreting evaluations of epidemiologic data, sperm production, reproductive endocrine system function, sexual behavior, and female reproductive cycle normality.

Risk assessment is defined by the National Research Council (152) as consisting of several components: hazard identification, dose-response assessment, exposure assessment, and risk characterization. The EPA uses these components as key determinants in their procedure for risk assessment.

Hazard characterization includes evaluation of all available experimental animal and human data to determine whether and under what conditions reproductive toxicity is caused in a specific species. This information can then be characterized as to whether it is sufficient or insufficient to use in risk assessment. The recommended approach is to include an evaluation of dose-response relationships, route, timing, and duration of exposure in studies used to identify hazard. As noted by Kimmel et al. (109), determining a hazard is often dependent upon whether a dose-response relationship is present. Thus, information important in comparing a chemical's toxicity to potential human exposures is included as part of the exposure assessment, minimizing inappropriate labeling of chemicals as "reproductive toxicants" or "developmental toxicants" on a purely qualitative basis.

Quantitative dose-response analysis includes determining a no-observed-adverse-effect-level (NOAEL) and/or the lowest-observed-adverse-effect-level (LOAEL) for each endpoint and study. When the data are sufficient, a benchmark dose, an alternate method considered to provide a more quantitative dose-response evaluation, may be used (42,43,109). This method accounts for the variability in the data and the slope of the dose-response curve when calculating the reference dose for developmental toxicity (RfD) or chronic exposure (RfC). When reproductive toxicity occurs at the lowest toxic dose, an RfD or RfC can be derived using either the NOAEL or the benchmark dose divided by uncertainty factors, which are used to account for interspecies differences in response, intraspecies variability, and database deficiencies. Uncertainty factors traditionally have been in units of 10, although mechanistic and pharmacokinetic evaluations can be used to reduce these values. Recently, the EPA interpreted the 1996 Food Quality Protection Act, Public Law 104-170 (229), and proposed an additional safety factor of 10 for use when there was evidence of developmental toxicity.

Exposure assessment includes the populations potentially exposed or actually exposed to an agent, as well as the type, magnitude, frequency, and duration of these exposures, some of which are unique for reproductive toxicity exposure assessments. Thus, exposures during certain critical points in the reproductive process may affect the outcomes observed in humans.

Risk characterization results in a statement of the potential for human risk and the consequences of exposure as the result of integration of the hazard characterization, quantitative dose-response analysis, and human exposure estimates. Included in this characterization are the strengths and weaknesses of each component of the risk assessment, as well as major assumptions, scientific judgements, and, when possible, qualitative descriptions and quantitative estimates of uncertainties. In 1995 (20), the EPA issued a new risk characterization policy and guidance refining the principles of the earlier 1992 policy (213).

Finally, risk assessment, in conjunction with risk management, is used in the overall regulatory process, which includes risk characterization, directives of the enabling regulatory legislation, and other factors regarding whether and the degree to which exposure to an agent should be controlled. Risk management

A: Animal studies and well-controlled studies in pregnant women failed to demonstrate a risk to the fetus.

B: Animal studies have failed to demonstrate risk to fetus; no adequate & well-controlled studies in pregnant women.

C: Animal studies showed adverse effect on fetus; no well-controlled human studies.

D: Positive evidence of human fetal risk based upon human data, but potential drug benefit outweighs risk.

X: Studies show fetal abnormalities in animals and humans; drug is contraindicated in pregnant women.

FIG. 29.20. FDA labeling requirements: Pregnancy categories.

decisions include socioeconomic, technical, and political factors that extend beyond scientific considerations. For example, acceptability of the margin of exposure (MOE) is a risk management decision, although the scientific basis used to generate this value fall into risk assessment.

FDA

The FDA considers risk on a risk/benefit basis; (i.e., the beneficial uses of the agent are compared with the risk of its use). The conclusion regarding this risk/benefit consideration is published in the labeling (the label is the official FDA-approved package insert of a drug or biologic). This system was established by law in 1979 and categorizes risk by assigning a pregnancy label category to drugs and biologics (see Figure 29.20); however, a new proposal, "Considerations in the Integration of Study Results for the Assessment of Concern for Human Reproductive and Developmental Toxicities," is presently being developed into a guidance document in accordance with the FDA's Good Guidance Practices, 62 FR 8961 (February 27, 1997).

At present, the FDA is reviewing these procedures and considering changing the labeling of drugs and biologics from categories (A–D, X) to text that would include each of the seven potentially affected reproductive and developmental endpoints. Conclusions regarding the animal data are to be based on an integrated analysis of all pharmacology, toxicology, and pharmacokinetic data. It is to be performed using "the wedge," a tool that is designed to assess each endpoint and the strength of its signal (effect), ultimately resulting in a quantification of the risk for human use of the agent. This decision tree process is to be used to integrate clinical and nonclinical data for therapeutic agents (drugs or biologics) and to attempt to assess the "probability" or "likelihood" of an adverse reproductive outcome in humans. It reduces the previously existing emphasis on malformations as the most important adverse outcome and is independent of the type of response and its reversibility; however, the nature of the risk, along with the severity and reversibility of the response, remain as considerations in the "clinical management" of therapeutic use (i.e., risk versus benefit).

In the new proposal, "positive signals" are broadly classified as reproductive or developmental toxicities. The three subclasses of reproductive toxicity, fertility and fecundity, parturition and lactation, include both structural and functional changes affecting the reproductive competence of male and/or female animals in the parental (Fo) generation. Developmental toxicity has four subclasses: developmental mortality, dysmorphogenesis, alterations to growth, and functional toxicity; these actually are more complex descriptions of the four endpoints originally described by Wilson and Warkany (235). Each signal, regardless of type or whether it is present in a reproductive, developmental or general toxicity study, is independently evaluated by using three flow charts (see Figures 29.21, 29.22, and 29.23) to estimate the concern for human risks.

Flowchart A is used to determine if animal or human reproductive or developmental studies were conducted, whether the test system and routes were relevant, and whether there were any positive signals. If there are no positive signals in any of the studies addressing a particular reproductive or developmental endpoint, the decision tree evaluation of risk ends with Flowchart B; however, when positive signals exist for reproductive or developmental endpoints, six factors (signal strength part A, signal strength part B, pharmacodynamics, metabolic/toxicologic concordance, relative exposure, class alerts) must be considered (see Flowchart C).

Signal strength has six contributory elements that should be evaluated independently and integrated into the overall risk evaluation: cross-species concordance, multiplicity of effects, and adverse effects as a function of time are assessed in part A; maternal toxicity, dose-response relationship, and rare effects are evaluated in part B. Unitary values of +1, –1, or 0 are assigned to each of the six factors if the factor is perceived as increasing, decreasing, or having no effect on the level of risk. Conclusions regarding the six factors are summed to produce an overall level of concern for human reproductive risk.

The sixth factor, class alert, needs a word of explanation. A class alert is based on the presence of a related chemical structure, reactive metabolic intermediate or pharmacologic effect, to one that has produced adverse effects in prior human experience. In general, concern is increased when reproductive toxicity in animals is caused by an agent from a class of compounds (structure or pharmacologic effect) known to produce adverse reproductive effects in humans. Concern is reduced only in those cases where a class of compounds has produced no adverse effects on human reproduction despite adverse effects in animals. In the absence of human reproduction data, the assessed level of concern remains unchanged.

When no signals exist in a specific reproductive or developmental subclass, a statement can be made that there is no predicted risk for adverse human effects regarding the named category of endpoints based on the animals studies; however, when adverse effects on other endpoints within the same category are identified, the evaluation should state that there was no effect on the incidence of the specific endpoint in animal studies.

To summarize the reproductive and developmental toxicity of a therapeutic accurately and concisely in

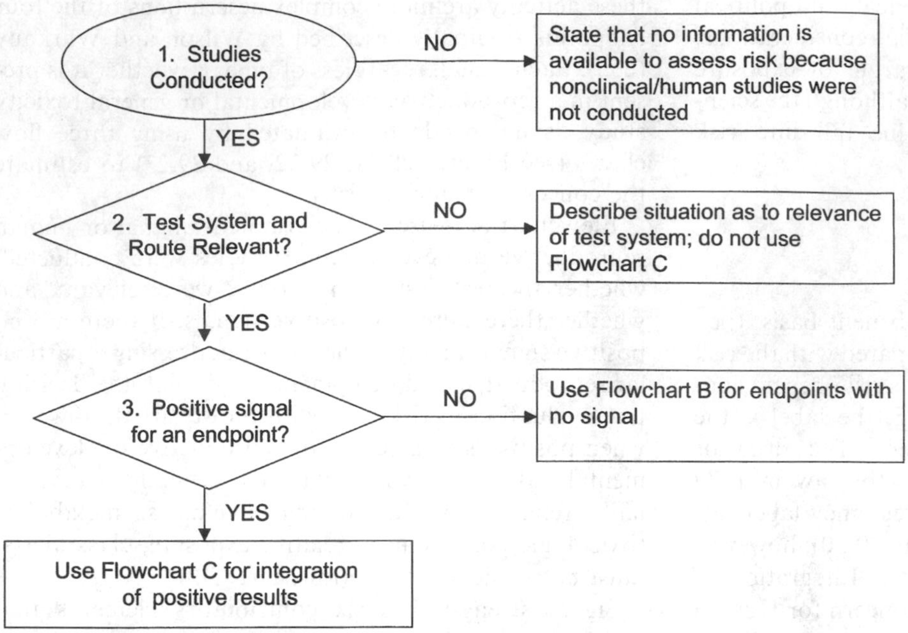

FIG. 29.21. Flowchart A. Overall decision tree for evaluation of repro/developmental toxicity risk from Wedge Document, 1999 distributed through *www.FDA.gov* (June, 1999).

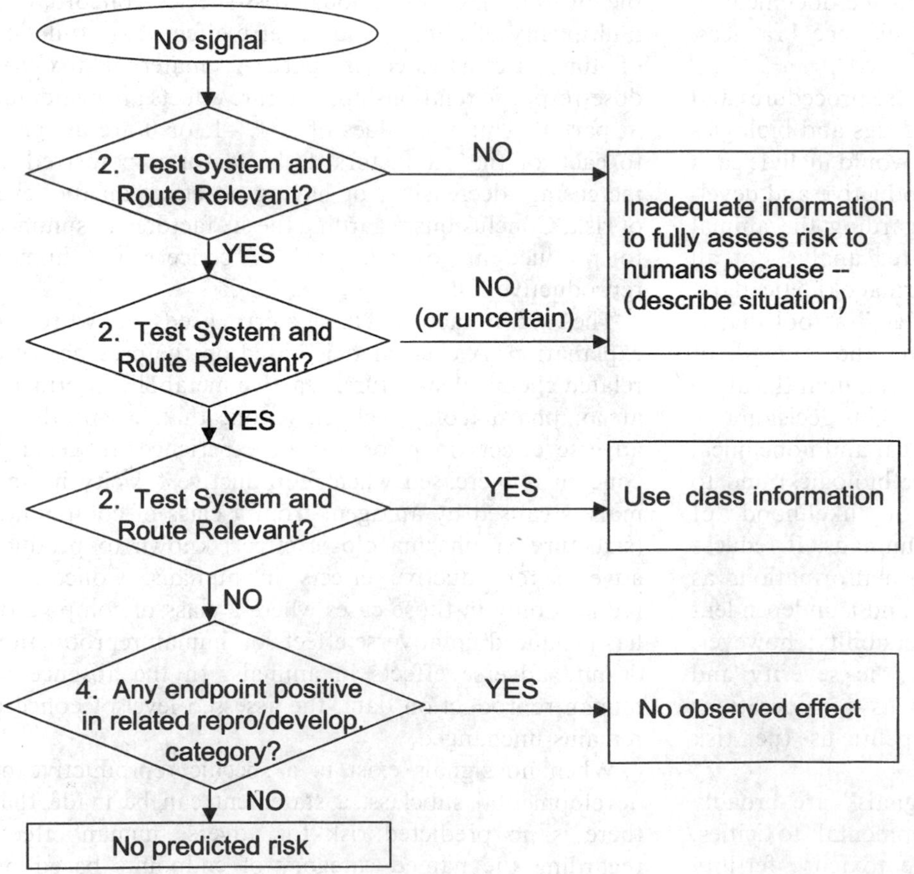

FIG. 29.22. Flowchart B. Decision tree for endpoints with no signal from Wedge Document, 1999 distributed through *www.FDA.gov* (June, 1999).

one or two paragraphs of a package insert is almost impossible. Therefore, it will be interesting to see if the "wedge" concept will withstand the test of time and effectively replace the present category system.

California—Proposition 65

Proposition 65 (California Safe Drinking Water and Toxic Enforcement Act of 1986) was enacted by

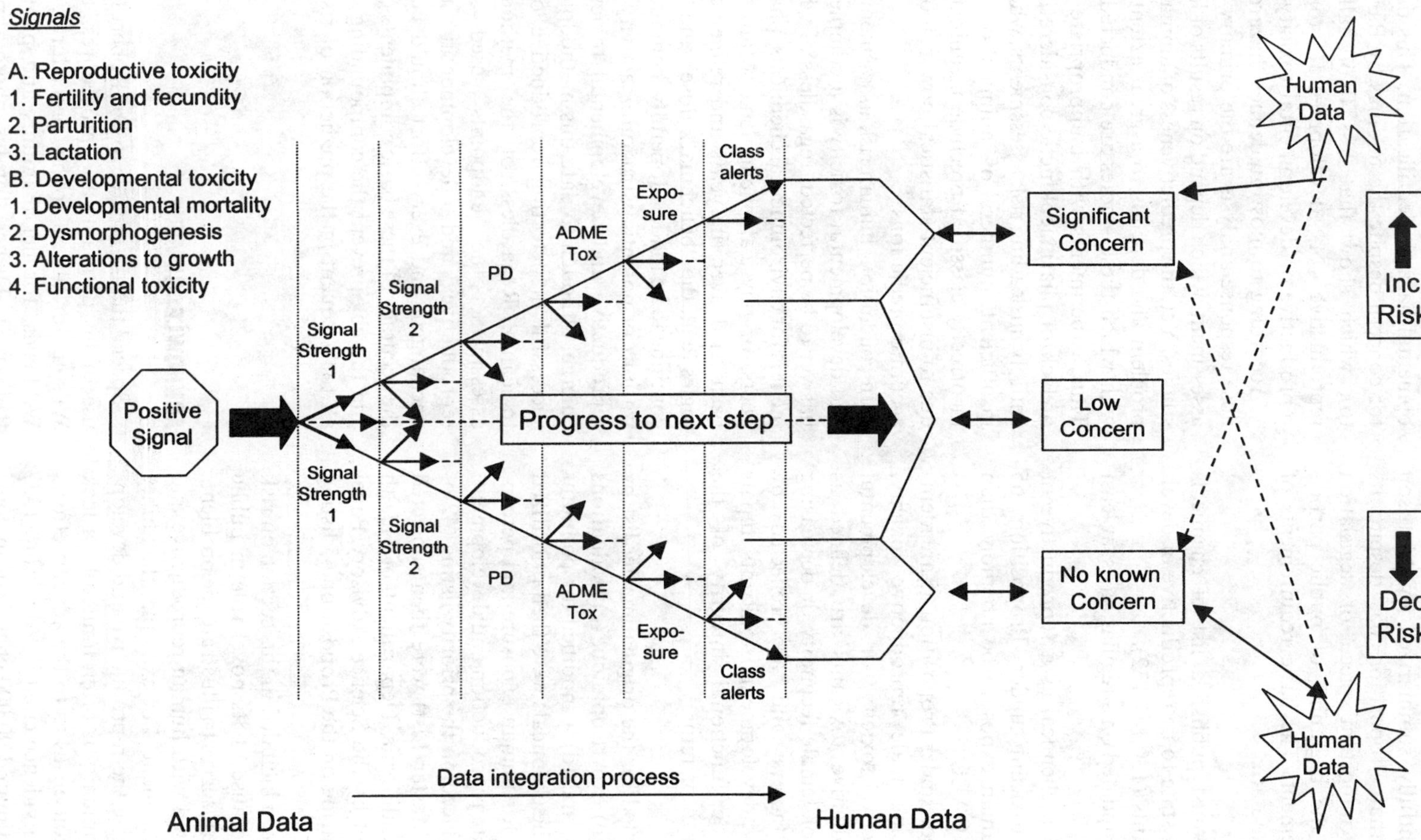

FIG. 29.23. Flowchart C. Integration of positive repro/ancillary study results from Wedge Document, 1999 distributed through www.FDA.gov (June, 1999).

California voters because of the perception that local, state, and federal regulatory agencies were not protecting them adequately against reproductive and developmental hazards (as well as carcinogens). The effect of this statute, and its implications on risk assessment and public health, are thoughtfully summarized by Mattison (133), who believes that Proposition 65, despite its imperfections, is an important piece of legislation because it represents the beginning of public participation in risk management. The basic requirements of this controversial statute are:

(1) The Governor must publish a list of chemicals "known" by the state to be reproductive or developmental toxicants (130,131,132).
(2) The list must be updated on a regular basis, at least annually.
(3) Identification of a chemical as a reproductive or developmental toxicant under Proposition 65 requires that human exposure be no more than 1/1000 of the NOAEL.
(4) Chemicals "listed" under Proposition 65 are identified as producing male reproductive toxicity, female reproductive toxicity, or developmental toxicity. Reproductive toxicants are defined as impairing male or female fecundity or decreasing couple-specific factors and are reflected by impaired fertility; developmental toxicants impair the structural or functional integrity of the developing embryo or fetus.

Chemicals were selected for the original master list by (a) literature reports, (b) expert opinion, (c) evaluations by regulatory agencies, and (d) a modified air pollutant prioritization screen. The chemicals were then prioritized according to potential for human exposure and perception of hazard for human reproduction and development. Substances that were placed on the priority listing (42 of 162 chemicals on the Master List) were then subjected to evaluation by the California Department of Health Services and considered by the Science Advisory Panel before ultimately appearing on the Proposition 65 listing (50).

Proposition 65 has been included in this section on risk assessment not only because of its novel role in public health, but also because it serves to illustrate the problems and difficulties associated with human reproductive and developmental risk assessment. For example, the ability to assess and characterize the reproductive and developmental health of a community is often limited by a lack of data and a lack of consensus as to the adverse effects of a specific chemical. Evidence cited by Mattison (133) indicates that of the estimated 90,000 chemicals in commerce in the United States, only 4000 have been tested in animals for reproductive or developmental toxicity, and up to one third of the tested substances may be reproductive or developmental toxicants. A study by the National Research Council (152) also concluded that only a small fraction of the chemicals tested contained enough toxicity information for reproductive and developmental hazard identification. This data gap is reason for concern despite the findings by Barlow and Sullivan (6), which show that less than half of the animal reproductive or developmental toxicants produce reproductive or developmental toxicity in humans.

According to most guidelines, hazard assessment and dose response analysis are the primary principles of risk assessment, which depend on results of laboratory animal studies. Yet, the predictiveness of animal studies is itself a problem and depends to a great extent on the expertise with which these studies are conducted and interpreted. Thus, experiments with inappropriate dosage regimens or lack of pharmacokinetic considerations may provide entirely misleading risk assessments, whereas studies with insufficient numbers of animals or effects that are incorrectly classified preclude meaningful interpretation due to insufficient statistical power upon which to make accurate predictions.

In conclusion, human risk assessment for reproductive and developmental toxicity is a complex procedure that has yet to be perfected, regardless of whether the assessment is for environmental chemicals, pharmaceutical products, or physical phenomena. Many procedures have been tried over the years and refinements in methodologies (e.g., the "benchmark dose" and the "wedge") will continue to be made. Hopefully, computerized characterizations of potential structure/ activity relationships for reproductive and developmental toxicity will someday emerge, although to date this methodology has not been successful in detecting reproductive or developmental toxicants. Regardless of the method used for risk assessment, the endpoints used to characterize reproductive and developmental toxicity remain unchanged, and every effort should be made to assure the accuracy of these basic components of risk assessment and thereby prevent the compounding of errors that are all too frequent in the prediction of risk.

ACKNOWLEDGEMENT

Special thanks are due to Dr. Robert E. Staples, for the use of his diagrams and procedures, to Dr. James G. Wilson, for access to his procedures, to Mrs. Donna W. Lewis, for her diagrams and photographs, to Dr. Robert M. Diener, for his photographs and editorial assistance, and to Mrs. Marjorie B. Vargo, for her assistance in developing and compiling this chapter.

QUESTIONS

1. Design the testing needs for a new drug entity that is to be used as a contraceptive agent.
2. A secretary was exposed to insecticide fumes used during office-cleaning procedures. Nine months later she delivered a child with a cleft palate. Identify whether there was a potential causal relationship of the insecticide fumes and the birth defect in the child.
3. A chemical company wants to develop a new herbicide. Design the testing paradigm that should be run.
4. A woman falls down the steps and breaks her leg. As part of the hospital examination, she undergoes an X-ray, and it is also discovered that she is about 2 months pregnant. She has read that exposure to radiation sometimes results in microcephaly and calls her physician to schedule an abortion. What counsel should the physician provide?
5. A new drug entity results in increased hematopoiesis and is administered weekly to humans. What are the expected adverse effects of pharmacotoxic doses of this agent in women of childbearing potential and their offspring? Design a testing paradigm that addresses these endpoints and results in registration of the agent.

REFERENCES

1. Agnish, N. D., and Keller, K. A. (1997): The rationale for culling of rodent litters. *Fund. and Applied Toxicol.*, 38:2–6.
2. Alison, M. R., and Sarraf, C. E. (1992): Apoptosis: A gene-directed programme of cell death. *J. Royal College of Physicians of London*, 26:25–35.
3. Antonov, A. N. (1947): Children born during the siege of Leningrad in 1942. *J. Pediatr.*, 30:250.
4. Astwood, E. B. (1939): Changes in the weight and water content of the uterus of the normal adult rat. *The Amer. Journal of Physiol.*, 126:162–170.
5. Baker, T. G. (1963): A quantitative and cytological study of germ cells in the human ovaries. *Proc. Roy. Soc. Lond. Biol.*, 158:417-433.
6. Barlow, S. M., and Sullivan, F. M. (1982): *Reproductive Hazards of Industrial Chemicals: and Evaluation of Animal and Human Data*. Academic Press, New York.
7. Barrow, M. V., and Taylor, W. J. (1969): A rapid method for detecting malformations in rat fetuses. *J. Morph.*, 127:291–306.
8. Beach, F. (1948): *Hormones and Behavior*. Hoeber, New York.
9. Beltrame, D., and Giavini, E. (1990): Morphological abnormalities in experimental teratology: Need for a standardization of the current terminology. *Cong. Anom.*, 3:187–195.
10. Biggers, J. D. (1975): Oogenesis. In: *Gynecologic Endocrinology*, edited by J. J. Gold, pp. 612–620, Harper & Row, New York.
11. Bold, R. J., Termuhlen, P. M., and McConkey, D. J. (1997): Apoptosis, cancer and cancer therapy. *Surgical Oncology*, 6:133–142.
12. Boué, J., Boué, A., and Lazar, P. (1975): Retrospective and prospective epidemiological studies of 1,500 karyotyped spontaneous abortions. *Teratology*, 12:11–26.
13. Brann, D. W., Mills, T. M., and Mahesh, V. B. (1995). Female reproduction: The ovulatory cycle. In: *Reproductive Toxicology, 2nd edition*, edited by R. J. Witorsch, pp. 23–44. Raven Press, New York.
14. Brent, R. L. (1964): Drug testing in animals for teratogenic effects: Thalidomide in the pregnant rat. *J. Pediatr.*, 64:762–770.
15. Brent, R. L. (1976): Environmental factors: Miscellaneous. In: *Prevention of Embryonic, Fetal and Perinatal Disease*, edited by R. L. Brent and M. I. Harris, pp. 211–218. M.I., DHEW, Pub. No. (NIH) 76-853, Bethesda.
16. Brent, R. L. (1980): The prediction of human diseases from laboratory and animal tests for teratogenicity, carcinogenicity and mutagenicity. In: *Controversies in Therapeutics*, edited by L. Lasagna. W. B. Saunders Company, Philadelphia.
17. Brent, R. L. (1985): The magnitude of the problem of congenital malformations. In: *Prevention of Physical and Mental Congenital Defects, Part A: The Scope of the Problem*, edited by M. Marois, pp. 55–68. Alan R. Liss, New York.
18. Brent, R. L. (1999): Utilization of developmental basic science principles in the evaluation of reproductive risks from pre- and postconception environmental radiation exposures. *Teratology*, 59:182–204.
19. Brinster, R. L. (1975): Teratogen testing using preimplantation mammalian embryos. In: *Methods for Detection of Environmental Agents That Produce Congenital Defects*, edited by T. H. Shepard, J. R. Miller, and M. Marois, pp. 113–124. American Elsevier, New York.
20. Browner, C. M. (1995): EPA risk characterization program. U.S. EPA Memorandum, March 21, 1995.
21. Burek, M. J., and Oppenheim, R. W. (1996): Programmed cell death in the developing nervous system. *Brain Pathology*, 6:427–446.
22. Byskov, A. G. (1978): Follicular atresia. In: *The Vertebrate Ovary*, edited by R. E. Joes, pp. 533–562, Plenum Press, New York.
23. Carter, C. O. (1976): Genetics of common single malformations. *Br. Med. Bull.*, 32:21–26.
24. Cassidy, A., Bingham, S., and Setchell, K. (1996): Biological effects of a diet of soy protein rich in isoflavones on the menstrual cycle of premenopausal women. *Am. J. Clin. Nutr.*, 60:333–340.
25. Challis, J. R. G., and Olson, D. M. (1988): Parturition. In: *The Physiology of Reproduction, Vol. 2*, edited by E. Knobil, and J. D. Neill, pp. 2177–2216. Raven Press, New York.
26. Chapin, R. E., and Heindel, J. J. (1993): Introduction. In: *Methods In Toxicology, Volume 3B. Female Reproductive Toxicology*, edited by J. J. Heindel and R. E. Chapin, pp. 1–15. Academic Press, San Diego.
27. Chernoff, N., and Kavlock, R. J. (1982): An in vivo teratology screen utilizing pregnant mice. *Toxicol. Environ. Health*, 10:541–550.
28. Christian, M. S. (1978): Postnatal functional teratology resulting from fetal insult. Dissertation, Thomas Jefferson University, Philadelphia.
29. Christian, M. S., and Voytek, P. E. (1982): In vivo reproductive and mutagenicity tests. In: *A Guide to General Toxicology*, edited by F. Homburger, J. A. Hayes, and E. W. Pelikan, pp. 294–325, Karger, Basel, Switzerland.
30. Christian, M. S. (1983a): Statement of Problem. In: *Advances in Modern Environmental Toxicology, Vol. 3: Assessment of Reproductive and Teratogenic Hazards*, edited by M. S. Christian, W. M. Galbraith, P. Voytek, and M. A. Mehlman, pp. 1–4. Princeton Scientific Publishers, Princeton, NJ.

31. Christian, M. S. (1983b): Postnatal alterations of gastrointestinal physiology, hematology, clinical chemistry, and other non-CNS parameters. In: *Handbook of Experimental Pharmacology: Teratogenesis and Reproductive Toxicology, Vol. 65*, edited by E. M. Johnson and D. M. Kochhar, pp. 263–286. Springer-Verlag, Berlin.
32. Christian, M. S. (1993): Problems in developmental toxicology caused by incorrectly used terminology. *J. Am. Coll. Toxicol.*, 12:323–328.
33. Christian, M. S., and Hoberman, A. M. (1996): Perspectives on the U.S., EEC and Japanese developmental toxicity guidelines, Chapter 18. In: *Handbook of Developmental Toxicology*, edited by R. D. Hood, pp. 551–596, CRC Press, Boca Raton, FL.
34. Christian, M. S., Hoberman, A. M., Bachmann, S., and Hellwig, J. (1998): Variability in the uterotrophic response assay (an in vivo estrogenic response assay) in untreated control and positive control (DES-DP, 2.5 μg/kg, bid) Wistar and Sprague-Dawley rats. *Drug and Chemical Toxicol.*, 21(Suppl. 1):51–100.
35. Chung, C. S., and Myrianthopoulos, N. C. (1975): Factors affecting risks of congenital malformations. In: *The National Foundation March of Dimes, Original Articles Series*, Vol. XI, No. 10; pp. 1–22.
36. Clarke, P. G. H. (1990): Developmental cell death: Morphological diversity and multiple mechanisms. *Anat. Embryol.*, 181:195–213.
37. Clark, R. L., Anderson, C. A., Prahalada, S., Robertson, R. T., Lochry, E. A., Leonard, Y. M., Stevens, J. L., and Hoberman, A. M. (1993): Critical developmental periods for effects on male rat genitalia induced by finasteride, a 5 α-reductase inhibitor. *Toxicol. Appl. Pharmacol.*, 119:34–40.
38. Collins, T. F. X. (1978): Reproduction and teratology guidelines: Review of deliberations by the National Toxicology Advisory Committee's Reproduction Panel. *J. Environ. Path. Toxicol.*, 2:141–147.
39. Collins, T. F. X., Sprando, R. L., Hansen, D. L., Schackelford, M. E., and Welsh, J. J. (1998): Testing guidelines for evaluation of reproductive and developmental toxicity of food additives in females. *International J. of Toxicol.*, 17:299–325.
40. Committee on the Safety of Medicines (CSM) (1974): *Notes for Guidance on Reproduction Studies*, Department of Health and Social Security, Great Britain.
41. Cooper, R. L., Goldman, J. M., and Vandenbergh, J. G. (1993): Monitoring of the estrous cycle in the laboratory rodent by vaginal lavage. In: *Methods In Toxicology, Volume 3B: Female Reproductive Toxicology*, edited by J. J. Heindel and R. E. Chapin, pp. 45–56. Academic Press, San Diego.
42. Crump, K. S. (1984): A new method for determining allowable daily intakes. *Fundam. Appl. Toxicol.*, 4:854–871.
43. Crump, K. S. (1995): Calculation of benchmark doses from continuous data. *Risk Analysis*, 15:79–89.
44. Culver, K. W. (1994): *Gene Therapy: A Handbook for Physicians*. Mary Ann Liebert Inc. Publishers, New York.
45. Cummings, A. M., and Perreault, S. D. (1990): Methoxychlor accelerates embryo transport through the rat reproductive tract. *Toxicology and Applied Pharmacol.*, 102:110–116.
46. Daston, G. P. (1994): Relationship between maternal and developmental toxicity. In: *Developmental Toxicology, 2nd edition*, edited by C. A. Kimmel and J. Buekle-Sam, pp. 189–212. Raven Press, New York.
47. DeSesso, J. M. (1997): Comparative Embryology. In: *Handbook of Developmental Toxicology*, edited by R. D. Hood, pp. 111–174. CRC Press, New York.
48. Dews, P. B. (1984): *Caffeine*. Springer-Verlag, Berlin.
49. Diczfalusy, E. (1964): Endocrine functions of the human feto-placental unit. *Fed. Proc.*, 23:791–798.
50. Donald, J. M., Monserrat, L. E., Hooper, K., Book, S. A., and Chernoff, G. F. (1991): Prioritizing candidate reproductive/developmental toxicants for evaluations. *Reprod. Toxicol.*, 5:99–108.
51. Edmonds, L., Hatch, M., Holmes, L., Kline, J., Letz, G., Levin, B., Miller, R., Shrout, P., Stein, Z., Warburton, D., Weinstock, M., Whorton, R. D., and Wyrobek, A. (1981): Report of panel II: Guidelines for reproductive studies in exposed human populations. In: *Guidelines for Studies of Human Populations Exposed to Mutagenic and Reproductive Hazards*, edited by A. D. Bloom, pp. 37–110. March of Dimes Birth Defects Foundations, White Plains, NY.
52. Ehrhardt, A. A., and Meyer-Bahlburg, H. F. L. (1981): Effects of prenatal sex hormones on gender-related behavior. *Science*, 211:1312–1318.
53. Elger, W., Beier, S., and Faehnrich, M. (1990): Interference with hormonal control of rodent reproduction and its implications for human risk assessment. In: *Proceedings of the Fifth International Congress of Toxicology*, edited by G. N. Valans, J. Sims, F. M. Sullivan, and P. Turner, pp. 445–456, Taylor & Francis, Philadelphia.
54. Erickson J. D. (1981): Epidemiology and developmental toxicology. In: *Developmental Toxicology*, edited by C. A. Kimmel and J. Buelke-Sam, pp. 289–301. Raven Press, New York.
55. Espey, L. L. (1978): Ovulation. In: *The Vertebrate Ovary*, edited by R. E. Jones, pp. 503–532. Plenum Press, New York.
56. European Economic Community (EEC), (1988): *The Rules Governing Medicinal Products in the European Community, Vol. III: Guidelines on the Quality, Safety and Efficacy of Medicinal Products for Human Use*. Office of Official Publications of the European Communities, Brussels.
57. European Economic Community (EEC) (1989): *Council decision on 28 July 1989 on the acceptance by the European Economic Community of an OECD decision/recommendation on compliance with principles of good laboratory practice*. Official Journal of the European Communities: Legislation, 32 (No. L 315; 28 October):1–17.
58. Faustman, E. M., Ponce, R. A., Seeley, M. R., and Whittaker, S. G. (1997): Experimental approaches to evaluate mechanisms of developmental toxicity. In: *Handbook of Developmental Toxicology*, edited by R. D. Hood, pp. 13–41. CRC Press, New York.
59. Favrot, M., Coll, J.-L., Louis, N., and Negoescu, A. (1998): Cell death and cancer: Replacement of apoptotic genes and inactivation of death suppressor genes in therapy. *Gene Therapy*, 5:728–739.
60. Feussner, E. L., Lightkep, G. E., Hennesy, R. A., Hoberman, A. M., and Christian, M. S. (1992): A decade of rabbit fertility data: Study of historical control animals. *Teratology*, 46:349–365.
61. Francis, B. M., Metcalf, R. L., Lewis, P. A., and Chernoff, N. (1999): Maternal and developmental toxicity of halogenated 4′-nitrodiphenyl ethers in mice. *Teratology*, 59:69–80.
62. Fraser, F. C. (1976): The multifactorial/threshold concept: Uses and misuses. *Teratology*, 14:267–280.
63. Fritz, M. A., and Fitz, T. A. (1991): The functional microscopic anatomy of the corpus luteum: The "small cell"—"large cell" controversy. *Clin. Obstet. Gynecol.*, 34:144—156.
64. Fujii, T., and Adams, P. M. (1987): *Functional teratogenesis: Functional effects on the offspring after parental drug exposure*. Teikyo University Press, Tokyo.
65. Gandelman, R. (1983): Gonadal hormones and sensory function. *Neurosci. & Behav. Rev.*, 7:1—17.
66. Garside, D. A., Charlton, A., and Heath, K. J. (1996): Establishing the timing of implantation in the Harlan Porcellus Dutch and New Zealand White Rabbit and the Han Wistar Rat. *Regul. Toxicol. and Pharmacol.*, 23:69–73.

67. Gelineau-Van Waes, J., Bennett, G. D., and Finnell, R. H. (1999): Phenytoin-induced alterations in craniofacial gene expression. *Teratology*, 59:23–34.

68. Generoso, W. M. (1980): Repair in fertilized eggs of mice and its role in the production of chromosomal aberrations. In: *DNA Repair and Mutagenesis in Eukaryotes*, edited by W. M. Generoso, M. S. Shelby, and F. J. De Serres, pp. 389–410. Plenum Press, New York.

69. George, J. D., Fail, P. A., Grizzle, T. B., Heindel, J. J., and Chapin, R. E. (1990): Mixed chemicals (MIX): Reproduction and fertility assessment in Swiss (CD-1) mice when administered in the drinking water: Final study report. (NTIS Publication PB91-158444).

70. Glücksman, A. (1951): Cell deaths in normal vertebrate ontogeny. *Biol. Rev. of the Cambridge Philos. Soc.*, 26:59–86.

71. Gondos, B. (1978): Oogonia and oocytes in mammals. In: The *Vertebrate Ovary*, edited by R. E. Jones, pp. 83–120. Plenum Press, New York.

72. Graham, A., Koentges, G., and Lumsden, A. (1996): A review: Neural crest apoptosis and the establishment of craniofacial pattern: An honorable death. *Molecular and Cellular Neuroscience*, 8:76–83.

73. Gregg, N. M. (1941): Congenital cataract following German measles in the mother. *Trans. Ophthalmol. Soc. Aust.*, pp. 3–35.

74. Gulati, D. K., Barnes, L. H., Chapin, R. E., and Heindel, J. (1991): Final report on the reproductive toxicity of a complex mixture of groundwater contaminants in Sprague-Dawley rats. (NTIS Publication PB91-184739).

75. Haanen, C., and Vermes, I. (1996): Apoptosis: Programmed cell death in fetal development. *European J. of Obstetrics and Gynecology and Reproductive Biology*, 64:129–133.

76. Hale, F. (1933): Pigs born without eyeballs, *J. Heredity*, 24:105.

77. Hale, F. (1935): The relation of vitamin A to anophthalmos in pigs. *Am. J. Ophthamol.*, 18:1087.

78. Hall, J. G. (1990): Genetic imprinting: Review and relevance to human diseases. *Ann. Hum. Genet.*, 46:857–873.

79. Haney, A. F. (1985): Effects of toxic agents on ovarian function. In: *Endocrine Toxicology*, edited by J. A. Thomas, K. S. Korach, and J. M. McLachlin, pp. 181–210. Raven Press, New York.

80. Hardin, B. D. (1987): Evaluation of the Chernoff/Kavlock test for developmental toxicity. *Teratogen. Carcinogen. Mutagen.*, 7:1–127.

81. Heindel, J. J., Thomford, P. J., and Mattison, D. R. (1989): Histological assessment of ovarian follicle number in mice as a screen for ovarian toxicity. In: *Growth Factors and the Ovary*, edited by A. N. Hirshfield, pp. 421–425. Plenum Press, New York.

82. Heindel, J. J., George, J. D., and Fail, P. A. (1990): Final report on the reproductive toxicity of a chemical mixture in CD-1 Swiss mice. Laboratory Supplement Volume 2., DEHP. (NTIS Publication PB91-158451).

83. Heinonen, O. P., Slone, D., and Shapiro, S. (1977): *Birth Defects and Drugs in Pregnancy*, pp. 127, 450. PSG, Littleton, MA.

84. Henderson, B. E., Ross, R. K., Judd, H. L., Krailok, M. D., and Pike, M. C. (1985): Do regular ovulatory cycles increase breast cancer risk? *Cancer*, 56:1206–1208.

85. Herbst, A. L., Ulfelder, H., and Poskanzer, D. C. (1971): Adenocarcinoma of the vagina: Association of maternal stilbestrol therapy with tumor appearance in young women. *New Eng. J. Med.*, (15). 284/878–81.

86. Hertig, A. T. (1967): The overall problem in man. In: *Comparative Aspects of Reproductive Failure*, edited by K. Benirschke, pp. 11–41. Springer-Verlag, Berlin.

87. Hoar, R. M., and Salem, A. J. (1961): Time of teratogenic action of trypan blue in guinea pigs. *Anat. Rec.*, 141:173–182.

88. Hoar, R. M. (1969): Resorption in guinea pigs as estimated by counting corpora lutea: The problem of twinning. *Teratology*, 2:187–190.

89. Hood, R. D., and Miller, D. B. (1997): Maternally mediated effects on development. In: *Handbook of Developmental Toxicology*, edited by R. Hood, pp. 61–90. CRC Press, Boca Raton, FL.

90. Hull, D., Dobbing, J., Miller, R. W., Naftolin, F., Ounsted, M. D., Rehder, H., Robinson, J. S., Tuge, C., and Usher, R. H. (1978): Definition, epidemiology, identification of abnormal fetal growth: Group report. In: *Abnormal Fetal Growth: Biological Bases and Consequences*, edited by F. Naftolin, pp. 69–83. Dahlem Konferenzen, Berlin.

91. Hurle, J. M., Ros, M. A., Garcia-Martinez, V., Macias, D., and Gañan, Y. (1995): Cell death in the embryonic developing limb. *Scanning Microscopy*, 9:519–534.

92. Inouye, M. (1976): Differential staining of cartilage and bone in fetal mouse skeleton by alcian blue and alizarin red S. *Cong. Anom.*, 16:171–173.

93. International Conference on Harmonisation (ICH) Harmonised Tripartite guideline (1993): *Detection of Toxicity to Reproduction for Medicinal Products* (Proposed Rule Endorsed by the ICH Steering Committee at Step 4 of the ICH Process, 24 June 1993). In: *Proceedings of the Second International Conference on Harmonization, Orlando, Florida*, edited by P. F. D'Arcy and D. W. G. Harron, pp. 557–586. IFPMA, 1994, Greystone Books, Ltd., Antrim, N. Ireland.

94. International Conference on Harmonisation (ICH) Harmonised Tripartite guideline (1995): *Male Fertility Studies in Reproductive Toxicology*. In: *Proceedings of the Third International Conference on Harmonization*, edited by P. F. D'Arcy and D. W. G. Harron, pp. 245–252. IFPMA, 1996, Greystone Books, Ltd., Antrim, N. Ireland.

95. Jackson, C. M. (1925): *Effects of Inanition and Malnutrition Upon Growth and Structure*. P. Blakiston's Son & Co., Philadelphia.

96. Jacobson, M. D., Weil, M., and Roff, M. C. (1997): Programmed cell death in animal development. *Cell Press*, 88:347–354.

97. Jaffe, R. B. (1981): *Prolactin*. Elsevier, New York.

98. Joffe, M. (1985): Biases in research on reproduction and women's work. *Int. J. Epidemiol.*, 4:118–123.

99. Johnson, E. M. (1964): A histologic study of postnatal vitamin B_{12} deficiency in the rat. *Am. J. Path.*, 44:73–83.

100. Johnson, E. M., and Armenti, V. T. (1978): Postnatal effects of prenatal insult on lung development in the rat. *Anat. Rec.*, 190:432–433.

101. Johnson, E. M., and Christian, M. S. (1984): When is a teratology study not an evaluation of teratogenicity? *J. Am. Coll. Toxicol.*, 3:431.

102. Johnson, E. M. (1986): The scientific basis for multigeneration safety evaluation. *J. Am. Coll. Toxicol.*, 5:197–201.

103. Karnofsky, D. A. (1965): Mechanism of action of certain growth-inhibiting drugs. In: *Teratology Principles and Techniques*, edited by J. G. Wilson and J. Warkany, pp. 185–194. University of Chicago Press, Chicago.

104. Kalter, H. (1968): *Teratology of the Central Nervous System*. University of Chicago Press, Chicago.

105. Kavlock, R. J., and Grabowski, C. T. (1983): *Abnormal Functional Development of the Heart, Lungs, and Kidneys: Approaches to Functional Teratology: Proceedings of a Conference held in Asheville, North Carolina*, May 11–13, 1983. Alan R. Liss, New York.

106. Khera, K. S. (1984): Maternal toxicity: A possible factor in fetal malformations in mice. *Teratology*, 29:411–416.

107. Khera, K. S. (1985): Maternal toxicity: A possible etiologic factor in embryo-fetal deaths and fetal malformations in rodent-rabbit species. *Teratology*, 31:129–153.

108. Kimmel, C. A. (1981): A profile of developmental toxicity. In: *Developmental Toxicology*, edited by C. A. Kimmel and J. Buelke-Sam, pp. 321–331. Raven Press, New York.
109. Kimmel, C. A. (1990): Quantitative approaches to human risk assessment for noncancer health effects. *Neurotoxicology*, 11:189–198.
110. Klinefelter, G., and Gray, L. E., Jr. (1993): The clinical relevance of animal models: Animal studies that assess the potential for drugs and environmental agents to cause reproductive disorders in humans. In: *Reproductive Toxicology and Infertility*, edited by A. R. Scialli and M. J. Zinaman, pp. 219–282. McGraw-Hill, New York.
111. Knight, D. C., and Eden, J. A. (1995): Phytoestrogens: A short review. *Maturitas*, 22:167–175.
112. Knight, D. C., and Eden, J. A. (1996): A review of clinical effects of phytoestrogens. *Obstet. Gynecol.*, 87:897–904.
113. Knudsen, T. B., and Wubah, J. A. (1998): Transgenic animal models: Functional analysis of developmental toxicity as illustrated with the p53 suppresor model. In: *Handbook of Developmental Neurotoxicology*, edited by W. Slikker, Jr., and L. W. Chang, pp. 209–221. Academic Press, New York.
114. Koebbe, M. J., Golden, J. A., Bennett, G., and Finnell, R. H. (1999): Effects of prenatal cocaine exposure on embryonic expression of *Sonic Hedgehog. Teratology*, 59:12–19.
115. Koos, B. J., and Longo, L. (1976): Mercury toxicity in pregnant women, fetus and newborn infant. *Am. J. Obstet. Gynecol*, 3:390–409.
116. Lamb, J. C. (1985): Reproductive toxicity testing: Evaluating and developing new systems. *J. Am. Coll. Toxicol.*, 4:163–171.
117. Lang, P. L. (1988): Embryo and Fetal Developmental Toxicity (Teratology) Control Data in the Charles River Crl : CD7BR Rat. Charles River Laboratories, Inc., Wilmington, MA 01887-0630. (Data base provided by Argus Research Laboratories, Inc.).
118. Lang, P. L. (1993a): Historical control data for development and reproductive toxicity studies using the New Zealand white rabbit. Compiled by MARTA (Middle Atlantic Reproduction and Teratology Association). Charles River Laboratories, Inc., Wilmington, MA 01887-0630. (Data base provided by Argus Research Laboratories, Inc.).
119. Lang, P. L. (1993b): Historical control data for development and reproductive toxicity studies using the Charles River Crl : CD7BR Rat. Compiled by MARTA (Middle Atlantic Reproduction and Teratology Association). Charles River Laboratories, Inc., Wilmington, MA 01887-0630. (Data base provided by Argus Research Laboratories, Inc.).
120. Leavitt, W. W. (1995): The female reproductive system during pregnancy, parturition, and lactation. In: *Reproductive Toxicology, 2nd edition*, edited by R. J. Witorsch, pp. 45–72. Raven Press, New York.
121. Lemasters, G. K., and Pinney, S. M. (1989): Employment status as a confounder when assessing occupational exposures and spontaneous abortion. *J. Clin. Epidemiol.*, 42:975–981.
122. Lenz, W. (1961): Kindliche micebildungen nach medikament wahrend der draviditat? *Deutsch. Med. Wochenschr.*, 86:2555.
123. McBride, W. G. (1961): Thalidomide and congenital abnormalities. *Lancet*, 2:1358.
124. McLaughlin, J. A. (1977): Prenatal exposure to diethylstilbestrol in mice: Toxicological studies. *J. Toxicol. Environ. Health*, 2:527–537.
125. McNeilly, A. S. (1988): Suckling and the control of gonadotropin secretion. In: *The Physiology of Reproduction, Vol. 2.*, edited by E. Knobil and J. D. Neill, pp. 2323–2349. Raven Press, New York.
126. Manson, J. M., and Kang, Y. J. (1994): Test methods for assessing female reproductive and developmental toxicology. In: *Principles and Methods of Toxicology, 3rd edition*, edited by A. W. Hayes, pp. 989–1037. Raven Press, New York.
127. Marr, M. C., Myers, C. B., George, J. D., and Price, C. J. (1988): Comparison of single and double staining for evaluation of skeletal development: The effects of ethylene glycol (EG) in CD rats. *Teratology*, 37:476.
128. Marr, M. C., Price, C. J., Myers, C. B., and Morrissey, E. (1992): Developmental states of the CD®(Sprague-Dawley) rat skeleton after maternal exposure to ethylene glycol. *Teratology*, 46:169–181.
129. Mattison, D. R., and Ross, G. T. (1983): Laboratory methods for evaluating and predicting specific reproductive dysfunctions: Oogenesis and ovulation. In: *Methods for Assessing the Effects of Chemicals on Reproductive Functions*, edited by V. B. Vouk and P. J. Sheehan, pp. 217–246. Wiley, New York.
130. Mattison, D. R., Kochar, D. M., and Rao, K. S. (1989): Criteria for identifying and listing substances shown to cause developmental toxicity under California's Proposition 65. *Reprod. Toxicol.*, 3:3–12.
131. Mattison, D. R., Plowchalk, D. R., Meadows, M. J., Al-Juburi, A. Z., Gandy, J., and Malek, A. (1990): Reproductive toxicity: Male and female reproductive systems as targets for chemical injury. *Med. Clin. North Am.*, 74:391–411.
132. Mattison, D. R., Working, P. K., Blazak, W. F., Hughes, C. L., Jr., Killinger, J. M., Olive, D. L., Rao, K. S., Hanson, J. W., and Kochar, D. M. (1991): Reply to: When scientists become policy makers: Shaping hazard identification under Proposition 65. *Reprod. Toxicol.*, 5:175–178.
133. Mattison, D. R. (1992): Protecting reproductive and developmental health under Proposition 65: Public health approaches to knowledge, imperfect knowledge, and the absence of knowledge. *Reprod. Toxicol.*, 6:1–7.
134. Mazarakis, N. D., Edwards, A. D., and Mehmet, H. (1997): Apoptosis in neural development and disease. *Archives of Disease in Childhood*, 77:F165–F170.
135. Mermelstein, R., Morrow, P. E., and Christian, M. S. (1994): Letter to the Editor: Organ or system overload and its regulatory implications. *J. Amer. Col. Tox.*, 13:143–147.
136. Meyer-Bahlburg, H. F. L., Ehrhardt, A. A., Feldman, J. F., Rosen, L. R., Veridiano, N. P., and Zimmerman, I. (1985): Sexual activity level and sexual functioning in women prenatally exposed to diethylstilbestrol. *Psychosom. Med.*, 47:497–511.
137. Midwest Teratology Association Historical Control Project: External and visceral malformations: 1988–1992. Sprague-Dawley CD® Rats, New Zealand White Rabbits (April, 1994).
138. Middleton, M. C., Milne, C. M., Moreland, D., and Hasmall, R. L. (1986): Ovulation in rats is delayed by a substituted triazole. *Toxicol. Appl. Pharmacol.*, 83:230–239.
139. Milligan, C. E., and Schwartz, L. M. (1997): Programmed cell death during animal development. *British Medical Bulletin*, 52:570–590.
140. Milne, C. M., Hasmall, R. L., Russell, A., Watson, S. C., Vaughan, Z., and Middleton, M. C. (1987): Reduced estradiol production by a substituted triazole results in delayed ovulation in rats. *Toxicol. Appl. Pharmacol.*, 90:426–435.
141. Ministry of Health and Welfare, Japan (MHW) (1975): *On Animal Experimental Methods for Testing the Effects of Drugs on Reproduction.* Notification No. 529 of the Pharmaceutical Affairs Bureau, Ministry of Health and Welfare, March 31, 1975.
142. Ministry of Health and Welfare, Japan (MHW) (1984): *Information on the Guidelines of Toxicity Studies Required for Applications for Approval to Manufacture (Import) Drugs.* Notification No. 118 of the Pharmaceutical Affairs Bureau, Ministry of Health and Welfare, February 15, 1984.

143. Moore, N. W., Adams, C. E., and Rowson, L. E. A. (1968): Developmental potential of single blastomeres of the rabbit egg. *J. Reprod. Fertil.*, 17:527–531.

144. Morrissey, R. E., Lamb, J. C., 4th, Morris, R.W., Chapin, R. E., Gulati, D. K., and Heindel, J. J. (1989): Results and evaluation of 48 continuous breeding reproduction studies conducted in mice. *Fund. Appl. Toxicol.*, 13:747–777.

145. Mosher, W. E. (1985): Reproductive impairments in the United States, 1965–1982. *Demography*, 22:415–430.

146. Mukherjee, A. B., Chan, M., Waite, R., Metzger, M. I., and Yaffee, S. J. (1975): Inhibition of RNA synthesis by acetyl salicylate and actinomycin-D during early development in the mouse. *Pediat. Res.*, 9:652–657.

147. Narayanan, V. (1997): Apoptosis in development and disease of the nervous system. 1: Naturally occurring cell death in the developing nervous system. *Pediatr. Neurol.*, 16:9–13.

148. Narotsky, M. G., Weller, E. A., Chinchilli, V. M., and Kavlock, R. J. (1995): Nonadditive developmental toxicity in mixtures of trichloroethylene, Di(2-ethylhexyl) phthalate, and heptachlor in a 5 × 5 × 5 design. *Fund. Appl. Toxicol.*, 27:203–216.

149. Nakatsuka, T., Horimoto, M., Ito, M., Matsubara, Y., Akaike, M., and Ariyuki, F. (1997): Japan Pharmaceutical Manufacturers Association (JMPA) survey on background control data of developmental and reproductive toxicity studies in rats, rabbits and mice. *Cong. Anom.*, 37:47–138.

150. Naruse, I., and Keino, H. (1995): Apoptosis in the developing CNS. *Progress in Neurobiology*, 47:135–155.

151. National Center for Health Statistics (NCHS) (1980): *Births, Marriages, Divorces and Deaths for 1979. Monthly Vital Statistics Report*. U.S. Department of Health, Education, and Welfare, Washington, DC.

152. National Research Council (1985): Toxicity testing: Strategies to determine needs and priorities. National Academy Press, Washington, DC.

153. Neubert, D., Barrach, H. J., and Merker, H. J. (1980): Drug-induced damage to the embryo or fetus: Molecular and multilateral approach to prenatal toxicology. *Curr. Top. Pathol.*, 69:241–331.

154. Newman, L. M., and Johnson, E. M. (1986): Teratogen-induced decrements of postnatal functional capacity. *J. Amer. Col. Tox.*, 5:517–524.

155. Niswander, K. R., and Gordon, M. (1972): *The Women and Their Pregnancies: The Collaborative Perinatal Study of the National Institute of Neurological Diseases and Stroke*. W. B. Saunders, Philadelphia (originally DHEW Publication No. (NIH) 73-379).

156. Numan, M. (1988): Maternal behavior. In: *The Physiology of Reproduction*, edited by E. Knobil and J. Neill, pp. 1569–1645. Raven Press, New York.

157. O'Connor, J. C., Cook, J. C., Craven, S. C., VanPelt, C. S., and Obourn, J. D. (1996): An in vivo battery for identifying endocrine modulators that are estorgenic or dopamine regulators. *Fund. Appl. Toxicol.*, 33:182–195.

158. Odum, J., Lefevre, P. A., Tittensor, S., Paton, D., Routledge, E. J., Beresfor, N. A., Sumpter, J. P., and Ashby, J. (1997): The rodent uterotrophic assay: Critical protocol features, studies with nonyl phenols, and comparison with a yeast estrogenicity assay. *Regulatory Toxicol. and Pharmacol.*, 25:176–188.

159. Organization for Economic Cooperation and Development (OECD) (1981): *Guidelines for Testing of Chemicals*. Section 4, No. 414: *Teratogenicity*, adopted 12 May 1981.

160. Organization for Economic Cooperation and Development (OECD) (1983a): *OECD Guidelines for Testing of Chemicals*. Section 4, No. 415: One-Generation Reproduction Toxicity, adopted 26 May 1983.

161. Organization for Economic Cooperation and Development (OECD) (1983b): *OECD Guidelines for Testing of Chemicals*. Section 4, No. 416: Two-Generation Reproduction Toxicity Study, adopted 26 May 1983.

162. Organization for Economic Cooperation and Development (OECD) (1995): *OECD Guidelines for Testing of Chemicals*. Section 4, No. 421: Reproduction/Developmental Toxicity Screening Test, adopted 27 July 1995.

163. Organization for Economic Cooperation and Development (OECD) (1996): *OECD Guidelines for Testing of Chemicals*. Section 4, No. 422: Combined Repeated Dose Toxicity Study with the Reproduction/Developmental Toxicity Screening Test, adopted 22 March 1996.

164. Organization for Economic Cooperation and Development (OECD) (1998): The Revised OECD Principles of Good Laboratory Practices [C(97) 186/Final].

165. Palmer, A. K., and Ulbrich, B. C. (1997): The cult of culling. *Fund. Appl. Toxicol.*, 38:7–22.

166. Pan, H., Yin, C., and Van Dyke, T. (1997): Apoptosis and cancer mechanisms. *Cancer Surveys*, 29:305–327.

167. Pederson, T., and Peters, H. (1968): Proposal for a classification of oocytes and follicles in the mouse ovary. *J. Reprod. Fertil.*, 17:555–557.

168. Peters, P. W. J. (1977): Double staining of fetal skeletons for cartilage and bone. In: *Methods in Prenatal Toxicology*, edited by D. Neubert, H. J. Merker, and T. E. Kwasigroch, pp. 153–154. Georg Thieme Publishing, Stuttgart.

169. Pfaff, D. W., and Schwartz-Giblin, S. (1988): Cellular mechanisms of female reproductive behaviors. In: *The Physiology of Reproduction*, edited by E. Knobil and J. Neill, pp. 1987–1568. Raven Press, New York.

170. Plowchalk, D. R., and Mattison, D. R. (1991): Phosphoramide mustard is responsible for the ovarian toxicity of cyclophosphamide. *Toxicol. Appl. Pharmacol.*, 107:472–481.

171. Plowchalk, D. R., Smith, B. J., and Mattison, D. R. (1993): Assessment of toxicity to the ovary using follicle quantitation and morphometrics. In: *Methods In Toxicology, Volume 3B: Female Reproductive Toxicology*, edited by J. J. Heindel and R. E. Chapin, pp. 57–68. Academic Press, San Diego.

172. Pharmaceutical Manufacturers Association (PMA) (1981): *PMA Guidelines: Reproduction, teratology and pediatrics*. Contributors: Christian, M., Diener, R., Hoar, R., and Staples, R.

173. Reel, J. R., Lamb, J. C., IV, and Neal, B. H. (1996): Survey and assessment of mammalian estrogen biological assays for hazard characterization. *Fund. Appl. Toxicol.*, 34:288–305.

174. Richards, J. S. (1980): Maturation of ovarian follicles. *Physiol. Ref.*, 60:51–89.

175. Richards, J. S., and Bogvich, K. (1980): Development of gonado-tropin receptors during follicular growth. In: *Functional Correlates of Hormone Receptors in Reproduction*, edited by Maresh, Muldoon, Saxena, and Sadler, pp. 223–244. Elsevier/North Holland, Amsterdam.

176. Ritter, E. J., Scott, W. J., Jr., Randall, J. L., and Ritter, J. M. (1987): Teratogenicity of di(2-ethylhexyl)phthalate, 2-ethylhexanol, 2-ethylhexanoic acid, and valproic acid, and potentiation by caffeine. *Teratology*, 35:41–46.

177. Rogers, J. M., Barbee, B. D., and Rehnberg, B. F. (1993): Critical periods of sensitivity for the developmental toxicity of inhaled methanol. *Teratology*, 47:395A.

178. Rogers, J. M., and Kavlock, R. J. (1996): Developmental toxicology. In: *Casarett and Doull's Toxicology: The Basic Science of Poisons, 5th edition*, edited by C. D. Klassen, pp. 301–331. McGraw-Hill Health Professions Division, New York.

179. Salewski, E. (1964): Färbemethode zum makroskopischen Nachweis von Implantationsstellen am Uterus der Ratte. *Arch. Pathol. Exp. Pharmakol.*, 247:367.

180. Sanders, S. A., and Reinisch, J. M. (1985): Behavioral effects on humans of progesterone-related compounds during development and in the adult. In: *Current Topics in Neuroendocrinology: Actions of Progesterone on the Brain, Vol. 5*, edited by D. Ganten and D. Pfaff, pp. 175–205. Springer-Verlag, Berlin, Heidelberg.

181. Sandler, M., (1985): *Mental Illness in Pregnancy and the Puerperium*. Oxford University Press, New York.

182. Sauders, J. W., Jr. (1966): Death in embryonic systems. *Science*, 154:604-612.

183. Schardein, J. L. (1992): *Chemically Induced Birth Defects, 2nd Edition*, Marcel Dekker, New York.

184. Schmidt, R. R. (1984): Altered development of immunocompetence following prenatal or combined prenatal-postnatal insult: A timely review. *J. Amer. Col. Tox.*, 3:57-72.

185. Schmidt, R. R., and Johnson, E. M. (1997): Principles of teratology. In: *Handbook of Developmental Toxicology*, edited by R. D. Hood, pp. 3–12. CRC Press, New York.

186. Shenefelt, R. E. (1972): Morphogenesis of malformations in hamsters caused by retinoic acid: Relation to dose and stage at treatment. *Teratology*, 5:103–118.

187. Shepard, T. H. (1995): *Catalog of Teratogenic Agents, 8th edition*. John Hopkins University Press, Baltimore.

188. Shield, M. A., and Mirkes, P. E. (1998): Apoptosis. In: *Handbook of Developmental Neurotoxicology*, edited by W. Slikker, Jr., and L. W. Chang, pp. 159–188. Academic Press, New York.

189. Shuler, C. F. (1995): Programmed cell death and cell transformation in craniofacial development. *Crit. Rev. Oral Biol. Med.*, 6:202–217.

190. Siiteri, P. K. (1966). Placental endocrine biosynthesis during human pregnancy. *J. Clin. Endocrinol.*, 26:751–761.

191. Simpson, J. L. (1980): Genes, chromosomes and reproductive failure. *Fertil. Steril.*, 33:107-116.

192. Smith, B. J., Mattison, D. R., and Sipes, I. G. (1990): The role of epoxidation in 4-vinylcyclohexene-induced ovarian toxicity. *Toxicol. Appl. Pharmacol.*, 105:372-381.

193. Smith, B. J., Plowchalk, D. R., Sipes, I. G., and Mattison, D. R. (1991): Comparison of random and serial sections in assessment of ovarian toxicity. *Reproductive Toxicology*, 5:379–383.

194. Smith, C. A. (1947): Effects of maternal undernutrition upon the newborn infant in Holland (1944–1945). *J. Pediatr.*, 30:229.

195. Smith, R. (1999): The timing of birth. *Scientific American*, 280(3) 68–75.

196. Snow, M. H. L., and Tam, P. P. L. (1979): Is compensatory growth a complicating factor in mouse teratology? *Nature*, 279:555–557.

197. Soloff, M. S. (1989): Endocrine control of parturition. In: *Biology of the Uterus, 2nd edition*, edited by R. M. Wynn and W. P. Jollie, pp. 559–607. Plenum Press, New York.

198. Speroff, L., Glass, R. H., and Kase, N. G. (1983): Investigation of the infertile couple. In: *Clinical Gynecologic Endocrinology and Infertility, 3rd edition*, pp. 467–492. Williams and Wilkins, Baltimore.

199. Spielmann, H. (1987). Analysis of embryotoxic effects in preimplantation embryos. In: *The Mammalian Preimplantation Embryo*, edited by B. D. Bavister, pp. 309–331. Plenum Press, New York.

200. Staples, R. E., and Schnell, V. L. (1964): Refinement in rapid clearing technic in the KOH-alizarin red s method for fetal bone. *Stain Technol.*, 29:61–63.

201. Staples, R. E. (1974): Detection of visceral alterations in mammalian fetuses. *Teratology*, 9:A37-A38.

202. Staples, R. E. (1993): Staples technique for evaluation of fetal soft tissue. Course presented for Center for Professional Advancement, New Brunsick, NJ, May 12–14.

203. Stuckhardt, J. L., and Poppe, S. M. (1984): Fresh visceral examination of rat and rabbit fetuses used in teratogenicity testing. *Teratogen, Carcinogen and Mutagen.*, 4:181.

204. Talamantes, F., and Ogren, L. (1988): The placenta as an endocrine organ: Polypeptides. In: *The Physiology of Reproduction, Vol. 2*, edited by E. Knobil, and J. D. Neill, pp. 2093–2144. Raven Press, New York.

205. Tanimura, T., Kameyama, Y., Shiota, K., Tanaka, S., Matsumoto, N., and Mizutani, M. (1989): Report on the review of the guidelines for studies of the effect of drugs on reproduction. Notification No. 118, Pharmaceutical Affairs Bureau, Ministry of Health and Welfare, Japan.

206. Thomas, J. (1996): Toxic responses of the reproductive system. In: *Casarett and Doull's Toxicology: The Basic Science of Poisons, 5th edition*, edited by C. D. Klaassen, pp. 547–581. McGraw-Hill, New York.

207. Treolar, A. E., Boynton, R. E., Behn, B. G., and Brown, B. W. (1967): Variation of the human menstrual cycle through reproductive life. *Int. J. of Fert.*, 12:77–126.

208. Tucker, H. A. (1988): Lactation and its hormonal control. In: *The Physiology of Reproduction, Vol. 2.*, edited by E. Knobil and J. D. Neill, pp. 2235–2263. Raven Press, New York.

209. Tyl, R. W., and Marr, M. C. (1996): Developmental toxicity testing: Methodology. In: *Handbook of Developmental Toxicology*, edited by R. Hood, pp. 175–225. CRC Press, New York.

210. U.S. Environmental Protection Agency: Federal Insecticide, Fungicide and Rodenticide Act (FIFRA); Good Laboratory Practice Standards; Final Rule. 40 CFR Part 160.

211. U.S. Environmental Protection Agency: Toxic Substances Control Act (TSCA); Good Laboratory Practice Standards; Final Rule. 40 CFR Part 792.

212. U.S. Environmental Protection Agency (EPA—Risk Assessment Forum) (1991): Guidelines for Developmental Toxicity Risk Assessment, Dec. 5, 1991. 56FR63798-63826.

213. U.S. Environmental Protection Agency (EPA) (1996): Guidelines for Reproductive Toxicity Risk Assessment, September, 1996, NTIS PB No. PB97-100098.

214. U.S. Environmental Protection Agency (EPA-FIFRA) (1985): *Hazard Evaluation Division Standard Evaluation Procedure*: Teratology Studies. Office of Pesticide Programs, Washington, DC, EPA-540/9-85-018.

215. U.S. Environmental Protection Agency (EPA-FIFRA) (1991): Pesticide Assessment Guideline. Subdivision F—Hazard Evaluation: Human and Domestic Animals, Addendum 10, Neurotoxicity, Health Effects Division, Office of Pesticide Programs.

216. U.S. Environmental Protection Agency (EPA-FIFRA) (1993): Health Effects Division Draft Standard Evaluation Procedure, Developmental Toxicity Studies, Office of Pesticide Programs, Washington, DC.

217. U.S. Environmental Protection Agency (EPA, OPPTS) (1998a): Health Effects Test Guidelines: Prenatal Developmental Toxicity Study. Office of Prevention, Pesticides and Toxic Substances (OPPTS) 870.3700, August, 1998.

218. U.S. Environmental Protection Agency (EPA, OPPTS) (1998b): Health Effects Test Guidelines: Reproduction and Fertility Effects. Office of Prevention, Pesticides and Toxic Substances (OPPTS) 870.3800, August, 1998.

219. U.S. Environmental Protection Agency (EPA, OPPTS) (1998c). Health Effects Test Guidelines: Developmental Neurotoxicity

Study. Office of Prevention, Pesticides and Toxic Substances (OPPTS) 870.6300, August, 1998.

220. U.S. Environmental Protection Agency (EPA-TSCA) (1985a): Subpart E—Specific Organ/Tissue Toxicity, No. 798.4900: Developmental Toxicity Study. 40 CFR Part 798—Toxic Substances Control Act Test Guidelines; Final Rules. 50FR39433-39434.
221. U.S. Environmental Protection Agency (EPA-TSCA) (1985b): Subpart E—Specific Organ/Tissue Toxicity, No. 798.4700: Reproduction and Fertility Effects. 40 CFR Part 798—Toxic Substances Control Act Test Guidelines; Final Rules. *Fed. Regist.*, 50:39432–39433.
222. U.S. Environmental Protection Agency (EPA-TSCA) (1997): Toxic Substances Control Act Test Guidelines (TSCA); [OPPTS-42193: FRL-5719-5]; Final Rule. 40 CFR Part 799.
223. U.S. Food and Drug Administration: Good Laboratory Practice Regulations; Final Rule. 21 CFR Part 58.
224. U.S. Food and Drug Administration (FDA) (1966): *Guidelines for Reproduction Studies for Safety Evaluation of Drugs for Human Use*.
225. U.S. Food and Drug Administration (FDA) (1982): Toxicological Principles and Procedures for Priority Based Assessment of Food Additives (Red Book), Guidelines for Reproduction Testing with a Teratology Phase. Bureau of Foods, U.S. Food and Drug Administration, Washington, DC, 1982, pp. 80–117.
226. U.S. Food and Drug Administration (FDA) (1993, 2000): Draft: Toxicological Principles for the Safety Assessment of Direct Food Additives and Color Additives Used in Food (Red Book II). Guidelines for Reproduction and Developmental Toxicity Studies, Center for Food Safety and Applied Nutrition, U.S. Food and Drug Administration, Washington, DC, 1993, pp. 123–134. Toxicological Principles for the Safety of Food Ingredients (Redbook 2000): Sections issued electronically July 7, 2000 at http:// vm.cfsan.fda.gov/ ~Redbook/Red-tcct.html.
227. U.S. Food and Drug Administration (FDA) (1994): International Conference on Harmonisation; Guideline on detection of toxicity to reproduction for medicinal products. *Federal Register*, Vol. 59, No. 183.
228. U.S. Food and Drug Administration (FDA) (1996): International Conference on Harmonisation; Guideline on detection of toxicity to reproduction for medicinal products; Addendum on Toxicity to male fertility. *Federal Register*, Vol. 60, No. 161.
229. U.S. Food and Drug Administration (FDA) (1996): Food Quality Protection Act (FQPA): Public Law 104-170, August 3, 1996.
230. Vermes, I., and Haanen, C. (1994): Apoptosis in programmed cell death in health and disease. *Advances in Clinical Chemistry*, 31:177–246.
231. Warkany, J., and Nelson, R. C. (1940): Appearance of skeletal abnormalities in the offspring of rats reared on a deficient diet. *Science*, 92:383.
232. Warkany, J., and Nelson, R. C. (1941): Skeletal abnormalities in offspring of rats reared on deficient diets. *Anat. Rec.*, 79: 83.
233. Warkany, J. (1965): Development of experimental mammalian teratology. In: *Teratology: Principles and Techniques*, edited by J. G. Wilson and J. Warkany, pp. 1–20. University of Chicago Press, Chicago.
234. Williams, B. O., Morgenbesser, S. D., DePinho, R. A., and Jacks, T. (1994): Tumorigenic and developmental effects of combined germ-line mutations in Rb and p53. *Gold Spring Harbor Symposia on Quantitative Biology*, 49:449–447.
235. Wilson, J. G., and Warkany, J. (1965): *Teratology: Principles and Techniques* (Lectures and demonstrations given at the First Workshop in Teratology, University of Florida, February 2–8, 1964). University of Chicago Press, Chicago.
236. Wilson, J. G. (1973): *Environment and Birth Defects*. Academic Press, New York.
237. Wilson, J. G., and Fraser, F. C. (1977): *Handbook of Teratology, Vol. 1–4*. Plenum Press, New York.
238. World Health Organization (1970): Spontaneous and induced abortion. *World Health Organization Technical Report Series*, Number 461, Geneva.
239. Young, W. C. (1961): The hormones and mating behavior. In: *Sex and Internal Secretions, 3rd edition, vol. 2*, edited by W. C. Young, pp. 1173–1239. Williams & Wilkins, Baltimore.
240. Zilva, S. S., Goulding, J., Brummond, J. C., and Coward, K. H. (1921): The relation of the fat-soluble factor to rickets and growth in pigs. *Biochem J.*, 15:427.

Principles and Methods of Toxicology, Fourth Edition, edited by A. Wallace Hayes.
Taylor & Francis, Philadelphia © 2001.

Chapter 30

Hormone Assays and Endocrine Function

Michael J. Thomas and John A. Thomas

Several drugs and chemicals can affect the endocrine system (61). The endocrine system can be defined as any glandular tissue or cells that release a hormone or chemical messenger to affect a target tissue or cells to produce a physiological response. Perturbation of endocrine homeostasis can produce consequences that can lead to metabolic derangements, developmental abnormalities, or reproductive dysfunction. Endocrine disruptor is a contemporary term to describe such effects.

Endocrine toxicology involves the study of chemicals and drugs that disrupt endocrine processes, leading to either augmentation or inhibition of a physiological response (64). In a broad sense, endocrine toxicology encompasses reproductive toxicology (72) (see chapters 28 and 29). In addition, endocrine toxicology can also include metabolic derangements that result from toxic injury to non-endocrine systems. For example, renal or hepatic toxicity may alter the rate of hormone catabolism.

This chapter reviews endocrine physiology and morphology, and evaluation of endocrine function as it relates to toxicology. Endocrine pharmacology involves the therapeutic and diagnostic use of hormones and other nonhormonally related agents. It can also encompass endocrine toxicology, as many of these medicinal products possess side effects that alter the biochemical activity of organs of internal secretion (58). Molecular biology continues to provide a number of techniques that are very useful in endocrinology (12).

While some endocrine organs appear to be more sensitive or vulnerable to toxicological agents than others, hormone–target organ interrelations often lead to the substance causing multiple disruptions in the hormonal balance of the organism. It is not uncommon to witness chemically induced changes in gonadal function along with alterations in thyroid gland activity. In some species, chemically induced changes in sex steroids can affect pancreatic secretion of insulin. Chemically induced stress leading to increased secretion of glucocorticoids can also affect insulin secretion, but more importantly it can affect adrenocorticotropin (ACTH) levels and hence alter the pituitary–adrenal axis.

The thalidomide tragedy of the 1960s led to the formulation of toxicological testing guidelines for the field of teratology. No such requirements have been invoked for the endocrine system. Pesticide-induced sterility (e.g., dibromochloropropane [DBCP]) has led to concern about the deleterious actions of such substances in both male and female reproductive systems. The inherent estrogenicity of *o*, *p*-DDT can affect the reproductive system, and concern has been expressed about the relation between diethylstilbestrol (DES) and the incidence of cervical cancer. Thus, numerous examples of chemical-induced changes in the endocrine system have been reported. Many of these agents represent reproductive hazards in the workplace. The endocrine system falls prey to many such agents. Polyhalogenated biphenyls, dibenzodioxins, and dibenzofurans interfere with thyroid hormone metaboism, and certain pesticides are toxic to the pancreatic beta cell.

Agents toxic to the endocrine system reach a relatively small number of individuals at the site of manufacture but gain access to entire communities when, for example, toxic wastes are released into the environment. Large geographic regions are exposed to natural goitrogens such as resorcinol that are derived from regional coal and shale deposits. Likewise, radioisotopes of iodine released during atmospheric nuclear weapons testing or reactor accidents disseminate in quantity over very large areas in detectable, if not clearly toxic concentrations, throughout the world (3).

Conceptually, the endocrine system is vulnerable to chemical toxicity at multiple points. Most, if not all tissues, are "target organs" of one or more hormones. Because of structural similarity to certain hormones, some toxic substances interfere with the hormones' metabolism or actions at the target organ. Still other toxic agents interfere directly with the glands that synthesize and secrete hormones. Compounding the chemical vulnerability of the endocrine system are the tier and feedback systems of many hormones. The effects of the thyroid hormone on a target organ are dependent upon the quantity of thyroid hormone secreted by the thyroid. Thyroid secretion is regulated by the serum concentration of the trophic hormone, thyroid-stimulating hormone (TSH), which is secreted by the pituitary thyrotroph cell. The function of the thyrotroph cell is likewise influenced by another trophic hormone, thyrotrophin-releasing hormone (TRH). Multi-level regulatory systems for thyroid and other hormones are counter-regulated in a negative fashion by the serum concentration of the hormone. A transient excess of circulating thyroid hormone would, for example, feed back upon the hypothalamus and pituitary thyrotroph to bring about a corrective reduction in TRH and TSH secretion. In effect, the glands producing the regulatory hormones are also target organs of the primary hormone.

Given this complexity of the endocrine system, it is not difficult to understand how the similar endocrine toxicities of relatively diverse compounds may in fact represent common manifestations of the compounds' interventions at very different points in a hormone's pathways of production, regulation, and action.

All chemically induced changes in the endocrine system cannot be considered undesirable. Indeed, synthetic steroids can be used to purposely inhibit pituitary gonadotropins, thereby providing a chemical method of birth control for millions of women. Chemical (or drug) suppression of target organ hormone secretion can also be therapeutically useful in such organs as the thyroid gland and the adrenal gland.

GENERAL PRINCIPLES

A fundamental concept of the endocrine system is that endocrine cells release a hormone that is transported to a receptor site in the target tissue, where the hormone binds and exerts its biological effect. Traditionally, endocrine systems have encompassed those tissues which release a hormone that is transported through the bloodstream to a target tissue. However, new techniques in tissue cell culture and molecular biology have permitted the identification of several intercellular signaling pathways that do not export hormones via the general circulation to target tissue. Paracrine effects are produced when an effector cell releases a hormone that acts on adjacent target cells to produce a local effect. Many examples of paracrine systems can be found among various growth factors and inflammatory mediators (such as arachadonic acid metabolites or complement factors).

Autocrine systems occur when a particular cell type releases a hormone that then acts on the same cell to augment a particular response. Several examples of autocrine systems exist in the nervous system, gastrointestinal system, and immune system.

Four main categories of hormones exist (see Table 30.1). Polypeptide hormones are composed of amino acid chains ranging in length from three amino acids (as in the

Table 30.1
Categories of hormones

Proteins (e.g., insulin, Growth Hormone, etc.)
Polypeptides (e.g., Thyroid-releasing hormone)
Biogenic amines (e.g., epinephrine)
Thyroid hormones (e.g., thyroxine)
Steroids (e.g., estrogens, androgens)

case of thyrotrophin-releasing hormone) to lengths of several hundred amino acids. They can be composed of two or more subunits (e.g., gonadotropins) or may be linked by disulfide bonds (e.g., growth hormone and insulin). Other post-translational modifications, such as glycosylation may occur, which can affect biological activity. Following synthesis in an endocrine cell, the hormone(s) may be stored in vesicles prior to stimulation of the endocrine system. Patterns of polypeptide hormone release can either be pulsatile or basal.

Biogenic amines are small, modified single amino acids, which also are stored in vesicles prior to their release into the circulation. In contrast to most polypeptide hormones, stores of biogenic amines can be quickly repleted by rapid synthesis. Biogenic amines include catecholamines (notably epinephrine, norepinephrine, and dopamine) as well as serotonin and related compounds found in the nervous system that can exert local effects in tissues such as the gastrointestinal tract.

Thyroid hormone is an intermediate molecular-sized group of compounds that fall in between biogenic amines and short polypeptides. They are composed of two iodinated tyrosine residues, which undergo further modification to enhance biological activity.

Steroid hormones have a characteristic four-ringed nucleus (cyclopentenophenanthrene) and are typically fat-soluble. The main categories of steroid hormones include the sex steroid hormones (e.g., testosterone, estrogen, and progesterone), corticosteroids, mineralocorticoids, vitamin D, and retinoic acid.

Transport of hormones from endocrine tissues to target tissues usually involves carrier proteins that bind the hormones with high affinity and specificity while the hormone is transported within the circulation. Although many of the carrier proteins possess high specificity and affinity, they often possess low capacity, so that the availability of binding sites is limited. Other non-specific carrier proteins, such as albumin, can bind hormones with a high capacity, but possess low specificity/characteristics unlike biogenic amines, steroid, thyroid, and some polypeptide hormones that have specific binding proteins.

After a hormone is transported to the target tissue, it must then interact with a receptor within the target tissue to exert a biological effect. An important concept of hormone action is that only the free, unbound hormone can interact with its receptor to exert a biological effect in the particular target tissue. Therefore, the hormone must become unbound from any carrier protein before it can interact with a receptor. Hormonal signal transduction occurs when the hormone interacts with the target tissue receptor, which in turn produces an intracellular change in the target tissue. Mechanisms of signal transduction depend on whether the target tissue receptor is bound to the cell membrane surface or present in the cytoplasm. Signal transduction by cell membrane-bound receptors is usually either via intracellular second messengers (e.g., cyclic AMP, calcium, or phosphatidylinositol metabolites) or through mechanisms such as phosphorylation of serine, threonine, or tyrosine residues of intracellular kinases and other enzymes (33).

Most polypeptide hormones interact with cell membrane surface receptors, although there is some evidence to suggest that hormonal receptor internalization may play a role in some processes. In contrast, steroid and thyroid hormones interact with intracellular receptors. Transport into the cell may be aided by cell membrane transporters, and once inside the cell, the steroid or thyroid hormone receptor complex is transported to the nucleus, where it may modulate gene expression by binding to certain DNA regulatory sequences.

ENDOCRINE REGULATION & COUNTER-REGULATION

Beyond the molecular biology of the endocrine system is a physiological hierarchy of control which regulates and counter-regulates the homeostasis of the endocrine system through a series of complicated feedback loops. Feedback is the modulation of output by an end product or by-product (such as a hormone or metabolite). A negative feedback loop inhibits an endocrine pathway, and a positive feedback loop enhances or augments an endocrine response (see Figure 30.1). Feedback loops can be further modulated by other endocrine systems that are either pulsatile, cyclical, or stimulated through other mechanisms. The integration of various feedback loops gives rise to a complex cascade of endocrine responses to particular stimuli.

BIOCHEMICAL ASSESSMENT

The diagnosis of endocrine disorders as well as an understanding of the mechanism(s) of hormonal action was significantly advanced when methods became avail-

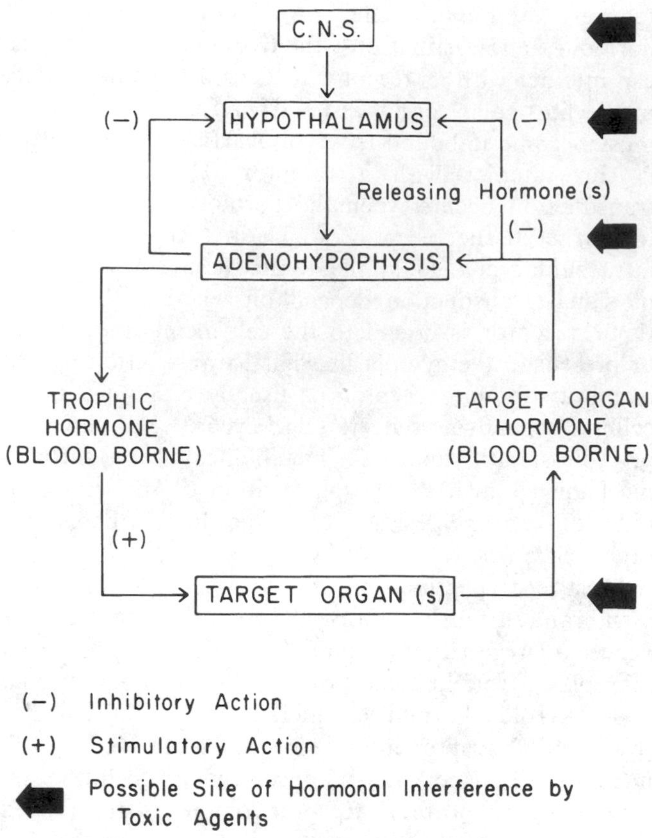

FIG. 30.1. Relation between adenohypophyseal–hypothalmic axis and hormone target organs.

able to measure them in the blood (50). Until about the 1960s, the measurement of hormones often involved in vivo bioassays. The discovery of monoclonal antibody techniques revolutionized the measurement of hormones. Subsequently, antibody-based competitive protein binding assays (i.e., radioimmunoassays or RIAs) were perfected with the availability of radioactive or "tracer" hormones. There are many appropriate endocrine methods available to the toxicologist (63). Molecular genetics has become increasingly important in reproductive endocrinology (30).

Evaluation of endocrine function is an important aspect in determining the mechanism of endocrine toxicity. Measurement of hormone and hormonal metabolite levels in the blood or urine can reveal important information regarding the site of endocrine toxicity. Potential sites of toxicity include the endocrine tissue (including hormone synthesis and release), the endocrine target tissue (including hormone receptor and intracellular signalling pathways), and the means of transport from the endocrine cell to the target cell to exert an endocrine effect (such as hormone carrier proteins). In addition, toxicity to feedback control mechanisms can augment or inhibit endocrine responses.

Even though such an appraisal of the endocrine system may reveal much about the pathophysiology of endocrine toxicology, biochemical assessment has limitations when studying toxicological mechanisms. For instance, derangement of other factors that may have modulatory effects on endocrine target cells cannot be identified by simple evaluation of hormone levels in the blood stream. Thus, biochemical assessment of the endocrine system offers a macroscopic survey of toxicology mechanisms, but study of molecular endocrine toxicity is difficult due to the interplay of several regulatory and counter-regulatory feedback loops.

Furthermore, application of biochemical assessment to physiological assessment can be confounded by several factors. Environmental factors, such as stress, or changes in the diurnal variation of sleep patterns, can affect biochemical assessment. Similarly, the female menstrual cycle can influence hormonal cycles in both the reproductive and nonreproductive organs. Lastly, the sensitivity and specificity of hormonal provocative testing varies greatly among different hormonal systems.

Bioassays

Bioassays provide a means of assessing endocrine status, and although more accurate measurements of hormonal levels are achieved with radioimmunoassay, bioassays are sometimes useful when radioimmunoassay is unable to distinguish active from inactive hormonal metabolites or precursors. An in vivo bioassay determines the biological activity of a hormone by noting its effect on a live animal or isolated organ preparation, compared to a known standard preparation. Historically, bioassays have used hypoglycemia to measure insulin, bone growth to measure growth hormone, and ovarian weight change to measure gonadotrophins. One of the main drawbacks to in vivo bioassays is that they are usually insensitive, nonspecific, and are imprecise comparisons to the dose-response curve for a "standard" preparation.

In vitro bioassays employ endocrine-responsive tissue cell culture lines that can assess the amount of biologically active hormone in sera. The hormonal activity of the sera can be determined by measuring a cellular response to a hormone. Classically, hormonally induced changes in adenylate cyclase activity (with changes in cAMP levels) have been used, but more recently, changes in intracellular calcium levels, phosphoinositol metabolites, and protein phosphorylation have been used to assess hormonal activity. Other in vitro bioassays examine changes more distal to the receptor/signal transduction mechanisms, and note changes in enzymatic activity or steroidogenesis. Some in vitro bioassays assess the mitogenic response to a given hormone. In all cases, addition of an antibody to the hormone receptor should blunt the cellular response.

A shortcoming to in vitro bioassays is that there may be co-existing stimulatory/inhibitory substances in the sera which affect the observed response. For this reason, it is difficult to design a valid bioassay without using fractionated serum, and full characterization of an endocrine-responsive cell line is thus required.

Radioimmunoassay

Measurement of endocrine values was revolutionized with the development of the radioimmunoassay to detect nanomolar concentrations of hormones in living subjects. Classic bioassays were surpassed in sensitivity, specificity, and facilitation with RIA. In addition, RIA allowed measurement of biological materials not previously detectable by chromatographic or spectrophotometric techniques.

RIAs can be used to measure hormones that cannot be radiolabeled to detectable levels in vivo. They are also used for hormones unable to fix complement when bound to antibodies, or they can be used to identify cross-reacting antigens that compete and bind with the antibody.

Competitive inhibition of radiolabeled hormone antibody binding by unlabeled hormone (either as a standard or an unknown mixture) is the principle of most RIAs. A standard curve for measuring antigen (hormone) binding to antibody is constructed by placing known amounts of radiolabeled antigen and the antibody into a set of test tubes. Varying amounts of unlabeled antigen are added to the test tubes. Antigen–antibody complexes are separated from the antigen and the amount of radioactivity from each sample is measured to detect how much unlabeled antigen is bound to the antibody. Smaller amounts of radiolabeled antigen–antibody complexes are present in the fractions containing higher amounts of unlabeled antigen. Usually, a standard curve is constructed that measures the percent of radiolabeled antigen bound with the concentration of unlabeled antigen present.

Although several methods exist for the separation of antigen–antibody complexes, two methods are most commonly employed in RIAs. The first, the double-antibody technique, precipitates antigen–antibody complexes out of solution by utilizing a second antibody, which binds to the first antibody. Although other means of antigen–antibody precipitation exist, they can sometimes chemically alter antigen–antibody binding properties. The drawback to the double-antibody technique is expense, which makes this technique uneconomical for RIA screening procedures.

The second most commonly used method is the dextran-coated activated charcoal technique. Addition of dextran-coated activated charcoal to the sample followed immediately by centrifugation absorbs free antigen and leaves antigen–antibody complexes in the supernatant fraction. Although most economical, some drawbacks to this technique are that it works best only when the molecular weight of the antigen is 30 kilodaltons or less. Also, sufficient carrier protein must be present to prevent adsorption of unbound antibody.

Once a standard curve has been constructed, the RIA can determine the concentration of hormone in a sample (usually plasma or urine). The values of hormone levels are usually accurate using the RIA, but certain factors (e.g., pH or ionic strength) can affect antigen binding to the antibody. Thus, similar conditions must be used for the standard and the sample.

Difficulties with RIAs include a lack of specificity. This problem is usually due to nonspecific cross-reactivity of the antibody. Despite the more complex and involved RIA and monoclonal antibody methodologies, they are of immense value for measuring various trophic hormones. RIA represents an analytical approach of great sensitivity, and such techniques have been applied to more than 200 biological substances, many of which cannot be assessed by other techniques. Unlike bioassays that often require large amounts of tissue (or blood), the greater sensitivity of the RIAs or monoclonal antibody techniques can be achieved using small samples of biological fluids. Some of these RIA methodologies are more useful than others and to some extent depend on the degree of hormonal cross-reactions or, in the case of monoclonal antibody methods, their degree of sensitivity.

Enzyme-Linked Immunosorbent Assay

Enzyme-linked immunosorbent assay (ELISA) is comparable to the immunoradiometric assay except that an enzyme tag is attached to the antibody instead of a radioactive label. ELISAs have the advantage of no radioactive materials and produce an end product that can be assessed with a spectrophotometer. The hormone is bound to the enzyme-labeled antibody, and the excess antibody is removed for immunoradiometric assays. After excess antibody has been removed or the second antibody containing the enzyme has been added (two-site assay), the substrate and cofactors necessary are added in order to visualize and record enzyme activity. The level of hormone present is directly related to the level of enzymatic activity. The sensitivity of the ELISAs can be enhanced by increasing the incubation time for producing substrate. Sometimes the substrate formed may yield a color change so that detection of the hormone being measured can be determined visually.

Immunoradiometric Assays

Immunoradiometric assays (IRMAs) are similar to RIAs in their use of a radiolabeled substance in an antibody–antigen reaction. The radioactive label, however, is attached to the antibody instead of the hormone. Further, excess of antibody, rather than limited quantity, is present in the assay. All the unknown antigen becomes bound in IRMA rather than just a portion, as in RIA; IRMA assays are more sensitive. In the one-site assay, the excess antibody that is not bound to the sample is removed by addition of a precipitating binder. In the two-site assay (i.e., "sandwich" technique), a hormone with at least two antibody- binding sites is adsorbed onto a solid phase, to which one of the antibodies is firmly attached (either the walls of the assay tube itself or beads that are added to the patient sample in assay buffer). After binding to this antibody is completed, a second antibody labeled with ^{125}I is added to the assay. This antibody reacts with the second antibody-binding site to form the so-called sandwich, composed of antibody–hormone-labeled antibody. In contrast to RIA and similar competitive protein-binding assays, the amount of hormone present is directly proportional to the amount of radioactivity measured in the assay (4).

Enzyme-Multiplied Immunoassay Technique

Using EMIT assays, enzyme tags are used instead of radiolabels. However, the antibody binding alters the enzyme characteristics, allowing for measurement of hormone without separating the bound and free components (i.e., homogeneous assay). EMIT assays are used in drug monitoring, but because of lack of sensitivity have not been used to assess hormones. The enzyme is attached to the hormone/drug being tested. This enzyme-labeled antigen is incubated with the sample and with the antibody to the hormone/drug. Binding of the antibody to the enzyme-linked hormone either physically blocks the active site of the enzyme or changes the protein conformation so that the enzyme is no longer active. After antibody binding occurs, the enzyme substrate and cofactor are added, and enzyme activity is measured. If the sample contains hormone, it will compete with enzyme-linked hormones for antibody binding, the enzyme will not be blocked by antibody, and more enzyme activity will be measurable.

Monoclonal Antibodies

Many hormones can now be assessed using monoclonal antibody techniques. Because hormones possess a number of antigenic determinants, it is possible to produce antisera containing a variety of polyclonal antibodies that recognize and bind many parts of the hormone. Antibodies against hormones have been used in many types of RIAs and radioreceptor assays; but polyclonal antisera can create some nonspecificity problems such as cross-reactivity and variation in binding affinity. Therefore, it is oftentimes desirable to produce a group of antibodies that selectively bind to a specific region of the hormone (i.e., antigenic determinant).

In the past, investigators produced antisera to antigenic determinants of the hormone by cleaving the hormone and immunizing an animal with the fragment of the hormone containing the antigenic determinant of interest (e.g., ACTH immunization with the 24-amino-acid N-terminal end of the hormone). This approach solved some problems with cross-reactivity of antisera with other similar antigenic determinants, but problems were still associated with the heterogeneous collection of antibodies found in polyclonal antisera.

The production of monoclonal antibodies offered investigators a homogeneous collection of antibodies that could selectively bind to a specific antigenic determinant with the same affinity. In addition to protein isolation and diagnostic techniques, monoclonal antibodies have contributed greatly to RIAs.

Because propagation of a single antibody-producing cell in vitro cannot occur, spleen cells from an immunized animal were fused with myeloma cells (malignant lymphocytes) using a reagent that causes the cells to fuse (e.g., Sendai virus in polythylene glycol). The fused cells, hybridomas, share characteristics of their antibody-producing cells from the spleen and can be propagated in vitro using tissue culture techniques.

Unfused spleen cells die in tissue culture medium. To separate unfused myeloma cells from hybridomas, the cells are placed in HAT medium (containing hypoxanthine, aminopterin, and thymidine). Myeloma cells used in the production of monoclonal antibodies lack the enzyme hypoxanthine–guanine–phosphoribosyltransferase (HGPRT), whereas hybridomas contain the enzyme (contributed by fused spleen cells). Because the main pathway of DNA synthesis is blocked by aminopterin, only cells containing HGPRT can utilize hypoxanthine and synthesize DNA to propagate. Thus, unfused myeloma cells die in HAT medium because they lack HGPRT. The hybridomas propagate to further isolate and separate variant myeloma cells that can overcome the aminopterin block (using thymidine kinase and exogenous thymidine), and the cells are subjected to 5-bromodeoxyuridine, a pyrimidine analog that kills cells using this pathway:

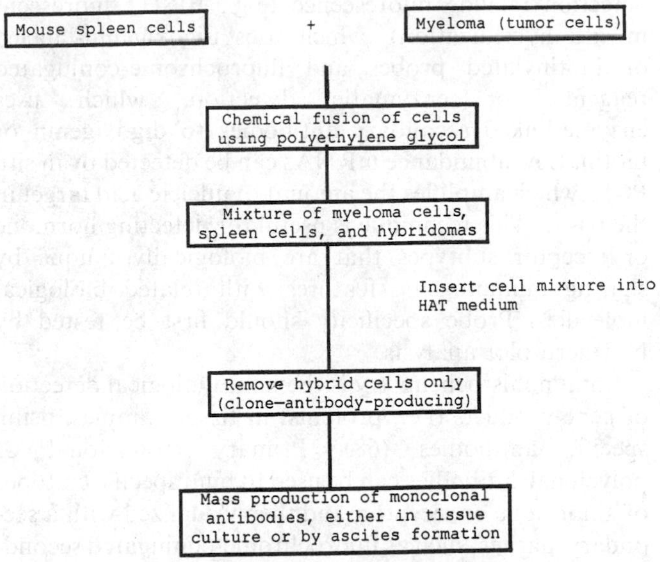

Once the hybridomas have been isolated from unfused cells, they are separated into individual colonies and the type of antibody they produce is characterized. Identification of a hybridoma clone that is producing a specific antibody to the antigen of interest allows for harvesting large quantities of the monoclonal antibody.

Although monoclonal antibodies offer a highly sensitive, specific method for detecting antigen, sometimes increasing monoclonal antibody specificity compromises affinity of the antibody for the antigen. In addition, there is usually decreased complement fixation, and costs are usually high for preparing and maintaining hybridomas that produce monoclonal antibodies (Table 30.2).

Monoclonal antibody techniques provide a means of producing a specific antibody for binding antigen. This technique is useful for studying protein structure relations (or alterations) and has been used for devising specific RIAs.

Table 30.2
Advantages and disadvantages of monoclonal antibodies compared to polyclonal antisera[a]

Advantages	Disadvantages
Sensitivity	Overly specific
Quantities available	Decreased affinity
Immunologically defined	Diminished complement fixation
Detection of neoantigens on cell membrane	Labor-intensive; high cost

[a] Modified from Reference 55.

Gene Expression

The effect of an endocrine modulator or disruptor can influence gene expression. Measurement of gene expression involves quantitating the amount of mRNA for a given gene (52). Because mRNA represents a small fraction of RNAs in the cell (the majority are rRNA and tRNA), methods that are sensitive and specific for detecting changes in mRNA levels have been developed. Northern blots employ total or poly A-enriched RNA that is electrophoretically separated on an agarose gel and then transferred to a matrix (e.g., nitrocellulose), where it is then allowed to hybridize to a labeled antisense riboprobe of interest. Though Northern blots are a standard molecular biology technique, they are sometimes not sensitive for low-abundance mRNAs or specific enough for RNAs derived from closely related genes or alternative splicing. RNase protection (solution hybridization) assays offer increased sensitivity and specificity over Northern blots, but are technically more difficult. A specific radiolabeled antisense riboprobe is permitted to hybridize with the RNA for several hours before digesting with RNase, which digests single-stranded, but not hybridized double-stranded RNA. The sample is then electrophoresed on a denaturing gel and subjected to autoradiography to detect specific bands (indicating the presence of "protected" RNA : RNA hybrids during RNase digestion). Quantitative RT-PCR is sometimes required for detection of low-abundance mRNA.

Subtractive hybridization can be used to identify mRNAs that are differentially expressed between tissue or cell types under different hormonal or environmental conditions (47). In this technique, poly A+RNA is isolated from the two sources and the cell or tissue expressing the mRNA of interest is converted into radiolabeled cDNAs using reverse transcriptase. After removing the RNA for the cDNA, the poly A+RNA from the second cell or tissue source is exhaustively hybridized to the radiolabeled cDNAs, and unhybridized cDNA is isolated and used to screen a cDNA library constructed from the cells or tissues expressing the sequences of interest. Differential display is a PCR-based technique that identifies mRNAs that are differentially expressed.

Polymerase Chain Reaction

Polymerase chain reaction (PCR) is a technique that permits the amplification of a small quantity of DNA template, using a pair of oligonucleotide primers (usually ranging from 10 to 40 nucleotides in length, flanking a DNA sequence of interest), and a thermostable DNA polymerase (an enzyme that catalyzes the elongation of DNA from a template) (24). Each "cycle" of PCR is comprised of an annealing step (annealing primer to template), an elongation step (elongation of the annealed primer by the thermostable DNA polyamerase), and a denaturation step (denaturation of elongated primers from template). Several cycles of PCR are performed in a machine called a DNA thermal cycler, which can be adjusted to optimize the amplification of DNA, depending on the length and nature of the DNA sequence, the source and quality of the DNA template, and the application of the procedure. Other critical parameters include the ionic conditions (most notably, Mg++ concentration), pH, and purity of reagents (i.e., absence of DNA contamination).

DNA templates can be derived from genomic DNA (e.g., human, animal, bacterial, or viral), or RNA that has been converted to a DNA template using reverse transcriptase (RT-PCR). This latter technique has been quantitatively adapted for measuring small amounts of mRNA (quantitative RT-PCR), or detecting differences in the amount of expressed mRNA (differential display). PCR can be employed to detect mRNA for hormones, growth factors, polypeptides, receptors, and other proteins involved with the endocrine system. Some PCR applications are listed in Table 30.3.

In Situ Hybridization and Immunohistochemistry

In situ hybridization is a technique that allows the detection and localization of mRNA in tissue samples with labeled nucleic acid probes (DNA or RNA) that specifically hybridize with cellular mRNA. Tissue samples (or cultured cells) are fixed and embedded and thinly sectioned prior to hybridization. Radiolabeled probes work well for abundant mRNAs, and can be detected using autoradiography. Other methods of signal detection include fluorescence (e.g., FISH, fluorescent in situ hybridization), which uses digoxigenin-labeled or biotinylated probes and fluorochrome-conjugated reagents; or enzymatic detection, which uses enzyme-linked secondary antibodies to digoxigenin or biotin. Low abundance mRNAs can be detected by in situ PCR, which amplifies the amount of nucleic acid target in the tissue. This technique is useful for detecting hormone or receptor subtypes that are biologically unique by sharing immunogenic features with related biological molecules. Probe specificity should first be tested by Northern blot analysis.

Immunohistochemistry is the immunological detection of gene products (i.e., proteins) in tissue samples, using specific antibodies (68). Primary monoclonal or polyclonal antibodies can be used to bind specific epitopes of a hormone or receptor, and then visualized with a secondary marker, such as fluorochrome-conjugated secondary antibody or streptavidin-biotin labels. Selection of a fluorochrome depends on microscopy wavelength and filters, the stability of the signal, the type of tissue being examined, and whether there is a need for double-labeling. Nonfluorescent markers, such as immunoperoxidase or immunogold conjugates, are suitable for bright-field microscopy, and offer increased stability over fluorochrome conjugates. Immunohistochemistry is a powerful complement to in situ hybridization, but limitations include the lack of antibody specificity, denaturation of the antigen during fixation, and cell membrane permeabilization (which permits the antibodies to bind to their respective antigens).

Table 30.3

Selected basic and clinical applications of the polymerase chain reaction

Basic
DNA Sequencing
Identification of DNA Polymorphisms
cDNA Cloning
DNA Mutagenesis
Expression and Quantitation of mRNA
In Vivo Footprinting (DNA/Protein Interactions)
Clinical
Detection of Infectious Agents
Diagnosis of Gene and Chromosome Defects
HLA Haplotyping
Legal and Forensic Applications

Analysis of Signal Transduction Pathways

The effects of a compound on hormone receptor signal transduction can be analyzed, depending on the nature of the signaling pathway and the generation of second messengers that mediate hormone action. Although a comprehensive review of signal transduction is beyond the scope of this chapter, several common endocrine signal transduction mechanisms are summarized in Table 30.4. A variety of techniques ranging from HPLC, Western immunoblotting, to protein kinase assays can be employed to examine the effects of a toxicant on a hormone signaling pathway. Besides affecting hormone receptor activation, some compounds can inhibit inactivation of signal transduction pathways, such as phosphodiesterase inhibitors. Some compounds also may be capable of directly traversing the cell membrane to bind to intracellular receptors without having an effect on signal transduction (e.g., phytoestrogens).

Table 30.4
Common endocrine signal transduction mechanisms

Activation of adenylate cyclase (cyclic AMP)
Activation of guanylate cyclase (cyclic GMP)
Activation of intracellular kinases
serine/threonine kinases
tyrosine kinases
Activation of phospholipases (phophoinositides)
Release of intracellular calcium
Receptor-operated ion channels

PITUITARY GLAND

Pituitary–Target Organ Relationships

Endocrine toxicology requires an understanding of hormonal feedback systems when attempting to predict the effects of potentially toxic agents on a particular target organ. Although measurement of specific hormone levels might not be feasible or economical for the general toxicological screening of a substance, some bioassays and microscopic techniques yield useful information. The reduction in animal growth rates, although in most instances caused by diminished nutritional intake, might be due to the suppression of pituitary growth hormone secretion. Similarly, a decrease in testicular weight following administration of certain chemicals can be due to interference with pituitary gonadotropins (59,60).

Chemically induced changes that affect pituitary–target organ relationships seldom are manifested after a single administration of a toxic substance. Rather, compounds that have the potential to exert deleterious effects on the endocrine system ordinarily require multiple administrations and longer durations of time before such changes are witnessed. Even though chemically induced stress could provoke a rapid response in catecholamine secretion and an outpouring of glucocorticoids, other hormonal responses would not be as immediate. Those chemicals causing the induction of hepatic microsomal enzyme systems that affect hormone metabolism (i.e., catabolism) would most certainly require close to a week before changes in the endocrine system are detected. Even those chemicals that are used as drugs and that are purposely designed to suppress a particular hormone target organ secretion (e.g., antithyroidal agents) exhibit an onset of action of several days.

To understand chemically induced changes in the endocrine system, it is important to understand some of the classic hormonal relations between the adenohypophysis and the respective endocrine target organs (Figure 30.1). Chemicals, including certain classes of therapeutic drugs, can interfere with the release of trophic hormones or can affect their synthesis. Still other toxic agents can exert inhibitory actions on the biosynthesis of target organ hormone secretions. Thus, there are several sites of action of chemicals on the adenohypophyseal-target organ feedback systems (Figure 30.1).

The site(s) of a chemical's action may differ in their respective sensitivities. Target organs such as the gonads are frequently sensitive to toxic substances, particularly because rapidly dividing cells are often vulnerable to chemicals. Furthermore, stress can affect the secretory activity of certain of the hypothalamic-releasing hormones and hence alter pituitary–target organ relationships. Oftentimes toxic agents bind to circulating blood proteins and alter the ratio of free to bound target organ hormones. Such changes in binding also can modify the pituitary–target organ relationship. Thus, several target organs can be affected by chemical perturbation.

Adenohypophysis

Hormones of the adenohypophysis and their hypothalamic-releasing hormones are depicted in Table 30.5. Because the trophic hormones are either protein or glycoprotein, they cannot be measured by standard spectrophotometric procedures. These hormones must be either bioassayed or measured using RIAs or by monoclonal antibody techniques. Although bioassays may be useful for certain of the adenohypophyseal hormones, such tests are often inaccurate or have been replaced by more sensitive methods. Bioassays, however, might be employed when there is only a secondary interest in determining if a particular toxicological agent is affecting trophic hormone levels. Sometimes a target organ known to be directly influenced by a particular trophic hormone can be measured and thus provide some general insight into the nature of the chemically induced alterations in the endocrine system.

Hormones of the adenohypophysis are either proteins or glycoproteins. Those trophic target organs whose secretions act back upon the adenohypophysis are usually small molecular weight hormones such as steroids (e.g., estrogens, androgens, or progesterones), or halogenated hormones such as thyroxine or triiodothyronine.

The glycoproteins include TSH, LH, FSH, and HCG. Each hormone is a heterodimer of two noncovalently associated subunits α and β, which are encoded by separate genes situated on different chromosomes. It is the β subunit that confers the unique biological specificity of each hormone. This biological activity is dependent

Table 30.5
Hormone assays and endocrine function
Trophic hormones of the anterior pituitary gland and their respective hypothalamic releasing hormones

Adenohypophyseal trophic hormone		Hypothalamic releasing hormone	
Abbreviation	Full name	Abbreviation	Full name
ACTH	Adenocorticotropic hormone	CRH	Corticotropic-releasing hormone
TSH	Thyroid-stimulating hormone	TRH	Thyrotopic-releasing hormone
FSH	Follicle-stimulating hormone	FRH	Follicle-stimulating releasing hormone
LH	Luteinizing hormone	LRH	Luteinizing-hormone releasing hormone
GH	Growth hormone, somatotropin	SRH,GRH	Somatotropin-releasing hormone
		SRIF[a],GIH	Somatotropin-inhibitory hormone
Prl	Prolactin	PIH	Prolactin-inhibitory hormone
		PRH	Prolactin-releasing hormone
MSH	Melanocyte-stimulating hormone	MRH	Melanocyte-stimulating releasing hormone
		MIH	Melanocyte-inhibiting hormone

[a] Somatostatin

upon the intact dimers; free subunits are biologically inactive.

MEASUREMENT OF ANTERIOR PITUITARY HORMONES

Adrenocorticotropin

Adrenocorticotropin (ACTH) exerts a number of physiological actions including maintenance of the adrenal gland and stimulation of adrenal cortical steroid secretion. Many pathological states can alter ACTH secretion. Stress, caused by a variety of environmental or chemical stimuli, can cause a rapid elevation in ACTH blood levels. ACTH and cortisol exhibit diurnal variations, with the highest levels occurring in the morning (about 8:00 a.m.) and the lowest levels in late afternoon.

Several methods are available for measuring ACTH (38), but most measurements have indirectly assessed adrenal gland secretions. A highly sensitive IRMA ACTH assay has been very useful in diagnosing adrenal deficiencies (65). Gravimetric assay of adrenal glands represents one of the simplest methods for indirectly evaluating ACTH activity. This assay uses hypophysectomized animals; injections of ACTH-like material maintain the weight of the adrenal glands. ACTH stimulates increases in plasma cortisol and corticosterone and elevates urinary 17-hydroxycorticosteroids and 17-ketosteroids. These steroid levels can be used to assess ACTH. ACTH causes involution of the thymus gland and deposition of hepatic glycogen, and leads to a decrease in circulating eosinophils in hypophysectomized rodents. ACTH can cause depletion of adrenal ascorbic acid.

In addition to those assays for ACTH that rely on adrenal gland responses (see section on adrenal glands), radioligand–receptor assays have been developed for ACTH. Often cortisol levels are used to assess ACTH. Cortisol can be determined using commercially available antibody-coated tube RIA kits.

Thyroid-Stimulating Hormone

Thyroid-stimulating hormone (TSH) is a glycoprotein capable of stimulating the growth and proliferation of cells of the thyroid gland. TSH can produce a number of biochemical and histological changes in the thyroid gland. The TSH receptor entails an extracellular domain as well as a transmembrane component (28). TSH assays have employed the uptake of ^{32}P in the thyroid glands of experimental animals. Like ACTH, and for routine toxicological assessment of TSH, tests often involve the measurement of target organ secretory responses. Thus, the evaluation of TSH in routine toxicological experiments often employs measurement of the thyroid hormones (i.e, thyroxine and triiodothyronine) (see section on the thyroid gland). Serum thyroid hormone concentrations alone do not explain the variability and severity of the range of symptoms observed in thyrotoxicosis (41).

Many chemicals, drugs, environmental factors, and pathological states can affect thyroid hormone section (9). Certain foodstuffs and plants contain chemicals that can act as antithyroidal agents. Most of these conditions or factors, however, seem to affect thyroid gland activity itself rather than impinge upon TSH secretion.

Immunochemistry assays are available for measuring TSH (21,54). A liquid-phase two-site immunoradiometric assay IRMA has been described for human TSH (hTSH). IRMA is based on the simultaneous addition of affinity purified sheep anti-hTSH IgG-^{125}I and rabbit anti-hTSH antiserum. This assay is specific for hTSH and exhibits no cross-reactivity with other pituitary glycoprotein (42). Thus, the IRMA assays for TSH may be more specific than current RIAs for TSH. The one-step IRMA method involves the use of monospecific antibody against two immunogenic sites on the TSH molecule (46). Other assays for thyrotropin involve a combination of bioluminescence and immunoassay techniques (51).

Growth Hormone (Somatotropin)

Human growth hormone (GH) is a peptide composed of 191 amino acids. GH exerts its actions on a variety of cells to stimulate lipolysis, protein anabolism, and hyperglycemia. Its actions on bone and cartilage are mediated through somatomedins (namely, IGF-1). A deficiency in GH leads to a reduction in the incorporation of amino acids into protein. GH causes a marked stimulation of cartilaginous growth at the epiphyses of long bones.

Many agents can affect GH secretion (Table 30.6). Hypoglycemia or insulin can cause a sudden and dramatic increase in serum GH. Starvation can affect GH levels; and cold, stress, or surgical trauma can lead to an increase in serum GH. Chemicals that affect catecholamine neurotransmission and the autonomic nervous system can influence GH secretion.

GH has been assessed using bioassays. Some GH assays simply use a 10-day body weight gain test in hypophysectomized female rats. The hormone has also been assayed by measuring the width of the tibial epiphysial growth plate.

Sensitive RIAs have been developed for experimental animals (e.g., rat) and for humans. Human GH concentrations can be measured with double-antibody RIAs.

Whether GH is assessed using bioassays or by the more accurate and sensitive RIA procedures, the experimental design of either acute or chronic toxicity tests must closely monitor the nutritional status of the animals. Several toxic agents can affect dietary intake and thus reduce body weight. Experimental designs using paired-feeding protocols are necessary for interpreting GH activity in any well-designed toxicology protocol.

Immunocytological assays for GH can also be performed on Epon-embedded, semi-thin sections of tissue using the avidin–biotin–peroxidase complex technique (23). Microdissection techniques (31) and other in vitro assays for the release of GH have been employed (1). An ultrasensitive immunofluometric assay (45) and a chemiluminescence-based GH assay (67) are now available.

Table 30.6
Effects of various agents on blood growth hormone (GH) levels

Increased GH levels	Decreased GH levels
Norepinephrine	Somatostatin
Epinephrine	
Serotonin	
TRH	
Vasopressin	
Substance P	
Endorphins	
Enkephalins	
Arginine[a]	
Prostaglandins	
Insulin (hypoglycemia)[a]	
α-Desoxyglucose	
Apomorphine	
L-DOPA[a]	
Clonidine[a]	

[a] Used as a provocative test for the diagnosis of GH disorders.

Gonadotropins

Follicle-stimulating hormone (FSH) and luteinizing hormone (LH) are both glycoproteins. These glycoproteins are composed of α and β subunits. There is some functional and immunological specificity with the β subunits of the gonadotropins, including human chorionic gonadotropin (HCG).

The adenohypophysis secretes FSH and LH, whose principal stimulatory actions are on the gonads. FSH stimulates follicular development in the ovary and spermatogenesis in the testes. LH, also referred to as interstitial cell-stimulating hormone (ICSH) in the male, causes luteinization of the ovary and stimulates androgen production in testicular Leydig cells. The gonads contain receptors for LH and FSH which are involved in intracellular signaling (33).

In the human female, blood levels of FSH and LH vary according to the phase of the menstrual cycle. In men, although there may be some diurnal fluctuation in FSH and LH, the blood levels are noncyclic. Unfortunately, there is a paucity of information about the direct effects of chemicals and drugs on the ovary (19).

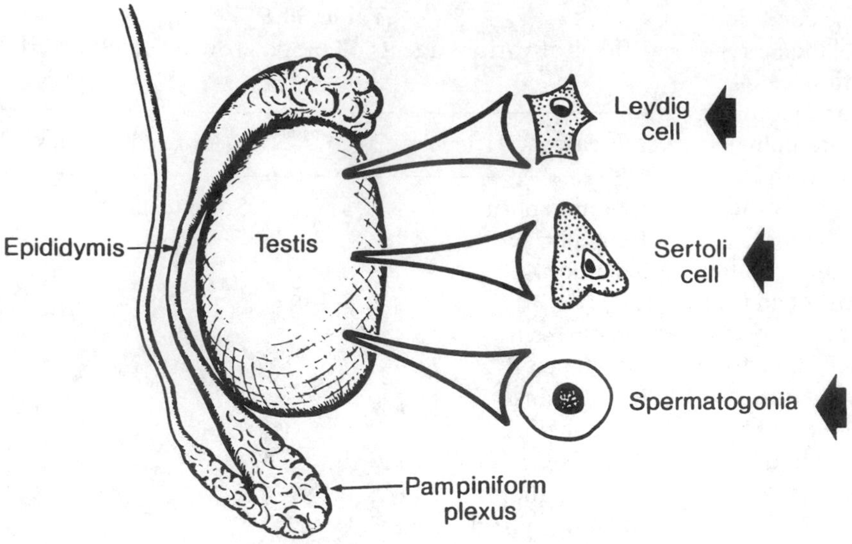

FIG. 30.2. Some possible sites of action of selected gonadotoxins.

Indeed, to evaluate it from a toxicological standpoint, gonadotropin secretion in women is more complex than in men. Conversely, the various secretory or cellular processes of the male gonad are more readily evaluated from the standpoint of toxicological assessment. Figure 30.2 shows the major cellular sites of testicular toxicants. In general, the Leydig cells (or interstitial cells) are comparatively resistant to chemical insult. However, the process of steroidogenesis is quite sensitive and can be used as an indicator of male sex steroid (e.g., testosterone, dihydrotestosterone) activity (see section on gonads). Methods have been devised to examine isolated Leydig cell cultures as well as testicular perfusion systems in an effort to study androgen secretion by the male gonad (5).

Spermatogenesis, on the other hand, is sensitive to chemical insult. Testicular sections (or biopsy) can be used to assess the degree of spermatogenic arrest as evidenced by the presence (or absence) of sterile or partially sterile seminiferous tubules. Electroejaculation methods and the use of an artificial vagina can be used for collecting semen for examination of sperm counts, morphology, and motility. Sertoli cells secrete a number of proteinaceous substances including androgen-binding protein (ABP) which has been used as an indicator of toxicological insult following the administration of potentially damaging chemicals.

FSH or LH levels can be assessed by direct measurement of the hormones or by indirect assays that reflect an influence of these hormones on their target tissues. RIAs are available to measure gonadotropins.

Earlier methods in classical endocrinology studies often employed bioassays. FSH has been bioassayed by assessing its ability to enhance ovarian weight in immature rats treated with a placental gonadotropin. A sensitive assay for LH once employed ovarian ascorbic acid depletion. The bioassay of gonadotropins has largely been abandoned because of low sensitivity and expense. The sensitivity of RIAs offers substantial advantages over bioassays even though the biological and immunological activities do not always correlate.

Indirect measurement of gonadotropins in women often includes the measurement of ovarian steroids or the study of vaginal cytology (see section on gonads). In men, indirect assays include the measurement of androgens or the histological assessment of spermatogenesis. Chromosome studies can also be of some value when assessing pituitary gonadal activity. Localization of FSH and LH and their receptors can be detected using immunoperoxidase techniques.

It is important that the appropriate separation system be employed when measuring FSH (14). Solid-phase RIAs have been developed that measure free alpha subunits of pituitary glycoprotein hormones (44). Semi-quantitative assays for LH are also available (8).

Inhibin

Inhibin is a proteinaceous substance found in the mammalian gonad that is involved in the negative feedback regulation of FSH secretion. Inhibin is a heterodimer with the α and β subunits linked by disulfide bonds. In men, inhibin can be detected in the testes, seminal plasma, rete testes fluid, and spermatozoa. The Sertoli cells are the only testicular cells that secrete an inhibin-like substance referred to as Sertoli cell factor (SCF). Inhibin, as well as SCF, can suppress the pituitary secretion of FSH. Inhibin (A or B) is synthesized in granulosa cells, and production is stimulated by FSH and by estradiol.

The biological activities of various inhibin preparations, including SCF, can be assessed in vitro using pituitary cell cultures (20,49). This in vitro assay consists of evaluating the degree of suppression of basal FSH release following an incubation with the test material relative to that of a control culture.

Prolactin

Prolactin is a protein hormone whose amino acid composition is quite similar to growth hormone. Prolactin causes initiation and maintenance of lactation in women. It has no known physiological function in men. In rodents, prolactin maintains the corpus luteum. In many species, milk ejection cannot be produced by suckling unless prolactin first stimulates the myoepithelial cells of the mammary glands.

Prior to the development of sensitive RIAs for prolactin, it was bioassayed. Prolactin has the ability to stimulate the crop sac of the pigeon. Prolactin can also be identified in tissues using in vitro immunoassays, but there are a number of test system conditions in vitro that can affect the detectable levels of prolactin (Table 30.7) (34). It is important to determine the optimal conditions for assessing tissue prolactin.

Many drugs or chemicals can affect blood levels of prolactin (Table 30.8). Several of the actions of these agents are mediated by dopaminergic mechanisms. Prolactin secretion can be increased by physical exercise, coitus, suckling, and surgical stress. Such factors must be taken into consideration when assessing prolactin levels in toxicological protocols.

Table 30.7
Conditions affecting immunoassay of prolactin and growth hormone

Duration of incubation
Incubation temperature
pH
Homogenate or tissue fraction
Concentration of test system constituents
Cysteamine
Reduce glutathione
EDTA
Urea
Sodium dodecyl sulfate
Iodoacetate

POSTERIOR PITUITARY HORMONES

Neurohypophysial Peptides

The posterior pituitary gland, or neurohypophysis, contains a number of peptides of which only oxytocin and vasopressin (antidiuretic hormone, ADH) have been thoroughly studied. This gland also contains a group of peptides known as the neurophysins. The neurophysins appear to be synthesized in the same hypothalamic neurons as the octapeptides oxytocin and vasopressin. The physiological function of oxytocin and vasopressin are well-established, but less is known about the biological function of the neurophysins. The supraoptic and paraventricular nuclei of the hypothalamus produce ADH and oxytocin, which traverse the pituitary stalk and are stored in the neurohypophysis.

The principal physiological function of vasopressin is conservation of fluids; it exerts its action on the renal tubule leading to the reabsorption of water. The release of vasopressin is mediated by neural impulses from osmoreceptors located in the hypothalamus.

Table 30.8
Effect of various agents on blood prolactin levels[a]

Increase prolactin levels	Decrease prolactin levels
Reserpine	Acetylcholine
Methyl-DOPA	Apomorphine
α-Methyl-p-trosine	Dopamine
Chlorpromazine	L-DOPA
Atropine	Iproniazid
Perphenazine (and other phenothiazines)	β-Hydroxy-GABA
	Somatostatin
Haloperidol	Bromocriptine
Tricyclic antidepressants	
Supiride	
Diethyl ether	
Nicotine	
Vasopressin	
Estrogens	
Thyroxine (and T_3)	
Histamine	
Prostaglandin E	
β-Endorphin	
Met-enkephalin	
Thyroid-releasing hormone (TRH)	
Opiates	

[a] Response may vary quantitatively depending on the dose and the particular species.

Table 30.9
Effects of various drugs on the release or action of neurohypophyseal hormones

Enhanced release	Inhibit release	Block peripheral action
I. Vasopressin		
Acetylcholine	Ethanol	Lithium
Nicotine		β-Adrenergic agonists
α-Adrenergic agonists		Tetracyclines
Vincristine		
Clofibrate		
II. Oxytocin		
Prostaglandin E_2	Ethanol	Propanolol
Prostaglandin F_{1_α}	Methalibure	Vasopressin analogues
		Oxytocin analogs

Oxytocin's principal physiological function is to stimulate uterine smooth musculature and to aid in the process of lactation. Oxytocin is released in response to suckling; it may also play a role in parturition.

Drugs and other hormones can affect the secretion of vasopressin or oxytocin (Table 30.9). Nonspecific stress also can stimulate the release of ADH and thus is an important variable to consider in any toxicological protocol involved with monitoring water balance. Some chemicals and drugs affect the central release of posterior pituitary hormones, whereas others block their peripheral action(s). Physiological factors also affect the secretory rate of oxytocin, and there are considerable differences among species. Suckling and mammary duct dilation lead to enhanced secretion of oxytocin. Estrogens and pregnancy enhance the sensitivity of the uterine smooth muscle to oxytocin.

Oxytocin

Oxytocin may be measured by RIA or bioassay. A solid-phase RIA for the direct measure of plasma oxytocin has been developed that is rapid, relatively sensitive, reproducible, and that does not require the prior extraction of plasma samples (6). Because oxytocin can stimulate the contraction of smooth muscles, several bioassays have been developed using isolated muscle strips. Oxytocin can be assayed employing a mammotonic activity of the hormone on strips of lactating rat mammary gland. The increment of tension developed by the muscle strip is used as an index of oxytocic activity. A four-point assay can be carried out using USP posterior pituitary standard as a reference.

Vasopressin (Antidiuretic Hormone)

Vasopressin (ADH), like oxytocin, is an octapeptide. In some species, ADH exerts a rather profound pressor action on vascular smooth muscle. Vasopressin acts by binding to cell surface receptors of at least two subtypes (V_1-vascular smooth muscle and V_2-renal epithelia). In humans and most other mammals, the actions of ADH are primarily on the renal tubules, exerting a body fluid-sparing action.

ADH can be measured by RIA or bioassay. With bioassay, ADH or extracts of posterior pituitary tissue can be measured for their antidiuretic activity in the rat using ether anesthesia and a constant water load; the diminution in urine flow is an index of antidiuretic activity. Unanesthetized trained dogs also have been employed in the bioassay, but stress must be minimized because it can affect urinary output and hence the ADH assay.

Simple and rapid radioimmunoassays for vasopressin are available (29). Because vasopressin is present in biological fluids in low concentrations (picograms), tests must be sensitive. It ordinarily has been difficult to measure basal levels or small fluctuations resulting from particular experimental designs.

THYROID GLAND

The thyroid gland secretes triiodothyronine (T_3) and thyroxine (T_4). This secretory process is modulated by the adenohypophysial–hypothalamic and is mediated by thyroid stimulating hormone (TSH). TSH stimulates the thyroid gland, leading to increased secretion and release of T_3 and T_4.

The primary secretions of the thyroid are thyroxine (T_4) and triiodothyronine (T_3). The initial step in the synthesis of these thyroid hormones is the uptake of iodide (derived from dietary iodine) into the follicular cells of the thyroid in response to the adenohypophyseal hormone thyrotropin (TSH). Once inside the cell, the iodide is oxidized, possibly through a free radical mechanism, and then chemically combined with the tyrosine components of a protein, thyroglobulin, to form either monoiodotyrosyl or diiodotyrosyl residues. Two molecules of the latter can combine to form triiodothyronine. Under normal conditions, T_4 predominates over T_3 in the thyroid, although the ratio can be altered by certain physiological states.

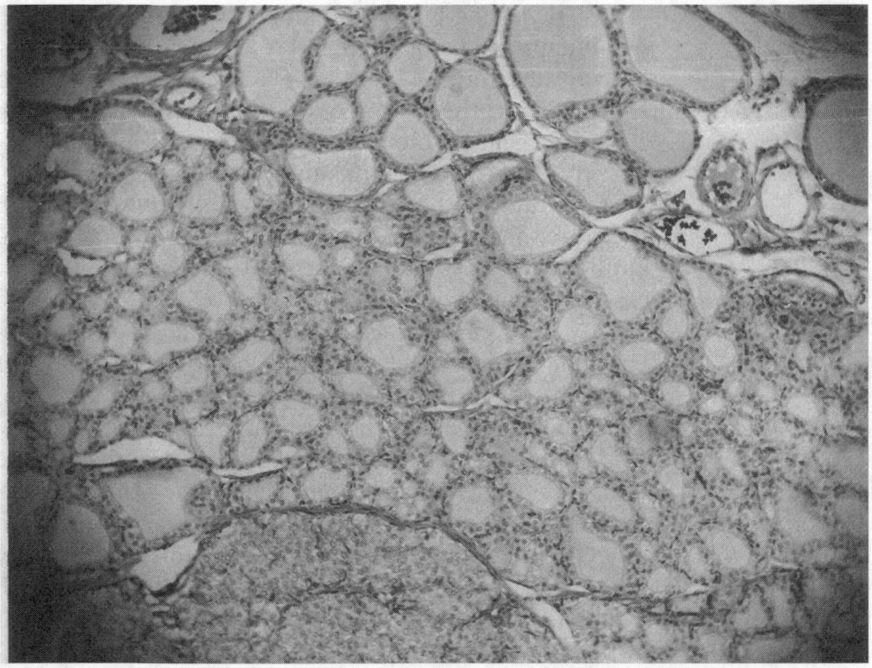

FIG. 30.3. Histology of rat thyroid gland. 125× magnification.

T_3 and T_4 remain incorporated in the thyroglobulin, which is stored in the follicular colloid material of the gland, until their release in response to TSH. The release, which involves lysosomes, results from the proteolytic cleavage of thyroglobulin into the thyroid hormones and component amino acids. Monoiodotyrosine and diiodotyrosine also are released at this stage; however, before reaching the circulation, they are enzymatically degraded, liberating iodide, which is eventually reincorporated into protein by the gland. Normally, thyroglobulin does not reach the circulation but remains inside the thyroid cell (Figure 30.3).

Once released into the circulation, T_3 and T_4 are transported in the plasma bound to specific proteins. Although there are species differences in the protein-binding patterns of the thyroid hormones, the primary binding protein in humans is thyroxine-binding globulin (TBG). TBG is an acidic glycoprotein (molecular weight 40,000) that binds T_4 with a relatively high binding affinity and T_3 with a lower binding affinity. A second transport protein, called thyroxine-binding prealbumin, although present in higher amounts than thyroxine-binding globulin, has a lower binding affinity for the thyroid hormones and is considered of secondary physiological importance. In humans and most other mammals, the thyroid hormones can also bind to albumin following occupation of the higher-affinity binding sites. As a consequence of this plasma protein binding, less than 0.1 percent of the total plasma thyroid hormones exist in a free or unbound form. Care must be exercised when monitoring thyroid function in a species such as the rat, which does not possess a thyroxine-binding globulin (i.e., high-affinity binding protein) and which therefore has lower plasma levels of protein-bound thyroid hormone. Also, because it is the free hormone that is available for degradation, it is not unreasonable to expect that the plasma half-life for T_4 would be longer in a species with a thyroxine-binding globulin than in a species without the protein. The T_4 plasma half-life in the human, which has a thyroxine-binding globulin, is 5 to 9 days. In the rat, which does not have a thyroxine-binding globulin, the T_4 plasma half-life is 12 to 24 h.

Various antithyroidal drugs can interfere with the biosynthesis of thyroid hormones. Some agents interfere with the uptake of iodine and some act by inhibiting thyroid peroxidase (TPO), resulting in a reduction in T_3 and T_4 levels. Furthermore, several other chemicals can affect thyroid hormone secretion (Table 30.10).

Table 30.10
Chemicals producing abnormal thyroid function

Blocks iodide trapping	Blocks iodide oxidation	Mechanism not established
Chlorate	Amphenone	Acetazolamide
Hypochlorite	Carbimazole	Chlorpromazine
Iodate	Cobalt	Chlortrimeton
Nitrate	Methimazole	Thiopental
Perchlorate	p-Aminosalicylate	Tolbutamide
Thiocyanate	Phenylbutazone	
	Phenylindanedione	
	Propylthiouracil	
	Resorcinol	

Table 30.11
Factors influencing TSH, T_3, and T_4 levels in rat plasma

Sex of animal
Age of animal
Time of day
Stage of estrous cycle
Strain of animal
Environmental temperature
Blood collection technique
Animal handling
Locomotor activity of animal

Industrial or environmental agents that affect thyroid function in humans typically do so by interfering with the intrathyroidal synthesis or secretion of thyroid hormone (i.e., "primary hypothyroidism") (3). Polychlorinated biphenyls (PCBs) affect thyroid hormone metabolism. Amiodarone, an antiarrhythmic drug, is an iodinated benzofuran derivative with a chemical structure similar to thyroxine. It may cause hyperthyroidism. They are goitrogenic in some animals. TCDD (2,3,7,8-tetrachlorodibenzo-p-dioxin) can reduce T_4 levels in experimental animals. DDT can produce avian hypothyroidism. Hydroxyphenols (e.g., resorcinol) and hydroxypyridines have been shown to inhibit TPO. Likewise, phthalates, known also as plasticizers, can be degraded by certain bacteria, producing dihydroxybenzoic acid (DHBA). DHBA can also inhibit TPO (3).

In addition to the different chemicals and environmental pollutants that can affect the thyroid gland, there are other factors that can influence the measurements of TSH, T_3, and T_4 levels (Table 30.11).

Measurement of Thyroid Hormones

Assays for thyroid hormones are used to monitor and confirm the extent of hyper- or hypothyroidism. There are a large number of laboratory tests that can be used to assess the function of the thyroid gland (Table 30.12). Assessment of laboratory tests can be divided into various categories including those that directly measure thyroid function (e.g., ^{131}I uptake), those that measure blood levels (free vs. bound), those that measure metabolic actions (e.g., cholesterol lowering), and those that provide insight into the modulations of thyroid function by the adenohypophysis (e.g., thyroid suppression test).

RIAs can be used to determine serum T_3 and T_4 levels. The RIA is based on the binding of endogenous hormone to a specific antibody, thereby displacing a proportional amount of radiolabeled hormone from that antibody. Obviously, the hormone-binding proteins in the sample (e.g., thyroxine-binding globulin, thyroxine-binding prealbumin, and albumin) tend to compete with the antibody for the hormone. This interference can be prevented by extracting the serum prior to the assay or adding chemical agents to block the binding of hormone to binding proteins. Another difficulty in measuring T_3 or T_4 by RIA is that the hormones are small and similar in structure, and it has been difficult to produce a specific antibody for T_3 and T_4 without the need for prior chromatographic separation.

T_3 and T_4 can be measured using a competitive protein-binding assay that is based on the displacement of radiolabeled hormone from thyroxine-binding globulin. The amount of label displaced is proportional to the amount of hormone added to the assay in the sample serum. T_4 can be effectively measured using the competitive protein-binding assay, but the hormone must first be extracted from the sample serum to eliminate any interference from endogenous binding proteins, which would tend to compete with the binding protein used in the assay.

Non-isotopic immunotechniques can also be used to measure thyroid hormones (e.g., EMIT). The principles of these tests are comparable to RIAs except that the labeled analyte may be an enzyme as in the ELISA (18). The EMIT is an enzymatic method that does not require separation of the free and bound portions of the hormone.

PARATHYROID GLAND

Parathyroid hormone (PTH) is synthesized as a prohormone consisting of 115 amino acids. PTH, containing 84 amino acids, is secreted by the chief cells within the parathyroid gland. The balance of endogenous calcium is maintained by several intrinsic factors that

Table 30.12
Laboratory assessment of the thyroid

Tests assessing metabolic effect of thyroid
Serum cholesterol
Basal metabolic rate
Cardiac rate (i.e., systolic time intervals)
Tests assessing thyroid function
TRH stimulation
Thyroid suppression test
Serum TSH
^{131}I uptake; T_3 uptake
Tests assessing blood levels (free and bound)
Serum total T_3 and total T_4
Serum free (unbound) T_4
Reverse $T_3(rT_3)$
TBG (thyroxine-binding globulin)

modulate the remodeling of bone and the absorption and excretion of calcium. PTH, vitamin D, and calcitonin are the principal factors involved in calcium homeokinesis (7). About 98 percent of endogenous calcium resides in skeletal tissue, with the remainder sequestered in soft tissues and extracellular fluids. About 50 percent of serum calcium exists in an ionized form; ionized calcium is the biologically active form of the cation. Hypocalcemia provokes secretion of PTH. While the direct involvement of PTH, calcitonin, and vitamin D are important in modulating calcium, other hormones such as thyroxine, GH, estrogens, and corticosteroids contribute to the maintenance of calcium homeostasis.

Parathyroid hormone was originally bioassayed using a hormone-induced elevation in serum calcium in dogs. Several commonly used in vivo assays employ the measurement of serum calcium in parathyroidectomized rats or in calcium-injected chicks or quail. A commonly used in vitro assay is based on determining the activation of renal adenylate cyclase in response to PTH.

PTH can be measured by immunoassay. The majority of assays are directed against the more stable C-terminal fraction (4). Assays for this N-terminal fragment are available and are better suited to detect rapid fluctuations in PTH levels. However, the C-terminal assay is the method of choice for assessing abnormal PTH function, particularly with concomitant hypercalcemia (13,18).

A monoclonal antibody assay for human vitamin D protein has also been reported (43). The anti-human vitamin-D-binding protein antibodies cross-react with monkey and pig vitamin-D-binding protein, but not with vitamin-D-binding protein from the rat, mouse, or chicken.

ADRENAL GLAND

The adrenal gland consists of an outer layer (adrenal cortex) and an inner layer (adrenal medulla). The inner and outer layers can be readily distinguished by histological preparations (Figure 30.4).

The adrenal medulla secretes epinephrine and norepinephrine in response to sympathetic nerve stimulation, and the release of these hormones produces systemic effects that, in turn, resemble generalized sympathetic nerve stimulation. The adrenal cortex produces two major groups of hormones, the mineralocorticoids and the glucocorticoids, as well as smaller amounts of androgenic hormones.

In humans, the main mineralocorticold is aldosterone, although deoxycorticosterone (DOCA) also exhibits mineralocorticoid activity. However, DOCA potency is reported to be only one-thirtieth that of aldosterone. Cortisol, the major glucocorticoid produced in humans, also possesses a small amount of mineralocorticoid activity. The basic physiological effect of aldosterone is on extracellular fluid volume. It promotes the renal reabsorption of sodium in the ascending portion of the loop of Henle, the distal tubule, and the collecting tubule. Sodium reabsorption is accompanied by reabsorption of the chloride anion. In addition to stimulating sodium reabsorption, aldosterone enhances the urinary excretion of potassium and hydrogen ions. The increased elimination of hydrogen ions can lead to alkalosis and an increased extracellular content of bicarbonate ions, that when combined with an increased extracellular sodium and chloride content, promotes tubular reabsorption of water.

The adrenal gland is essential for life, especially the salt-retaining properties of the mineralocorticoids. In the absence of mineralocorticoids, the extracellular fluid potassium concentration rises; sodium and chloride contents fall. Total lack of aldosterone secretion can cause the urinary elimination of 20 percent of the total body sodium in one day. The salt elimination can cause a life-threatening reduction in the extracellular and blood volume, that, if untreated, leads to diminished cardiac output and death.

The major glucocorticoid secreted in humans is cortisol, or hydrocortisone, although both corticosterone and cortisone do possess some glucocorticoid activity. The three major systems regulated by the glucocorticoids are carbohydrate, protein, and fat metabolism. With carbohydrate metabolism, the glucocorticoids stimulate gluconeogenesis and decrease glucose utilization by the cells, both of which lead to increased blood glucose levels. The glucocorticoids also produce a marked reduction in cellular protein content. An exception to this protein cata-

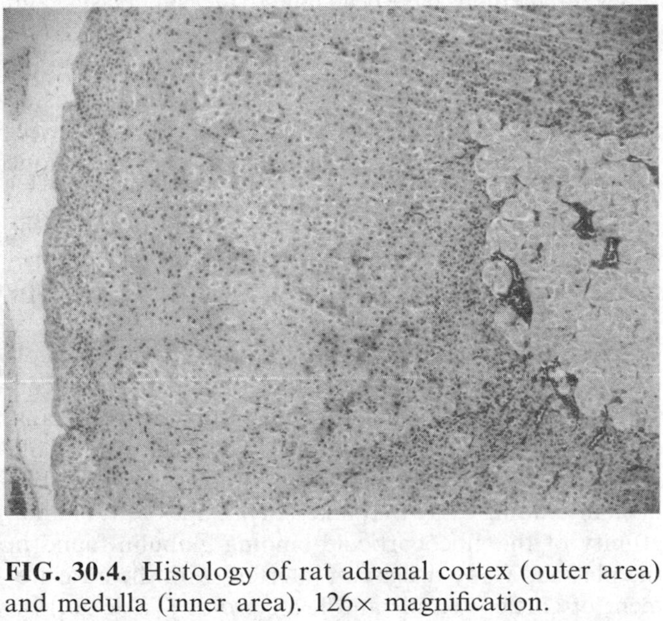

FIG. 30.4. Histology of rat adrenal cortex (outer area) and medulla (inner area). 126× magnification.

bolic action is the liver, where protein content increases as does the production of plasma protein by the liver.

Glucocorticoids probably interfere with the transport of amino acids into extrahepatic cells, and this action, combined with continuing protein catabolism in these cells, produces an increase in plasma amino acid content. Increased plasma amino acid levels and their subsequent transport into the liver probably promote gluconeogenesis (i.e., the conversion of amino acids to glucose). The glucocorticoids also promote mobilization of fatty acids from adipose tissue, which raises plasma fatty acid levels. This effect, plus increased oxidation of fatty acids in the cells, is probably involved in the switch from glucose utilization to fatty acid utilization as a source of energy during periods of stress.

Corticosteroids can bind to plasma protein fractions. A corticosteroid-binding globulin (CBG) has a high affinity but a low binding capacity. Plasma albumin, the second plasma protein, has a low affinity and a relatively high binding capacity. Under physiological conditions, most of the hormone is bound to CBG.

It is now recognized that many drugs and chemicals can produce lesions of either the adrenal medulla or the adrenal cortex (Table 30.13). Still other agents can specifically inhibit particular enzymatic steps involved in adrenal steroidogenesis (Figure 30.5). Metyrapone, aminoglutethimide and o,p′-DDD have been used not only as agents to aid in the diagnosis of adrenal cortical dysfunction, but some also have been used as adrenolytic drugs in treating adenocarcinomas of the adrenal gland.

Measurement of Corticosteroids

Several methods have been used to measure plasma and urinary aldosterone levels. Among them are double-isotope dilution techniques, gas-liquid chromatographic techniques and RIAs (4). A competitive immunoassay for cortisol reportedly is based on a capillary electrophoresis and laser-induced fluorescence technique (48).

Several analytical procedures have been used for the quantitation of glucocorticoids. One of the earliest procedures involved a colorimetric reaction between the glucocorticoid and a phenylhydrazine reagent. The Porter–Silber method and Zimmerman reactions are colorimetric assays used for measuring corticoids. Both cortisol, which is the primary glucocorticoid in humans, and corticosterone, which is the primary glucocorticoid in the rat, have also been measured using a competitive protein-binding assay that takes advantage of the binding affinity of the glucocorticoid-binding globulin found in the plasma. Many drugs can interfere with the measurement of corticosteroids and ketosteroids (Table 30.14).

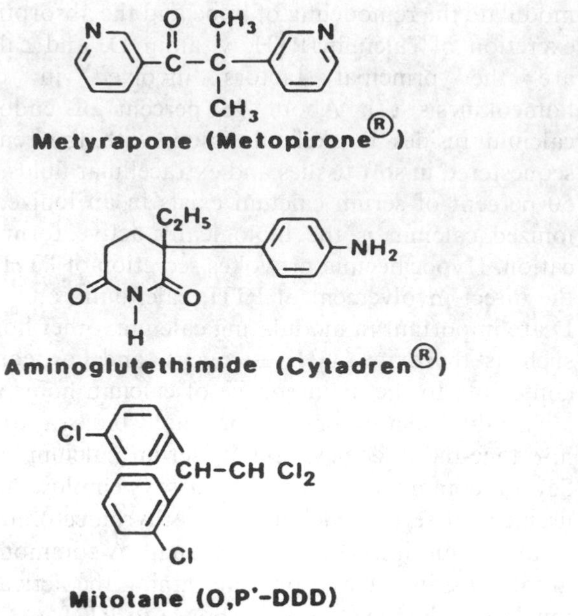

FIG. 30.5. Agents that inhibit adrenocortical steroid biosynthesis.

Table 30.13[a]
Agents causing lesions to the adrenal gland

Adrenal cortex	Adrenal medulla
Adriamycin	Acrylonitrile
Aminoglutethimide	ACTH
4-aminopyrazolo (3,4-d)pyrimidine	Alloxan
Cadmium	Blocadren
Carbon tetrachloride	Chlordecone
Chloramphenicol	o-Chlorobenzylidine
Chlordane	Malononitrile
Chloroform	Cysteamine
Chlorphentermine	Dichloromethane
Chlorpromazine	7,12-Dimethylbenzanthracene
Copper	Estrogens
Cyclosporin	Growth hormone
Cyproterone	Interleukin-2
o,p′-DDD	Lactitol
Danazol	Lactose
Dichlorvos	Malathion
7,12-Dimethylbenzanthracene	Mannitol
Etomidate	1-Methyl-4-phenyl-1,2,3,6-tetrahydropyrine (MPTP)
5-Fluorouracil	Neuroleptics
Kepone	Nicotine
Ketoconazole	Pyrazole
Nicotine	Reserpine
Phenobarbital	Retinol acetate
Polychlorinated biphenyls	Sorbitol
Spironolactone	Thiouracil
Tamoxifen	TSH
TCDD	Thyroid hormones
Tetrahydrocannabinol	1,1,2-Trichloroethane
Toxaphene	Xylitol

[a]From Reference 10.

Table 30.14
Drugs known to interfere with the measurement of corticosteroids and ketosteroids

Antibiotics/antibacterial agents
Nalidixic acid
Sulfamerazine
Triacetyloleandomycin
Sedatives/tranquilizers
Chloral hydrate
Chlordiazepoxide
Chlorpromazine
Ethinamate
Meprobamate
Phenaglycodol
Reserpine
Monoamine oxidase inhibitors
Etryptamine
Oral hypoglycemic agents
Acetohexamide
Miscellaneous drugs
Colchicine
Phenytoin (DPH)
Quinidine
Quinine
Spironolactone

With the development of immunochemical techniques, it was found that plasma glucocorticoids could be effectively measured using the RIA. A complicating factor was the existence of competition between the endogenous glucocorticoid-binding globulin and the added antibody for the radioligand.

Stress can produce a rapid increase in ACTH production, which, in turn, promotes the secretion of adrenocortical hormones. Thus, the conditions in which the animal is prepared for blood sampling can modify the corticoid levels. It has been demonstrated that under ether anesthesia, blood corticoid levels are higher than those found after pentobarbital administration, which are higher than those measured following decapitation. Likewise, the time elapsed following the administration of pentobarbital influences blood hormone levels. Stress can be a major problem affecting the interpretation of results. An additional related problem is that fairly large volumes of blood must be drawn for adrenocortical hormone measurement.

Adrenocortical function can be effectively monitored by measuring corticosteroid levels in 24-h urine samples. Major advantages to this approach are that

(a) the animals can be housed stress-free in metabolic cages during toxicity testing, and
(b) serial measurements can be conducted in the same animal by noninvasive techniques without killing of the animal.

However, this approach could not be used to measure urinary aldosterone in the rat because the primary site of degradation for aldosterone is the liver. Only about 1% of the secreted aldosterone is excreted unchanged in the urine. Nevertheless, relative changes in the urinary corticosteroid patterns could be of value as a screen for adrenotoxicity during chronic toxicity studies. RIA is the method of choice for the determination of urinary corticosteroids.

GONADS

Male Sex Hormones (Androgens)

Male reproductive toxicology endpoints can be assessed in several ways (Table 30.15). Androgens can be chemically measured or androgen-dependent end organs can be used to determine the endocrine status

Table 30.15[a]
End points used in assessment of male reproductive system

Sperm count
Sperm motility (reflectospermiograph)
Sperm head morphology
Testicular morphology
Sperm production rates
Epididymal sperm numbers and transit time
Spermatogenesis (dual-parameter flow cytometry)
Sperm membrane integrity
Viability (eosin Y exclusion)
Hypo-osmotic swelling
Nuclear maturity
Acid aniline blue stain
Nuclear Chromatin decondensation (SDS)
Acrosome assessment
Normal intact acrosomes
Acrosin activity
Objective motility assessment
Linearity (VSL/VCL)
ALH
Sperm-oocyte interraction
Sperm-zona pellucida binding ratio
Sperm-oolemma binding ratio
Serum follicle-stimulating hormone and luteinizing hormone
Serum testosterone and dihydrotestosterone
Gravimetric response (e.g., prostate, seminal vesicles)
Sex accessory organ biochemical constitutions (e.g., fructose)
Hemizona Assay (HZA)

[a] From Reference 61.

Table 30.16[a]
Possible sites of action of agents affecting the reproductive system

Anatomical site	Endocrine effect(s)
Central nervous system	
Cerebral cortex	Altered secretion of FSH/LH[b]
Median eminence	Altered releasing hormone secretion
Adenohypopysis	Changes in gonadotrophin secretion
Peripheral target organs	
Ovary	Altered secretion of estrogens
Testes	Altered secretion of androgens
Liver	Increased catabolism of steroids
Kidney	Increased excretion of steroids

[a] From Reference 61.
[b] FSH/LH, follicle-stimulating hormone/luteinizing hormone.

of male sex hormones. There are several anatomical sites wherein androgens and other steroids can be biotransformed (Table 30.16).

Some cell types of the testes are more sensitive to chemical insult than others. The various subpopulations of cells within the testes include the germ cells, the Sertoli cells, and the Leydig cells (interstitial cells) (Figure 30.2). Cross-sections of the mammalian testes reveal the seminiferous tubules containing the germinal epithelium and the Sertoli cells. Leydig cells lie outside these tubules and are located in the interstitium (Figure 30.6).

Gonadotoxicants may act directly on the testes or indirectly via the central nervous system (CNS) (Table 30.17). Relative to the germinal epithelium, the Leydig cells are not sensitive to the toxic effects of chemicals. A pig Leydig cell culture system has been devised to evaluate testicular toxicity (5). This in vitro system can test the ability of a compound to inhibit steroidogenesis. Some physiochemical characteristics of gonadotoxicants are shown in Table 30.18. The toxicity of a particular gonadotoxicant depends to some extent on its ability to penetrate the blood–testes barrier. In younger animals the testicular gap junctions are still relatively permeable and the germinal epithelium may be more vulnerable to chemicals and/or drugs than in the adult testes.

Androgens are steroids (Figure 30.7). They can be measured fluorometrically by chromatography and by RIA. They also can be bioassayed using various biological responses such as the stimulation of accessory sex organ weights in castrated animals (e.g., prostate gland or seminal vesicle weights). Still other androgen assessments can be made by measuring male sex accessory gland constituents (e.g., seminal vesicle fructose levels and zinc concentrations).

Androgens possess three main biological actions:

(a) virilizing or masculinizing actions;
(b) protein anabolic or myotropic actions; and
(c) antiestrogenic effects.

All of these biological effects can be bioassayed in experimental animals. Rodents are the most commonly used animal for the bioassay of androgens.

The actions of male sex hormones, that is, their masculinizing actions, are usually bioassayed on the basis of the response of male sex accessory organs. Generally, either the rat seminal vesicle or ventral lobes of the prostate gland are used to bioassay androgens. Figure 30.8 reveals the general anatomical relations of the rat sex accessory glands. For the bioassay, rats are castrated, and the sex accessory glands are allowed to regress for about seven days. Using testosterone as a standard, castrate rats are injected for several days, the animals killed, and either the seminal vesicles (empty) or the ventral prostate glands removed and weighed (Figure 30.9). Sometimes immature rats are used for the bioassay instead of castrated animals.

Another classical bioassay that has been used to assess androgenic activity is the weight or the size of the comb of the castrated cock or immature cockerel. The direct application of testosterone (or other androgenic substances) to the comb causes it to increase in size and weight. The rat levator ani muscle weight has been used to bioassay the protein anabolic actions of androgens. The levator ani bioassay was developed following observations of the myotropic and nitrogen-retaining activities of certain androgenic steroids. There is a lack of specificity of this test as a measure of protein anabolic activity. The levator ani test ordinarily uses immature castrate rats that have been treated for one week with the steroid. In addition to androgen bioassay methods using rodent sex accessory organs and muscles, as well as bird combs, the male sex hormones exert a renotropic action in mice. Androgens can stimulate the growth of the kidneys in castrate or immature mice.

Chemical indicator tests also have been used to assess androgen activity. Sex accessory organs contain several biochemical constituents that are androgen-dependent (36). For example, sex accessory fructose decreases following castration and can be restored by androgen administration. Sex accessory fructose has been used as a sensitive chemical indicator for testosterone and other androgens. Fructose can be measured spectrophotometrically by several colorimetric reactions. Similarly, sex accessory organ citric acid can be used to assess androgenic activity. These chemical indicator tests for androgens are more sensitive than the gravimetric responses used in bioassay procedures. A number of different endpoints to assess male reproductive function have been proposed for food and color additives (53).

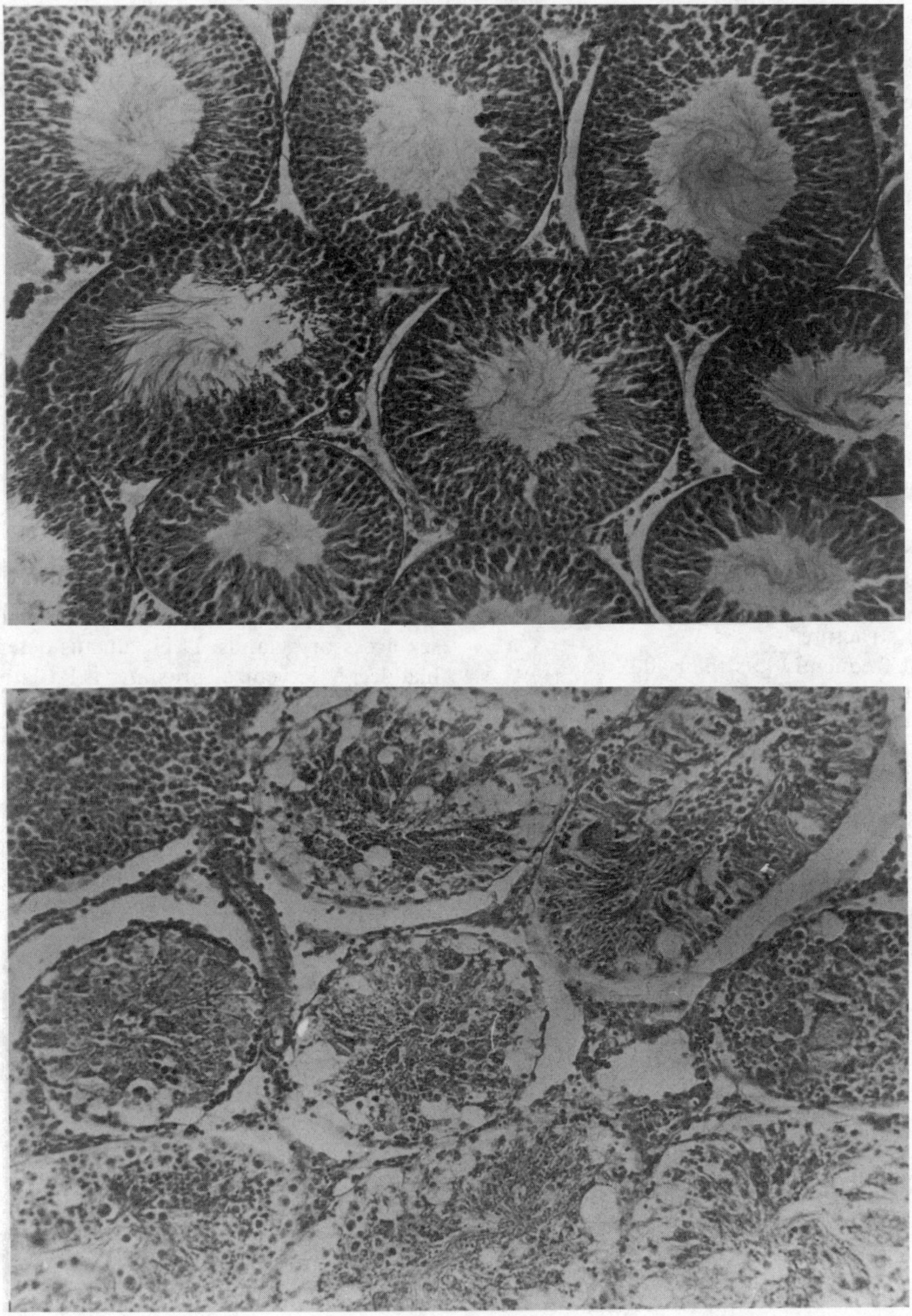

FIG. 30.6. Normal rat testes (top) and chemical-induced sterility in rat testes (bottom). Note the partially sterile seminiferous tubules.

Urinary creatine profiles have been used as a chemical indicator for testicular toxicity (40). Several chemicals have been assessed for their testicular toxicity as evidenced by increases in urinary creatine (Table 30.19). Creatine is associated primarily with cells of the seminiferous epithelium. Several chemicals destroy the germ cells and this is reflected by creatinuria. Chemicals that destroy primarily Leydig cells (e.g., EDS) do not produce creatinuria. EDS exerts a direct cytotoxic action on the Leydig cells. Creatinuria is related to testicular degeneration and a substantial portion of the testicular creatine is associated with the cells of the seminiferous epithelium.

Table 30.17
Sites of action of gonadotoxicants

Indirect-acting (e.g., CNS)
Hormonal
Nonhormonal
Direct-acting (e.g., testes)
Hormonal
Nonhormonal
Mixed (i.e., indirect and direct)
Hormonal
Nonhormonal

Table 30.18
Some physicochemical characteristics of gonadotoxicants

Usually lipophilic
Avidity for adrogen receptor
Can permeate the testes–blood barrier
Diverse chemical structure
Molecular weight frequently less than 400
Propensity for rapidly dividing cells

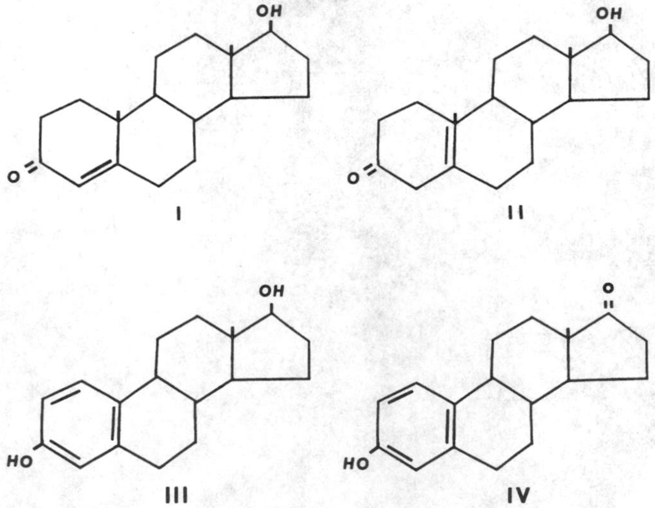

FIG. 30.7. I: Testosterone. II: Dihydrotestosterone. III: Estradiol-17β. IV: Estrone.

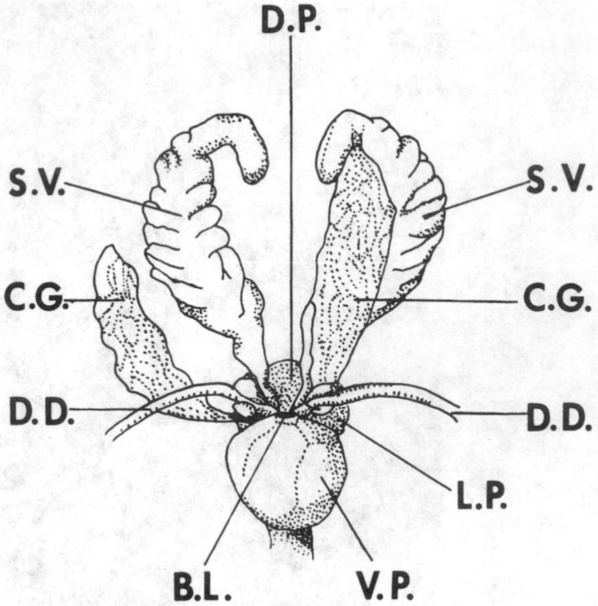

FIG. 30.8. Anatomical relation of components of rodent sex accessory glands. D.D., ductus deferens; B.L., bladder; V.P.,ventral prostate; L.P., lateral prostate; C.G., coagulating gland (also called anterior prostate); S. V. seminal vesicle; D.P., dorsal prostate.

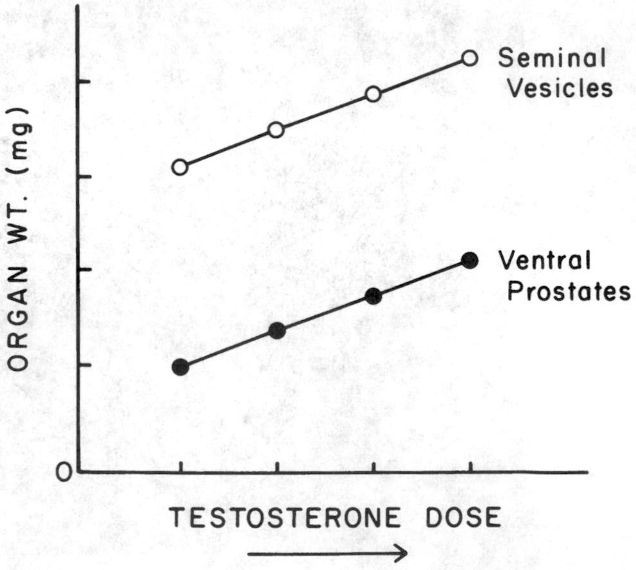

FIG. 30.9. Bioassay of adrogens using rat seminal vesicles or ventral prostate glands from castrated rats.

Testosterone levels have been determined using double-isotope derivative methods, gas liquid chromatography, and fluorometric procedures. Although these testosterone methods are specific and sensitive, elaborate purification is essential for accuracy, and routine application is often time-consuming.

Competitive protein binding assays and RIAs are available. In the RIA, antiserum against testosterone can be produced in rabbits immunized with testosterone-3-oxime-beef serum albumin. Biological samples must undergo solvent extraction and be eluted on microcolumns. If the extraction and purification of

Table 30.19[a]
Urinary creatine—a test for cell-specific testicular toxins

Agent	Urinary creatine	Site of toxicity
Cadmium (Cd)	↑	Vasculature
2-methoxyethanol (2-ME)	↑	Early & late stage Pachytene primary Spermatocytes
Methoxyacetic Acid (MAA)	↑	Germ cell
Di-n-pentyl phthalate (DPP)	↑	Initially Sertoli Cell; secondarily Germ cells
Dinitrobenzene (DNB)	↑	Initially Sertoli Cell; secondarily Germ cells
Ethane dimethane sulphonate (EDS)	↔	Leydig cell

[a]From Reference 40.

the samples are carried out appropriately, the RIA of testosterone is highly sensitive and accurate, capable of detecting testosterone in nanogram to picogram amounts.

Recently, a method has been described for assessing androgens under field or remote site conditions (22). Monoclonal antibody techniques can be used for assessing androgen receptors.

Male Infertility

The etiology of male infertility may be genetic or non-genetic. There may also be a psychological component. Both a neural or a hormonal element may be associated with male infertility. The hormonal factor can be affected by gonadotoxicants which cause spermatogenic arrest and degeneration of seminiferous tubules and their contents. Indeed, industrial chemicals (e.g., dibromochloropropane—DBCP), alkyling agents (e.g., nitrogen mustards), x-rays, and cryptorchidism can cause sterile tubules leading to infertility (57).

There are many useful tests that can aid in determining reproductive success, but such tests must be undertaken in both the male and the female (Table 30.20). Although the measurement of fertility is imprecise, it does have the advantage of integrating all reproductive functions from both the male and the female (71). Testicular histology is non-quantitative, but does provide some information about gonadal physiology (or pathology).

Through transgene technology, there are now several animal models in which to study male sterility (26). Gonadotropin-releasing hormone (GnRH) cell lines have been developed and can produce a transgenic mouse with hypothalamic hypogonadism (69). Thus, transgenic mouse models can be used to study mechanisms of spermatogenic arrest as well as altered neuroendocrine systems that interfere with gonadotropin secretion.

Female Sex Hormones

Estrogens are biosynthesized by the theca interna cells of the ovarian follicles, the corpus luteum, the placenta, and, in lesser amounts, the adrenal cortex and the testes. Estradiol-17β is the major estrogen secreted, although some estrone is present in blood. Estrone can be further metabolized to estriol by hepatic enzymes. Of these three main natural occurring estrogens, estradiol-17β is undoubtedly the most potent.

All of these naturally occurring estrogens are steroids. Synthetic estrogens such as diethylstilbestrol are not steroids. Although steroidal and nonsteroidal estrogens can be bioassayed using similar tests, their different molecular structures do not allow them to be measured by similar chemical methodologies. Testing guidelines for evaluating reproductive and developmental toxicity in the female have recently undergone some revisions (11).

The two methods once commonly used to bioassay estrogenic hormones involve either histological changes in the vaginal epithelium or an increase in the weight of the rodent uterus. Both assays require the use of ovariectomized animals.

The mouse vaginal smear bioassay uses ovariectomized animals with various standard doses of estradiol. To establish that the animals are responding, vaginal smears are characterized by nucleated epithelial cells or cornified cells. Vaginal responses characterized by epithelial cornification are considered positive responders to estradiol.

Estrogen bioassays also include using an increase in uterine weight in the ovariectomized rat or mouse. Uterine weight falls precipitously after ovariectomy. The fall in uterine weight can be restored by daily injections of estradiol. Ovariectomized mice are injected subcutaneously, killed, and the uteri removed and weighed. Like the vaginal smear bioassay, at least two dilutions of the unknown substance are run concurrently with the estradiol dose-response curve.

The immature chick can also be used to assess estrogenic potency. The immature chick bioassay is based on estrogens stimulating oviduct weights.

These bioassays (i.e., vaginal cornification, uterine weights, and oviduct weights), although quite sensitive

Table 30.20[a]

Potentially useful tests of male reproductive toxicity for laboratory animals and/or humans

Testis
Size in situ
Weight
Spermatid reserves
Gross and histological evaluation
Nonfunctional tubules (%)
Tubules with lumen sperm (%)
Tubule diameter
Counts of leptotene spermatocytes

Epididymis
Weight and histology
Number of sperm in distal half
Motility of sperm, distal end (%)
Gross sperm morphology, distal end (%)
Detailed sperm morphology, distal end (%)
Biochemical assays

Accessory Sex Glands
Histology
Gravimetric

Semen
Total volume
Gel-free volume
Sperm concentration
Total sperm/ejaculate
Total sperm/day of abstinence
Sperm motility, visual (%)
Sperm motility, vdeotape (%) (and velocity)
Gross sperm morphology
Detailed sperm morphology

Endocrine
Luteinizing hormone
Follicle-stimulating hormone
Gonadotropin-releasing hormone

Fertility
Ratio exposed: pregnant females
Number embryos or young per pregnant female
Ratio viable embryos: corpora lutea
Number 2–8 cell eggs
Number unfertilized eggs; abnormal eggs
Sperm per ovum

In Vitro
Incubation of sperm in agent
Hamster egg penetration test

Other tests considered
Tonometric measurement of testicular consistency
Qualitative testicular histology
Stage of cycle at which spermiation occurs
Quantitative testicular histology

Sperm Motility
Time-exposure photography
Multiple-exposure photography
Cinemicrography
Videomicrography
Sperm membrane characteristics
Evaluation of sperm metabolism
Fluorescent Y bodies in spermatozoa
Flow cytometry of spermatozoa
Karyotyping human sperm proneuclei
Cervical mucus penetration test

[a] From Reference 61.

to estrogen, have largely been abandoned for newer and more expedient and accurate assays. Nevertheless, cytology and histology of the female reproductive system remains important (Table 30.21).

Estrogens can be measured colorimetrically, by RIA, by monoclonal assays, and by other immunotechniques. Estrogen receptors can also be measured by monoclonal antibody techniques which employ enzyme immunoassays (EIA). Likewise, progesterone receptors can be measured with EIAs (15). The evaluation of techniques for the detection of functional estrogenicity has received renewed attention (27).

Ovarian Toxicity

In comparison to the known testicular toxicants, far less attention has been paid to ovarian toxicity. Some drugs are known to be toxic to the ovaries, such as the nitrogen mustards, chlorambucil, cyclophosphamide, busulfan, and vinblastine (19). The ovary is a site for chemical injury (37), and both the granulosa cells and the thecal cells can be targets for chemical injury (Table 30.22). Chemicals that are gonadotropin inhibitor antagonists, that damage gonadotropin receptors, or that uncouple the receptor from other molecules necessary for

Table 30.21[a]
Potentially useful tests of female reproductive toxicity

Ovary	*Cervix/Vulva/Vagina*
Organ weight	Cytology
Histology	Histology
Number of oocytes	Mucus production
Rate of follicular atresia	Mucus quality (sperm penetration test)
Follicular steroidogenesis	
Follicular maturation	
Oocyte maturation	*Fertility*
Ovulation	Ratio exposed: pregnant females
Luteal function	Number of embryos or young per pregnant female
	Ratio viable embryos: corpora lutea
Hypothalamus	Number 2–8 cell eggs
Histology	Number of unfertilized eggs; abnormal eggs
Altered synthesis and release of neurotransmitters, neuromodulators, and neurohormones	Number of corpora lutea
	In Vitro
	In vitro fertilization of superovulated eggs, either exposed to chemical in culture or from treated females
Pituitary	
Histology	
Altered synthesis and release of trophic hormones	
Endocrine	
Gonadotropin	
Choronic gonadotropin levels	
Estrogen and progesterone	
Oviduct	
Histology	
Gamete transport	
Fertilization	
Transport of early embryo	
Uterus	
Cytology and histology	
Luminal fluid analysis (xenobiotics, proteins)	
Decidual response	
Dysfunctional bleeding	

[a] From Reference 61.

hormone action, would be expected to adversely affect granulosa cells. Thecal cells provide precursors for granulosa cell steroidogenesis. Xenobiotics can alter either granulosa cells or thecal cells.

The oocytes are also targets for chemical insult or injury. Alkylating agents, lead, and mercury can be very destructive to the mammalian oocyte (37).

PANCREAS

The endocrine pancreas secretes two important hormones: insulin and glucagon. These hormones are synthesized in the islets of Langerhans by alpha cells (glucagon) and beta cells (insulin). The morphological arrangement of the rat pancreas is depicted in Figure

Table 30.22[a]
Ovarian cells as targets for chemical injury

	Granulosa Cells
Site of Action	*Mechanism of Action (Outcome)*
FSH/LH Receptors	Decreased receptor population
	Competition for receptors
	Uncoupling of receptors to secondary messenger
Steroidogenesis	Altered estrogen production (e.g., aromatase activity)
	Altered progesterone production (e.g., enzymatic inhibition)
	Insufficient androgens
	Inadequate luteinization (e.g., decreased progesterone)
Cell Proliferation	Cytotoxicity and mitotic inhibitors
	Reduction of growth factors
Thecal Cells	
LH Receptors	Decreased receptor population
	Competition for receptors
	Uncoupling of receptors to secondary messengers
Steroidogenesis	Inhibition of enzymes (e.g., decreased androgens)
	Insufficient substrate for granulosa cells
Cell Proliferation	Cytotoxicity and mitotic inhibitors
	Disrupted migration of stroma
	Reduction of growth factors

[a] From Reference 37.

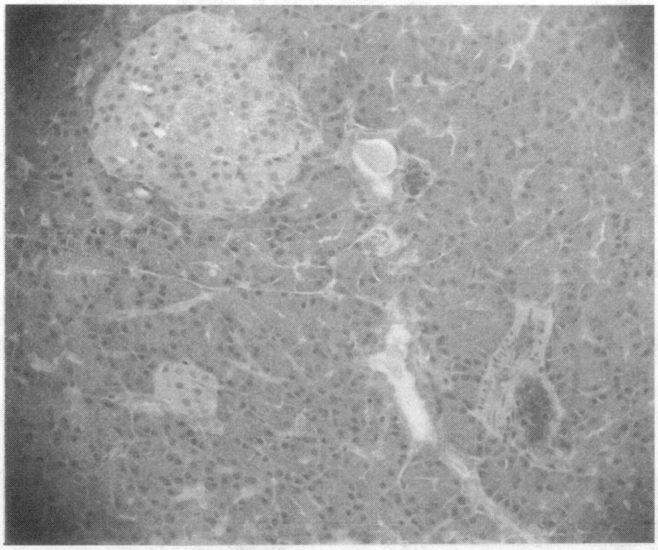

FIG. 30.10. Histology of rat pancreas. Note the acini ducts. 256× magnification.

30.10. A concern when testing for toxicity is the potential for the compound to interfere with the normal functioning of the pancreatic beta cells. The indicator that often alerts the toxicologist to a possible pancreatic side effect is hyperglycemia. Although this increased blood glucose level would usually be detected during routine clinical chemistry analyses, additional tests may be required to pinpoint specific pancreatic toxicity.

The interaction between insulin and carbohydrate, fat, and protein metabolism represents some of the complexities seen in diabetes mellitus. Hyperglycemia may result from impaired utilization of glucose by cells due principally to insufficient production of insulin. The failure of glucose to penetrate adipose tissue mobilizes fat, producing a rise in the free fatty acid and triglyceride content of plasma and the triglyceride content of the liver. A diabetic fatty liver can occur from the absence of lipoprotein synthesis due to accelerated gluconeogenesis. If glucose oxidation is impaired, fatty acids form the major source of energy. This condition generates an excess of intermediary metabolites, collectively described as ketone bodies (acetone, acetoacetic acid, and β-hydroxybutyric acid), which can lead to metabolic acidosis.

Hyperglycemia also can lead to presence of glucose in the urine (glycosuria) when the blood glucose levels exceed the renal threshold of approximately 180 mg/dl. At lower levels, all the filtered glucose is normally reabsorbed by the renal tubules. Blood glucose levels increased to the point of glycosuria also can be caused by emotional stress and the concomitant release of glucose from liver glycogen in response to epinephrine. Several drugs can affect blood glucose levels and can either increase or antagonize glucose levels (Table 30.23).

Table 30.23
Interaction of drugs with oral hypoglycemic agents and insulin

Enhanced effect (i.e., greater hypoglycemic action)	Antagonist effect
Ethanol	Acetazolamide
Anabolic steroids	D-Thyroxine
Chloramphenicol	Corticosteroids
Dihydoxycoumarin	Phenothiazines
Guanethidine	Epinephrine
Oxytetracycline	Phenytoin (DPH)
MAO inhibitors	Marijuana
Phenylbutazone	Oral contraceptives
Phenyramidol	Diuretics
K^+ salts	(e.g., chlorthalidone,
Propranolol	ethracrynic acid,
Probenecid	furosemide, thiazides,
Salicylates	triamterene)
Sulfonamides	
Sulfinpyrazone	

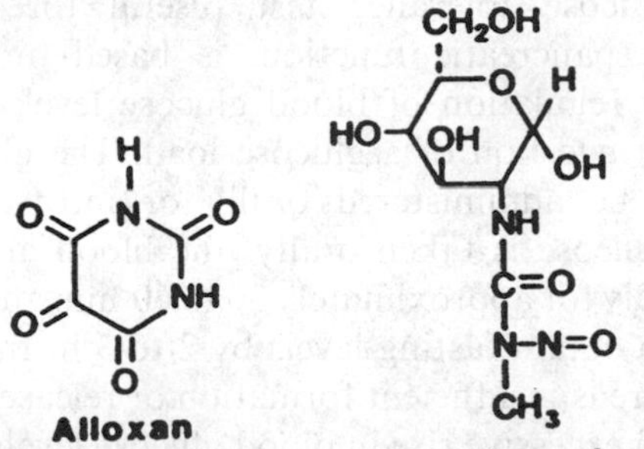

FIG. 30.11. Agents that inhibit pancreatic insulin and glucagon secretion.

Glycosuria also can be the consequence of impaired renal tubular function caused by compounds such as the glycoside phlorizin. Renal glycosuria can produce an osmotic diuretic effect that leads to dehydration and polydipsia. Glycogenolysis and gluconeogenesis are increased in diabetes, generating glucose, which in turn increases blood glucose levels.

As discussed earlier, the discovery of hyperglycemia during toxicity testing demands a more detailed investigation to determine the underlying mechanism(s). Such investigation focuses on the functional integrity of the pancreas and, in particular, of the beta cells. Experimental diabetes mellitus can be produced by destroying beta cell function with alloxan or streptozocin (Figure 30.11). In addition to chemically induced destruction of beta cells by alloxan and streptozocin, other chemicals can be diabetogenic (16,73). Alloxan, a cyclic urea analogue, can produce permanent hyperglycemia in the rabbit. Streptozotocin, a methylnitroso-urea analogue, has generally replaced alloxan to produce experimental insulin-dependent diabetes in laboratory animals. Both agents destroy pancreatic beta cells, but streptozotocin may involve the alkylation of critical cell components. Chlorozotocin, an analog of streptozocin, is lethal to beta cells in culture. Vacor (pyriminil), cyproheptadine, and pentamidine are all capable of causing pancreatic dysfunction.

In addition to chemically induced experimental models for diabetes mellitus, there are several genetic strains that are both diabetes-susceptible and diabetes-resistant (Table 30.24). Thus, experimental animal models for diabetes mellitus may exploit genetic susceptibility or may involve chemically induced destruction beta cells (32). Several inbred strains of mice are sensitive to *db* gene-induced diabetes with sexual dimorphism in some inbred strains, emphasizing the relationship between the obesity gene and sex. A major genetic regulator of inbred strain diabetogenic sensitivity is gender-related. In the rat, the BHE strain is an excellent animal model for the study of non-insulin-dependent diabetes mellitus (NIDDM). The Cdb : BHE stock is a subline of the parent BHE stock.

The NOD (nonobese diabetic) mouse is an ideal animal model of insulin-dependent diabetes mellitus (66). Spontaneous diabetes in the BioBreeding (BB) rat, like human Type I diabetes mellitus, results from the destruction of the pancreatic islets by autoreactive T lymphocytes recognizing beta cell-specific antigens.

Table 30.24[a]
Genetically altered rodents used to study diabetes mellitus

	Diabetes-Susceptible Strains
Mice	C57BLKsJ
	DBA/2J
	SWR/J
	C3H. SW/SnJ
	C3HeB/FeCHp (males only)
	CBA/Lt (males only)
	NOD (IDDM)
Rats	BB (IDDM)
	BHE
	BHE/cdb
	Diabetes-Resistant Strains
Mice	C57BL/6J
	129/J
	Ma/MYJ

[a] From Reference 62.

Table 30.25[a]
Drugs that have been implicated as causing acute pancreatitis

Definite	*Possible*
Azathiorine	Bumetanide
Cisplatin	Anticholinesterase
Colaspase	Carbamazepine
(L-asparaginase)	Chlorthalidone
Furosemide	Clonidine
Tetracycline	Colchicine
Thiazides	Corticosteroids
Sulphonamides	Co-trimoxazole
	Cyclosporin
	Cytarabine (cytosine arabinoside)
	Diazoxide
	Enalapril
Probable	Ergotamine
	ERCP contrast media
Cimetidine	Ethacrynic acid
Indomethacin	Isoniazid
Mefenamic acid	Isotretinoin
Estrogens	(13-cis-retinoic acid)
Opiates	Mercaptopurine
Paracetamol	Methyldopa
(acetaminophen)	Metronidazole
Phenformin	Nitrofurantoin
Valproic acid	Oxphenbutazone
Fonofos	Piroxicam
Diazinon	Procainamide
	Rifampicin
	Salicylates
	Sulindac

[a] From Reference 2.

Chemical insult is not unique to the endocrine pancreas. Indeed, many agents can cause acute pancreatitis (Table 30.25). Side effects resulting from a number of cytotoxic agents (e.g., colchicine), antibiotics (e.g., tetracyclines), antibacterial drugs (e.g., sulfonamides), and diuretics (e.g., thiazides) can produce irritation and inflammation of pancreatic cells.

Measurement of Insulin

Before RIAs, insulin was bioassayed using the rabbit hypoglycemia test. The biological potencies of porcine, bovine, and human insulin can be assessed using the rabbit bioassay. Insulin was the first protein hormone to be measured by RIA. Although the RIA techniques that are available are similar with regard to the interaction between antigen and antibody, there are numerous variations in the methods for separating free insulin from antibody-bound insulin: gel filtration, salt precipitation, alcohol precipitation, precipitation with anti-gamma-globulin serum, and absorption on anion-exchange resin, cellulose, dextran-coated charcoal, antibody-coated tubes, and Sephadex-coupled antibodies.

A radioreceptor assay has been developed for quantitation of plasma insulin levels. Plasma insulin levels may also be determined by enzyme-linked immunosorbent assay (ELISA). Generally, this procedure has a number of drawbacks that preclude its routine use for the measurement of insulin, including a lower sensitivity than is seen with the RIA. A hyperglycemic clamp can be used to assess insulin secretion and insulin sensitivity (39).

Insulin receptors can be isolated from a variety of sources, including placenta, rat liver plasma membranes, human lymphocytes, and guinea pig kidney.

Glucose Tolerance Tests

The glucose tolerance test, useful for evaluating endocrine pancreatic function, is based on the compensatory regulation of blood glucose levels by insulin following ingestion of a glucose load. The glucose load also can be administered orally or intravenously. If 50 g of glucose is taken orally, the blood glucose level rises rapidly for approximately 30 to 60 min and then falls rapidly to obtain fasting levels by 2 to 3 h. In situations where there is insufficient formation or release of insulin, there is an excessive rise in blood glucose levels following ingestion of the glucose load, and a slow, gradual fallback to pre-ingestion levels. Abnormal glucose tolerance curves are evident in diabetes mellitus, but may also be abnormal in other pathological states. Glucose oxidase methods involving colorimetric reactions are routinely used to measure blood sugar. Capillary blood glucose can be used to monitor diabetes mellitus (13).

Cytological Evaluation of Pancreatic Islet Cells

Alpha and beta cells can be differentiated using an aldehyde–fuchsin stain (Scott stain) following fixation of the tissue in Bouin's solution. The alpha cells stain light and the beta cells stain dark, permitting calculation of an alpha cell/beta cell ratio.

Pseudoisocyanic staining permits direct demonstration of insulin in the beta cells. The reaction involves the development of SO_2 groups formed by the oxidative splitting of the disulfide bridges of insulin with potassium permanganate.

Organ culture techniques for studying pancreatic islets have been investigated (35). The availability of suitably characterized dispersed islet cell preparation affords another in vitro test system to examine the effects of various drugs and chemicals on the pancreas (70). Monoclonal antibody methods are also available to assay for islet cell antibodies (55).

ACKNOWLEDGMENTS

The authors express their appreciation to Michelle Grigsby for her assistance in preparing this manuscript, and Barbara Thomas for her grammatical and editing diligence.

QUESTIONS

1. Define bioassay.
2. Describe the principle(s) involved in the measurement of hormone(s) using RIAs.
3. What is an ELISA test?
4. Discuss the importance of monoclonal antibodies in immunoassays.
5. Discuss chemical and nonchemical factors that can affect hormone levels.
6. How is androgen secretion affected by the adenohypopysis?
7. What are the principle factors involved in calcium homeokinasis?
8. Describe conditions or factors that affect insulin secretion.

REFERENCES

1. Badger, T. M., Millard, W. J., McCormick, G. F., Bowers, C. Y., and Martin, J. B. (1984): The effects of growth hormone (GH)-releasing peptides on GH secretion in perifused pituitary cells of adult male rats. *Endocrinology*, 115:1432–1438.
2. Banerjee, A. K., Patel, K. J., and Grainger, S. L. (1989): Drug-induced acute pancreatitis: A critical review. *Med. Toxicol. Adverse Drug Exp.*, 4:186–198.
3. Barsono, C. P., and Thomas, J. A. (1992): Endocrine disorders of occupational and environmental origin. *Occup. Med.*, 7:479–502.
4. Bennett, B. D., and Wells, D. J. (1992): Endocrinology. In: *Clinical Chemistry*, 2nd ed., edited by M. L. Bishop, J. L. Duben-Engelkirk, and E. P. Fody, pp. 317–352. J. B. Lippincott Company, Philadelphia.
5. Brun, H. P., Leonard, J. F., Moronvalle, V., Caillaud, J. M., Melcion, C., and Cordier, A. (1991): Pig Leydig cell culture: A useful in vitro test for evaluating the testicular toxicity of compounds. *Toxicol. Appl. Pharmacol.*, 108:307–320.
6. Burd, J. M., Weightman, D. R., and Baylis, P. H. (1985): Solid phase radioimmunoassay for direct measurement of human plasma oxytocin. *J. Immunoassay*, 6:227–243.
7. Capen, C. C. (1992): Pathophysiology and xenobiotic toxicity of parathyroid glands. In: *Endocrine Toxicology*, edited by C. K. Atterwill, and J. D. Flack. Cambridge University Press, Cambridge.
8. Chiu, T. T., Tam, P. P., and Mao, K. R. (1990): Evaluation of a semiquantitative urinary LH assay for ovulation detection. *Intern. J. Fertility*, 35:120–124.
9. Clark, F., and Hutton, C. W. (1985): The effect of drugs upon the assessment of thyroid function. *Adverse Drug React. Acute Poisoning Rev.*, 4:59–81.
10. Colby, H. D., and Longhurst, P. A. (1992): Toxicology of the adrenal gland. In: *Endocrine Toxicology*, edited by C. K. Atterwill, and J. D. Flack. Cambridge University Press, Cambridge.
11. Collins, T. F. X., Sprando, R. L., Hansen, D. L., Shackelford, M. E., and Welsh, J. J. (1998): Testing guidelines for evaluation of reproductive and developmental toxicity of food additives in females. *Intern. J. Toxicol.*, 17:299–325.
12. Davis, J. R. E. (1996): Molecular biology techniques in endocrinology. *Clin. Endocrin.*, 45:125–133.
13. Davis, M., and Walker, E. A. (1992): Capillary blood glucose monitoring for clinical decision making. *Lab. Med.*, 23:591–598.
14. Desai, M. P., Khatkhatay, M. I., Sankolli, G. M., and Joshi, U. M. (1991): Importance of selection of separation system in the development of enzyme immunoassay: An experience with follicle stimulating hormone (FSH) assay. *J. Immunoassay*, 12:83–98.
15. DiFronzo, G., Miodini, P., Brivio, M., Cappelletti, V., Coradini, D., Granata, G., Ronchi, E. (1986): Comparison of immunochemical and radioligand binding assays for estrogen receptors in human breast tumors. *Cancer Res.*, 46:4278s–4281s.
16. Fischer, L. J. (1985): Drugs and chemicals that produce diabetes. *TIPS* 2:72–75.
17. Gornall, A. G., Luxton, A. W., and Bhavnini, B. R. (1986): Endocrine disorders. In: *Applied Biochemistry of Clinical Disorders*, edited by A. G. Gornall, pp. 285–358. J. B. Lippincott, Philadelphia.
18. Guiles, H. J. (1992): Thyroid function. In: *Clinical Chemistry*, 2nd ed., edited by M. L. Bishop, J. L. Duben-Engelkirk, and E. P. Fody, pp. 509–525. J. B. Lippincott Company, Philadelphia.
19. Haney, A. F. (1985): Effects of toxic agents on ovarian function. In: *Target Organ Toxicology Series*, edited by J. A. Thomas, K. S. Korach, and J. A. McLachlan, pp. 181–193. Raven Press, New York.
20. Hasegawa, Y., Miyamoto, K., Iwamura, S., and Igarashi, M. (1988): Changes in serum concentrations of inhibin in cyclic pigs. *J. Endocr.*, 118:211–219.
21. Hermann, G. A., Sugiura, H. T., and Krumm, R. P. (1986): Comparison of thyrotropin assays by relative operating characteristic analysis. *Arch. Pathol. Lab. Med.*, 110:21–25.
22. Howe, C. J., and Handelsman, D. J. (1997): Use of filter paper for sample collection and transport in steroid pharmacology. *Clin. Chem.*, 43:1408–1415.
23. Hsu, S. M., Raine, L., and Fanger, H. A. (1981): Comparative study of the proxidase-antiperoxidase method for studying polypeptide antibodies. *Am. J. Clin. Pathol.*, 75:734.
24. Innis, M. A., Gelfand, D. H., Sninsky, J. J., and White, T. J. (1990): *PCR Protocols: A Guide to Methods and Applications*. Academic Press, Inc., San Diego.
25. Klee, D. G., Kao, P. C., and Heath, H., III. (1988): Hypercalcemia. *Endocrinol. Metab. Clin. N. Amer.*, 17:573–600.
26. Kobayashi, E., Kunieda, T., Ikadai, H., Imamichi, T., and Matsumoto, K. (1992): Genetic profiles of 11 inbred rat strains at 25 biochemical marker loci and five RFLP loci. *Lab. Anim. Sci.*, 42:86–88.
27. Korach, K. S., and McLachlan, J. A. (1995): Techniques for detection of estrogenicity. *Environ. Health Perspect.*, 103:5–8.
28. Kosugi, S., Sugawa, H., and Mori, T. (1996): TSH receptor and LH receptor. *Endocrine J.*, 43:595–604.

29. LaRose, P., Ong, H., and Du Souichm, P. (1985): Simple and rapid radioimmunoassay for the routine determination of vasopressin in plasma. *Clin. Biochem.*, 18:357–362.

30. Layman, L. C., and McDonough, P. G. (1995): Molecular genetics in reproductive endocrinology. In: *Reproductive Medicine and Surgery*, edited by E. E. Wallach, and H. A. Zacur. Mosby, St. Louis.

31. Leidy, J. W., and Robbins, R. J. (1986): Regional distribution of human growth hormone-releasing hormone in the human hypothalamus by radioimmunoassay. *J. Clin. Endocrinol. Metab.*, 62:372.

32. Leiter, E. H. (1989): The genetics of diabetes susceptibility in mice. *FASEB J.*, 3:2231–2241.

33. Leung, P. C. K., and Steele, G. L. (1992): Intracellular signaling in the gonads. *Endocrine Rev.*, 13:476–498.

34. Lorsenson, M. Y. (1985): In vitro conditions modify immunoassayability of bovine pituitary prolactin and growth hormone: Insights into their secretory granule storage forms. *Endocrinol.*, 116:1399–1407.

35. Mandel, T. E., Hoffman, L., Colier, S., Carter, W., and Koulmanda, M. (1982): Organ culture of fetal mouse and fetal human pancreatic islets for allografting. *Diabetes*, 3:39–47.

36. Mann, T. (1964): *The Biochemistry of Semen and of the Male Reproductive Tract*. Wiley, New York.

37. Mattison, D. R., Plowchalk, D. R., Meadows, M. J., Al-Juburi, A. Z., Gandy, J., and Malek, A. (1990): Reproductive toxicity: Male and female reproductive systems as targets for chemical injury. *Med. Clin. N. Amer.*, 74:391–411.

38. May, M. E., and Carey, R. M. (1985): Rapid ACTH test in practice. *Am. J. Med.*,.79:679–684.

39. Mitrakou, A., Vuorinen-Markkola, H., Raptis, G., Toft, I., Mokan, M., Strumph, P., Pimenta, W., Veneman, T., Jansen, T., and Bolli, G. (1992): Simultaneous assessment of insulin secretion and insulin sensitivity using a hyperglycemic clamp. *Clin. Endocrinol. Metab.*, 75:379–382.

40. Moore, N. P., Creasy, D. M., Gray, T. J. B., and Timbrell, J. A. (1992): Urinary creatine profiles after administration of cell-specific testicular toxicants to the rat. *Arch. Toxicol.*, 66:435–442.

41. Motomura, K., and Brent, G. A. (1998): Mechanisms of thyroid hormone action. *Endo. Metab. Clin. N. Amer.*, 27:1–23.

42. Piaditis, G. P., Hodgkinson, S. C., McLean, C., and Lowry, P. J. (1985): Thyroid stimulating hormone. *J. Immunoassay*, 6:299–319.

43. Pierce, E. A., Dame, M. C., Bouillon, R., Van Baelen, H., and DeLuca, H. F. (1985): Monoclonal antibodies to human vitamin D-binding protein. *Proc. Natl. Acad. Sci. USA*, 82:8429–8433.

44. Preissner, C. M., Klee, G. G., Scheithauer, B. W., and Abboud, C. F. (1990): Free alpha subunit of the pituitary glycoprotein hormones: Measurement in serum and tissue of patients with pituitary tumors. *Am. J. Clin. Path.*, 94:417–421.

45. Root, A. W., Duckett, G. E., Geiszler, J. E., Hu, C. S., and Bercu, B. B. (1997): Evaluation of the clinical utility of the ultrasensitive immunofluometric assay for growth hormone (GH) and of the cortisol secretory pattern in prediction of the linear growth response to treatment with GH. *J. Ped. End. Metab.*, 10:3–10.

46. Rosenfeld, L., and Blum, M. (1986): Immunoradiometric (IRMA) assay for thyrotropin (TSH) should replace the RIA method in the clinical laboratory. *Clin. Chem.*, 32:1.

47. Sambrook, J., Fritsch, E. F., and Maniatis, T. (1989): *Molecular Cloning: A Laboratory Manual*, 2nd ed. Cold Spring Harbor Laboratory Press, New York.

48. Schmalzing, D., Nashabeh, W., Yao, X. W., Mhatre, R., Regnier, F. E., Afeyan, N. B., and Fuchs, M. (1995): Capillary electrophoresis-based immunoassay for cortisol in serum. *Anal. Chem.*, 67:606–612.

49. Seethalakshmi, L., Steinberger, A., and Steinberger, E. (1984): Pituitary binding of ^{3}H-labeled Sertoli cell factor in vitro: A potential radioreceptor assay for inhibin. *Endocrinol.*, 115:1289–1294.

50. Segre, G. V., and Brown, E. N. (1998): Measurement of hormones. In: *Williams Textbook of Endocrinology*, 9th ed., edited by J. D. Wilson, D. W. Foster, H. M. Kronenberg, and P. R. Larsen, pp. 43–54. W. B. Saunders Co., Philadelphia.

51. Sgoutas, D. S., Tuten, T. E., Verras, A. A., Love, A., and Barton, E. G. (1995): AquaLite bioluminescence assay of thyrotropin in serum elevated. *Clin. Chem.* 41:1637–1643.

52. Shupnik, M. A. (1995): Measurement of gene transcription and messenger RNA. In: *Molecular Endocrinology: Basic Concepts and Clinical Correlations*, edited by B. D. Weintraub, pp. 41–58. Raven Press, New York.

53. Sprando, R. L., and Collins, T. F. X. (1998): Testing guidelines for evaluation of food additives' effects on male reproduction. *Int. J. Toxic.*, 17:327–336.

54. Squire, C. R., and Fraser, W. D. (1995): Thyroid stimulating hormone measurement using a third generation immunometric assay. *Ann. Clin. Biochem.*, 32:307–313.

55. Srikanta, S., Rabizadeh, A., Omar, M. A. K., and Eisenbarth, G. S. (1985): Assay for islet cell antibodies. *Diabetes*, 34:300.

56. Stites, D. P., Stobo, J. D., Fudenberg, H. H., and Wells, J. V. (1987): *Basic and Clinical Immunology*, 6th ed. Lange Medical Publications, Los Angeles.

57. Thomas, J. A. (1981): Reproductive hazards and environmental chemicals. *J. Toxic Subs.*, 2:318.

58. Thomas, J. A., and Keenan, E. J. (1986): Drugs affecting the endocrine system. In: *Principles of Endocrine Pharmacology*. Plenum Press, New York.

59. Thomas, J. A., and Ballantyne, B. (1990): Occupational reproductive risks: Sources, surveillance, and testing. *J. Occup. Med.*, 32:547–553.

60. Thomas, J. A. (1995): Gonadal-specific metal toxicology. In: *Metal Toxicology*, pp. 413–446. Academic Press, Inc., San Diego.

61. Thomas, J. A. (1996): Toxic responses of the reproductive system. In: *Casarett and Doull's Toxicology: The Basic Science of Poisons*, 5th ed., edited by C. D. Klaassen, pp. 547–581. Pergamon Press, New York.

62. Thomas, J. A. (1993): Transgenic animal models and genetically altered species. In: *Biotechnology and Safety Assessment*, edited by J. A. Thomas, and L. A. Myers. Raven Press, New York.

63. Thomas, J. A., editor (1996): *Endocrine Methods*, pp. 1–447. Academic Press, San Diego.

64. Thomas, J. A., and Colby, H. D., editors. (1996): *Endocrine Toxicology*, 2nd ed. Taylor & Francis, Philadelphia.

65. Thronton, P. S., Alter, C. A., Katz, L. E., Gruccio, D. A., Winyard, P. J., and Moshang, T., Jr. (1994): The new highly sensitive adrenocorticotropin assay improves detection of patients with partial adrenocorticotropin deficiency in a short-term metyrapone test. *J. Ped. Endo.*, 7:317–324.

66. Tochino, Y., Kanaya, T., and Makino, S. (1982): Genetics of NOD mice. In: *International Congress Series 597, Clinico–Genetic Genesis of Diabetes Mellitus*, edited by G. Miura, S. Baba, and Y. Goto, *Excerpta Medica*, 44:285–291.

67. Veldhuis, J. D., Liem, A. Y., South, S., Weltman, A., Weltman, J., Clemmons, D. A., Abbott, R., Mulligan, T., Johnson, M. L., Pincus, S., et al. (1995): Differential impact of age, sex steroid hormones, and obesity on basal versus pulsatile growth hormone secretion in men as assessed in an ultrasensitive chemiluminescence assay. *J. Clin. Endo. Metab.*, 80:3209–3222.

68. Watkins, S. (1998): Immunohistochemistry. In: *Current Protocols of Molecular Biology*, edited by F. M. Ausubel, R. Brent, R. E. Kingston, D. D. Moore, J. G. Seidman, J. A. Smith, and

K. Struhl, Ch. 14, sec. 6, pp. 1–13. John Wiley & Sons, Inc., New York.

69. Weiner, R. I., Wetsel, W., and Goldsmith, P. (1992): Gonadotropin-releasing hormone neuronal cell lines. *Front Neuroendo.*, 13.95–119.

70. Weir, G. C., Halban, P. A., Wollheim, C. B., Orci, L., and Renold, A. E. (1984): Dispersed adult rat pancreatic islet cells in culture; A, B, and D cell function. *Metabolism*, 33:447–453.

71. Wenk, R. E. (1992): Reproductive medicine and the clinical laboratory. In: *Clinics in Laboratory Medicine*, pp. 1–642. W. B. Saunders Co., Philadelphia.

72. Witorsch, R. J., editor. (1995): *Reproductive Toxicology*, 2nd ed. Raven Press, New York.

73. Yoon, J. W. (1990): The role of viruses and environmental factors in the induction of diabetes. *Curr. Topic Microbiol. Immunol.*, 164:95–123.

Principles and Methods of Toxicology,
Fourth Edition, edited by A. Wallace Hayes.
Taylor & Francis, Philadelphia © 2001.

Chapter 31

Immunotoxicology: Effects of, and Response to, Drugs and Chemicals

Jack H. Dean, Robert V. House, and Michael I. Luster

The immune system is a complex, multi-cellular organ system consisting of granulocytes, macrophages, lymphocytes, and dendritic cells with various functions and phenotypic characteristics, as well as various soluble mediators. These cells of hemopoietic origin are found in the peripheral blood, lymphatic fluid, and organized lymphoid tissues, including bone marrow, spleen, thymus, lymph nodes, tonsils, and mucosa-associated lymphoid tissue. The immune system is in a constant state of self-renewal involving cell proliferation, differentiation, and maturation. It exists to defend the body against invasion by infectious and opportunistic microorganisms, and spontaneously arising neoplasms. This network of cells and soluble factors is highly regulated and interdependent, must discriminate self from non-self, and can react to non-self with many different (pleiotropic) defensive responses (81).

IMMUNE MECHANISMS RESPONSIBLE FOR HOST DEFENSE

The host defense functions of the immune system are provided by two major mechanisms: a nonspecific (constitutive) mechanism that does not require prior sensitization with the inducing agent to elicit a response, and a specific (adaptive) mechanism directed against the eliciting agent to which the individual has been previously sensitized. Penetration of the skin or mucosal defense barriers by an invading microorganism results in nonspecific reactions by phagocytic cells (granulocytes and Mononuclear phagocytes [MØ]). If the microorganism is not controlled and persists, specific responses involving antibody production and the induction of effector lymphocytes follow. The effector lymphocytes respond through cytokine mediators to seek out and destroy the invading microorganism. Both antibody-producing lymphocyte responses (B-lymphocytes or B-cells) and thymus-dependent lymphocyte responses (T-lymphocytes or T-cells) are triggered by the presentation of foreign antigen to appropriate lymphocytes by MØ, dendritic cells, or other antigen-presenting cells. Following antigen-induced activation, B-cells proliferate and differentiate into plasma cells (PC), which subsequently produce large quantities of antigen-specific immunoglobulins (antibodies). Antibodies enter the plasma where they bind the foreign material and either neutralize, lyse, or facilitate phagocytosis of the agent. Antibody–antigen interactions are expanded by actions of the complement (C′) system and other inflammatory mediators (e.g., prostaglandins and leukotrienes). Fever, opsonization, and lytic factors released by activated lymphoid cells also contribute to this process of host defense.

Nonspecific and Specific Mechanisms of Immunity

Two categories of phagocytic leukocyte, the polymorphonuclear phagocyte (PMN) or granulocyte, and the MØ, are involved with nonspecific mechanisms of host resistance. Both cell types originate from myeloid progenitor cells in the bone marrow and normally pass through several maturation stages before entering the bloodstream. PMN readily traverse blood vessels and provide the primary defense against infectious agents. The inflammation associated with a splinter is typical of a nonspecific PMN and MØ response. Both PMN and MØ exhibit phagocytic activity toward foreign material, especially MØ in the presence of specific opsonic antibodies and complement, and can destroy most microorganisms. Macrophages are recruited to the site in the event that PMN either cannot contain or are destroyed by the infectious agent, as is the case with certain bacteria (e.g., Listeria). Macrophages can be activated to a state of enhanced bactericidal or tumoricidal activity by soluble lymphocyte products (e.g., cytokines) produced by T-lymphocytes sensitized to the invading microbe.

The immune responses that characterize adaptive host defense represent a series of complex events that occur following the introduction of foreign antigenic material into the body. There are two major types of specific immune response: cell-mediated immunity (CMI), which is initiated by specifically sensitized T-cells and is generally associated with delayed-type hypersensitivity (DTH), rejection of tumors or foreign grafts, and resistance to persistent infectious agents; and humoral immunity (HI), which involves the production of antibodies by cells following sensitization to a specific antigen.

Organization, Differentiation, and Function of Lymphoid Tissue

The cellular elements of the immune system arise from pluripotent stem cells, a unique group of unspecialized cells that have self-renewal capacity. The pluripotent stem cells are found in the blood islands of the embryonic yolk sac and in the liver of the fetus during fetal development, and later in the bone marrow. The pluripotent stem cell differentiates along several pathways, giving rise to either erythrocytes, myeloid series cells (i.e., MØ and PMN), megakaryocytes (platelets), or lymphocytes. Maturation generally occurs within the bone marrow, although lymphoid progenitor cells are disseminated through the blood and lymphatic vessels to the primary lymphoid organs where they undergo further differentiation under the influence of the humoral microenvironment of these organs (Figure 31.1).

The primary lymphoid organs include the thymus in all vertebrates and the bursa of Fabricius (in birds) or bursa-equivalent tissue in other vertebrates, the latter believed to be bone marrow and gut-associated lymphoid tissue in mammals (Table 31.1). Primary lymphoid organs are lymphoepithelial in origin, derived from ectoendodermal junctional tissue in association with gut epithelium. During the beginning of the second half of embryogenesis (days 12–13 in the mouse), stem cells migrate into the epithelia of the thymus and bursa-equivalent areas, where they differentiate independently of antigenic stimulation into immunocompetent T- and B-cells, respectively (Figure 31.1). The thymus, which is derived embryologically from the third and fourth pharyngeal pouches, is an organization of lymphoid tissue located in the chest, above the heart. Thymus development occurs during the sixth week of embryological development in humans and day nine of gestation in the mouse. The thymus reaches its maximum size at birth or shortly thereafter in most mammals and then begins a slow involution that is complete between the ages of 5 and 15 years in humans.

Histologically, the thymus consists of multiple lobules, each lobule containing a cortex (outer) and a medulla (inner). Lymphocyte precursors from bone marrow proliferate in the cortex of the lobules and then migrate to the medulla. In the medulla they further differentiate, under the influence of thymic epithelium and hormonal factors, into mature T-lymphocytes before emigrating to secondary lymphoid tissues. The neonatal/postnatal thymus has a significant endocrine function supported by non-lymphoid thymic epithelium cells. These cells produce a family of thymic hormones essential for T-lymphocyte maturation and differentiation. In contrast, B-cell differentiation occurs in the bursa of Fabricius in birds, a lymphoepithelial organ that develops from a diverticulum of the posterior wall of the cloaca. It is divided into a medullary region, containing lymphoid follicles and a cortical region. The mammalian bursa-equivalent is believed to be the fetal liver, neonatal spleen, gut-associated lymphoid tissue, and adult bone marrow, depending on age. Mature B-lymphocytes migrate from the bursa-equivalent tissue to populate the B-dependent areas of the secondary lymphoid tissues.

Neonatal removal or chemical destruction of primary lymphoid organs prior to the maturation of lymphocytes into T-or B-cells, or prior to their population of secondary

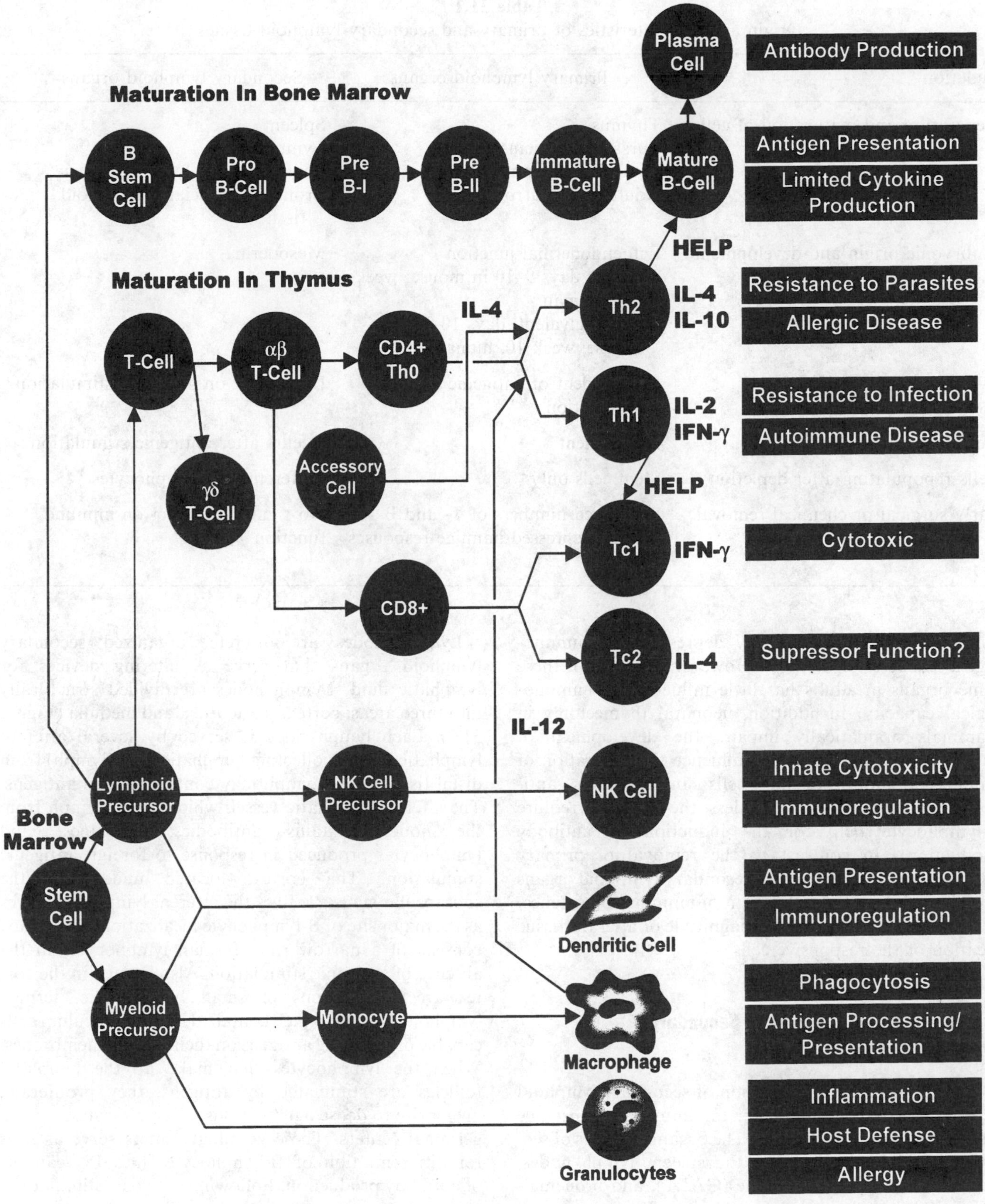

FIG. 31.1. Maturation and interaction of effector cells of the immune system.

Table 31.1
Origin and characteristics of primary and secondary lymphoid tissues

Function	Primary lymphoid organs	Secondary lymphoid organs
Generation and maturation of cells	Thymus Bursa of Fabricius (birds) Fetal liver (mammals) Adult bone marrow	Spleen Lymph nodes Gut-associated lymphoid tissue Bronchial-associated lymphoid tissue
Embryonic origin and development	Ectoendodermal junction Thymus: days 9–10 in mouse; week 6 in human Bursa-equivalent: days 10–13, mouse; week 10, human	Mesoderm
Lymphoid cell proliferation	Independent of antigenic stimulation	Dependent on antigenic stimulation
Germinal center formation	Nonexistent	Occurs after antigenic stimulation
Cells repopulating after depletion	Stem cells only	Differentiated lymphocytes
Early surgical or chemical removal	Depressed numbers of T- and B-cells; depressed immune responses	No significant effect on immune function

lymphoid tissue, dramatically depresses the immunological capacity of the host. However, removal of these same organs in adults has little influence on immunological capacity. In addition, neonatal thymectomy in mammals dramatically impairs the development of CMI but does not generally influence the generation of immunoglobulin-producing cells involved in antibody-mediated immunity (unless they strictly require T-lymphocyte help for the induction of antibody production). In contrast to the removal of primary lymphoid organs, removal of secondary lymphoid organs does not inhibit the development of immune competence, although it may suppress the magnitude or alter the tissue location of the responsive cells.

Organization and Function of Secondary Lymphoid Tissue

The organization and function of secondary lymphoid organs is extremely important for immune competence and host defense (Table 31.1). The organized areas of secondary lymphoid tissue are the spleen, lymph nodes, gut-associated lymphoid tissue (GALT), and bronchial-associated lymphoid tissue (BALT). The anatomical organization of these tissues provides a microenvironment for functional development of lymphoid cells and vital immune responses.

Lymph nodes are discrete, organized secondary lymphoid organs that serve as filtering devices for lymphatic fluid. Lymph nodes are divided structurally into three areas: cortex, paracortex, and medulla (Figure 31.2). Each lymph node is served by several afferent lymphatic vessels collecting lymphatic fluid (lymph) from distal tissue sites. Lymph may contain foreign antigens. The efferent lymphatic vessel, which drains lymph from the node, contains antibodies, cytokines, and lymphocytes produced in response to foreign antigenic stimulation. The cortex, located underneath the subcapsular sinus, receives the afferent lymph and serves as the major site of B-lymphocyte localization. The cortex consists of a narrow rim of small lymphocytes in the absence of antigenic stimulation. Also located in the cortex are aggregations of small lymphocytes, termed lymphoid follicles, which contain dendritic reticulum cells capable of retaining antigens on their plasma membranes. When the lymphocytes that make up the lymphoid follicles are stimulated by antigens, they proliferate, giving rise to dense aggregations of lymphocytes, termed germinal centers. These germinal centers serve as sites for differentiation of B-lymphocytes into PC capable of antibody production. Following antigenic stimulation, germinal centers are easily detectable as spherical or ovoid structures containing many large and medium-size lymphocytes, predominantly B-lymphocytes. The paracortex, lying between the cortex and the medulla,

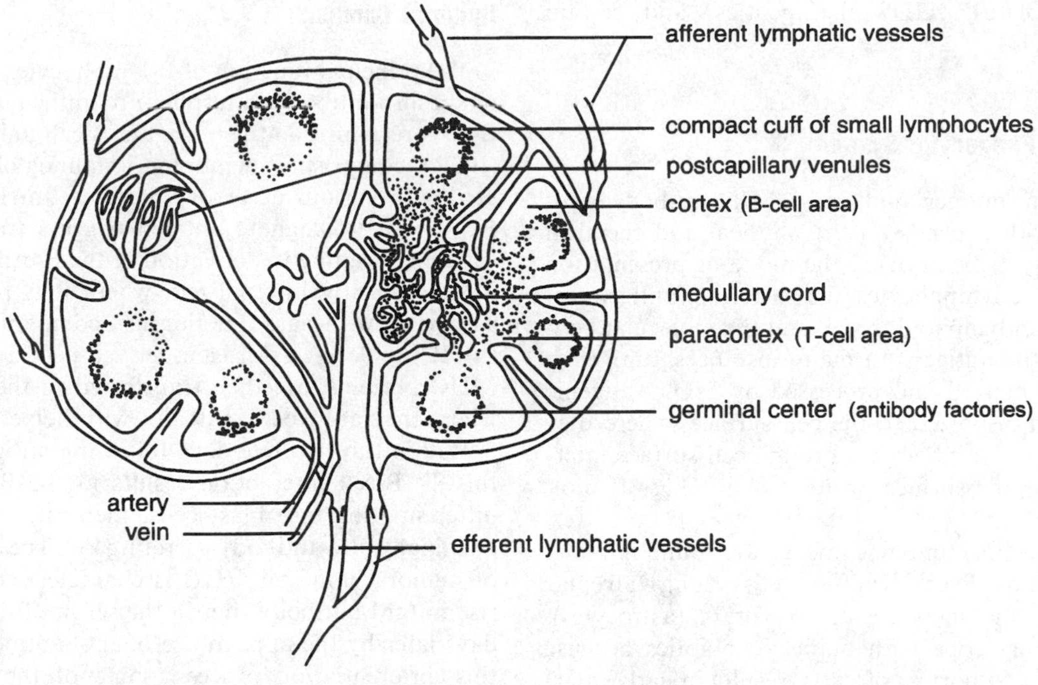

FIG. 31.2. Cross-section of a lymph node showing architectural organization.

is composed predominantly of T-cells and is a major site of MØ/T-cell interactions. Neonatal thymectomy or lymphocyte depletion by cytolytic drugs reduces the production of paracortical lymphocytes, leading to depressed immune capacity. In addition, the paracortex contains a specialized blood vasculature, termed postcapillary venules, that serves as a point of entry for recirculating lymphocytes from the bloodstream. The medulla of the lymph node is composed primarily of networks of cords and sinuses; it serves as an effective filter for removing particulate material from lymphatic fluid. Following antigenic stimulation, a majority of the antibody is produced by PC found within these medullary cords of nodes.

The spleen is the major filter of blood-borne antigens and the site of immunological responses to these antigens. In addition, the spleen is a site of extramedullary hematopoiesis (non-bone-marrow red blood cell production) and removal of damaged blood cells. There are two major histological regions within the spleen: the red pulp and the white pulp. These areas have been named for their colors in a freshly cut spleen. The white pulp consists of numerous white blood cell aggregates and lymphoid follicles. The red pulp contains cords and venous sinuses analogous to the medullary region of lymph nodes. The spleen has no afferent lymphatic vessels; thus, all antigenic material or cells enter the spleen through the blood vasculature. The marginal sinus in the spleen is structurally and functionally similar to the subcapsular sinus of the lymph node.

IMMUNE FUNCTION AND RESPONSES

Bone Marrow

The bone marrow functions as a primary lymphoid organ and serves as the principal source of uncommitted stem cells, including both myeloid and erythroid precursor cells. The bone marrow architecture is highly organized and complex, consisting of a matrix or cellular stroma derived from local mesenchymal cells, as well as cells of hemopoietic parenchyma that are descendants of circulating stem cells. The bone marrow matrix consists of reticular-dendritic cells, fibroblast-like cells, and immune cells within the bone marrow microenvironment.

Bone marrow stem and stromal cells have been shown to possess a significant capacity for metabolic activation because they contain cytochromes of the P450 and P448 families as well as peroxidases, and can generate reactive oxygen species, which could also activate xenobiotics via oxidant-dependent mechanisms (109). This metabolic activity is thought to contribute to the sensitivity of bone marrow elements to toxicants such as benzene, which is extensively metabolized within the bone marrow. In light of the cell proliferation and differentiation taking place within the marrow, this tissue is also one of the most sensitive to drugs or chemicals affecting cell division. Dose-limiting bone marrow toxicities are a significant problem with antiproliferative drugs including cytotoxic agents, antifolates, AIDS therapeutics, and certain cytokines (28,93).

Mononuclear Phagocytic System

Whether an antigen induces CMI, antibody production, or both depends on the physical and chemical characteristics of the antigen, the mode of presentation of the antigen to lymphocytes, the pattern of antigen distribution within lymphoid tissue, and the molecular configuration of the antigen. In many instances, antigen is initially phagocytized and processed by MØ. Antigenic peptides are transported to the cell surface, where they are presented to lymphocytes through cell surface interactions via specific surface proteins (e.g., Class II molecule antigens).

Cells of the MØ/monocyte lineage are found in many tissues, including liver (Kupffer cells), lung (alveolar MØ), skin (Langerhans cells), and brain (astrocytes). These cells must cope with many xenobiotics because their proximity to portals of entry results in early interaction with drugs, chemicals, and physical agents entering the organism via air, food, or blood. The capacity of cells of the mononuclear phagocytic system (formerly known as the reticuloendothelial system) to carry out these functions is associated with their state of activation, which in turn is a function of both endogenous (e.g., interferon-gamma, IFN-γ) and exogenous (e.g., bacterial lipopolysaccharide, LPS) stimuli. Responsive MØ obtained from the peritoneal cavity are relatively quiescent and require extracellular signals or "priming," followed by a second signal induced by triggers such as LPS, to be fully activated.

Although the mononuclear phagocyte system is designed to protect the host, once a xenobiotic has gained entry, extensive tissue damage can paradoxically result from MØ-mediated responses to the agent. Silicosis and asbestosis are two examples of diseases that may result from MØ-induced injury (117), possibly due to inflammation. In this condition, tissue damage from infectious organisms or other agents results in the influx of phagocytic cells such as PMN. In most instances, these cells effectively eliminate the agents by digesting them in internal vacuoles. However, if the foreign particles are insoluble (as, for example, with silica crystals or asbestos fibers), a chronic inflammatory process ensues in which monocytes/MØs are the predominant effector cells. These cells release a variety of active molecules (cytokines, nitric oxide, amines, lipid mediators, etc.) which damage tissue, as well as recruiting other inflammatory cells into the local environment. This sometimes leads to the development of a granuloma, a collection of inflammatory cells surrounded by fibrotic tissue (92).

Humoral Immunity

The principal function of B-lymphocytes is production of specific antibody in response to antigenic stimulation. B-cells recognize antigen via the B-cell antigen receptor (BCR), comprising membrane immunoglobulins associated with various accessory proteins. Interaction of the BCR with its cognate antigen triggers transmembrane signaling, leading to activation of the B-cell. The antigen is subsequently internalized, where it is processed and associated with class II major histocompatibility complex (MHC) molecules. Antigen-derived peptides, along with MHC proteins, are then transferred to the cell surface, where they are free to interact with helper T-cells.

Within three to five days following antigen exposure, this T-/B-cell interaction results in the B-lymphocytes differentiating into blast cells, then into immature PC, and finally into antibody-secreting PC. The establishment of humoral immunity (HI) is characterized by an early rise in IgM antibody titer in the serum, followed several days later by the appearance of IgG antibodies. During this differentiation process, some of the lymphocytes develop into long-lived or memory cells (sensitized but nonblast cells), so that subsequent antigen encounters result in an enhanced response. This secondary response is characterized by a shorter latency for antibody appearance, as well as an increased production of antibodies. Antibody molecules react with specific antigenic determinants (epitopes) on their target, facilitating its removal (e.g., lysis or enhanced phagocytosis).

Based on chemical structure and biological function, the five classes of antibody molecules in mammals are IgM, IgG, IgA, IgD, and IgE; some of the physical and biological characteristics of each of these classes are listed in Table 31.2. Antibodies operate via several mechanisms to protect the host from infectious agents. Some of these mechanisms include virus neutralization, in which antibodies bind and prevent virus particles from infecting target cells; opsonization, the process by which antibody molecules react with infectious agents and thus enhance their phagocytosis; and antibody-dependent cellular cytotoxicity, the process whereby antibody-coated target cells are killed by Fc receptor-bearing lymphocytes.

Cell-Mediated Immunity

Cell-mediated immunity (CMI) refers broadly to any host resistance mechanism in which cellular elements play a direct role. This is in comparison to HI in which there are certainly cellular interactions, but in which the final host resistance mechanism is mediated by soluble factors such as antibody or C′. There are a number of host defenses mediated directly by cells, including MØ-

Table 31.2
Biological properties of immunoglobulin classes

Class	Serum concentration (mg/dl)	Molecular weight	Placental transfer	Half-life (days)	Biological function	Abnormalities
IgG	670 ± 33	150,000	+	23	Primarily synthesized during secondary immune response. Readily diffuses into extravascular tissue. Fixes complement.	Increased in liver disease chronic infection. Reduced in B-cell depression.
IgM	61 ± 5	890,000	–	5	Produced early in immune response. Isoagglutinins. Fixes complement.	Increased in infection. Reduced in B-cell depression.
IgA	40 ± 4	170,000	–	6	Major Ig in seromucous secretions.	Increased in liver disease. Increased or decreased in sinopulmonary infection.
IgD	—	150,000	–	2.8	Lymphocyte receptor	Decreased following thymectomy.
IgE	0.02	196,000	–	1.5	Mediator of allergic reactions and atopic diseases.	Increased in parasitic and allergic diseases, homocytotropic.

mediated cytolysis, antibody-dependent cellular cytotoxicity, and natural killer cell cytotoxicity. More specifically, however, CMI refers to acquired immunity involving primary and secondary immune responses.

Functions associated with CMI are commonly considered the province of T-lymphocytes, although research within the past decade has shown that other immune cells (e.g., B-cells and MØ) as well as nonimmune cells (e.g., fibroblasts and dendritic cells) contribute to the development of CMI. As the primary effector cell in CMI, the T-cell represents one of the most complex and multifunctional of immune cells. Antigens that generally elicit CMI include tissue-associated antigens, chemicals and drugs that covalently bind to autologous proteins, and antigenic determinants on persistent intracellular microorganisms. The route of exposure also plays a major role in the type of response generated. For example, sheep erythrocytes elicit antibody production (but not CMI) when injected intravenously in humans, but elicit both when injected intracutaneously. The induction of CMI proceeds when small lymphocytes differentiate into large pyroninophilic cells and ultimately divide, giving rise to cells responsible for effector function as well as immunological memory.

T-cells can differentiate into populations responsible for either regulatory or effector function. Regulatory function is provided by the T-helper cells (CD3/CD4 phenotype). T-helper function facilitates antibody responses by B-cells and assists in other T-cell responses. For most antigens, B-cells require assistance from T-cells for differentiation into plasma cells. T-helper cells are integral in the B-cell response by participating in two distinct mechanisms: major histocompatibility locus-restricted B-/T-cell collaborations; and cytokine-mediated differentiation. Helper function is a result of interactions between surface molecules on T-helper cells and B-cells, as well as the production and secretion of immunoregulatory cytokines.

Effector functions take the form of cytotoxic activity (CD3/CD8 phenotype), the so-called cytotoxic T-lymphocyte (CTL). These cells are able to specifically lyse target cells via the release of various bioactive molecules. Another effector function is the ability of T-cells to mediate suppressor activity for both T-and B-cell responses. Suppressor activity is also mediated by cells bearing the CD3/CD8 phenotype, although recent studies suggest that this activity may be the result, at least in part, of differential cytokine production by this population (see Figure 31.1). This responsibility for both helper and suppressor activities indicates the crucial role of T-cells in normal immune function.

The T-helper 1/T-helper 2 Cell Paradigm

An important recent conceptual breakthrough in immunology has been the hypothesis of Type 1 and Type 2 immune responses mediated by T-helper cells. The concept was first established by Mosmann et al. (73), who demonstrated that cloned murine T-cells exhibited differential patterns of cytokine production. One population, designated T-helper-1 type cells (Th1), were found to produce interleukin-2 (IL-2), IFN-γ, and lymphotoxin. The second major population (designated Th2 cells) produces IL-4, IL-5, IL-10, and IL-13. Both populations of T-cells produce IL-3, granulocyte-macrophage colony-stimulating factor (GM-CSF) and tumor necrosis factor (TNF). Later, a third population, Th0, was described, and was found to exhibit an intermediate pattern of cytokine production. These cells are less well defined, but may be an early precursor of Th1 and Th2, or, alternatively, they may represent an intermediate stage in development of the other two populations.

Although there were initial doubts that human T-cells followed this paradigm, recent studies have demonstrated a similar (though not identical) pattern in human T-cells (89). The major differences appear to be in the profile of cytokine production, cytokine response (e.g., human Th1 and Th2 proliferate in response to IL-4), and cytolytic potential. Despite these differences, the human and rodent systems are similar enough to make experimental rodent models meaningful for understanding the human immune response.

Recent studies suggest that Th1 and Th2 cells may not necessarily represent distinct lineages descending from a common precursor, but rather may be seen as points in a continuum. For example, development of each population is influenced by type, location, and concentration of eliciting antigen and the cytokine milieu (see Figure 31.1). For example, the cytokines IL-12 and interferon gamma-inducing factor (from MØ) and IFN-γ (from NK cells) drive the development of Th1 cells, whereas IL-4 (from the ill-defined "T-accessory" cell, mast cells, or other sources) drives the development of Th2 cells (79). Interestingly, IL-4-driven development of Th2 appears to take precedence over IL-12-induced Th1 production; this may have ramifications in the etiology of some disease states.

The Th1/Th2 paradigm is especially important for immunotoxicology because certain immunopathologies have been associated with the predominance of one helper cell type over another, particularly in human disease states. For example, Th1 polarization has been associated with organ-specific autoimmune diseases such as multiple sclerosis and Hashimoto's thyroiditis, whereas systemic autoimmune conditions such as rheumatoid arthritis and Sjogren's syndrome lack a clear T-cell polarization (16). On the other hand, strong Th2-type responses appear to result in many hypersensitivity disorders. The extent to which cytokine polarization contributes to these pathologies, as opposed to being a sequela of other mechanisms, remains to be elucidated. It is possible, however, that assignation of Th1/Th2 patterns may eventually become much more important when designing and performing mechanistic immunotoxicology studies (99).

Natural Killer Cells

Natural killer (NK) cells are a population of non-B-, non-T-lymphocytes that exhibit cytotoxicity toward a variety of target cells, including tumor cells and virally infected cells. NK cells express a unique panel of cell surface markers and are morphologically distinct, being larger than other lymphocytes. In addition, they contain numerous granules, leading to their designation as large granular lymphocytes (LGL) (60). Unlike CMI, NK cell-mediated cellular cytotoxicity is MHC-unrestricted, and does not require prior exposure to the targets; thus, this form of cytotoxicity is generally referred to as "innate" or "natural" immunity.

NK cells have traditionally been seen principally as mediators of so-called "immune surveillance," the concept of a constant removal of spontaneously arising neoplastic cells (83,86). In fact, the standard methodology for assessing NK cell function relies upon the in vitro lysis of tumor target cells. However, an equally important, if not more important, role for NK cells is the control of infection (98,105).

In contrast to previous models in which NK cells were considered independent of the acquired immune response, recent studies have revealed an important role for these cells in the induction and regulation of acquired immunity (54,57,77). NK cells respond to, and produce, key immunoregulatory cytokines, and thus play an important role in the normal immune response. A more detailed understanding of these cells will certainly be crucial in future immunotoxicology study designs.

Other Immunoregulatory Circuits

Cytokines

Cytokines are glycoproteins which are generally produced in response to cellular activation. Most cytokines studied to date have multiple and overlapping actions, and they frequently function via cascading mechanisms referred to as the cytokine network, interacting with each other both synergistically and antagonistically. Two other important features of cytokines are that they usually act at a local level, and they are rapidly cleared

Table 31.3
The major classes of cytokines and chemokines

Class	Members	Functions
Interleukins (IL)	IL-1 (α and β), IL-1 receptor antagonist, IL-2, IL-4, IL-5, IL-6, IL-7, IL-9 through IL-18	Primarily immunoregulatory, act on immune system cells (generally lymphocytes) in either stimulatory or inhibitory fashion
Colony-stimulating factors (CSF)	Granulocyte (G-CSF), Macrophage (M-CSF), Granulocyte/Macrophage (GM-CSF), IL-3	Involved in the proliferation of leukocyte progenitors. GM-CSF and IL-3 have some immunoregulatory functions
Interferons (IFN)		
• Type I	IFN-α, IFN-β, IFN-δ, IFN-ω	Primarily antiviral activity, some immunoregulatory functions
• Type II	IFN-γ	Primarily immunoregulatory
Tumor necrosis factors (TNF)	TNF-α, TNF-β, TNF-related apoptosis-inducing ligand (TRAIL)	Immunoregulatory activities; anti-tumor effector functions; apoptosis growth regulation
Hematopoietins	Stem cell factor, stem cell growth factor, erythropoietin, thrombopoietin	Involved in the regulation of bone marrow function and the production of hematopoietic cells
Miscellaneous	Oncostatin M, leukemia inhibitory factor, transforming growth factor(s)	Various pleiotropic functions
Chemokines		
C	Lymphotactin	Chemotactic for lymphocytes
CC	C10, eotaxin, I-309, leukotactin-1, MARC, MCP, MIP-1, MIP-3, MPIF-1, PARC, RANTES, TARC, TECK	Primarily active on monocytes/macrophages
CXC	IL-8, 6Ckine (Exodus), BLC, CINC-1, CINC-2, CRG, ENA-78, gro, KC, MIG, MIP-2, NAP-2	Primarily active on neutrophils and T-cells
CX3C	Fractalkine	Modulates calcium flux; involved in cell adhesion

from the circulation. This combination of features helps ensure that cytokines remain compartmentalized, undoubtedly an important consideration given the potent bioactivity of these molecules (22,62).

Cytokines serve as primary immune system mediators. They are produced in the greatest proportion by T-helper lymphocytes, as discussed earlier. On the other hand, cytokines are certainly not exclusive to the immune system. In fact, certain of these molecules are phylogenetically ancient and highly conserved. Furthermore, both IL-1 and TNF are intrinsically involved in apoptosis and cellular proliferation, both fundamental biological processes. Thus, cytokines should be recognized for their role as conveyers of bioinformation, rather than as simple effector molecules involved in a single physiological process such as immunity and host resistance. For convenience, cytokines may be grouped into several classes (Table 31.3). These classifications are necessarily arbitrary because of the overlapping activity of these molecules.

Chemokines

Another, related group of molecules are the chemokines. Chemokines are small peptide molecules that (like cytokines) were originally associated primarily with the immune system, but which now are recognized as being produced by almost all cells of the body, and which are involved in a multitude of biological functions (Table 31.3). Chemokines play a role in modulating the Th1/Th2 balance associated with autoimmunity and hypersensitivity (72), as mediators of allergic inflammation (3), and modulating the function of

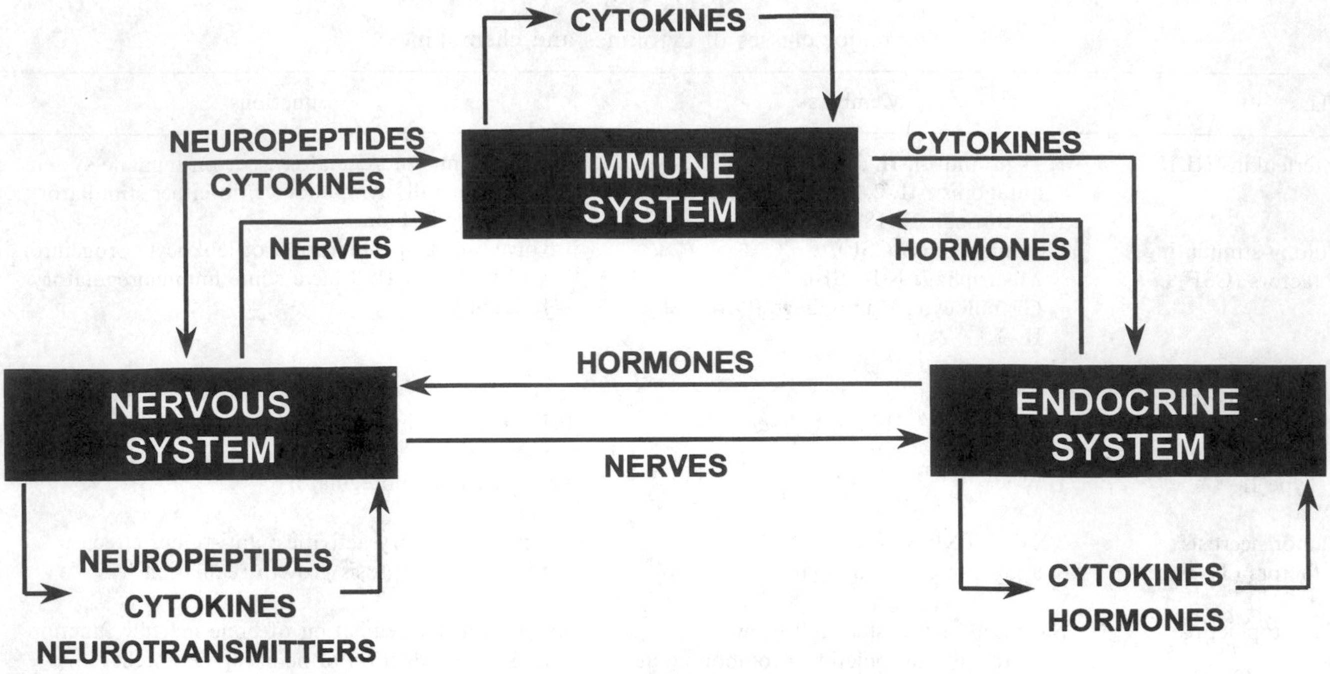

FIG. 31.3. Diagram of immune, nervous, and endocrine system axis.

leukocytes in disease states such as rheumatoid arthritis and asthma (104).

The Immune/Nervous/Endocrine System Axis

It has been recognized for some time that the nervous, immune, and endocrine systems, rather than being separate in function and structure, share many features and appear to cross-regulate each other's function (25,118). As illustrated in Figure 31.3, the soluble mediators used to regulate each of these systems (neurotransmitters, cytokines, and hormones) often serve multiple functions (31,84). The ramification for immunotoxicology of the existence of this neuro–immune–endocrine axis is that xenobiotics can affect the immune response indirectly by affecting other organ systems; conversely, modulation of the immune system may have secondary effects on other organ systems. To date, these interactions have not been extensively studied.

CONCEPTS AND APPROACHES FOR UNDERSTANDING DRUG- AND CHEMICAL-INDUCED IMMUNE DYSFUNCTION

Basic Considerations in Study Design

The value of incorporating immunological data for the toxicological evaluation of drugs, chemicals, and biologicals in human risk assessment has been increasingly accepted by regulatory agencies. For example, the U.S. Environmental Protection Agency (EPA) has established reference doses using immunotoxicity data for several compounds including 1,1,2-trichloromethane, 2,4-dichlorophenol, and dibutyltinoxide. The Agency for Toxic Substances and Disease Registry has derived "minimum risk levels" for arsenic, dieldrin, nickel, 1,2-dichloroethane, and 2,4-dichlorophenol from immune endpoints. More recently, this agency has established guidelines for testing chemical and biochemical agents.

On the other hand, rather than establish set guidelines, the U.S. Food and Drug Administration (FDA) has requested immunotoxicity testing of drugs and biologicals more on a case-by-case basis, with the recommended assays and testing approach suggested by the nature of the drug and its intended use (for previously untested agents), or based on the results of other toxicities observed during preclinical assessment (32,33). These guidance criteria have not been codified as yet for either drugs or biologicals, although much progress has been made for guidance on medical devices (2) and foods and food additives (36).

The sensitivity of the immune system to suppression by some drugs and environmental agents, that has been observed in experimental studies, is due as much to the general properties of the chemical (e.g., reactivity to macromolecules) as to the complex nature of the immune system (encompassing antigen recognition and processing; cellular interactions involving cooperation, regulation, and amplification; cell activation, proliferation, and differentiation; and mediator production by various cell types and their products). Because of this complexity, the initial strategies among immunologists working in toxicology and safety assessment have been to select and apply a tiered panel of assays to identify immunosuppression or, in rare instances, immunostimulatory agents in laboratory animals (17,75,114). Although the configurations of these testing panels vary by laboratory and species, they generally include measures for

(a) altered lymphoid organ weights or histomorphology;
(b) quantitative changes in cellularity of lymphoid tissue, peripheral blood leukocytes, and bone marrow;
(c) impairment of cell function at the effector or regulatory level; and
(d) increased susceptibility to infectious agents or transplantable tumors.

There are a number of advantages and limitations to using such test panels. For example, although the sensitivity of these batteries in detecting immune system changes is well recognized, it is difficult to establish the clinical significance of subtle immune changes on neoplasia or infectious diseases, particularly in humans. Furthermore, some of the tests require invasive procedures such as immunization. These tests are not usually feasible or ethical for inclusion in human studies and, therefore, limit the potential for animal–human comparisons, although several recent immunotoxicology studies in humans have included primary immunization (e.g., hepatitis B) as a test measure. In this respect, assays that require in vivo primary antigenic challenge are generally accepted as the most sensitive and predictive of all immune function tests.

A variety of factors must be considered when evaluating the potential of an environmental agent or drug to adversely influence the immune system. Assessment requires validation of the endpoints to be measured (quality control and biological relevance) as well as knowledgeable selection of animal models, exposure parameters, and consideration of general toxicological parameters, including metabolism, distribution, and toxicokinetics. Treatment conditions should take into account the potential route and level of human exposure, biophysical properties of the agent (including protein-binding properties and toxicokinetics), as well as any available information on the agent's mechanism of action. Dose levels should be selected that attempt to establish clear dose-response curves as well as a no-observable-effect level (NOEL). Even though in some instances it might be beneficial to include a dose level that induces overt toxicity, any immune change observed at such a dose level should be interpreted cautiously, because severe stress and malnutrition are known to impair immune responsiveness. It is often recommended that the highest dose used be considerably lower than the LD_{10}. Although laboratories routinely employ three dose levels, dose range-finding studies are recommended prior to a full-scale immunotoxicology evaluation.

The selection of the exposure route should parallel the most probable route of exposure in humans, which is most frequently oral, respiratory, or dermal. Other routes of exposure may include parenteral, subcutaneous, or intraperitoneal exposure. Because the major routes of exposure (i.e., skin, lung, or gut) are also associated with local immunity, attention has been directed to the development of methodology for assessment of local immune responses, particularly in the lung.

Selection of the most appropriate animal model for immunotoxicology studies has also been a matter of great concern. Ideally, toxicity testing should be performed in a species that will elicit chemical-related pharmacology and toxicities similar to those anticipated in humans (i.e., the test animals and humans will metabolize the chemical similarly and will have identical target organ responses and toxicity). For most immunosuppressive therapeutics, rodent data on target organ toxicities and comparability of immunosuppressive doses have generally been predictive of what was observed in the clinic. Exceptions to the predictive value of rodent toxicological data are seen infrequently, but have occurred—for example, in studies of glucocorticoids, which are lympholytic in rodents, but not in primates (34,63). Although certain compounds may exhibit different pharmacokinetic properties in rodents than in humans, rodents still appear to be the most appropriate animal model for examining immunotoxicity. This statement is based on the established similarities of toxicological profiles across these models, as well as the ease of generating host susceptibility challenge and immune function data.

Both the quantitative and qualitative susceptibility of an individual animal to an immunotoxic agent can be influenced by its genetic composition (genotype), indicating a need to consider not only species but also strain. Rao et al. (87) described two approaches to the selection of genotypes for rodent toxicity studies. The first approach is to select genotypes that are representative of the animal species, in the hope that the choice will also exhibit sensitivities similar to humans. This can be accomplished by using randomly bred rodents. However, due to the variability in immune responses associated with outbred animals, it may be necessary to use a large number of animals to identify a sensitive population. A second approach attempts to identify genotypes that are uniquely suitable for evaluation of a specific class of chemicals. This requires considerable knowledge of the mechanisms of toxicity for the particular compound. One compromise would be to use F1 hybrids that contain

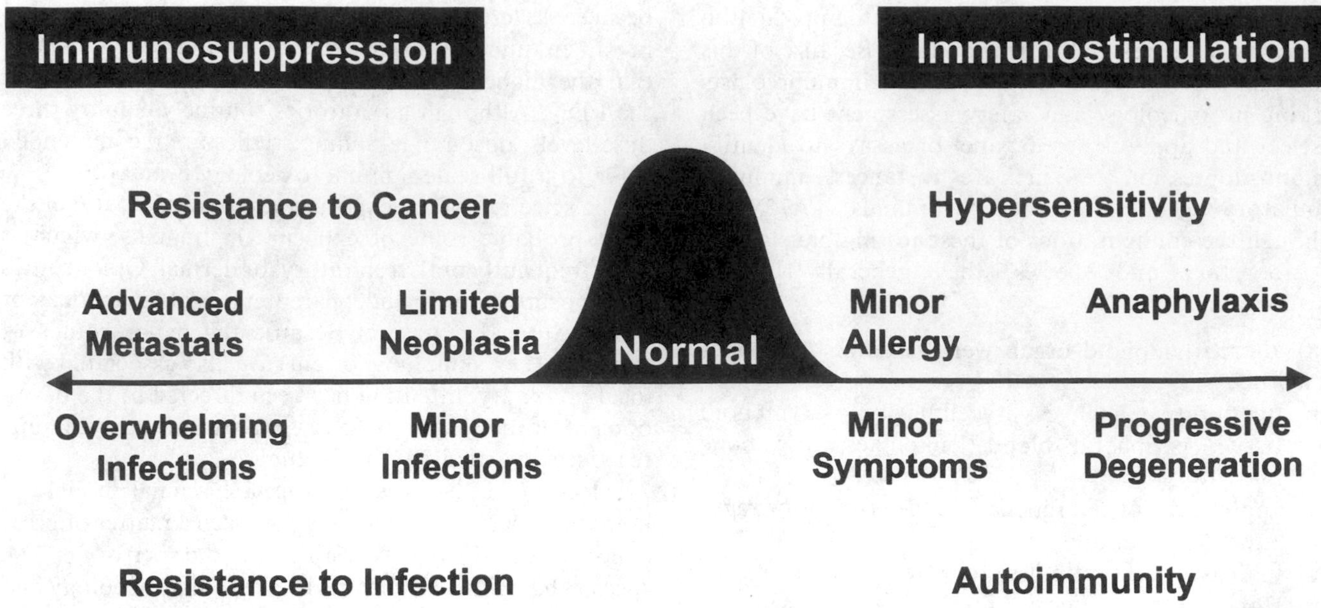

FIG. 31.4. Continuum of immune responsiveness and possible consequences.

the stability, phenotypic uniformity, and background information of an inbred animal, and yet have heterozygosity.

At present, it is impossible to determine how applicable these conclusions will be for immunotoxic compounds with different immune profiles. However, as more analyses become available, the ability to accurately estimate potential clinical effects from immunological tests should increase.

Immunosuppression

Introduction and Fundamental Concepts

Based on the preceding discussion of the important role that the immune system plays in protection of the host from infectious organisms and incipient neoplasia (Figure 31.4), it is logical to expect that disruption of this system following exposure to xenobiotics would have serious consequences. However, human exposure to many potential immunosuppressants is often difficult to assess given the uncertainties associated with dose, duration of exposure, and myriad other intervening variables. To better understand the potential for human effects following immunotoxic insult, it is instructive to examine a more controlled situation, namely the therapeutic use of agents designed specifically to suppress normal immune function.

Immunosuppressive therapy has been used to treat certain autoimmune, collagen, vascular, and chronic inflammatory diseases, as well as to prevent rejection of transplanted organs. However, therapeutic immunosuppression frequently causes complications from bacterial, viral, fungal, and parasitic infections. Another complication of immunosuppression observed in transplant patients has been a high frequency of secondary cancer. Partial or complete regression of the secondary cancers often occurs if the therapy is terminated. In a large sampling of renal transplant patients who survived 10 years, approximately 50% developed cancer (83). The types of tumors observed were heterogeneous and included skin and lip cancer (21-fold increase over the general population), non-Hodgkin's lymphoma (28- to 49-fold increase), Kaposi's sarcoma (400- to 500-fold increase), and carcinomas of the cervix (14-fold increase). Thus, it is clear that even controlled exposure to immunosuppressants may have severe consequences; this suggests that "uncontrolled" exposure to immunosuppressants (particularly when the mechanism of action is unknown) is of serious concern.

A large body of information has developed demonstrating that xenobiotic exposure can produce immune suppression and altered host resistance in experimental animals (Table 31.4) following acute or chronic exposure. Although only a limited number of reports indicate immune dysfunction following human exposure to xenobiotics, clinical data with a number of agents appear to demonstrate that immunotoxicity in rodents may form the basis for human risk assessment (115).

Given the complexity of the immune system (both natural and acquired) and the many potential target cells and molecules, it is impractical to enumerate all the potential targets of immunosuppressive agents. For this reason, a number of immune function assays have been developed

Table 31.4
Drugs and chemicals associated with immunosuppression

Pharmaceuticals	cytoreductive agents opiates	transplantation drugs AIDS therapeutics
Industrial Chemicals	organic solvents polychlorinated biphenyls glycol ethers	halogenated aromatic hydrocarbons polycyclic aromatic hydrocarbons
Environmental Agents	heavy metals ultraviolet light pesticides	air pollutants dusts (silica, asbestos)
Recreational Adjuncts	ethanol cannabinoids cocaine	tobacco (smoke) opiates

Table 31.5
Assays commonly employed to assess immunosuppression in laboratory animals

	Rodent	Nonhuman Primate
Initial Assessment ("Tier I")	Hematology	Hematology
	Bone marrow histomorphology	—
	Lymphoid organ weight and histomorphology	—
	Primary antibody response	Serum Ig level
	NK cell activity	NK cell activity
	Surface marker analysis	Surface marker analysis
Advanced Assessment ("Tier II")	CTL or DTH	—
	MØ function	MØ function
	Apoptosis	Apoptosis
	Cytokine analysis	Cytokine analysis
	Host resistance assays	–

Abbreviations: —: Not routinely performed; Ig = immunoglobulin; NK = natural killer; CTL = cytotoxic T-lymphocyte; DTH = delayed-type hypersensitivity.

and validated for evaluating immunotoxicity. These techniques and approaches are discussed in the following sections.

Techniques for Assessing Immunosuppression

The basic approach to immunotoxicity testing as it is currently practiced is based on the work of Luster et al. (64–66). This early work established the concept of the "tier" approach in which test materials are evaluated for effects on the immune system using a biphasic system of descriptive and functional assays. Tier I (screening) tests included hematology, body and selected organ weights, lymphoid organ cellularity and histology, evaluation of HI (using the IgM antibody-forming cell response and the B-cell proliferative response), evaluation of cellular immunity (T-cell proliferation in response to mitogens and alloantigens), and evaluation of NK cell activity. This group of tests provides a fairly comprehensive evaluation of immune structure and function (Table 31.5).

In situations where an effect was observed in one of the Tier I tests, the nature of the immune defect could be confirmed by using Tier II (comprehensive) tests. These included immunopathology (quantitation of T- and B-cell numbers), enumeration of IgG antibody response for HI, functional assessment of CMI using the cytotoxic T-lymphocyte (CTL) or DTH assays, and assessment of natural immunity using MØ assays. In addition, Tier II testing often included host resistance assays (bacterial, viral, parasite, or transplantable tumor) as a measure of whole-animal immune function.

Given the high predictive value of certain of these assays for immunotoxicity, as well as the time and expense involved in performing the entire battery of Tier I and Tier II tests, many practicing immunotoxicologists now use the AFC assay, in conjunction with more routine toxicological tests such as lymphoid organ weights and histomorphology, as an initial assessment for potential immunotoxicity of drugs or chemicals. In many cases, measurement of NK cell activity is also included in this initial assessment, since alterations in this effector of natural immunity would not normally be detected using the other assays. In the following section we, therefore, concentrate on these particular assays.

The following tests are commonly performed using the B6C3F1 mouse or the Fischer 344 rat, although they are readily applicable to other rodent strains. There are fewer well-developed immunotoxicology assays available for nonhuman primates at present, and even fewer tests available for use with canines.

Immunopathology. Routine histomorphology of bone marrow, thymus, spleen, and lymph node; a hemogram (complete blood count and differential); and determining spleen cellularity are useful for assessing the immunomodulatory activity of a drug or nondrug chemical, particularly when such data are combined with effects observed in lymphoid organ weights, such as the spleen, thymus, or lymph node (4,27,97). Because of the structural division of the spleen and lymph nodes into thymus-dependent and thymus-independent compartments, careful microscopic examination or immunocytochemical staining may indicate preferential effects for T- or B-cells. Likewise, microscopic examination of the thymus may reveal a compound that affects thymocyte viability.

IgM Antibody-Forming Cell Response. Within a few days following in vivo injection of a foreign antigen, antibody molecules of the IgM class are produced and released from PC into the systemic circulation. The antibody-forming cell assay (AFC, alternatively referred to as the plaque-forming cell, or PFC assay) quantitates the production of specific antibody through enumeration of antibody-producing cells in the spleen following a primary antigenic stimulus such as sheep red blood cells (SRBC). Although the AFC response to SRBC is a measure of B-cell function rather than T-cell function, it is an excellent functional parameter to examine, as this response requires cognate cell interaction and regulation by MØ, T-cells, and soluble regulatory molecules. The primary antibody response is currently measured using either a plaque-forming cell assay (15) or an ELISA (106). The steps involved in this assay are illustrated in Figure 31.5.

IgM Plaque Assay.

Materials and reagents required

- Earle's balanced salt solution (EBSS) supplemented with 25 mM HEPES buffer
- SRBC in Alsever's solution
- Guinea pig complement (GPC′)
- Dulbecco's phosphate-buffered saline (DPBS)
- DEAE dextran, 30 mg/ml in saline, pH 6.9
- Bacto-agar
- Petri dishes and cover slips

Procedure

1. Four days prior to assay, immunize animals with an intravenous injection of washed SRBC in sterile saline. Recommended inocula are approximately 1×10^8 SRBC for mice and approximately 2×10^8 SRBC for rats.
2. Euthanize the animals, remove the spleens, and prepare a single-cell splenocyte suspension in EBSS. Prepare two dilutions of the cell suspension in EBSS.
3. Wash SRBC three times by centrifugation. After the final wash, retain approximately 100 μl of SRBC, then adjust the remaining cells to a final density of 10% in EBSS. Add GPC′ to the reserved SRBC, mix well, and hold on ice until needed.
4. Prepare a solution containing 0.5% agar in DPBS, add DEAE-dextran (1.6 ml stock solution per 100 ml agar) and mix. Dispense the agar in 0.35 ml aliquots into polypropylene culture tubes, and maintain these tubes at 45°C.
5. For the assay, each tube contains 0.35 ml agar solution, 100 μl cell dilution(s), and 25 μl GPC′. Add SRBC first and then the cell suspension, and immediately remove the tube from the water bath. Add the GPC′ and mix the contents of the tube. Dispense the contents into a Petri dish, then drop the cover slip so that an even layer of fluid forms underneath.
6. Incubate the plates at 37°C for approximately 3 h, and number the plaques. While the plates are incubating, determine cell number and viability of the original splenocyte suspensions.
7. Calculate the results as follows:

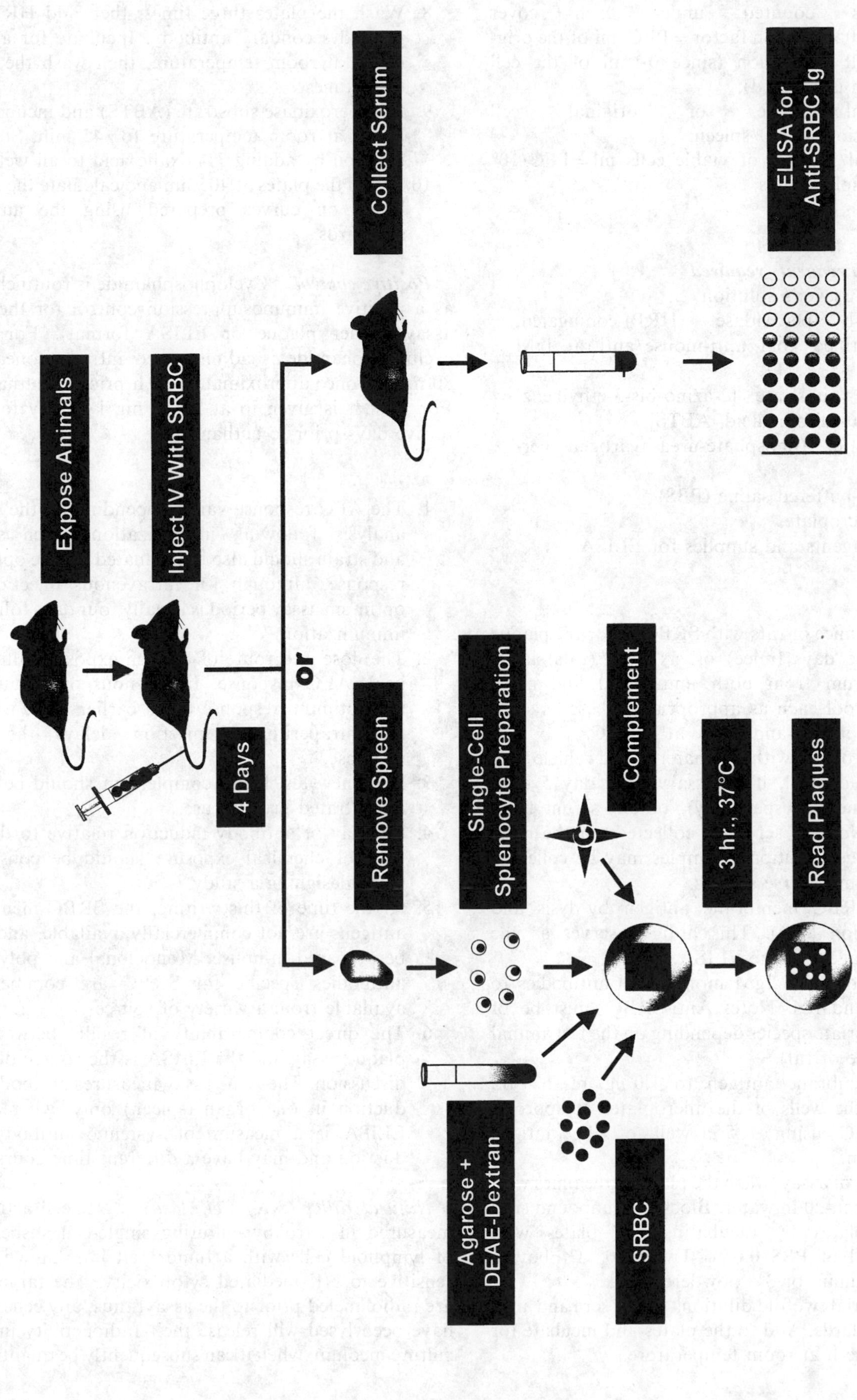

FIG. 31.5. Diagram of Antibody-Forming Cell (AFC) Assay.

a. Plaques counted under each cover slip × 10 × dilution factor = PFC/ml of the original cell suspension (since 0.1 ml of the cell dilution is counted);
b. PFC/ml × volume of original cell suspension = PFC/spleen;
c. PFC/ml/number of viable cells/ml = PFC/10^6 viable splenocytes.

Anti-SRBC IgM ELISA

Materials and reagents required

- SRBC in Alsever's solution
- Horseradish peroxidase (HRP)-conjugated, affinity-purified goat anti-mouse/anti-rat IgM antibody
- Peroxidase substrate [2-azino-bis-3-ethylbenzthiazoline-6-sulfonic acid, ABTS]
- ABTS buffer (phosphate-urea-hydrogen peroxide)
- Phosphate-buffered saline (PBS)
- 96-well microplates
- general reagents and supplies for ELISA

Procedure

1. Immunize mice or rats with SRBC as for the plaque assay. Five days (mice) or six days (rats) later, obtain serum from both immunized and naive animals. Pool each as appropriate to use as standards or controls and freeze at −20°C.
2. Treat mice or rats with test material and vehicle (and a positive control, if necessary). On day 5 or 6 post-treatment (respectively), obtain serum from animals. Note: If serum is collected via the retro orbital sinus, additional samples may be collected later for time-course studies.
3. Prepare SRBC membrane antigen by lysis and solubilization (106). This antigen serves as the capture reagent in the ELISA.
4. Obtain anti-SRBC IgM monoclonal antibodies to use as standards. Note: Anti-SRBC must be of the appropriate species depending on the test animal (i.e., mouse or rat).
5. Dilute membrane antigen to 1.0 μg/ml in PBS and coat the wells of the microplates at approximately 4°C using 125 μl/well of the antigen preparation.
6. On the day of assay, wash the plates three times with 0.01% Tween-20 in water. Block any unbound sites on the plates by incubating the plates with 200 μl/well of PBS/0.05% Tween-20, 3% bovine serum albumin, or 3% powdered milk.
7. Prepare serial twofold dilutions of test sera and antibody standards. Add to the plates and incubate for at least one h at room temperature.
8. Wash the plates three times, then add HRP-conjugated secondary antibody. Incubate for at least one h at room temperature, then wash the plates three times.
9. Add peroxidase substrate (ABTS) and incubate the plates at room temperature for 45 min. Stop the reaction by adding 3% oxalic acid to all wells.
10. Read the plates at 405 nm and calculate the results based on curves prepared using the antibody standards.

Positive control. Cyclophosphamide is routinely used as a positive immunosuppression control for the AFC assay (either plaque or ELISA format). For mice, cyclophosphamide is administered intraperitoneally at 80 mg/kg once approximately 24 h prior to euthanasia. For rats, it is given ip at 20–25 mg/kg daily for four to five days prior to euthanasia.

Notes

1. The AFC response varies depending on the day of analysis following immunization. Each species and strain should also be evaluated for the optimum response, although for intravenous injection the optimum assay period is usually four days following immunization.
2. The dose and route of antigen exposure alters the peak AFC response. Intravenous injections shift the optimum response to an earlier time, whereas an intraperitoneal injection delays the peak response.
3. Each new test lot of complement should be tested and titrated prior to use.
4. The day of antibody induction relative to the last dose of chemical exposure should be considered when designing a study.
5. At the time of this writing, the SRBC membrane antigens are not commercially available, and must be prepared in-house. Monoclonal and polyclonal antibodies specific for SRBC are commercially available from a variety of sources.
6. The direct comparability of results between the plaque assay and the ELISA is the source of some discussion. The AFC assay measures antibody production in one organ (spleen) only, whereas the ELISA is a measure of systemic antibody production and may have a different time course.

Natural Killer (NK) Cell Assay. NK cell activity is measured in vitro by culturing single-cell suspensions of lymphoid cells with a tumor cell line known to be sensitive to NK-mediated cytotoxicity. The target cells are radiolabeled prior to the assay; thus, any cells which have been lysed will release their radioactivity into the culture medium, when it can subsequently be quantitated.

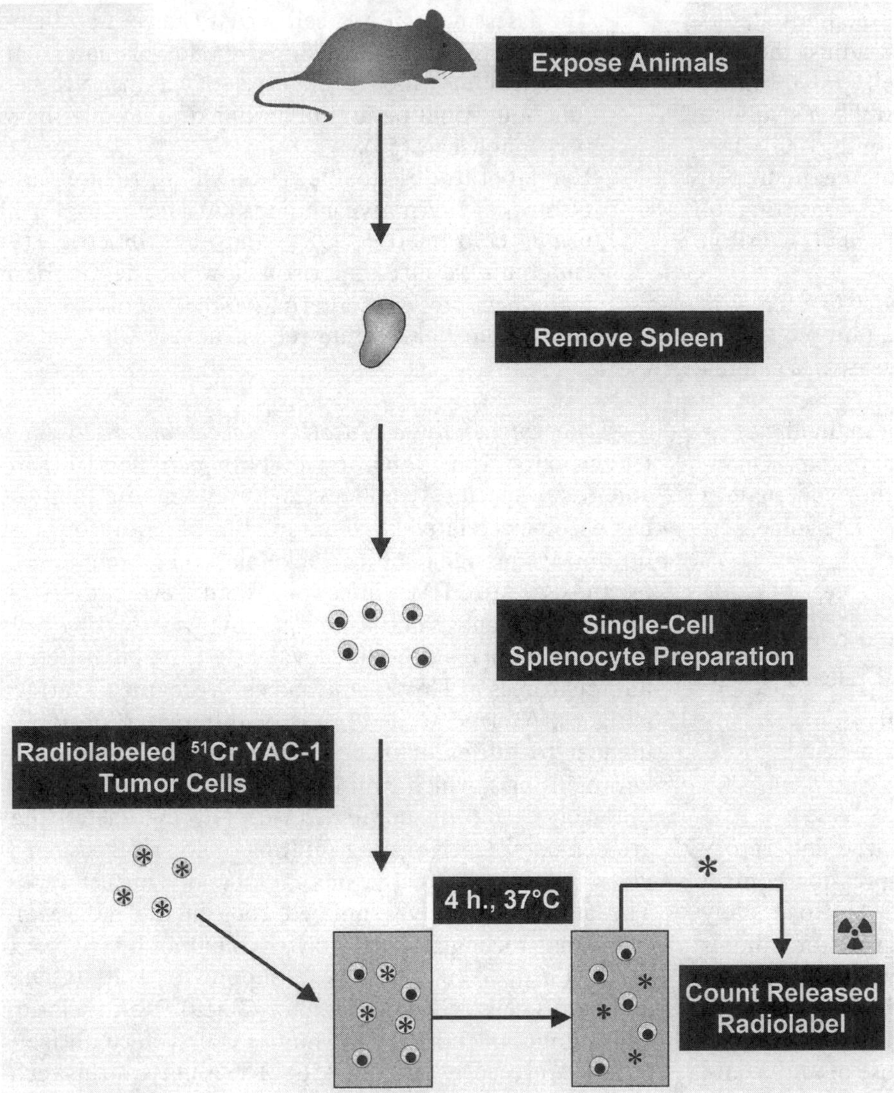

FIG. 31.6. Diagram of Natural Killer Cell Assay.

The procedure described below is modified from the microculture method described by Reynolds and Herberman (88), and is the standard approach for immunotoxicity assessment. The procedure for this assay is illustrated in Figure 31.6.

Materials and reagents required

- RPMI-1640 culture medium supplemented with 25 mM HEPES buffer, 10% FBS, 2 mM l-glutamine, and 50 μg/ml gentamicin
- Fetal bovine serum (FBS)
- DPBS
- Wash solution (DPBS/1% FBS)
- YAC-1 cell line (for rodent NK evaluation; ATCC #TIB 160) or K562 cell line (for primate NK evaluation; ATCC #243) maintained in log-phase growth in the culture medium described above
- 96-well round-bottom microculture plates
- 0.1% solution of Triton X-100 in distilled H_2O
- ^{51}Cr as sodium chromate in sterile saline; specific activity of 200–500 mCi/mg
- Supernatant collection system

Procedure

1. Prepare a single-cell suspension of the effector spleen cells, and adjust to a density of 5×10^6 viable cells/ml in culture medium.
2. Prepare two serial 1 : 3 dilutions of the cell suspension in culture medium. Dispense 100 μl of each dilution in quadruplicate wells of 96-well, round-bottom microculture plates.
3. Centrifuge a log-phase culture of target cells and suspend the cell pellet in 0.5 ml FBS. Add 200 μl ^{51}Cr to the cells, mix well, and incubate at 37°C for one h. Wash the cells three times.

4. Suspend the target cells in culture medium, determine cell number and viability, and adjust the cells to a final density of 5×10^4 viable cells/ml in culture medium. Add the target cells to all wells in a volume of 100 μl/well. Include a row containing 100 μl target cell suspension and 100 μl culture medium/well (spontaneous release) and one row consisting of 100 μl target cell suspension and 100 μl 0.1% Triton X-100/well (total release).
5. Incubate the plates at 37°C, 5% CO_2 for 4 h. Harvest all wells with a supernatant collection system, and determine radiolabel release in a gamma counter.
6. Harvest supernatant fractions either manually or by using a semiautomatic harvesting system. Quantitate radiolabel released into the supernatant fractions in a gamma counter, and determine percent cytolysis using the formula:

$$\text{Percent cytolysis} = (\text{experimental release} - \text{spontaneous release})/(\text{total release} - \text{spontaneous release}) \times 100$$

Positive controls

Immunosuppression control. Unless the laboratory has extensive experience, a positive suppression control of the NK response should be included. Approximately 24–78 h prior to euthanasia, a separate group of animals are injected intravenously with an optimum concentration of anti-asialo GM1 antibody. The exact amount to be given will vary from lot to lot, and between suppliers. Treatment with an optimum dose of anti-asialo GM1 will result in an essentially complete abrogation of the NK response in rodents (30).

Immunostimulation control. In some cases, it may be useful to include a positive control for NK cell augmentation. Although cytokines (IL-2 and IFN-γ) can enhance this response both in vivo and in vitro, an equally efficient, and more economical/reproducible option is the use of interferon inducers such as polyinosinic : polycytidilic acid (poly I : C) (23). Poly I : C is administered intraperitoneally at a concentration of 100 μg/mouse or 500–1000 μg/rat approximately 24 h prior to assay.

Notes

1. NK activity is highest in young mice, declining after 12 weeks of age. Basal NK activity may be highly variable or undetectable in mice over 20 weeks old.
2. The target cells must be in log-phase growth to achieve adequate labeling with ^{51}Cr. In addition, the target cell lines should be assessed for mycoplasma contamination at periodic intervals.
3. The assessment of NK cell activity has been utilized most extensively in rodents and primates. In instances in which evaluation of canine NK cell function would be useful, modified techniques have been published (53).
4. For laboratories unable or unwilling to use radioisotopes, alternative methods have been developed using colorimetric (78) and fluorometric (7) endpoints. A full comparison, however, has not been made between these alternative methodologies and the standard chromium-release assay.

Phenotypic Analysis of Cell Surface Markers by Flow Cytometry. The evaluation of both peripheral blood- and tissue-specific lymphocytes by cytometric analysis has become a relatively common clinical laboratory test for lineage assignment in leukemias and lymphomas, prognosis in HIV infection, and evaluation of immunodeficiency. The technique involves treating cells with monoclonal antibodies covalently bound to different fluorochromes. These antibodies recognize surface antigens, referred to as cluster of differentiation (CD), unique to different cell types. The availability of fluorochromes, which emit light at different wave lengths following excitation, combined with flow cytometers that are capable of performing multiple color analysis, provides a rapid and effective method of analyzing cell types. The most commonly examined CDs in the mouse are those that recognize pan T-cells (CD90 and TCR complex), T-helper cells (CD4), T-suppressor cells (CD8), and pan B-cells (CD45R/B220 or CD19). Nomenclature and immunophenotypes for mouse cell surface antigens have been recently updated (56). The ability of this technique to establish low-level immunodeficiency has not been established.

Materials and reagents required

1. Prepare single cell suspensions from the spleen (Ficoll-separated and whole blood have both been used occasionally). For washing and staining use DPBS (0.01 M).
2. Centrifuge conjugated reagents at $15 \times 10^3 \times g$ to remove aggregates.
3. Pipette desired concentration of antibody or control sera in 50 μl volumes to a small test tube or 96-well microtiter plates. For two-color analysis both conjugated antibodies can be added together.
4. Add 10^6 viable cells in a volume of 50 μl to the test tube or well containing the antibody.
5. Incubate 30 min on ice in the presence of 0.1% sodium azide.
6. Wash with 2.0 ml if in tubes or two 100 μl washes if in wells.

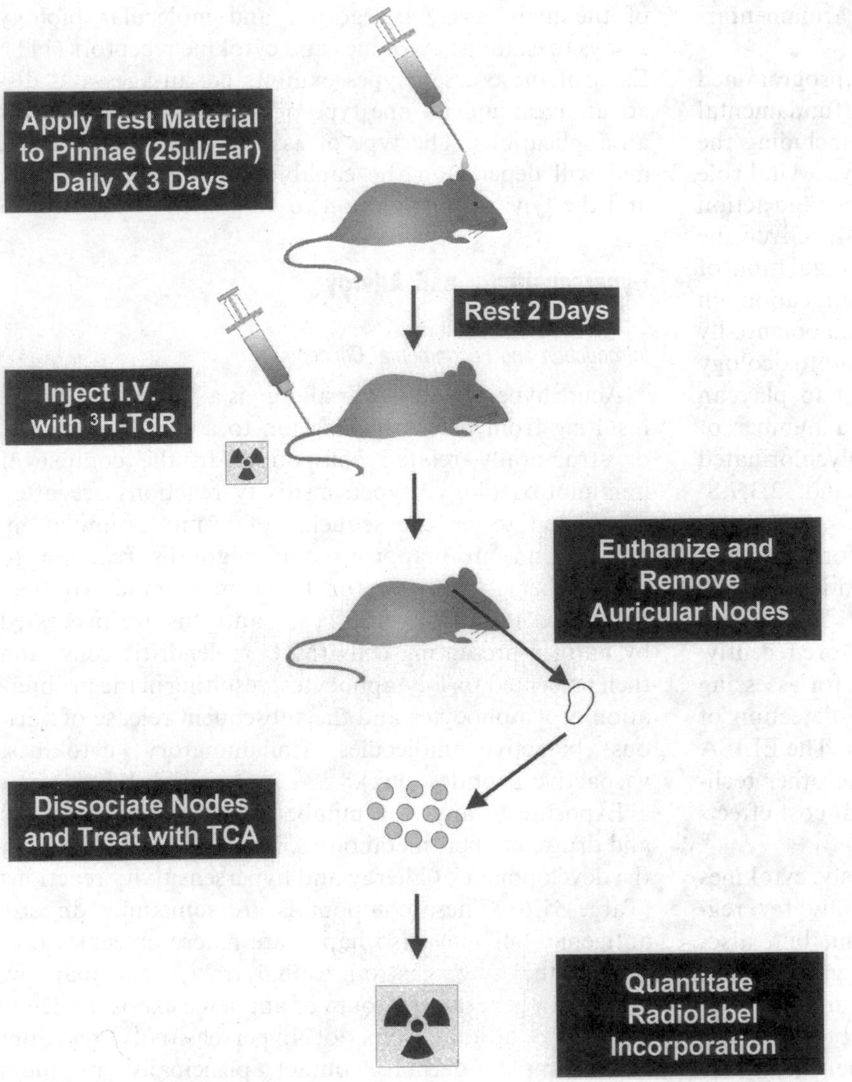

FIG. 31.7. Diagram of Murine Local Lymph Node Assay.

7. Suspend to a volume of 1–2 × 10^6 cells/ml in cold PBS containing 0.1% sodium azide and perform analysis.
8. Cell fluorescence and integrity can be preserved for up to five days by rapidly suspending the cell pellet in 50 μl cold PBS containing 1% paraformaldehyde.

Mechanistic Immunotoxicology Assays

From its beginnings, the discipline of immunotoxicology has constantly evolved and incorporated new techniques and paradigms to understand the nature of immunomodulation. The assays described previously in this section allow one to make a first-pass evaluation of drugs and chemical agents for generalized immunotoxicity. The assays will indicate that the immune system had been perturbed, although the cellular and molecular mechanisms involved will not necessarily be obvious. These assays are valuable for quick and relatively accurate identification of toxic agents.

The tools and concepts of immunotoxicology also are increasingly being utilized as research tools to understand the function of the immune system. For example, it may be useful to know not only whether or not an agent modulates the immune response, but why. This is especially important in the discovery and development of pharmaceutical agents, where therapeutic manipulation of the immune system may be a desirable goal. In response to these novel applications of immunotoxicology, assays are needed which will allow us to determine the precise mechanism of immunomodulation.

The methodology for Tier II-type assays such as T-cell-mediated immune function (CTL/DTH), MØ function, IgG antibody cell forming response, and host resistance models has been reviewed in detail elsewhere and will not be reiterated here (11,39,103,108). These assays are still valuable tools for understanding the mechanistic basis of immunotoxicity. In addition to these assays, several other methodologies are now being included in the immunotoxicology armamentarium.

Assessment of apoptosis. Apoptosis (programmed cell death) is increasingly recognized as a fundamental process in both health and disease states, including the response to toxic insult (14). Apoptosis plays a vital role in the immune response, regulating the number and action of immune cells such as lymphocytes (41,74). Given the important role apoptosis plays in normal regulation of the immune system, as well as its implication in immune-related disease (41), it is a logical and potentially valuable endpoint for mechanistic immunotoxicology evaluation (80). Apoptosis has been found to play an important role in the immunotoxicity of a number of compounds including organotins (85), polychlorinated biphenyls (119), methylmercury (102), and 2,3,7,8-tetrachlorodibenzo-p-dioxin (45).

Numerous techniques are available for assessing apoptosis, including analysis of DNA degradation, flow cytometry (10), morphological analysis, 3′-OH end labeling, and endonuclease analysis (101). More recently, a number of ELISAs have become available for assessing apoptosis; these ELISAs are based on the detection of Bcl-2 or histone-associated DNA fragments. The ELISA format offers a number of benefits over the other techniques including rapidity, simplicity, and cost-effectiveness.

Cytokine analysis. As described previously, cytokines represent an important mechanism not only for regulating the function of the immune system, but, also, for linking the immune system with other organ systems. Early studies employing cytokine analysis in immunotoxicology studies were more descriptive (38,67). However, as the intricacies of the cytokine/chemokine network become better understood, these assays are allowing us to assess the mechanisms responsible for a variety of immunomodulatory effects. As an example, a variety of nonbiological agents have been described which either specifically or nonspecifically alter cytokine production. These agents act via myriad mechanisms including direct toxicity to cytokine-producing cells (cyclophosphamide); inhibition of cytokine production (Cyclosporin, FK506, pentoxifylline); inhibition of cytokine release (pentamidine); induction of immunosuppressive factors (Leflunomide); alterations in cellular homeostasis (Tenidap); alterations in cellular activational or transcriptional mechanisms (Thalidomide); alteration of cell cycle progression (Rapamune); and miscellaneous or undefined mechanisms (glucocorticoids, phosphodiesterase isozyme inhibitors, metalloproteinase inhibitors, and p38 kinase inhibitors) (40).

There are currently four major types of cytokine assays: bioassays, immunoassays, mRNA gene expression, and flow cytometry. Sometimes used is what may be termed the "hybrid assay," employing elements of two or more of the main assay categories, and molecular biology assays to examine cytokines and cytokine receptors (111). Each of these assay types exhibits advantages and disadvantages, and no one type of assay is best suited for all applications. The type of assay chosen is subjective, and will depend on the capabilities of the laboratory, and the type of information to be gained.

Hypersensitivity and Allergy

Introduction and Fundamental Concepts

Acute hypersensitivity or allergy is a pathological state resulting from prior sensitization to a specific molecule or structurally related compound. In the context of immunotoxicology, hypersensitivity reactions are often considered to be the sequelae of immunostimulation, resulting in an inappropriately vigorous reaction to usually benign antigens or to chemical-modified (i.e., haptenated) self antigens. These antigens are processed by antigen-presenting cells (MØ or dendritic cells) and then presented to T-lymphocytes, resulting in the proliferation of lymphocytes and the subsequent release of various bioactive molecules (inflammatory cytokines, vasoactive peptides, etc.).

Exposure to any of a number of industrial chemicals and drugs, or their metabolites, has been associated with the development of allergy and hypersensitivity reactions (Table 31.6). These compounds are sometimes directly antigenic, but may also haptenate macromolecules present in the lung, gastrointestinal tract, bone marrow, or skin. In general, the route of antigenic exposure determines the ultimate type of hypersensitivity reaction; for example, dermal contact principally produces dermatological reactions (e.g., urticaria, rash, pruritus), whereas respiratory exposure results in airway reactions (e.g., bronchoconstriction). These reactions are not always localized, but may progress to systemic effects, with the most dramatic example being anaphylactic shock.

Individuals with potential occupational exposure (e.g., chemical manufacturing workers and farm workers) are at a higher risk than the general public for development of respiratory and cutaneous contact hypersensitivity to chemicals. Hypersensitivity is one of the most common and costly health problems in the United States, afflicting at least 35 million Americans. The indirect costs, such as wages lost because of illness, are estimated to be in excess of $800 million annually for asthma alone, with more than 35 million workdays lost to sickness each year (120).

Industrial processes utilize many materials capable of inducing occupational immunological lung disease or contact hypersensitivity in workers, and thus must be rigorously controlled to ensure worker safety. Studies

Table 31.6
Drugs and chemicals associated with hypersensitivity

Pharmaceuticals	phenylglycine acid chloride	ampicillin
	piperazine	spiramycin
	amprolium hydrochloride	antibiotic dust
	antihistamines	quinidine
	anesthetics	plasma substitutes
Foodstuffs	castor bean	pancreatic extracts
	green coffee bean	grain and flour
	papain	molds
Industrial Chemicals	ethylenediamine	phthalic anhydride
	diisocyanates (TMI, HDI, MDI)	trimellitic anhydride
	metallic salts	organic phosphorus
Miscellaneous Organics	cotton dust	animal products
	wood dusts	fragrance components

in the metal-refining industry, for example, suggested that many workers regularly exposed to the complex salts of platinum develop disorders of the respiratory tract. A study of workers exposed to toluene diisocyanate (TDI), a substance used in the manufacture of polyurethane, revealed that 5% of those surveyed developed occupational asthma in response to exposure to TDI. Studies of the detergent industry indicate that about 2% of employees exposed during manufacture developed asthma symptoms from inhaling enzymes used in detergents (120).

Drug allergy is also a significant problem and among the most common causes for new pharmaceuticals being withdrawn from the market after they are released. This allergic reactivity is not well predicted from the current battery of preclinical safety assessment methods (19). Drugs are unique in that they can provoke allergic and autoallergic reactions against blood cells including erythrocytes and platelets, as well as a variety of other antigens including the haptenated drug. Usually the reaction occurs to the drug or drug metabolites, in which case it is necessary for both the drug and the antibody to be present to produce the allergic or autoallergic reaction. The first observation of this type of drug reaction was made by Ackroyd, who observed thrombocytopenia purpura following administration of the drug Sedormid. Likewise, hemolytic anemias have been reported following the administration of a wide variety of drugs including penicillin, quinine, and sulphonamides. On rare occasions, drugs may induce allergic reactions where autoantibodies are raised that are directed against normal cellular constituents, as is seen against red blood cell antigens in 0.3% of patients given alpha methyl dopa. In addition to producing allergic manifestations or pathology under certain conditions, the presence of drug-specific antibodies can also alter the pharmacokinetics and clearance of the drug in plasma. Thus, drug-induced allergy reactions can come in many forms, producing either allergic or autoallergic phenomena. The autoimmune aspect of drug reactions is discussed in more detail in a later section.

Techniques for Assessing Contact and Respiratory Hypersensitivity

Given the potential economic and medical importance of hypersensitivity, the importance of sensitive and reliable assays for the detection of sensitizing potential for drugs and chemicals is obvious. For over 100 years, the guinea pig has served as the principal model for allergic reactions in humans because they demonstrate many similarities in their response to pulmonary hypersensitivity (response to histamine, demonstration of immediate and delayed allergic reactions, etc.), as well as dermal hypersensitivity. In addition, the lightly pigmented skin of albino guinea pigs, and their relatively small size and docile nature, make them manageable model animals. Thus, they have traditionally been used for assessing the human safety of drugs, as well as other chemicals, for contact and respiratory sensitization. Based on the specific experimental needs at hand, a variety of modifications have been described. In this section we will discuss only two, i.e., the Buehler assay and the guinea pig maximization test, which are probably the two most widely used tests for risk evaluation of contact sensitization at this time in the United States and Europe, respectively (70).

In recent years, the mouse has also been developed as an alternative model to the guinea pig. The impetus for this development has been the mouse's small size and reduced cost, more thoroughly understood immune system, and the perceived need of a more quantitative endpoint than the subjective degree of erythema that is the hallmark of most guinea pig assays. Two mouse models in particular have been developed: the mouse ear swelling test (MEST) of Gad (26), and the murine local lymph node assay (LLNA) first described by Kimber and Weisenberger (49). Of these two, only the LLNA has been fully validated and is described in this section.

As mentioned above, guinea pig models are also important for the assessment of potential respiratory sensitizers (95,112). The interested reader is directed to a number of excellent reviews of the use of these assays in risk assessment and drug development (13,69,112,113). In addition, a murine model for assessment of respiratory sensitizing potential, the Mouse IgE test, is currently being examined for its utility (21).

Buehler assay. The Buehler assay (8) was originally developed to evaluate strong and moderate contact sensitizers, leaving only negative or weakly positive compounds for testing in humans. The hallmark of the Buehler assay was the use of an occlusive patch to enhance or exaggerate exposure to test materials. This method also has the advantage of using an exposure method similar to the one that would be encountered in human exposure.

The specific technique for performing this assay is involved, and is only summarized below. A more detailed description of the assay is provided by Buehler (8,9).

Materials and reagents required

- young adult albino guinea pigs (Dunkin–Hartley strain)
- guinea pig restrainers
- patch delivery system (e.g., Hilltop chambers, Webril patch, PMP patch)
- dental dam

Procedure

1. On the day before induction exposure, clip the guinea pig's fur. Expose the skin to the selected test dose using a patch delivery system and then restrain the animal using a combination of guinea pig restrainer and dental dam. Duration of exposure, number of inductions, and induction regimens may vary, but are generally three 6-h induction exposures with an interval of 5–9 days.
2. Approximately 2 weeks after the last induction exposure the animals are exposed to the test material again, but at a different skin site that has not been previously exposed. Again, the timing and duration of exposure may vary.
3. If necessary, an animal may be rechallenged with test material between 6 and 14 days following the primary challenge.
4. The day after the challenge or rechallenge, depilate the animals using a commercial depilatory. Two h later the animals are ready to be scored.
5. Results are scored as 0 (no reaction), ± (slight patchy erythema), 1 (slight but confluent erythema), 2 (moderate erythema), and 3 (severe erythema, with or without edema). Scoring should be performed at 24 and 48 h after the challenge or rechallenge.
6. Scores of 1 or greater in the test group usually indicate that the test material is a sensitizer, if control scores are less than 1. Results of the challenge and rechallenge should be expressed as both incidence and severity.

Positive control. Dinitrochlorobenzene (DNCB) has been the traditional positive control for this assay. Suggested test concentrations are 0.3% DNCB in ethanol for induction and two concentrations of DNCB in acetone (0.05% and 0.01%) for challenge. Inclusion of two different challenge doses provides for a range of response (9).

Notes

1. An irritation screen is performed prior to the actual test. This assay requires an induction concentration that will not produce severe irritation or toxicity. The concentration used for challenge should produce only a slight degree of irritation.
2. Proper technique is essential to the success of this assay. In particular, animal restraint, test material occlusion, and consistency in scoring are all critical aspects. Whenever possible, it would be advisable to learn these techniques from a laboratory that has already demonstrated success with the assay.
3. Due to the relatively small number of animals and the nature of the readout, statistical analysis generally has not been practical for this assay. Rather, hazard assessment has been defined in terms of threshold levels.
4. It is important to maintain occlusion for the entire duration of the exposure in this assay. Proper use of the restraining devices is considered critical to obtaining consistent, meaningful results. Proper clipping and depilation of the animals are also important variables.

Guinea pig maximization assay. The maximization assay was described by Magnusson and Kligman in 1964 (68), and was developed to "maximize" the sensitivity

Table 31.7
Examples of drugs and chemicals implicated in autoimmune disease

Pathology	Agent	
Systemic lupus erythematosus/ Immune complex glomerulonephritis	Hydralazine Penicillamine Chlorpromazine Anticonvulsants Alfalfa sprouts (L. canavanine)	Heavy metals Isoniazid Organic solvents Procainamide
Hemolytic anemia	Methyldopa Penicillin Mefenamic acid	Diphenylhydantein Interferon α Sulfa
Thrombocytopenia	Acetazolamide Chlorothiazide Gold salts	p-amionsalicylic acid Rifampin Quinidine
Scleroderma-like disease	Vinyl chloride Silica	L-tryptophan
Pemphigus	Penicillamine	
Thyroiditis	PCBs Iodine	Lithium IL-2

of guinea pig tests. This was accomplished by intradermal injections of test material, inclusion of Freund's complete adjuvant, and the use of a pretreatment to irritate the skin at the site of exposure. These treatments enhanced the chance of a test material to penetrate the skin and subsequently produce allergic contact dermatitis (35).

Perhaps even more so than the Buehler assay, the Maximization assay is technically detailed, and only the basics of its performance are summarized below.

Materials and reagents required

- young adult albino guinea pigs (Dunkin–Hartley strain)
- Freund's complete adjuvant (FCA)
- Hilltop chambers or PMP patches
- hypoallergenic tape and elastic wrap
- dental dam

Procedure

1. Similar to the Buehler assay, a preliminary irritation/toxicity screen must be performed to determine the highest concentration of test material that can be tested. Both intradermal injection and occlusive patch tests are performed.
2. For the induction step, the animal's fur is clipped over the back on either side of the spine, and test material is injected intradermally in a volume of 0.1 ml. Each animal receives a total of six injections: two each of diluted adjuvant, two each of adjuvant containing test material, and two each of test material in vehicle. Control animals are treated similarly, but do not receive test material. Let the animals rest for 6 days.
3. If the test material being used is not an irritant, the injection sites should be treated with 10% sodium lauryl sulfate in petrolatum under an occluded patch for 24 h. This step may be skipped if the test material is a known irritant.
4. Place 0.8 ml of test material on a PMP patch (booster patch) and place this patch over the injection sites. Cover with dental dam and wrap the animal with elastic tape. Control animals should be treated with vehicle only. Remove the booster patch after 48 h.
5. Challenge the animals 10 days later by exposing to test material (or vehicle) under an occlusive patch (PMP patch or Hilltop chamber). Wrap the animals with dental dam and elastic tape. Note: animals

must be clipped prior to challenge, as the fur will have grown back.

6. Remove the patches 24 h later. Approximately 21 h later, remove any remaining fur with depilatory. Grade the reactions approximately 24 and 48 h after the challenge patches were removed.
7. Animals may be rechallenged with the same test material at the same or a different site within 2 weeks of the primary challenge. Naive test sites should be used on the animals.
8. The grading of this assay is similar to that of the Buehler assay.

Positive control. The positive control material generally used in the Maximization test is 1-chloro-2,4-dinitrobenzene, at a concentration of 0.1% in a vehicle of propylene glycol for the intradermal injections. The booster patch incorporates 0.1% (w/v) of test material in a 80:20 ethanol/water (vol/vol) vehicle.

Murine local lymph node assay. Although guinea pig models have proven exceptionally useful for assessing the potential of compounds to induce hypersensitivity reactions, they do have several drawbacks. For example, the endpoints are subjective and require skilled operators to evaluate the intensity of the reaction; in addition, this subjectivity precludes the use of statistical analysis. Moreover, the assays are relatively expensive and time-consuming. Finally, there are animal welfare issues regarding the use of agents such as adjuvant. Although none of these issues alone are major detriments, together they makes guinea pig assays less than ideal.

To address these concerns, Kimber and Weisenberger (49) reported the development of an alternative approach to assess potential contact hypersensitivity using the mouse as a model system; this model is known as the local lymph node assay (LLNA). The LLNA exhibits a number of advantages over guinea pig assays including a quantitative, objective endpoint, insensitivity to colored compounds, reduced turnaround time and cost, independence of specialized reagents or materials (adjuvant, wrapping material), and reduced animal welfare concerns. There is concern, however, that it loses predictability when weak sensitizers or irritants are tested.

The biological basis of the LLNA is simple. Test materials are applied epicutaneously to the dorsal surface of the pinna. From the skin, materials are transported by Langerhans cells to the draining (i.e., local) lymph node, where they are presented to T-lymphocytes. Contact sensitizers induce proliferation of these T-cells. By radiolabeling these proliferating cells in situ using a radioactive tracer, it is possible to determine the degree of proliferation. The LLNA does not utilize a secondary (challenge) exposure to the test material, as do the guinea pig assays. It differs fundamentally in that it evaluates only the induction phase of the hypersensitivity response.

The LLNA has been the subject of numerous validation studies, most recently a round of international validation studies employing a standardized protocol (51,52,61). The assay was consistently found to be robust, sensitive, and reproducible. In 1998, the LLNA was the first assay to be evaluated by the Interagency Coordinating Committee on the Validation of Alternative Animal Models (ICCVAM), and was found to provide an equivalent prediction of the risk for human contact dermatitis when compared to guinea pig assays (18,76).

The following protocol is the standard recommended by the ICCVAM Working Group (IWG):

Materials and reagents required

- Female CBA/J mice, 6–9 weeks old at initiation of assay
- Tritiated thymidine ([^{3}H]TdR), specific activity 5–10 Ci/mM
- Phosphate-buffered saline (PBS)
- Nylon mesh (100-micron opening size)
- 15 ml conical capped polypropylene centrifuge tubes
- 5 percent (w/v) trichloroacetic acid (TCA)
- Scintillation vials and scintillation mixture

Method

1. Apply vehicle, test compound, or positive control compound to the dorsum of each pinna (25 μl per ear), ensuring that the vehicle is evenly distributed on the pinna. Dose the animals daily for 3 consecutive days.
2. Rest the mice for 2 days, then inject each mouse iv with 20 μCi of [^{3}H]TdR in saline.
3. Five h following [^{3}H]TdR injection, euthanize the mice by CO_2 asphyxiation and remove the auricular lymph nodes. Place the nodes from individual mice in culture tubes containing 4 ml of PBS.
4. Transfer the nodes from the culture tubes to Petri dishes containing a 1-inch square of nylon mesh. Gently rub the lymph node cells through the mesh, then transfer the cell suspension back to the tube and allow it to settle for approximately 5 minutes.
5. Transfer the cell suspension to a 15 ml centrifuge tube containing 6 ml of PBS, taking care not to transfer the sedimented debris. Centrifuge the tubes for 10 minutes at approximately $200 \times g$. Wash the cells a second time in PBS.
6. After the second wash, suspend the cell pellet in 3 ml of 5% TCA and incubate at approximately 4°C for approximately 18 h.

7. Centrifuge the cell suspensions at approximately 200 × g for 10 min, discard the supernatant fluid, and suspend the pellet in 1 ml of 5% TCA. Transfer this suspension to a scintillation vial. Rinse the culture tubes with an additional 1 ml of TCA and add this to the scintillation vial. Mix the contents of the vial thoroughly.
8. Count the samples in a scintillation counter for 5–10 min, and record the counts as disintegrations per min (DPM).
9. Using the results obtained with the vehicle controls as baseline, calculate the stimulation index (i.e., mean experimental results divided by mean control results). Test compounds inducing a stimulation index of 3 or greater at any concentration evaluated in this assay, along with DPM values are statistically different from control DPM, are considered to be contact sensitizers.

Positive control. Hexylcinnamaldehyde (a contact sensitizer of moderate activity) in a solution of 20% serves as a useful positive control for this assay.

Notes

1. The LLNA is technically straightforward, and has been demonstrated to be forgiving of technical modifications (51,61). Perhaps the only difficulty a new investigator might have is in locating the lymph nodes draining the pinnae. A relatively simple way to determine this is to inject the ears with a dye (e.g., Evans Blue), and subsequently identify the nodes incorporating the dye.
2. Nonradioactive endpoints have been investigated, but at present their comparability to the radioactive endpoint has not been established.

Autoimmunity

Introduction and Fundamental Concepts

Autoimmunity comprises two processes. Initially, an immune response occurs to normal components of the host, and, second, a pathological condition may ensue in which the response causes structural or functional damage. As often noted by our colleagues in immunology, this immune response does not necessarily reflect disease, although it is a prerequisite for disease to occur, as autoimmune disease is multifactorial in nature. The autoimmune response can be cellular in nature, mediated by CD4 and/or CD8 T-cells. More often, however, it arises from antibody, mediated by specific B-cells that are driven by cytokines. Autoimmune disease is complicated by the fact that it is not a single disease, but rather represents more than 25 different diseases which can be either systemic or organ-specific. The most common autoimmune diseases are rheumatoid arthritis and those associated with the thyroid, such as Graves' disease (44). In total, they represent a significant and chronic morbidity problem, with recent estimates indicating that 1 in 31 individuals in the United States is affected, with women at 2.7 times greater risk than men (44).

The mechanisms responsible for autoimmune diseases are not clear. It is believed that the failure of any one of several immune processes can result in their development. However, the key process involves the loss of self-tolerance, such as the missed deletion or activation of autoreactive lymphocyte precursors. This process may be exacerbated by altered immunoregulation, such as over-expression of the immunoregulatory cytokine IL-4, or under expression of IFN-γ. Autoimmunity may also occur in the absence of an aberration in the immune system, such as when microbial agents express cryptic determinants (100). Although autoimmunity is a disease of the immune system, non-immunological genetic and epigenetic factors play a major role in disease development. For example, autoimmunity is influenced strongly by infectious agents, stress and diet (epigenetic), and polymorphisms in the T cell receptor and drug metabolizing phenotypes (genetic). The association of autoimmune diseases with certain haplotypes of the major histocompatibility complex (MHC), such as HLA-DR3 in systemic lupus, is striking. A detailed description of the potential mechanisms and the influential factors for autoimmune disease is beyond the scope of this section, and the reader is referred to recent reviews (59,90,100,107).

Autoimmune diseases have been associated with exposure to specific chemicals and, in particular, certain drugs. These diseases differ somewhat from their idiopathic counterparts in terms of their clinical spectrum or their specific immunological response (91). In addition, chemical/drug-induced autoimmune diseases normally remit when the agent is removed. In contrast to most agents, certain biologics, such as IFN-γ, while not themselves etiological agents for autoimmune disease, are believed to exacerbate preexisting disease (6). This occurs through their immunomodulatory properties rather than their ability to unmask novel antigenic determinants or to affect tolerance. The most common examples of drugs which produce autoimmune disease are those that cause hematological disorders such as neutropenia, thrombocytopenia, and immune hemolysis and include a variety of antibiotics as well as anticonvulsants such as phenytoin (Table 31.7). Another autoimmune disease commonly associated with drug exposure is systemic lupus erythematosus (SLE). Approximately 10–20% of patients receiving procainamide and 5–20% receiving hydralazine develop drug-induced SLE (6). Individuals with the low acetylator phenotypes are associated with

Table 31.8
Examples of potential experimental and screening models for autoimmunity

Experimental models to study autoimmunity
Organ-specific autoimmunity • Induced by immunization (EAE, AA) • Spontaneous mice (NOD, transgenics) • Toxicant-induced (streptozotocin, Cd) Systemic autoimmunity • Allogeneic reactions • Neonatal thymectomy • Spontaneous mice (NZM)
Models to evaluate the potential of xenobiotics to induce autoimmunity
• PLNA with reporter antigens • Increased titers of antibodies to self constituents • Examination of Ig complexes/deposits (immunohistochemical staining for immune complexes) • Spontaneous animal models

Abbreviations: PLNA: popliteal lymph node assay; Ig: immunoglobulin; EAE: experimental autoimmune encephalitis; AA: autoimmune arthritis; NOD: nonobese diabetic (develop immune diabetes); Cd: cadmium; NZM: New Zealand Mixed (prone to develop lupus).

drug-induced SLE and the relative risk for developing autoimmunity from gold salts increases 32-fold in individuals who possess the HL-A DR3 allele (for review see Miller [71]).

Although not as well demonstrated as for drugs, considerable evidence exists that autoimmune diseases can also be induced by substances found in food or the environment. Regarding food consumption, strong associations have been found to exist between the consumption of iodine and autoimmune thyroiditis, L-5-hydroxytryptophan and scleroderma, and alfalfa seeds and SLE. Exposure to occupational agents has also been linked to autoimmune diseases. Scleroderma-like skin diseases can result from exposure to vinyl chloride, silica, or aniline derivatives, the latter presumably the active agent resulting in the "toxic oil syndrome" (46). Agents such as heavy metals and nitrofurantoin and organic solvents such as trichloroethylene are associated with SLE or glomerulonephritis. Like their idiopathic counterparts, xenobiotic-induced autoimmune diseases are also associated with certain genetic backgrounds. Experimental studies of mercury-induced autoimmunity in the Brown–Norway rat and B.10 mice suggests the same genetic influences apply in animals as in humans (82).

Techniques for Assessing Autoimmunity

Although there is general consensus within the toxicology community that there is a major need to screen drugs or chemical agents for their potential to induce autoimmunity, suitable validated models do not, as yet, exist. This is despite the fact that a large number of experimental animal and in vitro models are available to study the mechanisms of autoimmune disease. The primary reason for the lack of validated assays probably stems from the complexity of the disease. First, and as mentioned earlier, autoimmune disease is not one disease but a group of over 25 diseases affecting distinct organs, often through different mechanisms. Unless a common early process is identified, a single test would be unlikely to provide an adequate degree of concordance to be useful for predictive risk assessment. Secondly, although almost all diseases are affected by genetic and epigenetic factors, the degree of influence in autoimmune diseases is such that it could drastically alter the outcome of a test. Lastly, when using animal models, there is some uncertainty regarding what actually constitutes autoimmunity. This is also reflected by a lack of well-defined diagnostic tests for identifying autoimmune disease in humans.

Despite these challenges, attempts to develop predictive screening assays for detecting xenobiotic-induced autoimmunity have been undertaken in several laboratories. Currently, four screening approaches, which are clearly different from those used for mechanistic studies, have been suggested, each having received varying levels of attention (Table 31.8). These include: (1) monitoring changes in the frequency or rate of autoimmune disease using autoimmune-prone rodents (55); (2) identifying immunoglobulin complexes or immunoglobulin deposits using immunohistological procedures; (3) monitoring for increased levels of serum autoantibodies; and (4) the use of the popliteal lymph node assay (PLNA) with reporter antigens (1).

The successful use of exacerbating disease by chemical exposure in autoimmune-prone rodent species has been illustrated by administering streptozotocin in diabetic mice (58) or $HgCl_2$ in glomerulonephritis-prone rodents (42). Less studied has been the monitoring of Ig deposits or autoantibody production (48). The approach that has received the most attention is the PLNA with reporter antigens (1). In this model, the "autoimmunogenicity" of chemicals, like GVH reactions, is determined by their ability to stimulate specific IgG responses to TNP–Ficoll and TNP–ovalbumin in the popliteal lymph node. Although more an indicator for adjuvancy than for disease, it may prove extremely valuable as a "first-tier" screen, as it is independent of the nature of the neo-antigens and eliminates many of the potential genetic

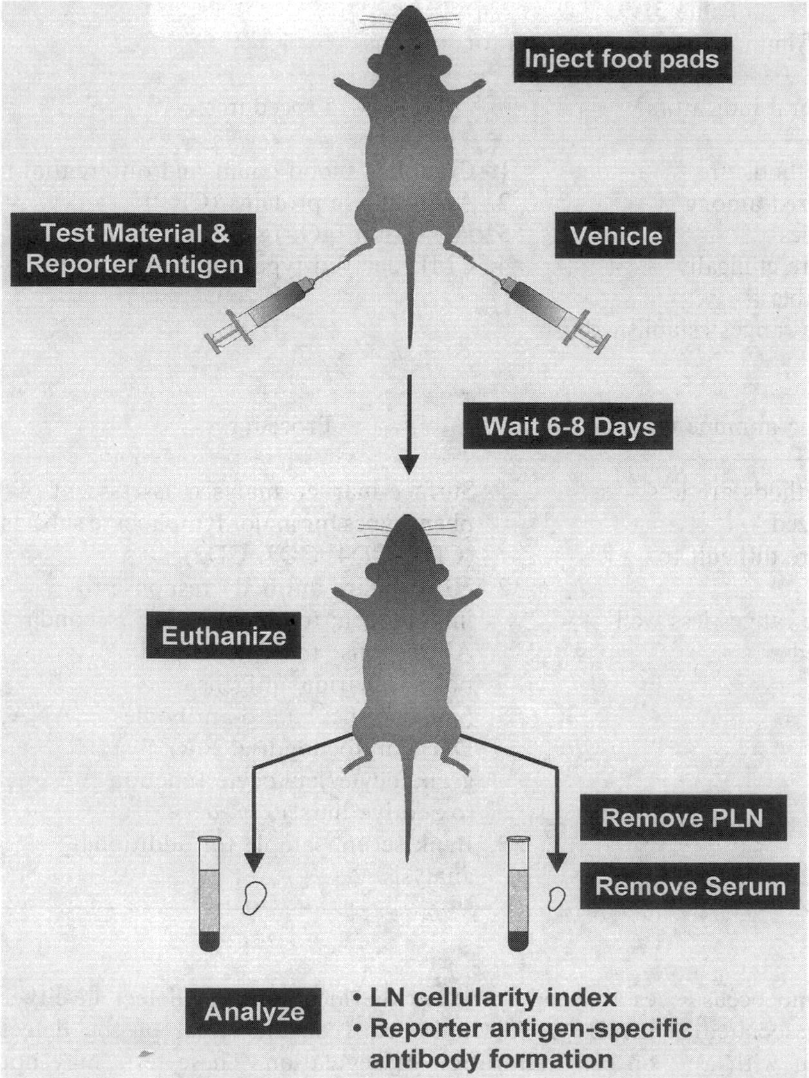

FIG. 31.8. Diagram of Popliteal Lymph Node Assay with Reporter Antigen.

confounders. In this assay the test compound is co-injected with 10 μg TNP-Ficoll or 10 μg TNP–ovalbumin subcutaneously into the right hind paw of BALB/c mice. The amount of test substance injected can be equimolar to a related compound or, if known, a concentration demonstrated to be stimulatory in the PLNA. Seven days following treatments, the thickness of the paw is measured using a micrometer and the draining popliteal lymph node (PLN) is isolated. Specific antibody-forming cells from the PLN are quantitated by any one of several methods such as ELISPOT. For memory responses, mice are similarly treated and then challenged in the right paw with 10 μg antigen, 4–5 weeks following the primary immunization, and antibody-producing cells from the PLN determined 6 days later. Serum samples can also be collected weekly following the primary immunization and serum antibodies determined using commercial procedures (illustrated in Figure 31.8).

EVALUATION OF IMMUNOLOGICAL CHANGES IN HUMANS

Introduction and Fundamental Concepts

Increased susceptibility to infectious disease, autoimmunity, and allergy is generally considered characteristic of altered immunity (116). In the case of increased susceptibility to infectious disease, the type of infectious agent or persistence of the infection often signals the nature of the immune defect. For example, individuals who suffer from recurrent infections with

Table 31.9
Classification of immune assessment tests for humans

I. Basic tests	General indicators	Procedures
Should be included with general health panels along with immune status questionnaire	• Assay methods are standardized among laboratories • Results are clinically interpretable • Reference ranges established	1. Complete blood count and differential 2. Acute phase proteins (CRP) 3. HI: serum IgG, IgA, IgM levels 4. CMI: delayed type skin test
II. Confirmatory tests	**More specific immune tests**	**Procedures**
Should be included when indicated by clinical findings or prior test results	• Assay methods are less standardized • Results are difficult to interpret • Reference ranges less well established	1. Surface marker analysis: assessment of phenotypes for major lymphocyte subsets (CD3, CD4, CD8, CD2). 2. HI: primary antibody response to immunogen; total serum IgE; secondary Ab response to proteins and polysaccharide antigens 3. Non-specific: auto-antibodies (ANA, DNA, mitochondria, RA); granulocyte/leukocyte function (oxidative burst) 4. Bank serum sample for additional analysis

encapsulated bacterial pathogens (e.g., Pneumococcus and *Haemophilus influenza*), often have associated B-cell deficiencies. These patients may present with a chronic sinopulmonary infection, bacteremia, or bacterial meningitis. In contrast, patients with defects in cellular immunity are predisposed to a wide variety of infections and opportunistic agents, including disseminated viral diseases caused by herpes simplex, varicella zoster, and cytomegalovirus; fungal agents such as mucocutaneous candidiasis; and parasitic agents including *Pneumocystis carinii*, an agent often associated with AIDS.

There are many clinical tests available to assess immune status in humans (91). A systematic approach based on simple screening procedures followed by more specialized tests of immune function usually provides the best overall assessment. This approach should include the functional evaluation of cellular immunity (T-cell), an antibody response (B-cell), and nonspecific resistance (e.g., PMN function). Recently, it has been suggested that immunization through vaccination, to elicit a primary immune response would, as in rodents, be the best criterion to establish immunotoxicity (110). Many of the screening tests employed in the past were established to define the location of a defect in either the B- or T-cell systems, or the effect of the defect on cell maturation or regulation. These tests may not be sufficiently sensitive or too specific to detect subtle or modest immune system changes that might result from exposure to toxic environmental agents. Sensitivity may also be impaired by the wide variation in test results in normal individuals. Therefore, a modest variation from the normal range in a single individual for one of these immunological tests might be expected in the normal population of subjects. Because of concern about individual variation, a confirmatory evaluation and a cross-sectional or longitudinal study design can be employed using randomized normal, non-exposed individuals. It is also imperative to document the nature of the exposure and to obtain a careful medical history that covers the clinical features of immune dysfunction.

The ability to identify individuals or populations affected by toxic compounds is also confounded ("assay confounders") by the signal-to-noise ratio of the test procedures, artifacts introduced by sample transportation, lack of well-established normative values for certain populations and age groups, lack of

Table 31.10
Comparative evaluation of the ICCVAM Peer Review Panel's revised LLNA database

Comparison	Number of comparisons	Sensitivity		Specificity		Accuracy	
		%	#	%	#	%	#
LLNA vs GPMT/BA	97	91	(62/68)	83	(24/29)	89	(86/97)
LLNA vs GPT	126	87	(81/93)	82	(27/33)	86	(108/126)
LLNA vs HUMAN	74	72	(49/68)	67	(4/6)	72	(53/74)
GPMT/BA vs HUMAN	57	70	(38/54)	100	(3/3)	72	(41/57)
GPT vs HUMAN	62	71	(42/59)	100	(3/3)	73	(45/62)

Abbreviations: LLNA = local lymph node assay; GPMT = guinea pig maximization test; BA = Buehler assay; GPT = nonstandard guinea pig tests; HUMAN = human maximization test (HMT) plus human patch test allergen (HPTA)

well-characterized or standardized reagents for some assays, different methods of data analysis between laboratories, and inherent interlaboratory variation. Clinical confounders for such studies include preexisting viral diseases, certain prescription and over-the-counter medications, alcohol and drug abuse, and preexisting HIV infection or AIDS.

Basic Test Panel

Complete Blood Count and Differential

The simplest screen to be included in the basic panel (Table 31.9) is a complete white blood cell count (WBC) and differential that is recommended for all individuals whose immune status is being evaluated. The data should be expressed as absolute lymphocyte count. Higher absolute lymphocytes counts should be expected in children than in adults and in certain ethnic groups. Lymphocyte counts consistently below $1500/mm^3$ are indicative of lymphocytopenia and may signal a defect in the T-cell system. Lymphocytopenia can be associated with primary immune deficiency disease, but also can occur secondary to viral infections, malnutrition, severe stress, autoimmune diseases, and hematopoietic malignancy. When lymphocytopenia is repeatedly observed, a bone marrow biopsy is recommended as an important adjunct for exclusion of other diseases and for identification of normal plasma cells, pre-B-cells, or diagnosis of bone marrow depression or dysplasia. Individuals with lymphocytopenia should be reevaluated and further assessed for changes in CMI.

Humoral Immunity

The assessment of humoral or antibody-mediated immunity should involve the measurement of the concentration of serum immunoglobulins (IgG, IgM, IgA, and IgE), the assessment of antibody formation following immunization (i.e., using a standard recall antigen or childhood immunogen), or the measurement of naturally occurring isohemagglutinins (blood type antibodies). However, as indicated previously, measurement of primary antibody would represent the gold standard (110).

Immunoglobulin concentration. As a screen for HI competence in the basic panel, it is recommended that the serum concentration of the major immunoglobulin classes IgG, IgM, and IgA be measured. There are several standardized laboratory methods and reagents available for measuring these major classes of immunoglobulin. These methods include single-radial diffusion, double diffusion in agar gel, immunoelectrodiffusion, radioimmunoassay, enzyme-linked immunoassay, and automated laser nephelometry. Single-radial diffusion is the most widely used method. As a screen for HI competence in the basic panel, it is recommended that the serum concentration of the major immunoglobulin classes IgG, IgM, and IgA be measured. Because serum Ig concentrations may vary with age, ethnic group, and environmental factors, appropriate norms must be used with any type of population assessment. Patients with humoral immunodeficiency can manifest a decrease in all Ig classes or only in a single class or subclass.

Cell-Mediated Immunity

A complete blood count with differential is one of the least expensive and most comprehensive ways to quickly survey for the presence of absolute number of PMN and lymphoid cells in the circulation. In addition, several tests are commonly used in clinical medicine to specifically assess cellular immunity. These include tests that identify delayed-type skin reactions, flow cytometry to enumerate T-cells, B-cells, and T-cell subsets, and quantitative cytokine production.

Delayed-Type Skin Testing. Skin testing is a commonly used procedure (Basic Tests Panel, Table 31.9) to assess cellular immune competence because delayed cutaneous hypersensitivity, a localized immunological skin response, depends on functional T-cells and the production of inflammatory cytokines. Antigens commonly employed to elicit a positive skin response include: purified protein derivative PPD of mumps, trichophyton, *Candida*, tetanus, or diphtheria. These antigens usually are employed in a panel and are administered by intradermal injection at the appropriate dilution. Skin responses are read at 48 and 72 h for maximal diameter of erythema and induration. The test is not considered very sensitive unless very severe immunosuppression is suspected, which is unlikely to occur.

Confirmatory Tests

Some of the tests that follow are less well established or not as well standardized for routine application, but may have utility for a confirmatory or research application.

Specific Antibody Assessment

In this procedure the antibody response is measured to a primary, novel antigenic challenge or to specific recall antigens to which most normal adults are commonly immunized following re-immunization (Confirmatory Tests, Table 31.9). Examples of recall antigens include diphtheria–tetanus and poliomyelitis. For diphtheria–tetanus vaccine and poliomyelitic vaccine it is recommended that blood be taken for antibody determination two weeks after the last immunization. Another approach is to measure the antibody response following a primary immunization with a novel antigen, such as the *Haemophilus influenza* capsular polysaccharide polyribose phosphate (PRP) or hepatitis B.

Phenotypic Analysis by Flow Cytometry

Modern flow cytometers have multiple photomultiplier tubes (four or more) and are capable of measuring three-color fluorescence, 90-degree light scatter, and forward light scatter. When highly specific fluor-labeled monoclonal antibodies are used in these instruments, very quantitative measurements can be made of T-, B-, and T-cell subsets. The most commonly used procedure for processing peripheral blood samples for immunofluorescence is first to stain an aliquot of whole blood with fluorescent-conjugated monoclonal antibodies, and then to lyse the erythrocytes. The proportion of circulating T-cells is then determined by immunofluorescence with fluor-labeled CD2 or CD3 monoclonal antibodies in a flow cytometer. Normally, T-cells constitute 55–80% of peripheral blood lymphocytes. Normal values reported for absolute numbers of circulating T-cells are 590–3090/mm^3 for individuals older than 18 months (24). If an immune defect is suspected, the ratio of CD4 to CD8 T-cells can also be beneficial. Although this method is quite quantitative, the ability of this test method to detect subtle immune changes in populations of individuals has recently been challenged (43).

Nonspecific Measurements

Neutrophil Function. Neutropenia may be observed and has many causes, often associated with bacterial abscesses and bacterial infections. Apart from neutropenia, there are also defects in PMN and monocyte function that contribute to increased susceptibility to bacterial infections. The measurement of nitroblue tetrazolium dye reduction by actively phagocytosing PMN is a method that should be considered if a PMN defect is suspected.

Autoantibodies. It is often stated that the immune system is established on a principle of self/non-self recognition. In some cases tolerance of self antigens breaks down and autoantibodies are produced which, in some cases, are manifested by autoimmune disease. Antibodies to cellular components and nuclear antigens (ANA, DNA, mitochondria) and to rheumatoid factor (RA) and their frequency in a population may reflect an immune alteration. Standardized diagnostic kits are available to detect the presence of these autoantibodies in sera. It is a good practice to establish a freezer bank of an aliquot of each test subject's sera for later evaluation when new research questions or test methods are developed.

RISK ASSESSMENT CONSIDERATIONS

Data used in risk assessment for immunotoxicology are derived primarily from animal toxicology studies. When data are available, epidemiological or controlled clinical exposure studies take precedence. The results obtained from in vitro studies, structure activity relationship (SAR), or mechanistic investigations are used normally as supportive information. Mechanistic studies, however, are important, as without them the "10-fold classical defaults" in the risk assessment process, such as inter-individual variability and species differences, are assumed valid (96). In toxicology, human clinical studies, of course, represent the gold standard. Questionnaires offer some value, particularly as they provide information on reportable diseases such as autoimmunity. They provide less utility in studies of immunosuppression. The National Institute for Occupational Safety and Health (NIOSH) has recently prepared questionnaires directed to immunotoxicology (5).

Animal studies that evaluate agents for immunosuppression are becoming increasingly more common in risk assessment. Because of the complexity of the immune system, the initial strategy devised by immunologists working in toxicology was to select and apply tiers of assays to identify hazardous agents (64). Among these are consideration of induced changes in the weight, composition, and histology of lymphoid organs, immunophenotyping, generally performed by cytometric analysis, and various functional assays. The latter were designed specifically to evaluate B-cell, T-cell, MØ and NK cell function to in vitro or in vivo antigen challenge. These tests were usually accompanied by an additional tier which included host resistance assays to help establish whether the immune changes observed translated into increased susceptibility to infectious or malignant diseases. This testing battery has been conducted in a number of laboratories and the results analyzed to improve the testing configuration in order to accurately identify immunosuppressive chemicals with the least number of tests and to help establish the quantitative relationship between immune function and host resistance (65,66).

Although a number of limitations exist, the following conclusions were drawn from these analyses:

(1) Examination of only two or three immune parameters is required to accurately predict an immunosuppressive agent. In particular, results from the T-cell-dependent antibody response appear to provide excellent concordance;
(2) Altered host resistance is closely associated with immune function although changes in immune function often occur at lower dose levels;
(3) No single immune test is predictive for altered host resistance although some tests showed relative good concordance (>70%);
(4) Logistic and standard modeling, using a single data set indicated most immune function-host resistance relationships follow a linear-quadratic model rather than a true threshold.

This would suggest that even very small changes in the immune system can alter host resistance, although due to the frank nature of most susceptibility tests, a large group size might be required to achieve statistical significance. Thus, at an individual level, small changes in immune function would likely have little impact in combating infectious disease. However, such changes may have significant impact when considering large populations or those already at increased risk such as the elderly or the very young. The consequence of an immune alteration may be difficult to definitively establish in humans because of the inability to detect small increases in the frequency or severity of infectious diseases resulting from the immune changes is exceedingly difficult.

As ethical considerations usually prevent the use of human patch testing for establishing the potential of agents to induce allergic contact dermatitis, animal models, particularly the Buehler occluded and Magnuson–Kligman maximization tests in guinea pigs have been used as predictive tests. Several graded doses of antigen may be examined simultaneously and an entire dose-response curve can be generated by comparing skin reactions in individual animals. However, it is expensive to purchase as well as maintain guinea pigs, there are few inbred strains, and immunological reagents are not widely available. Furthermore, there is some suggestion, although never fully substantiated, that these models are overly sensitive when compared to studies in humans and, thus, may present false positives.

A more quantitative and objective assay than the guinea pig tests, the LLNA (49) has successfully undergone a series of exercises which support its use as a "stand-alone" test to assess allergic contact hypersensitivity. Even though the strengths and weaknesses of this test have been discussed earlier (see section on murine local lymph node assay), much like tests for immunosuppression (64–66), the assay has undergone a series of examinations to provide technical refinement and assess inter- and intra-laboratory reproducibility, as well as relative sensitivity and specificity, referred to as concordance (50–52,76). Concordance for a new assay should be established to previously used test models as well as to available human data. Such data for the LLNA are shown in Table 31.10, where the assay is first compared to guinea pig tests and then to human studies. The analyses indicate that the LLNA is highly comparable to guinea pig tests (concordance almost 90%), but only about 70% accurate when compared directly to human studies. Because this is similar to results obtained when guinea pig tests are compared to human studies, in terms of risk assessment, the LLNA can be used in lieu of guinea pig tests, but an alternative assay which could provide higher concordance with humans would be desirable.

In contrast to predictive tests for allergic contact hypersensitivity, the identification of proteins and chemicals to induce respiratory hypersensitivity is in its infancy. As these tests are difficult to undertake, often involving respiratory exposure and lung function tests, efforts to develop and validate new methods are limited. Although the guinea pig has significant immunological differences compared to humans (e.g., IgG1 versus IgE reagenic antibodies), it appears to be a predictive model for humans given the limited comparative data available, and has been used to test for high and low molecular weight sensitizers. This test requires a systemic or inhalation sensitization phase and an aerosol challenge and both immediate and delayed-onset responses are measured, although this does not distinguish between nonspecific pulmonary hyperreactivity and specific immune responses (47). The latter can be established by examining sera for the presence of reagenic antibodies. An IgE test has been proposed for the prospective identification of chemical respiratory allergens in the mouse (20).

General agreement exists among the regulatory and pharmaceutical communities that predictive tests for autoimmunity or systemic allergy are in most need of development to improve risk assessment in immunotoxicology (19). Although many models exist to study autoimmune processes, they do not readily lend themselves to use in risk assessment because they do not consider the multifactorial nature of the disease. To improve the risk assessment process, screening models need to be developed and validated, not only incorporating mechanistic information into the assessment process, but allowing for the consideration of the genetic, physiological, and environmental influences that lead to the loss of self-tolerance, autoimmune disease, or systemic allergy. Despite the challenges in developing such screening tests, the considerable amount of data generated by immunologists and pharmacologists pertaining to basic mechanisms of chemical-induced autoimmune diseases have provided a conceptual framework which allows the establishment of potential structure–activity relationships. These structure–activity relationships are by no means definitive and, as the database increases, no doubt some will not be supported while others will be added. In all cases these relationships are supported by basic understanding of immunological and pharmacological processes. For example, estrogens are known to be a major factor in classical autoimmune diseases presumably due to their ability to stimulate certain components of the immune system (37), and, as such, agents of concern.

Laboratory studies have also shown that thymolytic chemicals, such as cyclophosphamide and cyclosporin A, can induce autoimmunity when given neonatally by altering normal patterns of autoreactive T-cell deletion (94). In this respect, the thymus has been shown to be a target for many toxic chemicals. As in the case of halothane, chemicals that form protein adducts or damage tissue in such a way to allow expression of cryptic determinants would provide novel host antigens which could now be recognized by T cells. Agents that have adjuvant activity, or biologicals which stimulate certain cytokines, may shift the balance of Th1 and Th2 cells and allow exacerbation of preexisting autoimmune disease (12). Common features associated with many drugs that induce autoimmune diseases are that they serve as myeloperoxidase substrates and/or cause changes in methylation (29). The explanation for the latter association is less clear, but may require identification of the specific antigenic epitopes responsible for the autoimmune response. In the case of the association with myeloperoxidase substrates, it has been suggested that many of the chemicals require metabolism in proximity to immune cells in order to be antigenic, and immune cells such as monocytes contain high levels of myeloperoxidase.

CONCLUSIONS AND FUTURE DIRECTIONS

The discipline of immunotoxicology has grown in importance in toxicology since its inception in the mid-1970s. It has progressed from the early identification of immunotoxic chemicals, through the validation of sensitive and quantitative assays that serve as biomarkers of immune system alterations in animals and humans. More recently, academic, industrial, and government scientists have taken a more mechanistic approach to define how therapeutic and environmental agents alter immune function at a cellular and molecular level. Immunotoxicity data (e.g., hypersensitivity) now play a key role in establishing health standards and defining permissible levels of toxic chemical exposure in humans. Most new pharmaceuticals are being studied for immunotoxicity on a case-by-case basis to define their margin of safety (19).

What is still needed is better correlation between animal data with known immunotoxicants and epidemiological or clinical studies to ascertain the predictive value of the immune evaluation methods for human populations that may be occupationally or environmentally exposed. Well-controlled studies are still needed in human subjects exposed to environmental chemicals to establish concretely the relationship between documented exposure and immune-mediated effects. With pharmaceuticals where exposure is well documented, the correlation of the prediction value of animal studies for immuno-alterations (e.g., immunosuppression or allergy) in humans are more clearly defined.

QUESTIONS

1. The immune system exists to protect the body against:
   a. Specific invading pathogens and microorganisms.
   b. Neoplastic cells.
   c. Non-self antigens.
   d. Transplanted foreign antigen.
   e. All of the above.
   f. A, B, and D.

Answer: e

2. Which of the following statements is false?
   a. Macrophages and leukocytes are types of phagocytic cells derived from the bone marrow.

b. Cell-mediated immunity represents a type of nonspecific immune response.
c. The two major mechanisms of immunity are nonspecific and specific.
d. Humoral immunity is associated with the production of antibody.
e. Pluripotent stem cells are found in the bone marrow and give rise to megakaryocytes and lymphocytes.

Answer: b

3. Which of the following statements are true?
   a. The primary lymphoid organs are represented by the thymus and bursa-equivalent tissues.
   b. Lymphoid tissue is derived from ectoendodermal junctional tissue.
   c. Secondary lymphoid tissue is found in the spleen, lymph nodes, gut-associated lymphoid tissue (GALT), and bronchial-associated lymphoid tissue (BALT).
   d. a and c
   e. all of the above

Answer: e

4. Autoimmunity is best defined as:
   a. an immune response to normal components of the host.
   b. being mediated by IgE.
   c. can best be measured in guinea pigs.
   d. reflects a single organ.

Answer: a

5. Immunotoxicity assessment is most often conducted using:
   a. epidemiology studies.
   b. in vitro studies.
   c. animal studies.
   d. combinations of SAR and clinical trials.

Answer: c

6. Chemical- or drug-induced autoimmunity differ from their idiopathic counterparts in that they:
   a. usually remit when the drug is withdrawn.
   b. only target the kidney.
   c. only target blood elements.
   d. are more common in females.

Answer: a

7. Validation of animal models for immunotoxicology studies requires:
   a. laboratory validation.
   b. establishment of specificity.
   c. establishment of sensitivity.
   d. reproducibility.
   e. all of the above.

Answer: e

8. The most appropriate animal model for evaluating immunotoxicity appears to be:
   a. rodents.
   b. mini-pigs.
   c. guinea pigs.
   d. nonhuman primates.

Answer: a

9. Allergic reactions to drugs may result from:
   a. direct antigenicity of the drug moiety.
   b. activation of complement proteins.
   c. haptenation of self proteins by the drug.
   d. bone marrow ablation.

Answer: a and c

10. Macrophages are an important potential target of immunotoxicants because:
    a. They are capable of metabolizing xenobiotics.
    b. They are potent immunoregulatory cells.
    c. They secrete large quantities of inflammatory antibodies.
    e. a and b.
    f. b and c.

Answer: e

REFERENCES

1. Albers, R., Broeders, A., van der Pijl, A., Seinen, W., and Pieters, R. (1997): The use of reporter antigens in the popliteal lymph node assay to assess immunomodulation by chemicals. *Toxicol. Appl. Pharmacol.*, 143:102–109.
2. Anderson, J. M., and Langone, J. J. (1999): Issues and perspectives on the biocompatibility and immunotoxicity evaluation of implanted controlled release systems. *J. Controlled Rel.*, 57:107–113.
3. Bacon, K. B., and Schall, T. J. (1996): Chemokines as mediators of allergic inflammation. *Int. Arch. Allergy Immunol.*, 109:97–109.
4. Basketter, D. A., Bremmer, J. N., Buckley, P., Kammuller, M. E., Kawabata, T., Kimber, I., Loveless, S. E., Magda, S., Stringer, D. A., and Vohr, H.-W. (1995): Pathology considerations for, and subsequent risk assessment of, chemicals identified as immunosuppressive in routine toxicology. *Food Chem. Toxic.*, 33:239–243.
5. Biagini, R. E. (1998): Epidemiology studies in immunotoxicity evaluations. *Toxicology*, 129:37–54.
6. Bigazzi, P. E. (1995): Autoimmunity caused by xenobiotics. Presented at the 4th Summer School in Immunotoxicology, Aix-les-Bains, France, October 18–20.
7. Blomberg, K., Hautala, R., Lövgren, J., Mukkala, V.-M., Lindqvist, C., and Åkerman, K. (1996): Time-resolved fluorometric assay for natural killer activity using target cells labelled with a fluorescence enhancing ligand. *J. Immunol. Meth.*, 193:199–206.
8. Buehler, E. V. (1965): Delayed contact hypersensitivity in the guinea pig. *Arch. Dermatol.*, 91:171.
9. Buehler, E. V. (1995): Prospective testing for delayed contact hypersensitivity in guinea pigs: The Buehler method. In: *Methods in Immunotoxicology, Volume 2*, edited by G. R. Burleson, J. H. Dean, and A. E. Munson, pp. 343–356. Wiley–Liss, Inc., New York.

10. Burchiel, S. W., Kerkvliet, N. L., Gerberick, G. F., Lawrence, D. A., and Ladics, G. S. (1997): Assessment of immunotoxicity by multiparameter flow cytometery. *Fundam. Appl. Toxicol.*, 38:38–54.
11. Burleson, G. R., Dean, J. H., and Munson, A. E. (1995): *Methods in Immunotoxicology, Vols. 1 and 2.* Wiley–Liss, New York.
12. Chazerain, P., Meyer, O., and Kahn, M. F. (1992): Rheumatoid arthritis-like disease after alpha-interferon therapy. *Ann. Intern. Med.*, 116:427–439.
13. Choquet-Kastylevsky, G., and Descotes, J. (1998): Value of animal models for predicting hypersensitivity to medicinal products. *Toxicology*, 129:27–35.
14. Corcoran, G. B., Fix, L., Jones, D. P., Moslen, M. T., Nicotera, P., Oberhammer, F. A., and Buttyan, R. (1994): Apoptosis: Molecular point control in toxicity. *Toxicol. Appl. Pharmacol.*, 128:169–181.
15. Cunningham, A. J., and Szenberg, A. (1968): Further improvement in the plaque technique for detecting single antibody-forming cells. *Immunology*, 14:599–600.
16. Del Prete, G. (1998): The concept of Type-1 and Type-2 helper T cells and their cytokines in humans. *Intern. Rev. Immunol.*, 16:427–455.
17. Dean, J. H., Padarathsingh, M. L., and Jeffells, T. R. (1979): Assessment of immunobiological effects induced by chemicals, drugs and food additives. I. Tier testing and screening approach. *Drug Chem. Toxicol.*, 2:5–17.
18. Dean, J. H., Twerdok, L. E., Tice, R. R., Sailstad, D. M., Haneke, R., and Stokes, W. S. (2000): ICCVAM: Evaluation of the murine local lymph node assay: Deliberation and conclusions of the peer review panel. *Toxicol. Sci.*, in preparation.
19. Dean, J. H., Hincks, J. R., and Remandet, B. (1998): Immunotoxicology assessment in the pharmaceutical industry. *Toxicol. Lett.*, 102–103:247–255.
20. Dearman, R. J., Basketter, D. A., and Kimber, I. (1992): Variable effects of chemical allergens on serum IgE concentration in mice. Preliminary evaluation of a novel approach to the identification of respiratory sensitizers. *J. Appl. Toxicol.*, 12:317–323.
21. Dearman, R. J., Basketter, D. A., Blaikie, L., Clark, E. D., Hilton, J., House, R. V., Ladics, G. S., Loveless, S. E., Mattis, C., Sailstad, D. M., Sarlo, K., Selgrade, M. K., and Kimber, I. (1998): The mouse IgE test: Inter-laboratory evaluation and comparison of BALB/c and C57BL/6 strain mice. *Toxicol. Meth.*, 8:69–85.
22. Dinarello, C. A. (1997): Role of pro- and anti-inflammatory cytokines during inflammation: Experimental and clinical findings. *J. Biol. Reg. Homeostat. Agents*, 11:91–103.
23. Djeu, J. Y., Heinbaugh, J. A., Holden, H. T., and Herberman, R. B. (1979): Augmentation of mouse natural killer cell activity by interferon and interferon inducers. *J. Immunol.*, 122:175–181.
24. Fleisher, T. A., Luckasen, J. R., Sabad, A., Gehrtz, R. C., and Kersey, J. H. (1975): T and B lymphocyte subpopulations in children. *Pediatrics*, 55:162–165.
25. Fuchs, B. A., and Sanders, V. M. (1994): The role of brain-immune interactions in immunotoxicology. *Crit. Rev. Toxicol.*, 24:151–176.
26. Gad, S. C. (1994): The mouse ear swelling test (MEST) in the 1990s. *Toxicology*, 93:33–46.
27. Gopinath, C. (1996): Pathology of toxic effects on the immune system. *Inflamm. Res.*, 45:S74–S78.
28. Greenberger, J. S. (1991): Toxic effects on the hematopoietic microenvironment. *Exp. Hematol.* 19:1101–1109.
29. Greim, P., Gleichmann, E., and Shaw, C. F. (1997): Chemically induced allergy and autoimmunity: What do T cells react against? In: *Comprehensive Toxicology*, edited by D. Lawrence, pp. 324–338. Elsevier, New York.
30. Habu, S., Fukui, H., Shimamura, K., Kasai, M., Nagai, Y., Okumura, K., and Tamaoki, N. (1981): In vivo effects of anti-asialo GM1. I. Reduction of NK activity and enhancement of transplanted tumor growth in nude mice. *J. Immunol.*, 127:34–38.
31. Haskó, G., and Szabó, C. (1998): Regulation of cytokine and chemokine production by transmitters and co-transmitters of the autonomic nervous system. *Biochem. Pharmacol.*, 56:1079–1087.
32. Hastings, K. L., Ahn, C.-H., Alam, S. N., Aszalos, A., Choi, Y. S., Jessop, J. J., and Weaver, J. L. (1997): Considerations in assessing the immunotoxic potential of investigational drugs. *Drug Information J.*, 31:1357–1361.
33. Hastings, K. L. (1998): What are the prospects for regulation in immunotoxicology? *Toxicol. Lett.*, 102–103:267–270.
34. Haynes, R. C., and Murad, F. (1985): Adrenocortical steroids and their synthetic analogs; inhibitors of adrenocortical steroid biosynthesis. In: *Goodman and Gilman's Pharmacological Basis of Therapeutics*, edited by A. G. Gilman, L. S. Goodman, T. W. Rall, and F. Murad, pp. 1459–1489. Macmillan, New York.
35. Hiles, R. A. (1988): Predicting hypersensitivity responses. In: *Product Safety Evaluation Handbook*, edited by S. C. Gad, pp. 107–142. Marcel Dekker, Inc., New York.
36. Hinton, D. M. (1995): Immunotoxicity testing applied to direct food and color additives: US FDA 'Redbook II' guidelines. *Hum. Exp. Toxicol.*, 14:143–145.
37. Homo-Delarche, F., Fitzpatrick, F., Christeff, N., Nunez E. A., Bach, J. F., and Dardenne, M. (1991): Sex steroids, glucocorticoids, stress and autoimmunity. *J. Steroid Biochem. Molec. Biol.*, 40:619–637.
38. House, R. V., Lauer, L. D., Murray, M. J., and Dean, J. H. (1987): Suppression of T-helper cell function in mice following exposure to the carcinogen 7,12-dimethylbenz(a)anthracene and its restoration by interleukin 2. *Int. J. Immunopharmacol.*, 9:89–97.
39. House, R. V. (1997): Immunotoxicology methods. In: *Handbook of Human Toxicology*, edited by E. J. Massaro, pp. 677–708. CRC Press, Boca Raton; Florida.
40. House, R. V. (1999): The theory and practice of cytokine assessment in immunotoxicology. *Methods*, 19:17–27.
41. Howie, S. E., Harrison, D. J., and Wyllie, A. H. (1994): Lymphocyte apoptosis—Mechanisms and implications in disease. *Immunol. Rev.*, 142:141–156.
42. Hultman, P., Turley, S. J., Enestrom, S., Lindh, A., and Pollard, K. M. (1996): Murine genotype influences the specificity, magnitude and persistence of murine mercury-induced autoimmunity. *J. Autoimmunity*, 9:139–149.
43. Immunotoxicity Technical Committee (1999): Application of Flow Cytometry to Immunotoxicity Testing: Summary of a Workshop. Report from an October 1997 workshop. ILSI HESI, Washington, DC.
44. Jacobson, D. L., Gange, S. J., Rose, N. R., and Graham, N. M. H. (1997): Epidemiology and estimated population burden of selected autoimmune diseases in the United States. *Clin. Immunol. Immunopathol.*, 84:223–243.
45. Kamath, A. B., Nagarkatti, P. S., and Nagarkatti, M. (1998): Characterization of phenotypic alterations induced by 2,3,7,8-tetrachlorodibenzo-p-dioxin on thymocytes in vivo and its effect on apoptosis. *Toxicol. Appl. Pharmacol.*, 150:117–24.
46. Kammuller, M. E., Bloksma, N., and Seinen, W. (1988): Chemical-induced autoimmune reactions and Spanish toxic oil syndrome: Focus on hydantoins and related compounds. *Clin. Toxicol.*, 26:157–174.
47. Karol, M. H. (1988): The development of an animal model for TDI asthma. *Bull. Euro. Physiopath. Respir.*, 23:571–576.
48. Kilburn, K. H., and Warshaw, R. H. (1992): Prevalence of symptoms of systemic lupus erythematosus (SLE) and of fluorescent antinuclear antibodies associated with chronic exposure to

trichloroethylene and other chemicals in well water. *Environ. Res.*, 57:1–9.

49. Kimber, I., and Weisenberger, C. (1989): A murine local lymph node assay for identification of contact allergens. *Arch. Toxicol.*, 63:274–282.
50. Kimber, I., and Basksetter, D. A. (1992): The murine local lymph node assay: A commentary on collaborative studies and new directions. *Food Chem. Toxicol.*, 30:165–169.
51. Kimber, I., Hilton, J., Dearman, R. J., Gerberick, G. F., Ryan, C. A., Basketter, D. A., Scholes, E. W., Ladics, G. S., Loveless, S. E., House, R. V., and Guy, A. (1995): An international evaluation of the murine local lymph node assay and comparison of modified procedures. *Toxicology*, 103:63–73.
52. Kimber, I., Hilton, J., Dearman, R. J., Gerberick, G. F., Ryan, C. A., Basketter, D. A., Lea, L., House, R. V., Ladics, G. S., Loveless, S. E., and Hastings, K. L. (1998): Assessment of the skin sensitization potential of topical medicaments using the local lymph node assay: An interlaboratory evaluation. *J. Toxicol. Env. Health*, 53:563–579.
53. Knapp, D. W., Leibnitz, R. R., DeNicola, D. B., Turek, J. J., Teclaw, R., Shaffer, L., and Chan, T. C. K. (1993): Measurement of NK activity in effector cells purified from canine peripheral lymphocytes. *Vet. Immunol. Immunopathol.*, 35:239–251.
54. Kos, F. J. (1998): Regulation of adaptive immunity by natural killer cells. *Immunol. Res.*, 17:303–312.
55. Lai, H., and Forster, M. J. (1991): Autoimmune mice as models for discovery of drugs against age-related dementia. *Drug Devel. Res.*, 24:1–27.
56. Lai, L., Alaverdi, N., Maltais, L., and Morse, H. C. (1998): Mouse cell surface antigens: Nomenclature and immunophenotyping. *J. Immunol.* 160:3861–3868.
57. Lanier, L. L., Corliss, B., and Phillips, J. H. (1997): Arousal and inhibition of human NK cells. *Immunol. Rev.*, 155:145–154.
58. Leiter, E. H. (1982): Multiple low-dose streptozotocin-induced hyperglycemia and insulitis in C57BL mice: Influence of inbred background, sex and thymus. *Proc. Natl. Acad. Sci.*, 79:630–634.
59. Liblan, R. S., Singer, S. M., and McDevitt, H. O. (1995): Th1 and Th2 $CD4^+$ T cells in the pathogenesis of organ-specific autoimmune diseases. *Immunol. Today*, 16:3–8.
60. Lotzova, E. (1993): Definition and functions of natural killer cells. *Nat. Immun.* 12:169–176.
61. Loveless, S. E., Ladics, G. S., Gerberick, G. F., Ryan, C. A., Basketter, D. A., Scholes, E. W., House, R. V., Hilton, J., Dearman, R. J., and Kimber, I. (1996): Further evaluation of the local lymph node assay in the final phase of an international collaborative trial. *Toxicology*, 108:141–152.
62. Lunney, J. K. (1998): Cytokines orchestrating the immune response. *Rev. Sci. Tech. Off. Int. Epiz.*, 17:84–94.
63. Luster, M. I., Germolec, D. R., Clark, G., Wiegand, G., and Rosenthal, G. J. (1988): Selective effects of 2,3,7,8-tetrachlorodibenzo-p-dioxin and corticosteroid on in vitro activation, proliferation and differentiation of murine B-lymphocytes. *J. Immunol.* 140:928–935.
64. Luster, M. I., Munson, A. E., Thomas, P. T., Holsapple, M. P., Fenters, J. D., White, K. L. Jr., Lauer, L. D., Germolec, D. R, Rosenthal, G. J., and Dean, J. H. (1988): Development of a testing battery to assess chemical-induced immunotoxicity: National Toxicology Program's guidelines for immunotoxicity evaluation in mice. *Fund. Appl. Toxicol.*, 10:2–19.
65. Luster, M. I., Portier, C., Pait, D. G., White, K. L. Jr., Gennings, C., Munson, A. E., and Rosenthal, G. J. (1992): Risk assessment in immunotoxicology. I. Sensitivity and predictability of immune tests. *Fund. Appl. Toxicol.*, 18:200–210.
66. Luster, M. I., Portier, C., and Pait, D. G. (1993): Risk assessment in immunotoxicology. II. Relationships between immune and host resistance tests. *Fund. Appl. Toxicol.*, 21:71–82.
67. Lyte, M., and Bick, P. H. (1986): Modulation of interleukin I production by macrophages following benzo(a)pyrene exposure. *Int. J. Immunopharmacol.*, 8:377–381.
68. Magnusson, B., and Kligman, A. M. (1964): The identification of contact allergens by animal assay. The maximization test. *J. Invest. Dermatol.*, 52:268.
69. Maurer, T. (1996): Guinea pig predictive tests. In: *Toxicology of Contact Hypersensitivity*, edited by I. Kimber and T. Maurer, pp. 107–126. Taylor & Francis, London.
70. Maurer, T., Arthur, A., and Bentley, P. (1994): Guinea-pig contact sensitization assays. *Toxicology*, 93:47–54.
71. Miller, F. W. (1998): Genetics of environmentally associated rheumatic disease. In: *Rheumatic Diseases and the Environment*, edited by L. D. Kaufman and J. Varga, Chapman and Hall, New York.
72. Montovani, A., Allavena, P., Vecchi, A., and Sozzani, S. (1998): Chemokines and chemokine receptors during activation and deactivation of monocytic and dendritic cells and in amplification of Th1 versus Th2 responses. *Int. J. Clin. Lab. Res.*, 28:77–82.
73. Mosmann, T. R., Cherwinski, H., Bond, M. W., Giedlin, M. A., and Coffman, R. L. (1986): Two types of murine helper T cell clone. I. Definition according to profiles of lymphokine activities and secreted proteins. *J. Immunol.*, 136:2348–2357.
74. Mountz, J. D., Zhou, T., Wu, J., Wang, W., Su, X., and Cheng, J. (1995): Regulation of apoptosis in immune cells. *J. Clin. Immunol.*, 15:1–16.
75. National Research Council (1992): *Biologic Markers in Immunotoxicology*. National Academy Press, Washington, DC.
76. National Toxicology Program. (1999): *The Murine Local Lymph Node Assay: A Test Method for Assessing the Allergic Contact Dermatitis Potential of Chemicals/Compounds*, NIH Publication No. 99-4494. National Institutes of Health, Bethesda, Maryland.
77. Naume, B., and Espevik, T. (1994): Immunoregulatory effects of cytokines on natural killer cells. *Scand. J. Immunol.*, 40:128–134.
78. Nouri, A. M. E., Mansouri, M., Hussain, R. F. Dos Santos, A. V. L., and Oliver, R. T. D. (1995): Super-sensitive epithelial cell line and colorimetric assay to replace the conventional K562 target and chromium release assay for assessment of non-MHC-restricted cytotoxicity. *J. Immunol. Meth.*, 180:63–68.
79. O'Garra, A. (1998): Cytokines induce the development of functionally heterogeneous T helper cell subsets. *Immunity*, 8:275–283.
80. Pallardy, M., Kerdine, S., and Lebrec, H. (1998): Testing strategies in immunotoxicology. *Toxicol. Lett.*, 102–103:257–260.
81. Paul, W. E. (1999): *Fundamental Immunology*, 4th edn. Lippincott–Raven, Philadelphia.
82. Pelletier, L., Ramanathan, S., and Druet, P. (1997): Autoimmune models. In: *Comprehensive Toxicology*, edited by D. Lawrence, pp. 365–380. Elsevier, New York.
83. Penn, I. (1985): Neoplastic consequences of immunosuppression. In: *Immunotoxicology and Immunopharmacology*, edited by J. H. Dean, A. Munson, M. I. Luster, and H. Amos. Raven Press, New York.
84. Peterson, P. K., Molitor, T., and Chao, C. C. (1998): The opioid-cytokine connection. *J. Neuroimmunol.*, 83:63–69.
85. Pieters, R. H., Bol, M., and Penninks, A. H. (1994): Immunotoxic organotins as possible model compounds in studying apoptosis and thymocyte differentiation. *Toxicology*, 91:189–202.
86. Pross, H. F., and Lotzová, E. (1993): Role of natural killer cells in cancer. *Nat. Immun.*, 12:279–292.

87. Rao, G. N., Birnbaum, L. S., Collins, J. J., Tennant, R. W., and Skow, L. C. (1988): Mouse strains for chemical carcinogenicity studies: Overview of workshop. *Fund. Appl. Toxicol.*, 10:385–394.
88. Reynolds, C. W., and Herberman, R. B. (1981): In vitro augmentation of rat natural killer (NK) cell activity. *J. Immunol.*, 126:1581–1585.
89. Romagnani, S. (1995): Biology of human TH1 and TH2 cells. *J. Clin. Immunol.*, 15:121–129.
90. Rose, N. R., and Caturegli, P. P. (1997). Autoimmune diseases of humans. In: *Comprehensive Toxicology*, edited by D. Lawrence, pp. 381–390. Elsevier, New York.
91. Rosen, F. S., Wedgwood, R. J., Eibl, M., Aiuti, F., Cooper, M. D., Good, R. A., Hanson, L. A., Hitzig, W. H., Matsumoto, S., Seligmann, M., et al. (1986): Primary immuodeficiency diseases: Report prepared for WHO scientific group. Immunodeficiency. *Clin. Immunol. Immunopathol.*, 28:450–475.
92. Rosenberg, H. F., and Gallin, J. I. (1999): Inflammation. In: *Fundamental Immunology*, 4th edn., edited by W. E. Paul, pp. 1051–1066. Lippincott–Raven, Philadelphia.
93. Rosenthal, G. J., and Kowolenko, M. (1994): Immunotoxicological manifestations of AIDS therapeutics. In: *Immunotoxicology and Immunopharmacology*, 2nd edn., edited by J. H. Dean, M. I. Luster, A. E. Munson, and I. Kimber, pp. 249–265. Raven Press, New York.
94. Sakaguchi, S., and Sakaguchi, N. (1989): Organ-specific autoimmune disease induced in mice by elimination of T cell subsets: Neonatal administration of cyclosporin A causes autoimmune disease. *J. Immunol.*, 142:471–480.
95. Sarlo, K., and Karol, M. H. (1994): Guinea pig predictive tests for respiratory allergy. In: *Immunotoxicology and Immunopharmacology*, 2nd edn., edited by J. H. Dean, M. I. Luster, A. E. Munson, and I. Kimber, pp. 703–720. Raven Press, New York.
96. Scala, R. (1991): Risk assessment. In: *Casarett and Doull's Toxicology: The Basic Science of Poisons*, 4th ed., edited by M. Amdur, J. Doull, and C. Klaassen, pp. 985–996. Pergamon Press, Elmsford, New York.
97. Schuurman, H.-J., Kuper, C. F., and Vos, J. G. (1994): Histopathology of the immune system as a tool to assess immunotoxicity. *Toxicology*, 86:187–212.
98. See, D. M., Khemka, P., Sahl, L., Bui, T., and Tilles, J. G. (1997): The role of natural killer cells in viral infections. *Scand. J. Immunol.*, 46:217–224.
99. Selgrade, M. K., Lawrence, D. A., Ullrich, S, E., Gilmour, M. I., Schuyler, M. R., and Kimber, I. (1997): Modulation of T-helper cell populations: Potential mechanisms of respiratory hypersensitivity and immune suppression. *Toxicol. Appl. Pharmacol.*, 145:218–229.
100. Sercarz, E. E., Lehmann, P. V., and Ametani, A. (1993): Dominance and crypticity of T cell antigenic determinants. *Ann. Rev. Immunol.*, 11:729–766.
101. Sgonc, R., and Wick, G. (1994): Methods for the detection of apoptosis. *Int. Arch. Allergy Immunol.*, 105:327–332.
102. Shenker, B. J., Guo, T. L., and Shapiro, I. M. (1998): Low-level methylmercury exposure causes human T-cells to undergo apoptosis: Evidence of mitochondrial dysfunction. *Environ. Res.*, 77:149–159.
103. Smialowicz, R. J., and Holsapple, M. P. (1996): *Experimental Immunotoxicology*. CRC Press, Boca Raton, FL.
104. Taub, D. D. (1996): Chemokine-leukocyte interactions: The voodoo that they do so well. *Cytokine Growth Factor Rev.*, 7:355–376.
105. Tay, C. H., Szomolanyi-Tsuda, E., and Welsh, R. M. (1998): Control of infections by NK cells. *Curr. Top. Microbiol. Immunol.*, 230:193–220.
106. Temple, L., Butterworth, L., Kawabata, T. T., Munson, A. E., and White, K. L. (1995): ELISA to measure SRBC specific serum IgM: Method and data evaluation. In: *Methods in Immunotoxicology, Volume 1*, edited by G. R. Burleson, J. H. Dean, and A. E. Munson, pp. 137–157. Wiley–Liss, Inc., New York.
107. Theofilopoulus, A. N. (1995): The basis for autoimmunity: Part II: Genetic predisposition. *Immunol. Today*, 16:150–159.
108. Thomas, P. T., and House, R. V. (1995): Preclinical immunotoxicity assessment. In: *CRC Handbook of Toxicology*, edited by M. J. Derelanko and M. A. Hollinger, pp. 293–316. CRC Press, Boca Raton, FL.
109. Twerdok, L. E., and Trush, M. A. (1988): Neutrophil derived oxidants as mediators of chemical activation in bone marrow. *Chem. Biol. Int.*, 65:261–273.
110. van Loveren, H., Germolec, D., Koren, H. S., Luster, M. I., Nolan, C., Repetto, R., Smith, E., Vos, J. G., and Vogt, R. F. (1999): Report of the Bilthoven Symposium: Advancement of epidemiological studies in assessing the human health effects of immunotoxic agents in the environment and the workplace. *Biomarkers*, 4:135–157.
111. Vandebriel, R. J., Van Loveren, H., and Meredith, C. (1998): Altered cytokine (receptor) mRNA expression as a tool in immunotoxicology. *Toxicology*, 130:43–67.
112. Verdier, F., Chazal, I., and Descotes, J. (1994): Anaphylaxis models in the guinea pig. *Toxicology*, 93:55–61.
113. Vial, T., and Descotes, J. (1994): Contact sensitization assays in guinea pigs: Are they predictive of the potential for systemic allergic reactions? *Toxicology*, 93:63–75.
114. Vos. J. G. (1980): Immunotoxicity assessment: Screening and function studies. *Arch. Toxicol.* [*Suppl.*], 4:95–108.
115. Vos, J. G., and Van Loveren, H. (1998): Experimental studies on immunosuppression: How do they predict for man? *Toxicology*, 129:13–26.
116. Waldmann, T. A. (1988): Immunodeficiency diseases: Primary and acquired. In: *Immunological Diseases, 4th ed., Vol. 1*, edited by M. Samter, D. W. Talmage, M. M. Frank, K. F. Austen, and H. N. Claman, pp. 411–466. Little, Brown, Boston.
117. Warheit, D. B., and Hesteberg, T. W. (1994): Asbestos and other fibers in the lung. In: *Immunotoxicology and Immunopharmacology*, 2nd ed., edited by J. H. Dean, M. I. Luster, A. E. Munson, and I. Kimber, pp. 363–376. Raven Press, New York.
118. Weigent, D. A., and Blalock, J. E. (1995): Associations between the neuroendocrine and immune systems. *J. Leukoc. Biol.*, 57:137–150.
119. Yoo, B. S., Jung, K. H., Hana, S. B., and Kim. H, M. (1997): Apoptosis-mediated immunotoxicity of polychlorinated biphenyls (PCBs) in murine splenocytes. *Toxicol. Lett.*, 91:83–89.
120. Young, P. (1980): Asthma and allergies: An optimistic future (Based on Report on the Task Force on Asthma and the Other Allergic Diseases). NIH Publ. No. M388. U. S. Government Printing Office, Washington, DC.

Principles and Methods of Toxicology,
Fourth Edition, edited by A. Wallace Hayes.
Taylor & Francis, Philadelphia © 2001.

Chapter **32**

Assessment of Behavioral Toxicity

Bernard Weiss and Deborah A. Cory-Slechta

LD50s, mainstays of quantitative toxicology a surprisingly short time ago, left little scope for functional assays such as those represented by behavior. Lethality may be a useful gauge for catastrophes, and is still embedded in some government regulations, but it is not the kind of metric featured in risk assessment. Pathological surveys simply extended the boundaries to locate the site and character of tissue damage. It was only when scientists and the general public finally came to recognize that disorders of function represented significant outcomes of toxic exposures that behavioral toxicology began to seep into the parent discipline. This chapter explains how that process evolved and how it is conducted. It recognizes the two major thrusts of the discipline: one component aimed at elaborating the behavioral impact of environmental and occupational chemical exposures and the behavioral mechanisms that underlie such changes, another occupying an important role in the discipline of risk assessment by achieving recognition of the significance of concerns over behavioral dysfunction.

Behavior is the primary means by which an organism interacts with its environment. Although, for example, fine adjustments to ambient temperature are carried out continuously by physiological regulatory mechanisms, the large-scale adjustments, such as seeking shelter or adjusting a thermostat, are behavioral responses. To survive, organisms must be sensitive to events occurring in their environments and respond appropriately. At the most elementary level, organisms must avoid hazards such as predators and other threats, must secure food, and, for species survival, must pursue reproduction. The nervous system is the site at which such transactions with the environment are processed. The nervous system also governs endogenous transactions such as controlling neuroendocrine secretions, and carries on commerce with the immune system, but such functions are processed in the background, so to speak. The nervous system crowns the hierarchy of biological systems because it governs behavior. Its integrity, paramount to both individual and species survival, is reflected predominantly by the integrity of behavior.

This chapter addresses the question of how to assess behavioral toxicity. For any facet of toxicity, analogous questions are never simple. For behavior, the complexities are multiplied manyfold. Some toxicologists viewing these complexities might ask: Why, if the nervous system is the target of behavioral assays, is it necessary to peer at it through the lens of behavior? Why not ask the question directly? Why not evaluate nervous system structure? Why not assay nervous system chemistry? The answer consists of two parts, the first of which is another question. Which aspects of nervous system structure or function should be assayed? If the answer is neurochemistry, then which among the dozens of neurotransmitter and neuromodulator systems and their chemical pathways should be emphasized? If the answer is morphology, then by which techniques and in which nervous system areas? The second part of the answer is less direct. It points to the variety of human behavioral disorders for which no definitive biochemical or morphological substrate has been identified; attention deficit disorder, schizophrenia, and learning disabilities are among them. Even most instances of mental retardation present no specific clues to the sites or indices of damage. The behavioral disorder itself is the issue.

The situation is similar in toxicology, where behavioral assessment provides a measure of functional competence and a compass to more specific, often more subtle measures. Simultaneously, it provides guidance to the possible substrates. Sometimes the guidance is in the form of a broad index such as elevated motor activity, which may indicate actions on specific neurotransmitter systems. Sometimes it uncovers specific deficits such as an inability to distinguish geometric forms, which would point to the visual cortex as a possible site of damage. Sometimes it is simply an indication of the dose or exposure levels at which substrate investigations require exploration. This is a critical issue because neurochemical and morphological questions are often pursued at dose levels so extreme that almost any neurotoxic index will be affected.

For these reasons, the assessment of behavioral toxicity, during the risk assessment process in particular, often proceeds in stages. Gross screening for lethality and identifiable systemic effects is undertaken for nearly all chemicals. Although the components of such a screen are predominantly neurotoxic in character anyway, they also provide little specificity. The first stage specific to neurotoxicity typically seeks a grasp of dose-response relationships based on systematic observations of a collection of responses such as those embodied in functional observation batteries (177).

More complex assays usually, though not always, come later. Such assays may probe for actions on processes such as simple learning, adaptation to startle stimuli, and somewhat more definition of sensory and motor function than can be derived by the simpler assays. These later stages of assessment are designed to yield more specific and quantitative measures than the preliminary assays and to help predict more clearly the scope of possible adverse effects in humans. Still, they remain assays designed more for breadth than for depth. Subsequent assessments may be undertaken if more comprehensive information about one or more of these functions is desired, such as if a specific impairment of learning or possible damage to the visual system is suspected. Questions of this kind may require complex experimental situations and instrumentation to achieve answers. Although such a sequence of questions is not formalized in regulatory guidance, it often occurs in practice, as when earlier assumptions about the basis for a regulatory standard become questionable. The requirements of the Food Quality Protection Act of 1996 represent one such instance.

Some observers make a distinction between what they call "naturalistic" behaviors, such as those scored on functional observation batteries, and the kinds of complex learned behaviors just described. But all behaviors are "naturalistic"; none exceeds the bounds of biological possibility. Using such a term simply implies that we lack understanding of its controlling variables. Even as apparently natural and spontaneous a behavior as self-grooming by monkeys can be brought under experimental control by reinforcing it with food (125). In the laboratory, when we study operant behavior, we simply limit the number of variables we have to explain. In the natural environment, we may study foraging by recording variables such as time spent at a particular site, the amount of food consumed there, the travel time from one site to another, and similar measures. In the laboratory, we convert the environment to one in which choices are more easily recorded and variables specifically controlled. For similar reasons, we bring a patient or worker to a clinic for neuropsychological assessment rather than assigning an observer to follow him or her on a daily schedule of activities.

Studies of exposed humans generally occur after an agent already has been documented as hazardous. Workplace exposures have stimulated the bulk of published human studies, but issues such as the neurobehavioral toxicity of lead in children also have generated a substantial literature. Human studies aim at a question that simpler laboratory animal experiments often ignore. They are designed to provide data from which risk evaluations and safety standards can be drawn. Many animal experiments continue only to address the risk assessment stage termed hazard identification because of their emphasis on acute, high-dose exposures.

The disparity between human and animal research goals is particularly evident in the special ways in which adverse behavioral effects erupt in human environments. Except for catastrophic accidents, they may appear as a progressive decline in function. Often the first clues are subjective disturbances such as nervousness (chlordecone) or personality changes (manganese), succeeded by more overt signs such as tremor (chlordecone) or akinesia (manganese). Regulatory standards aim for exposure levels providing enough of a margin to preclude even the early, nonspecific symptoms. Most animal laboratory investigations, however, have tended to adopt exposure levels likely to evoke a clearly visible toxic response. This strategy was defended by the need to develop methods responsive to neurotoxic agents and to acquire corresponding information about mechanisms of toxicity that will be applicable to lower levels. More recent animal studies now entail a greater concern with behavioral mechanisms and lower level exposures, and much of the work with humans grows out of the specific circumstances of exposure.

The high-dose strategy fails when the mechanisms of toxicity are different at the higher levels. For example, a metabolic pathway that detoxifies a particular substance may become saturated. Or, the gradual progression of toxicity, manifested at low exposure levels by a sequential unfolding of different signs, may be buried in the massive deterioration of function evoked by high acute exposures. Such phenomena are among the reasons that Golberg (100), in his speculations about the potential of in vitro methods, pointed to behavioral toxicology as a discipline whose objectives could be fulfilled only tangentially by such methods. Furthermore, it is virtually impossible to mimic complex human behavior in an in vitro preparation, particularly when we know that subtle behavioral differences can significantly influence neurobiology.

The chapter proceeds from the simpler techniques generally applied in the earliest steps of hazard identification, to the later steps that involve both hazard specification and confirmation and dose-response assessment, to the techniques designed to clarify specific endpoints and to understand both behavioral and neurobiological mechanisms. This is followed by a presentation of human evaluation techniques. The goals of the chapter are to provide enough familiarity with these techniques to enable most readers to approach the literature of behavioral toxicology with a more than elementary understanding of its content. The more elaborate techniques are more closely related to what we ultimately require of risk evaluation than to hazard identification. They are driven by parallels with human exposure conditions, in which the dominant questions arise from the modification of complex functional outcomes by modest or even minimal exposure levels, often of a chronic nature. An emphasis on these techniques would be warranted by their role in important policy decisions alone, but they also offer advantages in pursuing the biochemical and morphological substrates of their outcomes. In fact, they may identify such substrates more effectively than the contrasting strategy of high doses and crude endpoints because of their greater specificity and sensitivity.

Although much of the chapter features animal models, many of the techniques discussed are adaptable, with minimal changes, to human testing. In fact, some approaches were originally implemented in human subjects and subsequently modified for experimental animal use. In addition, an entire section is devoted to human testing in clinical and epidemiological settings. Inevitably, new techniques and modifications of existing ones will continue to proliferate, not only in behavioral toxicology itself but in fields that share common borders, such as the study of neurodegenerative diseases. For example, some of the speculations about the etiology of Parkinson's disease posit a chemical source in the environment, perhaps one related to the illicit drug contaminant MPTP (1-methyl-4-phenyl-1,2,3,6-tetrahydropyridine). Functional disabilities provoked in monkeys by MPTP, and therapeutic interventions as well, are assayed with behavioral tests. Some of the other degenerative processes related to aging, such as Alzheimer's disease, have spawned hypotheses about a possible link to substances in the environment such as aluminum and, correspondingly, a literature relating aluminum exposure in experimental animals to behavioral outcomes. Examples of this kind illustrate how profoundly the concept of behavioral toxicity now permeates views of the sources of disease and dysfunction. Two recent reports (180,190) aimed at the impact of neurobehavioral toxicants on public health demonstrate how behavior serves as the sentinel for less accessible endpoints. This widening scope of behavioral toxicology is certain to alter how it is practiced.

ORIGINS OF BEHAVIOR

The repertoire of behavior can be construed as varying along two dimensions: origin and modifiability. At one end of such a continuum are behaviors that are designated as innate or "hard-wired." These behaviors include unconditioned reflexes, fixed-action patterns, and instinctive behaviors that do not require learning on the part of the organism. The components of such innate behaviors may be unique to a particular species and may be insensitive to modification by the environment. For some such behaviors, once evoked, the behavioral process continues to completion even in the absence of the appropriate substrates.

On the other extreme of such a continuum are behaviors that are learned or acquired, and that are subject to modification by the environment. Such behaviors are based on voluntary emitted responses, which then are increased or decreased in strength, altered, or refined by environmental consequences. Falling between these

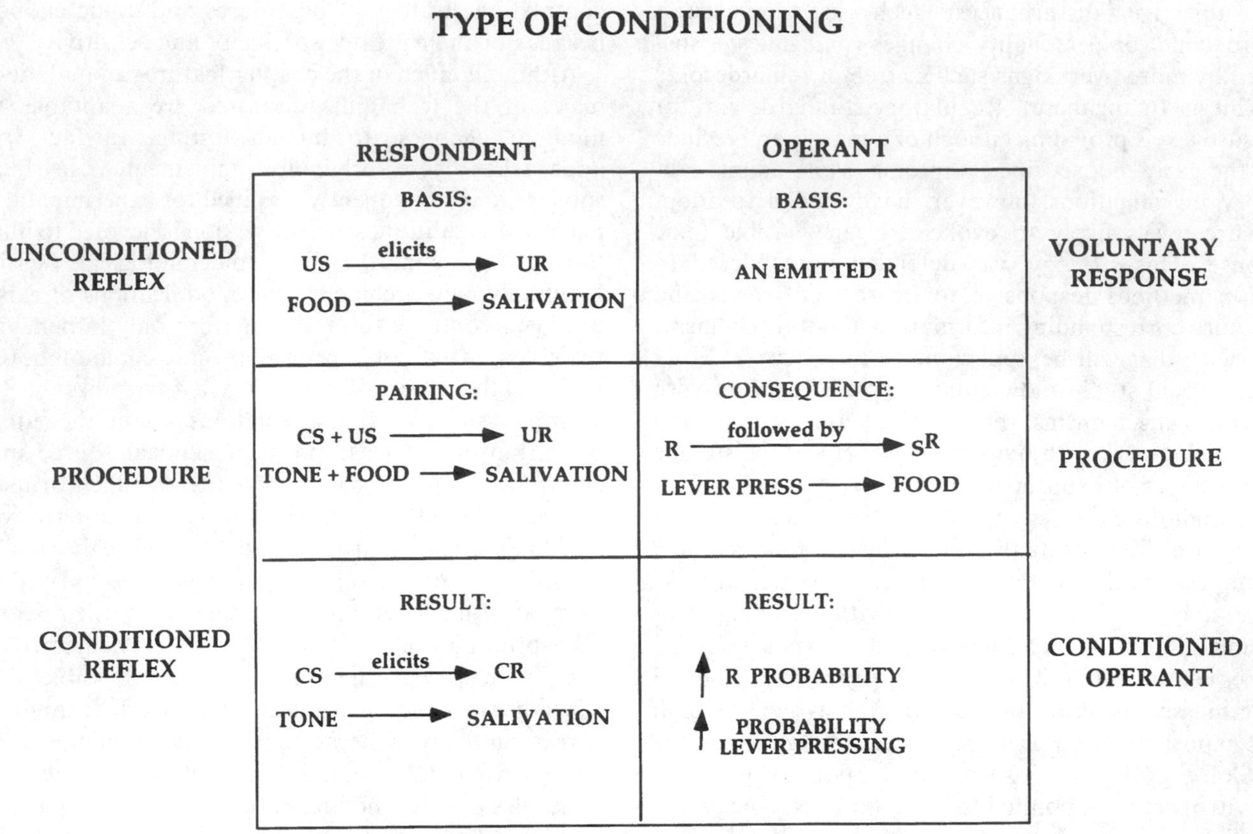

FIG. 32.1. The two types of behavioral conditioning are illustrated. Respondent conditioning (left column) is based upon unconditioned or innate reflexes in which an unconditioned stimulus elicits an unconditioned response. When an initially neutral stimulus is paired with the unconditioned stimulus (procedure), it acquires eliciting properties; that is, it becomes a conditioned stimulus capable of eliciting a conditioned response (result). Operant conditioning (right column) is based on voluntary responses emitted by the organism. If these responses are followed by a reinforcing stimulus (procedure), the frequency of the response will subsequently increase (result).

two extremes are instinctive behaviors such as fixed-action patterns that have components that can be modified by environmental circumstances. The extent to which the behavioral repertoire of an organism is comprised of learned versus unlearned behaviors is dependent on species, with a tendency for learned behaviors to predominate at the higher end of the phylogenetic continuum.

New behavior is generated by operant or respondent conditioning. The basis of the respondent conditioning paradigm, as shown in Figure 32.1, is an unconditioned response elicited, that is, evoked by an unconditioned stimulus, with the term *unconditioned* signifying the innate characteristics of the response and stimulus comprising the reflex. When the unconditioned stimulus is repeatedly paired with a neutral stimulus, the neutral stimulus acquires eliciting properties similar to those of the unconditioned stimulus; that is, the neutral stimulus becomes a conditioned stimulus that evokes a conditioned response typically, though not uniformly, similar to the unconditioned response. An example, also shown in Figure 32.1, is best exemplified by the studies carried out by the Russian physiologist I. P. Pavlov. In his experiments, meat powder, the unconditioned stimulus, evoked salivation, an unconditioned response, in dogs. Tones repeatedly paired with the meat powder eventually came to function as conditioned stimuli that elicited conditioned salivation. These pairings of the conditioned and unconditioned stimuli must occur at least intermittently for the conditioned stimulus to maintain its ability to elicit a conditioned response.

Operant conditioning does not rely on an elicited response. Instead, it is based on voluntary or emitted responses that occur at some baseline, or operant level, in the absence of any environmental influences. For example, newborn babies engage in voluntary skeletal muscle motions even at birth that can be modified by their environmental consequences and thus serve as the basis of later, more coordinated movements and precise motor functions. Operant conditioning refers to the process by which the frequency or strength of an operant (voluntary) response is modified by the consequences of that behavior. Reinforcement is the presentation of a stimulus contingent on a response that results in an increase in the frequency of that response. Reinforcers or reinforcing stimuli may be either positive or negative, a distinction that is purely procedural. Specifically, a positive reinforcer strengthens a response, that is, increases its probability, by its presentation, such as the delivery of food to a hungry organism, or perhaps the attention of a well-liked friend. With negative reinforcement, a response is strengthened by the removal or diminution of a stimulus event or the prevention of its onset, such as cessation of electric shock or loud noise contingent on a response, or prevention of a parent's scolding by cleaning one's room. Shock avoidance and escape procedures fit into this category.

Reinforcers cannot be classified intuitively or categorically, but only on the basis of the change in behavior subsequent to their presentation. Food may not serve as a positive reinforcer for someone with the stomach flu; attention and affection often fail to function as positive reinforcers for autistic children. Given the appropriate behavioral training conditions, electric shock presentation can actually maintain rather than suppress responding (160). As these examples indicate, a stimulus that serves as a reinforcer for one person may not so function for another. The sum total of an individual's interaction with the environment and reinforcement contingencies is deemed its behavioral history. Because all individuals could never simultaneously be in the same place, make the same responses, earn the same reinforcers, and so forth, each person's "behavioral history" is unique. This becomes particularly important because differences in behavioral history can radically modify the response to drugs (e.g., ref. 13), and thus, perhaps, to toxicants as well.

Reinforcers also are defined as primary (unlearned, SR) or secondary (conditioned, learned, Sr). Primary reinforcers function as effective reinforcers without any prior experience or training. Examples include food, water, and the opportunity to engage in sexual behavior. Conditioned reinforcers are stimuli that acquire their reinforcing efficacy only through pairing with other established reinforcers. Money serves as an extremely effective generalized conditioned reinforcer because of its pairing with many other reinforcers, both primary and conditioned. Conditioned reinforcers frequently are generated in an experimental setting by repeatedly pairing an initially neutral stimulus, such as a light flash or tone, with a primary reinforcer, such as food delivery. After repeated pairings, the light stimulus acquires reinforcing properties of its own and can maintain substantial operant responding itself. To retain its reinforcing efficacy, however, the conditioned reinforcer must be paired at least occasionally with the primary reinforcer.

Two operant procedures that decrease the frequency of learned responses are punishment and extinction. In punishment, a stimulus presented after a response decreases the frequency of that response. Spanking a child who has drawn on the wallpaper may constitute an example. Again, the stimulus must be classified only on the basis of the change in response frequency; if a promptly delivered spanking fails to decrease the frequency of writing on the wallpaper, then by definition spanking was not an effective punishing stimulus. In a clinical context, the presentation of ammonia to the nose contingent on self-abusive behavior often decreases the frequency of this response typically observed in autistic children. In extinction, the reinforcer for a response is withheld and the frequency of the response eventually (usually after an initial increase) declines. Withdrawing social attention from a child who has thrown a temper tantrum will in many cases decrease the future incidence of tantrums. Table 32.1 summarizes these terms, with respect both to the procedures involved and to the subsequent behavioral outcome.

A stimulus in the presence of which an operant response is repeatedly reinforced comes to acquire stimulus control over the response; in the presence of this and related stimuli, the probability of the response is increased. This stimulus that defines the occasion on which an operant response is followed by reinforcement is called a discriminative stimulus (S+ or SD). For example, the sight and/or smell of freshly baked cookies may be an SD setting the occasion for the response of reaching into the cookie jar to be reinforced with a cookie, whereas an empty cookie jar would be unlikely to occasion such a response. Similarly, a red light and a stop sign are discriminative stimuli that control the responses involved in stopping a vehicle. Braking at other times, that is, at a green light, may have disastrous consequences. It is important to remember that discriminative stimuli do not elicit or evoke responses as do unconditioned and conditioned stimuli in respondent conditioning procedures; they merely, but

Table 32.1
Consequences of responding

Stimulus condition	Change in response strength	
	Increased	Decreased
Presentation	Positive reinforcement	Punishment
Withdrawal	Negative reinforcement	Extinction

importantly, indicate the likelihood or probability of reinforcement for a given operant response.

The response of an organism may be explicitly reinforced in the presence of one stimulus (S+), such as a red light, while reinforcement is explicitly withheld in the presence of another stimulus, the S– (or S__), such as a green light. Using such a discrimination procedure, the organism soon comes to respond in a certain way only when the red light is on, that is, in the presence of the discriminative stimulus, and not in the presence of the S__, such that the behavior is said to be under stimulus control. When responding generalizes to other stimuli of the same or related stimulus classes, such as when a young child refers to all grown males as "daddy," responding has generalized across the stimulus class "adult male," and stimulus generalization has occurred. These processes of stimulus control and stimulus generalization are important aspects of such behavioral functions as concept formation and learning to learn.

In summary, a three-term contingency describes operant conditioning, as illustrated in Figure 32.2 (178). In the presence of antecedent discriminative stimuli, an operant response engenders some consequent event that alters the subsequent probability of that response, and also alters the future control of the antecedent stimulus (SD) over the response. It should be noted that discriminative and reinforcing stimuli need not be external events; internal stimuli, whether internal physiological changes such as headaches or our own nonvocal verbal behavior ("thinking"), can acquire such important behavioral functions.

Precise and operational definitions are critical in behavior because a toxic agent, like a brain lesion, may affect any stage in this three-term contingency. A goal of behavioral toxicology is to understand how toxic agents alter function, or, more precisely, the behavioral mechanism(s) of action of the compound. As discussed by Thompson and Schuster (268) and Thompson and Boren (264) in the context of behavioral pharmacology, attaining such a goal depends on a thorough knowledge of the variables that control behavior, just as the biologist must understand a biological system. Behavior is influenced by multiple factors: by antecedent factors, such as deprivation or motivational state; by antecedent stimulus conditions, such as the presence or strength of discriminative stimuli; by the nature of the response and response parameters, that is, its topography or physical characteristics; and by the consequences that serve to maintain the behavior. A toxicant may change behavior through its interaction with any or all such variables. That is, it may alter functional deprivation levels—for example, induce nausea—or it may interfere with the ability to discriminate among stimuli. Alternatively, it could modify the topography of the response, as by evok-

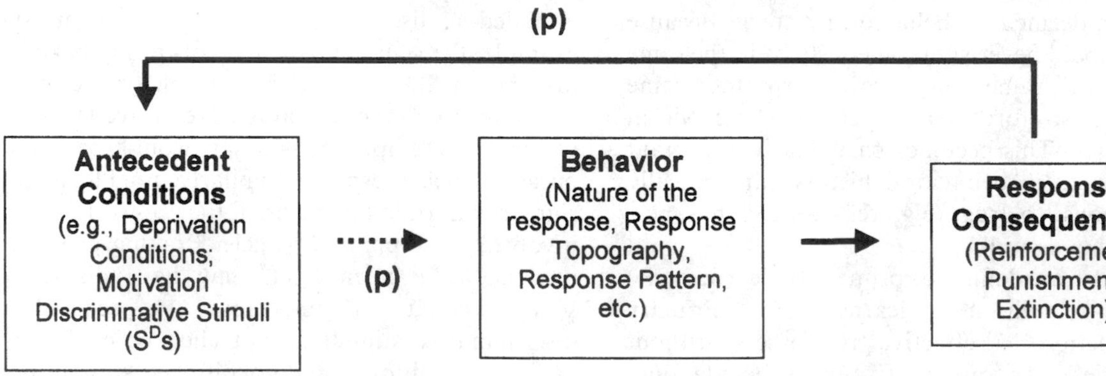

In the presence of antecedent conditions, a response occurs that engenders some consequence event. The nature of the antecedent conditions may alter the probability [(p)] of the response occurring. The nature of the consequence of the response determines its future probability, and may alter its characteristics. In addition, the response consequences may alter the strength of the discriminative stimuli that occasion the response.

FIG. 32.2. Three-term contingency describing operant behavior. A toxicant may act by altering the antecedent conditions such as the functional deprivation condition of the subject, or its ability to process information related to the probability of reward in the environment (discriminative stimuli). A toxicant may act by altering the characteristics of the response itself, such as its topography or duration. A toxicant may act to alter the response consequences, such as change the perceived magnitude of reward or punishment. Understanding how a toxicant interacts with these factors defines the behavioral mechanism of effect.

- **Home-cage and Handling**
  - posture
  - ease of handling
  - ease of removel
  - piloerection
  - vocalizations
- **Open Field**
  - time to first step
  - urination, defecation
  - gait
  - bizarre behavior
  - rearing behavior
- **Reflex and Physiological**
  - approach response
  - touch response
  - finger snap response
  - righting reflex
  - grip strength
  - catalepsy
  - forelimb grip strength

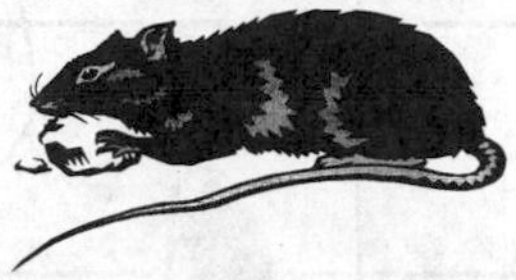

FIG. 32.3. Typical measures included in many functional observational batteries (FOBs). These include aspects of home cage and handling, behavior in an open field, and various reflex and physiological responses. Measurement of locomotor activity is also often included in an FOB.

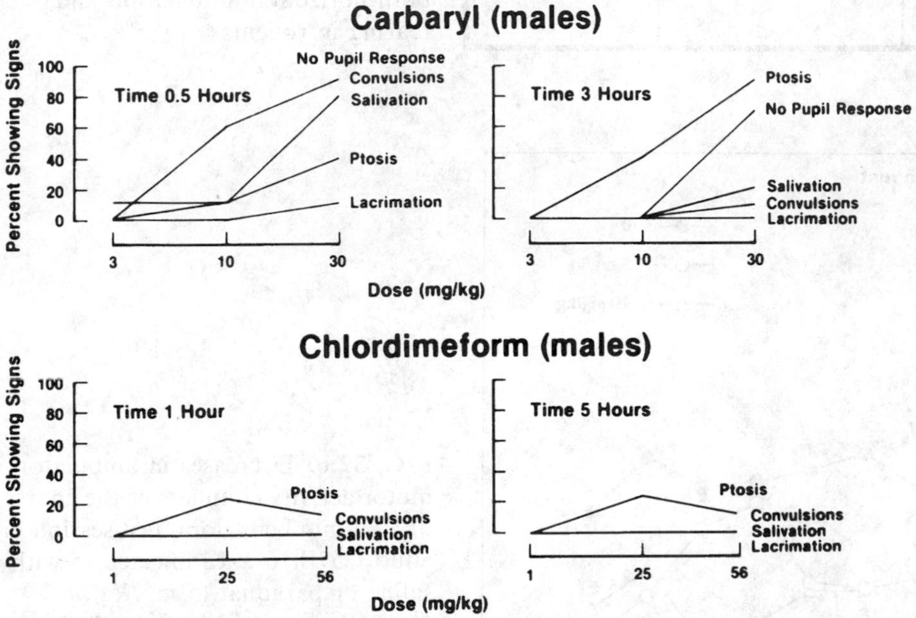

FIG. 32.4. Autonomic cholinergically mediated measures included in an FOB in response are increased in response to increasing doses of the anticholinesterase carbaryl (top row), as might be predicted, and not to the non-anticholinesterase pesticide chlordimeform. From Moser et al. (177).

ing incoordination, or it could interfere with the ability to associate the discriminative stimulus with the contingency, and so forth. Understanding the exact components of behavioral processes affected by toxic agents assists in understanding the underlying behavioral mechanisms as well as offering guidance to the neurobiological mechanisms of effect.

SCREENING BATTERIES

As pointed out earlier, one of the agendas that has emerged for behavioral toxicity involves the screening of new chemicals for potential neurotoxicity. The behavioral tests utilized for such purposes are often referred to as apical tests because they require the integrated function of several organ systems, including the nervous system. Such batteries typically have included two behavioral components: a functional observational battery (FOB) and an evaluation of motor activity. Figure 32.3 depicts the component tests of the FOB developed by Moser et al. (177), which include an array of measures of both unconditioned operant and respondent behaviors. Such batteries have been shown to exhibit utility for screening potential neurotoxicity, that is, hazard identification and elaboration, as exemplified in Figure 32.4. As it shows, those components of the FOB directed to cholinergic functions exhibited sensitivity to the effects of the anticholinesterase carbaryl, whereas few such signs of cholinergic disturbances were evident in the presence of the non-anticholinesterase pesticide chlordimeform. Further discussion of FOB measures by domain is provided by Moser et al. (177) and by Baird et al. (8a).

Motor activity is frequently included in screening batteries both as a measure of motor function and as an apical test (269a). Motor activity, generally considered an

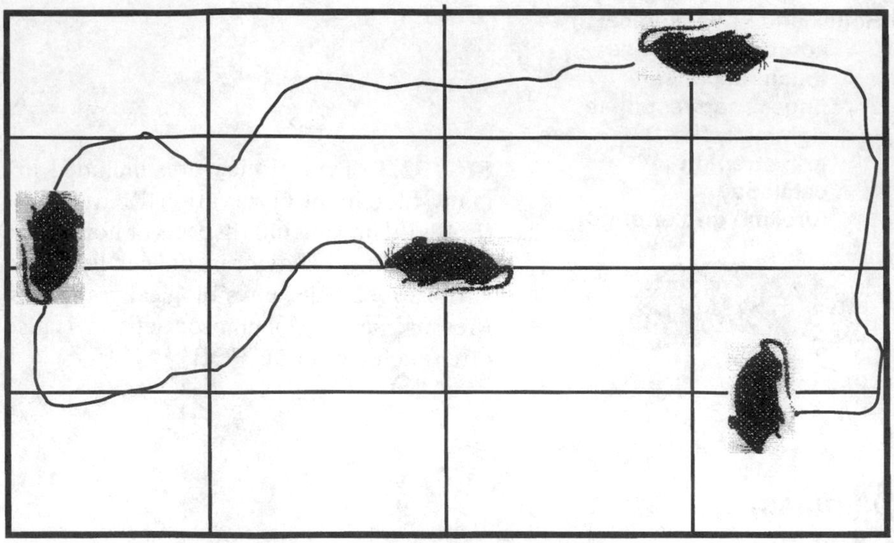

FIG. 32.5. Open field for the measurement of locomotor activity. In nonautomated procedures, the number of movements per unit time are recorded by an observer. Automated devices typically rely on computerized measurement of photobeam breaks by the movement of the subject to assess locomotor activity. Photobeams are typically positioned so as to measure aspects of both horizontal ambulation and rearing in rodents.

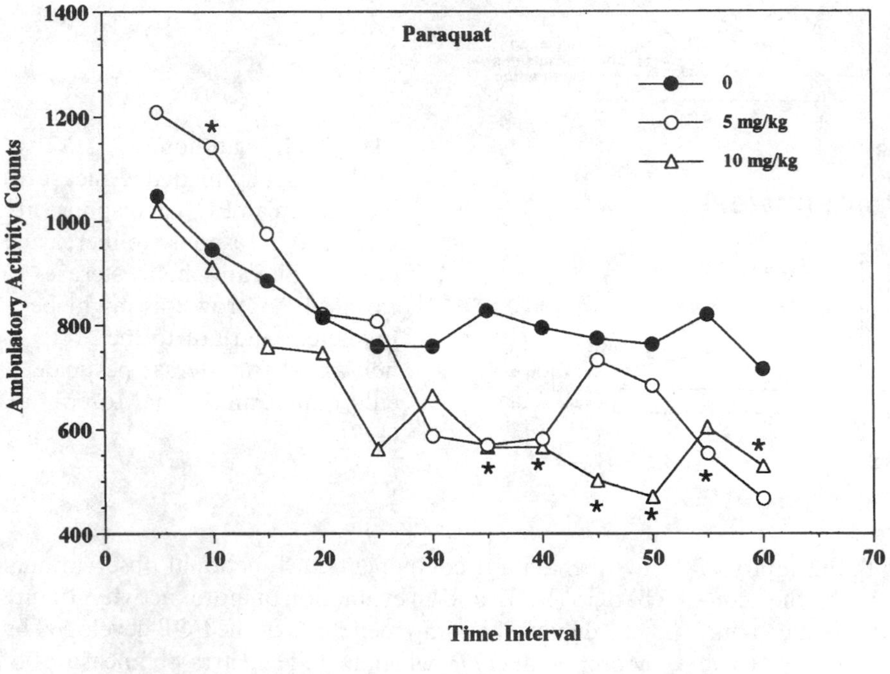

FIG. 32.6. Decreases in ambulatory motor activity counts over the course of a 60-min behavioral test session in adult C57Bl/6 mice injected ip with saline or paraquat (5 mg/kg or 10 mg/kg) one time per week for a total of 3 weeks. Motor activity was measured in an automated device using photobeam breaks. From Brooks et al. (24b).

unconditioned behavior, exists at some baseline level and is a complex behavior that includes numerous components such as ambulation, rearing, grooming, sniffing, etc. As discussed earlier, toxicants may alter motor activity by affecting any or all of its component behaviors.

Numerous devices have been designed to measure motor activity, which vary in complexity and in the component behaviors they measure. One such device that has been frequently employed is the figure 8 maze, which consists of a series of interconnected alleys converging on a central open area. Motor activity is detected by photobeams, and an activity count is registered each time a photobeam is interrupted by the animal. In a device such as the open field schematized in Figure 32.5, motor activity is instead quantified by counting the number of squares entered by the animal within some prescribed period of time. Figure 32.6 plots motor activity in mice treated with paraquat (24b). Over the past several years, these devices have become increasingly automated and locate photobeam devices in a manner that permits the separate detection of different types of motor activity, such as ambulation versus rearing, and measuring their occurrence in a time-course fashion. This is important since reliance on total counts may obscure toxicant-induced differences in patterns of activity. For example, in the open-field device, one could arrive at the same total number of squares entered in some period of time by very different patterns of behavior: The organism might show an initial period of rapid movement in the open field followed by immobility, or, alternatively, it could exhibit a continuous moderate rate of ambulation. Both patterns could result in the same total number of squares entered even though the underlying patterns of behavior are quite distinct. Thus, in the absence of a more detailed analysis of patterns of activity, a toxicant that alters motor activity primarily by altering its distribution in time could go undetected.

From the standpoint of screening and hazard identification, another notable point relating to the interpretation of data from FOB and motor activity studies is whether the effects observed in response to toxicant exposure represent a direct effect of the toxicant on the nervous system or are secondary to changes in other systems since such apical tests rely on the functional integrity of multiple systems. Under some circumstances, the fact that the toxic effect is ultimately expressed in behavior may minimize the importance of the direct versus indirect source of the effect. It also should be noted in the interpretation of toxicant-induced changes in FOBs and motor activity measures that the concurrent presence of body weight loss or decline in food or water intake does not by any means necessarily indicate that the behavioral changes are the result of malaise or sickness, as these measures may change independently of each other. Certain agents, such as volatile organic solvents, tend to enhance motor activity at low concentrations, so the problem of confounding with malaise is diminished with such results (303a).

BEHAVIORAL TERATOLOGY

Behavioral teratology is often presented as a separate component of behavioral toxicology, primarily because of its focus on behavioral modifications resulting from toxic exposures during early development. In general, such studies track the outcome of such exposures over the postnatal and possibly into the juvenile and early adult stages of the life cycle. Outcome measures almost invariably include the development of physical landmarks and reflexes, and also generally include assessment of one or more behavioral functions. Often attempts are made to evaluate multiple behavioral functions, such as motor function and activity, and sensory capabilities and learning, in the same experiment. In addition, testing for species-specific behaviors, such as aggression, play, and vocalization, may be included. Table 32.2 lists the criteria specified by the U.S. Environmental Protection Agency (EPA) for its developmental neurotoxicity guidelines.

Table 32.2
U.S. EPA developmental neurotoxicity criteria

Physical measures
—Body weights, sexually dimorphic indices
Brain weights
—Regional brain weights on days 4, 21
Neuropathology
—Postnatal (PN) days 4, 21, study termination, and GFAP
Locomotor activity
—PN days 13, 17, 21, 45, 60
Reactivity
—Auditory startle on PN days 22, 60
Learning and memory
—Olfactory discrimination on PN 21
—Active avoidance (or substitute) on PN 60

Testing during the infant, postnatal, and juvenile periods of development sometimes requires modifications of procedures that are utilized with adults or even the development of new paradigms. In other cases, behavioral paradigms identical to those used in more mature subjects may be employed, albeit with parametric modifications. One example of the former is a procedure that has been widely used in behavioral teratology studies to assess olfactory and motor capabilities and is referred to as *homing behavior,* a behavior used by rat pups to locate the nest should it be displaced. In such a test, a rat pup, the typical experimental subject for most experimental behavioral teratology studies, is placed in the center of a rectangular apparatus in which one side contains clean bedding material and the other side contains bedding from the pup's home-cage. The time taken for the pup to orient to or to reach the home-cage bedding constitutes the dependent variable of interest. Since this performance depends on both olfactory capabilities and the development of appropriate motor skills, it represents a type of apical evaluation (121a).

Other issues related to behavioral teratology, including appropriate fostering procedures to control for toxicant effects on the dam, statistical issues, and summaries of developmental effects of various toxicants, can be found in Buelke-Sam et al. (25), Voorhees (272), Riley and Voorhees (216), Yanai (304), Annau and Eccles (5), Ruppert (219), and Holson and Buelke-Sam (119). Because the central issue in behavioral teratology is the persistence or permanence of damage incurred during early development, the approaches to functional assessment described in this chapter generally do not differentiate the life-cycle stage at which exposure occurs.

COMPLEX OPERANT BEHAVIOR

The behavioral environment is a dynamic one in which multiple environmental contingencies are operating concurrently to produce, modify, refine, and eliminate aspects of learned operant behavior. The net result is a complex behavioral repertoire that includes a multitude of behavioral functions and processes, any or all of which may be the target of a toxic agent. Enumerating all such possibilities is beyond the scope of such a chapter and, indeed, constitutes a subject matter having spawned numerous volumes of its own.

Consequently, this section focuses on six particular behavioral functions that have evolved as primary interest areas in neurotoxicology: learning, memory, schedule-controlled behavior, stimulus and reinforcing properties of toxicants, sensory function, and motor function. One unique aspect of the experimental analysis of behavior is the enormous range and diversity of both apparatus and techniques designed to evaluate various aspects of complex learned behavior. Rather than enumerating all such possibilities for each behavioral function, this chapter emphasizes those procedures within each of these six categories that are the most widely used, as well as those that exemplify the range and scope of behavioral technology. It should become apparent that the increase in complexity of the latter classes of behavioral procedures is paralleled by a more selective and direct measurement of the behavioral function of interest.

Apparatus

The basic requirements for an assessment of complex performance must include a defined or specified unit of behavior to serve as the designated response. An environmental consequence or reinforcing event appropriate to the species and experimental parameters is arranged to follow the designated response. For some types of experiments, environmental stimuli of different modalities (visual, auditory, etc.) that can be varied along certain dimensions may be used as discriminative stimuli and/or conditioned reinforcers. The choice of the operant response, reinforcing consequence, and external or environmental stimuli should be congruent with the physical and behavioral capabilities of the experimental species. Teaching the chimpanzee to vocalize speech sounds proved impossible because of the physical limitations of its vocal apparatus. When the operant response was changed instead to sign language, however, experimental studies of the acquisition of verbal behavior proceeded successfully [reviewed by Ristau and Robbins (217) and Terrace (260)]. Similarly, under certain conditions, visual stimuli may prove inappropriate for rodents such as the mouse and rat, because of the poor visual capabilities of these species, which, instead, depend heavily upon olfactory information in their normal environment (113).

A broad spectrum of reinforcers has been used in behavioral experiments. The choice depends on the species and the aim of the particular experiment. These include the delivery of food, the delivery of liquid reinforcers such as water, fruit juice, or saccharin solutions, the opportunity to engage in wheel running, sexual behavior, or aggressive behavior, heat in a cold environment, the opportunity to self-administer a drug such as cocaine, electrical brain stimulation, and escape from or avoidance of electric shock. Such a breadth of choice in a standard experimental arrangement allows the experimenter enormous flexibility, such as to compare heat and food reinforcement in metabolically impaired animals (cf. ref. 137).

Many experiments on complex behavior are carried out in operant chambers such as that illustrated in Figure 32.7. In conventional chambers, response devices typically include levers (rat, mouse, monkey, human), disks (pigeons, monkeys, humans), running wheels (mouse, rat), and cones for snout insertion (mouse, rat, guinea pig). Typically, the execution of the response is defined by the closure of a switch or electrical circuit that can be recorded and acted on by a computer or by elec-

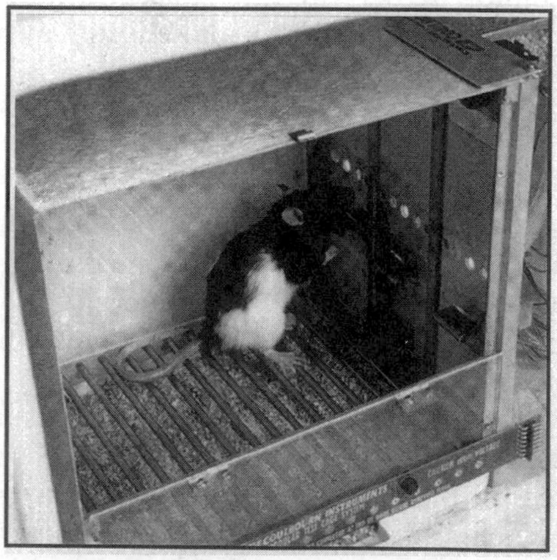

FIG. 32.7. Prototypical operant chamber (Skinner box) for use with the rat. This chamber is equipped with three response levers and a bank of lights above each lever. Also included are a sonalert for delivering tones, a speaker for the delivery of auditory stimuli, and a house light to utilize as a visual stimulus. Food deliveries used as rewards are delivered from a feeder outside the operant chamber through a plastic tube into a pellet trough located below the middle lever.

tromechanical devices. The operant chamber may contain multiple response devices, usually but not necessarily of the same type. In addition, stimuli of different modalities can be delivered to the chamber by lights, loudspeakers, and such, and the operant chamber may be adapted to utilize different reinforcers. Equally important are the ease and flexibility available to program experimental contingencies in the operant chamber and the precision and resolution with which data can be collected. Computer technology allows responses (and other events) to be measured and stored sequentially with millisecond resolution. This permits a more detailed analysis of behavior than was possible with the earlier electromechanical systems (280). For these reasons, an operant chamber equipped to deliver stimuli of various modalities, containing multiple response devices, and offering a choice of reinforcement delivery systems provides the maximal flexibility and versatility for behavioral studies. It similarly permits pursuit of scientific questions directed by research findings rather than having to be confined to research questions constrained by the apparatus, such as those specifically designed to measure a particular behavioral function.

In other cases, different types of devices, some automated and others not, have been used to measure specific aspects of behavior. Some are commercially available, while others have been designed to meet the requirements of a particular experiment. This has been the case particularly for the assessment of learning and memory functions, where mazes, including the more traditional mazes such as the T maze, the L maze, and the radial-arm maze, the latter consisting of a central area from which eight or more arms radiate like spokes, and more recently water mazes, have been used. The Wisconsin general test apparatus (WGTA) was used to study learning in primates, and modifications have since been made to accommodate other experimental species. The absence of automation of some such devices necessitates a far greater expenditure of personnel time, and thus ultimately costs, to carry out experiments and also introduces the possibility of experimental bias. While such devices can certainly provide in some cases a reasonable alternative to an operant chamber, as noted earlier, their limited utility for addressing a wide variety of other behavioral functions must also be considered when apparatus decisions are made.

Shaping an Operant Response

Before implementing a behavioral experiment, an effective reinforcer must be identified, one that can be presented immediately after the designated response occurs, because delayed reinforcement is less effective. In an operant chamber, a procedure known as magazine training is used to ensure the adequacy of the reinforcement contingency. Magazine training is accomplished by the presentation, at intermittent intervals, of the reinforcing stimulus, such as a food pellet, independently of behavior. After repeated presentations of food pellets in this manner, a slightly food-deprived organism will reliably approach the feeder and ingest the food whenever the appropriate noise is generated by the operation of the feeder. A stimulus such as a light is frequently paired with the food delivery and, along with the noise generated by the feeder, comes to serve as a conditioned reinforcer. These conditioned reinforcers are especially important because they provide the immediate reinforcement for responding given the delay necessarily imposed by the time required for the organism to approach and ingest the food. Once a reliable reinforcer is so established, "shaping" of the designated response can proceed. At this point, the reinforcing stimulus is presented only when the organism emits responses that more and more closely resemble the final designated response, such as a nose poke for a mouse, or the depression of a lever by a rat. For example, reinforcer delivery might first be contingent on touching the lever, then putting two paws on the lever, and eventually applying sufficient force to displace the lever downward. Reynolds (208) discusses these techniques in greater detail. In some cases, magazine training and shaping procedures can be automated (e.g., ref. 51), a major advantage when a large number of subjects must be used.

Shaping procedures also may be used in other types of apparatus to train the initial response. For example, in the WGTA, the monkey is first shaped to reach out and retrieve food from the food cups on the shelf in front of the enclosure. For other devices, such as mazes and running wheels, little overt shaping may be necessary, since exploring alleys and running usually occur spontaneously at a high enough frequency (high operant level) in rodents to ensure contact with the reinforcement contingency.

Once the organism is emitting the designated response at an adequate rate, it may still be necessary to progress through a series of training conditions before imposing a complex behavioral paradigm of experimental interest, just as a dancer must learn to connect the different steps of a choreographed performance. Likewise, a beginning reader could hardly be expected to tackle the plays of Shakespeare. In a similar way, requiring an organism to emit 100 responses for each food delivery will require intervening sessions with smaller response requirements to build up response strength and to prevent the behavior from undergoing extinction. It is the shaping process that creates new behaviors and pieces together responses to produce increasingly complex behavior.

Measures of Learning

Learning refers to the process of behavioral adaptation to changes in environmental contingencies, that is, behavior in transition. As Laties (136) pointed out, "There can be as many ways of studying learning as there are ways of confronting organisms with changed reinforcement contingencies and then watching them adapt to the new contingencies." The procedures and apparatus devoted to the study of learning are so diverse and numerous that an adequate description of their domain is beyond the scope of this chapter. As previously noted, this section includes those approaches that have been most frequently utilized, as well as those most promising for making understandable the behavioral and neurobiological mechanisms of toxicity. It also highlights some of the important methodological issues involved in a determination of changes in learning. Recent reviews describe in greater detail the effects of specific toxicants on learning, as well as other procedural issues (29,67,116).

The evaluation of learning processes frequently has been based on choice procedures from which accuracy and latency measures can be derived. Before the advent of more sophisticated technologies, the assessment of learning processes often relied on the use of mazes. For example, in a T maze, so named because of its shape, the subject was reinforced for choosing the arm of the maze that was designated as the correct side, whereas choosing the wrong arm of the maze resulted in no reinforcer delivery (extinction). Such procedures could be modified to some extent by the inclusion of external discriminative stimuli to signal which arm was the appropriate choice; for example, the black arm is the S+ and the white arm the S−. Typically, learning under such conditions was determined by the number of errors (entries into the wrong arm), the number of trials to some specified accuracy criterion, and the latency of the animal to enter the appropriate arm of the maze on each trial.

While such procedures were useful as potential indices of learning impairments, they have several disadvantages as well. Since such devices were not easily automated, after each trial the animal had to be replaced in the start box for initiation of the next trial. The necessity of handling animals, and experimenter intrusion into the recording of data, introduced the possibility of experimenter bias unless these procedures are carried out by personnel blind to all experimental conditions. Moreover, the demands on personnel time by nonautomated versions of mazes markedly increase the operational costs of such procedures and may limit the number of experiments that can be undertaken. Objections to automated procedures based on the expense of instrumentation often neglect to account for personnel costs incurred by procedures relying on human intervention, perhaps because the intervention is often conducted by graduate students. In addition, olfactory cues left by previous experimental animals and previous trials could be shown under some conditions to influence the performance of animals tested later. Such difficulties in controlling variables known to influence behavior may result in replication failures both within, and more probably across, laboratories. Moreover, the baselines were relatively simple learning tasks, decreasing the sensitivity of the baseline to drug or toxicant effects. The relative rapidity with which learning occurred also rendered such baselines ineffectual for assessing learning deficits following exposures to toxicants with delayed onset of action, or for tracking reversibility of any observed learning impairments. Finally, and perhaps most importantly, these dependent variables may be influenced by changes in other behavioral processes, limiting their ability to define a learning impairment. For example, the time to traverse the maze can be affected by changes in motor function; changes in sensory capabilities, particularly olfactory function, may likewise alter performance independently of changes in learning per se.

The radial-arm maze is a more complex learning task (Figure 32.8) that can be automated to some extent. It consists of a central area from which, typically, eight arms radiate like spokes, and a single food pellet is available in each arm. The subject then has access to eight reinforcer deliveries, one in each of the eight arms radiating from

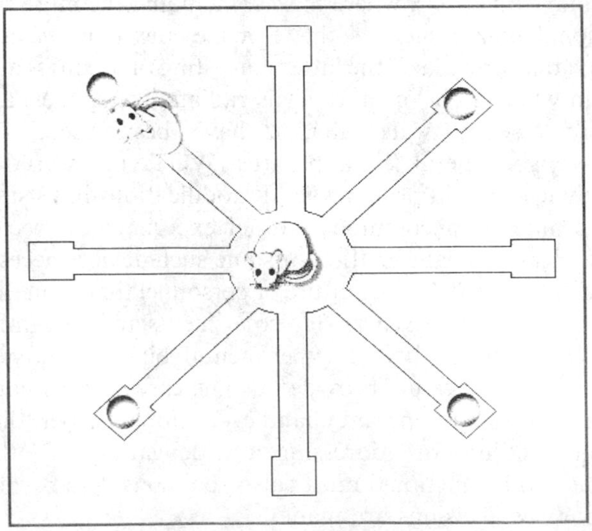

FIG. 32.8. Prototypical radial-arm maze for use with a rodent. The subject is typically placed in the center arena from which some number of arms radiate. Food reward is available under different configurations in various arms. Indices of performance include latencies to obtain rewards, number of arms visited to obtain rewards, and errors (e.g., returning to unbaited arms or arms in which the reward had already been obtained).

the central compartment. The accuracy, efficiency, and speed with which the organism learns to retrieve all eight food deliveries constitute the data of interest, with maximal efficiency requiring only eight arm entries to collect all eight food pellets. In addition, modifications of the standard procedures used with the radial-arm maze make it amenable to repeated learning. Peele and Baron (195) accomplished this by baiting only four of the eight arms, with the particular four baited arms changed during each successive experimental session.

The radial-arm maze has been shown to be sensitive to the effects of a wide variety of toxic agents and prenatal insults. For example, Walsh et al. (273) reported an impairment of reacquisition of radial-arm maze performance in rats that had been treated with trimethyltin, a toxicant that damages the hippocampus, a brain structure thought to play a prominent role in learning and memory functions. The problem presented to the animal in the radial-arm maze, because it is more complex than that embodied in the simpler mazes described earlier, offers a clear advantage with respect to sensitivity; however, it is also eventually solved, at which point the baseline ceases to provide a measure of learning. Thus, as is the case with the simpler maze procedures, neither long-term effects, delayed onset, nor reversibility can be easily addressed with this configuration. Also, in parallel with the simpler maze procedures is the possibility that changes in the baseline may reflect not changes in learning processes but rather the effects of the toxicant on motor function, sensory capabilities, etc. The water maze is a learning paradigm based on negative reinforcement procedures. In this particular paradigm, a rat or mouse is placed in a large tub of water that has been made opaque. The animal can escape from the water by finding a platform submerged so as to be invisible just under the surface. Again, the dependent variables include the number of trials to learn where the platform is hidden and the latency to find the hidden platform. This procedure has been employed widely in behavioral toxicology, in neuroscience, and in aging studies because of its ostensible simplicity and the lack of a training requirement or any food deprivation procedures. Performance on the maze has been reported to be influenced by a variety of manipulations, including lesions, toxicants, drugs, and aging. The procedure typically is nonautomated, rendering it a personnel-intensive approach to learning. Moreover, in the configuration described, it represents a relatively simple learning assay and thus may be of limited sensitivity and limited utility for studies of delayed onset of effect, reversibility, etc. This can be addressed to some extent by movement of the platform to new locations requiring learning of a new spatial site for escape. Like the maze procedures described earlier, its ability to define a selective effect on learning may be hindered by concurrent changes in motor function, body temperature, sensory alterations, and olfactory trails from prior subjects. Such possibilities require the use of additional probes (cued platform, swim speed and endurance, etc.) for evaluation. Furthermore, changes of as little as 1°C in water temperature may significantly alter performance and the procedure may prove stressful and effortful. In some studies involving genetically engineered mice, floaters are identified who must be eliminated from the experiment, thus enhancing the possibility of experimental bias.

Discrimination procedures in operant chambers represent another approach to the evaluation of learning processes. Technically, the discrimination paradigm reinforces the designated response in the presence of one stimulus (S+) but not in the presence of another (S−). As an example, a child's asking for a cookie after eating dinner is likely to pay off, whereas asking before dinner is not. Given such training, responding becomes confined to those periods during which the S+ is present, and has a low probability of occurrence during S− presentations. In an experimental situation, a lever-press response may be reinforced only when a red light is on, but never when the stimulus light is green. The dependent variable of primary interest using such procedures is the proportion of the total responses occurring on the correct (S+) lever (accuracy) and the number of sessions or session time until some specified accuracy criterion has been achieved. Such discrimination paradigms can be of two types: simultaneous or successive. In a simultaneous discrimination, the S+ and the S− are presented at the same time, each associated with a different response option. In a successive discrimination, only one of the stimuli is presented at any given time; if only a single response device is available, responding on this device is reinforced during S+ presentations but not during S− presentations.

Discrimination paradigms carried out in operant chambers offer the distinct advantage of being conducted as free operant rather than discrete trial procedures such as must be used in the maze techniques described earlier. In trials procedures, the time between each trial or opportunity to respond, that is, the intertrial interval, is determined by the experimenter, and a trial ends with a designated response. The necessity for an intertrial interval is imposed by the requirement of removing the animal from the reinforcement delivery site back to the start box. With free operant procedures, a response by the organism initiates a "trial" and no intertrial interval is necessarily imposed between responses. The advantage of this approach is that response rate can be used as a potential index of motivational and motor effects of a treatment, which may contribute to any presumed effect on discrimination learning (see also later discussion). Another advantage of the free operant procedure is that the initiation of the "trial" by the subject rather than by the experimenter assures its attention to the relevant environmental stimuli and improves accuracy (68).

A relatively simple operant discrimination procedure is exemplified by the study of Hastings et al. (114) examining the impact of neonatal lead exposure of rats. One experiment in this study that proved sensitive to lead exposure was a simultaneous visual discrimination task using lights as stimuli. In this discrete trial procedure, a trial was initiated by the insertion of two levers into the operant chamber. The light above one of these levers was illuminated, signaling it as the correct lever (S+), whereas the other light was not illuminated (S−). The choice of the correct lever was varied randomly from trial to trial. Criterion performance, defined as 90% correct responses during a daily test session, was reached significantly more slowly by lead-exposed rats.

An example of the kinds of complex problem that may be designed to confront the organism is a conditional discrimination procedure such as the matching-to-sample paradigm, shown by Rice (209) to be impaired in monkeys following lead exposure. One of three disks (the sample) was illuminated with one of three colors on this delayed matching-to-sample paradigm. A press on this sample disk darkened it. After a delay period, which was constant under some conditions and variable under others, all three disks were illuminated, each with one of the three colors. If the monkey pressed the disk with the color that had been presented on the sample disk, that is, if it matched the sample, a fruit-juice reward was delivered. The discrimination is described as conditional because the correct response for any trial is conditional on the sample stimulus for that trial. In this experiment, differences between control and lead-treated monkeys were not observed in the initial acquisition of the behavior, but appeared when delays were imposed between the conditional stimulus and matching stimuli, with shorter delay values in treated monkeys impairing performance to a greater extent than in controls. In the matching-to-sample paradigm, the response to the sample (conditional) stimulus itself is called an observing response; requiring a response to this sample stimulus ensures that the organism is attending to the relevant stimuli when a trial or experimental sequence begins, and improves the accuracy of performance (68). A variant of the matching-to-sample procedure, the oddity paradigm, requires the organism to choose the stimulus that does not match the sample.

Typically, a specified criterion defines learning, such as 8 correct responses in a block of 10 trials. In a discrete trials experiment with both a control and a treated group, the group mean total number of trials to reach the specific criterion can be compared. Using the free operant procedure, the proportion of the total responses occurring during the S+ presentations, (i.e., the correct responses), may be contrasted between the two groups. Alternatively, an organism can be used as its own control, in which case the accuracy of performance or the rate of learning can be compared before and after treatment. This approach has been made possible by the development of procedures that allow the repeated measurement of learning (discussed later).

As previously pointed out, one major limitation of many of the procedures described earlier is that once the correct response has been learned, performance rather than learning is being measured. To pursue issues such as time course of a toxicant's effects on learning, or the reversibility of toxicant effects, such procedures offer limited utility. They can, however, be modified to allow repeated measurements of learning. In a discrimination reversal task, for example, acquisition of the original discrimination is followed by a reversal of the S+ and the S−; that is, the stimulus-reward contingency is reversed until the learning criterion is met for the new discrimination problem. Multiple reversals of this sort can be carried out and behavioral adaptation evaluated by measuring the number of trials to criterion on each reversal. After a number of such reversals, however, organisms may acquire the concept "reversal" and effectively learn the discrimination in a single trial (111). Bushnell and Bowman (28) found that monkeys exposed to lead showed an increase in the number of trials to criterion and in the number of errors on the first reversal of a discrimination problem, but no effect on six subsequent reversals. Likewise, water maze procedures can be modified to permit repeated measurement of learning by moving the location of the submerged platform after the subject has successfully learned its location.

An automated paradigm designed specifically to provide a measure of repeated learning was originated for human subjects by Boren (21,22). This procedure requires the subject to learn a new response sequence or response chain during each experimental session and has since been widely used to study the effects of drugs on learning. In an experiment with pigeons (262), three stimulus keys in a chamber were all illuminated simultaneously by one of four colors. The pigeon's task was to peck the correct key in the presence of each color. For example, if the keys were yellow, peck the left key; if green, peck right; if red, peck center; if white, peck right. In such a case, if the sequence of light presentations was yellow, green, red, white, the correct sequence of responses would be left, right, center, right. The association between color and key position was changed during each successive session and the subject was required to learn a new four-response sequence. Each correctly completed sequence was followed by food delivery. With training, the number of errors (incorrect responses at any point in the sequence) per session stabilizes, yielding a steady baseline from which drug or toxicant effects on learning can be assessed repeatedly. Thompson and Moerschbacher (reviewed in ref. 263) have studied the effects of several drugs on this baseline in nonhuman primates.

Paule and McMillan (194) used a variant of this procedure to track the time course of trimethyltin (TMT) effects on learning in rats. In their incremental repeated acquisition procedure, the sequence length was incremented during the course of a session from one- to five-member sequences. By separating certain types of error classes in their analyses, they were better able to understand the particular behavioral processes affected by TMT. Their observations indicated a differential time course for TMT effects on various classes of errors and showed that acquisition of early responses in the sequence was disrupted to a greater degree than the later stages of the sequences, suggesting an effect on learning, while the recall necessary for the longer sequences remained intact. Another variant of the repeated acquisition procedure devised for rodents by Cory-Slechta and colleagues (38,40,47a) extended the explanatory power of this procedure. Through microanalyses of response patterns and patterns of errors, it could be shown that different drugs could achieve what appeared to be a similar effect, namely, decreases in overall accuracy, through very different patterns of errors. For example, the noncompetitive glutamatergic antagonist MK-801 decreased overall accuracy on the repeated acquisition paradigm by increasing the frequency of perseverative (repetitive) errors, while scopolamine, a cholinergic muscarinic antagonist, increased the frequency of errors composed of incorrectly skipping forward or backward through the sequence.

Before classifying the effects of a toxicant as one on learning, however, the critical issue of specificity raised earlier must be addressed. Changes in accuracy on learning paradigms may well arise from nonspecific performance effects such as changes in motor activity, sensory capacity, motivation, or other unrelated factors. For example, recent studies showed that aging-related impairments in performance by rats in a water maze can be attributed to hypothermia induced by the temperature of the water and inefficient body-temperature regulation (147). Odor trails can likewise affect performance in the water maze (163). The use of odor trails as a confounder of learning deficits in conventional mazes is a well-documented phenomenon. Attenuated motivation could increase latency in a maze, increasing the delay to reward, which, by itself would slow the rate of learning. For the maze procedures described earlier, the potential influence of changes in motor, sensory, and/or motivational functions and other influences such as temperature-related effects must be ruled out using an independent procedure, that is, carrying out additional experiments.

One approach that has been widely adopted for assessing the contribution of such nonspecific effects to learning with the repeated acquisition paradigm is to alternate the learning component with a performance component during each experimental session (technically a multiple schedule; discussed later). The learning or acquisition component, as previously described, requires the organism to learn a new response sequence during each session. In contrast, the response sequence reinforced during the performance component remains constant across sessions, with every occurrence of the correct sequence producing reinforcement, so that the organism is simply performing an already learned or rote response. By alternating the learning and performance components during each experimental session, such as after every tenth reinforcer delivery, the experimenter can separate, during the same session, drug- or toxicant-induced changes in learning from nonspecific changes in performance or motivation. This is based on the premise that if a compound selectively affects learning, then decreases in accuracy will only be manifest during the learning component of the schedule, since no learning is required in the performance component. Since intact motor, sensory, and motivational processes are required in both components, impairments of these functions would result in decreases in accuracy in both the learning and performance components.

This approach demonstrated selective effects of lead on learning as illustrated in an extreme case in Figure 32.9 (39), which compares the behavior of a typical control rat to that of a rat exposed to 250 ppm lead acetate from weaning. The particular session depicted began with a performance (P) component which was followed sequentially by the learning component (A), a return to the performance component, and a final presentation of the learning component. The control rat evidenced high levels of accuracy in the first performance component, generating a high rate of reinforcement delivery and a relatively low rate of errors. After the onset of the learning component, indicated to the subject by a change in illumination in the operant chamber, the rat was required to learn a new three-response sequence. As anticipated, the error rate initially increased producing a lower rate of reinforcement delivery. By the end of the learning component, however, the rate of errors had begun to decline and the rat was earning more food deliveries as it gradually learned the correct sequence. This pattern of behavior was even more pronounced during the second presentation of the learning component. The bottom record of Figure 32.9 shows the rather dramatic impact of lead exposure that was selective for the learning component of the schedule during which, in this particular session, the lead-exposed rat earned virtually no food deliveries during the learning component, emitting hundreds of incorrect responses over the course of both presentations of the learning component. By undertaking a microanalysis of the vari-

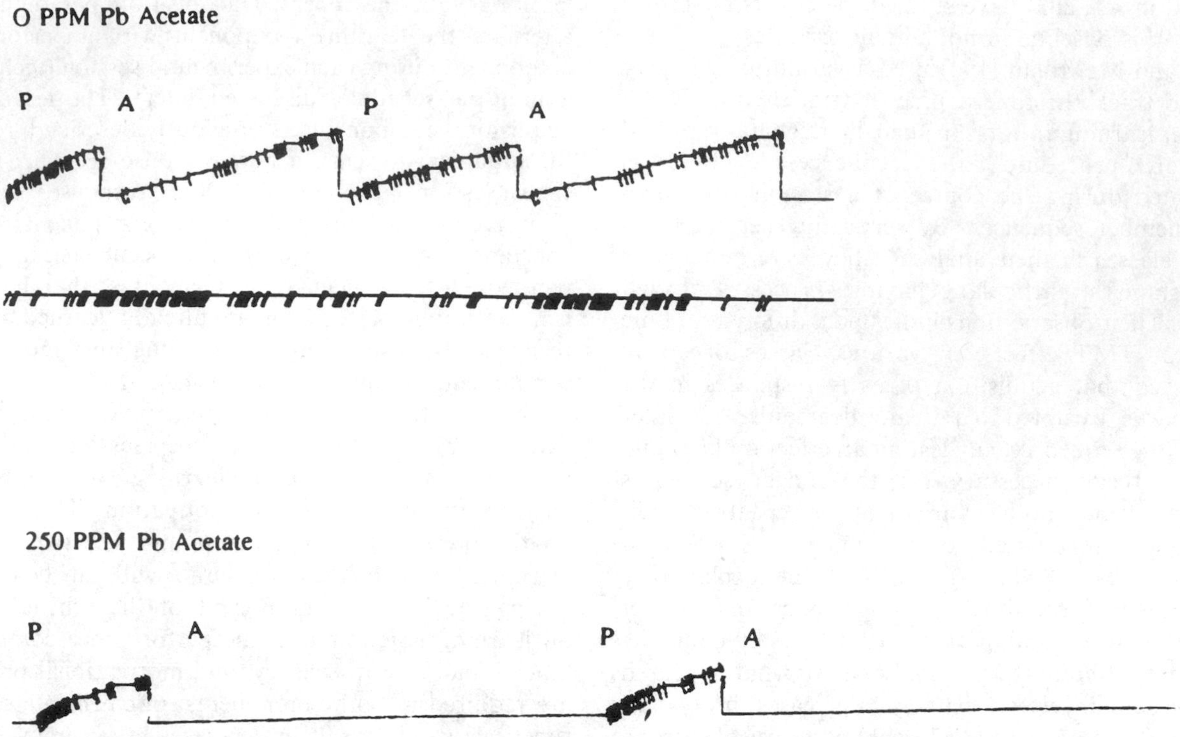

FIG. 32.9. Cumulative records of performance on a multiple schedule of repeated learning and performance in a rat exposed chronically to distilled water (top record) versus 250 ppm lead acetate drinking solutions over the course of a behavioral session from left to right. The multiple schedule involved a repeated learning component (A), which required learning a new three-response sequence during each behavioral session. These alternated with a performance (P) component in which the three-response sequence remained constant across sessions. The top tracing of each record shows correct responses, which cumulate vertically. Each pip depicts the delivery of a reinforcer for correctly completing the sequence of three responses required for reward. The pen reset to the baseline with each transition of the components between the performance and repeated learning components. The bottom tracing shows errors that occurred during the components. The lead-treated rat earned virtually no food deliveries, that is, completed no correct sequences, during the repeated learning components of the session despite normal performance under conditions where no learning was required (P component). From Cory-Slechta (unpublished data).

ous patterns of responses and classes of errors, it was found that the detrimental effect of lead on learning occurred via an increase in response perseveration, that is, repetitive responding on the same lever or repetitive iteration of the same sequence of responses.

Any learning assay also must consider the values of the experimental parameters and nature of the problem selected, because such factors influence the sensitivity of the task to disruption by chemical agents. For example, Winneke et al. (296a) investigated the effects of lead exposure on the acquisition by rats of both a form and a size discrimination. The form discrimination required rats to distinguish between vertical and horizontal stripes. On the average, only 8 training days were required by rats to reach criterion accuracy and the procedure did not differentiate the lead-exposed from the control groups. In contrast, the size discrimination, in which a small circle had to be distinguished from a larger circle, proved to be a much more difficult problem, requiring more than 20 training sessions, and revealed a substantial impairment due to lead. A similar effect was reported by Carlson et al. (31) in lead-exposed sheep. Such data demonstrate the important role of task complexity and difficulty in modulating sensitivity to disruption by chemical agents.

Often the degree of difficulty of the task can be equated with the degree of stimulus control over the performance, that is, the strength of the stimuli controlling the response. For example, Laties et al. (139) required rats to press a fixed number of times on one of two levers, then respond once on an alternate lever for reinforcement. During some parts of the session, a light and tone signaled that the criterion on the first lever had been met; in other parts of the session, no external stimulus signaled the completion of the response requirement. As would be expected, accuracy of performance was superior during the signaled components of the session, and much higher doses of *d*-amphetamine (139) or toluene (302a) were required to disrupt the signaled than the unsignaled performance (unlabeled, no SD) than the signaled component (SD), as can be seen in Figure 32.10. A similar example is exemplified by the data presented in Figure 32.9: Responding on the performance component represents a far less difficult discrimination and maintains higher overall levels of accuracy. These findings indicate that behavior strongly controlled by environmental stimuli, such as is the case during the signaled component, is less easily disrupted than behavior under weaker stimulus control. Thus, the degree of stimulus control over behavior can markedly influence its susceptibility to the effects of drugs or toxicants.

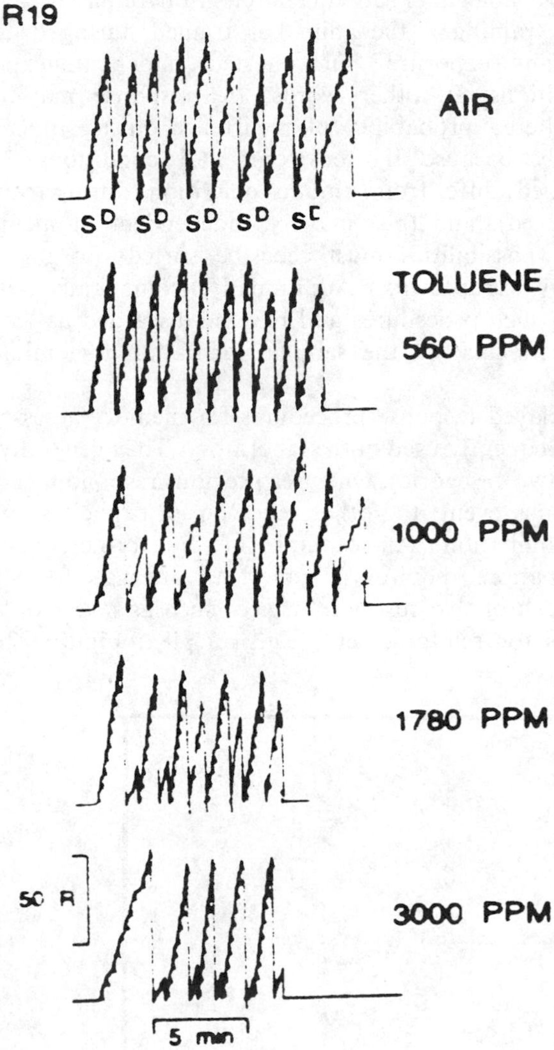

FIG. 32.10. Behavior of rats on a fixed consecutive number (FLN) schedule that required subjects to complete a specified number of responses on one lever before a single response on the second lever would produce reinforcement. This was carried out in a multiple schedule component in which during some FCN presentations, a discriminative stimulus was provided to signal the subject that the response requirement on the first lever had been met (SD component), whereas in the alternate components, no such stimulus was provided. Accuracy levels were higher in the SD component, and behavior in this component was also significantly less disrupted by toluene exposure. From Wood et al. (302a).

Memory

Memory is a term that has been used both to describe and to attempt to account for the behavior of recalling, or the influence on behavior of previous events. Experiences are said to be stored in memory, in encoded forms, such as neural engrams, or more recently as electrical fields, and later recalled from storage by some type of retrieval system. Many theorists have adopted the vocabulary of computer technology to describe memory processes, despite the lack of evidence of operational correspondence.

In a behavioral analysis, memory may be best understood and experimentally approached in terms of stimulus control. Increasing the accessibility of stored items, or remembering, is really another way to assert that the probability of certain responses is increased. Heise (116) referred to the fact that while learning is "manifested behaviorally by acquisition, an enduring change in behavior, ... memory may be defined as the preservation of the learned behavior over time." Experimentally, memory is indicated by the extent of the change in behavior that occurs as a consequence of a delay (retention interval) between the occasion for learning and the "test" or occasion for a recall response. A distinction is typically drawn between short-term memory, occurring over relatively short delay periods, and long-term or virtually permanent memory. Obviously, the temporal parameters of these two subclasses are species dependent.

As the preceding discussion suggests, the various techniques devised to assess memory typically involve the measurement of response accuracy following some stimulus event after various delay intervals have been imposed. Memory is measured as the difference between performance level in the absence of a delay and performance during retesting at longer delays. An effect of a drug or chemical on memory is suggested by an increased impairment of performance with lengthened delay values. Avoidance of an aversive stimulus, such as electric shock, is one frequently used measure of both learning and memory. Several different variants of these procedures have been employed; some are discrete trial procedures, and others are free operant procedures. The passive avoidance paradigm assesses the tendency of the subject to avoid the site of previous shock delivery. A mouse that

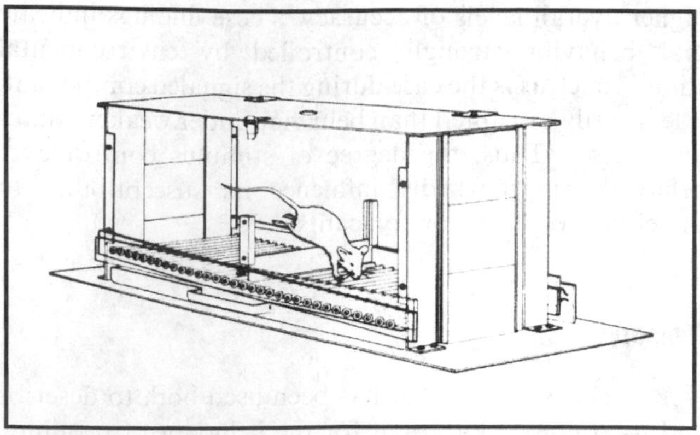

FIG. 32.11. Depicts a shuttle-box avoidance apparatus. In this active avoidance paradigm, the rat can avoid an impending shock or escape an ongoing shock by shuttling to the other side of the chamber, thus terminating an aversive stimulus.

avoids a dark (normally preferred) chamber where it previously has been shocked is said to be exhibiting a memory of that event. Active avoidance paradigms require a response to postpone shock onset. The usual situation is a two-compartment apparatus. The subject switches compartments at the appearance of a stimulus that signals impending shock (Figure 32.11).

There are several limitations of such avoidance procedures, especially the passive avoidance paradigm. Variability of response among animals tends to be high, often necessitating large groups of subjects. Besides learning or memory effects, a drug or toxicant might alter motivation by modifying shock sensitivity. The drug or toxicant may modify activity levels, for example, induce hypo- or hyperactivity, increasing the probability of returning to the shocked compartment independently of "remembering." Furthermore, state-dependent learning may alter subsequent retention for passive avoidance training if the animal is trained during drug or toxicant exposure but retested under nonexposed conditions. In other words, the response may have an altered probability of recurrence during the retest simply because the environmental conditions (nondrugged) differ from stimulus conditions during training (drugged), and thus may be independent of memory. Such possibilities must then be sorted out in additional experiments. Additionally, some rats fail to learn such procedures and may be discarded as "slow" learners, biasing the sample population for unknown reasons.

Delayed response procedures for memory assessment are frequently used in the laboratory. They generally fall into two categories: One uses previous responding as the stimulus event; the other relies on an explicit stimulus discrimination. An example of the former, delayed alternation, requires a subject to alternate responses on each of two response devices such as levers or nose cones for reinforcement (e.g., ref. 48a; Figure 32.12).

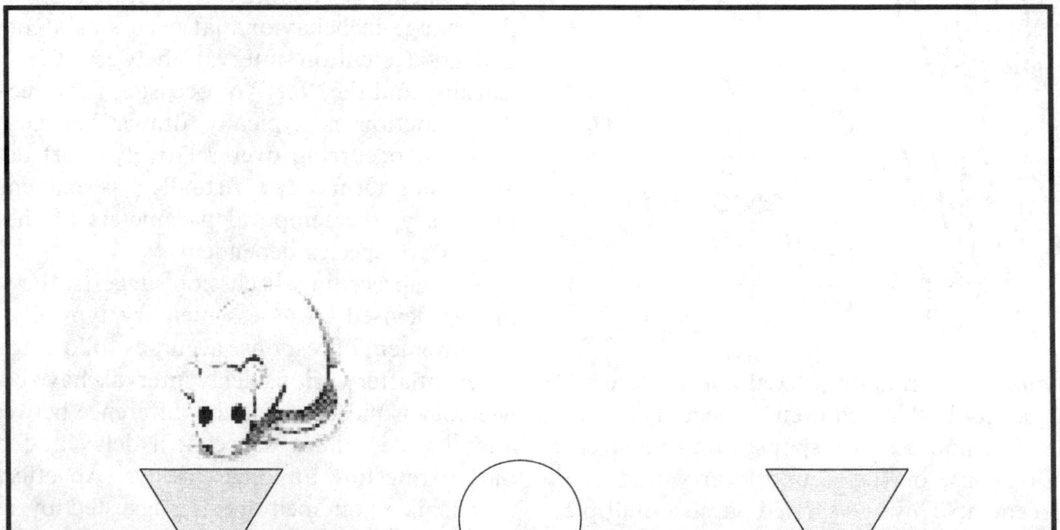

FIG. 32.12. Schematic of the delayed alternation procedure. This paradigm requires the subject to alternate responses between two response manipulanda for reward, that is, to nosepoke in this case first on the right manipulanda and then on the left manipulanda for reinforcement. The next reinforcement then requires a switch back to the right manipulanda. For the assessment of memory function, a delay between response opportunities is imposed, requiring the subject to "recall" on which manipulanda the previous response occurred and thus alternate accordingly.

That is, a response on device A followed by a response on device B produces a reinforcer, a return to device A, another reinforcer, and so on. After initial training, a delay requirement is interposed between the alternating responses, so that only alternations separated by at least the required delay interval are reinforced. Generally, the delay value varies randomly from trial to trial during an experimental session, allowing the collection of a complete delay function in a single session. A response occurring before the end of the delay period typically resets the time requirement, with the particular delay values specified dependent on the experimental species. On some trials, there is no delay. This no-delay condition is critical for evaluating the possible effects of the drug or toxicant on nonspecific performance factors independently of memory processes. Since no memory should be required in the absence of a delay value between alternating responses, accuracy values should not decline in the no-delay condition. Typically, one expects to see a decline in accuracy with increasing delay values. If a drug or toxicant impairs memory processes, an accelerated decline in the delay function would be anticipated. Using this procedure, Bushnell (27) reported that TMT could produce deficits in memory processes in rats, with TMT accelerating the decline in the delay function but not affecting accuracy on the zero-second delay trials. These data are consistent with the notion of a selective impairment of remembering.

The matching-to-sample procedure described earlier becomes a memory paradigm when delay intervals are imposed between the presentation of the sample stimulus and the later presentation of the matching stimuli. As with delayed response procedures, a range of delay values is presented in a semirandom manner throughout the course of an experimental session, allowing the experimenter to collect a complete delay function in every session. Taylor and Evans (257) reported impairments in delayed matching-to-sample performance in pigeons at an exposure concentration of toluene that maintains self-administration behavior (discussed later) in the primate (300). This impairment was not interpreted as an effect on memory, however, because accuracy was significantly impaired even when no delay was imposed.

As is the case for learning, then, changes in performance on a memory task may have little to do with memory but rather be an indirect result of other nonspecific behavioral effects such as changes in motivation, arousal, sensation and perception, etc. For example, a toxicant that increased the rate of responding might produce premature responding to the comparison stimuli in a matching-to-sample task and thereby increase error rates. Alternatively, decreased rates of responding might increase the latency to make the response in a choice situation and thus increase the functional delay interval. One efficient way in which to assess the contribution of nonspecific effects in free operant memory procedures is to examine changes in the rate of responding as well as changes in accuracy in the presence of a no-delay condition. With respect to the former, nonspecific effects on levels of arousal or motivation may be reflected in altered response rates. With respect to the latter, the no-delay condition permits drug or toxicant effects not related to memory to be determined since no remembering is required at the zero-second delay. For discrete trials procedures, alternative experiments or manipulations would have to be implemented to determine the specificity of the toxicant effect on remembering. A further condition for establishment of a true effect on memory requires that the magnitude of the effect on accuracy increase with increasing delay value (116) and that similar effects of the toxic agent can be demonstrated in other memory paradigms using other stimulus and response conditions. Automated procedures facilitate the incorporation of appropriate control procedures.

SCHEDULE-CONTROLLED BEHAVIOR

Every experimental procedure using operant behavior is based on the principle that behavior is generated, altered, refined, and eliminated by its consequences. Seldom, however, is every instance of a specific behavior in the natural environment followed by reinforcement. That is, continuous or invariant reinforcement is infrequent; intermittent, often unpredictable reinforcement is instead the rule. Paychecks are typically distributed on a weekly, semiweekly, or even monthly basis. Not every visit to the mailbox will be rewarded by the arrival of the letter we are awaiting. Often a string or chain of responses may be emitted before there is a reward, much as the pianist finishes playing an entire piece of music before the audience applauds. Similarly, the child may correctly put together several puzzle pieces or even the entire puzzle before the parent praises the child. In the wild, predation and foraging behavior are certainly maintained under conditions of intermittent reinforcement. Besides the economy achieved by intermittent presentation of reinforcement, behavior maintained under such conditions is actually considerably more robust than that maintained by continuous reinforcement (128). For example, a response that has been reinforced on every occurrence declines much more rapidly during an extinction procedure (withholding of reinforcement) than does behavior that has been intermittently reinforced. Put another way, continuously reinforced behavior is much less resistant to extinction than that maintained by intermittent payoff. Many parents have learned, to their distress, how occasional reinforcement of a temper tantrum (failure to ignore it) may subsequently increase the magnitude and persistence of the behavior (e.g., ref., 294).

In the human environment, reinforcement schedules, that is, the nature of the rules by which reinforcement is allocated, may be complex. The laboratory offers the experimenter direct control over such contingencies and allows a more precise analyses of the ways in which the scheduling of reinforcement controls various aspects of responding, including its temporal distribution, force, rate, resistance to extinction, and so on. The study of reinforcement schedules is a discipline in itself (82,96,231). Of most relevance to toxicology, an extensive body of literature has accrued describing the effects of a wide variety of central nervous system (CNS) drugs on schedule-controlled behavior (e.g., 126,131,132,159,161, 264,268; see also 129). This permits comparison of toxicant effects on schedule-controlled responding to those of CNS compounds whose mechanisms of action are often at least partially understood. More recently, the effects of numerous toxicants on schedule-controlled behavior have begun to be enumerated (e.g., 45–47, 97,151,210,290).

Schedules of reinforcement are especially important to behavioral toxicology since reinforcement schedules govern the rate and pattern of behavioral responding involved in different behavioral processes (see ref. 45). The rate of learning, for example, may well be influenced by the reinforcement schedule according to which the reinforcer is presented. The response may be only slowly acquired if initially reinforced only infrequently. Whether the response is learned at all may depend on the strength of competing responses, the magnitude of reinforcement, and the concurrent availability of competing schedules of reinforcement. In addition, changes in schedule-controlled behavior may actually underlie behavioral changes that are attributed to impairments of other behavioral processes. Decreases in rates of responding produced by a toxicant may be misidentified as a decline in the rate of learning in a discrimination procedure. Schedules of reinforcement can also be used as an index of learning processes, that is, whether treated subjects learn the behavioral patterns characteristic of the particular schedule under study, and whether changes in parametric values of the schedule produce corresponding changes in schedule-controlled performance at the same rate in treated and control subjects. To truly understand the behavioral effects of a toxicant, then, requires an understanding of its impact on schedule-controlled behavior, since behavior occurs at given rates and in particular patterns over time.

Simple Schedules

Although a virtually limitless number of ways to schedule reinforcement delivery is possible, most schedules are based on either number of responses or time. Four simple schedules have been defined: the fixed interval (FI) and the variable interval (VI), both of which are temporally based reinforcement schedules, and the fixed ratio (FR) and the variable ratio (VR), both of which are response-based schedules. Characteristic patterns of performance emerge on each of these schedules once steady-state performance is achieved (see ref. 265). The temporal pattern of responding, as well as drug effects on the performance, are frequently very similar across species (e.g., ref. 132), a feature providing confidence in cross-species extrapolation and the continuity of behavioral processes across species. One of the more attractive features of schedule-controlled behavior is that the pattern of performance is often remarkably stable over prolonged periods, a decided advantage for tracking the progression of toxicity and for assessing reversibility.

Training on simple reinforcement schedules generally begins with magazine training, followed by shaping of the designated response using conventional techniques. In most cases, the schedule of interest then is imposed directly, although it may reach its final parametric value only after a series of gradual changes from the initial parametric values. For example, in studying FR performance, the experimenter will most likely carry out several sessions at lower FR values before imposing a final value of 100. This prevents "ratio strain" [irregular pauses occurring between responses on an FR schedule, as described by Ferster and Skinner (82)] associated with high FR values and prevents extinction of the response. Interval schedules stipulate that a certain amount of time must elapse following a previous response before the next occurrence of the response will be reinforced. On an FI schedule, the time period is constant and typically is measured from the previously reinforced response. For example, an FI 5 min schedule reinforces the first response occurring at least 5 min after the preceding reinforced response; responses during the 5-min interval have no programmed consequence. The FI schedule typically generates a characteristic scalloped pattern of performance, as shown in Figure 32.13, which consists of a pause after reinforcement delivery (designated as the post-reinforcement pause, PRP) followed by a progressive increase in the rate of responding (running rate) as the time for the next food delivery approaches. In the human environment, studying for a scheduled exam has features resembling performance maintained by an FI schedule: normally, little or no studying occurs early in the semester, but as the time for the midterm approaches, the rate of studying begins to escalate. The species generality of the scalloped pattern of per-

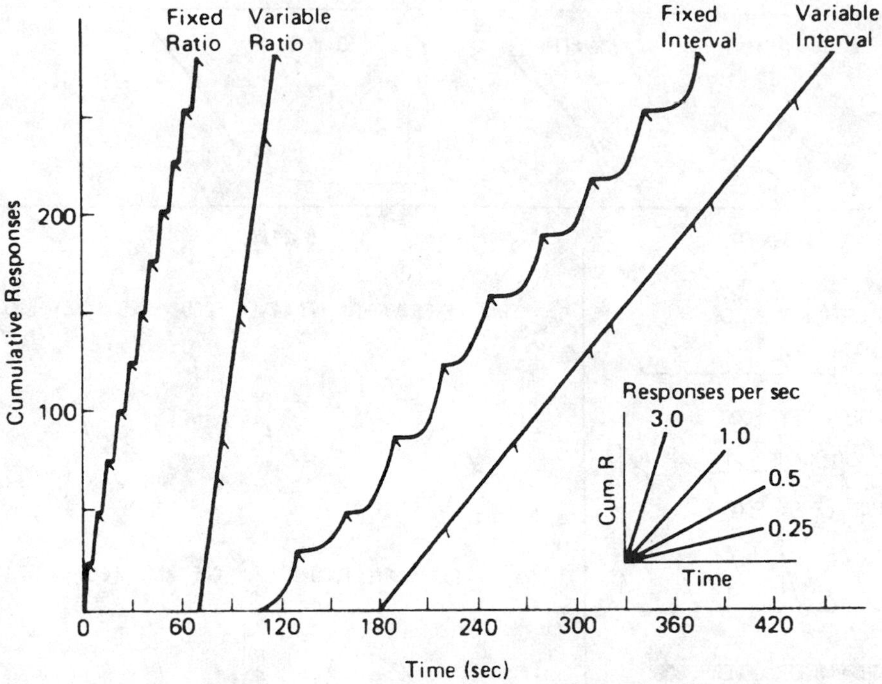

FIG. 32.13. Characteristic behavior on each of the four simple schedules of reinforcement: the fixed ratio, variable ratio, fixed interval, and variable interval. In these records, responses cumulate vertically, and the slope of the line indicates the rate of responding, with prototypical rates labeled in the inset. Each pip shows where a reinforcer was delivered according to schedule contingencies. The fixed ratio (FR) schedule generates a very high rate of responding, with short pauses (indicated by horizontal periods on the record) following each reinforcer delivery. The variable ratio (VR) schedule generates an even higher rate of responding with little or no pausing after reinforcement since the very next response may produce reward. The fixed interval (FI) schedule produces a "scalloped" pattern of responding characterized by pauses after reinforcement delivery followed by a gradually increasing rate of responding as the time of the next available reinforcer delivery approaches. The variable interval (VI) schedule generates a very stable moderate rate of responding with almost no pausing since the time to the next available reinforcement opportunity is unpredictable. From Reference 238.

formance is amply demonstrated in Figure 32.14, which illustrates the similarity of the behavior across species, type of response, and type of reinforcer.

Human FI performance shows a similar scallop under many conditions (e.g., refs. 138 and 261), although not all. Sensitivity of the FI schedule to a variety of toxicants has been demonstrated (e.g., ref. 46). The characteristic scalloped pattern of performance usually is described by one of two measures. The index of curvature (89) specifies the extent to which the scallop deviates from a straight line (a constant rate of responding throughout the interval); the quarter-life (117) is defined as that proportion of the interval required to emit the first 25% of the total responses in the interval.

The typical, though grossest, measure of schedule-controlled behavior is absolute or overall response rate, which is simply the total number of responses divided by total session time. Often a full understanding of chemical modification requires a microanalysis, which dissects the behavior into more elementary components. Like the separation of various classes of errors in a learning or memory experiment, schedule-controlled performance can be differentiated into component parts, which permits a more precise understanding of the manner in which the schedule controls performance. Such an analysis can suggest the possible behavioral processes that are altered by a chemical and point to directions for further analyses and manipulation.

FI performance provides an example. This schedule has been the focus of much experimental work partially because it exemplifies temporal control over behavior. As previously described, FI performance is characterized by a pause after reinforcement delivery (Figures 32.13 and 32.14). The length of this post-reinforcement pause time, or PRP (time from food delivery to the first response in the next interval), depends on the length of the fixed interval (239); the longer the interval, the longer is the pause. The PRP is followed by a long period of shorter pauses, interspersed with short bursts of responding.

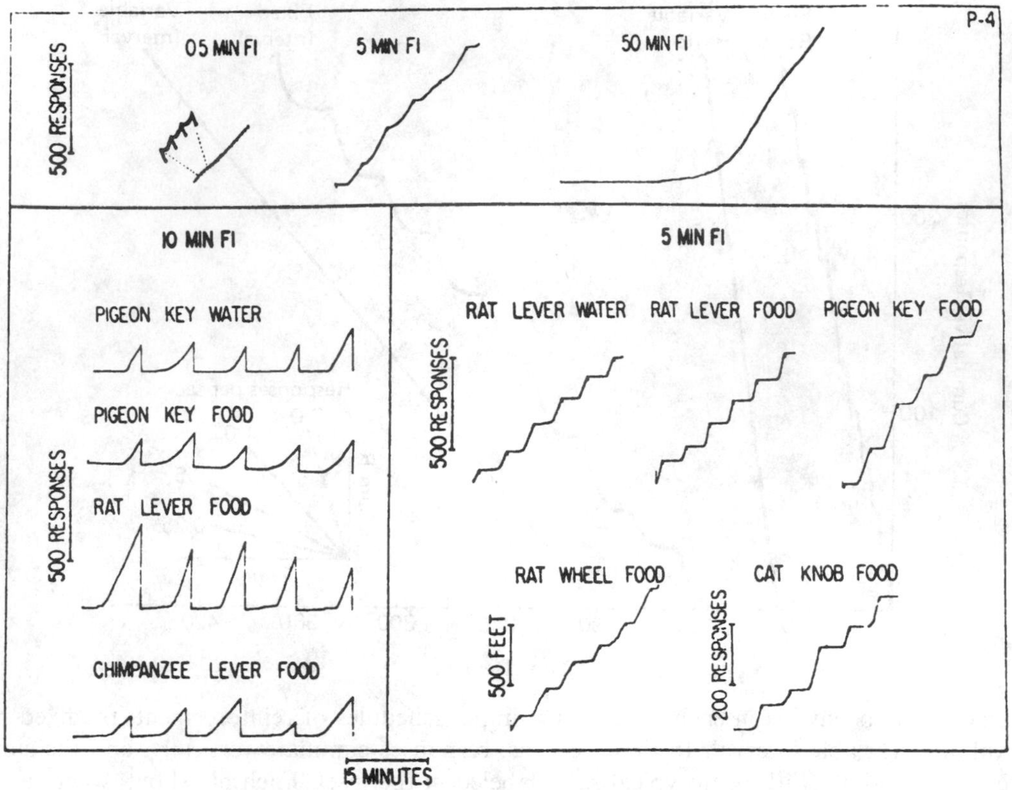

FIG. 32.14. Species generality of characteristic fixed interval (FI) schedule-controlled behavior. Responses cumulate vertically in these records, and time is represented horizontally. The top panel shows the behavior of an individual pigeon pecking a key for food at three different FI values, and the general scalloped pattern persists despite the 100-fold change in time value. Performance on an FI 5 min schedule is shown in the right panel with the pen continuing to accumulate responses up to 500. As can be seen, FI performance is remarkably similar for different species (rat, pigeon, cat) with different responses (lever press, key peck, wheel running, and knob pushing) and different reinforcers (water, food). The left panel shows performance on an FI 10 min schedule of reinforcement; in this case the pen was reset to the baseline after each reinforcer delivery. Again, comparable behavior is shown despite differences in species, response, and reinforcer. From Reference 131.

As the interval progresses, the long pauses cease and are replaced by alternating periods of moderate and high response rates until reinforcement delivery (94). The rate of responding during an interval, after the PRP is subtracted out, is referred to as running rate. With the aid of a computer, the actual times between each successive response, that is, the interresponse times (IRTs), can be collected, a frequency distribution of various length IRTs generated, and sequential patterns of IRTs reconstructed. It is these microanalyses that may permit detection of a toxicant effect and understanding of its behavioral mechanism of action. In the case of low-level lead exposure, for example, the proportion of "short" IRTs (0.5 s or less) is consistently increased by lead exposure (Figure 32.15) even while increases in overall response rate may be less impressive (see ref. 50). A similar effect has been reported in chronically exposed monkeys (210). Relatively higher lead exposure concentrations may initially produce the opposite effect, namely, a decreased proportion of short IRTs; with further exposure, short IRTs tend to rise substantially in frequency.

The type of effect produced by Pb exposure on FI schedule-controlled behavior might be viewed as loss of discriminative control by the schedule (reviewed in refs. 42 and 46). The behavioral mechanism might be explained as a failure of the FI schedule to exert temporal control over behavior; for example, lead-exposed subjects do not learn to discriminate interval length. This hypothesis earned further support from two additional experiments. In one (47), rats were required to hold down the lever for 3 s for each food delivery. Control rat median response durations were between 2.5 and 3 s, while some lead-exposed rats exhibited a much higher proportion of response durations too short to produce reinforcement, even when a tone stimulus was sub-

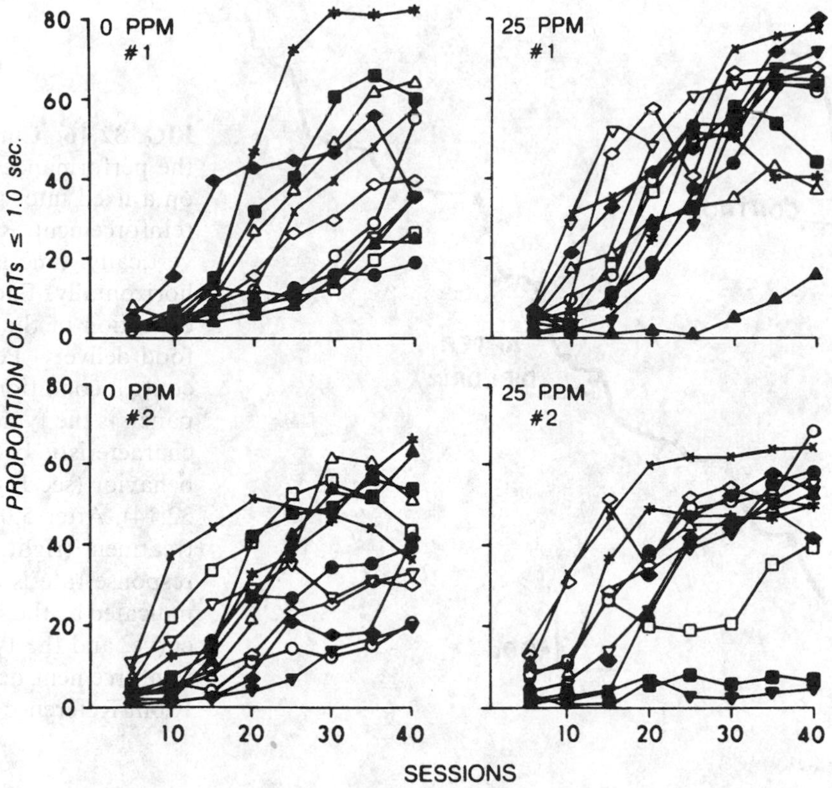

FIG. 32.15. Proportion of short interresponse times (IRTs less than or equal to 1.0 s) over the course of 40 experimental sessions on a fixed interval 1 min schedule of food reinforcement. Each curve represents the performance of an individual control (left panels) or lead-exposed (25 ppm lead acetate in drinking water from weaning; right panels) rat. Top row shows results of the first experiment; second row plots results from a replication experiment. Lead increases overall response rates by increasing the proportion of short IRTs. From Reference 50.

sequently added to signal that the required duration had been met. In another experiment (212), reinforcement depended on separation of responses by at least 30 s (a schedule known as DRL or differential reinforcement of low rate). Lead-treated monkeys acquired the performance more slowly than controls, as indicated by a higher frequency of nonreinforced responses during the initial sessions. It should be noted, however, that the findings with lead described earlier are consistent with other hypotheses regarding behavioral mechanisms of action that remain to be tested, since behavior can be altered through its interaction with antecedent discriminative (SDs) and controlling stimuli (SR), response parameters, or the nature of the consequences of the response.

In contrast to lead, certain pesticide classes alter both response rate and the temporal patterning of FI behavior, suggesting actions through different behavioral and neurobiological mechanisms (46). Both organochlorine pesticides (26) and formamidine compounds (140) have been shown to decrease rates of responding on the FI schedule and to disrupt the normal temporal pattern of responding. Such effects are shown in the cumulative records in Figure 32.16.

When relevant information about a toxic agent is scarce, the FI schedule offers several distinct advantages as an early test for behavioral toxicity. Because the schedule reinforces only the first response after the end of the interval, and because responses during the interval have no programmed consequence, response rates during the interval itself can vary quite broadly before the frequency of reinforcement is altered. This feature may explain in part why FI performance is often more sensitive to drugs than ratio-based schedules of reinforcement (57,130,241); a decrease in the rate of responding on the latter necessarily decreases reinforcement frequency (discussed later).

The patterns of behavior produced by the three other simple reinforcement schedules are shown in Figure 32.13. On a VI or variable interval schedule, the intervals between reinforcement availability are determined on the basis of time, with the specific value varying from interval to interval, and the mean of those values indicated by the schedule parameter value. For example, on a VI 30-s schedule, the specified interval between reinforcement opportunities will vary from one reinforcement delivery to the next, but the average of all the values

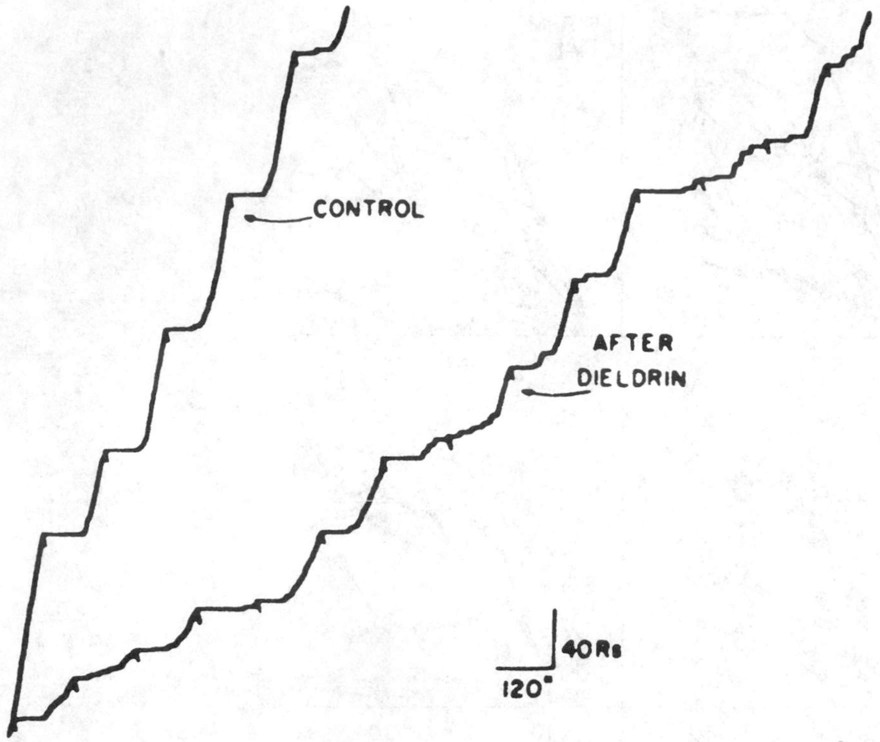

FIG. 32.16. Cumulative records of the performance of a Japanese quail on a fixed interval 2 min schedule of reinforcement. Responses cumulative vertically, time is represented horizontally. Each downward deflection of the pen (pip) indicates food delivery. Performance under control conditions, shown in the left panel, is the typical scalloped pattern characteristic of fixed interval behavior (see Figures 32.13 and 32.14). After 5.0 mg/kg of dieldrin treatment (right cumulative record), response rate is decreased, as indicated by the shallower slope of the curve, and the typical pause after reinforcement delivery is disrupted. From Reference 26.

will be 30 s. As indicated by Figure 32.13, the VI schedule generates a moderate but steady rate of responding, with little pausing evident after reinforcement, consistent with the lack of predictability of reinforcement availability. Reinforcement may be available immediately after the previous reinforcer delivery or may be delayed. Reynolds (208) cites as an example a busy signal on the telephone, with the caller continuing to make the response that is reinforced (by a ringing sound) on a VI schedule because of the variable length of telephone conversations. The steady persistent pattern of responding on the VI schedule would suggest its utility as a baseline for detecting toxic effects; however, little information in this regard is currently available, even though alterations in VI performance certainly are produced by CNS agents (59).

Ratio schedules require a specified number of responses for reinforcement. On the fixed ratio (FR) schedule, the requirement remains constant; for example, each completion of 100 responses produces food delivery on an FR 100 schedule. The piecework system that operated in the early factory production systems in this country serves as a classic example; salespeople working exclusively on a commission basis is another. The FR schedule typically generates a pattern of performance in which there is a characteristic pause (PRP) after food delivery, the length of which is related to ratio size, followed by a very rapid rate of responding until the ratio requirement is completed. The high, constant response rate on the FR schedule is the result of the relation between rate of reinforcement and rate of responding; the faster the ratio is completed, the sooner reinforcement delivery occurs. As a result, short IRTs tend to be differentially reinforced, amplifying the relationship. Figure 32.17 (102) plots the frequency distribution of IRTs for a pigeon maintained on an FR 30 schedule of reinforcement on the left and shows that short IRTs predominate. As shown in the right panel, a dose of 1.0 mg/kg of *d*-amphetamine produces marked changes in the IRT distribution, including a shift of the main peak to the right and a decline in the number of very short IRTs. As mentioned earlier, the rate of responding on the FI schedule can vary widely before affecting the frequency of reinforcement delivery; however, decreases in response rate on the FR schedule necessarily decrease the rate of reinforcement. It is precisely this difference in the contingencies controlling the two performances that generates the stark contrasts in FI and FR schedule-controlled performance.

Like all schedules, the FR schedule can be analyzed into its component parts, which generally include measurement of the length of the postreinforcement pause and the running rate, as well as an examination of the IRT distribution. Such a microanalysis reveals that the effect of chronic lead exposure on FR performance is to increase the median IRT, as can be seen in Figure 32.18 (43), and thus to decrease response rates. A variety of CNS agents have been shown to alter FR performance (e.g., refs. 57,59,192), as have various toxicants, including metals and pesticides (see ref. 46). Gentry

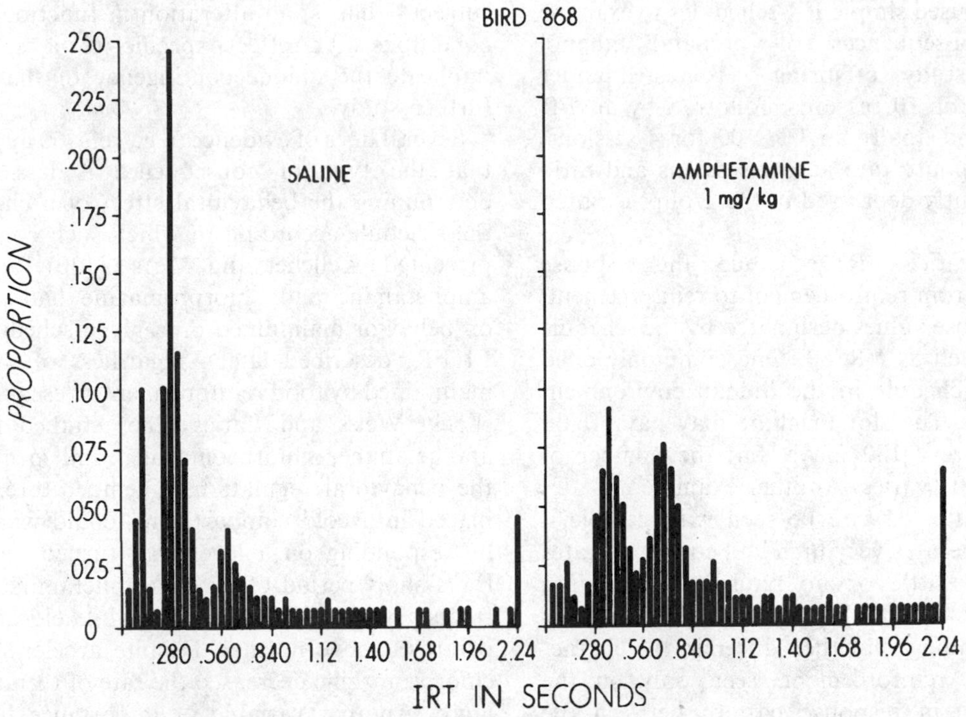

FIG. 32.17. Histogram of interresponse times (IRTs) from the performance of a pigeon on a fixed ratio (FR) of a 30 schedule of food reinforcement. The temporal resolution was 40 ms/bin on the abscissa and the distribution was based on a total of 1200 key-peck responses. Performance under saline control conditions is shown in the left panel. After treatment with 1.0 mg/kg of *d*-amphetamine, the distribution of IRTs changes with a decrease in the shortest IRT bins and an increase in the frequency of slightly longer IRTs. From Reference 102.

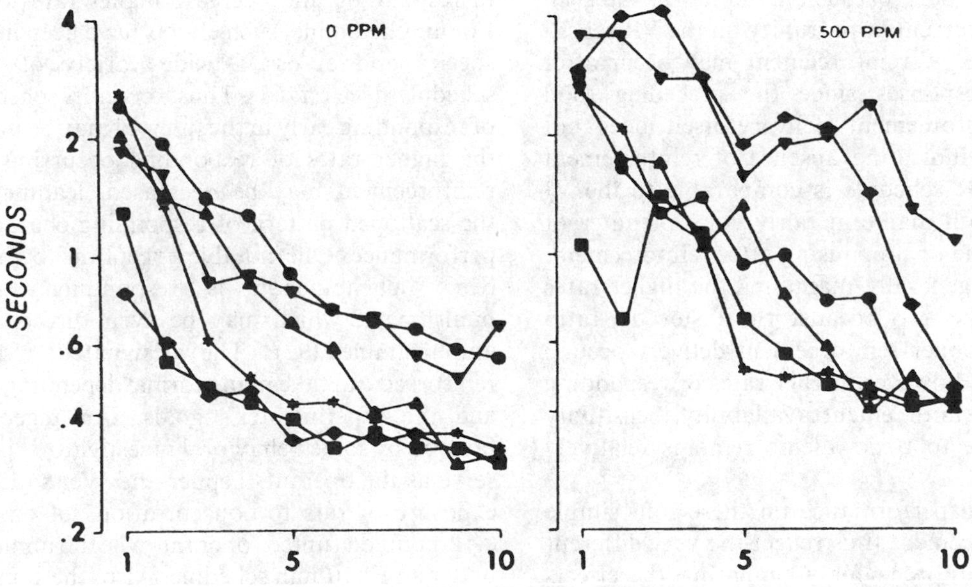

FIG. 32.18. Median interresponse time (IRT) values for individual control (left panel) and 500 ppm lead-treated rats (right panel) over the course of the first 10 experimental sessions on a fixed ratio (FR) of a 5 schedule of food reinforcement. Each data point on each curve represents the median IRT value of a subject for the indicated session. Median IRTs of lead-treated rats were considerably longer than controls, accounting for the decreased overall treatment rates that were observed in lead-exposed animals. From Reference 43.

and Middaugh (93) used simple FR schedules to examine the long-term consequences of prenatal ethanol exposure. In that study, offspring were tested under an FR 1 schedule for 10 sessions, followed by an FR 20 for 9 sessions and finally an FR 100 for 4 sessions. The increase in response rate across sessions and ratio values was significantly depressed in the groups exposed to ethanol prenatally.

On a variable ratio (VR) schedule, the response requirement varies from reinforcement to reinforcement, with the mean of those values designated by the schedule parameter value, such as VR 50. One commonly cited example of a VR schedule in the human environment is that of gambling. The slot machine may pay off on the average once every 100 plays, but the number of plays between payoffs varies. Another example includes the sale of real estate. As can be seen with gamblers, the VR schedule generates very high and consistent rates of responding with little or no pausing (see Figure 32.13). Both the VR and the FR schedule generate very high rates of responding, but they differ in the characteristic pause after reinforcement, seen only on the FR. This difference in response pattern between the two schedules derives from the fairly constant amount of time required to complete the fixed number of responses on the FR schedule. One hypothesis is that reinforcement delivery then becomes a stimulus associated with a subsequent period of nonreinforcement or extinction, decreasing response probability, since it represents the earliest part of such a temporal interval. In contrast, reinforcement opportunity on the VR schedule is unpredictable. A reinforcement may occur after any number of responses since the preceding food delivery; thus, reinforcement delivery itself does not become a stimulus indicating absence of reinforcement availability. The VR schedule is comparable to the VI schedule in that both maintain fairly constant rates of responding with little or no pausing after reinforcement. The VR, however, generally maintains the higher rates of responding of the two because the faster the ratio is completed, the sooner reinforcement delivery occurs. On the VI schedule, however, higher rates of responding cannot accelerate reinforcement availability. Sensitivity of the VR schedule to toxic agents remains relatively unexplored.

The differences in performance on these four simple schedules of reinforcement thus reflect the very different contingencies of reinforcement. Comparing the effects of a chemical agent on the various schedules can provide a better understanding of the mechanisms by which drugs modify behavior or the behavioral mechanism(s) by which drug effect is brought about. For example, suppression of response rate on all schedules might suggest a nonspecific effect of a treatment on antecedent factors, such as the motivational level of the subject—that is, an alteration in functional deprivation conditions. An effect specific to a schedule would implicate the unique contingency of that schedule for further study.

Several lines of evidence (e.g., refs. 60 and 132) indicate that the type of consequence is less important in determining the behavioral effect of a chemical than is the schedule according to which such consequences are presented. Kelleher and Morse (130) found that both amphetamine and chlorpromazine had similar effects on behavior maintained on a given schedule (a multiple FI FR, described later), regardless of whether it was maintained by food reinforcement or escape from electric shock. Weiss and Laties (286) studied the effects of amphetamine, chlorpromazine, and pentobarbital on the behavioral regulation of temperature. Shaved rats, placed in a cold compartment, could warm themselves by responding on a lever that turned on a heat lamp for a short period of time. Amphetamine increased the frequency of responding even while elevating skin temperature above normal. Despite accelerating heat loss, chlorpromazine decreased the rate of turning on the heat lamp. Another variable of importance in determining drug or toxicant effect is the baseline rate of responding (59). Many compounds, including stimulants, barbiturates, minor tranquilizers, and opiates, have been found on certain reinforcement schedules to increase the length of short IRTs and to decrease the length of long IRTs. In other words, many agents increase low rates of responding and decrease higher rates of responding. For amphetamine, such effects have been noted in several species and across a wide variety of reinforcement schedules (see ref. 63). Thus, on an FI schedule, low rates of responding early in the interval may be increased, while the higher rates of responding occurring just prior to reinforcement may be decreased, leading to a loss of the scalloped pattern of responding characteristic of FI performance. One notable exception to the rate dependency phenomenon is responding suppressed by punishment, which may be even further decreased by amphetamine (92). The designated response to be reinforced can take many forms, depending on the species and the experimenter's goals. For pigeons, a species favored by some behavioral investigators, pecks on a disk serve as the operant. Tepper and Weiss (258) found that exposure of rats to concentrations of ozone as low as 0.12 ppm disrupted operant wheel running reinforced under an FI 10 min schedule. Also, the simple lever press can be elaborated into a more complex requirement. For example, the response may consist of holding down the lever for a specified minimum duration, a performance disrupted by chronic lead exposure (47). A force requirement also can be specified. Or, the animal may be required to emit a series of responses with different topographies, such as a wheel run followed by a lever press. Another kind of complex response with an extensive literature in behavioral pharmacology specifies that only lever presses separated by a specified interval of time will be reinforced; that is, the differential reinforcement of low rate (DRL) schedule described earlier makes the pause part of the operant. For additional material, see the section on motor function.

Temporally based schedules of reinforcement also have been used to study processes analogous to retention (memory). Consider the fixed-interval schedule of reinforcement. Food delivery is programmed to follow the first response occurring after a specified interval since the event marking the start of the interval, such as the preceding food delivery. Responses emitted before the end of the interval carry no penalty. The DRL schedule previously described is another type of interval schedule but does prescribe a penalty for early responding in stipulating a minimum interval (and sometimes a maximum) between successive responses. Neither schedule conventionally provides external stimuli, such as lights or tones, to indicate the passage of time. Both schedules generate distinct temporal patterns of responding. FI schedules foster patterns in which little or no responding occurs at the beginning of the interval, which has become a stimulus for absence of reinforcement availability, but as the time of the next food delivery approaches, the rate of responding increases. Subjects experienced on the DRL schedule learn to separate successive responses by enough time to earn a high percentage of reinforcements. Increases in response rate on a DRL schedule, such as found by Colotla et al. (41) to be produced by solvent exposure, then decrease the rate of reinforcement.

One criticism leveled against the use of temporally defined schedules of reinforcement in a memory context is the inability to provide a within-session manipulation of the temporal intervals to be discriminated. Although multiple FI FI schedules (discussed later) represent an alternative approach (82), more direct psychophysical techniques for estimation of time intervals are available (54). In some duration estimation procedures, for example, a stimulus of specified length is presented and the subject makes a choice response to indicate whether the stimulus was short or long. Using a two-key procedure, Stubbs and Thomas (252) presented tone stimuli to pigeons that varied in discrete intervals from 1 to 10 sec. Tones 5 sec or less were defined as short and were reinforced after a response on a red key, whereas responding on a green key was rewarded after the presentation of long tones. Amphetamine increased the proportion of long tones that were discriminated as short. Using a variant of this procedure, Daniel and Evans (55) reported that acrylamide caused a significant decrement in duration discrimination accuracy, which recovered only gradually.

Complex Schedules

A major advantage of schedule-controlled performance is the flexibility of schedule combinations, so that more than one baseline can be studied concurrently in the same subject. This approach compounds the amount of information obtained in an experiment. In a multiple-schedule format, the most common combination, component schedules alternate during the course of an experimental session. Frequently, FI and FR schedules are used as the component schedules because of the marked differences in the contingencies of reinforcement on these two schedules (described earlier). On a multiple FI FR, the two schedules may alternate either on the basis of time (e.g., every 15 min) or after a certain number of reinforcers have been delivered (switch to the other schedule after every ten reinforcer deliveries). Different external stimuli are typically used to indicate to the organism which schedule component is in effect at a given time; for example, for pigeons, a red light might be illuminated throughout each FI component and a green light used to signal the FR component. After some training, each stimulus serves as a discriminative stimulus controlling the performance typical of the reinforcement schedule with which it is associated.

The multiple FI FR schedule for reinforcement has been used by several investigators to study a range of toxicants, such as mercury vapor (7) and methyl *n*-butyl ketone (4). In those studies, differential sensitivity of the two schedules was not demonstrated, indicating that these toxicants, at the doses used, produced a generalized impairment of performance. In contrast, Levine (145) demonstrated a greater sensitivity of FI than of FR performance in pigeons exposed to carbon disulfide, a difference similar to that reported for many drugs (Figure 32.19). A decline in FI rate, as indicated by the lower slope of the cumulative record, occurred after a single 8-h exposure (day 1), whereas the concurrent FR performance remained intact. A 2-day, 8-h exposure to carbon disulfide was required to disrupt FR responding. Similarly, Leander and MacPhail (140) studied the effects of the pesticide chlordimeform on a mult FI 1 min FR 30 schedule of reinforcement (Figure 32.20) and noted reductions in FI performance at doses lower than those required to disrupt FR performance. Wenger et al. (291) tracked the consequences of trimethyltin (TMT) exposure in C57B/6N mice responding on a mult FR 30 FI 10 min schedule of reinforcement. Rates of responding on the FI schedule had increased substantially within 3 h of the administration of TMT, whereas FR performance was as yet unchanged. Markedly divergent effects of TMT on these two schedules were observed 5–9 days after injection, with substantial rate increases on the FI and decreases on the FR. Such divergent drug or toxicant effects reflect the different reinforcement contingencies

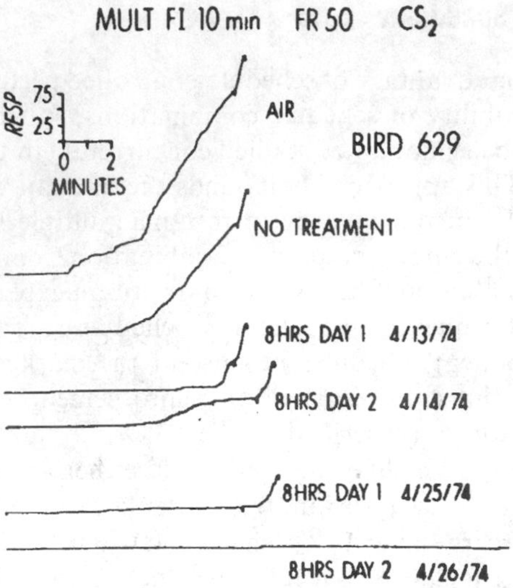

FIG. 32.19. Cumulative records of the performance of a pigeon on a multiple fixed interval (FI) 10 min fixed ratio (FR) 50 schedule of food reinforcement. Different stimuli signaled whether the FI and FR component was active. Records show a single FI followed by a single FR from the middle of each behavioral session with the exposures to vehicle or carbon disulfide as indicated. The diagonal slashes (pips) on each curve indicate reinforcement delivery. The first pip shows reinforcement delivery for the FI component and the second for the FR component. FI performance was disrupted even by a single 8 h carbon disulfide exposure whereas FR performance disruption only occurred after two 8 h exposures. From Reference 145.

of the two-component schedules and the very different behavioral performances they produce. These examples illustrate how the schedule of reinforcement itself may be a powerful determinant of the effect of a chemical agent.

Other complex schedules of reinforcement (see refs. 82 and 208 for further elaboration) include the mixed schedule, which operates identically to a multiple schedule but has no external stimuli to indicate which schedule component is in effect. The only stimuli available to the subject, then, come from its own behavior in relation to the reinforcement schedule contingencies. Thus, comparisons of drug or toxicant effects on multiple versus mixed schedules permit an assessment of the role of discriminative stimulus control over behavior. In that context, Leander and McMillan (141) compared the effects of chlorpromazine on the performance of pigeons under a multiple FR 30 FI 5 min schedule and a mixed FR 30 FI 5 min schedule of reinforcement. In this case, the contingencies of reinforcement were identical on the multiple and the mixed schedules; they differed only in the extent of stimulus control. On the multiple schedule, blue and red key lights were illuminated during the FR and FI components, respectively, while a white key light was illuminated during both components of the mixed schedule. A dose of 3.0 mg/kg chlorpromazine decreased FR response rates on the mixed schedule, whereas a dose of 100 mg/kg was required to produce an equivalent decrease in FR response rates on the multiple schedule. These results again demonstrate the modulation of the effects of a chemical agent by environmental conditions, in this case the degree and nature of the stimulus control over the performance. A toxicological example is provided by work using a fixed consecutive number (FCN) schedule of reinforcement (75). On this baseline, pigeons were required to peck eight or nine times on one key and then one time on a second key for reinforcement. Methylmercury exposure shortened the run of responses on the first key below the required level. When an external stimulus was added to signal the completion of the eight to nine required responses, however, the effects of methylmercury were eliminated. A return of the effects of methylmercury on the FCN baseline reemerged when the external stimulus was removed. Again, such an example illustrates how strong external stimulus control can overcome a toxicant-induced discriminative deficit.

A chained schedule of reinforcement also has different external stimuli associated with each component of the schedule, but it requires the completion of the entire sequence of schedule components for reinforcement delivery. For example, on a chained FI 5 min FR 30 schedule, an external stimulus first signals the FI component and the subject then is required to complete the FI with a response after 5 min elapses. This event produces a change to a different external stimulus, which acts both as a conditioned reinforcer (Sr) for the FI performance and a discriminative stimulus for the FR schedule component. After completing the FR requirement, the primary reinforcer is delivered, and the chain starts again. The tandem schedule of reinforcement is equivalent to the chained schedule, but no external stimuli indicate which component is in effect.

Wood et al. (302a) compared performances on FR 8 FR 1 chained and tandem schedules to determine whether the behavioral effects of toluene were modulated by stimulus control. Both schedules required the completion of the FR 8 on one lever, followed by a single response (FR 1) on the other lever for food delivery. During the chained schedule, the light above the first lever served as the discriminative stimulus for the FR 8 component. Completion of the FR 8 activated a tone and illuminated the light above the second lever, signaling the subject that a response on the alternate lever would now result in reinforcement delivery. The first of these two stimuli, then, served as the discriminative stimulus (SD) for FR 8 performance, while the second acted as both a con-

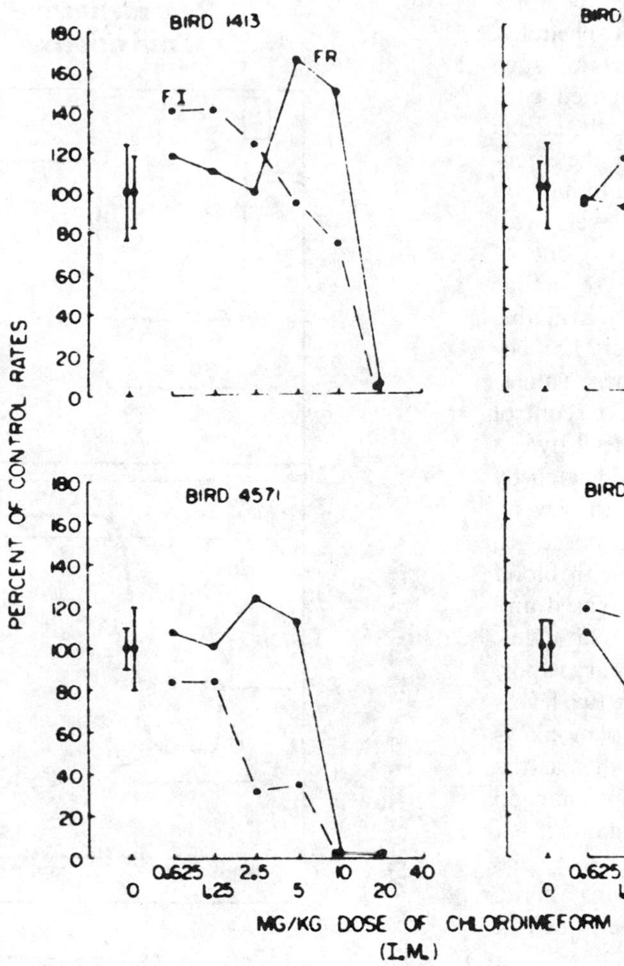

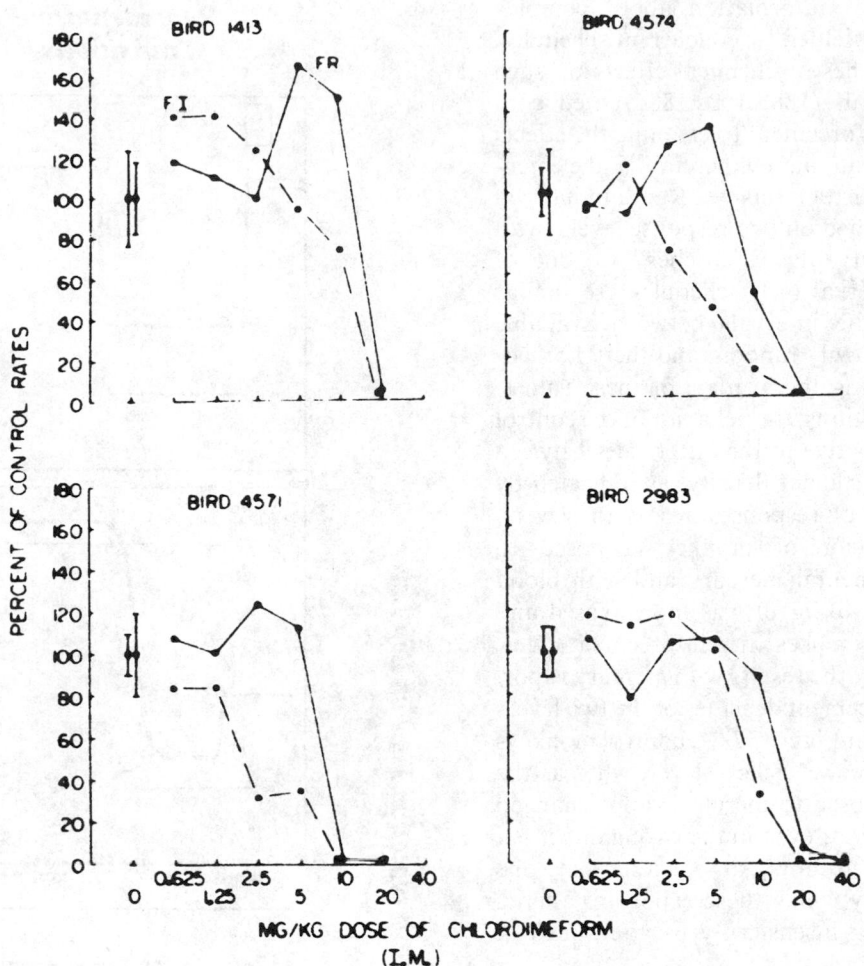

FIG. 32.20. Effects of acute administration of chlordimeform on a multiple fixed interval (FI) fixed ratio (FR) schedule of food reinforcement in pigeons. Changes in response rates (total responses divided by session time) are plotted in relation to increasing dose of chlordimeform separately for each component and for each of four subjects. Points and brackets above 0 indicate the mean±SE under control conditions. As is evident, overall response rates (ordinate) decreased with increasing dose of chlordimeform (abscissa). FI performance was generally more sensitive, however, declining at lower doses than those required to disrupt FR performance. From Reference 140.

ditioned reinforcer for FR 8 performance and the discriminative stimulus for the FR 1 component, completion of which was followed by food delivery. On the tandem schedule, only the house light was illuminated, and it remained illuminated during both the FR 8 and the FR 1 components. Clear differential effects of toluene were observed under these conditions, with performance on the chained schedule, which was under stronger external stimulus control, disrupted far less than the unsignaled tandem performance (see Figure 32.10).

In the complexity of the natural environment, we are routinely faced with many contingent relationships simultaneously, sometimes requiring choices among them. Concurrent schedules, an experimental simulation of such circumstances, facilitate a study of choice by making it possible to select among concurrently operative reinforcement schedules. In an experimental chamber, each is typically associated with a separate response device (for a review, see ref. 307). The choice of component schedules depends on the experimental question of interest. In addition to securing data about performance on the available reinforcement options, concurrent schedules permit analyses of the behavior of switching between the options, a category of responding under the control of the contingencies governing choice. Under some conditions (see ref. 32), schedule-controlled performance maintained by concurrent schedules differs from the performance observed under conventional schedule conditions.

Despite the wealth of information about complex behavior such as choice yielded by concurrent schedules, there are as yet few studies of chemical effects on such baselines. Newland et al. (188b,188c,188d) used concurrent schedules of reinforcement to examine the effects of in utero exposure to lead, methylmercury, and elemental mercury vapor in squirrel monkeys. Random interval schedules were programmed on two response levers, with the reinforcement density always "richer" on one of the levers. Random interval (RI) schedules are similar to VI schedules with the intervals between available reinforcement deliveries truly random and the RI schedule parameter representing the average of these values. Under steady-state conditions, the behavior of the control monkeys was indeed sensitive to the differences between the two levers in reinforcement density, as indicated by the relative distribution of responses across the levers. In contrast, the behavior of monkeys exposed to methylmercury and elemental mercury and with blood lead values in excess of 40 μg/dl was more biased and less sensitive to the differences in reinforcement rates. Further, as exemplified by the results with mercury vapor, when the relative reinforcement densities of the two levers were changed, as shown in Figure 32.21, control monkeys gradually shifted to the new "richer" lever, whereas the offspring of females exposed to mercury vapor changed more slowly, or not at all, or even in the wrong direction. These effects led the authors to suggest that one behavioral mechanism by which these exposures altered behavior was by causing insensitivity to alterations in reinforcement contingencies.

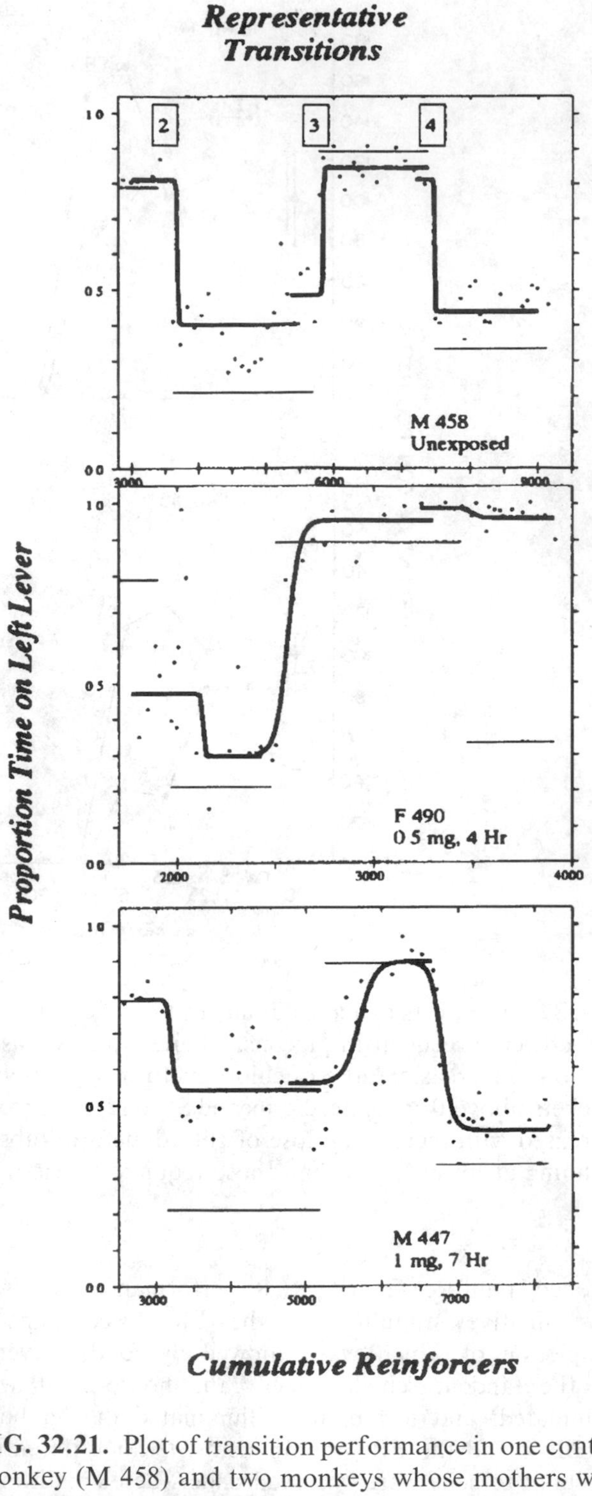

FIG. 32.21. Plot of transition performance in one control monkey (M 458) and two monkeys whose mothers were exposed to mercury vapor during gestation. The response allocations of the control monkey shifted rapidly when the proportion of reinforcers programmed for the left lever (shown by the unconnected horizontal lines) was changed. The two exposed monkeys proved less sensitive to the change in contingencies. The heavy black line shows the fit of a logistic equation to the plotted points. From Reference 188d.

STIMULUS PROPERTIES OF CHEMICALS

Chemical agents or drugs themselves may function as unconditioned stimuli, as discriminative stimuli, and as reinforcing stimuli (e.g., ref. 266). These roles correspond to those of conventional exteroceptive stimuli in controlling behavior. As reinforcing stimuli, they may pose the problem of dependence and the allied problem of abuse. Using compounds as discriminative stimuli in drug discrimination paradigms, subjects can be taught to report about the stimulus properties of the chemical by responding on one of two levers following an injection of the chemical, and on the other following injection of saline. In the same way, the organism can describe the comparative effects of drugs by responding on one lever after an injection of one of the agents, and the other lever if injected with a different agent or a different dose of the same agent. In this role, chemicals act as discriminative stimuli. Despite its potential, this area has as yet made little contact with toxicology.

Chemicals as Discriminative Stimuli

The capacity of a compound to act as a discriminative stimulus may be evaluated by a simple discrimination procedure. Before an experimental training session, an organism is injected with, or exposed to, a specified dose of an agent (drug, toxicant) or an appropriate vehicle. During the session, responding on one of two levers is reinforced if the vehicle was administered, but on the alternate lever if drug or toxicant administration preceded the session. The order of administering compounds across sessions is random, so that the organism is not trained to respond to the pattern of drug and vehicle administration. Typically, responding on the appropriate lever is reinforced according to an FR schedule, such as FR 10 or FR 20. Optimal training parameters of this procedure have been reported by Overton and Hayes (191). Accuracy of the discrimination within a session is typically based on the allocation of responses during the first ratio of the session, for example, 8 of 10 responses may be defined as the criterion for accuracy. This restriction of the accuracy determination to response allocation during the first ratio is necessary because the first food delivery indicates to the subject the appropriate lever for the session. The establishment of a discrimination between the agent and vehicle is arbitrarily defined, such as 8 of 10 consecutive sessions in which a 77% session accuracy criterion was met. The number of sessions required to establish such a discrimination depends on many factors, including parametric aspects of the procedure and training dose of the agent.

Once a discrimination is established, that is, once the subject has learned to accurately report whether it received a drug or vehicle injection, the dose of the agent is varied during test sessions that are typically short and designed to prevent any training to other doses of the agent. This procedure generates a dose-effect function relating proportion of responding on the drug lever to dose of the training drug; the ED_{50} value then can be extrapolated from this function. The procedure can be used to examine how toxicants induce changes in sensitivity of various neurotransmitter systems, information that can be further used to relate such changes in behavioral sensitivity to changes at more molecular levels of analysis and to a determination of the neurochemical basis of behavioral toxicity (46). For example, Cory-Slechta and colleagues (46,51) used this procedure to evaluate changes in dopaminergic and glutamatergic sensitivity as a function of Pb exposure. Rats were trained to discriminate either a D2 dopamine agonist from saline or a D1 agonist from saline using standard drug discrimination procedures. When the dose-effect curves depicting the proportion of drug lever responding to various doses of these agonists were determined, the ED_{50} values for postweaning (see Figure 32.22) and postnatally Pb-exposed rats were significantly shifted to the left of those of control, consistent with dopaminergic supersensitivity. A previous study also has shown a lead-induced subsensitivity to a *d*-amphetamine drug stimulus (306).

Such procedures also can be useful in delineating the neurochemical mediators of toxicant effects, as illustrated in a series of studies by Schechter and Rosecrans (227–230) examining the specificity of discriminative control by nicotinic versus muscarinic cholinergic compounds in rats. These authors reported that discriminative control by nicotine could be antagonized by pretreatment with the nicotinic cholinergic antagonist mecamylamine, but not by the muscarinic cholinergic antagonist atropine. Further, when the muscarinic cholinergic agonist arecoline was administered to rats trained to discriminate nicotine from saline, it evoked saline-appropriate responding. A discrimination based on nicotine versus arecoline was readily acquired, and pretreatment with mecamylamine before nicotine yielded chance responding, indicating that its administration produced a stimulus state dissimilar to both training drugs. Mecamylamine did not affect performance on arecoline test sessions. The stimulus properties of arecoline were antagonized by atropine in rats trained to discriminate arecoline from saline. This series of studies illustrates how the pharmacological specificity of such discriminations is determined, and the behavioral pharmacology literature, moreover, indicates pharmacological mediation of drug stimuli consistent with what would be expected on the basis of pharmacological classification.

These aspects of drug discrimination procedures can be used to examine the pharmacological and neurochemical properties and site of mediation of a toxicant. Rees et al. (205) noted that drug-appropriate responding of rats trained to toluene (either by injection or inhalation) generalized to pentobarbital, suggesting that toluene acts as a CNS depressant. These findings may help explain why toluene is so widely abused. Another example comes from Perkins et al. (197). These authors reported that the stimulus properties of the pesticide triadimefon were mimicked by methylphenidate and, conversely, the stimulus properties of methylphenidate were mimicked by triadimefon substitution. Together with other data, these findings indicate that triadimefon possesses psychomotor stimulant properties.

Chemicals as Reinforcing Stimuli

Operant techniques for experimentally evaluating the efficacy of drugs as reinforcers were developed in the 1960s for both rat (278) and monkey (267). Animals are often equipped with an intravenous catheter attached

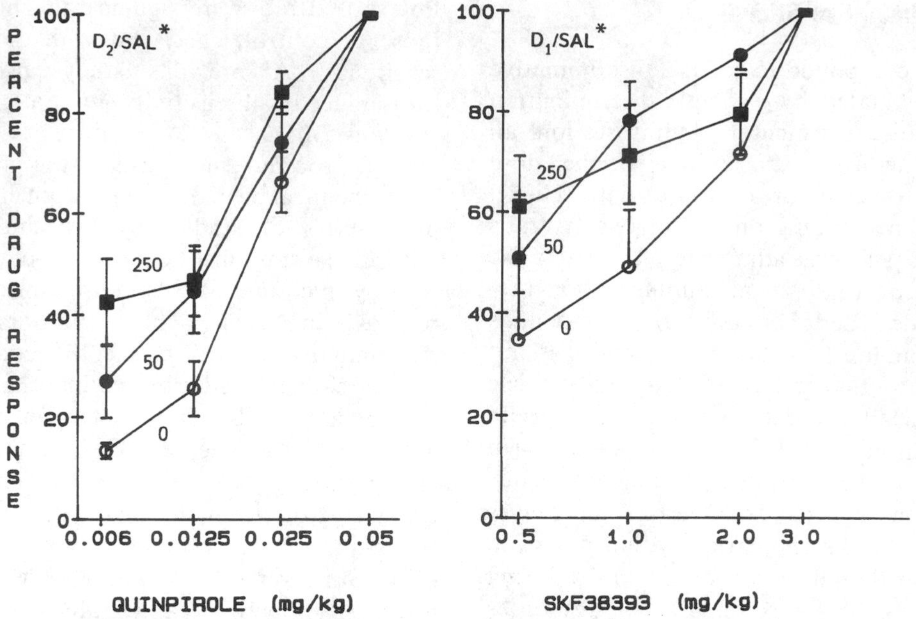

FIG. 32.22. Generalization dose-effect curves for control (0 ppm; open circles), 50 ppm lead-exposed (filled squares), and 250 ppm lead-exposed (filled triangles) groups trained to discriminate a dopamine D2 receptor agonist from saline (left panel) or a dopamine D1 receptor agonist from saline (right panel) using a drug discrimination paradigm that reinforced responding on one lever if the session was preceded by saline administration and on an alternate lever if agonist administration preceded the session. Test sessions involved administration of lower doses of the agonist. Each data point shows a group mean±SE based on $n = 10$. Ability to discriminate drug from saline declines with decreasing dose of the drug. These dose-effect curves were shifted to the left following lead treatment indicating supersensitivity to the dopamine agonists. From Reference 51.

to an infusion pump through which a specified amount of the drug is administered when a response requirement is met by the organism. The development of such procedures established the capability for an experimental analysis of drug dependence, and the resulting literature demonstrated unequivocally the correspondence between most of the substances self-administered experimentally and those abused by humans. Consequently, these techniques are commonly relied on today to evaluate the abuse liability of newly synthesized compounds. Frequently, animals first are trained to self-administer cocaine. The test compound then is substituted for cocaine and its efficacy in maintaining responding is determined.

Abuse potential is not, however, limited to drugs. Volatile materials and aerosols frequently encountered in occupational settings and also commercially available also are subject to abuse by inhalation. Using such procedures, Wood demonstrated in squirrel monkeys self-administration of toluene (300) and nitrous oxide (302), two substances that are also abused by humans. Other toxic compounds reported to engender self-administration in humans include *n*-hexane, gasoline, vinyl chloride, and other organic solvents and volatile agents.

Drugs or chemicals may function as negative reinforcers, and maintain escape or avoidance behavior. As shown in Figure 32.23, for example, mice will respond to terminate the flow of ammonia through a chamber (298). Response latency and incidence are directly related to the concentration of ammonia. In other studies, similar aversive properties of ozone (259), acetic acid (219), and formaldehyde (301) have been demonstrated. Also, Tepper and Weiss (258) found that rats working under an FR 20 schedule of reinforcement made fewer responses to release a brake on their running wheels, an avoidance of exercise that increased ozone flow into the lungs. Thus, such techniques can be used to assess both the pleasurable and aversive/irritating properties of chemical, properties previously considered subjective and consequently barred to experimental evaluation.

APPROACHES FOR GENETICALLY ENGINEERED MICE

The use of genetically engineered mice has become an important approach in toxicology as well as other disciplines in elaborating mechanisms of action. In neuroscience, these include both knock-out as well as

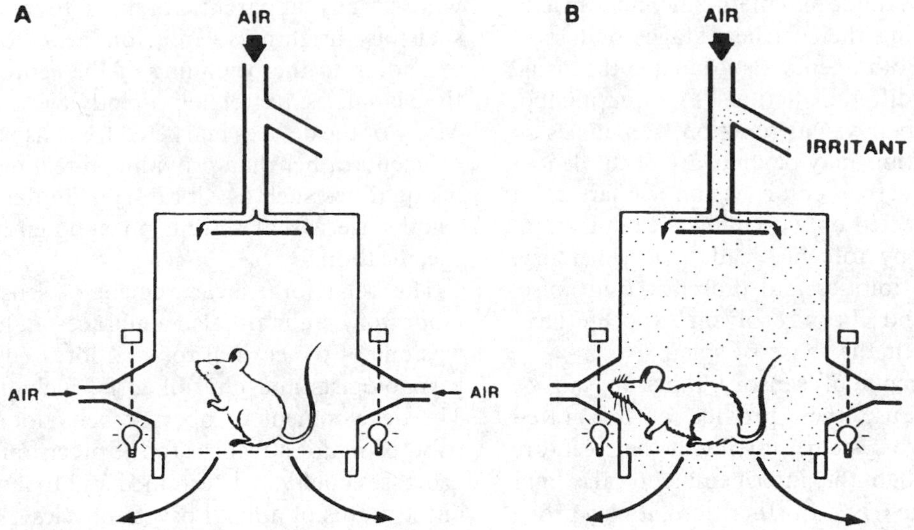

FIG. 32.23. Schematic drawing of an exposure chamber used to study the irritant properties of compounds. (A) Situation before irritant delivery. (B) During irritant delivery. The chamber atmosphere was introduced at the top and struck a baffle which ensured even mixing. The mouse stood on a perforated stainless steel platform through which the atmosphere exhausted. The irritant was added to the dilution air immediately above the chamber. Delivery of the irritant could be terminated by a mouse poke as shown in (B) that interrupted a light beam. Only one of the sensors shown was the active sensor for terminating irritant deliveries; the other served to measure the specificity of any behavioral changes. When the irritant exposure was terminated, either by a response or the end of the trial, a stream of clean humidified air was delivered through each cone to minimize the delay of irritant termination after a response had occurred. From Wood (298).

transgenic mice, plus newer technologies such as conditional transgenic mice in which a single gene product can be altered in a designated region of brain at a time point defined by the experimenter. The technique of somatic mosaic analysis (24a) illustrates one promising method. It exploits the unique properties of a gene-splicing enzyme called Cre recombinase, which performs site-specific recombination of DNA. Brooks et al. (24a) delivered a virus vector expressing Cre recombinase to increase NGF expression in a specific hippocampal region of adult mice. They subsequently displayed structural changes such as increases in ChAT-labeled cells. While some of the techniques described earlier can easily and readily be utilized in both mice and rats (e.g., motor activity, the functional observation battery, schedule-controlled behavior), differences between the two in operant level behavior necessitate some alterations in approach as well. In operant chambers, the higher overall activity levels of some strains of mice may, for example, mean that high levels of lever pressing occur in the absence of any shaping, so that additional procedures may have to be implemented to bring the high rates of behavior under appropriate control of the operant contingencies. This may necessitate implementing specific techniques to slow down response rates, such as time out for responding, or specific implementation of low rates of responding, or the use of response devices such as nose cones rather than levers (cf. Figure 32.12). In our experience, time-out lengths that are effective for mice must be substantially longer than those that are effective in eliminating behavior in most rat strains. Utilization of many of the specific behavioral procedures described here is possible in mice, however. Unpublished studies from our laboratories over the years have implemented multiple schedules of reinforcement, drug discrimination, and even delayed alternation procedures in operant chambers with mice. An accumulating literature attests to these possibilities. Nevertheless, differences between strains of mice may be much more marked than are observed in rats and engender the need for changes in behavioral training, parametric modifications of procedures, and experimentation with appropriate reinforcers.

SENSORY FUNCTION

Almost all behavioral processes depend ultimately on an organism receiving information from its environment. Many behavioral deficits can be traced to disturbances in the way this information is received or processed. Moreover, sensory systems seem to be special targets of certain agents. Acrylamide and methylmercury toxicity are characterized during their earliest stages by loss of sensitivity to touch. Both agents also damage the visual system, although by different actions. A large number of agents, in fact, impair visual function, sometimes so subtly that human victims may be unaware of the deficit. Individuals with defective color vision or areas of scotoma often are detected only on clinical examination. Hearing is degraded by toluene, lead, methylmercury, salicylates, certain antibiotics and diuretics, and noise. Cadmium exposure and chronic solvent exposure have been reported to impair the sense of smell.

Behavioral assessments of sensory function can be especially useful because they provide an integrated evaluation of the entire system, starting at the receptors and progressing through the intermediate to the final processing stages of the CNS. Furthermore, it may prove misleading to rely mainly on histopathology as the primary index of sensory system toxicity. The intactness of the visual system, for example, cannot be judged simply by examining the retina with a fundascope or by the gross histological appearance of the visual pathways. The ability to discriminate colors requires a verbal response in humans and some form of motor response in trained animals.

Psychophysics

Psychophysics describes the branch of psychology that studies the relationships between sensory stimuli and behavior (95). It began as an attempt to quantify sensation, viewed as a private event whose properties presumably depended on the physical properties of the stimulus, and its earliest procedures were devised by the physicist G. T. Fechner. From the publication of his book in 1860 to today, psychophysics has remained a vigorous component of experimental psychology, and in the early years of scientific psychology, its dominant activity. One of its central themes was the concept of a sensory threshold, or the limits of sensitivity for a particular sensory modality, defined as the minimum energy needed to produce a sensation. Even with the trained observers who typically served as subjects in such experiments, variation from trial to trial in sensitivity was apparent, leading to the development of procedures to cope with these fluctuations and to obtain precise estimates of thresholds. These methods became the staples of psychophysics, and have been refined and expanded since their introduction.

A crucial ingredient of sensory testing is precise specification of the stimulus and its properties. Such descriptions are often lacking in much of behavioral toxicology, as in the reaction-time literature discussed later in this chapter. Light and sound stimuli are used without any apparent attempts to measure properties such as brightness and loudness, despite evidence, extending to the beginning of the century, that reaction time latencies are related directly to stimulus amplitude. Many of the devices marketed for sensory testing are also deficient; rather than providing direct measures of stimulus qualities such as vibratory stimulus amplitude, they simply use a dial setting on a potentiometer, say, for specification.

The behavioral measurement of sensory processes in laboratory animals also embraces a long history and was one of the earliest topics addressed by experimental psychologists and physiologists, including I. P. Pavlov. The development of operant behavior technology contributed major advances to the precision with which such processes could be determined and to a marked elevation in the status of animal psychophysics. As Stebbins (249) noted, "Training and testing procedures based on the principles of operant conditioning have shown that animals can report on their sensory capabilities in as precise and reliable a fashion as humans." The basic technique in animal psychophysics is to reinforce responses to specified physical characteristics of the stimulus or stimuli. These stimuli serve no eliciting role. They exert control over behavior because they are associated with a particular history of reinforcement. This feature is of special relevance for extrapolation to humans, since many measurement techniques can be applied to animals and humans with equal facility.

Psychophysical Methods

During the extensive history of psychophysics, many procedures were developed for the collection of data (Table 32.3). Most of these have been effectively translated into procedures that can be used with animals. In most instances, the aim of psychophysical testing is to derive a threshold. Thresholds are not absolute values, but statistical functions of the techniques used to derive them. For example, if the subject is called on to designate the presence or absence of a stimulus, the threshold is typically defined as the stimulus value at which it is detected on 50% of the trials. If the subject is required, say, to discriminate a variable stimulus from a standard, the threshold is typically defined as the magnitude of the variable stimulus that can be differentiated from the standard on 75% of the presentations.

The traditional method of constant stimuli presents the observer with somewhere between five and nine different stimulus values presented repeatedly in a random sequence. The proportion of yes responses (indicating that the observer detected a stimulus event) to each stimulus intensity is calculated, a function drawn, and the threshold usually taken as the intensity yielding a 50%

Table 32.3
Basic psychophysical methods

Method of limits	
	Ascending and descending series of stimulus intensities from above and below thresholds, respectively
Method of constant stimuli	
	Equally spaced stimulus values presented in random sequence
Method of adjustment	
	Observer varies stimulus intensity to exceed and dip below detection limits
Adaptive methods	
	Stimulus intensity rises with failure of detection and falls with correct detection

incidence of such responses. The correspondence with dose-response functions and their analysis is obvious. For animals and nonverbal humans, such as the mentally retarded, the "yes" response is converted into an action such as a lever press. Even for capable adults, actions such as key presses are now preferred because they are compatible with computer-automated stimulus presentation and response recording. A modification of these traditional procedures known as a forced-choice paradigm requires the subject to choose between two stimuli presented either consecutively or simultaneously, and so has the advantage of less ambiguity about whether or not a stimulus has been presented, thus controlling for attempts at guessing. As noted earlier, the threshold in this situation is calculated as the stimulus magnitude corresponding to 75% correct detections because a 50% incidence corresponds to chance. In the method of limits, the observer is presented with a series of stimulus intensities that begin either well above or well below the presumed threshold. The limits of detection are approached in steps of either diminishing or increasing stimulus values. With alternating descending and ascending series of stimulus values, the transition intensities between "yes" and "no" responses in both directions become the values from which a threshold value is computed. An ascending series, for example, begins with a stimulus intensity well below the limits of detection. After each trial on which the observer fails to report detection, the intensity of the next stimulus is raised by a prescribed amount. Once the observer reports detection, the series is ended and the intensity recorded. A descending series is conducted in the same way, except that it begins with a stimulus intensity well above the detection limit. Thresholds are typically calculated as the average value or midpoint at which a transition between detection success and failure occurs.

In one variation of the method of limits, called variously the up-and-down or staircase or titration method, stimulus intensity is modulated in accordance with the responses of the subject, so that the threshold can be tracked continuously. A correct detection lowers the next stimulus amplitude, and an incorrect response raises it (Figure 32.24). This is the most efficient system for calculating thresholds, and was a clever variation introduced into audiometry by von Békesy (271). In the latter procedure, intensity rose or fell continuously. As the subject held down a switch, intensity rose; when it was released at the point where the subject could detect the stimulus, it reversed in direction. In this way, as intensity rose and fell, auditory thresholds for different frequencies could be traced continuously by a graphic recorder. For both human and animal testing, such continuous responses typically are replaced by discrete actions such

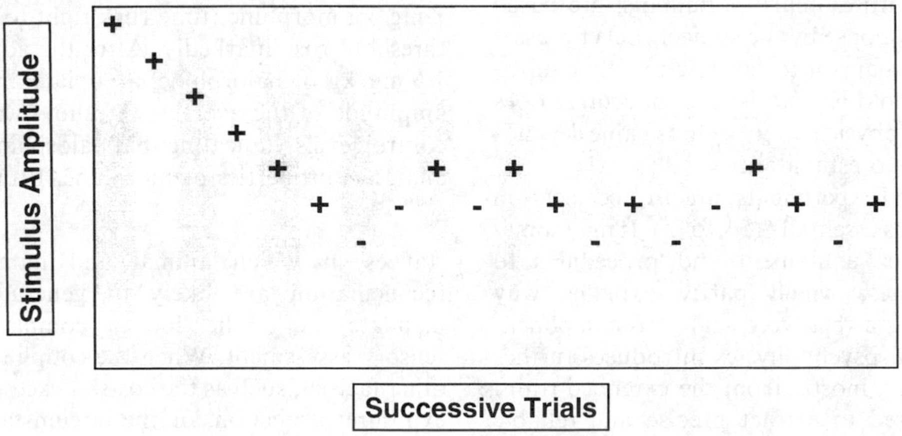

FIG. 32.24. Depiction of up–down (titration) psychophysical procedure. Stimulus amplitude typically begins at an intensity above the detection limit. Each successful detection (+) decreases the intensity setting for the next trial. Each failure (−) increases the intensity setting for the next trial or stimulus presentation.

as key presses, a feature that makes it easily adaptable for animal testing. With the availability of computer control, these adaptive methods are simple to carry out with maximum efficiency. Computer control also allows the use of PEST procedures (parameter estimation by sequential testing); these vary the sizes of the steps in up–down methods so that the threshold can be tracked to increasingly narrow boundaries.

Because titration procedures are designed so that the amplitude of the stimulus is governed by the behavior of the subject, they proved especially suitable for studies of analgesia (288), providing a means for tracing the impact over time of drugs such as morphine and aspirin on aversive thresholds (Figure 32.25). Alternative techniques would have required suprathreshold aversive stimuli to be applied to the animals, with inevitable behavioral disruption and unnecessary pain.

The theory of signal detection (256) first proposed in the 1950s introduced a new point of view into psychophysics. In essence, it conceived of the situation as one in which the task of the observer was to distinguish or detect the presence of a signal or stimulus against a background of random activity or noise. The notion of randomness reveals the origins of signal detection in the discipline of statistics, and the correspondence of noise and random error. Techniques derived from the theory permit the experimenter to take into account variables such as guessing habits or biases on the part of the observer that lead to false detections. Unlike classical psychophysics, these techniques can make explicit the consequences of correct detections and false reports, such as in the form of monetary gains and losses. By relying on explicit consequences, the concepts of signal detection theory may be translated into the terms of a stimulus discrimination experiment (183). For the purposes of the present chapter, however, it is essential only to recognize two principles. First, all psychophysical experiments, whether conducted with animals or humans, are based on a discriminative response by the subject. Lever presses and verbal responses happen to be functionally equivalent. Second, a threshold is a statistical concept. It does not imply an absolute physical limit, and its value depends on the methods used to estimate it.

In all psychophysical experiments, precise specification of stimulus attributes is essential (154,157a). It may sometimes require complex equipment and procedures to define these attributes, which partly explains why psychophysics remains a relatively neglected component of toxicology. Animal psychophysics introduces further complications, deriving mostly from the extended training sometimes required to extract precise and reliable data. Such investments in time and apparatus are worthwhile when the results are coupled closely to problems of human toxic exposure, as they almost surely would be if psychophysical studies were undertaken. Circumstances in which animal and human data require reconciliation are likely to generate questions that mandate the application of complex procedures for sensory assessment. When the coupling is more remote, other factors, such as the costs of excessive or insufficient exposure protection, or the circumstances of exposure, will determine feasibility. For this reason, as in the other sections, this section of the chapter accentuates the more advanced techniques. Descriptions of simpler approaches, such as reflex measures (cf. ref. 52), abound

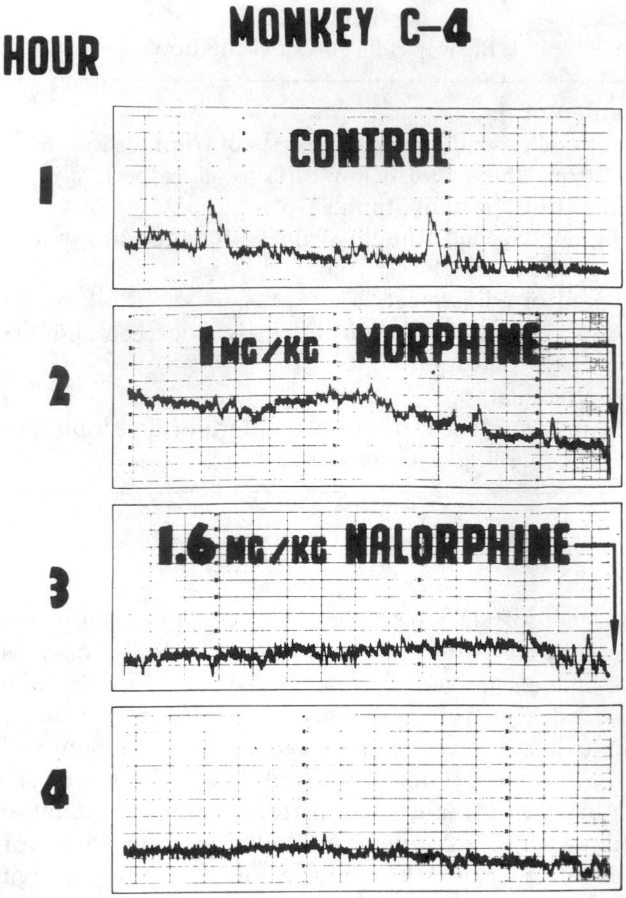

FIG. 32.25. Tracing of current amplitudes (aversive thresholds) maintained by monkeys. The current was delivered to the soles of the feet by electrodes. Every 2 s, the current rose by a small increment. Each lever press by the monkey caused an equivalent decrement in the current. A steady tracing, then, reflects the level of current tolerated by the monkey. Panel 2 shows the effects of 1 mg/kg morphine (time runs right to left); the aversive threshold rose markedly. After the administration of 1.6 mg/kg of nalorphine, an opiate antagonist, the amplitude of the aversive threshold was reduced to control levels, indicating that nalorphine antagonized the analgesic properties of morphine. From Reference 288.

in the toxicology literature. Explanations of the more complex procedures and the contexts in which they confer special virtues are less abundant.

Specific Sensory Systems

Vision

For humans and other primates, vision is the system through which most of the information about the external environment is transmitted. It correspondingly is the sensory system that has received the most attention from toxicology, where it is represented by two books (104,166) and by chapters in textbooks (e.g., ref. 198).

Toxic reactions can take place at many different sites in the visual system. Grant (104) has compiled a list of over 2800 agents that can induce visual system toxicity. Corrosive chemicals can damage the cornea, certain drugs can induce cataract formation in the iris, many different chemicals can damage the retina, and even that part of the cerebral cortex subserving vision can be a toxic target. Vision is unique in the way that information is transmitted along the system. The representation of the visual field on the retina, which contains the light receptors and constitutes what has been labeled a retinotopic map, preserves an analogous spatial distribution in the neuronal pathways ascending from the periphery to the final cortical map. Although ancillary influences may act on these pathways and the distribution of information in the cortex involves secondary projections, parallel and topographic segregation in the primary projection areas is preserved with remarkable fidelity. This feature of the visual system makes testing simple and complicated at the same time.

Color sensitivity, for example, is localized to the center of the visual field (the fovea), in receptor elements called cones, that are coded chemically to respond to light of different wavelengths. Deficits in color discrimination arise when the function of these receptors is impaired. Humans, however, are often unaware of such deficits because they learn to compensate by relying on brightness or other contextual cues, which is why specialized tests are used to detect color blindness. An illustration of how easily color discrimination deficits may be masked was provided by the experience with the monoamine oxidase inhibitor pheniprazine, which had been prescribed to treat depression. The treated patients developed red–green color blindness, a toxic effect of which neither the patients nor their physicians were aware. Only later, when normal visual function could be recovered in a relatively small fraction of the patients, did clinical investigators learn of this problem. Once they did, it was possible to demonstrate a corresponding effect in pigeons, whose color discriminative capacity is close to that of humans.

Hanson et al. (110) trained the pigeons to peck a translucent disk on which different colors could be projected. The birds were reinforced with grain, delivered by a magazine that was lifted into position by an electrical signal, for pecking the disk when it was illuminated by green and orange stimuli but not by blue, yellow, and red stimuli. Differential responding quickly appeared; few responses were made in the presence of the negative stimuli. After about a month of daily administration of pheniprazine, however, the birds apparently became unable to discriminate the different wavelengths and responded equally to all of them. (The experimenters took care to match brightness so that it could not be used as a cue.) Once treatment with pheniprazine ceased, the pigeons gradually recovered their ability to make the discrimination (Figure 32.26). This fairly simple discrimination procedure could have been used to preclude a serious, irreversible effect in humans had it been implemented.

Color vision deficits are recognized as one outcome of workplace exposure to organic solvents. Earlier, Raitta et al. (204) had noted such deficits among workers in the viscose rayon industry, where they are exposed to carbon disulfide. The investigators made use of the Farnsworth–Munsell 100 Hue Panel, which requires subjects to arrange a series of 85 reference caps representing incremental changes in hue. Color vision function is based on the ability of the subject to place the color caps in order of hue. Because the full test is tedious, a modification of the 100 Hue Test, the Farnsworth–Munsell Dichotomous D-15 Test, was devised for screening color vision defects. It requires the subject to arrange 15 numbered disks with different hues. A modification, the Lanthony D-15d desaturated hue panel, was later implemented and is claimed to be more sensitive. Geller and Hudnell (92a) noted the high incidence of errors sometimes made by control subjects and suggested revised test protocols to improve its diagnostic value.

Numerous studies, based on such techniques, have now been published in support of the claim that workplace organic solvent exposure impairs color vision. They implicate styrene, toluene, tetrachlorethylene xylene, methyl ethyl ketone, and others (e.g., refs. 30a, 97a, 164). A common finding in these studies is blue–yellow confusion, but red–green confusion seems to be a more specific marker for solvents.

Color vision deficits due to solvents are likely due to retinal damage or dysfunction. Toxicants that damage visual pathways at upstream sites in the central nervous system create other kinds of deficits that depend on the site of damage. Methylmercury is a potent CNS poison that in primates, including humans, tends to be most lethal to nerve cells buried deep in the folds of the cortex. The peripheral projections of the visual fields lie within the medial portions of the occipital cortex along the calcarine fissure, which is a principal site of damage

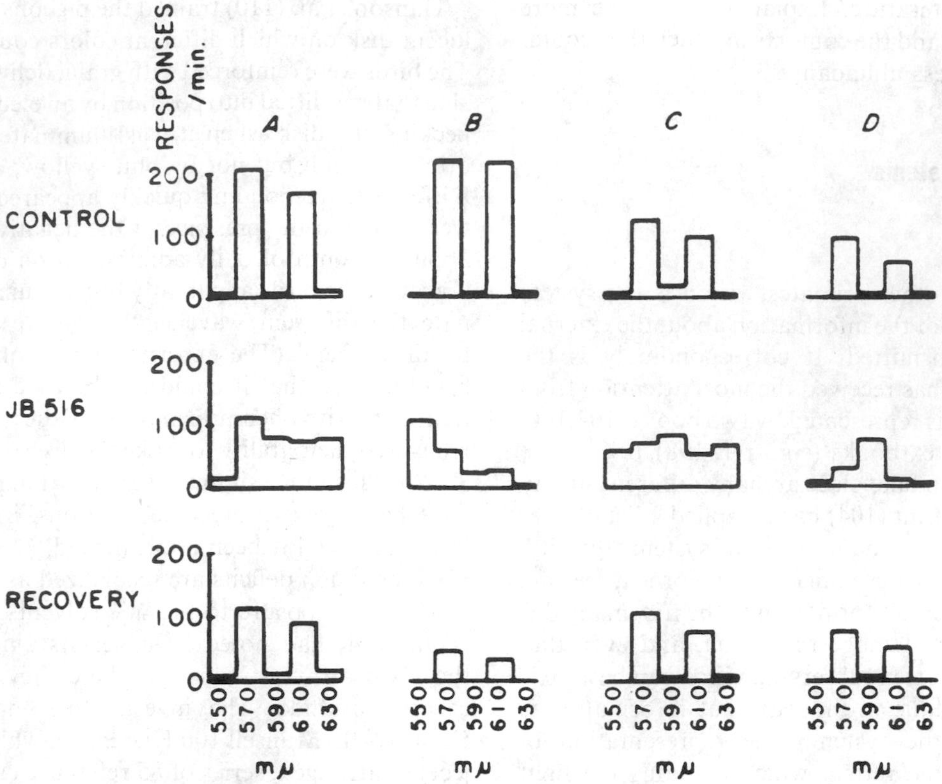

FIG. 32.26. Plots of color discrimination by pigeons after chronic administration of the monoamine oxidase inhibitor pheniprazine (JR 516) The four pigeons were first trained to respond differentially to wavelengths of 570 and 610 nm, as shown by rates of pecking at keys illuminated by different colors under control conditions. Pheniprazine treatment gradually obliterated the discrimination and the pigeons pecked at the keys irrespective of their color. Following drug withdrawal, discrimination performance tended to recover. From Reference 110.

induced by methylmercury. Humans who have undergone serious exposure show constriction of the visual fields, sometimes progressing to severe tunnel vision and, occasionally, blindness. Korogi et al. (133a) found, by magnetic resonance imaging, considerable atrophy in several brain regions, including the calcarine fissure, of Japanese victims of methylmercury poisoning. Evans et al. (76) sought to trace this progression in monkeys and to relate it to exposure and tissue levels of methylmercury. The monkeys were first accustomed to perching in a primate test chair. During testing, they faced a panel containing three Lucite disks illuminated from behind. Three geometric forms—a square, a circle, and a triangle—were projected on the disks. Pressing any one of the disks closed a circuit and allowed the experimenter to record the source of the response and to arrange certain consequences as a result. In this experiment, the monkeys were reinforced with a small amount of fruit juice for pressing the key with the square. The juice was delivered through a metal spout positioned next to the monkey's mouth (Figure 32.27).

The reasons for the choice of a geometric form discrimination to trace the progression of methylmercury toxicity illustrate how animal psychophysics is applied to toxicological questions. If methylmercury preferentially damages cortical cells receiving projections from the peripheral areas of the visual fields, then visual discriminations at low luminances should be differentially impaired. The periphery is represented in the retina by visual elements called rods, which are sensitive to low light levels. The cones in the center of the field, which are responsible for color vision and for fine acuity, function at high light levels. To detect a differential effect in the central and peripheral visual fields, the forms were illuminated on different occasions with a range of luminance values, the lowest of which made the forms visible only after the monkey had remained in the dark for at least 10 min so that the rods had become adapted. Monkeys treated chronically with methylmercury began to show deficits in visual function revealed earliest by diminished accuracy on the form discrimination at the lowest luminances. Only much later did damage progress far enough in the cortex to produce deficits in discrimination at the higher luminances (Figure 32.28).

What might be termed a systems approach to the evaluation of visual function has offered new infor-

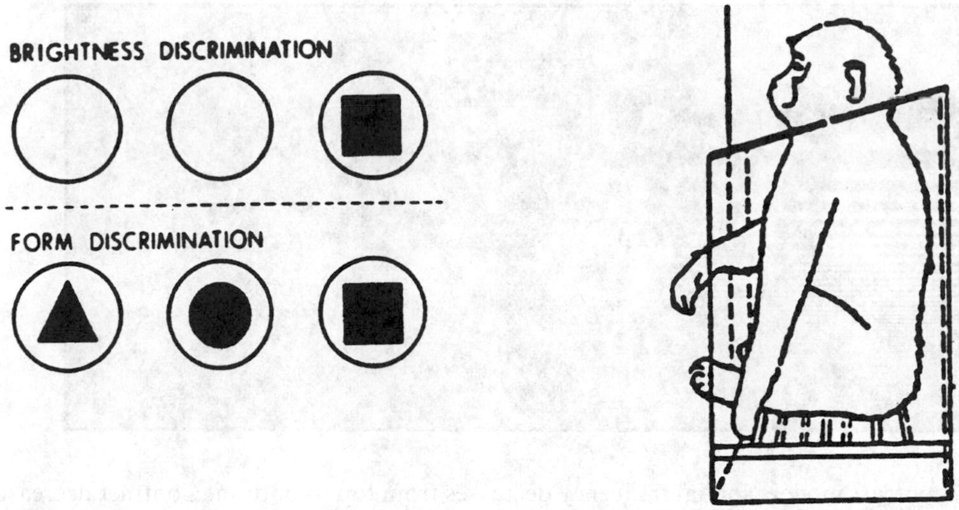

FIG. 32.27. Testing a geometric form discrimination in monkeys exposed to methylmercury. The monkey faced a panel of three disks. When examined for the ability to distinguish shape, the monkey was required to press the disk on which the square was projected. The position of the square varied randomly from trial to trial. When examined for its ability to perform a simple brightness discrimination, the monkey was required simply to indicate which disk contained the square. (On the figure, the light and dark areas are reversed for ease of presentation.) Correct responses were reinforced by pulses of fruit juice.

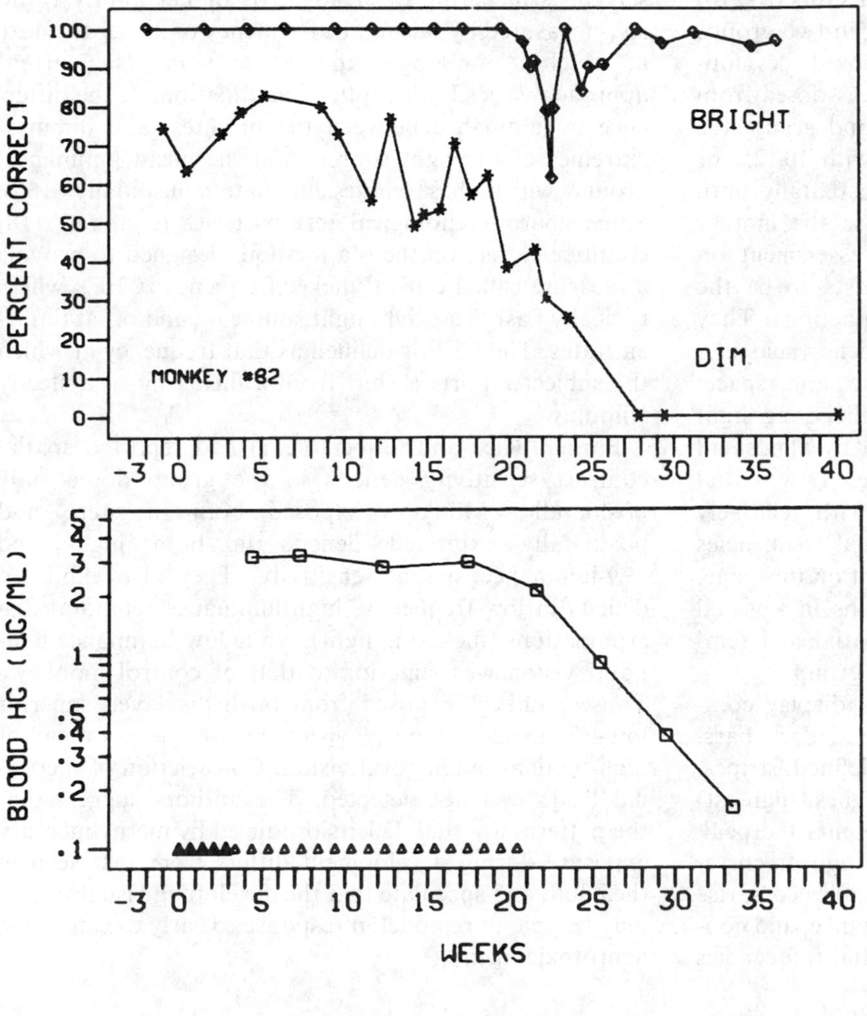

FIG. 32.28. Form accuracy (see Figure 32.27) of a monkey (*M. speciosa*) treated with methylmercury. The methylmercury was administered in doses of 0.5 mg/kg on occasions marked by small triangles on the tower graph. Resulting blood levels are traced by the connected squares. Performance under dim (scotopic) target luminances deteriorated before performance under bright (photopic) luminances and eventually reached zero, where it remained even after treatment ceased (76). Note the sharp fall in photopic accuracy beginning at about week 20. At this time methylmercury administration was discontinued, and was followed by recovery, but performance at scotopic luminances continued to deteriorate, suggesting that sensitive assays might help identify toxicity at a stage at which damage is still reversible. From Reference 74.

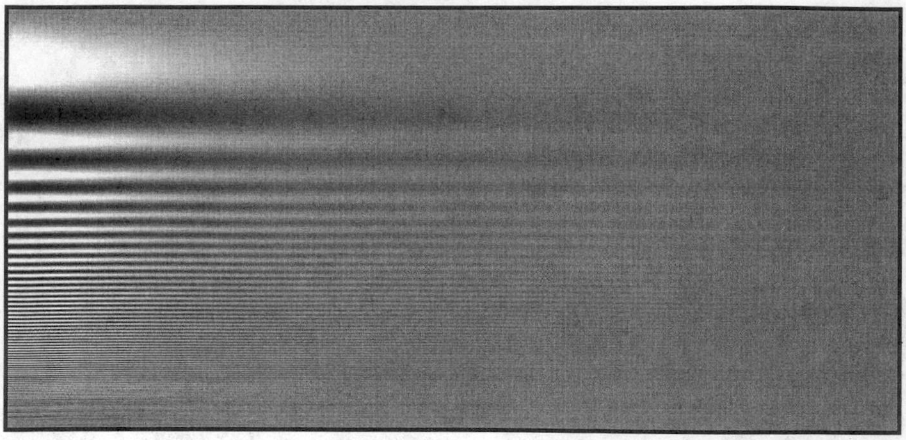

FIG. 32.29. Spatial contrast model. Spatial frequency decreases from top to bottom. Contrast decreases from right to left. A conventional contrast sensitivity plot would be based on the display of a grating with a specified visual angle, and would indicate the contrast level at which the grating appears uniform.

mation about the visual deficits induced by methylmercury. The primary health concerns aroused by methylmercury arise from its effects on brain development. Because visual deficits are such a conspicuous feature of adult poisoning, Rice and Gilbert (214) undertook to characterize visual function in two groups of monkeys (*Macaca fascicularis*) exposed developmentally to methylmercury. One group was dosed from birth onward with 50 μg/kg/day. A second group was exposed in utero by dosing the mother with 10, 25, or 50 μg/kg/day, and was then exposed postnatally until 4.0–4.5 years of age with the same dose the mother had received. The authors based their assessment on what is now conceived by vision scientists to be the principles on which the visual system functions. They view the visual system as basically a frequency analyzer, responding to variations in both time and space. Variations in time are exemplified by flickering light sources. Spatial variations are illustrated by almost all natural scenes containing different textures. Low spatial frequencies are represented by objects with relatively broad features, such as faces. High spatial frequencies correspond to fine details, such as the print on this page. Figure 32.29 shows the kinds of variations in a visual display defined by spatial frequency. Spatial and temporal visual function was tested in both groups.

For spatial testing, the subject views a display composed of gratings, or alternating light and dark bars. These bars typically are not sharply defined stripes, but are varied sinusoidally, so that the highest (lightest) luminance in the modulated signal represents the peak and the lowest (darkest) luminance the trough. In correspondence with temporal stimuli, the variables comprise spatial frequency (bar width), mean luminance, and contrast between peak and trough. High spatial frequencies are represented by narrow bars, which require intact visual acuity, and low frequencies by wide bars.

To assess temporal acuity, the human subject is asked to indicate whether a target, such as an oscilloscope screen, is flickering or steady. His or her ability to do so is measured by raising the frequency of flicker to a rate at which it no longer appears to vary. The current approach varies both depth of modulation, or the difference in luminance between the brightest and dimmest extremes of the light source, and the mean luminance, around which these values fluctuate sinusoidally (165). Some neuropsychological test batteries (e.g., ref. 118) continue to rely on the old method, designed to provide a measure called critical flicker frequency (CFF), which typically flashes a bright light source on and off at different rates. The CFF is defined as that frequency at which the subject reports a shift from a flickering to a steady stimulus.

Earlier, Rice and Gilbert (211) had reported spatial contrast sensitivity deficits in the group dosed only postnatally. Monkeys exposed both in utero and postnatally exhibited deficits in both high- and low-luminance spatial sensitivity. They also exhibited deficits in low-frequency, high-luminance temporal discriminations (flickering light), while low-luminance temporal vision was superior to that of control monkeys. Those monkeys exposed from birth displayed superior low-luminance temporal vision and no impairment of high-luminance temporal vision. Constriction of the visual fields was not detected. The authors suggest that the pattern of visual deficits produced by methylmercury exposure during development differs from that seen in the adult, and speculate that the developing visual system may be able to remodel in response to early damage by a neurotoxic agent.

Similar approaches indicate that the visual system is subject to damage from the axonopathic agent acrylamide. Until the report by Merigan et al. (167), it had been assumed that acrylamide neurotoxicity, expressed predominantly as a central–peripheral distal axonopathy, was largely reversible. Moreover, none of the previous publications, including those reporting cases of human poisonings, had mentioned visual deficits. Merigan et al., in a series of experiments with acrylamide (167,169,170), trained monkeys to choose between two targets, represented by two oscilloscopes. The monkeys sat in a special test stand positioned before a response panel that supported two pushbuttons and a spout for juice delivery. The oscilloscopes faced the monkeys at a distance of 114 cm. Before a test trial began, both screens were illuminated evenly. At the onset of a trial, a tone sounded and the test stimulus appeared on one of the oscilloscopes. For acuity testing, the test stimulus was a vertical grating. For tests of temporal resolution, it was a flickering screen. If the monkey pressed the pushbutton corresponding to the position of the test screen (left or right), it received a juice reward. Each response terminated the trial. An adjusting or titration procedure governed the stimulus parameters. Correct responses made the gratings finer on the next trial during acuity testing and raised flicker rate during flicker fusion testing. Incorrect responses drove the stimulus values in the other direction. The positions of the variable and steady targets shifted randomly from trial to trial and stimulus position and characteristics were controlled by a digital computer.

Treatment with acrylamide continued until the appearance of overt toxic signs; then it was stopped and recovery monitored. All measures of function recovered except for visual acuity, defined as the ability to resolve gratings at the highest contrast (Figure 32.30). Acuity recovered only to a level that remained below that of the original baseline. A subsequent series of histological studies (71,72,149) demonstrated that the source of this deficit was attributable to the destruction of a class of cells in the retina that project to a particular site in the lateral geniculate nucleus of the midbrain, which in turn projects to the visual areas of the cerebral cortex. The degree of persisting functional impairment noted in some of these studies, however, might go unnoticed by many, if not most, people, just like color blindness.

Merigan et al. (171) and Eskin et al. (73) adopted a similar approach to study the visual toxicity of carbon disulfide. Monkeys were exposed in inhalation chambers to 256 ppm for 6 h daily, 5 times each week, for 7 weeks. The visual acuity thresholds of the two exposed monkeys indicated severe functional losses after about 5 weeks. Further testing revealed a 7- to 10-fold loss of acuity from which only one of the exposed monkeys partially recovered. Flicker fusion thresholds, however, showed much smaller, reversible effects. Retinal examinations by fundus photography and fluorescein angiography showed no evidence of the kind of damage to the vasculature, such as microaneurysms, reported in exposed workers (253), nor was there any other clinical indication of damage. These results, like those of the acrylamide studies, argue that advanced psychophysical testing methods are the most dependable sources of information about the neurotoxic potential of agents acting on sensory systems. Color vision deficits, as noted above, have been observed among workers exposed to carbon disulfide (Raitta, ref. 204) and among those exposed to solvents such as toluene (18,164). These deficits were not accompanied by cogent evidence of ocular pathology.

It seems likely that advanced methods for testing color vision might also uncover early or incipient dysfunction. In fact, Merigan (172) later showed impaired color discriminations in monkeys exposed to acrylamide and confirmed that the class of retinal ganglion cells damaged by acrylamide carried color information. For these experiments, contrast sensitivity measures were based on red–green and yellow–blue contrasts as the grating components.

Hearing

The most frequent cause of hearing loss other than aging is exposure to excessive noise. Several classes of drugs also impair hearing and may interact with other sources of impairment. Some, like salicylates, produce transient effects such as tinnitus. Others, such as the aminoglycoside antibiotics (streptomycin and kanamycin), damage the hair cells in the cochlea, where the mechanical movements of sound are transformed into nerve impulses. Loop diuretics and quinine, especially with prolonged administration, can cause similar damage. It is now standard practice for such classes of drugs to be tested for auditory–system pathology, but behavioral testing may detect impairment at a stage when the cessation of treatment leads to recovery.

Stebbins and his co-workers have produced an extensive body of data on ototoxicity from which two important conclusions have emerged. First, they demonstrated that hearing can be assessed by many different behavioral methods and in many different species. Second, they established correlations between histopathology and the results of behavioral testing that yield valuable information about how the auditory system works. In a review of this work, Stebbins and Moody (250) noted the principles guiding their approach. Food delivery generally is used to train animals, by a process of successive approximations, to begin a trial by pressing a key or contact-sensitive plate, a response that activates a light. At a variable time after light onset, the acoustic stimulus, usually a pure tone, is presented. If the subject interrupts the manual response during the tone, the

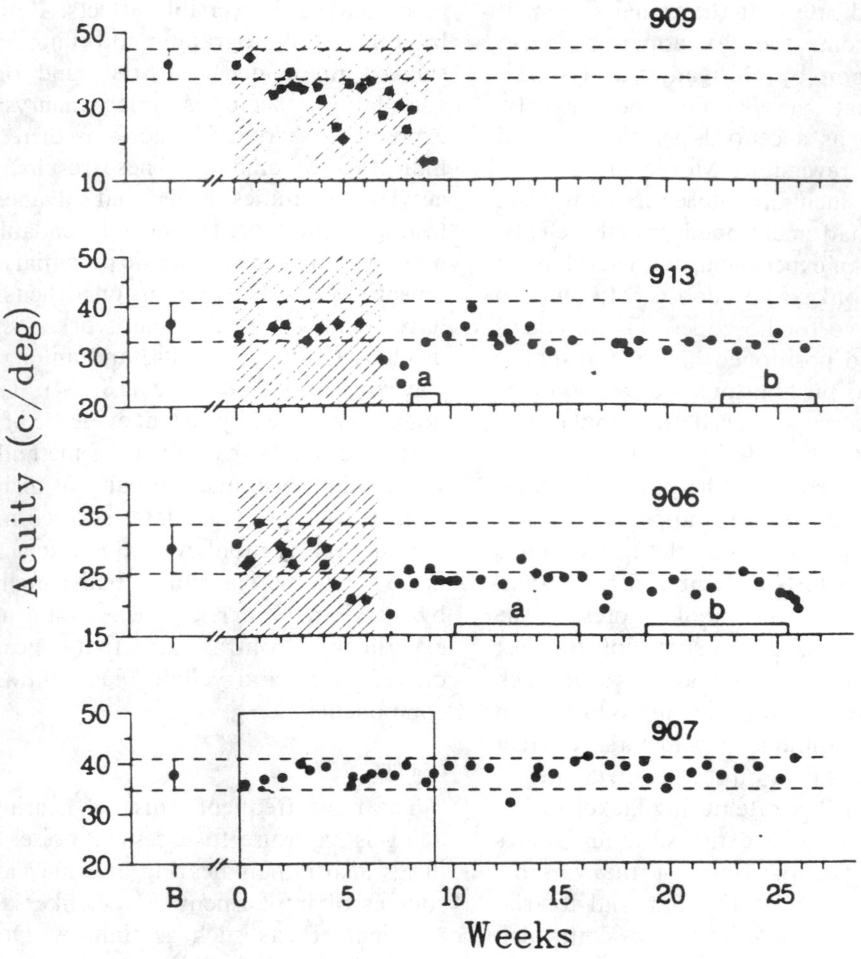

FIG. 32.30. Visual acuity plots of four monkeys (*M. nemestrina*) dosed with acrylamide. The monkeys faced two high-resolution oscilloscopes during testing; one displayed a grating and the other a uniform field, according to a randomly chosen sequence. For expressing acuity, grating contrast, which describes the differences between the brightest and dimmest areas of the vertical grating pattern, remained constant at 0 55. Spatial frequency, based on the width of light and dark bars of the grating, and expressed as cycles per degree of visual angle, was varied in steps according to an up–down procedure to obtain a threshold for the monkey's ability to distinguish a grating from a uniform display. Hatched areas show the period of acrylamide treatment. Acrylamide (10 mg/kg) was administered 5 times weekly until ataxia appears. Monkey 907 received only sham treatment. B, Mean of eight baseline sessions (±2SD), which was extended across the duration of the experiment (dashed tines). The intervals marked *a* and *b* for monkeys 913 and 906 designate collection of contrast sensitivity measures. Monkey 909 was killed at the end of dosing for neuropathology. Monkeys 913 and 906, despite some recovery, failed to reach predosing acuity. From Reference 169.

reinforcer is delivered immediately. Premature releases are followed by termination of the trial and a delay of 6–10 s before the next trial. Trials on which no tone is presented ("catch" trials) are interspersed among the tone trials to estimate the subject's tendency to guess. Training is continued until guessing is reduced to a low, stable rate. Both the method of constant stimuli and the up–down or titration method have been used in these studies.

Measurements of relative loudness, which involve stimulus intensities well above threshold, are made with a modification of these methods. The animals are trained, by differential reinforcement, to break manual contact quickly, say within 500 ms. This is basically a reaction-time situation, and, as noted earlier, because greater stimulus intensities produce shorter response latencies, loudness, which is a subjective variable, can be measured in animals. For example, response latency in monkeys falls from about 900 ms at a sound pressure level of 10 db to about 200 ms at a level of 90 db. With these techniques, in species as diverse as macaque monkeys, cats, guinea pigs, and chinchillas, these investigators have been able to demonstrate the effects of aminoglycoside antibiotics on the progression of hearing loss, and both the temporary and permanent consequences of exposure to noise. The earliest effects are seen at the high frequencies, a typical finding. Mattson et al. (153) note that such specificity makes it unlikely that ototoxicity would be detected with the usual elementary screening techniques because their stimulus dimensions tend not to be precisely described. With continued treatment, losses extend to lower and lower frequencies. Such a progression has its morphological counterpart in the hair cells attached to the basilar membrane, which stretches along the winding spiral structure of the cochlea.

If the cochlea is examined at an intermediate stage of hearing loss, when high- but not low-frequency discrimination is impaired, it shows damage to hair cells in the lower half of the cochlea, where high frequencies are represented, but no damage to the upper half of the cochlea, where the basilar membrane responds maximally to low frequencies. Given such correlations as a guide, it has become possible to largely confirm the notion that frequency is coded according to location along the basilar membrane from the base to the apex of the cochlea.

Lead and methylmercury have both been documented as ototoxicants. Schwartz and Otto (235,236) reported that thresholds to a 2-kHz tone rose almost linearly with blood lead levels in subjects 14–19 years of age. This function is based on conventional audiograms from more than 4000 individuals surveyed in the second National Health and Nutrition Examination Survey (NHANES II). In a more recent analysis, based on a subset of Hispanic subjects between 6 and 19 years of age, an increase in blood Pb level from 6 to 18 μg/dl was associated with a 2-db loss of hearing at all frequencies tested. Although a difference of such magnitude is of little consequence to an individual, it is significant to a population because of the great magnification it undergoes at the extremes of the distribution (cf. ref. 283). Complaints of hearing difficulties were voiced by individuals from Minamata, Japan, heavily exposed to methylmercury, but intensive testing beyond conventional audiometry has not been carried out. Rice and Gilbert (215) surveyed auditory function in *M. fascicularis* monkeys exposed to methylmercury from birth to 7 years of age. The testing was conducted at 14 years of age, after the monkeys were trained on an up–down detection procedure, as described earlier. The exposed monkeys, compared to controls, generally exhibited deficits at frequencies above 10 kHz. The age at which these deficits began to appear is not known because auditory testing did not begin until this experiment. Another group of monkeys was exposed beginning at gestation and continuing until they reached 4 years of age (215a). As in the postnatal group, both mothers and offspring received daily doses of 0, 10, 25, or 50 μg/kg. Pure-tone detection thresholds were determined at 11 and 19 years of age by the up–down psychophysical procedure. The difference in hearing thresholds between 11 and 19 years of age was striking. The degree of deterioration in the treated monkeys greatly exceeded that observed in the controls and supports speculations that accelerated impairment of function during aging is one possible consequence of developmental exposure to neurotoxicants.

Other instrumental techniques, as venerable as those used in Pavlov's laboratory, have been applied to questions of sensory function. Among the more recent applications in toxicology, a series of studies by Pryor and his associates should be noted because they established that hearing loss could be induced in rats by chronic exposure to common organic solvents such as toluene (200). These studies relied on conditioned avoidance for behavioral markers. The rats were trained to jump and grasp a pole upon presentation of a tone in order to avoid an aversive electric shock delivered through a grid floor in the chamber.

Most of the testing methods described above command extensive resources and time for their execution and limit the number of subjects that can be evaluated. They are not designed for inclusion in a preliminary screening battery designed simply to identify potential hazards. Their virtue lies in their ability to respond to questions arising at later stages of evaluation. Even so, there is constant speculation about how these methods might be replaced by less expensive and lengthy approaches. One of the most attractive alternatives is the paradigm known as reflex modulation. It is based on the ability of a low-intensity stimulus, delivered before a stimulus intense enough to elicit a startle response, to modify the amplitude of that response (124). The startle stimulus is typically a loud sound, and the response is measured in rats by confining them to a platform connected to a force or acceleration transducer. If a prepulse, such as a soft sound, appears at an appropriate interval, such as 80 ms, before the startle stimulus, the amplitude of the startle stimulus will be reduced. If the prepulse stimuli consist of pure tones of various frequencies and energies, it is possible to chart what in essence is a conventional audiogram because the amount of reduction is directly related to prepulse amplitude.

Applications of the auditory startle response technique have established the potency of solvents as ototoxicants. For example, rats exposed to trichlorethylene at 4000 ppm for 6 h/day for 5 days showed elevated thresholds at 8 and 16 kHz, perhaps due to a loss of spiral ganglion cells (81a). Startle also can be inhibited by cutaneous and visual stimuli and by brief gaps in a continuous auditory stimulus, but the reflex modification technique is limited to relatively simple questions. It would be unsuitable for plotting contrast sensitivity functions such as those reported by Merigan and his co-workers in their studies of acrylamide and carbon disulfide, or for evaluating disorders of color sensitivity. These studies demanded an extremely subtle form of stimulus discrimination that could be achieved only by highly trained and motivated animals. What seems most reasonable is to include reflex modulation in preliminary assessment batteries and to reserve the advanced psychophysical methods for advanced questions.

Somesthesis

The skin contains a heterogeneous population of receptors whose central representation is equally diverse. Mechanoreceptors are specialized to respond to deformations of the skin. Some respond on the basis of depth of displacement, some on the basis of velocity, and others on the basis of acceleration. Still others are activated by the movement of hairs. Additional receptors are responsive to temperature. Free nerve endings are thought to subserve pain. The pathways transmitting information from the skin travel to the CNS through the peripheral nerves and then, except for the head region, penetrate the spinal cord through the dorsal roots. The head region is supplied by the 12 cranial nerves. At the level of the cerebral cortex, the skin surface is represented in accordance with the density of receptors in various areas, so that the cortical areas devoted to the face and hands greatly exceed those devoted to the back, buttocks, and other low-density areas. A corresponding nonspecific system, which is less defined and which includes the reticular formation of the midbrain, makes a wider range of connections as it ascends and is thought to serve an arousal function.

Most disturbances of somesthetic function are attributed to impaired function of the peripheral nerves (i.e., peripheral neuropathy), although one prototypical agent, acrylamide, apparently exerts its earliest peripheral effects on the acceleration receptors known as Pacinian corpuscles. Damage anywhere along the pathways from receptor to cortex may produce such disturbances, but methylmercury is the only poison clearly documented to be involved at the cortical level. The other substances listed in Table 32.4, although some act as well at subcortical and cortical levels, seem to produce their somatosensory effects primarily through peripheral nerve damage. Note the breadth of chemical classes on the list. It includes metals, solvents, organophosphates, and other chemicals. A more complete list would include drugs from many different therapeutic classes. A satisfactory explanation of the mechanism of peripheral neuropathy that would accommodate such diversity in chemical structure has yet to be formulated (cf. ref. 105), making it difficult to predict, without either histological or functional data, whether a new chemical poses such a threat. Some current hypotheses seem to be converging on the cytoskeleton (36), although for at least one class of agents, the γ-diketones, protein cross-linking has been adduced as the toxic mechanism (103).

In assessing the scope of such a threat, histology will be of limited utility when the basic question is the risk to the health of a specific population such as workers. Sensitive methods for detecting incipient effects and tracing their progression to more serious consequences need to be developed or adopted if the coupling of exposure and hazard, which underlies estimates of risk, is to be a reasonable one. As demonstrated repeatedly, the typical clinical neurological examination is inadequate to the task because its aim is to uncover frank disease. Recall how such an examination seeks to evaluate deficits in touch sensitivity. The clinician may prick the skin with a pin, or draw a wisp of cotton across it, or ask the patient to judge whether a tuning fork is vibrating. Even the most controlled of these stimuli, the tuning fork, is a crude device held in a hand that itself has an oscillation of much greater amplitude than is discriminable at the skin. The threshold for vibration detection at a frequency of, say, 150 Hz lies close to 1 μm and requires precise instrumentation, calibrated to 0.1 μm, to determine. The simple vibration devices marketed by several producers and often used in clinical studies are too gross to yield useful data. Moreover, they tend to be used with improper psychophysical procedures (154,157a). A major flaw is their lack of direct specification of stimulus characteristics, particularly amplitude. Some of the commercial units express stimulus output as "volts," which refers to the setting on a dial. Others use unspecified "units," which are equally arbitrary.

Despite the requirements for precision, however, vibration sensitivity testing offers many advantages as a method for assessing sensory neuropathy. One reason is its underlying structural and functional diversity. It is thought to be mediated by at least two sets of large-diameter myelinated fibers originating from two kinds of receptors. One kind is the Pacinian corpuscles, presumed to be maximally responsive to stimulus frequencies from about 100 to 400 Hz. The other kind is maximally responsive to frequencies of about 50 Hz

Table 32.4
Response requirements for psychophysical assays

Forced-choice procedures
Subject must choose among alternatives
Yes–no procedures
Subject responds if stimulus is detected,refrains if it is not
Rating procedures
Subject reports likelihood of presence or absence using rating scale

and below and has been identified provisionally as Meissner corpuscles. As in the visual and auditory systems, then, vibration sensitivity can be evaluated by determining detection thresholds across a broad range of frequencies.

Monkeys and humans possess about the same degree of sensitivity to vibration and can be tested in essentially the same way. Maurissen and Weiss (155) tested monkeys perched in a primate chair, with one hand restrained by a plasticene mold fitted individually for each monkey. An electromagnetic vibrator drove a rod in contact with the middle finger and was positioned to indent the skin at a constant depth in the absence of vibration. It is essential to use a vibrator powerful enough to maintain its calibrated amplitude when opposing the mechanical resistance of the skin. (One flaw of some commercial instruments advertised for vibration testing is their sensitivity to pressure, which renders them unsuitable for precise measurement of displacement.) The monkey's other hand was free to respond on a key. The frequency and amplitude of stimuli were determined by function generators whose outputs, in turn, were governed by parameters entered into the computer program that controlled the sequence of experimental events and that stored the results.

One experiment with this system sought to trace the onset and development of sensory neuropathy induced by the axonopathic agent acrylamide (157). Six trained *Macaca nemestrina* monkeys served as the subjects. During training, they were first accustomed to the chairs and to the experimental setting. A training sequence then followed in which they learned to press and release the key to obtain a small amount of juice from a nearby dispenser, succeeded by a phase in which they learned to wait for the onset of vibration delivered to the other hand before releasing the key. In the final protocol, a tone signaled the beginning of a trial. The monkey then held down the key. After a foreperiod of variable length, a vibratory stimulus was presented. If the key were released during this period, juice delivery followed. On catch trials, inserted to discourage and compensate for random guessing and on which no vibration occurred, the monkey earned juice delivery by holding down the key during the tone and releasing it only after the tone ceased. Correct responses lowered the amplitude of the stimulus on the next trial and incorrect responses raised it, as in the vision experiments described previously.

Figure 32.31 shows the results of this experiment. After stable baselines were established, the monkeys were given 10 mg/kg acrylamide monomer in apple juice during each weekday of the treatment period. In addition to testing two vibration frequencies, 40 and 150 Hz, the monkeys also were tested, in a separate but identical apparatus, for electrical sensitivity. In this apparatus, the rod in contact with the monkey's finger was an electrode through which a 60-Hz electrical stimulus was delivered. As during vibration testing, correct detections lowered the amplitude of the stimulus on the next trial, and incorrect responses raised it. Gross motor deficits were assessed with an apparatus that allowed an observer to record the length of time required to retrieve marshmallows from a mesh grid. Body weights and the occurrence of standard clinical signs also were recorded.

As these charts show, vibration thresholds rose soon after dosing began. Once dosing ended, they fell slowly after a latency of several weeks. Electrical sensitivity remained stable, presumably because it is subserved by small, unmyelinated fibers that are not as sensitive to

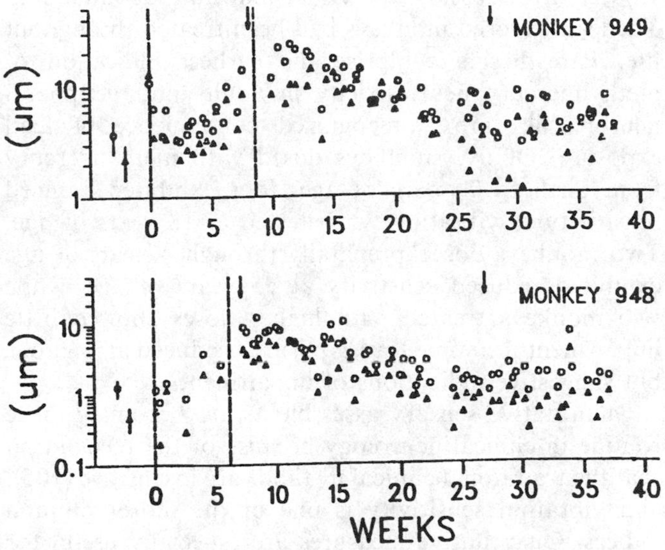

FIG. 32.31. Vibration sensitivity of two monkeys (*M. nemestrina*) assessed by determining thresholds to stimulation by a vibrating rod applied to a finger. The rod was driven by an electromagnetic vibrator controlled by a voltage determined by the computer program that managed the experiment. The monkey's paw was maintained in a stable position by a plasticene cast. The subjects were trained to press a telegraph key with the unrestrained hand when a vibratory stimulus was detected, and to respond only at the end of the trial period when a stimulus was not detected. Correct responses were reinforced by the delivery of fruit juice through a tube close to the monkey's mouth. Baseline thresholds (±2SD) are plotted in the area preceding acrylamide dosing at week 0 for vibration frequencies of 40 (circles) and 150 (triangles) Hz. Dashed vertical lines indicate the beginning and end of acrylamide treatment (10 mg/kg, 5 times weekly). Thresholds, given as vibration amplitude in grams on the ordinate, rose slowly for several weeks during treatment, then slowly declined. From Reference 157.

acrylamide as the large, myelinated nerve fibers that carry information from the Pacinian and other receptors that respond to vibration. A second course of acrylamide treatment, following the return to baseline sensitivity, duplicated the results obtained during the first course (156). What is especially notable about both sets of data is the absolute sensitivity to vibration. Note the baseline thresholds, which lie in the range of a few micrometers. As noted earlier, measuring such thresholds, which is required if early intervention is sought, requires instrumentation that can be calibrated to within tenths of micrometers. Rice and Gilbert (215b) used this method to determine the effects of methylmercury and lead on vibration sensitivity. The methylmercury-exposed monkeys consisted of the same group described previously in discussions of visual and auditory function. The lead-exposed monkeys had been treated throughout life. Paresthesias comprise the earliest indication of methylmercury neurotoxicity in adults and peripheral neuropathies are a recognized consequence of lead exposure. Of five monkeys dosed with methylmercury from birth to 7 years of age, four exhibited reduced sensitivity to vibration when tested at 18 years of age. Two monkeys dosed prenatally through 4 years of age exhibited reduced senstivity at 15 years of age, while two monkeys treated with higher doses showed little impairment. Lifetime lead exposure produced ambiguous but suggestive indications of impairment.

Quantitative sensory assessments are becoming more routine in clinical neurology because of the recognition that the traditional clinical methods are insensitive (105), and vibration sensitivity is one of the more common indices. Quantitative measures are especially useful for monitoring patients treated with drugs, such as cancer chemotherapeutic agents, that induce peripheral neuropathies, so that treatment can be interrupted before permanent damage is inflicted. A key problem remains, however. Despite the availability of instrumentation capable of the precise control of amplitude and frequency, considerable misunderstanding remains about the appropriate procedures. Many papers indicate that investigators are often confused about the difference between psychophysical methods for the presentation of stimuli and the type of responses with which they are used. Maurissen (157a) describes some of the typical errors made by investigators.

Smell

Olfaction is a primitive sense in the context of evolution. Its representation in the brain takes a different course than the senses already described because the olfactory pathways bypass the thalamus and travel directly to the piriform cortex. Recognition of odorants by the olfactory receptors comprises the first stage in odor discrimination, a process that is beginning to yield to a molecular understanding of odorant recognition. Only then do they link to subcortical structures in the limbic system, which includes the amygdala and hypothalamus. Because the limbic system is associated with behaviors such as those involved in reproduction, olfaction carries a crucial responsibility in species as well as in individual adaptation to the environment. Even in humans, the sense of smell, although not critical in meeting most environmental challenges, is nevertheless the source of both pleasant and unpleasant stimuli that contribute to the quality of life. Moreover, some chemicals announce the approach of dangerous ambient levels by stimulating olfactory receptors, so that diminished smell sensitivity might pose a danger.

Disorders of olfaction recently entered the argument about whether chronic, low-level exposure to volatile organic solvents inflicts neurotoxic consequences. Schwartz et al. (233) examined workers in the paint industry who had been exposed to a variety of solvents, all in settings well enough regulated that exposure concentrations did not exceed the threshold limit values (TLVs). The workers were tested by asking them to identify standardized odor patches produced by the Monell Center at the University of Pennsylvania. Compared to controls, the workers exhibited a lowered discriminative capacity. Such a test does not afford precise control over parameters such as concentration; it is a fairly blunt instrument designed for screening large groups. Precise control is achievable in both animal and human studies, although it requires specialized instrumentation, as shown by recent attempts to provide adequate precision for clinical use (133c). In animal studies, operant behavior, based on the use of odor as a discriminative stimulus, has proven successful (e.g., ref. 242). In the presence of one odor, responses are reinforced with food delivery; in the presence of another odor, or a neutral stimulus, responses are not reinforced. Similar experimental arrangements are discussed in an earlier section, Stimulus Properties of Chemicals. Differences in responding serve to index the ability of the subject to distinguish the specific odors at varying concentrations. A special reason for not neglecting olfaction is its exquisite elaboration in rodents, the most common laboratory species. Odor discrimination learning occurs rapidly in rats (69) and also seems sensitive to toxic intervention. Hastings (113) examined the effects of cadmium exposure in rats with a conditioned suppression procedure (cf. ref. 242). In this situation, a stimulus paired with a brief foot shock is occasionally introduced during stable lever pressing for food delivery, usually on a variable-interval schedule. The stimulus typically suppresses responding during its presence. Isoamyl acetate detection thresholds were not altered by cadmium exposure.

MOTOR FUNCTION

Movement disorders represent a major component of clinical neurology. Despite many clear examples, the full scope of contributions to such disorders by neurotoxic chemicals is necessarily vague. Part of the vagueness arises because the etiology may lie buried many years in the past. The emergence of clinical signs may simply reflect the diminished ability of compensatory mechanisms during advanced age to overcome the effects of earlier damage—that is, silent damage (289b). Part also may arise from an inability to identify a specific exposure period or chemical. Associations between Parkinson's disease and exposure to pesticides in agricultural settings have been reported by several authors (e.g., ref. 101a), but only for this general class of compounds.

Clear connections between exposure and neurological disease have been established for several metals. Wrist-drop afflicted many painters who were exposed occupationally to lead pigments. The cardinal sign of mercury vapor neurotoxicity is excessive tremor. One of methylmercury poisoning's primary signs is ataxia. Manganese miners display a condition best described as dystonia, but with some features of Parkinson's disease. Insecticides are designed as neurotoxicants, and the organophosphorous compounds produce axonopathies that impair both motor and sensory function. The industrial chemical acryamide also induces both motor and sensory neuropathies. Certain organic solvents produce central nervous system damage expressed as motor dysfunction. Many of the chemical classes described in this volume, in fact, even those not classifed primarily as neurotoxicants, can induce motor disorders.

Visible indications of toxic processes in the nervous system often take the form of abnormal movements, impaired coordination, slowing of responses, and complaints of weakness. Since any reduction in the capacity for coordinated movement reduces an organism's ability to cope with the demands of its environment, even subtle defects will influence how effectively it functions. Learned motor skills play an especially salient role in human activities. Even apart from the advanced skills of the surgeon or violinist, which are the culmination of years of practice, consider how much we rely on proficiencies in writing and driving as part of our daily activities.

The control of posture and movement is organized in the CNS as a collection of anatomically diverse motor centers. These centers are arranged hierarchically, from the least integrative, at the level of the spinal cord, through the basal ganglia and cerebellum, to the ultimate level of the cerebral cortex. Weaving through this basic hierarchical structure is a web of enormously complex pathways connecting the various motor centers and involving both afferent and efferent transmission. The total system depends on the functional integrity of many different components, all of which seem to present unique opportunities for the actions of toxic agents. Given such diversity, it might seem more fruitful to begin evaluations of motor function with the more elementary discrete elements such as muscle fibers and nerves. But the intricate integration of these elements by the nervous system hampers the utility of such an approach; it would imply a tedious step-by-step evaluation of progressively higher levels of organization. It makes more sense to begin with the integrity of the movements themselves before searching for causes in the separate system components. The selection of sensitive functional endpoints is the critical first step, and behavioral measures the premier tool.

The sources of movement disorders are as diverse as the nervous system itself and arise from many different sites and processes. Some may be due to damage in the peripheral nervous system, although most originate in central structures. Some are an expression of cell damage or loss, whereas others reflect neurochemical abnormalities. Some are manifested clinically as relatively blunt abnormalities, such as ataxia; others are as subtle as the inability to grasp small objects with thumb and forefinger. Because they represent a leading clinical problem, the neural basis of movement disorders is the subject of a vast literature, only a narrow portion of which has ever made contact with experimental toxicology. The considerable psychological literature on movement also has exerted little more than a rather tentative influence on toxicology, except for recent attempts to draw from it some techniques suitable for human functional assessment. The basic properties of movement, however, subsume only a few fundamental dimensions described by mass, time, and displacement, and by their joint expressions in measures such as force, duration, velocity, acceleration, momentum, amplitude, accuracy, and patterning in time. In this section, we feature operant behavior, although not exclusively. Our rationale is that most of the motor behavior that draws our interest in humans is skilled, learned, and voluntary. It is observed in a setting in which it occurs because of its consequences for the individual. This is not to deny the importance of observations based, say, on gait and balance measures, as used in the quantification of Parkinson's disease outcomes in clinical studies, and their analogs in the animal laboratory. However, they serve other functions in neurotoxicology, as in the study by Dick et al. (65).

Preliminary screening batteries often rely on single global indices, such as spontaneous locomotor activity, that are influenced by many variables independent of motor capacity. Some incorporate more specific assays of motor function such as the ability to maintain balance on a rotating rod. Because organisms effect change by producing patterns of muscular contraction, those measures of function likely to prove most sensitive to toxic impairment will typically be based on careful analyses of such patterns and will reflect the integration of the multiple systems that yield complex movements. Learned skills probably offer the most useful baselines for such an assessment because of the flexibility they offer to the experimenter for precise specification of the form of the response; however, because of their inherent capacity to compensate for incipient difficulties, they are especially challenging to evaluate. Mild ethanol intoxication, for example, is often accompanied by more watchful control over movement. Even locomotion, however, which usually is conceived of as an intrinsic skill, is profoundly influenced by its consequences, and some students of motor processes have urged greater attention by movement physiologists (292) to the analysis of behavior and the role of reinforcement contingencies. In either type of arrangement, learned or unlearned, it seems unlikely that minimal, early toxic effects could be detected except by a detailed quantitative analysis of movement topography, such as the system devised by Wolthuis and Vanwersch (297), described later, to study changes in the walking patterns of rats treated with organophosphate compounds, or the kind of kinematic analysis undertaken by Cohen and Gans (37) to describe the patterns of rat locomotion in running wheels. Kulig and Lammers (134) reviewed a wide range of techniques currently in use to investigate motor dysfunction.

Response Duration

The time occupied by a particular component of a movement can be studied either as an intrinsic variable, arising indirectly from contingencies applied to another response variable such as force, or as an explicit variable specified directly by the experimenter. Especially in the latter instance, the stimuli governing the response are almost wholly proprioceptive, arising from sources such as muscle spindle receptors. Assume a situation in which the operant is a lever press and the schedule specifies that response durations must exceed *t* seconds to produce reinforcement. If no external stimuli that change systematically with time are presented, the primary stimuli available to the organism are those arising from muscle and joint receptors. Since such proprioceptors are key elements in the control of movement, measures of response duration could prove useful in evaluating whether they have been damaged by agents such as acrylamide (148).

Shaping long response durations is a fairly straightforward process, as described earlier. Once the designated response, such as lever pressing, has been learned, the additional requirement of maintaining it for a specified minimum duration can be imposed. Early in training, the minimum is short enough that a substantial proportion of responses meet the criterion. The minimum, as in all shaping procedures, is then raised gradually until the final value is attained. Maxima can be imposed, so that a band of durations comes to serve as the criterion. Stevenson and Clayton (250a) trained rats to hold down a lever for at least 40 consecutive seconds. At the end of 40 sec, a white noise signal was sounded. Releasing the bar in the presence of the noise turned it off and triggered a feeder to deliver a pellet of food.

Relatively few experiments with neurotoxic agents have sought to exploit such possibilities. Cory-Slechta et al. (47) trained rats to respond on a schedule that reinforced only durations above a specified minimum value. After preliminary training, during which the rats were first trained to press a lever for food reinforcement, the experimenters imposed a schedule based on differential reinforcement of response duration. Each lever press that exceeded a specified duration was followed by food pellet delivery. These durations ranged from 0.5 sec at the beginning to 6.0 sec during later training. Lead treatment reduced durations and also expanded within-group variability. Several experiments with dogs have relied on response duration as the primary measure of performance. In the first (287), dogs were trained to press a button with their snouts for a food reward. The schedule did not specify response duration directly. Instead, it specified that reinforcement would be delivered when 60 s of responding had been accumulated. The dogs adjusted to this contingency by pressing the button between 10 and 20 times for each reinforcement; short responses predominated, as in a Poisson distribution. Response durations were longer under control conditions than after amphetamine, pentobarbital, or ethanol. Concurrent administration of pentobarbital or ethanol with amphetamine shortened durations even more sharply. In later experiments (279,281), response duration was made the criterion for a titration schedule; that is, the duration required for reinforcement changed in accordance with the dog's performance. Each session began with a specified minimum duration of 0.25 s. Each time the dog, this time pressing its snout against a panel, ended a response that exceeded the current minimum, the required duration was raised, by a computer program that controlled the experiment, to a higher level. In one variant of the program, the criterion also fell after a series of unsuccessful responses. The dogs learned the progression and, through a session, emitted longer and longer responses. Amphetamine reduced the rate of rise and alpha-methylparatyrosine (α-MPT), a tyrosine hydroxylase inhibitor, lengthened it even at doses as small as 3.12 mg/kg (Figure 32.32). Other studies with α-MPT, such as those based on avoidance performance, have identified it as a source of performance degradation. Under the conditions of the study just described, it might be viewed as a source of performance enhancement

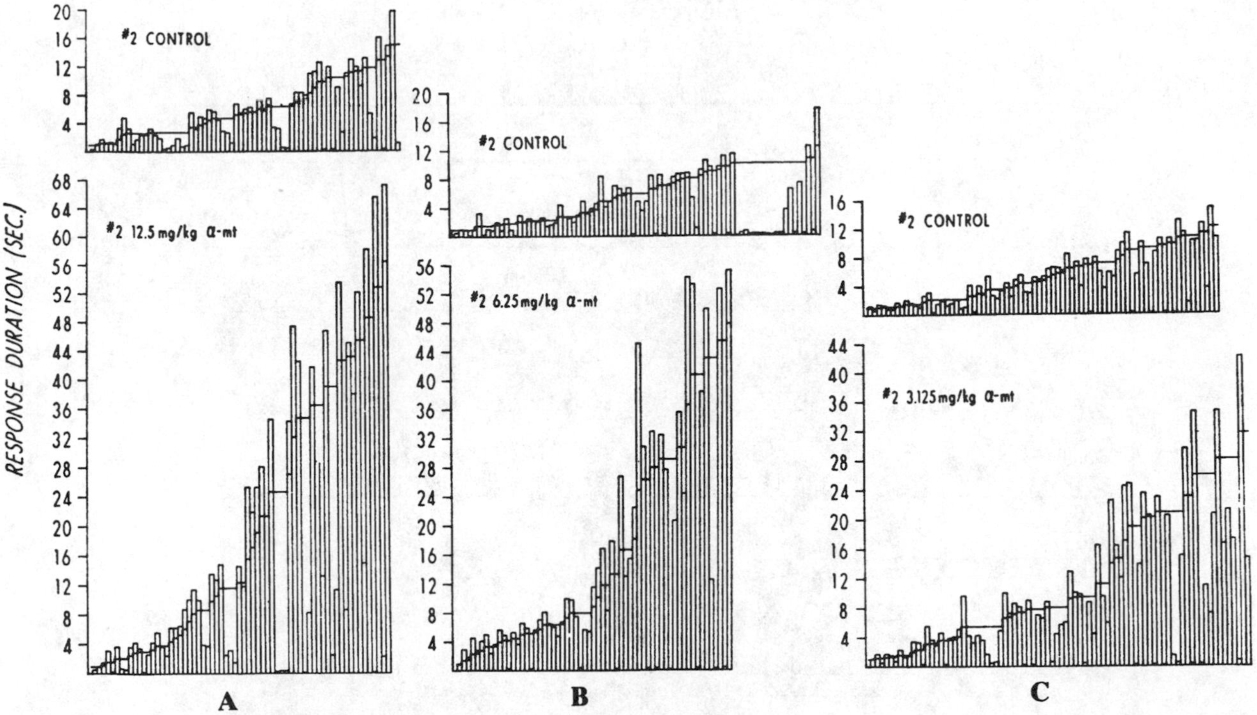

FIG. 32.32. Complex duration discrimination in a dog (Basenji). The dogs were trained to press a panel with their snouts. An experimental session began with a predetermined duration criterion of 0.25 s. Any response duration above the criterion produced delivery of reinforcement (dry dog food) and elevated the criterion by 25% of the difference between the old criterion and the new duration that had exceeded it. This proportion was chosen empirically. If the criterion were raised too quickly, the behavior would be lost, as it often is in shaping procedures that advance so rapidly that they lose contact with the behavior. Under control conditions, the dogs learned to produce longer and longer durations through the session. The compound α-methyltyrosine, which inhibits the rate-limiting step in the synthesis of catecholamines, enhanced the rate at which successive response durations rose, even at doses many times lower than those used in neuropharmacology experiments. Small doses of amphetamine (0.1 mg/kg) lowered the rate at which durations rose. From Reference 279.

and provides yet one more example of how much influence the chosen parameters of a behavioral assay exert on the results and interpretation of an experiment.

Precision

In the absence of clear visual cues, movement precision also is guided largely by proprioceptive information. A research program conducted by Falk and his associates exemplifies the rich variety of information that can be provided by the proper reinforcement schedule contingencies. Building on a technique developed by Notterman and Mintz (189), he trained rats to exert forces within a specified range, 15–20 g, for a duration of 1.5 sec (78). The rats responded on a lever that transmitted an electrical signal proportional to the applied force, and were reinforced by food pellets for responses meeting the joint force–duration criterion. Training was carried out by approaching the joint criteria of force and duration in small increments and required only 5- to 11-h-long training sessions. With this system, Falk demonstrated that several common CNS drugs exerted unique effects on this form of discriminative motor control. For example, the relative amount of time spent within the specified force band varied with the dose of amphetamine and pentobarbital, declining as dose was raised. Fowler et al. (86,87) extended Falk's methods to include other drugs and measures. Haloperidol, for example, raised peak force and lengthened response duration. The latter effect arose from a slowing in paw removal from the force-sensing device.

A similar device, adapted for monkeys (199), enabled Preston et al. to study deficits in fine motor control produced by various drugs. One side of a standard metal cage was modified with the addition of a Plexiglas tube through which the monkey could extend its arm and make contact with a conically shaped response device connected to a force transducer. The monkeys were trained to emit forces between 25 and 40 g for a continuous 3 s to obtain small

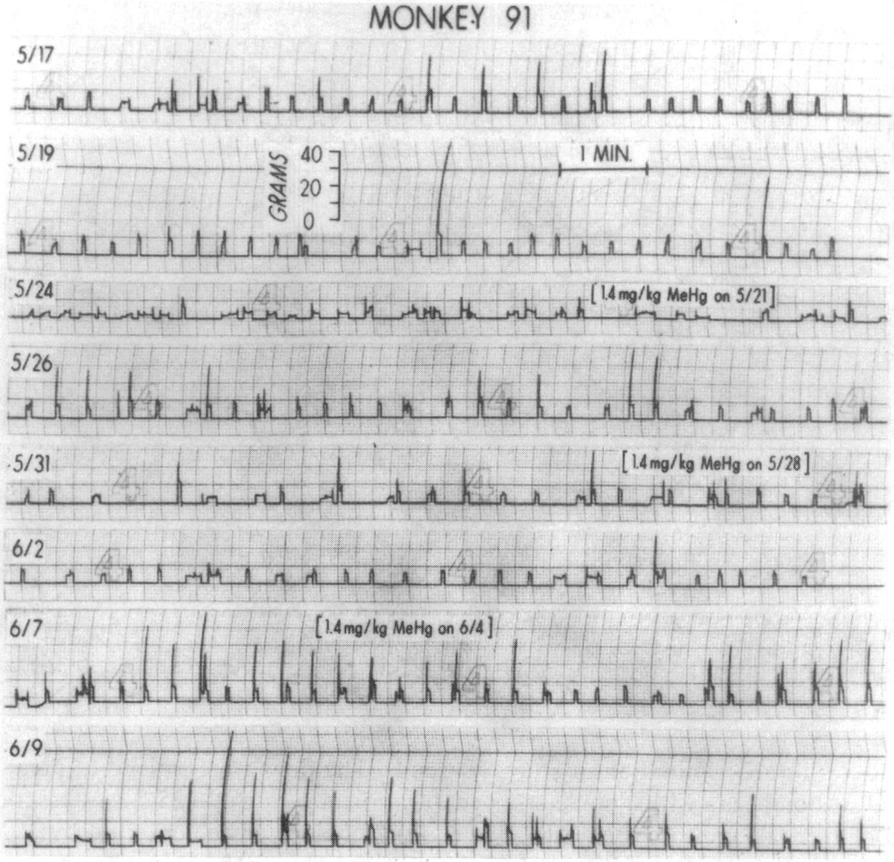

FIG. 32.33. Performance on a motor discrimination task of a monkey (*S. sciurea*) treated with methylmercury as labeled. The monkey was trained to insert a paw into a slot and to apply pressure on a force-sensitive plate connected to a computer. Applied forces of 25–40 g maintained continuously for 2 s triggered delivery of a sucrose pellet. The top two tracings show baseline performance, which was characterized by few overshoots or undershoots. After three weekly doses of methylmercury, most responses were initiated by sharp overshoots before settling into the reinforced zone. From Reference 282.

quantities of water. Various indices of performance demonstrated that the acute effects of methamphetamine, similar to the effects described earlier for rats, impaired performance after repeated high-dose treatment, the pattern of intake adopted by amphetamine abusers.

In another adaptation of this system (282), monkeys were trained to insert a paw through a slot and to touch a Lucite plate connected to a strain gauge. The strain gauge output was transmitted to an amplifier whose own output was coupled to the analog–digital converter inputs of a digital computer. The analog–digital converter transforms the continuously varying electrical signal from the amplifier into a form that can be processed by the computer. Computers are the ideal tool for such an arrangement because they can be programmed to specify variable parameter values such as the upper and lower bounds of the force that defined the response. With this system, the gradual dissolution of fine motor control produced by methylmercury could be traced. The typical pattern before treatment consisted of a precise emission of force within the 25- to 40-g range specified as the response criterion, maintenance in that range for the required 2 s, and release. After treatment, the first sign of coordination difficulty was overshoot at the beginning of the response, that is, a transient force above the specified ceiling (Figure 32.33). This early indication of impaired motor control was followed, after further dosing, by an increasing inability to maintain the force within the prescribed limits. Elsner (70) devised a somewhat similar system to study motor performance in rats, aiming to construct a model reflecting some of the characteristics of attention deficit disorder.

Since rodents clearly remain the most important species for routine toxicological testing, additional techniques for the measurement of movement precision in rats and mice, besides those mentioned above, are especially appealing. All require some investment of time or instrumentation, but can yield critical information about the dimensions of motor control. Lesion experiments designed to clarify the functional domain of certain brain areas are a useful source of approaches, and Newland (188a) has compiled a table showing which basic tests have shown motor effects of lesions in cerebral cortex, basal ganglia, cerebellum, and peripheral nerves and the neuromuscular junction. In a combination of operant and observational methods, Whishaw et al. (293) pointed their analysis at how normal rats compared with rats that underwent motor cortex lesions in their method of grasping food pellets. Before surgery, the rats were reduced to 90% of their initial body weight and trained to eat in a special filming box designed to capture their movements from various perspectives. Video records then were analyzed by a dance notation system adapted to describe animal motor behavior (98). Such an approach, applied frame by frame, requires considerable patience but revealed a spectrum of impairments that were not grossly obvious. A later study (293a) used the technique to evaluate motor skills required to reach for food located on a shelf and to manipulate and eat pieces of pasta. Both the pyramidal tract and the red nucleus are involved in skilled movements, but lesions in these sites suggested a greater role for the pyramidal tract in guiding limb movements.

Another technique designed to evaluate forelimb motor impairment was described by Schrimsher and Reier (237) in an evaluation of cervical spinal cord injury. They trained rats, in a special apparatus, to reach into a recessed tray to retrieve a food pellet. Training occupied 2 weeks after body weight had stabilized on a food deprivation schedule. Videotape recordings provided the raw data for analysis. Hypometria turned out to be the primary disability; it remained permanent in most of the rats, although other effects of the injury apparently recovered. Note that automation of procedures such as the two just discussed, with the potential to yield more accessible and quantitative data, requires little additional training (78).

Another situation devised for testing skilled movement in rats is the "staircase test" (175a). In the test, rats reach down from a central platform to retrieve food pellets located on each step of two adjacent staircases. The pellets are placed on the staircase and presented bilaterally at seven graded stages of reaching difficulty to provide measures of side bias, maximum forelimb extension, and grasping skill for each paw. Performance is measured by the number of food pellets obtained.

Wolthuis and Vanwersch (297) designed an ingenious procedure for recording and analyzing coordination deficits in rats. The traditional running wheel was modified with the addition of flanges spaced at 30-degree intervals around the interior surface. The wheel was driven at specified rates by a motor. The ability of rats to step from flange to flange as the wheel rotated was recorded on videotape and the analysis was performed by automated measures of the placement of the hind feet, which had been coded by color so that appropriate software could be used to measure their position in the video image. With this system, the experimenters could demonstrate that organophosphate treatment produced coordination deficits not readily detectable by common early screening techniques such as the rotarod and hindlimb foot splay.

Running wheels also served Cohen and Gans (37) in their detailed analysis of rat locomotion. Their studies arose from the observation that the locomation patterns of this common laboratory species had not been described adequately, even though its motor activity is frequently monitored to determine the effects of physiological and behavioral variables. To provide the data for their analysis, they trained adult male rats to run in an activity wheel. Photoflood lights provided the discriminative stimulus for running, and mild electrical stimuli delivered through an electrode provided a source of aversive reinforcement to encourage running. Electrodes implanted in forelimb muscles allowed the investigators to monitor muscle activity at the same time movement was being filmed.

The results of these studies are described in terms of what the authors label functional morphology. Running, they note, even in the circumscribed environment of a laboratory device, represents a "complex and highly adaptable grouping of motor sequences." When dissected with the thoroughness expended here, these sequences reveal that the rat's forelimb acts as a steering, propulsive, and supportive device with complicated temporal relationships defining their joint actions. The lesson to be drawn from this venture is that simple locomotor activity, which has been adopted widely as a component of screening batteries for neurotoxicology, or assays such as hindlimb foot splay, offer a misleading, perhaps even deceptive, simplicity about tests of motor activity.

Tremor

Excessive limb tremor accompanies many neurological disorders, is a product of many drug treatments, and can result from exposure to many different classes of toxicants (86). Tremor is associated with exposure to metals such as mercury and manganese; to insecticides such as chlordecone, dieldrin, and the organophosphates; and to solvents such as carbon disulfide. In a recent survey, Anger (1a) noted tremor as a response to 177 chemicals or chemical classes. Because of its pervasiveness as a marker of nervous system dysfunction, many techniques have been developed to measure tremor. The availability of relatively inexpensive digital computers and appropriate programs makes the task of recording and analyzing tremor much simpler now than in the past. Because abnormal tremor is a marker for many different neurological syndromes, and can be induced by damage at many sites in the nervous system, experimenters have to be wary of ascribing too much specificity to it. Newland (184) describes some of the characteristics of abnormal tremor associated with lesions or chemical exposures.

Several examples of how tremor can serve as an index of neurotoxicity come from the mercury literature because tremor is one of the cardinal signs of excessive mercury vapor exposure. Wood et al. (303) studied several women exposed to vapor in a factory workroom devoted to pipette calibration. When first seen clinically, the women exhibited visible tremor. After a prolonged absence from the factory, the pathological tremor faded. To follow the course of recovery, and especially to relate it to diminished blood levels, a system was devised to quantify the tremor. The system was built around a strain gauge to which was attached a Lucite slot in which the patient placed her finger. She was instructed to maintain a force within a range designated by lights to mark the upper (40 g) and lower (10 g) bounds. The output of the strain gauge was transmitted to the analog-to-digital converter of a digital computer, which recorded the successive samples and then processed them. The aim of this processing was to express the continuously varying electrical signal corresponding to the output of the strain gauge in the form of tremor frequency. Since physiological tremor is composed of many different frequencies, the analysis is designed to yield their relative contributions to the total signal. The algorithm by which this analysis is performed is called a fast Fourier transform.

Fast Fourier transforms demonstrated two features of the tremor induced by mercury vapor exposure (Figure 32.34). First, as expected, the total amount of tremor was greater than any seen with normal subjects. Second, and unexpected, the distribution of the relative amounts attributable to different frequencies showed multiple modes, indicating a very complex signal whose component could not be seen clinically. Eventually the amplitude of the tremor returned to normal levels, and at the same time the multiple modes collapsed into one dominant peak. Later, Langolf et al. (135) used a similar technique to monitor workers in a chloralkali processing plant who were exposed to mercury from the massive electrodes used in such plants. They found that as urine mercury rose, the distribution of tremor frequencies began to show multiple modes. With removal from exposure and a parallel decline in urinary concentrations of mercury, the secondary modes declined.

Several later studies have confirmed the usefulness of this method, called power spectral analysis, for monitoring workers exposed to mercury. Chapman et al. (34) compared battery workers exposed to mercury with controls by instructing them to maintain a steady force on a displacement transducer. All the battery workers were judged asymptomatic after interviews and clinical examinations. However, differences in power spectra were able to separate exposed from control workers. One distinguishing feature consisted of peak frequencies in the spectrum. The exposed workers generally showed a displacement toward the higher frequencies. The investigators noted that such subtle changes in tremor characteristics are not apparent in clinical examinations and are seen at relatively low exposure levels. Chapman et al. (34) noted similar findings in workers exposed to carbon disulfide in the grain industry, and concluded that frequency differences more effectively indicate neurotoxicity than amplitude differences.

Ethanol is surely the most venerable of neurotoxicants and surely the most easily recognized of its adverse effects is incoordination. "Easily recognized" also implies that less pronounced effects also might be measurable if the appropriate techniques are applied. Newland and Weiss (186) arranged a situation to try to quantify some of the less overt consequences of ethanol consumption (Figure 32.35). They trained squirrel monkeys to grip a rod attached to the hub of a rotary transformer whose output voltage was proportional to angular displacement. The monkeys received juice reinforcement for maintaining the rod within 15 degrees of horizontal for 8 s. The output voltage was sampled for 5.12 s.

Tremor analytical techniques are discussed extensively in Newland (1988). The primary method is power spectral analysis, which decomposes the power or variance in a continuously varying signal into its component frequencies. Figure 32.36 shows the basic signals produced by a monkey under control and ethanol conditions. Ethanol greatly reduced the amplitude of tremor, even at doses of 0.25 g/kg. It also tended to flatten the spectral distributions. Procedures such as those developed by Falk (78) and Fowler et al. (86) and described earlier can be used to obtain tremor indices in rats. Fowler et al. (88), in fact, showed that the neuroleptic haloperidol, which can induce a pseudoparkinsonism syndrome in patients, also elevates forelimb tremor in rats.

The virtues of tremor measures arise from their sensitivity to disturbances of motor function that may not be clinically apparent. However, as Beuter and de Geoffroy (7a) emphasize, the data yielded by tremor measurement techniques depend on the apparatus, the procedure, the data analysis techniques, and other variables. All of these must be weighed when comparing different reports, a far from unique precaution in science.

Simple tests of motor function almost always are included in comprehensive batteries. One of the most common is finger-tapping rate. Subjects or patients are asked to tap a key or button as rapidly as possible during a test period of several seconds. Both the preferred and alternate hand usually are tested. Chaffin and Miller

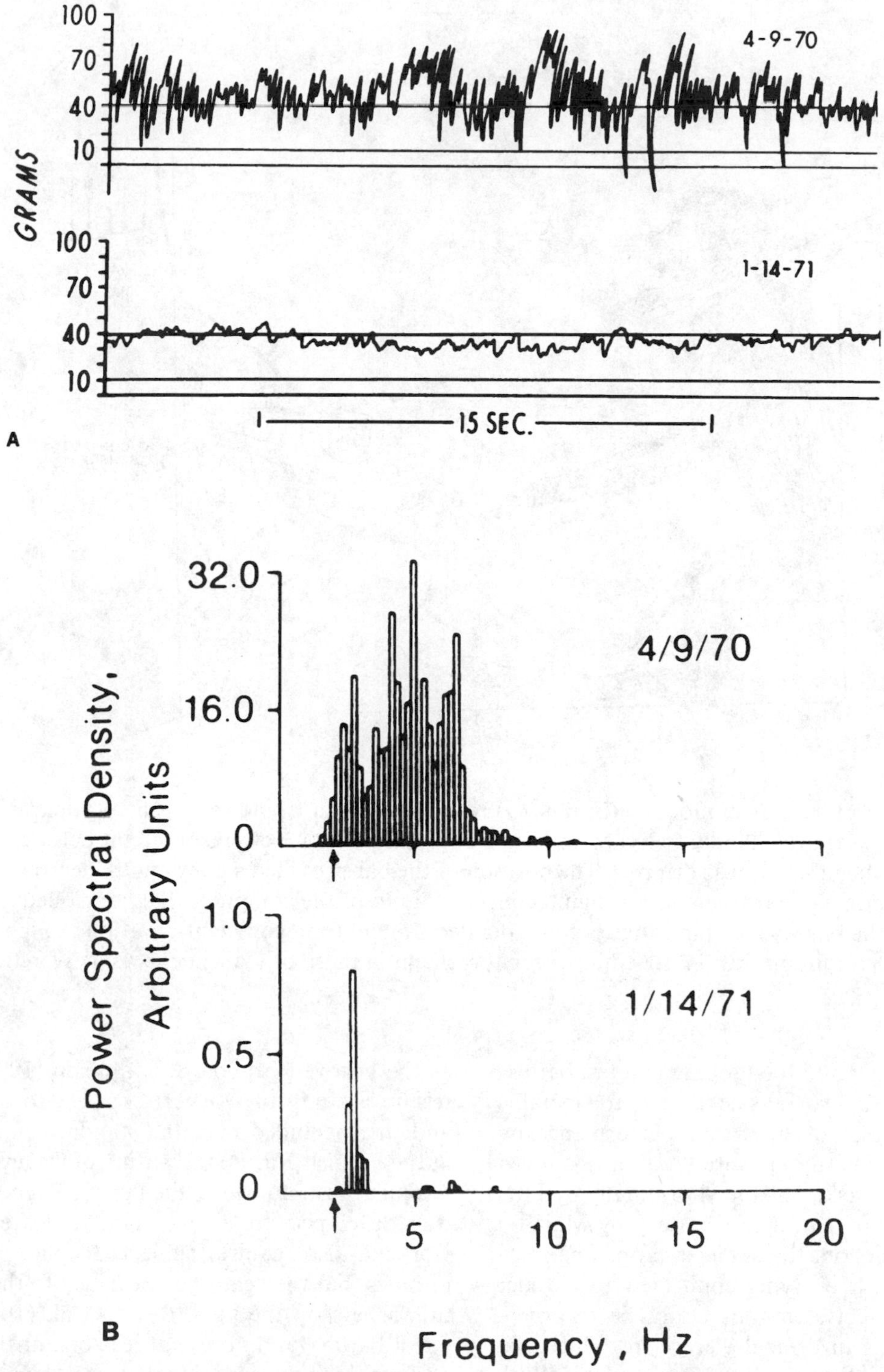

FIG. 32.34. (A) Tremor tracings from a female worker chronically exposed to mercury vapor in a factory area devoted to pipette calibration. The worker rested a forefinger in a Lucite slot attached to a strain gauge and was requested to maintain a force between 10 and 40 g, as signaled by lights. Strain gauge output was amplified and transfered to a digital computer for analysis. The upper tracing was recorded shortly after the worker entered the hospital for treatment. The lower tracing was recorded 9 months later, with no intervening workplace exposure and a marked decrease of mercury blood levels. (B) Power spectral density plots of tremor corresponding to tracings shown in (A). These plots show the amount of total power (variance) contributed by each component frequency in the tremor spectrum and were calculated by fast Fourier analysis. They emphasize the features of tremor, such as multiple modes, that cannot be evaluated by ordinary clinical examination. From Reference 303.

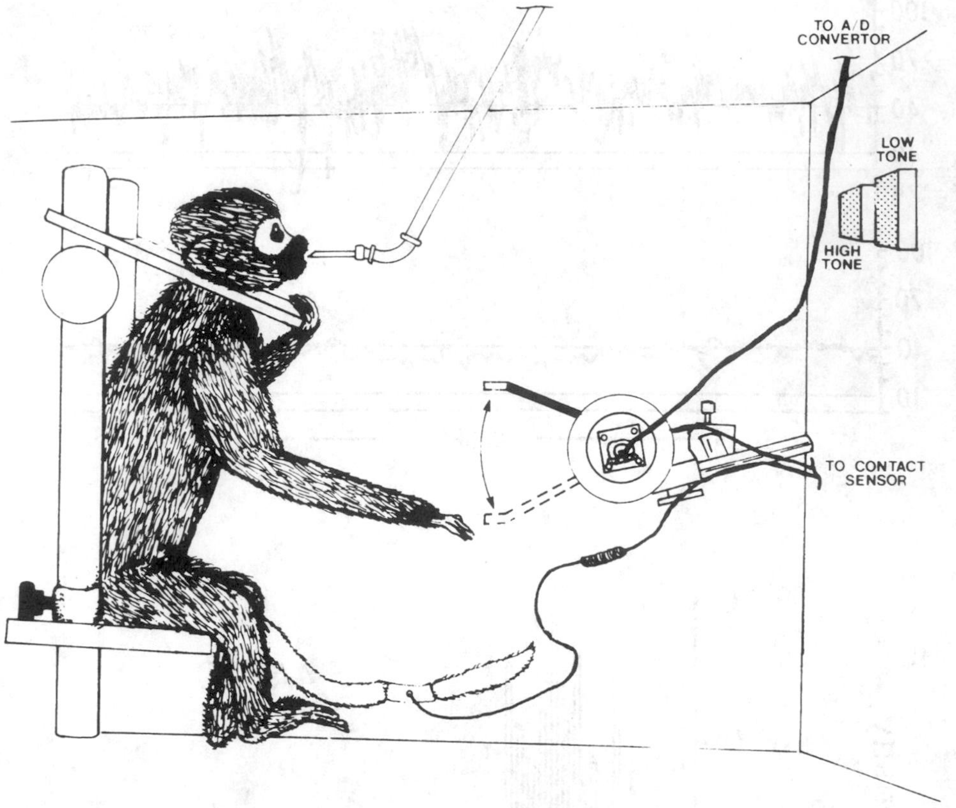

FIG. 32.35. Depiction of a squirrel monkey (*S. sciurea*) responding on a tremor assessment apparatus. The bar was insulated everywhere except the handle to limit response topography. A contact sensor circuit between the bar and the monkey's tail closed when the bar was gripped. The position of the bar provided a continuous electrical signal that was transformed into a digital code by the analog–digital converter input of the computer that controlled the experimental contingencies. When the bar was held in range, a tone sounded. If held for a sufficient duration, a high-frequency tone burst sounded, and on a random ratio 2 schedule of reinforcement, a pulse of fruit juice was delivered to the monkey. From Reference 186.

(33) included both finger and toe tapping in a test battery applied to chloralkali workers exposed to metallic mercury and were able to show that performance on the battery correlated with exposure. A more complex version of the tapping task, developed originally by Fitts (84), was included as part of a test battery by Maizlish et al. (152). In this version, the subjects tapped between two copper plates with a stylus connected to a timer so that the intervals between taps could be recorded. In addition, variations in difficulty were introduced by changing the size of or distance between the plates. With a similar technique, Sanes et al. (225) found slower rates in patients with Parkinson's disease than in controls.

Tests developed originally for assessing manual dexterity in workers also have been adopted for neuropsychology and, in turn, by behavioral toxicology. The Santa Ana test requires the subject to remove pegs from holes in a board, turn them 180 degrees, and reinsert them. The number rotated correctly within a specified time is taken as the score. It is similar to a test known as the grooved pegboard. Hanninen (109) first used the test in a study of workers exposed to carbon disulfide and then included it in the standard battery developed at the Finnish National Institute of Occupational Health. A similar test, known as the Purdue Pegboard, which also was developed to assess manual dexterity in factory workers, also requires subjects to place pins in a series of holes, but they can then be asked to then place collars or washers on the pins. Baker et al. (10) included it in a test battery and note that it is one of the tests deemed acceptable for occupational studies by a WHO–NIOSH expert committee.

Tests borrowed from the experimental psychology laboratory frequently are adopted by investigators. Studies of manganese-exposed workers by Roels et al. (218) tried to assess tremor by using a venerable device requiring the subject to hold a stylus in a hole without touching the sides. Small-diameter holes offer a greater challenge than large-diameter holes. Each contact is recorded as the completion of an electrical circuit. Workers with

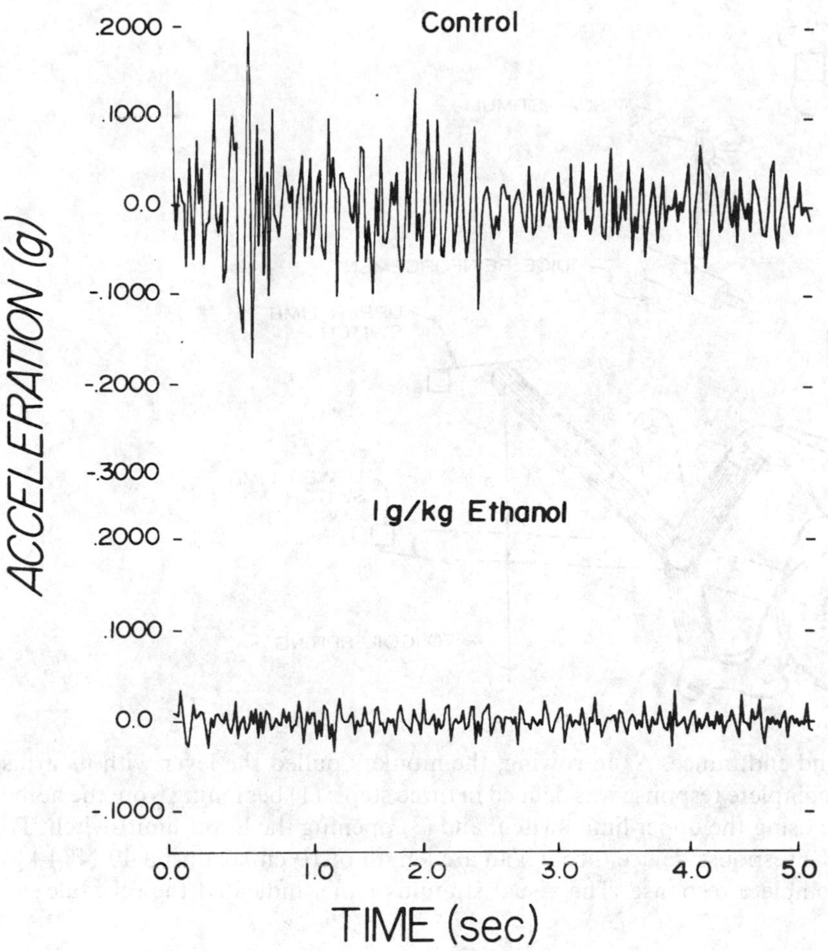

FIG. 32.36. Tracings of bar position (see Figure 32.33) after vehicle and after the oral administration of 1 g/kg ethanol to monkey SM834. Each tracing represents a 5.12-s sample of the second derivative of bar position. The ordinate is expressed as *g* values, or acceleration due to gravity. Differentiation of the position signal emphasizes frequencies important for tremor measures. The literature typically shows records of tremor with accelerometers. The contribution of slow or low-frequency undulations and position drift is accordingly reduced. Ethanol reduced peak-to-peak excursions in acceleration. From Reference 186.

higher urinary values of manganese produced a greater incidence of contacts. A much more extensive test battery was applied to another population of workers exposed to manganese (122); these data also indicate subclinical deficits in such populations. Both of these studies suggest that the methods used by Newland and Weiss (187) to study manganese neurotoxicity in monkeys might be directed to human assessment. Roels et al. (218), for example, found excessive fatigue to dominate the list of subjective complaints among the manganese workers but did not attempt more direct assays. Mergler and Baldwin (164a) also noted fatigue as a prominent complaint in their studies of manganese workers.

Strength

Complaints of weakness appear after exposure to acetylcholinesterase inhibitors, manganese, and other agents. In fact, weakness is one of the most frequent subjective indices of neurotoxicity. Although simple procedures for assessing strength in rodents, such as forcing them to pull against a spring (grip strength), have been devised, complex learned performance offers more direct answers to the kinds of questions likely to reflect human complaints or observations such as the relationship between blood pressure and effort (62). With an apparatus similar to a rowing machine, requiring simultaneous applications of force by the legs as well as the arms (Figure 32.37), Newland and Weiss (188) found that low doses of *d*-amphetamine and L-dopa reduced rates when the behavior was maintained by a multiple FR–FI schedule. Domperiodone, a peripheral dopamine-blocking agent counteracted the effects of L-dopa, suggesting that at least some of these effects arose peripherally. These techniques are readily adaptable to questions about complaints about weakness and fatigue arising from other agents and, since they are based on apparatus developed for human physical conditioning, could play a role in human toxic assessment as well.

Lead at high doses in adults produces neuropathies such as the syndrome of wrist-drop, due to radial nerve damage, in painters exposed to lead pigments. Newland et al. (188b) showed that prenatal lead exposure, at levels (21–70 μg/dl) insufficient to induce overt motor dysfunction, can cause deficiencies in strength. The

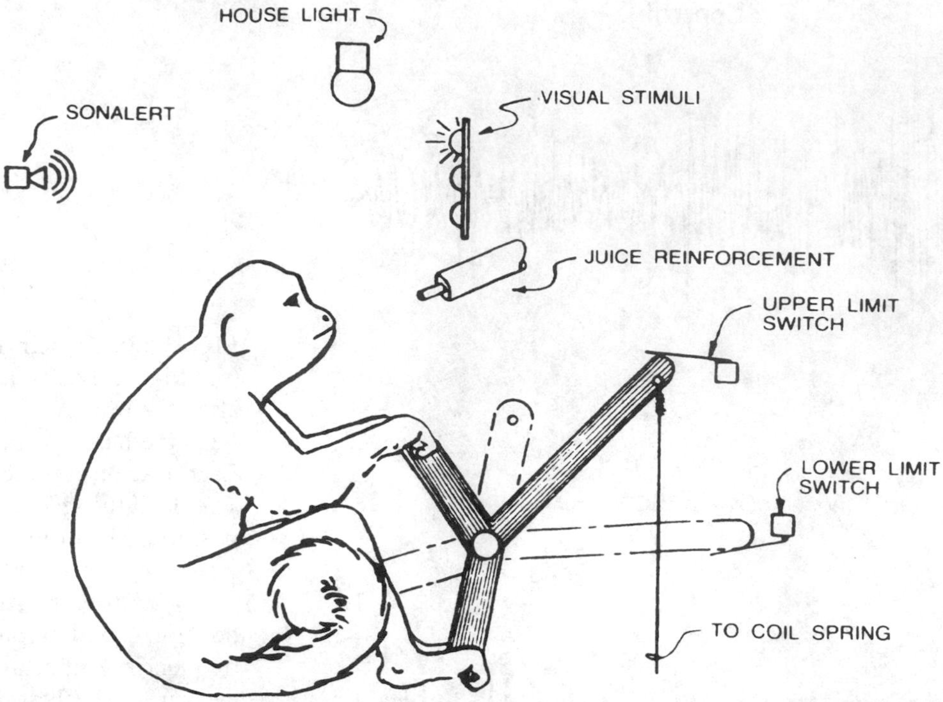

FIG. 32.37. Apparatus for testing strength and endurance. As in rowing, the monkey pulled the lever with its arms while simultaneously thrusting with its legs. A complete response was defined in three steps: (1) beginning from the home position by closing the lower limit switch, (2) closing the upper limit switch, and (3) opening the lower limit switch. To meet these criteria, the monkey had to move the response device through an arc length of 10 cm against a 40-N (4-kg) circular spring. A brief tone followed each complete response. The visual stimulus panel indicated the schedule component in effect. From Reference 188.

squirrel-monkey subjects, at 3–7 years of age, were trained to pull a T-shaped bar against a 1-kg spring through a distance of 1 cm. On FR schedules, which tend to evoke vigorous responding, the lead-exposed monkeys showed a higher incidence of incomplete responses than control monkeys. The authors concluded that in utero lead exposure at these levels produces subtle impairments in motor function detectable years after birth.

Studies such as those just described indicate how corresponding questions in toxicology may be approached. In its advanced stages, manganese intoxication exhibits signs sometimes interpreted as Parkinsonism but, as argued by Barbeau (12), more closely corresponds to dystonia. In its earlier stages, feelings of weakness and excessive fatigue predominate. As with many questions of neurotoxicity, tracking its progression provides the key both to the identification of the neural substrates and the appropriate measures on which to base quantitative risk estimates. The exercise device described earlier (188) offered a means to track progression (187).

After training, three monkeys were followed in a sequence of manganese treatments so that control performance could be measured in the monkey or monkeys that remained unexposed. A number of measures were recorded to reflect performance: number of missed or incomplete responses; response durations; and IRTs. Figure 32.38, depicting a history of more than 400 days, shows the effect on one index, number of misses, or failures to pull through the complete required arc. After the first manganese treatment (10 mg/kg iv), the frequency of misses on the FR component jumped sharply. Although this index occasionally drifted downward, it never reached a pretreatment baseline. Additional manganese treatments produced further variability. Overt signs, such as tremor and dystonias, appeared late in the course of the treatment. Even with the cumulative dosing regimen adopted for this experiment, total exposure amounted to a small fraction of the doses reported by Suzuki et al. (254) to induce overt signs of manganese toxicity.

Behavioral measures, in contrast to measures such as morphology and neurochemistry, which require the animal to be killed, permit the organism's status to be tracked continuously. Imaging techniques offer similar advantages that have been exploited to study manganese. Newland et al. (185) turned to magnetic resonance imaging (MRI) because manganese is paramagnetic. That study indicated that manganese accumulated in basal

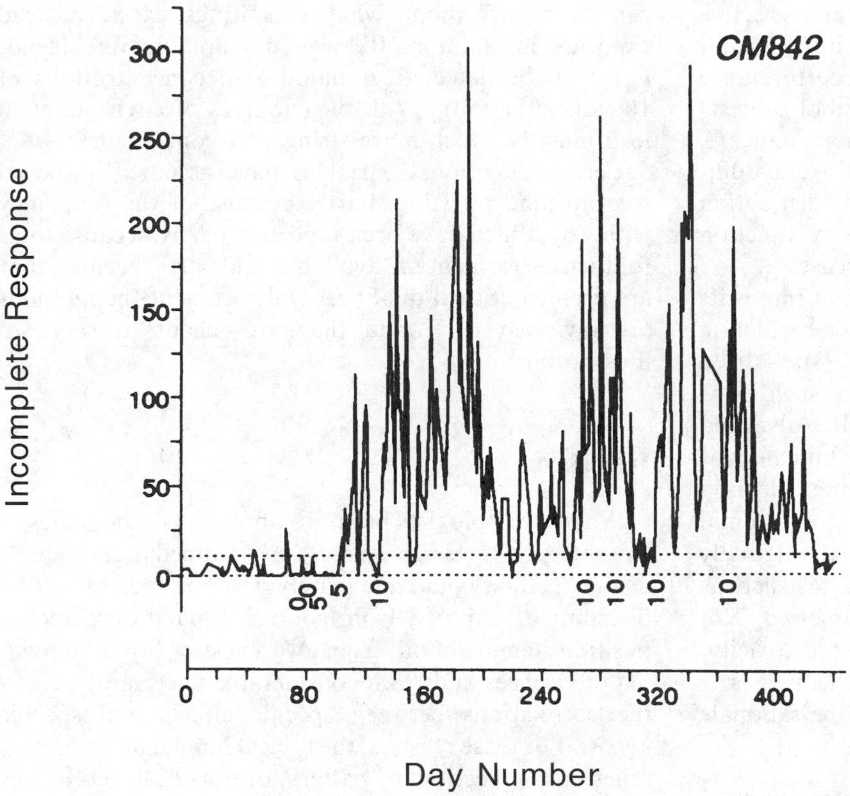

FIG. 32.38. Performance of a Cebus monkey on a device shown in Figure 32.35 during a course of manganese treatments. Incomplete responses designate those defaulting on the criteria listed in Figure 32.35, typically because of failure to operate the upper limit switch. The performance charted was maintained by the FR 20 component of the FR Fl multiple schedule of reinforcement. Manganese chloride was administered intravenously in doses of 5 or 10 mg/kg at times indicated on the baseline; saline infusions are represented by zeros. Dotted lines show 5th and 95th percentiles calculated from baseline sessions. From Reference 187.

ganglia structures, especially the globus pallidus and substantia nigra. The power of such techniques combined with behavioral assessments promises to shape new perspectives in neurotoxicology.

CLINICAL AND EPIDEMIOLOGICAL TESTING OF COMPLEX FUNCTIONS

With the recognition that toxic exposures in the workplace might lead to functional disturbances too subtle to be detected by ordinary clinical evaluation, an enlarging body of research based on psychological testing methods began to develop in the early 1970s. At the same time, awareness grew that equivalent problems in the community, such as the adverse consequences of excessive lead exposure in children, also required a greater reliance on quantitative behavioral methods rather than clinical examinations. The primary aim of the clinical examination is the detection of disease. The primary aim of toxicology is to establish exposure standards free of excessive risk. Psychological test methods, confined previously to clinic or laboratory settings, then were adapted to serve in field studies as well. These developments in behavioral toxicology occurred in parallel with attempts to develop laboratory animal methods for hazard prediction and for determining the biological substrates of behavioral effects.

Although in principle both streams of research flow from common tenets, there are marked differences in history and tradition. Laboratory animal testing is based on the traditions of experimental psychology and the technology refined by behavioral pharmacology. Much of human psychological testing is rooted in questions of diagnosis. Many of the tests most widely applied in occupational settings were designed to originally classify subjects or patients into various diagnostic categories or to characterize areas of deficit. The assessment of brain damage was the major focus of the specialty of neuropsychology, which has provided numerous tools now being turned to the evaluation of neurotoxicity. Lezak (146), one of its leading practitioners, sees the practice of neuropsychology as a response to "the practical problems of identification, assessment, and rehabilitation of brain damaged patients."

The aims and methods of neuropsychology, although overlapping with those of toxicology, originated in a different set of problems. Neuropsychology's emphasis on localizing brain damage and on focal effects contrasted with the aim of behavioral toxicology, which is to specify functional deficits generally arising from more diffuse processes. The recent surge of interest by neuropsychology in degenerative diseases such as Huntington's disease and Alzheimer's disease, which also involve diffuse damage, heightens its congruence with toxicology, however, and should help provide additional assessment tools. For these purposes, early and selective diagnosis also guides current research aims. Brandt and Butters (23) note, for example, that performance on the arithmetic, digit span, and digit-symbol subtests of the Wechsler Scale, discussed later, may indicate, during the early stages of Huntington's disease, modifications of concentration and freedom from distraction rather than a direct impairment of memory function during the early stages of Huntington's disease.

Another important role for psychological testing is its plethora of techniques for assessing and predicting achievement, such as the acquisition of specialized knowledge. Intelligence tests partly attain such aims and may serve diagnostic functions as well. Advanced tests of sensory and motor function in humans, as described earlier, are closer in design to those devised for animals, and in fact many of the laboratory animal methods are direct analogs of those created originally for humans. Disturbances of subjective state, such as depression and irritability, are frequently assessed. Not only may they sometimes foreshadow overt toxicity, but they can constitute important data in themselves.

Gamberale et al. (91) cogently described the rationale for behavioral testing:

> The growing interest in the measurement of performance is most probably due to the sensitivity shown by these methods in unveiling changes in the human organism that otherwise would not be detected. By now, the evidence that these changes are some of the earliest indicators of the occurrence of health effects has become unequivocal. As a consequence, the measurement of performance has come to be regarded by many as a device of major importance for monitoring hazards to health and safety in the work environment. (p. 359)

Some familiarity with human behavioral assessment is essential for toxicologists because so many of the questions and issues that make their way to the laboratory originate in human data. Such a situation is common in toxicology but is more complicated with behavioral endpoints compared, say, to cancer, because standard animal models so frequently are lacking. The result is that when a new observation in humans is reported, such as reduced scores on psychological tests persisting after an acute exposure, the data must be evaluated in the context of what is typically a complicated array of tests. Transforming such questions into those accessible to laboratory methods is an additional, perhaps even more tenuous step. A salient example of such an issue is the claim, advanced most consistently by Scandinavian investigators, of a syndrome, characterized by behavioral and neurological abnormalities, associated with chronic exposure to organic solvents (3,123a). Since the diagnosis of organic solvent syndrome or toxic encephalopathy makes a worker in those countries eligible for a disability award, official recognition of such a syndrome carries considerable economic implications. A similar point can be made about what constitutes excessive lead exposure in children. If lowered scores on intelligence tests can be detected at blood lead concentrations of 10 rather than 40 μg/dl, then sources of environmental lead must be much more stringently controlled.

Certain functional variables have assumed a special role in human testing, partly because of the frequency with which they have been reported, partly because tools for their assessment are available, and partly because they are deemed critical qualities. Only a few of the methods are reviewed here, and they are meant to serve as illustrations.

Test Choice

When psychologists began to apply their techniques to assess toxic effects in humans, they assumed that no single test or method could adequately describe such effects or discriminate exposed from control populations. Such a position stemmed both from awareness of broad individual differences and from considerable uncertainty about the correlations between specific effects and specific agents. For these reasons, the typical human investigation relies on a collection, or battery, of tests designed to survey many different aspects of function (2).

Decisions about which tests to include in such a survey vary widely from one investigation to another because for any specific function many choices are available. Among the criteria by which a test is selected, many investigators choose standardization, clinical evidence of sensitivity, and selectivity. Some may be chosen on theoretical grounds. Tests alleged to measure memory, for example, number in the dozens. A proper choice demands extreme care, especially in weighing two essential properties of tests. One is what psychologists call test validity, or the degree to which a test score reflects what the test was designed to measure. Validity can be determined in different ways because of its many dimensions, but all are defined essentially by the criterion just described. The other property is reliability, or reproducibility. A test that fails to yield consistent results from one administration to the next will bury true differences in excessive variability.

A related problem is standardization, which refers to the population from which the norms for certain kinds of tests are derived. The original Stanford–Binet intelligence test, for example, was developed and standardized on a white, middle-class sample of children, so that the intelligence quotient (IQ) scores calculated from it probably are misleading when the test is given to black children from other social strata.

Sensitivity and specificity may be weighed more carefully in epidemiological studies than other criteria considered in test choice, and as concepts are familiar to toxicologists. Sensitive tests reflect earlier manifestations of toxicity or those induced by low doses; tests with a high degree of specificity are less responsive to conditions not relevant to those the test was designed to detect. The mode of framing the question will also help guide choice. If the aim is screening, or determining whether toxicity is detectable at a particular exposure level, functional breadth is accorded more importance than selectivity. If the aim is to clarify the nature of the functional deficits or their mechanisms, selectivity will receive greater emphasis.

Sensitivity cannot be judged on an absolute scale in human studies, however. Only relative sensitivity, derived from a comparison of different measures, is within our grasp. Unlike the situation in animal studies, we rarely are in a position to exert control over exposure levels; studies with human volunteers are the exception. If one test instrument discriminates an exposed from an unexposed population more definitively than another, we may term it more sensitive. Such results do not indicate whether it could identify a population with lower exposures. One approach, advocated by Kennedy et al. (132a), calibrates the test battery by relating deficits in computerized performance tests to graded doses of alcohol.

Accumulated experience, coupled with theory and tradition, has led most investigators to select tests encompassing a fairly common set of categories. These may include tests of memory, of simple motor function, of complex cognitive performance, of attention and vigilance, and of mood or subjective state. Not all categories may appear in any single study because some investigations are directed at one or a small cluster of functions. When confronted with requirements for toxicity testing, the experience of psychologists with diagnostic tests induced many to rely most heavily on instruments designed to assess the consequences of brain damage or severe behavioral disorders such as psychosis (146). A common choice for inclusion in a test battery, because it was designed for those latter roles, has been the Wechsler Adult Intelligence Scale (WAIS), an attractive feature of which is its relatively careful standardization (275) and large body of accumulated experience. The WAIS is actually a battery of tests in itself and was designed to assess a broad sample of functions. It consists of 11 subtests, assigned to "verbal" and "performance" categories to yield two major subscores (Table 32.6). This division is somewhat arbitrary because the two categories show considerable functional overlap and high correlations. Many investigators have chosen certain WAIS subtests rather than the complete assemblage for incorporation into their own repertoire of tests.

Table 32.5
Chemicals impairing vibration sensitivity

Acrylamide
n-Hexane
Carbon disulfide
Arsenic
Methylmercury
Thallium
Methyl *n*-butyl ketone
Triorthocresyl phosphate
Lead
Cyanide
Chlorobiphenyl
Methyl bromide
Methamidophos

Table 32.6
Subtests of the Wechsler Adult Intelligence Scale (WAIS)–Revised

	Verbal
Information:	Questions of a general nature
Comprehension:	Interpretation, judgment
Arithmetic:	Numerical calculations
Similarities:	Comparisons of nouns
Digit span:	Repetition of digit sequences
Vocabulary:	Word definitions
	Performance
Digit-symbol:	Symbol–number coding
Picture completion:	Identify missing portions
Block design:	Duplication of patterns
Picture arrangement:	Construct narrative sequence
Object assembly:	Assemble jigsaw puzzle

Vocabulary tests are examples of the "verbal" category. An example of the "performance" category is the symbol-digit substitution test of the WAIS, which requires the patient or subject to enter, into appropriate blanks on a form, symbols paired with numbers according to a specified code. All the subscales can be combined to yield a full-scale IQ score, which correlates highly with academic achievement. The full-scale score, because it is a global score composed of the 11 subscale scores, is unlikely to provide much information about the areas of impaired function arising from exposure to a particular toxic agent. Brain-damaged persons typically reveal an uneven pattern of deficits (146) that in group comparisons might be masked and misinterpreted. For this reason, some investigators have simply adopted certain subscales of the WAIS to assay specific functions. However, the pattern itself is often useful for diagnosis, and techniques have been developed to explicitly relate the profile of performance to diagnosis (222).

Table 32.7
WHO neurobehavioral core test battery

Functional domain	Core test
Motor speed, steadiness	Aiming; placing dots in circle
Attention	Simple reaction time
Perceptual–motor	WAIS digit-symbol
Manual dexterity	Santa Ana test
Visual memory	Benton visual retention test
Auditory memory	WAIS digit span

Table 32.8
Neurobehavioral evaluation system (NES)

Psychomotor performance	*Memory and learning*
Symbol-digit	Digit span
Hand-eye coordination	Paired associate learning
Simple reaction time	Paired associate recall
Continuous performance test	Visual retention
Finger tapping	Pattern memory
	Memory scanning
Cognitive	Serial digit learning
Vocabulary	
Horizontal addition	*Perceptual ability*
Switching attention	Pattern ability
Grammatical reasoning	
Color word	*Affect*
	Mood test

Two of the most widely used test batteries in worksite research are shown in Tables 32.7 and 32.8. The World Health Organization (WHO) Neurobehavioral Core Test Battery consists of a small number of components selected because they already had gained wide popularity and because they were not reliant on instruments or techniques that would be unavailable in developing countries (Table 32.7, 32.8). To verify the applicability of the WHO battery in different settings, Anger (2) compared performance in ten countries representing diverse populations. In general, the results from country to country were remarkably consistent.

The Neurobehavioral Evaluation System (NES), devised originally by Letz and Baker (142) to exploit the potential of computer administration and scoring (10), is probably the most popular of the current batteries (Table 32.8). It embodies three main categories of tests: psychomotor, memory and learning, and cognitive. It is a much more ambitious battery than the WHO collection and has been translated into several languages other than English. In its current form, NES2 , it includes more than 15 tests of functions such as reaction time, motor coordination, and simple cognitive (143a). The next version, NES3, is a modification designed to make more optimal use of computer technology. Perhaps its most important property will be its ability to be used at the individual rather than at the population level. Other groups have devised batteries of their own, based on either personal preferences, theories, or unique aims, but the NES and WHO formats offer the most extensive databases. A major objection to the WHO battery, however, has been lodged by Gamberale et al. (91), who contend that its emphasis on traditional manual and paper-and-pencil tests, largely to avoid complicated technical equipment, especially computer-based administration and scoring, diminishes its sensitivity to neurotoxic effects. Even the more advanced batteries, however, exclude many of the higher level functions such as the complex monitoring and decision processes required of aircraft pilots.

One new development in computerized testing, pioneered by Anger and his colleagues (e.g., ref. 4a) expoits both computer technology and operant behavior principles to deliver instructions to subjects in novel ways. Reliance upon language to deliver instructions is an impediment to the use of neurobehavioral tests internationally because of the problem of translation. To avoid such problems, Anger and his colleagues program a set of preliminary instructions so that the subject's responses are shaped by techniques such as successive approximation to the criterion response, to conform to the test requirements. After the subject masters the test procedure, he or she is then ready for the actual test. Even under these circumstances, which are designed to minimize educational and cultural contributions, such variables still exert a pronounced effect. Another study (4b) compared samples of European descent with American Indian, African American, and Latin American populations on two consensus neurotoxicity test batteries. One was the WHO collection (cf. Table 32.7) and the other one was assembled by the ATSDR (Agency for Toxic Substances and Disease Registry). Education accounted for the most variance in the tests studied, followed by cultural group. Years of education and cultural group had 13–25% shared variance on the cognitive tests, suggesting that these factors should be controlled during the design phase of a study rather than in the statistical analysis. The authors stress that failure to adequately control and analyze these variables could lead to inaccurate conclusions about the association between poor performance and neurotoxic insult.

Memory

Complaints of impaired memory surface frequently in workers exposed to neurotoxic agents, and, according to a survey by Anger (2), are the functions most often assessed in work-site research. Memory disorders also appear in adults with focal brain damage and in patients suffering from degenerative neurological diseases. Given the prominence of such complaints in patients, and the central role accorded memory in psychological theory and in neuroscience, it is not surprising that numerous tests and techniques are available for the study of this function. Nor should it be surprising, because of the abundance of techniques, that there seem to be different varieties of memory function. A frequent distinction is made between immediate or working or short-term memory and remote or reference or long-term memory. Such distinctions, and the more elaborate ones offered by current workers, often are difficult to apply to specific experimental conditions, and it even has been argued that the term memory itself has grown too vague to be useful scientifically, as noted earlier in this chapter. Such vagueness and ambiguity are magnified by the tendency of many authors to apply terms borrowed from computer technology, such as storage and retrieval, to hypothetical processes alleged to account for memory. But if memory, as noted earlier, is defined by responses based on earlier experiences, this more neutral and empirical definition is a better platform from which to launch useful experiments. There is no need for toxicology to become enmeshed in doctrinal debates about models of memory. The examples that follow are presented from an empirical standpoint for that reason.

One of the most popular tests in clinical and epidemiological neurotoxicology is the WAIS assay of short-term memory known as digit span. In the traditional manner of administering the test, the examiner calls out a series of numbers that the patient or subject is asked to repeat. Smith et al. (243), like many other current investigators, adapted the digit-span technique to the digital computer and presented the numbers, one at a time, on a display terminal. Their subject population consisted of workers from two mercury-cell chloralkali plants whose urinary mercury concentrations had been monitored repeatedly. The lists of digits were presented with ascending length, beginning with three digits. If the worker then recited the list correctly, a list with four digits was presented, and so on. Errors on two successive presentations of the same list length halted the test, and the worker's score was noted as the length of the previously correct list. No relationship with mercury excretion was observed, primarily because the standard WAIS procedure proved to be unreliable, yielding a correlation between successive administrations of 0.36. To overcome this inherent flaw, the investigators modified the procedure so that they could use probit analysis to estimate the 50% threshold span. With this procedure, the reliability coefficient rose to 0.85, and regression analysis showed a significant correlation between this measure of digit span and urinary mercury concentration.

Hanninen (109) also noted that the digit span subtest of the WAIS may produce ambivalent results. Baker et al. (9), however, in a study of foundary workers exposed to lead, obtained a significant relationship between blood lead values and performance on a version of the digit span test that required the subjects to repeat the list backward. It is possible that this result arose not so much from the inability of workers to remember the list but from intruding factors such as the fatigue, depression, and confusion detected by an inventory of subjective state. Several authors have pointed out that complaints of cognitive difficulties and lowered scores on memory tests may stem from sources such as depression and the inability to concentrate (e.g., ref. 146). Variations of the digit-span procedure that are said to test verbal memory include letter span and word span. One contribution made possible by computer-based batteries is a restructuring of tests such as digit span to offer adaptive procedures in which the presentation of test items is contingent on the performance of the subject, as in programmed instruction. The Benton Visual Retention Test is a common component of many neuropsychological test batteries and seems to have been adopted widely for behavioral toxicology as well (e.g., ref. 10). The Benton procedure presents the subject with a three-figure design that he or she is asked to reproduce. Scoring systems have been developed to quantify the fidelity with which the designs are copied and to correlate the kinds of distortions that emerge with different kinds of brain damage. The test apparently is sensitive to brain lesions that lead to neglect of one side of the body (173), but such deficits are uncommon in neurotoxicology. The Benton test is representative of tests of nonverbal memory. The Graham–Kendall Memory-for-Designs Test (see ref. 146), for example, consists of a series of 15 geometric designs presented to the patient one at a time for 5 s. The patient is then asked to copy the design, and the reproduction is scored for various kinds of errors.

More complex tests of immediate memory may rely on the subject's ability to learn new material. The Wechsler Memory Scale (274) contains a paired associate learning task consisting of 10 word pairs. Some, such as baby–cries, are relatively simple; others, such as cabbage–pen, are less transparent. The list is read three times. After each repetition, a test trial is conducted during which the examiner calls out the first word and the subject is required to say the second word of the pair. This kind of learning paradigm has a long history in experimental psychology, and many different kinds of items, including pictures and nonsense syllables, have been used as materials. Swanson and Kinsbourne (255) demonstrated the adverse effects of food dyes on young children by paired associates learning of number and zoo (animal) combinations. The ability to memorize lists of words or nonsense syllables is commonly assessed in neuropsychological test batteries.

As part of their performance battery used to test lead workers, Williamson and Teo (295) also examined learning of paired associates. The experimenter presented five pairs of three-letter words followed by the first member of the pair. The subject's task was to write down the second member of the pair. This sequence was repeated until the subject was able to identify all five pairs. The lead workers performed much more poorly than the controls. They recalled fewer items than controls after the first presentation (mean of 0.72 versus 2.19); they required more trials to reach criterion (mean of 3.74 versus 2.81); and, in fact, more than half the lead group failed to reach criterion (64.2% versus 13.8%) of the controls.

Although it may have been sensible in the beginning to choose methods for assessing memory function that were based on widespread diagnostic acceptance, new concepts, data, and techniques are emerging at a rapid rate. Sahakian et al. (223) relied on complex matching-to-sample stimuli, presented by computer displays, to evaluate memory deficits in Alzheimer's disease. These emerging trends are bound to influence behavioral toxicology and eventually to displace or augment the traditional approaches that so far have dominated the literature.

Vigilance and Attention

These two categories are coupled because they often are assessed in the same or similar situations, and because performance on vigilance tasks assumes that the required motor responses are reasonably intact. Highway driving and piloting aircraft are situations that require competence in both. In other situations, vigilance predominates. Some examples are provided by power stations and chemical process plants. In these situations, remaining alert enough to respond to infrequent or slowly changing signals is critical, and is challenged by shift work schedules that induce chronic sleep disruption. In the laboratory, they can be examined in detail because of the available instrumentation and time. In field testing, where simpler, often portable equipment is mandated, and where workers must be allowed time from their jobs, performance assessment is usually directed to global screening for adverse effects rather than to definitive answers about the parameters of dysfunction.

Reaction-time measures are among the most common elements of test batteries in behavioral toxicology. Their popularity stems both from the relative simplicity with which they can be gathered, the relatively straightforward values they provide (which do not require elaborate clinical interpretation), and their long history in psychology. Also, the basic reaction-time situation can be modified to provide an immense range of complexity in the assessment of many kinds of stimulus variables. A frequent variation is to compare reaction times to simple stimuli such as light onset with reaction times when subjects are required to alter responses in accordance with the location or other properties of the stimulus. Reaction-time measures seem to reflect both acute and subchronic toxicity resulting from volatile organic solvent exposure. Cherry et al. (35) described a series of experiments with workers exposed to styrene, a solvent widely used in fabricating fiberglass boat hulls. The plan called for the experimenters to visit the plant on Friday, familiarize the workers with the reaction time situation, and deliver a questionnaire about work history and personal habits. On the succeeding Monday, simple reaction times were measured, with a portable device, at the beginning and end of the shift, and urine collected by each subject until bedtime. Blood samples were drawn at the end of the shift. Following the suggestions of Gamberale and Kjellberg (90), the rate of stimulus presentation was fairly high (16 trials per min), a decision based on findings that such high rates lead to a quicker decline in performance.

Those men exposed to styrene began the shift with slower reaction times than men in a reference group, but by the end of the day the groups did not differ. Within the exposed group, however, those men with the highest blood levels of styrene showed no improvement and displayed the greatest deterioration in ratings of alertness and exhaustion. In a subsequent study, the investigators observed substantial correlations between urinary mandelic acid (a styrene metabolite) and reaction-time performance on Monday morning, indicating that, even with a 60-h period away from the plant, the effects of exposure were still evident in performance. Exposure levels, it should be noted, did not exceed the British threshold limit value (TLV) of 100 ppm.

A study with volunteers exposed to 1,1,1-trichloroethane (methyl chloroform, MC), examined effects on both simple and complex reaction time (150). Simple reaction time was measured as the time required to respond to a stimulus light presented about eight times per minute during a 5-min test period. For complex reaction time measures, the subject faced a panel with four lights at the corners of a square and was instructed to respond on one of four buttons beneath the panel, arranged in the same way. The stimuli were flashed at a high rate; only 120 ms separated the next stimulus presentation from the previous response. These authors noted that the same arrangement had been used successfully to study the effects of sleep deprivation, antihistamines, alcohol, and styrene. All subjects were exposed to all treatments. These consisted of 0 ppm, 175 ppm (950 mg/m^3), and 350 ppm (1900 mg/m^3) of MC. The experimental sessions lasted for 2 h. MC exposure lengthened both simple reaction time and complex reaction time for those responses made on the correct button.

Needleman et al. (182) demonstrated that reaction time measures are sensitive to an important cumulative index of lead exposure. Their population consisted of children with levels of dentine lead in the highest and lowest deciles of a distribution obtained from two Boston suburbs and based on more than 2000 children. They also used simple reaction times, but varied the interval between the ready signal, which alerts the subject to the next stimulus, and the presentation of the stimulus. On two blocks of trials, the interval was specified as 3 s; on two other blocks, it was specified as 12 s. These values were chosen to probe for the possible influence of distractibility. The longer interval produced longer reaction times in both groups, but for both intervals the children with the higher lead levels responded less quickly than those with the lower levels. A subsequent study by Yule et al. (305) confirmed these results in British children with even lower lead levels. A study from Germany adds another dimension of support to these findings (296b). In addition to confirming the relationship between tooth lead and reaction time performance, these investigators also observed that when the children were categorized by social class, the data of those from the less advantaged group showed an even greater correlation with tooth lead than the group as a whole.

Despite a large number of publications featuring or including such measures, however, the power of reaction time measures to detect neurotoxicity remains only superficially exploited. Gamberale et al. (91) and Iregren and Gamberale (123) demonstrated that, with computerized testing and analysis, the sensitivity of such measures can be enhanced and can even contribute to the differentiation of various diagnostic groups, such as those suffering from solvent-induced deficits. One of the other limitations of reaction-time measures is the common practice of ignoring stimulus properties such as intensity. Almost never is the brightness of a stimulus light or the properties of a stimulus tone reported, even in studies of agents known to affect vision or hearing. Because reaction time is sensitive enough to stimulus intensity to be used as a psychophysical measure (176), ignoring stimulus characteristics can lead to the suspicion of confounding.

Vigilance includes elements of both motor performance and reaction time but is the subject of a considerable literature of its own. The prototype is the clock test devised by Mackworth, which has served as the criterion task in many studies with drugs (285). It is arranged so that a pointer on a clock face moves 1 degree every second, except for occasional deflections of two steps. The subject's task is to respond to these infrequent events by pressing a key. Typically, the frequency of detections falls sharply after the first 30 min, but can be counteracted by administering drugs, such as the amphetamines, that promote alertness. Dick et al. (64) included the clock test in a battery with which they evaluated experimental exposures to toluene, methyl ethyl ketone, and ethanol. Exposure to 100 ppm toluene (the TLV) for 4 h lowered the proportion of correct detections. Ethanol also impaired performance at a dose of 0.8 ml/kg.

More complex vigilance performance, which may demand a certain amount of coordination skills, also offers unexplored potential. In a series of now classic studies, Payne and Hauty (reviewed in ref. 285) reported the effects of various drugs and parametric variations on the School of Aviation Medicine Multidimensional Pursuit Test, which was designed originally as a tool for pilot selection. (Figure 32.39). The subject was seated in a simulated aircraft cockpit and asked to monitor four dials. The pointers on the dials drifted irregularly from their null positions, and the subject's task was to restore them to null by manipulating a control stick, rudder pedals, and a throttle control. With a typical group of subjects, total time at null reached asymptotic values after about 1 h of practice but with further testing began a gradual decline. The rate of decline was enhanced by drugs with sedative actions and retarded by drugs such as the amphetamines, even at remarkably low dose levels (Figure 32.40). The unusual sensitivity of this task to drugs suggests that it, or a contemporary analog based on computer technology, deserves to be evaluated in behavioral toxicology.

The Multidimensional Pursuit Test is not simply watchkeeping, because it also embodies the type of visually directed motor performance called tracking. The latter, too, is the focus of a large and unexploited literature, much of it aimed at the design of control systems in which a human operator is one of the components. Mackay et al. (150), referred to earlier in the section on reaction time, also examined the acute effects of carbon monoxide on a tracking task. The subjects controlled the position of a cross displayed on an oscilloscope screen by moving a small joystick. They were required to maintain the cross within a square target that moved continuously around the screen in random patterns. During a single test session, they performed on five 1-min trials. Carbon monoxide significantly increased error amplitude and decreased time on target during the 2-h exposure period. Tracking tasks are now included in a number of test batteries. For example, one of the tests used in studies of methylmercury-exposed children required the subjects to follow a sine-wave display by appropriate movements of a joystick (104a).

The quantitative methods developed by engineers for evaluating systems in which operators track complex displays, coupled with promising results from the experiments just described and several conducted with patients diagnosed with Parkinson's disease (e.g., 85),

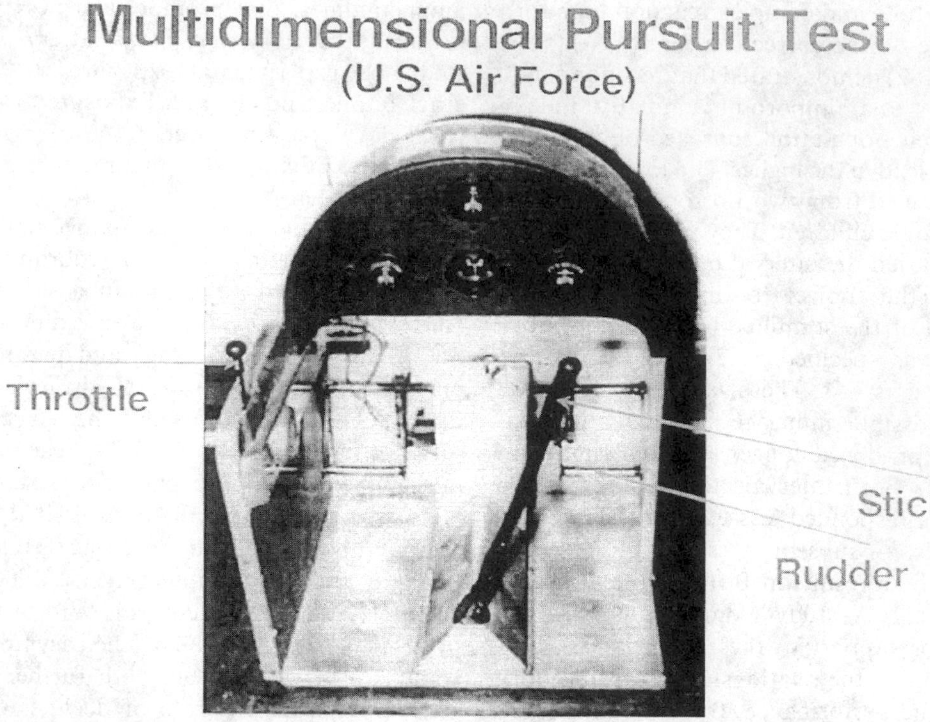

FIG. 32.39. United States Air Force Multidimensional Pursuit Test. The test was devised in WWII for aviation cadet selection. The four dial pointers drifted randomly from their null positions. The subject's task was to use the joy stick, throttle level, and rudder pedals to restore and maintain the pointers at their null positions simultaneously (163a).

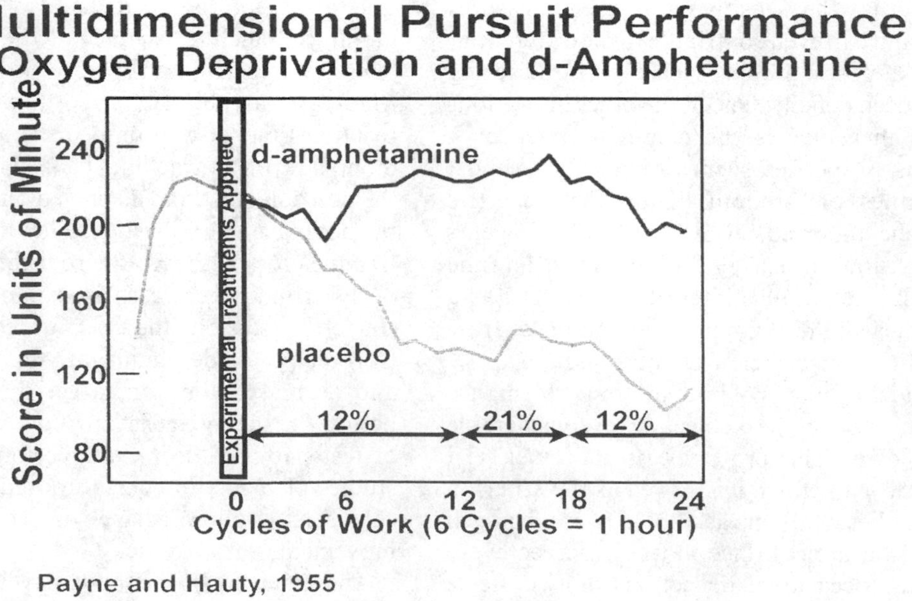

FIG. 32.40. Multidimensional Pursuit Test performance (see Figure 32.39) as a function of oxygen level (12 or 21%) and d-amphetamine administration (5 mg). Treatments were administered after 1 h of practice. Score refers to the times during which all four dial pointers were held simultaneously at their null positions (Reference 194a).

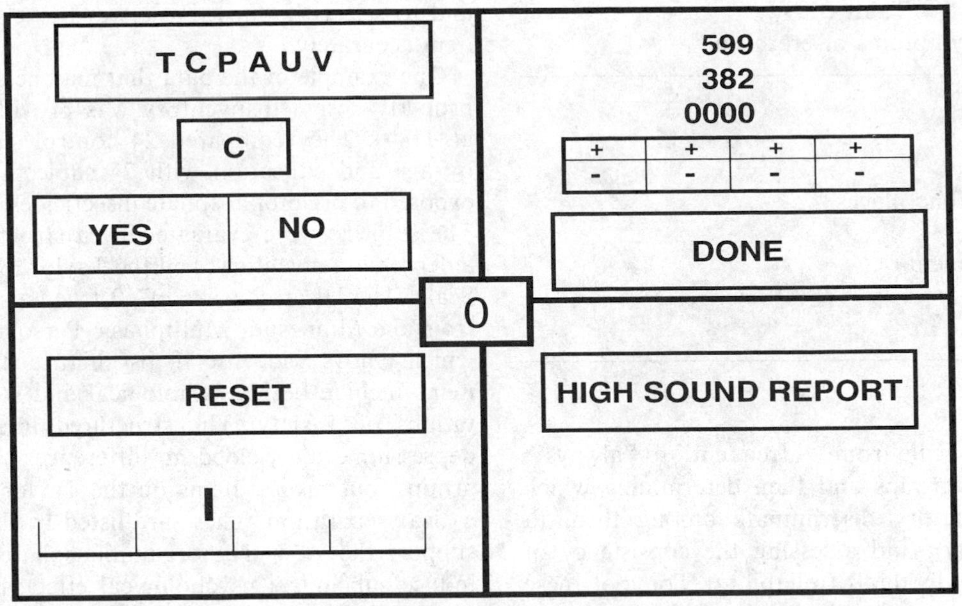

FIG. 32.41. Multitasking performance test (SYNWORK). Top left: a series of letters appears on the screen, then is removed. In the box below, letters are flashed in sequence, and the subject is required to indicate whether or not the letter belongs to the original set. Top right: the subject calculates the sum of the two upper numbers and, using the mouse, scans through the numerals 0-9 to place them in the appropriate positions in the third number. Lower left: the cursor drifts toward the end of the scale, and the subject is required, by mouse clicks, to prevent it from reaching the end. Lower right: a series of tones is presented through a headset. Intermittently, a louder tone is inserted. The subject is asked to respond when the louder tone is detected. The box in the center of the screen displays the subject's numerical score for that session. The SYNWORK task proved sensitive to toluene exposure in Reference 203a.

indicate that complex tracking performance should play a more significant role in behavioral toxicology than it has in the past. Particularly with tracking tasks that require predictive adjustments, as would be the case if the subject were instructed to minimize the lag in following a target moving according to a function such as simple harmonic movement, the impact of neurotoxicants on what are called executive processes might be assessed more directly.

More typically than not, performance demands occur in settings requiring more than one task to be monitored and responded to concurrently. Driving, piloting, air traffic control, and scanning and adjusting medical monitoring equipment provide examples. Most neurobehavioral test systems strive to examine one function at a time, making extrapolation to multitasking situations somewhat uncertain. A study conducted by Rahill et al. (203a) employed a multitasking scheme to evaluate the performance effects of exposure to 100 ppm of toluene. The display is shown in Figure 32.41. Significantly lower composite performance scores were obtained by the subjects during toluene exposure.

Subjective State

Certain clusters of symptoms seem to be characteristic of different toxic exposures. Mercury vapor induces a cluster so well known that it earned the label *erethism* (Table 32.9). Chronic solvent exposure is associated with complaints of tiredness, depression, and confusion. Measurement of such vague symptoms is not a task to be undertaken without an appreciation of the principles of psychometrics. The earlier discussion of validity and reliability probably applies more directly to symptom measurement than to almost any other criterion because accessory criteria are so difficult to define. Memory, for example, can be assessed by enough different techniques to provide some index of consistency. A complaint of depression is not as readily confirmed. To simply construct a questionnaire based on what the investigator believes are the most conspicuous symptoms associated with a particular exposure is a virtual guarantee of uninterpretable data. For this reason, neuropsychologists rely on standardized instruments such as the Beck Depression Inventory (14a).

An example of the arduous process required to design and develop a quantitative measure of specific symptoms is described by Goldberg (99), who aimed to construct a scale sensitive to minor psychiatric illness. The evolution of the questionnaire proceeded through several steps: selection of items, including careful editing of wording; decisions about the form of the response, that is, whether to ask for a yes–no response or to ask for some form

Table 32.9
Symptoms of erethism

Hyperirritability
Blushes easily
Labile temperament
Avoids friends, public places
Timid, shy
Depressed, despondent
Insomnia
Fatigue

of rating such as a scale from "infrequent" to "always"; selecting criterion groups and then determining which items of the inventory discriminate among them (a measure of validity); and assessing the consistency of responses within individuals (reliability). Some of these stages may be repeated, and items added, deleted, or modified. Some items may carry an excessive burden of social desirability and may not be answered with total candor. Several other well-designed inventories of subjective state are available that also offer considerable data about validity and reliability. Some were constructed, like the Goldberg questionnaire, to detect mild psychiatric dysfunction. Some were developed to measure the acute effects of drugs or to follow the course of drug therapy. The Profile of Mood States (POMS) is a self-rating scale designed to measure subjective responses to various therapeutic or experimental maneuvers (162). It consists of 65 adjectives that the subject judges on a 5-point rating scale at the time the inventory is given and have been tested on samples of both psychiatric patients and normals. A factor analysis yielded the following major factors: tension–anxiety, depression–dejection, anxiety–hostility, vigor–activity, fatigue–inertia, and confusion–bewilderment. Baker et al. (9) included the POMS in a battery given to lead foundary workers and observed marked elevations in several of these factors in workers with the higher blood lead levels. The SCL-90 (56) was devised as a self-report rating scale for psychiatric outpatients, and, like those already referred to, provides a set of dimensions (factors) extracted from the entire 90-item scale. Its designers cite it as particularly useful in clinical drug trials undertaken to evaluate psychoactive agents. Anyone contemplating the framing of an ad hoc questionnaire should note the care taken in the construction of the SCL-90. For example, to make the working of the items accessible to the widest variety of subjects, the designers of the inventory turned to the Thorndikc–Lorgc *Word Book* of 30,000 words, which provides frequency counts obtained from material such as newspapers. It allowed them to equate the vocabulary levels of the nine factors and to select the most basic word levels to express the item accurately.

One example of the data that may be extracted with a properly designed inventory was provided by Levin et al. (144). They compared 24 control subjects matched by age and education with 24 subjects who had been exposed to organophosphate insecticides in recent weeks. The subjects were evaluated by a structured interview, a depression inventory, and the Taylor Manifest Anxiety Scale. The latter consists of 50 true–false items derived from the Minnesota Multiphasic Personality Inventory, which enjoys wide use in psychiatric diagnosis. These items include both psychological and somatic manifestations of anxiety. The structured interview and the depression scale yielded no differences between the two groups, but several items on the Taylor scale provided a clear separation. These are listed in Table 32.10, and support the view that organophosphate exposure may induce subclinical psychological effects that would not be detected by conventional medical surveillance or even by inventories and questionnaires that did not contain specific kinds of symptom items. The 13 commercial applicators in the exposed group (the others were farmers) accounted for the bulk of the difference; their plasma cholinesterase levels, however, fell within the normal range, suggesting that this exposure measure is not an accurate reflection of central cholinergic status.

A more ominous legacy of organophosphate exposure is now undergoing examination. Earlier probes of the aftermath of acute organophosphate poisoning had suggested persisting neurotoxic consequences, but Savage et al. (226) were the first to combine well-documented exposures and neuropsychological measures. They reported on 100 individuals who had experienced a poisoning episode one year earlier and on 100 matched controls. Although clinical chemistries and medical examinations indicated normal function in the exposed group, psychological testing indicated residual deficits

Table 32.10
Items on the Taylor Manifest Anxiety Scale sensitive to differences in organophosphate insecticide exposure (144)

I work under a great deal of tension.
My sleep is fitful and disturbed.
I have periods of such restlessness that I cannot sit long in a chair.
I believe that I am no more nervous than most other people.
I feel anxiety about something or someone almost all the time.
I am usually calm and not easily upset.
It makes me nervous to have to wait.
I practically never blush.

Table 32.11
Persistent neurological sequelae of acute organophosphate pesticide poisoning (226)

Test name	100 Cases	100 Controls	*p* Value
WAIS Verbal IQ	105.40	111.86	.001
WAIS Performance	108.41	110.13	.242
WAIS Full Scale	107.50	111.77	.001
Impairment rating	1.07	0.91	.001
Halstead index	0.30	0.23	.020
Pegboard	148.34	137.96	.002
Card sorting	17.07	12.91	.001

as measured by several WAIS subtests and several other indices (Table 32.11). Subsequent reports by others (e.g., ref. 218a) confirm these findings.

Developmental Assessment

Most of the tests described earlier were devised to assess adults. Many questions about behavioral toxicity, however, arise from the possible impact on early development and involve testing during infancy or childhood. Methylmercury, lead, and polychlorinated biphenyls (PCBs) are examples of substances closely connected with developmental disturbances. Although the essential functions that need to be evaluated remain the same throughout the life cycle, early developmental stages pose several unique problems. One is that young children have not yet acquired or developed the full behavioral and functional repertoire of adults. Another is that early childhood is a period of rapid change with marked individual differences in rate of development, one of the factors that dilutes the ability of tests administered at that time to predict later capacities. For these and associated reasons, investigations of developmental toxicity have to adopt approaches that sometimes differ markedly from those suitable for adults. Infancy is the most difficult stage to evaluate because of the plasticity of infant behavior. The most common infant scale is the Brazelton Neonatal Behavioral Assessment Scale (24), which usually is administered within the first 3 days after birth. It consists of two subscales. One, of 27 behavioral items, includes items reflecting habituation, motor activity and control, stimulus responsiveness, and similar responses. The other comprises 21 neurological items based on elicited reflexes. Although Brazelton scores are not highly correlated with tests of later function, they have proven capable of reflecting the effects of obstetrical medications (238a).

One of the best examples of how the Brazelton scale might be used in a study of developmental toxicology is provided by Streissguth et al. (251). These investigators have been evaluating a cohort of about 500 children, selected at birth, to determine the consequences of various levels of maternal alcohol consumption. The mothers of these children were interviewed during the fifth month of pregnancy to obtain data on this and other relevant drug practices, and on social, educational, and demographic variables. Habituation in the infant was a special focus of this investigation because of observations indicating that neonates with a clinically overt fetal alcohol syndrome failed to display a response decrement to repeated auditory stimulation. A factor analysis of scores (a procedure that reduced the 27 original Brazelton scores to a smaller number of dependent variables) yielded six independent factors. After a multiple-regression analysis, which adjusted for possibly confounding contributions from smoking, caffeine, maternal nutrition, and so on, maternal alcohol consumption during pregnancy remained as a significant determinant of poorer habituation and increased low arousal in the infants. The care taken by these investigators to ensure that the examiners were kept uninformed of the other data, and in the efforts to train and preserve consistency in examiner ratings, can serve as a model for such studies.

The ultimate question for investigators is how well measures obtained during infancy predict later outcomes such as intelligence test scores or school status. One of the more promising techniques, the Fagan Test of Infant Intelligence, measures visual recognition memory (77). The infant is held so that it faces a display with two screens behind which an observer can record the amount of time the infant's gaze is directed to each screen. On an individual trial, a particular visual stimulus, such as a face, is projected on one of the screens. After the infant has had time to examine the stimulus, and after a brief interval, the previous stimulus and a new one are presented simultaneously. The observer measures the amount of time spent by the infant in examining the novel stimulus compared to the one displayed earlier. Infants who score higher on later developmental tests such as the Stanford–Binet tend to spend less time viewing the old stimulus. In studies exploring the developmental neurotoxicity of PCBs, the Fagan test revealed a significant relationship between umbilical cord PCB levels (attributed to maternal consumption of tainted Great Lakes fish) and psychological development (127). Gunderson et al. (107) found that infant monkeys exposed prenatally to methylmercury spent more time than controls gazing at the previously displayed stimulus.

The Fagan test has also been used in epidemiological studies of methylmercury neurotoxicity. Myers et al. (179a) have been conducting a prospective study of the relationship between measures of child development and prenatal exposure to methylmercury in the Seychelle Islands of the Indian Ocean. At 6 months of age, visual recognition memory was evaluated in the cohort of more than 700 children, but no association emerged between the maternal hair mercury level during pregnancy, a marker of maternal exposure, and scores on the Fagan test.

For later stages of infancy, encompassing a range from 2 to 30 months of age, the Bayley Scales of Infant Development (14) are among the most popular because of the care taken in their standardization and their ability to be used for repeated testing. The Bayley items are arranged chronologically and divided into three subscales: mental, motor, and behavioral. The mental scale is composed of 163 items, ranging from responses to visual and auditory stimuli to abilities such as naming objects. A notable application to toxicology was summarized by Bellinger et al. (16) in studies relating cord blood lead concentrations to performance. At 6, 12, 18, and 24 months of age, even after correcting statistically for many potential confounding variables such as maternal age and intelligence, a significant relationship between cord blood lead and scores on the mental development index emerged. Children in the group with the highest cord blood lead values (a mean of 14.6 μg/dl, compared to 6.5 for the middle group and 1.8 for the low group) attained the lowest scores at all ages tested. At 24 months of age, the difference between the lowest and highest groups reached 8% although by that time all three groups had converged toward the same mean blood level of about 7 μg/dl. Similar findings have now emerged from other prospective studies in Cincinnati (66) and Australia (8).

At later ages, the number and variety of instruments available for psychological assessment is overwhelming. Most investigators choosing a battery of tests will typically include one of the intelligence tests designed for children. The Wechsler Intelligence Scale for Children–Revised or WISC–R (277) is the dominant choice for children older than 6 years of age. In addition to its demonstrated reliability, it is attractive because, like the WAIS, it provides separate verbal and performance subscales that include several individual tasks. These offer a profile of the child's abilities across a variety of functional components. For younger children, the WPPSI, or Wechsler Preschool and Primary Scale of Intelligence (276), yields the same subscale advantages as the WISC and is basically an extension of the WISC to ages 4–6.5 years. Another instrument suitable for younger children, the McCarthy Scales of Children's Abilities (158), also extends into early school years, giving a span of 2.5–8.5 years of age. It provides five separate scales that can be combined into what is called a general cognitive index, similar to an IQ. All three of these, plus the older Stanford–Binet, have been used to assess the effects of lead. Needleman et al. (182) included the WISC–R in their landmark study, which indicated lowered performance on IQ tests in those children whose tooth lead concentrations fell at the upper portions of the distribution. Their results have since been confirmed by other investigators, including some from outside the United States who also used the WISC–R or an adaptation of it to measure intellectual function. This is one illustration of how reliance on a standardized test enabled different investigations to be combined with some degree of confidence.

Needleman (181) and Bellinger and Needleman (15), in two companion articles, discuss the strategy for using such scores in a context where many potential confounding variables should be considered. Some examples, besides obvious factors such as race, birth weight, and length of gestation, are maternal age, birth order, parental education, family social class, and quality of the rearing environment. Even when these and other variables were compensated for in the statistical analysis, cord blood lead values remained significantly associated with reduced scores on the mental development index of the Bayley scales. Parallel conclusions have been drawn by other groups.

As in adult epidemiological studies, most investigations try to assemble comprehensive test batteries to try to determine relationships between neurotoxic exposure and functional outcomes. For the evaluation of the cohort of another large prospective methylmercury study (104a), in the Faroe Islands of the North Atlantic, investigators chose a neuropsychological test battery for 7-year-olds consisting of the following components: Finger Tapping, Hand–Eye Coordination, Tactual Performance test (shape discrimination when blindfolded), Continuous Performance Test (vigilance and reaction time), Wechsler Intelligence Scale for Children–Revised (Digit Spans, Similarities, and Block Designs), Bender Visual Motor Gestalt Test, Boston Naming Test, California Verbal Learning Test (Children), and a pictorial analog of the Profile of Mood States survey. They also included a chart that is used to measure visual contrast sensitivity and several neurophysiological measures. Their analyses pointed to mercury-related deficits primarily in the domains of language, attention, and memory, but they also observed deficits in visuospatial and motor functions.

Evaluations of the Seychelles cohort have so far failed to demonstrate any adverse developmental outcomes due to methylmercury (e.g., ref. 55a). For this assessement, the test battery included the McCarthy Scales of Children's Abilities (the General Cognitive Index), the Preschool Language Scale for measuring expressive and receptive language, two subtests of the Woodcock–Johnson series designed to measure reading and arithmetic achievement, the Bender–Gestalt test, and the Child Behavior Checklist, designed to assess social and adaptive behavior.

These two groups of investigators selected somewhat different arrays of instruments for these two parallel investigations because they were pursuing somewhat different questions, in part because they were evaluating different age ranges and stages of maturity. All investigators agree that no one test battery will be suitable for all purposes or populations. Selection will be guided by the questions asked, the population studied, and the investigator's inclinations. Often, designers of test batteries attempt to provide researchers with a menu of tests, so to speak. One example is the battery assembled (1) to assist the Agency for Toxic Substances and Disease Registry (ATSDR), which is responsible for evaluating health risks at hazardous waste sites in the United States. The prototype test battery consists of the following components:

- Vineland Adaptive Behavior Scales.
- Parenting Stress Index.
- Personality Inventory for Children.
- Henderson Environmental Learning Processes Scale.
- Family Resources Scale.
- Visual acuity, contrast sensitivity.
- Contrast sensitivity pretest.
- Vibration II.
- Kaufman Brief Intelligence Test.
- Story Memory.
- Finger Tapping.
- Divided Attention Test.
- Visual–Motor Integration.
- Purdue Pegboard.
- Verbal Cancellation.
- Story Memory delay.

The entire battery, because it is designed for screening populations rather than for the intensive appraisal of small groups or individuals, consumes only about 1 h for the children. The first five items refer to information secured from the parent.

EMERGING ISSUES

Like other components of contemporary toxicology, behavioral toxicology is undergoing almost continuous change. Its literature has grown almost exponentially, and the range of techniques applied to its problems has expanded over a broader spectrum of behavioral and neuroscience. Compare, for example, the first U.S. book on the topic (289) with the most recent comprehensive survey (289a). The range of topics is not only broader but now more firmly based on a comprehensive literature. Especially for human assessment, however, greater efforts are needed to extend the range and relevance of test procedures. Although standardization and an extensive history are virtues, they should not limit investigators. Advances in test development are at least as crucial to behavioral toxicology as the analysis of toxic effects themselves. Contrast, for example, the relative crudeness of sensory and motor testing in most test batteries with the precise, elegant methods described in earlier sections of this chapter that have been applied to animals.

Even cognitive function, which has received the bulk of attention from neuropsychology, is only superficially addressed in most test batteries. Among the more promising advances in this area are those stemming from the translation of rigorous laboratory test procedures into practical test methods suitable for clinical and even field evaluations. For example, Paule et al. (193) devised an operant battery for measuring complex performance in children that, like the items on intelligence tests, reflects developmental maturity. Its advantage is its comparability with the techniques used for assessment in animals. Robbins and his collaborators (e.g., ref. 223) designed and refined a neuropsychological test battery that ingeniously exploits digital computer technology. Like the battery of Paule et al. (193), its components derive from animal laboratory methods. In addition, because of the flexibility afforded by computer technology, it can introduce increasingly difficult versions of the same basic test to avoid ceilings on performance. Finally, because it does not require verbal responses, it bypasses the problems of language translation and illiteracy.

The present chapter is designed as an introduction to the technology of behavioral testing. By itself, it is not sufficient as a manual for designing behavioral assays. Given the almost limitless variety of techniques available for such assays, it would have been foolish to pretend that such a manual could be embodied in a textbook. Far more important to the reader, it should serve as the basis for critically examining the literature and for communicating with specialists in the area. Rigor in behavioral toxicology is just as crucial as rigor in any other aspect of toxicology—perhaps even more crucial because so many scientists believe themselves capable of formulating behavioral investigations simply because they themselves are behaving creatures. Many misleading notions have appeared in print because of this unwarranted confidence. The material in this chapter, which was formulated to exemplify principles, should help readers who familiarize themselves with it to judge the validity of most of the publications in this field.

ACKNOWLEDGMENTS

The preparation of this chapter was supported, in part, by grants ES01247, ES08109, ES08958, ES05903, and ES05017 from the National Institute of Environmental Health Sciences.

QUESTIONS

1. New behavior can be generated in two basic ways: operant conditioning and respondent conditioning. They differ in (a) the type of response; (b) the con-

ditioning procedure; (c) the criteria for judging the strength of the conditioned response. How would you use each type of conditioning to test impaired learning capacity?

2. As a test of memory difficulties, design a procedure to test whether a rat can remember which of two levers (a left and a right, say) it had pressed 10 seconds earlier.
3. Workers in a machine shop, where tools are constantly being degreased, have been complaining that, away from work, their friends and families are telling them that they are confused about identifying colors. Could there be some validity to their complaints? How would you test them?
4. The Food Quality Protection Act of 1996 is a product of growing concern over vulnerability of children to environmental chemicals. What components of a neuropsychological test battery might be used to evaluate whether children living in a community located near a waste dump might be suffering adverse neurobehavioral effects?

REFERENCES

1. Amler, R. W., Gibertini, M., Lybarger, J. A., Hall, A., Kakolewski, K., Phifer, B. L., and Olsen, K. L. (1996): Selective approaches to basic neurobehavioral testing of children in environmental health studies. *Neurotoxicol. Teratol.*, 18:429–434.

1a. Anger, W. K. (1990): Worksite behavioral research: Results, sensitive methods, test batteries and the transition from laboratory data to human health. *Neurotoxicology*, 11:629–720.

2. Anger, W. K., (1992): Assessment of neurotoxicity in humans. In: *Neurotoxicology*, edited by H. A. Tilson and C. L. Mitchell, pp. 363–386. Raven Press, New York.

3. Anger, W. K., and Johnson, B. L. (1985): Chemicals affecting behavior. In: *Neurotoxicity of Industrial and Commercial Chemicals*, edited by J. O'Donoghue, pp. 51–148. CRC Press, Boca Raton, FL.

4. Anger, W. K., and Lynch, D. W. (1977): The effect of methyl *n*-butyl ketone on response rates of rats performing on a multiple schedule of reinforcement. *Environ. Res.*, 14:204–211.

4a. Anger, W. K., Rohlman, D. S., Sizemore, O. J., Kovera, C. A., Gibertini, M., and Ger, J. (1996): Human behavioral assessment in neurotoxicology: Producing appropriate test performance with written and shaping instructions. *Neurotoxicol. Teratol.*, 18:371–379.

4b. Anger, W. K., Sizemore, O. J., Grossmann, J., Glasser, J. A., Letz, R., and Bowler, R. (1997): Human neurobehavioral research methods: Impact of subject variables. *Environ. Res.*, 73:18–41.

5. Annau, Z., and Eccles, C. U. (1986): Prenatal exposure. In: *Neurobehavioral Toxicology*, edited by Z. Annau, pp. 153–169. Johns Hopkins University Press, Baltimore, MD.

6. Arcia, B., and Otto, D. A. (1992): Reliability of selected tests from the neurobehavioral evaluation system. *Neurotoxicol. Teratol.*, 14:103–110.

7. Armstrong, R. D., Leach, L. J., Belluscio, P. R., Maynard, E. A., and Hodge, H. C. (1963): Behavioral changes in the pigeon following inhalation of mercury vapor. *Am. Ind. Hyg. Assoc. J.*, 24:366–375.

8. Baghurst, P. A., McMichael, A. J., Wigg, N. R., Harleu, J. P., Niles, C. A., Dimsé, G. E., and Berkey, C. S. (1992): Environmental exposure to lead and children's intelligence at the age of seven years. *N. Engl. J. Med.*, 327:1279–1284.

8a. Baird, S. J., Catalano, P. J., Ryan, L. M., and Evans, J. S. (1997): Evaluation of effect profiles: Functional Observational Battery outcomes. *Fundam Appl Toxicol*. 40:37–51.

9. Baker, E. L., Feldman, R. C., White, R. A., Vimpani, G. V., Robertson, E. F., Roberts, R. J., and Tong, S. L. (1984): Occupational lead neurotoxicity: A behavioral and electrophysiological evaluation. Study design and year one results. *Br. J. Ind. Med.*, 41:352–361.

10. Baker, B. L., Letz, R. B., Fidler, A. T., Shalat, S., Plantamura, D., and Lyndon, M. (1985): A computer-based neurobehavioral evaluation system for occupational and environmental epidemiology: Methodology and validation studies. *Neurobehav. Toxicol. Teratol.*, 7:369–377.

11. Baker, B. L., White, R. F., and Murawski, B. J. (1985): Clinical evaluation of neurobehavioral effects of occupational exposure to organic solvents and lead. *Int. J. Ment. Health*, 14:135–158.

12. Barbeau, A. (1984): Manganese and extrapyramidal disorders. *Neurotoxicology*, 5:13–26.

13. Barrett, J. B. (1977): Behavioral history as a determinant of the effects of d-amphetamine on punished behavior. *Science*, 198:67–69.

14. Bayley, N. (1969): *Manual for the Bayley Scales of Infant Development*. Psychological Corporation, Berkeley, CA.

14a. Beck, A. T. (1978): *Beck Depression Inventory*. Psychological Corporation, San Antonio, TX.

15. Bellinger, D., and Needleman, H. L. (1985): Prenatal and early postnatal exposure to lead: Developmental effects, correlates, and implications. *Int. J. Ment. Health*, 14:78–111.

16. Bellinger, D., Leviton, A., Waternaux, C., Needleman, H., and Rabinowitz, M. (1987): Longitudinal analyses of prenatal and postnatal lead exposure and early cognitive development. *N. Engl. J. Med.*, 316:1037–1043.

17. Benignus, V. A., Muller, K. B., Smith, M. V., Pieper, K. S., and Prah, J. D. (1990): Compensatory tracking in humans with elevated carboxyhemoglobin. *Neurotoxicol. Teratol.*, 12:105–110.

17a. Beuter, A., and de Geoffroy, A. (1996): Can tremor be used to measure the effect of chronic mercury exposure in human subjects? *Neurotoxicology*, 17:213–227.

18. Blain, L., Lagace, J. P., and Mergler, D. (1985): Sensitivity and specificity of the Lanthony desaturated D-15 panel to assess chromatic discrimination loss among solvent-exposed workers. In: *Neurobehavioral Methods in Occupational and Environmental Health*, pp. 105–109. World Health Organization, Regional Office for Europe, Copenhagen.

19. Blakemore, C., and Vital-Durand, F. (1986): Effects of visual deprivation on the monkey's lateral geniculate nucleus. *J. Physiol.*, 380:493–511.

20. Bleecker, M. L., Bolla, K. I., Agnew, J., Schwartz, B. S., and Ford, D. P. (1991): Dose-related subclinical neurobehavioral effects of chronic exposure to low levels of organic solvents. *Am. J. Ind. Med.*, 19:715–728.

21. Boren, J. J. (1967): The study of performance enhancing drugs with a repeated acquisition technique. Presented at the Eastern Psychological Association, Boston, April.

22. Boren, J. J., and Devine, D. D. (1968): The repeated acquisition of behavioral chains. *J. Exp. Anal. Behav.*, 11:651–660.

23. Brandt, J., and Butters, N. (1986): The neuropsychology of Huntington's disease. *Trends Neurosci.*, 9:118–120.

24. Brazelton, T. B. (1973): *Neonatal Behavioral Assessment Scale*. Monograph of the National Spastics Society. Lippincott, Philadelphia.

24a. Brooks, A. L., Muhkerjee, B., Panahian, N., Cory-Slechta, D., and Federoff, H. J. (1997): Nerve growth factor somatic mosaicism produced by herpes virus-directed expression of cre recombinase. *Nat. Biotechnol.* 15:57–62.

24b. Brooks, A. I., Chadwick, C. A., Gelbard, H. A., Cory-Slechta, D. A., and Federoff, H. J. (1999): Paraquat elicited neurobehavioral syndrome caused by dopaminergic neuron loss. *Brain Res.* 823:1–10.

25. Buelke-Sam, J., Kimmel, C. A., and Adams, J. (1987): Design considerations in screening for behavioral teratogens: Results of the collaborative behavior teratology study. *Neurotoxicol. Teratol.*, 7:537–789.

26. Burt, G. A. (1975): Use of behavioral techniques in the assessment of environmental contaminants. In: *Behavioral Toxicology*, edited by B. Weiss and V. G. Laties, pp. 241–263. Plenum Press, New York.

27. Bushnell, P. J. (1988): Effects of delay, intertrial interval, delay behavior and trimethyltin on spatial delayed response in rats. *Neurotoxicol. Teratol.*, 10:237–244.

28. Bushnell, P. J., and Bowman, R. E. (1979): Reversal learning deficits in young monkeys exposed to lead. *Pharmacol. Biochem. Behav.*, 10:733–742.

29. Cabe, P. A., and Eckerman, D. A. (1982): Assessment of learning and memory dysfunction in agent-exposed animals. In: *Nervous System Toxicology*, edited by C. L. Mitchell, pp. 133–198. Raven Press, New York.

30. Camerino, D., and Arzuffi, E. (1983): Benton, V. R. T., and Raven, P. M. 38: Qualitative analysis of the answers. In: *Neurobehavioral Methods in Occupational Health*, edited by R. Gilioli, M. C. Cassitto, and V. Foa, pp. 183–190. Pergamon Press, New York.

30a. Campagna, D., Gobba, F., Mergler, D., Moreau, T., Galassi, C., Cavalleri, A., and Huel, G. (1996): Color vision loss among styrene-exposed workers neurotoxicological threshold assessment. *Neurotoxicology*, 17:367–373.

31. Carlson, R. L., Van Gelder, C. A., Karas, C. C., and Buck, W. B. (1974): Slowed learning in lambs prenatally exposed to lead. *Arch. Environ. Health*, 29:154–156.

32. Catania, A. C. (1966): Concurrent operants. In: *Operant Behavior: Areas of Research and Application*, edited by W. K. Honig, pp. 213–270. Appleton-Century-Crofts, New York.

33. Chaffin, D. B., and Miller, J. M. (1974): Behavioral and neurological evaluation of workers exposed to inorganic mercury. In: *Behavioral Toxicology*, edited by C. Xintaras, B. L. Johnson, and I. de Groat, pp. 214–239. Washington: US Department of Health, Education and Welfare, Publication No. 74-126.

34. Chapman, L. J., Sauter, S. L., Henning, R. A., Dodson, V. N., Reddan, W. C., and Matthews, C. C. (1990): Differences in frequency of finger tremor in otherwise asymptomatic mercury workers. *Br. J. Ind. Med.*, 47:838–843.

35. Cherry, N., Venables, H., and Waldron, H. A. (1983): The use of reaction times in solvent exposure. In: *Neurobehavioral Methods in Occupational Health*, edited by R. Cilioli, M. C. Cassitto, and V. Foa, pp. 191–195. Pergamon Press, New York.

36. Clarkson, T. W., Sager, P. R., and Syversen, T. L. M., eds. (1986): *The Cytoskeleton. A Target for Toxic Agents*. Plenum Press, New York.

37. Cohen, A. H., and Gans, C. (1975): Muscle activity in rat locomotion: Movement analysis and electromyography of the flexors and extensors of the elbow. *J. Morphol.*, 146:177–196.

38. Cohen, J., and Cory-Slechta, D. A. (1992): Differential effects in rats of MK-801, NMDA and scopolamine on learning in a four-member repeated acquisition paradigm. *Behav. Pharmacol.*, 3:403–413.

39. Cohn, J. C., Cox, C., and Cory-Slechta, D. A. (1993): The effects of lead exposure on learning in a multiple repeated acquisition and performance schedule. *Neurotoxicology*, 14:329–346.

40. Cohn, J. C., Ziriax, J., Cox, C., and Cory-Slechta, D. A. (1992): Comparison of the error patterns produced by scopolamine and MK-801 on a repeated acquisition and repeated transition baseline. *Psychopharmacology*, 107:243–254.

41. Colotla, V., Bautista, S., Lorenzana-Jimenez, M., and Rodriguez, R. (1979): Effects of solvents on schedule-controlled behavior. *Neurotoxicol. Teratol.*, 1(suppl.):113–118.

42. Cory-Slechta, D. A. (1984): The behavioral toxicity of lead: Problems and perspectives. In: *Advances in Behavioral Pharmacology*, Vol. 4, edited by T. Thompson, P. B. Dews, and J. E. Barrett, pp. 211–256. Academic Press, New York.

43. Cory-Slechta, D. A. (1986): Prolonged lead exposure and fixed-ratio performance. *Neurotoxicol. Teratol.*, 8:237–244.

44. Cory-Slechta, D. A. (1989): Behavioral measures of neurotoxicity. *Neurotoxicology*, 10:271–296.

45. Cory-Slechta, D. A. (1992): Schedule-controlled behavior in neurotoxicology. In: *Neurotoxicology*, edited by H. Tilson and C. Mitchell, pp. 271–294. Raven Press, New York.

46. Cory-Slechta, D. A. (1994): Neurotoxicant-induced changes in schedule-controlled behavior. In: *Basic Principles of Neurotoxicology*, edited by L. Chang, pp. 313–344. Marcel Dekker, New York.

47. Cory-Slechta, D. A., Bissen, S. T., Young, A. M., and Thompson, T. (1981): Chronic postweaning lead exposure and response duration performance. *Toxicol. Appl. Pharmacol.*, 60:78–84.

47a. Cory-Slechta, D. A., O'Mara, D. J., and Brockel, B. J. (1999): Learning versus performance impairments following regional administration of MK-801 into nucleus accumbens and dorsomedial striatum. *Behav Brain Res.* 102: 181–94

48. Cory-Slechta, D. A., Pokora, M. J., and Widzowski, D. V. (1993): Postnatal lead exposure induces supersensitivity to the stimulus properties of a dopamine D2–D3 agonist. *Brain Res.*, 598:162–172.

48a. Cory-Slechta, D. A., Pokora, M. J., and Widzowski, D. V. (1991): Behavioral manifestations of prolonged lead exposure initiated at different stages of the life cycle: II. Delayed spatial alternation. *Neurotoxicology*. 12:761–76.

49. Cory-Slechta, D. A., and Weiss, B. (1985): Alterations in schedule-controlled behavior of rodents correlated with prolonged lead exposure. In: *Behavioral Pharmacology: The Current Status*, edited by L. S. Seiden and R. L. Balster, pp. 487–502. Alan R. Liss, New York.

50. Cory-Slechta, D. A., Weiss, B., and Cox, C. (1985): Performance and exposure indices of rats exposed to low concentrations of lead. *Toxicol. Appl. Pharmacol.*, 78:291–299.

51. Cory-Slechta, D. A., and Widzowski, D. V. (1991): Low-level lead exposure increases sensitivity to the stimulus properties of dopamine D1 and D2 agonists. *Brain Res.*, 553:65–74.

52. Crofton, K. M. (1992): Reflex modification and the assessment of sensory function. In: *Neurotoxicology*, edited by H. A. Tilson and C. Mitchell, pp. 181–211. Raven Press, New York.

53. Crofton, K. M., Howard, J. L., Moser, V. D., Gill, M. W., Rector, L. W., Tilson, H. A., MacPhail, R. C. (1991): Interlaboratory comparison of motor activity experiments: Implications for neurotoxicological assessments. *Neurotoxicol. Teratol.*, 13:599–610.

54. Daniel, S. A., and Evans, H. L. (1984): Discriminative behavior as an index of toxicity. In: *Advances in Behavioral Pharmacology, Vol. 4*, edited by T. Thompson, P. B. Dews, and J. E. Barrett, pp. 257–283. Academic Press, New York.

55. Daniel, S. A., and Evans, H. L. (1985): Effects of acrylamide on multiple behavioral endpoints in the pigeon. *Neurotoxicol. Teratol.* 7:267–273.

55a. Davidson, P. W., Myers, G. J., Cox, C., Axtell, C., Shamlaye, C., Sloane-Reeves, J., Cernichiari, E., Needham, L., Choi, A., Wang, Y., Berlin, M., and Clarkson, T. W. (1998): Effects of prenatal and postnatal methylmercury exposure from fish consumption on neurodevelopment: Outcomes at 66 months of age in the Seychelles Child Development Study. *JAMA* 280:701–707.

56. Derogatis, L. R., Lipman, R. S., Rickels, K., Uhlenhuth, E. H., and Covi, L. (1974): The Hopkins Symptom Checklist (HSCL): A self-report symptom inventory. *Behav. Sci.*, 19:1–15.

57. Dews, P. B. (1955): Studies on behavior. I. Differential sensitivity to pentobarbital of pecking performance in pigeons depending on schedule of reward. *J. Pharmacol.*, 113:393–401.
58. Dews, P. B. (1956): Modification by drugs of performance on simple schedules of positive reinforcement. *Ann. NY Acad. Sci.*, 65:268–281.
59. Dews, P. B. (1958): Studies on behavior. IV. Stimuland actions of methamphetamine. *J. Pharm. Exp. Ther.*, 122:137–147.
60. Dews, P. B., and Morse, W. H. (1961): Behavioral pharmacology. *Annu. Rev. Pharmacol.* 1:145–174.
61. Dews, P. B., and DeWeese, J. (1984): Schedules of reinforcement. In: *Handbook of Psychopharmacology*, Vol. 7, edited by L. L. Iversen and S. D. Iversen, pp. 107–150. Plenum Press, New York.
62. Dews, P. B., and Herd, J. A. (1974): Behavioral activities and cardiovascular functions: Effects of hexamethonium on cardiovascular changes during strong sustained static work in rhesus monkeys. *J. Pharmacol. Exp. Ther.*, 189:12–23.
63. Dews, P. B., and Wenger, C. R. (1977): Rate-dependency of the behavioral effects of amphetamine. In: *Advances in Behavioral Pharmacology*, Vol. 1, edited by T. Thompson and P. B. Dews, pp. 167–229. Academic Press, New York.
64. Dick, R. B., Setzer, J. V., Wait, R., Hayden, M. B., Taylor, B. J., Tolos, B., Puts-Anderson, V. (1984): Effects of acute exposure of toluene and methyl ethyl ketone on psychomotor performance. *Int. Arch. Occup. Environ. Health*, 54:91–109.
65. Dick, R. B., Bhattacharya, A., and Shukia, R. (1990): Use of a computerized postural sway measurement system for neurobehavioral toxicology. *Neurotoxicol. Teratol.*, 12:1–6.
66. Dietrich, K. N., Kraftt, K. M., Bornschein, R. L., Hammond, P. B., Berger, O., Succop, P. A., Bier, M. (1987): Low-level fetal lead exposure effect on neurobehavioral development in early infancy. *Pediatrics*, 80:721–730.
67. Eckerman, D. A., and Bushnell, P. J. (1992): The neurotoxicology of cognition: Attention, learning and memory. In: *Neurotoxicology*, edited by H. A. Tilson and C. L. Mitchell, pp. 213–270, Raven Press, New York.
68. Eckerman, D. A., Lanson, R. N., and Cumming, W. (1968): Acquisition and maintenance of matching without a required observing response. *J. Exp. Anal. Behav.*, 11:435–442.
69. Eichenbaum, H., and Otto, T. (1993): Odor-guided learning and memory in rats: Is it "special?" *Trends Neurosci.*, 16:22–24.
70. Elsner, J. (1991): Tactile-kinesthetic system of rats as an animal model for minimal brain dysfunction. *Arch. Toxicol.*, 65:465–473.
71. Eskin, T. A., Lapham, L. W., Maurissen, J. P. J., and Merigan, W. H. (1985): Acrylamide effects on the macaque visual system. *Invest. Ophthalmol. Vis. Sci.*, 26:317–329.
72. Eskin, T. A., and Merigan, W. H. (1986): Selective acrylamide induced degeneration of color opponent ganglion cells in macaques. *Brain Res.*, 378:379–384.
73. Eskin, T. A., Merigan, W. H., and Wood, R. W. (1988): Carbon disulfide effects on the visual system. II. Retinogeniculate degeneration. *Invest. Ophthalmol. Vis. Sci.*, 29:519–527.
74. Evans, H. L. (1978): Early methylmercury signs revealed in visual tests. In: *Proc. International Conference on Heavy Metals in the Environment*, Vol. 3, edited by T. C. Hutchinson, pp. 241–256. University of Toronto Institute of Environmental Studies.
75. Evans, H. L. (1975): Scopolamine effects on visual discrimination: Modifications related to stimulus control. *J. Pharmacol. Exp. Ther.*, 195:105–113.
76. Evans, H. L., Laties, V. G., and Weiss, B. (1975): Behavioral effects of mercury and methylmercury. *Fed. Proc.*, 34:1858–1867.
77. Fagan, J. F., and McGrath, S. K. (1981): Infant recognition memory and later intelligence. *Intelligence*, 5:121–130.
78. Falk, J. L. (1969): Drug effects on discriminative motor control. *Physiol. Behav.*, 4:421–427.
79. Fallas, C., Fallas, J., Maslard, P., and Dally, S. (1992): Subclinical impairment of colour vision among workers exposed to styrene. *Br. J. Ind. Med.*, 49:679–682.
80. Farnsworth, D. (1993): The Farnsworth–Munsell 100-Hue and dichotomous tests for color vision. *J. Optical Soc. Am.*, 33:568–578.
81. Fechter, L. D., and Young J. S. (1983): Discrimination of auditory from nonauditory toxicity by reflex modulation audiometry: Effects of triethyl tin. *Toxicol. Appl. Pharmacol.*, 70:216–227.
81a. Fechter, L. D., Liu, Y., Herr, D. W., and Crofton, K. M. (1998): Trichloroethylene ototoxicity: Evidence for a cochlear origin. *Toxicol. Sci.*, 42:28–35.
82. Ferster, C. B., and Skinner, B. F. (1957): *Schedules of Reinforcement*. Prentice Hall, Englewood Cliffs, NJ.
83. Findley, L. J., and Capildeo, R. (1984): *Movement Disorders: Tremor*. Oxford University Press, New York.
84. Fitts, P. M. (1954): The information capacity of the human motor system in controlling the amplitude of movement. *J. Exp. Psychol.*, 47:381–391.
85. Flowers, K. (1976): Ballistic and corrective movement on an aiming task: Intention tremor and parkinsonian movements compared. *Neurology*, 25:413–421.
86. Fowler, S. C., Gramling, S. E., and Liao, R.-M. (1986): Effects of pinnozide on emitted force, duration and rate of operant response maintained at low and high levels of required force. *Pharmacol. Biochem. Behav.*, 25:615–622.
87. Fowler, S. C., LaCerra, M. M., and Ettenberg, A. (1986): Effects of haloperidol on the biophysical characteristics of operant responding: Implications for motor and reinforcement processes. *Pharmacol. Biochem. Behav.*, 25:791–796.
88. Fowler, S. C., Liao, R.-M., and Skjoldager, P. (1990): A new rodent model for neuroleptic-induced pseudo-parkinsonism: Low doses of haloperidol increase forelimb tremor in the rat. *Behav. Neurosci.*, 104:449–456.
89. Fry, W., Kelleher, R. T., and Cook, L. (1960): A mathematical index of performance on fixed-interval schedules of reinforcement. *J. Exp. Anal. Behav.*, 3:193–199.
90. Gamberale, F., and Kjellberg, A. (1983): Behavioral performance assessment as a biological control of occupational exposure to neurotoxic substances. In: *Neurobehavioral Methods in Occupational Health*, edited by R. Gilioli, M. C. Cassitto, and V. Foa, pp. 111–121. Pergamon Press, New York.
91. Gamberale, F., Iregren, A., and Kjellberg, A. (1990): Computerized Performance testing in neurotoxicology: Why, what, how, and whereto? In: *Behavioral Measures of Neurotoxicity*, edited by R. W. Russell, P. E. Flattau, and A. M. Pope, pp. 359–394. National Academy Press, Washington, DC.
91a. Garman, R. H., Weiss, B., and Evans, H. L. (1975): Alkylmercurial encephalopathy in the monkey (*Saimiri sciureus* and *Macaca arctoides*): A histopathologic and autoradiographic study. *Acta Neuropathol.* (*Berl.*), 32:61–74.
92. Geller, I., and Seifter, J. (1960): The effects of meprobamate, barbiturates, *d*-amphetamine and promazine on experimentally induced conflict in the rat. *Psychopharmacology*, 1:482–492.
92a. Geller, A. M., and Hudnell, H. K. (1997): Critical issues in the use and analysis of the Lanthony Desaturate Color Vision test. *Neurotoxicol. Teratol.*, 19:455–65.
93. Gentry, G. D., and Middaugh, L. D. (1988): Prenatal ethanol weakens the efficacy of reinforcers for adult mice. *Teratology*, 37:135–144.
94. Gentry, D. G., Weiss, B., and Laties, V. G. (1983): The microanalysis of fixed-interval responding. *J. Exp. Anal. Behav.*, 39:327–343.
95. Gescheider, G. A. (1976): *Psychophysics: Method and Theory*. Lawrence Erlbaum Associates, Hillsdale, NJ.
96. Gilbert, R. M., and Millenson, J. R. (1972): *Reinforcement: Behavioral Analyses*. Academic Press, New York.
97. Glowa, J. R. (1985): Behavioral effects of volatile organic solvents. In: *Behavioral Pharmacology: The Current Status*, edited by L. D. Seiden and L. S. Balster, pp. 537–552. Alan R. Liss, New York.

97a. Gobba, F., Righi, E., Fantuzzi, G., Predieri, G., Cavazzuti, L., and Aggazzotti, G. (1998): Two-year evolution of perchloroethylene-induced color-vision loss. *Arch. Environ. Health*, 53:196–198.

98. Golani, I., Wolgin, D. L., and Teitelbaum, P. (1979): A proposed natural geometry of recovery from akinesia in the lateral hypothalamic rat. *Brain Res.*, 641:237–267.

99. Goldberg, D. P. (1972): *The Detection of Psychiatric Illness by Questionnaire*. Oxford University Press, London.

100. Golberg, L. (1986): Charting a course for cell culture alternatives to animal testing. *Fundam. Appl. Toxicol.*, 6:607–617.

101. Goldberger, M. E., Bregman, B. S., Vierck, C. J., and Brown, M. (1990): Criteria for assessing recovery of function after spinal cord injury: Behavioral methods. *Exp. Neurol.*, 107:113–117.

101a. Gorell, J. M., Johnson, C. C., Rybicki, B. A., Peterson, E. L., and Richardson, R. J. (1998): The risk of Parkinson's disease with exposure to pesticides, farming, well water, and rural living. *Neurology*, 50:1346–1350.

102. Gott, C. T., and Weiss, B. (1972): The development of fixed-ratio performance under the influence of ribonucleic acid. *J. Exp. Anal. Behav.*, 18:481–497.

103. Graham, D. G., St. Clair, M. B., Amarnath, V., and Anthony, D. C. (1991): Molecular mechanisms of gamma-diketone neuropathy. *Adv. Exp. Med. Surg.*, 283:427–431.

104. Grant, W. M. (1986): *Toxicology of the Eye*, 3rd ed. Charles C. Thomas, Springfield, IL.

104a. Grandjean, P., Weihe, P., White, R. F., Debes, F., Araki, S., Yokoyama, K., Murata, K., Sorensen, N., Dahl, R., and Jorgensen, P. J. (1997): Cognitive deficit in 7-year-old children with prenatal exposure to methylmercury. *Neurotoxicol. Teratol.*, 19:417–428.

105. Grant-Webster, K. S., Gunderson, V. M., and Burbacher, T. M. (1990): Behavioral assessment of young nonhuman primates: Perceptual-cognitive development. *Neurotoxicol. Teratol.*, 12:543–546.

106. Griffin, J. W. (1992): Neurotoxicant-induced axonal degeneration. In: *Neurotoxicology*, edited by H. A. Tilson and C. M. Mitchell, pp. 51–65. Raven Press, New York.

106a. Gruener, G., and Dyck, P. J., (1994): Quantitative sensory testing: methodology, applications, and future directions. *Clin. Neurophysiol.*, 11:568–583.

107. Gunderson, V. M., Grant, K. S., Burbacher, T. M., Fagan, J. F., and Mottet, U. K. (1986): The effect of low-level prenatal methylmercury exposure on visual recognition memory in infant crab-eating macaques. *Child. Dev.*, 57:1076–1083.

108. Hanninen, H. (1971): Psychological picture of manifest and latent carbon disulfide poisoning. *Br. J. Ind. Med.*, 28:374–381.

109. Hanninen, H. (1983): Psychological test batteries: New trends and developments. In: *Neurobehavioral Methods in Occupational Health*, edited by R. Gilioli, M. G. Cassitto, and V. Foa, pp. 123–129. Pergamon Press, New York.

110. Hanson, H. M., Witoslawski, J. J., and Campbell, E. H. (1964): Reversible disruption of a wavelength discrimination in pigeons following administration of pheniprazine. *Toxicol. Appl. Pharmacol.*, 6:690–695.

111. Harlow, H. F. (1949): The formation of learning pets. *Psychol. Rev.*, 56:51–65.

112. Harris, J. E., and Morris, P. E., eds. (1984): *Everyday Memory, Actions and Absent-Mindedness*. Academic Press, London.

113. Hastings, L. (1990): Sensory neurotoxicology: Use of the olfactory system in the assessment of toxicity. *Neurotoxicol. Teratol.*, 12:455–459.

114. Hastings, L., Cooper, G. P., Bornschein, R. L., and Michaelson, I. A. (1979): Behavioral deficits in adult rats following neonatal lead exposure. *Neurotoxicol. Teratol.*, 1:227–231.

115. Hefferline, R. F., and Keenan, B. (1963): Amplitude-induction gradient of a small-scale (covert) operant. *J. Exp. Anal. Behav.*, 6:307–315.

116. Heise, G. A. (1984): Behavioral methods for measuring effects of drugs on learning and memory in animals. *Med. Res. Rev.*, 4:535–558.

117. Herrnstein, R. J., and Morse, W. H. (1957): Effects of pentobarbital on intermittently reinforced behavior. *Science*, 125:929–931.

118. Hindmarch, I., Alford, C., Barwell, F., and Kerr, J. S. (1992): Measuring the side effects of psychotrophics: The behavioural toxicity of antidepressants. *J. Psychopharmacol.*, 6:198–203.

119. Holson, R. R., and Buelke-Sam, J. (1992): Design and analysis issues in developmental neurotoxicology. Papers from a symposium on experimental design and statistical analysis. *Neurotoxicol. Teratol.*, 14:197–228.

120. Horak, F. B., and Anderson, M. E. (1984): Influence of globus pallidus on arm movements in monkeys. I. Effects of kainic acid-induced lesions. *J. Neurophysiol.*, 52:290–304.

121. Hore, J., and Vilis, T. (1980): Arm movement performance during reversible basal ganglia lesions in the monkey. *Exp. Brain Res.*, 39:217–228.

121a. Infurna, R., and Weiss, B. (1986): Neonatal behavioral toxicity in rats following prenatal exposure to methanol. *Teratology*. 33:259–65.

122. Iregren, A. (1990): Psychological test performance in foundry workers exposed to low levels of manganese. *Neurotoxicol. Teratol.*, 12:673–675.

123. Iregren, A., and Gamberale, F. (1990): Human behavioral toxicology. Central nervous effects of low-dose exposure to neurotoxic substances in the work environment. *Scand. J. Work Environ. Health*, 16(suppl. 1):17–25.

123a. Iregren, A., Gamberale, F., and Kjellberg, A. (1996): SPES: A psychological test system to diagnose environmental hazards. Swedish Performance Evaluation System. *Neurotoxicol. Teratol.*, 18:485–91.

124. Ison, J. R., and Hoffman, H. S. (1983): Reflex modification in the domain of startle: II. The anomalous history of a robust and ubiquitous phenomenon. *Psych. Bull.*, 94:3–17.

125. Iversen, I. H., Ragnarsdottir, A., and Randrup, K. I. (1984): Operant conditioning of autogrooming in vervet monkeys (*Circopithecus aethiops*). *J. Exp. Anal. Behav.*, 42:189–191.

126. Iversen, S. D., and Iversen, L. L. (1981): *Behavioral Pharmacology*, 2nd Ed., Oxford University Press, New York.

127. Jacobson, J. L., Jacobson, S. W., and Humphrey, H. E (1990): Effects of exposure to PCBs and related compounds on growth and activity in children. *Neurotoxicol. Teratol.*, 12:319–326.

128. Jenkins, W. O., and Stanley, J. C. (1950): Partial reinforcement: A review and critique. *Psychol. Bull.*, 47:193–234.

129. *Journal of the Experimental Analysis of Behavior* (*special issue on behavioral pharmacology*) (1991):56:167–423.

130. Kelleher, R. T., and Morse, W. H. (1964): Escape behavior and punished behavior. *Fed. Proc.*, 23:808–817.

131. Kelleher, R., and Morse, W. H. (1968): Determinants of the specificity of behavioral effects of drugs. *Ergebnisse der Physiol.*, 60:1–56.

132. Kelleher, R. T., and Morse, W. H. (1968): Determinants of the behavioral effects of drugs. In: *Importance of Fundamental Principles of Drug Evaluation*, edited by D. H. Tedeschi and R. E. Tedeschi, pp. 383–405. Raven Press, New York.

132a. Kennedy, R. S., Turnage, J. J., and Lane N. E. (1997): Development of surrogate methodologies for operational performance measurement: Empirical studies. *Human Perf.*, 10:251–282.

133a. Korogi, Y., Takahashi, M., Okajima, T., and Eto, K. (1998): M. R. findings of Minamata disease–organic mercury poisoning. *J. Magn. Reson. Imaging*, 8:308–16.

133b. Kovera, C. A., Anger, W. K., Campbell, K. A., Binder, L. M., Storzbach, D., Davis, K. L., and Rohlman, D. S. (1996): Computer-administration of questionnaires: A health screening system (HSS) developed for veterans. *Neurotox. Teratol.*, 18:511–518.

133c. Kremer, B., Klimek, L., and Mosges R. (1998): Clinical validation of a new olfactory test. *Eur. Arch. Otorhinolaryngol.*, 255:355–58.

134. Kulig, B. M., and Lammers, J. H. C. M. (1992): Assessment of neurotoxicant-induced effects on motor function. In: *Neurotoxicology*, edited by H. A. Tilson and C. L. Mitchell, pp. 147–179. Raven Press, New York.
135. Langolf, G. D., Chaffin, D. B., Henderson, R., and Whittle, H. P. (1978): Evaluation of workers exposed to elemental mercury using quantitative test of tremor and neuromuscular functions. *Am. Ind. Hyg. Assoc. J.*, 39:976–984.
136. Laties, V. G. (1978): How operant conditioning can contribute to behavioral toxicology. *Environ. Health Perspect.*, 26:29–35.
137. Laties, V. G., and Weiss, B. (1959): Thyroid state and working for heat in the cold. *Am. J. Physiol.*, 197:1028–1034.
138. Laties, V. G., and Weiss, B. (1963): Effects of a concurrent task on fixed-interval responding in humans. *J. Exp. Anal. Behav.*, 6:431–436.
139. Laties, V. G., Wood, R. W., and Rees, D. C. (1981): Stimulus control and the effects of *d*-amphetamine in the rat. *Psychopharmacology*, 75:277–282.
140. Leander, J. D., and MacPhail, R. C. (1980): Effect of chlordimeform (a formamidine pesticide) on schedule-controlled responding of pigeons. *Neurotoxicol. Teratol.*, 2:315–321.
141. Leander, J. D., and McMillan, D. E. (1974): Rate-dependent effects of drugs. I. Comparisons of *d*-amphetamine, pentobarbital and chlorpromazine on multiple and mixed schedules. *J. Pharmacol. Exp. Ther.*, 188:726–739.
142. Letz, R., and Baker, E. L. (1986): Computer-administered neurobehavioral testing in occupational health. *Sem. Occup. Med.*, 1:197–203.
143. Letz, R., Mahoney, F. C., Hershman, D. L., Woskie, S., and Smith, T. J. (1990): Neurobehavioral effects of acute styrene exposure in Fiberglas boatbuilders. *Neurotoxicol. Teratol.*, 12:665–668.
143a. Letz, R., Green, R. C., and Woodard, J. L. (1996): Development of a computer-based battery designed to screen adults for neuropsychological impairment. *Neurotoxicol. Teratol.*, 18:365–370.
144. Levin, H. S., Rodnitzky, R. L., and Mick, D. L. (1976): Anxiety associated with exposure to organophosphate compounds. *Arch. Gen. Psychiatry*, 33:225–228.
145. Levine, T. E. (1976): Effects of carbon disulfide and FLA-63 on operant behavior of pigeons. *J. Pharmacol. Exp. Ther.*, 199:669–678.
146. Lezak, M. D. (1976): *Neuropsychological Assessment*. Oxford University Press, New York.
147. Lindner, M. D., and Gribkoff, V. K. (1991): Relationship between performance in the Morris water task, visual acuity, and thermoregulatory function in aged F-344 rats. *Behav. Brain Res.*, 45:445–455.
148. Lowndes, H. E., Baker, T., Cho, E.-S., and Jortner, B. (1978): Position sensitivity of de-efferented muscle spindles in experimental acrylamide neuropathy. *J. Pharmacol. Exp. Ther.*, 205:40–48.
149. Lynch, J. J., Silveira, L. C., Perry, V. H., and Merigan, W. H. (1992): Visual effects of damage to P ganglion cells in macaques. *Visual Neurosci.*, 8:575–582.
150. Mackay, C. J., Campbell, L., Samuel, A. M., Alderman, K. J., Idzikowślei, C., Wilson, H. K., Gompertz, D. (1987): Behavioral changes during exposure to 1,1,1-trichloroethane: Time-course and relationship to blood solvent levels. *Am. J. Ind. Med.*, 11:223–239.
151. MacPhail, R. C. (1985): Effects of pesticides on schedule-controlled behavior. In: *Behavioral Pharmacology: The Current Status*, edited by L. S. Seiden and R. L. Balster, pp. 519–536. Alan R. Liss, New York.
152. Maizlish, N. A., Langolf, C. D., Whitehead, L. W., Fine, L. J., Albers, J. W., Goldberg, J., and Smith, P. (1985): Behavioral evaluation of workers exposed to mixtures of organic solvents. *Br. J. Ind. Med.*, 42:579–590.
153. Mattson, J. L., Boyes, W. K., and Ross, J. F. (1992): Incorporating evoked potentials into neurotoxicity test schemes. In: *Neurotoxicology*, edited by H. A. Tilson and C. M. Mitchell, pp. 125–145. Raven Press, New York.
154. Maurissen, J. P. J. (1988): Quantitative sensory assessment in toxicology and occupational medicine: Applications, theory, and critical appraisal. *Toxicol. Lett.*, 43:321–343.
155. Maurissen, J. P. J., and Weiss, B. (1980): Vibration sensitivity as an index of somatosensory function. In: *Experimental and Clinical Neurotoxicity*, edited by P. S. Spencer and H. H. Schaumbers, pp. 767–774. Williams & Wilkins, Baltimore, MD.
156. Maurissen, J. P. J., Weiss, B., and Cox, C. (1990): Vibration sensitivity recovery after a second course of acrylamide intoxication. *Fundam. Appl. Toxicol.*, 15:93–98.
157. Maurissen, J. P. J., Weiss, B., and Davis, H. T. (1983): Somatosensory thresholds in monkeys exposed to acrylamide. *Toxicol. Appl. Pharmacol.*, 71:266–279.
157a. Maurissen, J. P. J. (1995): Neurobehavioral methods for the evaluation of sensory functions. In: *Neurotoxicology. Approaches and Methods*, edited by L. W. Chang and W. Slikker, pp. 239–264. Academic Press, San Diego.
158. McCarthy, D. (1972): *The Manual for the McCarthy Scales of Children's Abilities*. Psychological Corporation, New York.
159. McKearney, J. W., and Barrett, J. E. (1978): Schedule-controlled behavior and the effects of drugs. In: *Contemporary Research in Behavioral Pharmacology*, edited by D. B. Blackman and D. J. Sanger, pp. 1–68. Plenum Press, New York.
160. McKearney, J. W. (1979): Interrelations among prior experience and current conditions in the determination of behavior and the effects of drugs. In: *Advances in Behavioral Pharmacology*, Vol. 2, edited by T. Thompson and P. B. Dews, pp. 39–64. Academic Press, New York.
161. McMillan, D. B., and Leander, J. D. (1976): Effects of drugs on schedule-controlled behavior. In: *Behavioral Pharmacology*, edited by S. D. Click and J. Goldfard, pp. 85–139. C. V. Mosby, St. Louis, MO.
162. McNair, D. M., and Kahn, R. J. (1983): Self-assessment of cognitive deficits. In: *Assessment in Geriatric Psychopharmacology*, edited by T. Crook, S. Ferris, and E. Bartus, pp. 13–143. Mark Powley Associates, New Canaan, CT.
163. Means, L. W., Alexander, S. R., and O'Neal, M. F. (1982): Those cheating rats: Male and female rats use odor trails in a water-escape "working memory" task. *Behav. Neural. Biol.*, 58:144–151.
163a. Melton, A. W., ed. (1947): Apparatus tests, AAF Aviation Psychology Research Reports, Rpt. No. 4. U.S. Government Printing Office, Washington, DC.
164. Mergler, D., and Blain, L. (1987): Assessing color vision loss among solvent-exposed workers. *Am. J. Ind. Med.*, 12:195–203.
164a. Mergler, D. (1987): Assessing color vision loss among solvent-exposed workers. *Am. J. Ind. Med.*, 12:195–203.
164b. Mergler, D., and Baldwin, M. (1997): Early manifestations of manganese neurotoxicity in humans: An update. *Environ. Res.*, 73:92–100.
165. Merigan, W. H. (1979): Effects of toxicants on visual systems. *Neurobehav. Toxicol.*, 1(Suppl. 1):15–22.
166. Merigan, W. H., and Weiss, B., eds. (1980): *Neurotoxicity of the Visual System*. Raven Press, New York.
167. Merigan, W. H., Barkdoll, B., and Maurissen, J. P. J. (1982): Acrylamide-induced visual impairment in primates. *Toxicol. Appl. Pharmacol.*, 62:342–345.
168. Merigan, W. H., Maurissen, J. P. J., Weiss, B., Eskin, T., and Lapham, L. W. (1983): Neurotoxic actions of methylmercury on the primate visual system. *Neurobehav. Toxicol. Teratol.*, 5:649–658.
169. Merigan, W. H., Barkdoll, B., Maurissen, J. P. J., Eskin, T. A., and Lapham, L. W. (1985): Acrylamide effects on the macaque visual system. I. Psychophysics and electrophysiology. *Invest. Ophthalmol. Vis. Sci.*, 26:309–316.

170. Merigan, W. H., and Eskin, T. A. (1986): Spatio-temporal vision of macaques with severe loss of P $\sim$3 retinal ganglion cells. *Vision Res.*, 26:1751–1761.

171. Merigan, W. H., Wood, R. W., Zehl, D., and Eskin, T. A. (1988): Carbon disulfide effects on the visual system. I. Visual thresholds and ophthalmoscopy. *Invest. Ophthalmol. Vis. Sci.*, 29:512–518.

172. Merigan, W. H. (1989): Chromatic and achromatic vision of macaques: Role of the P pathway. *J. Neurosci.*, 9:776–783.

173. Mesulam, M.-M. (1985): *Principles of Behavioral Neurology*. F. A. Davis, Philadelphia.

174. Millenson, J. R. (1967): *Principles of Behavioral Analysis*. MacMillan, New York.

175. Miller, J. M., Kimm, J., Clopton, B., and Fetz, B. (1970): Sensory neurophysiology and reaction time performance in nonhuman primates. In: *Animal Psychophysics: The Design and Conduct of Sensory Experiments*, edited by W. C. Stebbins, pp. 303–307. Appleton-Century-Crofts, New York.

175a. Montoya, C. P., Campbell, H. L., Pemberton, K. D., and Dunnett, S. B. (1991): The "staircase test": A measure of independent forelimb reaching and grasping abilities in rats. *J. Neurosci. Methods*, 36:219–228.

176. Moody, D. B. (1970): Reaction time as an index of sensory function. In: *Animal Psychophysics: The Design and Conduct of Sensory Experiments*, edited by W. C. Stebbins, pp. 277–302. Appleton-Century-Crofts, New York.

177. Moser, V. C., McCormick, J. P., Creason, J. P., and MacPhail, R. C. (1988): Comparison of chlordimeform and carbaryl using a functional observation battery. *Fundam. Appl. Toxicol.*, 11:189–206.

178. Moxley, R. (1982): Graphics for three-term contingencies. *Behav. Anal.*, 5:45–51.

179. Mutti, A., Mazzucchi, A., Frigeri, C., Falzoli, M., Arfini, C., and Franchini, I. (1983): Neuropsychological investigation on styrene exposed workers. In: *Neurobehavioral Methods in Occupational Health*, edited by R. Cilioli, M. C. Cassitto, and V. Foa, pp. 271–281. Pergamon Press, Oxford.

179a. Myers, G. J., Marsh, D. O., Davidson, P. W., Cox, C., Shamlaye, C. F., Tanner, M., Choi, A., Cernichiari, E., Choisy, O., and Clarkson, T. W. (1995): Main neurodevelopmental study of Seychellois children following in utero exposure to methylmercury from a maternal fish diet: Outcome at six months. *Neurotoxicology*, 16:653–664.

180. National Research Council Committee on Neurotoxicology and Models for Assessing Risk. (1992): *Environmental Neurotoxicology*. National Academy Press, Washington, DC.

181. Needleman, H. L. (1985): The neurobehavioral effects of low-level exposure to lead in childhood. *Int. J. Ment. Health*, 14:64–77.

182. Needleman, H. L., Gunnoe, C., Leviton, A., Reed, R., Peresie, H., Maher, C., Barrett, P. (1979): Deficits in psychological and classroom performance of children with elevated dentine lead levels. *N. Engl. J. Med.*, 300:689–695.

183. Nevin, J. A. (1970): On differential stimulation and differential reinforcement. In: *Animal Psychophysics: The Design and Conduct of Sensory Experiments*, edited by W. C. Stebbins, pp. 401–423. Appleton-Century-Crofts, New York.

184. Newland, M. C. (1988): Quantification of motor function in toxicology. *Toxicol. Lett.*, 43:295–319.

185. Newland, M. C., Ceckler, T. L., Kordower, J. H., and Weiss, B. (1989): Visualizing manganese in the primate basal ganglia with magnetic resonance imaging. *Exp. Neurol.*, 106:251–258.

186. Newland, M. C., and Weiss, B. (1991): Ethanol's effects on tremor and positioning in squirrel monkeys. *J. Stud. Alcohol*, 52:492–499.

187. Newland, M. C., and Weiss, B. (1992): Persistent effects of manganese on effortful responding and their relationship to manganese accumulation in the primate globus pallidus. *Toxicol. Appl. Pharmacol.*, 113:87–97.

188. Newland, M. C., and Weiss, B. (1990): Drug effects on an effortful operant: Pentobarbital and amphetamine. *Pharmacol. Biochem. Behav.*, 36:381–387.

188a. Newland, M. C. (1995): Motor function and the physical properties of the operant: Applications to screening and advanced techniques. In: *Neurotoxicology. Approaches and Methods*, edited by L. Chang, pp. 265–299. Academic Press, San Diego.

188b. Newland, M. C., Yezhou, S., Logdberg, B., and Berlin, M. (1996): In utero lead exposure in squirrel monkeys: Motor effects seen with schedule-controlled behavior. *Neurotoxicol. Teratol.*, 18:33–40.

188c. Newland, M. C., Yezhou, S., Logdberg, B., and Berlin, M. (1994): Prolonged behavioral effects of in utero exposure to lead or methyl mercury: Reduced sensitivity to changes in reinforcement contingencies during behavioral transitions and in steady state. *Toxicol. Appl. Pharmacol.*, 126:6–15.

188d. Newland, M. C., Warfvinge, K., and Berlin, M. (1996): Behavioral consequences of in utero exposure to mercury vapor: Alterations in lever-press durations and learning in squirrel monkeys. *Toxicol. Appl. Pharmacol.*, 139:374–386.

189. Notterman, J. M., and Mintz, D. B. (1965): *Dynamics of Response*. John Wiley, New York.

190. Office of Technology Assessment, U.S. Congress, (1990): *Neurotoxicity: Identifying and Controlling Poisons of the Nervous System*. OTA-BA-436. U.S. Government Printing Office, Washington, DC.

191. Overton, D. A., and Hayes, M. W. (1984): Optimal training parameters in the two-bar fixed ratio drug discrimination task. *Pharmacol. Biochem. Behav.*, 21:19–28.

192. Owen, J. B. (1960): The influence of *dl*-, *d*-, and *l*-amphetamine and *d*-methamphetamine on a fixed ratio schedule. *J. Exp. Anal. Behav.*, 3:293–310.

193. Paule, M. C., Cranmer, J. M., Wilkins, J. D., Stern, H. P., and Hoffman, B. L. (1988): Quantitation of complex brain function in children: Preliminary evaluation using a nonhuman primate behavioral test battery. *Neurotoxicology*, 9:367–378.

194. Paule, M. C., and McMillan, D. B. (1986): Effects of trimethyltin on incremental repeated acquisition. *Neurotoxicol. Teratol.*, 8:245–253.

194a. Payne, R. P., and Hauty, G. T. (1955): Factors affecting the endurance of psychomotor skill. *J. Aviat. Med.*, 26:382–389.

195. Peele, D. B., and Baron, S. P. (1988): Effects of scopolamine on repeated acquisition of radial-arm maze performance by rats. *J. Exp. Anal. Behav.*, 49:275–290.

196. Perino, J., and Ernhardt, C. B. (1974): The relation of subclinical lead level to cognitive and sensorimotor impairment in black preschoolers. *J. Learning Disabil.*, 7:26–30.

197. Perkins, A. N., Eckerman, D. A., and MacPhail, R. C. (1991): Discriminative stimulus properties of triadimefon: Comparison with methylphenidate. *Pharmacol. Biochem. Behav.*, 40:757–761.

198. Potts, A. M., and Conasun, L. M. (1980): Toxic response of the eye. In: *Casarett and Doull's Toxicology: The Basic Science of Poisons*, 2nd ed., edited by J. Doull, C. D. Klaassen, and M. O. Amdur, pp. 275–310. New York: McGraw-Hill.

199. Preston, K. L., Schuster, C. R., and Seiden, L. S. (1985): Methamphetamine, physostigmine, atropine and mecamylamine: Effects on force lever performance. *Pharmacol. Biochem. Behav.*, 23:781–788.

200. Pryor, C. T., Rebert, C. S., Dickinson, J., and Feeney, B. (1984): Factors affecting toluene-induced ototoxicity in rats. *Neurobehav. Toxicol. Teratol.*, 6:223–238.

201. Putz, V. R. (1979): The effects of carbon monoxide on dual-task performance. *Hum. Factors*, 21:13–24.

202. Putz, V. R., Johnson, B. L., and Setzer, J. V. (1979): A comparative study of the effects of carbon monoxide and methylene chloride on human performance. *J. Exp. Pathol. Toxicol.*, 2:97–112.

203. Putz-Anderson, V., Albright, B. B., Lee, S. T., et al. (1983): A behavioral evaluation of workers exposed to carbon disulfide. *Neurotoxicology*, 4:67–78.

203a. Rahill, A. A., Weiss, B., Morrow, P. E., Frampton, M. W., Cox, C., Gibb, R., Gelein, R., Speers, D., and Utell, M. J. (1996): Human performance during exposure to toluene. *Aviat. Space Environ. Med.*, 67:640–647.

204. Raitta, C. (1981): Impaired colour discrimination among viscose rayon workers exposed to carbon disuliphide. *J. Occup. Med.*, 23:589–592.

205. Rees, D. C., Knisely, J., Jordan, S., and Balseter, R. L. (1987): Discriminative stimulus properties of toluene in the mouse. *Toxicol. Appl. Pharmacol.*, 88:97–104.

206. Regan, D., Bartol, S., Murray, T. J., and Beverley, K. I. (1982): Spatial frequency discrimination in normal vision and in patients with multiple sclerosis. *Brain*, 105:735–754.

207. Repko, J. D., Jones, P. D., Garcia, L. S., Schneider, E. J., Roseman, E., and Corum, C. R. (1976): *Behavioral and Neurological Effects of Methyl Chloride*. NIOSH Publication No. 77-125. U.S. Government Printing Office, Washington, DC.

208. Reynolds, G. S. (1968): *A Primer of Operant Conditioning*. Scott Foresman, Glenview, IL.

209. Rice, D. C. (1984): Behavioral deficit (delayed matching to sample) in monkeys exposed from birth to low levels of lead. *Toxicol. Appl. Pharmacol.*, 75:337–345.

210. Rice, D. C. (1994): Testing effects of toxicants on sensory system function by operant methodology. In: *Neurobehavioral Toxicity. Analysis and Interpretation*, edited by B. Weiss and J. O'Donoghue. Raven Press, New York.

211. Rice, D. C., and Gilbert, S. G. (1982): Early chronic low-level methylmercury poisoning in monkeys impairs spatial vision. *Science*, 216:759–761.

212. Rice, D. C., and Gilbert, S. G. (1985): Low lead exposure from birth produces behavioral toxicity (DRL) in monkeys. *Toxicol. Appl. Pharmacol.*, 80:421–426.

213. Rice, D. C. (1985): Effects of lead on schedule-controlled behavior in monkeys. In: *Behavioral Pharmacology: The Current Status*, edited by L. S. Seiden and R. L. Balster, pp. 473–486. Alan R. Liss, New York.

214. Rice, D. C., and Gilbert, S. G. (1990): Effects of developmental exposure to methylmercury on spatial and temporal visual function in monkeys. *Toxicol. Appl. Pharmacol.*, 102:151–163.

215. Rice, D. C., and Gilbert, S. G. (1992): Exposure to methylmercury from birth to adulthood impairs high-frequency hearing in monkeys. *Toxicol. Appl. Pharmacol.*, 115:6–10.

215a. Rice, D. C. (1998): Age-related increase in auditory impairment in monkeys exposed in utero plus postnatally to methylmercury. *Toxicol. Sci.*, 44:191–196.

215b. Rice, D. C., and Gilbert, S. G. (1995): Effects of developmental methylmercury exposure or lifetime lead exposure on vibration sensitivity function in monkeys. *Toxicol. Appl. Pharmacol.*, 134:161–169.

216. Riley, E. P., and Voorhees, C. V. (1986): *Handbook of Behavioral Teratology*. Plenum Press, New York.

217. Ristau, C. A., and Robbins, D. (1982): Language in the great apes: A critical review. *Adv. Study Behav.*, 12:141–255.

218. Roels, H., Lauwerys, R., Buchet, J. P., Genet, P., Sarhan, M. J., Hanotiau, I., deFays, M., Bernard, A., Stanescu, D. (1987): Epidemiological survey among workers exposed to manganese: Effects on lung, central nervous system, and some biological indices. *Am. J. Ind. Med.*, 11:307–327.

218a. Rosenstock, L., Keifer, M., Daniell, W. E., McConnell, R., and Claypoole, K. (1991): Chronic central nervous system effects of acute organophosphate pesticide intoxication. The Pesticide Health Effects Study Group. *Lancet*, 338:223–227.

219. Ruppert, P. H. (1986): Postnatal exposure. In: *Neurobehavioral Toxicology*, edited by Z. Annau, pp. 170–192. Johns Hopkins University Press, Baltimore, MD.

220. Ruppert, P. H., Walsh, T. J., Reiter, L. W., and Dyer, R. S. (1982): Trimethyltin-induced hyperactivity: Time course and patterns. *Neurotoxicol. Teratol.*, 4:135–139.

221. Russell, R. W., Flattau, P. E., and Pope, A. M., eds. (1970): *Behavioral Measures of Neurotoxicity*. National Academy Press, Washington, DC.

222. Russell, E. W., Neuringer, C., and Goldstein, G. (1970): *Assessment of Brain Damage. A Neuropsychological Key Approach*. Wiley Interscience, New York.

223. Sahakian, B. J., Morris, R. G., Evenden, J. L., Heald, A., Levy, R., Philpot, M., and Robbins, T. W. (1988): A comparative study of visuospatial memory and learning in Alzheimer type dementia and Parkinson's disease. *Brain*, 111:695–718.

224. Samson, H. H., and Falk, J. R. (1974): Ethanol and discriminative motor control: Effects on normal and dependent animals. *Pharmacol. Biochem. Behav.*, 2:791–801.

225. Sanes, J. N., Colburn, T. R., and Morgan, N. T. Behavioral motor evaluation for neurotoxicity screening. *Neurobehav. Toxicol. Teratol.*, 7:329–337.

225a. Sanes, J. N., Colburn, T. R., and Morgan, N. T. (1985): Behavioral motor evaluation for neurotoxicity screening. *Neurobehav. Toxicol. Teratol.*, 7:329–337.

226. Savage, E. P., Keefe, T. J., Mounce, L. M., Heaton, R. K., Lewis, J. A., and Burcar, P. J. (1988): Chronic neurological sequelae of acute organophosphate poisoning. *Arch. Environ. Health*, 43:38–45.

227. Schecter, M. D., and Rosecrans, J. A. (1971): Behavioral evidence for two types of cholinergic receptors in the C.N.S. *Eur. J. Pharmacol.*, 15:375–378.

228. Schecter, M. D., and Rosecrans, J. A. (1971): C.N.S. effect of nicotine as the discriminative stimulus for the rat in a T-maze. *Life Sci.*, 10:821–832.

229. Schecter, M. D., and Rosecrans, J. A. (1972): Atropine antagonism of arecoline-cued behavior in the rat. *Life Sci.*, 11:517–523.

230. Schecter, M. D., and Rosecrans, J. A. (1972): Nicotine as a discriminative cue in rats: Inability of related drugs to produce nicotine-like cueing effects. *Psychopharmacology*, 27:379–387.

231. Schoenfeld, W. N. (1970): *The Theory of Reinforcement Schedules*. Appleton-Century-Crofts, New York.

232. Schuster, C. R., and Johanson, C. E. (1974): The use of animal models for the study of drug abuse. In: *Research Advances in Alcohol and Drug Problems*, Vol. 1, edited by R. J. Gibbins, Y. Israel, H. Kalant, R. E. Popham, W. Schmidt, and R. G. Smart. John Wiley, New York.

233. Schwartz, B. S., Ford, D. P., Bolla, K. I., Agnew, J., Rothman, N., and Bleecker, M. L. (1990): Solvent-associated decrements in olfactory function in paint manufacturing workers. *Am. J. Ind. Med.*, 18:697–706.

234. Schwartz, B. S., Doty, R. L., Monroe, C., Frye, R., and Barker, S. (1989): Olfactory function in chemical workers exposed to acrylate and methacrylate vapors. *Am. J. Public Health*, 79:613–618.

235. Schwartz, J., and Otto, D. (1987): Blood lead, hearing thresholds, and neurobehavioral development in children and youth. *Arch. Environ. Health*, 42:153–160.

236. Schwartz, J., and Otto, D. (1991): Lead and minor hearing impairment. *Arch. Environ. Health*, 46:300–305.

237. Schrimsher, G. W., and Reier, P. J. (1992): Forelimb motor performance following cervical spinal cord contusion injury in the rat. *Exp. Neurol.*, 117:287–298.

238. Seiden, L. S., and Dykstra, L. A. (1977): *Psychopharmacology: A Biochemical and Behavioral Approach*. Van Nostrand Reinhold, New York.

238a. Sepkoski, C. M., Lester, B. M., Ostheimer, G. W., and Brazelton, T. B. (1992): The effects of maternal epidural anesthesia on neonatal behavior during the first month. *Dev. Med. Child. Neurol.*, 34:1072–1080.

239. Shull, R. L. (1979): The postreinforcement pause: Some implications for the correlational law of effect. In: *Reinforcement and the Organization of Behavior*, Vol. 1, edited by M. D. Zeiler and P. Harzem, pp. 193–222. John Wiley, New York.

240. Small, L. (1973): *Neuropsychodiagnosis in Psychotherapy*. Brunner/Mazel, New York.

241. Smith, C. B. (1964): Effects of *d*-amphetamine upon operant behavior of pigeons: Enhancement by reserpine. *J. Pharmacol. Exp. Ther.*, 146:167–174.
242. Smith, J. (1970): Conditioned suppression as an animal psychophysical technique. In: *Animal Psychophysics, The Design and Conduct of Sensory Experiments*, edited by W. C. Stebbins, pp. 125–159. Appleton-Century-Crofts, New York.
243. Smith, P. J., Langolf, G. D., and Goldberg, J. (1983): Effects of occupational exposure to elemental mercury on short term memory. *Br. J. Ind. Med.*, 40:413–419.
244. Snapper, A. G., Kadden, R. M., and Inglis, G. B. (1982): State notation of the behavioral procedures. *Behav. Res. Methods Instr.*, 14:329–342.
245. Soule, A. B., Standley, K., Copans, S. A., and Davis, M. (1974): Clinical uses of the Brazelton Neonatal Scale. *Pediatrics*, 54:583–586.
246. Spear, L. P. (1990): Neurobehavioral assessment during the early postnatal period. *Neurotoxicol. Teratol.*, 12:489–496.
247. Squire, L. (1986): Mechanisms of memory. *Science*, 232: 1612–1619.
248. Standley, K., Soule, A. B., Copans, S. A., and Duchowny, M. S. (1974): Local-regional anesthesia during childbirth: Effects on newborn behaviors. *Science*, 186:634–635.
249. Stebbins, W. C. (1970): Principles of animal psychophysics. In: *Animal Psychophysics: The Design and Conduct of Sensory Experiments*, edited by W. C. Stebbins, pp. 1–19. Appleton-Century-Crofts, New York.
250. Stebbins, W. C., and Moody, D. B. (1979): Comparative behavioral toxicology. *Neurobehav. Toxicol.*, 1:33–44.
250a. Stevenson, J. G., and Clayton, F. L. (1970): A response duration schedule: Effects of training, extinction, and deprivation. *J. Exp. Anal. Behav.* 13:359–367.
251. Streissguth, A. P., Barr, H. M., and Martin, D. C. (1983): Maternal alcohol use and neonatal habituation assessed with the Brazelton scale. *Child Dev.*, 54:1109–1118.
252. Stubbs, D. A., and Thomas, J. R. (1974): Discrimination of stimulus duration and *d*-amphetamine in pigeons: A psychophysical analysis. *Psychopharmacology*, 36:313–322.
253. Sugimoto, K., and Goto, S. (1980): Retinopathy in chronic carbon disulfide exposure. In: *Neurotoxicity of the Visual System*, edited by W. H. Merigan and B. Weiss, pp. 55–71. Raven Press, New York.
254. Suzuki, Y., Mouri, T., Suzuki, Y., Nishiyama, K., Fujii, N., and Yano, H. (1975): Study of subacute toxicity of manganese dioxide in monkeys. *Tokushima J. Exp. Med.*, 22:5–10.
255. Swanson, J. M., and Kinsbourne, M. (1980): Food dyes impair performance of hyperactive children on a laboratory learning test. *Science*, 207:1485–1487.
256. Swets, J. A. (1992): The science of choosing the right decision threshold in high-stakes diagnostics. *Am. Psychol.*, 47:522–532.
257. Taylor, J. D., and Evans, H. L. (1985): Effects of toluene inhalation on behavior and expired carbon dioxide in macaque monkeys. *Toxicol. Appl. Pharmacol.*, 80:487–495.
258. Tepper, J. S., and Weiss, B. (1986): Determinants of behavioral response with ozone exposure. *J. Appl. Physiol.*, 60:868–875.
259. Tepper, J. S., and Wood, R. W. (1985): Behavioral evaluation of the irritating properties of ozone. *Toxicol. Appl. Pharmacol.*, 78:404–411.
260. Terrace, H. S. (1985): In the beginning was the name. *Am. Psychol.*, 40:1011–1028.
261. Tewes, P. A., and Fischman, M. W. (1982): Effects of *d*-amphetamine and diazepam on fixed-interval, fixed ratio responding in humans. *J. Pharmacol. Exp. Ther.*, 221:373–383.
262. Thompson, D. M. (1975): Repeated acquisition of response sequences: Stimulus control and drugs. *J. Exp. Anal. Behav.*, 23:429–436.
263. Thompson, D. M., and Moerschbaecher, J. M. (1979): Drug effects on repeated acquisition. In: *Advances in Behavioral Pharmacology*, vol. 2, edited by T. Thompson and P. B. Dews, pp. 229–260. Academic Press, New York.
264. Thompson, T., and Boren, J. J. (1977): Operant behavioral pharmacology. In: *Handbook of Operant Behavior*, edited by W. K. Honig and J. E. R. Staddon, pp. 540–569. Prentice Hall, Englewood Cliffs, NJ.
265. Thompson, T., and Grabowski, J. C. (1972): *Reinforcement Schedules and Multioperant Analysis*. Appleton-Century-Crofts, New York.
266. Thompson, T., and Pickens, R. (1971): *Stimulus Properties of Drugs*. Appleton-Century-Crofts, New York.
267. Thompson, T., and Schuster, C. R. (1964): Morphine self-administration, food-reinforced and avoidance behavior in rhesus monkeys. *Psychopharmacology*, 5:87–94.
268. Thompson, T., and Schuster, C. R. (1968): *Behavioral Pharmacology*. Prentice Hall, Englewood Cliffs, NJ.
269. Tilson, H. A. (1976): The neurotoxicity of acrylamide: An overview. *Neurobehav. Toxicol. Teratol.*, 3:445–461.
269a. Tilson, H. A. (1987): Behavioral indices of neurotoxicity: What can be measured? *Neurotoxicol. Teratol.*, 9:427–444.
270. Tuttle, T. C., Wood, C. D., and Grether, C. C. (1976): *Behavioral and Neurological Evaluation of Workers Exposed to Carbon Disulfide*. NIOSH Publication No. 75-184. U.S. Government Printing Office, Washington, DC.
271. von Bekesy, G. (1947): A new audiometer. *Acta Otolaryngol. (Stockh.)*, 35:411–422.
272. Voorhees, C. V. (1992): Developmental neurotoxicology. In: *Neurotoxicology*, Target Organ Toxicology Series, edited by H. A. Tilson and C. L. Mitchell, pp. 295–330. Raven Press, New York.
273. Walsh, T. J., Miller, D. B., and Dyer, R. S. (1982): Trimethyltin, a selective limbic system neurotoxicant, impairs radial-arm maze performance. *Neurotoxicol. Teratol.*, 4:177–183.
274. Wechsler, D. (1945): A standardized memory scale for clinical use. *J. Psychol.*, 19:87–95.
275. Wechsler, D. (1955): *Wechsler Adult Intelligence Scale. Manual*. Psychological Corporation, New York.
276. Wechsler, D. (1967): *Wechsler Preschool and Primary Scale of Intelligence*. Psychological Corporation, New York.
277. Wechsler, D. (1974): *Manual for the Wechsler Intelligence Scale for Children–Revised*. Psychological Corporation, New York.
278. Weeks, J. R. (1962): Experimental morphine addiction: Method for automatic intravenous injections in unrestrained rats. *Science*, 138:143–144.
279. Weiss, B. (1970): Amphetamine and the temporal structure of behavior. In: *International Symposium on Amphetamine and Related Compounds*, edited by E. Costa and S. Garratini, pp. 797–812. Raven Press, New York.
280. Weiss, B. (1973): Digital computers and the microanalysis of behavior. In: *Digital Computers in the Behavioral Laboratory*, edited by B. Weiss, pp. 99–140. Appleton-Century-Crofts, New York.
281. Weiss, B. (1981): Microproperties of operant behavior as aspects of toxicity. In: *Recent Developments in the Quantification of Steady-State Operant Behavior*, edited by C. M. Bradshaw, pp. 249–265. Elsevier, Amsterdam.
282. Weiss, B. (1983): Behavioral toxicology of heavy metals. In: *Neurobiology of the Trace Elements, Vol. 2, Neurotoxicology and Neuropharmacology*, edited by I. E. Dreosti and R. M. Smith, pp. 1–50. Humana Press, Clifton, NJ.
283. Weiss, B. (1988): Neurobehavioral toxicity as a basis for risk assessment. *Trends Pharmacol. Sci.*, 9:59–62.
284. Weiss, B., and Cott, C. T. (1972): A microanalysis of drug effects on fixed-ratio performance in pigeons. *J. Pharmacol. Exp. Ther.*, 180:189–202.
285. Weiss, B., and Laties, V. C. (1962): Enhancement of human performance by caffeine and the amphetamines. *Pharmacol. Rev.*, 14:1–36.

286. Weiss, B., and Laties, V. G. (1963): Effects of amphetamine, chlorpromazine and pentobarbital on behavioral thermoregulation. *J. Pharmacol. Exp. Ther.*, 140:1–7.
287. Weiss, B., and Laties, V. G. (1964): Effects of amphetamine, chlorpromazine, pentobarbital, and ethanol on operant response duration. *J. Pharmacol. Exp. Ther.*, 144:17–23.
288. Weiss, B., and Laties, V. G. (1970): The psychophysics of pain and analgesia in animals. In: *Animal Psychophysics: The Design and Conduct of Sensory Experiments*, edited by W. C. Stebbins, pp. 185–210. Appleton-Century-Crofts, New York.
289. Weiss, B., and Laties, V. G. (1975): *Behavioral Toxicology*. Plenum Press, New York.
289a. Weiss, B., and Elsner, J., eds. (1996): *Environ. Health Perspect.*, 104:suppl. 2:171–412.
289b. Weiss, B., and Reuhl, K., (1994): Delayed neurotoxicity: A silent toxicity. In: *Handbook of Neurotoxicology. Approaches and Methods for Neurotoxicology*, edited by L. Chang, pp. 765–84. New York: Dekker.
290. Wenger, C. R. (1985): The effects of trialkyl tin compounds on schedule-controlled behavior. In: *Behavioral Pharmacology, The Current Status*, edited by L. S. Seiden and R. L. Balster, pp. 503–518. Alan R. Liss, New York.
291. Wenger, C. R., McMillan, D. B., and Chang, L. W. (1984): Behavioral effects of trimethyltin on two strains of mice. II. Multiple fixed-ratio, fixed interval. *Toxicol. Appl. Pharmacol.*, 73:89–96.
292. Wetzell, M. C., and Howell, L. C. (1981): Properties and mechanisms of locomotion. In: *Handbook of Behavioral Neurobiology, Vol. 5, Motor Coordination*, edited by A. L. Towe and B. S. Luschel, pp. 567–625. Plenum Press, New York.
293. Whishaw, I. Q., Dringenberg, H. C., and Pellis, S. M. (1992): Spontaneous forelimb grasping in free feeding by rats: Motor cortex aids limb and digit positioning. *Behav. Brain Res.*, 48:113–125.
293a. Whishaw, I. Q., Gorny, B., and Sarna, J. (1998): Paw and limb use in skilled and spontaneous reaching after pyramidal tract, red nucleus and combined lesions in the rat: Behavioral and anatomical dissociations. *Behav. Brain Res.*, 93:167–183.
294. Williams, C. D. (1959): The elimination of tantrum behavior by extinction. *J. Abnorm. Soc. Psychol.*, 59:269.
295. Williamson, A. M., and Teo, R. K. C. (1986): Neurobehavioral effects of occupational exposure to lead. *Br. J. Ind. Med.*, 43:374–380.
296. Winneke, C. (1979): Behavioral effects of methylene chloride and carbon monoxide as assessed by sensory and psychomotor performance. In: *Behavioral Toxicology*, edited by C. Xintaras, B. L. Johnson, and I. deCroot. U.S. Department of Health, Education and Welfare, Washington, DC, Publication No. 74-126.
296a. Winneke, C., Brockhaus, A., and Baltissen, R. (1977): Neurobehavioral and systemic effects of long-term blood lead elevation in rats. I. Discrimination learning and open-field behavior. *Arch. Toxicol.*, 37:247–263.
296b. Winneke, C., and Kraemer, U. (1984): Neuropsychological effects of lead in children: Interactions with social background variables. *Neuropsychobiology*, 11:195–202.
297. Wolthuis, O. L., and Vanwersch, R. A. P. (1984): Behavioral changes in the rat after low doses of cholinesterase inhibitors. *Fundam. Appl. toxicol.*, 5:5195–5208.
298. Wood, R. W. (1979): Behavioral evaluation of sensory irritation evoked by ammonia. *Toxicol. Appl. Pharmacol.*, 50:157–162.
299. Wood, R. W. (1981): Determinants of irritant termination behavior. *Toxicol. Appl. Pharmacol.*, 61:260–268.
300. Wood, R. W. (1982): Stimulus properties of inhaled substances: An update. In: *Nervous System Toxicology*, edited by C. L. Mitchell, pp. 199–212. Raven Press, New York.
301. Wood, R. W., and Coleman, J. B. (1984): Behavioral evaluation of the irritant properties of formaldehyde. *Toxicologist*, 4:119.
302. Wood, R. W., Grubman, J., and Weiss, B. (1977): Nitrous oxide self-administration by the squirrel monkey. *J. Pharmacol. Exp. Ther.*, 202:491–499.
302a. Wood, R. W., Rees, D. C., and Laties, V. G. (1983): Behavioral effects of toluene are modulated by stimulus control. *Toxicol. Appl. Pharmacol.*, 68:462–472.
303. Wood, R. W., Weiss, A. B., and Weiss, B. (1973): Hand tremor induced by industrial exposure to inorganic mercury. *Arch. Environ. Health*, 26:249–252.
303a. Wood, R. W., and Colotla, V. A. (1990): Biphasic changes in mouse motor activity during exposure to toluene. *Fundam. Appl. Toxicol.*, 14:6–14.
304. Yanai, J. (1984): *Neurobehavioral Teratology*. Elsevier, Amsterdam.
305. Yule, W., Lansdown, R., Millar, I. B., and Urbanowicz, M. (1981): The relationship between blood lead concentrations, intelligence, and attainment in a school population: A pilot study. *Dev. Med. Child Neurol.*, 23:567–576.
306. Zenick, H., and Goldsmith, M. (1983): Drug discrimination learning in lead-exposed rats. *Science*, 212:569–571.
307. Ziriax, J. M., Snyder, J. R., Newland, M. C., and Weiss, B. (1993): D-amphetamine modifies the pattern of concurrent behavior. *Exper. Clin. Psychopharmacol.*, 1:1–12.

Principles and Methods of Toxicology, Fourth Edition, edited by A. Wallace Hayes.
Taylor & Francis, Philadelphia © 2001.

Chapter 33

Application of Isolated Organ Perfusion Techniques in Toxicology

Harihara M. Mehendale

The concept of employing organ perfusion for physiological and biochemical studies is not new. Early accounts of organ perfusion techniques in biochemical and physiological studies may be found in the descriptions of Baglioni (22) and Muller (219). More detailed accounts of the historical development of organ perfusion techniques may be found in the works of Brodie (41) and Embden and Glaüssner (81). Systematic early developments in organ perfusion techniques have been reviewed by Skutul (302) and Kapfhammer (142). Increasing interest in the application of the techniques of perfusing isolated organs and tissues in biochemical and physiological investigations is apparent in the more recent works of Ross (278), Diczfalusy (73), and Ritchie and Hardcastle (275). An interest in the applications of the isolated perfused organ techniques in the studies on the toxicological mechanisms (22,61,62,205–207,214,282,323) is apparent in the increasing number of reviews appearing in the literature. Some investigators have advanced the term "ex vivo perfusion" to refer to the technique of perfusing and maintaining functional isolated organs outside the animal body.

BACKGROUND

The rationale for experimental studies using perfused organs and for trying to improve the technology of organ perfusion lies in the following physiological and biochemical considerations. Homeostasis is recognized to be the outcome of many simultaneously occurring, interacting complex processes. It is recognized that when many simultaneously occurring processes interact, they may collectively take on functional properties that cannot be perceived in any of the individual component processes. In endocrine and metabolic systems, a basic experimental question arises at the organ level: How does the organ's uptake or output of some toxic substance depend on the composition of the arterial blood reaching the organ? The technique of organ perfusion can, if certain conditions are met, permit one to make controlled concentration changes in the perfusing blood while observing the time course of the organ's response in terms of its uptake or output of one or more substances. This kind of experimentation has several advantages. Mathematical models based on some convenient equations can be constructed relating the nature of a toxic compound(s) and its concentration in blood. The nature of the substances produced as a result of biotransformation can be investigated and related to the specific organ, and the role of that organ in converting a substance into either a more harmful, less harmful, or a biochemically inert species can be effectively evaluated. Quantitative input on these pathways of biotransformation into the appropriate mathematical models can lead to the understanding and development of predictable values.

In the simplest terms, the essentials of isolated organ perfusion techniques are (a) the desirability of separating individual organs from the whole animal to permit the study of one in the absence of complex interaction by others; (b) the need for the tissue to be physiologically compatible to the in vivo situation; and (c) the desire to simulate the natural circulation through an organ. In the latter regard, the composition of the medium changes constantly, as in the whole body, at least with respect to the experimental toxic substance: Not all substances reenter the perfusion medium, nor are all substances entirely removed by the organ. Finally, an analytical study of the organ itself can be undertaken; artificial means of stimulating organ function may aid in magnifying the physiological role of, or effect on, the organ, thus enabling determination of such an interaction. Although use of autologous whole blood would be considered ideal for homeostatic mechanisms, partial or complete substitution with artificial medium is often necessary for technical reasons; nonetheless, an attempt is made to maintain the cell structure and function by following as many viability criteria as possible.

Choice of Donor Animal

A variety of factors may influence the choice of organ donor animals in perfused organ studies. Often the nature of the particular problem being investigated is the determining factor when choosing the experimental animal. Susceptibility or refractoriness to the toxic agent to be tested and the presence or absence of biotransformation pathways govern the selection of a particular species and often a particular strain. Other factors may influence the final selection of the experimental animal as well. Availability of pertinent background information in a particular animal model may compel the investigator in favor of that species in the interest of savings in time and resources. Availability, cost of animals, and maintenance or unique genetic characteristics may become important considerations. The rat has been most popular in this regard as a donor for perfusion experiments. Thus perfused heart (13,82, 196,218,225), liver (5,40,197,207,211), lung (50,177,240, 241,245,253), kidney (23,26,181,182), brain (8,86,87, 160,321), and pancreas (110,146,246,247,348) obtained from the rat have been employed by many investigators for a variety of biochemical studies. Larger animals employed in perfusion experiments include the cat (9,68, 80,98,149,248), dog (9,80,133,169,339,347), rabbit (9, 57,169,178,205,229,245,266,268,277), and monkey (9). Among the larger animals employed for perfusion experiments are calves (179), chicken (194), dogs (121), goats (195), pigs (79), and sheep (79,317).

All small animals have the disadvantage of small blood vessels, which pose difficulties in surgical procedures. In many instances the experimenter is interested in using autologous blood for perfusion, and small animals may not yield sufficient blood supply to prime the perfusion apparatus. The trend has been to utilize either diluted or reconstituted blood or completely artificial perfusion medium composed of natural or synthetic ingredients. Nevertheless, in a few instances the necessity of using autologous whole blood as a perfusate essentially eliminates the use of small experimental animals in perfusion experiments. Additional factors to be considered are the volume and number of the perfusate samples needed to carry out necessary analytical tests during the course of the experiment. These difficulties are clearly overcome by using large experimental animals. Large animals, however, have the distinct disadvantage of increased cost, on the one hand, and requisite chemicals, equipment, space, and other supplies on the other. Use of expensive isotopically labeled chemicals or limited availability of valuable samples of newly synthesized or isolated test drugs may make it necessary to restrict the perfusion experiments to organs from smaller animals.

Large or small, other considerations may also be important. Much fat, particularly in the abdominal areas of large animals or old small animals contributes to surgical difficulties. The presence or absence of some tissues, such as the gallbladder, which is absent in rat and present in the rabbit, might be an additional consideration. For the purpose of acquainting oneself with the techniques of organ perfusion, the size of the animal per se matters little. However, considerations of economy of space, equipment, small apparatus, and animal costs might make the choice of a small animal a prudent one. In view of these and other considerations discussed above, whenever possible, the rat is considered the animal of choice. However, it is important to bear in mind that most procedural and other technical considerations remain the same with minor modifications when a particular perfusion technique is intended to be applied to a large animal or to an animal of similar, larger, or smaller size.

In Situ and Isolated Organ Perfusion System

Isolated organ perfusion may be defined as the maintenance of an organ in vascular isolation from the rest of the tissues and organs of the body by mechanically assisted circulation of a suitable fluid through its vascular bed. In most cases, special apparatus is required, and each investigator has invariably adopted an individual approach to solving the technical problems associated with maintaining a particular organ in viable condition for a particular toxicological investigation. The resulting scattered literature and many technical variations introduced in the techniques of organ perfusion have, to a large degree, contributed to the difficulty of a newcomer to the field of isolated organ perfusion to readily adopt the application of these techniques toward investigating the special problems of toxicology. Often it is difficult to assess the merits of the available methods. Given the complexity of the problem, there is often reluctance on the part of some toxicologists to embark on isolated perfused organ studies, even in those areas of biochemical toxicology where these techniques offer unique and definitive advantages over other in vitro or in vivo techniques. Establishment of a set of standards for each organ perfusion system by an internationally composed committee might alleviate many of the problems arising out of infinitely varied perfusion techniques and methodology introduced by individual investigators in a scattered body of diverse literature.

One rather obvious prerequisite for isolated organ perfusion studies is that the organ to be perfused is capable of vascular isolation from the neighboring tissues, although physical isolation is not obligatory. A separate vascular bed is sufficient to ensure that only one tissue or organ is perfused in isolation. For instance, an organ may be perfused in isolation but may remain in situ, as in the case of lung (174), liver (31,120), intestine (144,250), or kidney (23). A principal advantage of perfusing the organ in situ is the time saved in surgical removal of the organ, thereby reducing the time of interrupted perfusion. An additional advantage is that it reduces physical damage to the organ, which may be inflicted during surgical removal of the organ.

Alternatively, the organ to be perfused may be physically isolated from the animal, as in the case of lung (137,231), liver (43,197,211), kidney (180,228), heart (218,225,301), intestine (78), and pancreas (110). The principal advantage of physically isolating an organ is the elimination of interactions between the organ being perfused and other tissues and organs present in the body. Although the vascular bed of the organ being perfused may be totally isolated, the endogenous substances being secreted may seep out of other tissues and organs and might come in physical contact with the organ being perfused, resulting in uncontrollable or even unanticipated interactions. Similarly, the compound being studied in the perfused organ may be secreted and absorbed by other surrounding tissues and organs through physical contact and hence may introduce experimental errors in the quantitative and qualitative aspects of the disposition of the toxic chemical being studied. Accuracy and reliability of mass-balance studies of toxic chemicals and hence the accountability of the test chemical and possible metabolites are vastly superior with isolated organ perfusion systems.

Advantages of Isolated Perfused Organ Techniques

Isolated perfused organ preparations offer several advantages over experimentation with intact animals. Perfusion experiments lend themselves to a definitive evaluation of the role of a particular organ or tissue in the disposition of endogenous or exogenous chemicals. Although experimentation with whole animal preparations may provide clues implicating a possible role of a particular organ in regulating the levels of a test toxicant or an endogenous substance in response to a toxicant, decisive conclusions may not be feasible. A case in point is provided by the studies (89) that reported the presence of γ-aminobutyrate in the lungs of rats and mice after these animals were injected with radioactive putrescine. This finding cannot be taken as conclusive evidence for the formation of γ-aminobutyrate in the lungs, as it could have been transported from other sites of synthesis. Isolated, ventilated, and perfused lungs (268) and other tissue preparations were used to determine if rat and rabbit lungs were capable of metabolizing putrescine to γ-aminobutyrate (242), establishing that the lungs of these species are devoid of the diamine oxidase necessary for this metabolism. Isolated perfused organ studies provide opportunities to decisively ascertain or reject such possibilities.

Unlike the in vitro homogenate preparations, intact organ perfusion studies allow the experimenter to retain the structural and functional integrity of the organ in question during such experiments. Unlike in the intact animal, perfusion experiments allow the experimenter to retain control over several experimental parameters, for example, perfusion pressure and blood flow; in the intact animals these measurements are likely to change during the course of an experiment, especially in response to administration of the chemical. The concentrations of endogenous or exogenous stimulatory substances and other factors can be under experimental control in isolated perfused organ studies. The isolated perfused organ would lend itself to a broader range of concentrations of the experimental drug to be used in the study. That is, concentrations of drug at which the intact animal would not be expected to survive can be tested in isolated perfused organs. Determination of accurate and complete mass-balance of the toxic chemical in question is possible throughout the perfusion experiment, as the compound must either be in the perfusate or the tissue, or be excreted via excretory fluids such as bile and urine. Binding of the test drug to the glassware, tubing, and other components of the perfusion apparatus may occur, but this possibility can be explored in blank experiments, in which the perfusion experiment is conducted without the organ, from which appropriate correction factors are derived; moreover, removal of such interfering factors is often technically feasible. Another advantage of perfusion studies is the availability of large blood or perfusate samples; thus complete qualitative and quantitative analyses of minor and major biotransformation products of the test compound are feasible, as the volume of perfusate used in these experiments can be controlled. A further advantage of perfusion experiments in comparison with whole-animal experiments is the feasibility of tests with smaller quantities of chemicals. This point is particularly noteworthy, as limitations of either the availability of small quantities of the toxicants or the cost of isotopically labeled newly synthesized compounds can be formidable.

Another advantage of perfused organ studies is the maintenance of appropriate membrane barriers, not only between vascular and parenchymal sides but also between individual cells; hence the natural constraints of intact organs are retained throughout the experimental duration. Evidence has made it clear that one may not be able to predict the qualitative and quantitative aspects of biotransformation of a test drug by intact organ based only on the results of in vitro experiments with homogenate preparation (202). Factors governing the generation and availability of cofactors and transport of substrate to the site of biotransformation influence the final results in the intact perfused organ (130,202,322). These factors can remain operative in perfusion studies unlike with other in vitro techniques, thereby enabling realistic extrapolation of the results to in vivo situations. Finally, no matter how determined, experimental results have to be interpreted and extrapolated to the in vivo situation, where intact organs interact continuously; such interpretation and extrapolation are made easier by use of intact perfused organs in toxicological investigations.

Furthermore, the cell-to-cell interactions are preserved in an intact perfused organ, which might be either missing or at least compromised in isolated cells or other in vitro incubations. It is known that gap-junctioning plays an important role in the regulation of cellular and tissue homeostatic mechanisms. Gap junctions would be preserved in intact perfused organs. The collagenase trypsin or other proteases used in procedures to isolate cells might alter the plasma membrane, thereby altering the permeability and even receptor characteristics of isolated cells. For example, in freshly prepared hepatocytes, glutathione levels are only half of the normal values. Some essential and critical differences between the tissue slice experiments and perfusion studies are also of interest in this regard. Whereas the perfusion of intact organs allows entry of the chemical through the endothelium, which would be representative of what happens in the intact animal, tissue slice incubations permit entry of chemicals directly into the parenchymal cells through a direct contact. Studies using tissue slice incubations might not represent the in vivo situation, as some chemicals may not be taken up through the endothelial barrier altogether or be taken up to a smaller extent. Hepatocytes or liver slices incubated with the calcium-channel blockers do not have any influence on cellular calcium, whereas the perfused liver is responsive to these same calcium blockers. The latter would be clearly more representative of the in vivo situation than the former.

Limitations

The present day state of the art allows maintenance of isolated perfused organ preparations with adequate physiological and biochemical integrity for only short periods of time. Clinically, advances have allowed maintenance of the kidney for several days for later physical transplantation in patients. These procedures require subambient temperatures to preserve organ function. Such techniques are not generally useful in toxicological studies, as maintenance of the organ at optimal functional level is a prerequisite for most toxicological studies. Hence the principal limitation imposed by the isolated perfused organ preparations is the short duration of study. Critical and vital organ functions deteriorate in isolated perfused organs with time. For example, isolated perfused lung preparations can be maintained for a maximum of only 4 h (198). Often it is not possible to determine the effect of therapeutic agents on lung tissue in such a short period of time. Similarly, isolated perfused liver preparations cannot be maintained for longer periods without compromising liver function (126,166, 245). A practical consideration of interest in this connection may also be the level of expertise required for setting up the perfusion experiments. Setting up and conducting successful perfusion experiments requires specially trained personnel in surgical procedures and the technical aspects of associated instrumentation. Unavailability of such personnel requires that the investigator allows time for training.

Often a principal argument in favor of isolated perfused organ studies is the maintenance of natural membrane barriers, the integrity of the intact cells, and the complex and dynamic interrelations between individual and groups of cells. For certain studies this argument may represent a limitation. The complexity of a whole organ deprives the toxicologist of access to individual reactions that occur within the organ. Compartments and permeability barriers may prevent substrates and chemicals from exerting effects that are known to manifest when the particular toxic agent is allowed direct access to the enzyme or organelle of interest. In vitro experiments with homogenate preparations and tissue slice preparations would be the obvious choice of techniques when dissection of individual transport processes and biotransformation reactions is the principal objective. The size of a single experiment and the time required to perform it may make organ perfusion far less efficient from the point of time and resources than in vitro preparations that demonstrate the same effects with less investment of time and resources. Another consideration is the availability of the experimental tissue or organs. Although access to valuable human tissues might be available, such access might be infrequent; and in any event, the available tissue would be limiting. Clearly, isolated cell techniques or other in vitro techniques have the advantages of maximizing the use of such experimental material when designing and carrying out such studies. Schimmel and Knobil (292) pointed out the greater efficiency of establishing an experimental fact with tissue slices than with isolated perfused organ. Finally, despite all the refined techniques of maintaining the organ in vitro in as near a normal state as possible, the resulting preparation may differ in some highly significant manner from the organ in vivo, limiting the interpretation and application of results obtained in the organ perfusion system.

Scope of This Chapter

The principal purpose of this chapter is to acquaint the reader with general principles and methods for the isolation and perfusion of selected organs from experimental animals. Accordingly, the following discussion represents simplified and often idealized procedures, so that a novice could apply perfusion techniques to toxicological investigations. Sufficient references are included to benefit those who are already engaged in perfusion of isolated organs and who seek advanced information. The principles governing the choice of isolated perfused organ studies, the experimental protocols (including the composition of perfusion medium, duration of perfusion, considerations of recirculation, or single-pass circulation), and other related aspects are given in the examples of perfused organ studies employed in toxicology studies.

Considerations of pumps and mechanical devices (31) used in perfusion of organs, application and testing of pharmacokinetic concepts to isolated perfused organs (245), and the mathematical considerations of single-pass studies in isolated organs (75,218) are available elsewhere. Similarly, use of radiolabeled microspheres to determine intraorgan and regional blood flows (246) may also be considered in isolated perfused organ studies. Excellent reviews on the application of perfusion techniques to biochemical studies (240), to the studies of reproductive endocrinology (73), and to other general consideration of perfusion techniques, especially in large experimental animals (238), are available elsewhere for those seeking detailed considerations of organ perfusion techniques.

METHODOLOGY

Isolated Perfused Heart

Since Langendorff (169) described a procedure for isolation and perfusion of dog or rabbit heart, heart has been the model for studying the effects of toxic agents on metabolism in muscle. A succession of investigators (7,14,34,41,57,218,244) have demonstrated the stability and versatility of the preparation. The original method of Langendorff (169) has survived with only minor modifications and remains the standard preparation on which toxicological studies are performed (7,18,20,71,83,94, 147,152,154,155,168,173,190,194,286,301). The use of isolated heart preparations for toxicity studies has recently been reviewed (7). A wide variety of species have been employed for isolated perfused heart preparations. Chicken (194), ferret (152), guinea pig (190), rabbit (20,95), and rat (83,147,168,173,286,301,346) are representative examples.

Two procedures have been used for isolated perfused heart preparations. One uses the aortic perfusion described by Langendorff (169), and the other uses atrial perfusion, in which the left atrium is cannulated. The Langendorff preparation perfuses the muscle of both ventricles, although only the left ventricle produces any tension by contracting against the closed aortic valve. The atrial perfusion method gives a "working heart" preparation: It allows the left ventricle to fill, which results in normal systolic and diastolic cycles. The perfusion described by Morgan et al. (218) and later improvised by Neely et al. (225) provides for the working heart circulation (196,296). Several studies have compared the aortic perfusion of Langendorff and the atrial perfusion working heart preparation. One advantage in the working heart preparation is the ease and accuracy with which myocardial performance can be quantified. In the Langendorff preparation, coronary flow and heart rate are the only available physical parameters of function. The working heart, on the other hand, has aortic output as a quantifiable parameter of function, although it is dependent on the heart achieving an aortic pressure of at least 100 cm H_2O. Anoxia, lack of substrate, poison, and drugs may be qualitatively and quantitatively tested on this basis. Linearity of oxygen and substrate uptake is an additional means of assessing function in this preparation; and together with easily observed abnormalities of cardiac rhythm, which may also indicate failure of the

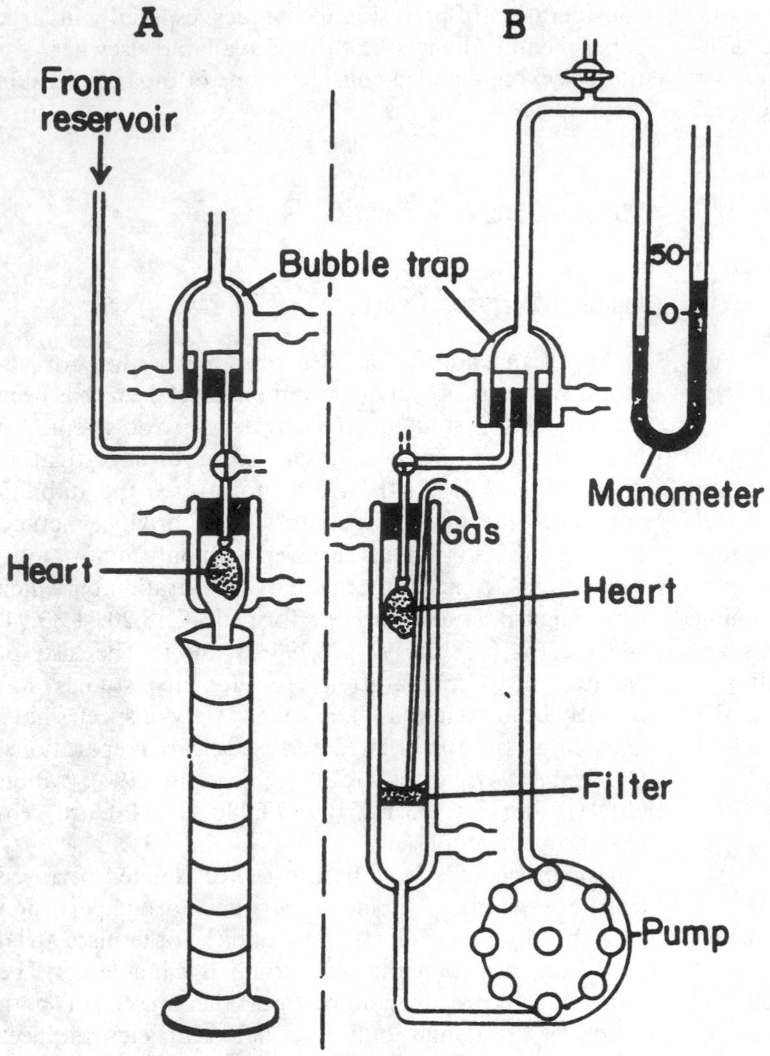

FIG. 33.1. "Langendorff" heart perfusion. **A:** Single-pass perfusion. **B:** Recirculating perfusion. From Reference 187, with permission.

preparation (82), the working heart preparation is easily and accurately assessed (168,196,296).

However, despite the completeness of description and advantages of the working heart, investigators in this field have experienced many difficulties in establishing a viable working heart preparation for significant lengths of time. Hence although quantitative differences do occur in many biochemical and functional measurements, the working and nonworking heart preparations are similar in many respects (158). Although with certain experimental protocols it is best to employ both preparations, it is doubtful if it will be necessary to carry out all toxicological tests on the heart in both Langendorff and working heart preparations. Because the former is so much simpler, its use will continue to be popular.

Aortic Perfusion

Apparatus. The heart is suspended in a water-jacketed cylindrical chamber of 3-cm diameter and 20-cm length with a coarse sintered-glass filter disk sealed into the lower portion (Figure 33.1). The aortic cannula is mounted in a Teflon stopper, through which pass the gas inlet tube and an outlet vent for the excess gases. The inflowing gas is delivered by means of a fine plastic tube extending into a small pool of perfusion medium, which collects on the surface of the sintered-glass filter. After passing through the filter, medium is recirculated by a peristaltic pump. This pumping arrangement results in a waveform applied to the heart, but it can be considerably dampened by passing the perfusate first through a bubble trap containing 1–2 ml of air so that the characteristics of the pump waveform may be eliminated.

Operation Procedure. Rats weighing approximately 250–300 g can be used for obtaining isolated heart preparations. The donor animal is killed by decapitation. It may be desirable to heparinize the animal by administering heparin intraperitoneally (5 mg) 1 h before decapitation to prevent formation of large clots. Within 20 s after decapitation, the thorax is widely opened by

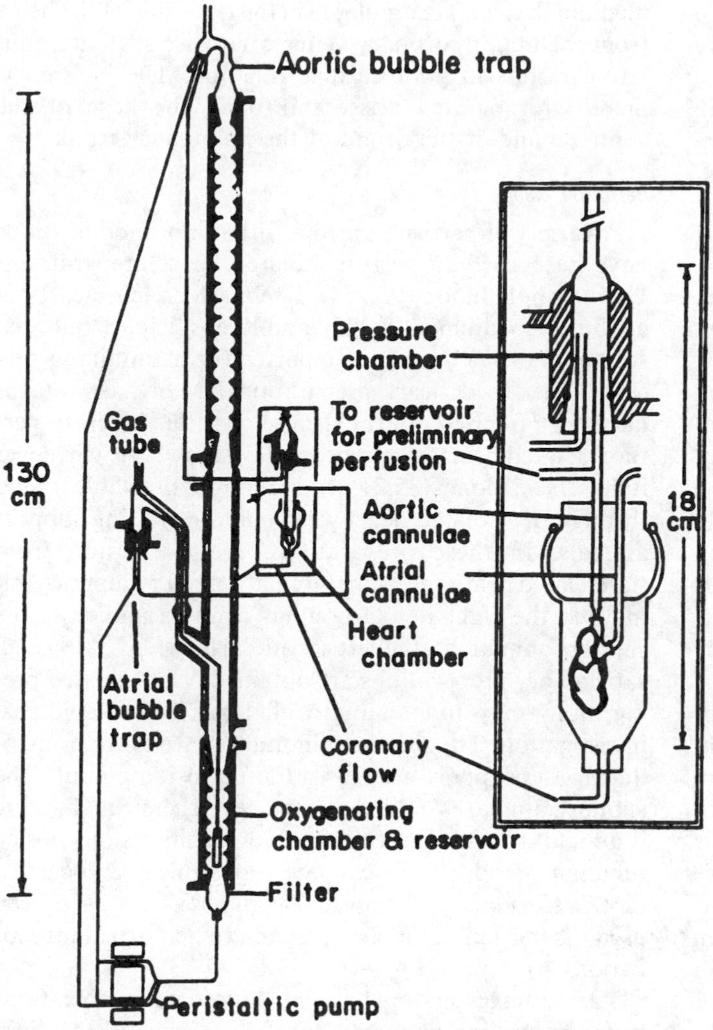

FIG. 33.2. Working rat heart preparation. Completely assembled apparatus is shown on the left. Heart chamber, cannula assembly, and pressure chamber are enlarged and illustrated on the right. The apparatus consists of the following components: The shaded portion of the glass apparatus indicates double-jacket arrangement for circulating warm water to facilitate warming the perfusate. Fluid in bubble traps and the pressure chamber is indicated by stippling. For other details refer to the text and Reference 192, with permission.

incisions to remove the anterior wall. The heart is removed immediately by means of a scissor cut across the great vessels about 5 mm from the heart. Earlier investigators (218) allowed a 1- to 2-min cooling period by immersing the heart in ice-cold Krebs–Ringer buffer solution. This step is not necessarily desirable, and in fact greater speed may help reduce the likelihood of anoxic damage to the heart. Ischemia and reperfusion give rise to the formation of toxic free-radical species that adversely affect the quality of heart preparations (143,157,346). After blotting the heart with filter paper and weighing it, a small glass cannula (or polyethylene tubing, PE-200) can be inserted into the aorta, with the tip of the cannula positioned just above the semilunar valves. The instantaneously beating heart is then perfused through the aortic cannula. The heart preparation is thus established may be allowed to equilibrate for 15–20 min by means of a setup in which the perfusate is allowed to recirculate (Figure 33.1). Oxygenation of the perfusate is accomplished using a mixture of oxygen and carbon dioxide (O_2/CO_2, 95 : 5) that is humidified by passing through water at 37°C before entering the apparatus to prevent loss of perfusate volume by evaporation.

Atrial Perfusion of the Working Heart

Apparatus. The apparatus for the atrial perfusion of heart (225) is shown in Figure 33.2. The glass components of the working heart perfusion apparatus are a double-jacketed oxygenator, a 100-cm bubble trap, a mixing column, connecting pieces, condensers, a 100-cm reservoir, a heart chamber, and a second bottle trap. The filter used is a closed Millipore system adapted from that used in ultrafiltration. For example, a Millipore in-line filter holder may be used. Whenever possible, tubing components are composed of glass; connections between glass tubings are made with flexible tubing, with the exception of the compression tubing used in the roller pumps, for which siliconized medical grade tubing may be used. The apparatus is assembled as illustrated in Figure 33.2.

Operating Procedures. A rat weighing approximately 250 g is lightly anesthetized with ether. Without preparation of the skin, the first incision is made with large, pointed scissors around the lower margin of the ribs. The first cut is made across the upper abdomen, taking care not to injure the liver. This cut is extended laterally, and for this purpose the rat may be held in the left hand. The point of the scissors is then directed toward the head, and a single cut is made through the layers of the thorax, including the ribs up to the clavicle. Cuts are made on the left side and the right side, producing a free flap of the anterior chest, which is removed with a cut transversely at the level of the second rib. At this time the heart is fully exposed. The heart is grasped firmly between the thumb and forefinger of the left hand and lifted, drawing it to the animal's right. This step exposes the pulmonary veins and the site of entry into the left atrium. The point of the scissors is passed horizontally and behind the left atrium, pulmonary veins, and aortic arch. Before closing the blades to cut, the instrument is drawn well over the animal's left to leave the maximum length of pulmonary vein in continuity with the atrium. After cutting the pulmonary vein, the scissors are pointed downward and away from the operator, and the aorta is cut about 0.5 cm from the ventricle. This length is adequate for cannulation. If the cut is made too near the heart, a hole is made in the left atrium, rather than through the pulmonary veins, which makes cannulation difficult.

The heart is thus removed and transferred rapidly to ice-cold Krebs–Ringer buffer, and aortic cannulation is carried out. The cannula is filled to the tip with oxygenated medium, making sure to avoid entrapping air bubbles. The aorta is grasped from opposite sides in two pairs of fine curved forceps and gently lifted over the straight cannula. The cannula may be retained by a single ligature around the aorta. It is important to watch that the tip of the cannula does not rest on the aortic valve because it is too far down the aorta. A flow of the medium at maximal rate is begun as soon as the ligature is tied, ending the unavoidable period of operative myocardial anoxia. The heart should begin to beat within 10–15 s of starting the perfusion.

Atrial cannulation may be conducted at leisure, as the heart is fully perfused via the aorta and is no longer at risk of anoxia. The atrial wall is grasped by forceps as it lies on either side of the cannula, and by turning the wrist outward the wall is slightly averted. The atrium is then drawn over the cannula itself. The cannula is positioned and retained in this position by means of a ligature. The final step is to incise the right ventricle and its pulmonary trunk, which allows drainage of the medium that has accumulated in the right side of the heart from the minor coronary veins; otherwise such accumulation results in poor cardiac function. The incision is made with pointed scissors through the base of the ventricle and at the origin of the pulmonary trunk.

Perfusion Media

A variety of perfusion media with minor modifications have been used to perfuse isolated heart preparations. Use of whole blood (95,254), Krebs–Henseleit bicarbonate buffer medium (218,225), and Krebs–Ringer buffered solution (14,57) have been reported for maintaining successful perfused heart preparations. Many advantages have been pointed out for the use of whole blood to perfuse isolated heart preparations (95). However, whenever it has been done (85,215), circulation of whole blood through the isolated heart was maintained using support animals. In these preparations, the circulation from the isolated heart enters the circulation of the support animal via the right jugular venous cannula and exits the support animal via the left carotid artery (95). Although satisfactory preparations are obtained, such isolated preparations may not adapt to all types of toxicological investigation. The principal limitation arises from introducing the support animal to the perfusion circuit. The support animal would clear the test chemical, making it difficult to correlate the effects of chemicals on cardiac function and to evaluate possible myocardial biotransformation. Hence artificial perfusates have been used most often in biochemical and toxicological investigations.

Various investigators have introduced minor variations in individual ion composition of the particular medium used in their own experimental setups. The medium of choice, however, seems to be the Krebs–Ringer bicarbonate-buffered solution of the following composition: NaCl 119 mM; KCl 4.75 mM; $CaCl_2 \cdot 2H_2O$ 2.54 mM; KH_2PO_4 1.19 mM; $MgSO_4 \cdot 7H_2O$ 1.19 mM; $NaHCO_3$ 25.0 mM; glucose 5.5 mM. The solution may be sterilized by ultrafiltration to avoid microbial contamination. If autoclaved, addition of glucose is withheld until later. Equilibration with O_2/CO_2 (95:5) for at least 30 min before using the perfusate increases the viability of the perfused preparation as well as the buffering capacity of the perfusate during perfusion. The pH of the medium is adjusted to 7.4 by means of a dilute solution of NaOH.

Viability Criteria

A number of functional, biochemical, and histological determinations have been used to ensure the viability and validity of the perfused heart preparation. Physical measurements of cardiac function include electrocardiogram (ECG) recordings of the left ventricular pressure and left ventricular end-diastolic pressure, and the perfusion pressure of the isolated heart preparations (95).

Table 33.1
Effect of perfusion on heart rate, coronary flow, and isometric systolic tension in the isolated perfused rat heart[a]

Perfusion time[b] (min)	Spontaneous No.[c]	Heart rate±*SE* (beats/min)	Coronary flow±*SE* (ml/min)	Isometric systolic tension (g)
0	32	285 ± 5.9	7.9 ± 0.4	13.8 ± 0.7
15	26	280 ± 5.2	7.8 ± 0.4	15.0 ± 0.9^d
30	26	270 ± 5.3^d	7.7 ± 0.4	14.3 ± 0.9
45	26	267 ± 5.0^d	7.8 ± 0.4	13.6 ± 0.9
60	26	270 ± 5.8^d	7.9 ± 0.5	12.6 ± 1.0^d
75	19	266 ± 6.0^d	7.9 ± 0.6	12.3 ± 1.2^d
90	19	263 ± 6.7^d	7.5 ± 0.6	11.4 ± 1.2^d
105	19	263 ± 6.7^d	7.3 ± 0.6	10.6 ± 1.2^d
120	19	262 ± 6.4^d	7.0 ± 0.5^d	9.6 ± 1.2^d
135	12	272 ± 8.6	7.2 ± 0.6	8.2 ± 1.4^d
150	12	272 ± 10.1	7.1 ± 0.5	7.7 ± 1.4^d
165	12	275 ± 11.0	7.3 ± 0.7^d	7.0 ± 1.4^d
180	12	265 ± 9.7^d	6.9 ± 0.5^d	6.4 ± 1.3^d
195	6	255 ± 10.2^d	6.2 ± 0.2^d	6.8 ± 2.0^d
210	6	245 ± 9.2^d	6.1 ± 0.6	6.0 ± 1.8^d
225	6	245 ± 9.2^d	5.7 ± 0.5^d	5.3 ± 1.7^d
240	6	245 ± 9.2^d	5.2 ± 0.5^d	4.8 ± 1.3^d

[a] Hearts obtained from untreated normal male animals.
[b] Duration of perfusion after initial 15-min equilibration period.
[c] Total number of measurements.
[d] Significant ($p < 0.05$) compared to zero perfusion time by paired variate Student's *t* test. From Reference 14 with permission.

Other functional parameters that can be continuously recorded include heart rate, isometric systolic tension, and coronary flow (14). Aronson and Serlick (14) examined the effect of perfusion time on a number of these parameters (Table 33.1). Changes in heart rate were evident 15 min after the end of the initial equilibration period. However, after being perfused for as long as 4 h, the heart rate was approximately 86% of the initial level, indicating the usefulness of the perfused heart preparation in toxicological studies. In contrast to the heart beat, coronary flow and isometric systolic tension (Table 33.1) appear to be more sensitive, as indicated by their decrease with perfusion time. A number of biochemical parameters can be examined in heart preparations as indices of viability (Table 33.2). Glycogen concentration was not significantly decreased until 3 h but decreased to 33% of the zero-time control values after 4 h of perfusion. Likewise, adenosine-5-triphosphate (ATP) concentrations remained stable for 3 h but significantly decreased in hearts perfused after 4 h. Creatine phosphate concentrations showed the greatest change during the lst hour of perfusion; it diminished to 51% of the amount present at zero time in the control group. After perfusion for 4 h, the creatine phosphate content of the tissue was 45% of the zero-time control value. Histochemical evaluation of heart preparations for viability can be useful initially in establishing the perfusion methodology (14). Tissues fixed by classical histological methods can be examined for evidence of inflammatory infiltrate, edema, or hemorrhage.

Applications

Although isolated perfused heart preparations have been used in a variety of ways to study the mechanism and interaction of various drugs and hormones (13–18,71,104,113), as well as in biochemical investigations (143,278), these preparations are not generally used to screen drugs or chemicals for potential cardiotoxicity. However, efforts (18,72,94,95,149,155, 157,196,209,264,265,296,346) have been directed toward using such preparations for toxicological investigations. For example, Autian (18) stressed the need for the development of reliable in vitro systems with which to screen large numbers of drugs and emphasized the advantages of using isolated perfused heart preparations. Gad et al. (94) used isolated perfused rat heart preparations to examine the inhibitory actions of the prooxidant butylated hydroxytoluene (BHT) on cardiac function.

Table 33.2
Effect of perfusion time on metabolite concentrations in the isolated perfused rat heart[a]

Metabolite	Concentration [b]$\pm SE$ (μM/g) at various perfusion times[c]				
	0 h	1 h	2 h	3 h	4 h
Glycogen	14.23 ± 1.25	11.83 ± 1.60	9.59 ± 1.60	5.44 ± 0.93[d]	4.75 ± 0.39[d]
D-Glucose-1-phosphate	0.0214 ± 0.0154	0.0142 ± 0.0141	0.0155 ± 0.0141	0.0018 ± .0	0.0062 ± 0
DGlucose-6-phosphate	0.0336 ± 0.0141	0.0480 ± 0.0109	0.0343 ± 0	0.0410 ± 0.0063	0.0532 ± 0.0134
D-Fructose-6-phosphate	0.0252 ± 0.0134	0.0096 ± 0	0[d]	0.0018 ± 0[d]	0.0052 ± 0
Fructose-1,6-bisphosphate	0.0380 ± 0.0161	0.0656 ± 0.0236	0.0248 ± 0.0091	0.0204 ± 0.0109	0.0258 ± 0.0118
D-Glyceraldehyde-3-phosphate	0.0750 ± 0.0218	0.0908 ± 0.0148	0.0626 ± 0.0276	0.0680 ± 0.0271	0.0732 ± 0.0373
Dihydroxyacetone phosphate	0.0438 ± 0.0271	0.0238 ± 0.0089	0.0320 ± 0.0091	0.0572 ± 0.0209	0.0134 ± 0.0077
Total triose phosphate	0.1188 ± 0.0223	0.1146 ± 0.0161	0.0946 ± 0.0294	0.1246 ± 0.0209	0.0866 ± 0.0313
L-(−)-Glycerol phosphate	0.1892 ± 0.0588	0.1764 ± 0.0331	0.2175 ± 0.0764	0.2326 ± 0.0399	0.4018 ± 0.1011
Pyruvate	0.0206 ± 0.0173	0.0146 ± 0.0099	0.0166 ± 0.0107	0	0.0300 ± 0.0299
L-(+)-Lactate	1.1458 ± 0.3296	0.6068 ± 0.1193	0.7733 ± 0.1505	0.6020 ± 0.0470	0.8980 ± 0.1961
Adenosine-5′-triphosphate	2.8882 ± 0.1258	2.4058 ± 0.2271	2.6448 ± 0.1670	2.3692 ± 0.1846	1.7400 ± 0.1290[d]
Adenosine-5′-diphosphate	0.1370 ± 0.0199	0.1688 ± 0.0503	0.1613 ± 0.0244	0.2118 ± 0.0354	0.2138 ± 0.0519
Adenosine-5′-monophosphate	0.0544 ± 0.0118	0.0776 ± 0.0138	0.0441 ± 0.0091	0.0364 ± 0.0126	0.0808 ± 0.0099
Total nucleotides	3.0796 ± 0.1174	2.6522 ± 0.1902	2.8503 ± 0.1650	2.6174 ± 0.1980	2.0346 ± 0.1140[d]
Creatine phosphate	3.7180 ± 0.1710	1.8866 ± 0.3085[d]	2.3355 ± 0.2002[d]	1.4494 ± 0.0885[d]	1.6766 ± 0.1698[d]

[a] Hearts were obtained from untreated control animals. Results are from five or six hearts in each group.
[b] Expressed per gram of tissue (wet weight).
[c] Duration of perfusion after initial 15-min equilibration period.
[d] Significant at 5% level when compared to zero perfusion time by an independent Student's t test. From Reference 11, with permission.

Cardiac contractility was depressed and leakage of creatine phosphate into the perfusate was found within 30 min of perfusion when BHT was included in the perfusion medium in concentrations ranging from 1–500 mg/L. Thus these investigations provided direct evidence that BHT depresses contractility and causes cellular damage of isolated heart as measured by the leakage of creatine phosphate from the myocardium.

Drug effects on myocardial contractile function are obviously of considerable practical importance for the toxicologist. The basic mechanism of such actions must reside at some point in the metabolism of cardiac muscle. Interference in the liberation of energy of the metabolic fuel utilized by the myocardial tissue may be implicated in many of the toxicological effects induced by drugs and other chemicals. For instance, chlorpromazine (50 ng/ml) decreased isometric systolic tension and prolonged the QT interval in the ECG of the perfused rat heart (18). Fructose-1,6-bisphosphate and pyruvate concentrations were elevated, suggesting aldolase inhibition and decreased pyruvate utilization. Anesthetic drugs that produce reversible depression of myocardial contractile function in a dose-dependent fashion have been shown to interfere with many of the mechanisms involving the generation and utilization of cellular energy in the heart tissue (209). Using ischemia and reperfusion injury model, 3 mM fructose-1,6-bisphosphate was recently shown to preserve higher concentrations of high energy bonds in the heart tissue, indicating the protective effects of this substrate (173). Use of isolated perfused heart preparations would be a valid and useful technique in toxicological investigations related to drug-induced heart disease (18,19,69).

De Wildt and Speijers (72) studied the effects of dietary rapeseed oil and pure erucic acid on the mechanical behavior of the isolated rat hearts after 24–26 weeks. Neither compound caused any effects on the ECG changes in comparison to the control sunflower seed oil diet. After inotropic intervention, only the rapeseed oil group showed less contractile reserve capacity. The authors concluded that a fat-rich diet might result in reduced myocardial function during a state of energy demand, and that the erucic acid effect must be on the peripheral vascular system.

A number of studies (83,85,154,157,173,222,346) have examined the role of oxyradicals on myocardial damage due to ischemia and reperfusion using perfused heart preparations. Koster et al. (157) demonstrated the release of malonaldehyde (MDA) in the coronary effluent of hearts perfused with cumene peroxide (0.5 mM), indicating susceptibility of the coronary vascular tissue preradical-induced lipid peroxidation. The possible role of oxygen free radicals in the development of reperfusion arrhythmias was investigated using a 10-min period of coronary ligation followed by reperfusion in the isolated rat heart (346). Glutathione (GSH) and a combination of superoxide dismutase, catalase, and mannitol reduced the incidence of reperfusion-induced ventricular fibrillation when given just prior to reperfusion. Because these oxyradical scavengers protected against the reperfusion-induced myocardial injury, such experiments have been employed to implicate the role of oxyradicals in reperfusion-induced arrhythmias (346). Ferrari et al. (85) induced ischemia in isolated, perfused rabbit hearts by reducing the coronary flow from 25 to 1 ml/min for 90 min. The effects of postischemic reperfusion were also followed for 30 min. These studies provided evidence that severe ischemia induces a reduction of the protective mechanisms, for example, GSH and protein SH groups and mitochondrial superoxide dismutase (SOD) activity. Reperfusion induces a massive release of reduced GSH, oxidized GSH (GSSG), and creatine phosphokinase (CPK), leading to a further decrease in tissue content of these important protective mechanisms, which in turn lead to loss of mechanical function. Interestingly, the CPK leakage associated with ischemia and reperfusion of the heart is augmented by arachidonic acid (143). In these studies the recovery of contractility was also suppressed by arachidonic acid (10 mg/ml). Arachidonic acid augmentation was protected by the antioxidant vitamin E, indomethacin, a prostaglandin synthesis inhibitor, and nordihydroguarietic acid, a lipoxygenase inhibitor, observations that are consistent with the preradical mediation of ischemia reperfusion injury of the myocardium. The studies demonstrated that isolated, perfused heart preparations have significantly advanced our understanding of the oxyradical involvement in myocardial injury.

Akahira et al. (4) employed the Langendorff preparation of the rat heart to study the effect of prazosin, an α_1 selective adrenergic antagonist, on H_2O_2-induced cardiotoxicity. H_2O_2 (600 μM) produced an increase in the left ventricular end-diastolic pressure, a decrease in ATP, and an increase in melonaldehyde levels. The mechanical and metabolic derangements were attenuated by 2.5, 5, and 10 μM prazosin, whereas the malonaldehyde formation was attenuated by 5 and 10 μM prazosin. Prazosin (up to 10 μM) had no adverse effects on the normal H_2O_2-nontreated perfused hearts. Nazeyrollas et al. (224) used the Langendorff constant pressure isolated rat hearts to test the protective effects of amifostine, known to possess free-radical scavenging properties, on doxorubicin cardiotoxicity. Amifostine at 10^{-5} and 10^{-4} M concentrations induced coronary dilation and protected against the cardiotoxic effects of doxorubicin (2.5×10^{-5} M).

Isolated, perfused heart preparations have also been employed to study mechanisms of specific chemicals (20, 83,147,154,168,194,196,220,222,286,301). McDonough et al. (196) employed the perfused working rat hearts to assess the intrinsic function after challenge with lethal or nonlethal doses of endotoxin to the rats. They concluded that the myocardial reserve was compromised by in vivo administration of endotoxin in a dose-dependent fashion. Bunc et al. (47) demonstrated direct cardiotoxic effect of equinatoxin II, a protein extracted from the sea anemone, *Actinia equina*.

Nahas and Trouve (220) employed Langendorff perfused rat heart preparations to assess the dose-response effects of cannabinoids on heart rate, coronary flow, and supra-aortic differential pressure (ΔP). Δ^9-Tetrahydrocannabinol produced a biphasic increase in heart rate without any change in coronary flow, but ΔP was increased. Studies of the toxicity of acetone (229), acrolein (263), allylamine (301), chronic alcohol consumption (266), dantrolene (103), cocaine (139), digitalis (149), doxorubicin (71,286), thioridazine-5-sulfoxide (113), *n*-hexane (147,265) and non-ionic as well as monomeric contrast media (20) have also been studied using perfused heart preparations.

For many toxicological studies it is necessary to determine the perfusate concentration of the experimental compound with time. It is also necessary to determine the appearance and disappearance kinetics of possible metabolites of the test chemical. As is true in the case of most perfused organ studies, these experiments can be carried out employing either recirculating perfusate or a single-pass mode. In most experimental protocols, it is prudent to determine in advance which mode of circulation will be used. It will also be necessary to determine the size of the perfusate sample needed to carry out the analyses and the time course and total duration of the experiment. As indicated in Table 33.1, many enzymatic determinations can be carried out in the perfusate and in the heart tissue itself.

Isolated Perfused Liver

The isolated perfused liver preparation has enjoyed the longest-standing attention in terms of functionally preserved isolated organs for biochemical, pharmacological, and toxicological studies. The views of Miller et al. (211) concerning the perfused liver is that functional performance of liver cells is best studied in the isolated liver perfused with continuously oxygenated whole, homologous blood under closely approximating physiological conditions. Earlier attempts to obtain viable, perfused liver preparations were marked by many problems, and in most cases the failure can be attributed to several factors (211): use of aqueous perfusion medium such as Ringer's solution in place of whole blood; lack of adequate filtering devices to remove tiny fibrin clots that plug the hepatic circulatory system; relative unavailability of effective, nontoxic anticoagulants such as heparin, which resulted in ominous failure to carry out perfusion for more than 1–2 h when whole blood was used as the perfusate. We have now witnessed the increased use of isolated liver preparations in a variety of pharmacological and toxicological investigations. Much credit for developing and standardizing isolated perfused liver techniques belongs to Miller et al. (211) and Schimassek (289).

There are two sources of blood supply to the liver: The portal vein supplies 80% and the hepatic artery 20% of the blood flow. Most workers have ignored the hepatic arterial supply when perfusing the rat liver. Although experiments confirm that the liver functions normally even in the absence of perfusion through the hepatic artery, techniques are now available that allow this small blood vessel to be perfused at normal arterial pressure, either under hydrostatic conditions (280) or by direct pumping (259). By and large, the rat has been the animal of choice for isolated perfused liver preparations (2,4,43, 44, 53,54,187,188,192,207,211,292,314,316,318,322, 324), although livers from other animals have been perfused for various investigations (9,54, 79,206,337).

Apparatus

In the technique of Miller et al. (211), the liver is perfused at a constant hydrostatic pressure using diluted rat blood as the perfusion medium, which passes through a glass multibulb oxygenator. The perfusate enters the portal vein via a filter and drains from the liver through the inferior vena cava either via an indwelling cannula or through a free cut of the vena cava; it collects in a bottom reservoir. From the reservoir it is pumped to the top of the oxygenator, which it enters through a filter. The liver is removed from the animal after the cannulation procedure, and perfusion is conducted by connecting the portal cannula of the liver to the preprimed circulation of the apparatus housed in an enclosed liver chamber.

The apparatus designed by Miller et al. has been almost universally adopted by workers using the liver perfusion technique, and the aparatus is also available commercially. The liver perfusion apparatus used in our laboratory (197) is based on the description of Miller et al. (211) and is illustrated in Figure 33.3. The perfusion chamber is kept warm by means of a heater–fan assembly that is thermostatically controlled. The original description of Miller et al. (211) noted use of a heating coil that traversed the inner surface of the chamber. Cleaning the chamber becomes difficult with this arrangement. Hence heating may be accomplished by installing a highly efficient heating coil inside a box, which would also house a fan (197). The glass multibulb oxygenator can be easily put together by connecting a series of 100-ml round-bottomed flasks (197). At the bottom of the multibulb glass oxygenator an inlet is provided for oxy-

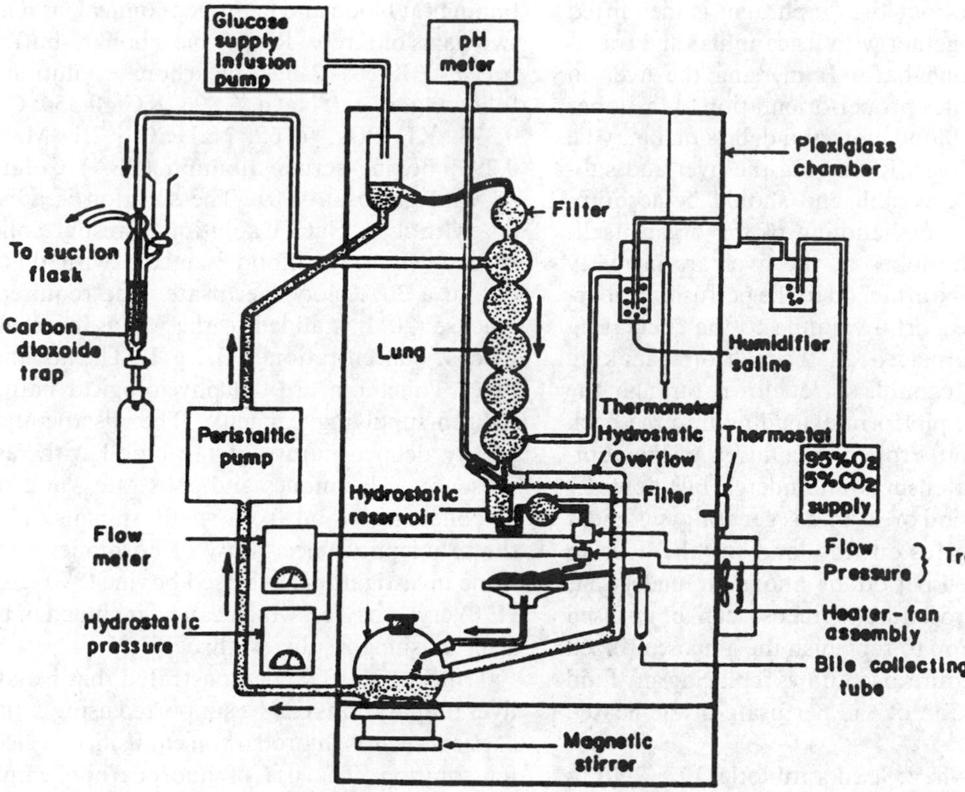

FIG. 33.3. Liver perfusion apparatus modified from that described by Miller et al. (181). The inside of the chamber is accessible via two overlapping sliding doors (not shown) in the front of the chamber. For other details refer to the text and Reference 168. From Reference 168, with permission.

gen supply, and at the top of the oxygenator a side outlet is provided for the carbon dioxide to escape. The bottom reservoir is provided with a number of side arms and a principal opening at the top to connect the platform that supports the liver. A magnetic stirrer can be introduced into the bottom reservoir, and a magnetic stirring device can be placed below the reservoir under the chamber. The perfusate can be pumped by means of a peristaltic pump to avoid hemolysis of red blood cells when either whole blood or diluted blood is used as the perfusate. O_2/CO_2 (95 : 5) is passed through a water trap to humidify the gas mixture. The expired gas escaping from the top of the multibulb glass lung is passed through a carbon dioxide trapping device. This phase is especially useful in studies in which either labeled carbon dioxide or other volatile metabolic products are expected to be formed. Efficient filtration of the blood perfusion medium is crucial for successful perfusion. Two disks of Lucite are compressed together to hold a disk of white silk (100 × 150 mesh per inch), and two such filters are introduced into the perfusate circulation to clear broken cells, tiny fibrin clots, and any other debris in the perfusate.

Surgical Procedure

Surgical removal of the liver from the rat should be performed under ether anesthesia. With the animal lying on its back, the limbs are fixed in extension on a surgical board. The anterior abdomen is cleaned with 75% alcohol, and a ventricle longitudinal midline incision is made extending from pubis to upper chest. The common bile duct is cannulated with PE-10 tubing. The animal is heparinized with 1000 units of sodium heparin by injecting the solution into the inferior vena cava anterior to the renal vein. Immediately after the injection the vena cava is ligated anterior to the site of injection. The portal vein is then cannulated with a PE-240 or a smaller cannula filled with the perfusate. An incision can be made in the thoracic vena cava using a PE-240 cannula. A loose ligature is placed around the inferior vena cava, and the outflow cannula is inserted through the right atrium. The inferior vena cava is cut between the heart and the cannula. The liver is then dissected together with the diaphragm. Some investigators have suggested an incision through the anterior diaphragm, leaving only a collar of the diaphragm attached to the inferior vena cava.

The liver with or without the diaphragm is then lifted free of the abdomen together with its cannulas and transferred to a warm saline bath. Immersing the liver in the warm saline facilitates proper orientation of the lobes as well as cleaning the blood clots and debris that may be on the surface of the liver. Removing the liver and subsequent handling requires skill and should be accomplished with a minimum of handling of the organ itself. After ensuring that the lobes of the liver are properly oriented, the liver may be attached to the perfusion apparatus by connecting the portal cannula to the circulating perfusate. The liver is placed on the platform, making sure that the outflow cannula is let down through the central porthole of the platform extending into the neck of the bottom reservoir. Proper orientation of the common bile duct cannula ensures unhindered bile flow.

An equilibration period of 30 min is generally sufficient to establish proper perfusion flow and for the liver to recover from the brief period of anoxia it underwent during the surgical procedure. Glucose can be infused throughout the perfusion to replenish the glucose utilized by the liver. This procedure also allows replacing any fluid losses due to evaporation of the perfusate in the heated chamber (187).

Earlier investigators have used antibiotics (211,290) to prevent bacterial growth in the perfusate during the course of the perfusion. In many toxicological studies, it is important to keep the perfusion system free of drugs in view of possible drug interactions. Most pieces of the perfusion apparatus can be autoclaved and sterilized. The perfusion chamber can be surface-sterilized using 75% ethanol. Other items that do not permit autoclaving can also be surface-sterilized with 75% ethanol. For instance, the perfusion flow transducer, pressure transducer, pH probe, and polyethylene cannulas and filters can be surface-sterilized using ethanol. Use of antibiotics to obtain viable preparations up to 6 h has not been necessary under these conditions (197).

Perfusion Media

Miller et al. (211) used a medium of fresh, heparinized rat blood diluted with Ringer's solution to a hematocrit of 25–40%. By far most variations introduced into a liver perfusion system are due to the differences in the composition of perfusate used. Whole rat blood would be the ideal physiological perfusate. Advantages of including whole blood are implicit in having hemoglobin and a natural oxygen carrier as well as natural protein and lipids to provide binding and carrier sites for experimental drugs. However, economic limitations often make use of whole rat blood as a perfusate impractical. Moreover, certain experimental protocols such as single-pass studies utilize large volumes of perfusate, and use of whole blood becomes exceedingly expensive and impractical. The following blood perfusate has the advantages of containing rat blood and being economical, as it is mixed with two parts of Krebs–Ringer bicarbonate-buffered solution (pH 7.4). Krebs–Ringer bicarbonate solution includes the following, in g/l: NaCl, 6.896; KCl, 0.354; $CaCl_2 \cdot 2H_2O$, 0.373; KH_2PO_4, 0.162; $NaHCO_3$, 2.1; $MgSO_4 \cdot 7H_2O$, 0.293; bovine serum albumin (BSA) Cohn fraction V 45; and glucose, 0.901. The solution is adjusted to pH 7.4 with 1 N NaOH solution. Freshly collected heparinized whole rat blood is mixed with this solution to obtain a 30% blood perfusate. The required volume of glucose (20%) is added to the perfusate to obtain a final glucose concentration of 3.2 g/L. The advantages of this type of medium are the physiological nature and high oxygen-supplying capacity. The disadvantages are the poorly defined nature of the blood with respect to the presence of hormones and substrates, and the difficulty of collecting blood from small animals. To circumvent the problem of uncertainty of hormones and substrates, some investigators have used bovine (290–292) or human (120) erythrocytes, which can be included in the perfusate after washing of the erythrocytes.

Triner et al. (328) demonstrated that isolated perfused liver preparations can be supported using artificial oxygen carriers such as fluorocarbon emulsified in electrolyte buffer solution. The use of fluorocarbon emulsion in the perfusion of isolated organs has a number of advantages over erythrocyte suspension. Avoidance of possible antigenicity from nonautologous erythrocytes and simpler, more standardized, less expensive preparations of perfusion media are among the advantages. In experiments comparing the adequacy of fluorocarbon emulsions to replace erythrocytes in the perfusate, three kinds of fluorocarbon were evaluated (107,236,328). Urea nitrogen, glucose, sodium, potassium, and alanine aminotransferase in the medium (and incorporation of ^{14}C-lysine into the liver proteins) were found to be either normal or above normal compared to perfusate containing erythrocytes (236) when fluosol-43 was used as the fluorocarbon oxygen carrier. Using fluorocarbon FC-47 emulsified in Krebs–Ringer bicarbonate-buffered solution, Goodman et al. (107) found that oxygen consumption, alanine aminotransferase level, gluconeogenesis, production of lactate and ketone bodies, and hepatic ATP concentrations were no different than when buffer or a medium containing suspended erythrocytes was used as perfusate. The cytosolic and mitochondrial redox states, as indicated by the hepatic lactate/pyruvate and β-hydroxybutyrate/acetic acid ratios, respectively, were also the same whether the medium contained erythrocytes or FC-47 (107).

Because of the varieties of perfusion media used for liver perfusion by various investigators (28,40,197, 207,211,322,323), it is prudent to select the most appropriate perfusion medium for a particular experimental protocol. The variables include the presence or absence of bovine or other serum albumin, erythrocytes, buffering agents, amino acids, glucose, vitamins, antibiotics, and heparin. These conditions in combination may or may not be appropriate for the particular experimental design. A study designed to examine the utilization of externally provided GSH may not be valid if bovine serum albumin (BSA) is included in the perfusion medium (138). GSSG is oxidized rapidly ($t_{\frac{1}{2}}$ 10 min) in Krebs–Ringer bicarbonate medium containing BSA (138). Replacing the albumin with high-molecular-weight dextran was found to preserve the GSSG. A perfusion system designed to study Ca^{2+} fluxes from the liver may not contain albumin or hemoglobin, as the ion-selective electrode used for measuring the change in perfusate Ca^{2+} might not be compatible with these constituents (207).

Viability Criteria

Certain viability criteria can be readily used to evaluate the perfused liver. For instance, bile flow can be used as a viability criterion. Here 1–1.5 μl/min/g of liver can be expected from a normal rat liver, which can change depending on the experimental conditions. Bile flow can be expected to drop with time of perfusion, as the endogenous bile acid pool would be depleted during bile collection. Some investigators have used an infusion of sodium taurocholate in the perfusate to maintain the bile flow throughout the perfusion.

Another easily recognizable viability criterion is the perfusion flow rate. At a hydrostatic pressure of 15–20 cm H_2O, a flow rate of up to 60 ml/min can be obtained using diluted (30%) blood as perfusate. Even after allowing for a lower viscosity of the perfusate, this flow rate would be judged to be beyond the normal physiological range. Hence the perfusion flow rate should be controlled by means of a suitable clamp placed between the portal cannula and the hydrostatic reservoir. Once a stable flow is attained, the flow rate through the liver can be used as a readily available criterion for evaluating the viability of the organ.

Another easily detectable criterion is visual examination of the liver. Inadequately perfused liver gives a reddish appearance, indicating anoxia, as well as a blotchy appearance on the surface of the liver. Often, if the liver is not secured on the platform, the liver moves in such a way as to impede proper, continuous, uniform perfusion through the organ. The liver may move such that the flow through the outflow cannula may be impeded, resulting in swelling of the liver. Visually, this problem is easily recognized by the tensile and anoxic appearance of one or more lobes of the liver.

Oxygen consumption by the liver can be used as another criterion for viability. For instance, Schimassek (289) reported that oxygen consumption by the perfused liver was 2.2 nmol/min/g of tissue after the 30-min equilibration period, and it was maintained at this level thereafter. Oxygen consumption can be measured by following the oxygen tension of the perfusate before it enters the liver and sampling the oxygen content of the perfusate after it effuses from the liver (197).

A number of biochemical parameters can be used for ascertaining the viability of the perfused liver. Schimassek (290) has shown that isolated perfused livers under standard conditions have glycolytic intermediate concentrations, a respiratory quotient, and adenine nucleotide levels close to those found in the liver fresh out of the animal (Table 33.3). Such measurements in the isolated perfused liver preparation have allowed investigators to determine normal conditions of perfusion. A variety of other biochemical parameters have also been determined in isolated perfused liver preparations to establish the physiological validity of using such a preparation (164). Miller et al. (211) determined incorporation of ^{14}C-lysine into hepatic proteins as a biochemical index of optimum macromolecular synthetic activity during perfusion. Bock et al. (36) measured a number of biochemical parameters associated with the microsomal mixed function oxidase (MFO) and cytochrome P450 (CYP) system and found satisfactory preservation of the hepatic MFO system after 4 h of perfusion when erythrocyte-containing perfusate was used. Biliary excretion of sulfobromophthalein (BSP) and indocyanine green have also been used as measures of functional status. The disadvantage of using these markers for functional status is that the same perfused livers cannot be used for toxicological investigations after establishing that these livers are indeed viable. These tests are helpful for evaluating isolated perfused liver preparations, establishing the procedure, and subsequently evaluating the functional status of the liver preparations after treating with an experimental toxic agent. Phenolphthalein glucuronide (PG) has been used as a marker of biliary excretory function (207). The advantages of using PG are that it requires no further metabolism, it can be used at low concentrations, and it is sensitive for detecting hepatobiliary dysfunction and so can be used in livers being perfused for toxicological investigations (201,207).

Although histological examination of perfused livers is not done routinely, the technique is useful for setting up a perfused preparation. Several authors (40,285,290) have reported results of histological examinations of perfused livers, indicating the general usefulness of morphological examination in ascertaining the viability of perfused liver preparations. However, one should be aware that morphological examinations may be of limited usefulness, as cells that appear abnormal morphologically may exhibit normal cellular function; and conversely, normal-appearing cells may exhibit abnormal cellular functions (40,211). Oomen and Chamalarun (243) reported an excellent correlation between biochemical

Table 33.3
Substrate content of isolated, perfused rat liver after various times of perfusion[a]

Metabolite	In vivo	Before perfusion	After 30 min perfusion	After 120 min perfusion
	Content (μmol wet wt. of liver) under various conditions			
Lactate (L)	1450	12,000	3570	3400
Pyruvate (P)	145	50	277	345
α-Glycero-P	253	1560	304	450
DAP	38	21	45	67
Malate (M)	443	750	281	280
Oxaloacetate (O)	7	<1	4.2	4
FDP	22	17	20	41
F-6-P	75	—	—	41
G-6-P	370	986	141	206
Glucose	8600	25,900	11,600	11,000
Glycogen	340,000	320,000	214,000	185,000
AMP	300	—	209	280
ADP	900	1853	684	620
ATP	2900	710	2270	2060
L/P	10	239	13	10
G/D	6.7	72	6.7	6.5
M/O	64	—	70	70
ATP/ADP	3.3	0.4	3.3	3.3

[a]Adapted from Reference 323.

and histological parameters in their isolated perfused rat liver preparations.

Applications

Depending on the experimental protocol, the isolated perfused liver preparation can be used in either a single-pass or a recirculating mode (197,207,326). Many examples can be cited for the use of isolated perfused liver preparations in the evaluation of toxic responses to a variety of chemicals. It is instructive to consider a few examples of isolated perfused liver preparations in toxicological investigations (27,41,44,96,105,132,150, 167,175,191,192,199,201,207,210,214,223,226,263,270, 274,283,287,304,316,318,320,322,334,337). Only a few of these will be discussed. Rice et al. (274) employed isolated perfused rat liver preparations to determine the effect of carbon tetrachloride (CCl_4) administered in vivo on the hemodynamics of the liver. Portal blood pressure and flow were recorded in perfused livers from either control or treated animals. The study concluded that although the primary lesion caused by CCl_4 was hepatocellular damage, subsequent effects included increased vascular resistance and enhanced response to norepinephrine. Masuda and Yamamori (192) employed the perfused liver to determine if bromotrichloromethane-induced cell necrosis can be differentiated from lipid peroxidation. Their study provided histological evidence for dissociation of lipid peroxidation from hepatocellular necrosis induced by this halomethane. Ambs et al. (6) investigated acute and chronic toxicity of aromatic amines in the isolated perfused rat liver. 2-Acetylaminofluorine (2-AAF) and its principal metabolites were not toxic in the range of 200–400 μM concentration in a 2-h exposure to perfused male Wistar rat livers. *N*-acetyl-2-AAF was, however, severely toxic. Chronic effects of feeding 2-AAF (0.02% in the diet) for up to 12 weeks were also studied. Excretion of glutathione in bile was drastically reduced after 5 or more weeks, increasingly less glucose was released in the perfusate, and O_2 consumption was constantly increased by 20% after 3 weeks of 2-AAF feeding. The authors suggested that these effects were adaptive responses to the toxicity of 2-AAF and may be related to the promoting properties of this carcinogen. Iwamoto et al. (132) used perfused rat liver to establish the decreased intrinsic hepatic clearance of propranolol in CCl_4-injured liver. Another study investigated the hepatic elimination of galactose in CCl_4-injured liver (334). Bullock et al. (46)

utilized isolated perfused rat liver preparations to examine the effects of two fungal toxins, sporidesmin and icterogenin, on the mechanisms of bile secretion. Electron microscopic examination of livers perfused with these two toxins indicated that the cholestatic reaction was due to changes in canalicular membranes, which included extrusion of material into the canalicular lumen and aggregation of lysosomes in the cytoplasm. Abraham et al. (1) examined the effect of hyperoxia on lysosomal enzymes using perfused liver preparations.

Colantoni et al. (60) investigated reoxygenation injury in isolated perfused rat livers. Employing 60 min of hypoxia followed by 30 min of reoxygenation, lactate dehydrogenase (LDH) release, protein and carbonyl content, and melondialdehyde production were significantly decreased in livers perfused with 2 mM salicylate. In another study (162), cold ischemia-reperfusion injury was investigated using isolated perfused rat liver preparations. The objectives were to investigate whether the inactivation of Kupffer's cells by gadolinium chloride modulates cold ischemia-reperfusion liver injury and whether cold storage of rat liver involves injury to biliary epithelial cells. The authors concluded that cold ischemia-reperfusion liver injury of rat liver is mediated by both Kupffer's cells-dependent and -independent mechanisms and cold storage of rat liver induces functional impairment of biliary epithelial cells.

Radwan and Henschler (263) employed isolated liver preparations to study the uptake and metabolism of the hepatocarcinogen, vinyl chloride. Using erythrocyte-suspension perfusion medium, they found that the solubility of vinyl chloride stayed constant at concentrations of 50–25,000 ppm. The amount metabolized, as determined by the difference between vinyl chloride concentration before and after passage through the liver, was constant at 14.6% of the 50–25,000-ppm concentrations. Ethanol (12 mM) and pyrazole (200 mM) decreased the metabolism of vinyl chloride, which was also modified by prior exposure of the animals to other inducing and inhibiting agents. It was concluded that vinyl chloride underwent a metabolic transformation via mixed function oxidation to reactive metabolites. This study represents how perfused liver preparations can be used to determine the metabolism of even volatile substances.

Lemaster et al. (175) used perfused liver to study hypoxic hepatocellular injury and concluded that shedding of cytoplasmic fragments resulting from the blebbing of centrilobular hepatocytes may represent a basis for the appearance of hepatic enzymes in the sera of patients with liver disease. Nastainczyk and Ullrich (223) used isolated perfused rat liver preparations to examine the effect of hypoxia on the metabolism of halothane. The study concluded that halothane was biotransformed via reductive in vivo metabolism to reactive intermediates when the oxygen concentration of the perfusate droped below a critical level (about 50 mM). These authors employed whole-organ spectrophotometry of isolated perfused livers to establish that a complex of a macromolecule and halothane was formed under slightly hypoxic conditions, and that metyrapone, an inhibitor of MFO reactions, abolished the formation of this complex.

Use of isolated perfused liver preparations in the metabolism of toxic substances as well as the effect of the toxic substances on hepatic function are illustrated by a series of studies in which the hepatobiliary function was examined after the animals had been exposed to toxic chemicals (199–201). In these studies the effects of exposure to the chlorocarbon pesticides, mirex and chlordecone (Kepone), were examined in isolated perfused liver preparations. Biliary excretion of the anionic model compounds, BSP and imipramine, was examined. These studies also illustrated the utility of isolated liver preparations in studying the biotransformation of chemicals. By assaying a series of perfusate samples as well as liver tissue at the end of a perfusion study, the metabolism of imipramine by control, as well as pretreated, livers was followed. Although both chlordecone and mirex were known to be inducers of hepatic MFOs, these experiments revealed that biliary excretion of endogenously formed metabolites of imipramine was suppressed by prior exposure to these chlorocarbons. The pattern of imipramine metabolism indicated that the suppressed biliary excretory function was not related to alterations in metabolism of imipramine.

Other experiments (199,200), in which readily excretable polar metabolites of imipramine were introduced into the perfusate of control and treated liver preparations, indicated that biliary excretion of these metabolites was also hindered by prior exposure to mirex and chlordecone. Thus such experimental manipulations using isolated liver preparations were useful for evaluating the role of drug metabolism in hepatobiliary function. Isolated liver preparations can also be used to examine the role of hepatic uptake and metabolism in the disposition of toxic chemicals (198). In these studies the uptake, metabolism, and biliary excretion of polychlorinated biphenyls was examined using isolated perfused rat liver preparations. Similar preparations were useful in discovering the inhibitory effect of mirex on biliary excretion of polar metabolites of monochlorobiphenyl (200).

Choo et al. (58) employed the isolated perfused rat liver in single-pass perfusion mode to study whether certain drug metabolizing pathways were affected more than the others in hepatic cirrhosis. Using *p*-nitrophenol as a substrate for glucuronidation and sulfation, and *d*-propranolol as substrate for oxidative metabolism, the authors concluded that in cirrhosis, oxidative metabolism and sulfation are significantly impaired whereas glucuronidation is spared. The decreased sulfation is attributed to a decrease in sulfotransferase as well as to decreased cofactor (PAPS) synthesis. Hoffmann et al. (127) examined ^{14}C-phenol in isolated perfused mouse livers. These studies were conducted to determine if metabolic fate of phenol produced during benzene metabolism was different in the absence of benzene. Administration of benzene produced bone marrow depression whereas administration of phenol, a major metabolite of benzene, did not. Mouse livers were perfused orthograde (portal vein to central vein) or retrograde (central vein to portal vein) direction to investigate the metabolic zonation of enzymes involved in phenol hydroxylation and conjugation. It was found that a larger percentage of radioactivity released from the liver was unconjugated hydroquinone after benzene perfusion than after phenol perfusion, indicating that enzymes involved in the *p*-hydroxylation of phenol were located nearer to the central vein than those involved in conjugation. The amount of radioactivity covalently bound to liver macromolecules was measured after each perfusion and determined to be the amount of hydroquinone glucuronide detected in the perfusate samples.

In other studies, pharmacokinetics (123) and acute toxic action of diclofenac (105) and troglitazone (262) were studied in isolated perfused rat livers. Livers were perfused for 2 h with Krebs–Henseleit bicarbonate buffer (250 ml) containing either 10.75 mg or 1.075 mg of diclofenac, representing 100 and 10 times the therapeutic level. At the higher concentration liver injury (LDH release) was observed at 90 min. Neither alanine aminotransferase nor aspartate aminotransferase were released. The lower concentration did not elicit liver injury. The authors concluded that the therapeutic level of diclofenac is unlikely to have any direct toxic effects even at 100 times the therapeutic levels. Preininger et al. (262) investigated the effect of troglitazone, a thiazolidinedione compound used as an antidiabetic agent in type II (adult-onset) diabetes. It is known to enhance insulin action and reduce plasma glucose concentrations when administered clinically to type II diabetic patients. Acute actions of troglitazone (0.61 and 3.15 μM) on hepatic glucose and lactate fluxs, bile secretion, and portal pressure under basal and insulin-and/or glucagon-stimulated conditions in isolated perfused rat livers were examined. During BSA-free perfusion, high-dose troglitazone increased basal, but inhibited glucagon-stimulated incremental, glucose production by 75% versus control. Low-dose troglitazone did not enhance the inhibitory effects of insulin on glucagon-stimulated glucose production but rapidly increased LDH release and portal venous pressure. The authors concluded that troglitazone exerted both insulin-like and non-insulin like hepatic effects that were blunted by the presence of albumin due to binding to albumin. In another study, Villanueva et al. (335) investigated the effects of bile acids on the transport of cisplatin in perfused rat liver. Enhancing the excretion of the cytostatic drug cisplatin from the body is envisaged as a way of decreasing cisplatin toxicity. The objective of the study was to investigate if bile acids could be used to enhance biliary excretion of cisplatin. Urodeoxycholic acid (a highly choleretic acid), glycocholic acid, and chenodeoxycholic acid, the latter two being the micelle-forming bile acids, were chosen for the study. The authors concluded that even though bile acids (1 mM) induced an enhancement in the transport of cisplatin from the hepatocyte to bile, the net excretion of cisplatin in the bile was reduced.

Hadasova et al. (112) investigated the influence of immunosuppression on *O*-demethylation of dextromethorphan in isolated perfused rat liver. They examined the effect of cyclophosphamide and dexamethasone on CYP2D1-dependent metabolism of detromethorphan in isolated perfused liver from male Wistar rats. Although cyclophosphamide and dextromethorphan both increased the *O*-demethylation of dextromethorphan to dextrorphan, only cyclophosphamide caused significant changes in the increased rate of conversion of dextromethorphan to dextrorphan. These findings suggest that CYP2D-dependent metabolism might be promoted in immunosuppressant therapy of autoimmune and other deseases.

Thurman et al. (322) studied the kinetics of *p*-nitroanisole *O*-demethylation in hemoglobin-free perfused rat liver preparations. These investigators demonstrate that the rates of *p*-nitroanisole metabolism were linear for 30 min in normal livers but only 1–2 min in phenobarbital-induced livers. This reduced rate of metabolism could be reversed by infusing additional glucose, suggesting an intimate relation between drug and carbohydrate metabolism in the intact liver. Alteration in the rate of *p*-nitroanisole metabolism with various inducing agents of the MFO system produced parallel changes in rates of hepatic lactate production, reflecting the action of *p*-nitrophenol to uncouple oxidative phosphorylation. Thus these investigators were able to demonstrate that the reduction in the rate of *p*-nitroanisole metabolism in induced liver preparations was due to reduced availability of NADPH for MFO-catalyzed substrate oxidation. Using a similar noncirculating liver perfusion system, Belinsky et al. (28) employed trypan blue to investigate the regiospecific hepatotoxic response of the liver. Periportal hepatocellular injury after allyl alcohol infusion to isolated perfused liver was evident from stained nuclei only in the periportal zone. Takano et al. (313) described a technique similar to the one described by Thurman et al. (322), in

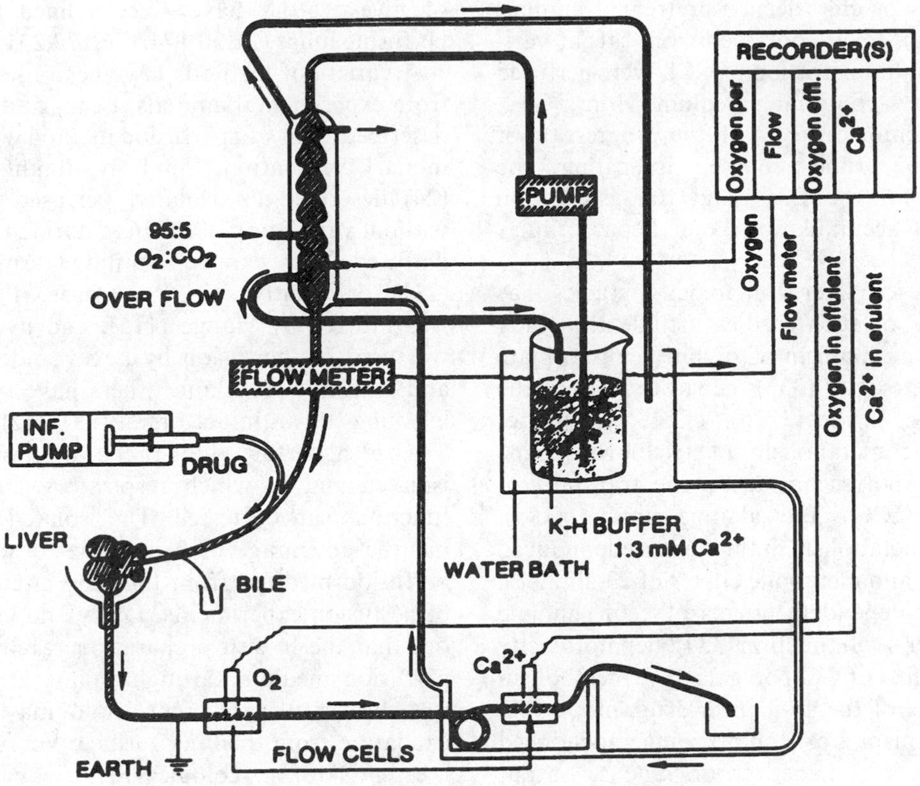

FIG. 33.4. Liver perfusion apparatus designed for on-line measurement of perfusate Ca^{2+} levels. From Reference 178, with permission.

which the dynamic effects of environmental agents on the hepatic drug-metabolizing system and on energy metabolism could be monitored in the perfused liver. Such experiments with intact liver preparations have provided valuable insights into what might be occurring in terms of drug metabolism under in vivo conditions. These results demonstrated that despite the induced status of the liver, enhanced drug metabolism may not necessarily be the end result, as other factors, for example, availability of cofactors, might become limiting and hence limit the quantitative aspects of drug metabolism.

There has been a significant interest in understanding the role of Ca^{2+} in chemical toxicity (287). Although it is generally agreed that a rising cytosolic Ca^{2+} level is detrimental to the cell, the source of the increased Ca^{2+} has been strongly debated (287,304). Because of the inherent disadvantages of working with isolated cells and organelles, intact perfused liver preparations offer the most suitable model. Such a perfusion setup, used by Mehendale et al. (207), is illustrated in Figure 33.4. Infusion of menadione elicited an increased oxygen utilization by the liver, followed by a decrease in the perfusate Ca^{2+}. Hepatic accumulation of Ca^{2+} was accompanied by stimulation of cytosolic phosphorylase a activity, indicating a rise in the cytosolic Ca^{2+} levels. A gradual recovery of perfusate Ca^{2+} to base levels was observed after cessation of menadione infusion. Leakage of LDH into the perfusate followed Ca^{2+} uptake, was not accompanied by a decrease in reduced pyridine nucleotide or ATP levels in the liver, as evidenced by measuring either during maximal Ca^{2+} uptake or after recovery. However, Ca^{2+} uptake was correlated with decreased GSH and increased GSSG levels in the liver, both of which reversed during recovery from Ca^{2+} uptake. The amount of protein-bound mixed disulfides showed a striking relation to Ca^{2+} uptake, reaching a maximal value during Ca^{2+} uptake and reversing toward normal during recovery from Ca^{2+} accumulation. Depletion of hepatic GSH with prior diethylmaleate treatment resulted in increased Ca^{2+} accumulation during menadione infusion. These findings suggested that menadione-induced Ca^{2+} uptake was due to plasma membrane dysfunction as a result of loss of protein thiol groups, which are critical for maintaining the plasma membrane Ca^{2+} extrusion mechanism. This perfused liver model is particularly useful for studying the mechanisms underlying toxic disturbances in Ca^{2+} homeostasis in intact liver, as Ca^{2+} fluxes can be monitored under conditions in which cellular control mechanisms are not obliterated by excessive toxicity. The perfused liver preparation have also been useful for establishing the extracellular origin of Ca^{2+} seen to accumulate in livers of chlordecone-pretreated animals treated with CCl_4 (2). Livers obtained from rats at various points after the administration of CCl_4 were perfused for 30 min with $^{45}Ca^{2+}$-containing medium. More $^{45}Ca^{2+}$ accumulation was demonstrated with the progression of toxicity during the time course, indicating the extracellular origin of the Ca^{2+} and the association between the Ca^{2+} accumulation and hepatocellular toxicity.

Use of the perfused liver for toxicity studies has increased. Examples of such studies include the study of hepatoprotective mechanism of silybin hemisuccinate on phenylhydrazine toxicity (333), hepatotoxicity of the hornet's venom sac extract (226), effect of ethanol pretreatment on the metabolism of trichloroethylene (338), effects of lipopolysccharide on the transport of indocyanine green (ICG) and alanine uptake (185), changes in nitrogen metabolism in thioacetamide-induced cirrhosis (193), toxic and metabolic effects of 23-aliphatic alcohols (308), dose-dependent effects of acute lindane treatment on Kupffer's cell function (334), hepatotoxicity of gossypol (187), effect of CCl_4 on galactose metabolism (336), hepatic uptake of the anticancer drug, mitomycin (188), the mechanism of chlorpromazine-induced cholestasis (5), effects of vanadate on glucose output by the liver (192), galactosamine (270,337), metabolism of acetaminophen by liver after overdosage (258), lipid peroxidation associated with acetaminophen toxicity (258), isolation and characterization of the metabolites of T-2 toxin (96), and the hepatotoxicity of several cytotoxic agents (210). One report (214) described a technique of in vivo isolated perfusion of the rat liver to study the effect of hyperthermochemotherapy with 5-fluorouracil for possible clinical application in treating unresectable liver cancer in patients. An example of the use of isolated perfused liver in evaluating the pharmacokinetics of drugs such as propranolol is also available (84,319). In recent studies, the uptake and excretion of taurocholate by isolated perfused neonatal sheep liver (109), kinetic modeling and toxicological implications of slow dissociation of bromosulfophthalein from albumin in perfused rat liver, (92) have been addressed.

Isolated Perfused Lung

The heart–lung preparation of Knowlton and Starling (153) has been used extensively to study the respiratory functions of the lung in small and large animals. However, refinement of the isolated perfused lung preparation technique was expedited only after the nonrespiratory functions of the lungs were recognized. Popjak and Beeckmans (255) employed a rabbit perfused lung preparation to examine oxygen and substrate incorporation into phospholipids of the lung tissue. A number of investigators have since refined the technique of perfusing lungs (21,50,174,176,177,231,237,238,239,307).

A variety of methods have been used to perfuse lungs from experimental animals. Leary and Ledingham (174) described an in situ perfusion method with or without pulmonary ventilation. Similarly, Bakhle and co-workers (24) described an isolated perfused lung preparation without ventilation of the lung during perfusion. Isolated perfused lungs can be ventilated using either negative (231) or positive (242) pressure. Pulsatile perfusion was utilized by Hauge (115), and hydrostatic pressure was used for perfusion by Levey and Gast (177). Gillis and Iwasawa (101) and others have perfused right and left lungs as an intact organ (231,242).

An ideal perfused lung preparation is one that is totally isolated and in which respiratory and nonrespiratory functions can be tested. The isolated lung preparation has the advantage of being able to account for all the perfusion medium from the lung circulation at the end of perfusion experiments. Levey and Gast (177) pointed out that the in situ preparation results in some loss of perfusion medium through collateral vessels supplying the chest wall, and some fluid may be lost through exudation from the lung surface. Ventilation of the lung is essential for toxicological investigations in which maintaining a physiological route of gas exchange is important. Ventilation is an integral part of lung function, and hence nonventilating lung preparations represent less than desirable conditions, regardless of whether respiratory or nonrespiratory functions are being investigated. Retaining the ability of testing certain experimental drugs through the gaseous phase to simulate inhalational exposure would also be an additional advantage of maintaining a ventilating perfused lung preparation (203). Two types of isolated lung preparation are described here, one that utilizes negative-pressure ventilation and another that utilizes positive-pressure ventilation.

Apparatus

The perfusion system developed by Niemeier and Bingham (231), with modifications (10,50,67,106, 206,239), is described (Figure 33.5). The apparatus consists of a combination of pumps for ventilation, a peristaltic pump to drive the perfusate, an assembly of tubing for carrying the perfusate to and from the lung, and an artificial thorax kept warm by heated, circulating water. The thorax is made of double-jacketed thick glass provided with an air-tight lid. Perfusate flow to the lung is from the upper reservoir connected to the central porthole of the lid. The bottom of the reservoir has an opening through which the perfusate can be directed to the peristaltic pump. A small-animal respirator and a vacuum pump are connected to two of the portholes on the lid; these parts provide alternating negative pressure

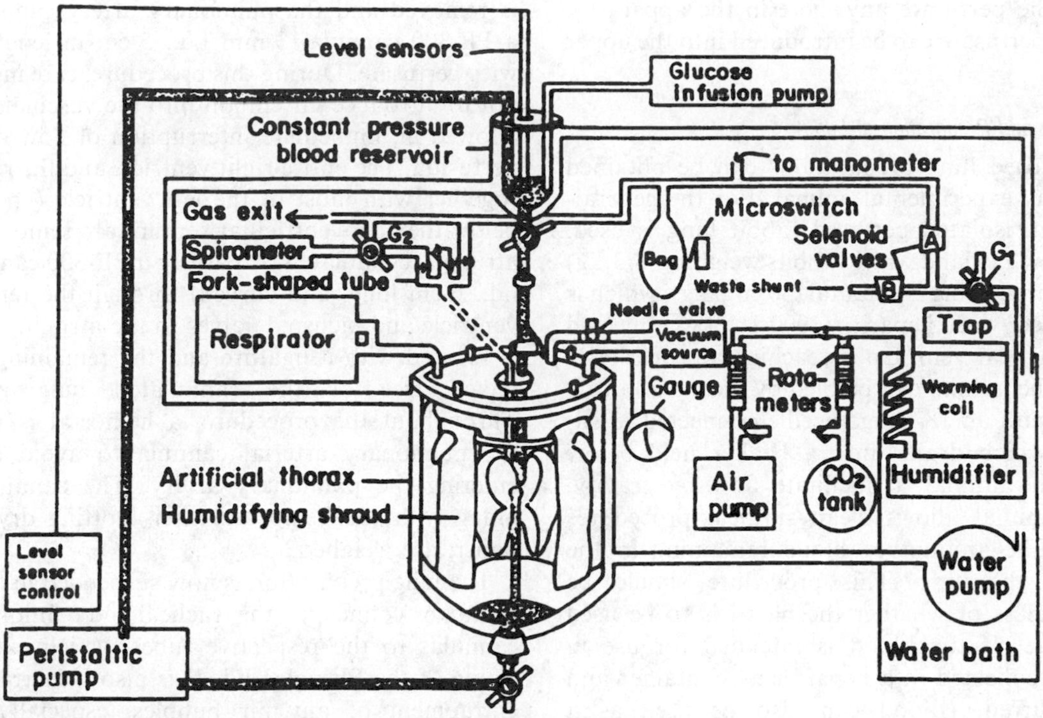

FIG. 33.5. Isolated perfused lung apparatus. This apparatus, originally developed by Niemeier and Bingham (198) for perfusion of rabbit lung, uses alternating negative pressure for ventilation. The apparatus can be scaled down to perfuse lungs from smaller animals (rats, guinea pigs) as well, using essentially the same procedure. From Reference 198, with permission.

as a means of ventilating the perfused lung preparation. A magnehelic gauge or a simple manometer can be connected to another porthole on the lid to monitor the negative pressure in the thorax. At the center of the lid there are two portholes, one for a tracheal cannula and another for a pulmonary arterial cannula. The upper reservoir, which is also double-jacketed, connects to the central pulmonary arterial cannula by means of a stop-cock arrangement and via pressure and flow transducers. The tracheal cannula is connected to a source of O_2/CO_2 (95:5), which is filtered and humidified by bubbling through warm saline. By means of appropriate one-way valves, provisions are made for inspiration and expiration of the ventilating lung. A spirometer is connected to measure the inspiration volume.

The perfusate from the upper reservoir passes through the assembly of transducers into the lung via the pulmonary arterial cannula. The perfusate empties into the bottom of the reservoir and is led to a peristaltic pump, which delivers it to the upper reservoir. A level-sensor controlling device can be introduced at the upper reservoir to maintain a constant level of the perfusate in the reservoir so as to provide constant hydrostatic pressure. This automatic sensing device regulates the peristaltic pump, maintaining a designated level of perfusate in the upper reservoir. An infusion pump can be used to infuse glucose, which replaces the glucose utilized by the lung. In the upper reservoir, a pH probe can be installed to monitor the pH of the circulating perfusate. The water bath, equipped with a heater and a circulating water pump, provides a means for maintaining the thorax and the upper reservoir at physiological temperature (37°C).

Almost all components that come in direct contact with the perfusate are composed of glass, with the exception of small pieces of medical grade Silastic tubing used in the peristaltic pump, which requires flexible tubing. The glass components and flexible tubing of the apparatus are coated with Siliclad or a similar liquid silicone avoid binding of chemicals to the tubing used for transporting the perfusate. The lid (thoracic roof) with a number of portholes is composed of Plexiglas fitted with a rubber "O" ring and sealed with silicone high vacuum grease; the lid is held in place on the ground-glass rim of the thorax by appropriate clamps. The small-animal respirator is connected in reverse to the porthole on the lid for the purpose of generating alternating negative pressure in combination with the vacuum pump.

Prior to the surgical procedure to remove the lung, the apparatus is thoroughly cleaned, assembled, and rinsed with physiological saline. A measured volume of perfusate can be introduced into the upper reservoir, and the entire perfusate line can be primed with the perfusate. Precaution is taken to avoid entrapment of any air emboli in the perfusate anywhere in the apparatus. The remaining perfusate can be introduced into the upper reservoir.

Surgical Procedure and Preparation of Lung

Isolated perfused lung preparations can be obtained from almost any experimental animal. For the generalized description, isolated perfused rabbit lung is used. The animal (New Zealand white rabbits weighing 2–3 kg) can be anesthetized using Nembutal (50 mg/kg), which is previously mixed with heparin (1000 IU/kg), injected into the marginal ear vein. Upon reaching a proper level of anesthesia, the animal can be bled by means of a cardiac puncture with an 18-gauge needle connected to silicone tubing, which drains into a beaker held below the plane of the animal to facilitate flow by gravity. Bleeding the animal allows clean surgical procedures and decreases the amount of blood remaining in the vasculature of the lung. This procedure should be followed regardless of whether the blood is to be used as the perfusate. If the blood is intended for use in perfusion, it is collected in a heparinized container and immediately stirred. (Blood can also be used as a perfusate upon proper filtration.) When carrying out cardiac puncture, care is taken to enter between the sixth and seventh ribs next to the sternum so as to not damage the lungs.

A midline incision is made from the neck to the abdomen to expose the trachea and rib cage. The liver is retracted and the sternum grasped by means of a curved hemostat. The sternum is lifted upward to facilitate inflation of the lungs, at which time the trachea can be clamped with a hemostat to entrap the proper amount of oxygen in the lungs. An incision in the diaphragm at the midline area facilitates cutting the diaphragm on both sides along the rib cage. The rib cage can be cut laterally on both sides, making sure that the lung tissue is detached from the roof of the rib cage. The lungs and heart are thus exposed through a midline sternotomy, and the rib cage is retracted. The lungs and heart can be removed from the animal en bloc and transferred to a Petri dish containing warm saline. All the subsequent operations can be carried out while the lungs rest in this Petri dish.

The trachea is first cannulated using PE-300 tubing (PE-200 for the rat). At this time, the lungs can be ventilated artificially by means of a 100-ml syringe attached to the tracheal cannula by silicone tubing. Alternatively, the tracheal cannula can be attached to a small-animal ventilator so that the lungs can be ventilated during the subsequent cannulation procedure. The trachea, lungs, and heart are dissected free from their attachments, connective tissue, and other extraneous material, taking care not to puncture the lungs, and then rinsed with warm physiological saline. The pericardium is removed and the pulmonary artery cannulated with a PE-300 cannula (3 mm i.d., 5 cm in length) prefilled with perfusate. During this procedure, care must be taken not to introduce air emboli into the vasculature; if air is allowed in, immediate interruption of flow occurs upon perfusion. The entire right ventricle and the right atrium, together with most of the left ventricle (up to 0.5 cm), below the atrioventricular septum are removed. The left atrium is cannulated by passing a PE-300 cannula (3 mm i.d., 6 cm long, and curved) through the remaining left ventricle and bicuspid valves to the atrium. The cannula is secured with a ligature and the remaining tissue dissected free of the cannulated lung preparation. Throughout the procedure, a hemostat is retained on the pulmonary arterial cannula to avoid air bubbles entering the pulmonary artery. The cannulated lungs along with the hemostat, after blotting dry with filter paper, are weighed.

The lung preparation is now suspended in the artificial thorax by connecting the tracheal and pulmonary arterial cannulas to the respective tubes, which extend to the inside of the Plexiglas lid. It is also important to avoid entrapment of any air bubbles, especially when the arterial cannula is connected to the perfusion apparatus. Flow is resumed through the arterial cannula after the lid is closed, and the perfusate line from the pump is connected to the top of the upper reservoir. Perfusion can be slowly established at this time, ensuring that no bubbles pass through into the pulmonary artery. The pumps can be activated to inflate the lung. The lungs are inflated by applying a negative pressure of 25–30 cm H_2O by activating the vacuum pump and increasing the vacuum. Once the collapsed lungs are inflated to a desired level, because the respirator is already turned on, the alternating negative–positive pressure automatically ventilates the lung. In the rabbit, the frequency is kept at 50 respirations per min. In the rat, respiration can be maintained at approximately 60 per min. Once the ventilation cycle is initiated, the apparatus is automatic, and perfusion and ventilation continue throughout the experiment. The perfusion flow rate increases quickly upon inflation of the lung and may steadily increase until steady-state ventilation is established. If the automatic level sensor is in operation, monitoring the perfusion flow rate is not necessary. However, if such an arrangement is not available, care must be exercised to maintain perfusate in the upper reservoir by manual control of the peristaltic pump. The lungs are usually allowed to equilibrate in the perfusion apparatus over a period of 15–20 min.

Positive-Pressure Ventilation Procedure

The perfusion apparatus developed by O'Neil and Tierney (242) can be used to illustrate perfusion of lungs from smaller animals and by using a positive-pressure

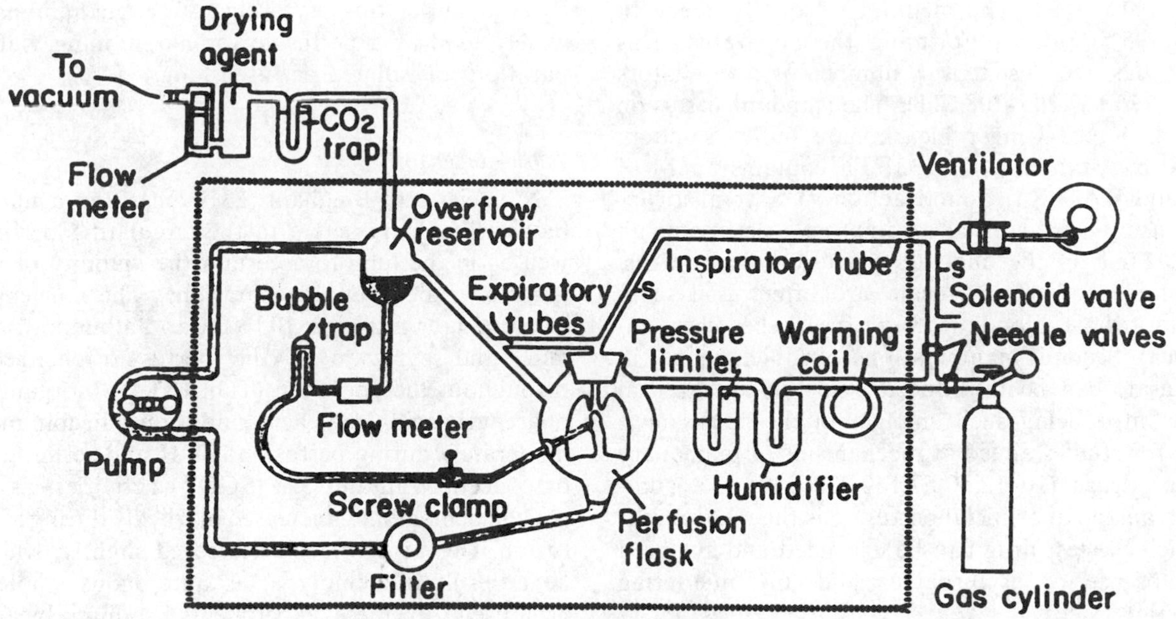

FIG. 33.6. Isolated perfused lung preparation of O'Neil and Tierney (208) This apparatus is used to perfuse lungs with positive-pressure ventilation. It can be scaled up to perfuse lungs from large animals as well. (S) solenid value; (O) needle valve. From Reference 208, with permission.

ventilation procedure. The apparatus and assembly are illustrated in Figure 33.6. The lungs are ventilated directly by means of an animal respirator that is attached to the tracheal cannula. This procedure avoids the need for the additional vacuum pump that is required in the negative alternating-pressure ventilation method. Two selenoid valves (Figure 33.6) are used to direct gas flow during the respiratory cycle. A tidal volume of approximately 3.5 ml is obtained for the rat and is adjusted to provide a maximum transpulmonary pressure of 12 cm H_2O. The end-expiratory pressure is set at 3.5 cm H_2O to keep the lung from collapsing during expiration. The rat lungs are perfused in this apparatus at a frequency of 13 respirations per minute. The procedure for isolating and cannulating the lung is essentially the same as described for the rabbit lung preparation, with the exception of smaller-diameter polyethylene cannulas. The procedure for maintaining isolated perfused rat lung using positive-pressure ventilation has been described adequately by O'Neil and Tierney (242) and Young (349), who may be consulted for additional details. Lungs can also be perfused using a setup similar to the one described for the negative-pressure ventilation procedure with simple modifications. The vacuum pump is deleted, and the ventilator is connected directly to the trachea in a forward direction instead of the reverse direction used in the negative-pressure ventilation procedure. The procedure described by Camus and Mehendale (50) may be consulted for other details.

Perfusion Media

Nicolaysen (229) studied the effect of perfusate composition on edema development and found whole blood to be the most suitable perfusate. The perfusion procedure described by Niemeier and Bingham (231) included the use of autologous whole blood as a perfusate. This perfusate was practical in the case of a rabbit, as 100 ml or more of whole blood can be obtained by cardiac puncture from a rabbit weighing 3 kg or more. Blood is collected in a heparinized container and filtered to remove any debris, dead cells, or small blood dots. The blood is heparinized once again prior to circulation in the apparatus to avoid clotting. Using autologous whole blood is impractical, however, for perfusing rat lungs or lungs of other small animals. Blood may have to be collected from several animals to supply an adequate volume of perfusate for a single perfusion experiment. Furthermore, for certain experimental protocols such as single-pass experiments, several liters of perfusate may be required. For these reasons, use of artificially constituted medium as perfusate has been popular.

The widely used lung perfusate is the one described by Junod (140), which has the following composition in millimolar concentrations: NaCl, 118; KCl, 4.75; $CaCl_2$, 2.54; KH_2PO_4, 1.19; $MgSO_4$, 1.19; and $NaHCO_3$, 25. BSA is added at a concentration of 4.5 g/L, and the final pH of the solution is adjusted to 7.4 with 1 N NaOH, so that the final Na^+ concentration of the standard medium is 161 mM. The medium is equilibrated with O_2/CO_2 (95:5) prior to priming the apparatus. This perfusate has been used by a number of investigators (50,58,92,176,177,205–208,211). The standard perfusion medium is Krebs–Ringer bicarbonate buffer solution, described by Umbreit et al. (331); it contains 5 mM of glucose and 4.5% BSA (Cohn fraction V). Several advantages of using this artificial medium as a perfusate can be cited. First, in the one-pass perfusion experiments, large volumes of the perfusate are often used (255) and using whole blood as a perfusate becomes uneconomical. Second, manipulations of ionic changes in the perfusate can be introduced easily in an artificial medium. Introducing such changes in the perfusate is essential for studies aimed at mechanisms of pulmonary uptake of drugs (10–12,50,67,140,238–242). An additional advantage of artificial perfusate is the relative ease with which the test drug can be extracted and analyzed in the absence of erythrocytes and any interfering hemoglobin.

For some studies the presence or absence of BSA in the perfusate may be critical. Albumin provides binding sites for drugs, which might be an important criterion for studies of uptake and metabolism. Including albumin in the perfusate allows simulation of conditions of blood plasma in vivo. The absence of albumin results in a proportionately greater fraction of the chemical being in a "free" state; consequently, drug uptake and metabolism might be expected to be greater. Studies have also indicated that albumin may interfere with GSH, cysteine, and similar thiol compounds (138,139). These thiol compounds are oxidized rapidly in the presence of albumin in Krebs–Ringer bicarbonate buffer (138,139). Replacing albumin with high-molecular-weight dextran ameliorated this particular difficulty. Other variations of the perfusion medium include the use of 4.5% Ficoll 70 instead of BSA (78) and Hepes buffer with only 2% BSA (29).

A combination of either autologous or mixed whole blood and the Krebs–Ringer bicarbonate buffer artificial medium as a perfusate can also be used for perfusing lung preparations. Such a preparation has the advantage of including the natural constituents of blood so natural binding sites can be provided for the test materials. Differences in the uptake of chemicals by the lung have been found between whole blood and artificial medium used as perfusate (10,245). Perfluorocarbons have not been used in the perfusate in isolated perfused lung preparations, although their successful usage in perfusing livers (107,236,289,290) suggests that fluorocarbon emulsions would also adequately support the isolated lung preparations. In the isolated lung preparations ventilated by positive pressure, Young (349) utilized Krebs–Ringer bicarbonate-buffered solution containing glucose and BSA, similar to the one described above. By and large, this erythrocyte-free medium has been widely used as a perfusate for maintaining viable preparations of isolated perfused lungs.

Viability Criteria

Niemeier and Bingham (231) measured a number of biochemical parameters in the circulating perfusate as well as in the lung to ascertain the viability of isolated perfused rabbit lung preparations. The concentrations of blood urea nitrogen (BUN), Ca^{2+}, albumin, total protein, and pyruvate in the perfusate changed little throughout the perfusion (Table 33.4). Inorganic phosphate, uric acid, lactic acid, and total bilirubin increased moderately during perfusion. LDH and serum glutamic oxaloacetic transaminase (SGOT) activities, as well as plasma hemoglobin, increased markedly during a 3-h perfusion. Hematocrit levels decreased slightly, which may be a result of hemolysis, as autologous whole blood was used. In these experiments, sodium bicarbonate was added periodically to maintain the blood pH at 7.4, and heparin and epinephrine were added to maintain proper perfusion flow rates. These additions might have contributed to the decrease in hematocrit. Glucose levels decreased (34.5 ± 4.1 mg/h) during perfusion, necessitating addition of glucose with an infusion pump at the rate of 30 mg/h in 0.3 ml of water. Thus when glucose was replenished, the glucose concentration in the perfusate did not decrease significantly over the 3-h period of perfusion. Cholesterol increased at a rate of approximately 11%/h, but when α-tocopherol was added to the perfusate, cholesterol increased markedly (53%/h).

Lungs can be examined visually during perfusion for the appearance of translucent areas, which would indicate development of edema. Niemeier and Bingham (231) found that the lungs gained weight on an average of 2.8%/h over the 3-h perfusion with autologous whole blood. Histopathological examination revealed no edema after 3 h of perfusion, and the integrity of the pulmonary ultrastructure was well preserved (231,245).

Often after prolonged perfusion of lungs, the lung preparation deteriorates, with the concomitant development of edematous areas characterized by a translucent appearance of the lung surface. After continued perfusion, the lung does not inflate and deflate with each respiratory cycle, and surfactant material might appear in the tracheal cannula. If the perfusion is continued after the lung appears to be edematous, large and copious flows of the surfactant material continue to appear through the tracheal cannula. Maintenance of perfusate pH can be a problem; Niemeier and Bingham (231) maintained the pH by adding 1 mM sodium bicarbonate to the perfusate. However, they used room air mixed with 5% CO_2 to ventilate the rabbit lung preparations. When O_2/CO_2 (95:5) was used for ventilating the isolated lungs and the lungs

Table 33.4
Biochemical changes and physiological values in the isolated perfused lung

Parameter	Average concentration in plasma prior to perfusion	Average change in concentration per h
Calcium (mg/dl)	13.8 ± 0.8	↓0.15 ± 0.29
Inorganic phosphate (mg/dl)	4.1 ± 0.4	↑0.78 ± 0.27
Glucose (mg/dl) adding 30 mg/h	236 ± 35	↓34 ± 4.1 ± 2.3
BUN (mg/dl)	17.5 ± 3.2	↑0.14 ± 0.22
Uric acid (mg/dl)	0.62 ± 0.18	↑0.20 ± 0.12
Cholesterol (mg/dl) with vitamin E	37 ± 13	↑4.2 ± 0.7 ↑19.5 ± 7.1
Total protein (g/dl)	5.7 ± 0.4	↑0.10 ± 0.15
Albumin (g/dl)	0.53 ± 0.07	↓0.04 ± 0.03
Total bilirubin (mg/dl)	0.14 ± 0.06	↑0.12 ± 0.16
Alkaline phosphatase (mU/ml) with vitamin E	55 ± 36	↑4.8 ± 2.1 ↑0.6 ± 1.1
Lactate dehydrogenase (mU/ml)	135 ± 42	↑485 ± 201
SGOT (mU/ml)	58 ± 23	↑121 ± 58
Plasma hemoglobin (mg/dl)	0.19 ± 0.12	↑2.3 ± 0.6
Lactic acid (mg/dl)	173 ± 17	↑19.8 ± 5.2
Pyruvic acid (mg/dl)	1.19 ± 0.06	n.c.[a] ± 0.01
Hematocrit (%)	35.0 ± 5.0	↓1.63 ± 0.34
Weight gain (% h)	↑2.81 ± 1.36	
Blood flow (ml/min)	160	—
Po_2 (mm Hg), typical values	118 ± 6; 121 ± 10	—
Pco_2 (mm Hg), typical values	39 ± 4; 34 ± 4	—
pH range	7.35–7.45	—
Tidal volume (ml)		
Typical values	11.7 ± 0.3; 11.0 ± 0.4	—
Normal values	23.9 ± 5.5 (16)	—

[a]No change.
From Reference 257, with permission.

are properly inflated, no problem was encountered in maintaining physiological pH of the perfusate (206).

An additional criterion of viability of the lung preparation is the evaluation of drug-metabolizing enzymes in the perfused lung (172). Various investigators have found that after 2–3 h of perfusion, microsomal drug-metabolizing activity of the lung remained unaltered, indicating satisfactory preservation of microsomal MFO activity of perfused lung preparation. ATP levels were measured in rat lungs perfused for 90 min by a positive-pressure ventilation procedure (349) and were found to be at or above the ATP levels in nonperfused lungs. By contrast, ATP content was decreased in lung slice incubations. Perfusion of rat (29) and rabbit (78,138) lungs resulted in only a slight decrease in the lung content of GSH, indicating that lungs can maintain GSH levels during perfusion.

Applications

Isolated perfused lung preparations have been used for a variety of studies, including drug uptake and metabolism and the disposition of various pharmacological and toxicological agents (205). Although rats and rabbits appear to be the species of choice, studies with mice (141), guinea pigs (137), and other species can be found in the literature. Rhoades (273) described a technique of using isolated perfused lungs ventilated by positive pressure for evaluating the effect of various gaseous environments on pulmonary biochemistry. Block and Cannon (35) investigated the effect of anoxia or hyperoxia on the ability of lungs to clear endogenous and exogenous chemicals. Use of isolated lung preparations has resulted in significant contributions to our understanding of the pulmonary role in uptake and metabolism of a variety of xenobiotics (37,50,55,67,125,131,167,171,203–207, 230,231,256,332,344). Examples of toxicological investigations using isolated perfused lung preparations include studies on the pulmonary uptake and disposition of aldrin and dieldrin (204,206); uptake of the herbicide paraquat (55); uptake and metabolism of trichloroethylene (66); pharmacokinetics and toxicity of doxorubicin (21); metabolism and toxicity of naphthalene oxide (141); metabolism of nitroaromatics (325); uptake, reactivity, and impairment of lung function by diisocyanates (145,170); nitrofurantoin toxicity (30); toxicity of H_2O_2 (111) and chlorine gas (208); modulation of 4-ipomeanol activation in the lung (327); effect of xanthine oxidase-induced lung injury on removal of 5-hydroxytryptamine by the lung (63); and uptake and metabolism of benzo(*a*)pyrene (32,332). Although this list is by no means a survey of toxicological investigations utilizing isolated perfused lung preparations, it shows that these preparations have been useful for determining the pulmonary contribution to the disposition of toxic chemicals.

Perfused lung preparations have been useful for demonstrating epoxidase activity in the lung tissue (202,205,206). Aldrin is a cyclodiene pesticide that is readily epoxidized to dieldrin and in the liver can be further metabolized by epoxide hydrase to dihydrodiol metabolites. In the lung, aldrin could be readily epoxidized to dieldrin, which is a stable epoxide and can be quantitated as a measure of aldrin epoxidase activity. This finding represented the first direct demonstration of epoxidase capability of lung tissue. Aldrin is metabolized to dieldrin irrespective of whether it enters via airways or through the vascular system, and the metabolite appears in the perfusate rapidly (202). In these studies, it was demonstrated that intact perfused lung preparations turned over aldrin to dieldrin at a slower rate than the in vitro incubations of lung homogenate preparations. These studies serve to illustrate the utility of perfusing intact organs to realistically evaluate the metabolic contribution by the organ to the metabolism and disposition of a test chemical. Turnover of aldrin to dieldrin was four to seven times greater in vitro preparations than in ex vivo preparations using perfused intact lungs (202). Although the reason for such a discrepancy between in vitro and intact organ perfusion systems is incompletely understood, Itakura et al. (130) demonstrated that the availability of necessary cofactors might be limiting in intact perfused lung preparations. They observed that demethylation of *p*-nitroanisole by the perfused rabbit lung preparations was limited by the availability of the cofactor NADPH, the generation of which could be stimulated by introducing glucose to the perfusion medium. Even in the presence of excessive glucose in the perfusate, aldrin epoxidation, a reaction requiring NADPH, was saturable (206), suggesting that the cofactor availability can be limiting in intact lungs, an observation that would not be apparent from the idealized in vitro incubations.

Perfused lung preparations of rat and rabbit (238–241) have been helpful in identifying a flavin monooxygenase capable of *N*-oxidizing chlorpromazine and imipramine. Most interestingly, these studies established that although the rat lung is capable of *N*-oxidation of both of these substrates, rabbit lung is devoid of this activity. Curiously, rabbit lung does contain a flavin monooxygenase capable of *N*-oxidizing *N,N*-dimethylaniline (204). These studies also established the absence of any significant cytochrome P450-mediated metabolism of these substrates. Furthermore, the remarkable species differences between rats and rabbits in pulmonary flavin monooxygenase activities became apparent from these perfusion studies (204,238–241).

Lessire et al. (176) investigated the toxicokinetics of parathion and paraoxon, metabolic activity, and cholinesterase inhibition in guinea pig and rabbit lungs using single-pass perfusion. Although lungs of both species extracted both compounds from the perfusate, extraction ratio was higher for guinea pig lungs. Cytochrome P450-related lung metabolic activity, inhibitable with inclusion of piperonyl butoxide, mediating the activation of parathion to paraoxon was demostrated in the lungs of both species. Cytochrome P450 activity was required for maximum inhibition of lung acetylcholineesterase activity.

The study of Dalbey and Bingham (66) illustrates the utility of isolated perfused lung preparations for studying the uptake and disposition of gaseous toxic substances. They studied the uptake and metabolism of trichloroethylene in isolated perfused rat lung preparations by introducing trichloroethylene vapors through the trachea. Perfused rat lung preparations metabolized trichloroethylene to trichloroethanol, and guinea pig lungs were even more active in the metabolism of trichloroethylene to the alcohol. In the future, it should be anticipated that more experimentation will be carried out utilizing isolated perfused lung preparations for such toxicological investigations (203).

Kennedy et al. (145) and Lastbom et al. (170) studied the reactivity and lung impairment by diisocyantes in isolated perfused guinea pig lungs. Perfused lungs were exposed to ^{14}C-labeled toluene diisocyante (TDI) at 0.2 and 0.7 ppm. Krebs–Ringer bicarbonate buffer only, with or without gunea pig albumin, human albumin, or diluted guinea pig plasma, was used to perfuse the lungs. The rate of TDI uptake was dependent on TDI concentration and composition of the perfusate. The percentage of conjugated products was higher when diluted guinea pig plasma was used as the perfusate (15% in buffer only versus 45% with diluted plasma). The authors concluded that perfused lungs could serve as a useful model to study the molecular mechanism of isocyanate-induced lung desease and metabolic activity. In another study (170), isolated perfused ventilated guinea pig lungs were exposed to 3.5 and 11 mg of hexamethylene diisocyanate (HDI) to induce lung impairment. There was a dose-dependent decrease in both airway conductance and compliance but no effects were noted on the pulmonary circulation. The reduction in lung function (with 11 mg/m^3) was abolished when 100 μM diclofenac, a cyclooxygenase inhibitor, was added to the perfusate. The thromboxane A_2 antagonist L-670,596 (20 μM) exerted only a partial protective effect. The authors concluded that HDI-induced bronchoconstriction was mediated via arachidonic acid release and thromboxane formation in isolated perfused guinea pig lungs.

The use of isolated perfused lung preparations to study the metabolism of carcinogenic chemicals such as benzo(*a*)pyrene is another example of the use of perfused lung preparations. Bingham and associates (32) studied the metabolism of benzo(*a*)pyrene and reported the formation of several metabolites of this chemical, including the formation of carcinogenic reactive epoxide and dihydrodiol metabolites in the lung. In addition to containing the enzymes for carrying out oxidative metabolism of these toxic chemicals, perfused lung preparations contain the enzyme systems that catalyze phase II reactions, such as epoxide hydrase, glucuronyl transferase, and GSH *S*-transferase. These reactions can be demonstrated using 1-chloro-2,4-dinitrobenzene as substrate (68,332).

The use of isolated lung preparations for demonstrating the effects of toxic chemicals mediated via endogenous hormone systems is illustrated by the studies of Seiler et al. (297). They examined the effect of certain anorexic agents, including chlorphentermine, on the clearance of 5-hydroxytryptamine (5-HT; serotonin) and observed that the anorexic agents enhanced the vasoconstrictor effects of 5-HT in the pulmonary circulation. Subsequent studies by Angevine and Mehendale in perfused rabbit (11) and rat (12) lungs suggested the mechanism. Chlorphentermine inhibited the pulmonary deactivation of 5-HT (11,12,204), consequently allowing the action of the vasoactive 5-HT to prevail. Another example of the use of isolated perfused lung preparations to evaluate the effect of foreign chemicals on pulmonary clearance of endogenous chemicals is the study of Gillis and Roth (102) in which they examined the turnover of endogenous hormones, such as 5-HT and norepinephrine.

Isolated perfused rabbit lungs were employed by Dunbar et al. (78) to examine the GSH status of the lung following perfusion with 420 μM paraquat or nitrofurantoin. Significant increases in lung GSSG were observed, which provided evidence for the proxidant nature of the lung injury caused by these agents. Possible utilization of externally provided GSH by rat (29) and rabbit (124) lungs was studied by determining the GSH status of the isolated, ventilated, and perfused lungs with or without prior GSH depletion. The rat lung appeared to be able to utilize external GSH (29), whereas the rabbit lung failed to do so (138). The question of whether externally provided GSH can be utilized by lung tissue is of significance for many toxicological considerations. The role of the GSH redox cycle as a defense system against H_2O_2-induced prostanoid formation and vasoconstriction was investigated in perfused rabbit lungs (295).

Bernard et al. (30) studied the toxicology of nitrofurantoin in the isolated perfused rat lung. Nitrofurantoin induced a decrease in tissue levels of glutathione but not protein thiols by the end of the 3-h perfusion. Tissue levels of angiotensin converting enzyme were not decreased. Electron microscopic analysis of the tissue revealed detachment of endothelial cells from the basement membrane, which may account for the edematogenic weight gain. The edema was matched by an increase in proteins content of the alveolar lavage fluid. Co-infusion of penicillamine, *N*-acetylcysteine, or *N*-(2-mercaptopropionyl)glycine failed to mitigate nitrofurantoin-induced edema. Allopurinol, an inhibitor of xanthine oxidase and a metal chelator, significantly decreased lung weight gain but did not prevent the loss of glutathione. The authors concluded that organ function was compromised more than the individual cells, and the allopurinol might be useful in modulating nitrofurantoin pulmonary toxicity. Oxyradicals generated by xanthine–xanthine oxidase also interfered with the endothelial removal of 5-HT in perfused rabbit lungs (63). The question of hydroxyl radical (·OH) involvement in granulocyte-mediated oxidant lung injury was examined in perfused rat lungs using dimethylthiourea (DMTU) as the radical scavenger (91). When isolated rat lungs were perfused with polymorphonuclear neutrophils (PMNs) activated by phorbol myristate acetate (PMA) to produce ·OH, lung weights were increased significantly. Because the increase in lung weight was preventable by 10 mM DMTU, the findings were supportive of the role for the ·OH radical in acute granulocyte-mediated lung injury. Evidence for a protective role of intact human erythrocytes against H_2O_2-mediated damage (287) and the finding that DMTU treatment might be helpful for treating acute edematous lung injury such as seen in adult respiratory distress syndrome have provided some insights into the origin and mechanism of such lung injury. Habib and Clements (111) employed isolated perfused rat lungs to investigate if treatment with H_2O_2 would result in measurable changes in exhaled ethane during early stages of capillary leakage. Exhaled ethane was not increased when perfused with 0.25 mM H_2O_2 in albumin containing Krebs–Ringer buffer perfusate. H_2O_2 caused a small but significant increase in capillary permeability coefficient and wet weight/dry weight ratio was increased. The authors concluded that small amounts of H_2O_2 may increase pulmonary capillary permeability without affecting exhaled ethane.

Additional examples of the use of perfused lungs are available (37,51,116,166,257,260,261,269,294). These studies include the effect of asbestos (51), chlorine gas (208), staphylococcal α-toxin (294), and the haloalkanes (257) on the pulmonary metabolism of vasoactive substances. Pulmonary uptake and release of morphine (67,116), metabolism and macromolecular binding of the carcinogenic nitropyrene (37), and cystamine uptake and metabolism (299) are additional examples of the applications of the perfused lung preparations. Lafranconi et al. (166) employed perfused rat lungs to investigate the toxic effects of equinatoxin, a peptide of 147 amino acid residues isolated from the venom of the sea anemone *Actinia equina*. In this study, equinatoxin adversely affected fluid regulation in lung tissue, suggesting that it might become an important tool for the investigation of fluid regulation in the lung.

Although the recirculation apparatus was illustrated above, simple modification allows one to perform experiments using a single-pass perfusion system. A number of investigators have utilized single-pass perfusion to investigate the mechanisms of drug uptake and release from the lung (101). For example, Junod (140) examined the mechanisms of pulmonary uptake of imipramine using a single-pass mode of perfusion. Likewise, single-pass kinetics were used to determine the uptake, metabolism, and release mechanism of aldrin and dieldrin in rabbit perfused lung preparations (206). Single-pass experiments can be expensive in terms of both materials (albumin used for preparing the perfusate) and the technical assistance required to conduct these experiments. An ideal single-pass experiment requires the assistance of three individuals to work in swift coordination and usually involves analyzing a large number of samples. Hence the information to be gained from such experimental protocols must be weighed against the expense involved. Often equally valuable information results from recirculating perfusion experiments at a fraction of the effort and resources expended. For additional information, the reader may wish to refer to Roth (282) for a review of the methodology and applications of perfused lung preparations.

Isolated Perfused Kidney

Although a number of methods for obtaining perfused kidney preparations from various mammalian species have been devised, use of isolated kidney preparations in toxicological studies has been infrequent. Historically, most workers in this field have been concerned with the study of autoregulation, excretion, and reabsorption functions of the organ (18,24). Isolated perfused kidney preparations have been used in such studies from the rat (23,26,39,70,156,279), dog (17,288,339,347), rabbit (89,277), pig (45), monkey (317) sheep (317), and human (163). Considerable variation has existed among the various investigators concerning the specific techniques used for perfusing kidneys. The kidney may be perfused via the dorsal aorta or the renal artery. Pulsatile or nonpulsatile perfusate flow can be used, and perfusion pressure may be exerted either with the pump (119) or by means of a hydrostatic pressure head (26).

As with other perfused organ systems, the most important variable has been the perfusion medium, and a considerable range of varying compositions has now been tested. Argument persists in the literature relating to whether pulsatile flow is preferred as a simulation of the in vivo situation (279). A second major problem has been vasoconstriction and deterioration of the kidney preparations associated with the use of whole blood as a perfusion medium. By and large, to circumvent this problem, investigators have used either diluted blood, a reconstituted blood perfusate, or an erythrocyte-free medium containing various electrolytes, glucose, and albumin. Most investigators are content with the use of a Krebs–Ringer bicarbonate-buffered solution containing albumin and glucose. As in the case of other organs, kidneys can also be perfused either in situ or in total isolation in chambers that can be kept warm for normothermic conditions. A further variation can be in the mode of perfusion; kidneys can be perfused either using recirculating perfusate or in a single-pass mode.

Apparatus

The apparatus used for perfusing kidney preparations is similar to the one described for perfusing livers (Figure 33.7). It includes the outer chamber used for perfusing the liver and is fitted with a heater–fan assembly for maintaining the desired temperature inside the chamber. A multibulb glass lung can be used to oxygenate the perfusate. Perfusate is led to a roller-type or peristaltic pump and is transported to the top of the oxygenator via glass tubing. A filter placed between the lung and the glass

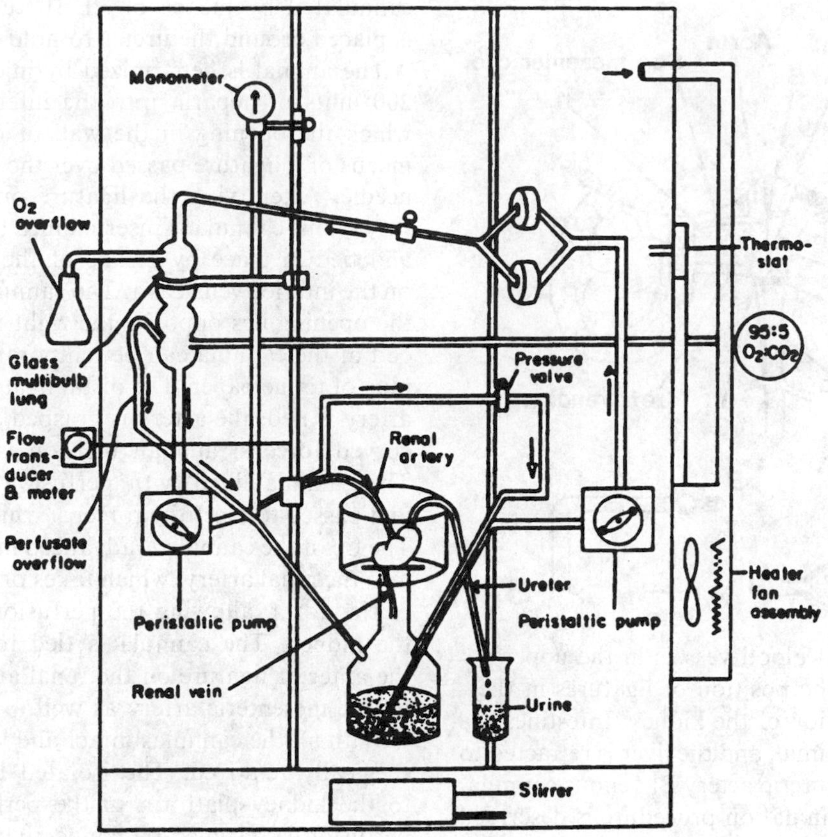

FIG. 33.7. Isolated perfused kidney apparatus (20). The entire perfusion assembly is housed in a Plexiglas chamber fitted with a heater-fan assembly (168). For other details refer to the text and Reference 168.

tubing ensures trapping fat droplets and any other particulate material, including cell debris, from the perfusate before it enters the kidney. A major difference between the liver and kidney is the higher (120 cm H_2O) hydrostatic pressure used for perfusing the kidney. Oxygenated blood by means of glass tubing then enters the renal arterial cannula. A set of perfusion pressure and flow transducers can be placed between the arterial cannula and the glass tubing to measure the perfusion pressure and flow rates. Similarly, electrodes can be placed before and after the kidney to monitor oxygen levels of the perfusate. A pH probe can be placed anywhere in the circulation to monitor pH continuously. The effusate from the kidney is guided back to the reservoir to complete the recirculation. An overflow arrangement from the hydrostatic reservoir to the central reservoir allows maintenance of a constant hydrostatic pressure. The kidney rests on a nylon mesh stretched over a ring approximately 7.5 cm in diameter. The stainless steel strip is mounted about 2.5 cm above the tray to support the arterial cannula. The temperature of the cabinet can be maintained at approximately 38°C, thereby allowing the kidney and the perfusate temperature to equilibrate at 37°C.

Most of the tubing used in the assembly of the apparatus can be replaced by glass to minimize binding of test drugs to rubber or plastic tubing used in earlier perfusion setups. The arterial cannula is composed of glass tubing (2.8 mm i.d.; 3.5 mm o.d.) drawn to a taper of 1.3 mm o.d. and 1 mm i.d. It is bent to a right angle 1.5 cm from the tip, and the short limb of the cannula has little or no taper. The tip of the cannula is leveled slightly to facilitate its insertion into the renal artery. The venous cannula, consisting of a 3 cm long PE-270 (2 mm i.d., 3 mm o.d.) cut off at an angle to form a short tip, is placed in the inferior vena cava. When the cannula is in position, its opening lies opposite the right renal vein. It might be advantageous to prepare several cannulas of varying sizes, as there is considerable variation in the renal artery from animal to animal. The renal arterial cannula is filled with heparinized perfusate to avoid any clots or air embolus during cannulation.

Surgical Procedure

The surgical procedure for isolating and perfusing the rat kidney is described here, as the rat appears to be the most popular experimental animal for toxicological investigation (62,227,279,280). Kidneys can be surgically

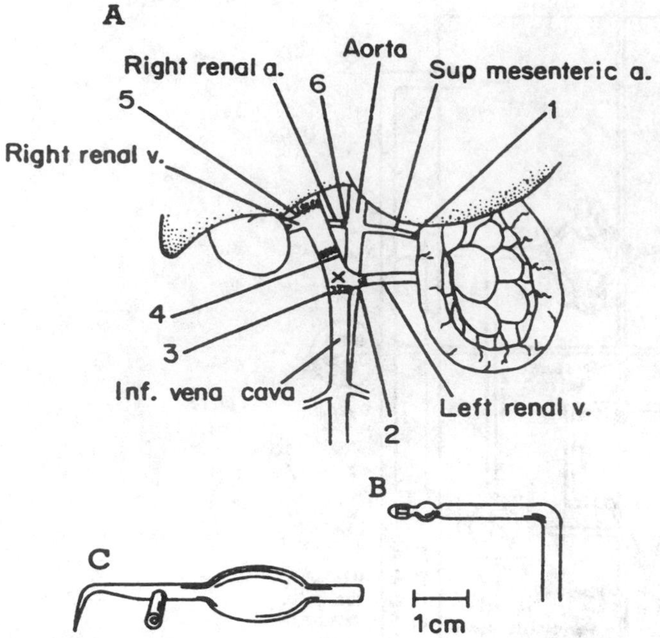

FIG. 33.8. **A:** Peripheral blood vessels in the upper abdomen of a rat with the position of ligatures in the preparation for cannulation of the kidney. Intestines are swept to the left of the animal, and the liver is retracted to expose the superior mesenteric artery **B:** venous cannula. **C:** Arterial cannula. Cannulation procedure is described in the text. From Reference 156, with permission.

removed from rats weighing 300–400 g, preferably starved overnight to decrease rates of gluconeogenesis and possibly reduce perinephric fat. After anesthetizing the rat with an injection of pentobarbital (50 mg/kg), an abdominal incision is made in the midline and extended laterally. The intestines can be swept to the animal's left to facilitate the next steps. Because of the anatomical advantage of the mesenteric artery arising from the aorta at the same level as the renal artery, the right kidney is used for perfusion. This technique facilitates passing the cannula through the aorta into the renal artery, with loss of little blood and no interruption of blood flow to the kidney. Figure 33.8 illustrates the principal blood vessels encountered in the cannulation and surgical preparation of the right rat kidney.

To expose the major abdominal vessels and the right kidney, fat and perivascular tissue are cleared away by teasing the tissues around the blood vessels. The adrenal branch of the right renal artery is ligated, and loose ligatures are placed around the vessels as follows: one on the inferior vena cava just distal to the liver, one on the aorta above the mesenteric artery, two on the mesenteric artery near the aorta separated by 0.5 cm, three on the inferior vena cava, one between the right and left renal vein, one distal to the left renal vein, and one further down on the inferior vena cava. Finally, a ligature is placed on the left renal vein. The ureter is cannulated by means of PE-10 tubing, and a ligature is placed around the ureter to hold the cannula in place.

The animal is heparinized by injecting approximately 200 units of heparin into the inferior vena cava, after which the opening in the wall of the vein is closed by means of a ligature passed over the point of the injecting needle. After tying the ligature on the left renal vein, the venous cannula is inserted into the inferior vena cava and tied in place by means of the two upper ligatures on the inferior vena cava. The cannula is turned such that the opening lies opposite the right renal vein. The other end of the cannula can be temporarily closed by a loose plug of tissue paper. The distal ligature on the mesenteric artery is tied, the artery is grasped at its origin with fine curved forceps, and an incision is made on the wall. The cannula filled with perfusion medium is inserted and passed to meet the forceps, which are then removed. The tip of the cannula is advanced into the aorta and then into the renal artery, which takes off on the opposite side of the aorta, allowing the perfusion medium to flow to the kidney. The cannula is tied in place by means of the anterior ligature on the renal artery and the ligature on the mesenteric artery as well.

With all the cannulas intact and in place, the kidney is surgically removed. The isolated kidney is transferred to the kidney platform in the perfusion chamber, and perfusion is resumed by connecting the arterial cannula to the perfusion flow of the preprimed apparatus. With practice, the total time required for the surgical procedure can be reduced to approximately 15 min, starting from the initial midline incision.

Perfusion Media

As indicated earlier, the perfusion medium of choice is a cell-free perfusion fluid with adequate buffering capacity and containing salts, glucose, and albumin (23,39,180,227,280). The perfusion medium described earlier for liver and lung, containing Krebs–Ringer bicarbonate-buffered solution, appears to be satisfactory for perfusing kidney preparations. Earlier attempts to utilize blood as a natural perfusate have met with problems relating to vasoconstriction, whether the blood was defibrinated (339) or heparinized (232). Another cause of impaired renal flow was found to be embolization of fat droplets, especially at later stages of perfusion using whole blood (232) as a perfusate. An additional disadvantage of using whole blood as a perfusate is the unavailability of a requisite volume of blood, especially in small experimental animals such as the rat. A volume of 100 ml of perfusate is often necessary to conduct an isolated perfused kidney experiment, and several animals would be required to obtain the volume of blood needed for perfusing the rat kidney. In addition to economic considerations, other problems may be encountered when mixing blood from several animals. One is the possibility of immunological interactions in blood pooled from several animals. Finally, in certain experiments it is essential to have one-pass circulation through the kidney. This method requires greater volumes of perfusate, and using blood would be impractical in such studies.

A major advance in the development of isolated perfused kidney preparations was made with the use of artificial, cell-free perfusion fluids such as buffered saline solutions supplemented with serum albumin (23,39, 61,180,227,281) or macromolecular plasma substitutes (93,293,310,340). A principal disadvantage of using a perfusion fluid devoid of red blood cells is the relatively high perfusate flow rates observed under these conditions (23) and the relative anoxia due to the limitation of oxygen-carrying capacity of the cell-free medium (93). Second, an absence of natural components of blood in perfusion medium devoid of whole blood may alter the disposition of the test chemical. Although Krebs–Ringer bicarbonate-buffered solution containing glucose and albumin can be used for perfusing kidneys, investigators have found it necessary to dialyze the BSA (Cohn fraction V) to obtain satisfactory kidney preparations that are perfused for longer durations (181). Third, Millipore filters must be used to filter out any cellular debris that may enter the circulation. Fourth, higher flow rates are necessary to ensure an adequate oxygen supply to the kidney when an artificial medium is used for perfusion.

In addition to the composition for artificial perfusate given above, Fonteles et al. (89) found that addition of GSH (500 mg/L) to the perfusate prevented depletion of endogenous cortical and medullary GSH. Furthermore, GSH supplementation of the perfusate decreased renal vascular resistance and increased perfusate flow. GSH extraction studies revealed a progressive decrease in renal extraction with time, ranging from complete extraction at 10 min to a value of 38% at 60 min (89). Including GSH in the perfusate might be especially relevant for toxicological investigations in view of the reports that many toxic agents deplete endogenous GSH levels in various tissues. Thus far, only kidney has been shown to use external GSH to any significant extent. As was pointed out earlier, rat lung is reportedly able to utilize external GSH (26) but rabbit lung cannot (138).

Viability Criteria

To date most of the isolated perfused kidney studies have dealt with the mechanism of autoregulation and physiological functions of the kidney. Techniques for evaluating adequacy and viability of the perfused kidney are abundant. Renal blood flow can be measured by placing a flow transducer prior to the kidney. Alternatively, a flow transducer can be placed after the perfusate exits the kidney. Blood flow through the kidney can reach 6–7 ml/min/g of tissue, depending on perfusion pressures, which vary from 90–130 mm Hg (232). With the artificial perfusate, flow through the kidney can reach as much as 30–60 ml/min/g of tissue. One problem associated with using perfusion flow rate as an index of viability is not knowing the intrarenal distribution of the flow. The regional distribution of the blood flow within the kidney can change markedly with artificial perfusion, with a striking increase in flow to the medulla and inner cortex (284). This fact is especially important for any toxicological investigations, as blood flow through an organ can either be shunted or altered in other ways as a result of toxic action of a test drug. Radiolabeled microspheres (10–15 μm) introduced into the circulation of a perfused organ may be used to assess the regional distribution of flow through the organ (284).

Another criterion for viability of perfused kidney preparations is the glomerular filtration rate (GFR). During the initial phase of perfusion, the GFR is at a lower limit (46–50 ml/min/100 g) of the normal range (232,339). Better rates (ml/min/100 g tissue) have been obtained with difibrinated blood (69). GFR decreases progressively after 2–3 h of perfusion. Often when blood is used as a perfusate, this decreased GFR has been attributed to the embolization of fat droplets in the glomeruli (339). In unsuccessful experiments, when the weight of the kidney increases, it is often due to retention of fluid in the tubules and interstitial edema (232,339).

Urine concentration and excretion of water are other criteria used for establishing the viability of perfused kidney preparations. During the first h, urine may reach an osmolality of 800 mosm, which is later reduced (60–150 mosm) because of increased urine flow. Water diuresis in the kidney preparation can be suppressed by administration of vasopressin in the perfusate. After 3–4 h the urine concentration approaches isotonicity (163,339,347). Loss of urine concentrating power is probably due to medullary edema and disturbances of deep cortical and medulla blood flow (232). Sodium excretion can be used as an additional parameter of viability. In contrast to frequent statements in the literature, the fractional reabsorption of sodium can be normal in perfused kidney preparations. In Berndt's experiments (unpublished data, 1980), sodium excretion exceeded 0.4% of the filtered load after 2 h of perfusion using the Krebs–Ringer bicarbonate buffer type of artificial medium. After prolonged perfusion, however, sodium rejection may develop (unless the perfusate is replaced) which may be due to accumulation of metabolic end products such as ammonia in the perfusate (163,339).

Acidification of urine is yet another functional viability criterion used for evaluating perfused kidney preparations. The loss of ability to excrete acidic urine represents a major functional abnormality of isolated kidney (163,339). An additional functional parameter that can be applied to perfused kidney preparations is the determination of insulin or *para*-aminohippurate (PAH) clearance values. A disadvantage of using these clearance values as determinants of viability is that, depending on the experimental conditions, these tests may or may not be compatible with the original intended use of the perfused preparation. Hence many functional tests may have to be carried out occasionally rather than routinely as an internal check of the perfused preparation.

Finally, kidney preparations can be sampled for electron microscopy and light microscopy, and morphological examination can be used as a determinant of functional abnormality. However, routine morphological examination at the light microscopic or ultrastructural level might not be practical for several reasons. Whether the preparation was viable cannot be determined until after the perfusion experiment. Facilities or expertise for routine morphological examination may not be available, and when available, might be prohibitively expensive for routine use. Often the validity of using morphological alterations as indicative of functional abnormality is questionable because other functional parameters might be optimal despite the morphological alterations at the cellular or subcellular level. Conversely, despite the normal morphological appearance, distinct functional aberrations may be observed. At least in part, such discrepancies can be explained on the basis of the relatively short time required for a functional abnormality to be detected, whereas longer periods may be required for the morphological alterations to develop. At any rate, as pointed out earlier for the liver and lungs, morphological observation should be helpful initially for establishing a viable perfused preparation in any laboratory (89,339,347). It is also useful for examining the effects of toxic chemicals on perfused kidney preparations (62,85).

Applications

Historically, the isolated perfused kidney preparation has not been utilized in pharmacological and toxicological investigations despite the availability of refined techniques (180,232,350). The bulk of the isolated perfused kidney work can be seen in physiological literature. One reason might be the increased attention devoted to establishment of physiological parameters such as GFR, autoregulation of blood flow through the kidney, absorption–reabsorption mechanisms in the kidney tubules, and hormonal regulation of renal tubular functions. However, the utility of isolated perfused kidney preparations can be demonstrated by the nature of the information obtained using this technique (203). For instance, control of GFR by an endogenously released humoral factor was definitively demonstrated using isolated kidney preparations (232).

Using isolated erythrocyte-free, perfused rat kidney preparations, Schureck et al. (293) demonstrated that sodium reabsorption can be increased by including glucose as the sole energy source of the kidney. The nature of glucose handling by the kidney has been investigated using perfused kidney (39). Because the tubular transport maximum (T_m) for glucose was proportional to GFR in the perfused kidney preparations, it was concluded that the T_m for glucose is not controlled by extrarenal factors.

Many physiological parameters of kidney function have been studied and are understood; and in many cases the renal control mechanism has been confirmed using isolated perfused kidney preparations (232). Use of the perfused kidney to investigate toxicological mechanisms has increased (62,135,180,189,212,213,216,217,271,281, 300,306,310,314,344), and these and other applications of the perfused kidney are briefly discussed.

Study of GSH extraction from the circulating perfusate by isolated perfused kidney preparations is an example of a biochemical study that can be useful in toxicological investigations (89). Including GSH in the circulating perfusate at a concentration of 500 mg/L resulted in the preservation of cortical and medullary GSH. Perfusion without the addition of GSH consistently resulted in depletion of tissue levels of this important tripeptide. In addition, including GSH in the perfusate resulted in decreased renal vascular resistance and increased perfusion flow. Whether the increased flow was due to intrarenal alterations in flow patterns is unclear. It appears that GSH storage in the kidney can level off, as indicated by the above study, in which complete extraction of added GSH was seen at 10 min; this uptake was reduced to 38% of administered GSH at 60 min. These studies of Fonteles et al. (89) indicated a high affinity of rabbit kidney for GSH and a relatively large net reabsorption of this important tripeptide. In view of the many toxicological molecular events being related to alterations in the endogenous pools of GSH, this observation might be important in toxicological studies using isolated perfused kidney preparations.

Another example lies in the studies of Dovrak et al. (76), in which they examined the effects of high doses of methylprednisolone on the isolated perfused dog kidney. They noted several histological changes in the kidneys perfused with methylprednisolone for 20 h or longer. The primary changes consisted in necrosis of capillary loops, inclusion of eosinophilic material in Bowman's space, thickening of the basement membrane, and endothelial cell damage. Arterial changes consisted primarily of inclusion of afferent arterioles with dense eosinophilic material. Tubular changes consisted in inclusion of tubular lumens and damage to tubular epithelial cells. These studies demonstrated that administration of high doses of methylprednisolone can produce irreversible hemodynamic and histological changes in the kidney. Trumper et al. (329) investigated effects of different concentrations of acetaminophen (APAP) on renal function in isolated perfused rat kidneys. Changes in fractional excretion of sodium, water, glucose, and GFR were measured. APAP (10 mM) increased fractional excretion of water (72%), sodium (79%), and glucose (55%), and these increases were associated with a decrease in GFR. Prostaglandin E_2 (PGE_2) prevented the decrease in GFR and glucose reabsorption induced by APAP, but did not change the fraction of water or glucose excretion. Verapamil prevented glomerular but not the tubular effects of APAP. The authors concluded that APAP exerts a direct effect on isolated perfused kidney, affecting hemodynamic and tubular function, and that the latter are not a consequence of hemodynamic alterations. Aiba et al. (3) investigated the renal handling of tobramycin (TOB), an aminoglycoside antibiotic, using a single-pass isolated perfused rat kidney. At trace concentration (7.4 μM), 32% of TOB remained in the lumen, but no TOB was found in the vein. This ratio of luminal uptake was reduced in a dose-dependent manner. Other aminoglycosides such as gentamycin inhibited this uptake, but tetramethyl ammonium and glucosamine had no effect. Alkalinization of urine led to a 67% decrease of TOB uptake. This indicated that TOB was mainly taken up by the epithelial cells from the luminal site and that this uptake process was saturable and specific for aminoglycosides, which have more than one cationic group.

Three studies (103,182,276) have investigated the toxicology of cyclosporin A (CsA) in isolated perfused kidneys. Roby and Shaw (276) studied the acute effect of CsA and its metabolites. Intralipid was used as a vehicle for CsA because ethanol, methanol, or Camphor caused significant effects on GFR. Intralipid enhanced the effects of CsA 25-fold, giving a CsA dose response comparable to human kidneys. This enhanced effect was due to vasoconstriction and not to vaso-obstruction and was specific to CsA, because enhancement of norepinephrine with intralipid did not occur. The primary metabolites (M1, M17, and M21) of cyclosporin A caused decreases in GFR comparable to or slightly less than the decrease in GFR induced by the parent compound CsA. Because CsA metabolites in human blood often exceed CsA concentration, the study suggested that CsA metabolites may contribute substantially to CsA nephrotoxicity. Longoni et al. (182) investigated the protective effects of L-propionyl carnitine (LPC) against CsA nephrotoxicity; their work with isolated perfused kidneys revealed that LPC protected against the toxic lipid peroxidation phenomenon induced by CsA. Giovannini et al. (103) found that LPC could restore CsA-induced decrease in intracellular ATP levels to normal and at the same time a decrease in the increased vascular resistence was not noted. Therefore, it was suggested that the protective effects of LPC included correcting biochemical alterations induced by CsA, thus explaining the pathogenesis of renal damage induced by CsA.

Herrero et al. (122) used isolated perfused kidney preparation to evaluate a new flushing solution (F–M) containing fructose-1,6-bisphosphate (g/de) and mannitol (2 g/de) with the University of Wisconsin (UW) solutions used to preserve kidneys intended for human transplantation. The kidneys were stored in hypothermia for 4 and 18 h after initial flushing with the solutions being tested and then reperfused at 37°C in an isolated perfused circulation for 90 min with Krebs–Ringer buffer containing 4.5% albumin. Plasma flow rate (PFR), renal vascular resistence (RVR), urine flow rate (UFR), GFR, fractional (FrNa) and net (TNa) sodium reabsorption were studied. Conventional histology and tissue malondialdehyde levels were also evaluated. After 4 and 18 h of cold ischemia, GFR, FrNa, and TNa were better and conventional histology worse in F–M- than UW-flushed kidneys. After 18 h of cold ischemia, F–M-flushed kidneys were better than the UW-flushed kidneys, although after 4 h they did not differ. After 18 h malondialdehyde was lower in F–M-campared to UW-flushed kidneys, although after 4 h there were no differences. The authors concluded that the newly developed flushing solution (F–M) showed promising results for renal preservation. Its ability to preserve was at least as good as the UW-solution, as assessed by isolated perfused kidney preparation.

Summerfield et al. (309) utilized isolated perfused kidney preparations to examine conjugating reactions involved in the elimination of certain bile acids in urine. These investigators demonstrated that lithocholic and chenodeoxycholic acids can be metabolized by the perfused kidney to their monosulfate conjugates; the disulfate metabolites of these bile acids were not detected in the urine. These findings supported the hypothesis that renal synthesis of monosulfate conjugates may account for at least some of the bile acid sulfates present in urine in the cholestatic syndrome of man. The results further suggested that in chemically induced hepatic injury the kidney may be able to conjugate some of the bile acids, and they demonstrated the presence of sufficient biochemical machinery within the renal tissue for conjugating endogenous substrates. The experiments also demonstrated the possibility of conjugation of foreign chemicals in renal tissue, facilitating their elimination in urine.

Jaffe et al. (135) employed perfused rabbit kidneys to evaluate the genotoxic potential of the *S*-(*trans*-1,2-dichlorovinyl)-L-cysteine (DDVC). The proposed mechanism of renal toxicity of this and other vinyl cysteine conjugates is activation by β-lyase, an enzyme in the renal brush border membrane of the renal tubular epithelial cells. This enzyme converts the halogenated vinyl cysteine conjugate to reactive thiovinyl intermediates, which alkylate subcellular macromolecules such as DNA. In these rabbit kidney perfusion studies, a dose-dependent (0.01–1.00 mM DDVC) effect of DDVC on DNA single-strand breaks was demonstrated.

The study of Tark et al. (315) is as an example of yet another use of the isolated perfused kidney in toxicological investigations. These investigators examined substrate metabolism in the isolated perfused dog kidney and established that free fatty acids (FFAs) and glucose serve as significant substrates for providing energy for sodium transport in the kidney. Their studies also suggested that glucose may substitute for FFAs as an energy source at times when FFAs are decreased. The effect of chemicals on substrate metabolism in the kidney can be examined using the methods described by Tark et al. (315). Johannesen et al. (136) employed perfused kidney preparations to study the renal energy metabolism inhibitor 2,4-dinitrophenol.

There has been a recent increase in the use of isolated perfused kidney preparations in toxicological investigations (62,156,180,189,212,213,216,281,300,310,314, 344,351). Perfused rat kidneys have been used to investigate the mechanism of gentamicin toxicity (62,212,213). Mitchell et al. (212) established that a specific effect of gentamicin on potassium secretion was responsible for clinically observed hypokalemia during gentamicin therapy. This study and those of Cojocel and associates (62) have established that reduced water and electrolyte reabsorption were the earliest effects of gentamicin on the kidney. Perfusion of the rat kidneys with gentamicin induced a dose-dependent decrease in reabsorption and metabolism of lysozyme (62). The basis of the sex differences in renal toxicity was the subject of additional inquiry (213). The sex differences could not be demonstrated in the perfused rat kidney exposed to gentamicin, suggesting that the sex differences in the susceptibility to this antibiotic in vivo might be due to some extrarenal factors. Koschier et al. (156) perfused rat kidneys to study the effects of bis-(*p*-chlorophenyl)acetic acid (DDA), the principal water-soluble metabolite of DDT. At a concentration of 1 mM DDA in the perfusate, the GFR, urine volume, and fractional excretion of sodium were decreased, suggesting a direct action of DDA on nephron function. Sumpio et al. (310) employed isolated perfused rat kidneys to characterize the renal toxicity of *cis*-diamminedichloroplatinum (CDDP) and to determine if treatment with ATP-$MgCl_2$ could prevent or reduce the nephrotoxic effect of CDDP. After 2 h of perfusion, CDDP (100 μg/ml) treatment led to marked inhibition of protein reabsorption with only a minimal decrease in sodium and water reabsorption. Despite a marked diuresis, GFR was not significantly altered. Post-treatment with ATP-$MgCl_2$ (2 mM) led to partial alleviation of the nephrotoxic effect of CDDP. After 1 h of perfusion, simultaneous treatment with ATP-$MgCl_2$ (0.3 mM), however, fully protected the protein reabsorptive capacity of CDDP-treated kidneys. Because the CDDP-induced toxicity simulates the acute renal failure seen clinically, these findings are suggestive of a potential therapeutic modality for clinical management.

Isolated Perfused Brain

Brain does not lend itself to simple and totally isolated perfusion, and all the preparations to date include more or less extraneural tissue. Perfusion has found little place in many of the biochemical and toxicological studies with brain tissue, as the technique presents great difficulty even when effort is not made to exclude extraneural tissue. In addition, the brain is heterogeneous, and the contribution by both neuronal and non-neuronal tissues of the brain to drug uptake and turnover in perfusion causes difficulties in duplicating the results. The blood–brain barrier is one aspect of brain metabolism in particular that remains noticeably obscure, and it has been the subject of studies with perfused brain preparations (8,87,98,100,321). The heterogeneity of the preparation together with the many neural tissues represented in the brain make perfusion a somewhat less valuable technique for toxicological investigations than other organs. Nevertheless, several investigators have been able to maintain a viable perfused brain preparation that can be utilized for drug metabolism and investigations on the effects of chemicals that may adversely affect the central nervous system. The difficulty of maintaining the isolated perfused brain preparation coupled with the readily available in vitro and in vivo techniques have resulted in underutilization of perfused brain preparations.

Comparatively simple techniques of perfusing the rat brain are described here. The "perfused rat head" preparation of Thompson et al. (321), in which the entire head is perfused with no attempt to limit the circulation to the brain, is not described in detail. However, such a technique may be useful in some toxicological investigations and may be considered before setting up more difficult preparations. Far more elaborate and therefore technically more difficult is the preparation described by Andjus et al. (8), which attempts to exclude the muscle of the head and neck from the perfusion circuit; this method is described because of the obvious superiority of the technique. The preparation is based on the more elaborate perfusion technique developed in the cat by Geiger and Magnes (98); that described by Chute and Smyth (59) may be consulted if larger animal models are used to meet a particular need. Readers may refer

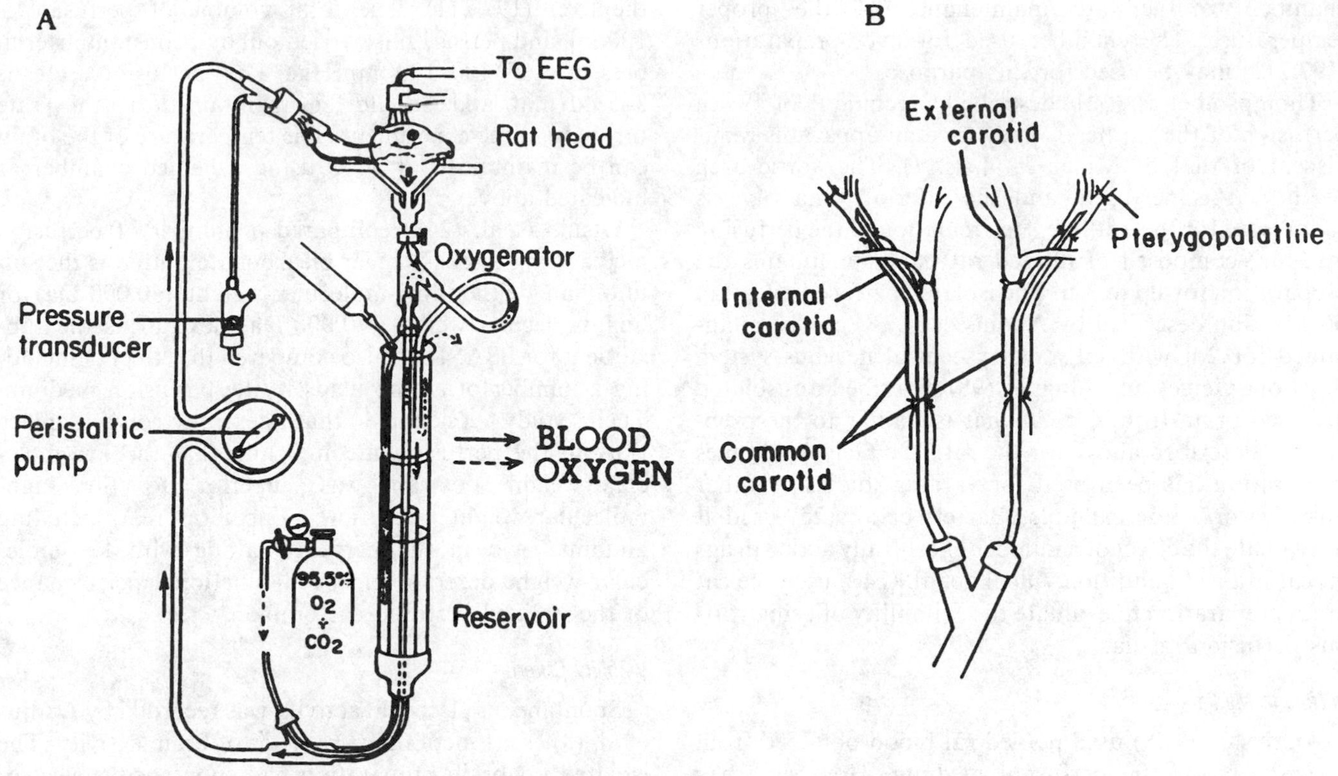

FIG. 33.9. A: Perfusion system for the isolated perfused rat brain preparation. **B:** Relation of the perfusion cannulas to the cannulated and adjacent arteries. For other details refer to the text and Reference 5. From Reference 5, with permission.

to White (341) for a total isolated, vascularly perfused monkey brain preparation or to Gilboe et al. (100) for a dog brain perfusion preparation.

Apparatus

Figure 33.9 shows the schematics of the equipment used for oxygenating the venous drainage from the brain and perfusion of the isolated rat brain as described by Andjus et al. (8). The bubble oxygenator and reservoir are made from two disposable plastic drug administration sets combined and fitted with connectors and plastic tubing. A small volume of recirculating fluid pumped by a peristaltic pump is used to perfuse the brain. The perfused brain preparation is held in a funnel from which the effluent perfusate drips to the oxygenator and passes through a filter to complete one circulation. If a single-pass circulation is desired, the peristaltic pump is disconnected, and a reservoir of perfusate is used at a height sufficient to provide satisfactory perfusion pressure and flow.

Surgical Procedures

After the animal is anesthetized using a proper anesthetic agent, both common carotid arteries are exposed, and the trachea is intubated via a tracheostomy. The animal is heparinized by injecting 500 IU sodium heparin through the jugular vein, which is then ligated by means of a suture. The external carotid and pterygopalatine arteries are ligated. In the rat the pterygopalatine artery is a branch of the internal carotid artery, which supplies blood to various extracranial structures. A plastic cannula filled with perfusion fluid is then inserted into each common carotid, advanced into the internal carotid artery, and tied in position so that its tip is near the origin of the previously ligated pterygopalatine artery. The arrangement of the vessels and the cannulas are illustrated in Figure 33.9.

A slow perfusion is initiated, and then the skin and the muscles of the head, face, and neck are removed together with the mandible. A sturdy ligature is placed around the vertebral column, which is transected just below the ligature. The transected vertebral canal is packed with a cotton or tissue paper plug, and the canal is sealed with melted wax. The completed preparation consists of the skull and its contents with the upper cervical vertebrae and small remnants of muscle tissue attached. Toward the end of the surgical procedure, the perfusion flow is gradually increased. After severing the vertebral column, the perfusion flow rate is adjusted to a desired value (1.4 ml/min). The cannulated preparation is then mounted above the collecting funnel. The entire preparation and the apparatus can be housed in a heating chamber to facilitate maintenance of the proper temperature. The chamber used for liver preparations (197,211) may be used for this purpose.

Thompson et al. (321) described a technique of in situ perfusion of the rat head. They used an apparatus reminiscent of that of Miller et al. (211). The aortic arch of the rat is perfused, and the inferior vena cava is cannulated for the outflow. Recirculation of the perfusion medium, composed of diluted rat blood, maintains the preparation for up to 3 h. The isolated perfused rat brain preparation described by Andjus et al. (8) can be maintained for 2 h with satisfactory central nervous system function. Geiger and Magnes (98) described an isolated perfused brain from the cat that is similar to the preparation described above for the rat. The Geiger–Magnes preparation has been used for various studies by other investigators. For example, Barrett et al. (25) used it to evaluate the effect of a number of centrally acting drugs on cat brain. In addition, Otsuki et al. (248) used the cat brain preparation to evaluate the suitability of using various perfusion media.

Perfusion Media

Andjus et al. (8) used pooled rat blood obtained from several rats as the perfusion medium. However, they found that when blood was used it did not support the spontaneous electrical activity of the isolated brain. After several trials they concluded that an artificial perfusion fluid similar to that described by Geiger (97) should be used.

The fluid portion of the artificial perfusate is Krebs–Ringer bicarbonate buffer solution, described earlier for perfusion of the liver, lung, and kidney. BSA (Cohn fraction V) is dissolved in distilled water and deionized by passing it through a column of Amberlite MB-3 before mixing it with the Krebs–Ringer bicarbonate-buffered solution. Erythrocytes obtained from dog blood were washed and used in this perfusion fluid. The cells are washed four times with cold, buffered (0.01 M, pH 7.4) isotonic sodium chloride solution and finally with isotonic Krebs–Ringer bicarbonate-buffered solution prior to use. The final perfusate contains 7–8% BSA, a hematocrit of 20–25%, with pH adjusted to 7.3. The perfusate is always best freshly prepared just prior to use. The glucose concentration of the blood for perfusion is adjusted to 200 mg/dl by adding a requisite volume of 5% glucose in normal saline solution.

The perfusate and the isolated brain preparation described by Andjus et al. (8) remained at room temperature (23–27°C) throughout the experiment; most of the perfusion experiments were conducted at 25°C. However, maintaining the entire perfusion at body temperature should be considered. It can be easily done by employing a heated chamber such as the one used for perfusing the liver (197,211). The total volume of perfusate is 100 ml, and perfusion is carried out at a constant arterial pressure of 100–120 mm Hg. The perfusion rate is 3–5 ml/min and should be maintained at this rate throughout the experiment. The temperature of the brain can be maintained at 30°C using a heated chamber as indicated above.

Otsuki et al. (248) compared a number of perfusion media using Krebs–Ringer bicarbonate buffer as the solution and either low-molecular-weight (40,000 Da) or high-molecular-weight (70,000 Da) dextran as the substituent for BSA. They also compared the effect of including a number of amino acids in the perfusion medium. Their study concluded that dextran could replace BSA in the perfusion medium and that the low-molecular-weight dextran was superior to the high-molecular-weight dextran. Furthermore, including glutamic acid in the perfusate along with low-molecular-weight dextran improved functional performance of the isolated perfused cat brain.

Viability Criteria

Spontaneous electrical activity was recorded by Andjus et al. (8) as a functional parameter of brain activity. The isolated rat brain preparation had spontaneous electroencephalographic (EEG) activity that persisted as long as 5 h with single-pass perfusion and about 2 h with recirculating perfusion. Although the reason for the shorter period of viability in a recirculation is not well understood, it is possible that endogenous biochemical products of intermediary metabolism may accumulate in the recirculating perfusion, to the detriment of the perfused brain. Addition of pentylenetetrazol to the perfusing blood evoked characteristic EEG signs of convulsive activity, either before or after spontaneous EEG activity had ceased. Otsuki et al. (248) carried out a similar study using EEG measurements to compare the suitability of altering the perfusion medium to perfuse cat brain. Response to loud sounds can be observed by EEG recordings and can be used as a viability criterion. After perfusion for 5 h, Andjus et al. (8) reported that the rat brain was nonresponsive to sound, indicating deterioration of the preparation. Thus, although EEG recordings indicated viability of the rat brain preparations, response to loud noise was lost after 5 h of perfusion (8), suggesting that not all the criteria were satisfied, especially during a perfusion that lasted several hours. Gilboe and associates (100) have used oxygen utilization and EEG pattern as satisfactory criteria for dog brain perfusion.

An additional criterion for viability is the rate of glucose utilization by the isolated brain preparation. It can be measured as the decrease in glucose concentration in the perfusing blood and should be linear during the 1st hour of the experiment; later it tends to decrease with the deterioration of the preparation. Lactate accumulates in the circulating perfusate, but the rate at which it accumulates does not appear to be directly related to glucose utilization (8). Otsuki et al. (248) also used rates of glucose utilization as a measure of viability for evaluating the various perfusion media to support isolated perfused cat brain preparations.

Applications

Although the use of isolated perfused brain preparations for toxicological investigations had been infrequent, examples can be cited where isolated perfused brain preparations have been used for such studies. The principal reason for the limited use of isolated perfused brain preparations seems to be the relatively slow development of the techniques (8,25,98,248). Hein et al. (118) investigated the effect of thiopental anesthesia on the energy metabolism of the isolated perfused rat brain. They perfused the rat brain in the presence and absence of 5.15 mM thiopental and investigated glucose turnover as well as a number of indicators of the glycolytic pathway. They noted that glucose uptake by brain preparation was increased when thiopental was included in the perfusate. However, the glycolytic pathway remained inhibited, indicating the sensitivity of the glycolytic pathway to thiopental. They also noted that this effect was not mediated via hindered uptake of glucose. In another study, Dirks et al. (74) investigated the effect of piracetam and methohexital on rat brain energy metabolism and conduded that piracetam had no acute effect on energy metabolism, and methohexital protected the rat brain from ischemic effects. These reports demonstrated the usefulness of the perfused brain preparation for studying intermediary metabolism (74,159) of the brain as affected by the presence of chemicals in the circulating perfusion medium. Similar preparations should be useful for studying the effect of centrally acting chemicals such as industrial solvents and gaseous substances as well as other neurotoxins. For example, Krieglstein and Stock (160) described the effect of chloral hydrate and trichloroethanol on cerebral intermediary metabolism. Fink et al. (86) used perfused rat brain to study the central activity of valtrate, following the EEG activity of brains perfused with or without valtrate. Fitzpatrick and Gilboe (87) used perfused dog brain to study the effects of nitrous oxide on the cerebrovascular tone, oxygen consumption, and EEG, and demonstrated that nitrous oxide reduced cerebral vascular tone but exhibited no effects on central oxygen metabolism.

The applicability of isolated rat brain preparations to study central neurological mechanisms can be illustrated by the study of Kilbinger and Krieglstein (148). They found that physostigmine caused a rise in the acetylcholine concentration of both the isolated perfused rat brain and the rat brain in vivo. Oxotremorine, on the other hand, produced an increase in acetylcholine content in the brain in vivo but was ineffective in the isolated rat brain at the same dosage. These investigations were carried out by recording the EEG as well as determining perfusate and brain levels of acetylcholine. These studies suggested the feasibility of using brain preparations to evaluate the effect of toxic chemicals on alterations of endogenous neurohormones and neurotransmitters.

Isolated guinea pig brain preparations were employed to investigate the influence of chronic amphetamine intoxication on the permeability of blood–brain barrier to inert and polar molecules (266). This study illustrates the use of isolated brain preparations to evaluate the effect of chronic drug treatment on vascular permeability. With a multiple-time brain analysis, the effects of repeated (14 and 20 days) amphetamine intoxication (5 mg/kg daily, IP) on the kinetics of ^{14}C-mannitol and ^{3}H-polyethylene glycol (PEG) into the forebrain of guinea pig were studied. Irrespective of their molecular weight or lipophilicity, these molecules were transferred across the blood–brain barrier progressively with the amphetamine treatment. The opening of the blood–brain barrier was associated with changes in behavior (increased locomotor activity, stereotypy, hypervigilance, social withdrawal, and loss of weight) with 14- and 20-day-treated animals. At 7 and 28 days after the withdrawal of the amphetamine treatment, bchavioral manifestations were absent and the opening of the blood–brain barrier to these inert molecules was not different from that in normal animals (266).

Although not isolated, in situ perfused rat brain was used to study drug metabolizing enzymes. Chikaoka and Tamura (56) employed the in situ perfused rat brain to study deethylation of 7-ethoxycoumarin (7-EC). Infusion of 7-EC through an internal carotid artery resulted in the formation of 7-hydroxycoumarin (7-HC) and its conjugates in the effluent perfusate collected from the superior vena cava. The rate of formation was 200 nmol h/g when 130 μM 7-EC was infused. This value was 100 times higher than the rate predicted from brain microsomal activity. Induction of drug metabolizing enzymes by phenobarbital and β-naphthoflavone increased the deethylation activity in the perfused brain, just as in the perfused liver.

The usefulness of brain perfusion for bridging in vitro and in vivo studies was demonstrated by Inagaki and Tamura (128). They employed a cannulation procedure for in situ preparation of a functionally intact hemoglobin-free isolated perfused rat brain without interrupting the brain circulation. The spontaneous distribution (8–25 Hz) and amplitude of a spontaneous EEG (50 μV) were kept within the normal ranges for up to 4 h after perfusion was started. The preparation gave characteristic flash-evoked EEG responses through the eyes. Administration of bicuculline elicited an epileptic seizure similar to that in normal rats. Redox behaviors of cytochrome oxidase a and a_3 in the brain were identical to those observed in normal brain tissue.

In addition to the studies mentioned above, the technique of perfusion has been used to aid histological fixation (249,324) of brains from experimental animals. For this purpose, the arch of the aorta is perfused with a balanced salt solution followed by a fixative. A distinct advantage of the perfusion technique to fix the brain preparation for histological examination is the delivery of oxygen through the oxygenated perfusion medium to the brain to achieve better preservation of the tissue.

Although the isolated perfused brain preparations described to date include extraneural tissue and many types of nerve centers within the brain itself, the perfusion technique should nevertheless be valuable for examining the specific effects of centrally active chemicals. The state of the art in this area has developed to a degree to which the technique should prove useful in toxicological investigations.

Isolated Perfused Intestine

Over the years there have been several attempts to study the mammalian intestine as an isolated tissue sustained by vascular perfusion. Mainly because of the nature of the tissue itself, there has been ambiguity in the use of the term "perfusion" in the field of intestinal research. Intraluminal circulation of fluid for the purpose of studying the transport of small molecules across the intestinal mucosa has often been referred to as intestinal perfusion (303,305). Intraluminal perfusion experiments can be performed in vivo for acute toxicity studies (183) or for short periods of time (272), or in vitro with excised segments of intestine (185). A full range of experimental techniques are available with intestinal tissue, and the topic has been reviewed (251), including vascular perfusion (134). No single experimental technique provides information about all phases of the absorptive processes involved in the removal of a substance from the lumen of the small intestine, its transport across the intestinal wall, and its entry into either blood or the lymphatic circulation. Techniques such as intraluminal perfusion and everted sac described by Wilson and Wiseman (343) are discussed elsewhere in this book (Chapter 26). This particular discussion deals with the vascular perfusion of the small intestine.

Isolated vascular perfusion of the intestine has not been prominent in gastrointestinal research because of the many problems encountered obtaining sustained viability (345). It is clear that vascular resistance, spasmodic bowel contractions, tissue edema, and progressive destruction of the mucosal epithelium were the principal problems encountered during earlier attempts to establish a vascularly perfused intestinal preparation. Furthermore, because most investigators were concerned with the mechanisms of intestinal absorption and were dealing with the mucosal layer, early investigators found it convenient to use intraluminal perfusion with fluid containing the experimental drug to study the intestinal absorption. In addition to supplying the experimental drugs through the intraluminal fluid, such fluid could also carry the necessary oxygen for supporting the mucosal layer (38). However, arguments can be made for developing a viable, vascularly perfused intestinal preparation (144,345). The role played by other layers of the intestinal wall such as muscle can be studied in a vascularly perfused intestinal preparation. Also, the disadvantages of the everted gut preparation, in which only transport across the wall is studied (rather than transport into the blood circulation), are overcome by utilizing an isolated vascularly perfused preparation. Thus anatomically and functionally distinct compartments, such as lumen, lymph, and bloodstream, are kept separated and can be studied individually. These arguments and the need to separate intestinal tissue to describe those absorptive, distributive, and metabolic functions of the tissue justify the development and use of the isolated, vascularly perfused intestinal preparation.

As has been observed for other isolated perfused organs, intestine can be perfused in situ (144,250,345) or in complete isolation (48,90,126). In addition, the perfused preparation can be used with an intraluminal flow maintained in the natural direction of peristalsis (77,144) or without the intraluminal flow (73,81). If the intestine is perfused without the intraluminal flow, two dynamic compartments (perfusion fluid and lymph) can be sampled for an experimental test chemical in addition to the intestinal tissue itself. If intraluminal flow is maintained, however, three dynamic compartments (perfusion fluid, lymph, intraluminal fluid) and the static compartment of intestine tissue can be sampled for the test chemical. For most practical purposes, maintaining intraluminal flow would introduce another dynamic variability in the experimental condition so that analysis and interpretation of the experimental results from analyzing all four compartments would be difficult if not impossible. The following description of an isolated perfused intestinal preparation is based on the procedure of Kavin et al. (144), later improved by Windmueller et al. (345).

Apparatus

An acrylic plastic box (75 cm high, 60 cm wide, 50 cm deep) houses the apparatus (Figure 33.10). Temperature in the chamber is maintained at 37°C by means of a heater and fan assembly that is thermostatically controlled. The chamber is kept humidified by a small jet of steam blown inside the chamber. The acrylic plastic cyclical

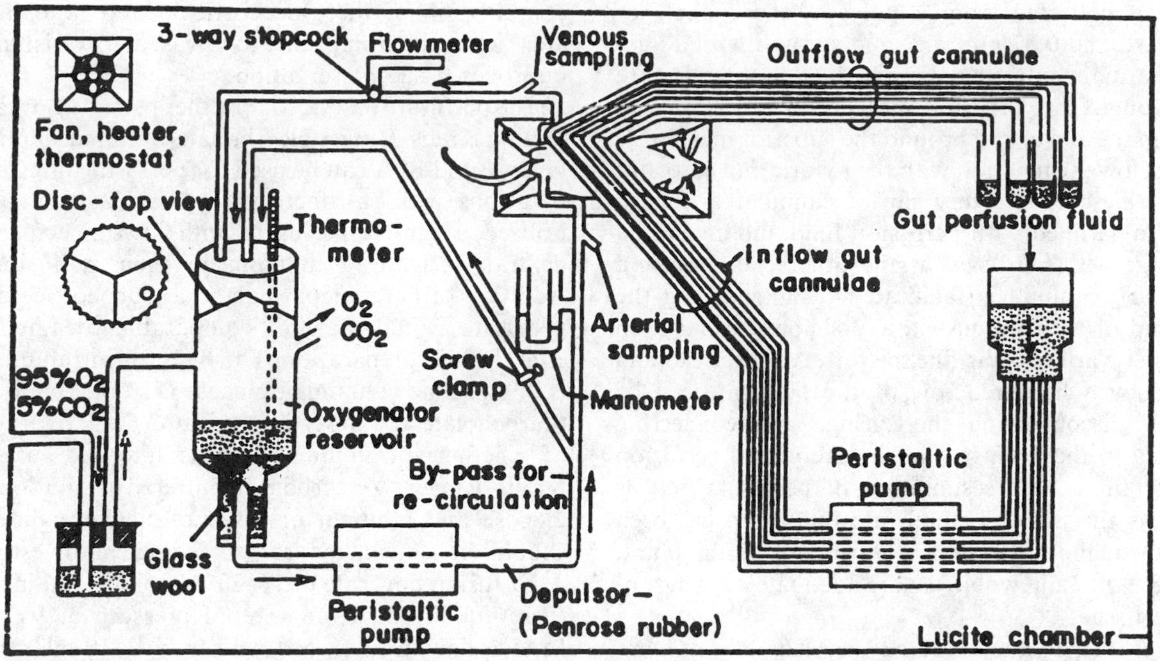

FIG. 33.10. Apparatus for vascular perfusion of small intestine. From Reference 123, with permission.

oxygenator–reservoir (7 cm diameter, 15 cm high) contains a thin acrylic disk with a gently sloping convex upper surface and separated edges supported by three equidistant flanges about 3.7 cm from the top. The tip of the Silastic tubing that carries venous and bypassed blood rests on the disk, so that the blood flows on the disk and spreads out to the serrated edges and finally down the inner wall of the cylinder as a thin film, thereby exposing a maximum surface area for oxygenation. O_2/CO_2 (95:5) is bubbled through distilled water and led into the gas inlet of the oxygenator–reservoir via the thin Silastic tubing. An appropriate blood filter can be placed at the bottom of the reservoir to filter out any broken cells or other debris before the blood circulation is pumped via a peristaltic pump to the animal. From the plastic filter, blood is led to a peristaltic pump via silicone tubing (4.60 mm o.d., 3.35 mm i.d.). A hydrostatic reservoir is maintained between the peristaltic pump and the animal to provide a constant perfusion pressure. A bypass flow from the hydrostatic reservoir to the central reservoir facilitates maintaining a constant hydrostatic head. Blood flow is determined by a transducer connected to the venous circuit by a three-way stopcock. Blood is sampled from the arterial and venous channel via polyethylene tubing, using Y connections near the arterial and venous cannulas. Thus blood is in contact with Silastic tubing, a hydrostatic reservoir, and polyethylene connections (Figure 33.10). Most of the silicone tubing can be replaced by glass in the apparatus, and use of the silicone tubing should be restricted to glass–tube connections and the peristaltic pump. If intraluminal flow is desired in the experimental protocol, an infusion pump can be used to introduce a fluid, with or without the test chemical, into the intestinal lumen. A peristaltic pump can be used for this purpose, giving a peristaltic wave motion for the intraluminal flow. Fluid effusing out of the intestine can be collected as desired or recirculated after sampling.

Perfusion Procedure

The rat is anesthetized with a mixture of ether and oxygen or an intraperitoneal injection of pentobarbital (50 mg/kg). Through an L-shaped abdominal incision, the small intestine, cecum, and proximal large intestine are gently exteriorized and supported on a plastic platform that is covered with gauze soaked in warm 0.9% NaCl. The intestine is covered with saline-soaked gauze in a plastic sheet and kept at 37°C by means of a heat lamp. Both ends of the intestine are ligated using an appropriate suture: proximally at the duodenum about 1.5 cm from the pylorus and distally near the midpoint of the descending colon. Included in the proximal ligature are the common bile duct and the mesentery between the duodenum and superior mesenteric vein. A PE-90 cannula is placed in the duodenal lumen and secured by the same ligature in those experiments in which intraluminal infusion is required.

Lymph is collected from a polyethylene cannula of 0.55 mm i.d. and 0.57 mm o.d. and secured with a ligature in the main intestinal lymph duct. Loose ties are placed around the superior mesenteric artery, about 5 mm from the aorta, and around the superior mesenteric vein just below the junction with the pyloric and coronary veins. The mesenteric artery can be cannulated using a PE-50 cannula filled with perfusion fluid and connected to a syringe with perfusate at the other end. Insertion of the PE-50 cannula is facilitated by introducing the beveled end of the cannula via a V-shaped cut made in the mesenteric artery using fine scissors. After the cannula is secured by a ligature, flow of the perfusate can be started by disconnecting the syringe and connecting the cannula to the perfusate of the preprimed perfusion apparatus. Immediate resumption of perfusate flow is essential, as the isolated small intestinal loop has been ischemic throughout the surgical procedure. At this point, a flow of 8–9 ml/min would ensure adequate oxygen supply to the tissue.

The rat is then exsanguinated by severing the left jugular vein and carotid artery. The superior mesenteric vein is cannulated by means of another PE-50 cannula in a manner analogous to the above procedure and secured by means of a suitable suture. The venous effluent is recycled through the perfusion apparatus to the oxygenator–reservoir. Once recirculation of the perfusate is established, arterial flow is increased until an arterial pressure of approximately 95 mm Hg is reached. The venous pressure is adjusted to 150 mm H_2O by an adjustable clamp on the outflow cannula. With experience, total surgical time can be minimized to 30 min or less. All of these procedures are easier with large animals; the isolated, vascularly perfused canine intestine is described in the literature (48,126,235).

Perfusion Media

The semiartificial perfusion medium consists of 80–120 ml fresh heparinized rat blood drawn by abdominal aortic puncture from an ether-anesthetized animal (345). The blood is heparinized with 10,000–25,000 IU sodium heparin. Windmueller et al. (345) used antibiotics in the blood (penicillin G, streptomycin), but often use of these compounds is undesirable as they may interfere with the test chemical. If the perfusion chamber and all of the components of the apparatus are sterilized, antibiotics have not been necessary for the perfusion of organs such as the lung and liver (197,205,207). Use of antibiotics should be avoided unless it becomes critical in a particular experimental protocol. Norepinephrine is used continuously at a rate of 1.0–2.2 ml/min as a 0.153-mg/ml solution to alleviate increased vascular resistance noted by earlier investigators. A glucocorticoid (dexamethasone, 6×10^{-7} M) is added in a single dose as a 25-mg/dl solution in the perfusate to the reservoir. A combination of the glucocorticoid and norepinephrine aids in maintaining the low vascular resistance and improves tissue preservation.

The perfusate described for other perfusate organs containing Krebs–Ringer bicarbonate-buffered solution with glucose and BSA can be used for perfusing intestinal preparations with satisfactory results. Kavin et al. (144) utilized a similar perfusate with low-molecular-weight dextran instead of albumin in their perfusion fluid. Addition of norepinephrine and a glucocorticoid to this perfusate would make it comparable to Windmueller et al.'s (345) preparation. The fluid for intraluminal flow is 0.9% saline containing glucose (220 mM) and sodium taurocholate (10 mM) infused at 2.6 ml/h. Regardless of whether intraluminal flow is intended, use of the Krebs–Ringer bicarbonate-buffered solution with glucose and albumin or low-molecular-weight dextran should be considered for toxicological investigations. A perfusion flow rate of 16–20 ml/min is obtained under these conditions at an arterial pressure of 95 mm Hg. In vivo flow in rats was found to be 8–10 ml/min (345), approximately half of that observed with the heparinized blood as perfusate. This rate is an indication of low vascular resistance; and when the intestinal vasculature is isolated, this resistance may persist during the remainder of the perfusion period.

Viability Criteria

Histological examination of the intestine after 5 h of perfusion (345) indicated that the integrity of the vascularly perfused tissue was well preserved. Cross-sections through the duodenum showed that the brush border of the intestinal wall and the base epithelium of the duodenum were well preserved after 5 h of perfusion (144,345). Additional parameters used for determining the viability of vascularly perfused intestinal preparations include the perfusion flow rate, uptake of glucose by tissue, production of lymph, and continued satisfactory oxygen consumption. In general, the preparation can be maintained viable for at least 5 h, as indicated by its gross and microscopic appearance and by the continued oxygen consumption, pelistaltic motility, water transport, and vascular responsiveness to norepinephrine. The perfused intestine is capable of glucose transport, and in most experiments, lymph flow continues without reduction for 5 h (345). The rate of lymph flow is increased by infusing intraluminal fluid and by increasing venous pressure. An additional parameter used for evaluating the perfused intestinal preparation is fat transport and lipoprotein biosynthesis (345). Morphological examination of the intestinal tissue by light and electron microscopy (144,345) is useful for ascertaining viability.

Applications

The effects of bolus intra-arterial doses of heroin and other stimulant drugs were studied (235) in vascularly perfused isolated segments of canine dog small intestine. Heroin caused dose-related increases in intraluminal pressure similar to those caused by morphine. Perfusion with Krebs bicarbonate solution containing naloxone selectively abolished intestinal responses to heroin. Perfusion with cinanserin, a 5-HT antagonist, decreased intestinal responses to 5-HT and heroin without affecting responses to dimethylphenylpiperazinium or bethanechol. Atropine antagonized the contractile responses. The authors concluded that heroin interacts with a conventional opiate receptor in the intestine and that the intestinal stimulatory effect of heroin is mediated by the release of endogenous 5-HT, which activates intramural cholinergic neurons. In other studies, perfused canine intestines were used to evaluate the proposed *k* receptor agonist such as ethylketoxyclazocine, nalorphine, and bremazocine (126) and concluded that *k* receptors did not appear to be involved in the contractile response of the canine small intestine to opioids.

The effects of hydrolytic products of food digestion on jejunal mucosal injury and restitution were assessed in anesthetized rats (161). Mucosal epithelial integrity was continuously monitored by measuring the blood-to-lumen clearance of ^{51}Cr-labeled ethylenediaminetetracctic acid (EDTA). Perfusion of the lumen with hydrolyzed casein (3%) or glucose (150 mM) did not affect ^{51}Cr-EDTA clearance compared with saline controls. By contrast, perfusion with emulsified lipids (20 mM sodium taurocholate and 10–40 mM oleic acid) increased ^{51}Cr-EDTA clearance in a dose dependent manner. This increase in clearance of ^{51}Cr-EDTA could be restored to normal if infusion of the lipid emulsion was terminated and saline infusion was resumed. Histological evaluation of jejunal mucosa indicated that the epithelial lining of the villous tips was damaged during lipid infusion and that restitution of the lining occurred within 50 min after the resumption of saline perfusion. Because the concentrations of the nutrients used in this study were similar to those measured in postprandial chyme, these findings suggest that the intestinal epithelium is injured and restitutes during the normal course of digestion and absorption of a meal. In another study (186), influence of cadaverine and aminoguanidine on uptake of histamine was studied in perfused intestinal segments of rats.

Nakai (221) employed isolated small bowel from the duodenojejunal junction to the ileocecal junction with intact small mesentic artery (SMA) and small mesenteric vein (SMV), was perfused with Krebs–Ringer buffer solution intraluminally in rat. After all the branches from the aorta and the portal vein were cannulated and perfused with Krebs–Dextran solution, the isolated perfused bowel was transferred immediately to a chamber equipped with constant temperature and humidity. B4 endotoxin (Difco) was added to the intravascular perfusate. Changes in the endotoxin-perfused bowel were compared to the control bowel perfused without the endotoxin. Active transport of D-glucose was decreased. Entry of water into the gut was not affected. Lactic acid level in the intravascular fluid was significantly higher, which was correlated with decreased pH of this fluid. Although oxygen consumption was not changed, carbon dioxide accumulation in the intravascular fluid was significantly higher.

Isolated vascularly perfused intestinal preparations have been used in toxicological investigations infrequently. It is not readily apparent as to why, but difficulty in developing the techniques for maintaining a viable perfused preparation and the requirement for elaborate equipment must have had some influence on the use of this technique. The preparation may prove useful in studies relating to drug absorption and the interaction of drugs during intestinal absorption and transport. It might also be useful for evaluating intestinal metabolism and overall disposition of chemicals. The preparation may also be useful for testing reported intestinal elimination of of chlorinated hydrocarbon compounds via the luminal surface. Finally, the effect of toxic chemicals on absorption of nutrients, generation and preservation of mucosal cell lining, and various drug-metabolizing enzymes can be evaluated using perfused intestinal preparations. The effect of chemicals on endogenous biochemical parameters that are related to intermediary metabolism of the intestine itself can also be investigated.

Isolated Perfused Pancreas

The pancreas is a highly vascular endocrine organ in which the anatomy of the blood supply lends itself to isolated vascular perfusion. Compared to the isolated islet incubation (165), pancreatic slices (179), and tissue fragments (64), the superfusion method of Burr et al. (49) for the isolated perfused pancreas is the most satisfactory and ideal approach to study the interrelations between pancreatic and other hormones and the effect of chemicals on pancreatic function. The isolated perfused pancreas is preferred over all the other tissue preparations for these studies in view of the following advantages (184). Superficial and deep islets are equally provided with oxygen, which is constantly replenished, and the substrates and effectors arrive at the cell in a physiologically normal way. The islets remain in anatomical relation with other cells and tissues of the organs, including blood vessels and nerves. Only extrinsic nerve control is lost, and many intrinsic factors that actively regulate the gland's function may be preserved in an isolated perfused pancreatic preparation. Maintenance of cellular integrity can be confirmed at the end of the experiment by light and electron microscopic examination. There is a possibility of a control and experimental period of study in the same pancreas preparation. Such control in other in vitro systems requires multiple incubations.

Of greater significance might be the ability to maintain the exocrine secretions of the pancreas from getting back into contact with the islet cells, as cannulation of the segment of duodenum into which the exocrine secretions drain allows separate collection of these secretions. Thus the enzymes and other secretions produced are kept separate from the cells that produce them, and the well-known digestive effect of pancreatic enzymes on the pancreatic tissue is avoided. Despite the overwhelming superiority of vascularly perfused pancreatic preparations, there has been a lag in the development of perfusion techniques with this endocrine tissue. The lag can be attributed to the technical difficulties encountered with surgical preparations and the heterogeneity of the tissue in the preparation.

The location of the pancreatic duct entering the duodenum might be of some significance, especially in studies related to exocrine function such as protein synthesis. The pancreatic ducts are multiple, and their entry into the intestine is variable (52). Doerr and Becker (75) reported the main pancreatic duct emptying into the bile duct rather than into the duodenum in the rat. In the guinea pig and rabbit (75), the main pancreatic duct enters the duodenal tract. The general rule is that in carnivores the ducts empty near or into the common bile duct, whereas in herbivores they empty more distally into the duodenum.

A limited literature is available on the technique of isolated perfused pancreatic preparation, although excellent descriptions of feline (52,80) and canine (121, 134,151) pancreas preparations are available. The principal descriptions are those of Grodsky et al. (110), Sussman et al. (311), and Loubatieres et al. (184). The following description is a combination of the best features of all three preparations.

Apparatus

The apparatus used by Sussman et al. (311) is adequate for perfusion of the isolated pancreas and is described here. The chamber of the perfusion apparatus is based on the original description of that used by Miller et al. (211). The details of the apparatus are given in Figure 33.11. Perfusate is pumped from the reservoir through Silastic tubing to a multibulb glass lung for oxygenation. The perfusate is then pumped by means of a peristaltic pump through a flow transducer, after which it courses

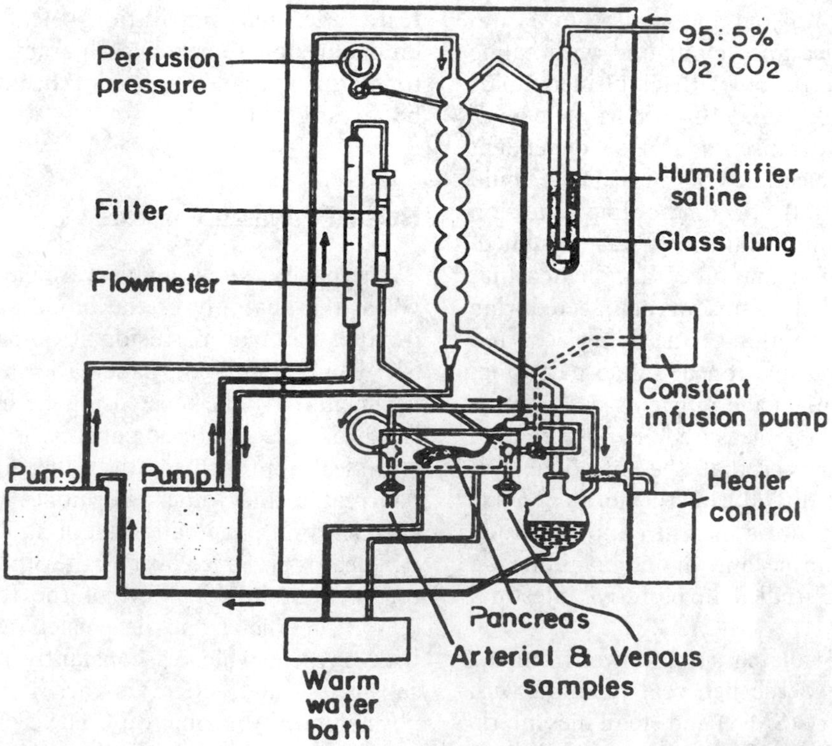

FIG. 33.11. Apparatus for perfusion of an isolated pancreas preparation, described by Sussman et al. (273). It is a modification of the apparatus described by Miller et al. (181) and adapted to the perfusion of the rat pancreas. From Reference 273, with permission.

through a filter to the enclosed perfusion chamber. The perfusate enters the pancreatic circulation through the arterial cannula, and the pressure is measured in millimeters of mercury using an ancroid manometer. The arterial blood may be sampled through another, similar arrangement (Figure 33.11) O_2/CO_2 (95:5) is directed to the lung after bubbling through a humidifier. The pancreas is kept moist with either the same solution used as perfusate or normal saline. The pancreas is perfused using Krebs–Ringer bicarbonate-buffered solution (pH 7.4) containing glucose and BSA, as described for the liver, which is circulated through the glass lung for oxygenation. A pediatric plastic cannula (1.5 mm o.d.) is used to cannulate the arterial side with an attachment for measuring intraluminal pressure. The venous cannula is polyethylene tubing (2 mm o.d.). The duodenal cannula, an arrangement similar to the one described earlier for perfusion of the intestine, is adequate.

Surgical Procedure

The animal may be starved overnight to facilitate the operation by depleting the omental fat. Although this method facilitates surgical procedures, the investigator may wish to avoid starving the animal as starvation is known to cause increased toxicity of some chemicals, which might also mean that pancreatic effects are altered. The animal is anesthetized by appropriate means (e.g., pentobarbital 50 mg/kg IP). A lateral incision and a midline incision through the skin and linea alba and through the skin over the inferior thorax are made as described for the surgical procedure to isolate the liver. The intestine is moved to the animal's left and covered with a wet saline gauze, and the aorta with the superior mesenteric branch is made clearly visible. The descending colon is easily identified as it remains attached to the lower posterior abdominal wall by a short mesentery. The fine layer of connective tissue is cut along the length of the colon in a plane in which no blood vessels are found, thereby mobilizing the lower gut, which is later removed. Using blunt-end dissection scissors, the pancreas is separated from the overlying colon. The jejunum is ligated and severed just behind its pancreatic attachment. This ligature will be useful for orientation later. The distal jejunum has a copious blood supply, and its vessels are tied for the last 1.2 cm of the distal segment to facilitate its later removal.

At this time the superior mesenteric vein, which runs into the portal vein, can be seen over the surface of the pancreas. The superior mesenteric vein is tied just below the pancreas with double ligatures and cut between them. Any other attachments of the pancreas to the descending colon are ligated and cut. At this stage the superior mesenteric artery and celiac axis can be identified and are preserved through the following dissection. The fine membrane covering the spleen and any other closely adherent tissue is carefully picked off with sharp forceps. The main splenic vessels, entering toward the upper pole, are tied twice and cut between the ligatures. A whole set of vessels curve through the mesentery to cross between the pancreatic tail and the spleen. If tied together, these pedicles can bunch the vessels in the tail of the pancreas. It is better to tie each of them individually with additional investments of time. A marker thread may be left to denote the tail of the pancreas for relative ease in orienting it upon its isolation.

The stomach is pulled downward, and the major left gastric artery, which runs into the upper and medial aspect of stomach near the esophagus, is tied. One ligature encloses both the vessels and the esophagus, and second and third ligatures include the vessel and esophagus separately and higher up. The vessels and esophagus are cut between ligatures. Lifting the stomach to the right exposes vascular connections to the posterior wall, which can be tied, using a single distal tie, and then cut. Finally, the pylorus is tied twice and cut between the ligatures, releasing the stomach, which can now be checked. At this stage the animal can be heparinized by means of an injection via the inferior vena cava. The right renal pedicle (containing artery, vein, ureter) is cleared with blunt dissection and a ligature passed behind the artery and vein with curved forceps. Double ligatures allow the vessels to be cut and the kidney removed.

By careful dissection, the aorta is exposed at this level to clear it from the inferior vena cava between the left renal artery and superior mesenteric artery. A ligature passed behind the aorta at this level can now be tied. Three loose ligatures are passed around the portal vein as it leaves the pancreas for the liver. The uppermost ligatures should include all structures of the portal tract (vein, hepatic artery, bile duct), whereas the other two include only the vein. Cannulation is delayed until the aorta has been cleared along its length, preserving the celiac and mesenteric branches. This step entails passing ligatures around and tying particularly the lumbar arteries. The aorta is free from the inferior vena cava from the level of the diaphragm to the ligature below the left renal artery. Loose ligatures are positioned around the aorta just below the diaphragm, avoiding the origin of the celiac artery.

The portal vein can be cannulated in a retrograde manner by tying the uppermost ligatures first and making an incision in the anterior wall of the vein. The cannula (made from PE-140 to PE-100 tubing) is filled with heparinized perfusion medium before insertion. When flow through a portal cannula is ensured, aortic cannulation is performed. The rat is turned around with the head toward the operator, and a midline incision is made through the thorax, cutting the diaphragm through the edge. The anoxic phase begins from the moment of

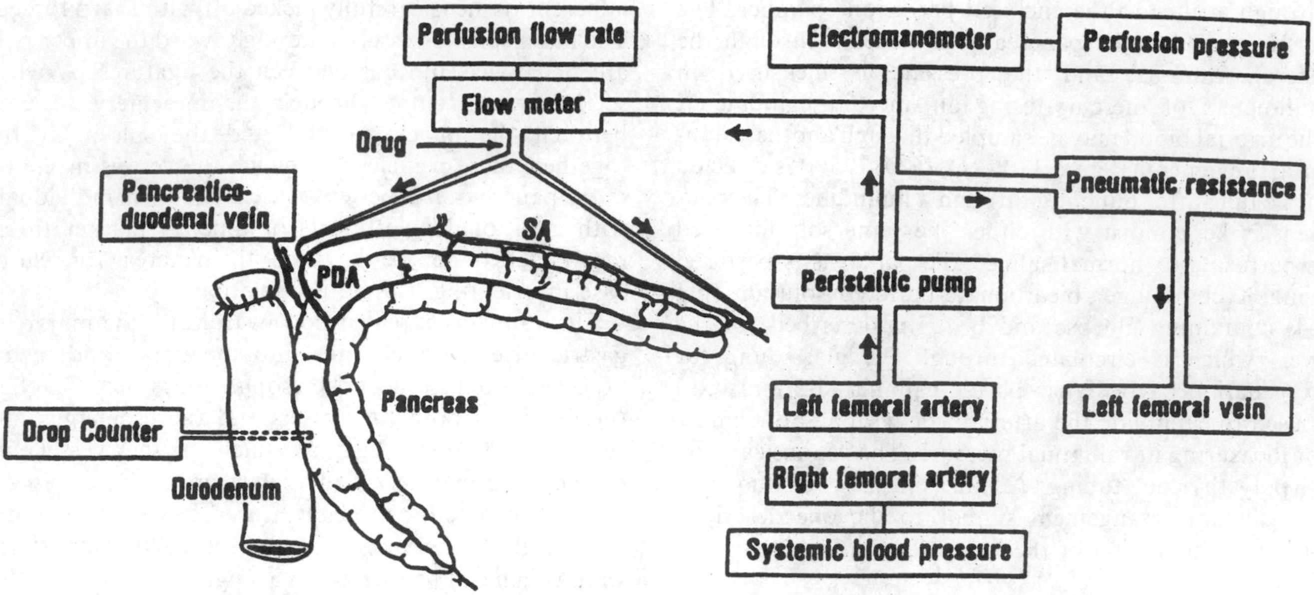

FIG. 33.12. Constant perfusion system of the blood-perfused canine pancreas preparation. Arterial cannulas are inserted into the pancreaticoduodenal (PDA) and splenic (SA) arteries. From Reference 112, with permission.

entering, and speed of surgical procedure is essential (it comes with practice). The thoracic walls are spread apart by means of appropriate retractors, and the thoracic aorta is separated from behind the esophagus. The cannula is inserted and advanced until its tip just passes the diaphragm. The abdominal aortic ligature is tightened, and with the cannula in place the flow should commence. The final step is to complete the isolation of the pancreatic circulation by tying the ligature, which has already been prepared, around the lower inferior vena cava.

The perfusing pancreas is now transported to the organ chamber. The inferior vena cava is cut distal to the last tied ligature, and removal of the cannulated pancreas should be possible by grasping the two cannulas and the loop of duodenum to lift the pancreas clear of the rat. The organ is oriented on the platform in the perfusion chamber by means of identifying ligatures that were placed during the preparation; successful uniform perfusion is obtained if this step is carefully undertaken. There should be a flow of 2 ml/min with a perfusion pressure of about 40 mm Hg. It may be wise to reject preparations if pressures above 80 mm Hg are obtained, as it usually results in further deterioration of the perfused pancreatic preparation. The entire surgical procedure takes roughly 60–75 min, assuming familiarity with surgical techniques (65).

With the method of Grodsky et al. (110), perfusion of the pancreas is performed together with perfusion of the stomach, spleen, and duodenum as a unit, which are removed from the rat through a vertical abdominal incision and transferred to the prewarmed chamber. The celiac axis is cannulated for the inflow and the portal vein for the outflow. A peristaltic pump supplies the perfusion medium to the celiac axis at a pressure of 40–100 mm Hg, and the flow is adjusted to 10 ml/min. The principal disadvantage of the procedure of Grodsky et al. is that it involves perfusion of additional tissues so that ascribing a particular biochemical function to the pancreas would be more difficult. The principal advantage is that the surgical procedure is much simpler. Procedures for the cannulation and perfusion of feline and canine pancreas are available. Figure 33.12 shows the constant perfusion system of the blood-perfused canine pancreas (133).

Perfusion Media

Grodsky et al. (110) used whole rat blood mixed with an artificial medium as a perfusate, but they, and others who utilized whole blood, encountered hemolysis of red blood cells, which resulted in complications of the perfusion. Hence the use of artificial medium has become more popular for perfusion of the pancreas. The medium containing 4% dextran in Krebs–Henseleit medium prepared and gassed with O_2/CO_2 (95:5) is satisfactory. This medium is the standard one mentioned in the subsequent work of Grodsky et al. as well as by many other investigators. Alternatively, 4% human serum albumin or BSA can be used instead of dextran with no apparent difference in insulin production, medium flow, and rate of circulation of perfusion (65). The pH is adjusted to 7.4, and the addition of sodium bicarbonate and adequate bubbling with the O_2/CO_2 ensures maintaining the appropriate pH. If the pH seems to fluctuate during the experiment, addition of sodium bicarbonate solution to the perfusate helps stabilize its pH.

Khayambashi and Lyman (146) used a medium containing fresh rat plasma diluted 1:1 with Ringer's saline or 0.9% saline with satisfactory results. Costiner et al. (65) used diluted heparinized rat blood as perfusate to support satisfactory pancreatic function. Advantages of perfusing pancreas with whole blood have been pointed out (114), and the advantage of the larger animal size has been noted by several investigators when using autologous blood (42,114,134,151).

Viability Criteria

Several parameters of physiological and biochemical function were reported by Grodsky et al. (110). Histological examinations at the end of the perfusion period indicated that well-preserved granules diminished in number roughly in proportion to the measured release of insulin into the medium (110). Oxygen consumption by the perfused pancreas can be used as a comparatively rough indicator of viability. However, in the preparation of Grodsky et al. (110), because other tissues are involved in the perfusion circulation, oxygen consumption may not be an exclusive indicator of viability of the perfused pancreas. In the preparation of Sussman and Vaughn (311), because less peripheral tissue is involved, oxygen consumption might represent a better viability criterion. In any case, production of insulin by the preparation, consumption of glucose, and the analysis of exocrine secretion collected through the duodenal cannula can be used as adequate criteria for the viability of the perfused pancreas. The pH of the circulating perfusate can be monitored and adjusted if necessary by regulating the O_2/CO_2 ratio when oxygenating the perfusate. Also, appropriate amounts of sodium bicarbonate solution can be added to adjust the pH of the circulating perfusate.

Amylase formation has been shown to be linear for 40 min in the preparation used by Khayambashi and Lyman (146), and an amylase assay might be a reasonable parameter for viability. However, they observed that the rate of amylase production fell beyond 40 min despite the linearity of the perfusion flow rate. This decrease may be a reflection of the discharge of existing enzymes rather than the inability for the isolated perfused organ to synthesize enzymes. In the work of Khayambashi and Lyman (146), the composition of the perfusion medium was demonstrated to have a definite effect on the secretion of the amylase type of enzymes by the pancreas. Hence such a criterion may have to be established in conjunction with other parameters of perfused preparation. Sampling of the tissue to demonstrate effects that may be reflected in the medium or related to a particular treatment of perfusion is clearly important in the assessment of the perfused organ. In this connection, it may be pointed out that the dendritic form of the rat pancreas lends itself to sampling when a single arm of the pancreas is tied off and perfusion is continued in the remaining tissue. However, if a portion of the organ is sampled, the biochemical study done with the same perfused organ may be compromised, especially with respect to later time points, as all of the organ would not be present at later times, especially if such sampling is carried out repeatedly.

Applications

The perfused pancreas has had limited use in toxicological investigations. The development of sensitive radioimmunoassays for insulin and glucagon in biological fluids has enabled quantitative measurement of their secretion and has led to the use of pancreas perfusion techniques in such studies (298). Inoue et al. (129) investigated the effects of amylin, a protein secreted by pancreatic beta cells, as well as a major constituent of the islet amyloid deposits in patients with non-insulin-dependent diabetes mellitus, on release of insulin and glucagon. Amylin (100 nM) did not alter glucose-stimulated secretion of insulin but significantly inhibited arginine-stimulated secretion of insulin. Amylin did not alter the release of glucagon from perfused rat pancreas in response to 16.7 mM glucose and 10 mM arginine. These findings suggest that amylin may modulate the secretion of insulin from pancreatic beta cells. Clearly, the perfused pancreas can be used to evaluate the effect of drugs and drug interactions that affect pancreatic function. Drugs not having exclusive action on the pancreas may mutually interact within the body to produce an action on pancreatic function (252). Yelich (348) studied the effect of epinephrine on insulin and glucagon secretion from endotoxin treated rats. Pancreases from control and endotoxin-treated rats were perfused with 240 mg/dl glucose in the presence or absence of 13.6 nM epinephrine.The absolute ability of epinephrine to inhibit glucose-induced immunoreactive glucagon secretion was similar for both control and treated pancreases. However, because endotoxic pancreases hypersecrete insulin, the relative ability of epinephrine to inhibit insulin secretion was reduced in endotoxic pancreas. Although epinephrine did not appreciably alter immunoreactive glucagon secretion, it prevented a progressive decrease in its secretion. The results partially explain endotoxin-induced hyperinsulinemia and also demonstrate a possible role for epinephrine with regard to the production of elevated glucagon levels during endotoxicosis. Blech et al. (33) tested the in vitro and in vivo effects of gold thioglucose on the insulin and glucagon secretion of the isolated perfused Wistar rat pancreas. The authors concluded that gold thioglucose reacts primarily on the hypothalamus and modulates the reactivity of the pancreas in a permanent manner via the nervous system. To elucidate the mechanism of insensitivity of hormone secretion to glucose in streptozotocin-induced diabetic rat islets, Ito et al. (131) investigated the effects of acetylcholine and norepinephrine on insulin and glucagon secretion to changes in glucose concentration in isolated perfused rat pancreas. Basal insulin secretion at a blood glucose level of 5.6 mmol/L was significantly higher and neither high (16.7 mmol/L) nor low (1.4 mmol/L) blood glucose concentrations influenced insulin or glucagon secretion. Addition of acetylcholine (10^{-6} mol/L) to the perfusate increased glucose-stimulated insulin secretion. Acetylcholine (10^{-6} mol/L) and norepinephrine (10^{-7} mol/L), or a combination of both, induced marked glucagon secretion, and was suppressed by high glucose levels. Histopathological examination revealed a marked decline in acetylcholinesterase and monoamine oxidase activities in the islets of streptozotocin-induced diabetic rats. The authors proposed that reduction of the potentiating effects of acetylcholine and norepinephrine lessen glucose sensitivity of islet beta and alpha cells in this rat model of diabetes.

Peterson and Fujimoto (252) have demonstrated increased pancreatic secretory activity after exposure to such agents as ethanol and CCl_4. The mechanism of such enhanced pancreatic secretory activity is not understood. Use of a perfused pancreatic preparation obtained from control and treated animals may be useful in the elucidation of the underlying mechanisms. Nordback et al. (233) investigated the role of acetaldehyde in the pathogenesis of acute alcoholic pancreatitis. They tested their hypothesis that acute alcoholic pancreatitis may be initiated by acetaldehyde in the presence of active xanthine oxidase in their experiments wherein xanthine dehydrogenase was converted to xanthine oxidase by a period of ischemia, and infusing acetaldehyde (250 mg/h after 2 h of ischemia). The authors concuded that in the presence of active xanthine oxidase acetaldehyde can initiate acute alcoholic pantcreatitis and that toxic oxygen metabolites play an important intermediary role.

Examples of the use of isolated perfused pancreas for a number of pharmacological (16,108,110,247), physiological (80,247), and toxicological (42,151) studies are available. The studies of Kimura et al. (151) provide one example of the utility of the perfused pancreas in mechanistic toxicological investigations. Although steroid administration has long been suspected of causing acute pancreatitis, clinical and experimental data have failed to firmly establish the association or to uncover a pathogenic mechanism. The acute effects of large doses of methylprednisolone on the pancreas were evaluated using an isolated, perfused canine pancreas (151). Using a dose of 200 mg of methylprednisolone, there were no significant differences between the control and steroid-treated preparations over a 4-h perfusion period. When the dose of methylprednisolone was increased to 400 mg, again there were no significant differences in gross appearance, weight gain, or serum amylase during a 3-h perfusion period. However, pancreatic secretion was initially depressed in the steroid-treated preparations. Following a maximal secretory stimulus (secretin), secretion markedly increased during the 4th hour of perfusion but again was significantly less in the steroid-treated glands. The viscosity of pancreatic secretions was significantly increased in the steroid-treated glands. These studies suggested a mild inhibitory effect of steroids on pancreatic secretion, which might be mediated through an increase in viscosity.

Another example is provided by the studies of Broe and Cameron (42). Controlled clinical trials have documented the development of acute pancreatitis in 5% of patients receiving azathioprine for Crohn's disease, by far the highest incidence of drug-induced pancreatitis recorded to date. The isolated, perfused canine pancreas was used to evaluate the effects of azathioprine on the pancreas. No significant changes in gross appearance, weight, or serum amylase were observed in azathioprine-treated glands compared to controls. Azathioprine administration, however, resulted in a twofold increase in secretory volume and bicarbonate output, as well as a profound depression of trypsin output, compared to controls. These preliminary studies demonstrate that azathioprine has a marked effect on pancreatic function in this model (42).

ACKNOWLEDGMENTS

This effort was supported by a U.S. Public Health Service grant (HL-20622) from the National Heart, Lung, and Blood Institute, by U.S. Environmental Protection Agency grant R-811072, and by a Starter grant from The Burroughs Wellcome Fund. The excellent assistance of Lillian Brown in the preparation of this manuscript is greatly appreciated. The contributions of former and present colleagues to the work referenced in this manuscript are appreciated.

QUESTIONS

1. Describe a technique for preparing an isolated perfused ventilated lung using positive pressure and negative pressure for ventilation. Which blood vessels are cannulated and why?
2. Describe the isolated perfused liver preparation. What are the advantages and disadvantages of in situ and isolated liver perfusion techniques?

3. Substantitate the statement that Langendorff preparation are useful for mechanistic studies in toxicology.
4. Why are isolated perfused organ techniques useful in toxicological investigations? Compare and contrast advantages and disadvantages of isolated vascularly perfused organ techniques and isolated cell incubations.
5. Describe three toxicological studies using isolated perfused brain preparations.
6. Using suitable examples illustrate how isolated perfused kidneys are useful in investigating mechanisms of toxicity.
7. Describe an isolated perfused pancreatic preparation. Design a study to investigate the mechanism of pancreatotoxic action of a suspected toxicant.
8. Design an investigation of toxicity of an intestinal toxicant using an isolated perfused rat intestine preparation.
9. What are the advantages and disadvantages of using artificial medium versus whole or diluted blood perfusate for toxicokinetic perfusion studies with isolated perfused organs?
10. Compare and contrast the use of one-pass versus recirculating perfusion systems for toxicokinetic and mechanistic studies.

REFERENCES

1. Abraham, R., Dawson, W., Grasso, P., and Goldberg, L. (1968): Lysosomal changes associated with hyperoxia in the isolated perfused rat liver. *Exp. Mol. Pathol.*, 8:370–387.
2. Agarwal, A. K., and Mehendale, H. M. (1986): Effect of chlordecone on carbon tetrachloride-induced increase in calcium uptake in isolated perfused rat liver. *Toxicol. Appl. Pharmacol.*, 83:342–348.
3. Aiba, T., Itoga, Y., Shimizu, H., Tanigawara, Y., and Hori, R. (1994): Renal handling of tobramycin in the isolated perfused rat kidney. *J. Pharm. Sci.*, 83:723–726.
4. Akahira, M., Hara, A., Hashizume, H., Nakamura, M., and Abiko, Y. (1998): Protective effect of prazocin on the hydrogen peroxide-induced derangements in the isolated perfused rat heart. *Life Sci.*, 62:1755–1766.
5. Akerboom, T., Schneider, I., Von Dahl, S., and Sies, H. (1991): Cholestasis and changes of portal pressure caused by chlorpromazine in the perfused rat liver. *Hepatology*, 13:216–221.
6. Ambs, S., and Neumann, H. G. (1996): Acute and chronic toxicity of aromatic amines studied in the isolated perfused rat liver. *Toxicol. Appl. Pharmacol.*, 139:186–194.
7. Anderson, P. G., Digerness, S. B., Sklar, J. L., and Boor, P. J. (1990): Use of the isolated perfused heart for evaluation of cardiac toxicity. *Toxicol. Pathol.*, 18:497–510.
8. Andjus, R. K., Suhara, K., and Stoviter, H. A. (1967): An isolated, perfused rat brain preparation, its spontaneous and stimulated activity. *J. Appl. Physiol.*, 22:1033–1039.
9. Andrews, W. H. H., Hecker, R., and Maegraith, B. G. (1956): The action of adrenaline, noradrenaline, acetylcholine and histamine on the perfused liver of the monkey, cat and rabbit. *J. Physiol. (Lond.)*, 132:509–521.
10. Angevine, L. S., and Mehendale, H. M. (1980): Chlorphentermine uptake by isolated perfused rabbit lung. *Toxicol. Appl. Pharmacol.*, 52:336–346.
11. Angevine, L. S., and Mehendale, H. M. (1980): Effect of chlorphentermine on the pulmonary disposition of 5-hydroxytryptamine in the isolated perfused rat lung. *Am. Rev. Respir. Dis.*, 122:891–898.
12. Angevine, L. S., and Mehendale, H. M. (1982): Effect of chlorphentermine treatment on 5-hydroxytryptamine disposition in the isolated perfused rat lung. *Fundam. Appl. Toxicol.*, 21:306–312.
13. Aronson, C. E. (1976): Effects of thyroxine pretreatment and calcium on the isolated, perfused rat heart. *Arch. Int. Pharmacodyn.*, 222:351–360.
14. Aronson, C. E., and Serlick, E. R. (1976): Effects of prolonged perfusion time on the isolated perfused rat heart. *Toxicol. Appl. Pharmacol.*, 38:479–488.
15. Aronson, C. E., and Serlick, E. R. (1977): Effects of chlorpromazine on the isolated rat heart. *Toxicol. Appl. Pharmacol.*, 39:157–176.
16. Arredondo, A. A., Chaudhuri, B., Kar, R., Crist, K. A., Thomford, M. R., and Chaudhuri, P. K. (1990): Isolated perfusion of pancreas with mitomycin C. *Am. J. Surg.*, 159:569–574.
17. Auda, S. P., Kesner, L., Butt, K., and Dountz, S. L. (1975): Continuous single pass perfusion of the isolated kidney. *Trans. Am. Soc. Artif. Intern. Organs*, 21:84–88.
18. Autian, J. (1975): In vitro toxicity testing gains strength. *Forum Advancement Toxicol.*, 8:1–2 (newsletter).
19. Aviado, D. M. (1975): Drug action, reaction, and interaction. II. Teratogenic cardiopathies. *J. Clin. Pharmacol.*, 15:641–655.
20. Baath, L., and Almen, T. (1989): Reduction of the risk of ventricular fibrillation in the isolated rabbit heart by small additions of electrolytes to non-ionic monomeric contrast media. *Acta Radiol.*, 30:327–333.
21. Baciewicz, F. A., Arredondo, M., Chaudhuri, B., Crist, K. A., Basilius, D., Bandyopadhyaah, S., Thomford, N. R., and Chaudhuri, P. K. (1991): Pharmacokinetics and toxicity of isolated perfusion of lung with doxorubicin. *J. Surg. Res.*, 50:124–128.
22. Baglioni, D. E. (1910): Stoffwecheseluntershuganagen and Uberlebenden organen. *Han. Biol. Arb. Meth.*, 3:364.
23. Bahlmann, J., Giebisch, G., Ochwady, B., and Schoeppe, W. (1967): Micropuncture study of isolated perfused rat kidney. *Am. J. Physiol.*, 221:77–82.
24. Bakhle, T. S., Reynard, A. M., and Vane, J. R. (1969): Metabolism of the angiotensins in isolated perfused tissues. *Nature*, 222:956–958.
25. Barrett, J. P., Ingenito, A. J., and Procita, L. (1969): A brain perfusion technique adapted for the study of drugs which may affect the peripheral circulation through a central action. *J. Pharmacol. Exp. Ther.*, 170:199–209.
26. Bauman, A. W., Clarkson, T. W., and Miles, E. M. (1963): Functional evaluation of isolated perfused rat kidney. *J. Appl. Physiol.*, 18:1239–1246.
27. Bautista, A. P., and Spitzer, J. J. (1990): Superoxide amion generation by in situ perfused rat liver: Effect of in vivo endotoxin. *Am. J. Physiol.*, 259:G907–G912.
28. Belinsky, S. A., Popp, J. A., Kauffman, F. C., and Thurman, R. G. (1984): Trypan blue uptake as a new method to investigate hepatotoxicity in periportal and pericentral regions of the liver lobule: Studies with allyl alcohol in the perfused liver. *J. Pharmacol. Exp. Ther.*, 230:755–760.

29. Berggren, M., Dawson, J., and Moldéus, P. (1984): Glutathione biosynthesis in the isolated perfused rat lung: Utilization of extracellular glutathione. *FEBS Lett.*, 176:189–192.
30. Bernard, C. E., Magid, A. A., Yen, T. S., and Hoener, B. A. (1997): Mitigation of nitrofurantoin-induced toxicity in the perfused rat lung. *Hum. Exp. Toxicol.*, 16:727–732.
31. Bernstein, E. F. (1971): Evaluation of mechanical systems used in perfusion. In: *Perfusion Techniques*, edited by E. Diszfalusy, pp. 44–73. Karolinska Institute, Stockholm.
32. Bingham, E., Warshawsky, D., and Niemeier, R. W. (1978): Metabolism of benzo(*a*)pyrene in the isolated perfused rabbit lung following N-dodecane inhalation. In: *Carcinogenesis: Mechanisms of Tumor Production and Carcinogenesis*, edited by T. J. Slaga, A. Sivak, and R. K. Boutwell, Vol. 2, pp. 509–516. Raven Press, New York.
33. Blech, W., Bierwolf, B., Weiss, I., and Ziegler, M. (1986): In vitro and in vivo effect of gold thioglucose on the insulin- and glucagon-secretion of the isolated perfused rat pancreas. *Biomed. Biochim. Acta*, 45:507–522.
34. Bleehan, N. M., and Fisher, R. B. (1954): The action of insulin on the isolated rat heart. *J. Physiol.*, (*Lond.*), 123:260–276.
35. Block, E. R., and Cannon, J. K. (1978): Effect of oxygen exposure on lung clearance of amines. *Lung*, 155:287–295.
36. Bock, K. W., Forhling, W., and Scholte, W. (1972): Activity and stability of microsomal mixed function oxidase and NAD glycohydrolase in isolated perfused rat liver. *Naunyn. Schmiedebergs Arch. Pharmacol.*, 273:193–203.
37. Bond, J. A., and Mauderly, J. L. (1984): Metabolism and macromolecular covalent binding of [^{14}C]-1-nitropyrene in isolated perfused and ventilated rat lungs. *Cancer Res.*, 44:3924–3929.
38. Boyd, C. A. R., Parsons, D. S., and Thomas, A. V. (1968): The presence of K^+ dependent phosphatase in intestinal epithelial cell brush borders isolated by a new method. *Biochim. Biophys. Acta*, 150:723–726.
39. Bowman, R. H., and Maack, T. (1972): Glucose transport by the isolated rat kidney. *Am. J. Physiol.*, 222:1499–1504.
40. Brauer, R. W., Pessotti, R. L., and Pizzolato, P. (1951): Isolated rat liver preparation: Bile production and other basic properties. *Proc. Soc. Exp. Biol. Med.*, 78:174–185.
41. Brodie, T. G. (1903): The perfusion of surviving organs. *J. Physiol.* (*Lond.*), 29:266–275.
42. Broe, P. J., and Cameron, J. L. (1983): Azathioprine and acute pancreatitis: Studies with an isolated perfused canine pancreas. *J. Surg. Res.*, 34:159–163.
43. Brown, P. C., Thurman, R. G., Belinsky, S. A., and Kauffman, F. C. (1991): Effect of allyl alcohol on xanthine dehydrogenase activity in the perfused rat liver. *Toxicol. Lett.*, 58:1–6.
44. Bruck, R., Prigozin, H., Krepel, Z., Rotenberg, P., Schechter, Y., and Bar-Meir, S. (1991): Vanadate inhibits glucose output from isolated perfused rat liver. *Hepatology*, 14:540–544.
45. Brull, L., and Louis-Bar, D. (1957): Toxicity of artificially circulated heparinized blood on the kidney. *Arch. Int. Physiol. Biochem.*, 65:470–476.
46. Bullock, G., Eakins, M. N., Sawyer, B. C., and Slater, T. F. (1974): Studies on bile secretion with the aid of the isolated perfused rat liver. I. Inhibitory action of sporidesmin and icterogenin. *Proc. R. Soc. Lond.*, 186:333–356.
47. Bunc, M., Drevensek, G., Budinha, M., and Suput, D. (1999): Effects of equinatoxin II from *Actinia equina* (L.) on isolated rat heart: The role of direct cardiuotoxic effects in equitoxin II lethality. *Toxicon*, 37:109–123.
48. Burks, T. F. (1974): Vascularly perfused isolated perfused intestine. In: *Proceedings of Fourth International Symposium on Gastrointestinal Motility*. Mitchell Press, Vancouver. Symposium held September 6–8, 1973, Banff, Alberta, Canada.
49. Burr, I. M., Stauffacher, W., Balant, L., Renold, A. E., and Grodsky, G. (1969): Dynamic aspects of proinsulin release from perfused rat pancreas. *Lancet*, 2:882–883.
50. Camus, P., and Mehendale, H. M. (1986): Pulmonary sequestration of amiodarone and desethylamiodarone. *J. Pharmacol. Exp. Ther.*, 237:867–873.
51. Cardieux, A., Masse, S., and Sirois, P. (1983): Effect of asbestos in the metabolism of vasoactive substances in isolated perfused guinea pig lungs. *Environ. Health Perspect.*, 51:287–291.
52. Case, R. M., Harper, A. A., and Scratcherd, T. (1968): Water and electrolyte secretion by the perfused cat pancreas. *J. Physiol.* (*Lond.*), 196:133–149.
53. Cesarone, C. F., Fugassa, E., Gallo, G., Voci, A., and Orunesu, M. (1984): Collagenase perfusion rat liver induces DNA damage and DNA repair in hepatocytes. *Mutat. Res.*, 141:113–116.
54. Chapman, N. D., Saint George, S., and Ishida, T. (1960): Small volume perfusion system of the isolated rat liver. *J. Appl. Physiol.*, 15:128–136.
55. Charles, J. M., Abou-Donia, M. B., and Menzel, D. B. (1978): Absorption of paraquat and diquat from the airways of the perfused rat lung. *Toxicology*, 9:59–67.
56. Chikaoka, Y., and Tamura, M. (1991): 7-Ethoxycoumarin deethylation activity in perfused isolated rat brain. *J. Biochem.* (*Tokyo*), 125:634–640.
57. Chiong, M. A., Berenzy, G. M., and Winton, T. L. (1978): Metabolism of the isolated perfused rabbit heart. I. Responses to anoxia and reoxygenation. II. Energy stores. *Can. J. Physiol. Pharmacol.*, 56:844–856.
58. Choo, E. F., Angus, P. W., and Morgan, D. J. (1999): Effect of cirrhosis on sulphation by the isolated perfused liver. *J. Hepatol.*, 30:498–502.
59. Chuté, A. L., and Smyth, D. H. (1939): Metabolism of the isolated perfused cat's brain. *Q. J. Exp. Physiol.*, 29:379–394.
60. Colantoni, A., de Maria, N., Caraceni, P., Bernardi, M., Floyd, R. A., and Van Thiel, D. H. (1998): Prevention of reoxygenation injury by sodium salicylate in isolated-perfused rat liver. *Free Radic. Biol. Med.*, 25:87–94.
61. Cohrs, P., Jaffe, R., and Meesen, H. (1958): *Pathologie der Laboratoriumstiere*, Vol. 1. Springer–Verlag, Berlin.
62. Cojocel, C., Docius, N., Maita, K., Smith, J. H., and Hook, J. B. (1984): Renal ultrastructural and biochemical injuries induced by aminoglycosides. *Environ. Health Perspect.*, 57:293–299.
63. Cook, D. R., Howell, R. E., and Gillis, C. N. (1982): Xanthine oxidase-induced lung injury inhibits removal of 5-hydroxytryptamine from the pulmonary circulation. *Anesth. Analg.*, 61:666–670.
64. Coore, H. G., and Randle, P. J. (1964): Regulation of insulin secretion studied with pieces of rabbit pancreas incubated in vitro. *Biochem. J.*, 93:66–78.
65. Costiner, E., Ghiea, D., Simionescu, L., and Oprescu, M. (1975): Modified technique of perfusion of isolated rat pancreas tested by insulin release after glucose administration. *Endocrinol. Exp.*, 9:197–204.
66. Dalbey, W., and Bingham, E. (1978): Metabolism of trichloroethylene by the isolated perfused lung. *Toxicol. Appl. Pharmacol.*, 43:267–277.
67. Davis, M. E., and Mehendale, H. M. (1979): Absence of metabolism of morphine during accumulation by isolated perfused rabbit lung. *Drug Metab. Dispos.*, 7:425–428.
68. Dawson, J. R., Vapakangas, K., Jernstrom, B., and Moldeus, P. (1984): Glutathione conjugation by isolated lung cells and isolated perfused lung: Effect of external glutathione. *Eur. J. Biochem.*, 138:439–443.

69. Deglin, S. M., Deglin, J. M., and Chung, E. K. (1977): Drug-induced cardiovascular diseases. *Drugs*, 14:29–40.
70. DeMello, G., and Maack, T. (1976): Nephron function of the isolated perfused rat kidney. *Am. J. Physiol.*, 231:1699–1707.
71. De Wildt, D. J., De Jong, Y., Hillen, F. C., Steerenberg, P. A., and Van Hoesel, Q. G. C. M. (1985): Cardiovascular effects of doxorubicin-induced toxicity in the intact Lou/M Wsl rat and isolated heart preparations. *J. Pharmacol. Exp. Ther.*, 235:234–240.
72. De Wildt, D. J., and Speijers, G. J. A. (1984): Influence of dietary rapeseed oil and erucic acid upon myocardial performance and hemodynamics in the rat. *Toxicol. Appl. Pharmacol.*, 74:99–108.
73. Diczfalusy, E. (1971): *Perfusion Techniques*. Karolinska Institute, Stockholm.
74. Dirks, V. B., Seibert, A., Sperling, G., and Krieglstein, J. (1984): Comparison of the effects of piracetam and methohexital on brain energy metabolism. *Azneimittelforschung*, 34:258–266.
75. Doerr, W., and Becker, V. (1958): Bauchspeicheldruse (pancreas). In: *Pathologie der Laboratariumstierre*, Vol. 1, edited by P. Cohrs, R. Jaffe, and Hm. Messen, p. 130. Springer–Verlag, Berlin.
76. Dovrak, K. J., Braun, W. E., Magnusson, M. O., Stowe, N. T., and Banowsky, L. H. W. (1976): Effect of high methylprednisolone on the isolated perfused canine kidney. *Transplantation*, 21:149–157.
77. Dubois, R. S., Vaughn, G. D., and Roy, C. C. (1968): Isolated rat small intestine with intact circulation. In: *Organ Perfusion and Perservation*, edited by J. C. Norman, pp. 863–868. Appleton–Century–Crofts, New York.
78. Dunbar, J. R., Delucia, A. J., and Bryant, L. R. (1984): Glutathione status of isolated rabbit lungs: Effects on nitrofurantoin and paraquat perfusion with normoxic and hyperoxic ventilation. *Biochem. Pharmacol.*, 33:1343–1348.
79. Eisman, B., Knipe, P., McColl, H., and Orloff, M. J. (1961): Isolated liver perfusion for reducing blood ammonia. *Arch. Surg.*, 83:356–363.
80. Elisha, E. E., Hutson, D., and Seratcherd, T. (1984): The direct inhibition of pancreatic electrolyte secretion by noradrenaline in the isolated perfused cat pancreas. *J. Physiol. (Lond.)*, 351:77–85.
81. Embden, G., and Glaüssner, K. (1902): Uber den ortder atherschwefelsaurebildung im tierkorpen. *Hoffmlisters Beituug 2 Chem. Phys. Band.*, 1:310–327.
82. Enser, M. B., Kunz, F., Borenstanjn, J., Opie, L. H., and Robinson, D. S. (1967): Metabolism of diglyceride fatty acids by perfused rat heart. *Biochem. J.*, 104:306–317.
83. Esser, E., Loschen, G., and Flohe, L. (1991): Phorbol ester cardiotoxicity: Are O_2-radicals involved? *Arch. Toxicol.*, 65:335–339.
84. Evans, G. H., Wilkinson, G. R., and Shand, D. G. (1973): The disposition of propranolol. IV. A dominant role of tissue uptake in the dose dependent extraction of propranolol by the perfused rat liver. *J. Pharmacol. Exp. Ther.*, 186:447–456.
85. Ferrari, R., Ceconi, C., Currello, S., Guarnieri, C., Caderara, C. M., Albertini, A., and Visioli, O. (1985): Oxygen-mediated myocardial damage during ischemia and reperfusion: Role of the cellular defenses against oxygen toxicity. *J. Mol. Cell Cardiol.*, 17:937–945.
86. Fink, V. C., Holzl, J., Riegger, H., and Kriegelstein, J. (1984): Effects of valtrate on the EEG of the isolated perfused rat brain. *Azneimittelforschung*, 34:170–174.
87. Fitzpatrick, J. H., Jr., and Gilboe, D. D. (1982): Effects of nitrous oxide on the cerebrovascular tone, oxygen metabolism, and electroencephalogram of the isolated perfused canine brain. *Anesthesiology*, 57:480–484.
88. Fogel, W. A., Bieganski, T., Schayer, R. W., and Maslinski, C. (1981): Involvement of diamine oxidase in catabolism of ^{14}C-putrescine in mice in vivo with special reference to the formation of γ-aminobutyric acid. *Agents Actions*, 11:679–684.
89. Fonteles, M. C., Pillion, D. J., Jeske, A. H., and Leibach, F. H. (1976): Extraction of glutathione by the isolated perfused rabbit kidney. *J. Surg. Res.*, 21:169–174.
90. Forth, W. (1968): Eisen und Kobalt-Resorption am perfundierten Dendarmasegment. In: *3 Konfder Gesellschaft fur Biologische Chemie*, edited by W. Staib and R. Scholz, pp. 242–254. Springer–Verlag, Berlin.
91. Fox, R. B. (1984): Prevention of granulocyte-mediated oxidant injury in rats by a hydroxyl radical scavenger, dimethylthiourea. *J. Clin. Invest.*, 74:1456–1464.
92. Foy, B. D., Toxopeus, C., and Frazier, J. M. (1999): Kinetic modeling of slow dissociation of bromosulphothalein from albumin in perfused rat liver: Toxicological implications. *Toxicol. Sci.*, 50:20–29.
93. Franke, H., and Weiss, C. (1976): The O_2 supply of the isolated cell-free perfused rat kidney. *Adv. Exp. Med. Biol.*, 75:425–432.
94. Gad, S. C., Leslie, S. W., and Acosta, D. (1979): Inhibitory actions of butylated hydroxytoluene on isolated ileal, atrial and perfused heart preparations. *Toxicol. Appl. Pharmacol.*, 49:45–52.
95. Gamble, W. J., Conn, P. A., Edalji-Kumer, A., Pleuge, R., and Monroe, R. G. (1970): Myocardial oxygen consumption of blood-perfused, isolated supported rat heart. *Am. J. Physiol.*, 219:604–612.
96. Gareis, M., Hashem, A., Bauer, J., and Gedek, B. (1986): Identification of glucuronide metabolites of T-2 toxin and diacetoxyscirpinol in the bile of isolated perfused rat liver. *Toxicol. Appl. Pharmacol.*, 84:168–172.
97. Geiger, A. (1958): Correlation of brain metabolism and function by the use of a brain perfusion in situ. *Physiol. Rev.*, 38:1–20.
98. Geiger, A., and Magnes, J. (1947): The isolation of the cerebral circulation and the perfusion of the brain in the living cat. *Am. J. Physiol.*, 149:517–537.
99. Gerber, G. B., and Remy-Defraigne, J. (1966): DNA metabolism in perfused organs. II. Incorporation in DNA and catabolism of thymidine at different levels of substrate by normal and x-irradiated liver and intestine. *Arch. Int. Physiol. Biochem.*, 74:785–794.
100. Gilboe, D. D., Betz, A. L., and Langebartel, D. A. (1973): A guide for the isolation of the canine brain. *J. Appl. Physiol.*, 34:534–537.
101. Gillis, C. N., and Iwasawa, Y. (1972): Technique for measurement of norepinephrine and 5-hydroxytryptamine uptake by rabbit lung. *J. Appl. Physiol.*, 33:404–408.
102. Gillis, C. N., and Roth, J. A. (1976): Pulmonary disposition of circulating vasoactive hormones. *Biochem. Pharmacol.*, 25:2547–2553.
103. Giovannini, L., Migliori, M., De Pietro, S., Taccola, D., Panichi, V., Bertelli, A. A., and Bertelli, A. (1999): L-propionyl carnitine reduces toxicity correlated to cyclosporine-induced intracellular ATP concentrations. *Drugs Exp. Clin. Res.*, 25:173–177.
104. Gollan, F., and McDermott, J. (1979): Effect of skeletal muscle relaxant dantrolene sodium on the isolated, perfused heart. *Proc. Soc. Exp. Biol. Med.*, 160:42–45.
105. Gonzalez-Martin, G., Dominguez, A. R., and Guevara, A. (1997): Pharmacokinetics and hepatotoxicity of diclofenac using an isolated perfused rat liver. *Biomed. Pharmacother.*, 5:170–175.
106. Gonmori, K., Prasada Rao, K. S., and Mehendale, H. M. (1986): Pulmonary synthesis of 5-hydroxytryptamine in isolated perfused rabbit and rat lung preparations. *Exp. Lung Res.*, 11:295–306.
107. Goodman, M. N., Parilla, R., and Toews, C. J. (1973): Influence of fluorocarbon emulsions on hepatic metabolism in perfused rat liver. *Am. J. Physiol.*, 225:1384–1388.
108. Goto, Y., Seino, Y., Note, S., and Imura, H. (1980): The dual effect of alloxan modulated by 3-O-methylglucose or somatostatin on

insulin secretion in the isolated perfused rat pancreas. *Horm. Metab. Res.*, 12:140–143.

109. Gow, P. J., Treepongkaruna, S., Ching, M. S., Ghabrial, H., Shulkes, A., Smallwood, R. A., Jin, C. J., and Morgan, D. J. (1999): Uptake and excretion of sodium taurocholate by the isolated perfused neonatal sheep liver. *J. Pharm. Sci.*, 88:445–449.
110. Grodsky, G. M., Batts, A. A., Bennett, L. L., Veella, C., McWilliams, N. B., and Smith, D. F. (1963): Effects of carbohydrates on secretion of insulin from isolated rat pancreas. *Am. J. Physiol.*, 205:638–644.
111. Habib, M. P., and Clements, N. C. (1995): Effects of low-dose hydrogen peroxide in the isolated perfused rat lung. *Exp. Lung Res.*, 21:95–112.
112. Hadasova, E., Charvatova, Z., Nerusilova, K., Hykosova, M., and Zelenkova, O. (1999): Influence of pretreatment with immunosuppressants on O-demethylation of dextromethorphan in isolated perfused rat liver. *Exp. Toxicol. Pathol.*, 51:330–334.
113. Hale, P. W., Jr., and Poklis, A. (1984): Thioridazine-5-sulfoxide cardiotoxicity in the isolated, perfused rat heart. *Toxicol. Lett.*, 21:1–8.
114. Hashimoto, K., Satoh, S., and Takeuchi, O. (1971): Effect of dopamine on pancreatic secretion in the dog. *Br. J. Pharmacol.*, 43:739–746.
115. Hauge, A. (1968): Conditions governing the pressor response to ventilation hypoxia in isolated perfused rat lungs. *Acta Physiol. Scand.*, 72:33–44.
116. Heaton, J. D., McAnalley, B. H., Gardiner, T. H., and Johnson, A. R. (1982): Uptake and release of ^{14}C-morphine by pulmonary endothelium and cultured pulmonary endothelial cells. *Gen. Pharmacol.*, 13:105–110.
117. Heavner, J. E., Shi, B., Inners-McBride, K., Asimakis, G., Wang, M. J., and Mcintyre, D. C. (1998): Cocaine cardiotoxicity differs markedly in isolated hearts of two strains of rats exhibiting phenolic differences in sensitivity to seizures. *Life Sci.*, 63:625–633.
118. Hein, H., Krieglstein, J., and Stock, R. (1975): The effects of increased glucose supply and thiopental anesthesia on energy metabolism of the isolated perfused rat brain. *Naunyn. Schmiedebergs Arch. Pharmacol.*, 289:399–407.
119. Hemingway, A. (1931): Some observations on the perfusion of the isolated kidney by a pump. *J. Physiol.* (*Lond.*), 71:201–213.
120. Hems, R., Ross, B. D., Berry, M. N., and Krebs, H. A. (1966): Gluconeogenesis in the perfused rat liver. *Biochem. J.*, 101:284–292.
121. Herman-Taylor, J. (1973): The isolated perfused canine pancreas. In: *Isolated Organ Perfusion*, edited by H. D. Ritchie and J. D. Hardcastle, pp. 171–190. University Park Press, Baltimore.
122. Herrero, I., Torras, J., Carrera, M., Castells, A., Pasto, L., Gil-Vernet, S., Alsina, J., and Grinyo, J. M. (1995): Evaluation of a preservation solution containing fructose-1,6-diphosphate and mannitol using isolated perfused rat kidney. Comparison with Euro-Collins and University of Wisconsin solutions. *Nephrol. Dial. Transplant.*, 10:519–526.
123. Hidaka, T., Furuno, H., Inokuchi, T., and Ogura, R. (1990): Effects of diethyl maleate (DEM), a glutathione depletor on prostaglandin synthesis in the isolated perfused spleen of rabbits. *Arch. Toxicol.*, 64:103–108.
124. Hilliker, K. S., Imlay, M., and Roth, R. A. (1984): Effects of monocrotaline treatment on norepinephrine removal by isolated, perfused rat lungs. *Biochem. Pharmacol.*, 33:2692–2695.
125. Hilliker, K. S., and Roth, R. A. (1985): Injury to the isolated, perfused lung by exposure in vitro to monocrotaline pyrrole. *Exp. Lung Res.*, 8:201–212.
126. Hirning, L. D., Porreca, F., and Burks, T. F. (1985): μ, but not k, opioid agonists induce contractions of the canine small intestine ex vivo. *Eur. J. Pharmacol.*, 109:49–54.
127. Hoffmann, M. J., Ji, S., Hedli, C. C., and Snyder, R. (1999): Metabolism of (^{14}C)phenol in the isolated perfused liver. *Toxicol. Sci.*, 49:40–47.
128. Inagaki, M., and Tamura, M. (1993): Preparation and optical characteristics of hemoglobin-free isolated perfused rat head in situ. *J. Biochem.* (*Tokyo*), 113:650–657.
129. Inoue, K., Hiramatsu, S., Hisatomi, A., Umeda, F., and Nawata, H. (1993): Effects of amylin on the release of insulin and glucagon from the perfused rat pancreas. *Horm. Metab. Res.*, 25:135–137.
130. Itakura, N., Fisher, A. B., and Thurman, R. G. (1977): Cytochrome P450-linked p-nitroanisole O-demethylation in the perfused lung. *J. Appl. Physiol.*, 43:238–245.
131. Ito, K., Hirose, H., Maruyama, H., Fukamachi, S., Tashiro, Y., and Saruta, T. (1995): Neurotransmitters partially restore glucose sensitivity of insulin and glucagon secretion from perfused streptozotocin-induced diabetic rat pancreas. *Diabetologia*, 38:1276–1284.
132. Iwamoto, K., Watanabe, J., Araki, K., Satoh, M., and Deguchi, N. (1985): Reduced hepatic clearance of propranolol induced by chronic carbon tetrachloride treatment in rats. *J. Pharmacol. Exp. Ther.*, 234:470–475.
133. Iwatsuki, K., Ikeda, K., and Chiba, S. (1982): Effects of nitroprusside on pancreatic juice secretion in the blood perfused canine pancreas. *Eur. J. Pharmacol.*, 79:53–60.
134. Jacobs, F. A. (1968): Continuous radioactivity monitoring of perfusion in the small intestine of the intact animal. *Adv. Tracer Methodol.*, 4:255–272.
135. Jaffe, D. R., Hassal, C. D., Gandolfi, A. J., and Brendel, K. (1985): Production of DNA single strand breaks in rabbit renal tissue after exposure to 1,2-dichlorovinylcysteine. *Toxicology*, 35:25–33.
136. Johannesen, J., Lie, M., and Kiil, F. (1977): Renal energy metabolism and sodium reabsorption after 2,4-nitrophenol administration. *Am. J. Physiol.*, 233:207–217.
137. Johnson, A., Phillips, P., Hocking, D., Tsan, M. F., and Ferro, T. (1989): Protein kinase inhibitor prevents pulmonary edema in response to H_2O_2. *Am. J. Physiol.*, 256:H1012–H1022.
138. Joshi, U. M., Dumas, M., and Mehendale, H. M. (1986): Glutathione turnover in perfused rabbit lung. *Biochem. Pharmacol.*, (in press).
139. Joshi, U. M., Prasada Rao, K. S., and Mehendale, H. M. (1987): Glutathione status in constituted physiological fluid containing albumin. *Int. J. Biochem.*, 19:1129–1135.
140. Junod, A. F. (1972): Accumulation of ^{14}C-imipramine in isolated perfused rat lungs. *J. Pharmacol. Exp. Ther.*, 183:182–187.
141. Kanekal, S., Plopper, C., Morin, D., and Buckpitt, A. (1991): Metabolism and cytotoxicity of naphthalene oxide in the isolated perfused mouse lung. *J. Pharmacol. Exp. Ther.*, 256:391–401.
142. Kapfhammer, J. (1927): Die leber im Stoffwechzel. In: *Handbuch der Biochemie*, edited by K. Oppenheimer, 2nd ed., Vol. 9, pp. 98–150. Jena, Germany. G. Fischer.
143. Karmazyn, M., and Moffat, M. P. (1985): Toxic properties of arachidonic acid in normal, ischemic and reperfused hearts: Indirect evidence for free radical involvement. *Prostaglandins Leukot. Med.*, 17:251–264.
144. Kavin, H., Levin, N. W., and Stanley, M. M. (1967): Isolated perfused rat small bowel technique: Studies of viability, glucose absorption. *J. Appl. Physiol.*, 22:604–611.
145. Kennedy, A. L., Lastbom, L., Skarping, G., Dalene, M., Ryrfeldt, A., Moldeus, P., and Brown W. E. (1995): Analysis of the reactivity of (^{14}C) toluene diisocyanate (TDI) in an isolated, perfused lung model. *Chem. Biol. Interact.*, 98:167–183.
146. Khayambashi, H., and Lyman, R. L. (1969): Secretion of rat pancreas perfused with plasma from rats fed soybean trypsin inhibitor. *Am. J. Physiol.*, 217:646–651.

147. Khedun, S. M., Maharaj, B., Leary, W. P., and Lockett, C. J. (1992): The effect of hexane on the ventricular fibrillation threshold of the perfused rat heart. *Toxicology*, 71:145–150.

148. Kilbinger, H., and Krieglstein, J. (1974): Applicability of the isolated perfused rat brain for studying central cholinergic mechanisms. *Naunyn. Schmiedebergs Arch. Pharmacol.*, 285:407–411.

149. Kim, D.-H., and Akera, T. (1984): Effects of myocardial hypoxia on digitalis-induced toxicity in the isolated heart of guinea pigs and cats. *Eur. J. Pharmacol.*, 104:303–312.

150. Kim, J. H., and Miller, K. L. (1969): The functional significance of changes in activity of the enzymes, tryptophan pyrrolase and tyrosine transaminase after induction in intact rats and isolated perfused rat liver. *J. Biol. Chem.*, 244:1410–1416.

151. Kimura, T., Zuidema, G. D., and Cameron, J. L. (1979): Steroid administration and acute pancreatitis studies with an isolated, perfused canine pancreas. *Surgery*, 85:520–524.

152. Kitakaze, M., Weisman, H. F., and Marban, E. (1988): Contractile dysfunction and ATP depletion after transient calcium overload in perfused ferret hearts. *Circulation*, 77:689–695.

153. Knowlton, F. P., and Starling, E. H. (1912): The influence of variations in temperature and blood pressure on the performance of the isolated mammalian heart. *J. Physiol.*, (*Lond.*), 44:206–219.

154. Komai, T., Yamamoto, F., Tanaka, K., Ichikawa, H., Shibata, T., Koide, A., Nakashima, N., Ohashi, T., and Kawashima, Y. (1991): Harmful effects of inotropic agents on myocardial protection. *Ann. Thorac. Surg.*, 52:927–933.

155. Kopp, S. J., Daar, A. A., Prentice, R. C., Tow, J. P., and Feliksik, J. M. (1986): ^{31}P-NMR studies of the intact perfused rat heart: A novel analytical approach for determining functional-metabolic correlates, temporal relationships, and intracellular actions of cardiotoxic chemicals nondestructively in an intact organ model. *Toxicol. Appl. Pharmacol.*, 82:200–210.

156. Koschier, F. J., Gigliotti, P. J., and Hong, S. K. (1980): The effect of bis(p-chlorophenyl)acetic acid on the renal function on the rat. *J. Environ. Pathol. Toxicol.*, 4:209–217.

157. Koster, J. F., Slee, R. G., Essed, C. E., and Stam, H. (1985): Studies on canine hydroperoxide-induced lipid peroxidation in the isolated perfused rat heart. *J. Mol. Cell. Cardiol.*, 17:701–708.

158. Kraupp, O., Adler-Kastner, L., Niessner, H., and Plank, B. (1967): The effects of starvation and acute and chronic alloxan diabetes on myocardial substrate levels and on liver glycogen in the rat in vivo. *Eur. J. Biochem.*, 2:197–214.

159. Krieglstein, G., Krieglstein, J., and Stock, R. (1972): Suitability of the perfused rat brain for studying effects on cerebral metabolism. *Naunyn. Schmiedebergs Arch. Pharmacol.*, 275:124–134.

160. Krieglstein, J., and Stock, R. (1973): Comparative study of the effects of chloral hydrate and trichloroethanol on cerebral metabolism. *Naunyn. Schmiedebergs Arch. Pharmacol.*, 277:323–332.

161. Krietys, P. R., Specian, R. D., Grisham, M. B., and Tso, P. (1991): Tejunal mucosal injury and restitution: Role of hydrolytic products of food digestion. *Am. J. Physiol.*, 261:G384–G391.

162. Kukan, M., Vajdova, K., Horecky, J., Nagyova, A., Mehendale, H. M., and Trnovec, T. (1997): Effects of blockade of Kupffer cells by gadolinium chloride on hepatobiliary function in cold ischemia-reperfusion injury of rat liver. *Hepatology*, 26: 1250–1257.

163. Kulatilake, A. E. (1967): Isolated perfusion of canine and human kidneys. *Br. J. Surg.*, 54:877–882.

164. Kvetina, J., and Guaitani, A. (1969): A versatile method for the in vitro perfusion of isolated organs of rats and mice with particular reference to liver. *Pharmacology*, 2:65–81.

165. Lacy, P. E., and Kostianowsky, M. (1967): Method for isolation of intact islets of Langerhans from the rat pancreas. *Diabetes*, 16:35–39.

166. Lafranconi, W. M., Ferlan, I., Russell, F. E., and Huxtable, R. J. (1984): The action of equinatoxin, a peptide from the venom of the sea anemone, *Actinia equinia*, on the isolated lung. *Toxicology*, 22:347–352.

167. Lafranconi, W. M., and Huxtable, R. J. (1984): Hepatic metabolism and pulmonary toxicity of monocrotaline using isolated perfused liver and lung. *Biochem. Pharmacol.*, 33:2479–2484.

168. Lambert, C., Mossiat, C., Tanniere, Z. M., Maupoil, V., and Rochette, L. (1990): Antiarrhythmic effect of amiodarone on doxorubicin acute toxicity working rat hearts. *Cardiovasc. Res.*, 24:653–658.

169. Langendorff, O. (1895): Untersuchungen am Uberleberden Saügertierzen. *Pflugers Arch. Ges. Physiol.*, 61:291–332.

170. Lastbom, L., Skarping, G., Moldeus, P., and Ryrfeldt, A. (1997): Hexamethylene diisocyanate(HDI)-induced lung impairment studies in isolated perfused and ventilated guinea pig lungs. *Pharmacol. Toxicol.*, 81:85–89.

171. Law, F. C. P. (1978): Metabolism and disposition of 4′-tetrahydrocannabinol by the isolated perfused rabbit lung. *Drug Metab. Dispos.*, 6:154–163.

172. Law, F. C. P., Eling, T. E., Bend, J. R., and Fouts, J. R. (1974): Metabolism of xenobiotics by the isolated perfused lung. *Drug Metab. Dispos.*, 2:433–442.

173. Lazzarino, G., Tavazzi, B., DiPierro, D., and Giardina, B. (1992): Ischemia and reperfusion: Effect of fructose 1,6-bisphosphate. *Free Radic. Res. Commun.*, 16:325–329.

174. Leary, W. P. P., and Ledingham, J. G. (1969): Removal of angiotensin by isolated perfused organs of the rat. *Nature*, 222:959–960.

175. Lemaster, J. J., Ji, S., Stemkowski, C. J., and Thurman, R. G. (1983): Hypoxic hepatocellular injury. *Pharmacol. Biochem. Behav.*, 18:455–459.

176. Lessire, F., Gustin, P., Delaunois, A., Bloden, S., Nemmar, A., Vargas, M., and Ansay, M. (1996): Relationship between parathion and paraoxontoxicokinetics, lung metabolic activity, and cholinesterase inhibition guinea pig and rabbit lungs. *Toxicol. Appl. Pharmacol.*, 138:201–210.

177. Levey, S., and Gast, R. (1966): Isolated perfused rat lung preparation. *J. Appl. Physiol.*, 21:313–316.

178. Levin, N. W., Ryan, W. G., Hayashi, J., and Kark, R. M. (1965): Studies on the isolated perfused rabbit kidney. *S. Afr. J. Med. Sci.*, 30:78–79.

179. Light, A., and Simpson, M. S. (1966): Studies on the biosynthesis of insulin. I. The paper chromatographic isolation of ^{14}C-labeled insulin from calf-pancreas slices. *Biochem. Biophys. Acta*, 20:251–261.

180. Linas, S. L., Whittenburg, D., and Repine, J. E. (1991): Role of neutrophil derived oxidants and elastase in lipopolysaccharide-mediated renal injury. *Kidney Int.*, 39:618–623.

181. Little, J. R., and Cohen, J. J. (1974): Effect of albumin concentration on function of isolated perfused rat kidney. *Am. J. Physiol.*, 226:512–517.

182. Longoni, B., Giovannini, L., Migliori, M., Bertelli, A. A., and Bertelli, A. (1999): Cyclosporine-induced lipid peroxidation and propionyl carnitine protective effect. *Int. J. Tissue React.*, 21:7–11.

183. Lorenz-Meyer, H., Roth, H., Elsässer, P., and Hahn, R. (1985): Cytotoxicity of lectins on rat intestinal mucosa enhanced by neuraminidase. *Eur. J. Clin. Invest.*, 15:227–234.

184. Loubatieres, A., Mariani, M. M., Chapal, J., and Portal, A. (1967): Action penetrice de faibles doses d'adrenaline et de noradrenaline sur l'insulin secretion etadiée sur le pancreas isolé et perfusé du rat. *C. R. Soc. Biol.* (*Paris*), 161:2578–2586.

185. Lund, M., Kang, L., Tygstrup, N., Wolkoff, A. W., and Ott, P. (1999): Effects of LPS on transport of indocyanine green and alanine uptake in perfused rat liver. *Am. J. Physiol.*, 277:G91–G100.

186. Lyons, D. E., Beery, J. T., Lyons, S. A., and Taylor, S. L. (1983): Cadaverine and aminoguanidine potentiate the uptake of histamine in vitro in perfused intestinal segments of rats. *Toxicol. Appl. Pharmacol.*, 70:445–458.

187. Manabe, S., Nuber, D. C., and Lin, Y. C. (1991): Zone-specific hepatotoxicity of gossypol in perfused rat liver. *Toxicon.*, 29:787–790.

188. Marinelli, A., Pons, D. H., Vreeken, J. A., Nagessen, S. K., Kuppen, P. J., Tjadew, U. R., and Van deVelde, C. J. (1991): High mitomycin C concentration in tumor tissue can be achieved by isolated liver perfusion in rats. *Cancer Chemother. Pharmacol.*, 28:109–114.

189. Martinus, A. M.,Monreiro, H. S., Junior, E. O., Menezes, D. B., and Fonteles, M. C. (1998): Effects of Crotalus durissus casacavella venum in the isolated rat kidney. *Toxicon*, 36:1441–1450.

190. Masini, E., Giannella, E., Palmerani, B., Pistelli, A., Gambassi, F., and Mannaioni, P. F. (1989): Free radicals induce ischemia-reperfusion injury and histamine release in the isolated guinea pig heart. *Int. Arch. Appl. Immunol.*, 88:132–133.

191. Masuda, Y. and Nakamura, Y. (1990): Effects of oxygen deficiency and calcium omission on carbon tetrachloride hepatotoxicity in isolated perfused livers from phenobarbital-pretreated rats. *Biochem. Pharmacol.*, 40:1865–1876.

192. Masuda, Y., and Yamamori, Y. (1991): Histological evidence for dissociation of lipid peroxidation and cell necrosis in bromotrichloromethane hepatotoxicity in the perfused rat liver. *Jpn. J. Pharmacol.*, 56:143–150.

193. Masumi, S., Moriyama, M., Kannan, Y., Ohta, M., Koshitani, O., Sawamoto, O., and Sugano, T. (1999): Changes in hepatic metabolism in isolated perfused liver during the development of thioacetamide-induced cirrhosis in rats. *Toxicology*, 135:21–31.

194. McCallum, T., Badylak, S. F., Van-Vleet, J. F., and Reed, R. M. (1989): Furazolidone-induced injury in the isolated perfused chicken heart. *Am. J. Vet. Res.*, 50:1183–1185.

195. McCarthy, R. D., Shaw, J. C., and Lakshmanan, S. (1958): Metabolism of volatile fatty acids by the perfused goat liver. *Proc. Soc. Exp. Biol. Med.*, 99:560–564.

196. McDonough, K. H., Brumfield, B. A., and Lang, C. H. (1986): In vitro myocardial performance after lethal and nonlethal doses of endotoxin. *Am. J. Physiol.*, 250:H240–H246.

197. Mehendale, H. M. (1976): Uptake and disposition of chlorinated biphenyls by isolated perfused rat liver. *Drug Metab. Dispos.*, 4:124–132.

198. Mehendale, H. M. (1976): Effect of preexposure to Kepone on the biliary excretion of polychloryinated biphenyl compounds. *Toxicol. Appl. Pharmacol.*, 36:369–381.

199. Mehendale, H. M. (1977): Mirex-induced impairment of hepatobiliary function: Suppressed biliary excretion of imipramine and sulfobromophthalein. *Drug Metab. Dispos.*, 5:56–62.

200. Mehendale, H. M. (1977): Effect of preexposure to Kepone on the biliary excretion of imipramine and sulfobropthalein. *Toxicol. Appl. Pharmacol.*, 40:247–259.

201. Mehendale, H. M. (1978): Pesticide-induced modification of hepatobiliary function; hexachlorobenzene, DDT and toxaphene. *Food Cosmet. Toxicol.*, 16:19–25.

202. Mehendale, H. M. (1980): Aldrin epoxidase activity in the developing rabbit lung. *Pediatr. Res.*, 14:282–285.

203. Mehendale, H. M. (1982): Use of isolated perfused lung in determining pulmonary disposition and potential toxicological significance of inhaled environmental pollutants. *J. Environ. Toxicol. Chem.*, 1:231–244.

204. Mehendale, H. M. (1984): Pulmonary disposition of pneumophilic agents and possible relationship to pulmonary hypertension. *Fed. Proc.*, 43:2586–2591.

205. Mehendale, H. M., Angevine, L. S., and Ohmiya, Y. (1981): The isolated perfused lung—a critical evaluation. *Toxicology*, 21:1–36.

206. Mehendale, H. M., and El-Bassiouni, E. A. (1975): Uptake and disposition of aldrin and dieldrin by isolated perfused rabbit lung. *Drug Metab. Dispos.*, 3:543–556.

207. Mehendale, H. M., Svensson, S. A., Baldi, C., and Orrenius, S. (1985): Accumulation of Ca^{2+} induced by cytotoxic levels of menadione in the isolated perfused rat liver. *Eur. J. Biochem.*, 149:201–206.

208. Menaouar, A., Anglade, D., Baussand, P., Pelloux, A., Corboz, M., Lantuejeul, S., Benchetrit, G., and Grimbert, F. A. (1997): Chlorine gas induced acute lung injury in isolated rabbit lung. *Eur. Respir. J.*, 10:1100–1107.

209. Merin, R. G. (1978): Myocardial metabolism for the toxicologist. *Environ. Health Perspect.*, 26:169–174.

210. Merker, G., Helling, H. J., Krahl, M., and Aigner, K. (1983): Ultrastructural changes in the dog liver cell after isolated liver perfusion with various cytotoxins. *Recent Results Cancer Res.*, 86:103–109.

211. Miller, L. L., Bly, C. G., Berry, M. N., and Krebs, H. A. (1951): The dominant role of the liver in plasma protein synthesis: A direct study of the isolated perfused rat liver with the aid of lysine-^{14}C. *J. Exp. Med.*, 94:431–453.

212. Mitchell, C. J., Bullock, S., and Ross, B. D. (1977): Renal handling of gentamicin and other antibiotics by the isolated perfused rat kidney: Mechanism of nephrotoxicity. *J. Antimicrob. Chemother.*, 3:593–600.

213. Miura, K., Pasino, D. A., Goldstein, R. S., and Hook, J. B. (1985): Effects of gentamicin on renal function in isolated perfused kidneys from male and female rats. *Toxicol. Lett.*, 26:15–18.

214. Miyazaki, M., Makowka, L., Falk, R. E., Falk, W., Venturi, D., Ambus, U., and Falk, J. A. (1983): Hyperthermochemotherapeutic in vivo isolated perfusion of the rat liver. *Cancer*, 51:1254–1260.

215. Monroe, R. G., Larfarge, C. G., Gamble, W. J., Honda, S., and Kevy, S. W. (1968): Ventricular performance and coronary flow of isolated hearts when perfused through isolated lungs and membrane oxygenators. In: *Organ Perfusion and Preservations*, edited by J. C. Norman, pp. 779–979. Appleton–Century–Crofts, New York.

216. Monteiro, H. S., Lima, A. A., and Fonteles, M. C. (1999): Glomerular effects of cholera toxin in isolated perfused rat kidney: A potential role for platelet activating factor. *Pharmacol. Toxicol.*, 85:105–110.

217. Moore, G. K., and Hook, J. B. (1978): Hemodynamic effects of furosemide in isolated perfused rat kidneys. *Proc. Soc. Exp. Biol. Med.*, 158:354–358.

218. Morgan, H. E., Henderson, M. J., Regen, D. M., and Park, C. R. (1961): Regulation of glucose uptake in muscle. I. The effect of insulin and anoxia on glucose transport and phosphorylation in isolated perfused heart of normal rats. *J. Biol. Chem.*, 236: 253–261.

219. Muller, F. (1910): Dir kunslitche Durchbluntung resp. durchspulung von organ. *Hand 6 Biol. Arb. Meth.*, 3:327.

220. Nahas, G., and Trouve, R. (1985): Effects of interactions of natural cannabinoids on the isolated heart. *Proc. Soc. Exp. Biol. Med.*, 180:312–316.

221. Nakai, T. (1984): Toxic effects of endotoxin perfusion on isolated rat bowel. *Nippon Geba Gakkai. Zasshi.*, 85:370–377.

222. Nakazawa, H., Arroyo, C. M., Ichimori, K., Saigusa, Y., Minezaki, K. K., and Pronai, L. (1991): The demonstration of DMPO superoxide adduct upon reperfusion using a law nontoxic concentration. *Free Radic. Res. Commun.*, 14:297–302.

223. Nastainczyk, W., and Ullrich, V. (1978): Effect of oxygen concentration of the reaction of halothane with cytochrome P450 in liver microsomes and isolated perfused rat liver. *Biochem. Pharmacol.*, 27:387–392.

224. Nazeyrollas, P., Prevost, A., Baccard, N., Manot, L., Devillier, P., and Millart, H. (1999): Effects of amifostine on perfused isolated rat heart and on acute doxorubicin-induced cardiotoxicity. *Cancer Chemother. Pharmcol.*, 43:227–232.

225. Neely, J. R., Liebermiester, H., Battersby, E. J., and Morgan, H. E. (1967): Effect of pressure development on oxygen consumption by isolated rat heart. *Am. J. Physiol.*, 212:804–814.

226. Neuman, M. G., Eshchar, J., Cotariu, D., Ben-Sason, R., Ziv, E., Baron, H., and Ishay, J. S. (1985): Hepatotoxicity of hornet's venom sac extract in isolated perfused rat liver. *Acta Pharmacol. Toxicol. (Copenh.)*, 56:133–138.

227. Newton, J. E., and Hook, J. B. (1981): Isolated perfused kidney. *Methods Enzymol.*, 77:94–105.

228. Nichiitsutsuiji–Uwo, J. M., Ross, B. D., and Dribs, H. A. (1967): Metabolic activation of the isolated perfused rat kidney. *Biochem. J.*, 103:852–862.

229. Nicolaysen, G. (1971): Perfusate qualities and spontaneous edema formation in an isolated perfused lung preparation. *Acta Physiol. Scand.*, 83:563–570.

230. Niemeier, R. W. (1976): Isolated perfused rabbit lung: A critical appraisal. *Environ. Health Perspect.*, 16:67–71.

231. Niemeier, R. W., and Bingham, E. (1972): An isolated perfused lung preparation for metabolic studies. *Life Sci.*, 11:807–820.

232. Nizet, A. (1975): The isolated perfused kidney: Possibilities, limitations and results. *Kidney Int.*, 7:1–11.

233. Nordback, I. H., MacGowan, S., Potter, J. J., and Cameron, J. L. (1991): The role of acetaldehyde in the pathogenesis of acute alcoholic pancreatitis. *Ann. Surg.*, 214:671–678.

234. Norman, J. C., ed. (1978): *Organ Perfusion and Perservation.* Appleton–Century–Crofts, New York.

235. Northway, M. O., and Burks, T. F. (1979): Indirect intestinal stimulatory effects of heroin: Direct action on opiate receptors. *Eur. J. Pharmacol.*, 59:237–243.

236. Novakova, V., Birke, G., Plantin, L. O., and Wretland, A. (1976): A perfluorochemical oxygen carrier (Fluosol-43) in a synthetic medium used for perfusion of isolated rat liver. *Acta Physiol. Scand.*, 98:356–365.

237. O'Brien, R. F., Makarski, J. S., and Rounds, S. (1985): Studies on the mechanism of decreased angiotensin. I. Conversion in rat lungs injured with alpha-naphthylthiourea. *Exp. Lung Res.*, 8:243–259.

238. Ohmiya, Y., Angevine, L. S., and Mehendale, H. M. (1983): Effect of drug-induced phospholipidosis on pulmonary disposition of pneumophilic drugs. *Drug Metab. Dispos.*, 11:25–30.

239. Ohmiya, Y., and Mehendale, H. M. (1979): Uptake and accumulation of chlorpromazine in the isolated perfused rabbit lung. *Drug Metab. Dispos.*, 7:442–443.

240. Ohmiya, Y., and Mehendale, H. M. (1980): N-Oxidation of imipramine by isolated perfused rat and rabbit lung. *Life Sci.*, 26:1411–1421.

241. Ohmiya, Y., and Mehendale, H. M. (1980): Uptake and metabolism of chlorpromazine by rat and rabbit lungs. *Drug Metab. Dispos.*, 8:313–318.

242. O'Neil, J. J., and Tierney, F. (1974): Rat lung metabolism, glucose utilization by isolated perfused lungs and tissue slices. *Am. J. Physiol.*, 226:867–873.

243. Oomen, H. A. P. C., and Chamalarun, R. A. F. M. (1971): Correlation between histological and biochemical parameters of isolated perfused rat liver. *Virchows Arch.*, 8:243–251.

244. Opie, L. H. (1965): Coronary flow rate and perfusion pressure as determinants of mechanical function and oxidative metabolism of isolated perfused rat heart. *J. Physiol. (Lond.)*, 180:529–541.

245. Orton, T. C., Anderson, M. W., Pickett, R. D., Eling, T. E., and Fouts, J. R. (1973): Xenobiotic accumulation and metabolism by isolated perfused rabbit lungs. *J. Pharmacol. Exp. Ther.*, 186:482–497.

246. Otsuki, M., Nakamura, T., Okabayashi, Y., Oka, T., Fuji, M., and Baba, S. (1985): Comparative inhibitory effects of pirenzapine and atropine on cholinergic stimulation of exocrine and endocrine rat pancreas. *Gastroenterology*, 89:408–414.

247. Otsuki, M., Sakamoto, C., Ohki, A., Akabayashi, Y., Suehiro, I., and Baba, S. (1983): Effect of acarbose on exocrine and endocrine pancreatic function in the rat. *Diabetologia*, 24:445–448.

248. Otsuki, S., Watanabe, S., Morimistu, J., and Edamatsu, N. (1967): Regulatory effects of blood constituents on the function and metabolism of the cat brain perfusion experiments. *Acta Med. Okayama*, 21:279–296.

249. Palay, S. L., McGee-Russell, S. M., Gordon, S., and Grillo, M. A. (1962): Fixation of neural tissues for electron microscopy by perfusion with solutions of osmium tetraoxide. *J. Cell Biol.*, 12:385–410.

250. Pang, K. S., Yuen, V., Fayz, S., Tekopple, J. M., and Mulder, G. J. (1986): Absorption and metabolism of acetaminophen by the in situ perfused rat small intestine preparation. *Drug Metab. Dispos.*, 14:102–111.

251. Parsons, D. D., and Prichards, J. S. (1968): A preparation of perfused small intestine for the study of absorption in amphibia. *J. Physiol. (Lond.)*, 198:405–434.

252. Peterson, R. E., and Fujimoto, J. M. (1976): Increased "bile duct-pancreatic fluid" flow in rats pretreated with carbon tetrachloride. *Toxicol. Appl. Pharmacol.*, 35:29–39.

253. Pickett, R. D., Anderson, M. W., Orton, T. C., and Eling, T. E. (1975): The pharmacodynamics of 5-hydroxytryptamine uptake and metabolism by the isolated perfused rabbit lung. *J. Pharmacol. Exp. Ther.*, 194:545–553.

254. Pitzele, S., Sze, S., and Dosell, A. R. C. (1971): Hypothermic plasma perfusion of the isolated heart. *Surgery*, 70:407–412.

255. Popjak, G., and Beeckmans, M. (1950): Extra-hepatic lipid synthesis. *Biochem. J.*, 47:233–238.

256. Post, C., Anderson, R. G. G., Ryfeldt, A., and Nilsson, E. (1978): Transport and binding of lidocaine by lung slices and perfused lung of rats. *Acta Pharmacol. Toxicol. (Copenh.)*, 43:156–163.

257. Post, C., and Hede, A. R. (1982): Trichloroethylene and halothane inhibit uptake or 5-hydroxytryptamine in the isolated perfused rat lung. *Biochem. Pharmacol.*, 31:353–358.

258. Poulsen, H. E., Lerche, A., and Skovgaard, L. T. (1985): Acetaminophen metabolism by the perfused rat liver twelve hours after acetaminophen overdose. *Biochem. Pharmacol.*, 34: 3729–3733.

259. Powis, G. (1970): Perfusion of rat liver with blood: Transmitter overflows and gluconeogenesis. *Proc. R. Soc. Lond.*, B174:503–515.

260. Prasada Rao, K. S., and Mehendale, H. M. (1987): Precursor utilization of 5–hydroxytryptophan for 5-hydroxytryptamine biosynthesis in isolated perfused rabbit and rat lungs. *Can. J. Physiol. Pharmacol.*, 65:2117–2123.

261. Prasada Rao, K. S., and Mehendale, H. M. (1986): Precursor utilization of [^{14}C]-L-tryptophan and [^{14}C]-5-hydroxytryptophan for pulmonary biosynthesis of [^{14}C]-5-hydroxythryptamine: A review. *Ind. J. Pharmacol.*, 18:186–196.

262. Preininger, K., Stingl, H., Englisch, R., Furnsinn, C., Graf, J., Waldhausl, W., and Roden, M. (1999): Acute troglitazone action in isolated perfused rat liver. *Br. J. Pharmacol.*, 126:372–378.

263. Radwan, Z., and Henschler, D. (1977): Uptake and rate of metabolism of vinyl chloride by the isolated perfused rat liver preparation. *Int. Arch. Occup. Environ. Health*, 40:101–110.

264. Raje, R. R. (1980): In vitro toxicity of acetone using coronary perfusion in isolated rabbit heart. *Drug Chem. Toxicol.*, 3:333–342.

265. Raje, R. R. (1983): In vitro toxicity of n-hexane and 2,5-hexanedione using isolated perfused rabbit heart. *J. Toxicol. Environ. Health*, 11:879–884.

266. Rakic, L. M., Zlokovic, B. V., Davson, H., Segal, M. B., Begley, D. J., Lipovac, M. N., and Mitrovic, D. M. (1989): Chronic amphetamine intoxication and the blood-brain barrier permeability to inert polar molecules studied in the vascularity perfused guinea pig brain. *J. Neurol. Sci.*, 94:41–50.

267. Rao, M. M., and Elmslie, R. G. (1970): A modified technic of isolated pancreatic perfusion. *J. Surg. Res.*, 10:357–362.

268. Rao, S. B., and Mehendale, H. M. (1987): Uptake and disposition of putrescine, spermidine, and spermine by isolated perfused rabbit lungs. *Drug Metab. Dispos.*, 15:189–194.

269. Rao, S. B., Rao, K. S. P., and Mehendale, H. M. (1986): Absence of diamine oxidase activity from rabbit and rat lungs. *Biochem. J.*, 234:733–736.

270. Rasenack, J., Koch, H. K., Lesch, R., and Decker, K. (1980): Hepatotoxicity of D-galactosamine in isolated perfused rat liver. *Exp. Mol. Pathol.*, 32:264–275.

271. Redgeld, F. A., Hofman, G. A., van de Loo, P. G., Koster, A. S., and Noordhoek, J., (1991): Nephrotoxicity of the glutathione conjugate of menadione (2-methyl-l,4-naphthoquinone) in the isolated perfused rat kidney. Role of metabolism by gamma-glutamyltranspeptidase and probenecid-sensitive transport. *J. Pharmacol. Exp. Ther.*, 256:665–669.

272. Reichelderfer, M., Pero, B., Lorenzsonn, V., and Olsen, W. A. (1984): Magnesium sulfate-induced water secretion in hamster small intestine. *Proc. Soc. Exp. Biol. Med.*, 176:8–13.

273. Rhoades, R. A. (1976): Perfused lung preparation for studying altered gaseous environments. *Environ. Health Perspect.*, 16:73–75.

274. Rice, A. J., Roberts, R. J., and Plaa, G. L. (1967): The effect of carbon tetrachloride administered in vivo on the hemodynamics of the isolated perfused rat liver. *Toxicol. Appl. Pharmacol.*, 11:422–431.

275. Ritchie, H. D., and Hardcastle, J. D. (1973): *Isolated Organ Perfusion*. University Park Press, Baltimore.

276. Roby, K. A., and Shaw, L. M. (1993): Effects of cyclosporine and its metabolites in the isolated perfused rat kidney. *J. Am. Soc. Nephrol.*, 4:168–177.

277. Rosenfeld, S., Sellers, A. L., and Katz, J. (1959): Development of an isolated perfused rabbit kidney. *Am. J. Physiol.*, 196:115–159.

278. Ross, B. D. (1972): *Perfusion Techniques in Biochemistry*. Clarendon Press, Oxford.

279. Ross, B. D., Epstein, F. H., and Leaf, A. (1973): Sodium reabsorption in the perfused rat kidney. *Am. J. Physiol.*, 225:1165–1171.

280. Ross, B. D., Hems, R., and Krebs, H. A. (1967): The rate of gluconeogenesis from various precursors in the perfused rat liver. *Biochem. J.*, 102:942–951.

281. Rossi, N. F., Churchill, P. C., McDonald, F. D., and Ellis, V. R. (1989): Mechanism of cyclosporine A-induced renal vasoconstriction in the rat. *J. Pharmacol. Exp. Ther.*, 250:896–901.

282. Roth, J. A. (1979): Use of the isolated perfused lung in biochemical toxicology. *Rev. Biochem. Toxicol.*, 1:287–310.

283. Rowland, M. (1972): Application of clearance concepts to some literature data on drug metabolism in the isolated perfused liver preparation and in vivo. *Eur. J. Pharmacol.*, 17:352–356.

284. Rudolph, A. M., and Hyemann, M. A. (1971): Measurement of flow in perfused organs using microsphere techniques. In: *Perfusion Techniques*, edited by E. Diczfalusy, pp. 112–117. Karolinska Institute, Stockholm.

285. Ryoo, H., and Tarver, H. (1968): Studies on plasma protein synthesis with a new liver perfusion apparatus. *Proc. Soc. Exp. Biol. Med.*, 128:760–772.

286. Sato, Y., Eddy, L., and Hochstein, P. (1991): Comparative cardiotoxicity of doxorubicin and a morpholino anthracyclic derivative. *Biochem. Pharmacol.*, 42:2283–2287.

287. Schanne, F. A. X., Kane, A. B., Young, E. E., and Farber, J. L. (1979): Calcium dependence of toxic cell death: A final common pathway. *Science*, 206:700–702.

288. Schermann, J., Stowe, N., Yarimizu, S., Magnusson, M., and Tingwald, G. (1977): Feedback control of glomerular filtration rate in isolated, blood perfused dog kidneys. *Am. J. Physiol.*, 223:217–224.

289. Schimassek, H. (1962): Perfusion of rat liver with a semisynthetic medium and control of liver function. *Life Sci.*, 1:629–637.

290. Schimassek, H. (1963): Metabolite des kohlendydrastoffwechels der isoliert perfundierten rattenleber. *Biochem. Z.*, 336:460–467.

291. Schimassek, H., and Gerok, W. (1965): Control of the levels of free amino acids in plasma by the liver. *Biochem. Z.*, 343:407–415.

292. Schimmel, R. J., and Knobil, E. (1969): Role of free fatty acid in stimulation of gluconeogenesis during fasting. *Am. J. Physiol.*, 217:1803–1808.

293. Schureck, J., Brecht, J. P., Lofert, H., and Hierholzer, K. (1975): The basic requirements for the function of the isolated cell free perfused rat kidney. *Pflugers Arch.*, 354:349–365.

294. Seeger, W., Bauer, M., and Bhakdi, S. (1984): Staphylococcal α-toxin elicits hypertension in isolated rabbit lungs: Evidence for thromboxane formation and the role of extracellular calcium. *J. Clin. Invest.*, 74:849–858.

295. Seeger, W., Suttrop, N., Schmidt, F., and Neuhof, H. (1986): The glutathione redox cycle as a defense system against hydrogen peroxide–induced prostanoid formation and vasoconstriction in rabbit lungs. *Am. Rev. Respir. Dis.*, 133:1029–1036.

296. Segel, L. D., Rendig, S. V., and Mason, D. T. (1979): Left ventricular dysfunction of isolated working rat hearts after chronic alcohol consumption. *Cardiovasc. Res.*, 13:136–146.

297. Seiler, K. U., Tamm, G., and Wasserman, O. (1974): On the role of serotonin in the pathogenesis of pulmonary hypertension induced by anorectic drugs: An experimental study in the isolated perfused rat lung. *Clin. Exp. Pharmacol. Physiol.*, 1:463–471.

298. Seiver, B. R., and Whitney, J. E. (1967): Biosynthesis of insulin by the isolated perfused dog pancreas. *Diabetes*, 16:647–651.

299. Sharma, R., Kodavanti, U. P., Smith L. L., and Mehendale, H. M. (1995): The uptake and metabolism of cystamine and taurine by isolated ventilated and perfused rat and rabbit lungs. *Int. J. Biochem. Cell Biol.*, 27:655–664.

300. Silva, P., Rosen, S., Spokes, K., and Epstein, F. H. (1991): Effect of glycine on medullary thick ascending limb injury in perfused kidneys. *Kidney Int.*, 39:653–658.

301. Sklar, J. L., Anderson, P. G., and Boor, P. J. (1991): Allylamine and acrolein toxicity in perfused rat hearts. *Toxicol. Appl. Pharmacol.*, 107:535–544.

302. Skutul, K. (1908): Uber durchstromunsapporate. *Pflugers Arch.*, 123:249–273.

303. Sladen, G. E. (1968): Perfusion studies in relation to intestinal absorption. *Gut*, 9:624–628.

304. Smith, M. T., Thor, H., and Orrenius, S. (1981): Toxic injury to isolated hepatocytes is not dependent on extracellular calcium. *Science*, 213:1257–1259.

305. Soergel, K. H. (1971): Intestinal perfusion studies: Values, pitfalls, and limitations. *Gasteroenterology*, 61:261–263.

306. Southard, J. H., Senzig, K. A., Hoffman, R. M., and Belzer, F. O. (1980): Toxicity of oxygen to mitochondrial respiratory activity in hypothermically perfused canine kidneys. *Transplantation*, 29:459–61.

307. Sperling, F., and Marcus, W. L. (1968): Turpentine-induced histological changes in isolated rat and guinea-pig lungs. *Arch. Int. Pharmacodyn. Ther.*, 175:330–338.

308. Strubelt, O., Deters, M., Pentz, R., Siegers, C. P., and Younes, M. (1999): The toxic and metabolic effects of 23 aliphatic alcohols in the isolated perfused rat liver. *Toxicol. Sci.*, 49:133–142.

309. Summerfield, J. A., Gollan, J. L., and Billing, B. H. (1976): Synthesis of bile acid monophosphates by the isolated perfused rat kidney. *Biochem. J.*, 156:339–345.

310. Sumpio, B. E., Chandry, I. H., and Baue, A. E. (1985): Reduction of the drug-induced nephrotoxicity by ATP-$MgCl_2$. I. Effects of the cis-diamminedichloroplatinum-treated isolated perfused kidneys. *J. Surg. Res.*, 38:429–437.

311. Sussman, K. E., and Vaughn, G. D. (1967): Insulin release after ACTH, glucagon and adenosine 3′,5′-phosphate (cyclic AMP) in the perfused isolated rat pancreas. *Diabetes*, 16:449–454.

312. Sussman, K. E., Vaughn, G. D., and Timmer, R. F. (1966): An in vitro method for studying insulin secretion in perfused rat pancreas. *Metabolism*, 15:466–476.

313. Takano, T., Miyazaki, Y., and Motohashi, Y. (1983): A method to evaluate the dynamic effects of environmental chemical agents on intracellular functions: The real time observations of changes in the spectra of mitochondrial cytochromes, cytochrome P450, and catalase and in the fluorescence or reduced pyridine nucleotides in perfused rat liver. *Jpn. J. Hyg.*, 38:649–656.

314. Takano, T., Nakata, K., Kawakami, T., Miyazaki, Y., Murakami, M., Seo, Y., and Suzuki, E. (1991): Validation of a toxicity testing model by evaluating oxygen supply and energy state in the isolated perfused rat kidney. *J. Pharmacol. Methods*, 25:195–204.

315. Tark, M., Randall, H. M., Jr., and Hoffer, T. L. (1976): Substrate metabolism in the isolated perfused kidney. *Invest. Urol.*, 14:132–136.

316. te Kopelle, J. M., Keller, B. J., Caldwell-Kenkel, J. C., Lemasters, J. J., and Thurman, R. G. (1991): Effect of hepatotoxic chemicals and hypoxia on hepatic nonperenchymal cells: Impairment of phagocytosis by Kupffer cells and disruption of the endothelium in rat livers perfused with colloidal carbon. *Toxicol. Appl. Pharmacol.*, 110:20–30.

317. Telander, R. L. (1964): Prolonged monothermic perfusion of the isolated primate and sheep kidney. *Surg. Gynecol. Obstet.*, 118:347–353.

318. Teo, S., and Vore, M. (1991): Mirex inhibits bile acid secretory function in vivo and in the isolated perfused rat liver. *Toxicol. Appl. Pharmacol.*, 109:161–170.

319. Terao, N., and Shen, D. D. (1985): Reduced extraction of l-propranolol by perfused rat liver in the presence of uremic blood. *J. Pharmacol. Exp. Ther.*, 233:277–284.

320. Thelen, M., and Wendel, A. (1983): Drug-induced lipid peroxidation in mice. V. Ethane production and glutathione release in the isolated liver upon perfusion with acetaminophen. *Biochem. Pharmacol.*, 32:1701–1706.

321. Thompson, A. M., Cavert, H. M., and Lifson, N. (1968): A rat head-perfusion technique developed for the study of brain uptake of materials. *J. Appl. Physiol.*, 24:407–411.

322. Thurman, R. G., Marazzo, D. P., Jones, L. S., and Kauffman, F. C. (1977): The continuous kinetic determination of p-nitroanisole O-demethylation in hemoglobin-free perfused rat liver. *J. Pharmacol. Exp. Ther.*, 201:498–506.

323. Thurman, R. G., Reinke, L. A., and Kauffman, F. C. (1979): The isolated perfused liver: A model to define biochemical mechanisms of chemical toxicity. *Rev. Biochem. Toxicol.*, 1:249–286.

324. Torack, R. M. (1969): Sodium demonstration in rat cerebellum following perfusion hydroxyadipaldehyde antimonate. *Acta Neuropathol. (Berl.)*, 12:173–182.

325. Tornquist, S., Moller, L., Gabrielsson, J., Gustafsson, J. A., and Toftgard, R. (1990): 2-Nitrofluorene metabolism in the rat lung. Pharmacokinetic and metabolic effects of beta-naphthoflavone treatment. *Carcinogenesis*, 11:1249–1254.

326. Toth, K. M., Clifford, D. P., Berger, E. M., White, C. W., and Repine, J. E. (1984): Intact human erythrocytes prevent hydrogen peroxide-mediated damage to isolated perfused rat lungs and cultured bovine pulmonary artery endothelial cells. *J. Clin. Invest.*, 74:292–295.

327. Trela, B. A., Carlson, G. P., Turek, J., Rebar, A., Mathews, J. M. (1989): Effect of carbon monoxide on the cytochrome P450-mediated activation of 4-ipomeanol by the isolated perfused rabbit lung. *J. Toxicol. Environ. Health*, 27:341–350.

328. Triner, L., Verosky, M., Habif, D. V., and Nahas, G. G. (1970): Perfusion of isolated liver with fluorocarbon emulsions. *Fed. Proc.*, 29:1778–1781.

329. Trumper, L., Monasterolo, L. A., Ochoa, E., and Elias, M. M. (1995): Tubular effects of acetaminophen in the isolated perfused kidney. *Arch. Toxicol.*, 69:248–252.

330. Tsuji, M., and Nakajima, T. (1978): Studies on the formation of γ-aminobutyric acid from putrescine in rat organic purification of its synthesis enzyme from rat intestine. *J. Biochem. (Tokyo)*, 83:1407–1420.

331. Umbreit, W. W., Burris, R. H., and Stauffer, J. F. (1972): *Manometric Biochemical Techniques*, 5th ed., p. 146. Burguess, Minneapolis.

332. Vähäkangas, K., Nevasaari, K., Pelkonen, O., and Karki, N. T. (1977): The metabolism of benzo(a)pyrene in isolated perfused lungs from variously treated rats. *Acta Pharmacol. Toxicol. (Copenh.)*, 41:129–140.

333. Valenzuela, A., and Guerra, R. (1985): Protective effect of the flavonoid silybin dihemisuccinate on the toxicity of phenyl hydrazine on rat liver. *FEBS Lett.*, 181:292–294.

334. Videla, L. A., Troncoso, P., Arisi, A. C., and Junquiera, V. B. (1997): Dose-dependent effects of acute lindane treatment on Kupffer cell function assessed in the isolated perfused rat liver. *Xenobiotica*, 27:747–757.

335. Villanueva, G. R., Mendoza, M. E., el-Mir, M. Y., Herrera, M. C., and Marin, J. J. (1997): Effect of bile acids on hepatobiliary transport of cisplatin by perfused rat liver. *Pharmacol. Toxicol.*, 80:111–117.

336. Vilstrap, H. (1983): Effects of acute carbon tetrachloride intoxication on kinetics or galactose elimination by perfused rat livers. *Scand. J. Clin. Lab. Invest.*, 43:127–131.

337. Wang, J. F., and Wendel, A. (1990): Studies on the hepatotoxicity of galactosamine/endotoxin on galactosamine/TNF in the perfused mouse liver. *Biochem. Pharmacol.*, 39:267–270.

338. Watanabe, M., Takano, T., and Nakamura, K. (1998): Effect of ethanol on the metabolism of trichloroethylene in the perfused rat liver. *J. Toxicol. Environ. Health.*, 55:287–305.

339. Waugh, W. A., and Kubo, T. (1959): Development of an isolated perfused dog kidney with improved function. *Am. J. Physiol.*, 217:227–290.

340. Welbourne, T. C. (1974): Ammonia production and pathways of glutamine metabolism in the isolated perfused rat kidney. *Am. J. Physiol.*, 226:544–548.

341. White, R. J. (1971): Preparation and mechanical perfusion of the isolated monkey brain. In: *Perfusion Techniques*, edited by E. Diczfalusy, pp. 200–216. Karolinska Institute, Stockholm.

342. Willinger, C. C., Moschen, I., Kulmer, S., and Pfaller, W. (1995): The effect of sodium fluoride at prophylactic and toxic doses on renal structure and function in the isolated perfused rat kidney. *Toxicology*, 95:55–71.

343. Wilson, T. H., and Wiseman, G. (1954): Use of sacs of everted small intestine for study of transference of subtrances from the mucosal to serosal surface. *J. Physiol.* (*Lond.*), 123: 116–125.

344. Winchell, R. J., and Halasz, N. A. (1989): Lack of effect of oxygen-radical scavenging systems in the preserved-reperfused rabbit kidney. *Transplantation*, 48:393–396.

345. Windmueller, H. G., Spaeth, A. E., and Ganote, C. E. (1970): Vascular perfusion of isolated rat gut: Norepinephrine and glucocorticoid requirement. *Am. J. Physiol.*, 218:197–204.

346. Woodward, B., and Zakaria, M. N. M. (1985): Effect of some free radical scavengers on reperfusion induced arrhythmias in the isolated rat heart. *J. Mol. Cell. Cardiol.*, 17:485–493.

347. Yamamoto, K., Hasegawa, T., and Ueda, J. (1968): Renin secretion in the perfused dog kidney. *Jpn. J. Pharmacol.*, 18: 1–8.

348. Yelich, M. R. (1993): The effect of epinephrine on insulin and glucagon secretion from the endotoxic rat pancreas. *Pancreas*, 4:450–458.

349. Young, S. L. (1976): An isolated perfused rat lung preparation. *Environ. Health Perspect.*, 16:61–66.

350. Youngman, R. C., Klugo, R. C., Cruickshank, R. D., and Cerny, J. C. (1976): A technique for isolated in vivo renal perfusion. *Invest. Urol.*, 14:187–190.

351. Zamlauski-Tucker, M. J., Morris, M. E., and Springate, J. E. (1994): Ifosfamide metabolite chloroacetaldehyde causes Fanconi syndrome in the perfused rat kidney. *Toxicol. Appl. Pharmacol.*, 129:170–175.

Principles and Methods of Toxicology,
Fourth Edition, edited by A. Wallace Hayes.
Taylor & Francis, Philadelphia © 2001.

Chapter 34

Organelles as Tools in Toxicology

Bruce A. Fowler, Mary L. Haasch, Kevin M. Kleinow, Katherine S. Squibb, and A. Wallace Hayes

Cells are composed of a number of organelle compartments that play crucial roles in facilitating metabolic processes essential to cellular viability (Figure 34.1). The effects of many toxic agents on cells are mediated via damage to one or more of these specialized subcellular compartments. Specific organelle systems may become damaged by toxic agents when they perform a primary role in the metabolism of a particular toxicant, when a toxicant is stored intracellularly, or as a result of an inherent sensitivity of some essential biochemical pathways in the organelle to perturbation. In terms of understanding the mechanisms of cellular toxicity, it is clear that evaluation of organelles as basic units of subcellular function may provide useful insights into the basis of toxicant action. It also should be obvious that the ability to detect damage within particular organelle systems depends on the sensitivity and nature of the parameters measured.

The following discussion examines some of the current ultrastructural and biochemical methods available for evaluation of specific organelles and reviews some of the ways in which these techniques have aided understanding the mechanisms of toxicity. A critical examination of these techniques is presented to aid the reader in assessing the potential value of a given procedure for delineating information about a specific toxic process.

MITOCHONDRIA

Mitochondria are essential organelles that play an important role in cell metabolism by mediating a number of metabolic functions (Figure 34.2). Enzymes involved in energy production, carbohydrate metabolism, heme biosynthesis, and the urea cycle are found in this organelle. These enzymes are not distributed randomly within the mitochondria but are localized within specific subcompartments, such as the outer and inner membranes, intermembrane space, and matrix (Table 34.1).

In terms of the effects of toxicants on this organelle, it is important to understand the relationship between par-

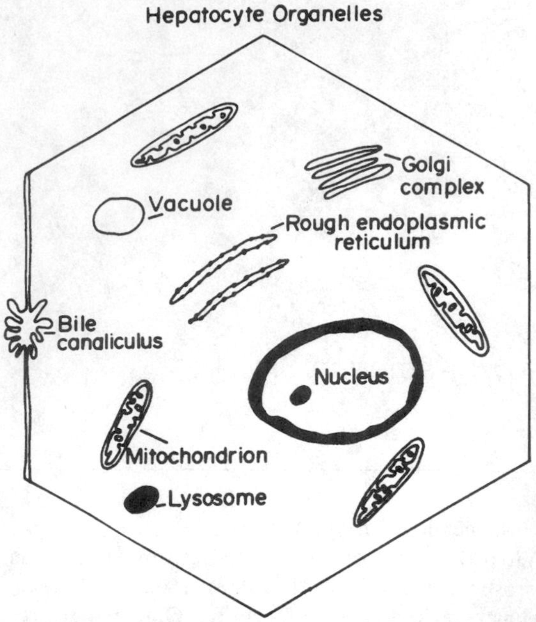

FIG. 34.1. Diagrammatic representation of a hepatocyte showing nucleus, mitochondria, lysosomes, peroxisomes, rough and smooth endoplasmic reticulum, and Golgi apparatus.

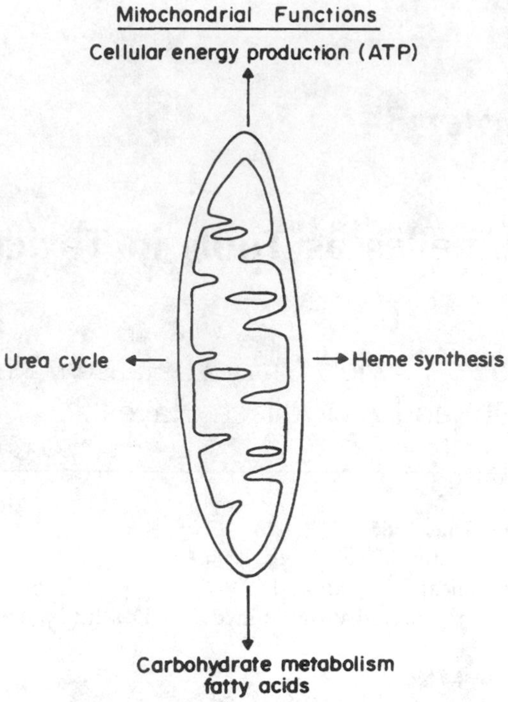

FIG. 34.2. Diagrammatic representation of a mitochondrion showing outer membrane, inner membrane with infoldings (cristae), and matrix. This multifunctional organelle has enzyme systems that are concerned with the production of ATP, carbohydrate metabolism, heme biosynthesis, and the urea cycle and that are specifically localized in the outer membrane, inner membrane or matrix. From Reference 54, with permission.

ticular metabolic functions and the physical integrity of the mitochondrion as a structure, because in vivo biochemical perturbations frequently result directly from structural damage. The following examination of ultrastructural and biochemical methods for mitochondrial evaluations uses examples of some well-known toxicants to illustrate how each technique aided in understanding the mechanisms of toxicity. More recently, the role of the mitochondria in releasing molecular factors involved in the initiation of apoptosis have added new insights into how this organelle may modulate basic processes of cell death. Over the last 5 years, great progress has been made in understanding the major roles played by this organelle in regulating the processes of cell injury and cell death through the regulation and control of a number of molecular factors and proteases which appear to be central factors in modulating programmed cell death or apoptosis.

Ultrastructural Techniques

Fixation and Embedding

Preservation of mitochondria within intact cells is carried out routinely by rapid chemical fixation using glutaraldehyde or glutaraldehyde-formaldehydc-based fixatives. Tissues may either be placed in these fixatives or perfused via the blood vasculature for optimal preservation of cellular structure. Electron density is imparted to the mitochondrial membranes by postfixation in a 1% solution of osmium tetroxide (OsO_4) followed by dehydration in a graded series of alcohol from 70%–100%. Dehydrated tissues are then placed in solutions of propylene oxide and embedded in plastic resins, such as Epon. A stepwise routine procedure for fixation and embedding of tissues for electron microscopy is as follows:

1. Place tissue blocks (1 mm^3) in fixative (2% glutaraldehyde, 2.6% formaldehyde in 0.07 M cacodylate buffer (pH 7.4), and 3% sucrose) for 2 h in a refrigerator.
2. Decant fixative and place blocks in cacodylate buffer overnight in a refrigerator.
3. Postfix blocks in 1% OsO_4 (Caution: volatile toxicant) in 0.1 M phosphate buffer (pH 7.4) for 2 h and then decant in a fume hood.
4. Dehydrate tissue blocks in 70%, 90%, 95% (two changes), and 100% alcohol at room temperature for 15 min at each step.
5. Decant final 100% alcohol solution and place blocks in two changes of propylene oxide.

Table 34.1
Activity and functions of enzymes and proteins in mitochondria

Enzyme Activities and Protcins	Function
Outer Membrane	
Fatty acid CoA synthetase	Fatty acid metabolism
Monoame oxidase	Catecholamine metabolism
Inter-Membrane Space	
I-AAA proteases	Regulation of mitochondrial protein metabolism
Inner Membrane	
NADH oxidase	Transport
Succinic dehydrogenase	TCA substrate
β-Hydroxybutyrate dehydrogenase	Oxidation
Mg^{2+}-ATPase	Ion transport
Coproporphyrinogen oxidase	
Ferrochelatase	Heme biosynthesis
ALA synthetase	
Anion and cation transport systems	Mitochondrial conformation
m-AAA proteases	Mitochondrial protein metabolism
Cytochrome c	Mitochondrial induction of apoptosis
Matrix	
Pyruvate dehydrogenase complex	
Malate dehydrogenase	
Isocitric dehydrogenase	Intermediary metabolism
Citrate synthetase	
Fumarase	
Glutamic dehydrogenase	
Glutamic transminases	Ammonia metabolism
Ornithine carbamoyltransferase	Urea synthesis
Carbamoyl PO_4 synthetase	
HSP 60	Protein refolding
Lon/PIM1 proteases	Regulation of mitochondrial protein metabolism
Clp proteases	

6. Place blocks in 50:50 propylene oxide plastic resin mixture overnight to infiltrate tissue blocks.
7. Place tissue blocks in final plastic resin mixture and embed in Teflon capsules.
8. Place in curing oven (60°C) to harden plastic before sectioning.

Ultrastructural Morphometry

This technique, which is essentially an approach to quantifying the dimensions of organelle compartments within intact cells based on evaluation of their surface area in a large number of electron micrographs, has been reviewed extensively (11,14,176,192). The method may be employed to determine the overall volume of organelles, such as mitochondria, within cells (volume density), but determinations of mitochondrial membrane surface area (surface density) and numbers of mitochondria (numerical density) require the application of correction factors that recently have undergone revision (11,14,176). The specific steps in this technique, as well as the equations necessary for evaluation of generated data, are given in articles by Weibel et al. (196) and Williams (201) and will not be repeated here.

The application of morphometry to evaluation of mitochondria following in vivo exposure to arsenate (52,55), cortisone (199), methyl mercury (51), and vitamin E deficiency (58) has been employed successfully to document increases or decreases in this organelle system and the relationship of these effects to observed biochemical changes.

The primary value of ultrastructural morphometry in delineating toxic mechanisms for organelles such as the mitochondrion rests with the ability to quantitatively assess changes in mitochondrial structure within the intact cell. Such data have proved to be invaluable not only in interpreting the results of biochemical studies on this organelle (53), but also in suggesting new and more integrative hypotheses that consider change in the biochemical functionality of the mitochondrion in relation to concomitant chemical-induced alterations in other organelle systems (e.g., the endoplasmic reticulum) within the same cells (49). In other words, this technique has provided a rigorous approach for simultaneously assessing whether changes are occurring in more than one organelle system and thereby minimizing the possibility of erroneously concluding that a chemical is acting at only one site within a target cell population, which is one of the great pitfalls in contemporary mechanistic toxicology. It should be noted (45,46) that the application of this technique to toxicology is extremely labor intensive and requires a serious commitment of resources for successful use. This aspect requires serious consideration by those contemplating use of this powerful morphological technique.

Ultrastructural Evaluation of Mitochondrial Fractions

Evaluation of mitochondria from tissues following homogenization and isolation in sucrose (discussed later) by electron microscopy provides one method for evaluating the purity of the samples and the degree of structural integrity. This technique also has been employed to examine changes in mitochondrial conformational behavior during respiration following in vitro exposure to uncoupling agents such as dinitrophenol (75) or in vivo following exposure to lead (62) or arsenate (55). The technique essentially involves using the chemical fixation and embedding process described previously to processed pellets of mitochondria and other organelles. A more quantitative approach to evaluation of isolated organelles has been described by Deter (39).

Negative Staining of Isolated Mitochondria

The technique of negative staining (80) involves uranyl acetate, phosphotungstic acid, or ammonium molybdate to stain the Formvar grid backing so that isolated organelles, such as mitochondria, stand out against the dark background. This method has proved to be extremely useful for high-resolution microscopy studies of mitochondrial membrane preparations and has been used to evaluate changes in mitochondrial membranes following in vitro exposure of these organelles to uncoupling agents (136). A general flowsheet for this technique follows, and a more complete discussion is given elsewhere (80). As with the other morphological techniques discussed in this section, the main value of this procedure rests with providing correlative structural information about changes in the internal structure of this organelle in relation to biochemical alterations within intramitochondrial compartments (46).

Technique

1. Isolate mitochondria (see Figure 34.3).

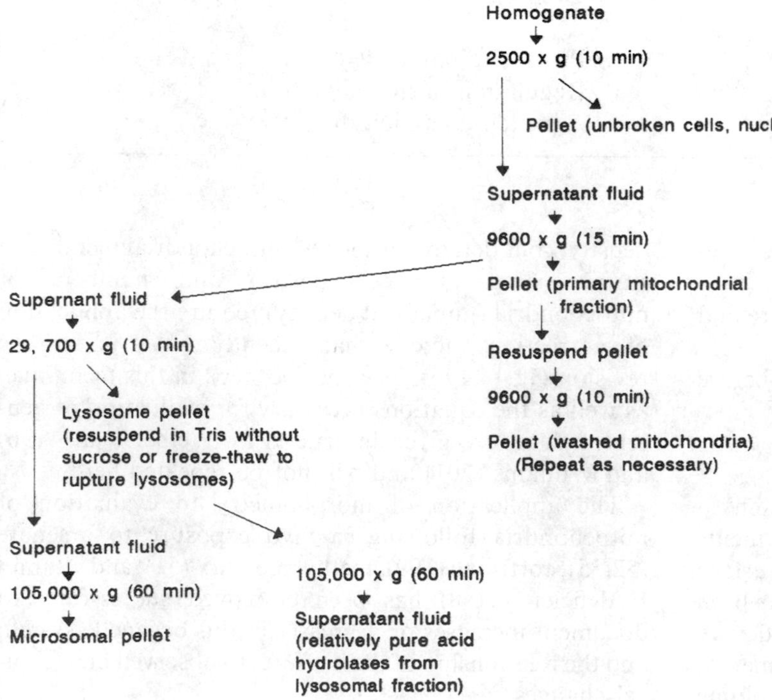

FIG. 34.3. Standard isolation procedure for mitochondria and other organelles such as lysosomes and microsomes by differential centrifugation in 0.25 M sucrose-0.05 M Tris buffer (pH 7.4).

2. Final dilution of mitochondria to 60 mg protein/ml.
3. Pipet sample on the Formvar-coated grids and allow to dry in covered dish.
4. Cover grids with a drop of negative stain (pH 7.4) at 1%–2% concentration.
5. Blot excess stain from edge of grid with filter paper.
6. Examine sample with transmission electron microscope.

Scanning Electron Microscopy

Application of scanning electron microscopy to evaluation of mitochondrial conformational behavior or the conformational behavior of the intact inner membrane (mitoplast) has been employed by Andrews and Hackenbrock (4) to confirm findings obtained by transmission electron microscopy.

Technique

1. Place mitochondrial or mitoplast sample (1 to 2 mg protein/ml) on Formvar-coated grids and cover with one drop 2% glutaraldehyde in 0.1 M phosphate buffer (pH 7.4).
2. Place grids in perforated vials and dehydrate in acetone; follow with critical point drying.
3. Coat samples with a 150-Å layer of palladium-gold in a vacuum evaporator.
4. Examine in a scanning electron microscope.

Freeze-Etch Analyses

The technique of freeze-etching has been employed to study the three-dimensional structure of mitochondrial membranes during different energy states (74,99) and their relationship to localization of protein complexes within the membrane. This method essentially involves chemical fixation and rapid freezing of biological samples in Freon prior to fracturing in a freeze-etch device (97). The fracture plane is believed to cleave primarily across the hydrophobic regions of the membranes, thereby exposing both inner and outer surfaces. The surfaces then are sputter-coated with metals, such as platinum and carbon, to form replicas that are floated off the tissue and collected on standard electron microscopy grids for evaluation in a transmission electron microscope. A detailed examination of the techniques and known artifacts has been given elsewhere (97). To date, this technique has not been applied to evaluation of toxicant action on mitochondria.

Technique

1. Fix tissue in the glutaraldehyde fixative described previously.
2. Incubate tissue in 10%–20% glycerol until tissue is impregnated.
3. Place specimen on specimen carrier and immerse in Freon 22 cooled to –165°C with liquid nitrogen.
4. Place specimen in freeze-etch device and fracture with steel blade.
5. Etch-clean surface of specimen by allowing ice to sublime from sample.
6. Shadow specimen surface with carbon-platinum to form replica and cover replica with carbon backing layer.
7. Remove specimen and replica from evaporator and place in an aqueous solution similar to original glycerol freezing solution to release replica from specimen surface.
8. Clean replica in 5% sodium hypochlorite solution.
9. Rinse replicas in several changes of water and mount on 150-mesh grids.

Overall Assessment

The primary value of the various ultrastructural techniques described in this section rests with delineating the organelle system within a target cell population that is being affected by a given toxicant within an intact tissue. These techniques may be extended further to provide information about changes in organelle infrastructure that may point to a molecular site of action, which may be approached by biochemical techniques. In this regard, these techniques also have proved highly useful in interpreting results of biochemical studies on various organelle systems following either in vivo or in vitro chemical treatment. Thus, although these procedures do not by themselves delineate mechanisms, they are extremely valuable techniques for detecting molecular sites of action and correctly interpreting biochemical studies that examine chemical mechanisms at those loci.

Biochemical Procedures

There are a variety of biochemical parameters that can be used to assess the effects of toxicants on mitochondrial function. In part, the effectiveness of these techniques depends on the procedures used to isolate mitochondria prior to evaluation. A relatively standard procedure is given in Figure 34.3 that essentially involves homogenizing in Tris (0.05 M)-sucrose (0.25 M) with subsequent pelleting of mitochondria by centrifugation. In addition to this basic procedure, resuspension and recentrifugation may be used to "wash" the mitochondria and to remove contamination by microsomes. In the process of reducing mitochondrial contamination, it should be noted that mitochondria from different tissues vary in their sensitivity to physical damage or chelating agents such as ethylenediaminetetraacetic acid (EDTA). This means that caution must be exercised in order to separate toxicant effects on these organelles from other effects derived from the isolation procedures. A more complete examination of problems encountered in the isolation of mitochondria and other organelles has been given by Deter (39).

In addition, mitochondria may be separated into the outer mitochondrial membrane and inner mitochondrial membrane plus matrix (mitoplast) by treatment with controlled digitonin digestion (159) or use of a pressure cell (65) with subsequent pelleting of membranes by centrifugation. This technique has been used successfully to identify the submitochondrial localization of a host of marker enzyme activities (Table 34.1).

General Mitochondrial Isolation Procedures

1. Homogenize tissues in 0.25 M sucrose or mannitol in 0.05 M Tris-HCl buffer (pH 7.4) at 1 g tissue/9 ml of Tris-sucrose. Agents such as EDTA may also be added to aid disruption of cells.
2. Place in centrifuge tubes and spin at 2500 × g for 10 min to remove nuclei and unbroken cells.
3. Decant supernatant fluid into centrifuge tubes and spin at 10,000 × g for 10 min to form primary mitochondrial pellet.
4. Decant supernatant fluid and gently resuspend pellet in 10 ml Tris-sucrose for washing. Recentrifuge pellet and decant supernatant fluid. This washing cycle may be repeated a number of times, depending on the tissue involved and the degree of mitochondrial purity desired.
5. Resuspend final mitochondrial pellet (1 ml Tris-sucrose/1 g of original sample).

Separation of Outer and Inner Mitochondrial Membranes

1. Place washed mitochondria (30–60 mg protein/ml) in a precooled French pressure cell and subject to 1500 psi. Extruded material is taken up in an equal volume of double-strength medium and centrifuged at 12,100 × g for 10 min.
2. Resuspend the resultant pellet in the previous volume and recentrifuge at 12,100 × g for 10 min.
3. Combine supernatant material from the above pellets and centrifuge at 27,100 × g for 10 min.
4. Supernatant fluid from this pellet is centrifuged at 144,000 × g for 90 min to obtain the outer membrane (pellet) and intermembrane fraction (supernatant fluid).

Respiratory Function

One of the primary functions of mitochondria within intact cells is the oxidation of substrates with subsequent generation of adenosine triphosphate (ATP). There are two major classes of oxidizable substrates that are capable of causing electron flow through the mitochondrial electron transport chain. The first of these involves those substrates (pyruvate, malate, and p-hydroxybutyrate) that use nicotinamide-adenine dinucleotide (NAD) as an acceptor of protons and is capable of generating 3 mol of ATP per molecule oxidized. Succinate is the other substrate type and generates 2 mol of ATP per molecule oxidized. Methods employed for the evaluation of mitochondrial respiratory function include Warburg respirometry and the oxygen electrode; each measures oxygen consumption by mitochondria in the presence of oxidizable substrates. The advantage of the first type of measurement rests with its ability to measure oxygen consumption within intact tissue slices, whereas the latter is capable of detecting changes in respiration during different states of respiration.

Technique (Oxygen Electrode)

1. Isolated mitochondria in Tris-sucrose medium (10–20 mg protein/ml) are placed into a 1- to 3-ml oxygen electrode cell with stirrer containing a reaction mixture composed of 40 mM Tris-HCl (pH 7.5), 5 mM K_2HPO_4, 5 mM $MgSO_4$, and 100 mM KCl with 1–2 mg mitochondrial protein per milliliter.
2. A stable recorder baseline is obtained and initial state 4 respiration is initiated by adding succinate or NAD-linked substrates to yield a final concentration in the cell of 5 mM.
3. After 1–2 min of state 4 respiration, state 3 respiration is initiated by adding 2 to 5 μmol adenosinediphosphate (ADP).
4. Following complete use of the added ADP, a return of state 4 respiration will be observed.
5. Respiratory control ratios (RCR) are calculated by dividing the state 3 rate by the state 4 rate. ADP/O ratios are calculated by dividing the amount of ADP added by the calculated amount of oxygen consumed as described by Estabrook (43).

As an approach to the toxicity assessment of mitochondria, respiratory function is an essential index of mitochondrial function that is easily damaged by many toxic agents. Toxic trace metals, such as arsenic (52,54,55), lead (62,65), mercury (44,51,165), and cadmium (91), inhibit mitochondrial respiration. For lead and arsenic, this inhibition is relatively specific for NAD-linked substrates, such as pyruvate/malate (50,54,55,62). This process is believed to be due to inhibition of mitochondrial dehydrogenases for these substrates, which are located in the mitochondrial matrix. In addition, alteration of mitochondrial conformation behavior has been reported in relation to these phenomena (55,62), indicating that the well-known energy-linked transformation (73–75) of these organelles also is altered. Organic toxicants, such as pesticides (140) and others (24,87), also damage mitochondrial respiratory function leading to diminished production of ATP.

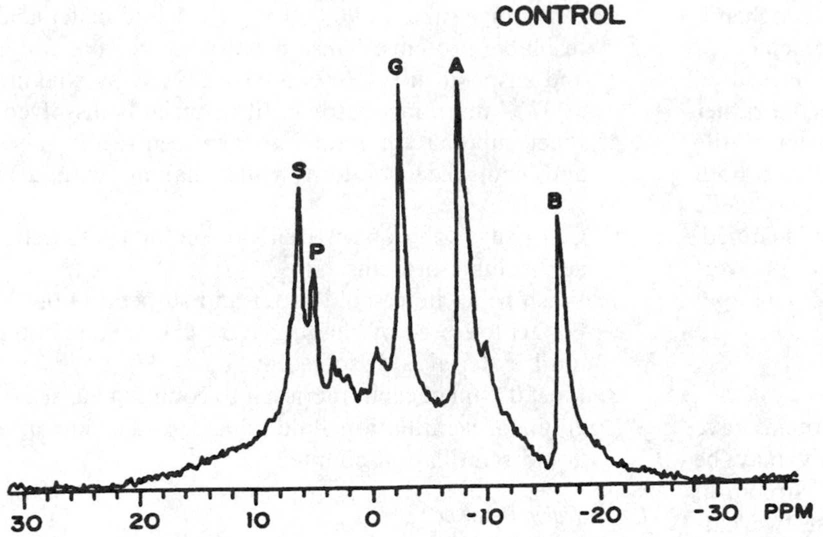

FIG. 34.4. *In vivo* ^{31}P-NMR spectra from a control rat liver showing three ATP peaks (G,A,B) and inorganic phosphorus (P) and sugar (S) compounds. (Courtesy of Dr. Benjamin Chen.)

Obviously, as the primary energy source for most cells, mitochondrial respiration and ATP generation are essential to cell survival. Although impairment of mitochondrial respiration implies the reduced availability of ATP for maintaining essential cellular processes, it should be noted that quantification of cellular ATP levels is essential to confirming such a mechanism, as ATP appears to be present in excess within cells. Chemical methods for quantifying ATP require an extraction process, which in our experience usually added to the variability in these measurements by such procedures. Such methodological problems increase standard deviations, which reduces the ability to discriminate effects between treatment groups on a statistical basis. More recently, the advent of in vivo ^{31}P-nuclear magnetic resonance (NMR) spectroscopy has permitted more specific measurement of the three ATP resonances as well as inorganic phosphorus, NAD, and sugar phosphates in other phosphorylated chemical species (Figure 34.4). A major advantage of this technique is the ability to monitor changes in ATP concentrations in major target organs, such as the liver, in real time without killing an animal by placing an NMR surface coil over the organ of interest (108) while the anesthetized animal rests inside the large-bore NMR magnet. We recently have employed this technique (25) to study the effects of acute arsenite (As^{+3}) treatment on hepatic ATP content following a single intravenous dose. The data demonstrate not only the expected decrease in hepatic ATP and rise in Pi, but the attendant increased phosphorylation of several other chemical species. These latter events would never have been appreciated via simple extraction and measurement of ATP.

Carbohydrate Metabolism

Many of the enzymes involved in intermediary metabolism are localized in the mitochondrial matrix. Dehydrogenases for pyruvate, malate, and glutamate are localized in this portion of the organelle. A typical assay procedure for malate dehydrogenase has been described extensively elsewhere (143). Toxicant damage to this aspect of mitochondrial function has been demonstrated for agents such as arsenic (52,54–56) and methyl mercury (115).

Heme Biosynthesis

Three of the key enzymes in the heme biosynthesis pathway are localized in the mitochondrion and are associated with the inner mitochondrial membrane. Ferrochelatase, coproporphyrinogen oxidase, and 8-aminolevulinic acid synthetase are highly sensitive to the action of toxic trace metals (203–206,208), with resultant increases in the urinary excretion of porphyrin precursors that have proved to be useful biological indicators of toxicity. Assay procedures for these mitochondrial enzymes also have been described extensively (203–206,208) and will not be described here.

The value of measuring mitochondrial heme biosynthetic pathway enzymes rests with determining enzymatic mechanisms for specific chemical-induced porphyrinuria patterns, which have widespread use as biological indicators for both organic (171) and inorganic (53) chemicals. Measurement of these enzymes in target tissues such as the liver (171,204,206) and kidney (203,205) has provided valuable insight into the tissue source of the excreted porphyrins, which are among the most useful biological indicators available for chemical exposure and toxicity. If other parameters of mitochondrial structure and function are measured (51–55) along with these enzyme activities, then a rather complete picture of the nature and mechanism of the mitochondrial toxicity emerges. In other words, both the biochemical mechanism and tissue/organelle localization of the chemical-induced injury are identified. Because these events usually precede the onset of overt clinical disease, they offer the prospect of detecting target tissue toxicity at an early stage.

Mitochondrial Protein Synthesis

Studies on the synthesis of mitochondrial proteins have been reviewed extensively (27) and generally may be regarded as divisible into two categories: structural and enzymatic. Beattie (5) showed that these two categories of protein could be separated biochemically on the basis of solubility in dilute acetic acid into (1) proteins synthesized within the mitochondria for structural purposes, and (2) those enzymes synthesized outside the mitochondria in the endoplasmic reticulum with subsequent incorporation into the mitochondria.

Mitochondrial protein synthesis studies are essential for determining whether changes in the specific activities of mitochondrial marker enzymes following in vivo chemical exposure are the result of a direct chemical-enzyme interaction, a change in the synthesis of that enzyme, or both. We have found these studies of value for interpreting structural changes in mitochondria delineated by ultrastructural morphometry. Thus, protein synthesis studies in this organelle are extremely valuable for interpreting the results of morphological and other biochemical studies.

Application of this technique to toxicology studies has shown that prolonged in vivo exposure of fetal rat liver mitochondria to methyl mercury produced preferential suppression of membrane but not enzymatic protein synthesis (51). In contrast, exposure of adult rats to arsenate (55) produced an increased synthesis of both protein compartments and morphometric increases in the surface density of the inner mitochondrial membrane. The changes in protein synthesis were associated with increases in the specific activities of the mitochondrial marker enzymes monoamine oxidase, cytochrome oxidase, and Mg^{+2}-ATPase.

Technique

1. Give the rat an intraperitoneal injection of [^{14}C]leucine (20 μCi) and kill 10 min later.
2. Liver tissue is excised and mitochondria are isolated as described previously.
3. Isolated mitochondria are placed in 1.4% acetic acid in capped ultracentrifuge tubes and shaken for 30 min in the cold (4°C).
4. Centrifuge tubes at 90,000 × g for 1 h to pellet acid insoluble proteins. Rinse pellet with ice-cold water and suspend in 0.4 N NaOH followed by shaking at 37°C in an incubator until material is dissolved.
5. Pipet supernatant fluid into new centrifuge tubes and neutralize solution while shaking with 2 N NaOH.
6. Centrifuge solutions at 105,000 × g for 1 h to pellet acid-soluble proteins.
7. Wash pellet in ice-cold water and suspend in 0.4 N NaOH followed by shaking at 37°C in an incubator until material is dissolved.
8. Pipet 0.2 ml of each fraction into counting vials, add 20 ml of scintillation fluid, shake, and count in a liquid scintillation counter.

Conformation Behavior

The technique of following mitochondrial swelling and contraction by measurement of light scattering in a spectrophotometer was developed by Tedeschi and Harris (176). This method is based on the increased optical density of mitochondria in a contracted state and decreased density in a swollen or orthodox configuration due to cation influx. Agents such as arsenic (55) and phosphate (117) produce detectable alterations of swelling and contraction behavior that can be detected by measurement of light scattering at 520 nm. Data from these studies are useful functional tests of mitochondrial membrane integrity following in vivo or in vitro exposure to a chemical agent. It is also useful for discriminating between high- and low-amplitude mitochondrial swelling.

Technique

1. Place a solution of 0.12 M KCl in 0.02 M Tris-Cl (pH 7.4) in spectrophotometer cuvettes and add isolated mitochondria to a final concentration of 2 mg/ml.
2. Mitochondrial swelling is measured as a decrease in optical density at 520 nm with time.
3. Maximal swelling usually is achieved within 15 min with liver mitochondria.
4. Initiate contraction of the mitochondria after about 15 min by adding Mg^{2+}-ATP (5 mM), which produces a corresponding increase in the optical density of the sample to near its original reading.

Ion Translocation by Specific Ion Electrodes

During mitochondrial respiration or changes in conformation, the transport of H^+, Na^+, K^+, or Ca^{2+} occurs (127,145,150). Movement of these cations between isolated mitochondria and the surrounding medium may be monitored by specific ion electrodes, as described in a review by Pressman (150) that contains specific details for application of this technique. Application of this approach to measuring mitochondrial membrane functionality following exposure to mercurials (13,102) and lead (147) has provided useful information about the nature of mercury-mitochondrial membrane interactions. Other studies have shown energy-dependent mitochondrial uptake of arsenic. Data from such investigations are highly useful in more specifically delineating which ion transport systems are altered by agents that affect mitochondrial membrane integrity.

Mitochondria and Programmed Cell Death (Apoptosis)

In recent years it has become clear that the mitochondria contain a number of factors that regulate the process of programmed cell death or apoptosis. This process appears to be controlled by a series of proteases known as caspaces, whose activities are regulated by a number of mitochondrial proteins, such as cytochrome c, which binds to a cytoplasmic protein identified as Apaf-1, and the combination of proteins to form a regulatory complex in turn activates caspace-9, which in turn activates other caspaces and results in the degradation of genomic DNA via DNAase activation. More recently (see Wallace (194,106) for a review), studies have shown that mitochondria can release an apoptosis-inducing factor (AIF) from the inter-membrane space. This protein has sequence homology with bacterial oxido-reductases. This factor is also capable of activating nuclear DNAase activity and producing the characteristic DNA laddering on sucrose gels, which is one hallmark of apoptosis.

The LON Family of Proteases

The LON proteases are ATP-dependent proteases found in bacteria, and related proteases have been found in the matrix of mitochondria (Table 34.1). These proteases are essential for mitochondrial respiration and maintenance of mitochondrial genomic integrity. Alteration of these enzymes by damage to the mitochondria results in increased cell injury.

Technique. Mitochondria are isolated as indicated previously and assayed according to the method of Wang et al. (193) using ^{3}H-alpha casein as the substrate. Protease activity is assayed at 37°C using a 50 mM Tris-HCl buffer at pH 8.0 with 10 mM $MgCl_2$ and 1 mM dithiothreitol in the presence or absence of 4 mM ATP. The unit of activity is defined as the degradation of 1 μg of casein/h released into a TCA-soluble form.

The Clp Family of Proteases

The Clp family of proteases represents a second class of ATP-dependent mitochondrial proteases that also appears to operate to regulate protein turnover in the mitochondrial matrix compartment (100). These proteins have both protease and chaperone-like activities that may be related to the yeast HSP 78.

The AAA Family of Proteases

This group of ATP-dependent proteases are localized in the mitochondrial inner membrane and exist in two main forms (m-AAA protease and i-AAA protease). The m-AAA protease acts on newly synthesized protein products at the mitochondrial inner membrane, whereas the i-AAA protease operates in the mitochondrial intermembrane space.

LYSOSOMES

Lysosomes are spherical structures that play a central role in the storage and catabolism of many substances. Biochemically, these organelles are characterized by the presence of several acid hydrolases. In terms of understanding the impact of toxicants on this organelle system, it is useful to discern the various categories of lysosomes by both ultrastructural and biochemical techniques.

Ultrastructural Techniques

Cytochemistry

Active lysosomes (secondary lysosomes) may be cytochemically distinguished from inactive (teleolysosomes) or autophagic vacuoles by the presence of acid phosphatase activity (Figure 34.5). This technique gives a clear demonstration of this enzyme's activity, provided development time of the reaction is monitored carefully to minimize spurious or nonspecific deposition of lead-phosphate reaction product. Though the technique is largely qualitative, it does provide essential information for delineating lysosomes from other subcellular structures.

Technique—Histochemical determination of acid phosphatase

1. Remove tissue under light ether anesthesia.
2. Cut into thick (2–3 mm) slices on plate of dental wax.
3. Fix at approximately 4°C for 2–3 h in 2.5% glutaraldehyde in 0.1 M Na-cacodylate buffer containing 7.5% sucrose (final pH 7.1) or standard glutaraldehyde-formaldehyde fixative described previously.
4. Rinse slices in cold Na-cacodylate buffer, pH 7.4, containing 0.33 M sucrose.
5. Transfer pieces to stage of tissue chopper and cut 10 50 μm sections.
6. Collect in cold Na-cacodylate, pH 7.4, containing 0.33 M sucrose.

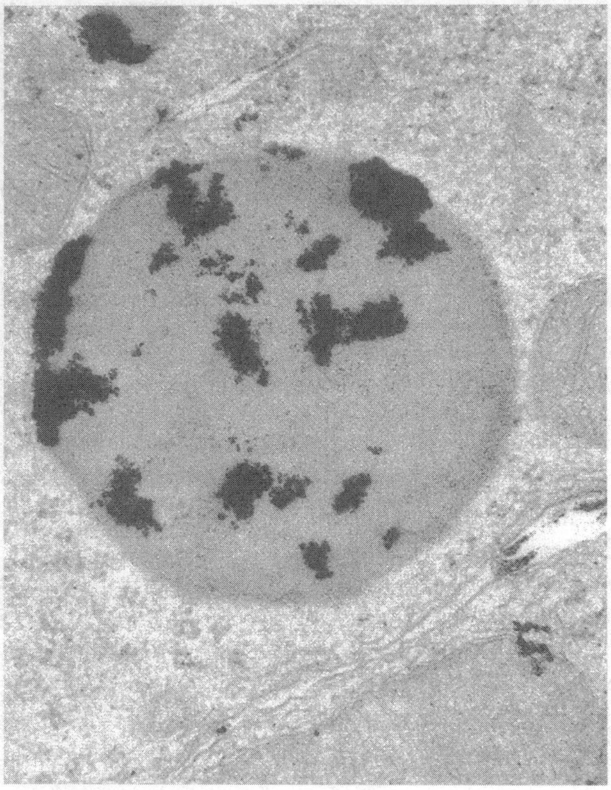

FIG. 34.5. Cytochemical demonstration of acid phosphatase activity at the electron microscope level showing positive (dense, lead phosphate precipitate) over a secondary lysosome in a renal proximal tubule cell of a rat exposed to methyl mercury in its drinking water. 46,000× magnification.

7. Rinse 20 min to 2 h in two changes of sucrose buffer.
8. Warm Gomori medium to 60°C for 1 h; cool to room temperature for 4 min, filter through one piece of Whatman #1.
9. Incubate sections 15 min to 2 h at 37°C in medium (depending on reactivity of tissue).
10. Rinse twice for 1 min in cold 0.05 M acetate buffer, pH 5.0, containing 7.5% sucrose and 4% formaldehyde.
11. For light-microscopic monitoring of reaction development, expose sections to $(NH_4)_2S$ (two drops of 45% $(NH_4)_2S$ in 10 ml H_2O).
12. Transfer to glass slides and mount in water-soluble embedding medium.
13. For electron microscopy: postfix for 30–60 min in 1% OsO_4 in acetate-veronal buffer, pH 7.4, containing 49 mg/ml sucrose.
14. Rapidly dehydrate starting with 70% ethanol.
15. Embed in plastic resin as described previously.

Gomori medium

1. 0.12 g $Pb(NO_3)_2$.
2. 100 ml 0.05 M NaAc buffer, pH 5.0, containing 7.5% sucrose.
3. Add slowly with gentle mixing, 10 ml of 3% sodium-β-glycerophosphate or cytidine monophosphate (CMP).

Glutaraldehyde fixative

1. 0.2 M cacodylate buffer, pH 7.4, 97.5 ml, containing 7.5% sucrose.
2. Ultrapure glutaraldehyde (70%), 2.5 ml.

Buffer rinse

1. 0.1 M cacodylate buffer, pH 7.4, containing 0.33 M sucrose (11.2%).

Formaldehyde rinse

1. 0.05 M acetate buffer, pH 5.0, 90 ml.
2. 37% Formaldehyde (formalin solution), 10 ml, 7.5 g sucrose.

Acetate buffer

1. 15 ml N HCl.
2. 50 ml N NaAc.
3. Adjust to pH 5.0; dilute to 1300 ml.

Localization of Substances Within Lysosomes

There are several ultrastructural techniques available for demonstrating the presence of particular substances within lysosomes of intact cells. X-ray microanalysis (Figure 34.6) has been used by several investigators (21,47,50,60,170) to demonstrate the presence of toxic trace metals within lysosomes following in vivo exposure. This method essentially uses the focused electron beam of the electron microscope to displace orbital electrons from the atoms present in the sample with resultant generation of characteristic x-rays from within the sample that are separated by wavelength- or energy-dispersive techniques. Major problems with the technique for analysis of biological samples are related to extraction or translocation of elements during tissue processing (78), volatilization of elements by specimen heating (21), and detection of elements within biological thin sections due to insufficient excitation or low concentrations of the elements within the tissue (78). The obvious chief advantage to this technique is that it provides a clear means of placing the toxic element of concern in structures such as lysosomes within target cell populations, thus providing evidence that could not be generated readily by subcellular fractionation studies:

1. Section blocks of tissue embedded for electron microscopy (as previously described) at 2500 Å or less using an ultramicrotome. Place on carbon-

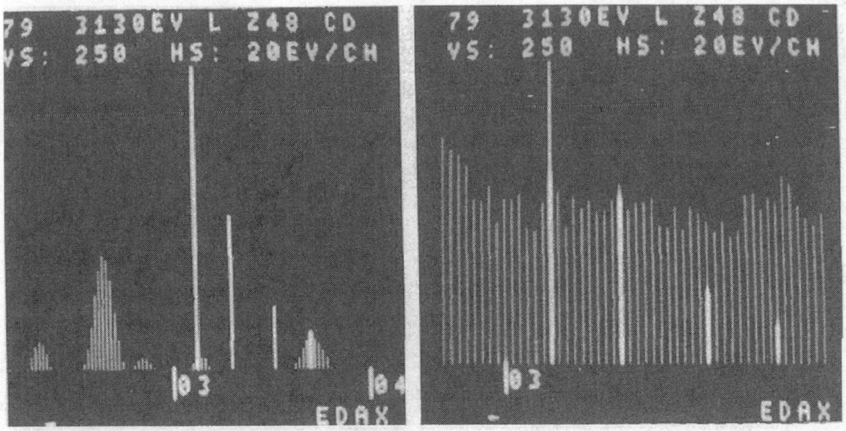

FIG. 34.6. Energy-dispersive x-ray spectrum from a renal proximal tubule lysosome of a rat injected with 0.6 mg/kg cadmium (Cd) as Cd-metallothionein before (right) and following (left) background subtraction. The presence of a Cd Lα x-ray peak (3.13 keV) is indicated by the first verticle marker bar.

coated grids made of carbon, beryllium, or some other element with x-ray emission lines different from those in the sample to be analyzed.

2. Place sample grid in specimen holder of transmission or scanning electron microscope fitted with energy-dispersive or wavelength-dispersive spectrometers.
3. Perform x-ray microanalysis of lysosomes (or other organelles of interest) by condensing the electron beam onto the site to be analyzed and monitoring the elemental x-rays generated.
4. Problems associated with extraction of elements from the tissue during fixation, dehydration, and embedding may be circumvented to some degree by use of cryosectioning of frozen samples and liquid nitrogen-cooled cold stages.
5. Vaporization of elements by specimen-heating from the condensed electron beam may be dealt with to some degree by altering the accelerating voltage of the electron microscope and reducing counting times.
6. A more complete description of this technique and the available instrumentation has been given elsewhere (78).

Ultrastructural Autoradiography

Autoradiography of compounds labeled with ^{125}I or ^{3}H is another sensitive tool that requires great care in application due to translocation of label and insufficient grain development. This technique has been applied successfully to detection of proteins within lysosomes of intact cells to show uptake into this cellular compartment. At the light microscope level, lysosomal uptake of fluorescent dyes has been demonstrated by fluorescence microscopy (2). Histochemical staining methods (15) also have been used to demonstrate lysosomal uptake of metals in cells of metal-exposed animals. These techniques, like x-ray microanalysis, provide useful approaches for localizing chemicals of interest in lysosomes of target cell populations.

Ultrastructural Morphometry

In terms of quantifying in vivo changes in the lysosomal compartment, ultrastructural morphometry has been employed to evaluate changes in the lysosome system with prolonged methyl mercury exposure (48), age (30), and cadmium metallothionein (169). Application of this method to lysosomes is subject to some of the same constraints and limitations noted previously for mitochondria.

Biochemical Procedures

Isolation procedures for lysosomes by centrifugation are given in Figure 34.3 and have been described extensively elsewhere (162). Changes in lysosomal sedimentation characteristics have been reported (39) following loading with metals such as iron. This effect, as well as alterations of lysosomal membrane stability (101), should be considered carefully when evaluating lysosomes in toxicity studies. In addition, consideration also should be given to distribution of lysosomes within different cell types within a given organ because not all cells will be affected equally.

Lysosomal Protein Degradation

Protein degradation by lysosomes has been monitored by following release of ^{125}I from labeled protein following either in vitro (120–123) or in vivo (114) incubations. In vitro exposure of lysosomes to agents such as toxic metals (114,120,122) or mycotoxins (123) has been found to alter the ability of lysosomes to perform this basic function.

Marker Enzyme Assays

Measurement of the various acid hydrolase activities found in lysosomes is another means for assessing lysosome functionality. As noted in Figure 34.3, these assays frequently are performed on lysed lysosomes so that activities of the lysosomal enzymes may be more clearly separated from those present in the microsomal fraction. Marker enzymes frequently measured are the cathepsins A, B, C, and D (162), acid phosphatase, aryl sulfatase, glycosidases, and acid RNAase. Exposure of animals by intravenous injection of protein (112,113) activates a number of the above enzymes in kidney lysosomes. As with the protein degradation procedure, these assays provide essential information about changes in lysosome functionality following chemical exposure. The metabolic consequences of lysosomal enzyme inhibition are varied but may include proteinuria or a number of lysosomal storage diseases.

Techniques

Acid Phosphatase Assay:

1. 0.1 ml 0.004 M Citrate buffer, pH 4.8.
2. 0.1 ml p-nitrophenylphosphate 100 mg/25 ml (kept frozen).
3. 0.1 ml enzyme extract.
4. Incubate at 37°C for various times.
5. Stop reaction by adding 5 ml of 0.2 M glycine, pH 10.4.
6. Centrifuge in tabletop centrifuge for 5 min.
7. Read optical density at 405 nm.
8. Report specific activity in terms of nmol/min/mg.
9. Prepare standard curve of OD_{405} versus nanomoles p-nitrophenol/5.4 ml of reaction mixture.

Cathepsin D Assay:

1. 1.0 ml 0.2 M acetate, pH 4.5.
2. 0.5 ml 2% hemoglobin.
3. Add 0.5 ml enzyme solution.
4. Incubate at 37°C for 1 h.
5. Stop reaction by adding 8 ml 5% TCA.
6. Centrifuge at 1400 rpm for 5 min.
7. Read absorbance at 280 nm.
8. Report specific activity as OD_{280}/mg protein.

RNAase Assay

1. 0.2 ml 0.03 M acetate—0.15 M NaCl, pH 5.8.
2. 0.1 ml enzyme solution.
3. 0.1 ml H_2O.
4. 0.2 ml 1% RNA.

The reaction mixture is shaken at 37°C for 20 min. After incubation the tubes are placed in ice. To precipitate the protein and RNA, add 0.9 ml of a mixture of 10 volumes of 76% ethanol in 1 N HCl and 1 volume of 0.75% uranyl acetate in 2.5 N $HClO_4$. After allowing the mixture to stand for 10 min, centrifuge at 1000 g for 10 min. The absorbance of a 1:10 dilution of each supernatant fraction is read at 260 nm. Specific activity is reported as OD_{260}/min/mg. *Caution: The RNA is unstable and needs to be prepared just before use to prevent high reading in the blank.*

B-Glucuronidase assay using p-Nitrophenyl-β-glucuronide as the substrate

1. 1.0 ml 0.2 M acetate, pH 5.0.
2. 0.6 ml p-nitrophenyl β-D-glucuronide (15 mM).
3. 0.2 ml lysosomal protein.
4. Incubate at 37°C for 15–30 min.
5. Stop the reaction by adding 3 ml 0.2 M glycine, pH 10.4.
6. Centrifuge in tabletop centrifuge for 5 min.
7. Read at 405 nm.
8. Obtain nanomoles of p-nitrophenol from standard curve.
9. Report activity in terms of nmol/min/mg of protein.

ENDOPLASMIC RETICULUM

The endoplasmic reticulum is comprised of a complex pattern of membranes or cisternae that permeates the cytoplasmic matrix. Two distinct forms of endoplasmic reticulum have been characterized by histological as well as biochemical and centrifugal techniques. The rough endoplasmic reticulum (RER) is a complex of granular basophilic membranes distinguished by extensive ribosomal units on the outer surface of the membrane. In mammals, the RER forms layered stacks of cisternae. The smooth endoplasmic reticulum (SER) is essentially agranular and forms a myriad of branching interconnecting tubules extending to all areas of the cytoplasmic matrix. In general, protein synthesis occurs in the RER, whereas the SER functions in protein transport and glycogen storage. Both the RER and SER function in drug metabolism, as evidenced by the detection of bioactivation/detoxification enzyme systems in both subfractions.

The heterogeneous microsomal fraction (centrifugal fraction containing fragmented endoplasmic reticulum) is commonly employed to assess the capacity of the endoplasmic reticulum to bioactivate and/or detoxify a variety of foreign chemicals as well as various endogenous compounds, such as fatty acids, eicosanoids, and the steroid hormones. The role that microsomal enzymes play in chemical toxicity is extremely difficult to evaluate because a single-enzyme system might activate or deactivate a chemical, depending on the molecular structure of the chemical, animal age (state of development or differentiation), site of metabolism (as related to organ-specific toxicity), and interactions with other chemicals (potentiation or antagonism). To study microsomal metabolism of chemicals, standard techniques are employed to prepare heterogeneous microsomal fractions or to separate SER and RER. Much of the information presented in this section deals with hepatic microsomal function because of the wealth of methodological information available for this tissue; however, the relative lack of time spent on extrahepatic tissues should not detract from the contribution of extrahepatic pathways to pharmacokinetics and toxic reactions.

Ultrastructural Techniques

Ultrastructural Morphometry

The surface area or, more precisely, the surface density (S_v) of smooth and rough endoplasmic reticulum may be estimated by application of morphometric techniques to intact cells (169,176,192). This approach has been used to quantify changes in the endoplasmic reticulum of hepatocytes following exposure of rats to phenobarbital (169). Studies of this type provide useful in situ correlations with the biochemical evaluation of microsomal enzyme preparations described later, as well as a means for estimating membrane recoveries from intact cells (10,13). The labor-intensive nature discussed earlier in reference to the mitochondria also applies to surface density (S_v) measurements of the endoplasmic reticulum, but the data generated have proved extremely useful in interpreting changes in microsomal enzyme activities produced by metals such as indium (49) and thallium (49,207,209).

Ultrastructural Evaluation of Microsomal Fractions

Ultrastructural examination of microsomal fractions may be conducted to assess the purity of the preparation in a manner similar to that previously described for mitochondria. Fixation, dehydration, and embedding procedures for microsomal pellets are essentially similar to those used for other organelle fractions. The value of these procedures for assessing relative microsomal purity and determining the efficiency of RER and SER centrifugal separations cannot be understated.

Biochemical Procedures

Preparation of Microsomes

Standard method. The most common method used to prepare microsomes from a variety of tissues involves tissue and cell disruption followed by differential centrifugation. A general procedure for rat liver is as follows:

1. Liver is removed, minced, and homogenized in 1.15% KCl buffered with 0.02 M N-2-hydroxyethylpiperazine-N-2-ethane-sulfonic acid (HEPES), pH 7.5, at 5°C to make a 20% (w/v) mixture. Homogenization is accomplished by using six strokes in a motor-driven Potter–Elvehjem homogenizer.
2. Nuclei and cell debris are removed by centrifugation at 670 × g for 10 min.
3. Mitochondria are removed by centrifugation of the 670 g supernatant fluid at 10,000 × g for 15 min.
4. Microsomes are pelleted by centrifugation of the postmitochondrial supernatant fluid at 105,000 g for 60 min, washed once with HEPES-KCl buffer, and finally resuspended in the buffer so that 1.0 ml of microsomal suspension contains material from 0.5 g liver (wet weight). The 10,000 × g pellet can be homogenized by hand and recentrifuged to avoid loss of microsomes in unbroken cells and sedimented microsomal vesicles.

There are some points that need to be considered when experimental protocols are being developed. For example, depending on the tissue, microsomal fragments may pellet with the nuclear or mitochondrial fraction. Researchers have mistakenly reported the subcellular distribution of microsomal enzymes because of tissue differences in fragmentation of the endoplasmic reticulum. Therefore, preliminary experimentation must include a thorough examination of the effect of various disruption techniques (homogenization, sonication, etc.) on the disruption of the endoplasmic reticulum. Furthermore, because of the variety of microsomal fractionation methods available, the optimum method for each specific purpose should be determined empirically.

Calcium aggregation method. An alternative method to prepare microsomes from rat liver involves the aggregation of microsomes following the addition of Ca^{2+} ions to the postmitochondrial supernatant fluid (96,157,158). In addition to eliminating the need for an ultracentrifuge, this method greatly reduces the time needed to prepare microsomes. The procedure is outlined as follows:

1. Liver is removed, minced, and homogenized in 10 mM Tris-HC1 containing 250 mM sucrose, pH 7.4, to make a 20% (w/v) mixture. Homogenization is accomplished by using six strokes in a motor-driven Potter–Elvehjem homogenizer.
2. Nuclei and cell debris are removed by centrifugation at 670 × g for 10 min.
3. Mitochondria are removed by centrifugation of the 670 g supernatant fluid at 10,000 × g for 15 min.
4. Solid $CaCl_2$ is added to the postmitochondrial supernatant fluid to achieve a final concentration of 8 mM. The suspension is stirred and the microsomes pelleted by centrifugation at 25,000 × g for 15 min.

5. The microsomal pellet is resuspended in 150 mM KCl-10 mM Tris-HCI, pH 7.4, and centrifuged at 25,000 g for 15 min, which sediments the washed microsomal pellet.

Many studies have compared the activities of microsomal enzymes prepared by the two methods. In general, specific activities of rat liver microsomes were similar in preparations derived by either method (158); however, the calcium aggregation method cannot be applied to all tissues or species. Researchers have found markedly different enzyme activities in preparations derived by the two methods as a function of the species and tissue. These findings emphasize the need to determine whether the calcium aggregation method is a viable method before applying it to preparation of microsomes from a source other than rat liver.

Preparation of Human Liver Microsomes

Human liver samples may be obtained from organ donors through the National Disease Research Interchange (NDRI) and should be considered biohazardous and handled accordingly. Samples should be removed within 30 min of death, and microsomes prepared immediately or, alternatively, samples can be quick-frozen in liquid nitrogen and stored at $-80°C$ until microsomes can be prepared (153).

1. Slowly thaw samples at 4°C in 100 mM Tris-HCl buffer, pH 7.4 containing 100 mM KCl, 1 mM ethylenediaminetetraacetic acid (EDTA), and 1 mM phenylmethylsulfonyl fluoride (PMSF).
2. Cut into small pieces and homogenize in 4 volumes of the same buffer using two 40 sec bursts in a prechilled Waring blender.
3. Pass the homogenate through cheesecloth or glass wool to remove capsule fibers.
4. Homogenize the filtrate using four strokes in a motor-driven Teflon/glass Potter–Elvehjem homogenizer.
5. Centrifuge at $10,000 \times g$ for 30 min at 4°C.
6. Filter the supernatant through cheesecloth or glasswool to remove lipid (which may be quite substantial).
7. Centrifuge at $100,000 \times g$ for 90 min at 4°C.
8. Resuspend the pellet in 100 mM sodium pyrophosphate buffer, pH 7.4 in a volume equal to the volume of the original homogenate (step 2).
9. Centrifuge at $100,000 \times g$ for 60 min at 4°C.
10. Resuspend the pellet in 50 mM potassium phosphate (KPO_4) buffer, pH 7.4 containing 0.1 mM EDTA, 0.1 mM dithiothreitol (DTT), and 20% glycerol. Freeze at $-80°C$ or use immediately.

Although many xenobiotics induce the specific activity of microsomal enzymes, these chemicals generally do not cause great changes in total microsomal protein content; however, some changes do occur in the relative distribution of SER and RER, and significant changes also occur in SER/RER-specific activity ratios of enzymes. For example, the potent inducing agent 2,3,7,8-tetrachlorodibenzo-p-dioxin (TCDD) reduces the SER/RER activity ratio for aminopyrine demethylation, benzo[a]pyrene hydroxylation, p-nitrophenol glucuronidation, and microsomal protein (111). These biochemical and pharmacological changes are associated with concomitant alterations in the cellular distribution of SER and RER in hepatocytes following in vivo exposure to TCDD as well as to a wide range of organohalogens, some of which are hepatotoxins.

The following discontinuous sucrose gradient method is commonly used to isolate SER from RER in liver (34):

1. Liver is homogenized in 0.25 M sucrose to make a 20% (w/v) mixture.
2. The postmitochondrial supernatant fluid is prepared as described earlier in this section.
3. 2.0 ml of 1.3 M sucrose (not containing CsCl) is added to a centrifuge tube.
4. 0.5 ml of 0.6 M sucrose (also not containing CsCl) is layered on the heavy sucrose.
5. The postmitochondrial supernatant fluid is made to 15 mM with respect to CsCl and 4.0 ml of the suspension layered above the 0.6 M sucrose. The three-layered system is then centrifuged at $105,000 \times g$ for 90 min. The RER is pelleted at the bottom of the centrifuge tube and the SER forms a band at the top of the 1.3 M sucrose.
6. The SER fraction can be aspirated off and pelleted by dilution with buffer and centrifugation at $105,000 \times g$ for 60 min.

Several other methods, including rate-differential centrifugation and isopycnic density gradient centrifugation, are available to further subfractionate SER and RER (34).

MICROSOMAL ACTIVATION/DEACTIVATION SYSTEMS

Microsomal Flavin-Containing Monoxygenases

In humans, the liver, kidney, and lung contain one or more flavin adenine dinucleotide (FAD) containing monoxygenases (FMO) that belong to a family of proteins that are important in the NADPH-dependent metabolism of hundreds of exogenous compounds (22,211) (Figure 34.7). Endogenous substrates of FMO

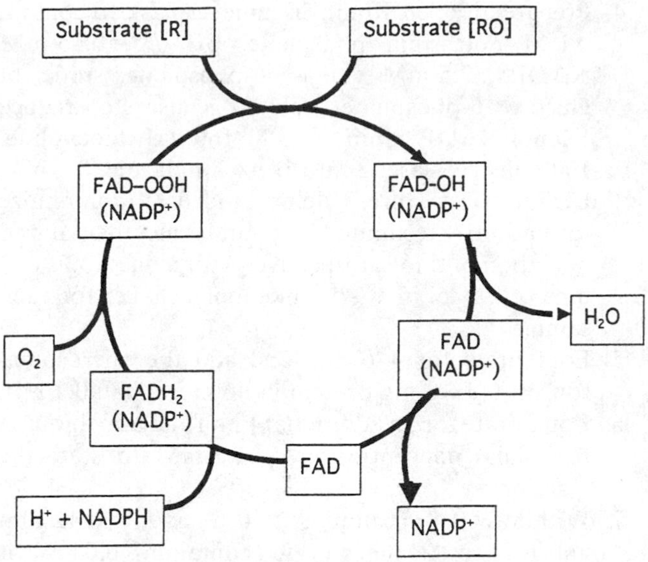

FIG. 34.7. Catalytic cycle and mechanism of action of flavin-containing monooxygenase (FMO). A single point of contact between the xenobiotic or endogenous substrate [R] and the terminal oxygen of the hydroperoxyflavin in all that is required for the formation of the oxygenated product [RO] by oxygen transfer to the nucleophile and immediate release of the product. The remaining steps, which do not require the presence of [R], simply regenerate the enzyme-bound oxygenating agent from NADPH and oxygen. Scheme adapted from Reference 211.

include cysteamine, cystamine, and trimethylamine. FMO catalyze the oxidation of nucleophilic tertiary amines to *N*-oxides, secondary amines to hydroxylamines, and oximes and sulfur or phosphorus-containing xenobiotics to *S*- and *P*-oxides, respectively. Hydrazines, iodides, selenides, and boron-containing compounds are also substrates for FMO. FMO are generally associated with detoxication reactions although several sulfur-containing xenobiotics (thiols, thioamides, 2-mercaptoimidazoles, thiocarbamates, thiocarbamides) are oxygenated to electrophilic reactive intermediates.

Humans and other mammals express five different FMO isoforms (FMO1–FMO5) in a species- and tissue-specific manner. Each FMO isoform appears to have arisen from one ancestral gene family with the five different members sharing 52% or more amino acid sequence identity. The major form of FMO in human liver has been designated FMO3 and is only 52%–57% identical to animal liver FMO1, whereas rabbit lung FMO2 is 55% identical to other FMOs. The various forms of FMO are distinct gene products with different physical properties and substrate specificities. Substrate stereoselectivity of *N*- or *S*-oxide product formation has been used in the development of isoform-selective catalytic methods. Species and tissue differences in the relative expression of FMO and cytochrome P450 (P450) isoforms (described later) account for species and tissue differences in the toxicity of several xenobiotics. Studies on FMO modulation have focused on developmental and hormonal changes or on decreases by dietary restriction. Most commercial laboratory chows contain enough xenobiotic soft nucleophiles to cause maximal induction of FMO. Therefore, demonstration of induction of FMO by specific xenobiotics requires specially formulated diets.

FMO require NADPH and oxygen to oxidize a variety of soft nucleophiles centered on nitrogen, sulfur, and phosphorus. In this regard, FMO are similar to P450 (described later), and several in vitro techniques have been developed to distinguish reactions catalyzed by FMO from those catalyzed by P450. In general, FMO are heat labile and can be inactivated in the absence of NADPH by warming microsomal preparations to 50°C for 1 min whereas P450 is inactivated with nonionic detergent, such as 1% Emulgen 911, which has a minimal effect on FMO activity.

A standard FMO enzyme assay has been described, and the mass spectral properties of various *N*- and *S*-oxides is included in Lomri et al. (107). Optimal conditions for these assays should be empirically determined for each FMO source and particular substrate.

FMO Enzyme Assays

1. Place 0.8–1.6 mg of microsomal protein in buffer (50 mM potassium phosphate, pH 8.4, 0.5 mM $NADP^+$, 2.0 mM glucose 6-phosphate, 1 IU glucose 6-phosphate dehydrogenase, 0.8 mM DETAPAC [diethylenetriaminepentaacetic acid]) and equilibrate for 1 min at 33°C.
2. Initiate reaction by the addition of substrate (various tertiary amines and sulfides) and incubate at 33°C for various time intervals.
3. Stop the reaction by the addition of 3 volumes of ice-cold methylene chloride, mix thoroughly, centrifuge to separate the aqueous and organic fractions, and analyze for product by High Pressure Liquid Chromatography (HPLC) or other appropriate method.

FMO activity can alternatively be assessed using the following modified protocol (16):

1. Obtain a microsomal source of FMO and use the described method to empirically determine optimal protein concentrations and time and temperature dependence of the reaction.
2. In a total reaction volume of 0.25 ml, add buffer: 50 mM potassium phosphate, pH 8.4 containing an NADPH-generating system (0.5 mM NADP,

2.0 mM glucose 6-phosphate, 2 IU glucose 6-phosphate dehydrogenase per ml of reaction), 0.8 mM DETAPAC (diethylenetriaminepentaacetic acid), and 0.001 mM FAD.

3. Add microsomes (0.4 mg of microsomal protein) and incubate with slow shaking for 2 min at 37°C (or empirically determined temperature).
4. Add methyl *p*-tolyl sulfide to a final concentration of 0.5 mM and incubate for 40 min (or previously determined time based on the activity of the samples).
5. Stop the reaction by the addition of 0.70 ml of ice-cold acetonitrile and briefly vortex the sample tube and immediately place on ice.
6. Add 20 mg of NaCl and extensively vortex each tube followed by centrifugation at 2,000 × g for 10 min at 4°C to separate the aqueous and organic phases.
7. Analyze the organic layer by isocratic HPLC using a mobile phase of 50% acetonitrile in water, flow rate of 1.0 ml/min, and UV detection at 220 nm on an Alltech C8 RSIL 250 × 4.6 mm HPLC column. The product of the reaction, methyl *p*-tolyl sulfoxide and parent compound, methyl *p*-tolyl sulfide, are quantified by comparison of the peak heights relative to those of reference standards of these two compounds.

Colorimetric FMO Assay

A convenient colorimetric method for measuring the activity of FMO in crude tissue fractions has been developed (69). The assay measures the thiourea-dependent oxidation of thiocholine. An alternative to preparing microsomes is to dilute the tissue homogenate about fivefold, followed by centrifugation at 40,000 × g for 45 min and resuspension of the pellet in 0.25 M sucrose containing 0.05 M potassium phosphate, pH 7.5. The assay can be performed without further tissue processing.

NOTE: To perform the measurements at pH 8.4, change the phosphate buffer to 0.03 M pyrophosphate and 0.1 M glycine.

1. Remove tissue and immediately place in 0.25 M sucrose on ice, mince, and rinse several times to remove excess blood.
2. Homogenize with a glass-Teflon homogenizer in six volumes of 0.25 M sucrose containing 0.05 M potassium phosphate, pH 7.5 and 0.1 mM butylated hydroxytoluene.
3. Prepare microsomes by differential centrifugation and wash once and resuspend in 0.25 M sucrose containing 0.05 M potassium phosphate to the original volume of the homogenate aliquot.
4. Prepare an open 10 ml Erlenmeyer flask to contain 0.1 M potassium phosphate, pH 7.5, 0.25 mM $NADP^+$, 2.5 mM glucose 6-phosphate, sufficient glucose 6-phosphate dehydrogenase to reduce 1 μmol $NADP^+$/min · ml, 80–160 μM thiocholine, 100 units catalase, 2 mM benzylimidazole, 0.4 mM EDTA (last three items added to minimize formation, accumulation, and metal-catalyzed oxidation of thiols, respectively) for a final total volume of 2.5 ml in a 37°C metabolic shaker for each sample.
5. Equilibrate for 4–6 min and add the microsomal source (0.5–10 mg protein in no more than 0.2 ml).
6. Equilibrate for an additional 1 min and add thiourea to a final concentration of 1.2 mM to start the reaction.
7. Withdraw 0.4 ml aliquots at 0, 3, 6, 9, and 12 min and transfer to tubes on ice containing 0.04 ml of 3.0 M trichloroacetic acid. After all the aliquots have been collected, separate the precipitated protein by centrifugation and transfer 0.35 ml of clear supernatant fluid to tubes containing 1 ml of 1.0 M phosphate, pH 7.5, 0.6 ml of water, and 0.05 ml of 10 mM DTNB.
8. Measure the concentration of thiocholine in each aliquot at 412 nm using a millimolar absorptivity of 13.6 cm^{-1} for 5-thio-2-nitrobenzoate.
9. The reduction of thiocholine disulfide can be determined by measuring the rate of thiocholine formation in aliquots of the completed reaction mixture containing 200–300 μM thiocholine disulfide in place of thiourea and thiocholine.
10. The rate constant for thiocholine disulfide reduction by glutathione (GSH) can be determined by the following procedure. In a 1 ml cuvette maintained at 37°C, add the reaction mixture consisting of 0.1 M potassium phosphate, pH 7.5, 150 μM NADPH, 1.0 mM EDTA, 18 units crystalline glutathione reductase, and 100–500 μM GSH. Record the reaction velocity after adding 100, 200, 300, 400, and 500 μM thiocholine disulfide and record the absorbance for 2–3 min after each addition.

Microsomal P450

P450 are not in fact cytochromes in the true sense, but belong to a large family of heme thiolate proteins consisting of multiple isozymes associated with the endoplasmic reticulum. Originally named for their absorption maximum at 450 nm (when bound with CO and reduced), these proteins serve as terminal oxidases in the membrane-bound electron transport system involved in biotransformation. Collectively, these heme protein

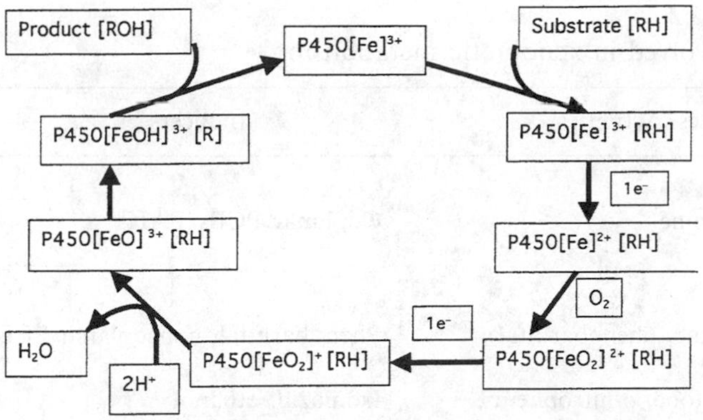

FIG. 34.8. Catalytic cycle and mechanism of action of cytochrome P450. The integral iron atom of the heme group at the active site is represented by Fe^{2+} or Fe^{3+} whereas RH represented the substrate and ROH the monooxygenation product of the reaction. This scheme is simplified for clarity and adapted from References 146 and 149.

catalysts participate in a variety of oxidative reactions with numerous lipophilic xenobiotics and many endogenous substrates, such as bile acids, fatty acids, eicosanoids, and steroids. Among these biotransformation reactions are included epoxide formation, N-hydroxylation, C-hydroxylation, N-dealkylation, 0-dealkylation, S-0 exchange, deamination, and S/N oxidations. For an in-depth overview of the versatility and regulation of P450, see the review by Ioannides (88).

The function of the cytochrome P450 system involves a series of sequential reactions (Figure 34.8): (a) the substrate combines with the oxidized P450 to form a substrate-ferric heme complex; (b) flavoprotein NADPH-P450 reductase mediates a reduction of this complex; (c) oxygen reacts with the reduced hemeprotein to form an oxycytochrome P450 substrate complex; (d) this complex accepts another electron from NADPH, activating oxygen for interaction with the organic substrate; (e) these reactions result in the introduction of one oxygen atom into the substrate whereas the other is reduced into water; and (f) the oxygenated substrate dissociates, regenerating the oxidized form of P450.

As a biological catalyst, P450 hemoproteins are unique in their multiplicity of isozymes, substrates, reactions, and regulatory mechanisms. Although individual isozymes may exhibit substrate overlap, each isozyme exhibits a unique overall profile of substrate selectivity. The substrate-heme binding domain appears to be structurally variable so that even a minor amino acid substitution at the critical positions will define the altered specificity. Another unique feature of P450 hemoproteins is the loosely isozyme-specific inducibility by a variety of chemicals, including phenobarbital, 3-methylcholanthrene, isosafrole, ethanol, clofibrate, and pregnenolone 16α-carbonitrile. The relative abundance of individual P450 isozymes is dependent on prior chemical exposure history and other factors, such as sex, age, species, and strain.

The nomenclature for individual isozymes is critical to understanding the scientific literature concerning P450-mediated biotransformation, regulation, and induction. Early on, almost every major laboratory developed its own nomenclature. For example, for what is now referred to as the CYP1A1 isozyme, the terms P450c, P450BNF, P450mc, PCB P448L, P_1450, P450MC, and P450 isozyme 6 were all used in the literature. The current nomenclature system was developed to alleviate confusion and is based on alignment of amino acid sequence data from proteins or deduced from cDNAs. As of 1996, the P450 gene superfamily consisted of 65 gene families, 14 of which exist in all mammals examined to date. Within a given family, the P450 protein sequences are more than 40% identical. Mammalian subfamilies are always more than 55% identical, but inclusion of other species drops this value to more than 46% identical. The gene is designated by the capitalized and italicized root symbol "*CYP*" (for human and all other species except mouse and *Drosophila* designated by "*Cyp*"), representing *CY*tochrome *P*450, followed by an Arabic number denoting the family, a letter designating the subfamily (when two or more exist), and an Arabic numeral representing the individual gene within the subfamily (e.g., *CYP1A1*). The cDNAs, mRNAs, and enzymes in all species (including mouse) is denoted by all capital letters without italics or hyphens (e.g., CYP1A1) (141). The primary hepatic drug metabolism enzymes currently comprise gene families 1 through 4. A brief outline of P450 nomenclature is given in Table 34.2.

The net action of the P450-dependent monoxygenase system is several-fold: (a) lipophilic compounds can be metabolized to more polar and therefore more excretable molecules; (b) lipophilic compounds may be metabolized such that the compounds are substrates for phase II reactions, such as glucuronidation, sulfation, glutathione conjugation, amino acid conjugation, and acetylation (these in turn are generally more polar); and (c) some P450 biotransformation products are electrophilic, reactive, and highly toxic metabolites.

A variety of methods are available to quantitatively and/or qualitatively study P450. Analytically, this system may be approached spectrophotometrically, enzymatically, immunologically, or by examination of specific gene or transcription products. Each approach has inherent strengths and weaknesses, as well as optimal applications. The approach selected is largely a function of the experimental goals, the biochemical level one is interested in (transcription, translation, activity), and the degree of specificity required.

Table 34.2
Selected gene families/subfamilies involved in xenobiotic metabolism

Gene Family	Synonyms	Substrates/Activities[a]	Inducers
CYP450 1 gene family			
1A1/1A2	P450c/P450d	PAH, arylamine	Coplanar PCBs/PAHs
CYP450 2 gene family			
CYP40 2B gene subfamily			
2B1/2B2	P450b/P450e	Benzphetamine, phenobarbital	Phenobarbital, noncoplanar PCBs
CYP450 2E gene subfamily			
2E1	P450j	Ethanol, acetone, p-nitrophenol	Isoniazid, ethanol
CYP450 3 gene family	P450 PCN	[a]Ethylmorphine N-demethylation [a]Erythromycin demethylation	Pregnenolone 16α-carbonitrile
CYP450 4 gene family		[a]Lauric acid hydroxylase	Clofibrate

[a] = activities of the enzymes.

Determination of P450 by Difference Spectra

A classical method of measuring the P450 content of a microsomal preparation is by the appearance of an absorbance band at 450 or 448 nm for the CO adduct of the reduced cytochrome (144). Animals induced with phenobarbital demonstrate P450 absorbance maxima at 450 nm whereas those exposed to 3-methylcholanthrene exhibit a hypochromic shift to 448 nm in the CO-reduced spectrum. Early on, other compounds that elicited an absorbance maxima at 450 nm were referred to as phenobarbital-type inducers whereas those at 448 nm were of the 3-methylcholanthrene type (61). These types of findings, along with enzymatic data, formed the early basis for the concept of P450 enzyme heterogeneity. Current applications of difference spectra are less oriented toward P450 heterogeneity as more specific immunological and cDNA methodologies are available. Difference spectra, however, are useful for determining total P450 content (inducible and constitutive), examining substrate interactions with P450, and to investigate mechanisms of inhibition of mixed-function oxidation reactions. Depending on the substrate or inhibitor, several types of spectral interactions can be detected in vitro: type I spectral change, which is characterized by a peak at 385 nm and a trough at 420 nm; reverse type I spectral change, which is the mirror image of type I spectral change; and type II spectral change, which is characterized by a broad trough between 390 and 410 nm and a peak between 425 and 435 nm (158). Heterogeneous microsomal preparations in which more than one isozyme interacts with the substrate or inhibitor may produce intermediate spectra. Therefore, it is recommended that purified isozymes be used to determine specific interactions. The procedure for determination of P450 by difference spectra is as follows:

1. Dilute the microsomal suspension with the homogenizing buffer to achieve a protein concentration of approximately 1.5 mg/ml.
2. The baseline of equal light absorbance is determined by placing equal volumes of diluted microsomal suspension into two cuvettes.
3. Gently gas the sample cuvette with CO (approximately 30 sec) and record the spectrum that quantifies oxyhemoglobin contamination.
4. Add sodium dithionite (about 1 mg solid) to the sample cuvette and record the difference spectrum of the CO adduct of the reduced P450.
5. Add sodium dithionite to the reference cuvette and record the difference spectrum of the CO complex of reduced P450 minus the spectral contribution of reduced P450.
6. Convert the change in absorbance at 450 nm relative to 490 nm to P450 concentration using a millimolar extinction coefficient of 91 mM^{-1} cm^{-1}.

Techniques for Identification and Quantification of P450 Isozymes

Techniques for the purification of microsomal P450 isozymes have been reviewed elsewhere (154,155). The large number of purified and characterized isozymes have allowed for a variety of inter-isozyme comparisons and reconstitution studies (68). Purified 450 proteins also have led to the production of specific antibodies providing an important set of reagents for the study of P450.

A number of techniques have been employed to assess the purity of isolated P450 isozymes. Sodium dodecyl sulfate-polyacrylamide gel electrophoresis (SDS-PAGE)

(98) providing resolution at about 5 kDa has demonstrated the multiplicity of the P450 proteins. Certain isozymes, such as P450b and P450e, however, have nearly identical minimum molecular weights, limiting the use of stained SDS-PAGE gels in examining isozyme purity. Techniques such as two-dimensional isoelectric focusing (190) have more clearly delineated highly homologous isozymes and also have provided insights into microheterogeneity resulting from polymorphisms. Other techniques, such as peptide mapping (29) and the use of monospecific antibodies, have provided further help in the examination and analysis of purified P450 isozymes (156).

Immunodetection of microsomal protein with specific antibodies is a technique widely used for the identification and quantification of individual P450 isozymes. This approach is contingent on the antibodies' specificity (181). This specificity may be lost on isolation of the antigen if it is not purified to homogeneity or if the antibodies' recognition site is found in more than one protein. Both polyclonal and monoclonal antibodies may lack specificity (57,181). Although monoclonals are highly specific for a single protein epitope, if that epitope exists on another P450, it will cross-react. Conversely, polyclonal antibodies are a group of antibodies directed at a variety of epitopes. Some may be specific for the isozyme of interest whereas others may be directed toward epitopes on other isozymes. A panel of techniques are required to screen the specificity of antibodies. Included on this list are enzyme-linked immunosorbent assay (ELISA), inhibition of enzymatic activity, immunodiffusion, immunoaffinity chromatography, and immunoblotting (181). These techniques can provide information on cross-reactions and specificity in purified and microsomal systems.

Once specificity of the antibodies is verified, they may be used for a variety of applications, including (a) as a reagent in recombinant DNA technology; (b) for immunoinhibition studies as a means to examine xenobiotic metabolism; (c) for immunocytochemistry as a means to localize P450 proteins; and (d) as a method for immunoquantification of P450 isozymes.

The following immunodetection technique encompasses gel electrophoresis, electrophoretic transfer to a membrane, and one of many available staining techniques.

SDS-PAGE of Microsomal Proteins

The sodium dodecyl sulfate, polyacrylamide gel electrophoresis (SDS-PAGE) technique as described by Laemmli (98) is the most common electrophoretic technique used for the separation of P450 proteins. In this technique, proteins are separated by molecular weight using polyacrylamide gels of varying acrylamide/Bis (N,N^1-methylene-bisacrylamide) percentages in an overlying stacking and lower resolving gel configuration. The stacking gel serves to concentrate the sample upon entry into the resolving gel. Cross-linking of the acrylamide and Bis upon initiation of polymerization with tetramethylethylene diamine (TEMED) and ammonium persulfate results in a characteristic porosity. Changing the acrylamide concentration, generally between 4% and 20%, results in differing mobility of low and high molecular weight proteins. For most applications, P450 separation can be accomplished with polyacrylamide concentrations of 3%–4% and 7.5% for the stacking and resolving gels, respectively. These percentages may vary depending on conditions and the application. A modification of the Laemmli (98) procedure is as follows:

1. Electrophoresis apparatus, spacers, and glass plates should be clean and dry. Set up casting apparatus avoiding contamination of glass plates with bare hands.
2. The following reagents should be mixed together for formulations of resolving gel:

   Tris-HCI pH 8.8 (0.375 M)
   7.5% acrylamide (w/v)
   0.02% bisacrylamide (w/v)
   0.10% SDS (w/v)

3. Degas the solution in step 2 under vacuum for 20 min.
4. Add ammonium persulfate (0.05%) and TEMED (0.04%) (v/v) to the components of the resolving gel (step 2).
5. Following gentle mixing, pipet resolving gel components along the internal edge of apparatus and glass plates. Avoid the introduction of bubbles in delivery of acrylamide solution. Cover gel with water and allow 1 h to polymerize (at 20°C).
6. Remove water after polymerization.
7. After placement of sample comb for stacking gel, follow same procedures as in steps 2, 3, 4, and 5 using the following reagents:

   Tris-HCl pH 6.8 (0.125 M)
   4.0% Acrylamide (w/v)
   0.01% Bisacrylamide (w/v)
   0.10% SDS (w/v)
   0.05% Ammonium persulfate (w/v)
   0.05% TEMED (v/v)

   Cover with water for polymerization
8. Dilute microsomal samples 1:5 with sample buffer as formulated below:

   Tris-HCl pH 6.8 (62 mM)
   2.0% SDS (w/v)
   10% Glycerol (v/v)
   5% 2-Mercaptoethanol
   0.001% (w/v) Bromophenol blue

(*Note*: Bromophenol blue marks the migration front of the proteins but may be omitted for immunodetection (Western blotting), as it will pass through the membrane during electrophoretic transfer. For immunodetection, Pyronin Y takes the place of the bromophenol blue as a dye front marker and is retained on the membrane as a check of transfer efficiency. Pyronin Y at 0.05% is diluted 1:20 with sample buffer just prior to dilution of the microsomal samples.

9. Heat buffered samples at 95°C for 2–4 min.
10. Remove the comb from stacking gel. Wash wells with electrode buffer (step 12), taking care to maintain well integrity.
11. Under a layer of electrode buffer, place 10–50 μg of microsomal protein in each well.
12. Place gels in the apparatus and fill with electrode buffer:

    25 mM Tris
    192 mM Glycine
    0.10% S DS (w/v)

13. With running conditions set according to apparatus instructions, run times range from 1–4 h for large gels or approximately 45 min for mini-gels.
    Note: Acrylamide is neurotoxic. Care should be taken to avoid dermal contact or inhalation.

Immunodetection of P450 Proteins

This procedure electrophoretically transfers the separated proteins from the SDS-PAGE gel to a membrane matrix, such as nitrocellulose or polyvinylidene difluoride (PVDF). The choice of membrane depends on the characteristics of the detection system and the type of analysis to be performed. Nitrocellulose is the most generally applicable and, with appropriate blocking (discussed later), compatible with most detection systems, whereas PVDF is often used when specific proteins will be submitted for automated solid phase protein sequencing. The following method is modified from the procedure of Burnette (20,93).

Reagents:
Transfer buffer:
25 mM Tris (pH 8.3);
192 mM Glycine;
20% v/v Methanol.

Electrophoretic transfer method. Specific manufacturer's directions should be followed, but a general method follows:

1. Equilibrate gel approximately 30 min in transfer buffer. This is to remove buffer salts and detergents from gel and allow for methanol-dependent shrinking of the gel.
2. With gloved hands, cut nitrocellulose (0.45 μm Schleicher and Schuell) to size of gel. Wet membrane for 30 min in transfer buffer, being careful not to trap air bubbles. PVDF membranes must be wet with methanol prior to buffer equilibration.
3. Soak filter paper (#470 Schleicher and Schuell) and fiber pads, removing any trapped air bubbles from pads.
4. Place presoaked fiber pad on the cathode panel of cassette. Place filter paper saturated with transfer buffer on top of fiber pad.
5. Flood filter paper with transfer buffer and place gel on filter paper, aligning gel with other components.
6. Saturate gel surface with transfer buffer and place equilibrated nitrocellulose on gel in a manner to exclude air bubbles from between nitrocellulose and gel (bubbles will prevent transfer).
7. Cover nitrocellulose with buffer. Complete the sandwich sequentially with saturated filter paper and fiber sponge. Close cassette and place cathode panel toward cathode in buffer chamber. Protein transfer occurs in a cathode to anode direction.
8. Fill the transblot chamber with transfer buffer. Maintain the temperature at 4°C for the duration of the transfer. For rapid miniblot transfer, allow 1 h at a constant 100 volts for transfer of P450 isozymes. Larger formats will require different settings with 200–400 mA (for 1–2 h) common constant amperage settings.

Immunological detection. A wide variety of immunodetection techniques are available. In general, for most procedures the membrane is incubated first with gelatin, casein, or albumin to block nonspecific binding sites. Then the transblot is placed in an antibody solution composed of the polyclonal or monoclonal antibody specific to the P450 isozyme or other enzyme of interest (primary antibody). After a suitable incubation period, the membrane is washed. At this point the nitrocellulose may be exposed to protein A or protein G conjugates (bacterial proteins bound to some detection modality, such as a radiolabel or enzyme) that bind directly to the Fc region (non-antigen binding fragments) of the primary antibody. Alternatively, a common technique uses a secondary antibody specific for the species IgG of the primary antibody. This secondary antibody is conjugated to an enzyme or metal colloid complex (such as gold) that mediates the detection (84,174). Other approaches require further specific colorimetric or chemiluminescent (such as with the antibody enzyme conjugates horseradish peroxidase or alkaline phosphatase), radiographic ([^{125}I]protein A), or enhanced (silver enhancement of gold colloids) (35) development. Chemiluminescent detection is becoming very popular, and detection reagents are available from a variety of vendors. Each detection technique offers inherent advantages and disadvantages that should be evaluated in terms of the particular purpose for using the method.

Protein A immunological staining. This staining procedure is useful when using primary antibodies from a variety of species or from an animal species for which a secondary antibody is not available. There is some variation in the binding of protein A to immunoglobulins from different species, so it is advisable to check this parameter. In addition, appropriate shielding and dosimetry are required for use of [^{125}I]Protein A. Protein A can be radioiodinated as described by Hunter (85). [^{125}I]Protein A immunological staining as described here is as modified by Williams et al. (200) from Burnette (20).

Technique
Reagents:
Buffer A: Blocking buffer
25 mM Tris-Cl pH 7.6
150 mM NaCl
25 mg/l Bovine serum albumin
.02% Sodium azide
Adjust to pH 7.5 with HCl
Store at 4°C
Buffer B:
25 mM Tris-Cl pH 7.6
150 mM NaCl
Adjust to pH 7.5 with HCl
Prepare fresh
Buffer C:
25 mM Tris-Cl pH 7.6
150 mM NaCl
0.05% Triton X-100
Adjust to pH 7.5 with HCl

Method

1. Incubate nitrocellulose transfer with albumin-containing blocking buffer A for 1 h at room temperature.
2. Replace buffer A in step 1 with new buffer A, which contains primary antibody at appropriate dilution. Incubate 1–3 h at room temperature with constant gentle agitation.
3. Wash with buffer B for 5 min with shaking.
4. Wash with buffer C for 5 min with shaking.
5. Wash with buffer C for 5 min with shaking.
6. Wash with buffer B for 5 min with shaking.
7. Prepare [^{125}I] Protein A solution in buffer A at 200,000 cpm/ml. Incubate nitrocellulose for 1 h at room temperature.
8. Wash as in steps 3, 4, 5, and 6.
9. Dry the nitrocellulose and fix protein with heat at 70°C for 30 min.
10. Mount and autoradiograph with Kodak (Rochester, NY) XR film with intensifying screen.
11. The resulting autoradiograph signal can be quantified on a densitometer relative to purified P450 standards of known concentrations.

ENZYME ACTIVITIES

P450-Dependent Enzymes

Phenoxazone-O-Dealkylation

The O-dealkylation of phenoxazone ethers is a commonly used method to examine P450 enzyme activity and induction. Methoxy (118), ethoxy (18), pentoxy (109), and benzyloxyphenoxazones (19) have received the greatest attention in regard to characterization and use. P450-mediated O-dealkylation of these R groups, for each of these substrates, results in the formation of resorufin. This metabolic product can be assayed directly by fluorimetric techniques.

Studies with ethoxyphenoxazone (EROD assay) and pentoxyphenoxazone (PROD assay) have indicated that a fair degree of selectivity exists between these substrates and the phenobarbital and polyaromatic hydrocarbon (PAH)-inducible isozymes. Burke et al. (19) demonstrated a 6-fold and 283-fold induction in a group of phenobarbitone-exposed rats while beta-naphthoflavone (BNF) administration resulted in a 74-fold and 8-fold induction when assayed with ethoxyphenoxazone and pentoxyphenoxazone, respectively. Studies with the purified CYP1A1 isozyme further indicate a substrate selectivity for ethoxyphenoxazone whereas pentoxyphenoxazone is metabolized preferentially by the CYP2B1 isozyme (19).

Other phenoxazone substrates, such as benzyloxyphenoxazone, appear to be much less specific. Although the O-dealkylation of benzyloxyphenoxazone is induced preferentially by isosafrole (43-fold), it also is a substrate for the phenobarbital and 3-methylcholanthrene–inducible isozymes.

The assay method is basically the same for each of the aforementioned phenoxazone ethers (19).

Technique
Reagents:

1. 0.1 M Phosphate buffer (Na-K salts) pH 7.6.2
2. 50 mM NADPH (in phosphate buffer).
3. 1 mM Substrate (in dimethylsulfoxide [DMSO]).
   (a) Methoxyphenoxazone
   (b) Ethoxyphenoxazone
   (c) Pentoxyphenoxazone

(d) Benzyloxyphenoxazone

4. 10 or 25 μM resorufin (in DMSO).

Fluorimeter settings:
1. Excitation and emission slit width 5–10 nm.
2. Excitation wavelength 530 nm.
3. Emission wavelength 585 nm.

Method:
To cuvette:
1. Add 5 μM of substrate (10 μl of stock).
2. Add 20–200 μg of microsomal protein (dependent on substrate and reaction rate).
3. Use phosphate buffer to bring reaction volume to 1990 μl.
4. Incubate reaction mixture 1–2 min at 37°C.
5. Add 10 μl of NADPH stock solution to start reaction (mix).
6. Allow reaction to run at least several minutes. Record linear reaction rate on chart recorder.
7. Add 10 μl of resorufin standard to cuvette and record increase (used as calibration standard).

Calculations:
1. Rate of increase in fluorescence (X units/min).
2. Y nM of resorufin = t fluorescence units.

$$\text{nM/unit} = \frac{\text{Y nM resorufin}}{t \text{ fluorescence units}}$$

3. X units/min × nM/unit = nM/min
4. $\text{nM/min} \times \frac{1}{[\text{protein}]} = \text{nM/min/mg protein}$

Notes:
1. Narrow bandpass slits (4–5 nm) on the fluorimeter will reduce the effect of microsomal turbidity on excitation light scatter.
2. Preparation of phenoxazones and resorufin in DMSO will afford greater stability of these reagents. Store both stocks in the dark.

Aminopyrine-N-Demethylation

One of the most common assays is oxidative demethylation using aminopyrine, ethylmorphine, or benzphetamine as the substrate. This method measures the production of formaldehyde, which is an intermediate in oxidative demethylation reactions (196). This assay is particularly useful with microsomes from animals induced with phenobarbital or other cytochrome CYP2B inducers. The assay for aminopyrine as the substrate is conducted as follows:

1. Add buffer (50 mM Tris-HCI, pH 7.5, 1.5 ml) to incubation tube.
2. Add saturating levels of NADPH (3.1 mM) in 0.5 ml Tris buffer.
3. The incubation medium is made 20 mM with respect to $MgCl_2$.
4. Add aminopyrine to achieve a substrate concentration of 2.5 mM.
5. After prewarming the incubation contents to 37°C, initiate the reaction by adding approximately 0.5–1.5 mg microsomal protein.
6. After a 10-min incubation, stop the reaction by adding 1.0 ml 10% trichloroacetic acid.
7. Sediment the protein by low-speed centrifugation and add 2 ml of supernatant fluid to 1 ml of NASH reagent (2 M ammonium acetate, 0.05 M acetic acid, 0.02 M acetylacetone).
8. Heat the solution for 8 min at 60°C. Measure the formaldehyde concentration at 405 nm and read against a standard curve. Blank values are obtained by omitting microsomes from the incubation medium.

The reaction rate is linear with respect to time and microsomal protein under these incubation conditions, although each investigator should assess these parameters as part of preliminary investigations. Ethylmorphine and benzphetamine demethylation rates can be determined using the same method. A radiolabel assay has been devised for aminopyrine demethylation that can be used when increased sensitivity is required to detect low enzyme activity as a function of tissue, developmental stage, toxicity, or disease state (148).

Benzo[a]pyrene Hydroxylase (Aryl Hydrocarbon Hydroxylase)

Benzo[a]pyrene (BaP), a polycyclic hydrocarbon, is metabolized by P450 as well as by a variety of conjugative enzymes (Figure 34.9). In this biotransformation process, a number of polar, water-soluble, and carcinogenic metabolites (epoxides) are formed. One of the first steps in this process is catalyzed by benzo[a]pyrene hydroxylase, a microsomal bound monoxygenase. More than 12 oxygen-containing polar metabolites are formed from this action, including 3-hydroxy and 9-hydroxy BaP. This enzyme system is inducible by a variety of compounds, including both phenobarbital and 3-methylcholanthrene.

A number of assays for measuring benzo[a]pyrene hydroxylase activity have been developed based on fluorimetric detection (37,137,138) or by isotopic detection through use of radiolabeled substrates (38,160,188). Often these techniques, while differing in detection modality, also differ in the number of metabolites available for detection. This is a function of the extraction protocol (188). Each of the techniques, however, takes advantage of the aqueous solubility of the metabolites versus the hydrophobicity of the parent benzo[a]pyrene.

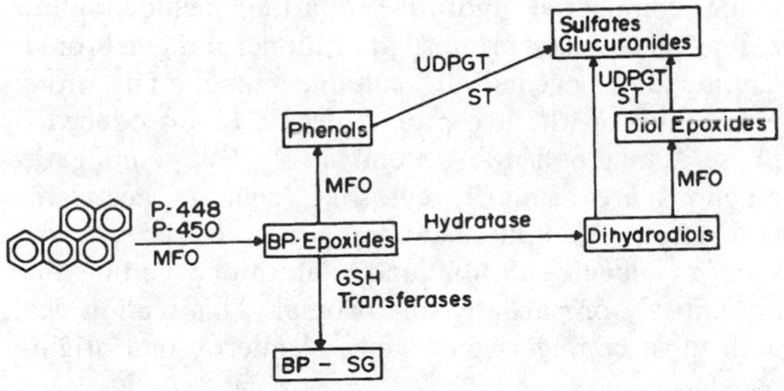

FIG. 34.9. Metabolic pathways for benzo[a]pyrene. BP—benzo[a]pyrene; MFO—mixed function oxidase; GSH—glutathionine; UDPGT—UDP-glucuronyl transferase; ST—sulfotransferase; BP-SG—glutathione conjugate of benzo[a]pyrene. From Reference 81, with permission.

The nature of these assays requires a pure BaP substrate in order to reduce background noise. BaP is photosensitive and can undergo chemical or radiochemical breakdown even upon prolonged storage under nitrogen at –70°C. A general extraction procedure for purification of BaP as described by Van Cantfort et al. (188) is as follows:

BaP Purification. Dissolve up to 50 mg of BaP or [^{3}H]BaP in 100 ml of hexane. Extract hexane/BaP solution 5 times with 50 ml of aqueous 1 M KOH/DMSO (65/85; v/v). Parent BaP should be retained in the hexane fraction, which can subsequently be blown down under nitrogen.

Another purification method uses a neutral alumina resin (M. O. James, personal communication). A slurry of resin (30 g) and hexane/methylene chloride (85/15) is loaded into a column. BaP dissolved in hexane/methylene chloride (85/15) is applied to the surface of the column bed. Fractions are collected through a solvent series of 85/15, 80/20, 75/25 hexane/methylene chloride. The column can be cleared with a 50/50 hexane/methylene chloride solution.

Fluorimetric Method

1. Add buffer (50 mM Tris-HCl, pH 7.5, 0.075 ml) to incubation vessel.
2. Add benzo[a]pyrene suspension (0.25 ml, 60 mM in 2.5% carboxymethyl-cellulose).
3. Add microsomes (0.25 ml) so that the final incubation medium contains approximately 1 mg protein/ml.
4. Equilibrate the reaction mixture at 37°C for 3 min and initiate the reaction by adding 0.25 ml NADPH solution to achieve a concentration of 3.1 mM in the incubation medium.
5. After 10 min stop the reaction by adding 2 ml ice-cold acetone.
6. Add hexane (20 ml) to stoppered 45-ml shaking tubes. Wash the incubation mixtures into the shaking tubes with water (three times with 0.5 ml).
8. Shake the tubes 10 min and store overnight at 4°C or freeze.
9. Centrifuge the tubes for 15 min at 600 × g.
10. Transfer the hexane layer (upper 15 ml) by pipet to a clean 45-ml shaking tube.
11. Add NaOH (5 ml, 0.1 M) and shake the tubes for 10 min followed by centrifugation for 10 min.
12. Read fluorescence of the aqueous layer (excitation 400 nm; emission 525 nm). Determine the concentration of phenolic metabolites by using 3-hydroxybenzo[a]pyrene as the standard.

Radiometric. The following is a radiometric BaP hydroxylase assay as described by Van Cantfort et al. (188).

1. Add Tris-HCl (pH 7.6) (50 mM), $MgCl_2$ (5 mM), NADP (0.37 mM), glucose-6-phosphate dehydrogenase (1 IU/ml), bovine serum albumin (0.8 mg/ml), [^{3}H]BaP (0.08 mM) (2×10^5 dpm) in acetone and glucose-6-phosphate (2.5 mM). All concentrations listed are final concentrations in a volume of 0.5 ml.
2. Incubate reaction mixture for approximately 3 min at 37°C.
3. The reaction is initiated with the addition of appropriate amounts of microsomal protein.
4. After a 10-min incubation, the reaction is stopped with 1 ml KOH (0.15 M in 85% DMSO).
5. The unmetabolized substrate in the aqueous phase is extracted with hexane (5 ml). The sample is centrifuged to form a clear interphase and the hexane is removed. This step is repeated.
6. The remaining aqueous phase is neutralized with HCl. An aliquot is used for radioactivity counting.
7. The total dpm in the aqueous phase and specific activity of [^{3}H]BaP are used to calculate the total nanomoles of BaP metabolized. This amount is placed on a per min and per mg microsomal protein basis.

In Vitro Methods for Evaluating Microsomal Function

Isolated Organs

Although the use of isolated microsomes has many advantages in the characterization of individual enzyme systems and the quantification of the response of these systems to inducers, inhibitors, or repressors, it is difficult to develop a good pharmacokinetic model using such preparations. Accordingly, many investigators have used isolated perfused organs to evaluate the complex interrelationships among heterogeneous cell types, different metabolic pathways, variations in substrate concentrations, and time-course relationships. This system represents an open metabolic system capable of generating important information on "steady-state" pharmacokinetics. Several organ systems have been used, including the liver, lung, intestine, kidney, and testis. Detailed methods for conducting isolated organ studies have been reviewed by Sies (163).

Isolated Cells

Isolated cells often are selected as an experimental model to study microsomal function because they provide a reasonable intermediate between perfused organ systems and preparation of organelle reconstituted systems. Isolated hepatocytes may be used to investigate the activity and products of complex bioactivation/detoxication enzyme systems. In addition, isolated cells allow one to investigate, in a more precise way, organelle interactions that might qualitatively and/or quantitatively alter the metabolic capacity of microsomal enzyme systems. References (66,128) are available that detail and summarize procedures for evaluating metabolism and toxicity in isolated cells.

Of particular importance for use of isolated cells is the requirement that (a) the cells remain viable for a sufficient period of time to evaluate a biochemical or pharmacological parameter, and (b) the isolated cells retain the characteristics and functions present in vivo. Cell viability commonly is determined by the trypan blue exclusion test or by leakage of cytosolic enzymes (indication of membrane dysfunction or damage), such as lactate dehydrogenase (128). Following the maintenance of isolated hepatocytes for relatively long periods of time (more than 2 days), liver cells have been reported to revert to a more fetal form (71,165). The relative contribution of fetal-type cells can be monitored by biochemical indicators, such as α-fetoprotein, alkaline phosphatase, and λ-glutamyl transpeptidase. A variety of techniques have been used to stabilize the function of P450 in culture, including altering the culture matrix (71), supplying additives (42), or co-culture with other cell types (187). Although most studies are conducted on liver cells, other organ systems can be investigated by analogous techniques.

Microsomal Conjugative Enzymes

In biotransformation, conjugation reactions refer to the enzymatically mediated addition of endogenous molecules to xenobiotics. Endogenous compounds undergoing conjugative biotransformation include sulfate, amino acids, acetyl groups, glutathione, and glucuronide. Conjugation occurs at suitable functional groups preexisting on the acceptor molecule or introduced by phase I metabolism. A number of these conjugation reactions are primarily cytosolic, such as acetylation and sulfate or amino acid conjugation. Other reactions, such as glucuronidation and glutathione conjugation, are entirely or partially microsomal. This section deals with those conjugative enzymes of microsomal origin.

UDP-Glucuronosyltransferase

Uridine diphosphate glucuronosyltransferase (UDP-GT) is a family of inducible microsomal isozymes associated with the liver, kidney, intestine, lung, and olfactory epithelium. These isozymes catalyze glucuronidation, the transfer of glucuronic acid from the high-energy nucleotide UDP-glucuronic acid (UDP-GA) to an electronegative group on a wide variety of endogenous and xenobiotic substrates. Endogenous substrates include steroid hormones, bilirubin, biogenic amines, and fat-soluble vitamins. Xenobiotic substrates include drugs, carcinogens, plant metabolites, and other environmental pollutants. Conjugation with alcohols, phenols, and carboxylic acids yield O-glucuronides, whereas N-glucuronides are formed with carbamates, amides, and amines. Substrates such as thiocarbamates and mercaptans form S-glucuronides.

Endogenous and xenobiotic compounds may serve as substrates for UDP-GT with or without prior metabolism by P450. Conjugation without other biotransformation steps is probably the rule rather than the exception, as many xenobiotics (eg., morphine, naphthols, and phenols) exist in forms suitable as substrates for UDP-GT. Structurally these 50- to 60-kDa UDP-GT isozymes exhibit a transmembrane region with a hydrophobic segment bordered on both sides by highly charged amino acid residues (17,89). Sequence, enzymatic, and antibody studies suggest that the active site of UDP-GT is in the lumen of the endoplasmic reticulum (ER). Cytosolic substrates and donors, such as UDP-glucuronic acid, appear to require transmembrane transport to the active site. Translocases embedded in the ER membrane are believed to be involved in this process. Substrates formed with the action of membrane-bound P450 and associated reductases appear to move vectorially to the closely located UDP-GT.

Multiple forms of UDP-GT appear to be present in most of the species thus far examined (177). The regulation of expression of this gene family is complex, giving rise to different isozyme patterns during development and following induction by xenobiotics. A 10-fold difference in the rates of drug glucuronidation is not uncommon in a healthy human population. Whether the variation is due to age, disease state, exposure to xenobiotics, or genetic background is yet to be determined (180). UDP-GT expressed in rat liver microsomes belong to two gene families (UGT1 and UGT2) differing from each other by more than 50% and each containing at least four members (eg., UGT1.1–UGT1.4). Members of UGT1 are formed by alternate splicing of a single gene whereas all members of UGT2 are distinct gene products. Similarly, UDP-GT isozymes of human liver microsomes are also products of either a single UGT1 gene locus generating at least six isozymes through alternative splicing or multiple UGT2B genes consisting of six distinct genes (146).

Glucuronidation generally detoxifies xenobiotics and potentially toxic endogenous compounds, such as bilirubin, and is therefore considered beneficial; however, glucuronidation of steroid hormone D-rings causes cholestasis, and induced glucuronidation may lead to abnormal decreases in serum thyroid hormone levels (33,119). In addition, glucuronidation can represent an important step in xenobiotic toxicity, such as with aromatic amine-mediated bladder cancer or colon tumor formation (146).

Considerable interlab variations in in vitro activities exist in the assay of microsomal UDP-GTs. In part this may be due to the fact that these enzymes are dependent on phospholipids for activity and are extremely labile. UDP-GT exhibits a latency in activity that is expressed upon membrane disruption. Lubrol-PX and other detergents have been demonstrated to effectively release latent UDP-GT activity. Accurate quantification of these activities requires measurement in the presence of optimal concentrations of detergent (17). This often necessitates a detergent titration curve to determine optimal transferase activity and incubation of detergent with the membrane preparation prior to use in enzyme assays. It has been reported with microsomal pellets (20 mg/ml) resuspended in 0.25 mM sucrose/5 mM HEPES, pH 7.4, that this latency, which may be as high as 95%, may be retained for as long as 2 months at –80°C (17). It has been postulated that disruption of the membrane barrier by detergents allows free access of the rate-limited donor substrate (UDP-GA) and reveals the full catalytic potential of the transferases.

Glucuronidation may be assayed by a variety of colorimetric, fluorometric, and radioisotopic methodologies. Many of these methods are substrate specific and require specific methods and/or specifically labeled substrates. Other methods, best described as multisubstrate assays, are based on quantification of the donated glucuronic acid moiety or by indirect reaction products. Often the former are based on the use of UDP [^{14}C]GA to produce labeled glucuronides that are separated by chromatography and quantified by liquid scintillation counting (32). Indirect reactions have been described that link the UDP-GT reaction to the NADH/NAD conversion through pyruvate kinase and lactate dehydrogenase (135).

Colorimetric Assay for p-Nitrophenol Glucuronidation

A reproducible simple colorimetric assay has been presented as a standard method for measuring p-nitrophenol glucuronidation (12).

Technique

1. Incubation mixture:
   (a) Liver microsomes (1 mg protein/ml) (0.10 ml)
   (b) 1 M Tris-HCl (pH 7.4) (0.05 ml)
   (c) Sodium cholate (0.25% w/v) or Triton X-100 (0.25% w/v) (0.02 ml)
   (d) 50 mM MgCl (0.05 ml)
   (e) H_2O (0.18 ml)
   (f) 5 mM p-Nitrophenol (0.05 ml)
   The total volume is 0.45 ml.
2. Preincubate mixture for 2 min at 37°C.
3. Add 30 mM UDP-GA (0.05 ml) to start reaction. Incubate for 10–30 min at 37°C.
4. Stop the reaction and precipitate protein with 1 ml 5% trichloroacetic acid.
5. Centrifuge to clear protein.
6. Add 0.25 ml 2 M NaOH to 1 ml of supernatant fluid.
7. Read supernatant OD at 405 nm.
8. p-Nitrophenol extinction coefficient is 18.1×10^3 cm^2/mol at pH >10.

Single Substrate Glucuronosyltransferase Assays (Radiometric)

A variety of radiolabeled single substrate assays have been developed for determination of UDP-glucuronosyltransferase activity. These methods often use radiolabeled substrates and some means to separate unreacted substrate from the respective glucuronide conjugates. The first of the methods described is a rapid radiometric method developed by Lucier and McDaniel (110). This method is particularly useful for the study of steroid conjugation reactions.

Rapid radiometric glucuronosyltransferase assay. The incubation system for glucuronidation measurements is added to liquid scintillation vials and consists of the following: 1.2 ml 75 mM Tris-HCI buffer (pH 7.4), 1.0 μm UDP-GA, 10.0 μmol unlabeled substrate in 50 μl methanol, and 1×10^5 dpm-labeled substrate in 50 μl methanol. This volume of methanol is used to ensure substrate solubilization and has no apparent effect on glucuronosyltransferase activity. The incubation contents are warmed at 37°C for 3 minutes, and then 0.4 to 0.6 mg microsomal protein is added. The incubation period is approximately 10 minutes. The reaction is stopped by the addition of 10 ml nonaqueous scintillation fluid prepared by mixing 43 ml liquifluor (New England Nuclear) per liter of toluene. Samples are capped, shaken for 10 seconds on a vortex mixer, and radioactivity is counted in the same vials in which the incubation reactions are performed. Addition of the toluene-based scintillation fluid results in a two-phase mixture (toluene on top and the aqueous fraction on the bottom). Unreacted substrate partitions into the toluene, and this radioactivity is detected in liquid scintillation counter equipped with an automatic quench analyzer. Glucuronides remain in the aqueous fraction, and because ^{14}C and ^{3}H in a water medium do not scintillate, radioactivity associated with glucuronides is not detectable by liquid scintillation spectrometry. This phenomenon enables steroid glucuronidation rates to be measured by substrate disappearance. Blank values are obtained by omitting UDP-GA from the reaction media. The incubation blanks represent 0% activity and correct for the amount of substrate remaining in the aqueous fraction (incubation medium). Glucuronides detected after addition of scintillation fluid to incubation media reflect the amount of radioactivity detected after 100% glucuronidation of substrate. Enzyme activity using 300 nmol substrate in the incubation medium is expressed by the equation:

$$1-\frac{\begin{matrix}\text{Radioactivity}\\ \text{after}\\ \text{incubation}\end{matrix} - \left[\begin{matrix}\text{Radioactivity}\\ \text{after}\\ \text{incubation}\end{matrix} \times \begin{matrix}\text{Fraction of respective}\\ \beta\text{-D-glucuronide}\\ \text{detected}\end{matrix}\right]}{\text{Radioactivity in black}}$$

$$\times 300\ \text{nmol} = \begin{matrix}\text{nmol}\\ \text{substrate}\\ \text{conjugated.}\end{matrix}$$

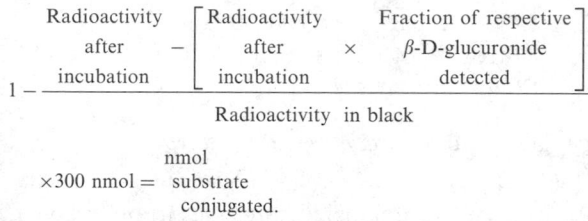

This assay procedure is applicable to a wide range of substrates and enzyme reactions in which the polarity of the product is significantly different from the substrates.

l-[1-^{14}C] naphthol glucuronidation. A commonly used assay for glucuronidation is similar to the technique described by Hazelton et al. (81). This technique uses radiolabeled 1-[1^{14}C]naphthol as the substrate and removes unreacted naphthol from the glucuronide conjugate by a chloroform extraction. The method is simple and sensitive.

Technique

1. Incubation mixture for liver microsomes:
   (a) Native: Microsome pellet is suspended in 0.25 M sucrose (0.33 g equivalent wet weight of liver/ml 0.25 M sucrose). This is then diluted with an equal volume of 0.25 M sucrose.
   (b) Activated: Similar as native microsomes; however, equal volume of sucrose contains 16 mM CHAPS and is agitated for 20 min at 4°C.
2. Incubation mixture: 0.2 M Tris-HCl, pH 7.5, 10 mM $MgCl_2$, 2.2 mM saccharic acid-1, 4 lactone, 0.5 mM 1-naphthol, and 1-[1^{14}C]naphthol (0.04 μCi) at 3°C. Total volume is 0.5 ml.
3. UDP-glucuronic acid is added to start reaction such that final concentration is 4 mM.
4. Reactions are terminated at desired time (10 min) by the addition of an equal volume of ice-cold ethanol.
5. Unreacted 1-naphthol is removed with an 8-ml chloroform extraction.
6. Remaining radioactivity in aqueous phase is determined in liquid scintillation counter.

Multisubstrate glucuronosyltransferase assay using UDP[^{14}C]GA. Assay of glucuronosyltransferase activity can be accomplished using a multisubstrate approach. This type of approach allows examination of multiple substrate interactions with the various isozymes for definition of UDP-GT isozyme catalytic boundaries. One such method, by Coughtrie et al. (32), through use of HPLC and incubation with UDP[^{14}C]GA, directly measures ^{14}C-labeled glucuronides of a range of model substrates. This method, as described later, has been used successfully with a variety of aglycone substrates, including 1-naphthol, 4-nitrophenol, androsterone, phenol, phenolphthalein, 2-hydroxybiphenyl, 4-hydroxybiphenyl, menthol, diethylstilbestrol, 1-hydroxybenzo[a]pyrene, 3-hydroxybenzo[a]pyrene, and 9-hydroxybenzo[a]pyrene. The glucuronides of these substrates were all resolved from precursors upon HPLC with this system.

Technique

Incubation:

1. The incubation mixture is comprised of 50 mM Tris-maleate buffer, 10 mM $MgCl_2$, pH 7.4, 2.7 mM UDP-GA, UDP[^{14}C]GA (0.25 μCi), and substrate such that the substrate is delivered in 5 μl of carrier vehicle and final concentration is 1 mM. Final volume of reaction mixture is 100 μl.
2. Add the detergent Lubrol-PX such that the detergent-to-protein ratio is 0.25.
3. Preincubate mixture for 2 min at 37°C. Start reaction by addition of 50 μl of microsomal protein (0.1–0.5 mg).
4. Incubate reaction 10–30 min with gentle shaking at 37°C. Time should be regulated such that the reaction rate is linear and no more than 10% of UDP[^{14}C]GA is used.
5. Stop reaction with 475 μl of 100% ethanol at –15°C.

6. Centrifuge in microfuge at 16,000 g for 3 min.
7. Filter supernatant fraction through a 0.45-μm filter.
8. Store samples up to 1 week in liquid nitrogen.

HPLC Analysis:

1. Analyses are performed on a Partisil 5 PAC (polar amino-cyano) bonded phase column (4.5 mm × 26 cm). The mobile phase consists of a linear gradient (1.5 ml/min) with acetonitrile and the ion pairing agent tetrabutylammonium hydrogen sulfate (TBAHS). Initially, the gradient runs from 100% acetonitrile to 100% 0.01 M TBAHS over 20 min. The gradient then is maintained at 100% 0.01 M TBAHS for 25 min before returning to 100% acetonitrile over 10 min.
2. Radioactivity measurements of HPLC eluent are taken at 20-second intervals over the 45-min gradient.

Multisubstrate Radiometric Assay for Glucuronidation in Intact Cells

In addition to microsomal preparations, glucuronidation may be studied in intact cells, such as those in tissue culture. As described earlier, glucuronidation often is studied with the radiolabeled UDP[^{14}C]GA as the measurable moiety in microsomal preparations. These types of studies are not possible in culture, as the radiolabeled UDP[^{14}C]GA is not permeable in intact cells. A novel method developed by Dawson et al. (36) bypasses this limitation by labeling GA in the cell by using permeable [^{14}C]fructose as a GA precursor. In this technique, donor animals are fasted so that endogenous GA is depleted. Because GA is derived from both glycogenolysis and gluconeogenesis, use of radiolabeled gluconeogenic substrates such as [^{14}C]fructose allows the radiolabel to be incorporated into UDP-GA and any subsequent glucuronides. The specific activity of the glucuronide is similar to that of the substrate. This method incorporates three major steps following cell procurement: (a) incubation, (b) HPLC of radiolabeled glucuronides, and (c) specific activity determinations. The method has been applied to the glucuronidation of a variety of substrates, including 4-nitrophenol and 1-naphthol.

Incubation:

1. To cell suspensions prepared from fasted animals, add 1-naphthol or 4-nitrophenol substrate dissolved in dimethylsulfoxide (final DMSO concentration is 1% v/v).
2. Add 200 μM [^{14}C] fructose (0.5% μCi).
3. Cap vials and gas with 95% O_2 and 5% CO_2.
4. Incubate mixture for 20–90 min in a shaking water bath set at 37°C.
5. Centrifuge (12,000 × g/30 sec) through 250 μl of silicone oil (Dow Corning 550 dinonylphthalate 2:1 v/v) to terminate incubation and separate cells from medium.
6. Heat supernatant fraction in boiling water bath for 5 min. Remove denatured protein by centrifugation at 12,000 × g for 1 min.
7. Store for glucuronide analysis.

HPLC Analysis:

1. Analysis is carried out on a 4.5 mm × 25 cm Partisil 5 PAC (polar amino-cyano) column.
2. Mobile phase consists of a linear gradient from 100% acetonitrile to 67% 0.01 M tetrabutylammonium hydrogen sulfate over 20 min. The gradient is maintained at 67% 0.01 M tetrabutylammonium hydrogen sulfate for 5 min before conditions are returned to 100% acetonitrile over the subsequent 10 min (1 ml/min flow rate).
3. HPLC fractions are collected at 0.5-min intervals.
4. Identify glucuronide peaks by hydrolysis with 1000 Units of P-glucuronidase (*Escherichia coli*).
   (a) 200 μl Supernatant fraction.
   (b) 40 μl 0.5 M Sodium phosphate buffer, pH 7.
   (c) Incubate for 2 h at 37°C.
   (d) Assay 0.1 ml of incubation mixture by HPLC, identifying glucuronide peaks by their disappearance.

Specific Activity Determination of [^{14}C]Glucose

1. Take 0.1 ml of boiled and centrifuged supernatant fraction from incubation procedure. Add 0.9 ml of 100 mM Tris buffer, with 1 mM magnesium acetate, 1.7 mM NAD^+, and 1.1 mM ATP.
2. Incubate mixture at 37°C in disposable cuvettes. Measure change in extinction at 340 nm following addition of 1 U hexokinase/1 U glucose 6-phosphate dehydrogenase, as well as following the addition of 0.1 U of 6-phosphogluconate dehydrogenase. Glucose concentrations are calculated using 6.22×10^3 M^{-1} cm^{-1} as the extinction coefficient for NADH (total glucose). (Hexokinase converts glucose to glucose 6-phosphate. Glucose 6-phosphate dehydrogenase then converts glucose 6-phosphate to 6-phosphoglucono-δ lactone, which is hydrolyzed to 6-phosphogluconate. This substrate is converted by 6-phosphogluconate dehydrogenase to ribulose 5-phosphate liberating CO_2.)
3. Under identical conditions, incubate another aliquot in 20-ml stoppered vial with center well. Add enzymes by syringe through stopper.

4. Add 0.1 ml of 20% $HClO_4$ (v/v) to end incubation and drive off $^{14}CO_2$.
5. The $^{14}CO_2$ released is absorbed by 2-phenethylamine/methanol (0.2 ml, 1:1 v/v) on a filter paper strip in center well. Allow $^{14}CO_2$ absorption to proceed 1 h with shaking at room temperature.
6. Remove wells to vials containing scintillation fluid for liquid scintillation counting (LSC).
7. Radioactivity in the original glucose is calculated as being six times that in the single carbon released as $^{14}CO_2$.

Microsomal Glutathione Transferases

Glutathione transferase, a multigene family of isoenzymes, catalyzes the nucleophilic attack of glutathione on a variety of electrophilic compounds. These enzymes may be found both in the soluble or membrane-bound cell fractions. Of the glutathione transferase that appears to be membrane bound, approximately 80% is associated with the endoplasmic reticulum whereas the remainder appears to be mitochondrial in origin (130). A number of cytosolic isozymes of glutathione transferase are found associated with membranes. It is not clear if these are truly membrane-bound isozymes rather than cytosolic contaminants. Additional evidence suggests that unique forms of glutathione transferase exist in microsomes (131). Glutathione transferase activity is expressed when the isozymes exist in the dimeric form. Within a gene family, the various subunits may form homodimers or heterodimers.

Microsomal glutathione transferase isozymes are capable of most of those reactions catalyzed by their cytosolic counterparts. For select substrates, such as chlorotrifluoroethylene (40) and hexachlorobutadiene (202), the microsomal form appears to be a better catalyst than the cytosolic glutathione transferase. 1-Chloro-2,4-dinitrobenzene, however, is the substrate of choice for assay of both cytosolic and microsomal glutathione transferases. Although inhibition is facilitated in both fractions by bromosulfophthalein and hematin, induction of activity varies substantially. Cytosolic glutathione transferase isozyme inducers, such as phenobarbital, 3-methylcholanthrene, or trans-stilbene oxide are ineffective on microsomal glutathione transferases (132,133). Other agents, such as 2(3)-tert-butyl 4-hydroxy anisole (7,8) and the peroxisome proliferator acetylsalicylic acid, have been shown to induce microsomal glutathione transferase effectively. N-ethylmaleimide has been identified as a potent and selective activator of the microsomal form of glutathione transferase (129).

Assay of glutathione transferase activity has been accomplished spectrophotometrically. This procedure is facilitated by substrates that change optical absorbance upon glutathione conjugation. A common procedure to assay glutathione transferase activity with 1-chloro-2,4-dinitrobenzene as modified from Habig et al. (72) and Morgenstern and DePierre (129) is as follows.

Technique

Reagents:
1. 10 mM Glutathione.
2. 20 mM 1-Chloro-2,4-dinitrobenzene in ethanol.
3. 0.1 M Potassium phosphate buffer.
4. Triton X-100.

Assay Conditions:
1. Final reaction volume 2 ml.
2. 30°C reaction temperature.

Incubation Mixture:
1. 1 mM 1-Chloro-2,4-dinitrobenzene/ethanol (50 μl).
2. Microsomes, washed twice with 0.15 M Tris-HCl, pH 8.0, to remove cytosolic contamination (20–100 μl, dependent on activity and protein content).
3. 0.1 M Potassium phosphate buffer pH 6.5 (pH 6.5 minimizes nonenzymatic reactions). Balance of reaction volume to 1 ml.
4. 0.1%–0.2% Triton X-100 (2 to 4 μl).
5. Add 1 mM glutathione (100 μl) to start reaction.

Analysis:
1. Read absorbance at 340 nm.
2. Molar extinction coefficient 9.6 mM^{-1} cm^{-1}.

Hydrolytic Enzymes

The endoplasmic reticulum also contains a variety of hydrolytic enzymes that exhibit a dual localization in that they are also active in lysosomes. These enzymes include β-D-glucuronidase (performs the reverse reaction of UDP-glucuronidase by liberating the free aglycone from β-D-glucuronic acid conjugates), acid and alkaline phosphatases, and aryl sulfatase. The function of these microsomal enzymes is not clear, although they appear to play a role in the regulation of steroid metabolism and, in some cases, may represent structural proteins of the endoplasmic reticulum. Bacterial β-glucuronidase plays an important role in the absorption and toxicity of many chemicals, including some carcinogens. One possible explanation for the dual localization of these enzyme systems is that they are synthesized in the RER, transported through the membranous cisternae of the SER, and fragments of the SER are incorporated into lysosomes. Reviews describing the potential role of these lysosomal/microsomal systems are available (76,192). Hydrolytic enzymes, such as β-glucuronidase, can be detected by histochemical or biochemical methods.

One simple method for measuring mammalian β-glucuronidase activity is as follows:

1. The incubation medium contains 1.0 mM substrate (β-D-glucuronide of p-nitrophenol, 4-methylumbelliferone, or phenolphthalein) in 50 mM acetate buffer, pH 4.5.
2. Warm the incubation mixture for 3 min at 37°C.
3. Initiate the reaction by adding 1.0 mg microsomal protein.
4. After a 10-min incubation period, stop the reaction by adding 5 ml glycine buffer (see p-nitrophenol glucuronidation assay).
5. Remove protein by low-speed centrifugation and measure the formation of the product spectrophotometrically (p-nitrophenol, 405 nm; phenolphthalein, 550 nm; and methylumbelliferone, 365 nm).

The value of measuring conjugation-deconjugation enzyme activities rests with assessing the potential capacity of a cell or organ to deactivate/activate potentially toxic reactive intermediates. Although these measurements are an indirect approach to assessing tissue/cell susceptibility to these highly toxic chemical species, the data generated from past studies have proved highly useful toward predicting cellular potential for injury.

PEROXISOMES

The peroxisomes are single, membrane-bound cytoplasmic organelles present in the cells of animals, plants, fungi, and protozoa. With the exception of mature erythrocytes, peroxisomes appear to be present in all eukaryotic cells. Studies by DeDuve and co-workers have shown that rat liver peroxisomes contain both hydrogen peroxide–generating oxidase enzymes and hydrogen peroxide–degrading catalase, causing the breakdown of hydrogen peroxide to oxygen and water. Peroxisomes are involved in lipid, sterol, and purine metabolism, as well as peroxidative detoxification. Peroxisomes contain a complete fatty acid β-oxidation cycle. In addition, peroxisomes are known to proliferate in response to both natural ligands, such as fatty acids, and a group of chemicals known as peroxisome proliferators or peroxisome proliferating agents (PPAs). PPAs are a very structurally diverse group of chemicals that include hypolipidemic agents, phthalate esters, perfluorocarboxy acids, solvents and phenoxyacetic acid herbicides; all considered to be nongenotoxic carcinogens because when tested they fail to cause DNA damage directly. Peroxisome proliferation consists of gross hepatomegaly associated with both hypertrophy and hyperplasia, with hepatocytes exhibiting a marked proliferation of peroxisomes and the endoplasmic reticulum. These morphological changes are associated with changes in the handling of fats (6). Extrahepatic tissues, including the kidney, intestine, testis, and adipose tissue, have also been shown to be susceptible to peroxisomal proliferation, but peroxisomes are most abundant in the liver and kidney. In rat liver it has been estimated that peroxisomes account for about 2.5% of total liver protein and occupy about 1.5% of the total cellular volume (116). Peroxisomal proliferation has been linked with reproductive and developmental toxicity, as well as hepatic and testicular cancers (31,189). A marked species-specific sensitivity to peroxisomal proliferation has been noted, with humans and apes considered refractory species whereas rats and mice are sensitive species; however, even in humans, peroxisomal dysfunction can result in severe disease states, including Zellweger syndrome, adrenoleukodystrophy, and Refsum syndrome (134).

By far the major portion of peroxisomal enzymes are lipid-metabolizing enzymes. Over 40 different enzymes have been identified, including enzymes involved in fatty acid activation, elongation, and β-oxidation, the oxidation of polyunsaturated fatty acids, carnitine acyltransferases, acyl Co-A hydrolases, bile acid synthesis, cholesterol and dolichol synthesis, glycerolipid synthesis, purine catabolism, polyamine catabolism, amino acid and glyoxylate metabolism, oxygen metabolism and reactive oxygen species, and nucleotide-binding proteins (116). The levels of the peroxisomal β-oxidation enzymes, such as acyl-CoA oxidase and the microsomal enzyme P450 4A1, are elevated between 10- and 30-fold in response to PPA administration. This is paralleled by an increase in the respective mRNAs, which is observed as early as 2 h post-administration. This coordinate and rapid increase in gene expression suggests a common mechanism of induction and peroxisome proliferation. The exact mechanism is, as yet, incompletely understood, but it is known that a nuclear receptor is involved (64).

The peroxisome proliferator-activated receptor (PPARα 52 kDa) is a member of the nuclear receptor family of ligand-activated transcription factors. Both peroxisomal proliferation and the induction of certain peroxisomal and microsomal enzymes require the expression of PPARα, as evidenced by the absence of response when PPARα expression is disabled by targeted disruption (103). Studies have shown that PPARα forms heterodimers with RXRα (retinoic acid X receptor; X = 9-*cis*-retinoic acid) and binds a peroxisome proliferator-activated receptor response element (PPRE) resulting in transcriptional activation of at least 15 different genes in response to PPAs or elevated levels of fatty acids and other endogenous compounds. Although it is suspected that the activation by PPARα reflects ligand binding, this has not been experimentally determined, and it may be that some product of altered metabolism rather than the PPA itself acts as the activating ligand (90).

The investigation of the myriad functional and structural features of peroxisomes requires the preparation of highly purified organelle fractions separated from microsomes and other contaminants, such as lysosomes and mitochondria. This is hampered by the fragility of peroxisomes and their relative paucity (2.5% of the total protein) within the cell. Thus, separation conditions must maintain the mechanical, hydrostatic, and osmotic integrity of the sample. Generally, three steps are employed in the purification of peroxisomes: (1) homogenization or tissue disruption, (2) subfractionation by differential centrifugation, and (3) isolation of the purified fraction by density gradient centrifugation (Figure 34.10). Purified peroxisomes can be used for enzyme assays, which are too numerous and varied to be covered in detail here, or for immunodetection of peroxisome-associated proteins using the methods covered under SDS-PAGE of microsomal fractions for P450. Several commercially available antibodies recognize catalase, PMP70, and any proteins containing certain peroxisomal membrane-targeting sequences. Fractions may also be observed for purity or structural features using electron microscopic evaluation to check for mitochondria or by staining with 3,3′-diaminobenzidine, which produces an electron dense reaction product with catalase found throughout the peroxisome. A method for the isolation of highly purified peroxisomes from rat liver follows (191).

Reagents:

Homogenization buffer: 250 mM sucrose, 6.717 mM MOPS (morpholinopropane sulfonic acid; free acid), and 1 mM EDTA.

0.9% Saline (NaCl).

Gradient Buffer: 6.717 mM MOPS, 1 mM EDTA, and 1 ml of ethanol per liter, adjust to pH 7.2 with NaOH. May be stored at 4°C. Just prior to use add per 100 ml: 0.2 ml of 0.1 M PMSF, 0.1 ml of 1 M ε-aminocaproic acid, and 20 μl of 1 M DTT.

Metrizamide Solutions: Stock Solution, 60% w/v (at 15°C density = 1.328 g/ml; 40% = 1.218 g/ml; 20% = 1.108 g/ml) in Gradient Buffer. To make one gradient, take 3.76, 3.38, 3.53, 2.06, and 3.2 ml of the Stock Solution and bring to total volumes of 10, 7, 6, 3, and 4 ml using Gradient Buffer, respectively. Resultant densities are 1.12, 1.155, 1.19, 1.225, and 1.26 g/ml.

Isolation of Purified Peroxisomes

1. Anesthetize the animal.
2. Open the abdominal cavity and perfuse the liver with 0.9% saline via the portal vein until all the blood is removed.
3. Remove the liver, cut into small pieces, and add 3 ml/g tissue (wet liver weight) of homogenization buffer. Place into ice-cold Potter–Elvehjem homogenizer and homogenize with a single up-and-down stroke using a motorized, loose-fitting pestle.
4. Decant into a 50 ml centrifuge tube and centrifuge at 70 × g for 10 min in a refrigerated centrifuge.
5. Collect the supernatant fraction and resuspend the pellet in 2 ml/g of ice-cold homogenization buffer, rehomogenize as before, and spin again under the same conditions. Collect the second supernatant fraction and combine it with the first to make up the postnuclear supernate. The remaining pellet is the nuclear fraction.
6. Centrifuge the postnuclear supernate at 1950 × g for 10 min in a refrigerated centrifuge.
7. Collect the supernate and resuspend the pellet manually in 1 ml/g of ice-cold homogenization buffer and spin again under the same conditions. Collect the second supernate and combine with the first to make up the postmitochondrial supernate. The final pellet contains the majority of mitochondria, large microsomal sheets, and some remaining nuclei.
8. Centrifuge the postmitochondrial supernate at 25,300 g for 20 min and, using suction, remove the supernate and the reddish fluffy layer. Resuspend the pellet in about 10 ml of ice-cold homogenization buffer using a glass rod and centrifuge again at 25,300 × g for 15 min. Resuspend the final pellet (enriched heavy peroxisomes) in 5 ml of ice-cold homogenization buffer using a glass rod. The supernate may be used to prepare a microsomal fraction with the supernatant fraction from that process constituting the cytosolic fraction. The postmitochondrial supernate may also be centrifuged at an integrated relative centrifugal force (RCF) of 4.47×10^5 g × min ($g_{max} = 39{,}000$), and the resulting pellet represents the enriched light peroxisomes. For highly purified peroxisomes, complete the density gradient fractionation described.

Isolation of Highly Purified Peroxisomes

1. Layer sequentially 4, 3, 6, 7, and 10 ml of the metrizamide solutions described above (1.26–1.12 g/ml) in a 40 ml Quick-Seal polyallomer centrifuge tube (Beckman) to form a discontinuous gradient.
2. Freeze the gradient in liquid nitrogen and store at –20°C. Prior to use thaw the gradient quickly at room temperature using a metallic stand to transform the discontinuous gradient into one with an exponential profile.

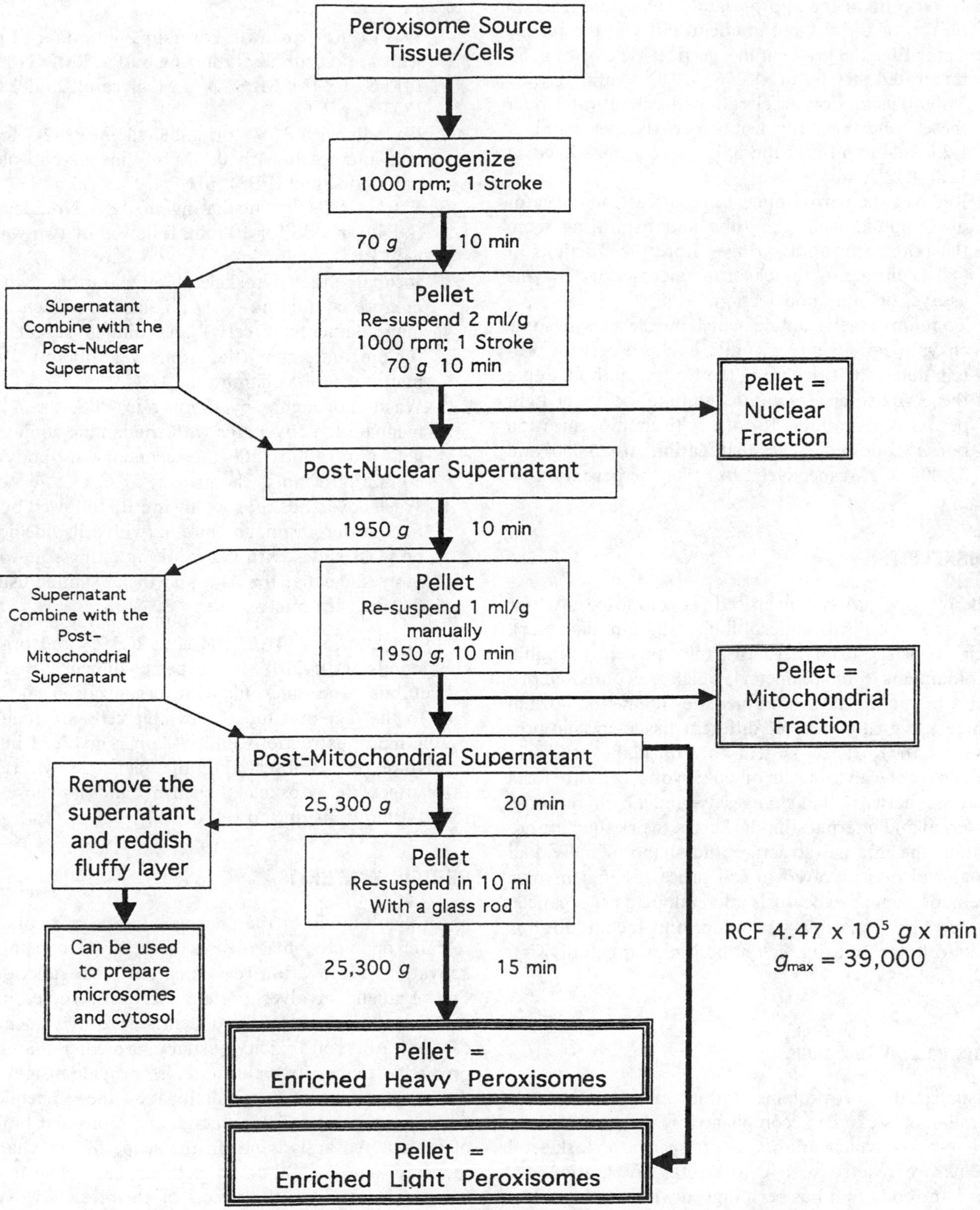

FIG. 34.10. Flow chart of the peroxisome isolation method. Rat liver peroxisomes prepared by differential centrifugation are purified to more than 95% of the total protein content with contributions of about 2% each from mitochondria and microsomes and 1% from lysosomes. Peroxisomal fractions prepared by density gradient centrifugation are highly purified (98%–99%), as confirmed by electron microscopy. Scheme adapted from Reference 191.

3. Layer 5 ml of the appropriate peroxisomal fraction on top of the thawed gradient and seal the tube.
4. Centrifuge the gradient in a vertical-type rotor at an integrated RCF of 1.256×10^6 g × min (g_{max} = 39,000) using slow acceleration/deceleration. Under these conditions the heavy peroxisomes band at 1.23–1.24 g/ml and the light peroxisomes band at 1.20–1.21 g/ml.
5. Recover the peroxisomes using a fraction collector or by puncturing the tube and aspirating from the bottom using a syringe. Store the fractions at –80°C until use for electron microscopy, enzyme assays, or immunodetection.
6. To remove metrizamide, which interferes with some enzyme activities (e.g., urate oxidase) or with protein determinations using the Lowry method, dilute the peroxisomal fraction containing heavy or light peroxisomes about 10-fold with homogenization buffer followed by centrifugation at 25,000 and 39,000 × g, respectively, to pellet the peroxisomes.

CYTOSKELETON

The cytoskeletal system in cells is composed of three main types of fibrils: microtubules (25 nm diameter), which consist primarily of the protein tubulin; microfilaments (6 nm diameter), which are composed primarily of actin; and intermediate filaments (10 nm diameter), which consist of different tissue-specific proteins (94,161). This system of fibrillar structures crisscrosses the cytoplasm of eukaryotic cells to form an internal network that changes dynamically in response to external and internal stimuli. This network functions to maintain the internal structure and shape of individual cells and also is involved in cell processes that involve movement such as exocytosis and endocytosis, organelle transport, protoplasmic streaming, and locomotion, as well as cellular polarity, cell adhesion, and cell division (1,59,77,82,95,124).

Ultrastructural Techniques

Visualization of proteins within microtubules and microfilaments can be accomplished by double antibody procedures in which antibodies to specific cytoskeletal proteins are reacted with cytoskeletal preparations. A second antibody that has been tagged with either a fluorescent dye molecule or a label visible by electron microscopy (e.g., colloid gold) is then allowed to react with the first immunoglobulin, and the structures are visualized by fluorescence or electron microscopy (9,63). The fluorescence microscopic technique developed by Zhao et al. (210) is as follows:

Technique

1. Wash cells grown on coverslips (12 mm × 12 mm) with a microtubule stabilizing buffer, PM2G (0.1 M PIPES, I MM $MgSO_4$, 2 M glycerol, and 2 mM EGTA, pH 6.9).
2. Fix cells with 3.7% formaldehyde in PM2G for 30 min and wash with 0.1 M glycine in phosphate-buffered saline (PBS), pH 7.4, for 5 min.
3. Extract cells by incubating in 0.3% Nonidet P40 (NP40) in PBS for 10 min, followed by two washes with PBS.
4. Incubate the cytoskeletal preparations with a mixture containing NBD-phallacidin (which labels microfilaments directly) and diluted rabbit anti-tubulin antiserum (the primary antibody) for 30 min in a moist chamber at 37°C.
5. Wash thoroughly by dipping in PBS, drain, and incubate the coverslips with rhodamine conjugated goat anti-rabbit IgG (the secondary antibody) for 30 min in a moist chamber at 37°C.
6. Wash coverslips thoroughly in PBS followed by distilled water, drain, and mount (with cells side down) on glass slides with Glevatol mounting solution.
7. Store slides flat for 24 h and then examine using a fluorescence microscope.

Both metal ions (41,63,104,125,126,151) and organic compounds (105,210) have been shown to affect microtubule and microfilament organization in cells. Due to the fact that most nonviable cells are removed by the many extractions and washings involved in this procedure, results observed on the final slides will reflect early effects on cytoskeletal elements and not those that reflect alterations due to cell death.

PROTEIN SYNTHESIS

Although much of the pharmacological/toxicological research on microsomes focuses on their role in metabolic activation/deactivation reactions, the main function of this organelle involves protein synthesis. Increasingly, researchers are attempting to identify sensitive biochemical indicators of toxicity (usually proteins) that have predictive/diagnostic value and also provide insight into the mechanisms of toxic actions of these chemicals. Although a survey of the genetics and molecular biology of protein synthesis is not in the scope of this chapter, there are some general useful methods that can be applied to investigations on the effects of chemicals on overall and/or specific protein synthesis. These methods involve injection of radiolabeled amino acids into intact animals (usually tail vein); the incorporation of radiolabel into specific organelles or specific proteins is then determined. Obviously, protein purification or immunochemical procedures must be undertaken to assess synthesis/

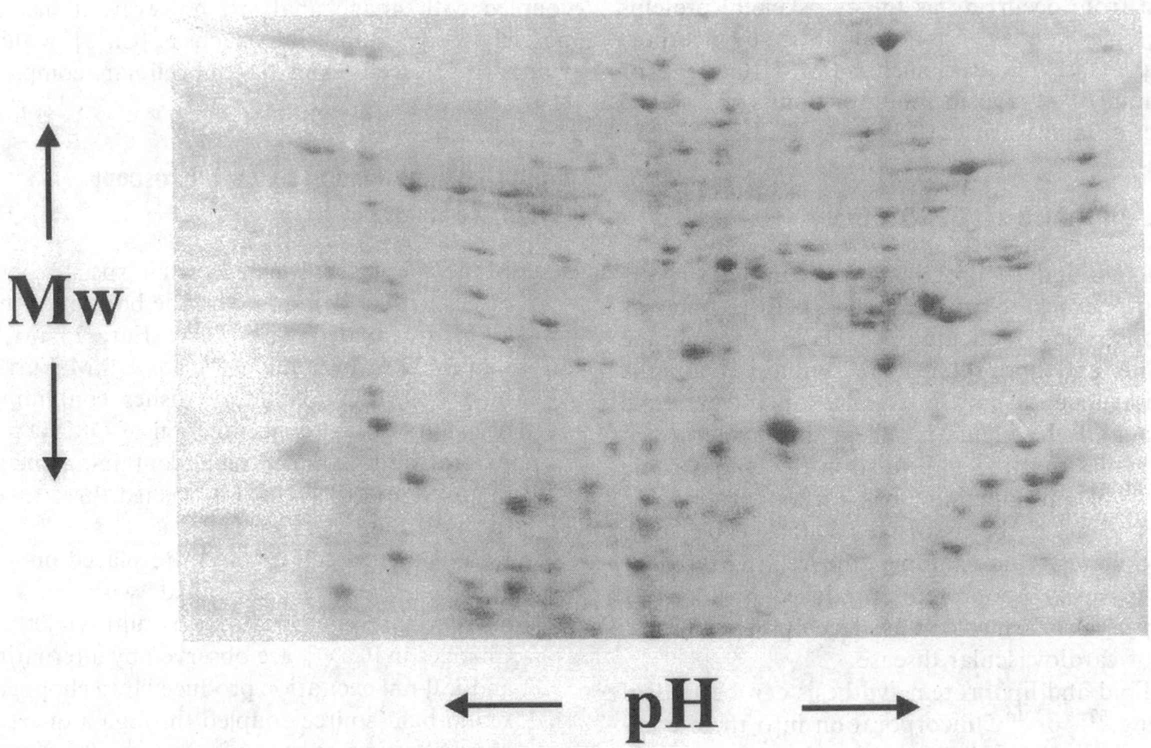

FIG. 34.11. Coomassie blue stained two-dimensional gel of rat kidney showing numerous gene product spots.

degradation of individual proteins. When conducting such pulse-label experiments, it is essential that samples are taken over a wide range of sample periods so that meaningful and valid conclusions can be made concerning alterations either in synthetic or degradative phases for a particular protein. For example, if a toxic chemical selectively alters protein degradation and a pulse label is conducted during the synthetic phase, the investigator could miss critical information. If possible, it is desirable to conduct pulse-label experiments with carbon rather than tritium in order to avoid nonspecific redistribution of the radiolabel.

Another method, termed two-dimensional gel electrophoresis, is being used to determine protein synthesis profiles (86). This procedure involves administration of high specific activity [^{35}S] methionine to intact animals or isolated cells, and the subsequent electrophoretic mapping of labeled proteins by SDS in one direction and isoelectric focusing in the second direction. This procedure is now commonly used in studies investigating the role of specific protein synthesis tissue differences in response to chemical exposure, "stress proteins," and in development and differentiation, and can resolve as many as 1000 proteins (Figure 34.11).

The synthesis of specific groups of proteins, such as cytoskeletal protein synthesis, can be measured by determining the amount of radiolabel incorporated into isolated fractions of cytoskeletal extracts from cells exposed to radioactively labeled amino acids (104,105). This can be accomplished by the following:

Technique

1. Plate cells at 1×10^5 cells/60 min dish and grow to subconfluency.
2. Replace medium with a serum-free Eagles' basal medium containing 1/20th of the normal concentration of amino acids plus ^{3}H-labeled amino acid mixture at 1.5 μCi/ml.
3. Incubate the cells for 1 h. Remove the labeled medium, rinse twice, gently scrape the cells from the plate, and centrifuge.
4. Wash the cell pellets once with PM2G buffer (0.1 M PIPES, 1 mM $MgSO_4$, 2 M glycerol, and 2 mM EDTA, pH 6.9). Extract cell pellets with 0.3% NP-40 in PM2G buffer containing 0.5 mM phenylmethyl sulfonyl fluoride (PMSF), microcentrifuge to pellet the cytoskeletal fractions, and wash twice with PM buffer (0.1 M PIPES, 1 mM $MgSO_4$, pH 6.9) containing 0.5 mM PMSF.
5. Extract the cytoskeletal fraction pellet with PM buffer containing 5 mM $CaCl_2$ and 0.5 mM PMSF to depolymerize the microtubules and release the cytoskeletal proteins.
6. Count an aliquot of the protein extract in a liquid scintillation counter and normalize to total cell protein. It is important to prevent protein degra-

dation from occurring as the cytoskeletal proteins are being isolated. This is accomplished by incorporating protease inhibitors such as PMSF (0.5 mM) or aprotinin (0.02 trypsin inhibitory units/ml) in the extraction and wash buffers.

PHOSPHOLIPIDS AND LIPOPROTEINS

Phospholipids and lipoproteins provide important permeability properties to membrane structures such as the endoplasmic reticulum. These membrane phospholipids and lipoproteins are synthesized on the endoplasmic reticulum and often play an integral role in enzyme activity by regulating the membrane environment of enzymes that are imbedded in the endoplasmic reticulum. The production of certain forms of lipoproteins seems to be associated with specific toxic and disease states. For example, the relative amount of very low density lipoproteins produced by the liver appears to play a critical role in the development and susceptibility of cardiovascular disease.

Phospholipid and lipoprotein synthesis can be studied by measuring ^{32}P or ^{14}C incorporation into these compounds as outlined earlier (see section on Protein Synthesis).

INTRACELLULAR IONS

Intracellular ions such as Na^+, K^+, Ca^{2+}, Mg^{2+}, and H^+ play important regulatory roles in normal cell processes and in the response of cells to injury. Sequential alterations in cellular ion concentrations have been shown to be an integral part of cellular repair and regeneration processes and in the sequelae of events leading to cell death (182,185,186). Direct effects of chemicals on ion regulation also can occur through direct effects on energy metabolism, plasma membrane integrity, and ion translocation systems.

Recent advances in instrumentation have made it possible to measure changes in ion concentrations in living cells following exposure to toxic compounds. Fluorescent probes sensitive to various ions are currently available and have been used to study effects of metals (167), oxidative stress (142), and chemical ischemia (186). These probes include Quin-2 AM and Fura-2 AM for $[Ca^{2+}]_i$, Mag-Fura-2 AM for $[Mg^{2+}]_i$, SBFI for Na^+, PBFI for K^+, BCECF for pH, and rhodamine-123 for mitochondrial membrane potential.

Initial studies of cellular ion concentrations were conducted in cell suspensions in which average changes occurring in cell populations were measured. These studies used standard fluorimeters to measure total fluorescence of the sample (3). With the development of digital imaging fluorescence microscopy (DIFM), coupled with image analysis, however, it has become possible to quantitate ions such as $[Ca^{2+}]_i$ within individual living cells and in subcellular compartments (175,183).

Digital Imaging Fluorescence Microscopy (DIFM) Technique

1. Monolayer cell cultures grown in specially prepared dishes with a "window" on the bottom of the plate (175) are loaded with 3 μM Fura-2 AM for 30 min at 37°C by adding 6 μl of 1 mM Fura-2 AM in dry DMSO to culture dishes containing 2 ml of medium (final concentration of DMSO is 0.3%). After loading, the Fura-2–containing medium is removed and the cells are washed three times with fresh medium.
2. Fura-2–loaded cell cultures are placed on a heated (37°C) stage and examined with an inverted microscope equipped with ultraviolet optics. Changes in $[Ca^{2+}]_i$ are observed by alternating 340- and 380-nm excitation produced by a chopper-based xenon light source coupled through a quartz bifurcated fiber optic to the microscope. The microscope is equipped with an Opelco KS1380 intensifier and a Dage 65 video camera.
3. Fluorescent images are acquired at an alternating rate of 5 frame-pairs/second, which are processed by a Tracor Northern 8502 image analyzer. The fluorescent images are corrected for camera and intensifier variations by subtracting background images collected when the port is closed. The images collected with the 340-nm excitation are divided on a pixel-by-pixel basis by the images collected with 380-nm excitation, and the mean value of pixel ratios for each "ratioed" image is obtained by histogram analysis.
4. Calibration of the ratioed images is accomplished using a calcium ionophore such as ionomycin or 4-bromo-A23187 to give fully Ca^{2+}-saturated Fura-2 (175). Ca^{2+} ion concentrations are calculated using the formula

$$\text{nM } Ca^{2+} = K_d(R - R_{min})/(R_{max} - R),$$

where $K_d = 224$ nM (67); R_{max} is the ratio obtained in a cell treated with a Ca ionophore; R_{min} is calculated from the ratio (R) obtained with normal cells in which the $[Ca^{2+}]$ was assumed to be 100 nm (166).

QUESTIONS

1. What are some of the advantages and disadvantages of studying the effects of toxic agents on subcellular organelles versus whole cells and intact organisms?

2. What measurements could one make to determine the purity of a sample of lysosomes isolated by differential centrifugation?
3. Why would it be advantagous to use both immunodetection and enzymatic assay measurements to study the effect of toxic chemicals on microsomal P450 enzymes?
4. What might be a possible benefit of not having a particular FMO isozyme?
5. Peroxisomes produce both catalase and hydrogen peroxide. What might be the possible adverse effects to a cell that could result from a toxic agent which perturbs production of either hydrogen peroxide or catalase activity?
6. What functional changes would lead you to suspect that a toxic agent was targeting the cytoskeleton and how could you assess this?
7. The combined ultrastructural and biochemical techniques described in this chapter provide powerful approaches to understanding mechanisms of cell injury from chemicals by helping to localize the primary organelle systems involved. Cell death via apoptosis or necrosis are major areas of current interest. How would you use the techniques described in this chapter to further basic knowledge about the underlying mechanisms which determine whether a cell dies by apoptosis or necrosis?

REFERENCES

1. Alberts, B., Bray, D., Lewis, J., Raff, M., Roberts, K., and Watson, J. D., eds. (1983): *Molecular Biology of the Cell*, pp. 549–668. Garland Press, New York.
2. Allison, A. C., and Young, M. R. (1964): Uptake of dyes and drugs by living cells in culture. *Life Sci.*, 3:1407–1414.
3. Ambudkar, I. S., Smith, M. S., Phelps, P. C., Regec, A. L., and Trump, B. F. (1988): Extracellular Ca^{2+}-dependent elevation in cytosolic Ca^{2+} potentiates $HgCl_2$-induced renal proximal tubule cell damage. *Toxicol. Ind. Health*, 4:107–123.
4. Andrews, P. M., and Hackenbrock, C. R. (1975): A scanning and stereographic ultrastructural analysis of the isolated inner mitochondrial membrane during change in metabolic activity. *Exp. Cell Res.*, 90:127–136.
5. Beattie, D. S. (1968): Studies on the biogenesis of mitochondrial protein components in rat liver slices. *J. Biol. Chem.*, 243:4027–4033.
6. Bell, D. R., and Elcombe, C. R. (1993): Peroxisome proliferation: Lipid metabolism and receptors. In: *Peroxisomes: Biology and Importance in Toxicology and Medicine*, edited by G. Gibson and B. Lake, pp. 137–147. Taylor & Francis, London.
7. Benson, A. M., Batzinger, R. P., On, S.-Y. L., Bueding, E., Cha, Y.-N., and Talalay, P. (1979): Elevation of hepatic glutathione S-transferase activities and protection against mutagenic metabolites of benzo(a)pyrene by dietary antioxidants. *Cancer Res.*, 38:4486–4495.
8. Benson, A. M., Cha, Y.-N., Bueding, E., Heine, H. S., and Talalay, P. (1979): Elevation of extrahepatic glutathione S-transferase and epoxide hydratase activities by 2(3)-*tert*-butyl-4-hydroxyanisole. *Cancer Res.*, 39:2971–2977.
9. Bershadsky, A. D., and Vasiliev, J. M. (1988): *Cytoskeleton*. Plenum Press, New York.
10. Billings, R. F., Tephly, T. R., and Tukey, R. H. (1978): The separation and purification of estrone and p-nitrophenol UDP glucuronyltransferase activities. In: *Conjugation Reactions in Drug Biotransformation*, edited by A. Aitio, pp. 365–367. Elsevier, Amsterdam.
11. Blouin, A., Bolender, R. P., and Weibel, E. R. (1977): Distribution of organelles and membranes between hepatocytes and nonhepatocytes in the rat liver parenchyma: A stereological study. *J. Cell Biol.*, 72:441–455.
12. Bock, K. W., Burchell, B., Dutton, G. J., Hanninen, O., Mulder, G. J., Owens, I. S., Siest, G., and Tephly, T. R. (1983): UDP-glucuronosyltransferase activities: Guidelines for consistent interim terminology and assay conditions. *Biochem. Pharmacol.*, 32:953–955.
13. Bogucka, K., and Wojtczak, L. (1979): On the mechanisms of mercurial induced permeability of mitochondrial membrane to K^+. *FEBS Lett.*, 100:301–304.
14. Bolender, R. P., Paumgartner, D., Losa, G., et al. (1978): Integrated stereological and biochemical studies on hepatocytic membranes. 1: Membrane recoveries in subcellular fractions. *J. Cell Biol.*, 77:565–583.
15. Brun, A., and Brunk, U. (1970): Histochemical indications for lysosomal localization of heavy metals in normal rat brain and liver. *J. Histochem. Cytochem.*, 18:820–827.
16. Brunelle, A., Bi, Y.-A., Russell, B., Luy, L., Berkman, C., and Cashman, J. (1997): Characterization of two human flavin-containing monooxygenase (form 3) enzymes expressed in *Escherichia coli* as maltose binding protein fusion. *Drug Metab. Dispos.*, 25:1001–1007.
17. Burchell, B., and Coughtrie, M. W. H. (1989): UDP-glucuronosyltransferases. *Pharmacol. Ther.*, 43:261–289.
18. Burke, M. D., and Mayer, R. T. (1974): Ethoxyresorufin: Direct fluorimetric assay of a microsomal O-dealkylation which is preferentially inducible by 3-methylcholanthrene. *Drug Metab. Dispos.*, 2:583–588.
19. Burke, M. D., Thompson, S., Elcombe, C. R., Halpert, J., Haaparanta, T., and Mayer, R. T. (1985): Ethoxy-, pentoxy- and benzyloxyphenoxazones and homologues: A series of substrates to distinguish between different induced cytochromes P450. *Biochem. Pharmacol.*, 34:3337–3345.
20. Burnette, W. N. (1981): Western blotting: Electrophoretic transfer of proteins from sodium dodecyl sulfate-polyacrylamide gels to unmodified nitrocellulose and radiographic detection with antibody and radioiodinated protein A. *Anal. Biochem.*, 112:195–203.
21. Carmichael, N. G., and Fowler, B. A. (1979): Effects of separate and combined chronic mercuric chloride and sodium selenate administration in rats: Histological, ultrastructural and x-ray microanalytical studies of liver and kidney. *J. Environ. Pathol. Toxicol.*, 3:399–412.
22. Cashman, J. R. (1995): Structural and catalytic properties of the mammalian flavin-containing monooxygenase. *Chem. Res. Toxicol.*, 8:165–181
23. Cashman, J. R., Olsen, L. D., Nishioka, R. S., Gray, E. S., Bern, H. A. (1990): *S*-oxygenation of thiobencarb (Bolero) in hepatic preparations from striped bass (*Morone saxatilis*) and mammalian systems. *Chem. Res. Toxicol.*, 3:433–440.
24. Cederbaum, A. L., Lieber, C. S., and Rubin, E. (1974): The effect of acetaldehyde on mitochondrial function. *Arch. Biochem. Biophys.*, 161:26–39.
25. Chen, B., Burt, C. T., Goering, P. L., Fowler, B. A., and London, R. E. (1986): In vivo ^{31}P nuclear magnetic resonance studies of arsenite-induced changes in hepatic phosphate levels. *Biochem. Biophys. Res. Commun.*, 139:228–234.

26. Chen, Y. C., and Smith, J. B. (1992): A putative lectin-binding receptor mediates cadmium-evoked calcium release. *Toxicol. Appl. Pharmacol.*, 117:249–256.
27. Christensen, E. L., and Madsen, K. M. (1978): Renal age changes: Observations on the rat kidney cortex with special reference to structure and function of the lysosomal system in the proximal tubule. *Lab. Invest.*, 39:289–297.
28. Chuha, N.-H., and Schmidt, G. W. (1979): Transport of proteins into mitochondria and chloroplasts. *J. Cell Biol.*, 8:461–483.
29. Cleveland, D. W., Fischer, S. G., Kirschner, M. W., and Laemmli, U. K. (1977): Peptide mapping by limited proteolysis in sodium dodecyl sulfate and analysis by gel electrophoresis. *J. Biol. Chem.*, 252:1102–1106.
30. Conney, A. M. (1967): Pharmacological implications of microsomal enzyme induction. *Pharmacol. Rev.*, 19:317–366.
31. Cook, J. C., Murray, S. M., Frame, S. M., Hurtt, M. E. (1992): Induction of leydig cell adenomas by ammonium perfluorooctanoate: A possible endocrine-related mechanism. *Toxicol. Appl. Pharmacol.*, 113:209–217.
32. Coughtrie, M. W. H., Burchell, B., and Bend, J. R. (1986): A general assay for UDP glucuronosyltransferase activity using polar amino-cyano stationary phase HPLC and UDP [U-^{14}C] glucuronic acid. *Anal. Biochem.*, 159:198–205.
33. Curran, P. G., and DeGroot, L. J. (1991): The effect of hepatic enzyme-inducing drugs on thyroid hormones and the thyroid gland. *Endocrin. Rev.*, 12:135–150.
34. Dallner, G. (1978): Isolation of microsomal fractions by use of density gradients. In: *Methods in Enzymology, Volume 52, Biomembranes, Part C*, edited by S. Fleischer and L. Packer, pp. 71–83. Academic Press, New York.
35. Danscher, G., and Norgaard, J. O. R. (1983): Light microscopic visualization of colloidal gold on resin-embedded tissue. *J. Histochem. Cytochem.*, 31:1394–1398.
36. Dawson, J., Knowles, R. G., and Pogson, C. I. (1992): Measurement of glucuronidation by isolated rat liver cells using [^{14}C]fructose. *Biochem. Pharmacol.*, 43:971–978.
37. Delmen, W., Tomingas, R., and Roos, J. (1973): A modified method for the assay of benzo(a)pyrene hydroxylase. *Anal. Biochem.*, 53:373–383.
38. DePierre, J. W., Moron, M. S., Johannesen, K. A. M., and Ernster, L. (1975): A reliable, sensitive and convenient radioactive assay for benzpyrene monoxygenase. *Anal. Biochem.*, 63:470–484.
39. Deter, R. L. (1973): Electron microscopic evaluation of subcellular fractions obtained by ultracentrifugation. In: *Principles and Techniques of Electron Microscopy: Biological Applications, Vol. 3*, edited by M. A. Hayat, pp. 199–235. Van Nostrand Reinhold, New York.
40. Dohn, D. R., Quebbemann, A. J., Borch, R. F., and Anders, M. W. (1985): Enzymatic reaction of chlorotrifluoroethene with glutathione: ^{19}F NMR evidence for stereochemical control of the reaction. *Biochemistry*, 24:5137–5143.
41. Elliget, K. A., Phelps, P. C., and Trump, B. F. (1991): $HgCl_2$-induced alteration of actin filaments in cultured primary rat proximal tubule epithelial cells labeled with fluorescein phalloidin. *Cell Biol. Toxicol.*, 7:263–280.
42. Engelmann, G. L., Staecker, J. L., and Richardson, A. G. (1986): Effect of sodium butyrate on primary cultures of adult rat hepatocytes. *In Vitro Cell. Dev. Biol.*, 23:86–92.
43. Estabrook, R. W. (1967): Mitochondrial respiratory control and the polarographic measurement of ADP:O ratios. In: *Methods in Enzymology, Vol. 10*, edited by S. Colowick and N. O. Kaplan, pp. 41–47. Academic Press, New York.
44. Fowler, B. A., and Woods, J. S. (1977): Ultrastructural and biochemical changes in renal mitochondria during chronic oral methyl mercury exposure: The relationship to renal function. *Exp. Mol. Pathol.*, 27:403–412.
45. Fowler, B. A. (1983): The role of ultrastructural techniques in understanding mechanisms of metal-induced nephrotoxicity. *Fed. Proc.*, 42:2957–2964.
46. Fowler, B. A. (1980): Ultrasturctural morphometric/biochemical assessment of cellular toxicity. In: *Proceedings of the Symposium on the "Scientific Basis of Toxicity Assessment,"* edited by H. P. Witschi, pp. 211–218. Elsevier, Amsterdam.
47. Fowler, B. A., Brown, H. W., Lucier, G. W., and Beard, M. E. (1974): Mercury uptake by renal lysosomes of rats ingesting methyl mercury hydroxide: Ultrastructural observations and energy dispersive x-ray analysis. *Arch. Pathol.*, 98:297–301.
48. Fowler, B. A., Brown, H. W., Lucier, G. W., and Krigman, M. R. (1975): The effects of chronic oral methyl mercury exposure on the lysosome system of rat kidney: Morphometric and biochemical studies. *Lab. Invest.*, 32:313–322.
49. Fowler, B. A., Kardish, R., and Woods, J. S. (1983): Alterations of hepatic microsomal structure and function by acute indium administration: Ultrastructural morphometric and biochemical studies. *Lab. Invest.*, 48:471–478.
50. Fowler, B. A., and Nordberg, G. F. (1978): The renal toxicity of cadmium metallothionein: Morphometric and x-ray microanalytical studies. *Toxicol. Appl. Pharmacol.*, 46:609–623.
51. Fowler, B. A., and Woods, J. S. (1977): The transplacental toxicity of methyl mercury to fetal rat liver mitochondria: Morphometric and biochemical studies. *Lab. Invest.*, 36:122–130.
52. Fowler, B. A., and Woods, J. S. (1979): The effects of prolonged oral arsenate exposure on liver mitochondria of mice: Morphometric and biochemical studies. *Toxicol. Appl. Pharmacol.*, 50:177–187.
53. Fowler, B. A., and Woods, J. S. (1987): Metal and metalloid-induced porphyrinurias: Relationship to cell injury. *Ann. N. Y. Acad. Sci.*, 514:172–182.
54. Fowler, B. A., Woods, J. S., and Schiller, C. M. (1977): Ultrastructural and biochemical effects of prolonged oral arsenic exposure on liver mitochondria of rats. *Environ. Health Perspect.*, 19:197–204.
55. Fowler, B. A., Woods, J. S., and Schiller, C. M. (1979): Studies of hepatic mitochondrial structure and function: Morphometric and biochemical evaluation of in vivo perturbation by arsenate. *Lab. Invest.*, 41:313–320.
56. Frenkel, R., and Cobo-Frenkel, A. (1973): Differential characteristics of the cytosol and mitochondrial isozymes of malic enzyme from bovine brain: Effects of dicarboxylic acids and sulfhydryl reagents. *Arch. Biochem. Biophys.*, 158:323–330.
57. Friedman, F. K., Park, S. S., Song, B. J., Cheng, K. C., Fujino, T., and Gelboin, H. V. (1986): Monoclonal antibody-directed analysis of cytochrome P450. *Adv. Exp. Med. Biol.*, 197:145–154.
58. Frigg, M., and Rohr, H. P. (1976): Ultrastructural and stereological study on the effects of vitamin E on liver mitochondrial membranes. *Exp. Mol. Pathol.*, 24:236–243.
59. Fuchs, E., and Cleveland, D. W. (1998): A structural scaffolding of intermediate filaments in health and disease. *Science*, 279:514–519.
60. Goldfisher, S. (1965): The localization of copper in the pericanalicular granules (lysosomes) of liver in Wilson's disease (hepatolenticular degeneration (1)). *Ariz. J. Pathol.*, 46:977–983.
61. Goldstein, J. A., Hickman, P., Bergman, H., et al. (1977): Separation of pure polychlorinated isomers into two types of inducers on the basis of induction of cytochrome P-450 or P-448. *Chem. Biol. Interact.*, 17:69–87.
62. Goyer, R. A., and Krall, R. (1969): Ultrastructural transformation in mitochondria isolated from kidneys of normal and lead intoxicated rats. *J. Cell Biol.*, 41:393–400.

63. Graff, R. D., Falconer, M. M., Brown, D. L., and Reuhl, K. R. (1997): Altered sensitivity of post translationally modified microtubules to methylmercury in differentiating embryonal carcinoma-derived neurons. *Toxicol. Appl. Pharmacol.*, 144:215–224.
64. Green, S., Issemann, I., Tugwood, J. D. (1993): The molecular mechanism of peroxisome proliferator action. In: *Peroxisomes: Biology and Importance in Toxicology and Medicine*, edited by G. Gibson and B. Lake, pp. 99–118. Taylor & Francis, London.
65. Greenwalt, J. W. (1979): Survey and update of outer and inner mitochondrial membrane separation. In: *Methods in Enzymology*, edited by S. Fleischer and L. Packer, pp. 88–98. Academic Press, New York.
66. Grisham, J. W., Charlton, R. K., and Kaufman, D. G. (1978): In vitro assay of cytotoxicity with cultured liver: Accomplishments and possibilities. *Environ. Health Perspect.*, 25:161–172.
67. Grynkiewicz, G., Poenie, M., and Tsien, R. Y. (1985): A new generation of Ca^{2+} indicators with greatly improved fluorescence properties. *J. Biol. Chem.*, 260:3440–3450.
68. Guengerich, F. P., Dannan, G. A., Wright, S. T., Martin, M. V., and Kaminsky, L. S. (1982): Purification and characterization of liver microsomal cytochromes P450: Electrophoretic, spectral, catalytic, and immunochemical properties and inducibility of eight isozymes isolated from rats treated with phenobarbital and P-napthoflavone. *Biochemistry*, 21:6019–6030.
69. Guo, W.-X. A., Ziegler, D. M. (1991): Estimation of flavin-containing monooxygenase activities in crude tissue preparations by thiourea-dependent oxidation of thiocholine. *Anal. Biochem.*, 198:143–148.
70. Guzelian, P. S., Bissel, D. M., and Meyer, U. A. (1977): Drug metabolism in adult rat hepatocytes in primary monolayer culture. *Gastroenterology*, 72:1232–1239.
71. Guzelian, P. S., Li, D., Schuetz, E. G., et al. (1988): Sex change in cytochrome P-450 phenotype by growth hormone treatment of adult rat hepatocytes maintained in culture system on Matrigel. *Proc. Natl. Acad. Sci. USA*, 85:9783–9787.
72. Habig, W. H., Pabst, M. J., and Jakoby, W. B. (1974): Glutathione S-transferases: The first enzymatic step in mercapturic acid formation. *J. Biol. Chem.*, 249:7130–7139.
73. Hackenbrock, C. R. (1972): States of activity and structure in mitochondrial membranes. *Ann. N. Y. Acad. Sci.*, 195:492–505.
74. Hackenbrock, C. R. (1972): Energy-linked ultrastructural transformations in isolated liver mitochondria and mitoplasts: Preservation of configurations by freeze-cleaning compared to chemical fixations. *J. Cell Biol.*, 53:450–465.
75. Hackenbrock, C. R., and Caplan, A. I. (1969): Ion-induced ultrastructural transformations in isolated mitochondria: The energized uptake of calcium. *J. Cell Biol.*, 42:221–234.
76. Hadd, M. E., and Blickenstaff, R. T. (1969): *Conjugates of Steroid Hormones*. Academic Press, New York.
77. Hall, A. (1998): Rho GTPases and the actin cytoskeleton. *Science*, 279:509–514.
78. Hall, T. A. (1971): The microprobe assay of chemical elements. In: *Physical Techniques in Biological Research, Vol. IA*, edited by G. Oster, pp. 157–275. Academic Press, New York.
79. Harris, E. J., and Achenjang, F. M. (1977): Energy-dependent uptake of arsenite by rat liver mitochondria. *Biochem. J.*, 168:129–132.
80. Haschemeyer, R. H., and Myers, R. T. (1973): Negative staining. In: *Principles and Techniques of Electron Microscopy, Vol. 2*, edited by M. A. Hayat, pp. 99–147. Van Nostrand Reinhold, New York.
81. Hazelton, G. A., Hjelle, J. J., and Klaasen, C. D. (1985): Effects of butylated hydroxyanisole on hepatic glucuronidation capacity in mice. *Toxicol. Appl. Pharmacol.*, 78:280–290.
82. Hirokawa, N. (1998): Kinesin and dynein superfamily proteins and the mechanism of organelle transport. *Science*, 279:519–526.
83. Holtzman, D., and Hsu, J. S. (1976): Early effects of inorganic lead on immature rat brain mitochondrial respiration. *Pediatr. Res.*, 10:70–75.
84. Hsu, Y.-H. (1984): Immunogold for detection of antigen on nitrocellulose paper. *Anal. Biochem.*, 142:221–225.
85. Hunter, W. M. (1967): In: *Handbook of Experimental Immunology*, edited by D. M. Weir, p. 608. F. A. H. Davis, Philadelphia.
86. Illsley, N. P., Lamartiniere, C. A., and Lucier, G. W. (1979): Analysis of sex-specific changes in rat hepatic cytosol protein patterns using two-dimensional electrophoresis. *J. Appl. Biochem.*, 1:385–395.
87. Inouye, B., Ogino, Y., Ishida, T., Ogata, M., and Utsumi, K. (1978): Effects of phthalate esters on mitochondrial oxidative phosphorylation in the rat. *Toxicol. Appl. Pharmacol.*, 43:189–198.
88. Ioannides, C. (1996): *Cytochromes P450: Metabolic and Toxicological Aspects*. CRC Press, Boca Raton, FL.
89. Iyanagi, T., Watanabe, T., and Uchiyama, Y. (1989): The 3-methylcholanthrene-inducible UDP-glucuronosyltransferase deficiency in the hyperbilirubinemic rat (Gunn rat) is caused by a-1 frameshift mutation. *J. Biol. Chem.*, 264:21302–21307.
90. Johnson, E. F., Palmer, C. N. A., and Hsu, M.-H. (1996): The peroxisome proliferator-activated receptor: Transcriptional activation of the *CYP*4A6 gene. In: *Peroxisomes: Biology and Role in Toxicology and Disease*, edited by J. K. Reddy, T. Suga, G. P. Mannaerts, P. B. Lazarow, and S. Subrami, pp. 373–386. Annals of the New York Academy of Sciences, Vol. 804, The New York Academy of Sciences, New York.
91. Jacobs, E. E., Jacob, M., Sanadi, D. R., and Bradley, B. (1956): Uncoupling of oxidative phosphorylation by cadmium ion. *J. Biol. Chem.*, 223:147–156.
92. Kagawa, Y., and Kagawa, A. (1969): Accumulation of arsenate-76 by mitochondria. *J. Biochem.*, 65:105–112.
93. Kleinow, K. M., Droy, B. F., Buhler, D. R., and Williams, D. E. (1990): Interaction of carbon tetrachloride with β-napthoflavone-mediated cytochrome P450 induction in Winter flounder (*Pseudopleuronectes americanus*). *Toxicol. Appl. Pharmacol.*, 104:367–374.
94. Kreis, T., and Vale, R. (1993): *Guidebook to the Cytoskeletal and Motor Proteins*. Oxford University Press, New York.
95. Kreis, T., and Vale, R. (19): *Guidebook to the Extracellular Matrix and Adhesion Proteins*. Oxford University Press, New York.
96. Kupfer, K., and Levin, R. (1972): Monooxygenase drug metabolizing activity in $CaCl_2$-aggregated hepatic microsomes from rat liver. *Biochem. Biophys. Res. Commun.*, 47:611–618.
97. Koehler, J. K. (1973): The freeze-etching technique. In: *Principles and Techniques of Electron Microscopy, Vol. 2*, edited by M. A. Hayat, pp. 51–98. Van Nostrand Reinhold, New York.
98. Laemmli, U. K. (1970): Cleavage of structural proteins during the assembly of the head of bacteriophage T4. *Nature*, 227:680–685.
99. Lang, R. D. A., and Bronk, J. R. (1978): A study of rapid mitochondrial structural changes in vitro by spray-freeze-etching. *J. Cell Biol.*, 77:134–147.
100. Langer, T., and Neupert, W. (1996): Regulated protein degradation in mitochondria. *Experientia*, 52:1069–1076.
101. Lauwerys, R., and Buchet, J. P. (1972): Study on the mechanism of lysosome labilization by inorganic mercury in vitro. *Eur. J. Biochem.*, 26:535–542.
102. Lee, M. J., Harris, R. A., and Green, D. E. (1969): Action of fluorescein mercuric acetate upon mitochondrial-energized processes. *Biochem. Biophys. Res. Commun.*, 36:937–946.

103. Lee, S. S.-T., Pineau, T., Drago, J., Lee, E. J., Owens, J. W., et al. (1995): Targeted disruption of the α isoform of the peroxisome proliferator-activated receptor gene in mice results in abolishment of the pleiotropic effects of peroxisome proliferators. *Mol. Cell. Biol.*, 15:3012–3022.

104. Li, W., and Chou, L.-N. (1992): Effects of sodium arsenite on the cytoskeleton and cellular glutathione levels in cultured cells. *Toxicol. Appl. Pharmacol.*, 114:132–139.

105. Li, W., Zhao, Y., and Chou, I.-N. (1987): Paraquat-induced cytoskeletal injury in cultured cells. *Toxicol. Appl. Pharmacol.*, 91:96–106.

106. Liu, X., Kim, C. N., Yang, J., Jemmerson, R., and Wang, X. (1996): Induction of apoptot program in cell-frcc extracts: Requirement for dATP and cytochrome c. *Cell*, 86:147–156.

107. Lomri, N., Yang, Z., and Cashman, J. R. (1993): Regio- and stereoselective oxygenations by adult human liver flavin-containing monooxygenase 3: Comparison with forms 1 and 2. *Chem. Res. Toxicol.*, 6:800–807.

108. London, R. E., Galvin, M. J., Thompson, M., Jeffreys, L., and Mester, T. (1985): An approach to NMR studies of the metabolism of internal organs using surface coils. *J. Biochem. Biophys. Methods*, 11:21–29.

109. Lubet, R. A., Mayer, R. T., Cameron, J. W., Nims, R. W., Burke, M. D., Wolff, T., and Guengerich, F. P. (1985): Dealkylation of pentoxyresorufin: A rapid and sensitive assay for measuring induction of cytochrome(s) P-450 by phenobarbital and other xenobiotics in the rat. *Arch. Biochem. Biophys.*, 238:43–48.

110. Lucier, G. W., and McDaniel, O. S. (1977): Steroid and nonsteroid UDP glucuronidation of synthetic estrogens as steroids. *J. Steroid Biochem.*, 8:867–873.

111. Lucier, G. W., McDaniel, O. S., Hook, G. E. R., et al. (1973): TCDD-induced changes in rat liver microsomal enzymes. *Environ. Health Perspect.*, 5:199–211.

112. Maack, T. (1967): Changes in the activity of acid hydrolases during reabsorption of lysozyme. *J. Cell Biol.*, 35:268–273.

113. Maack, T., Mackensie, D. D. S., and Kinter, W. D. (1971): Intracellular pathways of renal reabsorption of lysozyme. *Am. J. Physiol.*, 221:1609–1616.

114. Madsen, K. M., and Christensen, E. L. (1978): Effects of mercury on lysosomal protein digestion in the kidney proximal tubule. *Lab. Invest.*, 38:165–174.

115. Magnaval, R., Batti, R., and Thiessard, J. (1975): Methyl mercury effect on rat liver mitochondrial dehydrogenase. *Experientia*, 31:406–407.

116. Mannaerts, G. P., and Van Veldhoven, P. P. (1993): Metabolic role of mammalian peroxisomes. In: *Peroxisomes: Biology and Importance in Toxicology and Medicine*, edited by G. Gibson and B. Lake, pp. 19–62. Taylor & Francis, London.

117. Matlib, M. A., and Srere, P. A. (1976): Oxidative properties of swollen rat liver mitochondria. *Arch. Biochem. Biophys.*, 174:705–712.

118. Mayer, R. T., Jermyn, J. W., Burke, M. D., and Prough, R. A. (1977): Methoxyresorufin as a substrate for the fluorometric assay of insect microsomal O-dealkylases. *Pestic. Biochem. Physiol.*, 7:349–354.

119. McClain, R. M. (1989): The significance of hepatic microsomal enzyme induction and altered thyroid function in rats: Implications for thyroid gland neoplasia. *Toxicol. Pathol.*, 17:294–306.

120. Mego, J. L., and Barnes, J. (1973): Inhibition of heterolysosome formation and function in mouse kidneys by injection of mercuric chloride. *Biochem. Pharmacol.*, 22:373–381.

121. Mego, J. L., and Cain, J. A. (1973): The effect of carbon tetrachloride on lysosome function in kidneys and livers of mice. *Biochem. Biophys. Acta*, 297:343–345.

122. Mego, J. L., and Cain, J. A. (1975): An effect of cadmium on heterolysosome formation and function in mice. *Biochem. Pharmacol.*, 24:1227–1232.

123. Mego, J. L., and Hayes, A. W. (1973): Effects of fungal toxins on uptake and degradation of formaldehyde-treated ^{125}I-albumin in mouse liver phagolysosomes. *Biochem. Pharmacol.*, 22:3275–3286.

124. Mermall, V., Post, P. L., and Mooseker, M. S. (1998): Unconventional myosins in cell movement, membrane traffic, and signal transduction. *Science*, 279:527–533.

125. Mills, J. W., and Ferm, V. H. (1989): Effect of cadmium on F-actin and microtubules of Madin-Darby canine kidney cells. *Toxicol. Appl. Pharmacol.*, 101:245–254.

126. Mills, J. W., Zhou, J.-H. Cardoza, L., and Ferm, V. H. (1992): Zinc alters actin filaments in Madin-Darby canine kidney cells. *Toxicol. Appl. Pharmacol.*, 116:92–100.

127. Mintz, H. A., Youen, D. H., Safer, B., et al. (1967): Morphological and biochemical studies of isolated mitochondria from fetal neonatal and adult liver and from neoplastic tissues. *J. Cell Biol.*, 34:513–525.

128. Moldeus, P., Hogberg, J., and Orrenius, S. (1978): Isolation and use of liver cells. In: *Methods in Enzymology, Volume 52, Biomembranes, Part C*, edited by S. Fleisher and L. Packer, pp. 60–70. Academic Press, New York.

129. Morgenstern, R., and DePierre, J. W. (1983): Microsomal glutathione transferase: Purification in unactivated form and further characterization of the activation process, substrate specificity and amino acid composition. *Eur. J. Biochem.*, 134:591–597.

130. Morgenstern, R., and DePierre, J. W. (1985): Microsomal glutathione transferase. In: *Reviews in Biochemical Toxicology, Vol. 7*, edited by E. Hodgson, J. R. Bend, and R. M. Philpot, pp. 67–104. Elsevier/North-Holland, New York.

131. Morgenstern, R., DePierre, J. W., and Ernster, L. (1979): Activation of microsomal glutathione S-transferase activity by sulfhydryl reagents. *Biochem. Biophys. Res. Commun.*, 87:657–663.

132. Morgenstern, R., Meijer, J., DePierre, J. W., and Ernster, L. (1980): Characterization of rat-liver microsomal glutathione S-transferase activity. *Eur. J. Biochem.*, 104:167–174.

133. Morgenstern, R., DePierre, J. W., and Ernster, L. (1980): Reversible activation of rat liver microsomal glutathione S-transferase activity by 5,5′-dithiobis(2-nitrobenzoic acid) and 2,2′-dipyridyl disulfide. *Acta Chem. Scand.*, B34:229–230.

134. Moser, H. W., Moser, A. B. (1996): Peroxisomal disorders: Overview. In: *Peroxisomes: Biology and Role in Toxicology and Disease*, edited by J. K. Reddy, T. Suga, G. P. Mannaerts, P. B. Lazarow, and S. Subramani, pp. 427–441. Annals of The New York Academy of Sciences, Vol. 804, The New York Academy of Science, New York.

135. Mulder, G. J., and van Doorn, A. B. (1975): A rapid NAD^+-linked assay for microsomal uridine diphosphate glucuronyltransferase of rat liver and some observations on substrate specificity of the enzyme. *Biochem. J.*, 151:131–140.

136. Muscatello, U., Guarriero-Bobyleva, V., Pasquali-Ronchetti, L., and Ballotti-Ricci, A. M. (1975): Configurational changes in isolated rat liver mitochondria as revealed by negative staining III: Modifications caused by uncoupling agents. *J. Ultrastruct. Res.*, 52:2–12.

137. Nebert, D. W., and Gielen, J. E. (1972): Genetic regulation of aryl hydrocarbon hydroxylase induction in the mouse. *Fed. Proc.*, 31:1315–1325.

138. Nebert, D. W., and Gelboin, H. V. (1968): Substrate-inducible microsomal aryl hydroxylase in mammalian cell culture. 1: Assay and properties of induced enzyme. *J. Biol. Chem.*, 243:6242–6249.

139. Nebert, D. W., Nelson, D. R., Adesnik, M., Coon, M. J., Estabrook, R. W., Gonzalez, F. J., Guengerich, F. P., Gunsalus, I. C., Johnson, E. F., Kemper, B., Levin, W., Phillips, I. R., Sato, R., and Waterman, M. R. (1989): The P-450 superfamily: Update on listing of all genes and recommended nomenclature of the chromosomal loci. *DNA*, 8:1–13.
140. Nelson, B. D. (1975): The action of cyclodiene pesticides on oxidative phosphorylation in rat liver mitochondria. *Biochem. Pharmacol.*, 24:1485–1490.
141. Nelson, D. R., Koymans, L., Kamataki, T., Stegeman, J. J., Feyereisen, R., et al. (1996): P-450 superfamily: Update on new sequences, gene mapping, accession numbers and nomenclature. *Pharmacogenetics*, 6:1–42.
142. Nitta, N., Maki, A., Smith, M., Phelps, P., Elliget, K., Berezesky, L., and Trump, B. F. (1989): The effects of oxidative stress on rat proximal tubular epithelium (PTE): A role for cytosolic cadmium [Ca^{2+}]. *Circ. Shock*, 27:333–334.
143. Ochoa, S. (1955): Malic dehydrogenase from pig heart. In: *Methods in Enzymology, Vol. 1*, edited by S. Colowick and N. O. Kaptan, pp. 735–739. Academic Press, New York.
144. Omura, T., and Sato, R. (1964): The carbon monoxide-binding pigment of liver microsomes. I: Evidence for its hemoprotein nature. *J. Biol. Chem.*, 239:2370–2378.
145. Papa, S., Guerrieri, F., Simone, S., et al. (1973): Mechanisms of respiration-driven proton translocation by the inner membrane. *Biochem. Biophys. Acta*, 292:20–28.
146. Parkinson, A. (1996): Biotransformation of xenobiotics. In: *Casarett & Doull's Toxicology: The Basic Science of Poisons*, edited by C. D. Klaassen, pp. 113–186. McGraw-Hill, New York.
147. Parr, D. R., and Harris, E. J. (1976): The effect of lead on the calcium-handling capacity of rat heart mitochondria. *Biochem. J.*, 158:289–294.
148. Poland, A., and Nebert, D. W. (1973): A sensitive radiometric assay of aminopyrine N-demethylation. *J. Pharmacol. Exp. Ther.*, 184:269–277.
149. Porter, T. D., and Coon, M. J. (1991): Cytochrome P450: Multiplicity of isoforms, substrates, and catalytic and regulatory mechanisms. *J. Biol. Chem.*, 266:13469–13472.
150. Pressman, B. C. (1967): Biological applications of ion-specific glass electrodes. In: *Methods in Enzymology, Vol. 10*, edited by S. Colowick and N. O. Kaplan, pp. 714–726. Academic Press, New York.
151. Prozialeck, W. C., and Niewenhuis, R. J. (1991): Cadmium (Cd 12) disrupts intercellular junctions and actin filaments in LLC-PK1 cells. *Toxicol. Appl. Pharmacol.*, 107:81–97.
152. Randolph, M. L. (1972): In: *Biological Application of Electron Spin Resonance*, edited by H. M. Swartz, J. R. Bolton, and D. C. Borg, p. 119. Wiley-Interscience, New York.
153. Raucy, J. L., Lasker, J. M. (1991): Isolation of P450 enzymes from human liver. *Meth. Enzymol.*, 206:577–587.
154. Ryan, P., Lu, Y. H., and Levin, W. (1978): Purification of cytochrome P450 and P448 from rat liver microsomes. In: *Methods in Enzymology, Volume 52, Biomembranes, Part C*, edited by S. Fleischer and L. Packer, pp. 117–123. Academic Press, New York.
155. Ryan, D. E., and Levin, W. (1990): Purification and characterization of hepatic microsomal cytochrome P450. *Pharmac. Ther.*, 45:153–239.
156. Ryan, D. E., Ramanathan, L., Iida, S., et al. (1985): Characterization of a major form of rat hepatic microsomal cytochrome P450 induced by isoniazid. *J. Biol. Chem.*, 260:6385–6393.
157. Schenkman, J. B., and Cinti, D. L. (1972): Hepatic mixed function oxidase activity in rapidly prepared microsomes. *Life Sci.*, 11:247–257.
158. Schenkman, J. B., and Cinti, D. L. (1978): Preparation of microsomes with calcium. In: *Methods in Enzymology, Volume 52, Biomembranes, Part C*, edited by S. Fleisher and L. Packer, pp. 83–89. Academic Press, New York.
159. Schnaitman, C., Erwin, V. G., and Greenawalt, J. W. (1967): The submitochondrial localization of monoamine oxidase, an enzymatic marker for the outer membrane of rat liver mitochondria. *J. Cell Biol.*, 32:719–735.
160. Selkirk, J. K., Croy, R. G., Roller, P. P., and Gelboin, H. V. (1974): High-pressure liquid chromatographic analysis of benzo(a)pyrene metabolism and covalent binding of the mechanism of action of 7,8-benzoflavone and 1,2-epoxy-3,3,3-trichloropropane. *Cancer Res.*, 34:3474–3480.
161. Shay, J. W. (1986): *Cell and Molecular Biology of the Cytoskeleton*. Plenum Press, New York.
162. Shibko, S., and Tappel, A. L. (1965): Rat kidney lysosomes: Isolation and properties. *Biochem. J.*, 95:731–741.
163. Sies, H. (1978): The use of perfusion of liver and other organs for the study of microsomal electron-transport and cytochrome P-450 systems. In: *Methods in Enzymology, Volume 52, Biomembranes, Part C*, edited by S. Fleischer and L. Packer, pp. 48–60. Academic Press, New York.
164. Silbergeld, E. K., and Fowler, B. A. (1987): Mechanisms of chemical-induced porphyrinopathies. *Ann. N. Y. Acad. Sci.*, 514:1–352.
165. Sirica, A. E., Richards, W., Tsukada, Y., et al. (1979): Fetal phenotypic expression by adult rat hepatocytes on collagen gel/nylon meshes. *Proc. Natl. Acad. Sci. USA*, 76:282–287.
166. Smith, M. W., Ambudkar, I. S., Phelps, P. C., Regec, A. L., and Trump, B. F. (1987): $HgCl_2$-induced changes in cytosolic Ca^{2+} of cultured rabbit renal tubular cells. *Biochem. Biophys. Acta*, 931:130–142.
167. Smith, M. W., Phelps, P. C., and Trump, B. F. (1991): Cytosolic Ca^{2+} deregulation and blebbing after $HgCl_2$ injury to cultured rabbit proximal tubule cells as determined by digital imaging microscopy. *Proc. Natl. Acad. Sci. USA*, 88:4926–4930.
168. Southard, J. H., and Nitisewojo, P. (1973): Loss of oxidative phosphorylation in mitochondria isolated from kidneys of mercury poisoned rats. *Biochem. Biophys. Res. Commun.*, 52:921–927.
169. Squibb, K. S., Pritchard, J. B., and Fowler, B. A. (1984): Cadmium metallothionein nephropathy: Ultrastructural/biochemical alterations and intra-cellular cadmium binding. *J. Pharmacol. Exp. Ther.*, 228:311–321.
170. Stabuli, W., Hess, R., and Weibel, E. R. (1969): Correlated morphometric and biochemical studies on the liver cell. II: Effects of phenobarbital on rat hepatocytes. *J. Cell Biol.*, 41:92–112.
171. Strik, J. J. T. W. A. (1987): Porphyrins in urine as an indication of exposure to chlorinated hydrocarbons. *Ann. N. Y. Acad. Sci.*, 514:219–221.
172. Stuve, J., and Galle, P. (1970): Role of mitochondria in the handling of gold by the kidney: A study by electron microscopy and electron probe microanalysis. *J. Cell Biol.*, 44:667–676.
173. Suda, T., Horiuchi, N., Ogata, E., et al. (1974): Prevention by metallothionein of cadmium-induced inhibition of vitamin D activation reaction in kidney. *FEBS Lett.*, 42:23–26.
174. Surek, B., and Latzko, E. (1984): Visualization of antigenic proteins blotted onto nitrocellulose using the immuno-gold staining (IGS)-method. *Biochem. Biophys. Res. Commun.*, 121:284–289.
175. Swann, J. D., Smith, M. W., Phelps, P. C., Maki, A., Berezesky, I. K., and Trump, B. F. (1991): Oxidative injury induces influx-dependent changes in intracellular calcium homeostasis. *Toxicol. Pathol.*, 19:128–137.
176. Tedeschi, H., and Harris, D. L. (1958): Some observations on the photometric estimation of mitochondrial volume. *Biochem. Biophys. Acta.*, 28:392–402.

177. Tephly, T. R., and Burchell, B. (1990): UDP-glucuronosyltransferases: A family of detoxifying enzymes. *Trends Pharmacol. Sci.*, 11:276–279.
178. Tephly, T., Green, M., Puig, J., and Irshaid, Y. (1988): Endogenous substrates for UDP-glucuronosyltransferases. *Xenobiotica*, 18:1201–1210.
179. Tephly, T. R., Townsend, M., and Green, M. D. (1989): UDP-glucuronosyltransferases in the metabolic disposition of xenobiotics. *Drug Metab. Rev.*, 20:689–695.
180. Tephly, T. R., Burchell, B. (1990): UDP-glucuronosyltransferases: A family of detoxifying enzymes. *Trends Pharmacol. Sci.*, 11:276–279.
181. Thomas, P. E., Reik, L. M., Maines, S. L., Bandiera, S., Ryan, D. E., and Levin, W. (1986): Antibodies as probes of cytochrome P450 isozymes. In: *Biological Reactive Intermediates III: Mechanisms of Action in Animal Models and Human Disease*, edited by J. Kocsis, D. Jollow, C. Witmer, J. Nelson, and R. Snyder, pp. 95–106. Plenum Press, New York.
182. Trump, B. F., and Berezesky, I. K. (1989): Cell injury and cell death: The role of ion deregulation. *Comments Toxicol.*, 3:47–67.
183. Trump, B. F., Berezesky, I. K., and Morris, A. C. (1989): New technique for the assessment of cellular injury: Digital imaging fluorescence microscopy (DIFM). In: *The Applications of Histochemistry to Toxicology*, edited by J. Baker and P. Bach. Chapman and Hall, London.
184. Trump, B. F., Jones, T. W., Elligett, K. A., Smith, M. W., Phelps, P. C., Maki, A., and Berezesky, I. K. (1990): Relation between toxicity and carcinogenesis in the kidney: An heuristic hypothesis. *Renal Failure*, 12:183–191.
185. Trump, B. F., Jones, T. W., Berezesky, I. K., Elliget, K. A., Smith, M. W., Phelps, P. C., Miyashita, M., Harris, C. C., and Jones, R. T. (1990): Cell toxicity and ion regulation in the kidney and bronchus: An hypothesis. In: *Basic Science in Toxicology: Proceedings of the Vth International Congress of Toxicology*, pp. 636–650.
186. Trump, B. F., Berezesky, I. K., Smith, M. W., Jones, R. T., Phelps, P. C., Miyashita, M., and Harris, C. C. (1992): The role of cytosolic calcium ($[Ca^{2+}]_i$) in injury and recovery from anoxia and ischemia. *Md. Med. J.*, 41:301–304.
187. Utesch, D., Molitor, E., Platt, K., and Oesch, F. (1991): Differential stabilization of cytochrome P-450 isozymes in primary cultures of adult rat liver parenchymal cells. *In Vitro Cell Dev. Biol.*, 27:858–863.
188. Van Cantfort, J. V., Graeve, J., and Gielen, J. E. (1977): Radioactive assay for aryl hydrocarbon hydroxylase: Improved method and biological importance. *Biochem. Biophys. Res. Commun.*, 79:505–512.
189. Vanden Heuvel, J. P. (1996): Perfluorodecanoic acid as a useful pharmacologic tool for the study of peroxisome proliferation. *Gen. Pharmacol.*, 27:1123–1129.
190. Vlasuk, G. P., and Walz, F. G., Jr. (1980): Liver endoplasmic reticulum polypeptides resolved by two dimensional gel electrophoresis. *Anal. Biochem.*, 105:112–120.
191. Völkl, A., and Fahimi, H. D. (1998): Isolation of peroxisomes. In: *Cell Biology: A Laboratory Manual, Vol. 2*, edited by J. E. Celis, pp. 87–92. Academic Press, San Diego.
192. Wakabayashi, M. (1970): P-Glucuronidase in metabolic hydrolysis. In: *Metabolic Conjugation and Metabolic Hydrolysis*, edited by W. Fishman, pp. 520–592. Academic Press, New York.
193. Wang, N., Gottesman, Willingham, M. C., Gottesman, M. M. and Maurizi, M. R. (1993): A human mitochondrial ATP-dependent protease that is highly homologous to bacterial Lon protease. *Proc. Natl. Acad. USA*, 90:11247–11251.
194. Wallace, D. C. (1999): Mitochondrial diseases in man and mouse. *Science*, 283:1482–1488.
195. Weibel, E. R., and Paumgartner, D. (1979): Integrated stereological and biochemical studies on hepatocyte membranes. II: Correction of section thickness effect and volume and surface density estimates. *J. Cell Biol.*, 77:584.
196. Weibel, E. R., Staubli, W., Gnagi, H. R., and Hess, F. A. (1969): Correlated morphometric and biochemical studies on the liver cell. I: Morphometric model, stereologic methods, and normal morphometric data for rat liver. *J. Cell Biol.*, 42:68–91.
197. Welton, A. F., and Aust, S. D. (1974): Multiplicity of cytochrome P-450 hemoproteins in rat liver microsomes. *Biochem. Biophys. Res. Commun.*, 56:898–906.
198. Werringloer, J. (1978): Assay of formaldehyde generated during microsomal oxidation reactions. In: *Methods in Enzymology, Volume 52, Biomembranes, Part C*, edited by S. Fleischer and L. Packer, pp. 297–302. Academic Press, New York.
199. Wiener, J., Loud, A. V., Kimberg, D. V., and Sprio, D. (1968): A quantitative description of cortisone-induced alterations in the ultrastructure of rat liver parenchymal cells. *J. Cell Biol.*, 37:47–62.
200. Williams, D. E., Masters, B. S. S., Lech, J. J., and Buhler, D. R. (1986): Sex differences in cytochrome P-450 isozyme composition and activity in kidney microsomes of mature rainbow trout. *Biochem. Phamacol.*, 35:2017–2023.
201. Williams, M. A. (1977): Stereological techniques. In: *Practical Methods in Electron Microscopy, Vol. 6*, edited by A. M. Glauert, pp. 1–84. North-Holland, Amsterdam.
202. Wolf, C. R., Berry, P. N., Nash, J. A., Green, T., and Lock, E. A. (1984): Role of microsomal and cytosolic glutathione S-transferases in the conjugation of hexachloro-1,3-butadiene and its possible relevance to toxicity. *J. Pharmacol. Exp. Ther.*, 228:202–210.
203. Woods, J. S., Eaton, D. L., and Lukens, C. B. (1984): Studies of porphyrin metabolism in the kidney: Effects of trace metals and glutathione on renal uroporphyrinogen decarboxylase. *Mol. Pharmacol.*, 26:336–341.
204. Woods, J. S., and Fowler, B. A. (1977): Effects of chronic arsenic exposure on hematopoietic function in adult mammalian liver. *Environ. Health Perspect.*, 19:209–213.
205. Woods, J. S., and Fowler, B. A. (1977): Renal porphyrinuria during chronic methyl mercury exposure. *J. Lab Clin. Med.*, 90:266–272.
206. Woods, J. S., and Fowler, B. A. (1978): Altered regulation of mammalian hepatic heme biosynthesis and urinary porphyrin excretion during prolonged exposure to sodium arsenate. *Toxicol. Appl. Pharmacol.*, 43:361–371.
207. Woods, J. S., and Fowler, B. A. (1986): Alterations of hepatocellular structure and function by thallium chloride: Ultrastructural morphometric and biochemical studies. *Toxicol. Appl. Pharmacol.*, 83:218–229.
208. Woods, J. S., and Fowler, B. A. (1987): Metal alterations of uroporphyrinogen decarboxylase and coproporphyrinogen oxidase. *Ann. N.Y. Acad. Sci.*, 514:55–64.
209. Woods, J. S., Fowler, B. A., and Eaton, D. L. (1984): Studies on the mechanisms of thallium-mediated inhibition of hepatic mixed function oxidase activity: Correlation with inhibition of NADPH-cytochrome with (P450) reductase. *Biochem. Pharmacol.*, 33:571–576.
210. Zhao, Y., Li, W., and Chou, I.-N. (1987): Cytoskeletal perturbation induced by herbicides, 2,4-dichlorophenoxyacetic acid (2,4-D) and 2,4,5-trichlorophenoxyacetic acid (2,4,5-T). *J. Toxicol. Environ. Health*, 20:11–26.
211. Ziegler, D. M. (1993): Recent studies on the structure and function of multisubstrate flavin-containing monooxygenases. *Annu. Rev. Pharmacol. Toxicol.*, 33:179–199.

Principles and Methods of Toxicology, Fourth Edition, edited by A. Wallace Hayes.
Taylor & Francis, Philadelphia © 2001.

Chapter 35

Analysis and Characterization of Enzymes and Nucleic Acids

F. Peter Guengerich

CYTOCHROME P450 AS A PROTOTYPE OF A MULTIGENE ENZYME FAMILY INVOLVED IN XENOBIOTIC METABOLISM

Knowledge in the field of toxicology has been advanced by investigations at a number of levels of organism complexity, including whole animal, organ perfusion, single cell, subcellular organelle, and isolated enzyme studies. The purpose of this article is to review in vitro assay procedures as well as techniques associated with preparation and utilization of purified enzymes important in toxicology. There is an emphasis on detailed procedures, because the field contains many general reviews but few examples to individuals about how to do certain experiments. In all four editions of this chapter, there has been an emphasis on providing detailed protypic protocols. However, it should be emphasized that space restrictions do not allow presentation of all relevant procedures.

Highly purified and recombinant systems have been used to address a number of questions that could not have been definitively answered otherwise. For instance, while a number of early studies strongly suggested the existence of multiple forms of cytochrome P450 and other drug-metabolizing enzymes, isolation and characterization studies provided the strongest evidence for this hypothesis and demonstrated exactly how the individual enzymes differ. Moreover, isolated and recombinant enzyme systems have been used to define the roles of individual enzymes in various metabolic processes.

Nearly 50 years have elapsed since the concept of bioactivation of chemicals to ultimate toxic forms was first developed (293). Such activation is now widely accepted as the first step leading to the toxic and carcinogenic effects of many chemicals. By far the most common mechanism for such activation is mixed-function oxidation by cytochrome P450. This enzyme system was really discovered in the late 1950s and has attracted

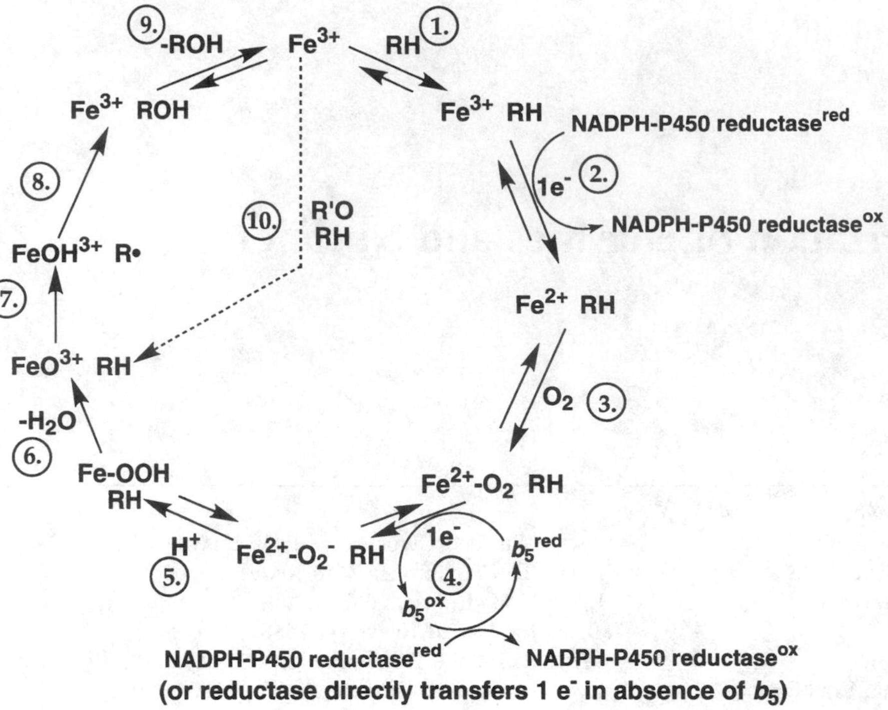

FIG. 35.1. Scheme of the catalytic mechanism of cytochrome P450. See references (141,143,161,162). Step 10 involves the use of artificial "oxygen surrogates" (e.g., iodosylbenzene, cumene hydroperoxide).

a great deal of interest ever since. A number of enzyme forms exist within each species; some are tissue specific as well as species specific. The different forms preferentially oxidize different substrates, and this specificity contributes to the preferential bioactivation and detoxication of chemicals by different enzyme forms.

With a general catalytic mechanism involving abstraction of electrons or hydrogen atoms followed by oxygen rebound (161), one can explain the apparently diverse oxidative reactions catalyzed by cytochrome P450, which can be classified as (a) carbon hydroxylation, (b) heteroatom oxygenation, (c) heteroatom release (dealkylation), (d) epoxidation, (e) oxidative group migration, and (f) suicidal inactivation by olefins (Figures 35.1 and 35.2). These basic mechanisms can also explain the suicidal inactivation observed with other substrates such as cyclopropyl heteroatoms and aminobenztriazole; variation of structural features has allowed the selective inactivation of individual enzymes by mechanism-based (suicide) inhibitors (321). Cytochrome P450 also reduces some compounds such as azo dyes, CCl_4, and *N*-oxides.

The total number of cytochrome P450 substrates easily runs into the thousands (460). The broad specificity is due in part to the existence of multiple forms, but even a single purified form (e.g., human P450 3A4) has been shown to oxidize >100 different substrates (145). The active site must be large enough to accommodate all of these. However, a number of larger substrates such as warfarin, testosterone, and debrisoquine and other drugs are stereo- and regioselectively oxidized, indicating that the binding sites do really have some distinct features. The smaller substrates apparently fit into these sites, and the sites of oxidation on them are probably governed more by chemical than spatial (physical) properties (Figure 35.3 and Table 35.1). The view is widespread that cytochrome P450 enzymes exist for the metabolism of specific endogenous substrates such as fatty acids, steroids, and eicosanoids; however, others feel that the purpose of these enzymes is the clearance of ingested foreign chemicals (terpenes, alkaloids, pyrolysis products, etc.) (207). There is validity in both viewpoints, and good cases for individual enzymes with each function may be found.

One of the major reasons for the widespread study of cytochrome P450 is that these enzymes are involved in the activation and detoxication of xenobiotics. However, much of the evidence has been circumstantial. The literature is filled with examples in which one can directly demonstrate covalent binding of a chemical to protein or DNA with a cytochrome P450 or produce mutations in bacterial strains. Known cytochrome P450-generated metabolites can be found bound to macromolecules in vivo, and in some cases administration of known products of cytochrome P450 oxidation can produce the toxicity observed with the parent substrate (e.g., fluoroxene and trifluoroacetic acid) (160). Often the administration of chemicals that are known to induce (or inhibit) forms of cytochrome P450 can increase or decrease the toxicity of a certain chemical in experimental animals. The usefulness of this approach is limited because of the ability of these chemicals to alter the levels of several cytochromes P450 concomitantly, alter the content of

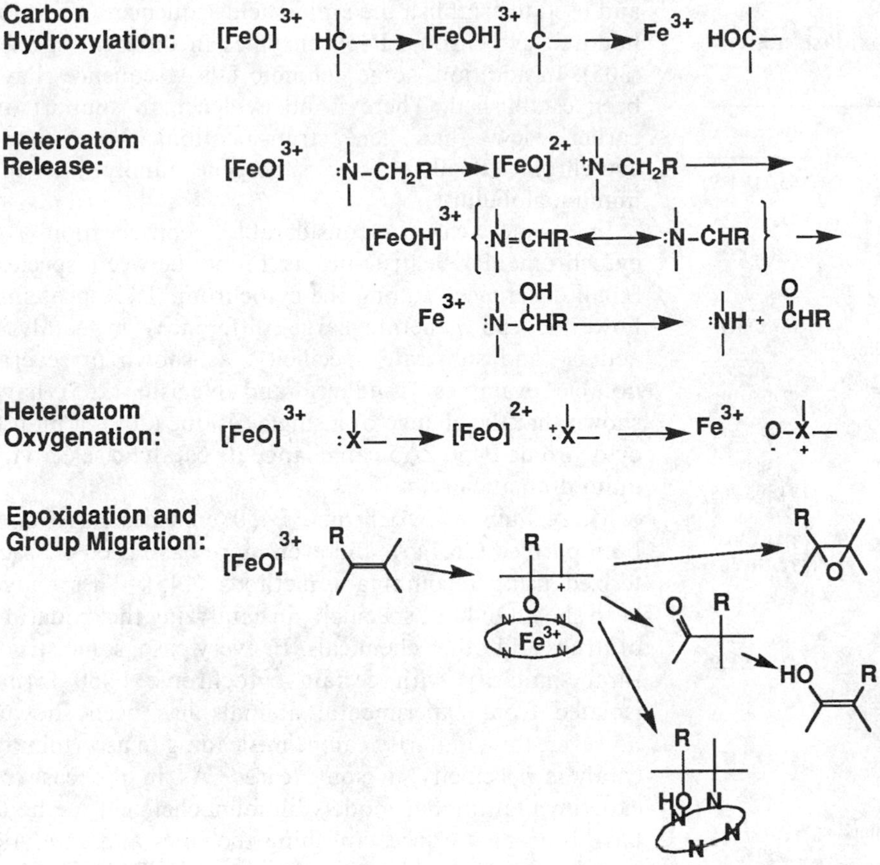

FIG. 35.2. Mechanisms of cytochrome P450 reactions rationalized by abstraction of electrons and hydrogen atoms (161). See text for discussion.

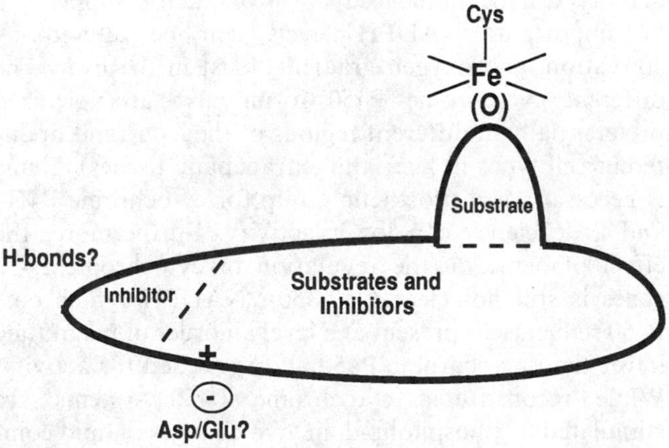

FIG. 35.3. Depiction of the active site of human cytochrome P450 2D6. Bufuralol is shown in the active center. The distance between the nonbonding electrons of the basic nitrogen and the site of hydroxylation of the substrate is ~5–7 Å (203,242,400,461). Evidence has been presented that the protein residue with the anionic charge is Asp-301 (97).

other enzymes, and affect physiological parameters (e.g., blood flow) that contribute to endpoints under consideration. The problem of not knowing exactly how metabolites exert toxic effects also obfuscates the problem. While cytochromes P450 do appear to play a role in the generation of ultimate toxicants and carcinogens, efforts to show the importance of changes in the composition of individual forms on the effects are still not very clear.

Today no doubt exists concerning the existence of distinct forms of cytochrome P450 in experimental animals or humans. More than 50 gene products have been characterized in rats and at least 40 in humans (307). See the internet sites http://drnelson.utmem.edu/nelsonhomepage.html and http://base.icgeb.trieste.it:80/p450 for more current information regarding cytochrome P450 genes and sequences. Consideration of the available sequences of the human genome argues that most (but not all) human cytochrome P450 genes are known. The purified proteins differ in electrophoretic properties, immunochemical aspects, primary sequence, and other criteria, including catalytic specificity. The assignment of the proteins as separate gene products has been done using recombinant DNA technology as well as amino acid sequencing. cDNAs have been cloned

Table 35.1
Survey of microsomal mixed-function oxidase activities and assays

Substrate	Methods	References
Acetanilide	Colorimetric	(163,243,419)
	Radiometric TLC	
	HPLC	
2-Acetylaminofluorene	Colorimetric	(34)
	Radiometric TLC	
	HPLC	
Aflatoxin B_1	HPLC	(348,349)
	Radiometric (covalent binding)	
Alkanes	Radiometric	(270,310)
	NADPH oxidation	
	GLC	
Aminopyrine	Radiometric	(342)
Aniline	Colorimetric	(184,196,268)
	Radiometric	
Benzo[a]pyrene	Fluorimetric	(81–83,304)
		(372,410,463)
	Radiometric	
	HPLC	
	Mutagenic	
Benzphetamine	Colorimetric	(147,310,359)
	Radiometric	
	NADPH oxidation	
	Oxygen uptake	
Biphenyl	Fluorimetric	(43,44,347)
	GLC	
	TLC	
Carbon disulfide	Radiometric (covalent binding)	(79)
Carbon tetrachloride	Radiometric (covalent binding)	(391)
Chlorcyclizine	Radioisotope derivative	(244)
Chloroform	GLC	(391)
Dimethylnitrosamine	Colorimetric	(55,70)
	Radiometric	
	Mutagenic	
7-Ethoxycoumarin	Fluorimetric	(126,429)
Ethanol	Colorimetric	
	Radiometric	(296)
	GLC	
	GC/mass spectrometry	(23)
Ethoxyresorufin	Fluorimetric	(43)
Furans	Radiometric (covalent binding)	(127,129)
Lauric acid	Radiometric	(101,270)
	HPLC	
Methyl azodyes	Colorimetric	(129,225,392)
	Radiometric (covalent binding)	
	GLC	
N-Methylchloroaniline	Fluorescent derivation	(431)
N-Nitrosopyrrolidine	HPLC	(52)
Parathion	Radiometric (TLC)	(226,227)
	Radiometric (covalent binding)	
Pyrroles	Radiometric (covalent binding)	(168)
Pyrrolizidine alkaloids	Colorimetric	(129)
	HPLC	
Terpenes	GLC	(263)
Testosterone	Radiometric	(64,415,446)
	TLC	
	HPLC	
Thioureas	TLC	(345)
	Oxygen uptake	
Vinyl chloride	Radiometric	(175)
	Mutagenic	(279)
Warfarin	HPLC	(103,228–230)
Zoxazolamine	Radiometric	(418)

and used to establish the amino acid sequences of several hundred cytochrome P450 enzymes in different species (305). In addition, some genomic DNA sequences have been established. There is no evidence to support an earlier view that gene translocations have made cytochrome P450 a huge supergene family like the immunoglobulins.

In some cases, considerable conservation of cytochrome P450 structure is found between species. Small differences among the cytochrome P450 proteins, however, can generate large differences in catalytic activity and substrate specificity, as shown in several notable examples. Lindberg and Negishi (265) have shown that the change of a single residue (209) of mouse cytochrome P450 2A5 can change its catalytic selectivity quite dramatically.

Many human cytochrome P450 enzymes have now been purified (86,145), and even more have been characterized using recombinant methods (145). These have been shown to have specificity in catalyzing the oxidation of drugs and other chemicals. In every case, some structural similarity with certain cytochrome P450 forms isolated from experimental animals has been shown; however, this similarity can be misleading in ascertaining catalytic specificity in some cases. As in the case of experimental animal models, immunochemical methods have been of use in establishing the roles and catalytic specificities of the human cytochromes P450. Probes for cytochromes P450 from experimental animals have been used to identify cDNAs for human cytochromes P450 and derive their sequences.

There are several levels at which overall catalytic activity can be influenced (137). Cofactor supply can be important: NADPH levels can be altered by starvation, and oxygen gradients exist in the liver. The different cytochrome P450 forms also are localized preferentially in different regions of the liver (and in different cell types in liver and extrahepatic tissues). Heme is necessary as a prosthetic group for cytochrome P450, and a deficiency can lower activity. Furthermore, the effect of heme on the regulation of cytochrome P450 genes is still not clear (212,350). NADPH-cytochrome P450 reductase is present at a level an order of magnitude lower than cytochrome P450 and is needed for activity. While reconstituted cytochrome P450 systems are stimulated by phospholipid, in vivo changes in lipid composition probably do not have any significant effect in most cases (301) with the very notable exception of the P450 3A family enzymes (179,200).

In experimental animals the major way in which activities, or at least rather specific catalytic activities, are modulated is via changes in the amounts of individual cytochrome P450 forms present (138,306). Such changes have been clearly demonstrated to involve de novo synthesis and often involve specific increases in rates of nuclear DNA transcription. The list of cytochrome P450 inducers is nearly as long as the list of substrates. Only in a few cases does one see induction of only one cytochrome P450; more commonly several are induced. In some cases the level of one of these proteins is depressed while others are induced (75,152). Several of the rodent liver cytochromes P450 are also regulated by steroid hormones. There are two aspects of such modulation (apparently by androgens in both sexes), neonatal imprinting and a later maintenance effect (77,446). Most of the cytochrome P450 proteins have similar half-lives (about 24 h); however, some evidence exists for a stabilizing effect of certain classic "inducers" on mRNA stability. In the case of some cytochromes P450 evidence exists for intracellular receptors (444).

Another aspect of regulation is polymorphism, which is observed with certain catalytic activities in both experimental animals and humans. While most of the catalytic activities associated with cytochromes P450 are affected at least somewhat by environmental factors, genetic polymorphisms are distinct and not as readily influenced by other factors. These can be produced by variations in structural genes (coding or regulatory regions) or by variations in other proteins which regulate expression. Several polymorphisms have been mapped to chromosomes in rats and mice, and structural details underlying the polymorphisms have been elucidated in many cases. In humans, genetic polymorphisms in the metabolism of certain drugs have been identified. Correlations have been made between individuals expressing individual phenotypes (or genotypes) and susceptibility to chemical carcinogenesis. Low activity of the steriodogenic P450s can lead to lethality or debilitating diseases (457).

While the cytochromes P450 have received considerable attention, one should realize that the existence of "isozymes" (or more appropriately, enzymes) in a family) is not unusual, nor is a multigene family. These probably occur with many enzymes, including some others which are involved in other aspects of metabolism of xenobiotic chemicals. For instance, at least 19 different forms of human glutathione (GSH) *S*-transferase exist and have been shown to be distinct gene products (8). Again, the catalytic specificities of these enzyme forms differ, and many are under differential regulatory control. Considerable evidence supports the view that many forms of UDP-glucuronosyl transferase exist (42), and the epoxide hydrolases are distinct gene products (180). Distinct forms of microsomal flavin-containing monooxygenase are found in different tissues, specifically the liver and lung (458). However, in some of the other instances only one gene appears to be involved [e.g., NADPH-cytochrome P450 reductase (343)].

ROLES OF CYTOCHROMES P450 AND OTHER ENZYMES IN BIOACTIVATION AND DETOXICATION

As mentioned above, cytochrome P450-catalyzed oxidation can result in either the bioactivation or detoxication of a potential toxicant. In general, reduction reactions catalyzed by either cytochrome P450 or NADPH-cytochrome P450 usually lead to more reactive products. Oxidations by other enzymes (i.e., microsomal flavin-containing monooxygenase, alcohol and aldehyde dehydrogenases) can also result in either bioactivation or detoxication. For instance, oxidation of allylic alcohols by alcohol dehydrogenase yields acrolein derivatives, which react rapidly with "soft" nucleophiles. In classical drug metabolism, oxidation–reduction reactions are usually considered Phase I and conjugation reactions, which usually follow after oxidation or reduction, are termed Phase II. The majority of these Phase II conjugation processes detoxicate chemicals, and, therefore, increases in the concentrations of the proteins that catalyze these reactions or increases in the concentrations of cofactors (cosubstrate) tend to render an organism at decreased risk to pro-toxicants. However, many exceptions to this generalism can be found. For example, epoxide hydrolase action on benzo[*a*]pyrene 7,8-oxide leads to formation of a substrate that is efficiently converted to 7,8-dihydroxy-7,8-dihydro-9,10-oxo-benzo[*a*]pyrene, which reacts rapidly with DNA and is a potent mutagen and carcinogen. GSH transferase, as indicated later, can activate *vic*-dihaloalkanes to yield DNA damage. Glucuronides formed by action of UDP-glucuronosyl transferase on hydroxylamines, which can break down in the acidic environment of the bladder to release nitrenium ions to alkylate DNA. Thus, we see that metabolic transformations must be viewed in a global manner to put the importance of individual steps into context.

What can studies on metabolic transformations tell us about the toxicity of chemicals? Comparison of the actions of a series of small industrial compounds provides some examples:

$$\text{A crylonitrile } CH_2 = CH - CN$$
$$\text{Vinyl chloride } CH_2 = CH - Cl$$
$$\text{Ethylene dibromide } Br - CH_2 - CH_2 - Br$$

The first, acrylonitrile, is acutely toxic and also causes several types of general toxicity problems when administered at high doses in chronic studies (i.e., nausea, weight loss, gastric disturbances, etc.). The compound is not particularly carcinogenic, causing only tumors of the forestomach, brain, and possibly Zymbal's gland at high doses. These actions can be understood when the various pathways for acrylonitrile are measured using in vitro

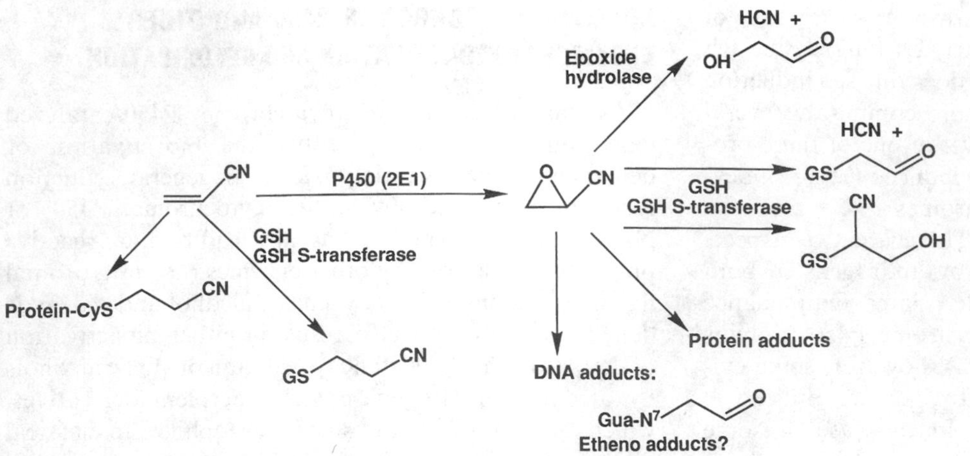

FIG. 35.4. Proposed scheme for metabolism of acrylonitrile (108).

assays. Acrylonitrile reacts rapidly and nonenzymatically with sulfhydryls, both in proteins and in GSH (Figure 35.4). Conjugation with GSH is the major fate of acrylonitrile and renders it inocuous. Reaction with proteins is considerable and probably accounts for the toxic effects of acrylonitrile. About 10% of acrylonitrile is oxidized by cytochrome P450 to its epoxide, which can (a) release cyanide (which does not appear to play a role in toxicity), (b) be conjugated with GSH, (c) alkylate proteins, or (d) alkylate nucleic acids. The extent of the latter reaction does not appear to be very great, consistent with the relatively low tumorigenic potential of acrylonitrile (108,154,188).

Vinyl chloride appears similar in structure to acrylonitrile at first glance but behaves quite differently. Only very high doses are acutely toxic, and this toxicity is probably unrelated to metabolism. However, vinyl chloride is carcinogenic, causing a peculiar hemangiosarcoma that is almost unique to vinyl chloride production workers and can be reproduced in laboratory animals. Unlike acrylonitrile, vinyl chloride does not react directly with thiols and its metabolism proceeds strictly through oxidation. The epoxide 1-chlorooxirane (2-chloroethylene oxide) can react with nucleic acids to form several lesions, including 1,N^6-ethenoadenine, N^3,4-ethenocytosine, 1,N^2-ethenoguanine, 7-hydroxy-1,N^2-ethanoguanine (5,6,7,9-tetrahydro-7-hydroxy-9-oxoimidazo[1,2-*a*]purine), N^2,3-ethenoguanine, and N^7-(2-oxoethyl)guanine (300). Which of these is most intimately related to tumorigenesis is yet unclear, although evidence favors the etheno adducts (19,252). The epoxide also spontaneously rearranges to form 2-chloroacetaldehyde (264,294), which is more like acrylonitrile, reacting rapidly and nonenzymatically with GSH and protein thiols. It reacts only slowly with nucleic acids and is probably not relevant to tumor initiation. The major site of vinyl chloride oxidation is the parenchymal cells of the liver. However, hepatic tumors originate in the reticuloendothelial cells, which have little if any oxidation capacity. A possible explanation is that the epoxide is formed in the parenchymal cells and is stable enough to migrate to other cells [some experimental evidence supports this view (167)]; the differential susceptivity to the alkylating agent may be explained by variations in rates of DNA adduct repair among the cell types.

The next compound to consider in this series is ethylene dibromide (1,2-dibromoethane). This compound causes kidney toxicity and is carcinogenic at a number of sites. Oxidation by cytochrome P450 (especially P450 2E1) (159) yields 2-bromoacetaldehyde, which behaves in the same way as 2-chloroacetaldehyde (vide supra) and depletes sulfhydryls. GSH transferase-catalyzed conjugation of ethylene dibromide with GSH also occurs; the ratio of ethylene dibromide metabolized through the oxidative and conjugative pathways is $\sim 4:1$ in rats (430). In this case the GSH conjugate is unstable, however, because of the leaving group still present (Br) (Figure 35.5). Nonenzymatic dehydrohalogenation produces an episulfonium (thiiranium) ion (336), which also has several fates. If it is hydrolyzed, *S*-(2-hydroxyethyl)-GSH is formed, and this inocuous product is degraded and excreted. The putative episulfonium ion can also react with another GSH to form the ethylene-bis-GSH adduct, which is also inocuous. Another possibility is elimination to yield GSSG (oxidized GSH) plus ethylene, another mode of detoxication (59). However, another reaction (of the episulfonium ion) occurs with DNA to yield *S*-[2-(N^7-guanyl)ethyl] GSH as the major product (322). This GSH pathway appears to be related to carcinogenesis because in vitro DNA binding and mutagenesis are much more dependent upon cytosolic than microsomal enzymes, and in vivo studies also support this view (202,241). Thus, we see here that GSH conjugation can become a major bioactivation pathway.

The three compounds just described share some apparent features of similarity, yet further analysis indicates that they differ widely in terms of their chemical

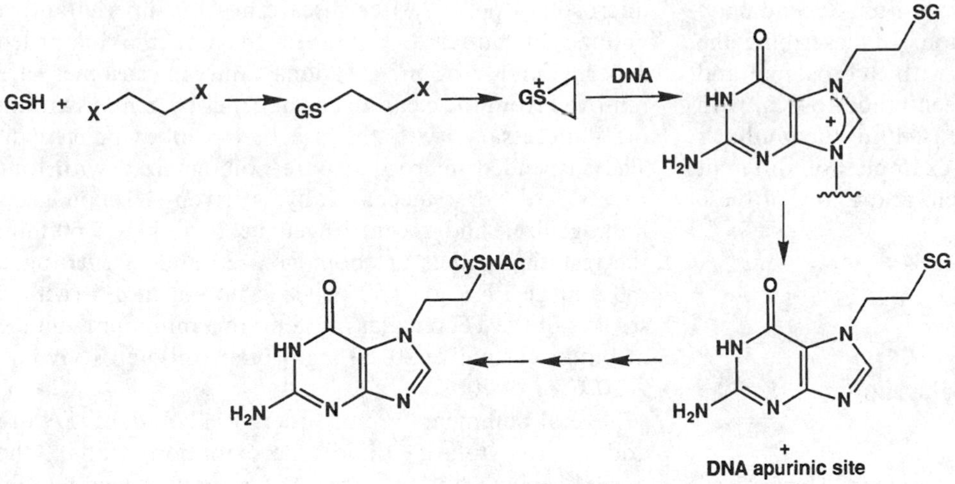

FIG. 35.5. Scheme depicting formation of the major DNA adduct from ethylene dihalides and the degradation of the adduct (202,236).

properties, the manner in which they are handled by the body, and the biological effects that are exerted. Much of our understanding of these chemicals has come from in vitro studies using assays of the type that are described here. But what can we learn from studies that focus on identification and quantitation of individual enzymes?

One example involves the suppression of a particular cytochrome P450 in rat liver. Polycyclic hydrocarbons such as 3-methylcholanthrene, β-naphthoflavone, and isosafrole induce increased synthesis of at least two forms of cytochrome P450 in rat liver, P450 1A1 and P450 1A2. Increases in microsomal catalytic activities following administration of such compounds have generally been held to support the involvement of these inducible forms in a particular transformation, and in many in vivo studies alterations in acute toxicity of compounds by these inducers has been interpreted in the same terms. The levels of a particular form of cytochrome P450, P450 2C11 (measured with a specific antibody), are decreased when compounds are given to rats that induce P450 1A1 and P450 1A2 (also measured immunochemically) (152). The decrease is as much as 10-fold when certain polybrominated biphenyl congeners are administered to rats (75). P450 2C11 is male specific (77,446) and is responsible for the bulk of certain catalytic activities, including testosterone 2α-hydroxylation (446) and (in rats) generation of the most toxic products of aflatoxin B_1 (383). If formation of a reactive metabolite is mediated by P450 2C11 and neither P450 1A1 nor P450 1A2 acts on the parent compound, then one might (without knowledge of the complexity of the situation) conclude that if administration of polycyclic hydrocarbons such as 3-methylcholanthrene to rats decreases toxicity and total cytochrome P450 levels, cytochrome P450 must have a detoxicating role in metabolism. As we see here, that view could be totally erroneous and lead to unsound predictions for other situations. The basic information underlying the phenomenon presented here, that is, the suppression of individual forms of cytochrome P450, could only have been obtained with the use of purification, enzyme reconstitution, and immunochemical techniques.

Do the identification and assay of individual enzyme forms have any relevance in clinical settings? The answer is yes, and several examples are given from the realm of drug toxicity and therapeutic effectiveness. The antituberculosis drug rifampicin is a potent enzyme inducer and appears to increase the cytochrome P450 form(s) that catalyzes the A ring hydroxylation of 17α-ethynylestradiol, the major estrogenic component of oral contraceptives. Such oxidation renders the drug ineffective, and cases have been reported where rifampicin administration to women has led to unanticipated pregnancies (33). In other clinical cases, genetic deficiency in cytochrome P450 2D6 has led to the accumulation of certain drugs and the production of undesirable side effects, such as the neuropathy associated with perhexiline and captopril-induced agranulocytosis (375). The suggestion has been made that dangers associated with chemicals in the environment may be affected by some of the same factors that influence drug clearance; for instance, individuals lacking cytochrome P450 2D6 have been suggested to be less prone to tumors related to aflatoxin B_1 and cigarette smoking (15,193), although the findings are controversial. The molecular basis of the cytochrome P450 2D6 polymorphism is now known (123). We can now understand some interindividual variations in response to potentially toxic chemicals at the level of specific sequence changes. Toward this end, methods in enzymology are necessary and need to be applied in the field of toxicology.

For many of the enzymes under consideration here, a number of purification techniques have been developed independently, and the reader is referred to the original literature for details. Different procedures for the purification of each enzyme have often been developed; the choice of the purification scheme will often depend upon the investigator's research situation. In describing the general assay procedures for use with microsomal and purified fractions, an effort has been made to deal with some of those most commonly used in the author's and other laboratories. Selected examples of different types of assay procedures are given, and many of these can be adapted to other uses.

ANALYTICAL PROCEDURES

Preparation of Microsomal and Cytosolic Fractions

Microsomal fractions have been prepared from a variety of tissues using procedures developed for use with rat liver. The following procedure (127,432) has been found to be useful in this laboratory for the preparation of microsomes and cytosol from a variety of animal and human tissues.

Reagents

1. 1.15% KCl (w/v).
2. Buffer A: 0.10 *M* Tris-acetate buffer (pH 7.4) containing 0.10 *M* KCl, 1.0 m*M* ethylenediamine tetraacetatic acid (EDTA), and 20 μM butylated hydroxytoluene (BHT).
3. Buffer B: 0.10 *M* potassium pyrophosphate buffer (pH 7.4) containing 1.0 m*M* EDTA and 20 μM BHT.
4. Buffer C: 10 m*M* Tris-acetate buffer (pH 7.4) containing 1.0 m*M* EDTA and 20% glycerol (w/v).

Rats are killed by CO_2 asphyxiation in a closed container, in line with current animal care regulations. Livers are excised and placed in cold 1.15% KCl. All subsequent steps are carried out at 0 to 4°C. The livers are trimmed of debris and washed with 1.15% KCl; if one desires, hemoglobin contamination can be lowered by perfusing livers with KCl via the portal vein. The livers are blotted and weighed, placed in four times that weight of buffer A, and minced with scissors. The method of homogenization depends upon the scale of the preparation. If only a few livers are used, a mechanically driven Teflon–glass homogenizer (four to five vertical passes) is preferred. For larger preparations, two 40-sec bursts in a Waring blender are more efficient.

The homogenate is centrifuged at $10^4 \times g$ for 20 min and the supernatant fraction is saved. If the yield of microsomes is a factor, the precipitate can be homogenized in buffer A again and recentrifuged to obtain additional supernatant fraction. The supernatant fraction is centrifuged for 60 min at $10^5 \times g$ (3.5×10^4 rpm in a Beckman 45 Ti rotor) to yield a microsomal pellet. After discarding the supernatant, a volume of buffer B equal to that of the discarded supernatant fraction is added and microsomes are removed from the clear glycogen pellet by gentle swirling or, if necessary, with the use of a rubber policeman. The suspended microsomes are homogenized with four passes of a mechanically driven Teflon–glass homogenizer and recentrifuged at $10^5 \times g$ for 60 min; the resulting pellets are homogenized and recentrifuged (60 min at $10^5 \times g$). The pellet is homogenized (with 4 strokes of the Teflon–glass system) in a minimum volume of buffer C (to give 20–50 mg protein/ml) and stored at −20°C or −70°C.

Several comments are in order. BHT and EDTA are added to retard lipid peroxidation, and the pyrophosphate buffer is useful in removing hemoglobin and nucleic acids (432). If proteases are a potential problem, as is often the case in extrahepatic tissues, phenylmethylsulfonyl fluoride (PMSF) or other protease inhibitors can be used. PMSF is unstable in water; a stock 0.10 *M* solution should be prepared in absolute ethanol or *n*-propanol, stored at −20°C, and added to buffers to give a final concentration of 0.10 m*M* immediately prior to their use. The use of dithiothreitol has also been reported to be necessary for the preparation of functional rat colon microsomes (102).

Buffers containing 0.25 *M* sucrose can be substituted for buffers A and B in the procedure. If an ultracentrifuge is not available, precipitation of microsomes can be done at lower speeds when 8 m*M* $CaCl_2$ is added to buffers (58). Alternatively, microsomes can be isolated using gel exclusion chromatography (216,406). More sophisticated techniques are available for the separation of rough and smooth endoplasmic reticulum and Golgi apparatus fractions. Some workers prefer to store microsomes as frozen pellets. For many enzyme activities, microsomes are functional for at least several months when stored either as pellets or frozen in buffer C.

Essentially identical procedures are routinely used to prepare microsomes and cytosol from livers of other animals, including humans (440). In work with human samples, it is advisable to have individual samples tested for human immunodeficiency virus (HIV) and hepatitis B (and other forms of hepatitis) if at all possible before proceeding. Personnel should be immunized against hepatitis B. In handling tissues, personnel should handle all samples as if a virus such as HIV or hepatitis might be present. Good hygiene is essential, and some key practices used in this laboratory include: (a) delivery of all residual tissue materials to the infectious diseases division of the institution for incineration or other disposal, (b) carrying out early steps that produce aerosols (homogenization, balancing of tubes containing crude fractions) in a fume hood, (c) absolutely *no* mouth pipetting, (d) prompt disposal of blotters over which all work has been done, (e) use of disposable plastic gloves and other protective clothing, (f) disinfection of glassware, knives, and so on in an appropriate detergent (e.g., O-Syl Disinfectant Detergent, National Laboratories, Lehn and Fink Industrial Products of Sterling Drug, Montvale, NJ—containing *o*-benzyl-*p*-chlorophenol-*o*-phenylphenol and isopropanol), and (g) above all, use of common sense in handling potentially dangerous material.

The same procedures used for livers of various animals may be adapted to extrahepatic tissues, although these are usually more resistant to homogenization. Cutting devices (e.g., Tissue-mizer) may be used, although caution is advised if catalytic activity is to be measured in samples. The effects of such procedures should be checked.

Protein Determination

A commonly used method for protein determination is probably that of Lowry et al. (266). The procedure that has been used in this laboratory is outlined next.

Reagents

1. Bovine serum albumin, 1 mg/ml (determined accurately using $E_{278}^{1\%} = 6.67$).
2. Solution A: Na_2CO_3 (20 mg/ml) and NaOH (4 mg/ml).
3. Solution B_1: 2.0% sodium potassium tartrate (w/v).
4. Solution B_2: 1.0% $CuSO_4 \cdot 7H_2O$ (w/v).
5. Folin reagent (2.0 *N* phenol solution).
6. Solution C: Mix 1 part each of solutions B_1 and B_2 and add to 100 parts solution A. Prepare just before use.

Clean test tubes contain 0, 10, 20, 30, 40, and 50 μg albumin (in duplicate) plus solution containing the same amount of each component (salt, glycerol, detergent, etc.) present in the sample. The total volume in each tube is brought to 0.10 ml, and 2.0 ml of buffer C is added while mixing the sample with a vortex device. After exactly 10 min at room temperature, 0.20 ml Folin reagent is added to each tube while mixing. After 30 min, the A_{750} of each tube is read and a standard curve is constructed.

All standards and samples should be done in duplicate, and samples are preferably done at more than one dilution. A standard curve should be constructed for each different set of samples.

In our own laboratory we have replaced the preceding procedure with the Pierce BCA method, using the manufacturer's instructions (Pierce, Rockford, IL). Specifically, samples are heated at 60°C for 30 min. This assay is considerably more sensitive than the first procedure and, perhaps more importantly, is not very subject to interference by salts, detergents, and so forth. It may even be done directly in a microtiter plate to facilitate reading and data handling.

The biuret procedure (258) is less sensitive to interfering materials but requires much larger amounts of sample. The Coomassie blue G-250 binding assay (37) can also be used; this assay gives values similar to the Lowry assay for microsomes but gives varying values for purified preparations of cytochrome P450 and other enzymes; it is rather sensitive to detergent interference. The fluorescamine assay (427) is very sensitive but has not been as widely used with the proteins under consideration. Another approach is to calculate an extinction coefficient ($E^{1\%}$ at a particular wavelength) based upon the individual amino acids, if known.

All of these assays yield results that are relative to albumin. If an absolute value is required for a purified protein, then quantitative amino acid analysis of the acid-hydrolyzed protein must be done.

Assay of Cytochrome P450

The most generally used method is that of Omura and Sato (319), which utilizes the reduced-CO versus reduced difference spectrum. The procedure used in this laboratory is outlined next.

Reagents

1. 0.10 *M* Potassium phosphate buffer (pH 7.4) containing 1.0 m*M* EDTA, 20% glycerol (v/v), 0.50% sodium cholate (w/v), and 0.40% Triton N-101 (Sigma Chemical Co., St. Louis, MO), Emulgen 913 (Kao-Atlas, Tokyo), or equivalent detergent (w/v).
2. $Na_2S_2O_4$ (sodium dithionite, sodium hydrosulfite), reagent grade (keep bottle tightly closed when not in use).
3. CO gas, reagent purity; store and use in fume hood.

Microsomes (or other preparations) are added to buffer to give a final concentration of 0.05 to 5 μM cytochrome P450, mixed, and divided into two 1.0-ml glass or (disposable) polystyrene cuvettes (10 mm pathlength). A baseline is recorded between 400 to 500 nm using a split-beam spectrophotometer. The sample cuvette is saturated with 30 to 40 bubbles of CO at a rate of about 1 bubble/sec. A few crystals of $Na_2S_2O_4$ (1–2 mg) are added to each cuvette; the cuvettes are covered with parafilm, inverted several times to mix the $Na_2S_2O_4$, and placed in the spectrophotometer again after checking for liquid on the sides of the cuvettes. Spectra are recorded (400–500 nm) until the 450-nm peak reaches a maximum.

The A_{490} (isosbestic point) serves as a reference point. Cytochrome P450 content is determined as follows (Figure 35.6):

$$[(A_{450-490})_{\text{baseline}}]/0.091 = \text{nmol cytochrome P450/ml}$$

Cytochrome P420 represents denatured forms of cytochrome P450 and is determined using the following formulas:

$$(\text{nmol cytochrome P450/ml}) \times (-0.041) = (A_{420-490})_{\text{theoretical}}$$

$$[(A_{420-490})_{\text{observed}} - (A_{420-490})_{\text{theoretical}} - (A_{420-490})_{\text{baseline}}]/0.110 = \text{nmol cytochrome P420/ml}$$

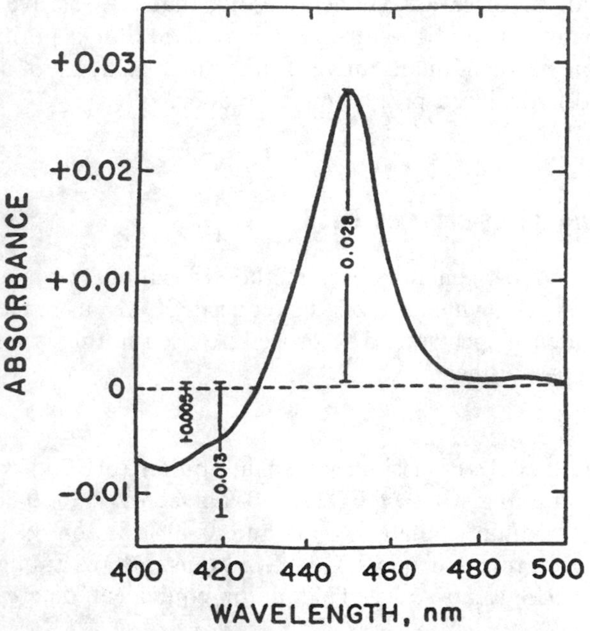

FIG. 35.6. Calculation of cytochrome P450 and P420 concentrations. A sample of rat liver P450 1A1 was diluted 10-fold with 0.1 *M* potassium phosphate buffer (pH 7.7) containing 1 m*M* EDTA, 40% glycerol (v/v), 0.2% Emulgen 913 (w/v), and 0.5% sodium cholate (w/v). The sample was divided into two cuvettes, which were balanced in a Cary 219 spectrophotometer using the automatic baseline correction mode. The corrected baseline was recorded (– – –). After addition of CO and $Na_2S_2O_4$ as indicated in the text the final difference spectrum was obtained. The calculations are as follow:
$0.028 \div 0.091 = 0.31$ nmol cytochrome P450/ml
$0.31 \times (-0.041) = -0.013$ (A_{420})
$-0.013 - (-0.005) = -0.008$
$0.008 \div 0.110 = 0.073$ nmol cytochrome P420/ml
$0.31 \times 10 = 3.1$ nmol cytochrome P450/ml
$0.073 \times 10 = 0.73$ nmol cytochrome P420/ml.
See text for further discussion.

The extinction coefficient ($\Delta\epsilon_{450--490}$) of 91 m$M^{-1}$ cm^{-1} has been verified using highly purified rat and rabbit liver cytochrome P450 preparations (183,360). The second set of formulas is based upon the observation that cytochrome P450 has an extinction coefficient of −41 mM^{-1} cm^{-1} ($\Delta\epsilon_{420-490}$) in the difference spectrum (i.e., the A_{420} of the reduced-CO complex is less than the A_{420} of reduced cytochrome P450) (320).

While rat liver microsomes can be routinely prepared with minimal hemoglobin contamination, this is not the case for many other preparations. The basic procedure of Matsubara et al. (288) for assaying cytochrome P450 in liver homogenates is then useful. In this method, two cuvettes are prepared as before but both are equilibrated with CO and the baseline is recorded. $Na_2S_2O_4$ is added only to the sample cuvette to obtain a reduced-CO versus oxidized-CO difference spectrum; the extinction coefficient ($\Delta\epsilon_{450-490}$) is 106 mM^{-1} cm^{-1}. Distinguishing between methemoglobin and cytochrome P420 is difficult, although Johannesen and DePierre (217) have reported that methemoglobin can be specifically reduced by ascorbate and phenazinemethosulfate.

Detergents are routinely used in the assay of cytochrome P450 in this laboratory, as these solubilize the microsomal membranes, reducing light scattering, and do not denature cytochrome P450 in the presence of glycerol (432). The buffer also helps prevent settling of any insoluble particles. However, some particular cytochrome P450 proteins may not necessarily be stable in the presence of these detergents (179). If one desires to carry out determinations in the absence of detergents, a spectrophotometer should be used that is capable of handling turbid solutions. The limit of detection of cytochrome P450 in extrahepatic tissues is influenced more by the presence of hemoglobin than instrumental considerations. In our own laboratory, we have used Varian 635 M and Cary 14, 210, and 219 spectrophotometers for such measurements. Other instruments are also suitable. The Aminco DW-2a instrument has historically been popular among investigators, and we currently use a computer-updated version (On-Line Instrument Systems, Bogart, GA) in our own laboratory; this is particularly useful with bacterial cells because of the ability to handle turbid samples.

Assay of NADPH–Cytochrome *c* Reduction

This enzyme is conveniently measured by its NADPH–cytochrome *c* reduction activity (338).

Reagents

1. Horse heart cytochrome *c* (0.50 m*M*) in 10 m*M* potassium phosphate buffer (pH 7.7).
2. 0.30 *M* Potassium phosphate buffer (pH 7.7).

3. 10 m*M* NADPH (fairly stable for <7 days at 4°C in the dark; however, for the most accurate work, solutions should be prepared fresh daily).

Pipette 80 μl cytochrome *c* solution, the enzyme sample, and sufficient 0.30 *M* phosphate buffer in a 1.0 ml cuvette (10 mm pathlength) to bring the total volume to 0.99 ml. The components are mixed and preincubated at 30°C in a recording spectrophotometer; the recorder is adjusted to zero absorbance at 550 nm (full scale 1.0; slit width 1.0 nm if possible, because of the narrow band being observed). After recording the baseline for 3 min, 10 μl NADPH is added and A_{550} is followed for about 3 min. Activity is calculated as follows:

$$\frac{\Delta A_{550}\ \text{min}^{-1}}{0.021} = \text{nmol cytochrome } c \text{ reduced min}^{-1}$$

An amount of enzyme should be used such that the initial ΔA_{550} does not exceed 0.2 min^{-1}. The assay is an indirect measure of NADPH–cytochrome P450 reductase activity; measurement of the actual NADPH–cytochrome P450 reductase activity requires anaerobic conditions and rapid reaction techniques (335). A small peptide of the reductase is required for efficient reduction of cytochrome P450 but not cytochrome *c*; if no proteolysis has occurred, the two activities are closely correlated (434).

NADPH–cytochrome *c* reduction activity is stimulated by the high salt concentration used in the assay (338). If activity is assayed in the presence of mitochondria (or in bacteria), KCN (1.0 m*M*) may be added as a precautionary measure to block nonmicrosomal activity. The reduction of several other compounds, such as dichlorophenolindophenol, ferricyanide (434), or a tetrazolium dye (356), may also be used to assay activity. Spectrophotometers with automatic sample positioners may be used to carry out multiple assays simultaneously.

Cytochrome P450-Linked Activities

Some classic and typical assays are presented, along wth prototypes of different types of methods and approaches.

Benzphetamine N-Demethylation

The assay of this activity (Figure 35.7) is popular because of its ease and sensitivity, especially with microsomes prepared from animals treated with barbiturates or similar inducers. At least three assays can be used. HCHO is released during the reaction and forms the basis for the first two of the assays.

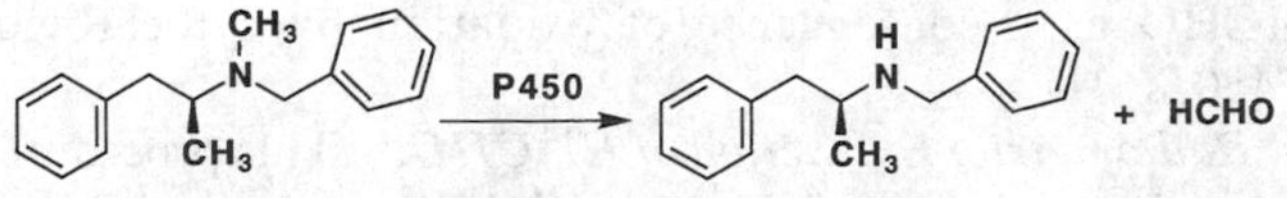

FIG. 35.7. *d*-Benzphetamine N-demethylation.

Colorimetric Measurement of HCHO. For studies on colorimetric measurement of HCHO and other carbonyls, see references (60, 277, and 303).

Reagents.

1. 1.0 *M* Potassium phosphate buffer, pH 7.7.
2. 10 m*M* $NADP^+$.
3. 10^3 IU Yeast glucose 6-phosphate dehydrogenase/ml [dissolved in 10 m*M* Tris-acetate buffer (pH 7.7) containing 1.0 m*M* EDTA and 20% glycerol (v/v)].
4. 0.10 *M* Glucose 6-phosphate.
5. 10 m*M* *d*-Benzphetamine-HCl.
6. 17% Aqueous $HClO_4$ (1/4 dilution of conc. $HClO_4$).
7. Nash reagent [300 g $NH_4CH_4CO_2$, 4.0 ml acetylacetone (2,4-pentanedione), and 6.0 ml glacial CH_3CO_2H per liter].

Incubations are carried out in 1.5 ml total volume and include 0.5 to 2 mg microsomal protein, 50 m*M* phosphate buffer, 0.50 m*M* $NADP^+$, 1.0 IU glucose-6-phosphate dehydrogenase/ml, and 1.0 m*M* benzphetamine-HCl (this should be added after the other components from a 10 m*M* aqueous stock). Tubes are preincubated for 3 min at 37°C and then glucose 6-phosphate is added to 10 m*M* to start incubations. After shaking the tubes (150 rpm) for 10 min at 37°C, the incubations are stopped by the addition of 0.50 ml of 17% $HClO_4$ and chilled on ice for 5 to 10 min. (Because of the short incubation time, it is convenient to start and stop individual tubes every 10 sec) Tubes are centrifuged at $3 \times 10^3 \times g$ for 5 min, and 1.0 ml of each supernatant is transferred to a new tube. To each of these tubes is added 0.40 ml Nash reagent. The tubes are heated at 60–70°C for 20 min in a water bath (covered to prevent evaporation). The tubes are cooled in tap water, and A_{412} values are read versus a water blank. Both minus benzphetamine and minus NADPH-generating system blanks should be included; the A_{412} values for these should be similar and are subtracted from the experimental values. A standard curve can be prepared using HCHO; we find that such curves routinely yield factors of 460 to 480, which, when multiplied by net A_{412}, give the total nanomoles of HCHO produced. If microcuvettes are used for reading A_{412}, the entire procedure can be scaled down 10-fold if an appropriate spectrophotometer is available. The same procedure is generally applicable to many substrates that release

HCHO as a consequence of oxidation by cytochrome P450.

Radiometric: Extraction of $H^{14}CHO$. This procedure necessitates the use of [*N*-methyl-^{14}C]-benzphetamine but offers increased sensitivity (147,360). This material can be synthesized from *d*-benzylamphetamine (available from Upjohn, Kalamazoo, MI). The synthesis has been carried out in this laboratory as follows (156).

Benzylamphetamine (free base, 1.0 mmol, 225 mg) is stirred with 1.1 mmol of $^{14}CH_3I$ (2 mCi, 156 mg) and 1.1 mmol of K_2CO_3 (152 mg) in 30 ml of $(CH_3)_2CO$ overnight. The solvent is removed in vacuo and the residue is suspended in water. The pH is adjusted to >10 with K_2CO_3 if necessary; the solution is extracted 3 times with CH_2Cl_2. The CH_2Cl_2 layers are combined, dried with anhydrous Na_2SO_4, and saturated with dry HCl gas. Solvent is removed in vacuo and the residue is crystallized from ethyl acetate to give [*N*-methyl-^{14}C]benzphetamine-HCl in ~50% yield. Purity can be checked by nuclear magnetic resonance (NMR) and mass spectrometry; the melting point (mp) appears to be sensitive to the crystallization procedure but should be sharp.[1]

Assays are set up as in the colorimetric procedure, but the volume is reduced to 0.75 ml and the protein concentration may be reduced to fit the situation. Incubations are stopped by the addition of 0.25 ml of 1 *N* NaOH and 5.0 ml $CHCl_3$ (or CH_2Cl_2). Tubes are mixed using a vortex device and centrifuged ($3 \times 10^3 \times g$ for 5 min). The aqueous upper layer is transferred to a clean tube, 5.0 ml of $CHCl_3$ is added, and the mixing, centrifugation, and transfer steps are repeated. The preceding step is repeated once more, and a 0.50-ml aliquot of the aqueous phase is transferred to a miniscintillation vial. The contents are neutralized by the addition of 0.50 ml of 0.10 M sodium citrate buffer (pH 6.5) to which has been added 0.060 *N* HCl; 5 ml of a water-miscible liquid scintillation mixture is added. Vials are capped, mixed, and counted (10 min will usually produce satisfactory counting deviation). Blanks contain all components except NADPH or protein.

The efficiency of extraction is >95%. HCHO remains in the aqueous phase and residual substrate is extracted in the $CHCl_3$ layers at the basic pH. A similar procedure may be used in the assay of any substrate that can be labeled with a labeled methyl group that is released following oxidation. An alternate method involves trapping the labeled HCHO product as the dimedone derivative (413) or as the 2,4-dinitrophenylhydrazone and doing high-performance liquid chromatography (HPLC) (470).

[1] The mp of a sample obtained from Upjohn was 152–154°C. The mp listed in the Merck Index is 129–130°C (crystallization from ethyl acetate). The mp found for material synthesized in this laboratory was 194–195°C (uncorrected).

Enhancement of NADPH Oxidation or O_2 Uptake. Because of high rates of endogenous oxidase activity, these procedures are more commonly used with reconstituted enzyme systems than with microsomes (276,310).

In the oxygen electrode procedure, experiments are set up as before and a background rate of O_2 uptake is observed. The differences in the rates obtained with substrates are measured; each nM of O_2 consumed corresponds to 1 nmol of substrate metabolized (310).

The NADPH oxidation assay is carried out in a similar way. The NADPH-generating system is deleted. Incubations, containing all components except NADPH, are preincubated for 3 min at 37°C in 1.0-ml cuvettes in a recording spectrophotometer set at 340 nm (1.0 full scale absorbance). NADPH (15 μl of a 10 m*M* solution) is added and the rate of decrease in A_{340} is observed. Blank incubations contain all components except benzphetamine. Rates are determined by dividing net ΔA_{340} min^{-1} by 0.00622 to obtain nmol NADPH oxidized/min. The benzphetamine demethylation rate determined by this procedure has been reported to be identical to that obtained by HCHO assay under some conditions (227) but not others (310) and should be checked before routine use.

Fluoresence: 7-Ethoxycoumarin O-Deethylation

This reaction (Figure 35.8) is an example of a fluorescence assay involving extraction; it is very sensitive, convenient, and applicable to a wide variety of samples (126,130).

Reagents.

1. 30 m*M* 7-Ethoxycoumarin (Aldrich Chemical Co., Milwaukee, WI), dissolved in CH_3OH (avoid exposure to light).
2. 1.0 *M* Potassium phosphate buffer (pH 7.4).
3. 10 m*M* $NADP^+$.
4. 10^3 IU Yeast glucose-6-phosphate dehydrogenase/ml [dissolved in 10 m*M* Tris-acetate buffer (pH 7.7) containing 1 m*M* EDTA and 20% glycerol (v/v)].
5. 0.10 *M* Glucose 6-phosphate.
6. 0.20 *M* Sodium borate (pH 9.6).
7. 1.0 m*M* 7-Hydroxycoumarin (Aldrich), dissolved in an aqueous solution of 0.10 *N* NaOH and 0.10 *M* NaCl (prepare fresh solution each day; avoid exposure to light).

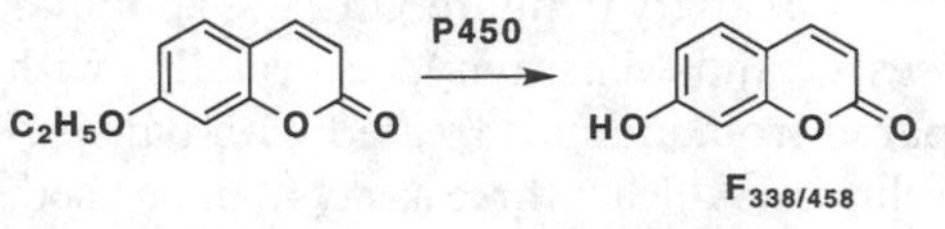

FIG. 35.8. 7-Ethoxycoumarin O-deethylation.

An appropriate amount of enzyme is placed in a test tube along with 50 m*M* phosphate buffer, 0.50 m*M* $NADP^+$, 1.0 IU glucose-6-phosphate dehydrogenase/ml, 0.30 m*M* 7-ethoxycoumarin, and water to bring the volume to 0.90 ml. After 3 min of preincubation at 37°C, glucose 6-phosphate is added to 10 m*M* to start incubations. (As in the case of benzphetamine, reactions are conveniently started and stopped each 15 sec) After 5 to 10 min, incubations are stopped by the addition of 0.10 ml of 2.0 *N* HCl and 2.0 ml $CHCl_3$. Tubes are mixed and centrifuged for 5 min at $3 \times 10^3 \times g$. One milliliter of the lower $CHCl_3$ phase (containing both substrate and product) is transferred to a clean tube and 2.0 ml of 0.20 *M* sodium borate buffer is added. The tubes are mixed and centrifuged 5 min at $3 \times 10_3 \times g$. The upper phase, containing the phenolic product, is transferred to a new tube and fluorescence is read versus a standard curve in a fluorimeter with the excitation wavelength set at 338 nm and the emission wavelength set at 458 nm.

Fluorescene: Benzo[a]pyrene Hydroxylation

This assay has been widely used because of its sensitivity, the widespread occurrence of this activity, and the interest in carcinogenic aspects of benzo[*a*]pyrene. This substrate is carcinogenic, light sensitive, and gives rise to many metabolites. The following procedure measures primarily the 3-hydroxy derivative (Figure 35.9) and, to a lesser extent, 9-hydroxybenzo[*a*]pyrene (304).

Reagents.

1. 1.0 *M* Potassium phosphate buffer (pH 7.4).
2. 10 m*M* $NADP^+$.
3. 10^3 IU Yeast glucose-6-phosphate dehydrogenase/ml [dissolved in 10 m*M* Tris-acetate buffer (pH 7.7) containing 1.0 m*M* EDTA and 20% glycerol (v/v)].
4. 8.0 m*M* Benzo[*a*]pyrene, dissolved in $(CH_3)_2CO$.
5. 6.0 m*M* Quinine, dissolved in 0.10 *N* H_2SO_4.
6. 1.0 m*M* 3-Hydroxybenzo[*a*]pyrene (this material can be obtained from the National Cancer Institute Chemical Carcinogen Reference Repository, c/o Midwest Research Institute, Kansas City, MO).

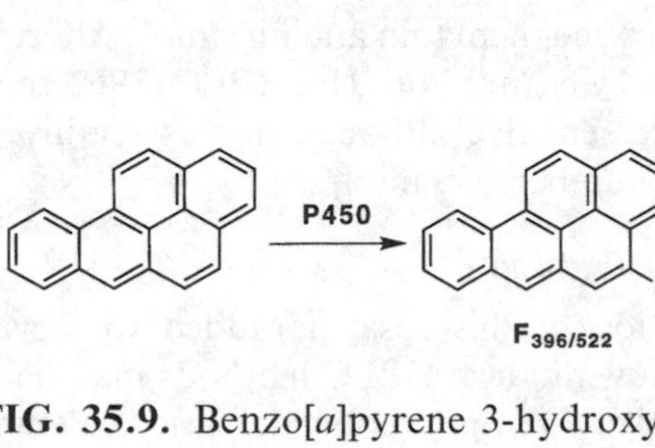

FIG. 35.9. Benzo[*a*]pyrene 3-hydroxylation.

An appropriate amount of enzyme is placed in a test tube along with 50 m*M* phosphate buffer (pH 7.4), 0.50 m*M* $NADP^+$, 10 IU glucose-6-phosphate dehydrogenase/ml, 80 μM benzo[*a*]pyrene, and sufficient water to bring the total volume to 1.0 ml. [All procedures should be carried out in dim light (or under yellow light). Alternatively, reactions may be done in amber glass vials. Appropriate precautions should be taken to prevent exposure of skin to benzo[*a*]pyrene or its metabolites. When solid material is being handled, precautions should be taken to avoid breathing dust.] After 3 min of preincubation at 37°C, glucose 6-phosphate is added to 10 m*M* to initiate reactions (this is conveniently done every 15 sec) After 5 to 10 min, reactions are stopped by the addition of 1.0 ml cold acetone and mixed. Hexane (3.25 ml) is added and mixing is repeated. Two milliters of the upper layer is transferred to a clean tube with a pipette and 4.0 ml of 1.0 *N* NaOH is added to this. After vortex mixing and centrifugation for 5 min at $3 \times 10^3 \times g$, the aqueous phase is carefully transferred to a clean tube.

Fluorescence is read with an excitation wavelength of 396 nm and emission wavelength of 522 nm. A standard curve is prepared in 0.10 *N* NaOH using 3-hydroxybenzo [*a*]pyrene. Since solutions of the standard are unstable, a convenient method involves setting up the standard curve, changing the wavelength settings to 350 nm (excitation) and 450 nm (emission) without adjusting other settings, and preparing a standard curve using serial dilutions of quinine sulfate. The quinine sulfate can then be used as a secondary standard in subsequent experiments and levels of 3-hydroxybenzo[*a*]pyrene can be calculated by reference to the original curves.

An alternative procedure devised by Dehnen et al. (81) is comparable in terms of convenience and sensitivity. Incubations are set up as before (1.0 ml volume) and stopped by the addition of 2.3 ml of a fresh aqueous mixture of 1.0 m*M* EDTA, 10% Triton X-100 (w/v), and 1.2% $(C_2H_5)_3N$ (w/v). After mixing, tubes are capped until fluorescence measurements are made. The excitation wavelength is set at 435 nm, and fluorescence emission is scanned (and a chart recorded) between 450 and 650 nm. Residual substrate gives a large peak near the 450 nm region of the chart and the product appears as a peak at 522 nm. A baseline is drawn between the trough [between benzo[*a*]pyrene and 3-hydroxybenzo[*a*]pyrene] and the point at which the 3-hydroxybenzo[*a*]pyrene peak tails into a baseline at about 575 nm. The distance between this slanted baseline and the top of the 522-nm peak can be calibrated against the quinine sulfate curve prepared as already described.

Other benzo[*a*]pyrene metabolism assays can be carried out with radioactive substrate to measure total polar metabolites (82), individual metabolites [after separation by HPLC] (21,372,410), or metabolites covalently bound to protein or added nucleic acids (83).

Thin Layer Chromatography: (S)-Mephenytoin 4-Hydroxylation

Many aromatic substrates are converted into phenols via hydroxylation by cytochrome P450 enzymes; in addition, many aryl ethers are *O*-dealkylated to form phenols. In many cases advantage can be taken of the increased polarity of the (deprotonated) phenolic product to aid in measuring its formation in in vitro assays. The general principle involves incubation of radioactive substrate with enzyme and separation of product from substrate by thin-layer chromatography (TLC) using a solvent containing NH_4OH to deprotonate the phenol, thus increasing its polarity and decreasing its mobility. Of course, more rigorous identification of the chemistry of the reaction products is usually necessary, particularly in the case of substrates that can be hydroxylated at any of several positions. However, in many cases essentially only *para*-hydroxylation occurs and the separation is relatively easy. We have utilized this general approach to measure rates of (*S*)-mephenytoin 4′-hydroxylation (Figure 35.10) (385), acetanilide 4-hydroxylation (163), and phenacetin *O*-deethylation (87). In practice the assays are set up in the same general manner as others involving cytochrome P450 enzymes (vide supra).

(*S*)-Nirvanol (20.4 mg, 0.10 mmol), synthesized as described elsewhere (186), is dissolved in a small amount of $(CH_3)_2CO$ (<1 ml) and 1 equivalent of KOH is added (0.10 ml of a methanolic 1.0 *N* KOH solution). The sample is mixed and dried under an N_2 stream and dissolved in ~1 ml of $(CH_3)_2CO$. $^{14}CH_3I$ (16 mg, 0.11 mmol; specific activity ~10 mCi/mmol; New England Nuclear, Boston) is added at 0°C, and the reaction is stirred at 0°C. The reaction is allowed to warm to 23°C and is nearly complete after about 1 h (as monitored by TLC, vide infra). The mixture evaporates to dryness under an N_2 stream, and the residue is dissolved in CH_2Cl_2 and washed with an equal amount of aqueous 1.0 *N* NaOH to remove residual starting material. The CH_2Cl_2 layer is dried with Na_2SO_4, filtered, and reduced to dryness under an N_2 stream. The resulting [methyl-^{14}C](*S*)-mephenytoin is redissolved in a small amount of $(CH_3)_2CO$ and crystallized by the careful addition of H_2O. The product is collected by centrifugation, washed with H_2O, and dried in vacuo over Drierite overnight. The typical yield of crystalline product (first crop) is 8–10 mg (~50%). Radiopurity is >99% as judged by TLC (Whatman LK6DF silica; $CHCl_3$–MeOH–conc. NH_4OH/90–10–1, v/v/v).

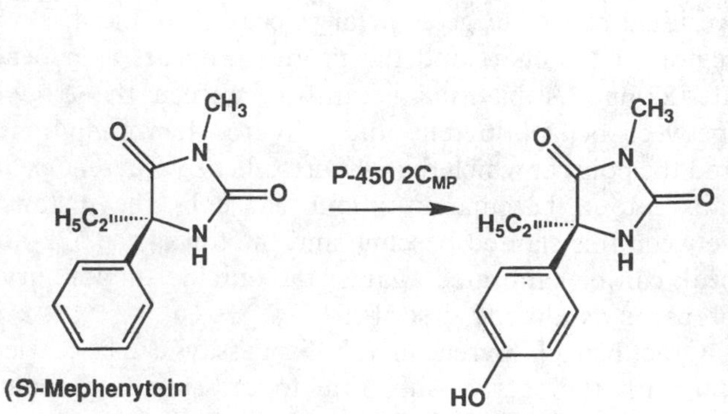

FIG. 35.10. 4′-Hydroxylation of (*S*)-mephenytoin (380,382).

The (*S*)-mephenytoin 4-hydroxylation activity of human liver microsomes is assayed as follows. The standard reaction mixture (final volume, 100 μl) contains liver microsomes (about 100 pmol cytochrome P450) or a reconstituted monooxygenase system containing 100 pmol of partially purified cytochrome P450, 100 pmol of NADPH–cytochrome P450 reductase, and 6 nmol of sonicated L-α-1,2-dilauroyl-*sn*-glycero-3-phosphocholine; an NADPH-generating system consisting of 50 nmol $NADP^+$, 1.0 μmol glucose 6-phosphate, and 0.20 IU yeast glucose 6-phosphate dehydrogenase; 10 μmol potassium phosphate buffer (pH 7.4); and 40 nmol *S*-[methyl-^{14}C]-mephenytoin. The reaction is started by the addition of glucose 6-phosphate to 10 m*M*, continued for 30 min at 37°C, and stopped with 50 μl of ice-cold tetrahydrofuran containing 0.20 m*M* unlabeled 4′-hydroxymephenytoin. An aliquot of the mixture (50 μl) is applied to the loading zone of a Whatman LK6DF chromatography plate using a plastic-tipped pipetting device. After separation by TLC in the solvent system used for analyzing the substrate purity (vide supra) and detection with 254-nm light, zones containing 4-hydroxymephenytoin are scraped from the TLC plate (alternatively, autoradiography under x-ray film can be used to locate the product zones). CH_3OH (1.0 ml) is added to elute the product. After 10 min, 4 ml of an appropriate liquid scintillation (nonaqueous) is added. Radioactivity is measured by liquid scintillation spectrometry. Enzyme activities are expressed as picomoles product formed per min per nM of cytochrome P450.

TLC analysis of (*S*)-[methyl-^{14}C]-mephenytoin and its 4′-hydroxy product after incubation with human liver microsomes (containing 100 pmol of cytochrome P450) for 0, 20, and 40 min at 37°C is shown in Figure 35.8. No radioactive metabolites of mephenytoin other than 4-hydroxymephenytoin were detected. Further, the only products detected using HPLC (247) of such incubates were 4-hydroxymephenytoin and nirvanol. Alternatively, the reaction may be monitored by HPLC (396); the HPLC assay is more sensitive although not as readily utilized with a large number of samples.

HPLC: Nifedipine Oxidation

A description of this assay is added to serve as an example of how modern HPLC methods may be utilized very effectively. Nifedipine is a widely used calcium chan-

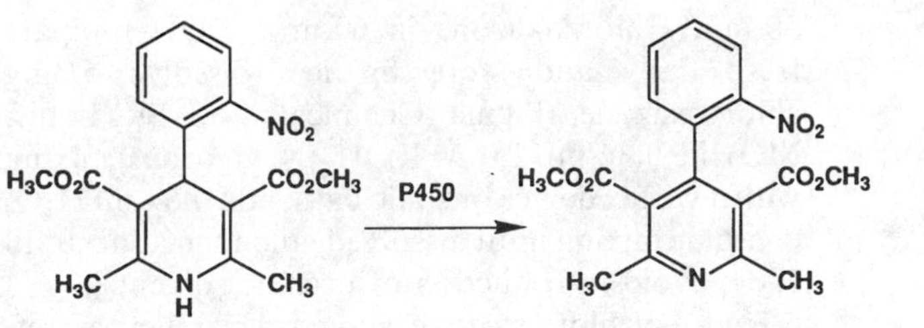

FIG. 35.11. Oxidation of nifedipine to the pyridine derivative (164).

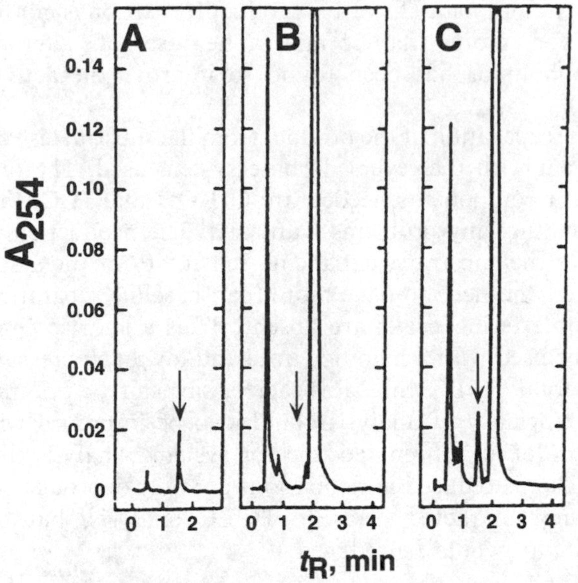

FIG. 35.12. HPLC separation of the oxidized (pyridine) product of nifipidine oxidation from human liver microsomes. A typical 10 min incubation with 100 pmol of human liver microsomal cytochrome P450 was done and 20 μl of the total extract was chromatographed as described. The t_R of the nifedipine oxidation product is indicated with an arrow. (A) Authentic standard of the metabolite (200 ng); (B) extract of an incubation devoid of NADPH; (C) complete incubation (164).

nel blocker, and oxidation by cytochrome P450 renders it inactive (164).

Nifedipine oxidation [from the dihydropyridine to the pyridine product (Figure 35.11)] is measured in the following manner. All incubation, extraction, and other handling of samples is done in amber vials because of the light sensitivity of nifedipine solutions. Amber glass vials are available from the Pierce Chemical Co., Rockford, IL. Typical incubations include liver microsomes containing 10–100 pmol of cytochrome P450, 0.10 *M* potassium phosphate buffer (pH 7.85), and 0.20 m*M* nifedipine (added from a stock solution of 20 m*M* in CH_3OH) in a final volume of 0.50 ml. The components are equilibrated for 3 min at 37°C and the reaction is initiated by the addition of an NADPH-generating system consisting of (final concentrations) 10 m*M* glucose 6-phosphate, 0.50 m*M* $NADP^+$, and 1.0 IU yeast glucose-6-phosphate dehydrogenase/ml. The reaction proceeds for 10 min at 37°C and is then quenched by the addition of 2.0 ml CH_2Cl_2. One hundred microliters of 1 *M* Na_2CO_3 buffer (pH 10.5, 1 *M*, 100 μl) containing 2.0 *M* NaCl is added to each vial. The contents of each vial are mixed using a vortex device and the two layers are separated by centrifugation at $3 \times 10^3 \times$ g for 10 min. From each lower organic layer, 1.4 ml is transferred to an amber Reacti-vial (Pierce Chemical Co., Rockford, IL). The total extract is reduced to dryness at 23°C under an N_2 stream. The residue is dissolved in 50 μl CH_3OH and 20 μl is injected onto an octyldecylsilane (C_{18}) reversed-phase HPLC column (e.g., 6.2×80 mm; Mac-Modd, Chadds Ford, PA) placed in series following a 1-cm-long octyldecylsilane guard column and 0.2-μm frit filter. The column is eluted with an isocratic mixture of 64% CH_3OH–36% H_2O (v/v) at a flow rate of 3.0 ml min^{-1}. Detection is at 254 nm (found to be optimal by previous scanning). Quantitation is usually done with external standards and by the use of peak heights. Alternatively, nitrendipine or another dihydropyridine (47,148) can be used as an internal standard. Typically a 20 ng sample of the metabolite (59 pmol) yields a maximal A_{254} of about 0.015 under these conditions (in the HPLC effluent). A typical chromatogram resulting from injection of a human liver microsomal incubation extract is shown in Figure 35.12.

Assay conditions were optimized with a human liver microsomal sample (164). Product formation was linear up to a time of 20 min, the pH optimum was 7.85 (Tris-HCl yielded lower rates than did potassium phosphate buffer), the rate of product formation per unit enzyme was constant over a range of 5–1000 pmol cytochrome P450/ml, and a substrate concentration of 200 μM was optimal ($K_m \sim 10$ μM; substrate inhibition observed at concentrations >500 μM; no evidence for multiphasic behavior observed over the concentrations range of 2–1000 μM).

When purified cytochrome P450 fractions are assayed for activity, the microsomes are replaced with 20–100 pmol cytochrome P450, 250 pmol rabbit NADPH–cytochrome P450 reductase, 250 pmol cytochrome b_5, and 15 nmol L-α-1,2-dilauroyl-*sn*-glyceryl-3-phosphocholine. These components are mixed and then incubated for 10 min at 23°C prior to addition of other materials. Examination of experimental conditions indicated that the NADPH–cytochrome P450 reductase, substrate, and phospholipid concentrations used are optimal. However, product formation is not linear for more than 5 min. The use of alternate phospholipids has been found to improve the activity (200).

The separation of the product from the substrate is very efficient with the reversed-phase system used. The only solvent components needed are CH_3OH and H_2O, thus eliminating any problems with salts. The product elutes before the substrate, enhancing sensitivity of the assay. There is no need to have more than baseline separation, and interfering peaks are absent. Thus a short column can be used with a high flow rate and low back pressure. The total HPLC time for each assay can be <3 min. The efficiency of analysis could also be improved with the use of an automated injector system. Analysis time can also be reduced if incubations are only deproteinized and not extracted prior to HPLC analysis, but the sensitivity would be reduced.

HPLC: Chlorzoxazone 6-Hydroxylation

Another HPLC-based assay of cytochrome P450 activity involves measurement of the 6-hydroxylation of chlorzoxazone (Figure 35.13). This reaction has been reported to be highly selective for cytochrome P450 2E1 in human liver (159,333). The assay presents considerable advantages of sensitivity, reliability, and specificity over many other traditional assays for the function of cytochrome P450 2E1 assays, such as *N,N*-dimethylnitrosamine *N*-demethylation and 4-nitrophenol 2-hydroxylation. Chlorzoxazone is used as a drug (ref. 333 and references therein) and this general procedure can be used to measure pharmacokinetic parameters in humans to assess their relative levels of cytochrome P450 2E1 (237,312).

Reagents.

1. 1 *M* Potassium phosphate buffer (pH 7.4).
2. $NADP^+$, 10 m*M*.
3. 10^3 IU Yeast glucose-6-phosphate dehydrogenase/ml [dissolved in 10 m*M* Tris-acetate buffer (pH 7.4) containing 1 m*M* EDTA and 20% glycerol (v/v)].
4. 0.1 *M* Glucose 6-phosphate.
5. 50 m*M* Chlorzoxazone in 60 m*M* KOH [prepare fresh daily and store on ice: dissolve 51 mg chlorzoxazone (Sigma Chemical Co., St. Louis, MO) in 0.36 ml 1.0 *N* KOH by vigorous mixing with a vortex device or sonic bath, add 0.64 ml H_2O, continue mixing until dissolved, and then add 5.0 ml H_2O; avoid introduction of organic solvents].
6. 6-Hydroxychlorzoxazone [standard product; see ref. 333 for synthesis].
7. Either 2-benzoxazolinone (Aldrich Chemical Co., Milwaukee, WI) or 5-flurobenzoxazolinone (333) dissolved in 2.0% aqueous propylene glycol 400 (internal standard).

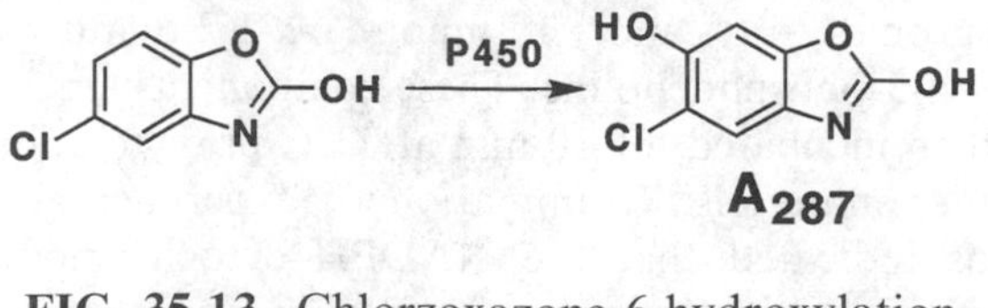

FIG. 35.13. Chlorzoxazone 6-hydroxylation.

An appropriate amount of enzyme is placed in a test tube along with 50 m*M* potassium phosphate buffer (pH 7.4), 0.50 m*M* $NADP^+$, 1.0 IU glucose-6-phosphate dehydrogenase/ml, and 0.50 m*M* chlorzoxazone (final incubation volume 0.50 ml). After 3 min of preincubation at 37°C, glucose 6-phosphate is added to 10 m*M* to start incubations. After 10 to 20 min at 37°C , reactions are stopped by the addition of 25 μl of aqueous 43% H_3PO_4 (w/v). An appropriate amount of the internal standard (5.0 nmol) is also added to each tube, followed by 2.0 ml CH_2Cl_2. The contents of each tube are mixed using a vortex device and the layers are separated by brief centrifugation ($3 \times 10^3 \times g$, 10 min). An aliquot (1.6 ml) of each lower (CH_2Cl_2) layer is transferred with a pipette to a clean test tube or conical vial (Reacti-vial, Pierce Chemical Co., Rockford, IL) and the solvent is removed under an N_2 stream of 23°C. The residue is dissolved in 50 μl CH_3CN (mixing on a vortex device), and 20 μl is injected onto a 6.2 × 80 mm Zorbax octylsilane (C8) HPLC column (3 μM, Mac-Modd, Chadds Ford, PA) utilizing a solvent mixture of 32% CH_3CN (v/v) and 0.5% H_3PO_4 (w/v) in H_2O, with ultraviolet (UV) detection at 287 nm (flow rate 3.5 ml min^{-1}) (Figure 35.14). Under these conditions each assay requires ≤5 min HPLC time. For more complex samples the CH_3CN concentration may need to be decreased to move the produce peak away from the solvent front. It is reasonable to use as little as 5 pmol microsomal cytochrome P450 in this assay and obtain reliable results.

GC-Mass Spectrometry: N,N-Dimethylaniline N-Demethylation

Amine *N*-dealkylations are catalyzed by a number of different oxidases and are important in the disposition of drugs and other chemicals. The cytochrome P450-dependent reactions have historically been of the most interest, although such reactions can also be catalyzed by peroxidases, flavoproteins, and other enzymes as well (141,438). The mechanism of the reaction has been a matter of considerable interest, and the reader

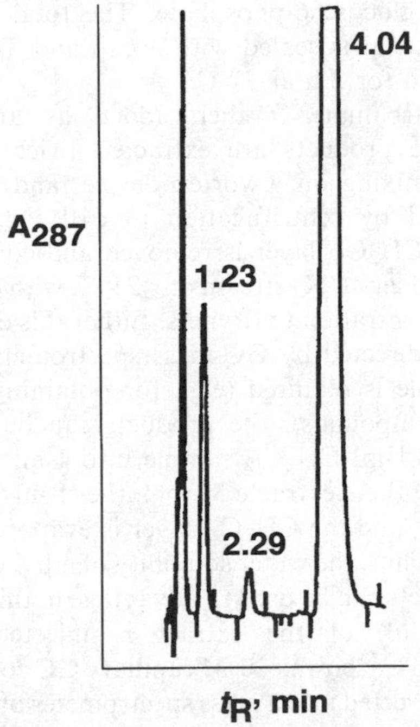

FIG. 35.14. HPLC separation of an extract of a chlorzoxazone incubation. See text for details. In this particular assay 0.27 nmol of human cytochrome P450 (in liver microsomes) was incubated for 10 min with 0.5 mM chlorzoxazone. The t_R values of the individual peaks are designated: 1.23 min, 6-hydroxychlorzoxazone; 2.29 min, 5-fluorobenzoxazolinone; 4.04 min, chlorzoxazone (333).

is referred to recent work on this topic (176,318). The *N*-demethylation of *N,N*-dimethylaniline (Figure 35.15) can be assayed by measurement of HCHO by other procedures (vide supra), but the assay is typical of many used for gas chromatography (GC) and GC-mass spectrometry. It was specifically used in our work to measure kinetic deuterium isotope effects (318).

Incubations contained enzyme, an NADPH-generating system (consisting of final concentrations of 0.50 mM $NADP^+$, 10 mM glucose 6-phosphate, and 1.0 IU glucose-6-phosphate dehydrogenase/ml), and 1.0 mM *N,N*-dimethylaniline in a final volume of 1.0 ml.

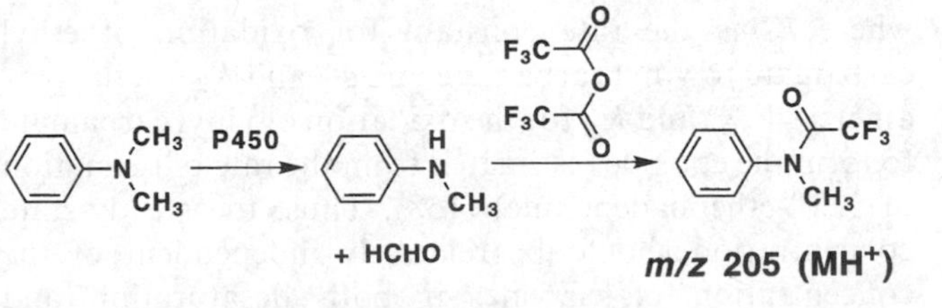

FIG. 35.15. *N,N*-Dimethylaniline N-demethylation assay (297,318).

Reactions proceed for 10 min in vials sealed with Teflon liners (to prevent evaporation of substrate) and are quenched by the addition of 0.40 ml of 17% $HClO_4$ (w/v). After 0.10 ml of 270 μM [N^2-H_3, ring-$^2H_5$]-*N*-methylaniline is added as an internal standard, the pH is made alkaline and the substrate, products, and perdeuterated internal standard are extracted into 2.0 ml CH^2Cl_2 by mixing with a vortex device (the internal standard may be prepared by reaction of [ring-$^2H_5$]aniline with C^2H_3I (318)]. The layers are separated by centrifugation ($3 \times 10^3 \times g$, 10 min) and the (lower) CH^2Cl_2 layer is removed, dried by adding anhydrous Na_2SO_4 and mixing, and then transferred to a clean vial. $(CF_3CO)_2O$ (50 μl) is added to each vial, and the vials are sealed with caps and Teflon liners and allowed to stand overnight at 4°C to form trifluoroacetanilide.

Most of the CH_2Cl_2 is removed under a stream of N_2 ($\leq$30°C) and aliquots ($\sim$2 μl) are injected onto a 0.5 mm × 3 m SPB-1 capillary GC column connected to a mass spectrometer operating in the chemical ionization mode with He as the carrier gas and CH_4 as the ionization gas. The column temperature is programmed from 100 to 280°C at 20°C/min. The ions at m/z 205 and 214 (both $[M+H^+]$) are monitored for the product and internal standard. Mixtures of varying ratios of trifluoroacetanilide and the perdeutero derivative are used to prepare a standard curve.

Another example of a procedure involving derivatization of product and GC-mass spectrometry involves the conversion of ethanol to acetaldehyde by human cytochrome P450 2E1 and derivatization as the hydrozone (23). Another example, without derivatization, is presented for ethyl carbamate (vide infra). In some cases it is impractical to use a heavy isotope as an internal standard, and product analogs must be considered. There are many procedures for GC-based methods involving flame ionization, electron capture, and other means of detection. Electron capture can be a very sensitive assay procedure when halides or nitro groups are present. The use of capillary GC columns has made packed columns nearly obsolete because of the superior resolution. However, the need to use very small injection volumes requires the need for internal standards except in cases where headspace analysis is done.

GC-Mass Spectrometry: Ethyl Carbamate Desaturation

Ethyl carbamate (urethane) desaturation is presented as another example of a reaction with an assay involving GC-mass spectrometry. The desaturation of ethyl carbamate to vinyl carbamate (Figure 35.16) had been suggested by Dahl et al. (71,72), but direct evidence for this view had been difficult to obtain. Now it is realized that the oxidation of ethyl carbamate to vinyl carbamate is a very slow process and that the succeeding

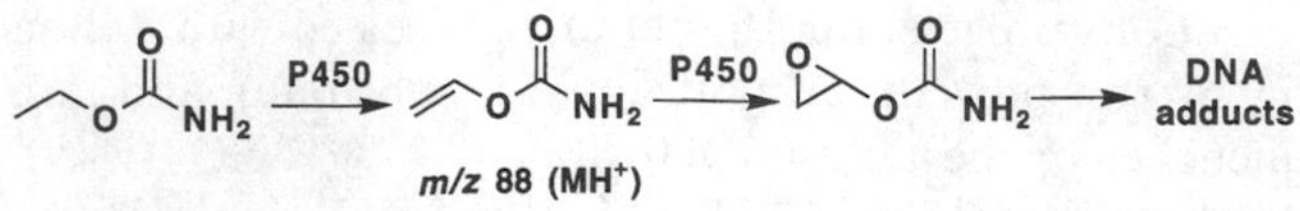

FIG. 35.16. Desaturation of ethyl carbamate and epoxidation of vinyl carbamate (158).

step, epoxide formation, is ~400 times faster (and is catalyzed by the same cytochrome P450 enzyme) (158). Thus, the steady-state level of vinyl carbamate is very low. The procedure described below can be used to estimate levels of several ethyl carbamate metabolites—vinyl carbamate, 2-hydroxyethyl carbamate, and *N*-hydroxyethyl carbamate (158). In the refrence cited, a major use was the qualitative demonstration of these products. With this procedure, it was possible to detect 1 part product in 10^4 parts substrate.

Reagents.

1. 1.0 *M* Potassium phosphate buffer (pH 7.4).
2. $NADP^+$, 10 m*M*.
3. 10^3 IU Yeast glucose-6-phosphate dehydrogenase/ml [dissolved in 10 m*M* Tris-acetate buffer (pH 7.4) containing 1.0 m*M* EDTA and 20% glycerol (v/v)].
4. 0.10 *M* Glucose 6-phosphate.
5. 0.10 *M* Ethyl carbamate (urethane, Aldrich Chemical Co., Milwaukee, WI; purify by sublimation—use house vacuum or a water aspirator to achieve ~15 mm Hg).
6. 2-Hydroethyl carbamate (Pfaltz and Bauer, Stamford, CT).
7. *N*-Hydroxyethyl carbamate (Aldrich).
8. Vinyl carbamate (72,259).
9. Methyl carbamate (Aldrich; purify by sublimation before use).

Note: These carbamates, particularly ethyl and vinyl, should be handled with care. They are carcinogenic and volatile. Use fume hoods, closed vials, and appropriate protective clothing.

The oxidation of ethyl carbamate is catalyzed primarily by cytochrome P450 2E1, so care should be taken to avoid adding organic solvents, which are inhibitory (469). The reaction is slow and a high concentration of microsomal protein is needed, so it is useful to remove glycerol (or sucrose) from microsomes by dialysis for 1–2 h versus 0.10 *M* potassium phosphate buffer (pH 7.4) at 4°C just prior to use. Microsomal protein (10–15 mg protein/ml) is mixed in a vial with 100 m*M* potassium or an equivalent amount of a reconstituted cytochrome P450 system, 10 m*M* ethyl carbamate, and an NADPH-generating system consisting of (final concentrations of) 0.50 m*M* $NADP^+$, 1 IU glucose-6-phosphate dehydrogenase/ml, and 10 m*M* glucose 6-phosphate. The total volume is 1.0 ml. Each vial is sealed with a cap and Teflon liner and incubated for 2 h at 37°C.

Methyl carbamate is then added as an internal standard, the products are extracted twice into 1 ml CH_2Cl_2 by mixing on a vortex device, and the layers are separated by centrifugation ($3 \times 10^3 \times g$, 10 min). The (lower) CH_2Cl_2 layer is removed and concentrated to ≤0.1 ml under an N_2 stream at ≤23°C, with care taken to avoid concentration to dryness. Either this extract can be analyzed directed by GC-mass spectrometry or, if a cleaner sample is required (e.g., for obtaining scans of individual compounds), the products can be extracted from the ~0.1-ml CH_2Cl_2 sample into 1 ml H_2O. The products are then extracted from the 1 ml H_2O into 2 ml CH_2Cl_2, and the CH_2Cl_2 layer is evaporated again to ~0.1 ml. Thus, the water solubility of ethyl carbamate and its products can be used to advantage in this case. An aliquot (1–2 μl) of the extract is injected onto a 0.1 mm × 9 m Carbowax 20 *M* capillary GC column with the effluent directed into a mass spectrometer operating in the chemical ionization mode with CH_4 as the carrier gas. The selectivity and sensitivity are enhanced in the chemical ionization mode, relative to electron impact, in this case. Total ion current and the ions at m/z 74, 88, and 106 are monitored as the column is heated with a linear temperature gradient. The actual t_R values depend upon the rate of heating, gas flow rate, and so on. Under typical operating conditions, methyl carbamate (m/z 74) eluted at ~4 min, vinyl carbamate (m/z 88) at 6.8 min, ethyl carbamate (m/z 90, not monitored) at 8.0 min, ethyl *N*-hydroxycarbamate (m/z 106) at 10.4 min, and 2-hydroxyethyl carbamate (m/z 106) at 12.9 min (158). Standard curves may be prepared by plotting the ratio of detector response relative to methyl carbamate versus the concentration of each product; such curves were linear over several orders of magnitude for each of the oxidation products under consideration (158).

The steady-state concentration of vinyl carbamate [VC], can be expressed as a function of the ethyl carbamate concentration, [EC]:

$$[VC] = \frac{(k_1 K_2)[EC]}{V_2}$$

where k_1 is the rate constant for oxidation of ethyl carbamate to vinyl carbamate and V_2 and K_2 are the parameters V_{max} and K_m for the oxidation of vinyl carbamate to form the epoxide (estimated from the rate of formation of 1,N^6-ethenoadenoxine) (158). Thus, the steady-state concentration should be relatively independent of the concentration of enzyme, if both desaturation and epoxidation are catalyzed by the same enzyme (i.e., P450 2E1 in this situation) (158).

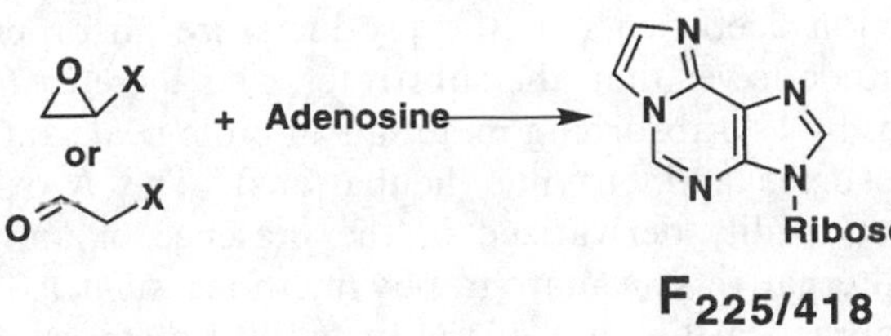

FIG. 35.17. Reaction of bifunctional electrophiles with adenosine.

HPLC-Fluorescence Assay: 1,N⁶-Ethenoadenosine Formation

Fluorescence assays have long been regarded for their high sensitivity (426). The discrimination of compounds provided by the use of selective excitation and emission wavelengths may be further enhanced by coupling to HPLC. In many cases the enzyme product has intrinsic fluorescence and may be monitored. In other cases, postcolumn derivatization can be used to render products fluorescent. The situation described here is somewhat different. A compound is present in the enzyme mixture (adenosine) that does not impede the reaction but reacts with the reaction product to generate a fluorescent product, that is, 1,N^6-etheno(ϵ)adenosine (Figure 35.17). The procedure has a deficiency in that it probably does not serve as a quantitative trap for any of the compounds under consideration. On the other hand, it is of considerable relevance to studies in toxicology and chemical carcinogenesis in that the same reaction serves to modify DNA to introduce a potentially mutagenic lesion. The procedure described here is based upon our own use (158,159) of methods described by Leithauser et al. (259) and Rinkus and Legator (355).

Reagents.

1. 1.0 *M* Potassium phosphate buffer (pH 7.4).
2. 50 m*M* Adenosine, dissolved in H_2O (heat in a bath of hot tap water or sonicate to dissolve).
3. Appropriate substrate, dissolved in H_2O (not organic solvent at ~10 × the concentration used in the assay).
4. 10 m*M* $NADP^+$.
5. 10^3 IU Yeast glucose-6-phosphate dehydrogenase/ml [dissolved in 10 m*M* Tris-acetate buffer (pH 7.7) containing 1.0 m*M* EDTA and 20% glycerol (v/v)].
6. Standard solutions of 1,N^6-ethenoadenosine dissolved in H_2O.
7. 0.60 *M* $ZnSO_4$ (in H_2O).

An appropriate amount of microsomes or purified enzyme system is placed in a glass vial (generally to provide ~2 mg microsomal protein/ml). Reagents are added to give 50 m*M* potassium phosphate buffer (pH 7.4), 0.50 m*M* $NADP^+$, 1.0 IU glucose-6-phosphate dehydrogenase/ml, and the substrate. Most of the substrates that generate products reacting with adenosine to produce 1,N^6-ethenoadenosine are small organic compounds (e.g., ethylene dibromide, ethylene dichloride, vinyl chloride, vinyl bromide, acrylonitrile, vinyl carbamate, ethyl carbamate, and some nitrosamines) (159). These are usually substrates for cytochrome P450 2E1 enzymes; since organic solvents are competitive inhibitors, they should be avoided (469). Although these compounds are considered to be organic solvents, most are actually reasonably soluble in H_2O (159) (see Merck Index and various handbooks of physical constants of chemicals). Many of these are rather volatile, so the vials may have to be sealed with screw caps and Teflon liners (rubber septa absorb these chemicals and should be avoided). Gases such as vinyl chloride can be added directly to the head space of such vials.

Incubations are initiated by the addition of glucose 6-phosphate to 10 m*M* and shaking at 37°C for a specified period of time. With some of the slower reactions (e.g., ethyl carbamate) we (158) and others (259) have found that reactions can proceed in a linear manner for up to 3 h. Reactions are stopped by the addition of $ZnSO_4$ to 30 m*M*. The protein is precipitated by centrifugation at $3 \times 10^3 \times g$ for 10 min, and aliquots of the supernatant fraction are injected onto an HPLC system [octadecylsilane (C_{18}), equilibrated with 11% CH_3CN (v/v) in 50 m*M* $NH_4CH_3CO_2$ (pH 5.0)]. With a 4.6 × 250 or a 6.2 × 80 m*M* column, as much as 250 μl of material may be injected; at a flow rate of 1.0]ml min^{-1}, the t_R of 1,N^6-ethenoadenosine is typically ~8 min. The effluent passes through the flow cell of a spectrofluorimeter designed for such monitoring, with the excitation wavelength set at 225 nm and using a 418-nm emission filter. The 1,N^6-ethenoadenosine peak follows a large negative peak of residual adenosine (Figure 35.18); if enough separation is not seen then the concentration of CH_3CN should be reduced. As little as 0.5 pmol of 1,N^6-ethenoadenosine can be detected using this method.

HPLC: Derivatization Assays—N-Oxide formation

HPLC is an extremely powerful method for resolving products from substrates. Under appropriate conditions, less than 1 part product in 10^4 parts substrate can be detected within a few min (e.g., ref. 164). However, in some cases the sensitivity of the detection system may not be sufficient for the problem. However, methods can often be developed to deal with the experimental situation without great difficulty, particularly if the number of samples is limited and there are no real alternative procedures.

The conversion of *N,N*-dialkylaniline derivatives to their *N*-oxides (Figure 35.19) by cytochrome P450

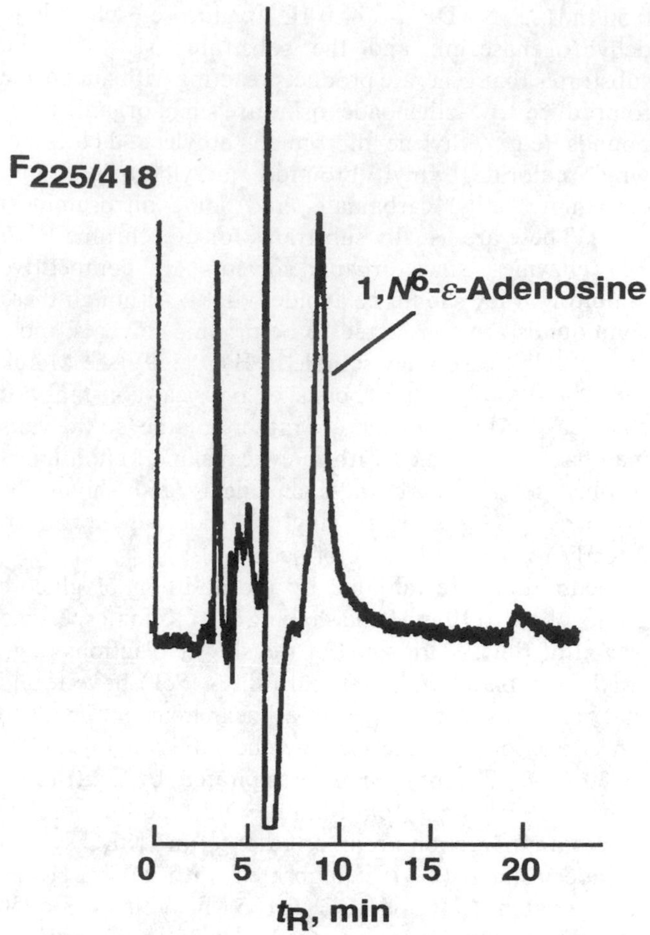

FIG. 35.18. Formation of 1,N^6-ethenoadenosine in a microsomal incubation. The incubation included 5 mg liver microsomal protein (prepared from isoniazid-treated rats/ml), 2.0 m*M* *N*-methyl,*N*-vinylnitrosamine, 10 m*M* adenosine, and an NADPH-generating system. After an incubation time of 120 min, a 100 μl aliquot was analyzed as described in the text (159).

enzymes has been examined (374). Little *N*-oxide is usually formed [in contrast to the flavin-containing monooxygenase (FMO) reaction] compared to the high rate of *N*-dealkylation, and a reliable procedure for analysis was required. The *N*-oxides are readily separated from the parent *N,N*-dialkylanilines by HPLC, but the extinction coefficients of the products are an order of magnitude lower than the substrates, and there is interference by UV-absorbing materials in biological samples (microsomes and enzyme incubations). The *N*-oxides are not readily derivatized in the presence of amines, and alternative chromatography methods such as GC are impractical because of the instability of these compounds. We developed a procedure in which the *N*-oxide fraction is separated by HPLC and reduced by $TiCl_3$ to the parent amine; the amine is then assayed by HPLC in a subsequent step (373). A prototype procedure is presented for *N,N*-dimethylaniline *N*-oxide formation; this assay was verified with the use of ^{14}C-labeled substrate (374).

Reagents.

1. 1.0 *M* Potassium phosphate buffer, pH 7.7.
2. *N,N*-Dimethylaniline-HCl, 10 m*M* in H_2O. Commercial *N,N*-dimethylaniline is purified by either (a) vacuum distillation with house vacuum (~15 mm Hg) or (b) applying ~5 g (in *n*-hexane) to a silicic acid column (2.2 × 25 cm) equilibrated with *n*-hexane and eluting with *n*-hexane (*n*-hexane is evaporated in vacuo). In either case the *N,N*-dimethylaniline is stored at −20°C under argon (Ar). A portion is dissolved in dry $(C_2H_5)_2O$ in a test tube and the solution is saturated with dry HCl gas (from a lecture bottle). The white precipitate (*N,N*-dimethylaniline-HCl) is collected by centrifugation; traces of $(C_2H_5)_2O$ are removed under an N_2 stream, and the hygroscopic material is stored over Drierite in a vacuum dessicator. Aliquots are dissolved in H_2O to prepare substrate solutions.
3. $NADP^+$, 10 m*M*.
4. Glucose 6-phosphate, 0.10 M.
5. 10^3 IU Yeast glucose-6-phosphate dehydrogenase/ml [in Tris-acetate buffer (pH 7.4) containing 1.0 m*M* EDTA and 20% glycerol (w/v)].
6. *N,N*-Dimethylaniline *N*-oxide (prepared according to ref. 68), mp 121–122°C (HCl salt), dissolve in H_2O to 0.10 *M* before use.

For this assay microsomes are unsuitable, since most of the *N*-oxide formation is the result of the FMO (vide infra). Also, in these experiments care must be taken

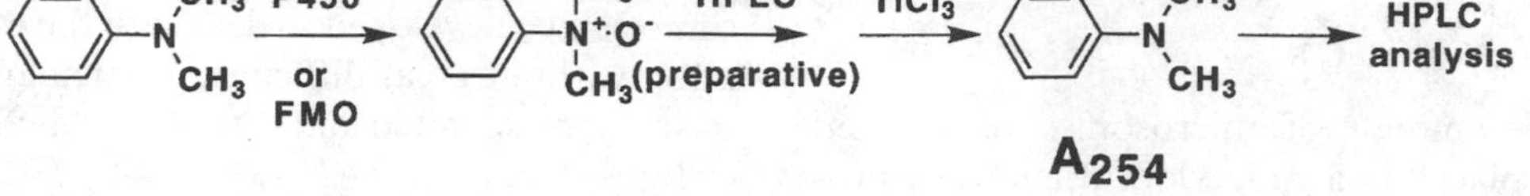

FIG. 35.19. Formation and assay of amine *N*-oxides (373,374).

to insure that N-oxide formation is not due to H_2O_2 produced by enzymes.

Rat liver cytochrome P450 2B1 (1 μM), rabbit liver NADPH–cytochrome P450 reductase (1 μM), and 30 μM L-α-1,2-dilauroyl-*sn*-glycero-3-phosphocholine are mixed and preincubated at 23°C for 10 min. Further additions include potassium phosphate buffer (to 50 mM), 1.0 mM N,N-dimethylaniline-HCl, catalase (bovine erythrocyte, Sigma Chemical Co., dialyzed to remove thymol, to 800 U ml^{-1}), 0.50 mM $NADP^+$, and 1.0 IU glucose-6-phosphate dehydrogenase/ml. The mixture is preincubated for 5 min at 37°C , and reaction is initiated by the addition of glucose 6-phosphate to 10 mM (total volume 5.0 ml).

After 10 min, each reaction is stopped by the addition of 1.7 ml of 17% aqueous $HClO_4$ (w/v) and chilled on ice to precipitate salts. The samples are centrifuged at $3 \times 10^3 \times g$ for 10 min, and part of the supernatant fractions (5.0 ml) is made alkaline by the addition of 0.32 ml of 5 N NaOH and applied to a Sep-Pak C18 cartridge [Waters-Millipore, Bedford, MA; previously washed with CH_3OH (v/v)]. The eluate is mixed with 100 μl of 1.0 M aqueous H_3PO_4 and evaporated to $\sim$250 μl under an N_2 stream at 40°C. Each sample (200 μl) is injected onto an HPLC column (10 × 250 mm Ultremex 5 C_{18}) using a mixture of CH_3OH and aqueous buffer [25 mM H_3PO_4, adjusted to pH 7.0 with $(C_2H_5)_3N$] (35–65, v/v). The N-oxide fraction (region previously found with standards) of the HPLC eluate is collected and acidified by the addition of 50 μl of 5.0 N aqueous HCl, concentrated to $\sim$2 ml under an N_2 stream at 40°C, and treated with 120 μl of a 30% $TiCl_3$ solution (w/v, dissolved in 5 N aqueous HCl) for 1 h. $TiCl_3$ quantitatively reduces all of the N,N-dimethylaniline N-oxide to N,N-demethylaniline (73), increasing the extinction coefficient 60-fold (from $\varepsilon = 240$ to $\varepsilon = 14{,}100$ M^{-1} cm^{-1}). To this material is added 200 μl of 5 N aqueous NaOH and 100 nmol of 4-methyl-N,N-dimethylaniline (N,N-dimethyl-p-toluidine) as an internal standard; the amines are extracted into CH_2Cl_2, to which is added 100 μl of 0.1 M aqueous H_3PO_4 prior to evaporation to dryness under N_2 at 40°C (added to prevent loss of amine). Dried samples are dissolved in a 1:1 mixture of CH_3OH and H_2O (v/v), and aliquots are analyzed on an analytical octadecylsilane (C18) HPLC column using a mixture of CH_3OH and buffer [25 mM H_3PO_4, adjusted to pH 7.0 with $(C_2H_5)_3N$], 75–25, v/v. Under these conditions N,N-dimethylaniline elutes at 6.6 min and 4-methyl-N,N-dimethylaniline at 9.7 min.

The procedure just described has been used to assay the N-oxidation of a number of different N,N-dialkylaniline derivatives (374). A colorimetric assay involving extraction of N,N-dialkylaniline N-oxides and derivatization by nitrosation at the *para*-position has been used to measure the reaction catalyzed by flavin-containing monooxygenase (475), but this assay is not particularly sensitive and of course is not applicable to the assay of *para*-substituted N,N-dialkylaniline N-oxides (374). A point to be made by presentation of this assay procedure is that many assays can be designed to circumvent analytical problems encountered in the assay of enzymatic reactions.

Tritium Release: Sparteine (Δ^5), Nifedipine, and 17β-Estradiol Oxidations

The measurement of sparteine Δ^5-oxidation activity (Figure 35.20) is an example of a tritium release assay. In the process of oxidation, a tritium atom is released from the substrate and partitions into H_2O. If the substrate is nonpolar, it can be extracted and the radioactivity in the H_2O can be determined. In addition to the measurement of sparteine Δ^5-oxidation activity, we have also utilized this assay to measure the 2- and 4-hydroxylation of 17β-estradiol (76,164) and the oxidation of nifedipine and its analogs (Figure 35.21).

Δ^5-Dehydrosparteine can be prepared from sparteine by mercuric acetate oxidation; reduction with NaB^3H_4 gives only the correct stereoisomer of sparteine (136,261). The 5-^3H material can be easily crystallized as the hydrosulfate or perchlorate salt. These salts are quite water-soluble and assays are set up in the general manner described earlier with 1.0 mM concentrations of the substrate. After 20 min at 37°C, the pH of the incubation (total volume 200 μl) is raised to >12 and the mixture is extracted 3 times with 1.0-ml aliquots of CH_2Cl_2, with brief intermediate centrifugation to separate the layers. One hundred microliters of the aqueous phase is counted in 5 ml of a scintillation cocktail designed to hold H_2O, with care taken to allow any chemiluminescence to decay in the dark.

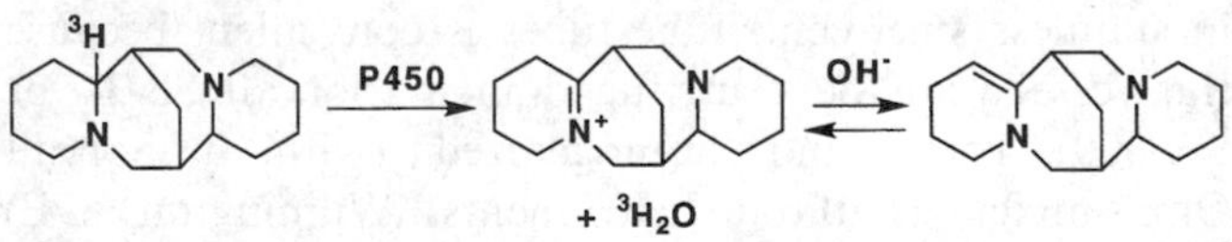

FIG. 35.20. Sparteine Δ^5-oxidation as an example of a tritium release assay (136).

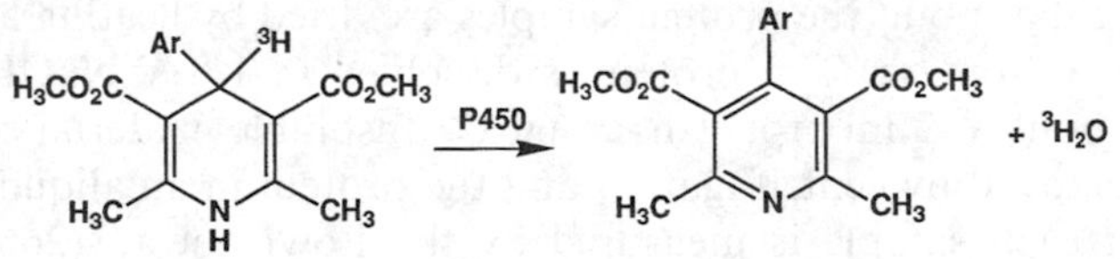

FIG. 35.21. Release of tritium from 2,6-dimethyl-4-phenyl-3,5-bis(carbomethoxy)-1,4-dihydropyridine during oxidation by cytochrome P450 (140,150).

In the case of 17β-estradiol hydroxylation a similar procedure can be used, except that acid is added prior to extraction to protonate the phenols (76).

When these approaches are used, the results should be corrected for the kinetic tritium isotope effect if one exists (261). One cannot be certain that this isotope effect is constant among different types of enzyme samples. In the cases of sparteine and nifedipine (and other 1,4-dihydropyridines) the intermolecular isotope effects are <3 (1361,140,150,318).

Covalent Binding of Metabolites to Protein

The irreversible binding of reaction products to protein was observed 40 years ago (293). Although no concensus is presently clear about the importance of individual targets or how such modification of proteins acutally leads to death of cells, in vitro binding of chemicals to protein provides an index of bioactivation processes and can be useful in the characterization of reactive intermediates.

In general the enzyme system under investigation is incubated with the radioactive substrate for a fixed amount of time, during which the rate of production of species binding covalently should remain constant. In practice this is usually less than 1 h. Incubations are terminated and binding to protein is measured. Several approaches are available for measuring binding.

One method involves precipitation of the protein with organic solvent (C_2H_5OH or CH_3OH, >2 volumes) or aqueous Cl_3CCO_2H (5% final concentration, w/v) and collection of the pelleted material after centrifugation in any case ($10^4 \times$ g, 15 min). The sensitivity of the residual substrate to the solvent must be considered, as well as the solubility. The supernatant fraction is decanted and more acid or solvent is added; the protein pellet is washed by vigorous mixing or homogenization. We have found that carrying out the entire procedure in stainless steel centrifuge tubes is convenient because the vessels can be centrifuged in a (Sorvall SS-34 or SA-600) rotor and homogenized (with a Sorvall Omni-mixer) (DuPont Instruments, Wilmington, DE) without the need to transfer contents. The process of homogenization, centrifugation, and decantation of supernatant fraction is repeated several times until significant radioactivity no longer appears in the wash fractions. At that point the protein samples are dried by heating at 60°C for 2 h. The protein is dissolved in 1.0 *N* NaOH (about 1–2 ml) for 1 h at 60°C. Insoluble material is removed by centrifugation and the protein in an aliquot of each sample is measured by the Lowry et al. (266) or Pierce bicinchoninic acid methods (vide supra), because the recovery is variable. A larger aliquot of each sample is added to 5–10 ml of a scintillation mixture capable of holding water and chemiluminescence is allowed to decay overnight at room temperature in the dark prior to counting. The results are expressed in terms of nanomoles adduct per mg protein, with subtraction of values obtained with an inactive enzyme (e.g., without NADPH in the case of mixed-function oxidases).

Another approach is extensive dialysis of protein samples against buffer containing sodium dodecyl sulfate (SDS) (401). We have utilized this method with hydrophilic materials such as acrylonitrile (108,154,188) but have not obtained as reliable results with more hydrophobic materials.

A third method involves the adsorption of protein to glass fiber filters, such as those used for in vitro protein translation experiments (437). These disks can be washed with organic solvents in a shaking device to remove unbound material. We have usually used 5–8 changes of the wash solvent, with wash times of 30 min per cycle (usually with C_2H_5OH as the solvent) (159,294). The capacity of these filters is limited, so that such an approach may not be satisfactory if considerable amounts of protein must be used. However, if satisfactory sensitivity can be achieved with the use of submilligram amounts of protein, then the method is considerably easier than the other approaches. In our experience with trichloroethylene, we have found that recovery of protein on the filters is nearly quantitative when $\leq$1 mg protein is used (checks on binding can be done with radiolabeled proteins) (159,294).

Covalent Binding of Metabolites to DNA

Like the binding of reaction products to protein, binding to DNA provides an index of bioactivation. One must remember that binding to naked DNA in such a system may be much higher than in vitro or in cells. Binding to protein is not to be equated with nucleic acid binding; notable examples demonstrate that different enzymes and pathways can be involved in the generation of the various types of adducts (cf. acrylonitrile, ethylene dibromide—vide supra) (151).

Calf thymus DNA has been used in many in vitro binding experiments. Herring sperm DNA is considerably cheaper and much more soluble; its fragmented nature should not really cause a problem in this type of work. In general, DNA is added to incubations, containing a radioactive substrate, at a concentration of ~2 mg/ml, with other components as used in standard procedures (vide supra).

Several methods can be used to purify the DNA for measurement of bound adducts, and the choice depends upon the situation.

One approach involves initial extraction of the aqueous solution with H_2O-saturated butanol to remove small compounds. Centrifugation ($3 \times 10^3 \times$ g, 10 min) is used to separate the layers after each step. The DNA solution is mixed with an equal volume of phenol solution [liquid phenol is first washed sequentially with equal volumes of 1.0 *M*, 0.50 *M*, and 0.02 *M* Tris-HCl (pH 7.4) and then 1 g of 8-hydroxyquinoline is added per liter of phenol]. After mixing (with a vortex device), the layers are separated by centrifugation; DNA remains in the lower phase. The step is repeated one or two more times. NaCl is added to the DNA layer to a concentration of 0.10 *M*. The DNA is precipitated by the addition of 5 volumes of cold (−20°C) C_2H_5OH and recovered by centrifugation; the material, dried under an N_2 stream, can be dissolved in any of a number of low ionic strength buffers, although shaking or other agitation may be necessary.

Another procedure that has been used as an alternative to the butanol and phenol extractions involves the sedimentation of DNA by ultracentrifugation (201). This process is usually done following the enzymatic incubation: SDS is added to a final concentration of 1% w/v, (from a stock 10% solution). The incubation buffer should not contain potassium ions because potassium dodecyl sulfate is rather insoluble. The preparations are centrifuged at $10^5 \times g$ for 16 h at 20°C to pellet the DNA. The recovery is generally good (>80%), and most proteins remain soluble and are decanted in the supernatant fraction. Although the procedure is limited by availability of rotor places in the ultracentrifuge, the effort involved in manipulations is minimal.

Sometimes these procedures do not completely remove unbound materials. A useful procedure for further purification is hydroxylapatite chromatography. A method used in this laboratory is outlined: For a sample containing 1 mg DNA, 1 g dry hydroxylapatite (Calbiochem DNA grade, Calbiochem, San Diego, CA) is suspended in 5 m*M* sodium phosphate buffer (pH 6.8) and swirled to hydrate the particles. The suspension is evacuated (at 40°C) to remove gas bubbles, using an aspirator, and is poured into a column (1.6 cm diameter), where 5 m*M* sodium phosphate buffer (pH 6.8) is pumped through the column at a flow rate of ~2 ml/min using a peristaltic pump. The DNA is applied to the column (using the pump) and the column is sequentially eluted with 100, 200, and 300 m*M* sodium phosphate buffers (pH 6.8). The eluate is monitored at 254 nm, and the elution buffer is not changed until A_{254} has decreased nearly to the baseline (eluted fractions are collected). Proteins are eluted with 100 m*M* phosphate, RNA with 200 m*M* phosphate, and DNA with 300 m*M* phosphate. Aliquots of fractions can be assayed for radioactivity after mixing with a solution containing a detergent and designed for aqueous samples. When large volumes of water and high phosphate concentrations are used, the conditions needed for formation of a stable gel should be checked carefully beforehand.

If concentration of peak fractions is necessary, this is conveniently achieved by removal of the salt from the pooled samples by extensive dialysis and subsequent lyophilization. In some cases further treatment of DNA with RNase (heating at 80°C for 10 min prior to use to destroy DNase) or pronase may be desired, with subsequent recovery of DNA by phenol extraction and ethanol precipitation. Analyses for RNA can be done using the orcinol procedure (84). Protein can be measured with any of several assays or, if necessary, by amino acid hydrolysis (188). (*Note*: Purine decomposition leads to abnormally high levels of glycine.) DNA itself can be estimated with the diphenylamine procedure (45), with Hoechst 33258 dye using a fluorimeter (49), or using the approximate relationship of $E_{260}^{1\%} = 200\ \text{cm}^{-1}$.

If major DNA adducts have been identified for a particular substrate, then the best approach is to hydrolyze the DNA and measure the adduct by a specific method, such as chromatography or immunoassay.

Other Cytochrome P450-Linked Activities

The assays just described are among the most widely used. However, the list of activities that have been examined is much more extensive. Some of these activities are presented in Table 35.1, along with appropriate references. This table (not intended to be totally inclusive) will acquaint the reader with the wide variety of cytochrome P450 substrates and the assays available for use. Many of these assays can be modified to permit the determination of almost any activity.

Microsomal Flavoprotein Oxidase

This mixed-function oxidase consists of a single flavoprotein (471,474), as opposed to a two-protein system, but recently the existence of multiple forms of the enzyme has been demonstrated (255,256,424,458). The best source of the enzyme appears to be porcine liver, and the activity appears to be less stable than cytochrome P450-linked activities (346). Several heterologous expression systems have been developed (48,204,257). The enzyme is often assayed by measuring the methimazole or *N,N*-dimethylaniline-stimulated rate of NADPH oxidation or oxygen uptake (345) (see section discussing benzphetamine); activity of some forms is stimulated by certain primary amines (471).

Polyunsaturated Fatty Acid Hydroperoxide-Dependent Oxidations by Peroxidases and Metal Complexes

Polyunsaturated fatty acid hydroperoxide-dependent oxidations provide an alternate to the mixed-function oxidase system for xenobiotic oxidation (96,285). Oxidations can be catalyzed by the peroxidase of prostaglandin endoperoxide (PGG_2) synthase or by metal complexes or certain metalloproteins (251,283).

Polyunsaturated fatty acid hydroperoxides are generated by the cyclooxygenase of prostaglandin H (PGH) synthase (often termed "COX" for "cyclooxygenase") or by lipid peroxidation (88,286). Assays are described for the quantification of hydroperoxide-dependent oxidations triggered by both pathways.

Guaiacol Oxidation

Principle. Addition of arachidonic acid to microsomal preparations of PGH synthase generates the hydroperoxide PGG_2, which is a substrate for the peroxidase activity (Figure 35.22). Formation of Compound I of the PGH synthase peroxidase leads to oxidation of the reducing substrate (251). A number of reducing substrates are oxidized by the peroxidase, including several chromogenic substrates (282,341).

Reagents.

1. Hematin, 0.50 m*M* in $(CH_3)_2SO$ (hematin—from bovine blood—Sigma, St. Louis, MO).
2. 9 m*M* Guiaicol (dissolve 50 μM in 50 ml of 0.12 *M* Tris-HCl buffer, pH 8.0); prepare on day of assay in amber glass container; keep at 4°C until assay begins; keep at room temperature throughout entire assay period.
3. 7 m*M* Sodium arachidonate. Add 2 mg arachidonic acid from a benzene stock solution to a test tube and evaporate the benzene under a stream of N_2. Dissolve the residue in 50 μl C_2H_5OH and add 100 μl of 0.10 *M* NaOH. Agitate the soapy solution and add 0.85 ml H_2O. Keep on ice throughout the assay period.
4. 0.12 *M* Tris-HCl buffer (pH 8.0 at room temperature). Dissolve 3.57 g in 250 ml water, adjust pH with HCl, keep at room temperature during assay, and store at 4°C.

Assay Procedure. Place the buffer (790 μl) into a cuvette, followed by hematin (2 μl), enzyme (microsomes or purified protein), and guaiacol (55 μl). The reaction is initiated by addition of 10 μl of the sodium arachidonate solution to the cuvette positioned in the spectrophotometer. The reference cuvette contains 0.12 *M* Tris buffer. Oxidation of guaiacol is monitored by the increase in absorbance at 436 nm.

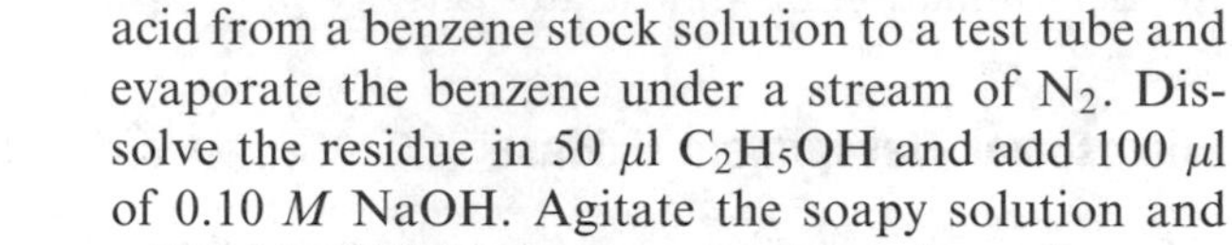

FIG. 35.22. Oxidation of arachidonic acid by PGH synthase.

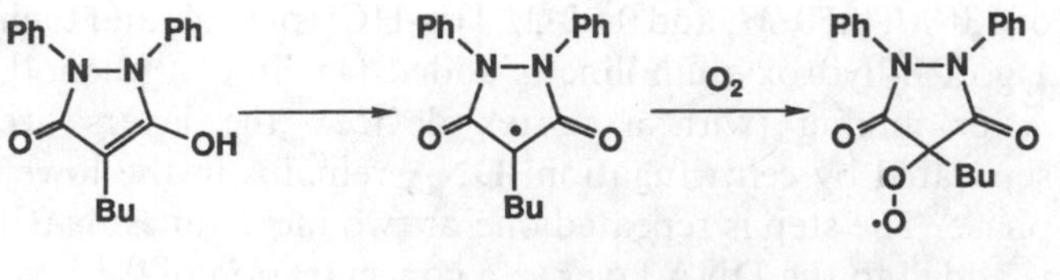

FIG. 35.23. Oxidation of phenylbutazone by PGH synthase.

Phenylbutazone Oxidation

Principle. Phenylbutazone is a nonsteroidal anti-inflammatory agent used for the treatment of rheumatoid disorders. It is cooxygenated by the peroxidase activity of PGH synthase to 4-hydroxyphenylbutazone (191,284). Arachidonic acid, PGG_2, 15-hydroperoxyarachidonic acid (284), or peroxide can affect oxidation. The source of the hydroxyl oxygen is the molecular oxygen state of the peroxidase, and the carbon-centered radical formed is the scavenged by O_2 (284) (Figure 35.23). The resultant peroxyl radical is eventually converted to a hydroxyl group (284). Since the source of the hydroxyl group is molecular oxygen, the uptake of O_2 from solution can be used to assay oxidation.

Reagents.

1. 0.10 *M* Potassium phosphate buffer (pH 7.8).
2. 50 m*M* Phenylbutazone (Sigma, St. Louis, MO) in CH_3OH.
3. 10 m*M* 15-Hydroperoxiarachidonic acid or H_2O_2 in CH_3OH or H_2O, respectively.
4. Enzyme preparation (e.g., ram seminal vesicle microsomes or recombinant PGH synthase).

Assay Procedure. Phenylbutazone (500 μM) is preincubated for 3 min with ram seminal vesicle microsomes or another PGH synthase preparation in the reaction cell of a Gilson oxygraph at 37°C. The hydroperoxide (100 μM) is added and the rate and extent of O_2 uptake are recorded. The initial velocity of phenylbutazone oxidation is calculated from the initial linear portion of the O_2 uptake curve.

Mixed-Function Oxidase- and Peroxyl Radical-Dependent Epoxidation of Benzo[a]pyrene-7,8-dihydrodiol

Principle. 7,8-Dihydroxy-7,8-dihydrobenzo[*a*]pyrene (BP-7,8-diol), a metabolite of the environmental pollutant benzo[*a*]pyrene (Figure 35.9), is converted by microsomal mixed-function oxidases and peroxyl free radicals to diastereomeric diol epoxides. The stereochemistry of oxygen insertion is a useful technique with which to distinguish cytochrome P450- and lipid peroxidation-dependent epoxidation. The formation of two enantiomeric pairs of diastereomeeric diol epoxides (BPDEs) formed from the racemic BP-7,8-diol is demon-

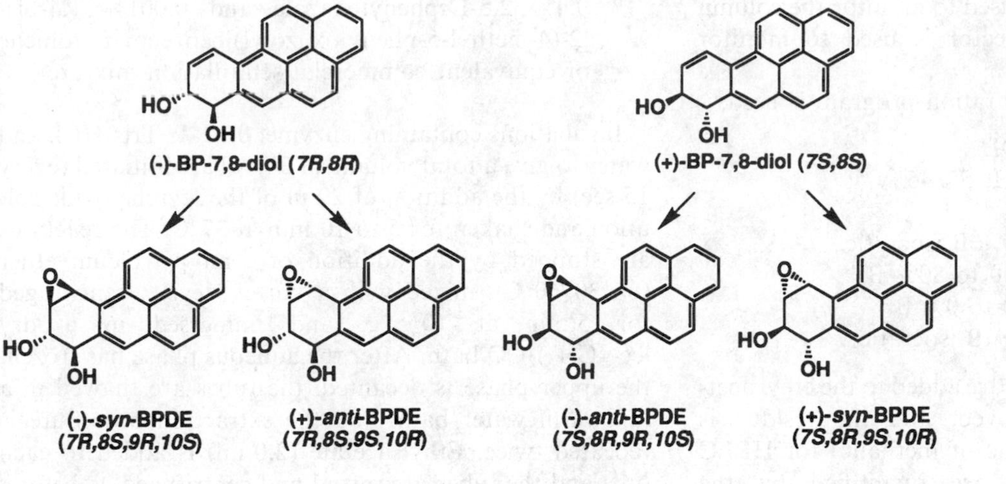

FIG. 35.24. Oxidation of benzo[a]pyrene 7,8-diol by cytochrome P450 and radical-mediated pathways to diastereomeric diol epoxide products.

strated in Figure 35.24. Mixed-function oxidase-dependent epoxidation of (±)-BP-7,8-diol by microsomes from uninduced rats results in approximately equal formation of *anti*- and *syn*-diol epoxides (ratio of 1.1±0.3) (409). In contrast, peroxidative epoxidation results in an excess of *anti*-diol epoxides (*anti*/*syn* ratio of 2.5±0.4) (324). The diol epoxides are unstable in aqueous media, so their formation is quantified from the yields of their stable tetraol hydrolysis products, separable by reversed-phase HPLC.

Resolved (+)-BP-7,8-diol is an especially useful probe for distinguishing mixed-function oxidase- and peroxyl radical-dependent metabolism. Microsomal and purified cytochromes P450 metabolize this enantiomer exclusively to the (−)-*syn*-diol epoxide (409), whereas peroxidative epoxidation gives predominantly (+)-*anti*-diol epoxide (88). Therefore the formation of *anti*-diol epoxide from (+)-BP-7,8-diol is diagnostic of peroxidative diol epoxidation.

Substrates.

1. Racemic and (+)-BP-7,8-diol, as well as (±)-*anti*- and *syn*-diol epoxides, are available from the National Cancer Institute Chemical Carcinogen Reference Standard Repository (NIH, Bethesda, MD).
2. *Trans*- and *cis*-tetraol standards are prepared by solvolysis of the *anti*- and *syn*-diol epoxides and characterized by UV spectroscopy and mass spectrometry of their tetraacetate derivatives, as described by Yagi et al. (465).

Reagents.

1. 50 m*M* Tris-HCl buffer (pH 7.5).
2. 1.0 m*M* BHT in ethyl acetate.
3. Rat liver microsomes, in 0.20 *M* KCl buffer (vide supra).
4. 0.10 *M* NADPH in buffer.
5. ADP (0.40 *M*) plus Fe^{3+} (1.5 m*M*), in buffer.
6. EDTA (10 m*M*) plus Fe^{2+} (10 m*M*), in deoxygenated buffer.
7. [^{14}C]BP-7,8-diol (1.2 m*M*, specific activity 5.7 mCi/nmol), in ethanol.
8. Thiobarbituric acid solution, prepared as described in ref. 40.

Incubation Procedure.

Mixed-Function Oxidase-Dependent Epoxidation. Microsomes (0.50 mg protein/ml) and 30 *μ*l of the [^{14}C]-BP-7,8-diol solution are added to the Tris buffer to give a final volume of 0.99 ml. Following a 3-min preincubation, reaction is initiated by the addition of 10 *μ*l of the NADPH solution and allowed to continue for 20 min at 37°C. Reaction is terminated by adding half of the incubation mixture to 1.0 ml of the thiobarbituric acid solution, while the remainder is extracted twice with 1.0 ml ethyl acetate containing BHT. The thiobarbituric acid-containing solution is mixed vigorously using a vortex device, heated at 100°C for 15 min, and analyzed for thiobarbituric acid-reactive material (indicative of lipid peroxidation), as described by Buege and Aust (40). The protein residue that remains after the ethyl acetate extraction may be analyzed for protein-bound metabolites (indicative of reactive intermediates), as described by Tunek et al. (422).

Peroxyl Radical-Dependent Epoxidation. Microsomes (0.50 mg protein/ml) and 30 *μ*l of the [^{14}C]-BP-7,8-diol solution are added to the incubation buffer to give a final volume of 0.97 ml. After preincubation, 10 *μ*l each of the NADPH, ADP/Fe^{3+}, and EDTA/Fe^{2+} solutions are added simultaneously to initiate the reaction. The termination and workup are as described earlier.

HPLC Analysis. HPLC separations have been performed using a Zorbax octadecylsilane colume (324). A UV detector is set at 344 nm (absorbance maximum for the tetraol products) and used to monitor the column effluent. A radioactivity detector is used to monitor radioactivity.

The following gradient separation program is used:

Reservoir: A = 100% CH_3OH
B = H_2O-CH_3OH, 55/45, v/v
Flow: 1.5 ml/min
Gradient: 0 to 20 min, 100% B isocratic
20 to 40 min, 100 to 80% B
40 to 50 min, 80 to 0% B
50 to 60 min, 0% B isocratic

Unlabeled tetraol standards are added to the ethyl acetate extract, solvent is removed, and the residue is dissolved in a minimal volume of methanol for HPLC injection. Tetraol products are quantified by the cochromatography of radiolabeled peaks with the unlabeled standards. Alternatively, unlabeled BP-7,8-diol can be used for the incubation and the tetraol formation estimated by the UV peak area ratios. The retention times of authentic standards of tetraols were *trans-anti* (20 min), *trans-syn* (25 min), *cis-anti* (28 min), and *cis-syn* (34 min). The sum of the tetraols derived from the *anti*- and *syn*-diol epoxides is an indication of the extent of epoxidation by peroxyl radicals and cytochrome P450, respectively (381).

Epoxide Hydrolase

This enzyme is active toward a wide variety of alkyl and aryl epoxides (134,180,289,313). There are at least three different epoxide hydrolase enzymes (134,180,412), but a single microsomal enzyme has a wide range of substrates (100,180). The most commonly used substrate is [7-^{3}H]-styrene oxide (Figure 35.25), which can be obtained from New England Nuclear, Boston, or Amersham-Searle, Des Plaines, IL.

Reagents.

1. [7-^{3}H]-Styrene oxide, 16 m*M* in tetrahydrofuran containing 0.1% $(C_2H_5)_3N$ (note: purity should be checked by TLC prior to use).
2. 0.5 *M* Tris-HCl buffer, pH 8.7 at 37°C (pH 9.0 at 25°C).

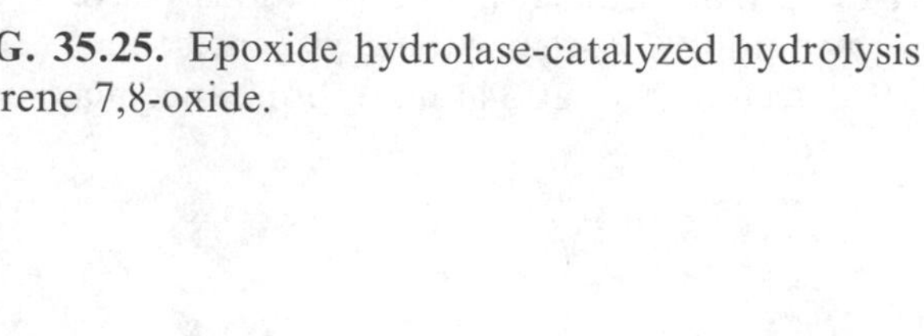

FIG. 35.25. Epoxide hydrolase-catalyzed hydrolysis of styrene 7,8-oxide.

3. 0.4% 2,5-Diphenyloxazole and 0.001% 1,4-bis-[2-(4-methyl-5-phenyloxazolyl)]benzene in toluene or equivalent commercial scintillation mixture.

Incubations containing enzyme, 0.17 *M* Tris-HCl, and water to give a total volume of 300 μl are initiated (every 15 sec) by the addition of 20 μl of the styrene oxide solution and shaken for 5 to 10 min at 37°C. The reactions are stopped by the addition of 5 ml petroleum ether (bp 30–60°C), mixed with a vortex device, centrifuged for 5 min at $10^3 \times g$, and immersed in a dry ice–$(CH_3)_2CO$ bath. After the aqueous phase has frozen, the upper phase is decanted, the tubes are thawed in a lukewarm water bath, and the extraction procedure is repeated twice. Ethyl acetate (2.0 ml) is added to each tube and the tubes are mixed and centrifuged as before. An aliquot (0.3 ml) of each ethyl acetate phase (containing the styrene glycol) is transferred to a mini-scintillation vial and 5 ml of scintillation mixture are added. Vials are counted (2–10 min is usually sufficient) and rates of glycol production are determined; blanks contain all components except enzyme (or enzyme boiled for 10 min) (315).

An alternative procedure is more convenient, especially if a large number of samples are involved (215). Incubations are scaled down to a total volume of 80 μl. Reactions are stopped by the addition of 25 μl of tetrahydrofuran containing 0.4 *M* styrene glycol (Aldrich) and placed on ice. A volume of 35 μl from each incubation is applied to the loading portion of a Whatman LK6DF TLC plate (Whatman, Clifton, NJ). Plates are dried briefly in air and developed in a 4 : 1 mixture of $CHCl_3$-ethyl acetate (v/v). When the solvent reaches the top of the plate, the styrene glycol zone ($R_f \sim 0.1$) is marked after visualization with short-wavelength (254 nm) UV light. The regions containing styrene glycol are scraped into mini-scintillation vials and shaken briefly after adding 1.0 ml of CH_3OH. Scintillation cocktail (4 ml) is added and the vials are counted. Chemiluminescence may be a problem, and raising the floor of the channel window is useful; alternatively, overnight decay in the dark may be necessary to give the best results.

The TLC procedure has been modified for a number of other radioactive substrates (215). Oesch has also described a generalized extraction procedure for a number of radioactive epoxides (27); we have found that this assay procedure can be used with these unlabeled epoxides when the diols are quantitated using fluorescence measurements (174). Assays based upon spectrophotometric measurement of residual substrate (safrole and 1-chlorooxirane) have been used, but these suffer from a lack of sensitivity (174,175,182,443). We have also devised an alternative spectrophotometric assay for the assay of epoxide hydrolase utilizing the reduction of NAD^+ by glycols in the presence of alcohol dehydrogenase (166).

Assays based upon spectrophotometric measurement of residual substrate (safrole and 1-chlorooxirane) have been used, but these suffer from a lack of sensitivity (174,175,182,443). One useful assay based on the disappearance of substrate utilizes phenanthrene 9,10-oxide (180,248).

Other Conjugating Enzymes

The methodology for assaying each of the enzymes will not be elaborated here. The reader should bear in mind that many of these also consist of families of related enzymes and that an assay for one may not be applicable to others.

A variety of assays for UDP-glucuronosyl transferase have been utilized and are reviewed by Burchell et al. (42) (see also refs. 41, 231, 407, and references therein). These include radiometric, colorimetric, fluorimetric, and chromatographic methods. This microsomal enzyme exhibits considerable latency; that is, its activity is increased considerably after solubilization of the membrane with detergent.

The most popular assays of GSH transferases are spectrophotometric, such as that involving conjugation of 1-chloro-2,4-dinitrobenzene (177) (Figure 35.26). Other spectrophotometric, titrimetric, and chromatographic assays have been developed and were reviewed by Jakoby and Habig (208) [see also refs. 8, 61, 235, and references therein). Some of the reactions catalyzed by GSH transferase occur at finite rates in the absence of the enzyme, and control reactions are needed in which enzyme is absent. In addition to the conjugating activities, some forms of the enzyme also catalyze steroid double-bond epimerization and peroxide reduction (208).

γ-Glutamyl transpeptidase cleaves the glutamate moiety of GSH and GSH conjugates. The enzyme is most abundant in the kidney and intestinal plasma membranes. The activity can be measured as described by Meister et al. (292).

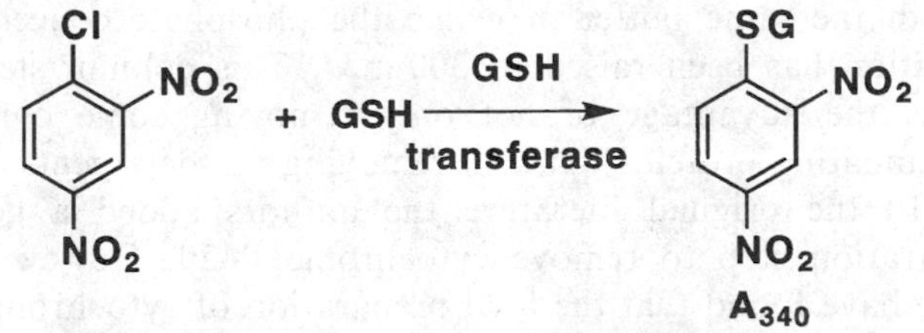

FIG. 35.26. Conjugation of glutathione (GSH) with 1-chloro-2,4-dinitrobenzene catalyzed by GSH transferase.

After the γ-glutamyl transpeptidase reaction occurs, hydrolysis of the glycine moiety then gives a cysteine conjugate. These cysteine conjugates can undergo β-elimination by a pyridoxal phosphate-containing enzyme found in liver and kidney, cysteine conjugate β-lyase. The assay is not very convenient: *S*-(2,4-dinitrophenyl)-L-[^{35}S]-cysteine is incubated with the enzyme and one of the products, 2,4-dinitrobenzethiol, is methylated with CH_3I and analyzed by TLC (404).

A number of enzymes form sulfate monoesters by transferring the sulfate group from 3′-phosphoadenosine-5′-phosphosulfate (PAPS) to a hydroxyl group. Since the acceptor substrates vary, so do the assays which can be used. One of the more common assays involves chromatographic separation after incubation with [^{35}S]-PAPS (1,210,371).

Methyltransferases are most conveniently assayed with radiolabeled methyl donors (14,35,453). Transfers can involve N, O, or S atoms. Other chromatographic, fluorometric, and spectrophotometric assays have also been used but are generally not as sensitive or rapid (35).

Another moiety that is often transferred in biological reactions of interest is the acetyl group (6,185,448). The physiological donor group is acetylcoenzyme A (acetylCoA), and a variety of colorimetric (451), fluorimetric (291), spectrophotometric (5,214,447,449), and radiometric (5,116,423) assays have been described.

ISOLATION OF ENZYMES

Cytochrome P450

Cytochrome P450 is the enzyme that has probably received most of the attention of those concerned with microsomal metabolism to date. Early studies on the role of the enzyme system and its inducibility in carcinogenesis and toxicology have been reviewed elsewhere (62,63,109,115) as well as more recently (138,460). Other reviews of progress in purification and reconstitution techniques have also appeared (133,138,271).

Liver microsomal cytochrome P450 was first solubilized and partially purified by Lu and Coon and their associates (267,270); since that time a number of advances have been made (306). Because various of forms of cytochrome P450 are found in various tissues of different animals, a number of procedures have been developed for purification of individual forms (152,183, 184,228–230,233,339,361). Major features of some of the purification schemes are presented here, and the reader is referred to the original literature for details [see ref. 306 and references therein]. The choice of a purification system depends upon the animal species of choice, whether simultaneous purification of other enzymes is desired, and other factors. Most of the procedures discussed here are carried out at 0–4°C in the presence of 20% glycerol (v/v) for stabilization. A number of different alkyl phenyl ether-based detergents have been used in purification, including Emulgens 911 and 913 (Kao-Atlas, Tokyo), Triton N-101 (Sigma), Renex 690, and Non-Idet NP40. Our work (130) and that of others (65,218–220) suggest that these and some additional nonionic detergents are relatively interchangeable, although some differences exist and may be significant in some cases (199). However, some of these detergents are actually substrates for cytochromes P450 and are also difficult to completely remove from the enzymes (189).

Rat Liver Cytochrome P450s

A general procedure for purification of rat liver microsomal cytochrome P450 was developed in our laboratory, a modification of earlier methods (129,130); the major inducible liver microsomal cytochromes P450 of phenobarbital- (P450 2B1) or β-naphthoflavone-treated (P450 1A1) rats can be highly purified in good yield using two basic chromatography steps (163). Details were provided in the last edition of this book (144). However, in the interest of space considerations, this has been deleted in favor of methods for use with recombinant P450 (P450 2E1 as a prototype).

Rabbit Cytochrome P450 1A2

The following procedure is an adaptation of the method of Alterman and Dowgii (2). The cytochrome P450 1A2 enzymes isolated from different animal species and humans are of interest because of their catalytic activities, particularly the *N*-hydroxylation of potentially carcinogenic aryl and heterocyclic amines, including those found in pyrolyzed food (46,467). The cytochrome P450 1A2 enzymes found in different species share a number of unusual physical properties, including their tendency to exist as high-spin iron complexes in the absence of substrates (135), their blue-shifted Fe^{2+}–CO complexes absorbing light at ~447 nm (135), and their tendency to precipitate in buffers containing low salt concentrations (87,135). We have utilized rabbit liver as an enzyme source in the past because of particular research needs for large amounts of enzyme and the applicability of this two-step purification procedure, which was subsequently adapted to use with recombinant human P450 1A2 (370).

Rabbits are administered 4 daily ip doses (80 mg/kg) of a corn oil suspension of 5,6-benzoflavone (β-naphthoflavone). The animals are killed by iv injection of pentobarbital and the livers are removed, trimmed of the gall bladders (take care not to open, or solubilizing bile acids will be released) and attached tissue, and washed in cold 1.15% KCl (w/v). When large amounts of material are processed (up to 12 rabbits), it is convenient to cut the livers into small pieces (~5 cm^3) and drop these pieces into liquid N_2 for rapid freezing. These frozen pieces may be stored at −80°C until preparation of microsomes, when they are thawed by adding them to cold 0.10 *M* Tris-acetate buffer (pH 7.4) containing 0.10 *M* KCl, 1.0 m*M* EDTA, and 20 μM BHT. Microsomes are prepared in the usual manner (vide supra).

Microsomes are suspended at a concentration of 10 mg protein/ml in cold 50 m*M* Tris-HCl buffer (pH 7.4) containing 1.0 m*M* EDTA, 1.0 m*M* dithiothreitol, and 20% glycerol (v/v). This and all subsequent steps are carried out at 4°C. Sodium cholate is added to a concentration of 0.625% (w/v, from a buffered aqueous 20% solution, not recrystallized) and Triton N-101 to 1.25% (w/v, from a 20% solution). With the columns described next, a typical preparation would begin with about 4500 mg microsomal protein. The clarified supension is stirred for 30 min at 4°C and subjected to centrifugation at $10^5 \times g$ for 60 min. The pellets are discarded and the soluble supernatant fractions are pooled and applied to a 5 × 30 cm column of DEAE-Sephacel (Pharmacia, Piscataway, NJ), which has been previously adjusted to pH 7.4 before pouring and washed with ≥2 l of the same buffer used for the solubilization (containing cholate and Triton N-101). Rabbit cytochrome P450 1A2 is eluted in the void volume of the column.

The material eluted in the void volume of the column is diluted twofold with a 20% aqueous solution of glycerol (v/v) and applied to a 2.5 × 20 cm column of CM Sepharose Fast Flow (Pharmacia), which has been adjusted to pH 7.4 and equilibrated with 20 m*M* potassium phosphate buffer (pH 7.4) containing 0.20 m*M* EDTA, 1.0 m*M* dithiothreitol, and 20% glycerol (v/v). The cytochrome P450 1A2 binds tightly to the top of the column in a dark brown band. We find it necessary in our experience to dilute the enzyme in order to get binding to the column, in contrast to the literature procedure (2). The column is washed with ~2 l of 50 m*M* potassium phosphate buffer (pH 7.4) containing 0.20 m*M* EDTA, 1.0 m*M* dithiothreitol, and 20% glycerol (v/v) and then with an equal amount of the same buffer in which the phosphate concentration has been raised to 100 m*M*. Cytochrome P450 1A2 is then eluted with the same buffer in which the phosphate concentration has been raised to 300 m*M*. This column step has the advantage of not only removing some contaminating proteins but also removing the detergents.

In the original literature the authors added a gel filtration step to remove cytochrome P420. However, we have found that the final preparation of cytochrome P450 contains very little cytochrome P420 if all buffers contain EDTA. The final preparations are routinely ≥95% pure as judged by SDS–polyacrylamide gel electrophoresis. The final preparation, which contains very little detergent (vide supra), is either diluted or dialyzed to a concentration of 100 m*M* phosphate [with 1.0 m*M* EDTA and 20% glycerol (v/v) present] and stored at −20°C. As with other cytochrome P450 1A2 enzymes, precipitation occurs when the phosphate concentration falls below ~100 m*M* in the absence of detergents. A typical yield of purified cytochrome P450 1A2 is ~4000 nmol (40% yield based on total cytochrome P450 in the microsomes).

Purification of Human Cytochrome P450 2E1 From E. coli *Membranes*

This procedure describes the chromatographic steps required to purify cytochrome P450 2E1 to electrophoretic homogeneity from a preparation of homogenized *Escherichia coli* membranes overexpressing cytochrome P450 2E1 (Figure 35.27). Prior to beginning chromatographic purification, membrane-bound cytochrome P450 2E1 must be solubilized from the membranes with a detergent solution (sodium cholate and Triton N-101) and the active site stabilized by the addition of 4-methylpyrazole, a tight binding inhibitor of cytochrome P450 2E1 (113). Cytochrome P450 2E1 is isolated through a series of ion-exchange steps utilizing both ionic and nonionic detergents, as well as the stabilizing ligand 4-methylpyrazole in order to maintain the structural integrity of the protein throughout purification. Binding and recovery at each step can easily be quantitated by spectrophotometric measurement of the ferrous CO-bound cytochrome P450 (vide supra). The purified protein can be stored for at least several months at −20°C in a stock solution of 100 m*M* potassium phosphate buffer (pH 7.4) containing 50 μ*M* NaEDTA and 20% glycerol (v/v).

A key to success with this procedure is careful equilibration of columns prior to protein loading. Additionally, binding is improved at lower loading rates, which can be achieved by protein dilution or by decreasing sample flow rates.

Escherichia coli membranes in which human cytochrome P450 2E1 has been expressed (113) are diluted to a concentration of 2 mg protein/ml in 50 m*M* Tris-HCl buffer (pH 7.4) containing 20% glycerol (v/v), 0.625% sodium cholate (w/v), 1.25% Triton N-101 (v/v), 1.0 m*M* EDTA, 1.0 m*M* DTT, and 50 μ*M* 4-methylpyrazole. Volumes will vary depending on the total amount of protein in the membrane preparation. For a bacterial membrane preparation containing ~3.5 g of total protein with a specific content of 0.4 nmol cytochrome P450/mg protein (i.e., 1400 nmol cytochrome P450), a DEAE Sephacel column packed to a volume of 75 ml (2.5 × 15 cm) is sufficient. (We do not suggest regeneration of the DEAE Sephacel column. A freshly prepared column is highly recommended for successful purification of cytochrome P450 enzymes.) The DEAE Sephacel column is equilibrated with a minimum of 5 column volumes of 50 m*M* Tris-HCl buffer (pH 7.4) containing 20% glycerol (v/v), 1.0 m*M* EDTA, 1.0 m*M* DTT, 0.6% sodium cholate (w/v), 1.2% Triton N-101 (v/v), and 50 μM 4-methylpyrazole at a flow rate of ~1 ml/min. Solubilized membranes are loaded onto column at a flow rate ~1 ml/min. [Remove membrane components from the solution of solubilized membranes by ultracentrifugation ($10^5 \times$ g, 60 min) prior to loading. Failure to do so will result in destruction of the chromatographic bed.] Cytochrome P450 2E1 elutes in the void volume. Often most, if not all, of the cytochrome P420 (representing any denatured cytochrome P450 plus noncytochrome P450 bacterial hemoproteins) will be

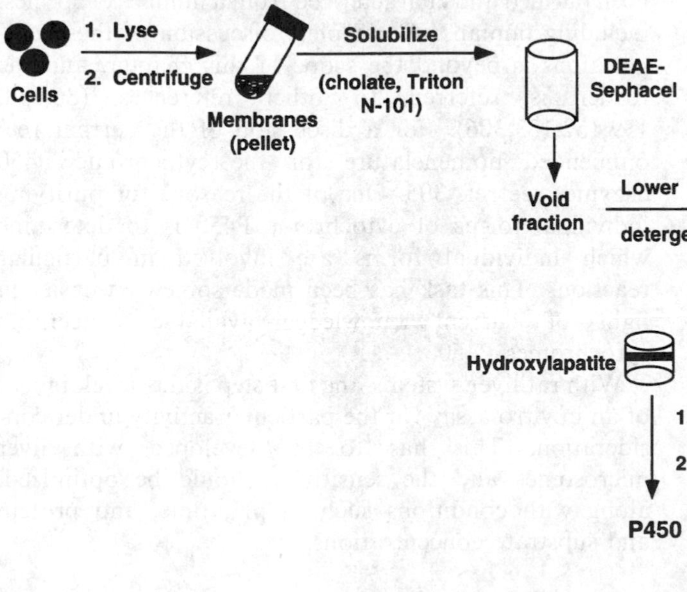

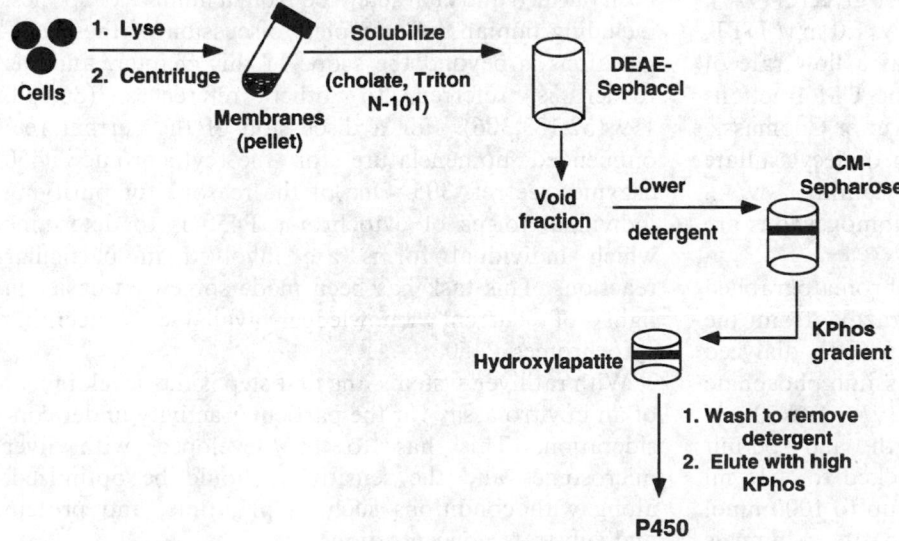

FIG. 35.27. Purification of recombinant human cytochrome P450 2E1 from *E. coli* membranes (25).

removed from the sample during this step. Following the solubilized membrane preparation, at least one column volume of the DEAE equilibration buffer is used to displace the cytochrome P450 from the column.

The next step is CM chromatography. A CM column packed to ~20 ml volume (1.5 × 10 cm) will typically bind up to 1000 nmol of cytochrome P450 2E1. Equilibrate a CM Sepharose Fast Flow column with a minimum of 5 column volumes of 20 m*M* potassium phosphate buffer (pH 6.5) containing 20% glycerol (v/v) and 0.2 m*M* EDTA. It is essential that the pH of this buffer be adjusted to 6.5. At pH >6.5, cytochrome P450 2E1 will not bind well to the column. If the pH is too acidic, the structural integrity of the cytochrome P450 may be compromised. Before loading the protein onto the column, dilute the DEAE Sephacel void volume pool threefold with a solution of 20% (v/v) glycerol and adjust the pH to 6.5 using 43% H_3PO_4 (w/v). The volume of the threefold-diluted DEAE void is substantial and may take up to 3 days to load completely onto the CM column. Because cytochrome P450 2E1 is slightly more stable at pH 7.4 than at 6.5, only fractions recovered from one DEAE column at a time should be diluted and applied to CM columns. Another batch can be diluted and pH adjusted to 6.5 when the previous batch has completed loading onto the CM column. The cytochrome P450 should bind tightly to the top of the column forming a visible, brownish-red zone. If the protein is not binding well, and if all of the solutions are properly adjusted to pH to 6.5, the flow rate is decreased (of the protein solution moving onto the column). After the protein has completely loaded, wash the column extensively with a minimum of 5 column volumes of 50 m*M* potassium phosphate buffer (pH 6.5) containing 20% glycerol (v/v), 0.2 m*M* EDTA, and 1.0 m*M* DTT. Elution of the protein is achieved using a linear potassium gradient increasing from 10 m*M* to 200 m*M* [250 ml each of potassium phosphate buffer (pH 7.4) containing 20% glycerol (v/v), 0.2% Triton N-101 (v/v), 0.2 m*M* EDTA, 1.0 m*M* DTT, and 50 μ*M* 4-methylpyrazole, elution at a flow rate of 1 ml/min, collect ~5-ml fractions]. The CM fractions are assayed for purity on the basis of silver or Coomassie brillant blue R-250 staining of sodium dodecyl sulfate SDS–polyacrylamide gels (7% acrylamide, w/v). Fractions that are electrophoretically homogeneous are pooled.

The purified protein must be further chromatographed to remove detergent and 4-methylpyrazole from the preparation. The pooled CM fractions are dialyzed against 3 × 2-L changes of 10 m*M* potassium phosphate buffer (pH 7.4) containing 20% glycerol (v/v) and 50 μ*M* EDTA to reduce the ionic strength and permit hydroxylapatite binding. A column packed to ~15 ml (1.5 × 8 cm) will usually accommodate up to 1000 nmol cytochrome P450 2E1. The hydroxylapatite column is equilibrated with 5 column volumes of 10 m*M* potassium phosphate buffer (pH 7.4) containing 20% glycerol (v/v) and 50 μ*M* EDTA. [Hydroxylapatite from different suppliers has yielded varying success at this step. Calbiochem (La Jolla, CA) hydroxylapatite has consistently provided the highest yield. Other preparations have proven resistant to protein elution.] The cytochrome P450 is loaded slowly onto the hydroxylapatite column (flow rate ≤0.5 ml min^{-1}). Again, the cytochrome P450 should bind forming a brownish-red zone at the top of the column. The column is washed extensively with 10 m*M* potassium phosphate buffer (pH 7.4) containing 20% glycerol (v/v) and 50 μ*M* EDTA to remove Triton N-101. In this case, as much as 10 column volumes or more may be required to completely remove the detergent. Detergent removal can be monitored by measuring absorbance at 280 nm. Absorbance should decrease to ≤0.01. The protein is eluted from the hydroxylapatite column using 300 m*M* potassium phosphate buffer (pH 7.4) containing 20% glycerol and 50 μ*M* EDTA. At this ionic strength, cytochrome P450 2E1 elutes in a very sharp band, which can easily be collected manually or with a fraction collector.

Dialyze the purified cytochrome P450 2E1 (using Spectrapor 12-14000 MWCO dialysis tubing) against 3 × 2 L of 100 m*M* postassium phosphate buffer (pH 7.4) containing 20% glycerol (v/v) and 50 μ*M* EDTA to decrease the concentration of potassium phosphate for long-term storage of the protein. The overall yield is ~50%, on the basis of the amount of P450 present in the solubilized membranes.

Use of Purified Cytochrome P450 Enzymes

Many individual forms of cytochrome P450 have now been purified and characterized from a number of species, including humans. A complete discussion of these preparations is beyond the scope of this chapter, and the reader is referred to other references (86,138, 139,152,153,306). For a discussion of the current recommended nomenclature for the cytochrome P450 enzymes see ref. 305. One of the reasons for purifying individual forms of cytochrome P450 is to determine which individual forms are involved in particular reactions. This task has been made somewhat easier in light of current knowledge available concerning cytochromes P450.

With rat liver systems, the first step is the development of an in vitro assay for the particular activity under consideration. This has to be developed with liver microsomes and the sensitivity should be optimized, along with conditions such as pH, time, and protein and substrate concentrations.

The next step involves comparison of rates of oxidation with microsomes isolated from (untreated) male and female rats and male rats treated with various inducing agents. A considerable body of knowledge now exists concerning the effects of gender and inducing agents on individual cytochrome P450 forms, and this information can be used to advantage (77,138,139,152,446). For example, male rats (adult) contain P450 2C11 and P450 3A2 but not P450 2C12. Phenobarbital administration induces P450 2B1, P450 2B6, P450 2B2, and P450 3A1. Pregnenolone 16α-carbonitrile and dexamethasone induce only P450 3A1 (and any closely related forms). Levels of P450 2C11 are suppressed by administration of any of several of the typical inducers, particularly polycyclic aromatic hydrocarbons. From information obtained in such experiments, one can begin to hypothesize which forms are involved.

The next step involves examination of the relative abilities of individual forms of cytochrome P450 to catalyze the reaction, if these are available. Reconstitution conditions are described elsewhere.

When specific inhibitors are known for individual forms of cytochrome P450 [e.g., 7,8-benzoflavone (α-naphthoflavone) for rat P450 1A1 and P450 1A2], these can also be used to advantage (vide infra) (67,178).

Another step involves using specific antibodies with microsomal preparations to determine which will inhibit the reaction. This approach is discussed later in this chapter. These results should agree with and confirm those obtained in the experiments just described.

The strategy is slightly different for studies with human enzymes, since induction and gender patterns are not involved. If some results are available on the catalytic selectivity of rat or other animal cytochrome P450 enzymes, this information may be of some use in predicting human enzymes, although there are many cases of catalytic selectivity jumping subfamilies when making such comparisons, particularly in the cytochrome P450 2C family (146,380).

One way to proceed is to first use diagnostic chemical inhibitors (67,178) (Table 35.2 and Figure 35.28). Because human samples are known to vary considerably in their cytochrome P450 composition, it is risky to rely only on a single human sample, particularly if there is little prior knowledge about its behavior. Usually several samples (≥3) should be used in initial screens. An alternative is to use a single experiment with microsomes proded on the basis of protein content (≥10 samples). The same strategy applies to human hepatocytes (here the number of samples available may be low).

Another useful strategy with microsomes is correlation analysis (22,170). A set of microsomal samples is compared for the new activity under consideration and also marker activities diagnostic of individual cytochrome

Table 35.2
Useful selective inhibitors of human P450 enzymes (67,308,387)

P450 1A1	7,8-Benzoflavone (but see refs. 290 and 387 regarding P450 1A2)
	Ellipticine
	1-(1-Propynyl)pyrene
	2-(1-Propynyl)phenanthrene
P450 1A2	7,8-Benzoflavone
	Furafylline
	Fluvoxamine
P450 1B1	7,8-Benzoflavone
	2-Ethynylpyrene
P450 2A6	Diethyldithiocarbamate (see ref. 466)
P450 2C9	Sulfaphenazole
	Tienilic acid
P450 2D6	Quinidine
P450 2E1	Aminoacetonitrile
	4-Methylpyrazole
	Diethyldithiocarbamate (see ref. 466)
P450 3A4	Troleandomycin
	Ketoconazole
	Gestodene

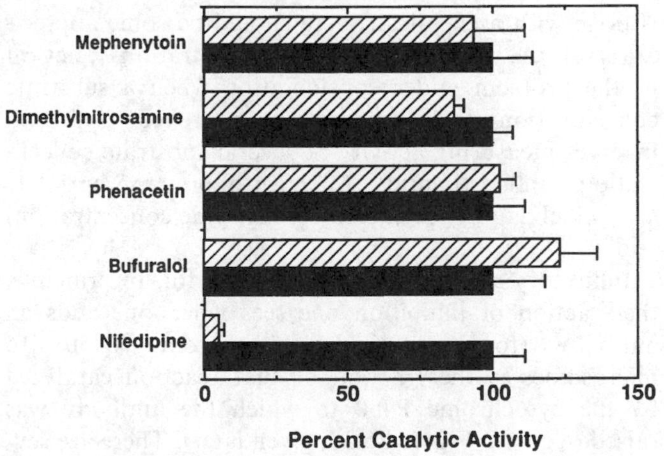

FIG. 35.28. Specificity of gestodene for inactivation of human cytochrome P450 enzymes. Human liver microsomes were incubated with (▨) or without (■) 100 μM gestodene in the presence of an NADPH-generating system for 20 min at 37°C; the microsomes were then diluted into buffers containing each of the indicated substrates for analysis of enzymatic activity (142).

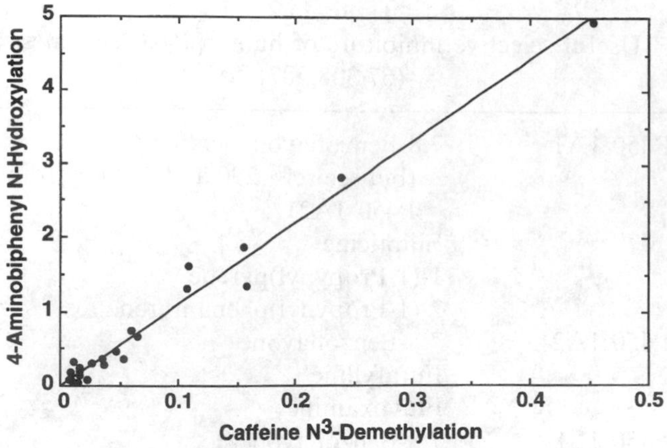

FIG. 35.29. Correlation of caffeine N^3-demethylation and 4-aminobiphenyl N-hydroxylation in different human liver microsomal samples, indicative of P450 1A2 variation and involvement in both reactions (46). All rates are expressed in nmol product formed/min/mg microsomal protein.

P450 enzymes (Figure 35.29). In general, $\geq$10 samples should be used. Correlation analysis can be done with either linear or Spearman rank methods (22,85). In principle, the parameter r^2 estimates the fraction of the variation accounted for by the relationship between two variables. Values of $r^2 \geq 0.5$ are generally judged to be significant (but p is dictated by sample size).

An additional approach is to utilize purified or, more likely, recombinant enzymes to assay the activity. If this is done with a chemical, there should be some appreciation of the plasma or tissue concentrations relevant to the problem under consideration when a substrate concentration is selected. An improved approach involves measuring activity at several substrate concentrations and estimating V_{max} (or more appropriately k_{cat}, which is V_{max} divided by the enzyme concentration) and K_m.

Inhibitory antibodies can also be useful. In principle, the fraction of inhibition one sees when one adds an antibody (to a particular cytochrome P450) to microsomes is the fraction of that reaction catalyzed by the cytochrome P450 to which the antibody was raised (e.g., see Figure 35.30, given later). There are several confounding problems. One is that antibodies generally do not distinguish between cytochrome P450 subfamily members, unless extensive cross-adsorption is done with the antibody. Despite early success in the area (230,415), not all anti-cytochrome P450 antibodies are inhibitory. Further, even antibodies raised against recombinant cytochrome P450 proteins have sometimes showed reactions with similar epitopes in different cytochrome P450 families (394). This cross-reactivity can vary with the individual rabbits. Although polyclonal antibodies raised against purified cytochrome P450 enzymes have been highly useful in development of the field, there are two prospects for improvements. One is the use of monoclonal antibodies, which have already been exploited for some uses (106,110,353,416). The other, more recent, is the use of anti-peptide antibodies. Some of these have shown impressive specificity (69,441) although sustained immunoinhibitory potency may still be a problem. An area for possible development in this area is phage display methods (16).

Two general points need to be made about use of such information (some points are also made later regarding heterologous expression systems). First, many of the parameters often cited for the in vitro systems used today are inappropriate, particularly with the recombinant systems. The expression of an activity of a recombinant system in terms of milligrams protein is not particulary helpful because no information is available about the level of expression. The concentration of the enzyme under consideration should be determined and used in the normalization. Such an analysis may be difficult if an immunochemical method is needed, since apoprotein or inactive enzyme will also be measured. Another common problem in cytochrome P450 work (and with most of the other enzymes of interest here) is the attachment of too much significance to the K_m value itself. Contrary to what is often conveyed in toxicology texts, K_m does not generally note substrate affinity, unless specifically proven so. The parameter K_m is an operational term, simply denoting the substrate concentration at which half-maximal reaction velocity occurs (246,438). It is a complex collection of microscopic rate constants, which are usually not known. In the case of cytochrome P450 2E1, K_m can be considered a function with k_{cat} appearing as a dependent variable (23).

Second, the ratio of k_{cat}/K_m (or V_{max}/K_m) is considered the most appropriate estimate of enzyme efficiency by enzymologists (246). In a plot of v versus S for an enzyme, this is the target to the plot at low substrate concentrations and has units of M^{-1} s^{-1} (or the equivalent). However, k_{cat}/K_m (or V_{max}/K_m) is *not* intrinsic clearance, which is an in vivo parameter with a distinct meaning. If blood flow is not rate-limiting and there are not complicating factors due to transport, then intrinsic clearance within a given organ might be a direct function of k_{cat}/K_m (352). However, the more proper term for the ratio k_{cat}/K_m is simply enzyme efficiency. This is not to demean efforts at physiologically based pharmacokinetic modeling, which can be very useful (3,4). However, these models must not make inappropriate assumptions about what they incorporate in the way of meanings of parameters, any more than they would incorporate the wrong pathways.

NADPH–Cytochrome P450 Reductase

Affinity procedures have been described by Yasukochi and Masters (468) and Strobel and Dignam (399) for purification of this enzyme from rat and hog liver using detergent extraction from microsomes, DEAE-cellulose chromatography, and 2′,5′-ADP- or $NADP^+$-agarose affinity chromatography. 2′,5′-ADP-agarose is commercially available from Pharmacia. Ion-exchange chromatography, or some other initial purification procedure, is often used to facilitate binding of the reductase to the affinity column (468). Alternatively, the *n*-octylamino-Sepharose 4B reductase fraction from rabbit, rat, or human liver cytochrome P450 purification procedures (128–130,163,195,197,439) can be directly applied to the affinity column. In our own laboratory we now produce the rat or human reductase in *E. coli* and isolate it from the membranes, using the methods of Hanna et al. (181). These expression vector systems are freely available upon request.

The column is washed with 0.25 *M* potassium phosphate buffer (pH 7.7) containing 0.10 m*M* EDTA, 20% glycerol (v/v), and 0.20% Triton N-101 (w/v) (or other nonionic detergent) to remove other proteins. The detergent is then removed by washing the column with 30 m*M* potassium phosphate containing 0.10 m*M* EDTA, 20% glycerol (v/v), and 0.10% sodium cholate (w/v). The reductase is eluted with the latter buffer containing 10 m*M* 2′-AMP or $NADP^+$ (and 0.10 m*M* phenylmethylsulfonyl fluoride) and dialyzed (48 h) versus 100 volumes of 10 m*M* Tris-acetate buffer (pH 7.4) containing 0.10 m*M* EDTA and 20% glycerol (v/v) to remove cholate and 2′-AMP (or $NADP^+$) (131,152, 163).

This procedure has been used to obtain NADPH–cytochrome P450 reductase in yields as high as 50%; specific activities for cytochrome *c* reduction range from 40 to 70 μmol/min/mg protein (131, 399,468). Spectra show the absence of nonflavin components; the $A_{455} : A_{380}$ ratios are 1.10 to 1.15 (131,163). The apparent monomeric M_r is 74 kD [the protein sequence has been deduced from cDNA and the actual weight is somewhat different (343)]. Sometimes proteolysis is a problem and results in cleavage of a peptide necessary for activity toward cytochrome P450 (but not cytochrome *c*). This problem can be avoided by adding phenylmethylsulfonyl fluoride (from a stock ethanolic solution) to 0.10 m*M* to buffers immediately prior to use to inhibit serine-active proteases. Some preparations appear to lose some flavin mononucleotide (FMN), as evidenced by stimulation by 10 μ*M* FMN. This problem can be minimized by including 1 μ*M* concentrations of FMN in buffers and minimizing exposure to light during dialysis (195).

Epoxide Hydrolase

Highly purified preparations of the rat, rabbit, and human liver enzymes have been prepared in a number of laboratories (26,174,240,272,274). In general, purification procedures are carried out at 0–4°C using nonionic detergents, and styrene-7,8-oxide hydrolase activity is usually monitored. The procedure presented next was developed in our laboratory and is based upon the original work of Knowles and Burchell (240); this procedure routinely yields apparently homogeneous enzyme in reasonably good yield (163,174).

Liver microsomes prepared from phenobarbital-treated rats (~4 g protein) are suspended at 4.0 mg protein/ml in 0.20 *M* potassium phosphate buffer (pH 7.4) containing 0.10 m*M* EDTA. Assays are described earlier in this chapter (Figure 35.25). A 20% aqueous solution of Lubrol PX (w/v, Sigma) is added dropwise while stirring at 0–4°C to yield a final detergent concentration of 1% (w/v). (The original Lubol PX is no longer available from Sigma or other suppliers; however, Sigma has a similar detergent termed polyoxyethylene ether W-1 available that can be substituted in this procedure.) After 30 min of additional stirring, the clarified solution is centrifuged for 60 min at $10^5 \times g$ (3.5×10^4 rpm in a Beckman 45 Ti rotor). The pellets are discarded and the combined supernatant fractions are dialyzed twice (8 h) against 15 volumes of 5 m*M* potassium phosphate buffer (pH 7.25) containing 0.05% Lubrol PX (w/v). The dialysate is applied to a 5 × 50 cm column of DEAE-cellulose (e.g., Whatman DE-52, Whatman, Piscataway, NJ) equilibrated with the dialysis buffer. The column is washed with the same buffer; no activity remains bound to the column. Since Lubrol PX does not absorb in the UV region, fractions are monitored at 280 nm and those fractions showing significant absorbance (>0.05) are pooled and dialyzed versus 10 volumes of 5 m*M* potassium phosphate buffer (pH 6.5) containing 0.05% Lubrol PX (w/v). The dialysate is applied to a 4 × 30 cm CM-cellulose (Whatman CM-52) column equilibrated with dialysis buffer. The column is eluted with 500 ml more dialysis buffer and then with a 1-L linear phosphate gradient (5–300 m*M*) containing 0.05% Lubrol PX (w/v). The void volume fractions are monitored for absorbance at 280 nm and contain epoxide hydrolase. The epoxide hydrolase in this fraction is nearly homogeneous as judged by $NaDodSO_4$–polyacrylamide gel electrophoresis and is devoid of colored proteins. Fractions are pooled and stirred with Amberlite XAD-2 (~0.5 g/mg protein) for 2 h; beads are removed by filtration through glass wool or nylon mesh. Alternatively, detergent can be removed using a hydroxylapatite column, with washing with buffer devoid of detergent and elution with 0.50 *M* phosphate buffer. Final preparations are concentrated by ultrafiltration using Amicon PM-30 membranes and stored at $-20°C$.

The overall yield is 10 to 20%; preparations are apparently homogeneous as judged by SDS–polyacrylamide gel electrophoresis and have varying activities toward a variety of epoxides. The human liver enzyme behaves quite differently and this procedure is not directly applicable (174). The rat enzyme can also be expressed in *E. coli* and purified using other methods (24,180,249, 425).

Other Enzymes

Microsomal flavin-containing monooxygenase has been isolated from porcine liver using detergent extraction, gel exclusion chromatography, and preparative electrophoresis (474). The enzyme is inherently less stable than the others already discussed. The enzyme has been purified from rat and mouse (362) liver and from rabbit lung (48,458), as well as heterologous expression systems (48). The lung enzyme appears to be different from that in the liver.

A number of transferases are involved in the overall metabolism of xenobiotics. Most of these are cytosolic enzymes and exist in multiple forms. References for the purification and characterization of the following enzymes are given: GSH *S*-transferase (8,61,177, 208,209,235,281,298), UDP-glucuronosyl transferase (41,42,358,407), *N*-acetyltransferase (6,433,450), metallothionein (actually more of a "sink" for trapping electrophiles and metals than an enzyme) (54,459), methyltransferases (7,260,453), sulfotransferase (93,210,452), and cysteine conjugate acetyl transferase (66,94).

Other redox-active enzymes of interest (and appropriate references) include alcohol dehydrogenase (95,194, 224), aldehyde and other carbonyl dehydrogenases (104,334), cysteine conjugate β-lyase (66,397,405), monoamine oxidase (48,368,454), quinone reductase (DT-diaphorase) (98,192,357), cytochrome b_5 (395), and NADPH–cytochrome b_5 reductase (323).

METHODS FOR USE OF ENZYMES

Methods for the Determination of Enzyme Purity

As in the case of other chemicals, no single technique can be used to establish purity; moreover, purity is always defined as a limit of given impurities in a given analytical system, and one can argue that nothing is really "pure." However, some techniques are more useful than others in ruling out heterogeneity and are discussed here. Some of the classical considerations about purity have been relaxed by the ability to express in recombinant systems, in that related enzyme family members are not expressed. However, for some purposes proteins must still hold to strict criteria (e.g., antibody production, certain enzymology experiments).

1. An obvious criterion of homogeneity is the absence of suspected contaminants. For instance, cytochrome P450 preparations should be devoid of NADPH–cytochrome *c* reduction activity, epoxide hydrolase preparations should be devoid of heme, and so on. Of course, such impurities must always be defined in terms of detectable limits of contamination. A point to be considered here is that an experimental situation may call for the absence of lipid or detergent contamination as well as protein contamination, and the limit of such impurity must be determined.[2]
2. Specific activity or specific content of the isolated enzyme is a guide to follow in purification. For instance, cytochrome P450 preparations should contain x nmol cytochrome P450/mg protein, where $x = 10^6/\text{subunit } M_r$ (i.e., $x = 16$–22), NADPH–cytochrome P450 reductase preparations should catalyze the reduction of 40 to 70 μmol cytochrome c/min/mg protein under optimal conditions, and epoxide hydrolase preparations should catalyze the hydrolysis of ~ 500 nmol styrene oxide/min/mg protein (26,240,274). However, such measurements are dependent on the accuracy of the protein estimation, which may be a problem. Specific activities are sometimes more variable than expected. In the case of cytochrome P450, some forms may exist in vivo without a full complement of heme (363) (these are issues regarding prosthetic group loss that involve expressed proteins as well as those purified from tissues). These general guidelines about activity and so forth are useful in evaluation of purity.
3. SDS–polyacrylamide gel electrophoresis (SDS-PAGE) (250) is routinely used as the main criterion for homogeneity. This technique has been quite useful in determination of homogeneity; moreover, the subunit M_r weight estimates appear to be reasonably valid for cytochrome P450 (30,130,156) and NADPH–cytochrome P450 reductase (238,343). However, even this powerful technique has its limitations. Evidence has been presented that

[2] Phospholipid can be determined by thoroughly dialyzing the enzyme versus Tris buffer and then H_2O to remove soluble phosphates; lipids are extracted as described by Bligh and Dyer (32), and phosphate is determined according to Chen et al. (53). Ethylene oxide-based detergents (including Emulgens 911 and 913, Renex 690, Triton N-101, and Lubrol PX) can be extracted and assayed as described by Garewal (107) and subsequently modified by Goldstein and Blecher (119). Alternatively, detergents can also be assayed by high-performance liquid chromatography (HPLC) (189).

different microsomal enzymes cannot always be distinguished by this technique (74,152). Furthermore, the results obtained with this technique are rather dependent upon the exact procedure used, and the methods vary in resolving abilities (130,152). Finally, apparent M_r values also vary depending upon the procedure and the standards used, and the reader is cautioned to compare results from different laboratories carefully and allow for as much as 3- to 4-kD differences. Further, it is well established that in some cases such a change may result from a single amino acid replacement regardless of the effect on the true M_r.

Isoelectric focusing offers a great potential for resolution of enzymes and has been used in studying cytochromes P450. However, a number of artifacts can be encountered in the use of this methodology, at least when used without specialized procedures (132,133,139,311,435).

Staining of electrophoretograms is usually done with protein stains. In the absence of SDS, NADPH–cytochrome P450 reductase can be stained using tetrazolium dyes (172) and cytochrome P450 can be stained using benzidine derivatives and H_2O_2 (173,417). The latter method has also been used to tentatively identify cytochrome P450 in SDS-PAGE. However, much of the heme leaves the enzyme, even in the absence of reducing agents. While others have claimed that heme does not bind to other proteins, Thomas et al. (417) found that heme was bound to albumin; thus, one must be cautious in interpreting data involving such a technique. Immunochemical techniques have been developed for the identification of cytochrome P450 separated from microsomal membranes by SDS; these methods proved useful in answering a number of questions about cytochrome P450 induction (vide infra).

4. N-Terminal amino acid analysis should produce single residues at each step of automated Edman degradation for homogeneous proteins (30,388). There has been considerable development in this area, and it is now common to be able to do this work with samples of <10 pmol (91,386).
5. Various immunochemical criteria have been used to assess homogeneity (26,80,152,171–173,230,240, 361). An antibody should produce a single precipitin line when diffused against the antigen, if the antigen is homogeneous. Immunoelectrophoresis of a crude preparation should show only the antigen (vide infra). Cross-reactivity of related proteins does exist, and many of the isolated microsomal and even recombinant proteins do not necessarily induce the production of monospecific antibodies (394).
6. Hydrodynamic criteria have been used in the past to assess the homogeneity of the various isolated microsomal proteins; because all of these proteins tend to aggregate, velocity and equilibrium studies carried out to examine homogeneity must be done in the presence of detergents or other strong denaturants (26,156). These techniques are not in very common use, but they are of great value in ascertaining aggregation properties.

Reconstitution of Enzyme Activity

Epoxide hydrolase activity toward a wide variety of substrates is observed with the purified enzyme. Many of the activities have slightly basic pH optima (269,274). The presence of phospholipid enhances activity of the purified enzyme toward some substrates but not others; these results have been interpreted in terms of a model in which the phospholipid micelles bind substrate (269).

Early work on reconstitution of mixed-function oxidase activity was reviewed by Lu and West (277). The following general statements can be made. The optimum rate of enzyme activity, based upon cytochrome P450, is obtained when NADPH–cytochrome P450 reductase is present at an equimolar concentration or slight excess. Phospholipid enhances the rates of most activities; this phospholipid can be in the form of a microsomal extract or synthetic L-α-1,2-dilauroyl-*sn*-glyceryo-3-phosphocholine. Some nonionic detergents will partially replace phosphatidylcholine at low concentrations (271,273,275). The activity toward some substrates can be further enhanced by small amounts of cholate or deoxycholate (277). The role of phospholipid is not completely understood, but a dual role has been postulated (105): L-α-1,2-dilauroyl-*sn*-glyceryo-3-phosphocholine increases the affinity of rabbit liver cytochrome P450 for both organic substrate and NADPH–cytochrome P450 reductase; all four components are complexed during catalysis. Several investigators have studied synthetic liposomal systems; however, no such system has been prepared to date that is more active in hydroxylation than a system reconstituted in the presence of subcritical micelle concentration levels of phospholipid. Neither cytochrome b_5 nor NADH is required for activity in many reactions, although some are definitely enhanced considerably by cytochrome b_5. The effect of the phospholipid appears to be kinetic and can, at least in some cases, be overcome with high protein concentrations and extended preincubation conditions (301). However, see also refs. 179 and 200.

A basic procedure for reconstituting mixed-function oxidase activity is outlined next. Equimolar concentrations of cytochrome P450 and NADPH–cytochrome

P450 reductase [both of which have been stripped of excess detergent by treatment with beads and/or calcium phosphate gel or hydroxylapatite (432)] are first mixed in the presence of 40 μM sonicated L-α-1,2-dilauroyl-*sn*-glyceryo-3-phosphocholine, and, after 5 min, an appropriate buffer (i.e., 50–100 mM potassium phosphate or other buffer, pH 7.0–7.7) is added plus a sufficient volume of water. The substrate is then added, preferably in water if possible. If not, the substrate should be dissolved in $(CH_3)_2CO$, $(CH_3)_2SO$, or CH_3OH such that the final concentration of organic solvent is $\leq 1\%$ (v/v) for the enzymes. Some forms of cytochrome P450 oxidize these compounds or are inhibited by them (e.g., P450 2E1) and caution must be exercised (469). See also ref. 51. The system is preequilibrated at 37°C for 3 to 5 min and the reaction is initiated by the addition of NADPH (0.15–0.5 mM) or, preferably, an NADPH-generating system. [The organic substrate should not be the last addition, as prior addition of NADPH will result in generation of H_2O_2, which can destroy cytochrome P450 (131).] The length of the time for which the reaction is linear depends upon the substrate; in general, rapidly metabolized substrates do not give long periods of linearity and some substrates are converted to metabolites that destroy cytochrome P450 rapidly.

Flavin-containing monooxygenase activity requires only the single protein, of course, but the enzyme is dramatically less heat-stable than others (471–473). The enzyme is stabilized by pyridine nucleotides, so NADPH should be added to the enzyme before incubation at 37°C, and then the organic substrate should be added. NADPH–cytochrome P450 reductase has other enzyme activities in the absence of cytochrome P450; many of these require no special conditions but may be stimulated, as is the case for lipid peroxidation, by high salt concentrations.

Use of Selective Cytochrome P450 Inhibitors

Chemical inhibitors offer considerable potential in the discrimination of enzymes involved in reactions. Unlike antibodies, they can readily be obtained by many laboratories by chemical synthesis or, in many cases, purchased directly. Further, they have the advantage that they can be used in vivo in many cases, even in humans. The approach of using chemical inhibitors with crude enzyme preparations to discern catalytic specificity has been most highly developed for the cytochrome P450 enzymes (Figure 35.28). Cytochrome P450 inhibitors have been known for some time, but many of the early compounds [e.g., SKF-255A (*N,N*-diethylaminoethyl-2, 2-diphenyl valerate) and metyrapone] are only partially selective. Newer and more specific compounds are now available. A list of those used for human cytochrome P450 enzymes is presented in Table 35.2 (67,308). For further example, evidence supporting the selectivity of the mechanism-based inactivator gestodene (P450 3A4) is presented in Figure 35.28 (142,464). A few comments are in order.

First, the specificity tends to carry over within each enzyme family (1A, 2A, 2B, 2C, etc.) between species, although some differences can be noted. For instance, quinine is a better inhibitor of rat cytochrome 2D enzymes than its diastereomer quinidine, while the opposite is true in humans. Some inhibitors are highly effective with more than one enzyme (e.g., diethyldithiocarbamate). Some inhibitors are irreversible and act by modifying the protein and/or prosthetic group. Ketoconazole is able to inhibit several cytochrome P450 enzymes but, many of its in vivo effects can probably be attributed to cytochrome P450 3A4. The same is probably true of cimetidine (239).

IMMUNOCHEMICAL TECHNIQUES

Antibodies have been raised to cytochrome P450, NADPH–cytochrome P450 reductase, epoxide hydrolase, and many of the other enzymes considered here. For instance, these antibodies have been used to show the involvement of cytochrome P450 (80,85, 218,226,228–230,414,415) and its reductase (172,287) in a number of reactions. Antibodies have also been used to examine the homogeneity of isolated enzyme fractions, the multiplicity of enzymes in microsomes, and the amounts of individual enzyme forms in microsomal preparations (26,74,75,80,152,219,220,240,361,414). The topical location of the enzymes in microsomal membranes has also been studied with immunological techniques (78,80,415), as have several aspects of enzyme biosynthesis. Antibodies have also been used to study the localization of the enzymes in various sections of individual organs (232,378).

Preparation of Antibodies

All three of the enzymes just mentioned are rather antigenic and antibodies have been raised in rabbits using less than 50 μg of protein. Sheep, goats, and guinea pigs have also been used for antibody production. A number of different immunization schedules can be used, depending upon the animal and the dose. Antisera can be used in some procedures, but immunoglobulin G (IgG) fractions are needed in some applications (80,230). To prepare these fractions, antisera are heated 20 min at 56°C and centrifuged at $10^4 \times g$ for 10 min. The supernatant fractions are mixed with equal volumes of 50% $(NH_4)_2SO_4$ (w/v) and recentrifuged. The pellets are washed with 25% $(NH_4)_2SO_4$ (w/v) to remove most of the color and then dissolved in 10 m*M* potassium phosphate buffer (pH 8.0) and dialyzed against the same buffer (at 4°C). The dialysates are passed through columns of DEAE-cellulose equilibrated with the same buffer. The void volume fractions (measured by absorbance at 280 nm) are pooled, retreated with $(NH_4)_2SO_4$ as above to remove color if necessary, concentrated by ultrafiltration (up to 50 mg/ml), and stored at −20°C. There are a number of alternative procedures available using Protein A affinity columns and others.

The list of immunochemical techniques that can be used with such antibodies is quite lengthy and the reader is referred to texts on the general subject (112); the procedures include double-diffusion analysis, radial diffusion quantitation, inhibition of enzyme activity, complement fixation, radioimmune assay, crossed gel electrophoresis, immunoprecipitation, immunoaffinity column chromatography, and immunohistochemical localization. These techniques should continue to be useful in future studies of the roles of individual forms of these microsomal enzymes in various processes.

Immunoinhibition of Catalytic Activity

In this approach, one adds an antibody to an enzyme preparation and determines if that antibody preparation can block catalytic activity (Figure 35.30). This approach is most useful with a crude enzyme system, such as a subcellular organelle preparation. Thus, one can ask what fraction of total activity is the result of the enzyme specifically recognized by the antibody (if the antibody completely inhibits the activity of the antigen itself). Such an approach has been useful in a number of cases in our own laboratory (85,87,139,382) as well as many others.

Antibodies to some proteins tend to be more inhibitory than others. In general, polyclonal antibodies raised against cytochromes P450 are usually inhibitory. However, inhibitory antibodies have not been reported for microsomal flavin-containing monooxygenase and only occasionally has inhibitory anti-epoxide hydrolase been prepared (314). Apparently antibodies raised against GSH transferases are not inhibitory. Some of the difference may be due to the size of the substrate or accessory protein that interacts with the antigen in catalysis. Thus, one would expect binding of an antibody to block binding of very large substrates (viz., other proteins) more readily than smaller compounds. In support of this view, anti-NADPH–cytochrome P450 reductase blocks reduction of cytochrome *c* but not ferricyanide or neotetrazolium blue (172). Another general trend is that only a limited fraction of monoclonal antibodies are inhibitory (327,328).

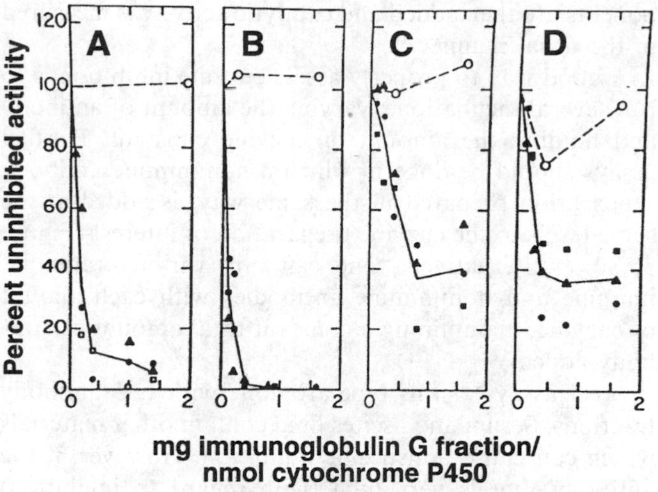

FIG. 35.30. Inhibition of mixed-function oxidation of debrisoquine, sparteine, encainide, and propranolol in human liver microsomes by anti-P450 2D1. Incubations were carried out with microsomes prepared from liver samples 17 (△), 25 (□), 31 (●), 32 (▲), 34 (■), 72 (◇), and 86 (◆), which contained 0.32, 0.55, 0.77, 0.50, 0.55, 0.61, and 0.30 nmol P450/mg protein, respectively. The microsomes were incubated with indicated amounts of anti-cytochrome P450 2D1 (IgG fraction) for 30 min at 23°C in the appropriate buffer and other incubation components were then added. Results are expressed as percent of the control activity (obtained in the absence of antibody) for debrisoquine 4-hydroxylation (A), formation of Δ^5-dehydrosparteine from sparteine (B), encainide O-demethylation (C), and propranolol 4-hydroxylation (D). The solid lines are drawn connecting the means of the values obtained with the various samples, and the broken lines connect the means of the values (○) obtained with IgG prepared from pre-immune antisera (individual values not shown). Control activities of debrisoquine 4-hydroxylation were 0.16, 0.060, and 0.19 pmol/min/nmol cytochrome P450 for samples 25, 31, and 32, respectively. Control activities of Δ^5-dehydrosparteine formation were 26.6, 20.4, and 2.0 pmol/min/nmol cytochrome P450 for samples 31, 32, and 34, respectively. Control activities of encainide O-demethylation were 0.044, 0.072, and 0.039 nmol/min/nmol cytochrome P450 for samples 31, 32, and 34 respectively. Control activities of propranolol 4-hydroxylase were 0.17, 0.12, and 0.081 nmol/min/nmol cytochrome P450 for samples 31, 32, and 34, respectively (85).

Analyzing for antibody inhibition is a relatively straightforward process. In general the enzyme preparation of interest is mixed with the antibody and incubated for 20 min at room temperature. Other components are then added and catalytic activity is measured in the usual manner.

A good way to properly assess enzyme inhibition is to run several incubations, varying the amount of antibody and holding the amount of enzyme constant. Parallel assays should be done in which a nonimmune antibody preparation prepared in the same way, is added at the same levels to the enzyme preparation of interest (Figure 35.30). (Alternatively, one can mix varying ratios of immune and nonimmune antibodies with each aliquot of enzyme, maintaining a constant total amount of antibody added.)

Most assays of this type are done with IgG antibody fractions. Serum and ascites fluid contain other materials which can cause nonspecific inhibition. However, if the antibody titer is very high (with regard to inhibition) or if the catalytic assay is so sensitive that little antibody is needed for inhibition, then such crude materials may be used.

In general, little can be said about inhibition of <15% of the total unless enough careful replicates are done and the difference between immune and nonimmune serum incubates is reproducible, concentration dependent, and statistically significant. To the first approximation, the percentage of inhibition is a reflection of the fraction of the total catalytic activity in the preparation that is due to the protein that reacts with the antibody. The antibody should completely inhibit the purified enzyme itself, however, for this analysis to be valid, because the possibility exists that non-inhibitory antibodies may hinder the binding of inhibitory antibodies and total inhibition may never be achieved.

Quantitation of Proteins by Immunoblotting

In many cases, the absolute concentration of a particular protein in a sample is derived, apart from its catalytic activity. The most direct way to obtain such measurements is with the use of specific antibodies. A variety of immunochemical techniques are available for use, including various types of radioimmune assays (RIA) and enzyme-linked immunoabsorbent assays (ELISA) (329). However, knowledge concerning the specificity of the antigen-antibody reaction must be available. Probably the single most reliable technique for evaluating specificity is coupled SDS-PAGE/immunoperoxidase staining, or immunoblotting (which often goes by the nickname "Western blotting"), where a crude mixture of protein is separated by electrophoresis and the resolved proteins are transferred to a thin sheet of nitrocellulose paper, where they can be detected after binding antibodies and antibodies coupled to enzymes with chromogenic substrates. In our early studies with this system, we found that the intensity of the staining of protein bands was proportional to the amount of antigen applied and that such a procedure could be utilized in making quantitative measurements (Figure 35.31). We continue to use such a system to quantify many proteins, for several reasons. Under appropriate conditions the method is accurate and quite sensitive. It provides a check on the specificity of antigen–antibody interaction in each individual antigen sample and provides data even when cross-reactive materials are present (if they can be resolved in a single electrophoretic dimension). The method is relatively rapid and straightforward, even when new systems are explored little optimization is required.

Samples of roughly 5 μg of microsomes or cellular homogenate protein are solubilized by heating with sodium dodecyl sulfate (SDS) and 2-mercaptoethanol. The samples are electrophoresed in a typical system based on the procedure of Laemmli (250)—a slab gel is used with up to 25 samples. Five or six lanes are used to prepare a standard curve for each gel; the lanes contain, for example, 0.5, 1, 2, 3, 5, and 10 pmol of the purified antigen. Crude protein samples to be analyzed are loaded into the wells for the other lanes. Typically, 1 to 50 μg of microsomal protein might be loaded per well for analysis of cytochrome P450 proteins. Protein samples are dissolved in a mixture of 63 m*M* Tris-HCl buffer (pH 6.8) containing 10% glycerol (v/v), 1.0% SDS (w/v), 0.001% pyronin Y (w/v), and 5.0% 2-mercaptoethanol (v/v) and heated for 60 sec at 95°C. Aliquots are loaded into the wells of a 1.5 mm × 16 cm × 20 cm gel (e.g., Hoefer, San Francisco, CA). The separating gel is poured from a mixture of 0.375 *M* Tris-HCl buffer (pH 8.8) containing 7.5% acrylamide (w/v), 0.03% tetramethylethylenediamine (TEMED) (w/v), 0.10% SDS (w/v), and 0.0425% $(NH_4)_2S_2O_8$ (w/v), and the stacking gel, in which the wells are formed, is poured from a mixture of 0.14 *M* Tris-HCl buffer (pH 6.8) containing 3.5% acrylamide (w/v), 0.057% TEMED (v/v), 0.65% sucrose (w/v), 0.11% SDS (w/v), and 0.045% $(NH_4)_2S_2O_8$ (w/v). The electrode buffer (pH 8.3) contains 190 m*M* glycine, 25 m*M* Tris, and 0.10% SDS (w/v). Power is applied to the system at a constant current setting of 25 mA per gel to move the samples through the separating gel. The electrophoresis takes ~4 h. When the pink dye front has moved to within about 1 cm of the edge of the gel, the power is turned off and the system is separated. One of the glass plates on the gel is removed and water is sprinkled on the surface. A wetted piece of nitrocellulose paper (0.45 μm, Scheicher and Schull, Keene, NH) is laid over the wet gel. Care should be taken (and enough water used) to avoid trapping air bubbles. Two sheets of Whatman number 3 paper, prewetted with water, are laid over the nitrocellulose. The glass plate is removed from the other side of the gel and replaced by a wet sheet of Whatman number 3 paper. The entire "sandwich" is placed between two wet sponges and then enclosed

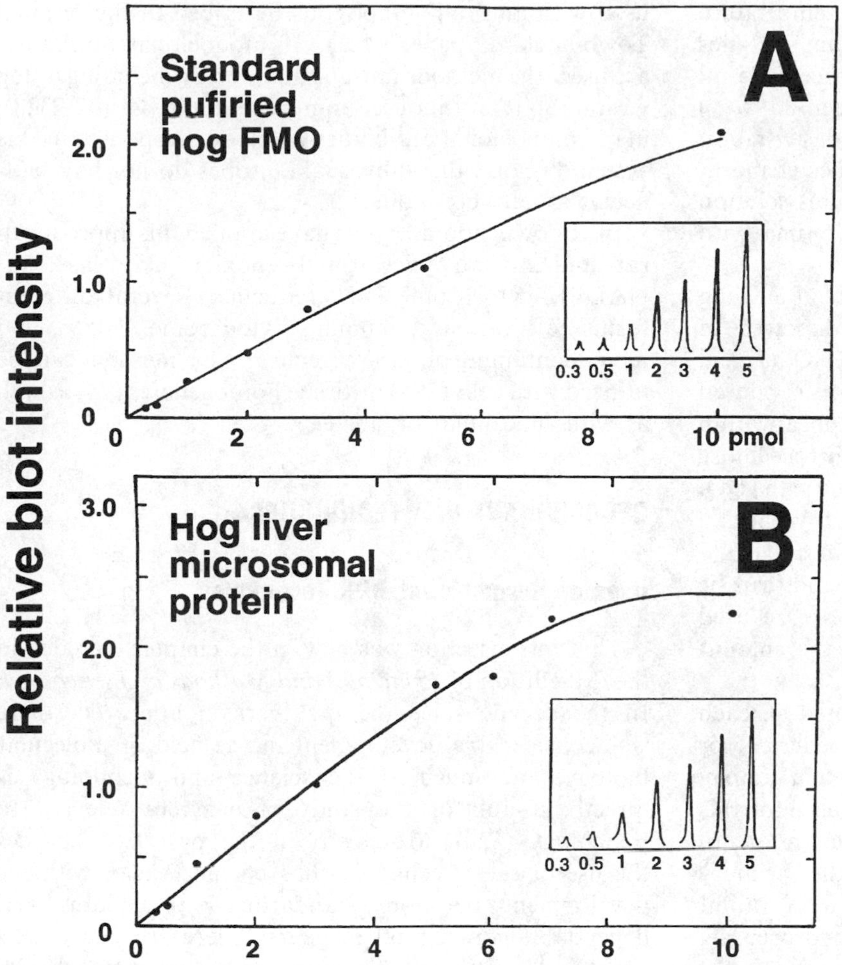

FIG. 35.31. Immunoelectrophoresis and densitometry of flavin-containing monooxygenase (FMO) in purified samples and porcine liver microsomes (74). A, Area under the densitometric peak as a function of the amount of purified porcine liver flavin-containing monooxygenase used for electrophoresis. The inset shows the actual densitometric traces. B, Area under the densitometric peak as a function of the amount of porcine liver microsomal protein electrophoresed (in μg). The inset shows the actual densitometric traces.

between the two electrode baffles of an electrotransfer apparatus (Hoefer), with the nitrocellulose closer to the anode than the cathode. The apparatus, with the gel and nitrocellulose between the baffles, is filled with 25 m*M* Tris-HCl buffer (pH 8.2) containing 190 m*M* glycine and 20% CH_3OH (v/v). Constant current (400 mA for 1 h or 200 mA for 2 h) is applied to the system. If a commercial electroblotting apparatus is not available, household sponges (Brillo, Purex Corp., Lakewood, CA) and a pair of stainless steel plates (attached to electrodes) can be substituted, with the device held by rubber bands and immersed in a beaker. Satisfactory results can be obtained (171,421), although the cathode plate tends to pit and corrode, especially if not washed thoroughly.

After the blotting operation, the polyacrylamide gel and the filter papers are discarded and the nitrocellulose sheet is placed in 25 ml of a solution of phosphate-buffered saline [PBS: 10 m*M* potassium phosphate buffer (pH 7.4) containing 0.9% NaCl (w/v)] containing 0.50% Tween 80 (w/v). The sheet is conveniently placed in a plastic box of only slightly larger dimensions (13 × 18 × 3 cm) with a lid. The gel is shaken in a 37°C water bath for 30 min to block reactive sites on the nitrocellulose sheet with serum proteins so that antibodies will not be bound in subsequent steps. After the blocking step, the nitrocellulose sheet is washed twice with 60 ml PBS at room temperature. In practice, the box is rocked on a platform rocker (Bellco Glass, Vineland, NJ) for 5 min, the buffer is decanted, and 60 ml of fresh PBS is added each time.

In the next step, 25 ml PBS containing 0.50% Tween 80 (v/v) and an appropriate dilution of the antiserum of choice is poured into the box over the nitrocellulose sheet. The system is shaken (or rocked) at 37°C for 30 min and then overnight at 4°C; alternatively, 37°C for 2 h is usually satisfactory. Typical antisera dilutions range from 1/100 to 1/2000 (some monoclonal antibodies have been successfully used at $1/10^6$ dilutions of ascites fluid). Then the nitrocellulose sheet is washed 6 times (5 min each, room temperature) with 60 ml PBS. The next addition is 25 ml PBS containing 0.50% Tween 80 (w/v) and 0.20% (v/v) goat anti-rabbit IgG antiserum (if the primary antiserum was made in rabbits). This solution is rocked or shaken with the nitrocellulose sheet at room temperature for 30 min, and the sheet is then washed again six times with PBS as before. The next addition to the sheet is 25 ml of a solution of PBS containing 0.50% Tween 80 (w/v) and 0.20% (v/v) horseradish peroxidase : rabbit anti-horseradish peroxidase complex (Miles Laboratories, Elkhart, IN). The sheet is rocked in this solution at room temperature for 30 min and washed 6 times with PBS as before.

Development of the stain is done in the following manner. 4-Chloro-1-naphthol (32 mg) is dissolved in 12 ml CH_3OH and diluted with 60 ml PBS. H_2O_2 (120 μl of a 30% solution) is added and the solution is poured over the nitrocellulose sheet; bands usually appear within a few minutes. The solution is removed; the nitrocellulose sheet is washed three times with PBS and twice with H_2O. Sheets can be dried between two layers of Whatman number 3 filter paper, with a uniform weight applied.

When the gel is dry (within 1–2 h), the bands can be scanned using a densitometer. The integrals are used to construct standard curves and estimate the amount of antigen in each sample (Figure 35.31).

In practice, a standard curve is constructed on each nitrocellulose sheet. An additional way to reduce error is to include an internal standard in each protein sample. Equine alcohol liver dehydrogenase can be used for this purpose, adding 0.2 μg to each sample prior to electrophoresis. The buffer containing the primary antisera is fortified with a 1/500 dilution of rabbit antisera raised against equine alcohol dehydrogenase. When the nitrocellulose sheets are visualized, the cytochrome P450 band in the 50–60 kD region is accompanied by a second band migrating with apparent M_r of 43 kD. The integrals of both bands are obtained from the densitometer. The ratio of the areas of the two bands can be compared to the ratios found with the standard antigen samples.

Even if the antigen–antibody system is not specific enough to visualize only a single electrophoretic band, useful information can be obtained, if the different antigens are electrophoretically separable. For instance, rat P450s 1A1 and 1A2 usually cross-react but can be separated and quantified (75,376). The same situation exists with human P450 2C enzymes (382).

Since the original immunoblotting work was done (421), a number of variations of the procedure have been reported. Many of these are cited in some recent reviews (111,420). For instance, different additives can be used in the buffers for blocking the sheets. Nylon membranes, such as Zeta-Probe (Bio-Rad, Richmond, CA), have increased capacity and can be used to increase the sensitivity of the methods. *Staphylococcus aureus* Protein A conjugates can be bound to the primary antibody. Other enzymes such as alkaline phosphate can replace peroxidase; alternatively, ^{125}I-labeled antibodies can be used with autoradiography, as described in the original Towbin et al. paper (421). If monoclonal antibodies are used, the methods must be adapted by including a step with rabbit anti-mouse immunoglobulin G (327,328); many monoclonal antibodies give poor responses in this system because the individual epitopes do not have sufficient affinity constants.

In our own laboratory we have applied this approach to rat and human microsomal epoxide hydrolase, rat NADPH–cytochrome P450 reductase, several different forms of rat and human cytochrome P450, and flavin-containing monooxygenase. The method can be utilized with cells (398) or tissue homogenates (74) as well as with subcellular organelles.

RECOMBINANT DNA TECHNIQUES

Uses of Recombinant DNA Techniques

This entire section was new in the chapter included in the 3rd edition of *Principles and Methods of Toxicology*. In the decade since the first version appeared, there was considerable development in the field of molecular biology, and much of the science and technology is directly useful for the study of enzymes relevant to toxicology (120). Moreover, in the past two decades the use of these techniques has become easier with the development of more standardized procedures and dependable commercial reagents. There are many texts and handbooks available in this field (e.g., refs. 13, 28, 369), and only a few procedures are specifically presented here. It should also be pointed out that a considerable body of commercial literature is available for the asking, and many commercial "kits" are now available to facilitate some of these techniques. Some of the approaches that are now routinely done include the analysis of levels of specific mRNA molecules in cells and tissues, measurement of rates of transcription from intact genes and from chimeric constructs in order to define regions critical to the process of gene expression, the binding of protein factors to specific regions of the genome involved in regulation, the detection of mutants responsible for abnormal phenotypes, the isolation of specific cDNAs, determination of nucleotide sequences of cDNAs and genomic DNA, the detection of specific mutations produced by chemical carcinogens (mutation spectra and site-specific mutagenesis), analysis of kinetic parameters associated with in vitro insertion of individual nucleotides opposite a damaged base and further extension, the production of proteins specifically modified at individual positions as a course to elucidation of catalytic function (site-directed mutagenesis), and the large-scale production of proteins through artificial vector systems. The availability of these approaches provides considerable help in efforts to understand the enzymes under consideration in toxicology and how their levels are regulated. Many of these techniqes are now even done in "high-throughput" modes with chip technology. Thc purpose of this chapter is to use protocols to help define the methods to individuals, regardless of what technology they actually use.

mRNA Isolation, Electrophoresis, and Blotting

Analysis of mRNA levels provides insight into regulatory mechanisms. In many cases, regulation of enzymatic activity is primarily at the level of transcription and mRNA levels are well correlated with levels of the protein. However, this is not always the case, and notable exceptions are documented in the case of some cytochrome P450 enzymes (389,393). Techniques of mRNA isolation and handling have now become relatively standardized and can be mastered without considerable difficulty. Moreover, the generation of highly specific probes can easily be done by synthesis of oligonucleotides or long probes developed by polymerase chain reaction (PCR) technology, in contrast to the production of antigens and antibodies for analysis of protein levels (vide supra).

The most widely used procedure for RNA isolation is that of Chomczynski and Sacchi (56). It is rapid, reliable, and adapted to large number of samples.

Reagents for RNA Isolation.

1. Stock guanidinium thiocyanate: 250 g of guanidinium thiocyanate (Fluka) is dissolved (at 65°C) in a mixture of 293 ml H_2O, 18 ml of 0.75 sodium citrate buffer (pH 7.0), and 26 ml of 10% sarcosyl (w/v). This solution can be stored $\geq$3 months at room temperature.
2. Denaturing solution: Add 0.36 ml of 2-mercaptoethanol per 50 ml of the solution just described (add before use—can be stored 1 month at room temperature if necessary).
3. Phenol (nucleic acid grade, available from several suppliers), preferably redistilled before use. Saturate with H_2O and store $\leq$1 month at 4°C.
4. 2 *M* Sodium acetate (pH 4.0).
5. $CHCl_3$/isoamyl alcohol (49:1, v/v).
6. All glassware and plasticware to be used should be previously treated with a solution of diethylpyrocarbonate (DEPC) (369, p. 190) and autoclaved, preferably in individual self-seal pouches (Baxter).
7. Whenever possible, solutions should be shaken with 0.1% DEPC (w/v) and then autoclaved to destroy excess DEPC, which can react with nucleic acids. For chemicals that react with DEPC (e.g., Tris buffers) or that cannot be autoclaved, filtration through 0.2-μm Nalge sterile filter units may reduce potential RNase contamination. Presterilized disposable pipettes, pipette tips, filter units, and so on may be used directly if individually wrapped as supplied.
8. Insofar as possible, all chemicals to be used in RNA isolation work should be reserved for this purpose and weighed out only with the use of DEPC-treated spatulas, and such.

First, one of the critical aspects of working with RNA is to avoid RNase. Even traces of the protein on glassware, dust, or fingertips are devastating. Disposable gloves should be used at all steps and, as mentioned earlier, glassware and plasticware should be treated with diethylpyrocarbonate, dried, and stored specifically for use with RNA procedures. The following procedure may be used for 100 mg tissue or an equivalent amount of cells.

The tissue is removed from the animal and minced on ice. If frozen material is to be used, the material should be ground with a mortar and pestle in liquid nitrogen (substantial RNA degradation can occur during this step). The material is homogenized in 10 ml of the denaturing solution per g tissue with the use of a Tissue-mizer (Tek-mar, Cincinnati, OH; probe is DEPC treated) in a 25-ml Corex or smaller polypropylene centrifuge tube. To this are added (sequentially, per 1.0 g tissue) 1.0 ml of 2 *M* sodium acetate buffer (pH 4.0), 10 ml of phenol, and 2 ml of the $CHCl_3$–isoamyl alcohol mixture, with thorough mixing by inversion after the addition of each reagent. The final mixture is shaken vigorously for 10 sec, cooled on ice for 15 min, and centrifuged at $10^4 \times g$ for 20 min at 4°C. The aqueous (upper) phase contains RNA and is transferred to a new tube, mixed with 10 ml of isopropanol (per 1.0 g tissue), and allowed to stand for $\geq$1 h at -20°C to precipitate RNA. The RNA is pelleted by centrifugation ($10^4 \times g$, 20 min, 4°C) and dissolved in 3.0 ml of the denaturing solution (per 1.0 g tissue), and precipitated with 1 volume of isopropanol at -20°C for 1 h. The RNA is collected as a pellet after centrifugation in a benchtop centrifuge ($\sim 3 \times 10^3 \times g$, 10 min, 4°C) and resuspended in 75% (aqueous) C_2H_5OH, resedimented in the same manner, and dried under vacuum. The material is dissolved in a minimum volume of 0.5% SDS (w/v) at 65°C for 10 min. This material may be used directly for preparation of mRNA (vide infra) or electrophoretic analysis. If the SDS is a problem for further procedures, the final pellet may be dissolved in H_2O or 1 m*M* EDTA (pH 8.0) treated with DEPC. The entire protocol may be scaled up or down accordingly. The (total) RNA concentration may be estimated by measuring absorbance at 260 nm ($A_{260} = 1.0$ for a solution of 40 μg/ml).

Reagents for mRNA Preparation

1. Oligo(dT)-cellulose is available from a number of suppliers.
2. Binding buffer: 10 m*M* Tris-HCl buffer (pH 7.5) containing 0.5 *M* NaCl, 1 m*M* EDTA, and 0.5% SDS (v/v) (also prepare a double-strength solution).
3. Wash buffer: 10 m*M* Tris-HCl buffer (pH 7.5) containing 0.1 *M* NaCl and 1 m*M* EDTA.
4. Elution buffer: 10 m*M* Tris-HCl buffer (pH 7.5) containing 1 m*M* EDTA.
5. Sodium acetate, 3 *M*.
6. Microfuge tube spin columns (Millipore-Waters, Bedford, MA—Ultra-free MC 0.45 μm filter unit, UFC3 OHVOO).
7. All glassware and plasticware are treated with diethylpyrocarbonate and autoclaved before use.

The basic procedure (206) can be varied depending upon the scale. Oligo(dT)-cellulose (0.1 g/mg total RNA) is suspended in 1–5 ml of the binding buffer and equilibrated for 60 min at room temperature with gentle agitation. The slurry is then pelleted, resuspended in fresh buffer, rewashed, and finally resuspended in binding buffer (50 mg/ml). The RNA is resuspended at 1–5 mg/ml elution buffer, heated at 65°C for 5 min, quickly chilled on ice, diluted with an equal volume of double strength binding buffer, and added to the oligo(dT) resin, from which excess binding buffer is removed by a brief spin immediately prior to loading. Binding is accomplished by 15 min incubation at room temperature, with gentle rocking, and then the mixture is loaded into microfuge spin columns (DEPC-treated and autoclaved). The flow-through (void) fraction is collected by a brief pulse spin in a microfuge; it is then reapplied to the column and the process is repeated. The column is then washed with 5–10 volumes of binding buffer and 5 volumes of wash buffer. The bound RNA is eluted with 2–3 column volumes of elution buffer and adjusted to 0.50 *M* NaCl with double-strength binding buffer; the entire procedure is repeated with the column (i.e., binding, washing, elution). RNA in the final eluate is recovered by the addition of 0.1 volume of C_2H_5OH and centrifugation.

Some protocols have procedures for regeneration of oligo(dT), but reuse is not recommended for best results.

Reagents for electrophoresis and blotting of RNA (316,436).

1. 5 × MOPS [3-(*N*-morpholino) propanesulfonic acid] running buffer (also prepare 1 ×): 0.20 *M* MOPS buffer (pH 7.0) containing 50 m*M* sodium acetate and 5.0 m*M* EDTA.
2. 37% HCHO (pH >4).
3. Formamide (deionized).
4. Loading buffer: 30% Ficoll (w/v), 1.0 m*M* EDTA, 0.25% bromphenol blue (w/v), and 0.25% xylene cyanol (w/v).
5. 1 × SSC buffer (also prepare 20 ×, 10 ×, and 0.25 ×): 15 m*M* sodium citrate buffer (pH 7.0) containing 150 m*M* NaCl.
6. Ethidium bromide, 5 mg/ml.
7. Prehybridization solution—Mix (187): 60 ml formamide, 3 ml of a sonicated solution of 10 mg salmon sperm DNA/ml, 12 ml of 100 × Denhardt's solution [2.0% Ficoll (w/v), 2.0% polyvinylpyrrolidine (w/v), and 2.0% bovine serum], 6 ml of a solution of 1 mg poly A/ml, 1.2 ml of 10% SDS (w/v), 30 ml of 20 × SSC buffer (vide supra), and 7–8 ml DEPC-treated H_2O.
8. SDS, 10% (w/v).
9. All H_2O should be treated with DEPC to inhibit RNase activity.

To pour a 20 × 20 cm gel, boil 3.0 g agarose in 186 ml DEPC-treated H_2O to dissolve and then let it cool to ~60°C. Add 60 ml of 5 × MOPS buffer and 54 ml of 37% HCHO. Pour the gel in the gel box, with the comb set such that slots are ~1 mm above the horizontal surface. Allow gel to set, remove the comb, and add 1 × MOPS buffer so that the gel is completely submerged.

Each sample should contain 2 μl of 5 × MOPS buffer, 3.5 μl of 37% HCHO, 10 μl formamide, and ≤20 μg RNA in 5 μl. Mix with a vortex device, spin 5–10 sec in a microcentrifuge, and incubate 15 min at 55°C or 5 min at 65°C. Add 2 μl of loading buffer to each sample, mix well, and spin 5–10 sec in a microcentrifuge. Load samples onto the gel and run the gel at a constant voltage of ~5 V/cm or until the bromphenol blue band has migrated halfway down the gel. It may be preferable to run a duplicate set of samples, so that one gel may be used for ethidium bromide staining and one for transfer/hybridization.

The duplicate gel to be used for staining is placed in a pan of 20 × MOPS buffer to which has been added a few drops of the ethidium bromide stock solution (5 mg/ml). After 45 min the gel is photographed with a ruler alongside it (it may be necessary to first destain the gel in H_2O if the stain is too intense). Two sharp bands—18S and 28S rRNA—should appear when total RNA is used in the electrophoresis. If the bands are not sharp, it is probably because of considerable degradation during the preparation.

The gel section to be transferred to nitrocellulose is cut out, placed in a large tray, and rinsed with 500 ml of 20 × SSC. A piece of nitrocellulose paper (~3 mm smaller on each side than the gel section), wet it 1 min in H_2O and equilibrate it 5–10 min in 20 × SSC buffer (use disposable gloves to handle nitrocellulose). Cut

3–5 sheets of chromatography paper (Whatman number 3 MM) into pieces ~3 mm smaller on each side than the sheet of nitrocellulose paper. To prepare a wick, cut a piece of chromatography paper ~2 cm larger than the gel with 4 tabs extending ~10 cm out each side. The gel is wet thoroughly with 20 × SSC buffer. Place a glass plate, slightly larger than the gel, on top of 4 petri dishes filled with 20 × SSC and the wick on top, with the ends of the wick hanging over the plate into the 20 × SSC buffer. Any air bubbles trapped between the wick and glass plate should be removed with a glass rod. Lift the gel out of the 10 × SSC buffer, allow most of the liquid to drip off, invert, and lay the gel on top of the chromatography wick, taking care to remove air bubbles as before. The nitrocellulose sheet (from the 20 × SSC buffer) is laid on top of the gel, with care to remove air bubbles (be sure that the nitrocellulose sheet does not overhang the gel). One piece of the stack of pieces of chromatography paper is wet in the 20 × SSC buffer, then placed on top of the sheet of nitrocellulose paper, again taking care to avoid trapped air bubbles and overhanging the nitrocellulose. On top of this place the rest of the chromatography sheets, a 5–10 cm stack of paper towels, a glass plate, and a weight. Cut long strips of Parafilm ~5 cm wide and place immediately alongside the gel, so as to cover the sides of the wick, which might come into contact with the towel stack as the gel contracts (prevents wicking at edges). The ends of the tray are covered with plastic wrap to minimize evaporation during transfer. Transfer to the nitrocellulose proceeds overnight.

Remove the materials to expose the nitrocellulose sheet and mark the upper right-hand corner and positions of the wells. A blunt-ended forceps is used to pick up the nitrocellulose sheet and place it between two sheets of chromatography paper. Bake this for 2 h at 80°C. Alternatively, RNA can be fixed to the wet membrane using a Stratalinker UV-linking device and then air-dried.

Hybridization of a labeled probe to the RNA present in the gel is carried out in the following way. The filter is baked as just described and placed in a sealable bag or box along with sufficient prehybridization solution to completely submerge the membrane; the bag is sealed and incubated for 2 h to overnight at the desired temperature (37–42°C). The appropriate probe is prepared by either (a) nick translation of a cDNA fragment, (b) random labeling, (c) polymerase chain reaction (PCR), or (d) oligonucleotide synthesis and end labeling. For discussion and details of these methods see ref. 28. The longer probes with higher levels of label incorporated are more sensitive; the shorter oligonucleotides are more specific if they are optimized for differences. The probe ($>5 \times 10^5$ cpm) is mixed with hybridization solution, heated at 95°C for 10 min, and added to the bag (added through a cut in the corner and spread over the sheet, and the bag is resealed) or box. Hybridization occurs overnight at the same temperature used for the prehybridization. On the following day, the bag or box is opened and the filter is removed. The filter is washed twice (1–2 min each) with 2 × SSC buffer at room temperature. Two similar washes are then done (45 min each) with 1 × SSC buffer containing 0.10% SDS (w/v). The hybridization may be changed by varying the temperature of the hybridization or wash and the salt concentration of the washing buffer, in order to increase the "stringency" of the wash and specificity of hybridization (e.g., see ref. 36). The filter is exposed to x-ray film. The time needed for an appropriate exposure will vary with the specific radioactivity of the probe, stringency of the hybridization, and concentration of mRNA.

Historically, most work has been done with ^{32}P-labeled probes. However, there are alternative procedures possible involving ^{33}P, avidin/biotin, immunochemical, and luminescence procedures (consult commercial vendors), and these will probably find increased use in the future because of decreased cost and increased restrictions on the disposal of radioactive waste.

Polymerase Chain Reaction (PCR) Technology

The basic principles of the method were developed in 1986 and are quite simple, and are depicted in Figure 35.32 for double-stranded DNA. The double-stranded DNA is heat denatured, and the two primers complementary to the ends of the target segment are annealed at a temperature close to the annealing temperature of the oligomers and then extended at a temperature optimal for the polymerase used. One set of these three consecutive steps is referred to as a cycle. Thus, the amount of the original sequence of interest is expanded in a geometric progression. Of course, this process could be accomplished with any polymerase by the addition of new enzyme in each cycle. The process is greatly facilitated by the use of a heat-stable polymerase isolated from a thermophilic bacterium; such polymerases function most effectively at relatively high temperatures (~72–78°C), so that the entire process is facilitated and many cycles can be carried out with the same enzyme. The cycle times are relatively short and commercial instruments are available that can be programmed to cycle through the steps automatically. DNA segments can be amplified 10^5 to 10^9-fold by this process, and several reports have appeared of the successful amplification of the genomic DNA of a single cell. Recently heat-stable polymerases of very high fidelity have become commercially available and can be used to reduce errors. The basic process (Figure 35.32) provides the opportunity for considerable innovation in the application to a wide variety of research problems, and only a few basic points are mentioned here. The reader is advised to consult cur-

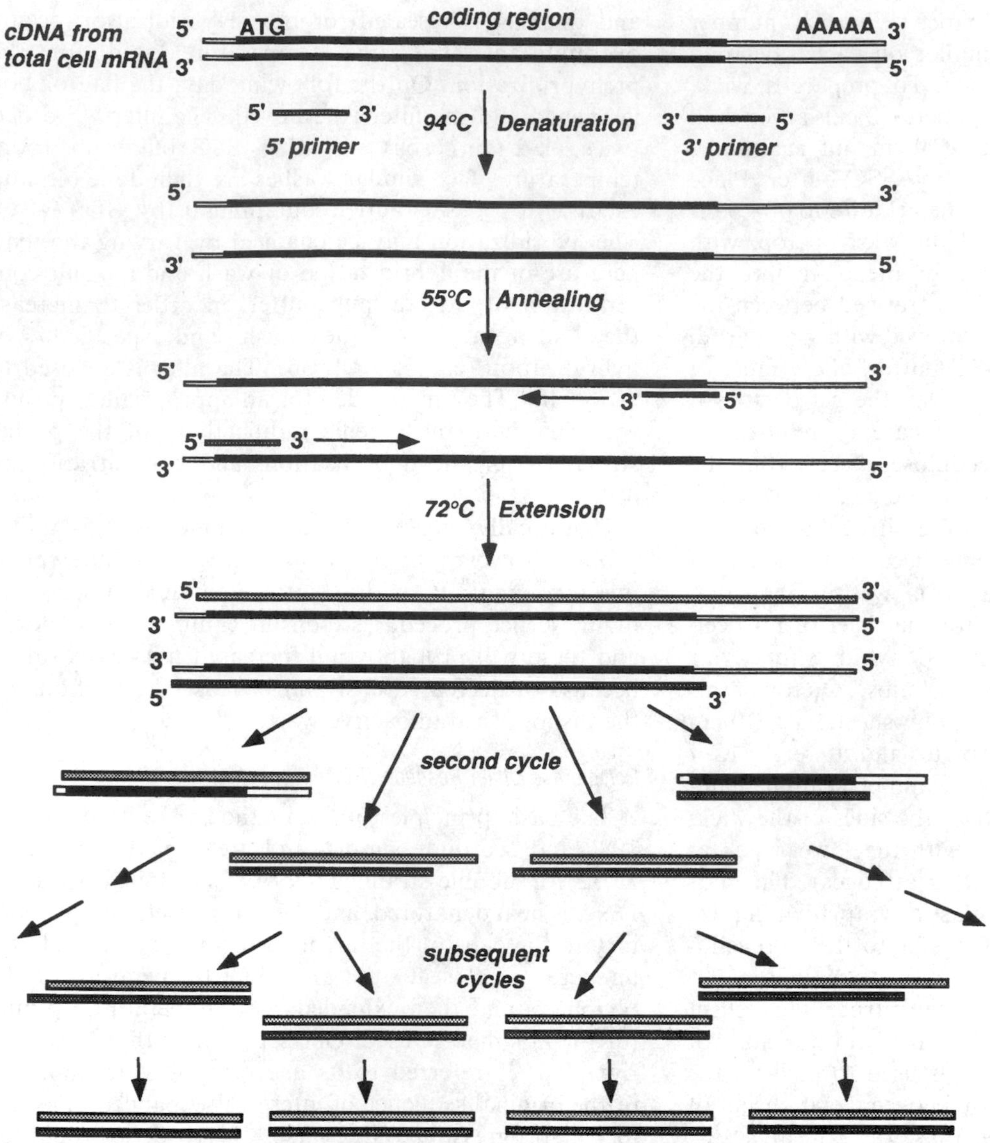

FIG. 35.32. General outline for polymerase chain reaction (PCR).

rent literature in this area, and there are numerous useful commercial technical reports.

Most PCR protocols are performed at the 100-μl scale in 0.5-ml microcentrifuge tubes. Because of the power of the system to amplify DNA, there is also considerable potential for generation of mistakes and false positives. Some of this is inherent in the infidelity of the polymerases and can be avoided by judicious choice of the enzymes, but it is imperative to minimize laboratory errors. Carryover of amplified sequences contributes to the majority of false positives, and appropriate precautions include physical separation of pre- and post-PCR reactions, aliquoting of reagents to minimize the number of repeated samplings, and careful use of positive placement pipettes. Other general precautions include changing (and washing) gloves frequently, careful uncapping of samples to prevent aerosol formation, minimization of sample handling, the addition of nonsample components (buffer, nucleotides, primers, and mineral oil) to the reaction mixture before addition of sample DNA (each tube should be capped after DNA addition before proceeding to the next sample), and the use of fresh pipette tips for each addition.

The PCR sample may be single- or double-stranded DNA or RNA. If the starting sample is RNA, reverse transcriptase is used to prepare the first strand cDNA prior to conventional PCR. Typically ng amounts of the template are used. PCR primers are oligonucleotides, typically 18–30 bases long, that are complementary to sequences defining the 3′ ends of the complementary template strands. Nontemplate-complementary 5′ extensions may be added to primers to allow a variety of useful postamplification operations on the PCR product (e.g., addition of restriction sites for insertion into vectors) without significant perturbation of the amplification itself. The two PCR primers should not contain substantial complementarity with each other (especially at the 3′ ends) to avoid the formation of an artifactual product termed "primer dimer." Internal secondary structure (e.g., hairpin loops) should be avoided in primers. A 40–60% G + C content is often recommended for both primers, without long stretches of any single base. If crude material such as total mRNA or generated cDNA is to be used for PCR, the primers can be checked in a sequence database for site of potential interference.

Optimal annealing temperatures must be determined empirically. *AmpliTaq* DNA polymerase (Perkin-Elmer/Cetus, Norwalk, CT) is a thermostable, 94-kD DNA polymerase encoded by a modified form of the *Thermus aquaticus* DNA polymerase gene, which has been inserted into an *E. coli* host. In general, an extension temperature of 72°C works well for *Taq*. A good annealing temperature from which to start optimizing the particular conditions for an amplification is 5–10°C below the T_m of the primers (primer T_m values should be well matched). Titration of the Mg^{2+} concentration over the range of 1.5–4 m*M* is needed to find the concentration producing the highest yield of a specific product. The fidelity decreases in the presence of high Mg^{2+} (this phenomenon can be used to advantage if a finite level of mistakes is desired, as in a random mutagenesis experiment). In most situations, where high fidelity is required, *Pfu* DNA polymerase (Stratagene, La Jolla, CA) is preferred to the *Taq* enzyme because of higher fidelity. The enzyme was originally isolated from the hyperthermophilic, murine archaebacterium *Pyrococcus furiosis* but is now supplied as a recombinant *E. coli* product. This multifunctional, thermostable enzyme possesses both 5′ to 3′ DNA polymerase activity and 3′ to 5′ exonuclease activity; this latter activity results in a 12-fold increase in fidelity of DNA synthesis over *Taq* DNA polymerase. The temperature optimum is near 75°C; at 35°C the enzyme has <8% activity, and the enzyme is reported to remain >85% active following 1 h of incubation at 95°C. *Vent* polymerase is also useful because of its high fidelity. Typically, *Pfu* reactions are performed in 100 μl of a mixture containing dATP, dCTP, dGTP, and dTTP (200 μM each), primer (0.25 μM), template (0.1–500 ng total), and 10 μl of a stock buffer containing 0.20 *M* Tris-HCl (pH 8.75), 0.10 *M* KCl, 0.10 *M* $(NH_4)_2SO_4$, 20 m*M* $MgCl_2$, 1.0% Triton X-100 (w/v), and 1.0 mg nuclease-free bovine serum albumin/ml (w/v). The tubes are mixed gently, centrifuged briefly, and overlaid with light mineral oil. The mixture is heated to 95°C for 5 min and then cooled to the desired annealing temperature in order to allow the primers to anneal to the template DNA. *Pfu* DNA polymerase (2.5 units) is added. Primer extension is allowed to proceed at 75°C. Cycles are then repeated as necessary to achieve adequate amplification. The products are checked by electrophoresis, with detection by ethidium bromide staining or hybridization to labeled probes as appropriate.

The uses of PCR technology are considerable, particularly in the high-specificity applications. For instance, specific probes can be constructed from crude samples such as total cellular mRNA and then labeled to use for quantitation of specific mRNAs. Also, full-length cDNAs for relatively large proteins (e.g., cytochrome P450 enzymes) can be made directly from cellular mRNA and inserted into vectors for expression (if this is done, sequence analysis should be used first for verification of the fidelity of amplification). There are numerous strategies for using PCR to detect mutations. For instance, a short section of a sequence can be specifically amplified by PCR and the product examined by restriction digestion/electrophoresis to determine if a change has occurred. Alternatively, primers can be selected such that only a particular variant will be amplified (e.g., allele-specific PCR).

Thus, with only a knowledge of sequences under consideration and crude biological samples (tissues, cells, etc.) it is possible to construct most of the reagents needed to analyze and express genes coding for individual proteins. The reader is referred to the literature in this area for examples of the use of these and other strategies (10).

Expression of Enzymes in Heterologous Vector Systems

This section briefly summarizes the current status of vector systems used for enzymes of interest in toxicology. The field is changing rapidly, and no specific protocols are presented. Some general comments are in order about the choice of an expression system. Some appropriate reviews of the subject have been published recently (13,117,445).

A number of different mammalian cell expression systems are available and have been used. These include systems for transient and stable expression. Transient systems [e.g., COS kidney cells (476)] usually give higher levels of expression but infection must be done each time cells are to be used; further, the level of expression must be analyzed with each use to permit appropriate conclusions to be reached. Even stable cell lines must be checked occasionally for expression levels; these systems generally produce much lower levels of enzymes. Mammalian cell systems have the advantage that the environment should be a reasonable facsimile of the mammalian environment to be modeled. Therefore such systems can be used with toxicity and mutagenicity as endpoints, within the cells containing the expressed enzyme. V79 and AHH-1 cell lines expressing certain cytochrome P450 enzymes and epoxide hydrolase are commercially available (89,121). Vaccinia-based expression systems produce fairly high levels of enzymes (20), although this system requires special containment procedures (e.g., immunization of laboratory personnel) and is not widely used. Mammalian cells are able to introduce posttranslational modifications, and if these are deemed necessary, they may be the only choice for expression work. However, the levels of expression are relatively low and not the choice if large amounts of enzymes are required. For instance, considerable amounts of COS (kidney origin) cells are required just in order to obtain weak cytochrome P450 Fe^{2+}-CO spectra. The level of expression is considerably higher in the vaccinia system, and spectra can be measured, but the costs of making large quantities of protein are considerable. For examples of use of other cell lines to express cytochrome P450, epoxide hydrolase, and UDP-glucuronosyl transferase, see ref. 445.

Baculovirus systems use cultured insect cells (122,211). The construction of vectors and the screening and use of these systems is technically more difficult than for many other cell lines, but the yield of protein can be considerably higher, to the point where this system is feasible to pursue structural studies. These systems have been used to express cytochrome P450 (12,122,317), NADPH–cytochrome P450 reductase (403), GSH transferase (190), epoxide hydrolase (9,124,180), and UDP-glucuronosyl transferase (9,309). The deficiency of heme synthesis is a problem for production of cytochrome P450 enzymes (12,317). The medium can be supplemented with heme (114,155,234) (although in no case has it been demonstrated that the expressed enzyme has a full complement of heme). However, this deficiency has been used to advantage to introduce abnormal and synthetic heme molecules (12). The ability of baculovirus systems to introduce posttranslational modifications varies. It should not be assumed that the system is a faithful mimic of mammalian cells in this regard, if this is considered to be an issue with a particular protein.

Yeast-based systems are capable of producing considerably more enzyme than most mammalian cell systems. Yeast are relatively easy to grow and do not require the expensive equipment and media that mammalian cells do. Moreover, the production volume can be scaled up without considerable difficulty (149). A number of cytochrome P450 enzymes have been expressed in *Saccharomyces cerevesiae* (149). Yeast systems can make some posttranslational modifications but cannot be expected to make all. Heme is apparently not limiting. Microsomal proteins such as cytochrome P450 are inserted into the endoplasmic reticulum, and NADPH–cytochrome P450 reductase and cytochrome b_5 are present there. Metabolism studies have been done with whole cells (366,367,379), with yeast microsomes (38,39,351), and with cytochrome P450 enzymes purified from yeast (39,198,223). With most mammalian cell systems, transformation of a drug must be measured in long incubations lasting for many hours, unless substrates of very high specific radioactivity are used (or extremely sensitive analytical techniques); incubations with yeast microsomes are usually done in a matter of minutes and used in a similar manner as liver microsomes. Although yeast appears to have many advantages as an expression system, there are some disadvantages as well. The level of production does have a limit, and very large amounts of enzyme cannot be produced; moreover, the cells are quite difficult to break and hydrolases must be used in addition to mechanical disruption. The level of yeast NADPH–cytochrome P450 reductase is relatively low and in some cases (e.g., human cytochrome P450 3A4) does not couple well for efficient reduction (39); Pompon and his associates have coexpressed human NADPH–cytochrome P450 reductase using the yeast genome to alleviate the problem (337).

Bacteria are capable of producing large amounts of enzymes. Constructions in inducible expression vectors are relatively easy. Of course, few posttranslational modifications are made by the bacteria. GSH transferases have been expressed in bacteria for some time (442) and so has NAD(P)H : quinone oxidoreductase (278). Initial efforts to express the intrinsic membrane proteins in bacteria were not very successful because of extensive proteolysis (344). However, more recent studies with other vectors indicate that the problems are not insurmountable, and NADPH–cytochrome P450 reductase (377) and several cytochrome P450 enzymes have now been expressed (17,18,253,254,262). The modification of the 5′ nucleotides of the coding region has been shown to be critical in some cases, apparently to decrease the energy due to RNA secondary structure and permit rapid translation (17,18). A significant fraction of the expressed cytochrome P450 may remain soluble, and the reasons are not yet clear (331,332). Enzymes expressed in bacteria may be used and crude fractions (membranes or soluble fraction) may be purified before use in assays. Conventional means have been used to purify the enzymes (165,253); it is also possible to attach oligomeric His residues to the enzymes to use metal–ligand chromatography for rapid purification (11,90,234). One disadvantage of bacterial expression systems is that care must be taken to avoid the formation of "inclusion bodies," which are very insoluble aggregates of protein sometimes encountered in high level expression. These may be avoided by choice of vectors and by lowering the incubation temperature. Actually, formation of these can be used to advantage in some cases, because they can be readily recovered in denatured form for use as antigens.

Bacterial expression systems have been used extensively for the expression of many of the individual enzymes of interest in this field (29,125,155,169,408).

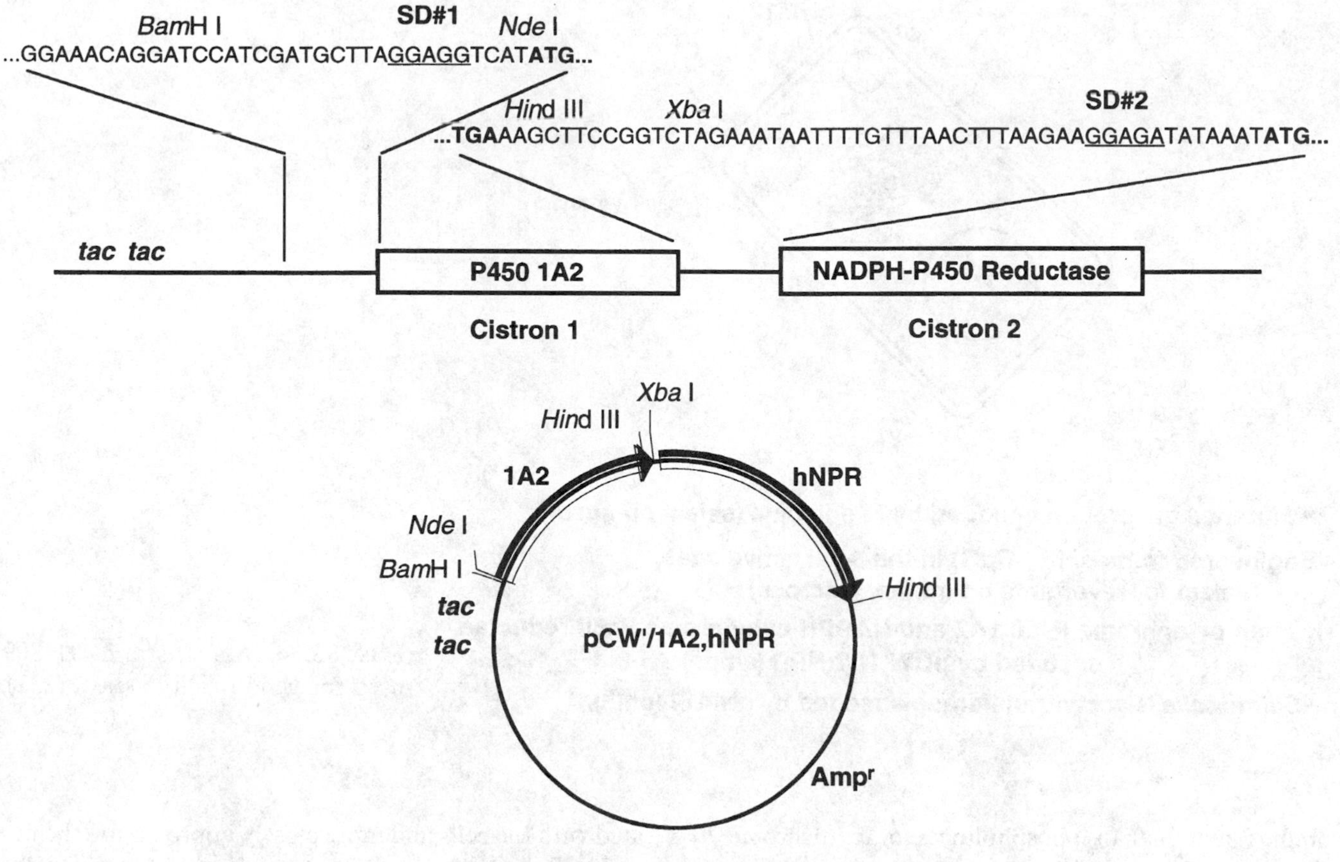

FIG. 35.33. Construction of bicistronic human cytochrome P450/NADPH-cytochrome P450 reductase plasmids (325). SD = Shine-Dalgarno sequence, 1A2-human cytochrome P450 1A2.

The only major exceptions have been proteins that require extensive posttranslational modification, such as monoamine oxidase and UDP-glycuronosyl transferase (169,245). Monoamine oxidase requires covalent attachment of FAD, a process for which the biochemical process is not yet clear. UDP-glycuronosyl transferase requires glycosylation and N-terminal processing in order to achieve its proper membrane orientation and catalytic activity. PGH synthases (cyclooxygenases) are also glycosylated enzymes and are generally expressed in mammalian cells or baculovirus-based systems, although it is not clear that the carbohydrates are essential for function. A historic problem with cytochrome P450 expression has been the low catalytic activity of the expressed protein in the absence of NADPH–cytochrome P450 reductase. Some activity is present due to electron transport from flavodoxins (213). Three methods have been used to improve the catalytic function of cytochrome P450 within bacterial cells. The first is the overexpression of flavodoxin. This is somewhat effective, but even at very high flavodoxin to cytochrome P450 ratios the activity of the cytochrome P450 is ~10% that seen with NADPH–cytochrome P450 reductase (92). The second method involves the use of cytochrome P450 : NADPH–cytochrome P450 fusion proteins. This concept has precedent in the natural fusion proteins of bacterial cytochrome P450 102 and the cytochrome P450 relative nitric oxide synthase (302,455) plus the initial work in this area by Ohkawa (299) and Estabrook (280) and their associates. Although some of these artificial fusion proteins have been reported to have high catalytic activity (364,365), others have not been particularly good (57,157,326) and the approach probably cannot be generally applied. The third approach is the use of constructs in which both a cytochrome P450 and NADPH–cytochrome P450 reductase are expressed from a single plasmid. A version developed in our laboratory uses a "bicistronic" construct in which a single promoter (*tac*/*tac*) is used to produce a single RNA that is translated to yield both individual enzymes (Figure 35.33) (325). Others have used plasmid systems with separate promoters (31,205). Relatively high catalytic activity is present in either the bacterial cells (supported by glucose) or the isolated membranes (supported by NADPH). The membranes can be handled like tissue microsomes, in that only substrate and NADPH need to be added. Apparently there is no essential need for

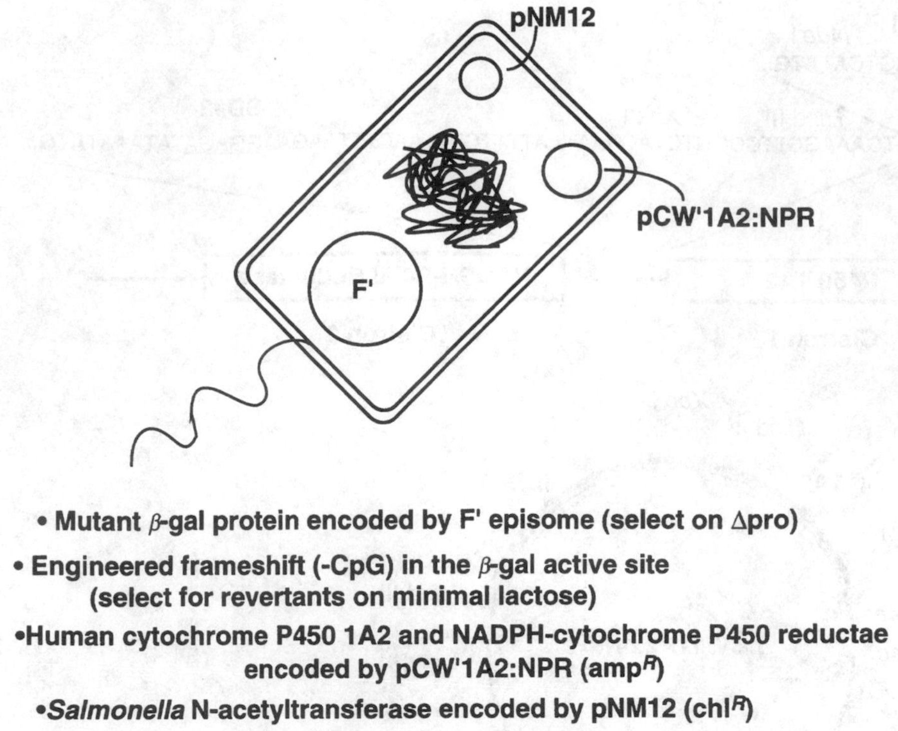

pNM12
pCW'1A2:NPR
F'
• Mutant β-gal protein encoded by F' episome (select on Δpro)
• Engineered frameshift (-CpG) in the β-gal active site (select for revertants on minimal lactose)
•Human cytochrome P450 1A2 and NADPH-cytochrome P450 reductae encoded by pCW'1A2:NPR (amp^R)
•Salmonella N-acetyltransferase encoded by pNM12 (chl^R)

FIG. 35.34. *E. coli* strain DJ4309 used for genotoxicity assays (222).

complex mammalian phospholipids or cytochrome b_5 (although these results do not mean that these molecules are without effect in the mammalian endoplasmic reticulum).

One use of the bacterial cytochrome P450 systems is development of convenient genotoxicity assays. This area is reviewed elsewhere (155), including the expression of human cytochrome P450 in *Salmonella typhimurium* (221). More recently, *E. coli* systems have been developed in which both cytochrome P450 and NADPH–cytochrome P450 reductase are expressed within the bacterial cell (and are catalytically active). The endpoint is *lac* protrophy (instead of the usual *his* in the Ames test.) A (bacterial) *N*-acetyltransferase can be concurrently expressed to increase sensitivity to aryl and heterocyclic amines (Figure 35.34). Such systems have been shown to respond to concentrations of some aryl amines as low as the classical *Salmonella typhimurium* systems (222). In addition, *S. typhimurium* systems have been used to express both human cytochrome P450 and NADPH–cytochrome P450 reductase for genotoxicity assays (402). These systems have several advantages. In other work, it has been possible to express rat and human GSH transferases (99,390,411) and *N*-acetyltransferase in *S. typhimurium* for use in genotoxicity assays. These systems have considerable potential, since bacterial systems will continue to be the mainstay of high-throughput, first-check genotoxicity screens in industry. In these systems, reactive products are generated with the cells and more closely approximate the normal cellular situation. One system that offers further potential is the *S. typhimurium umu* test (or the similar *E. coli* chromotest) (456), in which a reporter gene is linked to a promoter that responds to a cascade eminating from damage to bacterial DNA (384). These systems often have even faster readout than colony-counting systems (e.g., Ames test) with their colorimetric endpoints, which are seen within a few hours.

As pointed out before, the technology in this area is changing rapidly and the interested reader is encouraged to consult current literature before proceeding. The choice of an expression system is primarily a function of the specific problem at hand. The power of expressed systems is realized in studies where closely related enzymes are under consideration and it has not been clear from other studies exactly what the catalytic activities of individual enzymes are. For instance, in this laboratory we were able to use recombinant yeast and bacterial cytochrome P450 3A4 to demonstrate that the same enzyme (cytochrome P450 3A4) was able to catalyze both the 8,9-epoxidation and 3α-hydroxylation of aflatoxin B_1 and that these activities were differentially modified by the effector 7,8-benzoflavone (349,428). Also, (yeast and other) expression systems have been of use in delineating some of the catalytic activities [especially (*S*)-mephenytoin and tolbutamide hydroxylation] of the human cytochrome P450 2C family enzymes (39,118,354,396). Again, the other major advantage of expression systems is that they greatly facilitate the isolation of useful amounts of scarce enzymes. It is expected that such systems will find increasing use in the future.

Demonstration that a particular reaction can be catalyzed by an expressed or purified enzyme is a qualitative finding unless comparisons can be made with other enzymes suspected of catalyzing the same reaction (170). Therefore, findings regarding catalytic activities of expressed proteins must be placed in regard to other experiments involving chemical and immunoinhibition in crude tissue fractions, etc. For instance, in a number of reports, human cytochrome P450 2B6 has been reported to have appreciable catalytic activity (50). However, the level of expression of this enzyme in all human liver samples examined to date has been very low, as measured with both anti-monkey cytochrome P450 2B and anti-recombinant human P450 2B6 antibodies (295). One can roughly estimate the relative contributions of two enzymes from their in vitro kinetic activities, but a number of assumptions need to be made. For instance, in this case one must assume that the two enzymes compete equally for limiting amounts of NADPH–P450 reductase and so forth. This problem exists when using any recombinant enzyme or purified enzyme.

An even more complex problem arises when we consider the case of GSH transferases. Several GSH transferases catalyze the conjugation of GSH with ethylene dibromide (Figure 35.5) (59,340). Some alpha class enzymes are abundant in the liver. The mu and theta (5-5) class enzymes are present in many tissues. Apparently the theta class enzymes are present in erythrocytes (330). Ethylene dibromide causes rodent tumors at many sites, but the locus shifts to the liver when the oxidation of ethylene dibromide is inhibited by administration of disulfiram (462). One can raise the question of the role of GSH transferase theta in the blood cells. Does it protect? Activation of ethylene dibromide during its transit through the bloodstream might be an effective detoxication process in that there are no DNA targets there. However, if GSH transferase expression throughout the body tracks that in erythrocytes, increased transferase in target tissue could be detrimental. A similar situation can be considered with cytochrome P450 3A4, which is expressed in both human liver and small intestine. This enzyme activates aflatoxin B_1 to the *exo*-8,9-epoxide (428). Expression in the liver can be considered detrimental, although there is the caveat that the enzyme can also detoxicate aflatoxin B_1 by 3α-hydroxylation (349,428). Expression of more P450 3A4 in the small intestine may be considered beneficial in that oxidation of aflatoxin to either aflatoxin Q_1 (3α-hydroxylation) or the *exo*-8,9-epoxide can be considered a detoxication, in that DNA adducts formed in the small intestine are not considered detrimental in that they do not go on to form tumors (cells are sloughed rapidly). Thus, many factors need to be considered in putting enzyme studies in the context of diseases.

ACKNOWLEDGMENTS

The author's research has been supported by U.S. Public Health Service grants R35 CA44353 and P30 ES00267. Thanks are extended to Drs. E. M. J. Gillam and L. C. Bell-Parikh and Prof. L. J. Marnett for providing details of assay procedures.

QUESTIONS

1. Does Phase I always precede Phase II reactions in metabolism of individual chemicals? If not, provide examples.
2. Most assays for competitive inhibition of cytochrome P450 enzymes involve direct studies with assays of substrate oxidation. How could you develop a high-throughput screening strategy for identifying high-affinity inhibitors of a particular cytochrome P450 (e.g., 2D6) without the need to do assays of catalytic activity?
3. A new chemical of interest induces total hepatic cytochrome P450 (as measured spectrally) and is hepatotoxic (in rats). Are the two phenomena necessarily related? How would you establish the relationship?
4. An investigator tells you that he has found that a particular recombinant human cytochrome P450 enzyme catalyzes a reaction of interest to you. What other pieces of evidence are needed to put this information into the perspective of how much this enzyme contributes to the process in human liver?
5. The pathways shown next have been extended to demonstrate an example of situations often encountered in practical situations. Provide reasonable stepwise pathways to the products indicated.

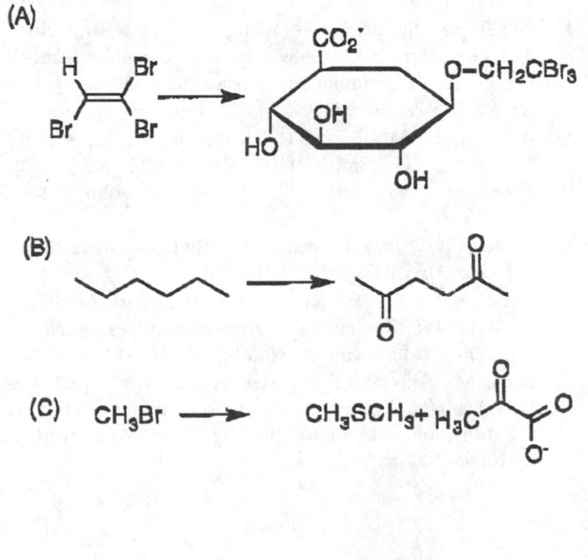

The number of steps is not specified. For each step provide the necessary cosubstrate(s) and name of enzyme (if enzymatic—only group name, no need for individual form).

REFERENCES

1. Adams, J. B., and Poulos, A. (1967): Enzymatic synthesis of steroid sulfates. III. Isolation and properties of estrogen suphotransferase from bovine adrenal gland. *Biochim. Biophys. Acta*, 146:493–508.
2. Alterman, M. A., and Dowgii, A. I. (1990): A simple and rapid method for the purification of cytochrome P450 (form LM4). *Biomed. Chromatog.*, 4:221–222.
3. Andersen, M. E., Clewell, H. J., and Frederick, C. B. (1995): Applying simulation modeling to problems in toxicology and risk assessment—A short perspective. *Toxicol. Appl. Pharmacol.*, 133:181–187.
4. Andersen, M. E., Clewell, H. J. III, Gargas, M. L., Smith, F. A., and Reitz, R. H. (1987): Physiologically based pharmacokinetics and the risk assessment process for methylene chloride. *Toxicol. Appl. Pharmacol.*, 87:185–205.
5. Andres, H. H., Klem, A. J., Szabo, S. M., and Weber, W. W. (1985): New spectrophotometric and radiochemical assays for acetyl-CoA: arylamine *N*-acetyltransferase applicable to a variety of arylamines. *Anal. Biochem.*, 145:367–375.
6. Andres, H. H., and Weber, W. W. (1986): *N*-Acetylation pharmacogenetics: Michaelis–Menten constants for arylamine drugs as predictors of their *N*-acetylation rates in vivo. *Drug Metab. Dispos.*, 14:382–385.
7. Ansler, S. S., and Jakoby, W. B. (1986): Amine *N*-methyltransferases from rabbit liver. *J. Biol. Chem.*, 261:3996–4001.
8. Armstrong, R. N. (1997): Glutathione transferases. In: *Biotransformation, Vol. 3, Comprehensive Toxicology*, edited by F. P. Guengerich, pp. 307–327. Elsevier Science, Oxford.
9. Armstrong, R. N., Lacourciere, G. M., and Vikharia, V. N. (1992): Expression of miscrosomal detoxication enzymes in a recombinant baculovirus system. The case of epoxide hydrolase and UDP-glucuronosyltransferase. *J. Basic Clin. Physiol. Pharmacol.*, 3(suppl.):170.
10. Arnheim, N., and Erlich, H. (1992): Polymerase chain reaction strategy. *Annu. Rev. Biochem.*, 61:131–156.
11. Arnold, F. H., and Haymore, B. L. (1991): Engineered metal-binding proteins: Purification to protein folding. *Science*, 252:1796–1797.
12. Asseffa, A., Smith, S. J., Nagata, K., Gillette, J., Gelboin, H. V., and Gonzalez, F. J. (1989): Novel exogenous heme-dependent expression of mammalian cytochrome P450 using baculovirus. *Arch. Biochem. Biophys.*, 274:481–490.
13. Ausubel, F. M., Brent, R., Kingston, R. E., Moore, D. D., Seidman, J. G., Smith, J. A., and Struhl, K. (1992): *Current Protocols in Molecular Biology, Vol. 2*, John Wiley & Sons, New York.
14. Axelrod, J. (1962): Catechol-*O*-methyltransferase from rat liver. *Methods Enzymol.*, 5:748–751.
15. Ayesh, R., Idle, J. R., Ritchie, J. C., Crothers, M. J., and Hetzel, M. R. (1984): Metabolic oxidation phenotypes as markers for susceptibility to lung cancer. *Nature*, 312:169–170.
16. Baca, M., Scanlan, T. S., Stephenson, R. C., and Wells, J. A. (1997): Phage display of a catalytic antibody to optimize affinity for transition-state analog binding. *Proc. Natl. Acad. Sci. USA*, 94:10063 10068.
17. Barnes, H. J. (1996): Maximizing expression of eukaryotic cytochrome P450s in *Escherichia coli*. *Methods Enzymol.*, 272:3–14.
18. Barnes, H. J., Arlotto, M. P., and Waterman, M. R. (1991): Expression and enzymatic activity of recombinant cytochrome P450 17α-hydroxylase in *Escherichia coli*. *Proc. Natl. Acad. Sci. USA*, 88:5597–5601.
19. Basu, A. K., Wood, M. L., Niedernhofer, L. J., Ramos, L. A., and Essigmann, J. M. (1993): Mutagenic and genotoxic effects of three vinyl chloride-induced DNA lesions: 1,N^6-ethenoadenine, 3,N^4-ethenocytosine, and 4-amino-5-(imidazol-2-yl)imidazole. *Biochemistry*, 32:12793–12801.
20. Battula, N. (1989): Transduction of cytochrome P_3-450 by retroviruses: constitutive expression of enzymatically active microsomal hemoprotein in animal cells. *J. Biol. Chem.*, 264:2991–2996.
21. Bauer, E., Guo, Z., Ueng, Y.-F., Bell, L. C., and Guengerich, F. P. (1995): Oxidation of benzo[a]pyrene by recombinant human cytochrome P450 enzymes. *Chem. Res. Toxicol.*, 8:136–142.
22. Beaune, P., Kremers, P. G., Kaminsky, L. S., de Graeve, J., and Guengerich, F. P. (1986): Comparison of monooxygenase activities and cytochrome P450 isozyme concentrations in human liver microsomes. *Drug Metab. Dispos.*, 14:437–442.
23. Bell, L. C. and Guengerich, F. P. (1997): Oxidation kinetics of ethanol by human cytochrome P450 2E1. Rate-limiting product release accounts for effects of isotopic hydrogen substitution and cytochrome b_5 on steady-state kinetics. *J. Biol. Chem.*, 272:29643–29651.
24. Bell, P. A. and Kasper, C. B. (1993): Expression of rat microsomal epoxide hydrolase in *Escherichia coli*: Identification of a histidyl residue essential for catalysis. *J. Biol. Chem.*, 268:14011–14017.
25. Bell-Parikh, L. C., Hosea, N. A., Martin, M. V., and Guengerich, F. P. (1999): Purification of cytochrome P450 enzymes. In: *Current Protocols in Toxicology*, Chaps. 1, 2, 4, John Wiley & Sons, New York.
26. Bentley, P., and Oesch, F. (1975): Purification of rat liver epoxide hydratase to apparent homogeneity. *FEBS Lett.*, 59:291–295.
27. Bentley, P., Schmassmann, H., Sims, P., and Oesch, F. (1976): Epoxides derived from various polycyclic hydrocarbons as substrates of homogeneous and microsome-bound epoxide hydratase. *Eur. J. Biochem.*, 69:97–103.
28. Berger, S. L., and Kimmel, A. R. (1987): *Guide to Molecular Cloning Techniques, Methods in Enzymology*, Vol. 152. Academic Press, Orlando, FL.
29. Bidwell, L. M., Gillam, E. M. J., Gaedigk, A., Zhu, X., Grant, D., and McManus, M. E. (1998): Bacterial expression of two human aryl sulfotransferases. *Chem. Biol. Interact.*, 109:137–141.
30. Black, S. D. and Coon, M. J. (1986): Comparative structures of P450 cytochromes. In: *Cytochrome P450*, edited by P. R. Ortiz de Montellano, pp. 161–216. Plenum, New York.
31. Blake, J. A. R., Pritchard, M., Ding, S., Smith, G. C. M., Burchell, B., Wolf, C. R., and Friedberg, T. (1996): Coexpression of a human P450 (CYP3A4) and P450 reductase generates a highly functional monooxygenase system in *Escherichia coli*. *FEBS Lett.*, 397:210–214.
32. Bligh, E. G., and Dyer, W. J. (1959): A rapid method of total lipid extraction and purification. *Can. J. Biochem. Physiol.*, 37:911–917.
33. Bolt, H. M. (1979): Metabolism of estrogens—Natural and synthetic. *Pharmacol. Ther.*, 4:155–181.
34. Booth, J., and Boyland, E. (1964): The biochemistry of aromatic amines. 10. Enzymic *N*-hydroxylation of arylamines and conversion of arylhydroxylamines into *o*-aminophenols. *Biochem. J.*, 91:362–369.

35. Borchardt, R. (1980): *N*- and *O*-methylation. In: *Enzymatic Basis of Detoxication*, Vol. 2, edited by W. B. Jakoby, pp. 43-62. Academic Press, New York.
36. Bork, R. W., Muto, T., Beaune, P. H., Srivastava, P. K., Lloyd, R. S., and Guengerich, F. P. (1989): Characterization of mRNA species related to human liver cytochrome P450 nifedipine oxidase and the regulation of catalytic activity. *J. Biol. Chem.*, 264:910–919.
37. Bradford, M. M. (1976): A rapid and sensitive method for the quantitation of microgram quantities of protein utilizing the principle of protein–dye binding. *Anal. Biochem.*, 72:248–254.
38. Brian, W. R., Sari, M.-A., Iwasaki, M., Shimada, T., Kaminsky, L. S., and Guengerich, F. P. (1990): Catalytic activities of human liver cytochrome P450 IIIA4 expressed in *Saccharomyces cerevisiae*. *Biochemistry*, 29:11280–11292.
39. Brian, W. R., Srivastava, P. K., Umbenhauer, D. R., Lloyd, R. S., and Guengerich, F. P. (1989): Expression of a human liver cytochrome P450 protein with tolbutamide hydroxylase activity in *Saccharomyces cerevisiae*. *Biochemistry*, 28:4993–4999.
40. Buege, J. A., and Aust, S. D. (1978): Microsomal lipid peroxidation. *Methods Enzymol.*, 52:302–310.
41. Burchell, B., and Coughtrie, M. W. H. (1989): UDP-Glucuronosyltransferases. *Pharmacol. Ther.*, 43:261–289.
42. Burchell, B., McGurk, K., Brierly, C. H., and Clarke, D. J. (1997): UDP-glucuronosyltransferases. In: *Biotransformation, Vol. 3, Comprehensive Toxicology*, edited by F. P. Guengerich, pp. 401–435. Elsevier Science, Oxford.
43. Burke, M. D., and Mayer, R. T. (1975): Inherent specificities of purified cytochromes P450 and P-448 toward biphenyl hydroxylation and ethoxyresorufin deethylation. *Drug Metab. Dispos.*, 3:245–253.
44. Burke, M. D., and Prough, R. A. (1978): Fluorimetric and chromatographic methods for measuring microsomal biphenyl hydroxylation. *Methods Enzymol.*, 52:399–407.
45. Burton, K. (1956): A study of the conditions and mechanisms of the diphenylamine reaction for the colorimetric estimation of deoxyribonucleic acid. *Biochem. J.*, 62:315–323.
46. Butler, M. A., Iwasaki, M., Guengerich, F. P., and Kadlubar, F. F. (1989): Human cytochrome $P450_{PA}$ (P450IA2), the phenacetin *O*-deethylase, is primarily responsible for the hepatic 3-demethylation of caffeine and *N*-oxidation of carcinogenic arylamines. *Proc. Natl. Acad. Sci. USA*, 86:7696–7700.
47. Böcker, R. H., and Guengerich, F. P. (1986): Oxidation of 4-aryl- and 4-alkyl-substituted 2,6-dimethyl-3,5-bis(alkoxycarbonyl)-1,4-dihydropyridines by human liver microsomes and immunochemical evidence for the involvement of a form of cytochrome P450. *J. Med. Chem.*, 29:1596–1603.
48. Cashman, J. R. (1997): Monoamine oxidase and flavin-containing monooxygenases. In: *Biotransformation, Vol. 3, Comprehensive Toxicology*, edited by F. P. Guengerich, pp. 69–96. Elsevier Science, Oxford.
49. Cerasone, C. F., Bolognesi, C., and Santi, L. (1979): Improved microfluorometric DNA determinations in biological material using 33258 Hoechst. *Anal. Biochem.*, 100:188–197.
50. Chang, T. K. H., Weber, G. F., Crespi, C. L., and Waxman, D. J. (1993): Differential activation of cyclophosphamide and ifosphamide by cytochromes P450 2B and 3A in human liver microsomes. *Cancer Res.*, 53:5629–5637.
51. Chauret, N., Gauthier, A., and Nicoll-Griffith, D. A. (1998): Effect of common organic solvents on in vitro cytochrome P450-mediated metabolic activities in human liver microsomes. *Drug Metab. Dispos.*, 26:1–4.
52. Chen, C. B., McCoy, G. D., Hecht, S. S., Hoffman, D., and Wynder, E. L. (1978): High pressure liquid chromatographic assay for alpha hydroxylation of *n*-nitrosopyrrolidine by isolated rat liver microsomes. *Cancer Res.*, 38:3812–3816.
53. Chen, P. S., Jr., Toribara, T. Y., and Warner, H. (1956): Microdetermination of phosphorus. *Anal. Chem.*, 28:1756–1758.
54. Cherian, M. G. (1997): Metallothionein and intracellular sequestration of metals. In: *Biotransformation, Vol. 3, Comprehensive Toxicology*, edited by F. P. Guengerich, pp. 489–503. Elsevier Science, Oxford.
55. Chin, A. E., and Bosmann, H. B. (1976): Microsome-mediated methylation of DNA by *N,N*-dimethylnitrosamine in vitro. *Biochem. Pharmacol.*, 25:1921–1226.
56. Chomczynski, P., and Sacchi, N. (1987): Single-step method of RNA isolation by acid guanidinium thiocyanate–phenol–chloroform extraction. *Anal. Biochem.*, 162:156–159.
57. Chun, Y.-J., Shimada, T., and Guengerich, F. P. (1996): Construction of a human cytochrome P450 1A1 : rat NADPH-P450 reductase fusion protein cDNA, expression in *Escherichia coli*, purification, and catalytic properties of the enzyme in bacterial cells and after purification. *Arch. Biochem. Biophys.*, 330:48–58.
58. Cinti, D. L., Moldeus, P., and Schenkman, J. B. (1972): Kinetic parameters of drug-metabolizing enzymes in Ca^{2+}-sedimented microsomes from rat liver. *Biochem. Pharmacol.*, 21:3249–3256.
59. Cmarik, J. L., Inskeep, P. B., Meyer, D. J., Meredith, M. J., Ketterer, B., and Guengerich, F. P. (1990): Selectivity of rat and human glutathione *S*-transferases in activation of ethylene dibromide by glutathione conjugation and DNA binding and induction of unscheduled DNA synthesis in human hepatocytes. *Cancer Res.*, 50:2747–2752.
60. Cochin, J., and Axelrod, J. (1959): Biochemical and pharmacological changes in the rat following chronic administration of morphine, nalorphine, and normorphine. *J. Pharmacol. Exp. Ther.*, 125:105–110.
61. Coles, B., and Ketterer, B. (1990): The role of glutathione and glutathione transferases in chemical carcinogenesis. *Crit. Rev. Biochem. Molec. Biol.*, 25:47–70.
62. Conney, A. H. (1967): Pharmacological implications of microsomal enzyme induction. *Pharmacol. Rev.*, 19:317–366.
63. Conney, A. H. (1971): Environmental factors influencing drug metabolism. In: *Fundamentals of Drug Metabolism and Drug Disposition*, edited by B. N. LaDa, H. G. Mandel, and E. L. Way, pp. 253–278. Williams & Wilkins, Baltimore, MD.
64. Conney, A. H., Levin, W., Jacobsson, M., and Kuntzman, R. (1969): Specificity in the regulation of the 6β, 7α, and 16α-hydroxylation of testosterone by rat liver microsomes. In: *Microsomes and Drug Oxidations*, edited by J. R. Gillette, pp. 279–301. Academic Press, New York.
65. Coon, M. J., van der Hoeven, T. A., Dahl, S. B., and Haugen, D. A. (1978): Two forms of liver microsomal cytochrome P450, $P450_{LM-2}$, and $P\text{-}405_{LM-4}$ (rabbit liver). *Methods Enzymol.*, 52:109–117.
66. Cooper, A. J. L., and Tate, S. S. (1997): Enzymes involved in processing of glutathione conjugates. In: *Biotransformation, Vol. 3, Comprehensive Toxicology*, edited by F. P. Guengerich, pp. 329–363. Elsevier Science, Oxford.
67. Correia, M. A. (1995): Rat and human liver cytochromes P450. Substrate and inhibitor specificities and functional markers. In: *Cytochrome P450: Structure, Mechanism, and Biochemistry*, 2nd ed., edited by P. R. Ortiz de Montellano, pp. 607–630. Plenum Press, New York.
68. Craig, J. C., and Purushothaman, K. K. (1970): An improved preparation of tertiary amine *N*-oxides. *J. Org. Chem.*, 35:1721–1722.
69. Cribb, A., Nuss, C., and Wang, R. (1995): Antipeptide antibodies against overlapping sequences differentially inhibit human CYP2D6. *Drug Metab. Dispos.*, 23:671–675.

70. Czygan, P., Greim, H., Garro, A. J., Hutterer, F., Schaffner, F., Popper, H., Rosenthal, O., and Cooper, D. Y. (1973): Microsomal metabolism of dimethylnitrosamine and the cytochrome P450 dependency of its activation to a mutagen. *Cancer Res.*, 33:2983–2986.

71. Dahl, G. A., Miller, E. C., and Miller, J. A. (1980): Comparative carcinogenicities and mutagenicities of vinyl carbamate, ethyl carbamate, and ethyl *N*-hydroxycarbamate. *Cancer Res.*, 40:1194–1203.

72. Dahl, G. A., Miller, J. A., and Miller, E. C. (1978): Vinyl carbamate as a promutagen and a more carcinogenic analog of ethyl carbamate. *Cancer Res.*, 38:3793–3804.

73. Damani, L. A., Patterson, L. H., and Gorrod, J. W. (1978): Thin-layer chromatographic separation and identification of tertiary aromatic amines and their *N*-oxides. *J. Chromatogr.*, 155:337–348.

74. Dannan, G. A., and Guengerich, F. P. (1982): Immunochemical comparison and quantitation of microsomal flavin-containing monooxygenases in various hog, mouse, rat, rabbit, dog, and human tissues. *Mol. Pharmacol.*, 22:787–794.

75. Dannan, G. A., Guengerich, F. P., Kaminsky, L. S., and Aust, S. D. (1983): Regulation of cytochrome P450. Immunochemical quantitation of eight isozymes in liver microsomes of rats treated with polybrominated biphenyl congeners. *J. Biol. Chem.*, 258:1282–1288.

76. Dannan, G. A., Porubek, D. J., Nelson, S. D., Waxman, D. J., and Guengerich, F. P. (1986): 17β-Estradiol 2- and 4-hydroxylation catalyzed by rat hepatic cytochrome P450: Roles of individual forms, inductive effects, developmental patterns, and alterations by gonadectomy and hormone replacement. *Endocrinology*, 118:1952–1960.

77. Dannan, G. A., Waxman, D. J., and Guengerich, F. P. (1986): Hormonal regulation of rat liver microsomal enzymes: role of gonadal steroids in programming, maintenance, and suppression of Δ^4-steroid 5α-reductase, flavin-containing monooxygenase, and sex-specific cytochromes P450. *J. Biol. Chem.*, 261:10728–10735.

78. De Lemos-Chiarandini, C., Frey, A. B., Sabatini, D. D., and Kreibich, G. (1987): Determination of the membrane topology of the phenobarbital-inducible rat liver cytochrome P450 isoenzyme PB-4 using site-specific antibodies. *J. Cell Biol.*, 104:209–219.

79. De Matteis, F. (1974): Covalent binding of sulfur to microsomes and loss of cytochrome P450 during the oxidative desulfuration of several chemicals. *Mol. Pharmacol.*, 10:849–854.

80. Dean, W. L., and Coon, M. J. (1977): Immunochemical studies on two electrophoretically homogeneous forms of rabbit liver microsomal cytochrome P450: $P450_{LM2}$ and $P450_{LM4}$. *J. Biol. Chem.*, 252:3255–3261.

81. Dehnen, W., Tomingas, R., and Roos, J. (1973): A modified method for the assay of benzo[a]pyrene hydroxylase. *Anal. Biochem.*, 53:373–383.

82. DePierre, J. W., Johannesen, K. A. M., Moron, M. S., and Seidegård, J. (1978): Radioactive assay of aryl hydrocarbon monooxygenase and epoxide hydrase. *Methods Enzymol.*, 52:412–418.

83. Deutsch, J., Leutz, J. C., Yang, S. K., Gelboin, H. V., Chiang, Y. L., Vatsis, K. P., and Coon, M. J. (1978): Regio- and stereoselectivity of various forms of purified cytochrome P450 in the metabolism of benzo[a]pyrene and (−)*trans*-7, 8-dihydroxy-7,8-dihydrobenzo[a]pyrene as shown by product formation and binding to DNA. *Proc. Natl. Acad. Sci. USA*, 75:3123–3127.

84. Dische, Z. (1955): Color reactions of nucleic acid components. In: *The Nucleic Acids*, Vol. 1, edited by E. Chargoff and J. N. Davidson, pp. 285–305. Academic Press, New York.

85. Distlerath, L. M., and Guengerich, F. P. (1984): Characterization of a human liver cytochrome P450 involved in the oxidation of debrisoquine and other drugs using antibodies raised to the analogous rat enzyme. *Proc. Natl. Acad. Sci. USA*, 81:7348–7352.

86. Distlerath, L. M., and Guengerich, F. P. (1987): Enzymology of human liver cytochromes P450. In: *Mammalian Cytochromes P450*, Vol. 1, edited by F. P. Guengerich, pp. 133–198. CRC Press, Boca Raton, FL.

87. Distlerath, L. M., Reilly, P. E. B., Martin, M. V., Davis, G. G., Wilkinson, G. R., and Guengerich, F. P. (1985): Purification and characterization of the human liver cytochromes P450 involved in debrisoquine 4-hydroxylation and phenacetin *O*-deethylation, two prototypes for genetic polymorphism in oxidative drug metabolism. *J. Biol. Chem.*, 260:9057–9067.

88. Dix, T. A., and Marnett, L. J. (1983): Metabolism of polycyclic aromatic hydrocarbon derivatives to ultimate carcinogens during lipid peroxidation. *Science*, 221:77–79.

89. Doehmer, J., Dogra, S., Edigkaufer, M., Molitor, E., Siegert, P., Friedberg, T., Glatt, H., Platt, K., Seidel, A., Thomas, H., and Oesch, F. (1989): Introduction of cytochrome P450 genes into V79 Chinese hamster cells to generate new mutagenicity test systems. *Arch. Toxicol.*, 13(suppl.):164–168.

90. Domanski, T. L., Liu, J., Harlow, G. R., and Halpert, J. R. (1998): Analysis of four residues within substrate recognition site 4 of human cytochrome P450 3A4: Role in steroid hydroxylase activity and α-naphthoflavone stimulation. *Arch. Biochem. Biophys.*, 350:223–232.

91. Dong, M.-S., Bell, L. C., Guo, Z., Phillips, D. R., Blair, I. A., and Guengerich, F. P. (1996): Identification of retained *N*-formylmethionine in bacterial recombinant cytochrome P450 proteins with the *N*-terminal sequence MALLLAVFL ...: Roles of residues 3–5 in retention and membrane topology. *Biochemistry*, 35:10031–10040.

92. Dong, M.-S., Yamazaki, H., Guo, Z., and Guengerich, F. P. (1996): Recombinant human cytochrome P450 1A2 and an N-terminal truncated form: Construction, purification, aggregation properties, and interactions with flavodoxin, ferredoxin, and NADPH-cytochrome P450 reductase. *Arch. Biochem. Biophys.*, 327:11–19.

93. Duffel, M. W. (1997): Sulfotransferases. In: *Biotransformation, Vol. 3, Comprehensive Toxicology*, edited by F. P. Guengerich, pp. 365–383. Elsevier Science, Oxford.

94. Duffel, M. W., and Jakoby, W. B. (1982): Cysteine *S*-conjugate *N*-acetyltransferase from rat kidney microsomes. *Mol. Pharmacol.*, 21:444–448.

95. Edenberg, H. J., and Bosron, W. F. (1997): Alcohol dehydrogenases. In: *Biotransformation, Vol. 3, Comprehensive Toxicology*, edited by F. P. Guengerich, pp. 119–131. Elsevier Science, Oxford.

96. Eling, T. E., Thompson, D. C., Foureman, G. L., Curtis, J. F., and Hughes, M. F. (1990): Prostaglandin H synthase and xenobiotic oxidation. *Annu. Rev. Pharmacol. Toxicol.*, 30:1–45.

97. Ellis, S. W., Hayhurst, G. P., Smith, G., Lightfoot, T., Wong, M. M. S., Simula, A. P., Ackland, M. J., Sternberg, M. J. E., Lennard, M. S., Tucker, G. T., and Wolf, C. R. (1995): Evidence that aspartic acid 301 is a critical substrate-contact residue in the active site of cytochrome P450 2D6. *J. Biol. Chem.*, 270:29055–29058.

98. Ernster, L., Davidson, L., and Ljunggren, M. (1962): DT diaphorase. I. Purification from the soluble fraction of rat-liver cytoplasm, and properties. *Biochim. Biophys. Acta*, 58:171–188.

99. Evans-Storms, R. B., and Cidlowski, J. A. (1995): Regulation of apoptosis by steroid hormones. *J. Steroid Biochem. Molec. Biol.*, 53:1–8.
100. Falany, C. N., McQuiddy, P., and Kasper, C. B. (1987): Structure and organization of the microsomal xenobiotic epoxide hydrolase gene. *J. Biol. Chem.*, 262:5924–5930.
101. Fan, L. L., Masters, B. S., and Prough, R. A. (1976): Microsomal lauric acid 11- and 12-hydroxylation: a new assay method utilizing high pressure liquid chromatography. *Anal. Biochem.*, 71:265–272.
102. Fang, W. F., and Strobel, H. W. (1978): The drug and carcinogen metabolism system of rat colon microsomes. *Arch. Biochem. Biophys.*, 186:128–138.
103. Fasco, M. J., Vatsis, K. P., Kaminsky, L. S., and Coon, M. J. (1978): Regioselective and stereoselective hydroxylation of *R* and *S* warfarin by different forms of purified cytochrome P450 from rabbit liver. *J. Biol. Chem.*, 253:7813–7820.
104. Flynn, T. G., and Kubiseski, T. J. (1997): Aldo-ketoreductases: structure, mechanism, and function. In: *Biotransformation, Vol. 3, Comprehensive Toxicology*, edited by F. P. Guengerich, pp. 133–147. Elsevier Science, Oxford.
105. French, J. S., Guengerich, F. P., and Coon, M. J. (1980): Interactions of cytochrome P450, NADPH-cytochrome P450 reductase, phospholipid, and substrate in the reconstituted liver microsomal enzyme system. *J. Biol. Chem.*, 255:4112–4119.
106. Fujino, T., Park, S. S., West, D., and Gelboin, H. V. (1982): Phenotyping of cytochromes P450 in human tissues with monoclonal antibodies. *Proc. Natl. Acad. Sci. USA*, 79:3682–3686.
107. Garewal, H. S. (1973): A procedure for the estimation of microgram quantities of Triton X-100. *Anal. Biochem.*, 54:319–324.
108. Geiger, L. E., Hogy, L. L., and Guengerich, F. P. (1983): Metabolism of acrylonitrile by isolated rat hepatocytes. *Cancer Res.*, 43:3080–3087.
109. Gelboin, H. V. (1967): Carcinogens, enzyme induction and gene action. *Adv. Cancer Res.*, 10:1–81.
110. Gelboin, H. V. (1993): Cytochrome P450 and monoclonal antibodies. *Pharmacol. Rev.*, 45:413–453.
111. Gershoni, J. M., and Palade, G. E. (1983): Protein blotting: principles and applications. *Anal. Biochem.*, 131:1–15.
112. Gill, T. J. III (1972): The chemistry of antigens and its influence on immunogenicity. In: *Imunogenicity*, edited by F. Borek, pp. 5–44. American Elsevier, New York.
113. Gillam, E. M. J., Guo, Z., and Guengerich, F. P. (1994): Expression of modified human cytochrome P450 2E1 in *Escherichia coli*, purification, and spectral and catalytic properties. *Arch. Biochem. Biophys.*, 312:59–66.
114. Gillam, E. M. J., Guo, Z., Martin, M. V., Jenkins, C. M., and Guengerich, F. P. (1995): Expression of cytochrome P450 2D6 in *Escherichia coli*, purification, and spectral and catalytic characterization. *Arch. Biochem. Biophys.*, 319:540–550.
115. Gillette, J. R. (1966): Biochemistry of drug oxidation and reduction by enzymes in hepatic endoplasmic reticulum. *Adv. Pharmacol.*, 4:219–261.
116. Glowinski, I. B., Radtke, H. E., and Weber, W. W. (1978): Genetic variation in *N*-acetylation of carcinogenic arylamines by human and rat liver. *Mol. Pharmacol.*, 14:940–949.
117. Goeddel, D. V., Ed. (1990): *Methods in Enzymology, Vol. 185, Gene Expression Technology*. Academic Press, San Diego.
118. Goldstein, J. A., and Demorais, S. M. F. (1994): Biochemistry and molecular biology of the human *CYP2C* subfamily. *Pharmacogenetics*, 4:285–299.
119. Goldstein, S., and Blecher, M. (1975): The spectrophotometric assay for the polyethoxy nonionic detergents in membrane extracts: A critique. *Anal. Biochem.*, 64:130–135.
120. Gonzalez, F. J. (1989): The molecular biology of cytochrome P450s. *Pharmacol. Rev.*, 40:243–288.
121. Gonzalez, F. J., Crespi, C. L., and Gelboin, H. V. (1991): cDNA-expressed human cytochrome P450s: A new age of molecular toxicology and human risk assessment. *Mutat. Res.*, 247:113–127.
122. Gonzalez, F. J., Kimura, S., Tamura, S., and Gelboin, H. V. (1991): Expression of mammalian cytochrome P450 using baculovirus. *Methods Enzymol.*, 206:93–99.
123. Gonzalez, F. J., and Meyer, U. A. (1991): Molecular genetics of the debrisoquin-sparteine polymorphism. *Clin. Pharmacol. Ther.*, 50:233–238.
124. Grant, D. F., Greene, J. F., Pinot, F., Borhan, B., Moghaddam, M. F., Hammock, B. D., McCutchen, B., Ohkawa, H., Juo, G., and Guenthner, T. M. (1996): Development of an in situ toxicity assay system using recombinant baculoviruses. *Biochem. Pharmacol.*, 51:503–515.
125. Grant, D. M., Josephy, P. D., Lord, H. L., and Morrison, L. D. (1992): *Salmonella typhimurium* strains expressing human arylamine *N*-acetyltransferases: metabolism and mutagenic activation of aromatic amines. *Cancer Res.*, 52:3961–3964.
126. Greenlee, W. F., and Poland, A. (1978): An improved assay of 7-ethoxycoumarin *O*-deethylase activity: induction of hepatic enzyme activity in C57BL/6J and DBA/2J mice by phenobarbital, 3-methylcholanthrene and 2,3,7,8-tetrachlorodibenzo-*p*-dioxin. *J. Pharmacol. Exp. Ther.*, 205:596–605.
127. Guengerich, F. P. (1977): Studies on the activation of a model furan compound: Toxicity and covalent binding of 2-(*N*-ethylcarbamoylhydroxymethyl)furan. *Biochem. Pharmacol.*, 26:1909–1915.
128. Guengerich, F. P. (1977): Preparation and properties of highly purified cytochrome P450 and NADPH-cytochrome P450 reductase from pulmonary microsomes of untreated rabbits. *Mol. Pharmacol.*, 13:911–923.
129. Guengerich, F. P. (1977): Separation and purification of multiple forms of microsomal cytochrome P450. Activities of different forms of cytochrome P450 towards several compounds of environmental interest. *J. Biol. Chem.*, 252:3970–3979.
130. Guengerich, F. P. (1978): Separation and purification of multiple forms of microsomal cytochrome P450. Partial characterization of three apparently homogeneous cytochromes P450 prepared from livers of phenobarbital- and 3-methylcholanthrene-treated rats. *J. Biol. Chem.*, 253:7931–7939.
131. Guengerich, F. P. (1978): Destruction of heme and hemoproteins mediated by liver microsomal reduced nicotinamide adenine dinucleotide phosphate-cytochrome P450 reductase. *Biochemistry*, 17:3633–3639.
132. Guengerich, F. P. (1979): Artifacts in isoelectric focusing of the microsomal enzymes cytochrome P450 and NADPH-cytochrome P450 reductase. *Biochim. Biophys. Acta*, 577:132–141.
133. Guengerich, F. P. (1979): Isolation and purification of cytochrome P450, and the existence of multiple forms. *Pharmacol. Ther.*, 6:99–121.
134. Guengerich, F. P. (1982): Epoxide hydrolase: properties and metabolic roles. *Rev. Biochem. Toxicol.*, 4:5–30.
135. Guengerich, F. P. (1983): Oxidation-reduction properties of rat liver cytochrome P450 and NADPH-cytochrome P450 reductase related to catalysis in reconstituted systems. *Biochemistry*, 22:2811–2820.
136. Guengerich, F. P. (1984): Oxidation of sparteines by cytochrome P450: Evidence against the formation of *N*-oxides. *J. Med. Chem.*, 27:1101–1103.
137. Guengerich, F. P. (1984): Effects of nutritive factors on metabolic processes involving bioactivation and detoxication of chemicals. *Annu. Rev. Nutr.*, 4:207–231.

138. Guengerich, F. P. (1987): Cytochrome P450 enzymes and drug metabolism. In: *Progress in Drug Metabolism*, Vol. 10, edited by J. W. Bridges, L. F. Chasseaud, and G. G. Gibson, pp. 1–54. Taylor & Francis, London.
139. Guengerich, F. P. (1987): Enzymology of rat liver cytochromes P450. In: *Mammalian Cytochromes P450*, Vol. 1, edited by F. P. Guengerich, pp. 1–54. CRC Press, Boca Raton, FL.
140. Guengerich, F. P. (1990): Low kinetic hydrogen isotope effects in the oxidation of 1,4-dihydro-2,6-dimethyl-4-(2-nitrophenyl)-3,5-pyridine-dicarboxy lic acid dimethyl ester (nifedipine) by cytochrome P450 enzymes are consistent with an electron–proton–electron transfer mechanism. *Chem. Res. Toxicol.*, 3:21–26.
141. Guengerich, F. P. (1990): Enzymatic oxidation of xenobiotic chemicals. *Crit. Rev. Biochem. Mol. Biol.*, 25:97–153.
142. Guengerich, F. P. (1990): Mechanism-based inactivation of human liver cytochrome P450 IIIA4 by gestodene. *Chem. Res. Toxicol.*, 3:363–371.
143. Guengerich, F. P. (1991): Reactions and significance of cytochrome P450 enzymes. *J. Biol. Chem.*, 266:10019–10022.
144. Guengerich, F. P. (1994): Analysis and characterization of enzymes. In: *Principles and Methods of Toxicology*, 3rd ed., edited by A. W. Hayes, pp. 1259–1313. Raven Press, New York.
145. Guengerich, F. P. (1995): Human cytochrome P450 enzymes. In: *Cytochrome P450*, 2nd ed., edited by P. R. Ortiz de Montellano, pp. 473–535. Plenum Press, New York.
146. Guengerich, F. P. (1997): Comparisons of catalytic selectivity of cytochrome P450 subfamily members from different species. *Chem. Biol. Interact.*, 106:161–182.
147. Guengerich, F. P., Ballou, D. P., and Coon, M. J. (1975): Purified liver microsomal cytochrome P450: Electron-accepting properties and oxidation-reduction potential. *J. Biol. Chem.*, 250:7405–7414.
148. Guengerich, F. P., Brian, W. R., Iwasaki, M., Sari, M.-A., Bäärnhielm, C., and Berntsson, P. (1991): Oxidation of dihydropyridine calcium channel blockers and analogues by human liver cytochrome P450 IIIA4. *J. Med. Chem.*, 34:1838–1844.
149. Guengerich, F. P., Brian, W. R., Sari, M.-A., and Ross, J. T. (1991): Expression of mammalian cytochrome P450 enzymes using yeast-based vectors. *Methods Enzymol.*, 206:130–145.
150. Guengerich, F. P., and Böcker, R. H. (1988): Cytochrome P450-catalyzed dehydrogenation of 1,4-dihydropyridines. *J. Biol. Chem.*, 263:8168–8175.
151. Guengerich, F. P., Crawford, W. M., Jr., Domoradzki, J. Y., Macdonald, T. L., and Watanabe, P. G. (1980): In vitro activation of 1,2-dichloroethane by microsomal and cytosolic enzymes. *Toxicol. Appl. Pharmacol.*, 55:303–317.
152. Guengerich, F. P., Dannan, G. A., Wright, S. T., Martin, M. V., and Kaminsky, L. S. (1982): Purification and characterization of liver microsomal cytochromes P450: Electrophoretic, spectral, catalytic, and immunochemical properties and inducibility of eight isozymes isolated from rats treated with phenobarbital or β-naphthoflavone. *Biochemistry*, 21:6019–6030.
153. Guengerich, F. P., Distlerath, L. M., Reilly, P. E. B., Wolff, T., Shimada, T., Umbenhauer, D. R., and Martin, M. V. (1986): Human liver cytochromes P450 involved in polymorphisms of drug oxidation. *Xenobiotica*, 16:367–378.
154. Guengerich, F. P., Geiger, L. E., Hogy, L. L., and Wright, P. L. (1981): In vitro metabolism of acrylonitrile to 2-cyanoethylene oxide, reaction with glutathione, and irreversible binding to proteins and nucleic acids. *Cancer Res.*, 41:4925–4933.
155. Guengerich, F. P., Gillam, E. M. J., and Shimada, T. (1996): New applications of bacterial systems to problems in toxicology. *Crit. Rev. Toxicol.*, 26:551–583.
156. Guengerich, F. P., and Holladay, L. A. (1979): Hydrodynamic characterization of highly purified and functionally active liver microsomal cytochrome P450. *Biochemistry*, 18:5442–5449.
157. Guengerich, F. P., and Johnson, W. W. (1997): Kinetics of ferric cytochrome P450 reduction by NADPH-cytochrome P450 reductase. Rapid reduction in absence of substrate and variation among cytochrome P450 systems. *Biochemistry*, 36:14741–14750.
158. Guengerich, F. P., and Kim, D-H. (1991): Enzymatic oxidation of ethyl carbamate to vinyl carbamate and its role as an intermediate in the formation of $1,N^6$-ethenoadenosine. *Chem. Res. Toxicol.*, 4:413–421.
159. Guengerich, F. P., Kim, D.-H., and Iwasaki, M. (1991): Role of human cytochrome P450 IIE1 in the oxidation of many low molecular weight cancer suspects. *Chem. Res. Toxicol.*, 4:168–179.
160. Guengerich, F. P., and Liebler, D. C. (1985): Enzymatic activation of chemicals to toxic metabolites. *Crit. Rev. Toxicol.*, 14:259–307.
161. Guengerich, F. P., and Macdonald, T. L. (1984): Chemical mechanisms of catalysis by cytochromes P450: A unified view. *Acc. Chem. Res.*, 17:9–16.
162. Guengerich, F. P., and Macdonald, T. L. (1990): Mechanisms of cytochrome P450 catalysis. *FASEB J.*, 4:2453–2459.
163. Guengerich, F. P., and Martin, M. V. (1980): Purification of cytochrome P450, NADPH-cytochrome P450 reductase, and epoxide hydratase from a single preparation of rat liver microsomes. *Arch. Biochem. Biophys.*, 205:365–379.
164. Guengerich, F. P., Martin, M. V., Beaune, P. H., Kremers, P., Wolff, T., and Waxman, D. J. (1986): Characterization of rat and human liver microsomal cytochrome P450 forms involved in nifedipine oxidation, a prototype for genetic polymorphism in oxidative drug metabolism. *J. Biol. Chem.*, 261:5051–5060.
165. Guengerich, F. P., Martin, M. V., Guo, Z., and Chun, Y.-J. (1996): Purification of recombinant human cytochrome P450 enzymes expressed in bacteria. *Methods Enzymol.*, 272:35–44.
166. Guengerich, F. P., and Mason, P. S. (1980): Alcohol dehydrogenase-coupled spectrophotometric assay of epoxide hydratase activity. *Anal. Biochem.*, 104:445–451.
167. Guengerich, F. P., Mason, P. S., Stott, W. T., Fox, T. R., and Watanabe, P. G. (1981): Roles of 2-haloethylene oxides and 2-haloacetaldehydes derived from vinyl bromide and vinyl chloride in irreversible binding to protein and DNA. *Cancer Res.*, 41:4391–4398.
168. Guengerich, F. P., and Mitchell, M. B. (1980): Metabolic activation of model pyrroles by cytochrome P450. *Drug Metab. Dispos.*, 8:34–38.
169. Guengerich, F. P., Parikh, A., Johnson, E. F., Richardson, T. H., von Wachenfeldt, C., Cosme, J., Jung, F., Strassburg, C. P., Manns, M. P., Tukey, R. H., Pritchard, M., Fournel-Gigleux, S., and Burchell, B. (1997): Heterologous expression of human drug-metabolizing enzymes. *Drug Metab. Dispos.*, 25:1234–1241.
170. Guengerich, F. P., and Shimada, T. (1991): Oxidation of toxic and carcinogenic chemicals by human cytochrome P450 enzymes. *Chem. Res. Toxicol.*, 4:391–407.
171. Guengerich, F. P., Wang, P., and Davidson, N. K. (1982): Estimation of isozymes of microsomal cytochrome P450 in rats, rabbits, and humans using immunochemical staining coupled with sodium dodecyl sulfate–polyacrylamide gel electrophoresis. *Biochemistry*, 21:1698–1706.
172. Guengerich, F. P., Wang, P., and Mason, P. S. (1981): Immunological comparison of rat, rabbit, and human liver NADPH-cytochrome P450 reductases. *Biochemistry*, 20:2379–2385.
173. Guengerich, F. P., Wang, P., Mason, P. S., and Mitchell, M. B. (1981): Immunological comparison of rat, rabbit, and human microsomal cytochromes P450. *Biochemistry*, 20:2370–2378.

174. Guengerich, F. P., Wang, P., Mitchell, M. B., and Mason, P. S. (1979): Rat and human liver microsomal epoxide hydratase. Purification and evidence for the existence of multiple forms. *J. Biol. Chem.*, 254:12248–12254.
175. Guengerich, F. P., and Watanabe, P. G. (1979): Metabolism of [^{14}C]- and [^{36}Cl]-labeled vinyl chloride in vivo and in vitro. *Biochem. Pharmacol.*, 28:589–596.
176. Guengerich, F. P., Yun, C.-H., and Macdonald, T. L. (1996): Evidence for a one-electron mechanism in *N*-dealkylation of *N,N*-dialkylanilines by cytochrome P450 2B1. Kinetic hydrogen isotope effects, linear free energy relationships with biomimetic models, comparisons with horseradish peroxidase, and studies with oxygen surrogates. *J. Biol. Chem.*, 271:27321–27329.
177. Habig, W. H., Pabst, M. J., and Jakoby, W. B. (1974): Glutathione *S*-transferases: The first enzymatic step in mercapturic acid formation. *J. Biol. Chem.*, 249:7130–7139.
178. Halpert, J. R., Guengerich, F. P., Bend, J. R., and Correia, M. A. (1994): Selective inhibitors of cytochromes P450. *Toxicol. Appl. Pharmacol.*, 125:163–175.
179. Halvorson, M., Greenway, D., Eberhart, D., Fitzgerald, K., and Parkinson, A. (1990): Reconstitution of testosterone oxidation by purified rat cytochrome P450p (IIIA1). *Arch. Biochem. Biophys.*, 277:166–180.
180. Hammock, B. D., Grant, D. F., and Storms, D. H. (1997): Epoxide hydrolases. In: *Biotransformation, Vol. 3, Comprehensive Toxicology*, edited by F. P. Guengerich, pp. 283–305. Elsevier Science, Oxford.
181. Hanna, I. H., Teiber, J. F., Kokones, K. L., and Hollenberg, P. F. (1998): Role of the alanine at position 363 of cytochrome P450 2B2 in influencing the NADPH- and hydroperoxide-supported activities. *Arch. Biochem. Biophys.*, 350:324–332.
182. Hanzlik, R. P., and Hilbert, J. M. (1978): Synthesis of epoxides with electronegative substituents: photometric substrates for epoxide hydrase. *J. Org. Chem.*, 453:610–614.
183. Haugen, D. A., and Coon, M. J. (1976): Properties of electrophoretically homogenous phenobarbital-inducible and *β*-naphthoflavone-inducible forms of liver microsomal cytochrome P450. *J. Biol. Chem.*, 251:7929–7939.
184. Haugen, D. A., van der Hoeven, T. A., and Coon, M. J. (1975): Purified liver microsomal cytochrome P450: Separation and characterization of multiple forms. *J. Biol. Chem.*, 250:3567–3570.
185. Hein, D. W. (1991): A new model for toxic risk assessments: construction of homozygous rapid and slow acetylator congenic Syrian hamster lines. *Toxicol. Methods*, 1:44–52.
186. Henze, H. R., and Isbell, A. F. (1954): Researches on substituted 5-phenylhydantoins. *J. Am. Chem. Soc.*, 76:4152–4156.
187. Hill, K. E., Lyons, P. R., and Burk, R. F. (1992): Differential regulation of rat liver selenoprotein mRNAs in selenium deficiency. *Biochem. Biophys. Res. Commun.*, 185:260–263.
188. Hogy, L. L., and Guengerich, F. P. (1986): In vivo interaction of acrylonitrile and 2-cyanoethylene oxide with DNA in rats. *Cancer Res.*, 46:3932–3938.
189. Hosea, N. A., and Guengerich, F. P. (1998): Oxidation of non-ionic detergents by cytochrome P450 enzymes. *Arch. Biochem. Biophys.*, 353:365–373.
190. Hsieh, J. C., Liu, L. F., Chen, W. L., and Tam, M. F. (1989): Expression of Y_{b1} glutathione *S*-transferase using a baculovirus expression system. *Biochem. Biophys. Res. Commun.*, 162:1147–1154.
191. Hughes, M. F., Mason, R. P., and Eling, T. E. (1988): Prostaglandin hydroperoxidase-dependent oxidation of phenylbutazone: relationship to inhibition of prostaglandin cyclooxygenase. *Mol. Pharmacol.*, 34:186–193.
192. Höjeberg, B., Blomberg, K., Stenberg, S., and Lind, C. (1981): Biospecific adsorption of hepatic DT-diaphorase on immobilized dicoumarol. I. Purification of cytosolic DT-diaphorase from control and 3-methylcholanthrene-treated rats. *Arch. Biochem. Biophys.*, 207:205–216.
193. Idle, J. R., Mahgoub, A., Sloan, T. P., Smith, R. L., Mbanefo, C. O., and Bababunmi, E. A. (1981): Some observations on the oxidation phenotype status of Nigerian patients presenting with cancer. *Cancer Lett.*, 11:331–338.
194. Ikuta, T., Fujiyoshi, T., Kurachi, K., and Yoshida, A. (1985): Molecular cloning of a full-length cDNA for human alcohol dehydrogenase. *Proc. Natl. Acad. Sci. USA*, 82:2703–2707.
195. Imai, Y. (1976): The use of 8-aminooctyl sepharose for the separation of some components of the hepatic microsomal electron transfer system. *J. Biochem.*, 80:267–276.
196. Imai, Y., Ito, A., and Sato, T. (1966): Evidence for biochemically different types of vesicles in the hepatic microsomal fraction. *J. Biochem.*, 60:417–428.
197. Imai, Y. and Sato, R. (1974): A gel-electrophoretically homogeneous preparation of cytochrome P450 from liver microsomes of phenobarbital-pretreated rabbits. *Biochem. Biophys. Res. Commun.*, 60:8–14.
198. Imai, Y., Uno, T., and Nakamura, M. (1990): Characterization of rabbit liver P450IIE1 synthesized in transformed yeast cells. *J. Biochem.*, 108:522–524.
199. Imaoka, S., and Funae, Y. (1986): Ion-exchange high-performance liquid chromatography of membrane-bound protein cytochrome P450. *J. Chromatogr.*, 375:83–90.
200. Imaoka, S., Imai, Y., Shimada, T., and Funae, Y. (1992): Role of phospholipids in reconstituted cytochrome P450 3A forms and mechanism of their activation of catalytic activity. *Biochemistry*, 31:6063–6069.
201. Inskeep, P. B., and Guengerich, F. P. (1984): Glutathione-mediated binding of dibromoalkanes to DNA: specificity of rat glutathione *S*-transferases and dibromoalkane structure. *Carcinogenesis*, 5:805–808.
202. Inskeep, P. B., Koga, N., Cmarik, J. L., and Guengerich, F. P. (1986): Covalent binding of 1,2-dihaloalkanes to DNA and stability of the major DNA adduct, *S*-[2-(N^7-guanyl)ethyl]glutathione. *Cancer Res.*, 46:2839–2844.
203. Islam, S. A., Wolf, C. R., Lennard, M. S., and Sternberg, M. J. E. (1991): A three-dimensional molecular template for substrates of human cytochrome P450 involved in debrisoquine 4-hydroxylation. *Carcinogenesis*, 12:2211–2219.
204. Itagaki, K., Carver, G. T., and Philpot, R. M. (1996): Expression and characterization of a flavin-containing monooxygenase 4 from humans. *J. Biol. Chem.*, 271:20102–20107.
205. Iwata, H., Fujita, K.-I., Kushida, H., Suzuki, A., Konno, Y., Nakamura, K., Fujino, A., and Kamataki, T. (1998): High catalytic activity of human cytochrome P450 co-expressed with human NADPH-cytochrome P450 reductase in *Escherichia coli*. *Biochem. Pharmacol.*, 55:1315–1325.
206. Jacobson, A. (1987): Purification and fractionation of poly(A)$^+$ RNA. *Methods Enzymol.*, 152:32768.
207. Jakoby, W. B. (1980): Detoxication enzymes. In: *Enzymatic Basis of Detoxication*, Vol. 1, edited by W. B. Jakoby, pp. 1–6. Academic Press, New York.
208. Jakoby, W. B. and Habig, W. H. (1980): Glutathione transferases. In: *Enzymatic Basis of Detoxication*, Vol. 2, edited by W. B. Jakoby, pp. 63–94. Academic Press, New York.
209. Jakoby, W. B., Ketterer, B., and Mannervik, B. (1984): Glutathione transferases: nomenclature. *Biochem. Pharmacol.*, 33:2539–2540.
210. Jakoby, W. B., Sekura, R. D., Lyon, E. S., Marcus, C. J., and Wang, J. L. (1980): Sulfotransferases. In: *Enzymatic Basis of Detoxication*, Vol. 2, edited by W. B. Jakoby, pp. 199–228. Academic Press, New York.

211. Jarvis, D. L., Oker-Blom, C., and Summers, M. D. (1990): Role of glycosylation in the transport of recombinant glycoproteins through the secretory pathway of lepidopteran insect cells. *J. Cell. Biochem.*, 42:181–191.

212. Jayarama Bhat, G., and Padmanaban, G. (1988): Heme is a positive regulator of cytochrome P450 gene transcription. *Arch. Biochem. Biophys.*, 264:584–590.

213. Jenkins, C. M., and Waterman, M. R. (1994): Flavodoxin and NADPH-flavodoxin reductase from *Escherichia coli* support bovine cytochrome P450c17 hydroxylase activities. *J. Biol. Chem.*, 269:27401–27408.

214. Jenne, J. W., and Boyer, P. D. (1962): Kinetic characteristics of the acetylation of isoniazid and *p*-aminosalicyclic acid by a liver enzyme preparation. *Biochim. Biophys. Acta*, 65:121–127.

215. Jerina, D. M., Dansette, P. M., Lu, A. Y. H., and Levin, W. (1977): Hepatic microsomal epoxide hydrase: A sensitive radiometric assay for hydration of arene oxides of carcinogenic aromatic hydrocarbons. *Mol. Pharmacol.*, 13:342–351.

216. Jernström, B., Capdevila, J., Jakobsson, S., and Orrenius, S. (1975): Solubilization and partial purification of cytochrome P450 from rat lung microsomes. *Biochem. Biophys. Res. Commun.*, 64:814–822.

217. Johannesen, K. A. M., and DePierre, J. W. (1978): Measurements of cytochrome P450 in the presence of large amounts of contaminating hemoglobin and methemoglobin. *Anal. Biochem.*, 86:725–732.

218. Johnson, E. F., and Muller-Eberhard, U. (1977): Multiple forms of cytochrome P450: Resolution and purification of rabbit liver aryl hydrocarbon hydroxylase. *Biochem. Biophys. Res. Commun.*, 76:644–651.

219. Johnson, E. F., and Muller-Eberhard, U. (1977): Purification of the major cytochrome P450 of liver microsomes from rabbits treated with 2,3,7,8-tetrachlorodibenzo-*p*-dioxin (TCDD). *Biochem. Biophys. Res. Commun.*, 76:652–659.

220. Johnson, E. F., and Muller-Eberhard, U. (1977): Resolution of two forms of cytochrome P450 from liver microsomes of rabbits treated with 2,3,7,8-tetrachlorodibenzo-*p*-dioxin. *J. Biol. Chem.*, 252:2839–2845.

221. Josephy, P. D., DeBruin, L. S., Lord, H. L., Oak, J., Evans, D. H., Guo, Z., Dong, M.-S., and Guengerich, F. P. (1995): Bioactivation of aromatic amines by recombinant human cytochrome P450 1A2 expressed in bacteria: a substitute for mammalian tissue preparations in mutagenicity testing. *Cancer Res.*, 55:799–802.

222. Josephy, P. D., Evans, D. H., Parikh, A., and Guengerich, F. P. (1998): Expression of active human cytochrome P450 1A2, NADPH-cytochrome P450 reductase, and *N*-acetyltransferase in *Escherichia coli*: Metabolic activation of aromatic amine mutagens. *Chem. Res. Toxicol.*, 11:70–74.

223. Juvonen, R. O., Iwasaki, M., and Negishi, M. (1991): Structural function of residue-209 in coumarin 7-hydroxylase (P450coh): Enzyme-kinetic studies and site-directed mutagenesis. *J. Biol. Chem.*, 266:16431–16435.

224. Jörnvall, H., Hempel, J., Vallee, B. L., Bosron, W. F., and Li, T. K. (1984): Human liver alcohol dehydrogenase: amino acid substitution in the b_2b_2 Oriental isozyme explains functional properties, establishes an active site structure, and parallels mutational exchanges in the yeast enzyme. *Proc. Natl. Acad. Sci. USA*, 81:3024–3028.

225. Kadlubar, F. F., Miller, J. A., and Miller, E. C. (1976): Microsomal *N*-oxidation of the hepatocarcinogen *N*-methyl-4-aminoazobenzene and the reactivity of *N*-hydroxy-*N*-methyl-4-aminoazobenzene. *Cancer Res.*, 36:1196–1206.

226. Kamataki, T., Belcher, D. H., and Neal, R. A. (1976): Studies of the metabolism of diethyl *p*-nitrophenyl phosphorothionate (parathion) and benzphetamine using an apparently homogeneous preparation of rat liver cytochrome P450: Effect of a cytochrome P450 antibody preparation. *Mol. Pharmacol.*, 12:921–932.

227. Kamataki, T., Lin, M. L., Belcher, D. H., and Neal, R. A. (1976): Studies of the metabolism of parathion with an apparently homogeneous preparation of rabbit liver cytochrome P450. *Drug Metab. Dispos.*, 4:180–189.

228. Kaminsky, L. S., Fasco, M. J., and Guengerich, F. P. (1979): Comparison of different forms of liver, kidney, and lung microsomal cytochrome P450 by immunological inhibition of regio- and stereoselective metabolism of warfarin. *J. Biol. Chem.*, 254:9657–9662.

229. Kaminsky, L. S., Fasco, M. J., and Guengerich, F. P. (1980): Comparison of different forms of purified cytochrome P450 from rat liver by immunological inhibition of regio- and stereoselective metabolism of warfarin. *J. Biol. Chem.*, 255:85–91.

230. Kaminsky, L. S., Fasco, M. J., and Guengerich, F. P. (1981): Production and application of antibodies to rat liver cytochrome P450. *Methods Enzymol.*, 74:262–272.

231. Kasper, C. B., and Henton, D. (1980): Glucuronidation. In: *Enzymatic Basis of Detoxication*, Vol. 2, edited by W. B. Jakoby, pp. 3–36. Academic Press, New York.

232. Kawabata, T. T., Guengerich, F. P., and Baron, J. (1981): An immunohistochemical study on the localization and distribution of epoxide hydrolase within livers of untreated rats. *Mol. Pharmacol.*, 20:709–714.

233. Kawalek, J. C., Levin, W., Ryan, D., Thomas, P. E., and Lu, A. Y. H. (1975): Purification of liver microsomal cytochrome P-448 from 3-methylcholanthrene-treated rabbits. *Mol. Pharmacol.*, 11:874–878.

234. Kempf, A., Zanger, U. M., and Meyer, U. A. (1995): Truncated human P450 2D6: Expression in *Escherichia coli*: Ni^{2+}-chelate affinity purification, and characterization of solubility and aggregation. *Arch. Biochem. Biophys.*, 321:277–288.

235. Ketterer, B., and Sies, H. (1988): *Glutathione Conjugation: Its Mechanisms and Biological Significance*. Academic Press, London.

236. Kim, D. H., and Guengerich, F. P. (1989): Excretion of the mercapturic acid *S*-[2-(N^7-guanyl)ethyl]-*N*-acetylcysteine in urine following administration of ethylene dibromide to rats. *Cancer Res.*, 49:5843–5851.

237. Kim, R. B., Yamazaki, H., Mimura, M., Shimada, T., Guengerich, F. P., Chiba, K., Ishizaki, T., and Wilkinson, G. R. (1996): Chlorzoxazone 6-hydroxylation in Japanese and Caucasians. In vitro and in vivo differences. *J. Pharmacol. Exp. Ther.*, 279:4–11.

238. Knapp, J. A., Dignam, J. D., and Strobel, H. W. (1977): NADPH-cytochrome P450 reductase: Circular dichroism and physical studies. *J. Biol. Chem.*, 252:437–443.

239. Knodell, R. G., Browne, D., Gwodz, G. P., Brian, W. R., and Guengerich, F. P. (1991): Differential inhibition of human liver cytochromes P450 by cimetidine. *Gastroenterology*, 101:1680–1691.

240. Knowles, R. G., and Burchell, B. (1977): A simple method for purification of epoxide hydratase from rat liver. *Biochem. J.*, 163:381–383.

241. Koga, N., Inskeep, P. B., Harris, T. M., and Guengerich, F. P. (1986): *S*-[2-(N^7-Guanyl)ethyl]glutathione, the major DNA adduct formed from 1,2-dibromoethane. *Biochemistry*, 25:2192–2198.

242. Koymans, L., Vermeulen, N. P. E., van Acker, S. A. B. E., te Koppele, J. M., Heykants, J. J. P., Lavrijsen, K., Meuldermans, W., and Donné-Op den Kelder, G. M. (1992): A predictive model for substrates of cytochrome P450-debrisoquine (2D6). *Chem. Res. Toxicol.*, 5:211–219.

243. Krisch, K., and Staudinger, H. (1961): Untersuchungen zur enzymatischen hydroxylierung: Hydroxylierung von acetanilid

und deren beziehungen zur mikrosomalen pyridinnucleotidoxydation. *Biochem. Z.*, 334:312–327.

244. Kuntzman, R., Tsai, I., and Burns, J. J. (1967): Importance of tissue and plasma binding in determining the retention of norchlorcyclizine and norcyclizine in man, dog and rat. *J. Pharmacol. Exp. Ther.*, 158:332–339.
245. Kwan, S. W., Lewis, D. A., Zhou, B. P., and Abell, C. W. (1995): Characterization of a dinucleotide-binding site in monoamine oxidase B by site-directed mutagenesis. *Arch. Biochem. Biophys.*, 316:385–391.
246. Kyte, J. (1995): *Mechanism in Protein Chemistry*. Garland, New York.
247. Küpfer, A., James, R., Carr, K., and Branch, R. (1982): Analysis of hydroxylated and demethylated metabolites of mephenytoin in man and laboratory animals using gas-liquid chromatography and high-performance liquid chromatography. *J. Chromatogr.*, 232:93–100.
248. Lacourciere, G. M., and Armstrong, R. N. (1993): The catalytic mechanism of microsomal epoxide hydrolase involves an ester intermediate. *J. Am. Chem. Soc.*, 115:10466–10467.
249. Lacourciere, G. M., Vakharia, V. N., Tan, C. P., Morris, D. I., Edwards, G. H., Moos, M., and Armstrong, R. N. (1993): Interaction of hepatic microsomal epoxide hydrolase derived from a recombinant baculovirus expression system with an azarene oxide and an aziridine substrate analogue. *Biochemistry*, 32:2610–2616.
250. Laemmli, U. K. (1970): Cleavage of structural proteins during the assembly of the head of bacteriophage T_4. *Nature*, 227:680–685.
251. Lambeir, A. M., Markey, C. M., Dunford, H. B., and Marnett, L. J. (1987): Spectral properties of the higher oxidation states of prostaglandin H synthase. In: *Advances in Prostaglandin, Thromboxane, and Leukotriene Research*, edited by B. Samuelsson, R. Paoletti, and P. W. Ramwell, pp. 25–28. Raven Press, New York.
252. Langouët, S., Mican, A. N., Müller, M., Fink, S. P., Marnett, L. J., Muhle, S. A., and Guengerich, F. P. (1998): Misincorporation of nucleotides opposite three 5-membered exocyclic ring guanine derivatives: 1,N^2-ethenoguanine, 5,6,7,9-tetrahydro-9-oxoimidazo [1,2-*a*]purine, and 5,6,7,9-tetrahydro-7-hydroxy-9-oxoimidazo [1,2-*a*]purine. *Biochemistry*, 37:5184–5193.
253. Larson, J. R., Coon, M. J., and Porter, T. D. (1991): Purification and properties of a shortened form of cytochrome P450 2E1: Deletion of the NH_2-terminal membrane-insertion signal peptide does not alter the catalytic activities. *Proc. Natl. Acad. Sci. USA*, 88:9141–9145.
254. Larson, J. R., Coon, M. J., and Porter, T. D. (1991): Alcohol-inducible cytochrome P450IIE1 lacking the hydrophobic NH_2-terminal segment retains catalytic activity and is membrane-bound when expressed in *Escherichia coli*. *J. Biol. Chem.*, 266:7321–7324.
255. Lawton, M. P., Gasser, R., Tynes, R. E., Hodgson, E., and Philpot, R. M. (1990): The flavin-containing monooxygenase enzymes expressed in rabbit liver and lung are products of related but distinctly different genes. *J. Biol. Chem.*, 265:5855–5861.
256. Lawton, M. P., Kronbach, T., Johnson, E. F., and Philpot, R. M. (1991): Properties of expressed and native flavin-containing monooxygenases: Evidence of multiple forms in rabbit liver and lung. *Mol. Pharmacol.*, 40:692–698.
257. Lawton, M. P., and Philpot, R. M. (1993): Functional characterization of flavin-containing monooxygenase 1B1 expressed in *Saccharomyces cerevisiae* and *Escherichia coli* and analysis of proposed FAD- and membrane-binding domains. *J. Biol. Chem.*, 268:5728–5734.
258. Layne, E. (1957): Spectrophotometric and turbidimetric methods for measuring proteins. *Methods Enzymol.*, 3:447–454.
259. Leithauser, M. T., Liem, A., Stewart, B. C., Miller, E. C., and Miller, J. A. (1990): 1,N^6-Ethenoadenosine formation, mutagenicity and murine tumor induction as indicators of the generation of an electrophilic epoxide metabolite of the closely related carcinogens ethyl carbamate (urethane) and vinyl carbamate. *Carcinogenesis*, 11:463–473.
260. Lennard, L. (1997): Methyl transferases. In: *Biotransformation, Vol. 3, Comprehensive Toxicology*, edited by F. P. Guengerich, pp. 437–454. Elsevier Science, Oxford.
261. Leonard, N. J., Thomas, P. D., and Gash, V. W. (1955): Unsaturated amines. IV. Structures and reactions of the dehydrosparteines and their salts. *J. Am. Chem. Soc.*, 77:1552–1558.
262. Li, Y. C., and Chiang, J. Y. L. (1991): The expression of a catalytically active cholesterol 7α-hydroxylase cytochrome P450 in *Escherichia coli*. *J. Biol. Chem.*, 266:19186–19191.
263. Licht, H. J., and Cosica, C. J. (1978): Cytochrome P450 LM_2 mediated hydroxylation of monoterpene alcohols. *Biochemistry*, 17:5638–5646.
264. Liebler, D. C., and Guengerich, F. P. (1983): Olefin oxidation by cytochrome P450: Evidence for group migration in catalytic intermediates formed with vinylidene chloride and *trans*-1-phenyl-1-butene. *Biochemistry*, 22:5482–5489.
265. Lindberg, R. L. P., and Negishi, M. (1989): Alteration of mouse cytochrome $P450_{coh}$ substrate specificity by mutation of a single amino-acid residue. *Nature*, 339:632–634.
266. Lowry, O. H., Rosebrough, N. J., Farr, A. L., and Randall, R. J. (1951): Protein measurement with the Folin phenol reagent. *J. Biol. Chem.*, 243:1331–1332.
267. Lu, A. Y. H., and Coon, M. J. (1968): Role of hemoprotein P450 in fatty acid ω-hydroxylation in a soluble enzyme system from liver microsomes. *J. Biol. Chem.*, 243:1331–1332.
268. Lu, A. Y. H., Jacobson, M., Levin, W., West, S. B., and Kuntzman, R. (1972): Reconstituted liver microsomal enzyme system that hydroxylates drugs, other foreign compounds and endogenous substrates. IV. Hydroxylation of aniline. *Arch. Biochem. Biophys.*, 153:294–297.
269. Lu, A. Y. H., Jerina, D. M., and Levin, W. (1977): Liver microsomal epoxide hydrase: hydration of alkene and arene oxides by membrane-bound and purified enzymes. *J. Biol. Chem.*, 252:3715–3723.
270. Lu, A. Y. H., Junk, K. W., and Coon, M. J. (1969): Resolution of the cytochrome P450-containing ω-hydroxylation system of liver microsomes into three components. *J. Biol. Chem.*, 244:3714–3721.
271. Lu, A. Y. H., and Levin, W. (1974): The resolution and reconstitution of the liver microsomal hydroxylation system. *Biochim. Biophys. Acta*, 344:205–240.
272. Lu, A. Y. H., and Levin, W. (1978): Purification and assay of liver microsomal epoxide hydrase. *Methods Enzymol.*, 52:193–200.
273. Lu, A. Y. H., Levin, W., and Kuntzman, R. (1974): Reconstituted liver microsomal enzyme system that hydroxylates drugs, other foreign compounds and endogenous substrates. VII. Stimulation of benzphetamine *N*-demethylation by lipid and detergent. *Biochem. Biophys. Res. Commun.*, 60:266–272.
274. Lu, A. Y. H., Ryan, D., Jerina, D. M., Daly, J. W., and Levin, W. (1975): Liver microsomal epoxide hydrase: Solubilization, purification, and characterization. *J. Biol. Chem.*, 250:8283–8288.
275. Lu, A. Y. H., Strobel, H. W., and Coon, M. J. (1969): Hydroxylation of benzphetamine and other drugs by a solubilized form of cytochrome P450 from liver microsomes: Lipid requirement for drug demethylation. *Biochem. Biophys. Res. Commun.*, 36:545–551.
276. Lu, A. Y. H., Strobel, H. W., and Coon, M. J. (1970): Properties of a solubilized form of the cytochrome P450-containing

mixed-function oxidase of liver microsomes. *Mol. Pharmacol.*, 6:213–220.

277. Lu, A. Y. H., and West, S. B. (1978): Reconstituted mammalian mixed-function oxidases: Requirements, specificities and other properties. *Pharmacol. Ther.*, 2:337–358.

278. Ma, Q., Cui, K., Wang, R. W., Lu, A. Y. H., and Yang, C. S. (1992): Site-directed mutagenesis of rat liver NAD(P)H: Quinone oxidoreductase: roles of lysine 76 and cysteine 179. *Arch. Biochem. Biophys.*, 294:434–439.

279. Malaveille, C., Bartsch, H., Barbin, A., Camus, A. M., and Montesano, R. (1975): Mutagenicity of vinyl chloride, chloroethylene oxide, chloroacetaldehyde and chloroethanol. *Biochem. Biophys. Res. Commun.*, 63:363–370.

280. Manchester, J. I., and Ornstein, R. L. (1995): Enzyme-catalyzed dehalogenation of pentachloroethane: why F87W-cytochrome P450cam is faster than wild type. *Protein Eng.*, 8:801–807.

281. Mannervik, B., Ålin, P., Guthenberg, C., Jensson, H., Tahir, M. K., Warholm, M., and Jörnvall, H. (1985): Identification of three classes of cytosolic glutathione transferase common to several mammalian species: Correlation between structural data and enzymatic properties. *Proc. Natl. Acad. Sci. USA*, 82:7202–7206.

282. Markey, C. M., Alward, A., Weller, P. E., and Marnett, L. J. (1987): Quantitative studies of hydroperoxide reduction by prostaglandin H synthase: Reducing substrate specificity and the relationship of peroxidase to cyclooxygenase activities. *J. Biol. Chem.*, 262:6266–6279.

283. Marnett, L. J. (1987): Peroxyl free radicals: potential mediators of tumor initiation and promotion. *Carcinogenesis*, 8:1365–1373.

284. Marnett, L. J., Bienkowski, M. J., Pagels, W. R., and Reed, G. A. (1980): Mechanism of xenobiotic cooxygenation coupled to prostaglandin H_2 biosynthesis. In: *Advances in Prostaglandin and Thromboxane Research*, Vol. 6, edited by B. Samuelsson, P. W. Ramwell, and R. Paoletti, pp. 149–151. Raven Press, New York.

285. Marnett, L. J., and Eling, T. (1983): Cooxidation during prostaglandin biosynthesis: A pathway for the metabolic activation of xenobiotics. In: *Reviews in Biochemical Toxicology*, Vol. 5, edited by E. Hodgson, J. R. Bend, and R. M. Philpot, pp. 135–172. Elsevier-North Holland, New York.

286. Marnett, L. J., Wlodawer, P., and Samuelsson, B. (1975): Co-oxygenation of organic substrates by the prostaglandin synthetase of sheep vesicular gland. *J. Biol. Chem.*, 250:8510–8517.

287. Masters, B. S. S., Baron, J., Taylor, W. E., Isaacson, E. L., and LoSpalluto, J. (1971): Immunochemical studies on electron transport chains involving cytochrome P450. I. Effects of antibodies to pig liver microsomal reduced triphosphopyridine nucleotide-cytochrome *c* reductase and the non-heme iron protein from bovine adrenocortical mitochondria. *J. Biol. Chem.*, 246:4143–4150.

288. Matsubara, T., Koike, M., Touchi, A., Tochino, Y., and Sugeno, K. (1976): Quantitative determination of cytochrome P450 in rat liver homogenate. *Anal. Biochem.*, 75:596–603.

289. Maynert, E. W., Foreman, R. L., and Watabe, T. (1970): Epoxides as obligatory intermediates in the metabolism of olefins to glycols *J. Biol. Chem.*, 245:5234–5238.

290. McManus, M. E., Burgess, W. M., Veronese, M. E., Huggett, A., Quattrochi, L. C., and Tukey, R. H. (1990): Metabolism of 2-acetylaminofluorene and benzo(a)pyrene and activation of food-derived heterocyclic amine mutagens by human cytochromes P450. *Cancer Res.*, 50:3367–3376.

291. Meisler, M. H., and Reinke, C. (1976): A sensitive fluorescent assay for *N*-acetyltransferase activity in human lymphocytes from newborns and adults. *Anal. Biochem.*, 75:596–603.

292. Meister, A., Tate, S. S., and Griffith, O. W. (1981): γ-Glutamyltranspeptidase. *Methods Enzymol.*, 77:237–253.

293. Miller, E. C., and Miller, J. A. (1947): The presence and significance of bound amino azodyes in the livers of rats fed *p*-dimethylaminoazobenzene. *Cancer Res.*, 7:468–480.

294. Miller, R. E., and Guengerich, F. P. (1983): Metabolism of trichloroethylene in isolated hepatocytes, microsomes, and reconstituted enzyme systems containing cytochrome P450. *Cancer Res.*, 43:1145–1152.

295. Mimura, M., Baba, T., Yamazaki, Y., Ohmori, S., Inui, Y., Gonzalez, F. J., Guengerich, F. P., and Shimada, T. (1993): Characterization of cytochrome P450 2B6 in human liver microsomes. *Drug Metab. Dispos.*, 21:1048–1056.

296. Miwa, G. T., Levin, W., Thomas, P. E., and Lu, A. Y. H. (1978): The direct oxidation of ethanol by a catalase- and alcohol dehydrogenase-free reconstituted system containing cytochrome P450. *Arch. Biochem. Biophys.*, 187:464–475.

297. Miwa, G. T., Walsh, J. S., Kedderis, G. L., and Hollenberg, P. F. (1983): The use of intramolecular isotope effects to distinguish between deprotonation and hydrogen atom abstraction mechanisms in cytochrome P450- and peroxidase-catalyzed *N*-demethylation reactions. *J. Biol. Chem.*, 258:14445–14449.

298. Morgenstern, R., and DePierre, J. W. (1983): Microsomal glutathione transferase: Purification in unactivated form and further characterization of the activation process, substrate specificity and amino acid composition. *Eur. J. Biochem.*, 134:591–597.

299. Murakami, H., Yabusaki, Y., Sakaki, T., Shibata, M., and Ohkawa, H. (1987): A genetically engineered P450 monooxygenase: construction of the functional fused enzyme between rat cytochrome P450c and NADPH-cytochrome P450 reductase. *DNA*, 6:189–197.

300. Müller, M., Belas, F. J., Blair, I. A., and Guengerich, F. P. (1997): Analysis of 1,N^2-ethenoguanine and 5,6,7,9-tetrahydro-7-hydroxy-9-oxoimidazo[1,2-*a*]purine in DNA treated with 2-chlorooxirane by high performance liquid chromatography/mass spectrometry and comparison of amounts with other adducts. *Chem. Res. Toxicol.*, 10:242–247.

301. Müller-Enoch, D., Churchill, P., Fleischer, S., and Guengerich, F. P. (1984): Interaction of liver microsomal cytochrome P450 and NADPH-cytochrome P450 reductase in the presence and absence of lipid. *J. Biol. Chem.*, 259:8174–8182.

302. Narhi, L. O., and Fulco, A. J. (1987): Identification and characterization of two functional domains in cytochrome P450BM-3, a catalytically self-sufficient monooxygenase induced by barbiturates in *Bacillus megaterium*. *J. Biol. Chem.*, 262:6683–6690.

303. Nash, T. (1953): The colorimetric estimation of formaldehyde by means of the Hantzsch reaction. *Biochem. J.*, 55:416–421.

304. Nebert, D. W., and Gelboin, H. V. (1968): Substrate-inducible microsomal arylhydroxylase in mammalian cell culture: Assay and properties of induced enzyme. *J. Biol. Chem.*, 243:6242–6249.

305. Nebert, D. W., Nelson, D. R., Coon, M. J., Estabrook, R. W., Feyereisen, R., Fujii-Kuriyama, Y., Gonzalez, F. J., Guengerich, F. P., Gunsalus, I. C., Johnson, E. F., Loper, J. C., Sato, R., Waterman, M. R., and Waxman, D. J. (1991): The P450 superfamily: Update on new sequences, gene mapping, and recommended nomenclature. *DNA Cell Biol.*, 10:1–14.

306. Nebert, D. W., Nelson, D. R., Coon, M. J., Estabrook, R. W., Feyereisen, R., Fujii-Kuriyama, Y., Gonzalez, F. J., Guengerich, F. P., Gunsalus, I. C., Johnson, E. F., Loper, J. C., Sato, R., Waterman, M. R., and Waxman, D. J. (1991): The P450 superfamily: Update on new sequences, gene mapping, and recommended nomenclature. *DNA Cell Biol.*, 10:397–398.

307. Nelson, D. R., Koymans, L., Kamataki, T., Stegeman, J. J., Feyereisen, R., Waxman, D. J., Waterman, M. R., Gotoh, O., Coon, M. J., Estabrook, R. W., Gunsalus, I. C., and Nebert, D. W. (1996): P450 superfamily: Update on new sequences, gene

mapping, accession numbers, and nomenclature. *Pharmacogenetics*, 6:1–42.
308. Newton, D. J., Wang, R. W., and Lu, A. Y. H. (1994): Cytochrome P450 inhibitors: Evaluation of specificities in the in vitro metabolism of therapeutic agents by human liver microsomes. *Drug Metab. Dispos.*, 23:154–158.
309. Nguyen, N., and Tukey, R. H. (1997): Baculovirus-directed expression of rabbit UDP-glucuronosyltransferases in *Spodoptera frugiperda* cells. *Drug Metab. Dispos.*, 25:745–749.
310. Nordblom, G. D., and Coon, M. J. (1977): Hydrogen peroxide formation and stoichiometry of hydroxylation reactions catalyzed by highly purified liver microsomal cytochrome P450. *Arch. Biochem. Biophys.*, 180:343–347.
311. O'Farrell, P. Z., Goodman, H. M., and O'Farrell, P. H. (1977): High resolution two-dimensional electrophoresis of basic as well as acidic proteins. *Cell*, 12:1133–1142.
312. O'Shea, D., Davis, S. N., Kim, R. B., and Wilkinson, G. R. (1994): Effect of fasting and obesity in humans on the 6-hydroxylation of chloroxazone: A putative probe of CYP2E1 activity. *Clin. Pharmacol. Ther.*, 56:359–367.
313. Oesch, F. (1973): Mammalian epoxide hydrases: Inducible enzymes catalyzing the inactivation of carcinogenic and cytotoxic metabolites derived from aromatic and olefinic compounds. *Xenobiotica*, 3:305–340.
314. Oesch, F., and Bentley, P. (1976): Antibodies against homogeneous epoxide hydratase provide evidence for a single enzyme hydrating styrene oxide and benz(a)pyrene 4,5-oxide. *Nature*, 259:53–55.
315. Oesch, F., Jerina, D. M., and Daly, J. (1971): A radiometric assay for hepatic epoxide hydrase activity with [7-^{3}H]styrene oxide. *Biochim. Biophys. Acta*, 227:685–691.
316. Ogden, R. C., and Adams, D. A. (1987): Electrophoresis in agarose and acrylamide gels. *Methods Enzymol.*, 152:61–87.
317. Ohta, D., Matsu ura, Y., and Sato, R. (1991): Expression and characterization of a rabbit liver cytochrome P450 belonging to P450IIB subfamily with the aid of the baculovirus expression vector system. *Biochem. Biophys. Res. Commun.*, 175:394–399.
318. Okazaki, O., and Guengerich, F. P. (1993): Evidence for specific base catalysis in *N*-dealkylation reactions catalyzed by cytochrome P450 and chloroperoxidase: Differences in rates of deprotonation of aminium radicals as an explanation for high kinetic hydrogen isotope effects observed with peroxidases. *J. Biol. Chem.*, 268:1546–1552.
319. Omura, T., and Sato, R. (1964): The carbon monoxide-binding pigment of liver microsomes. I. Evidence for its hemoprotein nature. *J. Biol. Chem.*, 239:2370–2378.
320. Omura, T., and Sato, R. (1967): Isolation of cytochromes P450 and P420. *Methods Enzymol.*, 10:556–561.
321. Ortiz de Montellano, P. R., and Correia, M. A. (1983): Suicidal destruction of cytochrome P450 during oxidative drug metabolism. *Annu. Rev. Pharmacol. Toxicol.*, 23:481–503.
322. Ozawa, N., and Guengerich, F. P. (1983): Evidence for formation of an *S*-[2-(N^7-guanyl)ethyl]glutathione adduct in glutathione-mediated binding of 1,2-dibromoethane to DNA. *Proc. Natl. Acad. Sci. USA*, 80:5266–5270.
323. Ozols, J., Korza, G., Heinemann, F. S., Hediger, M. A., and Strittmatter, P. (1985): Complete amino acid sequence of steer liver microsomal NADH-cytochrome b_5 reductase. *Carcinogenesis*, 260:11953–11961.
324. Panthananickal, A., and Marnett, L. J. (1981): Comparison of commercial reversed-phase high-performance liquid chormatographic columns for the separation of benzo[a]pyrene diolepoxide-nucleic acid adducts. *J. Chromatogr.*, 206:253–265.
325. Parikh, A., Gillam, E. M. J., and Guengerich, F. P. (1997): Drug metabolism by *Escherichia coli* expressing human cytochromes P450. *Nature Biotechnol.*, 15:784–788.
326. Parikh, A., and Guengerich, F. P. (1997): Expression, purification, and characterization of a catalytically active human cytochrome P450 1A2 : NADPH-cytochrome P450 reductase fusion protein. *Protein Express. Purif.*, 9:346–354.
327. Park, S. S., Fujino, T., Miller, H., Guengerich, F. P., and Gelboin, H. V. (1984): Monoclonal antibodies to phenobarbital-induced rat liver cytochrome P450. *Biochem. Pharmacol.*, 33:2071–2081.
328. Park, S. S., Fujino, T., West, D., Guengerich, F. P., and Gelboin, H. V. (1982): Monoclonal antibodies that inhibit enzyme activity of 3-methylcholanthrene-induced cytochrome P450. *Cancer Res.*, 42:1798–1808.
329. Paye, M., Beaune, P., Kremers, P., Frankinet-Collignon, C., Guengerich, F. P., Goujon, F., and Gielen, J. (1984): Quantification of two cytochrome P450 isoenzymes by an enzyme-linked immunosorbent assay (ELISA). *Biochem. Biophys. Res. Commun.*, 122:137–142.
330. Pemble, S., Schroeder, K. R., Spencer, S. R., Meyer, D. J., Hallier, E., Bolt, H. M., Ketterer, B., and Taylor, J. B. (1994): Human glutathione *S*-transferase theta (GSTT1): cDNA cloning and the characterization of a genetic polymorphism. *Biochem. J.*, 300:271–276.
331. Pernecky, S. J., and Coon, M. J. (1996): N-Terminal modifications that alter P450 membrane targeting and function. *Methods Enzymol.*, 272:25–34.
332. Pernecky, S. J., Larson, J. R., Philpot, R. M., and Coon, M. J. (1992): Composition of the NH_2-terminal region governs the targeting of expressed P450 to *Escherichia coli* cytosol or membranes. *J. Basic Clin. Physiol. Pharmacol.*, 3(suppl.):62–63.
333. Peter, R., Böcker, R. G., Beaune, P. H., Iwasaki, M., Guengerich, F. P., and Yang, C.-S. (1990): Hydroxylation of chlorzoxazone as a specific probe for human liver cytochrome P450 IIE1. *Chem. Res. Toxicol.*, 3:566–573.
334. Petersen, D., and Lindahl, R. (1997): Aldehyde dehydrogenases. In: *Biotransformation, Vol. 3, Comprehensive Toxicology*, edited by F. P. Guengerich, pp. 97–118. Elsevier Science, Oxford.
335. Peterson, J. A., Ebel, R. E., and O'Keefe, D. H. (1978): Dual-wavelength stopped-flow spectrophotometric measurement of NADPH-cytochrome P450 reductase. *Methods Enzymol.*, 52:221–226.
336. Peterson, L. A., Harris, T. M., and Guengerich, F. P. (1988): Evidence for an episulfonium ion intermediate in the formation of *S*-[2-(N^7-guanyl)ethyl]glutathione in DNA. *J. Am. Chem. Soc.*, 110:3284–3291.
337. Peyronneau, M. A., Renaud, J. P., Truan, G., Urban, P., Pompon, D., and Mansuy, D. (1992): Optimization of yeast-expressed human liver cytochrome-P450 3A4 catalytic activities by coexpressing NADPH-cytochrome P450 reductase and cytochrome b_5. *Eur. J. Biochem.*, 207:109–116.
338. Phillips, A. H., and Langdon, R. G. (1962): Hepatic triphosphopyridine nucleotide-cytochrome *c* reductase: Isolation, characterization, and kinetic studies. *J. Biol. Chem.*, 237:2652–2660.
339. Philpot, R. M., and Arinç, E. (1976): Separation and purification of two forms of hepatic cytochrome P450 from untreated rats. *Mol. Pharmacol.*, 12:483–493.
340. Ploemen, J. H. T. M., Wormhoudt, L. W., van Ommen, B., Commandeur, J. N. M., Vermeulen, N. P. E., and van Bladeren, P. J. (1995): Polymorphism in the glutathione conjugation activity of human erythrocytes towards ethylene dibromide and 1,2-epoxy-3-(*p*-nitrophenoxy)-propane. *Biochim. Biophys. Acta*, 1243:469–476.
341. Plé, P., and Marnett, L. J. (1989): Alkylaryl sulfides as peroxidase reducing substrates for prostaglandin H synthase: Probes for the reactivity and environment of the ferryl–oxo complex. *J. Biol. Chem.*, 264:13983–13993.

342. Poland, A. P., and Nebert, D. W. (1973): A sensitive radiometric assay of aminopyrine *N*-demethylation. *J. Pharmacol. Exp. Ther.*, 184:269–277.

343. Porter, T. D., and Kasper, C. B. (1985): Coding nucleotide sequence of rat NADPH-cytochrome P450 oxidoreductase cDNA and identification of flavin-binding domains. *Proc. Natl. Acad. Sci. USA*, 82:973–977.

344. Porter, T. D., Wilson, T. E., and Kasper, C. B. (1987): Expression of a functional 78,000 dalton mammalian flavoprotein, NADPH-cytochrome P450 oxidoreductase, in *Escherichia coli*. *Arch. Biochem. Biophys.*, 254:353–367.

345. Poulsen, L. L., Hyslop, R. M., and Ziegler, D. M. (1974): *S*-Oxidation of thioureylenes catalyzed by a microsomal flavoprotein mixed-function oxidase. *Biochem. Pharmacol.*, 23:3431–3440.

346. Poulsen, L. L., Sofer, S. S., and Ziegler, D. M. (1976): Properties and applications of an immobilized mixed-function hepatic drug oxidase. *Methods Enzymol.*, 44:849–856.

347. Raig, V. P., and Ammon, R. (1972): Nachweis einiger neuer phenolischer Stoffwechselprodukte des biphenyls. *Arzneim. Forsch. [Drug Res.]*, 22:1399–1404.

348. Raney, K. D., Meyer, D. J., Ketterer, B., Harris, T. M., and Guengerich, F. P. (1992): Glutathione conjugation of aflatoxin B_1 *exo* and *endo* epoxides by rat and human glutathione *S*-transferases. *Chem. Res. Toxicol.*, 5:470–478.

349. Raney, K. D., Shimada, T., Kim, D.-H., Groopman, J. D., Harris, T. M., and Guengerich, F. P. (1992): Oxidation of aflatoxins and sterigmatocystin by human liver microsomes: significance of aflatoxin Q_1 as a detoxication product of aflatoxin B_1. *Chem. Res. Toxicol.*, 5:202–210.

350. Rangarajan, P. N., and Padmanaban, G. (1989): Regulation of cytochrome P450b/e gene expression by a heme- and phenobarbitone-modulated transcription factor. *Proc. Natl. Acad. Sci. USA*, 86:3963–3967.

351. Renaud, J.-P., Cullin, C., Pompon, D., Beaune, P., and Mansuy, D. (1990): Expression of human liver cytochrome P450 IIIA4 in yeast: A functional model for the hepatic enzyme. *Eur. J. Biochem.*, 194:889–896.

352. Renwick, A. G. (1994): Toxicokinetics—pharmacokinetics in toxicology. In: *Principles and Methods of Toxicology*, 3rd ed., edited by A. W. Hayes, pp. 101–147. Raven Press, New York.

353. Reubi, I., Griffin, K. J., Raucy, J. L., and Johnson, E. F. (1984): Three monoclonal antibodies to rabbit microsomal cytochrome P450 1 recognize distinct epitopes that are shared to different degrees among other electrophoretic types of cytochrome P450. *J. Biol. Chem.*, 259:5887–5892.

354. Richardson, T. H., Jung, F., Griffin, K. J., Wester, M., Raucy, J. L., Kemper, B., Bornheim, L. M., Hassett, C., Omiecinski, C. J., and Johnson, E. F. (1995): A universal approach to the expression of human and rabbit cytochrome P450s of the 2C subfamily in *Escherichia coli*. *Arch. Biochem. Biophys.*, 323:87–96.

355. Rinkus, S. J., and Legator, M. S. (1985): Fluorometric assay using high-pressure liquid chromatography for the microsomal metabolism of certain substituted aliphatic to 1,N^6-ethenoadenine-forming metabolites. *Anal. Biochem.*, 150:379–393.

356. Roerig, D. L., Mascaro, L., Jr., and Aust, S. D. (1972): Microsomal electron transport: tetrazolium reduction by rat liver microsomal NADPH-cytochrome *c* reductase. *Arch. Biochem. Biophys.*, 153:475–479.

357. Ross, D. (1997): Quinone reductases. In: *Biotransformation, Vol. 3, Comprehensive Toxicology*, edited by F. P. Guengerich, pp. 179–197. Elsevier Science, Oxford.

358. Roy Chowdhury, J., Roy Chowdhury, N., Falany, C. N., Tephly, T. R., and Arias, I. M. (1986): Isolation and characterization of multiple forms of rat liver UDP-glucuronate glucuronosyltransferase. *Biochem. J.*, 233:827–837.

359. Ryan, D., Lu, A. Y. H., Kawalek, J., West, S. B., and Levin, W. (1975): Highly purified cytochrome P-448 and P450 from rat liver microsomes. *Biochem. Biophys. Res. Commun.*, 64:1134–1141.

360. Ryan, D., Lu, A. Y. H., West, S., and Levin, W. (1975): Multiple forms of cytochrome P450 in phenobarbital- and 3-methylcholanthrene-treated rats. *J. Biol. Chem.*, 250:2157–2163.

361. Ryan, D. E., Thomas, P. E., Korzeniowski, D., and Levin, W. (1979): Separation and characterization of highly purified forms of liver microsomal cytochrome P450 from rats treated with polychlorinated biphenyls, phenobarbital, and 3-methylcholanthrene. *J. Biol. Chem.*, 254:1365–1374.

362. Sabourin, P. J., Smyser, B. P., and Hodgson, E. (1984): Purification of the flavin-containing monooxygenase from mouse and pig liver microsomes. *Int. J. Biochem.*, 16:713–720.

363. Sadano, H., and Omura, T. (1983): Reversible transfer of heme between different molecular species of microsome-bound cytochrome P450 in rat liver. *Biochem. Biophys. Res. Commun.*, 116:1013–1019.

364. Sakaki, T., Kominami, S., Hayashi, K., Akiyoshi-Shibata, M., and Yabusaki, Y. (1996): Molecular engineering study on electron transfer from NADPH-P450 reductase to rat mitochondrial P450c27 in yeast microsomes. *J. Biol. Chem.*, 271:26209–26213.

365. Sakaki, T., Kominami, S., Takemori, S., Ohkawa, H., Akiyoshi-Shibata, M., and Yabusaki, Y. (1994): Kinetic studies on a genetically engineered fused enzyme between rat cytochrome P4501A1 and yeast NADPH-P450 reductase. *Biochemistry*, 33:4933–4939.

366. Sakaki, T., Oeda, K., Miyoshi, M., and Ohkawa, H. (1985): Characterization of rat cytochrome $P450_{MC}$ synthesized in *Saccharomyces cerevisiae*. *J. Biochem.*, 98:167–175.

367. Sakaki, T., Oeda, K., Yabusaki, Y., and Ohkawa, H. (1986): Monooxygenase activity of *Saccharomyces cerevisiae* cells transformed with expression plasmids carrying rat cytochrome P450MC cDNA. *J. Biochem.*, 99:741–749.

368. Salach, J. I. (1979): Monoamine oxidase from beef liver mitochondria: Simplified isolation procedure, properties, and determination of its cysteinyl flavin content. *Arch. Biochem. Biophys.*, 192:128–137.

369. Sambrook, J., Fritsch, E. F., and Maniatis, T. (1989): *Molecular Cloning. A Laboratory Manual*, 2nd ed. Cold Spring Harbor Laboratory Press, Cold Spring Harbor, NY.

370. Sandhu, P., Guo, Z., Baba, T., Martin, M. V., Tukey, R. H., and Guengerich, F. P. (1994): Expression of modified human cytochrome P450 1A2 in *Escherichia coli*: Stabilization, purification, spectral characterization, and catalytic activities of the enzyme. *Arch. Biochem. Biophys.*, 309:168–177.

371. Sekura, R. D., Marcus, C. J., Lyon, E. S., and Jakoby, W. B. (1979): Assay of sulfotransferases. *Anal. Biochem.*, 95:82–86.

372. Selkirk, J. K., Croy, R. G., Roller, P. P., and Gelboin, H. V. (1974): High-pressure liquid chromatographic analysis of benzo(a)pyrene metabolism and covalent binding and the mechanism of action of 7,8-benzoflavone and 1,2-epoxy-3,3,3-trichloropropane. *Cancer Res.*, 34:3474–3480.

373. Seto, Y., and Guengerich, F. P. (1993): Liquid chromatographic determination of *p*-substituted *N,N*-dialkylaniline *N*-oxides. *J. Chromatogr.*, 619:71–77.

374. Seto, Y., and Guengerich, F. P. (1993): Partitioning between *N*-dealkylation and *N*-oxygenation in the oxidation of *N,N*-dialkylarylamines catalyzed by cytochrome P450 2B1. *J. Biol. Chem.*, 268:9986–9997.

375. Shah, R. R., Oates, N. S., Idle, J. R., Smith, R. L., Dayer, P., Courvoisier, F., Balant, L., and Fabre, J. (1982): Beta-blockers and drug oxidation status. *Lancet*, 1:508–509.

376. Shaw, P. M., Reiss, A., Adesnik, M., Nebert, D. W., Schembri, J., and Jaiswal, A. K. (1991): The human dioxin-inducible NAD(P)H : quinone oxidoreductase cDNA-encoded protein expressed in COS-1 cells is identical to diaphorase 4. *Eur. J. Biochem.*, 195:171–176.

377. Shen, A. L., Porter, T. D., Wilson, T. E., and Kasper, C. B. (1989): Structural analysis of the FMN binding domain of NADPH-cytochrome P450 oxidoreductase by site-directed mutagenesis. *J. Biol. Chem.*, 264:7584–7589.

378. Shen, J., Moy, J. A., Green, M. D., Guengerich, F. P., and Baron, J. (1998): Immunohistochemical demonstration of β-naphthoflavone-inducible cytochrome P450 1A1/1A2 in rat intrahepatic biliary epithelial cells. *Hepatology*, 27:1483–1491.

379. Shibata, M., Sakaki, T., Yabusaki, Y., Murakami, H., and Ohkawa, H. (1990): Genetically engineered P450 monooxygenases: Construction of bovine P450c17/yeast reductase fused enzymes. *DNA Cell Biol.*, 9:27–36.

380. Shimada, T., and Guengerich, F. P. (1985): Participation of a rat liver cytochrome P450 induced by pregnenolone 16α-carbonitrile and other compounds in the 4-hydroxylation of mephenytoin. *Mol. Pharmacol.*, 28:215–219.

381. Shimada, T., Martin, M. V., Pruess-Schwartz, D., Marnett, L. J., and Guengerich, F. P. (1989): Roles of individual human cytochrome P450 enzymes in the bioactivation of benzo(a)pyrene, 7,8-dihydroxy-7,8-dihydrobenzo(a)pyrene, and other dihydrodiol derivatives of polycyclic aromatic hydrocarbons. *Cancer Res.*, 49:6304–6312.

382. Shimada, T., Misono, K. S., and Guengerich, F. P. (1986): Human liver microsomal cytochrome P450 mephenytoin 4-hydroxylase, a prototype of genetic polymorphism in oxidative drug metabolism. Purification and characterization of two similar forms involved in the reaction. *J. Biol. Chem.*, 261:909–921.

383. Shimada, T., Nakamura, S., Imaoka, S., and Funae, Y. (1987): Genotoxic and mutagenic activation of aflatoxin B_1 by constitutive forms of cytochrome P450 in rat liver microsomes. *Toxicol. Appl. Pharmacol.*, 91:13–21.

384. Shimada, T., Oda, Y., Yamazaki, H., Mimura, M., and Guengerich, F. P. (1994): SOS function tests for studies of chemical carcinogenesis in *Salmonella typhimurium* TA 1535/pSK1002, NM2009, and NM3009. In: *Methods in Molecular Genetics, Vol. 5, Gene and Chromosome Analysis*, edited by K. W. Adolph, pp. 342–355. Academic Press, Orlando, FL.

385. Shimada, T., Shea, J. P., and Guengerich, F. P. (1985): Convenient assay for mephenytoin 4-hydroxylase activity of human liver microsomal cytochrome P450. *Anal. Biochem.*, 147:174–179.

386. Shimada, T., Wunsch, R. M., Hanna, I. H., Sutter, T. R., Guengerich, F. P., and Gillam, E. M. J. (1998): Recombinant human cytochrome P450 1B1 expression in *Escherichia coli*. *Arch. Biochem. Biophys.*, 357:111–120.

387. Shimada, T., Yamazaki, H., Foroozesch, M., Hopkins, N. E., Alworth, W. L., and Guengerich, F. P. (1998): Selectivity of polycyclic inhibitors for human cytochromes P450 1A1, 1A2, and 1B1. *Chem. Res. Toxicol.*, 11:1048–1056.

388. Shively, J. E. (1986): Reverse-phase HPLC isolation and microsequence analysis. In: *Methods of Protein Microcharacterization*, edited by J. E. Shively, pp. 41–87. Humana Press, Clifton, NJ.

389. Simmons, D. L., McQuiddy, P., and Kasper, C. B. (1987): Induction of the hepatic mixed-function oxidase system by synthetic glucocorticoids: Transcriptional and post-transcriptional regulation. *J. Biol. Chem.*, 262:326–332.

390. Simula, T. P., Glancey, M. J., and Wolf, C. R. (1993): Human glutathione *S*-transferase-expressing *Salmonella typhimurium* tester strains to study the activation/detoxification of mutagenic compounds: Studies with halogenated compounds, aromatic amines and aflatoxin B_1. *Carcinogenesis*, 14:1371–1376.

391. Sipes, I. G., Krishna, G., and Gillette, J. R. (1977): Bioactivation of carbon tetrachloride, chloroform and bromotrichloromethane: role of cytochrome P450. *Life Sci.*, 20:1541–1548.

392. Sladek, N. E., and Mannering, G. J. (1969): Induction of drug metabolism. II. Qualitative differences in the microsomal *N*-demethylating systems stimulated by polycyclic hydrocarbons and by phenobarbital. *Mol. Pharmacol.*, 5:186–199.

393. Song, B. J., Gelboin, H. V., Park, S. S., Yang, C. S., and Gonzalez, F. J. (1986): Complementary DNA and protein sequences of ethanol-inducible rat and human cytochrome P450s: Transcriptional and post-transcriptional regulation of the rat enzyme. *J. Biol. Chem.*, 261:16689–16697.

394. Soucek, P., Martin, M. V., Ueng, Y.-F., and Guengerich, F. P. (1995): Identification of a common epitope near the conserved heme-binding region with polyclonal antibodies raised against cytochrome P450 family 2 proteins. *Biochemistry*, 34:16013–16021.

395. Spatz, L., and Strittmatter, P. (1971): A form of cytochrome b_5 that contains an additional hydrophobic sequence of 40 amino acid residues. *Proc. Natl. Acad. Sci. USA*, 68:1042–1046.

396. Srivastava, P. K., Yun, C.-H., Beaune, P. H., Ged, C., and Guengerich, F. P. (1991): Separation of human liver tolbutamine hydroxylase and (*S*)-mephenytoin 4′-hydroxylase cytochrome P450 enzymes. *Mol. Pharmacol.*, 40:69-79.

397. Stevens, J., and Jakoby, W. B. (1983): Cysteine conjugate β-lyase. *Mol. Pharmacol.*, 23:761–765.

398. Steward, A. R., Dannan, G. A., Guzelian, P. S., and Guengerich, F. P. (1985): Changes in the concentration of seven forms of cytochrome P450 in primary cultures of adult rat hepatocytes. *Mol. Pharmacol.*, 27:125–132.

399. Strobel, H. W., and Dignam, J. D. (1978): Purification and properties of NADPH-cytochrome P450 reductase. *Methods Enzymol.*, 52:89–96.

400. Strobl, G. R., von Kruedener, S., Stöckigt, J., Guengerich, F. P., and Wolff, T. (1993): Development of a pharmacophore for inhibition of human liver cytochrome P450 2D6: Molecular modeling and inhibition studies. *J. Med. Chem.*, 36:1136–1145.

401. Sun, J. D., and Dent, J. G. (1980): A new method for measuring covalent binding of chemicals to cellular macromolecules. *Chem. Biol. Interact.*, 32:41–61.

402. Suzuki, A., Kushida, H., Iwata, H., Watanabe, M., Nohmi, T., Fujita, K., Gonzalez, F. J., and Kamataki, T. (1998): Establishment of a *Salmonella* tester strain highly sensitive to mutagenic heterocyclic amines. *Cancer Res.*, 58:1833–1838.

403. Tamura, S., Korzekwa, K. R., Kimura, S., Gelboin, H. V., and Gonzalez, F. J. (1992): Baculovirus-mediated expression and functional characterization of human NADPH-P450 oxidoreductase. *Arch. Biochem. Biophys.*, 293:219–223.

404. Tateishi, M., and Shimizu, H. (1980): Cysteine conjugate β-lyase. In: *Enzymatic Basis of Detoxication*, Vol. 2, edited by W. B. Jakoby, pp. 121–130. Academic Press, New York.

405. Tateishi, M., Suzuki, S., and Shimizu, H. (1978): Cysteine conjugate β-lyase in rat liver: A novel enzyme catalyzing formation of thiol-containing metabolites of drugs. *J. Biol. Chem.*, 253:8854–8859.

406. Taugen, O., Jonasson, J., and Orrenius, S. (1973): Isolation of rat liver microsomes by gel filtration. *Anal. Biochem.*, 54:597–603.

407. Tephley, T. R. (1990): Isolation and purification of UDP-glucuronosyltransferases. *Chem. Res. Toxicol.*, 3:509–516.

408. Thabrew, M. I., and Ioannides, C. (1984): Inhibition of rat hepatic mixed function oxidases by antimalarial drugs: Selectivity for cytochromes P450 and P-448. *Chem. Biol. Interact.*, 51:285–294.

409. Thakker, D. R., Yagi, H., Akagi, H., Koreeda, M., Lu, A. Y. H., Levin, W., Wood, A. W., Conney, A. H., and Jerina, D. M. (1977): Stereoselective metabolism of benzo[a]pyrene and benzo[a]pyrene-7,8-dihydrodiol to diol-epoxides. *Chem. Biol. Interact.*, 16:281–300.

410. Thakker, D. R., Yagi, H., and Jerina, D. M. (1978): Analysis of polycyclic aromatic hydrocarbons and their metabolites by high-pressure liquid chromatography. *Methods Enzymol.*, 52:279–296.

411. Thier, R., Pemble, S. E., Taylor, J. B., Humphreys, W. G., Persmark, M., Ketterer, B., and Guengerich, F. P. (1993): Expression of mammalian glutathione *S*-transferase 5-5 in *Salmonella typhimurium* TA1535 leads to base-pair mutations upon exposure to dihalomethanes. *Proc. Natl. Acad. Sci. USA*, 90:8576–8580.

412. Thomas, H., Schladt, L., Doehmer, J., Knehr, M., and Oesch, F. (1990): Rat and human liver cytosolic epoxide hydrolases: evidence for multiple forms at the level of protein and mRNA. *Environ. Health Perspect.*, 88:49–55.

413. Thomas, P. E., Bandiera, S., Maines, S. L., Ryan, D. E., and Levin, W. (1987): Regulation of cytochrome P450j, a high-affinity *N*-nitrosodimethylamine demethylase, in rat hepatic microsomes. *Biochemistry*, 26:2280–2289.

414. Thomas, P. E., Koreniowski, D., Ryan, D., and Levin, W. (1979): Preparation of monospecific antibodies against two forms of rat liver cytochrome P450 and quantitation of these antigens in microsomes. *Arch. Biochem. Biophys.*, 192:524–532.

415. Thomas, P. E., Lu, A. Y. H., West, S. B., Ryan, D., Miwa, G. T., and Levin, W. (1977): Accessibility of cytochrome P450 in microsomal membranes: Inhibition of metabolism by antibodies to cytochrome P450. *Mol. Pharmacol.*, 13:819–831.

416. Thomas, P. E., Reidy, J., Reik, L. M., Ryan, D. E., Koop, D. R., and Levin, W. (1984): Use of monoclonal antibody probes against rat hepatic cytochromes P450c and P450d to detect immunochemically related isozymes in liver microsomes from different species. *Arch. Biochem. Biophys.*, 235:239–253.

417. Thomas, P. E., Ryan, D., and Levin, W. (1976): An improved staining procedure for the detection of the peroxidase activity of cytochrome P450 on sodium dodecyl sulfate polyacrylamide gels. *Anal. Biochem.*, 75:168–176.

418. Thomaszewski, J. E., Jerina, D. M., Levin, W., and Conney, A. H. (1976): A highly senstivive radiometric assay for zoxazolamine hydroxylation by liver microsomal cytochrome P450 and P-448: Properties of the membrane-bound and purified reconstituted system. *Arch. Biochem. Biophys.*, 176:788–798.

419. Thorgeirsson, S. S., Jollow, D. J., Sasame, H. A., Green, I., and Mitchell, J. R. (1973): The role of cytochrome P450 in *N*-hydroxylation of 2-acetylaminofluorene. *Mol. Pharmacol.*, 9:398–404.

420. Towbin, H., and Gordon, J. (1984): Immunoblotting and dot immunobinding—Current status and outlook. *J. Immunol. Methods*, 72:313–340.

421. Towbin, H., Staehelin, T., and Gordon, J. (1979): Electrophoretic transfer of proteins from polyacrylamide gels to nitrocellulose sheets: Procedure and some applications. *Proc. Natl. Acad. Sci. USA*, 76:4350–4354.

422. Tunek, A., Platt, K. L., Bentley, P., and Oesch, F. (1978): Microsomal metabolism of benzene to species irreversibly binding to microsomal protein and effects to modifications of this metabolism. *Mol. Pharmacol.*, 14:920–929.

423. Turesky, R. J., Lang, N. P., Butler, M. A., Teitel, C. H., and Kadlubar, F. F. (1991): Metabolic activation of carcinogenic heterocyclic amines by human liver and colon. *Carcinogenesis*, 12:1839–1845.

424. Tynes, R. E., and Philpot, R. M. (1987): Tissue- and species-dependent expression of multiple forms of mammalian microsomal flavin-containing monooxygenase. *Mol. Pharmacol.*, 31:569–574.

425. Tzeng, H.-F., Laughlin, L. T., Lin, S., and Armstrong, R. N. (1996): The catalytic mechanism of microsomal epoxide hydrolase involves reversible formation and rate-limiting hydrolysis of the alkyl-enzyme intermediate. *J. Am. Chem. Soc.*, 118:9436–9437.

426. Udenfriend, S. (1969): *Fluoresence Assay in Biology and Medicine*. Academic Press, New York.

427. Udenfriend, S., Stein, S., Böhlen, P., Dairman, W., Leimgruber, W., and Weigele, M. (1972): Fluorescamine: A reagent for assay of amino acids, peptides, proteins, and primary amines in the picomole range. *Science*, 178:871–872.

428. Ueng, Y.-F., Shimada, T., Yamazaki, H., and Guengerich, F. P. (1995): Oxidation of aflatoxin B_1 by bacterial recombinant human cytochrome P450 enzymes. *Chem. Res. Toxicol.*, 8:218–225.

429. Ullrich, V., and Weber, P. (1972): The *O*-dealkylation of 7-ethoxycoumarin by liver microsomes. *Z. Physiol. Chem.*, 353:1171–1177.

430. van Bladeren, P. J., Breimer, D. D., van Huijgevoort, J. A. T. C. M., Vermeulen, N. P. E., and van der Gen, A. (1981): The metabolic formation of *N*-acetyl-*S*-2-hydroxyethyl-L-cysteine from tetradeutero-1,2-dibromoethane. Relative importance of oxidation and glutathione conjugation in vivo. *Biochem. Pharmacol.*, 30:2499–2502.

431. van der Hoeven, T. (1977): A sensitive fluorometric method for the assay of microsomal hydroxylase: *N*-Demethylation of *p*-chloro-*N*-methylaniline. *Anal. Biochem.*, 77:523–528.

432. van der Hoeven, T. A., and Coon, M. J. (1974): Preparation and properties of partially purified cytochrome P450 and reduced nicotinamide adenine dinucleotide phosphate-cytochrome P450 reductase from rabbit liver microsomes. *J. Biol. Chem.*, 249:6302–6310.

433. Vatsis, K. P., and Weber, W. W. (1996): Acetyltransferases. In: *Biotransformation, Vol. 3, Comprehensive Toxicology*, edited by F. P. Guengerich, pp. 385–399. Elsevier Science, Oxford.

434. Vermilion, J. L., and Coon, M. J. (1978): Purified liver microsomal NADPH-cytochrome P450 reductase: Spectral characterization of oxidation–reduction states. *J. Biol. Chem.*, 253:2694–2704.

435. Vlasuk, G. P., and Walz, F. G., Jr. (1980): Liver endoplasmic reticulum polypeptides resolved by two-dimensional gel electrophoresis. *Anal. Biochem.*, 105:112–120.

436. Wahl, G. M., Meinkoth, J. L., and Kimmel, A. R. (1987): Northern and Southern blots. *Methods Enzymol.*, 572:581.

437. Wallin, H., Schelin, C., Tunek, A., and Jergil, B. (1981): A rapid and sensitive method for determination of covalent binding of benzo[a]pyrene to proteins. *Chem. Biol. Interact.*, 38:109–118.

438. Walsh, C. (1979): *Enzymatic Reaction Mechanisms*. W. H. Freeman, San Francisco.

439. Wang, P., Mason, P. S., and Guengerich, F. P. (1980): Purification of human liver cytochrome P450 and comparison to the enzyme isolated from rat liver. *Arch. Biochem. Biophys.*, 199:206–219.

440. Wang, P. P., Beaune, P., Kaminsky, L. S., Dannan, G. A., Kadlubar, F. F., Larrey, D., and Guengerich, F. P. (1983): Purification and characterization of six cytochrome P450 isozymes from human liver microsomes. *Biochemistry*, 22:5375–5383.

441. Wang, R. W., and Lu, A. Y. H. (1997): Inhibitory anti-peptide antibody against human CYP3A4. *Drug Metab. Dispos.*, 25:762–767.

442. Wang, R. W., Pickett, C. B., and Lu, A. Y. H. (1989): Expression of a cDNA encoding a rat liver glutathione *S*-transferase Y_a subunit in *Escherichia coli*. *Arch. Biochem. Biophys.*, 269:536–543.

443. Watabe, T. and Akamatsu, K. (1974): Photometric assay of hepatic epoxide hydrolase activity with safrole oxide (SAFO) as substrate. *Biochem. Pharmacol.*, 23:2839–2844.
444. Waterman, M. R. and Guengerich, F. P. (1997): Enzyme regulation. In: *Biotransformation, Vol. 3, Comprehensive Toxicology*, edited by F. P. Guengerich, pp. 7–14. Elsevier Science, Oxford.
445. Waterman, M. R., and Johnson, E. F. (1991): *Methods in Enzymology, Vol. 206, Cytochrome P450*. Academic Press, San Diego.
446. Waxman, D. J., Dannan, G. A., and Guengerich, F. P. (1985): Regulation of rat hepatic cytochrome P450: Age-dependent expression, hormonal imprinting, and xenobiotic inducibility of sex-specific isoenzymes. *Biochemistry*, 24:4409–4417.
447. Weber, W. W. (1971): *N*-Acetyltransferase (mammalian liver). *Methods Enzymol.*, 17B:805–811.
448. Weber, W. W. (1986): Commentary: The molecular basis of hereditary acetylation polymorphisms. *Drug Metab. Dispos.*, 14:377–381.
449. Weber, W. W., and Cohen, S. N. (1968): The mechanism of isoniazid acetylation by human liver *N*-acetyltransferase. *Biochim. Biophys. Acta*, 151:276–278.
450. Weber, W. W., and Hein, D. W. (1985): *N*-Acetylation pharmacogenetics. *Pharmacol. Rev.*, 37:25–79.
451. Weber, W. W., Miceli, J. N., Hearse, D. J., and Drummond, G. S. (1976): *N*-Acetylation of drugs. Pharmacogenetic studies in rabbits selected for their acetylator characteristics. *Drug Metab. Dispos.*, 4:904–911.
452. Weinshilboum, R. M., Otterness, D. M., Aksoy, I. A., Wood, T. C., Her, C., and Raftogianis, R. B. (1997): Sulfotransferase molecular biology: cDNAs and genes. *FASEB J.*, 11:3–14.
453. Weisiger, R. A., and Jakoby, W. B. (1979): Thiol *S*-methyltransferase from rat liver. *Arch. Biochem. Biophys.*, 196:631–637.
454. Weyler, W., and Salach, J. I. (1985): Purification and properties of mitochondrial monoamine oxidase type A from human placenta. *J. Biol. Chem.*, 260:13199–13207.
455. White, K. A., and Marletta, M. A. (1992): Nitric oxide synthase is a cytochrome P450 type hemoprotein. *Biochemistry*, 31:6627–6631.
456. White, P. A., and Rasmussen, J. B. (1996): SOS chromotest results in a broader context: Empirical relationships between genotoxic potency, mutagenic potency, and carcinogenic potency. *Environ. Mol. Mutagen.*, 27:270–305.
457. White, P. C., New, M. I., and Dupont, B. (1984): HLA-linked congenital adrenal hyperplasia results from a defective gene encoding a cytochrome P450 specific for steroid 21-hydroxylation. *Proc. Natl. Acad. Sci. USA*, 81:7505–7509.
458. Williams, D. E., Hale, S. E., Muerhoff, A. S., and Masters, B. S. S. (1985): Rabbit lung flavin-containing monooxygenase: Purification, characterization, and induction during pregnancy. *Mol. Pharmacol.*, 28:381–390.
459. Winge, D. R., Nielson, K. B., Zeikus, R. D., and Gray, W. R. (1984): Structural characterization of the isoforms of neonatal and adult rat liver metallothionein. *J. Biol. Chem.*, 259:11419–11425.
460. Wislocki, P. G., Miwa, G. T., and Lu, A. Y. H. (1980): Reactions catalyzed by the cytochrome P450 system. In: *Enzymatic Basis of Detoxication*, Vol. 1, edited by W. B. Jakoby, pp. 135–182. Academic Press, New York.
461. Wolff, T., Distlerath, L. M., Worthington, M. T., Groopman, J. D., Hammons, G. J., Kadlubar, F. F., Prough, R. A., Martin, M. V., and Guengerich, F. P. (1985): Substrate specificity of human liver cytochrome P450 debrisoquine 4-hydroxylase probed using immunochemical inhibition and chemical modeling. *Cancer Res.*, 45:2116–2122.
462. Wong, L. C. K., Winston, J. M., Hong, C. B., and Plotnick, H. (1982): Carcinogenicity and toxicity of 1,2-dibromoethane in the rat. *Toxicol. Appl. Pharmacol.*, 63:155–165.
463. Wood, A. W., Levin, W., Lu, A. Y. H., Yagi, H., Hernandez, O., Jerina, D. M., and Conney, A. H. (1976): Metabolism of benzo[a]pyrene and benzo[a]pyrene derivatives to mutagenic products by highly purified hepatic microsomal enzymes. *J. Biol. Chem.*, 251:4882–4890.
464. Wrighton, S. A., Brian, W. R., Sari, M. A., Iwasaki, M., Guengerich, F. P., Raucy, J. L., Molowa, D. T., and VandenBranden, M. (1990): Studies on the expression and metabolic capabilities of human liver cytochrome P450IIIA5 (HLp3). *Mol. Pharmacol.*, 38:207–213.
465. Yagi, H., Thakker, D. R., Hernandez, O., Koreeda, M., and Jerina, D. M. (1977): Synthesis and reactions of the highly mutagenic 7,8-diol 9,10-epoxides of the carcinogen benzo[a]pyrene. *J. Am. Chem. Soc.*, 99:1604–1611.
466. Yamazaki, H., Inui, Y., Yun, C-H., Mimura, M., Guengerich, F. P., and Shimada, T. (1992): Cytochrome P450 2E1 and 2A6 enzymes as major catalysts for metabolic activation of *N*-nitrosodialkylamines and tobacco-related nitrosamines in human liver microsomes. *Carcinogenesis*, 13:1789–1794.
467. Yamazoe, Y., Shimada, M., Maeda, K., Kamataki, T., and Kato, R. (1984): Specificity of four forms of cytochrome P450 in the metabolic activation of several aromatic amines and benzo[a]pyrene. *Xenobiotica*, 14:549–552.
468. Yasukochi, Y., and Masters, B. S. S. (1976): Some properties of a detergent-solubilized NADPH-cytochrome *c* (cytochrome P450) reductase purified by biospecific affinity chromatography. *J. Biol. Chem.*, 251:5337–5344.
469. Yoo, J. S. H., Cheung, R. J., Patten, C. J., Wade, D., and Yang, C. S. (1987): Nature of *N*-nitrosodimethylamine demethylase and its inhibitors. *Cancer Res.*, 47:3378–3383.
470. Yoo, J. S. H., Guengerich, F. P., and Yang, C. S. (1988): Metabolism of *N*-nitrosodialkylamines by human liver microsomes. *Cancer Res.*, 48:1499–1504.
471. Ziegler, D. M. (1980): Microsomal flavin-containing monooxygenase: Oxygenation of nucleophilic nitrogen and sulfur compounds. In: *Enzymatic Basis of Detoxication*, Vol. 1, edited by W. B. Jakoby, pp. 201–227. Academic Press, New York.
472. Ziegler, D. M. (1988): Flavin-containing monooxygenases: Catalytic mechanism and substrate specificities. *Drug Metab. Rev.*, 19:1–32.
473. Ziegler, D. M. (1993): Recent studies on the structure and function of multisubstrate flavin-containing monooxygenases. *Annu. Rev. Pharmacol. Toxicol.*, 33:179–199.
474. Ziegler, D. M., and Mitchell, C. H. (1972): Microsomal oxidase IV: Properties of a mixed-function amine oxidase isolated from pig liver microsomes. *Arch. Biochem. Biophys.*, 150:116–125.
475. Ziegler, D. M., and Pettit, F. H. (1964): Formation of an intermediate *N*-oxide in the oxidative demethylation of *N,N*-dimethylaniline catalyzed by liver microsomes. *Biochem. Biophys. Res. Commun.*, 15:188–193.
476. Zuber, M. X., Simpson, E. R., and Waterman, M. R. (1986): Expression of bovine 17α-hydroxylase cytochrome P450 cDNA in nonsteroidogenic (COS 1) cells. *Science*, 234:1258–1261.

Principles and Methods of Toxicology,
Fourth Edition, edited by A. Wallace Hayes.
Taylor & Francis, Philadelphia © 2001.

Chapter **36**

Modern Instrumental Methods for Studying Mechanisms of Toxicology

William S. Caldwell, Gary D. Byrd, J. Donald deBethizy, and Peter A. Crooks

The mechanisms underlying an organism's response to a toxic insult are usually complex, involving the toxicant itself, metabolites derived from it, and a host of tissue-derived endogenous compounds. A key to understanding these mechanisms lies in the ability to monitor the chemical changes that result from intoxication. In fact, the ability to monitor chemical changes associated with intoxication has often been the factor that limited our mechanistic understanding of toxicity. The development of gas chromatography in the 1950s and 1960s extended the lower range for detecting chemical changes in organisms and in the environment. The realization that exposure to chemicals such as DDT was widespread and that these chemicals could concentrate in the food chain fueled the development of modern toxicology. The result of this early development in instrumental analysis has been the subsequent development of a host of powerful instruments that have increased our ability to define the mechanism of toxicity better than ever before. However, each instrumental method has its strengths and limitations. It is important for toxicologists to have knowledge of these methods and an understanding of the types of studies for which each is suited.

This chapter is not intended to be a comprehensive survey of all modern instrumental methods. Rather, it focuses on those techniques that are likely to be most useful to toxicologists. Some of these techniques, such as mass spectrometry and nuclear magnetic resonance spectroscopy, are widely used in toxicology. Others, such as near infrared spectroscopy, are not commonly used but have tremendous potential for future studies. Emphasis has been placed on practical applications, not in-depth theoretical considerations. The discussion which follows serves as a starting point for further study and the interested reader is encouraged to make use of the references cited in the text to gain a more in-depth understanding of modern instrumental methods.

MASS SPECTROMETRY

Mass spectrometry is an analytical technique that determines the mass of ionized molecules and their fragments and adducts. It is perhaps the most generally applicable tool in chemical analysis and the method of choice for many specific analytical procedures. In addition to its application as a universal detector in qualitative analysis, mass spectrometry can be fine-tuned to quantify specific components at trace levels in complex mixtures. Mass spectrometers are often part of a hyphenated analytical system where chromatography (usually gas or liquid) precedes mass spectrometric detection.

Mass spectrometry has impacted biomedical, environmental, and toxicological research, including the study of toxic substances and their fate in the body. Considerable progress has been made in toxicology using mass spectrometry as an analytical tool. This section looks at the basic principles of mass spectrometry, new trends in the field, and some examples of where mass spectrometry has been applied to toxicology studies, such as elucidation of detoxification mechanisms and exposure assessment. This is not a comprehensive review of recent breakthroughs in the area as much as it is a starting point for the curious student of the art. A good text covering routine techniques in mass spectrometry with consideration of biochemical applications has been written by Johnstone and Rose (66).

Mass Spectrometers and Mass Spectra

There are many different types of mass spectrometers (35) but a few features are common to them all. Ions, unlike neutral compounds, can be manipulated by electromagnetic forces so that a separation by mass-to-charge (m/z) ratio is possible. A mass spectrometer is a device that creates ions from sample molecules, separates them by m/z, and determines the number of ions at each particular ratio. The mass spectrum is a plot of m/z ratio on the X-axis versus relative ion abundances (RA) on the Y-axis. The mass spectrum can give molecular weight and structural information about the compound that was ionized. Ions are normally produced with single charges ($z = 1$) so that the m/z ratio gives the mass in Daltons (Da) of intact molecules and fragments directly. A simple model of a molecule AB undergoing ionization is shown below:

$$AB \rightarrow \text{Ionization process} \rightarrow AB^{+\cdot} + A^{+} + B^{+}$$

The ionization process in this case produces a molecular ion $AB^{+\cdot}$ (usually designated as $M^{+\cdot}$) that is the sample molecule with an electron removed. Often, enough energy is imparted in the process so that a portion of the molecular ions decompose to form various stable fragment ions as shown by A^{+} and B^{+} above. The mass spectrum shows the mass and abundance of each of these fragments (see Figure 36.1). The spectrum is highly characteristic of a particular compound and has been likened to a "fingerprint" that can be used for identification purposes. Mass spectra of compounds with known structures are continuously reported and compiled so that patterns of fragmentation are established. This knowledge is useful

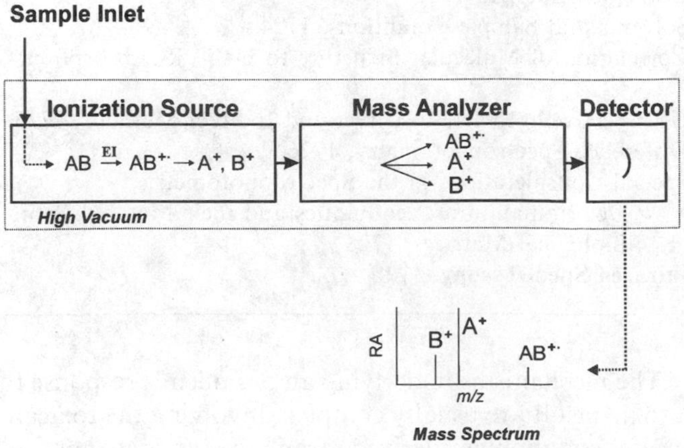

FIG. 36.1. Schematic of a basic mass spectrometer system interfaced to an inlet.

in interpreting spectra of unknown compounds. In addition, computerized searches of mass spectral databases can greatly facilitate compound identification. The sensitivity of conventional mass spectrometers permits good spectra to be obtained on less than 10 nanograms of material. So, although the ionization process destroys the sample, the mass spectrometer requires very small amounts of material for analysis.

Instrumental Design

Basic Configuration

There are many different types of mass spectrometers; they vary in size and complexity from small bench top units to large multiple-sector machines (35). Nevertheless, mass spectrometers can all be broken into a few basic components and their functions: sample introduction, ion production, mass analysis, and ion detection. These components are shown schematically in Figure 36.1. The hardware components from ion source to detector are housed in a high-vacuum chamber to provide the necessary mean free path for ions to travel from the source to the detector. Typical vacuum for a commercial mass spectrometer is less than 10^{-6} Torr.

Inlet Systems

Samples are introduced into the mass spectrometer vacuum housing via some type of inlet. The inlet selected depends on the sample, the nature of the sample matrix, and the type of ionization desired. Many mass spectrometers are designed with multiple inlets to accommodate a wide variety of samples with minimal time required for instrument reconfiguration.

For stable solid materials, the simplest means of introduction is to place the sample onto a long probe that is inserted directly into the ion source through a valve. This is commonly referred to as a direct-inlet probe or "DIP." Heating the probe volatilizes the sample into the gas phase where it can be ionized easily, usually by energetic electrons. The DIP method is very sensitive and can produce spectra from sub-microgram quantities of material; however, some materials such as glutathione conjugates are not easily volatilized and decompose on the probe. Analytes that occur in mixtures may require some separation before DIP analysis. Although some separation of components in time is achieved by heating the probe slowly, it is a crude means of separation and works best on reasonably pure samples. Probes are also used in conjunction with other ionization techniques where they serve merely to place the sample in a position to be ionized. Examples of this would be fast atom bombardment (FAB) or laser desorption (LD) which are described later in this chapter.

Chromatographic separation techniques coupled to the source add another dimension of analysis and most mass spectrometer systems used in biological sciences are configured in this manner. Gas chromatography–mass spectrometry (GC–MS) has worked very well in this regard, making GC–MS perhaps the most common hyphenated method for performing organic analysis (99,102). Although applications with packed gas chromatography columns are still reported with various types of interfaces, most GC–MS is performed with fused silica capillary columns. These columns use gas flows of 1–2 mL/min and the ends can be placed directly into the ionization source. High-resolution chromatography of reasonably volatile and thermally stable samples is possible with these columns.

Because many compounds will not pass through a gas chromatograph, liquid chromatography–mass spectrometry (LC–MS) has been developed as an alternative method for introducing analytes dissolved in solution into the mass spectrometer. In fact, because biological samples are usually aqueous-based and include thermally labile and polar substances, LC–MS now rivals GC–MS in popularity. This is due to the development and refinement of many reliable interfaces in the last two decades. High-performance liquid chromatography (HPLC) methods using a variety of columns and flow rates have used mass spectrometry as a detector. General procedures are well documented for LC–MS techniques (164,171).

A relatively new chromatographic technique now used with mass spectrometry is *capillary electrophoresis* (CE) (74). A high electrical field in a small-diameter capillary tube filled with aqueous solution is used to separate charged compounds. CE offers the advantages of high-resolution, low sample consumption, and short analysis times. It is well suited to the analysis of ions in solution. Interfacing to the mass spectrometer is often accomplished through electrospray ionization or continuous flow-fast atom bombardment, which are described below.

Ionization Sources For Volatile Compounds

This discussion of ionization sources is divided into two parts based on the volatility of the compound of interest. It might well be divided into the same parts based on two popular chromatography methods interfaced to mass spectrometers: GC and LC. Because mass spectrometry was originally limited to volatile samples, these types of ionization sources are considered "conventional." Volatile samples are introduced directly into the ion source using a leak valve for gases, a heated DIP described earlier for solids, or a GC. This section describes methods used in these types of applications.

The most established means of ionization for volatile samples is electron impact (EI) in which a sample is volatilized into the gas phase and passes through a beam of energetic (70 eV) electrons boiled from a filament.

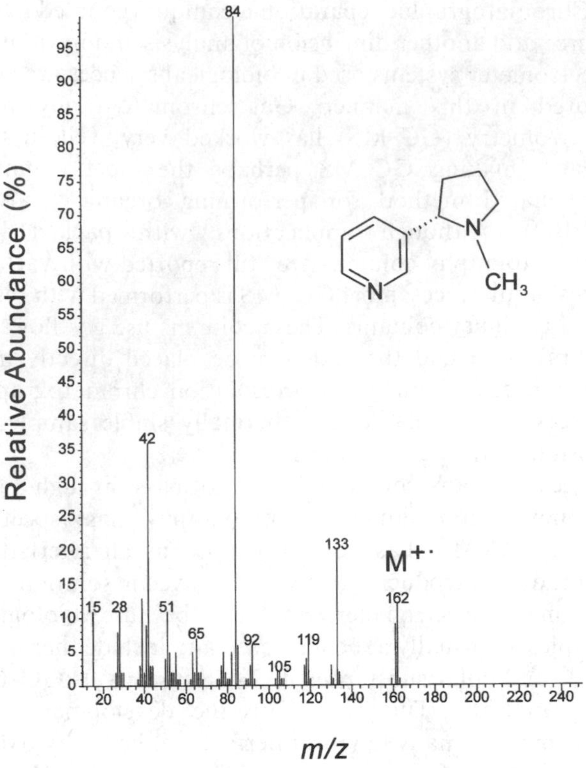

FIG. 36.2. Electron impact mass spectrum of nicotine. Data acquired on a quadrupole GC–MS system.

The process may be written as:

$$M + e^- \rightarrow M^{+\cdot} + 2e^-$$

The high-energy electron displaces an electron from molecule M, which may remain intact as the molecular ion $M^{+\cdot}$, and thus provide direct molecular weight information. The energetics of the process can also cause fragmentation of the molecule. Fragmentation patterns are related to the structure of the molecule and thus can be interpreted as representative of that compound. As an example, Figure 36.2 shows the EI mass spectrum of nicotine identified in an extract of urine from a smoker. The highest mass ion in the spectrum is m/z 162, which is the molecular ion. The most abundant peak in the spectrum (referred to as the base peak) is m/z 84 and results from cleavage of the bond between the two rings with the charge remaining with the pyrrolidine ring.

EI has several advantages. Both fragment and molecular ions are produced in most EI spectra. The mass spectra are fairly reproducible from one instrument to the next, which makes it possible to match sample spectra to reference EI mass spectra with some certainty. Several large mass spectral databases of compounds are available that can be readily searched against an EI spectrum produced on most types of mass spectrometers. Some disadvantages of EI include thc occasional lack of a molecular ion for some compounds, the difficulty of distinguishing between mass spectra of isomers, and limited application to samples with sufficient gas phase volatility and thermal stability.

An alternative ionization method called chemical ionization (CI) can be used in cases where the molecular ion is weak or not present in the EI mass spectrum. This process derives its name from the use of gas phase chemical reactions to produce ions from the sample (109). There are two types of chemical ionization, positive ion chemical ionization (PICI or PCI) and negative ion chemical ionization (NICI or NCI). In both cases, the ionization is softer than EI, resulting in less fragmentation. PICI is most often accomplished through a gas phase proton transfer reaction. The ion source is flooded with a reagent gas, usually methane, at a relatively high pressure (1 Torr). During electron bombardment under these conditions, a series of gas phase reactions occur as depicted below for reagent gas methane and sample molecule M:

$$CH_4 \rightarrow CH_4^{+\cdot}$$
$$CH_4^{+\cdot} + CH_4 \rightarrow CH_5^{+\cdot} + CH_3\cdot$$
$$CH_5^{+\cdot} + M \rightarrow CH_4 + (M + H)^+$$

Methane molecular ions formed in the high-pressure source collide with neutral reagent molecules (CH_4) and produce protonated methane. CH_5^+ acts as a strong Brönsted acid and transfers a proton to the sample molecule to produce the protonated molecular adduct $(M{+}H)^+$. PICI works best for samples with a relatively high proton affinity such as those containing a heteroatom. Fewer fragment ions and more abundant molecular ions characterize PICI mass spectra. In addition, sensitivity is enhanced relative to EI. The higher source pressure used, however, contaminates the instrument more rapidly and results in more frequent maintenance. Also, some modifications to the source are usually required when switching from EI to CI operation.

NICI sources operate under high-pressure conditions similar to those for PICI with voltages switched to detect negative ions. The underlying ionization processes, however, are somewhat different. Several processes can occur to form negative ions. A common method is "electron capture" which uses the reagent gas as a buffer to reduce the energy of electrons so that a molecule with a suitable electron affinity can capture an electron as shown below:

$$M + CH_4 + e^- \rightarrow M^{-}\cdot + CH_4$$

This process is rather selective because not every molecule will readily form a stable $M^-\cdot$.

Another process is adduct formation where a background anion such as Cl^- will attach to a molecule to form $(M + Cl)^-$. A variety of ion–molecule reactions are possible and some can be rather complex. Proton abstraction is common and works well for samples with an acidic proton. Negative ion formation can be enhanced using derivatization to form an analog with a high electron affinity. The sensitivity and selectivity of such assays can be very high. For example, one group reports conversion of nicotine using heptafluorobutyric anhydride to a stable electron scavenger derivative that can be detected at the femtogram (10^{-15} g) level on column (36).

Ionization Sources for Nonvolatile Compounds

This section describes ionization sources for compounds that cannot be volatilized sufficiently for EI ionization, particularly those that decompose upon heating. These include very polar and/or very large molecules such as those encountered in biological samples. For these types of samples, LC is preferred over GC for chromatographic separation. There are a number of interfaces that deal with samples in solution such as those that emerge from an HPLC column. Before introduction into the high vacuum of the mass spectrometer, most of the solvent molecules must be removed and the sample molecules ionized. Heat, nebulization with gas, and differential pumping are techniques used to remove the solvent. Ionization of the sample molecules can occur by a variety of different methods as described in this section. Some methods, like particle beam, have distinct ionization steps and others, like electrospray, have ion formation inherent in the process. With the exception of particle beam, LC–MS ionization methods are "soft" like chemical ionization and produce mostly molecular adduct ions.

Perhaps one of the more intriguing methods of ionization, electrospray (ES) simply transfers an existing ion from solution into the gas phase by using a high electric field (70). Figure 36.3 is a schematic of an ES interface. The LC effluent passes through a capillary needle that is maintained at a high applied voltage (2–5 kV). At low flows (1–10 μl/min), the high electrical field at the tip produces a mist of charged droplets at

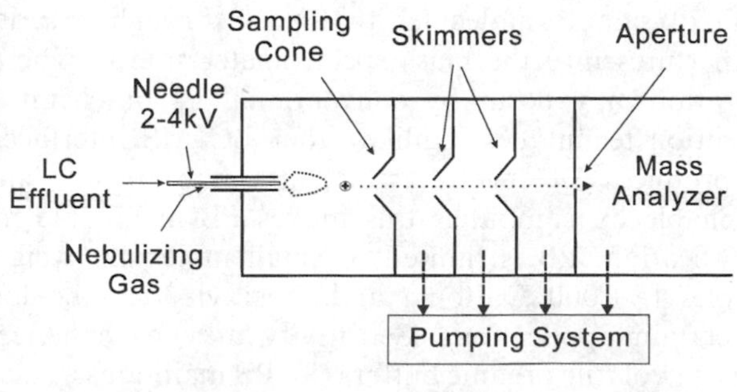

FIG. 36.3. Schematic diagram of ES ionization source interfaced to a mass spectrometer.

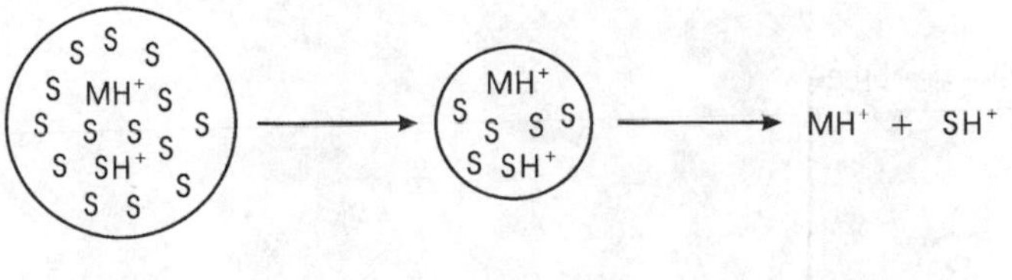

FIG. 36.4. The electrospray ionization process.

atmospheric pressure. For higher flow rates, a nebulizing gas delivered coaxially to the needle assists production of the mist. As evaporation decreases droplet size, ions are ejected as depicted for sample molecules M and solvent molecules S in Figure 36.4. Of course, the analyte must already exist as an ion in solution but this is easily accomplished by adjusting the pH. Positive ions are shown above, but the process works equally well for negative ions.

The ions are swept through a sampling cone and passed through a differential pumping system to remove solvent and nebulizing gas molecules before the ions enter the mass analyzer through a tiny aperture. ES is a very gentle ionization method and can be used with either small or large molecules. Figure 36.5 shows an ES spectrum of the glucuronide conjugate of cotinine, a phase II metabolite of nicotine. This thermally labile compound produces $(M + H)^+$ as the base peak at m/z 353. In comparison, a thermospray mass spectrum (discussed below) of this same compound yields mostly the protonated aglycon fragment (20,21). An interesting feature of ES is the ability to produce ions with multiple charges. Because mass spectra are plotted with m/z, this permits the available mass range of the analyzer to extend to thousands of Daltons. (For example, a compound with $(M + H)^+$ at m/z 5,000 would have $(M + 5H)^{+5}$ at nominal m/z 1,001). This feature is less useful for small molecules such as common pharmaceuticals and their metabolites but is very useful for macromolecules such as proteins. ES works well with aqueous mobile phases and some organic solvents. To achieve the low flows necessary with ES (usually <100 μL/min) when using conventional HPLC methods with high flows (0.5–2 mL/min), the effluent is split prior to the interface.

Atmospheric pressure chemical ionization (APCI) shares the same atmospheric pressure interface as ES but uses a different probe for producing ions (28). Instead of the capillary needle in Figure 36.3, APCI introduces the LC effluent to a heated tube (400–550°C) where the solvent and samples are volatilized at atmospheric pressure. A nebulizing gas (nitrogen) is used to assist with volatilization. A discharge needle after the heated tube creates a plasma where reagent ions and electrons are produced. Chemical ionization occurs in the gas phase to produce protonated and other molecular adducts. APCI is rugged, reliable, and very sensitive due to

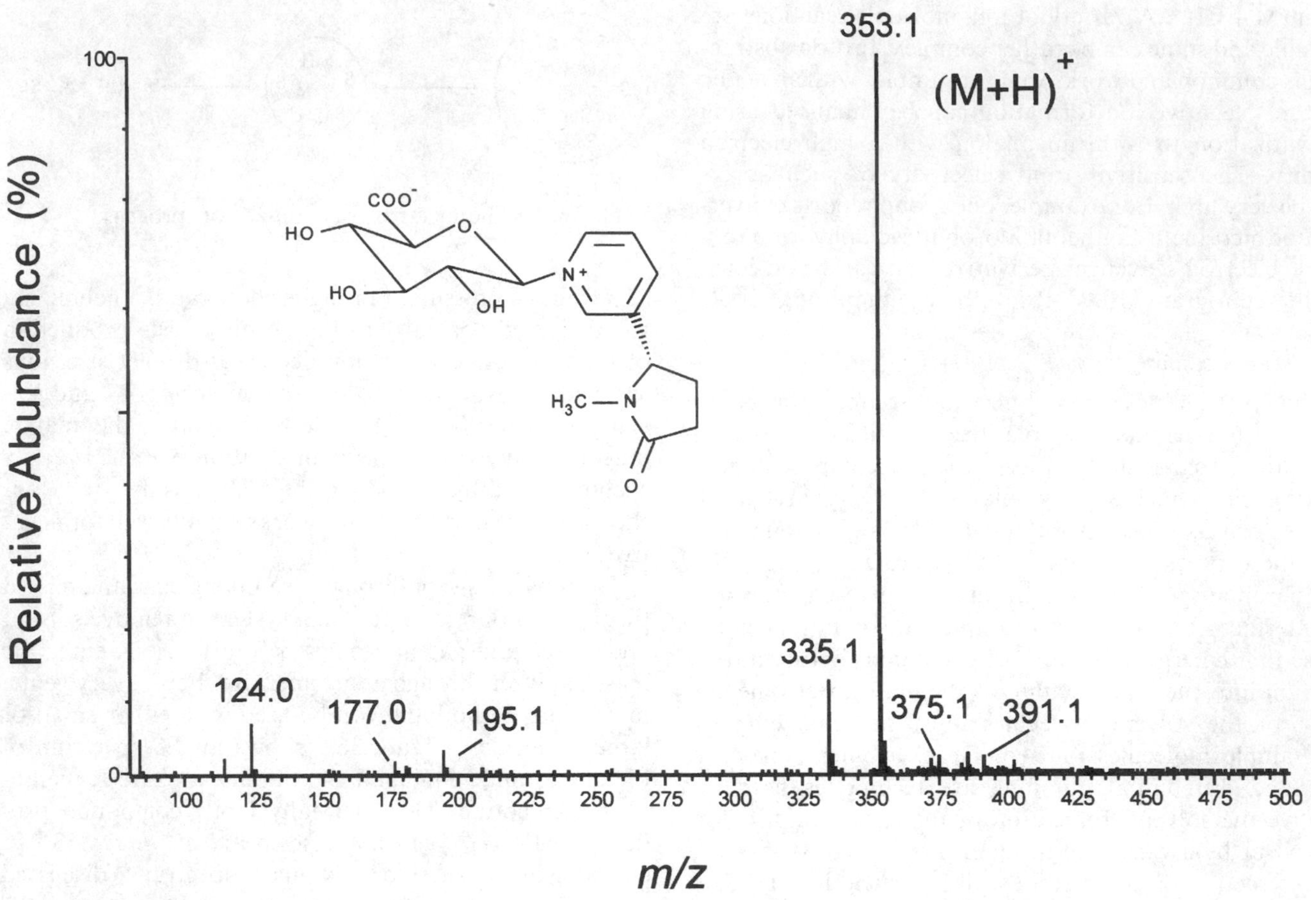

FIG. 36.5. ES mass spectrum of cotinine-N-glucuronide taken with a quadrupole mass analyzer.

efficient ionization, especially for molecules with heteroatoms. The rapid heating does produce some thermal degradation of labile species. APCI can accommodate HPLC flows of 2 mL/min and works well with most types of solvents.

One of the first widely applied interfaces developed for LC–MS was thermospray (TS) (12). The LC effluent passes through a narrow metal tube whose tip is maintained at a high temperature (100–200°C) by resistive heating. The heated liquid volatizes and forms a spray in a reduced pressure chamber. Ions in solution are desorbed from the shrinking droplet in the spray; some gas phase chemical ionization reactions also occur. The LC effluent must contain an ionizing buffer such as ammonium acetate to produce ions and precise temperature control of the probe is crucial for TS operation. An optional filament placed near the probe tip can be used to increase ionization in some cases. The spray passes a conical aperture where ions are directed into the mass analyzer. TS works best with aqueous mobile phases such as those used in reversed-phase HPLC. Numerous applications of TS LC–MS have been published (171). The strengths of TS are its simplicity and broad applicability to many types of samples. Like APCI, however, the high temperatures required for volatilization can degrade thermally labile samples. TS applications have decreased in the past few years due primarily to the success of APCI and ES techniques discussed previously.

The particle beam (PB) interface is not an ionization source as much as it is a solvent removal system prior to introducing the sample into a conventional EI source (24,163). The LC effluent is first mixed with a gas (usually helium) to create an aerosol in a heated chamber. Selective evaporation and removal of solvent leaves a beam of sample molecules that pass through a series of apertures into the mass spectrometer source. There, ionization may occur by conventional EI or chemical ionization techniques. Unlike other LC–MS interfaces, PB produces EI spectra, which are reproducible and searchable by computer; this makes PB invaluable for identification. PB is limited to small molecular weight samples (<1,000 Daltons) and sensitivity can be low for certain applications. Sensitivity may be enhanced by using volatile organic buffers (8). PB maintains a small market niche for certain industrial and environmental applications.

Continuous flow fast atom bombardment (CFFAB), sometimes called dynamic FAB or liquid secondary ion mass spectrometry (SIMS), allows the LC effluent to flow directly across the target area of a FAB probe (25). The target is bombarded with fast atoms or ions and the sample is ionized by a desorption process. The LC effluent enters the probe at a very low flow rate ($<10\ \mu$L/min). It is mixed with a matrix material such as glycerol to facilitate the ionization process. Like ES described above, it is a very gentle method of ionization. CFFAB is usually used on sector instruments with capillary LC columns for separation. CFFAB is not preferred as a general method because ionization of the sample depends on the matrix. It is good for certain classes of compounds such as peptides.

For all of these interfaces, an important consideration in coupling an HPLC method to a mass spectrometer is mobile phase compatibility. Popular LC–MS mobile phase solvents are water, methanol, and acetonitrile. They are good solvents for a wide range of samples and their low molecular weights reduce background ions in the mass spectrometer. Organic modifiers such as triethylamine, which are often used to improve chromatography, should be avoided because they can suppress ionization of sample molecules. Even though many of the interface/ionization sources listed here work best with a buffer at low concentrations (<20 mM), it must be a volatile organic buffer such as ammonium formate or ammonium acetate that will not leave deposits that block the apertures leading to the mass analyzer. Some recent work has been done on two-stage orthogonal sampling that permits "harsh" mobile phases like potassium phosphate buffers to be used (for example, the commercial "Z-spray" interface offered by Micromass, Manchester, UK). This is extremely useful when adapting existing HPLC methods to a mass spectrometer.

Other Ionization Sources

The bombardment of solid or liquid surfaces with intense light from a laser offers a soft means of ionizing nonvolatile, thermally labile compounds. This technique is called laser desorption. In matrix-assisted laser desorption ionization (MALDI) (69), the sample is suspended in a matrix material that absorbs light near the wavelength of the laser. Absorption of the energy desorbs and ionizes the analytes in the matrix resulting in molecular adducts such as $(M+H)^+$ or $(M+Na)^+$ with little fragmentation. MALDI is used with isolated samples rather than on-line chromatography.

In addition to organic and bioanalytical analyses, mass spectrometry used for elemental analysis figures prominently in toxicology (60). Unlike organic mass spectrometry, inorganic mass spectrometry is mostly concerned with atomic ions instead of molecular ions. Thus, methods have been developed for producing atomic ions of various elements from samples. A common ionization method used in inorganic mass spectrometry is thermal ionization, which takes place when an atom or molecule interacts with a heated surface. Samples are deposited directly on a filament and heated. Another method is the use of inductively coupled plasma (ICP), where the sample is volatilized, atomized, and ionized in a few milliseconds at plasma temperatures of 7000–8000 K.

An interesting field of expanding applications is accelerator mass spectrometry (AMS). Unlike the ion sources described above, AMS is a high-energy (MeV) nuclear physics technique that uses a Van de Graaf accelerator to measure very small amounts of rare and long-lived isotopes (6,156). For ^{14}C analysis, the sample is converted to graphite powder by oxidation followed by reduction. A cesium ion gun bombards the sample and the negative carbon ions produced are selected from the source and accelerated at 3–10 MeV. They pass through a thin foil or gas where electrons are stripped from C^- to create positive ions. These ions are then accelerated to several MeV, selected by a mass analyzer (quadrupole or magnet), and detected. AMS was first applied to geochemical and archeological samples, but it has seen growing biomedical applications, particularly in the monitoring of ^{14}C-labeled drugs. The high sensitivity of this method (10^{-18} mole) permits low doses of labeled materials to be monitored in humans.

Mass Analyzers

Mass analysis is the process by which a mixture of ions is separated according to their m/z ratios. There are several types of mass analyzers commonly used and these form the primary differences among various mass spectrometer systems. Each analyzer uses electric or magnetic fields or both for separating ions. Although there are many experimental combinations and variations, this section will briefly describe popular commercial models and the basis of their operation.

There are two basic modes of scanning for mass spectrometers: repetitive scanning and selected ion monitoring (SIM). In repetitive scanning, a mass range is covered in a fixed interval and constantly repeated. For example, a GC/MS system might be set to scan repetitively m/z 40 to 400 in 1 sec. This would detect any compound producing ions in this mass range every second, which is necessary for a high-resolution separation technique like capillary GC. The resulting plot of all responses versus time is called a total ion chromatogram (TIC). Wide-range repetitive scanning is very useful for screening samples like body fluid extracts for all types of compounds present. The mass range may be adjusted to detect only signals of interest or to exclude interferences such as low molecular weight solvents. This procedure offers less sensitivity than

SIM but provides much more information. In addition, ion chromatograms can be produced from the stored data file. Ion chromatograms are reconstructed responses for a particular ion and are useful in quantitation to exclude interferences in complex chromatograms.

For quantifying specific analytes, it is useful to restrict the ions detected to those of interest. In the SIM mode, the analyzer scans discontinuously, rapidly switching between only a few ions does this. Because more dwell time is spent on these ions, sensitivity is increased on the order of 10 to 100 times. This technique ignores ions from background materials and is useful in quantifying analytes in fairly complex matrices. Multiple-stage analyzers are capable of several more modes of scanning and these are described later in a separate section.

The earliest mass spectrometers used a magnetic sector to deflect ion currents into a detector system. Ions accelerated into a large electromagnet sector of radius R by a high voltage V are dispersed by the magnetic field B according to:

$$m/z = (constant)\frac{\mathbf{B}^2 R^2}{V} \quad (1)$$

A spectrum is normally produced by varying B and monitoring the ions with a detector at the end to convert the impinging ions to a signal. Early magnetic sector instruments were large, heavy, expensive, and relatively slow in scanning a large m/z range. When used in combination with an electrostatic sector, these instruments can provide high mass resolution.

The most popular analyzer system used today is the quadrupole mass analyzer. These compact systems are relatively cheap and durable, and can scan very rapidly. The quadrupole assembly consists of four parallel rods arranged equidistant around a central axis. DC and radio frequency (RF) voltages are applied to opposite pairs of rods to form a fluctuating electric field. Ions formed in the source are directed and focused into this field by electrostatic lenses. Only ions with a particular m/z ratio as determined by the DC and RF field strength can pass through to the detector. Thus, the analyzer scans for particular ions by ramping these parameters. Typically, a full mass spectrum of m/z 40 to 400 can be taken in less than 1 sec with good sensitivity. A detector is located at the end of the quadrupole assembly.

By using quadrupole analyzers in series (multiple-stage quadrupoles), tandem mass spectrometry (15) is possible. Although sector instruments with magnetic and electrostatic fields can be used as stages, quadrupoles are more often used for tandem mass spectrometry. These systems operate by selecting a particular ion from the first-stage analyzer and sending it into a second stage where the ion collides with an inert gas (such as argon) to produce further fragmentation. A third stage analyzes the resulting fragments, thus producing a mass spectrum from an ion in a mass spectrum. This technique is referred to as *MS/MS* or *collision-induced dissociation* (CID) and is often used with soft ionization such as CI, ES, or APCI to produce fragments from molecular adducts. An example is given below for a molecular adduct produced by PICI:

Source	Analyzer 1	Collision Cell	Analyzer 2
$M + CH_5^+ \rightarrow$	$(M + H)^+ \rightarrow$	Argon, eV $\rightarrow$	A^+, B^+
	"Precursor"		"Products"

The selected ion is usually referred to as the "precursor" or "parent" and its fragments as "products" or "daughters." Precursors and products can be linked to establish fragmentation pathways, thereby producing additional structural information. MS/MS systems can also be set to monitor specific fragmentation pathways, a process called multiple reaction monitoring or MRM. Setting the mass analyzer for a specific transition creates a very specific detector that can monitor an analyte in very complex samples. In this regard, it is analogous to selected ion monitoring. Even though the cost of an MS/MS system is much more than for a single-stage mass spectrometer system, the increased structural information and selectivity of these instruments is very attractive. They have become workhorse systems for identifying and quantifying metabolites, particularly when interfaced to LC.

A more recent development in mass analyzers that is increasingly found in analytical laboratories is the *ion trap* (30). These mass analyzers are a type of three-dimensional quadrupole composed of a doughnut-shaped ring and two end caps. Ions are contained in the circular electromagnet by a RF field until swept into a detector by an applied RF voltage amplitude ramp. Ions are ejected according to their resonance energy, which is related to their mass, and a spectrum is thus produced. A time sequence of events produces ions in the trap and then ramps the RF field to detect specific masses. Both GC–MS and LC–MS ion trap systems are commercially available. When coupled directly to a GC, ions are formed by EI just as for a quadrupole system and switching between EI and CI modes is simple. For LC–MS, ions are usually injected into the trap from an external source such as ES. Ion traps are similar to quadrupoles in sensitivity, size, and cost, but they are also capable of MS/MS analysis. MS/MS in the ion trap is performed in a timed series of events by colliding the ions while trapped either with themselves or a collision gas. The product ions are then detected. In addition, MS/MS on the product ions may be performed such that MS/MS/MS... (MS^n) is possible. For LC–MS interfaces that produce molecular adducts, the ion trap is a less expensive option over the triple stage systems described above to perform CID analyses.

Somewhat related to the ion trap but older in use is Fourier transform mass spectrometry (FT–MS) (33). Ions are produced by EI in a cubic cell consisting of opposing pairs of trapping plates, transmitting plates, and receiving plates. Ions may also be injected into the source from an external ionization source such as ES. A high constant magnetic field and electrostatic trapping plates trap the ions formed. Each ion undergoes cyclotron motion at a frequency determined by its m/z ratio. All the ions are excited (resulting in increased radius of motion) simultaneously by applying a burst of RF energy over a range of frequencies corresponding to the cyclotron frequencies of the ions. The ions are detected simultaneously by measuring the image current induced on the detection plates of the cell. The frequencies form a beat pattern and, by Fourier transformation, the individual cyclotron frequencies of the ions are determined and the m/z values produced. Many operational aspects of FT–MS are similar to FT–NMR. High mass resolution (discussed later) is possible with these systems as is MS^n described for the ion trap above.

Time of flight (TOF) analyzers work on the simple principle that ion velocity is mass-dependent (160). A high voltage accelerates ionized sample ions down a tube and the different m/z ratios are separated in time. The arrival time at the detector is based on m/z and a mass spectrum is produced. Naturally, scan speed is very fast and mass range is unlimited. Coupled with MADLI ionization sources described above, TOF analyzers have been applied to a variety of studies in biomedical research that require the mass analysis of very large molecules. TOF mass spectrometer systems have shown a growing popularity recently due to techniques that have improved their performance, including mass resolution. TOF has been recently interfaced with LC and GC systems (58).

High-resolution mass analyzers can measure masses to within a thousandth of a mass unit, 0.001 Da, or better. The utility of this feature is based on the fact that atomic masses, while close to integral values, are not truly integral. While ^{12}C is assigned 12.000000 Da, ^{16}O is actually 15.994915 Da, ^{1}H is 1.007825 Da, ^{14}N is 14.003074 Da, and so on. Thus, high-resolution mass measurements can lead to determination of elemental composition. For example, the exact mass of nicotine ($C_{10}H_{14}N_2$) is 162.115699. Using a high-resolution mass spectrometer, its molecular ion would be distinguishable from that of another compound with a nominal m/z 162 but a different molecular formula such as p-nitrobenzyl cyanide ($C_8H_6N_2O_2 = 162.042928$). As detectors, high-resolution mass spectrometers offer more selectivity than low-resolution mass analyzers by monitoring very narrow mass ranges and thus eliminating potential interferences. Quadrupole analyzers are not capable of resolving power much in excess of 0.1 mass unit and cannot produce high-resolution spectra. The most commonly used high-resolution system is a double-focusing instrument with an electrostatic sector to first select ions of a specific kinetic energy before analysis by magnetic sector. As mentioned earlier, FT–MS and some TOF systems are capable of high-resolution mass spectra.

Ion Monitoring

Conventional mass spectrometer systems (quadrupoles and magnetic sector instruments) focus the resolved beams of ions from the mass analyzer onto a detector. The most common detector is the electron multiplier, which is a series of electrodes. When an ion impinges on the first electrode, it releases a shower of electrons that impact a second electrode and so on. The cascading effect produces gains on the order of 10^6. Such high gain produces sensitivity so that a complete mass spectrum can be produced from a few nanograms or less of material.

Interpretation of Mass Spectra

Interpretation of mass spectra involves correlating the plots of ion abundance versus m/z ratio with structure. For unknowns, it is best performed with all auxiliary information possible regarding a compound, such as its origin and preparation, chromatographic behavior, and spectra from UV, IR, NMR, and so on, in order to assign structure with confidence. In this section, basic interpretation of EI mass spectra is reviewed followed by a discussion of mass spectra produced by softer ionization techniques.

EI Mass Spectra

Fragmentation in EI mass spectrometry can be complex but rich in information if correctly interpreted (100). It remains difficult to interpret all features in a mass spectrum but a few simple rules can be used to glean useful information.

The most significant datum in identifying an unknown compound is its molecular weight, thus, assignment of the molecular ion in the spectrum is the most important step in its interpretation. The molecular ion must be the highest mass ion in the spectrum and fragment ions must be logical neutral losses from this ion. Keep in mind that not all compounds will give a molecular ion. Fragmentation peaks in the spectrum result from one or more cleavages that may or may not involve rearrangements. The particular fragments produced are related to the strength and chemical nature of the bonds that held the fragment to the rest of the molecule. Thus, an understanding of organic chemistry is useful in assigning fragment ion structures and the associated neutral species lost. MacLafferty's book (100) remains a popular text on the interpretation of mass spectra.

EI mass spectra are very reproducible on different instruments, and assistance is available in the form of libraries of mass spectra that are searchable by computer. These are included with most data systems and are very straightforward to use. The data system suggests the best matches for one's compound and provides some number indicating its confidence in the assignment. These libraries are useful for quickly identifying known compounds and suggesting identities for others. The ability to create one's own library is an option in most data packages.

Soft Ionization Mass Spectra

These mass spectra are those produced by less energetic ionization methods such as CI, MALDI, and LC–MS interfaces like ES and APCI. They are all marked by the appearance of molecular adducts such as $(M + H)^+$. Other common adducts depend on the sample matrix and may include $(M + Na)^+$ and $(M + K)^+$. When using ammonium buffers in LC–MS, $(M + NH_4)^+$ is common along with adducts formed with solvent molecules such as $(M + H_2O + H)^+$ or $(M + CH_3CN + H)^+$. Also, dimers such as $(2M + H)^+$ may occur, especially when higher concentrations of analyte are present. These spectra serve primarily to verify the molecular weight of the compound.

CID Mass Spectra

Mass spectra produced by MS/MS are greatly influenced by different parameters such as collision energy and collision cell pressure (15). These conditions can vary from one compound to the next and also from one instrument to the next for the same compound. Thus, CID spectra are less quantitatively reproducible than EI mass spectra. Yet, CID spectra remain extremely useful for qualitative structure elucidation. Common neutral losses such as H_2O for hydroxyl groups or loss of glucuronic acid from a glucuronide conjugate are very informative and complement the soft ionization techniques.

Experimental Design

With such a variety of instruments and methods available, some thought must be given to designing a mass spectrometric analysis. This section provides some basic guidance for acquiring qualitative and quantitative information for a sample.

Method Selection

The nature of the sample determines the best approach. For example, if the sample is a large protein it is unlikely to volatilize intact from a DIP or pass through a GC. Another consideration is the complexity of the sample. Purified samples may not require chromatography but mixtures do. GC–MS and LC–MS are established techniques that perform separation and mass analysis and can rapidly identify unknowns and assess the relative composition of a sample. Samples that are thermally labile or nonvolatile must be ionized with a soft ionization method such as ES or APCI. MS/MS techniques are useful for providing structural information from soft ionization techniques. If high mass resolution is required, the mass analyzer must be a double-focusing sector instrument, an FT–MS, or one of the new TOF systems.

Qualitative Analysis

Qualitative analysis refers to correctly identifying an unknown substance. Although interpretation of mass spectra has already been discussed, other considerations must be mentioned. Many compounds have similar mass spectra and a single mass spectrum cannot give certain identification in every case. For example, there are at least three polycyclic aromatic hydrocarbons with molecular weight 252 (benzo[*a*]pyrene, benzo[*e*]pyrene, and perylene) and all have similar EI mass spectra. In these situations, using a separation technique such as GC or LC prior to mass analysis can assist identification. When an unknown gives a matching spectrum and coelutes with an authentic standard, then confidence in its identification is high. When no authentic standard is available, the use of two or more chromatographic techniques and ionization methods can be used to enhance confidence in the identity of an unknown. It should be emphasized that, even though mass spectrometry is a powerful tool in determining the identity of an unknown, auxiliary techniques outside of mass spectrometry should be used whenever possible to provide increased confidence in the identification of a compound.

Quantitative Analysis

The number of ions detected in the mass spectrometer is proportional to the amount of material introduced to the source making quantitative analysis possible. Using standard analytical calibration principles, mass spectrometers are capable of very precise, accurate, and sensitive determinations of analytes. The response of the mass spectrometer is calibrated using a series of standards that contain known amounts of the analyte or analytes of interest. External standard calibration plots are possible but prone to errors due to instrument response variation through the course of analyzing several standards and samples.

A preferred calibration system is the use of internal standards where a known amount of a reference compound is added to the samples and also to the standards. A response ratio of the analyte to internal standard is produced, which can partially offset variations in sample preparation and instrument sensitivity. The internal standard should be added to the sample prior to any mixing, extraction, derivatization, enzyme treatment, or chromatography to account for any sample losses during these processes. The instrument is usually calibrated with a series of standards that contain a fixed amount of the internal standard and varying amounts of the analyte of interest. The range of analyte concentrations in the standards must cover the values expected for the samples. A calibration plot can be produced from the response ratio versus analyte concentration. Analyte concentration can be obtained from this plot by interpolation. Most analysts prefer linear curves because the data are easier to process; however, many analytical software packages are available that will fit curves to nonlinear plots. There are good texts available for rigorous coverage of calibration plots, calculation of concentration, and limits of detection and quantitation (103,150).

A special case in quantitative mass spectrometry is the use of a labeled analog of the analyte as an internal standard; the procedure is referred to as isotope dilution. Isotope dilution provides a more accurate and precise means of calibration than either external standards or conventional internal standard methods. The isotopically labeled analog has physical, chromatographic, and mass spectral properties that are nearly identical to those of the analyte, and thus compensates in like manner for any losses due to sample preparation or instrument variability (32). Stable isotopes (such as ^{2}H and ^{13}C) are preferred to radioactive isotopes because of reduced hazards of handling the samples.

Sample Preparation

Investigations in toxicology involve the analysis of biological samples from in vivo and in vitro sources. Such samples include urine, blood, saliva, tissue extracts, and cell suspensions. The use of specific detection methods such as SIM or MRM coupled with chromatography permits these very complex samples to be analyzed directly with LC–MS; sample preparation is minimal (filter and inject, for example). As trace analysis becomes important, however, many samples require a preconcentration step prior to analysis so that adequate limits of detection can be obtained. Isolation and purification techniques commonly employed are solid- or liquid-phase extraction, preparatory HPLC, TLC, or a combination of these.

GC–MS analyses require the sample to be volatile and thermally stable. If the analyte of interest does not meet these requirements, derivatization of an analyte can assist in its analysis. Derivatization can enhance sensitivity, selectivity, and chromatographic performance in some cases. Thus, it should be considered as an alternative when difficulties with an analyte are discovered. Ideally, the mass spectrum of the derivative will provide an intense molecular ion or unique fragment ion. A common derivatization choice is trimethylsilation of hydroxyl or amine groups to increase volatility and thermal stability. Several commercial trimethylsilating reagents are available such as *bis*-trimethylsilylacetamide (BSA).

Applications

This section describes some recent examples of mass spectrometry applied to issues in toxicology. The first two examples employ GC–MS to identify potential carcinogens in biological fluids. Then, two different approaches for monitoring exposure to nicotine by determining metabolite concentrations with LC–MS are described. Finally, two examples are given where DNA adducts are determined using AMS and a combination of ICP and ES ion sources with LC–MS.

Determination of Toxic Metals Using Stable Isotope Dilution

Cadmium is highly toxic and comes from a variety of industrial and environmental sources. Aggarwal et al. (1) have developed an interesting stable isotope dilution GC–MS method for determining cadmium exposure. Their method determined cadmium in urine by using the chelating agent lithium bis(trifluoroethyl)dithiocarbamate, Li(FDEDTC), to form the chelate Cd $(FDEDTC)_2$ which was analyzed by GC/MS with EI ionization. $M^{+\cdot}$ was monitored for quantitation. The internal standard used was ^{106}CdO. Cd determination in urine was possible with this method at the 10-μg/L level with good precision and accuracy. The researchers note that the isotope dilution technique provides freedom from matrix effects so that precision and accuracy are not affected by incomplete recovery.

Determination of Aromatic Amines in Human Milk Using GC–MS

Aromatic amines come from several environmental pollution sources and have been associated with breast cancer in humans. The presence of these compounds in human breast milk was demonstrated in a straightforward manner by DeBruin et al. (42) using GC–MS. The method used solid-phase microextraction (SPME) (43) to sample the headspace over a heated milk sample. The SPME fiber was then inserted into the injector port of a GC–MS and desorbed onto the column. Aromatic amines identified were aniline, o-toluidine, and N-methylaniline. Two internal standards, aniline-d_5 and o-toluidine-d_9, were added to the milk samples prior to preparation. For quantitation, a quadrupole mass spectrometer was operated in the SIM mode with a base ion for each analyte selected. A qualifying ion was also used to confirm the identity. Using a calibration curve constructed from standards made in bovine milk, the authors quantified the three analytes in milk samples at the sub-ppb level.

Serum Cotinine by LC-MS/MS Using APCI

Serum cotinine is often used as a biomarker of exposure to nicotine. If methods have sufficient limits of detection, exposure to extremely low amounts of nicotine, such as those in environmental tobacco smoke, can be assessed. The analysis of low concentrations of analytes in complex matrices may be approached in different ways. One approach seeks to perform extensive sample clean-up to present a relatively clean sample to the instrument. Although this is labor-intensive and requires meticulous attention to the handling of the sample, it permits the analytical system to operate longer and more reproducibly between servicing. A good example of this approach is the determination of cotinine in serum by the method of Bernert et al. (11). They desired to measure exposure to nicotine for large numbers of samples from both smokers and nonsmokers. A rapid, sensitive LC–MS/MS method with APCI was developed for serum cotinine, utilizing sample extraction and concentration. Although sample preparation has many steps, the results of this method are impressive. The HPLC method had a retention time of less than one min for the analyte and internal standard, which permitted samples to be injected every two min. Under routine operation, 100 samples a day were analyzed. A detection limit of 0.05 ng/mL was achieved which was sufficient to monitor serum cotinine in nonsmokers exposed to environmental tobacco smoke.

Sample preparation began with the addition of the internal standard, methyl-d_3-cotinine, to 1 mL serum. The sample was acidified and centrifuged to remove protein. The supernatant was basified and extracted with methylene chloride, dried, redissolved for transferal to a microvial, evaporated to dryness again, and finally reconstituted in 20 μL of toluene. For LC–MS/MS analysis, 10 μL were injected onto a 4.6 mm $\times$ 3 cm C_{18} column for an isocratic separation with a flow rate of 1 mL/min of 80% methanol and 20% 2 mM ammonium acetate. The effluent was introduced to an APCI source on a triple-stage quadrupole mass spectrometer set to operate in the MRM mode. Ions monitored were m/z 177$\rightarrow$$m/z$ 80 for cotinine and m/z 180$\rightarrow$$m/z$ 80 for the internal standard. For a confirming transition for cotinine, m/z 177$\rightarrow$$m/z$ 98 was also monitored.

The key features of this method's performance were sample extraction and concentration followed by very specific detection. Recoveries were 60–70% and most background materials were removed. Reducing the final volume to 0.02 mL resulted in a greater than tenfold concentration of the sample. Highly specific MRM analysis and focusing on only one analyte reduced chromatography requirements so that retention time could be minimal and an isocratic method could be used. The latter eliminated column equilibration time after the run, which is necessary for gradient methods. Thousands of serum samples were analyzed by this method but only for cotinine. The mass spectral parameters of this method could be modified to include nicotine because it could be extracted by this same procedure. Extension to other more polar metabolites of nicotine such as *trans*-3′-hydroxycotinine would be problematic as the method now exists because they are more difficult than cotinine to efficiently extract into an organic phase.

Determination of Nicotine and Several Metabolites in Smokers' Urine Using LC–MS with TS

A different approach is to perform minimal sample preparation and let the specificity and sensitivity of the instrument work to measure the analyte. Keeping the sample close to its original state minimizes chances of analyte loss prior to detection, especially when numerous analytes are involved. An example of such a method is that of McManus et al. (101). Though neither as rapid nor as sensitive as the method above, it was ambitious in the scope of analytes it sought to determine. The objective of this method was to determine as many known urinary metabolites of nicotine as possible to assess nicotine exposure. The method used TS interfaced to a single quadrupole instrument. It permitted direct injection of urine from smokers and used a 10-min reverse-phase HPLC gradient method for separation. The $(M+H)^+$ for numerous known nicotine metabolites were detected by SIM and standards were used to establish retention times. Sample preparation was minimal with addition of methyl-d_3 cotinine as internal standard and filtration through a 0.2-μM mesh. Because no extractions were involved in this approach, extraction efficiency was not an issue and all identified metabolites could be reasonably determined. Only 4 of 17 known metabolites were detected in smokers' urine initially (*trans*-3′-hydroxycotinine, cotinine, nicotine-N′-oxide, and norcotinine).

The strength of this method is the determination of nicotine and several metabolites in a single run. By determining multiple metabolites at the same time, a better indication of nicotine absorption is provided because some individuals may produce more of one metabolite over another in their urine. The limit of detection of approximately 20 ng/mL makes this method useful for smokers but not for nonsmokers. Also, undiscovered minor nicotine metabolites would be difficult to find by this approach. The time and resources saved by it are offset partially by the introduction of many contaminants to the analytical system that damage columns and foul ionization sources so that performance is eventually compromised. Later applications of the method to urine samples from smokers used enzymatic hydrolysis to indirectly account for glucuronide conjugates of nicotine, cotinine, and *trans*-3′-hydroxycotinine (17–19). Further modification of this method has been reported using slightly faster chromatography and APCI tandem mass spectrometry (16). MRM detection of six metabolites was applied to saliva and serum samples from smokers, in addition to urine.

Determination of DNA Adducts

DNA adducts are believed to be biological dosimeters for exposure to chemical carcinogens. This is a developing area of mass spectrometry research and some impressive work has been done using radiolabeled compounds administered to animals and humans (50). Using AMS to detect ^{14}C has lowered detection limits to the point that ^{14}C-labeled carcinogens may be safely administered to humans at realistic exposure levels. Turtelbaum et al. (154) have studied the administration of ^{14}C-labeled heterocyclic amines to rodents in their diet at 100 ng/kg/day to mimic human exposure. Following isolation and purification of the DNA, adducts were detectable after 24 h in the liver and kidney. These data suggested that DNA adducts are formed at human exposure levels and are indicative of dose for this particular compound.

Another elegant approach for monitoring DNA adducts has been described by Siethoff et al. (140) using two different LC–MS methods. One of the problems with quantifying DNA adducts accurately is the lack of standards. This group has used ICP with a high-resolution sector mass spectrometer coupled to an HPLC to resolve the different adducts following digestion of the DNA sample to its monophosphate units. Each unit contains a phosphorus that is converted to P^+ by ICP. This ion occurs at m/z 30.97 but must be resolved from $^{15}N^{16}OH^+$ and $^{14}N^{16}OH^+$ interferences in the plasma background using high-resolution mass discrimination. Because ICP completely atomizes molecules, any phosphorous-containing molecule such as phosphoric acid may be used as an internal standard for quantitative purposes. Thus, ICP–MS is used to locate and quantify the DNA adducts. The authors then used the same LC method connected to a mass spectrometer with an ES source to elucidate the structure of the adducts from the molecular adduct $(M - H)^-$.

The Rationale for Choosing Mass Spectrometry for an Analysis

Contemporary mass spectrometry gives highly reliable analytical results and combines specificity and sensitivity. Determinations in the part-per-billion range (ng/mL) are now commonplace. The unique fingerprint identification provided by mass spectra gives a great deal of confidence that an analysis has been performed correctly.

Improvements in inlet systems, ionization sources such as ES and APCI, and mass analyzers such as multiple-stage quadrupoles for tandem mass spectrometry have greatly expanded the applicability of mass spectrometry. LC–MS has become the workhorse in modern bioanalytical laboratories. It is the method of choice for toxicokinetic and pharmacokinetic studies and is commonly used for metabolite characterization and quantification. Its high sensitivity makes it ideal for quantifying exposure to environmental toxins.

The analyst must keep in mind, however, that mass spectrometry is a technique that destroys the sample. This is particularly important in cases where sample sizes are very small and result from time-consuming and labor-intensive isolation and purification methods. Mass spectrometers are expensive, although the price of bench top systems is becoming attractive. Newer techniques in mass spectrometry are very powerful but do not work well for all samples. For example, if a sample could be one of several possible positional isomers, mass spectrometry may be inadequate for the unequivocal assignment of structure. Despite these limitations, mass spectrometry plays a very important role in studying mechanisms of toxicity.

NUCLEAR MAGNETIC RESONANCE SPECTROSCOPY

In 1946 Purcell, Torrey, and Pound of Harvard University and Bloch, Hansen, and Packard of Stanford University independently detected nuclear magnetic resonance (NMR) effects of the hydrogen nucleus in paraffin wax (Purcell) and water (Bloch). These first observations of nuclear magnetic resonance, although winning the Nobel Prize in Physics for Bloch and Purcell in 1952, would have remained of little interest to chemists if it had not been for the observation that the resonance frequency of a particular nucleus depends on its chemical environment. In 1951, Packard reported that the NMR spectrum of ethanol consisted of three distinct resonances and that these resonances arose from the three different chemical environments for the hydrogen nuclei in the molecule (CH_3, CH_2, and OH). This discovery quickly caught the attention of organic chemists who realized that NMR spectroscopy could be used as a tool for determining chemical structure (71,122).

Since those early observations, NMR spectroscopy has emerged as the most powerful technique for structural characterization of organic compounds. It has been used routinely to elucidate the structure and conformation of molecules so it is the method of choice for determining the identity of xenobiotic metabolites if they can be isolated in microgram to milligram quantities. In this regard, it is often used in conjunction with chromatographic and mass spectral methods. It can also be used to probe the structures of xenobiotic adducts to biological macromolecules such as DNA and proteins. NMR can be used to quantify xenobiotic exposure and changes in endogenous compounds in response to such exposure.

Due to its selectivity and the wealth of information that is available from NMR spectroscopy, it has found increasing application in pharmacology, toxicology, and biomedical research. Recent advances in NMR technology have enabled researchers and clinicians to study chemical and physiological changes within cell suspensions, isolated organs, and living organisms in a noninvasive manner. In vivo spectroscopic techniques have been used to measure cellular metabolism, intracellular pH, cytosolic sodium, magnesium and calcium levels, organ damage in response to toxicants, and a host of other toxicologically relevant phenomena.

NMR spectroscopy is a very powerful tool for studying mechanisms of toxicology. It has been successfully applied to a variety of problems and will almost certainly see increasing application in the years to come. It is important for toxicologists to have knowledge of the strengths and limitations of NMR spectroscopy and an appreciation of the types of studies for which it is suited.

The following sections include an overview of the theory of NMR and numerous examples of its application in toxicology and related disciplines. A detailed mathematical treatment of magnetic resonance is beyond the scope of this chapter; however, from time to time a mathematical formula will be used to describe and clarify the phenomena. It is assumed that the reader has encountered traditional proton and carbon NMR spectroscopy in an introductory organic chemistry course and very little discussion of the interpretation of NMR spectra will appear. A number of extremely good texts on the theory, application, and interpretation of NMR have appeared and the interested reader should refer to them for more detail (44,46,71,122,126,129).

Basic Theory of NMR Spectroscopy

Nuclear Spin

An understanding of the NMR phenomenon begins with a look at the atomic nucleus. Nuclei are composed of protons and (except for ^1H) neutrons; therefore, all atomic nuclei carry a positive charge. Many nuclei also rotate about the nuclear axis and the angular momentum of this spinning charge is described in terms of the spin quantum number, I. Spin numbers have values of 0, 1/2, 1, 3/2, and so forth. For our purposes, the most important spin-active nuclei are ^1H, ^{13}C, ^{31}P, and ^{19}F which all have $I = 1/2$.

Behavior of Nuclei in an External Magnetic Field

Since a spinning nucleus ($I>0$) is a charge in motion, it generates a magnetic field and behaves like a small bar magnet with a magnetic moment, μ. Just as a bar magnet will align itself with an external magnetic field, so to will any nucleus with $I>0$. For $I = 1/2$, the nuclei can adopt one of two orientations relative to the external magnetic field. They may be aligned with the field (low energy state) or against the field (high energy state).

A nucleus with $I>0$ exhibits another important property when placed in an external magnetic field. That property is precessional motion. We have all observed the behavior of a spinning top. As it spins, the top's axis slowly revolves around the vertical. The top is said to be precessing around the vertical axis, and this type of behavior is called precessional motion. A nucleus spinning in an external magnetic field also exhibits precessional motion, with the magnetic moment, μ, precessing around the axis of the applied magnetic field B_o (Figure 36.6). The frequency at which the magnetic moment precesses about B_o is called the precessional frequency, υ. While the spinning frequency of any given nucleus is constant, υ varies directly with the strength of the external magnetic field B_o:

$$\upsilon \propto \mathbf{B}_o$$

This proportionality is the most fundamental relationship of NMR spectroscopy and leads to the fundamental NMR equation:

$$\upsilon = \frac{\gamma \mathbf{B}_o}{2\pi} \tag{2}$$

The proportionality constant, γ, is the magnetogyric ratio and is a fundamental nuclear constant. It is related to the nuclear magnetic moment, μ, and the spin quantum number, I

$$\gamma = \frac{2\pi\mu}{hI} \tag{3}$$

where h is Planck's constant.

A proton (hydrogen nucleus) has a magnetogyric ratio of 2.6752×10^8 radians s^{-1} T^{-1}; therefore, in a magnetic field of 7.1 tesla (7.1 T) its precessional frequency is approximately 300 MHz. A proton in a magnetic field of 14.1 T will have $\upsilon \approx 600$ MHz. The magnetogyric ratio of ^{13}C is 6.727×10^7 radians s^{-1} T^{-1} so in a field of 7.1 T, $\upsilon \approx 75$ MHz. Table 36.1 lists the precessional frequencies at selected field strengths for several common magnetic nuclei. NMR spectrometers are most frequently classified by the precessional frequency of the ^1H nucleus at the field strength of the magnet. For example, a spectrometer with

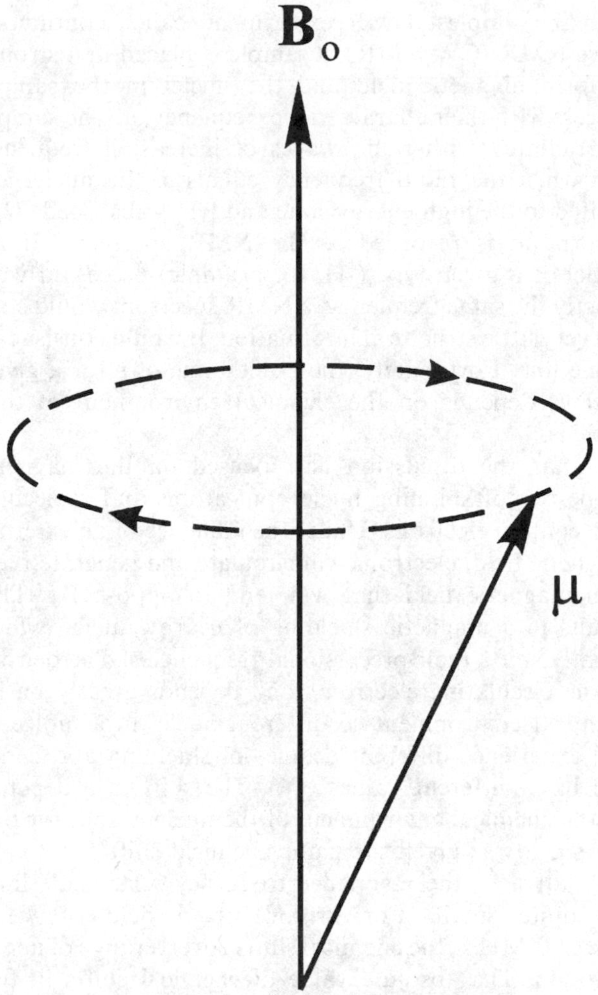

FIG. 36.6. Magnetic moment, μ, of a spinning nucleus precessing about the applied magnetic field, B_o, with precessional frequency υ.

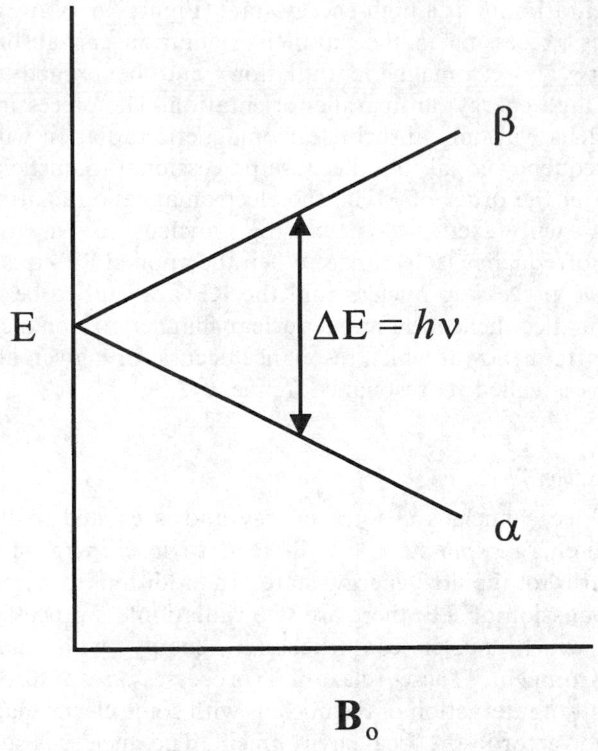

FIG. 36.7. Energy level diagram for a spin 1/2 nucleus in a magnetic field B_o.

a field strength of 7.1 T is commonly called a 300 MHz NMR.

A spin 1/2 nucleus in a magnetic field will have a precessional frequency, υ, and will be able to adopt one of two orientations, or spin states, relative to B_o. It will be aligned with (parallel) or against (antiparallel) the external field. The parallel orientation, α, is a low-energy state for the system and the antiparallel

Table 36.1
Precessional frequencies of several common nuclei at selected field strengths.

	Precessional Frequency (MHz) at Field Strength (T)									
Nucleus	1.4	2.3	4.7	7.1	9.4	11.7	14.1	17.6	18.8	21.1
^{1}H	60.0	100.0	200.0	300.0	400.0	500.0	600.0	750.0	800.0	900.0
^{2}H	9.2	15.4	30.7	46.1	61.4	76.8	92.1	115.1	122.8	138.2
^{13}C	15.1	25.1	50.3	75.4	100.6	125.7	150.9	188.6	201.2	226.3
^{14}N	4.3	7.2	14.4	21.7	28.9	36.1	43.3	54.1	57.8	65.0
^{15}N	6.1	10.1	20.3	30.4	40.5	50.7	60.8	76.0	81.0	91.2
^{17}O	8.1	13.6	27.1	40.7	54.2	67.8	81.3	101.6	108.4	122.0
^{19}F	42.4	94.1	188.2	282.2	376.3	470.4	564.5	705.6	752.6	846.7
^{23}Na	15.9	26.5	52.9	79.4	105.8	132.3	158.7	198.4	211.6	238.1
^{31}P	24.3	40.5	81.0	121.4	161.9	202.4	242.9	303.6	323.8	364.4

orientation, β, is a high-energy state (Figure 36.7). A nucleus precessing in the parallel orientation can absorb energy (electromagnetic radiation) and be excited to the high-energy, antiparallel orientation. The precessing nucleus will only absorb electromagnetic radiation with a frequency equal to υ. Because precessional frequencies are on the order of MHz, the electromagnetic radiation that will excite a precessing nucleus is in the radiofrequency (RF) range. When the applied RF equals υ, the precessing nucleus and the RF are said to be in resonance, hence the name nuclear magnetic resonance. The frequency at which resonance occurs for a given nucleus is called its resonance frequency.

Relaxation Times

Once a nucleus absorbs energy and is excited to the high-energy spin-state, it will tend to lose energy and return to the low-energy state. In addition to direct re-emission of RF, there are two radiationless processes by which nuclei can exchange energy with their environment. These relaxation processes are a direct result of interaction of the nucleus with some electromagnetic vector in the local environment. The nucleus is surrounded by solvent molecules and energy can be transferred to the solvent or other nearby atoms in a process called spin–lattice relaxation. The spin–lattice relaxation time, T_1, depends on such factors as temperature and solvent viscosity, with higher temperature and lower solvent viscosity slowing T_1 relaxation.

The nucleus can also transfer energy to nearby nuclei in a process called spin–spin relaxation. In spin–spin relaxation, one nucleus loses energy and the other one gains energy so there is no net change in the populations of the two spin states. The spin–spin relaxation time, T_2, depends on molecular mobility, and nuclei in large molecules that have highly constrained molecular motions have very efficient spin–spin relaxation (short T_2).

The magnitude of T_1 and T_2 determine the line widths of NMR spectral lines; short relaxation times lead to broad lines and long relaxation times lead to sharp lines. This means that NMR spectra obtained in viscous solvents (short T_1) will have broader lines than those obtained in nonviscous solvents. Also, NMR spectra of biological matrices, such as plasma or cell suspensions, will show many very broad resonances from proteins, nucleic acids, and other macromolecules which have very short T_2 relaxation times. These broad resonances can obscure the signals of small molecules of interest, such as xenobiotic metabolites. A variety of NMR techniques have been developed which enable the observation of low molecular weight compounds in the presence of macromolecules and the interested reader should refer to thc review by Rabenstein et al. (127).

Chemical Shifts

In the simplest NMR experiment, called continuous wave NMR (CW NMR), a sample is placed in a strong, uniform magnetic field and the nuclei in the sample precess with their characteristic frequency, υ. The sample is irradiated with radio waves of increasing frequency and when the radio frequency equals υ, the nuclei are excited to the high-energy state and RF is absorbed. This absorption is recorded as the NMR spectrum. If all nuclei of a given type (^1H, for example) precessed with exactly the same frequency, a NMR spectrum would convey very little structural information. It would consist of a single line. Fortunately, the exact value of υ for a given nucleus depends on the chemical environment of that nucleus.

So far the discussion has focused on the magnetic properties of spinning nuclei, but atoms and molecules also contain electrons. Under the influence of an external magnetic field, electrons will circulate and generate their own magnetic field that will tend to oppose B_o. This results in a magnetic shielding of nearby nuclei, which slightly shifts their precessional frequencies. The density of the circulating electron cloud depends greatly on its chemical environment so different nuclei in a molecule will experience different degrees of shielding and hence will have different values of υ. The shift in υ depends on the chemical environment of the nucleus and, for this reason, it was given the name chemical shift.

Relative to the resonance frequency, chemical shifts are quite small. For protons in a field of 7.1 T ($\upsilon \approx 300$ MHz), the chemical shifts cover a range of about 4000 Hz. The absolute value of chemical shifts in frequency units depends on the strength of the applied magnetic field. The greater the value of B_o, the greater the chemical shift range. This explains, in part, the desire to move to higher and higher field strengths for NMR spectroscopy. The higher the field, the greater the resolution of chemical shifts.

Chemical shifts are rarely (if ever) expressed in absolute frequency units. Instead, they are measured relative to a standard reference compound. For ^1H and ^{13}C NMR the universally accepted reference is tetramethylsilane (TMS). It is commonly added to samples as an internal standard at concentrations of less than 1%. TMS has several important properties that make it a near ideal reference standard. It contains 12 magnetically equivalent protons and 4 magnetically equivalent carbons so it gives a single, intense peak in the ^1H and ^{13}C NMR spectra. It is chemically inert, soluble in most organic solvents, and volatile (b.p. $= 27°C$) so it can be removed easily from the sample after analysis. The protons and carbons of TMS absorb at a lower frequency (are more shielded) than those of almost all other organic compounds so their chemical shifts can be arbitrarily set to 0 Hz and most other chemical shifts measured relative to them will be positive. TMS is not soluble in water so for aqueous solutions a suitable water-soluble internal standard must be chosen. The most widely used internal standard for aqueous samples is the sodium salt of 3-(trimethylsilyl)-propanoic acid (TSP).

Because chemical shifts vary with the strength of the applied magnetic field, their values in Hz vary from one NMR spectrometer to the next. Protons which absorb at 300 Hz relative to TMS in a field of 7.1 T (300 MHz instrument) will absorb at 100 Hz on a 2.3 T (100 MHz) instrument. To avoid confusion and enable comparisons of chemical shifts from instrument to instrument, chemical shifts are expressed in dimensionless units designated δ. The chemical shift in δ units is defined according to the following relationship:

$$\delta = \frac{\upsilon_s - \upsilon_{std}}{\text{operating frequency}} \times 10^6 \text{ ppm} \qquad (4)$$

where υ_s and υ_{std} are the resonance frequencies of the sample and standard, respectively.

Spin–Spin Coupling

A great deal of structural information may be obtained from the chemical shifts of nuclei in a molecule, but even more information is available from a NMR spectrum. Nuclei that are closely connected through bonding electrons are influenced by the spin-state of their neighbors. Consider two closely connected protons H_a and H_b:

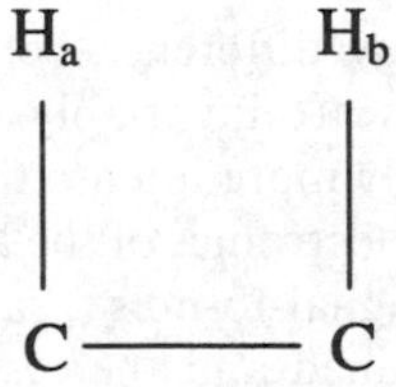

The bonding electrons in the H_a-C bond tend to align their spins with the spin of H_a, the C-C bonding electrons tend to align with the spin of the H_a-C bonding electrons, and the H_b-C bonding electrons tend to align with the spin of the C-C bonding electrons. H_b tends to align its spin with the spin of the H_b-C bonding electrons. In this way, the spin-state of H_a directly influences the spin-state of H_b. Because H_a can have two spin-states, parallel or anti-parallel, the resonance line of H_b is split into two closely spaced lines, a so-called doublet. H_b influences the spin-state of H_a in exactly the same way, so H_a also appears as a doublet. The spacing between the lines in the H_a doublet is the same as that in the H_b doublet. Figure 36.8 illustrates the appearance of the H_a and H_b NMR signals. This phenomenon, called spin–spin coupling (or simply coupling), results in characteristic splitting of NMR signals that is dependent on the number of neighboring spin-active nuclei, their geometrical arrangement, and the number of bonds between them.

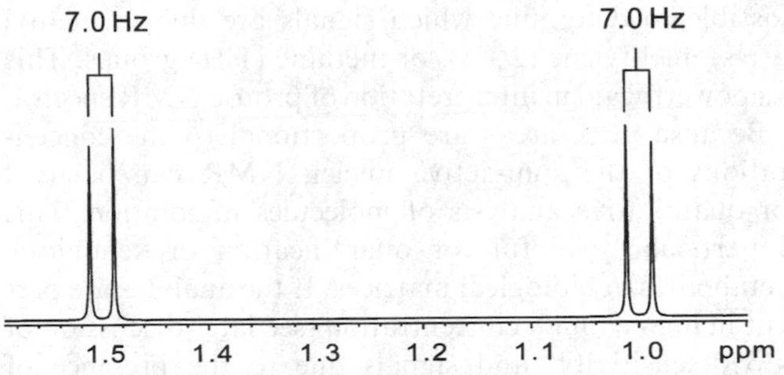

FIG. 36.8. Proton NMR spectrum of the H_a/H_b spin system. Note the coupling constant, *J*, is 7.0 Hz.

Coupling is usually not important beyond four bonds and magnetically equivalent nuclei do not show coupling. Unlike chemical shifts, coupling is independent of B_o.

The number of lines into which a NMR signal is split depends on the number of adjacent nuclei. The general rule is that n adjacent spin-active nuclei will split a signal into $2nI+1$ lines. For spin 1/2 nuclei such as ^1H, two adjacent nuclei will split a signal into three lines (a triplet), three adjacent nuclei will split the signal into four lines (a quartet), and so forth. The relative line intensities within a multiplet are determined by the coefficients in the binomial expansion. A triplet will have intensities of 1 : 2 : 1, a quartet will have intensities 1 : 3 : 3 : 1, and so on. The separation between spectral lines due to coupling is called the coupling constant, J (Figure 36.8). The magnitude of coupling constants depends on the number of intervening bonds and the bond geometry. The coupling constant for protons that are trans to one another in a rigid molecule is greater than that for protons that are *cis*.

Spin–spin coupling is most important in proton NMR spectroscopy since most organic molecules have adjacent protons and show extensive coupling. In ^{13}C NMR spectroscopy, proton coupling to the carbons is often undesirable because it leads to very complex spectra and reduced signal to noise ratio. For these reasons, it is usually suppressed by irradiating over the entire proton resonance frequency range to saturate the proton transitions. This so-called decoupling produces carbon spectra made up of only singlets.

Integral Areas

The area under a peak in a NMR spectrum is proportional to the total number of nuclei giving rise to that signal. In other words, the area of a peak can be used to gain information about the concentrations of the spin-active nuclei. All modern NMR spectrometers are capable of integrating peak areas and the resulting integrals can be plotted on the spectrum. In the case of a multiplet, the total area of the signal is integrated. By comparing integrals within a proton spectrum, it is possible to determine which signals are due to methyl (3 Hs), methylene (2 Hs), or methine (1 H) groups. This is a powerful aid in interpretation of proton NMR spectra.

Because peak areas are proportional to the concentrations of the spin-active nuclei, NMR can be used for quantitative analysis of molecules in solution. This is particularly useful for quantification of xenobiotic metabolites in biological matrices. If the analytes are present in high enough concentration (see later discussion of NMR sensitivity) and signals due to the presence of the analytes of interest can be distinguished in the spectrum, very little sample preparation is required. For quantitative analysis, analyte integrals are compared to integrals of an internal standard that is added to the sample at a known concentration. Quantitative analysis by NMR requires very careful calibration and attention to spectral acquisition parameters, so it should be carried out cautiously. Excellent discussions of quantitative analysis by NMR are available (122,152).

For heteronuclear NMR (such as carbon) where broadband proton decoupling is used, the peak areas do not always give an accurate estimate of the concentration of spin-active nuclei. Decoupling gives rise to nuclear Overhauser effects that complicate the interpretation of integral areas. For this reason, carbon spectra are rarely integrated; however, spectral acquisition parameters can be adjusted to correct for these effects if accurate integrals are required from a carbon (or other heteronuclear) NMR spectrum.

Sensitivity

For nuclei in an external magnetic field, the energy difference between spin states is quite small. This means that the two spin states are almost equally populated at room temperature, with the population of the low energy state exceeding that of the high energy state by only about 0.001%. The intensity of absorption (and, hence, the sensitivity of NMR) is proportional to the number of nuclei absorbing RF energy. As the population difference between spin states increases, there will be more nuclei to absorb RF energy and the sensitivity will increase. From Eq. (3) we see that the energy difference between spin states, $\Delta E = h\upsilon$, is proportional to the magnetogyric ratio, γ. This means that the sensitivity of NMR depends on the magnitude of γ. Detection of nuclei with relatively large magnetogyric ratios (such as ^{1}H and ^{19}F) will be fairly sensitive. The sensitivity of NMR also depends on the natural abundance of the spin-active nucleus under observation. Nuclei with a high natural abundance will be detected with greater sensitivity. Table 36.2 lists natural abundance, spin quantum number, magnetogyric ratio, and sensitivity for some selected nuclei.

The energy difference between spin states, $\Delta E = h\upsilon$, is also proportional to the magnetic field strength B_o. One way to increase the sensitivity of NMR is to increase the field strength. This approach has been somewhat successful; however, even at a field strength of 14.1 T, the energy difference between spin states is only on the order of 10^{-4} kJ mol^{-1}. NMR is (and is likely to remain) less sensitive than optical techniques such as electronic absorption spectroscopy, where ΔE is considerably larger. Even with the most sensitive high field instruments, tens to thousands of micrograms of sample are required.

FT NMR

Because the energy difference between spin states is small, NMR signals are invariably weak. In fact, they are often only slightly more intense than the background noise caused by the electronics of the NMR spectrometer. To improve the signal-to-noise ratio (S/N), several spectra can be obtained and the resulting collection of data averaged. The NMR signals in these spectra would always occur at the same frequencies; however, the ran-

Table 36.2
Selected NMR properties of several common nuclei.

Nucleus	Natural abundance (%)	Spin quantum number I	Magnetogyric ratio ($\times 10^{-7}$ radians s^{-1} T^{-1})	Relative sensitivity at constant field
^{1}H	99.985	1/2	26.752	1.000
^{2}H	0.015	1	4.107	9.65×10^{-3}
^{13}C	1.108	1/2	6.727	0.016
^{14}N	99.635	1	1.933	1.01×10^{-3}
^{15}N	0.365	1/2	2.711	1.04×10^{-3}
^{17}O	0.037	5/2	3.627	0.029
^{19}F	100	1/2	25.167	0.834
^{23}Na	100	3/2	7.076	0.093
^{31}P	100	1/2	10.829	0.067

dom noise would not. The desired signals would build up over time relative to the noise and the S/N would increase. It can be shown that for n repetitions, the signal increases by a factor of n and the noise increases by a factor of $\sqrt{n}$. As a result, signal averaging increases the S/N by a factor of $\sqrt{n}$.

If signal averaging were applied to the CW NMR experiment described previously, the spectrum would be scanned repetitively over the frequency range of interest and the resulting spectra averaged. This would result in an increase in S/N but the time required for the experiment would be quite long. Consider a proton spectrum covering 10 ppm at a field strength of 2.3 T. The sweep width (frequency range) of this spectrum is 1000 Hz. A sweep rate of 1 Hz/s is required to achieve a spectral resolution of 1 Hz so it would take 1000 sec to acquire one spectrum. Increasing the signal-to-noise ratio by a factor of 4 requires 16 repetitions (n) so this experiment would take almost 4 1/2 h. You can see that signal averaging in CW NMR is not very practical. How then is a significant increase in S/N achieved in a reasonable amount of time?

The solution to this problem is found in a technique called pulse NMR, in which the sample is irradiated with a pulse of RF energy containing all the frequencies required to excite the nuclei of interest. This pulse is applied for a very short period (on the order of μs) and the nuclei are allowed to relax to their equilibrium state with the emission of all the frequencies previously absorbed by the nuclei. This signal decays over time and is called a free induction decay (FID). The FID contains all the spectral information, including chemical shifts, coupling constants, and intensity.

To convert this information from the time domain to the frequency domain, which is the normal mode for a NMR spectrum, the FID is subjected to a mathematical operation called Fourier transformation. To achieve signal averaging, a series of FIDs are acquired and averaged prior to Fourier transformation. The resulting FT NMR spectrum is equivalent to a CW spectrum and is obtained in considerably less time. Figure 36.9 shows the FID and resulting proton FT NMR spectrum of a 0.1% solution of ethylbenzene. For this spectrum, 64 repetitions, or transients, were acquired requiring a total time of 4.7 min. Note the large TMS peak at 0 ppm and the presence of an impurity peak at about 1.55 ppm. Figure 36.10 shows the effect on S/N of increasing the number of transients. These proton spectra were obtained on the same ethylbenzene sample used to generate Figure 36.9 and only the quartet is plotted.

All modern NMR spectrometers are of the FT type. FT NMR has allowed insensitive nuclei like ^{13}C to be studied routinely and sensitive nuclei like ^{1}H and ^{19}F to be studied at much lower concentrations than previously possible. It has also opened up a multitude

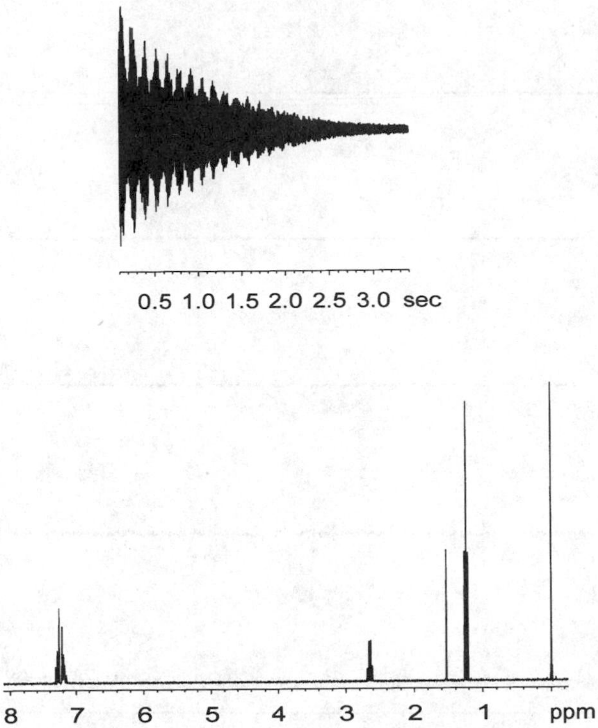

FIG. 36.9. FID and proton NMR spectrum of a 0.1% solution of ethylbenzene in $CDCl_3$. The data were collected at a frequency of 300 MHz and a field strength of 7.1 T.

of powerful new multipulse and two-dimensional NMR experiments, some of which will be discussed in a later section.

Instrumental Design

Although NMR spectrometer design and construction vary from one manufacturer to the next, all spectrometers share the same basic components. Figure 36.11 shows a schematic representation of the basic features of a high-field NMR spectrometer. The heart of the spectrometer is the NMR probe that sits inside the superconducting magnet. The probe contains coils that transmit the RF pulses to the sample and receive the NMR signals that are emitted. Specialized probes for a variety of NMR experiments are available and selection of the proper probe for the particular experiment is crucial to its success. They are exchangeable, and most NMR laboratories have more than one type. For in vivo spectroscopy, the probe may be surface coils placed in close proximity to the organ under study. The spectrometer contains a RF source for generating RF pulses and a RF detector for receiving and amplifying the NMR signal. A computer that is also used for storing, processing, and displaying data controls the RF source and detector.

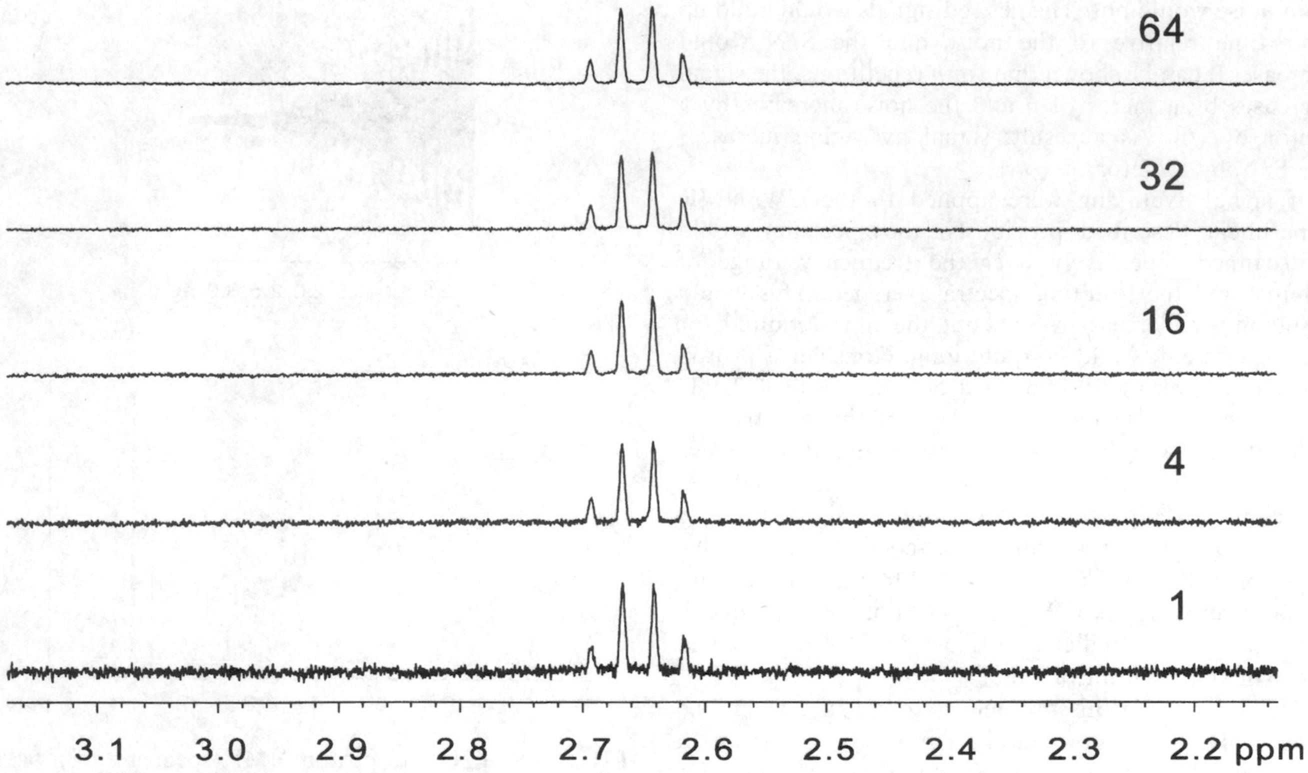

FIG. 36.10. The effect of increasing the number of transients on the S/N ratio of the proton NMR spectrum of ethylbenzene.

Experimental Design

The proper design of toxicological NMR studies depends on a number of factors. The first consideration when designing a NMR study is the nature of the sample. If the sample is a solution, cell suspension, or can be dissolved in a suitable solvent, then a host of liquid–state NMR experiments are possible. If the sample is alive (perfused organs, laboratory animals, or humans) then in vivo spectroscopy using surface coils or imaging techniques is required. The choice of nuclei, type of NMR experiment, probe, solvent (if liquid–state analysis is required), and method of sample preparation will all effect the outcome of the study. This section will provide some guidance to the researcher in designing NMR studies. Particular emphasis will be placed on liquid–state methods because spectrometers for liquid–state analyses are more readily available than those for in vivo spectroscopy, and liquid–state methods are by far the most commonly used for toxicology research.

Choice of Nucleus

The most useful NMR active nuclei for toxicology studies are ^{1}H, ^{13}C, ^{31}P, and ^{19}F. When the effects of heavy metal exposure are of interest, nuclei like ^{199}Hg or ^{113}Cd can sometimes be used, although examples of their successful application are quite limited. Biologically derived samples are often complex mixtures and NMR signals from the matrix can cause significant interference. This is particularly troublesome for ^{1}H and ^{13}C because these nuclei are ubiquitous. With proper sample cleanup and/or utilization of appropriate NMR techniques, these matrix effects can be overcome.

^{1}H is the most sensitive NMR active nucleus (in absolute terms) and is present in almost all organic compounds. If care is taken to minimize signal overlap from the matrix, it can provide qualitative and quantitative information on the metabolism and biochemical effects of xenobiotics. ^{1}H spectra can be obtained for compounds present in concentrations greater than about 50–100 μM in a reasonable amount of time. For these reasons, ^{1}H is the most commonly used NMR active nucleus for studying mechanisms of toxicology. A number of studies of crude urine or urine extracts have been reported; however, biological fluids are usually concentrated and fractionated by HPLC prior to ^{1}H NMR analysis. In some cases, two-dimensional NMR experiments such as COSY (discussed later) can adequately resolve signals of interest with little or no sample cleanup.

^{13}C is of very low natural abundance (about 1%) and its magnetogyric ratio is four times lower than ^{1}H . As a result, its absolute sensitivity is over 5000 times less than

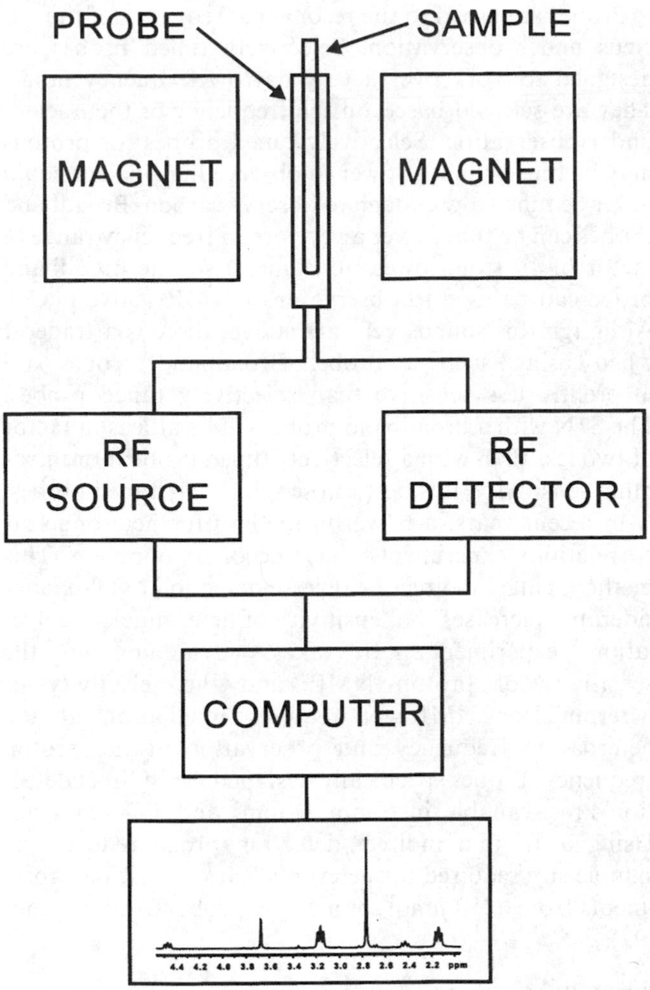

FIG. 36.11. Schematic representation of a NMR spectrometer.

^{1}H. Despite this low sensitivity, ^{13}C NMR spectra can be obtained for compounds present at concentrations greater than 10 mM in a reasonable amount of time. As in ^{1}H NMR studies, samples are most often concentrated and purified by HPLC prior to analysis. In some cases, isotopic enrichment with ^{13}C has been used to increase sensitivity. Enrichment to 90 atom-% ^{13}C results in a 90-fold increase in sensitivity, rendering direct analysis of crude urine for low molecular weight metabolites feasible. Combined with two-dimensional NMR experiments such as INADEQUATE, isotopic enrichment with ^{13}C is a powerful tool for metabolite characterization. Noninvasive in vivo ^{13}C NMR spectroscopy has been used to study the pharmacokinetics of ^{13}C-enriched xenobiotics in the rat (108). The high cost and limited availability of ^{13}C-enriched materials are the main disadvantages to isotopic enrichment.

^{31}P is a sensitive nucleus with a 100% natural abundance. As such, it is an attractive candidate for NMR studies. ^{31}P is one of the most commonly used nuclei for in vivo NMR spectroscopy and has been used extensively to determine the effects of xenobiotics on in vivo energy metabolism and intracellular pH (94). It is much less useful for studies of xenobiotic metabolism because very few xenobiotic metabolites contain phosphorus.

^{19}F is almost as sensitive as ^{1}H and because it is not normally found in biological samples, ^{19}F NMR signals from the matrix are not a problem. If the xenobiotic of interest contains fluorine, useful information such as quantitative determination of fluorinated metabolites and excretion rates can be obtained from ^{19}F NMR. Most fluorinated compounds contain only a few fluorine atoms (one to three), so structural characterization of metabolites by ^{19}F NMR is rare. ^{19}F is a very good tracer for in vitro and in vivo spectral determination of organ perfusion and has been used to determine cerebral, hepatic, and muscular blood flow (110).

In practice, NMR studies often utilize more than one type of NMR active nucleus. Characterization of metabolites is best accomplished with more than one type of NMR experiment. Typically, both one-dimensional ^{1}H and ^{13}C spectra and a variety of two-dimensional experiments are used.

Choice of NMR Experiments

A detailed discussion of modern NMR experiments is far beyond the scope of this chapter and a number of excellent books on the subject have been written (44,46,98,129). A brief description of those experiments which are likely to be most useful for studying mechanisms of toxicology is, however, appropriate. NMR experiments can be divided into two main categories—one-dimensional and multi-dimensional.

One-dimensional NMR experiments are of the type discussed in the earlier section on basic theory. The output of a 1D experiment is a spectrum of intensity versus frequency (or chemical shift in δ units). The ^{1}H spectrum of Figure 36.9 is a very good example. In principle, 1D spectra can be obtained for any spin-active nucleus. One-dimensional spectra are the type used most often for quantitative analysis.

For structural characterization of organic compounds, 1D proton and carbon spectra are almost always used. These spectra contain information about the chemical environments of the hydrogen and carbon atoms in the molecule. The proton spectrum, with its coupling information, also helps in assigning connectivities because coupling constants and peak multiplicity can assist the spectroscopist in determining which hydrogens are coupled. Coupling constants also help in assigning geometry in rigid systems (*cis* or *trans* isomers, for example). Although a great deal of structural information can be obtained from these 1D spectra, it is often useful to obtain 2D spectra as well.

For 2D experiments, two or more RF pulses with variable delay times between them are used to excite the nuclei. The variable delay times introduce a second time domain and, after two-dimensional Fourier transformation, a spectrum with two frequency domains is obtained. No attempt to explain the details of 2D NMR will be made here. The interested reader should refer to other texts for such detail (98). The 2D experiments, which are likely to be the most useful in toxicology research, are used to investigate spin–spin coupling by correlation spectroscopy. COSY spectra reveal ^{1}H-^{1}H spin–spin correlations and generate all connectivities between coupled protons. HETCOR (or HMQC and HMBC) spectra reveal proton–heteroatom correlations (usually ^{1}H-^{13}C correlations) and generate connectivities between protons and heteroatoms (like carbon). INADEQUATE spectra (which are used much less frequently and most often for ^{13}C-enriched compounds) are used to generate connectivities between carbons. Two-dimensional experiments are very useful for resolving signals of interest from overlapping matrix signals in biological samples, and examples of their application in metabolism studies will be presented in a later section.

Instrumental Considerations

In the best of all possible worlds (where money is no object), the instrument with the highest available field strength (frequency) should be used to obtain maximum resolution and sensitivity. Currently, the highest-field instrument commercially available is a 900 MHz NMR but advances in magnet design should make even higher-field instruments possible. In the real world, price is often important and must be considered when purchasing an instrument. As a very rough rule of thumb, NMR spectrometers cost about \$1000–\$1500 per MHz. For this reason, high-field NMR spectrometers are not ubiquitous. Fortunately, most academic NMR laboratories make instrument time available for a reasonable hourly rate.

In toxicology research, sample size is often quite limited. It may take many hours (or weeks) to isolate a few hundred micrograms of a xenobiotic metabolite, so sensitivity is a major concern. For a given field strength, the component which has the greatest influence on sensitivity is the probe. The most common probes are designed for 5-mm sample tubes and in many cases will give adequate sensitivity. Where sample size is limited, the smallest possible probe should be used. Microprobes designed for 3-mm sample tubes are available and recently a 1.7-mm probe has been developed (97).

Probes are tuned to the resonance frequency of the nucleus under observation. Selectively tuned probes are designed to work over a very narrow frequency range. They are selected based on the frequency of the nucleus under observation. Selectively tuned probes for protons may be tuned slightly lower to observe fluorine but could never be tuned low enough to observe carbon. Broadband probes can be tuned over a very broad frequency range (a factor of 10 from lowest to highest) so one broadband probe can be used to observe most NMR active nuclei. Although this sounds very attractive, there is a tradeoff when using such a probe. Broadband probes are inherently less sensitive than selectively tuned probes. The S/N with a broadband probe will be at least a factor of two less than with a selectively tuned probe. For maximum sensitivity, it is best to use selectively tuned probes.

In recent years, a powerful method for heteronuclear correlation experiments has become popular. This method, called indirect or reverse detection (38,96), considerably increases the sensitivity of heteronuclear correlation experiments. It takes advantage of the sensitivity of proton NMR and the selectivity of heteronuclear NMR. It requires irradiation at the heteroatom frequency and observation at the proton frequency. Probes specifically designed for indirect detection are available in 5-mm, 3-mm, and 1.7-mm sizes. Using a 1.7-mm indirect detection probe reduces the sample size required for heteronuclear correlation experiments from $\sim 50\ \mu$mol for a 5-mm probe to $<0.05\ \mu$mol (97).

Sample Preparation

Interference from the sample matrix and the dilute nature of many biological samples often require a purification and/or preconcentration step prior to NMR analysis. HPLC, solid or liquid phase extraction, and TLC have all been used to purify xenobiotic metabolites. The method of choice will depend on the nature of the matrix, the chemical properties of the metabolites, and the sample size. If organic solvents are used for the purification, it is very important to remove as much of the solvent as possible by evaporation prior to NMR analysis. Residual solvents can add very large signals to proton and carbon spectra. These large signals often obscure significant portions of the spectra and, if large enough, can make detection of small signals difficult or impossible due to the limited dynamic range of most spectrometers.

Liquid-state NMR requires the sample to be dissolved in a suitable solvent. Solvents used for most NMR analyses are deuterated, that is, they contain deuterium (^{2}H) instead of protium (^{1}H). Deuterium is required for the spectrometer frequency lock, which corrects for field drift during spectral acquisition. For proton NMR, deuterated solvents are also desirable because they cut down on the intense solvent resonance that would appear in the presence of protiated solvents. Common NMR solvents, commercially available in greater than 99 atom-percent deuterium, are $CDCl_3$, CD_2Cl_2, d_4-methanol, d_6-DMSO, d_6-acetone, and D_2O. If samples in H_2O are to be analyzed, a small amount of D_2O (10–20%) should be added for frequency locking and a suitable solvent suppression method (discussed later) should be used.

Once the sample is dissolved in a suitable solvent, it should be filtered to remove particulate matter. Even small particles can result in a loss of resolution, so filtration is particularly important when closely spaced signals or very small couplings are to be observed.

Solvent Suppression

Many biological samples are aqueous solutions. Acquisition of ^{1}H NMR spectra of such samples is complicated by the fact that the solvent water protons are present at a concentration of 110 M and the analytes of interest are often present in submillimolar concentrations. As a result of this very large dynamic range, weak solute signals are often obscured or not detectable in the presence of the very large solvent signal. It is essential to attenuate the water signal to observe weak signals in the ^{1}H NMR spectra of biological samples. A variety of so-called solvent suppression methods have been developed to reduce or eliminate the "water peak" in ^{1}H NMR spectra (63).

The simplest solvent suppression method is removal of H_2O by lyophilization. The sample is lyophilized to dryness and redissolved in D_2O. Typically, this is repeated several times to remove the last traces of H_2O prior to spectral acquisition. In practice, it is extremely difficult to eliminate the water peak completely because lyophilized biological samples such as urine are often quite hygroscopic and the sample invariably picks up moisture from the air. This method does, however, provide adequate reduction in the size of the water peak for most purposes. An additional advantage to this approach is that dilute samples can be concentrated to increase overall sensitivity.

A variety of instrumental methods are available for solvent suppression. Perhaps the simplest of these involves irradiation at the solvent resonance frequency to saturate the solvent signal. This irradiation may be continuous or it may be gated off during the pulse and acquisition. Suppression ratios of 1000 are possible for water, but, unfortunately, peaks close to it are often attenuated or distorted. To suppress the water peak with less distortion of other resonances, selective relaxation methods based on T_1 relaxation differences between solvent and solute, such as the water elimination Fourier transform (WEFT) method, have been used. Although adequate water suppression is often achieved with WEFT, if signals from the molecule of interest have slow relaxation times, their intensities may be attenuated. If accurate integration is required for signals with a range of relaxation times, other solvent suppression methods should be used.

A powerful method for water suppression takes advantage of rapid proton exchange between water and an added chemical agent such as ammonium chloride. Rapid proton exchange greatly reduces T_2 for the water signal, which is suppressed using a special pulse sequence called spin–echo. This pulse sequence allows the water signal to relax but still permits detection of the desired solute resonances which have longer T_2 relaxation times. This method, water attenuation by T_2 relaxation (WATR), can reduce the intensity of the water signal by factors of $>10^4$. A particularly impressive application of WATR was the determination of benzene and N-nitrosodimethylamine in aqueous solution by 500-MHz proton NMR with limits of detection of 35 and 510 ng/mL, respectively (49).

Recent advances in the theory and technology of NMR have led to the development of a host of pulse sequences designed specifically for solvent suppression. Fortunately, modern NMR computer control systems contain software for all common solvent suppression pulse sequences and they are now routinely used with a minimum of operator involvement. A very powerful method, based on the 2D experiment NOESY, is called NOESYPRESAT. This method results in attenuation of the water signal by a factor of 10^5 or more. Using NOESYPRESAT (for 1D spectra), a series of 2D experiments and a 750 MHz spectrometer, Nicholson et al. (111) were able to assign over 150 resonances in the ^{1}H spectrum of human blood plasma diluted with 10% D_2O.

Applications

Identification of Metabolites

To determine the structure of an organic compound, 1D and 2D spectra are often acquired on the same sample and the information obtained from the experiments is combined to reveal the structure. Caldwell et al. (21) used both 1D and 2D NMR spectra to fully characterize (S)-(−)-cotinine N-glucuronide, a previously unidentified metabolite of nicotine. The structure of this glucuronide was determined using 1D proton and carbon and 2D COSY and HETCOR spectra. The 1D spectra (Figure 36.12) were consistent with the proposed structure; however, complete assignment of the resonances in the spectra was difficult.

The COSY spectrum shown in Figure 36.13A was used to establish connectivities of the coupled protons, enabling the complete assignment of the proton resonances in the 1D spectrum. In COSY spectra, the contours that fall on the diagonal correspond to the 1D

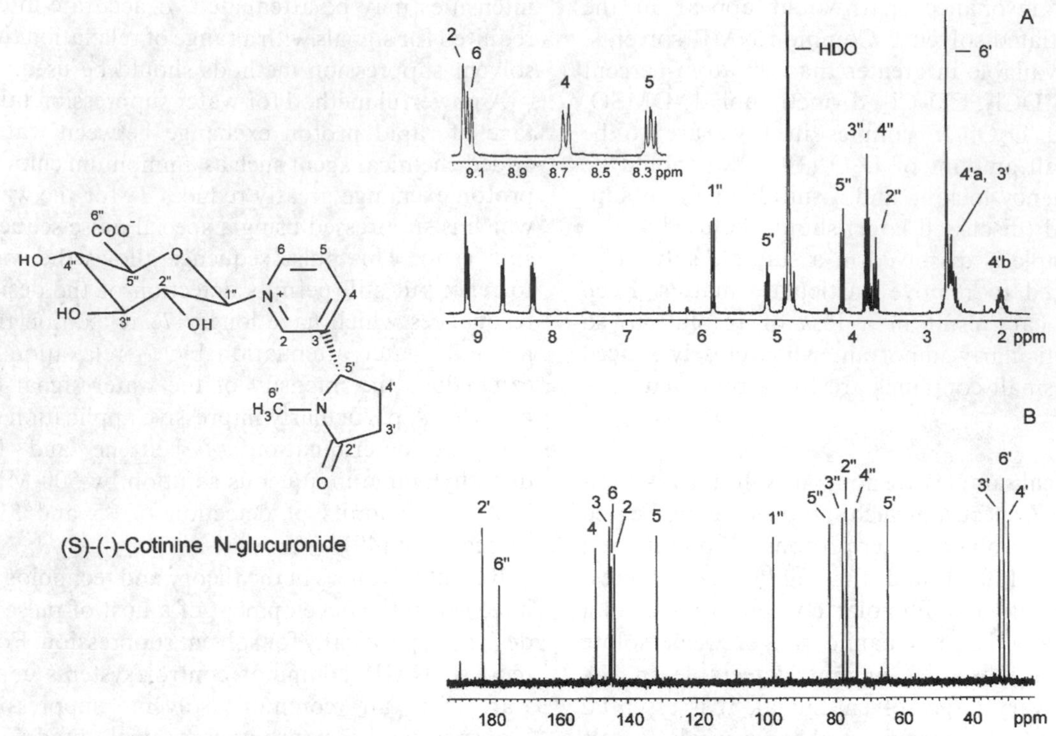

FIG. 36.12. One-dimensional proton (A) and carbon (B) NMR spectra of (S)-(−)-cotinine N-glucuronide.

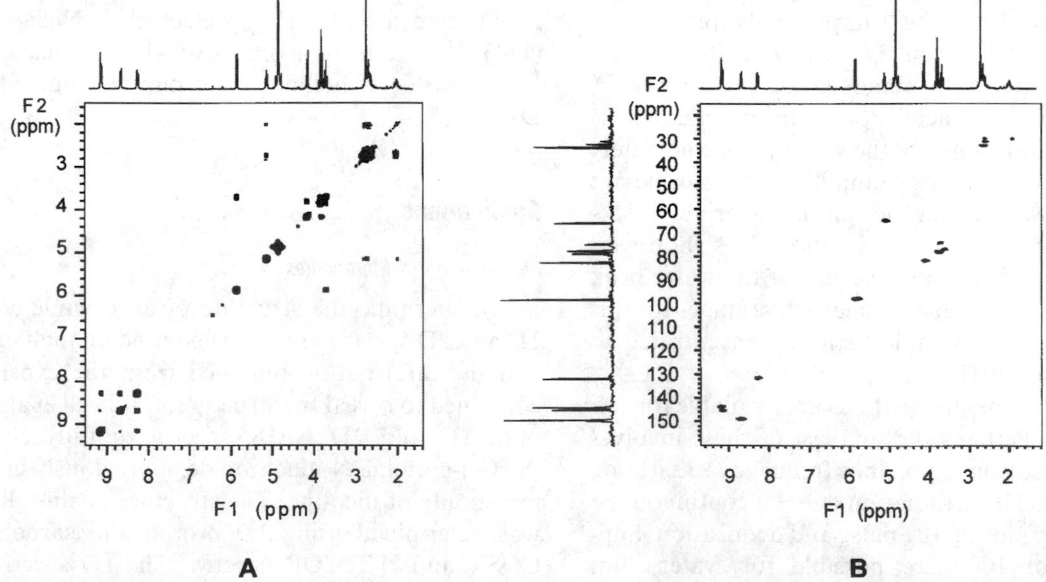

FIG. 36.13. COSY spectrum (A) and HETCOR spectrum (B) of (S)-(−)-cotinine N-glucuronide.

spectrum except they are seen as if the observer were looking down from above the spectrum. Contours that fall off the diagonal result from spin–spin coupling, so they reveal correlations between coupled protons. COSY spectra are usually presented with the 1D spectrum plotted on the top to facilitate interpretation. The HETCOR spectrum shown in Figure 36.13B was used to establish proton–carbon connectivities and enabled the complete assignment of the carbon resonances in the 1D carbon spectrum. HETCOR spectra may be thought of as a carbon spectrum plotted against a proton spectrum. Contours that appear in the HETCOR result from ^1H-^{13}C coupling and reveal proton–carbon connectivities, that is, which protons are bound to which carbons. This HETCOR spectrum is presented with the carbon spectrum (projection) plotted on the vertical axis and the proton spectrum plotted on the horizontal axis.

Perhaps the most common applications of NMR in toxicology research involve characterization of xenobiotic metabolites. Almost all issues of toxicology-related journals contain articles describing the isolation, purification, and NMR characterization of metabolites. Usually, NMR spectra of the purified metabolites are used in conjunction with mass spectral characterization and are included as final confirmation of the proposed structure. Such applications of NMR have contributed to the understanding of xenobiotic detoxification mechanisms, but even more information can be obtained using modern NMR techniques.

NMR analysis of crude or partially purified biological samples, although not frequently used, can be an extremely powerful tool for metabolic studies. Typically, 1D proton NMR spectra of crude biological samples are very complex, with many overlapping signals. Nicholson and Wilson (114) have demonstrated the utility of 2D COSY NMR spectroscopy of crude urine for the simplification of such complex spectra. They collected urine from a human volunteer before, and 3 h after, ingestion of 1 g paracetamol. The urine was lyophilized, reconstituted in D_2O, and examined directly by 1D proton and COSY NMR. The 1D spectrum revealed considerable signal overlap in the aromatic region; however, in the COSY spectrum, well-resolved cross peaks for five paracetamol metabolites were immediately evident. They pointed out that 2D techniques are costly in terms of instrument time but can be used quite successfully when a great deal of metabolic information is required from a few samples or spectral assignments are difficult from the 1D spectra alone.

When NMR spectroscopy is coupled with partial purification, structural characterization is often possible from 1D spectra alone. Solid phase extraction is a good method for the partial purification of biological samples on a moderately large scale and has been applied successfully to the characterization of ibuprofen metabolites by 1D proton and carbon NMR (114). For this study, a normal, healthy male volunteer was administered 400 mg ibuprofen and urine was collected pre-dose, 0–2 h, and 2–4 h. The urine was lyophilized, reconstituted in D_2O, and 1D proton spectra were acquired. The samples were next applied to a C-18 solid phase extraction column and eluted with a stepwise gradient of increasing methanol concentration. Fractions were collected, the solvent was evaporated, and the residue was redissolved in D_2O. Spectra of each fraction were acquired to follow the progress of metabolite elution. Using this method, three ibuprofen metabolites, essentially free of impurities, were obtained. Ibuprofen glucuronide was obtained in sufficient quantity for a good carbon spectrum to be acquired with 20,000 transients.

Mechanistic Studies of Xenobiotic Metabolism

To elucidate the mechanism of xenobiotic metabolism, detailed structural characterization of metabolites is required. Often, such detail is only available from NMR spectroscopic analysis. Because many metabolites are present in very small quantities, extremely sensitive NMR methods are required. A type of indirect detection called proton-detected heteronuclear multiple quantum coherence (HMQC) NMR provides detailed structural information (proton–carbon connectivities) with very good sensitivity. Using a novel 1D application of HMQC, Hackett et al. (55,56) have studied the microsomal hydroxylation of the herbicide triallate. They determined that cytochrome P450 catalyzed oxidation of triallate leads to the formation of an intermediate allylic radical (AR) which undergoes rearrangement leading to hydroxylation at two different positions (Figure 36.14). The structural characterization that led to such detailed mechanistic understanding was carried out on 20–45 μg of material isolated and purified by HPLC after microsomal incubation of ^{13}C-labeled triallate. Hackett et al. (55,56) used a 500 MHz NMR equipped with a 5-mm indirect detection probe. Even greater sensitivity could be realized with a higher-field NMR and/or a 1.7-mm probe. Their work has demonstrated the utility of 1D HMQC for mechanistic studies when sample size is quite limited and no other suitable analytical method is available.

Biochemical Changes Associated with Xenobiotic Toxicity

Exposure to toxicants invariably leads to certain biochemical changes. These biochemical effects often result

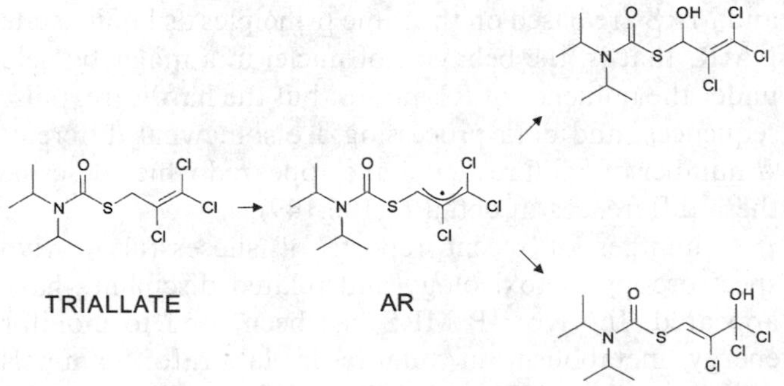

FIG. 36.14. Cytochrome P450 catalyzed oxidation of triallate showing the allylic radical (AR) intermediate.

in changes in the urinary excretion of endogenous compounds such as carbohydrates, amino acids, and carboxylic acids. Mercury is known to accumulate in the kidneys of experimental animals after injection, causing damage to the proximal tubular epithelium and severe kidney failure. Mercury-induced nephrotoxicity is characterized by increased urinary excretion of amino acids, glucose, calcium, phosphate, bicarbonate, and low molecular weight proteins. Nicholson et al. (113), by proton NMR, have studied changes in urinary and plasma levels of a large number of low molecular weight compounds in rats exposed to mercuric chloride, and correlated these changes with histopathology and enzyme excretion. They quantified metabolites in untreated urine and plasma and observed dose-dependent decreases in urinary excretion of creatinine and citrate and increases in glucose, glycine, alanine, α-ketoglutarate, succinate, and acetate. They observed increases in plasma levels of lactate and creatinine. The observed changes were consistent with Hg^{2+} inhibition of certain citric acid cycle enzymes and intracellular, tubular acidosis. Their NMR data provided not only a sensitive measure of Hg^{2+}-induced nephrotoxicity but mechanistic insight as well. Similar quantitative NMR techniques may also prove useful for studying the mechanism of action of other toxins.

In Vivo Spectroscopy and Imaging

In recent years, advances in NMR theory and hardware have enabled the study of morphological and metabolic changes in isolated organs and whole animals and humans based on NMR principles. Magnetic resonance imaging (MRI), which is widely used in clinical medicine, relies mainly on the detection of hydrogen nuclei in water and fat to construct high-resolution images. The contrast in these images results from different T_1 and T_2 relaxation times for hydrogen nuclei in different tissue environments. In vivo magnetic resonance spectroscopy (MRS) is used to obtain spectral information (such as chemical shift and intensity) on chemical compounds within living tissues and can be used to monitor metabolic changes resulting from disease or xenobiotic exposure. MRI and MRS are based on the same principles as liquid–state NMR, that is, the behavior of nuclei in a magnetic field under the influence of RF pulses, but the hardware, pulse sequences, and data processing are somewhat different. A number of good reviews have appeared which describe these differences in detail (7,106,149).

A number of recent reports of successful in vivo spectroscopy in toxicology and related disciplines have appeared. In vivo ^{31}P MRS has been used to monitor energy metabolism in tumors in laboratory animals during growth (147) and following hyperthermia (155) treatment with interleukin 1α (34) and endocrine therapy (146). In many cases, the changes seen in phosphorous metabolites (ATP, ADP, PCr, P_i, β-nucleoside triphosphate, phospholipids) correlate well with tumor growth. These results demonstrate the potential for noninvasive monitoring of tumor development by in vivo NMR spectroscopy.

MRI and MRS have been used very successfully to study liver damage induced by hepatotoxic halocarbons. Locke and Brauer (90) monitored the response of rat liver in situ to bromobenzene by proton MRI and ^{31}P MRS. They found that a sublethal dose of bromobenzene induced acute hepatic edema and decreased energy metabolism. Both effects had an onset of 15–20 h and were maximal at 25–60 h. These effects were blocked by Trolox C, a potent inhibitor of lipid peroxidation.

In vivo NMR spectroscopy has tremendous potential as a tool for studying mechanisms of toxicology. MRI and MRS techniques provide detailed information on the response of specific organs to toxicants and can also be used to monitor xenobiotic metabolism in vivo. In addition, they could greatly reduce the number of animals required for toxicology studies, because a single animal could be followed over an extended period of time to monitor internal changes. As spectrometers for in vivo NMR become more readily available to the practicing toxicologist, in vivo NMR spectroscopy will almost certainly become the method of choice for many toxicology studies.

LC–NMR

Hyphenated techniques coupling mass spectrometry and various separation methods such as GC, LC, and CE are now considered standard analytical tools widely used in toxicology research. Advances in the design of NMR probes and in methods for adequate solvent suppression together with the availability of high-field NMR spectrometers have enabled what is perhaps the most exciting recent development in NMR, the coupling of NMR with LC. This hyphenated method takes advantage of high-resolution liquid chromatographic separations and the wealth of structural information provided by 1D and 2D NMR spectra. This section will provide a brief overview of LC–NMR instrumentation, methods, and applications in toxicology research. For more detailed information the interested reader is referred to several very good reviews of the topic (87–89,112).

The complex nature of most biological samples makes direct analysis by NMR spectroscopy difficult. Spectra of crude biological samples typically contain many overlapping resonances, which greatly complicates their interpretation. One approach to the simplification of such samples is the removal of endogenous components and the separation of the compounds of interest. The use of solid phase extraction followed by 1D NMR analysis (SPE–NMR) for the isolation and characterization of ibuprofen metabolites from human urine has already been mentioned (114).

Although SPE–NMR can be quite effective, it suffers from several limitations. Solid phase extraction is a relatively low-resolution separation method. It is inadequate for very complex mixtures or mixtures of very similar compounds. SPE–NMR is a tedious and time-consuming technique involving collection of samples, solvent removal, and reconstitution of samples in an appropriate NMR solvent. It also requires a relatively large amount of sample. This is usually not a problem for analysis of human urine, but it can be limiting in some circumstances. These limitations are largely removed by hyphenation of NMR with high-performance liquid chromatography.

Although reports of successful LC–NMR experiments date back to the late 1970s, the limited sensitivity of NMR and the technical hurdles associated with suppression of signals from the protonated solvents commonly used for LC greatly limited the utility of LC–NMR. Only within the last decade, with the advent of micro NMR probes, the greater availability of high-field NMR spectrometers (>300 MHz) with increased dynamic range, and the development of truly effective solvent suppression methods, has LC–NMR come into its own as a widely used analytical technique. Hardware and software making LC–NMR a relatively routine method are now commercially available from major vendors.

Even though the configuration of LC–NMR systems varies from vendor to vendor and laboratory to laboratory, all systems share the same basic components. The design of a typical LC–NMR system is shown schematically in Figure 36.15. The LC pumps, injector, column, and detector are all standard equipment. From the detector the flow enters the LC–NMR interface which contains components for flow control and peak sampling. The LC–NMR interface can send the flow directly to the NMR probe, divert the flow to waste, or store peaks detected by the in-line detector for subsequent NMR analysis. The NMR probe contains a flow–cell that replaces the standard glass NMR tube and typically has a volume between about 50 μL and 250 μL. The probe can be of the selectively tuned type for direct detection of ^{1}H, ^{19}F, ^{31}P, and so on, or it can be of the indirect detection type. Broadband probes are inherently less sensitive than selectively tuned or indirect probes and, therefore, are rarely, if ever, used for LC–NMR.

The most commonly used LC–NMR probe is the dual indirect ^{1}H/^{13}C indirect probe. Instruments configured as in Figure 36.15 can be used in the continuous-flow mode where peaks eluted from the LC column pass through the LC–NMR interface to the flow–cell for detection in real time. This so-called "on-line" LC–NMR works well for fairly concentrated samples (mass detection limits >10 μg in the flow cell) but because the residence time in the flow cell is limited, it is difficult to obtain more than 32–64 transients and 2D experiments are not possible.

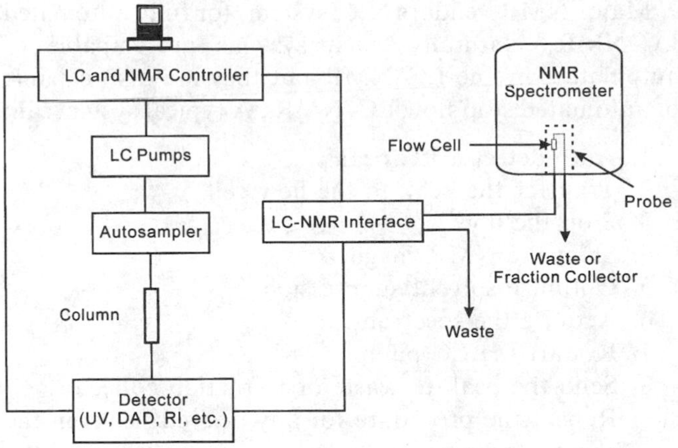

FIG. 36.15. Schematic representation of a LC–NMR system.

When higher resolution and/or sensitivity are required, the LC–NMR interface can be programmed to stop the flow once a peak of interest enters the probe. This "stop-flow" or "static" LC–NMR offers the opportunity to acquire as many transients as necessary for adequate signal-to-noise in 1D experiments and is compatible with 2D experiments as well. Using stop-flow, samples of ~1 μg or less can be analyzed. A variation of the stop-flow technique involves programming the LC–NMR interface to store peaks of interest in sample loops and then pass them one at a time to the probe. Once a peak enters the probe the flow is stopped and the peak is scanned.

A major development in the evolution of routine LC–NMR was in the area of solvent suppression. Because most LC separations of biological samples depend on reverse phase columns, they utilize solvent mixtures containing water and protonated organic solvents such as methanol or acetonitrile. The most common LC–NMR solvent mixtures are D_2O/acetonitrile or D_2O/methanol. The use of D_2O reduces the effective concentration of solvent protons and provides a source of deuterium for the instrument lock. D_2O is relatively inexpensive, and thus is a very good alternative to H_2O. As discussed previously, the use of protonated solvents (such as acetonitrile) requires attenuation of the solvent signals to observe the weak signals from solute molecules. Fortunately, LC–NMR control systems contain computer software for solvent suppression pulse sequences such as NOESYPRESAT. The suppression of signals from mixed solvents is now a routine operation requiring minimal operator involvement.

Major NMR vendors offer systems for fully automated LC–NMR. Naturally, such systems are capable of automated on-line LC–NMR but they are also capable of automated stop-flow LC–NMR . A typical system can:

1. Auto-detect a LC peak.
2. Transfer the peak to the flow cell.
3. Stop the flow.
4. Shim the NMR magnet.
5. Optimize solvent suppression.
6. Acquire the spectrum.
7. Restart the LC pump.
8. Send the peak to waste or a fraction collector.
9. Repeat the procedure for any desired peaks in the chromatogram.

Such a system can also automatically store peaks of interest in the LC–NMR interface for subsequent analysis.

The most common applications of LC–NMR involve the characterization of xenobiotic metabolites. An early example, reported by Spraul et al. (145) was the characterization of ibuprofen metabolites in human urine. For this study, a normal, healthy male volunteer was administered 400 mg ibuprofen and urine was collected 0–4 h after dosing. The urine was lyophilized and reconstituted in a D_2O d_3-acetonitrile mixture prior to LC–NMR analysis. Gradient elution LC was accomplished with

(a) potassium dihydrogen phosphate in D_2O and
(b) acetonitrile.

A linear gradient from 2–45% acetonitrile at a flow rate of 1 mL/min was used for stop-flow analysis. For on-line analysis, a flow rate of 0.5 mL/min was used. The 500 MHz NMR was equipped with a commercial selectively tuned ^1H flow probe with 60 μL flow–cell, and solvent suppression was accomplished using the NOESYPRESAT pulse sequence. For on-line analysis, a total of 16 transients were collected for each peak, giving a time resolution of 12 sec. For stop-flow analysis, both 1D (256 or 512 transients) and 2D TOCSY experiments were performed. Using on-line analysis, Spraul et al. (145) were able to identify five metabolites, including three glucuronide conjugates. The stop-flow analyses provided high-resolution 1D ^1H spectra and 2D TOCSY spectra which permitted unambiguous characterization of the five metabolites. On-column detection limits were 10 μg for the on-line analyses and 1 μg for the stop-flow. Using LC–NMR, the authors were able to identify one metabolite, the dicarboxylic acid metabolite of ibuprofen, which was not observed using SPE–NMR.

Glucuronic acid conjugates of carboxylic acids can undergo an isomerization reaction known as acyl migration, where the carboxylic acid moiety migrates from the 1 position of the glucuronic acid to the 2, 3, or 4 position. Such isomerizations can occur in vivo and in vitro at physiological pH and under mildly alkaline conditions. The resulting acyl migrated positional isomers can exist as either β or α anomers. Lenz et al. (86) used LC–NMR to characterize the glucuronic acid conjugates of the nonsteroidal antiinflammatory drug 6,11-dihydro-11-oxodibenz[*b,e*]oxepin-2-acetic acid in human urine and study the pH dependence of the acyl migration reaction in that matrix. They used a 400 MHz NMR with a 120 μL flow cell in the stop-flow mode to obtain ^1H spectra of the α and β anomers of all possible acyl migration products. For one metabolite, they used a 600 MHz NMR to obtain higher resolution spectra aiding in full characterization. This work is noteworthy because the α and β anomers were not separated by the LC, and yet using NMR as a detector allowed the unambiguous characterization of the metabolite anomers. The high resolution and rich information content of NMR spectra can often be used to characterize closely related metabolites that co-elute in the liquid chromatogram.

The use of very high-field NMR spectrometers (800 MHz) greatly increases spectral resolution and can aid tremendously in metabolite characterization by LC–NMR. Sidelmann et al. (139) used SPE–NMR at 400 MHz and stop-flow LC–NMR at 800 MHz to identify the major phase II metabolites of tolfenamic acid in human urine. They identified glucuronide conjugates of the parent compound and five metabolites, the first report of the direct identification of these phase II metabolites in biofluids. The 800 MHz NMR was particularly useful in determining the exact position of hydroxylation of the aromatic ring of tolfenamic acid. The increase in spectral dispersion obtained at ultra-high field provided very high resolution 1D ^1H spectra thus permitting unambiguous assignments.

LC–NMR has also been applied to studies of in vitro microsomal metabolism. Corcoran et al. (37) identified the metabolites of two phenoxypyridines obtained from incubation with rat microsomes using stop-flow LC–NMR at 750 MHz. They were able to characterize one metabolite that was 6% of the total and another that was only 0.6%. The unequivocal identification of these metabolites without the use of radiolabeled substrates or synthetic metabolite standards demonstrated that LC–NMR can be used for metabolite characterization in in vitro systems and could be used in a high throughput mode for lead optimization in drug discovery.

In an effort to further reduce the sample size required for hyphenated separation-NMR techniques, a number of laboratories have explored microbore or capillary LC as well as other separation methods such as capillary electrophoresis (CE) and capillary electrochromatography (CEC) coupled to NMR. Wu et al. (170) developed a theoretical model for predicting signal-to-noise ratio (SNR) as NMR flow cell volume is scaled down. Their model predicted only a twofold reduction in SNR for a 400-fold reduction in flow cell volume. They constructed a 50-nL flow cell by wrapping narrow-gauge copper wire around a fused silica capillary column. Using this microflow cell and a 300 MHz spectrometer, they realized a mass limit of detection of $\sim 1\ \mu g$ on-column in an on-line microbore LC–NMR analysis. The most serious limitation to their approach was the relatively broad line widths in the on-line NMR spectra. When the analysis was performed in the stop-flow mode, they were able to optimize the NMR shims and other instrument parameters and reduce the line widths to <1 Hz. As a result, 2D experiments such as COSY and NOESY were possible.

More recently, Pusecker et al. (125) constructed a 240-nL capillary flow cell coupled to a packed fused silica microbore column. This column could be used for CE, CEC, or capillary HPLC separations. Using a 600 MHz NMR, they realized a mass limit of detection of ~300 ng in the stop-flow mode. They also reported that in the on-line mode, the limit of detection was adequate for all three micro separation techniques. A major advantage to this system is the ease of changing from one separation method to another. When this micro flow cell was used in an on-line CE analysis of paracetamol metabolites in an extract of human urine (at 600 MHz) the mass limit of detection was ~10 ng (134). On-line CEC analysis afforded a similar mass limit of detection. This work clearly showed that identification of metabolites by NMR could be accomplished with nanoliter sample volumes. Improvements in flow cell and probe design are likely to reduce limits of detection even further and micro separation methods coupled to on-line NMR detection will almost certainly become routine tools for metabolite identification.

LC–NMR–MS

The hyphenated techniques of LC–MS and LC–NMR are both very powerful tools for characterization of xenobiotic metabolites but they both suffer from unavoidable limitations. Neither technique can, by itself, enable the unequivocal assignment of chemical structure in all cases. Mass spectrometry often cannot distinguish between positional isomers, but NMR is very good for this application. Certain functional groups do not contain NMR active nuclei and are invisible in NMR spectra. An example of an NMR-invisible functional group is the sulfate group of sulfate conjugates. In such cases, mass spectrometry can be used to characterize the sample. Because MS and NMR are complementary techniques and both have been successfully hyphenated with LC, it was inevitable that these techniques would be merged to form LC–NMR–MS.

The first report of successful LC–NMR–MS appeared in 1995 (123) and was soon followed by reports of its application for characterization and quantification of xenobiotic metabolites (14,40,62,130,131,132,138,166). The advantages of LC–NMR–MS are obvious in these reports. By capitalizing on the strengths of NMR and MS in one method, it affords rapid identification of unknown compounds in complex mixtures such as urine in a single chromatographic run. With the increasing availability of LC–NMR instruments that can be coupled to mass spectrometers, more reports of LC–NMR–MS in toxicology research are sure to appear.

Limitations

Even though NMR spectroscopy is a very powerful tool for studying mechanisms of toxicology, it is subject to a number of significant limitations. Perhaps the greatest limitation of NMR is its sensitivity. As discussed above, even the most sensitive spectrometers require nanograms of sample for NMR analysis. Recent advances in magnet, flow cell, and probe design have greatly reduced the amount of sample required for NMR, but it would be unrealistic to assume that NMR will be as sensitive an analytical technique as mass spectrometry in the foreseeable future.

Another limitation of NMR is cost, and, hence, availability. NMR spectrometers are quite expensive and their price goes up dramatically with field strength. High-field spectrometers are not common laboratory instruments so instrument time must be purchased from a local (or regional) NMR laboratory or acquired through collaboration.

NMR spectroscopy is a specialized discipline requiring a significant amount of expertise. Operation of NMR spectrometers and interpretation of spectra are not straightforward and require a great deal of training and experience. A toxicologist lacking this training and experience would do well to establish an active collaboration with a NMR spectroscopist to carry out sophisticated NMR studies.

ELECTRON PARAMAGNETIC RESONANCE SPECTROSCOPY

A free radical is a chemical species that contains an unpaired electron. Most free radicals are extremely reactive and there is increasing awareness of the role they play in the mechanism of tissue injury and the toxicity of a large number of chemicals (5,57,107). Free radicals are often formed during xenobiotic metabolism by enzymes such as cytochrome P450 and peroxidases. In the presence of ferrous iron, superoxide forms the extremely reactive hydroxyl radical (HO·) by the Haber–Weiss reaction.

It is the hydroxyl radical that is responsible for the toxic effects of iron overload. Free radicals are involved in the process of lipid peroxidation, which among other biological effects, leads to LDL oxidation and subsequent atherosclerosis.

Because free radicals are so reactive, they have short lifetimes and are present in biological systems at very low concentrations. As a result, they are usually difficult to detect. A number of indirect methods such as product analysis, inhibition by radical scavengers (e.g., antioxidants), and flash photolysis have been used to detect free radicals in biological systems but these methods provide little information on the nature of the radical. The most information-rich method for the determination of free radicals is electron paramagnetic resonance (EPR) spectroscopy, also called electron spin resonance (ESR) spectroscopy.

The following sections contain a very brief discussion of the theory of EPR spectroscopy and several examples of its application in toxicology. Because the basic phenomenon of magnetic resonance is common to both EPR and NMR, it is assumed that the reader is familiar with the preceding discussion of the theory of NMR spectroscopy. For a detailed description of the theory and instrumentation of EPR, the interested reader should refer to other texts (3,4,121).

Basic Theory of EPR Spectroscopy

Like a proton, an electron rotates about its axis and has a magnetic moment, μ. In an applied magnetic field, B_o, this magnetic moment will precess around the axis of B_o with a characteristic precessional frequency, υ. The spin quantum number of an electron (S) is 1/2 so, in a magnetic field, it exists in two energy states. The energy difference between these two spin states is given by:

$$E = h\upsilon = g\mathbf{B}_o \frac{eh}{4\pi m_e c} \qquad (5)$$

where m_e is the electron mass, e is the electronic charge, c is the speed of light, and h is Planck's constant. The proportionality constant, g, the spectroscopic splitting factor, is the ratio of the magnetic moment to the angular momentum with a value of 2.002319 for an unbound electron.

The exact precessional frequency (and position of the resonance signal) of an electron in a radical will depend on its chemical environment. In NMR spectroscopy, the position of the resonance signal is given by the chemical shift, δ, in EPR the resonance positions are expressed as g values. Tables of g values for common radicals are available (see pp. 336–337 of Gordon and Ford [51]).

The magnetic moment of an electron is about 700 times greater than that of a proton, so the energy difference between spin states is greater in EPR than in NMR. This means that EPR is more sensitive than NMR and EPR spectra can be recorded on radical concentrations in the low micromolar range. The larger energy difference between spin states also means that the energy required for EPR spectroscopy is greater than that for NMR. The frequencies used for EPR are in the microwave region of the electromagnetic spectrum. For a typical EPR spectrometer operating at a field strength of 0.34 T, the precessional frequency of an electron is approximately 9.5 GHz (9.5×10^9 Hz).

EPR signals are typically much broader than NMR signals. To facilitate assignment of resonance positions (g values), the spectra are virtually always plotted as first-derivative traces. NMR spectra are plotted as absorption versus frequency and EPR spectra are plotted as the rate of change of absorption versus frequency. Figure 36.16 shows these two different types of spectral traces. Because radicals have only one unpaired electron, an EPR spectrum of a single radical species will have only one signal. If a sample contains more than one radical species, then multiple signals will appear. The total area under a peak in an EPR spectrum is proportional to the number of unpaired electrons. For quantification of unknown radical concentrations, direct comparison is made to a standard of known concentration. The ratio of peak areas provides the concentration of the unknown. A commonly used standard is the commercially available diphenylpicrylhydrazyl (DPPH) with 1.53×10^{21} unpaired electrons per gram.

In a radical, the unpaired electron is not associated with only one atom. The electron spin is distributed over several atoms in the radical and can interact with any spin-active nuclei with which it is associated. This inter-

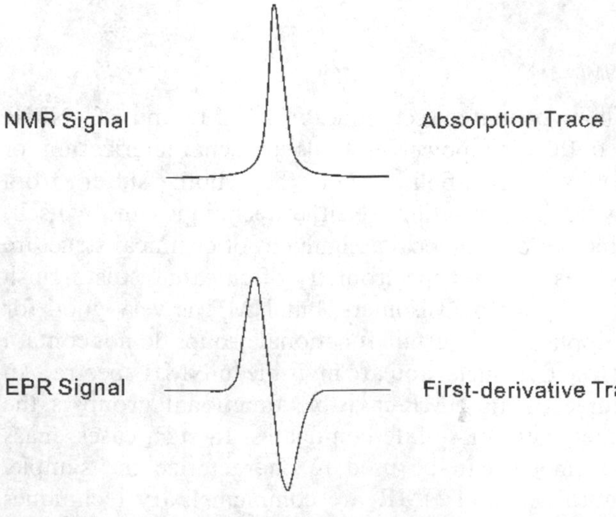

FIG. 36.16. NMR spectrum plotted as an absorption trace and an EPR spectrum plotted as a first-derivative trace.

action of electron and nuclear spins leads to spin–spin coupling called hyperfine splitting, reminiscent of the coupling seen in NMR spectra. An EPR signal will be split into $2nI+1$ peaks, where n is the number of equivalent nuclei of spin I. The hyperfine splitting constant is given the symbol a_i, where i is the atomic symbol of the nucleus to which the electron is coupled. Hyperfine splitting constants in EPR are typically measured in gauss (G), although in more recent literature they are sometimes reported in Hz. Figure 36.17 shows a computer-simulated EPR spectrum of the methyl radical. The unpaired electron is coupled to the three equivalent protons, so the signal appears as a quartet. The magnitude of the hyperfine splitting constant is directly proportional to the electron spin density at the coupled nucleus. In other words, it is related to the probability of finding the unpaired electron associated with the coupled nucleus. Hyperfine splitting constants are often used in the interpretation of EPR spectra and tables of a_i values have been compiled for easy reference (see pp. 337–339 of Gordon and Ford [51]).

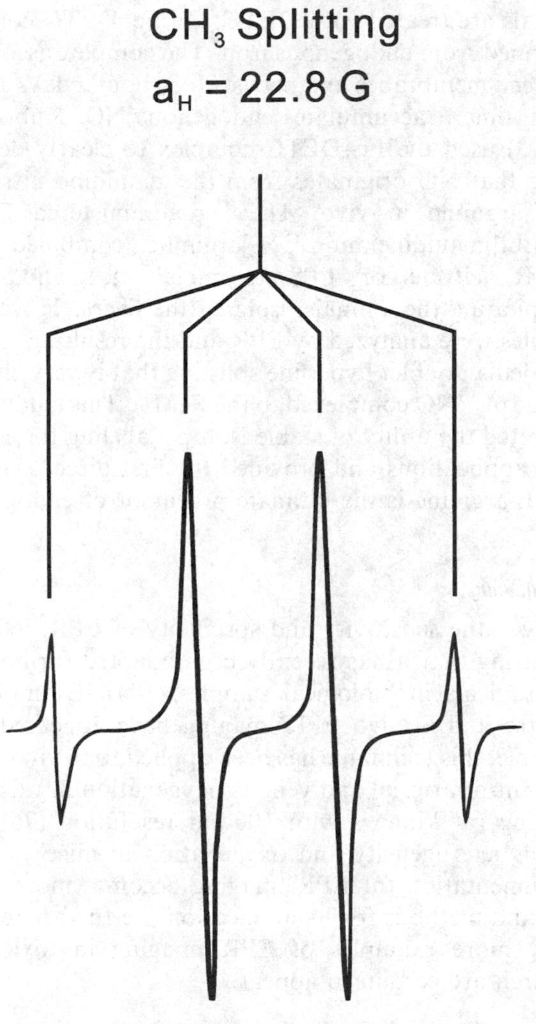

FIG. 36.17. Computer-simulated EPR spectrum of the methyl radical showing the 22.8 G hyperfine splitting caused by coupling of the unpaired electron to the three spin-½ protons.

Instrumental Design

EPR spectrometers contain the same basic components as NMR spectrometers: a probe, a magnet, a source of electromagnetic radiation (microwaves), a transmitter and receiver with associated amplifiers, and a system for data collection (usually a computer). In conventional EPR, the microwave frequency is typically held constant and the magnetic field is varied during spectral acquisition. Most conventional EPR spectrometers operate with a field strength of approximately 0.34 T and the field is swept over a several hundred G range. For a field strength of 0.34 T, the microwave frequency is about 9.5 GHz. In recent years, frequency pulse techniques and Fourier transform methods have been introduced in EPR. FT–EPR offers tremendous advantages over conventional EPR. Now multipulse 1D experiments and sophisticated 2D experiments are available. The use of frequency pulse techniques and Fourier transform methods will certainly revolutionize EPR just as they did NMR.

Spin Trapping

Some free radicals are stable enough in solution to be detected directly by EPR. Unfortunately, most free radicals of toxicological interest are quite unstable so an indirect method of detection is often required. The most commonly used indirect method for detecting free radicals is called spin trapping. The technique involves adding a spin trap (usually a nitrone or nitroso compound) to the sample prior to radical generation. When the radical is generated it reacts rapidly with the spin trap producing a secondary radical or spin adduct which is more stable than the parent free radical and can be detected by EPR. Even though the species that is detected is not the parent radical, it is often possible to determine the nature of the parent radical by studying model reactions between known radicals and the spin trap. For a detailed description of experimental methods for in vitro and in vivo spin trapping and subsequent EPR analysis the interested reader is directed to Brackett et al. (13).

Applications

Model Studies

An important approach to elucidating mechanisms of toxicology is the study of appropriate model systems, usually chemical or enzymatic reactions in aqueous solution. Such in vitro model systems often reveal the potential for a proposed in vivo reaction or pathway. This approach is often used to study free radical processes that are thought to play a role in xenobiotic toxicity.

Cobalt compounds have been reported to be genotoxic and carcinogenic in a variety of in vivo systems. Similar effects of other transition metals have been linked to the generation of free radicals by reaction of the metal ions with lipid hydroperoxides. Shi et al. (136) have studied the reaction of Co (II) with H_2O_2 and several lipid hydroperoxides in the presence of various biological ligands and the spin trap 5,5-dimethyl-1-pyrroline N-oxide (DMPO) to determine the potential for in vivo Co (II)-mediated free radical damage. They found that Co (II) did generate free radicals in the presence of reduced glutathione (GSH), cysteine, penicillamine, or N-acetylcysteine but not in the presence of oxidized glutathione or cystine. Histidine and histidyl oligopeptides did not promote Co (II)-mediated radical formation. They concluded that in the presence of certain biological ligands (those containing the—SH group) Co (II) can react with lipid hydroperoxides and H_2O_2 to generate free radicals which may be important in Co (II)-mediated toxicity and carcinogenicity.

In Vivo Spin Trapping

Through the application of spin trapping techniques, it is possible to obtain direct evidence for free radical generation in vivo in response to xenobiotic exposure. Ozone exposure is known to produce pulmonary damage as a result of lipid peroxidation of lung tissue. Indirect evidence has suggested the involvement of free radicals in this process; however, direct evidence of a radical pathway was lacking until Kennedy et al. (72) reported spin trapping and detection of free radicals produced in vivo during inhalation exposure of rats to ozone. They administered the spin trap α-(4-pyridyl-1-oxide)-N-*tert*-butylnitrone (4-POBN) ip to rats prior to ozone exposure and detected a 4-POBN spin adduct in lipid extracts from lungs after exposure. The concentration of the spin adduct in lung extracts correlated well with ozone dose and the lung weight/body weight ratio. Their results demonstrated that ozone exposure induced free radical production in rat lung and that the free radicals may be involved in the pulmonary toxicity of ozone.

Nitric oxide (NO) is an endogenous metabolite in many different organisms. It is a potent vasodilator and is important in the regulation of blood pressure and flow. It also inhibits blood clotting by platelets. In the CNS, it is an important signaling molecule involved in nerve-potentiation and short-term memory. These beneficial effects of NO are realized at low concentrations ($<1\ \mu M$). At higher concentrations, NO has cytotoxic effects and is important in the immune response to foreign cells.

Nitric oxide contains an unpaired electron and is relatively stable compared to many free radicals. It binds tightly to certain metal ions including Fe (II), forming stable complexes which are themselves EPR-detectable free radicals. NO binds to hemoglobin, myoglobin, and other Fe (II)-containing biomolecules such as mitochondrial iron–sulfur proteins, forming complexes that can be detected and quantified by EPR. A number of investigators have used EPR to study NO complexes with endogenous Fe (II)-containing biomolecules in response to environmental toxins and disease. Two very interesting recent reviews describe such studies (22,23).

Another method for detecting and quantifying NO in vivo is through the introduction of a suitable spin trap. Iron (II) forms a very stable complex with diethyldithiocarbamate (DETC) and the resulting free radical has a very characteristic EPR spectrum. When animals are treated with DETC, the Fe–DETC complex is formed from endogenous iron. The complex associates with cell membranes and persists for about a day, during which time it accumulates endogenous NO. Kubrina et al. (73) used the Fe–DETC complex to clearly demonstrate that NO originates from the guanidino nitrogens of L-arginine in vivo. They co-administered DETC and L-[guanidineimino-$^{15}N_2$]arginine combined with iron(II) citrate or LPS to male mice and, after decapitating the animals, isolated the livers. These liver samples were analyzed by EPR and the resulting spectra revealed a doublet hyperfine splitting that is very characteristic of ^{15}NO complexed to the Fe (II). This study demonstrated the utility of stable isotope labeling for certain EPR applications and provided the first direct evidence that L-arginine is the ultimate precursor of endogenous NO.

EPR Imaging

Given the sensitivity and specificity of EPR, it is not surprising that it has recently been adapted for imaging free radicals in biological samples (144). Examples of in vitro and in vivo EPR imaging have appeared. For example, this technique has been applied to in vivo measurement of arterial and venous oxygenation in rats (77), imaging rat kidneys with 100 μm resolution (76), and tumor heterogeneity and oxygenation in mice (78). As instrumentation for EPR imaging becomes more available and methods for its application are further refined, many more examples of EPR imaging in toxicology research are certain to appear.

Limitations

A significant limitation of EPR spectroscopy in toxicology research is a result of the species under study, the free radical. Because many free radicals are quite unstable, they are often detected indirectly by spin trapping techniques. This requires administration of a suitable spin trap that may have its own toxic effects. The spin adducts produced are secondary radicals and it is not always possible to determine the structure of the parent radical from EPR analysis of the spin adduct.

Despite these limitations, EPR spectroscopy has proven to be a very important tool for studying free radical mechanisms of toxicity. It is the method of choice for detecting the presence of radicals in vitro and in vivo.

UV AND VISIBLE SPECTROPHOTOMETRY

Principles

UV and visible (UV–VIS) absorption spectrophotometry have been principal methods of chemical analysis for over 40 years, and involve the measurement of light absorption by substances in the wavelength region from 190–380 nm for UV absorption and 380–900 nm for visible light absorption (39,47,135,143). Absorption in both these regions arises from electronic transitions within the molecule. The frequency of absorption depends on the energy difference between the normal or ground state of an electron versus that of the excited state (higher energy level). Absorption of UV or visible light is also accompanied by vibrational and rotational transitions which result in relatively broad bands that are characteristic of UV–VIS spectra.

A molecule containing electrons in σ, π, and n-orbitals (see Figure 36.18) may absorb light energy and be promoted from the ground state to higher energy states. Antibonding orbitals (σ^* and π^*) exist in the excited state for the bonding electrons, and n electrons may be associated in the ground state with heteroatoms that do not participate in bonding yet can absorb energy and be promoted to either σ^* or π^* orbitals. From a practical consideration, the $\pi \rightarrow \pi^*$ and $n \rightarrow \pi^*$ transitions are of most utility because these transitions occur in the useful

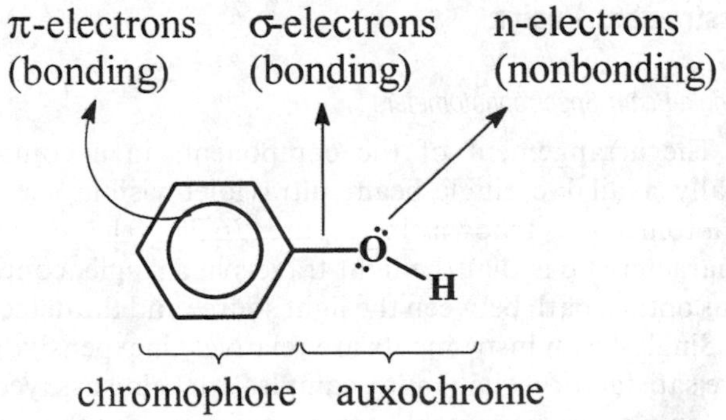

FIG. 36.18. Some basic terminologies in UV spectrophotometry.

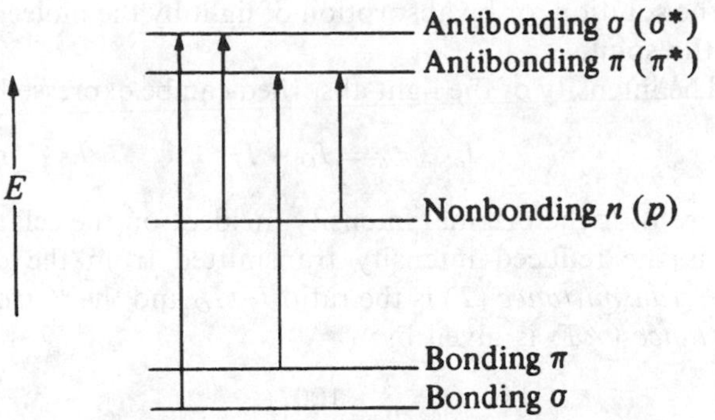

FIG. 36.19. Summary of electronic energy transitions.

range (200–750 nm) of the UV–VIS spectrum; $\sigma \rightarrow \sigma^*$ transitions require more energy and usually occur at wavelengths of less than 200 nm. Compounds that contain non-bonding electrons on oxygen, nitrogen, sulfur, or halogen atoms can undergo $n \rightarrow \sigma^*$ transitions, however, these are of lower energy than $\sigma \rightarrow \sigma^*$ transitions. The absorption due to $n \rightarrow \sigma^*$ transitions is of limited utility because it is very weak, and in most cases occurs at wavelengths too short to be easily measured on conventional instruments, for example, trimethylamine λ 277 nm, ϵ 227, and methanol λ 183 nm, ϵ 150. Molecules that contain oxygen, nitrogen, sulfur, or halogen atoms usually show an intense absorption around 200 nm due to $n \rightarrow \sigma^*$ transitions; this absorption is known as end absorption.

The energy required for the $\sigma \rightarrow \sigma^*$ transition is very high; consequently, compounds in which all valence shell electrons are involved in single-bond formation, such as saturated hydrocarbons, do not show absorption in the ordinary ultraviolet region. An exception is cyclopropane, which shows a wavelength of maximum absorption (λ_{max}) of about 190 nm (propane shows λ_{max} about 135 nm). Transitions to antibonding π^* orbitals are associated with unsaturated centers in the molecule such as alkenyl, carbonyl, imino, and azo groups. These transitions are of relatively lower energy requirement and occur in the useful part of the UV spectrum (e.g. C=O ~ 285 nm [low intensity, $n \rightarrow \pi^*$] and 185 nm [high intensity, $\pi \rightarrow \pi^*$]. $\pi \rightarrow \pi^*$ transitions lie between $n \rightarrow \sigma^*$ and $n \rightarrow \pi^*$ transitions in terms of energy content. Figure 36.19 illustrates in a non-empirical manner, the relative electronic excitation energies for the above electronic transitions.

Quantitative Aspects of UV–Visible Spectrophotometry—Beer–Lambert Law

When UV light traverses a cell containing an absorbing solute dissolved in a suitable solvent, the light intensity is diminished by either reflection at the inner and outer surfaces of the cell, by light scattering by any particles in the solution, or by absorption of light by the molecules of the solute.

The intensity of the light absorbed can be expressed as:

$$I_{absorbed} = I_O - I_T \quad (6)$$

where I_O is the original intensity incident on the cell and I_T is the reduced intensity transmitted from the cell. The *transmittance* (*T*) is the ratio I_T/I_O and the % *transmittance* (%*T*) is given by:

$$\%T = \frac{100 I_T}{I_o} \quad (7)$$

The *absorbance* (*A*) is the common logarithm of the reciprocal of *T*:

$$A = \log \frac{I_o}{I_T} \quad (8)$$

It can be shown that the intensity of a beam of parallel monochromatic radiation decreases exponentially as it passes through a medium of homogeneous thickness. Or, alternatively, the absorbance is proportional to the pathlength (*b*) of the solution. This is the basis of Lambert's Law.

Beer's Law states that the intensity of a beam of parallel monochromatic radiation decreases exponentially with the number of absorbing molecules, or, more simply, the absorbance is proportional to the concentration (*c*). A combination of the two laws yield the Beer–Lambert Law:

$$A = \log \frac{I_o}{I_T} = abc \quad (9)$$

The proportionality constant, *a*, is called the *absorptivity*.

The name and value of *a* depend on the units of concentration. When *c* is in moles per liter, the constant is called *molar absorptivity* or the *molar extinction coefficient* (ϵ). Thus:

$$A = \varepsilon bc \quad (10)$$

The molar absorptivity at a specified wavelength of a compound in solution is the absorbance at that wavelength of a 1 mol per liter solution in a 1-cm cell. The units of ϵ are therefore liter mol^{-1} cm^{-1}. Expressing the absorptivity in terms of a 1 mol per liter solution facilitates the comparison of the light-absorbing abilities of compounds with widely differing molecular weights. Substances that have ϵ values less than 100 are weakly absorbing; those with ϵ values above 10,000 are intensely absorbing. Many absorbing xenobiotics and drugs have an ε value at their wavelength of maximum absorption of $10^{3.5}$–$10^{4.5}$.

Another form of the Beer–Lambert proportionality constant is the specific absorbance, which is the absorbance of a specified concentration in a cell of specified pathlength. The most common form is the *A*(1%, 1 cm) value, which is the absorbance of a 1 g/100 ml (1% w/v) solution in a 1-cm cell. The Beer–Lambert equation therefore takes the form:

$$A = A^{1\%}_{1cm} bc \quad (11)$$

where *c* is in g/100 ml and *b* is in cm.

Whenever an analyte is involved in an equilibrium such as protonation or deprotonation, tautomerism, dimerization, or complex formation, the material added to the solution will be distributed among several forms and the apparent concentration (amount of material dissolved/volume) will not be proportional to the actual concentration of the parent substance. A deviation from Beer's Law will be observed under these circumstances unless the absorptivity is identical for all the species present or the equilibrium is controlled in some manner. If only two species are present and their spectra are not too different, useful measurements following Beer's Law can be made by measuring at the *isosbestic point* rather than at λ_{max}. The isosbestic point is the wavelength at which the UV spectra of the two species cross when measured at equal molarities or, equivalently, the wavelength at which their molar absorptivities are equal. Deviations arising from acid-base equilibria can be avoided by carefully buffering the solutions because the ratio of protonated to deprotonated analyte will be constant at constant pH. A variety of other equilibria can be controlled in a similar manner.

Absorption spectra of compounds with conjugated chromophores or aromatic moieties in their structure show maxima shifts to longer wavelengths (bathochromic shifts) when compared to the wavelength of individual chromophores. This is due to increased stability of the π-electron system which requires less energy for the $\pi \rightarrow \pi^*$ transition. This bathochromic shift is usually accompanied by an increase in intensity of the absorption (a hyperchromic shift).

Instrument Design

Single-Beam Spectrophotometers

The arrangement of the components in a commercially available single-beam ultraviolet–visible spectrophotometer is shown in Figure 36.20. The essential characteristic is that the light travels in a single, continuous optical path between the light source and the detector.

Single-beam instruments are relatively inexpensive and are satisfactory when many samples are being assayed by a simple measurement of absorbance at the same wavelength. A major disadvantage is the need to reset the 100% transmission value at each wavelength to com-

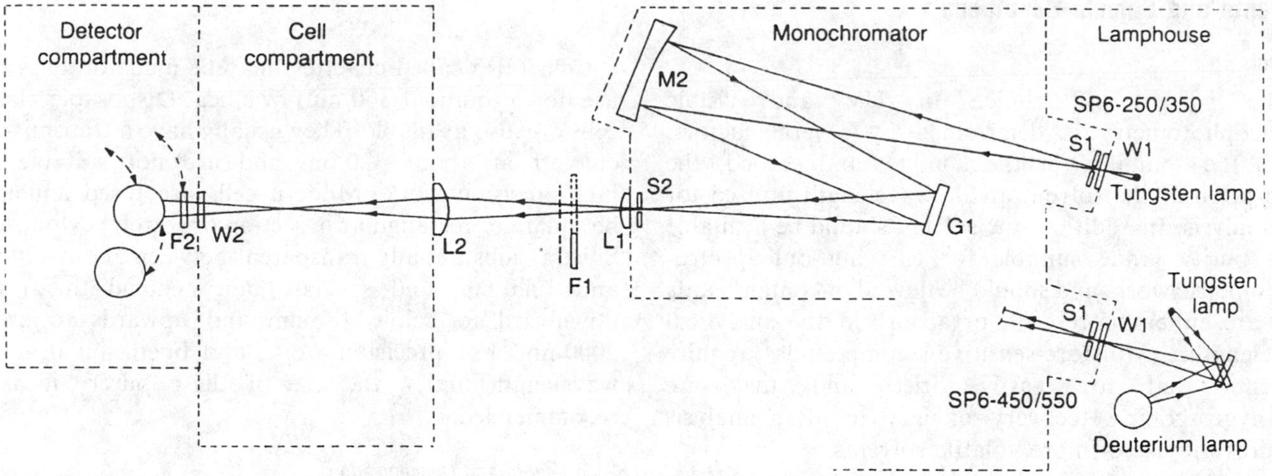

FIG. 36.20. Optical diagram of a single beam UV spectrophotometer; abbreviations: F = filter, G = grating, L = lens, M = mirror, S = slit, W = window (From Pye Unicam, Ltd., with permission).

pensate for the large variation of intensity of light from the lamp with wavelength.

Double-Beam Spectrophotometers

In this type of instrument (Figure 36.21), the monochromatic light is split by a rapidly rotating beam chopper into two beams which are directed alternately in rapid succession through a cell containing the sample and one containing the solvent only. If there is greater absorption of light in the sample cell than in the reference cell, the recombination of the beams at the detector produces a pulsating current that is converted into two direct current voltages proportional to the light intensities I_0 and I_T, transmitted by the reference solution and the sample solution, respectively. The ratio of voltages is recorded as a transmission. Double-beam optics therefore automatically compensate for variation of I_0 with wavelength. Recording spectrophotometers are double-beam instruments equipped with a wavelength scanning device which allows the rapid automatic scanning of spectra.

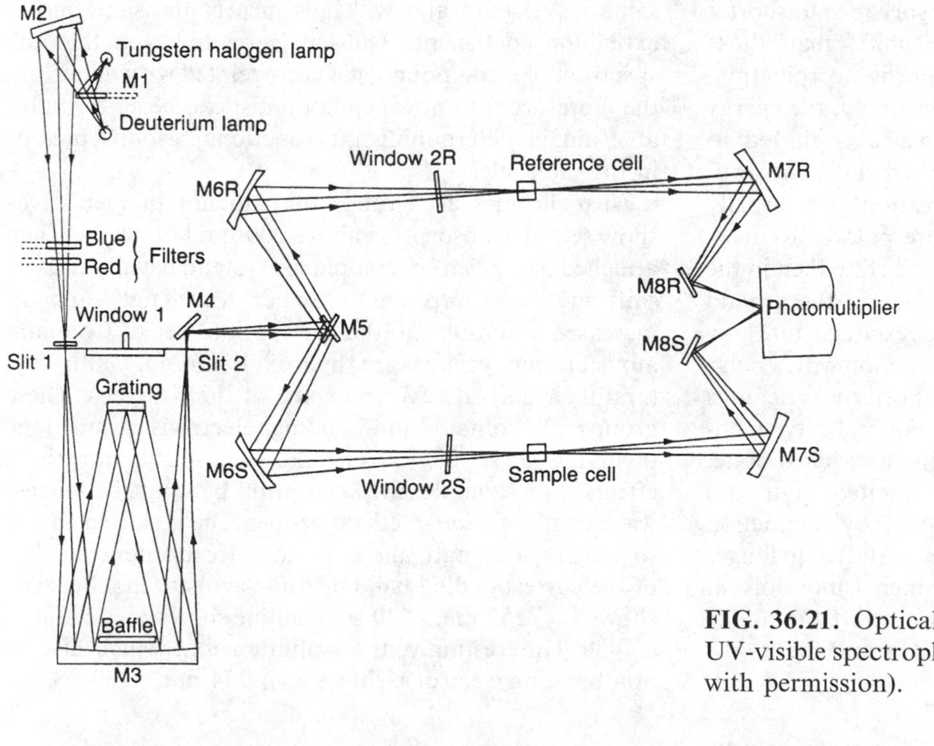

FIG. 36.21. Optical diagram of a double-beam UV-visible spectrophotometer. (From Pye Unicam, Ltd., with permission).

Solvents and Sample Conditions

Solvents

The solvent of choice in UV and visible spectrophotometry is determined by several factors: First, the solubility of the analyte, and second, the absorption of the solvent at the wavelength utilized for the analysis. In addition, the solvent should be available in a purity grade suitable for carrying out spectrophotometric work, and should be devoid of contaminants that are either fluorescent, or absorb at the analytical wavelength. Moisture-sensitive compounds require solvents that are easily dried and that are non-hygroscopic. Recovery of analyte after analysis requires the use of more volatile solvents.

It is important to note that the analyte may be sensitive to pH changes. For example, acid-base equilibria, tautomerism, complex formation, and other equilibria are often pH-dependent. Therefore, in such systems, a strongly acidic or basic solvent may be indicated to ensure that the analyte is present in solution as a single species. Non-absorbing buffers may also be used in UV analysis for this purpose.

The exact wavelength of a particular electronic transition depends not only on the chromophore, but also on the solvent, on substituents present on the chromophore, and on chromophore geometry. The solvent effect arises because solvation alters the electronic energy levels of a chromophore, and the degree of solvation is frequently different for the ground and excited states. If the ground state is solvated more strongly than the excited state, the energy difference between the levels is increased. The increase in energy difference is reflected in a shift of the absorbance to shorter wavelengths (hypsochromic or blue shift) than those observed in the gas phase where there is no solvation. If the excited state is solvated more strongly, the energy difference decreases and the absorbance is shifted to longer wavelength (bathochromic or red shift). Absorption due to $n \rightarrow \sigma^*$ and $n \rightarrow \pi^*$ transitions are usually shifted to shorter wavelengths in more polar solvents.

If a group is more polar in the ground state then in the excited state, the non-bonding electrons in the ground state are stabilized (relative to the excited state) by hydrogen bonding or electrostatic interaction with a polar solvent. The absorption is shifted to shorter wavelengths (higher energy) with increasing solvent polarity. Conversely, if the group is more polar in the excited state, the non-bonding electrons of the excited state are stabilized (relative to the ground state) by interaction with a polar solvent and the absorption is shifted to longer wavelength (lower energy) with increasing solvent polarity. Thus, polar solvents generally shift the $n \rightarrow \pi^*$ and $n \rightarrow \sigma^*$ bands to shorter wavelength and the $\pi \rightarrow \pi^*$ band to longer wavelength.

Cells

Cells (also called cuvettes) may be made of glass (for use down to about 360 nm) or silica. Disposable plastic cells are also available. They usually have a transmission cut off at about 320 nm and are not suitable for high-precision work. Modern cells are fused and may be square or rectangular in section or (rarely) cylindrical. Silica is substantially transparent between about 190 nm and 1000 nm, and special grades extend this range downward to below 180 nm and upwards to about 2000 nm. For precision work, and operation near the wavelength limits, the use of these purer silicas is recommended.

Path Length and Concentration

Optimum accuracy and precision in UV spectrophotometric analyses are obtained when the absorbance is about 0.9. However, in practice, absorbencies in the range 0.3–1.5 are sufficiently reliable, and the combination of cell pathlength and concentration of analyte should be adjusted to give an absorbance within this range.

Correlation of Molecular Structure to UV–VIS Absorption

An isolated functional group not in conjugation with any other group is said to be a chromophore if it exhibits absorption of a characteristic nature in the ultraviolet or visible region. If a series of compounds has the same functional group and no complicating factors are present, all the compounds will generally absorb at very nearly the same wavelength and will have nearly the same molar extinction coefficient. Thus, it is readily seen that the spectrum of a compound, when correlated with data from the literature for known compounds, can be a very valuable aid in determining the functional groups present in the molecule.

Auxochromes are groups that do not in themselves show selective absorption above 200 nm but which, when attached to a given chromophoric system, usually cause a shift in the absorption to longer wavelength and an increased intensity of the absorption peak. Common auxochromic groups are hydroxyl, amino, sulfhydryl (and their derivatives), and some of the halogens. These groups all contain non-bonding electrons; transitions involving these n electrons are responsible for these effects. For example, the absorption band at the longest wavelength of *trans-p*-ethoxyazobenzene is shifted 65 nm to longer wavelength and is about twice as intense as that of the corresponding band of *trans*-azobenzene. Benzene shows λ_{max} 255 nm, ϵ 230, and aniline shows λ_{max} 280 nm, ϵ 1430. (Interestingly, the anilinium ion, which has no non-bonding electrons, shows λ_{max} 254 nm, ϵ 160). Some functional groups that do not contain non-bonding electron—for example, alkyl groups—can also be considered auxochromes because of weak inductive or hyperconjugative effects.

If two or more chromophoric groups are present in a molecule and they are separated by two or more single bonds, the effect on the spectrum is usually additive; there is little electronic interaction between isolated chromophoric groups. However, if two chromophoric groups are separated by only one single bond (a conjugated system), a large effect on the spectrum results because the π electron system is spread over a least four atomic centers. When two chromophoric groups are conjugated, the high intensity ($\pi \rightarrow \pi^*$ transitions) absorption band is generally shifted 15–45 nm to longer wavelength with respect to the simple unconjugated chromophore.

Many colorimetric analyses developed for UV-absorbing drugs, xenobiotics, and metabolites have been based upon the formation of an analyte-specific multiple conjugated chromophoric system that readily absorbs in the visible range of the spectrum. This helps in avoiding interfering UV-absorption from impurities in the sample when the underivitized analyte is analyzed.

Compounds containing an extensively conjugated chromophore will appear colored to the eye if they absorb above 400 nm. As UV absorption peaks are frequently broad, the absorption of a peak with a λ_{max} of approximately 350 nm will generally extend into the visible region. Usually, if a compound appears to be colored, it will contain not less than four and usually five or more conjugated chromophoric and auxochromic groups.

Substitution of aromatic chromophores with auxochromic groups is worthy of mention. When benzene is substituted by halogen or alkyl groups, only a slight shift with a small increase in extinction coefficient is seen. However, substitution by groups carrying non-bonding electrons or π electrons (e.g., -OH, $-NH_2$, -CHO, etc.) causes a very pronounced shift and a greatly intensified absorption relative to benzene.

In aromatic and conjugated structures where an auxochromic group may function as an acid or base, the effect of pH on the absorption spectrum of the conjugated system can be qualitatively useful. For example, conversion of phenol (PhOH) to the phenolate ion (PhO^-) by addition of base, results in an additional electron pair and a formal negative charge being located on the auxochromic group; the interaction of these electrons with the conjugated system results in a bathochromic–hyperchromic shift when compared to the neutral phenol spectrum. Adjusting the pH of the solution reverses this process, so that the phenol is regenerated. Conversion of aniline ($PhNH_2$) to the anilinium ion ($PhNH_3^+$) by lowering the pH of the medium results in a hypsochromic–hypochromic shift that can be reversed by increasing the pH of the medium.

In polyaromatic compounds, as the number of fused rings increases, the absorption band is shifted to longer wavelength, and extensively conjugated polyaromatics, such as naphthacene (λ_{max} 480 nm, ϵ 11,000—yellow) and pentacene (λ_{max} 580 nm, ϵ 12,000—blue) absorb in the visible region of the spectrum. The spectra of simple heterocyclic aromatic compounds such as pyridine, pyrrole, indole, furan, thiophene, and their derivatives, generally resemble the spectra of analogous benzenoid or naphthalenoid structures.

UV Spectrophotometry—Direct and Indirect Methods

In a quantitative spectrophotometric assay, the analyte is dissolved in a solvent that is transparent in the wavelength region to be examined. The wavelength normally selected is that at which the analyte exhibits maximum absorption (λ_{max}). The usual procedure is to obtain the absorbance value of the solution under non-scanning conditions (i.e., with the monochromator set at the analytical wavelength). Alternatively, if a recording double beam spectrophotometer is used, the absorbance may be read from a recording of the spectrum. This latter procedure is generally utilized for qualitative purposes and in assays in which absorbances at more than one wavelength are required.

The measurement of absorbance is generally carried out using one of three methods:

(1) comparison with a standard absorptivity value,
(2) use of a calibration curve, and
(3) single- or double-point standardization.

Use of a standard absorptivity value is generally restricted to compounds that exhibit broad absorption bands and are not significantly affected by variation in instrumental parameters. An available value precludes the need to prepare a standard solution for absorptivity determination if the reference analyte is difficult to obtain.

The use of a calibration curve is a common procedure for carrying out quantitative spectrophotometric assays. Usually four to six standard solutions of the reference compound at concentrations above and below the expected concentration of the analyte are determined and a concentration versus absorbance graph is constructed. The concentration of the analyte in the sample solution is then read from the graph as the concentration corresponding to the absorbance of the solution. Calibration data are essential if the absorbance has a nonlinear relationship with concentration, if it is necessary to confirm the proportionality of absorbance as a function of concentration, or if the absorbance or linearity is dependent on the assay conditions. In certain visible spectrophotometric assays of colorless substances, based upon conversion to colored derivatives by heating the substance with one or more reagents, slight variation of assay conditions—for example, pH, temperature, and time of heating—may give rise to a significant variation of absorbance, and experimentally derived calibration data are required for each set of samples.

Single- or double-point standardization is often used in place of a calibration curve. In the single-point procedure, the absorbances of a solution of the sample and of a standard solution of the reference substance (the concentration should be close to that of the sample solution) are determined. The concentration of the test compound is calculated as follows:

$$C_{Test} = \frac{A_{Test} \times C_{std}}{A_{std}} \quad (12)$$

where C_{test} and C_{std} are concentrations in the sample and standard solutions, respectively, and A_{test} and A_{std} are the absorbances of the sample and standard solutions, respectively. This method is best suited for those compounds that obey Beer's Law and for which a reference standard of acceptable purity is readily available.

Occasionally, a linear but nonproportional relationship between concentration and absorbance occurs, and is indicated by a significant positive or negative intercept in a Beer's Law plot. A *two-point bracketing* standardization is therefore required to determine the concentration of the sample solutions. The concentration of one of the standard solutions is greater than that of the sample while the other standard solution has a lower concentration than the sample. The concentration of the substance in the sample solution is given by the equation:

$$C_{Test} = \frac{(A_{Test} - A_{std_1})(C_{std_1} - C_{std_2}) + C_{std_1}(A_{std_1} - A_{std_2})}{A_{std_1} - A_{std_2}} \quad (13)$$

where std_1 and std_2 refer to the more concentrated standard and the less concentrated standard, respectively.

Direct spectrophotometric analysis of a xenobiotic or metabolite may not be possible for several reasons. The natural absorption of the analyte may occur at too low a wavelength to be useful, the molar absorptivity may be too small to give the required sensitivity, or other materials contaminating the analyte may absorb at the same wavelength. These problems can be overcome in many cases by chemical modification of the analyte to change its absorption characteristics. Some examples of useful derivitization procedures for spectrophotometric utility are (1) the diazotization and coupling of primary aromatic amines, (2) condensation reactions (e.g., between amines or hydrazines and carbonyl compounds), (3) the reduction of tetrazolium salts in the present of an α-ketol group (-CHOH-C = O), (4) ion-pairing of amines with ionized acidic dyes, (5) oxidation of the side chains of weakly absorbing compounds containing an aromatic ring, and (6) metal-ligand complexation. It is also possible to measure a substance by the *change* in absorbance when a chromophore is destroyed.

Difference Spectrophotometry

This method of spectrophotometric analysis is useful for obtaining selective and accurate analytical data on solutions of analytes containing absorbing interferants. Basically, the technique measures a difference absorbance (ΔA) between two equimolar solutions of the analyte in different chemical forms which exhibit different spectral characteristics. The method is valid provided that reproducible changes are induced in the spectrum of the analyte by the addition of one or more reagents, and that the absorbance of the interfering substance(s) is (are) not altered by the reagents.

The simplest and most commonly employed technique for altering the spectral properties of the analyte is the adjustment of the pH by means of aqueous solutions of acid, alkali, or buffers. The UV–visible absorption spectra of many substances containing ionizable functional groups—for example, phenols, aromatic carboxylic acids, and amines—are dependent on the state of ionization of the functional groups and, consequently, on the pH of the solution.

The pHs chosen must quantitatively form single species with at least 99% spectral purity. This can be achieved with monofunctional analytes (e.g., aromatic amines or aromatic carboxylic acids and phenols) by simply working at a pH at least two pKa units above the pKa of the analyte. The difference spectrum is obtained by placing one form of the analyte in the sample cell of the spectrophotometer, and the other form in the reference cell, and plotting the observed absorbance against wavelength. The value of difference spectrophotometry is that it provides a reference solution that contains both analyte and interfering substances in the same concentrations but at a pH different from that of the analyte solution in the sample cell. Thus, interferants present in the sample should not be affected by the pH changes, and their contribution to the total absorbance is therefore canceled.

The absorption spectra of the drug benthiazide is shown in Figure 36.22 in both acidic and basic media (45). The difference absorption spectrum is plotted as the difference in absorbance between the basic solution and the acidic solution against pH. The spectrum may be generated automatically using a double-beam recording spectrophotometer with the basic solution in the sample cell and the acidic solution in the reference cell. At 255 nm

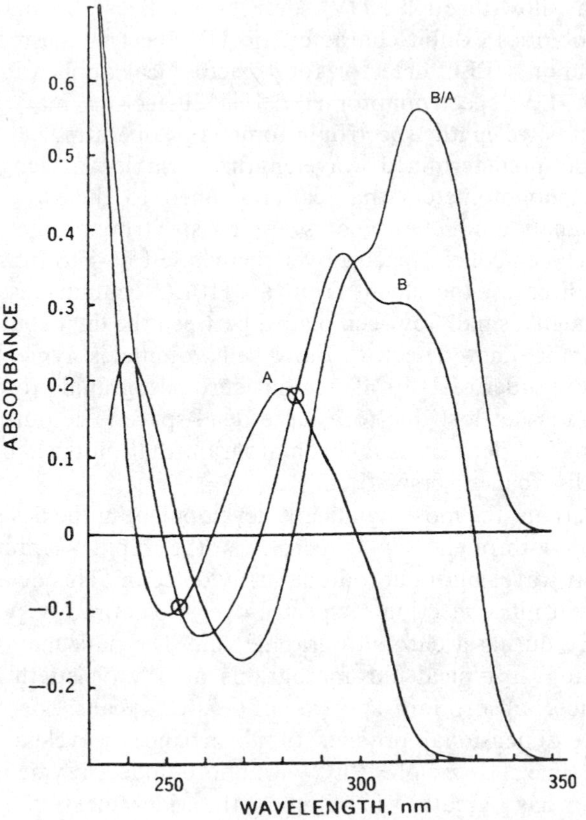

FIG. 36.22. Conventional and difference spectra of benzthiazide (15 g/mL) in acidic solution (A); and basic solution (B); and the difference spectrum of basic versus acidic solutions (B/A) (From American Pharmaceutical Association, with permission).

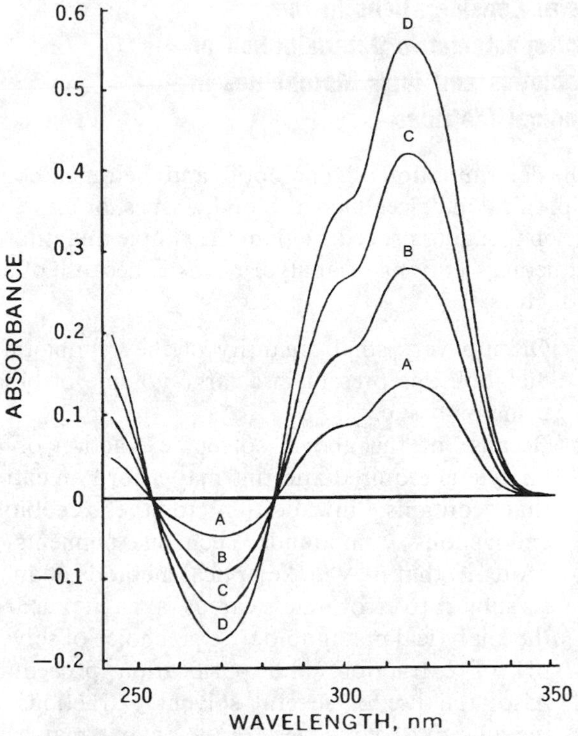

FIG. 36.23. Difference spectra used to verify Beer's Law for benthiazide. Plots are basic versus acid difference spectra for concentrations of 5 (A), 10 (B), 15 (C), and 20 g/mL (D) (From American Pharmaceutical Association, with permission).

and 287 nm both solutions have identical absorbance and consequently exhibit zero difference absorbance. Such wavelengths of equal absorptivity are the isosbestic or isoabsorptive points. Above 287 nm the basic solution absorbs more intensely than the acidic solution and the ΔA is positive. Between 255 and 287 nm ΔA has a negative value. There is a maximum in the difference spectrum at 313 nm and a minimum at 271 nm. The absorbance difference at these two wavelengths is termed the amplitude. A plot of absorbance differences versus drug concentration will obey Beer's Law and can be used for quantitative determinations. The isosbestic points are useful indicators of whether the absorbance of interferants in the sample are affecting the measurement of the absorbance of the drug. Figure 36.23 shows the isosbestic points for benzthiazide generated from several concentrations of the analyte. Any sample containing the drug or any standard curve concentration should show zero absorbance at the isosbestic wavelengths unless an interfering compound is present. If this is not observed, an alternative assay procedure, or removal of the interferant, is indicated.

Difference spectrophotometry is useful in the analysis of macromolecules such as proteins, peptides, and nucleic acids, because conformational effects are likely to be accompanied by changes in the environment of aromatic residues that will in turn lead to small wavelength shifts as well as other perturbations. A difference spectrum in a protein may be generated by unfolding or by proteolytic degradation, as well as by more localized changes engendered by conformational adjustments or subunit association or dissociation, or, in favorable cases, binding of a ligand, as well as a change in bulk solvent. The latter effect can be achieved simply by addition of a benign perturbant, such as glycerol, sucrose, or D_2O, or by a change of temperature below the region of denaturation. Such a change in solvent character will in general affect only those aromatic residues in contact with solvent, and provides, therefore, a means of determining, at least in a semi-quantitative way, what proportion of aromatic residues are so exposed, and of following any change in this degree of exposure.

Special Considerations in the Spectrophotometric Determination of Xenobiotics and their Metabolites in Biological Matrices

The determination of xenobiotics and their metabolites in biological matrices such as blood, tissues, or urine, is a more challenging procedure than the simple quantitation of aqueous solutions of analytes. This is because of several factors:

(1) Often a very small quantity of the xenobiotic or metabolite is present in a large volume of blood, urine or tissue.
(2) Because of the above, solvent extraction of the analyte is required and this may afford an extract that contains, in addition to the xenobiotic, endogenous compounds such as pigments or proteins, that may make optical methods of analysis subject to error unless care is taken in preparing the analytical methodology (e.g., choice of solvent, pH of extraction, and purification procedure). Also, the use of several solvent extractions for the quantitative recovery of the analyte may cause problems such as emulsification, and having to deal with large volumes of solvent for evaporation. These problems can usually be rectified by utilizing a large solvent:sample ratio, and by carrying out control analyses with biological matrices spiked with the analyte.
(3) The xenobiotic may be present both free and combined as conjugates such as glucuronide or sulfate, both of which are polar and water-soluble.
(4) A complicating factor for many drug molecules is protein binding. This can lead to poor recoveries of the drug and necessitates the inclusion of a protein denaturation step in the overall extraction procedure.

Thus, direct spectrophotometric procedures, even after purification of the sample by solvent extraction or chromatographic cleanup, often lack the sensitivity and selectivity required for the assay of low concentrations of drugs that are found in body fluids after the administration of therapeutic doses. However, modified spectrophotometric techniques—for example, those involving chemical derivatization, or difference spectrophotometry, are sufficiently discriminating and sensitive for the assay of therapeutic levels of certain drugs.

Flow-Through UV Detection

The difficulties associated with the spectrophotometric determination of xenobiotics and metabolites in biological matrices can often be overcome by the use of HPLC with flow-through UV detection. Because many xenobiotics exhibit characteristic UV spectra, the most common HPLC detector for toxicological applications is a UV spectrophotometer. UV detectors may be fixed-wavelength spectrophotometers, operating at a single predetermined wavelength, variable-wavelength spectrophotometers that can be tuned to the λ_{max} of the analyte of interest, or scanning spectrophotometers which can collect spectra over the whole UV–VIS range. In all cases, the eluent from an HPLC column passes through a small flow–cell placed between the light source and the photodetector. Flow–cell volume is typically on the order of 1–10 μL so that chromatographic resolution is not lost due to a large dead-space. The output of an UV detector is a chromatogram that plots change in absorbance versus time.

Perhaps the most significant development in the design of flow-through UV detectors is the rapid scanning multi-wavelength photodiode array detector. This detector permits collection of spectra over the entire UV–VIS range during a chromatographic run. The data may be plotted as typical chromatograms at a wavelength of choice, absorption spectra of eluted peaks, or as three-dimensional projects of absorbance, wavelength, and time. The use of HPLC with photodiode array detection has greatly facilitated the identification of xenobiotics and metabolites in biological samples.

INFRARED SPECTROSCOPY

Basic Technique

Infrared (IR) spectroscopy (116) deals with the absorption of electromagnetic radiation in the wavelength range 0.8 μm (800 nm) to 1000 μm (1 mm). This range can be subdivided into the near IR region (0.8–2 μm), the middle or fundamental IR region (2–15 μm), and the far IR region (15–1000 μm). The fundamental IR region is the one that provides the greatest information for the elucidation of molecular structure, and most IR spectrophotometers are designed to carry out measurements in this wavelength range.

When a molecule absorbs IR radiation, changes in the vibrational energy in the ground state of the molecule occur. All but the simplest of molecules have a large number of accessible vibrational and rotational energy levels with a correspondingly large number of allowed transitions. The energies of these transitions are extremely sensitive to the details of molecular structure. Thus, IR spectra are highly structured spectra with unique features that are ideally suited for the identification of xenobiotics, drugs, and other organic substances. A typical IR spectrum of the antibacterial drug sulfacetamide is illustrated in Figure 36.24.

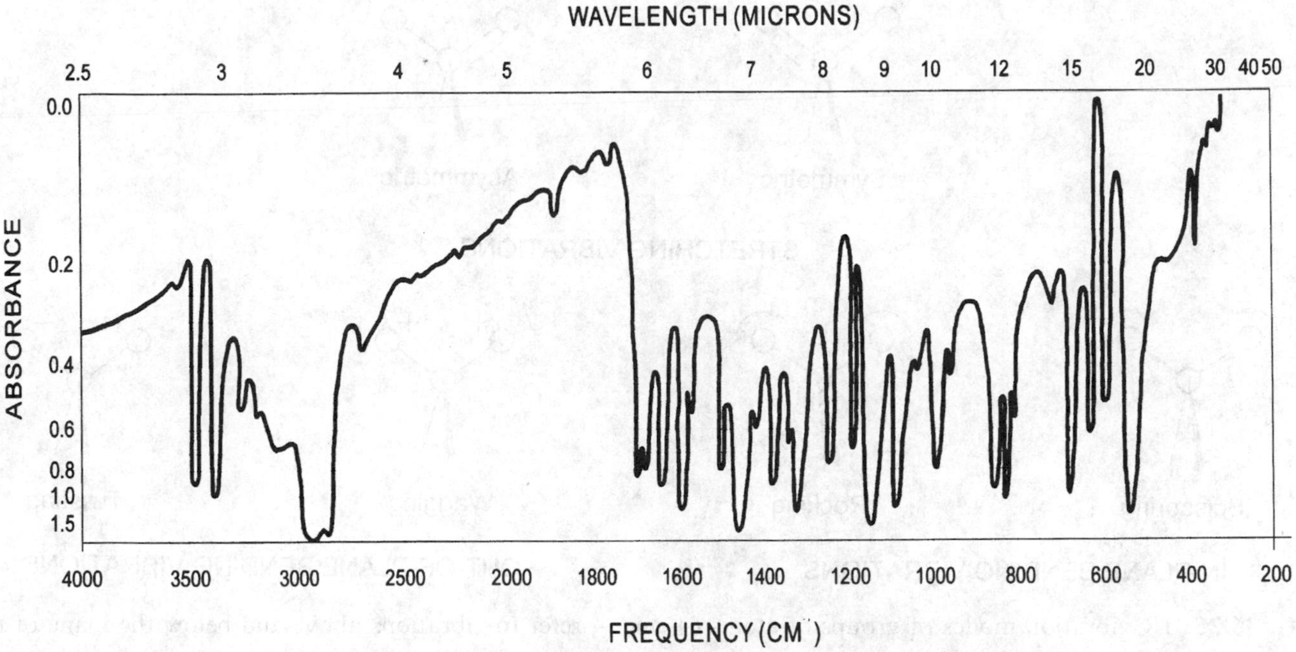

FIG. 36.24. IR spectrum of sulfacetamide.

For energy to be transferred from the IR source to the molecule, the frequency of vibration of both must coincide, and energy transfer must be accompanied by a change in the dipole moment of the molecule. Thus, molecules that contain certain symmetry elements will display more simplified spectra. For example, the C=C stretching vibration of ethylene and the symmetrical C-H stretching of the four C-H bonds of methane do not afford an absorption band in the IR region. For nonlinear polyatomic molecules, the number of fundamental modes of vibration is 3n–6 (3n–5 for linear molecules), where n = number of atoms. Certain groups within a molecule—for example, -OH, -C=O, $-NH_2$, -CN, -CC- —have characteristic absorption frequencies known as group frequencies. These frequencies are generally independent of the structure of the rest of the molecule, and can therefore be used diagnostically to confirm the presence of the functionality in a molecule of unknown structure.

In practice, it is usually not possible to observe the calculated number of peaks in the spectrum of a known compound. This may be due to the superimposition or coalescing of absorptions that are too close to be resolved, or a fundamental band may be too weak to be observed. Alternatively, additional (nonfundamental) bands may be observed that are either overtones and harmonics that occur with greatly reduced intensity, or combination and difference bands.

There are two kinds of fundamental vibrations for molecules—stretching, in which the distance between two atoms increases or decreases, but the atoms remain in the same bond axis; polyatomic molecules may be in-phase (symmetric) or out-of-phase (asymmetric) stretching vibrations (see Figure 36.25), and bending (or deformation), in which the position of the atom changes relative to the original bond axis.

The stretching frequency (υ) of a bond is related to the masses of the two atoms involved (M_a, M_b in g), the velocity of light (c), and the force constant of the bond (k, in dynes/cm). An approximate value for the stretching frequency can be calculated from the following equation:

$$\upsilon(\text{in cm}^{-1}) = \frac{1}{2\pi c}\sqrt{\frac{k}{M_a M_b/(M_a + M_b)}} \qquad (14)$$

Note the force constants for sp^3, sp^2, and sp bonds have values of 5, 10, and 15×10^5 dynes/cm, respectively.

IR spectra are usually recorded as a plot of sample absorbance (or % transmittance) versus wavelength or frequency in reciprocal cms (wavenumbers). The relationship between wavelength and wavenumber is:

$$\text{wavenumber (cm}^{-1}) = \frac{1 \times 10^4}{\lambda(\mu\text{m})} \qquad (15)$$

Unlike UV and visible spectra, IR spectra are by convention plotted with zero absorbance (or 100% transmittance) at the top of the spectrum, that is, in an inverted mode relative to UV-visible spectra.

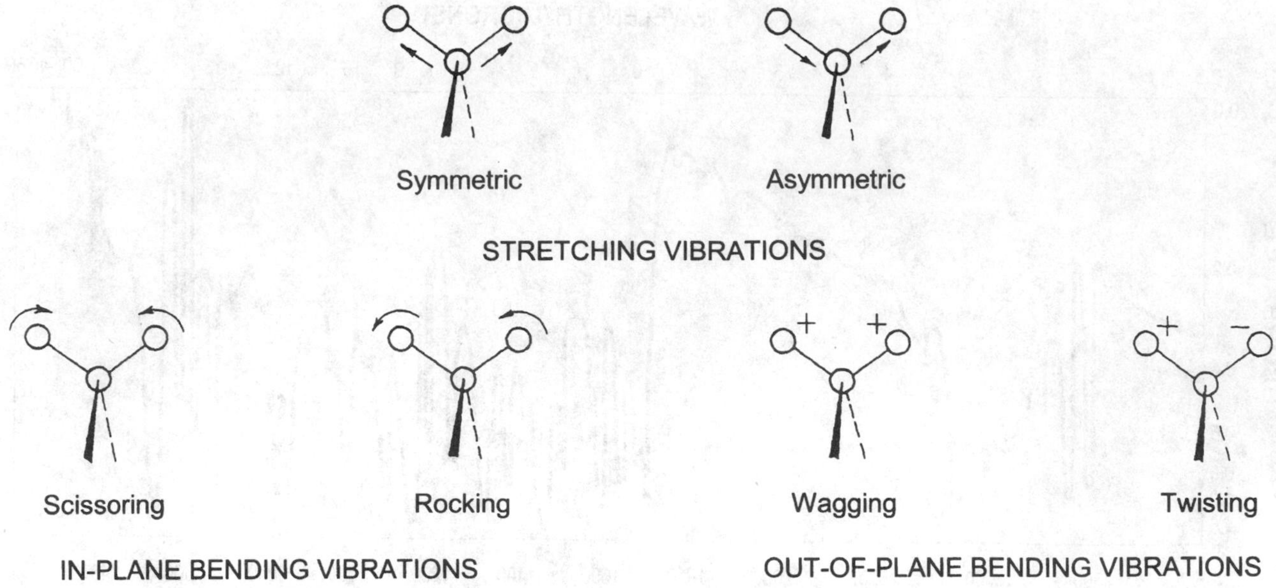

FIG. 36.25. IR vibration modes of groups of atoms (+ and − refer to vibrations above and below the plane of the paper, respectively).

Qualitative Uses and Interpretation of Spectra

The complexity in the IR spectra of organic molecules is a valuable tool that can be used for the unambiguous identification of unknown compounds if an authentic standard is available. If all the bands in the IR spectrum of the unknown structure are identical in all respects, that is, in their wavenumber value and their relative intensity, when compared with an IR spectrum of an authentic standard, then the two compounds are one and the same. The region 1430–910 cm^{-1} contains many absorptions caused by bending vibrations as well as absorptions caused by C-C, C-O, and C-N stretching vibrations. As there are many more bending vibrations in a molecule than stretching vibrations, this region of the IR spectrum is particularly rich in absorption bands and shoulders. Thus, it is termed the fingerprint region, and although similar molecules may show very similar spectra in the region 4000–1430 cm^{-1}, there will nearly always be discernible differences in the fingerprint region. Spectral comparisons are best carried out in the solution state. Compounds can often be prepared in different crystalline forms—that is, polymorphic forms—depending upon the conditions of crystallization. Polymorphic forms of the same compound may show significant differences in the fingerprint region of the spectrum. Therefore, if spectral comparisons are to be made in the solid state, then both unknown and authentic standard should be recrystallized from a specific solvent.

A second important use of qualitative IR spectroscopy is that it gives structural information about an unknown molecule. The previously mentioned group frequencies together with frequencies of other characteristic bands can be utilized in the form of comprehensive frequency correlation charts that have been compiled for easy reference (see pp. 185–203, Gordon and Ford [51]). This type of compilation is invaluable as a means of confirming the presence or absence of a particular functionality in an unknown structure. In this respect, the region between 4000 and 1500 cm^{-1} is probably easier to interpret than that between 1500 and 650 cm^{-1}, as a result of the latter including many skeletal vibrations which are not diagnostic because they are typical of molecules as a whole.

Instrumental Considerations

Dispersive IR Spectrophotometers

The arrangement of a typical double beam recording IR spectrophotometer is shown in Figure 36.26. The beam chopper, which is a rotating mirror, permits radiation passing alternately through sample cell and solvent cell to reach the IR detector. The difference in absorption by solute and solvent is measured as an alternating electric current from the thermocouple. The system operates on the optical null principle with the recorder pen linked mechanically to a "comb" (not shown), which is placed across the solvent cell beam and moved by a servomechanism to reduce or increase the solvent cell-beam intensity. The servomechanism is actuated by the amplified thermocouple output to make the solvent beam intensity equal to the solution beam intensity, which reduces the detector output to zero or the null point. The spectrum can be scanned through

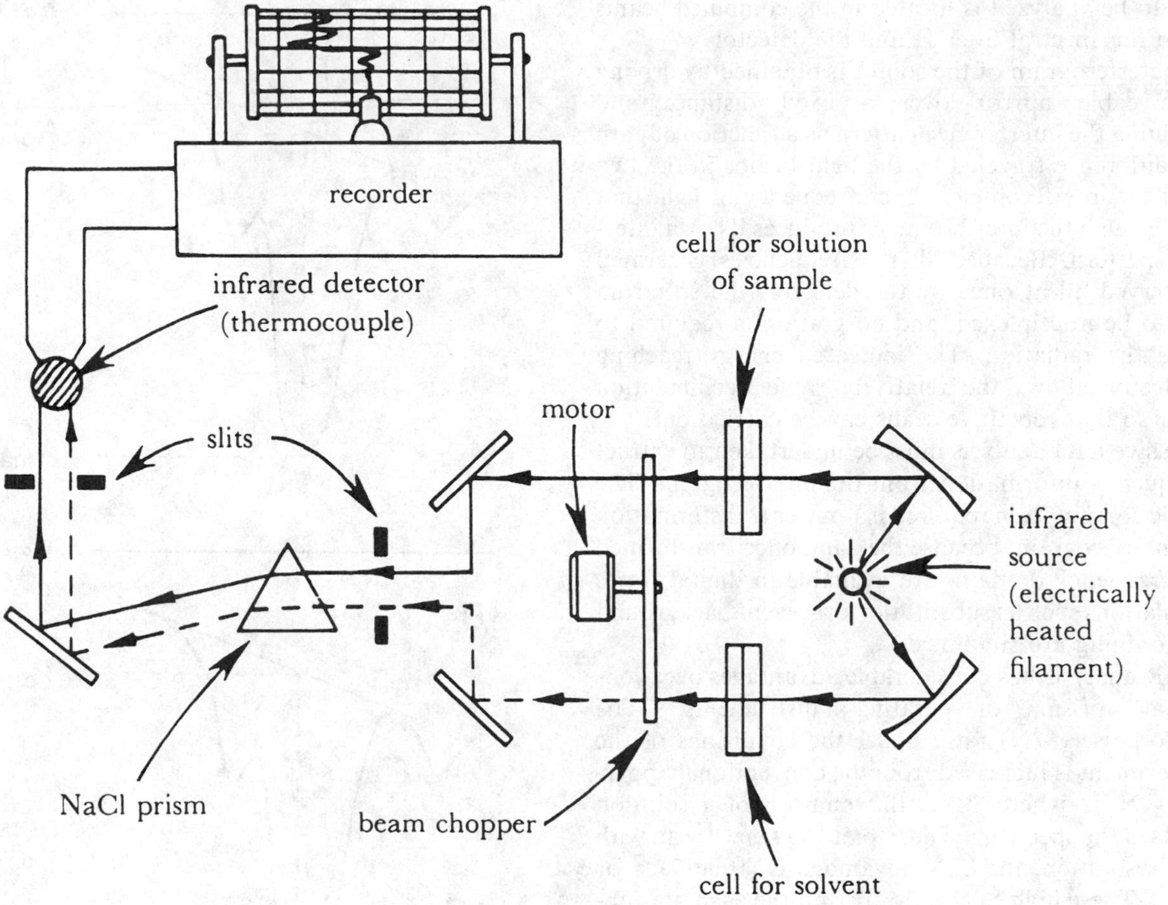

FIG. 36.26. Schematic representation of a double-beam recording infrared spectrophotometer.

the various wavelengths by rotation of the prism in synchronization with the motion of the recorder drum or chart. Most modern instruments now utilize a diffraction grating in place of the prism. Sodium chloride prisms can be used for the whole of the region from 4000–650 cm^{-1} but suffer from the disadvantage of low resolution at 4000–2500 cm^{-1} The use of a grating monochromator provides a better overall resolution throughout the range 4000–625 cm^{-1}.

Fourier Transform IR Spectrometers

Fourier transform (FT) IR spectrometers have gained rapid use over the past 25 years (2,54). This type of spectrometer is built around an interferometer rather than a monochromator (see Figure 36.27). The beam from the light source passes through the chopper and is collimated and directed to the beam splitter via mirror C. The beam splitter is a half-silvered mirror that reflects 50% of the incident light onto the movable mirror F and allows 50% to pass through fixed mirror E. The beams reflected from mirrors F and E are then combined at the beam splitter so that an interference pattern results, and this is focused by mirror G onto the detector J. The

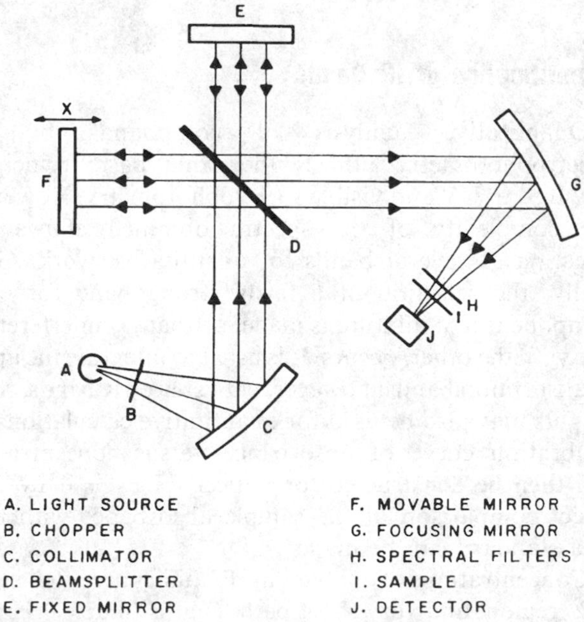

FIG. 36.27. Layout of the optics of a Fourier transform IR spectrometer.

sample to be analyzed is located in the combined beams between the spectral filter H and the detector.

The interferogram of the source is obtained by driving the moveable mirror over a fixed distance and determining the interference pattern as a function of path length difference traveled by the light beams in the two arms of the interferometer. Each frequency of light that passes through the interferometer produces its own interference pattern. Because all the frequencies generated are observed all at once by the detector, the spectrum is said to be multiplexed, and no grating is required to disperse the radiation. The increased energy reaching the detector allows the relatively rapid accumulation of data, so that repetitive scans can be carried out.

Extensive data analysis must be undertaken to extract the frequency information from the interferogram. The principle computation required is Fourier transformation of the interferogram; because the data, once transformed to the frequency domain, are available in digital form, manipulations such as substitution of solvent background and smoothing are simplified.

FT–IR analysis has considerable advantages over conventional prism or grating instruments. The signal-to-noise (S/N) ratio under the conditions of the FT experiment is increased from the conventional apparatus by $N^{1/2}$, where N is the number of resolution elements in the spectrum. Thus, for a 1000 cm^{-1} scan with 2 cm^{-1} resolution, the S/N advantage is $(1000/2)^{1/2}$ or about 22. These high S/N ratios permit the accurate subtraction of backgrounds due to liquid H_2O, thus, a principle application of FT–IR spectrometry is in the acquisition of protein spectra in aqueous media.

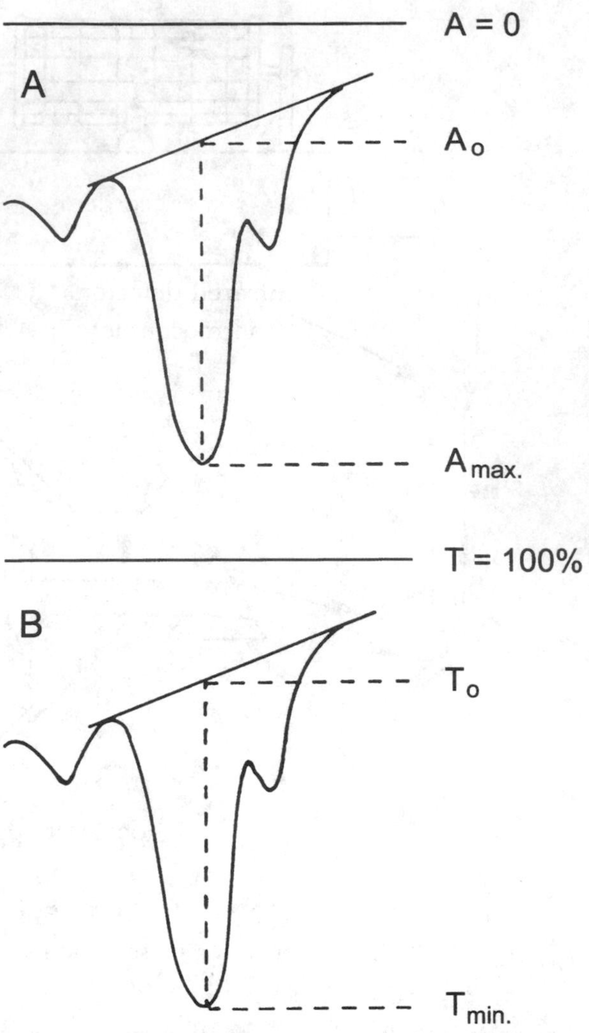

FIG. 36.28. Measurement of IR band intensities using the base-line technique. A: When the scale is linear in absorbance, peak absorbance $= A_{max} - A_o$. B: When the scale is linear in transmittance, peak absorbance $= -\log (T_{min}/T_o)$.

Quantification of IR Bands

Quantitative analysis of compounds by IR spectrophotometry utilizes the same basic principles involved in UV and visible spectrophotometry. However, the complexity of the spectra obtained allows the selection of several bands for quantitative work. Generally, the selection of a fairly strong band for each component in a mixture is made, so that no interference, one with the other, occurs. It is usual to integrate the areas of absorption bands; however, with sharp IR bands, peak heights may also be used for quantitative calculations. A calibration curve of absorbance versus concentration can then be constructed, or if Beer's Law is obeyed, a direct comparison of the sample absorbance with that of a standard can be made.

Concentrations of analytes in IR studies are often in the 10% region, and very short path lengths (0.025–0.1 mm) are used. Because there is a high concentration of solute, the accurate cancellation of solvent absorption (note, all solvents absorb in some part of the IR spectrum) is difficult to achieve. In this respect, the base-line technique is usually applied (see Figure 36.28), which assumes that absorption due to solvent (or a second component) is constant or varies linearly with wavelength over the region of the absorption band.

The determination of small amounts of impurities or low amounts of solutes in a preparation can also be improved by introducing the major component, or the solvent, into the reference beam of the spectrophotometer, thus compensating for the absorption of this component.

Deviations from Beer's Law are encountered much more frequently in IR spectrophotometry than in UV and visible spectrophotometry. This is due to the higher concentrations of samples required for IR analysis. Thus, significant intermolecular hydrogen-bonding effects may be observed, which increase as the concentration of the solute increases. The absorbance at the λ_{max} of a free-OH group actually decreases with increasing concentration of the analyte.

Sample Preparation and Sample Cells

Although IR spectra have been obtained on materials in every physical state from solids to gases, most analyses are carried out on the neat liquid analyte, solutions of the analyte in organic solvents, suspensions, Nujol suspensions, and KBr discs. Solution spectra are preferred for quantitative analysis because errors arising from sample inhomogeneity and path length are minimized. KBr discs are often used for qualitative analysis because subtle structural differences—for example, polymorphism—can often be observed in this sample form.

Cells for quantitative IR analysis of solutions consist of a pair of sodium chloride plates with a thin metal spacer between them. This unit is housed in a metal frame along with protective washers. The plate spacing is $\sim 10^{-2}$ cm. Considerable care in handling and storing the IR cells should be exercised, because the windows are easily fogged by traces of moisture, and are easily scratched. When not in use, cells should be stored in a desiccator.

Neat liquids and Nujol suspensions or mulls for qualitative analysis are usually placed as a drop on an unmounted circular sodium chloride plate, and a second plate is pressed on top until the liquid is spread into a thin film with a thickness on the order of 1×10^{-4} to 50×10^{-4} cm. The plates are held in a frame while the spectrum is scanned.

Nujol mulls are prepared by grinding the solid analyte in a small mortar with mineral oil until a milky emulsion is obtained. Other suspending agents such a perfluorokerosene, hexachlorobutadiene, or other heavy liquids can also be used. The spectrum obtained with mulls will consist of bands from the analyte superimposed upon bands from the mulling agent. The C-H regions of the spectrum will be obscured when mineral oil mulls are used, and the C-F or C-Cl regions will be obscured when the halogenated mulls are used.

Qualitative analysis of solid analytes is often accomplished using KBr discs. This involves grinding together the analyte (0.3–9 mg) with 300 mg of spectral quality KBr ($\sim$400 mesh). Between 100 and 300 mg of the grind is then pressed into pellets or discs at between 20,000 and 100,000 psig using a stainless steel die and a vacuum pump. The finished pellet is transparent and produces excellent spectra. KBr does not contribute extraneous bands in the IR spectrum, as do mulling agents. However, KBr is slightly hygroscopic and may pick up moisture during the disc preparation. This will lead to characteristic water bands at 3300 and 1640 cm^{-1}.

NEAR-IR SPECTROSCOPY—IN VIVO ANALYSIS

The combination of high signal-to-noise spectra achieved using FT–IR with the sophisticated data reduction techniques that are now available, has led to interesting advances in the acquisition of spectra from preparations such as monolayers and tissues, or from samples in situ, using FT–IR microspectroscopy or fiber optical wave-guides for beam handling.

Near-IR spectroscopy is a particularly useful emerging technique that holds great promise as a non-invasive in vivo analytical tool. Virtually every organic compound has a near-IR spectrum that can be measured. Near-IR spectra consist of overtones and combinations of fundamental mid-IR bands, giving near-IR spectra a powerful ability to identify organic compounds while still permitting good penetration of light into tissues. Figure 36.29 illustrates the structural moieties that can be determined by near-IR and their absorption characteristics.

The application of in vivo FT–IR microspectroscopy in the early diagnosis of disease has recently been reviewed (68,83). Several reports on the use of near-FT–IR spectroscopy in studying human arteries, cancers and tumors, and brain tissues from stroke and Alzheimer's disease patients have been published (84,85,95). Wetzel et al. (161) have utilized FT–IR microspectroscopy to investigate the metabolic activity in various layers of the cerebellum utilizing deuteration studies.

Some examples of the use of FT–IR spectroscopy in disease diagnosis follow.

Analysis of Solid Human Tumor Cells by FT–IR Microspectroscopy

Advanced forms of human tumors are characterized by a poor prognosis despite the therapeutic approach chosen. However, early detection often allows for a higher survival rate. Cells from normal and neoplastic human lung tissue have been analyzed by means of FT–IR microspectroscopy (9). This procedure makes it possible to obtain reliable spectra that can differentiate between normal and neoplastic cells. The latter cells show an increase in the intensity of the bands corresponding mainly to the PO_2^- symmetrical and asymmetrical vibrations (1080–1540 cm^{-1}) of DNA compared to normal cells. Thus, this analytical method may provide an approach for recognition of early neoplastic transformation that is usually not possible with traditional procedures. Similar results have been observed in the FT–IR spectra of microtomed sections of normal and malignant human colon tissues and in other malig-

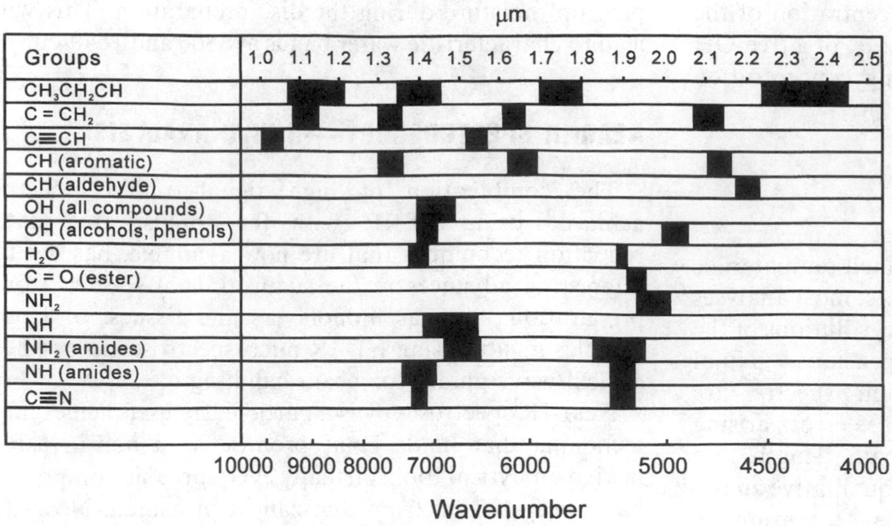

FIG. 36.29. Characteristic group frequencies in the near-IR spectrum.

nant tissues such as stomach, esophagus, skin, liver, cervix, and vagina (169). The results suggest that in all cancerous tissues and cells studied to date, most PO_2^- groups become hydrogen bonded and that the intermolecular packing among PO_2^- groups becomes closer. Indirect evidence points to nucleic acids as the molecules mainly responsible for the observed changes in the $\upsilon_s(PO_2^-)$ and υ_{as} (PO_2^-) bands.

Very recently, a new instrumental approach for performing spectroscopic imaging microscopy has been described (153). The instrument integrates an acoustic–optic tunable filter (AOTF) and charge-coupled device (CCD) detector with an infinity-corrected microscope for operation in the near-IR spectral regions. Images at moderate spectral resolution (2 nm) and high spatial resolution (1 μm) can be collected rapidly. Data can be presented containing 128×128 pixels. In operation, the CDD is a true imaging detector, with wavelength selection provided by the AOTF and quartz tungsten halogen lamp to create a tunable source. The instrument can be utilized for both absorption and reflectance spectroscopies. Such an instrument would appear to have good potential in the study of biological materials and processes.

Analysis of Stroke-Induced Changes by Near-IR Spectroscopy

Near-IR spectroscopy has historically been used to monitor fat and protein in agricultural products. Similar near-IR techniques have been employed more recently in the study of animal systems and have been used to examine stroke-induced changes in the lipids and proteins of whole gerbil brains (27). Near-IR spectroscopy is well suited for this work because tissue penetration by near-IR light is good, excellent S/N ratios can be obtained in near-IR measurements, and discrimination between various types of brain constituents is possible because the near-IR signals arise from combinations and overtones of the fundamental IR bands of these constituents. The gerbil brain is an established animal model of stroke. In addition, the gerbil brain is enriched in polyunsaturated fatty acids. There are dramatic changes in fatty acid metabolism during the ischemia and reperfusion stages. The changes parallel the hypothesized series of free radical and altered enzymatic events that occur during transient ischemia and reperfusion in the brain of humans. The skull of the gerbil is relatively thin, making near-IR spectroscopy of the brain readily achievable in vivo with common spectrometers of moderate light intensity.

To understand the early changes in lipid and protein metabolism following stroke and trauma, animal models have been developed to recreate these changes. The examination of whole brains has been made possible by a combination of hardware modifications and mathematical techniques designed to make the sample presentation to the spectrometer quite reproducible. A refrigerated sample compartment with dry nitrogen purge can be constructed for analysis of whole frozen brains. The cooled compartment enables repeated scans of frozen brains to be collected over time without thawing. The spectrophotometer itself can be purged with dry nitrogen gas, eliminating spectral artifacts associated with lipid/protein oxidation and atmospheric water vapor or other gases. A geometric noise filter removes spectral variations arising from positional variation of the brain. The BEST and extended BEST algorithms, which scale spectral vectors in multidimensional hyperspace with a directional probability, can be used with a supercomputer to analyze the spectra collected.

In addition to changes observed in stroke, there are age-related changes in the polyunsaturated fatty acid pool and in the state of protein oxidation within the central nervous system. The near-IR analytical method has many applications to this aging and stroke research, including:

1. Determination of age from brain spectra.
2. Prediction of short-term memory deficit from the spectra of injured brains.
3. Simultaneous multicomponent analysis of lipids and proteins.
4. Quantification of edema.
5. Transcranial scanning of the brain in vivo.

Near-IR scanning of brains in vivo simplifies the testing of antiepileptic drug candidates by reducing the number of subjects required, by allowing each subject to be used as its own control, and by eliminating variance due to outlier subjects (such as those that have had a stroke before the experiment).

Near-IR Fiber Optics as Arterial Probes for Studying Cardiovascular Disease

An exciting new application of near-IR spectroscopy, which has tremendous potential as a tool for studying mechanisms of toxicology, couples near-IR with fiber optic arterial probes. Fiber optic catheters have previously been used to locate atherosclerotic lesions, but the techniques merely distinguish lesions from healthy arterial tissue. Recently, a new method, based on near-IR fiber optics, has been developed to spatially map lesions *and* their chemical constituents (29). Chemical analysis of lesions in vivo permits the kinetic study of atherogenesis and contributes to the understanding of lesion formation and growth. The chemical imaging power of this technique permits the testing of important new hypotheses of lesion formation, growth, and regression.

RAMAN SPECTROSCOPY

Raman spectroscopy is closely related to infrared spectroscopy, because the information about molecular vibrational frequencies provided by the latter technique is of the same kind as that provided by the Raman vibrational spectrum (26,116). However, in molecules with a center of symmetry, vibrational transitions that are allowed in the IR spectrum are forbidden in the Raman effect, and vice versa, providing useful information about molecular symmetry. For example, structurally symmetrical diatomic molecules such as H_2 and O_2 are also electrically symmetrical and do not give IR absorption spectra. These molecules do afford Raman spectra due to excitation of symmetrical vibrations. In a molecule such as tetrachloroethylene ($CCl_2=CCl_2$), the double bond stretching frequency is symmetrical and the molecule does not show a double bond stretching frequency in the IR spectrum. However, this vibration appears strongly in the Raman spectrum of tetrachloroethylene and provides evidence of a symmetrical structure (see Figure 36.30). Thus, the two techniques are complementary.

The Raman effect is a scattering process in which the interaction between photon and the molecule occurs in a very short period of time and the Raman peaks obtained correspond to photons that have bounced inelastically off the molecule. The Raman spectrum arises as a result of the light photons being captured momentarily by molecules in the sample and giving up (or gaining) small increments of energy through changes in the molecular vibrational and rotational energies before being emitted as scattered light. The changes in the vibrational and rotational energies result in changes in wavelength of the incident light. The convention in Raman spectra is to quote the positions of vibrational peaks as the difference between the absolute wavenumbers of the exciting line and the absolute wavenumbers of the resulting scattered photons.

The Raman effect is extremely weak, and only a minute portion of the incident photons are useful emergent photons; thus, relatively high-power lasers must be used to create a high photon flux. Also, quite sophisticated optical and electronic equipment is required to detect the scattered photons.

One of the major advantages of Raman spectroscopy is that spectra may be obtained for molecules in aqueous solutions, because water has a weak Raman spectrum that interferes only minimally with the spectrum of the solute. Concentrations of analyte in the range 0.1 to 0.01 M in water are normally used, however, in resonance Raman spectroscopy, concentrations of chromophoric molecules in the range 10^{-4} to 10^{-6} M can be used, making this technique particularly useful for biochemical studies.

Basic Optics of the Raman Experiment

In a standard Raman experiment, intense monochromatic radiation provided by a continuous wave laser is focused onto or into the sample. Some of the resultant scattered light is collected by optics and directed to a dispersing system that is usually a monochromator. The monochromator separates the scattered light on the basis of frequency and these frequencies are then detected and recorded either by single-channel (scanning) or multichannel detection. Figure 36.31 illustrates the optics involved in a conventional Raman experiment.

Sampling Techniques and Problems

The preparation of samples for Raman spectroscopy requires some comment. Samples may be examined in

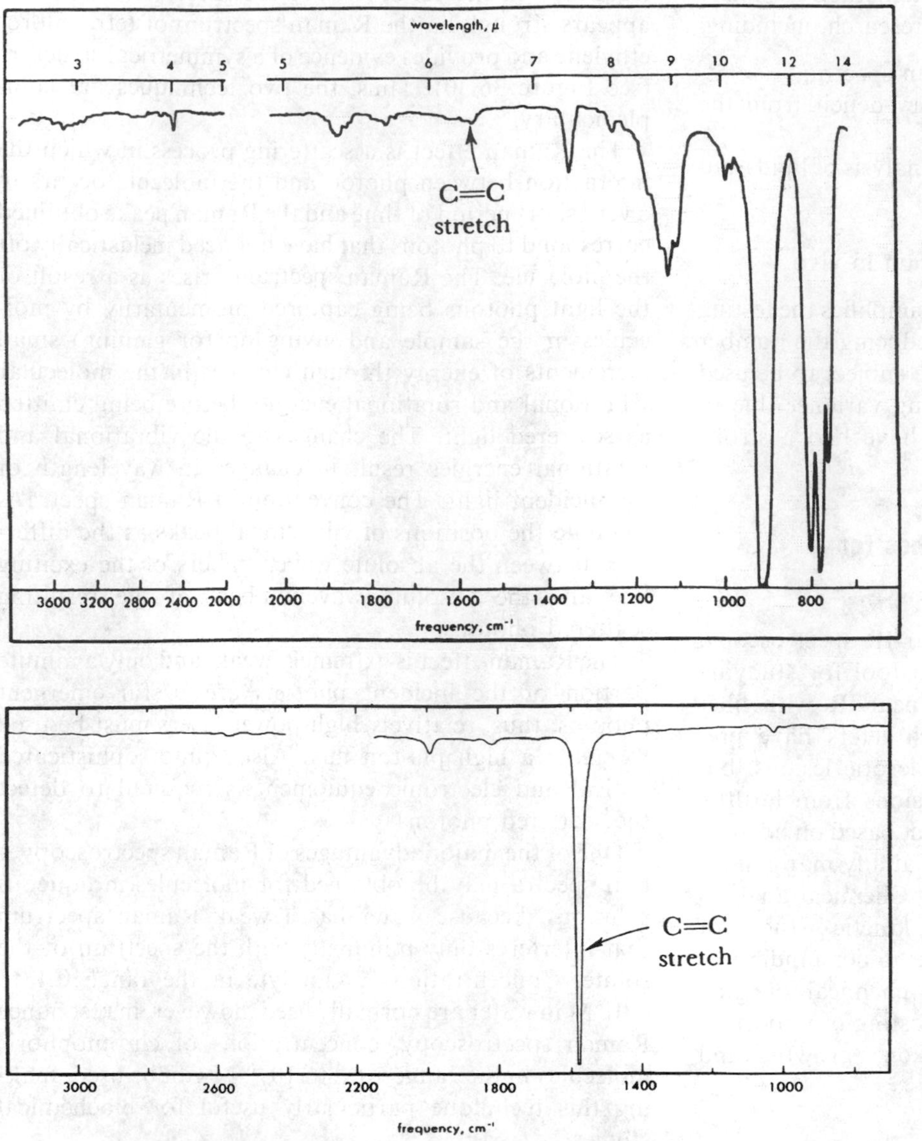

FIG. 36.30. Infrared (top) and Raman (bottom) spectra of tetrachloroethylene.

any physical state. Liquid samples are usually measured in a quartz (1-cm) cuvette similar to the type used in fluorescence spectroscopy, however, because the incident laser beam travels longitudinally down the length of the liquid column, the cell bottom must be transparent. Capillary cells are often used for biological samples, especially when material is limited in availability. Single crystals and fibers can be utilized by mounting on a goniometer head and solid crystalline or polycrystalline materials can be either pressed into pellets, prepared as KBr discs, or packed into capillary microprobes. Samples in the form of thin films can also be utilized. Major problems are usually the breakdown of photolabile analytes during laser irradiation. This can be reduced or eliminated for liquid samples by utilizing a spinning cell, a cell in which the liquid sample is continually moved through the laser beam, or a cell in which the liquid is continually stirred with a magnetic stirrer. These procedures reduce the buildup of degradation products usually observed with static sample analysis.

It is important in Raman spectroscopy that analytes are optically homogeneous (this is especially important for biological samples). Particulate matter in solutions should be removed either by centrifugation or filtration, because if present, hot spots may occur in the sample on irradiation, leading to possible degradation of the sample.

Luminescence, which may often obliterate the Raman effect, may often occur if the sample or an impurity in the sample has a chromophore. Luminescence can often be reduced or eliminated by changing the wavelength of excitation or adding a quenching agent such as KI.

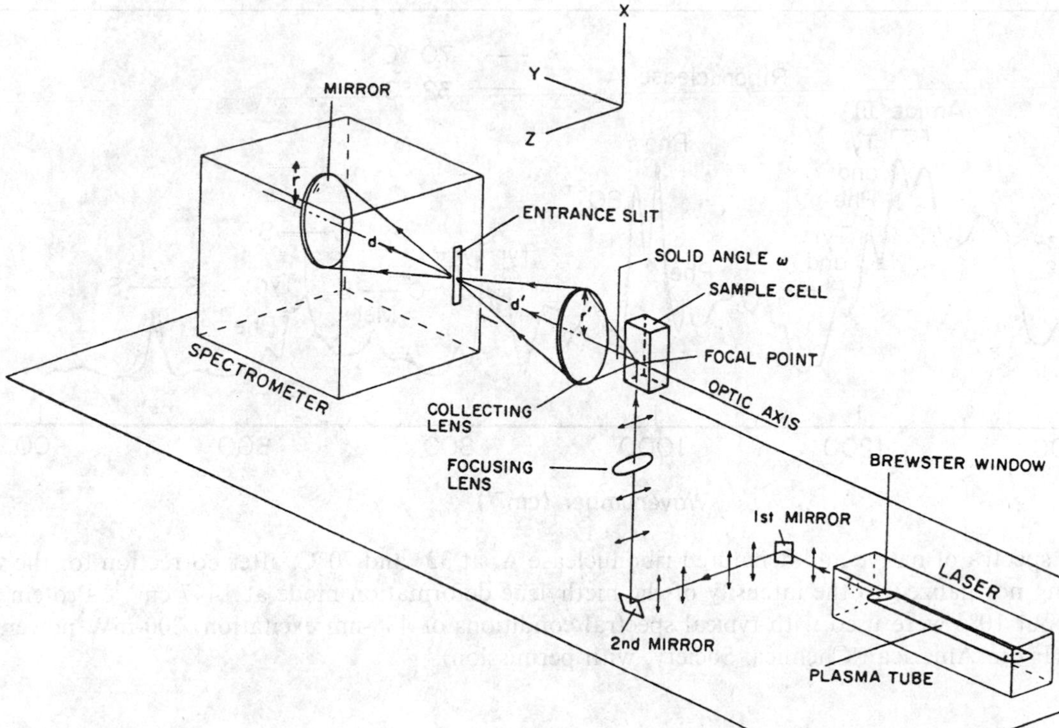

FIG. 36.31. The optics of a conventional Raman spectrometer.

Protein Conformation Determination

Protein molecules are classical examples of the application of Raman spectroscopy to biomolecules. This technique can probe structural details such as average peptide backbone conformation, and some amino acid side chains—for example, those of tyrosine and tryptophan can also be probed. Protein spectra are usually obtained in the 450–650 nm region; however, UV excited resonance Raman spectra of proteins containing aromatic amino acids of interest is often used with excitation below 300 nm. The normal Raman spectrum of proteins contains diagnostic amide I (C=O stretch) and amide III (N-H in-plane bending) bands that can be utilized to characterize the secondary structure of the protein or peptide backbone. Table 36.3 gives approximate positions for the amide I and amide III bands in both the IR and Raman spectra of various polypeptide conformations. Characterization of the secondary structure of a protein depends on the determination of characteristic amide I and III frequencies in the Raman spectrum for α-helical, β-sheet, and random protein conformations. This is often achieved by using polypeptide models and proteins of known conformation. Figure 36.32 illustrates

Table 36.3

Approximate positions (cm^{-1}) of the most intense Amide I and Amide III bands in Raman spectra, and the Amide I band in IR spectra for various polypeptide conformations

	Amide I		Amide III
Conformation	Raman	Infrared	Raman
α-Helix	1645–1660	1650.00	1265–1300
β-Sheet	1665–1680	1632.00	1230–1240
Unordered	1660–1670	1658.00	1240–1260

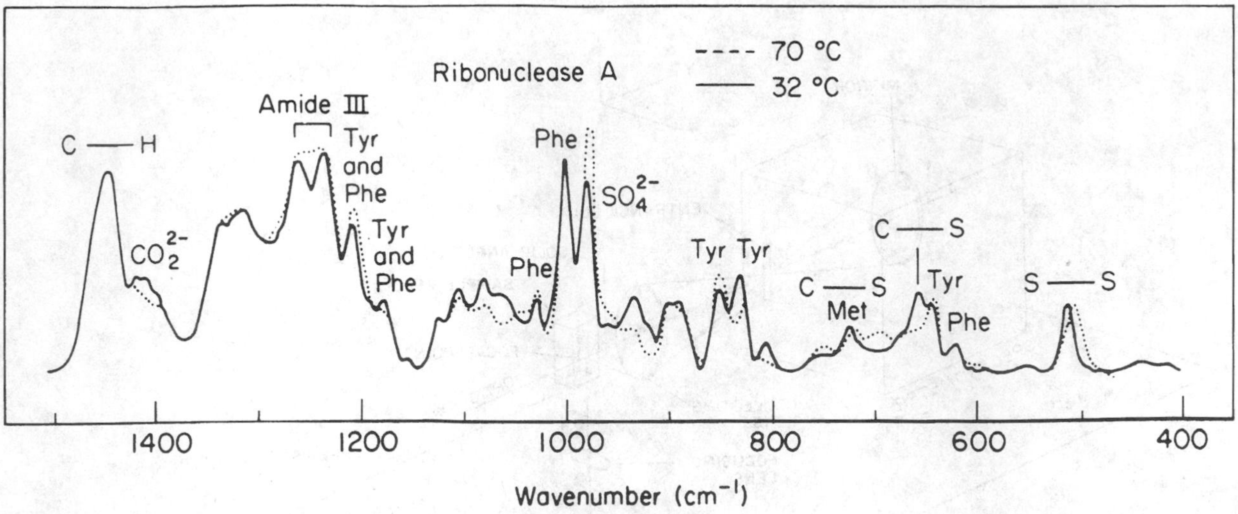

FIG. 36.32. Raman spectra of native and denatured ribonuclease A, at 32° and 70°C, after correction for the water background and being normalized to the intensity of the methylene deformation mode at 1447 cm^{-1}. Protein concentrations of about 10% were used with typical spectral conditions of 488-nm excitation, 200-mW power, and 7 cm^{-1} spectral slit (From American Chemical Society, with permission).

Raman spectra, run in water, of native and denatured ribonuclease A and shows the change in the amide III band in the disordered protein (31).

Resonance Raman Labels

Resonance Raman labels are chromophores that have been carefully designed to mimic natural biochemical components and are themselves biologically active molecules. They provide detailed vibrational and electronic spectral data when in the vicinity of a biologically important site. Extrinsic protein-bound chromophores—for example, methyl orange bound to bovine serum albumin—have been studied in detail. Protein-ligand interactions—that is, drug-enzyme and hapten-antibody complexes where the drug or hapten is the chromophoric resonance Raman label—are other systems that have been studied. This method is useful for studying enzyme–substrate complexes, and can provide vibrational spectra of the substrate during enzyme catalysis.

RNA and DNA Structural Analysis

Analysis of polynucleotides by Raman spectroscopy affords bands (~30) that are mainly attributable to purine and/or pyrimidine ring modes. In addition, the phosphate group shows interesting features in the spectrum. The sugar moieties in DNA and RNA molecules and the related polynucleotides are poor Raman scatterers. From the Raman spectrum it is possible to obtain a semiquantitative estimate of the relative population of bases in the polynucleotide molecule. Base protonation in DNA has been studied using Raman spectroscopy and metal–nucleotide binding has also been investigated. The mode of binding of ions such as Ca^{++}, Mg^{++}, Co^{++}, Cu^{++}, and Mg^{++} to adenosine triphosphate over a wide range of pH has also been studied. Raman spectroscopy can detect the disruption of base pairing and base stacking interactions (81). In Figure 36.33, raising the temperature of poly(rA) : poly(rU) from 32°C to 82°C results in thermal disruption of the helix. Important features in the difference spectra are the radical changes in the carbonyl region (1650–1700 cm^{-1}) due to the disruption of H-bonding in the Watson–Crick mode. Phosphate backbone conformation in nucleic acids has also been studied by monitoring the -O-P-O- symmetrical stretching vibration (800 cm^{-1}) and the $-PO^{2-}$ symmetrical stretch motion (1100 cm^{-1}).

The interaction of nucleic acids with proteins is an area of active study. For example, the stabilizing effect of the viral capsids on the secondary structure of the viral RNA has been investigated, and Raman data on DNA–histone interactions have indicated that the sites of DNA–protein interactions are probably located in the grooves running along DNA.

Lipids and Membranes

Raman spectroscopy is ideally suited for the study of lipids and membranes, and has some advantages over

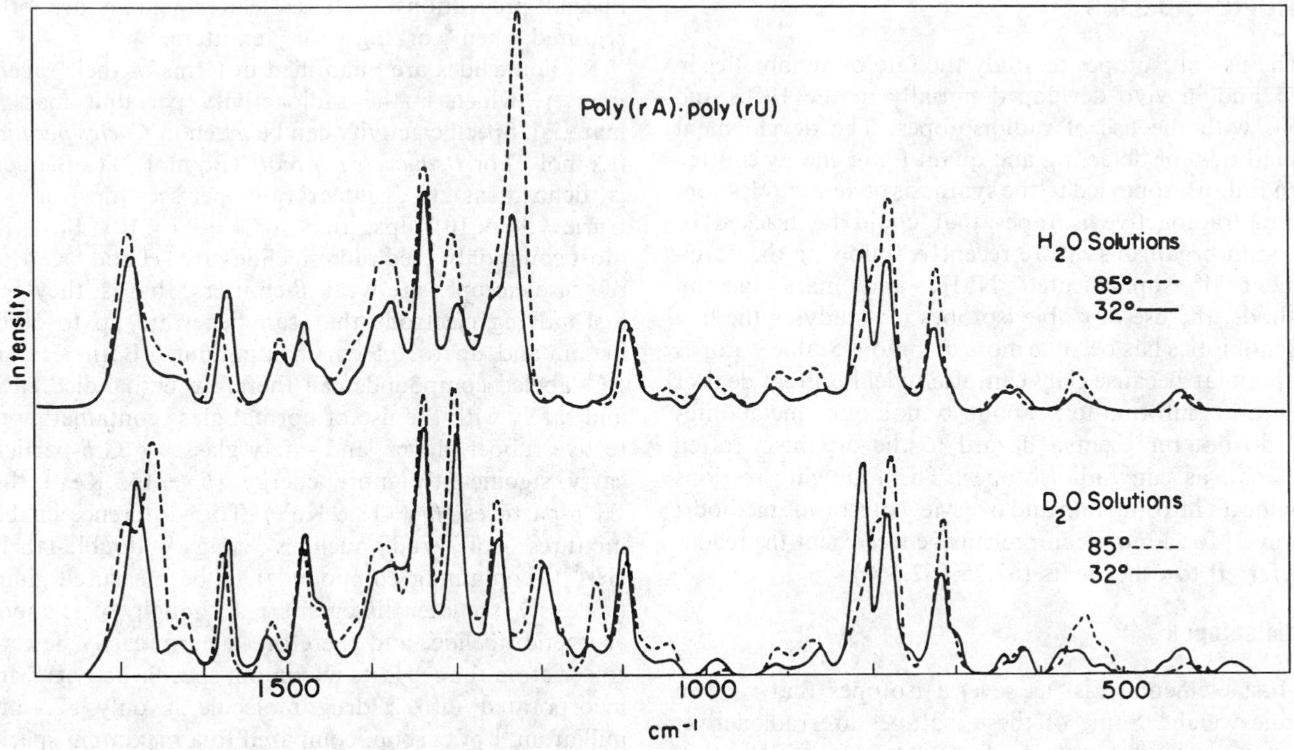

FIG. 36.33. Raman spectra of H_2O and D_2O solutions of poly(rA)poly(rU) at 32° and 85°C. The background of Raman scattering by the solvent has been subtracted from each spectrum. From Reference 81, with permission.

other techniques. The analysis time frame of fractions of a picosecond provides instant "snapshots," eliminating line broadening commonly seen in magnetic resonance spectra. Also, no probe molecule is required and both gel and liquid–crystal hydrocarbon regions can be monitored.

The most useful regions are the 1000–1150 cm^{-1} region (C-C "accordion" stretch) and the 2800–3000 cm^{-1} region (C-H stretching mode). Gel to liquid–crystal transitions in membranes are indicated by marked changes in the bands assigned to the C-C stretch mode, while the C-H stretch region is extremely sensitive to conformational change within the individual fatty acid chains.

Raman Microspectroscopy

The recent use of Raman microspectroscopy (124) to study single living cells and chromosomes has opened up this spectroscopic technique to the exploration of biological processes in cells and living tissues, with the possibility of in vivo diagnosis of certain diseases in their very early stages (137). Often, in vivo analyses can be performed relatively quickly, and several reports on the biomedical applications of in vivo Raman spectroscopy (IV–RS) have been published (68,82,137).

The potential use of IV–RS for diagnosing arterial disease and cancer in gynecological tissues, soft tissues, breast, colon, bladder, and brain has been discussed by Manoharan et al. (95). Lawson et al. (82) have recently reviewed the application of Raman spectroscopy in studying human arteries, tumors, gallstones, hair, and nails. Brain tissues have also been investigated using FT–Raman spectroscopy, and spectra from cerebral cortex, cerebral white matter, caudate–putamen, thalamus, synaptosomal fraction, and myelin fraction have been recorded (104,105). Brain tumors have also been studied using FT Raman spectroscopy (104).

More recently, Ong et al. (115) have studied the substantia nigra of the rostral mid-brain in monkeys, using Raman microspectroscopy to determine differences between white and gray matter. The laser spot size of 1 μm in Raman microspectroscopy, compared to 20 μm in IR microspectroscopy, afforded a much better spatial resolution in sample analysis than can be obtained using the latter technique. The white and gray matter could be clearly distinguished, and their relative proportions evaluated from the Raman frequencies in the 3000 cm^{-1} region. However, brain cells of monkeys suffering from Parkinson's disease did not show any clear differences compared to control cells from healthy monkeys.

ISOTOPIC LABELING

The use of isotopes to study the fate of xenobiotics in vitro and in vivo developed initially in the 1950s and 1960s with the use of radioisotopes. The development of methods for detecting and quantifying energy emitted from radioisotopes led to the synthesis of xenobiotics containing radioactive isotopes that could be tracked or traced in organisms. More recently, following the development of sophisticated NMR and mass spectral methods, the use of stable isotopes for studying the fate of xenobiotics has become more common. Stable isotopes are popular because they can often yield a great deal of structural information about xenobiotic metabolites and do not represent a hazard to the organism (often humans), as can radioisotopes. The following sections provide an introduction and overview of isotope methods; however, for a more comprehensive treatment the reader is referred to other texts (67,75,162,168).

Radioisotopes

Most elements exist as several isotopes that vary in atomic weight. Some of these isotopes are radioactive, spontaneously decaying to form an atom of another element. This decay is accompanied by the emission of radiation. The radiation emitted is of three distinct types: alpha (α), beta (β), and gamma (γ). Alpha particles are actually helium nuclei (^{4}He), β particles are electrons, and γ rays are high-energy electromagnetic radiation. Isotopes that emit β particles, so called β emitters, are less hazardous to laboratory workers than γ emitters because β particles do not possess sufficient energy to penetrate the skin. β emitters are only hazardous if ingested where they can come in contact with cells. In contrast, γ emitters are more hazardous to laboratory workers because γ rays are highly energetic and can easily penetrate the skin. Special precautions such as lead shielding are often required when working with γ emitters.

Radionuclides are quantified in terms of their *specific activity*, which is the radioactivity per unit mass of material. Specific activity can be given in *Curies per mole* (Ci mol^{-1}) or *Bequerels per mole* (Bq mol^{-1}) (a Bequerel is defined as 1 disintegration per sec [dps] and 1 Curie $= 3.7 \times 10^{10}$ dps, thus 1 Ci $= 3.7 \times 10^{10}$ Bq). The most commonly used radionuclides are ^{3}H and ^{14}C. Both of these isotopes are weak β-emitters, that is, they emit fast-moving electrons that can penetrate up to 50 cm in air, and up to 0.5 cm in aluminum. Both ^{3}H- and ^{14}C-labeled compounds can therefore be handled easily and safely with the use of normal glass containers, protective rubber gloves, and safety glasses. ^{14}C β-particles carry significantly more energy ($\beta^- = 155$ KeV) than ^{3}H β-particles ($\beta^- = 18.6$ KeV). This difference enables mixtures of radionuclides (e.g., double-labeled ^{3}H/^{14}C-containing compounds) to be measured simultaneously (see later disscussion). Although ^{14}C is a more energetic nuclide, and therefore a more easily detected tracer atom than ^{3}H, its maximum specific activity when incorporated into a drug molecule is only 62.4 mCi milliatom^{-1} of carbon, compared to a maximum specific activity for ^{3}H of 29.1 Ci milliatom^{-1} of hydrogen.

The energy emitted when radioactive isotopes decay can be easily traced because the radionuclide itself is not metabolically altered by the biological system under study. The radioisotopes most commonly used in biological systems are shown in Table 36.4.

Xenobiotic Disposition Studies using Radiolabeled Tracers

The most common use of radiolabeled xenobiotics in toxicology is the study of the fate of a chemical in animal

Table 36.4
Radioactive isotopes commonly used to study the fate of xenobiotics

Atomic number	Element	Atomic weight	Half-life	Radiation (MeV)
1	Hydrogen	3	12.33 y	β^- (0.019)
6	Carbon	11	20.4 min	β^+ (0.96)
		14	5730 y	β^- (0.156)
15	Phosphorus	32	14.28 d	β^- (1.71)
		33	25.3 d	β^- (0.25)
16	Sulfur	35	87.5 d	β^- (0.167)
17	Chlorine	36	3×10^5 y	β^- (0.71)
37	Rubidium	87	4.8×10^{10} y	β^- (0.272)
53	Iodine	125	60.14 d	γ (0.035)
		131	8.040 d	β^- (0.607, 0.336) γ (0.080, 0.284, 0.364, 0.637, 0.723)

models. In many toxicology research facilities these studies are often referred to as absorption, distribution, metabolism and excretion (often abbreviated ADME). The successful conduct of ADME studies requires:

1. A radiolabeled xenobiotic with the most appropriate isotope and position of the label.
2. An analytical method for separating the parent compound and its hypothesized metabolites.
3. Methods for quantifying the amount of radioactivity.

Choice and Location of Label

The radioisotope of choice for xenobiotic ADME studies is carbon-14 (^{14}C) because it is a radioactive form of the element that forms the backbone of most xenobiotics. In addition, ^{14}C has a very long half-life (over 5000 years) and is a weak β emitter so it poses few health risks to laboratory workers.

The position of the label must be carefully selected to ensure that the label is not lost upon metabolism. Often, researchers using ^{14}C will uniformly label one of the aromatic rings of a xenobiotic if it is thought not to undergo ring opening during metabolism. These positions are preferable to ^{14}C in a methyl group attached to an oxygen or a nitrogen, because both these carbons will undergo demethylation reactions catalyzed either by cytochrome P450 or flavin-containing monooxygenase (see chapter 3, Metabolism: A Determinant of Toxicity, by deBethizy and Hayes). Sometimes there are limitations for placing the label, based on synthetic concerns. Every effort should be made to locate the label in a chemically and metabolically stable position. Methods of general interest for synthesizing labeled xenobiotics are often published as stand-alone papers in the Journal of Labeled Compounds and Radiopharmaceuticals.

Tritium (^{3}H) is the radioactive form of hydrogen and is often used as a tracer because of the high specific activity that can be obtained with this isotope. High specific activity increases the researcher's ability to detect smaller amounts of the xenobiotic. Receptor binding assays typically use tritiated ligands for this reason. However, the use of tritium has some shortcomings including a relatively short half-life (12.33 y) that requires adjustment of the specific activity over time. In addition, because tritium is an isotope of hydrogen it undergoes exchange with nonradioactive protium (^{1}H) in solvents. This so-called solvent exchange must be taken into account when positioning a label on the xenobiotic. Positions that readily undergo solvent exchange are not good candidates for labeling. These positions are referred to as labile positions (for example, protons attached to oxygen, nitrogen, or sulfur atoms are labile). Tritium may also be lost due to metabolism of the xenobiotic, and an experienced investigator will usually avoid inserting labels at positions in the molecule where they may be lost during biotransformation. For example, ^{3}H-labeling at carbon adjacent to a heteroatom or at a hydroxylation site on a phenyl ring, or a ^{3}H-labeled N-methyl group, which may often be lost by oxidation, should generally be avoided.

Radiochemical Purity

The purity of labeled compounds is usually critical to the success of an experiment. When following (tracing) a radiolabeled compound, there is no specificity to the radioactivity emitted by the radioactive isotope. In other words, chemical impurities containing the radiolabeled isotope will be indistinguishable from the xenobiotic of interest. Therefore, the original material administered to the organism should be of the highest purity possible to ensure that the radioactivity detected is derived from the parent compound. Radiochemical purity should be confirmed by a suitable method, such as radiochromatography (discussed later), prior to using a radiolabeled compound for an ADME study.

In addition to radiochemical purity, it may be important to have enantiomeric purity. Many biological processes are stereoselective, with either the S or R enantiomer of a biologically active compound having the lion's share of the activity—that is, only one of the stereoisomers of a compound is active in the system under study. For example, the (S)-(−) enantiomer of nicotine is responsible for most of the pharmacological activity. The affinity of the (R)-(+) enantiomer for high-affinity nicotinic acetylcholine receptors is 60-fold less than the (S)-(−) enantiomer. In recent years with the recognition that many toxic responses are receptor-mediated, the enantiomeric purity of radiochemicals has become more important.

The solvent selected for storage of a radiolabeled compound can be very important. For example, radiolabeled peptides and proteins that have been stored in water undergo extensive degradation. Solvent exchange can also be a problem for tritiated compounds as described above. The selection of a solvent is usually a compromise between adequate solubility and a minimum of inherent reactivity with the radiolabeled compound.

Route of Administration

A primary consideration when conducting an ADME study with radiolabeled xenobiotics is the route of administration. The xenobiotic is usually administered to the animal model by a route appropriate to either the anticipated major route of exposure to the species of economic interest (usually humans), or by a route of administration that is consistent with the goals of the research. For example, if the xenobiotic of interest is a component of a consumer product applied to the skin, the appropriate route of delivery may be dermal administration. However, if the objective of the ADME experiment were to determine the pharmacokinetics of the xenobiotic in blood and tissues then an intravenous route of administration would be chosen over the dermal route. The solubility of the compound in a vehicle can also be a consideration when deciding on a route because some vehicles are not compatible with intravenous administration.

Liquid Scintillation Spectrometry

Total xenobiotic-derived radioactivity can be determined in all excreta, including urine, feces, and expired air, to quantify the routes of excretion for a xenobiotic and its metabolites. Total radioactivity in aqueous samples is relatively easy to quantify using liquid scintillation spectrometry. This method for quantifying radioactivity involves mixing an aliquot of the sample with liquid scintillation mixture (LSM) which uses an organic compound or mixture of compounds that are scintillators, compounds that give off light when they absorb radioactive energy. Traditionally, these scintillators were dissolved in toluene-based mixtures that allowed counting of both organic and aqueous samples. For aqueous samples, a mixture of two parts sample to eight parts LSM typically formed a gel that was counted. These LSMs could tolerate no more than about 20% water. In recent years, LSMs that are less hazardous, can tolerate higher water content, and can be discarded down the sanitary sewer have replaced toluene-based LSMs for most applications. The mixture of the radioactive sample and the liquid scintillation mixture is placed in special vials that are highly efficient at passing light and not absorbing radioactive energy. The vials are counted by placing them in a *liquid scintillation counter*, which uses two opposed photomultiplier tubes to detect light-emitting events triggered by the radioactive decay of the isotope. Coincidence circuitry is used to separate random events from radioactive-isotope-driven events. The counting region is lined with lead to shield the vial from extraneous environmental radiation. The sample is compared to a blank or background vial that contains everything but the radioisotope-containing sample. The radioactive counts from the background vial must be subtracted from the sample to obtain net radioactivity.

The liquid scintillation counter expresses data in counts per min (CPM) which must be corrected to disintegrations per min (DPM) to account for inefficiencies in capturing all the radioactive energy emitted. The method employed in most liquid scintillation counters today involves the use of external standard calibration. With this method, a radioactive source housed in the instrument is placed automatically near the vial containing the sample and the photomultiplier tubes detect the resulting light emitted from the scintillator within the sample vial. The CPMs detected by the instrument are then automatically compared to the known DPMs of the external standard source and a counting efficiency is determined. The counting efficiencies for ^{14}C are usually much higher than for the less energetic β emitter tritium.

In addition to the inefficiencies in transferring the energy of radioactive decay into light energy, there is also quenching of the light emitted from the scintillator. Many solvents and biological molecules can quench the light emitted by the scintillator. Therefore, the researcher must correct for the amount of quenching within the sample by comparing the expected DPMs to a quench curve and determining the actual DPMs present in the quenched sample. This is usually accomplished automatically by the liquid scintillation counter by first running a set of vials containing a known amount of radioactivity with increasing amounts of a quenching agent added to each vial. The resulting quench curve is stored in the computer memory of the counter and used to determine the DPMs of the sample.

Radioactive samples containing scintillant are often sensitive to external light, especially sunlight, which results in excitation and abnormally high CPMs on analysis. This phenomenon, called chemiluminescence, is usually more of a problem with ^{3}H-containing rather than ^{14}C-containing radiolabeled samples, and can usually be minimized or eliminated by storing scintillation fluids and samples containing scintillant in the dark for 30–60 min before analysis.

Combustion Techniques

Many samples are not amenable to liquid scintillation counting because they are either solids or not compatible with the LSMs. Total radioactivity in tissue samples and fecal samples can be determined by combustion of the sample to carbon dioxide and water. ^{14}C in the original sample is converted to $^{14}CO_2$ and tritium is converted to tritiated water. Instruments have been developed that automatically combust samples on a platinum electrode covered with a glass chimney. The resulting products of combustion are swept away by an airstream and trapped in appropriate solvents. Liquid scintillation mixture is added and the resulting samples are counted in a liquid scintillation counter.

Autoradiography

Autoradiography is the production of an image by the emission of radioactive decay energy from a radionuclide. It provides a qualitative visual image of the tissue distribution of a xenobiotic and in recent years has been used to provide quantitative distribution data as well. ^{14}C is probably the most often used radionuclide for autoradiography because of its long half-life and relatively high energy. Tritium is used when greater resolution is required because it is a weaker emitter. Radioisotopes of nitrogen and oxygen do not have sufficiently long half-lives to permit development of an image. Iodine, sulfur, chlorine, and phosphorus are also used for autoradiography.

Whole-body autoradiography is an excellent technique for visualizing the distribution of xenobiotic-derived radioactivity in an animal model. This technique involves administration of the xenobiotic to the animal and, following anesthesia, the animal is quick-frozen by immersion in hexane or acetone with dry ice. The time interval between administration and freezing must be selected based on some knowledge of the rate of elimination of the compound. After complete freezing, the animal is placed in a block of carboxymethylcellulose ice on the stage of a microtome. The microtome is an instrument that uses a sharp blade to shave thin sections off one side of the block. Sections varying in thickness from 5 to approximately 80 μm are captured from the microtome blade using a large piece of tape. The section is then placed on X-ray film that is allowed to stand in a freezer while the radiation emitted by the isotope exposes the film.

The resulting pictures (autoradiograms) illustrate where in the body the xenobiotic-derived radioactivity has distributed. The highly perfused organs such as kidney, liver, and heart are the first to "light up" with the compound (159). Over time it becomes obvious which tissues store the compound.

In recent years, digital imaging techniques have enabled quantitative analysis of whole-body autoradiograms providing absolute concentrations of xenobiotic-derived radioactivity in tissues. Zane et al. (172) have shown that autoradiography with quantitative digital image analysis compared extremely well with the more traditional combustion method. For this comparison, they treated rats with ^{14}C labeled CGS 18102A and sectioned the animals as described above. They also took 16 tissue samples from each animal for combustion analysis. The sections were placed on X-ray film along with a series of calibration standards of known radioactivity. After three weeks of film exposure, the autoradiograms were analyzed with a digital imaging system. The concentrations obtained from digital analysis of the autoradiograms compared very well to those obtained by combustion analysis. Jacob et al. (64) used quantitative whole-body autoradiography (QWBA) with digital image analysis to study the transplacental uptake and covalent binding of [^{14}C]-chloroacetonitrile (CAN) to various tissues in normal and glutathione-depleted pregnant mice. Their finding that covalent binding of CAN to maternal and fetal tissue was elevated in glutathione-depleted mice suggested a modulatory role of glutathione in CAN distribution and transplacental toxicity and demonstrated the utility of QWBA in mechanistic studies.

Even though X-ray film provides excellent resolution and has been used successfully for QWBA, it is not necessarily the medium of choice. For one thing, exposure times for X-ray film are typically weeks to months. Also, X-ray film often does not provide a linear calibration over the wide range of radioactivity (optical densities) common in QWBA. To avoid these limitations, many workers are now turning to storage phosphor screens instead of X-ray film for QWBA. Storage phosphor screens trap the energy released by radioactive samples. The energy is stored by the phosphor screen and is only released when the screen is scanned with a laser beam. The released energy appears in the form of blue light, which is detected by a photomultiplier tube and converted to a digital signal that is stored in a computer file. To quantify the levels of radioactivity in the whole-body sections, a series of standards are analyzed and the response of each is determined. A regression equation, derived for the standard responses, is used to determine the absolute concentration of radioactivity in the whole-body sections.

The autoradiograms can also be visualized by converting the digital data to a graphics file and printing the results. Fortunately, commercially available hardware and software are available for QWBA using storage phosphor screens. Storage phosphor screens overcome thc major limitations of X-ray film. They have a linear response over a five log-unit range and can be developed in hours to days. It has been estimated (165) that a two-week exposure to X-ray film is equivalent to a 24-h exposure to a storage phosphor screen. For a more comprehensive introduction to storage phosphors for QWBA, the reader is referred to the work of Wilson and Kraus (165) and Herman and Chay (59).

An interesting application of storage phosphor QWBA is illustrated in Figure 36.34. For this study, Sprague-Dawley albino rats were administered [^{14}C]-RJR-2403 at a dose of 15 mg/kg by gastric gavage. Animals were euthanized at specific time points and sectioned (30 μm) as described above. Sections were exposed to storage phosphor screens for seven days and data were collected using a PhosporImager SF (Molecular Dynamics). Figure 36.34A shows an autoradiogram obtained at 30 min and Figure 36.34B shows an autoradiogram obtained at 4 h after dosing. Table 36.5 lists the tissue concentrations by tissue for each time point. Note that radioactivity was extensively absorbed and distributed throughout the tissues of the rat at 30 min post dose. Tissue concentrations were highest in the kidney and liver with high levels also achieved in the stomach, heart, lung, and spleen. By 4 h post-dose, tissue concentrations decreased considerably, with high levels seen in tissues associated with metabolism and excretion such as the liver and kidney.

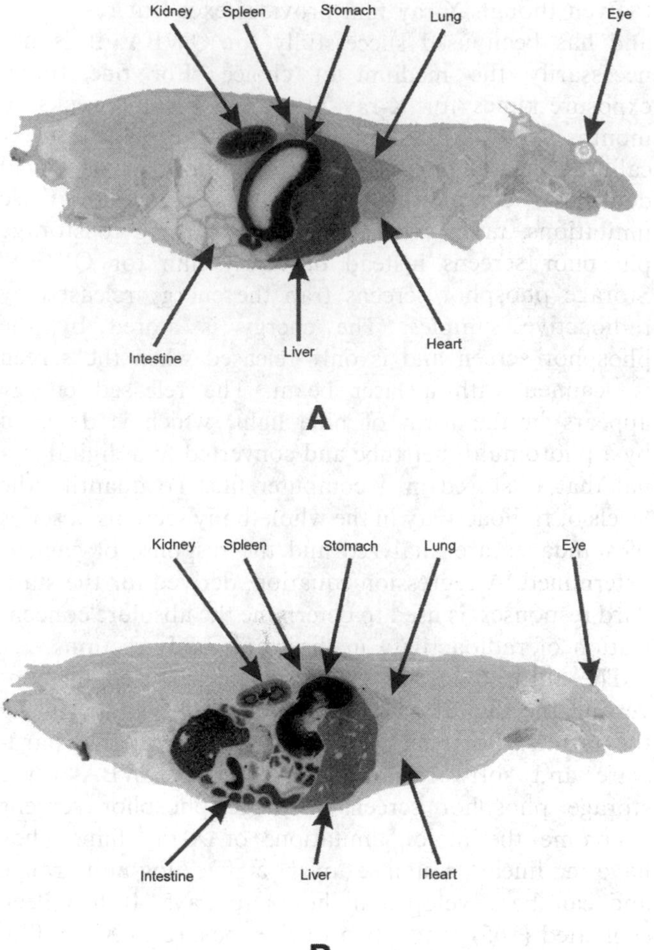

FIG. 36.34. Quantitative whole body autoradiograms of male albino rats after administration of [^{14}C]-RJR-2403 at a dose of 15 mg/kg by gastric gavage. A: 30 min after dosing, B: 4 h after dosing.

Analytical Methods for Determining Chemical Form

Total radioactivity data are of limited value because of their lack of specificity. Once major routes of excretion are determined, it is important to characterize the chemical form of the excreted radioactivity. For example, expired CO_2 can be selectively trapped in base (usually sodium hydroxide or an organic base such as ethanolamine) and provide valuable insight in how extensively a xenobiotic is metabolized. Acrylic acid and ethyl acrylate, two monomers used extensively in the plastics industry, are rapidly metabolized and 70% of the compounds eliminated from the body as CO_2 via normal catabolic biochemical pathways that degrade the carbon skeleton of the molecule (41). On the other hand, many xenobiotics are metabolized to polar compounds by selective metabolism of functional groups on the molecule without catabolic degradation of the carbon skeleton. High-pressure liquid chromatography (HPLC) has been very popular for quantifying metabolites in biological matrices because metabolites that are relatively hydrophilic and nonvolatile can be chromatographed easily. Other methods for separating metabolites from the parent compound include LC–MS, LC–NMR, thin layer chromatography, capillary zone electrophoresis, chemical reaction interface mass spectrometry, and gas–liquid chromatography.

Table 36.5
Tissue concentration of total radioactivity at 30 min and 4 h after a single oral administration of [^{14}C]-RJR-2403 to male albino rats. Target dose, 15 mg/kg. Results expressed as μg equivalents/g.

Tissue	30 min	4 h
Eye	1.01	0.67
Heart	5.39	2.46
Kidney	39.17	39.15
Large intestine wall	3.28	NM
Liver	26.12	17.53
Lung	6.49	3.52
Spleen	5.18	4.96
Stomach wall	15.38	7.53

NM = not measurable

The simplest approach to characterizing the radioactivity in excreta is to inject urine directly onto an HPLC. Usually the urine is filtered first by passing through a centrifugal ultra-filter with a small pore size (0.2–0.45 μm). Special HPLC guard columns can be used to protect the analytical column from the high concentration of other organics such as creatinine and salts that are found in urine.

The metabolites of the parent compound are "visualized" by achieving adequate separation of the radioactivity in excreta on the HPLC column. Radioactive peaks eluting from the HPLC column can be collected in scintillation vials as a series of fractions and the radioactivity counted in a liquid scintillation counter. A histogram of radioactivity in the fractions should reveal distinct peaks of radioactivity. The radioactive peaks can be coeluted with synthetic standards of putative metabolites by injecting the standards along with the sample onto the HPLC column. Radioactive effluent from the HPLC column can also be detected using a commercially available flow-through radioactivity detector (117). These detectors have improved in recent years to the point that they have replaced the more labor-intensive fraction collection method in many laboratories. Radioactive flow detectors use two types of flow-cells. Solid scintillator cells use glass beads, calcium fluoride, or yttrium silicate and permit the recovery of unadulterated effluent. Using this type of detector, peaks containing radioactivity can be collected and analyzed by some other method such as mass spectrometry to determine the identity of the radiolabeled metabolite. Liquid scintillator cells mix liquid scintillation cocktail with the column effluent prior to passing in front of the photomultiplier tubes where the radioactivity is detected. The mixture of effluent and LSM must be discarded in radioactive waste. The choice of the type and volume of the flow cell depends on the isotope and specific activity of the label. Optimization of these parameters permits rapid and accurate determinations.

Double-Label Techniques

The use of doubly labeled compounds in metabolic experiments is often necessary to obtain more in-depth information on metabolic pathways and biotransformation mechanisms. Thus, one part of a xenobiotic molecule may be labeled with ^{14}C and another group in the molecule may contain a ^{3}H-label. Because ^{3}H and ^{14}C have different maximal β-energies (see earlier discussion), this allows the quantitative measurement of both ^{3}H and ^{14}C within the same sample. Similarly, other β-emitting nuclides, such as ^{35}S, can also be measured in the presence of ^{3}H or ^{14}C. The determination depends upon the fact that there will be a region in the energy spectrum of the mixture where the β-particles from only one of the nuclides will be present, and by measuring this region and comparing it with a nuclide standard, the appropriate isotope content in the mixture can be obtained.

Some very elegant experiments have been conducted using doubly labeled xenobiotics. For example, Pool and Crooks (120) used ^{3}H and ^{14}C to determine the in vivo stability of (R)-(+)-[^{3}H-N′-CH^{3}; ^{14}C-N-CH$_3$]-N-methylnicotinium ion, a primary nicotine metabolite in the guinea pig.

Positron Emission Tomography

Positron-Emission Tomography (PET) was introduced in the early 1970s as a non-invasive diagnostic technique to study in vivo physiological processes in both animals and humans (128,151). The process is an imaging technique that provides quantitative, regional measurements and kinetics of specific biochemical and physiological processes in living animals or human subjects and is similar to X-ray CT (computerized axial tomography) and MRI (magnetic resonance imaging) in that images of cross-sectional slices of the body are produced. The technique involves the use of a substance with the desired biological activity containing a positron-emitting radioactive isotope. Positron-emitting nuclides are neutron-deficient compared to their stable isotopes and decay by spontaneous conversion of a proton to a neutron. This conversion is accompanied by release of a positron, which travels a small distance before encountering an electron resulting in antimatter–matter annihilation. This annihilation event releases energy in the form of two 511-KeV tissue penetrating gamma ray photons radiating at approximately 180 degrees from one another. A circular array of scanners consisting of scintillation crystals arranged so that opposing crystals are grouped in coincidence circuits are placed around the subject, and detect the paired gamma rays as they simultaneously arrive on opposite sides (see Figure 36.35) (48). The PET scanner's coincidence circuits enable the localization of the source of each annihilation and a computer then uses this information to reconstruct an image of the radionuclides' distribution within the body. Several million coincidences may be assimilated during a 1–15 min scan interval. In this way, a tomographic image can be obtained, illustrating the spatial distribution of the radionuclide.

When images are recorded at appropriate intervals after the administration of the radionuclide, quantitative measurements reflecting the dynamic process under study

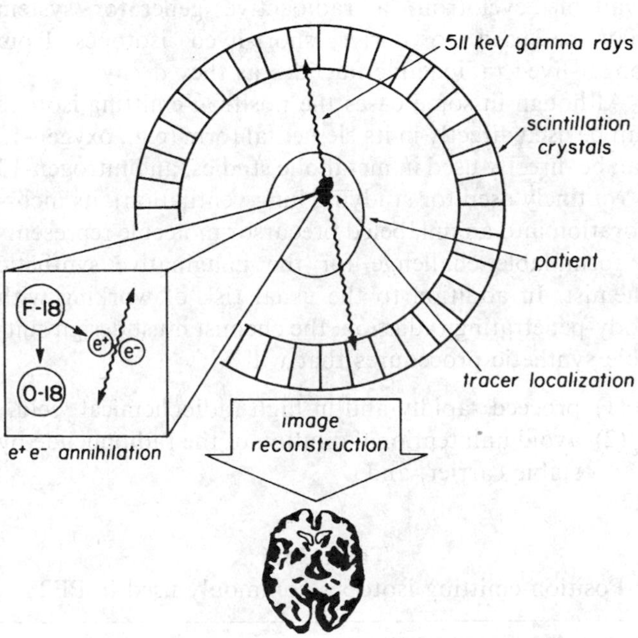

FIG. 36.35. Key features of a PET scan: radiopharmaceutical localization, radioisotope decay by positron emission and immediate positron-electron annihilation; detection of body penetrating 511-keV annihilation radiation by an external circular assay of scintillation crystals; reconstructed image of radioactivity distribution. (From Reference 48, with permission).

can be obtained. Images can also be color-coded to show differences in the levels of activity from one time point to the next.

Positron-Emitting Isotopes

The radionuclides most commonly used in PET are carbon-11, nitrogen-13, oxygen-15, and fluorine-18. All these isotopes decay exclusively by positron emission, producing readily detectable tissue-penetrating gamma ray photons, but have relatively short half-lives (see Table 36.6). Their brief existence means that they must be manufactured close to the detection site, and, more importantly, fast chemical reaction techniques and isolation procedures must be developed to ensure the production of a useful radionuclide. In addition, the use of such labeled compounds is limited to biochemical processes with rapid rates of turnover.

The production of positron-emitting isotopes is normally carried out using on-site medical cyclotrons immediately prior to use, via the transmutation of stable isotopes. For example, carbon-11 is usually prepared by irradiating nitrogen or boron with accelerated protons, oxygen-15 by irradiating nitrogen with deuterons, and nitrogen-13 by irradiating nitrogen with deuterons or irradiating carbon with deuterons. In the case of the longer-lived fluorine-18, stocks may be obtained from a regional distribution center. At sites remote from an available cyclotron, a radioactive generator system may be used to derive short-lived isotopes from longer-lived radioactive nuclides as they decay.

Although in some cases the positron-emitting isotope can be used directly in its elemental form (e.g., oxygen-15 can be directly used in metabolic studies, and nitrogen-13 is routinely used for studying lung ventilation), its incorporation into an unlabeled precursor molecule represents a formidable challenge for the imaginative synthetic chemist. In addition to the usual risk of working with body-penetrating radiation, the chemist must design suitable synthetic procedures that will

(1) proceed rapidly and in high radiochemical yield,
(2) avoid unintentional dilution of the radionuclide by stable carrier, and

Table 36.6
Position-emitting isotopes commonly used in PET.

Nuclide	Half-life (min)	Carrier-free specific activity (Ci/mol)
Carbon-11	20.40	9.22×10^3
Nitrogen-13	9.96	1.89×10^4
Oxygen-15	2.07	9.10×10^4
Fluorine-18	109.70	1.7×10^3

(3) avoid difficult and time-consuming separation procedures.

Thus, the number of steps in the synthetic process should be cut to a minimum to avoid working with large quantities of radioactivity, and to ensure compatibility with the half-life of the isotope.

A description of the successful synthesis of L-[^{13}N] tyrosine serves to illustrate the above points (48). A mixture of [^{13}N]-nitrate and [^{13}N]-nitrite obtained from an on-site cyclotron is converted to [^{13}N]-NH_3 by reduction with Devarda's alloy/NaOH reagent, the product collected by distillation and immediately reacted with α-ketoglutarate and NADH. The reaction mixture is then passed through a column containing glutamate dehydrogenase immobilized on a solid support, to give [^{13}N]-glutamate. Passage of this product down a second column containing immobilized glutamate oxaloacetate transaminase transfers the [^{13}N]NH_2 group from glutamate to *p*-hydroxyphenylpyruvate to give L-[^{13}N]-tyrosine in radiochemically pure form and 28% overall radiochemical yield. The total synthesis time is 25 min.

Instrument Design

A functional PET unit consists of a data-acquisition system and a computer. The acquisition system incorporates the radiation detectors, their associated circuitry, and, in some designs, a mechanical system that imparts a small motion to the detectors to obtain better sampling. Data from the acquisition system is assimilated in a fast computer, and a display system for immediate viewing and recording of the image is available, with interactive capabilities for the analysis of the image.

Specific Applications

PET is an extremely versatile method for probing fundamental biochemical processes in living systems. It will not be possible to cover all the biomedical applications in this review. However, some of the more important applications are in the areas of metabolism, drug disposition and pharmacokinetics, and physiological and neurochemical mechanisms. In the brain, PET has been used to measure regional blood flow (133), glucose utilization, blood volume, oxygen utilization, the oxygen extraction ratio, the permeability–surface area product for water, acid-base chemistry, protein synthesis, and the characterization of dopamine D_2, benzodiazepine, and opiate receptors.

PET measurement of regional rates of cerebral glucose metabolism utilizes [^{18}F]2-fluoro-2-deoxyglucose (FdG) as the tracer component (53,118). This procedure can determine quantitatively glucose utilization, since FdG, unlike dG, cannot be biotransformed further after its initial conversion to FdG-6-phosphate (FdG-6P) by hexokinase, due to the absence of an hydroxyl group at C-2. Thus, FdG-6P (and dG-6P) are metabolically trapped within the cell. Regional accumulation of FdG radioactivity is therefore proportional to blood glucose, and is a sensitive index of brain function. Regional blood flow and glucose utilization are established markers of local neuronal activity and PET measurement of these parameters has been used to identify regions of the brain that are activated during visual, auditory, and somatic sensations; limb and eye movements; the recognition of spoken and written words; speech; semantic associations, and pathological and normal forms of anxiety. Such parameters are also being used to identify regional brain abnormalities in patients with schizophrenia, panic disorders, epilepsy, Parkinson's and Huntington's diseases, obsessive–compulsive disorder, and clinical depression.

An FdG-PET study in acquired immune deficiency syndrome (AIDS) patients has focused on improving the diagnosis of the AIDS dementia complex (ADC), which is the major neurological outcome of AIDS, resulting in behavioral, cognitive, and motor disturbances (48). This study has shown that progressive development of ADC correlates well with regional rates of cerebral glucose metabolism, particularly in the basal ganglia and thalamus. PET studies have also indicated that patients with Alzheimer's disease exhibit characteristic patterns of cerebral blood flow and glucose utilization; glucose metabolism in such patients is significantly reduced in the posterial parietal temporal region of the brain, compared to control patients (65). PET images of cerebral glucose utilization have also been used to localize the epileptogenic foci in patients with intractable partial epilepsy.

The use of PET with radiolabeled synthetic drugs or radiolabeled analogs of naturally occurring neurotransmitters holds the promise for more reliable diagnoses of neurological disorders, or even presymptomatic diagnosis. N-methyl-[^{18}F]-spiroperidol (NMSP), a neuroleptic drug with high affinity for dopamine-D_2 receptors, has been used to visualize brain receptors in vivo in both normal and schizophrenic patients, and the effectiveness of the anti-Parkinson drug, L-deprenyl, as a monoamine oxidase inhibitor in the brain has been verified from PET studies with carbon-11 labeled L-deprenyl (119).

More recent studies (91,92) have shown that [^{18}F]-4′-fluoroclebopride ([^{18}F]-FCP) is a most promising candidate ligand for studying D_2 receptors with PET, and [^{18}F]-(+)-fluorobenzyltrozamicol ([^{18}F]-(+)-FBT) is a suitable ligand for studying cholinergic terminal density with PET via the vesicular acetylcholine transporter (93). [^{18}F]-FCP has been used recently in PET studies designed to measure synaptic dopamine levels and D_2 receptor numbers in rhesus monkeys after treatment with psychostimulants such as (−)-cocaine, d-amphetamine, methylphenidate, and d-methamphetamine (91). In these studies, psychostimulants caused an increase in the rate of washout of [^{18}F]-FCP from the basal ganglia. d-Methamphetamine and d-amphetamine had the greatest effect on washout kinetics of [^{18}F]-FCP relative to (−)-cocaine and methylphenidate, which was consistent with their ability to elevate synaptic dopamine levels. Thus, challenge studies with [^{18}F]-FCP may be a useful technique for studying the dynamics of interaction between psychostimulant-induced increases in synaptic dopamine and postsynaptic D_2 receptors.

[^{18}F]-FCP and PET analysis have also been utilized in chronic stress studies. Chronic stress results in heightened synaptic dopaminergic levels and a concomitant downregulation of D_2 receptors, analogous to the downregulation of dopaminergic receptors found following chronic cocaine exposure. Experiments with [^{18}F]-FCP in dominant and subordinate cynomologus monkeys showed a clearly greater uptake of the ligand in the basal ganglia by the dominant monkeys (52). The data provide strong evidence that stimuli controlling behavior/physiological consequences (stress) have a neurochemical correlate that can be imaged with PET techniques, and suggest that chronic stress results in heightened synaptic dopaminergic levels and a concomitant downregulation of D_2 receptors. Previous PET studies have found downregulation in dopaminergic receptors in human cocaine addicts (157,158) and alcoholics (61). PET may also be a powerful tool in addressing the etiology of complex behavioral disorders associated with stress.

[^{18}F]-(+)-FBT has high affinity for the vascular acetylcholine transporter and low affinity for σ_1 and σ_2 receptors (93). Its high uptake in the basal ganglia and reversible binding kinetics in vivo indicate that this tracer can provide quantitative measurements of vasicular acetylcholine transporter function in vivo with PET imaging. The vasicular acetylcholine transporter is a marker for cholinergic nerve terminals, and may be directly related to cholinergic neuronal density. An important goal in PET studies is relating cholinergic neuronal density to cognitive performance. Such studies may be able to correlate an individual's change in behavioral performance (i.e., cognition) with a change in (reduction in) cholinergic function.

The major usefulness of PET scanning of the torso is in the diagnostic evaluation of patients with certain disorders of the heart. Modeling metabolic processes in the heart is more complex than in the brain, because the heart draws energy from several substrate pools, such as fatty acids, carbohydrates, and lactate. FdG-PET studies and blood flow [^{13}N]-ammonia-PET measurements have been used to diagnose coronary artery disease with better than 95% accuracy. Other studies have utilized [^{11}C]-palmitate, which is accumulated homogeneously by the heart muscle, to diagnose cardiovascular abnormalities (48).

PET images of glucose utilization and amino acid uptake are now being used to examine patients with a variety of tumors throughout the body. PET images of labeled estradiol uptake are now being used to examine patients with primary and metastatic breast tumors.

PET has become an established technique in diagnostic medicine, and is routinely used for the neuroscientific investigation of normal and pathological human behaviors. The two main obstacles to more general utility of this technique are cost-effectiveness and the availability of appropriate radiotracers. The estimated cost of constructing, equipping, and generating a PET center is in the range of \$6 million to \$7 million (this includes building, PET system, cyclotron, and ancillary equipment), with an operating cost of more than \$1 million per year. The synthesis of novel positron-emitting drug molecules is an ever-challenging process for the radiochemist, requiring innovation and skill.

Nevertheless, PET has advantages over other functional imaging techniques such as single photon emission tomography (SPECT). Unlike magnetic resonance imaging, it has the potential to measure characteristics of biological compounds, such as neurotransmitters and neuroreceptors, that exist in minute concentrations. Improvements in the methodology for determining anatomical localization and data analysis, and the on-going improvement in the performance of PET systems, should ensure that this important analytical tool will continue to offer unique opportunities for medical and basic science researchers to study physiology, biochemistry, pharmacology, and toxicology.

Stable Isotopes

As mentioned above, most elements exist as several isotopes that vary in atomic weight. Some of the heavy isotopes are perfectly stable and do not decay with the emission of radiation. These so-called stable isotopes typically have a low natural abundance and chemical and physical properties that are nearly identical to those of their more abundant counterparts. Carbon exists naturally as a mixture of isotopes, ^{12}C, ^{13}C, and ^{14}C. ^{12}C is the most abundant isotope of carbon (98.89%), ^{13}C, the stable isotope of carbon, is much less abundant (1.11%), and ^{14}C is a radioisotope of carbon with a natural abundance so low as to be insignificant (except for its special application for carbon dating). Hydrogen also exists as a mixture of isotopes, ^{1}H, ^{2}H, and ^{3}H. ^{1}H (protium) is the most abundant isotope of hydrogen (99.985%), ^{2}H (deuterium), the stable isotope of hydrogen, is much less abundant (0.015%), and ^{3}H (tritium) is a radioactive isotope of hydrogen with insignificant natural abundance. Other stable isotopes which are useful for toxicology research are ^{15}N (0.37%), ^{17}O (0.037%), and ^{18}O (0.204%). A wide variety of chemicals specifically labeled with ^{2}H, ^{13}C, ^{15}N, ^{17}O, and ^{18}O at high atom-% enrichments are commercially available.

Stable isotopes with low natural abundance make ideal tracers for studying mechanisms of toxicology. Because they are stable, they pose no significant health risk to the researcher or the experimental subject. No special license is required for the acquisition and use of stable isotopes and no special precautions are necessary for their safe handling (other than the normal precautions used for handling the unlabeled compound). Because their chemical and physical properties are very similar to those of the more abundant isotope, their behavior in vivo is also quite similar. Compounds enriched in a stable isotope can be studied in the presence of natural abundance compounds with minimal background interference. A wealth of mechanistic information is available from stable isotope studies through the application of modern magnetic resonance and mass spectral techniques.

Choice and Location of Label

The stable isotope of choice for a toxicology study depends on the nature of the study (ADME, exposure assessment, mechanism of toxicity) and the instrumental method to be used for analysis. The most common stable isotopes for toxicology research are ^{13}C, ^{2}H, ^{15}N, and ^{18}O. Stable isotopes of heavy metals such as ^{199}Hg and ^{206}Pb have been used to study mechanisms of toxicity and clearance.

If NMR is used for analysis, it is best to use a spin 1/2 isotope for maximum sensitivity. For ^{13}C NMR analysis, uniform labeling offers distinct advantages in terms of metabolite characterization, as is discussed further below. For mass spectral analyses, the stable isotope that will give the greatest mass difference between natural abundance and labeled analytes is appropriate. Multiple sites of labeling are quite common and provide greater mass discrimination. If GC/MS is used, the optimum mass difference is 2–4u. A greater mass difference can lead to altered retention times and introduce uncertainty in quantitative analysis. Unlike radioisotopes where enrichments are quite low, stable isotopic enrichments are typically high, at least 90 atom-%. In general, the factors that govern the position of a radioisotopic label (stability and exchangeability) also govern the position of a stable isotopic label.

Applications

Pharmacokinetics of Isotopically Labeled Nicotine

Due to the widespread use of tobacco products, the pharmacokinetics of nicotine and its metabolites have been the subject of much study. Early studies focused on nicotine and its major metabolites cotinine and nicotine-1′-oxide. Recently, Kyerematen et al. (80) reported a pharmacokinetic study of nicotine and 12 of its metabolites in the rat. They administered ^{14}C-labeled nicotine in single intra-arterial doses of 0.1, 0.5, and 1.0 mg/kg and collected blood up to 30 h and urine up to 120 h. The authors were able to quantify nicotine and 12 of its metabolites by HPLC with radiometric detection. One of the longest-lived metabolites was previously unidentified so it was collected from the HPLC and further analyzed by EI mass spectrometry. This metabolite was identified as allohydroxydemethylcotinine. Plasma nicotine half-life, total body clearance, and apparent volume of distribution and half-lives of urinary excretion of cotinine, cotinine-N-oxide, and allohydroxydemethylcotinine were all determined. The use of radiolabeled nicotine enabled the convenient determination of nicotine and 12 of its metabolites with high sensitivity, demonstrating the power of this method for the study of nicotine pharmacokinetics.

In a further study of nicotine pharmacokinetics, Kyerematen et al. (79) determined the disposition of radiolabeled nicotine and eight of its metabolites in humans. The use of radiolabeled nicotine enabled detection of plasma and urinary nicotine and metabolites from a very low dose (190 μg per subject) so that a comparison of smokers and nonsmokers was possible. In this study, two new urinary metabolites, 3′-hydroxycotinine glucuronide and demethylcotinine $\Delta^{2',3'}$-enamine, were identified by mass spectral analyses.

Stable isotope labeling has also been applied successfully to the study of nicotine pharmacokinetics and bioavailability in humans (10). This study took advantage of the ability to distinguish labeled from unlabeled nicotine by GC/MS. After smoking a cigarette, smokers were administered nicotine labeled with deuterium in both 3′ positions (previously shown to be stable to metabolism). Plasma levels of both labeled and unlabeled nicotine were monitored by GC/MS with selected ion monitoring. The pharmacokinetic data obtained with this stable isotope method were of very high quality due to the sensitivity of the analytical method and the specificity of the labeled nicotine that eliminated background interference from unlabeled nicotine.

Characterization of Urinary Metabolites by ^{13}C NMR

Detection of ^{13}C resonances of natural abundance xenobiotic metabolites in a complex matrix such as urine is often very difficult due to interfering resonances of endogenous compounds. Appropriate use of ^{13}C-enriched xenobiotics can facilitate the characterization of metabolites in whole urine by ^{13}C NMR spectroscopy with little or no sample cleanup.

Sumner et al. (148) have studied the metabolism of [1,2,3-^{13}C]acrylamide in rats and mice using 1D and 2D ^{13}C NMR spectroscopic analysis of urine. Animals were administered the labeled xenobiotic at a dose of 50 mg/kg orally. Urine was collected for 24 h and centrifuged, then D_2O was added so that the final concentration was approximately 15 percent. INADEQUATE spectra were used to correlate all carbon signals and HET2DJ spectra revealed the number of protons attached to each carbon for all metabolites. These spectral data, along with calculated chemical shifts of proposed metabolites and spectra of synthetic standards, were used to identify five urinary metabolites of acrylamide. Quantification of the urinary output of acrylamide and the five metabolites was accomplished by integration of the carbons signals in 1D spectra relative to dioxane which was added as an internal standard. Approximately 50% of the administered dose of acrylamide was recovered as the five metabolites. This agrees well with a previous study that showed 62% of the administered dose of ^{14}C labeled acrylamide was recovered in urine within 24 h. This study clearly demonstrates the power of stable isotope labeling and ^{13}C NMR analysis for the study of xenobiotic metabolism. These methods enabled the characterization and quantification of metabolites in a complex matrix without thc need for tedious sample cleanup and chromatographic separation.

Determination of Toxic Metals Using Stable Isotope Dilution Mass Spectrometry

Use of stable isotopes is widely applied to elemental mass spectrometry studies of toxic elements. An excellent example is the study of detoxification of lead in humans. Smith et al. (141,142) have used stable lead isotopes to study the effectiveness of a chelating agent (DMSA) in removing lead from skeletal versus soft tissue and the redistribution of lead in other tissues. Lead has four naturally occurring isotopes: ^{204}Pb (1.4%), ^{206}Pb (24.1%), ^{207}Pb (22.1%), and ^{208}Pb (52.4%). By enriching drinking water given to rats in ^{206}Pb, the lead dose was distinguishable from the endogenous lead present in the animals. The mass spectrometer in this case used thermal emission to produce ions and measure the isotopic ratios that in turn reflected the ^{206}Pb dose.

Cadmium is another highly toxic metal, and environmental and industrial exposure are of great concern. In contrast to the previous thermal emission mass spectrometric method for lead determination, Aggarwal et al. (1) have developed a method for cadmium exposure that uses stable isotope dilution gas chromatography/mass spectrometry. This method determined cadmium in urine by using the chelating agent lithium bis-(trifluoroethyl)dithiocarbamate, Li(FDEDTC), to form the chelate $Cd(FDEDTC)_2$ which was analyzed by

GC/MS with EI ionization. $M^{+\cdot}$ was monitored for quantitation. Cd determination in urine was possible with this method at the 10-mg/L level with good precision and accuracy. The researchers note that the isotope dilution technique provided freedom from matrix effects so that precision and accuracy were not affected by incomplete recovery.

INTEGRATION OF TECHNIQUES IN TOXICOLOGY

The mechanism of toxicity of a xenobiotic is usually complex, involving not only the parent compound but also a broad array of metabolites and tissue-derived endogenous compounds. All these materials are produced in a dynamic process as the intoxicated organism responds to the toxic insult and attempts to maintain homeostasis. Modern instrumental methods are powerful tools that have their greatest utility when they are used in conjunction with one another in a synergistic fashion to characterize materials in complex mixtures. There are numerous examples in the literature of the use of multiple instrumental techniques to describe a variety of different chemical entities in complex mixtures. However, one study has merit as the example for this section because many of the techniques described in this chapter were used to confirm the identity of many compounds.

Wiltshire et al. (167) used diode-array ultraviolet spectrophotometry, mass spectrometry, NMR, radiolabeled tracers, open column chromatography, HPLC, and TLC to characterize the complex metabolic pathway of a calcium antagonist (Ro 40-5967) in the rat (Figure 36.36). A classic xenobiotic disposition study was conducted using Ro 40-5967 labeled with ^{14}C. Approximately 80% of the radiolabeled dose was recovered in all excreta including bile, urine, and feces. Thirty-seven percent of the dose was excreted in the bile so chemical characterization of the biliary radioactivity was carried out.

Bile was partially purified by passing through an open column of Amberlite XAD-2 resin. The fractions collected from the open column were evaporated to dryness and partitioned between ethyl acetate and water. Two of the fractions contained an insoluble gum that was taken up in ethanol. All fractions (aqueous and organic) were taken to dryness and then dissolved in aqueous methanol. These fractions were subjected to three sequential reverse phase HPLC purification steps to obtain material that was suitable for further characterization. It was readily apparent that there were a large number of radiolabeled metabolites with similar chromatographic properties. However, the compounds could be divided into six classes by diode-array UV spectrophotometry. The UV spectra were characteristic of major changes in the parent compound. For example, a λ_{max} at 280 nm is typical of oxygen substitution at

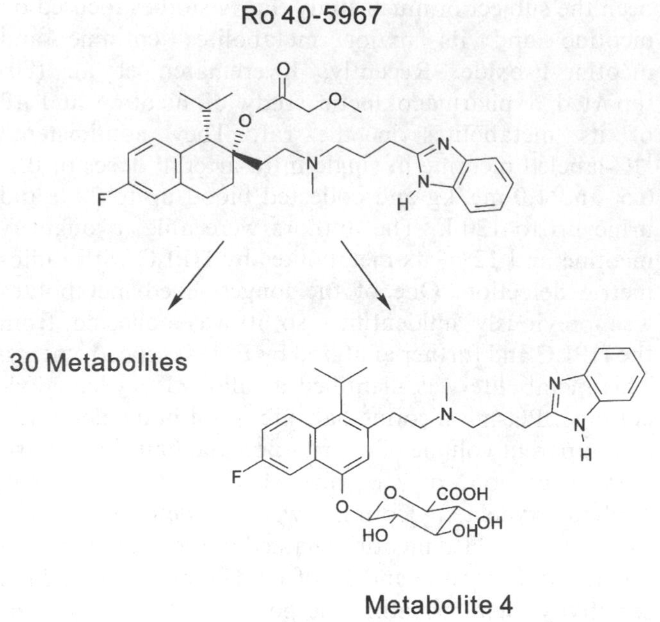

FIG. 36.36. Metabolism of the calcium antagonist Ro 40-5967 in the rat. Characterization of Metabolite 4 exemplifies the integration of modern instrumental techniques to study mechanisms of toxicology.

the 5 position of the parent compound. It was obvious that approximately four of the metabolites fell in this class.

Further characterization of the metabolites required NMR and mass spectrometry. Sufficient material from the HPLC purification was obtained from 11 of the XAD fractions. This represented approximately two-thirds of the radioactivity excreted in bile. The proton NMR spectrum of the parent compound possessed a number of characteristic features and it was possible to see similar features in the spectra of the fractions. A number of the metabolite fractions contained resonances characteristic of glucuronic acid conjugation.

Mass spectra were obtained from 45 subfractions of the original XAD fractions by thermospray LC–MS. As with the proton NMR spectra, features in the mass spectra were characteristic of the parent compound. For example, m/z 406 was characteristic of the loss of the side chain.

Rather than discussing the entire characterization which involved the description of 31 metabolites, it is instructive to describe the characterization of just one of the metabolites. Metabolite 4 was the major biliary metabolite and equivalent to about 25% of the total biliary radioactivity. It had a class 3 UV spectrum, indicating the presence of a substituted naphthyl group. Remember that the parent compound contains a tetrahydronaphthyl ring system where one of the rings of naphthylene is saturated. The very strong double peak at 240–250 nm is characteristic of a fully aromatic substituted naphthylene.

The proton NMR spectrum of this metabolite showed the presence of glucuronic acid as well as loss of the ester side chain. Evidence that the asymmetric center of the isopropyl side chain had been lost was obtained from a shift in the methyl resonances of the isopropyl group. Aromatization of the saturated ring was obvious by the addition of an aromatic singlet at 7.1 ppm. The metabolite structure was deduced to be an oxyglucuronide derivative of the parent compound in which the alicyclic ring had been aromatized. This was consistent with a mass spectrum containing a protonated molecular ion at $m/z = 596$, loss of the benzimidazole group ($m/z = 438$), and loss of glucuronic acid ($m/z = 262$).

The application of these instrumental techniques permitted a thorough characterization of metabolites that varied greatly in chemical structure and polarity. A total of 31 biliary metabolites, representing 67% of the excreted dose of Ro 40-5967, were characterized. Only through the integration of modern instrumental methods could this complex metabolic pathway be thoroughly elucidated.

QUESTIONS

1. Name two ways that mass spectrometry has been used to assess exposure to xenobiotics.

   Mass spectrometry has been used to determine metabolites of xenobiotics in biological fluids and to determine DNA adducts formed as a result of exposure.

2. An unknown compound in an organic extract of urine is sufficiently volatile to pass through a GC–MS system but fragments extensively under EI so that no $M^{+\cdot}$ is observed. Name at least two alternative approaches to determine the molecular weight of this compound using mass spectrometry.

   a. A GC–MS system with PICI could be used to form $(M+H)^+$.
   b. An HPLC method could be developed and the material analyzed by LC–MS, using a soft ionization method such as ES or APCI.
   c. If the compound contained a hydroxyl or amine group, derivatization with a common trimethylsilation reagent could form a compound with a more stable molecular ion.

3. An LC–MS method with an ES ionization source runs a binary gradient with mobile phase 1 = 2 mM ammonium acetate and mobile phase 2 = 90% methanol : 10% acetonitrile. There is a large background ion in the system at m/z 59. CID on this ion produces a fragment at m/z 42. What are likely assignments for these ions?

   m/z 42 is protonated acetonitrile. The mass difference of 17 Da (59-42) suggests ammonia, NH_3, as a neutral loss. Thus, m/z 59 is likely an ammonium adduct of acetonitrile, $(CH_3CN)(NH_4)^+$, produced from background mobile phase components.

4. EI mass spectrometers have several ions constantly present in the background mass spectrum at m/z 18, 28, 32, 40, and 44. Identify these components.

   These are all components of air with moisture present: m/z 18 = H_2O, m/z 28 = N_2, m/z 32 = O_2, m/z 40 = Ar, and m/z 44 = CO_2.

5. Using positive ES, a large protein is ionized under acidic conditions that create an $(M+4H)^{4+}$ ion in the mass spectrum at m/z 712.2. What is the molecular weight of this compound?

   Remember that four protons have been attached to this molecule so that: $m/z = 712.2 = (M+4H)/4$, $\rightarrow M = (712.2 \times 4) - 4$; $M = 2844.8$ Da.

6. $CDCl_3$ is a commonly used NMR solvent. Carbon NMR spectra of samples dissolved in $CDCl_3$ contain a residual solvent peak which is split due to ^{13}C-^{2}H coupling.

   a. Into how many lines is this signal split?

   ^{2}H has a spin quantum number (I) of 1. Applying the $2nI+1$ rule, the number of lines is $(2 \times 1 \times 1) + 1 = 3$.

   b. In most cases, carbon spectra are acquired with hydrogen decoupling. Why isn't the ^{13}C-^{2}H multiplet reduced to a singlet under the conditions of this decoupling?

   Decoupling is applied at the ^{1}H (protium) frequency. Deuterium (^{2}H) has a very different precessional frequency, therefore, it is not decoupled in the carbon NMR spectrum.

7. Why is ^{13}C-^{13}C coupling rarely seen in carbon NMR spectra?

   Coupling is only seen for closely spaced nuclei (<four–five bonds). To see ^{13}C-^{13}C coupling, two ^{13}C atoms would need to be in close proximity. The natural abundance of ^{13}C is only 1% so the likelihood of two ^{13}C nuclei being in close proximity is very low. Carbon spectra of molecules composed of natural abundance carbon do not show ^{13}C-^{13}C coupling. ^{13}C-^{13}C coupling is only seen with isotopically enriched molecules.

8. Sensitivity in NMR depends on what factors?

    a. Magnetic field strength
    b. Magnetogyric ratio
    c. Natural abundance of the spin-active nucleus

9. Describe three approaches for increasing sensitivity for a given nucleus in NMR?

    a. Using a higher-field-strength instrument (magnet)
    b. Using a smaller NMR probe and/or a selectively tuned probe
    c. Signal averaging (FT–NMR)

10. Why are chemical shifts expressed in dimensionless units designated δ?

    Chemical shifts vary with the strength of the applied magnetic field. To enable comparisons of chemical shifts from one instrument to the next, chemical shifts are expressed in δ units.

11. What factors limit time resolution in on-line LC–NMR?

    a. HPLC mobile phase flow rate
    b. Total time required to obtain one transient (scan)
    c. Total number of transients acquired per LC peak

12. Why is EPR inherently more sensitive than NMR?

    The magnetic moment of an electron is 700 times greater than that of a proton. This means that the energy difference between spin states is greater for electrons than for protons. This greater energy difference leads to higher sensitivity. It also means that the energy required for an EPR transition is higher than that required for a NMR transition. NMR uses energy in the radiofrequency range; EPR uses energy in the microwave range.

13. The EPR spectrum of the Fe–DETC complex with ^{15}NO shows doublet hyperfine splitting.

    a. Why?

    ^{15}N has a spin quantum number (I) of $\frac{1}{2}$. Applying the $2nI+1$ rule, ($n=1$, $I=\frac{1}{2}$) the number of lines is 2 (doublet).

    b. How was this used to distinguish between NO produced from ^{15}N-labeled arginine and NO produced from endogenous arginine?

    ^{14}N has a spin quantum number of 1, therefore, it splits electron signals into 3 lines (triplet hyperfine splitting). Endogenously formed NO is derived from natural abundance arginine. Natural abundance nitrogen is 99.6% ^{14}N so it leads to triplet hyperfine splitting. Any doublet splitting results from NO produced from added ^{15}N-labeled arginine.

14. Quantitative whole-body autoradiography is becoming a very popular method for determining xenobiotic tissue distribution.

    a. What is the major limitation of this technique?

    QWBA is used to determine total radioactivity. It cannot distinguish between different chemical forms of radioactivity. In other words, it cannot distinguish between xenobiotic metabolites. It determines the sum of parent compound plus metabolites and, therefore, yields no information on xenobiotic metabolism.

    b. In practice, how can this limitation be overcome?

    To overcome this limitation, follow-up studies must be performed. QWBA is used to determine the distribution of a xenobiotic. QWBA data reveal the tissues containing xenobiotic-derived radioactivity. The follow-up studies involve administration of the xenobiotic (radiolabeled or natural abundance) and isolation of tissues containing the parent xenobiotic and its metabolites. Extraction of these tissues provides solutions that can be analyzed for metabolites by suitable separation techniques like LC–MS or LC–NMR.

REFERENCES

1. Aggarwal, S. K., Orth, R. G., Wendling, J., Kinter, M., and Herold, D. A. (1993): Isotope dilution gas chromatography/mass spectrometry for cadmium determination in urine. *J. Anal. Toxicol.*, 17:5–10.
2. Alben, J. O., and Fiamingo, F. G. (1984): Fourier transform infrared spectroscopy. In: *Optical Techniques in Biological Research*, edited by D. L. Rousseau, pp. 133–179. Academic Press Inc., New York.
3. Alger, R. S. (1968): *Electron Paramagnetic Resonance, Techniquès and Applications*. Wiley-Interscience, New York.
4. Assenheim, H. M. (1967): *Introduction to Electron Spin Resonance*. Plenum Press, New York.
5. Aust, S. D., Chignell, C. F., Bray, T. M., Kalyanaraman, B., and Mason, R. P. (1993): Contemporary issues in toxicology: Free radicals in toxicology. *Toxicol. Appl. Pharmacol.*, 120:168–178.
6. Barker, J., and Garner, R. C. (1999): Biomedical applications of accelerator mass spectrometry-isotope dilution measurements at the level of the atom. *Rapid Commun. Mass Spectrom.*, 13:285–293.
7. Baudouin, C. J., Bryant, D. J., Collins, A. G., Goutts, G. C., Cox, I. J., Hajnial, J. V., Menon, D. K., Page, D. R., and Young, I. R. (1990): Aspects of chemical shift imaging which illustrate the cross-fertilization of methods and techniques in in vivo NMR imaging and spectroscopy. *Phil. Trans. R. Soc. Lond.*, 333:545–559.
8. Bellar, T. A., Behymer, T. D., and Budde, W. L. (1990): Investigation of enhanced ion abundances from a carrier process in high-performance liquid chromatography particle beam mass spectrometry. *J. Am. Soc. Mass Spectrom.*, 1:92–98.
9. Benedetti, E., Teodori, L., Trinca, M.L., Verhamini, P., Salvati, F., Mauro, F., and Spremolla, G. (1990): A new approach to the study

of human solid tumor cells by means of FT–IR microspectroscopy. *Appl. Spectrosc.*, 44:1276–1281.

10. Benowitz, N. L., Jacob, P. III, Denaro, C., and Jenkins, R. (1991): Stable isotope studies of nicotine kinetics and bioavailability. *Clin. Pharmacol. Ther.*, 49:270–277.
11. Bernert, J. T. Jr., Turner, W. E., Pirkle, J. L., Sosnoff, C. S., Adkins, J. R., Waldrep, M. K., Ann, Q., Covey, T. R., Whitfield, W. E., Gunter, E. W., Miller, B. B., Patterson, D. G. Jr., Needham, L. L., Hannon, W. H., and Sampson, E. J. (1997): Development and validation of sensitive method for determination of serum cotinine in smokers and nonsmokers by liquid chromatography/atmospheric pressure ionization tandem mass spectrometry. *Clin. Chem.*, 43:2281–2291.
12. Blakely, C. R., Carmody, J. J., and Vestal, M. L. (1980): A new liquid chromatograph/mass spectrometer interface using crossed-beam techniques. *Adv. Mass Spectrom.*, 8B:1616–1623.
13. Brackett, D. J., Wallis, G., Wilson, M. F., and McCay, P. B. (1998): Spin trapping and electron paramagnetic resonance spectroscopy. *Methods Mol. Biol.*, 108:15–25.
14. Burton, K. I., Everett, J. R., Newman, M. J., Pullen, F. S., Richards, D. S., and Swanson, A. G. (1997): Online liquid chromatography coupled with high field NMR and mass spectrometry (LC–NMR–MS): A new technique for drug metabolite structure elucidation. *J. Pharm. Biomed. Anal.*, 15:1903–1912.
15. Busch, K. L., Glish, G. L., and McLuckey, S. A. (1988): *Mass Spectrometry/Mass Spectrometry: Techniques and Applications of Tandem Mass Spectrometry*. VCH Publishers, Inc., New York.
16. Byrd, G. D. (1996): LC–MS/MS method for profiling nicotine and its metabolites in biological fluids. *44th Annual Conference on Mass Spectrometry and Allied Topics*, Portland, Oregon, May 12–16.
17. Byrd, G. D., Chang, K. M., Greene, J. M., and deBethizy, J. D. (1992): Evidence for urinary excretion of glucuronide conjugates of nicotine, cotinine, and trans-3′-hydroxycotinine in smokers. *Drug Metabol. Dispos.*, 20:192–197.
18. Byrd, G. D., Davis, R. A., Caldwell, W. S., Robinson, J. H., and deBethizy, J. D. (1998): A further study of FTC yield and nicotine absorption in smokers. *Psychopharmacology*, 139:291–299.
19. Byrd, G. D., Robinson, J. H., Caldwell, W. S., and deBethizy, J. D. (1995): Comparison of measured and FTC-predicted nicotine uptake in smokers. *Psychopharmacology*, 122:95–103.
20. Byrd, G. D., Uhrig, M. S., deBethizy, J. D., Caldwell, W. S., Crooks, P. A., Ravard, A., and Riggs, R. M. (1994): Direct determination of cotinine-N-glucuronide in urine using thermospray liquid chromatography/mass spectrometry. *Biol. Mass Spectrom.*, 23:103–107.
21. Caldwell, W. S., Greene, J. M., Byrd, G. D., Chang, K. M., Uhrig, M. S., deBithizy, J. D., Crooks, P. A., Bhatti, B. S., and Riggs, R. M. (1992): Characterization of the glucuronide conjugate of cotinine: A previously unidentified major metabolite of nicotine in smokers' urine. *Chem. Res. Toxicol.*, 5:280–285.
22. Cammack, R., and Shergill, J. K. (1998): Biomedical applications of EPR spectroscopy. In: *Modern Applications of EPR/ESR, From Biophysics to Material Science. Proceedings of the First Asia-Pacific EPR/ESR Symposium*, edited by C. Z. Rudowicz, P. K. N. Yu, and H. Hiraoka, pp. 66–73. Springer–Verlag, Singapore.
23. Cammack, R., Shergill, J. K., Inalsingh, V. A., and Hughes, M. N. (1998): Applications of electron paramagnetic resonance spectroscopy to study interactions of iron proteins in cells with nitric oxide. *Spectrochimica Acta, Part A*, 54:2393–2402.
24. Cappiello, A. (1996): Is particle beam an up-to-the-date LC–MS interface? *Mass Spectrom. Rev.*, 15:283–296.
25. Caprioli, R. M. (1990): Continuous-flow fast atom bombardment mass spectrometry. *Anal. Chem.*, 62:477A–485A.
26. Carey, P. R. (1982): *Biochemical Applications of Raman and Resonance Raman Spectroscopies*. Academic Press, New York.
27. Carney, J. M., Landrum, W., Mayes, L., Zou, Y., and Lodder, R. A. (1993): Near-IR spectrophotometric monitoring of stroke-related changes in the protein and lipid composition of whole gerbil brains. *Anal. Chem.*, 65:1305–1313.
28. Carroll, D. I., Dzidic, I., Horning, E. C., and Stillwell, R. N. (1981): Atmospheric pressure ionization mass spectrometry. *Appl. Spectrosc. Rev.*, 17:337–406.
29. Cassis, L. A., and Lodder, R. A. (1993): Near-IR imaging of atheromas in living arterial tissue. *Anal. Chem.*, 65:1247–1256.
30. Charles, M. J., and Glish, G. L. (1995): Review of modern ion trap research. In: *Practical Aspects of Ion Trap Mass Spectrometry, Vol. III*, edited by R. E. March and J. F. J. Todd, pp. 89–118. CRC Press, Boca Raton, FL.
31. Chen, M. C., and Lord, R. C. (1976): Laser Raman spectroscopic studies of the thermal unfolding of ribonuclease A. *Biochemistry*, 15:1889–1897.
32. Colby, B. N., Ryan, P. W., and Wilkinson, J. E. (1983): Strategies for compound identification and quantification using fused silica capillary column GC/MS. *J. High Resolut. Chromatogr. Chromatogr. Commun.*, 6:72–76.
33. Comisarow, M. B., and Marshall, A. G. (1996): The early development of Fourier transformation cyclotron resonance (FT-ICR) spectroscopy. *J. Mass Spectrom.*, 6:581–585.
34. Constantinidis, I., Braunschweiger, P. G., Wehrle, J. P., Kumar, M., Johnson, C. S., Furmanski, P., and Glickson, J. D. (1989): ^{31}P-Nuclear magnetic resonance studies of the effect of recombinant human interleukin 1α on the bioenergetics of RIF-1 tumors. *Cancer Res.*, 49:6379–6382.
35. Cooks, R. G., Hole, S. H. II, Morand, K. L., and Lammert, S. A. (1992): Mass spectrometers: Instrumentation. *Int. J. Mass Spectrom. Ion Proc.*, 118/119:1–36.
36. Cooper, D. A., and Moore, J. M. (1993): Femtogram on-column detection of nicotine by isotope dilution gas chromatography/negative ion detection mass spectrometry. *Biol. Mass Spectrom.*, 22:590–559ff594.
37. Corcoran, O., Spraul, M., Hofmann, M., Ismail, I. M., Lindon, J. C., and Nicholson, J. K. (1997): 750 MHz HPLC–NMR spectroscopic identification of rat microsomal metabolites of phenoxypyridines. *J. Pharm. Biomed. Anal.*, 16:481–489.
38. Crouch, R. C., and Martin, G. E. (1992): Micro inverse-detection: A powerful technique for natural product structure elucidation. *J. Nat. Prod.*, 55:1343–1347.
39. Davidson, A. G. (1988): Ultraviolet and visible absorption spectroscopy. In: *Practical Pharmaceutical Chemistry, 4th edition, Part Two*, edited by A. H. Beckett and J. B. Stanlake, pp. 275–337. The Athlone Press, London.
40. Dear, G. J., Ayrton, J., Plumb, R., Sweatman, B. C., Ismail, I. M., Fraser, I. J., and Mutch, P. J. (1998): A rapid and efficient approach to metabolite identification using nuclear magnetic resonance spectroscopy, liquid chromatography/mass spectrometry and liquid chromatography/nuclear magnetic resonance spectroscopy/sequential mass spectrometry. *Rapid Commum. Mass Spectrom.*, 12:2023–2030.
41. deBethizy, J. D., Udinsky, J. R., Scribner, H. E., and Frederick, C. B. (1987): The disposition and metabolism of acrylic acid and ethyl acrylate in male Sprague-Dawley rats. *Fund. Appl. Toxicol.*, 8:549–561.
42. DeBruin, L. S., Pawliszyn, J. B., and Josephy, P. D. (1999): Detection of monocyclic aromatic amines, possible mammary carcinogens, in human milk. *Chem. Res. Toxicol.*, 12:78–82.
43. DeBruin, L. S., Josephy, P. D., and Pawliszyn, J. B. (1998): Solid-phase microextraction of monocyclic aromatic amines from biological fluids. *Anal. Chem.*, 70:1986–1992.

44. Derome, A. E. (1987): *Modern NMR Techniques for Chemistry Research*. Pergamon Press, Oxford.
45. Doyle, T. D., and Fazzari, F. R. (1974): Determination of drugs in dosage forms by difference spectrophotometry. *J. Pharm. Sci.*, 63:1921–1926.
46. Dybowski, C., and Lichter, R. L., eds. (1987): *NMR Spectroscopy Techniques*. Marcel Dekker, New York.
47. Dyer, J. R. (1965): *Applications of Absorption Spectroscopy of Organic Compounds*. Prentice-Hall, Englewood Cliffs, New Jersey.
48. Feliu, A. L. (1988): The role of chemistry in positron emission tomography. *J. Chem. Educat.*, 65:655–660.
49. Fulton, D. B., Sayer, B. G., Bain, A. D., and Malle, H. V. (1992): Detection and determination of dilute, low molecular weight organic compounds in water by 500-MHz proton nuclear magnetic resonance spectroscopy. *Anal. Chem.*, 64:349–353.
50. Garner, R. C. (1998): The role of DNA adducts in chemical carcinogenesis. *Mut. Res.*, 402:67–75.
51. Gordon, A. J., and Ford, R. A. (1972): *The Chemist's Companion: A Handbook of Practical Data, Techniques, and References*. John Wiley & Sons, New York.
52. Grant, A. G., Shively, C. A., Nader, M. A., Ehrenkaufer, R. L., Line, S. W., Morton, T. E., Gage, H. D., and Mach, R. H. (1998): Effect of social status on striatal dopamine D_2 receptor binding characteristics in cynomolgus monkeys assessed with positron emission tomography. *Synapse*, 29:80–83.
53. Greitz, T., Ingvar, D. H., and Widen, L., eds. (1985): *Metabolism of the Human Brain Studied with Positron Emission Tomography*. Raven Press, New York.
54. Griffiths, P. R., and DeHaseth, J. A. (1986): *Fourier Transform Infrared Spectroscopy*. Wiley Interscience, New York.
55. Hackett, A. G., Kotyk, J. J., Fujiwara, H., and Logusch, E. W. (1990): Identification of a unique glutathione conjugate of trichloroacrolein using heteronuclear multiple quantum coherence ^{13}C nuclear magnetic resonance spectroscopy. *J. Am. Chem. Soc.*, 112:3669–3671.
56. Hackett, A. G., Kotyk, J. J., Fujiwara, H., and Logusch, E. W. (1991): Microsomal hydroxylation of triallate: Identification of a 2-chloroacrylate glutathione conjugate using heteronuclear multiple quantum coherence NMR spectroscopy. *Drug Metab. Dispos.*, 19:1163–1165.
57. Halliwell, B., and Gutteridge, J. M. C. (1985): *Free Radicals in Biology and Medicine*. Clarendon Press, Oxford.
58. Haufler, R. E., and Kerley, E. L. (1997): Miniaturized time of flight mass spectrometer for high-speed applications. *45th Annual Conference on Mass Spectrometry and Allied Topics*, Palm Springs, CA, June 1–5.
59. Herman, J. L., and Chay, S. H. (1998): Quantitative whole-body autoradiography in pregnant rabbits to determine fetal exposure of potential teratogenic compounds. *J. Pharmacol. Toxicol. Methods*, 39:29–33.
60. Heumann, K. G. (1987): Trace determination and isotopic analysis of the elements in life sciences by mass spectrometry. *Biomed. Mass Spectrom.*, 12:477–488.
61. Hietala, J., West, C., Syvalahti, E., Nagren, K., Lehikoinen, P., Sonninen, P., and Ruotsalainen, U. (1994): Striatal D_2 dopamine receptor binding characteristics in vivo in patients with alcohol dependence. *Psychopharmacology*, 116:285–290.
62. Holt, R. M., Newman, M. J., Pullen, F. S., Richards, D. S., and Swanson, A. G. (1997): High-performance liquid chromatography/NMR spectrometry/mass spectrometry: Further advances in hyphenated technology. *J. Mass Spectrom.*, 32:64–70.
63. Hore, P. J. (1989): Solvent suppression. In: *Methods in Enzymology, Vol. 176*, edited by N. J. Oppenheimer and T. L. James, pp. 64–77. Academic Press, New York.
64. Jacob, S., Abdel-Aziz, A. H., Shouman, S. A., and Ahmed, A. E. (1998): Effect of glutathione modulation on the distribution and transplacental uptake of 2-[^{14}C]-chloroacetonitrile (CAN) quantitative whole-body autoradiographic study in pregnant mice. *Toxicol. Ind. Health*, 14:533–546.
65. Johnson, K. A., Holman, L., Rosen, T. J., Nagel, J. S., English, R. J., and Growdon, J. H. (1990): Iofetame I-123 single photon emission computed tomography is accurate in the diagnosis of Alzheimer's disease. *Arch. Intern. Med.*, 150:752–756.
66. Johnstone, R. A. W., and Rose, M. E. (1996): *Mass Spectrometry for Chemists and Biochemists, 2nd ed.* Cambridge University Press, Cambridge.
67. Jones, J. R., ed. (1988): *Isotopes: Essential Chemistry and Applications II*. Royal Society of Chemistry, London.
68. Kalasinsky, V. F. (1996): Biomedical applications of infrared and Raman microscopy. *Appl. Spectrosc. Rev.*, 31:193–249.
69. Kaufmann, R. (1995): Matrix-assisted laser desorption ionization (MALDI) mass spectrometry: A novel analytical tool in molecular biology and biotechnology. *J. Biotechnol.*, 41:155–175.
70. Kebarle, P., and Liang, T. (1993): From ions in solution to ions in the gas phase. *Anal. Chem.*, 65:972A–986A.
71. Kemp, W. (1991): Nuclear magnetic resonance spectroscopy. In: *Organic Spectroscopy*, pp. 101–241. W. H. Freeman, New York.
72. Kennedy, C. H., Hatch, G. E., Slade, R., and Mason, R. P. (1992): Application of the EPR spin-trapping technique to the detection of radicals produced in vivo during inhalation exposure of rats to ozone. *Toxicol. Appl. Pharmacol.*, 114:41–46.
73. Kubrina, L. N., Caldwell, W. S., Mordvintcev, P. I., Malenkova, I. V., and Vanin, A. F. (1992): EPR evidence for nitric oxide production from guanidino nitrogens of L-arginine in animal tissues in vivo. *Biochim. et Biophys. Acta*, 1099:233–237.
74. Kuhr, W. G. (1990): Capillary electrophoresis. *Anal. Chem.*, 62:403R–414R.
75. Kuntzman, R. (1981): Applications of tracer techniques in drug metabolism studies. In: *Fundamentals of Drug Metabolism and Drug Disposition*, edited by B. N. La Du, H. G. Mandel, and E. L. Way, pp. 489–504. Robert E. Krieger Publishing Co., Malabar, FL.
76. Kuppusamy, P., Wang, P., Chzhan, M., and Zweier, J. L. (1997): High resolution electron paramagnetic resonance imaging of biological samples with a single line paramagnetic label. *Magn. Reson. Med.*, 37:479–483.
77. Kuppusamy, P., Shankar, R. A., and Zweier, J. L. (1998): In vivo measurement of arterial and venous oxygenation in the rat using 3D spectral-spatial electron paramagnetic resonance imaging. *Phys. Med. Biol.*, 43:1837–1844.
78. Kuppusamy, P., Afeworki, M., Shankar, R. A., Coffin, D., Krishna, M. C., Hahn, S. M., Mitchell, J. B., and Zweier, J. L. (1998): In vivo electron paramagnetic resonance imaging of tumor heterogeneity and oxygenation in a murine model. *Cancer Res.*, 58:1562–1568.
79. Kyerematen, G. A., Morgan, M. L., Chattopadhyay, B., deBethizy, J. D., and Vesell, E. S. (1990): Disposition of nicotine and eight metabolites in smokers and nonsmokers: Identification in smokers of two metabolites that are longer lived than cotinine. *Clin. Pharmacol. Ther.*, 48:641–651.
80. Kyerematen, G. A., Taylor, L. H., deBethizy, J. D., and Vesell, E. S. (1988): Pharmacokinetics of nicotine and 12 metabolites in the rat. Application of a new radiometric high performance liquid chromatography assay. *Drug Metab. Dispos.*, 16:125–129.
81. Lafleur, L., Rice, J., and Thomas, G. J. (1972): Raman studies of nucleic acids. VII. Poly A · poly U and poly G · poly C. *Biopolymers*, 11:2423–2437.

82. Lawson, E. E., Barry, B. W., Williams, A. C., and Edwards, H. G. M. (1997): Biomedical applications of Raman spectroscopy. *J. Raman Spectrosc.*, 28:111–117.
83. LeVine, S. M., and Wetzel, D. L. (1993): Analysis of brain tissue by FT–IR microspectroscopy. *Appl. Spectrosc. Rev.*, 28:385–412.
84. LeVine, S. M., and Wetzel, D. L. (1994): In situ chemical analysis from frozen tissue sections by Fourier transform infrared microspectroscopy: Examination of white matter exposed to extravasated blood in rat brain. *Amer. J. Pathol.*, 145:1041–1047.
85. LeVine, S. M., and Wetzel, D. L. (1994): In situ chemical analysis of brain tissue by Fourier transform infrared microspectroscopy. *Neuroprotocols*, 5:72–79.
86. Lenz, E. M., Greatbanks, D., Wilson, I. D., Spraul, M., Hofmann, M., Troke, J., Lindon, J. C., and Nicholson, J. K. (1996): Direct characterization of drug glucuronide isomers in human urine by HPLC–NMR spectroscopy: application to the positional isomers of 6,11-dihydro-11-oxodibenz[*b,e*]oxepin-2-acetic acid glucuronide. *Anal. Chem.*, 68:2832–2837.
87. Lindon, J. C., Nicholson, J. K., and Wilson, I. D. (1996): The development and application of coupled HPLC–NMR spectroscopy. *Adv. Chromatogr.*, 36:315–382.
88. Lindon, J. C., Nicholson, J. K., and Wilson, I. D. (1996): Direct coupling of chromatographic separations to NMR spectroscopy. *Prog. Nucl. Magn. Reson. Spectrosc.*, 29:1–49.
89. Lindon, J. C., Nicholson, J. K., Sidelmann, U. G., and Wilson, I. D. (1997): Directly coupled HPLC–NMR and its application to drug metabolism. *Drug Metab. Rev.*, 29:705–746.
90. Locke, S. J., and Brauer, M. (1991): The response of the rat liver in situ to bromobenzene—In vivo proton magnetic resonance imaging and ^{31}P magnetic resonance spectroscopy studies. *Toxicol. Appl. Pharmacol.*, 110:416–428.
91. Mach, R. H., Nader, M. A., Ehrenkaufer, R. L. E., Line, S. W., Smith, C. R., Gage, H. D., and Morton, T. E. (1997): Use of positron emission tomography to study the dynamics of psychostimulant-induced dopamine release. *Pharmacol. Biochem. Behav.*, 57:477–486.
92. Mach, R. H., Nader, M. A., Ehrenkaufer, R. L. E., Line, S. W., Smith, C. R., Luedtke, R. R., Kung, M.-P., Kung, H. F., Lyons, D., and Morton, T. E. (1996): Comparison of two fluorine-18 labeled benzamide derivatives that bind reversibly to dopamine D_2 receptors. *Synapse*, 24:322–333.
93. Mach, R. H., Voytko, M. L., Ehrenkaufer, R. L. E., Nader, M. A., Tobin, J. R., Efange, S. M. N., Parsons, S. M., Gage, H. D., Smith, C. R., and Morton, T. E. (1997): Imaging of cholinergic terminals using the radiotracer [^{18}F](+)-4-fluorobenzyltrozamicol: In vitro binding studies and positron emission tomography studies in nonhuman primates. *Synapse*, 25:368–380.
94. Malhotra, D., and Shapiro, J. I. (1993): Nuclear magnetic resonance measurements of intracellular pH: Biomedical implications. *Concepts Magn. Reson.*, 5:123–150.
95. Manoharan, R., Wang, Y., and Feld, M. S. (1996): Histochemical analysis of biological tissues using Raman spectroscopy. *Spectrochim. Acta, Part A*, 52:215–249.
96. Martin, G. E., and Crouch, R. C. (1991): Inverse-detected two-dimensional NMR methods: Applications in natural products chemistry. *J. Nat. Prod.*, 54:1–70.
97. Martin, G. E., Guido, J. E., Robins, R. H., Sharaf, M. H. M., Schiff, P. L. Jr., and Tackie, A. N. (1998): Submicro inverse-detection gradient NMR: A powerful new way of conducting structure elucidation studies with <0.05 μmol samples. *J. Nat. Prod.*, 61:555–559.
98. Martin, G. E., and Zektzer, A. S. (1988): *Two-Dimensional NMR Methods for Establishing Molecular Connectivity*. VCH Publishers, New York.
99. McFadden, W. A. (1973): *Techniques of Combined Gas Chromatography/Mass Spectrometry*. John Wiley & Sons, New York.
100. McLafferty, F. W. (1980): *Interpretation of Mass Spectra, 3rd ed.* University Science Books, Mill Valley, CA.
101. McManus, K. T., deBethizy, J. D., Garteiz, D. A., Kyerematen, G. A., and Vessel, E. S. (1990): A new quantitative thermospray LC-MS method for nicotine and its metabolites in biological fluids. *J. Chromatogr. Sci.*, 28:510–516.
102. McMaster, M., and McMaster, C. (1998): *GC/MS: A Practical User's Guide*. Wiley-VCH, New York.
103. Miller, J. C., and Miller, J. N. (1988): *Statistics for Analytical Chemistry, 2nd ed.* Ellis Horwood, Chichester.
104. Mizuno, A., Hayashi, T., Tashibu, K., Maraishi, S., Kawauchi, K., and Ozaki, Y. (1992): Near-infrared FT-Raman spectra of the rat brain tissue. *Neurosci. Lett.*, 141:47–52.
105. Mizuno, A., Kitajima, H., Kawauchi, K., Muraishi, S., and Ozaki, Y. (1994): Near-infrared Fourier transform Raman spectroscopic study of human brain tissues and tumors. *J. Raman Spectrosc.*, 25:25–29.
106. Moonen, C. T. W., van Zijl, P. C. M., Frank, J. A., Le Bihan, D., and Becker, E. D. (1990): Functional magnetic resonance imaging in medicine and physiology. *Science*, 250:53–61.
107. Moslen, M. T., and Smith, C. V., eds. (1992): *Free Radical Mechanisms of Tissue Injury*. CRC Press, Boca Raton, FL.
108. Muller, H. J., Lanens, D., de Cock Buning, T. J., Van de Vyver, F. L., Alderweireldt, F. C., Dommisse, R., Spanoghe, M., Mulder, G. J., and Lugtenburg, J. (1992): Noninvasive in vivo ^{13}C-NMR spectroscopy in the rat to study the pharmacokinetics of ^{13}C-labeled xenobiotics. *Drug Metab. Dispos.*, 20:507–509.
109. Munson, M. S. B., and Field, F. H. (1966): Chemical ionization mass spectrometry. I. General introduction. *J. Am. Chem. Soc.*, 88:2621–2630.
110. Neil, J. J. (1991): The use of freely diffusible, NMR-detectable tracers for measuring organ perfusion. *Concepts Magn. Reson.*, 3:1–12.
111. Nicholson, J. K., Foxall, P. J. D., Spraul, M., Farrant, R. D., and Lindon, J. C. (1995): 750 MHz ^{1}H and ^{1}H-^{13}C NMR spectroscopy of human blood plasma. *Anal. Chem.*, 67:793–811.
112. Nicholson, J. K., Holmes, E., Sidelmann, U., Lindon, J. C., and Wilson, I. D. (1996): HPLC–NMR spectroscopy: A powerful tool for the investigation of drug metabolism and metabolite reactivity. *Pharm. Sci.*, 2:127–130.
113. Nicholson, J. K., Timbrell, J. A., and Sadler, P. J. (1985): Proton NMR spectra of urine as indicators of renal damage: Mercury-induced nephrotoxicity in rats. *Molecular Pharm.*, 27:644–651.
114. Nicholson, J. K., and Wilson, I. D. (1987): High resolution nuclear magnetic resonance spectroscopy of biological samples as an aid to drug development. *Prog. Drug Res.*, 31:427–479.
115. Ong, C. W., Shen, Z. X., He, Y., Lee, T., and Tang, S. H. (1999): Raman microspectroscopy of the brain tissues in the substantra nigra and MPTP-induced Parkinson's disease. *J. Raman Spectrosc.*, 30:91–96.
116. Parker F. (1983): *Applications of Infrared, Raman and Resonance Raman Spectroscopy in Biochemistry*. Plenum Press, New York.
117. Parvez, H., Reich, A., Lucas-Reich, S., and Parvez, S. (1988): *Flow-Through Radioactivity Detection in HPLC*. VSP, Utrecht, The Netherlands.
118. Phelps, M. E., and Mazziotta, J. C. (1985): Positron emission tomography: Human brain function and biochemistry. *Science*, 228:779–809.
119. Philips, M., Mazziotta, J. C., and Schelbert, H. R., eds. (1986): *Positron Emission Autoradiography: Principles and Applications for the Brain and Heart*. Raven Press, New York.

120. Pool, W. F., and Crooks, P. A. (1988): Biotransformation of primary nicotine metabolites: Metabolism of R-(+)-[^{3}H-*N'*-CH_3; ^{14}C-*N*-CH_3] *N*-methylnicotinium acetate—the use of double isotope studies to determine the in-vivo stability of the *N*-methyl groups of *N*-methylnicotinium ion. *J. Pharm. Pharmacol.*, 40:758–762.
121. Poole, C. P. (1967): *Electron Spin Resonance, a Comprehensive Treatise on Experimental Techniques*. Wiley-Interscience, New York.
122. Popov, A. I., and Hallenga, K., eds. (1991): *Modern NMR Techniques and Their Application in Chemistry*. Marcel Dekker, New York.
123. Pullen, F. S., Swanson, A. G., Newman, M. J., and Richards, D. S. (1995): Online liquid chromatography/nuclear magnetic resonance mass spectrometry—A powerful spectroscopic tool for the analysis of mixtures of pharmaceutical interest. *Rapid Commun. Mass Spectrom.*, 9:1003–1006.
124. Puppels, G. J., de Mui, F. F. M., Otto, C., Greve, J., Robert-Nicoud, D., Arndt-Jovin, D. J., and Jovin, T. M. (1990): Studying single living cells and chromosomes by confocal Raman microspectroscopy. *Nature* (*London*), 347:301–303.
125. Pusecker, K., Schewitz, J., Gfrörer, P., Tseng, L.-H., Albert, K., and Bayer, E. (1998): On-line coupling of capillary electrochromatography, capillary electrophoresis, and capillary HPLC with nuclear magnetic resonance spectroscopy. *Anal. Chem.*, 70:3280–3285.
126. Rabenstein, D. L., and Guo, W. (1988) Nuclear magnetic resonance spectroscopy. *Anal. Chem.*, 60:1R–28R.
127. Rabenstein, D. L., Millis, K. K., and Strauss, E. J. (1988): Proton NMR spectroscopy of human blood plasma and red blood cells. *Anal. Chem.*, 60:1380–1390.
128. Reiman, E. M., and Mintan, M. A. (1990): Positron emission tomography. *Arch. Intern. Med.*, 150:729–731.
129. Sanders, J. K. M., and Hunter, B. K. (1987): *Modern NMR Spectroscopy: A Guide for Chemists*. Oxford University Press, Oxford.
130. Scarfe, G. B., Wilson, I. D., Spraul, M., Hofmann, M., Braumann, U., Lindon, J. C., and Nicholson, J. K. (1997): Application of directly coupled high-performance liquid chromatography–nuclear magnetic resonance–mass spectrometry to the detection and characterization of the metabolites of 2-bromo-4-trifluoromethylaniline in rat urine. *Anal. Commun.*, 34:37–39.
131. Scarfe, G. B., Wright, B., Clayton, E., Taylor, S., Wilson, I. D., Lindon, J. C., and Nicholson, J. K. (1998): ^{19}F-NMR and directly coupled HPLC–NMR–MS investigations into the metabolism of 2-bromo-4-trifluoromethylaniline in rat: A urinary excretion balance study without the use of radiolabeling. *Xenobiotica*, 28:373–388.
132. Scarfe, G. B., Wright, B., Clayton, E., Taylor, S., Wilson, I. D., Lindon, J. C., and Nicholson, J. K. (1999): Quantitative studies on the urinary metabolic fate of 2-chloro-4-trifluoromethylaniline in the rat using ^{19}F-NMR spectroscopy and directly coupled HPLC–NMR–MS. *Xenobiotica*, 29:77–91.
133. Schelbert, H. R. (1985): Positron emission tomography: Assessment of myocardial blood flow and metabolism. *Circulation*, 72(suppl. IV):122–133.
134. Schewitz, J., Gfrörer, P., Pusecker, K., Tseng, L.-H., Albert, K., Bayer, E., Wilson, I. D., Bailey, N. J., Scarfe, G. B., Nicholson, J. K., and Lindon, J. C. (1998): Directly coupled CZE–NMR and CEC–NMR spectroscopy for metabolite analysis: Paracetamol metabolites in human urine. *Analyst*, 123:2835–2837.
135. Schirmer, R. E. (1982): *Modern Methods of Pharmaceutical Analysis, Vol. 1.* CRC Press Inc., Boca Raton, FL.
136. Shi, X., Dalal, N. S., and Kasprzak, K. S. (1993): Generation of free radicals from model lipid hydroperoxides and H_2O_2 by Co(II) in the presence of cysteinyl and histidyl chelators. *Chem. Res. Toxicol.*, 6:277–283.
137. Shim, M. G., and Wilson, B. C. (1997): Development of an in vivo Raman spectroscopic system for diagnostic applications. *J. Raman Spectrosc.*, 28:131–142.
138. Shockcor, J. P., Unger, S. H., Wilson, I. D., Foxall, P. J. D., Nicholson, J. K., and Lindon, J. C. (1996): Combined HPLC, NMR spectroscopy, and ion-trap mass spectrometry with application to the detection and characterization of xenobiotic and endogenous metabolites in human urine. *Anal. Chem.*, 68:4431–4435.
139. Sidelmann, U. G., Braumann, U., Hofmann, M., Spraul, M., Lindon, J. C., Nicholson, J. K., and Hansen, S. H. (1997): Directly coupled 800 MHz HPLC-NMR spectroscopy of urine and its application to the identification of the major phase II metabolites of tolfenamic acid. *Anal. Chem.*, 69:607–612.
140. Siethoff, C., Feldmann, I., Jakubowski, N., and Linscheid, M. (1999): Quantitative determination of DNA adducts using liquid chromatography/electrospray ionization mass spectrometry and liquid chromatography/high resolution inductively coupled plasma mass spectrometry. *J. Mass Spectrom.*, 34:421–426.
141. Smith, D. R., and Flegal, A. R. (1992): Stable isotopic tracers of lead mobilized by DMSA chelation in low lead-exposed rats. *Toxicol. Appl. Pharmacol.*, 116:85–91.
142. Smith, D. R., Osterloh, J., Niemeyer, S. N., and Flegal, A. R. (1992): Stable isotope labeling of lead compartments in rats with ultra-low lead concentrations. *Environ. Res.*, 57:190–207.
143. Smith, R. V., and Stewart, J. T. (1981): *Textbook of Biopharmaceutical Analysis*. Leo and Febiger, Philadelphia.
144. Sotgiu, A., Colacicchi, S., Placidi, G., and Alecci, M. (1997): Water soluble free radicals as biologically responsive agents in electron paramagnetic resonance imaging. *Cell. Mol. Biol.*, 43:813–823.
145. Spraul, M., Hofmann, M., Dvortsak, P., Nicholson, J. K., and Wilson, I. D. (1993): High-performance liquid chromatography coupled to high-field proton nuclear magnetic resonance spectroscopy: Application to the urinary metabolites of ibuprofen. *Anal. Chem.*, 65:327–330.
146. Stubbs, M., Coombes, R. C., Griffiths, J. R., Maxwell, R. J., Rodrigues, L. M., and Gusterson, B. A. (1990): ^{31}P-NMR spectroscopy and histological studies of the response of rat mammary tumours to endocrine therapy. *Br. J. Cancer*, 61:258–262.
147. Stubbs, M., Rodrigues, L. M., and Griffiths, J. R. (1989): Growth studies of subcutaneous rat tumours: Comparison of ^{31}P-NMR spectroscopy, acid extracts and histology. *Br. J. Cancer*, 60:701–707.
148. Sumner, S. C. J., MacNeela, J. P., and Fennell, T. R. (1992): Characterization and quantitation of urinary metabolites of [1,2,3-^{13}C] acrylamide in rats and mice using ^{13}C nuclear magnetic resonance spectroscopy. *Chem. Res. Toxicol.*, 5:81–89.
149. Talangala, S. L., and Lowe, I. J. (1991): Introduction to magnetic resonance imaging. *Concepts Magn. Reson.*, 3:145–159.
150. Taylor, J. K. (1987): *Quality Assurance of Chemical Measurements*. Lewis Publishers, Chelsea.
151. Ter-Pogossian, M. M., Raichle, M. E., and Sobel, B. E. (1980): Positron-emission tomography. *Scientific Amer.*, 243:171–181.
152. Traficante, D. D. (1992): Optimum tip angle and relaxation delay for quantitative analysis. *Concepts Magn. Reson.*, 4:153–160.
153. Treado, P. J., Levin, I. W., and Lewis, E. N. (1992): Near-infrared acousto-optic filtered spectroscopic microscopy: A solid-state approach to chemical imaging. *Appl. Spectrosc.*, 46:553–559.
154. Turtelbaum, K. W., Frantz, C. E., Creek, M. R., Vogel, J. S., Shen, N., and Fultz, E. (1993): DNA adducts in model systems and humans. *J. Cell Biochem.*, 17F:138–148.

155. Vaupel, P., Okunieff, P., and Neuringer, L. J. (1990): In vivo ^{31}P-NMR spectroscopy of murine tumours before and after localized hyperthermia. *Int. J. Hyperthermia*, 6:15–31.
156. Vogel, J. S., Turteltaub, K. W., Finkel, R., and Nelson, D. E. (1995): Accelerator mass spectrometry. *Anal. Chem.*, 67:353A–359A.
157. Volkow, N. D., Fowler, J. S., Wang, G. J., Hitzemann, R., Logan, J., Schlyer, D. J., Dewey, S. L., and Wolf, A. P. (1993): Decreased dopamine D_2 receptor availability is associated with reduced frontal metabolism in cocaine abusers. *Synapse*, 14:169–177.
158. Volkow, N. D., Fowler, J. S., Wolf, A. P., Schlyer, D., Shuiue, C. Y., Alper, R., Dewey, S. L., Logan, J., Bendriem, B., and Christman, D. (1990): Effects of chronic cocaine abuse on postsynaptic dopamine receptors. *Am. J. Psychol.*, 147:719–724.
159. Waddell, W. J. (1981): Autoradiography in drug disposition studies. In: *Fundamentals of Drug Metabolism and Drug Disposition*, edited by B. N. La Du, H. G. Mandel, and E. L. Way, pp. 505–514. Robert E. Krieger Publishing Co., Malabar, Florida.
160. Weickhardt, C., Moritz, F., and Grotemeyer, J. (1996): Time-of-flight mass spectrometry: State-of-the-art in chemical analysis and molecular science. *Mass Spectrom. Rev.*, 15:139–162.
161. Wetzel, D. L., Slatkin, D. N., and LeVine, S. M. (1998): FT–IR microspectroscopic detection of metabolically deuterated compounds in the rat cerebellum: A novel approach for the study of brain metabolism. *Cell. Mol. Biol.*, 44:15–27.
162. Whateley, T. L. (1988): Radiochemistry and radiopharmaceuticals. In: *Practical Pharmaceutical Chemistry, 4th edition, Part Two*, edited by A. H. Beckett and J. B. Stanlake, pp. 501–534. The Athlone Press, London.
163. Willoughby, R. C., and Browner, R. F. (1984): Monodispersed aerosol generation interface for coupling liquid chromatography with mass spectrometry. *Anal. Chem.*, 56:2626–2631.
164. Willoughby, R., Sheehan, E., and Mitrovich, S. (1998): *A Global View of LC–MS*. Global View, Pittsburgh.
165. Wilson, A. G. E., and Kraus, L. J. (1995): Application of direct analytic and storage phosphor techniques in quantitating whole-body autoradiography data. *Toxicol. Methods*, 5:15–20.
166. Wilson, I. D., Lindon, J. C., and Nicholson, J. K. (1998): Liquid chromatography directly and jointly combined with nuclear magnetic resonance spectroscopy and mass spectrometry. *LC–GC*, 16:842–852.
167. Wiltshire, H. R., Harris, S. R., Prior, K. J., Kozlowski, U. M., and Worth, E. (1992): Metabolism of calcium anagonist Ro 40-5967: A case history of the use of diode-array u.v. spectroscopy and thermospray-mass spectrometry in the elucidation of a complex metabolic pathway. *Xenobiotica*, 22:837–857.
168. Wolfe, R. R. (1992): *Radioactive and Stable Isotope Tracers in Biomedicine: Principles and Practice of Kinetic Analysis*. Wiley-Liss, New York.
169. Wong, P. T. T., and Rigas, B. (1990): Infrared spectra of microtome sections of human colon tissues. *Appl. Spectrosc.*, 44:1715–1720.
170. Wu, N., Webb, A., Peck, T. L., and Sweedler, J. V. (1995): On-line NMR detection of amino acids and peptides in microbore LC. *Anal. Chem.*, 67:3101–3107.
171. Yergey, A. L., Edmonds, C. G., Lewis, I. A. S., and Vestal, M. L. (1990): *Liquid Chromatography/Mass Spectrometry, Techniques and Applications*. Plenum Press, New York.
172. Zane, P. A., O'Buck, A. J., Walter, R. E., Robertson, P., and Tripp, S. L. (1997): Validation of procedures for quantitative whole-body autoradiography using digital imaging. *J. Pharm. Sci.*, 86:733–738.

Principles and Methods of Toxicology,
Fourth Edition, edited by A. Wallace Hayes.

Chapter **37**

Methods in Environmental Toxicology

Anne Fairbrother, Michael A. Lewis, and Robert E. Menzer

Most testing of chemicals for their toxic effects has traditionally focused on concerns regarding the safety of humans. Such testing, however, invariably is conducted using surrogate species that are supposed to approximate the responses of the human. Over the years a body of literature has accumulated that provides a measure of confidence that such an approach, although with appropriate safety factors applied, has indeed provided data that can be extrapolated for the protection of human health. Most of that literature is based on testing chemicals with a variety of laboratory animal species that can be bred, reared, and maintained with confidence that results obtained will be comparable from one testing situation to another. Mice, rats, rabbits, dogs, and occasionally primates are the principal species used.

Recently, two important considerations have emerged in the discipline of toxicology that demand an extension of the limited testing protocols of the past. First, we have discovered that there are animal species that more closely mimic the human response than traditionally used laboratory animals (131). Secondly, we recognize today that there are important implications for human health in the response to xenobiotics of wild animals in their own environments. Thus, the subdiscipline of ecotoxicology has emerged today with its research emphasis on bioindicators of ecosystem health.

By expanding the number of species tested in assessing the toxicology of a chemical, one is able to gain considerable insight into its mechanism of action, biodegradability, organ-specific toxicity, and acute and potential chronic effects. The expansion of comparative toxicology from reliance on laboratory mammals to the inclusion of wild mammals, fish, birds, and some invertebrates is highly desirable in order to better understand the range of responses to a chemical in its interactions with the various target systems possible in different animals. With advances in understanding the physiology and biochemistry of different species, the possibility of a better understanding of toxic responses is enhanced.

With the inclusion of additional species in toxicity testing the need for the development of protocols to standardize approaches for the use of such new species has arisen. In this chapter, we provide some principles and examples of the development of such protocols.

ENVIRONMENTAL BEHAVIOR OF XENOBIOTICS

When testing the toxicity of chemicals to laboratory animals, the chemical is usually fed to or applied directly to the animal or directly into the medium in which the animal is living. However, when using wild mammals, fish, birds, or invertebrates, testing protocols must be designed to take into account the effects of the transport and fate of the chemical in the natural environment. Thus, the physical properties and chemical behavior of the test substance are important factors that must be understood. The most comprehensive and useful treatise on this subject is that of Lyman et al. (121).

Water Solubility and Lipophilicity

The most significant determinant of the transport and fate of a chemical in the environment is its water solubility. Highly soluble chemicals will be transported in large quantities through the hydrologic cycle and thus will be found widely distributed at large distances from their points of introduction into the environment. Conversely, hydrophobic compounds will tend to be more static and move little through the hydrologic cycle. Generally, the more water soluble the chemical, the less lipophilic, the less sorbed to soils and sediments and the less bioconcentrated it will be. Water solubility may be defined as the maximum amount of a chemical that may be dissolved in a given quantity of pure water at a particular temperature. It is important to note that even chemicals described as very insoluble may have sufficient water solubility to have a significant impact on their behavior in the environment.

A derivative property of a chemical's water solubility and lipophilicity is its octanol/water partition coefficient (K_{OW} or P), frequently reported as log K_{OW}. K_{OW} is defined as the ratio of the concentrations of a chemical in the water phase and the *n*-octanol phase after a chemical is equilibrated between equal volumes of the two solvents. It is a key property of a chemical from the environmental point of view because it is related to soil and sediment adsorption and bioconcentration of a chemical in aquatic organisms. In designing studies to assess toxicity of a chemical in model ecosystems, such as microcosms or mesocosms, the octanol/water partition coefficient must be known or experimentally determined so that the behavior of the chemical in the system can be predicted and the system designed appropriately.

Soil Adsorption

The extent of partitioning of an organic chemical between the solid and solution phases of a water-saturated soil or sediment is described by the soil sorption coefficient, K or K_d (120,175). It is determined experimentally using the Freundlich equation:

$$x/m = KC^{1/n},$$

where x/m is μg of chemical adsorbed/g of soil, C is μg of chemical/ml of solution, and K and n are constants for a particular soil type. The value of n must be experimentally determined, but is frequently assumed to be 1. K_{OC}, the soil sorption constant, is determined from K by dividing by the percent organic carbon in the soil and multiplying the result by 100. This constant is observed to be relatively independent of the type of soil or sediment and is the value most frequently used to describe the adsorption of a chemical to soil or sediment. Again, this property of a chemical is extremely important for the proper design of some ecological test systems.

Vaporization

The vaporization of a chemical from a solid surface or a solution is an important mass transfer process. Factors that control volatilization are diffusivity of the chemical, its water solubility, vapor pressure, the Henry's Law constant, and temperature. Diffusivity is the rate of diffusion of a chemical through a medium and depends on the nature of the chemical itself and the nature of the medium through which it moves. Vapor pressure is the tendency of a liquid to change from the liquid to the gaseous state and is highly dependent on temperature.

The air–water interface is an important factor in environmental analyses; the question of the ability of a chemical to diffuse across that interface is significant in evaluating its environmental behavior. The tendency of a chemical to escape from solution is described by the Henry's Law constant. Henry's Law states that the solubility of a gas in a liquid is directly proportional to the pressure of the gas above the liquid at equilibrium, $H = \mathrm{P}/\mathrm{C}$, where C is measured in mol/m^3 and P is in atm; that is, H is the ratio of the saturation vapor pressure and the water solubility of the chemical. Units of H are most often reported as atm m^3/mol. However, if C is expressed in mol/L and P is expressed in mol/m^3, H is dimensionless. Under these circumstances, the Henry's Law constant is sometimes referred to as the air/water partition coefficient.

Movement of chemicals in the environment occurs in the vapor state as well as in solution. The most important consideration in evaluating the extent of such movement is the Henry's Law constant, because in the environment most chemicals will eventually be found in water solution, and their tendency to move into the air will have an impact on their potential for toxic effects in organisms that may be exposed. In the design of toxicology test

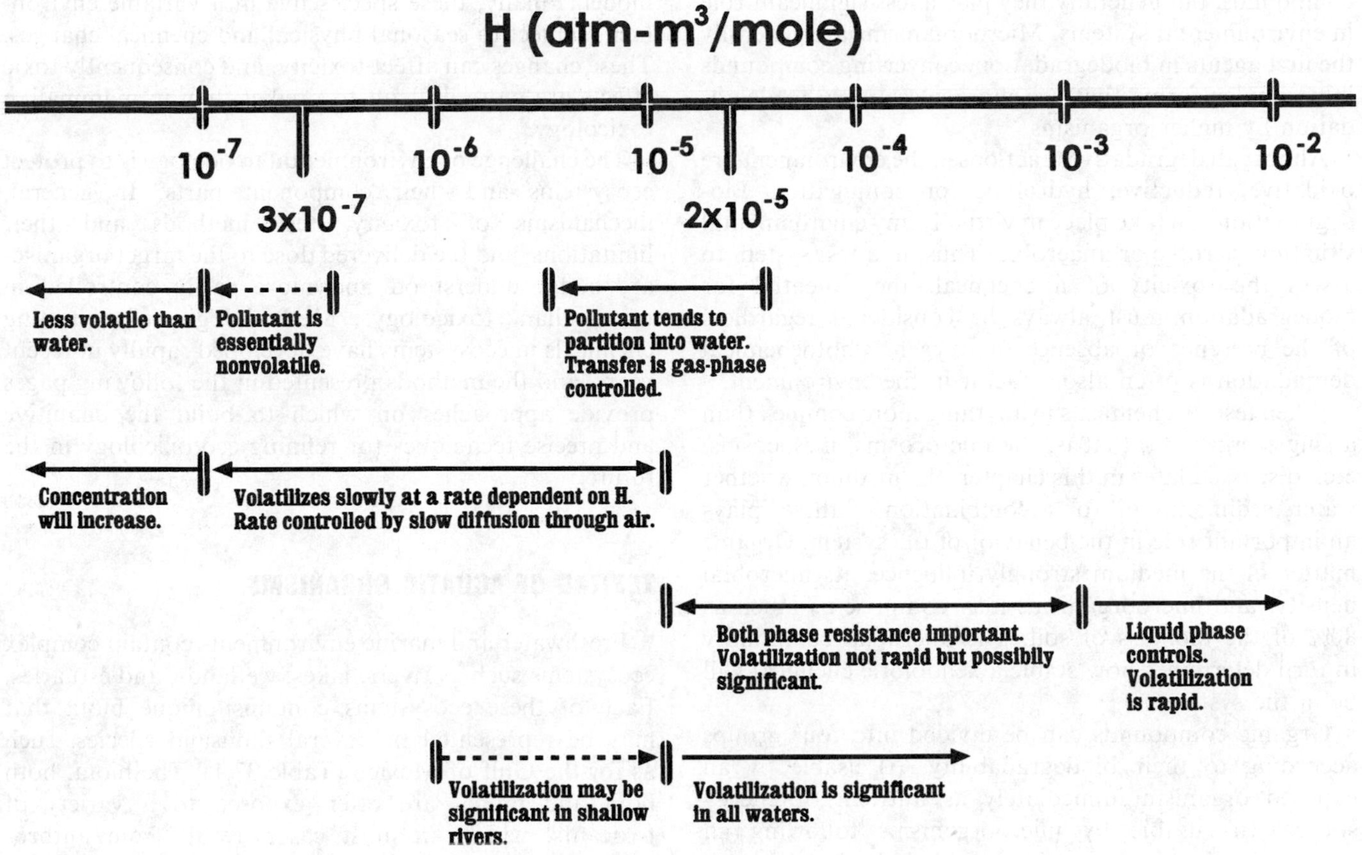

FIG. 37.1. Volatility characteristics associated with various ranges of Henry's Law constant. From Lyman et al. (121).

methods, such considerations must be taken into account. Their importance is illustrated in Figure 37.1 in which the relation of the Henry's Law constant of a chemical to its volatility characteristics is depicted.

Bioaccumulation

It is evident that certain chemicals accumulate in aquatic organisms exposed to them in their environments. There are now many well-known examples of chemicals being concentrated in feed webs to the point that toxic effects are exhibited in organisms that may have had no direct exposure to the chemical itself at its point of application, the insecticide DDT being an example. The tendency of a chemical to be more concentrated in an aquatic organism than the concentration in its environment is described by its bioconcentration factor (BCF). It is calculated by dividing the concentration of the chemical in the organism (wet weight) by the concentration of the chemical in the water. The units in both the numerator and denominator must be the same, for example, both μg/g. The BCF can be estimated from a chemical's water solubility, K_{OW}, or K_{OC}. A number of empirical equations specifically useful for calculating the BCF for particular chemical groups are found in Lyman et al. (121). Estimates of the BCF should be used in designing toxicity studies to understand the degree to which the test chemical will be taken up by and stored in aquatic biota being used as test organisms. However, bioaccumulation does not take into account the ability of an organism to metabolize the chemical. Thus, the use of a BCF without considering biodegradation may yield misleading conclusions.

Biodegradation

As chemicals move in the environment they are subjected to break down, primarily by microorganisms, termed biodegradation. This process represents a significant loss mechanism in soil, sediments, and aquatic systems, which leads ultimately to mineralization of the compound, that is, degradation to carbon dioxide, water, and the inorganic forms of other elements they may contain. Microorganisms are the primary converters of complex organic chemicals to inorganic substances. In many instances higher organisms are able to metabolize compounds, but generally they play a less significant role in environmental systems. Microorganisms are generally the first agents in biodegradation, converting compounds into simpler forms that are more susceptible to degradation by higher organisms.

Almost all degradative reactions in the environment are oxidative, reductive, hydrolytic, or conjugative. Biodegradation can take place in virtually any environmental situation, aerobic or anaerobic. Thus, in a test system to assess the toxicity of a chemical, the potential for biodegradation must always be considered regardless of the presence or absence of oxygen. Photochemical degradation is often also a factor in the environment.

When testing chemicals in anything more complex than a single organism, that is, the microcosms, mesocosms, etc., discussed later in this chapter, the medium, whether water, sediment, soil, or a combination of these, plays an important role in the behavior of the system. Organic matter in the medium strongly influences its microbial density, and microorganisms may comprise as much as 80% of the biomass of soil. The microbial community in turn determines how stable a xenobiotic chemical will be in the system.

Organic compounds can be divided into four groups according to their biodegradability: (i) usable by an exposed organism immediately as nutrient or energy source, (ii) usable by microorganisms following an acclimation period, and (iii) degraded slowly or not at all. In the fourth group, compounds are subject to cometabolic degradation wherein a compound that does not provide a nutrient or energy source for the degrading organism is broken down in conjunction with the degradation of other substances. Thus, ideally when evaluating the effect of a xenobiotic on complex systems, one needs to consider all aspects of the biology and chemistry of all of the organisms and chemicals present. The best design of such test systems demands the most complete knowledge possible of all the potential interactions of chemicals and organisms in the system.

Before presenting and discussing the various specific test methods used in environmental toxicology, it is important to note that there are several significant differences between the practice of toxicology using laboratory animals and methods that use wild animals, often located in their usual or at least simulated environmental conditions. Most importantly, the goal of environmental toxicology is considerably broader and more varied in that although the assessment of the impact of a test chemical on human health is important, an understanding of the impact of a chemical on whole ecosystems as well as their component parts is the paramount consideration. Furthermore, in ecotoxicology frequently the test organisms are the actual targets for a chemical pollutant and the test methodology thus utilizes the endpoint subjects of concern, rather than a surrogate animal model. Finally, these species live in a variable environment subject to seasonal physical and chemical changes. These changes can affect toxicity, and consequently toxic effects are more difficult to predict than in mammalian toxicology.

The challenge of environmental toxicology is to protect ecosystems and their component parts. In general, mechanisms of toxicity, test methods and their limitations, and the delivered dose to the target organism are better understood and more easily controlled in mammalian toxicology. Methodologies for testing chemicals in ecosystems have developed rapidly in recent years, and the methods presented in the following pages provide approaches on which to build the definitive and precise techniques for refining ecotoxicology in the future.

TESTING OF AQUATIC ORGANISMS

Freshwater and marine environments contain complex ecosystems such as rivers, lakes, wetlands, and estuaries. Each of these ecosystems contains unique biota that may be represented by several thousand species, such as for the Gulf of Mexico (Table 37.1). The biota, both flora and fauna, are often exposed to a variety of toxicants, which, in most cases, result from anthropogenic activities. As a result, toxicity and environmental damage may occur. The study of these adverse effects on freshwater and saltwater biota and on the ecosystems that contain them defines the aquatic toxicology discipline.

Aquatic toxicology differs from mammalian toxicology in several aspects. The primary goal of aquatic toxicology is to assess the effect of toxicants on the many diverse populations and communities of plants and animals

Table 37.1
Estimated number of species of fauna and flora in the Gulf of Mexico

Taxa	Species
Microalgae	30,000
Sea grasses	7
Molluscs	500
Polychaetes	600
Oligochaetes	200
Echinoderms	400
Cnidarians	600
Sponges	100
Fishes	800
Marine mammals	32

From Reference 70.

inhabiting saltwater and freshwater environments. The biota is usually cold-blooded and the physical and chemical characteristics of the aquatic environment have a significant effect on their sensitivity to toxicants. The aquatic test species of interest, unlike in mammalian studies, can be used directly. The objective of mammalian toxicology is to assess effects on humans whose sensitivity to toxicants is less affected by their environment than aquatic organisms. The dose of the toxicant used in mammalian toxicology can be measured more accurately, the mechanisms of toxic action are better understood and the test methods are more established.

Various species of aquatic life have been used in toxicity experiments for over 130 years. One of the earliest reported studies was conducted with fish in 1863 (155) and the first proposed standard test species was the goldfish in 1917 (158). Toxicity tests have been conducted with increasing frequency since the 1960s due to the numerous environmental regulations that have been enacted that require their use. An additional reason is the increasing availability of standardized test methods, the first of which were published in 1960 for animal test species and 1970 for algae. Hunn (92) provides additional detail on the development of aquatic toxicology as a field of study.

Many toxicity test methods are available for use. They differ in their cost, precision, complexity, and the skill needed to conduct them. Nevertheless, their objectives are similar: They are conducted to determine the relative potency among chemicals, the relative susceptibility among different species and life stages, and to identify other variables that influence the overall outcome of exposure. Toxicity tests are conducted usually to meet regulatory guidelines for the use and discharge of commercial chemicals such as pesticides (185) or nonpesticides (186). In addition, toxicity results have been used to derive national water quality standards to protect aquatic life (174) and to determine the environmental effects of municipal and industrial effluents (196,197).

Aquatic toxicologists do not use all of the available toxicity tests to determine the effects for any single toxicant. Instead, a tiered approach is used to provide a systematic and comprehensive process of deriving the toxicity data needed to assess the environmental hazard of a chemical. This approach consists of conducting short-term screening tests prior to using predictive studies that, are more complex and time consuming. This sequential evaluation provides an efficient use of resources and tends to eliminate unnecessary testing. The criteria used to determine the appropriate level of testing have been discussed in detail (9). The decision points and testing phase depend upon the quality and quantity of data needed for the test substance of interest. The types of toxicity tests used in this tiered approach are discussed briefly in this section. Key references on various types of aquatic toxicity testing methods are provided in Table 37.2.

Table 37.2
Sources of detailed information important to consult before conducting toxicity tests with marine and freshwater life

Tests	References
Single-species tests	6, 34, 95, 159, 170, 171, 172
Multispecies toxicity tests	107
Microcosms	38, 39, 54, 72
Outdoor ponds	49
Experimental streams	101
Phytotoxicity tests	
Algae	4, 144, 178, 210
Duckweed	112, 214
Rooted vascular plants	169
Effluent toxicity tests	73, 154, 196, 197, 211
Sediment toxicity tests	6, 36, 68, 77, 136, 179
Bioconcentration	76
Ecological risk assessment	41, 192, 194, 199

SINGLE-SPECIES TOXICOLOGY TESTS

Methodologies

There are two basic types of aquatic single-species toxicity tests, acute and chronic. Acute toxicity tests have been the "work horse" of aquatic toxicologists for many years (184). These tests are relatively simple, have short durations, and are cost effective. As a result, a large historical database exists for many chemicals, such as for detergent surfactants, metals, pesticides, and various other organic compounds (57,93,110,111,124,126,182, 183,207).

Acute toxicity tests are most often used to screen toxicity quickly or to determine the relative sensitivities of different test species. Mortality is the effect monitored during the test duration of 48 h (invertebrates) or 96 h (fish). In a typical acute toxicity test, 5–10 organisms are exposed under static conditions in glass test beakers to five test concentrations. A control is included. The test concentrations and control are conducted in triplicate. Daily observations are made on survival and dead organisms are removed. At test termination, the concentration that kills 50% of the test organisms (LC_{50} value)

Table 37.3
The availability of toxicity data for high volume commercial chemicals

Acute toxicity	90%
Repeat Dose toxicity	30%
Carcinogenicity	20%
Mutagenicity	50%
Reproductive toxicity	10%
Teratogenicity	30%
Acute toxicity (fish or daphnids)	50%
Short-term toxicity (green algae)	5%
Effects on soil organisms	< 5%

From Reference 206.

is determined using probit analysis or graphical interpolation. Unlike in chronic toxicity tests, there is no test solution renewal, the organisms are unfed and there is no analytical verification of the test concentrations. Furthermore, cumulative, chronic, and sublethal effects of a chemical are usually not evaluated in acute toxicity tests, although behavioral changes and lesions caused by a chemical can be determined.

Chronic toxicity tests are more complex and time consuming than acute studies and for these reasons are conducted less frequently (Table 37.3). The methodologies for these tests differ considerably, unlike for acute tests, because they are designed for the specific life histories of the various test species. Chronic toxicity tests may be for a full life cycle (egg–egg), partial life cycle (embryo–larval), and partial life history (egg–death). Full life cycle tests are uncommon with fish due to the long durations that are necessary, 1–2 years. Partial life cycle tests with fish can be as short as 7 days or as long as 60 days. The early life stage of fish (embryo/larvae) is usually the most sensitive period in a fish's life cycle (129), and consequently, partial life cycle tests are used as surrogates for the full life cycle studies. Chronic tests may be conducted for more than one complete life cycle if algal and invertebrate species are used, because their life cycles are shorter than those of fishes. Lethal and sublethal effects are monitored in chronic toxicity studies, and these effects include changes in growth, reproduction, behavior, physiology, and histology.

Fathead minnows and the freshwater invertebrate, *Daphnia magna*, are common species used in chronic toxicity tests to meet regulatory expectations for commercial chemicals. The results from two chronic studies of a detergent cationic surfactant conducted with these species appear in Table 37.4. A brief discussion of the study design used in the daphnid study follows. *D. magna* were exposed to the cationic surfactant in a 21-day static-renewal toxicity test. Ten 250 ml glass beakers containing 200 ml of the test solution were used for each of the five test concentrations and controls. A solvent was used in the study, which necessitated the use of a solvent control. Seven of the beakers at each concentration contained one daphnid (less than 24 h old) and the remaining three contained five organisms. Growth, survival, and reproduction were monitored in those beakers containing one daphnid, whereas only survival was monitored in the remaining test chambers. The test species were fed daily a combination of algae, trout chow, and alfalfa. The test solutions were renewed daily. Prior to renewal, survival and number of young were determined. Surviving adults were then transferred to test chambers containing "fresh" solution at the same levels of toxicant to which the organisms had been previously exposed. At test termination, the effects of the surfactant on growth, reproduction, and survival were compared for daphnids exposed to the various toxicant concentrations and those in the solvent control. It can be seen that the first significant effect level of the surfactant was 0.76 mg/L, based on changes in mean length, total young, and mean brood size.

Toxicity tests may be static, continuous flow, recirculating, or, as in the previous example, static renewal based on the toxicant dosing technique. The advantages and disadvantages of these designs have been summarized previously (34,197). Static and flow-through procedures are more widely used in toxicity tests conducted with pure chemicals and animal test species. Chronic toxicity tests conducted with effluents are usually static renewal, and those with algae, static. There is no change or renewal of the test substance and dilution water in a static test. This design is the simplest and least expensive; however, the toxicant concentrations may decrease due to adsorption and biodegradation. The test solutions and dilution water are renewed periodically, usually daily in a static-renewal test. In a continuous flow test, the dilution water and test substance are continuously renewed. The exposure concentrations remain fairly constant and the dose–response relationship can be well defined.

A variety of aquatic toxicity test methods have been published for single species and many have been standardized (Table 37.5). Test method development is an ongoing process, however, which continues to improve these methods by identifying more sensitive test species and effect parameters. These efforts often result in alternative study designs. For example, Blaise (27) summarizes several of the "microbiotests" developed recently to provide toxicity data more quickly. In addition, the use of genotoxicity as an effect parameter is becoming more common (219).

Table 37.4
Results of two chronic toxicity tests conducted with a cationic surfactant and a freshwater fish and an invertebrate[b]

Mean measured concentration (mg/l)	Embryos Mean% match	Larvae Mean% survival	Larvae Mean total length (mm)	Larvae Mean weight (mg)
Freshwater fish				
Solvent control	98	90	21	77
Control	99	95	20	73
0.006	99	97	21	77
0.013	94	97	21	77
0.024	98	97	21	75
0.053	98	90	21	78
0.090	98	44[a]	14[a]	31[a]

Mean measured concentration (mg/L)	Mean length (mm; ±SD)[a]	First day to reproduction	Total young	Mean brood	Adult mortality size
Invertebrate					
Solvent control	4.29 (±0.45)	6	2,234	45.6	1
control	4.49 (±0.56)	6	2,131	45.3	0
0.10	4.32 (±0.36)	6	2,261	45.2	1
0.19	4.25 (±0.20)	6	2,095	40.3	0
0.38	4.20 (±0.31)	6	1,932	42.0	1
0.76	3.71 (±0.15)[a]	7	1,195[a]	30.6[a]	0
1.55	2.92 (±0.21)[a]	8	320[a]	13.3[a]	5
3.10	—	—	—	—	22

[a] The exposures were for 35 and 21 days, respectively. Data from Lewis and Wee (114).
[b] Significantly different at 0.05 level.

Table 37.5
Examples of the availability of standardized toxicity test methods

APHA et al.[a]	ASTM[b]	USEPA effluent[c]	USEPA TSCA[d]	USEPA FIFRA[e]	OECD[f]
Toxicity tests	Toxicity tests	Toxicity Tests	Toxicity tests	Toxicity tests	Toxicity tests
• Protozoa	• Amphibians	Freshwater	Freshwater	Freshwater	• Algae
• Daphnia	• Invertebrates	• *Ceriodaphnia dubia*	• Algae	• Invertebrates	• Daphnia acute
• Annelids	• Fish	• *Daphnia pulex*	• Duckweed	• Fish (early life stage)	• Fish acute
• Crustaceans	• Rotifers	• Rainbow trout	• Daphnids	• Fish (life cycle)	• Fish prolonged
• Aquatic insects	• Molluscs	• Fathead minnow	• Fish (toxicity)	• Nontarget plants	• Fish early life stage
• Fish	• Microalgae	• *Selenastrum*	• Fish	• Daphnids	
• Algae		*capricornutum*	(bioconcentration)		
• Vascular plants					Bioaccumulation
• Bacterial	Microcosms	Saltwater	Saltwater	Saltwater	
bioluminescence	Bioconcentration	• *Mysidopsis bahia*	• Algae	• Mollusc	
	Teratogenesis	• *Cyprinodon variegatus*	• Fish (toxicity)	• Shrimp	
	Field sampling	• *Menidia* sp.	• Fish	• Oyster	
		• *Arbacia punctulata*	(bioconcentration)	• Fish (early life stage)	
Field sampling		• *Champia parvula*	• Fish (early life stage)	• Fish (life cycle)	
			• Oyster	• Nontarget plants	
			• Mysid shrimp		
			• Penaeid shrimp		

[a] American Public Health Association, American Public Works Association, Water Pollution Control Federation (2).
[b] American Society for Testing and Materials (6).
[c] U.S. Environmental Protection Agency (196,197).
[d] U.S. Environmental Protection Agency Toxic Substances Control Act (TSCA) (186,189).
[e] U.S. Environmental Protection Agency Federal Insecticide, Fungicide, Rodenticide Act (FIFRA) (185).
[f] Organization for Economic Co-operation and Development (146).

Experimental Conditions

In general terms, toxicity tests are conducted in a laboratory or a room controlled for light and temperature. The test solutions containing the test species are monitored for pH, temperature, dissolved oxygen, and hardness. The test organisms are exposed for a predetermined duration, which varies depending upon the type of test and test species. Daily observations on lethal and sublethal effects are made, and several calculations such as the LC_{50} value and the highest no observed effect (NOEC) and lowest first observed effect (LOEC) concentrations are determined based on the most sensitive effect parameter of interest. Although toxicity tests have similarities, as discussed below, variations among test animals, instrumentation, and methods influence the outcomes and utility of the assessments.

Test Chambers

The types of test chambers used in toxicity tests depend upon the test species. Various sizes of beakers, aquaria, jars, bowls, and Petri dishes have been used. The test chambers are usually constructed of materials such as glass, teflon, and certain plastics that minimize leaching of toxicants and adsorption of the test substance.

Test Concentrations

The test substances used in most toxicity tests in the past have been pure chemical compounds and municipal and industrial effluents. However, toxicity tests are being conducted more frequently with dredged soil materials, hazardous waste leachates, and contaminated sediments due to increasing regulatory concern for their potential environmental impacts.

Xenobiotic concentrations used in an acute toxicity test are routinely based on results obtained from a pretest or range-finding test. The test concentration range for a chronic test is based on the results of an acute test conducted prior to the chronic test. There are no standard guidelines for conducting these preliminary tests. Generally, 5–10 organisms are exposed to several test concentrations that are usually an order of magnitude apart. The dilution water and exposure conditions, that is, water temperature, hardness, and pH, in range-finding tests are usually similar to those in the definitive test.

The test organisms are exposed in the definitive test to five concentrations of the test compounds chosen in a geometric progression. The test concentrations and control are replicated at least threefold. The test compound is added to the dilution water, which may be well water, reconstituted water, dechlorinated tap water, uncontaminated river water, and natural or artificial seawater. The dilution water is well aerated and undesirable organisms are removed before use.

An organic solvent is used to dissolve substances with minimal water solubility. Several have been used and include triethylene glycol, dimethyl sulfoxide, acetone, and dimethyl formamide. The LC_{50} values for these solvents are between 9000 mg/L and 92,500 mg/L (156). The concentration of the solvent in the test water should not exceed 0.5 ml/L or should not be greater than 1/1000 of the LC_{50} value of the solvent. When a solvent is used, a solvent control is included in the study.

Toxicant delivery systems are used to deliver on a once-through basis the various test concentrations to the test chambers in continuous-flow toxicity tests. The serial proportional diluter (Figure 37.2) is the most common design (109,135) used to mix the dilution water with the test substance to produce the desired test concentrations. The construction materials in toxicant delivery systems, such as for the test chambers, should not be rubber, certain plastics, or metallic to prevent leaching of potentially toxic substances.

The test concentrations are analytically confirmed during chronic toxicity tests. Analyses are performed at least weekly for each test concentration and control for tests of 7-day duration or longer. In chronic tests of shorter duration, analyses are usually conducted on alternate days. Analytical verification of the test concentrations in range-finding and acute toxicity tests is seldom performed, and the results from these tests are generally based on nominal concentrations.

Test Species

Historically, animal test species have been used more frequently than plant species and freshwater species more frequently than marine species. This trend can be seen in Table 37.6.

Most toxicity tests are conducted with single cultured test species such as those listed in Table 37.7. The more commonly used freshwater species, particularly in tests used for regulatory compliance, are fathead minnows (*Pimephales promelas*), several daphnid species (*Daphnia magna, Ceriodaphnia dubia*), and green algae (*Selenastrum capricornutum*). Common marine species are sheepshead minnows (*Cyprinodon variegatus*), mysid shrimp (*Mysidopsis bahia*), and diatoms (*Skeletonema costatum*).

The species in Table 37.7 were selected based on several criteria, primarily ease of culture, commercial availability, and size. The test species are acclimated for a specific time prior to testing to eliminate diseased organisms. Generally, a minimum of 10 animals are exposed in static and static-renewal tests and 20 in a flow-through test to each test concentration and control. The recommended loading density for the test species is between 0.5–0.8 g/L in static tests and 1–10 g/L in continuous flow-through tests.

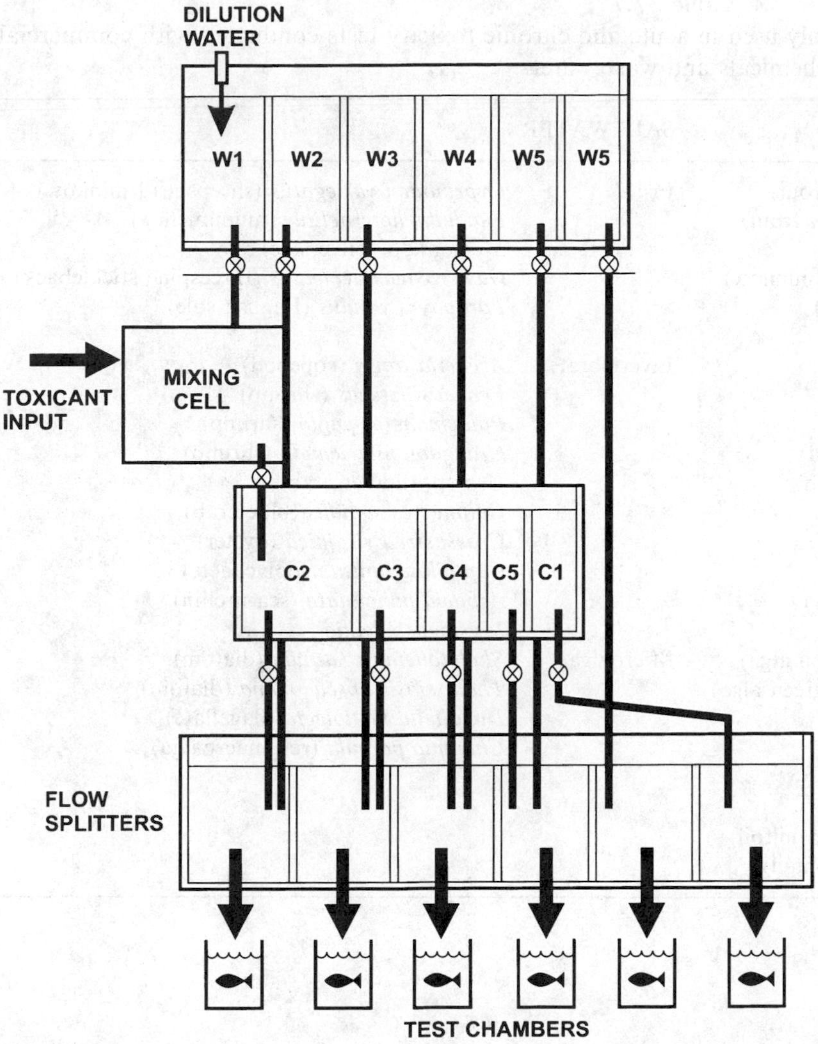

FIG. 37.2. Diagram of a proportional diluter designed to ensure that five concentrations of the toxicant are delivered to the test species in a toxicity test. Adapted from Landis and Yu (104).

Table 37.6
Most commonly reported test species in the AQUIRE database

Common name	Species	Percentage of reported data
Rainbow trout	*Salmo gairdneri*	8.6
Bluegill	*Lepomis macrochirus*	5.6
Fathead minnow	*Pimephales promelas*	4.9
Water flea	*Daphnia magna*	3.9
Carp	*Cyprinius carpio*	2.4
Coho salmon	*Oncorhynchus kisutch*	2.1
Goldfish	*Carassius auratus*	1.9
Channel catfish	*Ictalurus punctatus*	1.7
Mosquito fish	*Gambusia affinis*	1.5
Brook trout	*Salvelinus fontinalis*	1.0
Green alga	*Scenedesmus quadricauda*	0.9
Water flea	*Daphnia pulex*	0.8

Reference toxicants are often used to determine the "health" of the test species. There is no widely used reference toxicant; several that have been used include sodium dodecyl sulfate (anionic surfactant), sodium chloride, sodium pentachlorophenol, and cadmium chloride.

Sensitivity is a criterion that is also used in the choice of a test species. The sensitivities of the species in Table 37.7 relative to one another as well as to indigenous flora and fauna in the ecosystem is a matter of scientific contention (44). There is no single test species that is consistently most sensitive to toxicants or most reliable for extrapolation to all other organisms. Because toxicity is species specific, acute toxicity tests are conducted first with a variety of freshwater and marine test species to determine the most sensitive plant and animal. These sensitive species are then used in all subsequent chronic testing.

Table 37.7
Freshwater and saltwater test species commonly used in acute and chronic toxicity tests conducted with commercial chemicals and wastewaters

FRESHWATER		SALTWATER	
Fish	*Salvelinus frontinalis* (brook trout) *Oncorhynchus mykiss* (rainbow trout) *Carassius auratus* (goldfish) *Pimephales promelas* (fathead minnow) *Lepomis macrochirus* (bluegill) *Brachydanio rerio* (zebra fish)	Fish	*Cyprinodon variegatus* (sheepshead minnow) *Fundulus heteroclitus* (mummichog) *Menidia* sp. (silverside) *Gasterosteus aculeatus* (threespine stickleback) *Parophyrs vetulus* (English sole)
Invertebrates	*Daphnia magna* (daphnid) *Daphnia pulix* (daphnid) *Ceriodaphnia dubia* (daphnid) *Gammarus lacustris* (amphipod) *Gammarus fasciatus* (amphipod) *Ephemerella* sp. (mayfly) *Chironomus tentans* (midge) *Physa integra* (snail) *Brachionus calyciflorus* (rotifer)	Invertebrates	*Arcartia tonsa* (copepod) *Penaeus aztecus* (shrimp) *Palaemonetes pugio* (shrimp) *Crangdon migricauda* (shrimp) *Uca* sp. (fiddler crab) *Callinectes sapidus* (blue crab) *Crassostrea virginica* (oyster) *Capitella capitata* (polychaete) *Arbacia punctulata* (sea urchin) *Mysidopsis bahia*
Microalgae	*Selenastrum capricornum* (green alga) *Microcystis aeruginosa* (blue-green alga) *Navicula pelliculosa* (diatom)	Microalgae	*Skeletonema costatum* (diatom) *Thalassiosira pseudonana* (diatom) *Dunaliella tertiolecta* (flagellate) *Champia parvula* (red macroalga)
Aquatic vascular plant	*Lemna minor* (duckweed) *Lemna gibba* (duckweed) *Mysiophyllum spicatum* (water milfoil) *Ceratophyllum demersum* (coontail)		

Calculations

The results of acute toxicity tests are reported usually as the LC_{50} value and the corresponding 95% confidence interval. These calculations are determined using one of several statistical methods that are discussed in Stephan (173), such as probit analysis and moving average interpolation. Probit analysis (60) is the most commonly used statistical method to determine LC_{50} values. Graphical interpolation can be used also to estimate the LC_{50} value where the proportion of deaths versus the test concentration is plotted for each observation time.

The no observed effect concentration (NOEC) and lowest observed effect concentration (LOEC) are the usual calculations reported from chronic toxicity tests. The NOEC is the highest concentration in which the measured effect is not statistically different from that of the control. The LOEC is the lowest concentration at which a statistically significant effect occurred. These concentrations are based on the most sensitive effect parameter, that is, hatchability, growth, and reproduction. The statistical procedure for these calculations combines the use of analysis of variance techniques and multiple comparison tests. In some cases, the MATC (maximum acceptable toxic concentration) is reported from chronic toxicity results. The MATC is a concentration (x) that is within the range of the NOEC–LOEC, NOEC $< x <$ LOEC. The first-effect concentration can be expressed as the geometric mean of the two terms.

Variability/Precision

Laboratory toxicity tests conducted with freshwater and saltwater species are considered relatively precise and reliable based on current information from inter- and intralaboratory comparisons of toxicity results. Generally, the LC_{50} values from acute toxicity tests conducted under similar experimental conditions vary less than threefold. This has been observed for metals, effluents, reference toxicants, and different organic compounds (1,43,44,67,74,132,151,154,196,197). Coefficients of variation (CV) for acute and chronic toxicity tests conducted with daphnid species and chemicals and effluents are between 27–39% (51,74,164,218). The CV values for several reference toxicants and acute daphnid studies ranged between 10–72% (115) and from 47–83% for chronic

Table 37.8
Usefulness of toxicity tests

CONTAMINATED SEDIMENT	COMMERCIAL CHEMICALS	REFINERY WASTEWATER
• *Daphnia magna*	• Acute lethality	Larval bioassays
• *Ceriodaphnia dubia*	• Early life stage	• Sea urchins
• Fathead minnow, alga, midge	• Reproduction	• Molluscs
• Oliochaete	• Bioaccumulation	• Fish
• Amphipod	• Algal assay	
• Protozoa, mayfly	• Organoleptic	Algal tests
	• Behavioral	• Growth
	• Histological	• Photosynthesis
	• Physiological	• Macrophyte life stage
	• In vitro	
		Growth tests
		• Fish
		• Crustacean
		Life cycle tests
		• Shrimp
		• Copepods
		Physiological tests
		• Echinochrome synthesis
		• Bioenergetic measurements

Adapted from Reference 68 for contaminated sediments, from Reference 122 for commercial chemicals, and from the American Petroleum Institute (1) for refinery effluent testing. Test types listed in decreasing order of importance.

toxicity tests with algae (196). Gersich et al. (66) reported that the LC_{50} values for *D. magna* varied less than threefold when conducted repetitively with seven toxicants. Anderson and Norberg-King (17) reported the CV values for a variety of freshwater and marine species and found minimal variation. They concluded that biological tests can be conducted with a precision similar to that for chemical-specific measurements.

Data Utility

One measure of the usefulness of toxicity tests is their frequency of use. Based on a review of the PMN (premanufacture notification) submissions for TSCA (Toxic Substances Control Act), the more frequently conducted tests are, in decreasing order, acute fish, acute invertebrates, algal toxicity, chronic toxicity, and terrestrial toxicity. In addition, several judgements on the value of toxicity tests to the scientific and regulatory communities have been reported (Table 37.8). The acute toxicity test was judged the most useful for commercial chemicals with tests monitoring behavioral, histological, and physiological effects being less useful. Toxicity tests with daphnids (*D. magna* and *Ceriodaphnia dubia*) were judged to be of more value in monitoring sediment toxicity than those with other species and early life stage tests were judged most useful to determine the toxicity of refinery wastewaters.

MULTISPECIES TOXICITY TESTS

The results of the standard acute and chronic single-species toxicity tests conducted in the laboratory cannot be used alone, for several reasons, to predict effects on natural populations, communities, and ecosystems. First, the cultured species in laboratory tests are often different from those found inhabiting most ecosystems and conditions, and the size of the test species, its life stage, and nutritional state can have an effect, among others, on toxicity. Second, the laboratory tests conducted under controlled conditions cannot duplicate the complex interacting physical and chemical conditions of ecosystems, such as seasonal changes in water temperature, dissolved oxygen, and suspended solids.

Table 37.9
Advantages and disadvantages of single-species and multispecies toxicity tests

	TEST TYPES	SINGLE-SPECIES	MULTISPECIES
Advantages	Acute Chronic Short-term sublethal Early life stage	• Simple • Cost effective • Standard protocols available • Existing databases • Rapid • Reproducible	• Conducted under more realistic conditions • Can simultaneously study different trophic levels • Can use indigenous species • Can study effect of environmental modification
Disadvantages	Microcosms Mesocosms Outdoor ponds Enclosures (limnocorrals) Lake/stream closing In-situ bioassay	• Responses of only individuals determined • Use nonindigenous species • Controlled experimental conditions • Fate processes ignored • Recovery rate not considered • Cumulative effects not studied • Ecological interactions not considered	• Not cost effective • Standard protocols largely absent • Poor replication • Adaptation not considered • Stability of exposure concentration uncertain • Data interpretation difficult

Third, aquatic species are usually exposed simultaneously to numerous potential toxicants (mixtures). Although the toxicities of binary and ternary mixtures have been evaluated for some chemicals in laboratory toxicity tests (125), the resultant information has predictive limitations.

Because of the deficiencies of single-species toxicity tests, multispecies toxicity tests have been developed to address ecosystem structural and functional processes (194). These tests include the use of laboratory microcosms and mesocosms such as outdoor ponds, experimental streams, and enclosures. There are no standardized procedures for these tests. They can be conducted with plant and animal species either obtained from laboratory cultures, or with biota collected from natural sources. They can be conducted indoors or outdoors. The toxic effects, in addition to those determined in single-species tests, are determined for structural parameters such as community similarity, diversity, and density, and functional parameters such as community respiration and photosynthesis. Effects on these parameters are reported as the NOEC and LOEC.

A brief description of the major types of multispecies toxicity tests follows and their advantages and disadvantages relative to single-species studies are summarized in Table 37.9. More detail concerning specific test conditions, replicability, and regulatory usefulness is available from a number of reviews (38,39,72,79,80,105, 140,190).

Laboratory Microcosms

A laboratory microcosm is a small model or "piece" of an ecosystem contained in a test chamber. The use of microcosms provides an opportunity to study the effect of contaminants on a biotic community in a controlled environment. Microcosms are assumed to be functionally similar to the ecosystem they represent, but they may differ in origin and structure (54). The biotic component may be "constructed" from several cultured single species (artificial microcosms) or it may represent a sample of a natural ecosystem collected and placed in the test chambers. For example, a microcosm may contain sediment, water, and indigenous flora and fauna collected from a river, lake, or pond, or it may contain reconstituted water, artificial sediment, and a predetermined number of protozoa, plants, invertebrates, and fish obtained from laboratory cultures.

The SAM (standardized aquatic microcosm) method (177) has a set density of 15 species and is the only "standardized" microcosm test method that is currently available (14). Twenty-four 3-l microcosms are used in this method, which can be aquaria. They contain a well-defined medium of trace metals and vitamins and 200 g of sand (sediment) to which chitin and cellulose are added. The tests are conducted in the laboratory at 22°C with a 12-h period of light at 80 $\mu E\ m^{-2}\ s^{-1}$. Ten species of algae and five species of invertebrates are added to the microcosms, which are intended to represent a new pond ecosystem. The test species are exposed to three test concentrations of the contaminant for 63 days during which observations are made on a variety of parameters, including algal biovolume, species diversity and density, and dissolved oxygen concentrations. The toxicant concentrations are renewed periodically during the study and biological and chemical measurements are taken weekly or biweekly depending upon the parameter. In addition to the SAM method, a variety of other microcosms have been reported in which the volume has ranged from 0.1–19 l in various test chambers such as flasks, jars, and glass carboys.

Outdoor Ponds

Outdoor ponds have been used to investigate the fate and effects of several chemicals, but primarily pesticides on aquatic life (31,80,190). There is no universally accepted test design and examples of their use can be found in the references in Table 37.2. A variety of plant and animal life has been exposed in these systems. Ponds of various sizes and shapes have been utilized. The depth is usually 1 m or less. Volumes have ranged from 10–650 m^3; volumes of 10 m^3 or less are usually not suitable.

Experimental Streams

Experimental streams have been used to assess the effects of heat, nutrients, metals, insecticides, and effluents on natural biota in studies ranging in duration from several days to several years. Experimental streams may be flow through or recirculating and may be located indoors or outdoors. The streams have ranged in length from 1–1000 m and have been constructed from Plexiglas troughs, plastic lined wood flumes, concrete, and aluminum troughs. The depth of most streams is usually less than 1 m. The streams are colonized with organisms prior to use. Sources of organisms (periphyton, invertebrates, and fish) may be laboratory cultures or natural ecosystems. Time of colonization has varied from a month to over a year.

An example of a typical experimental stream design follows and is based on the report of Hansen and Garton (78). In this study, 10 indoor "streams" were used to determine the effect of the insecticide, diflubenzuron, on organisms representative of those found in a freshwater stream. Each 6.1 m long stream contained natural substrate and invertebrates and algae collected from a small creek in Oregon. Paddle wheels circulated the well water through the streams with a midstream surface current of 30 cm/s. The water depth was 10 cm. The biota in the streams was allowed to equilibrate for 3 months prior to the 5-month exposure to the toxicant. Eight streams were paired to deliver the four test concentrations and the remaining pair served as the control. Light intensity was 200 fc with a natural diurnal light cycle being used. The insecticide was continuously delivered to the streams, and effect on biomass and diversity of plant and animal life were determined monthly. Water chemistry such as pH, hardness, and temperature were determined at least weekly.

Enclosures

Enclosures isolate a portion of an ecosystem that can be dosed with the toxicant in such a way that significant con-

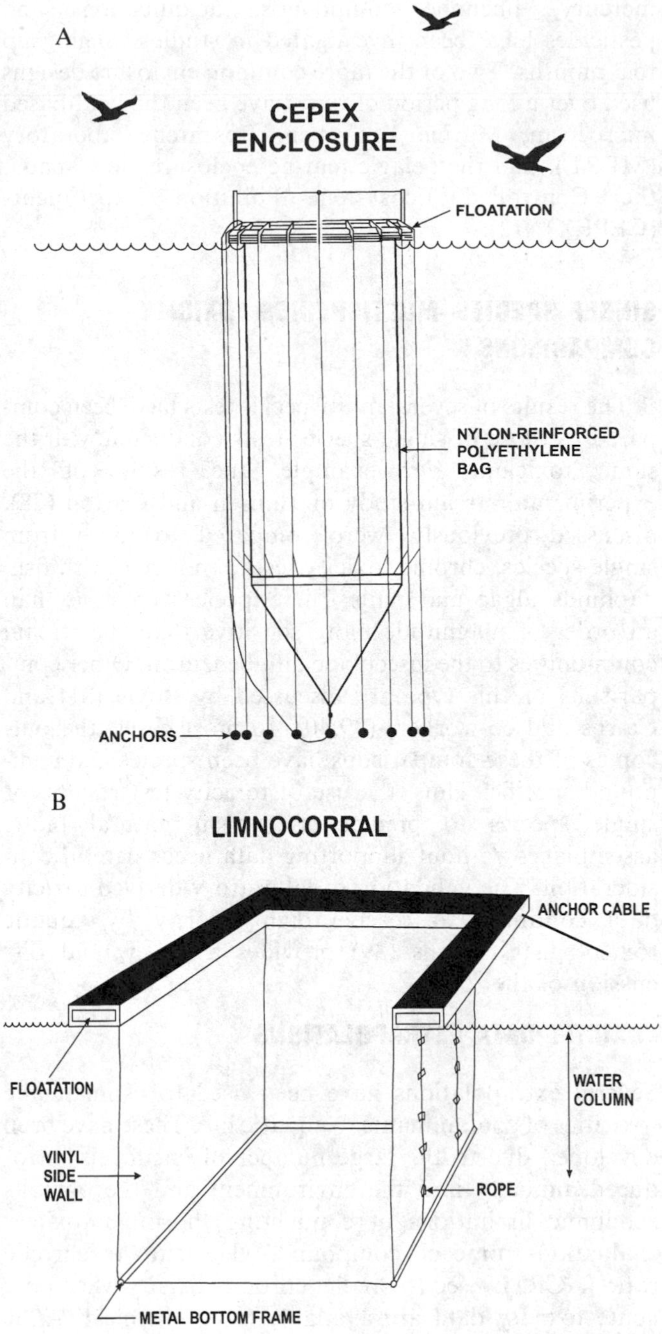

FIG. 37.3. Examples of enclosures used to expose natural biotic communities to toxicants. Enclosures represent those used in (A) the CEPEX program (72) and (B) a littoral design (limnocorral). See Reference 32 for more detail.

tamination beyond the limits of the enclosure will not occur (103). The size, shape, and volume of enclosures used have varied considerably. In freshwater experiments, the volumes have ranged from 8–300,000 l. Plastic tubes, carboys, plastic bags, and limnocorrals have been used to enclose the biota (Figure 37.3). The effects of oil, mercury, phenolic compounds, acidification, and pesticides have been investigated in studies ranging up to 3 months. Two of the more common enclosure designs used over a long period of time have been the land-based microcosm, Marine Ecosystem Research Laboratory (MERL), and the pelagic marine enclosures in Canada, the Controlled Ecosystem Pollution Experiments (CEPEX) (72).

SINGLE SPECIES–MULTISPECIES TOXICITY COMPARISONS

The results of several multispecies tests have been compared to those of single-species tests conducted with the same toxicant. For example, the results of the experimental stream study of Hansen and Garton (78), discussed previously, were compared to those from single-species, chronic toxicity tests conducted with fish, daphnids, algae, and snails. These species were more than an order of magnitude more sensitive than the stream communities to the insecticide diflubenzuron. Other comparisons of this type are discussed by Boyle (31) and Cairns and co-workers (39,40). In most cases, the outcomes of these comparisons have been species and compound specific. Thus, the use of toxicity test results for single species to predict effects on natural biotic assemblages without supporting data needs careful consideration. The validation of laboratory-derived toxicity data continues to receive high priority by aquatic toxicologists. Cairns (39) provides a review and discussion of the topic.

TOXICITY DATA EXTRAPOLATIONS

Several extrapolations have been used to estimate the toxicities of contaminants to aquatic life. These have been developed due to the large number of chemicals introduced annually into the environment and the obvious economic limitations of conducting thorough toxicity evaluations for each compound. The acute to chronic ratio (ACR) is used to predict chronic toxicity when only acute toxicity data are available for a chemical. ACR values have been reported for a variety of chemicals, particularly metals and pesticides, and most are 25 or less (96). Clements (47) reported several equations that can be used to estimate the acute and chronic toxicities of industrial chemicals such as surfactants based on their structure–activity relationships. Kenaga and Moolenaar (97), Maki (123), and LeBlanc (106) provide equations that can be used to predict acute toxicity of pesticides, metals, and nonpesticide organics to freshwater and marine algae, invertebrates, and fish based on interspecies relationships in sensitivity. McKim (129) discussed the relationship of results for partial and complete life cycle tests with fish.

As mentioned earlier, the results of single-species toxicity tests are often used to predict effects in the ecosystem with little known about the accuracy of the prediction. However, in some cases, multispecies toxicity test results are available and can be used with more confidence. In some cases, conservative "correction factors" are used to compensate for the limitations of the toxicity data. A variety of these correction techniques have been reported (145,208) and their usefulness reviewed (79,143). One of the more simple and common methods is the use of numerical "safety" or "uncertainty" factors to estimate "safe, concern, or risk" concentrations (53,188). Laboratory-derived chronic toxicity results, usually the NOEC, are divided by these factors, 1000, 100, and 10, to determine the concentration that, if exceeded in the ecosystem, may represent an environmental risk. The magnitude of the factor used depends upon the quantity and quality of the toxicity data available for the toxicant of interest. The greater the quality and quantity of data, the smaller the "safety" factor used. The technical validity and magnitude of these factors are largely unproven, although they are in general use. Consequently, this issue continues to be a subject of considerable debate within the scientific and regulatory communities.

SEDIMENT TOXICITY TESTS

In the past, toxicity tests have been conducted primarily with water column dwelling or planktonic organisms, with the objective of controlling water pollution. However, it has been realized that sediments act as "reservoirs" for chemicals that can adversely affect benthic aquatic life and, at times, also affect planktonic life. This concern has led to the development of sediment quality guidelines to protect benthic or bottom-dwelling life (46,120,166). Test methods have been developed to support the derivation of these criteria and to support other related regulatory activities, such as Superfund site evaluations and the disposal of dredged materials (45,193).

Sediment toxicity tests have been conducted in the laboratory with a variety of single species of freshwater and marine benthic organisms such as amphipods and midges, but planktonic species also have been used (Table 37.10). Most tests conducted to date have been acute and have been of 10-day duration or less. Sediment toxicity tests are conducted usually with the whole sediment (solid phase) or the pore water (interstitial water), although elutriates, sometimes solvent extracted, have also been used. An example of a whole sediment toxicity test is shown in Figure 37.4. In this test, an amphipod, such as that shown, is exposed to the field-collected sediment and mortality is recorded after 10 days of exposure.

Table 37.10
Several freshwater and salt water test species that have been used in sediment toxicity tests

Organism	Test duration (days)	Organism	Test duration (days)
Freshwater		Saltwater	
Hyalella azteca (amphipod)	28	*Rhepoxynius abronius* (amphipod)	10
Diporeia sp. (amphipod)	28	*Eohaustorius estaurius* (amphipod)	10
Chironomus riparius (midge)	14	*Ampelisca abdita* (amphipod)	10
Chironomus tentans (midge)	10	*Grandidierella japonica* (amphipod)	10
Hexagenia limbata (mayfly)	10	*Hyalella azteca* (amphipod)	28
Ceriodaphnia dubia (cladoceran)	7	*Leptocheirus plumulosus* (amphipod)	28
Daphnia magna (cladoceran)	10	*Neanthes* sp. (polychaete)	85
Lumbriculus variegatus	28	*Capitella capitata* (polychaete)	35
Tubifex tubifex	28	*Nereis virens* (polychaete)	12
		Sicyonia ingentis (prawn)	4
		Protothaca staminea (clam)	4
		Macoma nasuta (clam)	4
		Clevelanda ios (fish)	4
		Mytilus edulis (mussel)	2
		Crassostrea virginica (oyster)	2
		Strongylocentrotus purpuratus (sea urchin)	4
		Dendraster excentricus (sand dollar)	4
		Mysidopsis bahia (mysids)	4
		Menidia sp. (silversides)	4
		Atherinops affinis (top smelt)	4

Adapted from References 159 and 35. See Reference 179 for more detail.

Standard methods have been published describing the collection and preparation technique for sediments (3). Test guidelines for marine sediment (45,84) and freshwater sediment (35,36,69,136) have also been reported, as well as standardized test methods for freshwater invertebrates and freshwater and marine amphipods (9).

Recently, a chronic toxicity test has been developed for marine sediments (202). The results from such a test conducted with a sediment collected below a pulp mill outfall are shown in Table 37.11. Survival, growth, and reproductive effects of the amphipod, *Leptocheirus plumulosus*, were determined at the end of the 28-day toxicity test. Significant effects on the test species were noted at contaminated sediment concentrations of 10% (young production, fertility), 50% (survival), and 100% (length).

The availability of reliable test methods for contaminated sediments is relatively recent and the test method development process continues. A variety of issues remain to be solved before these types of studies will be considered as effective as those with planktonic species. Among the more important of these issues are validation of the single-species test results and determination of variations in species sensitivity.

EFFLUENT TOXICITY TESTS

Toxicity tests are used in the NPDES (National Pollutant Discharge Elimination System) permitting process to determine the toxicities of municipal and industrial effluents and storm water overflows on aquatic life. A summary of the experimental conditions in several of the available test methodologies appears in Table 37.12. The methodologies differ slightly from those used for pure chemicals. For example, the choice of the dilution water and effluent collection technique are important considerations. In most cases water collected from the receiving water above the outfall is used for dilution, and composite samples of effluent are used. The test species, an alga, invertebrate, or fish, is usually exposed to five effluent dilutions for 4–7 days. The tests are static renewal except those for algae, which are static. The calculations reported are the LC_{50} value, the NOEC, and the LOEC, which are expressed as percent effluent. The specific cause(s) of toxicity in the effluent can be identified using a toxicity identification evaluation (TIE) that consists of comparative toxicity testing and chemical fractionation techniques (133, 134).

Table 37.11
Results of a 28-day chronic sediment toxicity test conducted with the marine amphipod, *Leptocheirus plumulosus*

Test concentrations	Mean survival %	Young production (number of juveniles)	Fertility[a]	Mean length (mm)[b]
Control	97	91	59	5.83
10	93	32	31	5.31
25	92	30	19	5.45
50	83	8	6	4.95
100	9	0	0	3.06

Notes: The sediment was collected below a pulp mill-dominated wastewater discharge. Contaminated sediment was diluted with a noncontaminated reference sediment to obtain the test concentrations. For more detail on methodology see DeWitt et al. (52).

[a] $\text{Fertility} = \dfrac{\dfrac{\text{no. of juveniles } (F_1)}{2}}{\dfrac{2}{\text{surviving females } (F_0)}}$

[b] Of survivors.

The freshwater invertebrate, *Ceriodaphnia dubia*, is a test species commonly used in effluent toxicity evaluations and a brief description of its use in a typical test follows. *C. dubia*, obtained from a laboratory culture, are exposed to an effluent collected within 72 h from the source. The static-renewal test is usually conducted in a laboratory located off-site from the effluent source but the tests may be conducted on-site using a mobile bioassay facility. The test is conducted at 25°C, 10–20 $\mu E\ m^{-2}\ s^{-1}$, and under a photoperiod of 16 h light/8 h dark. The five test concentrations include undiluted effluent (100%) and four dilutions such as 50, 25, 12, and 6%. The effluent is diluted with either a high quality laboratory water or water collected from the receiving water above the effluent outfall. The control is comprised of 100% dilution water. For each test concentration and the control, 10 30-ml plastic test chambers containing 15-ml of the test solution are used. Each test chamber contains one daphnid and daily observations on mortality and young production are made during the 7-day test. The organisms are fed daily a combination of yeast, trout chow, and algae. Surviving organisms are transferred daily to renewed test solutions. The NOEC and LOEC values are determined based on the adverse effects on survival and reproduction occurring during the 7-day test.

The results of three wastewater toxicity tests are shown in Table 37.13. Three saltwater test species were exposed to a municipal wastewater for 4–7 days following standard procedures such as those in Table 37.12. The interspecific differences in response are obvious. It can be seen that the wastewater stimulated algal growth at a diluted concentration as low as 6%. The same wastewater concentration however, was not toxic to fish but did have an adverse effect on an estuarine invertebrate (mysid). For this species, a 63% mortality was observed after exposure to the 100% wastewater concentration.

PHYTOTOXICITY

The majority of aquatic toxicity tests has been conducted with animal test species because they were once thought to be more sensitive than plants. This generalization is not technically supported based on a review of the data for most toxicants (110). Nevertheless, only recently have phytotoxicity tests been routinely conducted with a limited number of species of algae and vascular plants.

A variety of test methods is available to determine the phytotoxic effects of chemicals and effluents (Table 37.14). The freshwater algal species most frequently used has been the green microalga, *Selenastrum capricornutum*, for which a relatively large database exists (108). Marine species used include the diatom *Skeletonema costatum*, the flagellate *Dunaliella tertiolecta*, and the red macroalga *Champia parvula*.

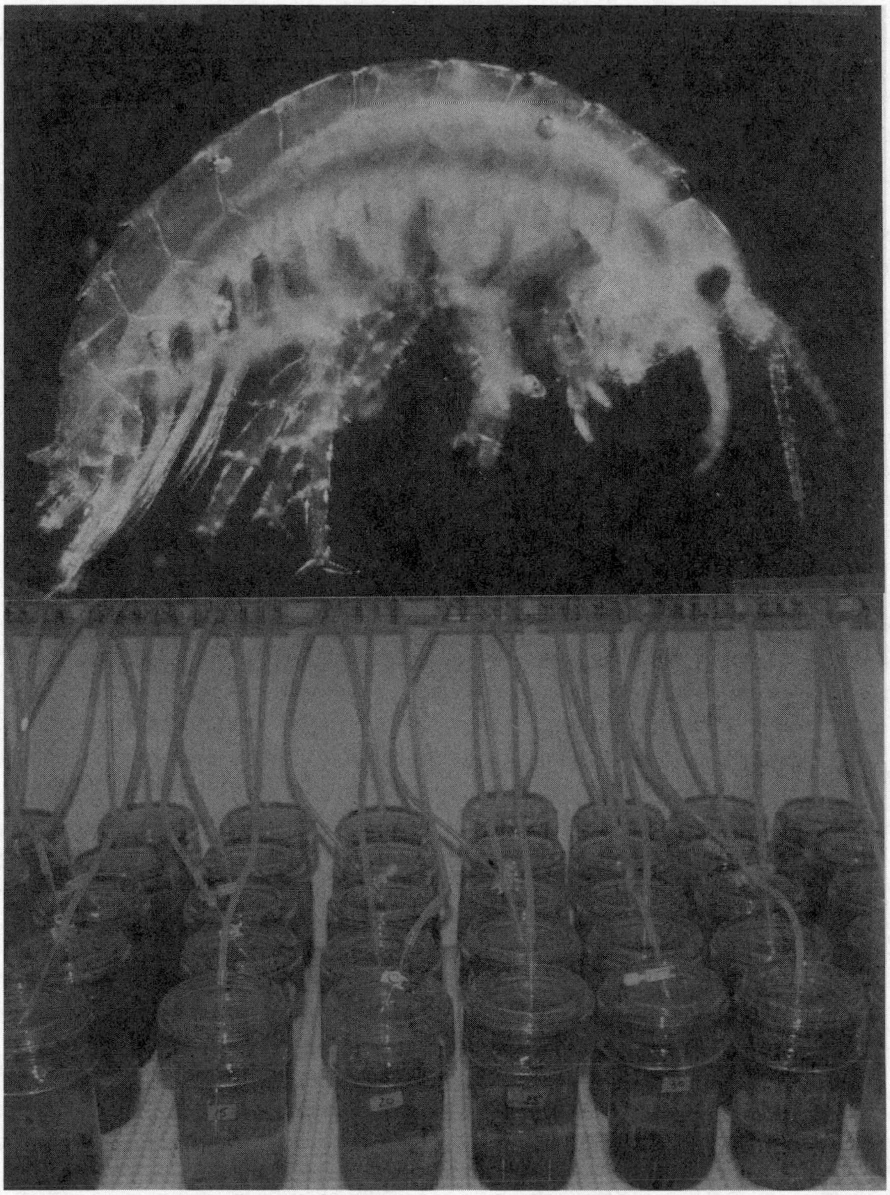

FIG. 37.4. An example of a solid-phase sediment toxicity test and a common benthic invertebrate test species.

Most toxicity tests conducted with algae are chronic. These tests are for 3–4 days duration, although exposures can be less than 1 day if effects on photosynthesis are measured. These static exposures occur in a liquid nutrient-enriched medium under conditions of controlled pH, temperature, and light. Inhibitory and stimulatory effects on population growth are monitored during the exponential growth phase. Five test concentrations and a control are included in each study. The most common calculation reported is the 96-h IC_{50} value (concentration that reduces the parameter of interest 50%), but algistatic (completely stops growth) and algicidal (lethal) concentrations have also been reported. In addition, the SC_{20} concentration (stimulatory concentration) is reported if growth stimulation is observed. The SC_{20} value represents that concentration that increases algal growth 20% above that of the algal population in the control.

Floating and rooted vascular plants are used less frequently in toxicity tests than algae. The duckweeds (freshwater floating species) are more commonly used than most due to their small size and rapid growth. Hillman (85) describes in detail the taxonomy and morphology of the duckweeds. Several published methods are available describing their use, particularly for *Lemna minor* and *L. gibba* (5,89,208,214,215). Tests

Table 37.12
Comparison of several experimental variables in chronic toxicity tests conducted with effluents

Test type	Duration (days)	No. of test concentrations	Test species	Age of test organisms	Total test species exposed[a]	No. of replicates	Temperature (°C)	Light intensity ($\mu E\ m^{-2}\ s^{-1}$)
Static-renewal	7	5	*Fathead minnow* (freshwater fish)	< 24 h	30–60	3–4	25 ± 1	10–20
Static-renewal	7	5	Sheepshead minnow (marine fish)	< 24 h	30–60	3–4	25 ± 2	10–20
Static-renewal	7	5	*Ceriodaphnia dubia* (freshwater invertebrate)	< 24 h	10	10	25 ± 1	10–20
Static-renewal	7	5	*Mysidopsis bahia* (marine invertebrate)	< 24 h	40	8	26–27	10–20
Static	4	5	*Selenastrum caricornutum* (freshwater) (green alga)	4–7 d	1×10^4 (initial density)	3	25 ± 1	86 ± 8.6
Static	4	5	*Skeletonema costatum* (marine) (diatom)	4–7 d	2×10^4 (initial density)	3	20 ± 2	60 ± 6

See USEPA (196,197) and Reference 154 for more information.
[a] Per test concentration.

Table 37.13

Response of an alga (*Dunaliella tertiolecta*), fish (*Cyprinodon variegatus*), and an invertebrate (*Mysidopsis bahia*) exposed in laboratory toxicity tests to a treated municipal wastewater

Species	Wastewater concentration (%)	Effect parameters					
Alga		Growth (% of control)					
	Control	100					
	6	160					
	12	144					
	25	222					
	50	178					
	100	756					
Fish		Mortality (%)	Mean Weight (mg)				
	Control	0	1.00				
	6	0	1.10				
	12	0	0.84				
	25	2	1.01				
	50	2	0.90				
	100	2	0.90				
				Reproductive Maturity			
Invertebrate		Mortality (%)	Mean weight (mg)	♀ Eggs	♀ No eggs	♂ Immature	♂ Mature
	Control	2	0.21	8	7	17	7
	6	4	0.30	8	7	18	6
	12	12	0.27	3	9	14	9
	25	8	0.32	6	7	17	7
	50	20	0.19	2	3	13	10
	100	63	0.25	1	5	9	19

Note: The test durations ranged from 4 to 7 days following USEPA procedure (196).

with these species are usually of 4–14 days duration, during which effects on frond number and chlorophyll content are monitored. The results are expressed as an EC_{50} value and the NOEC. The tests are conducted, like algae, in a nutrient-enriched medium. The test chambers can be jars, plastic cups, test tubes, and Erlenmyer flasks. The key research issue that remains to be investigated before the duckweeds will be more widely accepted as suitable tests species is their sensitivity relative to other aquatic plant and animal test species.

The use of rooted vascular plants such as pondweeds (*Potamogeton* spp.), waterweeds (*Elodea, Hydrilla*), the water hyacinth (*Eichhornia crassipes*), coontail (*Ceratophyllum demersum*), and water milfoil (*Myriophyllum* spp.) in toxicity tests is less common than that for algae and duckweed due to their large size and slow growth. There are no standard or commonly used test methods for these species. The experimental techniques that have been used vary considerably; examples of these can be found in Forney and Davis (63), Sortkjaer (169), and Guilizzoni (75). Recently, seeds from aquatic macrophytic vegetation have been used to assess the toxicities of chemicals and effluents. These studies are usually of 4–7 days duration, and the effect parameters are seed germination, root elongation, and early seedling growth. Seedlings of several species have been used to determine the effects of contaminated sediments (212,217). These studies may be up to 28 days in length. It has been found that plants do respond to phytotoxic substances in sediments (Figure 37.5) and therefore should be used in surveys for contaminated sediment.

In conclusion, the use of rooted macrophytes and their seeds in toxicity tests will increase in the future as the development of sediment quality criteria to protect aquatic life and wetlands increase in regulatory importance.

Table 37.14
Experimental conditions in several phytotoxicity tests conducted with algae and duckweed

Test Type	Duration (days)	No. of test concentrations	Test species[a]	No. of replicates	Temperature (°C)	Light intensity (μE m^{-2} s^{-1})
Algae						
Static	4	5	*Selenastrum capricornutum* (F) *Scenedesmus quadricauda* (F) *Chlorella vulgaris* (F) *Skeletonema constatum* (M)	3	20–24	300±25
Static	3	5	*Selenastrum capricornutum* (F) *Scenedesmus subspicatus* (F)	3	21–25	120±20%
Static	4	5	*Selenastrum capricornutum* (F) *Microcystis aeruginosa* (F) *Anabaena flos-aquae* (F) *Navicula pelliculosa* (F) *Skeletonema costatum* (M) *Dunaliella tertiolecta* (M)	3	20–24	30–90
Duckweed						
Flow-through	7	5	*Lemna minor*	4	22.8±.6	2700 lux
Static	14	5	*Lemna gibba*	3	25±2	100
Static	4	5	*Lemna minor*	3–6	27±2	6456 lux

Notes: Methods for algae are from OECD (148) and ASTM (5), respectively. Methods for duckweed are from References 209, 89, and 214.
[a] F = Freshwater, M = Marine.

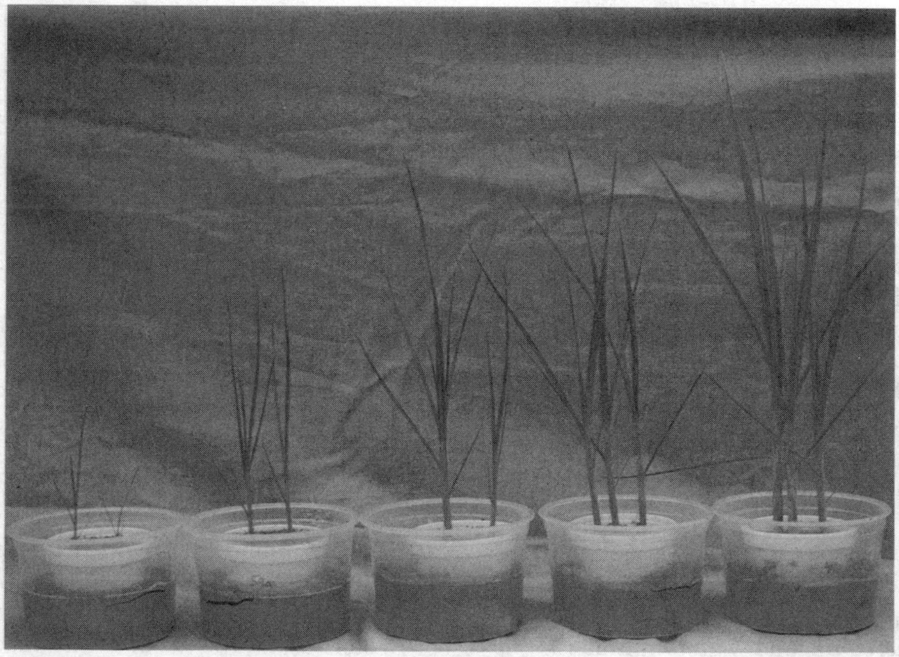

FIG. 37.5. The response of a rooted vascular plant (*Echinochloa crusgalli*) to several field-collected sediments. The differential growth of the species is obvious after the 14-d exposures.

Table 37.15
Several experimental conditions in a OECD bioconcentration test (147)

Test species	Carp (yearling)
Loading	8 g/L
Flow regime	Flow-through
Test concentrations	< .01 LC_{50} value
	< .001 LC_{50} value
Test duration	
Uptake	8 weeks
Steady state	Mandatory
Elimination	Mandatory
Dilution water	Well water/city water
Sampling frequency	Water—16 times
	Fish—8 times
Lipid content	Optional
Bioconcentration factor	C_{fish}/C_w

However, for this to occur test method development and validation and determination of species sensitivity will be needed.

BIOCONCENTRATION

A bioconcentration study is conducted to derive information on the ability of an aquatic species to concentrate a toxicant in its tissues (76). This uptake and accumulation can be hazardous to the organism as well as to other aquatic life utilizing the test species as a feed source. Bioconcentration tests are usually conducted with single chemicals and single species of algae, fish, and bivalve molluscs. A variety of fishes have been used, including the fathead minnow, bluegill, rainbow trout, and sheepshead minnow, and several species of oysters, scallops, and mussels. There are several test designs that can be used to estimate the bioconcentration potential of a compound, one of which is shown in Table 37.15. Typically, a group of the test species is exposed to the toxicant for an uptake and depuration phase. A control is included in which the test species is not exposed to the toxicant. In assessing the concentration of the test chemical in the organism, the literature contains examples of measuring total residues and measuring only the parent compound. The uptake phase is usually for 28 days or until a steady state is attained. The depuration period lasts until the concentration in the test species is 10% of the steady-state concentration in the tissue. During both phases, the test water and test species are analyzed daily for the test chemical. All results from a bioconcentration study are based on measured concentrations.

The uptake rate, depuration rate, and the bioconcentration factor (BCF) are typically reported. The relevance of the BCF value to the survival of the organism and to ecosystem dynamics is an issue that has received and continues to receive significant scientific attention. Recent reports provide important information on this and other technical issues related to tissue residues and their relevance to the individual and the ecosystem (48,198,201). Furthermore, reports are available that summarize the bioaccumulation potentials for polychlorinated biphenyls (PCBs) (196), polycyclic aromatic hydrocarbons (PAHs) (50), and pesticides (37).

TERRESTRIAL SYSTEMS

Standardization of toxicity testing for environmental problems in terrestrial systems lags behind that for aquatic systems. Risk-based soil quality guidelines have been developed by the Canadian Council of Ministers of the Environment (42) and selected Canadian provinces (e.g., ref. 26). No such guidelines exist in the United States, although the U.S. Environmental Protection Agency (EPA), Office of Solid Waste and Emergency Response, is in the process of developing ecological soil screening levels for contaminated site assessments, with the intent of having such values available by the year 2000. Several of the EPA regions have developed soil preliminary remediation goals (PRGs) for contaminated site clean-up for the protection of human health (e.g., ref. 200). The European countries, through an effort coordinated by the European Union, are in the process of developing procedures for contaminated site clean-up that likely will contain some form of soil screening values for protection of both human health and ecological receptors. This process, known as CARACAS (Concerted Action on Risk Assessment for Contaminated Sites), has completed one publication on the scientific basis of risk assessment for contaminated sites and is expected to be completed in 2002 following release of at least two additional publications.

Because of the lack of applicable soil quality criteria, and the difficulty in applying such criteria to specific sites within the heterogeneous soil ecosystem, terrestrial environmental toxicology still relies on standardized bioassays for assessing toxicity of new and existing chemicals to plants, wildlife, and soil ecosystem functions. These tests fall into one of two major categories: (i) a priori toxicity tests of single chemicals proposed for use or disposal in terrestrial systems and (ii) site-specific assessments of extant contamination. Both approaches utilize the same suite of tests for determining plant, wildlife, and soil toxicity and rely, to some extent, on data generated for human toxicology studies, although they differ significantly in their risk assessment approach

(58). All of the tests discussed below in detail have standard operating procedures published by the EPA and/or the American Society for Testing and Materials (ASTM) or the Organization for Economic Co-operation and Development (OECD). Many of these tests are under discussion for revision to incorporate up-to-date statistical designs and measurement of potential disruption of the endocrine system (e.g., ref. 150). However, at the time of this writing, no revisions have been formally accepted to the protocols as they are presented here. Additional tests are being developed and, where appropriate, references will be provided to direct the reader desiring further information.

Avian Tests

Laboratory Tests

Single chemical tests for acute, subchronic, and chronic reproductive toxicity have accepted standard methods. The EPA requires tests with bobwhite quail (*Colinus virginianus*) and mallards (*Anas platyrhynchos*) at a minimum for pesticide registration, so the largest database of toxicity information and testing experience for such compounds is available for these species, although relatively large databases also exist for Japanese quail (*Coturnix coturnix japonica*) and ring-necked pheasant (*Pahianus colchicus*) (82,83). However, the test methods are equally applicable to all other avian species, provided that appropriate adjustments are made in caging and feeding regimens (90,165).

The acute toxicity test (LD_{50}) is required when determining effects of ingestion of pesticide granules, seed treatments, or baits (181) or for comparative toxicology (90,165). A modified version of this test has been developed for testing potential toxicity of alternative shot pellets developed for waterfowl hunting (204). The LD_{50} test (185) requires the use of adult birds ($\geq$16 weeks old for bobwhite quail and mallards). Within a given test, all birds should be from the same hatch, unless the test is being conducted with wild birds. All birds should be of uniform weight and size and absent of obvious signs of disease. Birds should be housed under acceptable animal husbandry practices with a 10 h light/14 h dark cycle in order to avoid inducing a reproductive state. Animals should be acclimated to the test environment for a minimum of 2 weeks prior to starting the test. For pesticide testing, a minimum of six birds per dose level is required with the doses arranged by geometric progression such that at least one dose will be below the calculated LD_{50} and one dose above and one control group (administered carrier only). For nontoxic shot studies, 10 birds of each sex are dosed with 8 no. 4 shot, and a similar negative control (steel shot) and a positive control (lead shot) also are dosed. Birds should be fasted for 15 h prior to exposure; at all other times they should be allowed ad libitum access to feed and water. Chemical or shot should be administered through oral intubation into the crop or proventriculus, preferably in an encapsulated form, as birds frequently regurgitate liquid formulations or small pellets. The test animals should be observed for a minimum of 14 (pesticide) or 30 (shot) days postexposure, and all signs of intoxication and number and time of mortality recorded. For pesticide studies, if more than one bird from the control group dies during the 14-day period, the test may be considered invalid. Necropsies and histopathological studies of all birds that die during the test are encouraged. For studies of alternative shot, measurement of hematocrit, hemoglobin concentration, and other specified blood chemistries are required on days 15 and 30 postexposure, and histopathological analysis is required of liver and kidney at test termination. Additionally, analytical chemistry analysis of these or other tissues may be required to ascertain residue concentrations For pesticide studies, the LD_{50} value is calculated, along with the 95% confidence interval, using probit analysis (61) or other acceptable statistical method.

The subchronic avian toxicity test (LC_{50}) is conducted using 10- to 14-day-old bobwhite quail or 5- to 10-day-old mallards, although the test is not limited to these species (8,25,185). Birds used in the test should be either wild birds or pen-reared birds that are phenotypically indistinguishable from wild birds, preferably from colonies with known breeding history. If possible, all test birds should be from a single hatch and only birds free of obvious injury and disease should be used. Birds must be kept in brooders of appropriate dimensions and temperature (about 35°C for bobwhite quail and mallards). The standard protocol does not require a certain lighting regimen; however, because the length of the photoperiod influences daily feed consumption, it is recommended that a 10 h light/14 h dark or a 12 h light/12 h dark cycle be maintained. Water should be available ad libitum. A standard commercial game bird diet in mash or crumble should be used for mallard and bobwhite tests. Appropriate formulations should be developed as needed for other species. If possible, the test material should be added to the diet without the use of a vehicle. If a vehicle is needed, water is preferred but reagent grade evaporative material (acetone, methylene chloride) may be used if necessary and completely evaporated at room temperature prior to feeding. Other acceptable vehicles include table-grade corn oil, propylene glycol, carboxymethylcellulose, and gum arabic. The toxicant is added to feed in a ratio of 2 parts of solution to 98 parts of feed by weight, and subsampling should be done to confirm uniformity of mixing. Large batches may be mixed in mechanical feed mixers or similar devices. It is encouraged that feed batches be analyzed and actual concentrations be reported along with the nominal value. The chemical should be administered in at least four concentrations spaced geometrically to produce mortality ranging from 10–90%. A concurrent control group and a vehicle-control group (if appropriate) are required. A minimum of 10 birds is required for each dose and control group. Birds should be acclimated to the testing conditions and fed at least 2 weeks prior to presentation of treated feed. Birds are exposed to treated feed for 5 days, followed by an observation period on clean feed for at least 3 days or until mortality ceases. There must be at least 72 consecutive h without treatment-related mortality, and control mortality may not exceed 10% during this period for the test to be considered valid. Throughout the test, all signs of intoxication should be recorded, including time of onset and duration. Times of all mortalities must be recorded. Estimates of average feed consumption must be made for each pen of birds, with weighing of feed occurring at the beginning and end of the pretreatment, treatment, and observation periods. Provisions for minimizing spillage should be reported. Necropsies and histopathological examination of all dead birds are suggested. The LC_{50} and 95% confidence interval must be reported, along with the method used to determine these statistics.

Avian reproductive effects and chronic toxicity endpoints are determined according to methods described by the EPA (130,185) and in ASTM E1062 (10). The U.S. Fish and Wildlife Service (204) has modified these protocols for testing of alternative nontoxic shot to include a cold stress (ambient temperatures of -6.6–4.4°C) and dietary stress (a diet for mallards consisting of whole kernel corn). As with the subchronic toxicity test, birds should be pen-reared and phenotypically indistinguishable from wild birds. Additionally, it is recommended that the birds come from a colony that has maintained breeding records and that all birds be free of obvious disease or injury. Bobwhite quail should be at least 16 weeks old at the beginning of the test period and mallards should be at least 7 months of age. Ages of other bird species should correspond to known times of reproductive maturity. Birds should be acquired in a quiescent reproductive state, so onset of egg laying occurs in the test facility. Birds should be acclimated to the test environment for 2–6 weeks prior to the presentation of treated feed. Birds must be maintained in pens and/or rooms that conform to good husbandry practices (138), with minimum space being defined as the ability to stand upright and stretch the wings to the full extent possible. Birds may be housed as one pair per pen or in groups (one male and two females per pen for bobwhite quail or two males and five females for mallards). Generally, tests are conducted indoors; however, for some birds (e.g., kestrels) it is more appropriate to house them outside and the alternative shot study allows for this practice if the study is conducted in a cold weather environment. Photoperiod must be rigorously controlled, as the onset and maintenance of reproductive activity is determined by the length of the light period. During the acclimation period and for the first 8 weeks of a test conducted indoors, the photoperiod should be set at 7 or 8 h of light per day. The photoperiod should then be increased to 16 h of light per day, preferably by gradually increasing the day length over a 2-week period, and be maintained at this level for the remainder of the test. Lights should have an intensity of approximately 65 lux (6-ft candles) at each cage. For outdoor test environments, the tests should be initiated according to the phenology of the species tested, such that presentation of treated feed begins approximately 10 weeks prior to the anticipated onset of egg laying.

Feed preparation should follow the same guidelines discussed above for the subchronic test, with a minimum of one control and two test doses. Both test doses should be at sublethal concentrations and frequently represent known environmental concentrations. If a no-observable-adverse-effect level (NOAEL) determination is required, then three concentrations arranged in a geometric progression should be used in addition to the control group. The test chemical should be administered for at least 10 weeks prior to the onset of egg laying and continue until all control pens have produced 25 eggs, or 6 weeks after 50% of the control hens have laid one egg. For studies of nontoxic shot, birds are orally gavaged with one no. 4 lead pellet (positive control), or eight no. 4 pellets of either the test shot or steel shot (negative control), with a minimum of four pairs in the lead treatment group and 20 pairs in the other treatment groups. Shot is administered on 0, 30, 60, and 90 days after the start of the study.

Feed and water should be presented ad libitum for the entire test period and feed consumption should be recorded at least biweekly throughout the study. Eggs should be collected daily, marked according to the pen from which the eggs were collected, and stored at 16°C, 65% relative humidity. All eggs should be set in incubators once a week at a temperature and humidity suitable for the species being tested. Parental incubation and rearing of chicks may be used if suitable artificial husbandry parameters cannot be determined. Eggs should be candled on day 0 to look for cracks and on days 11 and 18 (bobwhite quail) or 14 and 21 (mallards) to determine fertility and embryo survival. Eggs collected on one day of weeks 1, 3, 5, 7, and 9 of the egglaying period should be opened at the equator, the contents washed out, and shells dried and measured for the thickness of the shell plus the membranes to the nearest 0.01 mm. Eggs should be transferred to a hatcher one day before expected pipping (day 21 for bobwhite quail and 23 for mallards). Hatchability for each egg batch is recorded and chicks are placed in brooders for 14 days and fed a control diet ad libitum. Survival at the end of 14 days is recorded. All birds should be weighed weekly prior to the onset of egg laying and at the termination of the experiment; handling should be minimized during the egg laying period to reduce disturbance. In addition to weight changes, reported endpoints include daily egg production per pen; type and frequency of abnormal eggs (including cracks and other gross defects); number of incubated eggs that are fertile (fertility); the number of fertile eggs that produce hatchlings that completely free themselves from the shell (hatchability); the number of normal young surviving to 14 days of age; weight of young at 1 day and 14 days of age; eggshell thickness; and chemical residue in tissues of adults, chicks, and eggs. Alternative shot studies also require measures of hematocrit, hemoglobin concentration, and appropriate blood chemistries. Standard appropriate statistical analyses should be conducted to determine if treated birds differ from controls or to ascertain the dose–response relationship.

Field Tests

Methods for examining effects of toxic substances on birds under field conditions have been developed by EPA Office of Pesticide Programs for use in obtaining pesticide registration data. A specific protocol for assessing reproductive effects using starlings (*Sturnus vulgaris*), representative cavity-nesting passerines, has been published (98) and is described here. Additional guidance for field determinations of mortality, behavioral effects, and territoriality changes will be presented briefly. Generally, field studies to determine effects of specific toxic substances are conducted only if preliminary laboratory studies indicate a potential hazard (e.g., high acute toxicity) and have been developed primarily for pesticide registration testing. However, these techniques are being adopted for use in determining individual level and population level effects of existing environmental pollution, such as at hazardous waste sites (216). Methods for field surveys of bird density, community composition, nesting success, and other ecologically relevant endpoints have a long history of use in biological assessments (30), but only recently have become widely used for ecotoxicological assessments. However, these methods are beyond the scope of this chapter and will not be discussed further here. Of more direct relevance are standardized controlled field studies, which are described below.

The starling nest box study (98) is one means of introducing standardized testing procedures into a field study. Nest boxes encourage starlings to nest within a study site and establish a large local population with readily accessible nests from which chemical-induced reproductive, behavioral, and biochemical perturbations can be documented. The full scale test is a 3-year procedure. The first field season serves as a pilot study in which 30 nest boxes are erected on each of 12 fields and occupancy and reproduction are documented. Pesticide application occurs in the definitive study during years 2 and 3 in a paired block design (i.e., each treated field is paired with a similar control field). The type of fields selected depend upon the pesticide (or other chemical) to be applied, although starlings prefer grasslands (e.g., hay fields), which should be selected in preference over other field types. Study fields are 16 hectares in size and should be located next to similarly cropped fields in order to keep starlings foraging on the test sites. Study sites must be located at least 3 km from each other to reduce the possibility that starlings will leave their initial study site and forage in another study area.

Nest boxes are constructed from utility grade lumber and measure $29 \times 23 \times 38$ cm ($l \times w \times h$). The back portion of the box, which attaches to the post, is 58 cm in length, centered so that 10 cm extends above and below the box. The box is attached to the top of a 10 cm × 10 cm × 3.67 m ($l \times w \times h$) post with aluminum sheet metal tubing placed around the post, starting immediately below the box and extending down about 75 cm to reduce predation. Nest boxes must be placed in the fields so that crop culture can occur with minimal disturbance. Therefore, boxes are placed in a single row down the middle of the field in the same orientation as the crop rows. Boxes are separated by 10 m and erected at least 2 months before the beginning of the breeding season.

Following the placement of the nest boxes, 7 days are allowed to pass before first observations are made. This allows time for the starlings to locate and utilize the nest boxes without disturbance. During the initial nest building stage (by males), observations are made every 4 days. When the females arrive and during the mating period, observations are made every 3 days. Once eggs are observed in the nest, observations are made every other day. Daily observations are made from the time hatching begins until fledging occurs. During all monitoring periods, observations are made between 11:30 AM and 3:00 PM, the time of least activity by the birds. Following are the reproductive information observed or calculated from nest box observations.

a. Date of nest box selection (based on the presence of some nesting material)
b. Notes on the development of the nest (amount of nest building material, quality of the nest, presence of a nest cup, etc.)
c. Date of the laying of the first egg (the previous day is designated the date of nest completion)
d. Interval of egg-laying

e. Clutch size
f. Number of eggs missing or broken
g. Number of eggs that hatch
h. Date of egg hatch
i. Number of missing or dead nestlings
j. Weight of 16-day-old nestlings (g)
k. Number of fledglings on each day
l. Date of fledging

Additional information collected includes weather data (maximum and minimum daily temperature, precipitation events, wind speed), observations of behaviors of adult starlings, and presence of predators in the study area. The study continues until all eggs and nestlings from the second clutch (starlings generally produce two clutches of eggs per breeding season) have hatched and fledged or died and at least 2 weeks have passed without any more eggs being laid. If none of the eggs hatch but remain in the nest box, the study is terminated when the last box occupied prior to the chemical application has been monitored for 12 days after the laying of the final egg in the clutch. All nestlings that are found dead in the box are analyzed for brain cholinesterase activity, liver enzyme induction, and/or tissue residues to verify cause of death (choice of assay is dependent upon the chemical being studied).

If the study being conducted is a pesticide safety study, the application rate of the pesticide should be the highest concentration proposed for registration. The timing of the application is dependent upon the age class of starling nestlings. The initial (or single) application to the fields should be performed when there is the greatest number of 1- to 14-day-old nestlings in the boxes. Pesticide application rates are verified through analysis of vegetation, spray cards, and subsampling of the pesticide holding tanks. For granular formulations, the deposition rate of the granules from the dispensing apparatus is measured. About 50 samples per field are required for an accurate representation of application rate.

The reproductive success of the starlings (as summarized by the number of fledglings per field) should be analyzed initially using a two-way analysis of variance (ANOVA) randomized block design, with the number of fledglings per field as the dependent variable, in order to determine differences between treatment groups. It is advisable to transform data using a square-root transformation prior to analysis. If this initial test shows significant differences, then inferential statistics should be used to identify which parameter(s) were affected.

Guidance for how to design and perform avian field studies for toxicity determinations is provided by Fite et al. (62). General guidelines are given for two kinds of studies: a general screening study to detect acute toxic effects resulting in mortality or obvious behavioral changes and a detailed, definitive study to quantify the magnitude of acute mortality, determine and measure reproductive impairment, and integrate indirect effects (e.g., feed reduction) that may influence the long-term survival of the subpopulation under study. The species and location for the study are determined primarily by the known or proposed location of the pollutant and the population densities and species diversity of the bird communities. The number of replicate study plots (both control and treatment) needed to make a determination of effect is based on the expected probability of occurrence of effect and the known variability of the system. True replicates are required and the tendency toward pseudoreplication must be avoided (91). Many statistical techniques are available for determining the minimum number of replicates required (66).

Information on population density, age and sex structure, and survival data can be acquired through a range of methods, including the use of mark-recapture techniques, radiotelemetry (33), line transects (for carcass searches), captures per unit effort, or counts of animal signs (30). Various models are available that utilize these types of data to determine probability of survival per unit time and intrinsic population growth rates (102). Reproductive success (from time of initiation of egg laying to fledging of young) is determined through visual observations of nests (egg and fledging counts), radiotelemetry of young, and behavioral observations (33,127).

In addition to documenting direct toxic effects to the species of concern, information also is gathered on the distribution and persistence of the chemical(s) in the environment. Relating harmful effects on animals to the degree of environmental contamination is dependent upon data establishing that a toxic dose has been reached for either the animal being studied or a second species upon which its survival depends on the environment being studied. These data can consist of tissue residues of the toxic chemicals or their metabolites, or through the use of markers of exposure, such as cholinesterase activity changes following exposure to organophosphorus or carbamate insecticides, or ALA-D (δ-aminolevulinic acid dehydratase) inhibition due to lead exposure. Both ALA-D and cholinesterase inhibition are legally acceptable indicators of harmful effects of exposure to environmental pollutants (139). Other biomarker responses have been developed and used in wildlife exposure studies for risk assessment purposes (e.g., cytochrome P450 induction), but are not yet standardized or legally acceptable endpoints (153). For persistent, bioaccumulative compounds, residues in feed sources and the lower portion of the feed web of the species of concern should also be measured in order to determine bioaccumulation and bioconcentration factors. It is important to recognize that for most chemicals, bioaccumulation is not a linear function of exposure concentration but rather attenuates at higher doses. Additional data about the effects of the chemical(s) on the feed source, competitors, or predators of the species of concern should also be gathered to ascertain whether indirect effects of feed reduction or changes in community composition may be affecting the endpoint species in addition to (or instead of) direct toxicology effects. These data must be interpreted in the context of what is known about the natural history and normal phenology of the species being studied.

Mammalian Tests

In environmental toxicology, mammalian effects data generally are gathered as part of human health impact studies. Both EPA (185) and ASTM (7,11) have published general guidelines for conducting acute and longer term toxicity studies with wild mammals and reference the avian and laboratory mammal protocols for more detailed approaches. For large or relatively scarce species, a single-dose regimen may be used where a group of three or more test animals are exposed to the chemical at a dose thought to be representative of expected environmental exposures and observed for at least 10 days for signs of intoxication. Additional doses may be tested sequentially if needed to develop a dose–response curve. This follows the method described for estimating acute oral toxicity in rats by the "up down method" (11) discussed in chapter 18.

Efficacy testing of anticoagulants in rodents (particularly rats and mice) is well developed as these animals are the target species (7). The tests present the animals with both contaminated feed and control feed simultaneously for a free-choice scenario, using a single concentration of chemical in the feed. Exposure times vary from 8–20 days, depending upon the species being tested, with a 7-day postexposure observation period. The higher the mortality, the greater the efficacy of the product.

Detailed protocols have also been developed for mink (*Mustela vison*) and the European ferret (*Mustela purotius furo*) as representative carnivores due to concern about compounds that bioconcentrate up the feed chain and those that might be expected to cause secondary poisoning due to high concentrations in the tissues of the target species. Both of these animals can be successfully propagated in the laboratory and stocks of known genetic origin are available. Additionally, the mink has been shown to be extremely sensitive to polychlorinated biphenyls (19), polybrominated biphenyls (20), hexachlorobenzene (28), aflatoxins (29), and 2,3,7,8-tetrachlorodibenzo-*p*-dioxin (86). Three protocols are available: dietary LC_{50}, reproduction, and secondary toxicity (162). For all three tests, animals should be of mature body weight (about 18–20 weeks of age). Either sex can be used in the subchronic dietary and secondary toxicity tests; however, the two sexes must be treated as separate subgroups due to significant size differences. Test animals may be obtained from commercial sources or reared in the laboratory and should be free from obvious disease or injury. It is recommended that mink be vaccinated against canine distemper, virus enteritis, infectious pneumonia, and botulism and that ferrets be vaccinated against canine distemper and botulism. Although space requirements for most carnivores have not been standardized, adherence to the guidelines of the Fur Farm Animal Welfare Coalition (64) should provide adequate husbandry guidance. Cages measuring $61 \times 76 \times 46$ cm ($l \times w \times h$) have proven adequate for housing individual mink or ferrets. Solid dividers should be used between adjoining cages to reduce aggression and a nest box containing straw, shredded wood, or marsh hay must be provided for females in reproduction tests prior to parturition. No specific photoperiod is required but the day length should not be altered from that in which the animals have previously been reared. A minimum of 7 days of acclimation is required during which time feed consumption should be measured and an initial body weight determined. Diets must be formulated to meet the requirements of the test species. Suggested composition of mink diets is provided by the National Research Council (141) and by Ringer et al. (162). Fresh feed and water must be provided daily ad libitum. Test diets are prepared by mixing the chemical directly into the feed or by dissolving or suspending in a solvent or carrier prior to mixing in the feed. If a solvent or carrier is used, it must also be added to the control group diet. If a volatile solvent is used (acetone or hexane), the diet should be air dried to evaporate the solvent prior to feeding. Sufficient diet should be mixed to provide feed for the entire exposure period and frozen in aliquots sufficient for 1 or 2 day feeding. All diets should be analyzed after mixing to determine actual concentrations and homogeneity of the test substance in the diet.

Dietary Toxicity Protocol for Ferrets or Mink

The doses for a definitive LC_{50} study (162) should be arranged in a geometric progression with the highest dose set so that an animal will consume the equivalent of an LD_{50} dose in 1 day's feed. The test concentrations should then be spaced to achieve at least two concentrations, yielding between 10–90% mortality. This generally can be achieved with four to six different concentrations. A minimum of eight animals per dose is required. If an LD_{50} value is not available, one may be determined from a range-finding procedure. A geometrically spaced series of doses is administered by gavage to two animals per dose and the LD_{50} is determined to be the dose at which one or two animals die during a 1-week observation period. Animals should be treated by gavage with a 3-in, 14-gauge, curved, stainless steel animal feeding needle. If a lethal dose is not found, the highest dietary concentration should be set at 5000 mg/kg, as concentrations above this value are considered nontoxic. It is recommended that the highest concentration to be tested be fed to two to four animals for several days prior to the start of the test to be sure that it is palatable. If it is not, the highest concentration should be reduced to a level that will be eaten. The test diet is then presented for 28 days. A withdrawal period when clean feed is given should be included if animals are still exhibiting signs of intoxication at the end of the exposure period but should not exceed 14 days. Body weights should be recorded at the beginning of the treatment period and weekly thereafter. Feed consumption should also be measured weekly. Mortality, behavioral abnormalities, and other signs of toxicity should be recorded daily. A test is considered invalid if more than 12.5% of the control animals die. It is recommended that a dietary concentration group be removed from the test when feed consumption values indicate that feed consumption has dropped to less than 10% of control values after the first 2 week's measurements or if animals lose 30% of their initial body weight. It is recommended that necropsies be performed on all animals at the time of death and on all test animals euthanized at the end of the observation period. Gross and histopathological examinations of all major organs should be conducted, including measurement of organ weight. Comparison of body and organ weight changes and feed consumption between control and treatment groups should be made by analysis of variance procedures with a posterior comparison of groups conducted by Dunnett's method (55). The LC_{50} value is calculated by probit analysis or other standard method.

Reproduction Test Protocol for Ferrets or Mink

This test (162) primarily measures female reproductive effects, because the male is used only for the period of time needed for insemination of the female. Proven breeders should be used if possible; otherwise, nulliparous animals may be used. A minimum of 12 females per treatment group is required. One male is needed for every three females in each treatment group; males should not service females in more than one treatment group. If proven breeders are used, the number of females per group can be reduced to eight and the number of males to two. Males are left with the females only for the duration of breeding. A minimum of two test concentrations and one control group are required. The highest dose must (i) produce an effect, (ii) contain at least 1000 mg/kg, or (iii) be at least 100 times higher than the known or expected environmental concentration. Animals are fed test diets for 8 weeks prior to breeding, during breeding, gestation, and parturition, and for 3 weeks of lactation (approximately 23 weeks in total). The test will be longer for mink than for ferrets because mink exhibit a variable delay in implantation of fertilized ova whereas ferrets do not. The gestation period for mink can range from 42–60 days, whereas the ferret has a more constant gestation period of 42 days. Under natural conditions, mating attempts begin at the first of March for mink and at the end of April for ferrets.

In breeding mink, a female is presented to a male (in his cage) and, if receptive, is allowed to mate. If not receptive, the female is removed and a mating attempt is tried again in 4 days. Successful mating is verified by the presence of viable spermatozoa in a vaginal aspiration taken after copulation. Following a successful mating, the female is given a second opportunity to mate to the same male either the next day or (preferably) 8 days later. In breeding ferrets, females are presented to males when in estrus (determined by extent of vulvar swelling) and left with the male overnight. They are not given the opportunity for additional matings.

Once the breeding period is over, animals should be left undisturbed except for daily feedings. Body weights should be measured weekly only during the 8 weeks prior to breeding. Feed consumption should be measured weekly throughout the duration of the test. Observations on behavioral changes, mortality, or other signs of toxicity should be recorded daily. During parturition (up to 3 weeks in length), females should be checked daily for newborn. Number, weight, and sex of all newborns are recorded within 24 h of birth. It may be necessary to remove the female from the nest box to check for newborns. Offspring should be weighed again at 3 weeks of age. After this time, they will begin eating the adult diet and should be fully weaned at 6 weeks of age, at which time the test is terminated. At the end of the test, all males and at least an equal number of females are euthanized (21) and necropsies performed for gross and histopathological examinations. A test is considered invalid if more than 20% of the control animals die during the test. The following reproductive parameters must be reported.

a. Length of gestation: time, in days, from last confirmed mating until parturition
b. Number whelped, not whelped: the number of females giving birth or not giving birth in a treatment group per number of females with confirmed matings; number whelped includes those females that die during parturition
c. Live newborns per females whelped: the average number of live newborns produced by all females that give birth in a treatment group; this does not include females that die during whelping
d. Average birth weight: the average weight within 24 h of birth of all live newborns within a treatment group

e. Average litter weight: the average weight of all litters (live newborns only) within each treatment group
f. Percent newborn survival to 3 weeks: the number of live newborn in a treatment group surviving to 21 days of age, expressed as a percentage of all live births in the treatment group
g. Average body weight at 3 weeks of age: the average weight of all live newborns in a treatment group on the 21st day after birth
h. Total newborns per female whelped: the average number of all newborn (alive and dead) produced by all females that give birth in a treatment group (including those females that die during whelping)
i. Percent newborn survival to 6 weeks: identical to 21-day survival, but extended to 42 days
j. Average 6-week body weight: identical to 21-day weights, but measured at 42 days of age

Number whelped and percent survival should be analyzed for differences among treatment groups using contingency tables and Bonferroni's chi-square test or similar statistical procedures. The remaining variables can be compared among treatment groups by analysis of variance techniques with Dunnett's method for comparison to controls.

Secondary Toxicity Protocol for Ferrets or Mink

This protocol (162) is used to determine the comparative toxicity of both a parent compound and its metabolites administered in the diet, such as might be ingested when consuming contaminated prey. The toxicity of the parent compound is determined following the procedures detailed above for dietary toxicity testing (LC_{50}). Secondary toxicity testing is conducted using the same protocol with the exception that the contaminated feed consists of mink and ferret prey items that have themselves been fed the test substance. Prey animals can be any species readily consumed by the test animals, including fish (salmon, perch, alewife, sucker, carp, and bloater chubs), birds (chickens), and mammals (beef, nutria, rabbits, voles, pocket gophers, rats, and mice). Prey animals may be contaminated by dietary, inhalation, or dermal routes and should be exposed to the same test substance (same source and lot number) as fed to the mink or ferrets in the primary toxicity test. The concentration of the test substance to which the prey are exposed should be sufficient to generate tissue residues of parent compound and/or metabolite at levels known to cause 10–90% mortality of the mink/ferret. This may need to be determined through a range-finder test with the prey species. The final body burden in the prey should allow for dilution of the tissues by the remainder of the dietary ingredients provided and for dilution by non-contaminated portions of the prey (e.g., if 10 mg/kg causes a 50% lethality in the mink or ferret and a diet consisting of 40% prey tissue is being fed, then a prey body burden of 25 mg/kg is needed to yield the final dietary concentration of 10 mg/kg). Prey animals that are not killed by the test substance should be euthanized in a manner that will not interfere with the test results. The gastrointestinal (GI) tract may be removed from the carcass if the test substance is known to accumulate in tissues. This will reduce the probability of direct poisoning from consumption of undigested material in the upper GI tract. However, some compounds do not readily accumulate in tissues (e.g., organophosphorus insecticides) and poisoning of carnivore species occurs primarily from ingestion of material in the GI tract. In these instances, the GI tract may be left intact. All prey animal carcasses should be frozen until being fed to the mink or ferret.

Honey Bees

Honey bees (*Apis mellifera*) are important economically, due to their use for pollination of many crops (e.g., fruit trees). Methods have been developed to evaluate the effects of pesticides on honey bees (187) and these tests have been adapted to determinations of environmental pollution in situ (216).

Toxicity to bees of residues on foliage is conducted using individual worker bees of uniform age (187). The compound of concern is applied to alfalfa foliage in the field and allowed to weather under natural conditions. Worker bees (either honey bees; the alfalfa leafcutting bee, *Megachile rotundata*; or the alkali bee, *Nomia melanderi*) are collected from the frames of established colonies and 50–100 individuals are introduced into each test cage. Cages are constructed by cutting wire screen into a 46 × 5 cm long strip and stapling the ends to form a cylinder. Tops and bottoms of 150 × 15 mm plastic Petri plates serve as the tops and bottoms of the cages. Fifty to 100 honey bees, 20–40 leafcutting bees, or 15–30 alkali bees should be placed in each cage. Ambient temperature during the 24-h test period should be 24–26°C (honey bee) or 29–31°C (leafcutting bee and alkali bee). Bees are fed during the test by providing cotton squares (5 × 5 cm) soaked with 50% sugar syrup and placed under the treated foliage.

The test compound is applied to 0.01-acre alfalfa plots in a randomized block design at applications simulating known environmental concentrations or proposed use patterns. The test may be designed to test a single dose; preferably, a geometrically spaced range of doses is used in order to determine an LC_{50} value. Foliage is harvested at 3, 8, and 24 h after application. If greater than 25% mortality of bees occurs when exposed to 24-h foliage, sampling should continue at 24-h intervals until mortality resulting from exposure to treated foliage is not significantly different from control groups. Foliage is chopped and mixed and 500 ml introduced to each cage. Mortality is determined after 24 h of exposure to the treated foliage. At least three cages of bees must be used per replicate and each treatment, including controls, must be replicated at least three times.

The honey bee acute contact LD_{50} test is based on the protocol developed by Atkins et al. (18) for screening pesticide dust and follows the same husbandry procedures detailed above. Worker bees of uniform age are exposed to the test substance through a dusting procedure. Twenty bees are transferred to the dusting cage and dusted for a period of 15 s. The dusted bees are then put in holding cages and observed for mortality over the next 24 h.

The honey bee subchronic test (187) is designed to test the effects of a chemical on the colony as a unit. The study is intended to identify those chemicals that may cause adverse reproductive, behavioral, or other effects that can be brought back to the hive by exposed foragers. This test is less developed than the tests described above for individual bee toxicity and, consequently, will not be detailed here. The general approach involves exposure of intact bee colonies to the test substance through feeding in pollen or sugar syrup (there is no consensus which component of the diet should contain the test compound). Through caging or location the colonies are restricted to feeding only on the treated feed provided. Periodic observations are made for 42 days to 4 months (42 days is the approximate time needed to complete two brood cycles). Measurements include: number of eggs, open brood or sealed brood, gross colony weight, estimated adult population, and amount of honey in storage. Other suggested observations are presence/absence of disease, discoloration, desiccation, egg and larvae abnormalities, and morphological or behavioral abnormalities in adults.

Soil Invertebrates

Soil invertebrates play a pivotal role in the terrestrial ecosystem, providing functions such as decomposition of organic matter as well as providing a prey base for many higher order organisms. A well developed, but infrequently applied, test determines an LC_{50} in soil for harvester ants (*Pogonomyrmex owyheei*) (65). Crickets (*Acheta domesticus*), isopods (i.e., *Porcellio scaber*), millipedes (*Brachydesmus superus*), centipeds (*Lithobius mutabilis*), collembola (e.g, *Folsomia* spp.), staphylinids (e.g., *Philonthus cognatus*), oribatid mites (e.g., *Platynothrus peltifer*), and soil nematodes also have been studied as possible bioassay organisms for soil toxicity determinations (119,213), but none of the protocols have yet been accepted by OECD, the European Union, or the United States for regulatory purposes.

Nevertheless, soil toxicity is an important parameter in terrestrial environmental assessments. Direct measures of chemical contamination of the soil can be, and frequently are, done following traditional analytical chemistry methods. However, these methods are costly and time consuming and do not provide information about the toxicity of the soil to terrestrial organisms, particularly because synergistic, antagonistic, and additive effects of the complex mix of compounds found in contaminated soils can occur. Furthermore, it has become recognized that chemicals in soil become bound to soil particles during the aging process and become progressively less bioavailable (118). Chemical assays that use harsh extraction procedures to extract all the chemical from the soil do not provide a realistic estimate of exposure to soil organisms. Models are being developed to calculate pore water concentrations for varying soil types (especially with reference to pH, organic matter, and clay content) in order to more closely estimate actual exposure regimes. However, even these methods cannot account for biological adaptations, behaviors, and micro-environment alterations. Therefore, bioassays have been developed to provide direct measures of toxicity. The amphibian bioassay (FETAX) described below can be conducted utilizing eluates from contaminated soils. Plant germination and growth tests also are available for determination of soil toxicity and will be described later in this chapter. A solid-phase version of the aquatic MICROTOX test has been developed and is used occasionally, and development indices of soil microbial biodiversity and function are underway (116). Soil microcosm tests also provide information on movement of chemicals through the soil and resulting toxic effects on plant communities. However, the earthworm (*Eisenia foetida*) survival and reproduction tests are the most widely accepted and conducted bioassay method for ascertaining toxicity of the biologically available fractions of chemicals of concern in soil ecosystems. Earthworms are found in nearly every soil type and play an important role in soil decomposition (81). Furthermore, they are composed of a high percentage of lipids and readily bioaccumulate contaminants from soils. As they are a significant feed item for many vertebrates, they often are an important first step in movement of soil contaminants into the above ground feed web.

The earthworm survival test (15,56,71) utilizes adult (>60 days old, 300–500 mg, with clitellum) *E. foetida* grown in a single culture chamber. Worms may be purchased from a commercial source or acquired from the environment. The identification must be verified (59) to ensure that the species is *Eisenia foetida*. Test soils are first homogenized using a blender and then mixed with artificial soil (10% 2.36-mm screened sphagnum peat, 20% colloidal kaolinite clay, and 70% grade 70 silica sand) to prepare 700 g each of a geometric series of test soil concentrations (e.g., 100, 50, 25, 12.5, 6.25, 3.13% *w*/*w*) plus a 100% artificial soil control. The total amount for each concentration is blended to ensure even mixing prior to dividing into aliquots for the test. After mixing, the soils are hydrated to 75% water holding capacity. Standard 1-pint canning jars with screw-top lids and rings are used as test chambers. Three replicate chambers are filled with 200 g (dry weight) of soil for each dilution. Ten earthworms are placed on the soil surface, the jars are capped, and incubated at 20±2°C under continuous light (540–1080 lux) for 14 days. Worms are not fed during the test. Soil pH is measured at the beginning and end of the test and temperature of the environmental control chamber is continuously monitored. The total organic carbon of the test soils should be measured in one test jar for each test concentration and the control. Jars are examined daily for dead worms (worms are considered dead when they do not respond to a gentle touch on their front end). At the end of the 14-day period, the soil is emptied into a tray and the jar thoroughly searched for worms. Dead worms decay very rapidly so all ten worms in a container may not be accounted for during the test and it is assumed that all missing worms have died. The percent mortality for each concentration is determined and the EC_{50} for mortality is calculated by probit analysis. Loss of earthworm biomass and behavioral and morphological endpoints such as coiling, segmental swellings or constrictions, lesions, rigidness, and flacidness also can be used as toxicity endpoints.

Growth and reproduction also can be used as biological endpoints in earthworm tests of longer duration, generally 140 days (15). Test conditions are the same as described for the 14-day study, although worms must be fed for any study with a duration greater than 28 days. Control of pH, temperature, and soil moisture content are very important, as variations in these environmental parameters have been shown to significantly affect the outcome of earthworm reproduction studies. Mortality and other sublethal observations are made at least weekly. At the conclusion of the test, the containers are emptied and the number of adult worms remaining is tabulated. The number of cocoons formed, cocoon mass, number and growth of young worms, and rate of clitellum development are measured as reproductive endpoints.

Amphibians

The frog embryo teratogenesis assay—Xenopus (FETAX) is a standardized bioassay developed for obtaining data on the developmental toxicity of test materials. Because amphibians usually are associated with wetlands, many of which are impacted from chemical pollution due to their distribution in low lying areas of the landscape and their connection to the surface and subsurface hydrology (113), FETAX primarily is used as a measure of the toxicity of environmental samples (water, sediments, and soil eluates to amphibians). However, results from this bioassay have an 85% correspondence with results from mammalian developmental toxicity tests, so the information can be extrapolated to other classes of animals with a high degree of certainty. The standard protocol, as described below, is a laboratory assay. A field application (by putting the egg masses in porous containers submerged in the water at the study site and following all other standard procedures) is being developed (117).

In FETAX (13), a range-finding and three replicate tests are performed. Each test includes both a negative control (no test material added) and a positive control (6-aminonicotinamide). The 96-h LC_{50} and 96-h EC_{50} (malformation) are determined and the teratogenic index (TI) is calculated by dividing the LC_{50} by the EC_{50}. The FETAX protocol is designed to use embryos of the South African clawed frog *Xenopus laevis* (Daudin). Other North American species can be used and are listed in the appendix of the protocol, although breeding times and methods would need to be adjusted to produce an appropriate egg mass for the test. For *Xenopus*, adult frogs that are proven breeders should be purchased and maintained in single pairs. The frogs should be bred in the same water in which the test is to be conducted (natural, nonchlorinated water known to be free of contaminants) and fed ground adult beef liver three times per week. Temperature should be kept at 23±3°C on a 12 h light/12 h dark photoperiod. Breeding is induced in the males and females by injection into the dorsal lymph sac 250–500 and 500–1000 IU, respectively, of human chorionic gonadotropin. Egg deposition usually occurs 9–12 h later. The eggs should be inspected for fertility which must be >75% for the egg mass to be used in a test. Eggs then are separated from the jelly coat by gently swirling them for 1–3 min in a 2% *w*/*v* -cysteine solution prepared in FETAX solution (625 mg NaCl, 96 mg $NaHCO_3$, 30 mg KCl, 15 mg $CaCl_2$, 60 mg $CaSO_4 \cdot 2H_2O$, and 75 mg $MgSO_4$ per liter of deionized or distilled water; final pH 7.6–7.9). Eggs should be removed from the dejellying solution and rinsed with clean water as soon as dejellying is completed or survival will be reduced. Only normally cleaving embryos should be selected for use in the test. The atlas of abnormalities (22) should be consulted in order to determine abnormalities during the assay. Each test must use embryos derived from a single mated pair.

FETAX is a 96-h test. Each test consists of at least five concentrations arranged in a geometric progression, three of which should fall within the 16–84% effect range on the mortality and malformation dose–response curves. A range-finding test should be conducted first, consisting of at least seven concentrations that differ by factors of 10. Each test concentration and the positive control should have two dishes, each containing 25 embryos and 10 ml of test solution. The negative control groups must have four dishes of 25 embryos each. The positive control (6-aminonicotinamide) consists of two dishes exposed to 2500 mg 6-aminonicotinamide/l and two dishes exposed to 5.5 mg/l. Dishes are placed in an incubator to maintain temperature at 24±2°C. The pH of the test solutions should be 7.7 (range: 6.5–9.0). The test material is renewed every 24 h during the test. Renewal should be done by removing the old test solution with a Pasteur pipette with the orifice enlarged and fire-polished to accommodate embryos without damage if they are picked up accidentally. Fresh solution is added quickly in order to minimize embryo desiccation.

Dead embryos are removed at the end of each 24-h period during the 96-h test (at the time the solutions are changed). Death at 24 h is ascertained by the embryo's skin pigmentation, structural integrity, and irritability. At 48, 72, and 96 h, the lack of heartbeat indicates death. Total number dead and numbers and types of malformations occurring at the end of 96 h are reported. The ability of the test material to inhibit growth is determined at 96 h by recording head to tail length. If the embryo is curved or kinked, the measurement should be made as if the embryo were straight (i.e., following the contour of the embryo). The minimum concentration of test material that significantly inhibits growth (MCIG) should be determined from these data using the *t* test to determine significance at $p = 0.05$. The LC_{50} and EC_{50} (malformation) should be determined using probit analysis.

Plant Tests

A standard guide for conducting terrestrial plant toxicity tests has been completed and published by ASTM (16). Included with the guide are standard protocols for seedling emergence, root elongation, woody plant assays, and a *Brassica* life cycle test. Additionally, a seed germination test is available (71,87,149,205) as is a test for vegetative vigor (88). These bioassays initially were developed to determine hazards due to soil contamination at hazardous waste sites or in sludge disposal areas (216). However, they also can be applied to a priori safety testing requirements. A comprehensive review of plant toxicity tests is available in Kapustka (94).

The seed germination test (71,87) is a 120 h static test and measures seed survival, germination, and seedling emergence. Lettuce (*Lactuca sativa*) is the most commonly used test species, although over 30 species have been accepted by regulatory agencies. Butter crunch lettuce seeds, and many other domestic plants, can be purchased from a commercial vendor. Only one lot should be used for each test and information on the germination percentage should be provided by the seed source. Alternatively, native seeds may be field collected. Regardless of source, only untreated seeds (i.e., no applications of fungicide, repellents, etc.) should be used. The seed lot should be examined to discard trash, empty hulls, and damaged seed. Seeds are sized by stacking four wire mesh sizing screens on top of each other with a collection pan underneath; the largest mesh screen should be on top. The seeds are poured in and the nest of screens is shaken until no more seeds fall through the screens. The size class containing the most seed is selected and used for all of the tests. Seeds can be stored in a dessicator at 4°C in airtight, waterproof containers until used.

Test soils are first homogenized using a blender and then mixed with artificial soil (commercially available, 20-mesh, washed silica sand) to prepare 400 g each of a geometric series of test soil concentrations (e.g., 100, 50, 25, 12.5, 6.25, 3.13% *w/w*) plus a 100% artificial soil control. ASTM requires (16) the use of boric acid as a positive control. The total amount for each concentration is blended to ensure even mixing prior to dividing into aliquots for the test. The soils are air dried and 100 g of each concentration is placed in each of three replicate 150-mm plastic Petri dishes labeled with the appropriate soil dilution. The Petri dishes are then randomized and 40 seeds are placed in each dish, at least 1.25 cm from the edge. The seeds are pressed into the test soil with a glass rod or beaker bottom. Soils are hydrated with deionized water to 85% of water holding capacity. Ninety grams of cover sand (commercially available 16-mesh sand, passed through a 20-mesh screen to remove fines) is poured over the top of the soil and leveled with a ruler. The dishes are then placed in an incubator for the duration of the test. They should be incubated at 24±2°C in the dark for 48 h, followed by 16 h of light and 8 h dark until termination of the test at 120 h. Light intensity should be 4300±430 lux. Soil pH should be measured at the beginning and end of the test (and should be between 4 and 10) and soil temperature should be measured every 24 h in one replicate of each concentration and the control. At 120 h, the number of germinated seeds in each dish is determined by counting each seedling that protrudes above the surface. The LC_{50} and its 95% confidence limits are determined by probit analysis.

The seedling emergence test (16) is very similar to the seed germination test. Seeds are placed in pots, rather than Petri dishes, and need not be stored in the dark for the first 48 h. Soil is hydrated to water holding capacity throughout the test. Test duration is twice the amount of time required to achieve acceptable germination for whatever test species is being used. In addition to counting number of emergent seedlings at the end of the test, optional measures include shoot and root growth. Shoot measurements are made from the transition point between hypocotyl and root to the tallest point on the shoot. Roots are measured from the same transition point to the tip of the root. If sufficient growth is present, dry weight measurements may be obtained. Material is harvested and placed in a preweighed drying vessel and dried at 70°C until constant weight is achieved (approximately 24 h). Weights are taken to the nearest 0.001 g.

Root elongation is a key component of the early stages of plant growth and development. The root elongation bioassay tests the toxicity of water or soil eluates (i.e., the water soluble constituents) to seed germination (16,160). It generally is used as a bioassay of hazards due to soil or water contamination at hazardous waste sites or in sludge disposal areas. However, as with the seed germination test, it also can be applied to a priori safety testing requirements. As a general rule, root elongation is more sensitive than seed germination. The test is a 120-h static test and measures seedling root growth. Butter crunch lettuce is the most commonly used and most sensitive species, but other plants have been used as well (e.g., cucumber, wheat, alfalfa, radish, red clover, and rape). Seeds are purchased, sorted, and sized as described for the seed germination assay. Soil eluates are prepared by mixing 4 ml of deionized water per g (dry weight) of soil. The slurry is mixed in total darkness for 48 h at 20±2°C . After mixing, the eluate is centrifuged and filtered through a 0.45-μm cellulose acetate or glass fiber filter. Water samples (or soil eluates) are diluted in deionized water to provide a geometrically spaced range of concentrations, generally using a 0.3 or 0.5 dilution factor and five concentrations. As with the seed germination study, boric acid should be used as a positive control. A sheet of Whatman no. 3 filter paper is placed in each of three replicate 100-mm plastic Petri dishes and 4 ml of the test solution is poured over the paper. Five seeds are placed in a circle on the filter paper, equidistant from the edge to the center and equally spaced from each other. The lid is placed on each Petri dish which are then set in layers in a black 33-gallon plastic garbage bag within a cardboard box. Moist paper towels are placed between layers of dishes to keep the humidity level elevated. The bag and box are sealed shut and placed in a controlled environmental chamber at 24±2°C for 120 h. The pH and hardness of the test solutions are measured at the beginning of the test, and temperature is recorded every 24 h. At the end of the 120-h period, root lengths are measured to the nearest millimeter by placing the seedling on a glass work surface and measuring the distance from the transition point between the hypocotyl and root to the tip of the root. Swellings or deformities at the transition area should be noted. Roots may be harvested, dried to a constant weight, and weighed to the nearest 0.001 g as an optional additional endpoint. The percent inhibition of the treated seeds as compared to the controls is calculated and an EC_{50} (the concentration that inhibits root growth to 50% of the control length) is calculated.

Whole plant toxicity is evaluated using a 5-day screening test (TOXSCREEN) conducted in hydroponic solutions (157) or a longer full-life-cycle test using vascular plants in soils, such as *Brassica* (16). TOXSCREEN uses whole plants such as soybean (*Glycine max*), barley (*Hordeum vulgare*), and woody perennials that have been grown in hydroponic culture for at least 28 days. Alternatively, known-age plants may be purchased commercially and adapted for hydroponic exposures (128). Regardless, exposures occur hydroponically when young plants are transferred from nursery containers to containers filled with exposure medium. Geometrically spaced dilutions of the exposure medium or chemical concentrations within the exposure medium are used in order to develop a dose–response curve. Soil eluates may be used in filling exposure containers. Tests are conducted under 16 h light/8 h dark photoperiod (light intensity of 350 μmol m^{-2} s^{-1} at the top of the canopy) at 25/21±2°C (light/dark) and relative humidity of 50–70% for 5 days. Following the exposure period, survival, root and shoot growth, and total biomass of the plants are measured. Probit analysis is used to calculate LC_{50} values.

An alternative procedure to TOXSCREEN is available in the woody plants test protocol (16). This is similar to the TOXCREEN test but woody plants are grown in either silica sand, a formulated soil, or a contaminated soil rather than in a hydroponic solution. Plants are obtained from the field or a horticulture source and the roots washed gently by dipping the root mass into deionized water. Plants are kept moist and sorted according to size and stage of development in order to begin the study with uniform sized plants in similar stages of root and shoot growth. The starting condition for all endpoints is measured and recorded. Plants are sorted randomly into treatment groups and placed in pots of sufficient dimension to contain test medium to a depth of approximately two times the root length of plants. Each replicate container should be planted with one test replicate; five replicates of each soil sample, sample dilution, and positive and negative control are required. Medium should be added to cover roots completely and to bring the level within 1–2 cm of the top of the container. Medium may be gently packed by hand but should not be compacted. Deionized water is used to bring the pots to water holding capacity.

A regular water application schedule should be followed thereafter for the duration of the test. Test duration should be approximately twice the length of time required to achieve amounts of shoot and root growth acceptable for statistical characterzation. Tests are conducted under 16 h light/8 h dark photoperiod (light intensity of 100–200 μmol m^{-2} s^{-1}) at 20–30°C and relative humidity of ≥50%. Measured endpoints include wet and dry shoot mass, number of new shoots or leaves, number of root initiation points and changes in total plant weight. Additional observations on general plant condition and leaf or root malformations also are noted. Plants may be harvested, dried at 85°C until constant weight (approximately 24 h), and weighed to the nearest 0.01 g.

The full-life-cycle plant test evaluates the effect of test materials on germination, growth of shoots and roots, photosynthetic systems, flower development, and reproductive capabilities of plants. It is conducted using either *Arabidopsis thaliana* (161) or *Brassica rapa* (16,167) exposed to the toxic substance for 25–36 or 36–44 days, respectively. Hydroponic exposures (161,167) occur in double-pot, static-replacement systems where a vermiculite-filled growth container (for *Arabidopsis*) or greenhouse potting soil (for *Brassica*) is nested above a second, larger pot that serves as a nutrient solution reservoir. Nutrients, toxics, and water move from the reservoir to the vermiculite or potting soil via polyester wicks that are draped between the two pots. Alternatively, *Brassica rapa* seeds (16) may be planted directly into test soil as described above for root elongation or woody plant tests. Dilutions and eluates of test substances are made as described above. Seeds are uniformly planted on the surface of the vermiculite or potting soil and incubated in the conditions described for TOXSCREEN and the woody plant test. Plants will germinate, grow, mature, and set seeds. Exposure to the test substance occurs from the time seeds are planted and continues until the mature plant drops its own seeds. Observations include leaf and flower structure, total biomass, vegetative and reproductive biomass (e.g., stems and leaves vs. seeds and reproductive structures), foliar height, initial flowering date, time to flowering, stunting, chlorosis, and survival. Probit analysis is used to calculate EC_{50} values for each endpoint. Analysis of variance techniques can be used to determine which test concentrations produce effects significantly different from control values.

Soil-core microcosms (12) can be used to develop site-specific or regional information on the probable chemical fate and ecological effects in a soil system resulting from release or spillage of chemicals into the environment. This test is most useful in the assessment process after preliminary knowledge of the chemical properties and biological activity of the compound(s) of interest have been obtained. The test is designed to determine impacts in agricultural or natural field soil ecosystems, and may not be applicable to forest soils. Specifically, the test will determine the effect of a chemical on growth and reproduction of either natural grassland vegetation or crops, nutrient uptake and cycling, potential for bioaccumulation in the plant tissues, and potential for and rate of transport of the chemical through soil to ground water.

Soil cores are extracted from the site or region of interest with a specially designed, steel extraction tube. The steel tube surrounds an ultrahigh-molecular-weight, high-density, nonplasticized polyethylene pipe to prevent the tube from warping or splitting during extraction. The tube is 60 cm deep by 20 cm diameter. In agricultural systems, the plowed topsoil is moved aside prior to coring, and backfilled into the upper 20 cm of the tube after collection. For the natural grassland system, the vegetation is clipped before the core is extracted. The polyethylene tube containing the soil core is removed from the steel coring device and placed within a specially designed wheeled cart that holds six to eight tubes packed within insulating styrofoam beads. The tube sits on a Buchner funnel that is covered by a thin layer of glass wool and connected by polyvinyl chloride tubing to a flask for collection of leachates. For the natural ecosystem, the natural plant cover collected with the soil core is suitable for the test. For agricultural systems, a mixture of grasses and broad leaves (e.g., legumes) that are typically grown together in the region of interest should be planted in the soil cores. The seed application rate should duplicate standard farming practices. Microcosms should be watered with purified water on a predetermined regimen, usually established on the basis of site history. Microcosms are leached once before dosing and once every 2 or 3 weeks after dosing. Microcosms that take longer than 2 days to produce 100 ml of leachate are not used in the test. The microcosms in their insulated carts are kept in a greenhouse or environmental chamber where temperatures and photoperiods are set to simulate outdoor conditions during a typical growing season in the region of interest.

If information is available, only one concentration of the test chemical above that known to cause at least a 50% change in plant growth or a 50% change in bacterial growth/respiration needs to be tested. Generally, three concentrations are used, choosing one that produced a 20–25% change in productivity. In any case, the lowest treatment level should not be less than 10 times greater than the analytical limits of detectability of the parent compound. A range-finding test utilizing concentrations of 0.1, 1.0, 10, 100, and 1000 μg/g in the upper 20 cm of topsoil can be used to determine the appropriate dose for the definitive test. The range finder should last a minimum of 4 weeks, whereas the definitive test lasts for 12 weeks. For aqueous compounds, the test solution is mixed with water and applied as single or multiple (daily, weekly) exposures in sufficient volume to bring the microcosm to field capacity. In no case should the exposure volume be sufficient to cause leaching in any of the microcosms. Frequency of application should reflect the situation encountered in the region of interest. The use of carriers should be avoided. If the test substance does not mix with water, it should be applied evenly to the top of the unplanted microcosm and mixed into the topsoil prior to planting. If the test substance is normally sprayed on growing plants, then it should be sprayed on the plants with a nebulizer when at the seedling stage. The number of replicate microcosms per dose is determined by the desired power of the statistical test and the variability between microcosms (determined in the range-finder). Individual microcosms should be assigned to treatment groups in a randomized block design, with the cart as a blocking variable.

The parent compound should be radiolabeled with ^{14}C, either in an appropriate aromatic, cyclic carbon group or in a linear chain in order to follow uptake and degradation rates. The following parameters are measured.

a. Primary productivity: the total yield or yield of harvestable portion (e.g., grain), reported as oven-dried weight
b. Physical appearance and abnormalities of plants
c. Amounts of nutrients in leachate (e.g., calcium, potassium, nitrate nitrogen, ammonium nitrogen, orthophosphate, and dissolved organic carbon)
d. Amounts of parent compound in all plant parts, soil horizons, and leachate (by measuring radioactivity of parent compound)
e. Amounts of chemical degradation products in plant material, soil, and leachate
f. Soil properties, including pedologic identity (according to the United States Department of Agriculture 7th Approximation Soil Classification System), percent organic matter, hydraulic characteristics, cation exchange capacity, bulk density, macro- and micronutrient content, organic matter content, inorganic mineral content, exchange capacity, particle-size distribution, and hydraulic characteristics

Data analysis should follow standard statistical techniques as appropriate, such as analysis of variance for comparing biomass data or regression analysis on sequential measures of productivity. The 5% level should be considered as the level of significance with a power of 0.90 or 0.95.

AIR POLLUTION

Air pollution has the potential to seriously injure plants and animals. A good example of air pollution effects is the change in the forest vegetation of the San Bernadino Mountains in southern California (23). Here, prolonged exposure to photochemical oxidants ("smog") resulted in a shift from ozone-sensitive pine trees to more ozone-tolerant oaks and shrubs. Ozone injury in pines results in decreased photosynthesis due to foliar injury and premature needle fall, reduced nutrient retention in needles, and decreased growth. In general, gaseous pollutants have the potential to disrupt plant-leaf biochemical processes through absorption by stomata or cuticle, whereas trace metals and organochlorine compounds tend to accumulate in humus and organic matter. Animals are affected either by uptake through the feed chain or direct exposure via inhalation (142). However, there has been little direct measurement of toxicity to wildlife from air pollutants other than studies of effects of smelter emissions and a documented reduction in small mammal diversity in the ozone-impacted San Bernadino Mountains. Many species of freshwater animals have been affected by wet deposition of sulfur dioxides, also known as "acid rain." In general, fish are most sensitive to acidification, followed by invertebrates, algae, and microbes (142). Certainly, the potential impact to biodiversity from global climate change is significant. Either the amount of production or the type of plant that will grow efficiently may change in response to increasing CO_2, to changes in the amount and timing of precipitation, or to the amount of available solar radiation. CO_2 enrichment alone would increase the rate of growth of plants, whereas higher temperatures would increase the rate of microbial decomposition of organic matter, adversely affecting soil fertility (152). On the other hand, higher temperatures generally hasten plant maturity in annual species, shortening the growth stages of some plants. At the same time, mid-latitude summer dryness is likely to reduce yields by 10–30% (163).

Air pollution levels generally are measured mechanically, through the use of biosensors or air sampling devices in situ. However, as with chemical analysis of soils and other media, this type of monitoring does not provide information about the toxicity of air pollutants to terrestrial organisms. Lichens are particularly sensitive to low levels of some forms of air pollution. Some are killed by pollutant levels that are too low to cause visible injury to other plants. Consequently, lichens are now used as qualitative indicators of air quality in parts of the United States and Europe, in particular for sulfur dioxide, hydrogen fluoride, acidic precipitation, ozone, nitrogen dioxide, heavy metals, and radioactive compounds (137). Lichen species in the area of study are identified, and species diversity, density, and frequency are recorded as is percent cover. Plants also are observed for obvious signs of damage. These parameters are compared with historical accounts of lichen communities to determine if airborne pollutants have affected the plants. Additionally, some compounds (e.g., heavy metals, organochlorines) are bioaccumulated by lichens without visible signs of damage to the plants. Residue analysis of lichens has been used to map the location and distribution of these pollutants.

ECOLOGICAL RISK ASSESSMENT

The toxicity tests described in this chapter ultimately become a component of the process of establishing the likelihood that adverse ecological effects are occurring or may occur as a result of exposure to one or more stressors. The process of ecological risk assessment has evolved rapidly since the EPA issued a framework for ecological risk assessment in 1992 (195). Since that time many workshops have been held by governmental entities and professional societies to refine the process, culminating in the publication of *Guidelines for Ecological Risk Assessment* in 1998 (203). The guidelines should be used for improving the quality and consistency of assessments of the impact of environmental stressors on components of an ecosystem. There are at least two books (24,175) that provide a wealth of information about ecological risk assessment.

Ecological risk assessment involves three stages in a continuous process: (i) problem formulation, (ii) the analysis of exposure and effects, and (iii) risk characterization. Because ecological risk assessment must consider effects at the population, community, and ecosystem levels as well as to the individual species, and the relevant assessment endpoints are not universally accepted, the process is generally more complex and protracted than are most human health risk assessments. Furthermore, ecological risk assessment frequently must consider the effect of mixtures of chemicals that interact in a complex chemical and physical environment rather than the single chemical focus of human health risk assessment. Three examples of comprehensive ecological risk assessments can be found in a special issue of the journal *Environmental and Toxicological Chemistry* (99,100,168).

The ecological risk assessment process is diagramed in Figure 37.6. The first, and most critical, phase of the process is problem formulation. It is during this phase that the affected environmental resource and the stressors of concern must be considered within the context of the overall situation that is to be evaluated. It is frequently useful at this stage to involve risk assessors, risk managers, and stakeholders in discussions about how to proceed so that the results of the assessment will be most useful to those who will have to use them. It is also worthwhile to spend some time modeling the problem, at least in a conceptual sense, so that assessment endpoints will be reasonable and achievable and that a sampling and analysis plan with appropriate measurement endpoints can be established. A quality assurance project plan should also be established at this stage.

During the analysis phase of the risk assessment, the exposure level or concentration of the stressor of concern on the environmental resource must be established and the effects assessed. The effects assessment should include both potential toxicological effects, as described in this chapter, and ecological effects. Although toxicological effects are usually measured on individual organisms using a variety of standardized tests and are relatively easily quantified, ecological effects involve predictions about changes in populations and communities of organisms in longer-term studies, which are more difficult to conduct and interpret. Studies in microcosms, mesocosms, small ponds, and streams are frequently required, as described earlier. Food web relationships may need to be determined. Finally, indirect effects of contaminants on the organisms of interest must be considered, such as changes in feed availability, habitat structure, or predator abundance. The analysis of exposure and effects also must include consideration of fate and transport of the stressors. As described earlier, exposure is dependent on the bioavailability of the stressor, which depends on its chemical, physical, and environmental characteristics, and effects are entirely dependent on exposure. Thus, knowledge of the physical/chemical behavior of stressors in the ecosystem is critical.

The final step in the risk assessment process is to integrate the exposure of the resource to the stressors with the observed or predicted effects within the context of the problem formulation to estimate the degree of risk and the probability of adverse environmental changes actually being observed. Very simple systems where statistical analyses can establish the confidence of the predicted result are rare in ecological risk assessment. The more usual cases involve a high degree of uncertainty, which in turn require the risk manager to establish the parameters within which regulation must be effected, frequently using a worst case scenario. Obviously, the more quantitative and precise the assessment results presented to the risk manager, the more effective the management of the ecosystem will be. In reality, as indicated on the diagram, ecological risk assessment is a continuous process in which risk managers and risk assessors must interact in concert with stakeholders to strive for continuous improvement in understanding the ecosystem and providing for optimum functionality.

More detailed analysis of the ecological risk assessment process will be found in the *EPA Risk Assessment Guide-*

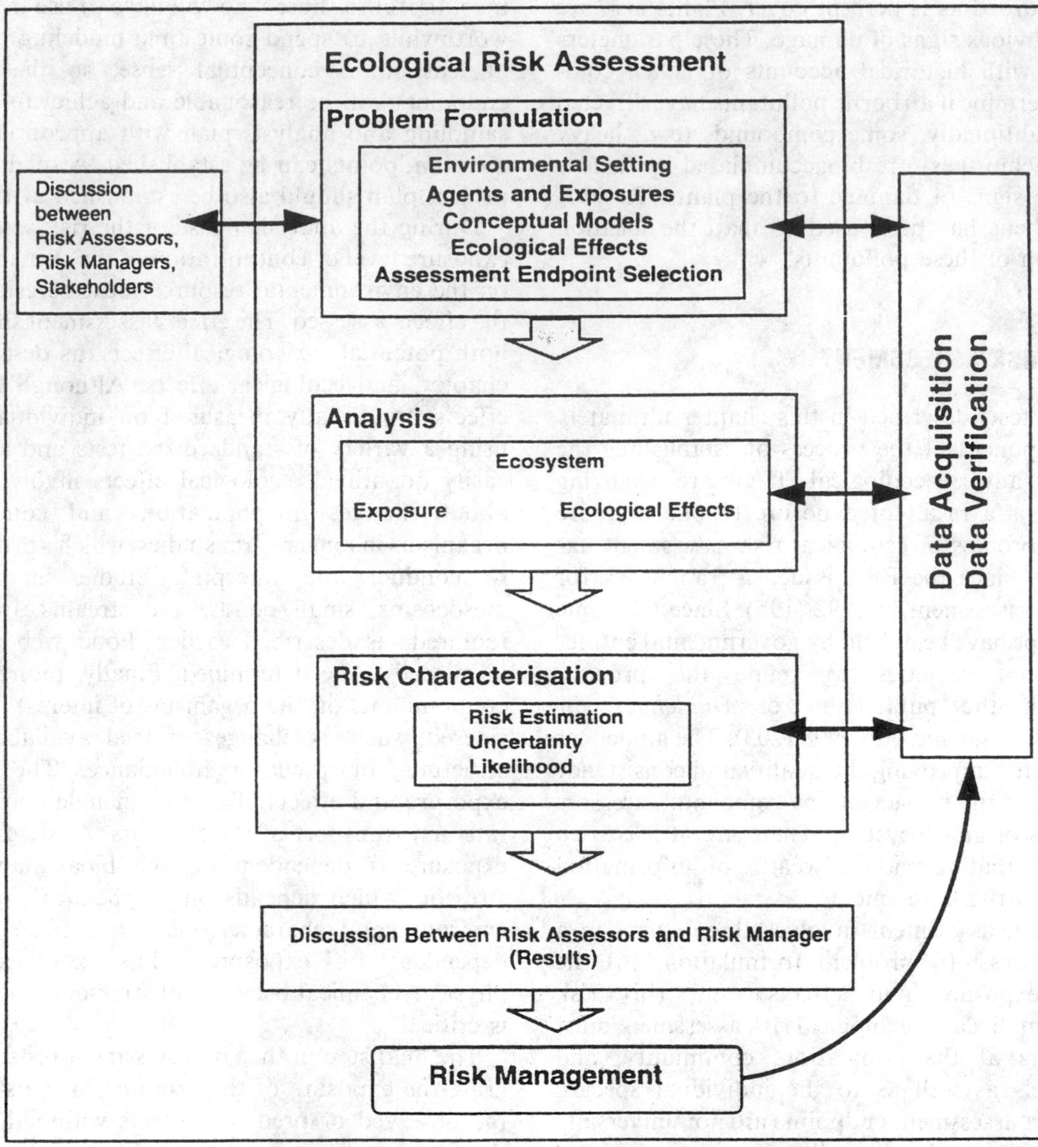

FIG. 37.6. The ecological risk assessment process. From UNEP (180).

lines (203) and in the several applications of the methodology that have been published (e.g., ref. 180).

CONCLUSION

Clearly, toxicity testing under realistic environmental conditions is a much more complex enterprise than determining the effects of single chemicals on single species under controlled laboratory conditions. However, the information obtained in a well-designed, well-executed environmental study provides a valuable supplement to the toxicity data obtained in more traditional laboratory studies. Understanding the impacts of a xenobiotic chemical upon the environment, including the organisms which live in it, requires these more complex studies.

Interactions of organisms with each other and with their environment are altered by the introduction of foreign chemicals. The impacts of such chemicals must be assessed in terms of these interactions as well as the effect on individuals if the overall health of an ecosystem is to be properly evaluated and understood. This is the essential difference between ecotoxicology and the discipline of toxicology as it relates to human health. Toxicologists have developed rigorous methods for assessing the effects of chemicals on single species under controlled conditions. However, effects on ecosystems in which many species are involved are much harder to identify and measure quantitatively. Great strides have been made in the development of controlled ecosystems, in the form of microcosms and mesocosms, for this purpose. There is still much work to be done, however, to perfect the methodology to the extent that effects can be truly assessed at the ecosystem level. The truism that "the whole is greater than the sum of its parts" definitely applies.

Much progress has been made by the various environmental regulatory authorities in systematically codifying procedures and requirements for the use of field-derived toxicology assessments for populations and communities to evaluate the impacts of chemicals on the environment (203). The guidance provided suggests not only community-level toxicological data, but also the requirement to understand the spatial and temporal scales of stress and the natural variability in biotic community dynamics.

Ultimately, the extra costs in terms of time and money for conducting environmental toxicology evaluations and ecological risk assessments will be returned many fold in our wiser use of natural resources and the protection of the environment in which we live.

QUESTIONS

1. Why are the chemical and physical properties of a chemical important in assessing its environmental toxicology?
2. How do toxicity tests differ? How are the appropriate ones selected? What is meant by a "tiered approach"?
3. What are the differences and cost/benefits of static, continuous-flow, recirculation, or static-renewal aquatic toxicity tests?
4. What is the primary goal of aquatic toxicology? How does it differ from mammalian toxicology?
5. How is toxicity information used in permitting waste water discharge?
6. Why do terrestrial toxicity assessments rely more heavily on bioassays as endpoints than do aquatic or mammalian toxicity assessments?
7. Why are honey bees and soil invertebrates important indicator species?
8. Why can results of single-species laboratory tests not be used alone to predict effects on natural populations, communities, or ecosystems? What has been developed to supplement these tests for such assessments?
9. What factors would affect the extrapolation of toxicity data derived for single species in the laboratory to populations, communities, and ecosystems?
10. Why is ecological risk assessment generally more protracted and contentious than human health risk assessments? What is the most critical phase of an ecological risk assessment?

REFERENCES

1. American Petroleum Institute. (1985): Fathead minnow 7 day test: Round robin study. No. 4468. Health and Environmental Sciences Department, Washington, DC.
2. American Public Health Association, American Water Works Association, and Water Pollution Control Federation. (1989): *Standard Methods for Examination of Water and Wastewater*, 17th ed., Suppl. Washington, DC.
3. American Society for Testing and Materials. (1989): Standard guide for collection, storage, characterization, and manipulation of sediments for toxicological testing, In: *Annual Book of ASTM Standards*, pp. 1105–1119. E1391. American Society for Testing and Materials, Philadelphia, PA.
4. American Society for Testing and Materials. (1990): Standard guide for conducting static 96-h toxicity tests with microalgae. E1218-90. In *Annual Book of ASTM Standards*, Vol. 11.04, pp. 168–179. American Society for Testing and Materials, Philadelphia, PA.
5. American Society for Testing and Materials. (1990): New standard guide for conducting static toxicity tests with *Lemna gibba*. In: *Annual Book of ASTM Standards*, E1415-91. American Society for Testing and Materials, Philadelphia, PA.
6. American Society for Testing and Materials. (1991): *Annual Book of Standards*, 1334 pp. American Society for Testing and Materials, Philadelphia, PA.
7. American Society for Testing and Materials. (1991): Standard test method for efficacy of a multiple-dose rodenticide under laboratory conditions. In: *Annual Book of ASTM Standards, Vol. 11.04, Pesticides; Resource Recovery; Hazardous Substances and Oil Spill Responses; Waste Disposal; Biological Effects*, pp. 238–243. E593. American Society for Testing and Materials, Philadelphia, PA.
8. American Society for Testing and Materials. (1991): Standard practice for conducting subacute dietary toxicity tests with avian species. In: *Annual Book of ASTM Standards, Vol. 11.04, Pesticides; Resource Recovery; Hazardous Substances and Oil Spill Responses; Waste Disposal; Biological Effects*, pp. 456–460. E857. American Society for Testing and Materials, Philadelphia, PA.
9. American Society for Testing and Materials. (1991): Standard guide for assessing the hazard of a material to aquatic organisms and their uses. In: *Annual Book of ASTM Standards*, pp. 624–640. E1022-84. Vol. 11.04. American Society for Testing and Materials, Philadelphia, PA.
10. American Society for Testing and Materials. (1991): Standard practice for conducting reproductive studies with avian species. In: *Annual Book of ASTM Standards, Vol. 11.04, Pesticides; Resource Recovery; Hazardous Substances and Oil Spill Responses; Waste Disposal; Biological Effects*, pp. 678–688. E1062. American Society for Testing and Materials, Philadelphia, PA.
11. American Society for Testing and Materials. (1991): Standard test method for estimating acute oral toxicity in rats. In: *Annual Book of ASTM Standards, Vol. 11.04, Pesticides; Resource Recovery; Hazardous Substances and Oil Spill Responses; Waste Disposal; Biological Effects*, pp. 741–746. E1163. American Society for Testing and Materials, Philadelphia, PA.
12. American Society for Testing and Materials. (1991): Standard Guide for conducting a terrestrial soil-core microcosm test. In: *Annual Book of ASTM Standards, Vol. 11.04, Pesticides; Resource Recovery; Hazardous Substances and Oil Spill Responses; Waste Disposal; Biological Effects*, pp. 819–831. E1197. American Society for Testing and Materials, Philadelphia, PA.
13. American Society for Testing and Materials. (1992): Standard guide for conducting the frog embryo teratogenesis

assay—Xenopus (FETAX). E1439-91. In: *Annual Book of ASTM Standards*, Vol. 11.04, pp. 1199–1209. American Society for Testing and Materials, Philadelphia, PA.

14. American Society for Testing and Materials. (1993): Practice for standardized aquatic microcosms: Fresh water. In: *ASTM Standards on Aquatic Toxicology and Hazard Evaluations*, E-1366-91. pp. 422–456. American Society for Testing and Materials, Philadelphia, PA.
15. American Society of Testing and Materials. (1996): Standard guide for conducting a laboratory soil toxicity test with lumbricid earthworm *Eisenia foetida*. In: *Annual Book of ASTM Standards*, Vol. 11.05, pp. 1093–1109. E1676-95. American Society for Testing and Materials, West Conshohocken, PA.
16. American Society of Testing and Materials. (1999): Standard guide for conducting terrestrial plant toxicity tests. In: *Annual Book of ASTM Standards*, E1963-98. Vol. 11.05, American Society for Testing and Materials, West Conshohocken, PA.
17. Anderson, S. L., and Norberg-King, T. J. (1991): Precision of short-term chronic toxicity tests in the real world. *Environ. Toxicol. Chem.*, 10:143–145.
18. Atkins, E. L., Anderson, L. D., and Tuft, T. O. (1954): Equipment and technique used in laboratory evaluation of pesticide dusts in toxicological studies with honeybees. *J. Econ. Entomol.*, 47:965–969.
19. Aulerich, R. J., and Ringer, R. K. (1977): Current status of PCB toxicity to mink, and effect on their reproduction. *Arch. Environ. Contam. Toxicol.*, 6:279–292.
20. Aulerich, R. J., and Ringer, R. K. (1979): Toxic effects of dietary polybrominated biphenyls on mink. *Arch. Environ. Contam. Toxicol.*, 8:487–498.
21. American Veterinary Medical Association, Panel on Euthanasia. (1986): 1986 Report of the AVMA Panel on Euthanasia. *J. Amer. Vet. Med. Assoc.*, 188:252–268.
22. Bantle, J. A., Dumont, J. N., Finch, R. A., and Linder, G. (1991): *Atlas of Abnormalities: A guide for the performance of FETAX*. Oklahoma State University Press, Stillwater, OK.
23. Barker, J. R., and Tingey, D. T. (1992): *Air Pollution Effects on Biodiversity*. Van Nostrand Reinhold, NY.
24. Bartell, S. M., Gardner, R. H., and O'Neill, R. V. (1992): *Ecological Risk Estimation*. Lewis Publishers, Chelsea, MI.
25. Bascietto, J. (1985): *Hazard Evaluation Division Standard Evaluation Procedure: Avian Dietary LC50 Test*. USEPA 540/9-85/008. USEPA. Washington, DC.
26. BC Environment. (1995): *Criteria for Managing Contaminated Sites in British Columbia*. Environmental Protection Department, Ministry of Environment, Lands and Parks, Victoria, British Columbia.
27. Blaise, C. B. (1991): Microbiotests in aquatic ecotoxicology: characteristics, utility and prospects. *Environ. Toxicol. Water Quality*, 6:145–155.
28. Bleavins, M. R., Aulerich, R. J., and Ringer, R. K. (1984): Effects of chronic dietary hexachlorobenzene on the reproductive performance and survivability of mink and European ferrets. *Arch. Environ. Contam. Toxicol.*, 13:357–365.
29. Bonna, R. J., Aulerich, R. J., Bursian, S. J., Poppenga, R. H., Braselton, W. E., and Watson, G. L. (1991): Efficacy of hydrated sodium calcium aluminosilicate and activated charcoal in reducing the toxicity of dietary aflatoxin to mink. *Arch. Environ. Contam. Toxicol.*, 20:441–447.
30. Bookhout, T. A., ed. (1994): *Research and Management Techniques for Wildlife and Habitats*, 5th ed. The Wildlife Society, Bethesda, MD.
31. Boyle, T. P., ed. (1985): *Validation and Predictability of Laboratory Methods for Assessing the Fate and Effects of Contaminants in Aquatic Ecosystems*, pp. 134–151. ASTM Special Publication, STP 865. American Society for Testing and Materials, Philadelphia, PA.
32. Brazner, J. C., Heinis, L. J., and Jensen, D. A. (1989): A littoral enclosure for replicated field experiments. *Environ. Toxicol. Chem.*, 8:1209–1216.
33. Brewer, L. W., and Fagerstone, K. A. (1998): *Radiotelemetry Applications for Wildlife Toxicology Field Studies*. SETAC Press, Pensacola, FL.
34. Buikema, A. L., Niederlehner, B. R., and Cairns, J., Jr. (1982): Biological monitoring Part IV—toxicity testing. *Water Res.*, 16:239–262.
35. Burton, G. A., Jr. (1991): Assessment of freshwater sediment toxicity. *Environ. Toxicol. Chem.*, 10:1585–1627.
36. Burton, G. A., ed. (1992): *Sediment Toxicity Assessment*. Lewis Publishers Inc., Boca Raton, FL.
37. Butler, P. A. (1973): Residues in fish, wildlife and estuaries. *Pesticides Monitoring J.*, 6:238–362.
38. Cairns, J., ed. (1985): *Multispecies Toxicity Testing*. Society of Environmental Toxicology and Chemistry, Special Publication Series, Pergamon Press, NY.
39. Cairns, J., ed. (1986): *Community Toxicity Testing*. ASTM-STP 920. American Society for Testing and Materials, Philadelphia, PA.
40. Cairns, J., Dickson, K. L., and Maki, A. W. (1978): *Estimating the Hazard of Chemical Substances to Aquatic Life*. ASTM-STP 657. American Society for Testing and Materials, Philadelphia, PA.
41. Cairns, J., and Niederlehner, B. R. (1993): Ecological fun and resilience: Neglected criteria for environmental impact assessment and ecological risk analysis. *Environ. Prof.*, 15:116–124.
42. Canadian Council of Ministers of the Environment. (1996): *A Protocol for the Derivation of Environmental and Human Health Soil Quality Guidelines*. The National Contaminated Sites Remediation Program. CCME-EPC-101E. ISBN 0-662-24344-7.
43. Canton, J. H., and Adema, D. M. M. (1978): Reproducibility of short-term and reproduction toxicity experiments with *Daphnia magna* and comparison of the sensitivity of *Daphnia magna* with *Daphnia pulex* and *Daphnia cucullata* in short-term experiments. *Hydrobiologia*, 59:135–140.
44. Chapman, G. A. (1983): Do organisms in laboratory tests respond like organisms in nature? In: *Aquatic Toxicology and Hazard Assessment: Sixth Symposium*, edited by W. E. Bishop, R. D. Cardwell, and B. B. Heidolph, pp. 315–327. STP 802. American Society for Testing and Materials, Philadelphia, PA.
45. Chapman, P. M. (1988): Marine sediment toxicity tests. In: *Chemical and Biological Characterization of Sludges, Sediments, Dredge Spoils and Drilling Muds*, edited by J. J. Lichtenberg, F. A. Winter, C. I. Weber, and L. Fradkin, pp. 391–402. STP 976. American Society for Testing and Materials, Philadelphia, PA.
46. Chapman, P. M. (1989): Current approaches to developing sediment quality criteria. *Environ. Toxicol. Chem.*, 8:589–599.
47. Clements, R. G., ed. (1988): *Estimating Toxicity of Industrial Chemicals to Aquatic Organisms Using Structure Activity Relationships*. EPA-500/6-8-001. Office of Toxic Substances, U.S. EPA, Washington, DC.
48. Crawford, J. K., and Luoma, S. N. (1994): *Guidelines for Studies of Contaminants in Biological Tissues for the National Water-Quality Assessment Program*. Open-File Report 92-494. U.S. Geological Survey, Lemoyne, PA.
49. Crossland, N. O., and Bennett, D. (1989): Outdoor ponds: Their use to evaluate the hazards of organic chemicals in aquatic environments. In: *Aquatic Ecotoxicology: Fundamental Concepts and Methodologies*, edited by A. Boudu and F. Ribeyre, pp. 273–296. CRC Press, Boca Raton, FL.

50. D'Adamo, R. D., Pelosi, S., Trotta, P., and Sansone, G. (1997): Bioaccumulation and biomagnification of polycyclic aromatic hydrocarbons in aquatic organisms. *Marine Chem.*, 56:45–49.
51. De Graeve, G. M., Cooney, J. D., Marsh, B. H., Pollock, T. L., and Reichenbach, N. G. (1992): Variability in the performance of the 7-d *Ceriodaphnia dubia* survival and reproduction tests: an intra- and interlaboratory study. *Environ. Toxicol. Chem.*, 11:851–866.
52. DeWitt, T. H., Redmond, M. S., Sewall, J. E., and Swartz, R. C. (1992): *Development of a Chronic Sediment Toxicity Test for Marine Benthic Amphipods.* Chesapeake Bay Program. CBP/TRS 89/93. U.S. Environmental Protection Agency, Office of Research and Development, Newport, OR.
53. Dourson, M. L., and Stara, J. F. (1983): Regulatory history and experimental support of uncertainty (safety) factors. *Reg. Toxicol. Pharmacol.*, 3:224–238.
54. Draggan, S., ed. (1980): *The Microcosm: Biological Model of the Ecosystem.* Report No. 19. Monitoring and Assessment Research Center, Chelsea College, University of London, London, England.
55. Dunnett, C. W. (1964): New tables for multiple comparisons with a control. *Biometrics*, 20:482–491.
56. Edwards, C. A. (1984): *Report of the Second Stage in Development of a Standardized Laboratory Method for Assessing the Toxicity of Chemical Substances to Earthworms.* Commission of the European Communities. EUR 9360 EN. Luxembourg.
57. Etnier, E. L., Meyer, R. E., Lewis, E. B., and Folmar, L. C. (1987): *Update of Acute and Chronic Aquatic Toxicity Data for Heavy Metals and Organic Chemicals Found at Hazardous Waste Sites.* ORNL-6392. Oak Ridge National Laboratory, Oak Ridge, TN.
58. Fairbrother, A., Kapustka, L. A., Williams, B. A., and Bennett, R. S. (1997): Effects-initiated assessments are not risk assessments. *Hum. Ecol. Risk Assessment*, 3:119–124.
59. Fender, W. M. (1985): Earthworms of the western United States. Part I. Lumbricidae. *Megadrilogica*, 4:93–129.
60. Finney, D. J. (1964): *Statistical Methods in Biological Assay*, 2nd ed. Hafner Publishing Company, NY.
61. Finney, D. J. (1971): *Probit Analysis*, 3rd ed. Cambridge University Press, Cambridge, England.
62. Fite, E. C., Turner, L. W., Cook, N. J., and Stunkard, C. (1988): *Guidance Document for Conducting Terrestrial Field Studies.* USEPA 540/09-88/109. USEPA, Washington, DC.
63. Forney, D. R., and Davis, D. E. (1991): Effects of low concentration of herbicides on submersed aquatic plants. *Weed Sci.*, 29:677–685.
64. Fur Farm Animal Welfare Coalition. (1988): *Standard Guidelines for Operation of Mink Farms in the United States*, 2nd ed. Fur Farm Animal Welfare Coalition, Ltd., St. Paul, MN.
65. Gano, K. A., Carline, D. W., and Roger, L. E. (1985): A harvester ant bioassay for assessing hazardous chemical waste sites. PNL-5434, UC-11. Pacific Northwest Laboratory, Richland, WA.
66. Gersich, F. M., Blanchard, F. A., Applegath, S. L., and Park, C. N. (1986): The precision of daphnid (*Daphnia magna* Straus, 1820) static acute toxicity tests. *Arch. Environ. Contam. Toxicol.*, 15:741–749.
67. Giesy, J., and Allred, P. M. (1985): Replicability of aquatic multispecies test systems. In: *Multispecies Toxicity Testing*, edited by J. Cairns, pp. 87–247. Society of Environmental Toxicology and Chemistry, Special Publications Series, Pergamon Press. Elmsford, NY.
68. Giesy, J. P., and Hoke, R. A. (1990): Freshwater sediment quality criteria: Toxicity bioassessment. In: *Sediments: Chemistry and Toxicity of In-Place Pollutants*, edited by R. Baudo, J. Giesy, and H. Muntau, pp. 265–348. Lewis Publishers, Chelsea, MI.
69. Giesy, J. P., Jr., Rosiu, C. J., and Graney, R. L. (1990): Benthic invertebrate bioassays with toxic sediment and pore water. *Environ. Toxicol. Chem.*, 9:233–248.
70. Gore, R. H. (1992): *The Gulf of Mexico.* Pineapple Press, Sarasota, FL.
71. Greene, J. C., Bartels, C. L., Warren-Hicks, W. J., Parkhurst, B. R., Linder, G. L., Peterson, S. A., and Miller, W. E. (1989): *Protocols for Short Term Toxicity Screening of Hazardous Waste Sites.* EPA/600/3-88/029. USEPA, Washington, DC.
72. Grice, G. D., and Reeve, M. R. (1982): *Marine Mesocosms: Biological and Chemical Research in Experimental Ecosystems.* Springer–Verlag, New York.
73. Grothe, D. E., Dickson, K. L., and Reed-Judkins, D. K. (1996): *Whole Effluent Toxicity Testing. An Evaluation of Methods and Prediction of Receiving System Impacts.* SETAC Press, Pensacola, FL.
74. Grothe, D. E., and Kimerle, D. R. (1985): Inter- and intra-laboratory variability in *Daphnia magna* toxicity test results. *Environ. Toxicol. Chem.*, 4:189–192.
75. Guilizzoni, P. (1991): The role of heavy metals and toxic materials in the physiological ecology of submersed macrophytes. *Aquatic Botany*, 41:87–109.
76. Hamelink, J. L. (1977): Current bioconcentration test methods and theory. In: *Aquatic Toxicology and Hazard Evaluation*, edited by F. L. Mayer and J. L. Hamelink, pp. 149–161. STP 634. American Society for Testing and Materials, Philadelphia, PA.
77. Hansen, P. D. (1996): Bioassays on sediment toxicity. In: *Sediments and Toxic Substances*, edited by W. Calmano and U. Forstner, pp. 179–194. Springer–Verlag, Berlin.
78. Hansen, S. R., and Garton, R. R. (1982): Ability of standard toxicity tests to predict the effects of the insecticide diflubenzuron on laboratory stream communities. *Can. J. Fish. Aquat. Sci.*, 39:127–128.
79. Harrass, M. C., and Sayre, P. G. (1989): Use of microcosm data for regulatory decisions. In: *Aquatic Toxicology and Hazard Assessment*: Vol. 12, edited by U. M. Cowgill and L. R. Williams, pp. 204–223, ASTM-STP 1027. American Society for Testing and Materials, Philadelphia, PA.
80. Heimbach, F., Pflueger, W., and Ratte, H. T. (1992): Use of small artificial ponds for assessment of hazards to aquatic ecosystems. *Environ. Toxicol. Chem.*, 11:27–34.
81. Hendrix, P. E., ed. (1995): *Earthworm Ecology and Biogeography.* CRC Press, Boca Raton, FL.
82. Hill, E. F., and Camardese, M. B. (1986): *Lethal Dietary Toxicities of Environmental Contaminants and Pesticides to Coturnix.* U.S. Fish and Wildlife Service Fish and Wildlife Technical Report 2. Washington, DC. US Fish and Wildlife Service, Washington, DC.
83. Hill, E. F., Heath, R. G., Spann, J. W., and Williams, J. D. (1975): *Lethal Dietary Toxicities of Environmental Pollutants to Birds.* U.S. Fish and Wildlife Service Special Scientific Report. Wildlife No. 191. Washington, DC. US Fish and Wildlife Service, Washington, DC.
84. Hill, I. R., Matthiessen, P., and Heinbach, F. (1993): Guidance document on sediment toxicity tests and bioassays for freshwater and marine environments. In: *Proceedings of "Workshop on Sediment Toxicity Assessment,"* Society of Environmental Toxicology and Chemistry, Renesee, Netherlands.
85. Hillman, W. S. (1961): The lemnaceae or duckweed: A review of the descriptive and experimental literature. *Botanical Rev.*, 27:221–287.
86. Hochstein, J. R., Aulerich, R. J., and Bursian, S. J. (1988): Acute toxicity of 2,3,7,8-tetrachlorodibenzo-p-dioxin to mink. *Arch. Environ. Contam. Toxicol.*, 17:33–37.
87. Holst, R. W. (1986): *Hazard Evaluation Division Standard Procedure Non-Target Plants: Seed Germination/Seedling Emergence—Tier 1 and 2.* EPA 5430/9-86-132. Office of Pesticides and Toxic Substances, USEPA, Washington, DC.

88. Holst, R. W. (1986): *Hazard Evaluation Division Standard Procedure Non-Target Plants: Vegetative Vigor—Tiers 1 and 2*. EPA 5430/9-86-133. Office of Pesticides and Toxic Substances, USEPA, Washington, DC.
89. Holst, R. W., and Ellwanger, T. C. (1982): *Pesticide Assessment Guidelines, Subdivision J., Hazard Evaluation: Nontarget Plants*. EPA-54019-81-020, USEPA, Washington, DC.
90. Hudson et al. (1984): *Handbook of Toxicity of Pesticides to Wildlife*, 2nd ed. U.S. Fish and Wildlife Service Resource Publication 153. USDI.
91. Hulbert, S. H. (1984): Pseudoreplication and the design of ecological field experiments. *Ecol. Monographs*, 54:187–211.
92. Hunn, Joseph B. (1989): *History of Acute Toxicity Tests with Fish, 1863–1987*. U.S. Fish and Wildlife Service Investigative Fish Control Publication 98.
93. Johnson, W. W., and Finley, M. T. (1980): *Handbook of Acute Toxicity of Chemicals to Fish and Aquatic Invertebrates*. U.S. Department of Interior, Resource Publication 137, Washington, DC.
94. Kapustka, L. A. (1997): Selection of phytotoxicity tests for use in ecological risk assessments. In: *Plants For Environmental Studies*, edited by W. Wang, J. W. Gorsuch, and J. S. Hughes, pp. 517–550. Lewis Press, Boca Raton, FL.
95. Keddy, C. J., Greene, J. C., and Bonnell, M. A. (1995): Review of whole-organism bioassays: soil, freshwater sediment and freshwater assessment in Canada. *Ecotoxicol. Environ. Safety*, 30:221–251.
96. Kenaga, E. (1982): Predictability of chronic toxicity from acute toxicity of chemicals in fish and aquatic invertebrates. *Environ. Toxicol. Chem.*, 1:347–358.
97. Kenaga, R., and Moolenaar, R. (1979): Fish and *Daphnia* toxicity as surrogates for aquatic and vascular plants and algae. *Environ. Sci. Technol.*, 13:1479–1480.
98. Kendall, R. J., Brewer, L. W., Lacher, T. E., Whitten, M. L., and Marden, B. T. (1989): *The Use of Starling Nest Boxes for Field Reproductive Studies: Provisional Guidance Document and Technical Support Document*. EPA-600/8-89/056. USEPA, Washington, DC.
99. Kendall, R. J., Lacher, T. E., Jr., Bunck, C., Daniel, B., Driver, C., Grue, C. E., Leighton, F., Stansley, W., Watanabe, P. G., and Whitworth, M. (1996): An ecological risk assessment of lead shot exposure in non-waterfowl avian species: Upland game birds and raptors. *Environ. Toxicol. Chem.*, 15:4–20.
100. Klaine, S. J., Cobb, G. P., Dickerson, R. L., Dixon, K. R., Kendall, R. J., Smith E. E., and Solomon, K. R. (1996): An Ecological Risk Assessment for the Use of the Biocide Dibromonitrilopropionamide (DBNPA) in Industrial Cooling Systems. *Environ. Toxicol. Chem.*, 15:21–30.
101. Kosinski, R. (1989): Artificial streams in ecotoxicological research. In: *Aquatic Toxicology: Fundamental Concepts and Methodologies*, Vol. II, edited by A. Boudou and F. Ribeyre, pp. 297–316. CRC Press, Boca Raton, FL.
102. Krebs, C. J. (1994): *Ecology: the Experimental Analysis of Distribution and Abundance*, 4th ed. Harper Collens College Publications, New York.
103. Kuiper, J. (1977): Development of North Sea coastal plankton communities in separate plastic bags under identical conditions. *Marine Biol.*, 37:97–107.
104. Landis, W. G., and Yu, M. H. (1995): *Introduction to Environmental Toxicology*. Lewis Publishers, Boca Raton, FL.
105. LaPoint, T. W., Fairchild, J. F., Little, E. E., and Finger, S. E. (1989): Laboratory and field techniques in ecotoxicological research: strengths and limitations. In: *Aquatic Ecotoxicology: Fundamental Concepts and Methodologies*, Vol. II, edited by A. Boudou and F. Ribeyre, pp. 240–255. CRC Press, Boca Raton, FL.
106. LeBlanc, G. A. (1984): Interspecies relationships in acute toxicity of chemicals to aquatic organisms. *Environ. Toxicol. Chem.*, 3:47–60.
107. Leffler, J. W. (1980): The use of self-selected, generic aquatic microcosms for pollution effects assessment. In: *Concepts in Marine Pollution Measurements*, edited by H. H. White, pp. 139–158. University of Maryland, College Park, MD.
108. Leischman, A. A., Greene, J. C., and Miller, W. E. (1979): *Bibliography of Literature Pertaining to the Genus Selenastrum*. EPA-600/9-79-021. U.S. Environmental Protection Agency, Corvallis, OR.
109. Lemke, A. D., Brungs, W. A., and Halligan, B. J. (1978): *Manual for Construction and Operation of Toxicity-Testing Proportional Diluters*. EPA-6003/3-78-072. U.S. Environmental Protection Agency, Washington, DC.
110. Lewis, M. A. (1990): Chronic toxicities of surfactants and detergent builders to algae: a review and risk assessment. *J. Ecotoxicol. Environ. Safety*, 20:123–140.
111. Lewis, M. A. (1991): Chronic toxicities of surfactants to aquatic animals: A review and risk assessment. *Water Res.*, 25:101–113.
112. Lewis, M. A. (1995). Use of freshwater plants in the environmental risk assessment process. *Environ. Pollut.*, 87:319–336.
113. Lewis, M. A., Powell, R. L., Nelson, M. K., Henry, M. G., Klaine, S. J., Dickson, G. W., and Mayer, F. L., eds. (1999): *Ecotoxicology and Risk Assessment for Wetlands*. SETAC Press, Pensacola, FL.
114. Lewis, M. A., and Wee, V. T. (1983): Aquatic safety assessment for a cationic surfactant. *J. Environ. Toxicol. Chem.*, 2:105–118.
115. Lewis, P. A., and Weber, C. I. (1985): A study of the reliability of *Daphnia* acute toxicity tests. In: *Aquatic Toxicology and Hazard Assessment: Seventh Symposium*. edited by R. D. Cardwell, R. Purdy, and R. C. Bahner, pp. 73–86. ASTM-STP 854. American Society for Testing and Materials, Philadelphia, PA.
116. Linder, G., Ingham, E., Brandt, C. J., and Henderson, G. (1991): *Evaluation of Terrestrial Indicators for Use in Ecological Assessments at Hazardous Waste Sites*. EPA/600/R-92/183. USEPA, Washington, DC.
117. Linder, G., Wyant, J., Meganck, R., and Williams, B. (1991): Evaluating amphibian responses in wetlands impacted by mining activities in the western United States. In: *Issues and Technology in the Management of Impacted Wildlife*, edited by R. D. Comer, P. R. Davis, S. Q. Foster, C. V. Grant, S. Rush, O. Thorne, and J. Todd, pp. 17–25. Thorne Ecological Institute, Boulder, CO.
118. Linz, D. G., and Nakles, D. V. (1997): *Environmentally Acceptable Endpoints in Soil: Risk-Based Approach to Contaminated Site Management Based on Availability of Chemicals in Soil*. American Academy of Engineers. Annapolis, MD.
119. Lokke, H., ed. (1998): *Handbook of Soil Invertebrate Toxicity Tests*. John Wiley & Sons, London.
120. Long, E. R., and Morgan, L. G. (1990): *The Potential for Biological Effects of Sediment-Solved Contaminants Tested in the National Status and Trends Program*. NOAA Technical Memorandum NOS ORCA 52. National Oceanic and Atmospheric Administration, Seattle, WA.
121. Lyman, W. J., Reehl, W. F., and Rosenblatt, D. H. (1982): *Handbook of Chemical Property Estimation Methods*. McGraw-Hill, New York.
122. Macek, K., Birge, W., Mayer, F., Buikema, A., and Maki, A. (1978): Discussion session synopsis. *Estimating the Hazard of Chemical Substances to Aquatic Life*, edited by J. Cairns, K. L. Dickson, and A. W. Maki, pp. 27–32. STP 657. American Society for Testing and Materials, Philadelphia, PA.
123. Maki, A. S. (1979): Correlations between *Daphnia magna* and fathead minnow (Pimephales promelas) chronic toxicity values for several classes of test substances. *J. Fish. Res. Board Can.*, 36:411–421.

124. Mance, G. (1994): *Pollution Threat of Heavy Metals in Aquatic Environments*. Elsevier Applied Science. New York.
125. Marking, L. L. (1977): Method for assessing additive toxicity of chemical mixtures. In: *Aquatic Toxicology and Hazard Assessment*, edited by F. L. Mayer and J. L. Hamelink, pp. 99–108. ASTM-STP 634. American Society for Testing and Materials, Philadelphia, PA.
126. Mayer, F., and Ellersieck, M. R. (1986): *Manual of Acute Toxicity: Interpretation and Database for 410 Chemicals and 66 Species of Freshwater Animals*. Resource Publication 160. U.S. Department of Interior, Washington, D.C.
127. Mayfield, H. F. (1975): Suggestions for calculating nest success. *Wilson Bull.*, 87:456–466.
128. McFarlane, J. C., Pfleeger, T. G., and Fletcher, J. S. (1990): Effect, uptake, and disposition of nitrobenzene in several terrestrial plants. *Environ. Toxicol. Chem.*, 9:513–520.
129. McKim, J. M. (1977): Evaluation of tests with early life stages of fish for predicting long-term toxicity. *J. Fish. Res. Board Can.*, 34:1148–1154.
130. McLane, D. J. (1986): *Hazard Evaluation Division Standard Evaluation Procedure: Avian Reproduction Test*. EPA/540/9-86/139. USEPA, Washington, DC.
131. Menzer, R. E. (1987): Selection of animal models for data interpretation. In: *Toxic Substances and Human Risk*, edited by R. G. Tardiff and J. V. Rodricks, pp. 133–152. Plenum Press, New York.
132. Morrison G., Torello, E., Comeleo, R., Walsh, R., Kuhn, A., Burgess, R., Tagliabue, M., and Greene, W. (1989): Interlaboratory precision of saltwater short-term chronic toxicity tests. *Res. J. Water Pollut. Contr. Fed.*, 61:1708–1710.
133. Mount, D. I., and Anderson-Carnahan, L. (1988): *Methods for Aquatic Toxicity Identification Evaluations. Phase I. Toxicity Characterization Procedures*. EPA-600/3-88-034. National Effluent Toxicity Assessment Center, USEPA, Duluth, MN.
134. Mount, D. I., and Anderson-Carnahan, L. (1989): *Methods for Aquatic Toxicity Identification Evaluations. Phase II. Toxicity Identification Procedures*. EPA-600/3-88-035. National Effluent Toxicity Assessment Center, USEPA, Duluth, MN.
135. Mount, D. I., and Brungs, W. A. (1967): A simplified dosing apparatus for fish toxicology studies. *Water Res.*, 1:21–29.
136. Munawar, M., and Munawar, I. F. (1987): Phytoplankton bioassays for evaluating toxicity of in-situ sediment contaminants. *Hydrobiologia*, 149:87–105.
137. Nash, T. H., and Wirth, V. (1988): Lichens, bryophytes and air quality. *Bibliotheca Lichenol.*, 30:231–267.
138. National Institutes of Health. (1985): *Guide for the Care and Use of Laboratory Animals*. U.S. Department of Health, Education, and Welfare Publication No. (NIH) 86-23.
139. National Oceanic and Atmospheric Administration. (1995): Natural Resource Damage Assessments: Proposed Rule. 15 CFR Part 990. *Fed. Register*, 60:39804–39836.
140. National Research Council. (1981): *Testing for Effects of Chemicals on Ecosystems*. National Academy Press, Washington, DC.
141. National Research Council. (1982): *Nutrient Requirements of Mink and Foxes. Nutrient Requirements of Domestic Animals Series*. National Academy of Sciences. Washington, DC.
142. Newman, J. R., Schreiber, R. K., and Novakova, E. (1992): Air pollution effects on terrestrial and aquatic animals. In: *Air Pollution Effects on Biodiversity*, edited by J. R. Barker and D. T. Tingey, pp. 177–233. Van Nostrand Reinhold, New York.
143. Norton, S., McVey, M., Colt, J., Durda, J., and Hegner, R. (1988): *Review of Ecological Risk Assessment Methods*. EPA-230/-10-88-041. U.S. Environmental Protection Agency, Office of Policy Analysis, Office of Policy, Planning, and Evaluation, Washington, DC.
144. Nyholm, N., and Källqvist, T. (1989): Methods for growth inhibition toxicity tests with freshwater algae. *Environ. Toxicol. Chem.*, 8:689–703.
145. Okkerman, P. C., v.d. Plassche, E. J., Sloof, W., Van Leeuwen, C. J. and Canton, J. H. (1991): Ecotoxicological effects assessment: A comparison of several extrapolation procedures. *Ecotoxicol. Environ. Safety*, 21:182–193.
146. Organization for Economic Cooperation and Development. (1979): *OECD Guidelines for Testing of Chemicals*. Paris, France.
147. Organization for Economic Cooperation and Development. (1981): Bioaccumulation: Sequential static fish test (305A). Bioaccumulation: Semi-static fish test (305B). Bioaccumulation: Test for the degree of bioconcentration in fish (305C). Bioaccumulation: Static fish test (305D). Bioaccumulation: Flow-through fish test (305E). In: *OECD Guidelines for Testing of Chemicals*. OECD, Paris, France.
148. Organization for Economic Cooperation and Development. (1984): Alga growth inhibition test, Test Guideline No. 201. In: *OECD Guidelines for Testing of Chemicals*, Paris, France.
149. Organization for Economic Cooperation and Development. (1984): Terrestrial plants growth test. Test Guideline No. 208. In: *OECD Guidelines for Testing of Chemicals*, Paris, France.
150. Organization for Economic Cooperation and Development (1996): *Report of the SETAC/OECD Workshop on Avian Toxicity Testing*. OECD/GD(96)166. Environmental Directorate, OECD, Paris, France.
151. Parkhurst, B. R., Forte, J. L., and Wright, G. P. (1981): Reproducibility of a life cycle toxicity test with *Daphnia magna*. *Bull. Environ. Contam. Toxicol.*, 26:1–8.
152. Parry, M. L. (1990): *Climate Change and World Agriculture*. Earthscan Publications, London.
153. Peakall, D. B., and Fairbrother, A. (1998): Biomarkers for monitoring and measuring effects. In: *Pollution Risk Assessment and Management*, edited by P. E. Douben, pp. 351–376. John Wiley & Sons, Chichester, England.
154. Peltier, W., and Weber, C. I. (1985): Methods for Measuring the Acute Toxicity of Effluents to Freshwater and Marine Organisms. EPA-600/4-85-013. U.S. Environmental Protection Agency, Cincinnati, OH.
155. Penny, C., and Adams, C. (1863): *Fourth Report, Royal Commission on Pollution of Rivers in Scotland, Vol. 2, Evidence*. H. M. Stationery Office, London.
156. Petrocelli, S. R. (1985): Chronic toxicity tests. In: *Fundamentals of Aquatic Toxicology*, edited by G. Rand and S. Petrocelli, pp. 96–110. McGraw-Hill International Co., New York.
157. Pfleeger, T., McFarlane, J. C., Sherman, R., and Volk, G. (1991): A short-term bioassay for whole plant toxicity. In: *Plants for Toxicity Assessment*: Vol. 2, edited by J. W. Gorsuch, W. R. Lower, M. A. Lewis, and W. Wang, pp. 355–364. ASTM Publication 04-011150-16. ASTM, Philadelphia, PA.
158. Powers, E. B. (1917): The goldfish (*Carassisus carassius*) as a test animal in the study of toxicity. *Ill. Biol. Monogr.*, 4:7–73.
159. Rand, G. M. (1995): *Fundamentals of Aquatic Toxicology*, 2nd ed., Taylor and Francis, Washington, DC.
160. Ratsch, H. (1983): *Interlaboratory Root Elongation Testing of Toxic Substances on Selected Plant Species*. NTIS, PB 83-226. U.S. Environmental Protection Agency, Washington, D.C.
161. Ratsch, H. C., Johndro, D. J., and McFarlane, J. C. (1986): Growth inhibition and morphological effects of several chemicals in *Arabidopsis thaliana* (L.) Heynh. *Environ. Contam. Toxicol.*, 5:55–60.
162. Ringer, R. K., Hornshaw, T. C., and Aulerich, R. J. (1991): *Mammalian Wildlife (Mink and Ferret) Toxicity Test Protocols (LC50, Reproduction, and Secondary Toxicity)*. EPA 600/3-91/043. USEPA, Washington, DC.

163. Rosenzweig, C., and Liverman, D. (1992): Predicted effects of climate change on agriculture: A comparison of temperate and tropical regions. In: *Global Climate Change: Implications, Challenges, and Mitigation Measures*, (Majumdar, S. K., Miller, E. W., Kalkstein, L. S., Yarnal, E. M., and Rosenfeld, L. M., eds.) pp. 342–361. The Pennsylvania Academy of Sciences, Philadelphia, PA.
164. Rue, W. J., Fava, J. A., and Grothe, D. R. (1988): A review of inter- and intralaboratory effluent toxicity test method variability. In: *Aquatic Toxicology and Hazard Assessment*: Vol. 10, edited by W. J. Adams, G. A. Chapman, and W. G. Landis, pp. 190–203. STP 971. American Society for Testing and Materials, Philadelphia, PA.
165. Schafer, E. W. (1972): The acute oral toxicity of 369 pesticidal, pharmaceutical, and other chemicals to wild birds. *Toxicol. Appl. Pharmacol.*, 21:315–330.
166. Shea, D. (1988): Developing national sediment quality criteria. *Environ. Sci. Technol.*, 22:1256–1261.
167. Shimabuku, R. A., Ratsch, H. C., Wise, C. M., Nwosu, J. U., and Kapustka, L. A. (1991): A new plant life-cycle bioassay for assessment of the effects of toxic chemicals using rapid cycling Brassica. In: *Plants for Toxicity Assessment*: Vol. 2, edited by J. W. Gorsuch, W. R. Lower, M. A. Lewis, and W. Wang, pp. 3365–3375. ASTM Publication 04-011150-16. ASTM, Philadelphia, PA.
168. Solomon, K. R., Baker, D. B., Richards, R. P., Dixon, K. R., Klaine, S. J., La Point, T. W., Kendall, R. J., Weisskopf, C. P., Giddings, J. M., Giesy, J. P., Hall, L. W., Jr., and Williams, W. M. (1996): Ecological risk assessment of atrazine in North American surface waters. *Environ. Toxicol. Chem.*, 15:31–76.
169. Sortkjaer, O. (1984): Macrophytes and macrophyte communities as test systems in ecotoxicological studies of aquatic systems. *Ecol. Bull. (Stockholm)*, 36:75–80.
170. Sprague, J. B. (1969): Measurement of pollutant toxicity to fish. I. Bioassay methods for acute toxicity. *Water Res.*, 3:793–821.
171. Sprague, J. B. (1970): Measurement of pollutant toxicity to fish. II. Utilizing and applying bioassay results. *Water Res.*, 4:3–32.
172. Sprague, J. B. (1971): Measurement of pollutant toxicity to fish. III. Sublethal effects and "safe" concentrations. *Water Res.*, 5:245–266.
173. Stephan, C. E. (1977): Methods for calculating an LC_{50}. In: *Aquatic Toxicology and Hazard Evaluation*, edited by F. L. Mayer and J. L. Hamelink, pp. 65–84. ASTM STP 634. American Society for Testing and Materials, Philadelphia, PA.
174. Stephan, C., Mount, D., Hansen, D., Gentile, J., Chapman, G., and Brungs, W. (1985): *Guidelines for Deriving National Water Quality Criteria for the Protection of Aquatic Organisms and Their Uses*. PB85-227049. U.S. Environmental Protection Agency, Office of Water Regulations and Standards, NTIS, Springfield, VA.
175. Suter, G. W., II, Barnthouse, L. W., Bartell, S. M., Mill, T., Mackay, D., and Paterson, S. (1993). *Ecological Risk Assessment*. Lewis Publishers, Chelsea, MI.
176. Swann, R. L., Laskowski, D. A., McCall, P. J., Vander Kuy, K., and Dishburger, H. J. (1983): A rapid method for the estimation of the environmental parameters octanol/water partition coefficient, soil sorption constant, water to air ratio, and water solubility. *Residue Rev.*, 85:17–28.
177. Taub, F. B. (1984): Synthetic microcosms as biological models of algal communities. *Algae as Ecological Indicators*, edited by L. E. Shubert, pp. 363–394. Academic Press, New York.
178. Thursby, G. B., Anderson, B. S., Walsh, G. E., and Steele, R. L. (1993): *A Review of the Current Status of Marine Algal Toxicity Testing in the United States*. In: *First Symposium on Environmental Toxicology and Risk Assessment: Aguatic, Plant, and Terrestrial, STP 1179*. American Society for Testing and Materials, Philadelphia, PA.
179. Traunspurger, W., and Drews, C. (1996): Toxicity analysis of freshwater and marine sediments with meio and macrobenthic organisms: A review. *Hydrobiologia*, 328:215–261.
180. UNEP International Environmental Technology Centre. (1996): *Environmental Risk Assessment for Sustainable Cities*. Technical Publication Series, Issue 3.
181. Urban, D. J., and Cook, N. J. (1986): *Hazard Evaluation Division Standard Evaluation Procedure: Ecological Risk Assessment*. USEPA 540/9-85/001. USEPA, Washington, DC.
182. U.S. Department of Interior. (1996): *Silver Hazards to Fish, Wildlife, and Invertebrates, a Synoptic Review*. Biological Science Report 32. National Biological Service, Washington, DC.
183. U.S. Department of Interior. (1998): *Copper Hazards to Fish, Wildlife, and Invertebrates, a Synoptic Review*. Biological Science Report, USGS/BRD/BSR Contaminant Hazard Reviews Report 33. U.S. Geological Survey, Washington, DC.
184. U.S. Environmental Protection Agency. (1975): *Committee on Methods for Acute Toxicity Tests with Aquatic Organisms: Method for Acute Toxicity Tests with Fish, Macroinvertebrates, and Amphibians*. EPA-660/3-75-009. USEPA, Washington, DC.
185. U.S. Environmental Protection Agency. (1978): *Pesticide Assessment Guidelines Subdivision E, Hazard Evaluation: Wildlife and Aquatic Organisms*. EPA/540/9-82/024. USEPA, Washington, DC.
186. U.S. Environmental Protection Agency. (1979): Toxic Substances Control Act premanufacture testing of new chemical substances. *Fed. Register*, 44:16240–16292.
187. U.S. Environmental Protection Agency. (1982): *Pesticide Assessment Guidelines Subdivision L, Hazard Evaluation: Nontarget Insects*. EPA/540/9-82/019. USEPA, Washington, DC.
188. U.S. Environmental Protection Agency. (1984): *Estimating "Concern Levels" for Concentrations of Chemical Substances in the Environment*. Environmental Effects Branch, Health and Environmental Review Division, USEPA, Washington, DC.
189. U.S. Environmental Protection Agency (1985): Toxic substances control act test guidelines; final rules. *Fed. Register*, 50:797.1050, 797.1075, and 707.1060 (includes technical support document).
190. U.S. Environmental Protection Agency. (1987): *Aquatic Mesocosm Tests to Support Pesticide Registrations*. EPA-EEB/HED/OPP. USEPA, Washington, DC.
191. U.S. Environmental Protection Agency. (1988): *Review of Ecological Risk Assessment Methods*. EPA/230-19-88-041. Office of Policy, Planning and Evaluation, USEPA, Washington, DC.
192. U.S. Environmental Protection Agency. (1991): *Summary Report on Issues in Ecological Risk Assessment*. EPA/626/3-91/018. USEPA, Washington, DC.
193. U.S. Environmental Protection Agency–U.S. Army Corps of Engineers. (1991): *Evaluation of Dredged Materials Proposed for Ocean Disposal. Testing Manual*. EPA-503/8-91-001. USEPA, Washington, DC.
194. U.S. Environmental Protection Agency. (1992): *Peer Review Workshop Report on a Framework for Ecological Risk Assessment*. EPA/625/3-91/022. Risk Assessment Forum, USEPA, Washington, DC.
195. U.S. Environmental Protection Agency. (1992): *Framework for Ecological Risk Assessment*. EPA/630/R-92/001. US EPA, Washington, DC.
196. U.S. Environmental Protection Agency. (1993): *Methods for Measuring the Acute Toxicity of Effluents and Receiving Waters to Freshwater and Marine Organisms*. EPA/600/4-90/027F. Office of Research and Development, Washington, DC.
197. U.S. Environmental Protection Agency. (1994): *Short-Term Methods for Estimating the Chronic Toxicity of Effluents and*

Receiving Water to Freshwater Organisms. EPA 600-4-91-002. Office of Research and Development, USEPA, Washington, DC.

198. U.S. Environmental Protection Agency. (1995): *Great Lakes Water Quality Initiative Technical Support document for the Procedure to Determine Bioaccumulation Factors*. EPA-820-B-95-005. Office of Water, Washington, DC.
199. U.S. Environmental Protection Agency. (1997): *Ecological Risk Assessment Guidance for Superfund: Process for Designing and Conducting Ecological Risk Assessments. Interim Final*. EPA 540-R-97-006. USEPA, Washington, DC.
200. U.S. Environmental Protection Agency. (1997): *Region 9 Preliminary Remediation Goals*. USEPA, San Francisco, CA. http://www.epa.gov/region09/water/sfund/prg/index.html.
201. U.S. Environmental Protection Agency. (1998): *National Sediment Bioaccumulation Conference Proceedings*. EPA 823-R-98-002. Office of Water, USEPA, Washington, DC.
202. U.S. Environmental Protection Agency. (1998): *Method for Assessing the Chronic Toxicity of Sediment-Associated Contaminants with Leptocheirus plumulosus*. USEPA, Office of Research and Development, Duluth, MN.
203. U.S. Environmental Protection Agency. (1998): *Guidelines for Ecological Risk Assessment*. EPA/630/R-95/002F. USEPA, Washington, DC.
204. U.S. Fish and Wildlife Service. (1997): Migratory bird hunting: Revised test protocol for nontoxic approval procedures for shot and shot coating; final rule. *Fed. Register*, 62:63608–63615.
205. U.S. Food and Drug Administration. (1987): Seed germination and root elongation, In: *Environmental Assessment Technical Handbook 4.06*. Center for Food Safety and Applied Nutrition, Center for Veterinary Medicine, Washington, DC.
206. Van der Zandt, P. T. J., and Van Leeuwen, C. J. (1992): A proposal for priority setting of existing chemical substances. Proposal prepared for the Directorate General for Environment, Nuclear Safety and Civil Protection of the Commission of the European Communities, Directorate General for Environmental Protection, The Hague, Netherlands.
207. Vittozzi, L., and De Angelis, G. (1991): A critical review of comparative acute toxicity data on freshwater fish. *Aquat. Toxicol.*, 19:167–204.
208. Wagner, C., and Lokke, H. (1991): Estimation of ecotoxicological protection levels from NOEC toxicity data. *Water Res.*, 10:1237–1242.
209. Wallbridge, C. T. (1977): *A Flow Through Testing Procedure With Duckweed* (*Lemna minor*). EPA-600/3-77-108. USEPA, Duluth, MN.
210. Walsh, G. E. (1988): Principles of toxicity testing with marine unicellular algae. *Environ. Toxicol. Chem.*, 7:979–987.
211. Walsh, G. E., and Merrill, R. G. (1984): Algal bioassays of industrial and energy process effluents. In: *Algae as Ecological Indicators*, edited by L. E. Shubert, pp. 329–360. Academic Press, New York.
212. Walsh, G. E., Weber, D. E., Simon, T. L., Brashers, L. K. and Moore, J. C. (1991): Use of marsh plants for toxicity testing of water and sediments. In: *Plants for Toxicity Assessment*, Vol. 2, edited by J. W. Gorsuch, W. R. Lower, W. Wang, and M. A. Lewis, pp. 341–354. STP 115. American Society for Testing and Materials, Philadelphia, PA.
213. Walton, B. T. (1980): Differential life-stage susceptibility of *Acheta domesticus* to acridine. *Environ. Entomol.*, 9:18–20.
214. Wang, W. (1986): Toxicity tests of aquatic pollutants by using common duckweed. *Environ. Pollut.* (*Series B*), 11:1–14.
215. Wang, W. (1990): Literature review on duckweed toxicity testing. *Environ. Res.*, 52:7–22.
216. Warren-Hicks, W., Parkhurst, B. R., and Baker, S. S. (1989): *Ecological Assessments of Hazardous Waste Sites: A Field and Laboratory Reference Document*. EPA/600/3-89/01. USEPA, Washington, DC.
217. Weber, D. E., Walsh, G. E., and MacGregor, M. A. (1995): Use of vascular aquatic plants in phytotoxicity studies with sediments. In: *Environmental Toxicology and Risk Assessment*, Vol. 3, edited by J. S. Hughes, G. R. Biddinger, and E. Mones, pp. 187–200. ASTM STP 1218. American Society for Testing and Materials, Philadelphia, PA.
218. Williams, L. R., Biesinger, W., Bentley, van der Schalie, R., and Suprenant, D. (1986): *Collaborative Study of Daphnia magna Static Renewal Assays*. EPA 600/3-86-115. USEPA, Las Vegas, NV.
219. Wong, P. T. S., Chau, Y. K., Ali, N., and Whittle, D. M. (1994): Biochemical and genotoxic effects in the vicinity of a pulp mill discharge. *Environ. Toxicol. Water Quality*, 9:59–70.

Appendix

University	Degree, Program	University website	Program website
Ashland University, Ohio	BS in Toxicology	www.ashland.edu	www.ashland.edu/tox.html
Case Western Reserve University	MS, PhD in Environmental Health Sciences with specialization in environmental toxicology or molecular toxicology	www.cwru.edu	www.cwru.edu/bulletin/Medicine/environmental_health.html#GRADUATE PROGRAMS
Clemson University	MS, PhD in Environmental Toxicology	www.clemson.edu	
Cornell University	MS, PhD in Environmental Toxicology	www.cornell.edu	www.gradschool.cornell.edu/grad/fields_1/env-tox.html
Dartmouth College	PhD in Pharmacology and Toxicology	www.dartmouth.edu	www.dartmouth.edu/dms/pharmtox/graduate_prog.html
Duke University	Master of Environmental Management in Environmental Toxicology, Chemistry, and Risk Assessment	www.duke.edu	www.env.duke.edu/degreeprof.html#3
	PhD in an Integrated Toxicology Program		pharmacology.mc.duke.edu/itp.html
Duquesne University	MS, PhD in Pharmacology-Toxicology	www.duq.edu	www.duq.edu/pharmacy/GraduateSchool/gradschoolhome.html
Emory University	PhD, Program in Molecular Therapeutics and Toxicology	www.emory.edu	www.biomed.emory.edu/MTT/MTT.html
Florida Agricultural and Mechanical University	PhD with a specialization in Pharmacology and Toxicology	www.famu.edu	www.famu.edu/gds/degree.html
The George Washington University	MS in Chemical Toxicology	www.gwu.edu	www.gwu.edu/~csas/chemtox.html
Harvard University	PhD in Biological Sciences in Public Health (Molecular and Cellular Toxicology)	www.harvard.edu	www.hsph.harvard.edu/Register/mct-int.html
Indiana University–Purdue University, Indianapolis	MS, PhD in Toxicology from Toxicology Graduate Program	www.iupui.edu	www.iupui.edu/~iutox/gradprogram.html
Iowa State University of Science and Technology	MS, PhD in Interdepartmental Graduate Major in Toxicology	www.iastate.edu	molebio.iastate.edu/~I_wild/toxhome.htm
Johns Hopkins University	PhD in Toxicological Sciences	www.jhu.edu	www.sph.jhu.edu/ehs/Education/degrees.htm
Long Island University, Brooklyn Campus	MS with specialization in Pharmacology/Toxicology	www.brooklyn.liunet.edu	www.liu.edu/cwis/pharmacy/phbut07/grad02.html#3
Massachusetts Institute of Technology	PhD, ScD or SM (Master's) in Toxicology	web.mit.edu	web.mit.edu/afs/athena.mit.edu/org/t/tox/www/
Medical College of Georgia	MS, PhD in Pharmacology and Toxicology	www.mcg.edu	www.mcg.edu/som/PhmTox/Index.html
Medical College of Wisconsin	PhD in Pharmacology and Toxicology	www.mcw.edu	www.mcw.edu/gradschool/Pharmtox.htm
Memorial University of Newfoundland	PhD in Biochemistry with research specialization in environmental biochemistry and toxicology	www.mun.ca	www.mun.ca/biochem/grad/gradinfo.html

University	Degree, Program	University website	Program website
Michigan State University	Multidisciplinary Master's Specialization or Doctoral Program in Environmental Toxicology	www.msu.edu	www.iet.msu.edu/gradprog.htm
New York University	PhD in Environmental Health Science with concentrations in molecular toxicology, systemic toxicology, aquatic toxicology or environmental toxicology	www.nyu.edu	www.nyu.edu/gsas/program/enviro/program/
North Carolina State University, Raleigh	MS, PhD in Toxicology, and Masters of Toxicology	www.ncsu.edu	www.cals.ncsu.edu/toxicol/academic.html
Northeastern University	PhD with specialization in toxicology from Bouvé College of Pharmacy and Health Science	www.northeastern.edu	www.neu.edu/bouvegrad/bio_ms_courses.html#biotoxicms
The Ohio State University	MS, PhD program in pharmacology/toxicology in College of Pharmacy	www.osu.edu	www.pharmacy.ohio-state.edu/homepage/program/graduate/pcol/pcolgrad.htm
Oregon State University	MS, PhD in Toxicology from College of Agricultural Sciences	www.orst.edu	www.orst.edu/Dept/grad_school/major_minor/majors/toxicology.htm
Pennsylvania State University	MS, PhD in Cellular and Molecular Mechanisms of Toxicity	www.psu.edu	www.cas.psu.edu/docs/CASDEPT/VET/moltox.htm
Philadelphia College of Pharmacy and Science	MS, PhD in Pharmacology and Toxicology	www.pcps.edu	www.pcps.edu/graduate/pharmtox.html
Queen's University at Kingston	MSc, PhD in Pharmacology and Toxicology	info.queensu.ca	meds-ss10.meds.queensu.ca/medicine/pharm/
Rutgers, the State University of New Jersey, New Brunswick	MS, PhD in a Joint Graduate Program in Toxicology (with University of Medicine and Dentistry of New Jersey)	www.rutgers.edu	www.eohsi.rutgers.edu/personel/creeden/jgpt.html
St. John's University, New York	MS in Toxicology from College of Pharmacy and Allied Health Professions PhD in Pharmacology/Toxicology from College of Pharmacy and Allied Health Professions	www.stjohns.edu	www.stjohns.edu/pahp/toxicology.html www.stjohns.edu/pahp/Phd.html#PHD
San Diego State University	MS, PhD with concentration in toxicology from School of Public Health	www.sdsu.edu	www-rohan.sdsu.edu/dept/gsphsdsu/web/degrees.html
Simon Fraser University	MS in Environmental Toxicology	www.sfu.ca	www.biol.sfu.ca/academics
State University of New York at Buffalo	PhD in Pharmacology and Toxicology	www.buffalo.edu	wings.buffalo.edu/academic/department/medicine/pmy/
Texas A&M University, College Station	PhD in Medical Pharmacology and Toxicology	www.tamu.edu	medicine.tamu.edu/pharm/gradprog.htm
Université de Montreal	DESS, Toxicologie et analyse due risque	www.umontreal.ca	alize.ere.umontreal.ca/gris/sp/dmthm/dmthm3a.html#desstox
University at Albany, SUNY	MS, PhD in Environmental Health and Toxicology, from School of Public Health	www.albany.edu	www.wadsworth.org/EHT/program.htm
The University of Alabama at Birmingham	PhD, Graduate Training Program in Toxicology	www.uab.edu	WWW.UAB.EDU/graduates/areas/toxicolo.htm
University of Arizona	MS, PhD in Pharmacology and Toxicology	www.arizona.edu	www.ahsc.arizona.edu/pharmacology/course.htm

University	Degree, Program	University website	Program website
University of Arkansas for Medical Sciences	PhD in interdisciplinary toxicology from Department of Pharmacology and Toxicology	www.uams.edu	www.uams.edu/pharmtox/tox.htm
University of California, Davis	MS, PhD from the Graduate Group in Pharmacology/Toxicology	www.ucdavis.edu	wdsroot.ucdavis.edu/caes/envtox/GRAD/ptxmain.html
University of California, Irvine	PhD in Environmental Toxicology	www.uci.edu	www.med.uci.edu/~env-tox/index.html
University of California, Riverside	MS, PhD in Environmental Toxicology	www.ucr.edu	cnas.ucr.edu/~etox/home.html
University of Connecticut, Storrs	MS, PhD specializing in toxicology from School of Pharmacy	www.uconn.edu	137.99.44.97/www.pharm/
University of Georgia	MS, PhD with major in toxicology from the Interdisciplinary Graduate Program in Toxicology	www.uga.edu	www.rx.uga.edu/info/depts/toxi.html
University of Guelph	MSc, PhD in Pharmacology-Toxicology from Department of Biomedical Sciences	www.uoguelph.ca	www.ovcnet.uoguelph.ca/BioMed/index.html
University of Kansas	PhD in Pharmacology or Toxicology from the Department of Pharmacology, Toxicology, and Therapeutics	www.ukans.edu	www.kumc.edu/igpbs/faculty/ResearchFacultyInformationPages-MTAEH.html
University of Kentucky	PhD from the Graduate Center for Toxicology	www.uky.edu	www.mc.uky.edu/toxicology/
University of Louisville	PhD in Pharmacology and Toxicology	www.louisville.edu	www.louisville.edu/medschool/pharmacology/
University of Maryland, Baltimore	MS, PhD from the Department of Pharmacology and Experimental Therapeutics	www.ab.umd.edu	graduate.umaryland.edu/Toxicology.html
	PhD from the Pharmaceutical Sciences Program		www.pharmacy.ab.umd.edu/webhome/PSC/guide.html
University of Maryland, College Park	MS, PhD from Toxicology Program	www.umcp.umd.edu	www.inform.umd.edu/EdRes/GradInfo/GradCat/GradProg/toxi.htm
University of Massachusetts Medical Center at Worcester	PhD in Pharmacology and Molecular Toxicology	www.ummed.edu	www.ummed.edu/dept/pharmacology/pharmac0.htm#I1
University of Michigan, Ann Arbor	PhD from the School of Public Health	www.umich.edu	www.sph.umich.edu/eih/tox
University of Minnesota Duluth,	PhD from the Toxicology Graduate Program	www.d.umn.edu	www.sph.umich.edu/eih/tox
University of Mississippi	MS, PhD in Pharmacology with emphasis on toxicology	www.olemiss.edu	www.olemiss.edu/depts/pharmacology/gprogrm.html
University of Mississippi Medical Center	PhD from the Department of Pharmacology and Toxicology	fiona.umsmed.edu	umc.edu/medicine/pharmacology/teaching/program.html
University of Nebraska Medical Center–University of Nebraska Lincoln	MS, PhD in various departments with emphasis on toxicology, from the Center for Environmental Toxicology	www.unmc.edu	www.unmc.edu/Eppley/ToxCenter/
University of New Mexico	MS, PhD from joint program with College of Pharmacy and Biomedical Sciences Graduate Program	www.unm.edu	hsc.unm.edu/pharmacy/tox.html

University	Degree, Program	University website	Program website
The University of North Carolina At Chapel Hill	PhD from the Curriculum in Toxicology	www.unc.edu	www.med.unc.edu/toxicology/
University of North Dakota	Undergraduate minor in Pharmacology and Toxicology, MS, PhD in Pharmacology and Toxicology	www.und.edu	www.med.und.nodak.edu/depts/pharmtox
University of Oklahoma	Oklahoma Center for Toxicology has a graduate program in Toxicology	www.ou.edu	www.cpb.uokhsc.edu/tox
University of Rhode Island	PhD in Pharmacology and Toxicology from the College of Pharmacy	www.uri.edu	nick.uri.edu/pharm/research.htm#BMS
University of Rochester	PhD in Toxicology	www.rochester.edu	www.envmed.rochester.edu/wwwrlp/niehsc/ur/tox.htm
University of Saskatchewan	Postgraduate Diploma, MSc and PhD programs in toxicology from the Toxicology Centre	www.usask.edu	www.usask.ca/toxicology/grad_index.shtml
University of Southern California	PhD in Molecular Pharmacology and Toxicology	www.usc.edu	www.usc.edu/hsc/pharmacy/graduate-programs.html
The University of Texas–Houston Health Science Center		www.uth.tmc.edu	gsbs.gs.uth.tmc.edu
The University of Texas Medical Branch at Galveston	MS, PhD from the Graduate Program in Pharmacology and Toxicology	www.utmb.edu	www.utmb.edu/phtox/educa/program/gradprog.htm
University of Toronto	Undergraduate Specialist Program in Toxicology; MA, MSc, MScF, MASc, or PhD from the Collaborative Graduate Program in Toxicology	www.utoronto.ca	www.library.utoronto.ca/www/pharm_tox/index.htm www.sgs.utoronto.ca/www/sgs/sgs%5Fdept%5Ftoxi.html
University of Utah	PhD in Pharmacology and Toxicology	www.utah.edu	lysine.pharm.utah.edu/phtx/phtxhome.html#Overview
University of Washington	MS, PhD from the Toxicology Graduate Program in the Department of Environmental Health	www.washington.edu	cucme.sphcm.washington.edu/DEHWeb/toxicology.html
University of Western Ontario	Honors BSc in Pharmacology and Toxicology Honors BSc in Toxicology with Environmental Sciences MSc, PhD in Pharmacology and Toxicology	www.uwo.ca	www.pharmtox.med.uwo.ca
University of Wisconsin–Madison	MS, PhD in Environmental Toxicology	www.wisc.edu	www.wisc.edu/etc
Vanderbilt University	MS, PhD from the Graduate Program in Toxicology and Carcinogenesis	www.vanderbilt.edu	www.toxicology.mc.Vanderbilt.Edu/grad.html
Virginia Commonwealth University	MS, PhD in Pharmacology and Toxicology	www.vcu.edu	views.vcu.edu/views/pharmtox/gen.html#1
Washington State University	MS, PhD in Pharmacology and Toxicology from the College of Pharmacy	www.wsu.edu	www.pharmtox.wsu.edu
West Virginia University	PhD in Pharmacology and Toxicology with research concentration in toxicology	www.wvu.edu	www.hsc.wvu.edu/som/pcol_tox/graduate.htm
Wright State University School of Medicine	Graduate Program in Pharmacology/Toxicology	www.wright.edu	www.med.wright.edu/som/academic/pharm/PHARM.HTML

Principles and Methods of Toxicology, Fourth Edition, edited by A. Wallace Hayes.
Taylor & Francis, Philadelphia © 2001.

Glossary

Absorbed Dose: Energy imparted to matter when radiation passes through. Measured in grays or rads.

Absorption: Uptake of the chemical from the site of administration into the general circulation. Absorption may involve a number of stages (e.g., dissolution) and diffusion through membranes. Chemicals may be changed during absorption due to metabolism or degradation, such that it is possible to have complete absorption and low bioavailability (see below).

Absorption Barrier: Any of the exchange barriers of the body that allow differential diffusion of various substances across a boundary. Examples of absorption barriers are the skin, lung tissue, and gastrointestinal tract wall.

ACB: Accelerated cancer bioassay.

Acceptable Daily Intake (*ADI*): Daily intake of a chemical (food additive, pesticide etc.) which, during the entire lifetime, appears to be without appreciable risk (affects 1 in 1 million people or less) on the basis of all known facts at the time.

Accessory Cells: Cells that support T or B cells in the induction of an immune response. These cells usually express MHC class II molecules.

Accuracy: A measure of the extent to which the mean estimate of a quantity approaches its true value.

ACTH: Adrenocortical tropic hormone.

Action Level: Level of unavoidable contaminants in foods and feeds considered as the upper limit of safety but are not subjected to regulatory control.

Acute: Characterized by a time period of short duration; commonly used to describe single-dose exposure in toxicity studies.

Acute Toxicity: The adverse effects occurring within a short time of administration of a single dose of a substance or multiple doses given within 24 hours.

Acute Toxicity Study: Usually, a single-dose study in which animals are observed for a 2-week period post-dose to determine overt signs of toxicity, normally including some form of assessment of the lethal dose.

Acute-to-Chronic Ratio (*ACR*): A ratio determined experimentally or mathematically for a chemical that is used to predict chronic toxicity when only acute toxicity data are available.

ADH: Antidiuretic hormone or vasopressin; an octapeptide.

Adjuvant: A material that enhances an immune response, it traditionally refers to a mixture of oil and mycobacterial cell fragments.

Ad libitum: Available with unrestricted access. This term is commonly used in toxicity studies to describe free access by the animals to feed or water.

ADME: Absorption, Distribution, Metabolism, and Excretion. The processes that determine the disposition and fate of an administered molecule.

Administered Dose: The amount of a substance given to a test subject (human or animal) in determining dose-response relationships, especially through ingestion or inhalation. In exposure assessment, because exposure to chemicals is usually inadvertent, this quantity is called potential dose.

Aerosol: A suspension of either microscopic liquid or solid particles dispensed in a gas, the particles of which have a negligible falling velocity. Also used to characterize a product or chemical form that contains particles that can enter the respiratory tract.

Aglycone: The xenobiotic substrate that is conjugated by glucuronosyltransferases.

Air Elutriation: A process in which particles are separated on the basis of size by pitting their settling velocity against the velocity of a current of air with which they move.

Air Shower: A device that uses high velocity, ultra-filtered air to remove particulates from the surfaces of the clothing worn by personnel.

AL: Ad libitum.

Aleveolar Macrophage: A motile, phagocytic cell found in the alveoli that plays an important role in the lung's cellular defense though the clearance and/or inactivation of inhaled particles and pathogens.

Alkaloids: Nitrogenous heterocyclic compounds that protect plants from attack by microorganisms, pests, and herbivores.

Allergic Contact Dermatitis: Chemically induced immunologic (delayed hypersensitivity) dermatitis.

Allergy: A state of altered immunity in which contact with an antigen (allergen) results in a hypersensitivity response.

Allogeneic: From a different genetic background. In the context of immunotoxicology, generally refers to the use of genetically dissimilar cells in in vitro assays to elicit a cell-medicated immune response.

Allometry: The study of the relationship between body size and various biological and physiological parameters, such as organ sizes, blood flow rates, and metabolic rates.

Alpha Particle: Nucleus of a helium atom emitted by certain radioisotopes upon disintegration. Contains two protons and two neutrons.

Alveoli: Air-filled sacs at the terminus of bronchioles in the mammalian lung which provide the surface for gas exchange and as a portal of entry and/or elimination for volatile chemicals.

Ambient Measurement: A measurement (usually of the concentration of a chemical or pollutant) taken in an ambient medium, normally with the intent of relating the measured value to the exposure of an organism that contacts that medium.

Amyotrophic Lateral Sclerosis: Fatal neurologic disease characterized by progressive degeneration of upper and lower motor neurons in the brain and spinal cord.

Analytic Study: A study designed to examine a priori hypothesized casual associations.

Anaphylaxis: An extreme, immediate immunologic reaction characterized by contraction of smooth muscle and dilation of capillaries due to release of pharmacologically active substances (e.g., histamine) in response to administration of a foreign material.

Androgens: Male sex steroids (e.g., testosterone).

Anemia: Reduction below normal of hemoglobin concentration; usually accompanied by a similar reduction of red blood cell count and hematocrit.

Anergy (*Tolerance*): Unresponsiveness to antigenic stimulation. Also referred to as tolerance.

ANOVA: Analysis of variance.

Antibody: Complex molecules produced by plasma cells that recognize specific antigens. Antibodies, also called immunoglobulins (Ig), consist of two basic units. The antigen-binding section (Fab) contains variable regions coding for antigen recognition. In mammals, the constant region of the molecule (Fc) may be grouped into several classes, designed IgA, IgD, IgE, IgG, and IgM, depending on the molecule's function. Cross-linking of antibody molecules on the surface of a target leads to activation of complement, usually resulting in the destruction of the target.

Antibody-forming Cell (*AFC*)/*Plaque-forming Cell* (*PFC*) *Assay*: An assay that measures the ability of animals to produce specific antibodies against a T-dependent or T-independent antigen following in vivo sensitization. Due to the involvement of multiple cell populations in mounting an antibody response, the AFC assay actually evaluates several immune parameters simultaneously. It is considered to be one of the most sensitive indicator systems for immunotoxicology studies.

Antigen: A molecule that is the subject of a specific immune reaction. Antigens are recognized in a cognate fashion by the T-cell antigen receptor, the B-cell antigen receptor, or immunoglobulins (antibodies). Antigens generally are proteinaceous in nature.

Antigen-presenting Cell (*APC*): Cells that are responsible for making antigens accessible to immune effector and regulatory cells. Following internalization and degradation of the antigen (generally by phagocytosis), a fragment of the antigen molecule is presented on the APC cell surface in association with an MHC molecule. This complex is recognized by either B cells via surface-bound immunoglobulin molecules or by T cells via the T-cell antigen receptor. Induction of a specific immune response then proceeds. APC include macrophages, dendritic cells, and certain B cells.

Antigenicity (*Immunogenicity*): The property of eliciting an immune response, characterized by an interaction of a foreign material with endogenous antibodies and/or immune cells, in a subject that has been previously exposed (sensitized) to that foreign material.

Anti-Mullerian Hormone (*also called Mullerian inhibiting substance*): A protein produced by fetal Sertoli cells that prevents formation of a female reproductive tract in male fetuses.

Aortic Perfusion: Aorta is cannulated for inflow of the perfusate through the heart and the perfusate exits through the left atrium.

Apoptosis: A series of biochemical events characterized by activation of a series of caspace enzymes that lead to the digestion of cellular DNA with the appearance of DNA laddering on agarose gels and morphological formation of intranuclear clumps in affected cells. This process is also known as programmed cell death, whereby cells die in a controlled, progressive manner that is regulated in part by the release of mitochondrial-initiating factors and cytochrome c.

Apparent Volume of Distribution: The volume of plasma (or blood) into which the body load appears to have been dissolved or distributed; equivalent to the body load, at any time, divided by the corresponding plasma (or blood) concentration. It is not a physiological volume, but is important, as it indicates the volume of plasma that has to be cleared of chemical; independent of concentration and dose under first-order conditions.

Applied Dose: The amount of a substance in contact with the primary absorption boundaries of an organism (e.g., skin, lung, gastrointestinal tract) and available for absorption.

Aquatic Toxicology: The study of adverse effects on freshwater and saltwater biota and on the ecosystems which contain them.

Arithmetic Mean: The sum of all the measurements in a data set divided by the number of measurements in the data set.

Atherosclerosis: Nodular sclerosis characterized by irregularly distributed lipid deposits in the intima of the large and medium-sized arteries; such deposits are associated with fibrosis and calcification.

Atophy: General systemic or local hypersensitivity (i.e., allergy), often related to genetic predisposition. May be thought of as "unwanted reactivity."

Atrail Perfusion: Right atrium is cannulated for inflow of the perfusate, which exits through the right ventricle via pulmonary arterial cannula or an open slit.

AUC: Area under the plasma concentration time course.

Autoimmunity: Immune reactivity toward self.

Autologous Blood Perfusate: Blood used as perfusate comes from the same animal from which the organ was removed for perfusion.

Autolysis: Enzymatic self digestion of cells or tissues that occurs after death. Autolysis complicates detection of pathologic changes in tissues or organs during necropsy and subsequent microscopic examination, and can make valid observations during these activities impossible.

Autoradiography: The production of an image by the emission of radioactive decay energy from a radionuclide. It provides a qualitative visual image of the tissue distribution of a xenobiotic and can provide quantitative distribution data as well. Quantitative whole-body autoradiography (QWBA) is becoming a standard tool for absorption, distribution, metabolism, and excretion (ADME) studies.

Autosome: A chromosome that is not a sex-determining chromosome.

Azotemia: Accumulation of nitrogenous wastes such as urea or creatinine in the blood.

Background Level (*Environmental*): The concentration of substance in a defined control area during a fixed period of time before, during, or after a data-gathering operation.

Basepair Substitution: A gene mutation characterized by the replacement of one nucleotide pair for another in a codon.

B Cell/B Lymphocyte: Lymphocytes that recognize antigen via surface-bound immunoglobulins. B cells that have been exposed to specific antigen differentiate into plasma cells that are responsible for producing specific antibodies. B cells differentiate in the bone marrow in mammals and in an organ known as the bursa in birds.

B-Cell Antigen Receptor: A membrane-bound molecular complex responsible for antigen recognition by B cells. It comprises membrane immunoglobulin (mIg) and several accessory molecules. Functionally analogous, but structurally dissimilar, to the T-cell antigen receptor.

Becquerel (*bq*): SI unit of radioactivity equaling one disintegration/second, approximately 2.7×10^{-11} curies (Ci).

Behavioral Teratology: The functional deficits arising from exposure to neurotoxic agents during early development.

Benchmark Dose: The lower confidence limit on a dose associated with a specified level of response.

Beer–Lambert Law: This law relates solute concentration and cell path length to UV absorbance. The law can be expressed by the following equation:

$$A = \log I_o/I_t = abc,$$

where A = absorbance, I_o is the original intensity incident on the cell, I_t, is the reduced intensity transmitted from the cell, a is a proportionality constant called the absorptivity, b is the path length of the solution, and c is the concentration of the analyte. When c is in moles per liter, the constant is called molar absorptivity or molar extinction coefficient. When c is a 1% solution and b is a 1 cm path length, the term specific absorptivity is used (a 1%/1 cm is the most common form used).

Bias: Systemic error as opposed to a sampling error. For example, selection bias may occur when each member of the population does not have an equal chance of being selected for the sample.

Bioaccumulation: The net uptake of chemicals from the environment from all sources.

Bioactivation: The enzymatic conversion of a chemical to a more toxic form (in the body, or in vitro by an enzyme as a model of a process in the body).

Bioassay: A functional assay that depends on the use of living cells or cell components as an indicator system.

Bioavailability: The fraction (or sometimes percentage) of the administered dose which enters the general circulation as the parent compound. A low bioavailability may be due to poor absorption and/or first-pass metabolism; independent of dose under first-order conditions.

Bioconcentration: The uptake of chemicals from water alone.

Bioconcentration factor (*BCF*): The tendency of a chemical to be more concentrated in an aquatic organism than the concentration in its environment, calculated by dividing the concentration of the chemical in the organism (wet weight) by the concentration of the chemical in the water.

Biocontainment: The process and equipment used for the purpose of preventing the unwanted release of hazardous material or organisms.

Biodegradation: The break down of chemicals in organisms or the environment, primarily by microorganisms.

Biodiversity: The variety of organisms considered at all levels, from genetic variants belonging to the same species through arrays of species to arrays of genera, families, and higher taxa; includes the variety of ecosystems, which comprise both the communities of organisms within particular habitats and the physical conditions under which they live.

Bioexclusion: The process of preventing the introduction of unwanted microorganisms into animals or their immediate environment.

Biologically Effective Dose: The amount of a deposited or absorbed chemical that reaches the cells or target site where an adverse effect occurs or where that chemical interacts with a membrane surface.

Biologically-Based Dose-Response Model: A mathematical expression of the relationship between the incidence of severity of a biological effect and dose that is based on the biological mechanism or mode of action.

Biomagnification: The increase in tissue contaminant concentrations in higher trophic levels as a result of dietary accumulation.

Biomarkers: Measurements that indicate exposure to a chemical, the effect of such an exposure, or susceptibility to effect, usually toxic, of such an exposure.

Biotransformation: The biochemical modification of a xenobiotic once it enters an organism. Chemical modification can be enzymatic or nonenzymatic and may result in either reduced or increased toxicity. This process generally gives rise to compounds that are more readily excreted in the urine and feces and thus serves as a detoxification process; however, some xenobiotics are activated to more toxic metabolites by these enzymatic conversions.

Birth Defect/Congenital Malformation: An abnormality identified in utero or within the first 2 years postnatal (i.e., death, growth or functional retardation or alteration or dysmorphogenesis).

Blackfoot Disease: A condition caused by long-term exposure to arsenic. The condition was first noted in Taiwan in regions containing high levels of arsenic in drinking water. The condition is characterized by poor circulation, leading to distal gangrene of the foot and other extremities.

Blood: A complex tissue composed of plasma and cellular elements with many different functions; the circulating tissue of the body; the fluid and its suspended form elements that are circulated through the heart, arteries, capillaries, and veins. The means by which oxygen and nutrient materials are transported to the tissues and carbon dioxide in various metabolic products are removed for excretion.

Body Burden: The amount of a particular chemical stored in the body at a particular time, especially a potentially toxic chemical in the body as a result of exposure. Body burdens can be the result of long-term or short-term storage; for example the amount of a metal in bone, the amount of a lipophilic substance such as polychlorinated biphenyl (PCB) in adipose tissue, or the amount of carbon monoxide (as carboxyhemoglobin) in the blood. Amount of radioactive material present in a human or animal.

Bolus Dose: A quantity of test material administered all at once. This term is commonly applied to the single daily administration of a test material by oral gavage in toxicity studies.

Bond Stretching Frequency: This frequency is related to the masses of the two atoms that form the bond (Ma, Mb in grams), the velocity of light ©, and the force constance of the bond (k, in dynes/cm). The frequency can be expressed approximately as:

$$\nu\,(\text{in cm}^{-1}) = \frac{1}{2\pi c}\sqrt{\frac{k}{M_a M_b/(M_a + M_b)}}.$$

The value of k is unique for a specific bond type (i.e., sp^3, sp^2, and sp bonds have values of 5, 10, and 15×10^5 dynes/cm, respectively).

Botulism: Fatal paralytic disease resulting from the consumption of food containing preformed toxin from *Clostridiun botulinum*.

Bounding Estimate: An estimate of exposure, dose, or risk that is higher than that incurred by the person in the population with the highest exposure, dose, or risk. Bounding estimates are useful in developing statements that exposures, doses, or risks are "not greater than" the estimated value.

Bowman's Membrane: An acellular layer of collagen and ground substance that provides a functional interface between the stroma and epithelium of the cornea.

Bursa of Fabricius: A structure located in the cloaca of avians, where bone marrow–derived lymphocytes mature into immunocompetent B cells prior to moving to the peripheral lymphoid organs.

Capture Velocity: Air velocity at any point in front of the hood or at the hood opening necessary to overcome opposing air currents and to capture the contaminated air at that point by causing it to flow into the hood.

Cascade Impactor: Instrument used to collect and sort aerosols by separating the particles by their aerodynamic size.

Case Control Study: A study in which the past histories of those with a specific disease (the cases) are compared with those who do not have the disease (the controls). The measure of association is the odds ratio (i.e., the odds of the cases having had some type of exposure compared to the odds of the controls having had that same exposure). In the context of exploratory data analysis, the case control approach has sometimes been called "a disease in search of an exposure."

Case Reports And Case Series: A description of a single individual or group of individuals with the same or similar disease. This type of work lacks controls, and therefore any conclusions derived from such anecdotal information must be viewed with caution. Nonetheless, case reports and case series sometimes are useful for generating hypotheses.

CBC: Corticosteroid-binding globulin.

CBI: Chemical-binding index.

CD (*Cluster Of Differentiation*): The CD series is used to denote cell surface markers (e.g., CD4, CD8). These markers, used experimentally as a means of identifying cell types, serve various physiological roles.

Centrilobular Cells: Collection of hepatic cells situated around the terminal hepatic venule (or central vein).

Centromere: A constriction along the length of a chromosome.

Chelating Agent: An organic compound that forms multiple coordinate covalent bonds with metal ions yielding stable compounds that can be excreted. Chelating agents are used in the treatment of metal toxicity. An example is dimercaptopropanol (British Anti-Lewisite) to treat arsenic poisoning.

Chemical Shift: The frequency at which a given nucleus absorbs in a nuclear magnetic resonance (NMR) spectrum. The precession frequency (ν) for a given nucleus depends on its chemical environment and the shift in ν from the standard value is given by the fundamental NMR equation.

$$\nu = \frac{\gamma_O^{btn}}{2\pi},$$

is called the chemical shift for that nucleus. Chemical shifts are rarely (if ever) expressed in absolute frequency units. Instead they are measured relative to a standard reference compound. For ^{1}H and ^{13}C NMR, the universally accepted reference is tetramethylsilane (TMS). The protons and carbons of TMS absorb at a lower frequency (are more shielded) than those of almost all other organic compounds, so their chemical shifts are arbitrarily set to O Hz and most other chemical shifts measured relative to them are positive. Chemical shifts are expressed in dimensionless units designated δ. The chemical shift in δ units is defined according to the following relationship:

$$\delta = \frac{\nu_s \nu_{std}}{\text{operating frequency}} \times 10^6\ \text{ppm}.$$

Chemokine: Small peptide molecules related to cytokines and associated with a variety of physiological states, such as inflammation and immunoregulation.

Chemotaxis: Directed movement of cells through a concentration gradient of an attractant molecule, such as chemokine.

Cholestasis: Diminution or cessation of bile flow, accompanied by decreased excretion, and enhanced retention, of normal constituents found in bile.

Chromatography: A process for separation of molecules on the basis of their affinities for a stationary phase and a mobile phase.

Chromophore: A structural moiety in an organic molecule, which absorbs light in the useful part of the UV spectrum. Common chromophores are aromatic moieties and conjugated double-bond moieties.

Chromophoric Resonance Raman Label: These labels provide detailed vibrational and electronic spectral data when they are incorporated into the vicinity of a biologically important site. They usually are designed to mimic natural biochemical components and are themselves biologically active compounds. These labels are useful for obtaining information on protein-ligand interactions and have been utilized for studying enzyme-substrate complexes, where vibrational spectra of the substrate during enzyme catalysis can be obtained.

Chromosome: Microscopically visible organelle composed of DNA and proteins.

Chronic: Characterized by a time period of long duration; commonly used to describe long-term (6–12 months) exposure in toxicity studies.

Chronic Toxicity Study: A multiple-dose study in which animals are treated for ≥6 months to comprehensively assess the potential toxicological effects of a compound following long-term exposure. Normally these studies are required prior to Phase II testing in humans.

Ciguatoxins: A group of colorless and heat-stable lipophilic polyether neurotoxins produced by 300 to 400 tropical reef and semipelagic marine animals.

Clastogen: An agent that causes chromosomal breakage.

Clastogenicity: Chromosome breakage and/or rearrangements.

Clearance: The volume of plasma (or blood) that is cleared of chemical per unit time; equivalent to the rate of elimination, at any time, divided by the corresponding plasma (or blood) concentration. Clearance may be dependent on the blood flow and/or the metabolic activity or extraction ratio (at steady state) of the organ(s) elimination; independent of concentration and dose under first-order conditions.

Cleft Phallus: See *hypospadia.*

C_{max}: Maximum achieved concentration.

CMI (*Cell-mediated Immunity*): Antigen-specific immune reactivity mediated primarily by T lymphocytes. Cell-mediated immunity may be expressed as immune regulatory activity (primarily mediated by CD4+ T-helper cells) or immune effector activity (mediated largely by CD8+ T-cytotoxic cells). Other forms of direct cellular activity (e.g., NK cells, macrophages) are generally not antigen specific (i.e., non-immune) and are more accurately described as natural immunity.

COD: Caloric optimization diet.

Codon: A DNA basepair triplet coding for an amino acid or stop signal.

Coefficient of Inbreeding: Refers to a mathematical relationship used to express the relatedness of an animal to other animals in a population and is expressed in mathematical values ranging between 0 and 1.

Cohort Study: This type of epidemiology study is conceptually quite similar to the approach used in most toxicology experiments. The health experience (incidence of disease or mortality) of those exposed to some agent is compared to that of a group not so exposed. In epidemiology, however, the results usually are presented in terms of a relative risk or Standardized Morbidity (or Mortality) Ratio. In the context of exploratory data analysis, the cohort approach also has been called "an exposure in search of a disease."

Collision-Induced Dissociation: A method where ions are collided with neutral molecules to produce fragmentation. This process is also called "MS/MS," as a mass spectrum is produced on an ion selected from a mass spectrum.

Commensal: An organism commonly found in association with animals or their environment that under normal circumstances does not produce disease.

Complement: A group of approximately 20 proteinase precursors that interact in a cascading fashion. Following activation, the various precursors interact to form a complex that eventually leads to osmotic lysis of a target cell.

Conditioned Response: Response to an originally neutral stimulus, such as a sound or light, that has acquired the ability to evoke the response because it was paired with an eliciting stimulus.

Confounding Variable, Confounder: A confounder is an alternative cause for the disease in question that is unequally distributed among those exposed and unexposed to the putative agent of interest. As a consequence, it can be confound or confuse the measure of association and any resulting interpretations of cause and effect.

Confidence Interval: A range of values (above, below, or above and below) about the midpoint of the sample (i.e., the mean, median, mode, etc.) that contain (with a specified level of probability, such as 95% or a standard deviation or error –67%) the true value of the population midpoint. The 95% confidence interval (also called the fiducial limit) is equivalent to the $p = 0.05$ region boundary.

Confidence Limit: A statistical estimate that considers the influence of experimental variation of a parameter.

Confocal Microscope: An instrument capable of producing high-resolution microscopic images that can be used to study ocular tissues. A confocal microscope with scanning capability can be used to determine area and depth of corneal injury.

Conjunctiva: The delicate membrane that lines the eyelid and covers the exposed surface of the eyeball. Histologically the conjunctiva is an aqueous nonkeratinized epithelium with numerous mucous-secreting cells. In the Draize eye test, effects to the conjunctiva represent a maximum of 20 out of 110 total points.

Conjugation: A common mechanism during phase II metabolism, where an endogenous compound is added to specific functional groups of a xenobiotic. Generally, this increases the excretion of the xenobiotic and decreases its potential to interact at critical sites to produce toxicity.

Coprophagy: The process of eating one's own feces.

Cornea: The transparent outermost covering of the anterior portion of the eye consisting of the epithelium, the stroma, and the endothelium. In the Draize eye test, effects to the cornea represent a maximum of 80 out of 110 total points.

Correlation: The relationship or interdependence between measurable varieties or ranks; that is, the extent to which as one set of values changes, another set also changes in the same (positive correlation) or an opposite (negative correlation) direction.

Cosmic Rays: Radiation of many sorts, mostly nuclei (protons) with very high energies, originating outside the earth's atmosphere.

Coupling Constant: The separation between NMR spectral lines due to coupling is called the coupling constant, *J*. The magnitude of coupling constants depends on the number of intervening bonds and the bond geometry. Coupling constants are expressed in units of Hz.

CPM: Comparative potency method.

Critical Temperature: Maximum temperature at which a gas may be liquefied by application of pressure alone. Above this temperature, the substance may only exist as a gas. The critical temperature for CO_2 is 31°C.

Cross-Sectional Study: A prevalence study (i.e., an epidemiology study) which examines the association between health status and other variables of interest as they exist in a defined population at one particular time. This type of research can also be useful for generating etiologic hypotheses, but these hypotheses then need to be tested in analytic studies. Conceptually, it is also the first step of the more rigorous cohort method.

Curie: Standard measure of rate of radioactive decay; based on the disintegration of 1 g of radium, or 3.7×10^{10} disintegrations/second.

Cyclone Separator: A process in which particle-laden air is introduced radially into the upper portion of a cylinder so that it makes several revolutions inside the cylinder. The particles in the air are accelerated outward to the cylinder walls, where they either stick and are retained (low particle loading) or are swirled down to a collection port at the bottom of the cylinder (high particle loading).

Cytochrome P450: Heme thiolate proteins associated with the endoplasmic reticulum originally named for their absorption maximum at 450 nm. These proteins, which serve as catalysts in a variety of oxidative reactions involving both endogenous and xenobiotic lipophilic compounds, are unique in their multiplicity of isozymes, substrates, reactions, and regulatory mechanisms.

Cytokine: Small peptide molecules that subserve a wide range of regulatory and effector mechanisms. Cytokines may be roughly grouped into nonexclusive categories, including interleukins, tumor necrosis factors, interferons, colony-stimulating factors, and miscellaneous other growth factors. Often referred to as "lymphokines" in the older literature.

Cytotoxic T Lymphocyte (*CTL*): A subset of T lymphocytes bearing the CD3/CD8 surface markers, CTL are able to kill target cells following induction of a specific immune response. The mechanism of this lysis appears to be a combination of direct lysis resulting from extrusion of lytic granules by the CTL, as well as the induction of apoptosis in the target cell. The target cells most frequently used for assessment of CTL activity are virally infected cells and tumor cells. Measurement of CTL activity provides an indication of cell-mediated immunity.

Datum: A single point of measurement. More than one point are data.

Default Value: A conservative value used for a model parameter or uncertainty (safety) factor when data are inadequate to justify a different value.

Definitive Test: A toxicity determination designed to provide an accurate quantitative result with low variability; a second-level test conducted following pretests or range-finding tests.

Delayed-type Hypersensitivity (*DTH*): A form of cell-mediated immunity in which recalled exposure to an antigen results in an inflammatory reaction mediated by T lymphocytes. Usually expressed as contact hypersensitivity.

Deposition: The amount of matter (either vapor, gas, or solid) that is absorbed into or onto a surface (usually described as the amount per unit area during a specified period of time).

Descemet's Membrane: An acellular layer which lies beneath the stroma and forms the basement membrane of the corneal endothelium.

Descriptive Study: A study designed to describe the distribution of certain variables (e.g., a health survey of a community which gathers data on disease status and presents the resulting information in the form of what disease was present when, where and among whom). Although not useful for etiologic research, it can be used to generate hypotheses.

Detoxication: The enzymatic conversion of a chemical to a less toxic form or, for these purposes, the conversion of a chemical to a form that can no longer be bioactivated (distinguished from "detoxification," which is the process of removing the chemical from the body by physical means).

Developmental Toxicology: The study of the causes, mechanisms, and sequelae of perturbed developmental events in species of animals that undergo ontogenesis; affected endpoints include death, delayed/retarded development, dysmorphology, and functional impairment.

Diastole: The dilation of the heart cavities during which they fill with blood.

Diffusion-limited Uptake: Tissue uptake is limited by the diffusion through the membranes rather than by the blood flow to the tissue.

Diploid: Two sets of chromosomes, one maternal and one paternal.

Discrimination Behavior: Behavior based on the ability of subjects to discriminate stimulus qualities. In the typical situation, because different stimulus properties require different behaviors, discrimination abilities can be measured by the type or location of responses.

Distribution: The reversible transfer of chemical from the general circulation into the body tissues.

DNA Adduct: A molecule which is covalently linked to a portion of the DNA helix.

DOCA: Deoxycorticosterone.

Donor Animal: Animal from which the organ or the blood was removed.

Dosage: A general term comprising the dose, its frequency, and the duration of dosing.

Dose: The amount of a substance available for interaction with metabolic processes or biologically significant receptors after crossing the outer boundary of an organism. The *potential dose* is the amount ingested, inhaled, or applied to the skin. The *applied dose* is the amount of a substance presented to an absorption barrier and available for absorption (although not necessarily having yet crossed the outer boundary of the organism). The *absorbed dose* is the amount crossing a specific absorption barrier (e.g., the exchange boundaries of skin, lung, and digestive tract) through uptake processes. *Internal dose* is a more general term denoting the amount absorbed without respect to specific absorption barriers or exchange boundaries. The amount of the chemical available for interaction by any particular organ or cell is termed the delivered dose for that organ or cell.

Dose Equivalent (*H*): Unit of biologically effective dose, defined as the absorbed dose in rads multiplied by the quality factor (Q). For all X-rays, gamma rays, beta particles, and positrons likely to be used in nuclear medicine, $Q = 1$.

Dose Rate: Dose per unit time (e.g., in mg/day), sometimes also called dosage. Dose rates are often expressed on a per-unit-body-weight basis, yielding units such as mg/kg/day (mg/kg-day). They are also often expressed as averages over some time period (e.g., a lifetime).

Dose Reconstruction: An approach to quantifying exposure from internal dose, which is in turn reconstructed after exposure has occurred, from evidence within an organism, such as chemical levels in tissues or fluids or from evidence of other biomarkers of exposure.

Dose-Response: "What is there that is not poison? All things are poison and nothing [is] without poison. Solely, the dose determines that which is not a poison." (Paracelsus)

The biological response to an agent is a function of the condition of exposure, including dose, duration, and route.

Dose-Response Model: A mathematical expression that relates the incidence or magnitude of a biological effect to the dose of a chemical.

Dosimetry: Estimating or measuring the quantity of material (mainly refers to particulate) at specific target sites at a particular point in time. The quantity can be measured in terms of mass number, surface area, or volume.

Dosimetry: Process of measuring or estimating dose.

DPA: Decision point approach.

DR: Diet restricted.

Duct Velocity: Air velocity through the duct cross section. When solid material is present in the air stream, the duct velocity must be equal to or greater than the minimum air velocity required to move the particles in the air stream.

Dust: Solid particles that are capable of temporary suspension in air or other gases. Usually produced from larger particles or masses through grinding, crushing, or other handling. Particles may be up to 300–400 μm, but those above 20–30 μm usually do not remain airborne.

Dysplasia: Abnormal tissue development.

Early Transient Incapacitation (*ETI*): Transient performance deficits observed in animals and humans after a large, rapidly delivered dose of ionizing radiation. Five to 10 minutes after radiation exposure, behavioral performance rapidly falls to near zero, followed by partial or total recovery 10–15 minutes later.

EC50 (Effection Concentration-50%): A statistically or graphically determined concentration of a chemical that reduces a sublethal response parameter of interest by 50%.

Ecological Risk Assessment: The process used to establish the likelihood that adverse ecological effects are occurring or may occur as a result of exposure to one or more stressors.

Ectopic or Cryptorchild Testis: Malposition or displacement of the testis outside the scrotum. Typically, such testes are found within the peritoneum or inguinal canal; however, abdominal sites outside the peritoneum have been observed.

ED_{50}: See *median effective dose*.

ED_{50} (*Effective Dose—50%*): The dose of radiation or a chemical agent that would result in a given response in 50% of the population.

Electrocardiogram: A bioelectric potential originating in the myocardium and recorded on the surface of the body; represents the sum of the electrical depolarizations of the myocardium syncytium as the wave of depolarization sweeps across the heart.

Electron Paramagnetic Resonance: An analytical technique that is used to study the structure and properties of free radicals. Electron paramagnetic resonance (EPR) spectroscopy is similar in principle and practice to NMR spectroscopy. Whereas NMR uses energy in the radiofrequency region of the electromagnetic spectrum, EPR uses energy in the microwave region.

Elimination: The irreversible transfer of the chemical from the circulation to the organs of elimination and its subsequent removal from the body by metabolism or excretion.

ELISA (*Enzyme-linked ImmunoSorbent Assay*): A type of immunoassay in which specific antibodies are used to both capture and detect antigens of interest. The most popular type is the "sandwich" ELISA, in which antibodies are bound to be a substrate such as a plastic culture plates. These antibodies bind antigenic determinants on molecules (or alternatively on whole cells). Unrelated material is washed away and the plates are exposed to an antibody of a different specificity; this antibody is coupled to a detector molecule.

EMIT: Enzyme-multiplied immunoassay technique.

Empirical Dose-Response Model: A mathematical model that is selected from plausible models based on agreement with experimental data.

Enantiomer: A type of stereoisomer, an enantiomer is one of a pair of isomers that are nonsuperimposable mirror images of each other. Although chemically identical (except for optical rotation), enantiomers may demonstrate widely different pharmacological and toxicological properties.

Endobiotics: Chemicals that are normally present in the biochemistry of a cell. These include chemicals that are normally found within the biochemistry of anabolic and catabolic metabolism.

Endoscopy: In vivo inspection of the internal surface of a hollow organ with an instrument.

Engineering Standards: Specifications which do not provide for interpretation and modification of prescribed methods or procedures, even if acceptable alternative methods are available or unusual circumstances occur. This term is most commonly used in conjunction with prescribing conditions for the care and use of laboratory animals.

Environmental Fate: The destiny of a chemical or biological pollutant after release into the environment. Environmental fate involves temporal and spatial considerations of transport, transfer, storage, and transformation.

Enzyme: A biological catalyst (for these purposes, proteins).

Epididymis: The duct that conveys sperm from the testis to the vas deferens. It consists of caput (Head), corpus (body), and cauda (tail) regions that support sperm transit, maturation, and storage prior to ejaculation.

Epitope: The portion of an antigen that is recognized by an antibody or T-cell antigen receptor. Also known as the antigenic determinant.

Epizootic: Refers to the initial period following introduction of a microorganism into a naïve population, during which time it undergoes rapid spread within the population and is often associated with a high incidence of clinical signs or disease.

EPR (*Early Phase Regeneration*): Tissue repair response, where arrested G_2 hepatocytes are activated to proceed through mitosis (see *SPR*).

Estrogen: Female sex steroid (e.g., estradiol).

Exon: Actively transcribed DNA in a eukaryotic gene.

Exposure: Contact of a chemical, physical, or biological agent with the outer boundary of an organism. Exposure is quantified as the concentration of the agent in the medium in contact integrated over the time duration of that contact.

Exposure Assessment: The determination or estimation (qualitative or quantitative) of the magnitude, frequency, duration, and route of exposure.

Exposure Concentration: The concentration of a chemical in its transport or carrier medium at the point of contact.

Exposure Pathway: The physical course a chemical or pollutant takes from the source to the organism exposed.

Extra Risk: (P-Po)(1-Po), where P is the total risk and Po is the background (spontaneous) risk in control animals or unexposed humans.

Exposure Route: The way a chemical or pollutant enters an organism after contact (e.g., by ingestion, inhalation, or dermal absorption).

Exposure Scenario: A set of facts, assumptions, and inferences about how exposure takes place that aids the exposure assessor in evaluating, estimating, or quantifying exposures.

Extrapolation: Using data or results from one set of conditions (e.g., animal experimental results) to predict results for a different set of conditions (e.g., humans).

Extravascular Hemolysis: Destruction of red blood cells by cells of the mononuclear phagocyte system (e.g., splenic macrophages); may be a normal process for removal of senescent red blood cells or part of a pathological process for removal of abnormal red blood cells or red blood cells coasted by immunoglobulin (i.e., immune-mediated hemolysis).

Eye Corrosion: Irreversible ocular tissue damage following exposure to a material. Eye corrosion represents gross tissue destruction, which generally occurs rapidly after exposure.

Eye Irritation: Reversible inflammatory changes in the eye and its surrounding mucous membranes following direct exposure to a material on the surface of the anterior portion of the eye.

Face Velocity: Air velocity at the hood opening.

Favism: A hemolytic disease in individuals deficient in glucose-6-phosphate dehydrogenase resulting from consumption of fava beans.

Fertility: The ability to conceive and produce a live offspring. The fertility index should be calculated separately for male and female animals and is generally calculated as the ratio of the number of animals pregnant divided by the number of animals inseminated.

Fetal Alterations (*Malformations, Variations, and Developmental Delays*): Any morphological change identified in a term conceptus, including frank malformation, minor deviations from normal development, and reversible delays or accelerations in development, regardless of the potential effect on subsequent viability or quality of life.

Fiber: A particle which has a length-to-width ratio of 3:1 and a length greater than 5 μ. These can be either naturally occurring, man-made mineral, or synthetic organic fibers.

Fibrosis: Accumulation of collagen.

First-Order Process: A process for which the rate of reaction is proportional to the available concentration; for example, diffusion, metabolism (at low concentrations) and filtration.

Fixation: Preparation of a histologic or pathologic specimen for the purpose of maintaining the existing form and structure of its constituent elements. Maintenance of the normal form and structure of tissues and organs is critical to the evaluation of pathologic effects during microscopic examination. Common fixatives, such as formaldehyde, result in the precipation of proteins. This "fixes" them in place and preserves the morphology of the specimen.

Flash-Point: The lowest temperature at which vapor is given off in sufficient quantity so that the air-vapor mixture above the surface of the solvent will ignite momentarily in a flame.

Flavin-Containing Monoxygenases (FMO): Flavin adenine dinucleotide-containing enzymes belonging to a family of proteins that are important in the NADPH-dependent metabolism of exogenous compounds. FMOs catalyze the addition of a single oxygen atom to nucleophilic nitrogen, sulfur, and phosphorus centers of a variety of xenobiotics.

Flavonoids: Phenolic plant pigments belonging to flavone, flavanone, isoflavone, anthocyanidin, chalcone, or aurone groups.

Food Poisoning: A predominantly gastrointestinal disease resulting from the consumption of food containing any of the ever-increasing number of toxigenic microorganisms and/or the performed toxins produced by them.

Fourier Transformation: A mathematical operation used to covert information from the time domain to the frequency domain. Fourier transformation (FT) can be applied to a variety of spectral techniques, including mass spectrometry, nuclear magnetic resonance, electron paramagnetic resonance, and infrared spectrascopy (IR).

Formication: The unpleasant sensation of tiny insects (L. *formica* ant) crawling on the skin.

Fractional Excretion: The excretion of a substance in urine relative to the rate it is filtered into the urine; an index of reabsorptive function.

Frameshift: A gene mutation characterized by the addition or deletion of one or more basepairs in a gene.

Free Radical: A molecule which is inherently unstable and highly reactive with other components of living systems and produced by sufficient exposure to ionizing radiation.

FSH: Follicle-stimulating hormone.

Fume: Small, solid particles created by condensation from the gaseous state, generally after volatilization or by chemical reaction such as oxidation.

Functional Observation Battery: A set of standardized observations, typically performed with rodents, that has been designed to assess neurobehavioral functions such as reflexes.

Functionalization: The addition to or uncovering of functional groups that are required for subsequent phase II metabolism. For example, hydroxylation of a hydrocarbon provides a functional group from which a conjugate can be formed during phase II metabolism.

Gametogenesis: Production of sperm or ova.

Gamma Rays: High energy, short wavelength electromagnetic radiation emitted from the nucleus of an atom.

Gas Chromatography–Mass Spectrometry: A method for introducing analytes volatized into the gas phase into the mass spectrometer through a chromatographic system where a carrier gas passes through a column packed with a solid phase material.

Gastrointestinal Transit: The rate of passage of the luminal contents of the gastrointestinal tract in the oral to anal direction, ordinarily measured with a nonabsorbable marker.

Gavage: Method of oral administration of a solution or suspension using a suitable stomach tube or feeding needle attached to a syringe. In toxicity studies, gavage is a common method of test material administration by the oral route.

Geometric Mean: The nth root of the product of n values.

Gene: Generally described as the smallest functional unit of an organism's genome.

Gene Pool: The total genetic information contained in the reproductive cells of a species.

Genome: The total number of genes contained in the hereditary material of an organism.

Genotoxic: Property of an agent making it capable of damaging or altering an organism's genetic composition.

Genotoxicity: Alteration of nucleic acids and associated components at subtoxic exposure levels, resulting in modified hereditary characteristics or DNA inactivation.

Genotype: The nucleotide composition of an organism's hereditary material.

Gestation/Pregnancy: The interval in a pregnant animal from conception (fertilization) to the beginning of parturition.

GH: Growth-hormone or somatotropin.

Glomerular Filtration Rate: The volume of plasma separated from the vascular space across the renal glomerulus, expressed per unit time; the filtrate is further modified by the nephron tubule to become the final urine that is eliminated from the body.

Glycone: The activated form of glucose used in glucuronidation. The term is sometimes used for other activated forms of the endogenous compound used in xenobiotic conjugation reactions.

Glycosides: Chemicals of varied structure linked to a mono- or disaccharide by a β-glycosidic linkage.

GNRH (*Gonadotropin-releasing Hormone*): A neuropeptide that regulates the release of the gonadotropins FSH (folicle stimulating hormone) and LH (luteinizing hormone).

GnRH: Gonadotropin-releasing hormone.

Gonadotropins: Usually considered to be follicle-stimulating hormone and luteinizing hormone.

Graded Response: A response to a stimulus or a treatment that can be determined quantitatively on a continuous scale. In acute toxicity studies, body weight and feed consumption are examples of measurements of graded responses.

Gray (*Gy*): SI standard unit of absorbed dose. One Gy equals 1 joule of energy per kilogram of absorber or 100 rads.

Haber's Rule: The hypothesis that equal values of ($C \times T$) produce equal biological effects, where C is the concentration of a chemical and T is the duration of exposures.

Half-Life: The time taken for the plasma (or tissue) concentration to change by 50%; half-life is a characteristic of first-order reactions and is independent of concentration and dose.

Half-Life, Biologic: Time it takes an organism to eliminate half of the radionuclide by biologic processes.

Half-Life, Effective: Time required for the activity of a radionuclide in a biologic system to be reduced to half its initial value as a consequence of both radioactive decay and biologic elimination.

Half-Life, Physical: The time necessary for a radionuclide to decay to half of its initial activity.

Haploid: A single set of eukaryotic chromosomes.

Hapten: Low molecular weight molecules that are not antigenic by themselves but are recognized as antigens when bound to larger molecules such as proteins.

Hazard: The inherent property of a single chemical or mixture to cause adverse effects if an organism is exposed to it.

Hazard Analysis And Critical Control Point (*HACCP*): A system designed to assess various stages of food processing critical in controlling microbial contamination and to propose and implement procedures aimed at minimizing the microbial burden in foods.

Hazard Identification: A qualitative assessment of the types of adverse effects caused by a particular chemical, including (but not limited to) an evaluation of quality of the studies, identification of susceptible subpopulations, and assessing the relevance of humans of the effects observed in animals.

Heinz Body: Irreversibly denatured hemoglobin attached to the inner cell membrane of the red blood cell; caused by oxidizing agents.

Henry's Law Constant: The relationship between the solubility of a gas in a liquid to the pressure of the gas above the liquid at equilibrium, which describes the tendency of a chemical to escape from solution.

Heterologous Blood Perfusate: Blood used as perfusate comes from another animal or another species than the source of the organ being perfused.

Heterologous Expression: Production of a recombinant protein in an artificial host system.

Heterozygous: Two different alleles on a chromosome pair.

Hexagonal Lobule: Classical morphological configuration of the functional unit of the liver as described by Kiernan in 1833.

High-End Exposure (*Dose*) *Estimate*: A plausible estimate of individual exposure or dose for those persons at the upper end of an exposure or dose distribution, conceptually above the 90th percentile but not higher than the individual in the population who has the highest exposure or dose.

High-End Risk Descriptor: A plausible estimate of individual risk for those persons at the upper end of the risk distribution, conceptually above the 90th percentile but no higher than the individual in the population with the highest risks. Note that persons in the high end of the risk distribution have high risk due to high exposure, high susceptibility, or other reasons, and therefore persons in the high end of the exposure or dose distribution are not necessarily the same individuals as those in the high end of the risk distribution.

Hippocampus: Radiosensitive area of the brain involved in learning and memory functions.

HMI (*Humoral-mediated Immunity*): Specific immune responses that are mediated primarily by humoral factors (i.e., antibodies and complement). The induction of humoral immune responses generally requires the cooperation of cellular immune mechanisms.

Homozygous: Two similar alleles on a chromosome pair.

Hormesis: A u-shaped dose response relationship in which adverse effects do not increase monotonically with dose, but decrease initially as dose increases and then rise with higher doses. (An inverted U-shaped dose response is observed with beneficial effects.)

Host Defense: The ability of an animal to protect itself against disease associated with exposure to infectious organisms, foreign tissues and chemicals, and neoplasia. Host defense may be either nonspecific or specific (immune) in nature.

Host Resistance: The ability of an organism to immunologically defend against infection. Host resistance may be decreased in response to an immunosuppressive insult.

HTE: Human time equivalents.

Hydroponic: Referring to a nutrient solution capable of supporting plant growth without the support of inert material.

Hyperplasia: A histopathologic finding characterized by an abnormal increase in the number of cells in a tissue or organ. Hyperplasia generally results from increased cell division but can result from decreased cell death.

Hypertrophy: A histopathologic finding characterized by an abnormal increase in the size of cells in a tissue or organ. For instance, accumulation of fat vacuoles within a cell can increase its size.

Hypospadia: In males, a congenial malformation in which the urethra remains open on the undersurface of the penis. An extreme expression of this malformation results in cleft phallus, which has a cleft running the entire length of the penis.

ICH: International Conference on Harmonization.

Immune Reserve: The concept that the immune response exhibits multiple redundancies capable of modulating acute reductions in certain immune functions. This reserve would theoretically prevent a severe reduction in host resistance following temporary immunosuppression of selected parameters (e.g., NK cell function, etc.).

Immunoassay: An assay that utilizes specific antibodies as reagents. Examples include ELISAs and RIAs.

Immunochemistry: The use of antibodies in analytical or preparative procedures.

Immunologic Contact Urticaria (*ICU*): Contact urticaria, "immediate type" reaction, on an immunologic basis, as in latex contact.

Immunostimulation: Enhancement of immune function above an established baseline (control) response. Immunostimulation may be beneficial (e.g., therapeutics designed to restore a depressed immune response) or detrimental (e.g., the induction of allergy/hypersensitivity or autoimmunity).

Immunosuppression: Depression of immune function below an established baseline (control) response. Immunosuppression may result from inadvertent exposure to immunosuppressive agents, deliberate (therapeutic) immunosuppression, or exposure to certain infectious agents. An important consideration in immunotoxicology is determining the degree or nature of immunosuppression necessary to alter host defense. Immunosuppression can be said to result in a state of immunodeficiency.

Immunotoxicity: The condition in which a drug, chemical, or physical agent alters the structure or function of the immune system.

Immunotoxicology: The discipline of synergistically applying cardinal principles of both immunology and toxicology to study the ability of certain materials to alter the normal immune response.

Incidence: The number of new cases of a particular disease in a defined population during a specified period of time. The term incidence is sometimes used synonymously with *incidence rate*. Note, in the medical literature, prevalence and incidence are often used incorrectly as equivalent terms.

Induction: As used in respect to xenobiotic metabolisms, induction refers to the process where exposure of an organism to a xenobiotic results in increased activity of specific biotransformation enzymes. Generally, but not always, induction results in more rapid metabolism of the inducing agent. Induction, as used in this context, does not require de novo protein synthesis but may result from other mechanisms.

Inflammation: A nonspecific host defense mechanism. It is characterized primarily by the infiltrating of leukocytes into the peripheral tissue, followed by release of various molecules that elicit nonspecific physiological defense mechanisms.

Inhalable: Materials that are capable of being deposited anywhere in the respiratory tract.

Inhibin: A glycoprotein produced by Sertoli cells and by the pituitary that acts as a negative regulator of FSH secretion.

Initiated Cell: A normal body (stem?) cell that has undergone the first transformation step in the process of cancer development to an intermediate state but that is not malignant.

In Situ: Perfusion—Vascularly isolated and perfused organs are left in the animal body with the neighboring tissues.

Instillation: Slow introduction of a fluid (or a fluid-containing particulate) directly into the trachea of an experimental animal; this is a surrogate method for the introduction of fluid/particulate into the lungs following inhalation.

Insufflation: Introduction of particulate (without fluid) directly into the trachea (or bronchioles) of an experimental animal; this is a surrogate method for the introduction of material into the lungs following inhalation.

Intake: The process by which a substance crosses the outer boundary of an organism without passing an absorption barrier (e.g., through ingestion or inhalation) (see *potential dose*).

Internal Dose: The amount of a substance penetrating across the absorption barriers (the exchange boundaries of an organism) via either physical or biological processes. This term is synonymous with absorbed dose.

International Conference on Harmonization of Technical Requirements for Registration of Pharmaceuticals for Human Use (*ICH*): An initiative intended to establish similar criteria to support the worldwide registration of drugs. Representatives from regulatory agencies and pharmaceutical companies from the United States, Europe, and Japan have been the primary participants.

Intravascular Hemolysis: Rupture or lysis of red blood cells within the vascular system causing release of intracellular substances (e.g., hemoglobin) into the plasma; if severe enough, may be recognized by hemoglobinema and/or hemoglobinuria.

Intron: Non-coding spacer DNA in a eukaryotic gene.

Intubation: Placement of a tube into a hollow organ. Intubation is used to place various materials into animals for toxicology studies. If the organ is in the stomach, the process is generally referred to as gavage.

Inulin: A polysaccharide (MW$\sim$5000) that is not metabolized by mammalian cells and is too large to enter cells. The clearance of inulin is used to measure glomerular filtration rate. Inulin is used in vitro as an indicator of extracellular space.

In Vitro Hemolysis: Rupture or lysis of red blood cells during blood collection or handling causing release of intracellular substances (e.g., hemoglobin, enzymes, electrolytes) into serum or plasma, if severe enough, may be responsible for artifactual test results.

In Vivo Nuclear Magnetic Resonnance (*NMR*) *Spectroscopy*: A technique of value for measuring alterations in specific P-31 species within cells in real time using a surface coil and large-bore, high-resolution NMR magnets.

IOCA: In ovo carcinogenicity assay.

Ionization: The formation of ions from neutral molecules. This is accomplished in mass spectrometry by a variety of methods, including bombardment with electrons, gas phase chemical reactions, and ion desorption methods.

Iris: The structure of the eye which is anatomically located posterior to the cornea. The iris forms the pupil of the eye and functions in regulating the amount of light that reaches the retina. In the Draize eye test, effects to the iris represent a maximum of 10 out of 110 total points.

IR Fingerprint Region: This frequency region of the infrared spectrum ranges from 910 cm^{-1} to 1430 cm^{-1} and contains bending and stretching absorptions of characteristic groupings in an organic molecule. The region is abundant in absorption bands, and their frequencies and intensities are unique for a specific compound. Hence, the absorption pattern in this region of the IR spectrum is utilized as a "fingerprint" for the recognition of an unknown molecule by comparison with the fingerprint frequencies of an authentic standard. It is important to note that polymorphic forms of the same compound may show significant differences in the fingerprint region. Therefore, comparisons should be made in the solution in the same solvent. If solid state spectra are utilized, the unknown and authentic standard should be crystallized from the same solvent under similar conditions.

IRMA: Immunoradiometric assay.

Irradiation: Exposure to radiation.

Irritant Dermatitis: Chemically induced, nonimmunologic contract dermatitis; complex syndrome has many types.

Ischemia: Local anemia due to mechanical obstruction (mainly arterial narrowing) of the blood supply.

Islet of Langerhans: Specialized cells (viz Beta cells) in the pancreas that secrete insulin.

Isoenzymes: Enzymatically active proteins that catalyze the same reactions and occur in the same species but differ in their physicochemical properties (also, isozymes or isoforms).

Isolated Perfused Organ: Vascularly perfused organ is physically removed from the donor animal and maintained in an artificial chamber usually kept at physiological temperature.

Isolated Perfused Ventilated Lung: Vascularly perfused isolated lungs are also ventilated using mechanical devices.

ITO Cells: Fat-storing cells found in the liver; also called lipocytes or stellate cells.

Juxtaglomerular Apparatus: A specialized area of the glomerulus where the distal tubule from the nephron has contact with the arterioles entering and leaving the glomerulus; one factor in control of renal blood flow.

LCB: Limited carcinogenicity bioassay.

LD_{50}: Lethal dose of radiation or chemical agent that has been determined to cause death in 50% of a defined population. Expressed in terms of weight of test substance per unit of test animal (mg/kg). See *median lethal dose*.

$LD_{50/30}$: Median lethal dose (MLD or LD_{50}) required to kill 50% of the population of organisms within 30 days.

Large Intestine: The region of the gastrointestinal tract from the ileum to the anus, which consists of the cecum, the colon, and the rectum.

Leukopenia: Any situation in which the total number of leukocytes in the circulation is less than normal.

Leydig Cell: Cells located in the interstitial compartment of the testes between the seminiferous tubules that synthesize testosterone. Androgen-secreting cells present in the interstitium of the testes.

LH: Luteinizing hormone.

Limit of Quantification (*LOQ*): The concentration of analyte in a specific matrix for which the probability of producing analytical values above the method detection limit is 99%.

Limit Study: A study in which a single, maximal dose level of test material is administered to the test animals. Limit studies are conducted when administration of test material at higher dose levels is not required either because exposure at higher levels is not physically possible or because the test material has been shown to be of extremely low toxicity.

Linear Energy Transfer (*LET*): The amount of energy transferred by a unit dose of radiation per unit pathway traveled through matter (keV/micro of path); varies with the type of radiation. Alpha particles are high LET radiation with 10 s to 100 s of keV/micron of path, whereas x-rays and gamma rays are low LET radiations (tenths to 10 keV/micron).

Linear Extrapolation: The process of estimating a value at conditions not directly measurable using a linear relationship between the biological effect and the dose or duration of exposure. (Technically, when a measure of the background effect is available, an *interpolation* is being performed.)

Linear Kinetics: With linear kinetics there is a linear relationship between dose and plasma concentrations and body loads. Linear kinetics are characteristic of first-order reactions because the rates of reactions increase as the concentration or body load increases; therefore, parameters such as bioavailability, clearance, apparent volume of distribution, and half-life are independent of dose (see definitions in text).

Linear Model: A model in which the change in a biological effect is proportional to the change in dose or duration of exposure.

Lipid Peroxidation: The chain reaction formation of the mediators of lipid degradation by ionizing radiation.

Lipophilicity: The tendency of a chemical to partition into a lipid medium or a fat solvent, such as hexane, from an aqueous medium.

Liquid Chromatography–Mass Spectrometry: A method for introducing analytes dissolved in solution into the mass spectrometer through a chromatographic system where a liquid mobile phase passes through a column packed with a solid phase material.

Liver Acinus: Functional unit of hepatocytes as defined by Rappaport; consists of a small parenchymal mass arranged around an axis consisting of a terminal portal venule, a hepataic arteriole, a bile ductule, lymph vessels, and nerves.

LOAEL: Lowest-observed-adverse-effect level.

Low-Dose Extrapolation Model: A model that uses information on observed dose-response relationships combined with mechanistic understanding to predict the dose-response relationship below the range of observable data.

Lymph: A clear, transparent, sometimes faintly yellow and slightly opalescent fluid that is collected from the tissues throughout the body. It flows into the lymphatic vessels and is eventually added to the venus blood circulation.

Lymphoproliferation: Proliferation of lymphocytes in response to stimulation with cellular activators, including antigens or mitogens. Because proliferation of lymphocytes is one of the initial consequences of cellular activation, lymphoproliferation is often used as a nonspecific in vitro measure of immunoresponsiveness. This assay is sometimes referred to as the *blastogenesis assay*.

Mab: Monoclonal antibodies.

Macrocirculation: Comprises the heart, the great vessels (both arterial and venous), and the larger arteries and veins.

Major Histocompatibility Complex (*MHC*): A complex of genes coding for tissue compatibility markers. Two major classes are recognized: Class I (present on all nucleated cells) and Class II (present on B cell, T cells, and macrophages). MHC molecules appear to direct the course of immune reactivity and are presented in association with antigen by antigen-presenting cells. The human equivalent is termed HLA, or human leukocyte antigen.

Malabsorption: Impairment in the uptake of ingested substances from the gastrointestinal lumen into the bloodstream because of defects in luminal digestion, mucosal transport, or gastrointestinal transit.

Malt (*Mucosa-associated Lymphoid Tissue*): Lymphoid tissue associated with the mucosal layer in various tissues, believed to act as a primary defense at secretory surfaces. It acts, to a limited extent, independently of the systemic response. Various tissues comprise this system, including gut-associated (GALT), nasal-associated (NALT), and bronchus-associated (BALT) lymphoid tissues.

MAP Kinase Pathway: The mitogen-activated protein kinase pathway is a key cellular signaling pathway resulting in transcriptional activation and mitogenic proliferation. It consists of several enzymatic activation steps and can be stimulated by a number of agents, including cytokines and radiation exposure. It is believed to account for the accelerated repopulation of cells occurring after radiation exposure, which can affect the success of radiation therapy.

Margin of Safety (*MOS*): The difference, normally expressed as fold-difference, between the dose (or exposure level) that results in toxicity and that which results in the desired pharmacological activity.

Mass Median Aerodynamic Diameter: Standard method of characterizing the size distribution of a particulate atmosphere—represents that size when 50% of the particles are larger (or smaller) than the stated size.

Mass Spectrometry: An analytical technique that determines the mass of ionized molecules and their fragments and adducts.

Mass Cell: A polymorphonuclear, granule-containing cell with a major role in hypersensitivity reactions.

Mating Performance: The ratio of mated (inseminated) animals to the number cohabited, generally expressed mathematically as the ratio of the number of female animals inseminated divided by the number cohabited with a cohort male.

Maximally Exposed Individual (*MEI*): The single individual with the highest exposure in a given population (also, most exposed individual). This term has historically been defined various ways, including as defined here and also synonymously with worst-case or bounding estimate. Assessors are cautioned to look for contextual definitions when encountering this term in the literature.

Maximum Tolerated Dose (*MTD*): The dose that causes no more than a 10% reduction in body weight and does not produce mortality, clinical signs of toxicity, or pathologic lesions that would be predicted to shorten the natural life span of an experimental animal for any reason other than the induction of neoplasms.

MCL: Mononuclear cell leukemia.

Mean: The average value. In a normally distributed sample, this has the same value as the median (the middle value) and the mode (the most frequent value).

Measure of Association: A term that represents the strength of association between variables. The relative risk, odds ratio, and standardized mortality ratio (SMR) are measures of association commonly used in epidemiology.

Median Effective Dose: A statistically derived single dose of a substance that can be expected to produce a particular effect in 50% of the study population (ED_{50}). The ED_{50} is expressed in terms of weight of test substance per unit weight of test animal (mg/kg).

Median Lethal Dose: A statistically derived single dose of a substance that can be expected to cause death in 50% of the study population (LD_{50}). The LD_{50} is expressed in terms of weight of test substance per unit weight of test animal (mg/kg).

Median Value: The value in a measurement data set such that half the measured values are greater and half are less.

Mee's Lines: Horizontal white lines on the fingernails that occur after exposure to arsenic. The lines appear after the exposed nail bed grows to the exterior.

Metabolic Activation: The process by which relatively stable substrates are converted to highly reactive, generally electrophilic products with the capability of producing damage to critical cellular macromolecules. The term is occasionally used to refer to the metabolism of therapeutically inactive pro-drugs to the active form of the drug.

Metal Fume Fever: An acute condition of short duration caused by exposure to fresh fumes of zinc and other metals. The condition is characterized by fever and chills, occurring 4 to 12 hours after exposure. Recovery usually is complete within 1 day.

Metalloid: Any element with both metal and nonmetal characteristics (e.g., arsenic, boron, tellurium).

Metallothionein: Any inducible low molecular weight, cytosolic protein with a high cysteine content (approx. 30%) and characteristically deficient in aromatic amino acids and histidine. Presence of numerous cysteinyl thiol groups permits high-affinity binding of several metals (e.g., cadmium, lead, mercury, or zinc).

Metals: A grouping of elements generally characterized by opacity, ductility, luster, being electropositive with a tendency to lose electrons, and having the property of conducting heat and electricity. Heavy metals may be further defined as any element having a density greater than 5 g/cm^{-3}, and those of toxicological significance preferentially bind to ligands containing sulfur or nitrogen (arsenic, cadmium, chromium, lead, and mercury).

Methemoglobin: A form of hemoglobin in which the ferrous ion (Fe^{2+}) of hemoglobin has been oxidized to the ferric state (Fe^{3+}); it is unable to carry oxygen.

Microcirculation: This is the business end of the circulation, where delivery of oxygen and nutrients and the removal of carbon dioxide and metabolites takes place.

Microcosm: A small model or "piece" of an ecosystem contained in a test chamber used to study the effect of contaminants on a biotic community in a controlled environment.

Microenvironment Method: A method used in predictive exposure assessments to estimate exposures by sequentially assessing exposure for a series of areas (microenvironments) that can be approximated by constant or well-characterized concentrations of a chemical or other agent.

Microenvironments: Well-defined surroundings, such as the home, office, automobile, kitchen, store, etc., that can be treated as homogeneous (or well characterized) in the concentrations of a chemical or other agent.

Microisolation Cage: An animal cage usually constructed of plastic that completely surrounds the animals contained therein such that air entering and exiting the cage must pass through an integrated filter designed to stop the passage of unwanted microorganisms or fomites. Most commonly, such caging is maintained using sterile techniques in order to prevent the introduction of unwanted microorganisms.

Micropuncture Technique: A method for measuring glomerular filtration and tubular reabsorptive capacity of a single nephron; it involves sampling urine from within the tubular lumen.

Microsomes: The operational definition of microsomes is the 105,000 × g pellet produced from a tissue homogenate after removal of nuclei, mitochrondria, and cell debris by centrifugation at 9000 × g. Microsomes are the remnants of the endoplasmic reticuluum after cellular disruption. The outer surface of microsomal vesicles represents the cytosolic side of the endoplasmic reticuluum.

Midzonal Cells: Collection of hepatic cells situated between the periportal area and the centrilobular area of the lobule.

Milk Sickness: Potentially fatal neurologic disease resulting from the consumption of unpasteurized milk containing the neurotoxin, trematol, derived from animals grazing on toxic plants, white snakeroot, or rayless goldenrod.

Misclassification: A type of bias in which an individual or attribute is assigned a value which is incorrect. The misclassification may be *nondifferential* (the same in all study groups) or *differential* (not equivalent across groups). Each type of misclassification may impact the results, the former usually underestimating the true measure of association and the latter often overestimating it.

Mitogen: Molecules capable of inducing cellular activation; may include sugars or peptides. The ability of a cell to respond to stimulation with mitogen (generally assessed by cellular proliferation) is believed to give an indication of the cells' immune responsiveness.

Mitogenesis: The induction of mitosis or cell transformation. The stimulation of cell proliferation, a natural recovery process in response to severe toxicologic insult that does not normally occur at reasonable multiples of human exposure levels, can account for the carcinogenic response toward nongenotoxic compounds that may not be meaningful in the clinical setting.

Mixed Lymphocyte Response/Reaction (*MLR*): An in vitro assay that measures the ability of lymphocytes to proliferate in response to exposure to allogeneic cells. This proliferation represents the initial stage in acquisition of CTL function; the assay thus serves as a measure of cell-mediated immune function. Sometimes referred to as *mixed lymphocyte culture* (MLC).

MOE: Margin of exposure.

Monocyte/Macrophage: Bone marrow–derived mononuclear cells that serve a wide variety of host defense needs, acting as both nonspecific phagocytic cells and as regulators of other immune and nonimmune host resistance mechanisms. A variety of forms exist, including monocytes (found in the blood), macrophages (found in peripheral tissue), Kupffer cells (liver), Langerhan cells (skin), microglia (brain), veiled cells (lymph), and others.

Monte Carlo Technique: A repeated random sampling from the distribution of values for each of the parameters in a generic (exposure or dose) equation to derive an estimate of the distribution of (exposures or doses in) the population.

Moribund Status: The condition of an animal as a result of the toxic properties of a test substance where death is anticipated. For toxicity determinations, animals killed for humane reasons are considered in the same way as animals that die.

Morphology: Pertaining to the form or structure of a cell, organ, or whole animal.

Motor Activity: Spontaneous locomotion in a specified enclosure designed to provide quantitative indices of movement.

MOU: Memorandum of understanding.

MRA: Mutual recognition agreement.

MSH: Melanocyte-stimulating hormone.

MTD: Maximum tolerated dose.

Mucociliary Transport: Mucous lining of the nasal passage extending from the respiratory epithelium to the pharynx whose purpose is to move waste solids up from the deeper lung to the pharyngeal area to be swallowed.

Multistage Model of Carcinogenesis: A model that describes the carcinogenesis process as a series of mutations or mutation-like events over time that result in a malignant growth.

Mutagenesis: The production of genetic alterations by exposure to chemicals or radiation. This can result in irreparable DNA damage and subsequent tumor development.

Mutation: A stable change in the nucleotide sequence of a gene.

Mycotoxins: A group of more than a hundred toxins produced by various fungal organisms in food and feed commodities.

Myocardium: The middle layer of the heart, consisting of cardiac muscle.

Nasopharyngeal: Region of the respiratory tract serving as the entry port for inspired air (includes the turbinates, epiglottis, glottis, pharynx, and larynx).

Natural Immunity: Host defense mechanisms that do not require prior exposure to antigen. Various effector mechanisms have been described, including cellular cytotoxicity mediated by macrophages or NK cells, complement, and activity of gamma-delta T cells.

Natural Killer (*NK*) *Cells*: A population of lymphocytes distinct from T and B lymphocytes; also referred to as large granular lymphocytes (LGL). NK cells exhibit cytotoxicity against virally infected cells and certain tumor cells. They are notable in that they do not require prior exposure to antigen to express cytotoxicity toward their targets. Assessment of NK activity provides a measurement of nonspecific host resistance.

Necropsy: Post-mortem examination of a nonhuman body. A similar term, autopsy, generally is used to refer to post-mortem examination of a human body. Necropsies are conducted in toxicology studies following spontaneous death or euthanasia of animals to detect potential pathologic effects of test material administration.

Neoantigen: A new antigen that appears on cells during malignant transformation, viral infection, or other process by which a naturally occurring antigen is modified.

Neoplasia: The pathologic process that results in the formation and growth of abnormal tissue (neoplasm). Neoplasms usually form a distinct mass of tissue (tumor) that may be benign or malignant.

Neuropsychology: A clinical discipline that specializes in the application of psychological tests to ascertain aberrations of neurobehavioral function.

Nictitating Membrane: An important ocular structure in many species of animals (but not humans or primates) that aids in protecting the cornea and conjunctiva when the eyeball is retracted. Also called the *third eyelid*.

NME: New molecular (chemical) entity.

NOAEL (No-observed-adverse-effect level): A number applied to the highest dose that did not elicit an adverse effect in a properly designed and executed toxicological study.

Nonimmunologic Contact Urticaria (*NICU*): Contact urticaria, "immediate type" reaction, on nonimmunologic basis.

Nonlinear Kinetics: With nonlinear kinetics there is not a linear relationship between dose and plasma concentrations or body loads. Nonlinear kinetics are typically due to saturation of absorption, and/or distribution, and/or elimination.

Nonparametric Statistical Methods: Methods that do not assume functional form with identifiable parameters for the statistical distribution of interest (distribution-free methods).

Nonregenerative Anemia: Anemia characterized by decreased production and delivery into circulation of newly formed red blood cells (reticulocytes).

No-Threshold Dose-Response Relationship: A dose-response relationship that assumes that any dose carries some probability of an effect.

Nose-Only Exposure: Experimental mode of inhalation exposure in which only the nose of the animal is placed in contact with the test atmosphere (variant is head-only).

NTEL: Nontumorigenic effect level.

Nuclear Magnetic Resonance Spectroscopy: An analytical technique that is used to study the structure of molecules. Nuclear magnetic resonance (NMR) spectroscopy takes advantage of the behavior of atomic nuclei in the presence of a strong magnetic field. When samples are placed in a magnetic field and irradiated with energy in the radiofrequency (RF) range, they absorb RF energy. The exact frequency absorbed by an atomic nucleus in the sample molecule differs depending on the environment of the nucleus (its position within the molecule). A plot of intensity of RF absorption versus frequency is called an NMR spectrum and is characteristic of the structure of the sample molecule.

Octanol-Water Partition Coefficient: (*Kow, P*): The ratio of the concentrations of a chemical in the water phase and the n-octanol phase after the chemical is equilibrated between equal volumes of the two solvents.

Odds Ratio: The ratio of two odds. In case-control studies, it is an *exposure odds ratio* (i.e., the odds of exposure among the cases as compared to the odds of that same exposure among the controls). Although less seldom used, an odds ratio is sometimes calculated for a cohort study, but it is a *disease odds ratio* (i.e., the odds of disease among the exposed versus the odds of that same disease among the unexposed).

Opportunistic Organism: Refers to an organism, most commonly a microorganism, that under the right set of biological conditions can cause disease when normally it coexists with its host without producing disease.

Organelle: A subcellular structure with a specialized function within the cell.

Orthologs: Genes that are believed to have evolved from a common ancestral gene. Orthologs may have a high degree of sequence homology, but their protein products do not necessarily have a high degree of functional homology.

Osteomalacia: Inadequate or delayed mineralization of bone, resulting in an increased softness of the bone. It is the adult equivalent of rickets.

Osteoporosis: A loss in both the mineral and matrix phase of bone; associated with an increased tendency to fracture.

Outlier: A value that is far separated from the other members of a sample. May be due to faulty sampling technique (the value actually belongs to a different population), an error in measurement, or may be "real" and very meaningful.

Oxidation: The net loss of electrons, which may also involve the addition of oxygen to a molecule.

Oxidative Stress: Imbalance between prooxidants and antioxidants.

Oxygen Enhancement Ratio (*OER*): The ratio of the dose of radiation required to produce a given biological effect in the absence of oxygen (anoxia or hypoxia) compared to the same dose of radiation exposure required in the presence of oxygen. The OERs for low LET radiation, such as x-rays or gamma rays, usually range from 2.8 to 3.0. Living systems are more radiosensitive when irradiated in the presence of oxygen.

p53: A 53,000 molecular weight tumor suppressor/trancriptional regulating protein that is commonly mutated in cancers. It participates in cell cycle regulation, transcription and apoptosis. Activation of p53 after radiation exposure leads to radiation-induced cell cycle delay.

Pachymetry: A means of obtaining quantitative measurements of corneal thickness using either optical or ultrasonic methods. Derived from the Greek words pachys (thick) and metry (the process of measuring).

Pancytopenina: Reduction of all three formed elements of blood: red blood cells, white blood cells, and platelets.

Paracelsus: The founder of modern toxicology.

Parenteral: Introduced into the body by a route other than the alimentary canal (e.g., subcutaneous intravenous, intramuscular injection).

Partition Coefficient: Ratio of concentration or relative distribution of a chemical in two matrices at equilibrium.

Parturition: The interval in a pregnant animal during which delivery of an offspring occurs; it is initiated at the first signs of labor and completed at the birth of the last offspring in the liter, in multiparous animals.

PCNA: Proliferating cell nuclear antigen.

PCR: Polymerase chain reaction.

Perfusion-limited Uptake: Tissue uptake is limited by the rate of blood flow to the tissue.

Performance Standard: A set of specifications that define an outcome in detail and provide criteria for assessing that outcome. The term is most commonly used in conjunction with prescribing conditions for the care and use of laboratory animals.

Peripheral Blood Leukocyte (*PBL*): Leukocytes derived from the peripheral circulatory system in humans. Due to the accessibility, these cells are often used in ex vivo assays of human immune function.

Periportal Cells: Collection of hepatic cells situated around the portal triad (branch of the portal vein, a hepatic arteriole, and a bile duct).

Peroxisome: Membrane-bound cell organelles present in cells of animals, plants, fungi, and protozoa that contain oxidative enzymes responsible for the formation and degradation of hydrogen peroxide. These organelles are involved in lipid, sterol, and purine metabolism, as well as peroxidative detoxification. Nongenotoxic chemicals that cause hepatic peroxisome proliferation can cause liver tumor development in rodents. This phenomenon has not been shown to be relevant to humans.

Persistent Light Eruption: Photoallergic contact dermatitis that flares with UV exposure continuing past cessation of photoallergen exposure.

Personal Measurement: A measurement collected from an individual's immediate environment using active or passive devices to collect the samples.

Phagocytosis: Process of ingestion by phagocytes whereby the cell membrane of the phagocyte engulfs bacteria and delivers them into the cell, where enzymatic digestion occurs.

Pharmacogenetics: The study of inherited differences in xenobiotic metabolism. This includes genetic mechanisms of species differences and inter-individual and interpopulation differences in the genotype and phenotype of cytochrome P450s and other xenobiotic metabolizing enzymes.

Pharmacokinetics: The study of the movement of a chemical (drug) in the body (absorption, distribution, metabolism, excretion).

Phase 1 Clinical Trial: The first stage of clinical testing, these single- and multiple-dose studies are normally conducted in healthy male volunteers to assess the safety and systemic exposure of new drug candidates.

Phase 2 Clinical Trial: The second stage of clinical testing, these trials are designed to assess safety and efficacy in the target patient population. The length of these trials is determined by the time required to demonstrate clinical endpoints suggestive of efficacy.

Phase 3 Clinical Trial: These are post-marketing trials that may be requested by regulatory agencies upon their review of the New Drug Application (NDA), or in response to effects that become evident as more patients become exposed to the drug. Sponsors may also choose to conduct these studies to support a line extension strategy (e.g. new formulations, expansion of the patient population).

Phase 4 Clinical Trial: These are post-marketing trials that may be requested by regulatory agencies upon their review of the New Drug Application (NDA) or in response to effects that become evident as more patients become exposed to the drug. Sponsors may also choose to conduct these studies to support a line extension strategy (e.g., new formulations, expansion of the patient population).

Photoallergic Contact Dermatitis: Allergic contact dermatitis dependent upon UV (typically UVA) exposure.

Photoirritant (*Phototoxic*): Acute irritant dermatitis dependent upon UV (typically UVA) exposure.

Physiological Leukocytosis: Increased white blood cell count associated with endogenous catecholamine release as a result of excitement, fear, or pain.

Physiologically-Based Pharmacokinetic (PBPK) Model: A mechanistic model that describes quantitatively the uptake, distribution, metabolism, and excretion of a chemical; the model can also be used to quantify the dose of active metabolite received by the target tissue.

Phytotoxin: A plant toxin.

Pica: Compulsive ingestion of nonnutritive items, such as dirt, flaking paint, plaster, ashes, or laundry starch. Individuals with pica often have greater exposure to toxicants (e.g., ingestion of lead in paint chips).

Pinocytosis: Cellular process of actively engulfing liquid.

Plenum Velocity: Air velocity in the plenum. For good air distribution with slot-type hoods, the maximum plenum velocity should be one half of the slot velocity or less.

Point-of-Control Measurement of Exposure: An approach to quantifying exposure by taking measurements of concentration over time at or near the point of contact between the chemical and an organism while the exposure is taking place.

Poison: Any substance (chemical, physical, biological) that is harmful or destructive to a biological (living) system.

Polymerase Chain Reaction: A method in which a region of a nucleic acid is selectively amplified by cycles of nucleotide polymerization.

Polymorphism: Multiple phenotypes of an organism determined by different alleles.

Polymorphisms: Two structurally distinct genes for the same protein. Polymorphic genes can be produced by mutations that result in nucleotide sequence differences. This can lead to the production of proteins which differ functionally or it may not alter functionality.

Polynomial Dose-Response Model: A dose-response model in which the response is expressed mathematically as the sum of quantities containing increasing powers of dose.

Polytocous: The production of litters of offspring.

Positron-Emitting Isotopes: These isotopes have relatively short half-lives (10–100 min) and decay exclusively by emission of a positron. They produce readily detectable tissue-penetrating γ-ray photons, and are thus commonly used in tomographic techniques (position emission tomography, PET). Examples of such isotopes are carbon-11, nitrogen-13, oxygen-15, and fluorine-18. Because of their brief existence, positron-emitting isotopes usually have to be manufactured close to the site where they are to be used.

Potential Dose: The amount of a chemical contained in material ingested, air breathed, or bulk material applied to the skin.

Power: The effect of the experimental conditions on the dependent variable relative to sampling fluctuation. When the effect is maximized, the experiment is more powerful. Power can also be defined as the probability that there will not be a type II error (1-Beta). Conventionally, power should be at least 0.07.

Precision: A measure of the agreement among replicate measurements of an analyte; reproducibility.

Prediction Model: In alternative methods development, the tool that is used to predict the endpoint of interest. The prediction model is an algorithm that defines how to convert results from the alternative method into a prediction of the in vivo toxicity.

Prevalence: The number of cases of a designated disease that exist at a particular point in time (*point prevalence*). There also are various types of *period prevalence* which represent the number of existing and new cases of a disease that are extant at the beginning of or anytime during a defined period of time. In the medical literature, both types of prevalence, particularly the latter, may erroneously be called incidence, especially if the data are presented as a *prevalence rate*.

Prevalidation: In alternative methods development, the preliminary phase to validation in which the purpose of a test, its capabilities, limitations, interlaboratory transferability, and predictability are determined.

Primary Enclosure: The cage, pen, or stall that forms the immediate limit of an animal's environment in a research facility.

Primary Response: The immune response following initial contact with an antigen, resulting in the establishment of immunologic memory. Synonymous with immunization.

PRL: Prolactin.

PTH: Parathyroid hormone.

Psychophysics: A group of methods formulated to guide the testing of sensory capacities.

Pulmonary: Region of the respiratory tract serving primarily as the air exchange region composed of respiratory bronchioles, alveolar ducts, and alveoli.

Quality Control: Procedures for monitoring and evaluating the quality of the testing process of each method to assure the reliability of test results for test subjects or patients.

Quantal Response: A response to a stimulus or a treatment that can be referred to as "all or none" (it either happens or it does not happen). In acute toxicity studies, mortality is an example of a quantal response.

Racemate: Compound containing a 50:50 proportion of enantiomers.

Rad: Radiation-absorbed dose of ionizing radiation. One rad = 100 erg/g.

Radiation: Energy propagated through space or matter or matter as waves (gamma rays, ultraviolet light) or as particles (alpha or beta rays).

Radionuclide: An element, either in the environment or internal, which emits ionizing radiation.

Radioprotective Agents: Chemical compounds that, when administered before irradiation, protect the organism against radiation damage.

Radiosensitizer: Substance that enhances the radiation response of biologic systems.

Radiotolerance: The eventual lack of sensitivity to radiation.

Random: Each individual member of the population has the same chance of being selected for the sample.

Randomization: Process used in toxicity studies to ensure a homogeneous population and to minimize errors due to sampling bias. Randomization can be done by assigning animals to treatment groups using computer-generated random numbers or through use of tables of random numbers.

Rate: An expression of the frequency with which an event occurs in a defined population. A measure of the *absolute risk* for the disease in that population. In a rate, the numerator is a subset of the denominator; therefore, all rates are ratios but not all ratios are rates. A rate usually also has a time dimension. For a prevalence rate, it is the implied or explicit time at which the data were collected. For an incidence rate, it is the time over which the new events took place. For convenience, the denominator of either type of rate usually is presented as some power of 10 (i.e., the number of cases per 100 or per 1000 or, for rare events, per 100,000 or even per 1,000,000).

Rate Difference: The difference between two rates. In the situation where etiology has been established, the rate difference between the disease incidence in the exposed and unexposed groups is sometimes called the *excess rate* or *attributable risk*.

Raw Data: Any laboratory worksheets, records, memoranda, notes, or exact copies thereof that are the result of original observations and activities from a study. This may include manually recorded information, printouts from automated instruments, computer printouts, photographs, microfilm or microfiche copies, and magnetic media (including dictated observations).

RCB: Rodent cancer bioassay.

Reasonable Worst Case: A semiquantitative term referring to the lower portion of the high end of the exposure, dose, or risk distribution. The reasonable worst case has historically been loosely defined, including synonymously with maximum exposure or worst case, and assessors are cautioned to look for contextual definitions when encountering this term in the literature. As a semiquantitative term, it is sometimes useful to refer to individual exposures, doses, or risks that, while in the high end of the distribution, are not in the extreme tail. For consistency, it should refer to a range that can conceptually be described as above the 90th percentile in the distribution, but below about the 98th percentile (compare maximum exposure range, worst case).

Receptor: The sensitive site for chemical-biological interaction.

Recirculating Perfusion: Perfusate flows from a reservoir through the organ being perfused and returns to the same reservoir.

Rederivation: Refers to a process that utilizes removal of term fetuses with subsequent cross-fostering onto mothers of the right microbiological status or the use of embryo transfer procedures to change the microbiological status of animals.

Reference Concentration: An air concentration of a chemical exposure expressed in mg/m^3, which is associated with minimal or no risk of adverse effects, even in susceptible subpopulations.

Reference Dose (*RfD*): An estimate of a daily exposure to a human population, including sensitive groups, that is likely to be without appreciable risk of deleterious health effects during a lifetime.

Reference Interval: The central interval of test values bounded by a lower reference limit and an upper reference limit for a designated percentile of a population (e.g., the central 95th percentile reference interval for an analyte includes the values that 95% of an apparently healthy reference population will have); frequently referred to as a reference range, historical range, or normal range.

Reference Toxicant: Chemicals of known toxicity that are used to determine the health of a population of a test species.

Regenerative Anemia: Anemia characterized by increased production and delivery of newly-formed red blood cells (reticulocytes) into circulation; typically associated with hemorrhage or hemolysis.

Reinforcement Schedule: A designated relationship between a specific behavior, such as pressing a lever in an experimental chamber, and the delivery of a reinforcer, such as a feed pellet.

Relative Biological Effectiveness (*RBE*): The ratio of a dose of a test radiation (neutron, gamma, x-ray, etc.) required to produce the same reference biological end point as the dose of a standard radiation of 250 KVP x-rays.

Relative Risk: The ratio of the absolute risk of disease or death (the incidence rate) among the exposed to the risk among the unexposed. A measure of association that sometimes is called the *risk ratio*, *rate ratio*, or *RR*.

Reproductive Toxicology: The study of the causes, mechanisms, and sequelae of adverse effects on the reproductive system including alterations to the reproductive organs, related endocrine system, or pregnancy outcomes, and manifested as adverse effects on sexual maturation, gamete production and transport, cycle normality, sexual behavior, fertility, gestation, parturition, lactation, pregnancy outcomes, premature reproductive senescence, or modifications in other functions dependent on the integrity of the reproductive system.

Residual Analysis: Analysis of the difference between experimental and simulated data as a function of time or other controllable variables. The residuals should be random if the model is adequate.

Residual Body: A lobe of cytoplasm containing residual organelles (e.g., mitochondria, Golgi appatus, endoplasmic reticulum, ribosomes, lipid droplets) that detaches from the elongated spermatid at spermiation. Residual bodies are eliminated from the seminiferous epithelium by Sertoli cell phagocytosis.

Respirable: Inhalable materials that are capable of (getting to and) being deposited in the gas-exchange region of the lung.

Respiratory System: Complex arrangement of organs designed primarily for the intake of oxygen and the elimination of carbon dioxide. Divided into the proximal or upper airway (nose, pharynx, larynx, trachea, nonalveolarized bronchioles) and the distal or lower airway (alveolar bronchioles, alveolar ducts, alveolar air sacs).

Retention: (of particulate material) quantity of particles present at specific respiratory tract sites that is the net difference between deposition and clearance processes.

RIA: Radioimmunoassay.

Ring Tail: A condition seen in rodents in which annular constructions of the tail occur which may lead to necrosis of all or part of the tail. This condition is presumed to be associated with abnormal environmental conditions.

Risk: Proportion or probability expressed on a scale of 0 to 1, or 0 to 100%, that individuals process or develop a specified biological effect by a given time for a defined set of exposure conditions.

Robust: Having inferences or conclusions little affected by departure from assumptions.

Rodent Lifetime: Generally taken to be 2 years for risk estimation.

Roentgen (*R*): Quantity of X- or gamma radiation/cubic centimeter of air that produces one electrostatic unit of charge.

Roentgen Equivalent Man (*REM*): Unit of dose equivalent. The absorbed dose in rads multiplied by Q of the type of radiation.

Route of Exposure: Portal of entry of a chemical into the body: oral, inhalation, dermal, or injection.

Safety Factor: A number/factor that considers inter- and intra-species variability, sensitivity, and extrapolatability and is applied to an NOAEL to establish an Acceptable Daily Intake (ADI). See *uncertainty factor*.

Safety Pharmacology: The study of the pharmacologic effects of a drug candidate that are unrelated to the desired pharmacologic effect. These studies are generally conducted at doses similar to the anticipated therapeutic dose.

SAM: (Standardized Aquatic Microcosm): A defined aquatic microcosm containing 15 species in a well-defined medium of trace metals and vitamins and 200 g of sand to which chitin and cellulose are added, contained in a 3-liter vessel.

Sample: In statistics, the collected set of data points which (if properly collected) are representative of the population (all the values there are).

Saponins: Steroidal or terpenoid glycosides from plants and animals capable of reducing surface tension and disruption of cell membranes.

Saturation Dose: Dose that overwhelms a toxification or detoxification mechanism such that no additional changes in the effect are incurred above that dose.

Schedule-Controlled Operant Behavior: An approach to the study of behavioral function that relies on manipulation of reinforcement schedules.

Scombroid Poisoning: An allergic fish poisoning resulting from the consumption of inadequately processed fish containing histamine and saurine formed from bacterial action.

Screening Tests: In acute toxicity testing, tests designed to define the range of toxicity using fewer animals per dose level or fewer dose levels.

Secondary Enclosure: The room or space in which a primary enclosure is located.

Secondary Response: The immune response that occurs after initial contact with an antigen (the primary response). The secondary response is quicker, of higher affinity, and more pronounced. For humoral-mediated immune reactions, the secondary response is associated with antibody class switching.

Secondary Toxicity: The toxicity of a chemical determined by feeding the test animals (especially ferrets or mink) with prey items that have themselves been fed the test chemical.

SEL: Safe exposure level.

Selection and Selection Bias: The process by which subjects are included in a study. If there are systematic differences between those who are selected for a study and those who are not, selection bias may occur. The bias may be introduced by the subjects themselves through self-selection (into or out of the study), as a result of the sources of the subjects, or by the study investigators.

Seminiferous Epithelium: The Sertoli cells and developing male germ cells within the seminiferous tubules in the testis.

Sensitivity: The number of subjects experiencing each experimental condition divided by the variance of scores in the sample.

Sensitivity Analysis: Evaluation of the effect of changes in the value of a particular parameter on the estimates of a state variable provided by a mathematical model. Sensitivity is expressed as the magnitude of change in the endpoint of interest (e.g., tissue dose) as a function of change in the value of a particular model parameter.

Sertoli Cell: A somatic cell present in the seminiferous epithelium of mammals. Solidly attached to the basement membrane of seminiferous tubules, it produces important regulatory glycoproteins, including anti-Mullerian hormone, inhibin, and androgen-binding protein, and is essential for male germ cell development.

Shuttle Vector: A DNA transfer agent capable of moving genes into or out of a cell.

Sievert (*Sv*): SI unit of dose equivalent. The absorbed dose in grays multiplied by the Q of the type of radiation. One Sv = 100 rems.

Significance Level: The probability that a difference has been erroneously declared to be significant, typically 0.05 and 0.01 corresponding to 5% and 1% chance of error.

Simulation: System behavior predicted for specific exposure conditions by solving the set of differential and algebraic equations of a model.

Single-Pass Perfusion: Pefusate flows from a reservoir through the vasculature of a perfused organ is collected and not reused so that the perfusate goes through only once.

SI Units: International system of units. SI refers to *Système International d'Unites*. Radiation units include joule/kilogram, gray, sievert, and becquerel.

Slit Lamp Biomicroscope: An instrument used to study ocular tissues that can detect lesions not observable by gross examination. It consists of a microscope and a high-intensity light source that allow the eye to be illuminated and observed from different angles.

Slope: The difference in the incidence or magnitude of an effect divided by the difference in dose that created the effect.

Slot Velocity: Air velocity through the openings in a slot-type hood. It is used primarily as a means of obtaining uniform air distribution across the face of the hood.

Small Intestine: The region of the gastrointestinal tract from the pyloric sphincter of the stomach to the cecum, which consists of the duodenum, the jejunum, and the ileum; the primary site of absorption of ingested substances.

S9 Mix: A 9000 × g supernatant fraction from a tissue homogenate (e.g., liver).

Soil Aging: The changes that occur in the interaction of chemicals with soil during which the chemicals are bound to soil particles and become less bioavailable.

Soil Sorption Constant (*Koc*): The extent of partitioning of an organic chemical between the solid and solution phases of a water-saturated soil or sediment.

Specific Activity: The radioactivity per unit mass of material. Specific activity is used to quantify radionuclides. Specific activity can be given in *Curies per mole* (Ci mol^{-1}) or *Bequerels per mole* (Bq mol^{-1}).

Specific Gravity: The ratio of the density of a substance to the density of a reference material at a specified temperature. Water is the reference standard for liquids and solids (density 1 g/ml at 4°C).

Spermatid: The haploid germ cell, arising from meiotic divisions of spermatocytes, that differentiates within the seminiferous epithelium into a spermatozoon.

Spermatocyte: Germ cells in the seminiferous epithelium that are derived from spermatogonia and subsequently undergo two meiotic divisions to form round spermatids.

Spermatogenesis: The process of germ cell division and differentiation that begins with the multiplication of spermatogonia and ends with the release of elongated spermatids into the lumen of the seminiferous tubules (spermiation).

Spermatogenic Cycle: A complete sequential progression of the cellular associations (or stages) of spermatogenesis. The stages follow one another though an entire cycle, returning to the original stage and repeating this cycle approximately 4.5 times until spermatogonia become elongated spermatids and undergo spermiation.

Spermatogonia: The diploid germ cells in adult males that divide by mitosis to produce additional stem cell spermatogonia and spermatocytes.

Spermiation: The process by which elongated spermatids are released from the germinal epithelium into the seminiferous tubule lumen.

Spermiogenesis: The last phase of spermatogenesis during which elongated spermatids are formed from round spermatids.

Spin Trapping: The most commonly used indirect method for detecting free radicals. The technique involves adding a spin trap (usually a nitrone or nitroso compound) to the sample prior to radical generation. When the radical is generated it reacts rapidly with the spin trap, producing a secondary radical or *spin adduct* which is more stable than the parent free-radical and can be detected by electron paramagnetic resonance (EPR).

SPR: Secondary phase regeneration; tissue repair response, where hepatocytes are mobilized from G_0/G_1 to proceed through mitosis (see *EPR*).

Standard Deviation: The most widely used measure of dispersion of the points in a frequency distribution about the midpoint (usually the mean). It is equal to the square root of the variance. For a normally distributed population, the region within one standard deviation of the mean contains 67% of the distribution.

Statistical Significance: An inference that the probability is low that the observed difference in quantities being measured could be due to variability in the data rather than an actual difference in the quantities themselves. The inference that an observed difference is statistically significant is typically based on a test to reject one hypothesis and accept another.

Steady-State: A situation in which the rate of change is equal to zero.

Steatosis: Accumulation of lipid within hepatocytes (fatty liver).

Stem Cell: A multipotential self-renewing cell in the bone marrow that serves as the precursor for all hematopoietic cell lineages, including those of the immune system.

Stereoisomers: A general term for isomers that differ only in the orientation of the atoms in space. Enantiomers, isomers that differ in their optical rotation, are a subclass of stereoisomers.

Stomach: The sac-like region of the gastrointestinal tract from the esophagus to the duodenum, consisting of the cardia, fundus, corpus, antrum, and pylorus; the site of hydrogen ion secretion from parietal cells of the gastric glands which activates pepsin-mediated proteolysis.

Subchronic: Characterized by a time period of intermediate duration; commonly used to describe exposure between acute and chronic duration in toxicity studies (usually 3 months).

Subchronic Toxicity Study: A multiple-dose study in which animals are treated for less than 6 months. These studies are intended to elucidate the target organs for toxicity and demonstrate dose-response relationships. They are normally required prior to any clinical testing.

Substrate Probe: Individual isozymes may show significant differences in substrate specificity. A substrate that is metabolized by a specific isozyme and does not show significant overlaps with other isozymes can be used to probe for the presence and activity of the isozyme. Substrate probes can be used in vitro and in vivo. Use of substrate probes may not be as accurate as certain other techniques for isozyme identification but are sometimes more practical.

Syncytium: A multinucleated protoplasmic mass formed by the secondary union of originally separate cells.

Systole: Contraction of the heart, especially of the ventricles, by which the blood is driven through the aorta and pulmonary artery to transverse the systemic and pulmonary circulation, respectively.

T_3: Triiodothyronine.

T_4: Thyroxine.

Tannins: Heterogeneous polyphenols of plant origin.

Target Tissue Dose: Concentration of a chemical in the tissue or organ where the biological effect occurs.

T Cell/T Lymphocyte: Lymphocytes primarily responsible for the induction and maintenances of cell-mediated immunity, as well as regulating humoral-mediated immunity and certain nonimmune effector mechanisms. A variety of T-cell subtypes have been described including T-helper cells, T-cytotoxic cells, T-suppressor cells, and T-inducer cells.

T-Cell Receptor (*TCR*): The heterodimeric surface molecule on T cells that serves to recognize antigen. It always occurs in conjunction with the CD3+ surface antigen, which is responsible for transmembrane signaling following antigen recognition.

TEF: Toxic equivalency factor.

TFM: Test facility manager.

Telomere: The terminal portion (end) of a chromosome.

T_{max}: Time to maximum achieved concentration.

Teratology: The study of the causes, mechanisms and sequelae of perturbed developmental events in species of animals that undergo ontogenesis; in the past, the definition was limited to malformation, but the term is now generally accepted to be synonymous with developmental toxicology.

Test Article: Any food additive, color additive, drug, biological product, electronic product, medical device, pesticide, or other chemical substance to be subjected to studies.

Test Material: Any chemical substance to be subjected to studies. This does not include electronic products or medical devices.

Test System: Any animal, plant, microorganism, subparts thereof (e.g., in-vitro organ systems) or physical matrix (e.g., soil or water) to which a test or control article is administered or added for study.

Testosterone: The primary male sex hormone produced by Leydig cells in the testis that, along with the metabolite dihydrotestosterone, is responsible for male reproductive tract development, maintenance of spermatogenesis, secondary sex characteristics, and sexual behavior.

Therapeutic Index (*TI*): The ratio of LD_{50}/ED_{50}. The therapeutic index is used to establish the safety margin of biologically active materials such as drugs. The higher the index, the greater the margin of safety.

Thermal Neutral Zone: The temperature or range of ambient temperatures at which an animal does not expend energy to heat or cool itself.

Threshold Dose: Dose below which a specified biological effect does not occur for specified exposure conditions.

Threshold Dose-Response Relationship: A dose-response relationship which assumes that adverse effects occur only once a threshold dose is exceeded.

Thrombocytopenia: A condition in which there is an abnormally small number of circulating platelets.

Thymus: A central lymphoid organ located in the thorax. Its function is the generation of immunocompetent T cells from lymphocytes originating in the bone marrow.

Tissue Time Constant: The product of partition coefficient and volume divided by blood flow rate.

Tolerance Level: The maximum legally permissible concentration of residues of a pesticide in food.

Toxicant: An agent that can result in the occurrence of a structural and/or functional adverse effect in a biological system.

Toxicodynamics: The process of interaction of chemical substances with target sites and the subsequent reactions leading to adverse effects.

Toxicokinetics: The process of the uptake of potentially toxic substances by the body, the biotransformations they undergo, the distribution of the substances and their metabolites in the tissues, and the elimination of the substances and their metabolites from the body. Both the amounts and the concentrations of the substances and their metabolites are studied. The term has essentially the same meaning as pharmacokinetics, but the latter term usually is restricted to the study of pharmaceutical substances.

Toxicology: The study of the adverse effects of chemical or physical agents on biological systems.

Toxin: A poison derived from a biological source.

Toxinology: The study of toxins.

Tracheobronchial: Region of the respiratory tract serving to deliver inspired air to deeper portions of the lung, comprised of a series of branching ducts beginning at the trachea and entry at the terminal bronchioles.

Transgenic: Referring to an organism in which new DNA is introduced into the genome. Some transgenic animal model have been suggested to complement the assessment of the potential for compounds to cause tumor development.

Translocation: Transfer of a portion of one chromosome to another chromosome.

TRH: Thyroid-releasing hormone; a tripeptide secreted by the hypothalamus.

TS: Test substance.

TSH: Thyroid-stimulating hormone.

Two-Dimensional Gel Electrophoresis: A series of electrophoretic techniques which separates proteins (gene products) on the basis of isoelectric points in one dimension followed by separation on the basis of molecular mass in the second dimension. This technique is useful for obtaining an overall assessment of both up- and down regulation of specific gene products as the result of cellular responses to chemical exposures.

Tyndall Phenomena: The abnormal cloudy appearance of the anterior chamber of the eye when light passes through the pupil; also called aqueous flair. It is the result of protein leakage from the iris into the aqueous humor causing the scattering of light and producing cloudiness.

Type I Error (*A False-Positive*): Concluding that there is an effect when there really is not an effect. Its probability is the alpha level.

Type II Error (*A False-Negative*): Concluding there is not effect when there really is an effect. Its probability is the beta level.

Ultrastructural Cytochemistry: A series of in situ techniques for localizing organelle-specific enzymes, such as acid phosphatase for lysosomes and peroxidase for peroxisomes, at the ultrastructural level.

Ultrastructural Morphometry: A series of techniques for quantitating changes in organelle systems from electron micrographs in situ. These techniques provide useful correlative information when used in combination with biochemical measurements of chemical-induced alterations in organelle system functionality.

Uncertainty Factor: A factor applied to a no-observed-adverse-effect-level or a lowest-observed-adverse-effect-level, which is used to derive a reference dose or reference concentration; the aim of the uncertainty factor is to account for lack of information on inter and intra-species variability, study deficiencies, and incomplete database.

Urticaria: Hives; an eruption of itching wheals.

UVR: Ultraviolet radiation.

Validation: In alternative methods development, the process whereby the reliability and relevance of a procedure are established for a particular purpose.

Variability: The range of values expected among individuals of a given population.

Vapor: Gaseous forms of substances that normally are in the liquid or solid state.

Vapor Pressure: The amount of pressure exerted by a saturated vapor above its own liquid in a closed container.

Vaporization: The transfer of a chemical from a solid surface or a solution as a gas, dependent upon the chemical's diffusivity, water solubility, and vapor pressure.

Vehicle: A substance to which a test material is added in order to confer a consistency or form suitable for its intended use. In toxicity studies, test materials are added to vehicles to prepare solutions (e.g., water), suspensions (e.g., methyl cellulose), ointments (e.g., petrolatum), triturates (e.g., milk, sugar), and other forms to facilitate administration to the animals.

Venom: An animal toxin.

Water Solubility: The maximum amount of a chemical that may be dissolved in a given quantity of pure water at a given temperature.

Whole-body Exposure: Experimental mode of inhalation exposure in which the entire animal is placed within the test atmosphere.

Wolffian Duct: Embryonic duct from which the male reproductive duct system, accessory sex glands and external genitalia are derived.

Xenobiotic: A substance that is foreign to a biological system.

X-ray Microanalysis: The in situ localization of trace elements within organelles at the ultrastructural level using the electron beam of either a transmission or scanning electron microscope to displace electrons from specific energy shells (K, L, M) with the resulting release of characteristic X-rays that may be monitored by energy-dispersive or wavelength-dispersive spectrometers.

Zero-order Process: A process for which the rate is constant and independent of dose or concentration; characteristic of enzymic processes under saturating concentrations.

Zonation, Hepatic Lobule: Quantitative (or qualitative) distribution of enzymes in liver lobule based on morphological configuration.

Zonation, Metabolic: Differences observed between enzymes activities in periportal and perivenous regions of the liver.

Zoonotic: Refers to the ability of an organism to be transmitted between species of animals and is most commonly used in reference to the ability of an organism to be exchanged between animals and man.

Principles and Methods of Toxicology, Fourth Edition, edited by A. Wallace Hayes. Taylor & Francis, Philadelphia © 2001.

Index

G

P